Textbook of Radiation Oncology

SECOND EDITION

Steven A. Leibel, MD

Chairman, Department of Radiation Oncology
Memorial Sloan-Kettering Cancer Center
New York, New York

Theodore L. Phillips, MD

Professor, Department of Radiation Oncology
University of California, San Francisco
San Francisco, California

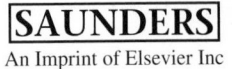

SAUNDERS

An Imprint of Elsevier Inc

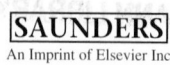

SAUNDERS
An Imprint of Elsevier Inc

The Curtis Center
Independence Square West
Philadelphia, Pennsylvania 19106-3399

TEXTBOOK OF RADIATION ONCOLOGY   ISBN 0–7216–0026–3

NOTICE

Radiation Oncology is an ever-changing field. Standard safety precautions must be followed but as new research and clinical experience broaden our knowledge, changes in treatment and drug therapy may become necessary or appropriate. Readers are advised to check the most current product information provided by the manufacturer of each drug to be administered to verify the recommended dose, the method and duration of administration, and contraindications. It is the responsibility of the treating physician, relying on experience and knowledge of the patient, to determine dosages and the best treatment for each individual patient. Neither the Publisher nor the authors assume any liability for any injury and/or damage to persons or property arising from this publication.

The Gamma-camera image on the cover appears courtesy of Dr. Sally DeNardo and is taken from DeNardo SJ, Kroger LA, DeNardo GL: A new era for radiolabeled antibodies in cancer? Curr Opin Immunol 11:563, 1999, with permission.

Library of Congress Cataloging-in-Publication Data
Textbook of radiation oncology/[edited by] Steven A. Leibel, Theodore L. Phillips.—2nd ed.
    p. ; cm.
    Includes bibliographical references and index.
    ISBN 0-7216-0026-3
    1. Cancer—Radiotherapy. 2. Medical physics. 3. Tumors—Radiography. 4. Radioisotope brachytherapy. I. Leibel, Steven A. II. Phillips, Theodore L.
    [DNLM: 1. Neoplasms—radiotherapy. 2. Health Physics—methods. 3. Radiation Oncology—methods. QZ 269 T355 2004]
    RC271.R3T45 2004
    616.99'40642–dc22
                                            2003069360

Executive Publisher: Susan Pioli
Acquisitions Editor: Dolores Meloni
Developmental Editor: Jennifer Shreiner
Senior Project Manager: Peter Faber

Printed in the United States of America.

Last digit is the print number: 9   8   7   6   5   4   3   2   1

To Margy and Joan.

This textbook is also dedicated to a colleague and friend,
Hideo "Dale" Kubo, Ph.D.,
who passed away during the production of this edition
to which he has contributed in an outstanding fashion.

Contributors

Andre A. Abitbol, MD
Clinical Professor of Radiation Oncology, University of Miami School of Medicine; Associate Director, Department of Radiation Oncology, Baptist Hospital, Miami, Florida
High Dose Rate Brachytherapy

David H. Abramson, MD
Attending Surgeon, Department of Surgery, Memorial Sloan-Kettering Cancer Center, New York, New York
Retinoblastoma

Judy Adams, CMD
Chief Proton Dosimetrist, Department of Radiation Oncology, Massachusetts General Hospital, Boston, Massachusetts
Skull Base Tumors: Chordomas and Chondrosarcomas

Oguz Akin, MD
Department of Radiology, Memorial Sloan-Kettering Cancer Center, New York, New York
Pelvis

Kaled M. Alektiar, MD
Assistant Attending Radiation Oncologist, Department of Radiation Oncology, Memorial Sloan-Kettering Cancer Center, New York, New York
Instruments and Techniques in Brachytherapy; Cancer of the Endometrium; Cancer of the Ovary

Howard I. Amols, PhD
Chief, Clinical Physics Service, Memorial Sloan-Kettering Cancer Center, New York, New York
Three-Dimensional Conformal Radiotherapy and Intensity-Modulated Radiotherapy

K. Kian Ang, MD, PhD
Professor of Radiation Oncology and Deputy Chairman, University of Texas M D Anderson Cancer Center, Houston, Texas
Fractionation Effects in Clinical Practice

John G. Armstrong, MD
Department of Radiology, St. Luke's Hospital, Dublin, Ireland
Tumors of the Salivary Gland

Barbara Asselin, MD
Associate Professor of Pediatrics and Oncology, University of Rochester School of Medicine and Dentistry; Pediatric Hematologist Oncologist, Golisano Children's Hospital at Strong, University of Rochester Medical Center, Rochester, New York
Pediatric Leukemias and Lymphomas

Mary Austin-Seymour, MD
Wootton Professor of Radiation Oncology, University of Washington School of Medicine; Professor and Vice Chair of Radiation Oncology, University of Washington Medical Center, Seattle, Washington
Skull Base Tumors: Chemodectomas – Nonchromaffin Paragangliomas

Ignacio Azinovic, MD, PhD
Oncología Radioterápica, Hospital San Jaime, Partida De La Lona, Torrevieja, Spain
Tumor-targeted Radioisotope Therapy

Joel S. Bedford, PhD
Professor, Department of Radiology and Health Sciences, Colorado State University, Fort Collins, Colorado
Radiobiological Principles

Adrian C. Begg, PhD
Professor, University of Nijmegen; Head, Division of Experimental Therapy, The Netherlands Cancer Institute, Amsterdam, The Netherlands
Prediction of Radiation Response

Luc M. Bidaut, PhD
Associate Attending Physician, Memorial Sloan-Kettering Cancer Center, New York, New York
Imaging in Radiation Oncology

Christopher Biggs, MD
Department of Radiation Oncology, Arizona Oncology Services, St. Joseph's Hospital and Medical Center, Phoenix, Arizona
Intraoperative Radiation Therapy

Eleanor A. Blakely, PhD
Senior Staff Biophysicist, Life Sciences Division, Lawrence Berkeley National Laboratory, Berkeley, California
Particle Radiation Therapy

Dmitry Bolkhovets, MD
Assistant Professor of Radiology, New York Medical College; Attending Physician of Radiology, Westchester Medical Center, Valhalla, New York
Thorax

Martin Brown, PhD
Professor, Radiation Oncology, Stanford University, Stanford, California
Chemical Modifiers of Radiation

Chandra M. Burman, PhD
Associate Attending Physicist, Department of Medical Physics, Memorial Sloan-Kettering Cancer Center, New York, New York
Immobilization and Simulation

Joseph R. Castro, MD, FACR
Professor of Radiation Oncology (Ret), University of California, San Francisco, School of Medicine, San Francisco; Participating Scientist, Lawrence Berkeley National Laboratory, Berkeley, California
Particle Radiation Therapy

Devron H. Char, MD
Director, The Tumori Foundation and Clinical Professor, Ophthalmic Oncology and Orbital Surgery, Department of Ophthalmology, Stanford University Medical School, Stanford, California
Uveal Melanoma

Lanceford M. Chong, MD
Associate Attending Radiation Oncologist, Department of Radiation Oncology, Memorial Sloan-Kettering Cancer Center, New York, New York
Tumors of the Salivary Gland

Fergus V. Coakley, MD
Associate Professor, University of California, San Francisco, School of Medicine; Section Chief, Abdominal Imaging, Department of Radiology, University of California, San Francisco, San Francisco, California
Abdomen

Louis S. Constine, MD
Professor of Radiation Oncology and Pediatrics and Vice Chair, Department of Radiation Oncology, James P. Wilmot Cancer Center, University of Rochester Medical Center; Radiation Oncologist and Section Chief, Pediatric Radiation Oncology, Strong Memorial Hospital, Rochester, New York
Pediatric Leukemias and Lymphomas

Richard L. Crownover, MD
Principal Investigator, CyberKnife Program, Chief of Breast and Musculoskeletal Tumor Services, Departments of Radiation Oncology and Neurological Surgery, Taussig Cancer Center, Cleveland Clinic Foundation, Cleveland, Ohio
Extracranial Stereotactic Radioablation

Bruce Culliney, MD
Assistant Professor of Medicine, Albert Einstein College of Medicine of Yeshiva University, Bronx; Attending Physician and Director, Infusion Suite, Cancer Center, Beth Israel Medical Center, New York, New York
Cancer of the Oropharynx

Inder K. Daftari, PhD
Senior Physicist, Department of Radiation Oncology, University of California, San Francisco, School of Medicine, San Francisco, California
Particle Radiation Therapy

Sally J. DeNardo, MD
Professor of Radiology and Internal Medicine, Division of Hematology and Oncology; Section of Radiodiagnosis and Therapy, Co-Director, Radiodiagnosis and Therapy, Department of Internal Medicine, University of California, Davis School of Medicine, Sacramento, California
Tumor-Targeted Radioisotope Therapy

William C. Dewey, PhD
Professor, Department of Radiation Oncology, University of California, San Francisco, School of Medicine, San Francisco, California
Radiobiologic Principles

Adam Dicker, MD, PhD
Associate Professor, Department of Radiation Oncology, and Director, Division of Experimental Radiation Oncology, Jefferson-Kimmel Cancer Center; Attending Physician, Thomas Jefferson University Hospital, Philadelphia, Pennsylvania
Cancer of the Oropharynx

Nancy Fischbein, MD
Assistant Professor of Radiology, University of California, San Francisco, School of Medicine, San Francisco, California
Head and Neck

Karen F. Fu, MD
Professor Emeritus, Radiation Oncology, University of California, San Francisco, California
Cancer of the Nasopharynx

Zvi Y. Fuks, MD
Professor of Radiation Oncology in Medicine, Weill Medical College of Cornell University, Attending Radiation Oncologist and Deputy Physician in Chief for Planning, Memorial Sloan-Kettering Cancer Center, New York, New York
Cancer of the Ovary

Dan P. Garwood, MD
Associate Professor and Clinical Director, Department of Radiation Oncology, University of Texas, Southwestern Medical Center at Dallas, Dallas, Texas
Cancer of the Testis; Extracranial Stereotactic Radioablation

Michelle S. Ginsberg, MD
Assistant Professor of Radiology, Weill Medical College of Cornell University; Director, General Radiology Section, Assistant Member, Department of Radiology, Memorial Sloan-Kettering Cancer Center, New York, New York
Thorax

Eli Glatstein, MD
Morton M. Kligerman Professor of Radiation Oncology, University of Pennsylvania School of Medicine and Hospital of the University of Pennsylvania, Philadelphia, Pennsylvania
Clinical Applications of Photodynamic Therapy

Brian J. Goldsmith, MD
Chairman, Radiation Oncology Centers, Radiological Associates of Sacramento, Sacramento, California
Meningeal Tumors

Alexander R. Gottschalk, MD, PhD
Assistant Professor, University of California, San Francisco, School of Medicine, San Francisco, California
Gene-Targeted Therapy

Sheryl Green, MB, BCh
Assistant Professor, Mount Sinai School of Medicine; Attending Physician, Mount Sinai Medical Center, New York, New York
Cancer of the Vagina

Daphne A. Haas-Kogan, MD
Assistant Professor, University of California, San Francisco, School of Medicine, San Francisco, California
Pediatric Central Nervous System Tumors; Gene-Targeted Therapy

Stephen M. Hahn, MD
Associate Professor, Department of Radiation Oncology, University of Pennsylvania, Philadelphia, Pennsylvania
Clinical Applications of Photodynamic Therapy

Francine E. Halberg, MD
Department of Radiation Oncology, Marin Cancer Institute, Greenbrae, California
Pituitary Tumors

Bilal Hameed, MD
Resident, University of Minnesota Medical School, Minneapolis, Minnesota
Abdomen

Louis B. Harrison, MD
Professor of Radiation Oncology, Albert Einstein College of Medicine of Yeshiva University, Bronx; Clinical Director, Continuum Cancer Centers of New York, New York, New York
Cancer of the Oropharynx

Richard T. Hoppe, MD
Henry S. Kaplan–Harry Lebeson Professor in Cancer Biology and Chair, Department of Radiation Oncology, Stanford University School of Medicine, Stanford, California
Hodgkin's Disease; Mycosis Fungoides

Hedvig Hricak, MD, PhD
Professor, Weill Medical College of Cornell University; Chairman, Department of Radiology, Memorial Sloan-Kettering Cancer Center, New York, New York
Pelvis

I-Chow Joe Hsu, MD
Assistant Professor and Radiation Oncologist, University of California, San Francisco, School of Medicine; Mount Zion Cancer Center, San Francisco, California
High Dose Rate Brachytherapy; Cancer of the Uterine Cervix

Kenneth Hu, MD
Assistant Professor, Albert Einstein College of Medicine of Yeshiva University, Bronx; Clinical Assistant Professor, State University of New York Downstate Medical Center; Attending Physician, Department of Radiation Oncology, Beth Israel Medical Center; Director of Radiation Oncology Programs, New York Eye and Ear Infirmary, New York, New York
Cancer of the Oropharynx

David Huang, MD
Radiation Oncologist, Valley Radiotherapy Associates Medical Group, Good Samaritan Hospital, Los Angeles, California
Pituitary Tumors

Melissa Hudson, MD
Professor of Pediatrics, University of Tennessee Health Science Center and College of Medicine; Member, Department of Hematology-Oncology, St. Jude Children's Research Hospital, Memphis, Tennessee
Pediatric Leukemias and Lymphomas

John L. Humm, PhD
Attending Physicist and Chief of Nuclear Imaging Physics, Memorial Sloan-Kettering Cancer Center, New York, New York
Imaging in Radiation Oncology

Madhu J. John, MD, FACR, FACRO
Clinical Professor, Department of Radiation Oncology, University of California, San Francisco, School of Medicine, San Francisco; Medical Director, Radiation Oncology Services, Sequoia Regional Cancer Center, Visalia; St. Agnes Cancer Center, Fresno, Fresno, California
Radiotherapy and Chemotherapy

Youn Kim, MD
Professor, Department of Dermatology, Stanford University School of Medicine, Stanford, California
Mycosis Fungoides

Lee M. Krug, MD
Assistant Professor, Weill Medical College of Cornell University; Assistant Attending, Memorial Sloan-Kettering Cancer Center, New York, New York
Tumors of the Lung, Pleura, and Mediastinum

Dale Kubo, PhD (deceased)
Professor and Chief Physicist, Department of Radiation Oncology, University of California, Davis, School of Medicine, Davis, California
Breathing Synchronized Radiotherapy

David A. Larson, MD, PhD
Professor of Radiation Oncology and Neurosurgery, University of California, San Francisco, School of Medicine, San Francisco, California
Radiosurgery

Steven Larson, MD
Professor of Radiology, Weill Medical College of Cornell University; Chief, Nuclear Medicine, Department of Radiology, Memorial Sloan-Kettering Cancer Center, New York, New York
Cancer of the Thyroid

Quynh-Thu Le, MD
Associate Professor, Stanford University School of Medicine, Stanford, California
Sarcomas of Soft Tissue

Nancy Lee, MD
Assistant Professor, Weill Medical College of Cornell University; Assistant Attending Radiation Oncologist, Memorial Sloan-Kettering Cancer Center, New York, New York
Head and Neck; Cancer of the Nasopharynx; Cancer of the Oral Cavity; Cancer of the Larynx

Steven A. Leibel, MD
Chairman, Department of Radiation Oncology, Memorial Sloan-Kettering Cancer Center, New York, New York
Primary and Metastatic Brain Tumors in Adults; Sarcomas of Soft Tissue

Alan A. Lewin, MD
Clinical Professor, University of Miami School of Medicine; Director, Department of Radiation Oncology, Baptist Hospital, Miami, Florida
High Dose Rate Brachytherapy

Gloria C. Li, PhD
Professor, Department of Biophysics and Physiology, Weill Medical College of Cornell University, Attending Biophysicist, Departments of Radiation Oncology and Medical Physics, Memorial Sloan-Kettering Cancer Center, New York, New York
Hyperthermia

Allen S. Lichter, MD
Professor of Radiation and Oncology and Dean, University of Michigan Medical School, Ann Arbor, Michigan
Cancer of the Breast

Norbert J. Liebsch, MD, PhD
Instructor, Department of Radiation Oncology, Harvard Medical School; Associate Radiation Oncologist, Massachusetts General Hospital, Boston, Massachusetts
Skull Base Tumors: Chordomas and Chondrosarcomas

Patricia Lillis-Hearne, MD
Consultant to the Surgeon General, US Army Medical Command, San Antonio, Texas
Cancer of the Pancreas

C. Clifton Ling, PhD
Chairman, Department of Medical Physics, Memorial Sloan-Kettering Cancer Center, New York, New York
Three-Dimensional Conformal Radiotherapy and Intensity-Modulated Radiotherapy

David E. Linstadt, MD
Assistant Clinical Professor of Radiation Oncology, University of California, San Francisco, School of Medicine, San Francisco; Chief, Radiation Oncology, Sutter Roseville Medical Center, Roseville, California
Spinal Cord Tumors

Jay S. Loeffler, MD
Andres Soriano Professor, Department of Radiation Oncology, Harvard Medical School; Chair, Department of Radiation, Massachusetts General Hospital, Boston, Massachusetts
Radiosurgery

Gikas S. Mageras, PhD
Member, Memorial Hospital, and Attending Physicist, Department of Medical Physics, Memorial Sloan-Kettering Cancer Center, New York, New York
Imaging in Radiation Oncology

Lynda R. Mandell, MD, PhD
Professor, Departments of Pediatrics and Radiation Oncology, Mount Sinai School of Medicine of the City University of New York; Attending Physician, Department of Radiation Oncology, Mount Sinai Medical Center, New York, New York
Pediatric Leukemias and Lymphomas

Lawrence W. Margolis, MD
Clinical Professor Emeritus of Radiation Oncology, University of California, San Francisco, School of Medicine; Mount Zion Hospital of UCSF, San Francisco, California
Cancer of the Skin

Beryl McCormick, MD
Associate Professor of Radiation Oncology in Medicine, Weill Medical College of Cornell University; Clinical Director and Attending Radiation Oncologist, Memorial Sloan-Kettering Cancer Center; Associate Attending Physician, New York Hospital, New York, New York
Retinoblastoma

Bruce D. Minsky, MD
Professor of Radiation Oncology, Weill Medical College of Cornell University; Vice Chairman, Department of Radiation Oncology, Memorial Sloan-Kettering Cancer Center, New York, New York
Cancer of the Esophagus; Cancer of the Stomach; Cancer of the Colon; Cancer of the Rectum; Cancer of the Anal Canal

John E. Munzenrider, MD
Associate Professor, Department of Radiation Oncology, Harvard Medical School; Associate Radiation Oncologist, Massachusetts General Hospital, Boston, Massachusetts
Skull Base Tumors: Chordomas and Chondrosarcomas

Subir Nag, MD
Professor, Ohio State University School of Medicine; Chief of Brachytherapy Service, Ohio State University Hospital, Columbus, Ohio
High Dose Rate Brachytherapy

Ashwatha Narayana, MD
Assistant Attending Radiation Oncologist, Department of Radiation Oncology, Memorial Sloan-Kettering Cancer Center, New York, New York
Primary and Metastatic Brain Tumors in Adults

Dattatreyudu Nori, MD, FACR, FACRO
Professor of Radiology, Weill Medical College of Cornell University; Chairman, Department of Radiation Oncology, New York–Presbyterian Hospital; Director of the Cancer Center, New York Hospital Queens, Flushing, New York, New York
Cancer of the Endometrium

Colin G. Orton, PhD
Professor Emeritus of Radiation Oncology, Wayne State University School of Medicine; Gershenson Radiation Oncology Center, Harper Hospital, Detroit, Michigan
High Dose Rate Brachytherapy

Paula L. Petti, PhD
Associate Professor, Department of Radiation Oncology, University of California, San Francisco, School of Medicine, San Francisco, California
Principles of Radiation Physics; Particle Radiation Therapy

Theodore L. Phillips, MD
Professor, Department of Radiation Oncology, University of California, San Francisco, School of Medicine, San Francisco, California
Intraoperative Radiation Therapy; Cancer of the Oral Cavity; Cancer of the Larynx; Sarcomas of Soft Tissue

Jean Pouliot, PhD
Associate Professor of Radiation Oncology, University of California, San Francisco, School of Medicine; Medical Physicist, Department of Radiation Oncology, UCSF Comprehensive Cancer Center, San Francisco, California
High Dose Rate Brachytherapy

David C. Price, MD
Professor of Radiology and Medicine and Chief, Clinical Nuclear Medicine, University of California, San Francisco, School of Medicine, San Francisco, California
Cancer of the Thyroid

Jeanne M. Quivey, MD
Professor, Radiation Oncology, University of California, San Francisco, California
Uveal Melanoma

Rachel Abrams Rabinovitch, MD
Associate Professor, Department of Radiation Oncology, University of Colorado Comprehensive Cancer Center, Aurora, Colorado
Cancer of the Kidney

Daniel R. Reed, DO
Resident Physician, University of Washington Medical Center, Seattle, Washington
Skull Base Tumors: Chemodectomas and Nonchromaffin Paragangliomas

Mark Roach III, MD
Professor of Radiation Oncology and Urology, Vice Chair, Radiation Oncology, Director of Clinical Research, University of California, San Francisco, San Francisco, California
Cancer of the Prostate

Jonathan E. Rosenberg, MD
Clinical Instructor, Department of Medicine, Division of Hematology/Oncology, University of California, San Francisco, Comprehensive Cancer Center, San Francisco, California, United States
Cancer of the Bladder

Seth A. Rosenthal, MD
Assistant Clinical Professor, Department of Radiation Oncology, University of California, San Francisco, School of Medicine, San Francisco, and University of California, Davis, School of Medicine, Davis; Chairman, Radiation Oncology, and Attending Radiation Oncologist, Radiological Associates of Sacramento, Sacramento, California
Benign Disease

Kenneth E. Rosenzweig, MD
Assistant Attending Radiation Oncologist, Department of Radiation Oncology, Memorial Sloan-Kettering Cancer Center, New York, New York
Thorax; Cancer of the Nasal Cavity and Paranasal Sinuses; Tumors of the Lung, Pleura, and Mediastinum

Lawrence N. Rothenberg, PhD
Associate Professor of Radiology, Weill Medical College of Cornell University; Attending Physicist, Memorial Hospital, and Clinical Member, Memorial Sloan-Kettering Cancer Center, New York, New York
Imaging in Radiation Oncology

Anthony H. Russell, MD
Associate Professor of Radiation Oncology, Harvard Medical School; Associate Radiation Oncologist and Head of Gynecologic Radiation Oncology, Massachusetts General Hospital and Boston Medical Center, Boston, Massachusetts
Cancer of the Vulva

Janice K. Ryu, MD
Associate Professor, Radiation Oncology, University of California, Davis, School of Medicine, Davis, California
Cancer of the Nasal Cavity and Paranasal Sinuses

Roberto Santiago, MD
Hospital of the University of Pennsylvania, Philadelphia, Department of Radiation Oncology, Pennsylvania
Clinical Applications of Photodynamic Therapy

Amy C. Schefler, MD
Weill Medical College of Cornell University; New York–Presbyterian Hospital, New York, New York
Retinoblastoma

Tracey Schefter, MD
Assistant Professor and Residency Program Director (Radiation Oncology), University of Colorado Comprehensive Cancer Center, Department of Radiation Oncology, Aurora, Colorado
Cancer of the Kidney

Karen Schupak, MD
Department of Radiation Oncology, Weill Medical College of Cornell University, New York, New York; Chief, Radiation Oncology, Memorial Sloan-Kettering at St. Clare's, Denville, New Jersey
Sarcomas of Bone

Roy B. Sessions, MD
Professor of Otolaryngology and Head/Neck Surgery, Albert Einstein College of Medicine of Yeshiva University, Bronx; Chairman, Otolaryngology – Head/Neck Surgery, Beth Israel Medical Center; Associate Director, Continuum Cancer Centers of New York, New York, New York
Cancer of the Oropharynx

Brenda Shank, MD, PhD, FACR
Clinical Professor, Department of Radiation Oncology, University of California, San Francisco, School of Medicine, San Francisco; Medical Director, J. C. Robinson, MD, Regional Cancer Center, Doctors Medical Center, San Pablo, California
Total Body Irradiation

Dennis C. Shrieve, MD, PhD
Professor and Chair, Department of Radiation Oncology, University of Utah School of Medicine, Salt Lake City, Utah
Radiosurgery

Eric J. Small, MD
Professor of Medicine and Urology, University of California, San Francisco, San Francisco, California
Cancer of the Bladder

Penny K. Sneed, MD
Professor in Residence, University of California, San Francisco, San Francisco, California
Hyperthermia

Marnee Spierer, MD
Resident, Department of Radiation Oncology, Memorial Sloan-Kettering Cancer Center, New York, New York
Neuroblastoma and Wilms' Tumor

Paul R. Stauffer, MSEE
Associate Adjunct Professor, Department of Radiation Oncology, University of California, San Francisco, School of Medicine, San Francisco, California
Hyperthermia

Gerard J. Stege, PhD
University of Nymegen Hospital, Nymegen, The Netherlands
Hyperthermia

Richard G. Stock, MD
Professor and Chairman, Department of Radiation Oncology, Mount Sinai School of Medicine and Medical Center, New York, New York
Cancer of the Vagina

Patrick S. Swift, MD
Medical Director of Radiation Oncology, Alta Bates Comprehensive Cancer Center, Berkeley, California
Cancer of the Thyroid; Cancer of the Uterine Cervix; HIV-Related Malignancies

Robert Takamiya, MD
Chief Resident, Department of Radiation Oncology, University of California, San Francisco, San Francisco, California
Uveal Melanoma

Welala Tereffe, MD
Resident, Memorial Sloan-Kettering Cancer Center, New York, New York
Neuroblastoma and Wilms' Tumor

Raul C. Urtasun, MD
Professor Emeritus, Department of Oncology, Cross Cancer Institute and University of Alberta Faculty of Medicine; Radiation Oncologist, Cross Cancer Institute, Edmonton, Alberta, Canada
Chemical Modifiers of Radiation

Lynn J. Verhey, PhD
Professor, Department of Radiation Oncology, University of California, San Francisco; UCSF Comprehensive Cancer Center, San Francisco, California
Principles of Radiation Physics

Raquel T. Wagman, MD
Assistant Attending, Radiation Oncology, Memorial Sloan-Kettering Cancer Center, New York, New York
Cancer of the Stomach; Cancer of the Liver, Bile Duct, and Gallbladder

Kent Wallner, MD
Associate Professor, Department of Radiation Oncology, University of Washington; Chief, Radiation Oncology, Veterans Affairs, Puget Sound Health Care System; Staff, Radiation Oncology, Group Health Cooperative, Seattle, Washington
Cancer of the Prostate

William M. Wara, MD
Professor and Chairman, Department of Radiation Oncology, University of California, San Francisco, San Francisco, California
Pediatric Central Nervous System Tumors

Michael D. Weil, MD
Manager, Sirius Medicine, LLC, Fort Collins, Colorado
Pediatric Central Nervous System Tumors

Moody D. Wharam Jr, MD, FACR
Professor of Radiation Oncology, Department of Radiation Oncology and Radiation Molecular Sciences, Johns Hopkins University School of Medicine; Sidney Kimmel Comprehensive Cancer Center at Johns Hopkins, Baltimore, Maryland
Pediatric Bone and Soft Tissue Tumors

Richard B. Wilder, MD
Department of Radiation Oncology, MD Anderson Cancer Center, Houston, Texas
Cancer of the Skin

Suzanne Wolden, MD
Assistant Professor, Weill Medical College of Cornell University; Assistant Member, Memorial Hospital, and Assistant Attending Radiation Oncologist, Memorial Sloan-Kettering Cancer Center, New York, New York
Neuroblastoma and Wilms' Tumor

Harvey B. Wolkov, MD
Associate Clinical Professor, Department of Radiation Oncology, University of California, Davis, Davis, California; Medical Director, Radiation Oncology Center, Sutter Cancer Center, Sacramento, California
Intraoperative Radiation Therapy

Ping Xia, PhD
Assistant Professor, Department of Radiation Oncology, University of California, San Francisco, School of Medicine, San Francisco, California
Three-Dimensional Conformal Radiotherapy and Intensity-Modulated Radiotherapy

Joachim Yahalom, MD
Professor of Radiation Oncology in Medicine, Weill Medical College of Cornell University; Member and Attending Radiation Oncologist, Memorial Sloan-Kettering Cancer Center, New York, New York
Non-Hodgkin's Lymphoma; Plasma Cell Tumors; Multiple Myeloma and Solitary Plasmacytoma

Yoshiya Yamada, MD
Clinical Assistant Radiation Oncologist, Department of Radiation Oncology, Memorial Sloan-Kettering Cancer Center, New York, New York
Cancer of the Male Urethra and Penis

Marco Zaider, PhD
Professor of Physics in Radiology, Weill Medical College of Cornell University; Attending Physicist, Department of Medical Physics, Memorial Sloan-Kettering Cancer Center, New York, New York
Aspects of Brachytherapy Physics

Michael J. Zelefsky, MD
Associate Professor of Radiation Oncology, Weill Medical College of Cornell University; Chief, Brachytherapy Service, Memorial Sloan-Kettering Cancer Center, New York, New York
Instruments and Techniques in Brachytherapy; Cancer of the Hypopharynx; Cancer of the Bladder

Foreword
to the First Edition

It is a great pleasure to have the opportunity to write the foreword for this excellent and much needed textbook. A textbook should be comprehensive to allow the formal study of a subject by the student. It should include the underlying principles, discuss the current state of our knowledge and practice, and provide the reader with information sufficient to understand new developments that will affect the future of our profession. This is a tall order indeed, but I believe this textbook fulfills these criteria in a fashion conducive either to easy reference or to complete reading.

The first section considers the principles of the sciences underlying radiation oncology. This includes basic radiobiology applied in clinical practice, as demonstrated by the chapters on fractionation and predictors of radiation response. Physics is a basic science required for the clinical practice of radiation oncology, and it is discussed in detail. Included are comprehensive sections on external beam treatment, which cover the topics of immobilization, simulation, and treatment planning. Specialized areas such as brachytherapy, total body radiation, intraoperative radiation, and the emerging importance of conformal radiotherapy are also covered.

All considerations of radiation oncology in the treatment of cancer should be presented in a multidisciplinary context. This requires that a textbook include the principles underlying such multidisciplinary treatment. These principles are covered in the chapters on chemotherapy and radiation and imaging in radiation oncology, and in the discussions on the use of the various diagnostic and treatment modalities in the disease site chapters.

The second section of the book is devoted to the specific cancers. Although this is a textbook on radiation oncology, it is important to understand the specific disease being discussed; therefore, epidemiologic considerations, molecular biology, and genetics as well as the anatomic nature of the disease are presented as prerequisites to defining the role of radiation therapy for each tumor type. This is accomplished with appropriate narrative and diagrammatic information on the nature and spread of the disease. The volume is rich in images necessary for understanding the principles related to radiation therapy.

The final section of the book is devoted to emerging areas of radiation oncology that have potential importance as future therapeutic approaches. These include particle radiation therapy, hyperthermia, gene therapy, the novel use of immunologic radioisotope carriers, and nonionizing focal energy deposition.

As a practicing radiation oncologist, I look forward to having this important reference source close at hand as I engage in the increasingly complex clinical care of cancer patients.

SAMUEL HELLMAN, MD

Preface

The second edition of the *Textbook of Radiation Oncology* is designed to emphasize changes in radiation physics, biology, and clinical radiation oncology that have occurred in the field over the past five years. This textbook has been the outgrowth of a long collaboration between the two editors and a shared recognition that a text was needed in our field that taught the reader how to treat for cure. We thought that this could be done best by presenting a reasonably uniform treatment philosophy. Thus, we have mainly chosen chapter authors who are on the faculty at our two institutions, were previously on the faculty, or were trained by us as residents and fellows.

Recent advances in physics and the introduction of three-dimensional conformal therapy and intensity-modulated therapy have been of key importance, and we have emphasized these approaches. A large number of color illustrations have been included to demonstrate these techniques. We have also stressed the importance of anatomic tumor spread so that the reader can make rational decisions about target volumes rather than memorize "classical" ports. Precise tumor targeting requires the use of imaging, including magnetic resonance imaging, helical computed tomography and positron emission tomography. We have emphasized the importance of these imaging modalities to our specialty with the introduction of new chapters on imaging, specific to anatomic tumor sites. Chapters on breathing synchronized radiotherapy and extracranial stereotactic radioablation have also been added to this edition.

Finally, advances in tumor genetics and molecular radiobiology are playing an ever increasingly important role in the practice of radiation oncology. This edition of the textbook highlights what is known today about these important topics. However, the field is moving ahead rapidly, and the reader is urged to pursue the basic science literature. Both of us hope that the second edition of the *Textbook of Radiation Oncology* meets your needs as a clinician studying or practicing the specialty.

STEVEN A. LEIBEL, M.D.

THEODORE L. PHILLIPS, M.D.

Acknowledgments

The task of assembling a major textbook requires the collective effort of many individuals. We wish to thank Dolores Meloni, Medical Editor; Jennifer Shreiner, Developmental Editor; Pete Faber, Production Manager, and Gene Harris, Designer, at Elsevier for bringing the second edition of our book to a reality. Special gratitude also goes to our administrative assistants, Eva DeVos, Francis Che, and Sam Mui who tirelessly managed the vast amount of correspondence and paperwork necessary to bring the work to fruition. We also thank Pam Akazawa who supplied many of the conformal and IMRT treatment plans contained in the disease site chapters.

STEVEN A. LEIBEL, M.D.

THEODORE L. PHILLIPS, M.D.

Contents

Color Plate Section Following Page xxii

Color Plates

PLATE 1

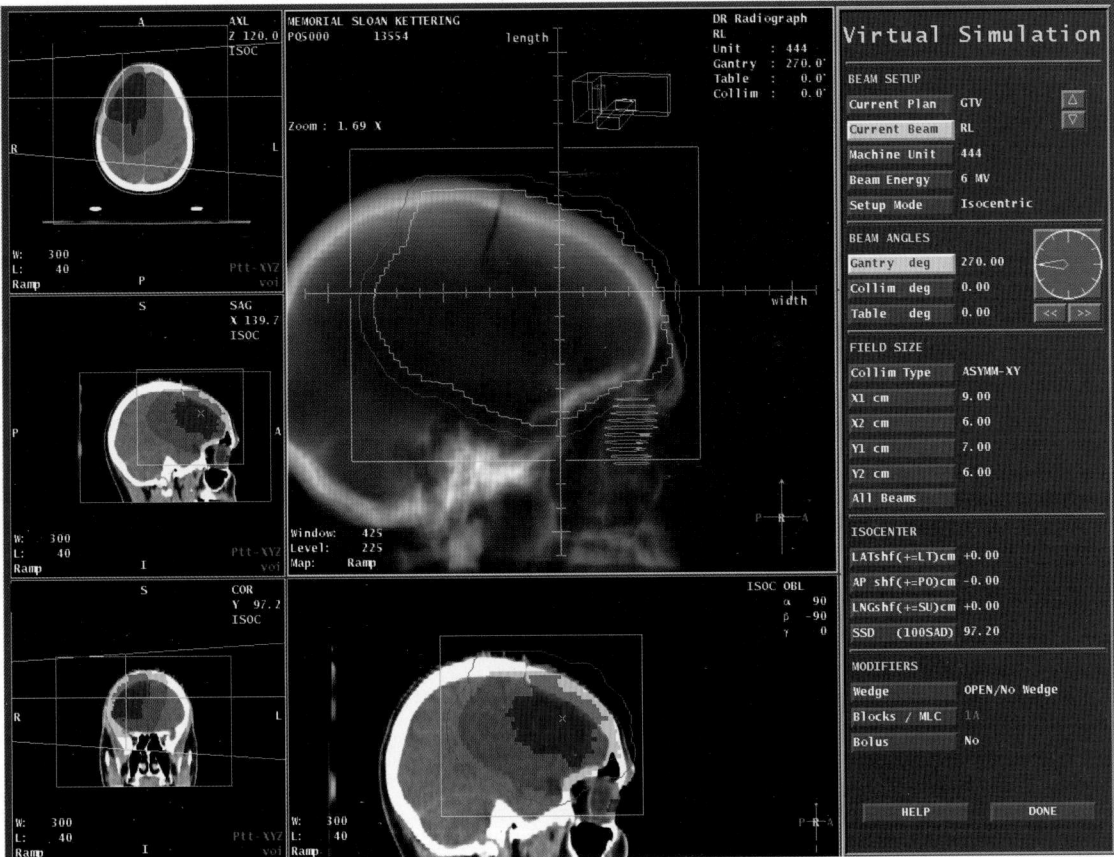

Figure 7–11. Example computed tomography simulation display (AcqSim, Philips Medical Systems, Andover, Mass.). Upper right image is a beam's eye view digitally reconstructed radiograph with planning target volume outlined in *yellow*, treatment field aperture in *blue*. Right panel shows simulated beam setup controls.

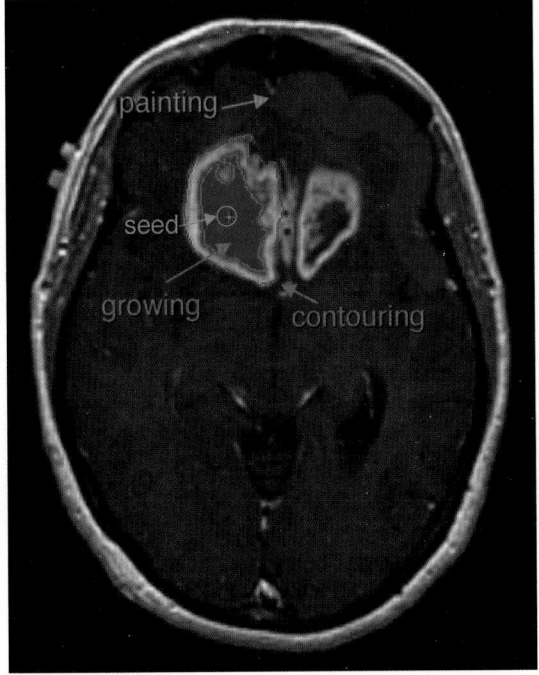

Figure 7–22. Segmentation of a magnetic resonance brain tumor image through contour, painting, and region growing.

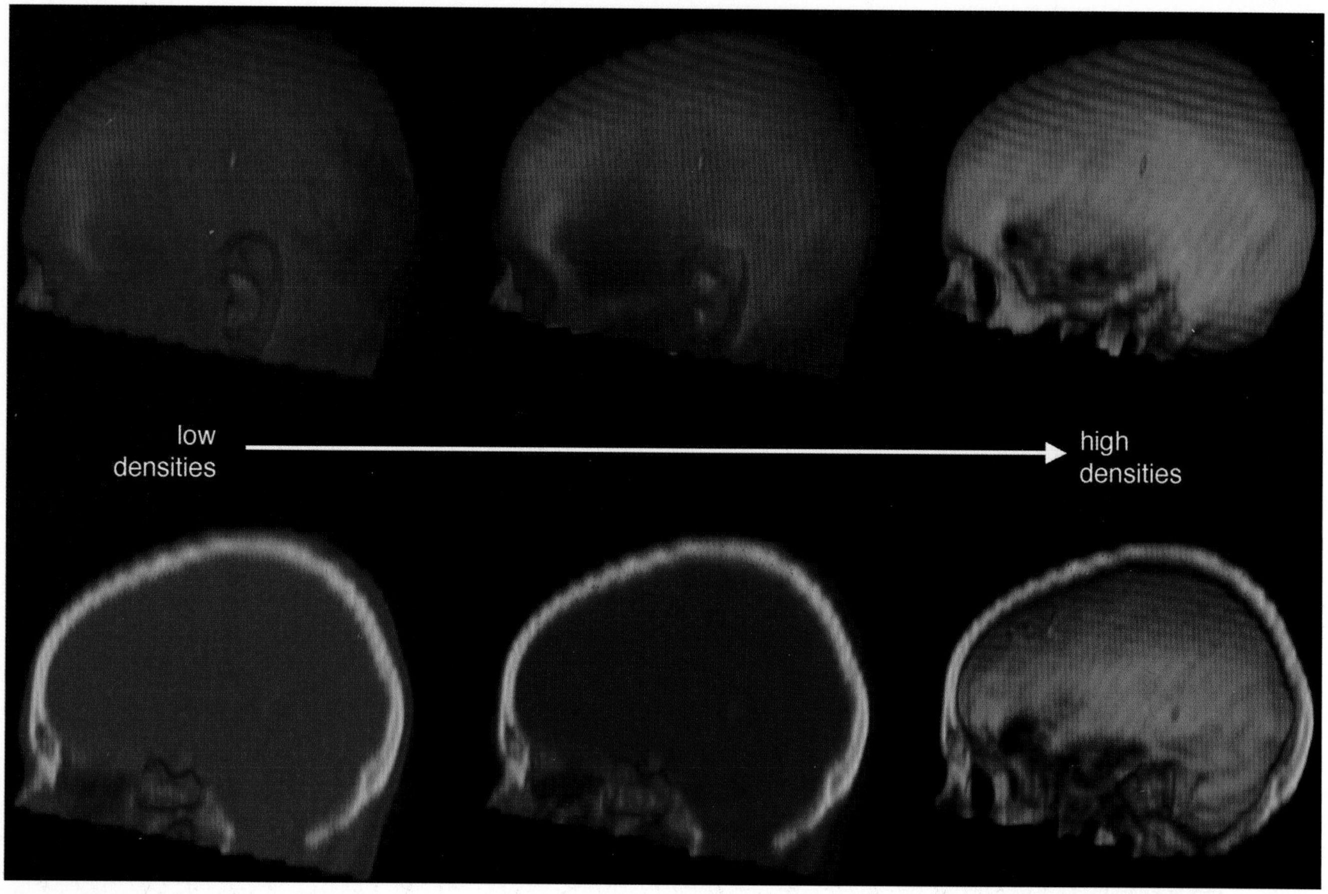

PLATE 2

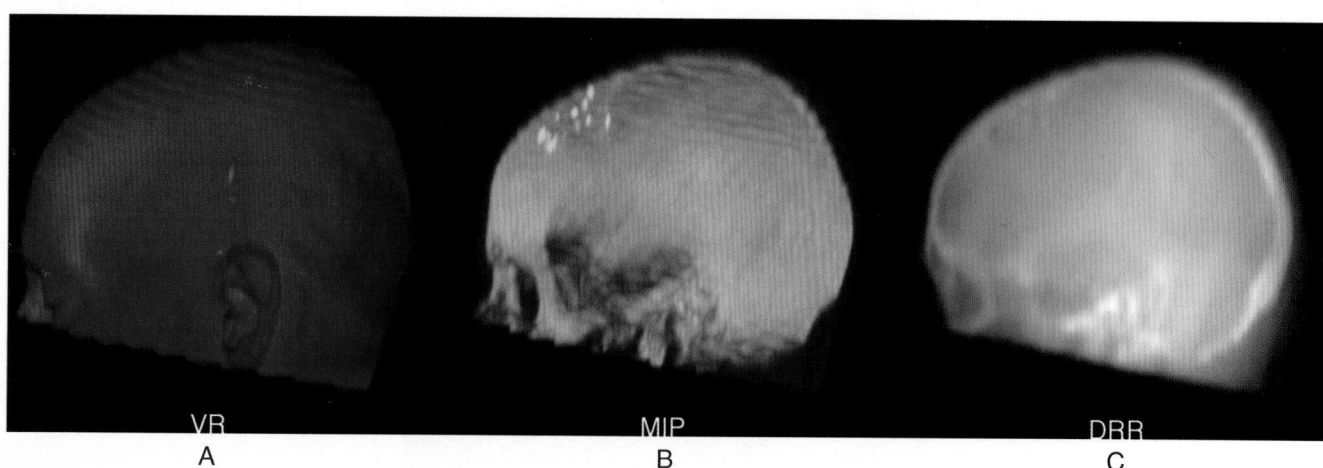

Figure 7–25. Volume rendering of a head computed tomographic image with variable transparency (full and cut head).

Figure 7-26. Comparison of VR (**A**) with maximum intensity projection (**B**) and digitally reconstructed radiograph (**C**).

PLATE 3

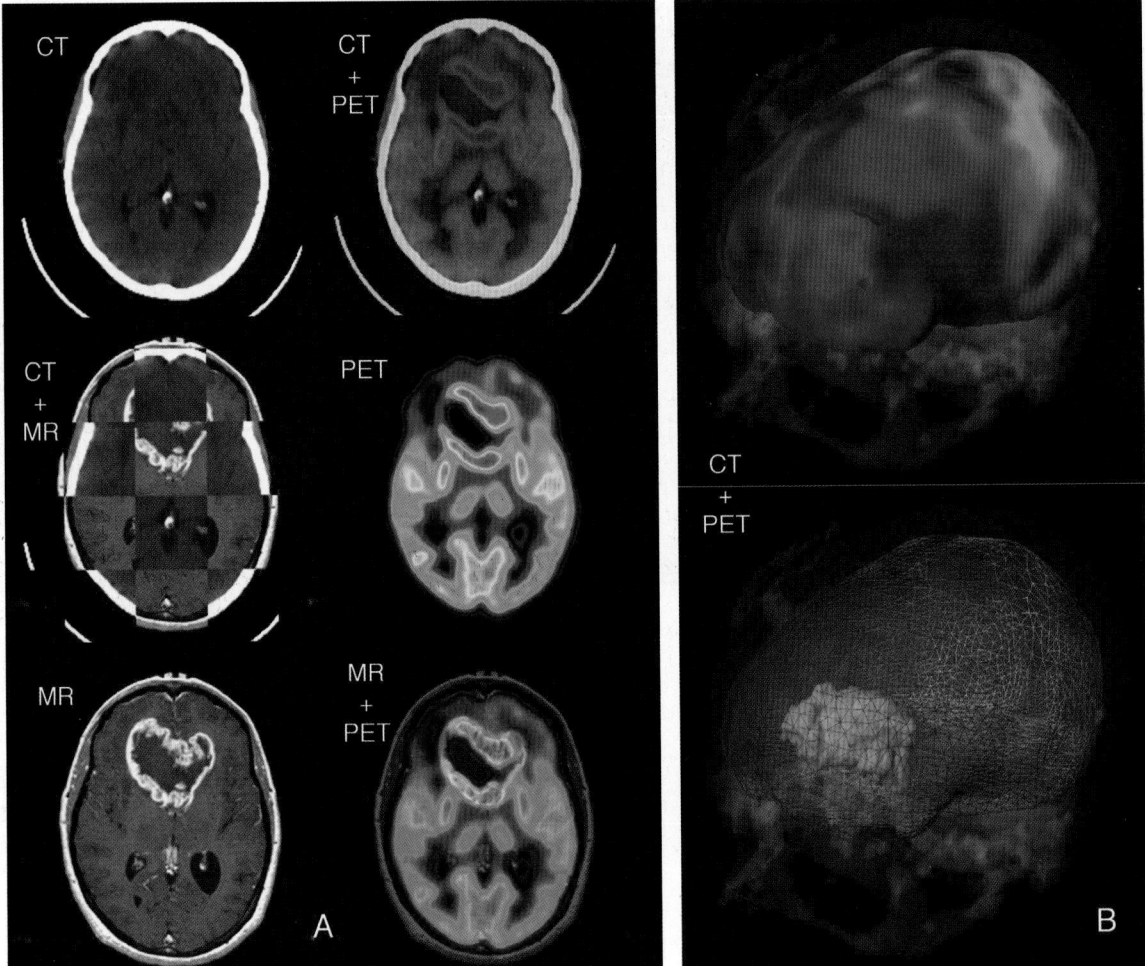

Figure 7–27. Multimodality (MM) visualization of a brain tumor. **A,** Multi-planar reconstruction (side-by-side, checkerboard and colorwash modes) of computed tomography (CT), magnetic resonance (MR), and positron emission tomography (PET) of the same patient after spatial registration. **B,** surface rendering of the skull and brain from CT, tumor from MR, and color from the PET. MM volume rendering can follow similar paradigms.

PLATE 4

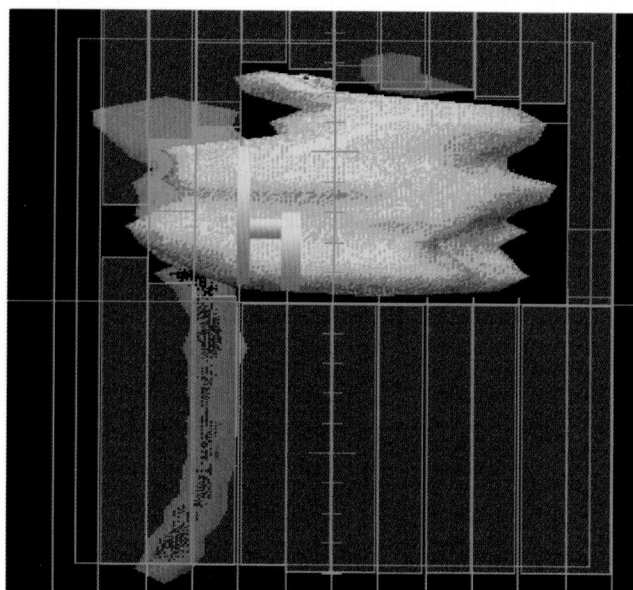

Figure 8–3. Beam's eye view of a right anterior oblique field for a head and neck patient in the supine position showing multileaf collimator (MLC) beam shaping. The planning target volume (PTV) is depicted in yellow, brainstem in green, cord in purple, and chiasm in red. Note how the MLC leaves (*transparent green*) are shaped to conform to the PTV.

Figure 8–5. A, An example of dose volume histogram (DVH)-based dose constraints for a commercial inverse planning system (Corvus, 4.0 NOMOS Corporation, Sewickley, Pa.).

Target Name		Type		Goal (Gy)	Vol Below Goal (%)	Min (Gy)	Max (Gy)	I
GTV-target		Basic		64.0	5	54.0	72.0	
CTV1-target		Basic		54.0	5	52.0	64.0	

Sensitive Structure Name		Type		Limit (Gy)	Vol Above Limit (%)	Min (Gy)	Max (Gy)	I
Tissue		Basic Tissue		54.0	0	0.0	54.0	
Spinal Cord		Basic Structure		35.0	5	20.0	40.0	
LT-Parotid		BU Structure		20.0	10	10.0	45.0	
RT-Parotid		BU Structure		20.0	10	10.0	45.0	
Other 1		Basic Structure		45.0	10	20.0	54.0	
LT-Eye		Basic Structure		45.0	10	20.0	54.0	
Brain-Stem		Basic Structure		35.0	10	20.0	45.0	
LT_TMJ		Basic Structure		30.0	10	20.0	40.0	
RT_TMJ		Basic Structure		30.0	10	20.0	40.0	
Mandible		Basic Structure		40.0	10	20.0	54.0	

A

PLATE 5

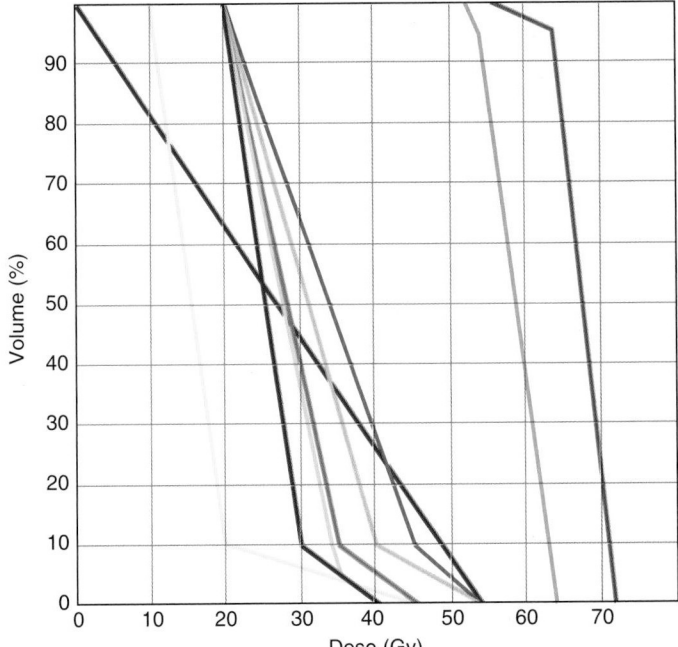

Figure 8–5. B, Simplified DVH based on three-point constraints.

B

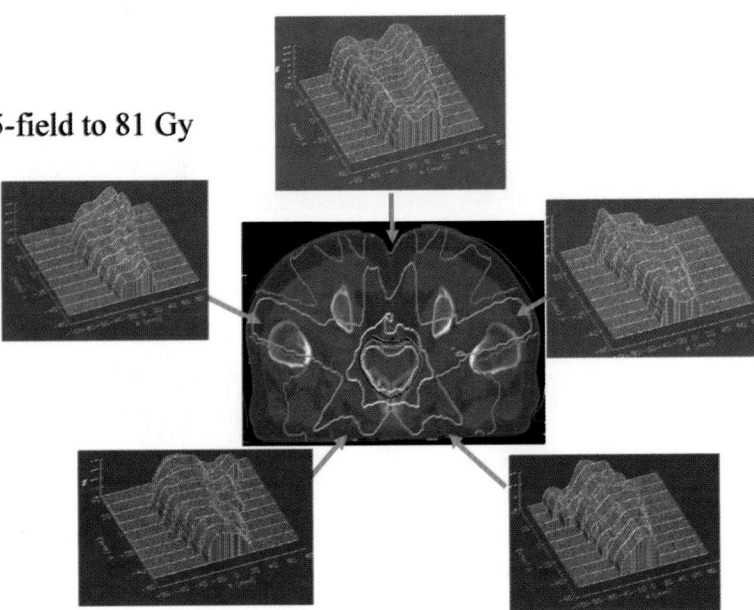

5-field to 81 Gy

Figure 8–6. The intensity profiles for all 5 beams in a typical IMRT prostate treatment to 81 Gy (patient is in the prone position). Note the decreased beam intensity in the center of the posterior field, designed to reduce dose to the rectum.

PLATE 6

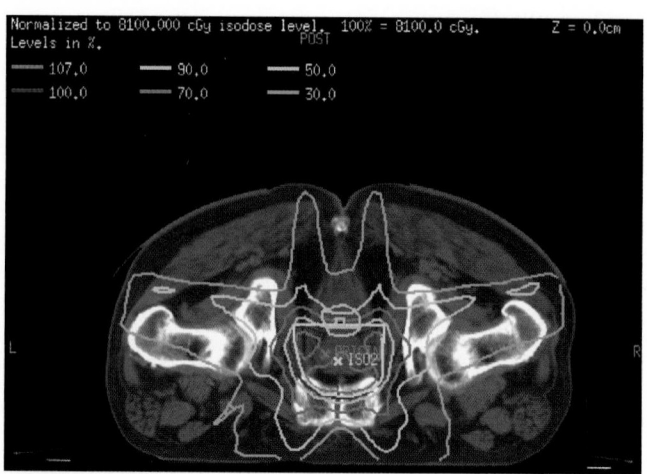

A

Figure 8–21. Typical dose distributions for a 5-field intensity-modulated radiotherapy prostate treatment to 81 Gy. See (**A**) transverse (axial) plane, (**B**) coronal plane, and (**C**) sagittal plane. The planning target volume is shown in yellow, and the rectal wall in blue.

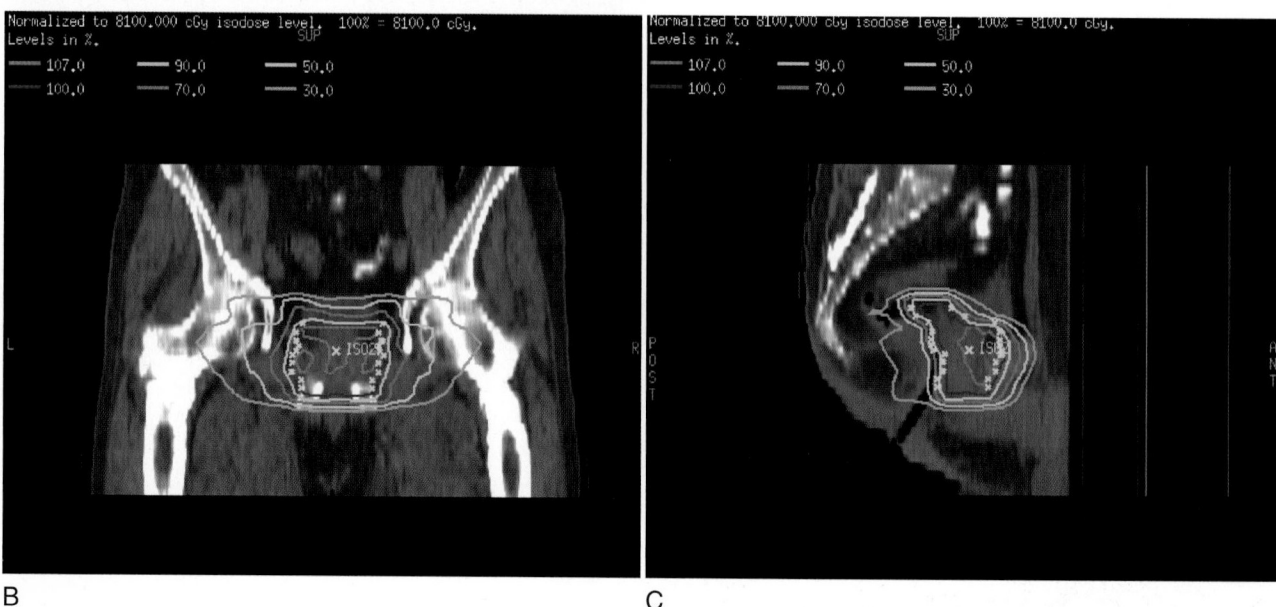

B

C

Figure 8–25. *Region of regret* plot showing the prescription isodose surface *(white)*, and regions of the planning target volume receiving less than the prescription dose *(red)* for traditional, 3DCRT, and IMRT plans. The brainstem and cord are shown in *blue*, and the eyes in *purple*.

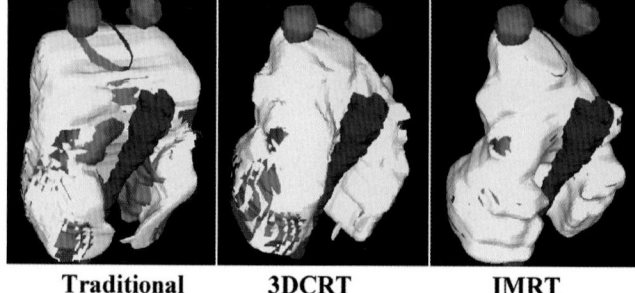

Traditional   **3DCRT**   **IMRT**

PLATE 7

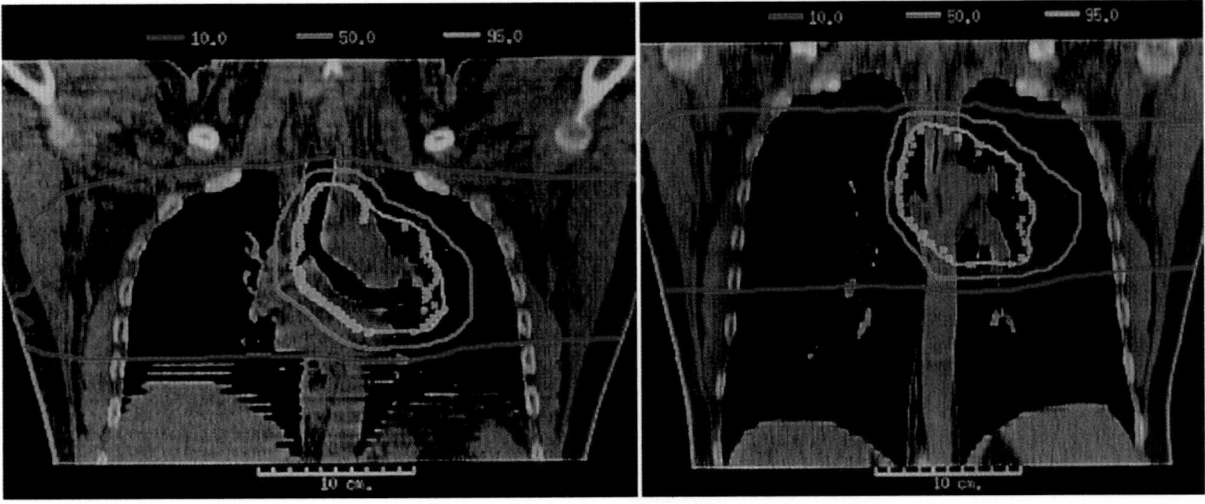

Figure 9–10. Comparison of (**A**) free-breathing and (**B**) deep inspiration breath hold (DIBH) treatment plans. Images are coronal planes through the isocenter for the same patient. Lines representing the 10%, 50%, and 90% isodose levels are in *red*, *green*, and *blue*, respectively. (From Rosenzweig KE, Hanley J, Mah D: The DIBH technique in treatment of inoperable non–small-cell lung cancer. *Int J Radiat Oncol Biol Phys.* 2000;48:81.)

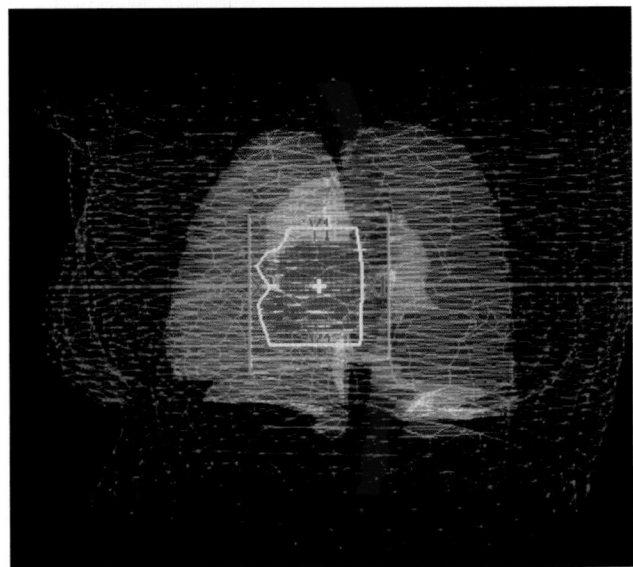

Figure 9–25. Beam's-eye view for a lung patient. In this oblique view, the outer contour (skin), lungs, spinal cord, and target volumes are visible. The aperture is drawn to cover the planning target volume but to exclude the cord.

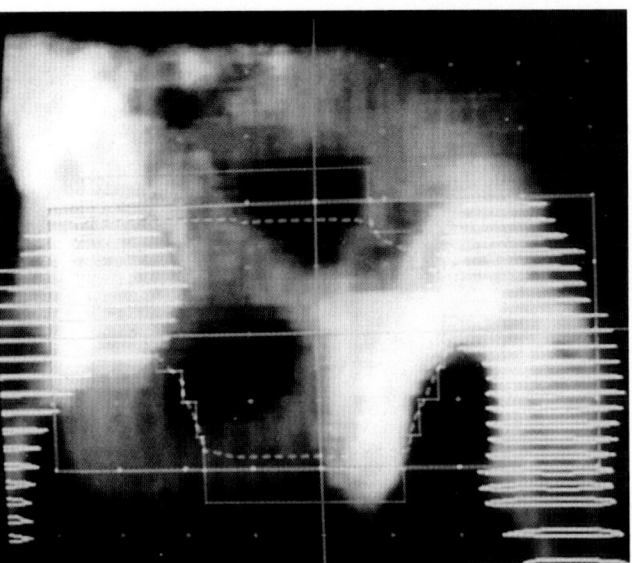

Figure 9–26. Digitally reconstructed radiograph for right-anterior-oblique treatment field for a prostate patient. The contours for the femurs (*in yellow*) have been projected to enhance the visibility of the femurs. The MLC aperture outline, collimators, cross hairs, and graticule points are also displayed.

PLATE 8

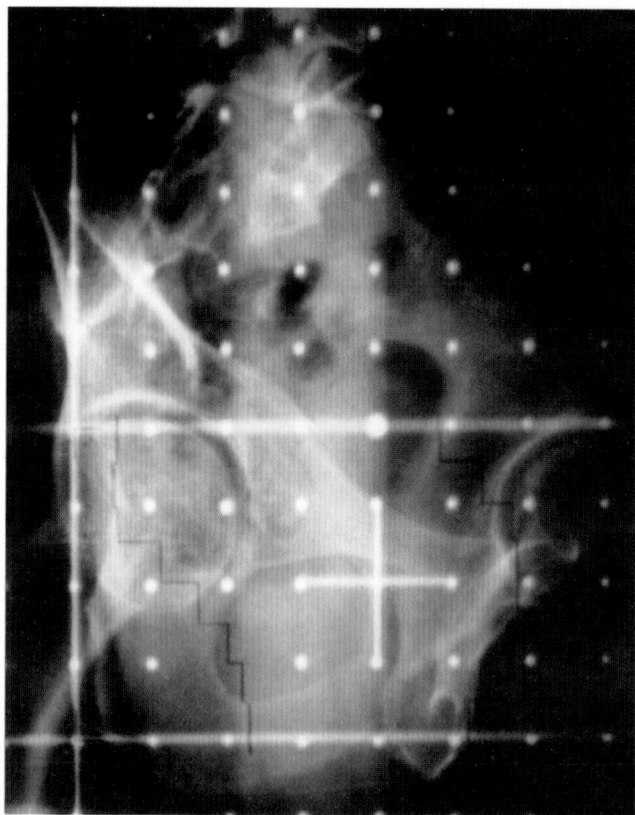

Figure 9–27. Simulation radiograph for the right-anterior-oblique beam on which the MLC aperture outline (shown in Figure 9-26) has been transferred.

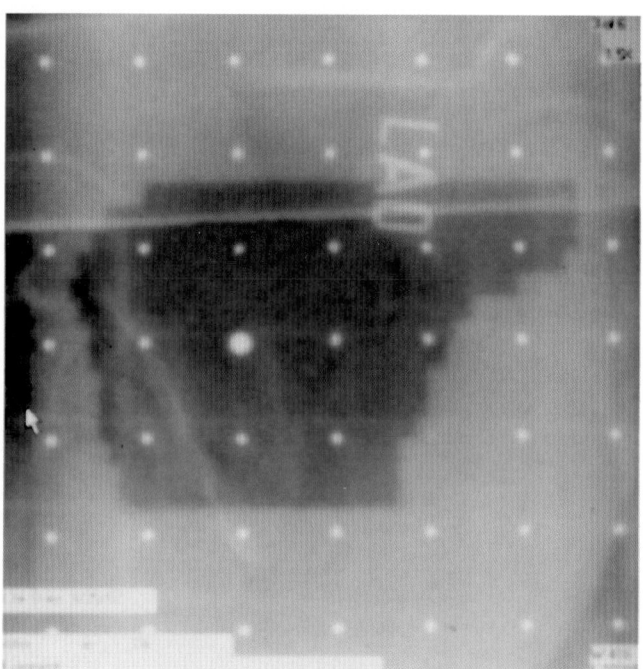

Figure 9–32. Portal image for an oblique beam for a prostate patient obtained with an amorphus silicon detector.

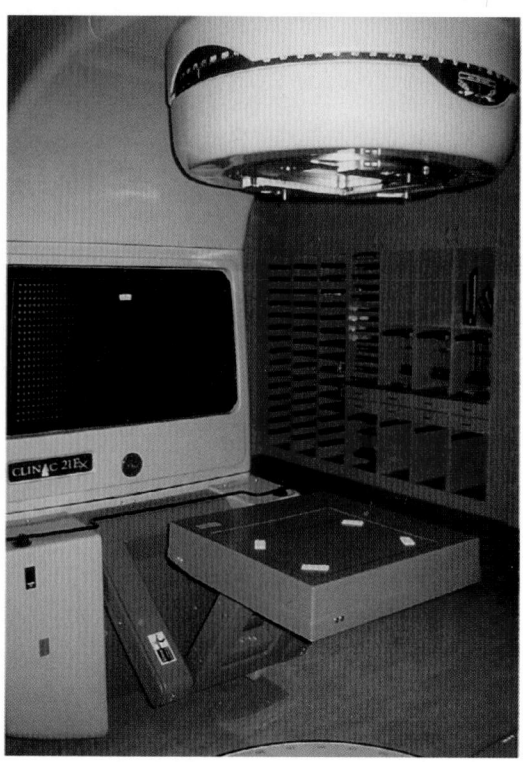

Figure 9–33. An amorphus silicon detector attached to a therapy machine. The motorized mount allows detector movement.

PLATE 9

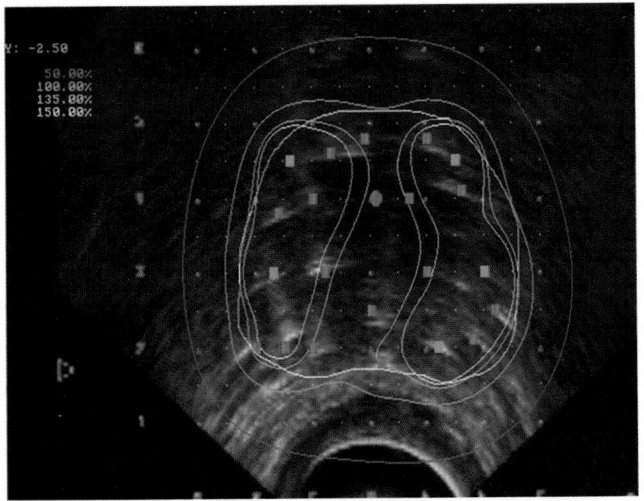

Figure 11–10. Planning for a permanent prostate implant. In this two-dimensional ultrasound image the *white line* delineates the prostate and the 100% isodose line (PD = 144 Gy) is shown in *green*. *Green dots* indicate occupied seeds and *red dots* show empty seed locations along needles.

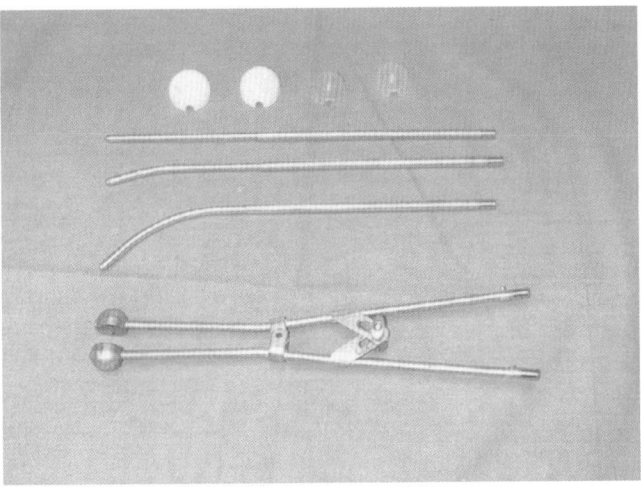

Figure 11–15. The Henshke applicator consists of an intrauterine tandem (three different shapes are shown) and two semi-spherical vaginal ovoids.

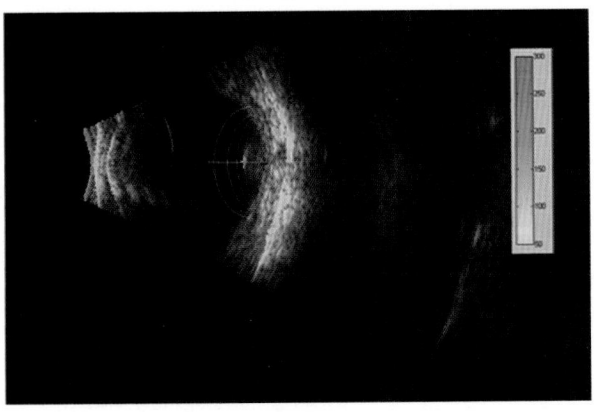

B

Figure 11–14. Schematic representation of an eye-plaque applicator (*left*, from[144]). The right panel (B) is an ultrasound image of an ocular tumor; also shown are isodose distributions. (Left panel, from Chiu-Tsao S-T: I-125 Episcleral ete plaque for treatment of intra-ocular malignancies. In Williamson JF, Thomadsen BR, Nath R, eds. *Brachytherapy Physics, AAPM Summer School 1994*. Madison, Wisc: American Association of Physicists in Medicine; 1994:451.)

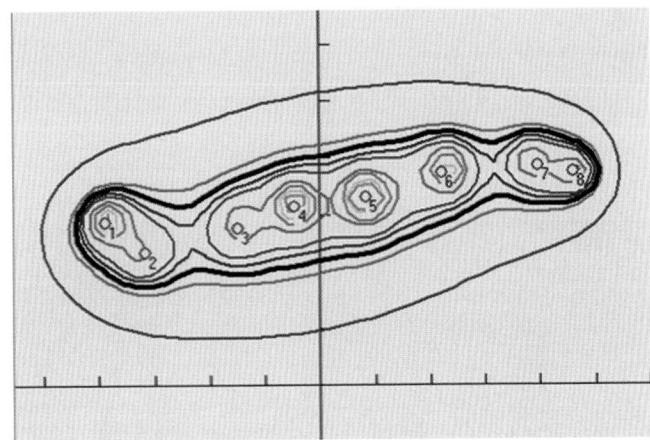

Figure 11–17. Planning for a sarcoma treatment: The heavy dark line surrounds all catheters and is taken as the prescription dose.

PLATE 10

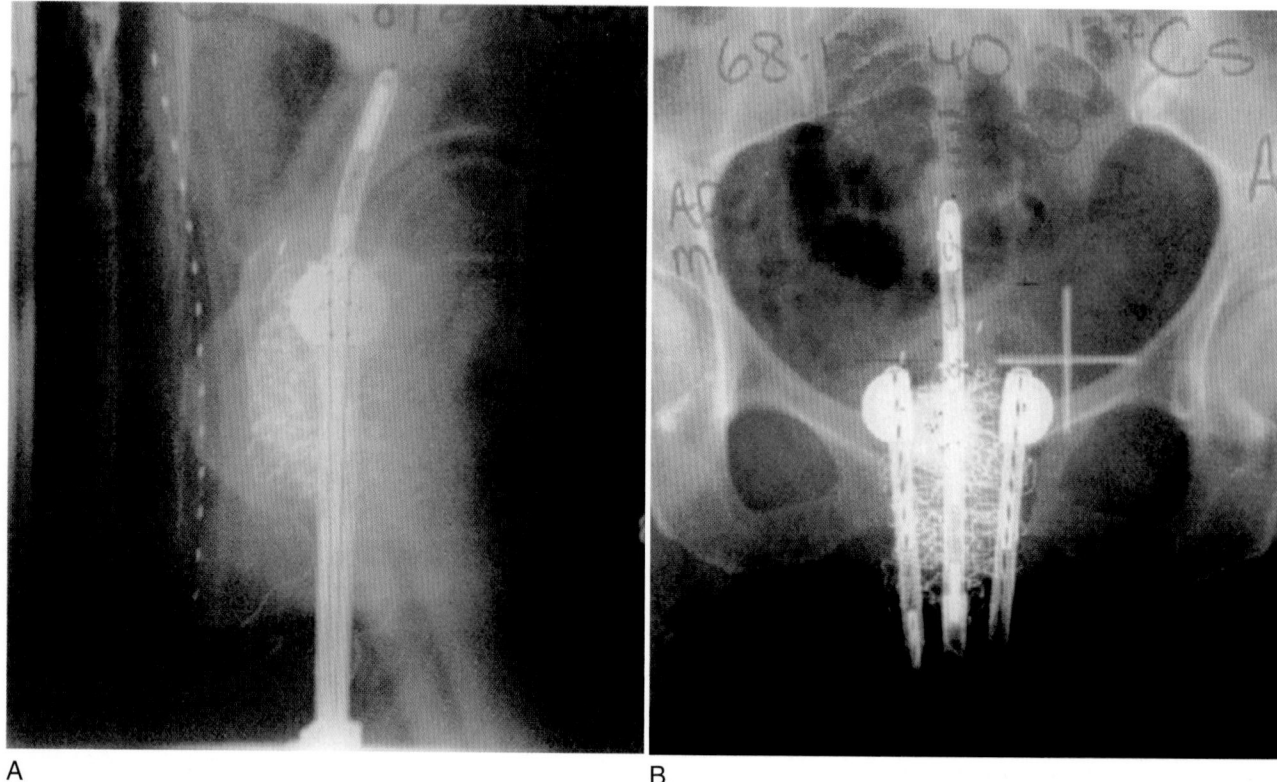

A   B

Figure 11–18. Lateral (*left*) and anterior-posterior localization films with ^{137}Cs dummy seeds for an implant with a Henshke applicator.

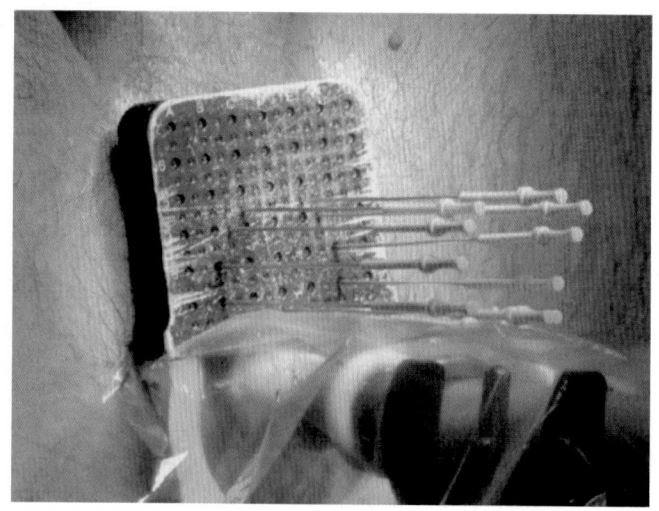

Figure 11–19. Template used in a prostate permanent implant. The template contains a rectangular pattern of holes. Needles are inserted through the template grid and seeds are placed along each needle at positions determined by the computer-generated plan.

PLATE 11

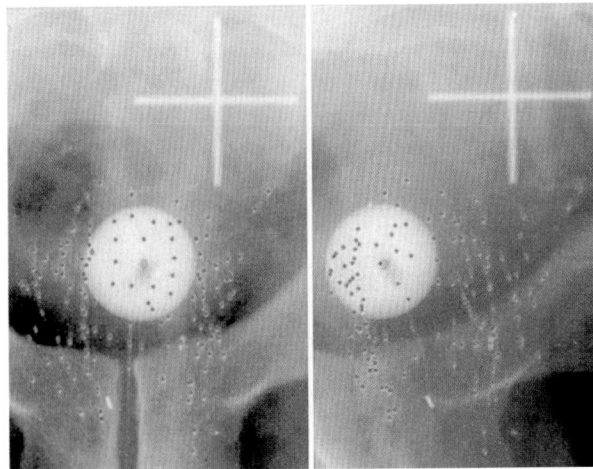

Figure 11–21. Matching seed projections in two different images is a difficult and time-consuming task, as illustrated in this (not atypical) patient data showing a ^{103}Pd implant with 134 seeds.

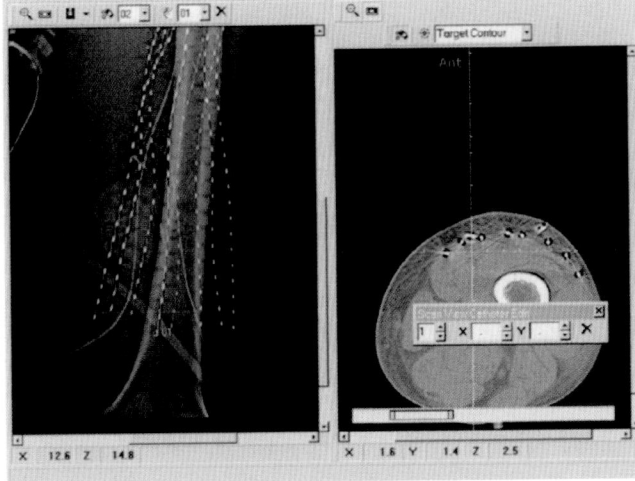

Figure 11–24. In this example, which illustrates planning for high-dose-rate (HDR) treatment of soft-tissue sarcoma, the trajectory of each catheter is digitized on each computed tomography cut and on the scout image.

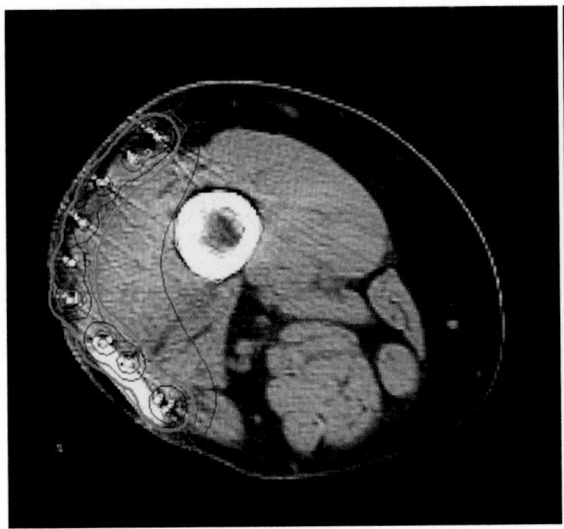

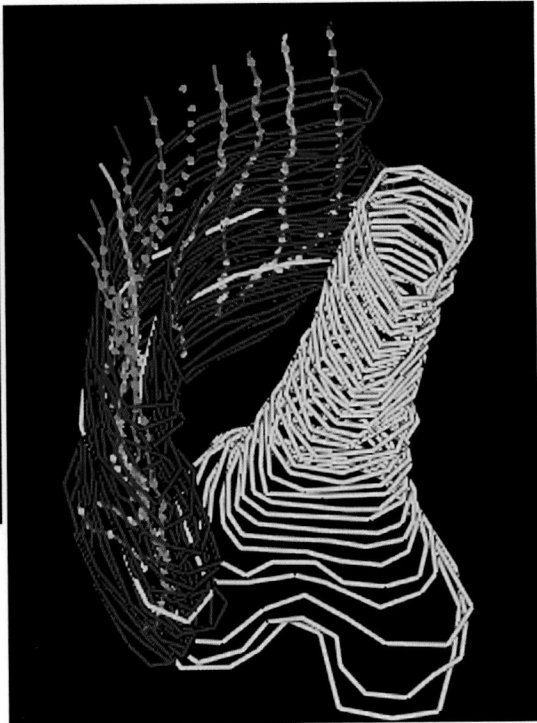

Figure 12–10. Computed tomography–based planning of an interstitial implant. **A,** Transverse view outlining the dose distribution in relationship to the target volume and adjacent normal structures (bone). **B,** Beam's-eye view of the catheters, target, and bone.

PLATE 12

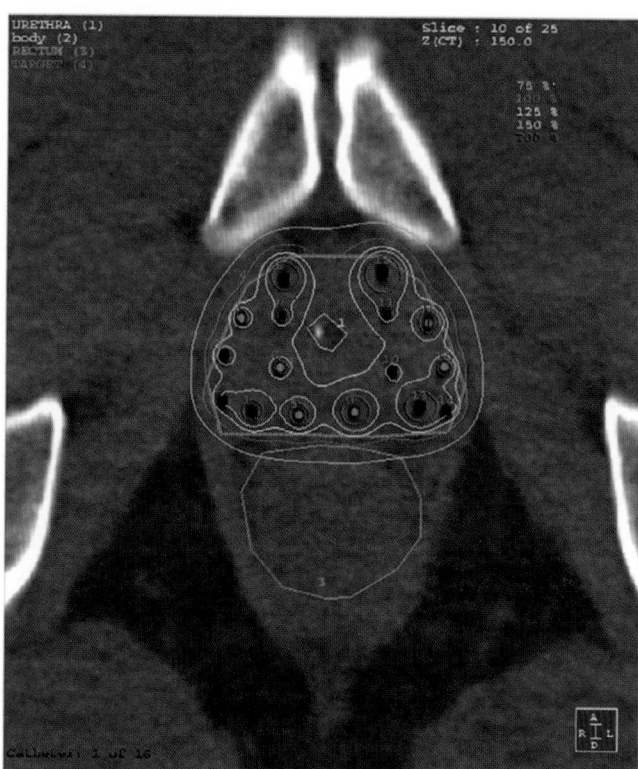

Figure 13–12. A three-dimensional brachytherapy planning system is an important part of modern brachytherapy. Critical organs such as the urethra, rectum, and bladder are contoured during the treatment planning process; in this way, the dose delivered to the critical organs can be accurately controlled.

Figure 13–13. Very conformal dose distribution can be delivered to the prostate using modern brachytherapy treatment system. A steep dose falloff outside of the implant volume decreases the dose and volume of radiated normal structures.

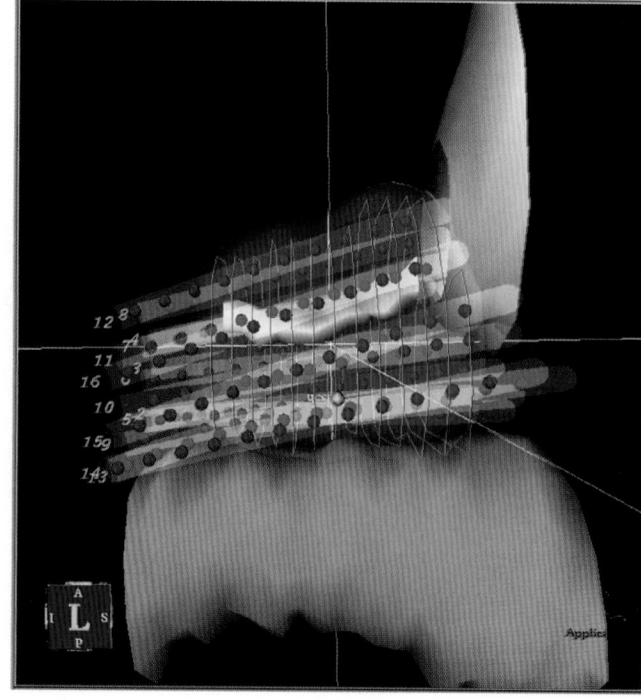

PLATE 13

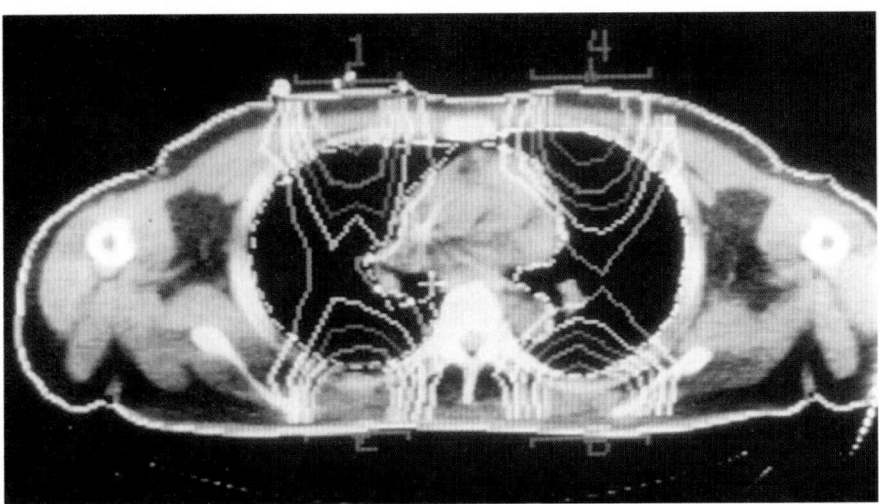

Figure 14–4. Example of electron boost planning for the chest wall after the use of lung blocks. The 90% isodose is at the inner chest wall; no more than 10% of the dose is delivered to the core of the lungs.

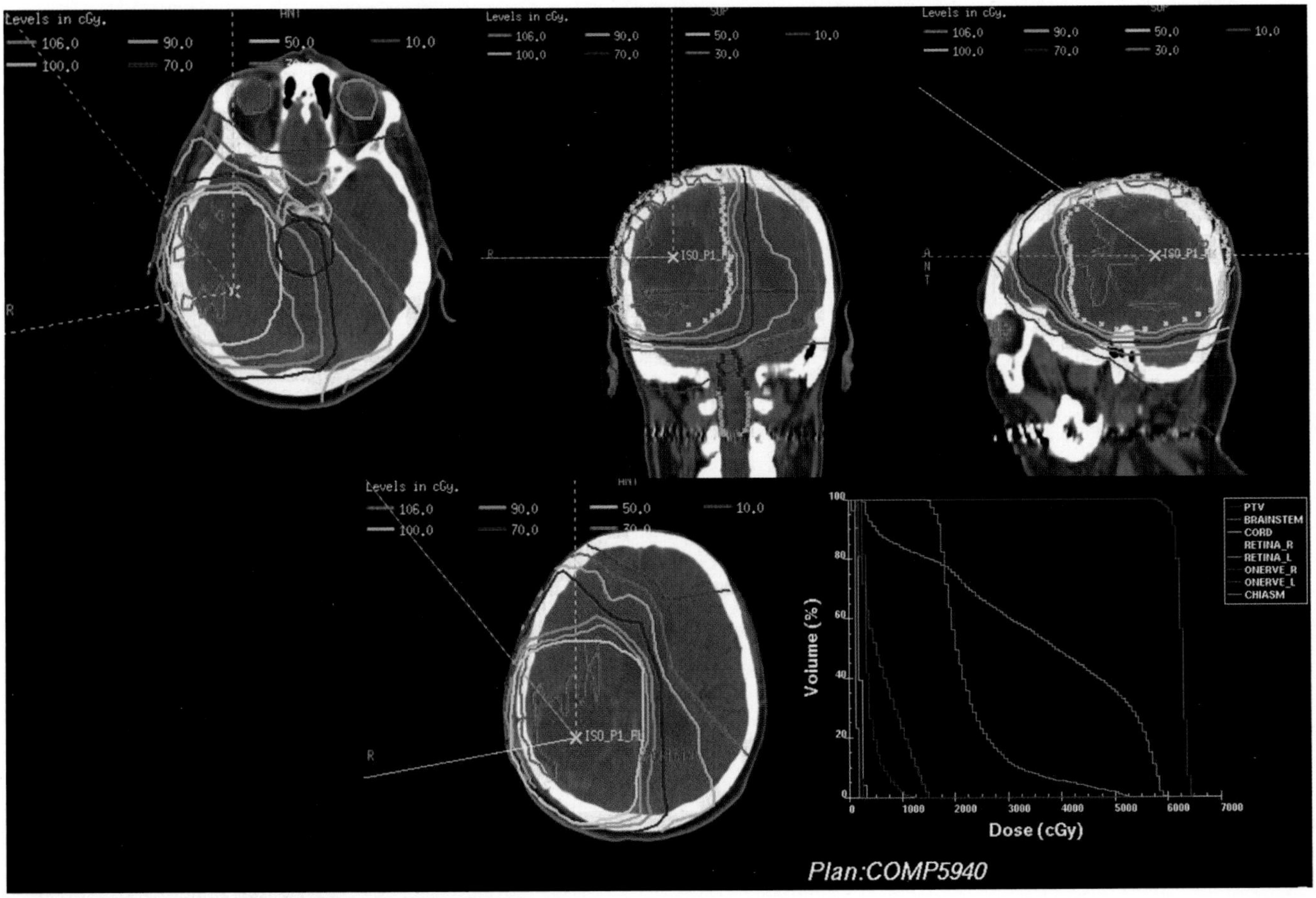

Figure 20–6. Intensity-modulated radiation therapy treatment plan for a patient with high-grade glioma of right parietal region.

PLATE 14

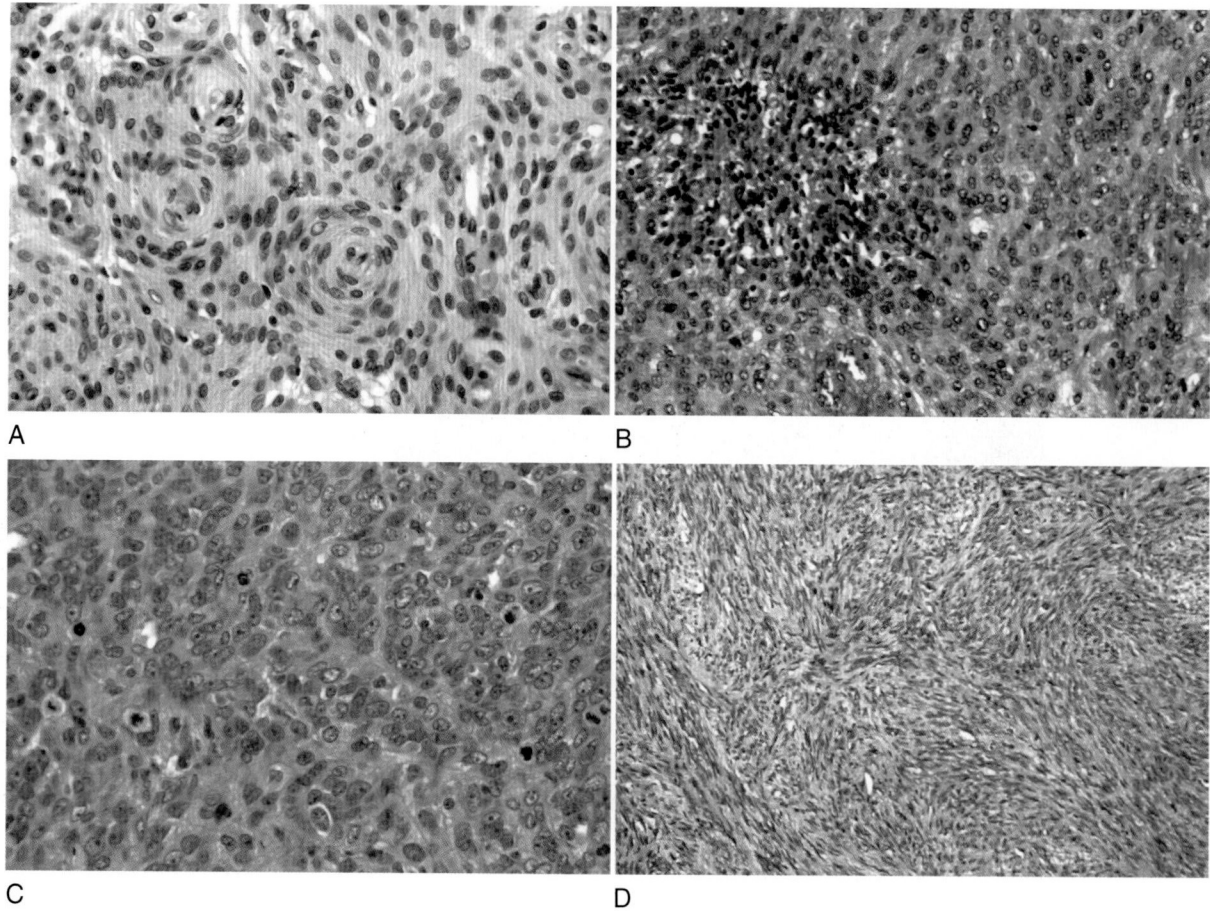

Figure 21–1. A (upper left), Grade I (benign) meningioma. This example exhibits meningothelial whorls and intranuclear pseudoinclusions. There is no mitotic activity. **B (upper right),** Grade II (atypical) meningioma. Focal necrosis (upper left) and isolated mitoses characterize this example. **C (lower left),** Grade III (anaplastic meningioma. A high mitotic rate and loss of differentiated meningothelial features are evident in this lesion. **D (lower right),** Grade III meningioma. shown here is a fibrosarcoma-like histologic presentation.

PLATE 15

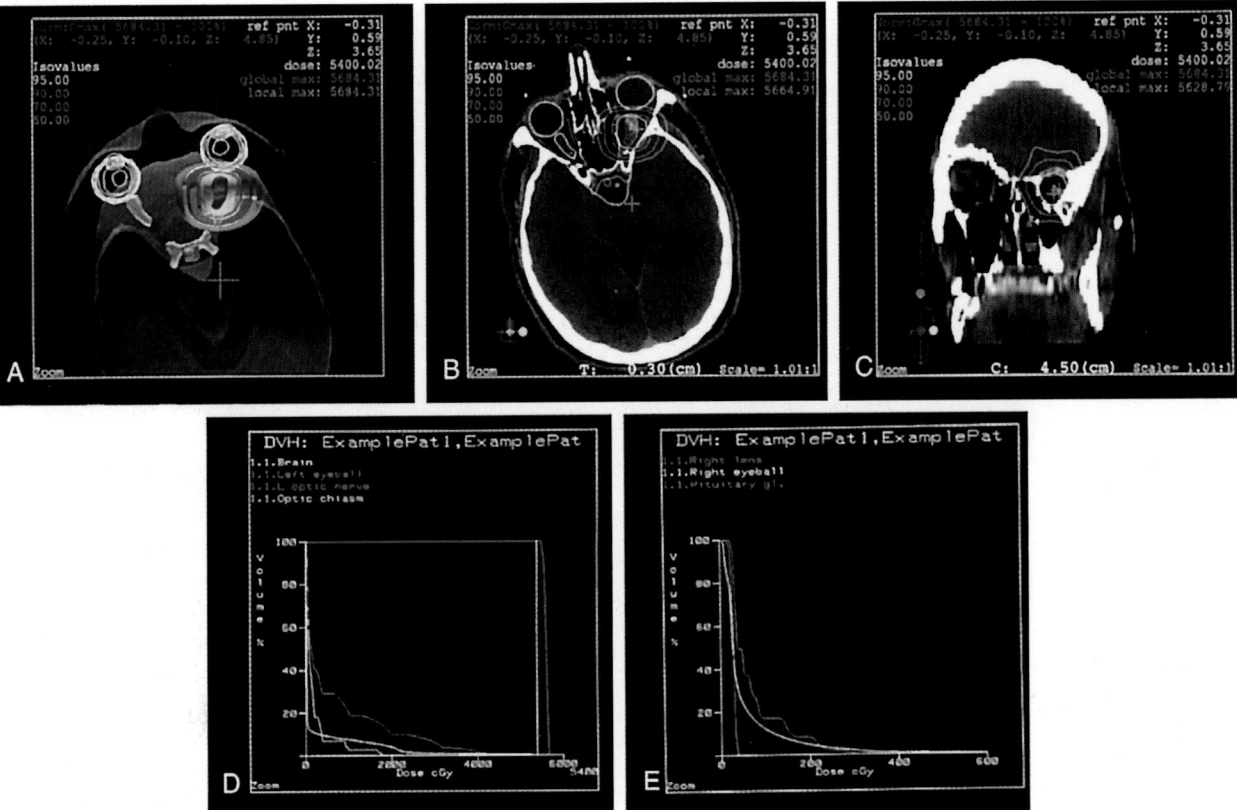

Figure 21–4. Precision conformal therapy technique for optic nerve sheath meningioma, example of 3D isodose plan (**A-C**), and dose volume histograms (**D-E**).

PLATE 16

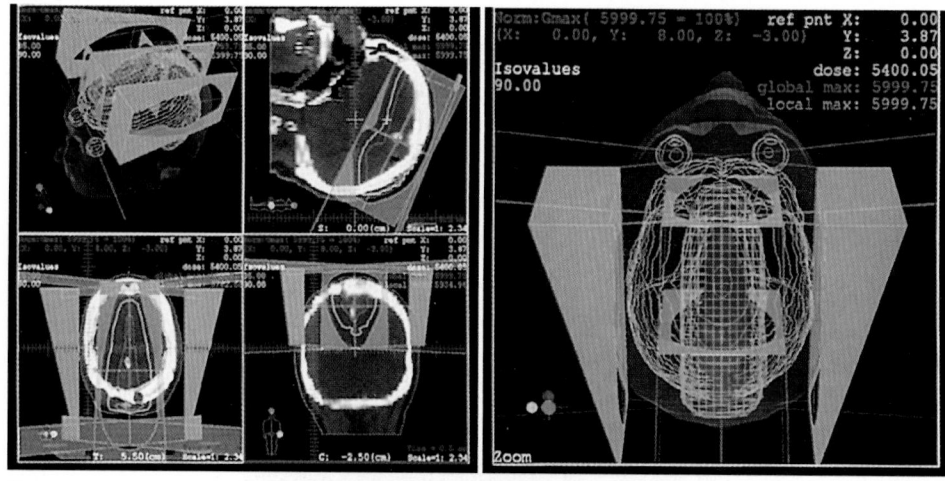

A   B

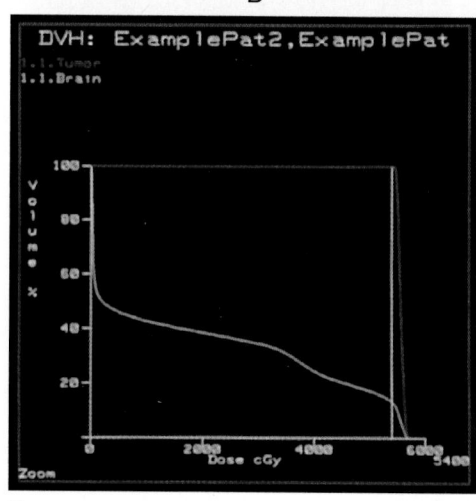

C

Figure 21–5. Example of three-field 3D isodose plan (**A** and **B**) and dose volume histogram (**C**) for a falx meningioma.

PLATE 17

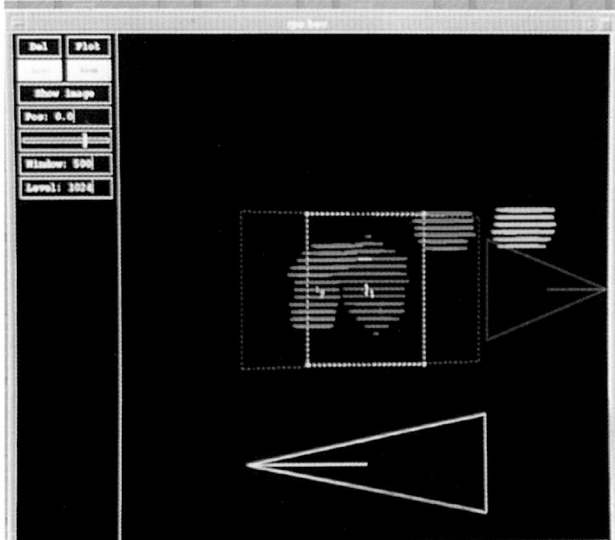

Figure 22–9. Beam's eye view of the right posterior oblique field shows the planning target volume, brainstem, and globes. Note that the left eye is excluded.

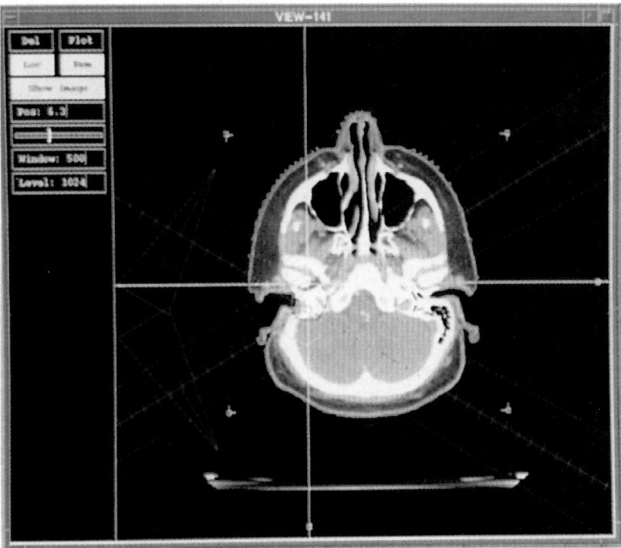

Figure 22–10. Dose distribution for treatment of a recurrent temporal bone paraganglioma. The 100% isodose line corresponds to 5040 cGy. The planning target volume and the 95% isodose line are also shown.

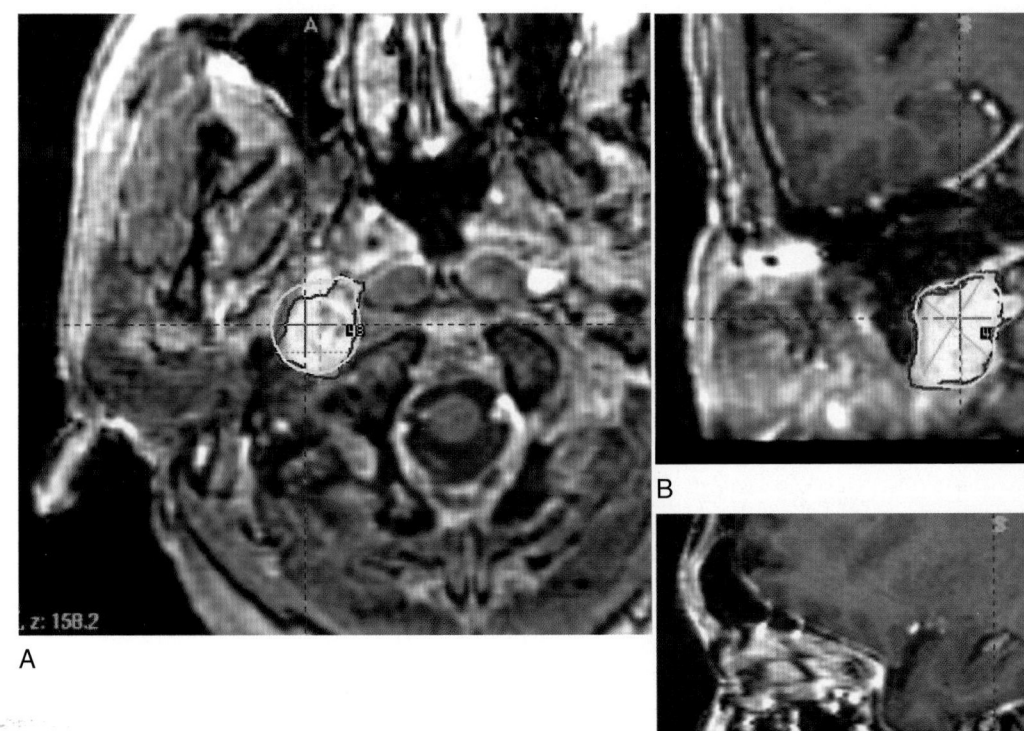

Figure 22–11. A, Axial stereotactic radiosurgery treatment planning magnetic resonance (MR) image of a 2.0 cm × 1.5 cm paraganglioma in the region of the jugular bulb (glomus jugulare) with posterior prominence and the carotid artery on the right. Gross tumor volume is blue and 50% isodose line is yellow. **B,** Coronal MR image. **C,** Sagittal MR image. (Courtesy of James G. Douglas, MD, MS.)

PLATE 18

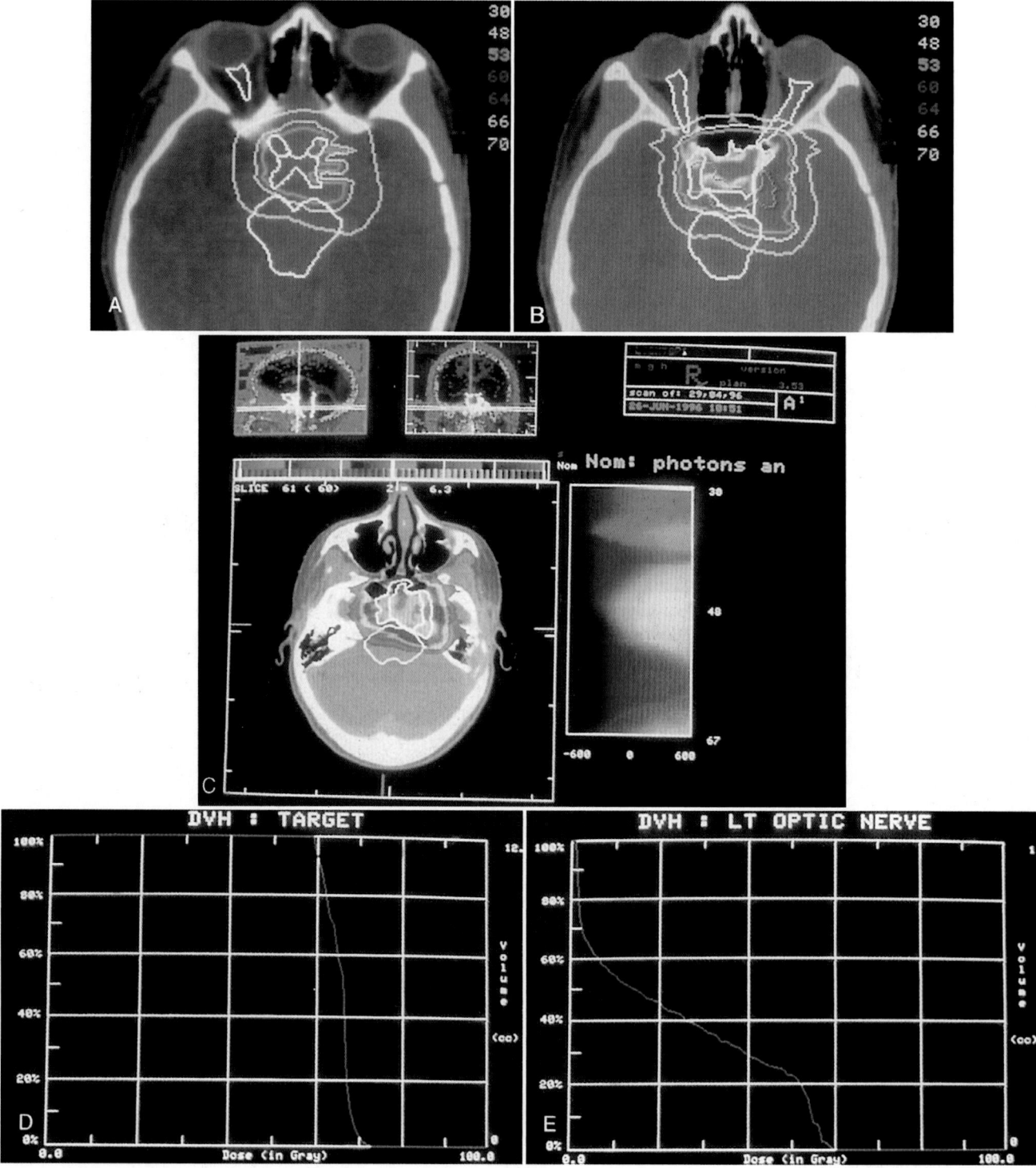

Figure 23–2. A, Section showing contours depicting the right optic nerve in the orbit, as well as both right and left optic nerves immediately anterior to the optic chiasm, which are also shown. Brainstem is also drawn. Dose distribution is shown in isodose lines. The entire chiasm and proximal optic nerves receive at least 53 Gy, but 60 Gy is not received by any structures at this level. **B,** A CT section 6 mm inferior to that shown in 2A shows both optic nerves, as well as both primary (smaller) and secondary (larger) target volumes, which include the entire sellar contents. Brainstem is also contoured. The posterior portion of the target volume receives a dose less than or equal to 60 Gy, while the anterior portion of the target volume receives a dose gradient from 60 to 53 Gy. **C,** At a level of 2.4 cm inferior to the chiasm, smaller and larger volumes both receive a uniform dose, as shown by the magenta color. A dose gradient exists across the brainstem from approximately 30 Gy (blue) up to 64 Gy (red-magenta transition at the edge of the brainstem). **D** and **E,** The dose volume histograms for the primary target (macroscopic disease) *(D)* and the left optic nerve *(E)*. Note that virtually all the target receives greater than 60 CGyEq, but the prescribed dose of 66.6 CGyEq is achieved in only 40% to 50% of the target. None of the left optic nerve receives greater than 60 CGyEq.

PLATE 19

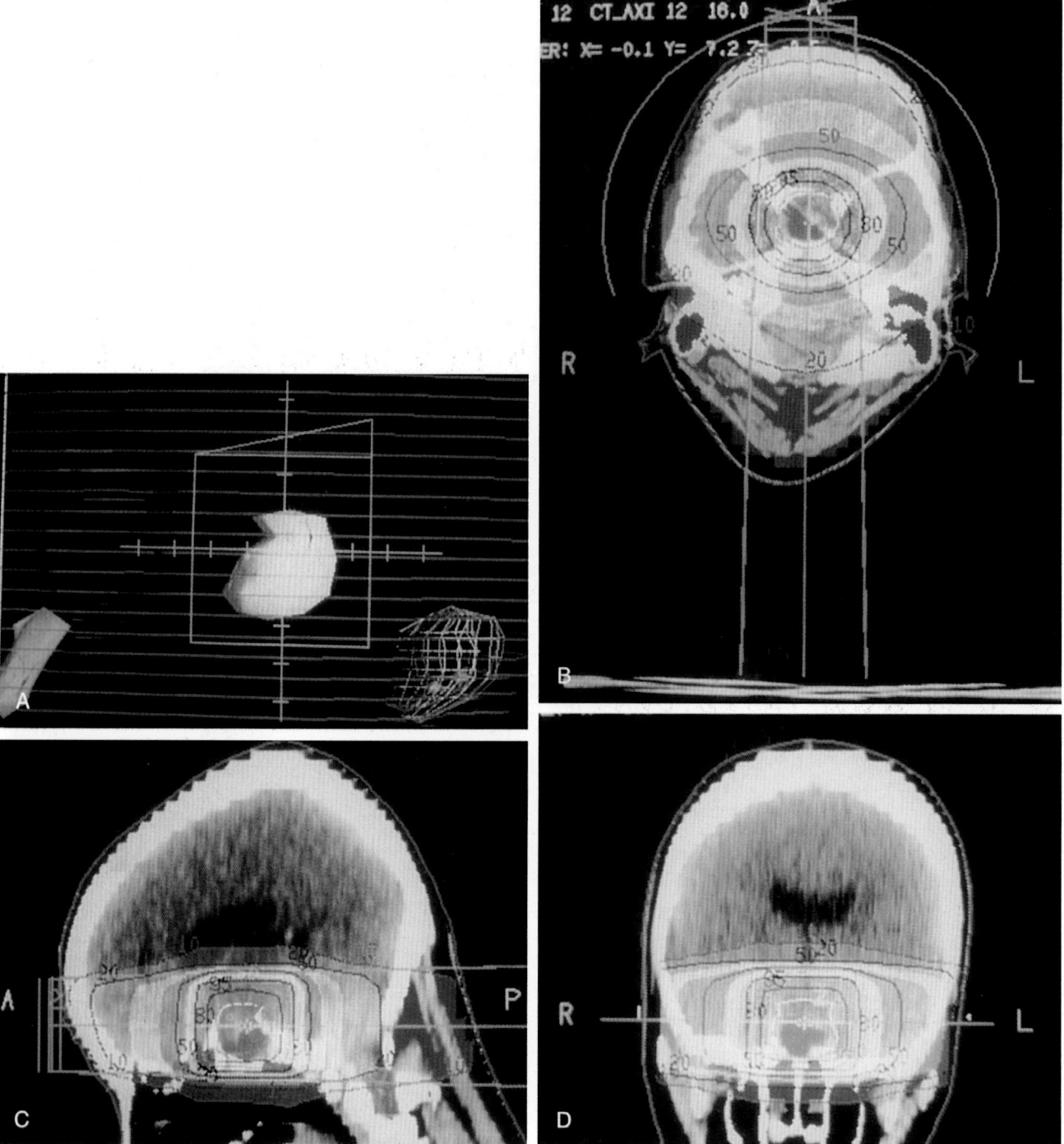

Figure 24–6. Isodose curves for a 5 cm diameter tumor volume:
18 MeV, bicoronal 110-degree arcs with moving 30-degree wedge filters. **A,** Lateral beam's-eye-view display showing the relationship of the target volume to the eyes and brainstem. **B,** Axial plane; **C,** sagittal plane; **D,** coronal plane.

PLATE 20

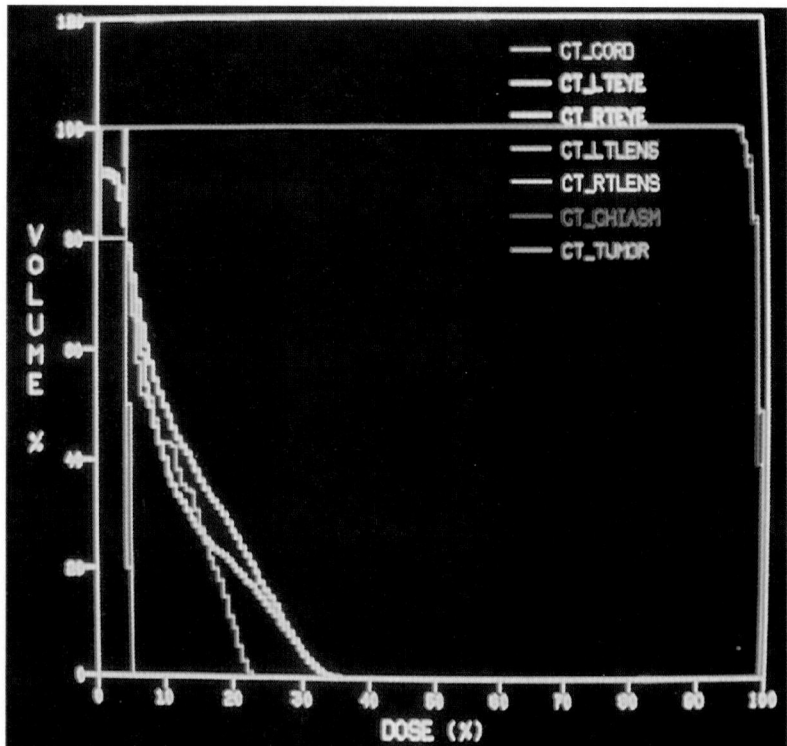

Figure 24–7. Dose volume histogram for bicoronal arc technique in the pituitary gland. The top 100% line is the tumor dose. Other normal structure doses are also shown.

PLATE 21

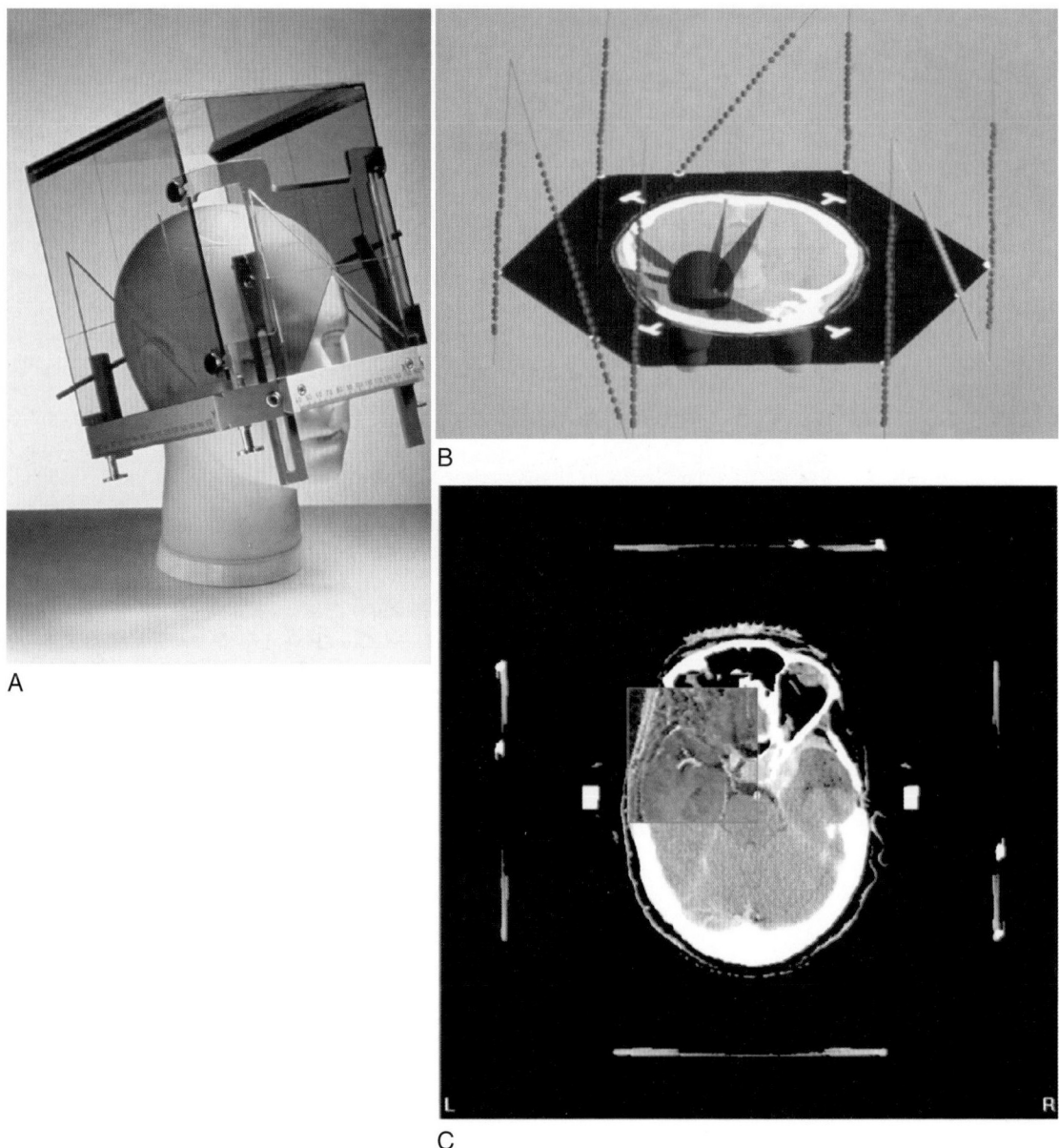

Figure 25–1. **A**, Leksell stereotactic frame with magnetic resonance (MR)-compatible localizer. Note "N"-shaped fiducial markers on localizer and scale on frame for patient positioning during treatment. **B**, Computer rendering of computed tomography (CT) slice depicting stereotactic space defined by "N"-shaped fiducials from linac radiosurgery planning system. Note projection of collimator (red) and paths of arcs for delivery of treatment (blue). **C**, Stereotactic CT of patient with left cavernous sinus meningioma with overlying "fused" MR (blue box). Note excellent fusion of images and fiducials, indicating they are level within stereotactic space.

PLATE 22

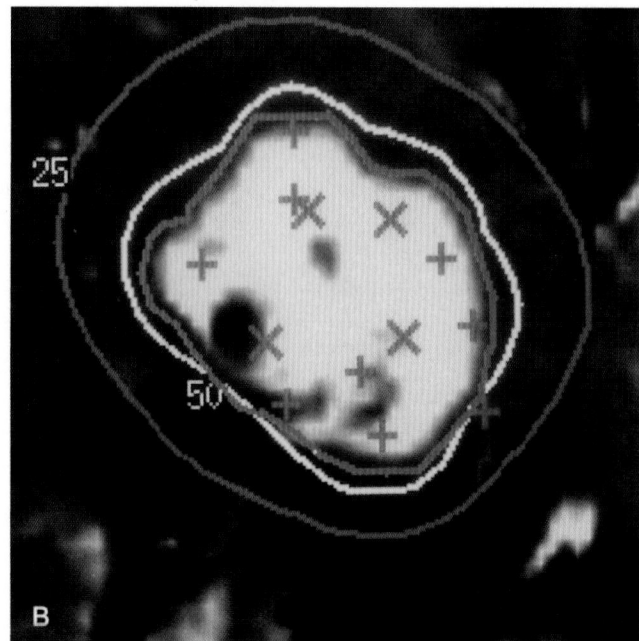

Figure 25–4. B, 13 isocenters were used to obtain conformity of 50% isodose line to tumor volume. Three different collimator helmets were employed (18 mm × 3, 14 mm × 7, 8 mm × 3). The target volume was 20.2 mL and a dose of 11 Gy was prescribed to the 50% isodose line representing the target periphery.

PLATE 23

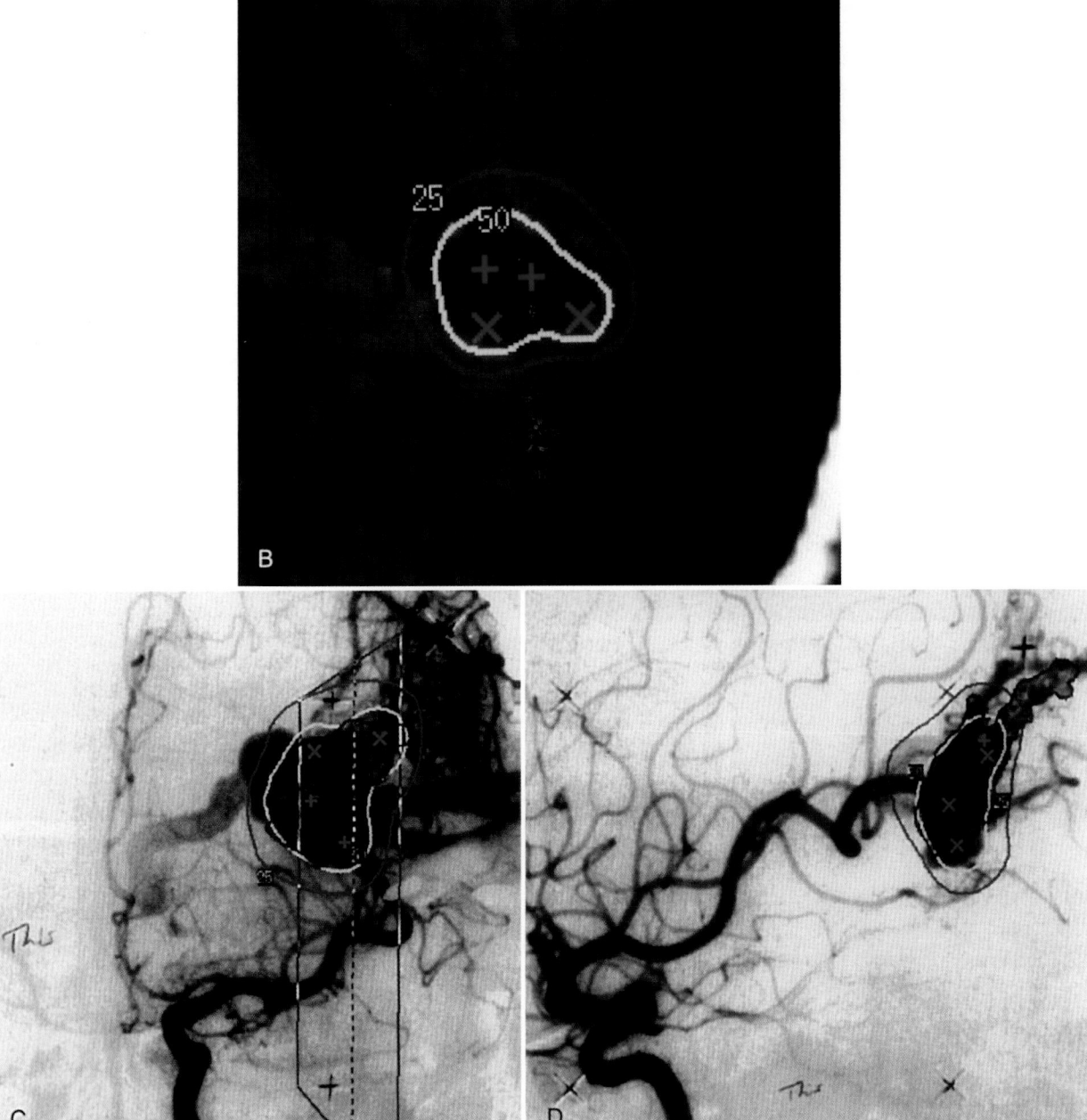

Figure 25–5. B, Four isocenters were used (14 mm x 1, 8 mm x 3) and 18.5 Gy was delivered to the 50% isodose line. **C** and **D**, Angiographic orthogonal views of the AVM with isodose distribution superimposed on anteroposterior [**C**] and sagittal (**D**) angiograms.

PLATE 24

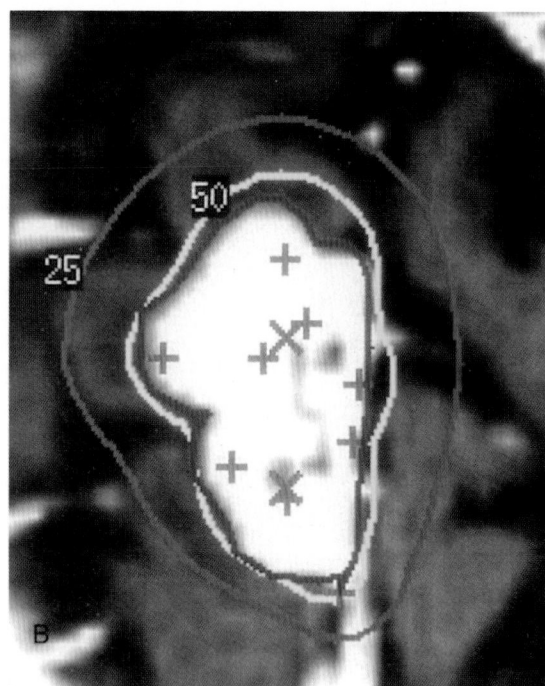

Figure 25–6. B, 11 isocenters (18 mm × 2, 14 mm × 5, 8 mm × 4) were used to cover the 13 mL target volume with the 50% isodose line. The clinician prescribed 16 Gy.

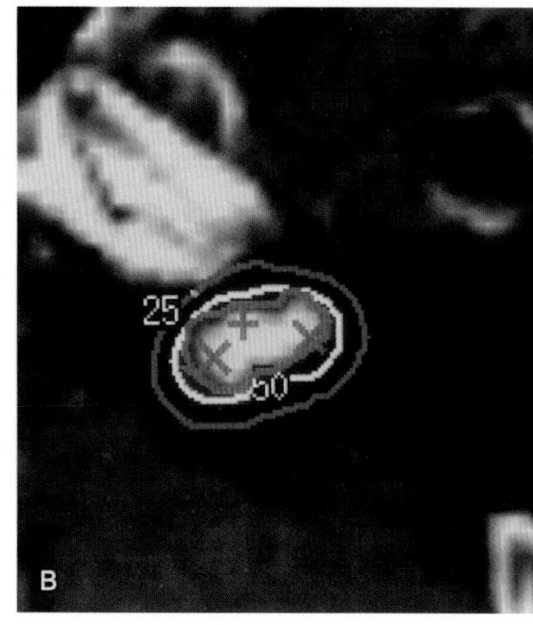

Figure 25–7. B, The Gamma Knife isodose plan. The patient received 14 Gy at the target periphery, delivered with three isocenters (8 mm × 3). The target volume was 0.4 cm^2.

PLATE 25

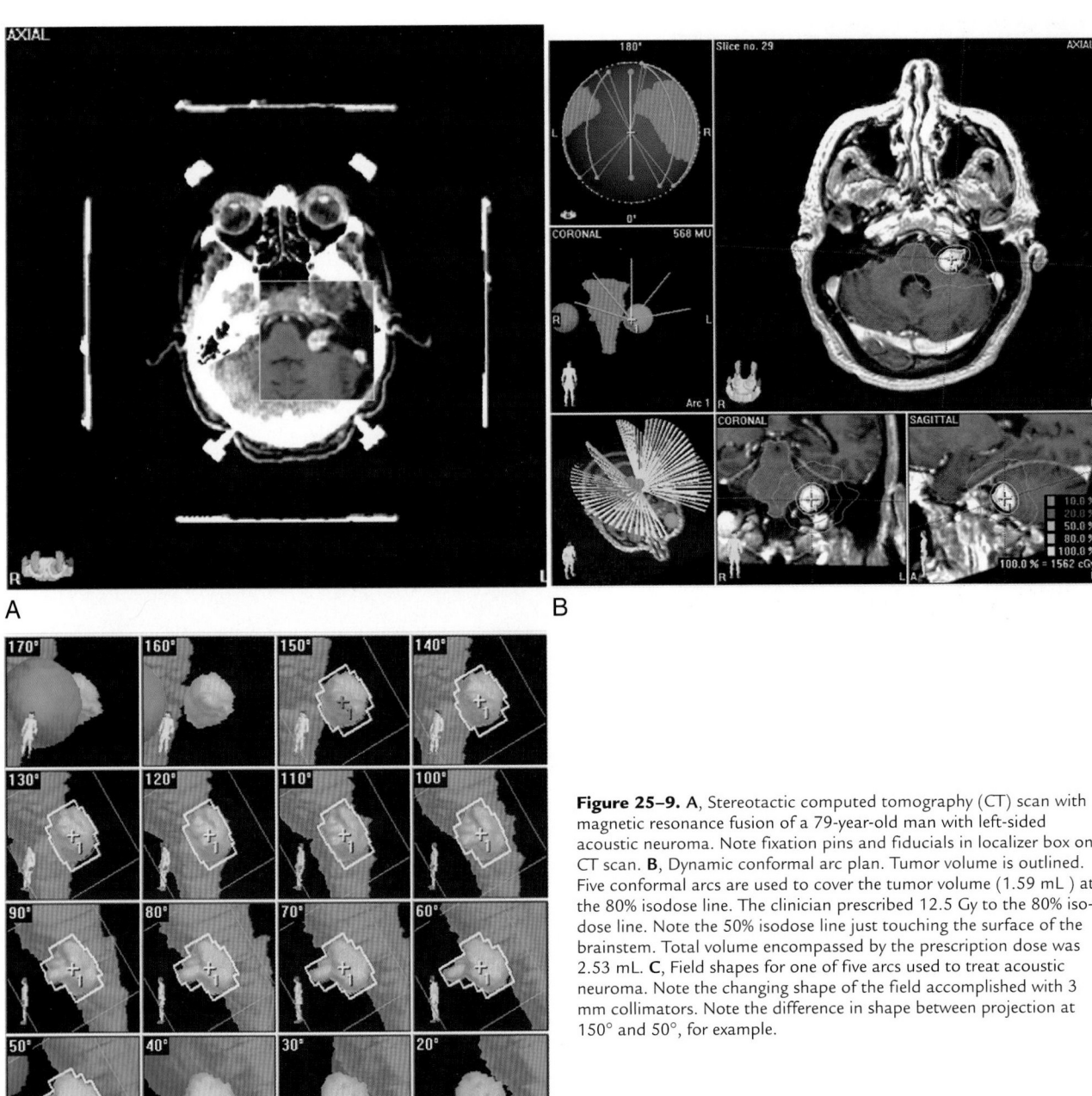

Figure 25–9. **A**, Stereotactic computed tomography (CT) scan with magnetic resonance fusion of a 79-year-old man with left-sided acoustic neuroma. Note fixation pins and fiducials in localizer box on CT scan. **B**, Dynamic conformal arc plan. Tumor volume is outlined. Five conformal arcs are used to cover the tumor volume (1.59 mL) at the 80% isodose line. The clinician prescribed 12.5 Gy to the 80% isodose line. Note the 50% isodose line just touching the surface of the brainstem. Total volume encompassed by the prescription dose was 2.53 mL. **C**, Field shapes for one of five arcs used to treat acoustic neuroma. Note the changing shape of the field accomplished with 3 mm collimators. Note the difference in shape between projection at 150° and 50°, for example.

PLATE 26

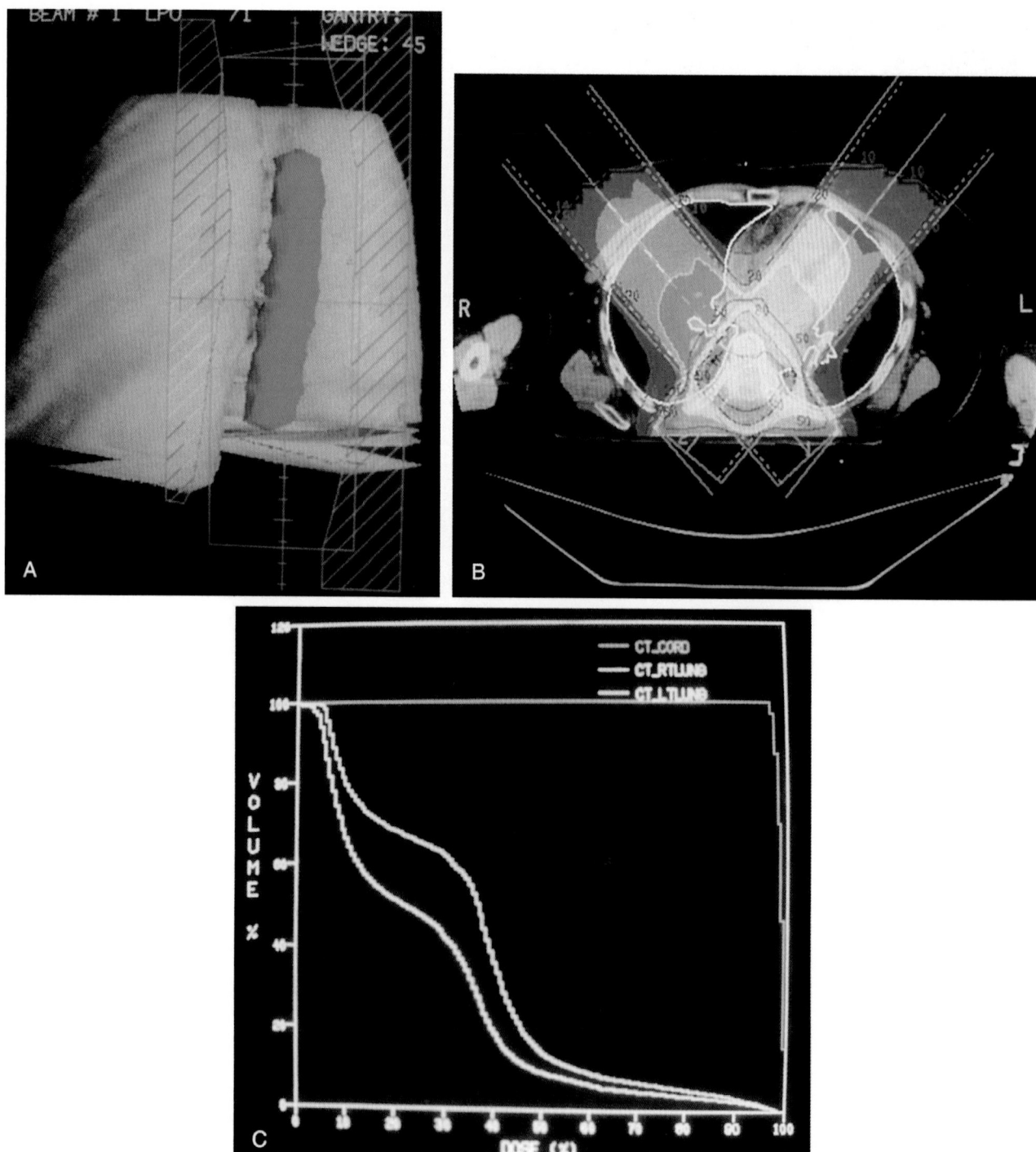

Figure 26–2. A, Beam's eye view achieved using
three-dimensional conformal reconstruction of a thoracic cord glioma target volume and adjacent lungs with a
posterior oblique wedged-pair irradiation technique. Custom low melting point alloy blocking is designed using the beam's eye view of the target volume.
B, Transverse section showing dosimetry from the treatment plan developed using the target volume derived from A. Note the substantial portion of lung
included in the beam's exit path at this level. **C,** Dose-volume histogram derived from the treatment plan shown in B using dosimetry information for the
entire treatment volume. Virtually the entire target volume receives 100% of the total dose of 50.4 Gy at 1.8 Gy per fraction. Despite the impressive
amount of lung included in the exit beam shown in B, the histogram shows that only 10% to 15% of each lung atually receives more than 25 Gy (50% of
the total dose) under this plan. Nonetheless, 40% of the left lung and 60% of the right lung receives a dose greater than 15 Gy (30% of the total dose).

PLATE 27

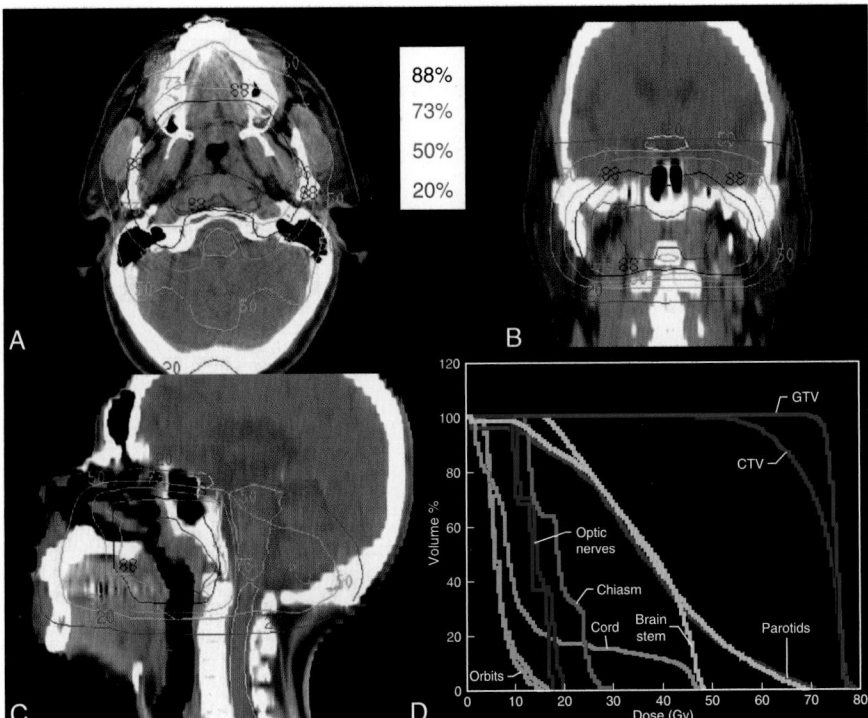

Figure 27–13. Isodose curves of a 10-field forward intensity-modulated radiotherapy plan for a patient with T1N1 carcinoma of the nasopharynx displayed on the axial (**A**), coronal (**B**), and sagittal (**C**) planes through the centroid of the primary tumor and the Dose Volume Histogram (**D**) for the relevant structures. (From Lee N, Xia P, Quivey JM, et al: Intensity-Modulated Radiotherapy in the Treatment of Nasopharyngeal Carcinoma: An Update of the UCSF Experience. *Int J Radiat Oncol Biol Phys*. 2002;53:15.).

PLATE 28

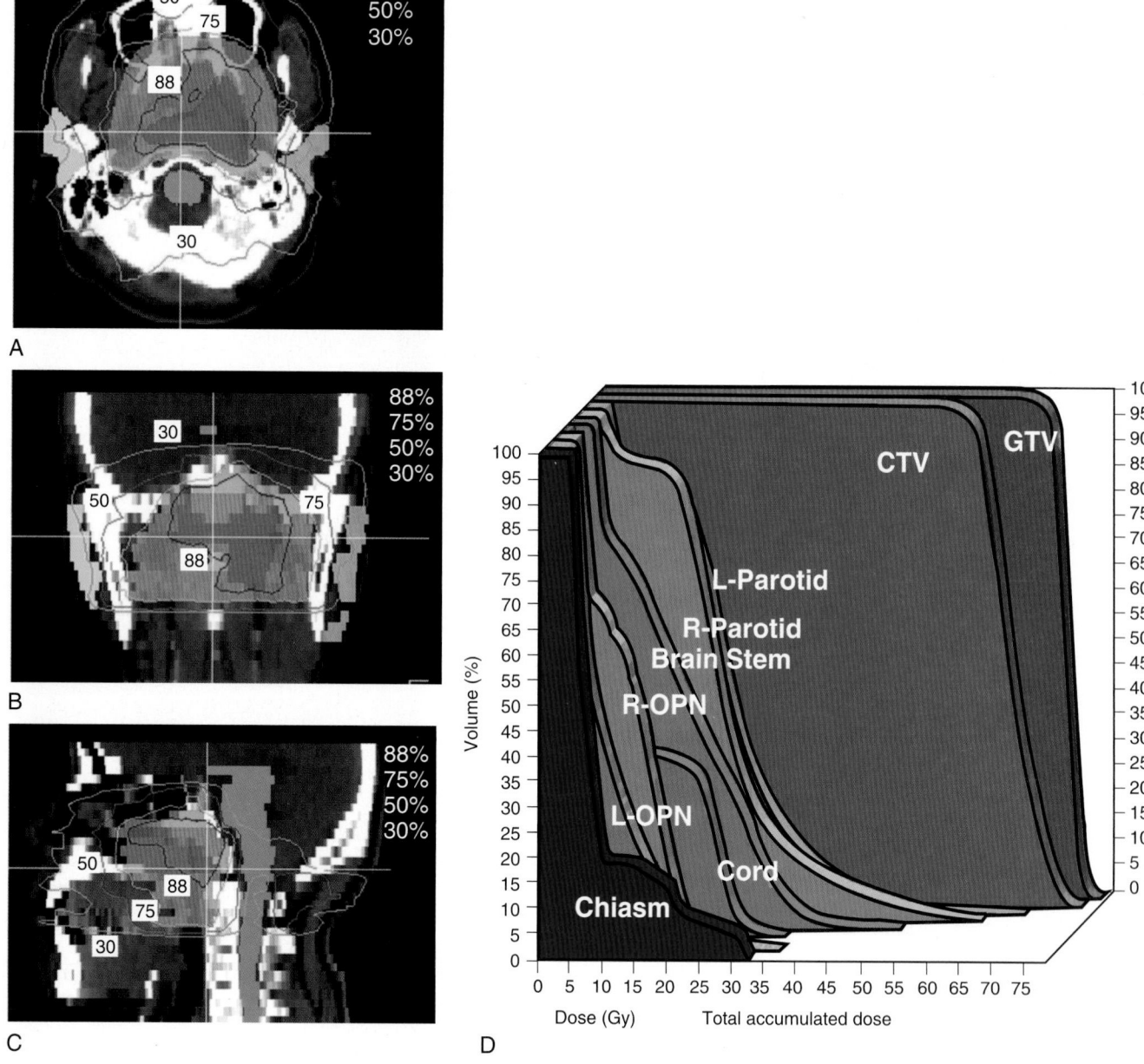

Figure 27–14. Isodose curves of an inverse IMRT plan delivered using multivane dynamic multi-leaf collimator (MIMiC) for a patient with T4N1 carcinoma of the nasopharynx displayed on the axial (**A**), coronal (**B**), and sagittal (**C**) planes through the centroid of the primary tumor and the Dose Volume Histogram for the relevant structures (**D**). The gross tumor volume is shown in red and the clinical target volume is shown in orange. (From Lee N, Xia P, Quivey JM, et al: Intensity-modulated radiotherapy in the treatment of nasopharyngeal carcinoma: An update of the UCSF Experience. *Int J Radiat Oncol Biol Phys.* 2002;53:16.)

PLATE 29

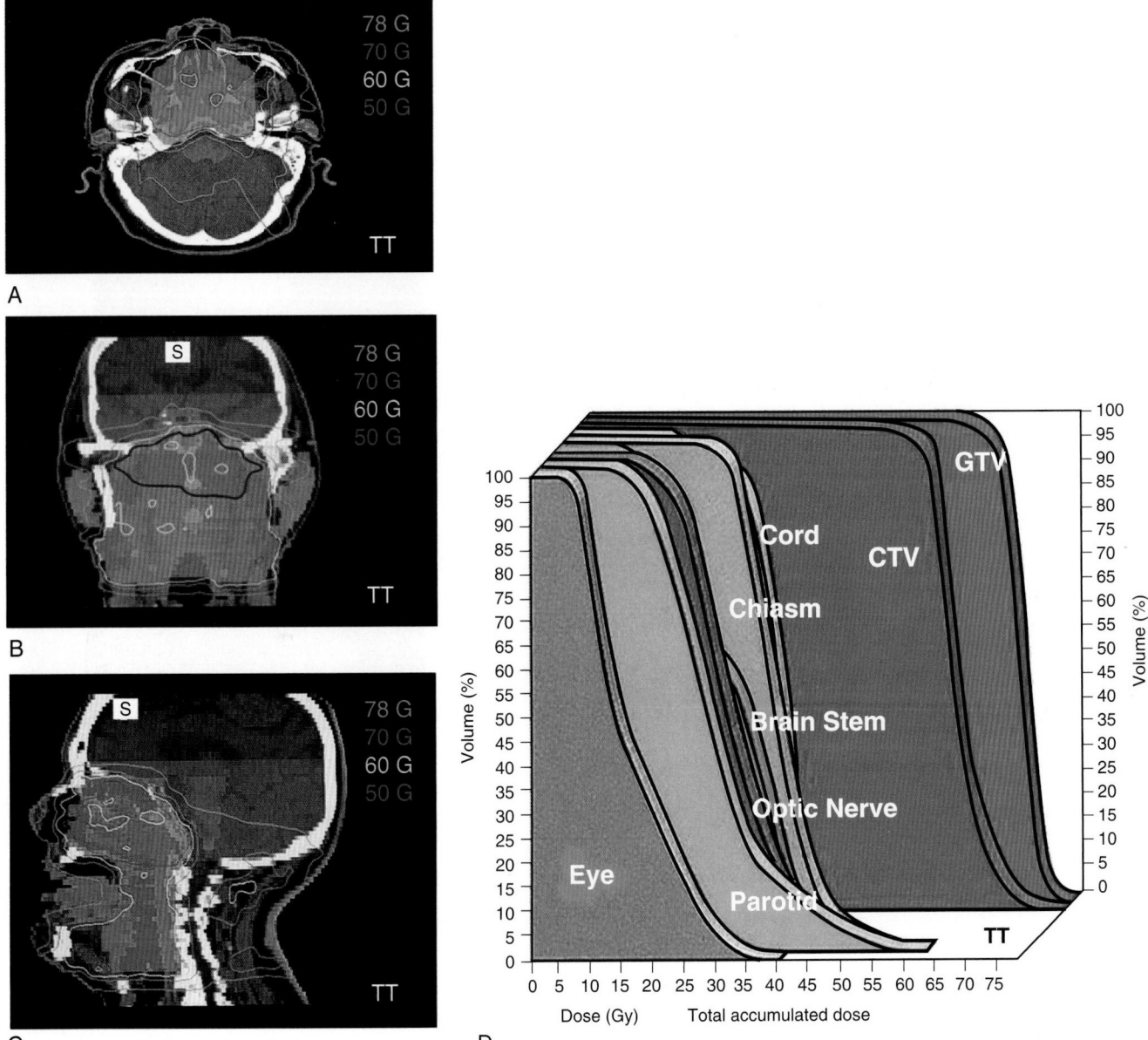

Figure 27–15. Isodose curves of an inverse IMRT plan using nine coplanar gantry angles delivered with conventional MLC for a patient with T3N0 carcinoma of the nasopharynx displayed on the (**A**) axial, (**B**) coronal, and (**C**) sagittal planes through the centroid of the primary tumor and the Dose Volume Histogram for the relevant structures (**D**). The GTV is shown in red and the CTV is shown in magenta. (From Lee N, Xia P, Fischbein N, et al: Intensity-modulated radiotherapy for head and neck cancer: The UCSF Experience focusing on target. *Int J Radiat Oncol Biol Phys.* 2003;57(1):49-60.)

PLATE 30

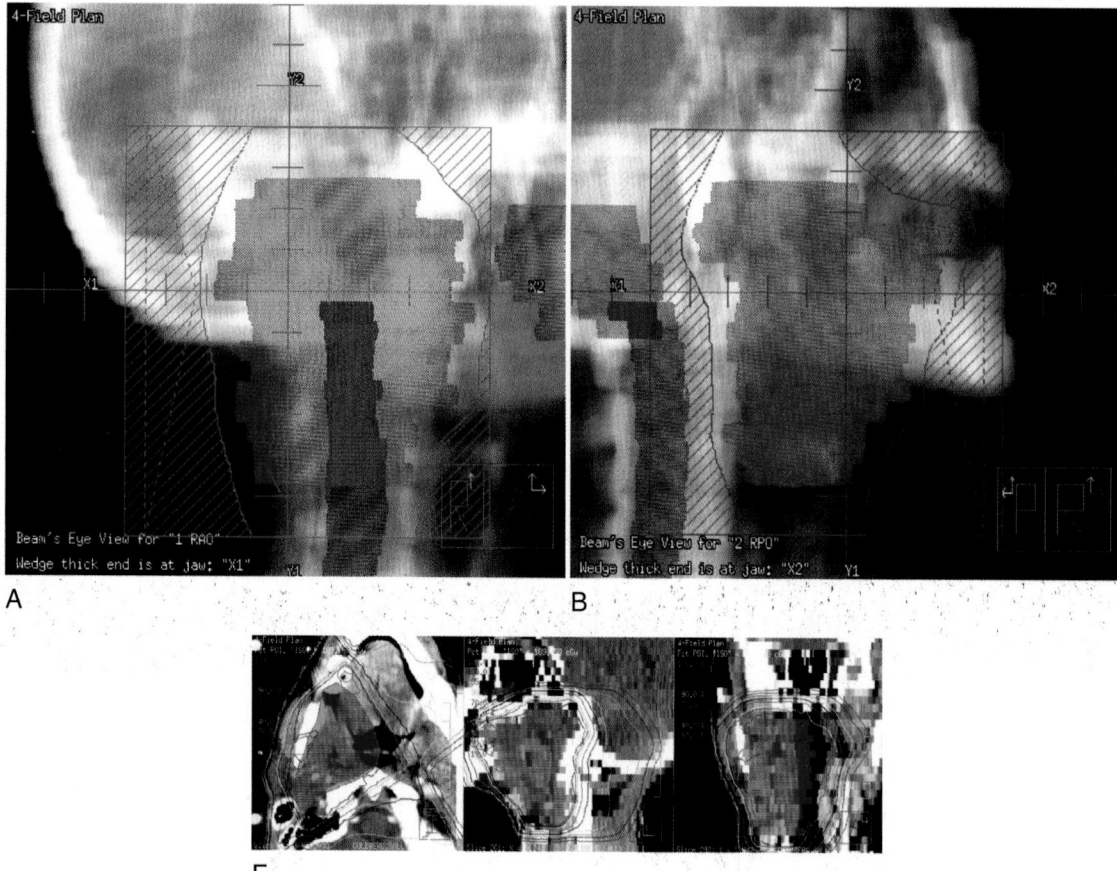

Figure 28–9. Simulation of an early-stage tonsil cancer with a wedge-pair technique and localization films of a tonsil cancer implant. The patient is a 43-year-old HIV-positive female who presented with a T2N0 right tonsillar carcinoma and was treated with an ipsilateral wedge-pair technique to cover the primary site. She was matched with an angled oblique field to treat the ipsilateral neck electively. The primary site received 70 Gy in 2-Gy fractions while the low anterior neck received 50 Gy in 2-Gy fractions. Fifteen months later, the patient presented with a metachronous left tonsillar squamous cell carcinoma with involved cervical lymph node. She underwent tonsillectomy and neck dissection. Margins were positive and multiple lymph nodes were involved. She was subsequently treated with a brachytherapy boost to the tonsillar site and wedge-pair technique to treat the contralateral neck and primary site. The brachytherapy boost was needed to treat the primary site for the positive margin as a full course of external beam radiation could not be given without exceeding normal tissue tolerance. **A–E,** 3D-planned wedge-pair field treating the initial primary lesion involving the right tonsil matched above the larynx to an ipsilateral low neck field. **F,** Dose to the contralateral parotid gland was limited to less than 5% of the total dose to the ipsilateral lesion.

PLATE 31

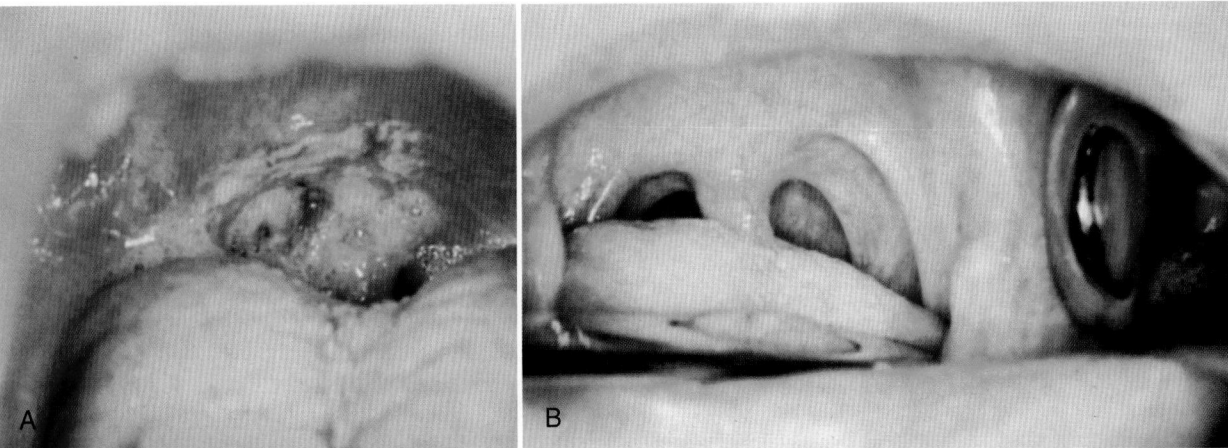

Figure 28–12. Results after treatment of a patient with a T2N0 squamous cell cancer of the soft palate, before (**A**) and after (**B**) radiation therapy. This patient was treated with external-beam radiation therapy to the primary site and both sides of the neck. Opposed lateral portals were used in conjunction with a low anterior neck field. Then the primary site and upper neck regions, including the retropharyngeal nodes, were treated to 54 Gy. The final dose to the primary site was 68.4 Gy. Fraction size is 1.8 Gy per day. The lower neck is treated with an anterior portal to 50 Gy over 5 weeks. The posterior neck regions are boosted with electrons to protect the spinal cord to 54 Gy. The patient currently has no evidence of disease.

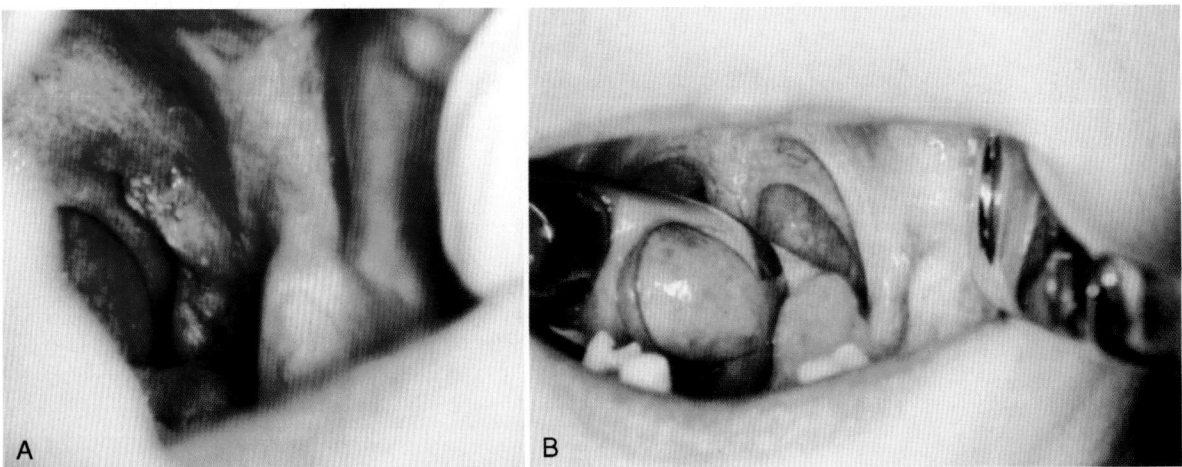

Figure 28–13. A patient with a T2N0 squamous cell cancer of the tonsil, before (**A**) and after (**B**) radiation therapy. The patient was treated with external beam radiation therapy to the primary site and ipsilateral neck using an ipsilateral wedge-pair beam arrangement in conjunction with an ipsilateral low anterior neck field. The final dose to the primary site was 70.2 Gy. Fraction size was 1.8 Gy/day. The lower neck was treated with an anterior portal to 50 Gy over 5 weeks.

PLATE 32

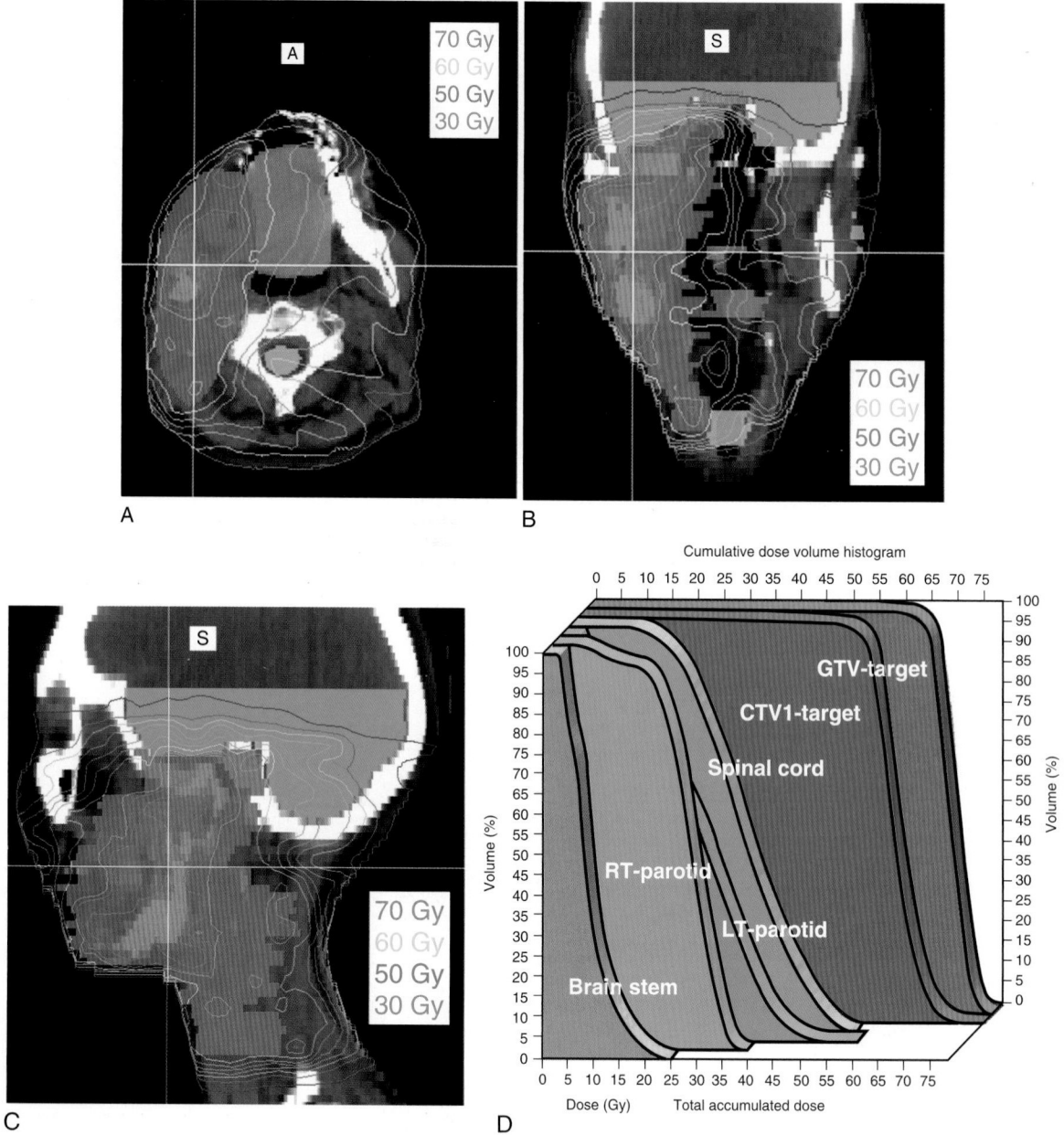

Figure 29–11. Isodose curves of an inverse intensity-modulated radiotherapy plan using seven coplanar gantry angles delivered with conventional multi-leaf collimator for a patient with recurrent carcinoma of the lip with perineural invasion displayed on the axial (**A**), coronal (**B**), and sagittal (**C**) planes through the centroid of the primary tumor and the Dose Volume Histogram for the relevant structures (**D**). The gross tumor volume is shown in red and the clinical target volume (including a margin for set-up errors) is shown in magenta.

PLATE 33

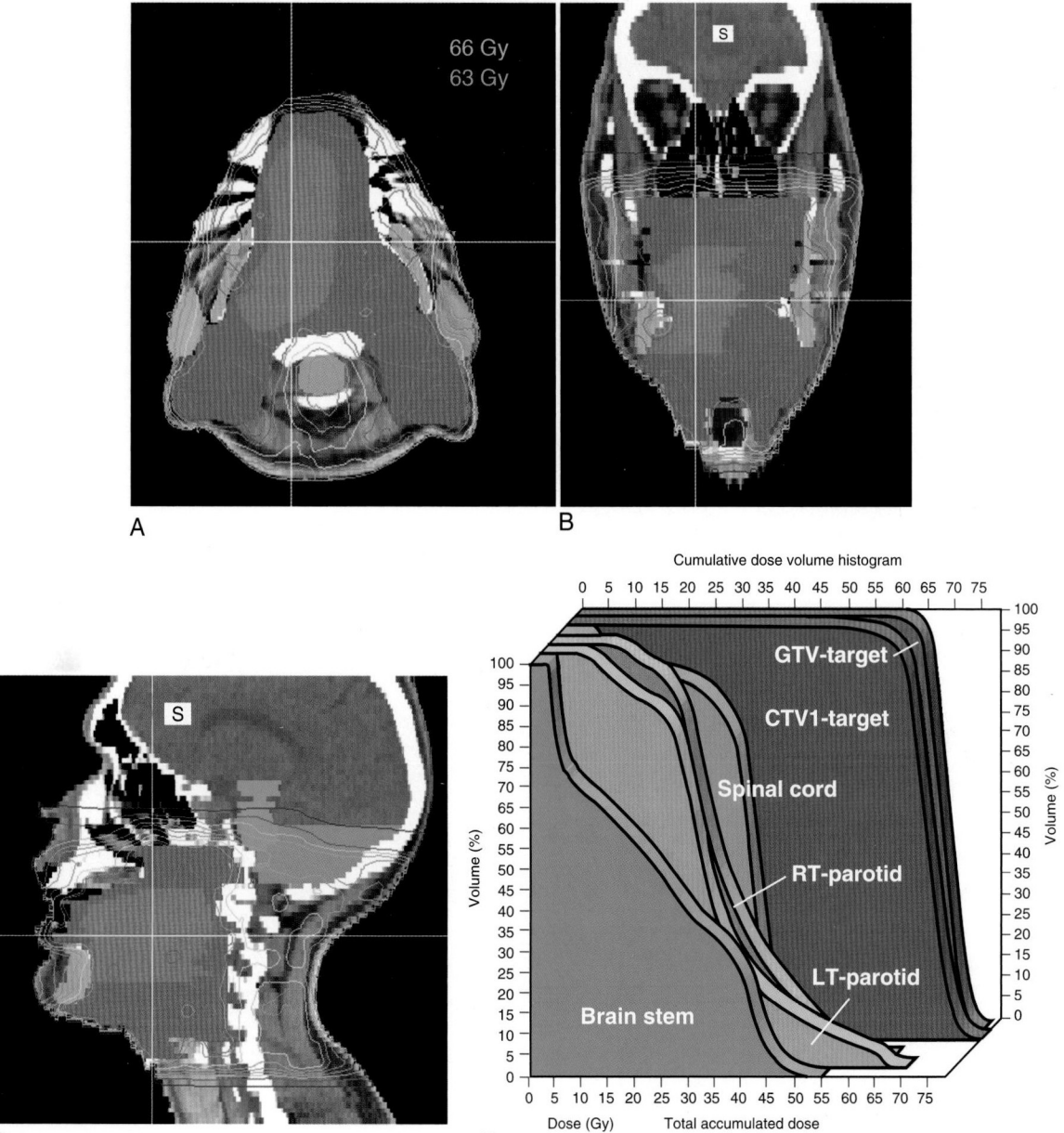

Figure 29–13. Isodose curves of an inverse intensity-modulated radiotherapy plan using seven coplanar gantry angles delivered with conventional multi-leaf collimator for a patient receiving post-operative radiotherapy for a T2N2b carcinoma of the oral tongue displayed on the axial (**A**), coronal (**B**), and sagittal (**C**) planes through the centroid of the primary tumor and the Dose Volume Histogram for the relevant structures (**D**). The gross tumor volume is shown in red and the clinical target volume (including a margin for set-up errors) is shown in magenta. A low neck/supraclavicular field is matched to the IMRT plan.

PLATE 34

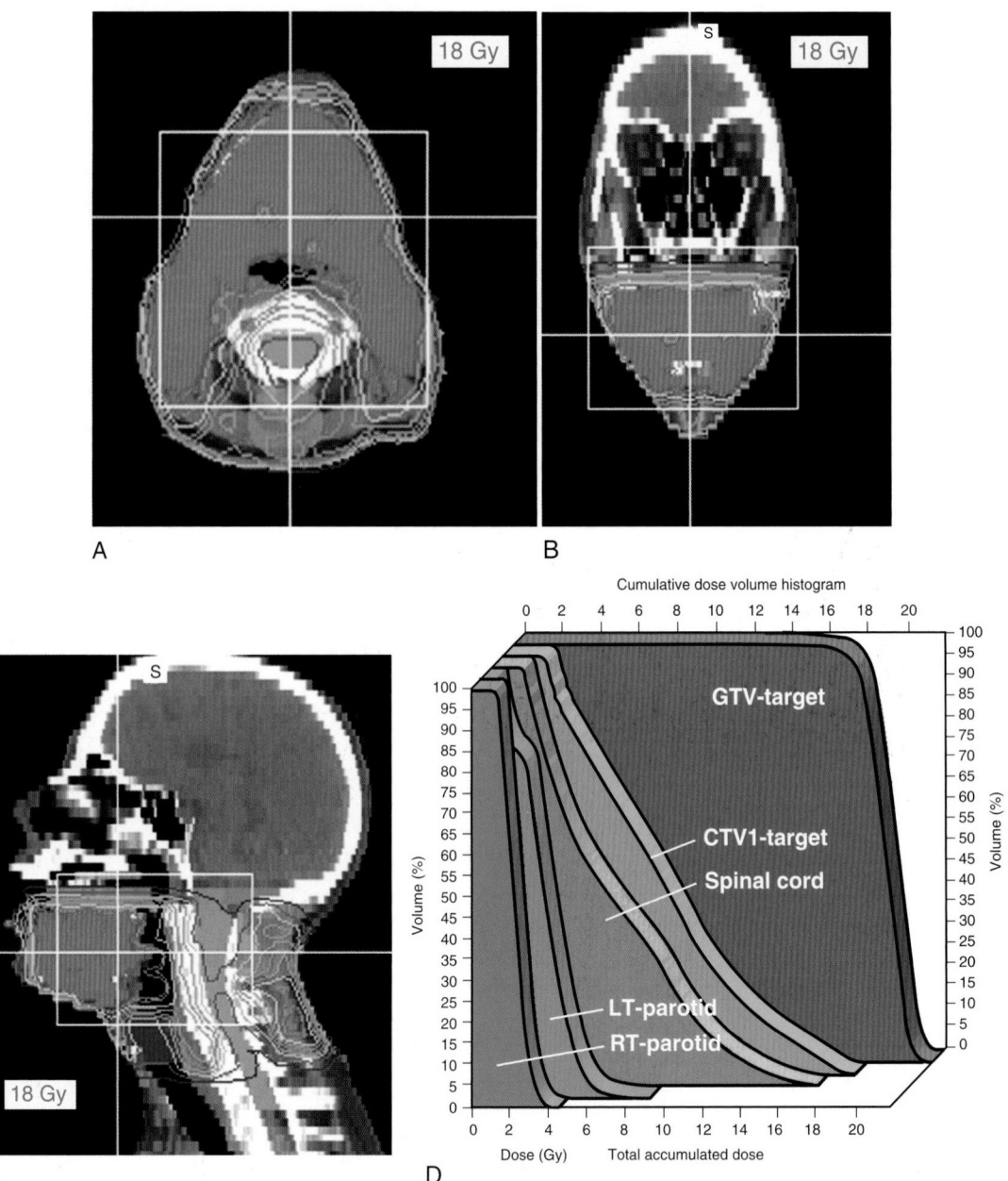

Figure 29–15. Isodose curves of an inverse intensity-modulated radiotherapy plan using seven coplanar gantry angles delivered with conventional multi-leaf collimator of a *boost plan* to the gross tumor volume (GTV) with a margin for a patient with T4N1 carcinoma of the floor of mouth displayed on the axial (**A**), coronal (**B**), and sagittal (**C**) planes through the centroid of the primary tumor and the DVH for the relevant structures (**D**). The GTV is shown in red and the clinical target volume (including a margin for set-up errors) is shown in magenta.

PLATE 35

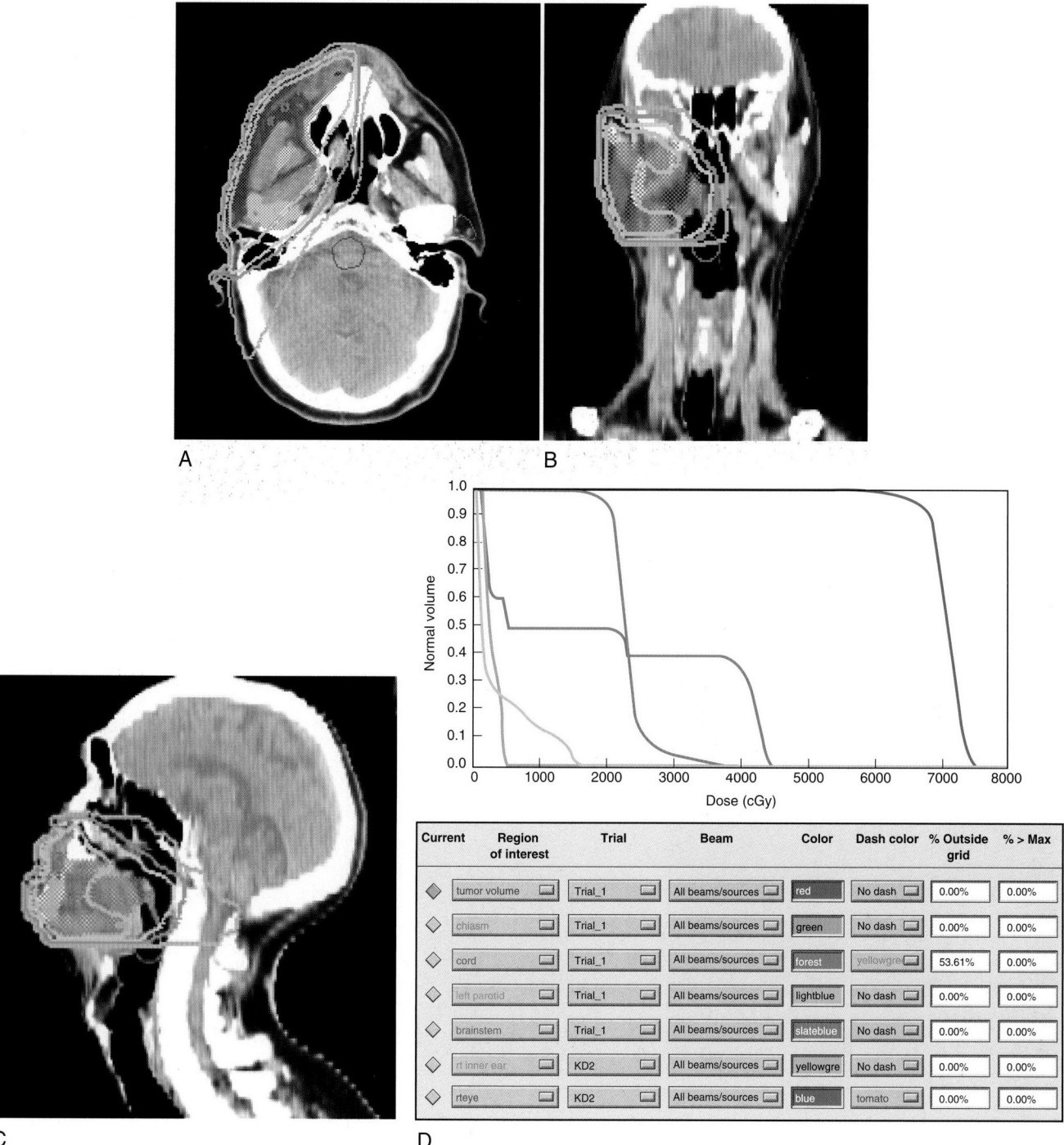

Figure 29–17. A, 3D treatment plan for buccal mucosal cancer, axial plane. **B,** 3D plan, coronal plane. **C,** 3D plan, sagittal view. **D,** Dose-volume histogram.

PLATE 36

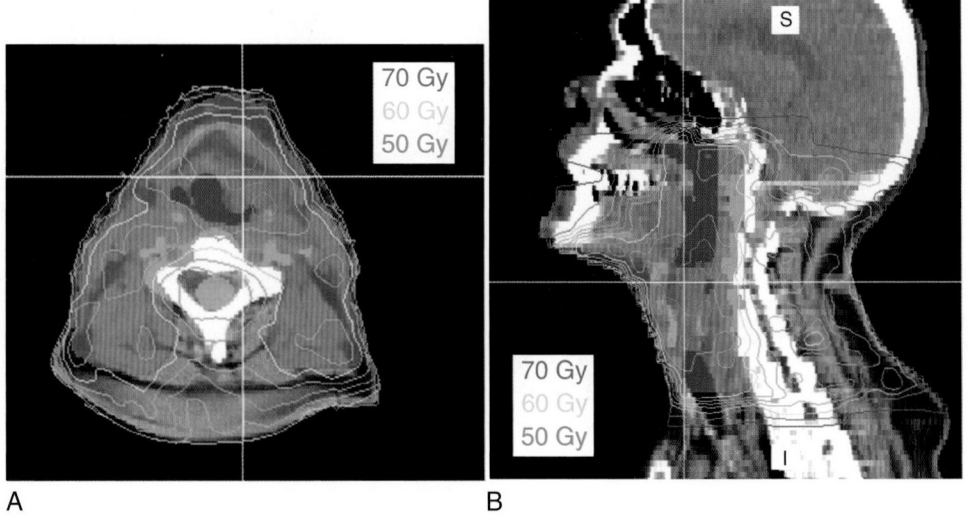

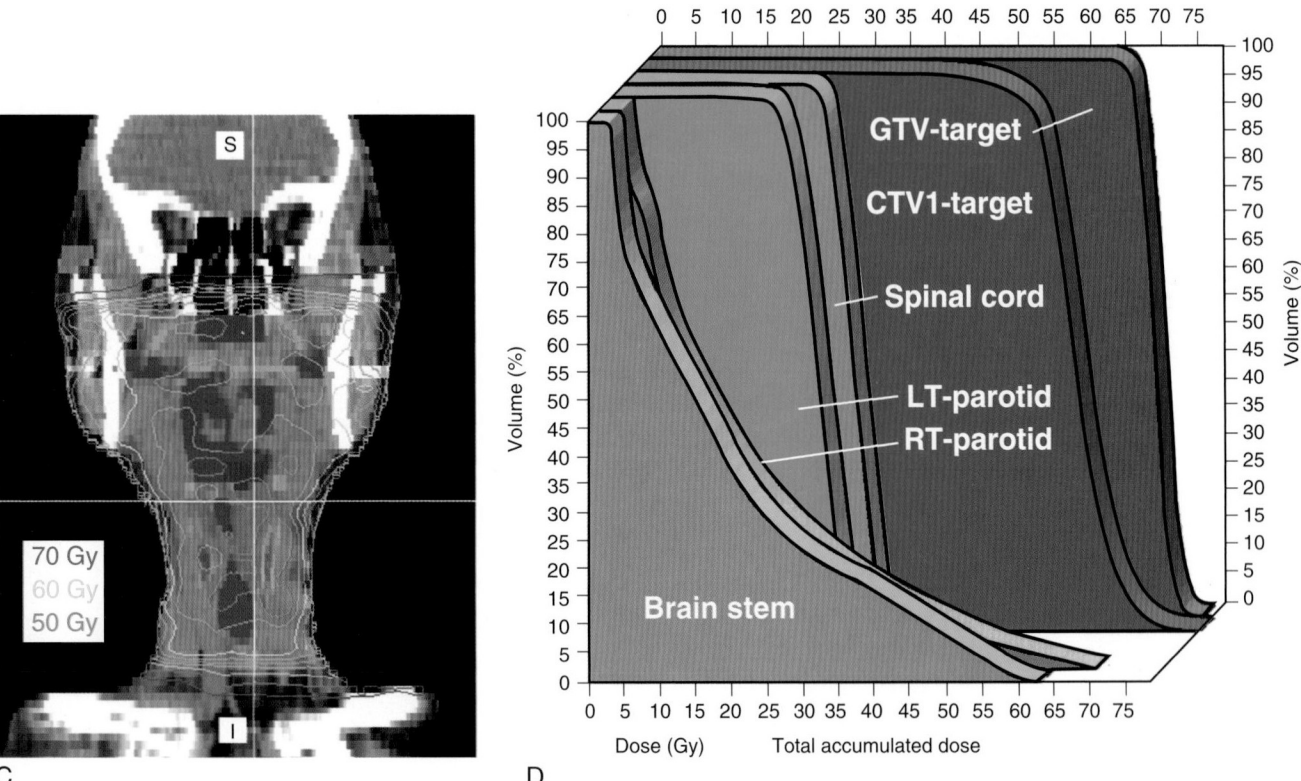

Figure 31–9. Three-dimensional treatment plan for supraglottic larynx cancer. Isodose distribution on the axial plane (**A**), sagittal plane (**B**), and coronal plane (**C**). **D**, Dose-volume histogram. Curves shown for external surface, spinal cord, and tumor as derived from CT scan.

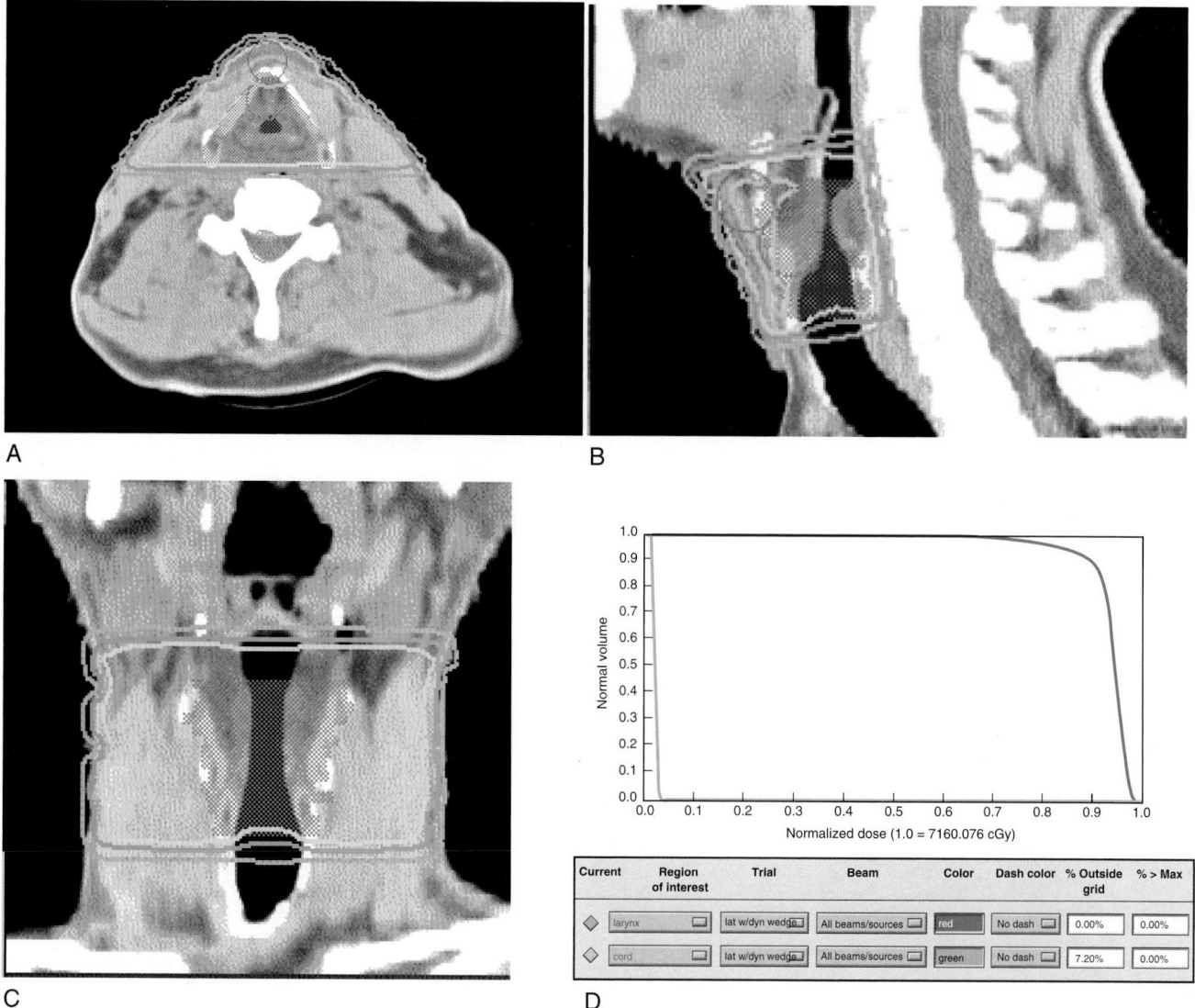

Figure 31–11. Isodose distribution on the axial plane (**A**), sagittal plane (**B**), and coronal plane (**C**). **D**, Dose-volume histogram for the tumor and spinal cord.

PLATE 38

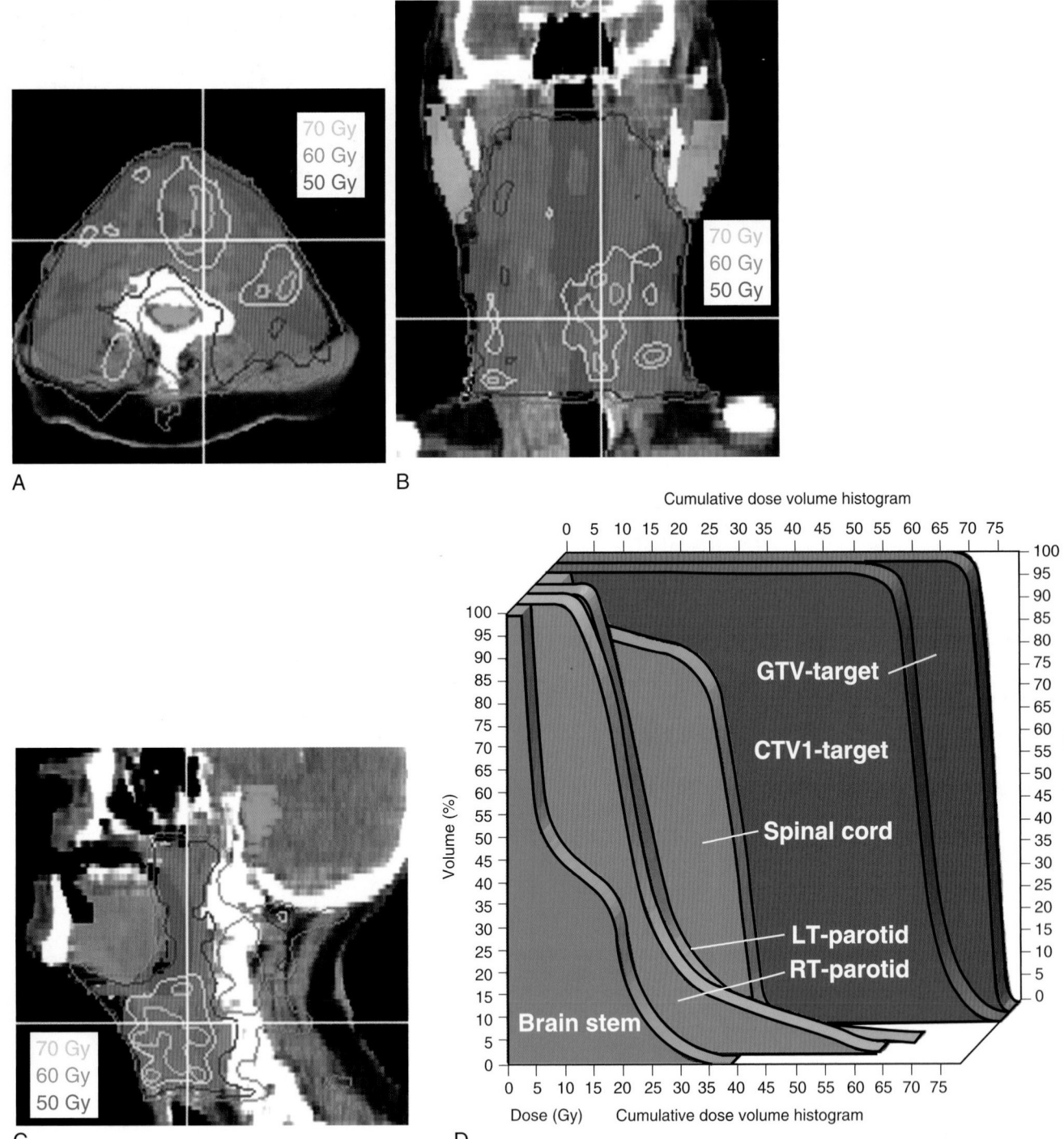

Figure 31–12. Isodose curves of an inverse intensity-modulated radiation therapy plan using seven coplanar gantry angles delivered with conventional multi-leaf collimators for a patient with T3N1 carcinoma of the larynx displayed on the axial (**A**), coronal (**B**), and sagittal (**C**) planes through the centroid of the primary tumor and the dose-volume histogram for the relevant structures (**D**). The gross tumor volume is shown in *red* and the clinical tumor volume (including margin for patient set-up errors) in *magenta*.

PLATE 39

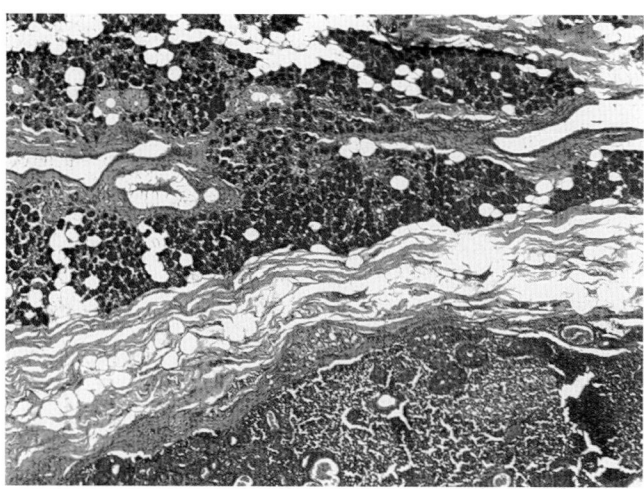

Figure 32–10. Mucoepidermoid carcinoma. There is no classic microscopic appearance as these salivary gland tumors have a wide variation in cellular composition. A predominance of "epidermoid cells" (closely resemble squamous cell carcinomas that form solid areas and nests) or "intermediate cells" (oval cells that contain a small, darkly staining nucleus), or both, is found. (Courtesy of Andrew Huvos, MD, Memorial Sloan-Kettering Cancer Center Department of Pathology.)

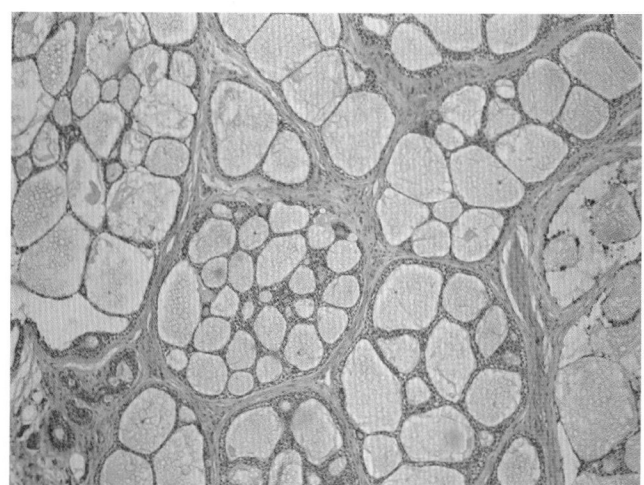

Figure 32–11. Adenoid cystic carcinoma. These are composed of a neoplastic epithelium composed of uniform basaloid cells that contain scant cytoplasm and which are arranged in cords or solid nests. This surrounds a stroma that contains hyaline eosinophilic material or a mucinous myxoid interstitium.

PLATE 40

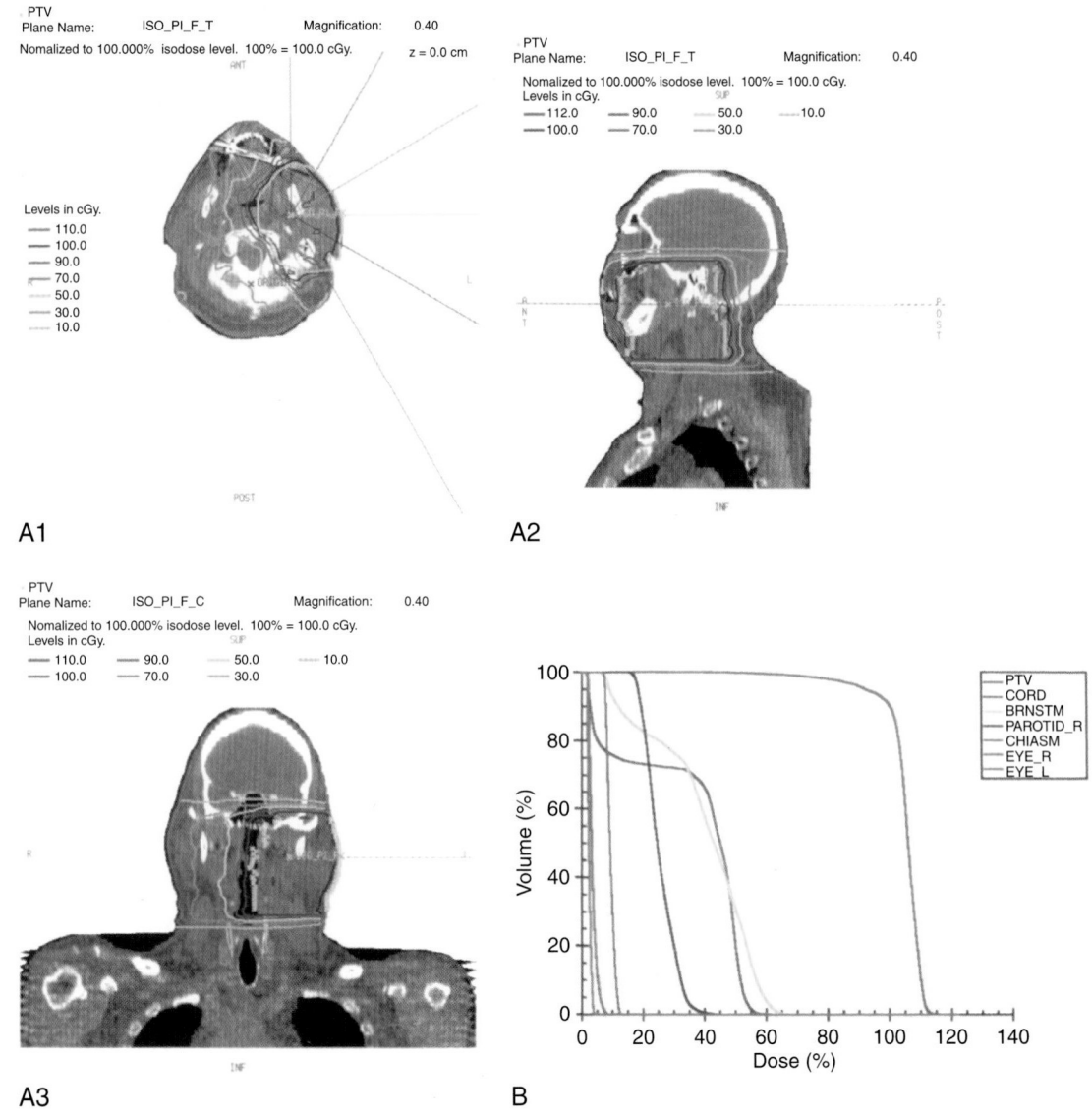

Figure 32–15. A 59-year-old man with an unresectable cT4N2aMO poorly differentiated carcinoma of the left parotid gland. He had progressive severe localized pain in the parotid gland and left facial nerve (CN VII) paralysis. This patient was treated with cisplatin chemotherapy concurrent with accelerated fractionation IMRT-based external beam radiation therapy with a delayed concomitant boost. The left parotid gland and cervical adenopathy were taken to 7000 cGy and the left cervical and supraclavicular nodes were taken to 5000 to 5400 cGy. A complete clinical response was achieved with resolution of all disease on examination and on computed tomography and positron emission tomography scans. **A**, Isodose distributions (A1, axial; A2, sagittal; A3, coronal). **B**, Dose volume histogram.

PLATE 41

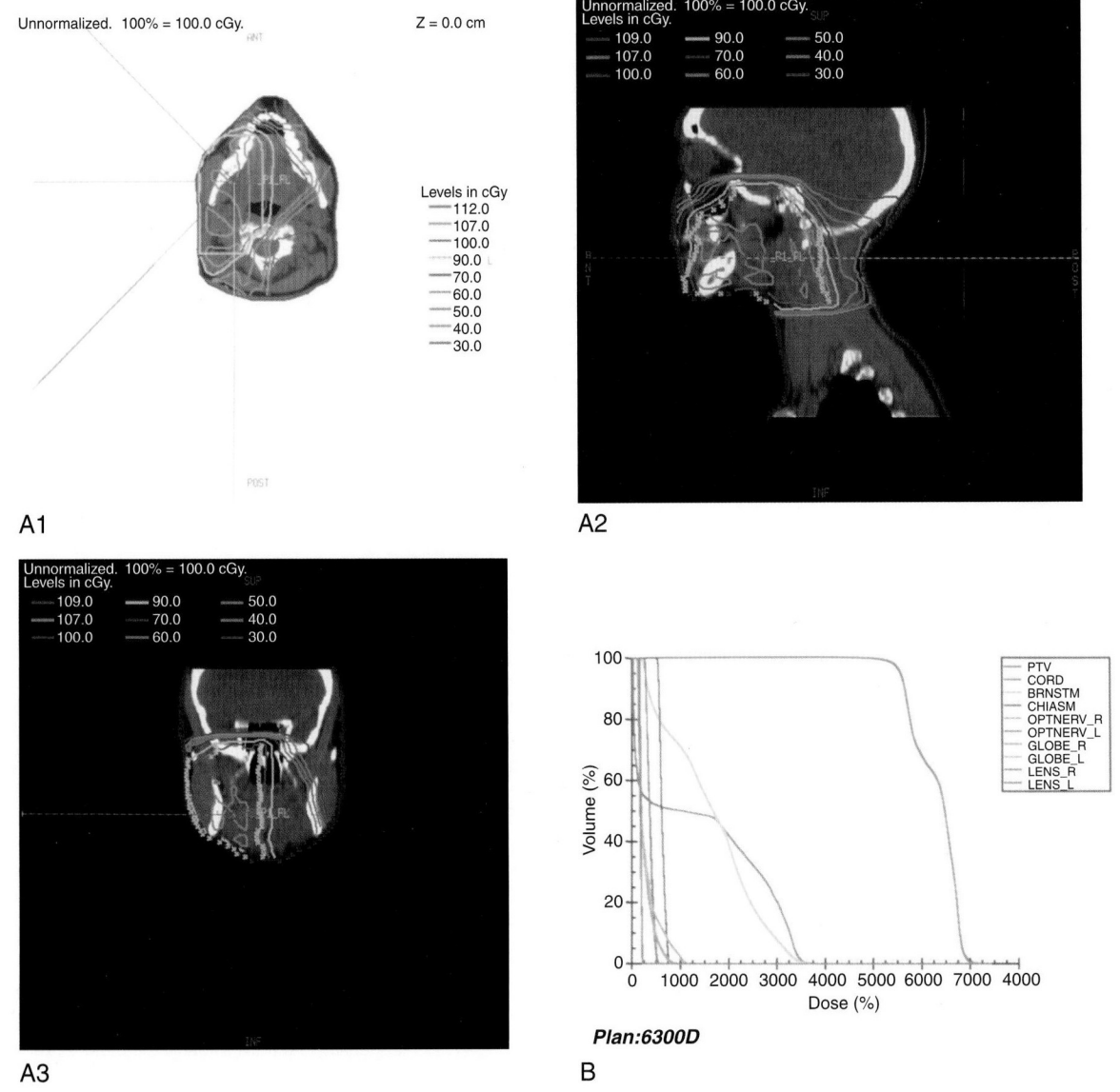

Figure 32–16. A 34-year-old woman with a pT1N0M0 adenoid cystic carcinoma of the right submandibular salivary gland. This patient underwent resection of the gland with pathology findings of positive surgical margins and perineural invasion. Postoperative intensity-modulated radiation therapy–based external beam radiation therapy was administered to a treatment volume consisting of the right submandibular gland area and the pathways of the adjacent lingual nerve (CN V3) and the hypoglossal nerve (CN XII) to the base of skull to a dosage of 5400 cGy. The postoperative bed in the submandibular area was then boosted to a total cumulative dosage of 6300 cGy. **A,** Isodose distributions (A1, axial; A2, sagittal; A3, coronal). **B,** Dose volume histogram.

PLATE 42

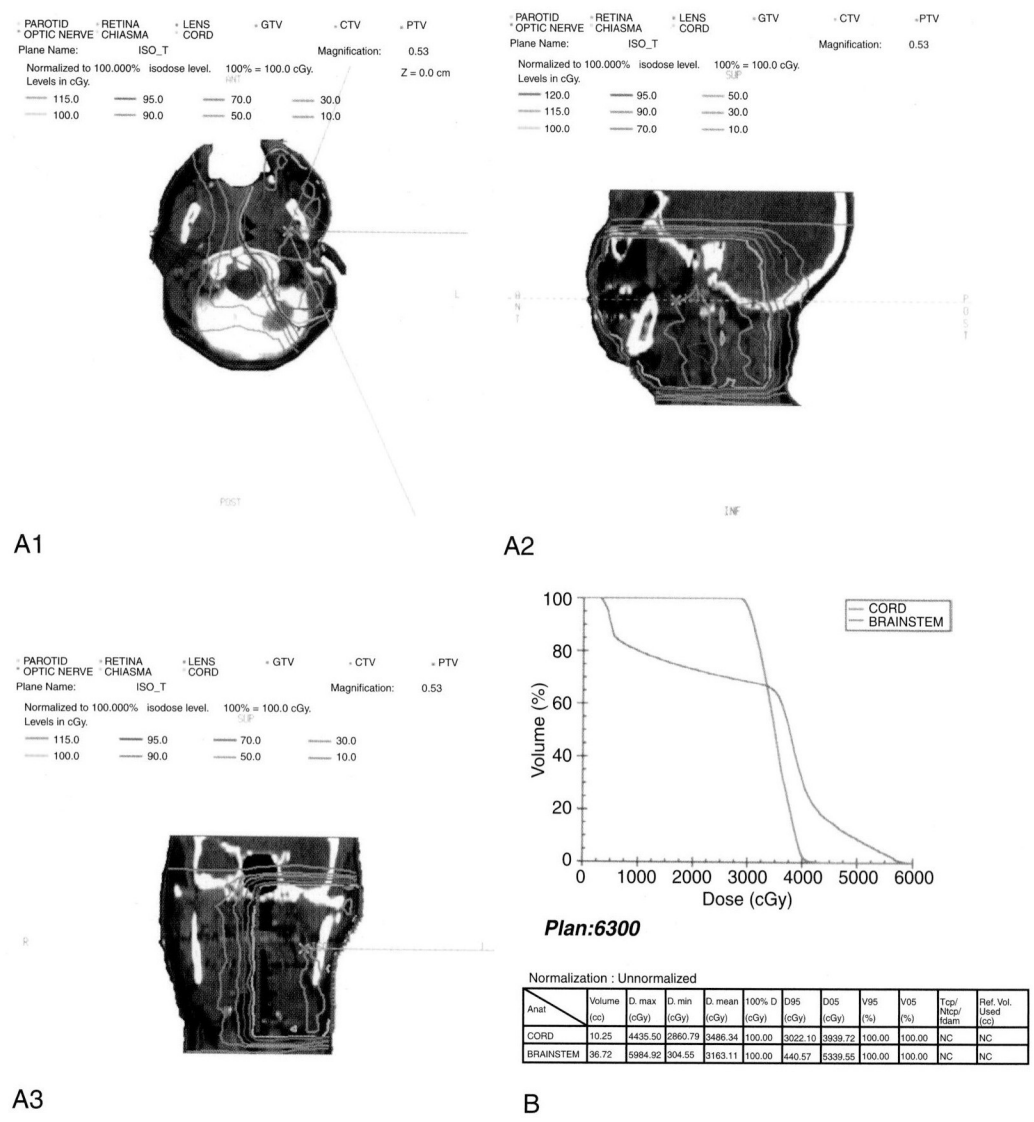

Figure 32–17. A 34-year-old man with a pT4B N0 M0 poorly differentiated mucoepidermoid carcinoma of the left parotid gland (deep lobe) with facial nerve (CN VII) paralysis. This patient underwent a left total parotidectomy with facial nerve sacrifice. A facial nerve graft with a facial sling was performed. The tumor extended superiorly to the left base of skull and had completely encased the facial nerve at the stylomastoid foramen. Pathology evaluation revealed a poorly differentiated mucoepidermoid carcinoma of the left parotid measuring 2.0 cm, which extended into the periparotid soft tissue and skeletal muscle. The carcinoma focally involved the inked resection margin. There was perineural invasion. All 13 lymph nodes were negative for metastatic disease. The patient was felt to be at high risk for local-regional recurrence, and therefore postoperative radiation therapy was administered to the left parotid gland–left base of skull, left retropharyngeal nodes–left upper cervical nodes using intensity-modulated radiation therapy–based external beam radiation therapy to 6300 cGy. The ipsilateral cervical and supraclavicular nodes (off spinal cord) were taken to 5000 cGy. **A,** Isodose distributions (A1, A2, A3). **B,** Dose volume histogram.

PLATE 43

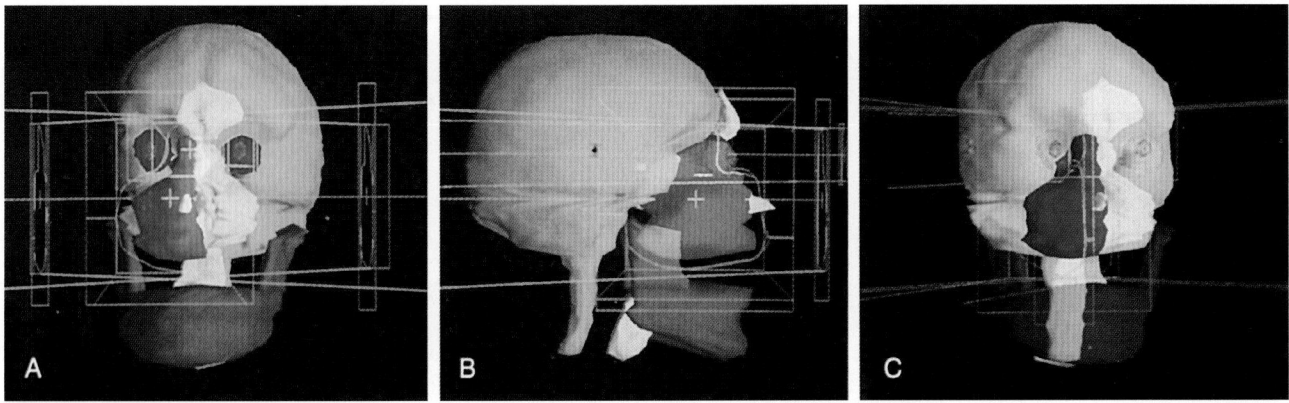

Figure 33–8. Three-dimensional beam's-eye views: four-field technique using opposed lateral portals, and anterior photon and electron portals. **A,** Anterior view. **B,** Lateral view. **C,** Oblique view.

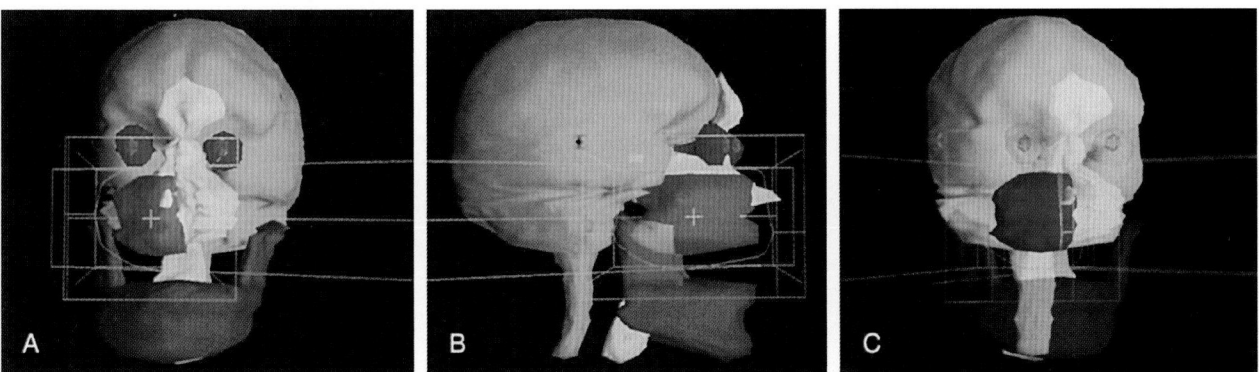

Figure 33–9. Three-dimensional beam's-eye views: wedged-pair portals. **A,** Anterior view. **B,** Lateral view. **C,** Oblique view.

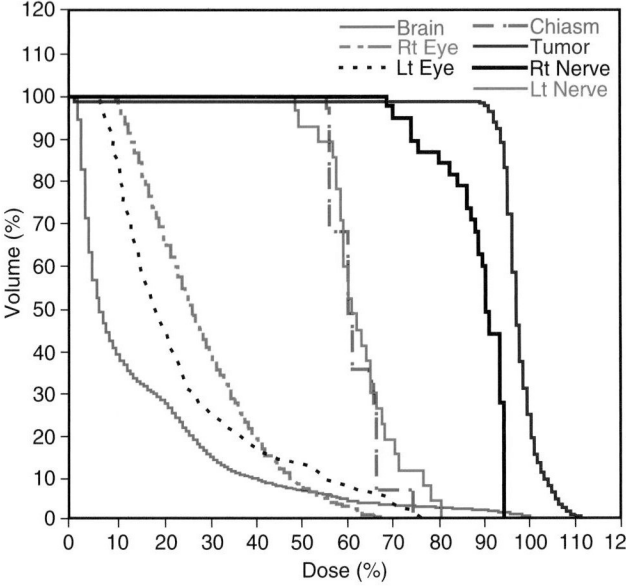

Figure 33–10. Three-dimensional dose-volume histogram. The optic chiasm and the contralateral optic nerve doses are limited to 65% to 70% of the prescribed dose while nearly 80% of the ipsilateral optic nerve receives greater than 90% of the prescribed tumor dose.

PLATE 44

Figure 33–11. Intensity-modulated radiation therapy isodose plans in axial planes (color-wash representations shown here in shades of gray) of a patient with locally advanced (stage T4NxM0) paranasal sinus undifferentiated carcinoma undergoing definitive radiotherapy. The plan was generated on Corvus planning system (Nomos Corp.) using 6 MV photons and MIMic multi-leaf collimator device with six table positions: **A,** At the level of the maxillary sinuses/parotid glands; **B,** at the level of the floor of the orbit/brainstem; **C,** at the level of ethmoid sinuses/mid-orbit. The bilateral eyes are nicely spared (<45 Gy isodose region) as are the brainstem (<45 Gy isodose region) and the parotid glands (<30 Gy isodose region).

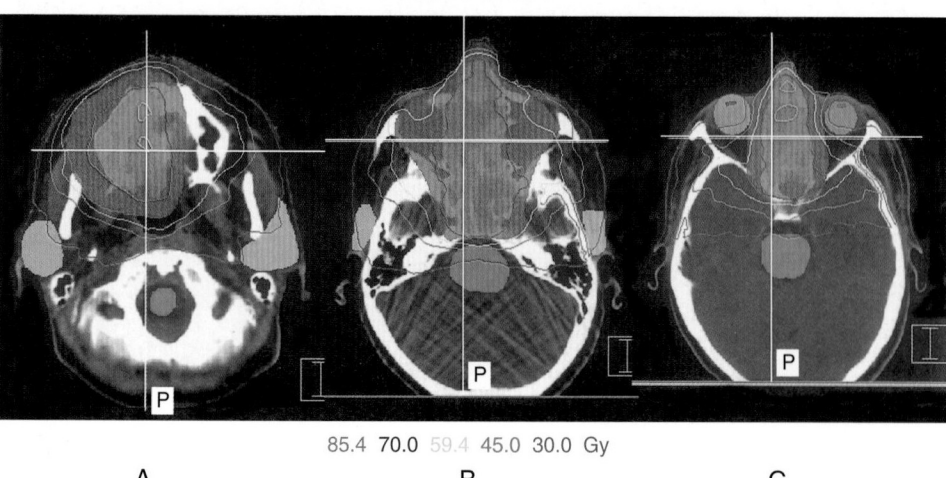

Paranasal Sinuses

85.4 70.0 59.4 45.0 30.0 Gy

A   B   C

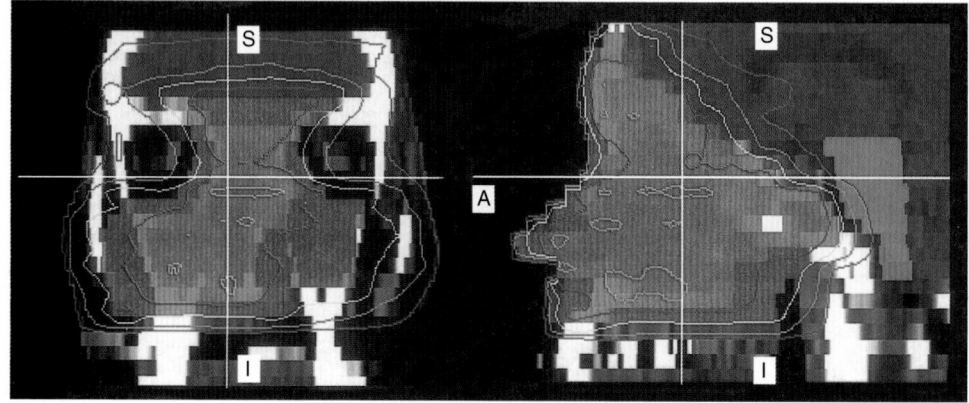

Paranasal Sinuses

85.4 70.0 59.4 45.0 30.0 Gy

A   B

Figure 33–12. Intensity-modulated radiation therapy isodose plans in sagittal and coronal planes: **A,** coronal view; **B,** sagittal view.

PLATE 45

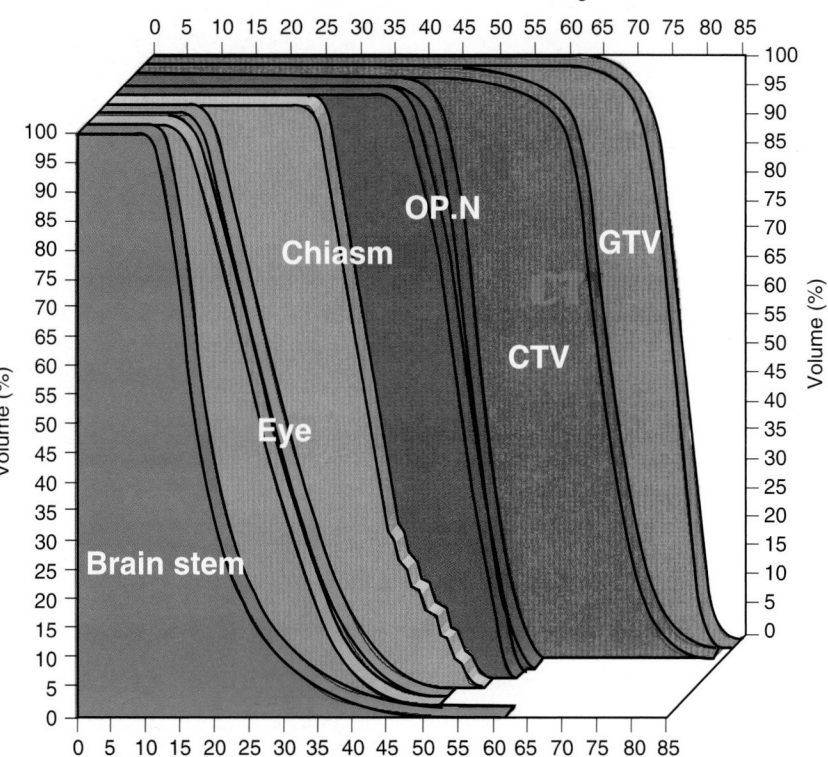

Figure 33–13. Intensity-modulated radiation therapy dose volume histogram. The gross target volume (GTV) receives 70 Gy and the clinical target volume (CTV) receives 59.4 Gy. Less than 10% of the optic chiasm receives greater than 55 Gy.

PLATE 46

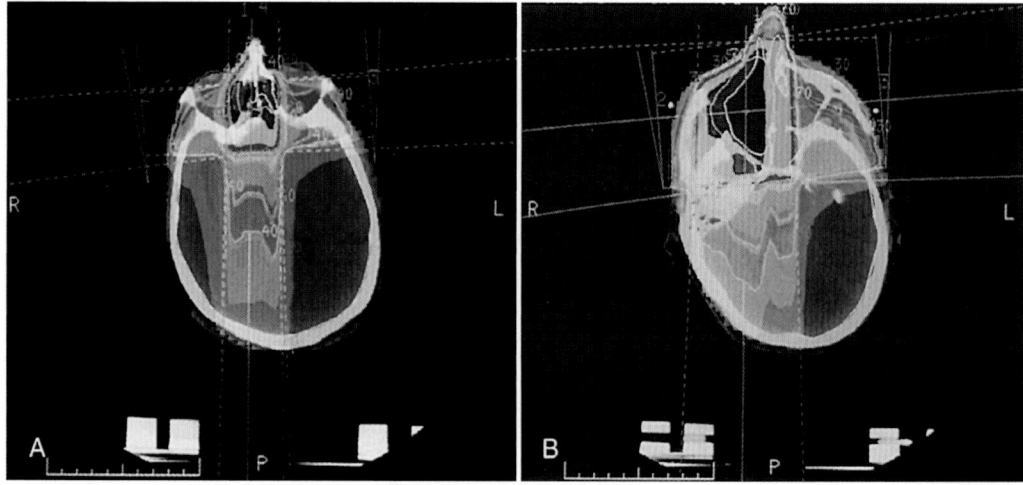

Figure 33–18. Three-dimensional isodose plans (color-wash representations shown here in shades of gray) of a four-field technique. Note the optic chiasm dose at the 60% to 70% region: **A,** At the level of the orbits and chiasm; **B,** at the level of the midantrum.

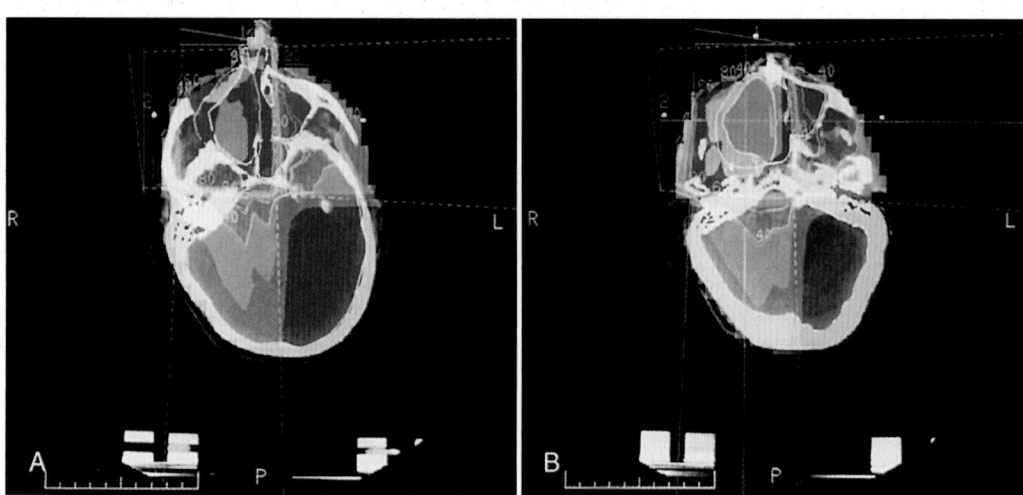

Figure 33–19. Three-dimensional isodose plans (color-wash representations shown here in shades of gray) of a wedged-pair technique: **A,** At the level of the midantrum; **B,** at the level of the lower antrum.

PLATE 47

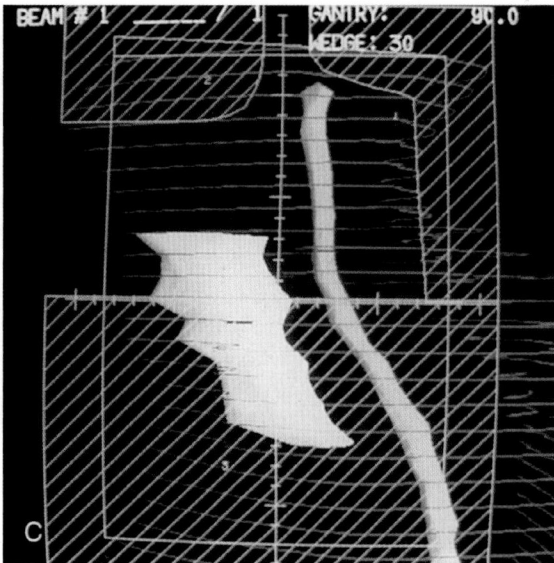

Figure 34–6. C, Beam's-eye view of lateral field, upper portion, with computed tomographically defined tumor volume, spinal cord, and blocks.

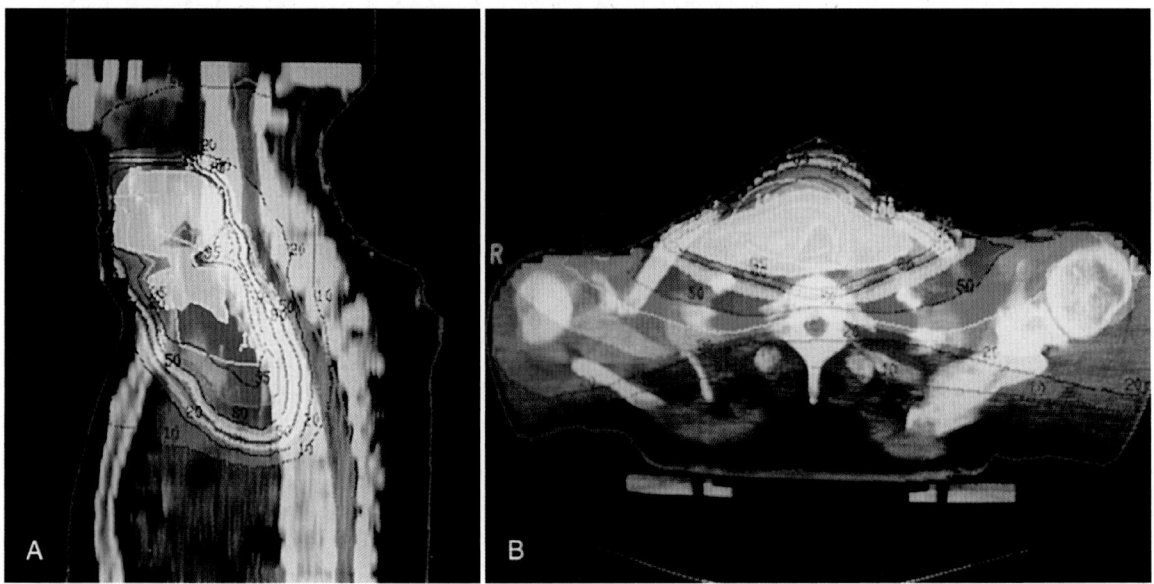

Figure 34–7. A, Sagittal reconstruction of the computed tomography (CT) scan used for treatment planning for the off-cord portion of therapy using the beam split approach, showing superimposed isodose distribution. **B,** Axial slice of CT scan with the superimposed isodose distributions in the lower half of the field for the two-field off-cord boost.

PLATE 48

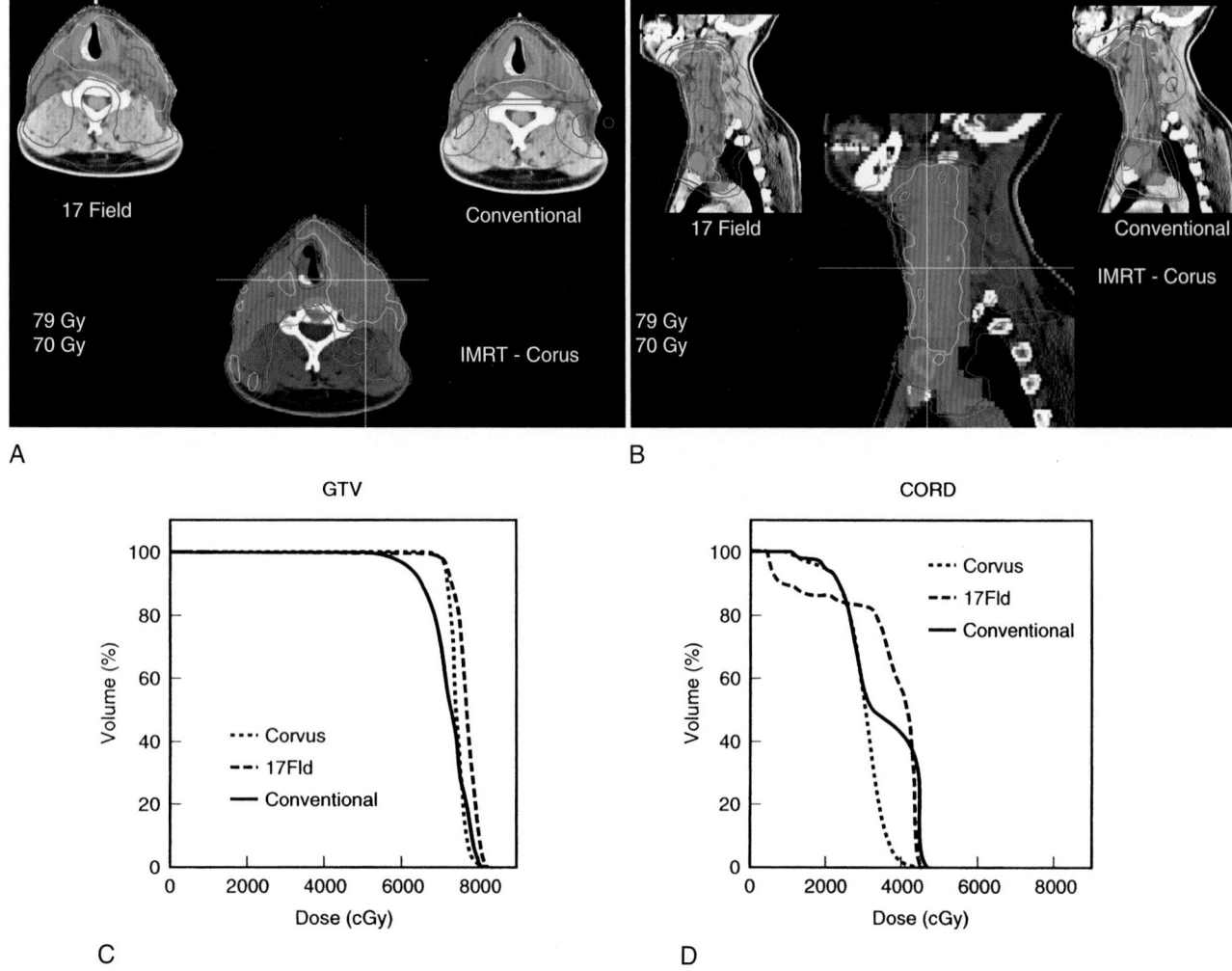

Figure 34–8. A, Axial dose distributions at the level of the larynx in a patient with locally advanced, left-sided anaplastic carcinoma—comparison of standard planning, 17-field three-dimensional treatment plan, and an intensity-modulated radiation therapy plan using the Corvus system. Note the differential dosing allowing laryngeal and cord dose reduction. **B,** Sagittal dose distributions. **C,** Dose-volume histogram comparison for these three plans. **D,** Dose-volume histogram comparison for the spinal cord with these plans

PLATE 49

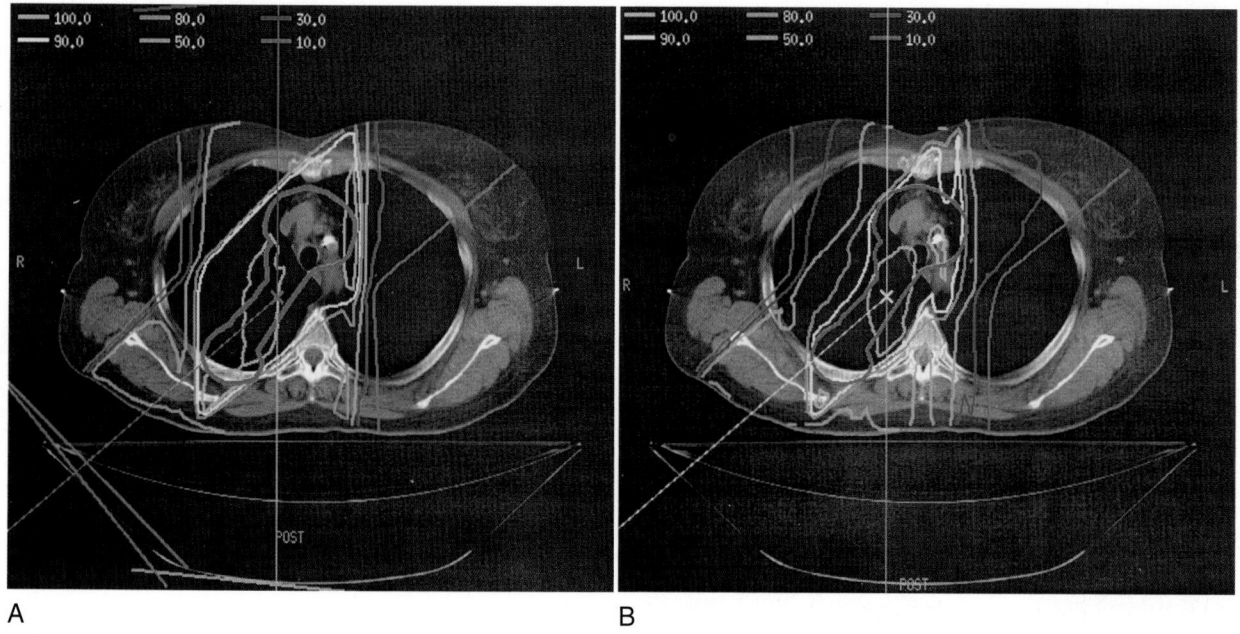

Figure 35–6. A, Dose distribution of a three-dimensional conformal radiation treatment (3D-CRT) plan. **B,** Dose distribution of an intensity-modulated radiation therapy plan. Note how the 90% isodose curve (*yellow*) is more conformal around the PTV (*pink*).

PLATE 50

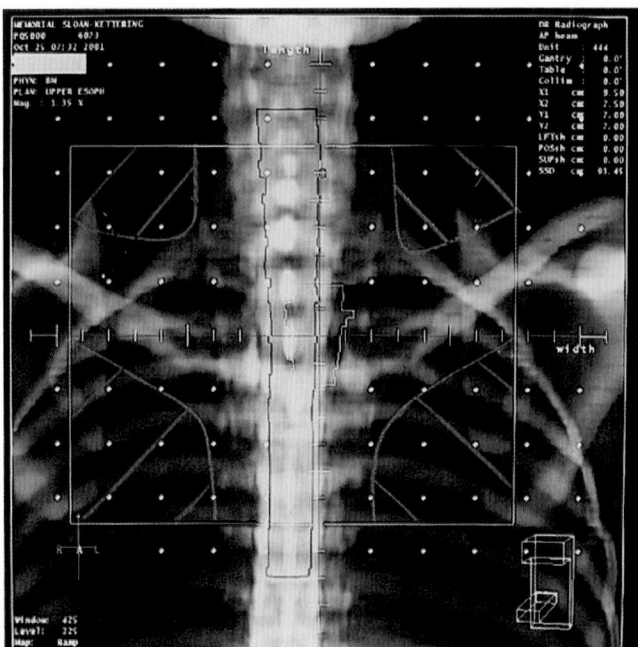

Figure 36-3. An example of the anterior-posterior–posterior-anterior (AP–PA) component for the treatment of a proximal esophageal cancer.

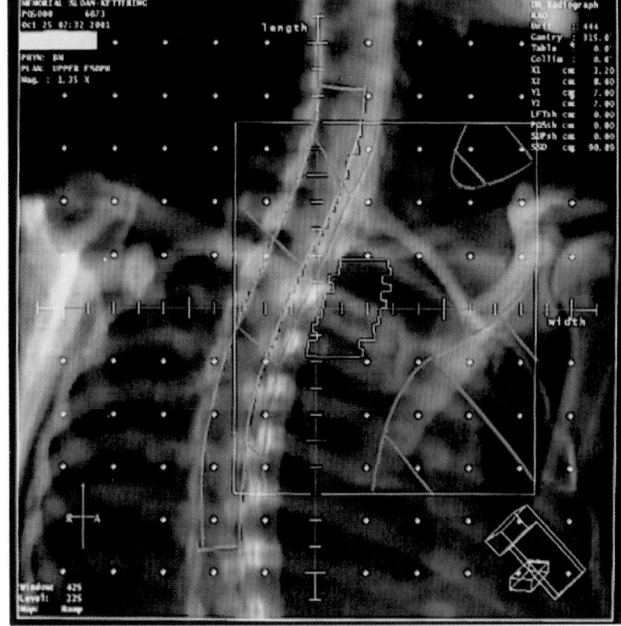

Figure 36-4. An example of the oblique component for the treatment of a proximal esophageal cancer.

PLATE 51

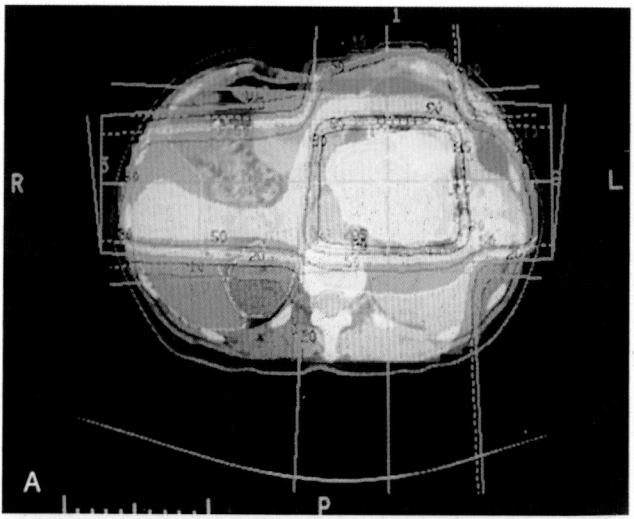

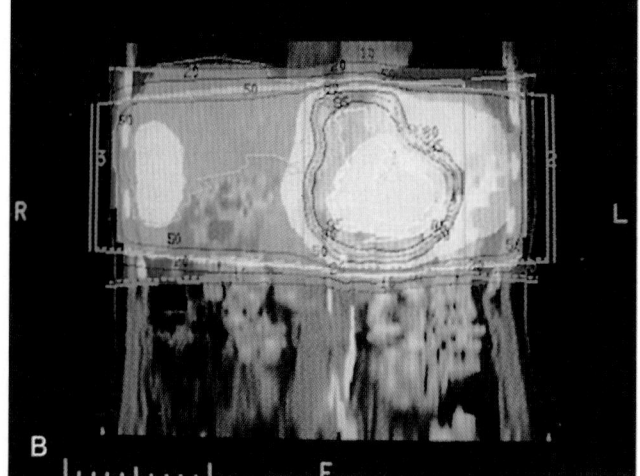

Figure 38–8. Axial (**A**), coronal (**B**), and sagittal (**C**) color-wash isodose distributions of three-field plan with lateral wedges. The tumor bed volume is covered in the 95% isodose line with a hot spot of 104%. The anterior field is weighted 40%, while the laterals have weighting of 30% each. Block margins for this T1N0M0 tumor are 1.0 to 1.5 cm.

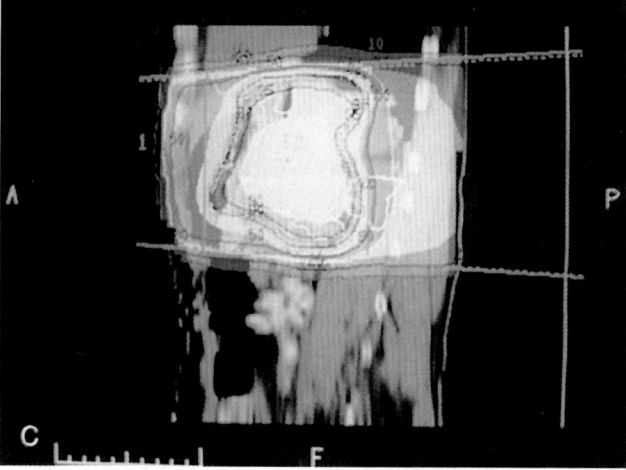

PLATE 52

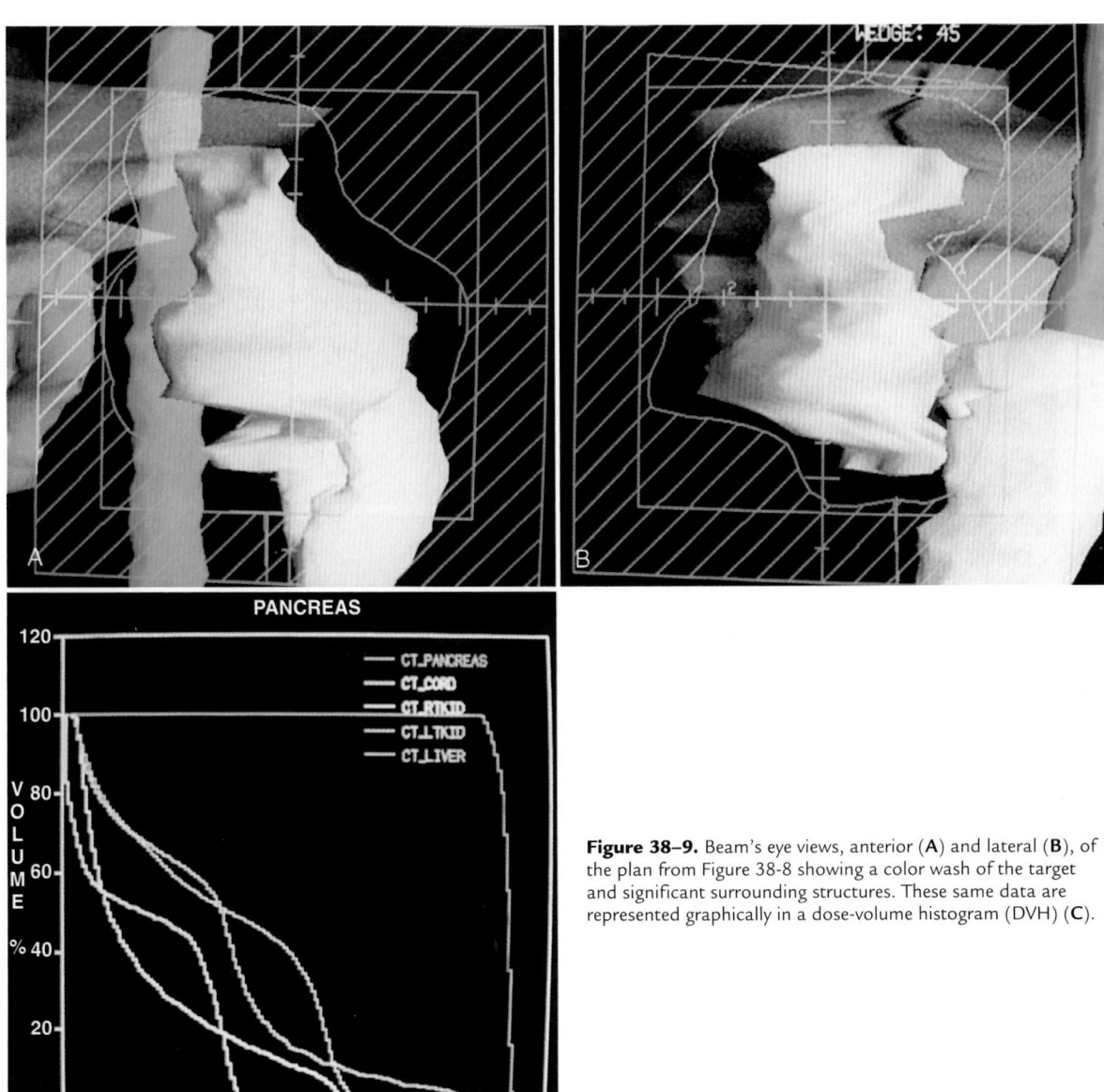

Figure 38–9. Beam's eye views, anterior (**A**) and lateral (**B**), of the plan from Figure 38-8 showing a color wash of the target and significant surrounding structures. These same data are represented graphically in a dose-volume histogram (DVH) (**C**).

PLATE 53

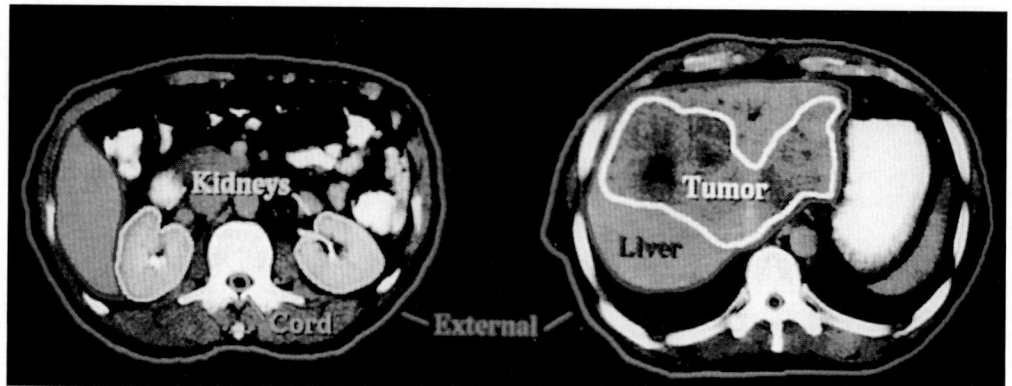

Figure 39–2. Contouring of critical structures for an external beam CT-guided radiotherapy plan (as used at the University of Michigan Medical Center). Contours are drawn on each computed tomography slice for tumor, liver, kidneys, spinal cord, skin, and, when appropriate, stomach and duodenum.

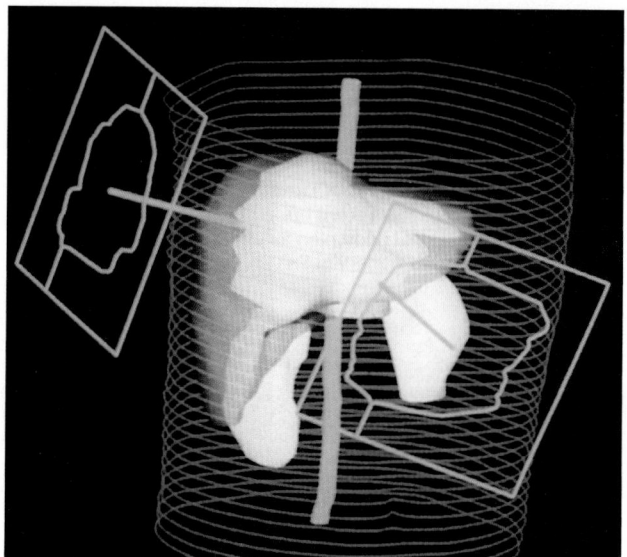

Figure 39–3. Multiple-beam conformal radiotherapy plan for hepatocellular carcinoma (as used at the University of Michigan Medical Center). A computer-generated plan showing varying angles and approaches to maximize tumor dose and minimize irradiation of the normal liver.

PLATE 54

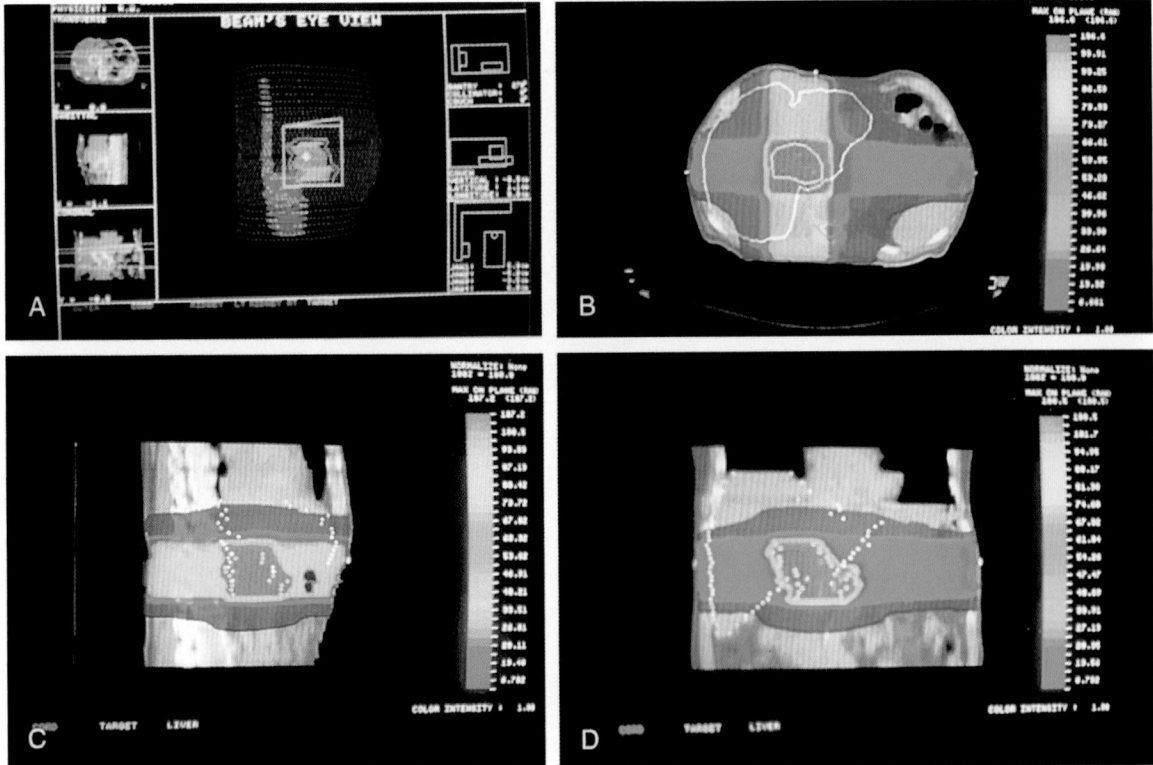

Figure 39–7. Boost portals for extrahepatic bile duct carcinoma (EHBDC) (external beam photons). The use of three-dimensional treatment planning allows for tight boosts and the potential for decreased morbidity. Shown are a beam's-eye view reconstruction (**A**), and axial (**B**), sagittal (**C**), and coronal (**D**) color-wash displays of a four-field, three-dimensional boost plan for a patient with an unresectable EHBDC of the junction of the right and left hepatic ducts and common hepatic duct (Klatskin tumor).

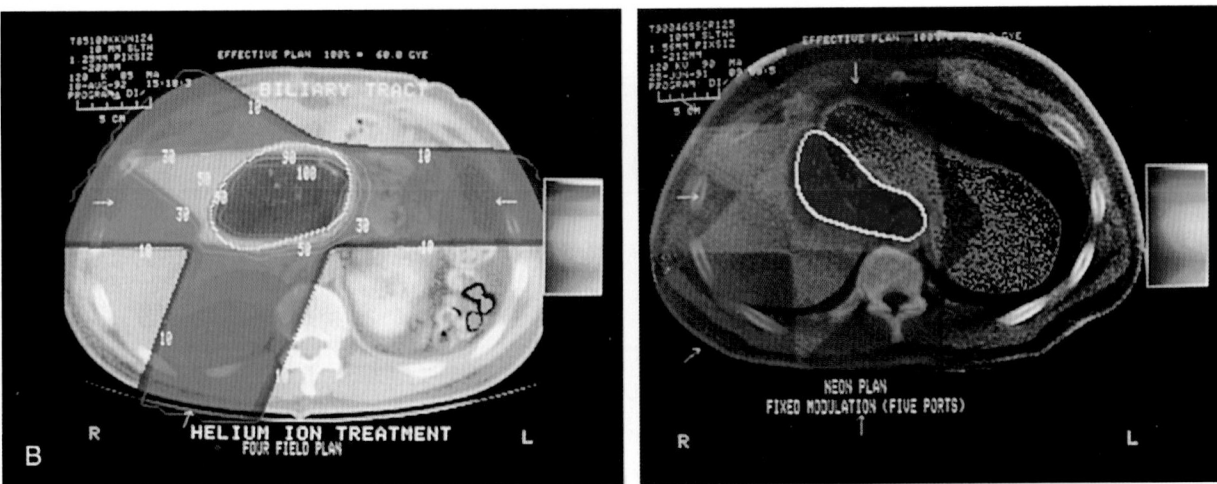

Figure 39–8. Specialized boost portals for extrahepatic bile duct carcinoma. Sophisticated treatment planning with charged particles (*left*, helium; *right*, neon) has resulted in some of the best results seen in the medical literature.

PLATE 55

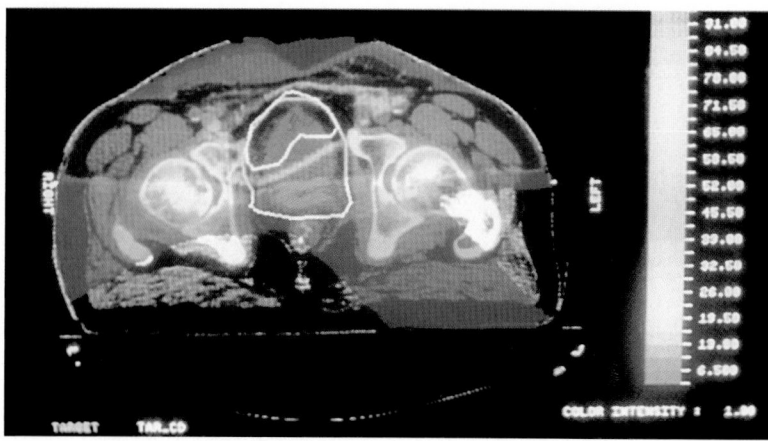

Figure 44–7. Three-dimensional conformal plan for the cone-down phase of therapy. Note the high-dose region confined to a small volume of bladder (site of known initial disease).

PLATE 56

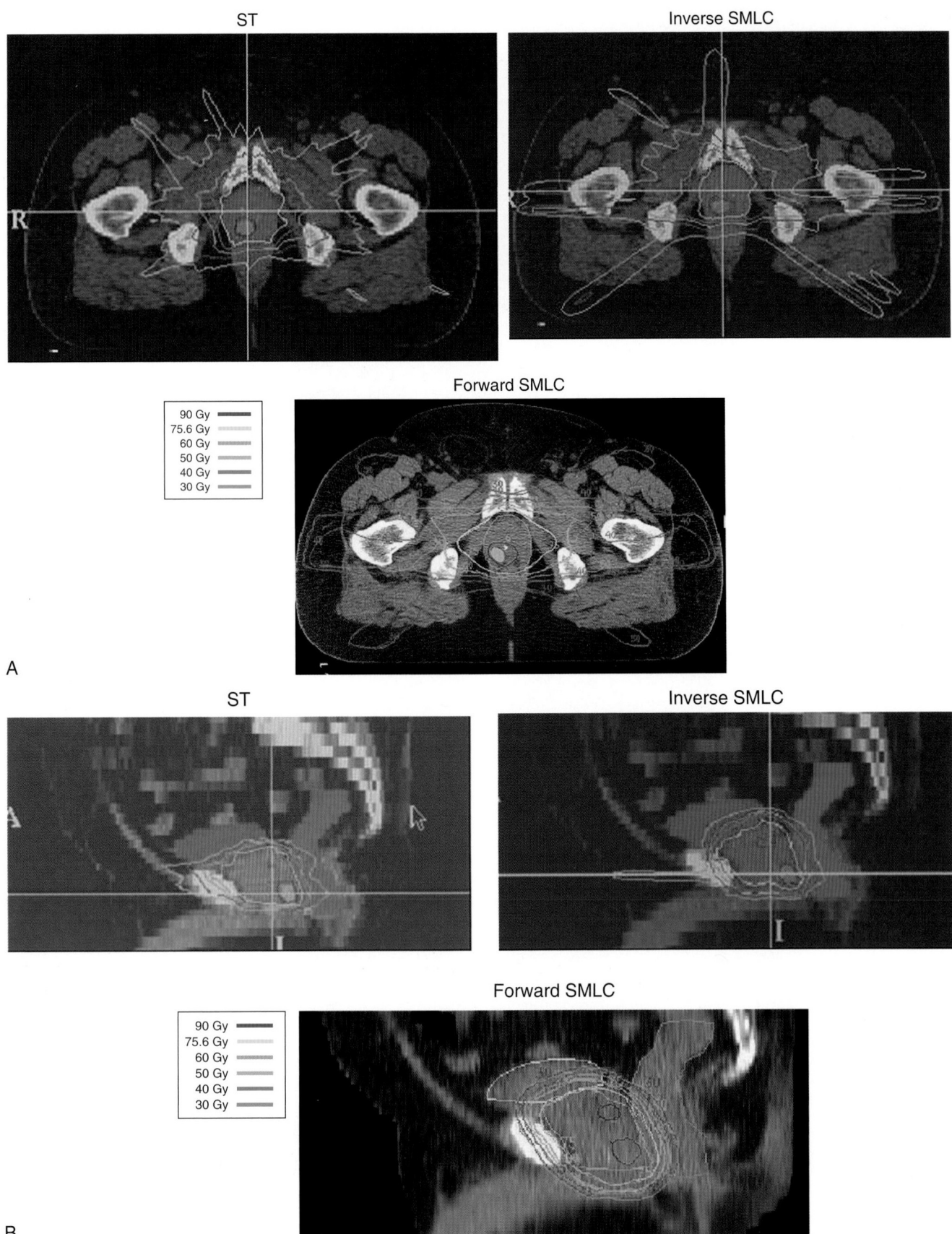

Figure 45–16. A, Axial, **B,** sagittal, and **C,** coronal distributions associated with tomotherapy, forward planned segmental multi-leaf collimator (SMLC) intensity-modulated radiotherapy (IMRT) and inverse planned SMLC IMRT, all targeting a dominant intra-prostatic lesion to 90 Gy while treating the entire prostate to 75.6 Gy. (From Xia P, Pickett B, Vigneault E, et al: Forward or inversely planned segmental multileaf collimator IMRT and sequential tomotherapy to treat multiple dominant intraprostatic lesions of prostate cancer to 90 Gy. *Int J Radiat Oncol Biol Phys.* 2001;51:244.)

PLATE 57

ST

Inverse SMLC

Forward SMLC

90 Gy
75.6 Gy
60 Gy
50 Gy
40 Gy
30 Gy

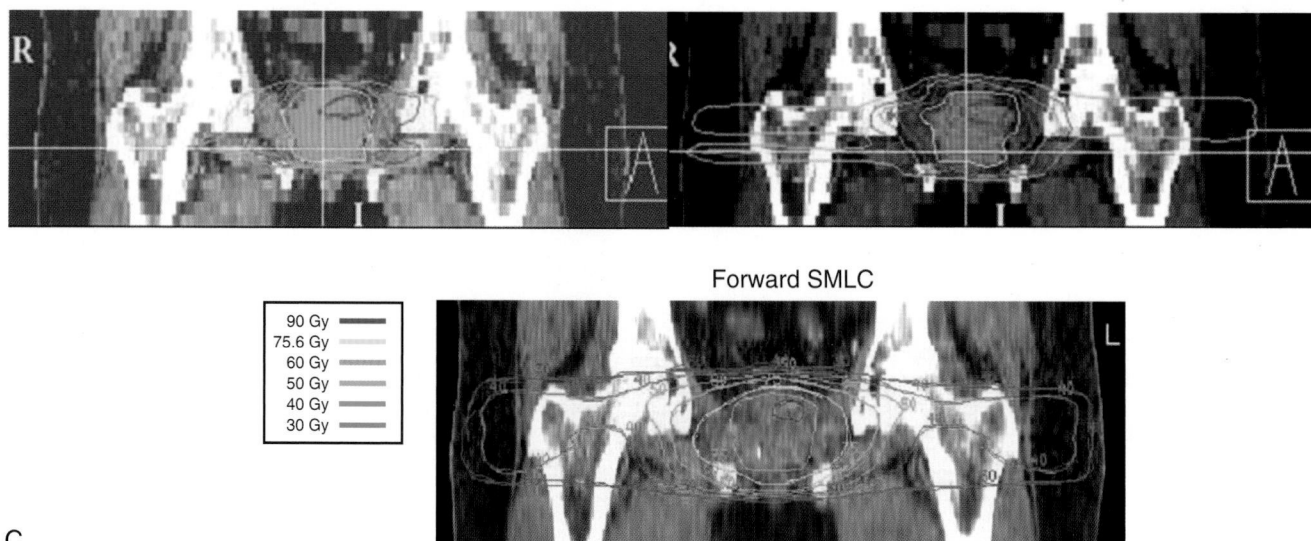

C

Figure 45–16. cont'd, For legend see previous page.

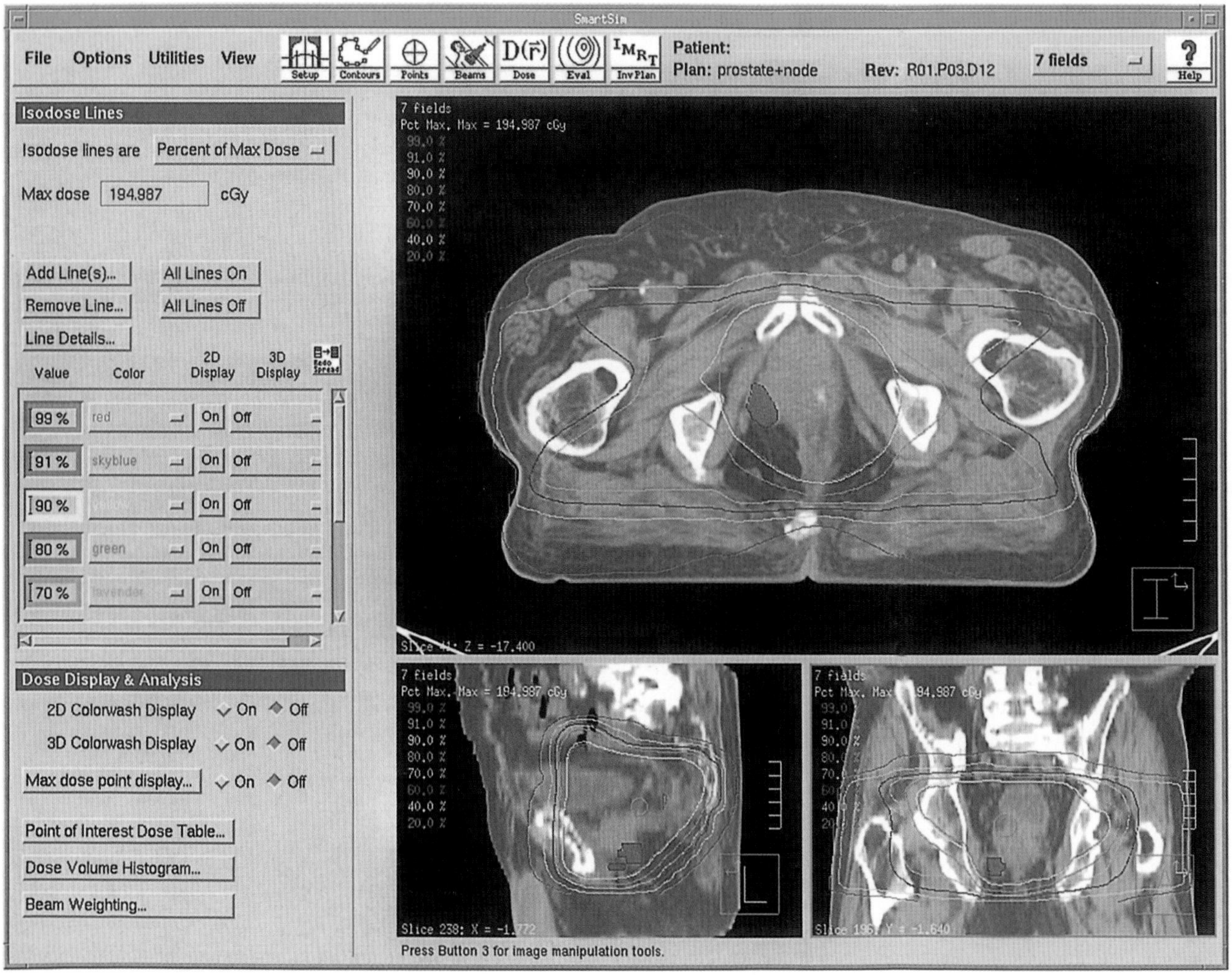

Figure 47–2. Conformal external beam radiotherapy for a lesion of the bulbo membrane urethra.

PLATE 58

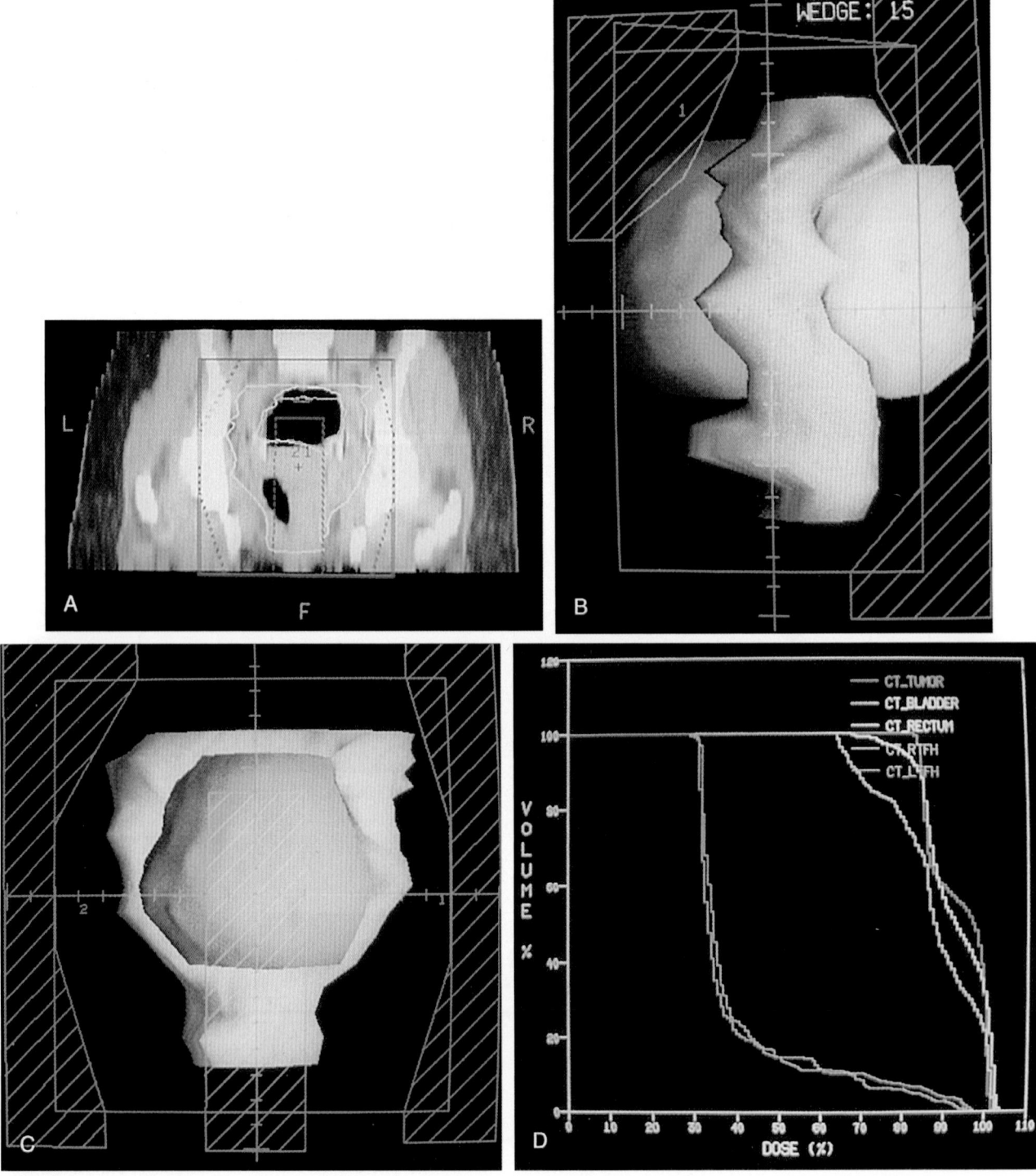

Figure 48–13. A, Field outline with blocks superimposed on coronal computed tomographic reconstruction; **B,** lateral three-dimensional (3D) reconstruction of bladder, rectum, and target volume of primary tumor plus regional nodes, with field and block outlines superimposed; **C,** Anterior-posterior 3D reconstruction of bladder and target volume (rectum concealed behind target) with superimposed field and block outlines; **D,** dose-volume histogram for initial 45 Gy (including addition of midline bar)-RTFH and LTFH indicate doses to femoral heads.

PLATE 59

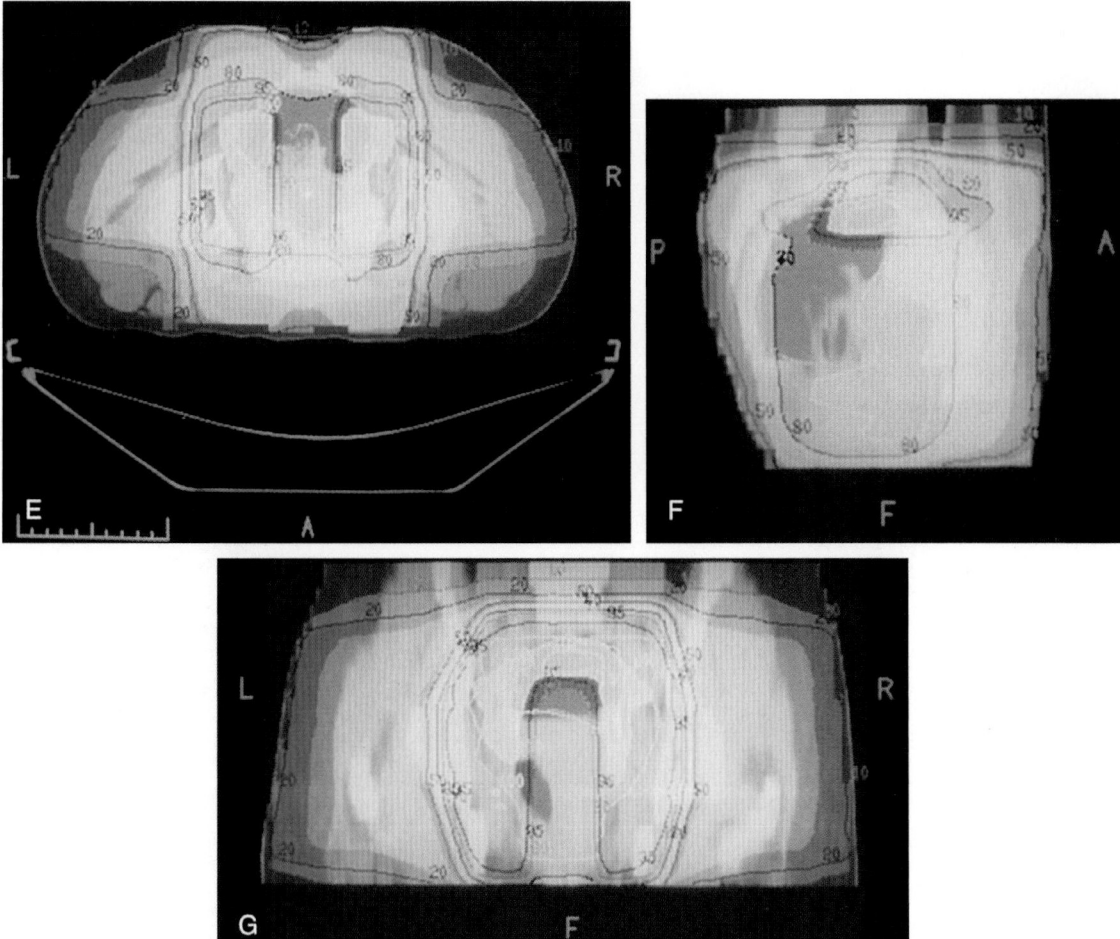

Figure 48–13. cont'd E, Composite axial isodose distributions of initial 45 Gy; **F,** sagittal isodose distributions; **G,** coronal isodose distributions.

PLATE 60

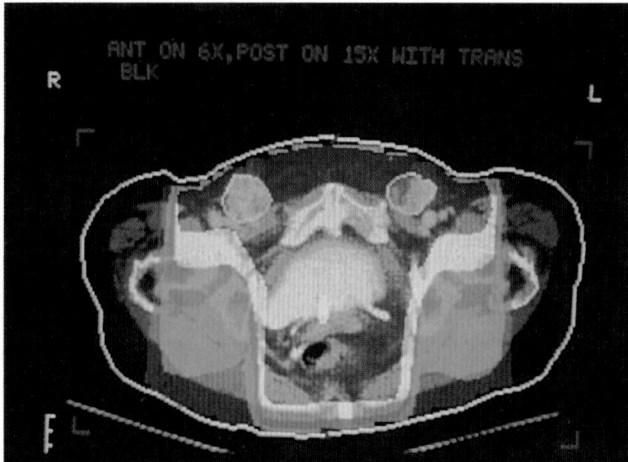

Figure 52–13. Computed tomography-based treatment plan of an alternative transverse dose distribution for the same patient as shown in Figure 52-3. This plan makes use of opposed anterior 6 MV and posterior 15 MV photon beams. Dose is prescribed at depth to the inguinal nodes from the anterior using the wider 6 MV photon field. Dose contribution to the midplane central axis is calculated and a partial transmission block is introduced in the beam over the central pelvis of sufficient thickness to reduce the central axis dose to 50% of the prescribed inguinal dose. A narrow, posterior 15 MV photon field, shaped to match the central partial transmission block and to exclude the femoral necks, is used to supplement the dose to the midplane central axis to a full, therapeutic level. Gradations in shade represent 10% increments in dose.

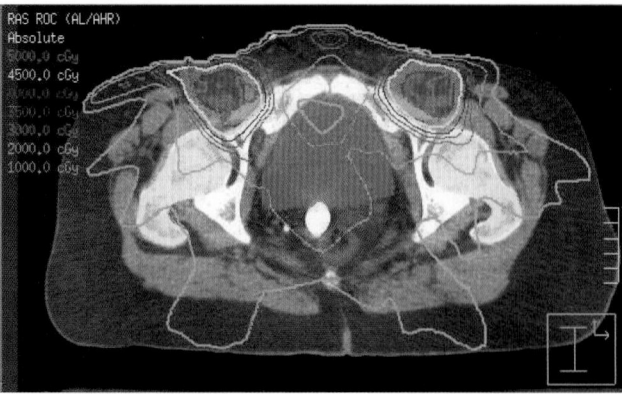

Figure 52–17. Transverse isodose distribution at the level of the urinary bladder (purple) and acetabulae. High dose volume is confined to the femoral vessels and associated lymph node tissue underlying the inguinal ligament.

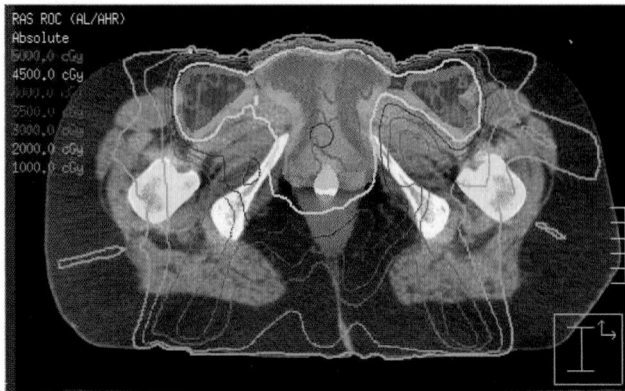

Figure 52–18. Transverse isodose distribution at the level of the anterior (superior) vulva at the level of the inferior ischial rami. High-dose volume is confined to the vulva and groin nodes and interconnecting skin.

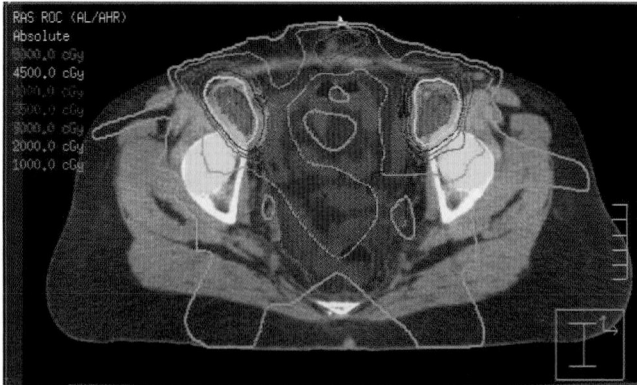

Figure 52–16. Transverse isodose distribution at the level of the mid-pelvis. Deep blue coloration corresponds to large and small bowel. High-dose volume is confined to caudal external iliac nodes.

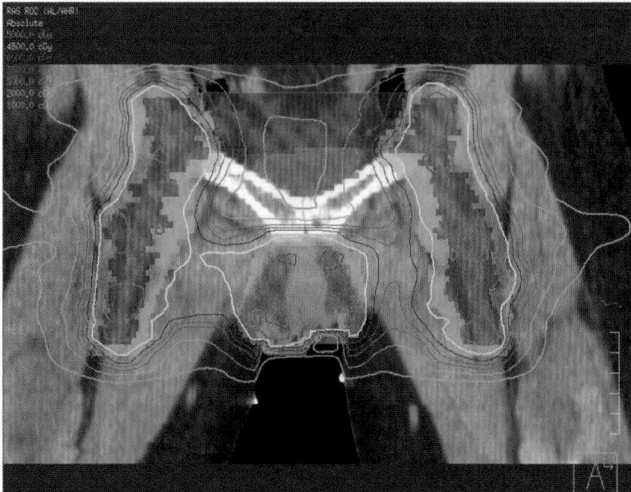

Figure 52–19. Coronal isodose distribution at the depth of the pubic symphysis illustrating selective dose deposition in the vulva, inguinofemoral, and caudal pelvic (external iliac) lymph nodes.

PLATE 61

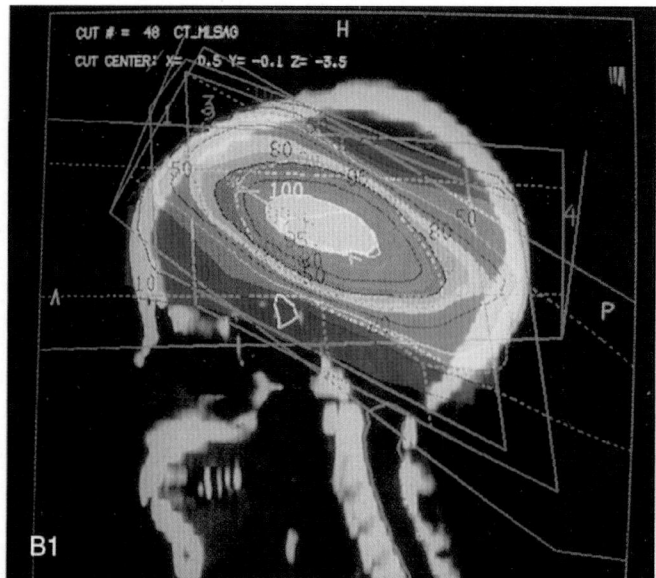

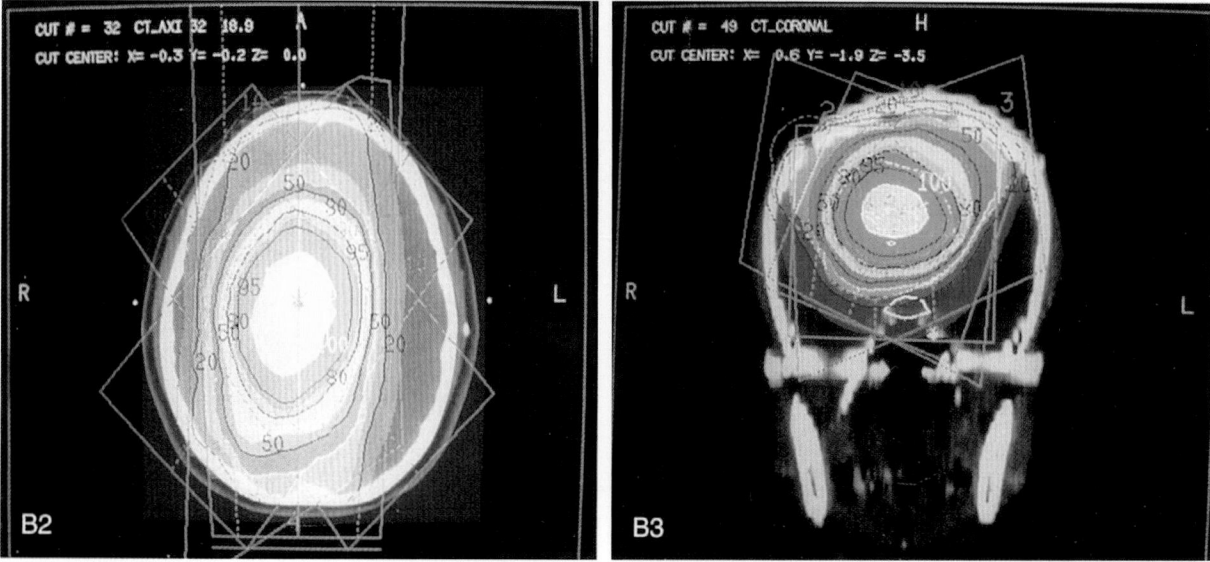

Figure 53–7. Three-dimensional conformal, noncoplanar treatment plan. The patient, a 21-year-old student, became increasingly disoriented over several days. Magnetic resonance imaging revealed a 5 cm intraventricular mass, which was subtotally resected because of involvement of the thalamus. Pathologic examination revealed an intraventricular neurocytoma. **B,** CT and MR images were merged to define the tumor volume, and a three-field, noncoplanar plan was devised, employing one posterior and two anterior, superior oblique beams. The plan's isodose curves are shown superimposed on the sagittal (*B1*), axial (*B2*), and coronal (*B3*) views.

PLATE 62

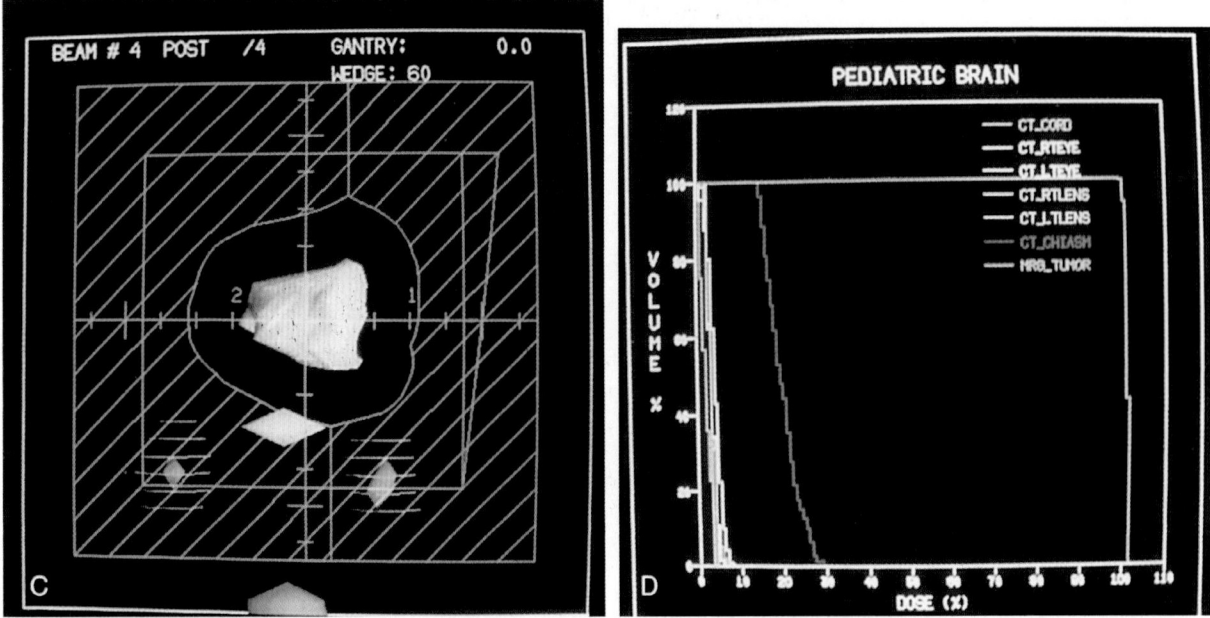

Figure 53–7. cont'd C, Beam's eye views were employed to design the blocking and to verify the plan. **D,** Dose-volume histograms were calculated and revealed satisfactory coverage of the planning treatment volume, and the dose to the chiasm was less than 30%.

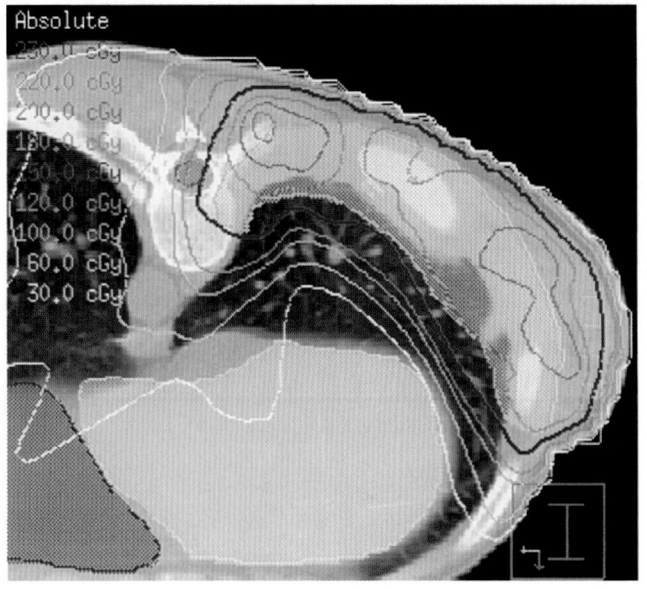

Figure 55–4. Imaging studies of a 19-year-old male with a primitive neuroectodermal tumor of the right thoracic wall. Following induction chemotherapy, chest wall resection (three ribs) was done and there was a positive margin. **B,** After receiving 18 Gy (1.5 Gy/fraction) to the right hemithorax postoperatively, a reduced volume for the tumor bed (prone position) was planned using 10 off-axis beams, which follow the curvature of the chest wall. The plan reduces dose to lung, liver, and spinal cord compared to an opposed oblique plan. Total dose to tumor bed: 49.5 Gy. (Courtesy of Diane Latronico, CMD.)

PLATE 63

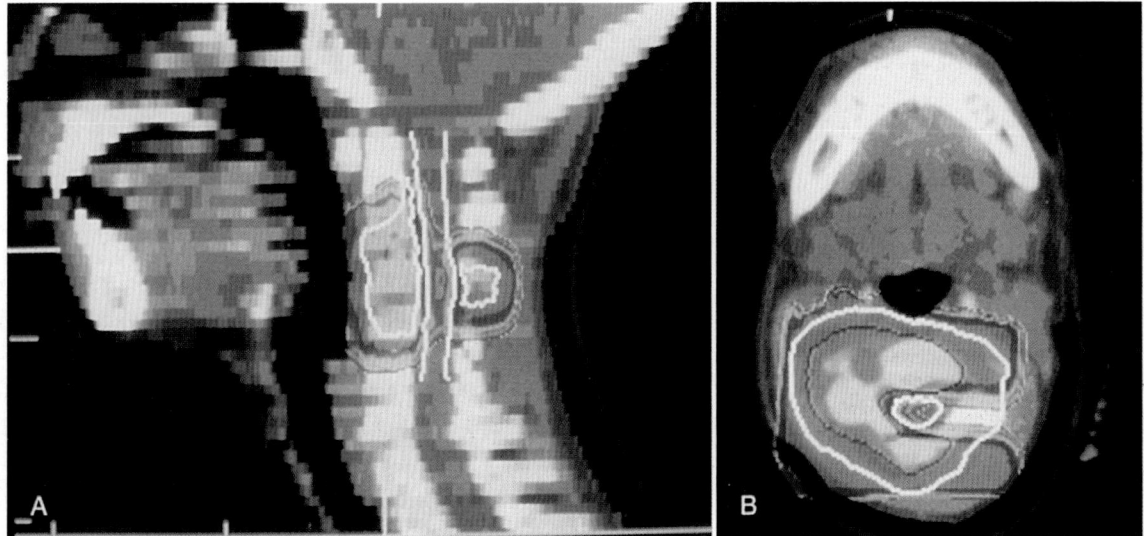

Figure 55–5. Isodose plan using proton beam therapy for Ewing's sarcoma of the third cervical vertebra in an 8-year-old boy. Sagittal (**A**) and axial (**B**) planes depict the volume receiving 55 cobalt GyEq. The majority of the cervical spinal cord received 50 cobalt GyEq or less. See also Color Figure 55-5. (Courtesy of Eugene B. Hug, MD, Department of Radiation Oncology, Massachusetts General Hospital, Boston.)

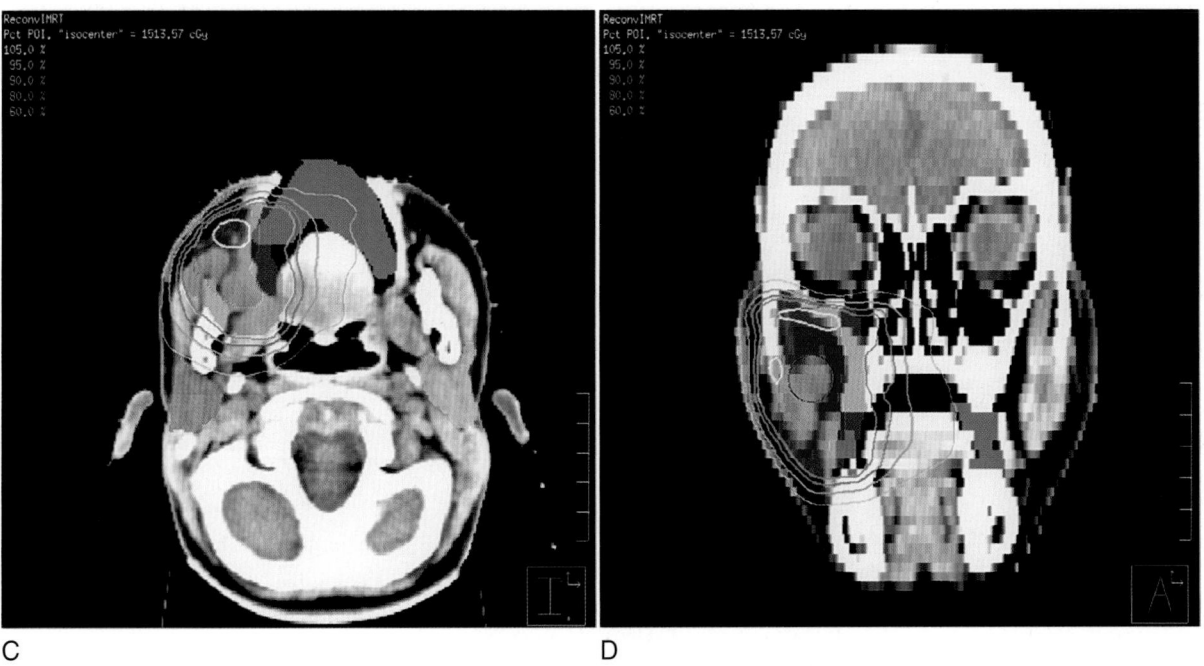

Figure 55–6. Eight-year-old male with a parameningeal rhabdomyosarcoma arising in the right pterygoid space. **C**, Reduced field plan (axial view) to the initial GTV plus 1 to 1.5 cm using intensity-modulated radiation therapy. A dental prosthesis pushes the tongue posteriorly. The child is immobilized in a plastic facial cast. **D**, Coronal dose distribution. The depicted isodose curves (central to peripheral) are: 95%, 90%, 80%, and 60%. Total dose, 50.4 Gy at 1.8 Gy/fraction. (**C** and **D**, courtesy Terrance Teslow, PhD.)

PLATE 64

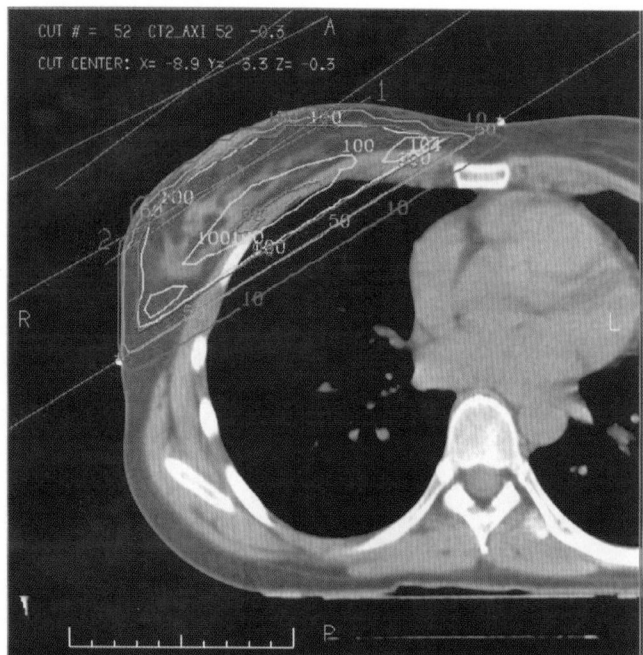

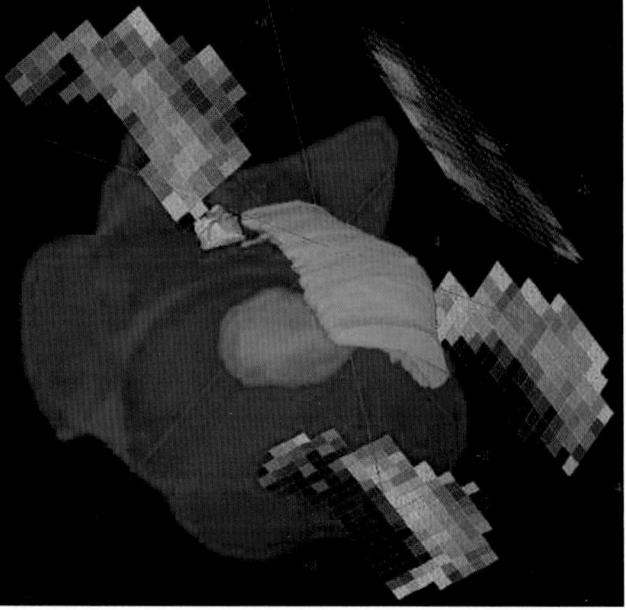

Figure 57–15. A typical treatment plan. The 100% line smoothly surrounds the breast except for a small cold area just above the lung. When lung density correction is used in breast treatment plans, this area just above the lung presents the greatest amount of tissue attenuation in the plan and thus often runs a few percentage points below the isocenter dose. The beams are weighted until the hot spots, in this case 104%, are equally balanced into the corners of the breast.

Figure 57–16. Example of intensity-modulated radiation therapy field arrangement. Each beam is divided into 1 × 1 cm beamlets of varying intensities. The breast (*violet*), supraclavicular region (*yellow*), internal mammary nodes (*green*), and heart (*red*) are shown.

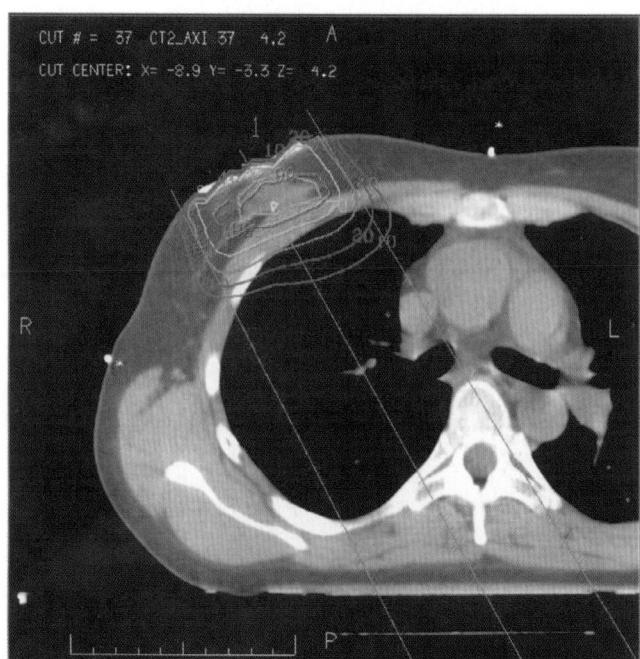

Figure 57–18. A suitable electron energy is used to cover the tumor bed with the 90% isodose line. Using electron energies of 16 MeV or greater can produce undesirable skin changes and such cases are often boosted with photons.

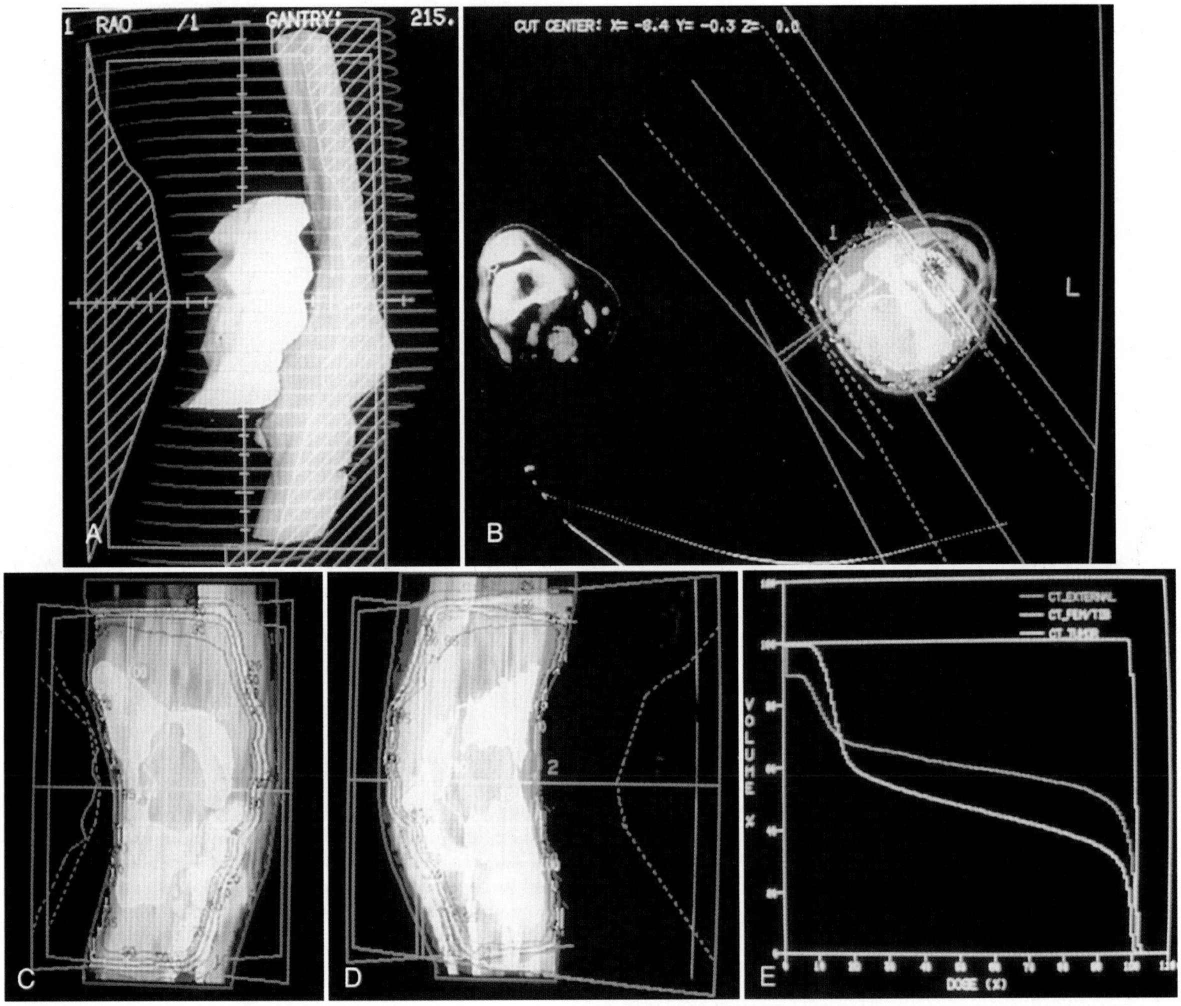

PLATE 65

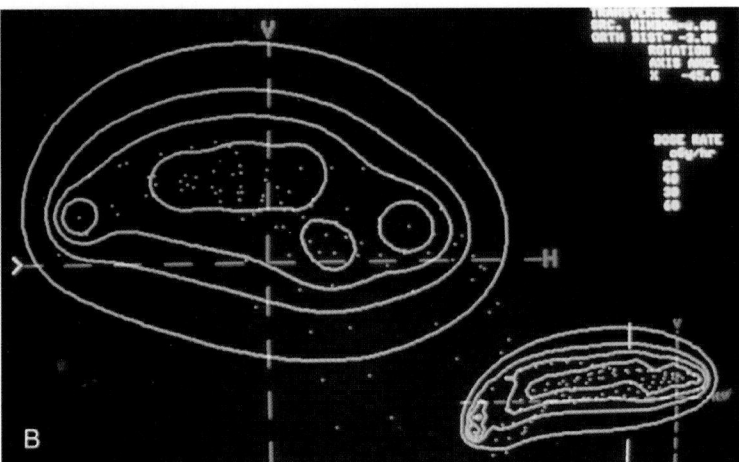

Figure 58–7. Computed tomography-based three-dimensional treatment plan using a right anterior oblique (RAO) and a left posterior oblique (LPO) field for the patient in Figure 58-6. **A,** Beam's eye view of the RAO field showing the tumor volume (*in pink*), the femur, the knee joint, the tibia (*in yellow*), and the computer-generated blocks (*in green*). **B,** Isodose distribution in relation to the tumor volume (*white line*) and surrounding structure—axial view, coronal view, and sagittal view. Note that the 95% isodose line (*in red*) encompasses all tumor volume. **C,** Dose volume histogram for the tumor volume (*white*), the surrounding skin (*green*), and adjacent bones (*yellow*) generated by three-dimensional computed tomography treatment planning. By using the plan, 40% to 60% of adjacent normal tissues will receive a full dose and the rest will receive 0% to 20% of the treatment dose from scatter radiation.

Figure 58–11. **B,** Isodose distribution in a transverse central plane (large inset), and a longitudinal plane (small inset) of the implant. The outermost line represents 20cGy/hr isodose line, the next line: 30cGy/hr, the third line: 40cGy/hr, and the innermost line: 60cGy/hr.

PLATE 66

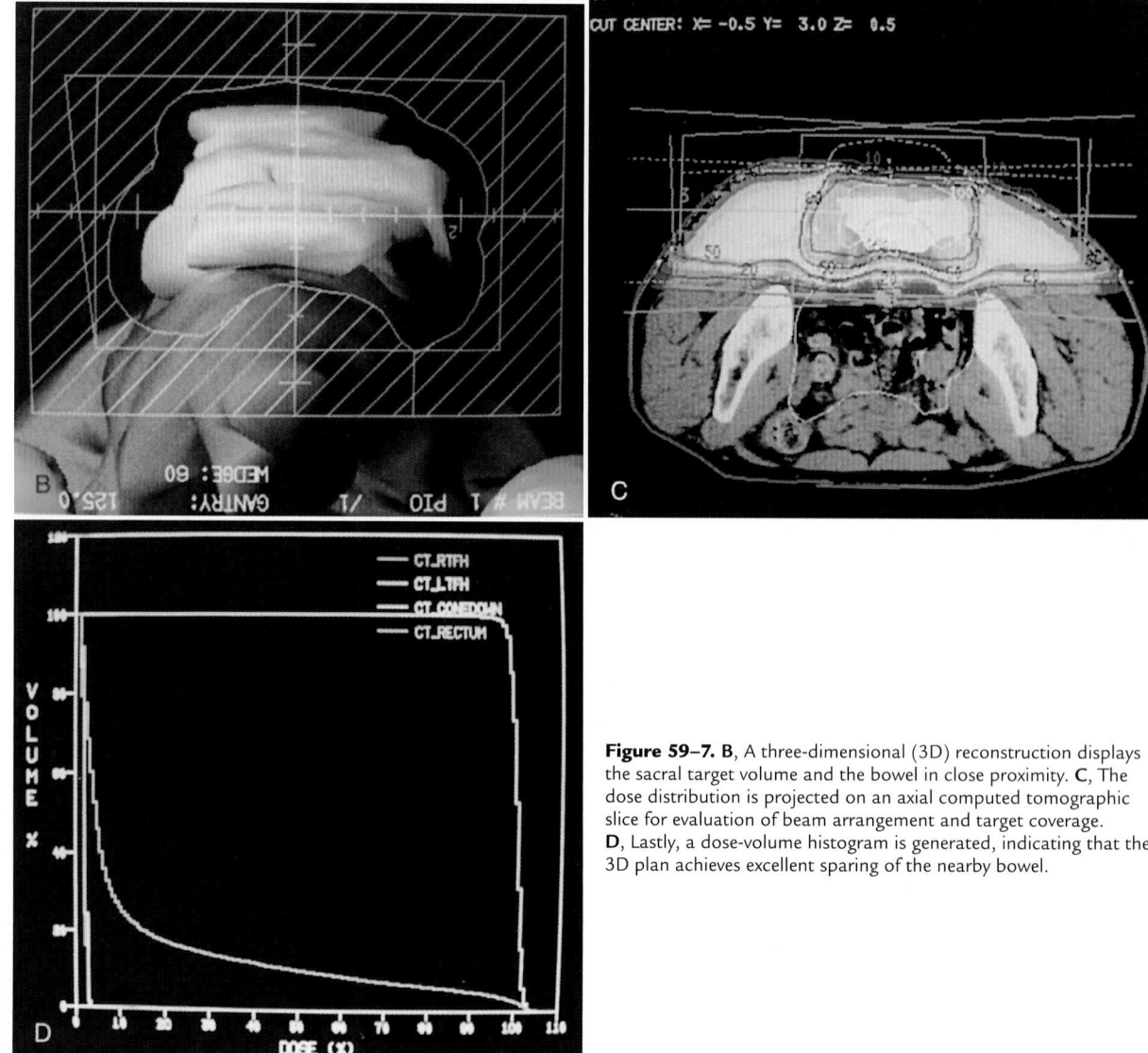

Figure 59–7. B, A three-dimensional (3D) reconstruction displays the sacral target volume and the bowel in close proximity. **C**, The dose distribution is projected on an axial computed tomographic slice for evaluation of beam arrangement and target coverage. **D**, Lastly, a dose-volume histogram is generated, indicating that the 3D plan achieves excellent sparing of the nearby bowel.

PLATE 67

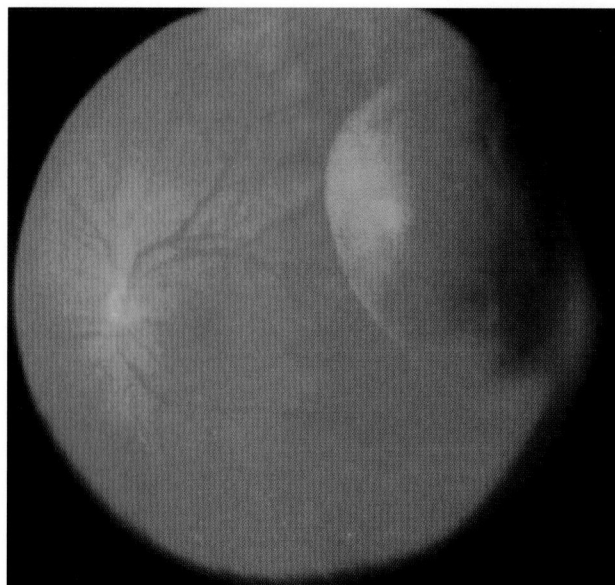

Figure 64–4. Fundus photo of a uveal melanoma.

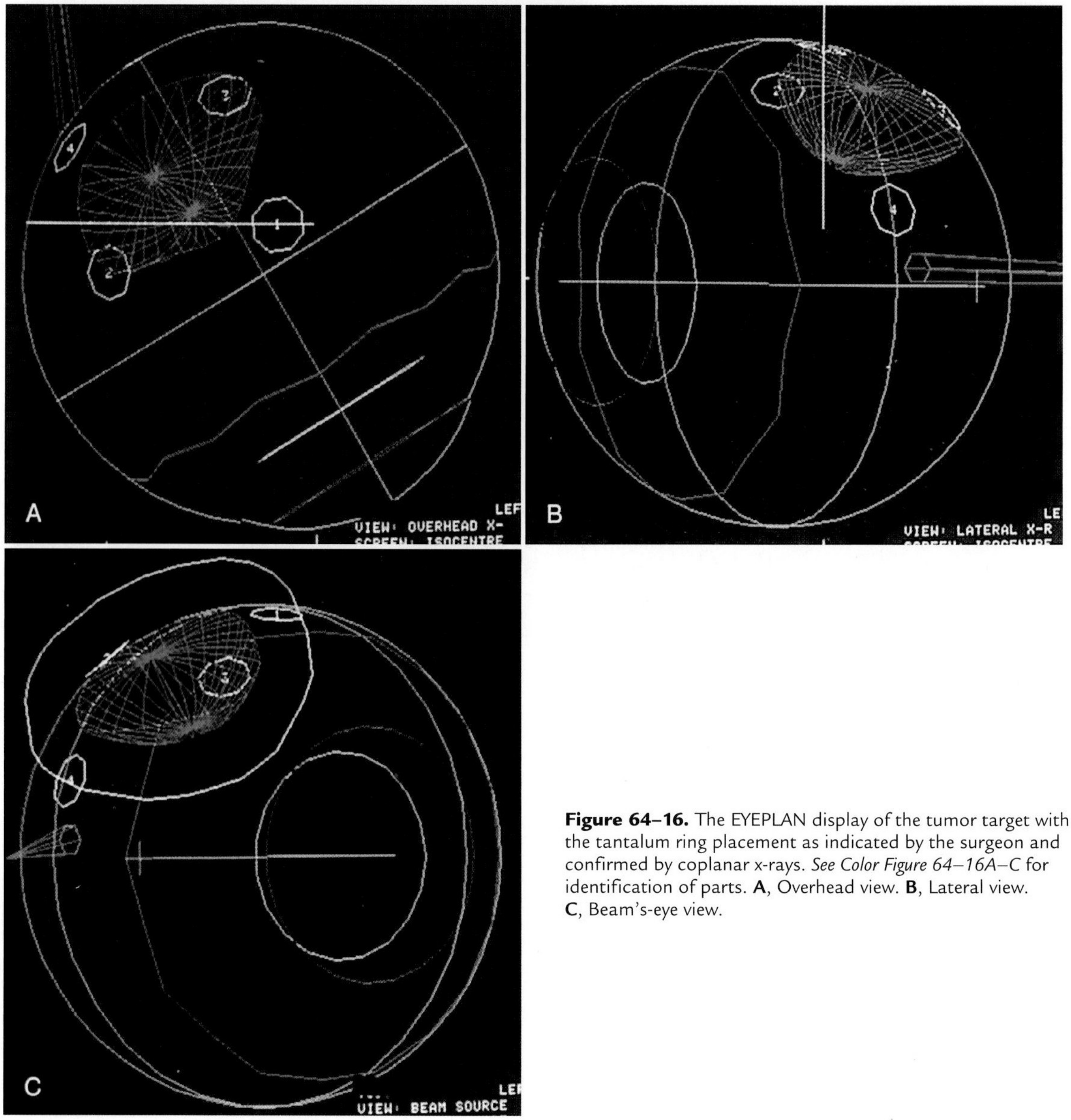

Figure 64–16. The EYEPLAN display of the tumor target with the tantalum ring placement as indicated by the surgeon and confirmed by coplanar x-rays. *See Color Figure 64–16A–C for identification of parts.* **A**, Overhead view. **B**, Lateral view. **C**, Beam's-eye view.

PLATE 68

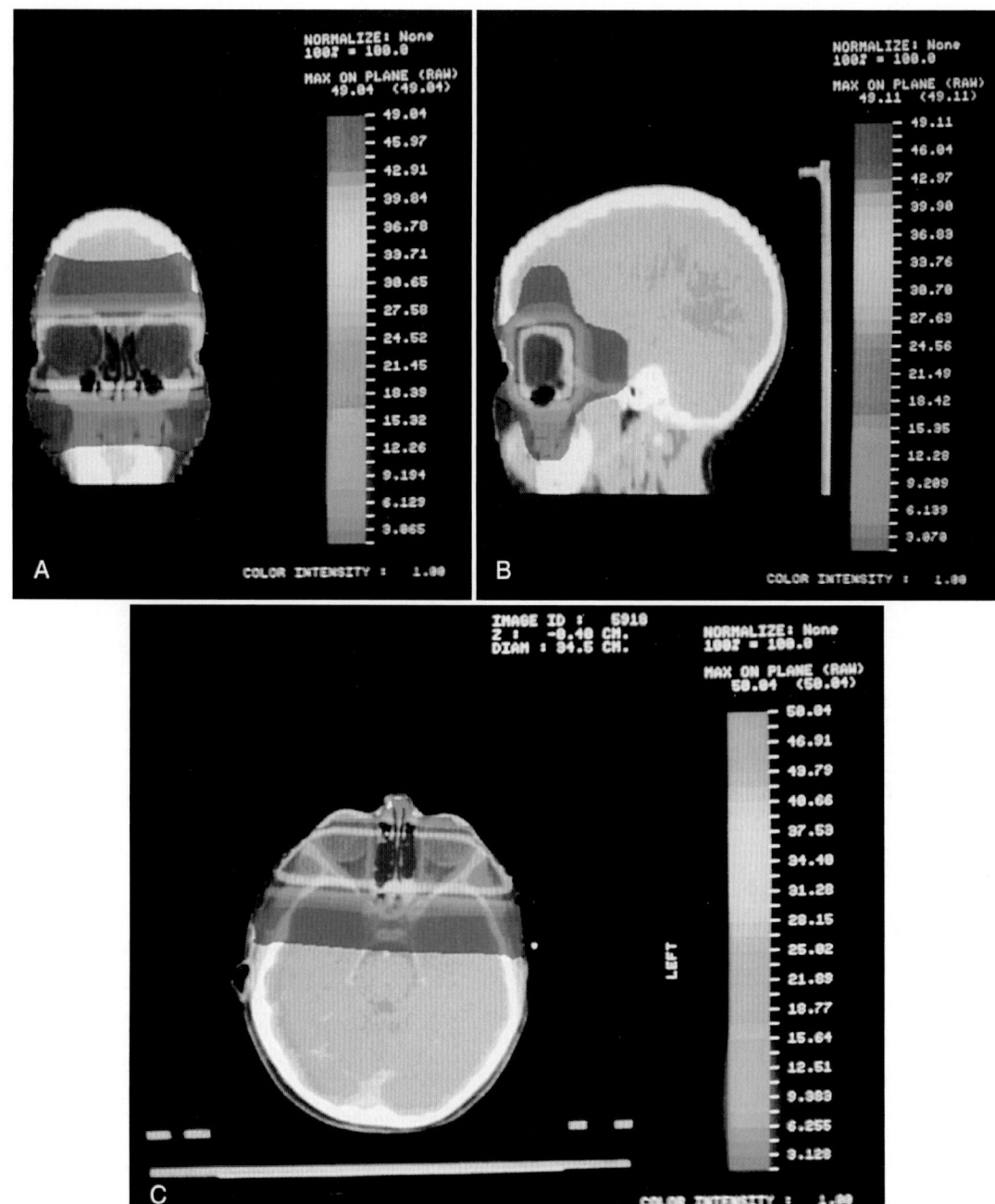

Figure 65–13. An isodose display for a patient with bilateral retinoblastoma located in each eye behind the equator. Parallel opposed fields with a D-shaped block are used to produce these isodose lines. The prescription is displayed in Gy in the coronal (**A**), sagittal (**B**), and transverse (**C**) directions.

PLATE 69

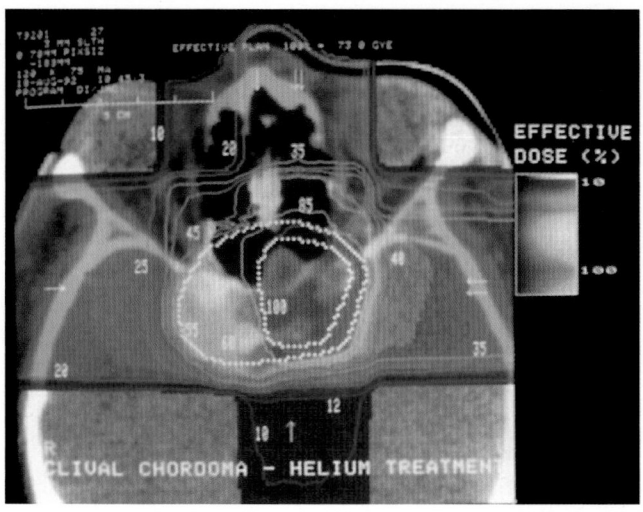

Figure 69–3. Clival chordoma isodose plan: a single slice through the tumor from a helium ion isodose plan for treatment of clival chordoma. Multiple coplanar portals are used. Isodose lines are in equivalent doses and corrected for relative biological effectiveness (RBE) to compensate for biological effects from the small amount of high linear energy transfer (LET) present in the helium beam. *Dotted lines* represent initial and cone-down tumor volumes as determined from magnetic resonance imaging and computed tomography scans. A total of 72 GyEq was given to the smaller target volume. Critical nearby normal tissues are also evaluated by use of three-dimensional dose-volume histograms, as are the target volumes.

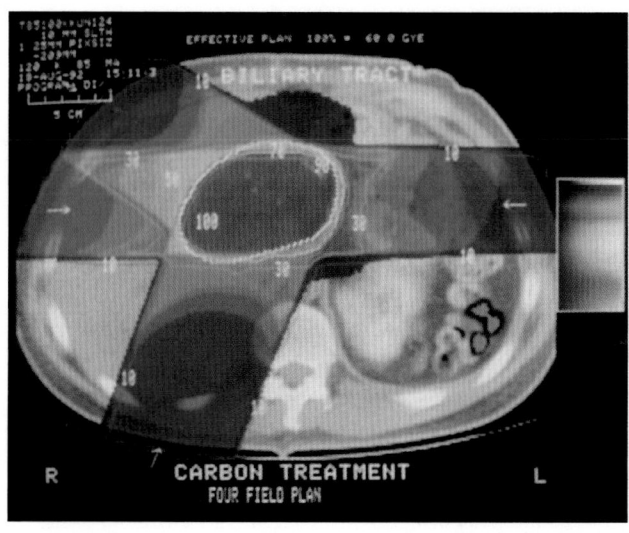

Figure 69–4. Heavy ion (carbon) treatment plan for biliary tract cancer consisting of four coplanar portals. The total dose was 60 GyEq. Isodose lines represent biologically (RBE) corrected doses. Three-dimensional dose-volume histograms were used to assess the dose to liver and stomach, as an aid in planning for this type of therapy, and to be certain that doses remain below the tolerance level to critical adjacent organs.

PLATE 70

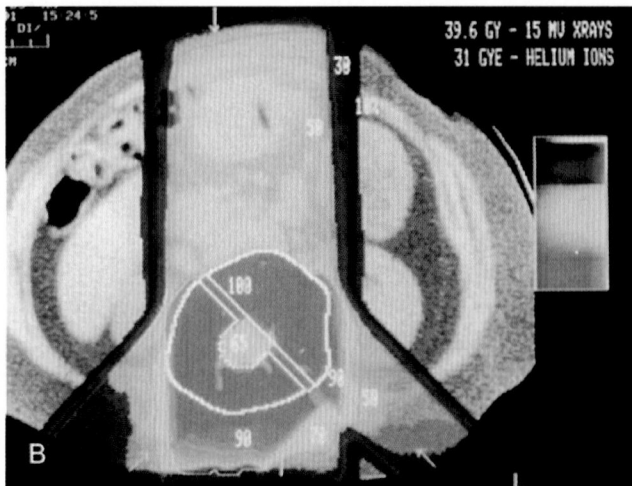

Figure 69–6. Divided target technique for irradiation of tumors of the para-central nervous system (CNS). Charged particles are used to irradiate a target volume wrapped around a critical structure such as the spinal cord. **A,** A large chondrosarcoma was present abutting and encircling the spinal cord and cauda equina and invading the vertebrae. **B,** After subtotal resection, a combined photon and charged-particle plan was devised to irradiate the target volume and minimize dose to the CNS. The target volume, indicated by the *heavy dotted line*, received a total of 70.6 GyEq, except for the inner region around the spinal cord, which received less than 46 GyEq. Computerized three-dimensional treatment planning based on metrizamide-enhanced CT scanning, together with precise immobilization and treatment delivery, is needed to accomplish this technique without CNS injury. A number of patients have been treated with this technique at Lawrence Berkeley Laboratory, with safe protection of the brainstem, spinal cord, and cauda equina.

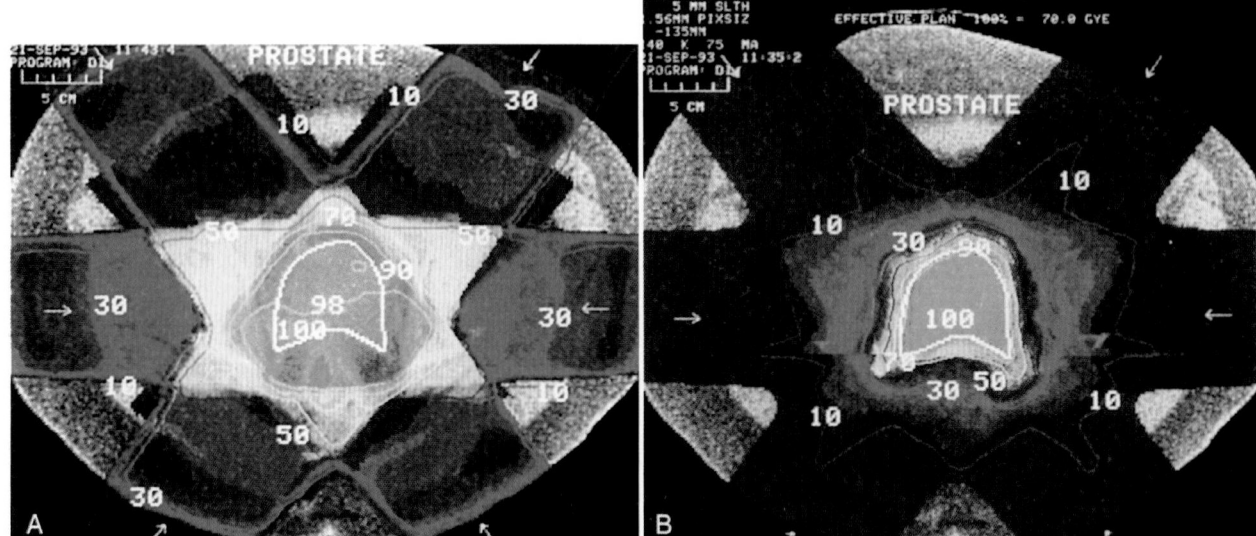

Figure 69–7. Prostate treatment plan comparison. **A,** Six-field coplanar 18 MeV x-ray conformal plan for irradiation of the prostate gland. **B,** A computer simulation of a plan using dynamic conformal proton therapy. Better conformation of the high-dose zone to the target volume is observed with conformal proton therapy. Evaluation of several target sites for proton and heavy ion therapy has suggested clinical gains when moving from static charged particle therapy to dynamic conformal charged particle therapy (Courtesy of I. Daftari, PhD.).

PLATE 71

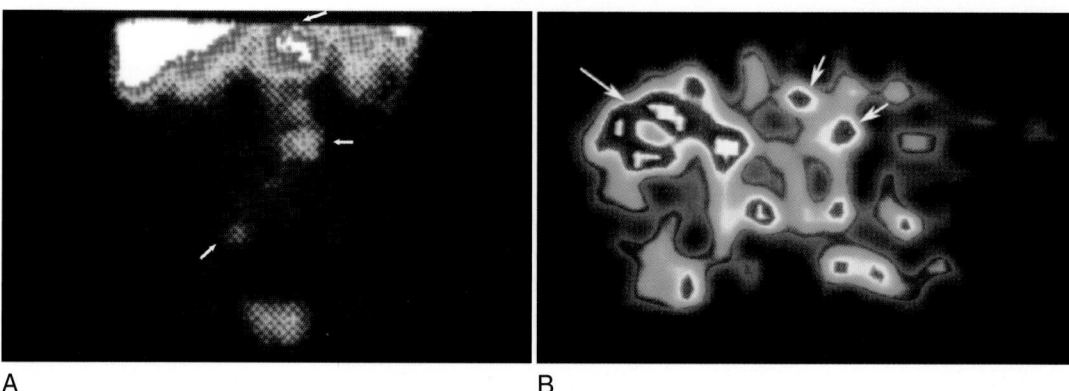

A   B

Figure 72–3. A, Gamma-camera image of the anterior pelvis of a patient with B cell lymphoma. The image was obtained 3 days after administration of ^{111}In-Lym-1 in order to derive pharmacokinetic data that can be used to calculate dosimetry for therapy with ^{90}Y-Lym-1. Excellent uptake in all known areas of lymphoma is demonstrated in the upper- and mid-abdomen and right iliac lymph nodes (*arrows*). Radioactivity in the bladder and liver demonstrates ^{111}In-Lym-1 metabolism and ^{111}In metabolite excretion. **B,** Gamma camera image of patient with metastatic breast cancer. Anterior (*A*) and posterior (*P*) aspects of the patient are indicated. The image was obtained 3 days after RIT with ^{111}In/90Y-DOTA-peptide-MAb. DOTA-peptide-MAb is a novel immunoconjugate with a catabolizable peptide linker. This three-dimensional, cross-sectional chest image was obtained by SPECT (single photon emission computerized tomography) and demonstrates uptake in metastatic disease in the right anterior chest wall, mediastinal lymph nodes, and lungs (*arrows*). No uptake is seen in normal tissues. The high therapeutic index for radiation dose in the tumor (compared with normal tissue) is evident. White is the most intense radiation, followed by red, yellow, and green. Blue/black indicates no radiation. (**A** from DeNardo GL, O'Donnell RT, Shen S, et al: Radiation dosimetry for 90Y-2IT-BAD-Lym-1 extrapolated from pharmacokinetics using [111]In-2IT-BAD-Lym-1 in patients with non-Hodgkin's lymphoma. *J Nucl Med.* 2000;41:952. **B** from DeNardo SJ, Richman CM, Goldstein DS, et al: Yttrium-90/Indium-111-DOTA-peptide-Chimeric L6: Pharmacokinetics, dosimetry and initial results in patients with incurable breast cancer. *Anticancer Res.* 1997;17:1735 and DeNardo SJ, Kroger LA, DeNardo GL: A new era for radiolabeled antibodies in cancer? *Curr Opin Immunol.* 1999;11:563.)

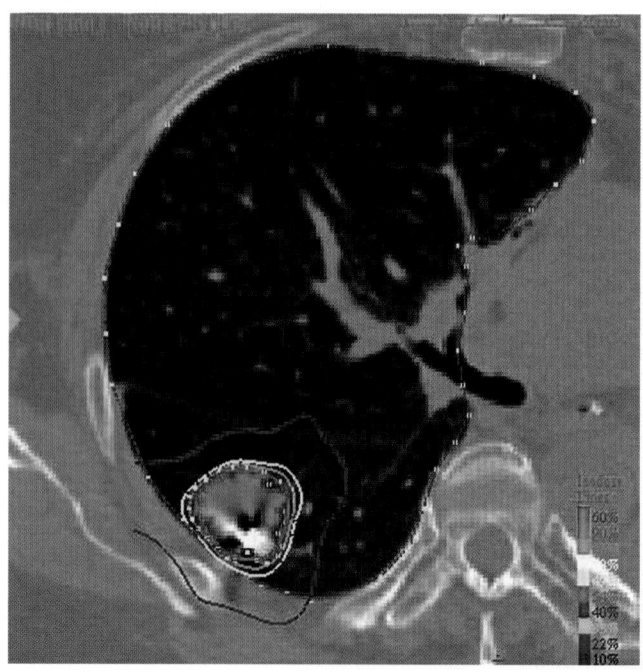

Figure 74–5. Radiosurgical dose distribution delivered using the CyberKnife with dynamic target tracking. *Red* outlines the gross target volume. *Yellow* is the prescription isodose line (IDL): 20 Gy in a single fraction at 49% IDL. *Blue* is the envelope that received 6 Gy or greater. Artifacts from the implanted gold fiducial are apparent. (Photo courtesy of Raymond Rodebaugh, Cleveland Clinic Foundation.)

Radiation Physics and Biology

Radiobiologic Principles

William C. Dewey, PhD and Joel S. Bedford, PhD

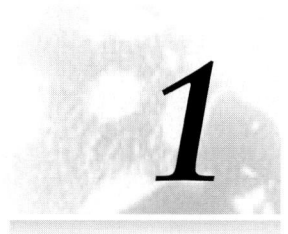

FUNDAMENTAL RADIOBIOLOGY

Ionizing x-rays and gamma-rays that interact with biologic material primarily by the Compton effect produce energetic electrons that traverse the cell and induce ionization events or ion pairs by removing orbital electrons, either from critical molecules in the cell (direct effect) or from water molecules located 3 to 5 nm from the critical molecules (indirect effect).[1] The direct and indirect effects produce highly reactive free radicals, which result in biologic damage. Studies on the various radiation syndromes in mammals following whole or partial body irradiation led Quastler,[2] by the mid-1950s, to conclude that these biologic effects resulted directly from damage to the reproductive capacity of individual stem cells that were responsible for cell renewal in the irradiated tissue. Earlier work on cell killing in bacteria, yeast, and protozoa had found that single acute x-ray doses in the range of tens to hundreds of Gy were required to destroy the reproductive integrity of approximately 50% of the cells. This finding led many investigators to conclude erroneously that a similar cell-killing process, involving the loss of reproductive integrity, was unlikely to account for tissue effects in mammals, including humans, because in mammals these effects were observed after a radiation dose of only a few Gy. If the radiosensitivities of mammalian cells were anywhere within the range of radiosensitivities displayed by microorganisms, hardly any mammalian cells at all would lose their reproductive integrity after a few Gy. However, Quastler deduced that this conclusion must be incorrect and that the radiosensitivity of mammalian cells with respect to loss of their reproductive integrity, that is, the ability to undergo multiple cell divisions to clonally repopulate a tissue, must be much greater than that of microorganisms and did, in fact, underlie those effects in tissues and tumors that are of interest for radiotherapy. Furthermore, it was recognized as early as 1906 that the manifestation of radiation-induced cell tissue injury was expressed much earlier and more severely in tissues with rapidly dividing cells than in those with slowly dividing cells. Cell death associated with dividing cells is called mitosis-linked death, and the increase in tissue response with an increase in mitotic activity is referred to as the Bergonié-Tribondeau law.[3] In fact, a wave of postmitotic cell death in the irradiated liver and thyroid is observed *in vivo* after the cells have been stimulated to divide and manifest chromosomal aberrations in the first division after irradiation.[4,5] Finally, for simplification of terminology, cell killing or cell lethality is defined as the loss of the cell's reproductive integrity; and conversely, cell survival is defined as the ability of the cell to undergo multiple cell divisions to form a macroscopic colony containing a large number of cells.

This chapter is devoted primarily to the cellular processes involved in mitosis-linked killing of mammalian cells and the phenomenon of apoptosis (programmed cell death). Much of the discussion is based on the assumption that DNA double-strand breaks (DSBs), or at least a sub-set of these, are the most important lesions in the cell responsible for lethality. Evidence that led to this assumption is as follows: Microbeam and other experiments that selectively irradiated different parts of the cell showed that the most critical targets reside in the nucleus;[1,6-8] cells are sensitive to killing by the induction of DSBs produced directly in the DNA following incorporation of (BrdU)[125] into DNA;[8] and cells are radiosensitized for both cell killing and chromosomal aberrations by incorporation of bromodeoxyuridine (BrdU) into DNA,[1,9,10] with the increase in aberrations occurring only where the BrdU is incorporated.[11] Details of radiation chemistry, the enzymology of DNA repair, and a discussion of the ongoing studies of cloning DNA repair genes are beyond the scope of this chapter, but there are several excellent reviews worth reading.[12-14] Likewise, the mutagenic and carcinogenic effects of radiation, which can cause secondary neoplasms after radiation therapy is completed, are not discussed, nor are important aspects of therapeutic gain, which is defined as a greater effect of radiation on tumor than on surrounding normal tissues (discussed elsewhere in this book as well as by Hellman[15]).

The First Survival Curves for Mammalian Cells

At about the same time Quastler reached the conclusions described in the preceding section, Puck and his coworkers[16-18] made several important observations about the radiosensitivity of mammalian cells. First, they demonstrated that mammalian cells in culture are at least an order of magnitude more sensitive to ionizing radiation than microorganisms, and that the doses required to kill 50% of the animals (LD_{50}) from bone marrow or gut damage might be expected to be killing 95% to 99% of the stem cells responsible for cell renewal in bone marrow and gut. Second, they showed that even though sterilized cells could not proliferate to form a macroscopic colony, virtually all the cells, after doses up to a few Gy, succeeded in completing at least one, often two or three, and sometimes even four or five abortive divisions before further proliferation stopped, often with the appearance of giant cells that were metabolically alive but reproductively dead. Third, they noted that functions other than reproductive capacity, such as the ability to metabolize nutrients or even the complex processes necessary to reproduce viruses, were largely unaffected by doses of even tens or hundreds of Gy. Fourth, they suggested that chromosomal aberrations induced by radiation were somehow responsible for the killing observed, based among other things on observations that these aberrations began to appear in some cells at the lowest doses at which killing first began to be measurable.

The first dose response curve for mammalian cell killing, shown in Figure 1-1A, was for HeLa cultured human cervical carcinoma cells.[16] In general, to obtain such curves, single cell suspensions are prepared and known numbers of cells are inoculated into Petri dishes containing the appropriate growth medium. These cells then settle to the bottom where they attach firmly to the dish. Without irradiation, inoculation of 100 cells into a dish yields nearly 100 macroscopic colonies, with each colony containing thousands of cells after incubation for 1 or 2 weeks. This fraction of colony-forming cells in unirradiated or untreated cells is known as the plating efficiency and is often expressed as a percentage rather than a fraction. Plating efficiencies for various tumor and normal cells are typically in the 40% to 90% range, although the system works reasonably well for plating efficiencies between 10% and 40%. (Below 10%, the cells surviving without any treatment may not be representative of the clonogenic population if the plating procedure either has sensitized the cells to radiation or has selectively killed a sub-population of cells.) Irradiated cultures show reduced fractional survival values relative to unirradiated control cultures. For high doses of irradiation corresponding to survival values of 1% or less, obviously no surviving colonies would be observed for 100 cells inoculated. Therefore, for high doses leading to low survival, the number of cells inoculated is usually increased, and the fraction surviving, S, is calculated as:

$$S = \frac{\text{Number of Colonies Counted}}{\text{Number of Cells Plated} \times PE}$$

where, in this case, the plating efficiency (PE) is expressed as the fraction of unirradiated cells that form colonies. Especially for large doses and low survival values or very low plating efficiencies for which large numbers of cells must be plated, appropriate controls using irradiated non-clonogenic feeder cells to maintain a constant cell density should be implemented to ascertain that variations in survival due to differences in the density of cells on the plates do not occur.[19] Note that the survival curve illustrated in Figure 1-1A, like many others that follow, has a characteristic shoulder in which, at low doses, the reduction in survival per unit dose (the slope) is less than the approximately constant slope for survival values below about 0.1.

An interesting finding from these and other studies was that cell populations derived from single cells surviving high radiation doses were not radioresistant, but had essentially the same radiosensitivity as the original parent populations. In fact, in many cases, populations from single cells surviving high doses of radiation have been found to be slightly more radiosensitive than the original population.[20,21] This finding may relate to the observation that progeny of cells surviving irradiation multiply at a reduced rate and have genetic instabilities[22,23] and reduced plating efficiencies.[20]

Subsequent to the studies that used cultured tumor cells, cells from human normal tissues were studied, and other techniques and methods were devised to measure survival of both normal and tumor cells *in vivo* in experimental animals. Hewitt and Wilson[24] devised an ingenious "dilution assay" method to determine the dose response for cell-killing in a transplantable murine lymphocytic leukemia of spontaneous origin. They found that, on average, only two cells were necessary to transplant the tumor to a recipient mouse. This corresponds to the inflection point on the titration curve relating the percent of injected animals that develop a tumor to the number of cells injected per animal. A convenient endpoint is the number, or "dose," of cells for 50% tumor take and is known as the TD_{50}. Hewitt and Wilson reasoned that if a radiation treatment killed half the cells, for example, then an injection of twice as many cells would be required to transplant the tumor. In other words, the inflection, or TD_{50}, of the titration curve would be shifted from two cells from an unirradiated tumor to four cells from the irradiated tumor in which half the cells were killed. Thus, a radiation dose survival curve could be constructed by dividing the TD_{50} for unirradiated tumors by the TD_{50} for tumor cells receiving various radiation doses. The survival curve the authors obtained for mouse lymphocytic leukemia cells,[24] shown in Figure 1-1B, was similar to the curve Puck and coworkers had obtained with cultured human cervical carcinoma (HeLa) cells.

What about normal cells? At about the same time the results of Hewitt and Wilson were published for mouse tumor cells *in vivo*, Till and McCulloch[25] reported an equally clever technique for assaying the survival of mouse normal hematopoietic stem cells. In the mouse, the spleen, as well as the bone marrow, is a major hematopoietic organ. The authors noticed in autopsies of mice sacrificed at various times after various doses of radiation that colonies arising from surviving cells could easily be seen as nodules in the spleen. For high enough doses, no such colonies could be seen, but injection of nucleated bone marrow cells from unirradiated mice could rescue the irradiated mice if the doses were not too high, and some of the injected cells were found to lodge in the spleen and form nodules. The number of these nodules was directly proportional to the number of cells injected. In a way then, spleens of the supralethally irradiated mice were acting like Petri dishes in which colonies could be counted, and if the *injected* cells were then irradiated, proportionally fewer colonies were counted. Survival curves constructed in this way for normal hematopoietic stem cells from mice were again similar to those for human HeLa cells or mouse leukemia cells, as shown in Figure 1-1B.

These early studies and several others immediately following pointed to a general conclusion that the radiosensitivities of mammalian cells were all about the same, at least of the same order of magnitude. Factors of about 2 were seen in doses to reach the same survival level for various cells but no systematic differences were observed in relation to tumor versus normal or rodent versus human cell origins. The range in which most high dose rate (20 to 2000 cGy/min) x-ray or gamma-ray survival curves fall for mammalian cells is shown by the dashed curves in Figure 1-1*B*. This general conclusion aside, it was recognized at a fairly early stage in the development of modern cellular radiobiology that cells of lymphoblast origin, either normal or tumor, appear to be somewhat more radiosensitive than cells from other tissues. It is also important to note that virtually all of the early studies focused on single acute (high-dose-rate) exposures, and "radiosensitivities" were judged largely by examination of survival curves in the 5 to 15 Gy range. Not until the past 20 years or so has it been widely appreciated that dose response curves over the first decade of survival and cellular responses for multiple-low-dose and low-dose-rate irradiations are not only most pertinent for radiotherapy but also show important systematic differences in cellular radiosensitivities. The surviving fraction after 2 Gy or SF_2 is an index of radiosensitivity that has been widely used.[26,27] Beyond this, and also in recent times, various mutant cell lines that are hypersensitive to ionizing radiation have been discovered or deliberately isolated following mutagenesis and selective screening procedures. These are discussed in more detail later.

Definitions and Descriptions of Radiosensitivity: N's, D_o's; α's and β's

As noted in relation to the typical mammalian cell survival curves depicted in Figure 1-1, when survival is plotted on a log scale against dose on a linear scale, the curves are characterized by an initial shoulder followed by a straight or relatively straight portion at higher doses. Much effort, thought, and ingenuity have gone into devising mathematical models to describe the shapes of cell survival curves based on certain assumptions as to mechanisms of cell killing. With appropriate adjustment of various parameters, many mutually exclusive models of radiation action adequately fit any given set of experimental data, so curve fits themselves tell us essentially nothing about radiobiologic mechanisms. Still, they are useful, principally in two ways: (1) These mathematical descriptions of survival curves provide a helpful way to catalog and compare radiosensitivities for different cells and different radiation conditions, so long as everyone, or most everyone, uses the same general mathematical description to fit the survival data; and (2) These mathematical survival curve descriptions are useful for analyzing and even predicting the outcome or the way survival changes following changes in radiation conditions. Such changes may lie in dose-rate or dose-fractionation, the chemical environment during irradiation, or radiation quality or the linear energy transfer (LET), or may occur because of alterations in the proportions of various subpopulations of cells in populations that are heterogeneous with respect to the radiosensitivity of individual cells comprising the population.

Historically, the mathematical description of dose-survival curves most widely used for mammalian cells was borrowed from "Target Theory," an analytical approach whose development began in the 1920s and whose aim was to deduce the size and number of critical targets in cells in which damage by the deposition of discrete ionizations led to a biologic effect. The need for a target concept in which damaging ionization events or packets of about 100 eV are deposited in critical structures, such

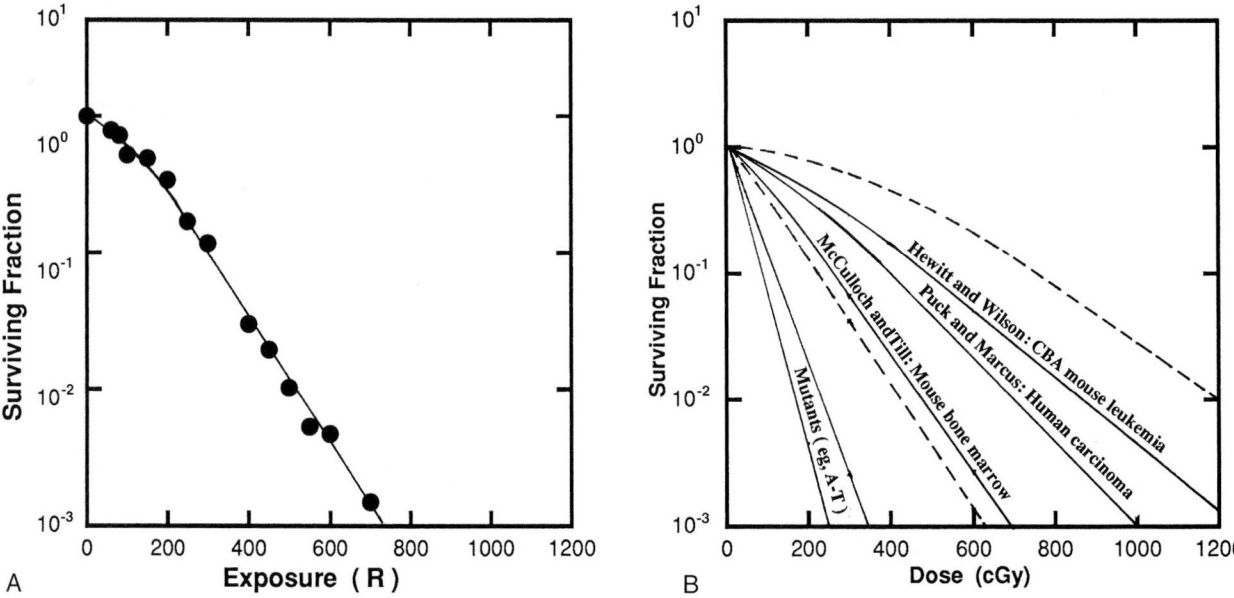

Figure 1–1. X-ray or gamma-ray dose-survival curves for mammalian cells. **A,** The first such survival curve reported in 1956 by Puck and Marcus.[16] **B,** A range of survival curves for other mammalian cells. The *dashed lines* encompass the range for "wild-type" cells of various origins. The steepest curves show a range typical of hypersensitive mutants, such as cells from patients with ataxia telangiectasia (AT). Note that in *part A,* the dose is expressed in roentgens (*R*), which, for the cells x-irradiated on glass, must be multiplied by ≈1.4 for the dose in cGy.

as DNA in chromatin structures, is evident in that the amount of energy deposited in a cell by 1000 cGy, which kills about 99% of the cells, is a very small amount of energy that would raise the temperature by only about 0.002°C.[1] Although it has been widely appreciated for 30 to 40 years that a number of complicating factors make these aims of classical target theory largely impractical and not very useful for mammalian cells, simplified mathematical dose survival expressions have been useful for the purposes mentioned previously. The simplest of these is of the form:

$$S = 1 - (1 - e^{-D/Do})^N \qquad (1)$$

where S is the fraction of cells surviving a dose, D. This curve is illustrated in Figure 1-2A. In this expression, D_o is the dose necessary on the straight-line portion of the log-linear survival plot to reduce the survival from some value S to $e^{-1} \times S$ or $0.37 \times S$. It is also sometimes called the "mean lethal dose" since it is the dose necessary to produce an average of one event per target in a cell containing N targets, all of which must be "hit" to kill the cell. If $N - 1$ of these targets have already been hit, as would be the case in virtually all the cells not yet killed after a dose corresponding to survival values below about 0.1, an *additional* dose of D_o would leave an average of one hit in the previously unhit targets and would thus reduce the survival from S to $e^{-1} \times S$. The number, N, which in this case is the number of targets, can be obtained by extrapolating the high-dose, low-survival portion of the curve to its intercept on the ordinate at zero dose. This value is perhaps more appropriately referred to as the *extrapolation number* rather than the target number, since the ideal situation in which the two are the same is seldom if ever seen in practice. It is easy to see, however, that the extrapolation number is a measure of the "size" or width of the shoulder of the survival curve. Another measure is the "quasi-threshold dose" or Dq, which is the intercept of the extrapolated high dose, low survival portion (below 0.1 survival) of the curve back to the dose axis drawn through the ordinate survival axis at a surviving fraction of 1.0. Another way to determine the Dq is to recognize that the equation for the high-dose portion of the curve approximates closely by:

$$S = N \, e^{-D/Do}$$

Thus, for a surviving fraction of 1.0 corresponding to the "Dq" dose

$$1.0 = N \, e^{-Dq/Do}$$

$$\log_e 1 = \log_e N - D_q/D_o$$

$$D_q/D_o = \log_e N$$

$$D_q = D_o \log_e N \qquad (2)$$

To actually determine the D_o from the straight-line portion of the curve fitted to a set of data, it is much easier to divide the dose (D_{10}) necessary to reduce survival by a factor of 10 (from ≈0.1 to 0.01) by 2.3 (where $\log_e 10 = 2.3$) than to attempt to work with the odd $e^{-1} = 0.368$ number (i.e., $\log_e 0.1 = -D_{10}/D_o$, $-2.3 = -D_{10}/D_o$, and $D_o = D_{10}/2.3$) Also, D_o values cannot be estimated well for data extending over only one log of survival

(to 0.1 or above) unless the curve has an extrapolation number near 1.0. Furthermore, for comparisons of radiosensitivities of different cells or different radiation conditions, survival data over the same dose range are often used for the comparisons, either as estimates of D_o or as ratios of survival for a given dose, when in fact, comparisons of D_os should be made over the same survival range. However, if one curve extends over only one log or decade of survival while the other extends over three logs, for example, the comparison should be focused on the first decade for *both* curves, ignoring the second and third decades; in this case, the comparison can be the ratio of doses, called a dose modifying factor for isosurvival, or survival values for 2 Gy, for example.

By far the biggest drawback to the use of the so-called simple multitarget expression (Equation 1) is the fact that it usually gives a poor fit to survival data in the shoulder region, that is, in the upper part of the first decade of survival. This is a problem because, as already mentioned, the first decade (in the shoulder region) is the *only* region of the curve for single acute (high-dose-rate) irradiations that is of interest for radiotherapy delivered in multiple 2-Gy fractions. The shape of the single acute dose survival curve below about the 0.1 survival fraction is of little interest for this purpose. The multitarget-type curve has zero slope at zero dose, and data indicating survival curves with large shoulders do not fit the multitarget expression well at low doses (below 2 to 3 Gy). One remedy has been to add a "single-hit" component to the expression, giving:

$$S_2 = e^{-D/D_1} [1 - (1 - e^{-D/D_n})^N] \qquad (3)$$

where $1/D_1 + 1/D_n = 1/D_o$, and D_o is still the reciprocal slope of the curve as defined above and N is still the extrapolation number. This expression provides a good fit to practically any set of data; it retains the "$N - D_o$" convention as an index of radiosensitivity and is also able to handle analyses involving changes in survival with dose rate, LET, and so on.

Another mathematical approach to the description of dose-survival relationships that lends itself to analyses involving changes in dose rate and so on is the so-called α-β model. In this model, survival follows the expression shown in Figure 1-2B:

$$S_2 = e^{-(\alpha D + \beta D^2)} \qquad (4)$$

One advantage of this model is that it readily derives from a mechanism of cell killing that we now know to be largely correct. The mathematics amounts to a simple description of the dose response for the formation of chromosomal aberrations, rather than some abstract targets of obscure identity and behavior. The model derives from the fact that cells die largely as a result of loss of genetic information in the progeny of cells bearing certain chromosomal aberrations induced by the radiation. This is not just one of a number of plausible mechanisms of cell killing, but there is a large body of evidence to support it.[17,18,28-34] Not only has quantitative agreement been found between aberration induction and cell killing,[17,18,28-33] but the strongest possible evidence is that provided by Revell and his associates,[35] who showed that virtually every diploid cell irradiated in G_1 reaching the first mitosis with a fragment-generating (micronucleus-generating) aberration

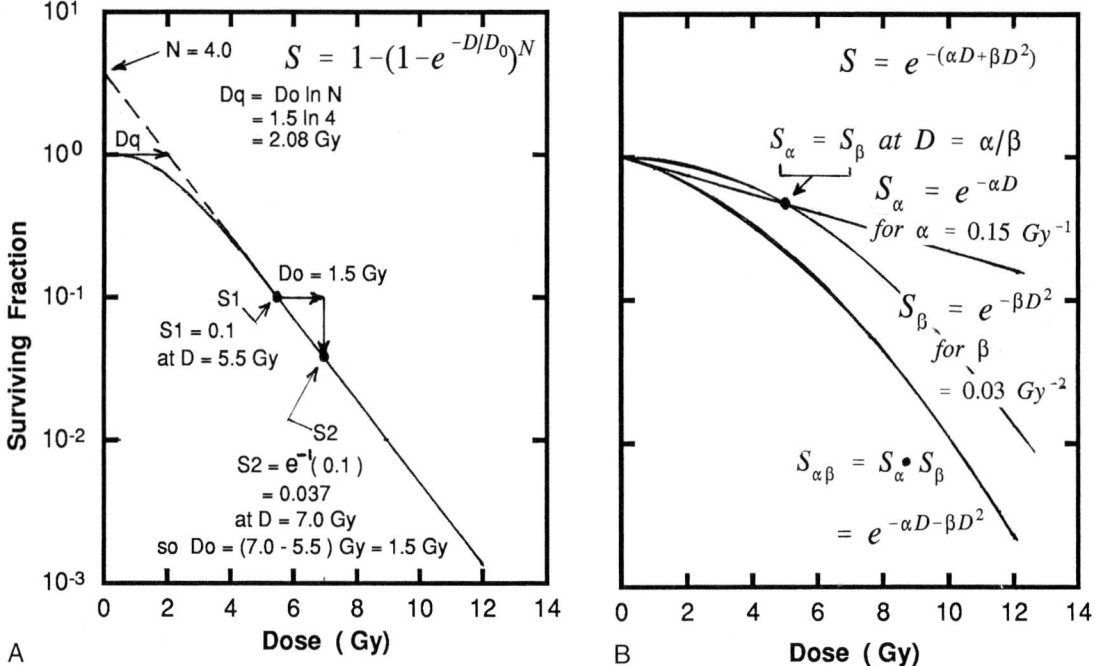

Figure 1–2. Different mathematical expressions relating radiation dose to cell survival and the parameters commonly used to characterize cellular radiosensitivity. **A,** Illustration of a form of the so-called N–D_o model and how N, D_o, and D_q are calculated or estimated from such a curve. **B,** Illustration of the α/β model in which killing occurs by either a single-event process or a double-event process such that the overall killing by either process is the product of the two, and the α/β ratio is the dose at which both processes contribute equally to the total killing, that is, the dose corresponding to the intersection of the two upper curves. Note that the *upper curve* is the survival value for the α component only, the *middle curve* is for the β component only, and the *lower curve* is for both the α and β components.

failed to form a colony, while every irradiated cell reaching the first mitosis without such an aberration did form a colony. If these aberrations and the lethal events were unrelated in a cause-and-effect sense, and some other unseen lesions with the same radiosensitivity for its production were actually the *lethal* lesion, then some cells with aberrations should have formed colonies while some cells without aberrations should not have formed colonies. Other mechanisms of cell killing, such as apoptosis, may contribute to cell killing to a greater or lesser extent depending on the circumstances. For some agents and particular hormonal induction processes, apoptosis may account for *all* of the cell death; but for exposure to ionizing radiation, most cells die principally as a result of the production of certain chromosomal aberrations. Apoptosis is such an important and currently topical subject that we have devoted a separate section of this chapter for a review and discussion of radiation-induced apoptosis.

Most chromosomal aberrations are exchange types requiring two chromosome breaks for their formation, with one event or electron track producing one break and another independent event or second electron track producing the other, or in some proportion of the cases, with one electron track producing both breaks (Figure 1-3). When two independent events must occur together or very near in space and time, the frequency of such double events increases as the square of the total number of separate single events. This is analogous to second order or bimolecular reaction kinetics in chemistry. The single break events are, of course, directly proportional to the radiation dose, so the exchanges from a "coincidence" of independent events will increase as the square of the dose.

However, when two breaks occur close enough together to form an exchange, they do not necessarily do so. Instead, they can "restitute" by joining the way they were, or they may fail to rejoin, which would result in a terminal deletion (rarely in human cells). The most interesting events are those that result from the closely spaced breaks that mis-rejoin to form either a symmetrical (nonlethal) or an asymmetrical (usually lethal) exchange. (When an exchange occurs between two chromosomes, the exchange is symmetrical if the exchange does not join the two centromeres together and is asymmetrical if the two centromeres are joined together) Thus, the initial break-pair forms what may be termed a potentially lethal break-pair or simply a potentially lethal lesion. This will be discussed in more detail in connection with a certain kind of repair process. As mentioned earlier, the yield of these independently produced lethal aberrations per cell, Y_2, increases as the square of the dose D, or

$$Y_2 = \beta D^2$$

where β is the proportionality constant relating to the fraction of potentially lethal break-pairs that are actually converted to lethal aberrations under a given condition. It is also possible, however, that two breaks could be produced along a single electron track, especially at the end of an electron track where the number of ionizations per unit track length (LET) increases.[1] In this case, the yield of such two-break single-track events would simply increase in direct proportion to dose D, rather than as the square of the dose, so the yield Y_1, would be

$$Y_1 = \alpha D$$

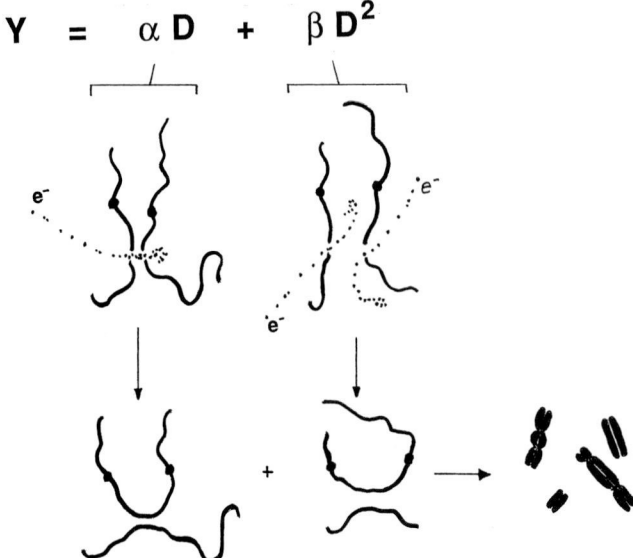

$$Y \; = \; \alpha D \; + \; \beta D^2$$

Figure 1–3. The α/β description of chromosome aberration production: $Y = \alpha D + \beta D^2$ where Y is the average yield per cell and D is the dose. The single-track α component of chromosome-type asymmetric interchange production (dicentric) is shown on the *left*, where a single electron track produces a break in each of two chromosomes, which (in some proportion of the cases) subsequently rejoin asymmetrically to produce a dicentric and acentric fragment. The same general type of exchange process occurring in the same chromosome can produce asymmetrical chromosome-type intrachanges yielding interstitial deletions. These types of exchanges also occur as a result of two independent electron tracks, as shown on the *right*. After high doses for which the two-hit β component predominates, most of the aberrations seen in the first mitosis after irradiation of G_1 or G_0 cells are of these kinds. After low doses or dose rates for which the one-hit α component predominates, there is an increase in the proportion of aberrations that are terminal deletions, in which a break simply fails to rejoin. In human cells, however, very few terminal deletions are observed, even after low doses of radiation.

where, again, α is a proportionality constant. The total yield of lethal aberrations, Y, per cell would then be the sum of $Y_2 + Y_1 = Y$ so

$$Y_1 = \alpha D + \beta D^2 \tag{5}$$

The total yield, Y, per cell is, of course, only an average; it does not mean that every cell has *exactly* Y. However, if the aberrations occur independently from one cell to the next and all cells have the same sensitivity, the probability that a cell *will* have exactly 0, 1, 2, 3, etc. lethal events can be calculated because such processes are well described by the Poisson distribution, which states that

$$P_x = \frac{e^{-\mu}\mu^x}{x!}$$

where P_x is the probability that exactly x events will occur for a given "trial" when the mean number of events over a large number of "trials" is μ. In our case $\mu = Y$, and the cell must have *no* lethal events (aberrations) to survive, so $x = 0$, and the probability of exactly *no* events is

$$P_0 = \frac{e^{-Y}Y^0}{0!} = e^{-Y} \tag{6}$$

and since for large numbers of cells or trials, $P_o \rightarrow S$ (the fraction surviving), and $Y = \alpha D + \beta D^2$, we can write

$S = e^{-(\alpha D + \beta D^2)}$, which is Equation 4 displayed earlier and plotted in Figure 1-2*B*. Curves of the form shown in Figure 1-2*B* fit experimental data well, especially over the first and second decades of survival. Recent studies have shown that a substantial fraction of aberrations for doses above 3 to 4 Gy are "complex," meaning they involve 3 or more breaks in 2 or more chromosomes.[36] The ways in which these form, and the impact on the mathematical description of dose responses from a mechanistic stand-point are not presently known, but there is still no doubt that the increase in lethal asymmetrical exchange aberrations closely follows a linear-quadratic function of dose. It has been argued that one flaw of this linear-quadratic model is that it gives a survival curve that continuously "bends" downward at higher and higher doses, whereas good experimental data for cell survival over 5 or more decades of cell killing tend to show a straight line on a log linear plot for the whole range of survivals below about 0.1. In fact, this is not a very good argument against the connection between aberrations and cell killing because these lethal aberrations *do not* actually increase as $\alpha D + \beta D^2$ at doses much higher than about 10 Gy; that is, they tend to saturate and approach linearity at high doses (at least up to 15 to 20 Gy). Another objection that is sometimes mentioned as a drawback for using Equation 4 is that it does not readily lend itself to a simple description of sensitivity in terms of constants that represent the shoulder and slope of the survival curve; that is, "these cells have a D_o of 1.5 Gy and an extrapolation number of about 4" description. Perceptually, some feel it is difficult or awkward to describe sensitivity as "these cells have an α of 0.2 Gy^{-1} and a β of 0.01 Gy^{-2}." What is an inverse Gy (i.e., a kilogram per joule)? Worse yet, what is a kilogram squared per joule squared? Actually, these questions do not represent a substantial objection, and what is sometimes done is to simply quote a D_{10} or the dose to yield a survival of 10% to give an estimate of radiosensitivity. For most purposes, the α/β description is probably the best one to use, but because many workers still use the $N - D_o$ description, we have included it in this chapter.

Cellular Processing of Radiation Damage

Cells can process radiation damage and are largely able to repair the molecular lesions that can lead to chromosomal aberrations and cell death. In some instances, however, the repair may be incomplete, or misrepair may occur. As mentioned previously, most of the lethal chromosome aberrations are exchanges (in human cells mostly asymmetric *intra*changes yielding interstitial deletions, or *inter*changes yielding dicentrics with an acentric fragment). Two events must occur close together for an exchange to occur, not only in space but also in time. Cells can repair or rejoin chromosome breaks, so if the entire radiation dose is delivered over a period of a few seconds or minutes, all the breaks that are ever going to be produced will occur together, or for practical purposes, simultaneously. After such a dose given in a short period ("acute" dose) there would be a certain number of break-pairs, each produced by two independent electron tracks close enough together for a possible exchange. However, if the same total dose were delivered over a period of several days (e.g., at a low dose rate), then there would be no such independent two-track break-pairs to form potential exchanges. Even though breaks occurred in the same proximity in the cell nucleus, the break-pairs would never (or rarely) exist together because the first break of the pair would have rejoined with itself and disappeared long before the second break of the pair ever arrived. Thus, the β, or dose-squared, component is very dose-rate dependent. There would, of course, still be the same number of break-pairs produced by the single-track mechanism; therefore, this "alpha" component of cell killing would be dose-rate independent and also important for very low acute doses for which the high LET track ends of electrons are expected to produce most of the lethal lesions.[1] These concepts are illustrated again by reference to Figure 1-3. Note also that the formation of complex aberrations may require a refinement of the mechanistic description, but this does not alter the established fact that aberrations for the most part underlie cell killing, and for all intents and purposes these increase as a linear-quadratic function of x-ray or gamma-ray dose.

The next topic for discussion is how this concept fits in with the well-studied cellular repair process known as sublethal damage repair (SLDR) and potentially lethal damage repair (PLDR).

Sublethal Damage

In 1957, Jacobson[37] presented some of the first evidence that x-irradiated cells (chlamydomonas) sustain sublethal damage (SLD) that can be repaired (SLDR). Jacobson showed that a radiation dose delivered in two separate fractions separated in time gave a higher survival than if the dose was given in one single fraction. In 1960, Elkind and coworkers[38] extended these observations and reasoned that the shoulder on survival curves for mammalian cells (or any other cells with similar survival curves having shoulders) by itself indicates that a damage accumulation process must be involved in cell killing.[21,38] Some arguments have arisen over this point because notions of "repair saturation" have been suggested, but even in this instance the putative saturation will still require damage accumulation. It also follows from this argument that cells surviving a radiation dose high enough that the survival would be "off the shoulder" (survival <0.1) must be sublethally damaged. In other words, they have accumulated damage that makes them more susceptible to killing by the next increment of dose than if they had not received any radiation. For this reason, such damage was termed SLD.[21,38] The question then asked was, if a population of sublethally damaged cells surviving one dose were allowed to incubate for various periods, would the cells be able to repair this SLD? If repair of all the sublethal damage occurred, a dose-survival curve determined for these surviving cells should have a shoulder similar to cells that had never been irradiated. If no repair occurred, the dose-survival response should be a simple exponential decrease continuing at the survival level corresponding to the initial dose and along the same curve as for the original cell population.

As illustrated in Figure 1-4A, the shoulder of the survival curve indeed returned, indicating that the cells had recovered from their sublethal injury and implying that the SLD had been literally "repaired," so the cells were in this respect "restored to their original condition." In further studies, Elkind and coworkers[21,38] found that this shoulder returned with the half-time for SLDR being of the order of half an hour. However, as discussed under cell cycle, a complete return of the shoulder does not necessarily mean that all sublethal damage has been repaired. Many other workers have obtained similar results for cells both *in vitro* and *in vivo*, and repair half-times range from about 0.5 to 1.5 hours. Typically, the way such studies are carried out is by the "split dose" technique, in which changes in survival are measured as a function of incubation time between two equal doses. The technique is illustrated in Figure 1-4B. Generally, for an *in vitro* experiment, a number of identical cultures would be set up, all with the same number of cells receiving the same total dose, 2D; the only difference is that for some cultures, the dose would be given all at once, while for others, the dose would be given in two fractions of D, each with various periods of time between the doses.

The concept of sublethal damage and its repair is readily apparent in the induction of fragment-producing exchange-type aberrations. One break by a single electron track is sublethal; by itself it almost always rejoins and is not lethal. After a certain dose, at which the survival is less than about 0.1, surviving cells will have many such single (sublethal) breaks and will, therefore, be more susceptible to killing by a further dose than if they had no previous irradiation. With incubation before a second dose, these sublethal single breaks will gradually disappear, and if the second dose is given much later, the survival of the cells will be much the same as if the cells had never been irradiated. *SLD, then, is damage that exists in surviving cells, by itself is not lethal, and is evident in the way it influences the response of cells to a second radiation dose.* The repair of sublethal lesions is responsible for the dose-rate and dose-fractionation effects so important as a fundamental process operating in radiotherapy.

According to this view, two breaks produced by a single electron track can also lead to a lethal exchange, and the number of such events is strictly proportional to the total dose; that is, it is dose-rate–independent. The contribution of this single-event, two-break process to the total lethal damage is given by the αD term of Equation 5. It is only the βD^2 term that governs dose-rate or dose-fractionation effects related to SLDR. In the simple case of the split dose experiment described earlier, if the total dose 2D is given all at once, the lethal aberration yield will be:

$$Y_{2D} = \alpha(2D) + \beta(2D)^2$$
$$Y_{2D} = 2\alpha D + 4\beta D^2 \tag{7}$$

If the total dose 2D is given as 2 doses of D separated by a time sufficient to allow complete repair of sublethal damage, the yield of lethal aberrations will be:

$$2\,Y_D = 2(\alpha D + \beta D^2)$$
$$2\,Y_D = 2\alpha D + 2\beta D^2 \tag{8}$$

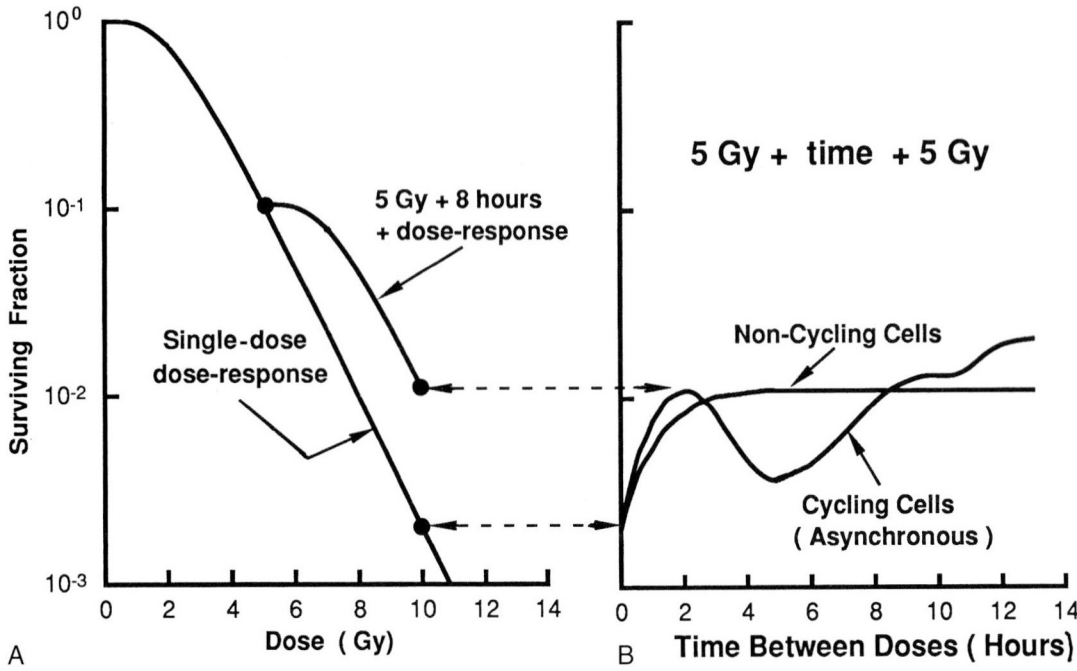

Figure 1–4. Illustration of sublethal damage and its repair (**A**) and the rate of repair (**B**). **A,** A single-dose dose-response curve (*lower curve*) and another curve obtained by first giving the cells a dose of 5 Gy and then incubating the cells (in this case 8 hours) before determining another survival curve for cells that survived the first dose. If these cells returned to their initial pre-irradiation state, they should respond (as they do) along the upper curve from 5 to 10 Gy, whereas if no change occurred during incubation in the cells surviving the first dose (i.e., no recovery from sublethal damage), the response would continue along the lower curve from 5 to 10 Gy. The increase in survival after 10 Gy for the 2 radiation doses amounts to a factor of ≈5 in this case. **B,** The rate at which this increase occurs. The complex curve for cycling cells results from the fact that there is a large difference in radiosensitivity for cells, depending on their position in the cell cycle (see text and Fig. 1-5).

Notice that the "αD" terms in Equations 7 and 8 are the same, but the βD^2 terms differ by a factor of 2, which translates to a survival for the split-dose treatment (using Equations 6, 7, and 8) that is higher by a factor of $e^{2\beta D}$ than for the single $2D$ dose. For many small doses, or in the limit of continuous irradiation at a sufficiently low dose rate, the βD^2 term disappears altogether, and the only remaining damage is that from the αD component. Thus, a "dose rate reduction factor," depending on the rate of rejoining of breaks and their rate of formation, can be applied to the βD^2 or "reparable" component of damage. This was first done by Lea[39] for the yield of chromosomal aberrations when doses were delivered over different periods of time, and by Kellerer and Rossi[40] in their theory of dual radiation action. Variations on this same theme[41-43] as well as other approaches[44] also have been described. The general case for different dose rates derived by Dale[43] is:

$$S = e^{-\zeta \alpha D} \qquad (9)$$

where

$$\zeta = 1 + 2R/\mu \times \beta/\alpha \times [1 - 1/\mu T \times (1 - e^{-\mu T})] \qquad (10)$$

and where R = dose rate in Gy/hr, μ = repair constant in hr^{-1} (with the half-time for repair equal to $0.693/\mu$), and T = total duration of irradiation in hours. For very low dose rates of ≈0.3 Gy/hr, $S = e^{-\alpha D}$.

There has been a great deal of discussion about the relative radiosensitivity and repair capacities of cells whose damage leads to early versus late effects in normal tissues, or effects in tumor versus late normal tissue damage.

This discussion generally has been placed in the context of the α/β cell survival expression.[45-48] The point in question is how the responses of these tissues change with dose fractionation and dose rate. Generally, there appears to be a greater dose fractionation sparing effect with late-responding normal tissues than with early-responding tissues. In terms of the α, β, and SLDR discussed, the radiosensitivity of the cells whose damage underlies late effects has a larger β component relative to the α component than the radiosensitivity of tumor cells or cells for early effects. Put another way, the α/β ratio is smaller for late effects than for early effects. The α/β ratio gives an index of the proportion of damage subject to the dose fractionation sparing effect. If α were zero, the ratio would be zero, and all the damage would be reparable; therefore, for low enough dose rates or a sufficiently low dose per fraction, the killing effect of radiation would disappear altogether. As β approaches zero, the ratio increases without bound, so no dose rate or fractionation effect at all would be seen; in fact, the survival curve would be linear without a shoulder and would be described by the α component only. Furthermore, as illustrated in Figure 1-2B, the α/β ratio corresponds to the dose for which there is an equal contribution to the damage from the α and β components. Thus, when

$$\alpha D = \beta D^2$$

$$\alpha = \beta D, \text{ and}$$

$$D = \alpha/\beta.$$

The relationship between survival and dose (using values of α and β in Equation 4) has been used to convert one fractionation scheme to another fractionation scheme that is calculated to give the same amount of radiation damage as the original scheme.[49] For example, n_1 fractions of dose d_1/fraction can be converted into n_2 fractions of dose d_2/fraction with the following equation:

$$n_2 \, d_2 = (n_1 \, d_1) \, [1 + d_1/(\alpha/\beta)]/[1 + d_2/(\alpha/\beta)] \quad (11)$$

Importance of Variations in Radiosensitivity Through the Cell Cycle

So far we have not mentioned an important factor complicating the interpretation of dose fractionation and dose-rate effects. This factor centers on the observation that the radiosensitivity of cells changes through the cell cycle. This was first discovered by Terasima and Tolmach[50] and has been studied extensively by many others.[10,51-53] Figure 1-5 shows dose-survival curves for synchronous cells irradiated at different stages of the cell cycle. Generally, cells in late G_2 and mitosis are most sensitive, cells in mid-to-late S phase (the portion of the cell cycle when DNA is replicated) and early G_2 are most resistant. Often, cells around the G_1/S border (late G_1/early S) are sensitive, and cells in mid G_1 are again resistant. The effect of this differential cell cycle radiosensitivity when asynchronous, randomly dividing cell populations are studied in dose fractionation experiments is

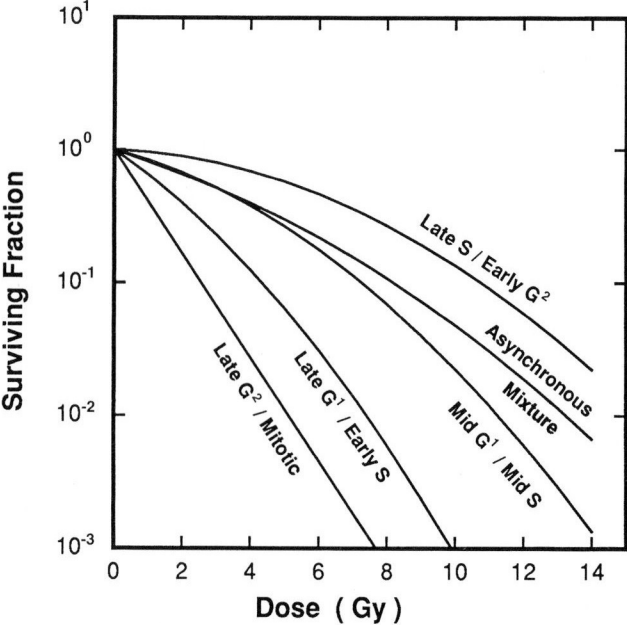

Figure 1–5. The cell cycle dependence of radiosensitivity. The figure shows typical survival curves for cells irradiated in various phases of the cell cycle. Also shown is the survival curve for an asynchronously dividing log phase culture, which is composed of a mixture of cells with the sensitivities shown. In this case, the curve labeled *asynchronous mixture* is a composite curve for a mixture consisting of 8% of cells responding as "late G_2/mitotic," 15% as "late G_1/early S," 50% as "mid G_1/mid S," and 27% as "late S/early G_2." This curve for asynchronous cells looks fairly homogeneous, and it would be difficult to suspect from a simple inspection of the curve that, in fact, it is derived from a mixture in which the subpopulations had very different radiosensitivities.

that the first dose selectively kills the more radiosensitive G_1 and G_2 cells in the population, so the S-phase cells surviving this dose not only have sublethal damage that they are repairing over time, but they also begin to progress toward the more sensitive G_2 and G_1 phases in the cell cycle. Both phenomena affect the way in which these cells will respond to the second dose. For example, after the first dose, the selective survival of radioresistant S-phase cells with a large shoulder on the survival curve complicates the interpretation of whether or not recovery of sublethal damage is complete, because for complete recovery, the shoulder of the survival curve for the second dose should be larger than the shoulder for the first dose delivered to the original asynchronous cells consisting of both radiosensitive G_1 and G_2 cells and radioresistant S-phase cells.[54] Because SLDR is usually faster than cell cycle progression, SLDR leads to the rapid early increase in survival in split dose experiments, while cell cycle progression leads to a gradual decrease over time (cell cycle redistribution or reassortment) followed by an increase in survival as the semi-synchronous surviving population divides (repopulates) (see Figure 1-4B). These three processes have been referred to by Withers as three Rs of radiotherapy: *repair, redistribution, and repopulation.*

Cell-cycle-dependent radiosensitivity and progression of cells in the cycle after irradiation can be important factors, both in comparing the radiosensitivities of different cell types and in determining the responses of cell populations in normal tissues and tumors when doses are fractionated or delivered continuously at low dose rates.[1,10,48,50-53] For example, accumulation of cells in the radiosensitive phase at the end of G_2 can, in certain instances, overshadow the dose-rate effect due to repair, such that the effect per unit dose actually increases rather than decreases with a reduction in dose rate.[55] In general, irradiated cells have the greatest cell cycle delay during G_2, with approximately 1 to 2 minutes per cGy for cells irradiated in late S and G_2[21] and about one-third less delay during G_2 when they are irradiated in G_1 or early S.[56] The delay from G_1 into S is usually only an hour or two, even for doses as high as 600 cGy,[56] but appears to increase in cells that express wild-type p53 (discussed by Murnane).[57] The accumulation of cells in G_1 that is observed approximately 16 hours after irradiation in cells expressing wild-type p53 is also associated with accumulation of cells in G_2,[58] and this reduction in the number of cells in the radioresistant S phase should cause a reduction in the shoulder of the survival curve for a second dose delivered ≈16 hours after the first dose (see Figure 1-5). A simple illustration of effects of heterogeneous populations on radiation survival curves, with explanatory equations, was presented years ago.[59] *Finally, the distribution of cells in the cell cycle must be considered when the radiosensitivities of different cell lines are being compared.* For example, if two cell lines, A and B, had *identical* radiosensitivities, but cell line A had its cells distributed primarily in G_1 at the time of irradiation, while cell line B had its cells primarily in S or distributed randomly (i.e., asynchronously) through the cycle, a comparison of the radiation responses of A and B would lead to the erroneous conclusion that cell line A is more radiosensitive than cell line B (compare G_1 with asynchronous or S cells in Figure 1-5 or in Dewey et al.[29]).

Potentially Lethal Damage

Cell survival also can be altered by the incubation conditions after irradiation. Many years before the work with mammalian cells, experiments showed that holding bacteria for a time after irradiation in a buffered salts solution and then plating for the survival assay gave a much higher survival than if the cells were kept in full nutrient broth after irradiation.[60] This phenomenon was called liquid holding recovery.

Similarly, if mammalian cells are held in suboptimal growth conditions for various times after irradiation, such as with metabolic inhibitors,[61] balanced salts solution,[62] reduced temperatures,[28,54,63] or in plateau phase confluent cell cultures with the cells in G_1/G_0,[64,65] survival is greatly enhanced. This is illustrated in Figure 1-6 for holding in plateau phase. In Figure 1-6A, survival curves are shown for normal human fibroblasts irradiated while they were in G_0 in plateau phase and then either subcultured immediately or 24 hours later to assay for survival by colony formation. In Figure 1-6B, the rate of PLDR is shown by an increase in survival as a function of the time delay between irradiation and subculture for the survival assay when all cultures received the same dose. The interpretation of such observations was that radiation produced lesions that were potentially lethal, and that under one set of incubation conditions, a "damage repair" process

operating in opposition to a "damage fixation" process resulted in a certain fraction of lesions being converted to nonlethal lesions while the remaining fraction was fixed into lethal lesions that killed the cells. If the conditions were changed, they may become more favorable to the repair process or less favorable to the fixation process or both, so that the end result would be a higher proportion of the potentially lethal lesions being converted into nonlethal lesions. This can be viewed from the perspective of chromosomal aberration formation by simply postulating that since similar incubation schemes affecting survival also affect the yield of aberrations in a way that quantitatively accounts for the killing, one set of incubation conditions favors restitution of breaks as opposed to formation of exchanges, while for another set, restitution is less favored.[28] The reason for this phenomenon is not known, although we know that certain "suboptimal" growth conditions, such as those accompanying plateau-phase confluent culture, favor restitution. Also, anisotonic salt treatment,[66-68] which inhibits PLDR and SLDR, greatly affects chromatin structure, which in turn could alter the proximity of lesions, such as DNA double-strand breaks, or in some other way affect the fixation versus repair processes that are involved in exchanges versus restitution.[68-70]

Chemical Modification of Radiation Damage

Details on modification of radiation damage by chemical sensitizers, such as oxygen or other electron affinic agents or chemical protectors such as sulfhydryl amines or

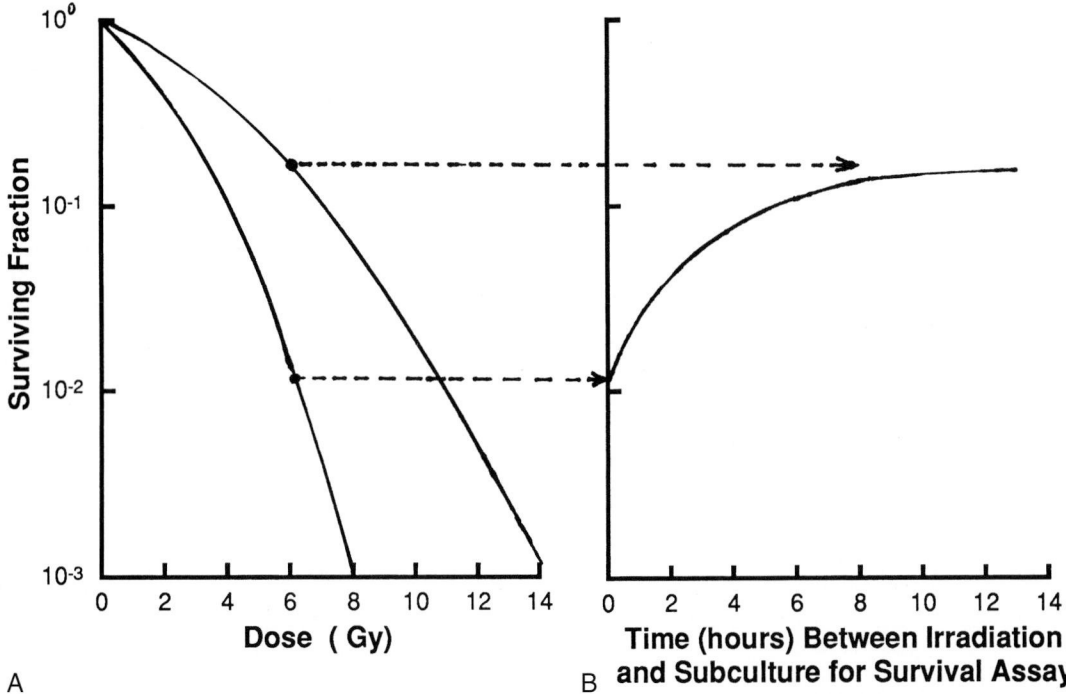

Figure 1–6. A, The effect of potentially lethal damage (PLD) and its repair (PLDR) on the dose-survival responses for immediate versus delayed subculturing. **B,** Survival increase due to PLDR after 6 Gy as a function of time of delay of subculturing. PLD is operationally different from sublethal damage (SLD). PLD is damage that is expressed or repaired depending on postirradiation conditions. Cells that may survive under one condition for a given dose may not survive the same dose under another condition. In contrast to SLDR, the increase in survival resulting from PLDR is not caused by a change in the response of cells surviving one dose to a second dose but, in this particular example, because of the fact that the balance between damage repair and misrepair or "fixation" shifts in favor of increased repair when cells are kept in a nongrowing, density-inhibited, plateau phase (delayed subculture) as opposed to starting to grow as a rapidly cell-cycling population (immediate subculture).

thiophosphates, are provided elsewhere in this volume, but it is appropriate to mention briefly the way they modify the parameters of dose-response relationships discussed earlier.

Most of these agents act as dose-modifying agents and alter the dose response by a simple dose modification factor (DMF). This is called a synergistic type of interaction between the modifying agent and radiation, which is distinctly different from an additive type of interaction that only reduces the shoulder of the survival curve. For an independent type of interaction, the shape of the radiation survival curve is unaffected other than the whole curve being shifted downward by an amount equal to the reduction in survival resulting from the modifying agent.[71] In fact, for independent interaction, if the population is synchronous, or asynchronous with no variation in cytotoxicity through the cell cycle for the modifying agent, the net survival for the two agents combined is simply survival for radiation multiplied by survival for the modifying agent. (See the publications by Dewey and coworkers[10,71] for these definitions and complications caused by variations through the cell cycle in sensitivities to the two agents.)

Oxygen is the classical example of a synergistic type of interaction. Oxygen sensitizes cells by reacting directly with damaged target radicals to "fix" them or render them less capable of repair by a competing, fast, hydrogen-donating reaction, which restores the target to its original condition. Other cellular species also can act in a way similar to oxygen by causing damage "fixation" (not repair). When the concentration of oxygen is reduced (e.g., to only about 1% to 2% of the concentration of O_2 in air), fewer oxidative radicals are present to fix the damage, so more fast repair by hydrogen donation occurs. Oxygen, therefore, simply increases the yield of "fixed" target radical species, producing essentially what could just as well be done by increasing the dose without the presence of oxygen.

The role played by oxygen in metabolic respiratory processes has nothing to do with its radiosensitizing effect. The "oxygen effect" disappears with increasing LET, the oxygen must be present during irradiation or within a few milliseconds after to produce the sensitization, and the oxygen effect is the same whether the irradiation occurs at 37°C or at 0°C, at which point oxygen-dependent respiration is greatly slowed.

When a sensitizing agent like oxygen acts as a simple dose modifying agent—and in this case, the DMF is around 3.0 for fully oxygenated versus anoxic conditions (the maximum oxygen enhancement ratio)—then only about one-third of the dose ($D/3$) is required to produce the same level of effect produced by the dose D in the absence of oxygen. The effect on the mathematical dose-response relationship and survival curve is then easy to calculate, as shown below.

For the N-D_o expression, if the survival under anoxic conditions, S_N, is

$$S_N = 1 - (1 - e^{-D/Do})^N$$

then, under oxygenated conditions the dose D would effectively be multiplied by 3 so

$$S_{ox} = 1 - (1 - e^{-3D/Do})^N$$

As can be seen by multiplying both the numerator and denominator of the exponent by 1/3 so that

$$S_{ox} = 1 - (1 - e^{-D/(Do/3)})^N$$

oxygen effectively reduces the D_o by a factor of 3 without changing the extrapolation number, N. A similar calculation applies for the N, D_1, and D_n expressions of Equation 3.

For the α/β expression, if the survival under anoxic conditions S_N is:

$$S_N = e^{-(\alpha D + \beta D^2)}$$

then, under oxygenated conditions

$$S_{ox} = e^{-[\alpha(3D) + \beta(3D)^2]}$$

or

$$S_{ox} = e^{-[3\alpha D + 9\beta D^2]}$$

so oxygen in this case increases the anoxic α constant by a factor of 3 and the anoxic β constant by a factor of 9.

This threefold increase in dose required for a certain amount of killing for irradiation under hypoxic conditions compared with irradiation under oxygenated conditions is thought to play an important role in radiotherapy. Many tumors contain a significant fraction of radioresistant hypoxic cells compared with primarily oxygenated cells in surrounding normal tissue. Thus, for one acute dose of irradiation, the dose required to cure about 90% of the tumors (e.g., a survival fraction of 10–13 for a tumor with 1012 clonogenic tumor cells) would have to be about 3 times larger than it would be if all of the cells in the tumor were oxygenated. However, the situation is not so bleak, because in most tumors considerable reoxygenation occurs during fractionated radiotherapy. This *reoxygenation* has been termed the fourth R of radiotherapy, which follows the three Rs (*repair, redistribution, and repopulation*).

Similar calculations can be made for radioprotective compounds that act as dose-modifying agents, except that to calculate the biological effect in the presence of the protector, doses in the absence of the protector must be divided by the DMF. Thus, cysteine has been shown to act as a dose-modifying radioprotector with a DMF of about 2. Effectively, α is reduced by 1/2 and β by 1/4.

Radiation Quality, Relative Biological Effectiveness, and Linear Energy Transfer

Radiation quality has long been known to affect biological responses to ionizing radiation. Densely ionizing radiations such as alpha particles are more effective in killing mammalian cells than sparsely ionizing x-rays or gamma-rays. This has nothing to do with "penetrating power" since the relative biological effectiveness (RBE) of radiations having different LETs (quality) is defined in terms of the amount of ionization energy absorbed in the cells (i.e., as the ratio of doses of two different types of radiation that are required to produce the same degree of the same biological effect. X-rays generated at 250 kV have been widely used in radiobiologic studies, so they have been the standard used for RBE comparisons. The RBE of a radiation in question is then defined as:

RBE = Dose of 250 kvp x-rays for a given level of a given effect

———————————————————

Dose of the radiation in question to produce the same level of the same effect

Naturally, other radiation conditions such as oxygenation, dose-rate, and so on must be equal. Similar equations can be used to express DMF, OER, and DEF.

An example of the dose-survival curves for mammalian cells for radiations associated with different LETs is shown in Figure 1-7. The aspect of radiation quality or LET that is, to a first approximation, most pertinent to the RBE is the LET that describes in a rough sort of way how the density of ionizations along the ionization track in irradiated material increases as the LET increases. Actually, sophisticated microdosimetric and nanodosimetric quantities are used for precisely relating RBE to radiation quality, but for our purposes LET is sufficient. Again very roughly, the higher the LET, the more ionizations occur along the charged particle tracks delivering the dose; namely, electrons with low LET (x-rays, gamma-rays, or beta particles) compared with atomic nuclei with high LET (neutrons, alpha particles, and accelerator-produced charged particles such as silicon and argon). It should be noted that protons used in therapy have an RBE close to 1.0, with the primary advantage being improvement in dose distribution.[1]

The relationship between RBE and LET can be viewed in terms of cell killing caused by the induction of chromosomal aberrations. At very low LETs associated with irradiation with high energy x-rays or gamma-rays, the distance between ionizations or ion clusters along the tracks of the electrons is almost always greater than the minimum interaction distance for two chromosome breaks to interact to form an exchange. Therefore, two or more tracks are necessary, and many ionizations that contribute to the dose are wasted because they are unlikely ever to be involved in a potential aberration-producing break-pair.

As the LET increases to the optimum, an RBE is eventually reached at which the optimum spacing of ionizations occurs for producing break-pairs with the maximum efficiency. This optimum RBE also probably includes a "repair" component, since the density of damage also appears to influence the processing of damage in the DNA; that is, after high LET of ≈100 keV/μ, more residual DNA double-strand breaks (DSBs) exist after several hours of repair than after low LET radiation.[72] The maximum RBE of 1.2 to 1.6 for DNA DSBs[72] and initial interphase chromosome breaks and ≈3 for chromosomal aberrations and cell killing occurs at an LET of ≈100 keV/μ. Then, with further increase in LET, the RBE declines because more energy is being deposited than necessary to produce the effect, while the wasted energy still contributes to increasing the dose; therefore, the efficiency per unit dose decreases. The relationship between RBE and LET is shown in Figure 1-8 for different endpoints of radiation damage. Also of importance is the observation that the oxygen enhancement ratio for cell killing that was discussed previously decreases from a maximum of ≈3 for low LET radiation to ≈1 as the LET increases to ≈100 keV/μ and above.[1] This probably occurs because the high LET events induce so much localized damage in the DNA that any additional effect from oxygen-generated free radicals at these damaged sites is unimportant.

Not only does an increase in LET cause an increase in the relative effectiveness per unit dose (up to a maximum),

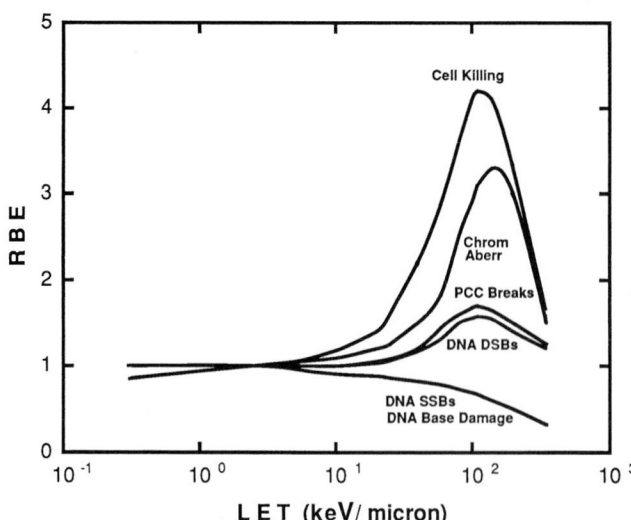

Figure 1–8. A semiquantitative illustration of the relationships between RBE and LET for different endpoints of biologic damage. Except for DNA base damage and single strand breaks (*SSBs*), the RBE versus LET curves are qualitatively similar, peaking at about 100 to 200 keV/μ for cell killing, chromosomal aberrations (*Chrom Aberr*), initial interphase chromosome breaks as seen in prematurely condensed chromosomes (*PCC breaks*), and DNA double strand breaks (*DSBs*). The peak RBEs are much higher for cell killing and chromosomal aberrations than for initial PCC chromosome breaks or DNA DSBs, presumably because there is an additional repair component that operates inefficiently at high LET for repairing DNA DSBs that result in chromosomal aberrations and cell killing. This repair component, of course, would not be present for initial damage yielding DNA DSBs or chromosome PCC breaks. The decline in RBE for LET over 200 keV/μ is the result of wasted energy (see text). For base damage and SSBs, the RBE decreases continuously with increasing LET over the entire range, again because of wasted energy.

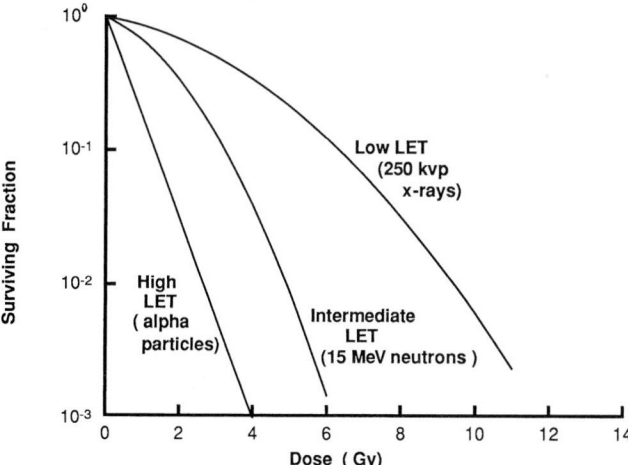

Figure 1–7. Dose-response curves for radiations with different associated linear energy transfers (LETs). The relative biologic effectiveness (RBE) of the neutrons or alpha particles relative to the x-rays is defined as a ratio of doses to produce the same level of effect, with the numerator of the ratio being the x-ray dose.

but an increase in LET also decreases repair of DNA damage, SLDR, PLDR, and often the sensitizing and protecting effect of chemical modifiers. Effectively, the dose response for high LET radiations, like alpha particles, is totally dominated by a dose-rate- and repair-independent alpha component of the expression

$$S_{OX} = e^{-(\alpha D + \beta D^2)}$$

Whereas the value of α for x-rays or gamma-rays might be of the order of 0.2 Gy^{-1}, the α parameter for 100 keV/μ alpha particles might be as much as 10 times higher or $\approx$2.0 Gy^{-1}, with the β parameter close to zero.

Ionizing Radiation–Sensitive Mutants

Our current understanding of DNA repair processes in microorganisms following treatment with agents such as ionizing and nonionizing radiations or other genotoxic chemical agents has been based in no small part on the availability and study of mutants that are hypersensitive to such agents. Progress in this area for mammalian cells has been slow but has accelerated in recent years. In 1961, Alexander and Mikulski[73] reported that a radiosensitive mouse lymphoma cell line, L5178Y, developed even greater radiosensitivity after prolonged culturing of the cells. These cells now have been more fully characterized.[74] Also, in the 1960s, Gotoff and coworkers[75] reported that patients with ataxia-telangiectasia undergoing radiation treatment for cancer uniformly showed "untoward responses" to x-irradiation. Taylor and his colleagues later showed that cells from such patients are very hypersensitive to ionizing radiation.[76] Ataxia-telangiectasia is thought to be a single gene defect whereby the phenotype for homozygous recessive individuals includes a hypersensitivity to ionizing radiation, immune deficiencies, and a predisposition to cancer. Heterozygotes are generally normal in this respect, although there have been recent suggestions that some heterozygotes have an increased incidence of breast cancer. About a dozen other ionizing-radiation-sensitive mutants of mammalian cells of rodent origin have been isolated during the past 20 years.[77-87] All of these, including human AT cells, are hypersensitive to ionizing radiation with respect to both cell killing and induction of chromosomal aberrations. The dose-survival response for some radiosensitive mutants is shown in Figure 1-1B where the x-ray or gamma-ray D_o is in the 0.4 to 0.5 Gy range compared to values of 1.5 to 2.0 Gy for the corresponding wild-types. Coupled with the fact that the dose response curves for the radiosensitive mutants generally show a greatly reduced shoulder, the relative radiosensitivities measured by the ratio of doses that yield a 10% level of survival is around 4 to 5 and is even greater for lower doses and higher survival levels.

There are some interesting differences among mutants and between mutants and their wild-type counterparts regarding chromosome breakage and their DNA repair properties as measured by rejoining of DNA double-strand breaks. Phenotypically, the radiosensitive mutants can be classified as either AT-like or L5178Y-S/S-like. The distinguishing L5178Y-S/S-like characteristics

include a radiosensitive inhibition of cell cycle progression and DNA synthesis and readily demonstrable deficiencies in rejoining DNA strand breaks, which leads to an increase in chromosomal aberrations.

The AT mutants differ from L5178Y-S/S-like mutants in that they are radioresistant for inhibition of cell cycle progression and DNA synthesis[88] and do not have a significant deficiency in the rate or amount of rejoining of DNA strand breaks. The AT gene, which apparently has four main complementation groups, has been cloned and mapped to chromosome 11q22-23.[89] It spans some 150 kb of genomic DNA, contains 66 exons, and produces a 13-kb transcript. ATM is a protein kinase related to the DNA-dependent protein kinase (DNA-PK) discussed later.[90] Following the breakage of the DNA double helix in both normal and AT cells, rejoining or restitution occurs most of the time, but in a certain proportion of the cases, interaction with a nearby break leads to mis-rejoining or exchange formation. About half of these exchanges are lethal in diploid cells irradiated in G_1 or G_o because half are asymmetrical, which generates an acentric chromosome fragment and leads to a large loss of genetic information in the progeny of cells bearing the acentric fragment. Ataxia cells and many other radiosensitive mutant cells show a large increase in aberration production per unit dose relative to wild-types. At least for the strains of AT fibroblast cells we have tested, this increase results from a much larger proportion, relative to normal cells, of initial chromosome breaks that rejoin incorrectly to yield an excess number of chromosome fragments.[91] This was studied by inducing premature chromosome condensation (PCC) in G_o human fibroblasts and measuring the number of PCCs and their fragments in many cells[91] that were held in plateau phase in G_1/G_o for up to 46 hours after irradiation before PCC was initiated. The same technique also has been used by many other investigators to study early breakage and rejoining of chromosomes.[92-95] The results for AT versus normal cells are shown in Figure 1-9. The initial number of chromosome breaks is apparently the same for normal and AT cells, although there is some uncertainty in estimating the number immediately after irradiation since the cell fusion and PCC process itself requires 15 to 20 minutes at 37°C. The rate of rejoining also is the same, but the residual number of excess fragments after 24 or even 46 hours while the cells remained in G_1 is much higher for AT cells than for normal cells. This difference fully accounts for the difference in radiosensitivity with respect to cell killing,[32] *and develops while the cells are in a non-cycling G_o state.* Specifically, the number of fragments observed in G_o/G_1 after repair was complete was the same as the number of aberrations observed in metaphase after the cells had traversed S phase and G_2. Furthermore, one lethal aberration per cell was observed for both AT cells and normal cells when survival was reduced to 37% by irradiation with 0.7 Gy or 4 Gy, respectively. Therefore, as discussed by Murnane,[57] the increased radiosensitivity of AT cells is not dependent on the failure of irradiated AT cells to arrest in G_1, which would result in the cells having less time to repair DNA damage before they enter S phase. In fact, the hypothesis that p53-induced G_1 arrest enhances radioresistance (discussed by Murnane[57])

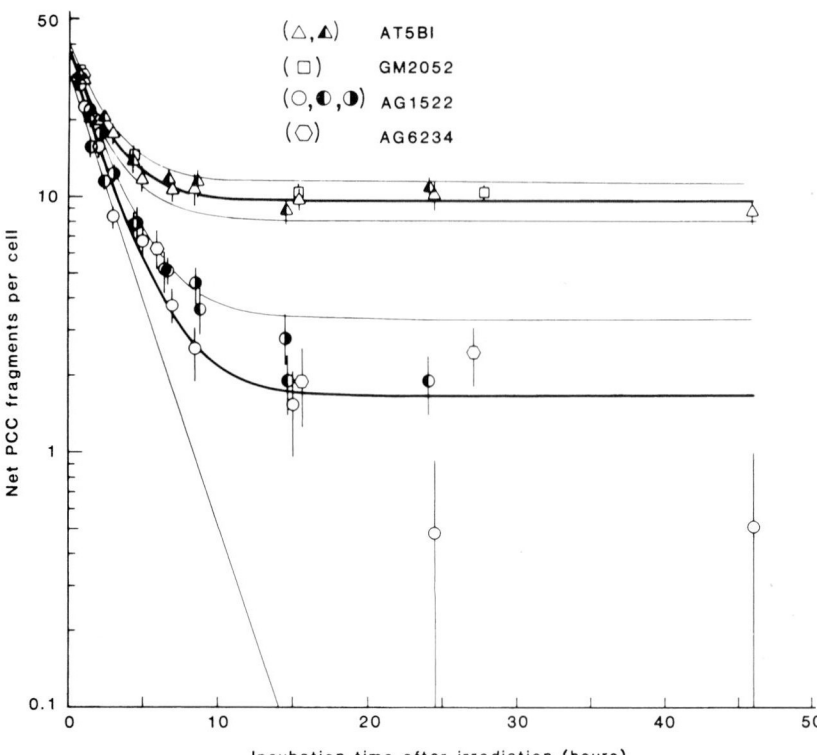

Figure 1–9. The initial breakage and rejoining during G_o of human chromosomes in normal and ataxia telangiectasia (AT) cells after an x-ray dose of 6 Gy. The initial break frequency and the rate of rejoining were determined by holding the cells in plateau phase in G_o while allowing the cells to incubate for various times before the chromosomes were condensed by fusing the G_o cells with mitotic cells (PCC). Note that the initial break frequency is the same for normal cells (*bottom curve*) and AT cells (*top curve*), but the residual frequency of excess chromosome fragments is much higher for AT cells. The magnitude of this difference quantitatively accounts for the difference in sensitivity to cell killing between normal and AT cells, and all the difference develops during a period when the cells are in a non-cycling G_o state. The difference is unrelated to a G_1 delay or to either repair or formation of DNA fragments during S or G_2 (see text). Apoptosis, at least before the cells enter mitosis, does not appear to contribute significantly to the killing of the cells. (From Cornforth MN, Bedford JS: On the nature of a defect in cells from individuals with ataxia telangiectasia. *Science.* 1985;227:1589, with permission of the publisher.)

could not apply for most asynchronous populations in which the radiosensitivity is determined by the radio-resistant cells that are usually in S phase and not G_1 (see Fig. 1-5 and Dewey et al.[29]). Finally, the suggestion that radiation-induced apoptosis is responsible for *AT* fibroblast cells being radiosensitive is unlikely because practically all of the cells irradiated in G_1 enter the first mitosis without the appearance of apoptotic (AP) cells (Bedford, unpublished data); however, the loss of chromosome fragments in subsequent generations following the production of excess fragments in *AT* cells might result in an AP death, a possibility that needs to be explored. The possibility of chromosome fragments leading to apoptosis will be discussed later under the section on apoptosis.

Related to the topic of radiosensitive mutants, experiments are under way to alter radiosensitivity by transfecting mammalian cells with oncogenes, mutant and wild-type p53 genes, and so on. These experiments have shown changes in radiosensitivity but have not delineated specific molecular pathways responsible for altering radiosensitivity (see Chapter 71, Gene Target Therapy for further details). Another related topic receiving considerable attention at this time is transient radiation-induced radioresistance observed after low doses of 50 cGy or less.[96,97] Certain genes are induced by these low doses, but no specific changes in RNA messages or unique enzymes or proteins have been identified as being responsible for the induced radioresistance that persists for only a few hours. Again, we emphasize that radiation has not been found to induce stable genetic changes that result in long-lasting radioresistance after a single large dose of radiation. Instead, only radiosensitive mutants have been isolated. However, radioresistant clones have

been isolated recently following fractionated irradiation.[98-100] Currently, many investigators are attempting to clone the genes involved in DNA repair pathways and to determine the specific molecular alterations responsible for the decreased and increased radiosensitivities. For example, rodent mutants (xrs-5) that are deficient in both repairing DSBs and V(D)J recombination appear to code for a protein (Ku-like) that is defective in binding to and repairing double-strand ends of DNA.[101,102] Furthermore, Ku 70 and 80 form a DNA targeting subunit that is part of a multiprotein complex containing a DNA protein kinase (DNA-PK) that also includes a large catalytic subunit (DNA-PK$_{cs}$) that co-segregates with the Scid mutation, resulting in immune deficiency and an increase in radiosensitivity.[103] Other recent evidence suggests that helicases and ligases are sometimes defective, and that defects in transcription machinery[102] can be associated with defects in DNA repair. All of these possibilities that probably involve a complex of enzymes and regulatory proteins that bind to DNA are actively being investigated, including alterations in chromatin structure such as changes in coiling of DNA and its attachment to the nuclear matrix. Finally, many investigators are attempting to identify the specific genes and molecular pathways that are involved in radiation-induced apoptosis that occurs in certain cell types.

APOPTOSIS

The phenomenon of apoptosis, or programmed cell death, was first described in 1972 by Kerr and associates[104] as a process occurring during normal development of organs and tissues and after certain toxic treatments. The term was derived from Greek ("falling off") and refers to leaves falling from a tree to emphasize the normal physiologic nature or programmed death of cells undergoing apoptosis. In 1982, the AP process was used to describe radiation-induced death observed in a small fraction of the cells in the crypt of the small intestine. Then, from 1986 to 1989, apoptosis was reported to play a primary role in radiation-induced death of post-mitotic cells in the salivary gland. Since 1990, radiation-induced apoptosis has been observed in several animal tumors and in several different cell lines in culture, and many investigators have been identifying molecular signals that control the induction of apoptosis in cells exposed to radiation or other toxic treatments. Although the information available in 2002 to describe and quantify radiation-induced apoptosis is incomplete, it has been reviewed[105-110] and will be summarized briefly.

An important consideration addressed in this section and illustrated in a model shown in Figure 1-10 is whether radiation-induced apoptosis (A) or necrosis (N) occurs: (1) early *pre-mitotically* during interphase (I)

without any requirement for cell division (IA or IN), or (2) late *post-mitotically* (MA or MN) in progeny of a cell that divides (M) but (3) only in progeny of a cell that had a *chromosomal aberration(s)* (MC), with the progeny dying by necrosis (MCN) if they are not stimulated to apoptose (MCA), or (4) *mitotically* by apoptosis or necrosis that usually occurs early during an *abortive mitosis* (FMA or FMN) or after a *failed division* (FDA or FDN). This last process is sometimes identified as *mitotic catastrophe* (i.e., associated with cells having multiple micronuclei).[111,112] Also, a *failed mitosis* (FM) is sometimes associated with nondisjunction between sister chromatids that can result in aneuploidy or endoreduplication that leads to an 8n content of DNA and diplochromosomes in the next mitosis. The other types of FD that result in multinucleated cells can also lead to aneuploidy or an 8n content of DNA. In addition,[5] a cell may be irreversibly arrested in the cell cycle, resembling *senescence* (ISn, MSn, MCSn), that is, reproductively dead, but continuing to be metabolically alive for days to weeks. For brevity in subsequent discussions, these definitions

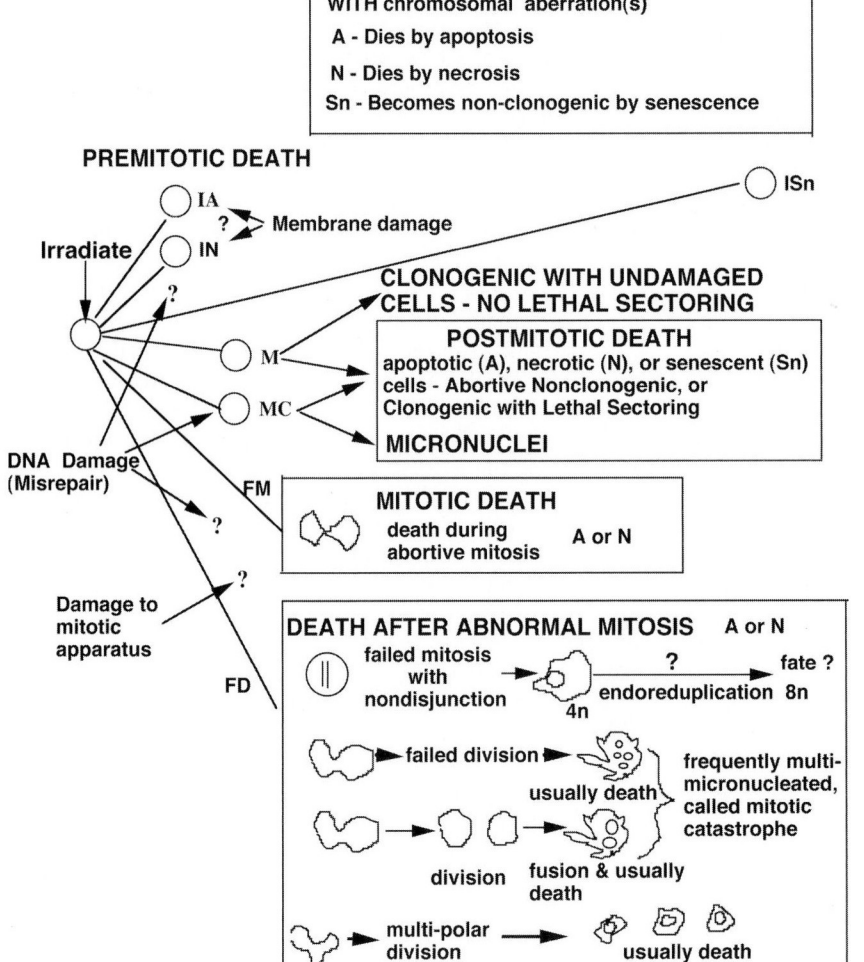

Figure 1–10. Schematic model for modes of death. See text for description.

and abbreviations will be used. *The model presented should serve as a framework for relating specific molecular alterations to particular cellular events that result in different types of cell death.*

Identifying Apoptotic and Necrotic Cells

Death of mammalian cells after being exposed to ionizing radiation has been described as due to either necrosis or apoptosis. Necrotic cells are characterized by loss of membrane integrity before DNA degradation, whereas AP cells are characterized as loss of membrane integrity after DNA degradation. In AP cells, the degradation of DNA is observed as nucleosome ladders of ≈50 kilobase pairs or fewer, but sometimes as large as 100 to 600 kilobase pairs. The DNA degradation that occurs later after necrosis is characterized by random DNA degradation into small molecules. Dewey and colleagues[105] offer a review of the histologic and flow cytometric methods used for identifying AP cells.

Observations of Radiation-Induced Apoptosis

In vivo, apoptosis is observed in individual cells that subsequently undergo phagocytosis by neighboring cells or macrophages, whereas necrosis is observed in tissues as clumps of cells involved in an inflammatory response resulting from the release of the contents of necrosing cells. In cell culture systems, apoptosis is observed in individual cells, and the AP cells are believed to persist for several hours with the AP characteristics described.[113-115] The necrotic process in cell culture systems is observed as a sudden rupture of the membrane of individual cells followed by their pyknosis, or lysis and disappearance from the culture.[115] An important question is the form of death occurring after two to six divisions following irradiation (i.e., the classical *postmitotic* death resulting from chromosomal aberrations (MC).[116] This death may be associated with either apoptosis or necrosis, and critical studies are needed to determine the circumstances, such as specific gene expression, that result in either apoptosis (MCA) or necrosis (MCN) being the cause of radiation-induced cell death that occurs *postmitotically in progeny of the irradiated cell.* As a corollary of this question, information is needed on whether or not apoptosis that occurs *postmitotically* occurs only in cells that have manifested chromosomal aberrations (MCA versus MA). For example, after x-irradiation of rat embryo fibroblasts (REC:myc), the probability of *postmitotic* apoptosis was much greater in progeny manifesting micronuclei (MCA) than in progeny not having any visible micronuclei (MA).[117]

Apoptosis was first recognized in vivo in normal cells. For example, the death of lymphocytes that occurs *premitotically* during interphase early after irradiation (IA) has been observed for many years and is most likely an AP type of death.[104] Studies have shown that in the intestinal crypt, a small percentage of the cells undergo *premitotic* apoptosis without cell division (IA) in 3 to 6 hr following ionizing radiation. This *premitotic* AP process,

which is very radiosensitive ($D_o \approx 0.2$ Gy) and apparently dependent on wild-type p53, is thought, however, to contribute little to the radiation damage in the crypt because only about 2% of the crypt cells become AP after radiation with 0.5 to 10 Gy.[118,119] Furthermore, controversial findings suggest that apoptosis of microvessel endothelial cells are the primary lesion initiating intestinal radiation damage.[120] Radiation-induced early death that was probably *premitotic* apoptosis (IA) was observed in 1961 in the bone marrow.[121] Also, the nondividing cells in the salivary gland manifest *premitotic* apoptosis (IA), which appears to be primarily responsible for the acute radiation injury observed in the salivary gland.[122] In addition, radiation induces apoptosis in proliferative immature cells in the cerebellum, kidney, intestine, and testis.[123] Recently, apoptosis has been observed in animal tumors, in particular those of the lymphoid and hematopoietic origin,[124] although tumors in the ovary and other sites also have been observed to have a considerable amount of apoptosis occurring both spontaneously and after ionizing radiation.[124] Finally, spontaneous apoptosis has been observed in 0% to 14% of the tumor cells scored in surgical specimens of human colon adenocarcinomas and cervical adenocarcinomas.[125] The clinical significance of these types of observations will be presented later.

Target for Radiation-Induced Apoptosis

The target for inducing apoptosis may be either the plasma membrane or nuclear DNA or both (See Dewey et al.[105] for references). For example, in the salivary gland, protection by treatment with lidocaine from radiation-induced *premitotic* apoptosis that occurs during interphase without any cell division (IA) suggests that the membrane is involved. Also, ionizing radiation appears to act directly on the plasma membrane to induce the hydrolysis of sphingomyelin to ceramide, which in turn causes apoptosis (probably *premitotic*, IA) of bovine aorta endothelial cells in vitro. However, ceramide is also produced in the nucleus by radiation activation of ceramide synthetase.[126] *Postmitotic* radiation-induced apoptosis (MA or MCA) in a murine T cell hybridoma cell line was enhanced significantly by incorporation of BrdU into the DNA, which suggests that the nuclear DNA is a target. This conclusion is supported by the observation that in several cell lines, a high incidence of apoptosis (IA and MA or MCA) was induced by DNA double-strand breaks caused by[125] disintegrations in the DNA (See Dewey et al.[105] for references). In addition, by irradiating different parts of the rodent cell (Rat 1: myc) with helium ions,[127] the nucleus was shown to be a critical target for radiation-induced *postmitotic* apoptosis (MA or MCA). Studies have shown that radiation-induced apoptosis has an oxygen enhancement ratio of ≈3 for x-irradiation and an RBE of 2.7 to 4 for 15 to 600 Mev neutrons, which could be associated with primary damage either in nuclear DNA or the membrane. Experiments are needed with ^{125}IdU to label and irradiate the nuclear DNA selectively or with ^{125}I-labeled concanavalin A to irradiate the cytoplasm selectively, and with a combination of the two, in order to determine the target for radiation-induced apoptosis in various cell types that apoptose either *premitotically* (IA), during an *abortive mitosis* (FMA), after a *failed division* (FDA), or *postmitotically* (MA or MCA).

Genes Controlling Apoptosis

Evidence exists that radiation-induced apoptosis can occur via p53 dependent and independent mechanisms[128] from damage in either the nucleus[127] or cytoplasm/membrane.[126] This damage can result in cells apoptosing either early *premitotically* during interphase (IA),[129] during or after an *aberrant mitosis* (FMA or FDA),[129] or *postmitotically* (MA or MCA) several hours after the irradiated cells and their progeny have divided a few times.[115] There is some evidence that early *premitotic* (IA) apoptosis is usually associated with the expression of wild-type p53, whereas late *postmitotic* apoptosis is independent of p53. The signal transduction pathways[130] resulting in radiation-induced apoptosis involve the nucleus and cytoplasm, with alterations in mitochondrial electron transport[131] and the release of cytochrome c from the mitochondria initiating caspase cleavage,[132] which terminates in activation of a nuclease responsible for internucleosomal digestion of DNA.[107] See publications by Rich et al.[109] and Hengartner[110] for excellent reviews of the major players in the AP pathways, including Bcl-2 and Bcl-X_L that reverse the AP effect of Bax on the mitochondria.[133]

Quantitative Comparisons of Apoptotic Death with Clonogenic Survival

Figure 1-11 illustrates the manner in which apoptosis is quantified both in vivo and in vitro. The upper two curves show that the AP percent for the lymphoid TK6 cells in culture reaches a constant or plateau value at about 20 hours after irradiation. This plateau level increases with dose, is assumed to represent the fraction of the cells susceptible to apoptosis, and is used to obtain a plot of AP percent versus dose.[113] In in vivo systems, however, apoptosis peaks and then declines, and the value for this peak is used to obtain a dose-response relationship.[134] Since, *in vivo*, apoptosis is occurring while the cells are being engulfed by neighboring cells, the absolute amount of apoptosis that could occur in the absence of elimination of the AP cells is unknown. However, investigators have used these peak values as estimates of the percent of the cells that apoptose after irradiation.

An example of radiation-induced apoptosis measured in the TK 6 human B lymphoblast cell line using the "comet" assay[113] is illustrated in Figure 1-12. *Panel A* shows the AP percent as a function of dose, as determined at 24 to 36 hours after irradiation when the plateau in percent apoptosis as a function of time after irradiation had been reached. The maximum of 90% AP cells observed for 10 to 15 Gy suggests that 90% of the population was susceptible to apoptosis. As a comparison, the lack of apoptosis is shown for the AP resistant CHO cells irradiated with 15 Gy (i.e., only 3% underwent apoptosis).

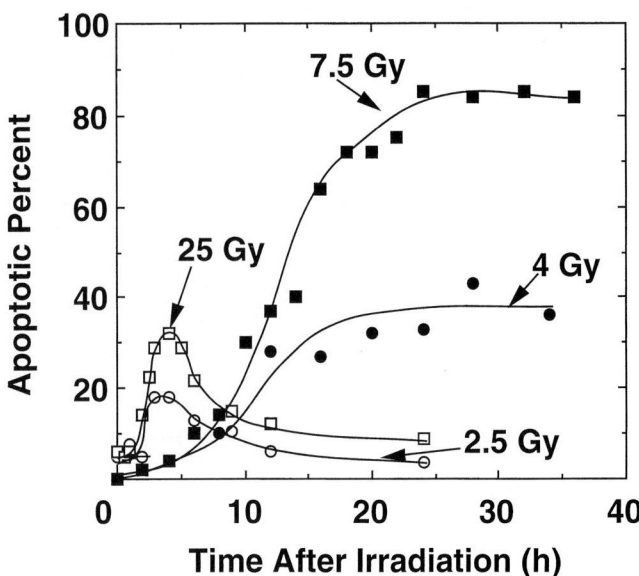

Figure 1–11. Percent of apoptotic cells plotted against time after irradiation. *Solid symbols* are for *TK6* human B lymphoblast cells in vitro assayed by the "comet" assay (data taken from Olive et al.[113]). *Open symbols* are for the murine ovarian carcinoma (*OCaI*) in vivo. The assay of the number of apoptotic bodies containing nuclear fragments per 100 nuclei was performed by microscopic examination of H&E-stained sections.[134] (From Dewey WC, Ling CC, Meyn RE: Radiation-induced apoptosis: Relevance to radiotherapy. *Int J Radiat Oncol Biol Phys.* 1995; 33:781, with permission of the publisher.)

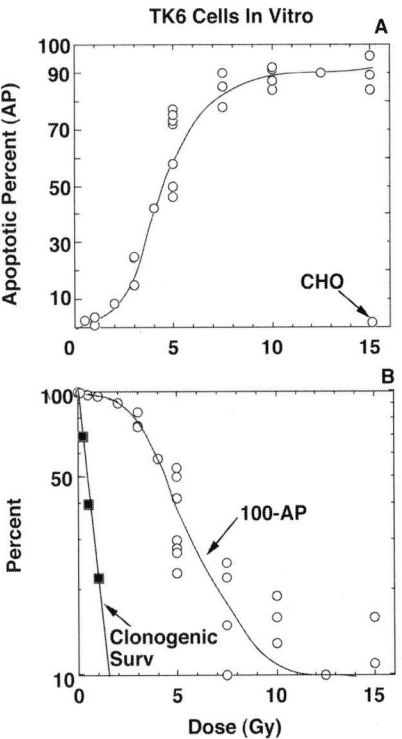

Figure 1–12. A, Percent of apoptotic cells (AP) plotted against radiation dose when *TK6* cells *in vitro* were scored as shown in Figure 1-11 at 24 hours after irradiation. For comparison, data are shown for Chinese hamster ovary cells (CHO) that were treated identically but which were not susceptible to apoptosis. (Data taken from Olive et al.[113]) **B,** Data in panel A were converted into a percent of the total population that survived apoptosis (i.e., *100–AP*). The line for *clonogenic survival* was obtained for the same *TK6* cell line.[180]

Panel B plots the same data for the percent of the TK 6 cells that have not undergone apoptosis (100 − AP) as a function of radiation dose. For comparison, the clonogenic survival also is shown for this same cell line. Note that although this cell line is classified as an AP sensitive cell line, only a small fraction of the loss of the reproductive integrity can be accounted for by the amount of apoptosis scored during the first 24 to 36 hours after irradiation before any significant amount of cell division should have occurred. For example, after 1 Gy, ≈90% of the cells apparently survived an AP death compared with only 10% of the cells that clonogenically survived a reproductive death. Therefore, either AP cells did not persist in the culture as they were being induced and scored during the 24- to 36-hour period after irradiation, or as illustrated in the next section, the true AP percentage was reduced because of cell proliferation.

A basic question concerning this study as well as other studies of apoptosis is whether the amount of apoptosis observed before any significant mitotic activity has occurred after irradiation can account for the loss of clonogenic survival. In practically all cases in which apoptosis has been quantified in cells both in culture and in vivo, the answer, as apoptosis has been measured, is no.[105,135] This is true for cells that manifest very little apoptosis and is usually true for cells that are classified as being AP sensitive. Then, most of the loss of clonogenic survival (i.e., loss of reproductive integrity) occurs later after mitotic activity has resumed, and is most likely caused by the typical *postmitotic* death (MCN or MCA) in which cells manifesting chromosomal aberrations during division divide and form nonclonogenic daughter cells[32] with micronuclei.[117] Many of these cells may divide a few times to form giant cells, abortive colonies, and reproductively viable colonies[116] with or without lethal sectoring.[21,115] This lethal sectoring is associated with cell death and formation of giant cells that are frequently multinucleated and may persist for several hours or days (Sn).[116] The cell death that occurs eventually may take place *postmitotically* either by the necrotic pathway (MCN) or by the AP pathway (MCA).

Cell Proliferation Must Be Considered When Quantitatively Comparing Apoptosis with Clonogenic Survival

The fates of irradiated cells and their progeny were determined by following individual cells in multiple fields by computerized video time lapse (CVTL) microscopy for as long as 6 days after irradiation.[115] With this method, clonogenic cells could be distinguished from nonclonogenic cells. Let us compare proliferation of irradiated *REC:myc* cells with proliferation of *REC:ras* cells after they received 9.5 Gy. In both cases, 97% to 99% of the cells were reproductively dead, that is, 97% to 99% nonclonogenic or 1% to 3% clonogenic. Both cell types apoptosed *postmitotically* (MA or MCA), but about 50% of the REC-ras cells underwent "senescent" events *postmitotically* (MSn). Figure 1-13 shows the time postirradiation (9.5 Gy) when the cells divided. For both *REC:ras* and *REC:myc* cells, the times of division for the different generations often overlapped (Figs. 1-13A and B). Therefore, cells from different generations were present at the same time, which is caused by the variation in generation times between individual cells in the progenies. As illustrated in Figure 1-13C, the generation times for *REC:myc* and *REC:ras* cells, respectively, increased

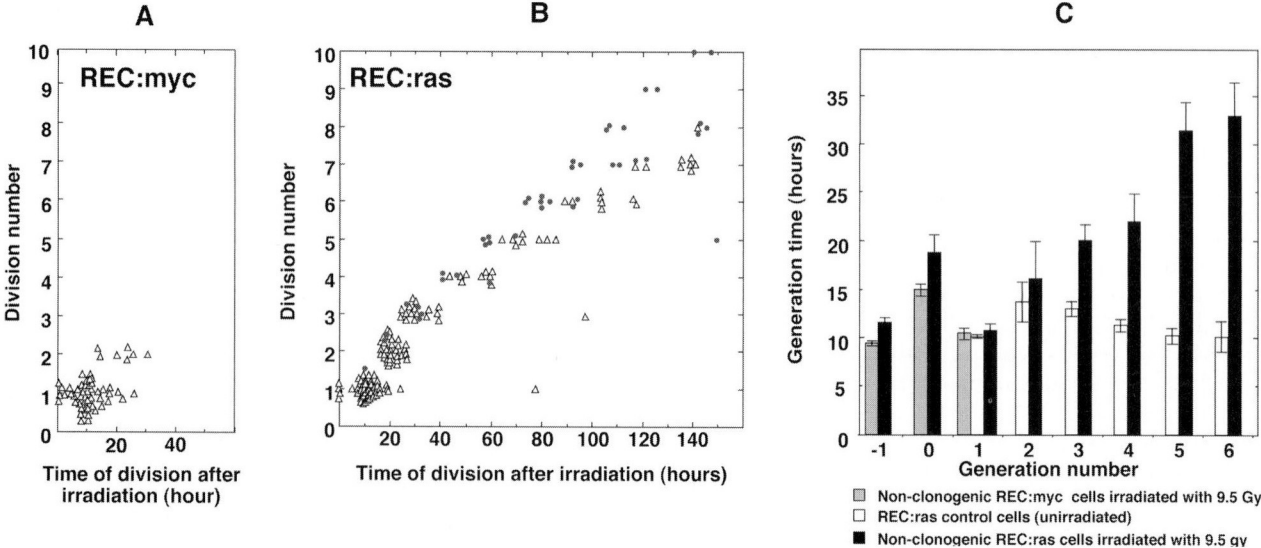

Figure 1–13. The times at which cells irradiated with 9.5 Gy completed their first, second, third, etc. divisions after irradiation. **A**, *REC:myc* cells, all of which were *non-clonogenic* due to *postmitotic* apoptosis (MA or MCA). **B**, *REC:ras* cells; the progeny of a cell that was *clonogenic* are indicated by the solid circles, and the progeny of 37 cells that were *nonclonogenic* are indicated by the open triangles. These nonclonogenic cells underwent *postmitotic* apoptosis (MA or MCA, or both) and *postmitotic "senescence"* (MSn). **C**, The mean generation times for both the unirradiated *REC:myc* and *REC:ras* cells (9.5 Gy) are shown for the generation before the cells were irradiated (gen -1), the generation in which irradiation occurred (gen 0), and the following 1 to 6 generations. None of the irradiated *REC:myc* cells survived beyond generation 2. Unirradiated *REC:ras* cells located in a shielded area of the irradiated flask were also followed, and the mean generation times for these cells are also presented. Standard error of means are indicated. (From Forrester HB, Vidair CA, Albright N, et al: Using computerized video time lapse for quantifying cell death of X-irradiated rat embryo cells transfected with c-myc or c-Ha-ras. *Cancer Res.* 1999;59:931, with permission of the publisher.)

from 10 to 12 hours for generation -1 (before irradiation) to 15 to 20 hours for generation 0 in which the cells were irradiated. In the following generation 1, the generation times for both the irradiated *REC:myc* and *REC:ras* cells returned to approximately the same time as for the unirradiated cells. The remaining *REC:myc* cells died in generation 2, so there were no generation times beyond generation 1. However, the generation times for the *REC:ras* cells gradually increased until by generations 5 and 6 they were almost three times that of the unirradiated cells, that is, a *senescent* (MSn) type of behavior (see pedigrees in Forrester et al.'s publication[115] for specific examples).

Figure 1-14 illustrates the kinetics of cell death by the *cumulative* percentage of the nonclonogenic cells that had apoptosed (MA or MCA identified by CVTL from morphological changes such as membrane blebbing,[136] nuclear fragmentation, and detachment from the surface). Note that from the mathematical definition of *cumulative* AP percentage in the legend of Figure 1-14,[115] any AP cells that lyse or disappear during the period when apoptosis is being observed by CVTL will not affect the *cumulative* percentage. The data show that after 9.5 Gy, there was much more AP death that occurred more rapidly for *REC:myc* cells than for *REC:ras* cells. For *REC:myc* cells, all 49 cells were nonclonogenic in this experiment (33 out of 34 in another experiment), and for *REC:ras* cells, 37 out of 38 cells were nonclonogenic. As shown by the solid circles in Figure 1-13B, the one clonogenic *REC:ras* cell caused a significant increase in cell number after 100 hours (also see cell number in Fig. 7B in Forrester et al.'s publication[115]). Also, as shown previously,[115] and illustrated in Figure 1-14, ≈50% of the progeny of nonclonogenic *REC:ras* cells were "*senescent*" and did not die

during the 140-hour duration of the experiment. These "*senescent*" cells must either persist for very long periods of time or eventually die because the 97% of the irradiated population that was classified as nonclonogenic, as determined by the CVTL analysis that included both AP and "*senescent*" events, corresponds closely to the 97% to 99% nonclonogenic determined by the standard clonogenic assay.[137] This figure illustrates clearly why determinations of the percentage of cells undergoing apoptosis at different times after irradiation, called single time-point assays, will not indicate the true percentage of cells that eventually apoptose if the progeny of the nonclonogenic cells are undergoing several divisions (illustrated in Dewey et al.'s publication[105]). Especially, if the AP cells rapidly disappear, such as from phagocytosis in vivo, single time-point assays will never yield AP percentages that approach the *cumulative* AP percentages. Only *cumulative* percentages will represent the true AP percentges, and if the progeny "*senesce*" or have prolonged generation times, the *cumulative* percentage will be less than the percentage undergoing a nonclonogenic death. Furthermore, if the proliferating clonogenic cells are not distinguished from the nonclonogenic cells, the *cumulative* AP percentage will be much lower than the percentage of cells that are nonclonogenic as determined in a clonogenic assay (illustrated in Figures 8 and 9 in Forrester et al.'s publication[115]).

Even when apoptosis occurs *premitotically* (IA) or *mitotically* (FMA or FDA), single time-point assays give AP percentages much less than nonclonogenic survival percentages[105]; however, the *cumulative* AP percentage approaches the nonclonogenic survival percentage. Figure 1-15 plots the *cumulative* AP percentages for radiosensitive human lymphoid cell lines—ST4, which undergoes early *premitotic* (IA) apoptosis, and L5178Y-S and MOLT-4, which undergo primarily *mitotic* (FMA or FDA) apoptosis (data taken from Endlich et al.'s publication[129]). For all of these cell lines irradiated with 4 Gy, the *cumulative* AP percentage approached 100%, which was similar to the nonclonogenic percentage of more than 90%.[105] In most cases, when apoptosis occurs early (within a few hours after irradiation), either *premitotically* (IA) or mitotically (FMA or FDA), the inability to identify and quantify proliferating clonogenic cells should not cause much of an error in quantifying the *cumulative* AP percentage.

Relevance of Radiation-Induced Apoptosis to Radiotherapy

Although AP killing may not appear to be the most important mode of cell killing by radiation in many cases in vitro and in vivo, including those in which cells are classified as AP susceptible, apoptosis occurring both spontaneously and after irradiation may play an important role in vivo. As stated previously, acute radiation effects on the salivary gland have been accounted for primarily by the appearance of *premitotic* AP cells. Also, in mice, a single dose required to cure 50% of the tumors (TCD_{50}) or to cause a given amount of growth delay showed a positive correlation with the level of both spontaneous apoptosis and radiation-induced apoptosis[124] (Fig. 1-16). Note that the TCD_{50}

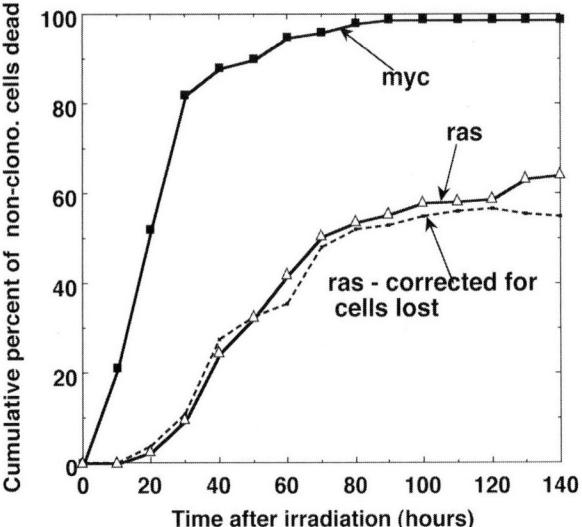

Figure 1–14. The cumulative percentage of *nonclonogenic* cells and their progeny that had died at various times after irradiation (the number of cells that had died divided by the number of cells still alive plus the number that had died). A correction[115] for lost *REC:ras* cells made little difference. *REC:myc* and *REC:ras* cells died by *postmitotic* apoptosis (MA or MCA, or both). However, ≈50% of the progeny of nonclonogenic *REC:ras* cells underwent prolonged "*senescent*" generations (see Fig. 1-13C) and had not died by 140 hours after irradiation; these were classified as nonclonogenic, however, which gave a nonclonogenic percentage of 97%. The figure was taken from[115] with permission of the publisher.

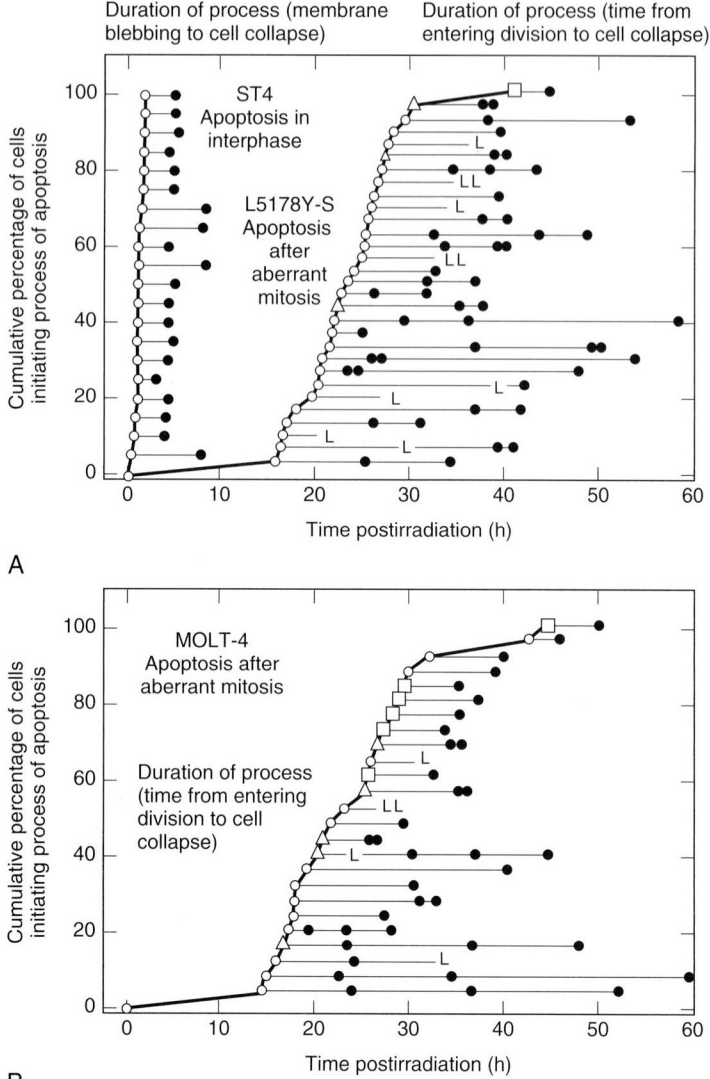

A

B

Figure 1–15. Time course of cumulative percentages of cells initiating apoptosis for populations of radiosensitive lymphoid cells. **A**, *ST4* and *L5178Y-S* cells irradiated with 4 Gy. **B**, *MOLT-4* cells irradiated with 4 Gy. All points are plotted for single cells as hours after irradiation. Initiation of *premitotic* apoptosis (IA) for *ST4* cells is defined as the time after irradiation that membrane blebbing commenced; 2 to 4 hours later, the cell collapsed (shown by horizontal lines ending with the solid circles). For *L51787-S* and *MOLT-4* cells, initiation of *mitotic* apoptosis (FMA or FDA) is defined as the time when the cells entered an abortive mitosis, or in the absence of mitosis, when membrane blebbing commenced. The cells collapsed at 3 to 23 hours after entering an abortive mitosis (shown by the horizontal lines); solid circles represent times at which different fragments of the cell collapsed for a given irradiated cell; "L" indicates that the cell fragment was lost from the field of view at the time shown. The aberrant mitosis occurred either when the cell entered the first division after irradiation or when it entered the second division after completing an apparently normal first division. For *L5178Y-S* cells and *MOLT-4* cells, respectively, 87% and 56% of the cells underwent *mitotic* apoptosis during the first division (open circles), 10% and 20% of the cells underwent *mitotic* apoptosis during the second division (open triangles), and 3% and 24% underwent *premitotic* (IA) apoptosis without division (open squares). In no case did *L5178Y-S* or *MOLT-4* cells complete a second division. (From Endlich B, Radford IR, Forrester HB, and Dewey WC: Computerized video time-lapse microscopy studies of ionizing radiation-induced rapdi-interphase and mitosis-related apoptosis in lymphoid cell lines. *Radiat Res.* 2000;153:36, with permission of the publisher.)

appears to be smaller by 20 to 30 Gy for tumors with a higher percent of radiation-induced apoptosis. However, for all of these tumors, less than 50 percent of the cells appeared to apoptose after high doses[134] (see Fig. 1-16). Therefore, the large change observed in TCD_{50} and growth delay was not expected because if only 50% of the cells were killed by apoptosis, this would lead to only ≈{1/2} log reduction in clonogenic survival. However, with the single time-point assays that were used, the absolute amount of apoptosis was not known because *cumulative* AP percentages were not determined.

Of great interest to radiotherapy is the effect of apoptosis observed after multiple clinically relevant doses of about 2 Gy. For example, after 2 Gy delivered to tumor cells, killing from apoptosis could contribute significantly to total cell killing. Specifically, a hypothetical survival value of 0.53 for cells with apoptosis compared with survival of 0.67 for cells without apoptosis[105] would result in a 100- to 1000-fold difference in survival after 20 to 32 fractions if the difference persisted for each fraction (i.e., determined by 0.53^{20} versus 0.67^{20}). This additional killing from apoptosis could conceivably result in a 20%

cure rate without apoptosis, increasing to 50% to 65% with apoptosis. This estimate is based on the calculation that one log decrease in survival of tumor cells in a heterogeneous group of tumors might result in the cure rate increasing by 15%.[15,49] However, an important question is whether all of the tumor cells would be: (a) susceptible to radiation-induced apoptosis, or (b) recruited into an AP susceptible fraction after each dose of irradiation. If neither (a) nor (b) occurs, ≈90% of the AP-susceptible cells would be eliminated after 12 Gy or six 2-Gy fractions, and after 20 fractions, survival with and without apoptosis might differ by only a factor of 0.3[105] (illustrated in Rupnow and Knox's publication).[108]

Experiments with *REC-myc* cells in culture suggest that some recruitment into an AP-sensitive S phase[117] could occur.[138,139] Also, experiments in vivo with the murine LY-TH lymphoma[140] and the ovarian *OCa-I* tumor[141] suggest that either: (a) all of the cells were susceptible to radiation-induced apoptosis or that (b) recruitment of AP-susceptible cells occurred after doses of 2.5 Gy. For the *OCa-I* mouse tumor, the maximum amount of *premitotic* apoptosis (15%) was observed 4 to

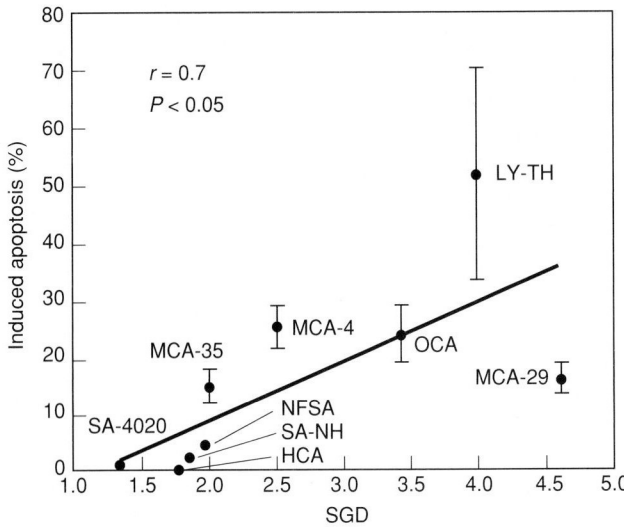

A

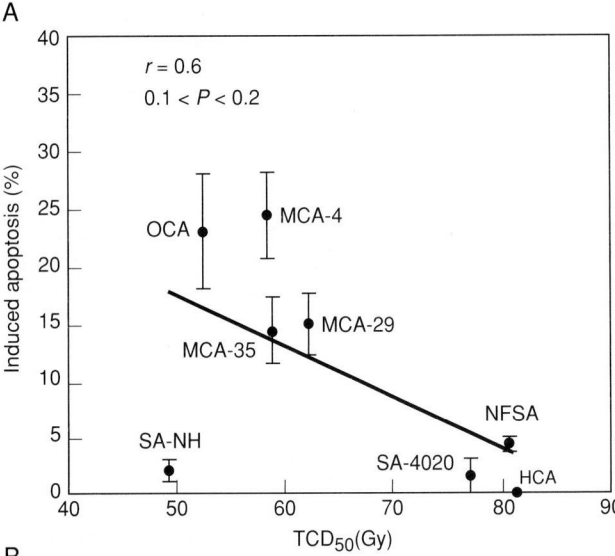

B

Figure 1–16. Apoptosis induced 3 hours after administration of 25 Gy for 9 different murine tumors is plotted against specific growth delay (SGD) (A) and TCD 50 (B). TCD50 is the dose required to give local tumor control in 50% of the animals. Specific growth delay, as determined for 20 to 30 Gy single doses, was based on the time required for the treated tumors to double their volume relative to the doubling time of the untreated tumors. In all cases, the tumors received only **one single** dose of irradiation when they were 8 mm in diameter. Apoptosis (probably premitotic) was scored histologically as described in the legend of Figure 1-11 for the *OCa-I* tumor, and the amount of apoptosis occurring spontaneously in unirradiated tumors (0.5% to 9%, which correlated with the amount induced) was subtracted. There were three mammary adenocarcinomas (MCA-4, MCA-29, and MCA-35), one ovarian adenocarcinoma (*OCA-I*, with data shown in Figure 1-11), three sarcomas (NFSA, SA-NH, and SA-4020), one hepatocarcinoma (HCA-I), and a lymphoma (LY-TH). (From Meyn RE, Stephens LC, Ang KK, et al: Heterogeneity in the development of apoptosis in irradiated murine tumours of different histologies. Int J Radiat Biol. 1993; 64:583, with permission of the publisher.)

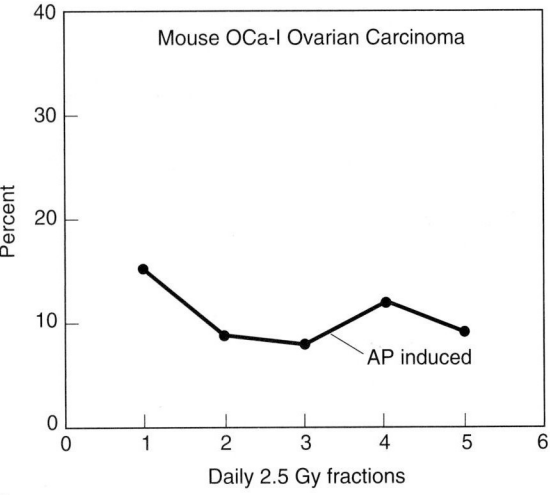

A

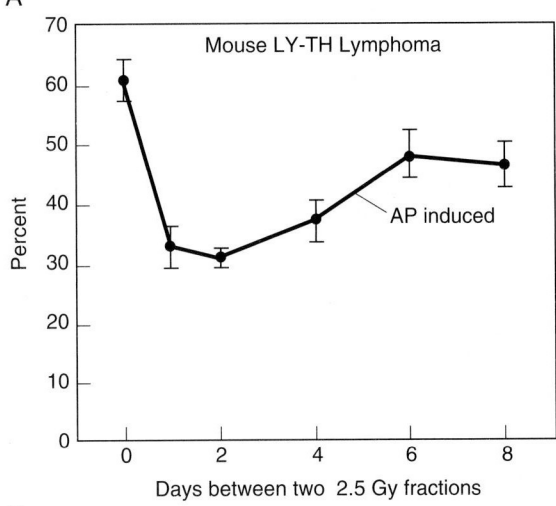

B

Figure 1–17. Percent of tumor cells induced by radiation to become apoptotic (AP induced) are plotted for fractionated radiation doses. Percent apoptosis (AP) was scored histologically as described in the legend of Figure 1-11 at the time of the peak in apoptotic response, which occurred at 4 hours after each dose; spontaneous values of 3% for panel *A* and 10% for panel *B* that were observed both in unirradiated tumors and at 24 hours after a single 2.5-Gy dose were substracted. **A,** Data taken from[141] are shown for the mouse *OCa-I* ovarian carcinoma, for which data also are shown in Figures 1-11 and 1-16. The tumors received a 2.5-Gy dose each day for a total of 5 days. **B,** Data taken from[140] are shown for the murine LY-TH lymphoma. The tumors received a 2.5-Gy dose on day 0 and a second 2.5-Gy dose from 1 to 8 days later.

5 hours after irradiation before any significant amount of cell division occurred, and then the amount of apoptosis decreased by 24 hours to the baseline of about 3%, which occurred spontaneously (Fig. 1-17A). Then, the amount of apoptosis increased to 10% to 13% by the time the next fraction was given 24 hours later. The percent of the population induced to become AP would not be expected

to remain at the observed level of 8% to 12% for the second through the fifth radiation doses unless either (a) or (b) mentioned earlier had occurred. Recruitment of cells into an AP-susceptible fraction could occur, for example, from cells killed preferentially in S phase by apoptosis[117] followed by recruitment of cells from G_1 and G_2 back into the sensitive S phase as mitotic activity resumed.[139] In addition, for the murine lymphoma LY-TH in vivo, which contained cells very sensitive to apoptosis,[141] the percent of *premitotic* apoptosis reached a maximum of 60% at about 4 hours after a dose of 2.5 Gy (IA) followed by a decline to the spontaneous level of 10% by 24 hours. Note (Fig. 1-17B) that at 2 to 4 days after 2.5 Gy, the apoptosis induced by a second dose of 2.5 Gy was 31% to 37%, and by 6 to 8 days, the apoptosis had increased to 46% to 48% compared with the initial value of 61%. This increase in apoptosis with time after irradiation suggests that there was either an increase in the fraction of the cells susceptible to radiation-induced apoptosis (probably *premitotic)* or that recruitment of cells into an AP sensitive phase had occurred. However, since *cumulative* AP percentages were not determined in these experiments, any interpretations are questionable. Indeed, carefully designed experiments are needed to distinguish between the two possibilities mentioned earlier.

Relationship Between Radiation-Induced Apoptosis and Clinical Responses

Reviews of the literature through 2001[106,108,142,143] indicate that the amount of spontaneous apoptosis before radiation therapy correlates both positively and negatively with tumor response that sometimes included patient survival. The review by Hendry and West[142] reported that elevated AP percentages had a positive correlation with prognosis in five studies (cervix adenocarcinoma, lymphoma, rectal cancer [also reported by Rodel et al.[143]], and bladder cancer, and a poor correlation in one (squamous cell cervix carcinoma). As discussed,[144] the opposite results for cervix carcinoma may be caused by hypoxia-induced apoptosis in squamous cell cervix tumors versus an AP increase in radiosensitivity in adenocarcinoma. In general, tumors arising from tissues in which the threshold for induction of apoptosis is relatively low (lymphoblastic leukemia and testicular cancer) are among the most curable malignancies, while carcinomas arising from epithelial tissues where the AP threshold is much higher (e.g., lung, prostate, stomach, and colon) are less amenable to therapy and require much higher doses for control.[108] However, a positive correlation between apoptosis and tumor response was reported for non–small cell lung carcinoma (NSCLC),[145] with a positive correlation for NSCLC squamous cell histology and a negative correlation for NSCLC adenocarcinomas and large cell lung carcinoma.[146] The bottom line is that the correlation between clinical results and levels of apoptosis are variable. As stated,[142] tumor apoptosis may be a reflection of intrinsic radiosensitivity, tumor cell proliferation, and tumor hypoxia, and that the importance of apoptosis will probably relate to tumor type, size, and stage. Possibly, apoptosis will play a most critical role in lymphoma tumors that are highly sensitive to anticancer therapy and die a rapid *premitotic* AP death (IA) that may be dependent on wild-type p53.[106,135]

Approaches for Enhancing Radiation-Induced Apoptosis with the Goal of Obtaining a Therapeutic Gain in Radiation Therapy

In this approach two factors must be recognized. First, any enhancement of apoptosis must render a therapeutic gain (i.e., more effect on the tumor than the normal tissue).

Second, an increase in apoptosis should result in a decrease in clonogenic survival. Several studies have indicated that an increase in radiation or etoposide-induced apoptosis had no effect on clonogenic survival.[135,147-150] This may have occurred because loss of clonogenic survival by *postmitotic* events such as necrosis (MN or MCN) or "senescence" (MSn) were converted into AP events (MA or MCA) (see Fig. 1-10). An example of converting MSn into MA or MCA without an effect on clonogenic survival is illustrated by the comparison of *REC:ras* and *REC:myc* cells in Figures-1-13 and 1-14. A similar phenomenon apparently occurred when *"senescence"* (ISn or Msn) in HCT116 cells expressing wild-type 21 was converted into apoptosis (FMA, FDA, MA, or MCA) in isogenic HCT116 cellsin which p21 had been knocked out.[149,150] Nevertheless, studies have been reported in which increasing radiation-induced apoptosis has resulted in a decrease in clonogenic survival[98,151-154] and in tumor response, especially with fractionated doses to mouse tumors.[153]

Various approaches are being considered to enhance radiation-induced apoptosis. These include use of antisense to inhibit anti-AP Bcl-2,[147,155,156] inhibition of cyclin-dependent kinases and caspases,[156-158] inhibition of NFkB signaling pathways,[108] anti-inflammatory ibuprofen sensitization of prostatic carcinoma cells,[108] upregulation of c-myc,[108] inhibition of 14-3-3 ligand interactions,[159] inhibition of cyclooxygenases,[160,161] farnesyl transferase inhibitors to block ras action,[162] inhibition of EGFR signaling,[163,164] inhibition of the anti-AP MAPK pathway,[165] and inhibition of protein kinase C.[166] Finally, as suggested by Piwnica-Worms[167] p53/14-3-3σ and cdc25C/14-3-3 pathways involved in the G2 to M transition could serve as therapeutic targets for drug development to enhance apoptosis, in particular (FMA and FDA).

In considering the approaches mentioned earlier, we emphasize again that cells can lose their reproductive integrity in various ways (see Figures 1-10, 1-14, and 1-15).[168] Therefore, a potential pitfall in increasing radiation-induced apoptosis by activating a target upsteam of caspases, for example, is that an increase in apoptosis might not enhance cell death. Instead, activating the AP pathway may merely cause cells to bypass another lethal pathway, such as *necrosis* or *senescence*, and die instead by *apoptosis*.[158] Strategically, we believe that converting a *postmitotic* death (MA, MN, or MSn) to *premitotic* (IA) or *mitotic* (FMA or FDA) apoptosis in tumors should have the greatest possibility of decreasing clonogenic survival and, in turn, increasing patient survival.

Considerations for Research Involving Radiation-Induced Apoptosis—Emphasis on Cellular and Molecular Mechanisms

In future studies, the amount of apoptosis or necrosis or both should be monitored as molecular pathways are modulated to determine specific molecular events that play a role in the expression of radiation-induced apoptosis or necrosis. Specifically, what are the molecular events that cause a cell to necrose or apoptose? Emphasis should be placed on the cell cycle, in terms of variations in sensitivity, the roles of different checkpoints, and the particular molecular and cellular events that occur in isogenic cell lines that differ in expression of certain genes (e.g., p53, p21, 14-3-3 sigma, Chk1). In these studies, (see Fig. 1-10) events that modulate apoptosis or necrosis that occurs early after irradiation during interphase *premitotically* (IA or IN) or *mitotically* as the cell attempts to divide (FM or FD) should be distinguished from events that occur before division to modulate misrepair of DNA damage. Misrepaired DNA damage results in chromosomal aberrations that are observed in mitosis (MC), which in turn results in loss of genetic information *postmitotically* and either apoptosis (MCA) or necrosis (MCN) in progeny of the dividing cells. As a first corollary, events should be identified that modulate the *postmitotic* occurrence of apoptosis in progeny of cells that have completed mitosis either with chromosomal aberrations (MCA) or without chromosomal aberrations (MA). As a second corollary, events should be identified that will cause an irradiated cell to stop indefinitely in the cell cycle, that is, *senesce* (IS_n or MSn), instead of dying by apoptosis or necrosis. As a third corollary, the modes of death should be determined for cells irradiated with fractionated doses (e.g., clinically relevant 2 Gy per day) because time lapse experiments have indicated that HeLa and V79 cells that undergo mostly *postmitotic* death (MCN and MSn) after a single dose behave differently after several fractionated doses.[53] After fractionated irradiation, they undergo primarily *mitotic* death (FM or FD) as they accumulate in G2/M. As a fourth corollary, experiments should be designed to determine if the events or signals that induce or modulate *apoptosis* or *necrosis*, as well as *senescence*, result from the deposition of ionization energy in the nucleus or cytoplasm or both, including the plasma membrane. In these experiments, *individual* cells and their progeny should be followed by time lapse photomicroscopy as molecular biology techniques are used with isogenic cell lines to modulate the expression of p-53 and other relevant genes (e.g., bcl-2 and bcl-X_L [repressors of apoptosis], and c-myc, bax, 14-3-3sigma,[112] and caspases [activators of apoptosis]). The questions should be addressed from the perspective of whether modulation of genetic expression: (1) alters the amount of apoptosis or necrosis with or without altering clonogenic survival, or (2) conversely alters clonogenic survival (e.g., by modifiying DNA repair mechanisms) independent of alterations in apoptosis or necrosis. Equally as important may be the effect of alterations in apoptosis (IA, FMA, FDA, MA, and MCA) on the *quality* of survival that may be observed as *genomic instability*[22,23] in progeny in surviving colonies that have lethal sectoring[115,169] caused by *postmitotic* apoptosis (MA or MCA)[115] or *postmitotic* necrosis (MN or MCN). Indeed, genomic instability may be responsible for resistance to radiation or drugs or both[98-100] that has been observed following several fractionated doses of radiation.

The "guardian of the genome" hypothesis has been proposed that either cell cycle arrest to allow time for repair of DNA damage, or apoptosis to eliminate damaged cells, prevents clonogenic progeny from manifesting genomic instability and ultimately carcinogenesis.[170-174]

In accord with the "guardian of the genome" hypothesis, mouse tumors undergoing apoptosis in a p53-independent manner manifested characteristics of genomic instability (i.e., abnormally amplified centrosomes, aneuploidy, and gene amplification).[175] Also, a decrease in radiation-induced apoptosis associated with nonfunctional p53 or expression of Bcl2 correlated with an increase in mutagenesis.[176-178] However, this last correlation might not be due to wild-type p53 enhancing radiation-induced apoptosis,[176] but instead to wild-type p53 suppressing homologous recombination,[179] which in turn might suppress genomic instability and a hypermutable phenotype.

In summary, mechanistic studies of radiation-induced apoptosis need to be directed toward understanding the role that apoptosis plays in both radiation therapy and carcinogenesis.

ACKNOWLEDGMENTS

This work was supported in part by NCI grants CA 31813, CA 31808, and CA 85610 to WCD and CA 18023 and CA 49501 to JSB.

REFERENCES

1. Hall EJ: *Radiobiology for the Radiologist*—4th ed. Philadelphia: JB Lippincott; 1994.
2. Quastler H: The nature of intestinal radiation death. *Radiat Res.* 1956;4:303.
3. Bergonie J, Tribondeau L: Intrepretation de quelques resultats de la radiotherapie et essai de fixation d'une technique rationnelle. *Compt Rend Acad Sci.* 1906;143:983.
4. Curtis HJ, Tilley J, Crowley C: The elimination of chromosome aberrations in liver cells by division *Radiat Res.* 1964;22:730.
5. Tubiana M, Dutreix J, Wambersie A: *Introduction to Radiobiology*—Translator: Bewley DK. London, Taylor & Francis; 1990:371.
6. Cole A, Humphrey RM, Dewey, WC: Low-voltage electron beam irradiation of normal and 5-bromouridine deoxyriboside-treated L-P59 mouse fibroblast cells in vitro. *Nature.* 1963;199:780.
7. Munro TR: The site of the target region for radiation-induced mitotic delay in cultured mammalian cells. *Radiat Res.* 1970;44:748.
8. Hofer KG, Harris CR, Smith JM: Radiotoxicity of intracellular ^{67}Ga, ^{125}I, and ^3H: nuclear versus cytoplasmic radiation effects of murine L1210 leukemia. *Int J Rad Biol.* 1975;28:225.
9. Erickson RL, Szybalski W: Molecular radiobiology of human cell lines V. Comparative radiosensitizing properties of 5 halodeoxycytidines and 5-halodeoxyuridines. *Radiat Res.* 1963;20:252.
10. Dewey WC, Stone LE, Miller HH, Giblak RE: Radiosensitization with 5-bromodeoxyuridine of Chinese hamster cells x-irradiated during different phases of the cell cycle. *Radiat Res.* 1971;47:672.
11. Dewey WC, Sedita BA, Humphrey RM: Radiosensitization of X chromosome of Chinese hamster cells related to incorporation of 5-bromodeoxyuridine. *Science.* 1966;152:519.
12. Hoeijmakers JHJ: Genome maintenance mechanisms for preventing cancer. *Nature.* 2001;411:366.
13. Thompson LH, Schild D: Homologous recombinational repair of DNA ensures mammalian chromosome stability. *Mutat Res Fundam Mol Mech Mut.* 2001;477:131.
14. Rothkamm K, Kuhne M, Jeggo PA, Lobrich M: Radiation-induced genomic rearrangements formed by nonhomologous end-joining of DNA double-strand breaks. *Cancer Res.* 2001;61:3886.
15. Hellman S: Principles of radiation therapy. In DeVita Jr VT, Hellman S, Rosenberg SA, eds. *Cancer—Principles and Practice of Oncology* 3rd ed. Philadelphia: JB Lippincott; 1989:247.

16. Puck TT, Marcus PI: Action of x-rays on mammalian cells. *J Exp Med.* 1956;103:653.

17. Puck TT: Action of radiation on mammalian cells. III. Relationship between reproductive death and induction of chromosome anomalies by X-irradiation of euploid human cells *in vitro*. *Proc Natl Acad Sci USA.* 1958;44:772.

18. Puck TT: Quantitative studies on mammalian cell in vitro. In Oncley JL, ed. *Biophysical Science—A Study Program.* New York: John Wiley & Sons, Inc.; 1959:433.

19. Highfield DP, Holahan EV, Holahan PK, Dewey WC: Hyperthermic survival of Chinese hamster ovary cells as a function of cellular population density at the time of plating. *Radiat Res.* 1984;97:139.

20. Sinclair WK: X-ray-induced heritable damage (small colony formation) in cultured mammalian cells. *Radiat Res.* 1964;21:584.

21. Elkind MM, Whitmore GF: *The Radiobiology of Cultured Mammalian Cells.* New York: Gordon and Breach; 1967:85.

22. Marder BA, Morgan WF: Delayed chromosomal instability induced by DNA damage. *Mol Cell Biol.* 1993;13:6667.

23. Kadhim MA, et al: Transmission of chromosomal instability after plutonium α-particle irradiation. *Nature.* 1992;355:738.

24. Hewitt HB, Wilson CW: A survival curve for mammalian leukaemia cells irradiated *in vivo* (implications for the treatment of mouse leukaemia by whole-body irradiation). *Brit J Cancer.* 1959;13:69.

25. Till JE, McCulloch EA: A direct measurement of the radiation sensitivity of normal mouse bone marrow cells. *Radiat Res.* 1961;14:213.

26. Fertil B, Malaise EP: Inherent cellular radiosensitivity as a basic concept for human tumor radiotherapy. *Int J Radiat Oncol Biol Phys.* 1981;7:621.

27. Deacon J, Peckham MJ, Steel GG: The radioresponsiveness of human tumours and the initial slope of the cell survival curve. *Radiother Oncol.* 1984;2:317.

28. Dewey WC, Miller HH, Leeper DP: Chromosomal aberrations and mortality of x-irradiated mammalian cells: Emphasis on repair. *Proc Natl Acad Sci USA.* 1971;68:667.

29. Dewey WC, Furman SC, Miller HH: Comparison of lethality and chromosomal damage induced by x-rays in synchronized Chinese hamster cells *in vitro*. *Radiat Res.* 1970;43:561.

30. Bedford JS, Mitchell JB, Griggs HG, Bender MA: Radiation-induced cellular reproductive death and chromosome aberrations. *Radiat Res.* 1978;76:573.

31. Carrano AV: Chromosome aberrations and radiation induced cell death. II. Predicted and observed cell survival. *Mutat Res.* 1973;17:355.

32. Cornforth MN, Bedford JS: A quantitative comparison of potentially lethal damage repair and the rejoining of interphase chromosome breaks in low passage normal human fibroblasts. *Radiat Res.* 1987;111:385.

33. Davies DR, Evans HJ: The role of genetic damage in radiation-induced cell lethality. In Lett JT, Adler H, eds. *Advances in Radiation Biology*, Vol 2, New York: Academic Press; 1966:243.

34. Joshi GP, Nelson WJ, Revell SH, Shaw CA: X-ray-induced chromosome damage in live mammalian cells and improved measurements of its effects on their colony forming ability. *Int J Radiat Biol.* 1982;41:161.

35. Revell SH: Relationship between chromosome damage and cell death. In Ishihara T, Sasaki MS, eds. *Radiation-induced Chromosome Damage in Man.* New York: Liss; 1983:215.

36. Cornforth MN: Analyzing radiation-induced complex chromosome rearrangements by combinatorial painting. *Radiat Res.* 2001; 155:643.

37. Jacobson BS: Evidence for recovery from X-ray damage in Chlamydomonas. *Radiat Res.* 1957;7:394.

38. Elkind MM, Sutton H: Radiation response of mammalian cells grown in culture. I. Repair of x-ray damage in surviving Chinese hamster cells. *Radiat Res.* 1960;13:556.

39. Lea DE: *Actions of Radiations on Living Cells*—2nd ed. London: Cambridge University Press; 1955.

40. Kellerer AM, Rossi HH: The theory of dual radiation action. *Curr Top Radiat Res.* 1972;8:85.

41. Bedford JS, Cornforth MN: Relationship between the recovery from sublethal X-ray damage and the rejoining of chromosome breaks in normal human fibroblasts. *Radiat Res.* 1987;111:406.

42. Thames HD, Hendry JH: *Fractionation in Radiotherapy.* London: Taylor and Francis; 1987.

43. Dale RG: The application of the linear-quadratic dose-effect equation to fractionated and protracted radiotherapy. *Br J Radiology.* 1985;58:515.

44. Lajtha LH, Oliver R: Some radiobiological considerations in radiotherapy. *Brit J Radiol.* 1961;34:252.

45. Thames HD, Withers HR, Peters JL, Fletcher GH: Changes in early and late radiation responses with altered dose fractionation: implications for dose survival relationships. *Int J Radiat Oncol Biol Phys.* 1982;8:219.

46. Fowler JF: Review: Total doses in fractionated radiotherapy—Implications of new radiobiological data. *Int J Radiat Biol.* 1984;46:103.

47. Withers HR, Thames HD, Peters LJ: Differences in the fractionation response of acutely and late responding tissues. In Karcher KH, Kogelnik HD, Reinartz G, eds. *Progress in Radio-Oncology*, Vol 2, New York: Raven Press; 1982:287.

48. Zeman EM, Bedford JS: Changes in early and late effects with dose per fraction: alpha, beta, redistribution and repair. *Int J Radiat Oncol Biol Phys.* 1985;10:1039.

49. Fowler, J.F. Review: The linear-quadratic formula and progress in fractionated radiotherapy. *Brit J Radiol.* 1989;62:679.

50. Terasima T, Tolmach LJ: X-ray sensitivity and DNA synthesis in synchronous populations of HeLa cells. *Science.* 1963;140:490.

51. Sinclair WK, Morton RA: Variations in x-ray response during the division cycle of partially synchronized Chinese hamster cells in culture. *Nature.* 1963;199:1158.

52. Bedford JS, Mitchell JB: Dose-rate effects in synchronous mammalian cells in culture. *Radiat Res.* 1973;54:316.

53. Mitchell JB, Bedford JS: Dose rate effects in synchronous mammalian cells in culture. II. A comparison of the life cycle of HeLa cells during continous irradiation or multiple dose fractionation. *Radiat Res.* 1977;71:547.

54. Winans LF, Dewey WC, Dettor CM: Repair of sublethal and potentially lethal x-ray damage in synchronous Chinese hamster cells. *Radiat Res.* 1972;52:333.

55. Mitchell JB, Bedford JS, Bailey SM: Dose rate effects in mammalian cell in culture. III. A comparison of the cell killing and cell proliferation during continuous irradiation for six different cell lines. *Radiat Res.* 1979;79:537.

56. Leeper DB, Schneiderman MH, Dewey WC: Radiation-induced cycle delay in synchronized Chinese hamster cells: Comparison between DNA synthesis and division. *Radiat Res.* 1973;53:326.

57. Murnane JP, Schwartz JL: Cell checkpoint and radiosensitivity. *Nature.* 1993;365:22.

58. Kastan MB, Onyekwere O, Sidransky D, et al: Participation of p53 protein in the cellular response to DNA damage. *Cancer Res.* 1991;51:6304.

59. Dewey WC, Cole A: Effects of heterogeneous populations on radiation survival curves. *Nature.* 1962;194:660.

60. Stapleton GE, Billen D, Hollaender A: Recovery of x-irradiated bacteria at suboptimal incubation temperatures. *J Cell Comp Physiol.* 1953;41:345.

61. Phillips RA, Tolmach LJ: Repair of potentially lethal damage in x-irradiated HeLa cells. *Radiat Res.* 1966;29:413.

62. Belli JA, Shelton M: Potentially lethal radiation damage repair of mammalian cells in culture. *Science.* 1969;1654:490.

63. Whitmore GF, Gulyas S: Studies on recovery processes in mouse L cells. *J Natl Cancer Inst Monogr.* 1967;24:141.

64. Little JB: Repair of sub-lethal and potentially lethal radiation damage in plateau phase cultures of human cells. *Nature.* 1969;224:804.

65. Hahn GM: Radiation and chemically induced potentially lethal lesions in noncycling mammalian cells: Recovery analysis in terms of x-ray and ultraviolet-like systems. *Radiat Res.* 1975;64:545.

66. Dettor CM, Dewey WC, Winans LF, Noel JS: Enhancement of x-ray damage in synchronous Chinese hamster cells by hypertonic treatments. *Radiat Res.* 1972;52:352.

67. Raaphorst GP, Kruuv J: Effect of toxicity on radiosensitivity of mammlian cells. *Int J Radiat Biol.* 1976;29:493.

68. Raaphorst GP, Dewey WC: Alterations in the radiosensitivity of CHO cells by anisotonic treatments: Correlations between cell lethality and chromosomal aberrations. *Radiat Res.* 1979;79:403.

69. Cornforth MN, Bedford JS: Ionizing radiation damage and its early development in chromosomes. In Lett JT, Sinclair W, eds. *Advances in Radiation Biology*, Vol 17. San Diego: Academic Press; 1993:423.

70. Dewey WC, Noel JS, Dettor CM: Changes in radiosensitivity and dispersion of chromatin during the cell cycle of synchronous Chinese hamster cells. *Radiat Res.* 1972;52:373.

71. Dewey WC: In vitro systems: Standardization of endpoints. *Int J Radiat Oncol Biol Phys.* 1979;5:1165.

72. Blocher D: DNA double-strand break repair determines the RBE of α-particles. *Int J Rad Biol.* 1988;54:761.

73. Alexander P, Mikulski B: Mouse lymphoma cells with different radiosensitivites. *Nature.* 1961;192:572.

74. Nagasawa H, Cox AB, Lett JT: The radiation responses of synchronous L5178Y S/S cells and their significance for radiobiological theory. *Proc R Soc London.* 1980;211:25.

75. Gotoff SP, Amirmokri E, Leibner E: Ataxia-telangiectasia, untoward response to X-irradiation and tuberous sclerosis. *Amer J Diseases of Children.* 1967;114:617.

76. Taylor AMR, et al: Ataxia telangiectasia: A human mutation with abnormal radiation sensitivity. *Nature.* 1975;258:427.

77. Jeggo PA, Kemp LM, Holliday R: The application of the microbial "tooth-pick" technique to somatic cell genetics, and its use in the isolation of X-ray-sensitive mutants of Chinese hamster ovary cells. *Biochemie.* 1982;64:713.

78. Stamato TD, Weinstein R, Giaccia AJ, MacKenzie L: Isolation of cell cycle-dependent gamma-ray-sensitive Chinese hamster ovary cell. *Somat Cell Genet.* 1983;9:165.

79. Jones NJ, Cox R, Thacker J: Isolation and cross-sensitivity of X-ray sensitive mutants of V79-4 hamster cells. *Mutat Res.* 1987; 183:279.

80. Zdzienicka MZ, Tran Q, van der Scans GP. Simons JW: Characterization of an X-ray-hypersensitive mutant of V79 Chinese hamster cells. *Mutat Res.* 1988;194:239.

81. Fuller LF, Painter RB: A Chinese hamster ovary cell line hypersensitive to ionizing radiation and deficient in repair replication. *Mutat Res.* 1988;193:109.

82. Whitmore GF, Varghese AJ, Gulyas S: Cell cycle responses of two X-ray sensitive mutants defective in DNA repair. *Int J Radiat Biol.* 1989;56:657.

83. Sato K, Hieda N: Isolation and characterization of a mutant mouse lymphoma cell sensitive to methyl methanesulfonate and X-rays. *Radiat Res.* 1979;78:167.

84. Thompson LH, Rubin JS, Cleaver JE, et al: A screening method for isolating DNA repair-deficient mutants of CHO cells. *Somat Cell Genet.* 1980;6:391.

85. Stackhouse MA, Bedford JS: An ionizing radiation-sensitive mutant of CHO cells: irs-20. I. Isolation and initial characterization. *Radiat Res.* 1993;136:241.

86. Stackhouse MA, Bedford JS: An ionizing radiation-sensitive mutant of CHO cells: irs-20. II. Dose-rate effects and cellular recovery processes. *Radiat Res.* 1993;136:250.

87. Stackhouse MA, Bedford JS: An ionizing radiation-sensitive mutant of CHO cells: irs-20. III. chromosome aberrations, DNA breaks and mitotic delay. *Int J Radiat Biol.* 1994;65:571.

88. Painter RB: Radioresistant DNA synthesis: An intrinsic feature of ataxia telangiectasia. *Mutat Res.* 1981;84:183.

89. Uziel T, et al: Genomic organization of the ATM gene. *Genomics.* 1996;33:317.

90. Lavin MF, et al: Relationship of the ataxia-telangiectasia protein ATM to phosphoinositide 3-kinase. *Trends Biochem Sci.* 1995;20:382.

91. Cornforth MN, Bedford JS: On the nature of a defect in cells from individuals with ataxia telangiectasia. *Science.* 1985; 227:1589.

92. Waldren CA, Johnson RT: Analysis of interphase chromosome damage by means of premature chromosome condensation after X-ray and ultraviolet irradiation. *Proc Natl Acad Sci USA.* 1974;71:1137.

93. Hittelman WN, Rao PN: Premature chromosome condensation. I. Visualization of X-ray induced chromosome damage in interphase cells. *Mutation Research.* 1974;23:251.

94. Iliakis GE, Pantelias GE: Production and repair of chromosome damage in an X-ray sensitive CHO mutant visualized and analysed in interphase using the technique of premature condensation. *Int J Radiat Biol.* 1990;57:1213.

95. Wlodek D, Hittelman WN: The relationship of DNA and chromosome damage to survival of synchronized X-irradiated L5178Y cells. II. Repair. *Radiat Res.* 1988;115:566.

96. Marples B, Joiner MC: The response of Chinese hamster V79 cells to low radiation doses—evidence of enhanced sensitivity of the whole cell population. *Radiat Res.* 1993;133:41.

97. Wolff S: Failla Memorial Lecture. Is radiation all bad—The search for adaptation. *Radiat Res.* 1992;131:117.

98. Russell J, Wheldon TE, Stanton P: A radioresistant variant derived from a human neuroblastoma cell line is less prone to radiation-induced apoptosis. *Cancer Res.* 1995;55:4915.

99. Li Z, et al: Effector genes altered in MCF-7 human breast cancer cells after exposure to fractionated ionizing radiation. *Radiat Res.* 2001;155:543.

100. Pearce AG, Segura TM, Rintala AC, Rintala-Maki ND, Lee H: The generation and characterization of a radiation-resistant model system to study radioresistance in human breast cancer cells. *Radiat Res.* 2001;156:739.

101. Rathmell WK, Chu GA: DNA end-binding factor involved in double-strand break repair and V(D)J recombination. *Mol Cell Biol.* 1994;14:4741.

102. Getts RC, Stamato TD: Absence of a ku-like DNA end binding activity in the xrs double-strand DNA repair-deficient mutant. *J Biol Chem.* 1994;269:15981.

103. Jackson SP, Jeggo PA: DNA double-strand break repair and V(D)J recombination: involvement of DNA-PK. *Trends Biochem Sci.* 1995;20:412.

104. Kerr JFR, Wyllie AH, Currie AR: Apoptosis: A basic biological phenomenon with wide-ranging implications in tissue kinetics. *Br J Cancer.* 1972;26:239.

105. Dewey WC, Ling CC, Meyn RE: Radiation-induced apoptosis: relevance to radiotherapy. *Int J Radiat Oncol Biol Phys.* 1995;33:781.

106. Held KD: Radiation-induced apoptosis and its relationship to loss of clonogenic survival. *Apoptosis.* 1997;2:265.

107. Wyllie A: An endonuclease at last. *Nature* 1998;391: 20-21.

108. Rupnow BA, Knox SJ: The role of radiation-induced apoptosis as a determinant of tumor responses to radiation therapy. *Apoptosis.* 1999;4:115.

109. Rich T, Allen RL, Wyllie AH: Defying death after DNA damage. *Nature.* 2000;407:777.

110. Hengartner MO: The biochemistry of apoptosis. *Nature.* 2000;407:770.

111. Ianzini F, Mackey MA: Delayed DNA damage associated with mitotic catastrophe following X-irradiation of HeLa S3 cells. *Mutagenesis.* 1998;**13**:337.

112. Chan TA, Hermeking H, Lengauer C, et al: 14-3-3 s is required to prevent mitotic catastrophe after DNA damage. *Nature.* 1999;401:616.

113. Olive PL, Frazer G, Banath JP: Radiation-induced apoptosis measured in TK6 human B lymphoblast cells using the comet assay. *Radiat Res.* 1993;136:130.

114. Chen CH, Zhang J, Ling CC: Transfected c-myc and c-Ha-ras modulate radiation-induced apoptosis in rat embryo cells. *Radiat Res.* 1994;139:307.

115. Forrester HB, Vidair CA, Albright N, et al: Using computerized video time lapse for quantifying cell death of X-irradiated rat embryo cells transfected with c-myc or c-Ha-ras. *Cancer Res.* 1999;59:931.

116. Okada S: Volume I: Cells. In Altman, K.I., Gerber, G.B, Okada S, eds. *Radiation Biochemistry*, Vol 1. New York: Academic Press; 1970:218.

117. Forrester HB, Albright N, Ling CC, Dewey WC: Computerized video time lapse (CVTL) analysis of apoptosis of REC:Myc cells x-irradiated in different phases of the cell cycle. *Radiat Res.* 2000;154:625.

118. Hendry JH, Potten CS: Intestinal cell radiosensitivity: A comparison for cell death assayed by apoptosis or by a loss of clonogenicity. *Int J Radiat Biol.* 1982;42:621.

119. Potten CS, Booth C: The role of radiation-induced and spontaneous apoptosis in the homeostasis of the gastrointestinal epithelium: A brief review. *Comp Biochem Physiol [B].* 1997; 118:473.

120. Paris F, et al: Endothelial apoptosis as the primary lesion initiating intestinal radiation damage in mice. *Science.* 2001;293:293.

121. Fliedner TM, Bond VP, Cronkite EP: Structural, cytological and radiographic (H³-thymidine) changes in the bone marrow following total body irradiation. *Am J Pathol.* 1961;38:599.

122. Stephens LC, et al: Acute and late radiation injury in Rhesus monkey parotid glands. *Am J Pathol.* 1986;124:469.

123. Allan DJ: Radiation-induced apoptosis: its role in a MADCaT (mitosis-apoptosis-differentiation-calcium toxicity) scheme of cytotoxicity mechanisms. *Int J Radiat Biol.* 1992;62:145.

124. Meyn RE, et al: Heterogeneity in the development of apoptosis in irradiated murine tumours of different histologies. *Int J Radiat Biol.* 1993;64:583.

125. Milas L, Stephens LC, Meyn RE: Relation of apoptosis to cancer therapy. *In Vivo.* 1994;8:665.

126. Haimovitz-Friedman A: Radiation-induced signal transduction and stress response. *Radiat Res.* 1998;150:S102.

127. Guo M, et al: Characterization of radiation-induced apoptosis in rodent cell lines. *Radiat Res.* 1997;147:295.

128. Strasser A, Harris AW, Jacks T, Cory S: DNA damage can induce apoptosis in proliferating lymphoid cells via p53-independent mechanisms inhibitable by Bcl-2. *Cell.* 1994;79:329.

129. Endlich B, Radford IR, Forrester HB, Dewey WC: Computerized video time-lapse microscopy studies of ionizing radiation-induced rapid-interphase and mitosis-related apoptosis in lymphoid cell lines. *Radiat Res.* 2000;153:36.

130. White E, Prives C: Cancer—DNA damage enables p73. *Nature.* 1999;399:734.

131. Voehringer DW, et al: Gene microarray identification of redox and mitochondrial elements that control resistance or sensitivity to apoptosis. *Proc Natl Acad Sci USA.* 2000;97:2680.

132. Finucane DM, Bossy-Wetzel E, Waterhouse NJ, et al: Bax-induced caspase activation and apoptosis via cytochrome c release from mitochondria is inhibitable by Bcl-xL. *J Biol Chem.* 1999;274:2225.

133. Nechushtan A, Smith CL, Lamensdorf I, et al: Bax and Bak coalesce into novel mitochondria-associated clusters during apoptosis. *J Cell Biol.* 2001;153:1265.

134. Stephens LC, Hunter NR, Ang KK, et al: Development of apoptosis in irradiated murine tumors as a function of time and dose. *Radiat Res.* 1993;135:75.

135. Brown JB, Wouters BG: Apoptosis, p53, and tumor cell sensitivity to anticancer agents *Cancer Res.* 1999;59:1391.

136. Mills JC, Stone, NL, Pittman RN: Extranuclear apoptosis: The role of the cytoplasm in the execution phase. *J Cell Biol.* 1999; 146:703.

137. Ling CC, Endlich B: Radioresistance induced by oncogenic transformation. *Radiat Res.* 1989;120:267.

138. Ling CC, Chen CH, Li WX: Apoptosis induced at different dose rates: implication for the shoulder region of cell survival curves. *Radiother Oncol* 1994;32:129.

139. Ling CC, Guo M, Chen CH, Deloherey T: Radiation-induced apoptosis: effects of cell age and dose fractionation. *Cancer Res.* 1995;55:5207.

140. Mirkovic N, Meyn RE, Hunter NR, Milas L: Radiation-induced apoptosis in a murine lymphoma *in vivo. Radiotherapy and Oncology* 1994;33:11.

141. Meyn RE, Stephens LC, Hunter NR, Ang KK, Milas L: Reemergence of AP cells between fractionated doses in irradiated murine tumors. *Int J Radiat Oncol Biol Phys* 1994; 30:619.

142. Hendry JH, West CML: Apoptosis and mitotic cell death: Their relative contributions to normal-tissue and tumour radiation response. *Int J Radiat Biol* 1997;71:709.

143. Rodel C, et al. Apoptosis as a cellular predictor for histopathologic response to neoadjuvant radiochemotherapy in patients with rectal cancer. *Int J Radiat Oncology Biol Phys* 2002;52:294.

144. Sheridan, MT, Cooper RA, West CML: A high ratio of apoptosis to proliferation correlates with improved survival after radiotherapy for cervical adenocarcinoma *Int J Radiat Oncol Biol Phys* 1999;44:507.

145. Hwang JH, et al: Apoptosis and bcl-2 expression as predictors of survival in radiation-treated non-small-cell lung cancer *Int J Radiat Oncol Biol Phys.* 2001;50:13.

146. Komaki R, et al: Apoptosis and mitosis as prognostic factors in pathologically staged N1 nonsmall cell lung cancer. *Int J Radiat Oncol Biol Phys.* 1996;36:601.

147. Lock, RG, Stribinskiene, L: Dual modes of death induced by etoposide in human epithelial tumor cells allow Bcl-2 to inhibit apoptosis without affecting clonogenic survival. *Cancer Res.* 1996;56:4006.

148. Voehringer DW, Story MD, ONeil RG, Meyn RE: Modulating Ca^{2+} in radiation-induced apoptosis suppresses DNA fragmentation but does not enhance clonogenic survival. *Int J Radiat Biol* 1997;71:237.

149. Wouters BG, Giaccia AJ, Denko NC, Brown JM: Loss of p21$^{Waf1/Cip1}$ sensitizes tumors to radiation by an apoptosis-independent mechanism. *Cancer Res.* 1997;57:4703.

150. Waldman T, et al: Cell-cycle arrest versus cell death in cancer therapy. *Nature Med* 1997;3:1034.

151. Haas-Kogan DA, et al: Inhibition of apoptosis by the retinoblastoma gene product *EMBO.* 1995;14:461.

152. Mitsuhashi N, et al: A quantitative study of radiation-induced apoptosis in two rat yolk sac tumour cell lines with different radiosensitivities in vitro. *Anticancer Res* 1997;17:3605.

153. Rupnow BA, Murtha AD, Alarcon RM, Giaccia AJ, Knox SJ: Direct evidence that apoptosis enhances tumor responses to fractionated radiotherapy. *Cancer Re.* 1998;58:1779.

154. O'Rourke DM, et al: Conversion of a radioresistant phenotype to a more sensitive one by disabling erbB receptor signaling in human cancer cells. *Proc Natl Acad Sci USA.* 1998;95:10842.

155. ZangemeisterWittke U, Ziegler A: Bcl-2 antisense therapy for cancer: The art of persuading tumour cells to commit suicide. *Apoptosis* 1998;3:67.

156. Nicholson DW, From bench to clinic with apoptosis-based therapeutic agents. *Nature* 2000;407:810.

157. Wolf BB, Schuler M, Echeverri F, Green DR: Caspase-3 is the primary activator of apoptotic DNA fragmentation via DNA fragmentation factor-45/inhibitor of caspase-activated DNase inactivation. *J Biol Chem* 1999;274:30651.

158. Bamford M, Walkinshaw G, Brown R: Therapeutic applications of apoptosis research. *Exp Cell Res* 2000;256:1.

159. Masters SC, Fu H, 14-3-3 proteins mediate an essential anti-apoptotic signal. *J Biol Chem* 2001;276:45193.

160. Grosch S, Tegeder I, Niederberger E, Brautigam L, Geisslinger G: COX-2 independent induction of cell cycle arrest and apoptosis in colon cancer cells by the selective COX-2 inhibitor celecoxib. *Faseb J* 2001;15:U300.

161. Liu XH, Yao S, Kirschenbaum A, Levine AC: NS398, a selective cyclooxygenase-2 inhibitor, induces apoptosis and down-regulates bcl-2 expression in LNCaP cells *Cancer Res* 1998;58:4245.

162. Muschel RJ, Soto DE, McKenna WG, Bernhard EJ: Radiosensitization and apoptosis. *Oncogene* 1998;17:3359.

163. O'Connor PM: Mammalian G1 and G2 phase checkpoints. *Cancer Surv* 1997;29:151.

164. Nasu S, Ang KK, Fan Z, Milas L: C225 antiepidermal growth factor receptor antibody enhances tumor radiocurability. *Int J Radiat Oncol Biol Phys* 2001;51:474.

165. Verheij M, vanBlitterswijk WJ, Bartelink H: Radiation-induced apoptosis—The ceramide-SAPK signaling pathway and clinical aspects. *Acta Oncol* 1998;37:575.

166. GarciaBermejo, M.L., et al: Diacylglycerol (DAG)-lactones, a new class of protein kinase C (PKC) agonists, induce apoptosis in LNCaP prostate cancer cells by selective activation of PKC alpha. *J Biol Chem* 2002;277:645.

167. Piwnica-Worms, H. Fools rush in. *Nature* 1999;401:535.

168. Fiers W, Beyaert R, Declercq W, Vandenabeele P: More than one way to die: apoptosis, necrosis and reactive oxygen damage. *Oncogene* 1999;18:7719.

169. Thompson LH, Suit HD: Proliferation kinetics of X-irradiated mouse L cells studied with time-lapse photography. II. *Int J Radiat Biol* 1969;15:347.

170. Lane, DP: Cancer.p53, guardian of the genome. *Nature* 1992; 358:15.

171. Levine, AJ: p53, the cellular gatekeeper for growth and division. *Cell* 1997;88:323.

172. White E, Chiou SK, Rao L, Sabbatini P, Lin HJ: Control of p53-dependent apoptosis by E1B, bcl-2, and ha-ras proteins. *Cold Spring Harb Symp Quant Biol* 1994;59:395.

173. Lengauer C, Kinzler KW, Vogelstein B: Genetic instabilities in human cancers. *Nature* 1998;396:643.

174. Kemp CJ, Wheldon T, Balmain A: p53-deficient mice are extremely susceptible to radiation-induced tumorigenesis. *Nat Genet* 1994;8:66.

175. Fukasawa K, Wiener F, VandeWoude GF, Mai SB: Genomic instability and apoptosis are frequent in p53 deficient young mice. *Oncogene* 1997;15:1295.

176. Xia F, et al: Altered p53 status correlates with differences in sensitivity to radiation-induced mutation and apoptosis in two closely related human lymphoblast lines. *Cancer Res* 1995; 55:12.

177. Cherbonnellasserre, C, Gauny S, Kronenberg A: Suppression of apoptosis by bcl-2 or Bcl-x(L) promotes susceptibility to mutagenesis. *Oncogene* 1996;13:1489.

178. Yu Y, Li C-Y, Little JB: Abrogation of p53 function by HPV 16 E6 gene delays apoptosis and enhances mutagenesis but does not alter radiosensitivity in TK6 human lymphoblast cells. *Oncogene* 1997;14:1661.

179. Sturzbecher HW, Donzelmann B, Henning W, Knippschild U, Buchhop S: p53 is linked directly to homologous recombination processes via RAD51/RecA protein interaction: *EMBO J* 1996;15:1992.

180. Evans HH, et al: DNA double-strand break rejoining deficiency in TK6 and other human B-lymphoblast cell lines. *Radiat Res* 1993; 134:307.

Fractionation Effects in Clinical Practice

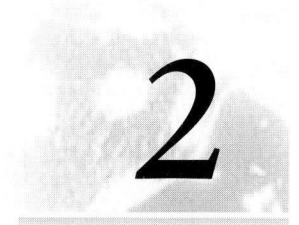

K. Kian Ang, MD, PhD

A biologic rationale for a therapeutic gain from fractionating radiation was first advanced by Schwarz in the first decade of the 20th century.[1] Then, fractionation strategies evolved gradually in different parts of the world, and what is now considered "standard" for the treatment of cancer still varies somewhat among centers. For example, in the Manchester School (United Kingdom), most definitive radiation treatments are delivered in 15 to 16 fractions over 3 weeks, whereas in the United States, they are usually administered in about 35 fractions over 7 weeks. Until recently, the evolution of "conventional" dose fractionation schedules was influenced mainly by logistics, economics, and resources rather than by clinical and biologic concepts. Careful clinical observations supported by a large body of experimental data emerging during the last few decades, however, established conclusively that changes in dose fractionation parameters differentially affect the response of tissues according to their organization and cell kinetics, that is, whether they manifest radiation reactions early (acutely) or late.[2] This knowledge underlies the development of radiobiologically based fractionation schedules of the modern era, which are often referred to as *altered fractionation schedules*.

To facilitate discussion we consider the radiation regimen administering 1.8 to 2.0 Gy on each treatment day, as commonly practiced in the United States, the conventional fractionation schedule. Although the possible permutations for altering the conventional schedule are infinite, this review focuses on regimens that use more than one dose fraction per day for all or part of the treatment course. The reason for this focus is that, for tumor types manifesting an acute (early) response to radiation, a sound radiobiological rationale can be developed for reducing the size of dose per fraction (hyperfractionation) or the overall time of treatment (accelerated fractionation), or both.

A summary of the data from published phase I to II clinical studies testing various altered fractionation schedules was presented at length in the previous edition of this textbook. In the interim, the results of many major phase III trials have been reported. Therefore, this update addresses biological rationales and clinical data of large prospective randomized trials with sufficient follow-up information. In cases where more than one report on a given trial was published, the most recent paper is presented.

BACKGROUND RADIOBIOLOGY AND NOMENCLATURE

Since the radiobiologic concepts of radiation therapy are addressed in Chapter 1, this section focuses on principles relevant for rational modifications of dose fractionation regimens.

Time-Dose-Fractionation Parameters

The time-dose-fractionation parameters that determine radiation response of tissues are total dose, overall duration of treatment, size of dose per fraction, and frequency of dose fractions. The latter two parameters determine the rate of dose accumulation, sometimes referred to as the "weekly dose rate." It is now well recognized that the relative impact of these parameters on radiation response varies with tissue characteristics.

The organizational structure and cytokinetics of tissues determine the timing of manifestation of radiation injury. Acute radiation reactions occur in tissues organized into stem cell, maturation, and functional compartments and are characterized by rapid cell turnover (such as in skin, mucous membranes, and bone marrow). The intensity of acute reactions reflects the balance between the rate of radiation cell killing and the pace of regeneration of surviving stem cells. This balance depends primarily on the rate of dose accumulation. The fraction size is also a factor in determining the severity of acute reactions (i.e., large fractions are more damaging than small ones for a given total dose), but to a lesser extent than is the case for late effects. Once an acute reaction has reached the peak, for instance, confluent mucositis over the whole treatment portal, further stem-cell killing cannot produce an increase in the *intensity* of the acute reaction (saturation) but will manifest as an increase in the healing time. If sufficient stem cells do not survive for tissue recovery, acute reactions may progress to chronic tissue injury, termed *consequential late effects*.[3,4] The concept of consequential late effects is important in that these reactions are governed by the time-dose parameters describing *acute reactions* and, as such, are likely to be more prevalent in altered fractionation schedules, which invariably induce more severe acute reactions.

Classic late reactions following radiation therapy occur in tissues characterized by slow cellular turnover, such as mature connective tissues and various organs. Because cellular depletion in these tissues usually does not manifest until after a typical course of radiation therapy, there is no opportunity for regeneration to occur during treatment. The rate of dose accumulation and overall duration of treatment are, therefore, of minor significance in determining the severity of late reactions, as time between fractions is sufficient for cellular repair processes to approach completion. As a result, such reactions depend mainly on total dose and fraction size.

REPAIR CAPACITY AND KINETICS

Both the capacity to repair sublethal lesions and the rate of repair vary among different cell lines and tissue types. Most quantitative information concerning these variables has been obtained from fractionation experiments in animals, mainly rodents. The general observation is that late-responding tissues have lower α/β ratios (2 to 5 Gy) and acutely responding tissues have higher α/β ratios (8 to 20 Gy). The α and β are the parameters of the linear-quadratic survival curve equation for the target cells determining the reaction.[1] This finding corresponds to the experimental observation that late-responding tissues exhibit more marked changes in radiation response with small changes in dose per fraction than do acutely responding tissues, and that late-responding tissues are preferentially spared by dose fractionation. To realize an increase in tolerance of late-responding tissues through dose fractionation, however, it is essential that the time interval between the dose fractions be sufficiently long to allow complete repair to take place. If doses are too closely spaced, unrepaired injury will accumulate between dose fractions, and successive doses will become increasingly more damaging. A dramatic clinical illustration of this phenomenon is the report of Nguyen and associates[5] in which a schedule of eight daily fractions of 90 cGy separated by 2 hours to a total dose of 60 to 72 Gy resulted in a high rate of severe late complications.

The kinetics of repair of sublethal injury has been estimated in a number of normal tissues in experimental animals in which either fractionated or low dose-rate irradiation was used. It is customary for repair kinetics to be quantitated in terms of the half-time for repair (usually in the range of 0.5 to 2.0 hours), although a simple monoexponential function does not adequately describe the process in certain tissues. Unlike repair capacity, there is no systematic difference in repair kinetics between acutely reacting and late-responding normal tissues in rodents. Of the tissues studied in animal models, half-times for repair tend to be longest (1 to several hours) in the skin, kidney, and spinal cord, shortest (about half an hour) in the jejunal mucosa, and intermediate in the lung and colon.[1,4,6-15]

Important is that some late-responding tissues (which one might hope to spare by hyperfractionation) have relatively long repair half-times, which limits the number of dose fractions that can be given per day. The kinetics of repair is of particular importance in the determination of the response of the spinal cord to fractionation schedules in which more than one daily fraction is used. In rats, experimental data showed that repair is best described by a biexponential function, in which the slower component has a half-time of 3.8 hours.[16] This would imply that any fractionation schedule delivering more than one fraction per day is associated with some degree of incomplete repair in the spinal cord. One clinical report of radiation myelopathy occurring in four patients whose spinal cord received 45 to 48 Gy in 28 fractions of 1.5 Gy, three times a day, with a 6-hour interfraction interval over 9 consecutive days supports this observation,[17] although incomplete repair cannot fully account for the observed frequency of injury.[18] Two reports from the Radiation Therapy Oncology Group (RTOG) have shown an increased rate of other late complications in patients who were treated on hyperfractionated protocols when the mean interfraction interval was less than 4.5 hours.[19,20] Although the authors interpret the data as evidence of incomplete repair, this conclusion must be regarded as tentative, since no dose-response relationship could be demonstrated for the risk of late complications in patients who received widely differing total doses with the *same* interfraction interval. Nonetheless, for clinical practice, it is prudent to account for the potential compounding effect of incomplete repair. Therefore, most protocols have stipulated a minimum 6-hour interval between dose fractions. A review of the clinical data suggests that this is adequate for normal tissues other than the spinal cord.[21]

A review of the human data relating to repair capacity and kinetics in normal tissues and tumors was published by Thames and colleagues[22] and recently updated by Ang and Thames.[23] Squamous cell carcinomas of the head and neck are characterized by high α/β ratios (>10 Gy), in agreement with rodent models. However, available data from melanomas and liposarcomas suggest somewhat lower α/β ratios for these tumor types. Studies based on both combining results from brachytherapy with results from external-beam therapy[24-26] and from external beam with brachytherapy boost[27] are consistent with the notion that α/β for prostate adenocarcinoma is low and in the range of approximately 1 to 1.5 Gy.

OVERALL TIME OF RADIATION

The importance of overall time in the determination of acute normal-tissue reactions has long been recognized, but the appreciation that the curability of many cancers (particularly squamous cell carcinomas) is also highly dependent on the duration of treatment came later. Although most common late radiation sequelae show little or no dependence on treatment duration (with 6 or more hours interfraction interval), overall time may be of significance for another class of late effects occurring with short, intensive-course regimens.[28-30] To understand the difference between these two classes of late effects, a distinction must be drawn between "generic" and "consequential" late reactions.[3] The latter occur as a consequence of severe and prolonged epithelial denudation (rather than direct radiation injury of the mesenchymal tissues normally associated with late reactions) and therefore have the same fractionation response as acute reactions.

With regard to tumors, the strong dependence of radiocurability of squamous cell carcinomas on duration of treatment implies that surviving clonogenic tumor cells must regenerate rapidly in response to depopulation occurring during a course of radiotherapy. Evidence for such accelerated regeneration came from three types of retrospective analyses: (1) time-to-recurrence data for tumors that are not sterilized by radiation therapy, (2) a comparison of split-course and continuous-course treatment regimens, and (3) an analysis of tumor-control doses as a function of time (with correction for fraction size differences).

TIME TO RECURRENCE. The great majority of recurrences of squamous cell carcinomas of the head and neck take place within 2 years of treatment. An example of time-to-recurrence data from patients with squamous cell carcinomas of the pyriform sinus was reported by El-Badawi and colleagues more than 2 decades ago.[31] This study showed that the median time to recurrence was approximately 6 months, and that 90% of all recurrences manifested clinically within 2 years. Since the recurrences stemmed from a population of tumors in which the majority were controlled, it follows that most recurrences must have arisen from one or a few surviving clonogenic cells. As it takes about 30 volume doublings for one surviving clonogen to produce a clinically detectable recurrence, the mean doubling time of nonsterilized tumor cells must have been only about 6 days.

SPLIT-COURSE VERSUS CONTINUOUS-COURSE TREATMENT. Million and Zimmerman[32] first reported inferior results with split-course versus continuous-course treatments for head and neck cancer when daily and total doses were not adjusted to compensate for the treatment interruption. Many subsequent studies have confirmed a poorer prognosis in patients whose treatment was intentionally or unintentionally interrupted. A review of the RTOG non–small-cell lung cancer database by Cox and coworkers,[33] for example, showed a significantly shorter survival time in patients whose treatment exceeded protocol specification by 5 days or more. Budhina and coworkers[34] calculated that the dose necessary to compensate for a split in treatment was approximately 50 cGy per day. A report from Overgaard and coworkers[35] established that to achieve equal probability of control of laryngeal cancers, a dose increment of 11 to 12 Gy was necessary to offset a treatment break of 3 weeks (i.e., 50 to 60 cGy/day). Assuming that 2 to 3 Gy in 2 Gy fractions is necessary to reduce the surviving fractions of clonogenic cells by half, these data imply that 4 to 6 doublings must have occurred during the 3-week treatment split, yielding a clonogenic cell doubling time of 3.5 to 5 days.

TUMOR CONTROL DOSE VERSUS TREATMENT TIME. Several retrospective clinical studies have demonstrated that overall treatment time is a significant independent prognostic factor in determining the outcome of treatment of squamous cell carcinomas of the head, neck, and cervix.[36-38] Analyses of the dose equivalent of regeneration occurring *during* fractionated radiotherapy show that after a variable lag period, each additional day of treatment requires approximately 60 cGy, on average, to achieve comparable tumor control rates. This value for the dose equivalent of regeneration during therapy is very similar to that obtained from analysis of the split-course data.[39,40]

It appears from all three types of analysis that after initiation of cytoreductive therapy, surviving clonogens in squamous cell carcinomas can regenerate with doubling times on the order of 3 to 5 days. Unfortunately, no reliable method is currently available to measure directly the proliferation kinetics of surviving clonogenic cells during treatment in humans.

Isoeffect Formulae

The importance of the duration of radiotherapy in determining the biological effect was already recognized during the first decade of this century. Many models have been proposed to estimate the biologically equivalent dose for treatments given in a specified number of days. Readers interested in the history of the development of isoeffect models can find details in *Fractionation in Radiotherapy*, edited by Thames and Hendry.[1] The origin and application of a few isoeffect formulas that have been used in the clinic are addressed briefly in this section to caution against careless use of mathematical models.

In 1944, Strandqvist[41] published clinical isoeffect curves that related total dose to overall time of treatment for the cure of skin cancers and different degrees of skin reaction. These isoeffect curves approximated straight lines on double logarithmic coordinates, suggesting a power function relationship between total dose and overall treatment time ($D \propto T^K$). When the time for a single dose treatment was taken as 0.35 days on the double-log plot, Strandqvist found the same time exponent (0.22) for recurrences and for various degrees of skin reactions. Subsequently, several authors applied similar time-dose formulas to different sets of clinical data and found time exponents ranging from 0.22 to 0.33.

In 1963, Fowler and Stern[42] provided experimental evidence from pig skin studies that the time factor represents contributions of two recovery mechanisms, that is, the effects of cellular repair of sublethal injury (also referred to as *Elkind repair*) between dose-fractions and proliferative response of surviving clonogens (repopulation). Their experimental data revealed that the main factor in determining the increase in isoeffective dose with extended fractionation was the size of the individual fractions. Between 5 and 28 days, the overall treatment time per se was relatively unimportant in determining the isoeffective dose. These results, together with Cohen's[43,44] and Cohen and Kerrich's analyses[45] of clinical data sets interpreted as showing a difference of 0.11 in the time exponents for acute skin reactions (0.33) and for cure of squamous cell carcinoma of the skin (0.22), led Ellis to formulate the *NSD formula*:

$$\text{Total Dose} = \text{NSD} \times N^{0.24} \times T^{0.11}$$

where *NSD* stands for nominal standard dose, *N* for number of fractions, and *T* for overall time. Subsequently, several derivative formulae were developed. A commonly used formula was the TDF (time, dose, and fractionation) factors introduced by Orton and Ellis,[46] which had the advantage of additivity of partial tolerances (PT). Hall[47] compiled tables of TDF factors that allow for rapid and accurate solution of NSD problems without recourse to lengthy calculations involving logarithmic tables.

The NSD-like formulae have had a significant impact on clinical practice for several decades in that they established a method for calculation of putative isoeffective treatment regimens with different numbers of fractions and overall times. This concept has facilitated the use of regimens that deliver fewer than five fractions per week to reduce the workload and treatment cost, which were important considerations, particularly in developing countries. Unfortunately, this practice has led to serious adverse consequences. For example, Singh[48] used five fractions of 5.8 Gy of external beam irradiation administered once a week (TDF, 66) as an alternative to 20 daily fractions of 2 Gy each (TDF, 66) before the intracavitary radium insertion to treat patients with stage III cervix carcinomas. The early skin and bowel reactions and tumor regression were similar between the two fractionation schedules; however, late severe rectal complications commencing 7 months after treatment developed in all surviving patients receiving weekly treatment. This study provided strong evidence that the NSD concept is inadequate for predicting isoeffective doses for late bowel complication.

The biological explanation for this deficiency is that the use of a power-law representation for the time factor implies that recovery is maximal in the first week or two of treatment and progressively decreases thereafter.[49] This contradicts biological data that show that proliferation begins only after a certain time lag, speeds up, and then gradually returns to equilibrium. In addition, it was recognized in the late 1970s that the exponents for *N* and *T* used in the NSD formula were not appropriate for all tissue types. In general, isoeffect curves for late-responding normal tissues were characterized by larger exponents of *N* and smaller exponents of *T* than isoeffect curves for acutely reacting normal tissues.

A different cell survival model was used by Douglas and Fowler[50] for interpretation of pig skin isoeffect doses for fractionated radiation. This was the so-called linear-quadratic (LQ) model for cell survival, which for fractionated doses with the assumption of equal effect per fraction reads:

$$\ln S = -n\cdot(\alpha d+\beta d^2)$$

where *S* stands for surviving fraction, *n* for number of fractions, and *d* for dose per fraction. The LQ model has grown in popularity for three reasons: (1) the discovery by Thames and colleagues[2] and Barendsen[51] that the fractionation sensitivity of tissues can be classified according to the ratio α/β; (2) the realization that the α/β ratio could be estimated from isoeffect data[2]; and (3) the simplicity and convenience of this cell survival-based mathematical model. A practical version of isoeffect formula based on the LQ model is

$$D/D_{ref.} = (\alpha/\beta+d_{ref.})/(\alpha/\beta+d).$$

If $D_{ref.}$ is the reference isoeffect dose given in fractions of size $d_{ref.}$, then the equivalent dose *D* for fractions of size *d* can be readily computed with this formula.[52] For example, the reference dose for a given tissue is 60 Gy when administered in 2 Gy fractions; assuming α/β for this tissue is 2 Gy, the equivalent dose (D_4) for 4 Gy fractions is

$$D_4/60 = (2+2)/(2+4),$$

$$D_4 = 60\cdot 4/6 = 40 \text{ Gy}.$$

This formula assumes complete repair of sublethal injury between fractions and ignores the potential contribution of tissue repopulation (the time factor). Therefore, this formula is valid only when the interfraction interval is long enough to allow sublethal injury repair to approach completion (e.g., daily fractionation) and when the isoeffect endpoint concerned is either not time-dependent (e.g., most late tissue complications) or the two schedules compared involve the same overall time. When short interfraction intervals are used or the overall time is drastically changed, proper corrections for incomplete repair and proliferation of target cells need to be introduced to account for these phenomena. As discussed earlier, a minimum of 6 hours between dose fractions appears to be adequate for sublethal injury repair in normal tissues other than the spinal cord.[21]

Isoeffect relationships based on the LQ model have now been tested in a large number of experimental animal systems for various tissue types and endpoints. In general, good agreement has been obtained for fraction sizes between approximately 1 Gy and 10 Gy. However, clinical application of the model for derivation of an unconventional fractionation scheme is limited by the uncertainty of the α/β ratios for various tissues in humans. Although the available human data are consistent with the α/β ratios determined in animal systems under closely controlled conditions, the confidence limits are very wide.[22] Therefore, caution must be exercised when this isoeffect formula is applied for designing new fractionation regimens. *It is thus very important to keep in mind that no isoeffect formula is sufficiently reliable to preempt clinical judgment, and each new fractionation schedule, particularly when combined with cytotoxic or biologic agents, must be tested carefully in the clinic to establish its safety.*

Nomenclature of Altered Fractionation

The terminology to be used in this chapter is first defined to facilitate discussion and categorization of the radiobiologic basis of different regimens in which multiple fractions per day are used.

Standard or conventional fractionation denotes a regimen delivering 1.8 to 2 Gy per fraction, once a day, 5 times per week to a total dose of 65 to 70 Gy in 6.5 to 7.5 weeks.

Hyperfractionation refers to schedules in which the size of dose per fraction is reduced, total dose is increased, the number of dose fractions is increased, and the overall time is relatively unchanged by administering two fractions a day. Regimens that resemble hyperfractionation but have no increase in the total dose have no biological rationale.

Accelerated fractionation describes a radiation regimen in which the overall time is reduced, but the number of dose fractions, total dose, and size of dose per fraction are either unchanged or somewhat reduced, depending on the extent of overall time reduction. Regimens that resemble accelerated fractionation but in which the overall time is not reduced because of introduction of a treatment interruption defeat the rationale of accelerated fractionation.

Accelerated hyperfractionation refers to a fractionation schedule that incorporates features of both hyperfractionation and accelerated fractionation. For this review, such regimens are classified as being predominantly hyperfractionated or predominantly accelerated, according to which rationale carries the greatest weight.

RATIONALES FOR ALTERED FRACTIONATION

Hyperfractionation

The basic rationale of hyperfractionation is that the use of small dose fractions allows higher total doses to be administered within the tolerance of late-responding normal tissues, and that this translates into a higher biologically effective dose to the tumor. For this rationale to hold, the α/β ratio for tumor cells must be greater than that for the dose-limiting normal tissues. As noted previously, acutely responding tissues as a class have higher α/β ratios than late-responding normal tissues. Because of the kinetic similarity between tumors and acutely responding normal tissues, it might be predicted that tumors would also tend to have large α/β ratios. This notion is supported by data for rodent tumors.[53] However, data for human tumors are sparse and imprecise.[22] As noted previously, most human tumors do appear to have large α/β ratios, but there are exceptions. This is important, since it would be inappropriate to use hyperfractionation in the treatment of tumors characterized by low α/β ratios, such as perhaps prostate adenocarcinoma.

There are two other rationales for hyperfractionation. First is the phenomenon of radiosensitization through cell cycle redistribution. With a larger number of fractions, cells in a radioresistant phase at the time of any given fraction administration are more likely to be caught in a more sensitive phase at the time of subsequent fraction administrations (i.e., sensitization by redistribution in the division cycle). Second is the lesser dependence on the oxygen effect. With small fractional doses, the influence of tumor cell hypoxia is reduced on two counts (i.e., the oxygen enhancement ratio is lower with small radiation doses[54]), and the smaller incremental cell kill produced by each dose fraction is less likely to expose a hypoxic "tail" on the survival curve.

Since the rationale for hyperfractionation depends on tumors behaving like acutely responding normal tissues, it is inevitable that the use of this strategy will be associated with more severe acute reactions relative to conventional fractionation, which is confirmed by a survey of the clinical data.[21]

Accelerated Fractionation

The basic rationale for accelerated fractionation is that reduction in overall treatment time reduces the opportunity for tumor-cell regeneration during treatment, and therefore increases the probability of tumor control for a given total dose. Since overall treatment time has little influence on the probability of late normal-tissue injury (provided that the size of dose per fraction is not increased and the interval between dose fractions is sufficient for complete repair to take place), a therapeutic gain should be realized.

Shortening of overall treatment time without reduction in total dose should always increase the therapeutic ratio, as long as acute reactions remain tolerable. However, when the overall duration of treatment is markedly reduced, it is necessary to reduce total dose to prevent excessively severe acute reactions. Under these circumstances, a therapeutic gain is realized only if the dose equivalent of regeneration of tumor cells exceeds the actual reduction in dose mandated by the maximum tolerated dose for acute reactions.

There are many approaches to accelerate radiation treatment, but the strategies used can be divided into two basic categories. The first group, referred to as *pure accelerated fractionation* regimens, reduces the overall treatment time without concurrent changes in the fraction size or total dose. This is accomplished, for instance, by delivering two fractions a day during some or all of the weekdays or once-daily fractions 6 to 7 days a week. The second group, referred to as *a hybrid accelerated fractionation*, reduces the overall treatment time in conjunction with changes in other parameter(s) such as the fraction size, total dose, time distribution, etc. Four forms of hybrid accelerated fractionation were designed, but only three approaches have been tested in randomized clinical trials. Type A consists of an intensive short course of treatment with drastic reduction of the overall duration with a corresponding substantial decrease in the total dose. Types B and C have more modest reductions of duration, but the total dose is in the same range as that of a conventional treatment. This is accomplished by using either a split-course or concomitant boost technique. These two types of regimens differ on the basis of the strategy for circumventing acute reactions (i.e., a dose reduction for type A, a break in treatment for type B, and a reduction in mucosal volume exposed to accelerated treatment for type C).

HYPERFRACTIONATION VERSUS ACCELERATED FRACTIONATION

As presented earlier, hyperfractionation and accelerated fractionation offer the prospect for improving the treatment outcome in a number of tumors. Since both strategies aim at improving the therapeutic differential between tumor control and late normal tissue injury, what considerations determine the choice of strategy? For any dose fractionation regimen, two major factors that influence tumor-cell kill are the radiosensitivity of the tumor cells at the dose per fraction used and the regenerative response of surviving cells during the treatment. Fowler[55] published an exhaustive comparison of different fractionation schedules as a function of clonogenic cell doubling time during treatment and its time of onset. The basic conclusion of this analysis is that tumor-cell kill is increased to much the same extent with the use of both high-dose hyperfractionation and accelerated fractionation of type C or D. Both techniques were significantly more effective than accelerated fractionation of type A unless the clonogen doubling time during treatment was less than approximately 2 days. The similarity of results modeled for the hyperfractionated and accelerated regimens considered is not surprising, since hyperfractionated treatment at 1.2 Gy twice a day incorporates a degree of acceleration, such that the overall time difference between the two strategies is minimized. Likewise, the accelerated fractionation schedules were based on fractional doses somewhat smaller than the conventional 2 Gy. This reflects a convergence of rationales toward the realization that the best therapeutic strategy is likely to result from delivering the maximum dose tolerated by late-responding normal tissues in the minimum time consistent with tolerable acute reactions.

One should not lose sight of the fact, however, that for tumors with a slow clonogen regeneration rate during treatment, pure hyperfractionation in order to maximize the total tumor dose may be preferable, but tumor-cell survival parameters also influence the choice of strategy. If the tumor α/β ratio is small, hyperfractionation is contraindicated. Under these circumstances, combined modality therapy, for example, with cytotoxic agents, radiosensitizers, or even hypofractionation should be considered.[56]

RESULTS OF CLINICAL TRIALS

Clinical research on altered fractionation (with or without chemotherapy) is approaching a closure as the data of 21 mostly large randomized clinical trials, enrolling more than 7000 patients, have either been published or presented in conferences. Therefore, this chapter focuses exclusively on summarizing phase III trial data with sufficient follow-up information. In cases where more than one report on a given trial was published, the most recent paper is presented.

Hyperfractionation

Hyperfractionation has been studied in patients with neoplasms of the head and neck, bladder, lung, and brainstem. Table 2-1 summarizes the patient characteristics, radiation regimens, and outcomes of seven reported prospective randomized trials.

HEAD AND NECK CARCINOMA. Three of the four head and neck trials accrued large numbers of patients. With regard to the eligibility criteria, the study of the European Organization for Research and Treatment of Cancer (EORTC)[57] enrolled patients with intermediate stage

(i.e., T2-3N0-1) oropharyngeal carcinomas whereas the other three trials accrued patients with more locally advanced, stage III to IV, carcinoma of various sites. Of note is that the control fractionation arm of the Princess Margaret Hospital (PMH) study[58] consisted of 51 Gy given in 2.55 Gy per fraction over 4 weeks rather than the more common regimen of 66 to 70 Gy given in 2-Gy fractions over 6.5 to 7 weeks used in the other three trials.[57,59,60] Consequently, the so-called hyperfractionation at PMH consisted of 58 Gy delivered in 1.45 Gy per fraction over 4 weeks instead of 70.4 to 81.6 Gy given in 1.1 to 1.2 Gy per fraction over 6 to 7 weeks. All four trials showed that hyperfractionation yielded significantly better local-regional tumor response or control than standard fractionation, and two trials[58,59] also yielded significantly higher overall survival in favor of hyperfractionation. With regard to normal tissue toxicity, all four studies showed that hyperfractionation induced more severe acute mucositis, but did not result in a detectable increase in late morbidity.

NON–SMALL-CELL LUNG CANCER. An intergroup trial[61] of the Radiation Therapy Oncology Group (RTOG), Eastern Cooperative Oncology Group (ECOG), and Southwest Oncology Group (SWOG) compared induction chemotherapy (cisplatin and vinblastine) plus 60 Gy in 2-Gy fractions or hyperfractionation (69.6 Gy in 1.2-Gy fractions) without chemotherapy with conventional fractionation (60 Gy in 2-Gy fractions) alone. This study showed a significant improvement of overall survival in favor of chemo-radiation. Hyperfractionation, though slightly better, did not significantly improve survival over the standard fractionation.

CHILDHOOD BRAINSTEM TUMOR. A trial of the Pediatric Oncology Group (POG)[62] compared the efficacy of 70.2 Gy given in 1.17 Gy per fraction to the standard 54 Gy in 1.8-Gy fractions, both combined with three cycles of cisplatin (100 mg/m^2 in 120-hour continuous infusions during weeks 1, 3, and 5). This study showed no difference in the median time to disease progression, median time to death, or survival at 1 and 2 years. There was also no significant toxicity reported in both arms.

BLADDER CANCER. Edsmyr et al.[63] conducted a study for patients with T2-4 tumors comparing three daily fractions of 1 Gy with 4-hour interfraction intervals to a total dose of 84 Gy with a single daily fraction of 2 Gy to a total dose of 64 Gy. Both treatments were given in a split course over a total time of 8 weeks. They found that the cystoscopic complete response rate was increased from 36% to 65% with hyperfractionation ($P < 0.001$), and the 5-year survival rate was also significantly increased. In this study, however, severe late treatment complications were higher in the hyperfractionated arm, indicating that the dose chosen might not be equivalent for late normal tissue injury. From these data, the lower bound of the α/β ratio for late reactions can be set at 2.2 Gy. Taking a more reasonable α/β ratio of 4 Gy would yield a dose of 77 Gy in 1-Gy fractions as being equivalent to 64 Gy in 2-Gy fractions. An updated analysis[64] revealed that the survival benefit persisted for 10 years and that

Table 2–1   Results of Randomized Trials Assessing Hyperfractionation

Tumor Site & Type	Patients, n	Fraction Size, Gy	Fractions/Day (Interval, h)	Total Dose, Gy	Overall Time, wk	Tumor Control Endpoints and Complications	Reference
Head and Neck Carcinomas							
Oropharynx Stage III-IV	98	1.1 2.0	2 1	70.4 66.0	6.5 6.5	Tumor response: 84% vs 64% (P = .02). 3.5-yr OS: 27% vs 8% (P = .03). Earlier onset of acute reactions with HF. Late complications: no details.	Pinto et al., 1991[59]
Oropharynx T2-3 N0-1	356	1.15 2.0	2 1	80.5 70.0	7 7	5-y LRC: 59% vs 40% (P = .02). Improved local control of T3 tumors. More acute mucositis with HF. No difference in late complication rate.	Horiot et al., 1992[57]
Various sites HNSCC. T3-4N0 or Any TN+	331	1.45 2.55	2 1	58.0 51.0	4 4	5-yr LRC: 45% vs 37% (P= .01). 5-yr OS: 40% vs 30% (P = 0.01). More acute mucositis with HF. 5-yr grade 3-4 late toxicity: 8% vs 14% (P = 0.31).	Cummings et al., 2000[58]
Various sites HNSCC. Stage III-IV, Stage II of tongue base, hypopharynx	1073	1.2 1.8* 1.6 2.0	2 1-2 2 1	81.6 72.0 67.2 70.0	6 7 6 7	LRC: higher with HF & CB (P = .045 & .05). DFS: trend in favor of HF & CB (P = .067 & .054) but no difference in OS. More acute mucositis with all altered fractionations. No difference in late complication rate.	Fu et al., 2000[60]
Non–Small-Cell Lung Cancer							
Stage II-III (surgically unresectable)	458	1.2 2.0	2 1	69.6 60.0	5.8 6	No significant difference in median or 5-year survival. (Cisplatin-vinblastine arm yielded better survival) Late toxicity not presented in detail	Sause et al., 2000[61]
Brainstem Tumors							
Age: 3-21 yr	130	1.17 1.80	2 1	70.2 54.0	6 6	No significant difference in time to disease progression and overall survival. Morbidity similar in both arms.	Mandell et al., 1999[62]
Bladder Transitional Cell Carcinomas							
T2-T4	168	1.0 2.0	3 1	84.0 64.0	8 8	Survival: higher with HF with an RH of 1.52 (95% C.I.: 1.10-2.09) No significant difference in bowel injury requiring surgical treatment.	Naslund et al., 1994[64]

CB, concomitant boost; DFS, disease-free survival; HF, hyperfractionation; HNSCC, head and neck squamous cell carcinoma; LC, local control; LRC, locoregional control; MST, median survival time; NSCLC, non–small-cell lung cancer; OS, overall survival.

there was a trend for higher bowel complications requiring surgery in the hyperfractionation group.

Pure Accelerated Fractionation

Pure accelerated fractionation has been studied in patients with carcinomas of the head and neck (four trials) and

those with NSCLC (one study). Table 2-2 summarizes the patient characteristics, radiation regimens, and outcomes of reported prospective randomized trials.

HEAD AND NECK CARCINOMA. Two trials compared a similar regimen (i.e., 6 fractions of 2 Gy per week, either by irradiating on Saturdays or giving twice-a-day irradiations on one of the weekdays) to the conventional

Table 2–2   Results of Randomized Trials Assessing Pure Accelerated Fractionation

Tumor Site & Type	Patients, n	Fraction Size, Gy	Fractions/Day (Interval, h)	Total Dose, Gy	Overall Time, wk	Tumor Control Endpoints and Complications	Reference
Head and Neck Carcinomas							
Various sites HNSCC, all stages	1485	2.0 / 2.0	1 / 1	66.0 / ~66.0	6 / 7	5-yr LRC: 66% vs 57% (P = .01). 5-yr DFS: 72% vs 65% (P = .04). No difference in OS. More acute mucositis with AF. No difference in late complication rate.	Overgaard et al., 2000[65]
Larynx carcinomas, T1-3N0	395	2.0 / 2.0	1-2 (≥6) / 1	66.0 / 66.0	5.5 / 6.5	LRC: higher with AF (P = .03). More acute reactions with AF. No difference in late complications except for telangiectasia.	Hliniak et al., 2000[66]
Various sites HNSCC. T2-4 N0-1	100	1.8-2.0 / 1.8-2.0	1 / 1	~70.0 / ~70.0	5 / 7	3-yr LC: 82% vs 37% (P <0.0001) & 3-yr OS: 78% vs 32% (P <0.0001). Severe mucositis: 62% vs 26%. Late complications: 10% vs 0%.	Skladowski et al., 2000[67]
Various sites HNSCC. Stage III-IV	82	2.0 / 2.0	2 (≥6) / 1	66.0 / 66.0	3.4 / 6.8	CR: 35% vs 29% (P = .18). No difference in 3-yr relapse-free survival. Grade 3-4 reactions: 27 vs 8 (P = .00005). Grade 4 late toxicity: 8 vs 2 (P = .10).	Jackson et al., 1997[68]
Non–Small-Cell Lung Cancer							
Inoperable non–small-cell lung cancer	204	2 / 2	2 / 1	60 ± Carbo / 60 ± Carbo	3 / 6	No significant difference in median survival time and 2-yr OS. Esophageal toxicity significantly greater in AF.	Ball et al., 1999[69]

AF, accelerated fractionation; Carbo, carboplatin; CR, complete response; DFS, disease-free survival; HNSCC, head and neck squamous cell carcinoma; LC, local control; LRC, local-regional control; OS, overall survival.

5 fractions per week.[65,66] Both trials showed that a 1-week reduction of treatment time yielded a significant improvement in local-regional tumor control, but not in overall survival. The accelerated regimen induced more severe acute mucositis, but no detectable increase in late complications.

One trial compared 7 fractions of 2 Gy per week given throughout weekends with the conventional 5 fractions per week.[67] The study showed that a reduction of treatment time by a total of 2 weeks resulted in a significant improvement of 3-year local-regional control and overall survival. However, the accelerated regimen induced more severe acute mucositis, which was reached 1.5 weeks earlier than the standard fractionation. The corresponding incidences of severe late complications were 10% and 0%, respectively. The late complications in the accelerated arm manifested between 8 and 12 weeks after completion of therapy in patients with the most severe and persistent mucositis. This type of late morbidity had been referred to as "consequential late effects."[3] Consequently, the investigators have abandoned this regimen.

Finally, one trial assessing 10 fractions of 2 Gy per week (i.e., 2 Gy per fraction, twice a day and five days a week)[68] showed that 66 Gy given in 3.5 weeks induced unacceptable acute mucositis leading to early termination

of the trial, which prevented proper assessment of the efficacy endpoints.

NON–SMALL-CELL LUNG CANCER. An Australian multi-center trial[69] applied double randomization, that is, 60 Gy in 3 weeks (2 Gy per fraction, twice a day and five days a week) versus 60 Gy in 6 weeks and both with or without carboplatin administered in a dose of 70 mg/m^2 per day for 5 days during week 1 for accelerated fractionation or weeks 1 and 5 for standard fractionation. With a sample size of 204 patients, this study did not show survival advantage associated with accelerated fractionation or concurrent carboplatin. It was found that 60 Gy in 3 weeks induced a significantly greater, but tolerable, esophagitis than 60 Gy in 6 weeks. In contrast, the head and neck cancer study[68] showed that 66 Gy given in 3.5 weeks induced unacceptable acute mucositis leading to early termination of the trial, which prevented proper assessment of the efficacy endpoints.

Hybrid Accelerated Fractionation

This type of accelerated fractionation has also been studied in patients with carcinomas of the head and neck (seven

Table 2–3   Results of Randomized Trials Assessing Hybrid Accelerated Fractionation Type A

Tumor Site & Type	Patients, n	Fraction Size, Gy	Fractions/Day (Interval, h)	Total Dose, Gy	Overall Time, wk	Tumor Control Endpoints and Complications	Reference
Head and Neck Carcinomas							
Various sites HNSCC, mainly stage II-IV	918	1.5 2.0	3 (6) 1	54.0 66.0	2.0 6.5	No difference in LRC, disease-free interval, & OS. More acute mucositis but less epidermis, telangiectasia, mucosal ulceration, & edema with AF.	Dische et al., 1997[70]
Various sites HNSCC. Stage III-IV	350	1.8 2	2 (≥6) 1	59.4 70	3.5 7	5-yr LRC: 52% vs 47% ($P = .30$). 5-yr DFS: 41% vs 35% ($P = .32$). 5-yr DSS: 46% vs 40% ($P = .40$). More severe acute mucositis ($P = .00008$) but reduced incidence of grade ≥2 late soft tissue effects ($P < .05$) with AF (except for mucosal late effect).	Poulsen et al., 2001[71]
Various sites HNSCC. Oropharynx—75%; T4—70%	268	2.0 2.0	2 1	~63 70	3.3 7	2-yr LRC: 58% vs 34% ($P < 0.01$). No difference in OS Grade 3-4 mucositis: 83% vs 28% ($P < 0.01$). No difference in late toxicity.	Bourhis et al., 2000[72]
Various sites HNSCC. T1-4 N0-3	188	1.65 2.0	2 1	55.3 70	2.4 7	V-CHART plus mitomycin-C yielded higher LRC ($P < 0.05$) and survival ($P < 0.03$) than V-CHART and CF V-CHART induced more mucositis than CF but not intensified by mitomycin-C. Late toxicity not reported.	Dobrowsky et al., 2000[80]
Non–Small-Cell Lung Cancer							
Locally advanced non–small-cell lung cancer	563	1.5 2.0	3 (6h) 1	54.0 60.0	2.0 6.0	2-yr OS: 29% vs 20% ($P = 008$). Lower risk of local progression ($P = .033$). No difference in short- or long-term morbidity	Saunders et al., 1999[73]

AF, accelerated fractionation; CB, concomitant boost (*boost dose given in 1.5-Gy fractions); DFMO, difluoromethylornithine; DFS, disease-free survival; DSS, disease-specific survival; HF, hyperfractionation; HNSCC, head and neck squamous cell carcinoma; LRC, local-regional control; OS, overall survival; PFS, progression-free survival.

trials) and those with non–small-cell lung cancer (one study). Table 2-3 summarizes the patient characteristics, radiation regimens, and outcomes of four randomized trials on head and neck carcinomas addressing type A regimens done by the British Medical Research Council (MRC), Trans-Tasman Radiation Oncology Group (TROG), a Vienna Group, and French Radiotherapy Oncology Group for Head and Neck Cancer (GORTEC). Relative to the standard fractionation arm, the British MRC (CHART) and TROG regimens for patients with mainly locally advanced head and neck cancer had a 4.5-week acceleration and 12-Gy (18%) dose reduction[70] and a 3.5-week acceleration and 10.6-Gy (15%) dose reduction,[71] respectively. These two regimens did not yield improvement in local-regional control and disease-free and overall survival. However, although both regimens induced more intense acute mucositis, late toxicity (i.e., telangiectasia, mucosal ulceration, edema, and soft tissue fibrosis). The Austrian study with median follow-up

of 48 months also showed no advantage of the Vienna variation of CHART, but the addition of mitomycin-C to V-CHART improved the local-regional control and survival significantly over 70 Gy in 7 weeks.

In contrast, the GORTEC regimen[72] for patients with locally advanced head and neck carcinoma with a 3.5-week acceleration and 7-Gy (10%) dose reduction significantly improved the local-regional control with no gain in the overall survival. This regimen also induced very severe acute mucositis but no detectable difference in late morbidity. Similarly, a British MRC trial[73] for locally advanced non–small-cell lung cancer showed that compared with 60 Gy in 6 weeks, CHART with a 4-week acceleration and 6-Gy (10%) dose reduction decreased the risk for local progression and improved the overall survival significantly without increasing short- and long-term morbidity.

Table 2-4 summarizes the patient characteristics, radiation regimens, and outcomes of three randomized trials on

Table 2–4   Results of Randomized Trials Assessing Other Hybrid Accelerated Fractionation and Accelerated Hyperfractionation

Tumor Site & Type	Patients, n	Fraction Size, Gy	Fractions/Day (Interval, h)	Total Dose, Gy	Overall Time, wk	Tumor Control Endpoints and Complications	Reference
Split-Course (Type B) and Concomitant Boost (Type C) Accelerated Fractionation							
Various sites HNSCC. T2-4 N0-1	500	1.6 2.0	3 1	72.0 70.0	5 7	5-yr LRC: 59% vs 46% (P = .02). Trend for higher 5-yr DFS (P =.08) but no difference in OS (P = .96) More severe acute mucositis & higher incidence of severe late morbidity (P <.001) with AF.	Horiot et al., 1997[74]
Various sites HNSCC. Stage III-IV, Stage II of tongue base, hypopharynx	1073	1.2 1.8* 1.6 2.0	2 1-2 2 1	81.6 72.0 67.2 70.0	6 7 6 7	LRC: higher with CB & HF (P = .045 & .05). DFS: trend in favor of HF & CB (P = .067 & .054) but no difference in OS. More acute mucositis with all altered fractionations. No difference in late complication rate.	Fu et al., 2000[60]
Various sites HNSCC, high-risk surgical-pathological features	151	1.8 1.8	1-2 1	63.0 63.0	5 7	A trend for higher LRC (P = .11) & OS (P = .08) with CB. Cumulative time was a significant prognostic factor for LRC (P = .005) & OS (P = .03) More acute mucositis with CB. No difference in late complication rate.	Ang et al., 2001[75]
Accelerated Hyperfractionation							
Glioblastoma multiforme	231	1.6 1.8	2 1	70.4±DMFO 59.4±DMFO	4.4 6.5	No difference in PFS (P = 0.32) and OS (P = 0.48). Cerebral necrosis was not observed. Morbidity more common in the DFMO arms.	Prados et al., 2001[78]

AF, accelerated fractionation; CB, concomitant boost (*boost dose given in 1.5-Gy fractions); DFMO, difluoromethylornithine; DFS, disease-free survival; DSS, disease-specific survival; HF, hyperfractionation; HNSCC, head and neck squamous cell carcinoma; LRC, local-regional control; OS, overall survival; PFS, progression-free survival.

head and neck carcinomas addressing type B and C regimens conducted by the EORTC,[74] RTOG,[60] and University of Texas M.D. Anderson Cancer Center (MDACC) Consortium.[75] The EORTC regimen consisted of 28.8 Gy given in three fractions of 1.6 Gy per day over 7 days followed by a 2-week break, then 43.2 Gy in 27 fractions over 11 days to a cumulative dose of 72 Gy in 45 fractions over 5 weeks. This 2-week acceleration was found to improve local-regional control, but not overall survival over standard fractionation (mainly 70 Gy in 7 weeks), probably secondary to twice as many grades 3 to 4 acute morbidities (including iatrogenic mortality) and a highly significant increase in the incidence of late toxicity (P <0.001). Severe neurological complications also occurred only in the accelerated arm consisting of seven cases of permanent peripheral neuropathy and two cases of radiation myelopathy. Consequently, the regimen tested has been abandoned.

The RTOG tested two types accelerated regimens. A split-course schedule designed at the Massachusetts General Hospital[76] delivers two fractions of 1.6 Gy per day to a total dose of 67.2 Gy in 6 weeks including a 2-week break in treatment after 38.4 Gy. The concomitant boost regimen designed at MDACC[77] administers 54 Gy of wide field irradiation in 1.8-Gy fractions over 6 weeks and 18 Gy of boost dose given in 1.5-Gy fractions as second daily fractions during the last 2.5 weeks. It was found that the split-course schedule with 1-week acceleration but a 3.8-Gy (5%) dose reduction increased the acute mucositis without improving the local-regional control rate. However, the concomitant boost with also 1-week acceleration but with 3% dose increment improved the local-regional control rate with a strong trend for a higher disease-free survival rate with more severe mucositis but no detectable increase in late complications. [60]

Concomitant boost type fractionation as an adjuvant postoperative radiotherapy was also tested in a phase III trial.[75] Patients with high-risk surgical pathological features were randomized to receive 63 Gy given in 35 fractions over either 5 weeks (daily fractions for 3 weeks, then two fractions per day for 2 weeks) or 7 weeks. This study showed that the cumulative time of the combined treatment was a significant determinant of local-regional control and overall survival. Concomitant boost partially offset the detrimental effect of a delay in initiating radiotherapy beyond 6 weeks after surgery without inducing a detectable increase in late complications.

Accelerated Hyperfractionation

A phase III trial was launched to assess the role of a combined accelerated, hyperfractionated regimen with a 2-week reduction of therapy duration and a dose increment of 11 Gy (18%) in the treatment of patients with glioblastoma multiforme.[78] This radiation regimen was evaluated (see bottom of Table 2-4), with or without difluoromethylornithine (DMFO), and was found to yield no better progression-free and overall survival than the conventional 59.4 Gy given in 1.8 Gy per fraction over 6.5 weeks.

SUMMARY AND CONCLUDING REMARKS

The role of biologically sound altered fractionation regimens in the management of various cancers has undergone stringent clinical testing. The results of 21 phase III trials enrolling more than 7000 patients have been reported. Careful examination of the data, mostly generated from patients with intermediate to locally advanced head and neck carcinomas, identifies the following observations useful for clinically practice:

1. **Head and neck carcinomas:** Two types of altered fractionation regimens consistently yield superior local-regional control of head and neck carcinomas without a detectable increase in late morbidity relative to conventional fractionation. These are hyperfractionation regimens with 10% to 15% dose increments and modestly accelerated fractionation with 1 week shortening of treatment duration, without total dose reduction or therapy interruption by delivering 6 fractions of 2 Gy per week or by a concomitant boost strategy. However, improvement in overall survival is not a consistent finding.

   Acceleration of radiotherapy by more than 3 weeks with a total dose reduction of no more than 6 to 7 Gy (10%) also improves the local-regional control. However, an additional 5% to 8% total dose reduction abrogates the gain in tumor control, but appears to reduce the severity of some late normal tissue complications, such as fibrosis and edema.

2. **Central nervous system neoplasms:** None of the altered fractionation regimens tested have been found to be better than standard fractionation in prolonging survival.

3. **Non–small-cell lung cancer:** CHART (Type A hybrid accelerated fractionation) regimen with no more than 10% dose reduction is found to yield improved survival. However, two other trials assessing hyperfractionation with 15% dose increment and pure accelerated fractionation without dose reduction, respectively, in relatively smaller sample sizes show no improvement in outcome.

4. **Transitional cell carcinoma of the bladder:** It is not straightforward to interpret the data of the single

study since the doses tested do not appear to be equivalent for late normal tissue injury. In other words, the trend toward a higher complication rate in the hyperfractionation arm may have resulted from relative overdosing.

These intensive clinical investigations have also generated the following human radiobiology data:

- Reducing the fraction size from 2 to 1.1 to 1.2 Gy permits a 7% to 17% total dose escalation without leading to a detectable increase in late normal tissue injury. This can be interpreted as indicating that late responding normal tissues in humans have low α/β ratios.
- Acute mucositis per se or its consequential late toxicity of the upper-aerodigestive tracts prevents delivery of more than 12 Gy per week, given in two fractions of 2 Gy per day, 5 days a week or daily fractions throughout weekends, to a total dose of 66 to 70 Gy.
- A three-fractions-per-day regimen without total dose reduction induces a significantly higher incidence of late normal tissue complications, which is partially attributable to compounding incomplete repair of sublethal radiation injury.
- To the extent that the magnitude of improvement in local-regional control achieved with hyperfractionation and moderately accelerated fractionation regimens without total dose reduction is similar, the cost of therapy to society and patients, workload, and logistic convenience should determine the choice between the two strategies.

With respect to refining the standard of care, however, one should integrate the results of altered fractionation with data of combinations of radiation and chemotherapy that have also undergone intensive investigation during the last few decades (see related chapters). A thorough analysis by the Meta-analysis of Chemotherapy on Head and Neck Cancer Collaborative Group,[79] for example, reveals that concurrent radiation, mainly given in conventional fractionation, and chemotherapy yielded in general larger survival benefit than that achieved with altered fractionation regimens. This benefit, however, has been detected mostly in patients with more locally advanced (i.e., stage IV) head and neck cancer and, unfortunately, has been achieved at the expense of increased late normal tissue toxicity. Therefore, many head and neck oncologists recommend radiation-chemotherapy for patients, mainly those with large T3 or T4 tumors or with N2 to N3 nodes, and choose altered fractionation for patients with T2 or exophytic T3 and with N0-1 disease and those with more advanced local-regional tumor but unfit to receive chemotherapy.

Advances in linear accelerator design, beam intensity modification, and in radiation planning-dosimetry technology, along with improvements in the accuracy of tumor delineation through progress in diagnostic imaging methodology, has introduced a new era of high-precision radiation therapy, referred to as conformal radiotherapy (see related chapters). This new technology has made it possible to deliver high radiation doses conforming to three-dimensional shape of the primary tumor and involved nodes and thereby reducing the dose to normal tissues such as parotid glands to prevent xerostomia. A new challenge is to conceive a creative approach to integrate knowledge gained from fractionation trials into the practice of IMRT given alone or in combination with chemotherapy or emerging biological therapies. Advances in the understanding of tumor biology have opened exciting new opportunities to develop specific molecularly targeted strategies to selectively enhance tumor response to radiation. Many of these strategies are being tested in preclinical models and clinical trials, which have already yielded encouraging results. There is little doubt that the pace of discovery will increase in the coming years.

REFERENCES

1. Thames HD, Hendry JH: *Fractionation in Radiotherapy*. London: Taylor & Francis; 1987.
2. Thames HD, Withers HR, Peters LJ, et al: Changes in early and late radiation responses with altered dose fractionation: Implications for dose-survival relationships. *Int J Radiat Oncol Biol Phys.* 1982;8:219.
3. Peters LJ, Ang KK, Thames HD: Accelerated fractionation in the radiation treatment of head and neck cancer: A critical comparison of different strategies. *Acta Oncol.* 1988;27:185.
4. Travis E, Thames H, Watkins T: The kinetics of repair in mouse lung after fractionated irradiation. *Int J Radiat Biol Rel Studies Physics Chem Med.* 1987;52:903.
5. Nguyen T, Demange L, Froissart D, et al: Rapid hyperfractionated radiotherapy: Clinical results in 178 advanced squamous cell carcinomas of the head and neck. *Cancer.* 1985;56:16.
6. Ang KK, Xu FX, Landuyt W: The kinetics and capacity of repair of sublethal damage in mouse lip mucosa during fractionated irradiations. *Int J Radiat Oncol Biol Phys.* 1985;11:1977.
7. Ang KK, Landuyt W, Xu FX: The effect of small radiation doses per fraction on mouse lip mucosa assessed using the concept of partial tolerance. *Radiother Oncol.* 1987;8:79.
8. Ang KK, Thames HD, van der Kogel AJ, et al: Is the rate of repair of radiation-induced sublethal damage in rat spinal cord dependent on the size of dose per fraction? *Int J Radiat Oncol Biol Phys.* 1987;13:557.
9. Down JD, Easton DF, Steel GG: Repair in mouse lung during low dose-rate irradiation. *Radiother Oncol.* 1986;6:29.
10. Fowler JF, Whitred CA, Joiner MD: Repair kinetics in mouse lung: A fast component at 1.1 Gy per fraction. *Int J Radiat Biol.* 1989;56:335.
11. Henkleman RM, Lam GKY, Kornelsen RO: Explanation of dose-rate and split-dose effects in mouse foot reaction using the same time factor. *Radiat Res.* 1980;84:276.
12. Huczkowski J, Trott KR: Jejunal crypt stem cell survival after fractionated gamma-irradiation performed at different dose rates. *Int J Radiat Biol.* 1987;51:131.
13. Rojas A, Joiner M, Ninis J: Rate of repair of radiation injury (kidney). *Gray Lab Ann Rep.* 1986;42.
14. Thames HD, Withers HR, Peters LJ: Tissue repair capacity and repair kinetics deduced from multi-fractionated or continuous irradiation regimens with incomplete repair. *Br J Cancer.* 1984;49(suppl VI):263.
15. Vegesna V, Withers HR, Thames HD: Multifraction radiation response of mouse lung. *Int J Radiat Biol.* 1985;47:413.
16. Ang KK, Jiang GL, Guttenberger R, et al: Impact of spinal cord repair kinetics on the practice of altered fractionation schedules. *Radiother Oncol.* 1992;25:287.
17. Saunders MI, Dische S, Grosch EJ, et al: Experience with CHART. *Int J Radiat Oncol Biol Phys.* 1991;21:871.
18. Guttenberger R, Ang KK, Thames HD: Is the experience with CHART compatible with experimental data? New model of repair kinetics and computer simulations. *Radiother Oncol.* 1992;25:280.
19. Marcial V, Pajak T, Chang C, et al: Hyperfractionated photon radiation therapy in the treatment of advanced squamous cell carcinoma of the oral cavity, pharynx, larynx, and sinuses, using radiation therapy as the only planned modality (preliminary report) by the Radiation Therapy Oncology Group (RTOG). *Int J Radiat Oncol Biol Phys.* 1987;13:41.
20. Cox JD, Pajak TF, Marcial VA, et al: ASTRO Plenary. Interfraction interval is a major determinant of late effects, with hyperfractionated radiation therapy of carcinomas of the upper respiratory and digestive tracts: Results from Radiation Therapy Oncology Group Protocol 8313. *Int J Radiat Oncol Biol Phys.* 1991;20:1191.
21. Thames HD, Peters LJ, Ang KK: Time-dose considerations for normal-tissue tolerance. In Vaeth J, Meyers J, eds: *Radiation Effects on Normal Tissues: Clinical Tolerance Levels. Frontiers of Radiation Therapy and Oncology.* Basel, Switzerland: Karger; 1989:113.
22. Thames HD, Bentzen SM, Turesson I, et al: Time-dose factors in radiotherapy: A review of the human data. *Radiother Oncol.* 1990;19:219.
23. Ang KK, Thames HD: Clinical trials in altered fractionation. In Perez CA, Brady LW, Halperin EC, Schmidt-Ullrich RK, eds: *Principles and Practice of Radiation Oncology.* 4th ed. Baltimore: Lippincott Williams & Wilkins; In press.
24. Brenner DJ, Hall EJ: Fractionation and protraction for radiotherapy of prostate carcinoma. *Int J Radiat Oncol Biol Phys.* 1999;43:1095.
25. Fowler J, Chappell R, Ritter M: Is α/β for prostate tumors really low? *Int J Radiat Oncol Biol Phys.* 2001;50:1021.
26. King CR, Fowler JF: A simple analytic derivation suggests that prostate cancer alpha/beta ratio is low. *Int J Radiat Oncol Biol Phys.* 2001;51:213.
27. Brenner DJ, Martinez AA, Edmundson GK, et al: Direct evidence that prostate tumors show high sensitivity to fractionation (low/ratio), similar to late-responding normal tissue. *Int J Radiat Oncol Biol Phys.* 2002;52:6.
28. Peracchia G, Salti C: Radiotherapy with thrice-a-day fractionation in a short overall time: Clinical experiences. *Int J Radiat Oncol Biol Phys.* 1981;7:99.
29. Svoboda V: Accelerated fractionation: The Portsmouth experience 1971-1984. Proceedings of Varian's Fourth European Clinic Users Meeting 70-75, 1984.
30. van den Bogaert W, van der Schueren E, Horiot JC, et al: Early results of the EORTC randomized clinical trial on multiple fractions per day (MFD) and misonidazole in advanced head and neck cancer. *Int J Radiat Oncol Biol Phys.* 1986;12:587.
31. El Badawi SA, Goepfert H, Fletcher GH, et al: Squamous cell carcinoma of the pyriform sinus. *Laryngoscope.* 1982;92:357.
32. Million R, Zimmerman R: Evaluation of University of Florida split-course technique for various head and neck squamous cell carcinomas. *Cancer.* 1991;35:1533.
33. Cox JD, Pajak TF, Asbell S, et al: Interruptions of high-dose radiation therapy decrease long-term survival of favorable patients with unresectable non-small cell carcinoma of the lung: analysis of 1244 cases from 3 radiation therapy oncology group (RTOG) trials. *Int J Radiat Oncol Biol Phys.* 1993;27:493.
34. Budhina M, Skrk J, Smid L, et al: Tumor cell repopulation in the rest interval of split-course radiation treatment. *Strahlentherapie.* 1980;156:402.
35. Overgaard J, Hjelm-Hansen M, Johansen LV, et al: Comparison of conventional and split-course radiotherapy as primary treatment in carcinoma of the larynx. *Acta Oncol.* 1988;27:147.
36. Bataini JP, Asselain B, Jaulerry CH, et al: A multivariate primary tumour control analysis in 465 patients treated by radical radiotherapy for cancer of the tonsillar region: Clinical and treatment parameters as prognostic factors. *Radiother Oncol.* 1989;14:265.
37. Barton MB, Keane TJ, Gadalla T, et al: The effect of treatment time and treatment interruption on tumour control following radical radiotherapy of laryngeal cancer. *Radiother Oncol.* 1992;23:137.
38. Fyles A, Keane TJ, Barton M, et al: The effect of treatment duration in the local control of cervix cancer. *Radiother Oncol.* 1992;25:273.
39. Withers HR, Taylor JMG, Maciejewski B: The hazard of accelerated tumor clonogen repopulation during radiotherapy. *Acta Oncol.* 1988;27:131.
40. Bentzen SM, Thames HD: Clinical evidence for tumour clonogen regeneration: Interpretations of the data. *Radiother Oncol.* 1991;22:161.
41. Strandqvist M: Studien über die kumulative Wirkung der Röntgenstrahlen bei Fraktionierung. *Acta Radiol.* 1944;55(Suppl):1.

42. Fowler JF, Stern BE: Dose-time relationships in radiotherapy and the validity of cell survival curve models. *Br J Radiol.* 1963;36:335.

43. Cohen L: Clinical radiation dosage. I. *Br J Radiol.* 1949;22:160.

44. Cohen L: Clinical radiation dosage. II. *Br J Radiol.* 1949;22:706.

45. Cohen L, Kerrich JE: Estimation of biological dosage factors in clinical radiotherapy. *Br J Cancer.* 1951;5:180.

46. Orton CG, Ellis F: A simplification in the use of the NSD concept in practical radiotherapy. *Br J Radiol.* 1973;46:529.

47. Hall EJ: *Radiology for the Radiologist.* Philadelphia: Harper & Row; 1978.

48. Singh K: Two regimens with the same TDF but differing morbidity used in the treatment of stage III carcinoma on the cervix. *Br J Radiol.* 1978;51:357.

49. Withers HR, Peters LJ: Biologic aspects of radiotherapy. In Fletcher GH, eds: *Textbook of Radiotherapy.* Philadelphia: Lea & Febiger; 1980:103.

50. Douglas BG, Fowler JF: The effect of multiple small doses of x-rays on skin reactions in the mouse and basic interpretation. *Radiat Res.* 1976;66:401.

51. Barendsen GW: Dose fractionation, dose rate and isoeffect relationships for normal tissue responses. *Int J Radiat Oncol Biol Phys.* 1982;8:1981.

52. Withers HR, Thames HD, Peters LJ: A new isoeffect curve for change in dose per fraction. *Radiother Oncol.* 1983;1:187.

53. Williams M, Denekamp J, Fowler J: A review of α/β values for experimental tumors: implications for clinical studies of altered fractionation. *Int J Radiat Oncol Biol Phys.* 1985;11:87.

54. Palcic B, Skarsgard LD: Reduced oxygen enhancement ratio at low doses of ionizing radiation. *Radiat Res.* 1984;100:328.

55. Fowler JF: The linear-quadratic formula and progress in fractionated radiotherapy. *Br J Radiol.* 1989;62:679.

56. Peters LJ, Brock WA, Travis EL: Radiation biology at clinically relevant fractions. In DeVita V, Hellman S, Rosenberg SA, eds. *Important Advances in Oncology.* Philadelphia: JB Lippincott; 1990:65.

57. Horiot JC, LeFur RN, Guyen T, et al: Hyperfractionation versus conventional fractionation in oropharyngeal carcinoma: Final analysis of a randomized trial of the EORTC cooperative group of radiotherapy. *Radiother Oncol.* 1992;25:231.

58. Cummings B, O'Sullivan B, Keane T, et al: 5-year results of a 4 week/twice daily radiation schedule—The Toronto trial. *Radiother Oncol.* 2000;56:S8.

59. Pinto L, Canary P, Araujo C, et al: Prospective randomized trial comparing hyperfractionated versus conventional radiotherapy in stages II and IV oropharyngeal carcinoma. *Int J Radiat Oncol Biol Phys.* 1991;21:557.

60. Fu KK, Pajak TF, Trotti A, et al: A radiation therapy oncology group (RTOG) phase III randomized study to compare hyperfractionation and two variants of accelerated fractionation to standard fractionation radiotherapy for head and neck squamous cell carcinomas: First report of RTOG 9003. *Int J Radiat Oncol Biol Phys.* 2000;48:7.

61. Sause W, Kolesar P, Taylor S IV, et al: Final results of phase III trial in regionally advanced unresectable non-small cell lung cancer: Radiation Therapy Oncology Group, Eastern Cooperative Oncology Group, and Southwest Oncology Group. *Chest.* 2000;117:358.

62. Mandell LR, Koadota R, Freeman C, et al: There is no role for hyperfractionated radiotherapy in the management of children with newly diagnosed diffuse intrinsic brainstem tumors: Results of a Pediatric Oncology Group phase III trial comparing conventional vs. hyperfractionated radiotherapy. *Int J Radiat Oncol Biol Phys.* 1999;43:959.

63. Edsmyr F, Andersson L, Esposti PL, et al: Irradiation therapy with multiple small fractions per day in urinary bladder cancer. *Radiother Oncol.* 1985;4:197.

64. Naslund I, Nilsson B, Littbrand B: Hyperfractionated radiotherapy of bladder cancer. A ten-year follow-up of a randomized clinical trial. *Acta Oncol.* 1994;33:397.

65. Overgaard J, Hansen HS, Grau C, et al: The DAHANCA 6 & 7 trial. A randomized multicenter study of 5 versus 6 fractions per week of conventional radiotherapy of squamous cell carcinoma (scc) of the head and neck. *Radiother Oncol.* 2000;56:54.

66. Hliniak A, Gwiazdowska B, Szutkowski Z, et al: Radiotherapy of the laryngeal cancer. The estimation of the therapeutic gain and the enhancement of toxicity by the one-week shortening of the treatment time. Results of the randomized phase III multicenter trial. *Radiother Oncol.* 2000;56:S5.

67. Skladowski K, Maciejewski J, Golen M, et al: Randomized clinical trial on 7-day continuous accelerated irradiation (CAIR) of head and neck cancer—Report on 3-year tumor control and normal tissue toxicity. *Radiother Oncol.* 2000;55:93.

68. Jackson SM, Weir LM, Hay JH, et al: A randomised trial of accelerated versus conventional radiotherapy in head and neck cancer. *Radiother Oncol.* 1997;43:39.

69. Ball D, Bishop J, Smith J, et al: A randomised phase III study of accelerated or standard fraction radiotherapy with or without concurrent carboplatin in inoperable non-small cell lung cancer: Final report of an Australian multi-centre trial. *Radiother Oncol.* 1999;52:129.

70. Dische S, Saunders M, Barrett A, et al: A randomised multicentre trial of CHART versus conventional radiotherapy in head and neck cancer. *Radiother Oncol.* 1997;44:123.

71. Poulsen MG, Denham JW, Peters LJ, et al: A randomised trial of accelerated and conventional radiotherapy for stage III and IV squamous carcinoma of the head and neck: A Trans-Tasman Radiation Oncology Group Study. *Radiother Oncol.* 2001;60:113.

72. Bourhis J, Lapeyre M, Tortochaux J, et al: Very accelerated versus conventional radiotherapy in HNSCC: Results of the GORTEC 94-02 randomized trial. *Int J Radiat Oncol Biol Phys.* 2000;48:S111.

73. Saunders M, Dische S, Barrett A, et al: Continuous, hyperfractionated, accelerated radiotherapy (CHART) versus conventional radiotherapy in non-small cell lung cancer: Mature data from the randomised multicentre trial. CHART Steering committee. *Radiother Oncol.* 1999;52:137.

74. Horiot JC, Bontemps P, van den Bogaert V, et al: Accelerated fractionation (AF) compared to conventional fractionation (CF) improved head and neck cancers: Results of the EROTC 22851 randomized trial. *Radiother Oncol.* 1997;44:111.

75. Ang KK, Trotti A, Brown BW, et al: Randomized trial addressing risk features and time factors of surgery plus radiotherapy in advanced head and neck cancer. *Int J Radiat Oncol Biol Phys.* 2001;51:571.

76. Wang CC: Local control of oropharyngeal carcinoma after two accelerated hyperfractionation radiation therapy schemes. *Int J Radiat Oncol Biol Phys.* 1988;14:1143.

77. Ang KK, Peters LJ, Weber RS, et al: Concomitant boost radiotherapy schedules in the treatment of carcinoma of the oropharynx and nasopharynx. *Int J Radiat Oncol Biol Phys.* 1990;19:1339.

78. Prados MD, Wara WM, Sneed PK, et al: Phase III trial of accelerated hyperfractionation with or without difluromethylornithine (DFMO) versus standard fractionated radiotherapy with or without DFMO for newly diagnosed patients with glioblastoma multiforme. *Int J Radiat Oncol Biol Phys.* 2001;49:71.

79. Pignon JP, Bourhis J, Domenge C, et al: Chemotherapy added to locoregional treatment for head and neck squamous-cell carcinoma: Three meta-analyses of updated individual data. *Lancet.* 2000;355:949.

80. Dobrowsky W, Naude J: Continuous hyperfractionated accelerated radiotherapy with/without mitomycin C in head and neck cancers. *Radiother Oncol.* 2000;57:119.

Chemical Modifiers of Radiation

Raul C. Urtasun, MD and J. Martin Brown, PhD

This chapter deals with chemical agents that have been used solely as modifiers of radiation response. For a discussion of the interaction of cytotoxic cancer chemotherapeutic agents with radiation (actinomycin D, 5-fluorouracil, doxorubicin [Adriamycin], hydroxyurea, and paclitaxel [Taxol]), the reader is referred to Chapter 5, Radiotherapy and Chemotherapy.

RATIONALE FOR THE USE OF RADIOSENSITIZERS AND RADIOPROTECTORS

There is a need in clinical practice to enhance the differential effects of radiation in tumor and normal tissues. This can be achieved by the use of chemical agents that either increase the damage to the tumor or protect normal tissues that are included in the radiation volume. However, to be effective in increasing the therapeutic ratio of radiotherapy, any radiosensitizing or radioprotective agent has to be specific for normal or malignant tissues. For example, an agent blocking the activity of any of the genes controlling double-strand break repair would be a radiation sensitizer, but to be effective, it would have to work *only* on the tumor cells. Even though radiotherapy focuses the radiation on the tumor mass, the dose that can be given is still limited by the cells of the surrounding and included normal tissue. Thus, any radiation sensitizer must be specific for the tumor cells, and any radiation protector must be specific for normal cells. Unless this is achieved, there will be no therapeutic gain. Unfortunately, this requirement is difficult to achieve. There has been considerable activity in this area in the past few years and several promising agents are in advanced clinical testing.

Radiosensitizers

Radiosensitizers are compounds that, when combined with radiation, achieve greater tumor inactivation than would have been expected from the additive effect of each modality (Fig. 3-1). The application of chemical agents that simply have an additive effect in normal tissues is equivalent to the administration of an increment of radiation dose with no differential benefit. The toxicities of the chemical agent and the radiation overlap with no major gain (Fig. 3-2).[1] The addition of a chemical modifier to a course of radiation in order to improve treatment results should be considered only in those tumor sites where there is already evidence that an increase in dose intensity by 20% to 30% will translate into an increase in tumor control, since most of the sensitizer enhancement ratios (SERs) are in the range of 1.2 to 1.3. Examples of such tumors are head and neck tumors and carcinoma of the cervix, where it has been recently demonstrated that there is a high fraction of hypoxic tumor cells and also a rapid cell turnover.[2,3]

Radioprotectors

Radioprotectors are compounds that protect against radiation damage to targeted normal cells but do not provide similar protection to tumor cells (Fig. 3-3).

CHEMICAL RADIOSENSITIZERS OF HYPOXIC CELLS AND THE TUMOR MICROENVIRONMENT

The role of the oxygen effect in promoting tumor cell inactivation by ionizing radiation has been well demonstrated in vitro and in animal tumor models for several decades. Mounting evidence of this influence in tumor control and patient survival has become available.[2-4] Clearly, the microenvironment, the nutritional state of the tumor, and the presence of hypoxia are only some of the many factors that contribute to tumor radioresistance, and it is likely that this resistance is multifactorial, that is, due to tumor hypoxia, proliferation rates, and inherent cell radioresistance as well as other biological microenvironmental factors, such as the presence of cytokines. Nonetheless, the clinical data that hypoxia, by conferring radiation resistance, is a prognostic indicator of poor response to standard radiotherapy, at least for some tumors, is reasonably clear. Hypoxia, however, has other consequences beyond conferring radiation resistance. First, hypoxia causes cells to slow their rate of proliferation. As most anticancer drugs are more effective against rapidly proliferating than slowly or nonproliferating cells, this slowing of cell proliferation will lead to decreased cell killing in the hypoxic cells. In addition, as

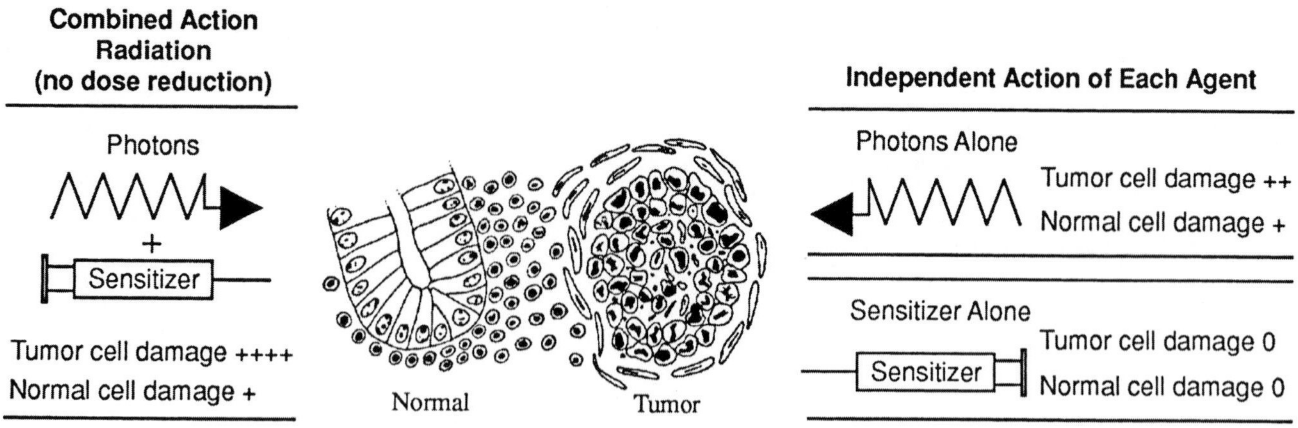

**Combined Action
Radiation
(no dose reduction)**

Photons

+

Sensitizer

Tumor cell damage ++++
Normal cell damage +

Normal   Tumor

Independent Action of Each Agent

Photons Alone

Tumor cell damage ++
Normal cell damage +

Sensitizer Alone

Sensitizer

Tumor cell damage 0
Normal cell damage 0

Figure 3–1. Tumor enhancement and sensitization. Greater tumor inactivation is achieved through the combination of modalities than would have been expected from the additive effect, based on the action of each agent alone.

the concentration of anticancer drugs will be higher closer to blood vessels than farther away, both as a consequence of geometry and the reactivity of the drugs, there will be less killing of the hypoxic cells that are invariably the farthest from the blood vessels.

In summary, numerous, well-established phenomena will cause a gradient of reduced cell killing by most anticancer agents as a function of distance from the vasculature (Fig. 3-4). Such a gradient has been shown in experimental tumors and in spheroids.[5,6]

Studies have also shown that hypoxia in solid tumors has an important consequence in addition to conferring a direct resistance to radiation and chemotherapy. Graeber and colleagues[7] have demonstrated that low oxygen levels cause apoptosis in minimally transformed mouse embryo fibroblasts, and by selecting for mutant p53, might predispose tumors to a more malignant phenotype. Clinical data support this conclusion: Studies with both soft tissue sarcomas[8] and carcinoma of the cervix[9,10] have shown that hypoxia is an independent and highly significant prognostic factor predisposing tumors to metastatic spread.

The rationale for developing hypoxic cell sensitizers is based on the assumption that sensitizing hypoxic cells to radiation killing would improve the outcome of radiotherapy. The possibility of doing this was based on pioneering studies by Adams and colleagues on the use of electron-affinic drugs to sensitize hypoxic bacteria and

mammalian cells in vitro.[11,12] The first drug of this class to show significant activity in sensitizing mouse tumors was the 5-nitroimidazole metronidazole, a drug that was already in clinical use.[13,14] Data on this and other such compounds are discussed as follows.

Nitroimidazole Compounds

Under hypoxic tissue conditions, electron-affinic nitroimidazoles bind to the radiation-induced free radicals on DNA, thereby mimicking oxygen for the fixation of DNA damage (Fig. 3-5).

The first compound to be investigated clinically in terms of oral and intravenous pharmacokinetics, toxicity, and efficacy in patients with solid tumors was metronidazole (a 5-nitroimidazole). The plasma β-half-life of the drug was 9.8 hours and the absolute oral availability was estimated to approximate 100%.[14] The dose-limiting toxicity was manifested in gastrointestinal and peripheral neuropathic effects; therefore, this compound reached an estimated SER of only 1.2. Given this limitation, the first efficacy study was performed with a human glioblastoma tumor model. This study demonstrated the relevance of tumor hypoxia in terms of patient survival, showing that the results with a less than optimal radiation fractionation regimen approached the level of the results obtained with conventional fractionation.[15]

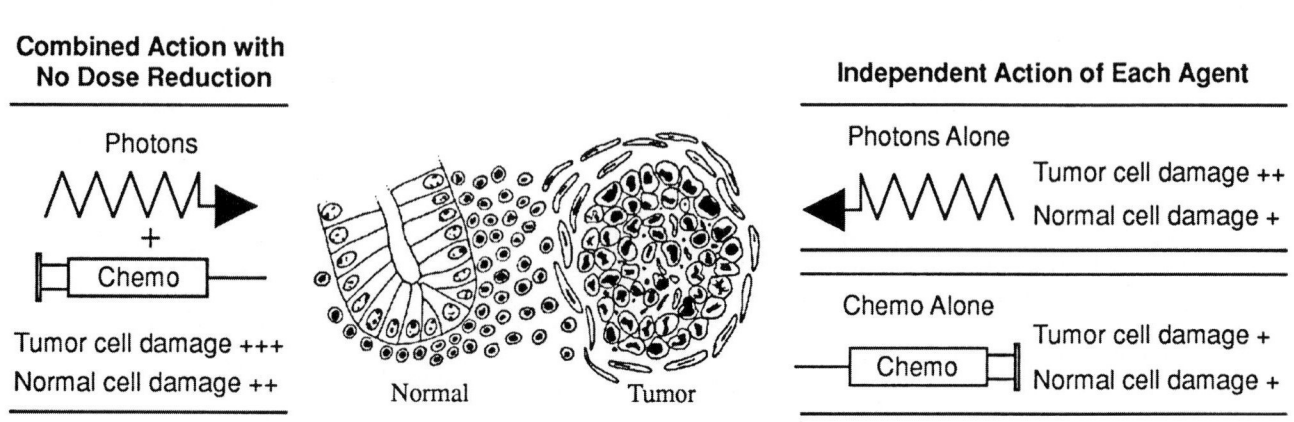

**Combined Action with
No Dose Reduction**

Photons

+

Chemo

Tumor cell damage +++
Normal cell damage ++

Normal   Tumor

Independent Action of Each Agent

Photons Alone

Tumor cell damage ++
Normal cell damage +

Chemo Alone

Chemo

Tumor cell damage +
Normal cell damage +

Figure 3–2. Simple addition of antitumor effects. Toxicities of chemicals and radiation could overlap with no major gain in tumor inactivation.

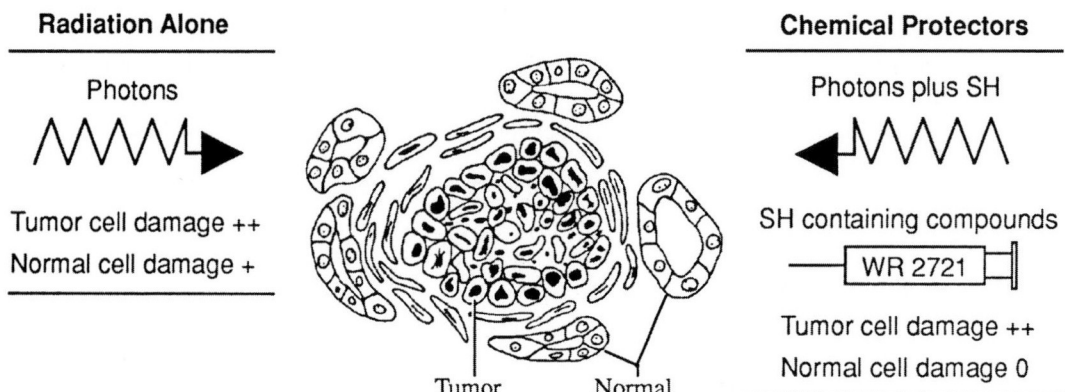

Figure 3–3. Radioprotectors of normal tissues. Chemicals that protect against radiation damage target normal cells but do not offer similar protection to tumor cells.

Of interest, a major spin-off of these early investigations with the pharmacokinetics of metronidazole, particularly the use of a high-dose intravenous route, was not in the field of oncology but in the practice of abdominal surgery and infectious diseases, in which the compound was used as a parenteral agent for anaerobic bacteria. These initial investigations prompted a level of high activity in the investigation of nitroimidazole compounds in human solid tumors and the search for new and better nitroimidazole compounds with less toxicity and higher SER. The first clinical studies of the second generation of these drugs, misonidazole, a 2-nitroimidazole, were initiated in both Europe and North America during the early 1980s (Table 3-1).

MISONIDAZOLE

Misonidazole, a 2-nitroimidazole, was developed as a more efficient radiosensitizer because of its known increased electron affinity. In the oral form, the dose-limiting toxicity was again manifested in gastrointestinal effects (nausea, vomiting) and peripheral neuropathy, which limits the effective SER.[16,17] Not surprisingly, almost all of the clinical trials of radiotherapy combined with misonidazole turned out to be null,[18] an outcome consistent with the small degree of radiosensitization expected with the clinically used low doses.[19] Once more the inability to deliver a sufficient dose may have been one of the reasons that a significant proportion of large

worldwide clinical trials showed no benefit to misonidazole (Table 3-2). However, it has been shown that select populations of patients with specific tumors did benefit by using this compound.[20] This observation was made in patients with head and neck cancers. Overgaard and colleagues[21] reported that not only with misonidazole but also with nimorazole (a 5-nitroimidazole) there was a significant benefit in a stratum of patients with stage T1 and T4 pharyn carcinoma in terms of local regional control (Fig. 3-6). Patients with hemoglobin levels below 9 mmol/L were particularly helped. These two studies also showed that the compounds had a similar benefit, despite the fact that fewer fractions of radiation were "sensitized" in the misonidazole groups than in the nimorazole groups, in which the drug was administrated with every fraction of radiation (first 30 fractions). The significant improvement of the effect of the radiotherapeutic management of supraglottic and pharynx tumors was again demonstrated on a randomized double-blind Phase III study of 414 patients receiving nimorazole or placebo in association with conventional primary radiotherapy (62–68 Gy, 2 Gy per fraction, 5 fractions per week).[22] Of interest is that in this study the nimorazole could be given without major side effects. The benefit of this treatment was not observed in another large clinical trial conducted in North America under the Radiation Therapy Oncology Group (RTOG) in patients

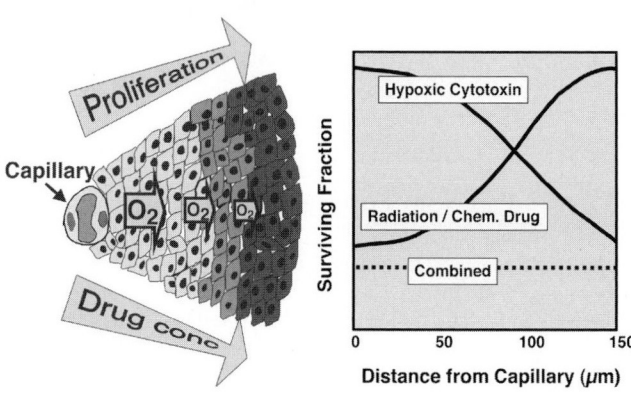

Figure 3–4. Gradient of reduced cell killing as a function of distance from the vasculature as seen in experimental tumors and spheroids.

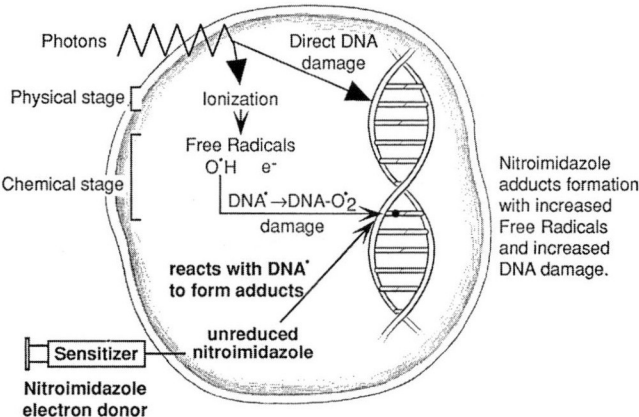

Figure 3–5. Hypoxic cell sensitizers increase DNA damage through free radical formation.

Table 3–1   The Evaluation of First- to Third-Generation Nitroimidazole Compounds Over the Past 25 Years

	Metronidazole (1st Generation)	Misonidazole (2nd Generation)	Etanidazole (3rd Generation)
Formulation	500 mg tablets 500 mg/100 mL solution	500 & 100 mg tablets & capsules 500 mg/20 mL solution	1000 mg/19.4 mL saline solution 50 mg/mL
Maximum Total Dose	Total cumulative dose not to exceed 54 g/m^2 Multiple doses 6 g/m^2 3 times/wk for 3-4 wk	Total cumulative dose not to exceed 12 g/m^2 Once or twice/wk for 5-6 weeks	Total dose not to exceed 40.8 g/m^2 at 1.7-2 g/m^2 3 times/wk for 6 wk Single dose 12 g/m^2 during IORT 48 h continuous infusion 20-21 g/m^2 during brachytherapy
Optimal Time for Administration	4 h before radiation	4 h before radiation	30 min before radiation
Main Toxicities	Gastrointestinal +4 Sensory peripheral neuropathy +1	Sensory peripheral neuropathy +4 Gastrointestinal toxicity +2	Sensory peripheral neuropathy +3 Gastrointestinal toxicity +1 Arthralgia +1, seen more often with 48 h continuous infusion
Sensitizer Enhancement Ratio(SER)	Estimated SER 1.15 with multiple doses of 6 g/m^2	Estimated SER 1.4 with multiple doses of 2 g/m^2 Estimated SER 1.15 with doses of 0.5 mg/m^2	Estimated SER 1.6 with multiple doses of 1.7-2 g/m^2 Estimated SER 2.5-3.0 with doses of 12 g/m^2
Comments	Not currently in use as a radiosensitizer	No longer in use as a first line radiosensitizer	No longer in use as a first line radiosensitizer

IORT, intraoperative radiotherapy.

with stage III and IV head and neck tumors, in which misonidazole was used with two of the five radiation fractions per week. In this study, the administration of the radiosensitizer was limited by neurological complications, and the use of efficient doses was prevented.[23] A prospective, randomized trial was initiated afterward in the same cooperative group with a newer third-generation compound, etanidazole. A significantly greater dose of etanidazole than misonidazole can be administered for a sensitizer effect with acceptable gastrointestinal and neurologic toxicity.[24]

ETANIDAZOLE

Etanidazole (originally known as SR2508) was developed by a team led by Brown and Lee with the aim of reducing the neurotoxicity seen with misonidazole.[25] It was postulated that since etanidazole is less lipophilic, it would be associated with a lower incidence of neuropathies. This was confirmed in a Phase I pharmacokinetic and toxicity study in which doses three times higher were delivered and fewer peripheral neuropathies were observed.[24]

Table 3–2   Summary of Efficacy of Clinical Trials with Nitroimidazoles, 1974-2001

Compounds	Trials, n	Significant Benefit	No Benefit
Metronidazole	1	1 (within the constraints of the study)	—
Misonidazole/ Nimorazole	38	5	33
Etanidazole (SR-2508)	7	—	7
Pimonidazole (Ro 03-8799)	1	—	1

Based on the encouraging results of the Danish Group in pharyn carcinoma with misonidazole and nimorazole, the RTOG initiated a two-part study in advanced head and neck cancer. The first part, a toxicity and logistic study in which etanidazole was used 3 times a week for 17 doses in combination with standard radiation, was completed with acceptable toxicity (although the 22% incidence of peripheral neuropathies still presented a problem). Subsequently, a Phase III study in a similar patient population and with the same frequency of sensitizer administration was initiated and completed in 1992. The results showed that adding

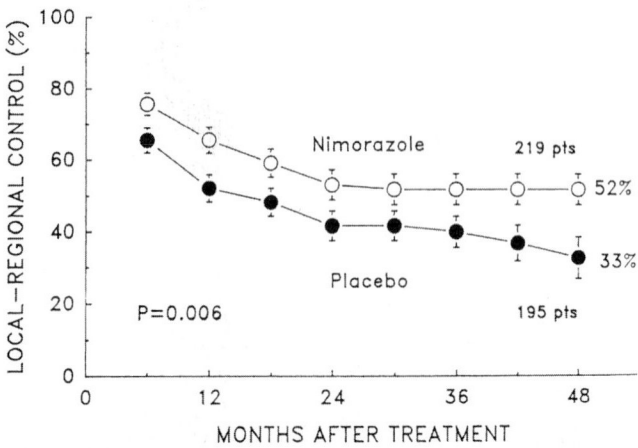

Figure 3–6. Results from the Danish Head and Neck Cancer Study Group 5 study. Patients with carcinoma of the pharynx and supraglottic larynx were randomly assigned to receive nimorazole or placebo in conjunction with radiotherapy. (From Overgaard J, Hansen SH, Overgaard M, et al: The Danish Head and Neck Cancer Study Group (DAHANCA) randomized trials with hypoxic radiosensitizers in carcinoma of the larynx and pharynx. In Dewey WC, Edington M, Fry MRG, et al, eds: *Radiation Research: A 20th Century Perspective.* Vol 2. Toronto: Academic Press; 1992:576.)

etanidazole to conventional radiotherapy produced no benefit for patients with advanced head and neck carcinomas, except for a suggestion of benefit in a subset of patients with early stages (N0-N1 disease).[26] A randomized study of 374 patients from 27 European centers conducted between 1987 and 1990 found that adding etanidazole to conventional radiotherapy did not afford any benefit for patients with head and neck carcinoma. Furthermore, the study failed to confirm the hypothesis of benefit for patients with early disease.[27]

A similar study in patients with locally advanced cancer of the prostate—T2b, T3, and T4—was also initiated in North America (RTOG). This study was designed to deliver the sensitizer with as many fractions of conventional radiation as possible. Nineteen doses of 1.8 g/m^2 were delivered 3 times a week during the course of radiation, with tolerable toxicity. The results of this trial with regard to prostatic specific antigen response and clinical disappearance of tumor are similar to those of historical control subjects and are not considered to represent an improvement.[28]

A single large dose of etanidazole (12 g/m^2) administered with intraoperative radiation was considered an ideal setting to assess hypoxic cell sensitizers in a Phase I study, which was also completed under the RTOG. The serum and tissue concentrations of etanidazole observed in the trial were 5 to 10 times higher than the levels seen when this compound was given with fractionated radiation. The estimated SER was 2.5 to 3. In 1993, a Phase III trial involving intraoperative radiation and single-dose etanidazole was initiated in patients with locally recurrent rectosigmoid carcinoma. This study was closed because of poor accrual. Also within the RTOG, a Phase II study was initiated to test the use of etanidazole in combination with stereostatic radiosurgery in recurrent malignant gliomas or central nervous system metastases.

There is evidence that prolonged exposure of hypoxic cells to nitroimidazoles can lead to increased sensitization beyond the oxygen effect, owing to the formation of reactive reduced metabolic species. Based on this evidence, an evaluation was made of etanidazole administered in 48-hour and 96-hour continuous intravenous infusions to patients undergoing brachytherapy.[29] The use of etanidazole under these particular conditions is considered worth pursuing.

Imaging studies that use ^{3}H-misonidazole and ^{123}I-iodoazomycin arabinoside show evidence of tumor hypoxia in more than 50% of patients with small cell carcinoma of the lung and indicate that tumor hypoxia could be one of the causes of chemoresistance and radioresistance in these patients. Therefore, a Phase I/II clinical prospective study was initiated in patients with all stages of small cell lung cancer, in which etanidazole was given in doses of 1.7 g/m^2 3 times a week with concomitant chemotherapy and thoracic irradiation. In patients with limited-stage disease, the median and crude rates of survival at 5 years with no evidence of disease were superior to the best results reported in the literature from similar radiotherapy and chemotherapy regimens in which etanidazole was not used.[30]

Pimonidazole (a 4-nitroimidazole) was developed in Europe at the same time that etanidazole was developed as a third-generation sensitizer, and was considered to be more potent than misonidazole because of its several-fold increase in tumor concentration. The maximum tolerated dose, when administered with a daily 20-fraction course of radiotherapy, was established at 750 mg/m^2. The dose-limiting toxicity is in the central nervous system, manifesting as disorientation and malaise. A randomized clinical trial in advanced carcinoma of the cervix was conducted by 16 centers in Western Europe under the guidance of the Medical Research Council of Great Britain. Patient accrual was completed in May 1989. Overall and disease-free survival rates were found to be poor among the patients who received pimonidazole in combination with external radiation.[31]

Conclusions

The current scene after 2 decades of clinical investigations with hypoxic cell sensitizers can be summarized by stating that these compounds are not yet ready for use in the standard practice of radiotherapy. The only patients who appear to have benefited significantly from this approach are those with advanced pharyngeal and supraglottic carcinomas treated with radiation and either misonidazole or nimorazole.[21,22] In the immediate future and with the advent of noninvasive markers of tumor hypoxia, it will be possible to select patients for the use of these agents.

POSSIBLE EXPLANATION FOR THE UNEXPECTED FAIR TO POOR THERAPEUTIC BENEFITS SEEN WITH NITROIMIDAZOLES

The failure to demonstrate a major improvement of the therapeutic ratio with these drugs could be related to the following:

1. It has been postulated that the response of tumors to multiple doses of radiation similar to those used in therapy is governed not by the most hypoxic cells in the tumor but by the more abundant cells at intermediate oxygenation.[32] Such cells require much higher concentrations of nitroimidazoles to give adequate radiosensitization, levels that are above clinically tolerated doses due to gastrointestinal toxicity and neurotoxicity.
2. Some of the tumor sites chosen did not have a steep radiation-dose response when a 10% dose increment could have made a difference in the results.
3. Patients with proven tumor hypoxic fractions were not preselected.
4. Many human tumors contain high levels of glutathione, which reduces the effectiveness of nitroimidazoles.

WHAT HAS BEEN LEARNED?

Clinicians have learned to predict, by the initial pharmacokinetics of the drug in individual patients, which patients could be at risk for drug-related neurotoxicity. We have learned that intravenous administration is preferable. We have learned to assess the characteristics of each tumor before the course of radiation by developing practical techniques to measure tumor hypoxia. We have learned that none of the hypoxic sensitizers developed to date can create more than an SER of 1.3 at tolerable doses with fractionated radiotherapy. It has also been recognized that sensitizers might be best tested in those tumors in which the dose response is sharp and which are known to contain hypoxic cells. Thus, to see a 20% to 30% improvement in local control, there is only a need to increase the dose by 5%.

The resistance of tumor hypoxic cells to conventional fractionated radiation in humans is a more complex problem than it appeared to be 25 years ago, when the first clinical investigations were initiated with these agents. We now know that in addition to the classically described state of chronic tumor hypoxia, there is intermediate acute hypoxia, and that both states can be influenced by manipulation of the tumor microenvironment. We also know drugs that kill rather than sensitize hypoxic cells might be a preferable way of dealing with, and indeed of exploiting, tumor hypoxia than the classic nitroimidazole radiosensitizers.

Current Status and Future Directions in Tumor Hypoxia

MICROINVASIVE METHODS OF MEASURING TUMOR HYPOXIA

Hypoxia in human solid tumors has been demonstrated invasively by measurement of intercapillary distance, oxygen tension, and intracapillary oxyhemoglobin[33] by microelectrodes with the well-established Eppendorf histograph,[34] by the binding of 2-nitroimidazole reduced adducts using the ^{3}H-misonidazole autoradiography in tumor biopsy material.[33] Most recently, pimonidazole has been bound to human tumor biopsies using an immunohistochemistry technique.[35] The absence of correlation between this quantitative immunohistochemical marker of hypoxia and VEGF expression has been demonstrated in humans.[36] It has also been demonstrated that the primary determinant of 2-nitroimidazole binding is related to low oxygen rather than to the nonhomogeneous distribution of nitroreductase activity.[37] Another well developed invasive method is the "comet" assay, which is based on the number of DNA strand breaks observed in tumor specimens obtained by needle biopsy and assessed by electrophoretic technique. Usually, well-oxygenated cells exhibit two to three times more DNA strand breaks than hypoxic cells. The aerobic cells exhibiting more damaged DNA will have a longer "tail" in the assay than the hypoxic cells. Through assessment of the "tails" or "comets" of a group of cells, the proportion of hypoxic cells can be determined.[38]

NONINVASIVE METHODS OF MEASURING TUMOR HYPOXIA

Methods of determining hypoxia that are noninvasive, easy to repeat during and after treatment, and capable of assessing deeply located tumors (e.g., lung cancers, malignant gliomas, sarcomas, abdominal tumors) are becoming available. These methods include study of tumor metabolic parameters by (1) oxygen utilization, (2) glucose metabolic rate, and (3) measurement of adduct formation of radiofluorinated fluoromisonidazole by positron emission tomography[39] or ^{123}I-IAZA by SPECT scan.[40] The radioiodinated azomycin nucleosides (^{123}I-IAZA) method can be combined easily with another available nuclear medicine scan to assess the level of tumor blood perfusion in the same patient by sequential imaging with ^{99m}Tc-hexamethylpropyleneamine oxime (^{99m}Tc-HMPAO).[41] To date, 40 patients with solid tumors have been studied by the ^{123}I-IAZA imaging technique. Half of the studied patients with squamous cell carcinoma of the head and neck and small cell lung cancer showed high levels of ^{123}I-IAZA avidity. Contrary to expectations, only 1 of 11 patients with the histologic diagnosis of glioblastoma had a positive scan, despite the fact that these tumors by definition have areas of necrosis.[40,41]

By the use of these techniques, patients can be selected for therapeutic manipulation of their tumor microenvironment. Currently, the most popular method used in the clinic to measure tumor hypoxia is computer-driven Eppendorf microelectrode histography. In this procedure, a microelectrode needle, 0.3 mm in diameter, is inserted into the tumor, and individual pO_2 measurements are made as the needle advances in a step-wise fashion through the tissue. Usually the step action involves an advance of 1.0 mm followed by a withdrawal of 0.3 mm just before the measurement. This is computer driven, and in any one tumor more than 200 measurements are made. The volume of tissue characterized by this method may be as large as 10 μL. The drawback of this technique, in addition to the pull-back action (which can cause considerable damage), is that the sampling volume means that the average oxygenation of possibly thousands of cells rather than individual cells is sampled. Obviously, microregional hypoxia cannot be measured, but multiple measurements obtained in this fashion through the tumor give a reliable average. This has been shown in head and neck tumors and carcinoma of the cervix, where hypoxia is correlated with poor local tumor control.[2,3]

MANIPULATION OF THE TUMOR MICROENVIRONMENT

Increasing the Oxygen-Carrying Capacity of Blood

HYPERBARIC OXYGEN AND FLUOSOL. Clinical studies have been completed in which hyperbaric oxygen,[42] carbogen,[43] packed red cell transfusions,[44,45] and oxygen-carrier substances such as perfluorocarbons (Fluosol-DA) have been used.[46,47] Although the use of the hyperbaric oxygen chamber at three atmospheres presented technical difficulties, such as barotrauma and the limitations of its use to only a few high-dose fractions of radiation, 3 of 10 clinical trials showed significant positive results. The beneficial effect was seen particularly in patients with advanced cancer of the head and neck and of the cervix.[48]

A Phase II study of Fluosol-DA and 100% oxygen in combination with radiotherapy in advanced head and neck tumors has shown promising results.[46,47] Investigators have also been assessing the compound RSR13, an allosteric hemoglobin modifier. Preliminary reports are encouraging.[49]

An alternative approach is to increase the level of hypoxia in tumor cells and to treat them with hypoxic cytotoxic agents. Previous attempts to reduce tumor perfusion by the use of agents like hydralazine have not proven valuable because of the potential systemic side effects. Another approach to increase the level of tumor hypoxia by modifying the oxyhemoglobin disassociation curve with a specific chemical agent such as BW12C is combining this approach with the hypoxic cytotoxic agent, mitomycin C. This approach was investigated in patients with advanced gastrointestinal cancer.[50]

Most recently the agent SU5416 (Sugen) has undergone initial clinical trials in metastatic colorectal cancer. Patients are randomized to receive treatment with 5-fluorouracil/leucovorin with or without SU5416. In addition, two clinical studies in low-grade and high-grade sarcoma using Sugen with radiotherapy are currently being undertaken within the RTOG.

Increasing Tumor Blood Flow

NICOTINAMIDE AND CARBOGEN/ARCON. Improvement in tumor pO_2 following carbogen breathing (95% + 5% CO_2) has been shown in both animal and human tumors. Tumor tissue oxygenation was measured in humans with the polarographic electrode system (Eppendorf) pO_2 histograph. In this particular study, in 12 of 17 patients with solid tumors there was a significant increase in median tumor pO_2 during the first 10 minutes of carbogen breathing. Measurements were taken in accessible superficial tumors, 15 of them epithelial tumors (most of them breast and lung carcinomas) and two soft tissue sarcomas.[51]

It is hypothesized that nicotinamide decreases the presence of acute intermittent hypoxia and that carbogen breathing reoxygenates the chronic hypoxic cells.[52,53] The benefit of this combination could be further enhanced in tumors with rapidly proliferating stem cells if accelerated radiotherapy schedules were used. This approach, accelerated radiotherapy with carbogen and nicotinamide (ARCON), was initiated originally in a pilot study by a European-Canadian working group (Gray Laboratory Annual Report, personal communication, 1992). A multiple institution ARCON Phase I trial was conducted under the EORTC (European Organization for Research and Treatment of Cancer). In this 3-step study, 115 patients with glioblastoma multiforme were registered. The overall survival was not different when compared with results of other series using radiotherapy alone.[54] Nicotinamide produced GI toxicity, necessitating dose reduction. Two other Phase I/II clinical trials using ARCON in non–small cell lung cancer[55] and 215 patients with advanced head and neck squamous cell carcinoma[56,57] were conducted recently with encouraging results regarding tumor responses, but continued to require a reduction in the dose of nicotinamide because of the incidence of gastrointestinal acute toxicity. Of interest, assessment of normal tissues and tumor perfusion using [99m]-HMPAO SPECT Nuclear Medicine studies

in glioblastoma demonstrated no perfusion changes[58] after administration of nicotinamide. So far, there have been no reports of Phase III studies with ARCON.

HYPOXIC CYTOTOXINS AND VASCULAR TARGETING

HYPOXIC CYTOTOXINS—TIRAPAZAMINE

The development of hypoxic radiosensitizers led to that of hypoxic cytotoxins, also known as bioreductive drugs. These are agents that can increase cell kill in a solid tumor by radiotherapy or by chemotherapy by killing, rather than sensitizing, the resistant hypoxic cells. Hypoxic cells in tumors are not only resistant to radiation, they are also resistant to most anticancer drugs. This is because hypoxic cells, by definition, must be those farthest from functioning blood vessels, and also, it is because cells at low oxygen levels divide much less rapidly than when fully oxygenated. These two factors lead to resistance to anticancer drugs, first because the majority of anticancer drugs are only effective against rapidly proliferating cells, and second because chemotherapy drugs must reach tumor cells from blood vessels. Thus, hypoxic cytotoxins are fundamentally different from conventional agents in that they target a different subpopulation of cells within the tumor. Typically, hypoxic cytotoxins have maximum cytotoxicity to the cells at maximum distance from tumor blood vessels, thereby complementing the pattern of cytotoxicity for both radiation and anticancer drugs, which is maximum for the cells immediately adjacent to the blood vessels (see Fig. 3-4). Thus, these agents can potentially overcome a major cause of resistance of solid tumors to conventional therapies—namely, that resulting from the inadequate oxygenation and drug delivery to tumor cells distant to blood vessels.

Mitomycin C, a quinone antibiotic that requires reductive metabolism for activity, is the prototype bioreductive agent. Introduced into clinical use in 1958, mitomycin C has demonstrated activity toward a number of different tumors in combination with other chemotherapeutic drugs and radiation. Some 30 years ago Sartorelli and colleagues suggested that what they thought would be the lower oxidation reduction (redox) potential of tumor relative to normal tissue might be exploited to obtain greater activation of this compound to its cytotoxic species.[59] Although tumor redox potential did not turn out to be key for the activity of mitomycin C, Sartorelli and Rockwell were able to show that this drug preferentially kills hypoxic compared to aerobic cells in vitro.[60] However, the differential toxicity is modest: The ratio of drug concentrations under aerobic to hypoxic conditions for the same level of cell kill (hypoxic cytotoxicity ratio, or HCR) is in the range of 1 (no differential) to 5.[61] Nonetheless, this can be sufficient to overcome the resistance of hypoxic cells in animal tumors, and clinical trials have reported higher cure rates for head and neck cancers by adding mitomycin C to radiotherapy compared with radiotherapy alone,[62] though as mitomycin C is a chemotherapy drug with toxicity toward all cells, it is unclear whether the improved cure rates over radiotherapy alone were the result of selective killing of hypoxic cells.

A second class of hypoxic cytotoxins was developed by Adams and colleagues,[12] who showed that nitroheterocyclic structures containing a side chain with alkylating properties were not only more active as radiosensitizers of hypoxic cells, they were also potent and selective killers of hypoxic cells, both in vitro and in vivo. The lead compounds of this group, RB 6145, have shown considerable activity in vitro and in animal tumors, but have proven too toxic to warrant clinical development.

A group led by Brown and Lee introduced a third class of bioreductive drugs in 1986. The compound introduced, SR 4233, now known as tirapazamine (TPZ), a benzotriazene di-N-oxide, had a hypoxic cytotoxicity ratio of 50:300 for different cell lines (Fig. 3-7),[63] and (unlike the classic hypoxic radiosensitizers) is active when combined with fractionated radiation at doses comparable to those used clinically.[64] The mechanism for the selective toxicity of TPZ (and other members of this class) toward hypoxic cells is that the drug is reduced (an electron is added) by intracellular reductases to form a highly reactive radical that produces both single- and double-strand breaks in DNA. However, under aerobic conditions oxygen removes the electron from the TPZ radical, thereby back-oxidizing it to the nontoxic parent with a concomitant production of superoxide radical. Thus, the differential hypoxic cytotoxicity results from the fact that the TPZ radical is much more cytotoxic than the superoxide radical. In addition to its toxicity to hypoxic cells, TPZ was shown to be remarkably efficient at enhancing the cytotoxicity of some chemotherapeutic agents, notably cisplatin, in experimental animal tumors.[65]

Following favorable results in Phase I and II studies with the combination of cisplatin and TPZ, a Phase III, multicenter, randomized clinical trial with TPZ combined with cisplatin in patients with advanced non–small cell lung cancer showed a doubling of the overall response when TPZ was combined with cisplatin compared to cisplatin only and a significant increase in the median survival time of the patients.[66] This increase of antitumor activity occurred without any evidence of increased systemic toxicity of the anticancer drug cisplatin as was also seen in experimental animal systems. More recently, promising results of Phase I-II trials of TPZ combined with both cisplatin and fractionated irradiation have been reported for cervix cancer[67] and for

head and neck cancer.[68] Currently there are two further Phase III trials under way with TPZ combined either with chemotherapy in NSCLC or with radiotherapy and cisplatin in head and neck cancer. A drawback to the use of TPZ is muscle toxicity.[69] Other hypoxic cytotoxins, such as AQ4N, are now just entering early clinical testing.

VASCULAR TARGETING

The concept that the vasculature could be a selective target in cancer therapy was first proposed by Denekamp based on the much more rapid proliferation rate of the endothelial cells in tumors compared to those in normal tissues.[70] However, it was not until experimental animal studies with the drug flavone acetic acid (FAA) were conducted that this concept become a reality. This and similar agents, such as the FAA analog DMXAA, and the tubulin-destabilizing agent combretastatin A-4, cause selective collapse of the vasculature in tumors with little or no effect on normal blood vessels.[71] This leads to an immediate increase in tumor hypoxia, extensive tumor cell killing, and tumor necrosis. The increased tumor hypoxia can be effectively combined with hypoxic cytotoxins[72] or can be combined with hyperthermia[73] or radiotherapy[74] to enhance tumor cell killing. The rationale for the efficacy of the latter combinations is that because the vascular targeting agents cause collapse of the neovasculature and necrosis of all the tumor cells supplied by these vessels, they kill all (or nearly all) of the tumor cells, leaving only a small rim of viable tumor cells at the tumor periphery. This rim is better oxygenated and therefore sensitive to radiation or anticancer drugs. Though early clinical results with FAA were negative, this was because the drug is only active with mouse tissues, whereas its analog DMXAA is also active in human tumors. Currently Phase I and II trials are being conducted with these agents, including DMXAA and combretastatin A-4.

MODIFIERS OF HEMOGLOBIN LEVELS

Erythropoetin

Erythropoetin is a growth factor that has been synthesized in the laboratory. It has shown efficacy in the treatment of anemia related to systemic chemotherapy,[75] as well as in combined chemoradiation. A significant increase in hemoglobin levels compared to controls has been shown in patients receiving radiotherapy.[76-77] These studies did not address the question of whether the increase in hemoglobin levels seen when administering erythropoetin results also in improvement in local tumor control. As of June 2000 a randomized Phase III trial to assess the effect of erythropoetin on local-regional control in anemic patients treated with radiotherapy for advanced carcinoma of the head and neck was initiated with the Radiation Therapy Oncology Group (RTOG). The sample size of this clinical protocol is expected to be 372 patients. Tumor response in the first 2 years and overall survival will be the endpoints. No results are yet available.

Glutathione Depletion

As shown in Figure 3–8, sulfhydryls are scavengers of free radicals, protecting chemical damage induced by

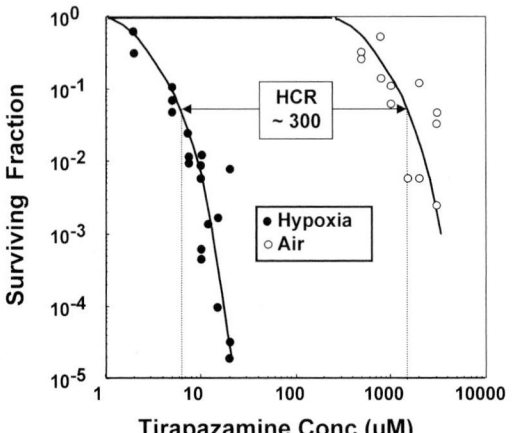

Figure 3–7. Effect of tirapazamine (TPZ) on tumor cells' surviving fraction under air and hypoxic conditions.

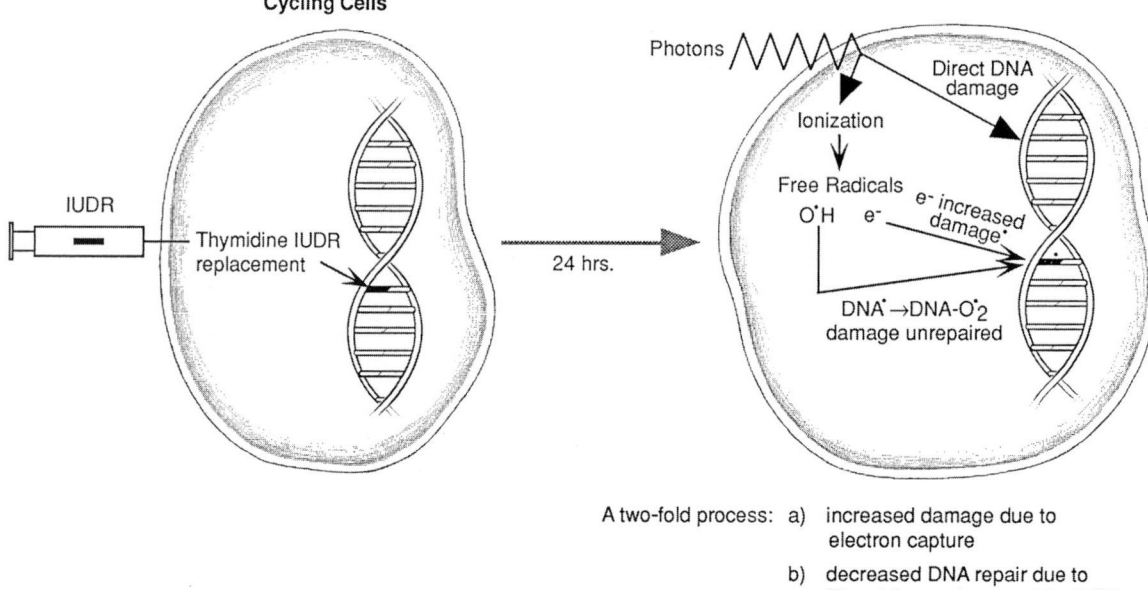

Figure 3–8. Sensitizers specific for proliferating cells. DNA repair is exploited through a specific cell cycle with specific agents. IUDR/BUDR shares similarities in molecular structure and topography with thymidine during repair processes.

either ionizing radiation or alkylating agents via glutathione S transferase. It has been postulated and demonstrated in the laboratory that one approach to increasing the efficacy of the nitroimidazoles as sensitizers is to decrease the levels of the competing endogenous sulfhydryls. Glutathione is one of the major endogenous sulfhydryls. Buthionine sulfoximine was developed as a specific inhibitor of glutathione. It has been shown to deplete glutathione levels in both in vitro and in vivo systems, therefore making misonidazole a more effective sensitizer.[78] Earlier studies in laboratory experiments showed little or no increase in the toxicity of misonidazole in normal tissue but showed an increased sensitizing efficacy in the tumor tissue.[79]

It is unlikely that depletion of the glutathione by itself could be a useful strategy to enhance the radiation effect without a chemical sensitizer.[80] Several investigators demonstrated that glutathione depletion can enhance the effectiveness of misonidazole and etanidazole,[81] as well as increase the effectiveness of bioreductive agents cytotoxic to hypoxic cells.[82] Therefore, the use of buthionine sulfoximine as a modulator for hypoxic cell sensitizers in combination with radiation and as a modulator of chemotherapeutic drugs such as alkylating agents and bioreductive hypoxic cytotoxics is of current interest and is being investigated actively.[83,84]

AN ALTERNATIVE TO NITROIMIDAZOLE HYPOXIC CELL RADIOSENSITIZERS

Nitric Oxide

The hypoxic cell radiosensitization properties and vasodilator effects on tumor vasculature of nitric oxide gas have been described, and there is continued laboratory interest on the possible practical therapeutic use of nitric oxide-releasing compounds (NONOATES) under specific physiologic conditions. Studies done in the laboratory

under in vitro conditions have shown a marked radiosensitizer effect under hypoxic conditions.[85] Further studies are being conducted in in vivo models. For the time being this approach is still limited to the laboratory level.

NONHYPOXIC CELL SENSITIZERS

The cancer chemotherapy agents hydroxyurea and 5-fluorouracil are not discussed in this chapter. The reader is referred to Chapter 5, Radiotherapy and Chemotherapy for descriptions of these agents as possible nonhypoxic cell radiosensitizers.

Halogenated Pyrimidine Analogues

5-BROMODEOXYURIDINE (BUDR) AND 5-IODODEOXYURIDINE (IUDR)

The pyrimidine analogues BUDR and IUDR are considered cell-cycle-specific radiosensitizers and act independently of the oxygen effect. As previously discussed, the radioresistance of human solid tumors could be multifactorial, where in addition to the microenvironment (nutrition oxygenation and presence of endogenous sulfhydryl compounds) tumor cell kinetics play an important role. The presence of rapidly proliferating clonogens may substantially influence the control of tumors by irradiation. Since BUDR and IUDR sensitize only rapidly proliferating cells, in such tissues either normal or tumor cells could be effectively sensitized. Rapidly proliferating tumor cells surrounded by slowly proliferating supporting normal tissue present the ideal scenario for an improved therapeutic ratio. However, this is often not the case, as will be discussed later.

Unlike the hypoxic cell sensitizers, these agents require extended exposure of the cells for the necessary incorporation into DNA, while the cells are undergoing DNA synthesis (see Fig. 3-8).

The pyrimidine analogue stands in for thymidine in DNA through the thymidine salvage pathway. The result of this substitution is that the physicochemical properties of DNA are altered. The basic mechanisms of radiosensitization are debatable and not clearly understood. Evidence from in vitro work suggests two components. One component (decreased repair) is related to the increase in the amount of DNA strand breakage induced by radiation in the presence of IUDR/BUDR substituting for thymidine. The second component (increased damage) is related to nonscavengeable aqueous electrons at sites of multiple damage. Together these two component mechanisms support the multiple damage site theory.[86]

Importance of Cell Labeling and DNA Incorporation

CLINICAL INVESTIGATIONS

The degree of incorporation and thymidine replacement and the sensitizer enhancement ratio are intimately related.[87] Therefore, measurements of thymidine replacement in individual human tumors by flow cytometry, to establish the potential doubling time, and assessment of thymidine replacement after short and long infusions is needed as part of the design of future clinical trials with these cell-cycle drugs.

The means of achieving an optimal incorporation of these compounds in the cell in the clinical situation has been extensively explored over the years, particularly the route of administration and length of drug exposure. Early on, BUDR was used intra-arterially both to avoid dehalogenation by the liver and to increase the tumor drug concentration.[88] However, the necessary prolonged use of this route in patients over several weeks was laborious and had a high incidence of complications. Although there have been reports of rapid debromination of halopyrimidines occurring after intravenous therapy, Goffinet and Brown[89] showed that following intravenous infusion, enough halopyrimidine apparently passes the hepatic vessels to permit tumor radiosensitization, despite dilution of the drug by the systemic circulation. This has also been shown in human studies. There has been a renewed interest over the past decade in the use of continuous intravenous infusion of halopyrimidines. It was observed that adequate steady-state arterial plasma levels could be maintained with this route of administration with acceptable systemic toxicities.[90] In 1987, continuous infusion of halopyrimidines were tested in patients who had malignant glioma (mixed population of glioblastomas and anaplastic astrocytomas), and a median survival of 13 months was reported.[91] A small pilot study was reported in 1990 in which intra-arterial BUDR was used in combination with external radiotherapy. The median survival for glioblastoma patients was 14 months.[92] Finally, a larger series was reported by the Northern California Oncology Group (NCOG) in 160 patients with glioblastoma treated with 96-hour infusion of BUDR at 800 mg/m² a day for a total of 6 weeks, in combination with 60 Gy irradiation directed to tumor plus a margin. The patients in this series received chemotherapy with PCV (procarbazine, lomustine [CCNU], and vincristine) for 1 year following radiotherapy. The median survival time was 12.8 months. Patients with anaplastic astrocytoma had a median survival time of almost 5 years, and the observation was made that the use of pyrimidine analogues in combination with radiation may be of greater benefit in this group of patients.[93] However, the most recent randomized study in anaplastic astrocytoma conducted by the RTOG using radiation and PCV chemotherapy compared to radiation and PCV plus BUDR was terminated earlier because of the inferior time to tumor recurrence and survival observed in the arm using BUDR.[94]

Although the generally accepted method of administering halogenated pyrimidines is intravenous infusion, there is controversy over both the length of the infusion and the dose intensity. Some investigators propose giving these drugs at relatively high doses with short infusions in an attempt to achieve maximum thymidine replacement in DNA.[92-95] Others, however, recommend using low doses of halopyrimidines, not only because the prolonged infusion can be better tolerated but also because more cells would be exposed to the drug.[96,97]

An experimental model using in vivo tumor xenografts and a mathematical model of continuous exposure to halogenated pyrimidines to assess the kinetics of cell labeling and DNA replacement was reported by Rodriguez and associates.[98] The results show that a relatively small DNA IUDR replacement is associated with significant sensitization and cell killing. Therefore, with this model, it has been claimed that a modest concentration of halogenated pyrimidines, as when a long infusion is used, gives adequate radiosensitization, provided that a high proportion of cells are labeled.

To address, in part, the controversy just described, a Phase I/II clinical study in patients with malignant gliomas was completed with the aim of assessing the toxicity and tumor efficacy of a "long" 96-hour intravenous infusion versus two "short" schedules of 24 and 48 hours at high-dose intensity. Despite hepatic and bone marrow toxicities and the fact that fewer patients received a minimum of 80% of the targeted dose, there was a trend toward improved survival in patients with anaplastic astrocytomas in the "long" infusion schedule. It was concluded that, owing on the one hand to the laborious continuous intravenous infusion and on the other to the toxicities and only fair tumor efficacy, the use of this drug with radiation was not warranted, at least in patients with glioblastoma.[99]

Intra-Arterial 5-Bromodeoxyuridne

The availability of a permanent implantable infusion pump for continuous intra-arterial infusions has revived the use of intra-arterial BUDR. Recently, the regional delivery of IUDR via the hepatic artery was considered for metastatic lesions in the liver.[100] As modulation of halogenated pyrimidines has been achieved in vitro, it has been postulated that the radiosensitization of these compounds could be enhanced with the addition of

5-fluorouracil,[101] which might increase analogue incorporation through blocking of the de novo synthesis of thymidine from pyrimidine, with increased analogue incorporation through the thymidine salvage pathway. This strategy was already attempted in a Phase I clinical trial without any therapeutic gain but with greater systemic toxicity.[102] Methotrexate also blocks the de novo synthesis of thymidine and has also been considered as a modulator.[98] Another approach to increasing the incorporation of these compounds into DNA is to combine them with leucovorin. The efficacy of this combination has been demonstrated in vitro, resulting in an enhanced IUDR incorporation and radiosensitization without increased cytotoxicity.[98]

CONCLUSIONS ON RADIOSENSITIZERS

After more than 2 decades of clinical investigations, the goal of using hypoxic cell or cell-cycle-specific radiosensitizers in everyday standard radiotherapy remains elusive. There is, however, a better understanding of the multifactorial cause of radiation resistance and current efforts are concentrated on the selection of specific tumor sites where one or two factors of resistance have been uncovered. Numerous studies indicate tumor hypoxia as one of the important factors in clinical radiotherapy. The application of radiosensitizers will not be universal in all solid tumors but could be specifically directed to tumor sites according to their characteristic cell kinetics and presence or absence of hypoxia using noninvasive markers of hypoxia.

CHEMICAL RADIOPROTECTORS

The first chemical radioprotector compounds intended for use on humans were developed to protect individuals from whole body irradiation, such as in the event of nuclear warfare. The sulfhydryl compounds, including β-mercaptoethylamine and thiophosphates, were considered. An extensive drug developmental program was initiated by the United States Department of Defense (Walter Reed Army Research Institute [WR]). Of 4000 screened compounds, the thiophosphate WR-2721 was the most promising. Clearly, these compounds were designed to protect all tissues, a very different requirement from their possible use in the field of oncology, in which protection of normal tissues to the exclusion of tumor tissues is essential to improve the therapeutic ratio. Therefore, there are still serious questions about whether these agents, to a lesser degree, also protect the tumor from the effects of radiation.[103,104]

The assumption that the tumor tissues are not protected to the same degree as normal tissues is based on the probability that there is poor drug penetration in tumors because of their poor blood perfusion, and that there is a higher concentration of the drug in normal tissues because of their higher pH. In addition, for WR-2721 to be active, the phosphate group must be cleaved by the enzyme alkaline phosphatase to form the dephosphorylated free thiol WR-1065. This enzyme is not as abundant in tumor tissues as in normal tissues;

therefore, the levels of alkaline phosphatase and pH in tissues determine the uptake of WR-2721. There is also a final assumption that thiol compounds could have less protective effect on tumor hypoxic cells. The mechanisms of *radioprotection* fit the competition-model, dual-action theory (Fig. 3-9). Once inside the cell, the active free thiol WR-1065 can scavenge oxygen-free radicals. It also takes part in the repair reaction of DNA damage. Of interest in the field of medical oncology and chemotherapy is the fact that dephosphorylated WR-2721 can bind to the active species of alkylating agents as well as prevent the formation of cisplatin-DNA adducts.[105]

Biological agents such as interleukin-1 have been shown to protect normal tissues in animal systems.[106]

Amifostine WR-2721 (Ethyol)

The dose-modifying factor (DMF) of amifostine WR-2721 for both normal and tumor tissues was studied in animals carrying solid tumors.[107,108] For normal tissues, the greatest protection is found in bone marrow, with a DMF of 2.7 to 3, and in the gastrointestinal tract, with a DMF of 1.6. The lowest DMF, at 1.2, is in lung tissue. However, this drug *also* protects tumor tissues, with DMFs ranging from 1.3 for cure of EMT-6 carcinoma to 2.2 for mean survival time of P-388 leukemia. Once more, the degree of protection to tumors appears to be related to the tumor blood perfusion, degree of hypoxia, the tissue pH, and the levels of alkaline phosphatase. A cautionary note is that most of these experiments were performed with single radiation doses. It is possible that the differential protective effect between normal and tumor tissues would be less if multiple daily small doses in combination with radiation were used.

Experimental work has also been done in which amifostine is used as a *chemoprotector* of normal tissues. Three studies performed with different animal tumor models showed protection of bone marrow and intestine

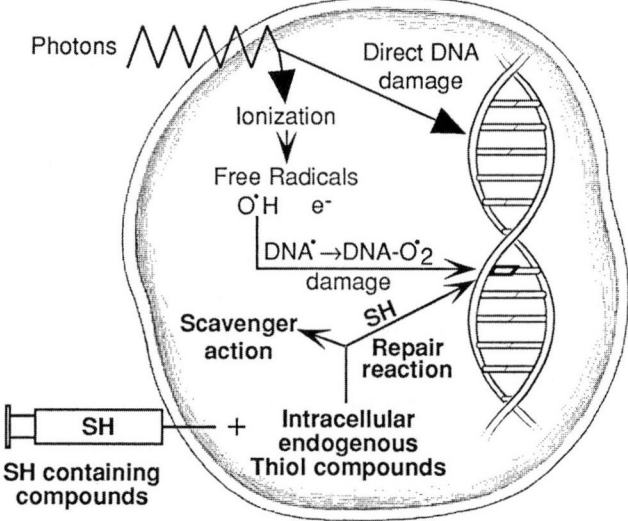

Figure 3–9. Chemical protectors: competition model. There is a dual action to chemical radioprotection: (1) thiols and sulfhydryl compounds act as repair compounds, and (2) they compete with free radicals (scavenging effect).

with no protection of the tumor when amifostine was used with melphalan[109] or in combined chemotherapy regimes with nitrogen mustard, cyclophosphamide, carmustine, cisplatin, and 5-fluorouracil.[110,111]

It should be noted that amifostine does not protect the central nervous system tissues from radiation effects because of the blood-brain barrier.[112]

CLINICAL EXPERIENCE

Amifostine has been approved for clinical use and is available for intravenous route in a sterile lyophilized powder mixture with mannitol, requiring reconstitution for intravenous administration. It is administered over a 15-minute period before radiation or chemotherapy. Initial single-dose toxicity and pharmacokinetic studies were performed in 1983. The plasma β-half-life is 9 minutes, and it is assumed that the protective concentrations are maintained in normal tissues for approximately 2 hours.[113,114]

The maximum tolerated dose for multiple doses is 340 mg/m² given 4 days a week for 5 weeks, 15 minutes before external radiation. Toxicities at this dose level are manifested as nausea, vomiting, anorexia, malaise, transient moderate hypotension, and occasional hypocalcemia. It is recommended that the amifostine infusion be interrupted if there is a 25% decrease in systolic blood pressure. The maximum tolerated dose with single doses is 740 mg/m², although the dose has been increased to 910 mg/m² given twice a week for at least 5 treatments, and this dose has been considered acceptable.[115]

The clinical effectiveness of amifostine as a radioprotector was subsequently studied using pelvic organs and bone marrow as normal tissue endpoints in patients receiving definitive radiation for advanced carcinoma of the cervix. External radiation and brachytherapy were combined to total 7760 cGy to the primary tumor and 5000 cGy to the parametrium (Table 3-3). The dose of amifostine was 75 mg/m² on a daily basis. In this study, there was no evidence of either normal or tumor tissue protection.[116] Another study, in which pelvic organs were the normal tissue endpoint, was a Phase III randomized study in patients with advanced rectal carcinoma. The whole pelvis received 4500 cGy 4 times a week for 5 weeks, with a boost of 1440 cGy to the primary tumor in 8 fractions for a total tumor dose of 5940 cGy, combined with amifostine at 340 mg/m² with each fraction of radiation. In this study, there was evidence of protection of mucous membranes, urinary bladder, and intestine, but not of tumor protection.[117] Bone marrow as a normal tissue endpoint was used in a Phase II study in patients

with miscellaneous solid tumors receiving palliative hemibody radiation. In this study, hemibody radiation was delivered in a single dose of 700 cGy, preceded 15 minutes by 600 to 900 mg/m² of amifostine. Protection against bone marrow toxicity was observed. Tumor effect was not assessed in this study (see Table 3-3).[118]

A Phase III randomized head and neck cancer clinical trial using radiation with or without amifostine was conducted using unstimulated saliva production and xerostomia as the endpoint. The incidence of grade 2 xerostomia was reduced from 78% to 51%.[119,120] In another lung cancer study, no tumor protection was found.[121]

Amifostine is therefore considered to reduce the natural toxicity related to cisplatin and the xerostomia related to radiation treatment of head and neck tumors.[122]

CHEMOPROTECTION

The clinical effectiveness of amifostine as a chemoprotector was assessed with the use of bone marrow as the normal tissue endpoint and cyclophosphamide as the chemotherapeutic agent (Table 3-4). Definitive evidence of bone marrow protection was observed. Tumor protection was not assessed.[123] In another study, renal damage and peripheral neuropathy were assessed as endpoints and cisplatin was used; normal tissue protection with no tumor protection was observed.[124] Another clinical study demonstrated the protective effect amifostine has in bone marrow, kidney, and peripheral nerves when cyclophosphamide is used in combination with cisplatin.[125] Protection of carboplatin myelotoxicity was observed in one study,[126] but findings were inconclusive in another preliminary study.[127] The use of amifostine in combination with chemotherapy or radiation or both is currently being used in clinical research protocols for both adult and pediatric patient populations.

A study was conducted within the RTOG in which esophageal mucosa was used as normal tissue endpoint in patients with limited stage small cell lung cancer receiving systemic chemotherapy and local thoracic radiation with no incidence of radiation esophagitis.[128]

Future Prospects

In view of the concern of systemic toxicity and possible tumor protection when thiol compounds are used, alternative agents are being explored, such as antioxidants (e.g., the nitroxide tempol), as well as inhibitors of prostaglandin synthesis. There is also interest in the use of

Table 3–3   Clinical Effectiveness of Amifostine (WR-2721) as a Radioprotector

Type of Trial	Endpoint	Tumor/Volume Radiation	Normal Tissue Protection	Tumor Protection	Reference
Phase II	Pelvic organs	Advanced cancer of cervix/Whole pelvic + brachytherapy	No	No	Mitsuhashi et al.[116]
Phase III, randomized	Pelvic organs	Advanced rectal cancer/ Whole pelvis + cone-down	Yes	No	Kligerman et al.[117]
Phase II	Bone marrow	Miscellaneous solid tumors/Palliative HBI	Yes	Not assessed	Constine et al.[118]

Table 3–4   Clinical Effectiveness of Amifostine (WR-2721) as a Chemoprotector

Type of Trial	Endpoint	Tumor/Volume Radiation	Normal Tissue Protection	Tumor Protection	Reference
Phase II	Bone marrow	Cyclophosphamide	Yes	Not assessed	Glick et al.[123]
Phase I	Renal damage, peripheral neuropathy	Cis-platinum	Yes (bone marrow)	No	Glover et al.[124]
Phase III	Bone marrow, renal damage, neuropathy	Cyclophosphamide combined with Cisplatinum	Yes (bone marrow)	No	Glick et al.[125]
Phase I/II	Bone marrow	Carboplatin and Cisplatin	Yes (bone marrow)	Not assessed	Muggia[126]

cytokine-releasing agents, such as endotoxin and glucan, and these are being considered for application, either alone or in combination with the thiol compounds.[129,130]

TEMPOL

This nonthiol nitroxide compound has been shown both in vitro and in vivo to be an effective radioprotector with the absence of tumor radioprotection. In addition, nitroxide compounds are known for their modest hypoxic cell radiosensitization. The potential of tempol as an aerobic cell radioprotector is attractive and has been recently highlighted.[131,132]

INHIBITORS OF PROSTAGLANDINS

Protection of hematopoietic tissue was observed in mice pretreated with indomethacin, an inhibitor of prostaglandin synthesis. This effect was found with the use of endogenous colony-forming unit-spleen assays. There is potential for a therapeutic application of this concept.[133] This agent does not protect tumor tissues in tumor-bearing animals. The mechanism of action does not involve free radical scavenging.

BIOLOGIC RESPONSE MODIFIERS

Endotoxin and Glucan

These biologic agents exert effects through physiological mechanisms by enhancing the recovery of the bone marrow or host immune system or both, possibly through macrophage activation and release of cytokines (interleukin-1, colony-stimulating factor, and tumor necrosis factor). The combination of thiol compounds with these less toxic biologic response modifier agents (e.g., glucan) has been proposed as an attractive therapeutic approach to be explored in the near future.[134] This concept is currently being evaluated by the Cancer and Leukemia Group B in which granulocyte-macrophage colony-stimulating factor and amifostine are being combined.

CONCLUSIONS ON RADIOPROTECTORS AND CHEMOPROTECTORS

As was the case with the hypoxic cell sensitizers, a spin-off of the work on radioprotectors is manifested in the increasing interest in the use of these compounds as chemoprotectors in the field of medical oncology.[135] The protective effects of amifostine have been seen in bone marrow during the use of alkylating and platinum compound agents. Phase III large clinical trials are ongoing to demonstrate conclusively normal tissue protection without tumor protection in esophageal mucosa, salivary glands, and bone marrow when these protectors are combined with radiation, and in kidney, peripheral nerves, and bone marrow when they are used with alkylating agents and platinum compounds.

An exciting evolving potential is in the combination of chemical protectors (amifostine or tempol) with biological stimulators (cytokines). Furthermore, the impact of thiol compounds might be even greater in the laboratory, based on their promising use as a probe in examining the mechanisms of radiation cell damage. It is likely that vital new information will be available in the near future on the molecular mechanisms of radiation protection.[135]

REFERENCES

1. Steel GG: Combined radiotherapy-chemotherapy: Principles. In Steel GG, Adams GE, Horwich E, eds: *The Biological Basis of Radiotherapy*. 2nd ed. Amsterdam: Elsevier; 1989:267.
2. Gatenby RA, Kessler HB, Rosenblum JS, et al: Oxygen distribution of squamous cell carcinoma metastases and its relationship to outcome of radiation therapy. *Int J Radiat Oncol Biol Phys*. 1988;14:831.
3. Hockel M, Knoop C, Schlenger K, et al: Intratumoral pO_2 predicts the survival in advanced cancer of the uterine cervix: Updated analysis of an open prospective clinical study. *Radiother Oncol*. 1992;26:45.
4. Bush RS, Jenkin RDT, Eltt WEC, et al: Definitive evidence for hypoxic cells influencing cure in cancer therapy. *Br J Cancer*. 1978;37:302.
5. Durand RE: Distribution and activity of antineoplastic drugs in a tumor model. *J Natl Cancer Inst*. 1989;81:146.
6. Durand RE: The influence of microenvironmental factors during cancer therapy. *In vivo*. 1994;8:691-702.
7. Graeber TG, Osmanian C, Jacks T, et al: Hypoxia-mediated selection of cells with diminished apoptotic potential in solid tumours. *Nature*, 1996;379:88.
8. Brizel DM, Scully SP, Harrelson JM, et al: Tumor oxygenation predicts for the likelihood of distant metastases in human soft tissue sarcoma. *Cancer Research*. 1996;56:941.
9. Hockel M, Schlenger K, Aral B, et al: Association between tumor hypoxia and malignant progression in advanced cancer of the uterine cervix. *Cancer Research*. 1996;56:4509.
10. Sundfor K, Lyng H, and Rofstad EK. Tumour hypoxia and vascular density as predictors of metastasis in squamous cell carcinoma of the uterine cervix. *Br J Cancer*. 1998;78:822.

11. Adams GE, Cooke MS: Electron-affinic sensitization. I. A structural basis for chemical radiosensitizers in bacteria. *Int J Radiat Biol.* 1969;15:457.

12. Adams GE, Asquith JC, Watts ME, Smithen CE: Radiosensitization of hypoxic cells in vitro: a water-soluble derivative of para-nitroacetophenone. *Nature* [New Biol]. 1972;239:23.

13. Foster JL, Willson RL: Radiosensitization of anoxic cells by metronidazole. *Br J Radiol.* 1973;46:234.

14. Rabin HR, Urtasun RC, Partington J, et al: Pharmacokinetics and bioavailability of metronidazole using an IV preparation and application of its use as a radiosensitizer. *Cancer Treatment Reports.* 1980;64:1087.

15. Urtasun RC, Band P, Chapman JD, et al: Radiation and high dose metronidazole in supratentorial glioblastomas. *N Engl J Med.* 1976;294:1364.

16. Urtasun RC, Chapman JD, Feldstein L, et al: Peripheral neuropathy related to misonidazole: Incidence and pathology. *Br J Cancer.* 1978;271.

17. Dische S, Saunders MI, Anderson P, et al: Neurotoxicity of misonidazole, pooling of data from five centers. *Brit J Radiol.* 1978;51:1023.

18. Dische S: Chemical sensitizers for hypoxic cells: A decade of experience in clinical radiotherapy. *Radiother Oncol.* 1985;3:97.

19. Brown JM: Clinical trials of radiosensitizers: what should we expect? *Int J Radiat Oncol Biol Phys.* 1984;10:425.

20. Overgaard J: Clinical evaluation of nitroimidazoles as modifiers of hypoxia in solid tumors. *Oncol Res.* 1994;6:509.

21. Overgaard J, Hansen SH, Overgaard M, et al: The Danish Head and Neck Cancer Study Group (DAHANCA) randomized trials with hypoxic radiosensitizers in carcinoma of the larynx and pharynx. In Dewey WC, Edington M, Fry MRG, et al, eds: *Radiation Research: A 20th Century Perspective.* Vol 2. Toronto: Academic Press; 1992:525.

22. Overgaard J, Sand Hansen H, Overgaard M, et al: A randomized double-blind phase III study on nimorazole as a hypoxic radiosensitizer of primary radiotherapy in supraglottic larynx and pharynx. *Results of the Danish Head and Neck Cancer Study (Dahanca). Radio and Oncol.* 1998;46:135.

23. Fazekas J, Pagak TF, Wasserman TH, et al: Failure of misonidazole-sensitized radiotherapy to impact upon outcome among stage III/IV squamous cancers of the head and neck. *Int J Radiat Oncol Biol Phys.* 1987;13:1155.

24. Wasserman TH, Lee DJ, Cosmatos D, et al: Clinical trials with etanidazole (SR-2508) by the Radiation Oncology Group (RTOG). *Radiother Oncol.* 1991;20:129.

25. Brown JM, Yu NY, Brown DM, Lee WW: SR-2508: A 2-nitroimidazole amide which should be superior to misonidazole as a radiosensitizer for clinical use. *Int J Radiat Oncol Biol Phys.* 1981;7:695.

26. Lee DJ, Cosmatos D, Marcial VA, et al: Results of an RTOG phase III trial (RTOG 85-27) comparing radiotherapy plus etanidazole with radiotherapy alone for locally advanced head and neck carcinomas. *Int J Radiat Oncol Biol Phys.* 1995;32:567.

27. Eschwege R, Sancho-Garnier H, Chassagne D, et al: Results of a European randomized trial of etanidazole combined with radiotherapy in head and neck carcinomas. *Int J Radiat Oncol Biol Phys.* 1997;39:275.

28. Lawton CA, Coleman CN, Buzydlowsky JW, et al: Results of a phase II trial of external beam radiation with etanidazole for the treatment of locally advanced prostatic cancer (RTOG protocol 90-20). *Int J Radiat Oncol Biol Phys.* 1996;36:673.

29. Coleman CN, Noll L, Howes AE, et al: Initial results of the phase I trial of the continuous infusion of SR-2508 (etanidazole). *Int J Radiat Oncol Biol Phys.* 1989;16:1085.

30. Urtasun RC, Palmer M, Kinney B, et al: Intervention with the hypoxic tumor cell sensitizer etanidazole in the combined modality treatment of limited stage small-cell lung cancer. A one-institution study. *Int J Rad Oncol Biol Phys.* 1998;40:337.

31. Dische S: Radiotherapy, carcinoma of cervix and the radiosensitizer Ro 03-8799 (pimonidazole). In Dewey WC, Edington M, Fry MRG, et al, eds: *Radiation Research: A 20th Century Perspective,* Vol. 2. Toronto: Academic Press; 1992.

32. Wouters BG, Brown, JM: Cells at intermediate oxygen levels can be more important than the "hypoxic fraction" in determining tumor response to fractionated radiotherapy. *Radiat Res.* 1997;147:541.

33. Urtasun RC: Tumor hypoxia, its clinical detection and relevance. In Dewey WC, Edington M, Fry MRG, et al, eds: *Radiation Research: A 20th Century Perspective,* Vol. 2. Toronto: Academic Press; 1992:725.

34. Vaupel P, Mueller-Klieser: Oxygenation and bioenergetic status of human tumors. In Dewey WC, Edington M, Fry MRG, et al, eds: *Radiation Research: A 20th Century Perspective.* Vol. 2. Toronto: Academic Press;1992:772.

35. Raleigh JA, Calkins-Adams DP, Rinker LH, et al: Hypoxia and vascular endothelial growth factor protein expression in human tumors. *Cancer Res.* 1998;58:3765.

36. Raleigh JA, Calkins-Adams DP, Rinker LH, et al: Hypoxia and vascular endothelial growth factor protein expression in human tumors. *Cancer Res.* 1998;58:3765.

37. Arteel GE, Thurman RG, Yates JM, Raleigh JA: Evidence that hypoxia markers detect oxygen gradients in liver: Pimonidazole and retrograde perfusion in rat livers. *Br J Cancer.* 1995;72:889.

38. Olive PL, Durand RE: Detection of hypoxic cells in a murine tumor with the use of the comet assay. *J Natl Cancer Inst.* 1992;84:707.

39. Koh WH, Rasey JS, Evans ML, et al: Imaging of hypoxia in human tumors with (F-18) fluoromisonidazole. *Int J Radiat Oncol Biol Phys.* 1992;22:199.

40. Parliament MB, Chapman JD, Urtasun RC, et al: Non-invasive assessment of human tumor hypoxia with ^{123}I-iodoazomycin arabinoside: Preliminary report of a clinical study. *Br J Cancer.* 1992;65:90.

41. Groshar D, McEwan AJB, Parliament MB, et al: Imaging tumor hypoxia and tumor perfusion. *J Nuclear Med.* 1993;34:885.

42. Hank JM: Does hyperbaric oxygen have a future in radiation therapy? *Int J Rad Oncol Biol Phys.* 1981;7:1125.

43. Rubin P, Hanley J, Keys HM, et al: Carbogen breathing during radiation therapy. Radiation Oncology Group study. *Int J Radiat Oncol Biol Phys.* 1979;5:1963.

44. Bush RS: The significance of anemia in clinical radiation therapy. *Int J Radiat Oncol Biol Phys.* 1986;12:2047.

45. Dische S, Saunders MI, Warvurton MF: Hemoglobin, radiation, morbidity and survival. *Int J Radiat Oncol Biol Phys.* 1986;12:1335.

46. Rose C, Lustig R, McIntosh LN, et al: A clinical trial of fluosol-DA 20% in advanced squamous cell carcinoma of the head and neck. *Int J Radiat Oncol Biol Phys.* 1988;12:1325.

47. Lustig R, McIntosh LN, Rose C, et al: Phase I/II, study of fluosol-DA and 100% oxygen as adjuvant to radiation in the treatment of advanced squamous cell tumors of the head and neck. *Int J Radiat Oncol Biol Phys.* 1989;16:1587.

48. Dische S: Hypoxia in local tumor control: Part 2. *Radiother Oncol.* 1991;20:9.

49. Amorino GP, Lee H, Holburn GE, et al: Enhancement of tumor oxygenation and radiation response by the allosteric effector of hemoglobin, RSR13. *Radiat Res.* 2001;156:294.

50. Ramsay JRS, Bleehan NM, Dennis I, et al: Phase I: A study of BW12C in combination with mitomycin C in patients with advanced gastrointestinal cancer. *Int J Rad Oncol Biol Phys.* 1992;22:21.

51. Falk SJ, Ward R, Bleehan NM: The influence of carbogen breathing on tumor tissue oxygenation in man evaluated by computerized pO_2 histography. *Br J Cancer.* 1992;66:919.

52. Rojas A: Radiosensitization with normobaric oxygen and carbogen. *Radiother Oncol.* 1991;20:65.

53. Horsman MR, Kristjansen PEG, Mizunom, et al: Biochemical and physiological changes induced by nicotinamide in a C3H mouse mammary carcinoma and CDF1 mice. *Int J Radiat Oncol Biol Phys.* 1992;22:451.

54. Miralbell R, Mornex F, Greiner R, et al: Accelerated radiotherapy, carbogen and nicotinamide in glioblastoma. *J Clin Oncol.* 1999;17:3143.

55. Bernier J, Denekamp J, Rojas A, et al: ARCON: Accelerated radiotherapy with carbogen and nicotinamide in non-small cell lung cancer: A phase I/II study by the EORTC. *Radiotherapy and Oncology.* 1999;52:149.

56. Bussink J, Kaanders JH, Van der Kogel AJ: Clinical outcome and tumor microenvironmental effects of accelerated radiotherapy with carbogen and nicotinamide. *Acta Oncologic.* 1999;38:875.

57. Kaanders JH, Pop LA, Marres HA, et al: ARCON experience into 115 patients with advanced head and neck cancer. *Int J Radiat Oncol Biol Phys.* 2002;1;769.

58. Hulshof MC, Rehmann CJ, Booij J et al: Lack of perfusion enhancement after administration of nicotinamide and carbogen in patients with glioblastoma: 99m-TcHMPAO SPECT study. *Radiotherapy and Oncology.* 1998;48:135.

59. Lin AJ, Cosby LA, Shansky CW, et al: Potential bioreductive alkylating agents. 1. Benzoquinone derivatives. *J Med Chem.* 1972;15:1247.

60. Rockwell S, Kennedy KA, Sartorelli AC: Mitomycin-C as a prototype bioreductive alkylating agent: In vitro studies of metabolism and cytotoxicity. *Int J Radiat Oncol Biol Phys.* 1982;8:753.

61. Brown JM, Siim BG: Hypoxia-specific cytotoxins in cancer therapy. *Seminars in Rad Onc.*1996;6:22.

62. Haffty BG, Son YH, Sasaki CT, et al: Mitomycin C as an adjunct to postoperative radiation therapy in squamous cell carcinoma of the head and neck: results from two randomized clinical trials [see comments]. *Int J Radiat Oncol Biol Phys,* 1993;27:241.

63. Zeman EM, Brown JM, Lemmon MJ, et al: SR-4233: A new bioreductive agent with high selective toxicity for hypoxic mammalian cells. *Int J Radiat Oncol Biol Phys.* 1986;12:1239.

64. Brown JM, Lemmon MJ: SR-4233: A tumor specific radiosensitizer active in fractionated radiation regimes. *Radiother Oncol.* 1991;1:151.

65. Dorie MJ, Brown JM: Tumor-specific, schedule-dependent interaction between tirapazamine (SR 4233) and cisplatin. *Cancer Research.* 1993;53:4644.

66. von Pawel J, von Roemeling R, Gatzemeier U, et al: Tirapazamine plus cisplatin versus cisplatin in advanced non-small-cell lung cancer: A report of the international CATAPULT I study group [In Process Citation]. *J Clin Oncol.* 2000;48:791.

67. Craighead PS, Pearcey R, Stuart G: A phase I/II evaluation of tirapazamine administered intravenously concurrent with cisplatin and radiotherapy in woman with locally advanced cervical cancer. *Int J Radiat Oncol Biol Phys.* 2000;48:791.

68. Rischin D, Peters L, Hicks R, et al: Phase I trial of concurrent tirapazamine, cisplatin and radiotherapy in patients with advanced head and neck cancer. *J Clin Oncol.* 2001;19:535.

69. Herscher LL, Krishna MC, Cook JA, et al: Protection against SR 4233 (tirapazamine) aerobic cytotoxicity by the metal chelators desferrioxamine tiron. *Int J Radiat Oncol Biol Phys.* 1994;30:879.

70. Denekamp J: Endothelial cell proliferation as a novel approach to targeting tumour therapy. *Br J Cancer.* 1982;45:136.

71. Tozer GM, Prise VE, Wilson J, et al: Combretastatin A-4 phosphate as a tumor vascular-targeting agent: Early effects in tumors and normal tissues. *Cancer Res.* 1999;59:1626.

72. Sun JR, Brown JM: Enhancement of the antitumor effect of flavone acetic acid by the bioreductive cytotoxic drug SR 4233 in a murine carcinoma. *Cancer Res.* 1989;49:5664.

73. Eikesdal HP, Bjerkvig R, Mella O, et al: Combretastatin A-4 and hyperthermia; a potent combination for the treatment of solid tumors. *Radiother Oncol.* 2001;60:147.

74. Murata R, Siemann DW, Overgaard J, et al: Interaction between combretastatin A-4 disodium phosphate and radiation in murine tumors. *Radiother Oncol.* 2001;60:155.

75. Bunn H. Recombinant erythropoietin therapy in cancer patients. *J Clin Oncol.* 1990;8:949.

76. Vijayakumar S, Roach N, Wara W, et al: Effects of subcutaneous recombinant human erythropoetin in cancer patients receiving radiotherapy: Preliminary results of a randomized, open-label phase II trial. *Int J Radiat Oncol Biol Phys.* 1993;26:721.

77. Lavey RS, Dempsey WH: Erythropoietin increases hemoglobin in cancer patients during radiation therapy. *Int J Radiat Oncol Biol Phys.* 1993;27:1147.

78. Brown MJ: Sensitizers in Radiotherapy. In Withers HR, Peters LJ, eds: *Innovations in Radiation Oncology.* Berlin: Springer-Verlag; 1988;247.

79. Yu NY, Brown JM: Depletion of glutathione in vivo as a method of improving the therapeutic ratio of misonidazole and SR 2508. *Int J Radiat Oncol Biol Phys.* 1984;10:1265.

80. Mitchell JB, Cook JA, DeGraff W, et al: Glutathione modulation in cancer treatment: Will it work? *Int J Radiat Oncol Biol Phys.* 1989;16:1289. Keynote address.

81. Kramer RA, Soble M, Howes AE: The effect of glutathione (GSH) depletion in vivo by buthionine sulfoximine (BSO) in the radiosensitization of SR2508. *Int J Radiat Oncol Biol Phys.* 1989;16:1325.

82. Giaccia AJ, Biedermann KA, Tosto LM, et al: Characterization of a CHO cell line resistant to killing by the hypoxic cell cytotoxin SR 4233. *Int J Rad Oncol Biol Phys.* 1992;22:681.

83. Allalunis-Turner MJ, Barrone GM, Day RS, et al: Heterogeneity in response to treatment with buthionine or sulfoximine or interferon in human malignant glioma cells. *Int J Radiat Oncol Biol Phys.* 1992;22:765.

84. Britten RA, Warenius HM, White R: BSO-induced reduction of glutathione levels increases the cellular radiosensitivity of drug-resistant human tumor cells. *Int J Radiat Oncol Biol Phys.* 1992;22:769.

85. Mitchell JB, Wink DA, DeGraff W, et al: Hypoxic mammalian cell radiosensitization by nitric oxide. *Cancer Res.* 1993;53:5845.

86. Webb CF, Jones GDD, Ward JF, et al: Mechanisms of radiosensitization in bromodeoxyurine substituted cells. *Int J Radiat Biol.* 1993;64:695.

87. Phillips TL, Prados MD, Bodell WJ, et al: Rationale for and experience with clinical trials for halogenated pyrimidines in malignant gliomas: The UCSF/NCOG experience. In Dewey WC, Edington M, Fry MRG, et al, eds: *Radiation Research: A 20th Century Perspective.* Vol 2.Toronto: Academic Press; 1992:601.

88. Bagsaw MA, Doggett RSL, Smith KC, et al: Intra-arterial 5-bromodeoxyuridine and x-ray therapy. *Radiology.* 1967;99:886.

89. Goffinet DR, Brown JM: Comparison of intravenous and intra-arterial pyrimidine infusion as a means of radiosensitizing tumors. *Radiology.* 1977;124:819.

90. Kinsella TJ, Collins J, Rowald J, et al: Pharmacology in phase I/II study of continuous infusions of iododeoxyuridine and hyperfractionated radiotherapy in patients with glioblastoma multiforme. *J Clin Oncol.* 1988;6:871.

91. Jackson D, Kinsella TJ, Rowlan J: Halogenated pyrimidines as radiosensitizers in the treatment of glioblastoma multiforme. *Am J Clin Oncol.* 1987;10:437.

92. Hegarty TJ, Thornton AF, Diaz RF, et al: Intra-arterial bromo-deoxyuridine radiosensitization of malignant gliomas. *Int J Radiat Oncol Biol Phys.* 1990;19:421.

93. Phillips TL, Levin VA, Ahn DK: Evaluation of bromodeoxyuridine in glioblastoma multiforme, a NCOG phase II study. *Int J Radiat Oncol Biol Phys.* 1991;21:709.

94. Prados M, Scott C, Sander H, Buchner J, et al: A phase III randomized study of radiotherapy with or without BUDR plus procarbazine, CCNU and vincristine (PCV) for the treatment of anaplastic astrocytoma: A preliminary report of RTOG 94-04 radiation and BUDR in malignant gliomas. *Int J Radiat Oncol Biol Phys.* 1999;45:1109.

95. Lawrence TS, Davis MA, Maybaum J, et al: The dependence of halogenated pyrimidine incorporation and radiosensitization on the duration of drug exposure. *Int J Rad Oncol Biol Phys.* 1990;18:1393.

96. Uhl V, Phillips TL, Ross GY: Iododeoxyuridine incorporation and radiosensitization in treating human tumor cell lines. *Int J Radiat Oncol Biol Phys.* 1992;22:489.

97. Speth PA, Kinsella TJ, Chang AE: Selective incorporation of iododeoxyuridine (IUdR) into DNA of human hematopoietic cells, normal liver and hepatic metastases in man as a radiosensitizer and a marker for cell kinetic studies. *Int J Radiat Oncol Biol Phys.* 1989;16:1247.

98. Rodriguez R, Ritter MA, Fowler JF: Kinetics of cell labeling and thymidine replacement after the continuous infusion of halogenated pyrimidines in vivo. *Int J Radiat Oncol Biol Phys.* 1994;29:105.

99. Urtasun RC, Cosmatos D, DelRowe J, et al: Iododeoxyuridine (IUdR) combined with radiation in the treatment of malignant glioma: A comparison of short vs long intravenous dose schedules (RTOG86-12). *Int J Radiat Oncol Biol Phys.* 1993;27:207.

100. Chung AE, Collins JM, Speth PA, et al: Phase I study of intra-arterial iododeoxyuridine in patients with colorectal liver metastases. *J Clin Oncol.* 1989;7:662.

101. Lawrence TS, Davis MA, Maybaum, et al: Modulation of iododeoxyuridine-mediated radiosensitization by 5-fluorouracil in human cancer cells. *Int J Radiat Oncol Biol Phys.* 1992;22:499.

102. Speth PA, Kinsella TJ, Belanger K, et al: Fluorodeoxyuridine modulation of the incorporation of iododeoxyuridine into DNA granulocytes: Phase I and clinical pharmacological study. *Cancer Res.* 1988;48:2933.

103. Yuhas MJ, Storer JB: Differential chemo protection of normal and malignant tissues. *J Nat Cancer Inst.* 1969;32:331.

104. Denekamp J, Rojas A, Stewart FA: Is radioprotection by WR-2731 restricted to normal tissues? In Nygaard OF, Simic MG, eds: *Radioprotectors and Anticarcinogens.* New York: Academic Press; 1983:655.

105. Tresher M, Nitjmans LG, Shepman A, et al: Effects of modulating agent WR-2721 and its main metabolites on the formation and stability of cisplatin/DNA adducts in vitro. *Bio Chem Pharmacol.* 1992;33:1013.

106. Neta R, Oppenheim JJ, Douche S: Interdependence of the radioprotective effects of human recombinant interleukin 1 alpha, tumor necrosis factor alpha, granulocyte colony-stimulating factor, and murine recombinant granulocyte-macrophage colony-stimulating factor. *J Immunol.* 1988;140:108.

107. Phillips TL, Kane L, Utley JF: Radioprotection of tumor and normal tissues by thiol phosphate compounds. *Cancer.* 1973;32:528.

108. Milas L: Improving radiotherapy by reducing normal tissue damage with radioprotectors. *Cancer Bull.* 1986;38:223.

109. Millar JL, McElwain TJ, Clutterbuck RD, et al: Demodification of melphalan toxicity as single agent in tumor bearing mice by WR 2721. *Am J Clin Oncol (CCT).* 1992;5:321.

110. Wasserman TH, Phillips TL, Ross G, et al: Differential protection against cytotoxic chemotherapeutic effects on bone marrow CFU's by WR-2721. *Cancer Clin Trials.* 1981;4:3.

111. Peters GJ, Vanderwilt CL, Gyergyay F, et al: Protection by WR-2721 of the toxicity induced by the combination of cisplatin and 5-fluorouracil. *Int J Radiat Oncol Biol Phys.* 1992;22:785.

112. Washburn LC, Rafter JJ, Hayes RL: Prediction of the effective radioprotective dose of WR-2721 in humans through an interspecies tissue distribution study. *Radiat Res.* 1976;66:100.

113. Kligerman MN, Glover DJ, Turrisi AT, et al: Toxicity of WR-2721 administered in single and multiple doses. *Int J Radiat Oncol Biol Phys.* 1984;10:1773.

114. Turrisi AT, Glover DJ, Hurwitz, et al: Final report of the phase I trial of single dose WR-2721. *Can Treat RTTS.* 1986;70:1389.

115. Coia L, Crigel R, Hanks G, et al: Phase I study WR-2721 in combination with total body radiation in patients with refractory lymphoid malignancies. *Int J Rad Oncol Biol Phys.* 1992;22:791.

116. Mitsuhashi N, Takahashi I, Takahashi M, et al: Clinical study of radioprotective effects of amifostine on long term outcome for patients with cervical cancer. *Int J Radiat Oncol Biol Phys.* 1993;26:407.

117. Kligerman MM, Liu T, Liu Y, et al: Interim analysis of a randomized trial of radiation therapy of rectal cancer with/without WR-2721. *Int J Radiat Oncol Biol Phys.* 1992;22:799.

118. Constine LS, Zagars G, Rubin P: Protection by WR-2721 of human bone marrow function following radiation. *Int J Radiat Oncol Biol Phys.* 1986;12:1505.

119. Brizel DM. Future directions in toxicity prevention. *Semin Radiat Oncol.* 1998;8:17.

120. Brizel DM, Wasserman TH, Strand V, et al. Final report of phase III randomized trial of amifostine as a radioprotectant in head and neck cancer. *Int J Radiat Oncol Biol Phys.* 1999;45:147.

121. Schiller JH, Store RB, Berlin J, et al: Amifostine, cisplatin and vinblastine in metastatic non-small cell lung cancer: A report of high response rates and prolonged survival. *J Clin Oncol.* 1996;14:1913.

122. Hensley ML, Schuchter LM, Lindley C, et al: American Society of Clinical Oncology clinical practice guidelines for the use of chemotherapy and radiotherapy protectants. *J Clin Oncol.* 1999;17:333.

123. Glick JH, Glover D, Weiler C, et al: Phase I controlled trials of WR-2721 and cyclophosphamide. *Int J Radiat Oncol Biol Phys.* 1984;10:1777.

124. Glover D, Glick JH, Weiler C, et al: Phase I/II trials of WR-2721 and cis-platinum. *Int J Radiat Oncol Biol Phys.* 1986;12:1509.

125. Glick J, Kemp J, Rose P, et al: A randomized trial of cyclophosphamide and cisplatin plus or minus WR-2721 in the treatment of advanced epithelial ovarian cancer. *ASCO.* 1992;11:122.

126. Muggia F, Parker R, Reed E, et al: WR-2721 pretreatment protects against the bone marrow toxicity of carboplatin and cisplatin. *ASCO.* 1992;11:132.

127. Luginbuhl W, Tester W, Shaw L, et al: One or two doses of WR-2721: Does it protect patients receiving carboplatin? *ASCO.* 1992;11:312.

128. Mehta MP. Protection of normal tissues from the cytotoxic effect of radiation therapy: Focus on amifostine. *Semin Radiat Oncol.* 1998;8:14.

129. Weiss JF, Kumar KS, Walden TL, et al: Advances in radioprotection through the use of combined agent regimes. *Int J Radiat Oncol Biol Phys.* 1990;57:709.

130. Goffman TE, Raubitschek A, Mitchell JB, et al: The emerging biology of modern radiation oncology. *Cancer Res.* 1990;50:7735.

131. Mitchell JB, DeGraff W, Kaufman D, et al: Inhibition of oxygen-dependent radiation-induced damage by nitroxide superoxide dismutase mimic, tempol. *Arch Biochem Biophys.* 1991;289:62.

132. Hahn SM, Tochner Z, Krishna CM, et al: Tempol, a stable free radical is a novel murine radiation protector. *Cancer Res.* 1992;52:1750.

133. Nishiguchi I, Furuta Y, Hunter N, et al: Radioprotection of hematopoietic tissues in mice by indomethacin. *Radiat Res.* 1990;122:188.

134. Murray D, Prager A, Meyn RE, et al: Radioprotective agents as modulators of cell and tissue radiosensitivity. *Cancer Bull.* 1992;44:137.

135. Coleman CN, Mitchell JB: Radiation modifiers. In: Chabner BA, Longo DL, (eds). Cancer chemotherapy and biotherapy: Principles and Practice. 3rd edition. Philadelphia: Lippincott Williams & Wilkins; 2001:707.

Prediction of Radiation Response

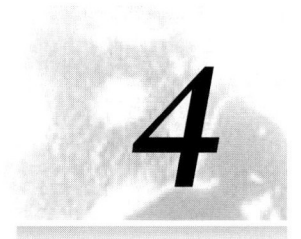

Adrian C. Begg, PhD

The prescription for clinical radiotherapy is usually based on such factors as tumor site, stage, and grade. All patients with tumors falling in the same category with regard to these clinical parameters receive the same radiation schedule, conforming to the department or center's current policy. An increasing body of evidence now shows that even for similar histological type and extent of tumor, wide variations exist in the response to fractionated irradiation. For example, the fractionation scheme (e.g., conventional, accelerated, hyperfractionated) has been shown to influence outcome in some clinical trials.[1-5] Total dose also influences outcome. These considerations together indicate that it is likely that a single radiotherapy prescription is not optimum for many patients, even those within the same clinical category. Some patients, but not all, may benefit from accelerated fractionation. Some, but not all, may benefit from hyperfractionation. Some may require higher doses; others may be overtreated with conventional doses; and for still others, conventional radiotherapy of 1.8 to 2 Gy per day for 6 to 7 weeks may be the best choice. A desirable goal would then be to give each patient a more tailored treatment. The probable consequence of this is improved local control and survival with reduced morbidity for the patient group as a whole.

Three main parameters are likely to influence outcome after radiation therapy: intrinsic radiosensitivity, the degree of tumor hypoxia, and the rate of repopulation of tumor cells. In addition, the radiosensitivity of normal tissues determines the dose that can be delivered safely. Current studies on predictive assay development have concentrated on these aspects.

PREDICTION OF RADIOSENSITIVITY

Cells in tissue culture exhibit wide variation in radiosensitivity despite being irradiated under standard conditions. This indicates the presence of inherent factors influencing the radiation response of mammalian cells, which was clearly illustrated by the discovery that both lymphocytes and fibroblasts from patients with the genetic disorder ataxia-telangiectasia (AT) were a factor of 2 to 3 times more radiosensitive than their normal counterparts.[6] Similar radiosensitivity phenotypes are seen in cells from patients with a number of other disorders, including Nijmegen Breakage Syndrome.[7] This indicates that mutations or deletions in a particular gene (or genes) can markedly influence radiosensitivity. Subsequent studies (e.g., creation of mammalian cell mutants exhibiting marked radiosensitivity) and the discovery of the identity and function of many of these genes confirm the genetically determined contribution to radiosensitivity.

This led to the concept of "inherent radiosensitivity" for a cell line. This is not a unique value since several environmental factors, such as oxygen concentration and cell-cell contact, influence radiosensitivity. In addition, cells in different phases of the cell cycle and in different growth stages (log or plateau) have different "inherent" radiosensitivities. Studies comparing different tumors must therefore keep these factors constant. Under such standard conditions, it is then not unreasonable to expect that tumors comprising cells that are found to be inherently resistant to radiation will be more difficult to cure with radiotherapy than those comprising radiosensitive cells. It is also likely that patients with radiosensitive tumors may be overtreated by "conventional" radiotherapy, undergoing the unnecessary risk of excessive complications to normal tissue, while some radioresistant tumors are undertreated, and would benefit either from a higher dose, an added therapy, or an alternative therapy. The goal of predicting inherent sensitivity is thus to select out tumors at the extremes of the radiosensitivity spectrum for adjusted or alternative therapies, with the aim of improving cure rates of the population as a whole.

Cell-Based Assays

Several methods that have been tested in human tumors for measuring radiosensitivity for predictive purposes are listed in Table 4-1. The most relevant measure of radiosensitivity is based on the fraction of cells surviving a particular radiation dose, defined as the ability of a cell to undergo at least six doublings, thus forming a clone of at least 50 cells. This is termed the *colony-forming*, or *clonogenic*, assay. Indications that intrinsic radiosensitivity measured in this way has clinical relevance came first from Fertil and Malaise,[8] who analyzed published studies of in vitro radiosensitivities of tumor cell lines from different histologic types and found a correlation with clinical curability. This work was supported by

Table 4–1   Clinical Studies Correlating Outcome After Radiotherapy with Intrinsic Radiosensitivity Measured on Cells Taken from Primary Tumor Material Before Treatment and Irradiated and Assayed in Vitro

Tumor	Assay*	No. pts	Treatment	p-value	Reference
Head and neck	Colony	84	RT	0.036	Bjork-Eriksson et al[189]
Head and neck	Colony	38	RT	ns	Stausbol-Gron and Overgaard[190]
Head and neck	CAM*	56	RT, post-op RT	0.001	Girinsky et al[191]
Head and neck	CAM	40	Post-op RT	ns	Brock et al[192]
Cervix	Colony	128	RT	0.0002	West et al[12]

*Colony: colony formation (clonogenic) assay; CAM: population growth assay using dishes coated with Cell Adhesive Matrix.
RT, radiotherapy; post-op RT, post-operative radiotherapy; ns, not significant.

subsequent observations of Deacon and coworkers.[9] Further support came from mouse tumor studies showing that surviving fraction after 2 Gy (SF_2) in vitro correlated well with the response of the tumors in vivo to multiple fractions of 2 Gy.[10] These correlations supported the idea that in vitro radiosensitivity measurements may be able to predict outcome. In addition, the large spread in sensitivities of cell lines within any one tumor category indicated the need for a predictive assay, since histology or site alone was clearly an insufficient guide to radiosensitivity.

A summary of predictive assay studies for radiosensitivity is shown in Table 4-1. Some were rather small studies or those that included treatments other than radiotherapy. Three of these five studies showed a significant correlation with outcome. The most convincing study is that of West and colleagues[11,12] on cervix carcinomas treated by radiotherapy alone. Tumor SF_2 values were found to correlate highly with outcome (Fig. 4-1). Patients with tumors exhibiting SF_2 values higher than the median value (radioresistant) had significantly worse local control and significantly worse survival rates than did those with tumors with SF_2 values below the median. This trend was the same for all tumor stages (I, II, and III). Absolute differences in local control and survival rates

between the high and low radiosensitivity groups were between 20% and 30% at 3 years. Two of the larger studies on head and neck tumors also showed a positive correlation of in vitro radiosensitivity with local control. These clinical studies support the notion that in vitro measurements of radiosensitivity, with all their potential limitations, have relevance to the response of tumors in situ.

Although these results are promising, it is unlikely that either the colony or CAM (cell adhesive matrix) assays could be used as predictors for routine clinical application. First, they take several weeks to complete. This is unacceptably long for many radiotherapy departments, which must wait for a result before planning the definitive treatment. Second, they require a highly skilled laboratory team with extensive experience. For these reasons, other assays that are more rapid and more suitable for a routine clinical laboratory have been sought. These alternative assays are indirect (i.e., they measure parameters that should correlate with cell kill). DNA is the primary target for cell killing by ionizing radiation. Studies using radiomodifiers indicated that DSBs were more closely correlated with cell kill than single-strand breaks (SSBs) or base damage.[13] Many subsequent studies therefore concentrated on double-strand breaks (DSBs) as the most important DNA lesion, attempting to validate its relevance as a predictor for cell kill. Filter elution or gel electrophoresis techniques used for this purpose can be completed within a few days rather than the few weeks necessary for colony assays. Results of studies correlating DSB induction or repair with cell kill have been variable, some showing good correlations, others not. These discrepant results suggest that DSBs are probably not a reliable predictor of radiation-induced cell kill. It is likely that DSBs are necessary for kill but that other factors also play a role.[14] These include the fidelity of repair, how much damage a cell can tolerate, and membrane damage.

The induction of chromosome aberrations has long been a recognized effect of ionizing radiation. Aberrations include chromatid and chromosome types, depending on whether the cell had duplicated its DNA or not at the time of irradiation. These are manifested as fragments, translocations (dicentrics or reciprocal), rings, chromatid exchanges, gaps, complex types, and micronuclei. All of these manifestations are dose related. Many studies have investigated the relationship between the incidence of aberrations and cell kill. A constant relationship under different radiation conditions and for

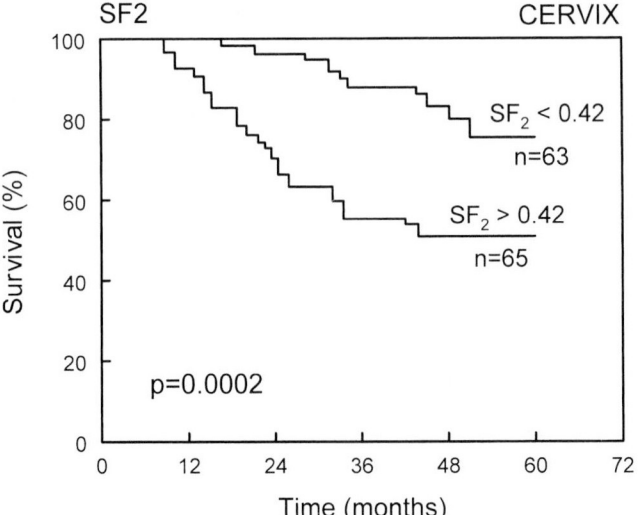

Figure 4–1. Prediction of radiotherapy outcome by intrinsic radiosensitivity measurements in vitro from pretreatment biopsies. Cells from cervix tumors in patients given radiotherapy were assayed for surviving fraction at 2 Gy (SF_2) by colony formation in soft agar. Patients with more sensitive tumors (lower than median SF_2) had significantly better survival.[12]

many different cell lines would mean that aberrations could be used to predict kill. This has therefore been proposed as a clonogenic assay alternative.[15] Chromosome aberrations, like DSBs, can be measured in a matter of days, satisfying the time requirement of a predictive assay. In addition, aberrations can be detected in cells after repair with doses markedly less than 1 Gy, making it a considerably more sensitive assay than those for DSBs.

Several studies have shown a good correlation between chromosome damage and cell kill,[16-20] supporting the notion that chromosome aberration frequencies could be used to predict radiosensitivity. Problems with conventional chromosome aberration assays include the need for metaphases and scoring by an experienced cytogeneticist. These could potentially be overcome by a combination of fluorescence in situ hybridization (FISH) and premature chromosome condensation (PCC).[15,21,22,23] PCC allows aberration detection in interphase cells, and FISH with a whole chromosome probe allows easy visualization of aberrations in a single chromosome. However, PCC yields from cells freshly extracted from human tumor biopsies are very low, rendering the technique impractical.[24] In summary, chromosome damage assays have many attractive features as predictors of radiosensitivity but are again unlikely to prove robust enough for routine clinical use.

Radiosensitivity Genes

The rapid growth in knowledge of oncogenes and tumor suppressor genes and in techniques for rapidly assessing gene expression and mutations has stimulated an ever increasing number of reports correlating these molecular parameters with prognosis. This raises the question of whether it would be possible to screen for expression or mutations of genes known to be involved in radioresistance. This would offer the possibility of a rapid test of radiosensitivity in individual tumors, which could easily be carried out between diagnosis and the start of treatment.

Numerous reports have looked at a specific gene or a small number of genes as predictors of outcome after radiotherapy. Two well-studied genes have been associated with radiosensitivity changes. The proto-oncogene *ras* has been found in some transfection studies to confer radioresistance on human cells.[25-28] Other studies have failed to show such an effect[29-31] and it has become clear that the genetic background of the cell—for example, which other oncogenes or suppressor genes are activated or mutated—plays an important role in determining the radiosensitivity phenotype when activated *ras* is introduced. Further studies point to the importance of the PI3 kinase pathway and Akt phosphorylation in the induction of radioresistance.[32] The tumor suppressor gene p53 has also been shown to influence the apoptotic response to agents including ionizing radiation, leading to the expectation that it would also influence radiosensitivity as measured in a colony assay. This has been found in some studies[33,34] but not in others.[35,36] While p53 can clearly influence the cell's response to radiation, the picture emerging from many preclinical and clinical studies is that p53 status alone is not an adequate predictor of the response of a tumor to radiation.[36,37] Many of these studies have used high levels of immunohistochemical staining as an indicator of mutant p53, although it has become clear that mutation analysis provides different and more accurate information[38-42] and often better prognostic information.[43,44]

The problem with the single gene approach is that multiple factors and pathways are known to influence the survival chance of a cell after irradiation. Complementation analysis with radiosensitive mutants shows that there are at least 11 complementation groups in mammalian cells[45-48] indicating the number of genes involved in rodent mutants screened so far. This is likely to increase as more studies are done, perhaps by several-fold. Indeed, the number of genes now known to be involved in the processes of the cell's handling of radiation damage has increased dramatically over the last few years. Genes include those involved in damage recognition and signaling, nonhomologous end-joining, homologous recombination, base excision repair, postreplication repair/translesion synthesis, apoptosis, cell cycle checkpoints, and others. Each of these involves multiple genes. It is likely that errors in some of these processes will dominate or occur more frequently than others, but accurate prediction of radiosensitivity from the expression or mutations in (subsets of) these genes or both will not be an easy task.

Repair of DNA DSBs is one of the most important processes determining survival after radiation. Nonhomologous end-joining is one of the main DSB repair pathways, involving the DNA-dependent protein kinase complex (comprising Ku70, Ku80, and DNA-PK$_{CS}$), XRCC4, and ligase IV genes.[49-52] In addition, the *ATM* gene (mutated in ataxia telangiectasia) is also a critical determinant of radiosensitivity, affecting checkpoint and DNA repair pathways.[53,54] Other genes involved in DSB repair are the Rad50/MRE11/NBS complex[55] and those involved in homologous recombination, including RAD51, RAD52, RAD54, BRCA2, and others.[56,57] Studies in tumor cell lines correlating expression of one or a few of these genes with radiosensitivity have shown mixed results, probably due to the many additional genes involved. Despite the obvious complexity, single gene studies related to radiosensitivity have shown predictive potential in the clinic (e.g., ku70[58]). However, using genetic data for radiosensitivity prediction is likely to become feasible only when the majority of relevant genes are simultaneously screened. This is now becoming a reality with array technology (see later).

PREDICTION OF REPOPULATION

Radiotherapy is not usually given as a single dose but rather as a series of fractions. These are usually separated by 1 day (daily fractionation), 3 days (weekends), or longer (planned or unplanned splits or gaps). During these gaps, cells that have survived the treatment up to that point have the opportunity to divide. This is good if it occurs in normal tissue, since the repopulation usually leads to tissue repair. It is bad if it occurs in a tumor, since more cells will need to be killed with subsequent radiation fractions. The consequence can be that some surviving tumor cells remain at the end of treatment, leading to a recurrence. Patients with tumors that are inherently rapidly dividing (short cell cycle, high growth fraction) are more at risk for failure than are slowly growing tumors, in which repopulation is small even over a conventional radiotherapy period of several weeks. Several clinical radiotherapy studies show that the chance of tumor control decreases with an increase in overall treatment time.[3-5,59-62] The obvious explanation lies in repopulation during treatment, in that a shorter treatment period means less repopulation. Patient selection influences some, but not all, of these studies, however, in that patients whose tumors have a worse prognosis are often treated with longer schedules.

A simple calculation illustrates the potential magnitude of the problem. Average potential doubling times of tumors (T_{pot}; doubling time of tumor cells in the absence of cell loss) are in the range of a few days. If the same rate occurred during radiotherapy, a T_{eff} (effective clonogen doubling time) of 3 days would allow approximately 13 doublings in a 6-week treatment, a factor of approximately 10^4. It is likely that the increase in cell number will be less than this since proliferation is inhibited by cell cycle progression delays induced by each fraction. There is also evidence of a lag time before maximum-rate repopulation begins, probably resulting from the time necessary for damage recognition after the process of cell death begins. However, it is clear that human tumor cells of many histological types have the capacity for doubling within a few days, and this could potentially reduce the chance of cure with therapies lasting many weeks.

The question is whether the tumors capable of rapid proliferation during treatment can be predicted and selected out before treatment begins. Several methods have been tried (Table 4-2). Counting the frequency of mitoses in tumor sections (the mitotic index, MI) is obvious and simple, although somewhat time consuming and subject to inaccuracies. MI and the labeling index (LI; fraction of thymidine or thymidine analogue-labeled cells) reflect the lengths of T_M and T_S (the mitotic and DNA synthesis times, respectively), relative to the total cell cycle, together with the proportion of cells in the cell cycle.[63]

Flow cytometry has advantages over counting cells under a microscope. It allows the measurement of many thousands of cells in less than 1 minute and can quantitatively measure cell properties using fluorescence and scatter properties. By using fluorescent dyes that bind to DNA, DNA histograms can be generated and analyzed for the fraction of cells in each cycle phase (G_1, S, and G_2/M). The flow cytometry parameter most frequently used for assessing tumor proliferation is the S phase fraction (SPF). Analogues of thymidine, bromodeoxyuridine (BrdU) and iododeoxyuridine (IdU), can also be used. They are incorporated into DNA during the S phase. Antibodies that recognize the small DNA structural distortions that occur when these analogues are incorporated have been developed.[64] Fluorescent conjugated antibodies allow the degree of analogue incorporation per cell to be rapidly measured by flow cytometry. Cell kinetics can be measured with this method in patients by injection or infusion of thymidine analogues at tracer doses showing no toxicity. The combination of thymidine analogues and flow cytometry allows rapid measurement of the LI. In addition, by taking samples a few hours after analogue administration, one can determine both the fraction of cells taking up the label (LI) and the rate of movement through the S phase (T_S).[65] The ratio of the two (T_S/LI) approximates the potential doubling time, T_{pot}, a parameter describing the cell number doubling time of a tumor population in the absence of cell loss.

The advantages of this method are first statistical, since tens of thousands of cells can easily be measured. Second, staining and measuring can be accomplished in 1 day. Third, a dynamic, or rate, parameter is derived rather than a static parameter such as an index, a theoretical advantage since tumors with the same MI or LI could have different proliferation rates due to a proportional increase in all phase lengths. Disadvantages include the inability to reliably distinguish malignant from nonmalignant cells in a biopsy. Aneuploidy often distinguishes the tumor population, but in the majority of

Table 4–2   Methods to Measure Tumor Cell Proliferation in Humans

Assay	Advantages*	Disadvantages
Mitotic index	Simple	Static parameter (MI)*
DNA histogram (FCM)	Rapid	Static parameters (phase fractions)
	Cell cycle phase fractions	
	Ploidy	
	SPF often poor correlation with LI	
BrdU/IdU (FCM)	Rapid	Analogue administration
	Direct measure of DNA synthesis	Poor distinction tumor/normal†
	LI, T_S, T_{pot} from one sample	
BrdU/IdU (IHC)	Rapid	Analogue administration
	Direct measure of DNA synthesis	Static parameter (LI)
	LI, Distinction normal/malignant	
Cell cycle markers (Ki67, PCNA, cyclin A, etc.) (IHC or FCM)	No drug administration	Static parameters

*Tumors with same MI or LI can have different cell cycle rates.
†Could be improved by using extra label specific or associated with tumor cells (e.g., cytokeratin)
BrdU, bromodeoxyuridine (thymidine analogue); FCM, flow cytometry; IdU, iododeoxyuridine (thymidine analogue); LI, labeling index (fraction of BrdU/IdU-labeled cells); MI, mitotic index (fraction of mitotic cells); SPF, S phase fraction (fraction cells with S phase DNA content); T_{pot}, potential doubling time ($\approx 0.8 \times T_S$/LI); T_S, DNA synthesis time.

cases an overlap remains, and in diploid tumors the overlap of tumor and nontumor cells is total. Possible solutions are to use a tumor cell-associated marker, such as cytokeratin antibodies, to distinguish the malignant cells,[66] or to count BrdU-labeled cells in tissue sections (morphologic distinction between normal and malignant cells) and combine it with a flow cytometric measurement of T_S.[67]

Finding a proliferation marker that does not require administration of a potentially toxic substance remains a worthwhile goal. Present markers include antibodies to Ki67 (cycle-specific), PCNA (S phase-specific),[68] cyclin A (S/G2 phase specific)[69,70] and DNA polymerase alpha (cycle-specific).[71] These all provide static, not rate, parameters and can be measured by either immunohistochemistry or flow cytometry. The rapidly increasing knowledge of cell cycle control gives hope that expression profiles that predict for proliferative capacity will be found.

There have been a few studies of sufficient magnitude to test cell kinetic measurements as predictors of outcome after radiotherapy. These have used T_{pot} measurements before the start of treatment as predictors. Only one Phase III randomized trial incorporating this predictor has been reported, a European EORTC study of accelerated versus conventional fractionation, in which approximately one-third of patients entered received the cell kinetic test. This study initially showed a significant difference between patients with short and long T_{pot} tumors who were given the conventional long (7.5 week) schedule.[72] Statistical significance was lost with greater patient numbers and longer follow-up, although the trend remained.[73] For patients treated with the accelerated (5 week) schedule, T_{pot} had no predictive value at all times tested. In a study of ultrashort fractionation, the 11-day CHART regimen, T_{pot} was found to have no predictive value, as expected in a schedule giving little chance for proliferation.[74] All these trials studied tumors in the head and neck region.

To obtain better statistics, data from T_{pot} studies in head and neck tumors in 11 different centers, including those described earlier, were pooled for 476 patients receiving radiotherapy alone given in an overall time of at least 6 weeks with a dose of at least 60 Gy.[75] A univariate analysis showed that only LI was significantly associated with local control (p <0.03; Fig. 4-2), with higher values correlating with a worse outcome. T_{pot} showed no trend (p <0.8). In a multivariate analysis of local control, LI lost its significance (p <0.16). Two potential confounding factors in this study are that each center carried out its own flow cytometry and analysis (rather than a standard reference center), and an adequate distinction between normal and malignant cells was not made in any of these data.

This multicenter analysis does not support the idea that the potential doubling time, T_{pot}, can predict repopulation during radiotherapy. However, one cannot conclude from these data that proliferation or repopulation are not important in determining outcome. Retrospective analyses of head and neck tumor data show that longer overall treatment times require the use of higher doses to achieve the same level of local

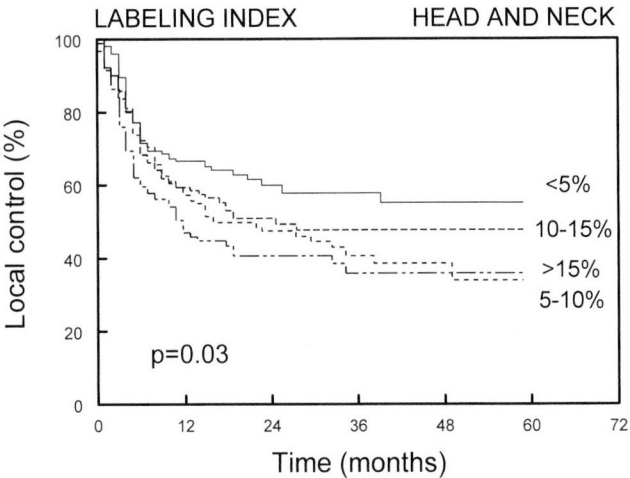

Figure 4–2. Predictive potential of labeling index (LI) measured by flow cytometry on biopsies from head and neck patients given IdU or BrdU. Data on 476 patients from a multicenter analysis of pretreatment cell kinetic parameters for conventional fractionation radiotherapy.[75] Patients with lower LI (slower proliferation) showed a significant trend for better local control (p=0.03), although significance was lost in a multivariate analysis (p=0.16). No other kinetic parameter did better, indicating present proliferation predictors are weak.

control.[59,62,76,77] Such analyses are subject to bias[61,78] and should be interpreted with caution. However, data from randomized trials of accelerated fractionation,[79,80] the Polish study of seven versus five fractions per week,[81] and a large RTOG study[3] support this notion by showing the value of shortening the overall treatment. It can therefore reasonably be concluded that repopulation of tumor cells during fractionated radiotherapy is an important negative factor influencing the chance of local control, but that we are not able to predict it with any certainty, either with T_{pot} or other single kinetic parameters. In addition to technical problems (inability to distinguish malignant and nonmalignant cells), possible reasons include the fact that pretreatment kinetics may not be directly related to kinetics during or after cytotoxic insults. For example, more differentiated tumors may have slow kinetics before treatment but be capable of rapid proliferation upon stimulation, similar to normal mucosa.[82] This would imply that differentiation must be taken into account together with proliferation parameter values to obtain accurate prediction. Prediction of the ability of a tumor to undergo accelerated proliferation in response to damage should also theoretically be feasible from expression profiles, including such genes as growth factor receptors and differentiation-related genes.

Ideally, measurements of proliferation during, and not before, treatment are desired, since this is when the damaging repopulation takes place. Labeling measurements can be made during treatment, but the data will be strongly dominated by doomed and dying cells that constitute the vast majority of cells after the first few 2 Gy fractions. Such measurements are therefore likely to be misleading, as shown in animal studies.[83] Until ways can be found to distinguish doomed but intact cells from surviving cells, measurements during treatment will remain unreliable at best, and often come too late to change treatment. It remains possible that changes in a cell kinetic parameter during treatment might correlate with outcome,[84] although this probably reflects less proliferation than radiosensitivity, for which more direct parameters are likely to be the more informative.

In summary, many studies have indicated the relevance and importance of predicting tumor proliferation for radiotherapy schedules 6 weeks or longer. Method improvements and better knowledge of the biology (e.g., role of cytokines and receptors in irradiated tissue) are now needed.

PREDICTION OF HYPOXIA

Hypoxia has a large influence on sensitivity to ionizing radiation, such that cells with oxygen concentrations below 1 to 2 mm Hg are 2 to 3 times more radioresistant. The importance of hypoxia in human tumors has been suggested by several findings, including the existence of tumor necrosis, known to be often associated with hypoxia[85] by direct measurement of hypoxia in human tumors using several techniques (see later), by the clinically observed correlation between anemia and outcome,[86-88] and by the success, albeit limited, of trials combining hyperbaric oxygen or hypoxic cell radiosensitizers with radiotherapy. A meta-analysis of such trials in which one of several methods to overcome hypoxia was employed has demonstrated an overall benefit compared with radiotherapy alone, indicating that tumor hypoxia can contribute to treatment failure after radiotherapy.[89] This is supported by a few trials in which oxygen measurements in individual patients' tumors have been correlated with radiotherapy outcome. This in turn suggests that oxygen measurement before treatment would aid the clinician in deciding whether or not to employ one of these antihypoxia methods. Examples of such methods would be the use of carbogen (95% oxygen + 5% CO_2) to overcome diffusion limited hypoxia,[90,91] nicotinamide to overcome transient hypoxia from blood vessel opening and closing,[92-94] hypoxic cell radiosensitizers such as nimorazole;[95] or bioreductive agents that selectively kill hypoxic cells;[96-100] increasing oxygen delivery by blood transfusions or fluorocarbons;[101-103] and, a future possibility, delivering gene-encoding toxins coupled to hypoxia-specific promoters.[96,104-107]

Table 4-3 lists methods that have been applied in the clinic, or are about to undergo clinical testing for measuring tumor hypoxia.[108] The most direct method is to use polarographic oxygen electrodes, which are thin probes that can be inserted into tumors and from which multiple measurements of oxygen tension can be made along a single electrode track. Median oxygen tension can be used as the parameter for comparison, or the fraction of values below 5 or 10 mm Hg (the "hypoxic fraction"). Such studies have been done on accessible tumors such as some head and neck tumors, neck node metastases, breast tumors, cervix tumors, and soft tissue sarcomas.[109-116] Nitroimidazoles have been shown to be selectively

Table 4–3   Methods to Measure Hypoxia in Human Tumors

Assay	Advantages	Disadvantages
Oxygen electrodes	Direct measure of O_2 tension	Invasive
		Accessible tumors only
		Influenced by necrosis and stroma
Nitroimadazoles: antibodies	Spatial information	Drug administration necessary
	IHC/IF or flow cytometry	Influenced by tumor enzyme levels
		Subject to sampling errors
Nitroimadazoles: radiolabeled*	Spatial information	Drug and radioactivity administration necessary
	IHC/IF flow cytometry	
	External scanning	Influenced by tumor enzyme levels
Endogenous markers† (e.g., HIF-1α, CAIX, VEGF)	No drug administration necessary	Can be subject to nonhypoxic regulation
		Subject to sampling errors
Comet assay	Measures radiobiological hypoxia	Requires at least 4 Gy-single dose in situ
	Individual cells	
Blood vessel parameters‡	Simple and cheap	Indirect
	Biopsy only	No distinction between functional and nonfunctional vessels
		Subject to sampling errors
Hemoglobin saturation	Biopsy only	Indirect
		No simple relationship with hypoxia fraction
MRS/MRI	Noninvasive	Resolution worse than IHC/IF
	Whole tumor measurement	BOLD measures changes, not absolute levels
PET§	Noninvasive	Resolution worse than IHC/IF
	Whole tumor measurement	
Bioluminescence	Spatial information	Indirect
		Energy status also nonoxygen dependent

*For example, ^{99}Tc for SPECT
†Genes up or down-regulated under hypoxia
‡Intercapillary distance, vascular density, diffusion limited fraction
§For example, with ^{18}F-nitroimidazoles
IHC, immunohistochemistry; IF, immunofluorescence; MRI, magnetic resonance imaging; MRS, magnetic resonance spectroscopy; PET, positron emission tomography.

reduced in and bind to hypoxic cells. Binding can be detected by the use of a labeled drug (such as in autoradiography,[117] SPECT,[118,119] or positron emission tomography for fluorinated drugs[120,121]) or by antibodies developed against bound products (immunohistochemistry/fluorescence, enzyme-linked immunosorbent assay, or flow cytometry[90,122-124]). A possible disadvantage is the dependence on enzymes responsible for nitro-reduction, which can vary between tumors and between normal tissues. Two of these nitroimadazoles, pimonidazole and EF5, are approved for human use and are undergoing predictive value tests.[124-126] Of interest is the report that the pimonidazole staining fraction in head and neck tumors does not appear to correlate with polarographic oxygen measurements in the same tumors.[125] Possible reasons include the influence of stroma and necrosis on the polarographic measurements, or that one method may be more influenced than the other by acute (fluctuating) hypoxia. Which will prove more useful or informative awaits the outcome of further clinical and preclinical tests.

There has been much recent interest and activity in endogenous hypoxia markers. Hypoxia affects the expression of various genes, both positively and negatively. The advantage of an endogenous marker is that it avoids the need to administer a drug. An example of such markers is HIF-1α (hypoxia inducible factor), which is a transcription factor component that is upregulated by protein stabilization under hypoxia.[127-129] In addition, there are various HIF1-dependent genes such as *VEGF* (vascular endothelial growth factor), *GLUT-1* and *-3* (regulating glucose transport), and *CAIX* (regulating pH).[130,131] These genes all contain a sequence in their promotors called a hypoxia responsive element (HRE), to which the HIF1 transcription factor binds, leading to expression of the target gene. There is much activity at the time of writing comparing intrinsic markers of hypoxia with both other methods for measuring hypoxia and radiotherapy outcome. Although no relationship has been seen between *VEGF* expression and measurements of hypoxia in human tumors,[132,133] promising data have been obtained using *CAIX*[134,135](Fig. 4-3) and *GLUT-1*.[136] In addition, measuring lactate levels in tumors (an endpoint of anaerobic glycolysis known to increase under hypoxia) has been shown to predict treatment outcome.[137]

The comet assay employs DNA electrophoresis of single cells and depends on the reduced radiation-induced DNA break induction in hypoxic cells.[138] For predictive purposes, a high enough single dose must be given to the patient, at least 4 Gy for good oxic/hypoxic discrimination, before the subsequently biopsied cells are assayed. The assay is fairly simple and quick to carry out and doesn't require drug or radioactivity administration. Three indirect methods for hypoxia involve blood vessels. The first measures the mean distance between capillaries in tumor sections.[139,140] The greater this distance, the greater the probability of development of diffusion-limited hypoxia. The second is the calculated fraction of tumor tissue greater than a typical diffusion distance away from the nearest vessel, called the Diffusion Limited Fraction.[141] The advantage of both is simplicity, although no distinction is made between functional (flowing) and nonfunctional vessels. The third method

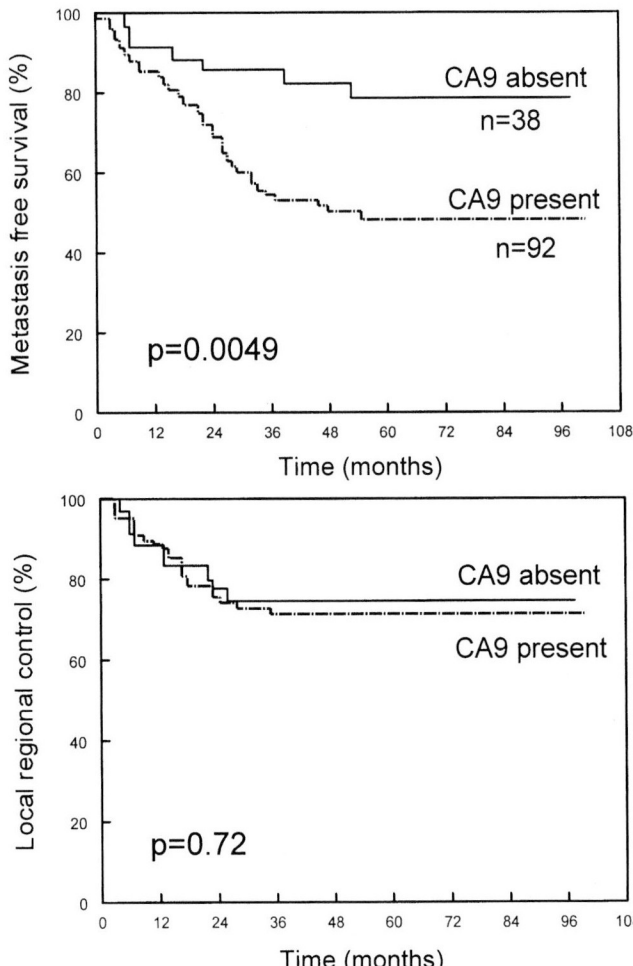

Figure 4–3. The presence or absence of the endogenous hypoxia marker carbonic anhydrase IX (CA9) significantly predicts metastasis-free survival but not local control in cervix tumors treated with radiotherapy.[135]

measures oxyhemoglobin saturation measured spectrophotometrically and requires quick-frozen material.[142] A disadvantage is that intertumoral variations in oxygen consumption and vascular density affect the relationship between oxyhemoglobin consumption and hypoxia.

Magnetic resonance imaging and spectroscopy have been used to indicate the degree of hypoxia. Measuring phosphorus energy state by adenosine triphosphate-inorganic phosphate (ATP/Pi) ratios using ^{31}P,[143] or lactate levels using ^{1}H[108] can give indirect information on oxygenation. More recently, the methods of BOLD (blood oxygen level dependent) and FLOOD (flow and oxygen dependent) contrast MR imaging have been tested in animals and patients to monitor changes in tumor oxygenation.[144-147] Accurate quantitation of hypoxia is not possible with these techniques although they could be useful in measuring relative changes occurring as a result of treatment, blood flow manipulation, carbogen breathing, etc.[144,148,149] Other methods being developed include fluorescence decay, near-infrared spectroscopy, electron spin resonance, and interstitial pressure.[108] Finally, it should be noted that none of the methods mentioned earlier can distinguish between clonogenic and nonclonogenic cells. Extrapolation from changes in the measured

Table 4–4   Eppendorf Polarographic Electrode Studies for Tumor Hypoxia

			Correlations of Pretreatment Measurements with Outcome			
Tumor Type	N	Treatment	Comments	Endpoint	p-value	Reference
Head/neck	35	RT		LC	0.018	Nordsmark et al[116]
	35	RT		S	ns	Eschwege et al[193]
	63	RT		LC/S	0.01/0.02	Brizel et al[194]
	35	RT		LC	0.04	Nordsmark et al*[187]
	134	RT/RT+CT		S	0.004	Rudat et al[195]
Cervix	89	RT, Su, CT		S	0.0039	Hockel et al[188]
	51	RT		DFS/LC	<0.02/0.053	Knocke et al[196]
	40	RT		DFS	0.006	Sundfor et al[197]
	106	RT	All pts	DFS	ns	Fyles et al[198]
	84	RT	Node neg pts	DFS	0.007	
Sarcoma	22	RT+HT		DFS	0.01	Brizel et al[199]
	28			DFS/S	0.05/0.01	Nordsmark et al[200]

*Independent confirmatory study of Nordsmark et al., 1996.
RT, radiotherapy; CT, chemotherapy; Su, surgery; HT, hyperthermia; DFS, disease-free survival; S, survival; LC, local control; ns, not significant.

hypoxia parameter occurring during treatment to reoxygenation patterns of the hypoxic, clonogenic cells cannot therefore be made with any degree of certainty.

Several studies have correlated results of direct or indirect measurements of pretreatment tumor hypoxia with outcome. Awwad and colleagues[140] used intercapillary distance as an indirect measure of hypoxia in carcinoma of the cervix uteri and found a significantly higher mean intercapillary distance in tumors that subsequently recurred after radiotherapy. Kolstad[139] measured human tumors using oxygen electrodes and found a good correlation between mean tumor oxygen tension and local recurrence after radiotherapy. Gatenby and coworkers[150] studied neck node metastases from squamous cell carcinomas of the head and neck using oxygen electrodes and correlated results with tumor volume response 3 months after completion of radiotherapy. They found a significantly lower mean oxygen tension in nonresponding tumors than in those showing a complete response.

Several studies have been performed with improved polarographic oxygen electrodes (Table 4-4; Fig. 4-4). The first of these was that of Höckel and colleagues,[113] who made up to 60 measurements along several tracks per tumor. They found a good correlation of pretreatment hypoxia (median oxygen tension above or below 10 mm Hg) with recurrence-free survival in cervix carcinoma patients treated with radiotherapy with or without another treatment modality. Other subsequent studies showed remarkable uniformity in that almost all found pretreatment oxygen tension to be a significant prognostic indicator. These include different tumor sites and all three major treatment modalities, although no sufficiently large series has been published for surgery alone or chemotherapy alone. However, when these two modalities are included, outcome correlations do not appear to worsen. Hypoxia could affect chemotherapy outcome through lower drug concentrations at hypoxic sites, and the fact that hypoxic cells tend to proliferate

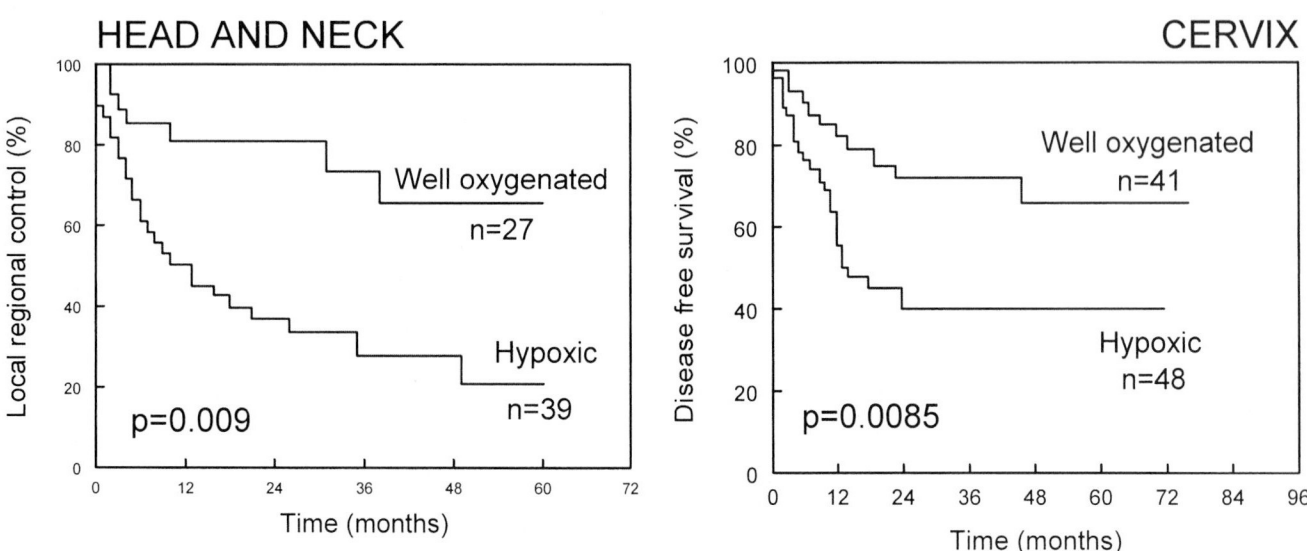

Figure 4–4. Predictive value of pretreatment hypoxia measurements made using Eppendorf oxygen electrodes in head and neck[187] and cervix[188] tumors. Both indicate that high pretreatment hypoxia is a significantly bad prognostic indicator.

slower, reducing the effectiveness of many drugs. Exposure to hypoxia can also lead both to selection of apoptosis-resistant cells[151,152] and consequently to malignant progression and an increase in metastatic capacity.[153-155] These may be contributing reasons why hypoxia is also a bad prognostic indicator for surgery.

In summary, these data collectively imply that hypoxia can limit cure of cancers by radiotherapy and other modalities in at least three sites, and that pretreatment hypoxia measurements with oxygen electrodes have prognostic significance. Results with more recently developed methods (e.g., exogenous and endogenous markers) are awaited with interest.

PREDICTION OF NORMAL TISSUE RADIOSENSITIVITY

Radiotherapy doses are unavoidably limited by the tolerance of normal tissues surrounding the tumor. In practice, doses are set at a level at which a small percentage of patients are expected to experience moderately severe treatment-induced complications. This small percentage may be, for example, the tail of a normal distribution of radiosensitivities within the patient population. Their unusual radiosensitivity may be determined genetically by the interplay of expression of the various genes, some known and some implied but not yet elucidated, that determine radiosensitivity. This would imply that the vast majority of patients could safely be given higher doses. In turn, this implies that if the sensitive subgroup could be detected by a simple test before treatment, doses could be lowered for this subgroup to reduce the risk of severe complications. More importantly, the dose for the rest of the patients could be increased, thereby increasing overall cure rates.[156,157] This forms the rationale for the search for predictors of normal tissue radiosensitivity.

Several studies have tested the relationship between the in vitro radiosensitivity of either fibroblasts or lymphocytes and the severity of normal tissue reactions. Burnet and colleagues[158] studied a small group of six patients from which fibroblasts were cultured from skin biopsies and tested for radiosensitivity in vitro by colony formation. A significant correlation was found between in vitro radiosensitivity and both early skin reactions and late reactions. Geara et al.[159] studied a series of 21 patients prospectively and found a significant correlation between fibroblast radiosensitivity and late reactions. Johansen and colleagues[160] similarly found a correlation between fibroblast radiosensitivity and late fibrosis. Begg and colleagues[161] found no correlation between in vitro fibroblast radiosensitivity and early reactions in a consecutive series of 24 patients. These and other studies indicated that colony survival of fibroblasts after in vitro irradiation may predict for late normal tissue damage, primarily fibrosis. However, two subsequent larger studies could not confirm the results of the smaller studies.[162,163] This does not, therefore, appear to be a robust predictor. In vitro radiosensitivity of lymphocytes, measured either by colony or cytogenetic assays, have been reported to predict normal tissue morbidity in some studies.[164,165]

Problems with cell-based assays include their technical difficulty and the long assay times. While they have been useful in showing that intrinsic radiosensitivity of somatic cells is probably a contributing cause to differences observed between patients in their reactions to radiotherapy, it is unlikely that they will be routinely useful as predictors for the two reasons just stated. In addition, intrinsic radiosensitivity is not the only determinant of radiation morbidity. Numerous biological factors influence treatment response, including the remodeling of tissues in vivo.[166] For several tissues (e.g., lung, skin, intestinal mucosa), the involvement of cytokine-mediated multicellular interactions are implicated,[167] including those mediated by interleukins 2 and 6 (IL-2, IL-6) and interferon alpha (IFN-α). Transforming growth factor beta (TGF-β) clearly also plays an important role in generating and modulating tissue fibrosis in many tissues and organs.[168,169] The renin-angiotensin system can also affect renal vasculature and its influence on the expression of radiation-induced renal damage, probably also involving TGF-β. Travis and colleagues[170,171] have shown that some mice strains have a greater genetic predisposition than others to develop radiation-induced lung and rectal fibrosis. Identification of the determinant genes will increase our understanding of the mechanism of radiation-induced fibrosis. These and similar studies are necessary for understanding the mechanisms of normal tissue radiation response other than the conventional radiobiological paradigm of target cell death and will ultimately lead to better prediction.

Analogous to tumors, response of normal tissues to radiation will be determined by multiple factors. With enough knowledge of the relevant genes and pathways, looking at expression or polymorphisms in a far wider range of genes than is now being done may provide a viable approach to predicting normal tissue morbidity (see later). Large microarray studies, analogous to those in tumors, have not yet been reported.

ARRAYS

One problem of most predictive assay studies to date is that they have usually been limited to the measurement of one, or at most, a few parameters. It is now abundantly clear that tumor and normal tissue responses are determined by the interplay of multiple factors. The expression of, or mutations in, a single gene, for example, is therefore highly unlikely to provide a robust predictor. The development of microarrays represents a major step forward in the ability to analyze the expression of thousands of genes simultaneously. mRNA extracted from biopsies is converted into cDNA, labeled with a fluorochrome and hybridized to an array (a matrix on a microscope slide of thousands of cDNAs or oligonucleotides representing known genes). Expression profiles of tumors generated in this way have provided greater prognostic power than classical clinical prognostic factors.[172,173] Expression profiles have also been developed to distinguish a high from a low chance of metastasis formation in young women with breast cancer (Fig. 4-5).[174] At the time of writing, no large study has been published demonstrating the value of expression profiles for predicting response of tumors to radiotherapy. However,

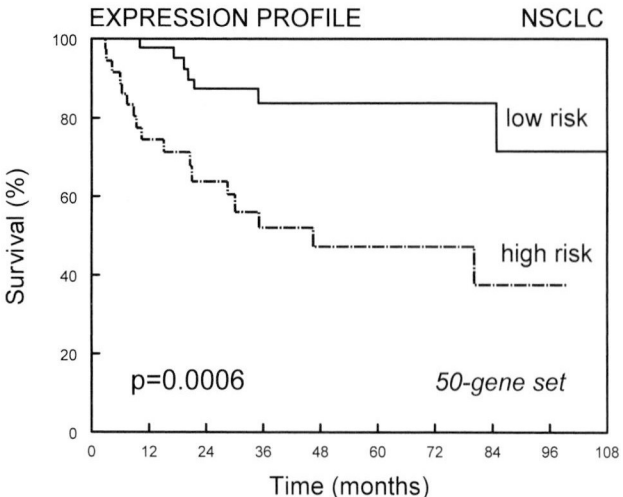

Figure 4–5. Gene expression profiles from oligonucleotide microarray analyses predict survival in stage 1 and 3 lung adenocarcinomas treated with surgery with or without adjuvant chemotherapy and radiotherapy.[173]

since these technologies allow the simultaneous study of genes associated with such characteristics as hypoxia, proliferation, radiosensitivity, and differentiation, it is feasible that expression profiles predicting radiation response will be found. Microarray technology is also applicable to normal tissues, as demonstrated by the studies of Quarmby[175] and Johnston.[176] Here, in addition to genes affecting radiosensitivity in terms of cell kill, those involved in various cytokine pathways are likely to be equally or more relevant. Other promising methodologies rapidly being developed for high throughput analysis are protein expression profiling (proteomics) and single nucleotide polymorphisms (SNP), the latter having the advantage that these DNA alterations will occur in all tissues, even readily accessible lymphocytes. Whether these methodologies will provide better predictive power than mRNA expression profiles remains to be seen.

ACTION BASED ON ASSAY RESULTS

The obvious question concerning the use of predictive assays is, what action should be taken based on assay result? It should be emphasized at the outset that prospective trials should be done only after an assay or assays have been sufficiently validated in retrospective trials, and this has so far not been done with the assays described. However, if assays for intrinsic radiosensitivity, proliferation, and hypoxia were validated and made sufficiently reliable and simple to use routinely, how should they influence the choice of treatment?

The answer is simplest for repopulation in which accelerated radiotherapy (shorter overall treatment time) is the obvious choice to minimize the number of possible divisions for rapidly proliferating tumors. Treatments shorter than 4 to 5 weeks must be accompanied by a dose reduction to reduce the chance of unacceptable early reactions in proliferating normal tissues such as buccal mucosa. Slowly proliferating tumors would be disadvantaged by any dose reduction accompanying acceleration

and could therefore be treated with conventional schedules, with or without concomitant chemotherapy (depending on institute policy), or with hyperfractionation to effectively increase the tumor dose.

For hypoxia, several options are available for high hypoxic fraction tumors. The main ones are the use of a chemical hypoxic cell radiosensitizer such as nimorazole,[95] or carbogen with or without nicotinamide, which is undergoing clinical testing.[177-180] An alternative approach to radiosensitizing the hypoxic cells would be to selectively kill them using a bioreductive agent. This approach is also undergoing extensive clinical testing.[97,181-185]

The question is more complicated for intrinsic radiosensitivity. If the tumor is radiosensitive, it is likely that a conventional fractionation scheme with conventional doses (e.g., 1.8-2.0 Gy per fraction, 60-70 Gy total) will be successful. If the tumor is extremely radiosensitive, there is also a possibility that the patient is genetically radiosensitive and a normal tissue test should be done (likely to be a rare event). If the tumor is resistant, adjuvant treatments could be considered, or highly conformal radiotherapy allowing an increased dose to the tumor. Changing the fractionation scheme is also a possibility, although usually no information on survival curve shape on which to base such a change is available. Even if a whole survival curve were carried out, translation of an in vitro curve shape (α/β ratio) to in vivo must be regarded as hazardous. If the tumor is extremely radioresistant, radiotherapy may not be the best treatment choice and an alternative modality should be considered.

For normal tissues, lower total doses could be considered for highly radiosensitive patients and somewhat increased doses for highly resistant patients. It must again be emphasized that the assays must be proven reliable if treatment choices are to be based on them.

THE FUTURE

Many assays tested to date have shown significant correlations with outcome in some studies, demonstrating proof of principle. Examples include SF_2 for radiosensitivity and oxygen electrode determinations for hypoxia. Most of these assays, however, have not proved robust, practical, or successful enough for use as routine assays on a wide scale. This is particularly true for cell-based assays (e.g., colony assays of tumor cells, fibroblasts or lymphocytes, chromosome damage assays). In addition, many assays suffer from the difficulty of distinguishing tumor cells from nonmalignant cells within the tumor volume. Often this can potentially be overcome by use of separation methods (analytical or physical).

However, a chief disadvantage remains, which is that most of the assays are limited to measuring one factor or parameter. This means that other biological factors known to affect outcome remain unexplored. The solution of applying multiple different assays to one patient is often impractical or impossible because of burden to the patient and the limited amount of tumor material available. Another factor to be considered is how biologically informative a predictive test is. For example, if a tumor were found to have a high SF_2, demonstrating resistance, this does not indicate why that tumor is radioresistant. The choice of therapy, therefore, remains somewhat arbitrary (although the patient could be considered for more aggressive or alternative treatments). The information gained in studies applying such a predictor is therefore limited, and will not ultimately provide a greater understanding of the response of tumors to therapy. What is needed for better prediction and ultimately improving therapy is a greater knowledge of the biology governing treatment response. This means harnessing all the powerful molecular, biochemical, and cell biological tools in the study of radiation damage to tumors and normal tissues.

Techniques such as microarrays are likely to play an important role, having the dual advantages of measuring multiple biological characteristics, and providing clues as to what genes are important in determining response. This may, in turn, provide potential leads for drug development. Protein expression and tissue array technologies are also undergoing rapid development, and may provide useful complements to cDNA or oligomer arrays in the near future. Analysis of such large data sets remains a challenging issue, but this area of bioinformatics is also undergoing rapid development and progress. Initial clinical studies will continue to employ tens of thousands of genes to look for a predictive expression profile for a particular disease and treatment. However, the profile itself may contain only tens or hundreds of genes. It can therefore be expected that once such an expression profile has been found, far simpler and cheaper "predictive chips" can be manufactured on a large scale for routine use. The few successes of array technology to date in the area of cancer prognostics give hope for the future, although this must be accompanied by good radio- and molecular-biologic studies aimed at a better understanding of tumor and tissue response. This will enable the development of strategies directed at intervention and modulation of tumor and normal tissue response, leading hopefully to improved therapeutic ratios for radiotherapy schedules given with curative intent.

For the "classical" biologic predictors, the immediate future is mixed. No rapid, robust assay for intrinsic radiosensitivity has yet been developed or tested. The future probably lies in gene profiling technology. Assays for proliferation have suffered mixed fortunes, with the simpler immunohistochemistry approaches with static markers appearing to be no worse than flow cytometry measurements and dynamic parameters. However, no parameter has yet proven to be a robust predictor. The rapidly increasing knowledge of cell cycle and growth factor control gives hope that not only pretreatment but also during-treatment proliferation will be predictable with suitable genetic tests or immunohistochemistry with multiple markers, or both. For hypoxia, the field continues to excite, with increasing knowledge of the biology, its importance for treatment outcome, and the genes involved, leading to a burgeoning choice of endogenous markers. This is running in parallel to successful application of exogenous markers, and considerable progress in the development of external scanning methods. In the future, gene expression profiling may deliver a "hypoxia signature," which could supersede present methods, but there is sufficient promise in the present methods to vigorously continue their testing.

For normal tissue response prediction, as with tumor response prediction, cell-based assays hold little promise for routine use, despite having provided useful information in the past (not rapid or robust enough; single parameter only; concentration on cell kill). Future efforts need to depend on progress in understanding the fundamental biology of radiation pathogenesis. For example, radiation can stimulate cytokine release from various cells, including endothelial cells, leading to increased vascular permeability, increased platelet adhesion, increased leucocyte adhesion, and invasion. These can, in turn, lead to short- and long-term disturbances in normal tissue function resulting from vascular damage. Prediction of specific types of normal tissue damage may therefore require more sophisticated tests in the future, concentrating on functional changes in different cell types rather than colony-forming ability. High throughput array technology may also help here (e.g., enabling single nucleotide polymorphisms [SNP] in a number of relevant genes in these processes to be simultaneously assessed).

SUMMARY

The four main factors likely to be relevant for predicting outcome after radiation therapy are intrinsic tumor cell radiosensitivity, normal tissue radiosensitivity, tumor hypoxia, and tumor cell proliferation. Positive correlations with outcome have been reported for all four parameters, measured by clonogenic assays, oxygen electrodes, and BrdU/IdU-flow cytometry, although large variability in results has been seen between studies for most parameters. The most consistent results have come from the oxygen electrode studies. Whatever the deficiencies of current assays or attempts to employ them, clinical and preclinical data strongly support the importance of all these factors in determining therapy outcome. The challenge remains to find rapid and robust ways to predict them in individual patients. In the future, emphasis will need to be on two aspects: (1) the multifactorial nature of the response to radiation, inevitably requiring evaluation of many factors concurrently, and (2) gaining a more fundamental knowledge of the molecular processes involved, facilitating the choice of factors to maximize the chance of accurate prediction. On a final note, it should not be forgotten that one of the most robust predictors of radiotherapy outcome is simply the size of the tumor.[186] This does not indicate the way ahead for biologists or clinicians in the future, but it should always be taken into account when assessing other potential predictive assays.

REFERENCES

1. Cox JD, Pajak TF, Asbell S, et al: Interruptions of high-dose radiation therapy decrease long-term survival of favorable patients with unresectable non-small cell carcinoma of the lung: Analysis of 1244 cases from 3 Radiation Therapy Oncology Group (RTOG) trials. *Int J Radiat Oncol Biol Phys.* 1993;27:493.

2. Horiot JC, Begg AC, Le Fur R, et al: Present status of EORTC trials of hyperfractionated and accelerated radiotherapy on head and neck carcinoma. *Recent Results Cancer Res.* 1994;134:111.

3. Fu KK, Pajak TF, Trotti A, et al: A Radiation Therapy Oncology Group (RTOG) phase III randomized study to compare hyperfractionation and two variants of accelerated fractionation to standard fractionation radiotherapy for head and neck squamous cell carcinomas: First report of RTOG 9003. *Int J Radiat Oncol Biol Phys.* 2000;48:7.

4. Peters LJ, Ang KK, Thames HD, Jr: Accelerated fractionation in the radiation treatment of head and neck cancer. A critical comparison of different strategies. *Acta Oncol.* 1988;27:185.

5. Skladowski K, Maciejewski B, Golen M, et al: Randomized clinical trial on 7-day-continuous accelerated irradiation (CAIR) of head and neck cancer—Report on 3-year tumour control and normal tissue toxicity. *Radiother Oncol.* 2000;55:101.

6. Taylor AM, Harnden DG, Arlett CF, et al: Ataxia telangiectasia: A human mutation with abnormal radiation sensitivity. *Nature.* 1975;258:427.

7. Gatti RA: The inherited basis of human radiosensitivity. *Acta Oncol.* 2001;40:702.

8. Fertil B, Malaise EP: Intrinsic radiosensitivity of human cell lines is correlated with radioresponsiveness of human tumors: analysis of 101 published survival curves. *Int J Radiat Oncol Biol Phys.* 1985;11:1699.

9. Deacon J, Peckham MJ, Steel GG: The radioresponsiveness of human tumours and the initial slope of the cell survival curve. *Radiother Oncol.* 1984;2:317.

10. Bristow RG, Hill RP: Comparison between in vitro radiosensitivity and in vivo radioresponse in murine tumor cell lines. II: In vivo radioresponse following fractionated treatment and in vitro/in vivo correlations. *Int J Radiat Oncol Biol Phys.* 1990;18:331.

11. West CM, Davidson SE, Roberts SA, et al: Intrinsic radiosensitivity and prediction of patient response to radiotherapy for carcinoma of the cervix. *Br J Cancer.* 1993;68:819.

12. West CM, Davidson SE, Roberts SA, et al: The independence of intrinsic radiosensitivity as a prognostic factor for patient response to radiotherapy of carcinoma of the cervix. *Br J Cancer.* 1997;76:1184.

13. Radford IR: Evidence for a general relationship between the induced level of DNA double-strand breakage and cell-killing after X-irradiation of mammalian cells. *Int J Radiat Biol Relat Stud Phys Chem Med.* 1986;49:611.

14. McMillan TJ, Tobi S, Mateos S, et al: The use of DNA double-strand break quantification in radiotherapy. *Int J Radiat Oncol Biol Phys.* 2001;49:373.

15. Brown JM, Evans J, Kovacs MS: The prediction of human tumor radiosensitivity in situ: An approach using chromosome aberrations detected by fluorescence in situ hybridization. *Int J Radiat Oncol Biol Phys.* 1992;24:279.

16. Carrano AV: Chromosome aberrations and radiation-induced cell death. II. Predicted and observed cell survival. *Mutat Res.* 1973;17:355.

17. Dewey WC, Miller HH, Leeper DB: Chromosomal aberrations and mortality of x-irradiated mammalian cells: Emphasis on repair. *Proc Natl Acad Sci U S A.* 1971;68:667.

18. Cornforth MN, Bedford JS: A quantitative comparison of potentially lethal damage repair and the rejoining of interphase chromosome breaks in low passage normal human fibroblasts. *Radiat Res.* 1987;111:385.

19. Bedford JS: Sublethal damage, potentially lethal damage, and chromosomal aberrations in mammalian cells exposed to ionizing radiations. *Int J Radiat Oncol Biol Phys.* 1991;21:1457.

20. Coco-Martin JM, Mooren E, Ottenheim C, et al: Potential of radiation-induced chromosome aberrations to predict radiosensitivity in human tumour cells. *Int J Radiat Biol.* 1999;75:1161.

21. Iliakis GE, Pantelias GE: Production and repair of chromosome damage in an X-ray sensitive CHO mutant visualized and analysed in interphase using the technique of premature chromosome condensation. *Int J Radiat Biol.* 1990;57:1213.

22. Evans JW, Chang JA, Giaccia AJ, et al: The use of fluorescence in situ hybridisation combined with premature chromosome condensation for the identification of chromosome damage. *Br J Cancer.* 1991;63:517.

23. Coco-Martin JM, Begg AC: Detection of radiation-induced chromosome aberrations using fluorescence in situ hybridization in drug-induced premature chromosome condensations of tumour cell lines with different radiosensitivities. *Int J Radiat Biol.* 1997;71:265.

24. Begg AC, Sprong D, Balm A, et al: Premature chromosome condensation and cell separation studies in biopsies from head and neck tumors for radiosensitivity prediction. *Radiother Oncol.* 2002;62:335.

25. McKenna WG, Weiss MC, Endlich B, et al: Synergistic effect of the v-myc oncogene with H-ras on radioresistance. *Cancer Res.* 1990;50:97.

26. Samid D, Miller AC, Rimoldi D, et al: Increased radiation resistance in transformed and nontransformed cells with elevated ras proto-oncogene expression. *Radiat Res.* 1991;126:244.

27. Sklar MD: The ras oncogenes increase the intrinsic resistance of NIH 3T3 cells to ionizing radiation. *Science.* 1988;239:645.

28. Ling CC, Endlich B: Radioresistance induced by oncogenic transformation. *Radiat Res.* 1989;120:267.

29. Mendonca MS, Boukamp P, Stanbridge EJ, et al: The radiosensitivity of human keratinocytes: Influence of activated c-H-ras oncogene expression and tumorigenicity. *Int J Radiat Biol.* 1991;59:1195.

30. Russell J, Khan MZ, Kerr DJ, et al: The effect of transfection with the oncogenes H-ras and c-myc on the radiosensitivity of a mink epithelial cell line. *Radiat Res.* 1992;130:113.

31. Garden AS, Meyn RE, Weil MM, et al: The influence of ras oncogene expression on radiation response in the Rat-1 cell. *Int J Radiat Biol.* 1992;62:307.

32. Gupta AK, McKenna WG, Weber CN, et al: Local recurrence in head and neck cancer: Relationship to radiation resistance and signal transduction. *Clin Cancer Res.* 2002;8:885.

33. McIlwrath AJ, Vasey PA, Ross GM, et al: Cell cycle arrests and radiosensitivity of human tumor cell lines: Dependence on wild-type p53 for radiosensitivity. *Cancer Res.* 1994;54:3718.

34. Bristow RG, Jang A, Peacock J, et al: Mutant p53 increases radioresistance in rat embryo fibroblasts simultaneously transfected with HPV16-E7 and/or activated H-ras. *Oncogene.* 1994;9:1527.

35. Slichenmyer WJ, Nelson WG, Slebos RJ, et al: Loss of a p53-associated G1 checkpoint does not decrease cell survival following DNA damage. *Cancer Res.* 1993;53:4164.

36. Brachman DG, Beckett M, Graves D, et al: p53 mutation does not correlate with radiosensitivity in 24 head and neck cancer cell lines. *Cancer Res.* 1993;53:3667.

37. Dahm-Daphi J: p53: Biology and role for cellular radiosensitivity. *Strahlenther Onkol.* 2000;176:278.

38. Kaserer K, Schmaus J, Bethge U, et al: Staining patterns of p53 immunohistochemistry and their biological significance in colorectal cancer. *J Pathol.* 2000;190:450.

39. Gao JP, Uchida T, Wang C, et al: Relationship between p53 gene mutation and protein expression: Clinical significance in transitional cell carcinoma of the bladder. *Int J Oncol.* 2000;16:469.

40. Oka T, Sarker AB, Teramoto N, et al: p53 protein expression in non-Hodgkin's lymphomas is infrequently related to p53 gene mutations. *Pathol Int.* 1998;48:15.

41. Top B, Mooi WJ, Klaver SG, et al: Comparative analysis of p53 gene mutations and protein accumulation in human non–small-cell lung cancer. *Int J Cancer.* 1995;64:83.

42. Kropveld A, Slootweg PJ, van Mansfeld AD, et al: Radioresistance and p53 status of T2 laryngeal carcinoma. Analysis by immunohistochemistry and denaturing gradient gel electrophoresis. *Cancer.* 1996;78:991.

43. Mineta H, Borg A, Dictor M, et al: p53 mutation, but not p53 overexpression, correlates with survival in head and neck squamous cell carcinoma. *Br J Cancer.* 1998;78:1084.

44. Alsner J, Sorensen SB, Overgaard J: TP53 mutation is related to poor prognosis after radiotherapy, but not surgery, in squamous cell carcinoma of the head and neck. *Radiother Oncol.* 2001;59:179.

45. Jeggo PA, Tesmer J, Chen DJ: Genetic analysis of ionising radiation sensitive mutants of cultured mammalian cell lines. *Mutat Res.* 1991;254:125.

46. Kraakman-van der Zwet M, Overkamp WJ, van Lange RE, et al: Brca2 (XRCC11) deficiency results in radioresistant DNA synthesis and a higher frequency of spontaneous deletions. *Mol Cell Biol.* 2002;22:669.

47. Zdzienicka MZ: Isolation of mutagen-sensitive Chinese hamster cell lines by replica plating. *Methods Mol Biol.* 1999;113:49.

48. Zdzienicka MZ: Molecular processes and radiosensitivity. *Strahlenther Onkol.* 1997;173:457.
49. Taccioli GE, Gottlieb TM, Blunt T, et al: Ku80: Product of the XRCC5 gene and its role in DNA repair and V(D)J recombination. *Science.* 1994;265:1442.
50. Blunt T, Finnie NJ, Taccioli GE, et al: Defective DNA-dependent protein kinase activity is linked to V(D)J recombination and DNA repair defects associated with the murine scid mutation. *Cell.* 1995;80:813.
51. Jeggo PA: DNA breakage and repair. *Adv Genet.* 1998; 38:185.
52. Critchlow SE, Jackson SP: DNA end-joining: From yeast to man. *Trends Biochem Sci.* 1998;23:394.
53. Jeggo PA, Carr AM, Lehmann AR: Splitting the ATM: distinct repair and checkpoint defects in ataxia-telangiectasia. *Trends Genet.* 1998;14:312.
54. Savitsky K, Bar-Shira A, Gilad S, et al: A single ataxia telangiectasia gene with a product similar to PI-3 kinase. *Science.* 1995;268:1749.
55. Carney JP, Maser RS, Olivares H, et al: The hMre11/hRad50 protein complex and Nijmegen breakage syndrome: Linkage of double-strand break repair to the cellular DNA damage response. *Cell.* 1998;93:477.
56. Karran P: DNA double-strand break repair in mammalian cells. *Curr Opin Genet Dev.* 2000;10:144.
57. Haber JE: Partners and pathways repairing a double-strand break. *Trends Genet.* 2000;16:259.
58. Wilson CR, Davidson SE, Margison GP, et al: Expression of Ku70 correlates with survival in carcinoma of the cervix. *Br J Cancer.* 2000;83:1702.
59. Withers HR, Taylor JM, Maciejewski B: The hazard of accelerated tumor clonogen repopulation during radiotherapy. *Acta Oncol.* 1988;27:131.
60. Overgaard J, Hjelm-Hansen M, Johansen LV, et al: Comparison of conventional and split-course radiotherapy as primary treatment in carcinoma of the larynx. *Acta Oncol.* 1988;27:147.
61. Bentzen SM, Thames HD: Clinical evidence for tumor clonogen regeneration: Interpretations of the data. *Radiother Oncol.* 1991;22:161.
62. Fowler JF, Lindstrom MJ: Loss of local control with prolongation in radiotherapy. *Int J Radiat Oncol Biol Phys.* 1992;23:457.
63. Steel GG, Adam K: Enhancement by cytotoxic agents of artificial pulmonary metastasis. *Br J Cancer.* 1997;36:653.
64. Gratzner HG: Monoclonal antibody to 5-bromo- and 5-iodo-deoxyuridine: A new reagent for detection of DNA replication. *Science.* 1982;218:474.
65. Begg AC, McNally NJ, Shrieve DC, et al: A method to measure the duration of DNA synthesis and the potential doubling time from a single sample. *Cytometry.* 1985;6:620.
66. Begg AC, Hofland I: Cell kinetic analysis of mixed populations using three-color fluorescence flow cytometry. *Cytometry.* 1991;12:445.
67. Bennett MH, Wilson GD, Dische S, et al: Tumour proliferation assessed by combined histological and flow cytometric analysis: Implications for therapy in squamous cell carcinoma in the head and neck. *Br J Cancer.* 1992;65:870.
68. Celis JE, Bravo R, Larsen PM, et al: Cyclin: A nuclear protein whose level correlates directly with the proliferative state of normal as well as transformed cells. *Leuk Res.* 1984;8:143.
69. Juan G, Li X, Darzynkiewicz Z: Correlation between DNA replication and expression of cyclins A and B1 in individual MOLT-4 cells. *Cancer Res.* 1997;57:803.
70. Oliver RJ, MacDonald DG: Comparison of BrdU and cyclin A as markers of the S-phase in oral precancerous lesions. *J Oral Pathol Med.* 2000;29:426.
71. Wahl AF, Geis AM, Spain BH, et al: Gene expression of human DNA polymerase alpha during cell proliferation and the cell cycle. *Mol Cell Biol.* 1988;8:5016.
72. Begg AC, Hofland I, Moonen L, et al: The predictive value of cell kinetic measurements in a European trial of accelerated fractionation in advanced head and neck tumors: An interim report. *Int J Radiat Oncol Biol Phys.* 1990;19:1449.
73. Begg AC, Hofland I, Van Glabbeke M, et al: Predictive value of potential doubling time for radiotherapy of head and neck tumor patients: results from the EORTC cooperative trial 22851. *Semin Rad Oncol.* 1992;1:22.
74. Lochrin CA, Wilson GD, McNally NJ, et al: Tumor cell kinetics, local tumor control, and accelerated radiotherapy: A preliminary report. *Int J Radiat Oncol Biol Phys.* 1992;24:87.

75. Begg AC, Haustermans K, Hart AA, et al: The value of pretreatment cell kinetic parameters as predictors for radiotherapy outcome in head and neck cancer: A multicenter analysis. *Radiother Oncol.* 1999;50:13.
76. Amdur RJ, Parsons JT, Mendenhall WM, et al: Split-course versus continuous-course irradiation in the postoperative setting for squamous cell carcinoma of the head and neck. *Int J Radiat Oncol Biol Phys.* 1989;17:279.
77. Taylor JM, Withers HR, Mendenhall WM: Dose-time considerations of head and neck squamous cell carcinomas treated with irradiation. *Radiother Oncol.* 1990;17:95.
78. Dubben HH: No clinical evidence for the influence of overall treatment time on TCD_{50} of head and neck tumours. *Radiother Oncol.* 1992;25:142.
79. Horiot JC, Bontemps P, Van Den Bogaert W, et al: Accelerated fractionation (AF) compared to conventional fractionation (CF) improves loco-regional control in the radiotherapy of advanced head and neck cancers: Results of the EORTC 22851 randomized trial. *Radiother Oncol.* 1997;44:111.
80. Saunders M, Dische S, Barrett A, et al: Continuous, hyperfractionated, accelerated radiotherapy (CHART) versus conventional radiotherapy in non–small cell lung cancer: Mature data from the randomised multicentre trial. CHART Steering committee. *Radiother Oncol.* 1999;52:137.
81. Chapman JD, Coia LR, Stobbe CC, et al: Prediction of tumour hypoxia and radioresistance with nuclear medicine markers . *Br J Cancer Suppl.* 1996;27:S204.
82. Hansen O, Overgaard J, Hansen HS, et al: Importance of overall treatment time for the outcome of radiotherapy of advanced head and neck carcinoma: dependency on tumor differentiation. *Radiother Oncol.* 1997;43:47.
83. Begg AC, Hofland I, Kummermehr J: Tumour cell repopulation during fractionated radiotherapy: Correlation between flow cytometric and radiobiological data in three murine tumours. *Eur J Cancer.* 1991;27:537.
84. Zackrisson B, Flygare P, Gustafsson H, et al: Cell kinetic changes in human squamous cell carcinomas during radiotherapy studied using the in vivo administration of two halogenated pyrimidines. *Eur J Cancer.* 2002;38:1100.
85. Thomlinson RH, Gray LH: The histological structure of some human lung cancers as the possible implications for radiotherapy. *Brit J Cancer.* 1955;9:539.
86. Dische S: Radiotherapy and anaemia—The clinical experience. *Radiother Oncol.* 1991;20 Suppl 1:35.
87. Bush RS: The significance of anemia in clinical radiation therapy. *Int J Radiat Oncol Biol Phys.* 1986;12:2047.
88. Vaupel P, Thews O, Hoeckel M: Treatment resistance of solid tumors: role of hypoxia and anemia. *Med Oncol.* 2001;18:243.
89. Overgaard J, Horsman MR: Modification of hypoxia-induced radioresistance in tumors by the use of oxygen and sensitizers. *Semin Radiat Oncol.* 1996;6:10.
90. Rojas A, Joiner MC, Hodgkiss RJ, et al: Enhancement of tumor radiosensitivity and reduced hypoxia-dependent binding of a 2-nitroimidazole with normobaric oxygen and carbogen: A therapeutic comparison with skin and kidneys. *Int J Radiat Oncol Biol Phys.* 1992;23:361.
91. Suit HD, Marshall N, Woerner D: Oxygen, oxygen plus carbon dioxide, and radiation therapy of a mouse mammary carcinoma. *Cancer.* 1972;30:1154.
92. Chaplin DJ, Horsman MR, Trotter MJ: Effect of nicotinamide on the microregional heterogeneity of oxygen delivery within a murine tumor. *J Natl Cancer Inst.* 1990;82:672.
93. Chaplin DJ, Horsman MR, Siemann DW: Further evaluation of nicotinamide and carbogen as a strategy to reoxygenate hypoxic cells in vivo: Importance of nicotinamide dose and pre-irradiation breathing time. *Br J Cancer.* 1993;68:269.
94. Laurence VM, Ward R, Dennis IF, et al: Carbogen breathing with nicotinamide improves the oxygen status of tumours in patients. *Br J Cancer.* 1995;72:198.
95. Overgaard J, Hansen HS, Overgaard M, et al: A randomized double-blind phase III study of nimorazole as a hypoxic radiosensitizer of primary radiotherapy in supraglottic larynx and pharynx carcinoma. Results of the Danish Head and Neck Cancer Study (DAHANCA) Protocol 5-85. *Radiother Oncol.* 1998;46:135.
96. Brown JM, Giaccia AJ: Tumour hypoxia: The picture has changed in the 1990s. *Int J Radiat Biol.* 1994;65:95.

97. Zeman EM, Brown JM, Lemmon MJ, et al: SR-4233: a new bioreductive agent with high selective toxicity for hypoxic mammalian cells. *Int J Radiat Oncol Biol Phys.* 1986;12:1239.

98. Stratford IJ, O'Neill P, Sheldon PW, et al: RSU 1069, a nitroimidazole containing an aziridine group. Bioreduction greatly increases cytotoxicity under hypoxic conditions. *Biochem Pharmacol.* 1986;35:105.

99. Brown JM, Giaccia AJ: The unique physiology of solid tumors: opportunities (and problems) for cancer therapy. *Cancer Res.* 1998;58:1408.

100. Rischin D, Peters L, Hicks R, et al: Phase I trial of concurrent tirapazamine, cisplatin, and radiotherapy in patients with advanced head and neck cancer. *J Clin Oncol.* 2001;19:535.

101. Teicher BA: Use of perfluorochemical emulsions in cancer therapy. *Biomater Artif Cells Immobilization Biotechnol.* 1992;20:875.

102. Evans RG, Kimler BF, Morantz RA, et al: Lack of complications in long-term survivors after treatment with Fluosol and oxygen as an adjuvant to radiation therapy for high-grade brain tumors. *Int J Radiat Oncol Biol Phys.* 1993;26:649.

103. Koch CJ, Oprysko PR, Shuman AL, et al: Radiosensitization of hypoxic tumor cells by dodecafluoropentane: A gas-phase perfluorochemical emulsion. *Cancer Res.* 2002;62:3626.

104. Liu SC, Minton NP, Giaccia AJ, et al: Anticancer efficacy of systemically delivered anaerobic bacteria as gene therapy vectors targeting tumor hypoxia/necrosis. *Gene Ther.* 2002;9:291.

105. Nuyts S, Van Mellaert L, Theys J, et al: *Clostridium* spores for tumor-specific drug delivery. *Anticancer Drugs.* 2002;13:115.

106. Wouters BG, Weppler SA, Koritzinsky M, et al: Hypoxia as a target for combined modality treatments. *Eur J Cancer.* 2002;38:240.

107. Shibata T, Giaccia AJ, Brown JM: Hypoxia-inducible regulation of a prodrug-activating enzyme for tumor-specific gene therapy. *Neoplasia.* 2002;4:40.

108. Stone HB, Brown JM, Phillips TL, et al: Oxygen in human tumors: Correlations between methods of measurement and response to therapy. Summary of a workshop held November 19-20, 1992, at the National Cancer Institute, Bethesda, Md. *Radiat Res.* 1993;136:422.

109. Okunieff P, Hoeckel M, Dunphy EP, et al: Oxygen tension distributions are sufficient to explain the local response of human breast tumors treated with radiation alone. *Int J Radiat Oncol Biol Phys.* 1993;26:631.

110. Terris DJ, Dunphy EP: Oxygen tension measurements of head and neck cancers. *Arch Otolaryngol Head Neck Surg.* 1994;120:283.

111. Lartigau E, Le Ridant AM, Lambin P, et al: Oxygenation of head and neck tumors. *Cancer.* 1993;71:2319.

112. Vaupel P, Schlenger K, Knoop C, et al: Oxygenation of human tumors: evaluation of tissue oxygen distribution in breast cancers by computerized O_2 tension measurements. *Cancer Res.* 1991; 51:3316.

113. Höckel M, Knoop C, Schlenger K, et al: Intratumoral pO_2 histography as predictive assay in advanced cancer of the uterine cervix. *Adv Exp Med Biol.* 1994;345:445.

114. Brizel DM, Sibley GS, Prosnitz LR, et al: Tumor hypoxia adversely affects the prognosis of carcinoma of the head and neck. *Int J Radiat Oncol Biol Phys.* 1997;38:285.

115. Brizel DM, Rosner GL, Harrelson J, et al: Pretreatment oxygenation profiles of human soft tissue sarcomas. *Int J Radiat Oncol Biol Phys.* 1994;30:635.

116. Nordsmark M, Overgaard M, Overgaard J: Pretreatment oxygenation predicts radiation response in advanced squamous cell carcinoma of the head and neck. *Radiother Oncol.* 1996;41:31.

117. Urtasun RC, Chapman JD, Raleigh JA, et al: Binding of 3H-misonidazole to solid human tumors as a measure of tumor hypoxia. *Int J Radiat Oncol Biol Phys.* 1986;12:1263.

118. Hoebers FJ, Janssen HL, Valdes Olmos RA, et al: Phase 1 study to identify tumor hypoxia in patients with head and neck cancer using technetium-99m BRU 59-21. *Eur J Nucl Med Mol Imaging.* 2002;In press.

119. Chapman JD, Schneider RF, Urbain JL, et al: Single-photon emission computed tomography and positron-emission tomography assays for tissue oxygenation. *Semin Radiat Oncol.* 2001;11:47.

120. Rasey JS, Koh WJ, Evans ML, et al: Quantifying regional hypoxia in human tumors with positron emission tomography of [18F]fluoromisonidazole: A pretherapy study of 37 patients. *Int J Radiat Oncol Biol Phys.* 1996;36:417.

121. Koh WJ, Rasey JS, Evans ML, et al: Imaging of hypoxia in human tumors with [F-18]fluoromisonidazole. *Int J Radiat Oncol Biol Phys.* 1992;22:199.

122. Raleigh JA, Zeman EM, Rathman M, et al: Development of an ELISA for the detection of 2-nitroimidazole hypoxia markers bound to tumor tissue. *Int J Radiat Oncol Biol Phys.* 1992;22:403.

123. Hodgkiss RJ, Jones G, Long A, et al: Flow cytometric evaluation of hypoxic cells in solid experimental tumours using fluorescence immunodetection. *Br J Cancer.* 1991;63:119.

124. Evans SM, Hahn S, Pook DR, et al: Detection of hypoxia in human squamous cell carcinoma by EF5 binding. *Cancer Res.* 2000;60:2018.

125. Nordsmark M, Loncaster J, Chou SC, et al: Invasive oxygen measurements and pimonidazole labeling in human cervix carcinoma. *Int J Radiat Oncol Biol Phys.* 2001;49:581.

126. Raleigh JA, Chou SC, Calkins-Adams DP, et al: A clinical study of hypoxia and metallothionein protein expression in squamous cell carcinomas. *Clin Cancer Res.* 2000;6:855.

127. Wang GL, Jiang BH, Rue EA, et al: Hypoxia-inducible factor 1 is a basic-helix-loop-helix-PAS heterodimer regulated by cellular O_2 tension. *Proc Natl Acad Sci U S A.* 1995;92:5510.

128. Carmeliet P, Dor Y, Herbert JM, et al: Role of HIF-1alpha in hypoxia-mediated apoptosis, cell proliferation and tumour angiogenesis. *Nature.* 1998;394:485.

129. Salceda S, Caro J: Hypoxia-inducible factor 1alpha (HIF-1alpha) protein is rapidly degraded by the ubiquitin-proteasome system under normoxic conditions. Its stabilization by hypoxia depends on redox-induced changes. *J Biol Chem.* 1997;272:22642.

130. Gleadle JM, Ratcliffe PJ: Induction of hypoxia-inducible factor-1, erythropoietin, vascular endothelial growth factor, and glucose transporter-1 by hypoxia: evidence against a regulatory role for Src kinase. *Blood.* 1997;89:503.

131. Semenza GL: HIF-1 and tumor progression: Pathophysiology and therapeutics. *Trends Mol Med.* 2002;8:S62.

132. Raleigh JA, Calkins-Adams DP, Rinker LH, et al: Hypoxia and vascular endothelial growth factor expression in human squamous cell carcinomas using pimonidazole as a hypoxia marker. *Cancer Res.* 1998;58:3765.

133. West CM, Cooper RA, Loncaster JA, et al: Tumor vascularity: A histological measure of angiogenesis and hypoxia. *Cancer Res.* 2001;61:2907.

134. Wykoff CC, Beasley NJ, Watson PH, et al: Hypoxia-inducible expression of tumor-associated carbonic anhydrases. *Cancer Res.* 2000;60:7075.

135. Loncaster JA, Harris AL, Davidson SE, et al: Carbonic anhydrase (CA IX) expression, a potential new intrinsic marker of hypoxia: Correlations with tumor oxygen measurements and prognosis in locally advanced carcinoma of the cervix. *Cancer Res.* 2001;61:6394.

136. Airley R, Loncaster J, Davidson S, et al: Glucose transporter glut-1 expression correlates with tumor hypoxia and predicts metastasis-free survival in advanced carcinoma of the cervix. *Clin Cancer Res.* 2001;7:928.

137. Walenta S, Wetterling M, Lehrke M, et al: High lactate levels predict likelihood of metastases, tumor recurrence, and restricted patient survival in human cervical cancers. *Cancer Res.* 2000;60:916.

138. Olive PL, Durand RE, Le Riche J, et al: Gel electrophoresis of individual cells to quantify hypoxic fraction in human breast cancers. *Cancer Res.* 1993;53:733.

139. Kolstad P: Intercapillary distance, oxygen tension and local recurrence in cervix cancer. *Scand J Clin Lab Invest Suppl.* 1968;106:145.

140. Awwad HK, el Naggar M, Mocktar N, et al: Intercapillary distance measurement as an indicator of hypoxia in carcinoma of the cervix uteri. *Int J Radiat Oncol Biol Phys.* 1986;12:1329.

141. Haustermans K, Hofland I, Van de Pavert L, et al: Diffusion limited hypoxia estimated by vascular image analysis: comparison with pimonidazole staining in human tumors. *Radiother Oncol.* 2000;55:325.

142. Mueller-Klieser W, Schaefer C, Walenta S, et al: Assessment of tumor energy and oxygenation status by bioluminescence, nuclear magnetic resonance spectroscopy, and cryospectrophotometry. *Cancer Res.* 1990;50:1681.

143. Steen RG: Characterization of tumor hypoxia by 31P MR spectroscopy. *AJR Am J Roentgenol.* 1991;157:243.

144. Al Hallaq HA, Zamora M, Fish BL, et al: MRI measurements correctly predict the relative effects of tumor oxygenating agents on hypoxic fraction in rodent BA1112 tumors. *Int J Radiat Oncol Biol Phys.* 2000;47:481.

145. Howe FA, Robinson SP, McIntyre DJ, et al: Issues in flow and oxygenation dependent contrast (FLOOD) imaging of tumours. *NMR Biomed.* 2001;14:497.

146. Robinson SP, Howe FA, Rodrigues LM, et al: Magnetic resonance imaging techniques for monitoring changes in tumor oxygenation and blood flow. *Semin Radiat Oncol.* 1998;8:197.

147. Robinson SP, Collingridge DR, Howe FA, et al: Tumour response to hypercapnia and hyperoxia monitored by FLOOD magnetic resonance imaging. *NMR Biomed.* 1999;12:98.

148. Rijpkema M, Kaanders JH, Joosten FB, et al: Effects of breathing a hyperoxic hypercapnic gas mixture on blood oxygenation and vascularity of head-and-neck tumors as measured by magnetic resonance imaging. *Int J Radiat Oncol Biol Phys.* 2002;53:1185.

149. Hermans R: Estimation of tumour oxygenation levels with dynamic contrast-enhanced magnetic resonance imaging. *Radiother Oncol.* 2000;57:1.

150. Gatenby RA, Kessler HB, Rosenblum JS, et al: Oxygen distribution in squamous cell carcinoma metastases and its relationship to outcome of radiation therapy. *Int J Radiat Oncol Biol Phys.* 1988;14:831.

151. Graeber TG, Osmanian C, Jacks T, et al: Hypoxia-mediated selection of cells with diminished apoptotic potential in solid tumours. *Nature.* 1996;379:88.

152. Kim CY, Tsai MH, Osmanian C, et al: Selection of human cervical epithelial cells that possess reduced apoptotic potential to low-oxygen conditions. *Cancer Res.* 1997;57:4200.

153. Cairns RA, Kalliomaki T, Hill RP: Acute (cyclic) hypoxia enhances spontaneous metastasis of KHT murine tumors. *Cancer Res.* 2001;61:8903.

154. Hasan NM, Adams GE, Joiner MC, et al: Hypoxia facilitates tumour cell detachment by reducing expression of surface adhesion molecules and adhesion to extracellular matrices without loss of cell viability. *Br J Cancer.* 1998;77:1799.

155. Young SD, Marshall RS, Hill RP: Hypoxia induces DNA over-replication and enhances metastatic potential of murine tumor cells. *Proc Natl Acad Sci U S A.* 1988;85:9533.

156. Norman A, Kagan AR, Chan SL: The importance of genetics for the optimization of radiation therapy. A hypothesis. *Am J Clin Oncol.* 1988;11:84.

157. Tucker SL, Geara FB, Peters LJ, et al: How much could the radiotherapy dose be altered for individual patients based on a predictive assay of normal-tissue radiosensitivity? *Radiother Oncol.* 1996;38:103.

158. Burnet NG, Nyman J, Turesson I, et al: Prediction of normal-tissue tolerance to radiotherapy from in-vitro cellular radiation sensitivity. *Lancet.* 1992;339:1570.

159. Geara FB, Peters LJ, Ang KK, et al: Prospective comparison of in vitro normal cell radiosensitivity and normal tissue reactions in radiotherapy patients. *Int J Radiat Oncol Biol Phys.* 1993;27:1173.

160. Johansen J, Bentzen SM, Overgaard J, et al: Evidence for a positive correlation between in vitro radiosensitivity of normal human skin fibroblasts and the occurrence of subcutaneous fibrosis after radiotherapy. *Int J Radiat Biol.* 1994;66:407.

161. Begg AC, Russell NS, Knaken H, et al: Lack of correlation of human fibroblast radiosensitivity in vitro with early skin reactions in patients undergoing radiotherapy. *Int J Radiat Biol.* 1993;64:393.

162. Russell NS, Grummels A, Hart AA, et al: Low predictive value of intrinsic fibroblast radiosensitivity for fibrosis development following radiotherapy for breast cancer. *Int J Radiat Biol.* 1998;73:661.

163. Peacock J, Ashton A, Bliss J, et al: Cellular radiosensitivity and complication risk after curative radiotherapy. *Radiother Oncol.* 2000;55:173.

164. West CM, Davidson SE, Elyan SA, et al: Lymphocyte radiosensitivity is a significant prognostic factor for morbidity in carcinoma of the cervix. *Int J Radiat Oncol Biol Phys.* 2001;51:10.

165. Barber JB, Burrill W, Spreadborough AR, et al: Relationship between in vitro chromosomal radiosensitivity of peripheral blood lymphocytes and the expression of normal tissue damage following radiotherapy for breast cancer. *Radiother Oncol.* 2000;55:179.

166. Sassi M, Jukkola A, Riekki R, et al: Type I collagen turnover and cross-linking are increased in irradiated skin of breast cancer patients. *Radiother Oncol.* 2001;58:317.

167. Herskind C, Bamberg M, Rodemann HP: The role of cytokines in the development of normal-tissue reactions after radiotherapy. *Strahlenther Onkol.* 1998;174 Suppl 3:12.

168. Border WA, Noble NA: Transforming growth factor beta in tissue fibrosis. *N Engl J Med.* 1994;331:1286.

169. Franko AJ, Sharplin J, Ghahary A, et al: Immunohistochemical localization of transforming growth factor beta and tumor necrosis factor alpha in the lungs of fibrosis-prone and "non-fibrosing" mice during the latent period and early phase after irradiation. *Radiat Res.* 1997;147:245.

170. Haston CK, Travis EL: Murine susceptibility to radiation-induced pulmonary fibrosis is influenced by a genetic factor implicated in susceptibility to bleomycin-induced pulmonary fibrosis. *Cancer Res.* 1997;57:5286.

171. Skwarchuk MW, Travis EL: Changes in histology and fibrogenic cytokines in irradiated colorectum of two murine strains. *Int J Radiat Oncol Biol Phys.* 1998;42:169.

172. Alizadeh AA, Eisen MB, Davis RE, et al: Distinct types of diffuse large B-cell lymphoma identified by gene expression profiling. *Nature.* 2000;403:503.

173. Beer DG, Kardia SL, Huang CC, et al: Gene-expression profiles predict survival of patients with lung adenocarcinoma. *Nat Med.* 2002;8:816.

174. van't Veer LJ, Dai H, van de Vijver MJ, et al: Gene expression profiling predicts clinical outcome of breast cancer. *Nature.* 2002;415:530.

175. Quarmby S, West C, Magee B, et al: Differential expression of cytokine genes in fibroblasts derived from skin biopsies of patients who developed minimal or severe normal tissue damage after radiotherapy. *Radiat Res.* 2002;157:243.

176. Johnston CJ, Williams JP, Okunieff P, et al: Radiation-induced pulmonary fibrosis: examination of chemokine and chemokine receptor families. *Radiat Res.* 2002;157:256.

177. Falk SJ, Ward R, Bleehen NM: The influence of carbogen breathing on tumour tissue oxygenation in man evaluated by computerised pO_2 histography. *Br J Cancer.* 1992;66:919.

178. Martin L, Lartigau E, Weeger P, et al: Changes in the oxygenation of head and neck tumors during carbogen breathing. *Radiother Oncol.* 1993;27:123.

179. Kaanders JH, Pop LA, Marres HA, et al: ARCON: Experience in 215 patients with advanced head-and-neck cancer. *Int J Radiat Oncol Biol Phys.* 2002;52:769.

180. Bernier J, Denekamp J, Rojas A, et al: ARCON: Accelerated radiotherapy with carbogen and nicotinamide in non–small cell lung cancer: A phase I/II study by the EORTC. *Radiother Oncol.* 1999;52:149.

181. Brown JM: Hypoxic cytotoxic agents: A new approach to cancer chemotherapy. *Drug Resist Updat.* 2000;3:7.

182. Craighead PS, Pearcey R, Stuart G: A phase I/II evaluation of tirapazamine administered intravenously concurrent with cisplatin and radiotherapy in women with locally advanced cervical cancer. *Int J Radiat Oncol Biol Phys.* 2000;48:791.

183. von Pawel J, von Roemeling R, Gatzemeier U, et al: Tirapazamine plus cisplatin versus cisplatin in advanced non–small-cell lung cancer: A report of the international CATAPULT I study group. Cisplatin and Tirapazamine in Subjects with Advanced Previously Untreated Non–Small-Cell Lung Tumors. *J Clin Oncol.* 2000;18:1351.

184. Lee DJ, Trotti A, Spencer S, et al: Concurrent tirapazamine and radiotherapy for advanced head and neck carcinomas: A Phase II study. *Int J Radiat Oncol Biol Phys.* 1998;42:811.

185. Treat J, Johnson E, Langer C, et al: Tirapazamine with cisplatin in patients with advanced non-small-cell lung cancer: A phase II study. *J Clin Oncol.* 1998;16:3524.

186. Dubben HH, Thames HD, Beck-Bornholdt HP: Tumor volume: A basic and specific response predictor in radiotherapy. *Radiother Oncol.* 1998;47:167.

187. Nordsmark M, Overgaard J: A confirmatory prognostic study on oxygenation status and loco-regional control in advanced head and neck squamous cell carcinoma treated by radiation therapy. *Radiother Oncol.* 2000;57:39.

188. Hockel M, Schlenger K, Aral B, et al: Association between tumor hypoxia and malignant progression in advanced cancer of the uterine cervix. *Cancer Res.* 1996;56:4509.

189. Bjork-Eriksson T, West C, Karlsson E, et al: Tumor radiosensitivity (SF2) is a prognostic factor for local control in head and neck cancers. *Int J Radiat Oncol Biol Phys.* 2000;46:13.

190. Stausbol-Gron B, Overgaard J: Relationship between tumour cell in vitro radiosensitivity and clinical outcome after curative radiotherapy for squamous cell carcinoma of the head and neck. *Radiother Oncol.* 1999;50:47.

191. Girinsky T, Bernheim A, Lubin R, et al: In vitro parameters and treatment outcome in head and neck cancers treated with surgery and/or radiation: cell characterization and correlations with local control and overall survival. *Int J Radiat Oncol Biol Phys.* 1994;30:789.

192. Brock WA, Baker FL, Wike JL, et al: Cellular radiosensitivity of primary head and neck squamous cell carcinomas and local tumor control. *Int J Radiat Oncol Biol Phys.* 1990;18:1283.

193. Eschwege F, Bourhis J, Girinski T, et al: Predictive assays of radiation response in patients with head and neck squamous cell carcinoma: A review of the Institute Gustave Roussy experience. *Int J Radiat Oncol Biol Phys.* 1997;39:849.

194. Brizel DM, Dodge RK, Clough RW, et al: Oxygenation of head and neck cancer: changes during radiotherapy and impact on treatment outcome. *Radiother Oncol.* 1999;53:113.

195. Rudat V, Stadler P, Becker A, et al: Predictive value of the tumor oxygenation by means of pO₂ histography in patients with advanced head and neck cancer. *Strahlenther Onkol.* 2001;177:462.

196. Knocke TH, Weitmann HD, Feldmann HJ, et al: Intratumoral pO₂-measurements as predictive assay in the treatment of carcinoma of the uterine cervix. *Radiother Oncol.* 1999;53:99.

197. Sundfor K, Lyng H, Trope CG, et al: Treatment outcome in advanced squamous cell carcinoma of the uterine cervix: Relationships to pretreatment tumor oxygenation and vascularization. *Radiother Oncol.* 2000;54:101.

198. Fyles A, Milosevic M, Hedley D, et al: Tumor hypoxia has independent predictor impact only in patients with node-negative cervix cancer. *J Clin Oncol.* 2002;20:680.

199. Brizel DM, Scully SP, Harrelson JM, et al: Tumor oxygenation predicts for the likelihood of distant metastases in human soft tissue sarcoma. *Cancer Res.* 1996;56:941.

200. Nordsmark M, Alsner J, Keller J, et al: Hypoxia in human soft tissue sarcomas: adverse impact on survival and no association with p53 mutations. *Br J Cancer.* 2001;84:1070.

Radiotherapy and Chemotherapy

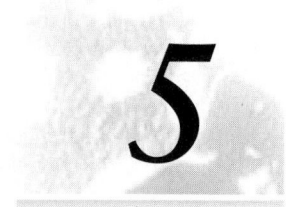

Madhu J. John, MD

DEFINITIONS

The oncology world of today is awash with recent discoveries of newer pathways of tumorigenesis, metastatic spread, development of resistance to treatment modalities, and the availability of several classes of drugs with unique modes of action. These changes have had major effects on the manner in which oncology is researched today. The surgical oncologist sees the futility and morbidity of extensive carve-outs and dedicates his or her unique skills toward preservation of anatomy and function. The medical oncologist realizes the transient nature of remissions brought about by so-called primary chemotherapy and the potential toxicity of prolonged chemotherapeutic courses. And the radiation oncologist, after 4 decades of attempts to increase dose delivery, is painfully aware of the limitations of treating essentially systemic or advanced locoregional disease with local radiotherapy.

Combining radiotherapy and systemic therapy is, in essence, a pragmatic response to the needs of today's cancer patient and the progressive awareness of oncologists of the confines of their adopted modality. Thus, *chemoradiation* is the science of combining the local discipline of radiotherapy with systemic therapy in the treatment of cancer. The term refers to the combination of various types and techniques of irradiation with systemic agents that may be conventional chemotherapeutic agents or even protectors, antagonists, cytokines, hormones, and modifiers. In chemoradiation, the drugs used may be infused over several days or given by bolus administration. They may be administered by oral, intramuscular, or intravenous routes. Radiotherapy may be delivered externally or through intracavitary, interstitial, or other brachytherapy methods. Finally, the discipline of chemoradiation indirectly emphasizes the judicious and tempered use of surgery to achieve cosmetic and functional integrity.

HISTORICAL PERSPECTIVE

Anticancer medications, mostly metal compounds, have been used for many hundreds of years. Chemoradiation, in its crudest form, probably began in 1905 with the treatment of leukemia with benzene and radiotherapy,

based on the rationale that both agents were myelotoxins. Colloidal lead, distilled water, and vitamin K are some of the systemic agents used to influence radiation effect on human cancer.[1] Modern chemoradiation began with the combined use of radiotherapy with the antimetabolite 5-fluorouracil (5-FU) in the late 1950s.[2] Halogenated pyrimidines (idoxuridine and 5-bromodeoxyuridine); antibiotics such as bleomycin, mitomycin C, and doxorubicin; and antimetabolites such as cisplatin and methotrexate have either been tested or used frequently in combination with radiotherapy for several diverse cancers.[1] One of the first studies initiated by the Radiation Therapy Oncology Group (RTOG) was a prospective randomized study comparing radiotherapy alone versus radiotherapy in combination with methotrexate in the treatment of head and neck cancers.[3] Pediatric cancers such as Wilms' tumor and rhabdomyosarcoma were the first to benefit from the combination. Systematic national studies honed the best and least toxic combinations of drugs and radiotherapy for various stages of these diseases.[1] The major impetus for the widespread use of chemoradiation today, however, came from an observation by Nigro that a preoperative course of chemoradiation with 5-FU, mitomycin C, and radiotherapy resulted in pathologically verified absence of disease at surgery on patients with anal cancer.[4] Cummings and colleagues[5] and Flam and colleagues[6] subsequently suggested that in their experience, a modified version of the 5-FU plus mitomycin C plus radiotherapy regimen could very well serve as definitive treatment in patients with anal cancer and thereby avoid colostomies. Adult cancers that have benefited from the chemoradiation liaison to date are legion, notably including numerous gastrointestinal (GI), head and neck, cervical, lung, prostate, and bladder cancers; lymphomas; and soft-tissue sarcomas.

RATIONALE

The increasing use of drugs with radiotherapy has been instigated by long-stagnant cure rates of many locally advanced tumors treated traditionally with radiotherapy alone, surgery alone, or chemotherapy alone. Examples are surgically treated head and neck cancers and esophageal, lung, bladder, and central nervous system (CNS) cancers; diseases treated primarily by radiotherapy such as cervical and non–small cell lung cancers and Hodgkin's lymphoma; and diseases treated primarily by chemotherapy such as small cell lung cancer and non-Hodgkin's lymphoma.

The reasons for these unchanging cure rates in the case of patients treated with radiotherapy are varied and may include the presence of tumor outside the confines of traditional radiation fields, the inability to deliver higher than standard doses without unacceptable side effects, and the presence of a subpopulation of tumor cells that are, for various reasons, inherently partially resistant to radiotherapy. In diseases traditionally treated by surgery alone, the lack of improved cure rates may again be due to the presence of disease just outside the realm of "reasonable" resection or, as has been realized in the case of breast cancer, a disease long considered a local problem may often be a systemic condition.[7] In the case of primary chemotherapy, probable reasons for failure may include unacceptable toxicities and the presence (or subsequent development) of resistant subpopulations of tumor cells during the generally long course of combination chemotherapy.

Another provocative factor has been the increasing demand for organ preservation. Radical surgery, used hitherto for anal canal, esophageal, laryngeal, breast, head and neck, and bladder cancers, is being replaced, in some instances, by chemoradiation, the latter having shown improved or similar cure rates compared with surgical resection.

A third and particularly significant population of patients that may be considered for chemoradiation is that of inoperable or unresectable patients, either with advanced disease or with comorbid conditions that preclude the attendant risks of anesthesia and surgery but not those of radiotherapy or chemotherapy. In actual clinical practice, these patients probably receive a wide spectrum of interventions, depending on the vagaries and the philosophical bents of primary clinicians, oncologists, the patients themselves, and their relatives. Treatments may range from the exclusive use of complementary or alternative medicine to a premature allocation to hospice care. A common example seen in oncologic practice is a patient with locally advanced esophageal cancer who can be cured with definitive chemoradiation, but who, nevertheless, is offered supportive care at best.

PRINCIPLES

Why Standard Treatment Fails

The primary rationale for chemoradiation is the established limitations of single-modality treatments and the desire to improve results of such therapy. Therefore, it might be worthwhile to examine the biologic and clinical reasons that treatments fail. Table 5-1 is a list of the potential obstacles faced by the oncologist when treating patients with solid tumors, particularly those with locally advanced cancers. Possible counter-interventions or counter-strategies for each factor are also listed; that they are sometimes contradictory is a reflection of the complexity and variability of tumor growth and host characteristics.

Table 5–1 Possible Reasons for Treatment Failure, Particularly in Patients with Locally Advanced Cancers, and Corresponding Counter-Strategies

Obstacles to Cure	Potential Counter-Strategies
Inaccessibility	
Decreased vascularity	Fractionated RT, sequential CRX
Postradiation/surgical fibrosis	Perioperative or concurrent CRX
Circulating tumor cells	Add chemotherapy to local therapy
Insensitivity	
Inherent or developed resistant subpopulations	Multiple drugs
	Shorten treatment time; concurrent/alternating CRX
Hypoxic cells	Hypoxic cell sensitizers
Tumor with high "n" number	Hypofractionation
Increased Tumor Burden	
Accelerated proliferation	Expeditious postoperative CRX
	Late intensification, accelerated RT fractionation, hyperfractionation
	Concurrent/alternating CRX
	High-medium dose pulse chemotherapy
Metastatic phenotypes	Maintenance chemotherapy following RT or CRX
	Shortened treatment time
Increased Toxicity	
Wide anatomic tumor extent	Sequential CRX; split-course RT
Agents having overlapping toxicities	Prophylactic biologic modifiers/cytokines/antibiotics
	Alternate effective drug combinations
	Low-dose infusion chemotherapy
	Hyperalimentation; temporary colostomy, PEG tubes
Host Intolerance	
Comorbid conditions	Avoid surgery; use "tight" RT fields
Advanced age	Sequential/split-course CRX
	Low-dose infusion chemotherapy
Inhibition of Apoptosis	
Enzyme/oncogene/protein overexpression, angiogenesis, tumor suppressor deactivation	Adding agents modifying these various molecular pathways to CRX or using them in maintenance therapy after definitive therapy

CRX, chemoradiation; PEG, percutaneous endoscopic gastrostomy; RT, radiotherapy.

INACCESSIBILITY

Tumor cells may exist and thrive outside the reach of conventional treatment, be it localized (surgery or radiotherapy) or systemic (chemotherapy). For example, the tendency for locally advanced human solid tumors to develop hypoxic areas is well established and has two major implications. First, hypoxic cells are more resistant to radiation. Second, the poor vascular access that made these cells hypoxic means that they are less likely to be affected by drugs in circulation.[8] Fractionated radiotherapy might improve vascular access of the initially large tumors, as will the sequential use of chemotherapy and irradiation and vice versa.

Also, chemotherapeutic access to residual tumor cells after radiotherapy or surgery may be impeded by fibrosis. Using preoperative concurrent chemoradiation or perioperative chemotherapy may prevent such inaccessibility. Another partial solution may be to decrease the time interval between surgery and postoperative chemotherapy, allowing less time for consolidative fibrosis.

The presence of subclinical disease just outside the surgical bed or the radiation field may be the reason for eventual failure in many cases. To accommodate this situation, instead of extending conventional surgical or radiation fields, the addition of specific systemic therapy may be less likely to increase morbidity and mortality.

Finally, a sizable proportion of patients with certain cancers, such as breast and prostate cancers, may experience treatment failure systemically, even when the primary tumor has been eradicated. These failures are attributed to the presence of potentially clonogenic tumor cells circulating outside the reach of surgical dissection or tolerable radiation fields. This forms the rationale for maintenance systemic chemotherapy or hormonal therapy after successful elimination of the primary tumor by radiotherapy or surgery or both.

INSENSITIVITY

Through in vivo and in vitro studies, as well as considerable clinical evidence, it is evident that even within a histologically homogeneous tumor, wide variations in response to irradiation and chemotherapy occur.[9] The cause of the development of resistance or insensitivity to irradiation and chemotherapy can be similar but are generally different. Chemoradiation with multiple drugs offers the potential to eradicate subpopulations within a tumor that might be resistant to one modality and not the other or resistant to one drug and not others.

The development of metastatic phenotypes in a tumor has been experimentally shown to be proportional to time. The obvious strategy to counteract the evolution of such phenotypes is to diagnose and treat early in the growth of the tumor, as well as to shorten the overall treatment time. This may translate into using alternating and concurrent chemoradiation rather than the sequential mode.

The mechanisms of development of resistant or metastatic phenotypes in a tumor may be genetic or environmental. If hypoxia is the major reason for this resistance to treatment, then fractionated radiotherapy may be the suitable strategy employed. On the other hand, tumors with high "n" numbers, or those "inherently" resistant to radiotherapy, may require hypofractionation or large individual doses of radiation to overcome this resistance.

INCREASED TUMOR BURDEN

Although radiotherapy and some chemotherapies kill cancer cells exponentially, the fact remains that larger tumors are more difficult to eradicate than smaller ones and that a dose relationship exists between most solid tumors and therapeutic agents. Thus, locally advanced tumors, besides being difficult to extirpate surgically, are also difficult to control with maximally tolerated doses of radiotherapy or chemotherapy. Also, such locally extensive tumors are imminently on the verge of sending out a "cascade" of metastatic phenotypes.

For these reasons, it is almost imperative to combine radiotherapy and chemotherapy in some fashion in the treatment of these advanced tumors. Also, because time is of paramount importance, a concurrent course of chemoradiation is preferable. When concurrent chemotherapy is not feasible for some reason or another, alternating or sequential chemoradiation is the adopted treatment in which irradiation is preferentially given first, followed by chemotherapy.

Hyperfractionation has proven to be an effective and generally tolerated means of exploiting the dose relationship of radiotherapy on solid tumors; therefore, it should be used when a large tumor burden is at hand.[10] Similarly, in the case of chemotherapeutic agents, high- to medium-pulsed doses are preferable to low-dose infusions because higher drug concentrations are achieved, albeit for a shorter duration of time.[11]

The phenomenon of *accelerated proliferation* of a tumor is frequently cited as the reason for incomplete response to current therapeutic intervention. This phenomenon of decreased doubling time in residual tumors that have been incompletely excised, or have been treated with the initial dose of chemotherapeutic agent or radiation, has been established in the laboratory and often clinically manifested (recurrent tumors appear to grow faster than the original tumor).[12] Late intensification treatment regimens with hyperfractionation or accelerated fractionation, expeditious perioperative chemotherapy, or concurrent chemoradiation are some of the means by which accelerated proliferation by tumor cells can be countered.

INCREASED TOXICITY

Radical treatment is often hampered by the wide anatomic extent of locally advanced cancers. Adequate irradiation (or surgery) in these cases invariably results in excessive morbidity and sometimes mortality. In such cases, most oncologists resort to sequential chemoradiation, which with rare exceptions has been shown to have no impact on survival in clinical studies. Others employ split-course radiotherapy with the implicit understanding that any survival advantage obtainable with standard continuous radiotherapy is in jeopardy.

Another situation in which oncologists often acquiesce to giving patients less than optimal therapy is when the effective agents for a particular tumor have overlapping toxicities. For example, both ifosfamide and pelvic radiotherapy are effective against cervical cancer and both can result in considerable bone marrow toxicity. A possible strategy to avail of their combined effect would be to use ifosfamide during intracavitary irradiation, the latter having little myelotoxicity.

Other means of avoiding an expected and excessive toxicity would be the use of aggressive and prophylactic supportive therapy while pursuing the most effective treatment regimen. This could include the use of prophylactic antibiotics, biologic modifiers, or cytokines, creating a temporary colostomy during pelvic chemoradiation and using intravenous or percutaneous endoscopic gastrostomy

(PEG) alimentation during the treatment of head and neck and mediastinal tumors.

Finally, evidence is increasing that one can modulate radiation fields and dose as well as chemotherapy dose to decrease toxicity while using concurrent chemoradiation without affecting cure rates. In several current chemoradiation regimens used to treat anal and esophageal cancers, *both* radiation and chemotherapeutic doses are reduced compared with optimal doses of the two when they are used alone. The use of low-dose continuous infusion of certain chemotherapeutic agents during radiotherapy is another means of decreasing toxicity.

HOST INTOLERANCE

One of the most common reasons for not offering definitive curative treatment to a cancer patient is the presence of comorbid medical conditions and advancing age. In many cases no treatment is offered initially and far more attention is paid to palliative treatment at a later stage after disease progression.

Several strategies might be employed with such patients to achieve a reasonable chance at cure. They include the use of nonstandard radiation fields covering only grossly involved areas of disease and the use of low-dose infusion chemotherapy. Sequential or alternating chemoradiation or concurrent split-course chemoradiation may be used as a concession to host vulnerability without altogether abandoning the possibility of cure.

INHIBITION OF APOPTOSIS

We now know that many human cancers are induced, develop, and metastasize by the means of mutations, which are changes in gene expression. These mutations sometimes consist of changes in purine or pyrimidine sequence in the DNA molecule or, more commonly, by DNA methylation. A few mutations may be inherited, but the vast majority are acquired through the course of a lifetime. The activation of oncogenes, the deactivation of tumor suppression genes, the overexpression of certain proteins, and angiogenesis are some of the most important molecular pathways that are responsible for tumor cells having the capability for unmitigated growth, the ability to metastasize or spread, and the capability to avoid programmed cell death or apoptosis.

The Bcl-2 protein, a regulator of apoptosis, is overexpressed in many human cancers such as breast, colorectal, and prostate cancers as well as in lymphomas, myelomas, and malignant melanoma. Bcl-2 acts by blocking signals that usually trigger apoptosis. Agents that block the Bcl-2 protein (such as oblimersen sodium or Genasense) are currently being used in clinical trials combining them with conventional treatments (surgery, radiotherapy, and chemotherapy) in human trials.

The enzyme COX-2, which is overexpressed in a large number of human cancers, including lung, head and neck, GI, gynecologic, and bladder cancers, is known to inhibit immune function (by regulating the synthesis of the prostaglandin PGE_2), block apoptosis, and enhance angiogenesis. COX-2 inhibitors, such as celecoxib, have shown some promise when combined with radiotherapy

or chemotherapy or both in trials involving patients with colon and lung cancer.

Drugs with anti-angiogenesis activity (thalidomide) and gene therapies that were initially heralded as major breakthroughs and since found wanting are now more realistically being employed in conjunction with other therapies such as chemotherapy and radiotherapy in clinical trials. Other novel therapeutic agents now being actively investigated include signal transduction inhibitors such as ZD1839 and hypoxic cytoxins such as Tirapazimine in conjunction with standard anti-neoplastic agents (cisplatin[13,14] and radiotherapy[14]).

Mechanics of Interaction

TYPES OF INTERACTION

Steel and Peckham[15] were the first to categorize various theoretical scenarios of drug and radiotherapy interactions. The first process described was *spatial cooperation,* in which each of the two modalities was aimed at disease in different sites. The classic example of this process is seen in the treatment of childhood leukemia when chemotherapy is used to treat systemic disease while cranial radiotherapy is used to treat subclinical disease at a sanctuary site, the brain. No interaction is intended between the two modalities.

Conceptually, with this interaction, full doses of both modalities can be delivered with impunity because no enhancement of toxicity is expected. However, even in the example just given, radiation doses to the brain are reduced owing to the additive effects of systemic chemotherapy and cranial radiotherapy on the brain. Thus, *independence of toxicity* is an important corollary of spatial cooperation whereby the two modalities may address cell kill in different anatomic areas but do not enhance each other's toxicities. The combination of androgen suppressors, such as flutamide and goserelin acetate (Zoladex), with local radiotherapy is a good example in which systemic hormonal agents are used to decimate potentially clonogenic cells in the systemic pool, and radiotherapy is used to eradicate or diminish the localized bulk of tumor in the prostate. No enhancement of toxicity takes place here. Even so, this example is flawed because the hormonal agents used here do indeed have a marginal but very definite effect on the primary site (i.e., the prostate). In other words, in this example, besides spatial cooperation, the process of enhancement is taking place at the same time.

Clinically, improved tumor response is the primary intention of most chemoradiation regimens. This increased response or *enhancement* is superior to that achieved by either radiotherapy or chemotherapy alone. The term enhancement can, however, be used to denote an increased effect on normal tissues as well.

Types of enhancement are described by the terms *supra-additivity, additivity,* and *subadditivity,* which refer to responses (in tumor or normal tissues) that are greater than, equal to, and less than the sum response of radiotherapy and systemic agents. Even a subadditive interaction on a tumor system is a beneficial one. If the effect of radiotherapy on a tumor is 3+ and the chemotherapy effect on the same tumor is 2+, a net effect of 4+ is subadditive yet better than with either modality alone. An additive effect in this example would be 5+; a supra-additive effect would be 6+.

Diminution is the term used to describe the interaction between radiotherapy and systemic therapy, in which the observed tumor response is less than that observed with either modality alone. When the combined response of both modalities is less than that with the more active of the two modalities, the interaction is described as *inhibition*. *Antagonism* is the term used when the combined effect is less than that of the less active of the two modalities.

Although these terms are generally used to describe effects on tumor and less often to describe effects on normal tissues, the term *protection* is used primarily for effects on normal tissues. Cyclophosphamide (Cytoxan), etoposide, and methotrexate are some of the more commonly used cytotoxic drugs in chemoradiation that have been shown to have a protective effect on bone marrow stem cells against the effects of radiotherapy and even other drugs.[16] Sulfhydryl compounds such as glutathione, which have radioprotective and chemoprotective effects by scavenging free radicals, provide "pure" protection, because they do not have any specific effects on tumor or normal tissues.

BIOLOGIC MECHANISMS OF INTERACTION

There are several mechanisms by which radiotherapy and systemic agents effect changes in tumor cells and normal cells. Most of these mechanisms overlap. Yet it is useful to remember in general that radiotherapeutic effects take place mainly in a confined area where the bulk of the known tumor cells are present. Systemic agents, however, have whole-body effects with some proclivity on the part of their metabolites to affect proliferative systems such as the hematopoietic and GI systems.

INHIBITION OF SUBLETHAL AND POTENTIAL LETHAL DAMAGE REPAIR. Radiation effect on tumor and normal tissues may be enhanced by several drugs that inhibit DNA repair or sublethal radiation damage. Several common drugs such as cisplatin, hydroxyurea, and nitrosoureas have shown such enhancement in in vivo and in vitro studies.[17] In vitro studies have also shown doxorubicin, cisplatin, and topoisomerase I inhibitors (e.g., irinotecan) to inhibit the repair of potentially lethal damage caused by irradiation.

CELL PHASE DISTRIBUTION CHANGES. Radiotherapy has been known to be more toxic to cells in the mitotic phase as well as the early part of the S phase.[18] Several drugs such as 5-FU, methotrexate, *Vinca* alkaloids, and bleomycin are known to interact with radiotherapy through disruption of cell kinetics. The classic example of exploiting cell phase-specific activity of drugs and irradiation is the one of hydroxyurea and radiotherapy in the treatment of CNS tumors and early cervical cancers.[17,19] Hydroxyurea kills cells in the S phase, leading to synchronization and blockage in the S/G_1 phase of the cell

cycle. As the cells emerge through this block into the M phase, they can be said to have been "primed" for radiation-induced death by hydroxyurea.

EFFECTS ON TUMOR SIZE AND VASCULAR SUPPLY. The effect of both radiotherapy and chemotherapy on a tumor is inversely proportional to tumor size. For example, the tumor that has been reduced by radiotherapy is more likely to be successfully cured by a subsequent course of chemotherapy than the original bulky tumor. Another reason for the increased efficiency of chemotherapy in this example is that the decreased tumor volume by radiotherapy is likely to result in greater vascular access for subsequent chemotherapy, resulting in greater concentrations of the drug in the tumor cell. This, in turn, can lead to recruitment of tumor cells from a quiescent to a proliferative state, rendering them more vulnerable to chemotherapy or radiotherapy.

EFFECT ON REPOPULATION. During the course of several cycles of chemotherapy or a fractionated course of radiotherapy, repopulation by tumor cells that are in a proliferative state occurs. Radiotherapy and certain drugs such as 5-FU and actinomycin D are known to suppress repopulation specifically.[17,18]

EFFECT ON HYPOXIC AND LOW pH CELLS. Hypoxic cells are said to be one of the primary reasons for failure to cure a locally confined tumor by radiotherapy.[20] Solid tumors in animals as well as humans tend to develop areas of hypoxia within their volume. Mitomycin C and cisplatin have been shown to have selective cytotoxic effects on hypoxic cells. This possibly explains why, with the single exception of 5-FU, the drugs mitomycin C and cisplatin are most frequently used in chemoradiation treatment regimens in the clinic today. In addition, both of these drugs have shown supra-additive or additive effects on tumors in vitro and in vivo when combined with radiotherapy.[21] Because hypoxic cells produce lactic acid by the process of anaerobic glycolysis, they may exist in conditions of low pH. Selective activity against low pH cells and sparing of cells of normal or near-normal pH have been demonstrated in mammalian cells. Agents such as amiloride analogues show potential for such pH-based cell kill and may provide an additive or supra-additive effect with radiotherapy.

There is now evidence by meta-analysis that hypoxic cell radiosensitizers such as nimorazole increase survival in many human cancers, particularly head and neck tumors.[22] More importantly, considerable laboratory evidence has shown that bioreductive agents such as quinones (mitomycin C, porfiromycin, and EO9), N-oxides such as Tirapazimine, and mitroaromatics (RSU1069) are efficient hypoxic-sensitive cytotoxins, particularly when combined with standard radiotherapy and some chemotherapeutic agents such as cisplatin and other alkylating agents. Many of these are being studied in phase I and II trials.[21,22]

ALTERATION OF CELL SURVIVAL CURVES. In radiobiology, most survival curves of normal and tumor cells are sigmoid or nonexponential curves. This verifies the "multitarget, single hit" concept used to explain the mechanism of radiation damage. In a tumor system, this sigmoid curve can be divided into two parts: a curved shoulder or slope representing the "resistant" subpopulation of a heterogeneous tumor and a straight exponential portion representing a predictable sensitive subpopulation of the tumor.[23] Both radioenhancers and radioprotectors can alter the slope of these cell survival curves in vitro. Byfield's pioneering work showed that exposure of human tumor cells to 5-FU after irradiation altered the survival curve, as shown in an increase in the slope (or reduction in the shoulder) of cell survival curves. In other words, radiation damage in this case was being enhanced by 5-FU.[24] Similar changes in radiation cell survival curves have been shown with the drugs cisplatin, paclitaxel, and actinomycin D.[25-27]

MODIFICATION OF APOPTOSIS. Apoptosis is the dynamic process by which cells undergo an orderly series of intracellular events that lead to their death. The p53 tumor suppressor gene and the Bcl-2 protein are important mediators in the apoptotic pathway. Their presence or absence plays a vital role in the ability of drugs and ionizing radiation to induce or resist apoptosis in both normal and malignant cells. In the presence of a normal p53 gene, the drugs doxorubicin, etoposide, and 5-FU and irradiation have been shown to increase cell kill through apoptosis.[28] Similarly, its absence can lead to resistance to these same drugs and radiotherapy. Other drugs that have elicited programmed cell death in various human tumors include the taxanes, anthracyclines, and cyclophosphamide.[29]

TIMING OF ADMINISTRATION

The integration of radiotherapy and chemotherapy in a clinical schedule has evolved empirically. The general aim is to combine a conventionally fractionated course of radiotherapy: for example, 2 Gy daily five times per week for 7 weeks with standard dose schedules of chemotherapy, such as 1 g/m² per 24 hours of 5-FU given for 5 days every 3 to 4 weeks.

For maximal effect on a hypothetical patient with a tumor that is sensitive to radiation and 5-FU, the 7-week course of radiotherapy would be given simultaneously with three cycles of 5-FU infusion. This schedule, however, would likely cause an excess in toxicity quite intolerable to this hypothetical patient. Depending on the volume of irradiated tissue and host tolerance, one could either (1) reduce radiation fraction size or total dose, or increase the overall period of irradiation such as by split-course irradiation; (2) reduce the chemotherapeutic dose per cycle, the number of days of infusion, or the number of cycles; or (3) temporally separate radiotherapy and chemotherapy with either sequential or alternating chemoradiation.

In clinical oncology, the easiest way to temporize the combination toxicity would be to choose the third option; that is, separate the administration of radiotherapy and chemotherapy. And that is exactly how clinical investigations using chemoradiation were empirically designed initially—with sequential chemoradiation. It became increasingly clear, during the past several years especially, that temporally separating the two modalities resulted in no practical gain in cure or survival. This was most dramatically evident with advanced head and neck tumors; although induction chemotherapy yielded exceptional response rates, the eventual survival of these patients was no different than that from radiotherapy alone. Moreover, as a result of newer laboratory and clinical data, it became increasingly evident that the first two options were more likely to achieve a cure advantage. Temporizing radiotherapy and chemotherapy administration, but with the least temporal separation possible, is more likely to achieve superior results. Although enhancement of toxicity was evident, it was more manifest in acutely responding tissues such as the skin, which healed rapidly, as well.

Timing of administration of systemic agents and radiotherapy can be classified as remote, sequential, alternating, and simultaneous. They are best described schematically as shown in Table 5-2.

At the outset, two generalizations can be made regarding the importance of timing or scheduling of chemoradiation. First, despite the often contradictory results of radiobiologic studies with regard to the timing of various chemotherapeutic agents in relation to various radiotherapy schedules, there should be no question about the ultimate importance of scheduling modalities. The various strategies in timing have implications for both tumors and normal tissues. The skepticism that often greets experimental data concerning chemotherapy and radiotherapy delivery is based on the lack of satisfactory animal tumor model systems that are compatible with clinical reality. Until the work of Kallman and colleagues,[30] for example, most studies involved single doses of radiation, compared with multifractionated courses of radiotherapy that are the clinical norm. Human tumors differ from experimental tumors in their cellular heterogeneity; their microenvironment, including blood supply, hypoxic components, and pH; and the normal tissues that envelop them. They differ greatly from human tumors in their sensitivity to chemotherapy. Yet on both the experimental and clinical levels, evidence is irrefutable that some schedules are more effective than others in various solid tumors.[30-32]

Table 5–2 Chemoradiation Schedules

Schedule						
1. Remote:						
a) Adjuvant:	R → → C	C	C			
b) Neoadjuvant:	C	C	C → → R			
2. Sequential:	C	C	C	R		
or	R	C	C	C		
or	C	C	RC	RC		
3. Alternating:	C	R	C	R		
or	R	C	R	C		
4. Simultaneous:						
a) Continuous:	RC	R	RC	R	R C	
b) Intermittent:	RC		RC		R C	
c) Variant:	RC	R	RC	R	R C	C C

R, radiotherapy; C, chemotherapy.

Second, it is also quite clear that each of the different types of scheduling outlined in Table 5-2 has relevance or importance in different clinical situations. For example, the remote adjuvant use of systemic chemotherapy after primary treatment with local treatment by surgery, radiotherapy, or both has been found to be an effective treatment regimen for early breast cancer. At the other end, the concurrent use of chemotherapy and radiotherapy has been established as being superior to remote or adjuvant use of chemotherapy for esophageal cancers.

A newer type of chemoradiation schedule currently in vogue is the use of induction chemotherapy with two or more cycles followed by concurrent chemoradiation. This sequence is being investigated in trials of head and neck and lung cancers. The rationale of this sequencing is similar to the sequential chemoradiation model: induction chemotherapy will induce marked tumor cell regression, reducing residual disease for radiotherapy (and chemotherapy) kill. The criticisms that might be leveled against this approach are that, in effect, this is just a variation of the sequential model and provides the opportunity (time wise) of a subpopulation of tumor cells to develop resistance to the drugs to be used in the concurrent chemoradiation phase of the treatment and perhaps to radiation itself. These objections are perhaps validated by the poor results of the large number of clinical trials using sequential chemotherapy followed by radiotherapy in head and neck cancers.

THE MAXIMAL THERAPY–MINIMAL TIME CONCEPTUAL MODEL

Having stated these two universalities, it may also be ventured that the preponderance of theoretical reasoning in clinical oncology points to the potential superiority of simultaneous chemoradiation over the other ways of temporally separating the two modalities. This proposition has been elaborated in the past, the gist of it being that in locally advanced cancers, it is critical to combat all subpopulations in the heterogeneous tumor within the shortest period of time possible.[32]

Figure 5-1A elaborates the basic principles of clinical tumor growth. Initially, there is a period of growth before a tumor becomes clinically manifest and diagnosed. The variabilities in the length of this time period depend on the type of tumor, its biologic and kinetic properties, as well as the efficiency with which it is diagnosed. Presuming no treatment is instituted, the tumor proceeds to expand over a variable period of time, during which three incidents with catastrophic implications can take place: (1) the development of drug- and radiotherapy-resistant phenotypes; (2) the development of metastatic phenotypes; and (3) the achievement of the tumor of a critical size, mass, or state and the dispatch of metastatic phenotypes to distant sites. Figure 5-1B shows that even when treatment is instituted quickly, before the tumor reaches the critical size just described, the potential for development of resistant phenotype increases as the treatment regimen is stretched over a period of time. Figure 5-1C illustrates that this resistant subpopulation of cells would then proliferate to reach that critical status

when metastasis can begin. Figure 5-1D shows treatment regimens that address both basic issues of potential treatment failure. The treatment here is characterized by the use of all agents or combinations that effectively address all subpopulations of a heterogeneous tumor and by its expeditious use during the "window of curability" before the development of resistant phenotypes and before the tumor reaches that critical state before metastasis. In other words, all advanced tumors are "best" treated with simultaneous or concurrent use of local and systemic agents.

In this conceptual model, two matters pertaining to chemotherapy delivery must be addressed. Is infusion chemotherapy to be preferred over bolus administration? Is low-dose continuous infusion of chemotherapy throughout a radiotherapy course preferable to high-dose pulse infusion (for 4 to 5 days every 3 to 4 weeks) in conjunction with radiotherapy?

Lokich[27] and Byfield[33] have reviewed their own results and the experiences of others at considerable depth regarding infusion schedules. In clinical chemoradiation schedules, the decision regarding the mode of chemotherapy delivery is based on toxicity consideration rather than effectiveness. In their conclusions, Lokich[27] and Byfield[33] state that the continuous infusion schedule does not compromise their therapeutic effect, does change their toxicity profile, and, in some cases, increases the spectrum of their antitumor activity.

Although a number of factors influence drug activity, the most useful classification may be the drug cell cycle-specific or cycle phase-specific activity. In lung, breast, and some GI tumors, for example, in which at any one time only a small percentage (<5%) of cells are in cycle and the rest are in G_0 phase, antimetabolites, antibiotics, and *Vinca* alkaloids are more effective, especially when given in continuous infusion schedules. In pediatric and germ cell tumors, lymphomas, and small cell lung cancer in which a larger percentage of cells are in cycle, alkylating agents given in bolus injections may be more effective.

Examples of toxicity influencing the mode of administration of a drug are (1) 5-FU given by infusion with pelvic radiotherapy when myelotoxicity is of concern and by bolus injections when stomatitis is the dose-limiting toxicity and (2) ifosfamide not being used with external pelvic radiotherapy because of overlapping myelotoxicity but given with intracavitary radiotherapy because it has considerable activity in cervical cancers.

The principal obstacle to this *maximal therapy-minimal time* (MT^2) concept is, of course, the greater potential for acute and intolerable toxicity. On the basis of earlier laboratory data and clinical observations of enhanced acute toxicity, several investigators suggested that simultaneous radiotherapy and chemotherapy should be avoided.[31,34] However, more recent clinical trials and radiobiologic studies suggest that even though acute toxicity is enhanced, it occurred primarily in proliferative normal tissues that heal or reverse changes quickly enough that results are clinically acceptable. The toxicity of nonproliferative or late-responding normal tissues was not increased.

An example would be that of patients with anal cancers treated with simultaneous 5-FU, mitomycin C,

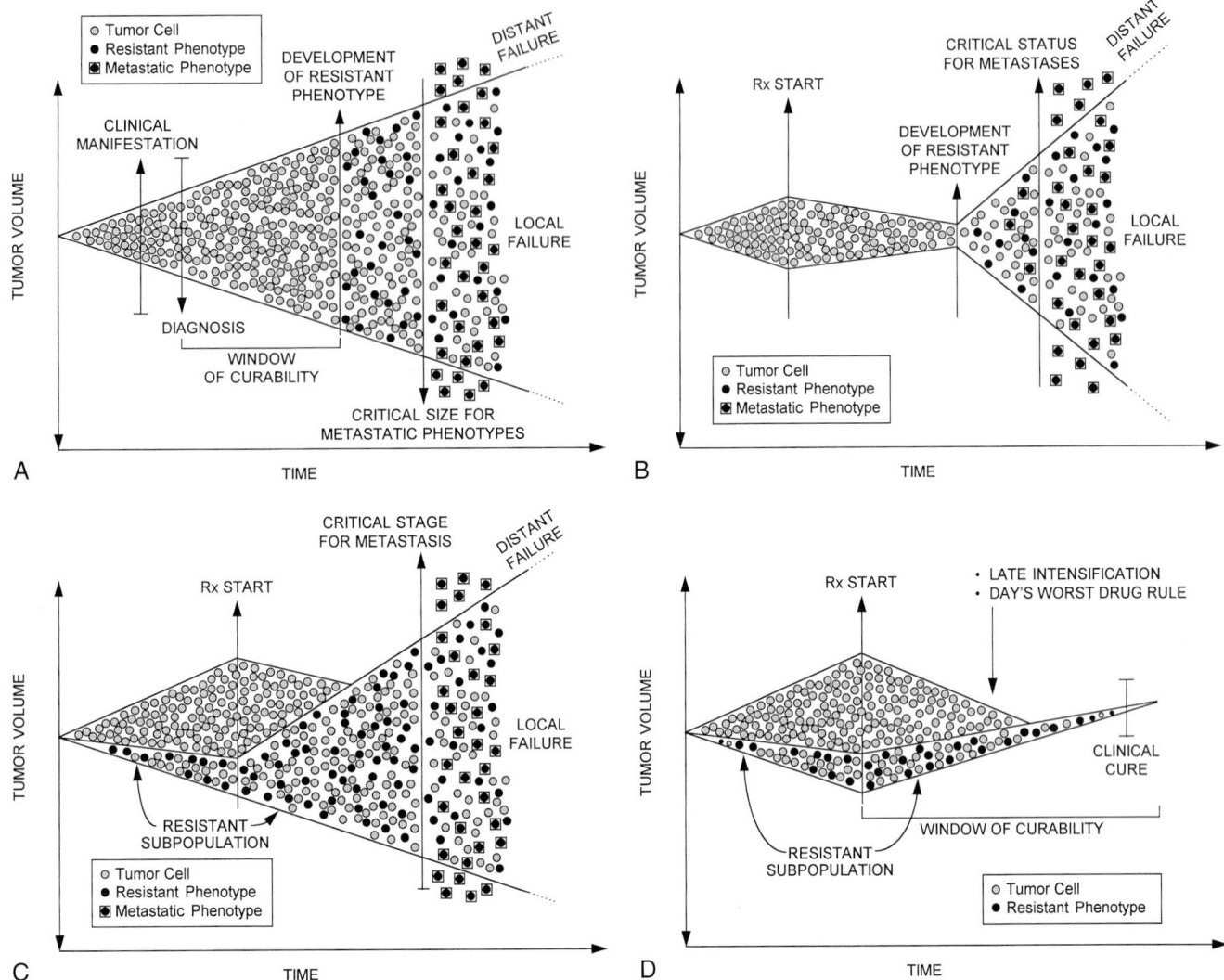

Figure 5-1. Graphic representation of the maximal therapy–minimal time conceptual model of cancer treatment. **A,** The clinical course of untreated tumor. Resistant or metastatic phenotypes are variables related to time. **B,** The development of treatment-resistant and metastatic phenotypes takes place eventually, irrespective of tumor type or volume. **C,** When suboptimal treatment is given, resistant subpopulations within the heterogeneous tumor increase in number to eventually metastasize or manifest as local failure. **D,** Effect of maximal treatment within the "window of curability." The resistant subpopulation issue is addressed by using the best available drugs last (when overall treatment volume is reduced and when microcirculation is improved) and by intensification of radiotherapy schedule (hyperfractionation, accelerated fractionation, or hypofractionation).

and radiation in whom perineal dermatitis is markedly, but transiently, increased, but in whom long-term chronic toxicity has not been increased.[35] Another example would be the overall experience with patients with head and neck cancers. A large number of clinical trials for this disease site have employed sequential induction chemotherapy followed by irradiation. An equal number of clinical trials have employed concurrent chemoradiation either in continuous or interrupted fashion. An overview of these controlled clinical trials has shown that intensive induction chemotherapy before radiotherapy has not provided improved cure rates or survival.[36] Simultaneous chemoradiation, with tolerable doses of chemotherapeutic agents, on the other hand, appears to increase local control and survival without affecting distant failure rates, as shown in two meta-analyses.[37,38]

Another important parameter to consider in the MT[2] model is the manner in which chemotherapy or other systemic agents are administered. Should chemotherapy

be given in the traditional manner every 3 weeks or should it be given in continuous (low) doses throughout the radiotherapy course? The answer to that question is nearly as complex as anything about cancer itself.

The reasons for delivering optimal courses of chemotherapy during radiotherapy (i.e., every 3 weeks) are: (1) in quantitative dose responsiveness of tumors in general (increased log kill) and (2) the possibility that prolonged use of low doses of a drug is likely to induce mutations in cancer cells that confer on them a resistance to that drug as well as future drugs. A clinical example of this may be the results of the recent National Cancer Institute of Canada (NCIC) trial for cervical cancer, where weekly cisplatin during radiotherapy did not increase survival over radiotherapy alone.[39]

The objection against using optimal or high doses of a drug during radiotherapy is the potential for increased toxicity. There are, however, several methods by which one could sidestep this problem. The most popular means is by decreasing doses to between one third and two thirds of the standard dose of the drug or drug combination. A second way is by using a drug/drug combination that has no major overlapping toxicity with radiotherapy. Cisplatin used concurrently with radiotherapy in head and neck cancer is a good example of this method. Finally, the best means of combining effective drugs in full doses with concurrent radiotherapy is to alternate effective drugs or drug combinations during radiotherapy. This has the triple benefit of achieving maximal quantitative and qualitative cell-kill, the avoidance of overlapping toxicity, and engaging the tumor effectively within the "window of *curability*." On the other hand, a drug such as the ubiquitous 5-FU may be given effectively in lower doses and continuous infusion in anal cancer.[40]

There are clearly certain clinical situations in which treatment time is not as critical, such as in malignant lymphomas, where the daily radiotherapy dose and overall treatment time are not as important as in other solid tumors. In other instances, certain tumor responses might be highly dose dependent, in which case dose modifications of radiotherapy or chemotherapy would be inappropriate. Most of all, it appears that in many locally advanced cancers, parameters of optimal chemoradiation regimens have yet to be established. In all these instances, in which concurrent chemoradiation is not feasible, it might be worthwhile to use alternating, sequential, or remote chemoradiation regimens in the hope that the window of curability in these situations is wide enough to allow for various degrees of temporal separation of the modalities.

When sequential chemoradiation is the chosen mode of delivery of treatment, two general rules can be applied to decide which modality should be preferentially given first. Goldie[41] has suggested that it depends on the predominant site of treatment failure (i.e., local versus distant). According to his model on combined modality therapy, in the clinical situation in which distant failure is common, radiotherapy should be given early in the treatment regimen. In situations in which there are large tumors, it may make intuitive sense to use chemotherapy first to shrink them to a size that can be easily eradicated by radiotherapy. However, most solid tumors that are visible clinically have a high likelihood of containing drug-resistant cells. If chemotherapy is given first in these cases, the drug-resistant cells are likely to convert to metastatic phenotypes, which soon proceed to transport themselves outside the confines of the subsequent radiation field. If radiotherapy is given first, then the drug-resistant population is likely to be killed in tandem with drug-sensitive cells, but the chances of drug-resistant cell metastasizing are reduced.

A second general rule that may be applied to reach a decision about sequentially administered modalities can be based on the nature of the cancer itself—locoregional cancer versus "systemic" cancers. Cancers that are often systemic, such as malignant lymphomas and breast cancers, are probably best handled with systemic therapy followed by consolidation radiotherapy to areas of "bulky" disease. Cancers that tend to remain confined to a particular region (e.g., cervical and head and neck cancers) are best treated by initial radiotherapy or better concomitant chemoradiation followed by consolidation, maintenance, or adjuvant chemotherapy.

NORMAL TISSUE EFFECTS

Acute Effects

The effect of a chemoradiation regimen on normal tissues is often equally important as its effect on a malignant tumor. Phillips and Fu[42,43] first described this effect in 1978 and have reported their extensive experimental work on chemoradiation effects on normal tissues. They also introduced the term *dose effect factor,* or DEF, which is the ratio of the radiation dose required to produce a particular effect without chemotherapy divided by the radiation dose required to produce the same effect with chemotherapy.[42] A number of factors such as type of chemotherapy, drug dose, duration of exposure, radiotherapy fraction size and total dose, the type of normal tissues involved, and the scheduling of the two modalities have important repercussions on acute and late toxicities. Table 5-3 outlines these factors and their influence in toxicity.

Besides increasing total radiation dose or treatment volume, alteration of fractionation by using

Table 5-3 Factors Influencing Chemoradiation Toxicity

Factor	Effect on Tissue
Radiotherapy	
Hypofractionation	↑ Late effects
Hyperfractionation	↑ Acute effects, ↓ late effects
↑ Total RT dose	↑ Acute and late effects
Large field	↑ Acute effects
Chemotherapy	
↑ Dose	↑ Drug-specific acute and late toxicity
	↑ Acute toxicity of radiotherapy
Duration of exposure:	
Bolus	↑ Toxicity of proliferative tissues
Infusion	↓ Acute toxicities in general
	Possible ↑ radiotherapy interaction on tumors and normal tissues
Type of Drug	
Cell-cycle dependent	↑ Toxicity of proliferating tissue (e.g., alkylating agents, 5-fluorouracil, bleomycin)
Cell-cycle independent	↑ Toxicity in all tissues (e.g., anthracyclines, actinomycin D)
Limited organ interaction	Vincristine—neuropathy
Multiple organ interaction	Doxorubicin—cardiac, gastrointestinal effect
	Bone marrow and pulmonary toxicity
Normal Tissue Type	
Critical	Central nervous system, lung, heart, kidney, and liver toxicities
Noncritical	Skin, bladder, esophagus toxicities
Timing/Scheduling of Modalities	
Concurrent (simultaneous)	↑ Acute effects
Sequential/remote	↓ Side effects

hyperfractionation or hypofractionation can result in increased acute toxicity and affect late toxicity as well. Hypofractionation of radiotherapy with chemotherapy generally is to be avoided because the resultant acute toxicity can be excessive and possibly prevent appropriate total doses of radiation from being delivered. Hyperfractionated radiotherapy, while allowing greater local control of disease and diminishing long-term toxicity, also increases acute toxicity, making concurrent chemotherapy potentially hazardous.[10] Studies have shown that concurrent chemoradiation with conventional daily radiotherapy, as well as hyperfractionated radiotherapy, has yielded superior local control, as well as survival, over conventional radiotherapy in inoperable non–small cell carcinoma of the lung.[44,45] Therefore, it is likely that the next generation of trials for locally advanced lung cancers will involve hyperfractionated radiotherapy with concurrent chemotherapy. Because increased acute toxicity is a certainty, these trials can be expected to use various doses and schedules of both radiotherapy and chemotherapy to settle the issue of which particular combinations achieve superior cure rates with the least increase in toxicity.

One of the most common objections to chemoradiation regimens is that the optimal/maximal radiotherapy dose was not given and that the end result from maximal doses of radiotherapy alone would be equal to that achieved by chemoradiation. This argument is specious at several levels. One of the major reasons for using chemotherapy with radiotherapy is to improve on the results obtained by a standard radical course of radiotherapy. The standard optimal radiotherapy dose for inoperable esophageal cancer was the equivalent of 60 Gy in 6 weeks, yielding a cure rate of about 5% by meta-analysis.[46] An identical dose given with concurrent chemotherapy in these patients has achieved a fivefold to sixfold increase in survival with identical toxicity except for acute and reversible hematologic toxicity.[47]

The second major raison d'être for chemoradiation is anatomic or function preservation. In treatment of anal cancers, chemoradiation has replaced definitive radiotherapy (and surgery) because it achieves a superior colostomy-free or sphincter preservation rate. Moreover, there is ample empirical evidence that a radiation dose of 45 Gy with concurrent 5-FU and mitomycin C achieves an equal or perhaps superior overall survival rate compared with 60 Gy of radical radiotherapy alone in anal cancers.[48] The matter of using "suboptimal" doses of radiotherapy in chemoradiation regimens is a moot one. There will be human tumors that require "full" doses of radiation in spite of combining it with chemotherapy, and there will be tumors that *do not* require such doses.

The same principles hold true for modification or non-modification of chemotherapy doses. Almost all successful concurrent chemoradiation regimens require dose modification of drugs. In chemoradiation protocols for lung cancers, for example, the doses of cisplatin and etoposide are about half the standard doses of these drugs when they are given alone. Even in sequential chemoradiation regimens, modifications of doses of either radiation or chemotherapeutic agents are often required. In Hodgkin's disease, for example, only 25 to 30 Gy (instead of 36 to 40 Gy) of radiation to the noncontiguous para-aortic region is required after mantle radiotherapy when alternated with systemic chemotherapy.[49]

Late Effects

Because of the relatively long history of radiotherapy, its extensive use for benign disease in the not-too-distant past, or perhaps the worldwide notoriety of the nuclear bombing of Hiroshima and Nagasaki and its aftermath, the lay public is somewhat familiar with the late effects of irradiation. Only recently have the late effects of prolonged chemotherapy come into focus. An increased incidence of late effects when radiotherapy and chemotherapy are combined is not only theoretically possible but also has been realized in long-term results of chemoradiation in Hodgkin's disease.[50]

The biologic basis of late radiation damage is its effect on microcirculation and fibroconnective tissues leading to organ hypoplasia and dysfunction. The corresponding effect of chemotherapy is on cellular parenchymal components causing, for example, stem cell depletion. Thus, both radiotherapy and chemotherapy can have late effects manifesting in the same organ system through different pathophysiologic mechanisms.[51]

Table 5-4 shows various drugs that have been associated with late, and sometimes acute, toxicities manifested in various critical and subcritical organ and tissue systems.

Table 5–4 Late Effects of Chemoradiation on Various Organs and Tissue Systems

Organ	Toxicity	Drugs
Heart	Cardiomyopathy	Doxorubicin, mitomycin C, carmustine (e.g., vincristine and etoposide)
	Ischemia/Infarction	5-fluorouracil, plant derivatives
Bone marrow	Leukopenia	Almost all current drugs; notable exceptions: bleomycin, vincristine,
	Thrombocytopenia	prednisone, 5-fluorouracil by infusion
Liver	Elevated enzyme levels	Carmustine
	Cirrhosis	Methotrexate
Kidney	Tubular damage	Cisplatin, high-dose methotrexate, carmustine
Lung	Pneumonitis or fibrosis	Bleomycin, carmustine, mitomycin C, cyclophosphamide, taxanes
Intestinal system	Esophagitis	Cyclophosphamide, doxorubicin
	Enteritis	5-fluorouracil, cisplatin, methotrexate, hydroxyurea, gemcitabine
Central nervous system	Encephalopathy	Intrathecal and high-dose methotrexate
	Necrotizing leukoencephalopathy	Procarbazine, carmustine, cisplatin
Spinal cord	Peripheral neuropathies	*Vinca* alkaloids, cisplatin, etoposide

When radiation therapy is followed by chemotherapy, subclinical damage from irradiation can be uncovered and clinically manifest as a *recall phenomenon*.[52] Most commonly seen in the skin, this effect of radiotherapy-chemotherapy interaction can be seen acutely in the small bowel and clinically in several critical organs, such as the breast and lung.

When the processes are reversed and chemotherapy is followed by radiotherapy, the same subclinical damage caused by chemotherapy can become clinically manifest during radiotherapy. On the skin, this process can be termed *reverse recall* and has been reported with the drug busulfan.[53] On other tissue systems and organs, however, the critical changes outlined in Table 5-4 can become evident. Small doses of radiation directed to lung parenchyma after administration of actinomycin D can result in pneumonitis.[52] Intrathecal methotrexate followed by cranial irradiation is known to increase the incidence of acute encephalopathy. After even medium doses of chemotherapy, radiotherapy appears to deplete bone marrow reserve faster than when it is the sole means of therapy.

When chemoradiation is given sequentially, the choice of modality for induction therapy tends to be quite arbitrary in clinical practice. Either due to acute or late toxicity, the second modality is invariably given in reduced doses. In the treatment of advanced Hodgkin's disease, for example, giving six cycles of MOPP (mechlorethamine, vincristine, procarbazine, prednisone) chemotherapy generally damages the hematopoietic system to the extent that full doses of total nodal irradiation may not be possible. With "full" doses, the reason for this excessive sensitivity to irradiation is that, aside from direct damage of stem cell population by this chemotherapy, the remaining stem cell population becomes hyperactive and hyperplastic, causing it to be increasingly sensitive to subsequent irradiation. This results in hematologic depression to the point that a so-called complete course of irradiation would cause significant morbidity and even mortality. Fortunately, noncurative or suboptimal doses of total nodal irradiation are sufficient to achieve long-term cures in these cases.[49]

GUIDELINES TO MINIMIZING TOXICITY

There are several means to reduce normal tissue toxicity when combining radiotherapy and chemotherapy. Generally, radiotherapy fields should cover clinically evident disease only and not attempt to cover areas where subclinical disease is likely to be present. Also, daily fractions should generally not exceed 1.8 Gy. The principles of modifying radiotherapy parameters in chemoradiation protocols have been employed successfully in the treatment of esophageal and lung cancers.[54,55] The use of hyperfractionated or hypofractionated radiotherapy with chemotherapy is fraught with the possibility of excess acute toxicity, and major dose and other modifications of chemotherapy delivery might be necessary.

Bolus administration of chemotherapeutic drugs is more often being replaced by infusion, particularly when chemotherapy is used with radiotherapy. 5-FU is generally given by intermediate- or low-dose infusion when combined with radiotherapy to reduce myelotoxicity, particularly when sizable portions of bone marrow are covered by the radiotherapy field (e.g., pelvic irradiation). The interaction of several drugs such as 5-FU, cisplatin, and anthracyclines with radiotherapy is enhanced by the duration of exposure (area under the curve) when radiotherapy is given.

Cell cycle–dependent drugs tend to increase the toxicity of acutely responding tissues such as the skin and mucous membranes. Examples include alkylating agents such as cisplatin and others such as 5-FU and bleomycin. These drugs are generally preferred over cell cycle–independent drugs (anthracyclines) because their enhanced toxicity is generally transient and reversible. Drugs such as doxorubicin tend to deposit their metabolites in a wide range of tissues, such as the heart, small bowel, and skin and are to be generally avoided when radiotherapy is being considered to the mediastinum, abdomen, or large areas of skin. When critical organs are being irradiated, care must be taken to avoid the use of drugs that have similar organ toxicity. Thus, bleomycin, actinomycin D, and taxanes are to be avoided when irradiating lung tumors; vincristine should not be used with CNS irradiation; anthracyclines should be avoided with mediastinal (cardiac) irradiation; and cisplatin should not be administered with abdominal (kidney) radiotherapy. When necessary, these drugs can be used in smaller doses in combination with other drugs and irradiation, particularly when they have specific activity against the tumor in question.

The advantages and disadvantages of combining radiotherapy and chemotherapy simultaneously have been discussed. When drugs with proven efficacy in the treatment of a cancer are combined with radiotherapy concurrently, there is a reasonable chance that the net effect on the cancer will be enhanced, be it a subadditive, an additive, or a supra-additive effect. At the same time, if the drugs used here are toxic to the same site as radiotherapy, then an enhancement effect (again, subadditive, additive, or supra-additive) can be expected on that normal tissue site or organ. This scenario is best described by the results of trials using bleomycin and radiotherapy concurrently for head and neck cancers. Both bleomycin and radiotherapy are effective against well-oxygenated proliferative cells and have similar cell cycle–sensitivity (M and G_2 phases).[56] High concentrations of the drug remain in tissues, such as the lungs, skin, and mucous membranes, long after administration. These are the reasons that bleomycin is used in small doses of 5 to 15 U per week with irradiation but has generally been replaced in the chemoradiation regimens for head and neck cancers by drugs such as cisplatin and 5-FU.

When the drug that is effective against a "radiosensitive" tumor has similar toxicity to radiotherapy (e.g., the myelotoxicity secondary to ifosfamide and pelvic radiotherapy for cervical cancer), the oncologist has recourse to several alternatives:

1. Drop the dose of the drug during concurrent chemoradiation.
2. Combine the drug with other effective drugs in similar reduced doses (e.g., ifosfamide with cisplatin and etoposide [the so-called *ICE regimen*] in reduced doses with radiotherapy).
3. Alternate different and effective drug combinations during the course of radiotherapy (e.g., use 5-FU and

cisplatin during week 1, 5-FU and mitomycin C during week 4 or 5 of external radiotherapy for a stage IIIB cervical cancer, and the ICE regimen during intracavitary application.

4. Use drugs and radiotherapy in alternating or sequential fashion.

Theoretically, the third option offers the best means of achieving maximal combined effect while reducing the opportunity for additive normal tissue effect. However, in many cases effective drugs may not be available in sufficient number to avail of this technique and the other three options may have to do.

CLINICAL RESULTS

The use of systemic treatment with radiotherapy has burgeoned in the past 10 years as a direct response to the realization that cure rates have stagnated for several years with unimodality treatment of locally advanced cancers at many sites. In still other sites, chemoradiation is being used in lieu of surgery to achieve organ and function preservation and in situations for which surgery is not possible or is contraindicated.

In individual chapters in the clinical section of this textbook, the role of chemoradiation is addressed in respective primary sites. What follows is a brief description of chemoradiation in select tumor sites with emphasis on the rationale for its use, the high points of progress to date, and a brief overview of studies under way. Disease categories such as pediatric cancers, sarcomas, and malignant lymphomas and certain primary sites such as the CNS, female breast, and hepatobiliary tract are not addressed here because the chemoradiation experience is either far too complex to be abbreviated or just very limited at this point.

Head and Neck Cancers

RATIONALE. An estimated two thirds of patients with head and neck cancers present with locally advanced cancer (stages III and IV). The so-called standard treatment for these patients was until recently either surgery with preoperative or, more commonly, postoperative radiotherapy or primary radiotherapy followed by surgery. The reasons for combining radiotherapy and chemotherapy in head and neck cancers are myriad. In patients with inoperable or unresectable stage III and IV disease, chemoradiation is primarily an attempt to increase cure rates over radiotherapy alone. In cancers of the larynx and pharynx and base of tongue tumors, the purpose of using definitive chemoradiation is to preserve vocal cord function. The added advantage in these cases is the improved cosmesis and function that result compared with a combined resection operation or a laryngopharyngectomy for advanced head and neck cancers of the sites just listed. Finally, in many cases when surgery or radiotherapy has been used alone, or even in tandem, the cure rates have remained virtually unchanged for decades. In

these cases, chemoradiation offers a chance for improved cure rates.

RESULTS OF CHEMORADIATION. In the past quarter-century, a large number of phase II and III studies employing chemoradiation in head and neck cancers have been reported.[36] Almost all the studies are in agreement that combining chemotherapy with irradiation results in increased toxicity, sometimes acceptable, sometimes not. With regard to survival results, there is wide variability, with a few studies reporting worse survival and others reporting either no difference or increased survival with chemoradiation compared with radiotherapy alone.

It is difficult to arrive at any definite conclusion from these studies, even when they are prospective randomized ones, owing to the heterogeneity of the tumors, the short periods of follow-up, the lack of uniformity in radiotherapy dose and technique, the different single drugs and drug combinations used, and the differences in mode of chemoradiation delivery (i.e., in sequential, simultaneous, or maintenance form with relation to radiotherapy). Nevertheless, there is increasing consensus among clinicians that simultaneous or concurrent chemotherapy and radiotherapy holds the most promise in terms of future research in the treatment of head and neck cancers. There is no such consensus as to the nature of the drug or drug combinations that are to be combined with the radiation.

Concurrent chemoradiation with cisplatinum-based chemotherapy has been shown to yield superior survival rates over radiotherapy alone in randomized clinical trials involving the nasopharynx[57] and oropharynx, including lesions in the tonsillar fossa, oropharyngeal wall, or base of tongue.[58,59] Two randomized trials have demonstrated statistically improved results with hyperfractionated and accelerated radiotherapy combined with mitomycin C[60] or cisplatin.[61]

In their analysis of chemoradiation studies, Taylor and Murthy[36] conclude that induction chemotherapy (or sequential chemoradiation) has failed to produce any survival or local control benefit in head and neck cancers and that concomitant chemoradiation has improved locoregional control and survival but has not had an impact on metastatic disease. Also, El-Sayed and Nelson,[38] in a meticulous analysis of 25 prospective randomized trials, concluded that a statistically significant improvement in survival was found when chemotherapy and local definitive treatment were given simultaneously. Two recent meta-analyses of trials combining chemotherapy and radiotherapy continue to show improved survival and quality of life measurements in patients receiving combined and concurrent therapy over those receiving radiotherapy alone or sequential induction chemotherapy followed by radiotherapy.[62,63]

The recent availability of intensity modulation of radiation should have a profound effect on decreasing toxicities of accelerated radiotherapy and concurrently intensified chemotherapies. Other promising means of intensifying combined modality treatment while still increasing the therapeutic ratio are the increasing use of amifostine, biologic modifiers such as epoetin, alimentary support during treatment, chemo prevention with retinoids, anti-angiogenesis agents, and the possible emergence of newer and more effective chemotherapy with taxanes and irinotecan.

Lung

NON–SMALL CELL LUNG CANCER

RATIONALE. The role of chemoradiation in non–small cell lung cancer (NSCLC) is in the definitive treatment for patients with stage I, II, and III surgically resectable disease but who are medically inoperable and for stage III patients with locally advanced and unresectable disease. About 50,000 patients present with locally advanced or stage III NSCLC annually. The large numbers of patients affected by this disease are why small improvements in cure rates translate to sizable numbers of saved lives. Radiotherapy alone can obtain 2- and 5-year progression-free survivals of 28% and 9%, respectively, in medically inoperable patients.[45]

CHEMORADIATION EXPERIENCE. Multiple phase II and III studies have used various drug combinations with sequential or concurrent radiotherapy in medically inoperable/unresectable non–small cell lung cancer. Dillman and coworkers[64] randomized patients with stage III disease to receive sequential cisplatin plus vinblastine followed by radiotherapy versus radiotherapy alone. The 2-year (26% vs. 13%) and 5-year (19% vs. 7%) survival rates were statistically superior with the chemoradiation group.

Sause and colleagues[65] reported on a randomized phase III study on patients with stage III non–small cell lung cancer comparing standard radiotherapy versus hyperfractionated radiotherapy versus induction chemotherapy with cisplatin plus vinblastine followed by concurrent radiotherapy plus cisplatin. The chemoradiation arm showed a statistically superior 2-year survival over radiotherapy alone.[65] Two other randomized studies have shown that concurrent chemoradiation is superior to sequential chemoradiation in terms of survival in NSCLC.[66,67] Furuse et al. employed cisplatinum, vindesine, and mitomycin in their trial, whereas the RTOG trial reported by Curran et al. used vinblastine and cisplatinum.

The case for neoadjuvant chemoradiation (followed by surgery) was made by Albain and associates for the Southwest Oncology Group (SWOG),[68] using cisplatin plus etoposide plus 45 Gy of radiation in 5 weeks concurrently followed by surgical resection. A 2-year survival of 39% and 37% was reported for patients with stage IIIA (N2) and IIIB disease, respectively.

Thus, there appears to be a trend toward using concurrent chemoradiation for stage III NSCLC in general and for all patients with nonmetastatic (M0) cancer that is deemed to be unresectable or medically inoperable. Future trials are likely to compare chemoradiation with and without surgery for patients with stage III disease and to introduce newer drugs such as paclitaxel, taxotere, gemcitabine and irinotecan into chemoradiation regimens.

Newer treatment paradigms in NSCLC include the incorporation of signal transduction inhibitors, anti-angiogenesis agents, and targeted gene therapies such as *p53* and *Bcl-2* into chemoradiation regimens.

SMALL CELL LUNG CANCER

RATIONALE. When treated by chemotherapy alone, patients with limited small cell lung cancer have local failure rates from 60% to 100%. This is reduced to approximately 30% by the addition of thoracic radiotherapy. Whether the addition of sequential thoracic radiotherapy increases disease-free or overall survival is debatable.[69]

CHEMORADIATION EXPERIENCE. The results of combined chemoradiation protocols for limited small cell lung cancer are inconsistent owing to several variants in their design and reports: the use of cyclophosphamide-based versus cisplatin-based chemoradiation combinations; the early (concurrent) or late (sequential) use of thoracic radiotherapy; the dose, volume, and fractionation used in thoracic radiotherapy; and the use or nonuse of prophylactic cranial irradiation.[69,70] As in several solid tumors described in this chapter, there appears to be increasing consensus toward the use of cisplatin-based chemotherapy and toward the early concurrent use of thoracic radiotherapy in the treatment of limited-stage small cell lung cancer.

A good example of a chemoradiation protocol for small cell lung cancer is the prospective randomized trial reported by the National Cancer Institute of Canada clinical trials group.[71] These patients were randomly assigned to receive thoracic radiotherapy early (after one chemotherapy cycle) or late (after five chemotherapy cycles) with alternating cisplatin-based chemotherapy (cisplatin + etoposide) and cyclophosphamide-based chemotherapy (cyclophosphamide + doxorubicin + vincristine). Prophylactic cranial irradiation was used in both arms of the study. The early or concurrent use of thoracic radiotherapy resulted in statistically improved disease-free survival (26% vs. 19%), overall survival (20% vs. 11% at 5 years), and lowered risk of brain metastasis (18% vs. 28%).

Three cooperative research groups—the Japanese Clinical Oncology Group (JCOG), Southwest Oncology Group (SWOG), and Eastern Cooperative Oncology Group (ECOG)—have completed randomized clinical trials, addressing questions regarding timing of radiotherapy vis-à-vis chemotherapy and fractionation of radiotherapy.[72,73,74] Both JCOG and SWOG studies showed 2-year survival rates superior with concurrent versus sequential chemoradiation. The ECOG results implied the superiority of accelerated radiotherapy within a concurrent chemoradiation regimen.

Other promising combinations of chemoradiation include alternating chemotherapy with radiotherapy as reported by Arriagada and coworkers[75] (17% survival at 5 years) and accelerated radiotherapy concurrent with chemotherapy as reported by Turrisi and associates (36% survival at 4 years).[76]

FUTURE TRENDS

The next decade of studies will probably involve the use of newer and more effective chemotherapeutic agents, specifically those crossing the blood-brain barrier; variations in radiotherapy fractionation and dose; and the use of biologic modifiers to shorten overall treatment time and to allow "full" doses of drugs and radiotherapy to be delivered. Or, perhaps a drug such as amifostine or the use of IMRT may be found to effectively prevent or treat esophagitis, the foremost toxic effect of these chemoradiation protocols.

Gastrointestinal System

ESOPHAGUS

RATIONALE. It was recognized in the early 1980s that conventional treatment of esophageal cancer, which was a one-stage esophagectomy for more than 40 years, had a sizable morbidity and mortality, with 5-year cure rates of about 5%.[77] Patients with unresectable but non-metastatic disease and those who could not undergo surgery because of medical conditions received definitive radiotherapy with minimal morbidity and mortality but with cure rates also of about 5%. When the two modalities were combined, there was no increase or only marginal increase in cure rates and some increase in morbidity and mortality.[78] With all three treatment techniques, the major site of failure was still local or regional, with rates between 20% and 85%.[79]

The activity of most chemotherapeutic drugs against esophageal cancer is limited both in response rate and period of response. Single-agent activity with vindesine, mitomycin C, and cisplatin ranges from 22% to 32%, and combination chemotherapy, usually including cisplatin, has a 50% to 60% response rate.[80] Despite these limitations, the addition of chemotherapy to local modalities such as radiotherapy and surgery has turned around the prognosis of esophageal cancer in just the past 2 decades.

CURRENT TREATMENT APPROACHES. The occasional T1N0M0 esophageal cancer is generally subjected to en bloc esophagectomy, which appears to be the surgical procedure of choice in the United States.[64] The standard treatment for all other patients with nonmetastatic disease can be said to be preoperative chemoradiation or definitive chemoradiation. Two large randomized studies on preoperative chemoradiation have shown somewhat conflicting results. Walsh et al. reported on 113 patients randomized to receive surgery alone or concurrent 5-FU and cisplatin with radiotherapy given before surgery. The 3-year cure rates were 32% for the preoperative group and 6% for surgery alone ($P = 0.01$).[82] Bosset et al. reported on 282 patients randomized to similar treatments.[83] Although median survival was identical in the two groups, disease-free survival in the preoperative chemoradiation group was significantly superior over that of surgery alone ($P = 0.003$).

CHEMORADIATION TRENDS. Two randomized prospective trials comparing preoperative chemotherapy with surgery alone have shown no difference in median survivals and an increase in operative morbidity and mortality in the preoperative chemotherapy arms.[84,85]

Three major reports have set the trend for future trials in the management of esophageal cancer. Forastiere and colleagues[86] reported a 5-year survival of 34% and a 29-month median survival using a fairly intensive preoperative chemoradiation course of continuous infusion of 5-FU and cisplatin with 45 Gy of radiation in 3 weeks. The surgical procedure used in this University of Michigan study was a transhiatal esophagectomy, which is widely considered not to be true cancer surgery but that nevertheless is far less toxic than an en bloc esophagectomy.

On the nonsurgical front, Al-Sarraf and associates[47] updated the landmark randomized RTOG study comparing radiotherapy alone versus chemoradiation. The 5-year results were 0% and 30%, respectively. The RTOG study established chemoradiation as the standard treatment of locally advanced cancers of the esophagus that are unresectable or inoperable owing to comorbid medical conditions. By inference, these excellent results in patients believed to have inoperable disease are further credence to those who question the value of esophagectomy in patients with esophageal cancer.[54,87] Mantravadi and colleagues[88] reported a 4-year survival of 43% with patients treated with chemoradiation alone. The ECOG conducted a randomized study of patients treated with 5-FU and mitomycin C concurrently with radiotherapy versus radiotherapy alone.[89] The 2-year survival in favor of chemoradiation was 27% versus 12%. Also, an intergroup trial comparing induction chemotherapy (cisplatin) followed by chemoradiation versus chemoradiation alone showed no difference between the two groups.[90]

STOMACH

RATIONALE. To examine the role of chemoradiation in stomach cancer, it is best to evaluate it in light of two basic categories: (1) the need and effectiveness of adjuvant chemoradiation in completely excised cancer and (2) the preoperative or definitive role of chemoradiation in unresectable or inoperable gastric cancer. An overview of published data suggests that there is no conclusive proof that chemoradiation in both these scenarios is helpful, but some phase II and III data point to its potential benefit.[91] The rationale for chemoradiation in managing stomach cancer is based on the limitation on surgical resection and regional node dissection as required and on the high incidence (20%) of locoregional failure.[92]

CHEMORADIATION RESULTS. A prospective randomized trial at the Mayo Clinic compared surgery alone versus surgery followed by chemoradiation consisting of 37.5 Gy over a 4- to 5-week period with a bolus of 5-FU for 3 days.[93] The study was methodologically flawed, but when patients with equally poor prognostic features were compared, there was a statistically significant improved 5-year survival for the chemoradiation arm (20% vs. 4%; $P < 0.05$). Sixteen years later, McDonald et al.[94] reported on the results of an Intergroup (INT-0116) trial evaluating the role of concurrent bolus 5-FU and 45 to 55.8 Gy of radiotherapy in postgastrectomy patients. A survival advantage (52% to 61%) was seen in patients given postoperative chemoradiation.

For patients with unresectable gastric tumors or those who undergo resection but have residual disease, most trials suggest a survival advantage for chemoradiation over radiotherapy alone or chemotherapy alone. A prospective randomized study from the Gastrointestinal Tumor Study Group (GITSG) showed patients treated with 5-FU, semustine, and radiation having superior survival rates compared with patients treated with 5-FU and semustine alone.[95] More recently, another GITSG trial on incompletely resected gastric cancer treated with chemotherapy alone versus split-course chemoradiation was abandoned early due to treatment-related toxicity.[96] However, a significant (26% vs. 6% $P < 0.01$) advantage was seen in patients receiving chemoradiation.

FUTURE TRENDS

As a result of the previously mentioned studies, the standard treatment for resectable gastric cancer now includes 5-FU–based chemoradiation. Numerous single- and multi-institutional studies are under way to address issues such as preoperative, postoperative, and definitive chemoradiation with newer drugs such as taxanes and gemcitabine.

PANCREAS

RATIONALE. The overall 5-year cure rate for pancreatic cancer has slightly improved from 1% to around 3% in the past 3 decades.[97] This minimal improvement is primarily due to a decrease in operative mortality from around 25% to less than 5%.[98] Other reasons may include increased resectability with improved diagnostic tests such as dynamic computed tomographic scans, endoscopic retrograde cholangiopancreatography, percutaneous cholangiography, and laparoscopy. Radiotherapy has been found to be an effective palliative tool, and chemotherapy has shown little value as primary therapy. Chemoradiation offers some hope for subpopulations of patients with resectable small tumors without spread to contiguous structures or nodes and is often effective in palliating locally advanced disease.

TRADITIONAL TREATMENT APPROACHES. Local factors that preclude surgical resection of pancreatic cancer are local extension of disease to the inferior vena cava or the aorta or involvement or encasement of the superior

mesenteric artery and vein and the portal vein. Whereas pancreaticoduodenal nodal involvement is not a contraindication to resection, involvement of para-aortic or celiac nodes is considered distant disease. Pancreaticoduodenectomy or its modification is the surgical treatment of choice in pancreatic cancer, and pancreaticojejunostomy is used to restore GI continuity most often. Two studies on patients with unresectable pancreatic cancer formed the basis of current chemoradiation protocols for neoadjuvant/adjuvant or palliative purposes. First, Moertel and coworkers,[99] in a randomized study, showed that radiotherapy plus 5-FU was superior to radiotherapy plus placebo (10 vs. 6 months; $P < 0.05$). Second, Haslem and colleagues[100] used 60 Gy of radiation given over 10 weeks (20 Gy in two double-split courses) to obtain a 34% 1-year survival compared with less than 10% 1-year survival in a historical series of untreated patients.

CHEMORADIATION RESULTS. A concurrent combination of radiotherapy and 5-FU can be considered standard treatment in the following situations (Table 5-5):

1. After pancreaticoduodenectomy as *adjuvant* treatment: The GITSG randomly assigned patients with pancreatic cancer undergoing radical surgery to no adjuvant treatment versus chemoradiation consisting of 40 Gy given split course as two doses of 20 Gy with 5-FU given in 500 mg/m² bolus on days 1 through 3 of each of two radiotherapy courses, followed by weekly maintenance 5-FU at the same dose indefinitely or until recurrence was demonstrated. The median survival for the chemoradiation group was 20 months versus 11 months ($P = 0.03$) for the untreated control group.[101] Similar results were reported in a more recent study by the European Organization for Research and Treatment of Cancer (EORTC).[102]

2. In the treatment of locally unresectable disease for *palliation:* Chemoradiation with radiotherapy 40 to 60 Gy plus 5-FU has been shown in GITSG randomized studies to be superior to radiotherapy alone as well as combination chemotherapy alone.[103,104] The first study compared patients treated with 60 Gy of radiation given in three double split courses or 20 Gy each versus 40 Gy (single split course) and a 500 mg/m² bolus of 5-FU on days 1 through 3 of each course versus 60 Gy (double split course) and 5-FU given as a 500 mg/m² bolus on days 1 to 3 of each of three radiotherapy courses. The median survival with both

Table 5–5   Standard Chemoradiation Regimens for Pancreatic Cancer

Purpose	Study	Chemoradiation (CR)		
		RT	Chemotherapy*	Median Survival CR vs. Control (mo)
Definitive (postop)	Kalser (GITSG)[101]	40 Gy	5-FU 500 mg/m²	20 vs. 11
Palliative	Moertel (GITSG)[103]	40/60 Gy	5-FU 500 mg/m²	10.5 vs. 5.7
	GITSG[104]	40/60 Gy	Streptozocin + mitomycin C + 5-FU†	10.5 vs. 8

*Chemotherapy given concurrently with RT followed by maintenance for 2 years or until tumor recurrence.
†SMF regimen noted to be more toxic than 5-FU alone.
RT, radiation therapy.

chemoradiation arms (10.5 months with 40 Gy, 10 months with 60 Gy) was superior to radiotherapy alone (5.7 months).[103] The second study compared SMF (streptozotocin, mitomycin C, and 5-FU) combination chemotherapy alone every 8 weeks for 2 years or until progression versus chemoradiation consisting of radiotherapy with 54 Gy in 6 weeks and a bolus of 5-FU on the first and last 3 days of radiotherapy followed by SMF maintenance chemotherapy as described.[104] The median survival with chemotherapy alone was 8 months, compared with 10.5 months with chemoradiation. The GITSG concluded that chemoradiation with 40 to 60 Gy of radiation and 5-FU could offer as many as 25% of patients with unresectable pancreatic cancer a chance of survival of 2 years or more.

FUTURE PROSPECTS. It is evident that for any progress from here on, innovative methods of early diagnosis, improved methods of radiotherapy delivery, newer and more effective systemic agents, and the maturation of molecular approaches will be required. Phase II chemoradiation studies of some promise include those employing combinations of 5-FU and gemcitabine[105]; 5-FU, cisplatin, and gemcitabine[106]; and cisplatin and gemcitabine.[108]

COLON AND RECTUM

RATIONALE. There are three clinical situations, particularly with rectal cancer, in which chemoradiation has a definitive role to play: (1) resectable primary rectal cancers at high risk for local recurrence, in which chemoradiation reduces local recurrence and improves survival, as well; (2) unresectable primary rectal cancers in which chemoradiation improves resectability and thereby cure, and possibly local recurrence, as well; and (3) local recurrences in which chemoradiation provides local control occasionally and prolonged palliation often.

The role of chemoradiation in these cases has evolved with multiple studies over just the past decade. For colon cancers, there is no proven role for chemoradiation. Nevertheless, there are instances (Gunderson's modified Astler-Coller stages B2/B3 and C2/C3) in which local recurrence rates after surgery range from 11% to 49%.[109] Certain sections of the colon that have limited mobility and are partially retroperitoneal are at similar risk as the rectum for local failure.

CHEMORADIATION EXPERIENCE. Postoperative randomized chemoradiation trials from GITSG and the National Surgical Adjuvant Breast and Bowel Project (NSABP) reported between 1985 and 1992 showed decreased local recurrence, disease-free survival, and overall survival in patients with stage T3 (B2) rectal cancer or above.[110-113] Whereas the initial studies used 5-FU and semustine with or without vincristine in the chemoradiation arms, the final study (1992) showed no additional benefit to adding semustine to 5-FU.[113] In another randomized study, the North Central Cancer Treatment Group (NCCTG) showed statistically improved local recurrence rates (14% vs. 25%), distant failure rates (29% vs. 46%), disease-free survival rates (58% vs. 38%), and overall survival

rates (53% vs. 38%) in patients receiving chemoradiation over those receiving radiotherapy alone.[114] The standard of treatment for stage B2 and C rectal cancers is postoperative 45 to 50.4 Gy in about 5 weeks to the pelvis with a bolus or infusion of 5-FU during the first and fourth weeks of radiotherapy.

For high-risk colon cancers (e.g., stage B2/B3 and C2/C3 cancers of the cecum, hepatic and splenic flexure, and the distal sigmoid colon), studies are being done to test the feasibility and efficacy of local radiotherapy in addition to systemic treatment with 5-FU and levamisole.

Preoperative chemoradiation is now increasingly used in rectal cancer. The rationale for its use is to preserve the anal sphincter in distal cancers (by avoiding abdominoperineal resection), downstage disease by sterilizing regional lymphatics as well as reducing T stage, and reduce bowel toxicity. Three recent studies of preoperative chemoradiation with bolus or infusion 5-FU with 45 Gy of radiotherapy have shown: (1) 15% to 30% complete response at surgery, (2) downstaging rates between 30% and 85%, and (3) sphincter preservation rates of 58% to 85%.[115-117]

ANAL CANAL

RATIONALE. Before the establishment of definitive chemoradiation for anal cancers, the initial provocation for using drugs and radiotherapy was to increase resectability. Currently, chemoradiation is proven to increase cure rates over abdominoperineal resections by meta-analysis, as well as to decrease colostomy rates from 100% to about 20%.[48]

CHEMORADIATION EXPERIENCE. Evolving from a preoperative regimen to a definitive one, the combination of 5-FU plus mitomycin C plus pelvic radiotherapy has now been established as the treatment of choice for anal cancers in Europe and the United States at least. Several studies of the efficacy of this combination have been reported in recent years.

In the first such randomized study on anal cancers, the EORTC showed a statistically improved colostomy-free and overall cure rate for patients treated with chemoradiation over those treated by radiotherapy alone.[118] Flam and colleagues,[119] reporting on a randomized RTOG trial, noted that the mitomycin C plus 5-FU plus radiotherapy combination was superior to the 5-FU plus radiotherapy combination in terms of colostomy-free survival rates in spite of increased but still acceptable toxicity. The same study also showed that approximately 50% of those who failed initial chemoradiation could be salvaged by additional 5-FU plus cisplatin plus radiotherapy without resorting to abdominoperineal resection.[119]

Another large randomized trial from the United Kingdom comparing radiotherapy alone to chemoradiation with bolus 5-FU and mitomycin C showed an increased local recurrence rate (59% vs. 36%) in the radiotherapy-alone group.[120]

John and associates,[35] reporting on long-term toxicity and survival, noted that long-term survival was possible (83% in 10 years) with the 5-FU plus mitomycin C plus radiotherapy schedule and that there was no significant increase in late toxicity.

Table 5-6   5-Year Survival Results of Various Treatments for Clinical Stages A-D1 or T1-T4 Bladder Cancer

Clinical Stage	Rad. Cyst., %	External RT, %	RT & Rad. Cyst., %	Interst/IOP RT, %
A/T1	70–80	60–70*	NA	70–96
B$_1$/T2	45–50	40	NA	55–60
B$_2$-C/T3	32	20–30	50	48
D$_1$/T4	0	10	NA	NA

*With salvage cystectomy.

Interst, interstitial; IOP, intraoperative; NA, not available; Rad. Cyst., radical cystectomy; RT, radiation therapy.

Current investigations are those studying the impact of high radiotherapy doses on larger (T3 and T4) anal cancers in terms of colostomy-free survival and toxicity. Other investigations are comparing the efficacy and toxicity of 5-FU plus mitomycin C plus radiotherapy versus 5-FU plus cisplatin plus radiotherapy.

Genitourinary System

BLADDER

RATIONALE. In spite of technical improvements in staging techniques, decreased anesthetic and surgical mortality, and improvements in delivery of radiation, more than half of patients with muscle-invading bladder cancers eventually develop metastatic disease. Radical cystectomy involves the removal of the bladder, prostate, and seminal vesicles in the male and the bladder, uterus, and upper vagina in the female. The procedure has a significant impact on the social and sexual activities of both sexes.[121,122] The impetus for the large number of phase II and III chemoradiation regimens being tested today is a reflection of the need to improve cure rates that are now being achieved with radical cystectomy in the United States, and with radical radiotherapy in Europe, as well as the desire to improve the quality of life in these patients by bladder preservation.

CURRENT TRADITIONAL MANAGEMENT. Just as with carcinoma of the prostate, there is no universal agreement about the most appropriate radical treatment for carcinoma of the bladder. Table 5-6 summarizes available results of purely *clinically* staged tumors subjected to various treatments.[121,122] Results for radical cystectomy alone and interstitial/intraoperative radiotherapy in the early stages of the disease (stages A and B) are roughly equivalent. Yet radiotherapy for such disease is virtually unheard of in the United States. As a rule, most

patients in the United States undergo radical cystectomy with or without preoperative radiotherapy, whereas most patients in Europe undergo radical external-beam radiation or interstitial irradiation with salvage cystectomy. Two randomized studies comparing these two approaches have not shown statistical difference in overall survival.[122,123]

Patients with T2 to T4 lesions appear likely to benefit from the addition of combination chemotherapy. Because most patients with bladder cancer are between 60 and 75 years of age, they may not be candidates for surgery, owing to unresectable disease, poor medical condition, or nodal metastases. On the other hand, the optimal chemoradiation course for such patients would have to be generally tolerable with minimal mortality and reversible morbidity to make it worthwhile.[124,125]

CHEMORADIATION RESULTS. There are now five chemotherapeutic agents—cisplatin, methotrexate, doxorubicin, taxol, and gemcitabine—that have individual significant activity in bladder cancer with response rates higher than 20%.[126-128] Others with less activity, such as 5-FU and vinblastine, may be used in combination with other drugs, especially when they are known to have additional effects when combined with radiotherapy.

Combination chemotherapy with methotrexate, vinblastine, doxorubicin, and cisplatin (MVAC) has been shown to be superior to cisplatin in the treatment of metastatic and recurrent bladder cancer.[129] Table 5-7 lists selected published series that used drug combinations with concurrent radiotherapy; the data show long-term (4 to 5 years) follow-up and salvage of the bladder in a significant percentage of patients.[130-134] On review of these reported series, it is evident that chemoradiation in its various forms is generally both efficacious and tolerable in this older population of patients with invasive bladder cancer. As such, it should be offered to all such patients as an alternative to cystectomy, and in particular

Table 5-7   Long-Term Results of Patients Treated with Chemoradiation for Invasive (T2-T4) Bladder Cancer

Study	Patients, *n*	Chemoradiation	Bladder Preservation, %	Overall Survival, % (yr)
Kaufman et al (1993)[130]	53	MCV Π (RT + cisplatin)	59	55 (4)
Dunst et al (1994)[131]	139	Cisplatin + RT	83	50 (5)
Tester et al (1996)[132]	91	MCV Π (RT + cisplatin)	60	62 (4)
Fellin et al (1997)[133]	56	MCV Π cisplatin	41	59 (5)
Shipley et al (2002)[134]	190	Cisplatin	65	54 (5)

to those who are in poor medical condition and to those who absolutely refuse surgery.

FUTURE TRENDS

If the past is any indication, there is very little likelihood that there will be a prospective randomized study comparing cystectomy and chemoradiation for bladder cancer. In the immediate future, it is likely that multi-institutional studies will compare chemoradiation with neoadjuvant chemotherapy plus concurrent chemoradiation regimens for efficacy measured by overall survival and bladder preservation as well as toxicity.

PROSTATE

RATIONALE. Androgen deprivation has been the standard form of therapy for metastatic prostate cancer for more than half a century. With newer and more effective synthetic hormones available recently, the concept of achieving total androgen blockade has been extended to its use with local treatment, be it prostatectomy or radiotherapy for nonmetastatic but locally advanced prostate cancer. The combination of antiandrogens such as flutamide (Eulexin) and luteinizing hormone-releasing hormone agonists such as goserelin acetate serves to ablate gonadal *and* adrenal precursors of testosterone. The intent of using neoadjuvant or adjuvant systemic hormonal therapy with local therapy is to reduce tumor volume and to increase local control, disease-free survival, and, possibly, overall survival.

RESULTS. Pilepich and coworkers[135] reported one prospective randomized RTOG study that was initiated a decade ago in which patients with locally advanced prostate cancer were randomly assigned to receive definitive radiotherapy with and without neoadjuvant and concurrent androgen deprivation by systemic hormonal treatment. At 5 years, local progression of disease was decreased (45% vs. 71%) and progression-free survival was significantly improved (30% vs. 15%) with combined modality treatment over radiotherapy alone, but no significant difference was found in overall survival. A recent update of the study showed similar results and even noted a survival benefit for patients having Gleason scores of 2 to 6.[136]

Another RTOG study (#85-31) studied patients with high-risk disease treated with radical external-beam radiotherapy or prostatectomy and who were randomized to receive androgen ablation versus no additional treatment.[137,138] This trial also showed decreased local failure, distant metastases, and biochemical failure in those receiving androgen therapy. In addition, a subset of patients with Gleason scores of 8 to 10 had improved survival rates. An EORTC randomized study[139] where goserelin was given for 3 years showed that androgen therapy added to radiotherapy improved local control, disease-free survival, and overall survival as well, compared to radiotherapy alone.

FUTURE TRENDS

Studies under way and those awaiting mature data include those testing the timing of administration of androgen ablation with regard to radiotherapy, the duration of androgen ablation required for various subsets of patients, and the role of such combined treatment on patients with lymph node metastases. The combination of drugs, such as estramustine, with radiotherapy is also being tested.

Gynecologic System

CERVICAL CANCER

RATIONALE. Conventional radiotherapy or surgery produces excellent long-term cure rates in early cervical cancer (International Federation of Gynecology and Obstetrics [FIGO] stages I to IIB) in general. Owing to limitations of the FIGO staging system, certain subsets of these stages have less than favorable prognosis. These subsets and more advanced disease (stages III to IVA) have been the target of several phase II studies using chemoradiation. Recurrent cervical cancer after hysterectomy, generally treated with radiotherapy alone, has also been the subject of chemoradiation trials. Vaginal and vulvar cancers are generally managed with radical surgery as primary treatment. Here, too, chemoradiation has been used to limit surgical resection, particularly since the patients who are affected by these diseases tend to be older women with comorbid conditions that might preclude surgery.

CHEMORADIATION EXPERIENCE. A large number of phase II studies have used chemoradiation as primary treatment for the patient populations just described.[107] These studies used either sequential chemoradiation or concurrent chemoradiation. Just as with head and neck cancers, sequential chemoradiation resulted in high response rates in cervical cancers with no ultimate benefit in survival.

Until 1999, chemoradiation experience in general could have been categorized into four groups: (1) the hydroxyurea experience mostly reported by Piver and coworkers and the Gynecology Oncology Group (GOG); (2) the Princess Margaret Hospital experience; (3) the Northern California Oncology Group (NCOG)-RTOG experience; and (4) miscellaneous phase II studies from diverse sources that used either 5-FU and mitomycin C or 5-FU and cisplatin combinations.[19,140,141] The NCOG and RTOG experience appeared to indicate that the 5-FU plus mitomycin C plus cisplatin combination was possibly superior to radiotherapy alone in stage III and IVA disease but not in poor prognostic stage IIB disease.[142] The multiple phase II studies using concurrent chemoradiation generally showed good tolerance and "promising" disease-free survival rates, although for minimal follow-up periods.

In February 1999, the National Cancer Institute (NCI), in an extraordinary clinical announcement, advised that cisplatinum-based chemotherapy administered concurrently with radiotherapy exhibited a marked superiority over standard radiotherapy alone in cervical cancer and that, furthermore, concurrent chemoradiation was the new standard of treatment for this disease. This was based on the results of five randomized prospective trials (four GOG, one RTOG) that consistently showed that cisplatin given concurrently with radiotherapy decreased the risk of recurrence by 40% to 60%.[144-148] These studies are discussed in detail in Chapter 48. A worthwhile point to make here is that the weekly cisplatin regimen (40 mg/m^2) reduced recurrence by 48% and the 3-weekly regimen of 75 mg/m^2 given with 5-FU achieved a 40% reduction.[144,145]

VULVAR CANCER

Chemoradiation as primary management of locally advanced cancer of the vulva has been reported sporadically in the past decade.[149] It appears to be a potentially curative method of treating women with locally advanced cancers without radical surgery. See Chapter 52, Cancer of the Vulva, in this text.

FUTURE TRENDS

Chemoradiation trials under way include those addressing special circumstances, such as involved para-aortic nodes or bulky cervical cancer unsuitable for hysterectomy; sarcomas of the uterus and cervix; and for recurrent disease after surgery in cervical, vaginal, vulvar, and ovarian cancers.

STRATEGIES FOR COMBINING RADIOTHERAPY AND CHEMOTHERAPY

In considering future modes of combining radiotherapy and systemic therapy in the treatment of cancer, one needs to revisit the basic rationale of such combined use. Briefly, chemoradiation is a science that has been engendered by stationary cure rates that are achieved with unimodality treatment. There is also the increasing realization that extensive surgery can be tempered, that organs and their function can be preserved, and that morbidity can be decreased by treatment with chemoradiation without jeopardizing cure rates that are achieved with radical surgery or radiotherapy. And finally, we have alluded to a silent but sizable minority of elderly cancer patients with multiple medical conditions who are not given the benefit of any significant attempt at cure because they are not considered surgical candidates.

As remarked on at the very outset, the success of many chemoradiation regimens, particularly for purposes of organ and function preservation, is markedly dependent on the skill of the surgeon. For example, a woman with early breast cancer who wishes to undergo breast preservation treatment relies on the surgeon's capability of removing the primary tumor with adequate margins without distorting the contour or shape of the breast significantly; the type of chemotherapy used or the radiotherapy technique will have less bearing on the ultimate cosmetic effect.

A conceptual model for the use of chemoradiation has been described before and elaborated on earlier in this chapter as the *maximal therapy–minimal time* model.[32] Variations of this model may be used for a wide spectrum of patients with various cancers.

SCENARIO A

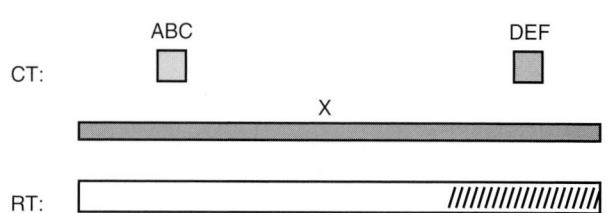

Here the radiotherapy course is characterized by treatment of the gross primary tumor and first station of regional (generally nodal) disease. Daily single doses of 180 cGy or less are preferred. At least one reduction of field size is necessary. The last 1 or 2 weeks of radiotherapy may be intensified by using hyperfractionated (external) or hypofractionated radiotherapy (e.g., high dose rate [HDR] brachytherapy).

If two drug combinations, ABC and DEF, are known to have significant activity against the tumor in question (even better if they happen to have additive effects with radiotherapy), they are to be used during this phase of treatment. When given concurrently with radiotherapy, the individual drug doses are reduced generally by 25% to 75% of the dose normally used when only chemotherapy is used. The more active of the two combinations, DEF, is used in the late intensification part of the combined course, because the remaining tumor population at that time is likely to contain the more resistant subpopulations and because fractionated radiotherapy earlier has caused previously hypoxic and resistant cells to be more oxygenated, accessible, and vulnerable to the best drug combination.

Another advantage of using two drug combinations, ABC and DEF, rather than two courses of DEF, is that the chances of overlapping toxicity among the individual drugs, as well as the additive effects, on normal tissues with radiotherapy are reduced. For example, using one to two courses of 5-FU or bleomycin rather than three or four during radiotherapy for a head and neck tumor is less likely to cause dose limitations or the splitting of the radiotherapy course secondary to oral mucositis. The drug X given in low-dose infusion throughout in the previous scenario may be used instead of or in addition to the drug combinations of ABC and DEF, depending on the nature of the primary tumor in question (low-cycling cell population requires a prolonged exposure to drug), the drug's efficacy against the specific tumor, and its capability of adding to the radiotherapy effect on that particular tumor. For example, 5-FU in a low-dose infusion can be given throughout a radiotherapy course for rectal cancers and is known to enhance the radiotherapy effect on that tumor.

SCENARIO B

If Scenario A is too toxic, one may then resort to the continuous intermittent schedule:

SCENARIO C

Less preferably, a concurrent split schedule can be used:

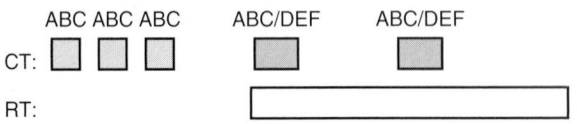

In this last concurrent but split schedule, the radiotherapy schedule could be intensified by hyperfractionation or hypofractionation as described previously, along with the most effective drug combination (DEF) during the last phase of the treatment course. Scenario A should always be preferred to scenarios B and C. All the toxicity that is likely to prevent scenario A from being carried out should be addressed preemptively whenever possible. For example, if myelotoxicity is the limiting toxicity with pelvic radiotherapy and concurrent therapy with paclitaxel, it may be useful to use cytokines that expedite bone marrow regeneration up front, along with the administration of the myelotoxic drug. If esophagitis is the limiting toxicity with thoracic radiotherapy and methotrexate, then a combination of topical emollients and antibiotics such as the "Stanford solution" may be used prophylactically along with the first radiotherapy treatment itself. As an alternative, a temporary gastrostomy tube may be considered.

SCENARIO D

When the previously discussed concurrent scenarios are just too toxic, one can then resort to an alternating regimen:

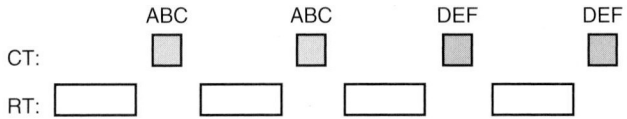

Here the effective drug regimens are given in closer to full doses than in the concurrent scenarios during scheduled breaks in the radiotherapy course. If this also is too toxic, the preemptive steps to reduce toxicity as suggested earlier may be taken before abandoning this approach altogether. The chemoradiation schedule with the least chance of success in the locally advanced tumor would be the sequential mode (scenario E), for reasons that are graphically shown in Figure 5-1.

SCENARIO E

This form of sequential chemoradiation may be appropriate therapy for some patients, particularly those alluded to earlier as the "silent minority"—those who, owing to their age or comorbid medical conditions, are unable to undergo surgery and are unlikely to tolerate an extensive course of concurrent or alternating chemoradiation.

Some of them may prefer the small chance of cure and the reasonable chance of prolonged palliation this approach could offer over a "wait-and-see" approach, symptomatic management, or a premature allotment to a hospice.

SCENARIO F

A newer mode of chemoradiation delivery now being piloted in a few institutions and with multi-institutional research groups for head and neck and esophageal cancers is a combination of the sequential and concurrent schedules:

Here neoadjuvant chemotherapy is used and followed by concurrent chemoradiation and invariably concluded with surgical resection. According to the construct of our conceptual model, this mode of treatment would increase the treatment time possibly beyond the window of curability. The extended time period without maximal therapy (during the period of neoadjuvant chemotherapy) would allow the development of drug and radiotherapy-resistant phenotypes or of metastatic phenotypes.

EXEMPLARY CHEMORADIATION REGIMENS

The theoretical scenarios described for combining radiotherapy and chemotherapy can be applied to most locally advanced solid tumors for purposes of improving cure rates, for organ preservation, to maintain functional integrity, and to treat an elderly population of patients who cannot undergo a surgical procedure. A practical example of a model chemoradiation regimen attempting to do all of this could be suggested for locally advanced (T2 to T4) carcinoma of the bladder.

Three chemotherapy regimens (among others) have been separately seen to be effective when combined with pelvic radiotherapy in bladder cancer. These included 5-FU plus mitomycin C plus cisplatin alone, and the MVAC (methotrexate, vincristine, doxorubicin, and cisplatin) combination. Thus, the main treatment course could be graphically represented as follows:

If not tolerated well, or if significant dose modification is necessary, scenarios B and C could be used, thus

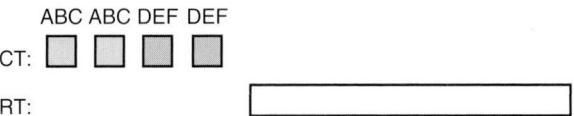

or somewhat similar to the Massachusetts General Hospital bladder preservation approach:

By alternating three known effective chemotherapy combinations, the chances of excessive toxicity would be reduced compared with repeating three or four cycles of the very same drug combination. Also, the chances of delivering unmodified doses of these drug combinations are improved and the possibility of development of drug resistance is also reduced. The drug combination of MVAC is used last because it is known to have the most activity against bladder cancer. Finally, with the different modes of individual action, as well as their interaction with radiotherapy, the different drug combinations would likely reduce the presence of resistant subpopulations in a heterogeneous tumor. If none of these three methods works, either due to excessive toxicity or the need to modify radiotherapy and drug doses, then the other scenarios (D to F) should be attempted. However, in increasing the overall treatment time period, the individual doses of drugs and radiotherapy should also be progressively increased to be effective.

The previous discussion represents, in brief, various strategies of combining radiotherapy and chemotherapy in the clinic. Numerous ancillary drugs that affect the milieu of interaction between the two modalities are being studied extensively in the laboratory, and some have made their way to single and multi-institutional phase I and II studies. These include drugs that reduce the development of multiple-drug resistance, those that reduce angiogenesis, hypoxic cell antagonists, drugs that sensitize the hypoxic cancer cell to radiotherapy, and drugs that affect tumor and normal tissue pH. Drugs such as cytokines, processes such as hyperalimentation, and surgical diversionary procedures such as a temporary colostomy are all required to be considered at the very least when planning a definitive chemoradiation regimen.

The science of chemoradiation is truly a multidisciplinary development, and improvements in its use in the treatment of several cancers depends not only on a clear understanding of medical and radiation oncology but also on a practical overview of developments in surgical technique and in the biology laboratory. In spite of developing technologies, the combined use of chemotherapy and radiotherapy is likely to play a dominant role in cancer therapy for several decades.

REFERENCES

1. D'Angio GJ: Historical perspective. In John M, Flam M, Legha S, Phillips T, eds. *Chemoradiation: An Integrated Approach to Cancer Treatment*. Philadelphia: Lea & Febiger; 1993:36.
2. Heidelberger C, Chaudhari NK, Dannenberg P, et al: Fluorinated pyrimidines, new class of tumor-inhibiting compounds. *Nature*. 1957;179:663.
3. Kramer S: Use of methotrexate and radiation therapy for advanced cancer of the head and neck. *Front Radiat Ther Oncol*. 1969;4:116.
4. Nigro ND, Vaitkevicius VK, Considine B Jr: Combined therapy for cancer of the anal canal: A preliminary report. *Dis Colon Rectum*. 1974;17:354.
5. Cummings BJ, Rider WD, Haywood AR, et al: Combined radical radiation therapy and chemotherapy for primary squamous cell carcinoma of the anal canal. *Cancer Treat Rep*. 1982;66:489.
6. Flam M, John M, Lovalvo L, et al: Definitive non-surgical therapy of epithelial malignancies of the anal canal: A report of 12 cases. *Cancer*. 1983;51:1378.
7. Fisher B, Redmond C, Fisher ER, and participating NSABP investigators: The contribution of recent NSABP clinical trials of primary breast cancer therapy to an understanding of tumor biology: An overview of findings. *Cancer*. 1980;46:1009.
8. Gray LH, Couger AD, Ebert M, et al: The concentration of oxygen dissolved in tissues at the time of irradiation as a factor in radiotherapy. *Br J Radiol*. 1953;26:638.
9. Tannock IF: Tumor growth and cell kinetics. In Tannock IF, Hill RP, eds. *The Basic Science of Oncology*. New York: Pergamon Press; 1987:14.
10. Komaki R, Cox JD: Multiple radiotherapy fractionation schedules. In John M, Flam M, Legha S, Phillips T, eds. *Chemoradiation: An Integrated Approach to Cancer Treatment*. Philadelphia: Lea & Febiger; 1993:609.
11. Kramer AM, Legha SS: Continuous venous infusion chemotherapy: An overview. *Cancer Bull*. 1986;38:179.
12. Tannock IF: Potential for therapeutic gain from combined modality treatment. *Front Radiat Ther Oncol*. 1992;26:1.
13. von Pawel J, von Roemeling R, Gatzemeier W, et al: Tirapazimine plus cisplatin versus cisplatin in advanced non-small cell cancer. A report of the international CATAPULT I study group. *J Clin Oncol*. 2000;18:1351.
14. Rischin D, Peters L, Hicks R, et al: Phase I trial of concurrent tirapazimine, cisplatin and radiotherapy in patients with advanced head and neck cancer. *J Clin Oncol*. 2001;19:535.
15. Steel CG, Peckham MJ: Exploitable mechanisms in combined radiotherapy-chemotherapy. *Int J Radiat Oncol Biol Phys*. 1979; 5:85.
16. Millar JL, Blackett NM, Hudspith BN: Enhanced post-irradiation recovery of the haematopoietic system in animals pretreated with a variety of cytotoxic agents. *Cell Tissue Kinetics*. 1978;11:543.
17. Fu KK: Interactions of chemotherapeutic agents and radiation. *Front Radiat Ther Oncol*. 1992;26:16.
18. Phillips TL, Fu KK: Basic mechanisms of radiation cell injury. In John M, Flam M, Legha S, Phillips T, eds. *Chemoradiation: An Integrated Approach to Cancer Treatment*. Philadelphia: Lea & Febiger; 1993:67.
19. John MJ, Flam MS: Gynecologic system. In John M, Flam M, Legha S, Phillips T, eds. *Chemoradiation: An Integrated Approach to Cancer Treatment*. Philadelphia: Lea & Febiger; 1993:374.
20. Hockel M, Schlenger K, Mitze M, et al: Hypoxia and radiation response in human tumors. *Semin Radiat Oncol*. 1996;6:3.
21. Brown M, Siim BG: Hypoxia-specific cytotoxins in cancer therapy. *Semin Radiat Oncol*. 1996;6:227.
22. Overgaard J, Horsman MR: Modification of hypoxia-induced radioresistance in cancers by the use of oxygen and sensitizers. *Semin Radiat Oncol*. 1996;6:10.
23. Hall EJ: *Radiobiology of the Radiologist*, 3rd ed. Philadelphia: JB Lippincott; 1988.
24. Byfield JE, Chan PYM, Seagren SL: Radiosensitization of 5-FU: Molecular origins and clinical scheduling implications. *Proc Am Assoc Cancer Res*. 1977;18:74. Abstract.
25. Calabres F: Drug resistance: Lonidamine. *Principles Pract Oncol Updates*. 1994;8:1.
26. Donehower RC, Rowinsky EK: Paclitaxel. *Principles Pract Oncol Updates*. 1994;8:1.
27. Lokich JJ: Principles and practice of infusional chemotherapy. In Lokich JJ, Byfield JE, eds. *Combined Modality Cancer Therapy: Radiation and Infusional Chemotherapy*. Chicago: Precept Press; 1991:49.
28. Lowe SW, Ruley HE, Tacks T, et al: P53-dependent apoptosis modulates the cytotoxicity of anti-cancer agents. *Cell*. 1993; 74:957.
29. Bresnick E: Biochemistry of cancer. In Holland JF, Frei E, Bast RC, et al, eds. *Cancer Medicine*, 3rd ed. Philadelphia: Lea & Febiger, 1993;121.

30. Kallman RF, Bedarida G, Rapacchietta D: Experimental studies on schedule dependence in the treatment of cancer in a combination of chemotherapy and radiotherapy. *Front Radiat Ther Oncol.* Basel: Karger; 1992;26:31.

31. Looney WB, Hopkins HA: Experimental and clinical rationale for alternating chemotherapy and radiotherapy in human cancer management. In John M, Flam M, Legha S, Phillips T, eds. *Chemoradiation: An Integrated Approach to Cancer Treatment.* Philadelphia: Lea & Febiger; 1993:27.

32. John MJ: A model for concurrent chemoradiation in clinical trials. In John M, Flam M, Legha S, Phillips T, eds. *Chemoradiation: An Integrated Approach to Cancer Treatment.* Philadelphia: Lea & Febiger; 1993:53.

33. Byfield JE: Clinical basis for radiation and infusional chemotherapy. In Lokich JJ, Byfield JE, eds. *Combined Modality Cancer Therapy—Radiation and Infusional Chemotherapy.* Chicago: Precept Press; 1991:15.

34. Tubiana M, Arriagada R, Cosset JM: Sequencing of drugs and radiation, the integrated alternating regimen. *Cancer.* 1985; 55:2131.

35. John MJ, Flam MS, Palma N: Ten year results of chemoradiation for anal cancer: Focus on late morbidity. *Int J Radiat Oncol Biol Phys.* 1996;34:65.

36. Taylor SG, Murthy AK: Head and neck. In John M, Flam M, Legha S, Phillips T, eds. *Chemoradiation: An Integrated Approach to Cancer Treatment.* Philadelphia: Lea & Febiger; 1993:181.

37. Munro AJ: An overview of randomized controlled trials of adjuvant chemotherapy in head and neck cancer. *Br J Cancer.* 1995;71:83.

38. El-Sayed, Nelson N: Adjuvant and adjunctive chemotherapy in the management of squamous cell carcinoma of the head and neck region: A meta-analysis of prospective and randomized trials. *J Clin Oncol.* 1996;14:838.

39. Pearcey RG, Brundage MD, Drouin P, et al: A clinical trial comparing concurrent cisplatin and radiation therapy versus radiation alone for locally advanced squamous cell carcinoma of the cervix carried out by the NCIC Clinical Trials Group. *Proceed ASCO.* 2000;19:378. Abstract.

40. Rich T, Ajani JA, Morrison WH, et al: Chemoradiation therapy for anal cancer. Radiation plus continuous infusion of 5-fluorouracil with or without cisplatin. *Radiother Oncol.* 1993;27:209.

41. Goldie JH: Neoadjuvant combined modality therapy. In John M, Flam M, Legha S, Phillips T, eds. *Chemoradiation: An Integrated Approach to Cancer Treatment.* Philadelphia: Lea & Febiger, 1993:18.

42. Phillips TL, Fu KK: The interaction of drug and radiation effects on normal tissues. *Int J Radiat Oncol Biol Phys.* 1978;4:59.

43. Phillips TL: Effects of chemotherapy and radiation on normal tissues. *Front Radiat Ther Oncol.* 1992;26:45.

44. Komaki R: Combined chemotherapy and radiation therapy in surgically unresectable regionally advanced non–small cell lung cancer. *Semin Radiat Oncol.* 1996;6:86.

45. Dosoretz DC, Katin MJ, Blitzer PH, et al: Medically inoperable lung carcinoma: The role of radiation therapy. *Semin Radiat Oncol.* 1996;6:98.

46. Earlam R, Cunha-Melo JR: Esophageal squamous cell carcinoma: I: A critical review of radiotherapy. *Br J Surg.* 1980;67:451.

47. Al-Sarraf M, Martz K, Herskovic A, et al: Superiority of chemo-radiotherapy (CT-RT) vs radiotherapy (RT) in patients with esophageal cancer: Final report of an intergroup randomized and confirmed study. *J Clin Oncol.* Proceedings of ASCO. 1996;15:206.

48. Cummings BJ, Keane TJ, O'Sullivan B, et al: Epidermoid anal cancer: Treatment by radiation alone or by radiation and 5-FU with or without mitomycin C. *Int J Radiat Oncol Biol Phys.* 1991; 21:1115.

49. Hoppe RT, Horning SJ, Hancock SL, et al: Current Stanford clinical trials for Hodgkin's disease. *Recent Results Cancer Res.* 1989;117:182.

50. Tucker MA, Coleman CN, Cox RS, et al: Risk of second cancers after treatment for Hodgkin's disease. *N Engl J Med.* 1988;318:76.

51. Rubin P, Constine LS, Nelson DF: Late effects of cancer treatment: radiation and drug toxicity. In Perez CA, Brady LW, eds. *Principles and Practice of Radiation Oncology.* Philadelphia: JB Lippincott; 1992:124.

52. D'Angio GJ, Farber S, Maddock C: Potentiation of x-ray effects by actinomycin-D. *Radiology.* 1959;73:175.

53. John MJ, Rochford R: Skin and soft tissue toxicity. In John M, Flam M, Legha S, Phillips T, eds. *Chemoradiation: An Integrated Approach to Cancer Treatment.* Philadelphia: Lea & Febiger; 1993:502.

54. John MJ, Flam MS: Esophagus. In John M, Flam M, Legha S, Phillips T, eds. *Chemoradiation: An Integrated Approach to Cancer Treatment.* Philadelphia: Lea & Febiger; 1993:285.

55. Emami B, Scott C, Byhardt R, et al: The value of regional nodal radiotherapy (dose/volume) in the treatment of unresectable lung cancer. *Int J Radiat Oncol Biol Phys.* 1996;36:209.

56. Overgaard J, Grau C: Interactions between bleomycin and x-irradiation. In Hill BT, Bellamy AS, eds. *Antitumor Drug-Radiation Interactions.* Boca Raton, Fla: CRC Press; 1990:53.

57. Al-Sarraf M, LeBlanc M, Givi S, et al: Chemoradiotherapy versus radiotherapy in patients with advanced nasopharyngeal cancer: Phase III randomized intergroup study 0099. *J Clin Oncol.* 1998; 16:1310.

58. Calais G, Alfons M, Bardet E, et al: Radiation alone (RT) versus RT with concomitant chemotherapy (CT) in stages III and IV oropharynx carcinoma. Final results of the 94-01 GORTEC randomized study (Abstract). Presented at the 43rd Annual Meeting of ASTRO. Nov 2001; San Francisco.

59. Brizel DM, Albers ME, Fisher SR, et al: Hyperfractionated irradiation with or without concurrent chemotherapy for locally advanced head and neck cancer. *N Engl J Med.* 1998;338:1798.

60. Dorrowsky W, Nande J: Continuous hyperfractionated accelerated radiotherapy with/without mitomycin C in head and neck cancers. *Radiother Oncol.* 2000;57:119.

61. Jeremic B, Shibamoto Y, Milicic B, et al: Hyperfractionated radiation therapy with or without concurrent low-dose daily cisplatin in locally advanced squamous cell carcinoma of the head and neck: a prospective randomized trial. *J Clin Oncol.* 2000; 18:1458.

62. Broadman GP, Hodson DI, Mackenzie RT, et al: Choosing a concomitant chemotherapy and radiotherapy regimen for squamous cell head and neck cancer: A systematic review of the published literature with subgroup analysis. *Head Neck.* 2001;23:579.

63. Nguyen NP, Sallah S, Karlsson U, Antoine JE: Combined chemotherapy and radiation therapy for head and neck malignancies; quality of life issues. *Cancer.* 2002;94:1131.

64. Dillman RO, Seagren SL, Herndon J, et al: Randomized trial of induction chemotherapy plus radiation therapy vs radiation therapy alone in stage II non-small cell lung cancer: Five year follow-up of CALGB 84-33. *Proc Am Soc Clin Oncol.* 1993;12:329.

65. Sause WT, Scott C, Taylor S, et al: Radiation Therapy Oncology Group 88-08 and Eastern Cooperative Oncology Group 4588: Preliminary results of phase III trial in regionally advanced unresectable non–small cell lung cancer. *J Natl Cancer Inst.* 1995;87:198.

66. Furuse K, Fukuoka M, Kawahara M, et al: Phase III study of concurrent versus sequential thoracic radiotherapy in combination with mitomycin, vindesine and cisplatin in unresectable Stage III non–small cell lung cancer. *J Clin Oncol.* 1999;17:2692.

67. Curran WJ, Scott C, Langer C, et al: Phase III comparison of sequential vs. concurrent chemoradiation for patients with unresected stage III non–small cell lung cancer (NSCLC): Initial report of Radiation Therapy Oncology Group (RTOG) 9410. *Proceed ASCO.* 2000;19:484a.

68. Albain KS, Rusch VW, Crowley JJ, et al: Concurrent cisplatin/ etoposide plus chest radiotherapy followed by surgery for stages IIIA (N$_2$) and IIIB non–small cell lung cancer: Mature results of Southwest Oncology Group Phase II study 8805. *J Clin Oncol.* 1995;13:1880.

69. Komaki R, Cox JD: The lung and thymus. In Cox JD, ed. *Moss' Radiation Oncology. Rationale, Techniques, Results,* 7th ed. St. Louis: CV Mosby; 1994:320.

70. Holmes EC, Livingston R, Turrisi A: Neoplasms of the thorax. In Holland JF, Fred E, Bast RC, et al, eds. *Cancer Medicine,* 3rd ed. Philadelphia: Lea & Febiger; 1993:1285.

71. Murray N, Coy P, Pater JL, et al: Importance of timing for thoracic irradiation in the combined modality treatment of limited-stage small cell lung cancer. *J Clin Oncol.* 1993;11:336.

72. Goto K, Nishiwaki Y, Takada M, et al: Final results of a phase III study of concurrent versus sequential thoracic radiotherapy (TRT) in combination with cisplatin (P) and etoposide (E) for limited-stage small cell lung cancer (LD-SCLC): the Japanese Clinical Oncology Group (JCOG) study. *Proceed ASCO.* 1999;18:468a.

73. McCracken JD, Janaki LM, Crowley JJ, et al: Concurrent chemotherapy/radiotherapy for limited small cell lung carcinoma: A Southwest Oncology Group Study. *J Clin Oncol*. 1990;8:892.

74. Turrisi AJ, Kim K, Blum R, et al: Twice-daily compared with once-daily thoracic radiotherapy in limited small cell lung cancer treated concurrently with cisplatin and etoposide. *N Eng J Med*. 1999;340:265.

75. Arriagada R, Kramer A, Le Chevalier T, et al: Competing events determining relapse-free survival in limited small cell carcinoma. *J Clin Oncol*. 1992;10:447.

76. Turrisi AT, Glover DJ, Mason B, et al: Long term results of platinum etoposide (PE), thoracic radiotherapy (TRT) for limited small cell lung cancer: Results on 32 patients with 48 months minimum follow-up. *Proc Am Soc Clin Oncol*. 1992;11:975.

77. Guili R, Gignoux M: Treatment of carcinoma of the esophagus: Retrospective study of 2400 patients. *Ann Surg*. 1980;192:44.

78. Gignoux M, Roussel A, Paillot B, et al: The value of preoperative radiotherapy in esophageal cancer: Results of a study by the EORTC. *World J Surg*. 1987;11:426.

79. Aisner J, Forastiere A, Aroney R: Patterns of recurrence for cancer of the lung and esophagus. In Wittes RE, ed. *Cancer Treatment Symposia: Proceedings of the Workshop on Patterns of Failure After Cancer Treatment*, vol 2. Washington, DC: US Department of Health and Human Services; 1983:87.

80. Kelsen DP: Chemotherapy for loco-regional and advanced esophageal cancer. *Cancer Updates*. 1988;2:1.

81. Skinner DB: En-bloc resection for neoplasm of the esophagus and cardia. *J Thorac Cardiovasc Surg*. 1983;85:59.

82. Walsh TN, Noonan N, Hollywood D, et al: A comparison of multimodal therapy and surgery for esophageal adenocarcinoma. *N Eng J Med*. 1996;335:462.

83. Bosset JF, Gignon M, Triboulet JP, et al: Chemoradiotherapy followed by surgery compared with surgery alone in squamous cell cancer of the esophagus. *N Eng J Med*. 1997;337:161.

84. Roth JA, Pass H, Flanagan MM, et al: Randomized clinical trial of preoperative and postoperative adjuvant chemotherapy with cisplatin, vindesine and bleomycin for carcinoma of the esophagus. *J Thorac Cardiovasc Surg*. 1988;96:242.

85. Schlag P, for the CAO Study Group: Preoperative chemotherapy in localized squamous cell carcinoma of the esophagus: Results of a prospective randomized trial. *Eur J Cancer*. 1991;27 (suppl 2):S76.

86. Forastiere AA, Orringer MB, Perez-Tamayo C, et al: Preoperative chemoradiation followed by transhiatal esophagectomy for carcinoma of the esophagus: Final report. *J Clin Oncol*. 1993;11:1118.

87. Coia LR: Esophageal cancer: Is esophagectomy necessary? *Oncology*. 1989;3:101.

88. Mantravadi RVP, Bajpai D, Crawford JN, et al: Combined chemotherapy and radiotherapy for carcinoma of the esophagus without surgery. Proceedings of ASCO. *J Clin Oncol*. 1996;15:223.

89. Smith TJ, Ryan LM, Douglass HOJ, et al: Combined chemoradiotherapy vs. radiotherapy alone for early stage squamous cell carcinoma of the esophagus: A study of the Eastern Cooperative Oncology Group. *Int J Radiat Oncol Biol Phys*. 1998;42:269.

90. Minsky BD, Neuberg D, Kelsen DP: Final report of intergroup trial 0122 (ECOG PE-289, RTOG 90-12) phase II trial of neoadjuvant chemotherapy plus concurrent chemotherapy and high-dose radiation for squamous cell carcinoma of the esophagus. *Int J Radiat Oncol Biol Phys*. 1999;43:517.

91. Rich TA, Ajani JA: Stomach, pancreas, biliary system. In John M, Flam M, Legha S, Phillips T, eds. *Chemoradiation: An Integrated Approach to Cancer Treatment*. Philadelphia: Lea & Febiger; 1993:303.

92. O'Connell MJ, Gunderson LL, Moertel CG, et al: A pilot study of intensive combined therapy for locally unresectable gastric cancer. *Int J Radiat Oncol Biol Phys*. 1985;11:1827.

93. Moertel CG, Childs DS, O'Fallon JR, et al: Combined 5-fluorouracil and radiation therapy as a surgical adjuvant for poor prognostic gastric carcinoma. *J Clin Oncol*. 1984;2:1249.

94. McDonald J, Smalley S, Benedetti J, et al: Post-operative combined radiation and chemotherapy improves disease free and overall survival in resected adenocarcinoma of the stomach and GE junction. *Proceed ASCO*. 2000;19:1a. Abstract.

95. Schein PS, Nourk J (per GITSG): Combined modality therapy (xrt-chemo) versus chemotherapy alone for locally unresectable gastric cancer. *Cancer*. 1982;49:1771.

96. Gastrointestinal Tumor Study Group: Comparison of combination chemotherapy and combined modality therapy for locally advanced gastric carcinoma. *Cancer*. 1982;49:1771.

97. Wingo PA, Tang T, Bolden S: Cancer statistics 1995. *CA Cancer J Clin*. 1995;45:8.

98. McGrath PC, Sloan DA, Kenady DE: Surgical management of pancreatic carcinoma. *Semin Oncol*. 1996;23:200.

99. Moertel CG, Childs DS, Reitemeier RJ, et al: Combined 5-fluorouracil and supervoltage radiation therapy of clinically unresectable gastrointestinal cancer. *Lancet*. 1969;2:865.

100. Haslam JB, Cavanaugh PJ, Stroup SL: Radiation therapy as the treatment of unresectable adenocarcinoma of the pancreas. *Cancer*. 1973;32:1341.

101. Kalser MH, Ellenberg SS: Pancreatic cancer adjuvant combined radiation and chemotherapy following curative resection. *Arch Surg*. 1985;120:899.

102. Klickenbijil JH, Jeekel J, Sahmoud T, et al: Adjuvant radiotherapy and 5-fluorouracil after curative resection of cancer of the pancreas and periampullary region: Phase III trial of the EORTC Gastrointestinal Tract Cancer Cooperative Group. *Ann Surg*. 1999;230:776.

103. Moertel CG, Frytak S, Hahn RG, et al, and the Gastrointestinal Tumor Study Group: Therapy of locally unresectable pancreatic carcinoma: A randomized comparison of higher dose (6000 rads) radiation, moderate dose radiation (4000 rads + 5-fluorouracil), and high dose radiation + 5-fluorouracil. *Cancer*. 1981;48:1705.

104. Gastrointestinal Tumor Study Group: Treatment of locally unresectable carcinoma of the pancreas: Comparison of combined modality therapy (chemotherapy plus radiotherapy) to chemotherapy alone. *J Natl Cancer Inst*. 1988;80:751.

105. Wilkowski R, Heinemann V, Rau H: Radiochemotherapy including gemcitabine and 5-fluorouracil for treatment of locally advanced pancreatic cancer. *Proceed ASCO*. 2000;19:1078a. Abstract.

106. Harris W, Landry J, Staley C, et al: A phase I study of gemcitabine, cisplatin and 5 fluorouracil with radiation for patients with advanced GI malignancies. *Proceed ASCO*. 2000;19:1205. Abstract.

107. Eifel PJ: The uterine cervix. In Cox JD, Ang KK, eds. *Radiation Oncology: Rationale, Technique, Results*. St. Louis: CV Mosby; 2003:681.

108. Brunner T, Grabenbauer G, Kasti S, et al: A phase I trial of simultaneous gemcitabine/cisplatin and radiotherapy in patients with locally advanced pancreatic cancer. *Proceed ASCO*. 2000;19:1109a. Abstract.

109. Higgins GA, Donaldson RC, Humphrey EW, et al: Adjuvant therapy for large bowel cancer. Update of VASOG trials. *Surg Clin North Am*. 1981;61:1311.

110. Gastrointestinal Tumor Study Group: Prolongation of the disease-free interval in surgically treated rectal carcinoma. *N Engl J Med*. 1985;312:1465.

111. Gastrointestinal Tumor Study Group: Survival after postoperative combination treatment of rectal cancer. *N Engl J Med*. 1986;315:1294.

112. Fisher B, Wolmark N, Rockette H, et al: Postoperative adjuvant chemotherapy or radiation therapy for rectal cancer: Results from NSABP protocol RO 1. *J Natl Cancer Inst*. 1988;80:21.

113. Gastrointestinal Tumor Study Group: Radiation Therapy and 5-FU with and without semustine for the treatment of patients with surgical adjuvant adenocarcinoma of the rectum. *J Clin Oncol*. 1992;10:549.

114. Krook JE, Moertel CG, Gunderson LL, et al: Effective surgical adjuvant therapy for high-risk rectal carcinoma. *N Engl J Med*. 1991;324:709.

115. Bosset JF, Magnin V, Maingon P, et al: Preoperative radiochemotherapy in rectal cancer: Long-term results of a phase II trial. *Int J Radiat Oncol Biol Phys*. 2000;46:323.

116. Pucciarelli S, Friso ML, Toppan P, et al: Preoperative combined radiotherapy and chemotherapy for middle and lower rectal cancer: Preliminary results. *Ann Surg Oncol*. 2000;7:38.

117. Janjan NA, Crane CH, Feig BW, et al: Prospective trial of pre-operative concomitant boost radiotherapy with continuous infusion 5 fluorouracil for locally advanced rectal cancer. *Int J Radiat Oncol Biol Phys*. 2000;47:713.

118. Roelofsen F, Bosset JF, Eschwege F, et al: Concomitant radiotherapy and chemotherapy superior to radiotherapy alone in the

treatment of locally advanced anal cancer. Results of Phase III randomized trial of the EORTC radiotherapy and gastrointestinal group Proceedings of ASCO. *J Clin Oncol*. 1995;14:194. Abstract 454.

119. Flam MS, John MJ, Pajak T, et al: The role of mitomycin C in combination with 5-fluorouracil and radiotherapy and of salvage chemoradiation in the definitive nonsurgical treatment of epidermoid carcinoma of the anal canal. Results of phase III randomized intergroup study. *J Clin Oncol*. 1996;14:2527.

120. Epidermoid anal cancer: Results from the [UK Coordinating Committee on Cancer Research] UKCCCR [Anal Cancer Trial Working Party] randomized trial of radiotherapy alone versus radiotherapy, 5 fluorouracil and mitomycin: *Lancet*. 1996;348:1049.

121. Parsons JT, Millan RR: Bladder. In Perez CA, Brady LW, eds. *Principles and Practice of Radiation Oncology*, 2nd ed. Philadelphia: JB Lippincott; 1992:1036.

122. Bloom HJG, Hendry WF, Wallace DM, et al: Treatment of T3 bladder cancer: Controlled trial of preoperative radiotherapy and radical cystectomy versus radical radiotherapy. *Br J Urol*. 1992;54:136.

123. Sell A, Jakobsen A, Nerstrom B: Treatment of advanced bladder cancer category T_2, T_3, T_4a. *Scand J Urol Nephrol Suppl*. 1991;138:193.

124. Mommsen S, Jakobsen A, Sell A: Quality of life in patients with advanced bladder cancer. *Scand J Urol Nephrol Suppl*. 1989; 125:115.

125. Lynch WJ, Jenkins BJ, Fowler CG, et al: The quality of life after radical radiotherapy for bladder cancer. *Br J Urol*. 1992; 70:519.

126. Yagoda A: Systemic chemotherapy for curative and unresectable disease. In Alderson AR, Oliver RT, Hanham IW, Bloom HJ, eds. *Urological Oncology Dilemmas and Developments*. New York: John Wiley & Sons; 1991.

127. Moore MJ, Tannock IF, Ernst DS, et al: Gemcitabine: A promising new agent in the treatment of advanced urothelial carcinoma. *J Clin Oncol*. 1997;15:3441.

128. Raghavan D: Systemic chemotherapy for metastatic cancer at the uroepithelial tract. In Hall RR, ed. *Clinical Management of Bladder Cancer*. London: Arnold Publishing; 1999.

129. Loehrer PJ Sr, Elson P, Kueble JP, et al: Advanced bladder cancer: A prospective intergroup trial comparing simple agent cisplatin (CDDP) versus M-VAC combination therapy (INT0078). Proceedings of the American Society of Clinical Oncology. *J Clin Oncol*. 1990;9:132.

130. Kaufman DS, Shipley WU, Griffin PP, et al: Selective preservation by combination treatment of invasive bladder cancer. *N Engl J Med*. 1993;329:1377.

131. Dunst J, Sauer R, Schrott KM, et al: Organ-sparing treatment of advanced bladder cancer: A 10 year experience. *Int J Radiat Oncol Biol Phys*. 1994;30:261.

132. Tester W, Caplan R, Heaney J, et al: Neoadjuvant combined modality program with selective bladder preservation for invasive bladder cancer: Results of RTOG Phase II trial 8802. *J Clin Oncol*. 1996;14:119.

133. Fellin G, Gratter U, Bolner A, et al: combined chemotherapy and radiation with selective organ preservation for muscle-invasive bladder carcinoma; a single-institution phase II study. *Br J Urol*. 1997;80:44.

134. Shipley WU, Kaufman DS, Zehr E, et al: Selective bladder preservation by combined modality protocol treatment: Long-term outcomes of 190 patients with invasive bladder cancer. *Urology*. 2002;60:62.

135. Pilepich MV, Krall JM, Al-Sarraf M, et al: Androgen deprivation with radiation therapy compared with radiation therapy alone for locally advanced prostatic carcinoma: A randomized comparative trial of the Radiation Therapy Oncology Group. *Urology*. 1995;45:616.

136. Pilepich MV, Winter K, John MJ, et al: Phase III Radiation Therapy Oncology Group Trial 86-10 of androgen deprivation adjuvant to definitive radiotherapy in locally advanced carcinoma of the prostate. *Int J Radiat Oncol Biol Phys*. 2001;50:1243.

137. Pilepich MV, Caplan R, Byhardt RW, et al: Phase III trial of androgen suppression using goserlin in unfavorable-prognosis carcinoma of the prostate treated with definitive radiotherapy. Report of the Radiation Therapy Oncology Group protocol 85-31. *J Clin Oncol*. 1997;15:1013.

138. Lawton CA, Winter K, Murray K, et al: Updated results of the phase III Radiation Therapy Oncology Group (RTOG) trial 85-31 evaluating the potential benefit of androgen suppression following standard radiation therapy for unfavorable carcinoma of the prostate. *Int J Radiat Oncol Biol Phys*. 2001;49:937.

139. Bola M, Gonzalez D, Warde P, et al: Improved survival in patients with locally advanced prostate cancer treated with radiotherapy and goserelin. *N Engl J Med*. 1997;337:295.

140. Sikic BI: Combined chemotherapy and radiotherapy for advanced stage carcinoma of the cervix. *Front Radiat Ther Oncol*. 1992; 26:153.

141. Piver MS, Krishnamsetty RM, Emrich LJ: Survival of nonsurgically staged patients with negative lymphangiograms who had stage IIB carcinoma of the cervix treated by pelvic radiation plus hydroxyurea. *Am J Obstet Gynecol*. 1985;151:1006.

142. John M, Flam M, Caplan R, et al: Final results of a phase II chemoradiation protocol for locally advanced cervical cancer: RTOG 85-15. *Gynecol Oncol*. 1996;61:221.

143. National Cancer Institute: Concurrent chemoradiation for cervical cancer. Clinical announcement. Feb 1995. Available at http:/www.nci.nih.gov/clinical trials/developments/cervical-cancer_alert0600.

144. Morris M, Eifel PJ, Lu J, et al: Pelvic radiation with concurrent chemotherapy compared with pelvic and para-aortic radiotherapy for high-risk cervical cancer. *N Engl J Med*. 1999;340:1137.

145. Rose PG, Bundy BN, Watkins J, et al: Concurrent cisplatin-based chemotherapy and radiotherapy for locally advanced cervical cancer. *N Engl J Med*. 1999;340:1144.

146. Keys HM, Bundy BN, Stehman FB, et al: Cisplatin, radiation and adjuvant hysterectomy for bulky stage IB cervical carcinoma. *N Engl J Med*. 1999; 340:1154.

147. Whitney CW, Sause W, Bundy BN, et al: A randomized comparison of fluorouracil plus cisplatin versus hydroxyurea as an adjunct to radiotherapy in stages IIB-IVA carcinoma of the cervix with negative para-aortic lymph nodes. A Gynecology Oncology Group and Southwest Oncology Group study. *J Clin Oncol*. 1999;17:1339.

148. Peters WA III, Liu PY, Barrett RJ, et al: Concurrent chemotherapy and pelvic radiation therapy compared with pelvic radiation alone as adjuvant therapy after radical surgery in high-risk early-stage cancer of the cervix. *J Clin Oncol*. 2000;18:1606.

149. Eifel PJ, Morris M, Burke TW, et al: Prolonged continuous infusion of cisplatin and 5-fluorouracil with radiation for locally advanced carcinoma of the vulva. *Gynecol Oncol*. 1995;59:51.

Principles of Radiation Physics

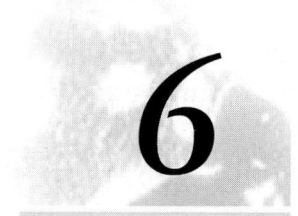

Lynn J. Verhey, PhD and Paula L. Petti, PhD

In this chapter, we present the basic radiation physics that is needed for the practice of radiation oncology. Many of the specific applications of these basic physics principles, such as brachytherapy and treatment planning, are presented elsewhere in this textbook. Since the primary audience for this textbook is assumed to be practicing radiation oncologists and resident clinicians, many topics are not treated in the detail that would be required by radiation physicists. Excellent physics textbooks that present the topics in more depth are available.[1-3]

BASIC CONCEPTS

Atomic and Nuclear Structure

Matter is composed of individual elements that are distinguishable from each other on the basis of their physical and chemical properties. The fundamental building block for these elements is the individual atom, which consists of a small central core, called the nucleus, surrounded by diffuse clouds of electrons. The nucleus, containing almost all the mass in the atom, consists of uncharged neutrons (mass of 1.675×10^{-27} kg) and positively charged protons (mass of 1.673×10^{-27} kg), bound together by the strongly attractive nuclear force. The electrons (mass of 0.911×10^{-31} kg) are negatively charged particles with the same absolute value of charge as the protons. Since the atoms have the same number of electrons and protons, they are electrically neutral. The radius of the atom is about 10^{-10} m, whereas the radius of the nucleus is about 10^{-14} m.

The atom is completely specified by the atomic number Z, which is the number of protons in the nucleus (or electrons in the atom), and the mass number A, which is the number of neutrons plus protons in the nucleus. Obviously, the number of neutrons in the nucleus, N, is just A – Z. Element X is specified as $_ZX^A$. *Isotopes* of an element have the same Z but different A and, therefore, have the same chemical properties but can have different physical properties. *Isobars* are atoms with the same A but different Z, and *isotones* are atoms with different A and Z but the same N.

In the planetary model of the atom, first described by Niels Bohr, the electron orbits make up discrete concentric shells, with a different binding energy associated with each shell. The shells are labeled K, L, M, . . . from the innermost to the outermost shell. The maximum number of electrons allowed in each shell is $2n^2$, where $n = 1$ for the K shell, $n = 2$ for the L shell, and so on. Therefore, there are up to 2 electrons in the K shell, 8 in the L shell, 18 in the M shell, and so on. A simple schematic drawing of the Bohr model is shown in Figure 6-1.

The electrons are bound to the protons in the nucleus by the attractive electromagnetic force; therefore, the inner K orbit electrons are bound most tightly because they are closest. The electrons in the outer orbit are called *valence* electrons and they are typically bound very loosely. The process of *excitation* is the movement of an electron from an inner orbit to an outer orbit. This requires the addition of energy to the atom. If an electron is completely removed from an atom, the process is called *ionization*. The energy required to just barely remove an electron from an atom is called the *binding energy*. In a heavy atom such as tungsten, the binding energy of K shell electrons is about 70,000 electron volts (eV), whereas the valence electrons have binding energies of a few eV, where 1 eV

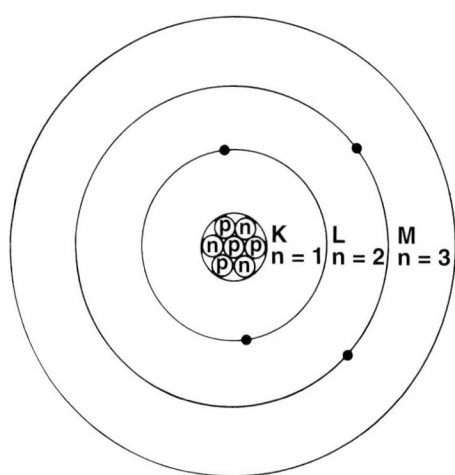

Figure 6–1. Schematic drawing of the Bohr model of the atom. The nucleus contains neutrons and protons, bound together by the attractive nuclear force. The nucleus is surrounded by electrons that are moving in specific orbits with discrete energy levels. By convention the orbits are labeled K, L, M, . . . from inside out. (From Perez CA, Brady LW: *Principles and Practice of Radiation Oncology.* 2nd ed. Philadelphia: JB Lippincott; 1992:184.)

is the energy acquired by an electron accelerated through a potential difference of 1 volt.

Electromagnetic Radiation

Electromagnetic radiation is energy transmitted at a fixed velocity through sinusoidally varying electric and magnetic fields. The frequency of variation of this energy, represented by the Greek letter ν, is the number of oscillations per second, measured in hertz (Hz). The wavelength, λ, is the distance in meters between two crests of the sine wave. The velocity of propagation of the radiation is the product of the wavelength and the frequency, which, in a vacuum, is equal to the speed of light, $c = 3 \times 10^8$ m/sec.

The range of wavelengths encountered in conventional physics is from 10^5 m for AM radio waves, to 10^{-7} m for visible light, to 10^{-12} m for x-rays and cosmic rays. Although electromagnetic radiation is conventionally described as waves of energy, quantum physics tells us that it is equally valid to describe the radiation as particle-like packets of energy called *photons*. Experiments that scatter x-rays off particles have been used to validate this concept. In general, the shorter wavelength radiation is more "particle-like" than the longer wavelength radiation. The energy of a photon is directly proportional to the frequency of the radiation, with a constant of proportionality called *Planck's constant*. That is, $E = h\nu$, where $h = 6.626 \times 10^{-34}$ J/s and the energy is in joules.

Nuclear Transformations

Henri Becquerel discovered natural radioactivity in 1896 when he observed the blackening of wrapped photographic plates when they were placed in contact with certain elements. This event was preceded by the discovery of an invisible form of energy, dubbed *x-rays*, by Röntgen, who observed the glowing of fluorescent material placed near a gas discharge tube.

We now understand that Becquerel observed the natural decay of radioactive nuclei into one of three types of radiation: positively charged alpha particles (α), which we now know are helium nuclei; negatively charged beta particles (β), which are electrons; and uncharged gamma-rays (γ), which are a type of electromagnetic radiation emitted from nuclei. It is entirely possible that Becquerel also observed other types of elementary particles that can exist in the nucleus, or can be produced in nuclear decay processes.

The explanation of nuclear decay depends on understanding the interplay between the very strong, attractive nuclear force that binds the neutrons and protons together in the nucleus, and the moderately strong repulsive electromagnetic force between the protons. As the protons and neutrons move about within the nucleus, there is some probability that one of them will acquire enough kinetic energy to escape from the nuclear potential energy "well." Large nuclei with many neutrons and protons tend to be less stable because of the increasing repulsion of the protons. For large nuclei to be stable, an excess of

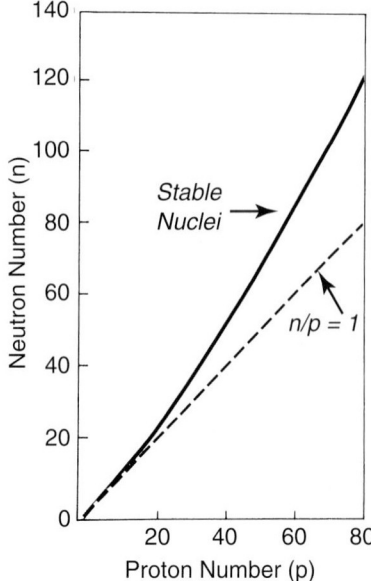

Figure 6–2. Plot of numbers of neutrons and protons in stable nuclei. (From Khan FM: *The Physics of Radiation Therapy.* 2nd ed. Baltimore: Williams & Wilkins; 1994:2.)

neutrons is required to provide the nuclear attraction to keep the protons from escaping. Figure 6-2 shows the line of stable nuclei for the range of known elements.

DECAY CONSTANT

The decay of a large collection of nuclei can be described as a statistical phenomenon. At any moment in time, the number of nuclei disintegrating per unit of time is proportional to the number of nuclei available. Mathematically,

$$(dN/dt) = -\lambda N$$

where N is the number of radioactive nuclei and λ is the *decay constant*. The minus sign indicates that the number of nuclei is decreasing with time. Integration of this differential equation leads to the following equation:

$$N(t) = N_0 e^{-\lambda t}$$

where N_0 is the number of radioactive nuclei initially present, $N(t)$ represents the number remaining at time t, and e is the base of the natural logarithm (2.71828).

The rate of decay, previously referred to as dN/dt, is also called the *activity* of a radioactive substance, referred to by the symbol A. Then $A = -\lambda N$ and

$$A(t) = A_0 e^{-\lambda t}$$

where A_0 is the initial activity and $A(t)$ is the activity at time t. The unit of activity is the curie (Ci) or the becquerel (Bq), which is 1 disintegration per second.

$$1 \text{ Ci} = 3.7 \times 10^{10} \text{ disintegrations per second}$$
$$= 3.7 \times 10^{10} \text{ Bq}$$

The Ci was originally defined to be the activity associated with 1 g of radium, although the number of disintegrations per second from 1 g of radium is now known to be somewhat less than 3.7×10^{10}.

HALF-LIFE AND MEAN LIFE

The *half-life* ($T_{1/2}$) of a radioactive substance is the time required for a population of atoms to decay to half the original number. That is,

$$0.5 = 1.0 \times e^{-\lambda T_{1/2}}$$

Solving this equation,

$$T_{1/2} = (\ln 2)/\lambda = 0.693/\lambda$$

The *mean* or *average life* (T_λ) is the time for the number of atoms to decay to 1/e of the initial number, so

$$T_\lambda = 1/\lambda = 1.44 \ T_{1/2}$$

The mean life can also be thought of as the time required for all the atoms to decay if the decay rate could be maintained at its initial value.

MODES OF RADIOACTIVE DECAY

Just as electrons have energy levels related to the orbit or shell they occupy, nucleons (protons and neutrons) are thought to occupy shells that represent discrete energy levels within the nucleus. When nucleons are excited into higher levels, they can subsequently decay back to their initial energy level, emitting a photon in the process. This process is called *gamma decay*. Due to the very strong nature of nuclear forces, these excited states are very short-lived, with half-lives on the order of 10^{-15} seconds. If, in the process of leaving the nucleus, the gamma-decay photon transfers enough energy to an inner shell electron to eject it from the atom, the process is called *internal conversion*. The subsequent cascade of an outer shell electron into the vacated hole in the inner shell releases a *characteristic x-ray* photon with energy equal to the difference between the energy levels of the inner and outer shells. In some situations, the characteristic x-ray is absorbed and re-emitted by the atom in the form of an ejected orbital electron. Such electrons, emitted in lieu of x-rays, are called *Auger electrons*.

The decay of a nucleus accompanied by the ejection of an electron (e^-) or positron (e^+) is called *beta decay*. In beta (−) decay, a nucleus that has an excess of neutrons can reduce its energy by converting a neutron into a proton, an electron, and an antineutrino (which has energy but no mass). In beta (+) decay, a neutron-deficient nucleus can become more stable by converting a proton into a neutron, a positron, and a neutrino. The typical disintegration energy of 1 to 3 MeV is shared between the emitted particles, the neutrino (antineutrino), and positron (electron). For heavy nuclei, the average binding energy of the nucleons inside the nucleus may be less than 10 MeV. Half-lives for beta decay can range from a few seconds to many years.

A second way in which neutron-deficient nuclei can gain stability is by the process of *electron capture*. In this process, an electron in one of the inner shells is captured by the nucleus, thus transforming a proton into a neutron. That is, a proton plus the captured electron is converted to a neutron plus a neutrino. In general, the inner electron orbital vacancy is quickly filled with an electron from an outer shell, resulting in the emission of characteristic x-rays or Auger electrons.

Very heavy nuclei with Z > 82 frequently decay with the emission of an *alpha particle*, which is identical to the helium nucleus and is composed of two protons and two neutrons tightly bound together. The binding energy of this configuration is particularly high, making this decay mode a very efficient way to decrease the energy and increase the stability of a heavy nucleus. From a specific nuclide, the alpha decay is monoenergetic, that is, the α particle is emitted with a single, well-defined energy. Typically, α particles are emitted with kinetic energies of between 5 and 10 MeV.

RADIOACTIVE DECAY SERIES AND EQUILIBRIUM

A total of 106 elements are known. Of these, the first 92 occur naturally; that is, they are either stable or radioactive with half-lives long enough that they can still be found naturally in trace amounts on the earth. Elements 93 to 106 are very unstable and can only be produced artificially in accelerators with heavy ion bombardment of heavy nuclei. Lead, with Z = 82 is the heaviest known element that has completely stable isotopes. All naturally occurring isotopes of elements with Z between 83 and 92 are members of one of three *radioactive series* referred to as the uranium (Z = 92) series, the actinium (Z = 89) series, and the thorium (Z = 90) series. The name of each series refers to the *parent*, a long-lived nuclide that decays into a *daughter* nuclide, that then decays into another daughter, followed by successive transformations that continue until a stable isotope of lead is reached.

In each series, the half-life of the parent is longer than any of the half-lives of any of the daughter nuclides. This phenomenon leads to a state of *transient* or *secular equilibrium*. Since each daughter is less stable than the original parent, the activity of the daughter will increase with time, until it approaches the activity of the long-lived parent. If the half-lives are very different, the activities will become essentially identical after a number of daughter half-lives, and this is called secular equilibrium. An example is shown in Figure 6-3. If the half-lives of the parent and daughter are very similar, transient equilibrium is reached in a few half-lives, after which the daughter has an activity in excess of the parent activity but decays with the same rate as the limiting parent decay rate. An example of this phenomenon is shown in Figure 6-4. For either case, after a time that is long compared to the half-life of the shorter-lived nuclide,

$$A_d/A_p = T_p/(T_p - T_d)$$

where A_i and T_i refer to the activity and half-life of the daughter (d) or parent (p).

X-Ray Production

Most radiotherapy is delivered with beams of x-rays that are produced as a result of the interactions of accelerated electrons with matter. This can be either through excitation or ionization of the atom via interactions of the accelerated electrons with target electrons leading to the emission of *characteristic x-rays*, mentioned earlier, or through direct interaction between the electrons and the

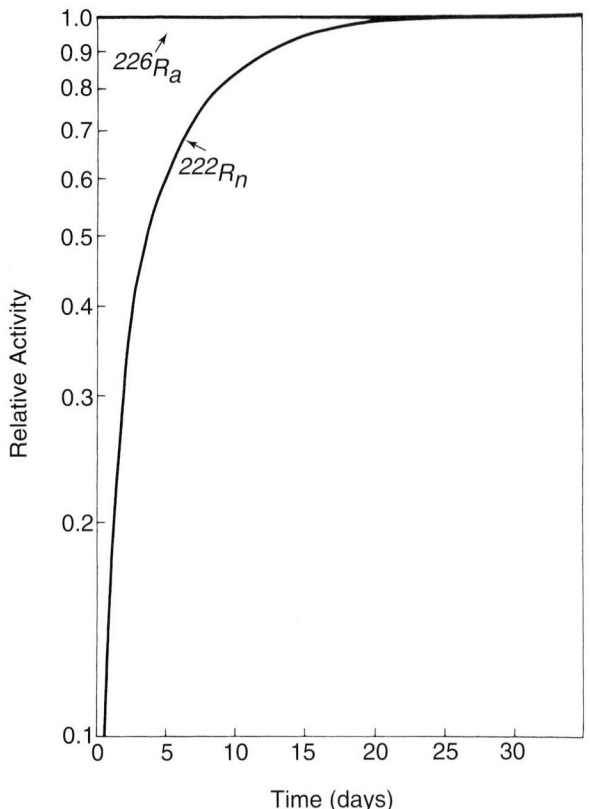

Figure 6–3. Example of secular equilibrium in the decay of ^{226}Ra to ^{222}Rn. (From Khan FM: *The Physics of Radiation Therapy.* 2nd ed. Baltimore: Williams & Wilkins; 1994:25.)

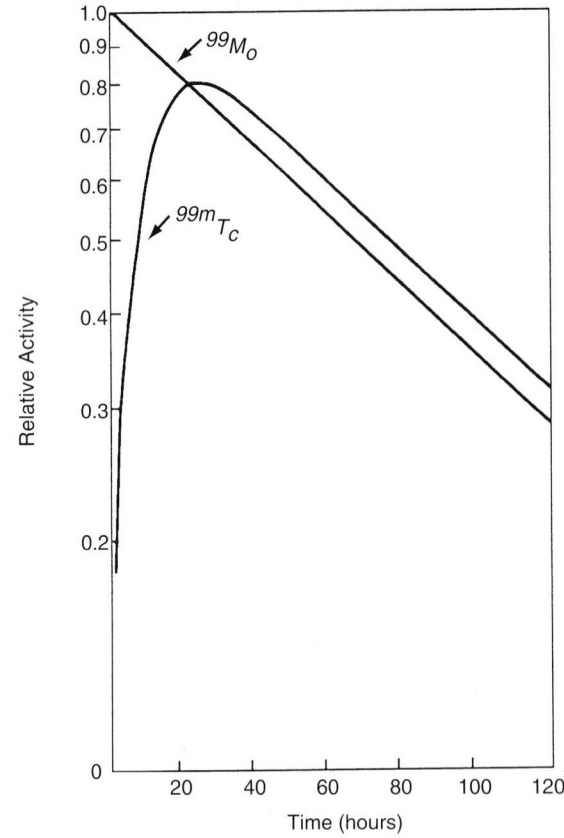

Figure 6–4. Example of transient equilibrium in the decay of ^{99}Mo to ^{99m}Tc. (Redrawn from Khan FM: *The Physics of Radiation Therapy.* 2nd ed. Baltimore: Williams & Wilkins; 1994:20.)

electromagnetic field of the target nuclei, leading to *bremsstrahlung x-rays*.

CHARACTERISTIC X-RAYS

When electrons are incident on target atoms, they can ionize those atoms by depositing sufficient energy to eject an inner shell electron. The inner shell vacancy is subsequently filled by an outer shell electron, causing the emission of a characteristic x-ray with energy equal to the difference between the binding energies of the inner and outer shells. This process is diagrammed in Figure 6-5. Although this process can take place in both low-Z and high-Z atoms, only for high-Z atoms are the binding energies sufficient to produce radiation in the x-ray portion of the electromagnetic spectrum. For example, the binding energy of K-shell electrons in tungsten, a common target for x-ray tubes and accelerators, is about 70 keV, whereas for aluminum, it is only about 1.5 keV. As mentioned earlier, the characteristic x-ray energy is occasionally transferred directly to an orbital electron, leading to the production of an Auger electron.

BREMSSTRAHLUNG X-RAYS

When high-energy electrons interact directly with the electromagnetic field of a target nucleus, they are deflected

and lose a portion of their energy due to deceleration. The energy lost is then emitted in the form of radiation called *bremsstrahlung* (literally, "braking radiation").

Since the incident electron can lose any portion of its energy in this process, the energy of these bremsstrahlung x-rays can vary continuously from nearly zero to the full energy of the incident electron. The angle of the x-rays,

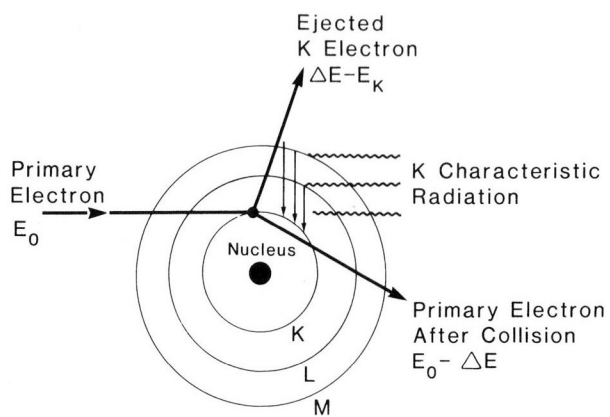

Figure 6–5. Illustration of the production of characteristic radiation. (From Khan FM: *The Physics of Radiation Therapy.* 2nd ed. Baltimore: Williams & Wilkins; 1994:41.)

relative to the beam direction, depends on the energy of the electron. At low energies typical of those used for diagnostic radiology, the x-ray has equal probability of being emitted in any direction, whereas at high energies typically used for radiotherapy, the x-rays are emitted preferentially in the forward direction. These facts explain the use of thick targets and 90-degree angles between electrons and x-rays for diagnostic applications and thin transmission targets for radiotherapy.

The probability of bremsstrahlung production varies with Z^2 of the target material, whereas the efficiency of x-ray production depends on the product of Z and E, the energy of the electrons. At 100 keV in a tungsten target, only about 1% of the incident energy of the beam is converted into x-rays, the remainder ending up in heat.

In general, both bremsstrahlung and characteristic x-rays are present when electrons strike a target. Figure 6-6 shows x-ray spectra for a thick tungsten target for electron energies of from 65 keV to 200 keV. Note the appearance of the characteristic x-rays on top of the bremsstrahlung spectrum once the electron energy is in excess of the K-shell binding energy of 70 keV. Any material in the x-ray beam, including the target itself, will absorb some of the energy of the beam. The effect of such absorption is to preferentially *filter out* the low energy portion of the bremsstrahlung spectrum. Intentional filtering of the beam can lead to *beam hardening*, increasing the average energy of the x-rays at the expense of reduced intensity.

INTERACTION OF X-RAYS AND PARTICLES WITH MATTER

X-Ray Interactions

As described earlier, x-rays can be considered as packets of energy, called photons, for purposes of considering their interactions with matter. There are a number of different interaction processes that the photons can experience, and each of these has a probability described by an *attenuation coefficient*. Mathematically, this can be written as:

$$dN = -\Sigma\mu_i\, N\, dx$$

where dN is the reduction in the number of photons due to interactions in a thickness dx of an absorber, N is the number of incident photons, and μ_i is the attenuation coefficient for the ith interaction process. After integration over the thickness, this equation becomes:

$$N(x) = N_0\, e^{-\Sigma(\mu_i/\rho)\rho x} = N_0\, e^{-(\mu_{tot}/\rho)\rho x}$$

where $N(x)$ is the number of photons left in the beam (without interaction) as a function of the thickness x of material traversed and μ_{tot} is the sum of the individual attenuation coefficients. This equation is written with (μ_i/ρ) being a *mass*-attenuation coefficient for process i, with ρ is the density of the material. Dividing the conventional attenuation coefficients by density removes the dependence on the physical density of materials and results in mass attenuation coefficients that are approximately equal from material to material. The corresponding thickness, ρx, is in units of grams per square centimeter (g/cm^2). The total mass attenuation coefficients as a function of energy are shown for water and lead in Figure 6-7. There are five different processes through which the photon can interact, including coherent scattering, photoelectric effect, Compton scattering, pair production, and photodisintegration. These will be discussed in turn.

The thickness of material that reduces the number of transmitted photons to one-half the initial value is referred to as the half-value layer (HVL) and depends on the nature of the material and the energy of the photons. This occurs when

$$N/N_0 = 1/2 = e^{-\mu_{tot}\times HVL}$$

implying that

$$HVL = (\ln 2)/\mu_{tot} = 0.693/\mu_{tot}$$

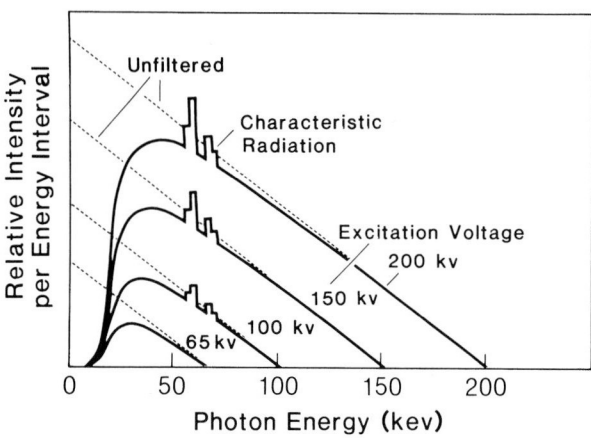

Figure 6–6. Spectral distribution of x-rays calculated for a thick tungsten target. Dotted curves are for no filtration and solid curves are for a filtration of 1 mm aluminum. Note the characteristic radiation peaks on top of the continuous bremsstrahlung spectra. (From Khan FM: *The Physics of Radiation Therapy*. 2nd ed. Baltimore: Williams & Wilkins; 1994:42.)

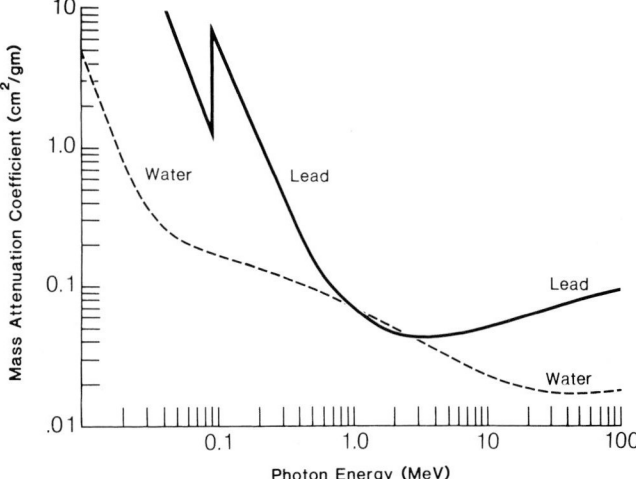

Figure 6–7. Mass attenuation coefficients for lead and water. The sharp discontinuities in the lead curve are due to absorption edges. (From Johns HE, Cunningham JR: *The Physics of Radiology*. 4th ed., 1983. Courtesy of Charles C. Thomas, Publisher, Springfield, Ill.)

Although not constant with depth, HVL is often used to describe the quality of the beam or its ability to penetrate material.

COHERENT SCATTERING

Coherent scattering, also called classical scattering, is a low-energy phenomenon in which the electromagnetic field of the incident photon interacts with the field of a bound electron in the atom without any transfer of energy. The bound electron is set into oscillation by the passing photon, but then reirradiates the energy of oscillation back to the outgoing photon. The net effect is only a change in direction for the photon. Since there is no transfer of energy, this process is of little importance to radiotherapy.

PHOTOELECTRIC EFFECT

In the *photoelectric effect*, the energy of the photon is totally absorbed by the atom and subsequently transferred to an orbital electron, which is then ejected from the atom with an energy equal to the original energy of the photon minus the binding energy of the electron. The vacancy created by the ejection of the photoelectron from a shell gets filled by an electron from a shell with lower binding energy, followed by the emission of a characteristic x-ray with energy equal to the difference in binding energies of the two shells. Again, an Auger electron can be emitted in lieu of the x-ray in some cases.

The most likely angle of ejection of the photoelectron relative to the incident photon direction is 90 degrees for low-energy photons (50 keV or less), becoming smaller (more forward) as the photon energy increases. The mass attenuation coefficient for the photoelectric effect is proportional to Z^3/E^3 where Z is the atomic number of the target atom and E is the energy of the photon.

The photoelectric effect is important at diagnostic x-ray energies of 100 keV and is the basis for the radiographic contrast of bone versus soft tissue. However, due to the $1/E^3$ energy dependence, the photoelectric effect is relatively unimportant at typical radiotherapy energies of several MeV.

COMPTON SCATTERING

Compton scattering is a process in which the incident photon interacts with an orbital electron as if it were a free particle, since the binding energy is small compared to the photon energy. The dynamics of the interaction can be described as a typical particle–particle scattering interaction whereby the photon transfers some of its energy to the electron and is scattered at an angle ϕ relative to the incident direction. The electron is ejected at an angle θ relative to the forward direction. The energy of the outgoing Compton-scattered photon is equal to the difference between the incident photon energy and the energy transferred to the electron. A diagram of the Compton process is shown in Figure 6-8.

As with any particle–particle scattering process, energy and momentum conservation can be applied to obtain relationships between energy and angle.
From conservation of energy:

$$h\nu_0 = E + h\nu'$$

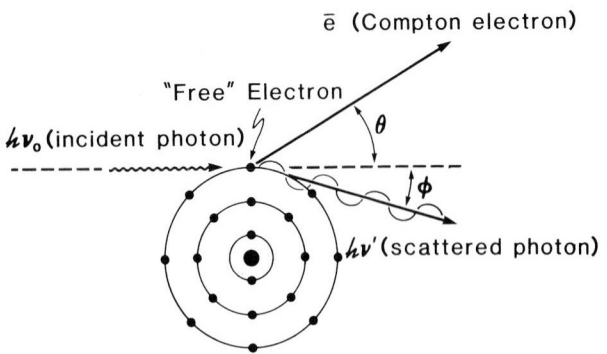

Figure 6–8. Illustration of the Compton effect. (From Khan FM: *The Physics of Radiation Therapy.* 2nd ed. Baltimore: Williams & Wilkins; 1994:82.)

From conservation of momentum:

$$\gamma m_0 v \sin \theta = (h\nu'/c) \sin \phi$$

and

$$(h\nu_0/c) = (h\nu'/c) \cos \phi + \gamma m_0 v \cos \theta$$

where v is the velocity of the electron, m_0 is the rest mass of the electron, c is the speed of light, and $\gamma = (1 - v^2/c^2)^{1/2}$. Solving these three simultaneous equations, we obtain the following relationships:

$$E = h\nu_0 [\alpha f / (1 + \alpha f)]$$

$$h\nu' = h\nu_0 [1/(1 + \alpha f)]$$

$$1/\tan \theta = (1 + \alpha) \tan (\phi/2)$$

where $\alpha = h\nu_0 / m_0 c^2$ and $f = (1 - \cos \phi)$.

From these equations, we can examine several limiting cases of the Compton effect. A grazing hit corresponds to $\theta = 90$ degrees, in which case the photon is undeflected, and continues in the forward direction. A direct hit corresponds to $\theta = 0$ degrees, meaning that $\phi = 180$ degrees, or in other words, the photon comes off backwards. For intermediate situations, for example, when the photon goes off at 90 degrees, the angle and energy of the electron depend on the energy of the photon. When α is much greater than 1 (high energy), θ is small and E is essentially equal to $h\nu_0$. When α is much less than 1 (low energy), the photon energy remains nearly unchanged and the Compton process approaches that of coherent scattering.

The mass attenuation coefficient for Compton scattering is independent of Z, decreases slowly with photon energy, and is directly proportional to the number of electrons per gram, which varies by only 20% from the lightest to the heaviest elements (with the exception of hydrogen). Therefore, in the energy region where Compton processes dominate, the attenuation of the beam will vary according to the integrated density of the material traversed. This fact is responsible for the relatively poor contrast observed in portal verification films exposed with megavoltage x-rays exiting from the irradiated patient.

PAIR PRODUCTION

Pair production is an interaction of a photon with the electromagnetic field of a nucleus in which the energy of the photon is converted into an electron (e⁻) and a positron (e⁺). Since the rest mass of each of these particles is 0.511 MeV, the threshold energy for pair production is 1.02 MeV. The total shared kinetic energy of this pair of particles is just the photon energy minus 1.02 MeV. The mass attenuation coefficient for pair production increases logarithmically with energy above the threshold, and is proportional to Z^2. Subsequent to the production of the electron-positron pair, the positron has a high probability of combining with a free electron during the process of energy loss in the medium and converting the combined e⁺-e⁻ mass into a pair of annihilation photons, each of energy 0.511 MeV, that will leave the annihilation region in opposite directions.

PHOTODISINTEGRATION

At very high energies, the photon can deposit so much energy into the nucleus that partial or complete disintegration of the nucleus takes place. Since the binding energies of nucleons within the nucleus tend to be typically 7 MeV or higher, this process is of little importance at therapy energies. However, photodisintegration is a source of low-level neutron production that must be considered when designing radiation shielding around high-energy linear accelerators.

RELATIVE IMPORTANCE OF INTERACTION TYPES

The total mass absorption coefficient is the sum of the coefficients for coherent, photoelectric, Compton, and pair production. For low-Z targets such as tissue (average Z = 7), Compton processes are overwhelmingly dominant throughout the range of energies used in therapy. Figure 6-9 shows the relative importance of photoelectric, Compton, and pair production as a function of photon energy and the atomic number of the target material.[4] For tissue, Compton dominates between approximately 30 keV and 30 MeV, whereas for lead, photoelectric dominates up to approximately 800 keV and pair production above

about 5 MeV. Because of its calcium content, bone has a higher absorption by photoelectric and pair production. This leads to high bone doses for orthovoltage and kilovoltage and for higher energy accelerator beams.

Electrons and Other Charged Particles

The interaction of electrons with matter has been discussed as a way of understanding the creation of x-ray beams for radiation therapy. The processes by which the electron energy is lost to the medium can be divided into ionization and radiation. Ionization processes are interactions with the atomic electrons, whereas radiation losses are interactions with the field of the nucleus, leading to bremsstrahlung x-ray production. While the microscopic interactions are well understood, the macroscopic description of the energy and range of the particles at any point in the medium is not simple. This is because the electrons are very light—obviously, the same mass as the atomic electrons and very much lighter than the nuclei. Therefore, the electron can lose a very large fraction of its energy in a single process and can be deflected by very large angles. This means that even if the electron beam is monoenergetic when entering a medium, there will be a large amount of *range-straggling*, or a large variation from electron to electron as to where, in the phantom, the electron will stop. Figure 6-10 shows a plot of absorbed dose as a function of depth for monoenergetic electrons incident on water. There is a depth beyond which the dose is almost zero, where all the incident electrons have been stopped and where the remaining dose is due to bremsstrahlung x-rays produced by the electrons in the medium. This is in sharp contrast to the exponential falloff of dose for x-rays. This "ranging out" of electrons in matter is responsible for the popularity of electrons for treatment of superficial disease.

PROTONS AND HEAVIER IONS

Beams of both protons[5-8] and heavy ions[5,9-14] have been used in radiotherapy. Similar to electrons, protons lose

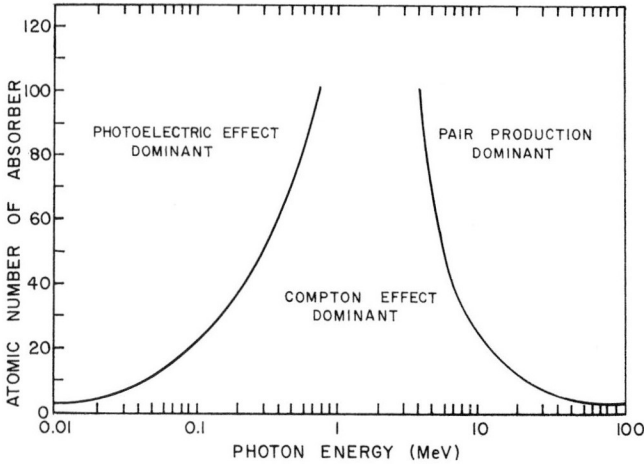

Figure 6–9. Relative importance of the three main modes of energy loss for photons as a function of energy and atomic number of the medium. (From Hendee WR: *Medical Radiation Physics: Roentgenology, Nuclear Medicine and Ultrasound*. Chicago: Year Book Medical Publishers; 1979:115 with permission from Mosby.)

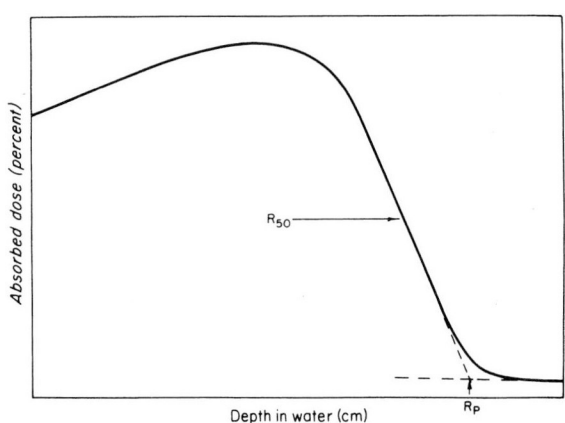

Figure 6–10. Depth-dose curve for monoenergetic electrons incident on water. R_{50} is the mean range and R_p is the extrapolated or practical range. (From Johns HE, Cunningham JR. *The Physics of Radiology*. 4th ed., 1983:197. Courtesy of Charles C. Thomas, Publisher, Springfield, Ill.)

energy primarily by electromagnetic interactions with the atomic electrons. A major difference between protons and electrons is that protons are much heavier than electrons and therefore lose only a very small fraction of their energy in an individual interaction, scattering minimally in the process. Protons lose energy at an increasing rate as they slow down, yielding an enhanced region of energy deposition called the *Bragg Peak* just before they stop. One can predict very accurately the depth at which the protons will come to rest if the initial energy of the protons and the electron density of the material traversed are known. The absence of exit dose beyond the intended target makes protons nearly ideally suited for optimal physical dose delivery. A typical depth dose distribution for a clinical, energy-modulated proton beam, compared to that of a 10 MV bremsstrahlung x-ray beam, is shown in Figure 6-11. A small percentage of proton interactions is via nuclear interactions with the nucleus. These rare interactions are qualitatively different than electromagnetic interactions and are thought to be responsible for enhancing the cell kill per unit dose by about 10% to 20% over that of x-rays.[15]

Heavy ions such as helium, carbon, neon, and argon nuclei have also been used in radiotherapy.[10,12,14,16,17] Similar to protons, they lose energy by interacting with the atomic electrons. Being even heavier than protons, they scatter even less and have even more rapid dose falloff outside the central beam and even faster falloff of dose beyond the end of range. In addition to these electromagnetic interactions, heavy ions have a probability of interacting with the nucleus via nuclear interactions that increases with the mass of the incident ion. In particular, as the heavy ions begin to slow down, they tend to suffer nuclear interactions in which they lose a very large amount of their energy in a single event. This high density of deposited energy kills cells in a far more efficient way per unit dose than x-rays. These particles are said to have a high *radiobiological efficiency (RBE)*. For more information on these particles, the reader is referred to the literature.[13]

Neutrons

Neutrons have also been used in clinical treatments.[18-22] These particles are neutral so they cannot lose energy by any means other than the nuclear interaction. All of their interactions are "catastrophic" since a significant portion of their energy is deposited in an individual event. Their primary interactions are with protons within the nucleus. These nuclear events result in recoil protons and charged nuclear fragments that have rather low energy and deposit large amounts of energy very close to the site of the original interaction. The falloff of neutron dose with depth is exponential and similar to that of low energy x-rays, with the depth of the 50% dose being around 10 cm for typical treatment energies. Neutrons are very efficient in producing cell kill per unit dose (high RBE) relative to x-rays for both tumor tissue and normal tissues. Clinical trials have been conducted to investigate the areas where neutrons might have an advantage over x-rays. A summary of the physical characteristics and results of early clinical results is available.[13]

In addition, clinical trials are under way to investigate the use of slow neutrons, either thermal or epithermal in energy, to treat boronated tumor cells in patients.[23-25] The clinical efficacy of these neutrons for cancer therapy depends on the very high cross section for neutron capture by Boron and on a high ratio of Boron in the tumor cells to that in the surrounding normal cells.

RADIATION THERAPY TREATMENT MACHINES

Before about 1950, external beam radiation therapy was primarily carried out with x-ray beams produced in evacuated x-ray tubes by electrons accelerated with an electric field, impinging on a target and interacting with the nuclei of target atoms. The details of the interactions and the properties of the resulting x-ray beams are described elsewhere in this chapter. The maximum energy of these electrons and the photon beams that they produced was about 400 kV. Therefore, this period of radiation therapy history is called the *kilovoltage era*. Although most of these machines have been replaced in the intervening years with ^{60}Co teletherapy machines and electron linear accelerators, low-energy x-ray generators still play a limited role in the treatment of superficial disease.

Kilovoltage Units

A schematic diagram of an x-ray tube suitable for radiation therapy is shown in Figure 6-12. Since a high-voltage supply is used to generate the accelerating potential for the electron beams, a maximum energy of approximately

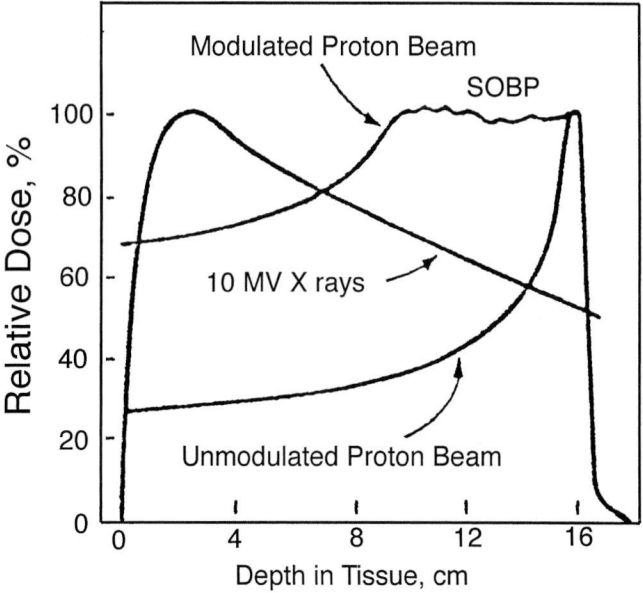

Figure 6-11. Depth-dose curve for a modulated proton beam of 160 MeV compared to that for a 10 MV bremsstrahlung x-ray beam. The region of the flat dose is referred to as the spread-out bragg peak (SOBP).

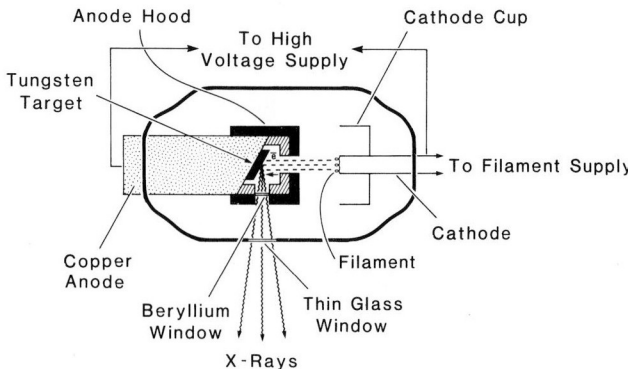

Figure 6–12. Schematic diagram of an x-ray tube that could be used for radiation therapy. (Khan FM. *The Physics of Radiation Therapy*. 2nd ed. Baltimore: Williams & Wilkins; 1994:33.)

300 kV is achievable with this design. The resulting x-ray beams have a spectrum of photon energies with a maximum equal to the energy of the electron beam.

CONTACT THERAPY MACHINES

X-ray machines that operate at potentials of 40 to 50 kV are referred to as *contact units*. They typically operate at tube currents of 2 mA and the beams are usually filtered with 0.5 to 1.0 mm aluminum in order to remove the very low energy x-rays in the beam—a process often referred to as "hardening" the beam. Treating at a typical source-to-skin (SSD) distance of 2 cm, the dose in this beam drops off to 50% of its surface value in less than 5 mm of water or soft tissue. Such a beam would be useful only for the most superficial of targets.

SUPERFICIAL THERAPY MACHINES

Units with x-ray beams produced by electrons with energies between 50 and 150 kV are usually referred to as superficial therapy units. These units normally are filtered with 1 to 4 mm aluminum and treated at distances of 20 cm SSD. The 50% depth in water or soft tissue in this energy range would be typically 1 to 2 cm. By using thicker filters, it is possible to further harden the beam and move the 50% dose somewhat deeper with a reduction in dose rate. Superficial units can be very useful for treatment of skin lesions, using either regular fields defined by interchangeable cones or irregular fields defined with custom lead cutouts.

ORTHOVOLTAGE THERAPY MACHINES

Orthovoltage x-ray units are defined as those that operate in the 150 to 300 kV range. Typical SSDs are 50 cm, field sizes up to 20 × 20 cm and filters of 1 to 4 mm of copper. Depths of 50% are usually between 5 and 7 cm depending on filter thickness and field size. Regular fields are defined with detachable cones or adjustable collimators and irregular fields with lead cutouts or special hand blocking. Before 1950, these units were the workhorses of radiation therapy. Although useful for treating disease in thin sections of the body such as the neck, in thicker areas of the body, where tumors may lie 10 to 15 cm below the surface, the dose to normal tissue can be quite

high when using beams in this energy range. Very few of these machines remain in current use in radiation therapy centers.

Megavoltage Units

X-ray and gamma-ray beams of energy greater than 1 MV are classified as *megavoltage beams*. In the 1930s a number of transformer-based and van de Graaff generator–based units working in the 800 KeV to 2 MeV range were installed around the world. However, it was not until the introduction of the ^{60}Co teletherapy machine and the linear accelerator that the routine use of megavoltage x-ray and gamma-ray beams occurred, significantly changing the practice of radiotherapy and leading to substantial improvements in clinical results.[26]

TELETHERAPY MACHINES

The megavoltage era really began with the introduction of the ^{60}Co teletherapy machine into radiotherapy clinics beginning in 1951.[27,28] The development of nuclear reactors in the late 1940s made possible the production of small ^{60}Co sources with specific activities (in curies per gram) high enough to produce clinically acceptable dose rates of more than 1 Gy per minute at a typical treatment distance of 80 cm from the source. These machines quickly became the standard of radiotherapy due to their simplicity of design and operation, low cost, and availability. The two photons produced by the decay of ^{60}Co have energies of 1.17 and 1.33 MeV, yielding a depth-dose curve that falls to 50% of maximum in about 10 cm of water or tissue. In addition, the relatively high energy of the photons leads to "skin sparing" due to a reduced entrance dose that builds up for a distance of 5 mm (the maximum range of the secondary electrons from ^{60}Co photons) to a maximum value. The half-life of ^{60}Co is 5.28 years, making the source change a relatively infrequent requirement. With the highest specific activities currently achievable, dose rates of at least 1.5 Gy per minute for a field size of 40 cm × 40 cm can be achieved at 80 cm source-to-treatment distance.

Aside from the requirement to replace the sources every few years, additional disadvantages to ^{60}Co isotope machines include the need to shield against continuous leakage radiation and the lack of field flatness for the largest field sizes. In addition, the physical size of the source capsule, typically 1.5 cm to 2.0 cm in diameter, is much larger than the effective source size available on any machine that uses an electron beam (typically 4 mm or less for linear accelerators). This large source size contributes to a geometric penumbra (the penumbra is the area at the edge of the beam where the dose falls from high dose to low dose) that can be significantly wider than with accelerators.

Before the development of ^{60}Co isotope machines, both radium and cesium sources were used for teletherapy treatments. However, the limitations of low specific activity for radium and low energy and limited specific activity for cesium limited their usefulness for general radiotherapy.

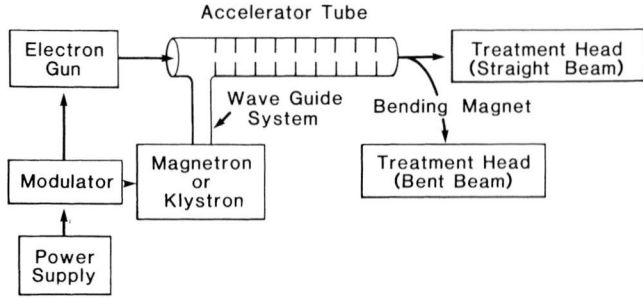

Figure 6–13. A block diagram of a typical medical linear accelerator. (From Khan FM: *The Physics of Radiation Therapy*. 2nd ed. Baltimore: Williams & Wilkins; 1994:51.)

BETATRONS

The next chronological development in treatment machines is the betatron, first developed by D. W. Kerst at the University of Illinois[29] primarily for physics experimentation. Electrons with energies of up to 45 MeV have been produced in betatrons for radiotherapy and used either directly or to produce bremsstrahlung x-rays beams. The massive size of these machines, their high cost, and relatively low dose rate combined to limit their usefulness in radiation therapy.

LINEAR ACCELERATORS

The use of microwaves to accelerate electrons to high energies for radiotherapy was first demonstrated in Great Britain in 1953.[30] This became possible primarily because of the development of high-power microwave generators for military radar use during World War II. The major components of a typical medical linear accelerator (linac) are shown in a block diagram in Figure 6-13. The acceleration of the electron beam takes place in the accelerator wave guide, consisting of a stack of cylindrical cavities with a hole through the center, into which resonant electromagnetic waves of frequency in the microwave range

(≈3000 MHz) have been coupled. The electron beam is created and preaccelerated to approximately 50 keV in a conventional electrostatic electron gun, injected into the resonating waveguide, spatially bunched and accelerated through interactions with the electromagnetic field in the individual cavities, and then emerges from the accelerating structure as a narrow pencil beam that can be magnetically bent or focused onto a scattering foil (for electron treatments) or a bremsstrahlung target (for x-ray treatments) in the treatment head of the linac. For low energies of 6 MeV or less, the beam can be magnetically focused in the forward (vertical) direction onto the axis of the treatment head, whereas at higher energies, the beam is usually bent through a 90-degree or 270-degree angle before entering the treatment head since the accelerating structure is much longer for high energies and is frequently oriented horizontally to save space. For more details about the acceleration process, the reader is referred to several excellent review articles in the literature.[31-33]

Although the details of the acceleration process can be quite technical, the shaping of the beam in the treatment head is both important and conceptually easy to understand. Figure 6-14 shows a schematic diagram of the head of a typical linear accelerator in x-ray and electron treatment mode. In the x-ray mode, the beam first strikes an x-ray target made of high-Z material such as tungsten and produces a bremsstrahlung beam that is forward peaked—the higher the electron energy, the more forward the angular distribution of the resulting x-rays. After primary collimation, the beam strikes a flattening filter made of high-Z material that is thick in the center and thin toward the outside, thereby flattening the angular distribution of the x-ray beam. Although the beam can be made precisely flat only for one particular field size and at one particular depth in a patient, the filters are selected to produce beams that have acceptable flatness over the entire range of field sizes and depths normally used in therapy. If the accelerator is designed to deliver x-ray bremsstrahlung beams produced by electrons of more than one energy, a second flattening filter, optimized for

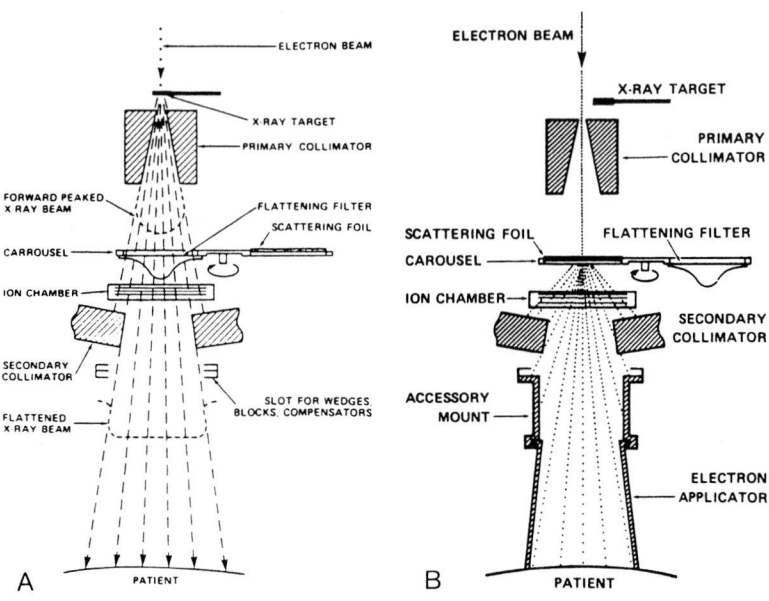

Figure 6–14. Schematic diagram showing the basic components of the treatment head of a modern linear accelerator. **A,** Components in place for x-ray therapy. **B,** Components in place for electron therapy. (From Khan FM: *The Physics of Radiation Therapy*. 2nd ed. Baltimore: Williams & Wilkins; 1994:56.)

that energy, will be rotated into position on the carousel. Following the flattening filter, the beam encounters the transmission ion chamber used to monitor the beam intensity (and, if segmented, the beam position), and then a secondary collimator that, along with the primary collimator, defines the rectangular field size. Patient-specific collimators and compensators, as well as wedges, if required, are placed beyond the secondary collimator as shown. In all contemporary machines dual ion chambers are used.

In the electron mode the x-ray target is out of position and the beam first strikes a thin scatterer that is rotated into position on the multi-element carousel. This scatterer is designed to produce flat electron beams when used in combination with a field size–specific combination of secondary collimator settings and electron applicators as shown in Figure 6-14. The scatterer is commonly a dual system of lead foils, with the second foil thicker in the center to remove the forward peaking prevalent at high energies. Bremsstrahlung x-rays will inevitably be produced in the scattering foils, but since the foils are thin, they will typically account for less than 5% of the dose received by the patient. The transmission monitor ion chamber remains in the beam as for x-ray therapy.

In the 1990s a new X-band linear accelerator was developed for medical applications. This accelerator operates at $\approx$9000 MHz frequency, resulting in a smaller diameter wave guide. X-band linacs capable of accelerating electrons to 6 or 12 MeV are relatively compact and are now being used with a robotic delivery system[34]; a portable IORT device; and a tomotherapy device, which mounts it on a computed tomography gantry.[35]

MICROTRONS

The microtron is an electron accelerator that combines the linear acceleration principle of the linac with a fixed magnetic field to confine the electrons, similar to a cyclotron (see later). The electrons move in circular orbits of increasing radii as they repeatedly recirculate through a resonant accelerating cavity. A moveable deflection tube can be placed in any location inside the magnet to select the desired electron energy for extraction. The advantages of the microtron over a linear accelerator are its simplicity, compact size, and ease of energy selection. In addition, compared to a linac, the energy spread, beam divergence, and beam size are all small, simplifying subsequent beam transport. The first example of a microtron in clinical use was a 10 MeV unit, described in 1972.[36] The first commercial unit, manufactured by AB Scanditronix in Sweden, was a 22 MeV unit installed at the University of Umeå, Sweden.[37] Currently, microtron units of up to 50 MeV are installed at various facilities in Europe and the United States.

Cyclotrons

Cyclotrons are used to accelerate heavy charged particles such as protons, deuterons, and heavier ions. The cyclotron was invented by Ernest Lawrence in the 1930s as a tool for physics research and isotope production. It has been used to produce protons for radiotherapy since the 1960s at several physics laboratories around the world including locations in the United States, the former Soviet Union, Europe, and Japan. Cyclotrons have also been used to produce therapeutical neutron beams through the interaction of accelerated proton or deuteron beams with beryllium or other light targets.

In its simplest form, the cyclotron is composed of two conducting D-shaped half-cylinders that are evacuated and placed between the poles of a direct current magnet. An alternating potential difference is applied between the two Ds such that when protons are injected into the center of the Ds, they are accelerated toward the negative potential. Under the constant magnetic field, they travel in circular orbits, experiencing acceleration each time they reach the gap. Energies of 200 MeV or more are needed for proton therapy if all areas of the body are to be reached. Deuteron energies of approximately 50 MeV are adequate for the production of neutron beams for therapy. Proton and deuteron beams of these energies can be produced in appropriately designed cyclotrons.

A 225 MeV proton cyclotron is now being used for therapy at the Northeast Proton Treatment Center at Massachusetts General Hospital in Boston. This cyclotron, developed by IBA[38] from Belgium, began treating patients in 2001. A 200 MeV cyclotron has also been converted for proton radiotherapy at the Paul Scherrer Institute (PSI) in Switzerland.[39]

Synchrotrons

Whereas cyclotrons use a fixed magnetic field and variable radius orbits as the particles increase energy, synchrotrons use a variable magnetic field and a fixed radius orbit to confine the protons or other heavy charged particles. The synchrotron consists of a ring of magnets with interspersed resonating structures that together can confine and accelerate the charged particles to high energy. Loma Linda University Medical Center has the world's first dedicated proton facility that uses a synchrotron to produce proton beams that are used in any of several treatment rooms.[8] Synchrotrons have also been used to create heavy ion charged particle beams for radiotherapy at Lawrence Berkeley Laboratory in California and at the National Institute for Radiological Sciences in Chiba, Japan.[16]

RADIATION DOSIMETRY

Biological damage depends on how much energy is absorbed from the radiation beam and deposited in the tissue. The absorbed dose is defined as the energy absorbed per unit mass of material and can be used to describe the interactions of all types of ionizing radiation with matter—both directly ionizing (charged particles such as electrons and protons) and indirectly ionizing (neutral particles such as photons and neutrons). Since it is difficult to measure absorbed dose in tissue-like material directly, radiation dosimetry is typically performed by measuring ionization in air and then converting this measurement into absorbed dose.

Radiation Exposure

When ionizing radiation passes through a volume of air, some of the atoms of the air are ionized by interactions of the beam with the atoms. Exposure is defined as the ratio of the number of ions of either sign created by the passage of a beam through a sample of air, divided by the mass of that volume of air from which the ions are produced, assuming all of the ions are completely stopped in the air volume. The unit of exposure is the Roentgen (R) defined as[2]

$$1 \text{ R} = 2.58 \times 10^{-4} \text{ coulombs per kilogram}$$
$$\text{(C/kg) of air}$$

Although this definition is difficult to use operationally, the free-air chamber that can directly measure exposure for photons of energy less than approximately 3 MeV has been constructed and used in standards laboratories for absolute measurements.[1] The difficulty with satisfying the definition for higher energies is that the mean free path length in air for electrons produced by high energy photons is several meters, and therefore the free air chamber, which must be large enough to stop these electrons, is not practical above a few MeV. As a result, exposure is not a valid concept at energies above 3 MeV.

In practice, thimble ionization chambers are used to measure exposure. These chambers, either cylindrical or spherical in shape, typically contain less than 1 mL of air and, in combination with an electrometer, can be used conveniently and reproducibly to measure the quantity of charge produced when ionizing radiation passes through those volumes. National standards laboratories, using either free-air chambers or other methods, can provide calibrations of these chambers in units of R/C (i.e., exposure per unit of collected charge in a ^{60}Co beam that can then be converted to dose per unit collected charge in beams of other energies and in phantoms of various materials). A schematic diagram of a typical cylindrical thimble ionization chamber is shown in Figure 6-15.

Absorbed Dose

Whereas exposure, as defined earlier, is a property of the beam, absorbed dose is a measure of the energy deposited by the beam and absorbed by the target and is assumed to be closely related to the observed biological effects. The units of absorbed dose are: 1 Gy = 1 J/kg, that is,

1 Gray, (Gy) is the dose associated with the absorption of 1 Joule of energy per kg of the medium of interest. Clinical doses are often described in units of centigray (cGy), which is equal to the historical unit rad. That is,

$$1 \text{ Gy} = 100 \text{ cGy} = 100 \text{ rad} = 1 \text{ J/kg}$$

Another useful concept is *kerma*, an acronym for kinetic energy released in the medium. Although it has the same units as dose, the distinction is that kerma refers to energy *transferred to* the medium, whereas dose refers to energy *absorbed by* the medium. As a beam of photons enters a medium, there is an initial distance in which secondary electrons are being produced more rapidly than they are being stopped (the "buildup region") due to the interactions of the photons with the material. In this region, the absorbed dose is increasing with depth, whereas the kerma is decreasing with depth due to the exponential attenuation of the beam in the medium. After a distance that corresponds approximately to the path length of the highest energy secondary electron that can be produced by a photon in the beam, the number of electrons produced per unit pathlength becomes approximately equal to the number that come to the end of their range. From this depth on, the photons are said to be in "electronic equilibrium" with the secondary electrons and kerma is approximately equal to dose. Figure 6-16 shows the relationship between kerma and dose as a function of depth.

DOSE DETERMINATION

Absolute dose determinations are difficult. They require a detector that responds linearly to deposited energy and that has an absolute calibration factor in units of response per unit dose that is known or that can be determined independently. As will be seen, most dosimetry is performed using exposure measurements that are then converted to absorbed dose using a number of conversion factors that are detector-specific and beam-specific. A third class of useful detector is used only for relative dose measurements.

Absolute Dose Measurements

CALORIMETERS

The most widely used direct dose measuring device is the calorimeter. The calorimeter can be used to determine absorbed dose by measuring a change in temperature in an irradiated material since, for most materials, energy

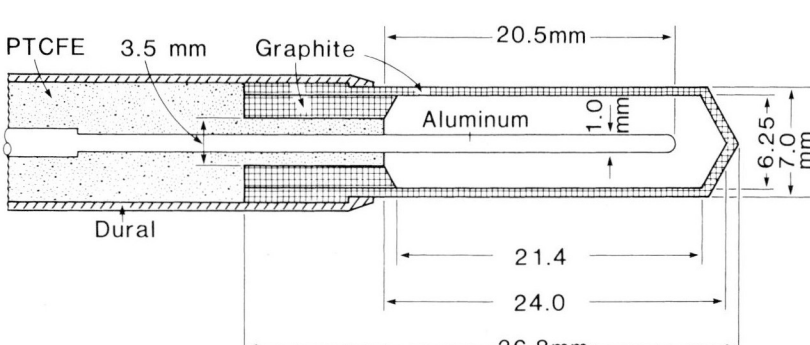

Figure 6-15. Diagram of Farmer thimble ionization chamber. (From Khan FM: *The Physics of Radiation Therapy*. 2nd ed. Baltimore: Williams & Wilkins; 1994:107.)

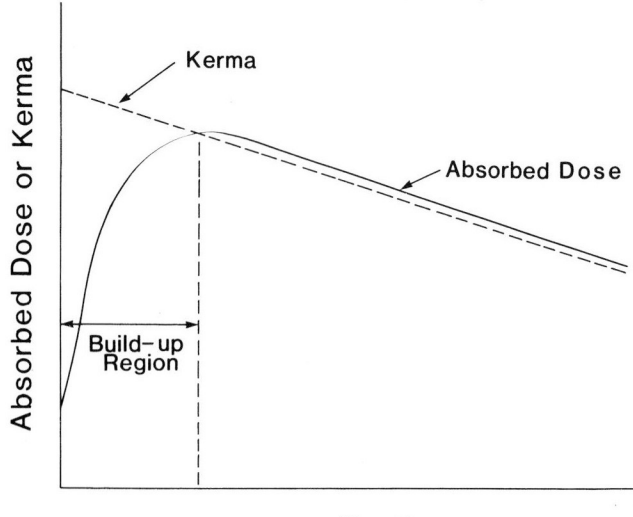

Figure 6–16. Schematic plot of absorbed dose and kerma as functions of depth. (From Khan FM: *The Physics of Radiation Therapy*. 2nd ed. Baltimore: Williams & Wilkins; 1994:182.)

deposited eventually appears as heat within the material, although for some materials a small portion of the absorbed energy (called the *thermal defect*) may be lost due to lattice deformations or chemical changes. The primary detector in the calorimeter is a thermistor embedded in the absorbing phantom. A thermistor is a solid state device that has a rapidly varying resistance with temperature. In carefully controlled situations, a thermistor can measure a change in temperature of as little as 10^{-5}°C. This corresponds to a deposited dose of approximately 4 cGy in water. To accurately measure clinically relevant doses delivered at achievable dose rates, the thermistor needs to be very well isolated from the outside environment so that temperature changes due to atmospheric conditions are much smaller than those produced by the energy absorbed from the beam during the time required to make a single measurement. Successful calorimeters have been constructed out of carbon,[40] water,[41-43] and tissue-equivalent conducting plastic.[44] An excellent review of the field of calorimeters can be found in Attix's textbook on radiation dosimetry.[45] Although calorimeters are the most direct method of directly measuring dose, they are generally expensive, bulky, and difficult to use. Therefore, they are rarely used for routine clinical dosimetry, although water calorimetry is becoming close to a standard for calibrations laboratories worldwide.[46]

FRICKE DOSIMETRY

The Fricke dosimeter[47] is based on the conversion of ferrous sulfate ions in a solution to ferric sulfate ions due to the deposition of energy by ionizing radiation. It is not truly a direct dosimeter because there is no a priori way of knowing the calibration constant in units of molecules of ferric ion produced per unit of absorbed dose. This calibration factor, called the *G value*, is dependent on both energy and modality. However, since the dosimeter response is proportional to absorbed dose, it can be a useful device, particularly since the solution is tissue-equivalent and the dosimeter is very small.

Exposure-based Dosimetry

Much of the practical dosimetry of clinical x-ray beams is based on ionization measurements made with thimble ionization chambers. The number of ion pairs produced by interactions of the beam in the gas of the chamber is first converted to exposure using an exposure calibration factor N_x that is obtained from a standards laboratory and is appropriate for a particular energy x-ray beam (typically Co^{60}) and a particular set of measurement conditions. In general,

$$X = M \times N_x \times C$$

where
X = exposure in roentgens
M = meter reading in coulombs
N_x = calibration factor for the energy of interest in roentgens/coulombs
C = correction factor to account for any differences in measurement technique between the calibration condition and the experimental condition

The corrections that must be made to obtain exposure include, most importantly, a correction for differences in temperature and pressure between the calibration condition (normally N_x is valid for a temperature of 22°C and atmospheric pressure of 760 mm Hg) and the experimental condition.[1] If the walls of the chamber are assumed to be made of condensed air-equivalent material and are thick enough to produce electronic equilibrium, then the dose to the air of the chamber can be obtained from the exposure as:

$$D_{air} = 0.873 \times X \times A_{eq} \text{ cGy}$$

since 1R of exposure (1.61×10^{15} ion pairs per kilogram) deposits .00873 J of energy per kilogram of air (33.85 eV per ion pair) if electronic equilibrium has been established. The term A_{eq} is a small correction that accounts for the attenuation of the photon beam in the condensed air walls needed to produce the electronic equilibrium. If we wish to know the dose at the point of measurement to a small mass of some material other than air, this is:

$$D_{med} = [0.873 \times \frac{(\mu/\rho)_{med}}{(\mu/\rho)_{air}} \times X \times A_{eq}]$$
$$= f_{med} \times X \times A_{eq} \qquad (1)$$

where f_{med}, the term in brackets in this equation, was referred to historically as the roentgen-to-rad conversion factor.[2] It must be realized that since the roentgen is only defined for energies 3 MeV or less, this exposure-based dosimetry method is also valid only in this low-energy region. The variation of f_{med} with energy and material is shown in Figure 6-17. Further corrections are necessary if an exposure determination in free space, such as just described, is to be used to predict the dose to a finite phantom rather than a small mass, due to the effects of scatter.[2]

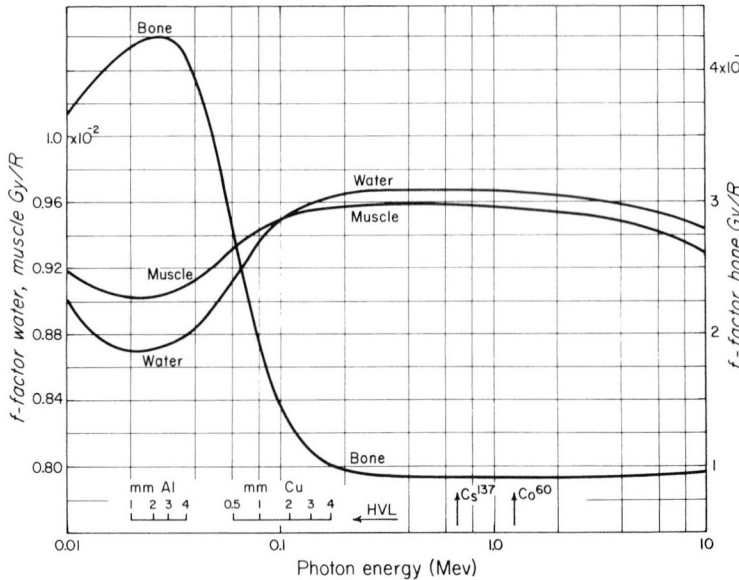

Figure 6–17. The ratio of exposure to dose for bone, muscle, and water as a function of photon energy. (From Johns HE, Cunningham JR: *The Physics of Radiology*. 4th ed, 1983. Courtesy of Charles C. Thomas, Publisher, Springfield, Ill.)

DOSE DETERMINATION USING BRAGG-GRAY CAVITY THEORY

As mentioned, the exposure-based calibration method cannot be used above 3 MeV photon energies, so another technique must be used to evaluate dose at higher energies. The Bragg-Gray cavity theory is designed to directly relate the charge measured in a small air cavity in a phantom to the dose that would be delivered to the same point in the phantom in the absence of the air cavity. Figure 6-18 shows a schematic drawing of the geometry of such a measurement. The Bragg-Gray theory[2] states that if the air cavity is so small that it does not interfere with either the photons or their associated secondary electrons (an assumption that cannot be exactly true unless no ionizations are produced in the cavity) and if the cavity is located in a place where electronic equilibrium has been established, then

$$D_{med} = \frac{(s/\rho)_{med}}{(s/\rho)_{air}} \times \frac{Q}{m_{air}} \times \frac{W}{e} \qquad (2)$$

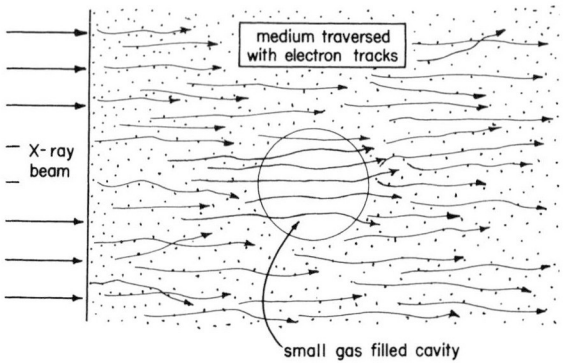

Figure 6–18. Schematic drawing of a Bragg-Gray cavity in a medium exposed to an x-ray beam. (From Johns HE, Cunningham JR: *The Physics of Radiology*. 4th ed, 1983. Courtesy of Charles C. Thomas, Publisher, Springfield, Ill.)

where

D_{med} is the dose to the medium in the absence of the cavity (in Gy)

$(s/\rho)_x$ is the mass stopping power for the secondary electrons in substance x in units of MeV–cm^2/g[48]

Q is the quantity of charge of either sign released by ionizations in the gas in units of coulombs (C)

m_{air} is the mass of air in the cavity in kg

W/e is the average energy required to create an ion pair in air (= 33.97 J/C for dry air)[49]

It should also be noted that

$$D_{air} = [Q/m_{air}] \times [W/e]$$

that is, the product of the last two bracketed factors in Equation 2 is just the dose absorbed by the air in the cavity due to the interactions of the secondary electrons with the air. Note that because the cavity is very small, it is assumed that there are no direct interactions of the passing photons with the air molecules in the cavity, only the secondary electrons.

If we now replace the theoretical small air cavity with a realistic thimble ionization chamber as shown in Figure 6-19, then we must assume that the chamber has a finite wall thickness of a material that may be different than the medium of the phantom. In this case, we have to modify the previous formula to account for electrons that are produced in the wall as well as in the phantom material and for a possible difference in the attenuation of the photons in the wall material versus the phantom. The Bragg-Gray theory, modified to account for this situation, leads to the following expression:

$$D_{med} = \left[\alpha \times \frac{(\mu/\rho)_{med}}{(\mu/\rho)_{wall}} \times \frac{(s/\rho)_{wall}}{(s/\rho)_{air}} \right.$$

$$\left. + (1 - \alpha) \times \frac{(s/\rho)_{med}}{(s/\rho)_{air}} \times \frac{Q}{m_{air}} \times \frac{W}{e} \times A \right] \qquad (3)$$

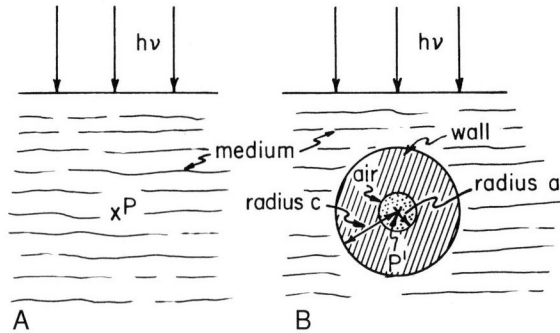

Figure 6–19. Determination of absorbed dose in a medium with a practical ion chamber. **A,** Homogeneous phantom showing the point *P* at which the absorbed dose is desired. **B,** Practical ion chamber with outer radius *c* and inner radius *a* shown centered at position *P′*, which is identical in position to *P*. (From Johns HE, Cunningham JR: *The Physics of Radiology.* 4th ed., 1983. Courtesy of Charles C. Thomas, Publisher, Springfield, Ill.)

where

α is the fraction of electrons crossing the air cavity that come from the wall

$(\mu/\rho)_x$ is the mass attenuation coefficient for photons of this energy in material x^2 and

A accounts for the perturbation of the beam by the chamber wall (probably very close to 1.00 for thin, low-Z walls)

The first term in Equation 3 corresponds to electrons produced in the wall that interact in the air of the chamber and the second term to electrons that are produced in the medium. Obviously, if the wall is very thin, α is very close to zero and *A* is very close to 1.0, in which case Equation 3 becomes nearly identical to Equation 2.

PRACTICAL DOSIMETRY WITH THIMBLE IONIZATION CHAMBERS

In practice, dosimetry is performed at a variety of photon and electron energies with thimble ionization chambers that have been calibrated by a standards laboratory at one or a few photon energies. In fact, in the United States, the practice is still to obtain an exposure calibration constant for each chamber obtained in a ^{60}Co beam. In Europe and elsewhere, it is common practice to obtain a direct dose calibration factor for ^{60}Co. In reality, this dose or exposure calibration factor can be thought of as a determination of the effective mass of the gas in the chamber that is available for ionizations.

In 1983, the American Association of Medical Physicists published a new formalism for photon and electron dosimetry based on existing exposure or dose calibrations at ^{60}Co energies.[50] This formalism, called TG21, defines a new parameter called $N_{gas} = D_{air}/M_c$ (dose to the air of the chamber per unit meter reading in the calibration beam) that contains all the chamber-specific and calibration beam-specific parameters, including the ^{60}Co exposure constant (N_x) or dose calibration constants. Knowledge of N_{gas} is equivalent to knowledge of the effective mass of air in the chamber. The quantity N_{gas}/N_x

is a function of only the geometry of the chamber and the well-known properties of ^{60}Co photons and is tabulated for specific thimble ionization chambers in the literature.[50] This ratio can also be calculated from a knowledge of the materials and dimensions of the chamber. Once the N_{gas} for a chamber is known, the above formalism of Equation 3, based on Bragg-Gray cavity theory, can be used to obtain the dose to a medium for photons or electrons of arbitrary energy. That is, for photons of energy λ,

$$D_{med} = M_\lambda \times N_{gas} \times \left[\alpha \times \frac{(\mu/\rho)_{med}}{(\mu/\rho)_{wall}} \times \frac{(L/\rho)_{wall}}{(L/\rho)_{air}} \right.$$
$$\left. + (1 - \alpha) \times \frac{(L/\rho)_{med}}{(L/\rho)_{air}} \right] \times P_\lambda$$

$$(4)$$

where

M_λ is the meter reading in this photon beam and

P_λ is a factor to account for the perturbation of the beam by the presence of the chamber

L/ρ is the *restricted* mass stopping power, only accounting for those electrons with energy large enough to cross the air cavity

Similarly, for electrons of energy *E*

$$D_{med} = M_E \times N_{gas} \times \left[(L/\rho)_{med}/(L/\rho)_{air} \right] \times P_E \quad (5)$$

since one normally assumes that the electron beam will not be modified by the wall material so the equation is simplified.

Although this discussion does not display all of the details associated with routine ion chamber dosimetry, the reader should appreciate the relative simplicity of the concepts that is made possible by the application of the Bragg-Gray cavity theory.

Thermoluminescent Dosimetry

Certain crystalline materials display a property called *thermoluminescence* (TL) that can be exploited for dosimetry. When such a crystal is irradiated, a portion of the absorbed energy can be stored in the lattice and recovered later in the form of visible light emission if the material is heated. If the emission of light after radiation is spontaneous, the phenomenon is called *fluorescence*.

In a crystal lattice, discrete electron energy levels are perturbed by the interactions between atoms, forming both allowed and forbidden energy bands. In the presence of certain impurities, energy traps can be formed in the forbidden region, and when irradiated, electrons can be excited out of their ground states into one of these forbidden energy traps. Since they are in the forbidden region, spontaneous decays back to the ground state are rare and the imprint of the absorbed dose remains until extra energy is provided to force the transition. This extra energy can be externally applied heat. By observing the heated TL material with a light-sensitive phototube, an electronic signal can be created that is proportional to the number of electrons in forbidden traps, which is, in turn, related to the energy absorbed by the TL material due to irradiation. Over a restricted range of absorbed dose, the response can be linear.[51]

The TL materials most commonly used for dosimetry are lithium fluoride, lithium borate, and calcium fluoride. They can be prepared in the form of powders, solid chips, and solid rods. By careful handling procedures, 3% to 5% reproducibility can be achieved after individual calibration of dosimeters with a photon beam.[1,51] Due to their small size (typically <1 mm³ in volume) they are very conveniently used to attach to patient surfaces or place in patient cavities as in vivo dosimeters to verify dose calculations.

Solid State Detectors

Silicon diodes and other semiconductors can also be used to produce signals that are proportional to radiation dose. In a typical diode, there is a "p" region having an excess of positively charged "holes" and a depletion layer, or "n" region that has an excess of electrons. Radiation to the depletion layer produces electron-hole pairs that can cause current to flow across the junction between the layers if the diode has a reverse bias across it. The amount of current flow is proportional to the energy deposited by charged particles passing through the depletion layer.[45] Silicon diodes have the great advantage of small size and a low-energy threshold for producing an ion pair, resulting in a high sensitivity. The disadvantage of the diode is that radiation damage causes a decrease in sensitivity with radiation dose.

Another solid state detector is the so-called "MOSFET" which is an acronym for metal oxide semiconductor field effect transistor. A MOSFET detector for radiation dosimetry consists of two MOSFETs operating at different voltages. The difference in the threshold voltage shifts of the two MOSFETs is proportional to absorbed dose. Like diodes, these detectors are very small and sensitive and are now being used clinically at some institutions to evaluate dose in a phantom for highly complex dose distributions.[52] They have been shown to be very linear over the range of doses of interest for radiotherapy verification. However, they have an angular dependence to radiation sensitivity that can limit their accuracy in clinical situations.

Film Dosimetry

Radiographic film consists of an emulsion of fine silver bromide crystals on a transparent film base. When the film is exposed to ionizing radiation, a chemical reaction takes place within the exposed crystals, forming what is called a latent image. The development process reduces the exposed crystals to small grains of metallic silver that remain attached to the base during the fixing process, which removes all of the unexposed crystals of silver bromide. The degree of blackening of an area of the film depends on the amount of free silver deposited; therefore, it is related to the radiation energy absorbed by the film. A densitometer can be used to measure the optical density of the film, defined as:

$$OD = \log(I_o / I_t)$$

where I_o is the amount of light transmitted through an unexposed portion of the film and I_t is the amount of light transmitted through the exposed portion of interest. By carefully exposing and developing film to a series of known doses using the same photon energies as will be used for the test exposure, it is possible to obtain curves of optical density versus dose for specific emulsions from which absolute dose information can be subsequently extracted with some substantial uncertainty. This uncertainty is due to the fact that the silver in the emulsions strongly absorbs radiation below about 150 keV by the photoelectric process. For electrons, the information is much more trustworthy.

In spite of the dose uncertainties in photon beams, films are very useful for measuring relative dose distributions in phantoms and can be used with high-energy photon beams to obtain absolute information with only about 3% to 5% uncertainty. Computer-controlled densitometers can be used to quickly scan complex films and convert the information into dose contours.

DOSE DISTRIBUTION IN MEDIA

The clinical use of radiation in patients requires the specification of dose at any point within the irradiation field. In general, if the dose at a reference point is known, the dose at any other point can be calculated if the field size, distance to source, field shape, depth of point of interest, and energy of the beam are known, as well as the constituents of the irradiated medium. In this section, we consider methods of determining the dose at any point of interest, relative to a reference point dose.

Phantoms

Since it is seldom possible to measure dose distributions directly in patients, phantoms have been developed. These phantoms have absorption and scattering properties that mimic those in human patients. The phantoms can be constructed to have the same geometry as humans and are then said to be anthropomorphic. An example of such a phantom is the Alderson Rando Phantom (Alderson Research Laboratories, Inc., Stamford, Conn.), which is sectioned transversely for dosimetric studies and incorporates materials to simulate specific body tissues including muscle, bone, lung, and air. To be equivalent to a given tissue in terms of the interactions of photons and electrons, the phantom material must have the same electron density (in electrons per gram or electrons per gram per square centimeter) as the tissue to be simulated. Basic dose distribution data are frequently measured in a water phantom that closely approximates the radiation absorption and scattering properties of soft tissue.

Percentage Depth Dose

The percentage depth dose is a way of characterizing the change in dose with depth along the central axis of the beam. The definition for any beam is:

$$P(d, \text{ref}, r, f, E) = (D_d / D_{\text{ref}}) \times 100$$

where d is the depth of the point of interest below the surface and ref corresponds to the reference depth. This definition is described schematically in Figure 6-20. In general, P depends on the depths d and ref, on the distance (f) from the source to the surface (often referred to as SSD), the field size on the surface (r), and the beam energy (E). The definition assumes that the field is square, so corrections must be made if rectangular or irregular field shapes are used.

In the absence of scattering effects, the dose to any point in space varies as the inverse of the square of the distance from the source to the point (the so-called inverse square law). Using this assumption, if we compare the percentage depth dose for different SSDs, one would expect that:

$$\frac{P(d, \text{ref}, r, f_1, E)}{P(d, \text{ref}, r, f_2, E)} = \frac{(f_1 + d_{\text{ref}})^2}{(f_2 + d_{\text{ref}})^2} \cdot \frac{(f_2 + d)^2}{(f_1 + d)^2}$$

The term on the right-hand side of the equation is called the *Mayneord F factor*. This factor is greater than 1 for $f_1 > f_2$. Therefore, the percent depth dose is seen to increase with increasing SSD.

Percentage depth dose also increases with increasing field size due to the increasing contribution, with field size, of scatter to the dose on the central axis. As the field size is increased from zero, where we have only primary radiation, to a finite field size of radius r, the dose at all depths will increase due to the contribution of scatter. At deeper depths, where the field size is larger, the increase in dose will be larger than for shallower depths. For low energies and for small field sizes, the rate of change of the percent depth dose with field size will be fairly rapid. This variation of percent depth dose with field size for various energies is displayed in Figure 6-21.

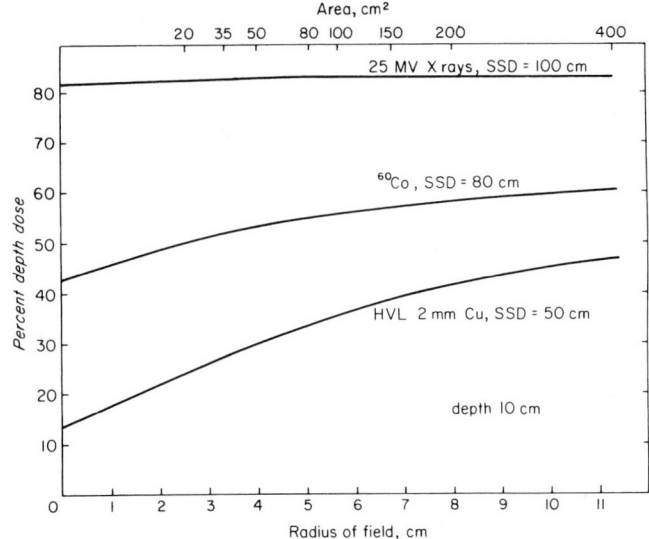

Figure 6–21. Plot showing variation of percentage depth-dose with field size for three photon beams, at a depth of 10 cm. HVL, half-value layer; SSD, source-to-skin distance. (From Johns HE, Cunningham JR: *The Physics of Radiology*. 4th ed., 1983. Courtesy of Charles C. Thomas, Publisher, Springfield, Ill.)

Compilations of central axis depth dose for various energies have been published[53,54] and are summarized, for a few energies, in Figure 6-22 for a fixed-field size of 10×10 cm. Of interest in this figure is the buildup of dose from the surface to a maximum value at a depth of d_{max} for high energy photons, and an increasing percentage depth dose with energy, for a fixed depth. The so-called buildup region near the surface for high-energy photon beams is due to the increase of secondary electron fluence with depth from the surface to a depth that corresponds approximately to the maximum range of the

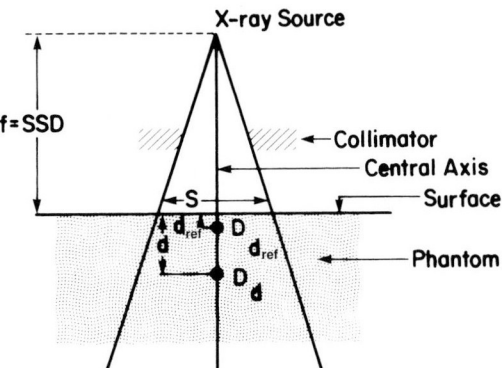

Figure 6–20. Schematic drawing illustrating the definition of percentage depth-dose. D_d, dose at the depth d; D_{ref}, dose at the point on the central axis which is at dept ref; S, field size at the surface of the phantom; SSD, source-to-surface distance. (From Perez CA, Brady LW: *Principles and Practice of Radiation Oncology*. 2nd ed. Philadelphia: JB Lippincott; 1992:198.)

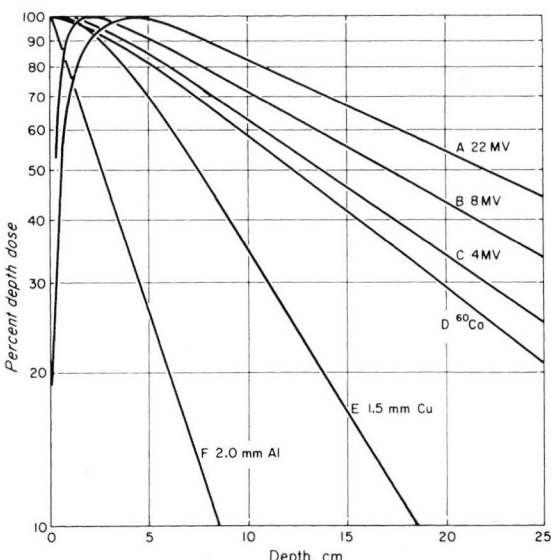

Figure 6–22. Plot showing variation of dose with depth for 6 different energy photon beams. (From Johns HE, Cunningham JR: *The Physics of Radiology*. 4th ed., 1983. Courtesy of Charles C. Thomas, Publisher, Springfield, Ill.)

secondary electrons produced by the photons in the material of the phantom. The photon fluence, on the other hand, is exponentially decreasing with depth starting from the surface itself. The combination of these two effects yields a dose that is low at the surface, builds up to a maximum value at a depth that increases with the energy of the beam (and the maximum range of the secondary electrons), and then falls exponentially with depth beyond d_{max}. The rate of the exponential falloff in dose with depth beyond d_{max} is determined by the mean attenuation coefficient μ such that

$$P(d, m, r, f, E) = 100 \times \frac{(f + d_m)^2}{(f + d)^2} \times e^{-\mu(d - d_m)} \times K_s$$

where m is the depth of d_{max}, and K_s is the contribution of scatter to the dose on the central axis at depth d. It should be noted that the exact value of the dose in the buildup region and the depth of d_{max} are critically dependent on the design of the treatment head of the machine and the field size. The addition of any material near the surface of the patient or phantom, such as special blocks, produces electrons and thereby increases the surface dose[55] and potentially changes the depth of maximal dose. For low-energy photons the buildup region is vanishingly small due to the combined effects of backscatter in the phantom and the short ranges of the secondary electrons produced in the phantom.

Correction of the PDD for rectangular fields (or irregular fields) requires that the integrated scatter from all points along the periphery of the field be calculated. The "equivalent square" field is that field, of radius r, that has the same integrated scatter as the field of interest. Tables of equivalent square fields corresponding to various rectangular fields are available in the literature.[53]

Tissue-Air Ratio

The use of PDD depends on SSD, as discussed earlier. This makes its use rather cumbersome, since in practical circumstances, the SSD may vary substantially across the field and from field to field. The tissue-air ratio (TAR) was introduced to allow dosimetry for rotational therapy, where the gantry moves around a fixed point in the patient.[56] The TAR is defined as:

$$\text{TAR}(d, r_d, E) = D_d / D_{fs}$$

where D_d is the dose at depth d in a phantom for field size r_d defined at that depth and D_{fs} is the dose in free space at the same point. The TAR concept is schematically represented in Figure 6-23. The D_{fs} is measured with a small equilibrium mass around the point of interest to provide dose buildup. Since the point in the phantom and in free space are at the same distance from the source, TAR depends only on scatter and attenuation in the phantom. To the extent that phantom scatter is nearly independent of divergence of the beam, TAR is usually considered to be independent of SSD, an assumption that has been shown correct to within about 2% over the range of SSDs used clinically.[57]

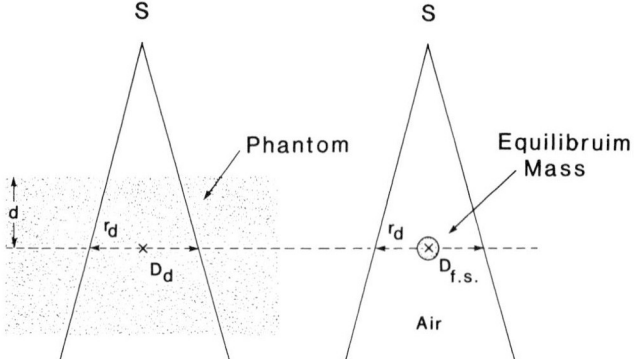

Figure 6–23. Illustration demonstrating the definition of tissue-air ratio (TAR). d, depth; D_d, dose at depth d; D_{fs}, dose in free space; r_d, field size depth d; S, source. (From Khan FM: *The Physics of Radiation Therapy*. 2nd ed. Baltimore: Williams & Wilkins; 1994:189.)

The TAR at d_{max} is given the special name *backscatter factor* (BSF), since the variation of this TAR from unity is a measure of the importance of scatter dose at d_{max}. As might be expected, BSF increases with increasing field size and decreases with increasing energy. The variation of BSF with HVL and field size is shown in Figure 6-24. Above about 8 MV, the scatter contribution to the dose at d_{max} for all field sizes becomes negligibly small and BSF approaches unity.

Scatter-Air Ratio

The scatter-air ratio (SAR) is that portion of the TAR that is due to scatter. That is,

$$\text{SAR}(d, r_d, E) = \text{TAR}(d, r_d, E) - \text{TAR}(d, 0, E)$$

where $\text{TAR}(d, 0, E)$ is the TAR for zero field size and represents the primary component of the TAR. The SAR concept is useful in calculating the net scatter dose to a point inside an irregular field.[58] In this method, referred to as Clarkson's method,[59] radii are drawn at regular angular intervals from a point of interest inside an irregular field to the periphery of the field. The $(SAR)_{avg}$ is then calculated as the average SAR for all the intersections of these radii with the field edge, using the appropriate circular field SARs for each radial distance. Finally, the average TAR for the point of interest can be calculated as

$$(\text{TAR})_{avg} = \text{TAR}(0) + (\text{SAR})_{avg}$$

More information on this technique can be found in textbooks on medical physics.[1,2]

Tissue-Phantom Ratio and Tissue-Maximum Ratio

The concept of TAR was developed partially to overcome the difficulty created by the dependence of PDD on SSD. As we go to higher photon energies, we encounter a difficulty with TAR due to the requirement of measuring a dose in free space. At low energies, the free space dose can be measured with a small buildup cap placed around

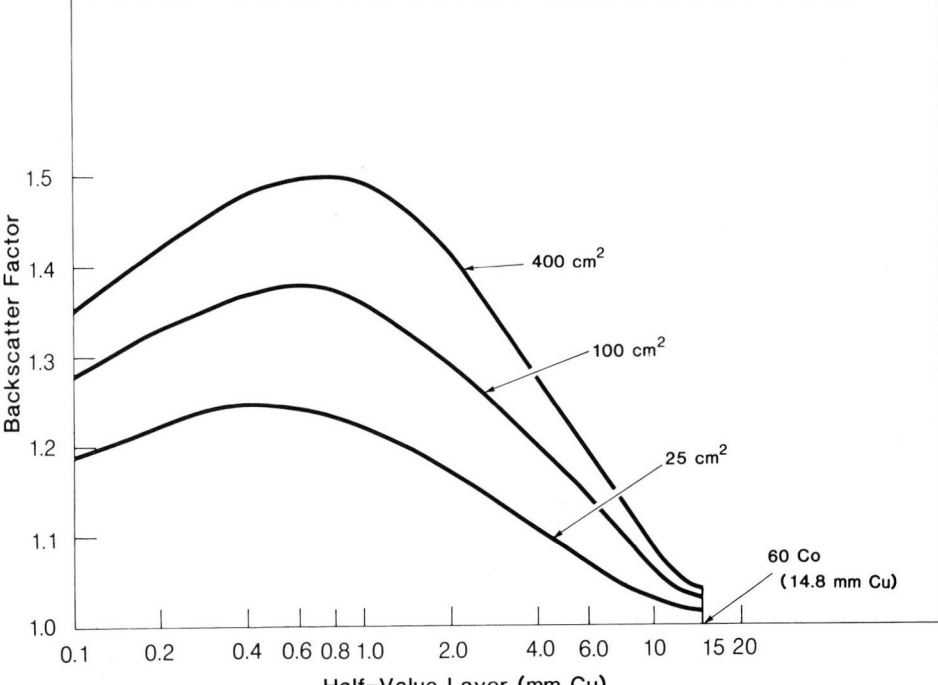

Figure 6–24. Variation of backscatter factor with beam quality for circular fields of different sizes. (From Khan FM: *The Physics of Radiation Therapy.* 2nd ed. Baltimore: Williams & Wilkins, 1994;191.)

the ion chamber to provide electron equilibrium. At high energies, however, this buildup cap becomes very thick and the attenuation of the beam in the cap as well as the effect of different materials in the cap and the wall must be considered. To avoid these difficulties, the concepts of tissue-phantom ratio (TPR)[60] and tissue-maximum ratio (TMR)[61] were developed. For both concepts, the reference dose and the dose of interest are measured in the phantom, thus overcoming the difficulty of measuring a dose in free space. Like TAR, however, TMR and TPR are considered to be independent of SSD. The definitions are given by:

$$\mathrm{TPR}(d, d_{\mathrm{ref}}, f_{\mathrm{d}}, E) = D_{\mathrm{d}} / D_{\mathrm{ref}}$$

and

$$\mathrm{TMR}(d, d_{\mathrm{max}}, f_{\mathrm{d}}, E) = D_{\mathrm{d}} / D_{\mathrm{max}}$$

where D_{d} is the dose on the central axis of the beam at the depth d for field size f_{d} and D_{ref} is the dose at the reference depth for the same field size. For the case of TMR this depth is d_{max}, whereas for TPR, the depth is some standard depth greater than d_{max}. One difficulty with TMR is created by the fact that the depth of d_{max} is a function of field size and SSD, thereby presenting a measurement problem.

In a manner analogous to SAR, a scatter-maximum ratio (SMR) or scatter-phantom ratio (SPR) can be defined:

$$\mathrm{SPR}(d, f_{\mathrm{d}}, E) = \mathrm{TPR}(d, f_{\mathrm{d}}, E)$$
$$\times S_p(f_d) / S_p(0) - \mathrm{TPR}(d, 0, E)$$

where $S_p(f_d)/S_p(0)$ is the ratio of the phantom scatter at the reference depth for the field size f_{d} to that for zero field size and where the reference depth is either d_{max} or d_{ref} for SMR or SPR. The phantom scatter factor ratio can be considered the same as the ratio of backscatter factors.

Dose Distributions

To this point, we have considered methods for determining the absolute dose at a point in free space and in a phantom, and then methods for determining the ratio of doses on the central axis to doses at a reference point. We now consider the distribution of dose outside the central axis as a way of evaluating the dose at any point of interest in an irradiated phantom.

An *isodose curve* connects points of equal dose in a single plane. Frequently, one of the axes of the isodose curve display is the central axis of the beam, in which case the curves represent the variation in dose as a function of depth and transverse distance from the central axis. Figure 6-25 shows two such displays for a 4 MV x-ray beam, one normalized to the maximum dose and the other to the depth of the isocenter, that is the axis of rotation for an isocentric therapy unit. The shape of the isodose curves is affected by the beam parameters such as SSD, field size, and beam filter characteristics, as well as the shape of the entrance surface. Such curves are normally reconstructed after measuring at a large number of fixed points in a water phantom with an ionization chamber or diode. Computer-driven scanning probes are commercially available to help with this task.

A *dose profile* is a display of dose at a fixed depth along a single axis transverse to the central axis. These displays are useful as a way to characterize beam flatness and beam penumbra (the rate of lateral dose falloff) as a function of field size and depth.

Compensators

Most linear accelerators and Co[60] machines contain flattening filters designed to produce beam profiles that

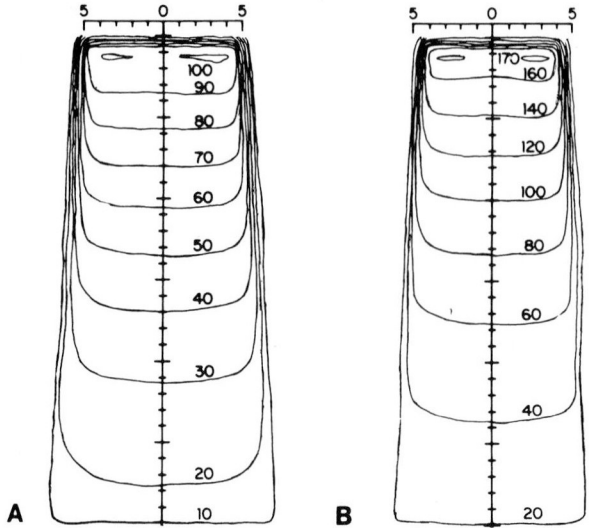

Figure 6–25. Examples of isodoses for a 4MV x-ray beam. **A,** 80 cm SSD with field size 10 cm × 10 cm at the surface. **B,** 80 cm SAD with field size 10 cm × 10 cm at isocenter. (From Perez CA, Brady LW: *Principles and Practice of Radiation Oncology.* 2nd ed. Philadelphia: JB Lippincott; 1992.)

The wedge angle is defined as the angle between the isodose curve and a perpendicular to the central axis at some reference depth, often 10 cm. Wedges are normally furnished with commercial linear accelerators to produce wedge angles of 15, 30, 45 and 60 degrees. Examples of wedge isodose curves are shown in Figure 6-26. When a wedge is used, a *wedge factor* must be defined, that is, the ratio of the dose at d_{max} on the central axis with the wedge in place to that with the wedge removed.

Patient-specific compensators are frequently made to compensate for rapid variations in the patient surface over the field.[62] These can be made of cells of high-density metal distributed so as to attenuate the beam where the patient surface is far from the source, relative to those areas where the patient surface is closer.

The presence of any high-density beam filter in the beam, beyond the usual flattening filter, can lead to *beam hardening.* This phenomenon is caused by differential attenuation of the low-energy photons in the beam, thereby increasing the average energy of the transmitted photons. Beam hardening can lead to significant changes in the percent depth dose, particularly for low-energy beams.

are flat at a typical depth for a typical field size. These filter designs assume that the patient entrance is flat and that the patient tissues have uniform electron density. Special compensating filters can be used when this is not the case or when nonflat isodose contours are desired, to shape the isodose curves at depth.

The most common form of compensator is the *wedge filter.* These wedges are normally constructed of brass, steel, or lead. When placed in the beam, they cause the isodose curves to be angled relative to the central axis.

Output Factor

The final dosimetric factor that needs to be defined is *output factor.* This factor is defined as the ratio of the dose in air at a reference source-to-calibration (SCD) distance for a given field size to that for the reference field size (usually 10 × 10 cm). For field sizes greater than the reference field size, the output factor will be greater than 1.0 due to the increased scatter from the collimator for the

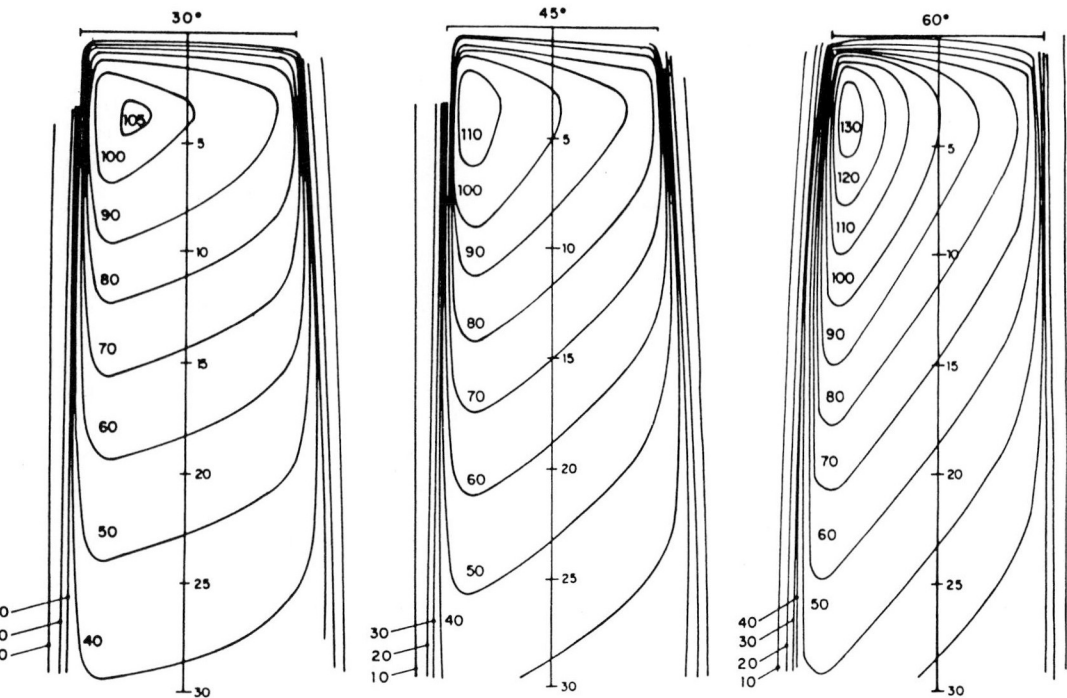

Figure 6–26. Wedged isodose curves for 30-, 45- and 60-degree wedges for a 10 cm × 10 cm field size. (From Abrath FG, Purdy JA: Wedge design and dosimetry for 25-MV x-rays. *Radiology.* 1980;136:757.)

larger fields. This factor is sometimes called the *collimator scatter factor*. For rectangular fields, the equivalent square field must be found using published tables[53] or by using the approximation:

$$S = (2 \times L \times W)/(L + W)$$

where S is the side of the equivalent square and L and W are the sides of the rectangle.

DOSE CALCULATIONS AND MONITOR UNIT SETTINGS

Before the late 1980s, photon dose calculations were based primarily on interpolations of measured depth dose data. Since these data are measured in homogeneous water phantoms for standard field sizes, corrections have to be made to account for tissue heterogeneities, sloping patient surfaces, and irregular field shapes. Mackie[63] has characterized this type of dose calculation as "correction-based." Cunningham[64] has described several commonly used tissue heterogeneity correction algorithms.

Advances in imaging and computing technologies have made it possible to incorporate sophisticated model-based dose calculation algorithms in clinical treatment planning systems. In model-based dose calculations, the treatment parameters, including the setup and patient geometry, are simulated from first principles by taking into account the physics of radiation transport. Measured relative dose quantities (e.g., percent depth dose and tissue phantom ratios) are used to verify the results of the model-based dose calculations, but they are not used directly to perform the calculation. Salient aspects of model-based photon dose calculation algorithms can be found in the review article of Ahnesjo and Aspradakis.[65]

Dose Calculations Based on Correction Methods

The most general method of dose calculation by correction methods would be for irregularly shaped fields and for off-axis points of interest. In any field, it is necessary to be able to calculate the effects of scatter and primary separately. In general, the TAR and SAR formalisms are used in conjunction with the Clarkson calculation method described earlier. The dose at an arbitrary point in an irregular field can be calculated in the following way:

$$D_p = D_{fs} \times OF \times f_{ssd} \times OAF \times [TAR(d, 0) + SAR_{avg}(d)]$$

where

D_p is the dose to the arbitrary point p at depth d in the phantom

D_{fs} is the dose in free space as described in the TAR discussion earlier

OF is output factor for the collimator opening compared to 10×10 cm

$f_{ssd} = [(SSD_c + d_{max})/(SSD_p + d_p)]^2$ (the inverse square factor), SSD_c and SSD_p are the source-to-skin distances

on the central axis and to the skin above point p, respectively

OAF is the off-axis factor measured with dose profiles in air

$TAR(d, 0)$ is the TAR for zero field size (primary dose fraction), and

$SAR_{avg}(d)$ is the average SAR to point p from the periphery of the irregular field (scatter dose fraction)

Further information on this can be found in the standard textbooks on Medical Physics.[1,2]

Dose Calculation Corrections

In the earlier dose calculation discussions, we assumed that the beam was normally incident on a uniform medium of unit density. For real patients, these assumptions are never exactly correct and we must therefore deal with corrections to our dose calculation formalism to account for this fact.

Correction for Non-Normal Beam Incidence

EFFECTIVE SOURCE-TO-SKIN METHOD

Figure 6-27 illustrates the effective SSD method of correcting for surface obliquity. In this figure, S represents the patient surface, which is at a distance F from the source on the central axis, at a distance $F + h'$ above point p' and a distance $F - h''$ above point p''. In this case, the dose on the central axis, D_c, gets modified at p' and p'' due to the decrease or increase in the overlying tissue relative to the central axis. However, an inverse square

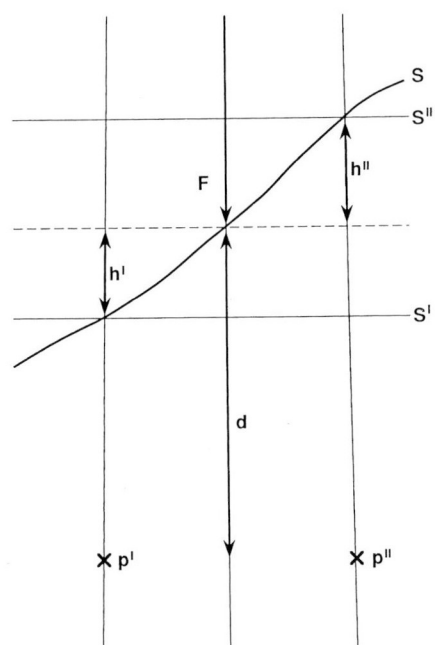

Figure 6–27. Demonstration of the missing tissue method of calculating the effect of surface obliquity. (From Williams JR. Thwaites DI: *Radiotherapy Physics in Practice.* By permission of Oxford University Press; 1993.)

correction must be made because the points of interest are still at a distance of $F + d$ from the source. The complete correction is:

$$D_{p'} = D_c \times (F + d_{\max})^2 / (F + h' + d_{\max})^2$$

and

$$D_{p''} = D_c \times (F + d_{\max})^2 / (F - h'' + d_{\max})^2$$

This correction is appropriate for SSD treatment techniques, and is simple enough to be done either manually or by computer treatment-planning programs. Note that in general, there is an additional modification to the dose at points such as p' due to changes in scatter, but this technique adequately corrects the primary dose component and is a good approximation to the total dose at such points.

TISSUE-AIR RATIO CORRECTION METHOD

For isocentric treatments, a better approach involves the use of TARs, which are independent of SSD. For this reason, we can simply calculate

$$D_{p'} = D_c \times \mathrm{TAR}(d - h', r) / \mathrm{TAR}(d, r)$$

Again, this corrects only the primary component of the dose but for most situations is sufficiently accurate.

Corrections for Inhomogeneities

The presence of tissues with electron densities different than water leads to a further modification of dose to points in the irradiated medium. The primary component of dose to any point is modified by any change in attenuation properties of overlying tissues. In addition, the scatter component of the dose will be influenced by the presence of neighboring inhomogeneities. This latter effect will be reduced for greater distances from the inhomogeneities and for higher energies. There are a number of ways of correcting for the presence of inhomogeneities from very simple and fast approximations to more complex three-dimensional methods that are more accurate but much more computation-intensive. We discuss a few of these methods and refer the interested reader to other sources for more detailed information.[3,66]

EFFECTIVE DEPTH METHOD

The simplest method of correcting for inhomogeneities involves simply calculating an effective depth, d_{eff}, for the point of interest, which is defined as the depth in unit density material that would result in the same net attenuation as the depth d in the phantom. Referring to Figure 6-28, the effective depth of point p would be

$$d_{\mathrm{eff}} = d_1 + (d_2 - d_1) \times 0.3 + (d_p - d_2)$$

Since the distance of point p from the source has not changed, the dose at p would also have to be corrected by an inverse square factor, so

$$D_p = D_{\mathrm{ref}} \times \mathrm{PDD}(d_{\mathrm{eff}}) / 100 \times (F + d_{\mathrm{eff}})^2 / (F + d)^2$$

This method does not take account of the proximity of the inhomogeneity to the point of interest but is sufficiently

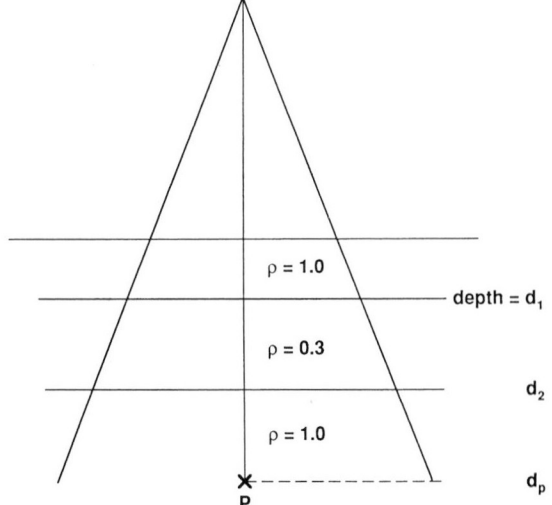

Figure 6–28. Illustration of the power law tissue-air ratio method of correcting for inhomogeneity beneath a slab of material of density 0.3. (From Williams JR, Thwaites DI: *Radiotherapy Physics in Practice*. By permission of Oxford University Press; 1993.)

accurate for many applications and simple enough to be calculated manually.

TISSUE-AIR METHOD

For isocentric techniques, a correction to the dose at point p can be calculated with TARs using d_{eff} as defined earlier:

$$D_p = D_{\mathrm{fs}} \times \mathrm{TAR}(d_{\mathrm{eff}}, r)$$
$$= D_{p, \mathrm{uniform}} \times \mathrm{TAR}(d_{\mathrm{eff}}, r) / \mathrm{TAR}(d, r)$$

where $D_{p, \mathrm{uniform}}$ is the dose that would be measured at a true depth of d in a uniform phantom of water-equivalent material. This method considers both the beam size and the depth of the point of calculation and is probably more accurate than the effective depth method.

EQUIVALENT TISSUE-AIR (ETAR) METHOD

A further improvement to the tissue-air method can be accomplished by using an effective field size as well as an effective depth.[67] In this case,

$$D_p = D_{\mathrm{fs}} \times \mathrm{TAR}(d_{\mathrm{eff}}, r_{\mathrm{eff}})$$
$$= D_{p, \mathrm{uniform}} \times \mathrm{TAR}(d_{\mathrm{eff}}, r_{\mathrm{eff}}) / \mathrm{TAR}(d, r)$$

where r_{eff} is the radius of a circular field that, when incident on unit density material, produces the same scatter dose to the point of interest as is observed for the inhomogeneous medium. For a uniform phantom of non–unit density material, the value of r_{eff} has been shown to scale directly with the density of the medium.[68]

POWER LAW TISSUE-AIR RATIO METHOD

In this method, the thickness and composition of overlying inhomogeneities are accounted for as well as the position of the calculation point relative to the inhomogeneity,[69,70] although the lateral extent and shape of the inhomogeneity are not. Under the assumption that the calculation point is not very close to a boundary between two tissues of varying composition, the dose at point P in Figure 6-28 can be written as:

$$D_p = D_{p,\,uniform} \times [\mathrm{TAR}(d_p - d_2, r)]^{(1.0 - 0.3)}$$
$$\times [\mathrm{TAR}(d_p - d_1), r)]^{(0.3 - 1.0)}$$

for the general case where the point of interest is imbedded in the nth layer of tissues,

$$D_p = D_{p,\,uniform} \times \prod_{i=1}^{n-1} \mathrm{TAR}\left(d_n - d_i, r\right)^{\rho_{i+1} - \rho_i}$$

where ρ_i is the density of the ith layer.

OTHER METHODS OF CORRECTING FOR INHOMOGENEITIES

The specific methods discussed to this point have been relatively simple approximations of the effect of inhomogeneities on the dose at an arbitrary point in a phantom. The most exact method would need to account for all the scatter contribution to the dose at the point of interest with and without the inhomogeneities.

Computed tomography is now routinely used as a basis for treatment planning. It provides the basis for target and normal tissue identification and location as well as a three-dimensional array of computed tomography numbers that are directly related to the electron density of the tissues. This array of electron densities can be used to calculate, the dose at each point, corrected for scatter from all other points in the phantom. It has been shown that such an approach yields only a marginal improvement in accuracy relative to the simpler methods, described above.[71]

Model-Based Dose Calculations

CONVOLUTION/SUPERPOSITION METHODS

At present, model-based dose calculation methods can be divided into two categories, those that use convolution/superposition principles to calculated dose[63,72,73] and those that rely purely on Monte Carlo methods. The beam energy spectrum is required as input for both of these dose calculation methods. Convolution/superposition calculations are defined by the basic equation:

$$D(\bar{r}) = \iiiint T_E(\bar{s}) h(E, \bar{r} - \bar{s}) d^3 s \, dE$$

In this equation, D represents the dose at some point $\bar{r}$, $T_E(\bar{s})$ represents the *total energy released* by primary photon interactions per unit mass (or terma), and $h(E, \bar{r} - \bar{s})$ is the point-spread function (also called the energy deposition kernel). The point-spread function represents the fraction of the energy deposited (per unit volume) at point $\bar{s}$ that is subsequently transported to the calculation point, $\bar{r}$. The dose at point $\bar{r}$ is, thus, computed by adding together (i.e., integrating over all

space) the contributions from photons and electrons produced at all other points in the phantom or patient.

Ahnesjö[74] found that the point-spread function, $h(E, \bar{r} - \bar{s})$, changes only slightly as a function of energy (beam hardening), and that, in the convolution integral from earlier, can be replaced by $h(\bar{r} - \bar{s})$, the average dose-spread function weighted by the spectral components of the beam. Dose-spread functions for mono-energetic photons are generally pre-computed using Monte Carlo methods.[74] The energy dependence of the terma, $T_E(\bar{s})$, can be expressed by applying the inverse-square law and exponential attenuation to the photon fluence at the surface of the phantom or patient.

Once the energy dependence of the terma in the convolution equation has been simplified, the four-dimensional integral in this equation reduces a three-dimensional integral over all space. This evaluation is usually divided into two parts. First, it is necessary to compute the energy fluence at the phantom or patient surface. This requires that the treatment planning program models specific aspects of the linear accelerator including the finite source size, the primary collimator, the flattening filter, dynamic or physical wedges, multileaf collimators or cerrobend blocks, and compensators. Secondly, one must apply the inverse square law and exponential attenuation to this incident fluence to determine the terma, $T_E(\bar{s})$, at each point within the phantom or patient and convolve the result with the point-spread function, $h(\bar{r} - \bar{s})$. Essentially, the first part of the calculation takes into account the properties of the accelerator (including any beam-modifying devices used for the treatment), and the second part of the calculation takes into account the patient anatomy.

The convolution equation given earlier is strictly valid only for homogeneous media (i.e., $h(\bar{s})$ must be spatially invariant). One way to model the effects of tissue heterogeneities is to replace all physical distances in the convolution integral with radiological distances, where radiological distance is defined as the physical distance multiplied by the average density along the line in question. Many investigators have used this approximation.[63,74,75] Details of this and other approximations that allow the convolution/superposition integral to be evaluated efficiently under many different conditions are not discussed here, but an excellent review is found in Webb's book.[76]

The convolution/superposition algorithm can account for the effects of non–unit density material anywhere in the vicinity of the calculation point because it requires a three-dimensional integral over the entire radiation field. In contrast, most correction-based dose-calculation techniques require only a simple one-dimensional evaluation of radiological path length, and can thus account for the effects of only those tissue heterogeneities that lie along a ray connecting the radiation source to the calculation point. For example, consider a patient with lung cancer, and consider a point somewhere in the mediastinum where the tissue density is unity, but the density of the surrounding lung tissue is less than one. For the same number of monitor units (MUs), the convolution/superposition algorithm will predict a lower dose to this point than a correction-based dose calculation using the ratio-of-TAR method. The reason for this is that the convolution/superposition method accounts for the fact that fewer photons (and hence fewer electrons) are scattered in the low-density lung material than would be scattered in unit-density tissue. The ratio-of-TAR method cannot predict this reduction in scattered dose.

Ahnesjö[77] has tested the convolution method against Monte Carlo–generated data for layered and mediastinum-like phantom geometries and found that the convolution model predicted the buildup dose and penumbra in the low-density regions fairly accurately. Lydon[78] has tested the convolution model for clinical beams in homogeneous media and also obtained generally good results.

MONTE CARLO METHODS

Photon and electron doses are most accurately calculated with Monte Carlo techniques. This method uses the known cross sections for electron and photon interactions in matter and follows individual photons and their associated electrons through the entire phantom. By calculating the trajectories and interactions of a very large number of photon and electrons, one can accurately model the dose to all points within the heterogeneous phantom or patient. Recently, several Monte Carlo codes have been developed for radiotherapy treatment planning. These are discussed by a number of authors.[79-88]

MONITOR UNIT CALCULATIONS

Monitor Unit Calculations for Correction-Based Dose Calculations

We have now defined all the parameters needed to calculate the number of MUs (or timer setting) as well as the dose to any point of interest in the irradiated field. The dose normalization for each field is usually done with one of two techniques. The first, for a fixed SSD, normalizes the dose from each field to be 100% on the central axis at the depth of d_{max}. The second method, often called the source-to-isocenter (SAD) or isocentric technique, normalizes the dose for each beam to be 100% at the isocenter, that is, the point about which the gantry (and possibly the couch) rotates from field to field. We now consider how to calculate the number of MUs required to give a desired dose at the depth of interest, for these two techniques.

Fixed Source-to-Skin Distance Technique

Since by definition there is a fixed SSD distance for this technique, PDD is the appropriate choice of parameterizations for the dose variation along the central axis. PDD is normalized to be 100% at the depth of the maximum dose, d_{max}. The number of MUs is then calculated as follows, where r is the equivalent square field size defined at the surface:

$$MU = \frac{D}{CF \times OF \times (PDD/100) \times S_p(r) \times f_{ssd} \times f_{mod}}$$

where

MU = monitor unit setting on console
D = dose prescribed at depth d (cGy)
CF = calibration factor for machine in cGy/MU at d_{max} in phantom
OF = output factor for collimator field size r compared to 10 × 10 cm
PDD = percent depth dose for equivalent square field size r at surface, for SSD and depth d of treatment
$S_p(r) = BSF(r)/BSF(10 \times 10)$, that is, the phantom scatter factor
$f_{ssd} = [SCD/(SSD + d_{max})]^2$ (the inverse square factor)
f_{mod} = product of transmission factors of beam modifiers not in the calibration (e.g., wedge factor, blocking tray)

The reader should note that the product CF × OF in the above equation is simply the effective calibration factor for the treatment at d_{max} for the actual field size used in units of cGy/MU. Also, the product PDD × $S_p(r)$ is the PDD at depth d corrected for the actual field size r at the surface. The product of all four terms CF × OF × (PDD/100) × $S_p(r)$ is the dose per MU at depth d for the equivalent square field size r (defined at the surface) in units of cGy/MU. The dose at any other depth on the central axis for the same field size can be calculated by multiplying D by the ratio of the PDD at the new depth, to the PDD at the old depth.

Isocentric (Source-to-Isocenter) Technique

For the SAD technique, the SSD might be changing across the field, so an appropriate choice of variables to describe the change in dose with depth on the central axis is one that is independent of SSD. The best choice seems to be TPR, since it can be specified at a fixed depth for all field sizes. For this technique, the MUs can be calculated as follows:

$$MU = \frac{D}{CF \times OF \times TPR \times S_p(r) \times f_{sad} \times f_{mod}}$$

where

D = dose prescribed at depth d_{iso} (cGy)
CF = calibration factor for machine in cGy/MU at d_{ref} in phantom
OF = output factor for collimator field size r compared to 10 × 10 cm
TPR = tissue-phantom ratio evaluated at d_{iso} where the field size is of an equivalent square of side r (defined at d_{iso})
$S_p(r) = BSF(r)/BSF(10 \times 10)$, which is the phantom scatter factor and where r is defined at d_{iso}
$f_{sad} = [SCD/SAD]^2$ (SCD is the source-to-calibration distance and SAD is the source-to-isocenter distance) (usually $f_{sad} = 1$)

Note that CF × OF is the dose/MU at d_{ref} corrected for the actual collimator field size; TPR × $S_p(r)$ is the TPR (corrected for phantom scatter) at depth d_{iso} for equivalent square field size r defined at d_{iso}; and CF $\times$ OF $\times$ TPR $\times$ $S_p(r)$ is the dose/MU at depth d_{iso} for field size r at d_{iso}. The dose at any other depth on the central axis can be calculated as follows:

$$D(d) = D(d_{iso}) \times$$

$$\frac{TPR(d, r_d) \times (SAD)^2 \times BSF(r_d)}{TPR(d, r_{iso}) \times [SAD - (d - d_{iso})]^2 \times BSF(r_{iso})}$$

Monitor Unit Calculations for Convolution/Superposition Dose Calculations

If the convolution/superposition model is used for the dose calculations, then the MUs for a given beam may be calculated from the following equation (Pinnacle, 1999, Philips Medical Systems, Andover, Mass.):

$$MU = \frac{D_Q}{ND \times OF_C \times TTF \times CF}$$

where D_Q is the dose at the dose-specification point Q (usually isocenter). The calibration factor, CF, is the measured dose per MU at the reference point for the calibration field. For convolution/superposition calculations, this reference point is typically selected to be sufficiently large (e.g., 10 cm) such that the effects of electron and photon contamination from the treatment head are negligible. ND is the normalized dose, defined as the dose per unit energy fluence at point Q relative to the dose per unit energy fluence at the reference point for the calibration field (i.e., the point at which CF is measured). TTF is the tray transmission factor, and OF_C is the collimator output factor.

OF_C is determined from the relationship between phantom scatter and collimator scatter proposed by Khan[1]; that is, the total scatter factor, $S_{c,p}$ is the product of the phantom scatter, S_p, and the collimator scatter factor, S_c. The total scatter factor is easily measured and is simply the ratio of the dose in a phantom at the reference point for field size r to the dose measured at the reference depth for the standard field size (typically 10 cm $\times$ 10 cm). That is, $S_{c,p} = D(r, d_{ref})/D(r_{ref}, d_{ref})$. The phantom scatter, $S_p(r, d_{ref})$, represents the dose contributed from scattered radiation generated in the phantom or patient divided by the dose due to phantom scatter measured at the reference point for a standard field size. This quantity may be calculated directly for each field using the convolution/superposition model. The factor OF_C may then be obtained by dividing the measured $S_{c,p}$ value by the calculated S_p value.

Comparing the MU equation for the convolution/superposition model to that used for standard correction-based dose calculations, we see that, for a water phantom with normally incident beam in an SAD treatment setup, the term ND corresponds to:

$$ND = TPR \times OAR \times S_p \times f_{SAD}$$

Thus, ND may be thought of as a patient-specific, treatment-field-specific TPR. All of the correction terms

that must be included in the standard MU equation (i.e., the OAR, S_p, and f_{SAD}) are implicitly included in the value of ND, which is calculated by the convolution/superposition method for each treatment field.

REFERENCES

1. Khan FM: *The Physics of Radiation Therapy*. 2nd ed. Baltimore: Williams & Wilkins; 1994:542.
2. Johns HE, Cunningham JR: *The Physics of Radiology*. 4th ed. Springfield, Ill: Charles C Thomas; 1983:796.
3. Williams JR, Thwaites DI: *Radiotherapy Physics in Practice*. Oxford: Oxford University Press; 1993:280.
4. Hendee WR: *Radiation Therapy Physics*. 2nd ed. Chicago: Yearbook Medical Publishers; 1979:517.
5. Amaldi U: Cancer therapy with particle accelerators. *Nuclear Physics*. 1999;A:375c.
6. Austin-Seymour M, Munzehrider JE, Goitein M, et al: Progress in low-LET heavy particle therapy: Intracranial and paracranial tumors and uveal melanomas. *Radiation Res*. 1985;104:S219.
7. Miller D: A review of proton beam radiation therapy. *Med Phys*. 1995;22:Part 2.
8. Slater JM, Miller DW, Archambeau JO: Development of a hospital-based proton beam treatment center. *Int J Radiat Oncol Biol Phys*. 1988;14:761.
9. Castro JR, Chen GTY, Blakeley EA: Current considerations in heavy charged-particle radiotherapy: A clinical research trial of the University of California Lawrence Berkeley Laboratory, Northern California Oncology Group and Radiation Therapy Oncology Group. *Radiat Res*. 1985;104:S263.
10. Castro J, Phillips T, Prados M, et al: Neon heavy charged particle radiotherapy of glioblastoma of the brain. *Int J Radiat Oncol Biol Phys*. 1997;38:257.
11. Futami Y, Kanai T, Fujita M, et al: Broad-beam three-dimensional irradiation system for heavy-ion radiotherapy at HIMAC. *Nuclear Instr Meth Physics Res*. 1999;A:143.
12. Kraft G, Arndt U, Becher W, et al: Heavy ion therapy at GSI. *Nuclear Instr Meth Physics Res*. 1995;A:66.
13. Raju MR: *Heavy Particle Radiotherapy*. New York: Academic Press; 1980:500.
14. Orecchia R, Zurlo A, Loasses M, et al: Particle beam therapy (Hadrontherapy): Basis for interest and clinical experience. *Eur J Cancer*. 1998;34:459.
15. Verhey L, Koehler A, McDonald J, et al: The determination of absorbed dose in a proton beam for purposes of charged-paraticle radiation therapy. *Radiat Res*. 1979;79:34.
16. Kanai T, et al: Biophysical characteristics of himac clinical irradiation system for heavy-ion radiation therapy. *Int J Radiat Oncol Biol Phys*. 1999;44:201.
17. Kraft G: Tumortherapy with ion beams. *Nuclear Instr Meth Physics Res*. 2000;A:1.
18. Douglas J, Laramore G, Austin-Seymour M, et al: Neutron radiotherapy for adenoid cystic carcinoma of minor salivary glands. *Int J Radiat Oncol Biol Phys*. 1996;36:87.
19. Douglas J, Laramore G, Autin-Seymour M, et al: Treatment of locally advanced adenoid cystic carcinoma of the head and neck with neutron radiotherapy. *Int J Radiat Oncol Biol Phys*. 2000; 46:551.
20. Huber P, Debus J, Latz D, et al: Radiotherapy for advanced adenoid cystic carcinoma: Neutrons, photons or mixed beam? *Radiother Oncol*. 2001;59:161.
21. Raymond J, Vuong M, Russell K: Neutron beam radiotherapy for recurrent prostate cancer following radical prostatectomy. *Int J Radiat Oncol Biol Phys*. 1998;41:93.
22. Schwartz D, Einck J, Bellon J, et al: Fast neutron radiotherapy for soft tissue and cartilaginous sarcomas at high risk for local recurrence. *Int J Radiat Oncol Biol Phys*. 2001;50:449.
23. Sauerwein W, Zurlo A: The EORTC Boron Neutron Capture Therapy (BNCT) Group: Achievements and future projects. *Eur J Cancer*. 2002;38:S31.
24. Scalliet P, Remouchamps F, Lhoas M, et al: A retrospective analysis of the results of p(65) + Be neutrontherapy for the treatment of prostate adenocarcinoma at the Cyclotron of Louvain-la-Neuve.

Part 1: Survival and progression-free survival. *Cancer/Radiother.* 2001;5:262.

25. Palmer M, Goorley T, Kiger W, et al: Treatment planning and dosimetry for the Harvard-Mit phase I clinical trial of cranial neutron capture therapy. *Int J Radiat Oncol Biol Phys.* 2002;53:1361.

26. Allt WE: Supervoltage radiation treatment in advanced cancer of the uterine cervix: A preliminary report. *J Can Med Assoc.* 1969; 100:792.

27. Johns HE, Bates LM, Watson TA: 1,000 curie cobalt units for radiation therapy. 1. The Saskatchewan cobalt 60 unit. *Br J Radiol.* 1952;25:296.

28. Green DT, Errington RF: Design of a cobalt 60 beam therapy unit. *Brit J Radiol.* 1952;25:309.

29. Kerst DW: The betatron. *Radiology.* 1943;40:115.

30. Miller CW: Travelling-wave linear accelerator for x-ray therapy. *Nature.* 1953;171:297.

31. Purdy JA, Goer DA: Dual energy x-ray beam accelerators in radiation therapy: An overview. *Nucl Inst Method Phys Res.* 1985; 10/11:1090.

32. Karzmark CJ, Pering NC: Electron linear accelerators for radiation therapy: History, principles and contemporary developments. *Phys Med Biol.* 1973;18:321.

33. Karzmark CJ, Morton RJ: *A Primer on Theory and Operation of Linear Accelerators in Radiation Therapy.* Rockville, Md: US Bureau of Radiological Health; 1981.

34. Adler J, Murphy MJ, Chang SD, et al: Image-guided robotic radiosurgery. *Neurosurgery.* 1999;44:1299.

35. Mackie T, Balog J, Ruchalak K, et al: Tomotherapy. *Semin Radiat Oncol.* 1999;9:108.

36. Reistad D, Brahme A: *The Microtron, a New Accelerator for Radiation Therapy. In 3rd International Conference on Medical Physics.* Gøtenberg, Sweden: Chalmers University of Technology; 1972.

37. Svensson H, Jonsson L, Larsson LG, et al: A 22 MeV mictrotron for radiation therapy. *Acta Radiol Ther Phys Biol.* 1977;16:145.

38. Jongen Y, Beeckman W, Cohilis P: The proton therapy system for MGH's NPTC: Equipment description and progress report. *Bull Cancer Radiother.* 1996;82(Suppl):219s.

39. Pedroni E, Bohringer T, Coray A, et al: Initial experience of using an active beam delivery technique at PSI. *Strahlenther Onkol.* 1999;175(suppl 2):18.

40. Domen SR, Lamperti PJ: A heat-loss compensated calorimeter: Theory, design and performance. *J Res NBS.* 1974;78A:595.

41. Schulz RJ, Wuu CS, Weinhous MS: The direct determination of dose-to-water using a water calorimeter. *Med Phys.* 1987;14:790.

42. Domen SR: A sealed water calorimeter for measuring absorbed dose. *NIST J Res.* 1994;99:121.

43. Domen SR: Absorbed dose water calorimeter. *Med Phys.* 1980; 7:157.

44. McDonald JC, Domen SR: A-150 plastic radiometric calorimetry for charged particles and other radiations. *Nucl Instr Meth Phys Res.* 1986;752:35.

45. Attix F: *Introduction to Radiological Physics and Radiation Dosimetry.* New York: John Wiley and Sons; 1986:607.

46. Seuntjens J, Palmans H: Correction factors and performance of a 4°C sealed water calorimeter. *Phys Med Biol.* 1999;44:627.

47. Fricke H, Hart EJ: *Chemical dosimetry,* In Attix FH, Roesch WC, eds. *Radiation Dosimetry.* New York: Academic Press; 1966.

48. ICRU: *Stopping Powers for Electron Beams with Energies Between 1 and 50 MeV.* International Commission on Radiation Units and Measurements, 1984.

49. ICRU: *Average Energy Required to Produce an Ion Pair.* International Commission on Radiation Units and Measurements, 1979.

50. AAPM: American Association of Physicists in Medicine, A protocol for the determination of absorbed dose from high-energy photon and electron beams. *Med Phys.* 1983;10:741.

51. Cameron JR, Suntharalingam N, Kenney GN: *Thermoluminescent Dosimetry.* Madison, Wisc: University of Wisconsin Press; 1968.

52. Chuang C, Verhey L, Xia P: Investigation of the use of MOSFET for clinical IMRT dosimetric verification. *Med Phys.* 2002;29:1109.

53. Cohen M, Jones DEA, Greene D: Central axis depth dose data for use in radiotherapy. *Br J Radiol.* 1972;11(suppl):1.

54. Health Physics Association: Depth dose tables for use in radiotherapy. *Br J Radiol.* 1961;10(suppl):1.

55. Velkley DE, Manson DJ, Purdy JA: Build-up region of megavoltage photon radiation sources. *Med Phys.* 1975;2:14.

56. Johns HE, Whitmore G, Watson T, et al: A system of dosimetry for rotation therapy with typical rotation distributions. *J Can Assn Radiol.* 1953;4:1.

57. Johns HE, Bruce WR, Reid WB: The dependence of depth dose on focal skin distance. *Br J Radiol.* 1958;31:254.

58. Cunningham JR: Scatter-air ratios. *Phys Med Biol.* 1972;17:42.

59. Clarkson JR: A note on depth doses in fields of irregular shape. *Br J Radiol.* 1941;14:265.

60. Karzmark CJ, Deubert A, Loevinger R: Tissue-phantom ratios—An aid to treatment planning. *Br J Radiol.* 1965;38:158.

61. Holt JG, Laughlin JS, Moroney JP: The extension of the concept of tissue-air ratios (TAR) to high energy x-ray beams. *Radiology.* 1970;96:437.

62. Ellis F, Hall EJ, Oliver R: A compensator for variations in tissue thickness for high energy beams. *Br J Radiol.* 1959;32:421.

63. Mackie T, Scrimger J, Battista J: A convolution method for calculating dose for 15-MV x rays. *Med Phys.* 1985;12:188.

64. Cunningham J, ed. Tissue inhomogeneity corrections in photon-beam treatment planning. In Orton C, ed. *Progress in Medical Radiation Physics.* New York: Plenum; 1982:45.

65. Ahnesjö A, Aspradakis M: Dose calculations for external photon beams in radiotherapy. *Phys Med Biol.* 1999;44:99.

66. Coffey CW, Hines HC: Inhomogeneity corrections in treatment planning of the thorax. *Am Assoc Med Dosimetrists J.* 1983;8:6.

67. Sontag MR, Cunningham JR: The equivalent tissue-air ratio method for making absorbed dose calculations in a heterogeneous medium. *Radiology.* 1978;129:787.

68. O'Connor JE: The variation of scattered x-rays with density in an irradiated body. *Phys Med Biol.* 1957;1:352.

69. Young MEJ, Gaylord JD: Experimental tests of corrections for tissue inhomogeneities in radiotherapy. *Br J Radiol.* 1970;43:349.

70. Batho HF: Lung corrections in cobalt 60 beam therapy. *J Can Assoc Radiol.* 1964;15:79.

71. Parker RP, Hobday PA, Cassell KJ: The direct use of CT numbers in radiotherapy dosage calculations for inhomogeneous media. *Phys Med Biol.* 1979;24:802.

72. Boyer A, Mok E: A photon dose distribution model employing convolution calculations. *Med Phys.* 1985;12:169.

73. Mohan R, Chui C, Lidofsky L: Differential pencil beam dose computation model for photons. *Med Phys.* 1986;13:64.

74. Ahnesjö A, Andreo P, Brahme A: Calculation and application of point spread functions for treatment planning with high energy photon beams. *Acta Oncol.* 1987;26:49.

75. Nilsson M, Knöös T: Application of the Fano theorem in inhomogeneous media using a convolution algorithm. In *1st Biennial ESTRO Meeting on Physics in Clinical Radiotherapy.* Budapest: European Society for Therapeutic Radiology and Oncology; 1991.

76. Webb S: *The Physics of Three-Dimensional Radiation Therapy. Medical Science Series.* Bristol and Philadelphia: IOP Publishing, Ltd. 373; 1993.

77. Ahnesjö A: Collapsed cone convolution of radiant energy for photon dose calculation in heterogeneous media. *Med Phys.* 1989;16:577.

78. Lydon J: Photon dose calculations in homogeneous media for a treatment planning system using a collapsed cone superposition convolution algorithm. *Phys Med Biol.* 1998;43:1813.

79. Ma C-M, Faddegon B, Rogers DWO, et al: Accurate characterization of the Monte Carlo beams for radiotherapy. *Med Phys.* 1997; 24:401.

80. Ma C-M, Mok E, Kapur A, et al: Clinical implementation of a Monte Carlo treatment planning system. *Med Phys.* 1999;26:2133.

81. Ma C-M, Li J, Pawlicki T, et al: A Monte Carlo dose calculation tool for radiotherapy treatment planning. *Phys Med Biol.* 2002; 47:1671.

82. Hartmann-Siantar C, Walling R, Daly T, et al: Description and dosimetric verification of the PEREGRINE Monte Carlo dose calculation system for photon beams incident on a water phantom. *Med Phys.* 2001;28:1322.

83. Faddegon B, Blogh J, Mackerzie R, et al: Clinical considerations of Monte Carlo for electron radiotherapy treatment planning. *Radiat Phys Chem.* 1998;35:217.

84. DeMarco J, Solberg T, Smathers J: A CT-based Monte Carlo simulation tool for dosimetry planning and analysis. *Med Phys.* 1998;25:1.

85. Wang L, Chui C, Lovelock M: A patient-specific Monte Carlo dose-calculation method for photon and electron radiotherapy treatment planning dose calculations. *Med Phys*. 1998;25:867.

86. Sempau J, Wilderman S, Bielajew A: DPM, a fast, accurate Monte Carlo code optimized for photon and electron radiotherapy treatment planning dose calculations. *Phys Med Biol*. 2000;45:2263.

87. Kawrakow I, Fippel M, Friedrich K: 3D electron dose calculation using voxel based Monte Carlo algorithm. *Med Phys*. 1996;23:479.

88. Chetty I, Moran J, Nurusher T, et al: Experimental validation of the DPM Monte Carlo code using minimally scattered electron beams in heterogeneous media. *Phys Med Biol*. 2002;47:1837.

Imaging in Radiation Oncology*

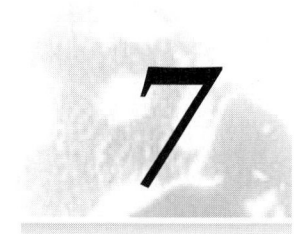

*Luc M. Bidaut, PhD, John L. Humm, PhD,
Gikas S. Mageras, PhD, and
Lawrence N. Rothenberg, PhD*

Accurate, patient-specific anatomic information is a prerequisite for planning and implementing the delivery of radiation to the entire extent of the malignancy while minimizing exposure to critical structures. For this reason, anatomic images are of utmost importance in radiotherapy. In fact, most of the significant recent advances in radiation oncology have resulted from developments in imaging modalities such as computed tomography (CT), magnetic resonance imaging (MRI), magnetic resonance spectroscopy imaging (MRSI), positron emission tomography (PET), and digital planar image receptors. With information from the new imaging modalities, it is now possible to define treatment volumes and critical structures with great precision, thus reducing marginal misses and irradiation of normal tissues. Such capabilities may permit higher tumor doses, potentially leading to improved local control, while maintaining the same level of normal tissue morbidity or even reducing it.[1-4]

Images of various types are employed at virtually every step of the radiation treatment process, including diagnosis, assessment of the extent of disease, treatment planning, treatment delivery, follow-up, and outcome evaluation. These images may be classified in several ways. Images may be cross sectional or projectional. The former category includes CT, MRI, MRSI, PET, and single-photon emission computed tomography (SPECT); examples of the latter are simulation and portal films and CT scout views. In some cases, useful projectional images (e.g., digitally reconstructed radiographs [DRRs]) can be reconstructed from the cross-sectional data. The acquired image data may be in either analog or digital format. Conventional images captured on photographic film are analog, whereas most tomographic images like CT and MRI are acquired as digital data. In general, analog images have better spatial resolution but a smaller dynamic range. Digital images can be mathematically processed (e.g., filtered and enhanced). Analog images can be similarly manipulated, provided that they are converted into digital format with the use of such devices as a "frame-grabber," which consists of a video camera connected to the digitizer. (Of course, the spatial resolution is reduced in the conversion process.) No one imaging modality has all the information required for radiotherapy. The attributes of various imaging modalities and their application in radiation oncology are discussed under Generation of Images.

The use of different digital images depends not only on their intrinsic content but also on the software tools available to facilitate their use. Specifically, tools are needed to extract the maximal information, to integrate the data from different modalities, to aid in the interpretation of data, and to present the results in an effective format. The various functions of these tools can be categorized as follows:

- Image data acquisition, communication, and storage
- Image data analysis
- Image processing and enhancement
- Image segmentation
- Image registration, correlation, and fusion
- Image presentation

The functional and technical aspects of image processing tools are discussed under Image Acquisition and Processing. How information from different sources is pooled and integrated into a complete data set is also discussed.

Many aspects of medical imaging have benefited from the substantial and sustained developments in computer technology, both in hardware and in software. A direct consequence is the increased use of digital images relative to analog images. This trend is likely to continue as methodologies based on computer technology and digital imaging advance further. The development of computed radiography, electronic portal imaging, and picture archiving and communication systems (PACSs) are important examples.

*This chapter is an update and expansion of material presented in the First Edition by C. C. Ling, R. Mohan, L. E. Reinstein, and L. N. Rothenberg

GENERATION OF IMAGES

Computed Tomography

PRINCIPLES OF OPERATION

CT is an x-ray imaging technique used to visualize thin slices of the body. The first commercial CT scanner was developed by Sir Godfrey Hounsfield of the EMI Corporation in 1972. Alan Cormack developed an accurate mathematical technique to reconstruct images from x-ray projections. Hounsfield and Cormack received the 1979 Nobel Prize in medicine for their efforts. Modern scanners employ a pure rotation motion and require only 0.4 to 1.0 second per rotation to acquire the data (Fig. 7-1). Multi-slice detector arrays allow as many as 16 slices to be acquired in one rotation.

A thin beam of x-rays of about 120 kV, in the fan-beam geometry, is incident on the patient transversely. The transmitted x-rays are detected by an array of many solid-state detectors. Concomitantly, the x-ray source and the detector array are rotated through an angular range from 180 to 360 degrees. The detected x-ray transmission factors are input data to a computer program, the so-called reconstruction algorithm, which produces an output matrix (usually 512 × 512) of digital values. Current scanners using workstations and the filtered-back projection algorithm can reconstruct an image in a fraction of a second. Each element of the matrix represents a small area, or pixel; the product of a pixel area and the slice thickness constitutes a volume element, or voxel (Fig. 7-2). The digital value reconstructed for each

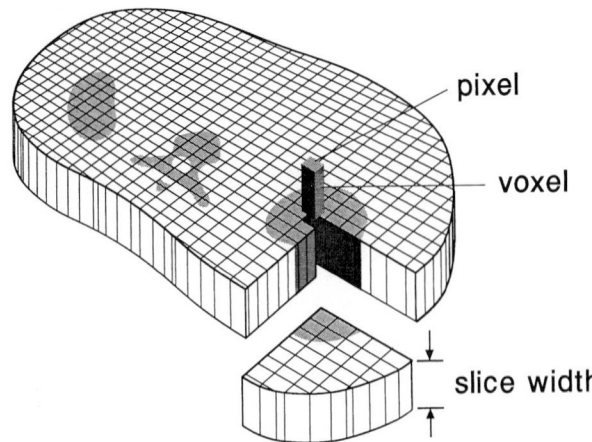

Figure 7–2. Pixel value in a computed tomographic image represents the linear attenuation coefficient of a right square prism volume element, or voxel (i.e., pixel area × slice width). (Figure and legend borrowed from Barnes GT, Lakshminarayanan AV: Computed tomography: Physical principles and image quality considerations. In Lee JKT, Sagel SS, Stanley RJ, eds. Computed Body Tomography with MRI Correlation. 2nd ed. New York: Raven Press; 1989:4.)

pixel (or voxel) represents the linear attenuation coefficient (approximately equivalent to the electronic density) of that volume. The digital values are converted to gray-scale levels for display on a video monitor screen or are used as input to a PACS workstation or to a laser imager for hard copy output on film. The contrast of the image may be adjusted by window and level settings that determine the range of attenuation values displayed within the gray-scale range of the output device.

The linear attenuation coefficients of the pixels can be expressed as *CT numbers* and defined in Hounsfield (H) units as

$$\text{CT number (H)} = 1000 \, (\mu_t - \mu_w) / \mu_w \text{, or}$$
$$\text{CT number (H)} = 1000 \, (\mu_t / \mu_w) - 1000$$

where μ_t is the linear attenuation coefficient of the tissue element in that pixel, and μ_w is the linear attenuation coefficient of water at the effective energy of the x-ray beam. With this definition, water has a CT number of 0 H, air of −1000 H, and dense bone of more than 1000 H. In general, CT values for soft tissues range from −100 to +100 H.

For therapy-planning dosimetry, the value of 1000 is not always subtracted; then the CT value scale runs from 0 (air) to more than 2000 (dense bone) and negative values are avoided. CT images can show attenuation differences of less than 0.5% with high-contrast resolution of 10 line pairs per centimeter or more. Each image typically consists of a 512 × 512 matrix of numbers, each of which can be displayed at 256 gray levels.

USES IN RADIATION ONCOLOGY AND LIMITATIONS

Computed tomographic images initially gained widespread use in various areas of radiation oncology including (1) the delineation of the target volume, (2) the determination of the relative geometry of critical structures, (3) the optimal placement of beams and the shaping of apertures, (4) the calculation of dose distribution, and

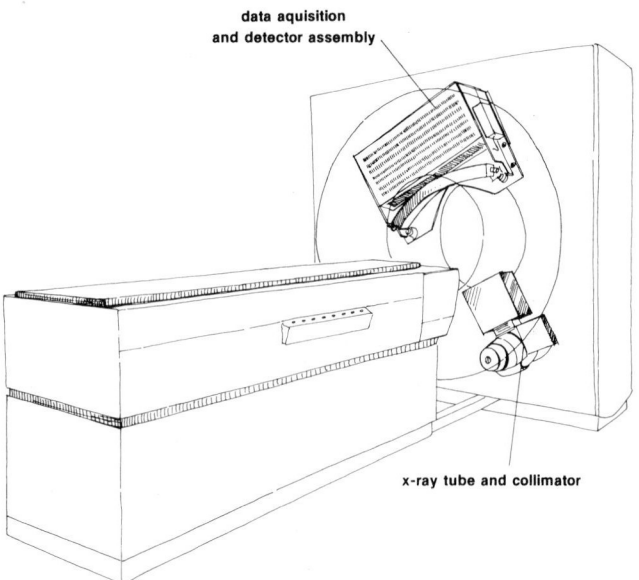

data aquisition and detector assembly

x-ray tube and collimator

Figure 7–1. Schematic drawing of a third-generation scanner showing the x-ray tube, collimator, detector array, and data acquisition system. The four subsystems are rigidly attached and go through a single rotational movement during a scan. Their weight typically is on the order of 2000 pounds. Also shown are outline drawings of the patient couch and gantry. (Figure and legend borrowed from Barnes GT, Lakshminarayanan AV: Computed tomography: Physical principles and image quality consideration. In Lee JKT, Sagel SS, Stanley RJ, eds. *Computed Body Tomography with MRI Correlation.* 2nd ed. New York: Raven Press; 1989:7.)

(5) follow-up evaluation of treatment outcome. Currently, the process of CT simulation has received increased clinical adoption; see the section on CT Simulation. Some centers have reported on using repeat CT scans during treatment as a means of measuring and reducing target positioning errors.[5-7] A commercial system is now available that combines a linear accelerator and conventional CT scanner in the treatment room.

Computed tomographic images are usually acquired with a 120 to 140 kV x-ray beam (an effective energy of 70 to 80 keV), which undergoes a significant number of photoelectric interactions, particularly in bone. Therefore, a nonlinear conversion table must be used to obtain electron densities for dose calculations relevant to the much higher energy treatment photons that undergo mainly Compton interactions. Several authors have developed an empiric relationship between CT numbers in H units and electron densities normalized to 1.0 for water. An example of this relationship is given in Fig. 7-3. Phantoms that contain multiple objects of a known electron density for converting CT numbers are commercially available.

Computed tomography provides cross-sectional images, which are ideal for radiation oncology treatment planning; however, there are several limitations. First, although CT images show exquisite cross-sectional anatomy, in some cases they do not allow one to differentiate diseased from normal tissue. Typical commercial scanners have a gantry opening of less than 70 cm in diameter, which can be restrictive for setting up patients with immobilization devices. To simulate the patient treatment position, a flat insert is needed for the standard imaging couch that has a concave surface in the transverse plane.

Artifacts arising from various sources can have a significant impact on the accuracy of CT numbers. The boundary of an object occupying only a portion of a voxel may not be accurately represented in the CT image, an effect known as partial volume averaging. Motion from respiration can affect the apparent shape and extent of organs. Streak artifacts can occur as a result of highly attenuating objects such as dense bone or metallic implants; there may also be darkened regions between or behind highly attenuating objects. Additionally, when contrast agents with high attenuation coefficients are used to provide improved visualization of certain tumors or structures, the CT numbers (H units) in the affected portions of the image are artificially high and will introduce errors in dose calculations. Editing of the image (e.g., by substituting soft tissue values in the affected region) is usually performed, but distortions in the organ shapes are difficult to correct.

The modern CT gantry is capable of tilting up to 30 degrees from the vertical, although the majority of CT images for radiotherapy application are in the transverse plane. Therefore, sagittal or coronal images, or DRRs (see sections on CT Simulation and Image Reconstruction), if desired, must be reconstructed from sequential and preferably contiguous axial images. The resolution of such reconstructed images depends on the slice thickness and spacing. The availability of helical scanners has made practical the acquisition of larger data sets in a few minutes (i.e., 50 to 100 axial images spaced 2 mm to 3 mm apart), thus improving the quality of images reconstructed along non-axial planes.

RECENT DEVELOPMENTS

Faster and more accurate CT examinations have become possible with the introduction first of the single-slice and then of the multi-slice spiral, or (more properly) helical, scanners. Volumetric scan data is acquired by having the table move continuously relative to the gantry, concomitant with the continuous rotation of the x-ray tube and detector array around the patient. Multi-slice units may acquire the data for as few as 4 or as many as 16 slices during a single rotation. State-of-the-art multi-slice CT scanners can obtain isotropic data sets with voxels of dimension as small as 0.5 mm. These scanners can acquire the data for a full set of images in times well below 1 minute, usually during one breath hold. For radiotherapy application, however, one must consider the possibility that patient anatomy during a breath hold may not be in its "average" location during radiation treatment.

To address the limitations of CT gantry aperture on the ability to set up patients with immobilization devices, a commercial scanner with an 85 cm aperture has become available. In connection with respiration-gated radiation therapy, in which dose delivery from the treatment accelerator occurs at a preselected interval in the respiratory cycle while the patient breathes normally, different means of synchronizing CT acquisition with respiration have been introduced. In one method (Fig. 7-4), a respiration monitor system triggers the scanner to acquire a single axial image while the patient breathes normally, followed by indexing of the table to the next position; the process is repeated until the volumetric set of images is obtained.[8] An emerging development is the acquisition of volumetric

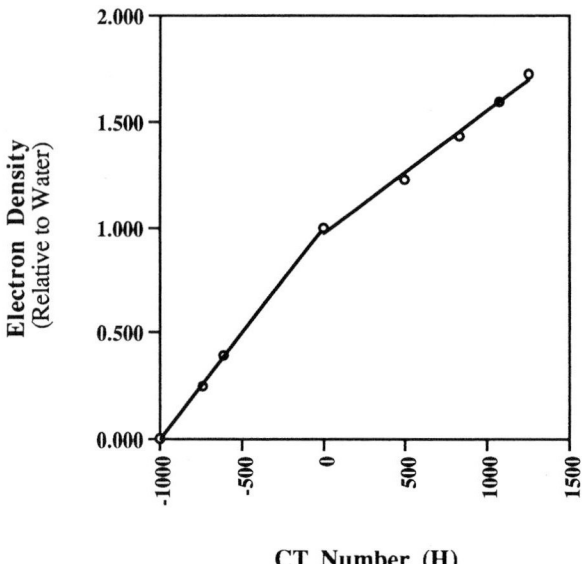

Figure 7–3. Conversion of computed tomographic number to electron density. (From Mohan R, Chui C, Miller D, et al: Use of computerized tomography in dose calculations for radiation treatment planning. *CT.* 1981;5:273.)

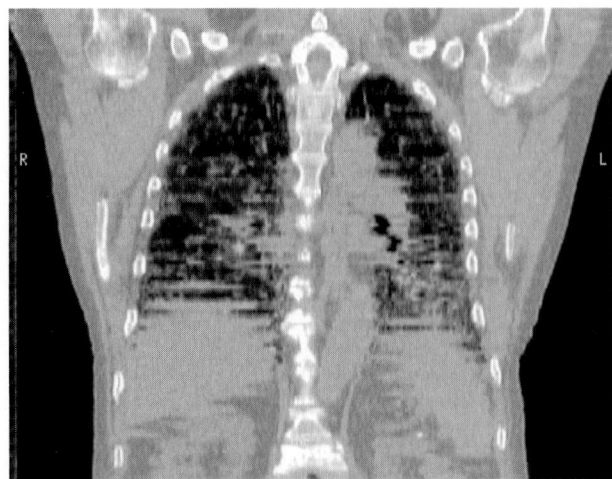

A

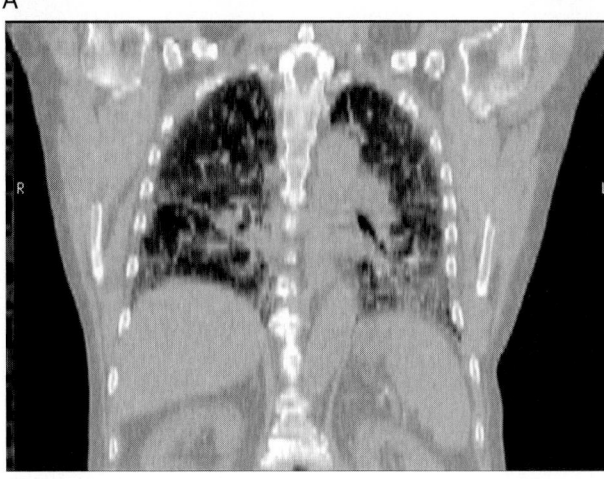

B

Figure 7–4. **A,** Sagittal section of a computed tomographic scan not synchronized with respiration; note motion artifacts. **B,** Computed tomographic scan (Philips PQ5000) in which a respiration-gated radiotherapy system (Varian Medical Systems) triggered acquisition of axial images at end expiration.

data concurrently throughout the respiration cycle, for the purposes of obtaining information on anatomical motion and more accurately accounting for it in the treatment plan.[9] In this approach, axial images are acquired continuously while the respiration signal is simultaneously recorded; the images are then retrospectively sorted according to the respiration phase to form volumetric sets at different phases.

USE AND LIMITATIONS OF COMPUTED TOMOGRAPHIC SCOUT VIEW

Digital projection images, the so-called *scout view*, can be obtained from CT scanners by translating the patient relative to the x-ray tube and detector array (Fig. 7-5). Although the x-ray tube may be oriented at any angle, the most common arrangement is in either the anterior-posterior (AP) or the lateral direction. The data obtained are a 2-D matrix of relative transmission values in an arbitrary numeric range that may differ from one type of scanner to another. Adjustment of the window and level controls provides an image of appropriate brightness and contrast. The scout view is often useful in determining the extent and spacing of axial scans. In addition, in the hard copy output, the positions of the axial images can be annotated on the scout views, relative to a reference position selected during the patient setup.

The CT scout view differs from conventional projection radiographs in that the x-ray beam diverges only in the direction across the patient table, but not in the direction along the patient table. In addition, the shape of the CT detector array is concave. Thus, CT scout views cannot be directly compared with conventional projection images used in radiation oncology such as the simulator films. Furthermore, although window and level adjustment allows the scout view images to have excellent contrast, the spatial resolution of the CT scout view is significantly less than that of simulation images, by almost an order of magnitude.

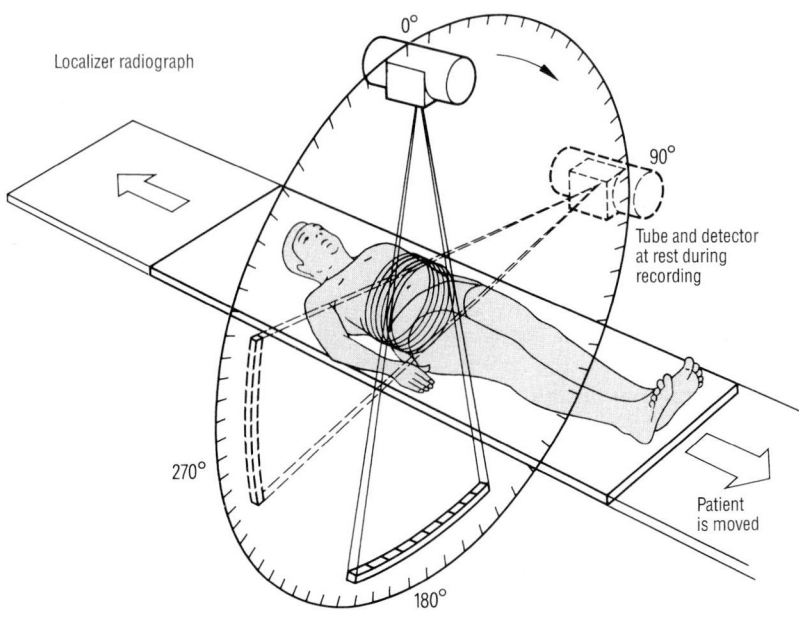

Figure 7–5. Schematic drawing illustrating the acquisition of a localizer radiograph, or scout view. (From Krestel E, ed. *Imaging Systems for Medical Diagnostics: Fundamentals and Technical Solutions.* Berlin: Siemens; 1990:434.)

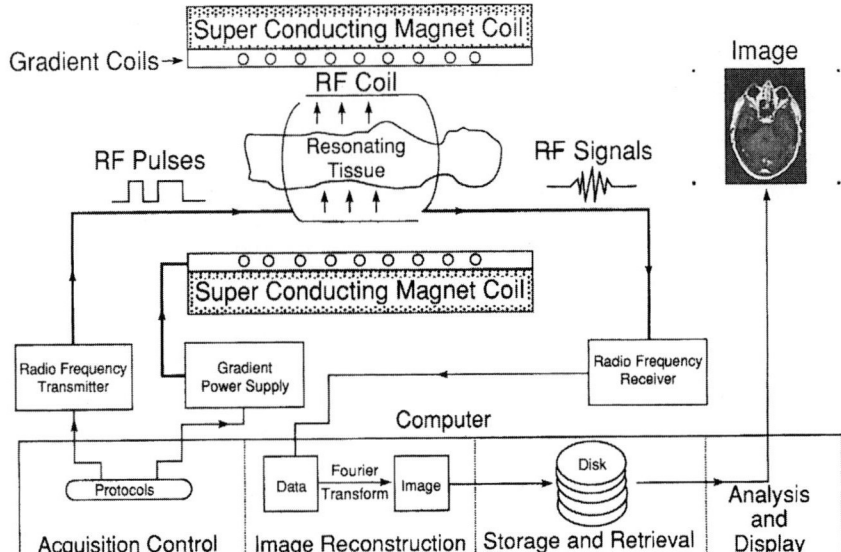

Figure 7–6. Typical magnetic resonance imaging system. RF, radiofrequency. (From Sprawls P: *Physical Principles of Medical Imaging.* 2nd ed. Madison, Wisc: Medical Physics Publishing; 1993.)

Magnetic Resonance Imaging

PRINCIPLES OF OPERATION

The phenomenon of nuclear magnetic resonance (NMR) was first described by Purcell and Bloch, the 1952 winners of the Nobel Prize in physics. Early work on the use of NMR for imaging was done by Lauterbur, Damadian, and others. Nuclei with a magnetic moment, usually those with odd numbers of protons or neutrons, when placed in a strong magnetic field, can be excited from their ground or lowest energy state to a higher state by a pulse from a second and weaker magnetic field that is varying in radiofrequency. When these nuclei return to the ground energy state, they emit radiofrequency energy that can be detected by very sensitive wire coils and appropriate electronics. Many commercial MRI units use a 0.5 to 1.5 tesla (T) magnetic field produced by a super-conducting magnet and radiofrequency signals of 20 to 65 MHz for studies of the distribution of hydrogen nuclei (protons) in the body. Additional electromagnets are used to localize the region where resonance takes place (x-, y-, and z-gradient coils) and remove inhomogeneities in the main magnetic field (shim coils) (Fig. 7-6).

Typical magnetic resonance (MR) images contain a matrix of 256 × 256 values, a factor of 2 less than CT images in each dimension. Each pixel contains a complex combination of information about hydrogen nuclei density (ρ), spin-lattice relaxation time (T_1), and spin-spin relaxation time (T_2). The relaxation times are a measure of the time required for the disappearance of the signal due to nuclei returning from an excited to the unperturbed energy state, or for dephasing of the initially aligned and precessing nuclear spins. Radiofrequency pulse sequences can be designed to enhance the dependence of the image on the values of any of the three parameters and improve the contrast for various tumors or other abnormal tissue variations. The appearance of MR images may be further affected by blood flow or by injection of contrast agents such as gadolinium compounds. MR image data may be obtained for a three-dimensional (3-D) volume or for any arbitrary plane within the volume. MRI offers the possibility of excellent discrimination of certain tumors with high contrast, the ability to select arbitrary planes for imaging, and good resolution (Fig. 7-7).

USES AND LIMITATIONS IN RADIATION ONCOLOGY

MR images often provide better soft tissue contrast than CT, thus improving discrimination between tumor and normal tissue in some disease sites. Small differences in T1 and T2 can be exploited by manipulating imaging parameters to enhance the contrast among different tissues. In addition, by using the three orthogonal field gradients independently or in combination, the image plane can be orientated in a direction that best displays

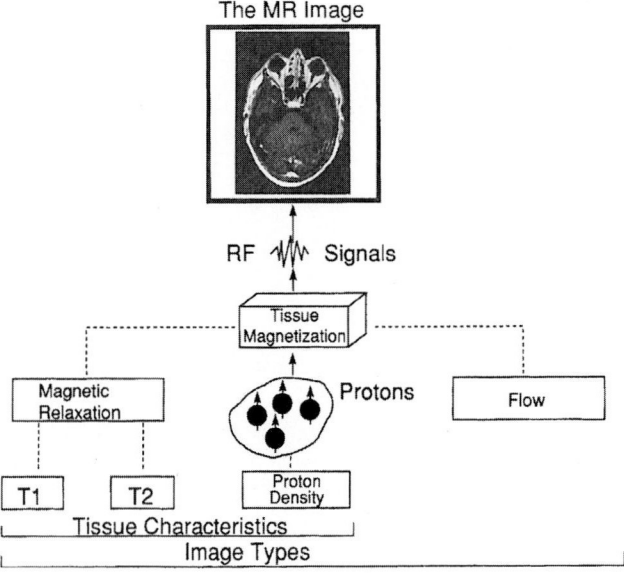

Figure 7–7. Physical characteristics of tissue that are displayed in the magnetic resonance image. MR, magnetic resonance; RF, radiofrequency; T_1, spin-lattice relaxation time; T_2, spin-spin relaxation time. (Figure and legend borrowed from Sprawls P: *Physical Principles of Medical Imaging.* 2nd ed. Madison, Wisc: Medical Physics Publishing; 1993.)

the extent of a particular tissue. Functional MRI of the brain can identify speech, visual, and sensory areas to avoid when treating intracranial lesions.[10]

Several characteristics have limited the applicability of MR images alone for treatment planning. One is the lack of signal from cortical bone: Although bone location can be inferred in some disease sites, it is not possible to distinguish bone-air interfaces such as sinuses. Pixel intensities do not correlate with electron density as they do in CT, thus they cannot be used directly in dose calculations. Intensity variations occur across the images, such as those arising from falloff in sensitivity toward the ends of the receiver coil. The images may be distorted by variations in local magnetic fields caused by imperfections in the machine itself and by the presence of metal objects in the environment and within the patient. Because of these limitations, MR images are usually registered to CT, and the information MRI provides is transferred to the CT study for treatment planning purposes. The registration of CT and MR images is described in another section. MRI has been effectively used for treatment planning of brain, head and neck, liver, pelvis, and prostate tumors (Fig. 7-8). Other disadvantages include the high cost of equipment and site preparation, examination times that are 1.5 to 2.0 times those required for CT, a limited diameter of the patient tunnel opening in the magnet, and magnetic and radio frequency shielding problems.

MRSI of ^{1}H nuclei in combination with MRI is receiving increased clinical adoption for evaluating tumor extent and necrosis in brain tumors and potential staging and evaluation of prostate cancer, and thus as an aid to external beam and brachytherapy planning.[11-13] The relative concentrations of metabolites choline, creatine, and citrate, specifically elevated values of the ratio (choline + creatine)/citrate, have been hypothesized to be

an indicator of malignant prostatic tissue (Fig. 7-9).[14-15] A present limitation of MRSI for radiation treatment planning of the prostate is that it requires an endorectal radio frequency coil to achieve a sufficiently large signal. The coil pushes the prostate anteriorly and deforms it, thus limiting the accuracy with which the suspected tumor regions can be identified in the planning CT, which is performed without the coil. Development of algorithms for registering MR-to-CT and MR-to-ultrasound image sets that account for prostate organ deformation is currently under investigation.[16]

The use of polymer gels with MRI for measurement of complex 3-D dose distributions has received increased attention, particularly for application to brachytherapy, intensity modulated radiotherapy, and stereotactic radiosurgery.[17] The gel is poured into a phantom and exposed to radiation; the molecules polymerize to a degree proportional to absorbed dose. The phantom is then measured using MRI or optical tomography to obtain a 2- or 3-D dose distribution.

RECENT DEVELOPMENTS

Several recent developments may increase the use of MRI, MRS, and MRSI in radiation oncology. Self-shielded magnets, and very specialized, low-cost permanent magnet systems will make MRI more available in the radiation oncology clinic.

The introduction of new fast-pulse sequences and greater computer power for data manipulation make it possible to track the uptake of gadolinium diethylenetriamine pentaacetic acid, Gd-DTPA, dynamically to measure tissue perfusion quantitatively with high resolution. Dynamic contrast enhanced imaging can also be used to measure cerebral blood volume, blood-brain barrier permeability, necrotic fraction, extracellular

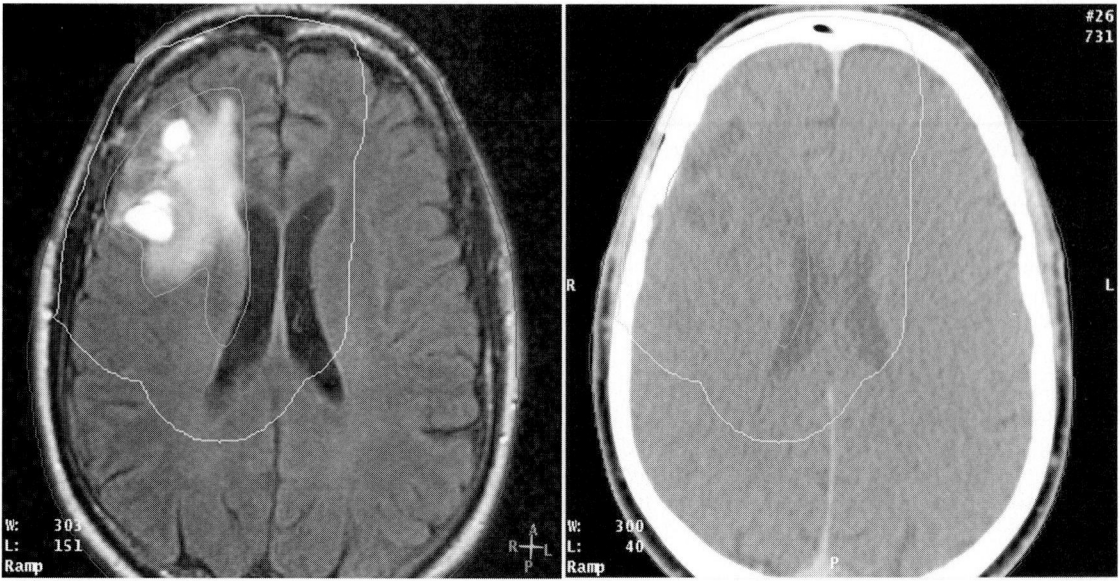

Figure 7–8. *Left*: Axial magnetic resonance image of the brain. Malignant tissue appears as brighter areas in the upper left. Gross target volume and planning target volume are outlined in light blue and yellow, respectively. *Right*: Axial computed tomographic image of the same patient. The computed tomographic and magnetic resonance image sets have been registered by alignment of the patient surface and the target volume contours transferred to the computed tomographic image (AcqSim, Philips Medical Systems, Andover, MA).

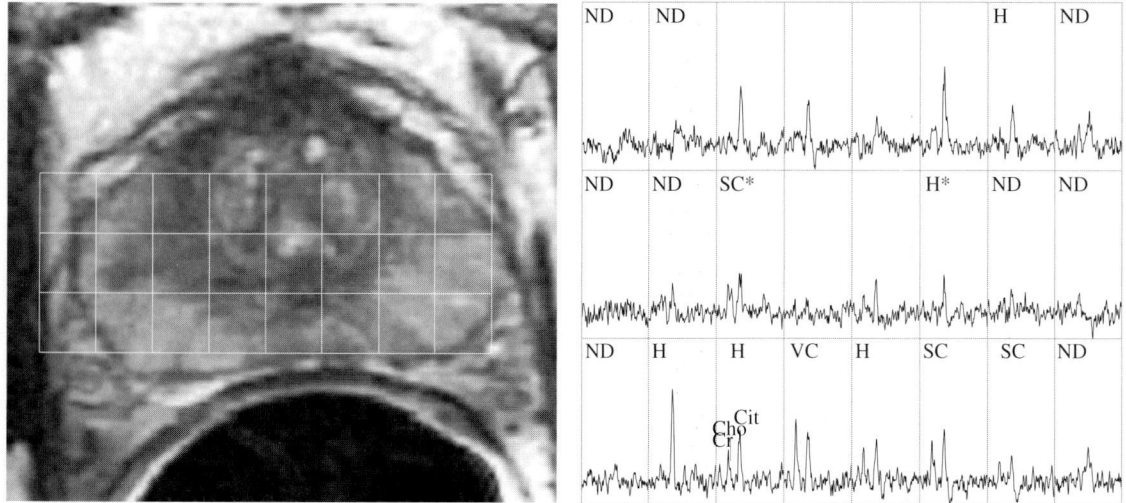

Figure 7–9. A single plane of ¹H magnetic resonance spectroscopy imaging (MRSI) data from a prostate cancer patient (Gleason score 7, PSA 8ng/mL). *Left*: MRSI grid shown on the T2-weighted magnetic resonance image. *Right*: spectra corresponding to the voxels shown on the grid. *H* = healthy peripheral zone, *SC* = suspicious for cancer. (From Zaider M, Zelefsky MJ, Lee EK, et al: Treatment planning for prostate implants using magnetic-resonance spectroscopy imaging. *Int J Radiat Oncol Biol Phys.* 2000;47:1085.)

space, and permeability surface area product. This technique is being used to study osteosarcoma and to attempt to predict necrotic fraction after treatment.

The in vivo mobility of water molecules depends on the properties of the diffusing medium and the presence of physical barriers. Diffusion weighted imaging (DWI) is being used to provide information on bone marrow cellularity and changes in hematopoiesis resulting from chemotherapy in leukemia patients.

Rapid imaging techniques such as echo-planar imaging (EPI) that allow images to be obtained in a fraction of a second are allowing functional MRI (fMRI) studies of sensory and motor stimulation, vision, and language. These techniques are also being used to study angiogenesis in tumors and healing of wounds.

The availability of high field (≥3.0 T) clinical MRI systems will provide images with increased signal-to-noise ratio (SNR), increased separation of spectrum peaks, and enhanced susceptibility effects. The increased SNR can reduce acquisition time or enhance resolution for fMRI studies. The improved image spectroscopic resolution might also provide the opportunity to obtain new biochemical information.

There is also a new class of MRI contrast agents, which are capable of gene transfection into cells. These agents will allow gene therapy to be monitored by MRI through co-transported MRI contrast agents. Additional refinements include MRI contrast agents that will enable the MRI signal to be greatly amplified through association of the site-directed contrast agent with its target.[18]

Ultrasound Imaging

PRINCIPLES OF OPERATION

Medical ultrasonography is a direct descendant of sonar techniques developed during World War II to search for submarines. Short bursts of sound are sent out into the ultrasound transmission medium at regular intervals. Between bursts, sound echoes return from reflecting objects or interfaces. A knowledge of the speed of sound in the medium and the time of the roundtrip travel to the reflector enable one to calculate the distance from the sound source and detector to the reflecting object.

Medical ultrasound imaging requires the production and detection of mechanical pressure waves within the tissues of the body. It normally uses sound frequencies in the 3 to 10 MHz range. Ultrasound beam production and detection are accomplished with piezoelectric materials. When placed in a varying electric field, such substances vibrate and produce ultrasound. And when they are deformed by mechanical pressure, for example, because of the reflected ultrasound, they produce electric fields that are detected as the signals in ultrasound scanners. Manufactured ceramic piezoelectric crystals are incorporated in the transducer, the component of the ultrasonographic system that is placed against the patient. The transducer produces the initial ultrasound energy and detects reflected energy. Some of the ultrasound energy sent into the body is reflected from tissue interfaces and returns to the transducer. The total time between the production and the detection of the sound waves, which move at an approximately constant velocity of 1540 m/s through soft tissue, is a measure of the roundtrip distance from the transducer to the tissue interface. Ultrasonographic image resolution depends on the ultrasound frequency, transducer size, and focusing characteristics of the system. In general, resolution increases with increasing frequency and decreasing transducer size. Medical ultrasound-imaging systems have resolution capabilities of 1 to 10 mm. At the higher frequencies, imaging becomes more difficult at depth, because of increasing absorption of the ultrasound energy in the tissue. The ultrasound energy is not ionizing.

The images produced show interfaces and variations in acoustic impedance. The acoustic impedance of a given tissue is equal to the product of the tissue density (mass/volume) and the velocity of sound in that tissue. The images can show tomographic views in almost any orientation.

USES AND LIMITATIONS IN RADIATION ONCOLOGY

Early medical ultrasound B-scan units provided some of the first cross-sectional images for treatment planning; however, current CT and MRI units, although 5 to 10 times more expensive, produce images with better resolution and contrast that are more desirable for treatment planning. The major exception is the use of high-resolution images of the prostate obtained with an ultrasound imager that employs a special rectal probe. Transrectal ultrasound has become the predominant image modality for planning and delivery of prostate implants using transperineal template-guided insertion; Chapter 11, Aspects of Brachytherapy Physics, provides a more extensive description. Intraoperative ultrasound has been also applied to evaluate high dose rate prostate brachytherapy implants.[19] Most intravascular brachytherapy studies have included intravascular ultrasound analyses for assessing restenosis.[20] A commercially available device allows ultrasound-guided patient positioning for external beam radiation therapy; several centers have reported on its application to daily localization and correction of prostate position.[21-22]

Ultrasound beams cannot penetrate bone or gas-filled cavities. This limits the use of ultrasonography. Furthermore, ultrasonographic images are much more difficult to interpret than those from CT or MRI.

RECENT DEVELOPMENTS

Imaging systems consisting of multi-element transducers can produce ultrasonographic images in a slice at rates fast enough to show smooth motion on a video screen (≈30 pictures per second). All modern ultrasonographic units use a digital scan converter to produce digital images. Individual pictures, or frames, can be transferred to PACS or to film with a laser imager.

The Radiotherapy Simulator

The radiotherapy simulator is the mechanical analog of an isocentric therapy unit (Fig. 7-10). It serves several functions, but its primary purpose is to help establish the optimal beam and setup parameters for a patient before the first treatment. These parameters may include the gantry angle, collimator angle, field size, target-to-skin distance (TSD), isocenter, and treatment couch position for each beam. The patient setup position, fiducial skin marks, and immobilization devices can also be determined during the treatment simulation. With the increasingly widespread use of CT simulation and high-quality DRRs as reference images (see section on CT simulation), the role of the radiotherapy simulator for CT-scanner–based planning has diminished. [For a more detailed description of the radiotherapy simulator and its fluoroscopic and radiographic subsystems, see the First Edition of this text.]

RECENT DEVELOPMENTS

In connection with respiration-gated radiotherapy, one commercial system enables recording and playback of fluoroscopic images from the image intensifier of a simulator, synchronized with the waveform from the respiration monitor. The operator can examine anatomical motion in the playback to evaluate and optimize the choice of treatment interval in the respiratory cycle.[23] A recently introduced commercial simulator has replaced the image intensifier with an amorphous silicon flat panel detector (see the section on Electronic Portal Imaging Devices), providing distortion-free radiographic and fluoroscopic digital images. The detector is mounted on a retractable arm that allows imaging of a larger range of patient setup positions compared to an image intensifier unit. Such systems will also be capable of obtaining 3-D image sets through cone beam image reconstruction; see the section on Other Applications of Electronic Portal Imaging Devices in Radiation Oncology.

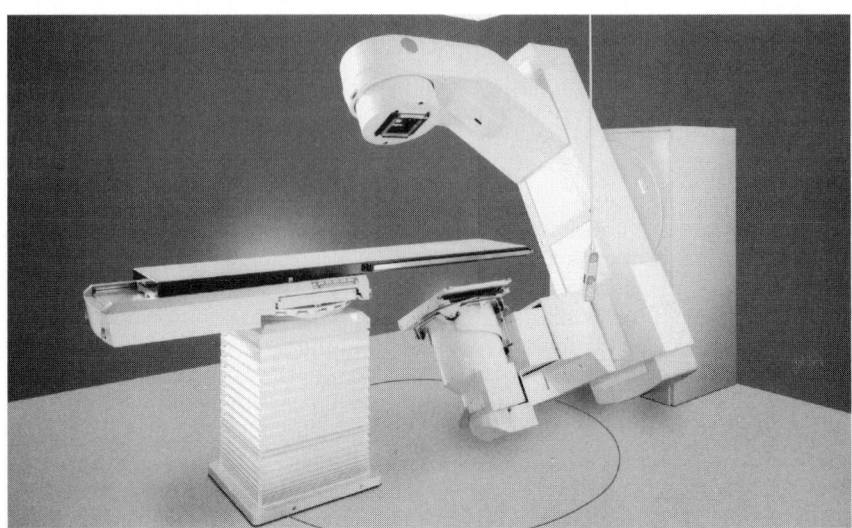

Figure 7–10. The radiotherapy simulator "head" (containing the x-ray tube) as well as the image intensifier (supported on the opposite side of the gantry arm) can be remotely positioned to provide variable target-to-axis distances and magnifications. (Courtesy of Siemens Medical Systems.)

QUALITY ASSURANCE

Quality assurance measurements are as important for radiotherapy simulators as for therapy accelerators. All important mechanical parameters of the simulator should be tested regularly and corrective actions be taken if needed, per the report of the American Association of Physicists in Medicine (AAPM) Task Group 40.[24]

A quality assurance program for the imaging components (x-ray and fluoroscopic) should also be established in accordance with national guidelines and state/local regulations (National Council on Radiation Protection and Measurement Report 99).[25] Quality assurance of the automatic film processor should also be included.

COMPUTED TOMOGRAPHY SIMULATION

In recent years, software systems for performing CT simulation have become available. These systems provide treatment simulation functions with volume representation from a CT image set. CT simulation has become a widely accepted standard for pretreatment simulation in a wide range of disease sites. CT simulation functions include:

- Patient alignment from scout view images.
- Target and normal organ localization by defining contours on axial CT images, or by virtual fluoroscopy.

- Virtual fluoroscopy, which allows definition of a treatment portal without requiring contour segmentation of the target on all axial CT slices. The computer displays AP and lateral DRRs, and mimics the movement of a conventional fluoroscopic simulator in the vertical, transverse and longitudinal directions, and symmetric or asymmetric collimation as well as collimator rotation.
- Definition of reference isocenter points directly from the volumetric CT data, followed by CT table positioning such that alignment lasers indicate triangulation points for marking on the patient surface.
- Treatment portal design including entry of block or MLC outlines.
- Generation of DRRs for comparison to portal films or electronic portal images. The DRR display may include a treatment field outline, graticule tray, and outlines of organs (Fig. 7-11).
- 3-D displays (e.g., for viewing beam intersections with the patient surface or internal organs).
- Transfer of CT images and associated simulation data to a radiation treatment planning system for dose calculation and plan evaluation.

With earlier CT systems that placed practical limits on the CT slice spacing and thus limited DRR quality, many radiotherapy centers used CT simulation in combination

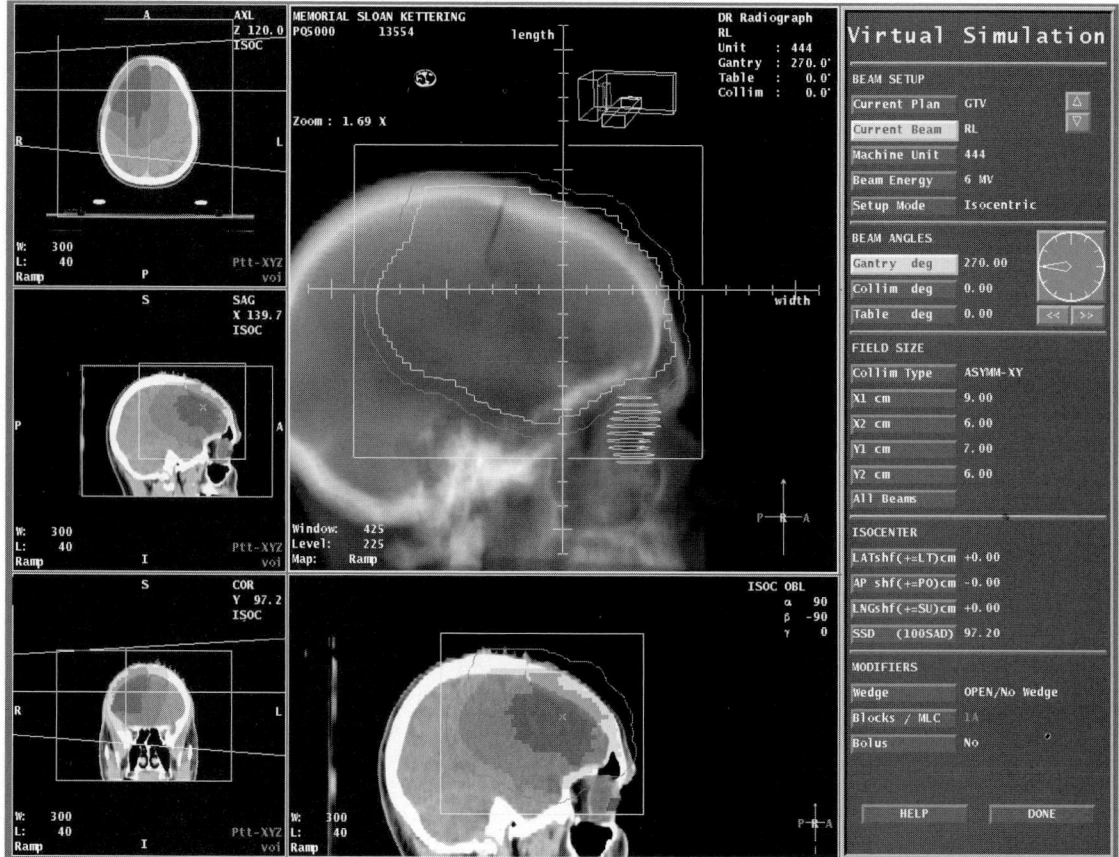

Figure 7–11. Example computed tomography simulation display (AcqSim, Philips Medical Systems, Andover, Mass.). Upper right image is a beam's eye view digitally reconstructed radiograph with planning target volume outlined in *yellow*, treatment field aperture in *blue*. Right panel shows simulated beam setup controls. See also Color Figure 7-11.

with the conventional simulator, by aligning DRRs with the simulator radiographs and transferring the beam apertures to them. The advent of helical scanners has made feasible smaller slice spacing (≤3 mm), thus improving DRRs' quality for use directly as reference images and thereby eliminating the necessity for conventional simulation.

Portal Radiographs

Portal radiographs are a fundamental part of the clinical quality assurance program. They provide a *beam's eye view* (BEV) record of the patient treatment volume, radiographically revealing the relationship between anatomical structures and the treatment field. There are three types of imaging systems available for acquiring portal radiographs: film, electronic portal imaging devices (EPIDs), and computed radiography; each system is described in later sections. The AAPM Task Group 28[26] defines a portal radiograph as "a radiograph produced by exposing the image receptor to the radiation beam which emanates from the portal of a therapy unit." The report describes three types of radiographs (within the context of acquisition with film):

- *Localization*: A portal radiograph produced by an exposure that is short compared with the daily treatment of that field (generally called localization films, beam films, or port films).
- *Verification*: A film exposed for an entire treatment field.
- *Double exposure*: A localization film composed of two sequential exposures; the first is that of the shaped treatment field, and the second of a larger rectangular field, superimposed on the first. The double-exposure portal makes it easier to relate the treatment field to the surrounding anatomy and is particularly useful for relatively small field sizes.

The importance of portal radiography as a quality assurance tool is supported by numerous published studies, which have made it clear that portal radiographs are essential to accurate radiotherapy and that frequent imaging is desirable for difficult patient setups or highly conformal treatments.[27]

PORTAL FILMS

The films traditionally used for portal imaging are the TL (therapy localization) film and the V (verification) film, both manufactured by Kodak. The former has a high silver content and is properly exposed by only a few centigray. The latter is a relatively slow industrial film, making it more useful for a full-treatment exposure. Several different films by other manufacturers have been successfully used for portal imaging with optimal exposure techniques determined through trial and error.

The image quality of either type of film is reduced in part by high-energy secondary electrons that exit from the patient onto the film. Portal film quality is improved with specialized radiotherapy cassettes that provide metal front screens in uniform and close contact with the film and thick enough to absorb the shower of secondary electrons exiting the patient. The thickness of these screens is determined by measurements of scatter-to-primary ratios (S/P) for large fields.[28] Thicknesses are generally 1 to 4 mm, depending on the beam energy and on the screen material (usually lead or copper). A rear metal screen is also often used to improve the overall sensitivity, or *speed*, of the system. The use of rear screens may cause some reduction in image resolution; however, in practice no significant degradation of image quality is observed. A second important function of the film cassette is to provide good film-screen contact. Thin plastic or cardboard cassettes fail in this respect and result in poor-quality images. Even rigid cassettes may warp over time and may exhibit nonuniform film-screen contact. Periodic testing of all radiotherapy cassettes for adequate film-screen contact and mechanical stability is recommended.

In recent years Kodak has introduced the EC/L film system, which provides higher display contrast in portal radiographs compared to previous metal-screen-film combinations. The cassette consists of the same 1 mm copper front screen, but two fluorescent intensifying screens have been added and the back lead screen has been removed. The film has very low speed and inherently high contrast, and is exposed primarily by light from the fluorescent screens.[29]

To improve the readability and accessibility of portal films, various film digitizing and image processing systems are available. The most commonly used film digitizers are either charge coupled device (CCD)-based or combination laser-photomultiplier tube. The resultant images can be stored, accessed over a computer network, and enhanced and processed similarly to electronic portal or computed radiography images; see section on Use of Portal Radiographs in Radiation Oncology.

COMPUTED RADIOGRAPHY

Photostimulable phosphors (PSP), also called storage phosphors, are compounds that are capable of absorbing and storing energy from x-rays. They can be stimulated subsequently to release energy in the form of visible light. The term *computed radiography* (CR) refers to the process of image acquisition and readout of PSP plates, then conversion to a digital image. Absorbed x-ray energy excites electrons in the PSP plate to semi-stable higher energy levels, producing a latent image. The plate is read out with a helium-neon (red) laser, which stimulates the semi-stable electrons to drop down to their ground energy state while emitting visible (blue) light. The light is sensed by a photomultiplier tube and converted to an electrical signal, which is digitized. In a commercial system designed specifically for simulator and portal radiographs, the PSP plate is exposed in a standard film cassette and processed by a computed radiography reader. The exposure requirements are similar to those for conventional simulator or portal localization films; however, the exposure flexibility reduces the likelihood

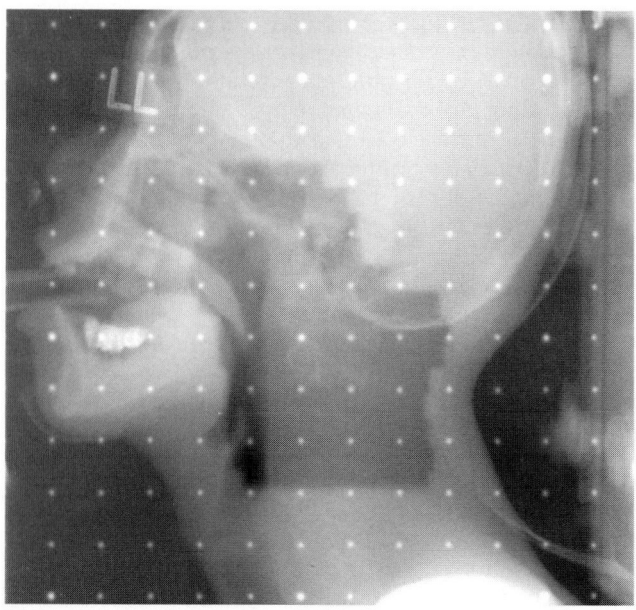

Figure 7–12. Portal radiograph made with a computed radiography system (Kodak 2000RT) using double-exposure technique. Note the projected grid scale (graticule) indicating the field central axis and calibrated in 2 cm intervals in the isocenter plane.

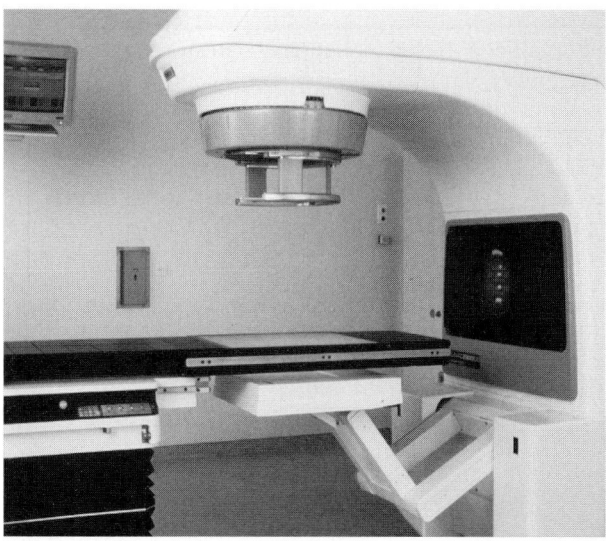

Figure 7–13. Electronic portal imaging device (matrix ionization chamber system or amorphous silicon flat panel detector) is supported by a robotic arm, which allows imaging at all gantry angles as well as removal (retraction) from the radiation beam. (Courtesy of Varian Medical Systems.)

of under- or over-exposure, thus reducing the number of retakes (Fig. 7-12).

ELECTRONIC PORTAL IMAGING DEVICES

EPIDs have received more widespread clinical use in recent years due to advances in detector technology and hence image quality, and to the availability of commercial picture archiving and communication systems (PACS) specifically designed for radiation oncology. Several features make EPIDs attractive for portal radiography. One is the ability to acquire and display an image in seconds. When combined with a computer-controlled accelerator fitted with an MLC, field setup and image acquisition can be performed remotely, obviating the need to re-enter the treatment room each time. This allows for more frequent treatment verification, or to acquire a series of images during a single treatment for examining patient movement. Another powerful feature is that the images are in digital form, which allows for application of software tools to extract information relevant to treatment verification.

The EPID is attached to the gantry of an isocentric radiation treatment machine so that it may intercept the exiting photon beam at all gantry angles (Fig. 7-13). The ideal support system must be sturdy and capable of precise repositioning, yet easily retracted or removed to facilitate patient access. First-generation commercial EPIDs have been either video-based or matrix ionization chamber-based systems.[30] In video-based systems, the image is formed by the interaction of the radiation with a fluorescent screen assembly consisting of a metal (e.g., copper or tungsten) plate onto which the phosphor is

deposited. The metal plate is upstream relative to the phosphor and absorbs scattered electrons emanating from the patient, as well as interacting with the photons to generate high-energy electrons that, in turn, produce the fluorescent image in the phosphor. A front-silvered mirror, placed diagonally, reflects the fluorescent light by 90 degrees into a video camera. The analog output of the video camera is converted into a digital image with an analog-to-digital converter, typically 512×512 pixels ($\approx$0.8 mm pixel size for a 40×40 cm^2 detector area), where the brightness information of each pixel is described by 1 byte (of 8 bits), capable of specifying 256 different gray levels. In the matrix ionization chamber system, electrode strips on two printed circuit boards form an array of ionization chambers; the strips run horizontally on one board and vertically on the other. A 1 mm gap between the boards is filled with iso-octane liquid, which serves as an ionization medium for the x-rays. An image consisting of 256×256 pixels (32.5×32.5 cm^2 detector area) is obtained by switching on the high voltage to one row, collecting the currents from each of the 256 column electrodes, and repeating the process for each of the 256 rows. An electronic circuit performs the rapid switching and analog-to-digital conversion; acquisition time is about 3 seconds per image.

The first-generation systems, while more convenient than film, have a number of limitations. The camera-based systems are bulky and image quality is reduced due to the poor optical transfer system, while the matrix ionization chamber system requires long irradiation times and is especially sensitive to small changes in dose rate, resulting in line and band artifacts.

The current commercially available EPIDS take advantage of the large industrial development of flat display panel technology, and provide faster acquisition and superior image quality than their predecessors. Variously referred to as active matrix flat panel imagers or amorphous silicon flat panel image detectors, the array of electronic circuitry comprising the pixels is fabricated on panels of hydrogenated amorphous silicon (Fig. 7-14). Each pixel comprises a light-sensitive photodiode attached to a thin-film transistor acting as a switch. The physical buildup of the detector array consists of a metal plate (typically 1 mm copper) and phosphor screen to convert x-rays to visible light; the metal layer also serves to attenuate scattered radiation. The light is converted to electron-ion pairs in the photodiode, and collected by application of a bias voltage onto a storage capacitor. The charges stored in the pixels are transferred to the readout electronics by activating the pixel switches row-by-row and reading out all columns simultaneously. It is possible to design arrays capable of 30 frames per second, thus being applicable to fluoroscopy as well as radiography; the present limitation is in the electronics that control image acquisition ($\approx 1/2$ second per image) and transfer of the images to the viewing workstation. For portal imaging applications, several frames are averaged together to reduce image noise. Panel sizes of 30×40 cm^2 are available in arrays of 512×384 or 1024×1024 pixels, although the associated clinical significance of the latter is unclear, given spatial resolution limitations caused by the x-ray source size and thickness of the overlying scintillator.

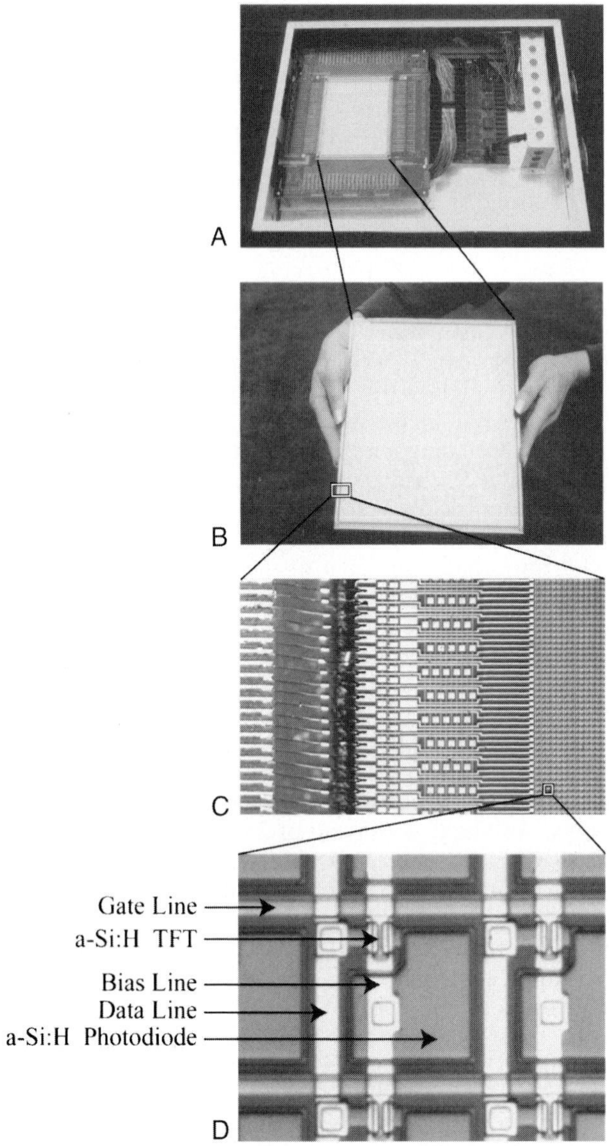

IMAGE PROCESSING

The digital nature of electronic radiographs facilitates processing to make the image more "readable" in evaluating and comparing the delivered treatment with a reference (e.g., simulation or DRR) image. Improvement of image quality through control of the display *window* and *level* or with more sophisticated digital filtering techniques can be quite helpful for locating anatomical landmarks and other reference points. High-pass filtering or Sobel edge detection may help to determine bony anatomy such as the pelvic sidewall or the femoral head, as well as surgical clips. Histogram equalization and adaptive histogram equalization methods can improve contrast and readability throughout an image. Other image manipulation features include the ability to rotate, zoom and pan the image; annotate (i.e., add text to) the image; draw and overlay graphics; and measure distances with an "electronic" ruler.

USE OF PORTAL RADIOGRAPHS IN RADIATION ONCOLOGY

Image Registration

Portal radiography is a primary tool for quality assurance in radiation delivery. The portal image from the first treatment is compared with the corresponding reference image (a digitized simulator film or digital image, or digitally reconstructed radiograph from CT) to ensure correct patient setup and proper block construction and placement or MLC programming. Since portal (and simulator) radiographs of oblique fields are confusing and difficult to interpret because of their nonstandard view of radiographic anatomy, AP and lateral portal films are generally used to verify the isocenter location. Side-by-side comparison of the simulator and portal images can be facilitated with the use of a graticule, a device that projects a cross-hair shadow and centimeter scale in the portal film; the device is supplied by several vendors.[24] The use of such a device is recommended since the cross hairs of the linear accelerator or cobalt-60 fields do not appear on the portal image. If field adjustments are needed, this tool facilitates the quantification and communication of the desired changes (see Fig. 7-12).

Besides the side-by-side manual procedure, various algorithms have been developed to enable computer-assisted comparison of images for detection of field placement errors. This is usually accomplished in several

Figure 7–14. Prototype amorphous silicon flat panel detector. **A,** Housing containing detector and readout electronics; **B,** detector array; **C,** a portion of the array near the peripheral contacts; **D,** a single pixel showing the photodiode, thin film transister (TFT) switch, gate line for controlling the switch, data line, and bias line for applying bias voltage to the photodiode. (From Antonuk LE, El-Mohri Y, Siewerdsen JH, et al: Empirical investigation of the signal performance of a high-resolution indirect detection, active matrix flat-panel imager [AMFPI] for fluoroscopic and radiographic operation. *Med Phys.* 1997;24:51.)

Gate Line
a-Si:H TFT
Bias Line
Data Line
a-Si:H Photodiode

steps: (1) information about the positions of the patient anatomy and radiation field are extracted from both portal and reference images; (2) a common reference frame for both images is established by registration of the radiation fields; and (3) setup error is determined by registering the patient anatomy in both images, then measuring the resulting displacement between the portal and reference radiation field edges.

Two of the most common methods of interactive, or manual, image registration are the line drawing or template technique, and point pair registration. Point-pair registration involves identifying the positions of corresponding anatomical landmarks in the reference and portal images; the portal image is then transformed (i.e., translated, rotated, and scaled) such that the selected points align with those in the reference image. Although the methodology is simple, point pair registration is error prone, due to the difficulty in correctly identifying corresponding fiducial points, particularly when reference and portal images are of different image quality (i.e., kilovoltage vis-à-vis megavoltage beam quality). The template method involves drawing (graphically, by means of a mouse or trackball) lines or curves indicating the field edge and patient anatomy on the reference image, which is then overlaid and aligned with the portal image (Fig. 7-15). Semi-automatic extensions of the template method are those that automatically extract anatomical features in the portal image and align them with the reference template. A third category of registration methods uses automated pixel-by-pixel, grayscale intensity-based image correlation. This approach assumes similar quality images for matching; thus, it requires registration of a first-day portal image to the reference image by some other means, then uses the first-day portal image as reference for subsequent treatment sessions.

As previously indicated, portal radiographs are part of the overall quality assurance program for ongoing verification of treatment accuracy. Portal images can reveal errors in the patient setup position, field size and orientation, or placement and shaping of shielding blocks. Thus they should be taken during the initial treatment setup and weekly thereafter, as recommended by the AAPM Task Group on Radiotherapy Portal Imaging Quality and the recent AAPM Task Group on Comprehensive Clinical Quality Assurance.[24] The actual frequency may be modulated depending on other factors such as:

- Treatment site. (What degree of precision and reproducibility is needed?)
- Patient weight. (Is the patient obese? Are the skin marks fixed relative to internal anatomy?)
- Patient age.
- Patient ability to maintain a fixed position.

Portal images may be taken for all treatment fields or only for a subset. Whatever the case, the frequency of portal radiographs should be clearly defined and included in the department's policy and procedures manual. Regular review takes place at the weekly chart (film) rounds; the current week's portal films are compared side by side with the appropriate reference image. Alternatively, electronic images can be displayed by means of a computer monitor or LCD projector. Approved portal images should be signed (on the film electronically via a radiotherapy PACS) and dated for medicolegal documentation purposes, and discrepancies should be investigated and rectified. Note that altering the patient setup position or skin marks based on a small discrepancy (e.g., <0.5 cm) observed in a single portal image may *not* be appropriate. Rather, it may be more

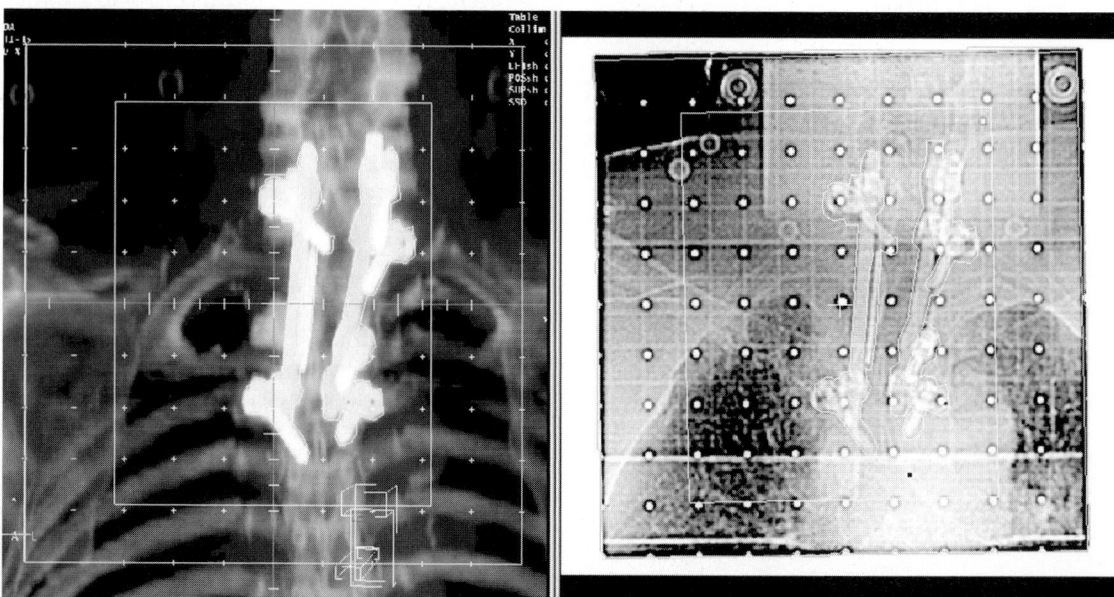

Figure 7–15. Example of template-based portal image registration (Portal Vision, Varian Medical Systems, Palo Alto, Calif.) as applied to treatment of a paraspinal tumor. *Left*: Digitally reconstructed radiograph in which a template is drawn around a surgical metallic (titanium) implant; localization field edge is represented by the outer squared lines. *Right*: portal image (from an amorphous silicon flat panel detector) in which the template has been aligned to the observed implant; differences between the position of the software-detected field edge in the portal image and reference field edge from the DRR indicate the patient setup error.

appropriate to take a repeat image on the subsequent day before effecting a change.

Other Applications of Electronic Portal Imaging Devices in Radiation Oncology

A number of patient position monitoring systems have been developed, including at least one commercial system, that use one or more image detectors together in combination with diagnostic x-ray sources in the treatment room (Fig. 7-16).[31-34] The diagnostic quality radiographs facilitate automatic image registration and beam alignment just before treatment or in real time during treatment. The use of EPIDs for detecting radiopaque markers implanted in the target has received increasing attention as a means of correcting errors in target position from internal organ motion.

An active area of development is to obtain kilovoltage or megavoltage quality 3-D image sets through cone beam image reconstruction.[33,35-37] The cone beam geometry is actually pyramidal in shape, diverging both in longitudinal and lateral directions with its apex at the x-ray source. The source-detector pair moves around the patient to collect a set of 2-D projection images, which are then processed with a cone-beam reconstruction algorithm to obtain a 3-D image set.

Another application that has received increased interest is to verify intensity-modulated treatment fields delivered with a multileaf collimator (MLC). With present algorithms, this is usually accomplished by irradiation of a flat phantom before actual treatment.[38] The images of the subfields comprising the intensity-modulated field are summed in the computer to obtain a 2-D intensity pattern (Fig. 7-17), which is compared to the intended pattern from the treatment planning system. Other uses of EPIDs include *transit dosimetry* to measure the accuracy of dose delivery during treatment, and in accelerator quality assurance procedures.

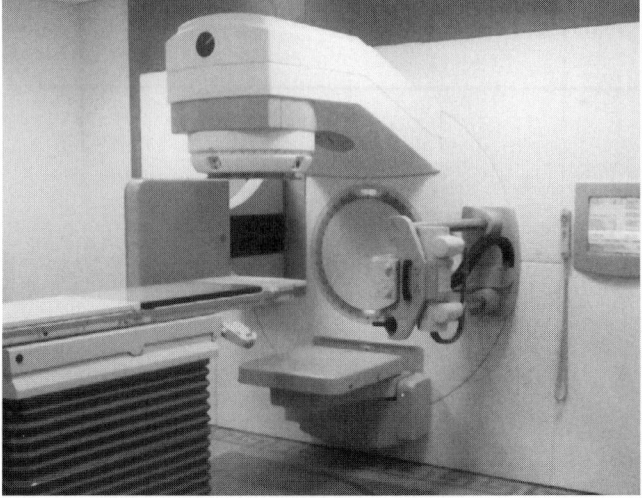

Figure 7–16. Linear accelerator (Elekta Oncology Systems, Norcross, Ga.) fitted with two amorphous silicon flat panel detectors, one for imaging with the megavoltage beam, the other mounted 90 degrees to the treatment head and opposite to a kilovoltage x-ray source. (From Elekta Oncology Systems: Christie hospital among first to evaluate new Elekta technology. *Wavelength*. 2002;6:3.)

LIMITATIONS

Portal radiograph quality is limited primarily by the predominance of Compton scattering at megavoltage energies. Since there is no strong dependence on atomic number (Z), there is very little differential absorption, as is the case at diagnostic x-ray energies. Blurring of structures is caused by a relatively large radiation source (focal spot) and by patient movement during radiation exposure.

There appears to be a systematic degradation of portal image quality with increasing accelerator beam energy. This is attributable to a reduction in subject contrast and in resolution, although the relative importance of these factors is uncertain. Although the decrease in contrast with photon energy, changing from the kiloelectron volt to megaelectron volt range, is a result of the reduced probability of photoelectric interaction, the reduction in image quality with sources above 1 MeV cannot be similarly explained and may be due in part to the increased range of Compton electrons generated in the front screen for film, or in the conversion plate and phosphor screen for CR and electronic portal imaging systems.[39] At the high end of megavoltage photon energies, the situation is further complicated by increased multiple photon scattering and some increase in pair production. Additional degradation of cobalt-60 beam images is due to blurring caused by the relatively large cobalt-60 source size.

The PSP plates used in CR systems are sensitive to ambient light, which can erase the latent stored image. Care must be taken to use dimmed ambient light near the CR reader and to minimize the time between removing the plate from its cassette and scanning it in the reader. EPIDs have a more limited field of view relative to film or PSP plates; in addition, care must be taken not to irradiate the readout electronics outside the detector sensitive area, as radiation damage can shorten detector lifetime.

PORTAL RADIOGRAPH QUALITY ASSURANCE

A quality assurance program for portal films should include regular inspection of radiotherapy film cassettes for repair or replacement; periodic image quality testing and evaluation using a standard phantom; and monitoring and preventive maintenance of the automated film processor. Quality assurance of a computed radiography system should include inspection of both PSP plates and cassettes; periodic image quality testing; monitoring and preventive maintenance of the computed radiography reader; monitoring of available disk space on the viewing workstation; and database maintenance. The images should also be checked for spatial distortions by periodically scanning a geometric test pattern with the reader.

Most EPIDs require a calibration process to correct for inherent systematic artifacts (e.g., variations in sensitivity across the detecting device). For video-based systems, such variations may be caused by the lens characteristics, the geometric configuration, nonuniformity of the phosphor screen, or the camera itself. For matrix ionization chamber or amorphous silicon EPIDs, the sensitivities of the individual chambers or photodiode pixels can vary with time. The AAPM Task Group 58 has reported on acceptance testing, commissioning, and periodic quality assurance of EPIDs.[30] The recommended quality assurance

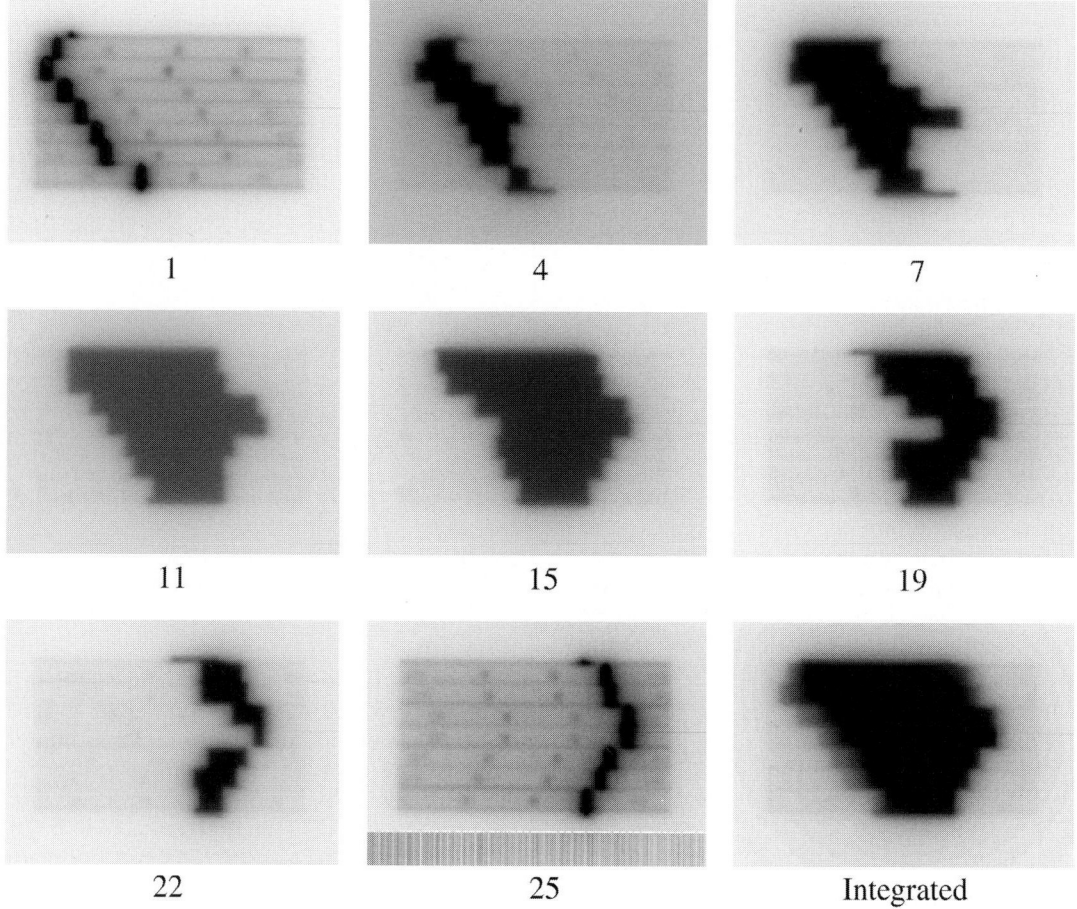

Figure 7–17. Electronic portal images of an intensity-modulated treatment field delivered with a multileaf collimator. Eight images are shown out of a total of 25. Each image is converted into an array of dose values, and summed to obtain an integrated dose map. (From Chang J, Mageras GS, Chui CS, et al: Relative profile and dose verification of intensity-modulated radiation therapy. *Int J Radiat Oncol Biol Phys.* 2000;47:231.)

tasks include tests of the collision interlock system that prevents collision of the EPID with the couch or patient, accuracy of the EPID positioning relative to the isocenter, image artifacts, image resolution and noise using phantoms designed for this purpose, and geometric localization accuracy.

Nuclear Medicine Imaging in Radiation Oncology

Radiation treatment planning has relied on the definition of target volumes from CT (or simulation x-ray films), where the location of the treatment volume is related to the bony anatomy. Nuclear medicine imaging provides supplementary information about the tumor in terms of: extent of metabolic spread (often not readily observed by CT), metabolic activity (frequently equated with cell viability), microenvironmental information (blood flow/hypoxia), and potential properties of the tumor biology and genetics. In addition to potentially assisting in the tumor definition (tumor extent) and radiation treatment prescription (dose painting), there is also a foreseeable role of nuclear medicine imaging in determining tumor response in metabolic rather than geometric terms. A third area of interest is in measures of physiological function for

several normal organs frequently associated with dose limiting toxicity in radiotherapy treatment (e.g., lung).

The strength of nuclear medicine imaging is that it is several orders of magnitude more sensitive than other imaging modalities. How sensitive depends upon the radiotracer used. For example, the typical concentration of ^{18}F-fluorodeoxyglucose (FDG) uptake in a lesion is 0.5 pmole (i.e., almost 9 orders of magnitude lower than the mmole concentrations required for ^{19}F-FDG NMR).[40] Nuclear medicine operates by the "tracer principle," in which a bio-molecule is labeled, is injected into the body, and serves as a precursor for the bio-molecule it mimics. Some tracers are chemically identical to the bio-molecules they mimic (e.g., ^{11}C-glucose or ^{11}C-methionine). Others are synthetic precursors such as ^{18}F-FDG and ^{123}I, ^{124}I, or ^{131}I-iododeoxyuridine, which are not chemically identical, but sufficiently similar to participate in the biochemical process of interest, albeit with slightly altered metabolic rates. The number of possible tracers for nuclear medicine imaging is potentially infinite.

Nuclear medicine imaging is usually divided into two branches: (1) single photon emission gamma camera imaging, including SPECT and (2) PET. The difference between these two modalities is defined by the selection of isotope used for the radiotracer. The following discussion consists of a short section on single photon gamma camera imaging followed by a much larger section on PET. This focus reflects the recent greater interest in PET, because of its greater sensitivity, resolution, and quantitative accuracy (due to the smaller scatter fraction and exact attenuation correction), resulting in higher-definition images.

Single Photon Emission Gamma Camera Imaging

PRINCIPLES OF OPERATION

Most radionuclides emit gamma rays or x-rays and can therefore be imaged by a gamma camera. A gamma camera consists of a detector, usually thallium-activated sodium iodide (NaI:Tl), the purpose of which is to stop the incident photon and convert the energy deposited in the crystal into light quanta and finally an electronic pulse, the amplitude of which is proportional to the energy of the radionuclide emission. In order to determine the direction of the photon emerging from the body, and thereby produce a sharp high-resolution image of the radionuclide distribution within the patient, a collimator is required. The resolution of single photon emission images is optimal between 100 and 250 keV. Both lower and higher energies result in lower sensitivity, due in the first instance to greater self-attenuation in the patient, and in the latter instance to the necessity of thicker collimator septa. More than 90% of conventional nuclear medicine studies use ^{99m}Tc, which emits a single 140 keV gamma ray. Other isotopes in regular use include ^{67}Ga, ^{111}In, ^{123}I, ^{131}I, and ^{201}Tl. The energy resolution of NaI:Tl is 9%, allowing a multi-window acquisition of more than one isotope simultaneously (e.g., ^{99m}Tc and ^{131}I) and the spatial resolution between 7 and 12 mm. Gamma camera imaging is frequently used in whole body mode, where the camera heads produce anterior-posterior projections of the body, to produce spot views, or in SPECT mode, where the heads rotate around the patient to produce a full set of angular projections for tomographic reconstruction (Fig. 7-18).

USES AND LIMITATION OF SINGLE PHOTON EMISSION GAMMA CAMERA IMAGING IN RADIATION ONCOLOGY

Nuclear medicine studies are rarely the primary method of choice for the diagnosis of tumors, with the exception of the role of radioiodine in thyroid cancer, where it also plays an important role in therapy.[41] Nuclear medicine is a sensitive method for the detection of metastatic spread of disease, the most widely used of which is the bone scan agent technetium-99m methylene diphosphate (Tc-99m MDP), for determining the extent of metastatic spread to the bone.[42] A methodology to quantitatively track the progression of bone metastases has been proposed by Imbriaco et al.[43] and is called the "bone scan index." A broader class of tumor diagnostic (and therapeutic) tracers include the somatostatin binding peptides, with selective binding to neuroendocrine cancers.[44] Several groups have evaluated the use of ^{99m}Tc-sestamibi for the detection of breast cancer. One example is Lumachi et al.,[45] who reported that the sensitivity of sestamibi scintimammography reaches 100%

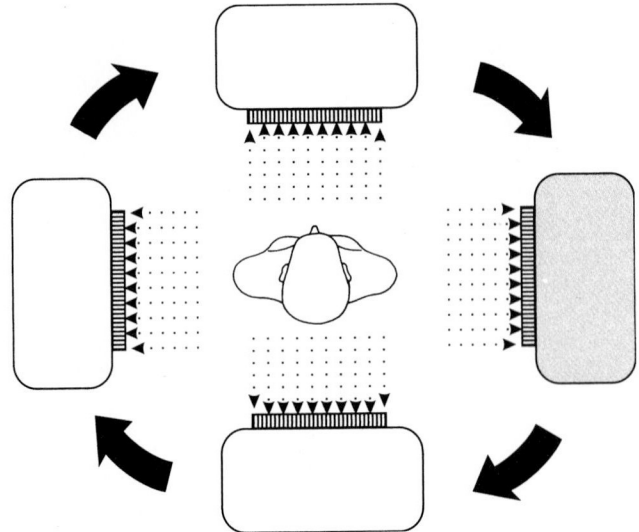

Figure 7–18. Single photon emission computed tomography system. (From Sprawls P: *Physical Principles of Medical Imaging.* 2nd ed. Madison, Wisc: Medical Physics Publishing; 1993.)

in patients with breast lesions ≥8 mm, and that the predictive value of mammography, sestamibi scintimammography, and mammography+sestamibi scintimammography together were 63.4%, 95.1%, and 97.6%, respectively. Lymphoscintigraphy is a procedure in which a radiotracer, ^{99m}Tc sulfur colloid, is injected subcutaneously into sites providing lymphatic drainage to the nodes of interest. Spot views are then taken with a gamma camera at two angles for stereoscopic localization of the nodes. The use of lymphoscintigraphy is the precise localization of the internal mammary/axillary lymph nodes, information from which can be used in the design of radiotherapy portals for breast radiotherapy and in guiding sentinel node biopsy. ^{123}I and ^{131}I- MIBG have been widely used for the diagnosis and therapy of neuroblastoma and pheochromocytoma.[46-47] Gallium-67 citrate has been widely used for detection of cancer, in particular lymphoma,[48] through targeting, internalization, and retention via the over-expressed ferritin receptor. The usefulness and complementarity of ^{67}Ga SPECT and CT in the management of patients with lymphoma have been extensively demonstrated.[49] Gallium-67 SPECT has also been reported to be an essential addition to chest x-ray and CT for radiation treatment planning of mantle cell lymphoma.[50] Another general cell tumor viability tracer, ^{201}Tl, has been used to diagnose tumors as well as measure residual tumor, such as in the brain, post radiation therapy.[51] Others have used ^{201}Tl SPECT imaging in addition to blood flow images with ^{99m}Tc-HMPAO to assist in the differentiation between viable tumor and necrosis in the target definition for stereotactic radiosurgery.[52] A new SPECT imaging agent has emerged to complement ^{67}Ga and ^{201}Tl, which focus on tumor cell viability. This is ^{99m}Tc-annexin V, which can be used to noninvasively measure apoptotic cell death.

Radiolabeled monoclonal antibodies are a generic class of tumor targeting agents of greater specificity and selectivity, but have not gained widespread use, in part due to their complexity and expense. Whether antibodies will achieve their potential status as the ideal tumor-specific imaging agents still remains a question that is reviewed by Bischof Delaloye.[53] The attempt to use antibodies as carriers of therapeutic levels of radionuclide into tumors is called radioimmunotherapy (RIT). Yet, in spite of 25 years of development, RIT has had limited success, with the exception of non-Hodgkins lymphoma, where more durable responses have been achieved relative to all alternative treatment modalities.[54-55]

Evaluation of Normal Tissue Toxicity

Nuclear medicine methods are routinely used to assess normal tissue function (e.g., lung, cardiac, stomach, renal). Although some nuclear medicine tests (e.g., gastric emptying) have not been shown to be sensitive predictors of radiation damage,[56] others may be more useful. The most studied of these, in the context of radiation therapy, have been ventilation and perfusion studies of the lung. Boersma et al.[57-58] and Damen et al.[59] performed perfusion (^{99m}Tc-MAA) and ventilation (^{81}Kr) studies in patients before radiotherapy for patients with Hodgkin's lymphoma to determine the dose-effect relations for regional lung-function changes after radiotherapy. Pulmonary function of 25 patients was re-evaluated 3 to 4 months after irradiation for malignant lymphoma from the 3-D dose distribution, looking at relative reduction of local perfusion and ventilation. By combining the 3-D dose distribution with the average dose-effect relations for local perfusion or ventilation, an overall response parameter was calculated before irradiation, which is predictive for the radiation-induced change in the overall pulmonary function, and possibly for the incidence of radiation pneumonitis, in this group of patients. Valdes Olmos et al.[60] demonstrated that ^{111}In-pentetreotide SPECT scans can delineate areas of radiation pneumonitis, through correlation with areas of decreased ventilation/perfusion and x-ray abnormalities, and may be a potential method of assessing radiation damage. Work is ongoing to evaluate perfusion-weighted optimization in radiotherapy treatment plans for patients with non–small-cell lung cancer. Seppenwoolde et al.[61] compared treatment plans in which the beam weights directed through the hypo-perfused lung regions were increased versus geometrically optimized plans. For patients with one hypo-perfused hemi-thorax, an estimated gain of 6% of the prescribed dose compared to the geometrically optimized plan was reported. No advantage was found in patients with small perfusion defects.

Positron Emission Tomography

The radionuclides required for positron emission tomography are those that undergo β^+ decay. There are numerous positron emitters in the table of nuclides, at least one for almost every element in the periodic table. Whereas at least 95% of current PET procedures use FDG, several other isotopes can and have been used clinically (e.g., ^{11}C, ^{13}N, ^{15}O, ^{82}Rb, ^{124}I). Positrons lose energy on their passage through tissue until they subsequently undergo annihilation with an orbital electron of one of the atomic constituents of tissue. This electron-positron annihilation results in two almost collinear (180 degrees ± 0.3 degrees) photons of 511 keV (the rest mass energy of an electron-positron pair). The coincident detection of these two photons forms the basis of PET. A collimator is not required in PET and so its sensitivity is between 1 and 2 orders of magnitude greater than SPECT. PET scanners can operate in 2-D or 3-D mode. The term 2-D is a misnomer. All modern PET scanners acquire 3-D multiple slice image sets, regardless of 2-D or 3-D mode of operation. The difference lies in whether the acquisition is performed using septa (2-D) or without septa (3-D). The septa serve to restrict the lines of response from the individual (and adjacent) detector rings. In 3-D acquisition mode, no septa are used and oblique lines of response are accepted between several rings of detectors.

Positron emission tomography was developed in the 1970s, but remained practically a research tool until the year 1997, when the Health Care Financing Administration (HCFA) recommended reimbursement of fluorodeoxyglucose (FDG) PET exams for the staging of solitary pulmonary nodules. The HCFA decision was based on the increased number of clinical studies showing the high sensitivity and specificity of FDG relative to CT. HCFA extended its recommendations to: non–small-cell lung, esophageal, colon, melanoma, lymphoma, head and neck (2000), and breast (2002) tumors. Reimbursement, together with the widespread commercial availability of the PET tracer FDG, thereby no longer necessitating that hospitals purchase a cyclotron, has fueled the explosive growth in the number of PET scanners in the industrialized world. Two additional forces have driven the interest in PET: (1) the term "molecular imaging," which broadly includes MR spectroscopy image, optical imaging, and nuclear medicine imaging as modalities capable of imaging the biochemical and molecular processes of cells; and (2) the commercial availability of combination PET/CT units, greatly easing the interpretation of PET exams through precise anatomical registration.

PRINCIPLES OF OPERATION

PET scanners (Fig. 7-19) are typically operated in one of three imaging protocol types: (1) whole body, (2) single field high-count density, and (3) dynamic. In whole body mode, the clinician determines the region of the body to be scanned. This can be limited to the head and neck, thorax, abdomen, and pelvis, but more frequently includes the entire torso from the bottom of the ear to the bladder, dependent upon type of cancer and the known sites of metastases. In some cases (e.g., melanoma), the entire body from head to feet is scanned. PET scans are acquired in a different manner from modern helical CT, where the data are acquired while the patient is translated through the detector ring. PET scanners require a much longer dwell time over each section of the body in order acquire sufficient counts to form a diagnostic quality image. Although PET scanners use a CT couch, the couch remains stationary during the image acquisition time. The length of the patient, which can simultaneously be acquired, is called the field of view. For commercial dedicated PET scanners, the axial field of view is approximately

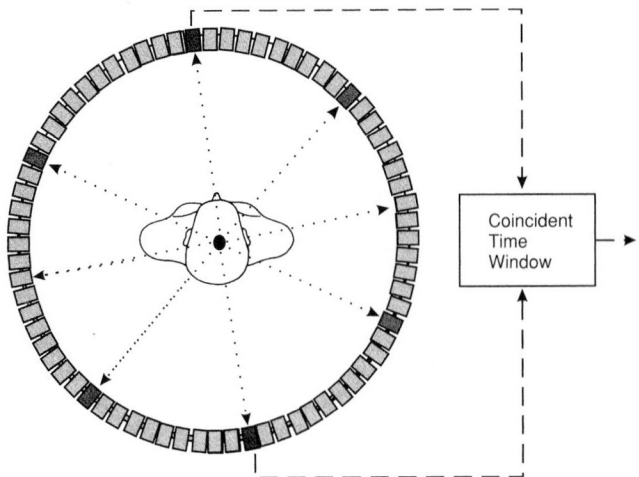

Figure 7–19. Positron emission tomographic imager. (From Sprawls P: *Physical Principles of Medical Imaging.* 2nd ed. Madison, Wisc: Medical Physics Publishing; 1993.)

15 cm. A whole body patient PET scan is obtained piecewise, the couch being moved to the next bed position at the completion of each 15 cm body segment. In 2-D view, the bed is moved by an amount such that the first slice of the new position overlaps with the last slice of the previous bed position. In 3-D view, the amount of overlap is greater (i.e., usually between 15% and 30% of the field length). This required overlap compensates for longitudinal variation in camera sensitivity, which exhibits a triangular response due to the diminishing contribution of oblique coincidence events at the end detector rings of the scanner. The number of bed positions in a whole body PET scan can range from 3 or 4 fields of view up to more than 12 with melanoma patients. The time to acquire each field of view varies from institution to institution, and depends upon the amount of activity injected, patient size, whether it's 2-D or 3-D, and detector material. The shortest emission scan times have been 1 minute per bed position with the latest LSO (Lutetium Oxyorthosilicate)-based PET/CT called REVEAL RT (CTI, Knoxville, Tenn.), but more typical scan times range from 3 to 6 minutes per bed position.

The second mode of acquisition is high-count density studies, for which a single field of view is acquired for 20 to 60 minutes. The improved count statistics of this type of image allow lower contrast features to be observed. This mode of acquisition is mostly used in imaging the brain or heart.

The third type of scan is dynamic mode. A dynamic acquisition also provides a single field of view, except that the full duration of the scan is divided into numerous successive time frames (or bins) that allow the kinetics of the tracer to be observed. Dynamic data, gleaned from the images of successive time frames, are frequently used in compartmental models to generate parametric images (i.e., metabolic rate images). One example is dynamic FDG images of the brain, which, using the Sokoloff compartmental model and measurement of the arterial input function, can be converted to a regional glucose metabolic rate.[62] Dynamic imaging is also useful when establishing the optimal imaging time for a new radiopharmaceutical.

The modes of acquisition discussed earlier all constitute the emission component of a PET scan. When the emission data are reconstructed, it results in a tomographic image set that has not been corrected for attenuation of the 511 keV photons in the patient. Such images exhibit a characteristic hot periphery relative to the central body organs, which appear cold. To rectify this bias, an attenuation map of the patient is used to correct the emission data. On dedicated PET scanners this map is obtained by a transmission scan of the patient, using either a long-lived (270 day half-life) positron generator ($^{68}Ge \Rightarrow {}^{68}Ga$) or a ^{137}Cs singles source, where the linear attenuation coefficient of 662 keV is scaled to 511 keV. Transmission scans take from 1 to 4 minutes per field of view and can therefore constitute a significant fraction of the overall scan time. The recent introduction of PET/CT units replaces the transmission scan by the CT scan, which serves the dual purpose of providing functional/anatomical fusion, as well as the attenuation map for PET reconstruction. The CT obtains the whole body attenuation map in approximately 1 minute, reducing the time of the overall PET examination by 30% to 40%.

FDG Positron Emission Tomography

FDG is an almost ubiquitous cancer-imaging agent for PET. The basis for tumor visualization by PET is the elevation of glucose metabolism by most malignancies. Most PET studies performed today are diagnostic FDG scans. An excellent book that summarizes FDG PET within different tumors is one edited by Wahl.[63] A second is regarding the collaborative effort between University Hospital in Liege, Belgium and the Memorial Sloan-Kettering Cancer Center (MSKCC). This book provides an atlas of FDG case studies on a disease site basis.[64] The increased level of glucose metabolism by cancer cells is frequently reported in clinical practice by the standardized uptake value (SUV). This is a quantitative measure of FDG uptake defined by the ratio of the activity per cc in tumor (per gram assuming unit density tissue) to the administered activity per unit patient mass:

$$SUV = (\text{activity per gram in tumor})/(\text{activity administered per gram of body weight})$$

Clinical scanners are routinely equipped with an SUV tool, which allows clinicians to draw a region of interest (ROI) around the tumor from which the SUV is automatically calculated. SUV has been used to differentiate between benign and malignant disease. For lung nodules an SUV > 2.5 is commonly indicative of malignant lung cancer, although other factors, such as size, shape, and location may reinforce the nuclear medicine clinician's judgment. The magnitude of the SUV is often thought to be correlated with tumor aggressiveness, and there is some animal tumor model data to support this.[65] The most direct clinical evidence for the association between FDG uptake with tumor aggressiveness comes from comparative lesion by lesion analysis in thyroid cancer, which exhibits an inverse correlation between radioiodine and FDG uptake.[66] The variability among tumor types, patients, and even among lesions in the same patient suggests a large variability of glucose metabolism within tumors.[67] Nevertheless, there are reports of the usefulness of SUV in the staging of cancers. One such example is the correlation of SUV in 125 non–small-cell lung cancer patients with survival.[68] Clearly, for any SUV analysis to be meaningful, it is essential in comparative studies that the patient be imaged at the same time post FDG injection, in the same fasted and relaxed state to minimize competitive uptake by the brain, heart, and muscle.

Combination Positron Emission Tomography/Computed Tomography

The current PET/CT scanners are just emerging as fully integrated units, and not just independent CT and PET units, coupled together using a common patient transport assembly (couch). The system is integrated in the sense that the PET and CT image data are physically registered (i.e., the isocenter of one scanner is related to the other by a longitudinal [z-axis] shift). When the CT data is used for attenuation correction, it is reformatted to the same matrix size (128 × 128) and slice thickness as the PET data. For display, the CT data are shown in its original 512 × 512 pixel size, but also at the PET slice thickness (usually 2.125 to 4.25 cm corresponding to the specific manufacturer of the detector size). This is essential if clinicians are to sequentially view corresponding PET/CT slices in a paired or fused format. The acquisition is further integrated in that the PET (like the CT) scan limits are defined from the scout view (topogram), ensuring appropriately matched scan lengths.

The display of the PET and CT image sets assumes that the patient does not move in between the two scans. Since the duration of the PET scan is 20 to 40 minutes relative to the 1 to 2 minute duration of the CT scan, comfortable patient immobilization is essential. It further assumes that the palette, on which the patient lies is rigid upon translation through both CT and PET gantries. The advantages and difficulties of PET/CT were first described in a series of articles on the prototype PET/CT at the University of Pittsburgh.[69-71] From this experience, companies have designed special couch support systems to eliminate couch sag over the extended couch travel required to traverse both CT and PET scanners. The variants of these couches currently include (1) a support pick-up in between the CT and PET to remove sag; (2) moving the entire couch support assembly (instead of the palette), thereby providing a constant sag associated with the palette load through both scanners; and (3) a couch support with two stationary states, equivalent to the longitudinal separation of the two scanners. All current PET/CT systems operate with couch sag differences between the two modalities of <2 mm, according to the manufacturers. For radiation oncology, special flat surface palettes that have holes for the attachment of radiotherapy immobilization devices are available.

Although the benefits of PET/CT scanners, such as improved throughput and diagnosis due to automatic image registration, are apparent, there are drawbacks of these new instruments relative to dedicated PET scanners. The principal drawbacks are: (1) CT attenuation correction and (2) respiration mismatch (discussed in the next section). The first pertains to the inaccuracies in

performing the attenuation correction of the 511 keV emission image from a 40 to 140 kV x-ray source. Patient studies on the GE Discovery PET/CT, which allows both CT and transmission rod attenuation correction, showed average overestimates of about 10% when CT attenuation correction is performed.[72] Additional difficulties have been reported when CT contrast agents are used, where the high linear attenuation coefficient for iodine or barium can result in reconstruction artifacts at sites of contrast pooling. In a study of 60 patients (30 of whom received oral Gastrografin 45 minutes and 30 no contrast agent before PET data acquisition), Dizendorf et al.[73] concluded that oral contrast agent can be used for co-registered PET/CT without the introduction of artifacts in PET. This conclusion may hold for the majority of patients, but not for all.

USES AND LIMITATIONS OF POSITRON EMISSION TOMOGRAPHY IN RADIATION ONCOLOGY

Relatively little work has been performed by radiation oncologists in PET until very recently, principally because of the lack of availability of PET scanners and the image transfer and registration obstacles of incorporating PET images into the radiation treatment planning systems. These hurdles have now been overcome due to the recent appearance of PET DICOM transfer protocols and the commercial availability of PET/CT scanners. It now remains for radiation oncologists to decide how to use PET images in the treatment planning process.

The visualization of FDG images requires considerable care, because the viewing windows are less well defined than for CT. Therefore, the PET window in fused PET/CT displays may be set to provide the best match between PET and CT.[74] This practice can result in a misleading complacency. Erdi et al.[75] defined the PET window setting based on phantom studies, in which spheres of known size, representing lesions, were imaged within different ^{18}F background levels. This study concluded that to accurately define the lesion size, the optimum window setting should set the upper window level to the maximum intensity voxel and the lower level set at a value of 42% of the upper level for spherical lesions of size greater than 4 cc. For smaller lesions, where partial volume effects become significant, the optimum threshold level increased above 42% due to the resolution constraints of the camera. Furthermore, the lower level threshold is not independent of the contrast (lesion–background ratio). Lower contrast necessitated elevating the lower threshold level, if accurate lesion volumetrics were to be obtained. Such empirical methodologies are effective at accurately determining lesion size within a homogeneous background (such as the lung) where the methodology has been validated, but become problematic when attempting to unambiguously define the boundaries of a lesion within a nonuniform background (e.g., the prostate due to the close proximity of the bladder).

The first efforts have focused on using PET to verify coverage of the tumor, especially in lung[76] and head and neck cancers.[77] Numerous reports have been published[78-82] indicating that a significant percentage of patients would have their planned target volume (PTV) altered after the inspection of PET images, principally due to the detection of malignant lymph nodes identified through the PET scan. A future application may be to use the map of FDG uptake (voxel to voxel variation) for intensity-modulated treatment planning. One of the difficulties in using an FDG tomographic image in this way is the uncertainty in the meaning of FDG intensity in a PET image. The FDG uptake in a voxel can depend on many factors: cell number, fraction of tumor/stroma, cell type, distance from capillary supply, pO_2, mitotic index, inflammation, etc. Until the dependence on these factors is well understand, extreme caution is advised if FDG is to be used for dose painting.

Currently, the largest problem associated with PET/CT scanners (and also SPECT/CT) is the misregistration between the PET and the CT image in the thorax, caused by respiratory (and also cardiac) motion. Whereas high-speed CT can acquire images of the whole thorax within one breath-hold, this cannot be accomplished by PET. Any radionuclide imaging modality is count-rate limited, and therefore to obtain images of adequate diagnostic quality, images must be acquired for a minute to several minutes per field of view ($\approx$15 cm). Whereas increasing this field of view to perhaps 30 cm could be beneficial from a radiation oncology perspective, in order to avoid performing the PET scan of the treatment area in two or more axial fields, the cost increases proportionally with the number of detector rings, and so does the length of the tunnel, which may then become claustrophobic to the patient. Despite using state-of-the-art 3-D PET units, it is unlikely that sufficiently short scan times will ever be achieved so as to allow the acquisition of a PET scan in a single breath-hold. For this reason, respiratory gating approaches are under development to reduce/correct motion image blurring (Nehmeh et al., 2002a) and recover the quantitative accuracy of PET.[83]

Respiratory gating, as well as the more standard cardiac gating, divides the acquisition into n individual bins (usually from 4 to 10). Data are acquired in a cyclical manner, with a trigger signal sent to the scanner to initiate the return of data capture to the initial bin 1. For respiratory gating, this trigger can be derived from a number of sources: a spirometer, nasal thermistor, or the respiratory management system (RPM) of Varian, Palo Alto, Calif. In cardiac gating, the trigger is generated from an electrocardiogram (ECG). Since both the respiratory and cardiac cycle can affect tumor motion, dependent on the position of the lesion, either type of gating may be required. Although gating requires slightly longer acquisition times, to compensate for reduced counting statistics, it can result in improvements in volume estimation, fusion with the CT, and quantitation of tracer activity within the tumor.[83-84]

At the present time, no commercial PET/CT radiotherapy simulator is available. However, such instruments are in development. Their design will model the CT simulator, the only difference being that behind the CT scanner (on the same gantry) exists a PET scanner. The primary function of the simulator is to establish an initial treatment-planning reference coordinate, using orthogonal directed lasers for triangulation, determination of the isocenter, as well as the optimum beam configuration and setup parameters for treatment. By integration of the above-mentioned treatment planning software tools, coupled with digitally reconstructed radiographs (with co-registered PET), and a fixed association of the combined PET/CT image display to a laser triangulation system, a PET/CT radiotherapy simulator is readily feasible. Adaptation of the display software to allow digitally reconstructed PET image data to follow the co-registered CT data will be required, where a question remains how the lower resolution PET image data, typically 128×128 pixels versus 512×512 pixels for CT, will affect diagnostic quality when viewed in beam's eye view.

EVALUATION OF TREATMENT RESPONSE

PET provides an alternative perspective relative to CT and MRI in measuring treatment response. Several centers perform FDG scans pre- and postchemotherapy and radiation therapy. The ability to discern viable from necrotic tissue has been an important application of PET, and was first used to assess response after stereotactic radiosurgery.[85] However, the difficulty of separating viable tumor post therapy from inflammation has reduced the reliability of FDG as a quantitative index of response. The potential use of FDG in measuring radiation response has been expressed by Oku et al.,[86] who reported, for rectal carcinoma, a change in the mean value of SUV from 7.6 to 4.2 before and after radiotherapy. There was a significant difference in SUV reduction between the groups with and without recurrence, suggesting SUV to be a good prognostic indicator for long-term prognosis of rectal cancer patients. Allal et al.[87] and Greven et al.[88] have assessed the value of PET FDG in predicting the outcome of radiation therapy for head and neck cancers, concluding that there is little use in early scans 4 weeks post treatment, but improved predictive capacity at several months post therapy.

ALTERNATIVE POSITRON EMISSION TOMOGRAPHY TRACERS

FDG PET has been so successful in diagnostic oncology that it has overshadowed the development of alternative tracers for cancer detection. But not all tumors image well with FDG, because of either low glucose metabolism or proximity to hot structures such as the prostate, unless they are high-grade tumors with metastatic spread.[89] However, which tracers are useful for imaging tumor biology is a big unanswered question and a large area of active research. Some of the PET tracers that have been clinically used for tumor imaging include: ^{11}C-methionine,[90-91] ^{11}C-thymidine,[92] ^{124}I-iododeoxyuridine,[9318] F-FLT,[94] ^{11}C-choline,[95] ^{11}C-acetate,[96] and ^{68}Ga-DOTATOC.[97]

The limited success of FDG in imaging prostate and brain tumors has led to the investigation of new ^{11}C-based tracers for these sites: ^{11}C-methionine,[90-91] ^{11}C-acetate,[96] and ^{11}C-choline.[95] Although ^{11}C has only a 20-minute half-life, limiting the use of these tracers to hospitals with in-house cyclotrons and radiochemistry facilities, the rapid (10-minute) uptake and plateau of ^{11}C-methionine within cancers, due to incorporation within cellular proteins, allows whole body PET imaging with decay correction.[90] The low metabolic amounts accumulated in the bladder result in prostate images of excellent contrast for all three of these tracers relative to FDG. The high rate of glucose metabolism of normal brain limits the application of FDG for the detection of brain tumors. Weber et al.[98] showed that ^{11}C-methionine is superior for the detection of brain tumors, relative to FDG. ^{11}C-choline offers a potential method for distinguishing more aggressive versus less aggressive prostate tissue on the basis of differential incorporation of ^{11}C-choline into cell membrane.[99] This approach may offer an alternative to choline-citrate nuclear magnetic spectroscopy. Studies have also reported potential advantages of ^{11}C-choline over FDG for imaging of the brain[100] and mediastinum.[101] The use of thymidine analogs offers the potential to image cell replication directly, rather than a metabolical process inferring viability, which is especially important when measuring post-therapeutic response.[93,102] Blasberg has used [124]I-iododeoxyuridine with PET to measure the proliferative capacity of brain tumors. The low 0.24 positron abundance of [124]I has led others to investigate fluorinated thymidine ^{18}F-FLT.[94]

The optimum tracer appears also to depend on the unique patient tumor biology. For patients with multiple lesions, visualized by FDG, the relative uptake may vary from site to site. In some cases, when the same patient is scanned with a different tracer, there is imperfect concordance between the two. Examples for this observation include thyroid cancer patients imaged with ^{131}I and FDG[66] and with ^{11}C-methionine and FDG for metastatic prostate cancer.[91] These differences reflect the differing tumor biology and level of differentiation between the individual lesions.

Another class of nuclear medicine imaging agents, which may provide measures of the level of tumor differentiation, are the hormonal receptor binding tracers such as ^{18}F-fluoro-17beta-estradiol (FES) for estrogen levels in breast cancer[103] and ^{18}F-fluorodihydrotestosterone for androgen receptors in prostate cancer,[104] which are now involved in preliminary clinical trials. Alternatively, antibodies with binding specificity for tumor-associated antigens, labeled with a long-lived PET tracer, such as [124]I,[105] [64]Cu,[106] and [86]Y,[107] will provide the ability to perform serial PET imaging for tumor-specific antibodies for several days post administration, with the benefits of greater quantitative accuracy needed for tumor and normal organ dosimetry with radioimmunotherapy trials.

One subject that has preoccupied radiobiologists for more than 30 years is the phenomenon of tumor hypoxia, known to increase the radioresistance of tumors. Methods to noninvasively quantitate the magnitude and fraction of tumor hypoxia are currently being developed. The earliest nuclear medicine studies of tumor hypoxia imaging agents in patients include PET studies with ^{18}F-MISO,[108] and SPECT studies with ^{123}I-IAZA.[109] Since that time, others have been explored: ^{18}F-EF1,[110] [124]IAZG,[111] and [60]Cu-ATSM.[112] In the latter work, Chao and colleagues used the PET images of [60]Cu-ATSM, acquired between 30 and 60 minutes post injection, for the selective targeting of regions of tumor hypoxia by intensity-modulated radiotherapy. Hypoxia tracers, and any other tracer that may potentially provide spatial maps of tumor radioresistance, offer the prospect of dose painting based on 3-D maps of the tumor's radiobiologic attributes, rather than anatomic information alone.[113]

RECENT DEVELOPMENTS

Gene Imaging

A major development driving molecular imaging in nuclear medicine is the development of *SPECT/PET* reporter genes. This technology offers the promise of noninvasive imaging of gene expression and protein transcription. The first systems both relied on transfection of tumor host cells with the herpes simplex thymidine kinase gene *HSV-1-tk*, which selectively phosphorylates, and thus entraps, a thymidine analog within the transduced cell. The first nuclear medicine demonstration of the reporter gene system was published by Tjuvajev, who used an RG2 glioma rat model, which was first imaged by SPECT and later by PET using [131]I-[114] and [124]I-labeled FIAU.[115] Morin[116] and Gambhir et al.[117-118] used a different radioiodinated nucleoside analog, (E)-5-(2-iodovinyl)-2'-fluoro-2'-deoxyuridine, and obtained microPET images using ^{18}F-fluoro GCV as a PET imaging probe. These studies demonstrated the feasibility of using PET for clinically monitoring gene incorporation and expression in gene therapy for cancer.

Further advances in in vivo gene imaging have demonstrated that *p53* activity could be imaged by PET, using the same *HSV1-tk* reporter gene expression and [[124]I] FIAU, but where the *HSV1-tk* reporter gene is placed under the control of an artificial *p53*-promoter, which was retrovirally incorporated into the tumor cell DNA.[119] The ability to noninvasively image *p53* activity provides a means to monitor the effect of radiation and drug efficacy through the activation of *p53*-signaling pathways. The development of several new fusion reporter genes is already under way and will open an entire new horizon of noninvasive tumor imaging. Although most studies to date have been proof-of-principle in rodent model systems, in which viral transfection was performed in vitro or through intratumor injection, human trials are already under way. Jacobs et al.[120] have used liposomal/plasmid-mediated gene delivery of *HSV1-tk* and [124]I-FIAU and successfully imaged patients with high-grade brain tumors by PET.

IMAGE ACQUISITION AND PROCESSING

Image Acquisition, Communication, and Storage

While all relevant modalities have already been described elsewhere in this book, their respective main characteristics can be summarized as follows. CT provides information about the absolute density of tissues as measured by the attenuation of x-rays. By design, CT is better for visualizing dense (i.e., hard) tissues such as the bones, etc. MRI relates to proton (i.e., water) density and relaxation mechanisms while MR spectroscopy (MRS) relates to the finer chemical contents of the tissues. MR is therefore more suited for evaluating tissues containing water (i.e., soft tissues) such as the brain and cartilage. SPECT and PET demonstrate the in vivo metabolism of specific labeled tracers through the detection of radioactive decay.

For any given modality, various information can also be acquired through different protocols: injection of contrast agents in CT or MR, various tracers in SPECT and PET, dynamic acquisitions, etc. All these data may provide different viewpoints for a given anatomical or physiological process. This complementary nature is further discussed and exploited in the multimodality portion of this text.

PICTURE ARCHIVING AND COMMUNICATION SYSTEM

In modern hospitals and radiology departments, all imaging equipment produces and handles digital images and data and is interconnected through a comprehensive picture archiving and communication system (PACS).[121] In a standard PACS design, imaging modalities and equipment such as computed radiography (CR), ultrasound, CT, MR, SPECT, PET, workstations, archive servers, and film printers are all connected together through a backbone/network. By design and function, a PACS encompasses only the physical links and communication protocols between the imaging equipment (production, visualization, and printing) and the archival systems. Image production (e.g., individual modalities) and high-level processing and visualization are independent components that communicate through the PACS but are based on different technical principles. A PACS interacts with hospital information systems (HIS) and radiological information systems (RIS). While the HIS handles the demographics of a patient and his or her global management within the hospital mainly for administrative purposes, the RIS is targeted at radiology's specific needs and deals with workflow management, including modality booking and reporting. By natural extension in the age of the Internet, PACSs often include connections to the outside world for teleradiology and telemedicine applications.

Though the PACS concept initially suffered from a relatively closed proprietary approach of most manufacturers, PACSs now benefit from the widespread acceptance and deployment of the DICOM (Digital Imaging and Communication in Medicine) standard from the American College of Radiology-National Electrical Manufacturers Association (ACR-NEMA).[122] This standard provides a realistic foundation for the exchange—and storage—of all medical imaging data across and between compatible equipment. Through its relative openness, DICOM has standardized access to most scanners' data and has provided a means for independent companies or universities to develop archival and imaging systems that can nicely complement the ones proposed by the major manufacturers.

RADIOTHERAPY PACS

An essential condition for the successful use of electronic portal radiographs in the clinic is that they be a part of a PACS specifically designed for radiotherapy departments. Several such systems are commercially available and provide the various tools that are needed for portal image acquisition and verification, integrating this information with that from other parts of a patient's treatment (i.e., from treatment simulation, planning, and delivery). Radiotherapy PACS functions include transfer of reference images from the simulator, CT simulation, or treatment planning system; portal image acquisition; convenient selection and display of portal and reference images and related patient data; tools for image processing and registration; clinician approval of images; and means of communicating messages related to images among clinicians, therapists, and other radiotherapy staff.

Image Processing

Image processing relates to everything that can modify an image either to enhance its appearance or to extract information from its content. While the following operations will be described for a 2-D image, they can generally be extended to 3-D and more.

WINDOWING

Most digital display systems have historically had a depth of 8 bits (also called a byte). This depth produces 256 (2^8) gray levels or monochrome luminance values from 0 to 255 (= 2^8-1), which is enough dynamic range for the gray nuances that can be differentiated by the human eye. In medical imaging, images generally have a depth of 12 bits (2^{12} > values from 0 to 4095 = $2^{12}-1$, e.g., for CT) or more. From this discrepancy came the need to optimally convert a 12 bit data set to an 8 bit representation. For this conversion, a simple proportional scaling ([0,4095] > [0,255]) would be the most obvious solution. Because of the undersampling it implies, though (16 input values would produce only one output value), it would then become very difficult to assess the subtle density variations actually contained within the initial 12 bit data range. As the full spectrum of 12 bit values is seldom of interest to radiologists, the concept of value windowing was introduced to expand the full contrast of the output/display range over the input density range actually useful for the investigation. For CT, absolute density (or H units, as described earlier) windows are either defined by minimum and maximum values or by center and width in absolute units. Most often on clinical systems, preset windows are used to increase the contrast of specific tissue types as the examples in Figure 7-20A show. Combining several windows on a single representation also allows enhancement of the contrast of several disjoint density ranges (see Fig. 7-20A).

LOOK-UP TABLES

In actual display systems, the conversion between a digital image and the display screen occurs through what is called a *look-up table* (LUT).[123] An LUT simply converts an index derived from the input image data to an output value. This output value is then used to drive the luminance input on the display screen to produce a point whose brightness will be proportional to the incoming signal at the corresponding image location (Fig. 7-20B).

HISTOGRAM EQUALIZATION

The appearance and contrast of images can be enhanced by other means than display window or LUT shape. One method commonly used is to redistribute the pixel values so that they optimally cover the complete available

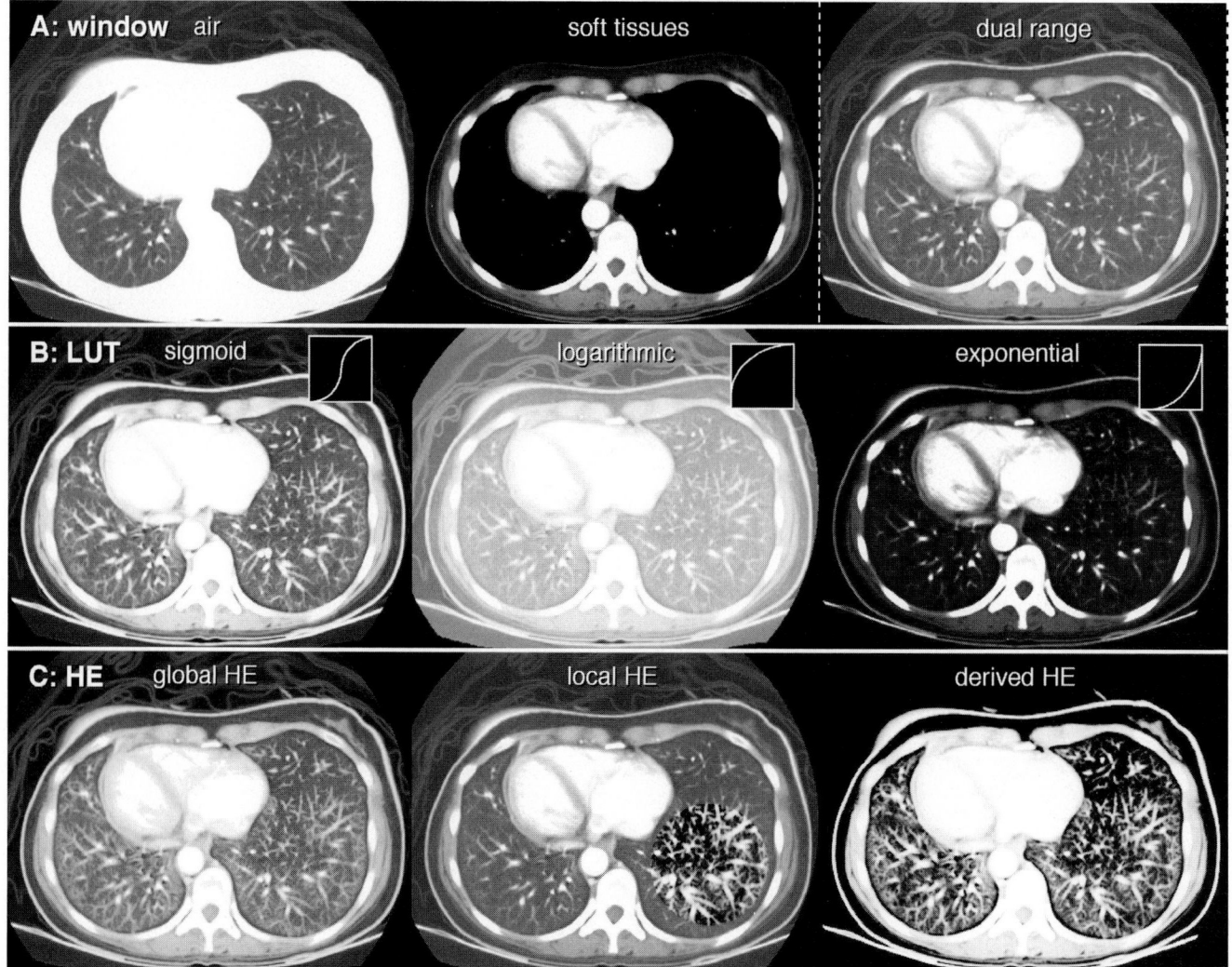

Figure 7–20. Contrast enhancement of a chest computed tomographic image through (**A**) Hounsfield windows, (**B**) various LUT shapes, and (**C**) histogram equalization (global and local). The images in **B** and **C** are based on the dual range image in **A**.

display range of gray levels or intensities. The most common processing of this type relies on the histogram of the initial image. A histogram is a curve that shows, for each possible value in an image, the total number of all pixels at this value. Histogram equalization[124-125] ends up redistributing the initial image values so that the new image's histogram becomes uniform or linear. This spreading, which can be confined to only select parts of the image, produces an optimal contrast in the image (Fig. 7-20C), but, as with changing the shape of the LUT, will suppress the direct linear relationship between displayed and original values.

DIGITAL FILTERING

Space vs. Frequency

As with standard photography, digital images can be processed through various filters to modify, suppress, or enhance some of their characteristics. In biomedical imaging, the application of most digital filters is generally empirical and aims at enhancing visual perception to improve detection of a particular lesion. The user should

always evaluate whether the improvement dangerously distorts the image presentation.

Any 2-D image can be described both in the spatial domain as a collection of pixels, or in the frequency domain as a collection (i.e., spectrum) of frequency components after a 2-D Fourier transform (FT).[126] Because of the space/frequency duality of images through the FT, frequency-based filters can generally be defined and applied in either of these two domains (Fig. 7-21): (1) on spatial images, a kernel (2-D arrays of values used as a filter) is convoluted with the image: every pixel of the original image 2-D array is mathematically combined (i.e., convoluted) with the kernel to produce a new image; (2) on frequency representations, a filter function (frequency window, etc.) is multiplied with the 2-D frequency spectrum representing the FT of the original image. The result is then transformed by the inverse FT to go back to the original 2-D spatial domain in which the new image can be displayed.

In the spatial domain, the main parameter of a filter is the size of the kernel that directly relates to the size of the features to be preserved or affected. Because simple multiplications in the frequency domain take less time

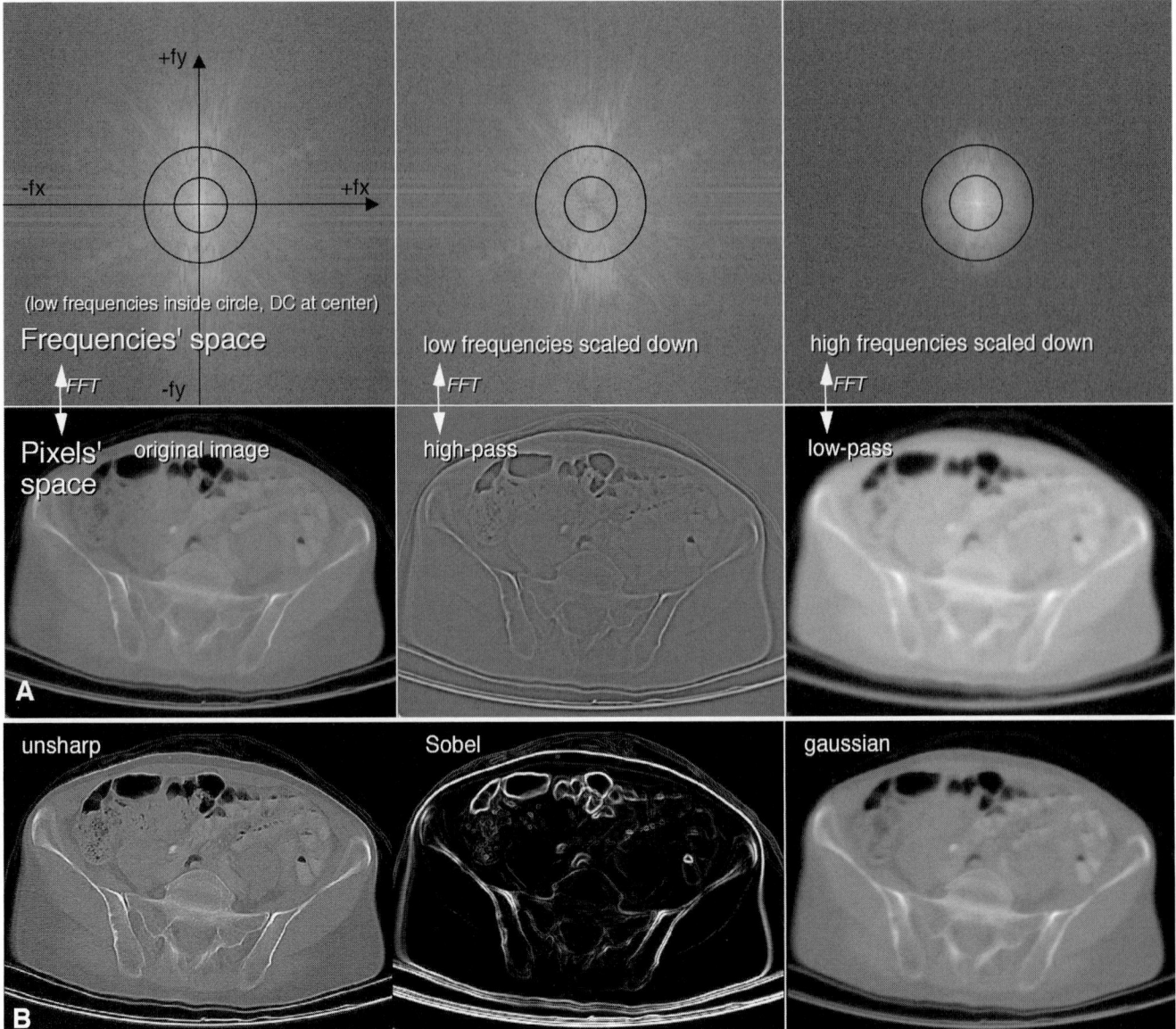

Figure 7–21. Fourier transform and filtering of an abdominal computed tomographic image in (**A**) the frequency and (**B**) the spatial domain.

than 2-D (or 3-D) matrix operations in the spatial domain—and despite the need for a forward and reverse FT to get in and out of the frequency domain—there is generally a significant reduction in computing cost between spatial- and frequency-based convolutions. For this reason, under suitable conditions and although space is intuitively simpler to comprehend than frequencies, Fourier filtering is often used to speed up processing times.

Smoothing Images

Images are smoothed to get rid of small details (irrelevant texture) or some of the noise (e.g., high-frequency components). Such low-pass filtering preserves larger structures (characterized by low frequencies in the frequency domain) while strongly reducing the visibility of smaller ones (see Fig. 7-21).[124-125] Smoothing is most commonly performed through direct averaging of neighbor pixels through a kernel containing only 1s and 0s.

If the values in the kernel are weighted by factors proportional to the distance from the center location, a weighted mean filter is produced. When the weighting coefficients assume a gaussian shape centered at the middle of the kernel, the filter produces a gaussian smoothing.

Median filtering extracts the median value of all pixels overlapped by the kernel after they have been value ordered. This filter produces actual values from the image and preserves edges better than simpler averaging. Median filtering is a type of rank filtering that includes minimum and maximum filters.

Enhancing Details and Edges

Several filters are designed to enhance or extract small features (i.e., high-frequency components) from images (see Fig. 7-21).[124-125] High-pass and first or second derivative filters are generally based on the detection and enhancement of differences and discontinuities (characterized by high frequencies in the frequency domain) within the images. The major problem with such filters is their sensitivity to noise, which generally lies in the high-frequencies. Therefore, enhancing small details and edges often results in increasing noise. To reduce this effect, the output of the filters can be further combined with the original—smoother—image such as in the LoG (Laplacian-of-Gaussian) and unsharp masking filters.

IMAGE SEGMENTATION

In biomedical imaging, segmentation is the extraction from the images of simple features (e.g., points, lines, measurements, etc.) or of complete regions or volumes of interest (e.g., organs, structures). As for image processing, most segmentation operations will be described for 2-D images, but they can generally be easily extended to 3-D and more. Besides the simple visualization of multiplanar reconstruction (MPR) slices (see Visualization later), distances and angles can be computed from 3-D data sets to provide accurate absolute measurements of complex structures. 3-D volumes can also be used to extract (i.e., segment) complete structures of interest and visualize or manipulate them in 3-D.

CONTOURING

A volume of interest (VOI) can be segmented from a volume of data with different techniques depending on the volume or the data characteristics, and on the requirements of the user.[127] Contours can be drawn around a structure of interest on every slice that shows a part of it (Fig. 7-22). At the end of the process, these contours can be displayed on a workstation and interactively

manipulated (translations, rotations, zooms) in real-time to provide a crude 3-D representation of the corresponding structure (see Visualization later).

By preprocessing the initial image through edge filters, contouring can be made to track edges and further help the user define accurate outlines of the objects of interest. So-called active contours or snakes[128] can be seen as a more automated version of edge tracking. An initial contour is modified (e.g., inflated) iteratively to maximize contents while preserving edges and minimizing the contour's energy.

TAGGING/PAINTING, REGION GROWING

Another manual way of extracting a structure is to paint/tag its pixels in every slice that contains a part of it (see Fig. 7-22). A semi-automated variation of the painting approach is the thresholding of data that will extract only the voxels whose value falls within a user-defined value range.

Another variation of tagging is region growing, where all voxels falling into some kind of user-defined condition (e.g., a combination of value range, texture, continuity, topology, gradient, shape) are joined together from a seed in the volume.[129-130] Providing that a good growing criterion can be defined, region growing is a very powerful semi-automated segmentation tool. The seed can either be any specific location inside the 3-D volume, or the result of a previous segmentation. Tagging or growing produces a 3-D mask over the structure of interest. The resulting mask can then be used to apply further processing on the data representing the structure inside the full 3-D data set. Such a mask is generally more comprehensive than contouring as it may include finer and more complex details that are not always easy, or possible, to extract with contours alone.

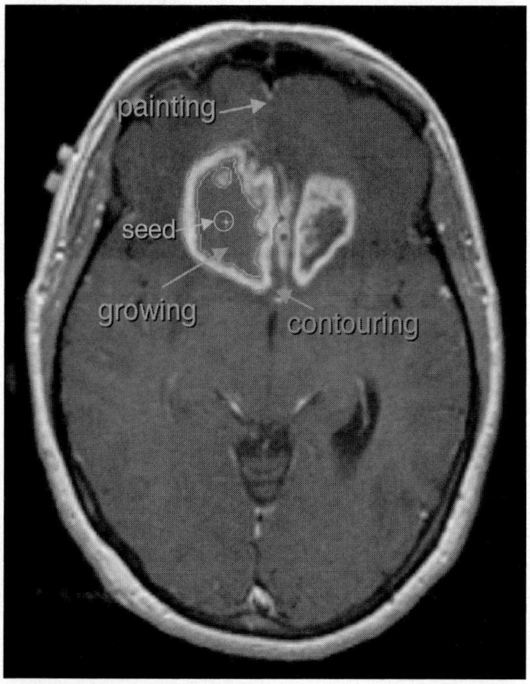

Presentation of Multidimensional (>2-D) Image Data

Digital images can be 2- or 3-D arrays of elements, referred to as pixels (for picture elements) or voxels (for volume elements), respectively. Four-dimensional (e.g., 3D + time) and higher-dimensional data sets can also be generated in the course of an investigation, but they are not addressed in detail here. Because most display systems present images in a 2-D format, multi-dimensional entities (3-D and more) need to be formatted to accommodate and exploit this situation. With the advent of modern hardware and standards [OpenGL], more of these capabilities are actually performed on sophisticated graphical boards and require fewer software developments.

2.5-D DISPLAY OF 3-D DATA SETS: SLICES AND MULTI-PLANAR RECONSTRUCTION

All tomographic modalities produce cross-sectional slices presented as 2-D images (called source images). Window-based display systems allow the screen space to be partitioned between various images, which can be either from the same study or from different ones. Each data set can be displayed with its own parameters (value windowing, color scale, zoom, etc.).

Figure 7–22. Segmentation of a magnetic resonance brain tumor image through contour, painting, and region growing. See also Color Figure 7-22.

For tomographic modalities, source images can be stacked together to recreate the volume in the field of view (FOV) at the time of the acquisition. This volume can then be cut along orthogonal planes (standard multi-planar reconstruction, or MPR)[131] in order to produce images with orientation other than those of the source images (Fig. 7-23A). Such a representation can be very useful to display structures that are not "well oriented" in regard to the original acquisition's main axis. A natural extension of the classical orthogonal MPR approach is the oblique plane extraction and display, which shows a cut of the reconstructed volume along any arbitrary plane (Fig. 7-23B).[132] Another extension of MPR is the curved plane extraction and display, which shows a bi-dimensional nonplanar cut along a 3-D curved path inside the reconstructed volume (Fig. 7-23C).

Because tomographic volumes are generally anisotropic (the elementary voxels do not have the same absolute size on all three axes), the initial data most often need to be interpolated to produce adequately reconstructed images in orientations other than that of the acquisition.

3-D DISPLAY OF 3-D DATA SETS

As previously mentioned, tomographic data sets are made up of 2-D slices that are discrete cuts through a 3-D volume considered as static during the whole acquisition. Under this assumption, these data can be used to extract and visualize information or objects in volumetric rendering or anatomical rendering that are more realistic than 2-D slices alone. These 3-D renderings can be assessed in direct relation to the patient's actual morphology.

Contour, Wireframe Display

For a simpler approach, contours can be drawn manually or (semi-) automatically on the source images (see Image Segmentation earlier). Contours from the same structure can then be grouped together across slices and rendered by using the spatial parameters (e.g., pixel size and slice spacing) of the source images (Fig. 7-24A). When the contour points of the same structure are joined across slices, the final display makes up a wireframe enclosing the structure of interest (Fig. 7-24B), which can be manipulated interactively on a screen (see 3-D Manipulation later).

Surface Rendering

DEFINING SURFACES. To further refine the representation of objects, their defining voxels (contour points, mask elements, etc.) —which can simply be specified by a given threshold—can be joined together by small triangular/polygonal surfaces or tiles, which will be merged to represent the outer shell of the structure of interest.[135]

SURFACE VISUALIZATION. Once a digital surface has been extracted, it can be given various properties regarding its representation, color, transparency (or opacity), and response to external lighting.[133] The easiest way to understand how a digital object is represented on a screen to an observer is through the ray tracing paradigm (Fig. 7-24C).[133] In ray tracing, rays extend from infinity through the object and toward the observer (ray casting being the opposite).

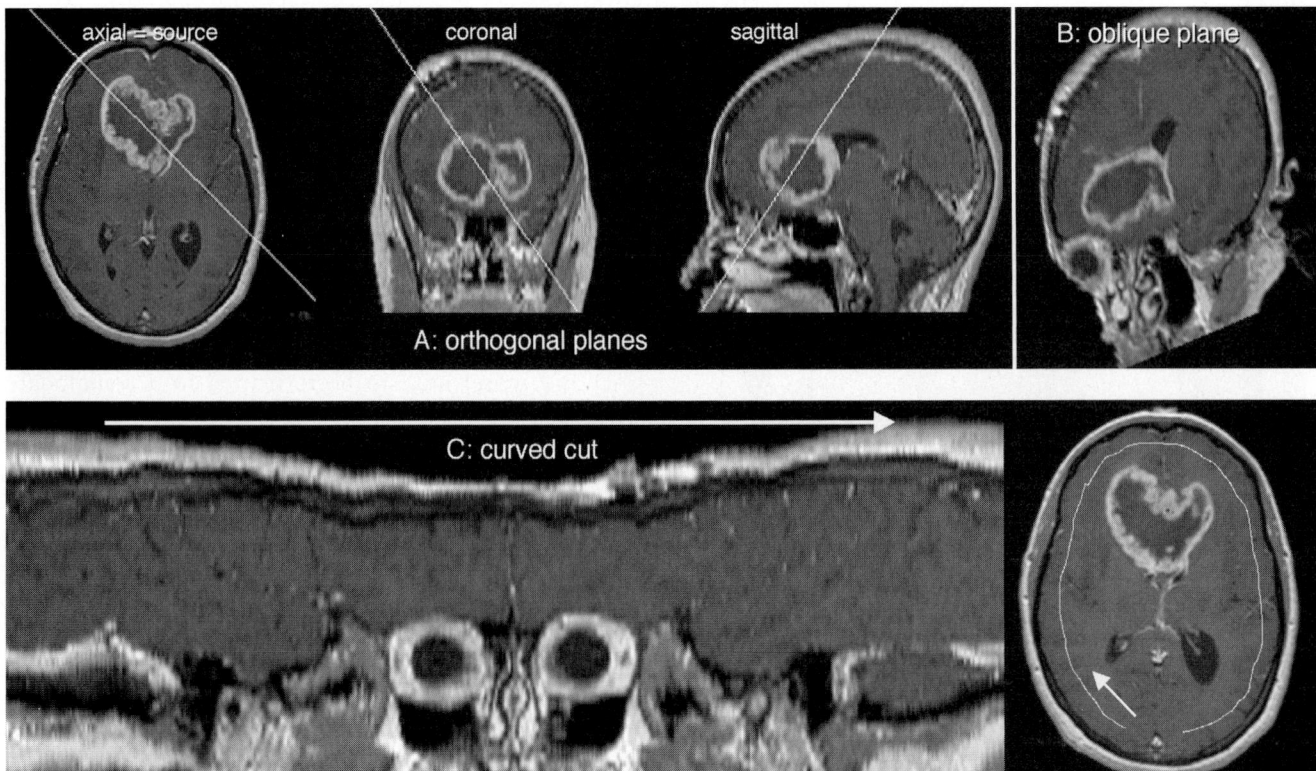

Figure 7–23. A, orthogonal; **B,** oblique; and **C,** curved multi-planar reconstruction from a head magnetic resonance volume.

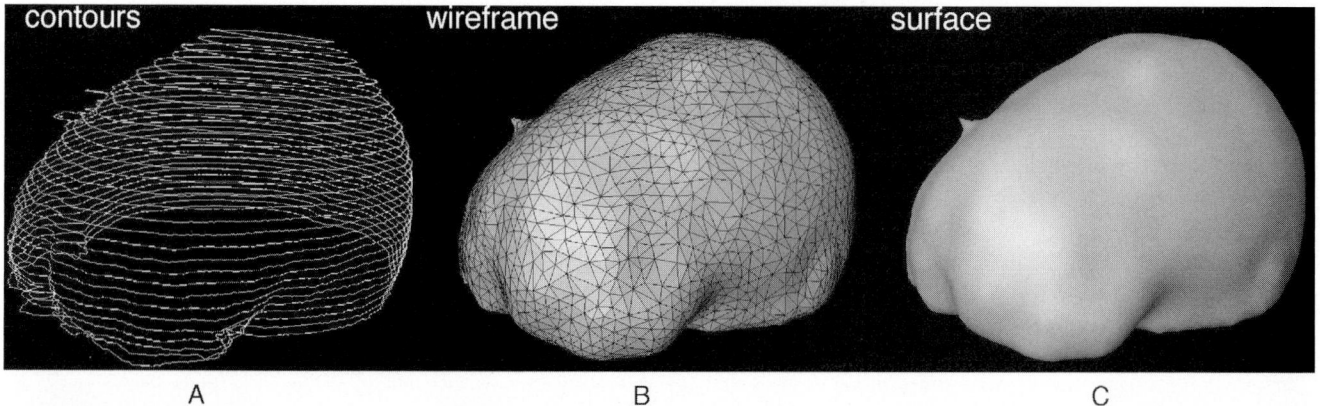

Figure 7–24. Segmented brain from a head computed tomographic image: **A,** contours; **B,** wireframe; and **C,** surface.

3-D MANIPULATION. A successful concept for 3-D manipulation is the virtual trackball, which assumes that the object (i.e., its contour/wireframe/surface representation) is at the center of a sphere. The user can then rotate and translate the sphere/object by simple manipulation of a standard input device such as a mouse. More sophisticated 3-D input devices can also be used to track motion (such as breathing) or instruments and persons in a surgical setting.

Volume Rendering

Compared to surface rendering, volume rendering (VR)[127,133] does not intrinsically require the segmentation of structures, but uses all the voxels from the volume simultaneously. For VR, voxels are assigned a color and an opacity/transparency that can be linked to their value (e.g., through an LUT scheme) or to other characteristics (Fig. 7-25). The volume is then represented to the user/observer through the same ray tracing (or casting) paradigm as the one described before for rendering surfaces. A special (simplified) mode of VR is maximum intensity projection (MIP), where only the highest value on a ray is projected to the observer (Fig. 7-26*B*). This technique is mainly used for rendering isolated, high contrast objects such as bones or vascular structures in CT or MR angiography. Because there is no binary decision

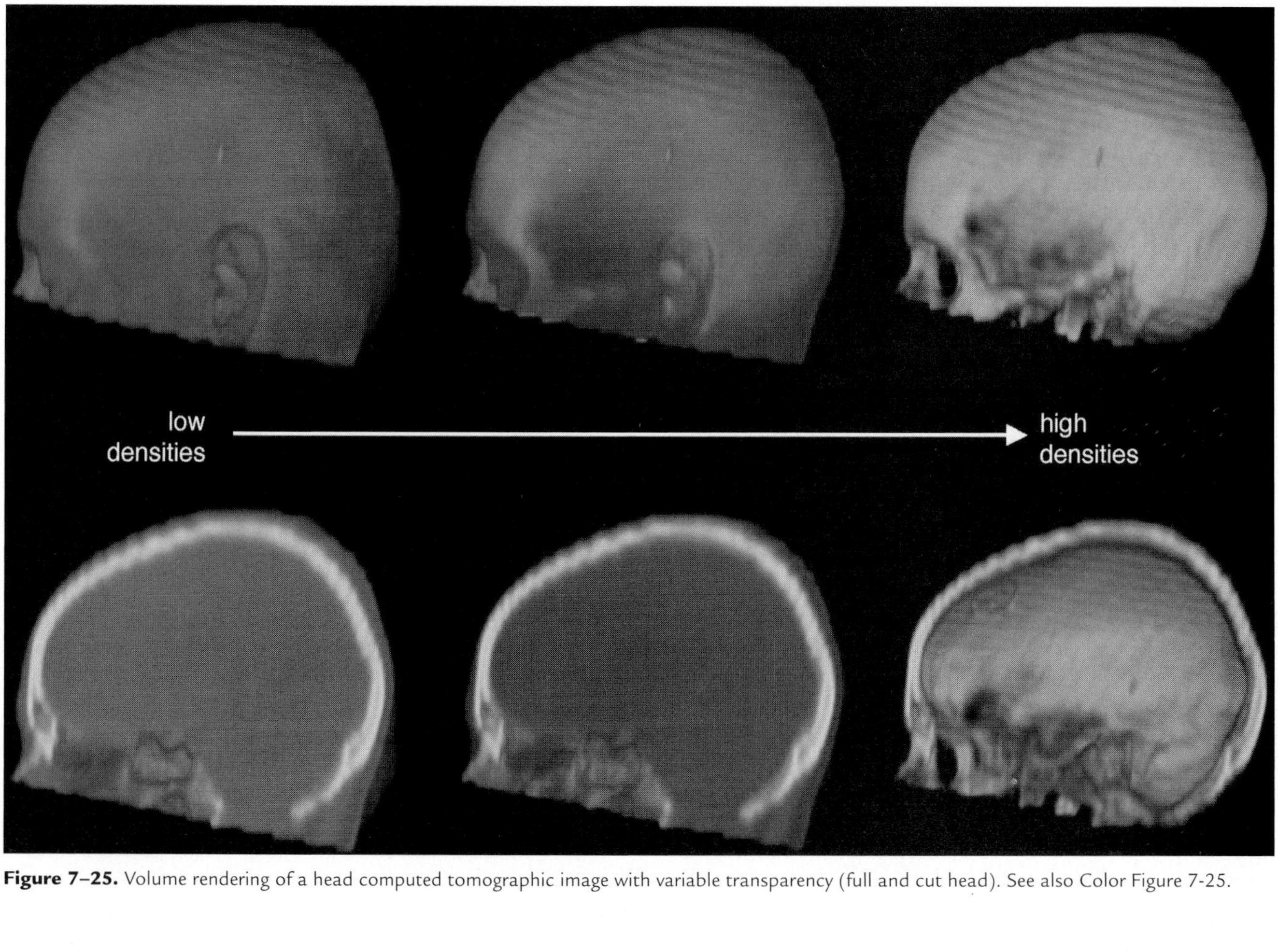

low
densities

high
densities

Figure 7–25. Volume rendering of a head computed tomographic image with variable transparency (full and cut head). See also Color Figure 7-25.

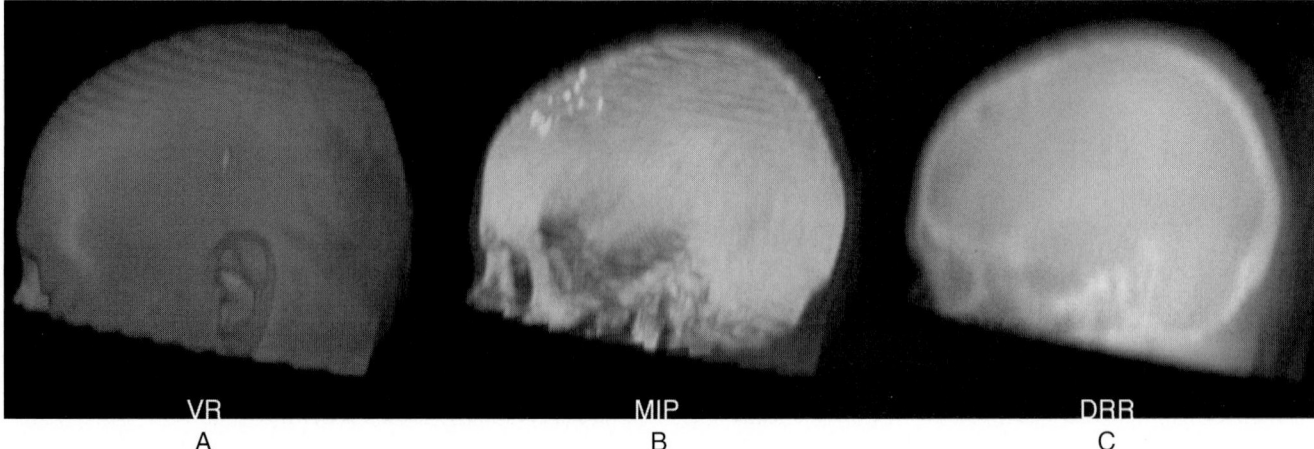

Figure 7-26. Comparison of VR (**A**) with maximum intensity projection (**B**) and digitally reconstructed radiograph (**C**). See also Color Figure 7-26.

such as when setting a surface threshold, VRs generally look more realistic and convey more textural information than surface renderings. A VR approach also allows arbitrary cuts to be performed through the whole volume and rendered to the user in relation to the 3-D VR.

Digitally Reconstructed Radiographs

DRRs (discussed previously) are a special application of VR. They simulate a standard 2-D projection x-ray image (such as on a film or from a portal system) from the original CT volume data. By applying strict models based on the absolute H units of the CT image, on the properties of the x-rays, and on the response of the detector (e.g., film, phosphor, EPID) to be simulated, DRRs can be made to look very realistic. By tuning intensity and transparency, and selecting among various combination techniques (direct integration, weighed integration, etc.) of CT voxels along the rays, DRRs can also look many different ways, including realistic (Fig. 7-26C). Radiation energies that mimic simulator or mimic 6 MV can be simulated when generating the DRR. An obvious plus when compared to traditional x-ray planar projections (e.g., from film or C-arm) is that the DRR orientation can be totally arbitrary and linked to any given geometric transformation. This feature can be used, for example, when trying to align a planning data set to the patient during treatment. An important characteristic of DRRs that sets them apart from traditional VR is that they use a cone beam geometry for the simulation of a point x-ray source. Perspective imaging, which has not been addressed here but can simply be added to the viewing transformation during ray tracing, actually relates to such geometry.

IMAGE CORRELATION AND FUSION

As most imaging modalities are based on different principles, they provide different viewpoints (such as anatomy and metabolism) on the same reality: the patient. The synthetic data sets produced by registering and combining modalities—or computed parameters—can therefore be used for improving diagnosis and the targeting and planning of therapy.

Similar registration approaches can also be used to correct for a patient's motion or repositioning.

PARAMETRIC IMAGING

Besides doses calculated by computerized planning systems, relevant parameters for RT targeting or assessment may be extracted from dynamic data sets (either PET or MR). For MR or PET, a contrast agent or tracer, respectively, is injected and rapid imaging provides a dynamic sequence of the flow and uptake of the material in the body. Image-based dynamic parameters such as time of arrival, maximum uptake slope, or time of maximum contrast can be extracted and mapped onto the anatomic image. Subtle variation in the dynamics of the contrast or tracer may provide added information for the identification of tumors or other structures.[134-135] Slightly more complex compartmental modeling approaches indirectly estimate metabolic parameters.[136]

MULTIMODALITY IMAGING

Because of different technical principles and responses to specific protocols, data coming from various modalities or protocols—and the parameters that can be extracted by further processing—are most often complementary when it comes to evaluating in vivo morphology or metabolism.[137-139] The goal of multimodality imaging is therefore to merge all information at hand to better synthesize and assess its global content.[138] This approach can be used either for visualizing information of a complementary nature simultaneously, or for enhancing information from one modality with data or parameters extracted from another one.[137]

MULTIMODALITY REGISTRATION

Although the data sets of interest should all represent the same volume (or a reasonable overlap of it), they seldom do it at the exact same spatial location and therefore need to be registered together before direct comparison can take place.

The simpler way to align images with enough similar features is through the interactive manipulation of the geometric transformation (e.g., translations and rotations about the three axes; also scales for affine transformations) with direct feedback from the overlaid images.[140] Although rather tedious at times, particularly with low-resolution data sets, this technique can achieve reasonably good results. Because it is the only interactive technique that can be implemented in clinical applications, it also is a necessary component of any registration system either as a preliminary step (e.g., to get near the optimal solution) or as a final correction step for more complex, sensitive but still error-prone techniques.

Other simple registration techniques align paired landmarks (either fiducial markers or anatomic landmarks) between two data sets.[141] While the most common way is to select the landmarks by hand—or semi-automatically when their geometry is known enough—automated methods attempt to select the best landmarks through a given criterion. For example, ridge-based techniques[142] would select as registration landmarks the points of greater spatial change.

Various geometric landmarks—such as significant points, lines, curves, and surfaces—can also be combined and paired (e.g., through an iterative distance minimization algorithm).[143,144] For iterative algorithms based on

Euclidean distance, precalculating 3-D distance maps from the features to be aligned[145-146] can drastically speed up calculations. As a general rule, the more distributed the landmarks, the more robust is the result of an alignment. This rule obviously puts a heavier weight on the landmark selection process, which therefore needs to be objective and accurate.

Unsupervised (i.e., fully automatic) volume-based registration techniques can help to relieve this burden. These techniques rely on the fact that even if the data to align are complementary, they still "look" similar enough to a given iterative registration algorithm. At each iteration, a similarity measure between the reference volume and the match volume (the volume to be realigned, which is transformed by the current geometric transformation) is calculated, and a new transformation is calculated through a given minimization technique.[147-148] The similarity measure is analog to a distance or an alignment cost and can take several forms depending on the registration paradigm.[149-151] For intra-modality registration or similar enough modality pairs (e.g., CT-CT, MR-MR, PET-PET), voxel differences, ratios, or image correlation can be used as costs. For dissimilar modalities (e.g., CT-PET, CT-MR,

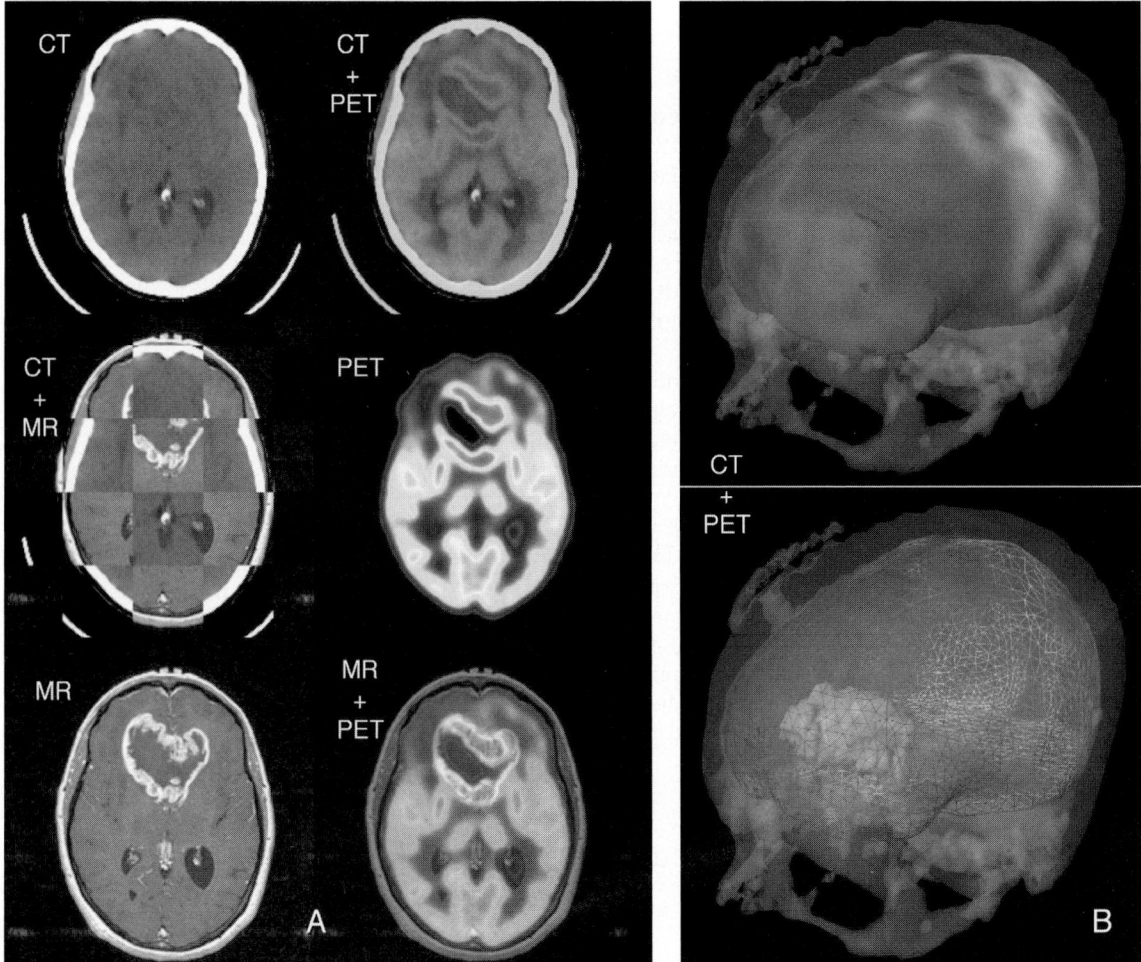

Figure 7–27. Multimodality (MM) visualization of a brain tumor. **A,** Multi-planar reconstruction (side-by-side, checkerboard and colorwash modes) of computed tomography (CT), magnetic resonance (MR), and positron emission tomography (PET) of the same patient after spatial registration. **B,** surface rendering of the skull and brain from CT, tumor from MR, and color from the PET. MM volume rendering can follow similar paradigms. See also Color Figure 7-27.

MR-PET), voxel ratio or entropy-based measures (joint entropy, mutual information) are generally more relevant.[152,153]

While the hybrid modality concept (e.g., PET/CT or SPECT/CT) appears to solve the registration issue in the best manner, it is worth mentioning that, in the current design, the modalities are still acquired sequentially. To compensate for possible motion or physiology or both between the two acquisitions, registration techniques still need to be available and used whenever necessary.

Visualizing Multimodality Data Sets

Once registered, two data sets can be represented as two side-by-side 2-D sets of MPR images, with or without a coupled cursor. Another way is to blend both images—with different color scales and a varying blending ratio—into a single one. When dealing with 3-D objects, objects extracted from one data set can be visualized along objects extracted from the other one. Finally, information from one data set (e.g., the "functional" one) can be projected on the surface of objects from the other one (e.g., the "anatomical" one) (Fig. 7-27). Such merging of information[140] can obviously also take place with volume-rendering techniques.

SUMMARY AND CONCLUSIONS

The importance of imaging in radiation oncology cannot be overemphasized. With the advent of CT and MRI, our ability to "see" inside the patient and obtain geometrically accurate information has been significantly improved. Development of tools to incorporate this information in treatment planning and delivery has been in progress and has contributed to improved radiotherapy, and will likely continue to do so. Nevertheless, advances in a number of important areas are needed.

Perhaps the most needed improvement, and the most difficult to achieve, is *the ability to better define the extent of disease*, including regions of microscopic extensions. Related to this is the substantial variability in delineating target volumes.[154] Another deficiency is the poor contrast of portal images (due to the high photon energies), which negatively affects treatment delivery verification. The use of low-energy photons for portal imaging is being explored to circumvent this problem. A related issue, the uncertainty introduced by organ motion during treatment, which compromises the valid comparison of planning images and treatment verification images, is being actively studied.

REFERENCES

1. Fuks Z, Leibel SA, Wallner KE, et al: The effect of local control on metastatic dissemination in carcinoma of the prostate: Long-term results in patients treated with 125-I implantation. *Int J Radiat Oncol Biol Phys.* 1991;21:537.
2. Leibel SA, Kutcher GJ, Mohan RM, et al: Three-dimensional conformal radiation therapy at the Memorial Sloan-Kettering Cancer Center. *Semin Radiat Oncol.* 1992;2:274.
3. Leibel SA, Ling CC, Kutcher GJ, et al: The biological basis for conformal three-dimensional radiation therapy. *Int J Radiat Oncol Biol Phys.* 1991;21:805.
4. Leibel SA, Heimann R, Kutcher GJ, et al: Three dimensional-conformal radiation therapy in locally advanced carcinoma of the prostate: Preliminary results of a phase I dose escalation study. *Int J Radiat Oncol Biol Phys.* 1994;20:55.
5. Lattanzi J, McNeely S, et al: Daily CT localization for correcting portal errors in the treatment of prostate cancer. *Int J Radiat Oncol Biol Phys.* 1998;41:1079.
6. Mackie TR, Balog J, et al: Tomotherapy. *Semin Radiat Oncol.* 1999;9:108.
7. Yan D, Lockman D, et al: An off-line strategy for constructing a patient-specific planning target volume in adaptive treatment process for prostate cancer. *Int J Radiat Oncol Biol Phys.* 2000;48:289.
8. Ford E, Mageras GS, et al: Evaluation of respiratory movement during gated radiotherapy using film and electronic portal imaging. *Int J Radiat Oncol Biol Phys.* 2002;52:522.
9. Ford EC, Mageras GS, et al: Respiration-correlated spiral CT: A method of measuring respiratory-induced anatomic motion for radiation treatment planning. *Med Phys.* 2003;30:88.
10. Hamilton RJ, Sweeney, PJ, et al: Functional imaging in treatment planning of brain lesions. *Int J Radiat Oncol Biol Phys.* 1997;37:181.
11. Pickett B, Vigneault E, et al: Static field intensity modulation to treat a dominant intra-prostatic lesion to 90 Gy compared to seven field 3-dimensional radiotherapy. *Int J Radiat Oncol Biol Phys.* 1999;44:921.
12. Zaider M, Zelefsky MJ, et al: Treatment planning for prostate implants using magnetic-resonance spectroscopy imaging. *Int J Radiat Oncol Biol Phys.* 2000;47:1085.
13. DiBiase SJ, Hosseinzadeh K, et al: Magnetic resonance spectroscopic imaging-guided brachytherapy for localized prostate cancer. *Int J Radiat Oncol Biol Phys.* 2002;52:429.
14. Kurhanewicz J, Vigneron DB, et al: Three-dimensional H-1 MR spectroscopic imaging of the in situ human prostate with high (0.24-0.7-cm³) spatial resolution. *Radiology.* 1996;198:795.
15. Zakian KL, Koutcher JA, et al: Developments in nuclear magnetic resonance imaging and spectroscopy: Application to radiation oncology. *Semin Radiat Oncol.* 2001;11:3.
16. Bharatha A, Hirose M, et al: Evaluation of three-dimensional finite element-based deformable registration of pre- and intraoperative prostate imaging. *Med Phys.* 2001;28:2551.
17. McJury M, Oldham M, et al: Radiation dosimetry using polymer gels: Methods and applications. *Br J Radiol.* 2000;73:919.
18. Hricak H, Humm J, Ling C, et al: Innovations in oncologic imaging. In DeVita VT, Hellman S, Rosenberg SA, eds. *Principles and Practice of Oncology.* vol. 15, no. 11. Philadelphia: Lippincott, Williams & Wilkins; 2001:1.
19. Kini VR, Edmundson GK, et al: Use of three-dimensional radiation therapy planning tools and intraoperative ultrasound to evaluate high dose rate prostate brachytherapy implants. *Int J Radiat Oncol Biol Phys.* 1999;43:571.
20. Mintz GS, Weissman NJ, et al: Intravascular ultrasound assessment of the mechanisms and results of brachytherapy. *Circulation.* 2001;104:1320.
21. Lattanzi J, McNeeley S, et al: A comparison of daily CT localization to a daily ultrasound-based system in prostate cancer. *Int J Radiat Oncol Biol Phys.* 1999;43:719.
22. Mohan DS, Kupelian PA, et al: Short-course intensity-modulated radiotherapy for localized prostate cancer with daily transabdominal ultrasound localization of the prostate gland. *Int J Radiat Oncol Biol Phys.* 2000;46:575.
23. Mageras GS, Yorke E, et al: Fluoroscopic evaluation of diaphragmatic motion reduction with a respiratory gated radiotherapy system. *J Applied Clin Med Phys.* 2001;2:191.
24. Kutcher GJ, Coia L, et al: Comprehensive QA for radiation oncology: Report of AAPM Radiation Therapy Committee Task Group 40. *Med Phys.* 1994;21:581.
25. (NCRP), N. C. o. R. P. a. M.: *Quality Assurance for Diagnostic Imaging Equipment.* (Report 99). Bethesda, Md., NCRP, 1988.
26. Reinstein LE, Amols HI, et al: *Radiotherapy Portal Film Quality.* (AAPM Technical Report No. 24). Madison, WI, Medical Physics Publishing, Reinstein, LE, Amols HI, 1987.
27. Hurkmans CW, Remeijer P, et al: Set-up verification using portal imaging; review of current clinical practice. *Radiother Oncol.* 2001;58:105.
28. Droege RT, Bjarngard BE: Influence of metal screens on contrast and megavoltage x-ray imaging. *Med Phys.* 1979;6:487.

29. Haus AG, Dickerson RE, et al: Evaluation of a cassette screen-film combination for radiation therapy portal localization imaging with improved contrast. *Med Phys.* 1997;24:1605.

30. Herman MG, Balter JM, et al: Clinical use of electronic portal imaging: Report of AAPM Radiation Therapy Committee Task Group 58. *Med Phys.* 2001;28:712.

31. Murphy MJ: An automatic six-degree-of-freedom image registration algorithm for image-guided frameless stereotaxic radiosurgery. *Med Phys.* 1997;24:857.

32. Schewe JE, Lam KL, et al: A room-based diagnostic imaging system for measurement of patient setup. *Med Phys.* 1998;25:2385.

33. Jaffray DA, Drake DG, et al: A radiographic and tomographic imaging system integrated into a medical linear accelerator for localization of bone and soft-tissue targets. *Int J Radiat Oncol Biol Phys.* 1999;45:773.

34. Shirato H, Shimizu S, et al: Four-dimensional treatment planning and fluoroscopic real-time tumor tracking radiotherapy for moving tumor. *Int J Radiat Oncol Biol Phys.* 2000;48:435.

35. Cho PS, Johnson RH, et al: Cone-beam CT fo radiotherapy applications. *Phys Med Biol.* 1995;40:1863.

36. Mosleh-Shirazi MA, Evans PM, et al: A cone-beam megavoltage CT scanner for treatment verification in conformal radiotherapy. *Radiother Oncol.* 1998;48:319.

37. Ford EC, Chang J, et al: Cone-beam CT with megavoltage beams and an amorphous silicon electronic portal imaging device: Potential for verification of radiotherapy of lung cancer. *Med Phys.* 2002;29:2913.

38. Chang J, Mageras GS, et al: Relative profile and dose verification of intensity-modulated radiation therapy. *Int J Radiat Oncol Biol Phys.* 2000;47:231.

39. Amols HI, Reinstein LE, et al: A quantitative assessment of portal film contrast as a function of beam energy. *Med Phys.* 1986;13:711.

40. McSheehy PM, Leach MO, Judson IR, Griffiths JR: Metabolites of 2'-fluoro-2'-deoxy-D-glucose detected by 19F magnetic resonance spectroscopy in vivo predict response of murine RIF-1 tumors to 5-fluorouracil. *Cancer Res.* 2000;60:2122.

41. Maxon HR: Detection of residual and recurrent thyroid cancer by radionuclide imaging. *Thyroid.* 1999;9:443.

42. Krasnow AZ, Hellman RS, Timins ME, et al: Diagnostic bone scanning in oncology. *Semin Nucl Med.* 1997;27:107.

43. Imbriaco M, Larson SM, Yeung HW, et al: A new parameter for measuring metastatic bone involvement by prostate cancer: The bone scan index. *Clin Cancer Res.* 1998;4:1765.

44. Weiner RE, Thakur ML: Radiolabeled peptides in the diagnosis and therapy of oncological diseases. *Appl Radiat Isot.* 2002;57:749.

45. Lumachi F, Zucchetta P, Marzola MC, et al: Positive predictive value of 99mTc sestamibi scintimammography in patients with non-palpable, mammographically detected, suspicious, breast lesions. *Nucl Med Commun.* 2002;23:1073.

46. Brisse H, Edeline V, Michon J, et al: Current strategy for the imaging of neuroblastoma. [Article in French]. *J Radiol.* 2001;82:447.

47. Monsieurs M, Brans B, Bacher K, et al: Patient dosimetry for (131)I-MIBG therapy for neuroendocrine tumours based on (123)I-MIBG scans. *Eur J Nucl Med Mol Imaging.* 2002;29:1581.

48. Anderson KC, Leonard RC, Canellos GP, et al: High-dose gallium imaging in lymphoma. *Am J Med.* 1983;75:327.

49. Chajari M, Lacroix J, Peny AM, et al: Gallium-67 scintigraphy in lymphoma: Is there a benefit of image fusion with computed tomography? *Eur J Nucl Med Mol Imaging.* 2002;29:380.

50. Jochelson MS, Herman TS, Stomper PC, et al: Planning mantle radiation therapy in patients with Hodgkin disease: Role of gallium-67 scintigraphy. *AJR Am J Roentgenol.* 1988;151:1229.

51. Lorberboym M, Mandell LR, Mosesson RE, et al: The role of thallium-201 uptake and retention in intracranial tumors after radiotherapy. *J Nucl Med.* 1997;38:223.

52. Alexander E III, Loeffler JS, Schwartz RB, et al: Thallium-201 technetium-99m HMPAO single-photon emission computed tomography (SPECT) imaging for guiding stereotactic craniotomies in heavily irradiated malignant glioma patients. *Acta Neurochir (Vienna).* 1993;122:215.

53. Bischof Delaloye A: Radioimmunoimaging and radioimmunotherapy: Will these be routine procedures? *Semin Nucl Med.* 2000;30:186.

54. Press OW: Radiolabeled antibody therapy of B-cell lymphomas. *Semin Oncol.* 1999;26(Suppl 14):58.

55. Meredith RF, Knox SJ: Radioimmunotherapy of B-cell NHL. *Curr Pharm Biotechnol.* 2001;2:327.

56. Makrauer FL, Oates E, Becker J, et al: Does local irradiation affect gastric emptying in humans? *Am J Med Sci.* 1999;317:33.

57. Boersma LJ, Damen EM, de Boer RW, et al: Estimation of overall pulmonary function after irradiation using dose-effect relations for local functional injury. *Radiother Oncol.* 1995;36:15.

58. Boersma LJ, Damen EM, de Boer RW, et al: A new method to determine dose-effect relations for local lung-function changes using correlated SPECT and CT data. *Radiother Oncol.* 1993;29:110.

59. Damen EM, Muller SH, Boersma LJ, et al: Quantifying local lung perfusion and ventilation using correlated SPECT and CT data. *J Nucl Med.* 1994;35:784.

60. Valdes Olmos RA, van Zandwijk N, Boersma LJ, et al: Radiation pneumonitis imaged with indium-111-pentetreotide. *J Nucl Med.* 1996;37:584.

61. Seppenwoolde Y, Engelsman M, De Jaeger K, et al:. Optimizing radiation treatment plans for lung cancer using lung perfusion information. *Radiother Oncol.* 2002;63:165.

62. Phelps ME: Positron computed tomography studies of cerebral glucose metabolism in man: Theory and application in nuclear medicine. *Semin Nucl Med.* 1981;11:32.

63. Wahl RL, ed: *Principles and Practice of Positron Emission Tomography.* Philadelphia: Lippincott Williams & Wilkins; 2002.

64. Hustinx R, Paulus P, Rigo P, et al: *Clinical PET in Oncology.* France: GE Medical Systems and Mallin-krodt Medical; 1996: 96361-E.

65. Burt BM, Humm JL, Kooby DA, et al: Using positron emission tomography with [18F]FDG to predict tumor behavior in experimental colorectal cancer. *Neoplasia.* 2001;3:189.

66. Grunwald F, Kalicke T, Feine U, et al: Fluorine-18 fluorodeoxyglucose positron emission tomography in thyroid cancer: Results of a multicentre study. *Eur J Nucl Med.* 1999;26:1547.

67. Huang SC: Anatomy of SUV. Standardized uptake value. *Nucl Med Biol.* 2000;27:643.

68. Vansteenkiste JF, Stroobants SG, Dupont PJ, et al: Prognostic importance of the standardized uptake value on 18F-fluoro-2-deoxy-glucose-positron emission tomography scan in non–small-cell lung cancer: An analysis of 125 cases. Leuven Lung Cancer Group. *J Clin Oncol.* 1999;17:3201.

69. Martinelli M, Townsend D, Meltzer C, Villemagne VV: Survey of results of whole body imaging using the PET/CT at the University of Pittsburgh Medical Center PET facility. *Clin Positron Imaging.* 2000;3:161.

70. Charron M, Beyer T, Bohnen NN, et al: Image analysis in patients with cancer studied with a combined PET and CT scanner. *Clin Nucl Med.* 2000;25:905.

71. Beyer T, Townsend DW, Brun T, et al: A combined PET/CT scanner for clinical oncology. *J Nucl Med.* 2000;41:1369.

72. Burger C, Goerres G, Schoenes S, et al: PET attenuation coefficients from CT images: Experimental evaluation of the transformation of CT into PET 511-keV attenuation coefficients. *Eur J Nucl Med Mol Imaging.* 2002;29:922.

73. Dizendorf EV, Treyer V, Von Schulthess GK, Hany TF: Application of oral contrast media in coregistered positron emission tomography-CT. *AJR Am J Roentgenol.* 2002;179:477.

74. Israel O, Keidar Z, Iosilevsky G, et al: The fusion of anatomic and physiologic imaging in the management of patients with cancer. *Semin Nucl Med.* 2001;31:191.

75. Erdi YE, Mawlawi O, Larson SM, et al: Segmentation of lung lesion volume by adaptive positron emission tomography image thresholding. *Cancer.* 1997;80(12 Suppl):2505.

76. Erdi YE, Rosenzweig K, Erdi AK, et al: Radiotherapy treatment planning for patients with non-small cell lung cancer using positron emission tomography (PET). *Radiother Oncol.* 2002;62:51.

77. Schechter NR, Gillenwater AM, Byers RM, et al: Can positron emission tomography improve the quality of care for head-and-neck cancer patients? *Int J Radiat Oncol Biol Phys.* 2001;51:4.

78. Mah K, Caldwell CB, Ung YC, et al: The impact of 18FDG-PET on target and critical organs in CT-based treatment planning of patients with poorly defined non–small-cell lung carcinoma: A prospective study. *Int J Radiat Oncol Biol Phys.* 2002;52:339.

79. Rosenman J: Incorporating functional imaging information into radiation treatment. *Semin Radiat Oncol.* 2001;11:83.

80. Nestle U, Walter K, Schmidt S, et al: ^{18}F-deoxyglucose positron emission tomography (FDG-PET) for the planning of radiotherapy in lung cancer: High impact in patients with atelectasis. *Int J Radiat Oncol Biol Phys.* 1999;44:593.

81. Rahn AN, Baum RP, Adamietz IA, et al: Value of 18F fluorodeoxyglucose positron emission tomography in radiotherapy planning of head-neck tumors. *Strahlenther Onkol.* 1998;174:358. German.

82. Kiffer JD, Berlangieri SU, Scott AM, et al: The contribution of ^{18}F-fluoro-2-deoxy-glucose positron emission tomographic imaging to radiotherapy planning in lung cancer. *Lung Cancer.* 1998;19:167.

83. Nehmeh SA, Erdi YE, Ling CC, et al: Effect of respiratory gating on reducing lung motion artifacts in PET imaging of lung cancer. *Med Phys.* 2002;29:366.

84. Nehmeh SA, Erdi YE, Ling CC, et al: Effect of respiratory gating on quantifying PET images of lung cancer. *J Nucl Med.* 2002;43:876.

85. Mogard J, Kihlstrom L, Ericson K, et al: Recurrent tumor vs radiation effects after gamma knife radiosurgery of intracerebral metastases: Diagnosis with PET-FDG. *J Comput Assist Tomogr.* 1994;18:177.

86. Oku S, Nakagawa K, Momose T, et al: FDG-PET after radiotherapy is a good prognostic indicator of rectal cancer. *Ann Nucl Med.* 2002;16:409.

87. Allal AS, Dulguerov P, Allaoua M, et al: Standardized uptake value of 2-[^{18}F] fluoro-2-deoxy-D-glucose in predicting outcome in head and neck carcinomas treated by radiotherapy with or without chemotherapy. *J Clin Oncol.* 2002;20:1398.

88. Greven KM, Williams DW III, McGuirt WF Sr, et al: Serial positron emission tomography scans following radiation therapy of patients with head and neck cancer. *Head Neck.* 2001;23:942.

89. Morris MJ, Akhurst T, Osman I, et al: Fluorinated deoxyglucose positron emission tomography imaging in progressive metastatic prostate cancer. *Urology.* 2002;59:913.

90. Macapinlac HA, Humm JL, Akhurst T, et al: Differential metabolism and pharmacokinetics of L- [1-[11]C-] methionine and 2-[^{18}F] fluoro-2-deoxy-D-glucose (FDG) in androgen independent prostate cancer. *Clin Positron Imaging.* 1999;2:173-181.

91. Nunez R, Macapinlac HA, Yeung HW, et al: Combined ^{18}F-FDG and ^{11}C-methionine PET scans in patients with newly progressive metastatic prostate cancer. *J Nucl Med.* 2002;43:46.

92. Wells P, Gunn RN, Alison M, et al: Assessment of proliferation in vivo using 2-[^{11}C]thymidine positron emission tomography in advanced intra-abdominal malignancies. *Cancer Res.* 2002;62:5698.

93. Blasberg RG, Roelcke U, Weinreich R, et al: Imaging brain tumor proliferative activity with [[124]I]iododeoxyuridine. *Cancer Res.* 2000;60:624.

94. Vesselle H, Grierson J, Muzi M, et al: In vivo validation of 3′deoxy-3′-[^{18}F]fluorothymidine ([^{18}F]FLT) as a proliferation imaging tracer in humans: Correlation of [^{18}F]FLT uptake by positron emission tomography with Ki-67 immunohistochemistry and flow cytometry in human lung tumors. *Clin Cancer Res.* 2002;8:3315.

95. De Jong IJ, Pruim J, Elsinga PH, et al: Visualization of prostate cancer with ^{11}C-choline positron emission tomography. *Eur Urol.* 2002;42:18.

96. Kato T, Tsukamoto E, Kuge Y, et al: Accumulation of [^{11}C]acetate in normal prostate and benign prostatic hyperplasia: Comparison with prostate cancer. *Eur J Nucl Med Mol Imaging.* 2002;29:1492.

97. Hofmann M, Maecke H, Borner R, et al: Biokinetics and imaging with the somatostatin receptor PET radioligand ^{68}Ga-DOTA-TOC: Preliminary data. *Eur J Nucl Med.* 2001;28:1751.

98. Weber WA, Wester HJ, Grosu AL, et al: O-(2-[^{18}F]fluoroethyl)-L-tyrosine and L-[methyl-^{11}C]methionine uptake in brain tumours: Initial results of a comparative study. *Eur J Nucl Med.* 2000;27:542.

99. DeGrado TR, Coleman RE, Wang S, et al: Synthesis and evaluation of ^{18}F-labeled choline as an oncologic tracer for positron emission tomography: Initial findings in prostate cancer. *Cancer Res.* 2001;61:110.

100. Hara T, Kosaka N, Shinoura N, Kondo T: PET imaging of brain tumor with [methyl-11C]choline. *J Nucl Med.* 1997; 38:842.

101. Kobori O, Kirihara Y, Kosaka N, Hara T: Positron emission tomography of esophageal carcinoma using ^{11}C-choline and

[18]F-fluorodeoxyglucose: A novel method of preoperative lymph node staging. *Cancer.* 1999;1;86:1638.

102. Krohn KA, Mankoff DA, Eary JF: Imaging cellular proliferation as a measure of response to therapy. *J Clin Pharmacol.* 2001;(Suppl):96S. Review.

103. Van de Wiele C, De Vos F, Slegers G, et al: Radiolabeled estradiol derivatives to predict response to hormonal treatment in breast cancer: A review. *Eur J Nucl Med.* 2000;27:1421.

104. Bonasera TA, O'Neil JP, Xu M, et al: Preclinical evaluation of fluorine-18-labeled androgen receptor ligands in baboons. *J Nucl Med.* 1996;37:1009.

105. Daghighian F, Pentlow KS, Larson SM, et al: Development of a method to measure kinetics of radiolabelled monoclonal antibody in human tumour with applications to microdosimetry: positron emission tomography studies of iodine-124 labelled 3F8 monoclonal antibody in glioma. *Eur J Nucl Med.* 1993;20:402.

106. Cutler PD, Schwarz SW, Anderson CJ, et al: Dosimetry of copper-64-labeled monoclonal antibody 1A3 as determined by PET imaging of the torso. *J Nucl Med.* 1995;36:2363.

107. Lovquist A, Humm JL, Sheikh A, et al: PET imaging of [86]Y-labeled anti-lewis y antibodies in a nude mouse model; Comparison between [86]Y and ^{111}In radiolabels. *J Nucl Med.* 2001;42:1281.

108. Rasey JS, Koh WJ, Evans ML, et al: Quantifying regional hypoxia in human tumors with positron emission tomography of [^{18}F] fluoromisonidazole: A pretherapy study of 37 patients. *Int J Radiat Oncol Biol Phys.* 1996;36:417.

109. Urtasun RC, Parliament MB, McEwan AJ, et al: Measurement of hypoxia in human tumours by non-invasive spect imaging of iodoazomycin arabinoside. *Br J Cancer Suppl.* 1996;27:S209.

110. Koch CJ, Hahn SM, Rockwell K Jr, et al: Pharmacokinetics of EF5 [2-(2-nitro-1-H-imidazol-1-yl)-N-(2,2,3,3,3-pentafluoro-propyl) acetamide] in human patients: Implications for hypoxia measurements in vivo by 2-nitroimidazoles. *Cancer Chemother Pharmacol.* 2001;48:177.

111. Chapman JD, Schneider RF, Urbain JL, Hanks GE: Single-photon emission computed tomography and positron-emission tomography assays for tissue oxygenation. *Semin Radiat Oncol.* 2001;11:47.

112. Chao KS, Bosch WR, Mutic S, et al: A novel approach to overcome hypoxic tumor resistance: Cu-ATSM-guided intensity-modulated radiation therapy. *Int J Radiat Oncol Biol Phys.* 2001;15;49:171.

113. Ling CC, Humm JL, Larson SM, et al: Towards multidimensional radiotherapy (MD-CRT): Biological imaging and biological conformality. *Int J Radiat Oncol Biol Phys.* 2000;47:551.

114. Tjuvajev JG, Finn R, Watanabe K, et al: Noninvasive imaging of herpes virus thymidine kinase gene transfer and expression: A potential method for monitoring clinical gene therapy. *Cancer Res.* 1996;56:4087.

115. Tjuvalev J, Avril N, Oku T, et al: Imaging herpes virus thymidine kinase gene transfer and expression by positron emission tomography. *Cancer Res.* 1998;58:4333.

116. Morin K, Knaus E, Wiebe L: Non-invasive scintigraphic monitoring of gene expression in a HSV-1 thymidine kinase gene therapy. *Nucl Med Commun.* 1997;18:599.

117. Gambhir SS, Barrio JR, Wu L, et al: Imaging of adenoviral-directed herpes simplex virus type 1 thymidine kinase reporter gene expression in mice with radiolabeled ganciclovir. *J Nucl Med.* 1998;39:2003.

118. Gambhir SS, Barrio JR, Phelps ME, et al: Imaging adenoviral-directed reporter gene expression in living animals with positron emission tomography. *Proc Natl Acad Sci U S A.* 1999;96:2333.

119. Doubroven M, Ponomarev V, Berensten T, et al: Imaging transcriptional regulation of p53-dependent genes with positron emission tomography in vivo. *Proc Natl Acad Sci U S A.* 2001; 98:9300.

120. Jacobs A, Voges J, Reszka R, et al: Positron-emission tomography of vector-mediated gene expression in gene therapy for gliomas. *Lancet.* 2001;358:727.

121. Ratib O, Ligier Y, Scherrer J-R: Digital image management in medicine. *Comput Med Imaging Graph.* 1994;18:73.

122. American College of Radiology, National Electrical Manufacturers Association: *Digital Imaging and Communications in Medicine (DICOM)*: Version 3.0. Washington, D.C.: Draft Standard of the ACR-NEMA Committee Working Group VI; 1993.

123. Lutz RW, Pun T, Pellegrini C: Colour displays and look-up tables: Real time modification of digital images. *Comput Med Imaging Graph.* 1991;15:73.
124. Gonzalez RC, Wintz P: Digital image processing. Boston: Addison-Wesley; 1987.
125. Russ JC: The image processing handbook. Boca Raton, Fla.: CRC Press; 1994.
126. Oran BE: Fast Fourier transform and its applications. Upper Saddle River, N.J.: Prentice Hall; 1988.
127. Robb RA: Three dimensional biomedical imaging. New York: VCH Publishers, Inc.; 1995.
128. Kass M, Witkin A, Terzopoulos D: Snakes: Active contour models. *Int J Comp Vision.* 1987;321.
129. Castleman KR: Digital Image Processing. Upper Saddle River, N.J.: Prentice Hall; 1996.
130. Sonka M, Hlavac V, Boyle R: Image Processing, Analysis, and Machine Vision. London: Chapman and Hall Computing; 1993.
131. Peters TM: Multi-planar transformations of CT images. *J Can Assoc Radiol.* 1980;31:126.
132. Rhodes ML, Glenn WV, Azzawi YM: Extracting oblique planes from serial CT sections. *J Comput Assist Tomogr.* 1980;4:649.
133. Watt A: 3D computer graphics. Boston: Addison-Wesley; 1993.
134. Semelka RC, Shoenut JP, Kroeker MA, et al: Focal liver disease: Comparison of dynamic contrast-enhanced CT and T2 weighted fat suppressed, FLASH, and dynamic gadolinium-enhanced MR imaging at 1.5T. *Radiology.* 1992;184:687.
135. Whitney WS, Herfkens RJ, Jeffrey RB, et al: Dynamic breath-hold multiplanar spoiled gradient-recalled MR imaging with gadolinium enhancement for differentiating hepatic hemangiomas from malignancies at 1.5T. *Radiology.* 1993;189:863.
136. Jacquez JA: Compartmental analysis in biology and medicine. Ann Arbor, Mich.: The University of Michigan Press; 1988.
137. Bidaut LM: Composite PET and MRI for accurate localization and metabolic modeling: A very useful tool for research and clinic. SPIE Medical Imaging. 1991;1445:66.
138. Bidaut LM, Pascual-Marqui R, Delavelle J, et al: Three- to five dimensional biomedical multisensor imaging for the assessment of neurological (dys)function. *J Digit Imaging.* 1996;9:185.
139. Ferris JV, Marsh JW, Little AF: Presurgical evaluation of the liver transplant candidate. *Radiol Clin North Am.* 1995;33:497.
140. Pietrzyk U, Herholz K, Fink G, et al: An interactive technique for three-dimensional image registration: Validation for PET, SPECT, MRI and CT brain studies. *J Nucl Med.* 1994;35:2011.
141. Arun KS, Huang TS, Blostein SD: Least square fitting of two 3D point sets. *IEEE Trans Pattern Mach Intell.* 1987;9:698.
142. Bruce J, Giblin P, Tari F: Ridges, crests and sub-parabolic lines of evolving surfaces. *Int J Comp Vision.* 1996;18:195.
143. Pelizzari CA, Chen GTY, Spelbring DR, et al: Accurate three-dimensional registration of CT, PET, and/or MR images of the brain. *J Comput Assist Tomogr.* 1989;13:20.
144. Meyer CR, Leichtman GS, Brunberg JA, et al: Simultaneous usage of homologous points, lines and planes for optimal 3D linear registration of multimodality imaging data. *IEEE Trans Med Imaging.* 1995;14:1.
145. Mangin J-F, Frouin V, Bloch I, et al: Fast nonsupervised 3D registration of PET and MR images of the brain. *J Cereb Blood Flow Metab.* 1994;14:749.
146. van Herk M, Kooy HM: Automatic three-dimensional correlation of CT-CT, CT-MRI, and CT-SPECT using chamfer matching. *Med Phys.* 1994;21:1163.
147. Nelder JA, Mead R: A Simplex method for function minimization. *Comput J.* 1965;7:308.
148. Powell MJD: Restart procedure of the conjugate gradient method. *Math Programming.* 1977;12:241.
149. Woods R, Mazziotta JC, Cherry S: MRI-PET registration with automated algorithm. *J Comput Assist Tomogr.* 1993;17:536.
150. Maes F, Collignon A, Vandermeulen D, et al: Multimodality image registration by maximization of mutual information. *IEEE Trans Med Imaging.* 1997;2:187.
151. Meyer CR, Boes JL, Kim B, et al: Demonstration of accuracy and clinical versatility of mutual information for automatic multi-modality image fusion using affine and thin plate spline warped geometric deformations. *Med Image Anal.* 1997;3:195.
152. Loew MH: Issues in multimodality medical image registration. *J Digit Imaging.* 1997;10:24.
153. West J, Fitzpatrick JM, Wang MY, et al: Comparison and evaluation of retrospective intermodality brain registration techniques. *J Comput Assist Tomogr.* 1997;21:554.
154. Austin-Seymour M: Interinstitutional comparison of defining target volumes. *Int J Radiat Oncol Biol Phys.* 1994;30(suppl 1): 117. Abstract.

SUGGESTED READING

1. Sprawls P: *Physical Principles of Medical Imaging.* 2nd ed. Gaithersburg, Md: Aspen Publishers; 1993.
2. Bushberg JT, Seibert JA, Leidholdt EM, Boone JM: *The Essential Physics of Medical Imaging.* 2nd ed. Philadelphia: Lippincott William & Wilkins; 2002.

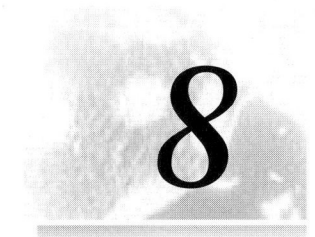

Three-Dimensional Conformal Radiotherapy and Intensity-Modulated Radiotherapy

Ping Xia, PhD, Howard I. Amols, PhD, and C. Clifton Ling, PhD

It is well accepted that local tumor control and normal tissue complications have sigmoidally shaped dose response curves.[1] For normal tissue complications, radiation response also depends on the volume of tissue irradiated, with some tissues (such as the lung, liver, and kidney) having greater volume dependence than others (such as the spinal cord and brainstem). The success of radiotherapy is therefore highly dependent on the radiosensitivity of the particular tumor being treated relative to that of the surrounding normal tissues. For tumor sites, where the tumor control curve is less steep than the normal tissue complication curve, the high doses required for tumor cure may cause unacceptable normal tissue complications. The goal in radiation therapy therefore is to sufficiently separate the dose response curves of local tumor control and normal tissue complications. The only physical or dosimetric means for achieving this is to configure the radiation portals so as to reduce both the dose and the total volume of normal tissues irradiated.

During the past 2 decades, advances in radiologic imaging and computer technology have significantly enhanced our ability to achieve this goal through the development of three-dimensional image-based conformal radiotherapy (3DCRT), which permits better conformity between the irradiated high-dose volume and the geometric shape of the tumor while minimizing the radiation dose delivered to surrounding normal tissue. Intensity-modulated radiation therapy (IMRT) is an especially advanced form of 3DCRT that incorporates sophisticated computer controlled radiation beam delivery and computer-optimized treatment plan design. This is achieved by varying the beam intensity within each beam portal, as opposed to the uniform beam intensities used in conventional 3DCRT. Both 3DCRT and IMRT use sophisticated strategies for patient immobilization and positioning, image-guided treatment planning, and computer-enhanced treatment verification. At the heart of these techniques is advanced computer technology, and in particular, 3D patient imaging with computed tomography (CT), and more recently magnetic resonance (MR) and positron emission tomography (PET). Many treatment planning comparison studies have demonstrated the dosimetric advantages of 3DCRT, especially its advanced form of IMRT.[2-7] Early results have shown the improvement of local tumor control for prostate cancer, and for head and neck cancer.[8-10]

In this chapter, we describe the rationale and processes for 3DCRT and IMRT, including patient imaging and simulation, treatment planning, dose calculation algorithms, plan evaluation, treatment delivery, and quality assurance issues. We will identify the similarities and differences between 3DCRT and IMRT and emphasize those features and benefits unique to IMRT.

3DCRT AND IMRT TREATMENT PLANNING PROCESS

Conventional radiation therapy entails irradiation of the patient from multiple beam directions (as the accelerator rotates about the patient), using beam configurations such as shown in Figure 8-1, which depicts a five-field isocentric treatment of the prostate. Usually all beams are aimed at a single point denoted as the isocenter, which geometrically represents the intersection of the axes of rotation of the linear accelerator gantry head, the collimator assembly, and the treatment couch. Most often the geometric center of the tumor is purposely positioned at the isocenter. Even though for each individual beam the intervening superficial tissues receive higher radiation doses than does the tumor, the summation of all beams results in a higher dose to the tumor. 3DCRT entails more sophisticated shaping of the dose distribution than does conventional radiation therapy because the collimation design (or shaping of fields) and the selection of beam directions is based on 3D images of the patient (usually CT, but often augmented with MR, PET, or other functional imaging studies). IMRT goes a step beyond 3DCRT by also enabling variations of the *radiation intensity* within each beam. This intensity modulation can be achieved via several different approaches including fabrication of complex physical compensators using computer-controlled milling machines, or via use of a multileaf collimator (MLC) capable of dynamic or static beam

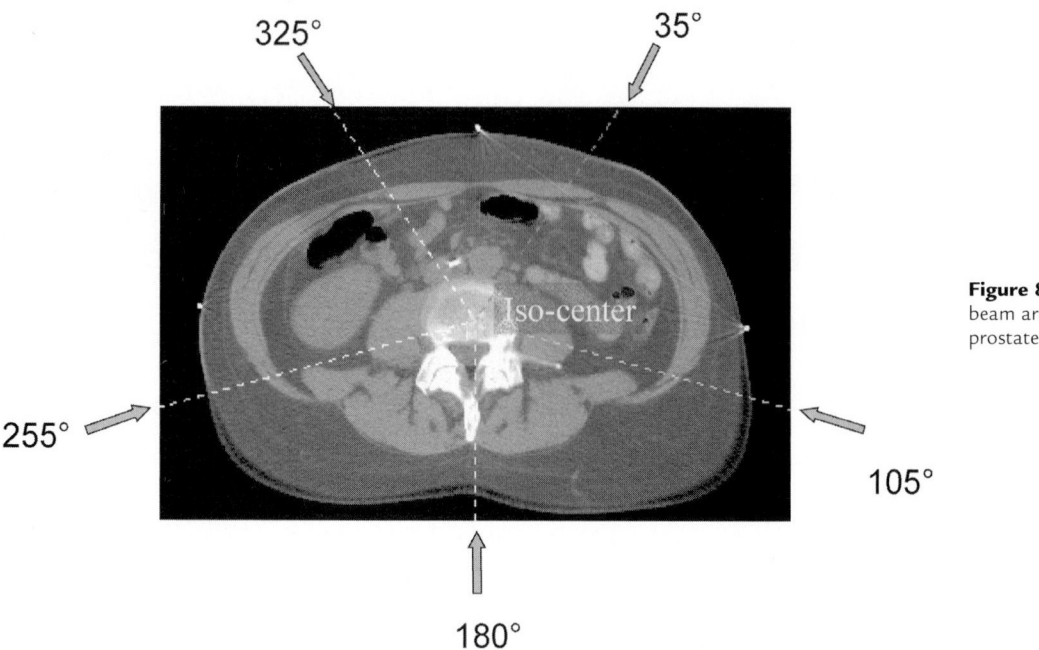

325°   35°

255°

Iso-center

105°

180°

Figure 8–1. A typical five photon beam arrangement for treatment of prostate.

delivery. This chapter focuses mainly on the latter (i.e., MLC) approach, which is by far more commonly used.

Let us first briefly describe the process of 3DCRT and IMRT, after which we present details of each step in the process. The treatment planning steps for IMRT and for 3DCRT are similar during the initial and final steps, but diverge in the middle. In particular, patient imaging and simulation are identical for both processes. IMRT differs from 3DCRT in some key steps of treatment planning and delivery, which we will discuss along the way.

The treatment planning process begins with "treatment simulation," which entails setting up the patient on the conventional simulator or on the CT unit in the treatment position. The first step in simulation is fabrication of custom-designed body molds, or partial body molds to facilitate accurate reproduction of patient position during both CT image acquisition and multi-fraction treatment delivery. Please see Chapter 9, Immobilization and Simulation. With the patient thus immobilized in the treatment position, CT images are acquired. From these images the radiation oncologist, medical physicist, and dosimetrist delineate both target and nontarget structures. More and more frequently patient CT imaging is being augmented with MRI, PET, and other functional imaging studies to better define the tumor and target volume. The delineation of anatomical volumes is usually done directly on a computer display of transverse CT images using standard computer graphics options.

Once all relevant tissues have been delineated, and beam directions specified, the radiation oncologist must specify the desired doses to tumor and normal tissues. From these specifications the medical physicist or dosimetrist or both adjust beam directions, shapes, and beam intensities to best meet these dose criteria. The design of treatment portal shapes and selection of radiation beam directions are usually determined via a specialized type of computer display denoted as beam's eye view (BEV), which shows the patient anatomy from any desired beam direction.

For 3DCRT, the optimization of treatment beams is performed via "manual" iteration, and flexibility is constrained by time and by the fact that x-ray beam intensities within each individual beam are uniform (or, if wedges are added, monotonically variable in one dimension). Once beam directions, shapes, and intensities are specified, the computer calculates the resulting dose distribution, which one compares to the radiation oncologist's specifications. If there are discrepancies, beam intensities, shapes, and directions are iteratively adjusted (based primarily on the physicist's experience and intuition) and dose distributions recalculated. In practice, only a few parameters can really be adjusted, and each iteration is time consuming. Hence the ability to truly optimize a dose distribution with 3DCRT techniques is often quite limited. This type of iteration is also referred to as "forward planning." For IMRT, the optimization of treatment beams is usually performed via computerized iteration as opposed to the manual adjustment described earlier. Here, the computer performs hundreds, or even thousands of iterations in less time than a human could perform a few iterations. This type of optimization is referred to as "inverse planning."

Whether it be forward or inverse optimization, once a treatment plan or dose distribution has been calculated, the radiation oncologist and physicist must evaluate the plan to determine how well it meets the original criteria, or dose constraints. This is typically done via analysis of dose distributions and Dose Volume Histograms (DVHs). When a treatment plan has finally been accepted, all planning data describing beam configurations and intensities are transferred to the linear accelerator, and patient treatment proceeds using the beams designed during the treatment planning process. For IMRT, the data transferred includes information on dynamic multileaf collimator (DMLC) motion files or multiple static MLC shapes for each field required to deliver the desired x-ray intensity profiles. Finally, the physicist must perform dosimetric and QA tasks to verify that all equipment is functioning properly, and that the specifics of the dose prescription and treatment plan are accurately delivered to the patient daily.

The following sections address each of these treatment planning steps in greater detail.

Patient Setup, Immobilization, and Image Acquisition

The minimization of patient setup uncertainty is more important in 3DCRT than in conventional radiotherapy because of the improved conformity of the dose distribution (i.e., smaller field margins). This becomes even more critical in IMRT because IMRT often produces higher dose gradients. Thus, immobilization devices and precise patient positioning procedures must be used throughout the process of image acquisition, simulation, and treatment. Many different techniques and devices are in use to achieve this, including conventional items such as vacuum cradles, plaster casts, and face masks. More elaborate devices specific to IMRT are also being introduced, such as immobilization devices that attach directly to the treatment couch to ensure that patients are positioned in the same location during each daily treatment. The same "index positioning method" is also used during the CT image acquisition. Stereotactic body frames (SBF) have also been developed to achieve setup accuracy approaching that of stereotactic radiosurgery.

With the use of 3DCRT and IMRT, the utility of conventional radiation therapy simulators is greatly decreased as treatment planning and so-called *virtual simulation* can now be based entirely on 3D CT images instead of conventional 2D simulation films. A conventional simulator may still be used for an initial (pre-CT) simulation carried out in conjunction with patient immobilization to establish fiduciary skin marks, to define a tentative treatment isocenter, and to obtain anterior-posterior (AP) and lateral radiographic films. A second simulation (also called verification simulation) may also be performed, after the treatment plan has been accepted, to position the patient at the established treatment isocenter and to acquire reference radiographs of each field for comparison with the corresponding digitally reconstructed radiographs (DRRs) obtained from the CT images. Such films can also be used for comparison with verification portal images taken on the linear accelerator during treatment.

Continued reliance on conventional simulators for 3DCRT, however, is becoming something of an anachronism, as CT virtual simulation provides more flexibility by permitting changes to be made to beam directions and shapes after the patient has left the simulation suite. In addition, DRRs can be used in lieu of conventional 2D films. DRRs are computer-rendered 2D projection images similar to conventional x-ray films, that enable the planner to "view" the patient from any beam direction. These images are generated electronically (i.e., digitally), and can easily be manipulated on the computer to enable contrast and image enhancement, plus automatic comparison with digital port films obtained during patient treatments with electronic portal imaging devices (EPIDs). Figure 8-2 shows a typical AP DRR for a prostate patient.

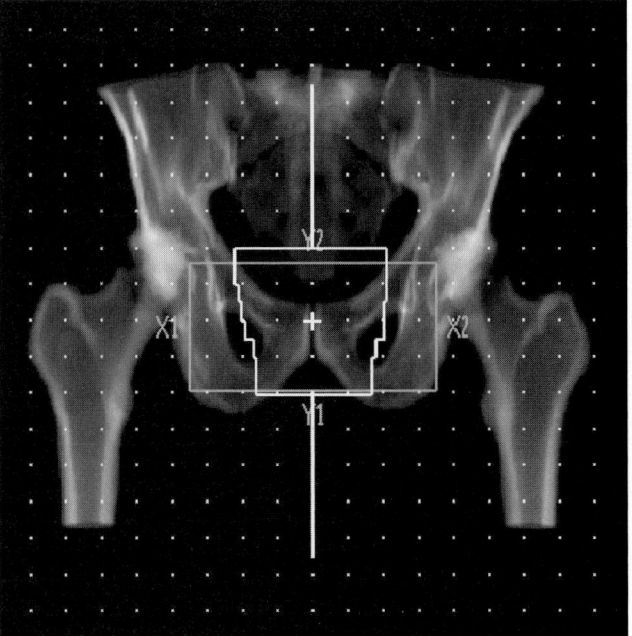

Figure 8–2. A posterior-anterior digitally reconstructed radiograph for a prostate field showing multileaf collimator settings superimposed on 2D patient anatomy.

Thus the entire sequence of initial simulation, CT simulation, and verification simulation can often be completely replaced by a single CT-based "virtual simulation."[11] This CT-simulator is essentially a CT scanner with capabilities for spiral (or helical) scanning and volumetric data acquisition, combined with a laser localization system similar to the laser system on a conventional simulator or linear accelerator, plus a high-speed graphic workstation that emulates a treatment planning computer. The laser localization system permits marking the treatment isocenter with fiduciaries on the patient skin, as in conventional simulation. It is important that the CT image set be obtained with the patient in the treatment position on a flat couch that is geometrically identical to the couch on which the patient will ultimately be treated. The high-speed computer workstation provides capabilities for rapid image reconstruction, target volume and normal tissue delineation, and three-dimensional beam geometry display. During the virtual simulation, patient anatomy is reconstructed from the CT data and displayed in BEV according to the specific treatment setup parameters. Digitally reconstructed simulation-type fluoroscopic images plus DRRs are used for viewing, decision making, and documentation. One current limitation of DRRs, however, is their degraded image quality as compared to conventional simulation films because of the relatively large size of the CT pixels (typically 0.6×0.6 mm^2), and more importantly the slice thickness (typically 3 to 5 mm). Newer CT scanners, however, can rapidly produce full sets of images with slice thickness of 1.5 mm or less, which greatly improves the quality of DRRs, but at a cost of increased file sizes.

In addition to improved efficiency and flexibility, CT simulation permits electronic format and transfer of all required information (e.g., target volume and normal tissue contours, isocenter coordinates) directly to the treatment planning computer system. In theory, data transfer between computers occurs seamlessly using computer programs or database systems or both, all conforming to an international standard format known as DICOM. In practice, however, it is not uncommon to find small differences in file formats between different manufacturers (even though all claim to be DICOM compatible) that require modification.

Delineation of Treatment Volume and Critical Organs

Treatment volumes are defined on the CT images according to the ICRU Report 50 nomenclature[12] with the gross target volume (GTV) defined as the visible tumor as seen on CT or other imaging studies; the clinical target volume (CTV) being the visualized tumor plus regions at risk such as microscopic extension of disease and nodal chains; and planning target volume (PTV) being an expanded CTV to include setup errors, patient motion, linear accelerator alignment errors, and other uncertainties. The manual delineation of CTV, PTV, plus adjacent critical organs is time consuming. Many virtual simulation and treatment planning systems now incorporate various software tools for performing autocontouring of tissue structures, but these are of limited use as current algorithms are accurate only for outlining external body contours and internal contours of very high contrast such as bone, lung, and air cavities. While these tools are often useful, and are constantly being improved, human intervention will likely remain a necessary and important component for defining the GTV, CTV, PTV, and other critical structures for the foreseeable future.

With IMRT, accurate delineation of the tumor volume and critical organs is even more important than in 3DCRT—with inverse planning optimization, the delineated contours are used as direct input to the computer optimization algorithm (discussed later) as it attempts to produce dose distributions conforming to the prescribed dose constraints of the delineated tumor and sensitive normal structures. For similar reasons, it is often necessary with IMRT and inverse treatment planning to contour many normal tissues in the vicinity of the PTV that would not normally be contoured for 3DCRT treatment planning. This is necessary to "advise" the optimization algorithm as to where it is permissible or not permissible to deposit moderate or high doses. For example, in a typical head and neck case, in addition to the structures commonly contoured when performing 3DCRT planning (such as the spinal cord and brainstem) it may also be necessary to contour parotid glands, optical structures, tongue, mandible, inner and middle ears, the tissues behind the spinal cord, etc., lest the optimization algorithms "unwittingly" deposit large doses to these volumes to meet dose constraints placed on other structures.

Selection of Treatment Beams

Various display schema have been developed for 3DCRT to represent the PTV and the adjacent critical organs in

3D perspective on a 2D computer display monitor. The objective is to facilitate the selection of beam angles and field shapes based on the relative positions of these various anatomic structures. The anatomic structures are often displayed as wire frames or solid structures, using colors to differentiate among them and intensity to indicate depth below the surface (so-called *color wash display*). The treatment geometry is usually best visualized in BEV when the anatomy is viewed from the perspective of the radiation source.[13,14] Figure 8-3 illustrates a BEV display of a single right anterior oblique field for a head and neck patient in the supine position. Note in Figure 8-3 that the brainstem (green), spinal cord (purple), and chiasm (red) are all partially or totally shielded by the MLC whereas the PTV is completely covered by the radiation field. (*Note:* User design of MLC field shapes as shown in Figure 8-3 is done only for 3DCRT forward planning. With inverse planning, the computer optimization algorithms design the actual field shape). BEV display can be depicted in 2D form such as a DRR as shown in Figure 8-2, or in pseudo 3D using wire frames and color wash to represent the various structures as in Figure 8-3.

Beam orientations are chosen by observing the patient in BEV from various beam directions and selecting those directions for which the PTV appears to be best separated from the normal tissues. That is, one tries to select beam angles that minimize the volume of irradiated normal tissue. Once the beam orientations have been chosen, their shapes (apertures) can be determined, again facilitated by the BEV display as shown previously in Figure 8-3. Selection of beams is based on a combination of experience, (sometimes) standard protocols, and patient-specific anatomy. For example, the relatively small variations from patient to patient in the anatomic relationship between the prostate and its nearby critical structures (most

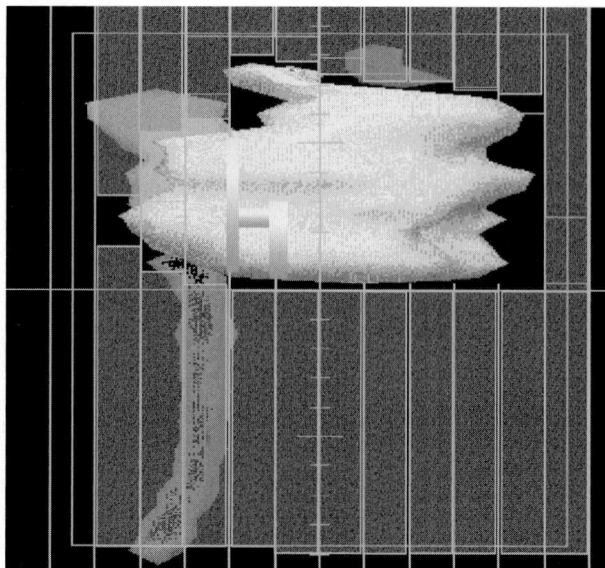

Figure 8–3. Beam's eye view of a right anterior oblique field for a head and neck patient in the supine position showing multileaf collimator (MLC) beam shaping. The planning target volume (PTV) is depicted in yellow, brainstem in green, cord in purple, and chiasm in red. Note how the MLC leaves (*transparent green*) are shaped to conform to the PTV. See also Color Figure 8-3.

importantly rectum, bladder, and urethra) enable IMRT prostate treatment plans to follow a more or less standard protocol with regard to beam selection. For brain and head and neck tumors, on the other hand, beam selection is highly dependent on patient-specific anatomy and the individual planner's experience.

The selection of the number of beams and their orientations can often make the difference between an acceptable plan and an unacceptable plan. Perhaps not surprisingly, the selection of beam angles is sometimes more critical for 3DCRT than for IMRT.[15,16] This is because the many degrees of freedom in IMRT computer optimization permits compensation (via intensity modulation of individual beamlets) if a less than optimum choice of beam directions has inadvertently been made. Nonetheless, determining optimum beam directions in IMRT may reduce the complexity of intensity profiles (i.e., the magnitude of intensity gradients within the field), thus improving delivery accuracy and efficiency.

In particular, IMRT fields with large fluctuations in intensity require higher velocities and accelerations of MLC leaves (when using dynamic or sliding-window IMRT) during beam delivery, which can be impractical to actually deliver. Similarly, for delivery of static IMRT fields (or "step and shoot"), large-dose fluctuations require more beam segments, which will also increase delivery time. Also, as the complexity of an intensity profile increases, so does the total number of monitor units, and hence the contribution of scatter and leakage dose,[17] which at best can be calculated only approximately by most dose calculation algorithms.[18,19] The selection of optimum beam directions is often critical when treating concave-shaped PTVs or where there is minimal separation between the PTV and a critical normal structure. Unfortunately, no available IMRT treatment planning systems can effectively determine optimum beam directions. This must still be done based primarily on the treatment planner's experience and intuition.

Plan Optimization

MANUAL OPTIMIZATION

In forward 3DCRT planning, the starting point for dose calculations (by the computer) is the number of beams, their directions and shapes, inclusion or exclusion of hard or dynamic wedges (wedges modulate beam intensity monotonically along a selected wedge direction), and the *static* beam intensities *selected by the planner*. Thus, in forward planning the computer merely calculates the resulting dose distribution from the beam intensities and shapes selected by the treatment planner. This is fundamentally different than inverse planning (described more fully later) in which the treatment planner specifies the desired dose to the PTV plus dose limits to various sensitive structures, and the computer optimization generates beam intensities and shapes to best meet the specified doses.

In either case, after the computer calculates the resultant dose distribution, the planner may choose to make adjustments in order to improve the plan. In forward planning the planner adjusts the beam intensities (or weights), possibly field shapes or directions or both, and then asks the computer to recalculate the dose distribution. This process, called manual optimization, is repeated until an "optimal" dose distribution is obtained. The experience of the individual planner is critical in manual planning. Even for a skilled planner, the quality of the plan may be limited by the restricted number of degrees of freedom one has, particularly the constraint that intensity within each field must be uniform. Further, the number of iterations one can perform within the allotted time is clearly limited. For inverse planning, as we will describe in section 1.4.3, the philosophy of plan optimization is completely reversed.

PARTIAL OPTIMIZATION

Slightly more sophisticated than manual optimization (but not as sophisticated as inverse planning) is so-called *aperture-based optimization*, where the planner designs one or more beam shapes for each beam direction, and the computer optimizes the intensities (or weights) of each beam shape.[20] The beam shape for each beam direction could be partial fields or fields within fields. Another variation of the aperture-based optimization, so-called *partial optimization*, entails the planner selecting the number of segments (subfields) allowed for each beam with the computer optimizing the shape of each segment and its associated intensity or weight.[21] The advantage of this partial optimization method is that the planner can control the complexity of a treatment. For tumor sites that are not adjacent to sensitive normal tissues, such as the breast, the relative simplicity of this approach may have advantages as compared to plans produced by inverse planning.

INVERSE PLANNING

The process of inverse treatment planning was first proposed by Brahme in 1988.[22] With inverse planning, the planner does not directly attempt to optimize or readjust beam intensities. Instead, after defining the orientation and energies of all beams (but *not* their intensities), the planner specifies the *desired* dose limits for the GTV and CTV and all tissues of interest. To achieve this, the *computer* optimization algorithm first divides each beam into many small beamlets (or rays, or pencil beams). It then iteratively alters the intensities of beamlets until the composite 3D dose distribution best conforms to the specified dose objectives. After the optimal beam intensities and resulting dose distribution have been determined, the computer then calculates the sequence of MLC leaf motions that will achieve this. The details of the various steps in this process are described.

Central to the success of any optimization schema is the specification of an objective or cost function. The cost function is a mathematical definition of the "goodness" of a treatment plan, which the computer optimization algorithm attempts to minimize as it adjusts the beam weights from one iteration to the next. Objective functions can be based on biologic criteria,[23] or more often dose-based criteria.[24] Biologic-based objective functions (OFs) use a calculated radiobiologic response as a measure of the merit of a plan (with calculations based on some model that relates radiation dose plus volume of irradiated tissue to predicted biologic response). The use of biologically weighted OFs is in principle more relevant because treatment outcome is determined by the biologic response. However, a universally accepted biologic model that predicts treatment outcome is yet to be developed. Hence, most inverse planning algorithms currently rely on dose-based cost functions.

The numerical value of a dose-based objective functions (OF) is calculated from a weighted average of the differences between delivered and prescribed doses for every voxel in every tissue defined in the treatment plan (i.e., the PTV plus all normal tissues for which a dose constraint has been specified). The prescription dose to the PTV, specified tolerance doses to normal tissues, and weighting factors for each tissue are designated as the *constraints*. For the PTV, one (of many) possible OFs is given by the algebraic expression:

$$OF = \Sigma_i \; w_i \; {}^* \; (d_{cal} - d_{pres})_i^2 \qquad (1)$$

where Σ_i represents a summation over all voxels in the PTV; w_i equals the weighting (or penalty) factor for the ith voxel; d_{cal} equals the calculated dose (using the current beam parameters) for the ith voxel; and d_{pres} equals the prescribed dose for the ith voxel.

The exact formulation for the objective, however, could take many other algebraic forms. For example, the absolute value of $(d_{cal} - d_{pres})_i$ could be used rather than its square. Or, one could include $(d_{cal} - d_{pres})_i$ in the summation only if $(d_{cal} - d_{pres})_i$ is negative; that is, assign a penalty only if the calculated dose is less than the prescribed dose. Conversely, when calculating the contribution to the OF for a normal tissue, one would usually assign a penalty only if d_{cal} is greater than d_{pres}. The total OF is then the sum of the OFs for each tissue, weighted by the w_i values, which will likely differ for each tissue. For example, one would often assign a higher penalty or weighting factor to the spinal cord than rectum or bladder, as the former is a more radiosensitive structure with more disastrous consequences if overdosed.

For many tissues, however, acceptable doses cannot be specified by a single dose value, and dose volume effects are often incorporated into the OF. A typical dose volume constraint may be stated as "no more than q% of the particular organ is to receive a dose greater than d." This is equivalent to specifying a single point on a DVH with the constraint that the value of the DVH at a dose value of d must be less than q%. Most inverse treatment planning algorithms allow the planner to define multiple such points for each tissue, with different penalties assigned to each point if desired. DVH-type constraints, rather than a single-dose limit, can also be assigned to the PTV if desired.

Several OFs are illustrated graphically in Figure 8-4. For the PTV, the graph illustrates the concept of the "allowable inhomogeneity." That is, if the dose is between a lower limit P_l and an upper limit P_u, no penalty is assessed. Also, a larger weight can be assigned to penalize underdose as opposed to overdose (or vice versa). For the normal tissue, a penalty can be applied if the dose exceeds a certain critical value (D_c) or the OF can be based on dose volume considerations, as represented schematically in the rightmost panel of Figure 8-4.

Figure 8-5a is an example of DVH-based dose constraints from a commercial inverse planning system (Corvus, 4.0 NOMOS Corporation, Sewickley, Pa.). In the Corvus system, the dose constraints for each

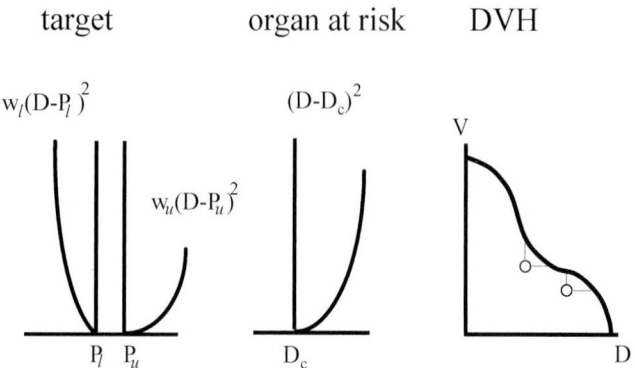

Figure 8–4. Examples of possible objective functions, illustrated graphically. Planning target volume (*leftmost graph*) doses within the "allowable inhomogeneity" receive no penalty, but different penalties are assessed for underdose as opposed to overdose. For the normal organ, a penalty can be applied if the dose exceeds a certain critical value (D_c) (*middle graph*), based on dose volume considerations (*rightmost panel*).

structure are described by three points, a dose goal or limit, a minimum dose point, and a maximum dose point. The PTV and sensitive structures are listed separately and are not interchangeable. For the PTV, the dose goal is the prescribed dose. The parameter "volume below goal" is used to describe the allowable volume of the target that can receive a dose less than the prescription dose. Similarly, for sensitive structures, the parameter "volume above limit" describes the allowable volume of sensitive structures that can exceed the dose limit. The three dose points, along with the volume parameter, depict a simplified desired DVH, as shown in Figure 8-5b. The column "I" defines the importance of the structure, if any of the three dose point constraints must be violated.

The choice of OFs and the specification of dose constraints are key components in inverse planning. For most inverse planning systems the user has only one choice of OF. The only direct input from users in an inverse planning system, therefore, is the specification of dose constraints. The resultant inverse plan is highly dependent on the algebraic form of the OF and also on the specification of dose constraints. Specification of physically unrealistic dose constraints may lead the computer optimization to produce an inferior plan. For example, prescribing 100% dose to a paraspinal tumor with large penalty for underdose, plus 5% dose to an adjacent section of spinal cord with large penalty for overdose, may resultant in an inverse plan that is worse than a conventional plan. The reason for this seemingly incongruous result is that the optimization algorithm may attempt to adjust beamlet weights to extreme values in a futile attempt to meet dose constraints that it does not "know" are physically impossible.

To specify realistic dose constraints, users need to learn the relationship between the dose constraints and the resulting dose distributions for the specific inverse planning system they are using, and also have some familiarity with basic radiation dosimetry concepts. This learning process is one of trial and error, and is less intuitive than the trial and error planning process involved in forward planning. Once the treatment planner has gained this experience, it becomes possible to develop disease-specific templates that can be used as starting point dose constraints for

Target Name		Type		Goal (Gy)	Vol Below Goal (%)	Min (Gy)	Max (Gy)	I
GTV-target		Basic		64.0	5	54.0	72.0	
CTV1-target		Basic		54.0	5	52.0	64.0	

Sensitive Structure Name		Type		Limit (Gy)	Vol Above Limit (%)	Min (Gy)	Max (Gy)	I
Tissue		Basic Tissue		54.0	0	0.0	54.0	
Spinal Cord		Basic Structure		35.0	5	20.0	40.0	
LT-Parotid		BU Structure		20.0	10	10.0	45.0	
RT-Parotid		BU Structure		20.0	10	10.0	45.0	
Other 1		Basic Structure		45.0	10	20.0	54.0	
LT-Eye		Basic Structure		45.0	10	20.0	54.0	
Brain-Stem		Basic Structure		35.0	10	20.0	45.0	
LT_TMJ		Basic Structure		30.0	10	20.0	40.0	
RT_TMJ		Basic Structure		30.0	10	20.0	40.0	
Mandible		Basic Structure		40.0	10	20.0	54.0	

A

Figure 8–5. A, An example of dose volume histogram (DVH)-based dose constraints for a commercial inverse planning system (Corvus, 4.0 NOMOS Corporation, Sewickley, Pa.). **B,** Simplified DVH based on three-point constraints. See also Color Figure 8-5.

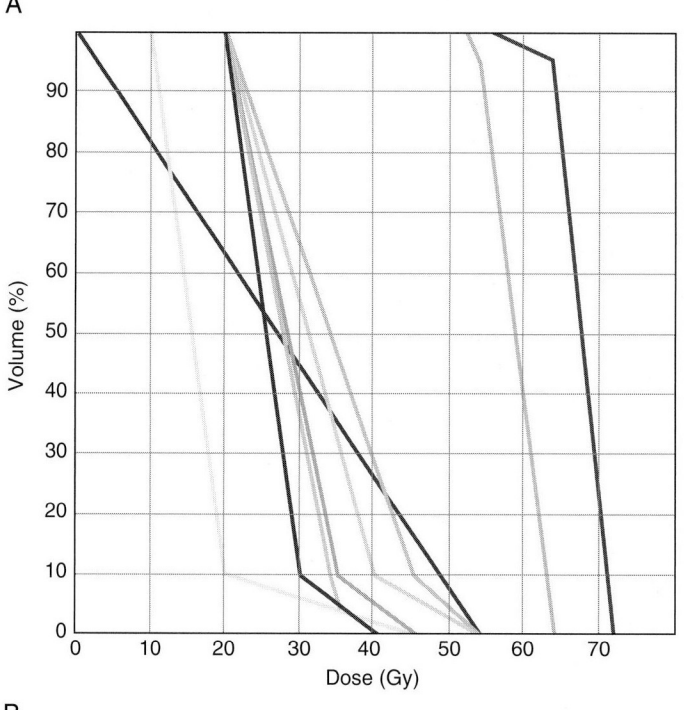

B

commonly treated tumor sites such as prostate, nasopharyngeal and oropharyngeal cancers. Patient-to-patient anatomic variations obviously limit the use of standard dose constraints, but they can be good starting points.

PLAN EVALUATION

The process of treatment plan evaluation continues to evolve, particularly for IMRT and inverse planning. The tools used for plan evaluation are similar for 3DCRT

and IMRT, although the schema for adjusting plans based on this evaluation is quite different, as discussed earlier. Evaluation tools include 2D dose distributions superimposed on CT images, 3D volumetric or color wash rendering of dose distributions overlayed on the PTV and critical organs or both, structure specific DVHs, and biological indices. Additionally, for IMRT plans, inspection of the intensity profiles is often useful for evaluating an individual beam's contribution to the dose distribution. Inspection of beam intensity distributions can be made using the so-called *observer's view*, which is similar to a relief map (Fig. 8-6), or by the projection of "isointensity" lines on a BEV.

In the forward process of 3DCRT, the planner and the clinician evaluate the initial treatment design with a view toward improvement by altering beam parameters (e.g., directions, weights, shapes, wedges). The identification of deficiencies and the devising of remedies rely very much on the experience and intuition of the planner. The effort-intensive nature of this approach limits the practical number of iterations of evaluation and alteration. On the other hand, the application of class solutions to some disease sites (e.g., prostate) minimizes the alterations needed and facilitates convergence to an acceptable solution within a few cycles.

Improving an unacceptable inverse IMRT plan can often be difficult for several reasons. First, without a good deal of IMRT experience, one usually does not know a priori whether the calculated plan is "bad" because of inappropriately chosen beams, dose volume constraints, penalties, etc., or because the dose parameters requested are physically impossible to achieve. Second, unlike forward treatment planning where corrective action for an unacceptable plan involves the very intuitive process of adjusting beam parameters, for inverse IMRT planning the treatment planner must adjust the dose constraints and penalties for the different anatomical structures. The relationship, however, between changes made to dose constraints and the resultant changes to the ensuing dose distribution are difficult to predict, often unintuitive, and may depend strongly on the exact algebraic form of the particular cost function programmed into the optimization algorithm.

Sometimes the treatment planner finds it necessary to resort to "artificial methods" of adjusting an IMRT dose distribution when attempts at altering dose constraints are unsuccessful. For example, if a resultant IMRT treatment plan has an undesirable hot spot in a specific region of the PTV that cannot be eliminated by adjusting, say, the penalty weight for overdosing the PTV, one could deceive the computer by contouring the overdosed section of the PTV separately, defining it as a new structure, and assigning different dose constraints to that structure than to the rest of the PTV. Similarly, one can define subvolumes within normal structures, and assign different dose constraints than have been assigned to the rest of the structure. In prostate treatments, for example, the anterior wall of the rectum that is closest to the prostate (assuming the prostate is the PTV) can be assigned different dose constraints than the rest of the rectal wall. A more reasonable set of dose constraints may then permit the optimization algorithm to find a better plan, rather than futilely search for a physically impossible plan. Defining subvolumes is a user strategy to better control specific regions of the dose distribution. Resorting to such tricks is a recognition of the fact that DVH-based OFs such as Equation 1 make no account of the spatial distribution of "hot" or "cold" dose regions (i.e., according to Equation 1, a hot or cold dose region is of equal importance no matter where it is located). In reality, of course, this is not always clinically realistic, hence the need sometimes to define substructures.

GENERATION OF LEAF MOTION FILES

The "leaf sequencer" is an algorithm within the IMRT planning system. It converts the beam intensity pattern calculated by the planning system into an instruction set specifying how the MLC leaves must move during beam delivery in order to deliver said intensity pattern. In practice, a separate computer algorithm (independent of the inverse planning algorithm), sometimes referred to as the "leaf sequencer," is used to calculate these files. The files created, or MLC instruction set, are sometimes referred to as DMLC files. Depending on the specific inverse planning system and beam delivery system being used, this optimized intensity pattern may be either continuously variable within each treatment portal (deliverable with

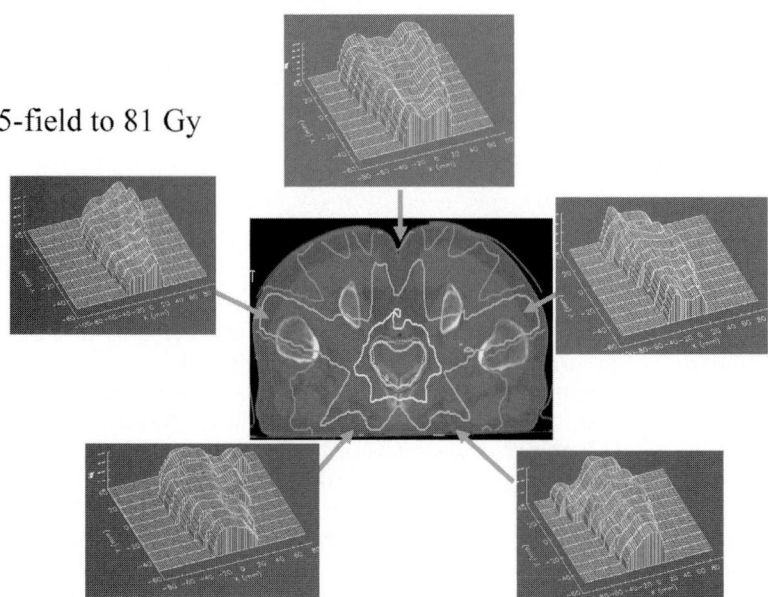

5-field to 81 Gy

Figure 8–6. The intensity profiles for all 5 beams in a typical IMRT prostate treatment to 81 Gy (patient is in the prone position). Note the decreased beam intensity in the center of the posterior field, designed to reduce dose to the rectum. See also Color Figure 8-6.

sliding-window technique) or discretized (for step-and-shoot beam delivery). When using discretized intensity profiles, one must specify the size of both the spatial steps (such as 10 mm × 10 mm step sizes in x and y) and the intensity steps (such as 10% or 20% intensity difference between intensity levels). For step-and-shoot beam delivery, x, y, and intensity must all be discretized. For sliding-window beam delivery, intensity plus one spatial dimension can be continuous. The second spatial dimension—the one perpendicular to the direction of leaf motion—must be discretized because the MLC leaf widths are finite (usually 5 or 10 mm leaf width).

For both sliding-window and step-and-shoot methods, there are many possible sequences of leaf motion capable of delivering the desired pattern. For a selected delivery method, determining the optimum leaf sequence for efficient delivery must take into account the number of segments, the number of total monitor units (MUs), restrictions on MLC leaf motion and speed, and the total delivery time.[25-31] Descriptions of two basic leaf sequencing techniques follow.

The first leaf sequencing method[31] described is designed for sliding-window beam delivery. It divides the 2D intensity distributions into a number of 1D intensity profiles, with each profile being delivered by one pair of leaves. The leaf paths are illustrated schematically in Figure 8-7. The dotted lines represent the positions of a leaf pair (x-axis) as a function of beam on time (y-axis). Both leaves start at the extreme left edge of the intended treatment field. As the beam is turned on (point a), both leaves move, with different speeds, from left to right. Initially the right leaf moves more rapidly than does the left leaf. The point P begins to receive radiation when the right leaf edge moves past it (point b), and continues to receive radiation until the left leaf passes over it (point c). By controlling the position and speed of the leaves, the computer can effectively control the beam on time (i.e., the duration between b and c) for every point in the beam, and thus deliver any desired dose intensity pattern.

Dynamic Delivery

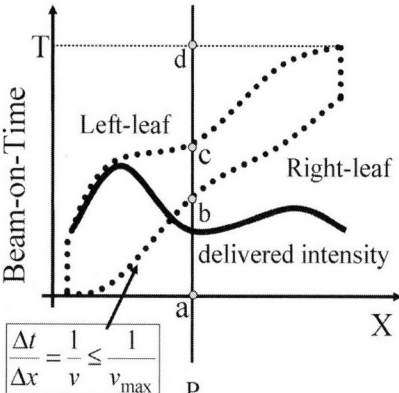

$$\frac{\Delta t}{\Delta x} = \frac{1}{v} \leq \frac{1}{v_{max}}$$

Figure 8–7. Schematic representation of radiation delivery using the sliding-window method. The dotted lines represent the positions of a leaf pair (x-axis) as a function of beam on time (y-axis), and the solid line depicts the total integrated beam intensity to all points underneath the strip of tissue being treated by this leaf pair. See text for details.

The solid line in Figure 8-7, for example, depicts the total integrated beam intensity to all points underneath the strip of tissue being treated by this leaf pair.

By extending this concept to multiple pairs of leaves, any desired 2D intensity modulation pattern can be produced with properly designed sequences of leaf positions. Since each leaf pair must deliver a different intensity profile, the speed and position of each leaf as a function of monitor units (MU) delivered must be individually controlled. For maximum efficiency in beam delivery (i.e., shortest possible treatment times) it is necessary to be able to move all leaves simultaneously. This requires modulation of leaf speeds as well as modulation of accelerator dose rate. Ideally one would always treat at the maximum dose rate of the accelerator, but if a particular leaf is required to move a large distance in a short period, it might require a speed exceeding the maximum mechanical leaf speed, and in such cases the dose rate must be reduced.

Unfortunately, not all desired intensity profiles are exactly achievable because of the constraints on leaf motion imposed by the design of the MLC and the clinical dose rate of the machine. The multileaf collimator manufactured by Varian Medical Systems, for example, is constrained by a maximum leaf speed (v_{max}) of 2.5 cm/sec. Thus, if one were running the accelerator at 600 mu/min, and the DMLC file instructed a leaf to move more than 0.25 cm per MU (i.e., [2.5 cm/sec]/[600 mu/min]) there would have to be a beam holdoff. There is also a constraint on the maximum DMLC field width of 14.5 cm (fields larger than 14.5 cm width require a carriage movement). These MLC design limitations are discussed more fully in "Characteristics of MLCs" later in this chapter.

The second leaf sequencing method described[27] is designed for step-and-shoot delivery in which a continuous 2D intensity distribution must be approximated by a discretized matrix delivered by superposition of a finite number of fixed field shapes. The number of intensity-level steps, and hence the number of fixed fields required can be selected by the treatment planner. The greater the number of intensity levels used, the larger the number of segments required, and the closer the delivered dose will be to the intended dose. That is, step-and-shoot technique, by its very nature, cannot deliver exactly the intensity plan calculated by the optimization algorithm (and thus introduces some error into the delivered dose). Some treatment planning systems overcome this delivered dose error by purposely designing a discretized "optimum" intensity (again, with a user-selected number of intensity levels) before the optimization. In this case, the finite number of intensity levels affects the delivery time and plan quality, but does not introduce any error between calculated and delivered dose.

The concept of step-and-shoot leaf sequencing is illustrated in Figure 8-8a, where we represent a planned, or desired, intensity pattern having a maximum intensity of 8 dose units. The algorithm first determines the maximum contiguous field shape that can be exposed to an intensity level equal to one half of the maximum intensity (i.e., 4 units). This area would be the first field shape. Subsequent field shapes, or steps, must have decreasing intensity levels, and decreases must be by powers of 2. In this case, the decrements are 4, 2, and 1. Due to the

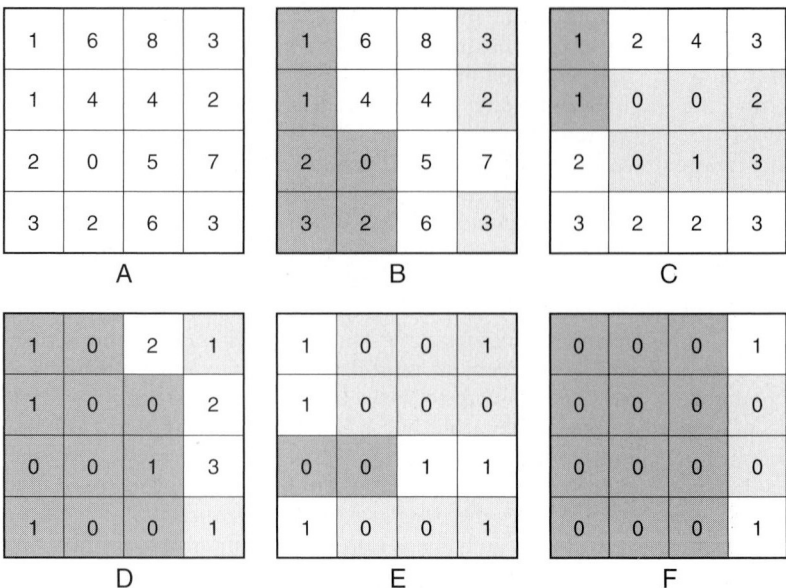

Figure 8–8. Example of an intensity-modulated radiotherapy treatment using five step-and-shoot beam segments. The desired final intensity map is shown in panel **A**. Panels **B–F** depict 5 separate multileaf collimator-shaped fields (*open portion of field in white, blocked portions of field in dark and light gray*) with beam intensities of 4, 2, 2, 1, and 1, respectively, used to deliver the desired total intensity pattern. (From Xia P, Verhey LJ: MLC leaf sequencing algorithm for intensity-modulated beams with multiple static segments. *Med Physics.* 1998;25:1424.)

limitation of MLC motion constraints, it may sometimes be necessary to deliver one exposure intensity level more than once with different MLC shapes. In this example, the exposure intensities are in an order of 4, 2, 2, 1, 1, and the corresponding MLC shapes are shown in Figure 8-8b through 8f. The shaded areas are covered by MLC leaves (the dark area is covered by the left set of MLC leaves and the gray area is covered by the right set of leaves) and open areas are to be exposed. In Figure 8b, for example, the open area receives 4 dose units. In Figure 8c the open area receives 2 units, etc. These MLC shapes need not be contiguous, and each shape is associated with a given MU. Each segment shown in Figures 8b through 8f can be considered as an individual conventional field.

DELIVERY OF INTENSITY-MODULATED TREATMENT

Delivery of forward planned 3DCRT treatment beams is similar to conventional treatment delivery except for the fact that plans often require an increased number of treatment fields. Even without an MLC, IMRT can be delivered via the use of custom-designed 3D physical compensators fabricated on a computer-controlled milling machine. The milling machine can be used to cut either the compensator itself or a negative mold of the compensator to be filled with Cerrobend or similar type material. This approach can be implemented without a significant capital investment, as it does not require an MLC. There is, however, additional personnel time required for fabricating the filters and for inserting them unto each field during treatment. Physical compensators also harden the beam, generate scattered radiation, and increase skin doses and doses outside the field. Nonetheless, this technique is capable of delivering dose distributions comparable to more exotic MLC-based

beam delivery systems. This technique is not, however, commonly used.

Much more commonly, IMRT is delivered by using a computer-controlled MLC, shown schematically and in photographs (from several different manufacturers) in Figures 8-9 through 8-13. MLC-based IMRT, as described previously, follows one of two basic approaches: multiple static fields (step-and-shoot technique) or dynamic fields (sliding-window technique). Both techniques require computer-controlled MLCs, but differ in that the latter approach uses continuously moving MLC leaves (while the radiation beam is on), whereas the former approach uses a sequence of multiple fixed-field shapes, each with its own predetermined incremental radiation dose. In the step-and-shoot technique, after the dose from the first subfield is delivered, the beam is turned off, the MLC field shape reset by the computer, the second incremental dose delivered, etc. The number of steps or field shapes in the sequence can be as small as a few, or as large as 100 or more.

A technologically different approach to IMRT beam delivery is so-called *tomotherapy*, wherein a rotating fan beam (broad in the transverse direction, but narrow in the superior-inferior direction—approximately 1.0–2.0-cm beam width in this direction) is intensity modulated with a bimodal MLC. The bimodal MLC has multiple leaf pairs similar to a more conventional MLC, but differs in that each leaf pair has only two positions—completely open or completely closed. Two different approaches to IMRT tomotherapy have been proposed, one being a truly dedicated tomotherapy system, the heart of which is a machine that is a hybrid between a spiral CT scanner and a linear accelerator.[32] The second approach uses a custom-designed MLC attached to a conventional linear accelerator and requires axial stepping of the linear accelerator treatment couch.

The first type of tomotherapy machine, being developed at the University of Wisconsin,[32] functions much the same way as a conventional spiral CT scanner,

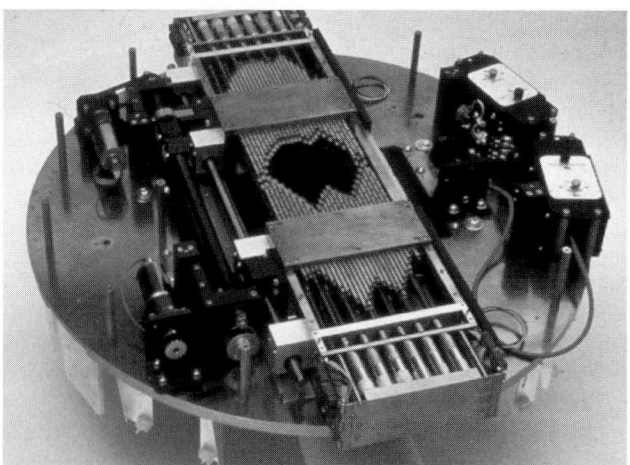

Figure 8–9. Varian multileaf collimator

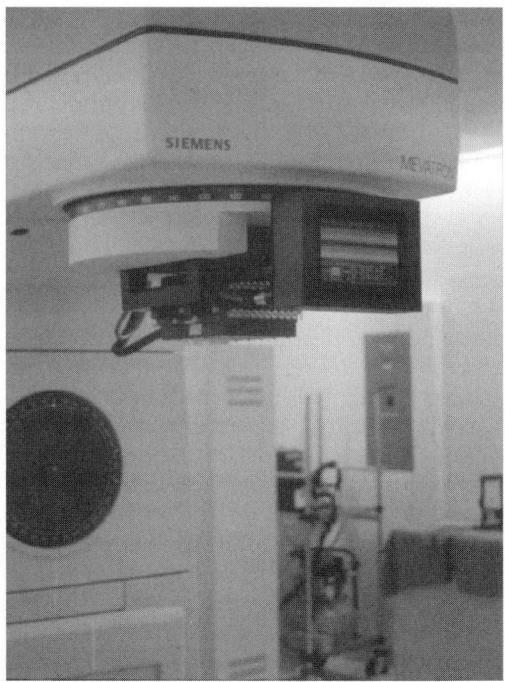

Figure 8–10. The MIMiC mounted on a linear accelerator

wherein a 6MV fan beam x-ray source rotates around the patient, modulated by the opening and closing of MLC leaf pairs. Simultaneous with the beam rotation and MLC leaf openings and closings, the treatment couch translates through the treatment gantry donut to facilitate 3D dose delivery. The dedicated, spiral type design incorporates a small 6MV electron linear accelerator that has been modified to replace a conventional kV x-ray tube in a spiral CT machine. Thus, a 6MV photon fan beam rotates around the patient in synchrony with a translating treatment couch, and the patient is irradiated with a spiral fan beam. A specially designed MLC (similar to the device shown in Fig. 8-10) opens and closes in synchrony with the beam rotation and couch translation to produce a 3D intensity-modulated beam.

The second type of tomotherapy system, developed commercially (the Mimic collimator, NOMOS Corp., Sewickley, Pa.), is shown in Figure 8-10. It is designed as an add-on to a conventional linear accelerator and greatly reduces the capital expense required for tomotherapy treatment. With this system, as in CT, the radiation beam is delivered in narrow slices as the linear accelerator beam rotates around the patient, aimed at a single isocenter. This technique uses a special short-stroke MLC (trade name, MIMiC) to produce an intensity-modulated slit (or fan) beam that rotates about the patient. The MIMiC consists of two banks of 20 stubby tungsten vanes with a leaf length of 1 cm or 2 cm and leaf width of 1 cm when projected 100 cm from the x-ray target to the isocenter.

Figure 8-10 illustrates the MIMiC mounted on a linear accelerator. The vanes are rapidly driven via an electro-pneumatic system to either an open or a closed position in synchrony with the gantry rotation. The beam intensity is usually modulated every 5 or 10 degrees of gantry rotation by moving leaves into and out of the beam. The beam intensity produced at each leaf position is proportional to the fraction of time the leaf is held in the open position. The leaves in the MIMiC have a tongue-and-groove design (described more fully in the next section, Characteristics of MLCs) that limits beam transmission between adjacent leaves to less than 0.5%. Each leaf end is shaped to match the radiation beam divergence in the array's long dimension. The nominal maximum field size

is 2 × 20 cm for a single arc when projected to the 100-cm isocenter. Depending on the beam penumbra and the distance from the radiation source to the block tray slot, the thickness of each treatment slice is 0.84 cm depending on the particular accelerator design.

The MIMiC collimator is mounted on a custom slot installed in the faceplate of the linear accelerator with its long axis oriented along the patient's transaxial direction. Since a rotation about the patient treats only two 1-cm slices through the patient, the treatment couch is successively indexed craniocaudally when treating targets with dimensions greater than 2 cm. A special device called the Crane controls the treatment couch movement with submillimeter precision. Two treatment slices can be delivered at each index position. With multiple indices, the treatment slices from different indices are matched at the isocenter. Due to the beam divergence, the field match is imperfect at any depth other than the isocenter, but rotational beams effectively average out hot and cold regions of dose in the overlap regions, with a net result of dose homogeneity typically being better than ±10%.[33] However, this method of delivery requires more stringent patient immobilization since an error of 1.0 mm in a couch position can cause up to a 25% dose error.[34]

Another pseudo-tomotherapy system, a cross between the step-and-shoot and sliding-window techniques, has been dubbed as intensity-modulated arc therapy (IMAT). It entails the delivery of multiple radiation arcs (i.e., beam delivery with a rotating accelerator gantry), with each arc consisting of a different pattern of dynamically changing 2D radiation field shapes.[35] Unlike the "regular" step-and-shoot technique, with IMAT the MLC leaves move continuously while the beam is on and while the gantry is rotating, and in this respect it is similar to the sliding-window technique. The actual creation of an intensity-modulated radiation dose, however, is created by the superposition of different field shapes (rather than by modulation of MLC leaf speeds), and in this regard it is similar to the step-and-shoot technique. As pointed out earlier, there are many possible permutations of decomposition patterns for the 2D beams, and therefore the design of the most efficient MLC position sequence in the arc therapy is a challenging problem.

Characteristics of MLCs

To better understand some of the technical details of MLC-based IMRT delivery, we review the basic physical and geometric characteristics of multileaf collimator design, as implemented by three major manufacturing companies: Elekta, Norcross, Ga.; Siemens Medical Systems, Concord, Calif.; and Varian Medical Systems, Palo Alto, Calif. The three designs differ in many ways including the location of the MLC relative to the conventional jaws, whether MLC leaves are single- or double-focused, the physical characteristics or shapes of leaves, leaf movement restriction, and maximum achievable field sizes. These design features all affect IMRT beam delivery and dosimetry characteristics.

The MLC can be installed within the accelerator gantry head either above the upper set of secondary collimator jaws or below the lower set of secondary collimator jaws as a tertiary collimator. In the Elekta linear accelerator, for example, the MLC replaces the upper (Y) jaws, although it is augmented with an additional 3-cm thick Y jaw to reduce the radiation leakage from the MLC. A schematic drawing of the location of the Elekta MLC collimator in relationship to the other jaws is shown in Figure 8-11. In the Siemens linear accelerator, the MLC completely replaces the lower (X) jaws, as shown schematically in Figure 8-12. In the Varian linear accelerator the MLC is a tertiary collimator located below and in addition to the conventional X and Y secondary collimators, as shown schematically in

Figure 8-13 (see also Figure 8-9). Placing the MLC below both sets of secondary collimators places it closer to the patient, which in principle improves the geometric penumbra, but at the expense of a physically larger device with less clearance between the MLC and the patient. Placing the MLC above the secondary collimators (as in the Elekta design) produces a poorer geometric penumbra, but also results in a smaller and lighter MLC design with increased physical clearance between the accelerator head and the patient. The Siemens design obviously takes a middle course in this unavoidable tradeoff of geometric penumbra versus MLC size.

Complicating design considerations is the fact that adjacent leaves must be able to slide smoothly across each other with minimal gaps between leaves to reduce radiation leakage and transmission. Most MLC designs accomplish this by cutting so-called *tongues and grooves* into the sides of the leaves. The side of one leaf has an extended portion called the tongue, while the abutting side of the adjacent leaf has an indented portion called the groove. Two adjacent leaves are coupled together as the tongue of one leaf slides within the groove of the adjacent leaf. Each leaf has a tongue on one side, and a groove on the opposite side. The manufacture of precise tongues and grooves into extremely small individual leaves is an exacting process that places a lower limit on the size of individual MLC leaves.

While this tongue-and-groove design reduces radiation leakage, it also complicates treatment-planning dose calculations because the transmission through any leaf depends on whether the beam passes through the tongue, the center, or the groove portion of the leaf. When two adjacent leaves have different degrees of extension, the tongue side of the more extended leaf produces an underdose region near the leaf edge. This phenomenon is called the tongue-and-groove effect. This effect is more predominant in IMRT than in conventional 3DCRT because IMRT often requires adjacent leaves to be set far apart from each other.

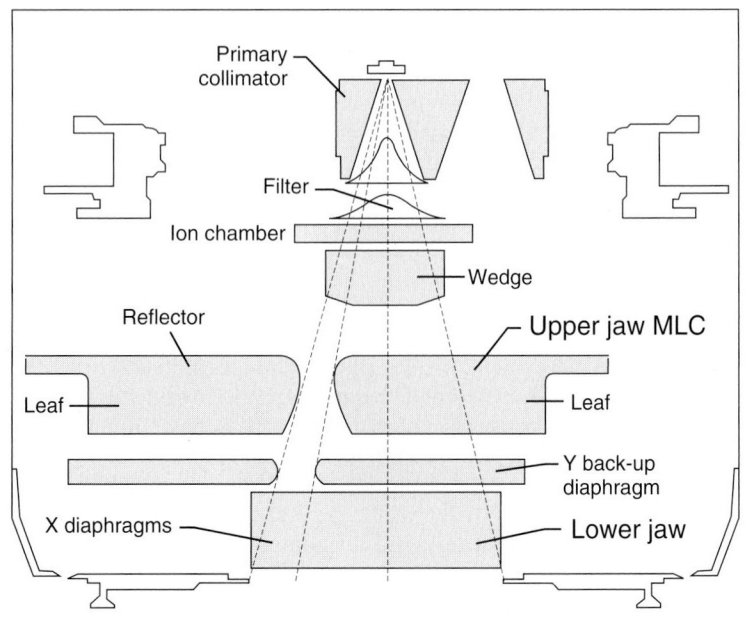

Figure 8–11. A schematic drawing of the Elekta multileaf collimator. (From Van Vyk J, ed: *The Modern Technology of Radiation Oncology*. Madison, Wisc.: Medical Physics Publishing; 1999.)

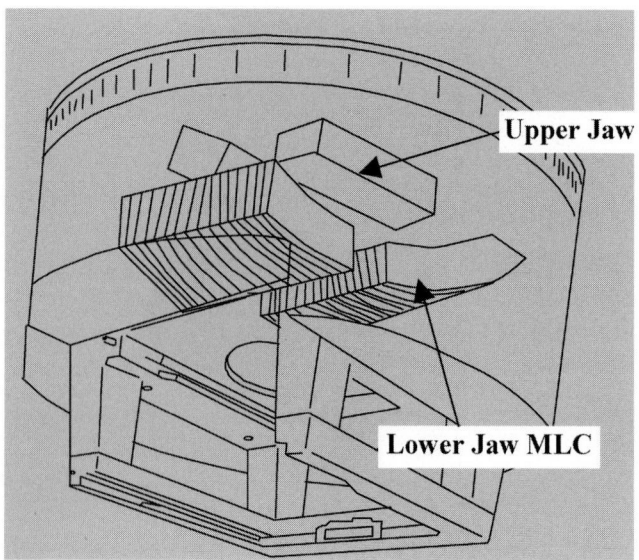

Figure 8–12. A schematic drawing of the Siemens multileaf collimator

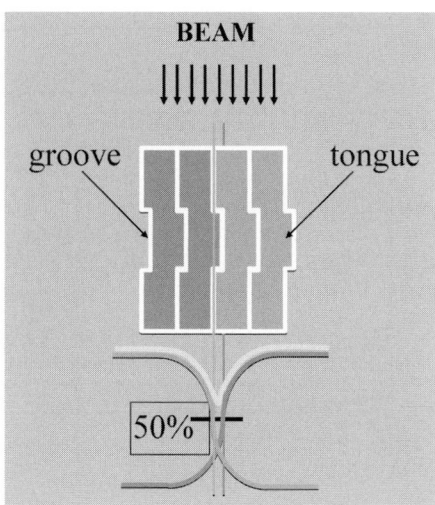

Figure 8–14. Schematic "end-on" view of multileaf collimator showing tongue and groove design and approximate resulting beam transmission.

Figure 8-14 shows schematically a "head-on" view of the MLC leaves, illustrating how adjacent leaves have interlocking tongues and grooves,[36,37] plus the variations in transmission dose that result. The differences in beam transmission through tongues and grooves is demonstrated in Figure 8-15, where we show a sheet of radiographic film (center panel, Fig. 8-15b) that was doubly exposed to two matched MLC shapes, shown in panels 8-15a (left) and 8-15c (right), respectively. The two MLC shapes are complementary to each other as suggested by Sykes et al.,[38] wherein leaves that were open in Figure 8-15a were closed in Figure 8-15c, and vice versa. The resultant exposed film (Fig. 8-15b) clearly shows underdose regions at the match lines where the tongue is exposed to radiation. The magnitude of the dose reductions in these match line areas is about 17% and 25% for Siemens (MXE) and Varian (CL2300 C/D) linear accelerators, respectively, and similar results have been reported for the Elekta design.[38]

Another important design consideration is focusing the ends of MLC leaves to match the radiation field beam divergence. This is, of course, a 2D problem as the beam diverges in both the direction along MLC leaf motion and in the direction perpendicular to MLC leaf motion (designated as the X and Y directions, respectively). Focusing MLC leaves in the Y direction can be accomplished in the same manner as in a conventional secondary collimator. Namely, the width of each MLC leaf is designed to be slightly narrower at the top of the leaf (nearer the radiation source) than at the bottom of the leaf (nearer the patient), as shown in Figure 8-16a. MLCs focused only in the Y direction are called single-focused MLCs.

Double-focused MLCs are also focused in the X direction, which is parallel to the leaf motion. This is a more difficult problem because in the X direction the beam divergence is a function of the leaf position, and to be perfectly focused in the X direction the divergence angle at the end of each leaf must be equal to the arctangent of the ratio of leaf position divided by the distance of the MLC from the source. Of the three manufacturer designs discussed here, only the Siemens MLC is double-focused.

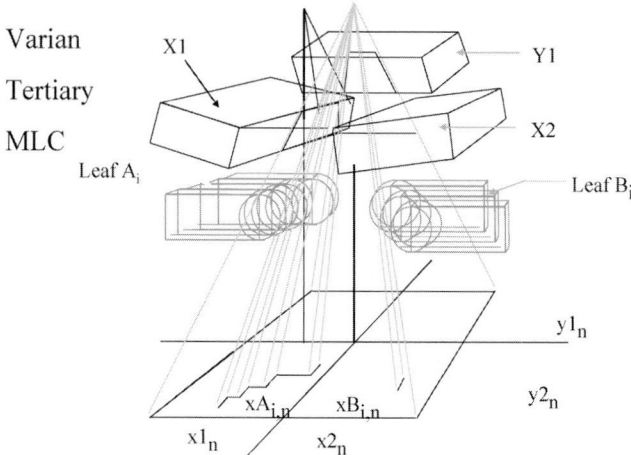

Figure 8–13. A schematic drawing of the Varian multileaf collimator. (From Van Vyk J, ed: *The Modern Technology of Radiation Oncology.* Madison, Wisc.: Medical Physics Publishing; 1999.)

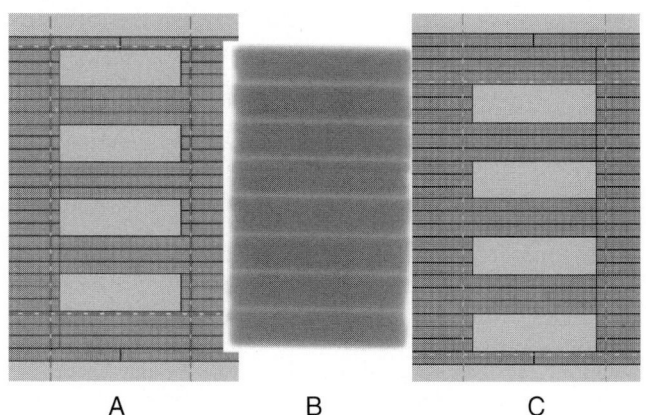

Figure 8–15. Dosimetric demonstration of tongue-and-groove effect using a doubly exposed film (*panel* **B**) with two matched multileaf collimator shapes, shown in (**A**) and (**C**), respectively.

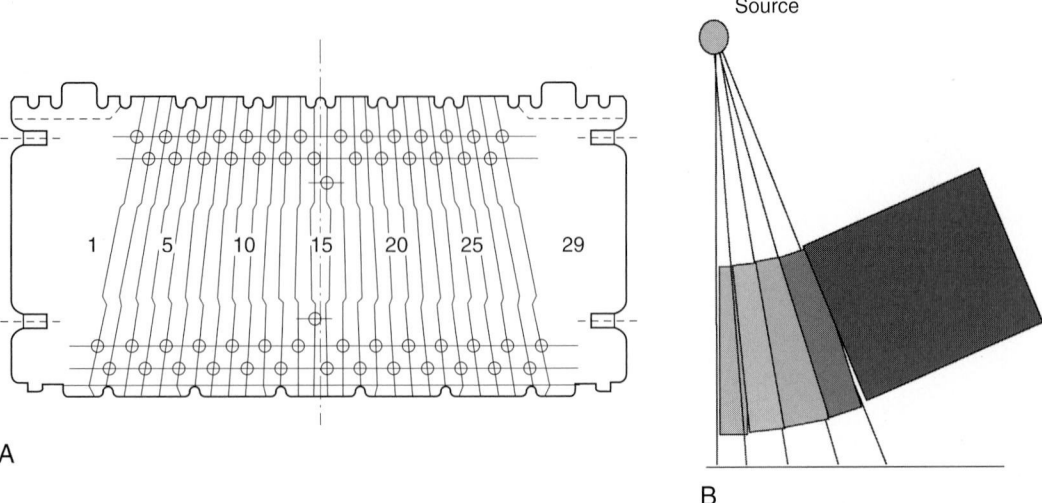

A

Figure 8–16. **A,** Multileaf collimator (MLC) leaves are arranged to follow the radiation divergence in Y direction. **B,** MLC leaves move along a spherical surface centered at the radiation source to follow the radiation divergence in X direction. (From Xia P, Verhey LJ: Delivery systems of intensity-modulated radiotherapy using multi-leaf collimators. *Med Dosim.* 2001;26:169.)

This is achieved by having the leaves move along a spherical surface centered at the radiation source (as shown in Fig. 8-16b)—a feat readily accomplished in the Siemens design since the MLC essentially replaces the secondary X collimator.

Both the Elekta and Varian MLCs are single-focused and the leaf motion is in the plane perpendicular to the beam direction, rather than along a spherical surface as in the Siemens design. This precludes the possibility of true 2D focusing, but in both the Elekta and Varian designs there is "pseudo" focusing in the X direction achieved by machining the ends of the leaves with a slight convex curvature rather than as flat surfaces (Fig. 8-17, and see also Fig. 8-11). This convexly curved leaf end greatly reduces (but does not eliminate) the variations in beam penumbra that would otherwise result if the leaf ends were perfectly flat. Even with a rounded leaf end design, the radiation field still passes through slightly differing thicknesses of material with different field sizes, resulting in second-order effects on penumbra. Also, the coincidence between the radiation and light fields can be leaf-position dependent. The offset between the radiation field and light field can be corrected using either an internal correction file (provided by the vendor) or an external correction file created by the end user.[39] The rounded-leaf end design, while improving penumbra variations, significantly increases radiation leakage to as high as 20% or more[40] when opposing leaves abut each other (i.e., zero field size).

The number of leaves and leaf thicknesses and widths vary among manufacturers. The Elekta MLC consists of 40 pairs of tungsten alloy leaves with 7.5-cm thickness. Each leaf projects as 1.0 cm wide and 32.5 cm long at the isocenter (the physical dimensions of the leaves are of course <1/2 this size). The maximum leaf speed, also a factor in total treatment time, projects to 2.0 cm/second at the isocenter. The Siemens MLC consists of 29 pairs of tungsten alloy leaves of 7.6-cm thickness. The inner

27 pairs of leaves project a 1.0-cm leaf width and 31-cm leaf length at the isocenter, while each outer pair of leaves (called *mage leaves*) projects a 6.5-cm leaf width at the isocenter. Combining the two pairs of mage leaves plus

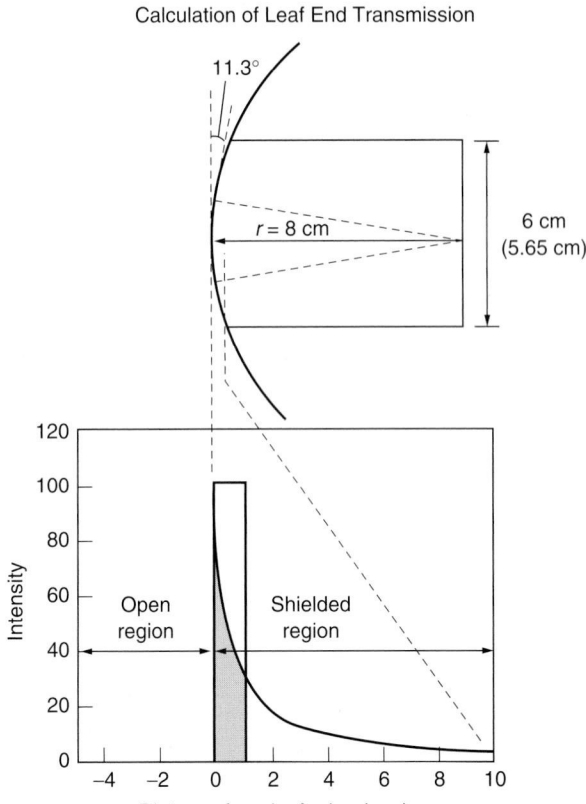

Figure 8–17. Schematic of a typical rounded leaf end design of a multileaf collimator. Note that the variable beam transmission affects the shape of the beam dose penumbra, and that both penumbra and coincidence of light and radiation fields are functions of leaf position.

the inner 27 leaf pairs yields a maximum field size of 40×40 cm^2 (but only 40×27 cm^2 with the inner leaves alone). A new Siemens design includes 40 leaf pairs, each projecting a 1-cm width at the isocenter. Also in this design the central beam axis projects through the central leaf (rather than between two leaf pairs), substantially reducing radiation leakage in the center of the beam. The over-travel distance for any leaf is 10.0 cm past midfield. The maximum leaf speed projects to 2.0 cm/second at the isocenter, although the speed of each individual leaf cannot be independently controlled. To minimize the radiation leakage, the upper jaws always automatically follow the shape of the MLC and are positioned no more than 0.5 cm beyond the boundary of the MLC shape, but can be positioned any distance inside the boundary of the MLC shape.

Several different Varian MLC designs exist. They incorporate 26, 40, or 60 pairs of tungsten alloy leaves with 5-cm thickness. In the 26- and 40-pair designs all leaves project to 1-cm width at the isocenter (the maximum MLC field size therefore being 26×40 cm^2). In the 120-pair design the central 40 leaves project to 0.5-cm width at the isocenter, and the outer 20 pairs of leaves project to 1-cm width (total field size 40×40 cm^2). The leaves are attached to leaf carriages, which can each be retracted up to 20 cm from the beam axis and can travel up to 1 cm beyond the axis. Leaves can, in turn, travel up to 15 cm beyond the end of the carriages. The maximum leaf speed is 2.5 cm/second as projected to the isocenter, and leaf speeds can be independently controlled. There is no restriction on the upper or lower jaw locations relative to the MLC shape, but the recommended jaw position is 0.5 cm beyond the boundary of the MLC shape for conventional treatment. For IMRT delivery, the upper or lower jaws are kept stationary. Because the leaf length is 16 cm, the distance between the most leading leaf and the most retracted leaf from the same bank is limited to 14.5 cm to avoid the radiation leakage through the tail of the most leading leaf or the tip of the most retracted leaf.

Additional leaf motion restrictions affect the delivery, efficiency, and dose accuracy of IMRT. Figure 8-18 shows three such types of leaf motion restrictions. In Figure 8-18 all left bank leaves are denoted in gray, and right bank leaves in black. Figure 8-18a shows a design where there is a minimum gap width, such that opposing leaves cannot be closer than a preset minimum distance apart. Figure 8-18b shows a design that prohibits interdigitation, wherein one (black) leaf end cannot extend beyond the tips of its two neighboring opposing (gray) leaves. Figure 8-18c shows a design that prohibits any leaf from extending more than a fixed distance past field center. Such restrictions of one sort or another exist for all currently manufactured MLC designs.

Maximum achievable IMRT field sizes are limited by the over-travel distance (past field center) of MLC leaves, which in turn is related to the length of the leaves, as a leaf extending farther past field center than its own length will leave the beam unblocked at its other end. As a result, the maximum usable field in IMRT is always smaller than the maximum field size for conventional beam delivery. For example, for the Elekta MLC, the field width for IMRT is twice the over-travel distance in the leaf motion direction (i.e., 25×40 cm^2). In the Siemens MLC, the maximum field size for IMRT is 21×29 cm^2. However, if a field length is greater than 20 cm, some IMRT fields may not be deliverable with the Siemens MLC since some segments may require a Y jaw over-travel of more than 10 cm.

The maximum field size in IMRT delivery can be increased if the secondary jaws can be moved to cover the region behind the most extended MLC leaves, as is the case for Varian's MLC. Thus, a combination of carriage moves plus secondary jaw moves can sometimes be used to increase the maximum field size for IMRT, but in effect this is being achieved via use of multiple fields. Various combinations of carriage motion, backup with the secondary jaws, and leaf extensions can therefore yield a total IMRT treatment field size of 34×26 or 40 cm^2 (depending on the number of leaf pairs), although a single IMRT field is limited to 14.5 cm in width (15-cm width for later design). The limitation of a single IMRT field to 14.5 cm (or 15-cm width with more recent designs) is partly because of the projected leaf length of 16 cm and partly because the MLC carriages and secondary jaws are restricted from moving during IMRT delivery. With the Varian system, therefore, IMRT field width greater than 14.5-cm width must be split into two or three fields. This field splitting in IMRT delivery can potentially cause over- or underdosing at match lines, although some treatment planning systems[41] purposely add dose feathering at these match lines.

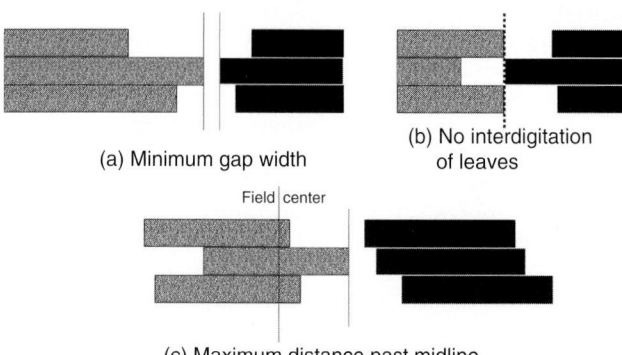

(a) Minimum gap width

(b) No interdigitation of leaves

(c) Maximum distance past midline

Figure 8–18. Three types of leaf motion constraints: (**A**) no leaf end can come closer than a fixed distance (typically 2-5 mm) to the tip of its directly-opposing leaf or to the tips of its two neighboring opposing leaves; (**B**) a design that prohibits interdigitation (i.e., a leaf traveling beyond the tips of its opposing neighbors); and (**C**) leaves cannot extend more than a fixed distance (usually about 10 cm) beyond field midline.

More on Static versus Dynamic Multileaf Collimator Delivery

As discussed earlier, there are two conceptually different ways to deliver MLC-based IMRT: static (or step-and-shoot delivery) and dynamic (or sliding-window delivery). All MLC designs can deliver the former, but the latter requires dynamic control of leaf motions. In principle, static IMRT treatments can be "forward planned," although they are more commonly "inverse planned." Dynamic treatments, on the other hand, must be inverse planned. Static MLC delivery can, in principle, be delivered using many sets of conventional Cerrobend blocks instead of an MLC with each segment being considered as a conventionally delivered individual field. This, however, would be extremely tedious and time consuming, as many sets of blocks would be required for each beam direction, not to mention that executing a treatment plan dose calculation with dozens (or even hundreds) of individual fields would be highly impractical. Dynamic IMRT cannot, even in theory, be delivered without an MLC.

For both dynamic and static IMRT, all treatment parameters and fields are usually monitored using a record and verify (R/V) system. Such an R/V system is almost essential, as the volume of data describing beam parameters and MLC settings is too large to be checked or monitored manually. R/V systems also usually incorporate so-called *autosequencing software* that can be used to automatically deliver each segment of the treatment with little or no human intervention. This can be particularly useful for step-and-shoot treatments requiring many subfields, although even with autosequencing the overhead time required for downloading, setting up, and verifying each beam segment can be 5 to 7 seconds. For a complex intensity pattern delivery, this overhead time can be a significant portion of the total treatment time. R/V and autosequencing software also permit relatively easy resumption of an interrupted treatment.

The advantages of static MLC-based IMRT are that it is conceptually simple, there are no requirements to control the individual leaf speeds (thus simplifying the MLC control system) or delivery dose rate, an interrupted treatment is easy to resume, it is easy to verify an intensity pattern for each subfield, and fewer monitor units are required in comparison with the dynamic MLC delivery. The disadvantages are that it may require prolonged treatment time, particularly for complex intensity patterns, and that very complex intensity patterns can only be approximated, which could compromise dose optimization and the accuracy of delivered dose. Some treatment planning systems (such as Corvus/Nomos), however, incorporate discretized (rather than continuous) intensity patterns in their optimization routines and dose calculations, which eliminates differences between intended and delivered intensity patterns, but still does not solve the limitations of discretized intensity levels.

The advantage of dynamic or sliding-window MLC delivery is that it can deliver a smoothly varying intensity profile, which enables greater flexibility in treatment plan design. There is also only one field (i.e., no subfields) per beam direction. The disadvantages are that the delivery mechanism is more complicated, involving leaf speed and dose rate modulation; precise control of individual leaf speeds is required; and small errors in the calibration of leaf position could (for highly modulated fields) result in significant errors in delivered doses (leaf position calibration is also a problem for static IMRT, but less so). Thus, careful quality assurance tests are required for dynamic IMRT. Finally, intensity patterns designed to have regions with zero dose intensity, such as for a cord block, cannot be easily delivered. This is because leaves generally cannot be completely closed when in dynamic mode, and even if they could, the rounded leaf ends still permit as much as 20% leakage.[40] In such a situation one must

either split the IMRT treatment field into two separate beam segments or augment the IMRT treatment with the addition of a Cerrobend block.

DOSE CALCULATION ALGORITHMS

Dose calculation models for IMRT are not fundamentally different than those used for conventional forward planning. This is because the dose calculations and the actual optimization processes are decoupled. That is, first the computer divides each treatment field into multiple pencil beams and calculates the dose distribution for each individual pencil beam. These dose distributions are stored in memory (or on disk) and need only be done once. The optimization algorithm then adjusts the weight of each pencil beam so that the dose distribution resulting from the summation of all pencil beams best matches the dose prescription specified by the treatment planner. But the initial pencil beam dose calculation algorithm need not be fundamentally different from calculation algorithms used for conventional treatment planning.

Having said that, we must note that there are still some complications associated with MLC IMRT dose calculations that are not normally present when calculating doses for conventional static fields. First, when delivering IMRT dose, only a portion of the entire field is exposed at any given time. As a result, the total beam on time (or monitor units) required can be two to four times longer than for conventional treatments. In general, the more complex the intensity modulation, the more monitor units required. Thus factors such as variable beam transmission through rounded leaf ends or through tongues and grooves, which are usually ignorable in conventional dose calculations, must be more accurately calculated with IMRT. Total leakage dose through MLC leaves can amount to several percent of the total IMRT dose as opposed to less than 1% for conventional treatments. Extremely variable effective field sizes during IMRT beam delivery also complicate calculation of the output factor, as the relationship between collimator scatter factor (CSF) and phantom scatter factor (PSF) becomes more complicated than for conventional dose calculations.

One accurate method of dose calculation developed at Memorial Sloan-Kettering Cancer Center (MSKCC)[19] entails a one-time Monte Carlo (MC) calculation of pencil beams, or dose kernels to describe the transport of photons and electrons in homogeneous and inhomogeneous media. Patient treatment planning then incorporates a convolution of pencil beams. In this dose model, inhomogeneity effects are accounted for by the traditional method of equivalent path length (or similar algorithm), and pencil beam convolution is used only as a correction factor to account for the variation of intensity relative to a flat, uniform field. However, in a highly heterogeneous media such as the lung, this method of calculation can result in errors of 3% to 4% or more, although methods are being developed to improve accuracy without greatly increasing computation times. Incorporating full-scale MC dose calculations for each patient treatment plan can provide the most accurate dose calculation, but because of the lengthy computation time, the routine use of MC awaits faster computer speeds and more efficient algorithms. Nevertheless, the MC method is relied upon to derive an accurate pencil beam kernel and the source function (which predicts the incident-intensity pattern), with detailed accounting for the finite source size, extra-focal radiation (from the flattening filters, primary and secondary collimators), beam spectrum, etc.

A good quality assurance program requires an independent, or so-called *second check*, calculation of beam on time and total monitor units for IMRT treatments. Such calculations, however, are too difficult to perform manually. They must be made with a second, completely independent computer program. Commercial versions of such software are only now becoming available. In the absence of commercial independent dose-check software, many institutions have developed in-house software for this purpose. The process for such calculations requires downloading the leaf sequence files calculated for the patient treatment to a second computer program, completely independent of the original treatment planning program, which then recalculates the dose independently for comparison to the original treatment plan.

Such independent-check programs, however, are still not widely available and most institutions rely on physical measurements to confirm IMRT dose calculations. This is performed typically by having the treatment planning system recalculate the dose to points or planes in a geometric (usually flat) phantom using the exact beam-intensity profiles that will be used for patient treatment. Direct measurements of doses are then made in the phantom, usually with ion chambers, diodes, or film, and are compared to computer calculations. If agreement is satisfactory, one then *assumes* that the dose distribution within the patient was also calculated correctly. Obviously, this is a tedious and time-consuming process that requires not only dose measurements, but also a second dose calculation for the phantom.

QUALITY ASSURANCE FOR IMRT DELIVERY

In this section, we focus on QA issues related to static and dynamic MLC delivery, including recommended "routine" mechanical and dosimetric tests, plus tests specific to each patient's treatment plan.

Mechanical Tests

The geometric accuracy of leaf positions is critically important for both static and dynamic IMRT, much more so than are collimator settings for conventional radiotherapy. For conventional beam delivery, a systematic error in collimator or leaf position affects only the width of the beam and therefore either increases or decreases slightly the volume of tissue being irradiated. For static IMRT, however, there are many subfields, and thus many beam edges within each field. Consequently, the same systematic error in leaf position affects the dose at many different locations within the field. For dynamic IMRT the dose delivered to each strip of tissue is proportional to the gap width of the leaf pair passing

over it, and small errors in average gap width can result in significant dose errors. Consider, for example, an MLC field for which the average gap width is intended to be 1 cm, but for which one or the other leaf has a systematic positional error of 1 mm. The resulting gap, and consequently the delivered dose to that strip, would therefore be in error by 10% (i.e., 1 mm/1 cm) everywhere within the strip of tissue covered by that leaf, and not just at the field edge as would be the case for conventional static beam delivery.

Thus, precise calibration and verification of leaf position is much more important for IMRT than for conventional therapy or for 3DCRT, and somewhat more important for sliding window than for step and shoot. Mechanical calibration of the leaf positions can be tested using procedures and software supplied by the manufacturers, although independent physical verification methods such as caliper/micrometer measurements of leaf positions are also recommended. Several MLC test patterns have been designed and used for MLC leaf position quality assurance. One such test pattern, shown in Figure 8-19,[42] is specifically designed to test for small errors in DMLC leaf position. In this test, a leaf motion file is generated, instructing the MLC to deliver five narrow vertical bands of radiation. The left panel shows a film exposure in which the MLC functioned properly, as indicated by the fact that all five dark strips are of equal intensity and thickness (lighter horizontal bands and streaks are the result of normal MLC leakage). In the right panel, however, several individual leaves have been intentionally miscalibrated by −.5, −.2, +.2, and +.5 mm (top to bottom of film, respectively). Note the narrow spots in all five vertical bands for the −.5 and −.2 mm errors in calibration, and the broad spots for the +.5 and +.2 mm errors. This demonstrates that a simple daily film QA test can detect MLC positioning errors of a fraction of a millimeter.

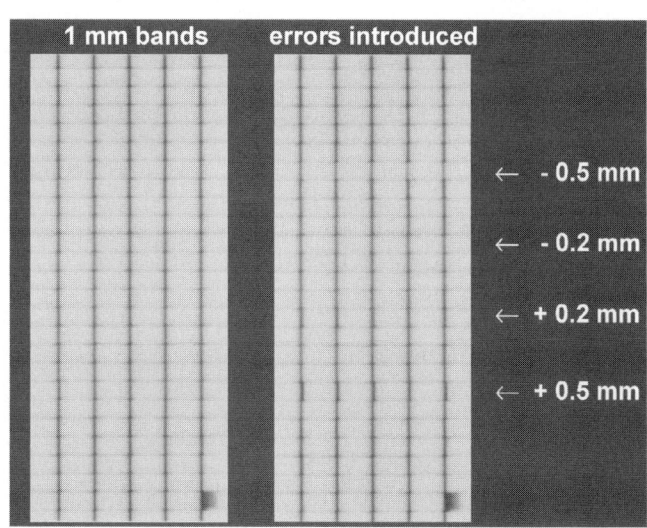

Figure 8–19. Multileaf collimator film test pattern in which leaves are programmed to deliver 5 separate 5-mm wide dose strips. Note that in the rightmost film certain leaf pairs were intentionally programmed to improper gap widths of ±.2 and ±.5 mm, respectively, which are clearly visibly lighter or brighter on the films.

Another important consideration for IMRT is monitoring MLC performance during treatment. While the beam is on, the Varian MLC control computer, for example, checks all leaf positions every 55 msec, compares them to the planned leaf positions in the DMLC file, and records them in a DMLC "log file." If any leaf deviates from its planned position beyond a preset tolerance, the control computer invokes a beam holdoff, and radiation delivery is withheld until all leaves are again within tolerance. Deviations that invoke beam holdoff should occur infrequently, as the leaf sequencer algorithm incorporates MLC leaf speed limitations and accelerator dose rates when calculating DMLC files. Our experience has been that leaf deviations greater than 1 mm occur less than 1% of the time. The DMLC control software permits the user to preset the tolerance for invoking a beam holdoff, and we have found 2 mm to be a good compromise between ensuring against a true hardware failure (such as a stuck leaf) and an unreasonably small tolerance that would result in a large number of unnecessary beam holdoffs.

Dosimetric Tests

Dosimetric characterization of the MLC, using film or ion chambers or both, includes measurements of radiation transmission through the leaves and their rounded ends, and the contribution of scatter radiation for different leaf settings. The dosimetric contribution of these factors can amount to as much as 15% for large, highly modulated fields. Periodic dosimetric and geometric verification of IM fields must therefore be part of the physics QA program. For example, image patterns of predesigned fields, such as shown in Figure 8-19, can be used on a regular basis to provide a quick visual assessment that the MLC is functioning properly. Ion chamber and diode array measurements at different gantry and collimator angles should be performed monthly by a physicist to ensure constancy of the DMLC output and to track long-term stability.

Additional tests must be made of dose linearity plus field symmetry and flatness. The step-and-shoot IMRT technique in particular often introduces delivery of many small dose segments, sometimes as low as a fraction of 1 mu. At such low doses the normal internal accelerator feedback dosimetry systems designed to ensure beam symmetry and flatness may not function properly, and special dosimetry tests must be performed to quantify any such errors.

Patient-Specific Issues

Specific tests should be performed to ensure the accuracy of each patient's IMRT treatment field. This includes verification that all field/file names are correct, and that the proper DMLC leaf motion files or sequence of static MLC segments has been downloaded to the linear accelerator through the R/V system. Before patient treatment, the shapes and intensity patterns of each treatment field should be verified. One technique for performing this test is to attach a sheet of radiographic

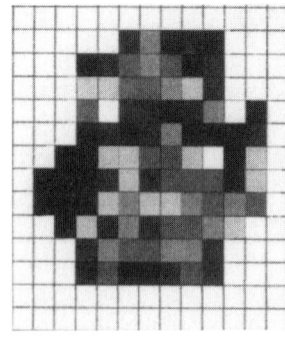 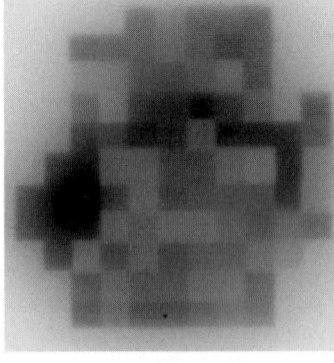

Print Out   **EDR Film**

Figure 8–20. Comparison between a radiographic film mounted and exposed in the blocking tray and an intensity pattern calculated by the treatment planning system.

film (e.g., EDR2, Kodak, Rochester, N.Y.) to the blocking tray of the accelerator, expose it to an entire fraction of dose, and compare the developed film to the expected intensity pattern calculated by the treatment-planning system. An example is shown in Figure 8-20. From such films a simple visual inspection can reveal gross errors in treatment delivery or field identification. More accurate comparisons could of course be done by scanning the film and recording true dose values. Such techniques work well for both static and dynamic IMRT.

For each IMRT plan, a dosimetric check at multiple specific points in a phantom is currently required to ensure that each treatment portal of each treatment plan is correct. If one has an independent computer program to recalculate these doses, it can be used in lieu of actual dosimetric measurement. If dose confirmation is being made by actual measurement, a phantom plan must be created with the treatment-planning system wherein the exact modulated beam intensities calculated for the patient are used to calculate dose in the phantom geometry—a feature now found in most IMRT treatment-planning systems. These in-phantom dosimetry measurements are usually made with ionization chambers, diodes, thermoluminescent dosimeters (TLDs), or film. Such measurements are best made in regions with relatively uniform dose intensity to prevent apparent errors caused by small displacements in dosimeter position. For film measurements of IMRT fields, one should be particularly cognizant of possible film calibration errors due to the large amounts of low-energy scatter radiation that are present in large, highly modulated IMRT fields (radiographic film overresponds to low energy x-rays because of its high silver content). Finally, in vivo dosimetry measurements can be made in the patient using diodes or TLDs, but again, measurements should be made in regions with relatively uniform dose.

CLINICAL EXPERIENCE

As IMRT is both expensive and time-consuming, it is important to focus effort on tumor sites for which IMRT offers the most potential benefit. Clearly not all patients or tumor sites will require IMRT. In general, only patients requiring exceptional dose escalation or normal tissue dose sparing or both will benefit from IMRT. At our institutions (MSKCC and University of California at San Francisco [UCSF]), IMRT was first applied to the treatment of prostate, head and neck, thyroid, and breast. Now other treatment sites are being treated with IMRT. Following are brief descriptions of the dosimetric and treatment-planning aspects of IMRT for prostate and for head and neck, as examples of IMRT's potential benefits.

Prostate Cancer

Since 1996 more than 1000 patients with prostate cancer have been treated with IMRT at MSKCC. In one clinical trial 40 patients were treated to 86.4 Gy prescription dose using a five-field IMRT technique. The "standard" IMRT treatment to the prostate at MSKCC is now 81.0 Gy.[43] Patients are immobilized in the prone position using modified alpha cradles, which are used both for CT simulation and treatments. CT data are transferred electronically to the treatment planning system, and the PTV, bladder, rectum (inner and outer rectal wall), bowel, femurs, and pelvis are contoured. A standard five-field treatment technique is used with the patient prone and accelerator gantry angles of 0, 75, 135, 225, and 285 degrees (Fig. 8-21), a photon beam energy of 15 MV is used. The starting criteria for optimization of the 81Gy prescription dose include these dose volume constraints[2]:

1. dose uniformity within the PTV of 12% or better,
2. less than 34% of the rectal wall to receive greater than 75 Gy,
3. less than 58% of the bladder wall to receive greater than 81 Gy.

The overlap region between the PTV and the rectal wall is defined as a separate structure with its own dose constraint of 76 Gy to permit greater control of the dose optimization, and to avoid falling into the previously-alluded-to trap of obtaining a poor quality plan because one specified (for the optimization algorithm) physically

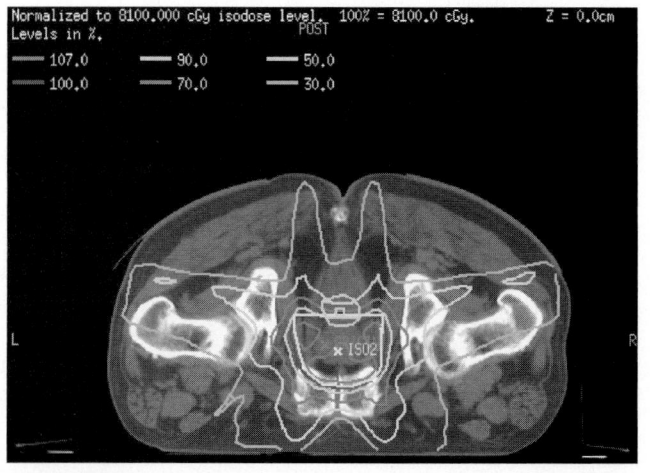

A

Figure 8–21. Typical dose distributions for a 5-field intensity-modulated radiotherapy prostate treatment to 81 Gy. See (**A**) transverse (axial) plane, (**B**) coronal plane, and (**C**) sagittal plane. The planning target volume is shown in yellow, and the rectal wall in blue. See also Color Figure 8-21.

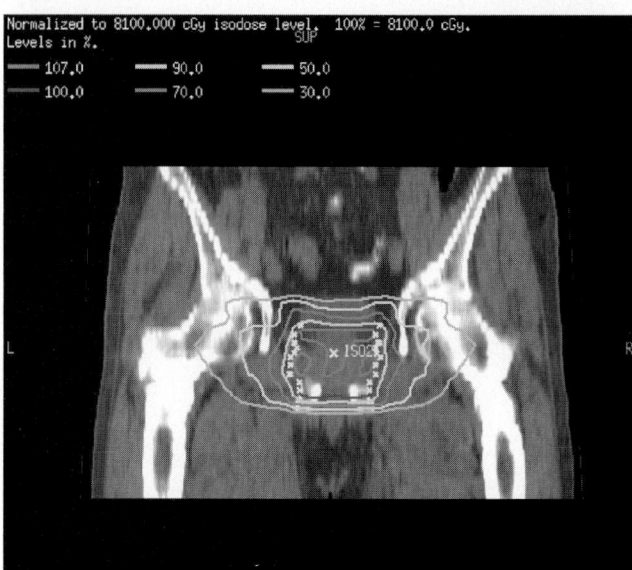

B

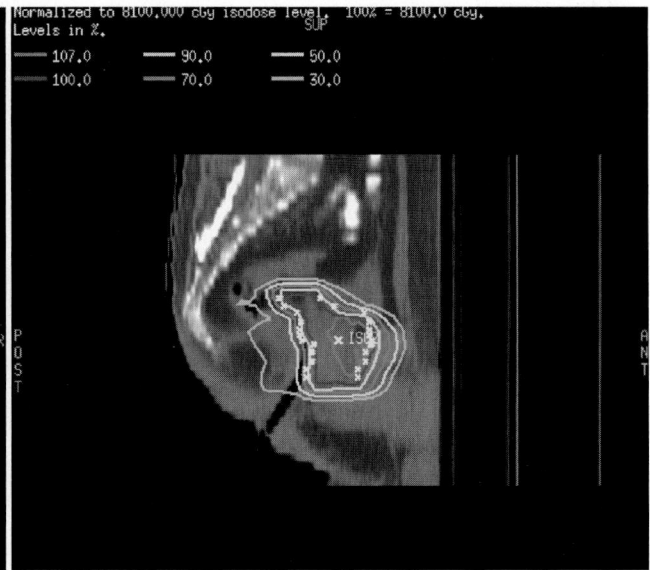

C

impossible dose constraints (e.g., specifying 81 Gy to the PTV, but <75 Gy to the rectal wall).

Figures 8-21*A* through *C* show typical dose distributions for such a plan in the axial (transverse), coronal, and sagittal planes respectively. The PTV (yellow) and rectum (light blue) are outlined. Note how the dose distribution conforms to the PTV and restricts the volume of rectal tissue irradiated to high doses (i.e., the 100% isodose contour, dark blue, scallops around the rectum). The cumulative dose volume histograms shown in Figure 8-22 reinforce this point.

Head and Neck Cancer

Treatment of nasopharyngeal tumors with IMRT often results in significant clinical advantage as compared to 3DCRT because IMRT is particularly well suited to delivering conformly shaped *concave* dose distributions for PTVs in close proximity to radiation-sensitive normal tissues—as is often the case for these tumors. At MSKCC a particularly useful, although somewhat anti-intuitive, beam geometry is used for such treatments. It consists of seven coplanar equi-spaced intensity-modulated beams directed from the *posterior* and lateral directions, as shown in Figure 8-23. The use of mostly posterior fields, aimed directly through the brainstem and spinal cord, actually produces the desired concave isodose profiles. This treatment geometry often requires a complicated dose intensity pattern such as shown in Figure 8-24 for a left, posterior, oblique IMRT beam. Note in Figure 8-24 the area of minimum beam intensity overlying the spinal cord and brainstem with increased intensity on either side to improve coverage of the base of skull. The overall intensity is quite irregular and could not be easily simulated using standard beam modulators such as blocks or wedges.

Often these beams exceed 14.5 cm in width (which, because of mechanical limitations of the MLC, is the maximum IMRT field width) and must be divided into two narrower fields. Whenever possible, the junction of

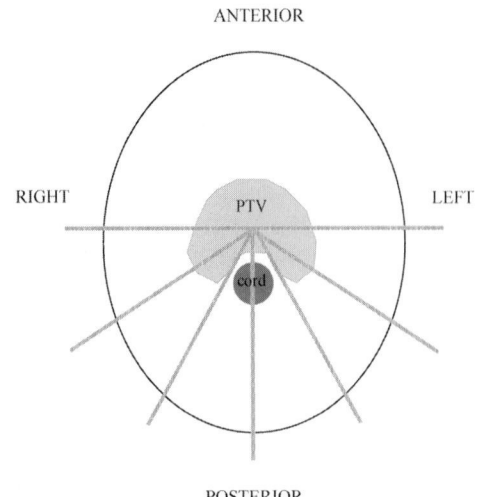

Figure 8–23. The seven-field beam arrangement used for intensity-modulated radiotherapy treatment of the nasopharyngeal cancer at Memorial Sloan-Kettering Cancer Center.

the two fields is placed at the level of the spinal cord and brainstem, where the beam intensity is designed to be minimal. A second delivery issue in the design of these treatment fields is the need to extend the field edges laterally beyond the patient's skin surface in the area of the neck. This will ensure an adequate margin and account for patient motion and breathing. Under normal circumstances, the intensity profile created by the inverse planning algorithm ends at the patient skin surface. A modification to the algorithm allows the intensity profile to extend into the nodal regions by a user-defined amount, typically at least 2 cm beyond the skin surface.

Treatment planning dose constraints for these plans include the specifications of a minimum PTV dose equal to the prescription dose, with a maximum dose less than 120%. Maximum spinal cord and brainstem doses are constrained to 40 and 45 Gy, respectively. Doses to

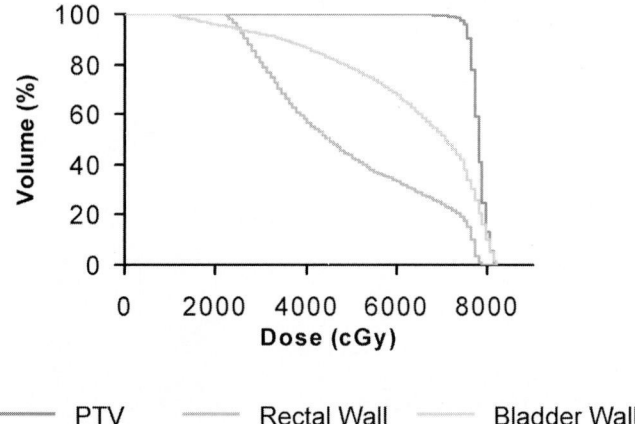

Figure 8–22. The cumulative dose volume histograms (DVHs) for the 81 Gy intensity-modulated radiotherapy plan illustrated in Figure 8-21. The DVHs for the planning target volume, rectal wall, and bladder wall are shown.

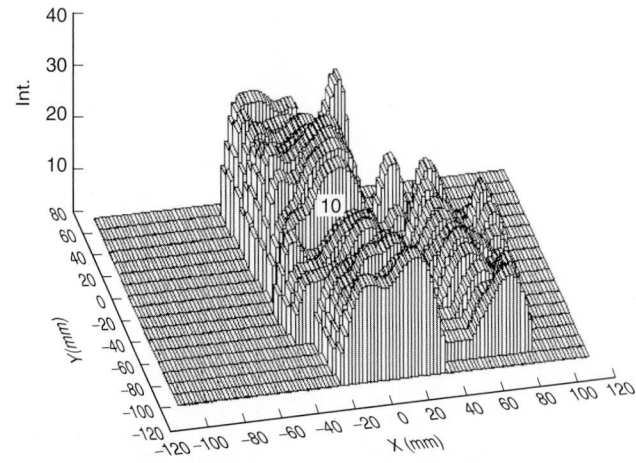

Figure 8–24. Intensity profile for a left posterior oblique dynamic multileaf collimator field.

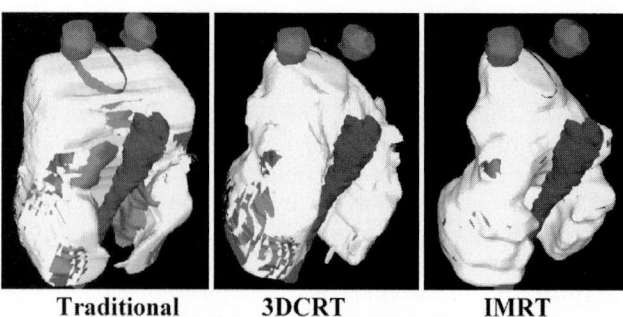

Traditional   **3DCRT**   **IMRT**

Figure 8–25. *Region of regret* plot showing the prescription isodose surface *(white)*, and regions of the planning target volume receiving less than the prescription dose *(red)* for traditional, 3DCRT, and IMRT plans. The brainstem and cord are shown in *blue*, and the eyes in *purple*. See also Color Figure 8-25.

parotids, the mandible, temporal lobes, spinal cord, and brainstem are often 10% to 20% lower using IMRT, even when these tissues are not given explicit dose constraints. IMRT treatments can yield improved PTV coverage as compared to 3DCRT as shown in a so-called *region of regret* plot in Figure 8-25. In this type of plot, the prescription isodose contour is plotted in white, and regions of the PTV receiving less than the prescription dose are plotted in red. A detailed comparison among conventional, 3DCRT, and IMRT treatment plans is available in the literature.[6,44]

The UCSF approach for treatment of nasopharyngeal cancer differs slightly from the MSKCC approach. Typically seven to nine coplanar beam directions are used, shown schematically in Figure 8-26. An anterior beam is always used while a direct posterior beam is avoided. The different solutions found for selection of optimum beam angles between the two institutions may reflect, in part, the use of different inverse planning systems employing different optimization algorithms. At UCSF, a commercial inverse planning system (NOMOS Corporation, Sewickley, Pa.) is used, whereas MSKCC uses an in-house planning system.[18,19,31]

Three treatment techniques, dependent on patient-specific clinical criteria, have been used at UCSF for IMRT of the nasopharynx. The first technique uses IMRT to treat only the primary tumor, with the IMRT fields being matched to larger conventional fields. The second technique treats the primary tumor and upper neck nodes with IMRT fields matched to a conventional supraclavicular field. The third technique treats the entire PTV with IMRT. More than 100 nasopharyngeal patients have been treated using these techniques.

Two standard sets of dose constraints are used, one for early-stage nasopharyngeal patients, and the other for advanced stage. The treatment goal in either case is to deliver 70 Gy at 2.12 Gy/fraction to more than 95% of the GTV and, simultaneously, 59.4 Gy at 1.8 Gy/fraction to more than 95% of the CTV (akin to a field within a field). For early-stage nasopharyngeal cancer, the maximum doses to spinal cord, brainstem, chiasm, and optic nerves are limited to 38, 51, 28, 24 Gy, respectively. The mean doses to parotid glands, T-M joints, and middle/inner ears are limited to 27, 34, and 42 Gy, respectively. For advanced-stage nasopharyngeal cancer, where the increased size of the CTV renders such conservative dose limits unrealistic, the maximum normal tissue doses for cord, brainstem, chiasm, and optical nerves are relaxed slightly to 43, 55, 43, and 42 Gy, respectively. The mean doses to parotid glands, T-M joints, and middle/inner ears are relaxed to 28, 38, and 50 Gy, respectively.

Initially, increased acute skin reactions occurred in many IMRT nasopharynx patients. Several causative factors were identified, including a bolus effect from the use of head-neck-shoulder masks, the use of multiple tangential beams with IMRT plans, and the inclusion of neck skin as part of the CTV.[45] This latter factor forces the inverse planning system to drive up the skin dose to levels not normally prescribed when treating with conventional opposed lateral fields. To reduce skin toxicity, therefore, we now exclude the skin from the CTV (unless it is clinically contraindicated) and instead identify it as a "sensitive structure" with a dose constraint of 55 Gy. In addition, special care is taken to minimize the thickness of our polystyrene face masks. Subsequently, skin toxicity has been reduced.

DEVELOPMENT AND RESEARCH ISSUES

IMRT can be considered an advanced form of 3DCRT. Both begin with, and would not exist without, 3D patient imaging. To date, imaging has commonly been based entirely on CT, but more and more, it is being augmented by MR, PET, and other functional imaging studies. 3D patient imaging enables the clinician to accurately contour the PTV plus normal tissues of interest. Coupled with BEV design of treatment portals, this permits delivery of dose distributions that conform to the shape of the PTV and to spare normal tissues to levels not approachable during the era of conventional plain film simulation.

While most institutions have used 3DCRT treatment planning for at least several years, IMRT is still very

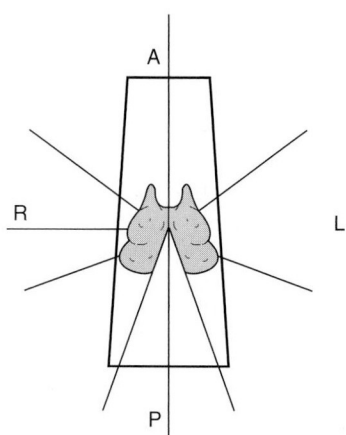

Figure 8–26. The eight-field beam arrangement used for intensity-modulated radiotherapy treatment of nasopharyngeal cancer at the University of California at San Francisco.

much in the developmental phases. It only recently moved from an experimental procedure available at a few large hospital centers to the radiotherapy community at large. Within the next few years, IMRT will likely become the standard of care for many types of radiotherapy treatments.

The first major decision when starting an IMRT program is whether to implement static- or dynamic-mode IMRT (the advantages and disadvantages of each are discussed throughout this chapter). Whatever choice is made, if the experiences at our centers are in any way typical, centers new to IMRT will begin using it first for the most commonly treated sites, such as prostate and head and neck. There will be a significant learning curve, as clinicians, physicists, and dosimetrists become comfortable with the philosophical differences between forward planning and inverse planning (really, the only significant difference between 3DCRT and IMRT with regard to treatment planning). Commissioning a new IMRT system also requires a significant amount of physics effort, as extensive dosimetric tests of MLC operation are required, as is verification of the accuracy of IMRT dose calculations and beam delivery. Compared to forward-planned 3DCRT, IMRT planning is at first more time-consuming, but with practice becomes equal to or even less labor intensive than conventional treatment planning. The length of daily patient treatment sessions is also comparable for IMRT and 3DCRT plans, even though the MUs required for IMRT are about two to three times higher. An excellent knowledge of normal anatomy, the location of potentially involved lymph nodes, and close coordination with diagnostic imaging are required for IMRT.

Once the treatment planning team becomes familiar with IMRT techniques for prostate and head and neck, IMRT will begin to be applied to other disease sites. Each new application of IMRT, however, will represent a challenge, requiring adaptation or new custom features or both, plus a better understanding of the use of optimization criteria for inverse planning. Expect much "trial and error," as inverse treatment planning strategies differ for different disease and for different treatment planning systems.

As for future developments, one area of great interest is the use of biological models of tumor and normal tissue radiation response as criteria for plan optimization,[46-48] either in addition to, or instead of, dose volume-based plan optimization. In general, biology-based score functions consist of some weighted combinations of biologic indices such as normal tissue complication probability (NTCP)[49] and tumor control probability (TCP).[50] These indices condense structure-specific dose-distribution data to yield relative figures of merit for the respective objects of interest. However, all such indices are based on rather rudimentary models with simplistic assumptions, complicated by the fact that clinical data for validating the models and deriving model parameters have been heretofore lacking.

Nevertheless, the increasing number of patients who have been treated with 3DCRT and IMRT over the past 10 years is now providing a database from which DVH data can finally be correlated with clinical outcome. Analysis of such data is now being reported for several normal tissues including liver, prostate, lung, and optic pathways.[51-53] Such studies offer the possibility of significantly improving the predictive power of these models to the point where they could be used for treatment plan optimization. It is hoped that the iterative process of generating clinical data and refinement/validation of the models will incrementally improve the predictive power of the biological indices and facilitate the quantitative evaluation of 3D treatment plans.

Much work is also being focused on methods to improve computational algorithms and dosimetric verification techniques for IMRT. For example, current computer algorithms for treatment plan optimization are themselves far from optimum. Commonly used optimization algorithms such as gradient-based optimization, simulated annealing, and genetic algorithm all have shortcomings. Some are slow and all occasionally get trapped in so-called *global minima*. The latter term refers to the computer's finding only the best plan close to the treatment planner's starting point rather than the absolute best plan. A demonstration of this effect can be seen by having the computer calculate several treatment plans using slightly different beam angles or slightly different dose constraints or both. Often one will find such tests yield quite different final results! Related to this is the problem of finding the optimum number and orientation of intensity modulation beams—something that still must be done manually (i.e., none of the existing treatment planning systems find optimum beam directions).

There is also significant interest in developing better methods for verification of IMRT dose calculations and beam delivery. Dosimetric verification of IMRT, in particular, is quite labor intensive, and currently available dosimeters all have limitations. Radiographic film, for example, has a significant energy response and is labor intensive. Diodes and ion chambers have limited spatial resolution and can measure dose only one point at a time. Newer dosimetric techniques (e.g., GEL dosimetry, TLD sheets) are still very much in the developmental stage. Real time (i.e., as the patient is being treated) verification of IMRT dose delivery may soon become possible as a result of the maturation of EPID technology, in particular amorphous silicon (ASi) detectors, which are faster (i.e., more sensitive) and have better spatial resolution than previous generation detectors.

Finally, in recent years there has been growing interest in the application of functional and biological imaging to radiation therapy treatment planning.[54] In contrast to CT images that provide only anatomical information, biological images such as magnetic resonant spectroscopy (MRS) and PET provide information on cell metabolism and genotypic and phenotypic data. Such imaging modalities thus present the possibility of identifying subvolumes within tumors that may be more or less radiosensitive than other subvolumes. Such information, coupled with the ability of IMRT to deliver nonuniform dose patterns, brings to fore the possibility of "dose painting," or "sculpting," akin to "field-within-a-field" techniques. Incremental to the concept of GTV, CTV, and PTV is the possibility of identifying a "biological target volume" (BTV) that may improve target delineation and treatment plan design.

SUMMARY

In conclusion, IMRT is a powerful technique that provides new degrees of freedom in customizing the dose distribution for photon radiotherapy. With the development of computer-controlled treatment machines equipped with multileaf collimators, it is now possible to deliver these treatments reliably. The clinical implementation of inverse planning and treatment delivery is complex and involves a substantial developmental effort. However, once accomplished, the process is efficient and capable of providing the dual benefits of improved dose distribution and cost savings. It is likely that this new modality will become widely accepted and applied in the future.

REFERENCES

1. Hall EJ: *Radiobiology for the Radiologist*. 4th ed. Philadelphia: Lippincott-Raven Publishers; 1994.
2. Burman C, Chui CS, Kutcher G: Planning, delivery, and quality assurance of intensity modulated radiotherapy using dynamic multileaf collimator: A strategy for large scale implementation for the treatment of carcinoma of the prostate. *Int J Radiat Oncol Biol Phys*. 1997; 39:863.
3. Ling CC, Burman C, Chui CS: Conformal radiation treatment of prostate cancer using inversely planned intensity modulated photon beams produced with dynamic multileaf collimation (see comments). *Int J Radiat Oncol Biol Phys*. 1996;35:721.
4. Posner, MD, Quirey JM, Akazawa PF: Dose optimization for the treatment of anaplastic thyroid carcinoma: A comparison of treatment planning techniques. *Int J Radiat Oncol Biol Phys*. 2000; 48:475.
5. Hong L, Hunt M, Chui CS: Intensity modulated tangential beam irradiation of the intact breast. *Int J Radiat Oncol Biol Phys*. 1999;44:1155.
6. Xia P, Fu KK, Wong GW: Comparision of treatment plans involving intensity modulated radiotherapy for nasopharyngeal carcinoma. *Int J Radiat Oncol Biol Phys*. 2000;48:329.
7. Xia P, Pickett B, Vigneault E: Forward or inversely planned segmental multileaf collimator IMRT and sequential tomotherapy to treat multiple dominant intraprostatic lesions of prostate cancer to 90 Gy. *Int J Radiat Oncol Biol Phys*. 2001;51:244.
8. Zelefsky MJ, Cowen D, Fuks Z: Long term tolerance of high dose three dimensional conformal radiotherapy in patients with localized prostate carcinoma. *Cancer*. 1999;85:2460.
9. Lee N, Xia P, Quivey JM: Intensity modulated radiotherapy in the treatment of nasopharyngeal carcinoma: An update of the UCSF experience. *Int J Radiat Oncol Biol Phys*. 2002;53:12.
10. Chao KS, Low DA, Perez CA, Purdy JA: Intensity modulated radiation therapy in head and neck cancers: The Mallinckrodt experience. *Int J Cancer*. 2000;90:92.
11. Sherouse GW, Bourland JD, Reynolds K: Virtual simulation in the clinical setting: Some practical considerations. *Int J Radiat Oncol Biol Phys*. 1990;19:1059.
12. ICRU-50: *Prescribing, Recording and Reporting Photon Beam Therapy*. Washington, D.C: International Commission on Radiation Units and Measurements; 1993.
13. McShan DL, Fraass BA, Lichter AS: Full integration of the beam's eye view concept into computerized treatment planning. *Int J Radiat Oncol Biol Phys*. 1990;18:1485.
14. Goitein M, Abrams M, Rowell D: Multidimensional treatment planning. II: Beam's eye view, back projection and projection through CT sections. *Int J Radiat Oncol Biol Phys*. 1983; 9:789.
15. Stein J, Mohan R, Wang XH: Number and orientations of beams in intensity modulated radiation treatments. *Med Phys*. 1997;24;149.
16. Pugachev A, Li JG, Buyer AL: Role of beam orientation optimization in intensity modulated radiation therapy. *Int J Radiat Oncol Biol Phys*. 2001;50:551.

17. Mohan RA, Arnfield M, Shidong T: The impact of fluctuations in intensity patterns on the number of monitor units and the quality and accuracy of intensity modulated radiotherapy. *Med Phys*. 2000;27:1226.
18. Spirou SV, Fournier-Bidot N, Jie Y: Smoothing intensity modulated beam profiles to improve the efficiency of delivery. *Med Phys*. 2001;28:2105.
19. Chui CS, LoSasso T, Spirou S: Dose calculation for photon beams with intensity modulation generated by dynamic jaw or multileaf collimations. *Med Phys*. 1994;21:1237.
20. Xiao Y, Galvin J, Hossain M: An optimized forward planning technique for intensity modulated radiation therapy. *Med Phys*. 2002;27:2093.
21. Shepard DM, Earl MA, Li XA: Direct aperture optimization: A turnkey solution for step and shoot IMRT. *Med Phys*. 2002;29:1007.
22. Brahme A: Optimization of stationary and moving beam radiation therapy techniques. *Radiother Oncol*. 1988;12:129.
23. Brahme A: Optimized radiation therapy based on radiobiological objectives. *Semin Radiat Oncol*. 1999;9:35.
24. Bortfeld T: Optimized planning using physical objective and constraints. *Semin Radiat Oncology*. 1999;9:20.
25. Budgell GJ: Temporal resolution requirements for intensity modulated radiation therapy delivered by multileaf collimators. *Phys Med Biol*. 1999;44:1581.
26. Que W: Comparison of algorithms for multileaf collimator field segmentation. *Med Phys*. 1999;26:2390.
27. Xia P, Verhey LJ: Multileaf collimator leaf sequencing algorithm for intensity modulated beams with multiple static segments. *Med Phys*. 1998;25:1424.
28. Galvin JM, Chen XG, Smith RM: Combining multileaf fields to modulate fluence distributions. *Int J Radiat Oncol Biol Phys*. 1993;27:697.
29. Ma L, Buyer AL, Ma CM: Synchronizing dynamic multileaf collimators for producing two dimensional intensity modulated fields with minimum beam delivery time. *Int J Radiat Oncol Biol Phys*. 1999;44:1147.
30. Bortfeld TR, Kahler DL, Waldron TJ: X-ray field compensation with multileaf collimators. *Int J Radiat Oncol Biol Phys*. 1994; 28:723.
31. Spirou SV, Chen-Shou C: Generation of arbitrary intensity profiles by combining the scanning beam with dynamic multileaf collimation. *Med Phys*. 1996;23:1.
32. Mackie TR, Balog J, Ruchalak: Tomotherapy. *Sem Radiat Oncol*. 1999;9:108.
33. Low DA, Mutic S: Abutment region dosimetry for sequential arc IMRT delivery. *Phys Med Biol*. 1997;42:1465.
34. Carol M, Grant WH 3rd, Bleier AR: The field matching problem as it applies to the peacock three dimensional conformal system for intensity modulation. *Int J Radiat Oncol Biol Phys*. 1996;34:183.
35. Yu CX, Li XA, Ma L, et al: Clinical implementation of intensity modulated arc therapy. *IJROBP* 2002;53:453.
36. Webb S, Bortfeld T, Stein J: The effect of stair step leaf transmission on the 'tongue and groove problem' in dynamic radiotherapy with a multileaf collimator. *Phys Med Biol*. 1997;42:595.
37. van Santvoort JP, Heijmen BJ: Dynamic multileaf collimation without 'tongue and groove' underdosage effects. *Phys Med Biol*. 1996;41:2091.
38. Sykes JR, Williams PC: An experimental investigation of the tongue and groove effect for the Philips multileaf collimator. *Phys Med Biol*. 1998;43:3157.
39. Graves MN, Thompson AV, Martel MK: Calibration and quality assurance for rounded leaf end MLC systems. *Med Phys*. 2001;28:2227.
40. Galvin JM, Smith AR, Lally B: Characterization of a multileaf collimator system. *Int J Radiat Oncol Biol Phys*. 1993;25:181.
41. Wu Q, Arnfield M, Tony S: Dynamic splitting of large intensity modulated fields. *Phys Med Biol*. 2000;45:1731.
42. LoSasso T, Chen-Shou C, Ling CC: Comprehensive quality assurance for the delivery of intensity modulated radiotherapy with a multileaf collimator used in the dynamic mode. *Med Phys*. 2001;28:2209.
43. Leibel SA, Fuks Z, Zelefsky MJ: Intensity modulated radiotherapy. *Cancer J*. 2002;8:164.
44. Hunt MA, Zelefsky M, Wolden S: Treatment planning and delivery of intensity modulated radiation therapy for primary nasopharynx cancer. *Int J Radiat Oncol Biol Phys*. 2001;49:623.

45. Lee N, Chuang C, Quivey JM: Skin toxicity due to intensity modulated radiotherapy for head and neck carcinoma. *Int J Radiat Oncol Biol Phys.* 2002;53:630.

46. Wang XH, Mohan R, Jackson A: Optimization of intensity modulated 3D conformal treatment plans based on biological indices. *Radiother Oncol.* 1995;37:140.

47. Niemierko A: Reporting and analyzing dose distributions: A concept of equivalent uniform dose. *Med Phys.* 1997;24:103.

48. Niemierko A, Urie M, Goitein M: Optimization of 3D radiation therapy with both physical and biological end points and constraints. *Int J Radiat Oncol Biol Phys.* 1992;23:99.

49. Lyman JT: Complication probability as assessed from dose volume histograms. *Radiat Res.* 1985;8:104.

50. Niemierko A, Goitein M: Modeling of normal tissue response to radiation: The critical volume model. *Int J Radiat Oncol Biol Phys.* 1993;25:135.

51. Levegrun S, Jackson A, Zelefsky MJ: Analysis of biopsy outcome after three dimensional conformal radiation therapy of prostate cancer using dose distribution variables and tumor control probability models. *Int J Radiat Oncol Biol Phys.* 2000;47:1245.

52. Jackson A, Ten Haken RK, Robertson JM: Analysis of clinical complication data for radiation hepatitis using a parallel architecture model. *Int J Radiat Oncol Biol Phys.* 1995;31:883.

53. Martel MK, Sandler HM, et al: Dose volume complication analysis for visual pathway structures on patients with advanced paranasal sinus tumors. *Int J Radiat Oncol Biol Phys.* 1993;38:273.

54. Ling CC, Humm J, Larson S: Towards multidimensional radiotherapy (MD-CRT): Biological imaging and biological conformality. *Int J Radiat Oncol Biol Phys.* 2000;47:551.

Immobilization and Simulation

Chandra M. Burman, PhD

9

External beam radiation therapy is one of the treatment arms of cancer management. During radiotherapy the patients are treated with high-energy x-rays, gamma-rays, electrons, or protons. The treatment machines that provide the radiation are capable of generating collimated ionizing radiation beams. The aim of the radiation therapy is to deliver a specific dose of radiation to the target volume while minimizing the dose to the surrounding healthy tissues. The prescribed dose depends on the site, stage, and histologic state of the tumor.

Multimodality imaging such as computed tomography (CT), magnetic resonance imaging (MRI), and positron emission tomography (PET) plays an important role in accurately identifying the diseased and the normal tissues. CT images are generally used for the treatment planning, whereas magnetic resonance images provide better soft-tissue definition. PET images are useful in identifying the disease at the metabolic level even before it is visible on the CT or MRI scans. Image registration is a valuable tool for transferring the information about the disease from MRI and PET to CT scans for treatment planning purposes.

For radiobiologic reasons, the dose is delivered in single or multiple daily fractions over a period of several weeks.[1] During radiation therapy it is important to ensure that on a day-to-day basis, the patient is treated in a reproducible manner and that the same volume is irradiated during each fraction. Particularly with the modern conformal techniques,[2] in which the planned isodose line tightly surrounds the target volume, a mismatch between the planned dose distribution and the delivered dose causes an underdose to the target and overdose to the surrounding normal tissues. This results in a suboptimal outcome for the patient. Furthermore, for treatment sites such as the lung and liver, where larger margins are needed to account for the respiratory motion, techniques such as deep inspiration breath hold (DIBH),[3] robot tracking, and respiratory gating (RG)[4] are being developed to spare more healthy tissues.

Radiotherapy simulation plays a crucial role in planning the strategy for the proper delivery of radiation dose. Important issues are decided during the simulation (e.g., how the patient will be positioned and immobilized, how the treatment beams will be directed). The flow chart in Figure 9-1 shows several steps involved before treatment delivery. The simulation is carried out on a simulator or a virtual simulation is carried out on a CT-simulator. To help with the patient's alignment, the room also contains wall-mounted laser lights.

SIMULATOR

The purpose of a radiation therapy simulator is to mimic a radiation treatment unit, but instead of a high-energy therapy beam, it produces low-energy x-rays for radiographs and fluoroscopy. Most preparation for the treatment is done at a therapy simulator, which saves valuable treatment machine time. A simulator has most of the functionality of a treatment unit; the relevant components of a modern therapy simulator are shown in Figure 9-2. The simulator head contains a diagnostic x-ray tube, which is mounted at one end of a rotating gantry. At the other end are a film cassette holder and a fluoroscopic unit.

Housed in the simulator head is the collimator, which has movable delineator (cross) wires and blades (jaws). On a radiograph, the delineator wires are projected as straight lines that define the field size. The blade positions determine the image size. A field localization light in the head projects the cross hair and the delineator wires on the patient's skin, which help in positioning the patient. The optical distance indicator measures the depth of the isocenter. The collimator includes an accessory mount that allows the treatment accessories, such as the block tray or the electron cones, to be mounted on the simulator. A gridded graticule tray with radiopaque markers provides a scale for measurement on the film. Figure 9-3 shows a lateral head-and-neck radiograph on which the delineator wires, the cross hairs, and the graticule markers are projected. Figure 9-4 is an anterior-posterior simulation film for a lung patient.

The simulator couch looks like a treatment couch, but is modified to produce optimal images. It has three degrees of freedom for translational motion and rotates in a horizontal plane about the isocenter and the pedestal. The fluoroscopic unit contains an image intensifier and a video camera. The fluoroscope can move longitudinally, laterally, and radially. A collision sensor on top of the image intensifier senses potential collisions with the patient or the couch and stops the motion, preventing patient injury or machine damage. On a video monitor, fluoroscopic images are viewed in real time. An electronic storage unit to save images is often provided. A radiographic film cassette holder on top of the fluoroscopic unit is used for taking permanent simulation radiographs.

A hand pendant allows the operator to adjust the couch and simulator settings from inside the simulator room. The operator can adjust the gantry angle and move the couch while watching closely for possible collision. The simulator settings and the couch position can also be

1. **Positioning**

2. **Immobilization**

3. **Simulation or CT-simulation**

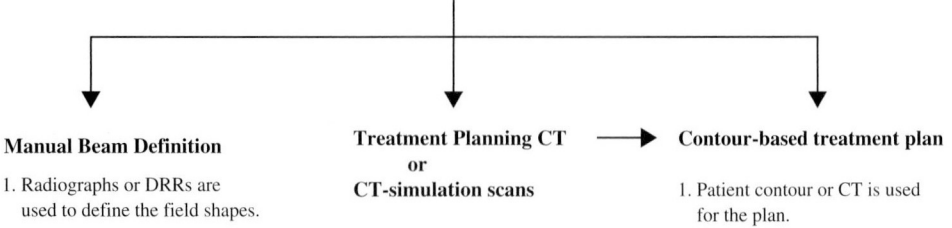

Manual Beam Definition

1. Radiographs or DRRs are used to define the field shapes.

2. Depth of the isocenter is used to determine the monitor units.

Treatment Planning CT
or
CT-simulation scans

1. If needed, a plan check is done to obtain additional radiographs.

2. Beam apertures are transferred To the radiographs or DRRs.

Contour-based treatment plan

1. Patient contour or CT is used for the plan.

2. If needed, a plan check is done obtain additional radiographs.

3. Field shapes are drawn on x-rays or radiographs.

Figure 9–1. Flow chart showing some of the procedures required before external beam radiotherapy. The positioning, immobilization, and external contour measurements of the patient are carried out during the simulation or computed tomography simulation.

adjusted from the console outside the shielded room. This is particularly useful during fluoroscopic imaging, when the delineator wires and the isocenter position can be adjusted interactively. A lead glass window separates the console from the simulator to shield the operating personnel from radiation exposure.

ALIGNMENT LASERS

The wall-mounted alignment laser system provides beams of laser lights. With the help of a lens system, each beam is spread out in a plane. The beams pass through the isocenter of the simulator. On the patient's skin, these beams project as fine lines along three major planes—transverse, sagittal, and coronal. The intersections of these light beams

on the patient's skin help in marking triangulation points on the skin. Generally, at the end of the simulation, the triangulation points are tattooed. Similar laser systems in the CT and therapy rooms are helpful in placing the patient in the treatment position. Although the lasers used in the localization system are low power, they can nevertheless cause retinal damage. It is advisable not to stare at the laser lights or their reflections from a shiny surface.

COMPUTED TOMOGRAPHY SCANNER AND SPIRAL COMPUTED TOMOGRAPHY SCANNER

Since the first CT images were obtained by Hounsfield[5] in 1980, CT imaging has undergone rapid development.

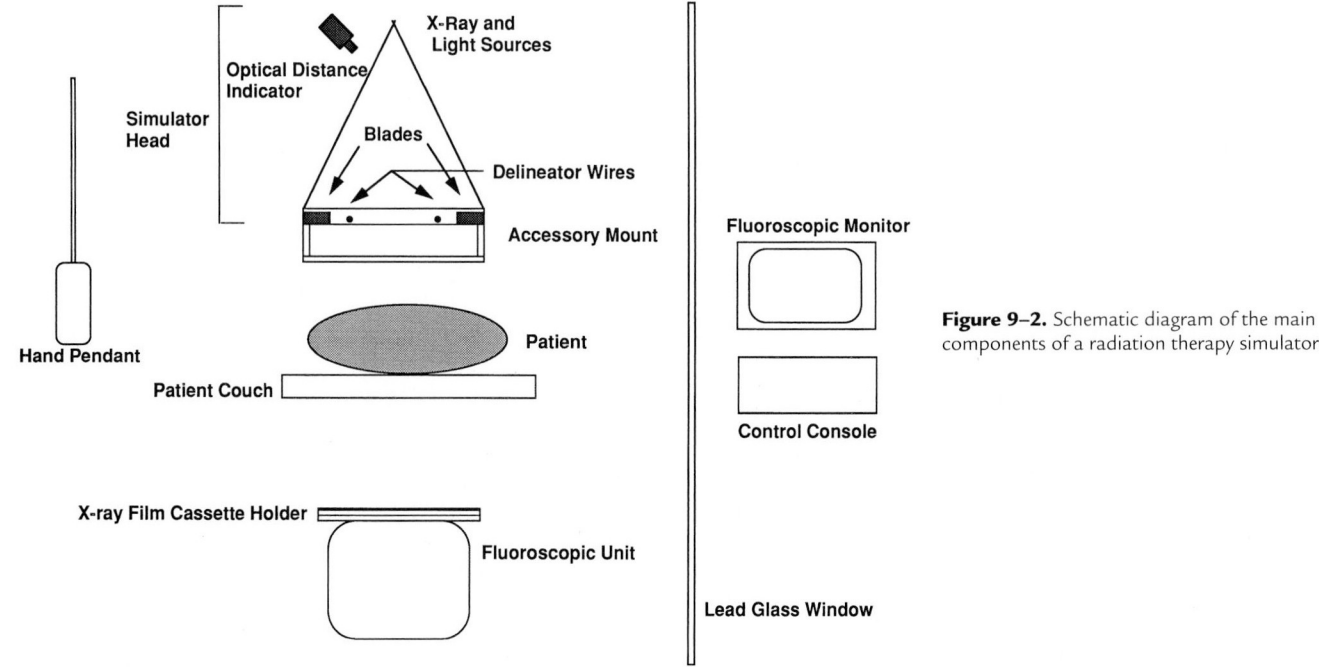

Figure 9–2. Schematic diagram of the main components of a radiation therapy simulator.

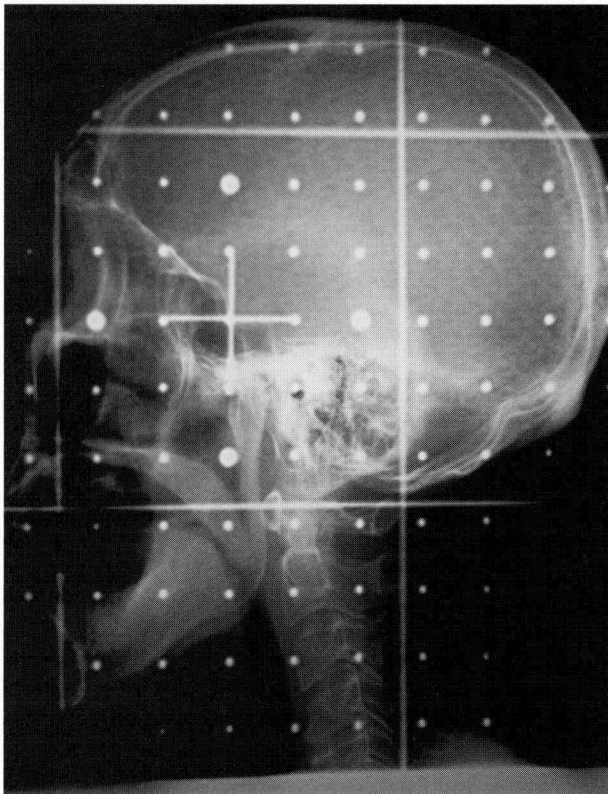

Figure 9–3. Left-lateral simulation radiograph for a head-and-neck patient. The delineator wires, cross hair, and graticule marks are projected on the x-ray film.

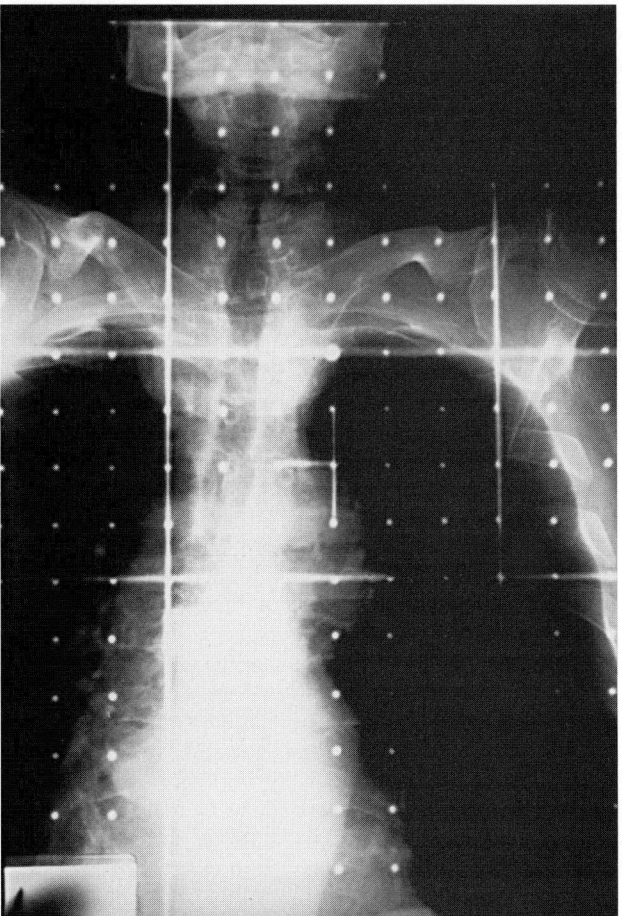

Figure 9–4. Anterior-posterior simulation film for a lung patient.

The major advancements have been in the areas of image quality and scan time reduction. A fourth-generation CT scanner is shown schematically in Figure 9-5. The x-ray tube and collimator assembly rotate around the patient, and the intensities of the transmitted radiation reaching the detectors are recorded. Either a solid scintillation detector (e.g., bismuth germanate, cesium iodide, cadmium tungstate) array or a gas-filled (e.g., xenon, xenon-krypton) array is used for the detection. Transmission data are stored in the computer, and the image is reconstructed based on the attenuation information. The linear attenuation coefficients are converted into CT numbers, and the image is displayed on a video monitor. The CT numbers for the pixels are expressed in Hounsfield numbers and are related to linear attenuation coefficients:

$$H = \frac{\mu - \mu_w}{\mu_w} \times 1000$$

where H is the CT number, μ is the linear attenuation coefficient for the pixel under analysis, and μ_w is the linear attenuation coefficient of water. The CT numbers in a scan range from −1000 to approximately +1000, with the CT number for water set at zero. A CT number of −1000 corresponds to air, and a CT number of +1000 is for very dense bone.

In a conventional CT scanner, an x-ray source mounted on a gantry rotates 360 degrees to collect the data for one CT slice. The slice thicknesses available depend on the scanner. Generally, they are of the order of 1, 3, 5, and 10 mm. A smaller thickness results in better resolution.

To obtain the volumetric data on a conventional CT scanner, after each scan the patient couch is translated to the new scan position. Because of the patient's breathing and involuntary movement of the internal organs, unless special precautions are taken, motion artifacts are present. In a spiral or helical CT scanner, the patient is transported through the gantry in synchrony with continuous data acquisition over a multitude of circular (360-degree) scans. Mathematical schemes[6] have been developed to reconstruct axial scans similar to the scans obtained with a conventional scanner.[7] On a spiral scanner a volume or a subvolume can be scanned in a short time, on the order of 30 seconds. The data for the whole study can be acquired with single breath hold, resulting in images without interscan motion. From the diagnostic point of view, this is significant for locating small structures such as small pulmonary nodules, with which respiratory motion can cause detection problems.[8] From the radiation therapy point of view, the advantages of the spiral CT scanning compared with standard scanning are the ability to collect CT data with the patient in the immobilized treatment position for a shorter time and to create coronal and sagittal reconstructions with finer detail.

The requirements for a therapy CT scan are different from those for a diagnostic scan.[9,10] Some requirements are: (1) the patient should be scanned in the treatment position. The couch top should be flat, similar to a

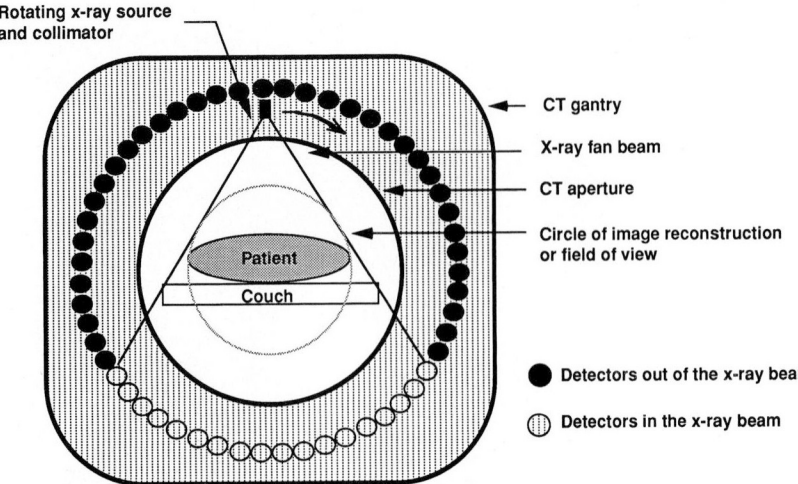

Rotating x-ray source
and collimator

CT gantry

X-ray fan beam

CT aperture

Circle of image reconstruction
or field of view

Patient

Couch

● Detectors out of the x-ray beam

◍ Detectors in the x-ray beam

Figure 9–5. Schematic diagram of fourth-generation computed tomography scanner. A circular array of x-ray detectors remain fixed, and a rotating x-ray source with fan-shaped beam scans the patient.

treatment couch. The physical CT aperture diameter and circle of reconstruction (field of view) should be large enough to accommodate the patient in the treatment position. If an immobilization device will be used during the treatment, the patient should be scanned immobilized, but the device should be made of materials that do not cause CT artifacts. The anterior and lateral isocentric lines and other landmarks are marked on the skin by taping radiopaque catheters or lead beads. (2) CT scans should be of high quality so that the disease, tissue at risk, and surrounding normal tissues can be identified clearly. (3) Particularly for three-dimensional (3D) treatment planning, a volume scan is required in order to delineate the treatment volume in three dimensions. In the region of treatment volume, a contiguous set with 5-mm spacing or smaller should be used to make sure those small tumor extensions and normal structures are not missed. Closely spaced scans also allow better image reconstruction. (4) Anterior-posterior and lateral scout views should be obtained with the CT images indexed to these. These views are helpful in comparing CT data with conventional simulation radiographs. (5) The CT scanning should be completed in a short time so that the patient remains adequately immobilized during the CT data collection. (6) For the treatment-planning scans in the thoracic region, the patient should be scanned under shallow-breathing conditions. Although the breathing introduces some motion artifacts in the images and the image quality may be degraded slightly, the scans represent the condition of the patient during treatment. However, using interventional techniques, such as active breathing control, deep inspirational breath-hold, and respiratory gating, can minimize the effect of respiratory motion, as discussed later.

Virtual Simulation

During a simulation the oncologist relies on the x-ray radiographs for designing the treatment ports. At times, even with the help of MRI, CT, and other diagnostic information, it is difficult to draw these ports accurately on plain radiographs. In the mid-1980s, Sherouse and colleagues[11-13] introduced the term *virtual simulation* to describe a computer-based simulation. They developed a software package that allowed the user to carry out simulation at a computer monitor instead of at a real simulator. The advantage of this method compared with plain radiographs is that the target volumes and anatomical structures, outlined on the CT scans, are used to make the decision about the position of the isocenter, field sizes, beam directions, and shielding blocks. CT scans provide better visualization of the disease and normal tissues, resulting in better target coverage and normal tissue shielding. The virtual simulator system has the ability to display and execute all the functions of a conventional radiotherapy machine, including gantry, couch, and collimator control.

The CT data are obtained by scanning the patient in the immobilized treatment position. The CT scans are transferred to the planning system, and the skin, target, dose-limiting organs, and bony landmarks are contoured on the CT scans. The planner can view a 3D display of the patient model that consists of the skin, target, and other anatomical structures abstracted from the CT data. The contoured structures use different surface rendering and variable degrees of transparencies to enhance the visualization. Figure 9-6 shows a typical virtual simulator screen. Like a physical simulator, the virtual simulator allows the planner to adjust treatment parameters, such as the gantry angle and field size. The beam's-eye view (BEV) provides images that are similar to fluoroscopic images. The planner can select the treatment beam direction by watching projections of the target and surrounding structures in the BEV. The fields are then shaped by drawing the beam apertures using a mouse or other pointing device. At the end of the virtual simulation, digitally reconstructed radiographs (DRRs) are produced for each treatment field. A DRR[14] is similar to a radiograph, but is designed by the computer based on the attenuation information derived from CT numbers in the original data set. The image quality of a DRR depends on the CT slice spacing—a smaller spacing results in a better DRR. The divergence of anatomical structures projected on a DRR is similar to that in the projection on a radiograph. The magnification of a DRR can be adjusted to

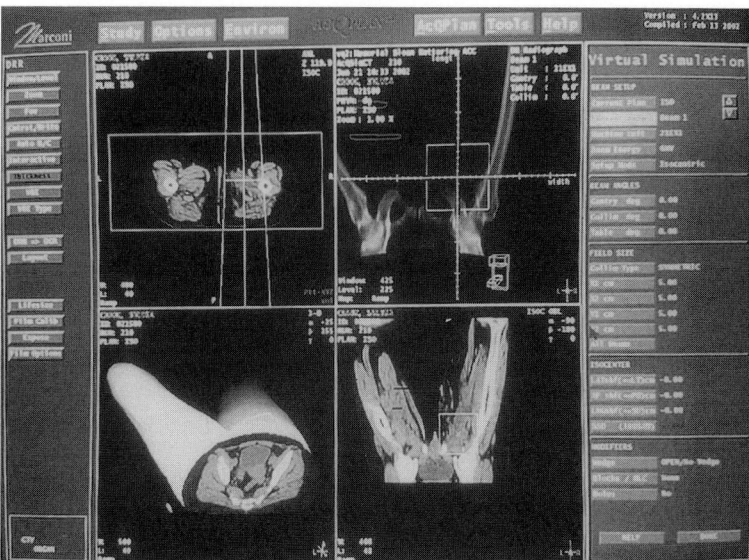

Figure 9–6. Typical virtual screen. The beam's-eye view and simulator controls are displayed on the screen.

match the simulation x-ray film. Along with the beam aperture and collimator, the target and other structures of interest are projected onto it. A list of beams, table parameters, and the templates for the beam modifiers are generated. Before the treatment, to verify the treatment ports, the localization port films can be compared directly with DRRs. Or, if the DRR quality is not good, the simulation radiographs in the treatment position can be taken and compared with the corresponding DRR. In many planning systems the beam's energy can be altered so that the DRR will look like a high-energy radiograph, making comparison to the port film simpler.

Computed Tomographic Simulator

The CT simulator is a whole-body CT scanner designed for radiation therapy simulation.[15,16] It consists of three basic components: (1) a CT scanner, (2) an interactive workstation capable of virtual simulation, and (3) a mechanism for marking the beam portals on the patient's skin. The patient is scanned in the treatment position and the CT images are transferred directly to a virtual simulation workstation. The target volume and relevant critical structures are outlined on the CT scans, the beam geometries are optimized, and DRRs are produced for the block definition and treatment verification.

Lasers for patient alignment and marking are similar to those used in conventional simulators, except that the sagittal laser can be moved laterally with respect to the longitudinal axis of the couch. The wall-mounted lasers are mounted at a longitudinal distance from the gantry to facilitate marking the patient reference point for setup.

Advantages of a CT simulator over a conventional simulator include: (1) The CT simulator allows for the visualization of treatment volumes for the portal design. On a conventional simulation radiograph it is difficult to identify the target volume. (2) On DRRs the target volume and critical structures can be superimposed, based on which the treatment ports can be designed. If needed, the margins can be added around the target

before outlining the shielding block. (3) The DRRs for the boost phase of the treatment can be produced from the same CT data set, without the need for the patient to return. (4) Conventional simulators have physical limitations; for example, radiographs for the vertex field cannot be obtained, whereas virtual simulation software *can* produce these DRRs. (5) Generally, virtual simulation software packages include software to enhance the DRRs by adjusting the window and contrast levels. For example, the AcQsim package (Philips Medical Systems, Cleveland, Ohio) includes a digital composite radiograph (DCR), which groups CT numbers into ranges corresponding to bone, fat, muscle, etc. The CT numbers in each category are modified by a weighting factor and re-displayed to provide greater enhancement of the specified tissue range.[17] Figure 9-7(*A,B,C*) shows the regular DRR, DCRs for the bone and skin, respectively, for a head-and-neck patient; (6) The DRRs corresponding to each treatment field are generated. The magnification of the DRRs can be adjusted. Cross hairs and grid points can also be projected onto DRRs for direct comparison with the portal images.

However, there is a limitation of the CT simulator compared to the conventional simulator. Due to the finite bore size of the CT gantry, typically 65 to 70 cm, it is impossible to accommodate all patients. For example, extremely large patients, some breast patients, and patients requiring special immobilization devices may not be able to enter the 65- to 70-cm opening without compromising the position. A larger opening, 85-cm-bore, scanner has the potential to eliminate these problems. The image quality and doses for the larger bore have been found comparable to the 70-cm-bore size scanner.[18] Figure 9-8 shows an AcQsim CT-simulator with 85-cm-bore gantry.

Interventional Strategies

With the use of 3D conformal radiation therapy (3DCRT) and intensity-modulated radiation therapy (IMRT), dose distributions have become highly conformal. Great care must be taken to ensure that the dose is delivered as

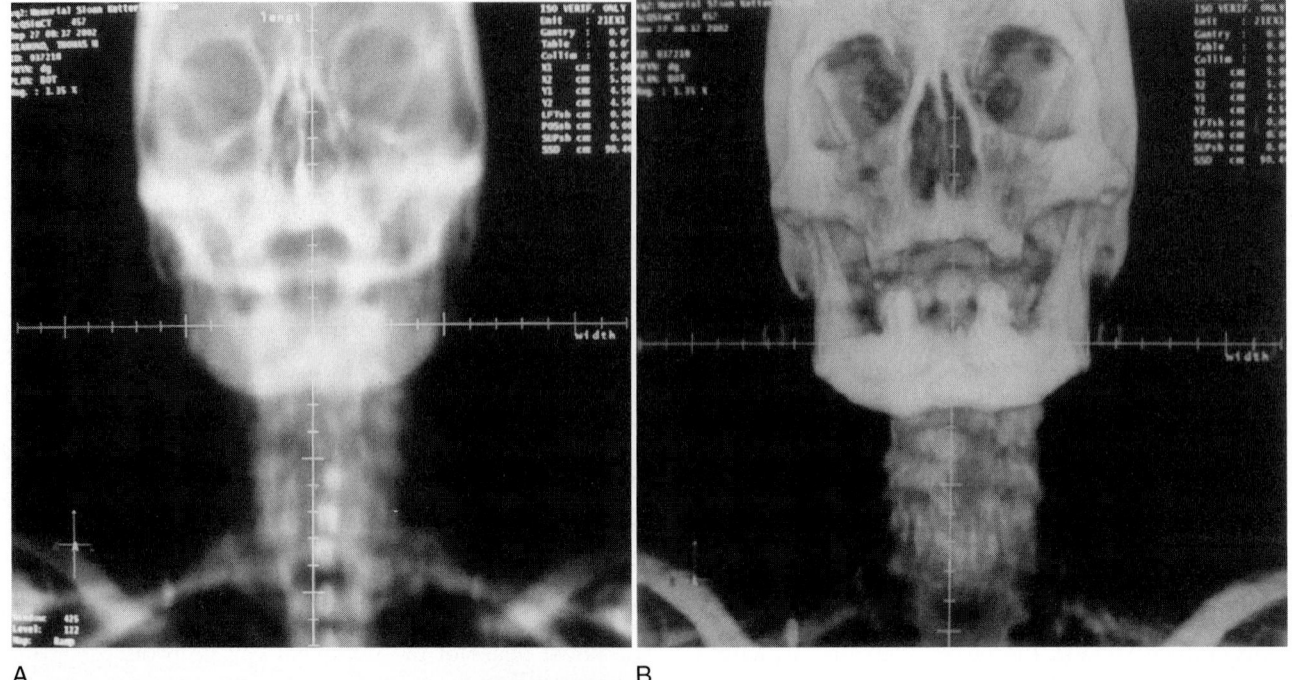

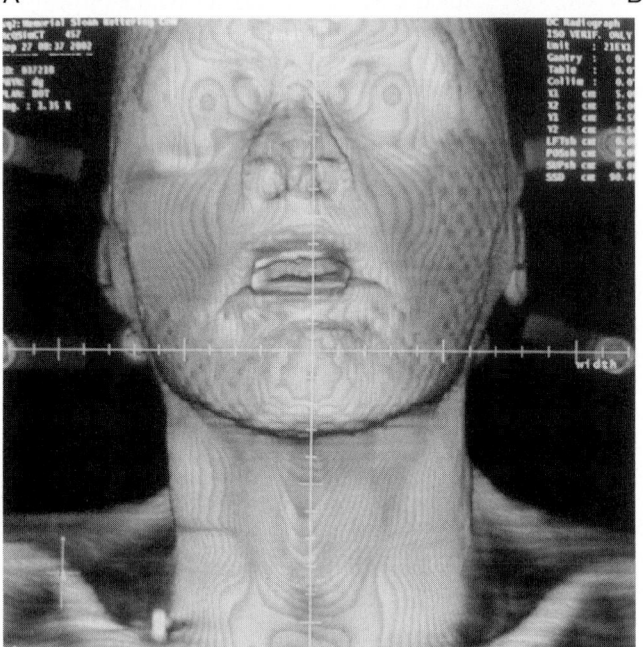

Figure 9–7. A, Digitally reconstructed radiograph. **B**, Digital composite radiograph for bone. **C**, Digital composite radiograph for the skin for a head-and-neck patient.

planned; otherwise, the risk of marginal failure increases. Two main causes of treatment inaccuracy are: (1) uncertainty in defining the clinical target volume (CTV) and (2) variation in treatment geometry during treatment. If other imaging modality data sets, such as MRI or PET, are available, the image registration or fusion[19] can be used to increase the accuracy of the CTV.

Variations in treatment geometry for sites such as the thorax and abdomen are significant due to breathing motion. Larger margins are required in these regions to define the PTV. Currently, several techniques are being investigated to reduce the uncertainty due to respiratory

motion. These include active breathing control (ABC), DIBH (mentioned earlier), and respiratory gating (RG). These techniques are used during simulation, CT, and treatment delivery. The three interventional techniques are discussed briefly here and RG is described in more detail in Chapter 10, Respiratory Gating.

Active Breathing Control

In this method a patient's nose is clamped and he or she breathes through an ABC apparatus via a mouthpiece as

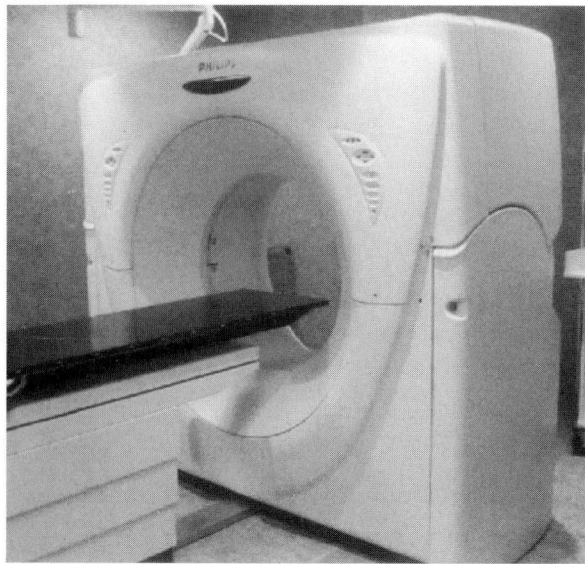

Figure 9–8. AcQsim computed tomography scanner with 85 cm-bore gantry.

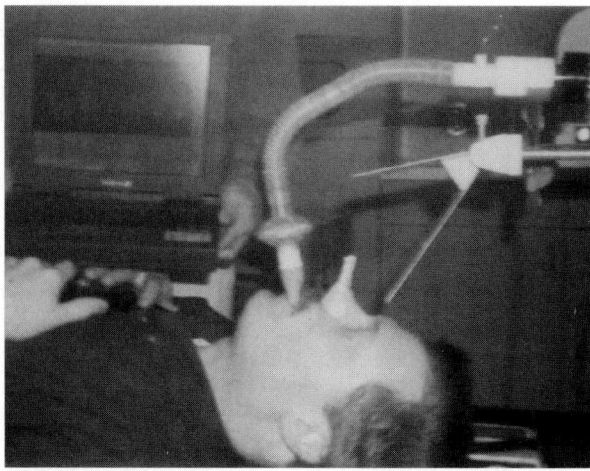

Figure 9–9. A patient breathing into the active breathing control (ABC) apparatus. A nose clip is used to make sure that the breathing is through the ABC unit. (From Wong JW, Yan D, et al: Interventional strategies to optimize the delivery of radiation therapy. In Bragg DG, Rubin P, Hricak H, eds. *Oncologic Imaging.* 2nd ed. Philadelphia: WB Saunders; 2002:116.)

shown in Figure 9-9. The signal from the flow monitor is processed and a trace on the computer monitor displays the lung volume. During a particular sequence of breathing cycle, at a predetermined flow direction and lung volume, a valve is activated to stop the airflow temporarily, resulting in the suspension of the breathing motion.[20-22] The duration of the breath hold is such that the patient can easily tolerate it. The amount of breath-hold a patient can tolerate depends on the disease site. For example, patients with lung disease can easily tolerate a breath hold of 15 seconds near the end of normal inspiration, whereas for patients with Hodgkin's disease and liver cancer, the breath hold ranges from 35 to 50 seconds when ABC is applied during inspiration.[22] ABC can substantially reduce the treatment margins without the need to modify the therapy accelerator.

Deep Inspiration Breath Hold Technique

In this method the patient is coached on the technique of reproducible deep inspiration through the various phases of treatment planning and delivery.[3,23,24] The DIBH uses a modified version of slow vital capacity maneuver[25] to bring the patient to approximately 100% vital capacity, followed by a breath hold, which maintains the patient at that level for a prescribed period, during which the patient is simulated, CT scanned, treated, and port filmed. The patient breathes through a mouthpiece connected to a spirometer control unit. A nose clip is used to ensure that the patient breathes through the mouth. The spirometer measures the airflow and it is interfaced to a computer. The airflow is integrated to yield the lung volume as a function of time and is displayed on a computer monitor. The DIBH maneuver begins with quiet tidal breathing, followed by a slow deep inspiration, slow deep expiration, then a slow deep inspiration to the maximum limit and breath-hold. A training session is held to familiarize the

patient with the spirometer and to measure patient parameters, such as the tidal volume, vital capacity, and comfortable breath-hold duration. Some patients are unable to follow the directions and are unsuitable for DIBH.

The technique has two advantages. First, the breath-hold minimizes tumor motion due to breathing. Second, it expands the patient's lung to its maximum volume, pushing the healthy lung tissue out of the primary radiation field and consequently reducing the fraction of the lung in the treatment beam. Figure 9-10 compares the free breathing and DIBH treatment plans for a patient. The images are coronal planes through the isocenter for the same patient. Hanley et al.[3] found that DIBH can reduce the volume of the lung receiving more than 25 Gy by 30%, compared to free-breathing plans. They found it to be highly reproducible. Patients could perform 10 to 13 breath holds in one session, with comfortable breath-hold duration of 12 to 16 seconds.

Respiratory Gating

Commercially available systems (e.g., Real Time Position Management Respiratory Gating, Varian Medical Systems, Palo Alto, Calif.) permit breathing-synchronized fluoroscopy on a treatment simulator, acquisition of breathing-synchronized CT-imaging, and gated treatment on a linear accelerator.[4,26] The Varian system consists of a charge-coupled-device (CCD) video camera attached to an infrared illuminator (Fig. 9-11) that tracks a patient's respiratory motion by detecting reflected infrared light from two reflective markers on a lightweight block (Fig. 9-12). The block is placed on the patient's chest or abdomen. The upper marker tracks the respiratory motion, while the lower marker, separated from the upper marker by 3 cm, calibrates the system. The camera signal is processed by software running on a personal

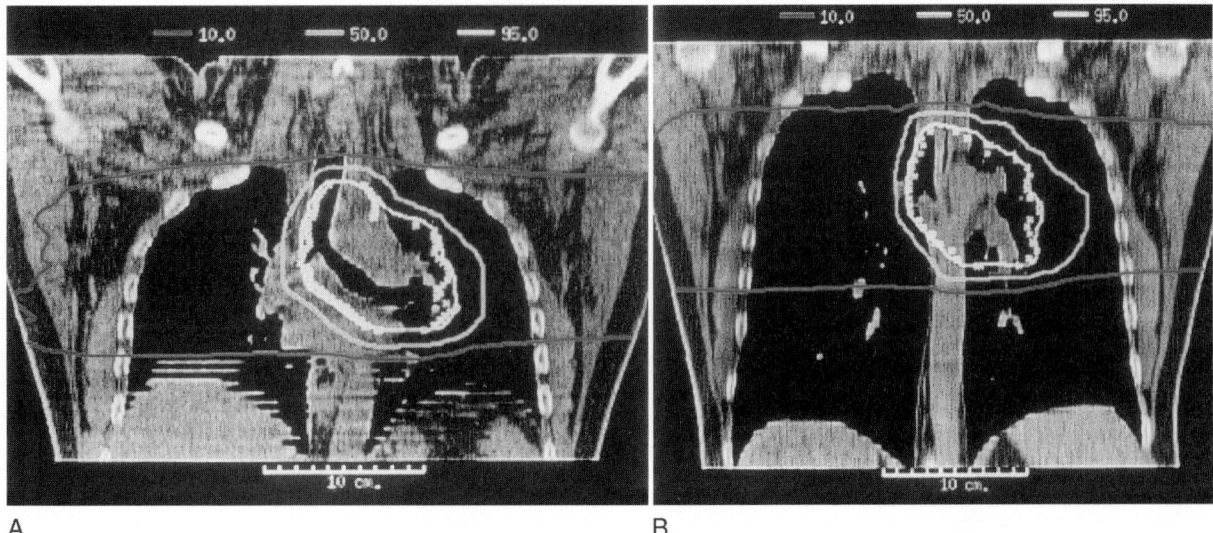

A   B

Figure 9–10. Comparison of (**A**) free-breathing and (**B**) deep inspiration breath hold (DIBH) treatment plans. Images are coronal planes through the isocenter for the same patient. Lines representing the 10%, 50%, and 90% isodose levels are in *red, green,* and *blue,* respectively. (From Rosenzweig KE, Hanley J, Mah D: The DIBH technique in treatment of inoperable non–small-cell lung cancer. *Int J Radiat Oncol Biol Phys.* 2000;48:81.) See also Color Figure 9-10.

computer. At the start of any session, whether simulation, CT, or treatment, the operator places the system into tracking mode for a few breathing cycles. This allows the system to determine the minimum and maximum vertical position of the upper marker. These values establish the scale of marker motion for subsequent display and for setting a gating threshold, as described later. At simulation, either amplitude or phase gating can be selected. For amplitude gating, the user adjusts the threshold levels that appear as two horizontal lines.

OPERATION DURING SIMULATION. The system allows synchronization of fluoroscopy with the breathing. The user selects the gating threshold for the breathing waveform. Only those fluoroscopy frames occurring during the gate intervals are played back. The operator then examines the anatomic motion in the playback to evaluate and optimize the choice of gating thresholds.

OPERATION ON A CT SCANNER. Scan acquisition can be synchronized with the normal breathing motion. The CT is operated in axial mode. The images are acquired only when the respiratory motion enters the selected gate. The breathing-synchronized images are used as the planning scans for the gated treatments. The breathing trace recorded during the planning scan is saved as a reference trace and is recalled before each gated treatment.

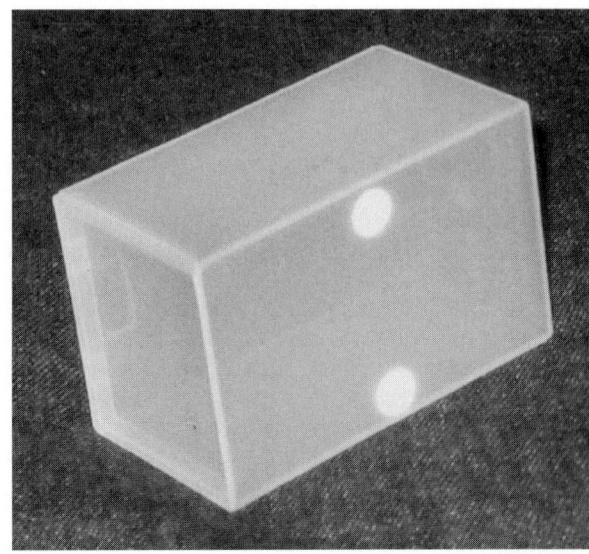

Figure 9–11. Charge-coupled-device video camera attached to infrared illuminator for tracking the respiratory motion.

Figure 9–12. Lightweight plastic block with reflective markers.

OPERATION DURING TREATMENT. During treatment, similar thresholds are selected. The beam is turned on only during the window defined by the threshold. Verbal breathing instructions have been found useful to improve the reproducibility and regularity in breathing.

SIMULATION PROCESS

Once the radiation oncologist has decided to treat the patient with external beam radiation therapy, the objective is to treat the target volume, diseased tissue plus a margin, to a tumoricidal dose while minimizing the dose to the surrounding normal tissues. If critical tissues are located nearby, the aim is to keep the dose to these organs to a level within the acceptable limit of complication. To determine the target volume, the radiation oncologist relies on the physical examination, radiographs, and other diagnostic tests, such as CT, MRI, and ultrasonography. Most patients treated with external beam radiation therapy undergo a treatment simulation before radiotherapy.

Planning for the simulation starts well before the patient is brought in for the actual procedure. Generally, the clinician has a reasonably good idea about the treatment volumes based on the physical examination and other diagnostic tests. Ideally, a team consisting of the radiation oncologist, the treatment planner, and the simulation therapist chalks out a tentative treatment approach beforehand. During the simulation, a strategy to treat the patient in a reproducible manner on a daily basis is developed. This includes decisions about the treatment position, the use of immobilization devices, the number of fields, gantry angles, collimator angles, field sizes, and field shapes. Appropriate points are tattooed on the patient's skin to ensure that the patient can be brought back to the treatment position rapidly each day for treatment. If the target volume is located near critical structures—for example, the nasopharynx target volume wraps around the spinal cord or the target volume extends between the retinas or is close to the optical chiasm—then intricate treatment planning is required to limit the dose to the critical organs. In these cases customized plans are developed, and an outline of the patient's external contour is needed. The outline is obtained either by a CT scan or by using one of the methods discussed later. To obtain the treatment-planning CT scans, the patient is placed in the treatment position on the CT couch; special attachments are available to ensure that the couch top is similar to that of a treatment couch. The clinician outlines the target volumes and the critical structures on these scans, and the treatment plans are designed based on these data.

Positioning of the Patient

Many issues are involved in deciding the treatment position. The most important factor is that the patient be able to lie comfortably in the treatment position for the duration of the treatment. Otherwise, it may be necessary to have the patient sit in a chair or in some other comfortable position during treatment. Depending on the site to be treated and the technique to be used, various institutions have preferred protocols for patient positioning. For example, to treat prostate patients, some institutions use a prone position,[27] whereas others prefer a supine position.[28] The next factor is that the position be such that the treatment beams avoid unnecessary tissue irradiation. For example, for the treatment of lung patients, if lateral fields will be used, an arms-over-the-head position is preferable so that the treatment beams do not pass through the arms. For brain patients, if the treatment volume is located posteriorly, a prone position may be preferable. Relative positions of the internal organs, such as esophagus and bowel, change depending on how the patient is lying on the couch. One position may offer better normal tissue sparing than the other. Fluoroscopic images can be helpful in making the decision.

To help in positioning the patient, many commercial devices are available. These include head-and-neck supports, a breast board, pillows, and various types of straps. Head-and-neck supports (Fig. 9-13) are made of polyurethane foam or clear plastic, offering minimal attenuation for megavoltage x-rays. Various sizes provide different head angulations and neck extensions. Use of the same support during each treatment helps in day-to-day reproducible positioning of the patient. At times, to solve a specific problem it may be necessary to develop a positioning device locally. A head-and-neck board (Fig. 9-14) was developed to treat nasopharynx patients with the conformal technique, which requires treatment with multiple posterior-lateral beams.[2] The board is made of low-density wood, and the patient can be treated through the board with megavoltage x-rays. The patient's head is supported at the smaller section of the board, which extends beyond the edge of the couch. This position allows treatment with posterior-lateral beams without interference from the couch-support bars. Similarly, a prostate board, made of low-density wood (Fig. 9-15), helps in positioning and immobilizing of the prostate patient. The board is placed atop a tennis racket or on the open section of the couch. With the help of this board the patient can be treated without any sag. The clamps at the side hold the thermoplastic mold in place. For any nonroutine treatment situation, the radiation oncologist, the treatment planner, and the radiation therapist should discuss the positioning of the patient beforehand.

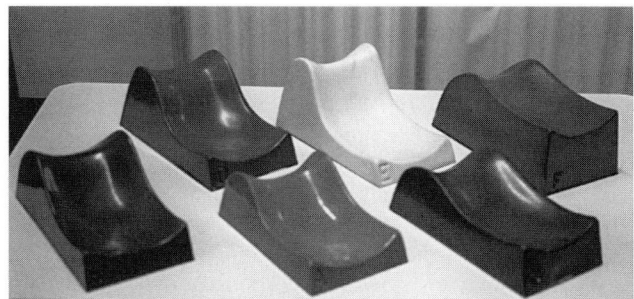

Figure 9–13. Commercially available set of head-and-neck supports. Different size supports allow various degrees of head angulation and neck extension.

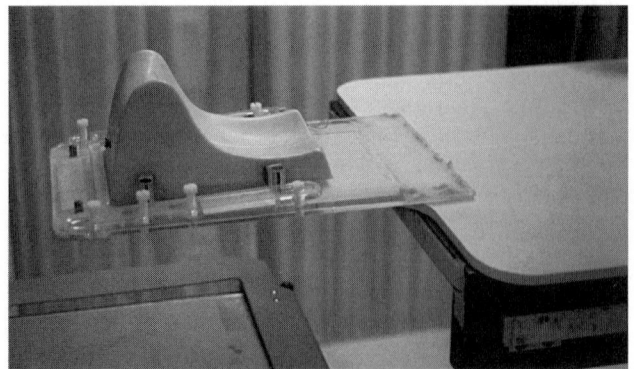

Figure 9–14. Head-and-neck board. The patient is supported at the thin section of the board that extends beyond the edge of the treatment couch. On the board, the patient can be treated with posterior-lateral beams without interference from couch support bars.

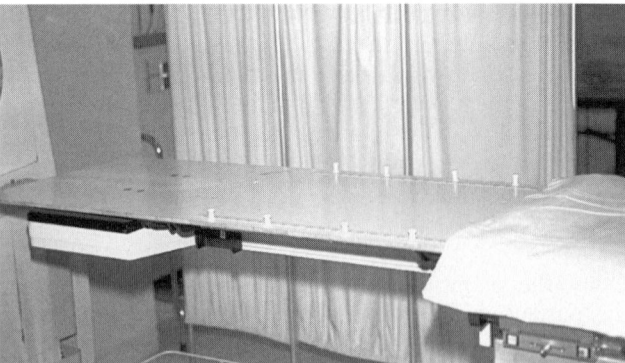

Figure 9–15. Prostate board. This low-density wood board is placed on top of a tennis racket or on the open section of the couch. It allows positioning of the patient without any sag. Clamps on the side are for attaching a thermoplastic mold.

Immobilization of the Patient

IMMOBILIZATION DEVICES

Once a treatment position has been determined, it may be necessary to use an immobilization device to ensure that the patient stays in the treatment position during the course of treatment and can be set up in the treatment position easily on a day-to-day basis. If the immobilization device is also used during CT scans, ensure that the material used to fabricate the device does not cause CT artifacts.

Different types of materials are available for immobilization. The selection depends on the site and preference of the oncologist and radiation therapist. Some materials that can be used are described in the following sections.

PLASTER CASTS. The patient is placed in the treatment position. Wet plaster of Paris bandages are used to create a cast around the body section to be immobilized. Within 10 to 15 minutes the cast hardens. To allow the patient to be removed from the cast, if necessary, a knife is used to divide the cast into two sections. When the pieces are completely dry, clamps are used to join the pieces. On the day of the treatment, the patient is immobilized by being placed in the treatment position and the two sections clamped together. The casts designed this way are heavy and opaque. If the cast is in the treatment beam, an opening is made by cutting away a piece of the cast.

THERMOPLASTICS. Thermoplastic sheets are available in different sizes and thicknesses, as perforated or solid sheets. Thermoplastic is rigid at room temperature, but when heated in a pan of water to temperatures in the range of 55°C to 70°C the material softens and becomes malleable.[29] The softened sheet can be molded around the body part to be treated and the flared ends of the mask clamped to the supporting board. When thermoplastic cools down, it hardens and forms a rigid mask. Figure 9-16 shows a commercially available system (Postfix, Sinmed, Reeuwijk, The Netherlands) to immobilize brain and head-and-neck patients. Patients in a

supine position on a headrest are immobilized with a thermoplastic mask that attaches to a carbon fiber base plate fixed to the treatment couch. The combination of a base plate and mask provides a system of accurate patient immobilization. Gilbeau et al.[30] analyzed the setup accuracy of three different types of thermoplastic masks. The first type of mask (Fig. 9-16A) fastens the head of the patient with three fixation points, two on both sides of the head and one on top of the head. The second type of mask (Fig. 9-16B) has four fixation points, two on the sides of the head and two around the shoulder. As shown in Figure 9-16C, the third type has five fixation points. Gilbeau et al. found that for the isocenter located in the head and neck, there was no substantial difference in the setup deviation between the three masks. The setup reproducibility was found to be better at the shoulder level with four- and five-fixation point masks. A body cast to immobilize a prone prostate patient is shown in Figure 9-17.

Another method of making the masks is the vacuum-forming technique.[31] First, a plaster cast is made as described previously. Then a positive plaster mold is constructed from the negative cast. Finally, the plastic cast is produced by "vacuum forming" over the positive mold. This results in a strong, clear lightweight mask that can be attached to a base plate.

POLYURETHANE FOAM. In this case a cast is made by mixing two liquids, a bottle of polyol and a bottle of papi (available under the trade name Alpha Cradle mold maker), in a plastic bag. The patient is positioned on top of this bag in the treatment position. As the two chemicals mix, foam forms and fills up the bag. The bag conforms to the patient's body shape. In about 15 minutes the foam hardens, providing a body cast. These casts are lightweight and provide rigid body support. For megavoltage x-rays, they produce little attenuation of the incident radiation. Figure 9-18 shows a foam mold for immobilizing a lung patient.

VACUUM-FORMING MOLD. This device consists of a lightweight plastic mattress that is loosely filled with radiolucent polystyrene (Styrofoam) beads. This flexible

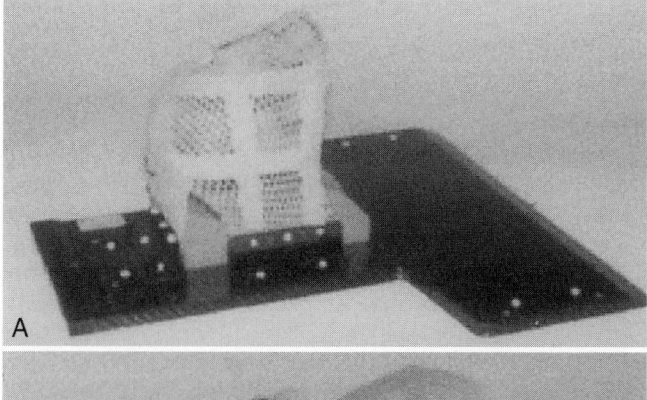

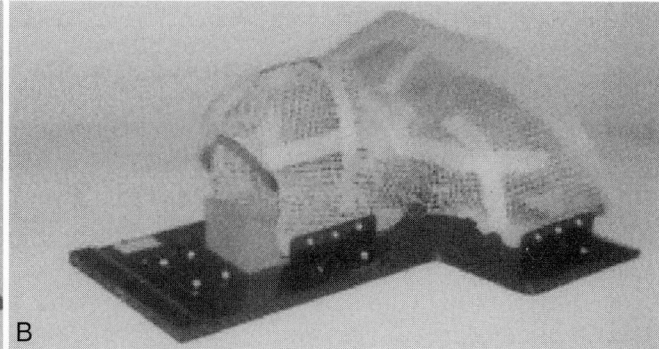

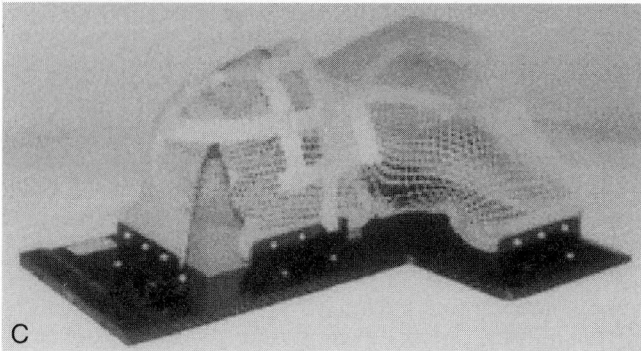

Figure 9–16. Three types of masks for the head and neck: **A**, three fixation points; **B**, four fixation points; **C**, five fixation points. (From Gilbeau L, Octave-Prignot M, Loncol T: Comparison of setup accuracy of three different thermoplastic masks for the treatment of brain and head and neck tumors. *Rad Ther Oncol.* 2001;58:155.)

mattress can be molded around the patient, and then as the air is removed from the bag by means of a vacuum pump, the beads are drawn together and form a rigid mold around the patient. As long as the vacuum is maintained, the mold retains its shape. After completion of the treatment, the bag is cleaned and recycled for the use of other patients.

Use of an immobilization device during treatment may create a situation in which the immobilization device is in the treatment beam. If the thickness of the material in the beam is significant, the material acts as a bolus and reduces the skin sparing. If this is not acceptable, cutting away a piece of the immobilization device can create an entrance port for the treatment beam.

At the same time it is necessary to make sure that the rigidity of the immobilization device is maintained. If a treatment beam passes through the support board or the body cast, it is necessary to know the attenuation due to the device and, if needed, adjust the beam-on time accordingly.

Immobilization of Pediatric Patients

Special boards with straps that immobilize small children are commercially available. Vacuum-forming molds in small sizes that can hold the patient in the treatment position are also available. If a situation arises in which the use of these devices is unsuitable and the child is too young to cooperate, it may be necessary to use anesthesia during the simulation, CT, and treatment.

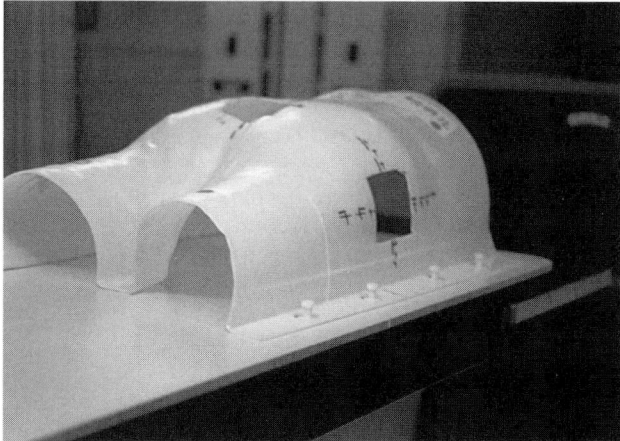

Figure 9–17. Thermoplastic body cast to immobilize a prostate patient in prone treatment position.

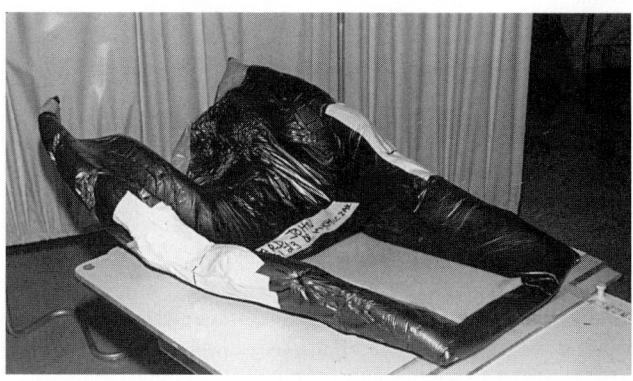

Figure 9–18. Polyurethane foam mold for immobilizing a lung patient.

Use of Contrast Material During Simulation

Radiopaque compounds with high atomic numbers, such as iodine and barium, and low-density materials, such as air, are used to enhance radiographic contrast. The use of contrast material helps in identifying and isolating anatomic structures and diseased tissue in radiographs and CT scans. Contrast materials are available in various forms. Agents such as Renografin and Omnipaque can be administered intravenously. As the bloodstream carries the contrast material to different organs, the radiographic contrasts of the organs change. Radiographic compounds such as Polibar and Gastrografin can be given orally to enhance the contrast of esophagus, stomach, and bowel. To increase the contrast of the rectum compared with the surrounding tissue, either a radiopaque compound or air is administered using a rectal catheter. A urinary Foley catheter with an inflatable balloon is used to visualize the bladder and urethra on the x-ray films. Figure 9-19 shows an anterior-posterior simulation film for a pelvic patient. An oral contrast agent is used to enhance the visibility of the bowel, and a Gastrografin-soaked tampon is used for localizing the vagina on the radiograph.

The concentrations of the contrast material and timing of its administration are important factors. Depending on the need, contrast material is used either during simulation or during the CT scan or both. If a contrast material with a high atomic number is present in high concentration during CT, it can give rise to artifacts that interfere with the localization of disease and normal organs. When a CT scan follows a simulation, the contrast material administered during simulation may be present during the CT scan, causing artifacts. Before the administration of a contrast material, the pros and cons of its use should be considered.

Localization of the Disease

After the patient has been placed in the treatment position, aligned, and if necessary immobilized, a tentative isocenter and the treatment field sizes are selected based on clinical information about the location and extent of the disease. Radiopaque catheters, wires, or lead beads are taped to the patient's skin to help identify any anatomical landmark, diseased tissue, or scar on the skin. Either a pair of orthogonal radiographs is taken or the patient is imaged fluoroscopically. These images are reviewed for coverage of the disease; if necessary, the isocenter and the field sizes are adjusted. A complete set of radiographs that includes an orthogonal pair and x-ray films for each treatment field is obtained. In order to set up the isocenter reproducibly on a daily basis, the triangulation points for the isocenter and a few alignment points are tattooed on the patient's skin. The alignment points are selected judiciously so that the patient can be brought back to treatment position without too much day-to-day variation. More emphasis is given to the bony anatomical landmarks, compared to the skin marks, particularly if the skin is flabby.[32] The relevant beam parameters, such as the gantry angles and field sizes, are recorded in the patient's chart along with the set-up depth. Polaroid photographs of the patient's setup, obtained during the simulation, are helpful in day-to-day positioning of the patient for radiotherapy.

CT SIMULATION

During CT simulation, a CT data set in the treatment position is obtained and a virtual simulation is carried out. Instead of radiographs, the DRRs are created from the CT data. Otherwise, the process is similar to that of a conventional simulation. Some of the main steps follow.

PATIENT IMMOBILIZATION. This is an essential part of precision radiotherapy. Devices such as thermoplastic molds, Alpha Cradles, and vacuum-forming molds can be used. However, when the patient is immobilized, these devices should fit through the CT bore. It may be necessary to either modify patient position or the immobilization device for this purpose. The devices should be free of large metallic pieces, which can cause artifacts on the CT images.

PATIENT ALIGNMENT. Once the patient is placed in the treatment position on the CT couch, the AP and lateral scout (pilot) images are taken to make sure the patient is properly aligned. With the help of the alignment lasers, provisional marks are placed on the patient to monitor the position throughout the procedure.

USE OF CONTRAST MATERIAL. The contrast materials suitable for CT scans should be used. Some material used for conventional simulation may not be suitable because it may cause CT artifacts.

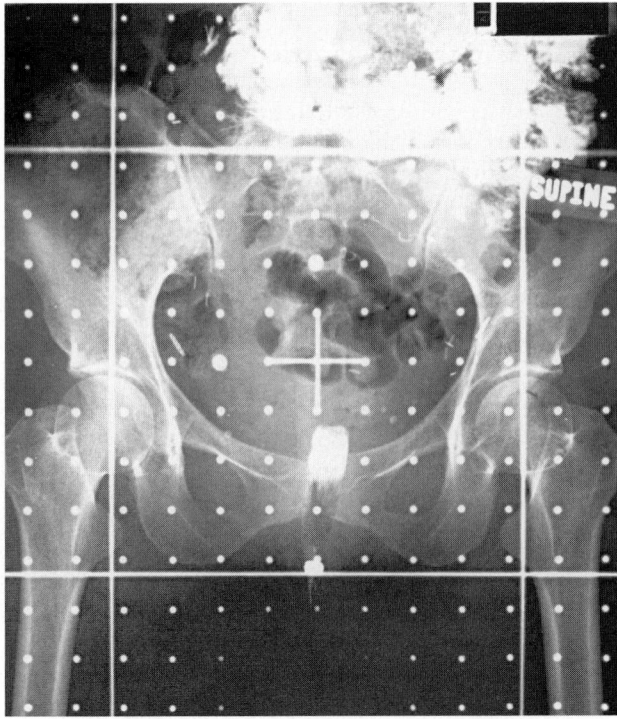

Figure 9–19. Simulation radiograph for pelvic treatment. An oral bowel contrast agent is used to enhance the visibility of the bowel, and a Gastrografin-soaked tampon is used for localizing the vagina.

SURFACE MARKERS. If some areas are of special interest, such as scars, previously treated area, and skin nodules, they can be highlighted with solder wire or lead beads. These may not be so easily visible on the DRRs, but DCRs in which skin is highlighted show these skin markers clearly. Figure 9-20A shows the DRR for a breast patient and Figure 9-20B is the DCR, in which the skin is highlighted and the markers are clearly visible.

CT SCANNING. The extents of the superior and inferior borders are decided based on many factors (e.g., these should include the disease with adequate margins so that the DRRs produced have anatomic information for the surrounding areas). If the beams are directed from a noncoplanar direction, the entrance port of the beam should be within the scanned region (e.g., if a vertex beam is used for the brain treatment, then the apex of the skull should be included). Smaller CT spacing and thickness are desirable for better-quality DRRs, but this requires a larger number of CT scans, resulting in longer scan times and time delays due to tube heating, during which it may be difficult for the patient to stay in the treatment position. A large number of scans requires more computer storage space and longer time for data processing. Usually 3 mm spacing and thickness are adequate. However, if it is a large field, 5 mm spacing and thickness may be used. In some cases a combination of different spacings—3 mm in the region of high definition and 5 mm in the surrounding area—may be desirable.

ISOCENTER LOCALIZATION. After the CT scan, virtual simulation software is used for localization. In the simplest case the isocenter location can be selected based on the patient's anatomy. For this purpose, CT images, DRRs, or DCRs are used. For cases where the disease is located in the soft tissue and it is difficult to determine the isocenter location based on the DRRs, the clinician outlines the GTV, CTV, or PTV on the CT images and the CT-simulation software automatically positions the isocenter in the middle of the target volume.

ISOCENTER MARKING. Once the isocenter location is determined, it is printed. The patient couch is moved longitudinally and the sagittal laser is shifted laterally to the location specified in the printout. Triangulation points are tattooed on the skin. At this point the patient can leave and the rest of the simulation is carried out.

VIRTUAL SIMULATION. Depending on the complexity of the situation, the patient's bony anatomy can be used to decide the beam orientation, field size, and block shape, as during a conventional simulation, but in place of radiographs, DRRs are used. The image quality of the DRRs can be adjusted by changing the window and contrast. Figure 9-21 shows the right lateral treatment port for a whole brain case.

Soft tissues are difficult to identify on the DRRs. In these cases the target and the normal tissues are contoured on the CT scans. The virtual software package contains the tools to help draw these contours. For example, if

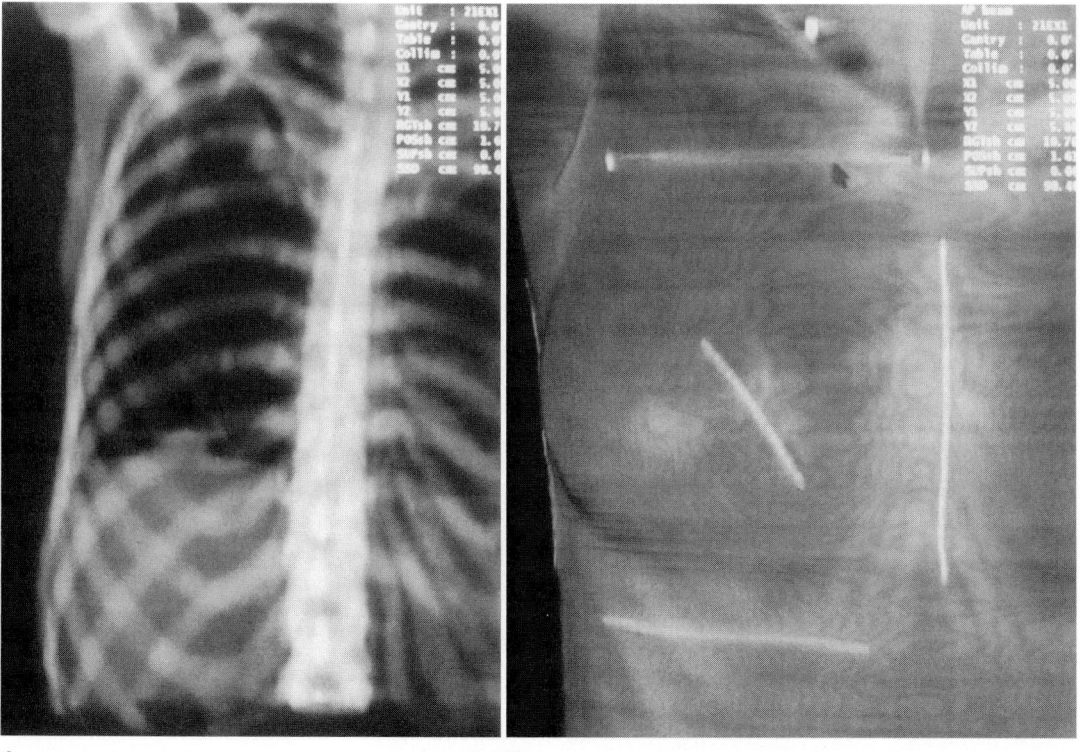

A   B

Figure 9–20. A, Digitally reconstructed radiograph for a breast patient, in which bones are visible. **B**, Digital composite radiograph in which skin is highlighted and markers are visible.

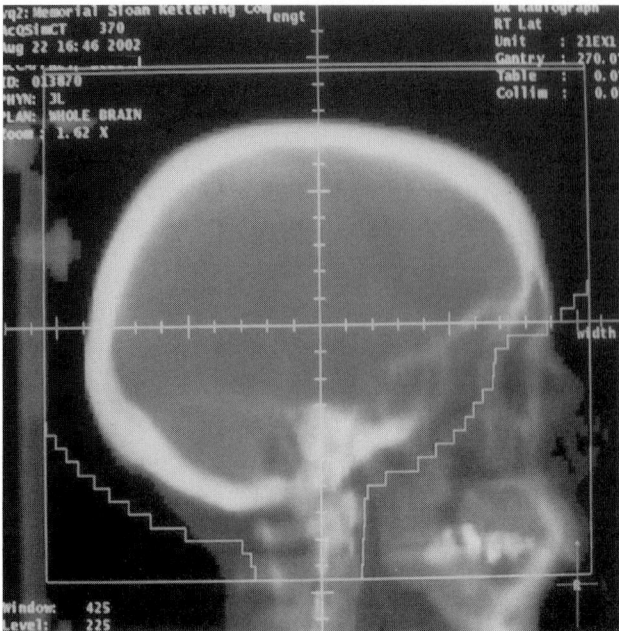

Figure 9–21. Digitally reconstructed radiograph for right-lateral beam for a brain patient. The multileaf collimator aperture outline, collimator, and graticule points are also displayed.

the CTV is drawn then a predetermined margin can be added to define the PTV. Figure 9-22 shows the anterior-posterior DRR for a pelvis field for a bladder patient.

For more complex cases the CT data are transferred to the treatment planning system, and the beams are optimized to give a satisfactory dose distribution. The DRRs are generated for the final beams.

Another advantage of the CT simulation is that for the cone-down plans there is no need to bring the patient back. The same data can be used for the next phase of

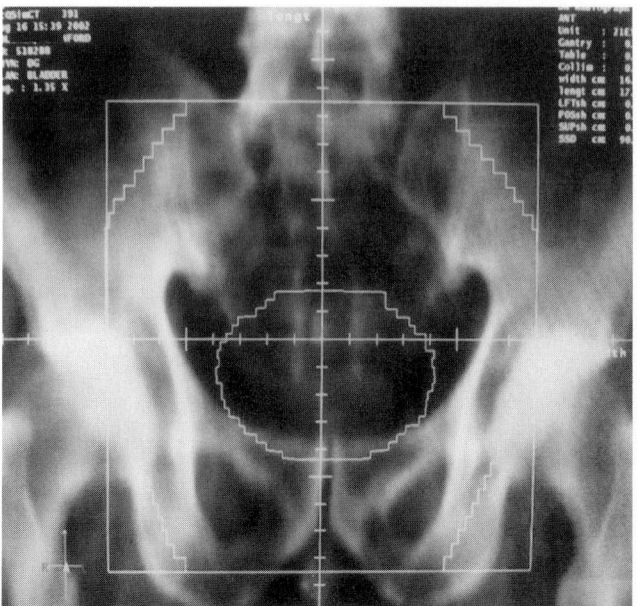

Figure 9–22. Digital composite radiograph for anterior-posterior treatment field for a bladder patient. The multileaf collimator aperture shape and bladder are shown.

the treatment, provided that there is no significant change in the patient's anatomy during the treatment.

METHODS FOR OBTAINING EXTERNAL PATIENT CONTOURS

If a treatment plan is needed for radiation therapy, the external contours are obtained. Usually, the contour is taken through the central axis of the beam. If the patient's thickness changes significantly within the treatment field, contours in more than one plane are taken. The best method for obtaining patients' external contours is the treatment-planning CT. A CT scan provides the external contour and the location of the disease and internal organs. If a treatment-planning CT is not available, various methods and devices can be used for obtaining the contours. Some devices are available commercially, whereas others have been described by researchers and can be constructed locally. The devices use mechanical,[33] optical,[34] ultrasonographic,[35] and electromechanical methods.[36]

Among the mechanical devices that are commercially available is the *pentograph*. A plotter pen is linked to a stylus; as the stylus is moved on the patient's body, the pen traces the contour on the plotter paper.

The external contour information can also be obtained easily with the help of a flexible solder wire and a caliper. This is a widely used method. The solder wire is placed on the patient's body and molded in the shape of the external contour. With a felt tip pen the important points are marked on the wire; these include the patient's midline, the tattoo locations, and anatomic landmarks. The wire is carefully lifted, and the contour shape and points are transferred onto paper. The contour dimensions are verified by measuring the anterior-posterior and lateral patient separations with a caliper. A horizontal line representing the tabletop is drawn as a reference for measuring the beam angles. Instead of a solder wire, a long thermoplastic contour tube or strip can also be used. The low-temperature thermoplastic is heated in a pan of water and shaped in the patient's contour; as the thermoplastic cools, it hardens and the contour shape is retained. The plaster of Paris bandage provides an alternative method of obtaining the external contour. Sufficient length of the bandage to obtain the contour and reach the tabletop on both sides is taken. It is folded along the width to a strip approximately 1 cm wide and thick enough to provide rigidity. The bandage is wet with water and molded along the patient's skin. Sufficient time is allowed for the strip to harden, the relevant points are marked, and then the strip is removed carefully. With a pencil, the shape outline is transferred to a sheet of paper. Figure 9-23 shows a contour obtained with the help of a thermoplastic strip.

TREATMENT DECISION

Depending on the location of the disease, the extent of the disease, and whether the treatment is palliative or curative, the patient can be treated in one of the following ways.

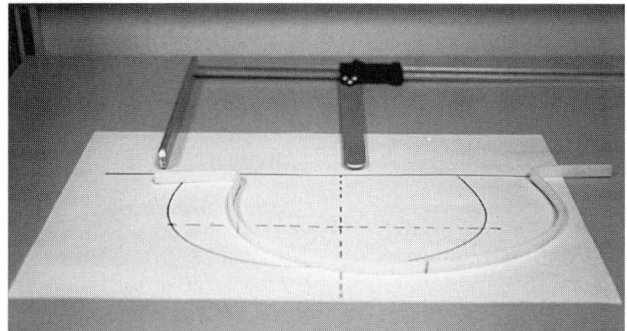

Figure 9–23. Thermoplastic strip and a contour obtained with it.

Manual Beam Definition

With manual beam definition, the clinician draws the aperture outlines for the blocks or Multileaf Collimators (MLCs) on the radiographs obtained during the simulation or DRRs during the CT simulation. Using the machine data table, beam-on times are calculated based on the field size, isocenter depth, extent of blocking, and prescribed dose. Examples of this type of calculation are treatment with parallel-opposed beams, the four-field "box" technique, and "enface" electron treatment.

Treatment Planning from Contours

If the target volume is close to critical organs and the intent is to limit the dose to these organs during radiation therapy, it may be necessary to design a treatment plan. The contours necessary for the plan are obtained either during the simulation or by a treatment-planning CT scan. The information about the location of the disease and critical structures is provided by the clinician on the simulation radiographs or on the treatment-planning CT images or both. A digitizer can be used to enter the information about the contours into the treatment-planning system. Generally, the external contours obtained using one of the mechanical methods are life-size and can be digitized directly. The small hard copies of the CT images can be enlarged to true size using an enlarger. The outer

contour, internal organs, and target volume can be projected and traced onto paper and then digitized into the treatment-planning computer. A magnification grid on a CT image is valuable for treatment planning. It can be used for alignment and verifying the magnification along the horizontal and vertical directions. If a treatment-planning system has the option of digitizing at a lower magnification, contours can be digitized directly from the CT hard copies using a light box (Fig. 9-24). Sometimes, a magnifying lens with cross hair helps in entering the data accurately. Most treatment-planning systems allow planning with the CT images; the external contour and the internal structures can be outlined directly on a video monitor by means of a light pen or some other pointing device.

The beams' parameters are selected by the planner. They include the type of radiation (electrons or photons) and its energy, field sizes and shapes, gantry angles, collimator angles, couch angles, wedges, and thicknesses of the bolus materials. The planning process is described in more detail in Chapter 8, Three-Dimensional Conformal Radiotherapy and Intensity-Modulated Radiotherapy. If the planned isocenter is different from the original isocenter or if the treatment plan uses beams for which x-rays were not obtained during the first simulation, then it may be necessary to bring the patient back to the simulator for a plan check or resimulation. However, if the patient was CT-simulated, it is not necessary for the patient to return. The virtual simulation can be done using the original CT data. During the plan check, the treatment isocenter is localized according to the planner's instructions, and radiographs for all of the treatment beams are taken. Sometimes it is impossible to radiograph certain beams (e.g., a vertex field). In such cases, a pair of orthogonal x-rays can be used for verification. The block outlines are drawn on the radiographs, and field-shaping blocks are constructed from the aperture outlines. Currently available are treatment machines equipped with MLCs. The beam apertures are digitized on a separate workstation. A computer program generates apertures designed by MLC leaves based on the digitized outlines. The MLC settings are transferred to the treatment machine by computer network or a disk.

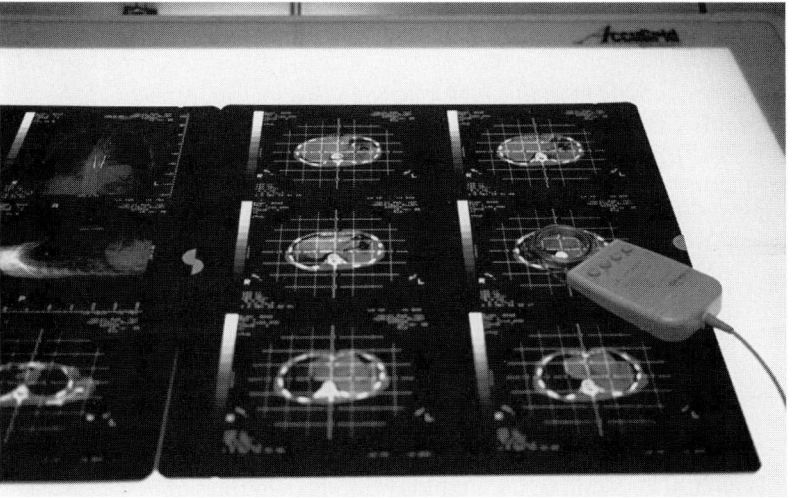

Figure 9–24. Digitizer with light box for digitizing the contours directly from CT scans.

IMAGE REGISTRATION

In radiation therapy CT images are generally used for treatment planning. High-resolution CT images provide excellent visualization of bony structures and MR images give detailed soft tissue information. Sometimes the abnormalities that are not visible on the CT scans can be clearly seen on the MR studies. Functional images such as single photon emission computed tomography (SPECT) and PET (described earlier) provide valuable metabolic information at the cellular level. But these studies do not contain enough anatomic information. Different imaging modalities provide complementary information. The process of image registration (or fusion) brings into spatial registration the principal components of different imaging modalities, thus providing a much better evaluation of the clinical situation. Before the development of the dedicated tool for image registration, the oncologist performed the same process mentally.

The process of image registration is based on the definition of the transformation of an image from one modality to the other modality. The end result of the image registration is the alignment of the two image data sets. Commercial systems that employ different methods of image registration are available. Some of the basic techniques follow.

CONTROL POINT–BASED REGISTRATION. In this method either externally placed point landmarks or internal anatomic landmarks on both primary and secondary data sets are used. The image registration consists of defining the transformation, which maps the control points of the primary data set to the secondary data set. The use of internal anatomic landmarks requires considerable operator expertise. The registration process can be carried out automatically, manually, or semiautomatically. Usually the semiautomatic approach—automatic followed by the manual registration—gives satisfactory results.

INTERACTIVE REGISTRATION. In this method the two studies are overlaid—one on top of another in different color in different images: axial, sagittal, and coronal. The operator manipulates the secondary image set to best match the primary study. Rotation and translation controls are available.

CONTOUR MATCHING REGISTRATION. In this method, the contours that can be identified on both image sets (e.g., the skin surface, bone) are drawn. Then the software automatically manipulates the studies using multiple image shifts and rotations, until the best registration between the two data sets is found.

COMBINING OPTION. Once the two image sets are registered, fusing the two can generate a third data set. This is usually the way to deal with combined anatomical-functional studies from sources such as CT or MR and PET or SPECT.

Recently combined units have become commercially available. These units can obtain CT and PET in the same treatment position. The advantage of these types of units is that the images are automatically registered.

Computed Tomography–Based Three-Dimensional Planning

3D treatment-planning systems use a set of CT scans for the treatment planning,[37-41] compared with a contour for the traditional plan. These systems offer more flexibility in planning, and the dose calculations are more accurate. Investigators have compared the 3D plans with the traditional two-dimensional (2D) plans and have found that the 3D plans can offer better target coverage and reduced dose to normal tissues.[42] For 3D treatment planning, the CT data are transferred to the planning system, and the relevant structures including the skin, bony landmarks, and critical structures are outlined. Once the structures have been entered, they can be viewed from the BEV perspective. The BEV for a lung patient is shown in Figure 9-25. Some of the normal structures, including the skin, and the target volume are shown as wire frames. The aperture outline (*in white*) has been drawn to cover the target but to exclude the spinal cord. As the gantry and the couch angles are varied, the view changes interactively. The planner can select the beams that treat the target while minimizing the dose to the surrounding tissues. Because the CT number is proportional to the electron density, the dose calculations for the plans can use the CT numbers to correct for the tissue inhomogeneities. Planning with noncoplanar beams is easier on a 3D treatment-planning system. For a 3D plan, if the isocenter is moved or if there are treatment beams for which no radiographs were initially taken, a plan check or resimulation is carried out to obtain a complete set of radiographs. However, if the DRRs are used instead

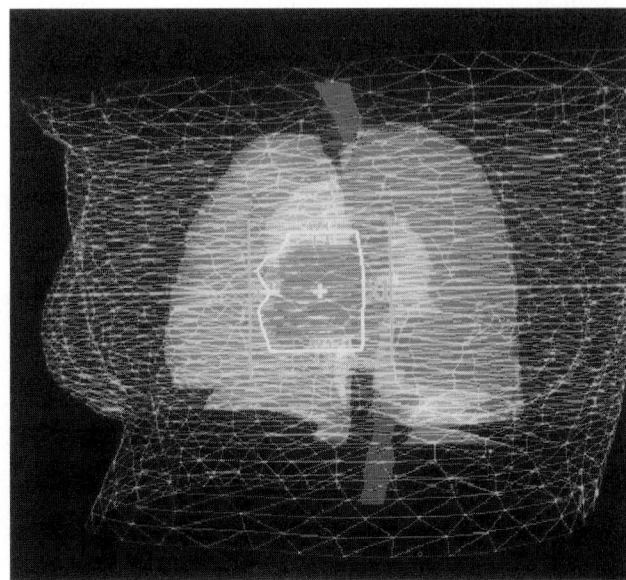

Figure 9–25. Beam's-eye view for a lung patient. In this oblique view, the outer contour (skin), lungs, spinal cord, and target volumes are visible. The aperture is drawn to cover the planning target volume but to exclude the cord. See also Color Figure 9-25.

of the radiographs, there is generally no need to bring the patient back.

PLAN CHECK OR RESIMULATION

To design a complex plan, it may be necessary to move the isocenter, change the number of treatment beams, or adjust the gantry angles, field sizes, and other beam parameters to achieve an acceptable plan. If the isocenter has been changed or beams have been used for which the radiographs were not taken during initial simulation, the patient is brought back to the simulator for a plan check. The patient is set up in the treatment position, and the original isocenter is verified radiographically. The isocenter is shifted as determined by the plan, and all the required radiographs, which include an orthogonal pair and x-ray films for all the treatment beams, are taken with the appropriate gantry angles and field sizes.

Volumetric CT data are used for 3D treatment planning. Based on these data, DRRs can be constructed. Figure 9-26 shows the DRR for a right-anterior-oblique treatment field for a prostate patient on which the contours for the femurs (*in yellow*) have been projected. For this treatment, MLC apertures were used. Projected also are the cross hair, graticule markers, MLC field shape, and collimators. The dashed outline in red is the aperture based on which the MLC aperture was created. The DRRs are compared with the corresponding simulation radiograph, and the treatment aperture can be transferred onto the x-ray films. Figure 9-27 shows the corresponding radiograph onto which the MLC aperture outline has been transferred.

If Cerrobend (a low-temperature melting alloy) blocks are used for the treatment, the blocks are fabricated based on the aperture outlines. Before the patient's

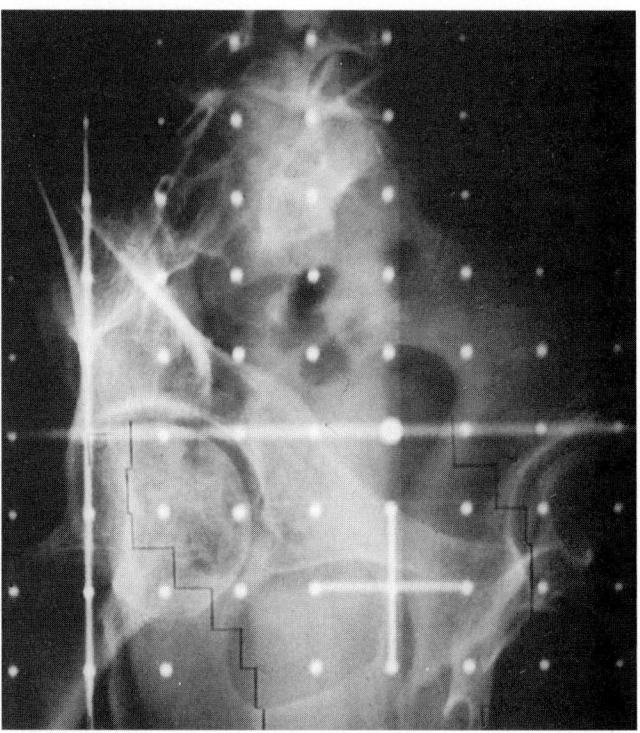

Figure 9–27. Simulation radiograph for the right-anterior-oblique beam on which the MLC aperture outline (shown in Figure 9-26) has been transferred. See also Color Figure 9-27.

treatment, either double-exposure localization port films are obtained or portal verification films are taken on the first day of the treatment. Portal verification is discussed in a later section. These films are compared with the corresponding simulation radiographs. The placement of the radiation field and aperture shapes are verified.

In some cases a DRR can be constructed, but it is not feasible to obtain a simulation radiograph (e.g., it is impossible to radiograph a vertex field). In such cases, one of the orthogonal films can be used for verification of the aperture shape. An anterior simulation radiograph can be used to draw the block shape for a vertex field. The orthogonal pair of films verifies the treatment isocenter, and the aperture shape is verified on the anterior localization port film. This film is just for verification; the beam pointing in the vertex direction delivers the actual treatment. Reisinger and colleagues[43] describe a verification technique for the vertex field. In this technique, the exposures from a lateral field and the vertex fields are superimposed on a localization port film. First, a double-exposure localization port film for one of the lateral fields is obtained. Then, without moving the film or the patient, one sets up the vertex field by rotating the treatment couch by 90 degrees. The table is moved laterally so that the film in the cassette holder is in the radiation axis plane. The couch is shifted inferiorly to obtain the same magnification as for the lateral field. The final film exposure is made so that the vertex field is superimposed on the film. The isocenter position and field size for the vertex fields are verified by this method.

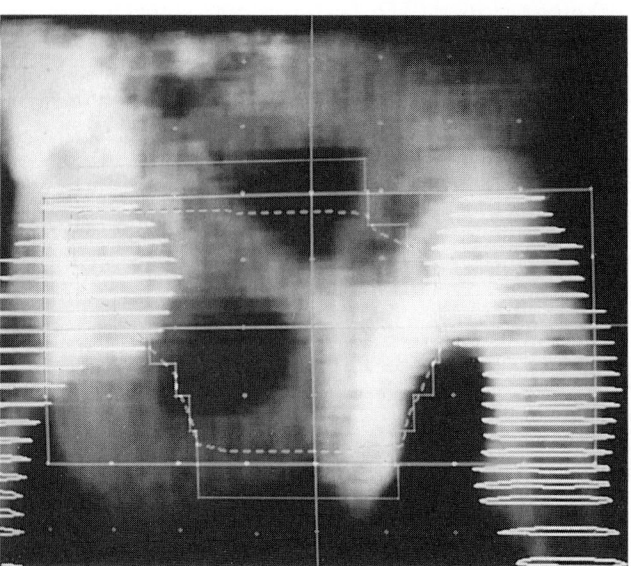

Figure 9–26. Digitally reconstructed radiograph for right-anterior-oblique treatment field for a prostate patient. The contours for the femurs (*in yellow*) have been projected to enhance the visibility of the femurs. The MLC aperture outline, collimators, cross hairs, and graticule points are also displayed. See also Color Figure 9-26.

TRANSFER OF TREATMENT INFORMATION TO THE THERAPY MACHINE

The information needed for the patient's treatment is produced during the simulation, treatment planning, and plan check. These include the instructions about positioning, immobilization, and tattoo marks on the skin for setting the isocenter. Polaroid pictures are taken to show the patient's positioning and tattoo marks. This information is documented in the patient's chart.

For each treatment beam all necessary parameters are recorded. These include the type of radiation; the beam energy; the beam-on time; the couch angle; the gantry angle; the collimator angle; the collimator jaw settings; the presence of a field-shaping block; if a wedge is used, its angle and orientation; the presence of a tissue compensator; and the type of bolus and its thickness.

For the treatment machines equipped with MLCs, the MLCs rather than Cerrobend blocks define field shapes. The MLC configuration for each beam is either designed on a treatment-planning computer or on a dedicated workstation. The information about the MLC leaf settings is loaded onto a computer disk and transferred to the therapy machine's MLC computer. On each day of the treatment, the aperture shape is defined by the MLC.

In some modern computer-controlled therapy machines, treatment parameters for the beams can be downloaded directly from the treatment-planning computer to the treatment machine's computer.[44] These machines can automatically set each beam and deliver the whole treatment without operator intervention. It has been suggested that a virtual treatment or "dry run" be carried out before actual treatment delivery to ensure patient safety during the automatic gantry and couch motion. During the virtual treatment the patient is placed in the therapy position, and the operator takes the machine through the whole treatment sequence but without radiation, while keeping the motion-enable switch depressed. This ensures that a collision situation does not exist during the machine and couch movement.

TREATMENT VERIFICATION

On the basis of instructions generated during the simulation and treatment planning, the patient is placed in the treatment position. To verify the correctness of the setup, the patient is imaged directly on the treatment machine with the shielding blocks or MLCs in place. This process is carried out before treatment. It serves two purposes. First, it confirms that the patient is set up correctly and the shielding blocks are protecting the normal structures as planned. Second, it documents the patient's position for future reference. It has also been shown that frequent treatment verification reduces localization errors.[45]

Portal Imaging with Films

High-energy therapy beams are used for portal radiographs. These could be either portal localization images or portal verification images. The quality of these images is generally poor compared with that of simulation radiographs.

PORTAL LOCALIZATION

A portal localization radiograph is obtained by exposing a radiographic film in a specially designed cassette with a metal screen. Only a fraction of the treatment beam-on time is used for the exposure. Droege and Bjarngard[46] investigated the screen-film combinations for portal imaging. Figure 9-28 shows a screen-film combination. The purpose of the front metal screen is to prevent the electrons generated within the patient from reaching the film and to generate electrons for the radiographic image production. The purpose of the high-atomic-number back screen, if used, is to serve as an intensifier and to provide additional film exposure. The use of a back screen results in higher speed at the cost of slight reduction in resolution. To expose a portal localization film, a double-exposure technique is used. The first exposure is given with the treatment field size and shielding blocks in place. For the second exposure, a graticule tray replaces the blocks, and an open field is used. The resulting image contains the

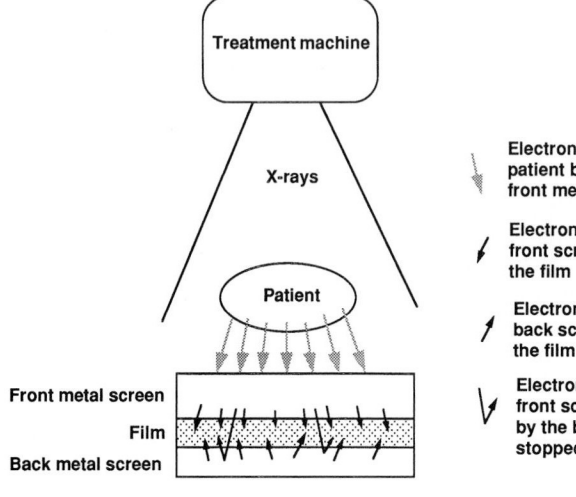

Electrons generated within the patient but stopped by the front metal screen

Electrons generated within the front screen and stopped in the film

Electrons generated in the back screen and stopped in the film

Electrons generated by the front screen, backscattered by the back screen and stopped in the film

Figure 9–28. Screen-film combination for portal localization imaging.

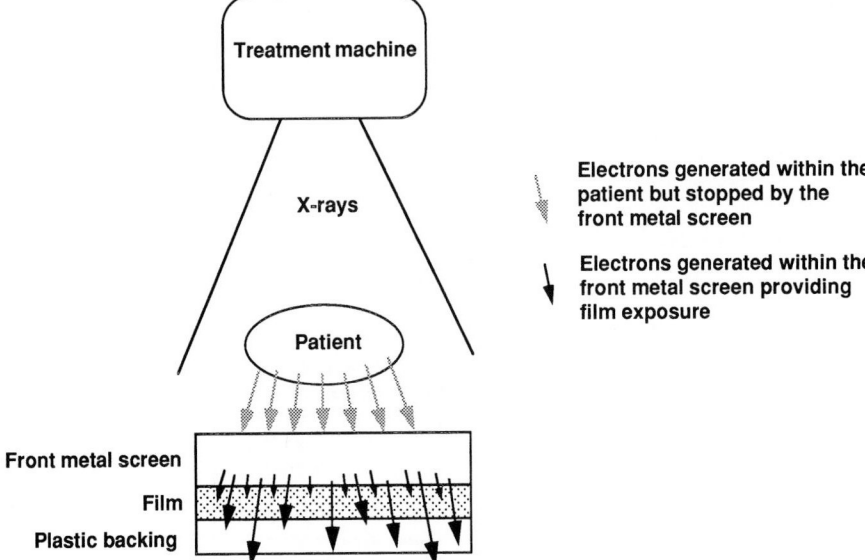

Figure 9–29. Screen-film combination for portal verification imaging.

image of the shaping block, the surrounding anatomical structures, and grid points that serve as the cross hair and scale for measurement. These films are compared with the simulation films to verify the treatment port shape and its location with respect to the patient's anatomy.

PORTAL VERIFICATION

For portal verification, a slow film with or without a screen is used. To obtain the radiograph, one exposes the film to the exit radiation for the duration of the treatment. Figure 9-29 schematically shows the film-screen combination for portal verification. In this case the function of the front metal screen is the same, to stop the electrons generated within the patient from reaching the film and to produce electrons for the radiographic image. A second metallic back screen is not used; instead, a plastic backing is used to provide support for the film and to eliminate artifacts from backscattered radiation. These radiographs image only the treatment area; the surrounding anatomical structures are not imaged.

Electronic Portal Imaging

For electronic portal imaging, an electronic portal imaging device (EPID) instead of a film is placed in the exit beam to produce the image. The images are captured and displayed on a video screen. Boyer and colleagues[47] reviewed the existing EPIDs. EPIDs produce images almost instantaneously and store them digitally on a computer. The images can be processed on the computer to enhance their various attributes.[48] Work is in progress to automatically compare these images with the simulation films and determine the placement differences.[49] The patient can be monitored throughout the treatment, and motion during the therapy can be detected. One of the commercial video-based systems is shown schematically in Figure 9-30[50] as the x-ray beam passes through the patient; its intensity is modulated by the inhomogeneity of the

patient's anatomic structures. The exiting photon beam strikes the metal plate coated with phosphorous material to produce fluorescence. A video camera and computer combination digitally record the resulting light and display the images on a video monitor. A mirror inclined at a 45-degree angle allows the video camera to be out of the direct radiation beam. The whole system is packaged in a collapsable housing. When the device is not in use, it can be retracted.

Another type of EPID uses a matrix of liquid ion chambers as detectors (Fig. 9-31).[51-52] This system consists of a 256×256 matrix of ionization chambers. An organic liquid serves as the ionizing medium between the electrodes.

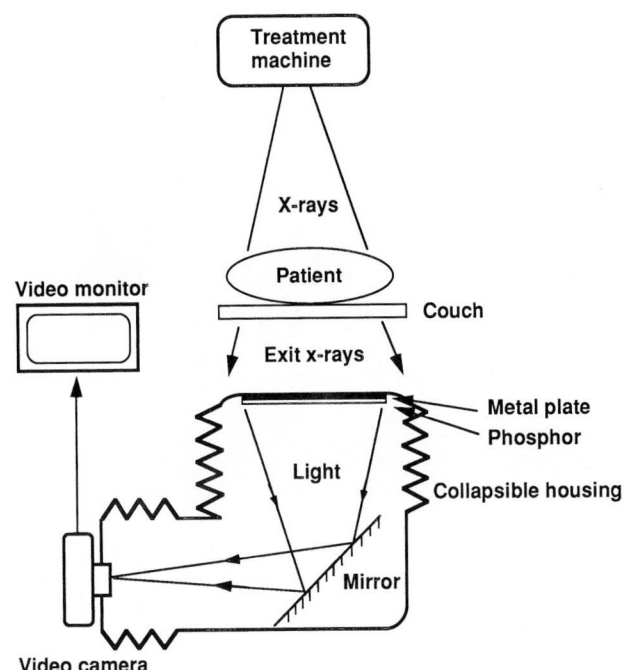

Figure 9–30. Schematic diagram of the components of a (commercially available) video-based electronic portal imaging device.

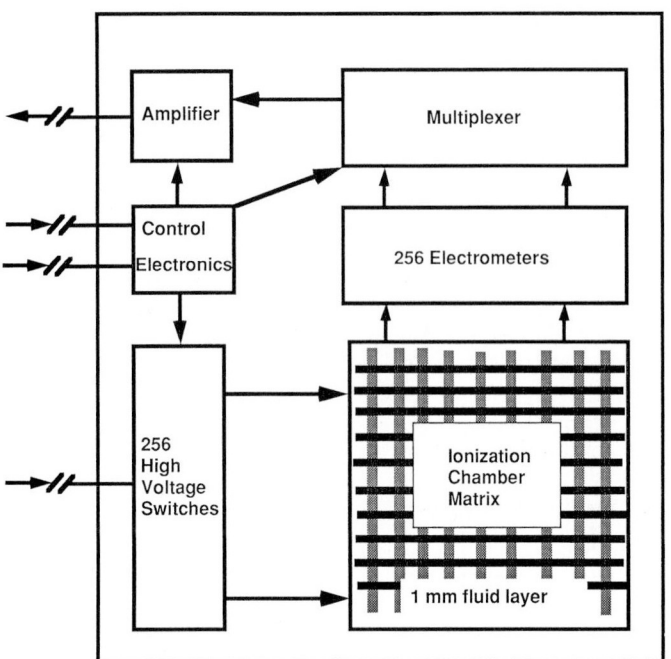

Figure 9–31. Schematic diagram of a matrix-ionization chamber electronic portal imaging device. (Redrawn from Boyer AL, Antonuk L, Fenster A, et al: A review of electronic portal imaging devices (EPIDs). *Med Phys.* 1992;19:1.)

The ionization current in each chamber is measured with a current-to-voltage converting electrometer. An analog-to-digital converter, providing the intensity information for the pixel corresponding to the ionization chamber, then digitizes the collected charge. The matrix ion chambers, metal screens, and support electronics are packaged in a compact cassette form, which can be mounted on the gantry. Recently, amorphous silicon detectors have become available. These detectors have 512 × 384 resolution, and better corresponding image quality. Figure 9-32 shows the image for a prostate patient obtained with an amorphous silicon imager. Figure 9-33 shows an amorphous silicon detector attached to a therapy machine. A motorized mount allows variable source-to-detector distance and movement along lateral and longitudinal directions.

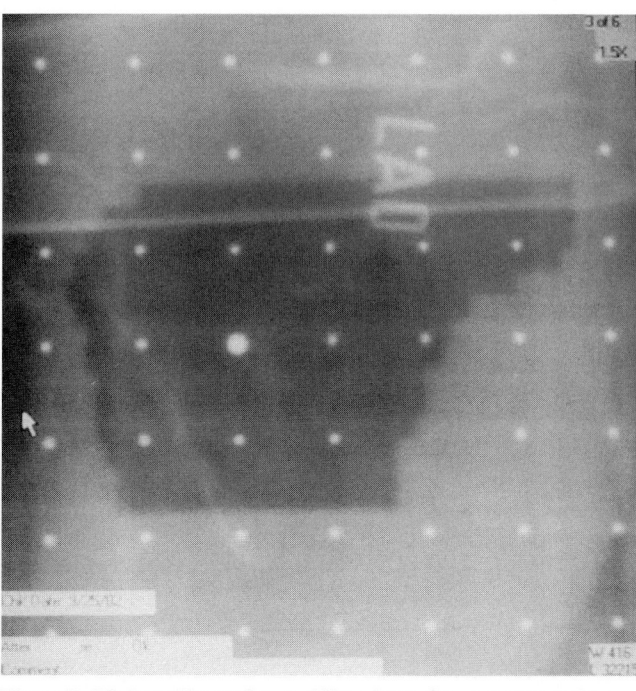

Figure 9–32. Portal image for an oblique beam for a prostate patient obtained with an amorphus silicon detector. See also Color Figure 9-32.

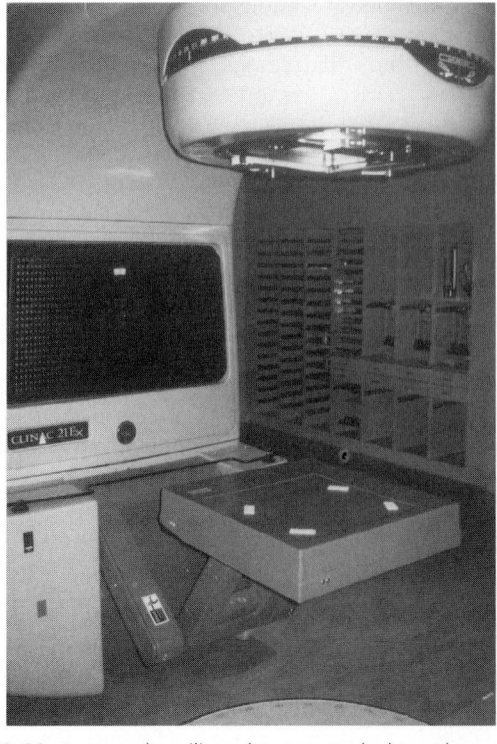

Figure 9–33. An amorphus silicon detector attached to a therapy machine. The motorized mount allows detector movement. See also Color Figure 9-33.

REFERENCES

1. Hall EJ: *Radiobiology for the Radiologist.* 4th ed. Philadelphia: JB Lippincott; 1994:211.
2. Leibel SA, Kutcher GJ, Harrison LB, et al: Improved dose distribution for 3D conformal boost treatments in carcinoma of the nasopharynx. *Int J Radiat Oncol Biol Phys.* 1991;20:823.
3. Hanley J, Debois MM, Mah D, et al: Deep inspiration breath-hold technique for lung tumors: The potential value of target immobilization and reduced lung density in dose escalation. *Int J Radiat Oncol Biol Phys.* 1999;45:603.
4. Mageras GS, Yorke E, Rosenzweig K, et al: Fluoroscopic evaluation of diaphragmatic motion reduction with respiratory gated radiotherapy system. *J Appl Clin Med Phys.* 2001;2:191.
5. Hounsfield GN: Computed medical imaging. *Med Phys.* 1980;7:283.
6. Crawford CR, King KF: Computed tomography scanning with simultaneous patient translation. *Med Phys.* 1990;17:967.
7. Arkadiusz P, Kalender W, Brink J, et al: Measurement of slice sensitivity profiles in spiral CT. *Med Phys.* 1994;21:133.
8. Vock P, Soucek M, Daepp M, et al: Lung: Spiral volumetric CT with single-breath-hold technique. *Radiology.* 1990;176:864.
9. Goitein M: Computed tomography in planning radiation therapy. *Int J Radiat Oncol Biol Phys.* 1979;5:445.
10. Lichter AS, Fraass BA, van de Geijn J, et al: An overview of clinical requirements and clinical utility of computed tomography based radiotherapy treatment planning. In Ling CC, Rogers CC, Morton RJ, eds. *Computed Tomography in Radiation Therapy.* New York: Raven Press; 1983:1.
11. Sherouse GW, Mosher CE, Novins K, et al: Virtual simulation: Concept and implementation. In Bruinvis IAD, van der Giessen PH, van Kleffens HJ, Wittkamper FW, eds. *The Use of Computers in Radiation Therapy.* Amsterdam: Elsevier Science; 1987:433.
12. Sherouse GW, Bourland JD, Reynolds K, et al: Virtual simulation in the clinical setting: Some practical considerations. *Int J Radiat Oncol Biol Phys.* 1990;19:1059.
13. Sherouse GW, Chaney EL: The portable virtual simulator. *Int J Radiat Oncol Biol Phys.* 1991;21:475.
14. Sherouse GW, Novins K, Chaney EL: Computation of digitally reconstructed radiographs for use in radiotherapy treatment design. *Int J Radiat Oncol Biol Phys.* 1990;18:651.
15. Goitein M: CT Simulation: An overview. In Jani SK, ed. *CT Simulation for Radiotherapy.* Madison, Wisc.: Medical Physics; 1993:161.
16. Wen BC, Pennington E, Jani S: Clinical applications of CT simulators in unconventional radiation therapy techniques. In Jani SK, ed. *CT Simulation for Radiotherapy.* Madison, Wisc.: Medical Physics; 1993:129.
17. Butker EK, Helton DJ, Keller JW, et al: Practical implementation of CT-simulation: The Emory experience. In Purdy J, Starkschall G, eds. *A Practical Guide to 3-D Planning and Conformal Radiation Therapy.* Middleton, Wisc.: Advanced Medical Publishing, Inc.; 1999:57.
18. Garcia-Ramirez JL, Mutic S, Dempsey JF, et al: Performance evaluation of an 85-cm-bore x-ray computed tomography scanner designed for radiation oncology and comparison with current diagnostic CT scanner. *Int J Radiat Oncol Biol Phys.* 2002;52:1123.
19. Chen GTY, Pelizzari, Hamilton RJ, et al: Image processing and integration in oncologic imaging. In Bragg DG, Rubin P, Hricak H, eds. *Oncologic Imaging.* 2nd ed. Philadelphia: WB Saunders; 2002:92.
20. Yan D, Wong J, Vicini F, et al: Adaptive modification of treatment planning to minimize the deleterious effect of treatment setup error. *Int J Radiat Oncol Biol Phys.* 1997;38:197.
21. Wong JW, Sharpe MB, Jaffray DA, et al: The use of active breathing control (ABC) to reduce margin for breathing motion. *Int J Radiat Oncol Biol Phys.* 1999;44:911.
22. Wong JW, Yan D, Jaffray DA, et al: Interventional strategies to optimize the delivery of radiation therapy. In Bragg DG, Rubin P, Hricak H, eds. *Oncologic Imaging.* 2nd ed. Philadelphia: WB Saunders; 2002:116.
23. Rosenzweig KE, Hanley J, Mah D, et al: The deep inspiration breath hold technique in treatment of inoperable non–small cell lung cancer. *Int J Radiat Oncol Biol Phys.* 2000;48:81.
24. Mah D, Hanley J, Rosenzweig KE, et al: Technical aspects of deep inspiration breath-hold technique in the treatment of thoracic cancer. *Int J Radiat Oncol Biol Phys.* 2000;48:1175.
25. American Thoracic Society: Standardization of spirometry. *Am J Respir Crit Care Med.* 1994;152:1107.
26. Ford EC, Mageras GS, Yorke E, et al: Evaluation of respiratory movement during gated radiotherapy using film and electronic portal imaging. *Int J Radiat Oncol Biol Phys.* 2002; 52:522.
27. Leibel SA, Heimann R, Kutcher GJ, et al: Three-dimensional conformal radiation therapy in locally advanced carcinoma of the prostate: Preliminary results of a phase I dose-escalation study. *Int J Radiat Oncol Biol Phys.* 1994;28:55.
28. Ten Haken RK, Perez-Tamayo C, Tesser RJ, et al: Boost treatment of the prostate using shaped, fixed fields. *Int J Radiat Oncol Biol Phys.* 1989;16:193.
29. Gerber RL, Marks JE, Purdy JA: The use of thermal plastics for immobilization of patients during radiotherapy. *Int J Radiat Oncol Biol Phys.* 1982;8:1461.
30. Gilbeau L, Octave-Prignot M, Loncol T, et al: Comparison of setup accuracy of three different thermoplastic masks for the treatment of brain and head and neck tumors. *Rad Ther Oncol.* 2001;58:155.
31. Devereux C, Grundy G, Littman P: Plastic molds for patient immobilization. *Int J Radiat Biol Phys.* 1976;1:553.
32. Khan FM: *The Physics of Radiation Therapy.* 2nd ed. Baltimore: Williams & Wilkins; 1994:307.
33. Stern BE, Hodges GB: A pentograph for body contours. *Br J Radiol.* 1957;30:613.
34. Clayton CB, Thompson DJ: An optical apparatus for reproducing outlines of body cross-section. *Br J Radiol.* 1970;43:489.
35. Day MJ, Harrison RM: Cross-sectional information and treatment simulation. In Bleehen NM, Glatstein E, Haybittle JL, eds. *Radiation Therapy Planning.* New York: Marcel Dekker; 1983:87.
36. Doolittle AM, Berman LB, Vogel G, et al: An electronic patient contouring device. *Br J Radiol.* 1977;50:135.
37. Fraass BA, McShan DL: 3-D Treatment Planning: I. Overview of a clinical planning system. In Bruinvis IAD, van der Giessen PH, van Kleffens HJ, Wittkamper FW, eds. *The Use of Computers in Radiation Therapy.* Amsterdam: Elsevier Science; 1987:273.
38. Purdy JA, Wong JW, Harms WB, et al: Three-dimensional treatment planning system. In Bruinvis IAD, van der Giessen PH, van Kleffens HJ, Wittkamper FW, eds. *The Use of Computers in Radiation Therapy.* Amsterdam: Elsevier Science; 1987:277.
39. Mohan R, Barest G, Brewster L, et al: A comprehensive three-dimensional radiation treatment planning system. *Int J Radiat Oncol Biol Phys.* 1988;15:481.
40. Sailer SL, Chaney EL, Rosenman JG, et al: Treatment planning at the University of North Carolina at Chapel Hill. *Semin Radiat Oncol.* 1992;2:267.
41. Photon Treatment Planning Collaborative Working Group: State-of-the-art of external photon beam radiation treatment planning. *Int J Radiat Oncol Biol Phys.* 1991;21:9.
42. Armstrong JG, Burman C, Leibel S, et al: Conformal three-dimensional treatment planning may improve the therapeutic ratio of high dose radiation therapy for lung cancer. *Int J Radiat Oncol Biol Phys.* 1993;26:685.
43. Reisinger SA, Palta J, Tupchong L: Vertex field verification in the treatment of central nervous system neoplasms. *Int J Radiat Oncol Biol Phys.* 1992;23:429.
44. Mageras GS, Podmaniczky KC, Mohan R: A model for computer-controlled delivery of 3-D conformal treatments. *Med Phys.* 1992;19:945.
45. Marks JE, Haus AG, Sutton HG, et al: The value of frequent treatment verification films in reducing localization error in the irradiation of complex fields. *Cancer.* 1976;37:2755.
46. Droege RT, Bjarngard BE: Influence of metal screens on contrast in megavoltage x-ray imaging. *Med Phys.* 1979;6:487.
47. Boyer AL, Antonuk L, Fenster A, et al: A review of electronic portal imaging devices (EPIDs). *Med Phys.* 1992;19:1.
48. Leszczynski KW, Shalev S, Ryder S: A study of efficacy of digital enhancement of on-line portal images. *Med Phys.* 1992;19:999.

49. Bijhold J, Gilhuijs GA, van Herk M: Automatic verification of radiation field shape using digital portal images. *Med Phys.* 1992;19:1007.

50. Munro P, Rawlinson JA, Fenster A: A digital fluoroscopic imaging device for radiotherapy localization. *Int J Radiat Oncol Biol Phys.* 1990;18:641.

51. Van Herk M, Meertens H: A digital imaging system for portal verification. In Bruinvis IAD, van der Giessen PH, van Kleffens HJ, Wittkamper FW, eds. *The Use of Computers in Radiation Therapy.* Amsterdam: Elsevier Science; 1987:371.

52. Meertens H, van Herk M, Bijhold J, et al: First clinical experience with a newly developed electronic portal imaging device. *Int J Radiat Oncol Biol Phys.* 1990;18:1173.

Breathing Synchronized Radiotherapy

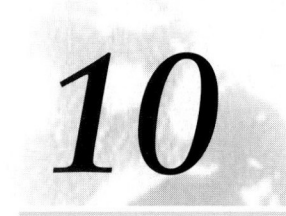

Dale Kubo, PhD

A golden rule of radiation therapy may be expressed as "delivering as much dose as possible to tumor while sparing the dose to the surrounding normal tissue." To achieve this golden rule, three-dimensional conformal radiation therapy (3DCRT), intensity-modulated radiation therapy (IMRT), and breathing synchronized radiotherapy (BSRT) have been tested and have shown encouraging results. The main topic of this chapter, BSRT, includes both nongated and gated methods and occupies a very unique spot in the history of radiation therapy in North America. For the sake of simplicity, gated radiotherapy may be defined as a method of radiation therapy whereby the on-off status of the treatment beam is controlled by signals that are produced whenever the breathing signal falls in the preset gating window while the nongated BSRT is manually controlled.

Gated radiotherapy in North America began around 1995 and is receiving a great deal of attention for two reasons. First is the goal of higher precision radiotherapy for greater patient benefit. Many publications support the concept that for a smaller planning target volume (PTV), higher dose can be prescribed to the target, thereby leading to better tumor control probability with less or equivalent normal tissue complication probability. Moving targets such as tumors in the lung, liver, and stomach have frustrated radiation oncologists and physicists because the PTV should include the total extent of target motion due to normal breathing. Thus, contrary to the golden rule of radiotherapy, we are forced to increase the radiation field size to encompass the extended target. The accuracy of PTV definition, including margins around the gross tumor volume (GTV), depends on several fac-tors including disease extension, beam penumbra, extent of organ motion during beam-on and positioning setup error. As image guidance methods improve patient positioning over the next several years, setup error due to positioning is expected to decrease. With organ motion synchronized with beam delivery, the irradiated volume can be reduced as illustrated in Fig. 10-1.

The second reason is somewhat related to the first one in that a cutting edge of 3DCRT is IMRT. Optimal use of the dose-sculpting capabilities of IMRT requires precise knowledge of anatomy for both treatment planning and beam delivery. Since the target organ is moving in time and space, the radiation beam must be delivered

at the right time to the right place to prevent tumor underdose or normal tissue overdose. This problem can be exacerbated, in particular, with IMRT because IMRT is often used to produce high dose gradients, which require more precise definition of anatomy in time and space. The intent of IMRT is to reduce the treatment volume by better dose conformity to the target, thus sparing normal tissue. Then one may be able to dose-escalate according to the golden rule. However, the moving target partially defeats this goal of IMRT. Ideally, one should turn on a beam only when the target is within a predetermined volume or the beam should move and track the tumor, so that the target gets a sufficiently high dose to kill the tumor while sparing the surrounding normal tissue. Therefore, a combination of IMRT and BSRT is considered essential in dealing with moving targets in the steep dose gradient regions. For the same reason, the accuracy of target positioning (or patient positioning) is crucial in performing accurate IMRT + BSRT.[1,2] Thus, gated radiotherapy has become a critical element of modern 3DCRT. However, up to this point, there have been few reports on accounting for moving organs in treatment planning.

This section reviews various BSRT techniques that were developed in North America. Since BSRT was originally developed in Japan in late 1989 to early 1992,[3,4] this is included in the review. Recently, many exciting developments with BSRT have been reported—in particular, tumor tracking systems. Due to the extensive use of imaging in combination with IMRT and

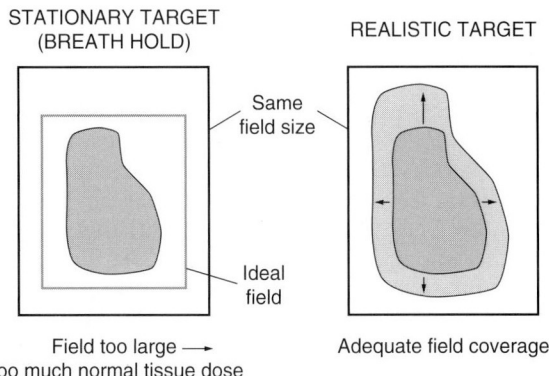

Figure 10–1. Stationary target and target with motion included.

BSRT, many of these methods are considered to be a part of *image-guided radiotherapy (IGRT)*. Therefore, in this section we focus only on the audio-gated radiation treatment (ART) system developed at the University of California Davis Cancer Center (UCDCC),[1,5-13] the active breathing control (ABC) system developed at William Beaumont Hospital,[2,14,15] deep inhalation breath hold (DIBH) method and the Varian Real-Time Position Management (RPM) system (Palo Alto, Calif.) in use at Memorial Sloan-Kettering Cancer Center (MSKCC),[16-23] and a highly technical tumor tracking system developed at Hokkaido University Hospital[24-27] and Tohoku University Hospital,[28] both in Japan. A tracking method that uses a robot-mounted linear accelerator (LINAC) is discussed in Chapter 74, Extracranial Stereotactic Radioablation.

BRIEF REVIEW OF BREATHING SYNCHRONIZED RADIATION THERAPY

Since BSRT is relatively new in this country, its effect on clinical outcome is not yet established. Therefore, we review mainly its technical aspects.

BSRT in radiation therapy was discussed by Henkelman and Mah[29] in 1982. Just before and after their paper, numerous papers dealing with "gating" for diagnostic purposes were published. These papers reported on cardiac, liver, and pancreatic organ motion. Most of this work is based on CT imaging,[30-39] but some is based on magnetic resonance imaging (MRI) scans[40-42] and there is one publication on ultrasound.[43] Gating studies in diagnostic radiology continue, as indicated by further publications.[44-51] In the mid-1980s, some of the tools and methods devised for diagnostic imaging were considered in the domain of radiation therapy. Specifically, Rekonen and Toivonen[52] discussed the possibilities of and need for breathing gated radiotherapy in 1985. Peltola[53] proposed a method for implementing patient breathing into gated radiotherapy. In 1987, Willett et al.[54] mentioned respiration gating but did not take any action. Moreland et al.[55] discussed the effect of kidney motion on the accuracy of radiotherapy treatment planning.

The first report on truly gated radiotherapy was published in 1989 by a group of radiation oncologists and medical physicists at Tsukuba University Proton Therapy Center.[3] Initially, they implemented their gating technique on a LINAC. Their method was based on monitoring the signal from a combination of an airbag and a strain gauge taped on the patient's abdomen. This signal was then fed into a LINAC for 6 MV and 10 MV x-ray treatment. This historical paper was followed by another publication. In 1992[4] they reported a similar but improved gating method, which was adapted to an energy-degraded proton beam from the 500 MeV nuclear physics proton accelerator. They pointed out that the average excursion of the diaphragm in seven patients was 1.0 to 2.5 cm in quiet respiration and 3.0 to 7.0 cm in deep inhalation. They set the gate window at the expiratory end phase of quiet respiration, where the diaphragm was most relaxed and its position was most reproducible.

In 1995 Kubo and Hill[11,56] reported the first gated radiotherapy system in North America at the annual American Association of Physicists in Medicine (AAPM) summer meeting, followed by a publication.[12] They discussed the feasibility of gating and the dosimetry of short beam duration using the Varian 2100C LINAC. They confirmed that the beam's on- and off-mechanism initiated by gating did not cause any dosimetry differences from normal continuous beam operation. This fact was further verified by Ramsey et al.[57] Kubo and colleagues published several papers in the domain of technical improvement.[1,5-13] Their studies are focused on gating the LINAC during a breath-hold at the end of the exhalation phase of breathing cycles. They confirmed by the use of an amorphous silicon detector that the breath-hold was maintained during the treatment.[6] They also verified that gating did not interfere with the operations of enhanced dynamic wedge (EDW) and IMRT.[1] In other words, EDW or IMRT and BSRT can be combined without sacrificing dosimetric accuracy. The introduction of time-sequence gating, audio-gated radiotherapy (or ART), should further reduce organ motion during breath-hold.[9,13] The latest work on ART by Kubo[13] was to examine the correlation between the actual organ motion and the breath-hold signal. Their study also shows that a point in the breathing cycle corresponds to a specific point of diaphragm location within 2 mm accuracy.

In the mid-1990s, the Michigan group[58-65] initiated a series of studies dealing with the implementation of organ motion into treatment planning. Soon after the Michigan study, MSKCC started patient treatment with a deep inhalation breath hold BSRT method in 1998 and a commercial gating system designed by Varian (RPM, Palo Alto, Calif.).[16-23] At about the same time, another method of BSRT was reported by a group from William Beaumont Hospital in Detroit. Their device, termed the *ABC system*, controls the patient breathing patterns by computer commands. At the time of publication,[14] ABC focused on controlling the patient's breathing and did not have automatic LINAC gating capability. However, the output of the ABC could be used to gate a LINAC. Since its first publication, clinical results of the ABC have been published.[2,15]

Yet another major advance in BRST came from Japan in 1999, where a group of radiation oncologists in Hokkaido University headed by Shirato reported use of a real-time tumor tracking method in radiation therapy.[24-27] They insert radiopaque markers in the target. Four sets of x-ray tubes and fluoroscopic imagers are located around the gantry of the treatment unit to capture the marker motion. The x-ray tubes were embedded under the treatment floor and the fluoroscopic units were mounted on the ceiling. While only two sets of tube-fluoro unit pairs are needed to identify markers embedded in the tumor, two more sets were added in case the target was obscured at certain angles by the gantry head or couch. Real-time tumor tracking is a new feature in gated radiotherapy and opens up a new era of gated radiotherapy. Their publications detail the merits of their system. Takai et al.[28] reported at the 2002 ASTRO meeting that target tracking can be complimented by the motion of multi-leaf collimator (MLC) leaves so that the field shape changes continuously to adequately cover the moving target. Before Takai's work, a more comprehensive investigation using laboratory equipment was published by Keall et al.[65] This method is yet to be tested in the clinic. However, both methods have an advantage in that the beam can be delivered continuously as long as the leaf motion does not get delayed. Since both methods involved an addition to the usual 3D domain, they are sometimes referred as *four-dimensional.*

Other notable developments have been reported during the past decade. For example, Accuray (Sunnyvale, Calif.) has developed the CyberKnife,[67,68] which is also capable of target tracking. CyberKnife is being tested clinically in North America and Japan. This device, which uses two sets of fluoroscopic imagers, was originally designed for the treatment of tumors rigidly located in the brain or spine but can also be used as a real-time tumor tracking system. At this point there is no published report of clinical use of this device as a tumor tracking and treatment system, but such publications are expected. Other publications on aspects of BSRT include Kutcher et al.,[69] Morrill et al.,[70] Sontag et al.,[71] Crawford et al.,[72,73] Jacobs et al.,[74] Killoran et al.,[75] and Ahmad et al.[76] National Institute of Radiological Sciences (NIRS) reported a gating system developed for their heavy-ion medical accelerator in Chiba (HIMAC).[77,78] Li and Xing attempted to incorporate the organ motion into inverse treatment planning,[79] and Medical College of Virginia has been investigating theoretical and experimental aspects of gated radiotherapy.[66,80,81] Many other reports on BSRT and gated radiotherapy have been published.[82-106]

BSRT methodology is rapidly combining three elements of accurate 3DCRT (i.e., patient positioning, BSRT, and IMRT) for treatment of tumors in the thorax. For IMRT, the first test of the technical compatibility of BSRT and IMRT was reported by Kubo for the Varian 2100C clinical accelerator.[1] There are, of course, many publications on patient setup accuracy. These studies are often focused on electronic portal imaging devices (EPIDs) and are somewhat isolated from BSRT and IMRT. Many of these studies have been pursued outside North America.[82-85] Since setup errors are beyond the scope of this section, this topic and IMRT are only briefly discussed except as they directly relate to BSRT.

In the remainder of this section, clinical and theoretical approaches to BSRT are presented together with the future outlook.

NONGATED SYSTEMS

Clinical Experience at Memorial Sloan-Kettering Cancer Center

Two methods of respiratory motion control have been clinically implemented at MSKCC: (1) DIBH and (2) automatic respiration gating using the Varian RPM system (Palo Alto, Calif.). In DIBH, both the patient and the therapist are active participants; the therapist, guided by spirometer output, trains the patient into a reproducible state of maximum inhalation and then turns the beam on. In automatic respiratory gating, the patient and the therapist are nominally passive participants; the patient breathes "normally" and the beam is electronically turned on only when the patient's respiration—as monitored by an external marker—is within a user-chosen range. MSKCC's DIBH experiences are summarized in the next section. Since the technical aspects of the RPM system are the same as those reported by Kubo et al.,[5] the clinical implementation of this method is discussed later in Video Camera and Respitrace-Based System.

Deep Inhalation Breath Hold

The DIBH technique was developed at MSKCC and implemented clinically in 1998.[16-18] Fig. 10-2 shows a typical patient setup. The patient breathes through a spirometer and is trained through a "modified slow vital capacity maneuver" consisting of a deep inhalation, deep exhalation, second deep inhalation, and breath hold. The trainer (typically by a therapist) is guided in this process by a computer display of the spirometer output, as shown

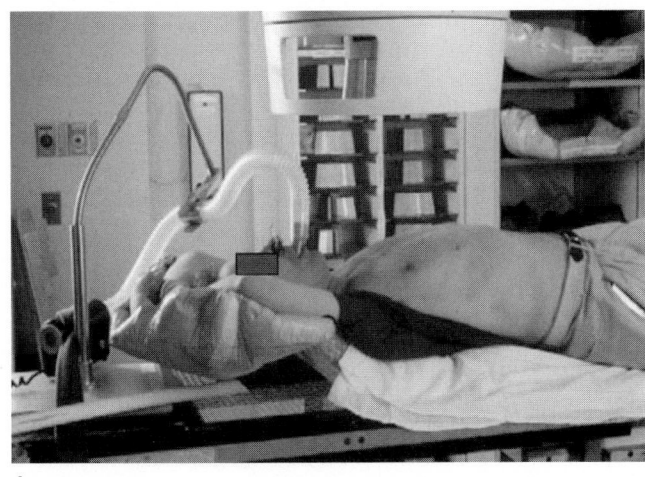

A

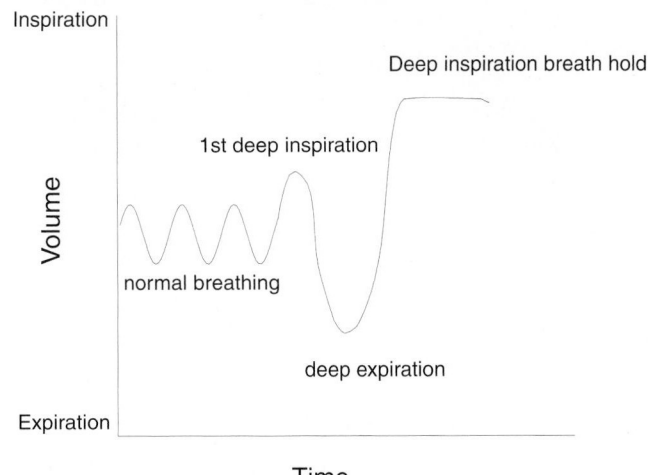

B

Figure 10–2. Patient setup for deep inhalation breath hold.

in the lower panel of Fig. 10-2. For patients who can comply with the training, this maneuver has been shown to result in a reproducible state of maximum inhalation that can be maintained for 10 to 20 seconds (patient-specific). The therapists are instructed to turn on the treatment beam only when the target breath-hold level has been achieved and to stop treatment if the level has fallen outside a preset tolerance. For static 3DCRT treatments at 2 Gy/fraction on LINACs operated at 500 to 600 MU/minute, a single breath hold is usually sufficient for each field. Because IMRT beams require a longer delivery time, DIBH is used mostly for static fields. For selected patients, MSKCC has started to use IMRT and DIBH. Simulation must also be performed with the patient performing DIBH. For this purpose, CT acquisition is broken up into 4 to 6 separate single-breath-hold segments. An additional normal breathing scan is acquired for reference and a scan at end-normal-inhalation is acquired to assess gross tumor volume (GTV) mobility and determine the deep-inhalation tolerance levels. Thus, simulation is longer than an ordinary, normal breathing simulation, particularly as the patient is encouraged to rest between acquisitions.

In a pilot study, fluoroscopy, simulator, and port films showing the position of the diaphragm relative to fixed vertebral anatomy were analyzed to assess the reproducibility achieved with DIBH.[16,18] Intrabreath hold reproducibility of 1.8 + 1.0 mm and interbreath hold reproducibility of 1.3 + 5.3 mm were found. In addition to the reproducible reduction of diaphragmatic (and presumably *f* tumor) motion, there is a large, patient-specific increase in lung volume. For some patients, lung volume approximately doubles in going from normal breathing to DIBH. This is a major benefit of the DIBH technique in the treatment of lung cancer. Normal lung tissue moves out of the treatment beams while the volume of the GTV remains largely unchanged, thus reducing the estimated risk of normal lung complications and allowing treatment to higher total doses,[16,23] even with the same margin (1 to 2 cm) of expansion from GTV to PTV for DIBH

as for normal breathing treatments. Larger gains would be realized if GTV to PTV expansion margins were reduced.[16] However, currently, MSKCC does not reduce margins for DIBH treatments. This decision is based on two considerations: The margins protect against a possible expansion of microscopic disease outward from the GTV under DIBH, and the decreased lung density exacerbates the potential for underdose due to electronic disequilibrium at edges of the PTV within lung.[23]

The applicability of DIBH is limited by patient compliance. Approximately 60% of lung cancer patients cannot perform the maneuver reproducibly enough to permit its use. It also calls for special therapist effort as therapists must be trained to advise the patients, and the treatment sessions usually take 5 to 10 minutes longer than a similar beam arrangement for a normal breathing patient. In addition to the usual weekly beam films, an anterior-posterior (AP) localization film showing the entire lung is taken at least weekly to confirm the constancy of lung inflation. Because DIBH is relatively demanding for patients, it is used only for compliant patients in whom the significant lung inflation allows treatment to a higher total dose than is possible with normal breathing.

Active Breathing Control System

Another approach to reduce the margin for breathing motion was reported by a group of physicists and radiation oncologists at William Beaumont Hospital headed by John Wong.[14] Unlike MSKCC's method of audio-controlled voluntary breathing and manually supervised breath hold, the Beaumont method controls the level of breath hold by a reproducible computer control called an *ABC system*. The length and level of breath hold can be preprogrammed depending on the comfort of the patient. The principle of their approach is the following: In the original publication, they used two air flow control valves: one to control intake flow and the other to control outflow as shown in Fig. 10-3. These valves can be

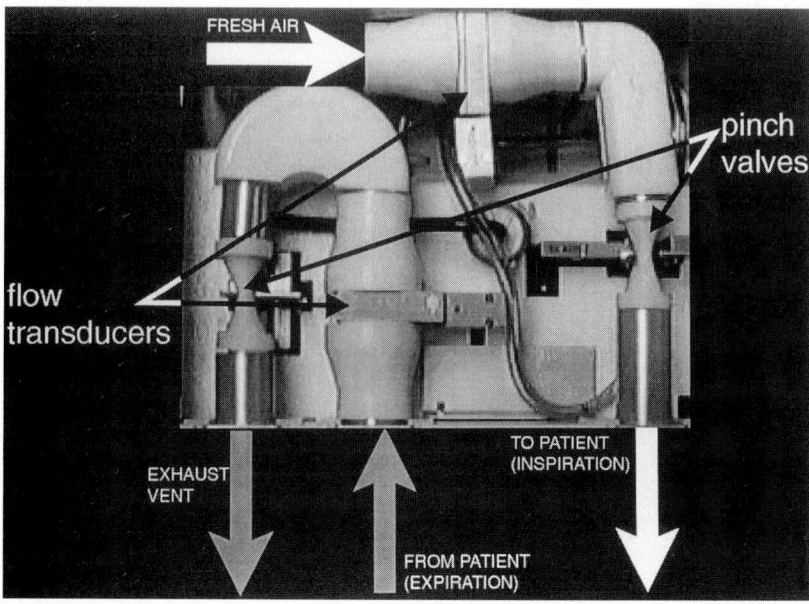

Figure 10–3. An active breath control system. (From Fig. 1, *Int J Radiat Oncol Biol Phys.* 1999;44:912.)

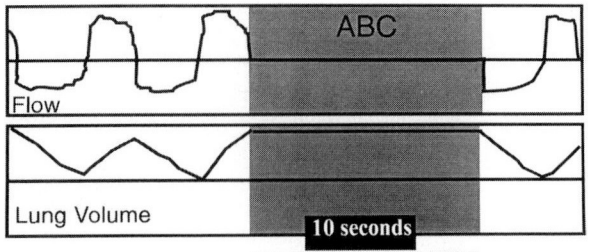

Figure 10–4. The flow and volume display extracted from the active breathing control system. (From Fig. 1, *Int J Radiat Oncol Biol Phys.* 1999;44:913.)

opened or closed by a computer command at a preset level of the total lung volume. In addition, ABC uses a mouthpiece and nose clip similar to the Memorial DIBH method. Fig. 10-4 shows when, where, and how long breathing was held using ABC. Due to computer control, both the level and length of breath hold are expected to be more reproducible per session (i.e., smaller intratreatment deviations) than with voluntary breathing systems. The operational procedure of this device is that at the beginning of a session, the patient's breathing is monitored continuously with ABC. When the airflow from and to the lung is matched at the preset level, the airflow is temporarily blocked, thus immobilizing breathing motion. As shown in Table 10-1,[14] the data are quite good: the reproducibility of the apex of diaphragm (intratreatment variation) is 2.6 + 2.0 mm during one session, a portion of which is attributed to patient positioning problems. The intertreatment reproducibility was reported to be 2.0 + 2.2 mm. They reported that some patients can hold their breath in excess of 40 seconds. Typically, the active breath hold duration was 15 to 20 seconds for lung cancer patients and at least 20 seconds for other patients. The CT spiral scan and LINAC treatment were done during this active breath hold by manually turning on and off the beam. The entire beam delivery for a typical 2 Gy/fraction at 4 Gy/minute can be completed within no more than two to three breath holds. For more than three fields, each field can be treated with one breath hold.

Clinical Results of Active Breathing Control

Using hepatic microcoils, the ABC device was extensively studied in the clinical setting for treatment of unresectable hepatic cancer by Dawson et al.[2] Patients were positioned supine in a customized immobilization cast. The patient's breathing was blocked by ABC for the planning CT scan and treatment as described.[14] During

Table 10–1   Average Excursion Between Edge Profiles of 2 ABC Scans

Region	*n* Data Points	Intra-fraction (mm)	Inter-fraction (mm)
Diaphragm	60	1.5 ± 1.8	4.0 ± 3.3
Mid-thorax	20	2.1 ± 1.7	3.9 ± 3.1
Apex	36	2.6 ± 2.0	2.0 ± 2.2

From Fig. 1, *Int. J. Radiol Oncol Biol Phys.* 1999;44:912

hepatic artery catheter placement, one to four radiopaque platinum embolization microcoils (5 mm × 0.5 mm) were deposited intra-arterially in the liver by an interventional radiologist. The breath hold trigger was adjusted to block the airflow at the end-exhalation of the breathing cycle. They reported that the original ABC was somewhat uncomfortable for some patients and speculated that this discomfort may lead to changes in liver position with repeat breath holds. Therefore, they acquired a more comfortable device, ABC2 (Vmax22LV, SensorMedics, Yorba Linda, Calif.). The major difference between the original ABC (ABC1) and ABC2 is the method of determining the trigger for breath holds. With ABC, the breath hold trigger was possible only after the breathing becomes reproducible. Each patient's parameters, including the position of the breath hold in the breathing cycle, the phase of the breathing, and the length of comfortable breath hold were determined in the same manner as described by other groups throughout this chapter. Eight of 13 patients were entered into an Institutional Review Board (IRB)-approved protocol (5 did not go on due mainly to preexisting diseases). The total time to deliver a daily fraction was approximately 25 to 30 minutes.

The results for the reproducibility and maximum excursion of diaphragm and hepatic microcoils relative to bony landmarks in the superior-inferior (SI) direction are summarized in Table 10-2.[2] For example, the maximum intra-treatment variations of microcoil excursion averaged over six of the eight protocol patients was 5.8 + 2.3 mm. The maximum diaphragm excursion averaged over eight patients was 5.5 + 2.5 mm. The corresponding intertreatment average maximum diaphragm excursions were 14.1 + 4.4 mm. There were no data for the average maximum microcoil excursions, but the standard deviation was noted to be 4.3 mm. The maximum normal breathing diaphragm excursion relative to bony landmarks was 14.3 mm ranging from the minimum of 12 mm to the maximum of 30 mm. The larger intertreatment standard deviation of diaphragm in comparison to intratreatment is indicative of the change of diaphragm position during breath hold between different treatment days. They noted that two patients showed a larger maximum excursion under the ABC control than under normal breathing. The intertreatment variability in the position of the liver relative to bony landmarks was large. Therefore, they concluded that without daily imaging of the liver, the ABC system does not substantially improve intertreatment variability, leading to no substantial reduction in PTV. They speculate that the observed poor intertreatment reproducibility in the SI direction is mostly due to physiologic change in breathing pattern over the relatively long course of radiotherapy. The authors suggest the need for target imaging immediately before or during the treatment, combined with repositioning of the patient in order to safely reduce the treatment margin. This issue is common to all static BSRT systems that have been developed up to now. The main reason for the necessity of extra imaging is that the static BSRT methods do not have instantaneous and continuous organ visualization capability. However, the dynamic tumor tracking systems discussed later in Merit of Reducing PTV by Gating use two or more sets of fluoroscopic imagers for

Table 10–2 Reproducibility (Standard Deviation [σ]) and Maximal Excursion of Diaphragm and Hepatic Microcoils Relative to Skeleton in CC Direction for Each Patient and Free Breathing CC Diaphragm Excursions Relative to the Skeleton

| | Intra-fraction (mm) | | | | Inter-fraction (mm) | | | Free breathing (mm) |
| | Coils | | Diaphragm | | Coils | Diaphragm | | |
Patient	σ	Maximal excursion	σ	Maximal excursion	σ	σ	Maximal excursion	Maximal excursion
1	3.7	4.8	3.2	5.6	5.1	5.1	9.8	10.0
2	1.5	3.5	1.8	2.3	5.7	3.5	9.4	10.0
3	2.4	6.5	2.5	7.9	4.5	4.0	9.3	10.0
4	1.2	6.1	2.0	5.9	3.1	4.4	11.1	12.0
5	1.9	3.8	2.0	3.7	3.1	3.0	14.7	30.0
6*	3.3	9.8	2.5	6.5	3.7†	3.8	25.9	12.0
7			3.0	2.8		5.4	10.4	15.0
8			3.7	9.3		6.1	21.9	15.0
Average	2.3	5.8	2.5	5.5	4.3	4.4	14.1	14.3

*This patient had a substantial change in the shape of the liver after the 2-week break in radiation treatment. One microcoil was placed in the anterior inferior tip of the liver.
†This is the average σ (from σ before 2-week break and σ after 2-week break), because there was a substantial change in liver shape after the break in radiation.
From *Int J Radiat Oncol Biol Phys.* 2001;51:1410.

visualization and tracking of the tumor or of implanted markers.

Another factor that compromises intertreatment reproducibility is the residual volume of air in the lung, on which ABC's breath hold level is added. If the residual volume of air varies day by day, intertreatment uncertainty increases accordingly. Similar types of uncertainty are common to all static BSRT systems, including a video camera–based system discussed in the next section. This fact, in combination with patient positioning uncertainty, contributes to larger intertreatment variations. The intertreatment variation can be reduced by adjusting the target location at breath-hold either by fluoroscopic or EPID images. The use of diagnostic quality images that can be obtained from the gantry-mounted fluoroscopic imagers for both patient positioning and accurate determination of organ motion is an approach of current interest, though the cost of such devices cannot be ignored.

VIDEO CAMERA– AND RESPITRACE-BASED SYSTEM

The very first gated radiotherapy system developed at the Tsukuba Proton Therapy Facility used a combination of air bag and strain gauge as an indirect organ motion detector.[3,4] However, their system, and the RPM system developed jointly between the University of California Davis Cancer Center (UCDCC) and Varian are similar in principle.[5,6] Currently, UCDCC uses their own plethysmographic system, where the Respitrace by NIMS (North Bay Village, Fla.) was used instead of a video camera .[5-11,13] These three systems, as well as a video camera–based system developed at the heavy-ion medical accelerator in Chiba (HIMAC),[77,78] are described together here. Two minor differences among the UCDCC system, the two Japanese systems, and the RPM system are: The UCDCC system (1) takes full advantage of breath hold by audio command, thereby increasing the beam duty cycle; and

(2) integrates a time-sequence gating method or audio-gated radiation treatment (ART) to further reduce the organ motion. The second item is discussed further in the following section.

At Tsukuba University Hospital, a combination of air bag and strain gauge taped on the patient trunk produced the electrical signal caused by the piezoelectric effect.[3,4] The piezoelectricity produced by the strain gauge in response to breathing motion corresponds to internal organ motion. Whenever the strain gauge signal falls between the preset levels of a gating window, an electronic circuit produces a pulse corresponding to the duration of the signal within the gate window. This pulse is used to trigger a treatment machine to control beam on and off conditions. To assess the validity and performance of their gating system, they calculated dose volume histograms (DVHs) with and without gating. For example, for treatment of a 50.9 cc liver cancer with a minimum dose of 80 Gy, the normal tissue volume irradiated to over 60, 40, and 20 Gy without gating are approximately 41, 83, and 119 cc, respectively. The corresponding volumes with gating were 4.7, 11, and 19 cc, demonstrating substantial reduction of the irradiated normal tissue when gating was used. It is remarkable to note that they even discussed the possibility of gating by beam or collimator scans in coincidence with respiratory organ motion. They further discussed moving the patient couch in synchrony with organ motion as an alternative gating method. Unfortunately, the proton machine is used mainly for high-energy physics research and is not flexible for daily radiation therapy treatment. However, this is the first reported implementation of gated radiation therapy.

At the National Institute of Radiological Sciences (NIRS), a video camera detects the position of infrared light emitted from a light source placed on the patient's upper torso.[77,78] The location of the light source is correlated with the patient's breathing and corresponds indirectly to internal organ motion. In this position-sensitive detector, or PSD, system, the vertical motion of the light

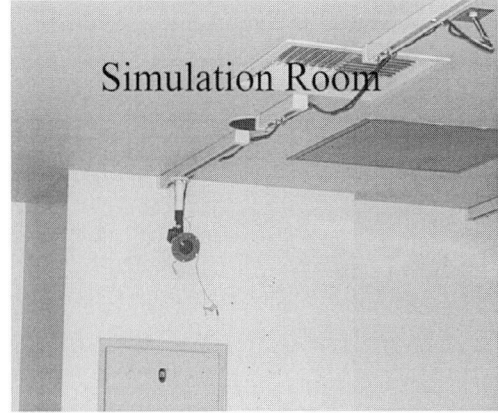
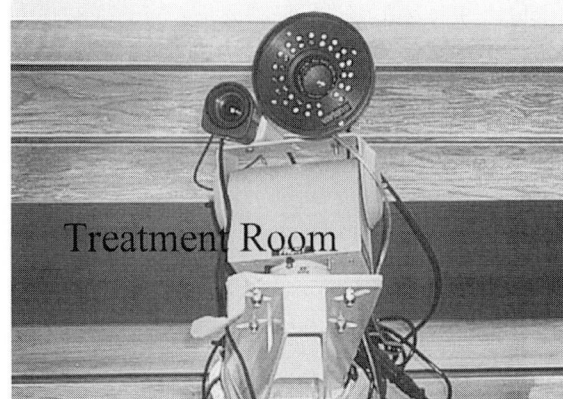
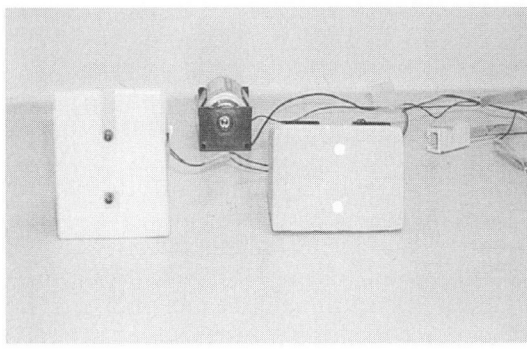
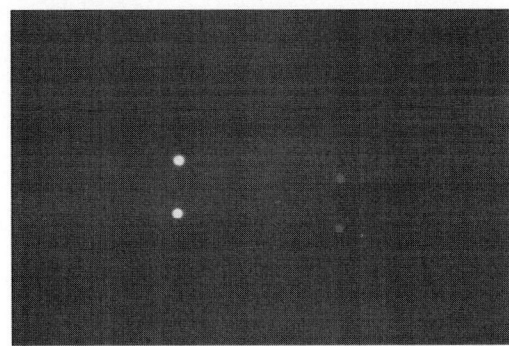

Figure 10–5. A video camera looking down at the patient in a treatment room. A calibration block with two reflective markers on the computer screen is shown.

source is converted to digital signals just as in the case of the strain gauge signal. When the video signal falls between the preset levels of the gate window, an electronic circuit produces a pulse whose length corresponds to the duration of the signal within the gate window. The gate pulse was used to trigger the HIMAC beam on and off.

At the University of California, Davis Cancer Center (UCDCC), Kubo et al.[5,6] developed a video camera–based BSRT system, which works basically the same way as the two systems at NIRS and Tsukuba. Two notable differences are (1) the UCDCC system emits the light from the circular array of infrared light sources surrounding the video camera as shown in Fig. 10-5. This light is reflected by a two-marker block placed on the patient's upper torso (e.g., the upper trunk inferior to the rib). The two markers on the marker block are separated by 30 + 0.2 mm. When the video camera starts capturing the vertical motion of the block, the system calibrates the size of the motion with respect to the 3 cm separation, allowing the subsequent marker block motion amplitude to be determined absolutely. For the past 3 years, Kubo et al. have perfected the use of Respitrace, which is strapped around the trunk as seen in Fig. 10-6. The breathing signal is created by the expansion and shrinkage of the area covered by the strap. This method, plethysmography, is commonly used in the critical pulmonary and pediatric ward to monitor patient breathing. The principle is the same as the video camera method except that the breathing signal is generated by plethysmograph. One advantage of this method is that the system stabilizes quickly for data taking while the radiation therapist is

setting up the patient in the treatment position. Another minor advantage is that the entire system can be easily transported from one place to another when a laptop computer is used (Fig. 10-7). Contrary to plethysmography, the video camera system is based on an image grabber and requires a desktop computer. Additionally, the video camera itself is either mounted on a tripod and carted around, or several cameras must be purchased to

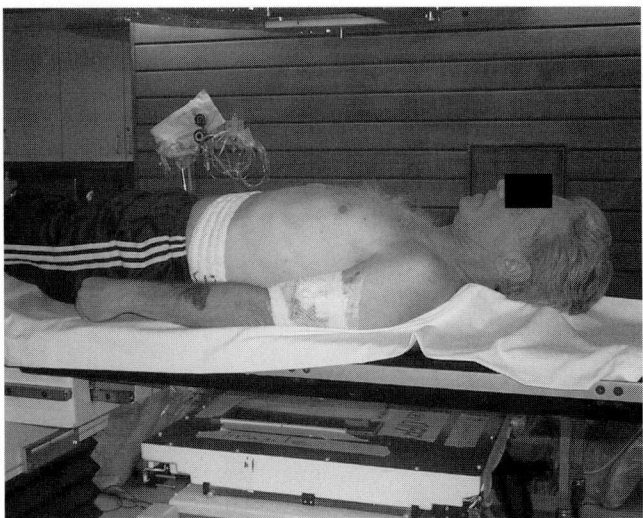

Figure 10–6. A patient in the treatment position. A Respiband is wrapped around the patient. Below the treatment couch, a beta-test silicon electronic portal imaging device is shown.

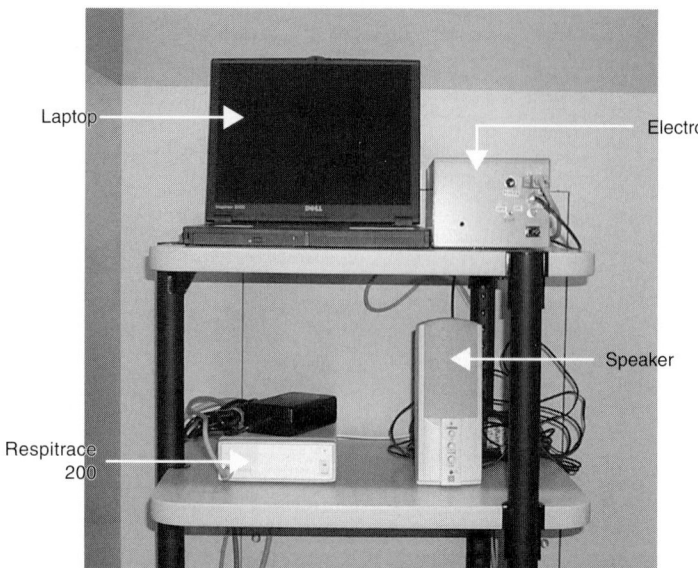

Figure 10–7. The University of California, Davis Cancer Center plethysmography system. A VCR used for fluoroscopic image capture is not shown.

mount one on the wall in each procedure room (e.g., the training room, fluoroscopic examination room, CT room, and each treatment room).

At both Japanese institutions, the patient was instructed to breathe normally and the gate window was set at the exhalation phase of the breathing cycle. When gating is activated during normal breathing, irradiation occurs only during part of each breath and the resulting lower duty cycle prolongs the treatment time. Occasionally, the amplitude of the breathing signal decreases as the patient becomes comfortable. This is particularly noticeable on a system where both the duty cycle and the beam intensity are low. It is difficult to achieve both a high beam-on duty cycle and smaller organ motion during normal breathing since the two factors are incompatible. To alleviate some of these problems, UCDCC has taken a different approach. UCDCC implemented audio instruction including breath hold in the system so that the beam duty cycle can be increased. In addition, the audio instruction keeps the patient alert.

Clinical Implementation of Automatic Respiratory Gating at MSKCC

In late 1999, MSKCC initiated clinical studies of automatic respiratory gating using the Real-time Position Management (RPM) system (Varian Medical Systems, Palo Alto, Calif.), which is based on the UCDCC camera-based system described earlier. The camera and infrared illumination source are mounted on a wall in the conventional simulator, in the treatment rooms, and at the foot of the couch at the CT simulator. If the RPM system is used with "normal" breathing (versus breath hold), regular and reproducible breathing is important for efficient, accurate gated simulation and treatment since the beam-enable or CT trigger signal is not issued with irregular breathing. Several publications[1,21] report negligible dosimetric effects of gated operation for both static and sliding window IMRT fields. Nonetheless, it is recommended that users independently commission their own

RPM (or similar) system. Currently, MSKCC has used the RPM system for gated static and IMRT treatments of more than 30 lung cancer and liver cancer patients.[20] RPM is well tolerated by patients and technical staff. However, clinical implementation of this form of BSRT requires considerable care and patient-specific quality assurance. This is because the RPM system—like all gating systems based on signals generated outside the tumor—makes two assumptions. First, there is assumed to be a one-to-one correspondence between the external signal (the motion of the markers on the patient's chest) and the patient's internal anatomy (tumor and critical normal tissues). Second, it is assumed that this relationship, once determined at simulation, is maintained over the entire course of treatment. While studying the validity of these assumptions, we also adopt measures to keep the breathing motion as reproducible as possible from session to session, verify this with frequent portal imaging of internal anatomy, and make field adjustments as necessary.

Simulation—Conventional and Computed Tomography

Traditionally, simulation establishes the treatment position, immobilizes the patient to maintain it, and acquires reference and planning images. For RPM-gating simulations, the breathing period and amplitude (as indicated by the marker-motion trace) are also determined and the gating portion of the breathing cycle—the range of amplitudes or phases for planning image acquisition and treatment—is chosen. Because the marker-motion trace recorded during simulation is the reference session for the treatments (analogous to simulator films or Digitally Reconstructed Radiographs [DRRs]), MSKCC takes steps at simulation to assure regular and reproducible breathing.

Fig. 10-8 shows a typical motion trace display for a patient treated at end-expiration. The gating thresholds are indicated by horizontal lines. Respiration-triggered CT slice acquisition starts each time the motion trace

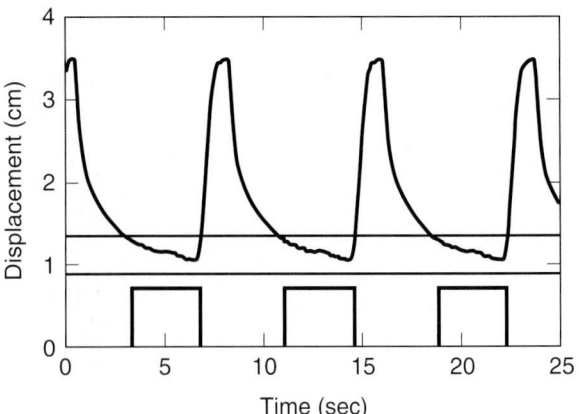

Figure 10–8. Simulated breathing signal and voltage gate window. The resulting pulse shown below will enable the accelerator intensity-modulated radiation therapy beam delivery. (From *Med Phys.* 2000;27:1734, Figure 2.)

enters the gate. The choice of gating thresholds is a compromise between large respiratory motion (large duty cycle) and long treatment (small duty cycle). The time for single slice acquisition affects the range of motion included in the planning images and is also a consideration in threshold choice (and possibly patient selection). For example, if it takes 1 second to acquire a CT slice and the breathing period is 3 seconds, setting the RPM duty cycle lower than 33% guarantees out-of-gate contribution to the image.

Irregular marker motion compromises the efficiency of CT acquisition and treatment. Worse, it can cause image acquisition or beam delivery, or both, at the wrong phase of the breathing cycle. To reduce breathing irregularity, many institutions usually set the gating thresholds around end-expiration (which is more stable and provides a longer duty cycle per marker displacement). Also, simple verbal coaching instructions ("breathe in … breathe out"), customized to the patient's breathing pattern, have been shown to improve regularity[5,9,22] and are used for the majority of BSRT patients. In a combined immobilization and training session at a conventional RPM-outfitted simulator, customized recorded audio instructions are used so that the patient can follow them comfortably. Fluoroscopic movies including the diaphragm, isocenter, and, if it is visible, the tumor, help with gate-width determination and later troubleshooting. The marker block corners are tattooed for reproducible repositioning.

The same audio instructions are played during the planning CT scan and treatments. Even with regular breathing, respiration-triggered image acquisition (which is done in axial mode) takes slightly longer than with normal breathing because only part of the breathing cycle is used. For example, if the breathing period is 5 seconds, acquiring a 60-slice study at the rate of one CT image per breathing cycle (e.g., only at end-expiration) on a single slice scanner requires 5 minutes under ideal conditions of regular breathing—compared to 1 minute for helical, normal-breathing acquisition at 1 slice/second. Despite the vocal coaching, it is not uncommon for some irregular breathing to occur at CT simulation, causing out-of-phase slices and motion artifacts. A physicist operates the

RPM system during CT simulation and records the "bad slices," which can be deleted if desired or reacquired when regular breathing resumes. MSKCC does a repeat respiration-triggered scan (same gate) to assess GTV and organ position reproducibility within the simulation session and help in deciding adequate margins.

The session at the conventional simulator includes an RPM system test, immobilization, isocenter selection, audio instruction customization and training, fluoroscopic movies, gated radiographs, and patient marking. The CT simulation includes system test, two respiratory-triggered CT scans and final patient tattooing. The combined sessions take approximately 2 hours (a nongated immobilization/CT simulation session is approximately 1 hour).

Treatment and Patient-Specific Quality Assurance

Although the RPM system turns on the linac beam only when the marker motion is within the gate, this does not necessarily prevent beam delivery at the wrong phase of the breathing cycle. Well-trained therapists are a vital component of RPM-gated treatments. They must watch the displayed motion trace and turn the beam off if they see serious irregularity or drift, then re-track the marker or talk to the patient before proceeding, or both. The RPM display shows the trace amplitude achieved at the CT simulation and the therapists encourage the patient to maintain this amplitude. They report patient compliance problems to a designated physicist. Recently, visual feedback to the patient has been implemented and its benefits in improving breathing amplitude consistency are being evaluated.

Studies of fluoroscopic movies of the first eight patients treated with RPM at MSKCC[19] indicate that gated treatment is capable of reducing the patient-averaged standard deviation of the diaphragm position (i.e., intrafractional motion) from 6.9 + 2.1 mm (no gate) to 2.6 + 1.7 mm (gated). AP portal images (at least weekly) of these patients showed a mean deviation of the diaphragm position relative to bony anatomy (i.e., interfractional variation) of 2.8 + 1.0 mm. However, for four of the eight patients, the diaphragm position on port films showed a systematic shift of more than 4 mm relative to its position on the DRR constructed from the planning CT simulation.

Studies of subsequent patients confirm the initial findings that systematic differences between the diaphragm position at simulation and at treatment occur for a significant fraction of patients. Currently MSKCC takes three diaphragm films during each of the first 2 weeks of treatment. If no systematic differences are observed, they reduce the frequency (biweekly, then weekly). For systematic errors over 4 to 5 mm, the clinician decides whether to adjust the fields. To date, they have made field adjustments for 5 of 30 patients. Techniques for convenient visualization of tumor location through the course of treatment or deciding whether the diaphragm is as acceptable a surrogate for lung tumor position as for liver[2] would be a helpful adjunct to RPM gating—or any form of gating based on an external marker. Benefits of gating in improving uncomplicated tumor control remain to be explored.

BSRT AT UNIVERSITY OF CALIFORNIA, DAVIS CANCER CENTER

Kubo and Wang[1] tested the compatibility of Varian 2100C gated operations with EDW and IMRT dose delivery to determine whether the dose distribution was changed when a gating signal controlled the EDW or IMRT dose delivery. They exposed films to dose delivery by IMRT leaf sequencing under five conditions: (1) a static film; (2) a film moving parallel to the leaf motion with no gating; (3) a film moving parallel to the leaf motion with gating; (4) a film moving perpendicular to the leaf motion with no gating; and (5) same as (4) except with gating. Fig. 10-8 shows the simulated breathing signal and the gate pulse generated by the voltage gating window, which is set by the two horizontal lines. The total breathing signal was 24 mm high and the gate was applied at 9.4% of total breathing signal, thus the total excursion of breathing signal during the gating was approximately 2.3 mm. A breathing cycle was approximately 7.5 seconds. Using these parameters, films were exposed for the five cases mentioned earlier. The resulting film scans are shown in Figs. 10-9 and 10-10. Fig. 10-9 shows the results of film motion parallel to the motion of the leaves, and Fig. 10-10 the results for perpendicular film motion. Figs. 10-9*A* (10-10*A*), 10-9*B* (10-10*B*), and 10-9*C* (10-10*C*) are the images of static film, film motion without gating, and film motion with gating, respectively. As expected, the intensity in Fig. 10-9*B* is expanded in the left and right directions and that in Fig 10-10*B* is expanded in the up and down direction. However, when Figs. 10-9*A* and 10-9*C*, and 10-10*A* and 10-10*C* are compared, the differences between them become almost unnoticeable. It is, therefore, concluded that gating does not interfere with the IMRT dose distribution, except that the images can be blurred depending on the amount of motion permitted within the width of the gate window. It was also found that BSRT does not interfere with the EDW dose distribution.

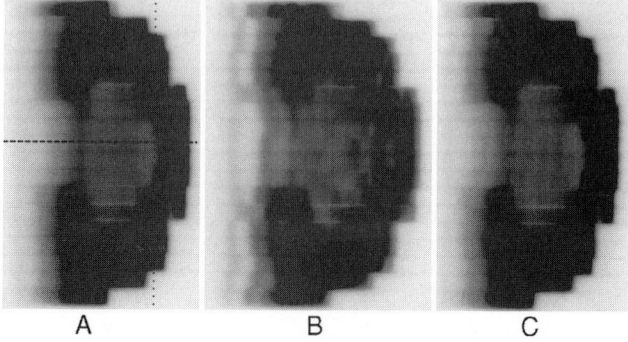

Figure 10–9. A combination of breathing synchronized radiotherapy and intensity-modulated radiation therapy. **A,** Stationary image. **B,** Images obtained according to the breathing signal shown in Fig. 10-8 with a film moving parallel to the leaf direction. **C,** The result of gating on the film moving in the same manner as Figure 10-9**B**. (From Kubo HD, Wang L: Compatibility of varian 2100C gated operations with enhanced dynamic wedge and IMRT dose delivery. *Med Phys.* 2000;27:1736.)

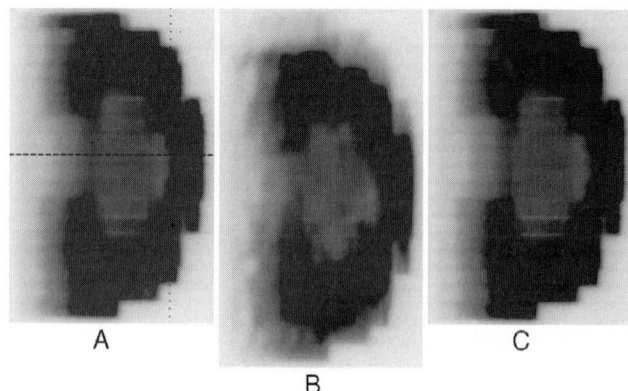

Figure 10–10. Same as Figure 10-9 except that the film moves perpendicular to the motion of the leaves. (From Kubo HD, Wang L: Compatibility of varian 2100C gated operations with enhanced dynamic wedge and IMRT dose delivery. *Med Phys.* 2000;27:1736.)

UCDCC AUDIO-GATED RADIOTHERAPY SYSTEM

One common feature of the existing breath monitoring systems, except for the tumor tracking system,[24-28,66] is that the breathing-induced signal is displayed on the vertical axis of a monitor screen, whereas the elapsed time is on the horizontal axis. Therefore, the voltage gate window is selected by two horizontal levels indicated by, for example, dotted lines (*A*) in Fig. 10-11. Whenever the breathing signal falls between these two levels, the voltage gate pulses A_i (i = 1, 5) are produced. Assuming that the voltage gate window is set near the end-exhalation, it cannot remove sharp rises and falls seen near the end of exhalation or the beginning of inhalation. The fluoroscopic examinations show that the diaphragm moves rapidly, corresponding to these sharp rises and falls, and that they should be avoided in gated radiotherapy. This can be contrasted to the flat regions achieved by audio-gating shown by *B* (i.e., time-sequence gate pulse). In addition, there may be a delay between the actual organ motion and the corresponding breathing signal,[9,13,78] which contributes to the organ motion uncertainty. By adjusting the beginning of the audio gate trigger level, one can avoid the phase difference of 0.25 seconds between the breathing signal and the actual organ motion. Also, even if the instruction says " … hold breath," the breathing signal does not normally drop to the steady reproducible signal level immediately simply because there is patient lag time in response to the instruction. Therefore, the beginning of the audio gate window is set at the level where the breathing signal becomes steady. By the same token, when the patient hears the beginning of the next "breathe in …," the patient does not react to the instruction immediately. Therefore, the end gate window in audio-instructed breath hold is typically set at the time of the next cycle.

The audio (or time-sequence) gate is designed to avoid such regions of sharp rises and falls by selecting an appropriate gate window *B* in the time domain of breath-hold phase of the breathing cycle. The essence of this new gating mechanism is based on the observation that the patient follows a reproducible, repetitive breathing instruction as described earlier. During the breath hold,

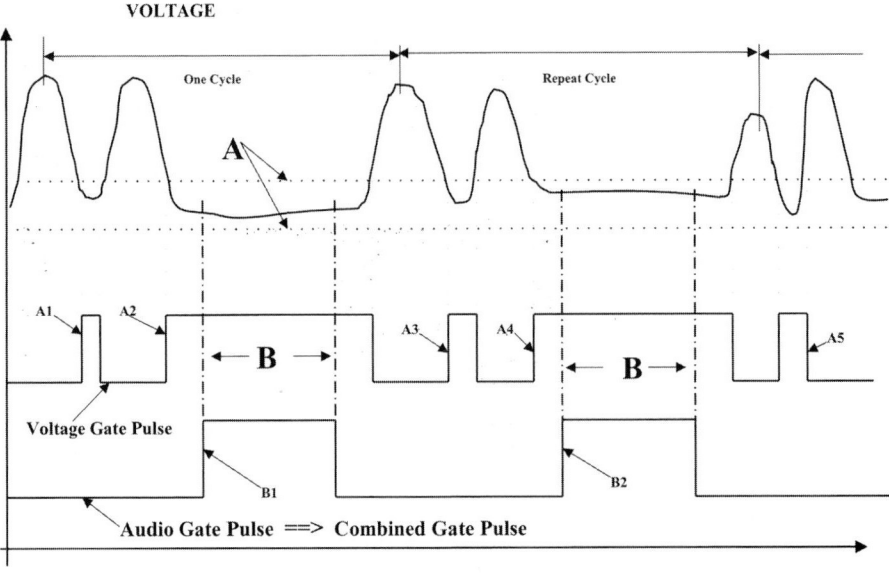

Figure 10–11. Audio gating diagram. The patient's breathing response to audio instruction is depicted on the top. The diagram in the middle shows the resulting beam enable pulse by voltage gate alone. The bottom diagram shows results of a combination of voltage and audio gate. The audio gate can easily allow the operator to adjust the beginning and end of the gate to take care of time delay between the breathing signal and actual organ motion. (From *Med Phys*. 2002;29:346, Figure 1.)

very little organ motion is reported.[5,6,9,13] The gate window *B* is set during the training session. Except for occasional minor changes, the same gate window is maintained throughout the procedures including CT scan, fluoroscopic examinations, and treatment. A Boolean AND between the voltage gate A_i (i = 1, 2, ... n) and audio gate pulses B_j (j = 1, 2, ... m) will result in the final gate pulses, which happen to be identical to B_j (j = 1, 2, ... m) in this example. This section describes some advantages that can be realized by a combination of voltage- and audio-gating.

The top half of the screen in Fig. 10-12 shows a typical view of the breathing signal and the AND gate (or beam enable) pulses. The figure shows the entire sequence of events (i.e., from time t = 0 to 50 seconds) the

patient is breathing normally. At approximately t = 46 seconds, the audio instruction is initiated by the operator. At the same time, the audio gate pulse is generated and is combined with voltage gate to generate an AND gate pulse, enabling the beam delivery. The actual beam will not be delivered until t = 100 seconds, as seen at the bottom of Fig. 10-12. Blue and orange horizontal lines in the top half of the screen are the voltage gate levels finalized at t = 65 seconds. When the breathing signal falls between these two lines, the software controller requests a beam. It should be noted that in this example, there is no difference between the beam enable pulse and audio gate pulse.

The instructed breathing signal reflects the reaction of the patient to the audio instruction. For example,

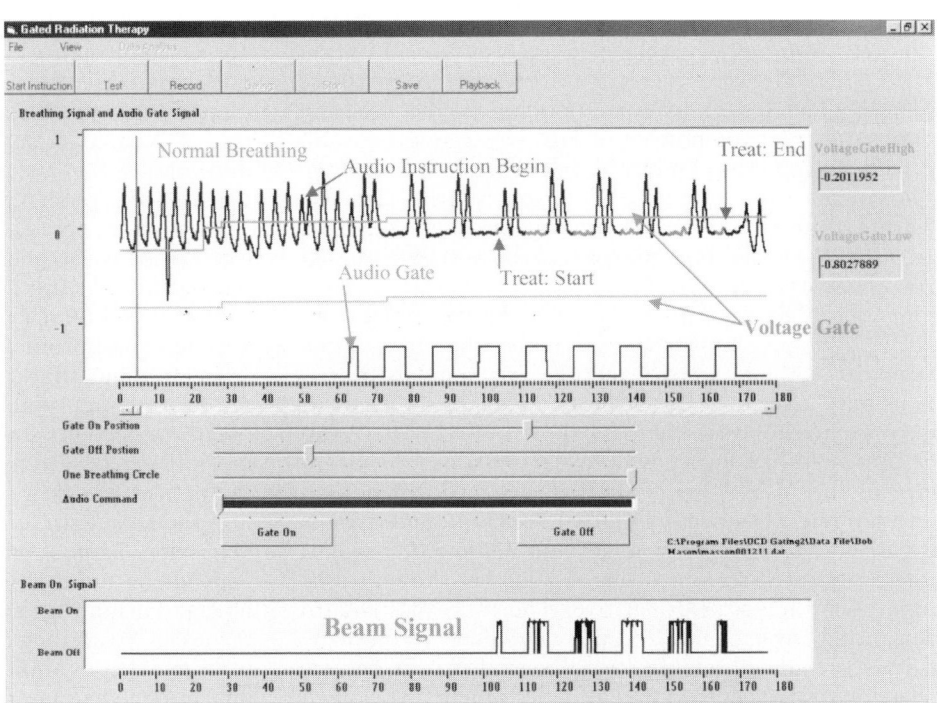

Figure 10–12. A computer screen of the University of California, Davis Cancer Center plethysmograph. The red regions indicate where the beam is delivered and correspond to the beam-on signal shown at the bottom.

"breathe in, breathe out, breathe in, breathe out and hold (for 5 seconds)" is one cycle, and is approximately 13 seconds long as seen in Fig. 10-12. After several 13-second intervals, the ART system operator observes that the patient has reached a steady breathing pattern. The operator will determine if the audio gate window needs modifications from those obtained earlier. If so, the operator will move the "Gate On" and "Gate Off" sliders to the appropriate points to change gate-on and -off times. Since the instruction is repeated, the subsequent gate window and the duration of breath hold are automatically repeated. The numeric voltage gate window levels at the point indicated by a green vertical line (time indicator) are shown to the right of the screen.

Included in the ART system is a simple method to capture the actual beam-on signal from the Varian machine (Palo Alto, Calif.) since such information is currently lacking. With our new system the beam-on signal is simultaneously collected with the breathing signal.[9] The usefulness of the beam-on signal can be explained as follows: One needs to know exactly when the beam was delivered (beam-on signal in red at the bottom of Fig. 10-12), not when the accelerator was enabled by the gate pulse, so that one can perform retrospective statistical analysis of organ motion during normal breathing and gated breathing periods. The breathing signal shown in Fig. 10-12 is a typical pattern obtained from many physically fit patients. With these patients, the therapists may manually interrupt the beam temporarily during the course of treatment or the beam may be withheld because the breathing signal is outside the gate window setting. Therefore, knowing exactly when the beam is delivered becomes valuable information for data analysis. The ART system can easily switch from one breathing pattern to another by selecting the appropriate breathing instruction files. At any rate, patient selection is important in BSRT, in particular, the system that uses breath hold.

Results of the average value of breathing signal data and one standard deviation are displayed in the "Data Analysis" window when the data analysis request button is pushed. The average voltage of breathing signal over the red painted regions corresponding to the beam-on signal shown at the bottom of Fig. 10-12 and one standard deviation is automatically calculated. Also the average voltage over any selected region and its standard deviation can be calculated by the operator. For example, the average normal breathing signal size is 0.098 + 0.085 volts, whereas it is −0.018 + 0.006 volts during beam-on (or gating). The standard deviation of breathing variations during gating is almost 14 times smaller than that during normal breathing. Knowledge of these standard deviations may become useful when one compares intertreatment organ motions. The data shown in Fig. 10-12 can be presented in another way to demonstrate the advantage of the ART system. The first 10 cycles of normal breathing signal shown in Fig. 10-12 are reproduced to the left of Fig. 10-13. The voltage- and audio-gated signals (the red painted regions in Fig. 10-12) are shown to the right. The time scale is relative. The ratio of standard deviation between gated and nongated depends on many factors, including breathing signal reproducibility and the selection of gate levels. One difficulty of gated treatment

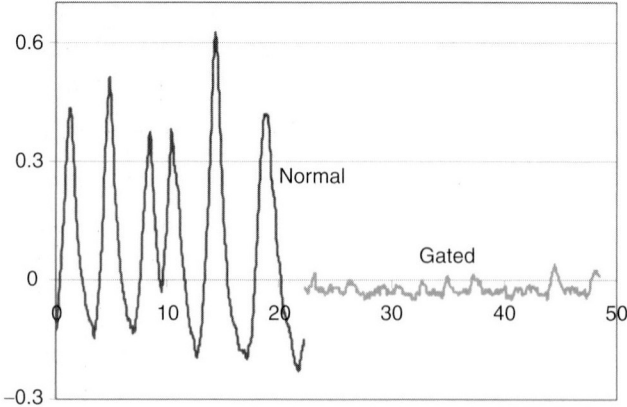

Figure 10–13. The first 10 cycles of normal breathing signal and breathing signal during gating. The results are taken from Figure 10-12.

may be that one has to set the limits as to when to stop gating or beam delivery when the breathing signal starts drifting more than expected.

Simulation to Treatment Process

The typical breath hold is set at approximately 5 seconds. By creating different instructions, it is possible to make the breath hold longer or shorter and to hold breath at any point in a breathing cycle. Since in our case the breath hold is immediately after end-exhalation, the breath hold duration is intentionally made short compared to the published values of more than 20 seconds[2,14,19,78] so as to compensate the lack of oxygen. When an appropriate candidate for the gated radiotherapy is referred, the patient is taken for a breathing training session before fluoroscopic examination begins. During this session, length of breath hold, levels of gate window, and speed of instruction are adjusted for the patient's comfort. This session will take 20 to 30 minutes. Since the breath hold occurs immediately after the exhalation phase of the breathing cycle, the patient tends to want the air immediately after the breath hold. This tends to make the patient breathe harder than normal. For this reason, one important verbal instruction before and during the training is to keep reminding the patient to breathe in and out as normally as possible. The repeat of "breathe in, breathe out" twice is designed to give the patient a chance to recover from breath hold. When the level of breath hold is reproduced for at least 10 times, the patient is enrolled in the internal protocol and is sent to simulation.

In the simulation room, the patient will listen to his or her specific audio instruction. After the instructed breathing becomes stable, the AP and lateral fluoroscopic images are recorded for three to four breath holds. Unless the patient has clear landmarks that move with breathing, the actual size of the organ motion is very hard to determine. Some results indicate that organ motion size depends on the location of the organ. For example, the lung and diaphragm motion is quite visible during breathing cycles. According to our limited studies of the motion of brachytherapy dummy markers in the lung[11] and the images of a stent inserted into the lower esophagus,[13] the maximum dummy markers and stent motions are on the order of 1.5 to 3 cm. From the same brachytherapy dummy markers, it is found that the upper lung motion is rather small. The lower lung motion, diaphragm motion, and upper gastro-intestinal motion including the lower esophagus motion are almost equal in size. As expected, as the distance from the diaphragm to moving organ increases, the organ motion amplitude decreases. It is to be noted that the fluoroscopic images are first collected without gate, so that one can establish the correlation between the signal size and the size of the organ motion during normal breathing. This size can be compared to the organ motion during the breath hold. This approach is also applied before the treatment. An advantage of the breath hold gating is that the beam duty cycle increases to almost 50%[2,5,6,13] from a typical 25%[22,26] reported for normal breathing gating.

It is important to note that organ motion is not linear and is complex.[2,11,14] In general, the SI motion is larger than the AP motions. The lateral organ motion seems to be the smallest. The fluoroscopic images stored at the rate of 10 to 30 frames per second are replayed off-line to determine the amplitude of the diaphragm motions in three orthogonal directions. Typical SI and AP motion sizes are shown in Table 10-3. In the same table, the intratreatment variations of the diaphragm during three to four breath holds are shown. This variation includes image analysis uncertainty due partly to the poor resolution of the fluoroscopic images collected under the automatic brightness control. The system uncertainty can be reduced to 2 mm if the image collection conditions are optimized.

Computed Tomography Scan

A CT scanner can be gated in the same manner as a LINAC so that the scan proceeds only when the gate pulse is present. One major difference between the CT gating and LINAC gating is the camera position. In the case of a LINAC, the camera and reflector are kept in the same geometrical configuration throughout the session. The same configuration can be achieved for a CT scan if the camera is mounted on the couch. This is a not an issue with plethysmography, since it does not depend on the geometry. Needless to say, the ABC system does not depend on the geometry either. One example of CT scan images taken during the audio-instructed breathing is shown in Fig. 10-14. The scan was obtained only when the breathing signal fell between the preset gate windows. In this particular case, the CT scanner was manually turned on during the 5 second breath hold and off otherwise. This process was repeated until the desired length

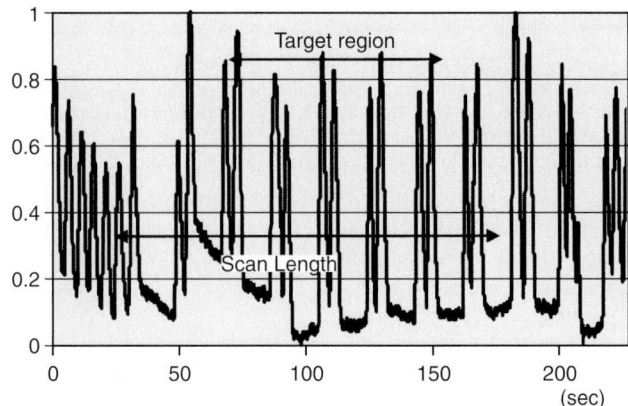

Figure 10–14. The breathing signal during a CT scan.

of anatomy was completely scanned (i.e., approximately $t = 55$ seconds to 190 seconds for a whole scan and $t = 95$ seconds to 160 seconds for a target). From this figure, one can say that the target scan is completed after 4 to 6 breath holds. The slightly larger variations of breathing signal for the first few breath holds are due to the anxiety this particular patient exhibited. The rest of the scans were obtained relatively smoothly.

CASE PRESENTATION

Patient

A 57-year-old male with a T2N0M0, moderately differentiated GE junction adenocarcinoma. The patient was treated with concurrent chemotherapy, Taxol/Carboplatin, and radiation followed by surgical resection. His radiation prescription was to give 45 Gy parallel opposed at 1.8 Gy per fraction to the distal esophagus. He was treated with 18 MV x-ray beams using MLC-shaped fields. The jaw size was 10.7 cm × 14 cm (width × length). The total MUs per beam were 98. The treatment beam was gated by ART during the instructed breath hold breathing. The lack of diaphragm motion was detected by a silicon electronic (si)-EPID for AP images only.

Fluoroscopic Image Analysis

By examining the images of this patient frame by frame, the location of the diaphragm was identified and traced. It is found that there is a one-to-one correspondence between the apex location and the location of audio-gated breath hold signal in such a way that the breath hold position can predict the location of the diaphragm within 2 mm.

Table 10–3   Standard Deviations of Distance Measurements*

	Positioning (A)	Positioning (B)	Positioning Plus Breath Hold (C)	Breath Hold (D)
Intratreatment	Less than 1	Less than 1	Less than 3	Less than 3
Intertreatment	3.6	4.5	4.9	1.5

*Units are mm.

PORTAL IMAGE ANALYSIS

Amorphous Silicon Electronic Portal Imaging Device

The si-EPID used in this work was a beta-test prototype developed by Varian (Palo Alto, Calif.). Its effective area of image capture was approximately 26 cm × 26 cm.[6] Since the sensitive region of the detector was placed approximately 130 cm from the source, the maximum image object size was limited to 20 cm × 20 cm at the isocenter. For each treatment session, two to five analyzable images were obtained.

With ART, the portal images are taken when the beam is on. The detector can bring up one image every 5 seconds or so. Therefore, it is possible to obtain one decent image during one breath hold. Treatment of 1.8 to 2 Gy per fraction, at say 400 MU/minute, requires approximately five breath holds. The purpose of using the si-EPID is to ensure that intratreatment variation is kept small. Comparison of breathing signal with the portal images during the treatment will give a good clue as to the effectiveness of the breath hold. Unfortunately, the actual organ motion size during treatment is not measurable due to the slow image capture rate of our prototype si-EPID. However, as discussed later in Fluoroscopic Image Analysis, a point in the breathing cycle corresponds to the diaphragm location within 2 mm, so that the exact measurement of diaphragm location may not be needed once it is established. The two-dimensional AP images are sensitive to the SI and lateral setup errors. They are not sensitive to AP/PA setup errors. Since the imager could not be used from the lateral direction, no discussion was made on the accuracy of AP/PA setup errors. The organ motion in this section is limited in the SI direction.

Fig. 10-15 shows a typical portal image. Note that three types of measurements are presented in this figure. A and B represent the distances between the bony markers and field edges. Their variations indicate the accuracy of patient positioning. The variation of distance D between the apex of diaphragm and bony markers indicates the accuracy of the breath hold. The third one is the distance C between the apex of the diaphragm and the field edge. This information provides the combined uncertainty of patient positioning and the breath hold. These distances are measured on the EPID portal images taken during each session and over the entire course of treatment.

Image Analysis

The average distance and the standard deviation (STD) of the mean were obtained from daily images (or intra-treatment analysis) as well as the images from an entire course of treatment (intertreatment analysis). Altogether, 50 images were used for this distance analysis. Table 10-3 illustrates the results of the analysis. Distance D has the smallest intertreatment STD of 1.5 mm, followed by A of 3.6 mm. Since D depends only on breath hold accuracy, the standard deviation of breath hold accuracy throughout the analyzable treatment period is approximately 1.5 mm. Distance C has the largest STD of 4.9 mm with

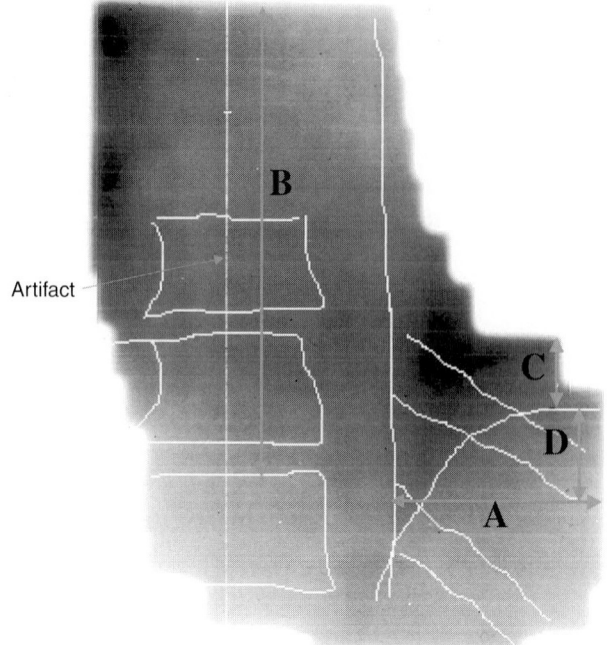

Figure 10–15. A portal image. **A** and **B,** Distances between the field edge and bone structure. **C,** Distance between the field edge and the apex of diaphragm. **D,** Distance between the bony marker and the apex of diaphragm.

B being 4.5 mm. For 11 daily intratreatment STDs, A and B are less than 1 mm and the smallest, whereas C and D are comparable to each other and are less than 3 mm. Since the patient is presumably stationary throughout each treatment day, any intratreatment STD should depend only on breath hold accuracy. Therefore, the positioning independent intratreatment STDs of A, B, and C are expected to be smaller than the positioning dependent intertreatment STDs of A, B, and C. Since D does not depend on positioning, its results are expected to be the same between intra- and intertreatment STD. Due to breath hold uncertainty, the intratreatment STDs of C and D are expected to be slightly larger than those of A and B. When the breath hold and setup errors are added as with C, the combined intertreatment STD becomes the largest among all four distances. A much larger intertreatment STD of C (combination of position and breath hold accuracy) than that of D (a breath hold accuracy) shows the dominance of setup errors with this patient. This table shows that the patient's daily setup uncertainty is the main contributing factor to the larger intertreatment STDs.

The intertreatment variation certainly includes the contributions from the uncertainty of the residual lung volume even though the exhalation phase of breathing cycle is reproducible, and from the poor image quality that renders image analysis more difficult. Again, if the imaging device has a higher resolution such as fluoroscopic images, the distance and its variations can be more accurately determined. Improvement in high-energy portal imagers or the application of diagnostic x-ray units in conjunction with the high-energy photon beam treatment is highly desirable.

ART with breath hold technique proves to be useful because (1) the instruction will keep the patient alert and (2) using approximately a 5-second breath hold, the beam duty cycle is increased from the reported non–breath hold technique of 20% to 30% to almost 50%. The actual number of breath holds needed to deliver a daily fraction is typically 5. It takes approximately an additional five breath holds to get the patient ready and obtain some preliminary results. It has been found that good communication and coordination among the radiation therapists, physicist, and patient are crucial for successful implementation of gated radiotherapy. Daily ART treatment needs no more than a conventional 15-minute time slot. In addition, any phase delay between the organ motion and the breathing signal can be easily incorporated into the audio gate window (e.g., delaying a beam delivery by 0.5 seconds) with a minor reduction in the beam duty cycle. Contrary to breath hold, the beam duty cycle in the normal breathing treatment will be further reduced if the gate window is narrowed by 0.5 seconds to accommodate the phase delay.

One difficult issue is how to delineate the target organ and the surrounding tissues on fluoroscopic images, since they tend to be transparent to x-rays. Even CT images are not always good enough to distinguish between the target and the surrounding tissue. Sometimes one becomes fortunate in that the esophagus can be seen during barium swallow, or lung nodules can be seen due to tissue density differences. The same can be said about the liver. But in general these organs may need to be identified by implanted markers or x-ray opaque landmarks. Otherwise, the whole concept of 3DCRT, including gated radiotherapy and IMRT, may fail due in part to poor organ visualization.

CLINICAL CONSIDERATIONS

Even though a typical daily treatment can be completed in five or so breath holds at mid-range dose rates, the patient usually undergoes nearly a dozen breath hold cycles before the treatment is completed. Each fraction can be longer for various reasons such as a longer patient treatment setup, non-stable treatment beam, unintentional beam holds, or any problems associated with lower performance status. Under these circumstances, some patients have difficulty in maintaining reproducible breath hold. For these patients, some distress toward the end of the course of treatment should be anticipated in deciding how to handle the problem. It may be wise to implement a shorter breath hold toward the final fractions. If the breathing signal before beam delivery shows somewhat erratic behavior, it may come to a point where one has to make a decision as to relax the gate window intentionally to complete the daily session or postpone the treatment 1 day. The patient's medical status needs to be taken into account for any precision radiotherapy including BSRT and IMRT. The ART system allows us to easily modify the breathing patterns to the patient's needs, though most of the UCDCC patients felt comfortable with the standard breath hold breathing instruction.

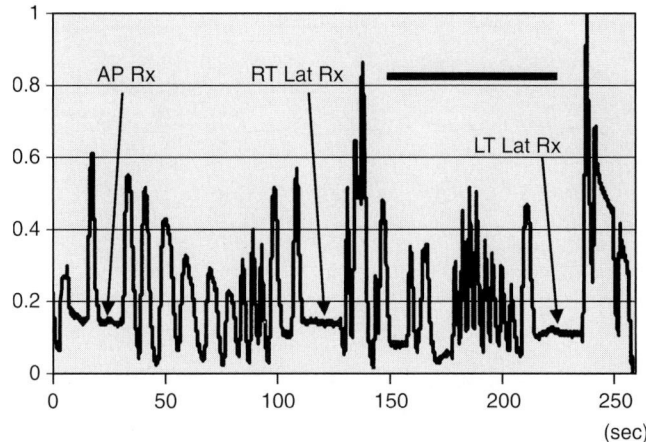

Figure 10–16. An entire course of breathing signal on one treatment day. Anterior-posterior, right lateral, and left lateral treatment are indicated. This patient was able to hold his breath reproducibly for 20 seconds or more at the inhalation phase of the breathing cycle. Each field is treated within one breath hold. The breathing instruction was given verbally when the treatment was ready.

For those slightly erratic breathing behaviors, one needs to carefully study each patient independently, hoping to come to some consensus as to how to give BSRT to each patient. To deal with these problems, BSRT may require stricter protocol eligibility criteria. The criteria not only include the breath hold parameter determination but also estimates of the merit of BSRT in reducing GTV, clinical target volume (CTV), or PTV before the patient is put on the gated treatment. However, some patients can hold their breath long enough to finish one field, as seen in Fig. 10-16.

TUMOR TRACKING RADIATION THERAPY

Gated radiation therapy took a new turn when the motion of a marker embedded in the target was tracked by four fluoroscopic units.[24-27] When the marker is located within the boundaries of acceptable tolerance, the LINAC is gated and the beam is directed to the target. The acceptable tolerance is the parameter that dictates how tightly one wants to surround the target with the radiation field. This value ranged from 1.0 mm to 9.0 mm and was determined during treatment planning. The major factors that influence this parameter are the radiosensitivity of nearby organs, the distance of critical organs from the radiation field, the volume of the normal tissue within the field, and the prescribed dose. The patient, who has been implanted with a 2 mm diameter gold marker, is positioned on the treatment couch using a laser-tattoo three-point method. The insertion of the gold markers is performed under spinal anesthesia with pelvic diseases and local anesthesia with disease in other locations.

Shirato and the group at Hokkaido University were the first team to use the tracking method in gated radiation therapy. This method is a major deviation from earlier systems in two respects: (1) this system fully uses fluoroscopic imagers for the marker visualization and (2) the system can be quite expensive compared to all

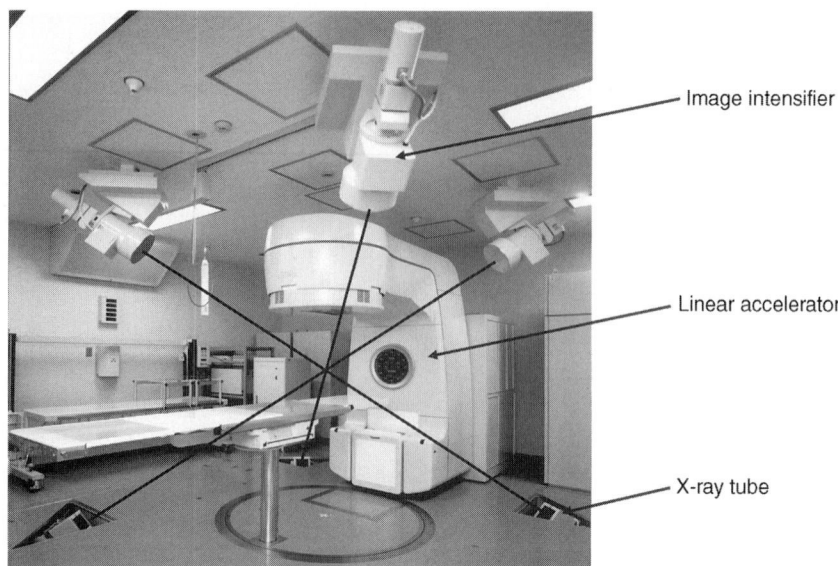

Image intensifier

Linear accelerator

X-ray tube

Figure 10–17. A tumor tracking system developed by Shirato et al. at the Hokkaido University Hospital. Four pairs of fluoroscopic imagers are integrated into the linear accelerator gating system. 1. A current commercial model presumably produces almost one image display per second. 2. The conventional gross tumor volume (GTV), as defined by ICRU 50,[111] is independent of motion, though it may depend on other diagnostic images or biopsy information not directly seen on the computed tomography scan. The same is true of the clinical target volume—it's only the planning target volume that incorporates information about motion. To avoid confusion, the motion-influenced GTV is termed a GTV$_{eff}$. (From *Int J Radiat Oncol Biol Phys.* 2000;48:436, Figure 1.)

other earlier systems. It is an exciting new approach and other similar methods are expected to follow soon. At Hokkaido University (Fig. 10-17), four x-ray tubes are mounted under the floor and the corresponding fluoroscopic imagers are mounted on the ceiling. The central axis of an x-ray tube and the corresponding fluoroscopic imager intersect with the isocenter of the LINAC. The distance between the image intensifier and the isocenter is 280 cm and the distance between the x-ray tube and the isocenter is 180 cm. Because of these rather large distances, x-ray tubes with high heat ratings are used. Theoretically, only two x-ray tube-imager pairs are needed to locate the coordinates of a target marker. However, these pairs are permanently fixed. Therefore, at certain gantry angles, one or two x-ray tubes may be blocked by the gantry. To circumvent such problems, they use four x-ray image-intensifier combinations. The LINAC is turned on and the diagnostic imager is turned off whenever the gold marker falls within the predetermined allowed dislocation or vice versa. This on-off mechanism reduces the background noise in the image intensifier created by the scattered radiation from the LINAC. This tracking method is based on normal patient breathing. The organ motion is characterized by calculating each target marker coordinate continuously using the target image information from at least two pairs of x-ray tube-image intensifiers. The target markers are displayed on the monitor screen and the region of acceptable tolerance is digitized and circumscribed on the screen. The patient couch top is made of carbon fiber reinforced plastic and is transparent to diagnostic x-rays. They reported no complications in 14 patients they enrolled in this protocol. The beam duty cycle was approximately 26% to 57% for lung and liver tumors. For a study of principle, another set of test measurements were made with a static phantom to characterize the system accuracy. The localization accuracy of the target marker was better than 1.5 mm. Both systematic and random errors in positioning the target caused by setup errors and organ motion uncertainty are corrected by observing the fluoroscopic images on the monitor screens. With their tumor tracking system, they were able

to reduce the marker motion from 9.6 to 38.4 mm to 2.5 to 5.3 mm.[26] The chief disadvantage they observed for this system is the invasive procedure needed for insertion of the gold marker. Despite this disadvantage, they state that the gain of gated radiotherapy can be visualized from the precision required in the treatment. In 2000 there was a report by Chung, who indicated an approach to track the motion of a gold marker implanted in the target.[106] This idea was expanded upon by the Tohoku University Hospital in Japan.[28] There, two x-ray tubes are mounted on the side of a LINAC gantry head and are separated by 90 degrees. A corresponding pair of amorphous si-EPID fluoroscopic imagers are mounted on the gantry. The x-ray tubes and EPIDs are rigidly mounted on arms extended from gantry in a cross-fire configuration, intersecting the LINAC's isocenter. The images are digitized by diagnostic quality EPIDs. The Elekta[107] LINAC and Varian's new LINAC have one diagnostic x-ray tube and a si-EPID for better visualization of anatomy. These units can easily accommodate on-site cone-beam CT scan capability. In summary, the fluoroscopic real-time tumor tracking system has a potential of improving the accuracy of treatment for moving tumors by reducing the tumor margin.

The use of a tracking system for a CyberKnife has been reported.[66,108] This system is somewhat similar to that of the Hokkaido University Hospital. The CyberKnife treats with a 6 MV x-ray beam from an accelerator mounted on a robotic arm. For the image-guided radiotherapy, they use two pairs of diagnostic x-ray tubes mounted on the ceiling and the corresponding fluoroscopic imagers mounted on the floor. The cross hairs of these pairs intersect with the beam axis. The latest report[109] at the ASTRO meeting in 2002 indicated a treatment time of 2 to 8 hours per patient. As the CyberKnife becomes familiar to physicists and clinicians, the treatment time is expected to decrease. The principle of this system is to predict target location after several cycles of breathing patterns. The computer-controlled robotic arm will, then, move to the next position almost continuously. Since the beam can be directed to the target continuously during treatment, the beam duty cycle can be as high as 100%. The largest beam-shaping circular collimator is reported to be 5 cm. Any target larger than 5 cm in any direction needs to use a multi-collimator configuration.

The most exciting image-guided radiotherapy system was reported at the ASTRO meeting in 2002 by Tohoku University Hospital in collaboration with Varian. As predicted in the 1992 paper[4] by the Tsukuba University Hospital and in the 2000 presentation by Ulsan University Hospital in Korea,[106] Tohoku University Hospital perfected the tracking of a marker in the target by the dynamic MLC sequences. That is, the moving target is tracked by fluoroscopic images, which in turn dictate the MLC motion. One major advantage of this method is that the beam duty cycle is theoretically 100% unlike any other tracking method. There may be some limitations in that the MLC shape changes may not be fast enough to accommodate ideal field shapes in high-dose-rate modes. One will need to slow down the beam delivery rate. At any rate this method can be used for any breathing patterns except sudden changes caused by, for example, coughing. Needless to say, this problem is universal for all BSRT systems and not limited to the tracking systems. In a few years, this type of system will be perfected and perhaps may become prevalent if the costs become reasonable.

For all the tracking systems, one may have to consider how the CT scan is incorporated into the treatment planning and how IMRT can be incorporated into the beam delivery. Despite some concerns, these systems are expected to raise the level of 3DCRT to the next level.

MERIT OF REDUCING PLANNING TARGET VOLUME BY GATING

PTVs defined for gated and ungated treatment can be used to calculate dose distributions, which are then put into normal tissue complication probability and tumor control probability calculations for control and study groups, respectively. Even though these calculations are associated with large uncertainties, they can be useful to gauge the merit of gated radiotherapy over conventional treatment. The differences in tumor control probability and normal tissue complication probability between the gated and ungated groups will provide a guideline as to whether or not the gating is worth pursuing for a particular patient. For example, with the ART method, the prerecorded audio instructions are used to CT scan the patient in a breath hold mode at the same setup position as in the training and fluoroscopic examinations. Then, the radiation oncologist will define the target and surrounding organs in 3D. The information obtained from fluoroscopic exams (i.e., the organ motion variations [1σ standard deviations] during breath hold) are added to generate an effective GTV. Understanding that the conventional GTV_{eff} is defined as (stationary GTV + 1σ of motion, S0), the PTV can be defined as a sum of the GTV_{eff} plus margins (S0) for microscopic disease (CTV), and the patient setup uncertainties (S1). In short, a total linear dimension that needs to be added to the conventional GTV_{eff} (BH = breath-hold) is (S0 + S1). The sum in

the bracket is the total margin for gated radiotherapy for the study group. The PTV for the normal breathing (or control) group can be expressed as a sum of GTV_{eff} = the stationary GTV(BH) + normal breathing organ variation ($\Sigma 0$). The total margin for the normal breathing PTV is the sum of the conventional GTV(BH) plus the linear dimension of (S0 + S1). The only difference between the control and study groups is the size of organ motion variation due to normal breathing. It should be noted that one needs to do a CT scan only once during the breath hold, assuming that the clinical target margin S0 is 5 mm and the patient's positioning accuracy S1 is 5 mm, which, in reality, depends on the anatomic site, patient size, and beam direction. The positional accuracy should be improved by the use of diagnostic quality x-ray imagers. The beam penumbra S2 is, say, 5 mm at both high- and low-photon energies. These values are the same between normal breathing and breath hold. Let's assume that the organ variation during breath hold is 2 mm and the normal breathing organ variation is $\Sigma 0 = 20$ mm. If the diameter of the GTV target is 50 mm, the breath hold PTV and normal breathing PTV are the volumes of a diameter 67 mm and 85 mm, respectively, or 157 and 322 cc.

SUMMARY

Two types of breathing synchronized radiation therapy systems are currently under investigation. The first type includes static systems that are derived from the system developed by the Tsukuba University Medical Center.[3,4] These systems are relatively low cost, user friendly, and simple. They include the Varian RPM system, the UCDCC TV camera or a RespiTrace system, or both, and the position-sensitive detector system at the National Institute of Radiological Sciences (NIRS) in Chiba. Though automatic gating was not used, the ABC system and the DIBH method also belong to this group. Many other systems can also be traced to the Tsukuba University Medical Center system.

The second type is represented by the tumor tracking system, which was developed at Hokkaido University Hospital[24-27] and is currently only available there. But it is not hard to imagine that similar systems will go into clinical use soon. The tracking system is rather complex and expensive. It is also dynamic in that the treatment beam is delivered only when the marker is within the "acceptable tolerance." The acceptable tolerance can be made larger toward noncritical organs and tightened near the critical organs. A further refined tracking system by the Tohoku University Hospital is indeed exciting.[28] Similar systems include the robot-controlled LINAC and the dynamic following of target with MLC.

The accuracy of the static group depends mainly on (1) the reproducibility of the lung residual volume and (2) the reproducibility of patient positioning. Some systems in this group use fluoroscopic imaging just before or during treatment. Therefore, patient positioning errors can be substantially reduced. It is likely that fluoroscopic units will soon be mounted on the treatment machine or placed in the room. Therefore, the remedy for large patient positioning inaccuracy will easily be reduced by using bony landmarks or implanted radiopaque markers. Yet the lung day-to-day residual volume variations can be substantial as reported by Dawson et al.[2] Unfortunately, there are not enough data to assess all these systems. However, the dynamic system represented by the tracking system comes with fluoroscopy as an integral part of the gating process. Therefore, patient positioning error can be substantially reduced since the target marker will clearly be visualized on the monitor. By appropriate delineation of the acceptable tolerance, one can dynamically adjust the accuracy of the tumor treatment.

3DCRT is facing yet another watershed. At this point IMRT is used even at small community hospitals. As more institutions introduce IMRT, the process of IMRT including treatment planning and quality assurance is becoming streamlined and easier to implement. However, for moving targets, the conformality of IMRT dose distributions may work against the intent of the treatment, because current IMRT planning assumes a static anatomy. To avoid potential problems related to moving organs, BSRT must be incorporated with IMRT. This problem is discussed by Kubo et al.[1] Another problem of precision treatment is the lack of patient positioning accuracy. There is a long list of publications whereby the on-line EPIDs have been used both in North America and Europe. Some improvements have been reported, in particular, by the introduction of an amorphous silicon flat panel detector. However, at this time, the image quality of conventional EPIDs including si-EPID is still not quite adequate to delineate relative target organs. Even if the metallic marker is used, the conventional EPID's uncertainty is substantially larger than that of the diagnostic images. In addition, the development of the marker tracking software for EPID may be difficult due to (1) inferior image quality in comparison to the fluoroscopic images and (2) a slow refresh rate on the monitor screen.

Future BSRT development may have to include accurate tumor and normal tissue delineation in combination with IMRT treatment planning and a higher beam duty cycle. It is an exciting time to be in radiation oncology when so many new diagnostic tools such as PET scans, CT/PET image fusion, and CT/MRI fusion are readily available. Ten years ago, many of these opportunities were unimaginable. Against tightening budgets and increasing medical costs, one must carefully analyze which area of radiation oncology is meritorious and which is not. By solving the concerns of each element, one wishes to come up with a winning combination.

REFERENCES

1. Kubo HD, Wang L: Compatibility of Varian 2100C gated operations on enhanced dynamic wedge and IMRT dose delivery. *Med Physics*. 2000;27:1732.
2. Dawson LA, Brock KK, Kazanjian S, et al: The reproducibility of organ position using active breathing control (ABC) during liver radiotherapy. *Int J Radiat Oncol Biol Phys*. 2001;51:1410.
3. Ohara K, Okumura T, Akisada A, et al: Irradiation synchronized with respiration gate. *Int J Radiat Oncol Biol Phys*. 1989;17:853.
4. Inada T, Tsuji H, Hayakawa Y, et al: Proton irradiation synchronized with respiratory cycle. *Nippon Acta Radiol*. 1992;52:1161 (in Japanese).
5. Kubo HD, Len P, Minohara S, Mostafavi H: Breathing-synchronized radiotherapy program at the University of California Davis Cancer Center. *Med Phys*. 2000;27:346.
6. Kubo HD, Shapiro EG, Seppi EJ: Characteristics and role of a prototype amorphous silicon array electronic portal imaging device in breathing gated radiation treatment. *Med Phys*. 1999;26:2410.
7. Kubo HD, Wang L: New breathing gating mechanism and its potential clinical advantages. *Med Phys*. 2001;28,1285.
8. Kubo HD, Wang L: Preliminary results of organ motion during instructed breath-hold in gated radiotherapy. *Med Phys*. 2001; 28:1219.
9. Kubo HD, Wang L: Introduction of audio gating to further reduce organ motion in breathing synchronized radiotherapy. *Med Phys*. 2002;29:345.
10. Kubo HD, Len PM, Wang L, et al: Clinical experience of breathing synchronized radiotherapy procedure at the University of California Davis Cancer Center. *Int J Radiat Oncol Biol Phys*. 1999;45:204.
11. Kubo HD, Hill BC: Use of brachytherapy dummy seeds for measurement of lung motion caused by respiration. *Med Phys*. 1995; 22:905.
12. Kubo D, Hill BC: Respiration gated radiotherapy treatment: A technical study. *Phys Med Biol*. 1996;41:83.
13. Kubo HD: Breathing signal as reference standard in monitoring organ motion in breath-hold gated radiotherapy. (In preparation)
14. Wong JW, Sharpe MB, Jaffray DA, et al: The use of active breathing control (ABC) to reduce margin for breathing motion. *Int J Radiat Oncol Biol Phys*. 1999;44:911.
15. Stromberg S, Sharpe MB, Kim LH, et al: Active breathing control (ABC) for Hodgkin's disease: Reduction in normal tissue irradiation with deep inspiration and implications for treatment (in process citation). *Int J Radiat Oncol Biol Phys*. 2000;48:797.
16. Hanley J, Debois MM, Mah D, et al: Deep inspiration breath-hold technique for lung tumors: The potential value of target immobilization and reduced lung density in dose escalation. *Int J Radiat Oncol Biol Phys*. 1999;45:603.
17. Rosenzweig KE, Hanley J, Mah D, et al: The deep inspiration breath-hold technique in the treatment of inoperable non-small-cell lung cancer. *Int J Radiat Oncol Biol Phys*. 2000;48:81.
18. Mah D, Hanley J, Rosenzweig K, et al: Technical aspects of the deep inspiration breath-hold technique in the treatment of thoracic cancer. *Int J Radiat Oncol Biol Phys*. 2000;48:1175.
19. Ford EC, Mageras GS, Yorke E, et al: Evaluation of respiratory movement during gated radiotherapy using film and electronic portal imaging. *Int J Radiat Oncol Biol Phys*. 2002;52:522.
20. Wagman R, Yorke E, Giraud P, et al: Reproducibility of organ position with respiratory gating for liver tumors: Use in dose-escalation. *Int J Radiat Oncol Biol Phys*. 2003;55:659.
21. Yorke E, Mageras G, LoSasso T, et al: Respiratory gating of sliding window IMRT, CD-ROM. Proceedings of the World Congress on Medical Physics and Biomedical Engineering, July 23-28, 2000.
22. Mageras GS, Yorke E, Rosenzweig KE, et al: Fluoroscopic evaluation of diaphragmatic motion reduction with a respiratory gated radiotherapy system. *J Appl Clin Med Phys*. 2001;2:191.
23. ED Yorke, Wang L, Rosenzweig KE, et al: Evaluation of deep inspiration breath-hold lung treatment plans with Monte Carlo dose calculation. *Int J Radiat Oncol Biol Phys*. 2002;53:1058.
24. Shirato H, Shimizu S, Shimizu T, et al: Real-time tumor tracking radiotherapy. *Lancet*. 1999;353:1331.
25. Shimizu S, Shirato H, Aoyama H, et al: High-speed magnetic resonance imaging for four-dimensional treatment planning of conformal radiotherapy of moving body tumors. *Int J Radiat Oncol Biol Phys*. 2000;48:471.
26. Shirato H, Shimizu S, Kitamura K, et al: Four-dimensional treatment planning and fluoroscopic real-time tumor tracking radiotherapy for moving tumor. *Int J Radiat Oncol Biol Phys*. 2000;48:435.
27. Shirato H, Shimizu T, Kunieda K, et al: Physical aspects of real-time tumor-tracking system for gated radiotherapy (in process citation). *Int J Radiat Oncol Biol Phys*. 2000;48:1187.
28. Takai Y, Mitsuya M, Nemoto K, et al: Development of real-time tumor tracking system with cMLC with dual x-ray fluoroscopy and amorphous silicon flat panel on the gantry of linear accelerator. *Int J Radiat Oncol Biol Phys*. 2002;54S:193.
29. Henkelman RM, Mah K: How important is breathing in radiation therapy of the thorax? *Int J Oncol Biol Phys*. 1982;8:2005.

30. Kuhns LR, Thornbury J, Seigel R: Variation of position of the kidneys and diaphragm in patients undergoing repeated suspension of respiration. *J Comput Assist Tomogr.* 1979;3:620.

31. Jones KR: A respiration monitor for use with CT body scanning and other imaging techniques. *Br J Radiol.* 1982;55:530.

32. Morehouse CC, Brody WR, Guthaner DF, et al: Gated cardiac computed tomography with a motion phantom. Radiology. 1980; 134:213.

33. Kivasaara L, Makela P, Aarimaa M: Pancreatic mobility: An important factor in pancreatic computed tomography. *J Comput Assist Tomogr.* 1982;6:854.

34. Moore SC, Judy PF, Garnic JD, et al: Prospectively gated cardiac computed tomography. *Med Phys.* 1983;10:846.

35. Suramo L, Paivansal M, Myllyla V: Cranio-caudal movements of the liver, pancreas and kidneys during respiration. *Acta Radiol Diagn.* 1984;25:129.

36. Moore SC, Judy PF: Cardiac computed tomography using redundant-ray prospective gating. *Med Phys.* 1987;14:193.

37. Mayo R, Muller NL, Henkelman RM: The double-fissure sign: A motion artifact on thin-section CT scans. *Radiology.* 1987;165:580.

38. Frohlich H, Dohring W: A simple device for breath-level monitoring during CT. *Radiology.* 1985;156:235.

39. Tarver RD, Conces DJ, Godwin JD: Motion artifacts on CT simulate bronchiectasis. *Am J Roentgenol.* 1988;151:1117.

40. Amoore JN, Ridgway JP: A system for cardiac and respiratory gating of a magnetic resonance imager. *Clin Phys Physiol Meas.* 1989;10:283.

41. Runge M, Clanton JA, Partain CL: Respiratory gating in magnetic resonance imaging at 0.5 Telsa. *Radiology.* 1984;151:521.

42. Ehman RL, McNamara MT, Pallack M, et al: Magnetic resonance imaging with respiratory gating: Techniques and Advantages. *Am J Roentgenol.* 1984;143:1175.

43. Bryan PJ, Custar S, Haaga JR, Balsara V: Respiratory movement of the pancreas: An ultrasonic study. *J Ultrasound Med.* 1984;3:317.

44. Ross CS, Hussey DH, Pennington EC, et al: Analysis of movement of intrathoracic neoplasms using ultrafast computerized tomography. *Int J Radiat Oncol Biol Phys.* 1990;18:671.

45. Hedley M, Yan H, Rosenfeld D: Motion artifacts correction in MRI using generalized projections. *IEEE Trans Med Imaging.* 1991;10:40.

46. Korin HW, Ehman RL, Riederer SJ: Respiratory kinematics of the upper abdominal organs: A qualitative study. *Magn Reson Med.* 1992;23:172.

47. Liu YL, Riederer SJ, Rossman P III, et al: A monitoring, feedback, and triggering system for reproducible breath-hold MR imaging. *Magn Reson Med.* 1993;30:507.

48. Davies SC, Hill AL, Holmes RB, et al: Ultrasound quantification of respiratory organ motion in the upper abdomen. *Br J Radiol.* 1994; 67:1096.

49. Mori M, Murata K, Takahashi M: Accurate contiguous sections without breath-holding on chest CT: Value of respiratory gating and ultrafast CT. *Am J Roentgenol.* 1994;162:1057.

50. Jackson PC, Davies SC, Zananiri FV, et al: The development of equipment for the technical assessment of respiratory motion induced artifacts in MRI. *Br J Radiol.* 1993;66:132.

51. Ritchie CJ, Hsieh J, Gard MF, et al: Predictive respiratory gating: A new method to reduce motion artifacts on CT scans. *Radiology.* 1994;190:847.

52. Rekonen A, Toivonen J: Breathing gated radiation therapy—Possibilities and need. XIV International Conference on Medical and Biological Engineering and VII International Conference on Medical Physics, Espoo, Finland, 1985.

53. Peltola S: Gated radiotherapy to compensate for patient breathing. Proceedings of 11th Varian User Meeting, Florida, 68. 1986.

54. Willett CW, Linggood RM, Stracher MA, et al: The effect of respiratory cycle on mediastinal and lung dimensions in Hodgkin's disease. *Cancer.* 1987;60:1232.

55. Moerland MA, van den Bergh AC, Bhagwandien R, et al: The influence of respiration induced motion of the kidneys on the accuracy of radiotherapy treatment planning: A magnetic resonance imaging study. *Radiother Oncol.* 1994;30:150.

56. Kubo HD, Hill BC: Respiration gated radiotherapy treatment: Technical study. *Phys Med Biol.* 1996;41:83.

57. Ramsey CR, Cordrey IL, Oliver AL: A comparison of beam characteristics for gated and nongated clinical x-ray beams. *Med Phys.* 1999;26:2086.

58. Ten Haken RK, Lam KL, Balter JM, et al: Assessment of liver and lung motion for conformal therapy using radiopaque markers. *Med Phys.* 1993;20:1293.

59. Balter JM, Ten Haken RK, Lam KL: Assessment of margins for ventilatory motion during radiotherapy. *Med Phys.* 1994;21:913.

60. Balter JM, Ten Haken RK, Lawrence TS, et al: Uncertainties in CT-based radiation therapy treatment planning associated with patient breathing. *Int J Oncol Biol Phys.* 1996;36:167.

61. Ten Haken RK, Balter JM, Marsh LH, et al: Potential benefits of eliminating planning target volume expansions for patient breathing in the treatment of liver tumors. *Int J Oncol Biol Phys.* 1997; 38:613.

62. Balter JM, Lam KL, McGinn C, et al: Improvement of CT-based treatment planning models of abdominal targets using static exhale imaging. *Int J Radiat Oncol Biol Phys.* 1998;41:939.

63. Balter JM, Kwok LL, Cornealus JM, et al: Improvement of CT-based treatment-planning models of abdominal targets using static exhale imaging. *Int J Radiat Oncol Biol Phys.* 1998;41:939.

64. Lujan AE, Balter JM, Larsen EW, et al: A method for incorporating organ motion due to breathing into 3D dose calculations. *Med Phys.* 1999;26:715.

65. Keall PJ, Kini V, Vedam SS, Mohan R: Motion adaptive x-ray therapy: A feasibility study. *Phys Med Bio.* 2001;46:1.

66. Adler J: Image-guided robotic radiation therapy with Cyberknife and its indication for extracranial radiosurgery. *Gatedradiotherapy 2000.* The third Japanese body stereotactic irradiation meeting, Sapporo, Japan, July 2000.

67. Cihat O, Martin M: Issues in respiratory motion compensation during external-beam radiotherapy. *Int J Radiat Oncol Biol Phys.* 2002;52:1389.

68. Murphy M, Martin D, Whyte R, et al: The effectiveness of breath holding to stabilize lung and pancreas tumors during radiosurgery. *Int J Radiat Oncol Biol Phys.* 2002;53:475.

69. Kutcher GJ, Mageras GS, Leibel SA: Control, correction, and modeling of setup errors and organ motion. *Semin Radiat Oncol.* 1995;5:134.

70. Morrill SM, Langer M, Lane RG: Real-time couch compensation for intratreatment organ motion: Theoretical advantages. *Med Phys.* 1996;23:1083.

71. Sontag MB, Lai ZW, McRoy BW, Waters RP: Characterization of respiratory motion for pediatric conformal 3D Therapy. *Med Phys.* 1996;23:1082.

72. Crawford CR, King KF, Ritchie CJ, Godwin JD: Respiratory compensation in projection imaging using a magnification and displacement model. *IEEE Trans Med Imaging.* 1996;15:327.

73. Ritchie CJ, Crawford CR, Godwin JD, et al: Correction of computed tomography motion artifacts using pixel-specific back-projection. *IEEE Trans Med Imaging.* 1996;15:333.

74. Jacobs I, Vanregemorter J, Scalliet P: Influence of respiration on calculation and delivery of the prescribed dose in external radiotherapy. *Radiother Oncol.* 1996;39:123.

75. Killoran HM, Kooy DJ, Gladstone FJ, et al: A numerical simulation of organ motion and daily setup uncertainties: Implications for radiation therapy. *Int J Radiat Oncol Biol Phys.* 1997;37:213.

76. Ahmad R, Huq MS, Corn BW: Respiration-induced motion of the kidneys in whole abdominal radiotherapy: Implications for treatment planning and late toxicity. Radiother Oncol. 1997;42:87.

77. Report on the clinical investigation of cancer therapy using heavy-ion medical accelerator in Chiba, NIRS Annual Reports, 1996-1998 (in Japanese).

78. Minohara S, Kanai T, Endo M, et al: Respiratory gated irradiation system for heavy-ion radiotherapy. *Int J Radiat Oncol Biol Phys.* 2000;47:1097.

79. Li JG, Xing L: Inverse planning incorporating organ motion. *Med Phys.* 2000;27:1573.

80. Kini VR, Keall Ph, Vedam SS, et al: Preliminary results from a study of a respiratory motion tracking system: Underestimation of target volume with conventional CT simulation. *Int J Radiat Oncol Biol Phys.* 2000;48:164.

81. Vedam SS, Keal PJ, Kini VR, Mohan R: Determining parameters for respiration-gated radiotherapy. *Med Phys.* 2001;28:2139.

82. Booth JT, Zavgorodni SF: Set-up error and organ motion uncertainty: A review. *Australas Phys Eng Sci Med.* 1999;22:29.

83. Stroom JC, Kroonwijk M, Pasma KL, et al: Detection of internal organ movement in prostate cancer patients using portal images. *Med Phys.* 2000;27:452.

84. Zavgorodni SF: Treatment planning algorithm corrections accounting for random setup uncertainties in fractionated stereotactic radiotherapy. *Med Phys.* 2000;27:685.

85. Engelsman M, Damen EMF, De Jaeger K, et al: The effect of breathing and set-up errors on the cumulative dose to a lung tumor. *Radiother Oncol.* 2001;60:95.

86. Bkberg L, Holmberg O, Wittgren L, et al: What margins should be added to the clinical target volume in radiotherapy treatment planning for lung cancer? *Radiother Oncol.* 1998;48:71.

87. Yamashita Y, Yokoyama T, Tomiguchi S, et al: MR imaging of focal lung lesions: Elimination of flow and motion artifact by breath-hold ECG-gated and black-blood techniques on T_2-weighted turbo SE and STIR sequences. *J Magn Reson Imaging.* 1999; 9:691.

88. Uematsu M, Shioda A, Suda A, et al: Intra-treatment tumor position stability during computed tomography (CT)-guided frameless stereotactic radiation therapy for lung or liver cancers with a fusion of CT and linear accelerator (focal unit). *Int J Radiat Oncol Biol Phys.* 2000;48:443.

89. Aruga T, Itami J, Aruga M, et al: Target volume definition for upper abdominal irradiation using CT scans obtained during inhale and exhale phases. *Int J Radiat Oncol Biol Phys.* 2000;48:465.

90. Seiler PC, Blattmann H, Kirsch S, et al: A novel tracking technique for the continuous precise measurement of tumor positions in conformal radiotherapy. *Phys Med Biol.* 2000;45:N103.

91. Schweikard A, Glosser G, Bodduluri M, et al: Robotic motion compensation for respiratory movement during radiosurgery. *Comput Aided Surg.* 2000;5:263.

92. Ozhasoglu C, Murphy MJ, Glosser O, et al: Real-time tracking of the tumor volume in radiotherapy: A novel approach to compensate for respiratory motion. *Proc. 14th Int. Conf. on Computer Assisted Radiology and Surgery (CARS 2000, San Francisco).* Amsterdam: Elsevier Science BV; 2000:691.

93. Dhanantwari AC, Stergiopoulos S, Lakovidis I: Correcting organ motion artifacts in x-ray CT medical imaging systems by adaptive processing. I. Theory. *Med Phys.* 2001;28:1562.

94. Dhanantwari AC, Stergiopoulos N, Zamboglou D, et al: Correcting organ motion artifacts in x-ray CT systems based on tracking of motion phase by the spatial overlap correlator. II. Experimental study. *Med Phys.* 2001;28:1577.

95. Negoro Y, Nagata Y, Aoki T, et al: The effectiveness of an immobilization device in conformal radiotherapy for lung tumor: Reduction of respiratory tumor movement and evaluation of the daily setup accuracy. *Int J Radiat Oncol Biol Phys.* 2001;50:889.

96. Balter J, Dawson L, Kazanjian S, et al: Determination of ventilatory liver movement via radiographic evaluation of diaphragm position. *Int J Radiat Oncol Biol Phys.* 2001;51:267.

97. Oin-Sheng Chen MS, Weinhous FC, Deibel JR, et al: Fluoroscopic study of tumor motion due to breathing: Facilitating precise radiation therapy for lung cancer patients. *Med Phys.* 2001; 28:1850.

98. Pemler R, Besserer J, Lombriser N, et al: Influence of respiration-induced organ motion on dose distributions in treatments using enhanced dynamic wedges. *Med Phys.* 2001;28:2234.

99. Sixel KE, Aznar MC, Ung YC: Deep inspiration breath hold to reduce irradiated heart volume in breast cancer patients. *Int J Radiat Oncol Biol Phys.* 2001;49:199.

100. Barnes EA, Murry BR, Robinson DM, et al: Dosimetric evaluation of lung tumor immobilization using breath hold at deep inspiration. *Int J Radiat Oncol Biol Phys.* 2001;50:1091.

101. Stevens CW, Munden RF, Forster KM, et al: Respiration-driven lung tumor motion is independent of tumor size, tumor location, and pulmonary function. *Int J Radiat Oncol Biol Phys.* 2001;51:62.

102. Giraud P, de Rycke Y, Dubray B, et al: Conformal radiotherapy (CRT) planning for lung cancer: Analysis of intrathoracic organ motion during extreme phases of breathing. *Int J Radiat Oncol Biol Phys.* 2001;51:1081.

103. Yan D, Lockman D: Organ/patient geometric variation in external beam radiotherapy and its effects. *Med Phys.* 2001;28:593.

104. Lange KM, Jones DT: Organ motion and its management. *Int J Radiat Oncol Biol Phys.* 2001;50:265.

105. Nehmeh SA, Erdi YE, Ling CC, et al: Effect of respiratory gating on reducing lung notion. *Med Phys.* 2002;29:366.

106. Gatedradiotherapy by Korean group headed by W.K. Chung. P28. This abstract does not contain the MLC motion synchronized with the marker motion, but they discussed and presented some results.

107. Jaffray DA, Siewerdsen JH, Wong JW, et al: Flat-panel cone-beam computed tomography for image-guided radiation therapy. *Int J Radiat Oncol Biol Phys.* 2002;53:1337.

108. Crownover RL, Rodebaugh RF, Weibhous MS, et al: Dynamic radiosurgery by tracking lung tumors during relaxed breathing. *Int J Radiat Oncol Biol Phys.* 2002;53:194.

109. Kubo HD, Pappas C, Wilder RB: A comparison of arc-based and static mini-multi leaf collimator-based radiosurgery treatment plans. *Radiother Oncol.* 1997;45:89.

110. ICRU 50. Prescribing, Recording and Reporting Photon Beam Therapy. 1993.

Aspects of Brachytherapy Physics

Marco Zaider, PhD

The two problems of brachytherapy physics are these: (1) given a distribution of radiation sources, evaluate the dose at some point in tissue, and (2) given a prescription dose, construct a spatial distribution of sources—consistent with anatomic constraints—that best generates it. These two problems are known as *direct* and *inverse* treatment planning, respectively. There is, of course, a mass of work relating treatment planning to its practical implementation in the clinic and—as advertisers used to say—much, much more.

Direct planning is a matter of radiation physics. Since the physics of radiation transport in tissue matter is largely a closed subject, dosimetric calculations are merely a matter of performing complicated transport calculations (typically with the aid of Monte Carlo techniques) or obtaining empirical data. Inverse planning belongs to the field of applied mathematics and concerns making use of optimization algorithms to search for a source configuration that results in a specified dose distribution in tissue. It comes without saying that the advent of computers (especially inexpensive personal computers) made this approach practical and brought it into the clinic.

Traditionally, treatment planning in brachytherapy appears to have been inspired by the work of the artillery officer, that is to say, consisted of precalculated plans presented in the form of tables and nomograms. With computers unavailable, the idea was to save time and effort, yet still provide a reasonable treatment plan. Although often treated as historical relics, these so-called classical systems of implantation remain in use because of tradition and as quick and efficient means of verifying (at the level of 10% to 20% accuracy) computer-based plans. Commercial planning systems also include various implementations of these classical systems.

Concerning dosimetry, full transport calculations are not performed routinely. Although ready-to-use Monte Carlo transport codes are available commercially, cross sections for the interaction of radiation with condensed matter (liquid water included) are poorly known—which brings up the need to complement calculations with empirical data. An example of a pragmatic response to this state of affairs is a dosimetric formalism (colloquially known as *TG-43*).[1] TG-43, recommended by a task group of the American Association of Physicists in Medicine (AAPM), makes use of both theoretical and experimental data to evaluate the dosimetry of interstitial brachytherapy sources.

This chapter is intended to provide the reader with a clear presentation of both the theory and application of the fundamental principles of brachytherapy physics. Because the effort has been focused on transparency of exposition, most results are given with no derivation and must be taken on trust. Whenever the usual "it can be shown that ... ," or worse, "it is readily evident that ..." appear, the reader must go to the original papers for the elaborations of various mathematical equations.

The first part of this chapter emphasizes the need to grasp fundamental principles and their mathematical formulation and deals with the topics of radiation sources, dosimetry, and microdosimetry. The second part covers the practical matters of dose prescription and treatment planning. Each section is preceded by a synopsis covering its essential features. Certain subsections require more concentration from the reader than others. To alleviate the tedium of being exposed to concepts that may be beyond the reader's knowledge and to aid those interested primarily in one aspect of the subject, the chapter was written in a way that allows, without loss of continuity, selection of individual sections.

It has not, of course, been possible in a chapter of this size to deal exhaustively with all applications. Many topics of practical importance were either omitted or did not receive the serious attention they merit. Then again, to quote Voltaire's line: "The way to be a bore is to say everything."

Synopsis

Radioactive nuclei are the sources of radiation in brachytherapy. Only certain combinations of protons and neutrons constitute stable nuclei. Unstable nuclei, also known as *radionuclides* or *radioisotopes*, disintegrate in a process known as *radioactivity*. If the number of neutrons in the nucleus is too large, a high-energy electron

Continued

S y n o p s i s—cont'd

(*beta particle*) is emitted. If the number of protons is too large, the particle emitted is generally the *positron*. In heavy elements a form of radioactivity exists whereby the nucleus emits an *alpha particle*, which is the nucleus of a helium atom. In a population of unstable nuclei, the number of radionuclides decreases exponentially. Thus, the remaining number of nuclei at time t, N(t) is given by N(t)/N(0) = exp(−λt). The quantity λ—termed the *decay constant*—is the fraction of nuclei that decay per unit time. A quantity equivalent to λ is the *half-life*, $T_{1/2}$, which is the time required, on average, to halve the number of radionuclides. Mathematically, λ = 0.693/$T_{1/2}$. The average number of disintegrations per unit time is termed *activity*, A, of that amount of radionuclide. The activity is measured in becquerels (Bq) or curies (Ci) and may be calculated from A(t) = λN(t). The main radionuclides used in brachytherapy are: ^{137}Cs, ^{192}Ir, ^{125}I, and ^{103}Pd.

RADIATION SOURCES

Radioactive Decay

Nuclei are *stable* only when there cannot be any separation of the nucleus into two fragments, the sum of the masses of which is less than the mass of the nucleus. Unstable (or *radioactive*) nuclei decay, often in more than one step, into stable nuclei—a process known as *disintegration*. The type of particles emitted determines the mode of decay. Atoms containing radioactive nuclei are termed *radionuclides* or *radioisotopes*. Three types of radioactivity are known to exist: alpha, beta, and gamma decay.

ALPHA DECAY

In this process a nucleus disintegrates by emitting an α particle (the nucleus ^{4}He$_2$):

$$^{A}X_{Z} \rightarrow {}^{A-4}Y_{Z-2} + {}^{4}\alpha_{2} + Q \qquad (2.1)$$

In this notation, $^{A}X_{Z}$ represents a nucleus (chemical element X) of atomic number Z and mass number A, and Q is the difference between the total mass of the radioactive nucleus and its decay products:

$$Q = m\left(^{A}X_{Z}\right) - \left[m\left(^{A-4}Y_{Z-2}\right) + m\left(^{4}\alpha_{2}\right) \right] \quad (2.2)$$

The α particle has a fixed energy, characteristic of the radioactive nucleus.

BETA DECAY

Three elementary processes are classified as beta decay. In β⁻ *decay* a neutron inside the atomic nucleus transforms into a proton and, as a result, an *electron* (a β⁻ particle) is emitted from the nucleus. The second process, known as β⁺ *decay*, results when a nuclear proton turns into a neutron, and a *positron* (β⁺) is emitted from the nucleus. The third process, *electron capture* (EC), occurs when the nucleus absorbs one of the atomic electrons. Thus, the three elementary processes that occur during beta decay are:

$$n \rightarrow p + e^{-} + \bar{v}_{e} + 0.782\,MeV \quad (\beta^{-})$$
$$p \rightarrow n + e^{+} + v_{e} - 1.803\,MeV \quad (\beta^{+}) \quad (2.3)$$
$$e^{-} + p \rightarrow n + v_{e} - 0.782\,MeV \quad (EC)$$

β decay is accompanied by the emission of a neutral particle named the *electron neutrino* (v_e, mass <3 eV) or

its antiparticle, $\bar{v}_e$. Because the last two reactions are endothermic, they must occur inside the nucleus to balance the energy required. The *nuclear* β decays are:

$$^{A}_{Z}X \rightarrow {}^{A}_{Z+1}Y + e^{-} + \bar{v}_{e} + Q \quad (\beta^{-})$$
$$^{A}_{Z}X \rightarrow {}^{A}_{Z-1}Y + e^{+} + v_{e} + Q \quad (\beta^{+}) \qquad (2.4)$$
$$^{A}_{Z}X \rightarrow {}^{A}_{Z-1}Y + v_{e} + Q \qquad (EC)$$

GAMMA DECAY

Following α or β decay, the nucleus Y (see Equations 2.1, 2.4) may be left in an excited state, Y*. In this case Y* will decay to a lower energy state by emitting a photon—a process known as γ *decay*. In *internal conversion*, an alternative mode of deexcitation, Y* gives its energy to an atomic electron that is ejected.

In a population of unstable nuclei, the number of radionuclides decreases progressively. The following empirical law governs this process*: "The average fraction of radioactive nuclei, ΔN/N, that decay in a fixed time interval, Δt, is constant." The mathematical expression of this statement is:

$$\frac{dN(t)}{N(t)} = -\lambda\, dt \qquad (2.5)$$

where λ—the *decay constant*—is a positive number characteristic for each radioactive nucleus. The negative sign in front of λ indicates that dN(t) = N(t + dt) − N(t) <0. A more familiar form of Equation 2.5 is:

$$N(t) = N(0)e^{-\lambda t} \qquad (2.6)$$

which gives the average remaining number, N(t), of radioactive nuclei at time t, when the initial number is N(0).

There are two equivalent representations of the decay constant. The *half-life*, $T_{1/2}$, is the time required, on average, to halve the number of radionuclides. Thus:

$$N(T_{1/2}) = N(0)\frac{1}{2} = N(0)e^{-\lambda T_{1/2}} \qquad (2.7)$$

---

*Here, and in subsequent definitions, reference is made to average (or expected) quantities. It should be evident that the actual number of, say, disintegrations per unit time interval is a stochastic quantity—the average measure of which is activity.

Elementary manipulations lead to:

$$T_{1/2} = \frac{\ln(2)}{\lambda} \approx \frac{0.693}{\lambda} \qquad (2.8)$$

The *mean life*, $\overline{T}$, of a radioactive nucleus is the average lifetime until it disintegrates. Mathematically:

$$\overline{T} = \frac{1}{\lambda} = \frac{T_{1/2}}{\ln(2)} \qquad (2.9)$$

If there are several decay modes, each with decay constant λ_i (i = 1, 2, ...) then the total decay constant is additive with respect to these partial quantities:

$$\lambda = \lambda_1 + \lambda_2 + ... \qquad (2.10)$$

a property that its equivalent quantities ($T_{1/2}$ or $\overline{T}$) obviously do not possess.

The average number of disintegrations per unit time of an assembly of radioactive nuclei is termed the *activity*, A, of that amount of radionuclide:

$$A(t) = -\frac{dN(t)}{dt} = \lambda N(t) \qquad (2.11)$$

The unit of activity is the *becquerel* (Bq), defined as one disintegration per second. Another unit of activity* is the curie, Ci. It represents 3.7×10^{10} Bq.

The average number of nuclei that disintegrate during a time interval t is:

$$N(0) - N(t) = N(0)\left(1 - e^{-\lambda t}\right) = \frac{A(0)}{\lambda}\left(1 - e^{-\lambda t}\right) \qquad (2.12)$$

an equation that is useful for estimating the dose in temporary (or permanent) implants (see Equations 6.1 and 6.2).

---

*The becquerel is invariably too small a unit, and the curie is too large. Common activities in brachytherapy are of the order of mCi.

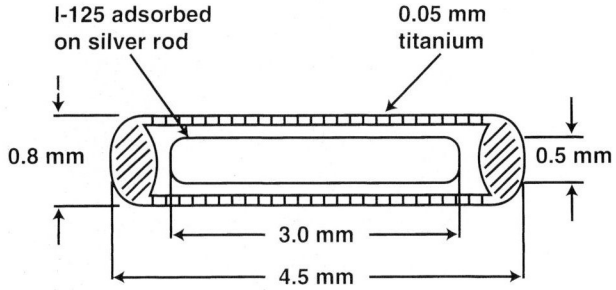

Figure 11–1. The ^{125}I 6711 seed consists of a welded titanium capsule containing ^{125}I adsorbed on a silver rod. These seeds are used primarily in permanent implants, at strengths of 0.4 to 1.0 U (see the following section on dosimetry for the definition of U). The radio-opaque marker is useful in source localization, which is one of the reasons this type of source is used in permanent implants where adequate source localization is needed for dosimetric calculations. (Courtesy of Amersham Medi-Physics, Inc. Arlington Heights, Ill.)

RADIONUCLIDES

Before the advent of nuclear technology, the only significant use of radioactive material in medicine involved radium (Ra) and its decay products. Radium has been essentially replaced by radioisotopes produced in nuclear reactors in (n,γ) reactions:

$$^{A}X_Z + n \rightarrow {}^{A+1}X_Z + \gamma \qquad (2.13)$$

Nearly all radionuclides produced in reactors emit γ and β radiation.

The physical characteristics of the main radioactive sources currently used in brachytherapy are given in Table 11-1.

Some common features of these radioisotopes are: (a) high specific activity needed for a small size source; (b) low photon energy, necessary for radiation protection and conformal dose distribution; and (c) appropriate half-life for permanent or temporary implants. The physical design of several commonly used sources is shown in Figs. 11-1 to 11-5 (many other sources are available, especially for low-energy isotopes; see, for instance, the AAPM/ Radiological Physics Center Registry of Low Energy Brachytherapy Seeds at http://rpc.mdanderson.org/rpc/ htm/Home_htm/Low-energy.htm).

Table 11–1   Physical Characteristics of Radioactive Sources Currently Used in Brachytherapy*

Isotope	$\overline{E}_\gamma$/MeV	E_β(max)/MeV	$T_{1/2}$	Air kerma rate constant/ (cGy/h) (cm²/mCi)	HVL$_{Pb}$ or Range†
^{137}Cs	0.662	1.17	30 y	2.87	0.65
^{198}Au	0.412	0.96	2.7 d	2.08	0.33
^{192}Ir	0.380	0.67	74.2 d	4.11	0.3
^{125}I	0.028	—	60.2 d	1.32	0.002
^{103}Pd	0.021	—	17 d	1.296	0.002
^{131}I	0.364	0.61	8.06 d	1.93	0.30
^{90}Sr/^{90}Y	—	2.27	28.9 y	—	1.1†
^{32}P	—	1.71	14.3 d	—	0.8†
^{106}Ru/^{106}Rh	—	3.55	367 d	—	1.8†

*Air kerma rate constant is defined in Equation 3.10. HVL stands for half value layer and represents the thickness of material that will reduce the fluence of uncharged particle to half; units: cm.
†The range of electrons (in units of g/cm²) is given at the maximum electron energy.

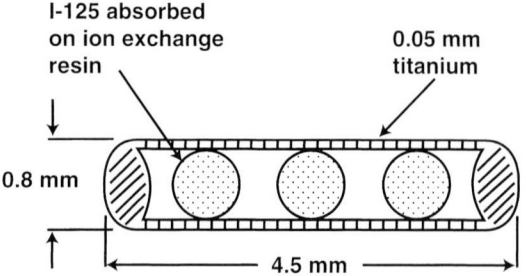

Figure 11–2. The ^{125}I 6702 seed consists of a welded titanium capsule containing ^{125}I absorbed on resin spheres. These seeds are used at strengths of 10 to 30 U. These sources are often used in ribbons, and thus the lack of a radiomarker is not an impediment as seed localization can be performed with ribbons containing equidistant nonradioactive (dummy) seeds. (Courtesy of Amersham Medi-Physics, Inc. Arlington Heights, Ill.)

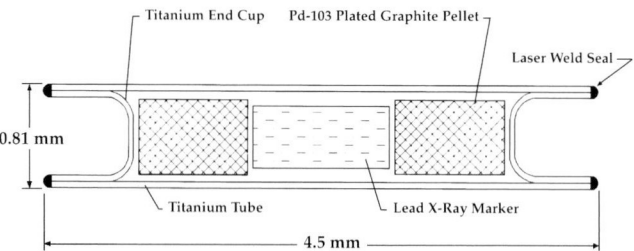

Figure 11–3. The TheraSeed ^{103}Pd model 200 seed consists of a laser-welded titanium tube containing two ^{103}Pd graphite pellets and a lead x-ray marker. Typical source strengths are 1.0 to 3.0 U. (Courtesy of Theragenics Corporation, Norcross, Ga.)

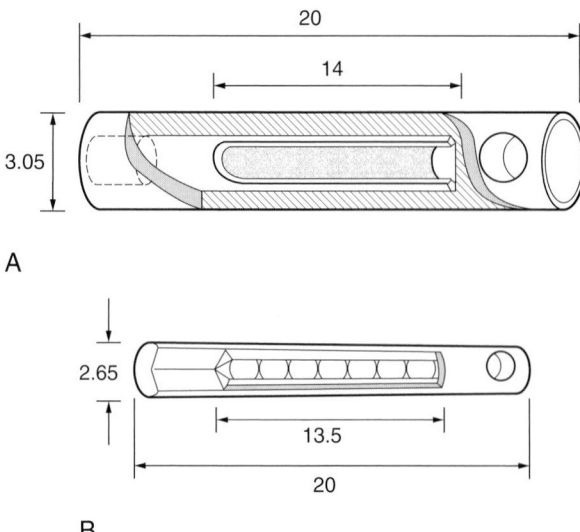

A

B

Figure 11–4. ^{137}Cs intracavitary sources. **A,** The 3M model with a core of ceramic microspheres. **B,** The Amersham J-type source with a core of glass beads. Dimensions are in mm. (From Meli JA: Dosimetry of some interstitial and intracavitary sources and their applicators. In Williamson JF, Thomadsen BR, Nath R, eds. *AAPM Summer School 1994.* Madison, Wisc: Medical Physics Publishing Company; 1995:185.)

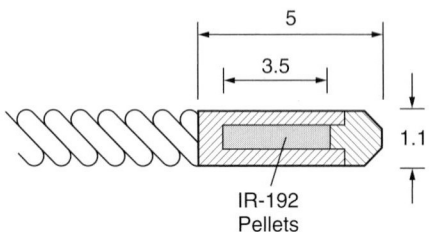

Design of the HDR iridium source.
All dimensions in mm.

Figure 11–5. Cable-mounted ^{192}Ir source used for high-dose-rate treatments. A typical initial activity is 10 Ci. (From Meli JA: Dosimetry of some interstitial and intracavitary sources and their applicators. In Williamson JF, Thomadsen BR, Nath R, eds. *AAPM Summer School 1994.* Madison, Wisc: Medical Physics Publishing Company; 1995:185.)

DOSIMETRY

Synopsis

The central quantity in radiologic physics is the *absorbed dose* (or simply *dose, D*), which is the average energy absorbed per unit mass at a point in the irradiated matter. The quantity *kerma*, K, refers to the first step of energy transfer to matter and is defined as the average energy transferred from uncharged to charged particles per unit mass of the material at a point in matter. The older quantity, the *exposure*, is equivalent to kerma but is restricted to photons; it represents the total charge of the ions of one sign produced per unit mass of air. If the fluence of charged particles does not depend on position—a condition known as *charged particle equilibrium* (CPE)—then D = K. This expression is important because dose is easy to measure but difficult to calculate, while kerma is easy to calculate but difficult to measure. CPE cannot exist in a medium irradiated externally with charged particles. For uncharged particles CPE obtains if their mean free path is significantly larger than the range of charged particles that result from their interactions.

Continued

Synopsis—cont'd

A simple expression for evaluating the dose rate at distance r from of a photon-emitting source is:

$\dot{D}(r) = S_K \dfrac{1}{r^2} T(r) \left(\dfrac{\mu_{en}}{\rho}\right)^{tissue}_{air}$. Here S_K (the *air kermastrength*) is a measure of the amount of activity in the

source and is provided by the source manufacturer, and $\left(\dfrac{\mu_{en}}{\rho}\right)^{tissue}_{air}$ is the ratio of *mass absorption coefficients* for

tissue and air (use 1.01 for ^{125}I and ^{103}Pd and 1.11 for ^{137}Cs and ^{192}Ir). For ^{137}Cs and ^{192}Ir and $r < 5$ cm by taking $T(r) = 1$, the error made in the calculated dose rate will be smaller than 10%. However, for low-energy sources, such as ^{103}Pd or ^{125}I, $T(r)$ changes significantly with distance and the so-called *Meisberger polynomials* (see Equation 3.20) must be used.

The absorbed dose rate at distance r from an isotropic radioactive source (activity A) emitting n(E) *charged particles* of energy E per disintegration is given by:

$$\dot{D}(r)_{Gy/h} = 1.7 A_{Ci} \frac{n(E)}{r^2_{cm}} \left(\frac{S}{\rho}\right)_{MeV\ cm^2/g}$$

If the *fluence rate*, $\dot{\Phi}$, is known, then:

$$\frac{\dot{D}}{Gy/h} = 5.76 \ 10^{-13} \frac{\dot{\Phi}}{particles/cm^2,\ sec} \frac{S/\rho}{MeV\ cm^2/g} \dot{\Phi}$$

where S/ρ is the *mass stopping power* of the medium. For *permanent implants* the total dose delivered by a source with initial dose rate, $\dot{D}(0)$, is given by: $D_{total} = 1.44\ T_{1/2}\ \dot{D}(0)$. For a *temporary implant* (treatment time t):

$$D(t) = \dot{D}(0) \frac{1}{\lambda} \left(1 - e^{-\lambda t}\right)$$

$$= 1.44\ T_{1/2}\ \dot{D}(0) \left(1 - e^{-0.693 \frac{t}{T_{1/2}}}\right)$$

Conceptual Matters*

The *absorbed dose*, D, is defined[2] as the quotient of $d\bar{\varepsilon}$ by *dm*:

$$D = \frac{d\bar{\varepsilon}}{dm} \quad (3.1)$$

where $d\bar{\varepsilon}$ is the *average* energy imparted by ionizing radiation to matter of mass dm. The qualifier "average" recognizes the fact that energy is imparted in random and discrete energy deposition events. This can be made more precise with reference to the quantity *specific energy*, z, which is the stochastic counterpart of absorbed dose. By definition:

$$z = \frac{\varepsilon}{m} \quad (3.2)$$

In this expression ε is the energy imparted to the *finite* volume, V, which contains the mass m. Unlike dose, which is measured at a point, $\vec{r}$, and is therefore a *field* quantity[†], the specific energy is measured always in nonzero volumes. The relationship between dose and specific energy is:

$$D(\vec{r}) = \lim_{V \to 0,\ \vec{r} \in V} \bar{z} \quad (3.3)$$

In general $D(\vec{r})$ changes with $\vec{r}$, and this is termed the *dose distribution* in the irradiated object.

To evaluate the dose at a point (in practice, a small volume), one needs information on the distribution in number, energy, angle, and type of the ionizing particles that enter or leave the volume. For instance, for a radiation field with only one type of charged particle of energy E, and no transport of energy by secondary particles:

$$D(\vec{r}) = \Phi(\vec{r})\left[-\frac{1}{\rho} S(E)\right] \quad (3.4)$$

The quantity in the square bracket is the mass stopping power of the medium (density ρ) and $\Phi(\vec{r})$ is the particle *fluence* at position $\vec{r}$. If the field consists of particles with a spectrum of energies, Equation 3.4 becomes:

$$D(\vec{r}) = \int_0^\infty dE\ \Phi(\vec{r}, E)\left[-\frac{1}{\rho} S(E)\right] \quad (3.5)$$

where $\Phi(\vec{r}, E)$ is the *distribution of fluence in energy*. Again, this equation is valid only when energy transport by secondary particles (e.g., electrons set in motion by the

---

*For definitions of various quantities, see Appendix A.

†There is no such thing as the "dose to an organ."

primary particles) can be neglected, because only then the energy lost by the particles (to which the stopping power, S(E), refers) equals the energy absorbed in the medium (to which the dose refers).

For a field containing both charged (subscript c) and uncharged (subscript u) particles, but where radiation sources emit only uncharged particles, the corresponding equation for the absorbed dose is[3]:

$$D(\vec{r}) = \int_0^\infty dE_u\, E_u\, \Phi_u(\vec{r}, E_u) \left(\frac{\mu_{en}(E_u)}{\rho} \right)$$
$$- \int_0^\infty dE_u\, E_u \int_0^\infty dE_c\, \Phi_c(\vec{r}, E_c)\, \frac{\mu_s(E_c \to E_u)}{\rho}$$
$$+ \frac{1}{\rho} \int_0^\infty dE_c\, E_c \int_0^\infty d\,\vec{u}_c \left[-\vec{u}_c \nabla \Phi_c(\vec{r}, E_c) \right] + \frac{\partial Q_c}{\partial m}$$

$$(3.6)$$

In the expression, Equation 3.6, $\mu_{en}(E)$ is the *energy transfer coefficient* of uncharged particles of energy E_u and is defined as the fraction of energy E_u transferred to kinetic energy of the charged particles per unit distance traversed; $\mu_s(E_c \to E_u)dE_u$ is the probability per unit distance traveled that a charged particle (moving in the direction $d\vec{u}_c$ about $\vec{u}_c$) with energy E_c will produce, as a result of an interaction at $\vec{r}$, an uncharged particle of energy E_u; and $\partial Q_c/\partial m$ the change in rest mass per unit mass.

The second and fourth terms on the right-hand side of Equation 3.6 are usually small compared to the first term. If the fluence of charged particles, Φ_c, does not depend on $\vec{r}$—a condition known as* *charged-particle equilibrium (CPE)*[†]—then

$$D(\vec{r}) \approx K(\vec{r}) \qquad (3.7)$$

where $K(\vec{r})$, called the *kerma* of the uncharged particles, represents the average initial kinetic energy of charged particles created by the uncharged particles per unit mass (see Appendix A):

$$K(\vec{r}) = \int_0^\infty dE_u\, E_u\, \Phi_u(\vec{r}, E_u) \left(\frac{\mu_{en}(E_u)}{\rho} \right) \qquad (3.8)$$

The quantity *kerma* (more precisely, *air kerma*) is replacing an older quantity, *exposure*, which is defined[2] as "the quotient of dQ by dm, where dQ is the absolute value of the total charge of the ions of one sign produced in air when all the electrons and positrons liberated or

created by photons in air of mass dm are completely stopped in air." Thus, exposure (X) is given by:

$$X = \frac{dQ}{dm} \qquad (3.9)$$

and is measured in C/kg. A special unit of exposure is the *roentgen* (1 R = 2.58 10[−4] C/kg). The mass of air to which the definition of exposure refers can be in free space or inside a material (e.g., tissue).

For each radionuclide one can define a quantity, the *air kerma rate constant* (Γ_δ), which relates the activity, A, to its kerma rate. Specifically, Γ_δ of a radionuclide emitting photons is "the quotient of $l^2 \dot{K}_\delta$ by A, where $\dot{K}_\delta$ is the air kerma rate due to photons of energy greater than δ, at a distance l in vacuo from a point source of this nuclide"[4]:

$$\Gamma_\delta = \frac{l^2 \dot{K}_\delta}{A} \qquad (3.10)$$

where Γ_δ is measured in units of $m^2 Gy\, s^{-1}\, Bq^{-1}$. Numerical values of Γ_δ for selected nuclides are given in Table 11-1. Because the air kerma–rate constant refers to a point source, its numerical value is independent of the distance l.

A quantity closely related to Γ_δ is the *exposure rate constant*, $\Gamma_{X,\delta}$, which is defined as

$$\Gamma_{X,\delta} = \frac{l^2 \dot{X}_\delta}{A} \qquad (3.11)$$

$\dot{X}_\delta$ being, in analogy to $\dot{K}_\delta$, the exposure rate due to photons of energy greater than δ. The common unit of $\Gamma_{X,\delta}$ is R/h cm[2]/mCi. To convert $\Gamma_{X,\delta}$ to Γ_δ, one makes use of the fact that K and X are related by:

$$K = \frac{W}{e} X \qquad (3.12)$$

In this equation W/e is the average energy imparted to air per ion pair created by photons (W/e = 33.97 J/C = 33.97 eV/ion pair = 0.876 cGy/R).

The expressions, Equations 3.6 to 3.8, illustrate the point that in order to calculate the dose, one needs information on the distribution of fluence in position, energy, etc. at the position of interest. This is accomplished with the aid of transport equations (deterministic or stochastic) where the configuration of sources as well as the penetration, scattering, and slowing down of ionizing radiation in the medium is explicitly taken into account. Transport calculations are complex and time consuming to implement, and often simplifications are necessary. An important example is the case of *radiation equilibrium* (not to be confused with charged-particle equilibrium), where sources of radiation are uniformly distributed in an infinite and homogeneous medium; as a result, the fluence will not depend on position. If, furthermore, the energy loss can be described in terms of stopping power, S(E), the fluence of charged particles of energy E is given by:

$$\Phi(E) = \frac{1}{S(E)} \int_E^\infty dE'\, n_0(E') \qquad (3.13)$$

---

*Charged-particle equilibrium is defined by the condition $\nabla \Phi_c = 0$. The more general condition termed *radiation equilibrium* is defined as $\nabla(\Phi_u + \Phi_c) = 0$.

†Charged-particle equilibrium (CPE) cannot exist in a medium irradiated externally with charged particles. For uncharged particles, CPE obtains if their mean free path (1/μ) is significantly longer than the range of the charged particles (R) that result from their interactions; thus Rμ<<1. Under the weaker condition, Rμ<1, dose and kerma are not equal anymore; however, the ratio D/K is independent of penetration distance—a case known as *transient* CPE.

Table 11–2   Coefficients Used to Represent the Function T(r)

	A	B/cm⁻¹	C/cm⁻²	D/cm⁻³	r_{lim}/cm	μ_0/cm⁻¹	R/cm
^{192}Ir	1.0128	5.019 10⁻³	–1.178 10⁻³	–2.008 10⁻⁵	10	0.03	7.41
^{137}Cs	1.0091	–9.015 10⁻³	–3.459 10⁻⁴	–2.817 10⁻⁵	10	0.03	4.83
^{60}Co	0.9942	–5.318 10⁻³	–2.610 10⁻³	1.327 10⁻⁴	10	0.03	3.09
^{125}I	0.9357	–5.530 10⁻²	–4.280 10⁻²	5.598 10⁻³	5	0.25	0.035

$n_0(E)dE$ is a source term representing the expected number of particles produced per unit volume with energy in the interval dE about E. For a monoenergetic source (energy E_0):

$$n_0(E) = n_0\, \delta(E - E_0) \qquad (3.14)$$

and

$$\Phi(E) = \begin{cases} 0 & if\ E > E_0 \\ \dfrac{n_0}{S(E)} & if\ E \le E_0 \end{cases} \qquad (3.15)$$

A similar equation is valid for photons:

$$\Phi(E) = \begin{cases} 0 & if\ E > E_0 \\ \dfrac{n_0}{E\mu_{en}(E)} & if\ E \le E_0 \end{cases} \qquad (3.16)$$

In practical situations the conditions or radiation equilibrium are rarely (if ever) rigorously satisfied. A condition of interest that approximates radiation equilibrium for uncharged particles occurs when their charged secondaries have ranges that are much shorter than the distance over which they are significantly attenuated. Photons with energies up to tens of MeV satisfy this condition, termed *transient equilibrium*.

From Equations 3.7, 3.8, and 3.16, it follows that for monoenergetic photons:

$$D(\vec{r}) = \int_0^{\infty} dE\ E\ \Phi(\vec{r}, E)\ \frac{1}{\rho}\ \mu_{en}(E)$$

$$= \frac{n_0(\vec{r})}{\rho} \int_0^{E_0} dE = \frac{n_0(\vec{r})}{\rho}\ E_0 \qquad (3.17)$$

which is, of course, the kerma at $\vec{r}$.

This conceptual framework forms the basis for the practical implementation of a system describing the dosimetry of brachytherapy sources.

Practical Matters: Analytic Formalisms

Day-to-day dosimetric calculations in brachytherapy make use of a formalism based on a single measurable quantity—the source strength (essentially, a surrogate for the amount of activity in the source). As well as avoiding detailed theoretical calculations or full dosimetric measurements for each type of source, the main advantage of this formalism is that dosimetry is traceable to calibrations made at a single institution (in the United States, the National Institute of Standards and Technology, NIST*). This is accomplished by characterizing each source in terms of a quantity, *air kerma strength*, S_K, which refers to the product of air kerma rate in free space, $\dot{K}(d) = dK(d)/dt$, and d^2, where d is a fixed (given) distance from the source along the transverse axis of the source†:

$$S_K(d) = \frac{dK(d)}{dt}\ d^2 \qquad (3.18)$$

The distance d (taken, by convention, as 1 m) is assumed to be sufficiently large to justify treating the source as a point. The unit of S_K, termed U, is defined as 1 µGy/h m². Other specifications of source strength in brachytherapy, and their relation to S_K, are given in Appendix B.

Dosimetric calculations may be performed at different levels of accuracy. For an unencapsulated *isotropic point source*, which is the simplest case, the dose in water at distance r from the source is given by:

$$\dot{D}_w(r) = \underbrace{\frac{S_K(d)}{r^2} \left(\frac{\mu_{en}}{\rho}\right)_a^w}_{\dot{K}_w(r)} T(r) \qquad (3.19)$$

Here $\left(\dfrac{\mu_{en}}{\rho}\right)_a^w$ is shorthand for the ratio of the mass energy-transfer coefficients of water and air; it is 1.11 for ^{192}Ir, ^{137}Cs and ^{60}Co, and 1.01 for ^{125}I. T(r), the *tissue attenuation factor*, is defined as the ratio of $D_w(r)$ to the water-kerma in free space, $K_w(r)$. Analytic expressions for T(r) have been calculated for different radioactive sources[5,6] as given in Table 11-2 and Equation 3.20:

$$T(r) = \begin{cases} A + Br + Cr^2 + Dr^3 & for\ r < r_{lim} \\ \exp\left[-\mu_0(r - R)\right] & for\ r \ge r_{lim} \end{cases} \qquad (3.20)$$

---

*Presently, NIST provides dosimetric calibrations (air kerma strength) for the following radioactive photon emitters: ^{103}Pd, ^{125}I, ^{192}Ir, ^{137}Cs, and ^{60}Co. Calibrations provided by NIST, or equivalently by NIST-Accredited Dosimetry Calibration Laboratories (ADCL), are transferred to users who establish calibration factors for their local instruments (e.g., re-entrant ionization chambers).

†There is something peculiar about air kerma strength, namely that—unlike other physical quantities, which can be expressed at will in any units—S_K becomes meaningless (or better, incorrect) if instead of µGy/h m² one uses, say, cGy/hour cm². This was noticed by the Comité Français pour le Mésure des Rayonnements Ionisants (CFMRI),[190] and by others, who suggested instead the quantity reference air kerma rate (see Appendix B).

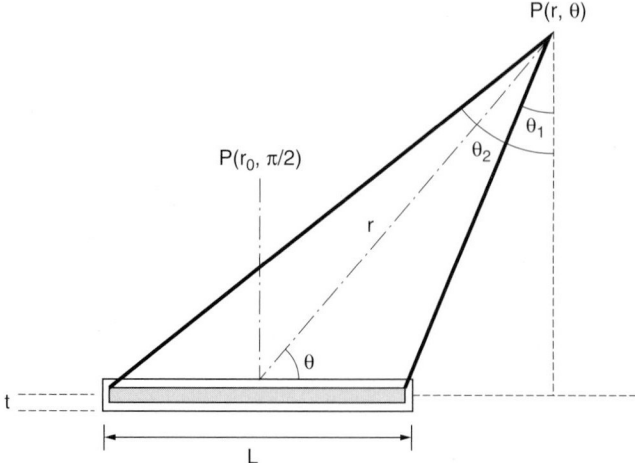

Figure 11–6. The geometry of the linear source used in the Sievert integral, Equation 34. (From Nath R: Physical properties and clinical uses of brachytherapy radionuclide. In Williamson JF, Thomadsen BR, Nath R, eds. *AAPM Summer School 1994.* Madison, Wisc: Medical Physics Publishing Company; 1995:7)

Table 11–4 Recommended Dose Rate Constants in Water[1]

Source	Λ/cGy h^{-1} U^{-1}
^{192}Ir (Fe clad)	1.12
^{125}I (model 6702)	0.93
^{125}I (model 6711)	0.98
^{103}Pd (model 200)	0.68

A more realistic dosimetric treatment must take into account the effects of the spatial extension of the radioactive material (typically, a line source) as well as absorption of the primary radiation in the source itself and its sheath. For a source of length L and thickness t (Fig. 11-6) one can readily obtain[7]:

$$\dot{D}_w(r, \theta) = \frac{S_K(d)}{L\, r \sin(\vartheta)} \left(\frac{\mu_{en}}{\rho}\right)_a^w$$

$$\times\, e^{\mu t} \int_{\theta_1}^{\theta_2} e^{-\mu t \sec \theta'}\, T\big((r \sin \vartheta - t) \sec \theta'\big)\, d\theta'$$

$$(3.21)$$

where μ is the effective attenuation coefficient for the encapsulation material.

The model, Equation 3.21, has been successfully applied to ^{137}Cs and ^{226}Ra sources.[8,9] However, for low energy sources the application of the Sievert model may lead to significant errors.[10]

A recommended protocol exists for the dosimetry of sources used in interstitial brachytherapy.[1] It proceeds as follows: Assuming cylindrical symmetry about a two-dimensional source, let $\dot{D}(r, \vartheta)$ represent the dose rate in water at position P(r, θ) (see Fig. 11-6). Formally, one can express this quantity as the product of two factors: (1) G(r, θ), describing the dose falloff with distance (r) and polar angle (θ) for a given distribution of radioactive material in the source, and (2) S(r, θ), accounting for absorption of radiation in the source material, filtration

through the encapsulating material, and scattering and absorption in the medium separating the source from point P. Thus:

$$\dot{D}(r, \theta) = S(r, \vartheta)\, G(r, \theta) \tag{3.22}$$

The function G(r, θ) is given by:

$$G(r, \theta) = \frac{\int \rho(\vec{r}\,') \big/ \left|\vec{r} - \vec{r}\,'\right|^2 d\,\vec{r}\,'}{\int \rho(\vec{r}\,')\, d\,\vec{r}\,'} \tag{3.23}$$

Here $\rho(\vec{r})\, d\vec{r}$ represents the amount of radioactivity in volume $d\vec{r}$ about $\vec{r}$. For a point source one obtains the "inverse squared" relationship:

$$G(r, \theta) = \frac{1}{r^2} \tag{3.24}$$

For a line source of length L (see Fig. 11-6) straightforward integration (see Equation 3.21) yields:

$$G(r, \theta) = \frac{\theta_2 - \theta_1}{Lr \sin(\theta)} \tag{3.25}$$

Let further P(r$_0$, θ$_0$) be a reference point (see Fig. 11-6) and $\dot{D}_0$ the dose rate in the medium of interest (commonly, water) at P(r$_0$, θ$_0$). The following sequence of identities defines the functions g(r) and F(r, θ):

$$\dot{D}(r, \theta) \equiv \dot{D}_0\, \frac{\dot{D}(r, \theta)}{\dot{D}_0} \equiv \dot{D}_0\, \frac{S(r, \theta)G(r, \theta)}{S(r_0, \theta_0)G(r_0, \theta_0)}$$

$$\equiv \dot{D}_0\, \frac{G(r, \theta)}{G(r_0, \theta_0)} \underbrace{\left[\frac{S(r, \theta_0)}{S(r_0, \theta_0)}\right]}_{g(r)} \underbrace{\left[\frac{S(r, \theta)}{S(r, \theta_0)}\right]}_{F(r,\theta)} \tag{3.26}$$

The interpretation of these new quantities is straightforward: g(r) describes the effect of absorption and scattering along the transverse axis (Table 11-3); and F(r, θ) accounts for anisotropy.

One then proceeds to define a ratio, Λ, of $\dot{D}_0$ to $S_K(d)$. Λ—the *dose rate constant*—is a number characteristic to each type of source (Table 11-4).

Table 11–3 Coefficients of $g(r) = a_0 + a_1 r + a_2 r^2 + a_3 r^3 + a_4 r^4 + a_5 r^5$(1)

Source	a_0	$a_1 \times 10^2$	$a_2 \times 10^2$	$a_3 \times 10^2$	$a_4 \times 10^3$	$a_5 \times 10^4$
^{125}I (6711)	1.01376	12.2747	−17.3025	4.02378	−3.85227	1.34283
^{125}I (6702)	1.02307	8.63751	−13.7155	3.07795	−2.86946	0.987558
^{192}Ir (Fe clad)	0.989054	0.881319	0.351778	−0.146637	0.092437	0
^{103}Pd	1.62891	−76.8559	15.4272	−2.27185	3.39330	−2.67215

Table 11–5   Average Anisotropy Factors, $\overline{\phi_{an}}$

^{103}Pd (Model 200)	^{125}I (Model 6711)	^{125}I (Model 6702)	^{192}Ir (Best Industries)
0.90	0.93	0.95	0.98

With this one arrives at:

$$\dot{D}(r, \theta) = S_K \ \Lambda \ \frac{G(r, \theta)}{G(r_0, \theta_0)} \ g(r) \ F(r, \theta) \quad (3.27)$$

The structure of this equation separates out in the evaluation of $\dot{D}(r, \vartheta)$ a factor (S_K) that is measured in a way traceable to a single calibration standard (at NIST) and which is proportional to the amount of radioactive material in each source, and a series of functions uniquely determined for each type of source. A report by a task group of AAPM[1] advocates using Equation 3.25 for $G(r, \theta)$ and offers recommended tabulated values for $F(r, \theta)$ and polynomial expressions for $g(r)$ (see Table 11-3).

In situations where a large number of randomly oriented seeds are implanted, it is feasible to further simplify Equation 3.27 by averaging $\dot{D}(r, \theta_0)$ over the polar angle θ. This results in the one-dimensional expression:

$$\dot{D}(r) = S_K \ (d) \ \Lambda \ \frac{G(r, \theta_0)}{G(r_0, \theta_0)} \ g(r)\phi_{an}(r) \quad (3.28)$$

where $\phi_{an}(r)$ is the quotient of the average dose rate (with respect to θ) at distance r by $\dot{D}(r, \theta_0)$. Because $\phi_{an}(r)$ depends only weekly on r, one can go a step further and replace $\phi_{an}(r)$ with its average value, $\overline{\phi_{an}}$ (Table 11-5).

If one makes use of the *tissue attenuation factor*, $T(r)$, then (see Equation 3.19):

$$\dot{D}_w(r, \theta_0) = \dot{K}_w(r, \theta_0)T(r) = \underbrace{\dot{K}_a(r, \theta_0)\left(\frac{\mu_{en}}{\rho}\right)_a^w}_{\dot{K}_w(r, \theta_0)} T(r)$$

$$\approx \underbrace{S_K(d) \ G(r, \theta_0)}_{\dot{K}_a(r, \theta_0)}\left(\frac{\mu_{en}}{\rho}\right)_a^w T(r) \quad (3.29)$$

where K_a stands for air kerma in vacuo. This expression is only an approximation because $G(r, \theta_0)$ refers to a bare source in air. With this:

$$\dot{D}_w(r, \theta) = S_K(d)\left(\frac{\mu_{en}}{\rho}\right)_a^w T(r) \ \left[G(r, \theta)F(r, \theta)\right]$$

$$(3.30)$$

Polynomial fits to the data on $g(r)$, $F(r, \theta)$ or $T(r)$ are available for a variety of sources.[1,5,6,11-20]

Measurement of Absorbed Dose in Brachytherapy

Although, strictly speaking, absorbed dose is not a measurable quantity, measurements of dose distribution are performed because, at least in principle, the only quantity one needs is a calibration factor (dosimeter signal per unit dose) for the detector employed. Experimental dosimetry is problematical for a number of reasons, for instance:

a. The dose is defined at a point, yet the sensitive volume of any detector has finite dimensions. Unless one knows that the measurement takes place in a region where the dose does not depend on position, the quantity determined is the average dose in that site. In situations where there are sharp spatial gradients in dose, this may not be a satisfactory situation. Low-energy brachytherapy sources are, of course, a classical example: for instance, in the point-source approximation the dose rate 1 cm away from a ^{125}I seed will vary by a factor of almost 5 per cm.

b. The size of the sensitive volume (ideally, negligibly small) is limited by the requirement that it yield a measurable signal. This becomes a problem (again, in brachytherapy) for low-dose-rate sources. The infrequent use of ionization chambers in brachytherapy is a direct result of this dilemma.

c. The dose depends on the local energy fluence of ionizing particles, Equations 3.5 and 3.6. But the dosimeter, unless manufactured from a material that matches the medium of interest (tissue or water), may change the particle fluence at the point of interest.

d. The detector response (D_{det}) must be converted to dose to water, D_{water}, (or tissue) in the absence of the detector. This creates a problem when the ratios*:

$$\frac{D_{water}}{D_{det}} = \left\{\int_0^\infty dE_u \ E_u \ \Phi_u(\vec{r}, E_u)\left(\frac{\mu_{en}(E_u)}{\rho}\right)\right\}_{detector}^{water}$$

$$(3.31)$$

---

*A more general expression is[191]

$$\frac{D_{det}}{D_{water}} = (1 - d)\left\{\int_0^\infty dE_u E_u \Phi_u(\vec{r}, E_u)\left(\frac{\mu_{en}(E_u)}{\rho}\right)\right\}_{water}^{det}$$

$$+ d\left\{\int_0^\infty dE \ \Phi(\vec{r}, E)\left[-\frac{1}{\rho} S(E)\right]\right\}_{water}^{det}$$

where *d* is a parameter that represents the fraction of detector response due to secondary charged particles originating in the medium and which depends on the cavity size.
†This equation is applicable under the continuous slowing down approximation (CSDA).
‡The detector must also be small relative to the range of the charged particles present in the radiation field.

for a detector large enough to satisfy the conditions of charged-particle equilibrium, or[†]

$$\frac{D_{water}}{D_{\text{det}}} = \left\{ \int_0^\infty dE \, \Phi(\vec{r}, E) \left[-\frac{1}{\rho} S(E) \right] \right\}_{air}^{water} \quad (3.32)$$

for a Bragg-Gray detector (a detector that, by definition, does not change the fluence of charged particles in the surrounding medium[‡]; e.g., a small air cavity), depend on $\vec{r}$, in which case one has to know the energy fluence at each location $\vec{r}$. This problem is solved (or, more precisely, avoided) with the aid of an energy correction factor, $E(\vec{r})$, which gives—as a function of distance and source type—the detector response, $DR(\vec{r})$, relative to the dose in water, $D_w(\vec{r})$ at the same location. In practice, one calculates $E(\vec{r})$ for a given source relative to $E(\vec{r})$ for a calibration beam (e.g., ^{60}Co). Thus:

$$E_{rel}(\vec{r}) = \frac{\left[E(\vec{r}) \right]_{brachy}}{\left[E(\vec{r}) \right]_{calibr}} = \frac{\left\{ DR(\vec{r}) \, / \, D_w(\vec{r}) \right\}_{brachy}}{\left\{ DR(\vec{r}) \, / \, D_w(\vec{r}) \right\}_{calibr}}$$
$$(3.33)$$

$E_{rel}(\vec{r})$ can be measured or calculated.[21] The calibration factor, $\left\{ DR(\vec{r}) \, / \, D_w(\vec{r}) \right\}_{calibr}$, is determined experimentally and the dose to water for the brachytherapy source is obtained from:

$$D_w(\vec{r}) = \frac{DR(\vec{r}) \, / \, E_{rel}(\vec{r})}{\left\{ DR(\vec{r}) \, / \, D_w(\vec{r}) \right\}_{calibr}} \quad (3.34)$$

e. Some detectors have additional problems such as anisotropic response or dose-rate and temperature dependence of the signal.

Dosimeters commonly used in brachytherapy include solid-state detectors (thermoluminescent chips, semiconductor junctions), radiographic film, GAF-radiochromic film and small-volume ionization chambers. Some of their properties are now described.

THERMOLUMINESCENT DETECTORS (TLD)

Thermoluminescent dosimeters are being extensively used for the dosimetry of practically all brachytherapy sources. This includes ^{192}Ir,[22-26] [125]I,[27-37] [103]Pd,[38,39] and [137]Cs.[40]

Spatial resolution: TLD chips come in various sizes, for instance cubes ($1 \times 1 \times 1$ mm³), ribbons ($3.1 \times 3.1 \times 0.2$ mm³), or disks (of 0.13 mm thickness), and thus provide good spatial resolution.

Sensitivity (relative to an air-filled ion chamber)[41]: 0.12

Energy response (TLD dose relative to water dose): changes from 1.4 at 30 keV to 1 at 300 keV[41]; this is due to the predominance of photoelectric effect at low energies and the subsequent sensitivity to the effective atomic number of the detecting material (for TLD, $Z_{eff} = 5.7$). There is no variation with energy outside this range of energies. For ^{125}I, the interactions of which are dominated by photoelectric effect, E_{rel} is independent of distance and

equal to 1.40. For ^{192}Ir, $E(\vec{r})$ changes from 1.008 at 1 cm to 1.08 at 10 cm.[21,24]

SILICON DIODE

Because of their rather sharp (see below) energy response, silicon diodes have been used mostly for low-energy sources[42,43] (^{125}I and [103]Pd) for which the energy spectrum does not change as a function of distance.[44]

Spatial resolution: The active volume of a Si diode can have a thickness as small as several tens of μm, with total thickness of 1 mm or less and diameters of the order of mm.

Sensitivity (relative to an air-filled ion chamber)[41]: 17,000.

Energy response (diode dose relative to water dose): Because of its comparatively large atomic numbers ($Z_{eff} = 14$), the silicon diode response at low energies ($\approx$30 keV) relative to ^{137}Cs is larger by a factor of 7 to 8 (for ^{192}Ir this ratio is $\approx$1.5).[41] As reported by Perera et al. (*loc cit*), at 100 keV there is a difference of 100% in the energy response at 1 cm and at 10 cm; and this difference remains as high as 62% at ^{192}Ir energies. Thus, the Si diode cannot be used for relative dosimetry for intermediate-energy sources.

PLASTIC SCINTILLATOR

The use of plastic scintillators in brachytherapy is a relatively new development.[45-49] Dosimetric measurements have been reported for eye plaques (^{125}I or [106]Ru)[49] and [192]Ir.[50]

Spatial resolution: on the order of 1 mm³.
Sensitivity (relative to an air-filled ion chamber)[41]: 2.6
Energy response (plastic scintillator dose relative to water dose): The response of commercially available plastic scintillators (PS) matches quite closely the response of water at energy larger than 100 keV. At lower energies, polyvinyl toluene (PTV)–based PS under-respond by 30% to 60%; however, recent studies[47] indicate that the addition of compounds that contain elements with higher atomic numbers than PTV make the energy response of the PS constant within 10% over the 10 keV to 1 MeV range. A similar result obtains for $E(\vec{r})$.

RADIOCHROMIC FILM/GAFCHROMIC FILM

Radiochromic film (also known as GafChromic film) is a polymer containing radiosensitive dye bonded to a Mylar base. Radiochromic film dosimetry has been reviewed by the AAPM Radiation Therapy Committee Task Group No. 55.[51] Recent applications of this technique include dosimetric measurements of [125]I[52,53] and [192]Ir.[54,55] The main advantages of radiochromic film are: high spatial resolution, two-dimensional dose mapping, no postirradiation development processing necessary, low sensitivity to room light, and near tissue equivalence for higher energy photons and electrons (>100 keV). Known shortcomings are sensitivity to thermal history, time between exposure and densitometry and densitometer readout wavelength, as well as nonuniform distribution of the sensitive material over the Mylar base.[56]

Spatial resolution: sub-millimeter.

Energy response: The response of radiochromic film is about 30% to 40% lower at the energy of ^{125}I than at higher energies (e.g., ^{60}Co).[57-59]

IONIZATION CHAMBERS

The need to obtain a measurable signal sets a lower limit to the size of the air cavity in ionization chambers, and this in turn requires correction factors that take into account the nonuniform charged-particle fluence inside the cavity. Corrections can be made by referring the dose measurement to an *effective point of measurement* (different from the cavity center) or by correcting the dose measurement to represent the dose in water at its center. An example of this latter approach, as applied to dosimetric measurements for a ^{192}Ir source, can be found in Tolli and Johansson.[60]

Calculation of Absorbed Dose Distributions

Many problems that may affect dose measurements (in particular, the need to establish charged-particle equilibrium when the Bragg-Gray conditions do not obtain) can be avoided by resorting to calculated dose distributions. To perform dose calculations, one needs information on the geometry and physical composition of radiation sources and absorbing material, as well as on the relevant interaction cross sections. Other than using simplified theoretical assessments (e.g., the Sievert integral), dose calculations are being performed with the aid of two methods, termed *deterministic* and *stochastic*.

In the *deterministic* approach, given sources and boundary conditions, a transport equation is solved to obtain the phase space density of particles (at any point in space) with respect to energy and angle. For instance, the classical form of the transport equation for a single type of particle is[3,61]:

$$\frac{1}{v}\frac{\partial \varphi}{\partial t} + \vec{u} \cdot \vec{\nabla}\varphi + \mu_T \varphi$$

$$= \int_0^\infty dE' \int_{4\pi} d\vec{u}' \left[\mu_s(E' \rightarrow E, \vec{u}' \rightarrow \vec{u}) \cdot \varphi \right] + s \quad (3.35)$$

where: $\varphi(\vec{r}, E, \vec{u}, t)$ is the flux density distribution with respect to energy, E, and direction (unit vector $\vec{u}$) at position $\vec{r}$ and time t; $\mu_T(\vec{r}, E)$ is the probability per unit path length of a particle at $\vec{r}$ and with energy E to have an interaction; $\mu_s(E \rightarrow E', \vec{u} \rightarrow \vec{u}')dE'd\vec{u}'$ is the probability per unit distance traveled that a particle with E and $\vec{u}$ will produce, as a result of interaction at $\vec{r}$, a particle (including the primary one itself, i.e., scattering) with energy E' and direction $\vec{u}'$. It is important to remember that this equation refers only to average values and is simply a mathematic expression of the balance between different mechanisms by which particles are gained or lost from the volume of interest.

Results of deterministic calculations by Berger[62] and Loevinger[63] have been used, for instance, by Meisberger et al.[5] to obtain polynomial fits to the tissue attenuation factors, T(r), of Equation 3.30. Equation 3.6, to give

another example, was obtained by solving a transport equation such as the expression, Eq (3.35).

The other (and more popular) approach is *stochastic simulation* of particle trajectories using *Monte Carlo techniques*. Essentially, this method is preferred to the deterministic one (which is simpler) because of the difficulty in the latter of treating complicated source-receptor geometries. The Monte Carlo approach is a collection of mathematic techniques for sampling values of a random variable, x, given its cumulative distribution function, F(x).[64,65] By way of illustration, the simplest such method proceeds as follows*:

1. Select a random number, ξ, between 0 and 1 (a random number generator is standard software on most computers),
2. From $F(x) = \xi$, calculate $x = F^{-1}(x)$.

A notable application of this algorithm is the calculation of the free-flight distance, s, of a particle interacting with a medium, which is a standard step in any Monte Carlo transport code. The probability distribution of s is:

$$f(s)\,ds = \sum_{tot} e^{-\Sigma_{tot} s} ds \quad (3.36)$$

where Σ_{tot} is the total *macroscopic interaction cross section* (= volume density of scattering centers multiplied by the cross section). Thus:

$$F(s) = 1 - e^{-\Sigma_{tot} s} \quad (3.37)$$

and $s = [\log(\xi)]/\Sigma_{tot}$.

Complete information on particle transport obtains in the so-called *event-by-event simulation*, where the positions of all scattering events (elastic or inelastic) are recorded for each ionizing track. Such information is needed for microdosimetric calculations.[66-68] Dosimetric calculations, on the other hand, do not need such complete information, and are usually performed by making certain simplifications, for instance by treating energy loss by charged particles within the continuous slowing down approximation (CSDA), or the angular deflection with multiple-scattering formulae. The medium is divided into sub-volumes (e.g., slabs) and the energy deposited in each segment is recorded.

Of the many computer codes available for photon-electron transport calculation by Monte Carlo methods [e.g., ETRAN,[62,69] MCNP,[70] EGS,[71] GEPTS[72]], we shall briefly discuss here only one—MCNP.

MCNP (which stands for Monte Carlo N-Particle) was developed at Los Alamos National Laboratory to simulate coupled neutron/photon/electron particle transport, primarily as a computational tool for weapon

---

*This algorithm obtains as follows: Let f(x) represent the density probability function of x. If f(x) is normalized to 1, the random variable

$$y = \int_{-\infty}^{x} f(x')dx'$$

is uniformly distributed in [0, 1]. Indeed, by definition, y = F(x) = Prob[X ≤ x]. Because F(x) is a monotonically non-decreasing function of x, it follows that Prob[F(x) ≤ F(x')] = Prob[x ≤ x'] = F(x'). Thus Prob[Y ≤ y] = y.

design. The latest version of this code (4b2) is applicable to photon and electron transport in the energy range of [1 keV-100 GeV] and [1 keV-1 GeV], respectively. Photon transport includes photoelectric effect, Thomson scattering, Compton scattering, and pair production. Bremsstrahlung photons are also included. Electron transport, which is simulated essentially in the same manner as in the ERTRAN code, occurs in a series of major and minor steps. Major steps are predetermined such that their path lengths (s_n, $n = 1, 2, \ldots$) satisfy $E_n/E_{n-1} = 1/2^{1/8}$; here E_n is the electron energy at the end of the nth step. A major step is further divided into a number of (user-selected) substeps. Electrons lose energy at a rate determined on the basis of the Landau energy-loss straggling; the energy loss is determined for each major step and is assumed to be equally distributed among substeps. Angular deflections are sampled (for each substep) from calculated multiple-scattering distributions. In a typical simulation one sets lower energy cutoffs (on the order of several keV), and particles below these energies are no longer transported. The code is attractive for brachytherapy simulations (and other medical physics applications) because it allows straightforward modeling and visualization of complicated geometrical structures (sources, applicators); for this purpose it makes use of intersections and unions of planes, cones, spheres, and cylinders. MCNP is equipped with software that calculates various quantities of interest. For instance, photon kerma is obtained by taking advantage of the fact that the fluence, $\Phi(\vec{r})$, (Equation A1, Appendix A) can be expressed as the sum of the track lengths, $\Sigma(l_i)$, of all particles that traverse a small volume, ΔV, centered at $\vec{r}$, per unit volume[73]:

$$\Phi(\vec{r}) = \frac{\sum_i l_i}{\Delta V} \qquad (3.38)$$

Thus, the code keeps score of the fluence distribution in energy of the photons, $\Phi(\vec{r}, E_u)$, and obtains kerma using its definition, Equation 3.8.

There is extensive literature describing the use of Monte Carlo transport techniques to evaluate dosimetric distributions in brachytherapy.[9,23-25,40,42,74-85] They are also used to determine calibration factors (detector response relative to absorbed dose) as a function of photon or electron energy and distance, for instance $E(\vec{r})$ of Equation 3.33. Other applications include the calculation of dose rate constants and radial dose functions (the TG-43 recommendations[1] are based, in part, on Monte Carlo calculations performed by Williamson.[74]

Calculation of the Mean Absorbed Dose

The formalism described so far refers to the dose *at a point* in matter. Quite generally, in radiation treatments the dose distribution in the human body is nonuniform. In certain situations (for instance, therapy with unsealed radionuclides such as ^{131}I, ^{32}P) the quantity of interest is the *average* dose in an organ in which the radioisotope is distributed *uniformly*, or in an adjacent healthy tissue. Methodology for such calculations is the subject of this section. We draw here on the treatment given to this subject in section 9 of the NCRP Report No. 108.[3]

Consider a source domain, S, of volume V_S and a target domain, T, of volume V_T, both embedded in an extended medium of density ρ. ("Extended" refers to the situation where boundaries do not affect the dosimetry in T.) Next, let E(r) represent the average energy imparted, *per decay*, by a point source to a spherical volume of radius r centered at the source. With the aid of this quantity, termed *integral isotropic point source kernel*, the average dose rate in V_T can be formally calculated from:

$$\overline{\frac{dD_T(t)}{dt}} = \frac{\alpha(t)}{V_T} \int_{V_T} dV_T \int_{V_S} \frac{dE(r)}{dr} \frac{dV_S}{4\pi r^2} \qquad (3.39)$$

In this expression $\alpha(t)$ is the specific activity (activity per unit mass) in S at time t, and r is the distance between dV_S and dV_T. Because the integrand depends only on r, it is possible to reduce the double (six-dimensional) integral to a single-dimensional integral over r:

$$\overline{\frac{dD_T(t)}{dt}} = \alpha(t)V_S \int_0^\infty \frac{dE(r)}{dr} \frac{p_{ST}(r)}{4\pi r^2} dr \qquad (3.40)$$

The function $p_{ST}(r)$ is the *point-pair distance distribution* of V_S relative to V_T; it is the probability that two random points—one in S and the other in T—are separated by a distance in [r, r + dr]. A related quantity is the geometric reduction factor[62,86]:

$$U_{ST}(r) = V_T \frac{p_{ST}(r)}{4\pi r^2} \qquad (3.41)$$

Typically, point-pair distribution functions are calculated using Monte Carlo techniques.[87-89] However, for a number of simple volumes, analytic expressions exist.[3,90,91] For instance, if S and T are spheres of radius R and if they coincide:

$$U(r) = 1 - \frac{3r}{4R} + \frac{r^3}{16R^3} \quad r \in [0, 2R] \qquad (3.42)$$

Calculations of isotropic point-source kernels for photons and electrons have been published.[69,86]

As a simple illustration, consider the problem of evaluating the average dose in a sphere (radius R) containing low-energy photon emitters (energy E_γ), and let α represent the specific activity. Assume further that:

$$\frac{dE(r)}{dr} = \mu E_\gamma e^{-\mu r} \qquad (3.43)$$

where μ is the linear attenuation coefficient. From Equations 3.40-3.42, one obtains:

$$\overline{\frac{dD(t)}{dt}} = \alpha(t)E_\gamma \left[1 - \frac{3}{4}\frac{1}{(\mu R)} + \frac{3}{8}\frac{1}{(\mu R)^3} \right. $$
$$\left. - e^{2(\mu R)}\left(\frac{3}{8}\frac{1}{(\mu R)^3} + \frac{3}{4}\frac{1}{(\mu R)^2} \right) \right] \qquad (3.44)$$

This expression can be used for an electron-emitting source (energy E_e) provided that the electron range is much smaller than R. Thus, by taking the limit of $\mu \to \infty$:

$$\frac{\overline{dD(t)}}{dt} = \alpha(t)E_e \qquad (3.45)$$

The total average dose delivered in the time interval [0, t] is obtained in the usual manner:

$$\overline{D(t)} = \frac{1}{\lambda_{eff}} \frac{\overline{dD(0)}}{dt}\left(1 - e^{-\lambda_{eff}t}\right) \qquad (3.46)$$

where λ_{eff} is the effective decay constant (the sum of the physical, λ, and biological, λ_B, decay constants). This is not the place for a detailed account of the biodistribution kinetics responsible for the value of λ_B; however, the interested reader is referred to the MIRD Primer for Absorbed Dose Calculations[92] and related publications.[93-102]

MICRODOSIMETRY

Synopsis

The absorbed dose represents the *average* energy imparted per unit mass to a cell, but the *actual* energy deposited is a random *(stochastic)* quantity. If the biological effect were proportional to the energy absorbed, the average energy (and thus, dose) would be sufficient to determine the average effect. However, for most radiation-induced biologic effects proportionality does not obtain and thus—in order to correlate properties of the radiation field to biologic effect—one must know the probability distribution of energy deposition in cells. *Microdosimetry* is the study and quantification of the spatial and temporal distribution of absorbed energy in irradiated matter. The two basic concepts of microdosimetry are the *event* (energy deposition by a charged particle and its statistically correlated particles, e.g., δ rays from the same track), and *specific energy* (z), which is the energy deposition occurring in a volume within irradiated matter per unit mass.

An important result of microdosimetric theory is the *linear-quadratic (LQ) equation*, $E(D) = \alpha D + \beta D^2$, which relates probability of effect, $E(D)$, to the delivered dose, D. The ratio α/β can be calculated *ab initio* if the geometry of the sensitive site and the microdosimetric spectrum of the radiation field are known. Within the LQ formulation the *relative biologic effectiveness (RBE)* of radiation H (α_H, β_H) relative to radiation L (α_L, β_L) is given by:

$$RBE(D_H) = \frac{\alpha_L}{2\beta_L D_H}\left[\sqrt{1 + \frac{4\beta_L(\alpha_H D_H + \beta_H D_H^2)}{\alpha_L^2}} - 1\right]$$

Another consequence of microdosimetry is the result that the magnitude of the quadratic term in dose (βD^2), but not the linear one, depends on dose rate. This is formalized as $E(D) = \alpha D + q(t)\beta D^2$ where the function q(t), termed *dose-rate factor*, can be calculated for any temporal pattern of dose delivery. For instance, for irradiation at a constant dose rate over time t: $q(r) = \frac{2}{r} - \frac{2}{r^2}\left(1 - e^{-r}\right)$, where r = t/$t_0$ and t_0 represents a characteristic repair time for sublethal damage (typically 0.5 to 1 hour).

Brachytherapy physics is concerned with electrons (whether primary or secondary), and at low doses or low dose rates the RBE of low-energy photons relative to ^{60}Co radiation may exceed 2.

The use of the quantity *absorbed dose* in radiologic physics—brachytherapy included—is predicated on the notion that when its numerical value is the same, irradiation of equal objects results in equal effects. In fact, most biologic effects of radiation depend on the (highly nonuniform) macroscopic pattern of energy deposition,* and the absorbed dose is merely the expected value (microscopic average of energy deposited per unit mass. That the same

dose of radiation may result in vastly different effects, when delivered by different types of radiation, is well documented. For instance, at low doses the RBE of neutrons relative to gamma rays (see Fig. 11-7 for the definition of RBE) to induce a cell to become malignant is on the order of 100, which means that the ratio of absorbed doses of gamma rays and neutrons causing equal effects is about 100.[103-112]

Brachytherapy physics is concerned with electrons, whether primary or secondary as in the case of photon sources, but even in this case at low doses or low *dose rates*, the RBE of 100 keV photons relative to, say, 1-MeV photons may exceed 2.[76,77] For instance, the RBE for ^{125}I

---

*It may be helpful to emphasize that, unlike pharmacology, where "dose" refers to the amount of agent administered to the patient, the physical quantity absorbed dose relates to the energy actually *deposited* in the biologic receptor.

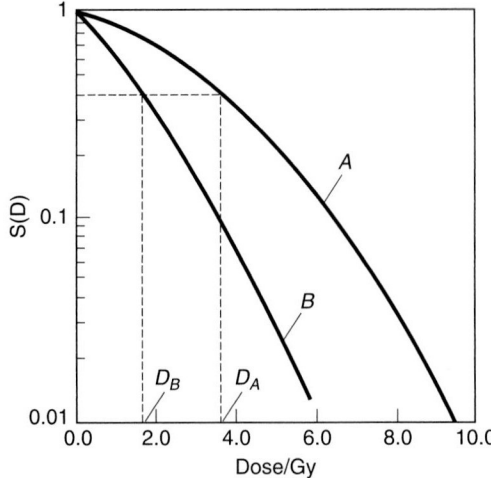

Figure 11–7. The relative biologic effectiveness (RBE) is used to compare the effects of two radiations. Let D_A and D_B represent, respectively, doses of radiations A and B that result in the same probability of cellular effect—in this figure, survival probability S(D). Then, by definition, RBE of radiation B relative to the reference radiation A (usually high-energy photons) is given by: RBE = D_A/D_B. (From Zaider M, Rossi HH: *Radiation Science for Physicians and Public Health Workers*. New York: Kluwer Academic/Plenum Publishers; 2001)

has been extensively studied and results of 1.2 to 2 have been reported for the dose-rate range of 0.03 to 9 Gy/h.[113] Similarly, for [103]Pd a study performed at 0.07 to 0.8 Gy/h reported RBE values of 1.9 ± 0.7.[113-116] While considerably lower RBE values apply to the much higher doses or dose rates usually employed in external radiotherapy, differences in biologic effectiveness on the order of 10% to 15% remain.

Fundamentally, RBE ≠ 1 because the radiation effect on cells is not proportional to the energy deposited in the radiation-sensitive site. Indeed, if

$$Effect \propto z \qquad (4.1)$$

[z = specific energy (see Equation 3.2)], it would follow that, on average:

$$\overline{Effect} \propto \overline{z} = D \qquad (4.2)$$

On the other hand, if, for instance:

$$Effect \propto z^2 \qquad (4.3)$$

then:

$$\overline{Effect} \propto \overline{z^2} \neq (\overline{z})^2 = D^2 \qquad (4.4)$$

This means that in order to obtain a physical predictor of biologic effect, one needs information on the distribution of specific energy, z. *Microdosimetry* is the study and quantification of the *spatial* and *temporal* distribution of absorbed energy in irradiated matter.[117-121] One makes a distinction between *regional microdosimetry*— the object of which is the study of microdosimetric distributions, *f(z)—and* structural *microdosimetry*, a mathematically more advanced approach that is concerned with characterizing the spatial distribution of individual energy deposition events (ionizations, excitations, or both). Regional microdosimetry asserts that the effect is entirely determined by the amount of specific energy deposited

in the relevant site (typically, a cell nucleus). The two "kinds" of microdosimetry, *regional* and *structural*, were shown, in fact, to be mathematically equivalent—once the sensitive site is judiciously determined.[122] In the following, the aim is to give a brief summary of the principles of microdosimetry, and some examples applicable to brachytherapy.

Spatial Elements

The basic concept of microdosimetry is the *microdosimetric event* (or simply, *event*), which is energy deposition by a charged particle and its statistically correlated particles (e.g., secondary electrons from the same particle track). Events are important because they are statistically independent entities. The principal microdosimetric quantity, specific energy, z, was defined earlier in this chapter, in *Dosimetry, Conceptual Matters* and Appendix A. A second (physically equivalent) quantity is the *lineal energy*, which is the quotient of ε by l, where ε is the energy imparted to matter in a volume of interest by an energy deposition event, and l is the mean chord length in that volume:

$$y = \frac{\varepsilon}{\overline{l}} \qquad (4.5)$$

In this definition ε refers to energy deposition imparted in a *single event*, a restriction that does not apply to z.

In matter of mass density ρ, the relationship between z (in a single event) and y is:

$$z = \frac{4y}{\rho S} \qquad (4.6)$$

This follows from a theorem by Cauchy,[123] according to which the mean chord length, $\overline{l}$, in a convex site is given by $4V/S$, where V and S are, respectively, the volume and surface area of the site. For a spherical site of diameter d:

$$\overline{l} = \frac{2}{3}d \qquad (4.7)$$

and thus:

$$z = \frac{4y}{\pi d^2 \rho} \qquad (4.8)$$

which, for ρ = 1 g/cm³ and with units as indicated, becomes:

$$\frac{z}{Gy} = \frac{0.204}{\left(\dfrac{d}{\mu m}\right)^2}\frac{y}{keV/\mu m} \qquad (4.9)$$

The probability that the lineal energy delivered in *single* events is in the interval [y, y + dy] is f(y)dy. The corresponding distribution in z is $f_1(z)dz$, where the subscript makes explicit the fact that this distribution refers to single events only. The distributions f(z), $f_1(z)$, and f(y) depend on the geometry of the site where specific energy is determined. Two moments of these distributions that are often invoked are the *frequency average*, y_F

(or z_F), and the *dose average*, y_D (or z_D). They are defined as follows:

$$y_F = \int_0^\infty y f(y) dy \qquad z_F = \int_0^\infty z f_1 dz$$

$$z_D = \frac{1}{y_F} \int_0^\infty y^2 f(y) dy \qquad z_D = \frac{1}{z_F} \int_0^\infty z^2 f_1(z) dz \qquad (4.10)$$

The first and second moments of the multi-event distribution, $f(z)$, are denoted $\bar{z}$ and $\overline{z^2}$, respectively. Because, by definition, $D = \bar{z}$, the average number of events, n, at dose D is:

$$n = \frac{D}{z_F} \qquad (4.11)$$

At a given dose, D, or equivalently n, the distribution $f(z)$ is determined uniquely by $f_1(z)$. This can be understood from the following argument: The probability of exactly v events is given by the Poisson distribution:

$$p(v, n) = e^{-n} \frac{n^v}{v!} \qquad (4.12)$$

If we denote by $f_v(z)$ the distribution of z in *exactly* v events then, because by definition events are statistically independent, $f_v(z)$ can be evaluated by successive iterations:

$$f_0(z) = \delta(z)$$

$$f_1(z) \equiv f_1(z)$$

$$f_2(z) = \int_0^\infty f_1(z') f_1(z - z') dz' \qquad (4.13)$$

$$\cdots$$

$$f_v(z) = \int_0^\infty f_1(z') f_{v-1}(z - z') dz'$$

The distribution $f(z)$ becomes:

$$f(z) = \sum_{v=0}^\infty p(v; n)\, f_v(z) \qquad (4.14)$$

In order to obtain a quantity that relates to biologic effect, one must postulate a functional dependence of effect probability on specific energy. One such approach, the Theory of Dual Radiation Action,[124] takes as its starting point the empirical observation that for numerous effects, the yield of *lesions* (alterations responsible for the end point observed) depends quadratically on specific energy:

$$E(z) = \beta z^2 \qquad (4.15)$$

where β is a positive constant found to be only weakly dependent on radiation quality. The form of this equation obtains by postulating that a lesion is the result of two molecular *sublesions*, produced each at a rate proportional to z. On average

$$\overline{E(D)} = \beta \overline{z^2} = \beta(z_D D + D^2) \qquad (4.16)$$

The last step follows from Equations 4.13 and 4.14.[120] The expression, Equation 4.16, is the familiar *linear-quadratic equation*; in a more familiar notation:

$$\overline{E(D)} = \alpha D + \beta D^2 \qquad (4.17)$$

Thus:

$$z_D = \frac{\alpha}{\beta} \qquad (4.18)$$

Although not strictly valid,[125] it is possible to extend this formulation to the probability of cellular survival [reproductive inactivation, S(D)] by making the assumptions that (a) one lesion inactivates the cell, and (b) the number of lesions produced is Poisson-distributed. When valid (mostly for low-LET radiation) it leads to:

$$S(D) = e^{-\alpha D - \beta D^2} \qquad (4.19)$$

Examples of sublesions are single chromosome breaks that combine to produce a dicentric aberration (Fig. 11-8), or single-strand DNA breaks that, when in close proximity, result in double-stranded DNA breaks. The expression, Equation 4.18, provides the link between the microdosimetric quantity, z_D, and the dose-effect coefficients, α and β.

Within the linear-quadratic formulation, the RBE of radiation $H(\alpha_H, \beta_H)$ relative to radiation $L(\alpha_L, \beta_L)$ is given by[126-128]

$$RBE(D_H) = \frac{\alpha_L}{2\beta_L D_H}\left[\sqrt{1 + \frac{4\beta_L(\alpha_H D_H + \beta_H D_H^2)}{\alpha_L^2}} - 1\right] \qquad (4.20)$$

Note that the RBE is a decreasing function of D_H. If $\beta_H \cong \beta_L$, and taking Equation 4.20 into account, one obtains the simplified expression:

$$RBE = \frac{1}{2D_H}\left[\sqrt{z_{D,L}^2 + 4D_H(z_{D,H}^2 + D_H)} - z_{D,L}\right] \qquad (4.21)$$

If, furthermore, $\beta_H = \beta_L \approx 0$, the RBE is independent of dose:

$$RBE = \frac{\alpha_H}{\alpha_L} \approx \frac{z_{D,H}}{z_{D,L}} = \frac{y_{D,H}}{y_{D,L}} \qquad (4.22)$$

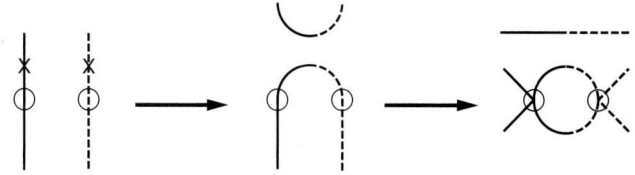

Figure 11-8. Illustration of the mechanism that leads to the formation of a dicentric chromosome aberration. The ends left by the two breaks *(left)* join to form a structure with two centromeres *(center)*. The other two pieces remain acentric. Following chromatid duplication, the chromosome takes the shape shown on the right. The dicentric is the easiest aberration to score and, not surprisingly, the best studied. (From Zaider M, Rossi HH: *Radiation Science for Physicians and Public Health Workers.* New York: Kluwer Academic/Plenum Publishers; 2001.)

The efficacy of radiotherapy is generally considered to depend on the probability of cell killing, 1-S(D). Because RBE depends nonlinearly on absorbed dose, both the absorbed dose and (through z_D) the microdosimetric properties of the radiation field must be known at locations in the tumor and in the surrounding healthy tissues.

Temporal Elements

The temporal pattern of dose delivery, an important parameter in radiotherapy, further changes the expressions derived thus far. To fix ideas, consider the archetypical lesion, a chromosomal dicentric aberration (see Fig. 11-8), which obtains when two single-chromosome breaks (sublesions) misjoin. A pair of sublesions can be produced by a single track (single event) or by two independent tracks. The yield of lesions that result via the first mechanism (termed *intratrack* action) is proportional to dose because the number of events is proportional to dose. In contrast, and for analogous reasons, the second mechanism (*intertrack* action) generates lesions at a rate proportional to D^2. The two mechanisms are represented in Equations 4.17 and 4.19 by the linear (αD) and quadratic (βD^2) terms, respectively.

An important consequence of this interpretation is the fact that the magnitude of the quadratic term (but not the linear one) depends on dose rate. Indeed, in most cases sublesions undergo repair, and thus the lower the dose rate (i.e., the larger the [average] time interval that separates the formation of the two sublesions), the lower the yield of inter-track lesions. With this, the linear-quadratic equation becomes:

$$\overline{E(D)} = \alpha D + \beta\, q(t)D^2 \qquad (4.23)$$

where q(t) is a function—termed *dose-rate factor*—that modifies the quadratic term to account for the temporal distribution of dose.[129] The effect of q(t) on survival probability is illustrated in Fig. 11-9.

Mathematic expressions for the function q(t) can be obtained for practically any temporal pattern of dose delivery.[130] It is commonly assumed that during the time interval, t, repair eliminates sublesion damage according to $\exp(-t/t_0)$, with t_0 being a characteristic time required for repair (typically on the order of 1 hour). For instance[126]:

a. For irradiations at a constant dose rate:

$$q(r) = \frac{2}{r} - \frac{2}{r^2}\left(1 - e^{-r}\right) \qquad (4.24)$$

where $r = t/t_0$. In particular, when $t \gg t_0$:

$$q \cong \frac{2t_0}{t} \qquad (4.25)$$

b. For *f* well-separated fractions (complete sublesion repair in between fractions):

$$q = \frac{1}{f} \qquad (4.26)$$

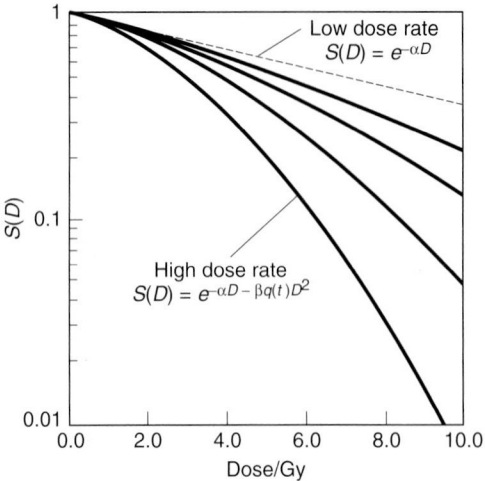

Figure 11–9. As the dose rate is progressively lowered, the term quadratic in dose, $\beta q(t)D^2$, grows smaller. Accordingly, the survival curve becomes increasingly less concave. At the limit of very low dose rates, only the term linear in dose, αD, remains *(dashed line)*. (From Zaider M, Rossi HH: *Radiation Science for Physicians and Public Health Workers.* New York: Kluwer Academic/Plenum Publishers; 2001.)

In a typical *low-dose-rate* (LDR) treatment in brachytherapy, the total irradiation time is on the order of several days and therefore $q \approx 0$. It follows that the probability of cell survival, $S(D)$, is quasi-exponential, and the RBE is determined by the linear (α) coefficient—or in microdosimetric terms, by z_D.

In *high-dose-rate* (HDR) brachytherapy the dose rate is on the order of 1.5 Gy/min; for a prescription dose of, say, 6 Gy and taking $t_0 = 60$ minutes, one obtains q = 0.978. Thus, both terms, linear (αD) and quadratic (βD^2), contribute significantly. HDR brachytherapy, which has the advantage of increased cell killing, is now used for treatment of various clinical sites[131-141] (e.g., the cervix, vagina, endometrium, rectum, esophagus, bronchus, head and neck, bile duct, brain, skin, prostate, breast, or for treatment of sarcomas and for intraoperative radiation therapy).

Microdosimetric Distributions

A compilation of microdosimetric distributions for radiations commonly employed in brachytherapy appears in Appendix C. Dose-averaged lineal energies, y_D, and RBE relative to ^{60}Co radiation for the spectra shown in Fig. 11-C2 (see Appendix C) are summarized in Table 11-6 (see above, *Practical Matters: Analytic Formalisms*).

Table 11–6 Dose-Averaged Lineal Energy for the Distributions Shown in Appendix C, Figure 11-C2

Radionuclide	y_D (keV/µm)	Relative Biological Effectiveness
^{103}Pd	3.8	2.3
^{125}I	3.5	2.1
^{241}Am	3.5	2.1
^{192}Ir	2.0	1.3
^{60}Co	1.6	1.0

DOSE PRESCRIPTION IN BRACHYTHERAPY

Synopsis

There is no generally accepted system of dose prescription in brachytherapy. As a result, dose prescription remains a vaguely defined notion and is often decided jointly by the clinician and physicist team during (rather than before) treatment planning. Three modalities of dose prescription are currently in use: (a) relative to the actual target, (b) relative to fixed-geometry applicators, and (c) relative to catheters placed in the target. Understanding the process of dose prescription also has legal implications because *misadministration* is defined relative to the *ordered dose*.

There appears to be no unanimously accepted system of dose prescription in brachytherapy. Methods of dose prescription vary with the site treated, the treatment modality, and often with the personal preferences of the medical team in charge. Strictly speaking, dose specification should not be a matter that belongs to this chapter; one would assume that the physicist is provided with directions as to the dose that must be delivered at any treatment location. In practice, dose prescription is a vaguely defined notion and is often decided jointly by the clinician and physicist team during (rather than before) the planning process. Understanding the process of dose prescription also has legal implications because misadministration is defined with respect to the "ordered dose." Unavoidably, the methodology for dose specification described as follows reflects, on occasion, accepted practice at my institution (Memorial Sloan-Kettering Cancer Center [MSKCC]).

Dose Prescription Relative to the Actual Target

Representative of this modality of dose prescription is the *minimum peripheral dose* (mPD), which is the largest dose isodose surface that completely surrounds the clinical target (Fig. 11-10). This approach has been endorsed by the American Brachytherapy Society.[142] A problem with using mPD is its sensitivity to minor variations in the planned dosimetry. The mPD for a target that is, say, 99.9% covered by the prescription dose, is still given by the dose delivered to the remaining 0.1% of the volume (if lesser than the prescription dose), however small. This problem may be avoided by relaxing the requirement that the prescription isodose surface covers 100% of the target; instead, one may adopt the so-called *Dx method*, which means that x% of the target volume will be treated to a dose of at least Dx. A typical value is D95 (D100 is, of course, the same as mPD).

The determination that mPD or, say, D95 were indeed achieved is made with the aid of *dose-volume histograms* (DVH), which tabulate as a function of dose, D, the probability that a randomly selected voxel volume receives a dose of at least D (this is, of course, the cumulative probability distribution of dose in the target volume). An example is given in Fig. 11-11, which shows the dose volume histogram as planned for a HDR prostate implant

with a ^{192}Ir source. In this instance D100 is 96% of the prescription dose (5.5 Gy) and D95 is 106% of the PD. (Note that for this plan mPD = 2.5 Gy.)

Dose Prescription Relative to a *Fixed-Geometry* Applicator

In this method an applicator in contact with the target is taken as system of reference for specifying the dose reference points. Examples are: (a) vaginal treatments with a HDR afterloader where the target surface points are defined relative to a plastic cylinder (Fig. 11-12), (b) postexcisional treatments of the tumor bed with a HAM applicator, where prescription points are at 0.5 cm from the applicator surface (Fig. 11-13), or (c) the treatment of ocular melanomas and pediatric retinoblastomas with eye plaques (prescription point is 3 to 10 mm along the central axis of the plaque, Fig. 11-14).

Another case in point is the Manchester system for the treatment of uterine cervix cancer. The applicator (Fig. 11-15) consists of an intrauterine tandem and two vaginal ovoids in which tubular sources (^{137}Cs) are

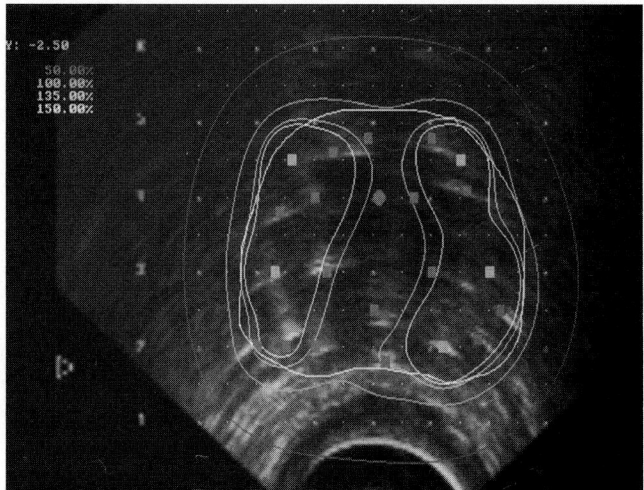

Figure 11–10. Planning for a permanent prostate implant. In this two-dimensional ultrasound image the *white line* delineates the prostate and the 100% isodose line (PD = 144 Gy) is shown in *green. Green dots* indicate occupied seeds and *red dots* show empty seed locations along needles. See also Color Figure 11–10.

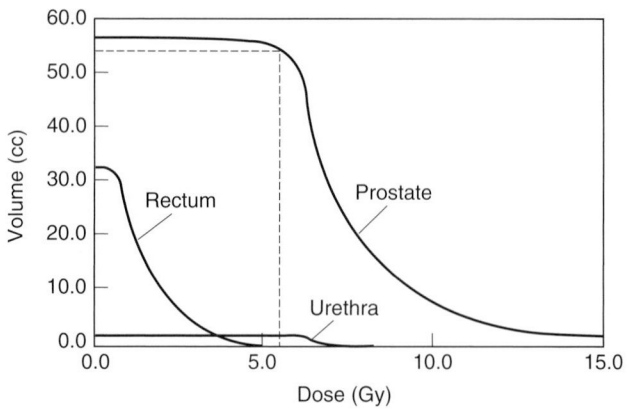

Figure 11–11. An example of dose volume histogram for a prostate high-dose-rate permanent implant.

Volume (cc) 52.9   Dose 5.5 Gy   100.0% Prescription

Structure	Volume (cc)	Max Dose (GY)	Min Dose (Gy)	Avg Dose (Gy)
Target	55.0	96.1	2.9	8.1
Urethra	2.0	14.7	5.5	6.7
Rectum	32.0	4.9	0.5	1.7

inserted. Planning is performed (in part) in relation to the dose rate at several points, which, in the so-called *New York Memorial system* (one of several such prescription methods) are defined as follows (Fig. 11-16): points A (labeled REF_L and REF_R) are 2 cm above the cervical os along the central axis of the uterus and 2 cm lateral (perpendicular) to this line; the uterine surface points (UTE) are 1 cm inferior to the tip of the tandem and 2 cm laterally; cervix points (CVX) are taken 1 cm above the cervical os and 1 cm laterally; the vaginal surface points (VG_1) on the surface of the ovoids. The average dose rate at point A (left and right), which determines the treatment time, should be between 55 and 60 cGy/hour. The plan, as performed at MSKCC with a Henshke applicator, includes obturator node points (OBT, close to the so-called B *point*); five rectal points (R_{1-5}) that are most nearly centered about the cervix longitudinally ($\approx$20 cGy/hour); a sigmoid colon point, SC, (halfway between the top of the tandem and the sacral promontorium); bladder center ($\approx$25 cGy/hour); bladder surface (closest to the cervical os, $\approx$45 cGy/hour); and vaginal mucosa, as delineated by the Foley balloon.

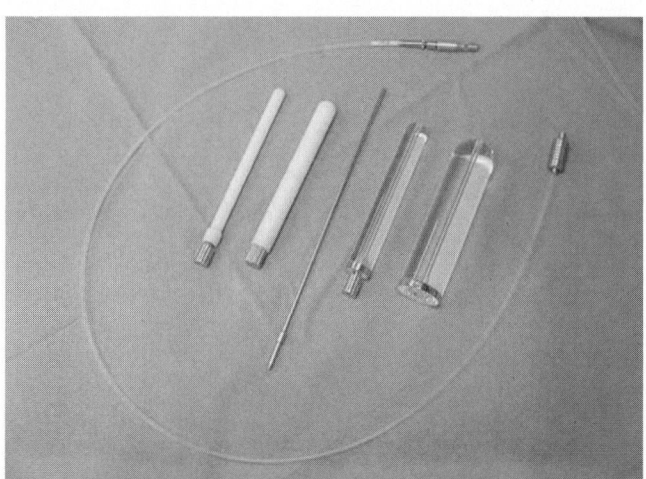

Figure 11–12. Cylindrical applicators used for high-dose-rate vaginal treatments. The hollow cylinders shown *(two on the right and two on the left)* are built to accommodate along their central axis a metal tube, or tandem *(shown in the middle)*, which is connected, via the source guide tube shown, to the remote afterloader.

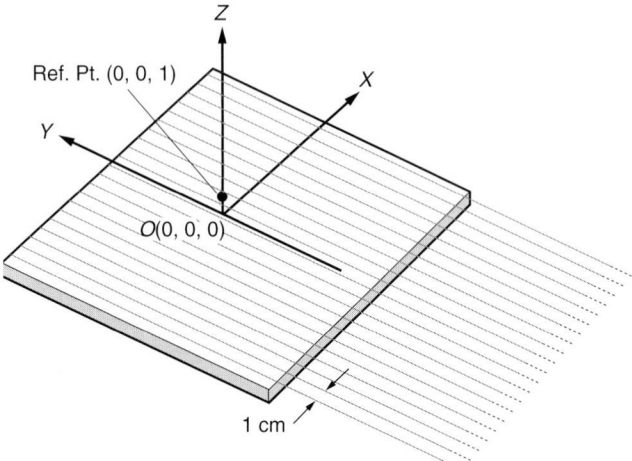

Figure 11–13. HAM applicator[143] used for high-dose-rate intraoperative radiation treatments. For further details, see the earlier section on temporal elements in dosimetry. (From Cohen G, Amols HA, Zaider M: An independent dose-to-point calculation program for the verification of high-dose-rate brachytherapy treatment planning. *Int J Radiat Oncol Biol Phys.* 2000;48:1251.)

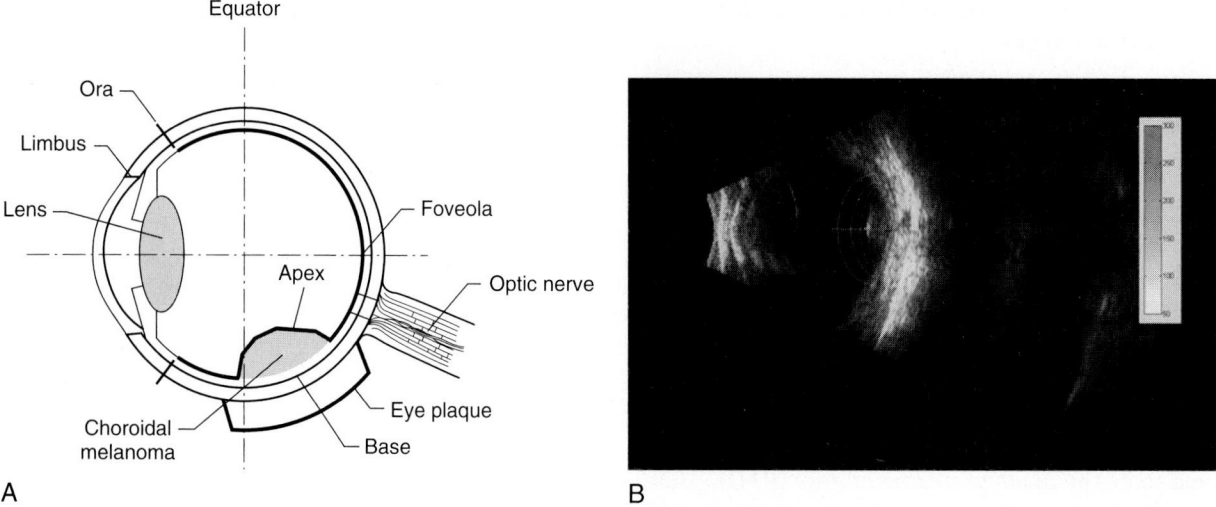

Figure 11–14. Schematic representation of an eye-plaque applicator (*left*, from 144). The right panel is an ultrasound image of an ocular tumor; also shown are isodose distributions. See also Color Figure 11–14B. (Left panel, from Chiu-Tsao S-T: I-125 Episcleral eye plaque for treatment of intra-ocular malignancies. In Williamson JF, Thomadsen BR, Nath R, eds., *Brachytherapy Physics, AAPM Summer School 1994.* Madison, Wisc: American Association of Physicists in Medicine; 1994:451.)

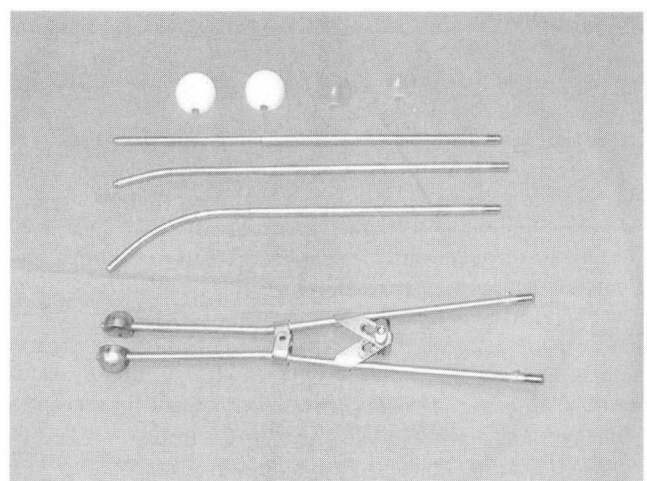

Figure 11–15. The Henshke applicator consists of an intrauterine tandem (three different shapes are shown) and two semi-spherical vaginal ovoids. See also Color Figure 11–15.

Figure 11–16. Reference prescription points for an intracavitary application of ^{137}Cs sources in a cervix applicator with shielded ovoids. (From Anderson LL, Nath R, Olch AJ, et al: American Endocurietherapy Society recommendations for dose specifications in brachytherapy. *Endocurietherapy Hypertherm Oncol.* 1991;7:1. **A,** adapted from Rosenstein LM: A simple computer program for optimization of source loading in cervical intracavitary applicators. *Br J Radiol.* 1977;50:119. **B,** from Anderson LL: Physical optimization of afterloading techniques. *Strahlentherapie.* 1985;161:264.)

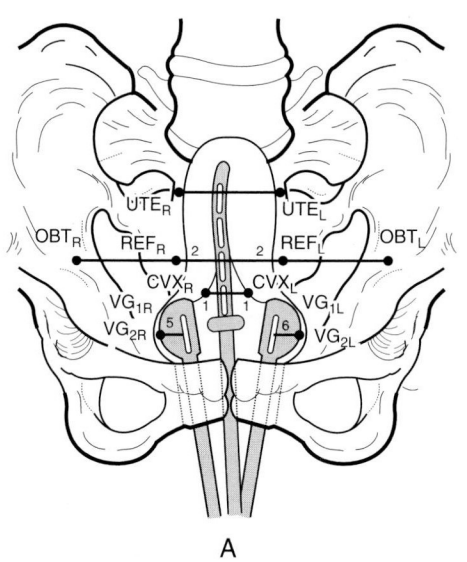

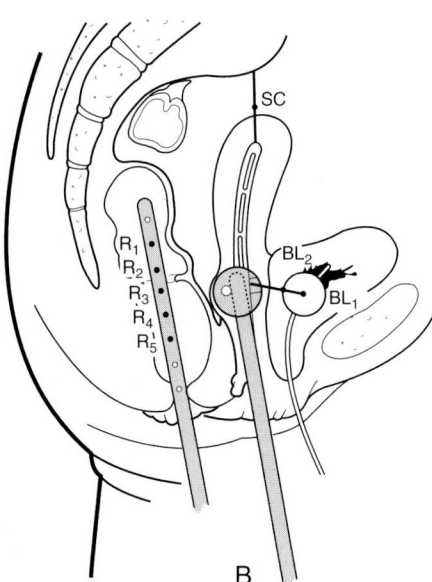

Dose Prescription Relative to Catheters Placed in the Target

When volume anatomic images of the target are not obtainable, it is helpful to take advantage of the fact that catheters placed in the patient at the time of surgery can be used to define the target volume relative to them. For instance, in an LDR treatment of soft tissue sarcoma the planning target (anatomically, the tumor bed) is delineated by a hull 0.5 cm away from the curvilinear plane defined by the mesh of catheters implanted in the OR (Fig. 11-17).

A plan is evaluated by considering on each slice (slices are roughly perpendicular to the catheter plane) the largest-dose continuous contour that covers the target volume adequately. These doses are quite likely different from slice to slice and their median value may be accepted to be the *planned treatment dose* (PTD). This is a reasonable (and accepted) approach to the treatment of sarcoma with radiation.[146]

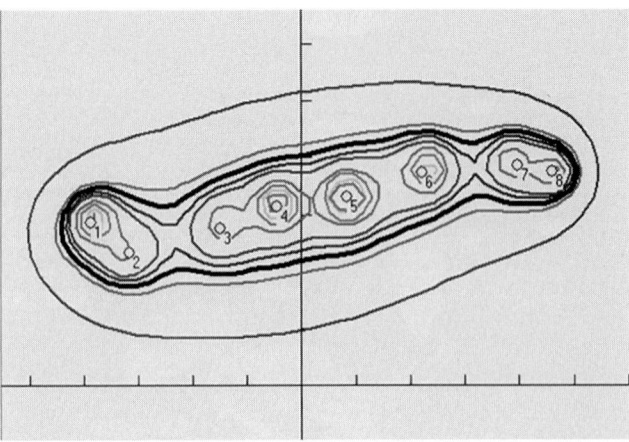

Figure 11–17. Planning for a sarcoma treatment: The heavy dark line surrounds all catheters and is taken as the prescription dose. See also Color Figure 11–17.

TREATMENT PLANNING

Synopsis

The treatment-planning sequence includes the following steps: (a) selection of appropriate sources, (b) localization of sources and catheters, (c) treatment plan design and evaluation, and (d) treatment plan verification. There are two criteria used in the selection of radioactive sources: (a) the particle energy and (b) the decay rate of the isotope. Low-energy sources are better from the radiation protection perspective and also in terms of flexibility in achieving the desired dose distribution. The main advantage of high-energy sources is that fewer of them may be needed to cover large volumes. A common procedure for source localization is to place inactive seeds into an applicator or catheters that were placed in the patient and then reconstruct the three-dimensional coordinates of the seeds from localization images. A second method consists of identifying potential source positions with respect to a template (e.g., for prostate implants).

Four treatment-planning methods are used in brachy-therapy: (a) nomograms, (b) precalculated plans, (c) trial-and-error (iterative methods), and (d) computer-based optimization. *Nomograms* are tables that, together with empirical implantation rules, indicate the total source strength needed to produce a particular dose distribution. Several systems are described as follows. The *Manchester system* is useful for sources with energy greater than 200 keV. It prescribes a pattern of sources claimed to result in 10% dose nonuniformity over the treatment volume. The *Quimby system* is applicable to high energy sources. It is a volume implant where source strength is distributed uniformly. The *Memorial system* is for low-energy photon sources (basically, ^{125}I and ^{103}Pd). The *Paris system* is a recipe for placing ^{192}Ir wires in the target volume in order to achieve a predictable level of dose uniformity. *Precalculated plans* are performed with fixed-geometry applicators (e.g., intravaginal tandem or intraoperative radiation therapy with HAM applicators). The *iterative method* entails finding—via successive adjustments—source strengths that generate the desired dose distribution. The most advanced treatment planning methodology makes use of *optimization algorithms* that automatically find optimal source positions which satisfy dosimetric constraints.

Overview

The process of treatment planning has two interconnected aspects: (a) defining and prescribing minimum doses in the target volume and the maximum dose in organs at risk, and (b) finding a source configuration that achieves, as closely as possible, the doses prescribed to these structures. The former is the role of the clinician, while the physicist carries out the latter. The treatment planning sequence includes the following steps:

a. Placement of applicator in patient (if needed)
b. Selection of appropriate sources (*)
c. Localization of sources or catheters (*)
d. Target volume and organs-at-risk designation
e. Dose prescription
f. Treatment plan design and evaluation (*)
g. Treatment plan verification
h. Post-treatment evaluation

The items marked with an asterisk are discussed as follows.

Selection of Suitable Radioactive Sources

Brachytherapy has four forms:

a. *Interstitial*, where sources are surgically placed into the malignant tissue; the implant can be permanent (sources: ^{125}I, ^{103}Pd) or temporary (sources: ^{125}I, ^{192}Ir).
b. *Intracavitary*, where sources are placed in applicators positioned inside body cavities, for instance in the

treatment of cancer of the cervix (tandem and ovoid applicators, see *Dose Prescription Relative to a Fixed-Geometry Applicator*), nasopharynx, endometrium or esophagus; this type of implant is always temporary and the radionuclides commonly used are ^{137}Cs or ^{192}Ir.

c. *Surface implants*, for instance for eye plaques, which are applicators with radioactive sources embedded in them and which are placed in direct contact with a body surface. Examples of sources used for surface applicators are: ^{90}Sr, ^{125}I, or ^{106}Ru.

d. *Intraoperative radiation therapy* uses HDR afterloaders connected to flab applicators or catheter arrays to treat the tumor bed immediately after cancer resection.

Two main criteria are used in the selection of appropriate radioactive sources: (a) the energy of the ionizing particle, and (b) the decay rate of the radionuclide.

Low-energy sources are better from the radiation protection perspective. In terms of achieving the desired dose distribution, they offer more flexibility (but more sources are needed) as well as improving on the avoidance of healthy critical structures. High-energy sources are typically used in interstitial implants where fewer sources may cover a larger volume.

Sources that have short half-lives (^{125}I, ^{103}Pd, ^{192}Ir) deliver—for the same total dose—a larger initial dose rate. Indeed, from Equation 2.12 it follows that:

$$D(t) = \dot{D}(0)\frac{1}{\lambda}\left(1 - e^{-\lambda t}\right) = \frac{T_{1/2}}{ln(2)}\dot{D}(0)\left(1 - e^{-ln(2)\frac{t}{T_{1/2}}}\right)$$

$$(6.1)$$

In particular, for a permanent implant (t → ∞):

$$D_{total} = \frac{T_{1/2}}{ln(2)}\dot{D}(0) \qquad (6.2)$$

For instance, the initial dose rate in a typical permanent implant of the prostate (prescription dose: 144 Gy) is 6.4 cGy/hour for ^{125}I and 22.5 cGy/hour for ^{103}Pd. A higher dose rate means a larger dose-rate factor (see Equation 6.2) and, accordingly, enhanced cell killing. A practical disadvantage of short-lived radionuclides is the need to order sources for a specific treatment day; sources not used must be discarded. In contrast, long half-life sources (e.g., ^{137}Cs) are usable over long time intervals.

Source Localization

In a brachytherapy implant the accuracy of the dose calculation depends on the physicist's ability to correctly localize the radioactive seeds. A familiar approach is to place "dummy" (nonradioactive) source substitutes (seeds) into an applicator that was previously positioned in the patient and then reconstruct the three-dimensional coordinates of the seeds from localization images (Fig. 11-18). A second method consists of identifying potential source positions with respect to a template that is placed in a fixed, and identifiable, position vis-a-vis the treatment region.

An example of template-based source localization is the jig used in permanent prostate implants (Fig. 11-19).

The template contains a rectangular pattern of holes and is attached to a rectal ultrasound transducer.

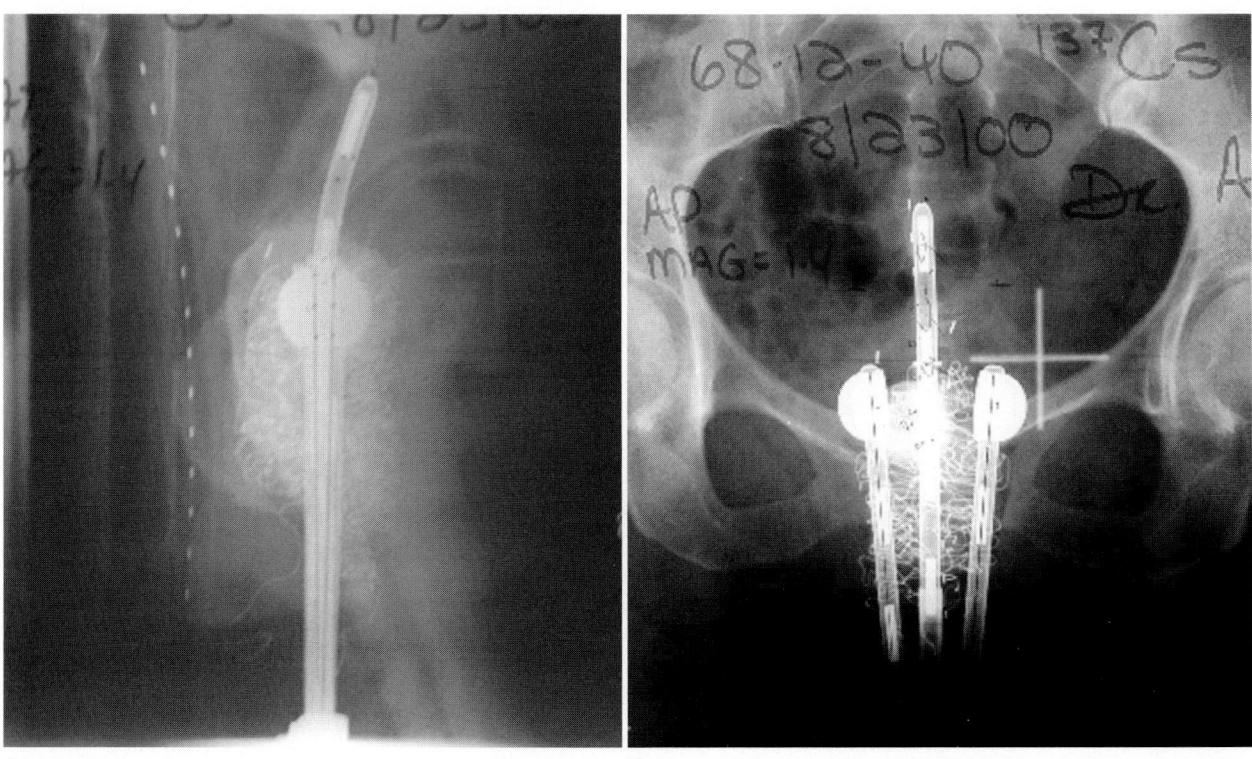

A   B

Figure 11–18. Lateral *(left)* and anterior-posterior localization films with ^{137}Cs dummy seeds for an implant with a Henshke applicator. See also Color Figure 11–18.

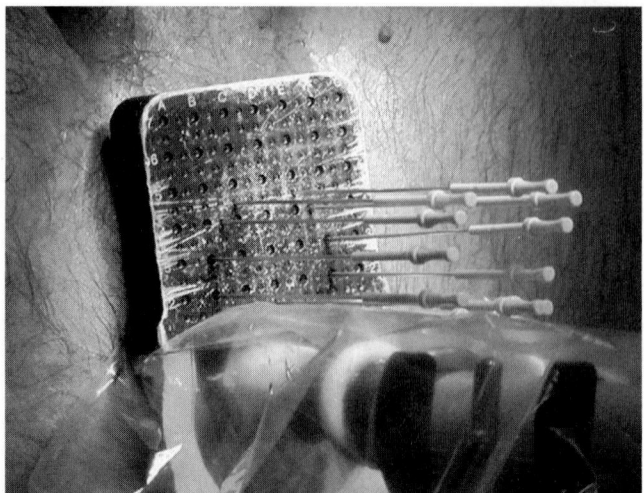

Figure 11–19. Template used in a prostate permanent implant. The template contains a rectangular pattern of holes. Needles are inserted through the template grid and seeds are placed along each needle at positions determined by the computer-generated plan. See also Color Figure 11–19.

Implantable needles are inserted through the template grid and seeds are placed along each needle at positions (typically, in multiples of 0.5 cm intervals) predetermined by the computer-generated plan. A series of parallel ultrasound images is taken through the prostate, and firmware in the ultrasound unit overlays a grid of dots onto these images that correspond to the template holes. The grid coordinates on the template and the distance of the ultrasound image away from the template uniquely identify the three-dimensional coordinates of each potential seed position relative to the gland anatomy.

The general question of localizing sources using radiographic films amounts to a transformation of coordinates between a reference system associated with the patient (S_P) and a system of coordinates (S_I) linked to the imaging system (film and x-ray source). S_P may be defined in different ways: For an isocentric imaging system (e.g., a therapy simulator) one may take the isocenter as origin and two of the axes along the gantry axis of rotation and the source-to-axis (SAD) direction, respectively (the third axis is automatically determined). For a nonisocentric system (for instance, a C-arm fluoroscopic unit), S_P can be defined by four noncoplanar markers (reference points) attached to the patient. Without any loss of generality, one may take the origin at one of these markers (call it O) and the other three (A, B, C) at unit distance along three perpendicular directions. The origin of S_I could be placed at the center of the imaging plane (e.g., film) with the z-axis perpendicular to this plane and directed toward the x-ray source, and the other two axes set at fixed (but otherwise arbitrary) positions in the plane. The problem is reduced to finding the parameters that define the transformation from the two-dimensional projections of seeds or reference points, or both. (The source-to-film distance is assumed known.)

A rotation-translation transformation is defined by six parameters: the coordinates of the origin of S_I in the system of reference $S_P(x_0, y_0, z_0)$ and three angles (for instance, the Euler angles). The projections of the markers (A, B, C) on the film plane (two equations each) provide a system of equations, the solution of which are the transformation parameters wanted. For a single seed, the two equations obtainable from projection on the film plane are obviously insufficient for determining its three coordinates in S_P, and thus a second image is required.

Localization with a nonisocentric imaging system is used in situations where the patient cannot be transported to a more conventional setting (e.g., when it is desirable to reconstruct seed positions intraoperatively). In the following, these difficulties are avoided, and the more common condition, in which source localization is performed with an isocentric unit, is assumed.

The next level of complication concerns the fact that implants contain more than one seed. The localization of sources with *two* radiographic films requires that each seed be identified in both images.

The nature of this problem may be understood from Fig. 11-20: A_1 and B_1 are the projections of two sources, A and B, when the x-ray source occupies position S_1. Similarly, A_2 and B_2 are projections that obtain with the source at S_2.

When back-projected, the points A1, B1 and A2, B2 generate four intersections, only two of which correspond to real seeds. Unless one can determine *a priori* that, say, projections A_1 and A_2 represent the same seed, a third image must be used to remove this ambiguity.

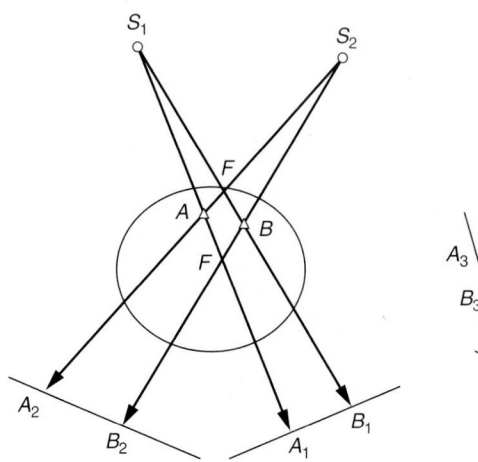

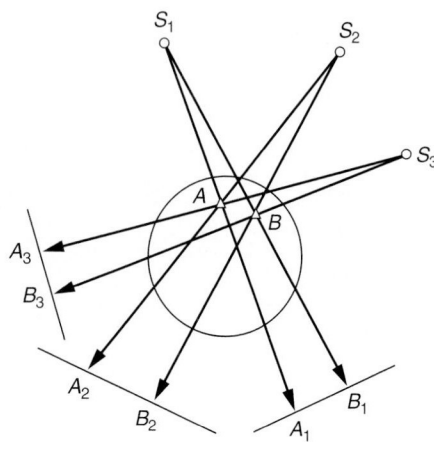

Figure 11–20. Two films *(left)* cannot resolve seed positions. When back-projected, [A_1, B_1] and [A_2, B_2] generate two real seeds *(triangles)* and the two false seeds *(F)*. In theory, three-film seed reconstruction *(right)* removes this ambiguity. (From Todor DA, Cohen GN, Amols HI, Zaider M: Operator-free, film-based 3D seed reconstruction in brachytherapy. *Phys Med Biol.* 2002;47:2031.)

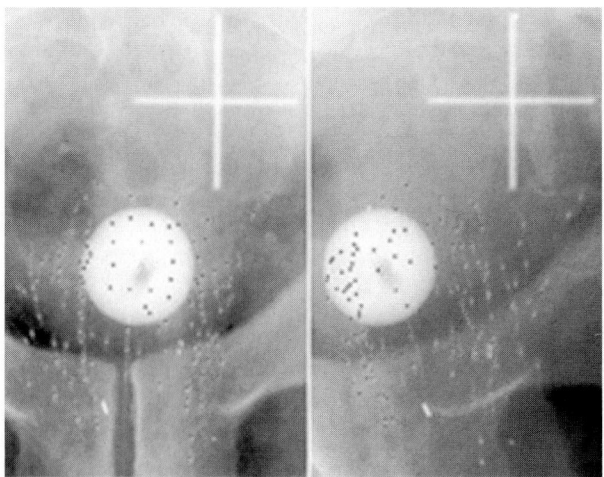

Figure 11–21. Matching seed projections in two different images is a difficult and time-consuming task, as illustrated in this (not atypical) patient data showing a ^{103}Pd implant with 134 seeds. See also Color Figure 11-21.

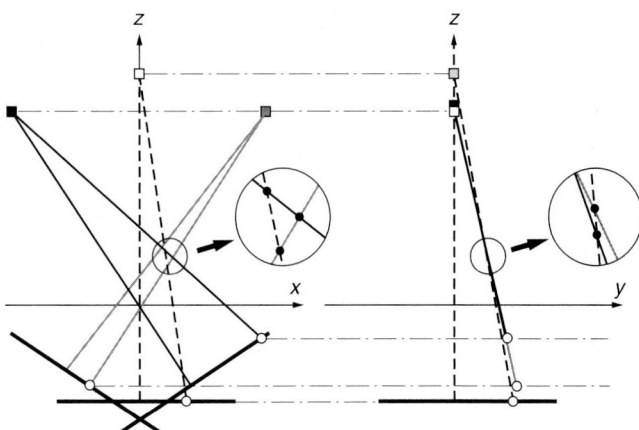

Figure 11–22. Three-film seed reconstruction may be affected by errors, with the result that two-dimensional projections of the same seed may not meet—when back-projected—at a point. The projections in the planes zx and zy are shown separately. (From Todor DA, Cohen GN, Amols HI, Zaider M: Operator-free, film-based 3D seed reconstruction in brachytherapy. *Phys Med Biol.* 2002;47:2031.)

Except for plans that have small numbers of sources, matching seed projections in two different images is a difficult and time-consuming task, often prone to errors (Fig. 11-21).

Additional sources of uncertainty come from patient movement during and in between radiographs or the limited precision with which seeds can be localized on the films. A number of algorithms that make use of three or more images, and which have in common the fact that seeds need be only digitized but not cross-identified among images, have been developed.[147,148-151] The prototype of this approach is a method suggested by Amols and Rosen:[147] three images (one with the gantry vertical at 0° and the other two symmetric with respect to this axis, at angles ±θ) are taken with the film cassette raised at the isocenter and kept horizontally at a fixed position. To fix the notation, assume that the film cassette is in the (x, y) plane and that the gantry rotates about the y axis in the (x, z) plane. The coordinates of the x-ray source are $(SAD \sin(\theta_i), 0, SAD \cos(\theta_i))$, where $\theta_1 = -\theta$, $\theta_2 = \theta$, and $\theta_3 = 0$. The two-dimensional coordinates $(x_i, y_i, i = 1, 2, 3)$ of the projections of a seed $A(x_0, y_0, z_0)$ on films taken at $+\theta$, $-\theta$ and 0°, respectively, must satisfy:

$$\begin{cases} x_{1,2} = x_0 + \dfrac{z_0(\pm SAD \sin \theta + x_0)}{SAD \cos \theta - z_0} \\ y_{1,2} = y_0 + \dfrac{z_0 y_0}{SAD \cos \theta - z_0} \end{cases} \begin{cases} x_3 = \dfrac{SAD\, x_0}{SAD - z_0} \\ y_3 = \dfrac{SAD\, y_0}{SAD - z_0} \end{cases}$$

$$(6.3)$$

The solution of the first set of (three independent) equations provides seed coordinates x_0, y_0, z_0, which, if real, must satisfy the second set of equations as well. In this arrangement $y_1 = y_2$ and, at least in principle, this condition can be used to identify in images 1 and 2 projections that belong to the same seed (the obvious exceptions are seeds that have different x coordinates but identical y and z). In practice, the determination of the projections y_1, y_2, y_3 can be inexact (Fig. 11-22) and one must consider all projection triplets (one from each film) that have their y values within a band of values Δy, typically several mm (Fig. 11-23). Triplets are examined in order with the goal of finding unique assignments for all seed projections.

The capability of algorithms, such as this one, to correctly identify sources lessens substantially as the number of seeds increases. Recently, more advanced methods have been proposed with the goal of achieving closer to 100% reconstruction efficiency.[152-154] These methods, one of which is briefly described, are based on heuristic rules implemented to minimize seed position misclassification that results from patient motion and the finite tolerances of the systems used. A system, proposed by Todor et al.,[152] works as follows:

a. Seeds are segmented (i.e., detected) in any random order on the three films.
b. A seed, i, is selected from one film and possible candidates (seed projections with y values within Δy = 0.75 cm, see Fig. 11-23) are extracted from the other two films.
c. A triplet is a set of assumed projections of a given seed on films. Using expressions such as Equation 6.3, coordinates (x_{ij}, z_{ij}) are calculated for each triplet by using pairs of films denoted $(i, j) = (1, 2)$, $(2, 3)$, and

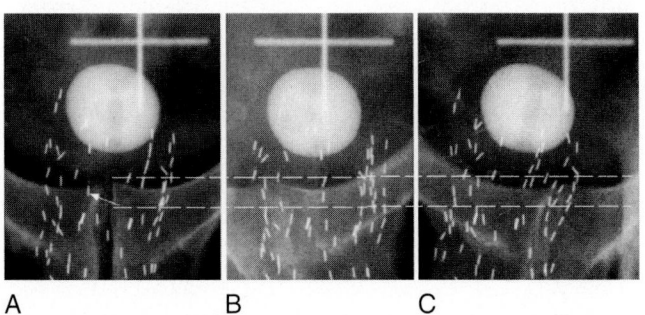

Figure 11–23. Seeds with their y coordinate within a band, Δy, *(dashed lines)* are candidates for triplets that represent (potentially) the same seed.

(1, 3). For a real seed the three sets of coordinates thus obtained would be expected to coincide. Because of the unavoidable experimental artifacts discussed earlier, one calculates instead the Euclidean distance in the (x, z) plane between these three points:

$$d = \sqrt{(x_{12} - x_{13})^2 + (z_{12} - z_{13})^2} \\ + \sqrt{(x_{23} - x_{13})^2 + (z_{23} - z_{13})^2} \\ + \sqrt{(x_{12} - x_{23})^2 + (z_{12} - z_{23})^2} \quad (6.4)$$

and sorts the first 20 candidates according to the value of d.

d. Equation 6.3 is used again to obtain three y coordinates and a similar distance, d′, is computed, this time with the y and z coordinates rather than x and z. A new ranking is produced. Each triplet will generally be associated with three virtual seeds, either because the triplet does not correspond to a real seed or because of errors in the 2D coordinates. The average coordinates of these three virtual seeds are taken to represent an *average virtual seed*.

e. The average virtual seed is back-projected on the films and the Euclidean distance between reconstructed and digitized seeds are evaluated. This provides a third sorting criterion.

f. The triplet with the best overall ranking is selected to represent the "true" seed.

g. This process is repeated sequentially for all the seeds.

h. Seeds that have been used more than once are being re-evaluated separately and those triplets are reshuffled.

Reconstruction based on computed tomography (CT) and magnetic resonance imaging (MRI), when practicable, avoids some of the problems described earlier; as well, they make possible identifying the target volume in the image—an additional benefit relative to conventional radiographic films. For instance (Fig. 11-24), a HDR treatment-planning modality (developed at MSKCC) makes use of CT images obtained immediately after

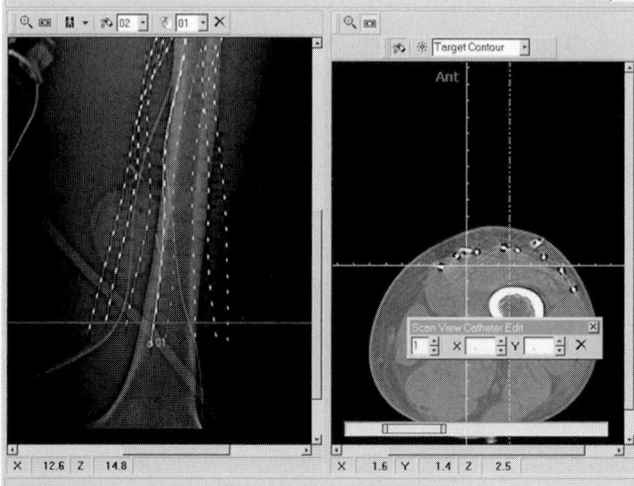

Figure 11–24. In this example, which illustrates planning for high-dose-rate (HDR) treatment of soft-tissue sarcoma, the trajectory of each catheter is digitized on each computed tomography cut and on the scout image. See also Color Figure 11-24.

catheters with dummy ribbons have been placed in the patient. The trajectory of each catheter is digitized concurrently on each CT cut and on the scout image. The program reconstructs the path of each catheter and then calculates dwell times that produce an optimal dose distribution (in the least-squares sense) in the outlined structures.

A comprehensive review of the subject of source localization may be found in *AAPM Summer School 1994*.[155]

Planning

Brachytherapy planning means: (1) defining a target volume and prescribing the dose to it and (2) outlining healthy organs at risk and stipulating the maximum dose in them. The physicist's role is to find a source configuration that achieves the prescribed doses. There are essentially four treatment-planning methods. They are set apart by what they use to calculate a plan, namely:

a. Nomograms
b. Pre-calculated plans
c. Trial and error (iterative) methods
d. Computer-based optimization

Examples of each planning technique are given in the following.

Nomograms

Nomograms, presented as tables or in graphical format, are empirical working rules to determine (within the stated accuracy) the total source strength needed to produce a specific dose distribution.

THE MANCHESTER SYSTEM[156]

Because it was originally designed for radium and radon sources (thus neglecting the effects of scattering and absorption), this planning method—also referred to as the Patterson-Parker system—is useful only for photon sources with energy larger than approximately 200 keV, for instance ^{192}Ir. When used for treatment planning, the Manchester system prescribes a pattern of source distribution that will result in a dose nonuniformity of only ±10% in the treatment volume (excluding the HDR region immediately adjacent to the sources).

For a rectangular *planar* implant, sources are placed equidistantly along parallel lines. The Manchester formalism is essentially a table (see Equation 6.5) that gives the total source strength as a function of the implanted area, A. Several ad hoc rules are pertinent to this approach:

a. The peripheral sources define the dimension of the implantation region.

b. The total source strength of the peripheral sources should be two thirds of the total strength for an implant area, A, less than or equal to 25 cm², one half for A∈[25,100] cm², and one third for A greater than 100 cm².

c. The total source strength should be increased by 5% for an elongation E = 2:1, by 9% for E = 3:1, and by 12% for E = 4:1.

d. For two-plane implants separated by distance h, the area A is taken as the arithmetic average of the areas of the two planes. The total source strength is increased by 25% for h = 1.5 cm, by 40% for h = 2 cm, and by 50% for h = 2.5 cm.

With this, the total air kerma strength, $S_K(A;h)$, needed to deliver (over time t) dose D at distance h from an implanted area, A, of elongation E is given by:

$$S_K(A; h) = S_K\left(A\left(\frac{0.5}{h}\right)^2; 0.5\right)\left(\frac{h}{0.5}\right)^2 \quad (6.5a)$$

where (Gilad Cohen, personal communication)

$$S_K(A; 0.5) =$$
$$\frac{D(Gy)}{10.} \frac{1}{t_{eff}} 7.227\left(39.2 A^{0.734} + 37.8\right)e^{0.05(E-1)^{0.75}}$$

$$(6.5b)$$

and:

$$t_{eff} = \frac{T_{1/2}}{\ln(2)}\left[1 - e^{\frac{\ln(2)}{T_{1/2}}t}\right] \quad (6.6)$$

In this expression the units are as follows: S_K in U, h in cm, and A in cm^2.

As in the case of a planar implant, the *volume* implant is defined by peripheral sources. The basic rule of this type of implant is to divide the volume into two approximately equal regions (the core and the outer shell) and then to place three times as much source strength in the outer shell relative to the core. The total air kerma strength, S_K, necessary to deliver dose D (±10%) to a volume, V, can be calculated as follows:

$$S_K(U) = \frac{D(Gy)}{10.} \frac{1}{t_{eff}} 258 \, V^{2/3}(cm^3)e^{0.07(E-1)} \quad (6.7)$$

Here E is the elongation.

The expressions, Equations 6.6 and 6.7, may be used to calculate the total dwell time in HDR brachytherapy by solving them for t_{eff} (and then for the total nominal time t, via Equation 6.6) and using for S_K the appropriate air kerma strength of the source, usually around 10 Ci (^{192}Ir).

THE QUIMBY SYSTEM

A volume implant where the source strength is distributed uniformly conforms to the so-called *Quimby system*. As in the case of the Manchester system, this method is applicable only to high-energy (>200 keV) photon sources. The total air kerma strength needed to deliver over a treatment time, t, a minimal dose D (minimum peripheral dose) to a volume V (cm^3) can be calculated as follows (Gilad Cohen, personal communication):

$$S_K(U) = \frac{D(Gy)}{10.} \frac{1}{t_{eff}}$$
$$\times 7.227\left(81.92 + 43.916V^{0.7} - 0.196V^{1.4}\right)e^{0.07(E-1)}$$

$$(6.8)$$

which is applicable for $V \in [5, 300]$ cm^3. In the Quimby system sources are placed 1 to 2 cm apart. Elongation corrections are the same as for the Manchester method.

VOLUME AND PLANAR IMPLANTS WITH LOW-ENERGY PHOTON SOURCES

Nomograms for permanent volume implants are tools designed to predict the total air kerma strength, S_K, necessary to deliver a stated (minimal) dose to a known tumor volume. More precisely, they stipulate the total source strength, S_K, such that the isodose surface corresponding to the prescription dose has a stated volume. The volume nomograms were obtained in connection with permanent prostate implants and thus, strictly speaking, the volume in question refers to the geometry of this particular organ; this should be kept in mind when applying the expressions given below to volumes of considerably different shape. Additionally, the implants assumed a uniform spatial distribution of sources.[157,158] However, if a uniform dose distribution in the treatment target is desired, the seeds must be placed predominantly peripherally; it has been shown[159] that within a good approximation (about 10%) the equations given below are insensitive to the details of source positioning in the target (peripheral or uniform).

For a ^{125}I *permanent* implant and a prescription dose of 144 Gy[159]:

$$\frac{S_k}{U} = \begin{cases} 5.709\left(\dfrac{d_{avg}}{cm}\right) & d_{avg} \leq 3\,cm \\[2mm] 1.524\left(\dfrac{d_{avg}}{cm}\right)^{2.2} & d_{avg} > 3\,cm \end{cases} \quad (6.9)$$

For a ^{103}Pd *permanent* implant and a prescription dose of 140 Gy:

$$\frac{S_k}{U} = \begin{cases} 29.41\left(\dfrac{d_{avg}}{cm}\right) & d_{avg} \leq 3\,cm \\[2mm] 5.395\left(\dfrac{d_{avg}}{cm}\right)^{2.56} & d_{avg} > 3\,cm \end{cases} \quad (6.10)$$

The quantity d_{avg} refers to the average of three orthogonal dimensions of the volume to be implanted.[160] In a typical application of these equations one evaluates d_{avg} and then calculates the total number of radioactive sources needed by dividing the total required source strength, S_K, by the single-seed strength. The equations provided earlier can be scaled to any other doses. For temporary implants that are removed after time t, the required source strength, $S_{K, temp}(t)$, may be estimated using S_K of Equations 6.9 and 6.10 and:

$$S_{K, temp}(t) = \frac{S_K}{1 - e^{-\lambda t}} \quad (6.11)$$

The corresponding equation for a *planar permanent* implant (^{125}I, prescription: 150 Gy at 0.5 cm from the implant plane) is:

$$\frac{S_K}{U} = 0.93\frac{Area}{cm^2} + 4.78 \quad (6.12)$$

THE PARIS SYSTEM

Although not strictly a nomogram, the implantation method known as the *Paris system*[161-163] provides a practical recipe for placing [192]Ir (or nuclides of similar energy) wires in the target volume with the goal of achieving a predictable level of dose uniformity. The general approach for placing sources follows three rules:

1. Wires should be rectilinear and parallel, and with the centers located in a plane perpendicular to the wires. This is the *central plane* of the implant.
2. The wires must have a uniform linear density of air kerma strength (μGy/h m²/m), identical for all wires.
3. Wires are placed equidistant from each other. There are single-plane and double-plane configurations, the latter with wires intersecting the central plane at points that form squares or equilateral triangles.

Dosimetrically, the key element of the method is obtaining the average *basal dose* (BD); this results—when the implant is performed according to the stated rules—in a peripheral dose (i.e., prescription dose) of approximately 0.85(BD). Basal doses are calculated in the central plane of the implant. For a single-plane implant, the basal doses are calculated midway between each source. For a double-plane implant, the basal doses are calculated at points in the middle of the squares or triangles formed by the wires. Specific rules on the spacing and active length of wires, the number of source planes to be used (one or two), or the spacing between planes are listed in Table 1 of Gillin et al.'s publication.[164]

PRECALCULATED PLANS

For many procedures performed with fixed-geometry applicators, such as single-channel intra-vaginal tandem, endobronchial, esophageal, or gynecologic ring applicators, it is convenient to have a collection of precalculated plans. A representative example is intraoperative radiation therapy (IORT) with HDR brachytherapy. It makes use of rectangular plastic applicators (Fig. 11-13), embedded with parallel catheters 1 cm apart, to treat the tumor bed immediately after cancer resection. The device, known as a *flab*[165] or *HAM* (Harrison-Anderson-Mick) applicator,[143] is connected to a remote afterloader and a dose of 10 to 17.5 Gy is delivered at a distance of 1 cm away from the source plane, or 0.5 cm from the applicator surface. The variable parameters for this type of treatment are the dimensions of the region to be treated (which translates into number of catheters and length along each catheter to be used for the treatment) and the total dose. Because prompt planning is of essence for an anesthetized patient, at our institution an atlas of more than 5000 precalculated plans for arrays from 2 × 2 to 24 × 20 cm² is stored in the computer and used for IORT brachytherapy.[143]

ITERATIVE (TRIAL AND ERROR) COMPUTER-AIDED PLANNING

This method entails finding—based on previous experience and successive adjustments—source strengths that generate the desired dose distribution. Given a particular

set of source strengths, a computer program is used to evaluate rapidly the resulting dosage. Shortcomings of this approach are best understood by considering an example of such semi-manual planning. LDR brachytherapy for soft-tissue sarcoma is administered to the tumor bed, which for planning purposes is defined by catheters placed in the site at the time of surgery. Although the intention is to place catheters in a regular coplanar configuration, the resulting arrangement is typically nonuniform, and this makes the use of ribbons with single-strength sources and accompanying nomograms (Manchester or Quimby) unsuitable (Fig. 11-25). The solution adopted at MSKCC is to use a combination of several source strengths, with each ribbon having three to four different-activity segments, essentially achieving a Manchester-type uniform dose distribution.[146] Planning proceeds as follows: Several days after surgery, dummy (inactive) sources are placed in ribbons, and the patient is sent for radiographic localization of potential source positions. The prescription (typically 45 Gy) is given to a target defined relative to ribbons, namely a hull that surrounds the catheters approximately 0.5 to 1 cm away. For manual planning this target volume is not actually outlined but kept in mind during plan evaluation. Typically, 5 to 10 catheters are used and

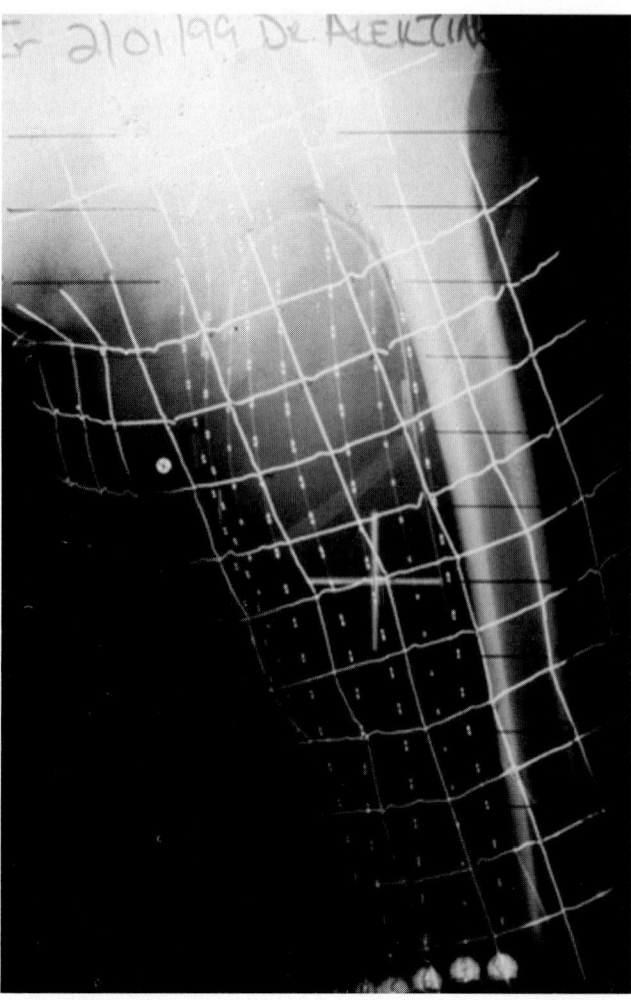

Figure 11–25. Radiographic localization film of a soft-tissue sarcoma implant with dummy seeds.

the total number of available source positions, spaced 1 cm apart, is on the order of 200. In principle, up to 20 different source strengths may be available from the manufacturer, and therefore the total number of source configurations becomes astronomically large ($\approx 20^{200}$).

As a result, and at the risk of eliminating potentially superior plans, one must restrict the number of different activities for each ribbon to two or three strengths. The plan that results from a particular source configuration is evaluated by examining two-dimensional cuts (as best as possible perpendicular to the catheter plane) to ascertain whether the prescribed isodose indeed conforms to the desired target volume. Manual planning takes—even for experienced workers—on the order of 3 to 6 hours and there is no guarantee for 100% target coverage. In contrast, computer-based optimization (described in the following section) produces a plan of similar or better quality in several minutes.

COMPUTER-BASED OPTIMIZATION

In computer-based optimization the problem at hand is formulated as follows: consistent with certain dosimetric constraints, find a set of binary variables (0/1) that record the presence or absence of sources on a prespecified grid of potential locations. The search for the optimal source configuration is guided by an *objective function*, which is a mathematical construct that quantifies the "distance" between the desired and the attained dosimetric distributions. Numerical search algorithms used in brachytherapy treatment planning include simulated annealing,[166,167] genetic optimization,[146,168,169] and integer programming.[170-172]

The following formulation, proposed by Lee et al. for the treatment of permanent prostate implants,[171] illustrates the general features of an optimization model. Let x_j be the 0/1 indicator for recording the placement of a source at grid position j. The total dose, D(P), at point P is given by:

$$D(P) = \sum_{j=1}^{n} D\big(\|P - R_j\|\big)x_j \qquad (6.13)$$

Here *n* is the number of potential source positions, R_j is a vector that gives the coordinates of grid position j, $\|P - R_j\|$ is the Euclidian distance between P and R_j, and D(r) is the dose contribution to P from a source at distance r away (to simplify the presentation, the point source approximation is used here). For each point of interest one can define upper (U_P) and lower (L_P) limits that D(P) must satisfy:

$$\sum_{j=1}^{n} D\big(\|P - R_j\|\big)x_j \leq U_P$$
$$\sum_{j=1}^{n} D\big(\|P - R_j\|\big)x_j \geq L_P \qquad (6.14)$$

Quite generally, it is not possible to have all points P satisfy these constraints, in which case there will be no solution [x_j] to this problem. The next best thing is to attempt to maximize the number of points that satisfy Equation 6.14. This is achieved in the following manner. Let $U_P + M_P$ denote the absolute maximum acceptable dose at point P, and similarly $L_P - N_P$ for the absolute minimum dose. Finally, let v_P, w_P be binary (0/1) variables that indicate whether Equation 6.14 satisfied (when equal to 1) or not (when equal to 0). With this, the constraints, Equation 6.14, are replaced with:

$$\sum_{j=1}^{n} D\big(\|P - R_j\|\big)x_j \leq U_P + M_P(1 - w_P)$$
$$\sum_{j=1}^{n} D\big(\|P - R_j\|\big)x_j \geq L_P - N_P(1 - v_p) \qquad (6.15)$$

and the sum:

$$F(x_1, x_2, \ldots, x_n) = \sum_{P} (v_P + w_P) \qquad (6.16)$$

which depends on the configuration [x_j], gives the total number of points P that satisfy the original constraints, Equation 6.14. The optimization problem consists of maximizing the objective function, F.

All points *P* need not have the same clinical importance; for instance, avoiding urethral toxicity (a common side effect) may be more important than satisfying the condition of dose uniformity across the target. This is addressed by assigning different weights, α_P and β_P, to v_P and w_P, respectively, and maximizing instead:

$$F'(x_1, x_2, \ldots, x_n) = \sum_{P} (\alpha_P v_P + \beta_P w_P) \qquad (6.17)$$

In mathematical parlance, the problem described by the expression, Equation 6.17, and constraints, Equation 6.15, is known as a *linear integer programming (IP) problem* because the objective function is linear in the unknown variables and since these variables can take only integer (here 0 or 1) values. We shall proceed to describe, in the simplest possible terms, some algorithms commonly used for solving this problem. For this purpose we shall rewrite the problem in the following schematic way:

$$\begin{aligned} &\textit{Maximize: } c^T x \\ &\textit{Subject to: } Ax \leq b; \quad x \in \{0, 1\} \end{aligned} \qquad (6.18)$$

where x, c, and b are column vectors of order n and A is a rectangular array of order (n, m).

Branch-and-Bound Algorithm

Consider the IP problem, Equation 6.15, but with the integrality condition relaxed, that is, allow *x* to take any value in [0, 1]. This new problem, known as *linear relaxation (LR)*, has two important properties that form the basis of the branch-and-bound approach. They are:

a. The optimal objective function of LR is greater than or equal to that of the IP problem, and
b. If LR is not feasible (no solution exists), so is IP.

These statements follow from the fact that LR has fewer constraints than IP.

The algorithm starts out by generating the LR solution. In the unlikely case that all components of x are integers, this solution is the IP solution as well and the search is finished. Otherwise, a tree search starts at this (zero) node by selecting one of the (still noninteger) components of x, say x_j, and branching on that variable to create two new problems, one with $x_j = 0$ and the other one with $x_j = 1$. Components of x that are already integers are kept fixed on this and any subsequent branchings. For each of the two new problems, LR solutions are generated (relaxed in the noninteger variables); an LR solution may be either IP-compatible (all x are integers, no further branching) or unfeasible (the constraints are not satisfied; no further branching) or still LR—in which case new branching occurs. If a feasible IP solution is found, the resulting value of the objective function is a *lower bound* on all other solutions that may result from branching at different nodes. This means that any time an *LR* solution yields an objective value *less* than the current lower bound, that node needs no further exploration (in the botanical lingo used in connection with this algorithm, one calls this process *turning nodes into leaves and also pruning the tree*). This solution is the best so far. If another *LR* solution has a larger objective value than the best-so-far solution, the lower bound (and the best so far solution) are correspondingly updated. An inactive node is said to be *fathomed*. The tree search ends when all nodes are fathomed (i.e., turned into leaves).

Genetic Algorithm

A genetic algorithm is an optimization method modeled after the biological mechanism of natural selection and evolution.[173-176] Genetic algorithms, like their natural counterparts (chains of DNA nucleotides) represent potential solutions as streams of binary symbols. Given an initial population of individuals, a subset of the population is selected to parent offspring for the next generation. Parent selection is random but weighted by the relative fitness (as judged from the objective function) of each individual (stream).

When parents mate, the genetic makeup of the two new members of the next generation is determined by: (a) crossover (exchange of subsections of streams between the two parents), and (b) mutation (alteration of a randomly selected symbol in the stream). An exception is made for the stream with the highest fitness (objective value), which is transferred unchanged to the next generation. This strategy is known as *elitism*.

An implementation of the genetic algorithm to the planning of permanent prostate implants proceeds as follows[168]: Initially, 600 sets of streams [x_j] are generated, each with the same number of 1−s (an initial estimate of the number of sources in the implant). For each source configuration, one calculates doses, D(P), on a three-dimensional grid of points that cover all structures of interest (here, prostate, urethra, and rectum) and obtains a score using the following steps (D_0 = prescription dose):

a. Prostate score: number of prostate points, P, with D_0 less than D(P) less than 1.6D

b. Urethral score: number of urethral points with D(P) less than 1.3 D_0

c. Rectal score: number of rectal points, P, with D(P) less than 0.8 D_0

d. Raw score: (Prostate score) + 35(Rectal score) + 40 (Urethral score)

e. Final score: A*(Raw score) + B

Here, A and B are positive constants, and the coefficients that appear in the raw score equation were chosen to indicate the relative weight given to each structure in the optimization process as performed in this particular application.

The top (distinct) 15 scoring streams are selected for the next generation, with 14 streams paired up for crossover and mutation, and the top scorer (no. 15) allowed to go to the next generation without any further alteration.

A peculiarity of genetic algorithm is that no test for optimality is embedded in it. The algorithm terminates either after a preset number of generations (e.g., several thousands) or after changes in the objective score from one generation to the next become sufficiently small.

Simulated Annealing

The method of simulated annealing,[177,178] also known as the Metropolis algorithm,[179] rests on the analogy with the process of slow cooling (annealing) of a liquid in which an ordered crystal is formed and therefore a state of minimum energy is attained. At a given temperature, T, the energy of domains of equal volume in the melt is distributed according to Boltzmann's probability distribution (k_B = Boltzmann's constant):

$$P(E) \propto \exp\left(-E/k_B T\right) \qquad (6.19)$$

With probability $\exp(-\Delta E/k_B T)$ each domain can change energy from E_1 to $E_1 + \Delta E$. Because at ΔE less than 0 the exponential is larger than 1, the change occurs with unit probability. The system thus tends to the lowest energy state consistent with T.

By analogy one can take the objective function, say χ^2 of the planned treatment to represent its "energy" and measure "temperature" ($k_B T$) in units of χ^2. For instance:

$$\chi^2 = \sum_i \left[D(P_i) - D_i\right]^2 \qquad (6.20)$$

where $D(P_i)$ is the calculated, and D_i the prescribed dose at point P_i. At a given temperature, a random trajectory in the parameter space (i.e., a sequence of source configurations [x_i]) is generated by taking random steps with probability proportional to $p = \exp(-\Delta\chi^2/T)$ calculated for each consecutive pair of displacements. The step is always taken if $\Delta\chi^2$ less than 0, but otherwise with probability p. After a sufficient large number of steps it is assumed that the lower "energy" state has been attained, the temperature is lowered, and a new trajectory is generated.

An example of optimization of dose distribution in brachytherapy using simulated annealing can be found in an article by Sloboda.[166]

WHERE ARE WE HEADED?

This chapter gives an account (by necessity, superficial, although—one would hope—not shallow) of the main topics and present trends in brachytherapy physics. This leaves us with the traditional end-of-the-chapter question, *quo vadis?*

Dosimetric calculations have reached an unprecedented level of accuracy. The current (and, in the view of this writer, too restrictive) recommendation is that dose be determined to better than 2% accuracy in order to obtain 5% uncertainty for the entire planning treatment process.[180] An uncertainty of 5% in dose calculation appears to be quite comfortably within the realm of presently available experimental and theoretical dose models, and consequently treatment planning algorithms. Delivering the dose to the patient within 5% of the intended value remains a questionable issue. The two main physical factors responsible for this state of affairs are uncertainties in imaging applicators and potential locations of radiation sources, and (possibly the main factor) errors in the implementation of the plan. Further efforts in this direction will have to be preceded by the demonstration that they are clinically justified. Perhaps dosimetry is reaching the end of the road.[181]

Dosimetric questions are intimately linked to the process of treatment planning. It seems to be the case that in the (hopefully, near) future, functional imaging and biologic dose will replace absorbed dose to become the two ingredients that will govern the thinking of the medical physicist who designs treatment plans. *Biologic dose* refers to an index (e.g., RBE) that quantifies the biologic effect of a given dose delivered by a specific radiation type. This is discussed briefly in the previous section, Microdosimetry.

Functional imaging concerns our ability to detect and treat selectively only those subvolumes of the target that contain clinically significant cancer. The simplest definition is tumor as defined by contrast CT and by multiple MRI sequences. This type of localization has now been introduced into brachytherapy with inverse planning. Optimization based on true tumor location will replace all previous systems. To this can be added more specific functional imaging. This means localizing tumor cells that are radioresistant, fast proliferating, or both. That functional imaging is desirable derives from the notion that it is the behavior of these cells that ultimately determines the success or failure of a particular modality of disease management. An imaging tool that will provide information on the *location* and *number* of these particular types of tumor cells may be referred to as *functional imaging*. It entails the ability to obtain the spatial distribution of any cellular property that determines—directly or indirectly—tumor response to radiotherapy. The position of cells in the cell cycle or their levels of oxygenation, which are both factors that determine the intrinsic radiosensitivity of a tumor, are examples of such properties.

Brachytherapy (perhaps more than intensity-modulated radiation therapy, IMRT) is well suited to take advantage of these innovative tools because, by necessity, it delivers nonuniform doses to the target volume. The question left for the planner is to place the dosimetric "hot spots" at locations in the target identified to contain "significant" cancer, while maintaining target coverage and dose restrictions to the healthy tissues.

Biological imaging is currently in use at our institution, MSKCC, in a planning system that employs magnetic resonance spectroscopy (MRS) information to escalate the dose at prostate volumes identified as having increased choline/citrate ratios.[172] MRS, as applied to prostate cancer, is based on the observation that in regions of cancer the choline/citrate ratio is elevated.[182-186] On biochemical grounds this ratio is expected to reflect an increased rate of cell proliferation, although no direct proof exists yet. The prostate as a whole is treated to 100% to 150% of the prescription dose (144 Gy for ^{125}I seeds); however, denser tumor regions are prescribed 200% of the prescription dose with no upper limit. The resulting plans are sufficiently flexible to produce these dose levels while keeping the urethral dose under 120%.

In this, as in the more traditional aspects of brachytherapy physics, there is certainly room for further improvement.

APPENDIX A: FUNDAMENTAL QUANTITIES AND UNITS

The definitions of quantities and units given here follow the conventions adopted by ICRU[187]; the reader is referred to this document for additional details.

Radiometric Quantities

Particle fluence, Φ, is defined by:

$$\Phi = \frac{\Delta N}{\Delta a} \qquad (A1)$$

where ΔN is the number of particles incident on a sphere of cross sectional area Δa. The fluence is a characterization of radiation at a point P in the center of Δa, either in free space or within irradiated matter. The area Δa must be sufficiently small with respect to fluence changes with location. In the International System of units (SI) Φ is specified in m^{-2}.

Radiance, R, is the energy transmitted in a beam of N particles, each with energy E:

$$R = NE \qquad (A2)$$

If there is a spectrum of particle energies, the radiance is:

$$R = \sum_E n(E)E \qquad (A3)$$

Here $n(E)$ is the number of particles with energy E [$N = \Sigma n(E)$]. Unit: J

Energy fluence, Ψ, is:

$$\Psi = \frac{\Delta R}{\Delta a} \qquad (A4)$$

where ΔR is the radiance falling on a sphere of cross sectional area Δa. Unit: Jm^{-2}.

Particle flux:

$$\dot{N} = \frac{\Delta N}{\Delta t} \tag{A5}$$

Unit: s^{-1}.

Energy flux:

$$\dot{R} = \frac{\Delta R}{\Delta t} \tag{A6}$$

Unit: W.

Fluence rate:

$$\dot{\Phi} = \frac{\Delta \Phi}{\Delta t} \tag{A7}$$

Unit: $m^{-2}s^{-1}$.

Energy fluence rate:

$$\dot{\Psi} = \frac{\Delta \Psi}{\Delta t} \tag{A8}$$

Unit: Wm^{-2}.

Interaction coefficients

The *cross section* is defined by:

$$\sigma = \frac{P}{\Phi} \tag{A9}$$

where P is the probability of interaction when a target entity is subjected to the particle fluence Φ. Unit: m^2.

The *attenuation coefficient*, μ, is the fraction of uncharged particles interacting in absorption or scattering in traversing a distance Δx in a material:

$$\mu = \frac{\Delta N}{N} \frac{1}{\Delta x} \tag{A10}$$

Unit: m^{-1}. The quantity μ/ρ (unit: m^2kg^{-1}) is the *mass attenuation coefficient*, with ρ the mass density of the material traversed.

The *mass energy transfer coefficient*, μ_{tr}/ρ, is the fraction of the radiance of uncharged particles that is transferred to the kinetic energy of charged particles in traversing a distance Δx in a medium of density ρ:

$$\frac{\mu_{tr}}{\rho} = \left(\frac{\Delta R}{R} \right)\left(\frac{1}{\rho \, \Delta x} \right) \tag{A11}$$

Unit: m^2kg^{-1}.

The *mass stopping power* is the kinetic energy, ΔT, lost when charged particles traverse a distance Δx in a medium of density ρ:

$$\frac{S}{\rho} = \frac{\Delta T}{\rho \, \Delta x} \tag{A12}$$

Unit: Jm^2kg^{-1}. The *stopping power* is $S = \Delta T/\Delta x$. When nuclear interactions may be neglected, one may write S as the sum of a collision term, S_{coll}, (collision stopping power) and radiative term, S_{rad}, (radiative stopping power): $S = S_{coll} + S_{rad}$.

The linear energy transfer or restricted linear collision stopping power, L_E, of a material is the mean energy, ΔE, lost by a charged particle in traversing a distance Δx; only collisions with electrons in which the energy loss is less than E are considered:

$$L_E = \left(\frac{\Delta E}{\Delta x} \right)_E \tag{A13}$$

Unit: Jm^{-1}. It is common to express the energy cutoff, E, in eV (i.e., L_{50} refers to 50 eV). The notation LET designates L_∞, which is the same as S_{coll}.

Dosimetric quantities

Specific energy, z, is:

$$z = \frac{\varepsilon}{m} \tag{A14}$$

where ε is the energy imparted by ionizing radiation to matter of mass m. Unit: $Gy = Jkg^{-1}$.

The *absorbed dose*, D, is the average energy imparted, per unit mass, by ionizing radiation. Formally:

$$D(\vec{r}) = \lim_{V \to 0, \, \vec{r} \subset V} \bar{z} \tag{A15}$$

where $\bar{z}$ is the average specific energy in a domain of volume V centered at $\vec{r}$, and the limit is taken at constant density ρ. Unit: Gy.

The *kerma*, K, is the average total kinetic energy, ΔT_{kin}, of all charged particles liberated, per unit mass Δm, by interactions of uncharged ionizing particles in Δm:

$$K(\vec{r}) = \lim_{V \to 0, \, \vec{r} \subset V} \frac{\Delta T_{kin}}{\Delta m} \tag{A16}$$

Unit: Gy.

APPENDIX B: SPECIFICATIONS OF SOURCE STRENGTH IN BRACHYTHERAPY

Air kerma strength, S_K, is the quantity currently recommended by the AAPM for specifying source strength in brachytherapy.[188] Its definition is discussed in Dosimetry, Practical Matters: Analytic Formalisms, Equation 3.18. In this appendix several related quantities, some of which have only historic interest, are introduced. In each case, their relationship to S_K is given.

a. *Reference air kerma rate,* $\dot{K}_{ref}$: is the kerma rate to air (in air) at a reference distance of 1 meter, corrected for air attenuation and scattering. This quantity is numerically equal to S_K; however, it has different units (μGy/hour instead of μGy/hour m^2).

b. *Equivalent mass of radium* (mg-Ra-Eq): is the mass of radium filtered by 0.5 mm Pt, which leads to the same exposure rate as that from the source of interest at the same distance (usually large enough that each source can be considered a point source). Thus:

$$S_K(d) = \dot{K}_{air}(d)d^2 = \left(\frac{W}{e} \right)\dot{X}d^2$$

$$= \left(\frac{W}{e} \right)\frac{\Gamma_X A}{d^2} d^2 = \left(\frac{W}{e} \right)\Gamma_X A \tag{B.1}$$

Since equivalent mass of radium is defined at the same exposure rate at the same distance (*d*), $\Gamma_X A(mCi) = \Gamma_{Ra} M_{Ra}(mg)$ (By definition, 1 mg of ^{226}Ra has an activity of 1 mCi.) With this:

$$S_K(d) = \left(\frac{W}{e}\right) \Gamma_{X,Ra} M_{Ra}(mg) \qquad (B.2)$$

For a point source containing 1 mg of radium at 0.5 mm Pt filtration $\Gamma_X = 8.25$ R h^{-1}cm^2, and it follows that $S_K(U) = 7.227$ M$_{Ra}$ (mg-Ra-Eq).

c. *Apparent activity*, A_{app}: is the activity of an unfiltered isotropic point source that has the same source strength, S_K, as that of the radioactive source of interest (exposure rate constant: Γ_X). From Equation B.1:

$$S_K(d) = \left(\frac{W}{e}\right) \Gamma_X A_{app} \qquad (B.3)$$

APPENDIX C: A COMPILATION OF MICRODOSIMETRIC DISTRIBUTIONS

Microdosimetric distributions have been determined for a wide range of photon energies, including those of the photon sources quoted in Table 11-6. Kliauga and Dvorak[189] measured lineal-energy spectra for photon energies in the range of 12 to 1250 keV and for site diameters of 0.24 to 7.7 μm. Fig. 11-C1 shows these spectra as a function of photon energy.

Microdosimetric distributions for ^{103}Pd, ^{125}I, ^{241}Am, and ^{192}Ir encapsulated sources were published by Wuu et al.[77] and are shown in Fig. 11-C2.

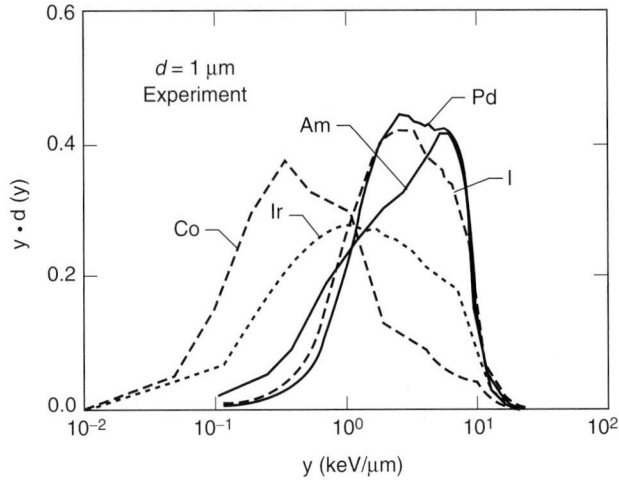

Figure 11–C2. Microdosimetric distributions for several photon radiations commonly used in brachytherapy. (From Wuu CS, Kliauga P, Zaider M, Amols HI: Microdosimetric evaluation of relative biologic effectiveness for 103Pd, 125I, 241Am, and 192Ir brachytherapy sources. *Int J Radiat Oncol Biol Phys.* 1996;36:689.)

For various technical reasons,[120] the empirical determination of microdosimetric spectra is not always possible, particularly for site sizes significantly smaller than 1 μm or for volumes of irregular shape. In these situations calculations may be used instead. A key element that facilitates this approach is the possibility of regarding the spectrum of energy deposition as resulting from the random overlap of two "objects": the charged-particle track (essentially, a collection of energy transfer points), and the sensitive site.[117-121] Theoretical microdosimetric distributions are generated by randomly placing a site on a Monte-Carlo generated track. In a sense, this is the opposite of what happens in experiments where the detector (a fixed object) is traversed by random tracks. To the extent that accurate cross sections for the interaction of the ionizing particles with the medium are known, theoretical calculations represent the best procedure for obtaining microdosimetric quantities.

Because a full description of computational techniques in microdosimetry is beyond the charter of this chapter, the interested reader may consult the textbook by Rossi and Zaider.[120] Briefly, the calculation proceeds along the following lines:

a. For a given source one generates, at each point in space, the electron distribution in energy (slowing down spectrum), n(E); commercially available codes are available for this purpose.

b. For each electron energy, E, the interactions with tissue (frequently represented by liquid water) are simulated event by event, which means that one obtains a detailed description of the geometric coordinates, energy locally deposited, and type of energy transfer (ionization or excitation) for each interaction point, primary or secondary.

c. Microdosimetric spectra, f(y;E), for electrons of energy E are generated by randomly placing the volume of interest (commonly, spheres or cylinders) on each track and then evaluating—at each instance—the total energy deposited in it.

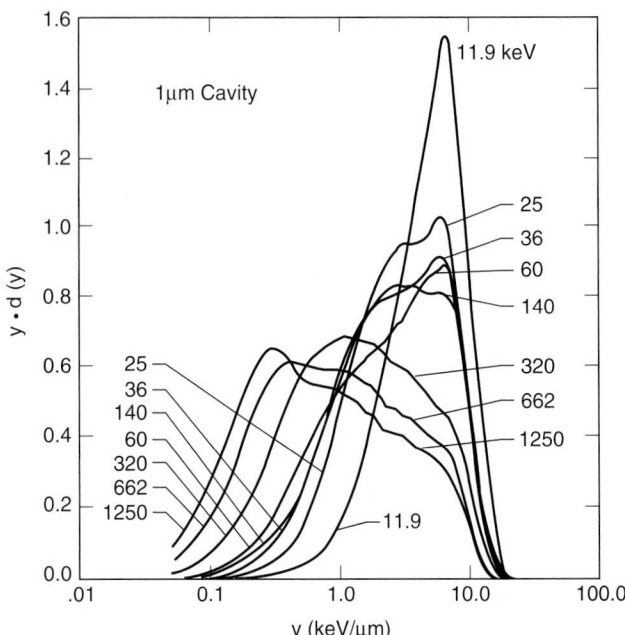

Figure 11–C1. Microdosimetric distributions for photons of different energies. The spectra were measured in a 1-μm diameter spherical cavity. (From Kliauga P, Dvorak R: Microdosimetric measurements of ionization by monoenergetic photons 1199. *Radiat Res.* 1978;73:1.)

d. The lineal energy spectrum of the brachytherapy source is evaluated from:

$$f(y) = \frac{\int_0^\infty \frac{n(E)\,E}{y_F(E)} f(y; E)dE}{\int_0^\infty \frac{n(E)\,E}{y_F(E)} dE} \tag{C.1}$$

REFERENCES

1. Nath R, Anderson LL, Luxton G, et al: Dosimetry of Interstitial Brachytherapy Sources—Recommendations of the AAPM Radiation-Therapy Committee Task Group No 43. *Med Physics.* 1995; 22:209.
2. International Commission on Radiation Units and Measurements: *Fundamental quantities and units for ionizing radiation* Bethesda, Md: International Commission on Radiation Units and Measurements, 1998.
3. National Council on Radiation Protection and Measurements: *Conceptual basis for calculations of absorbed-dose distributions.* Bethesda, MD: National Council on Radiation Protection and Measurements, 1991.
4. International Commission on Radiation Units and Measurements: *Fundamental quantities and units for ionizing radiation* Bethesda, Md: International Commission on Radiation Units and Measurements, 1998.
5. Meisberger LL, Keller RJ, Shalek RJ: The effective attenuation in water of the gamma rays of gold 198, iridium 192, cesium 137, radium 226, and cobalt 60. *Radiology.* 1968;90:953.
6. Nath R, Meigooni AS, Meli JA: Dosimetry on Transverse Axes of I-125 and Ir-192 Interstitial Brachytherapy Sources. *Med Physics.* 1990;17:1032.
7. Sievert RM: Die Intensitaetsverteilung der Primaren Strahlung in der Naehe medizinisher Radiumpraeparate. *Acta Radiol.* 1921;1:89.
8. Breitman KE: Dose-Rate Tables for Clinical Cs-137 Sources Sheathed in Platinum. *Br J Radiol.* 1974;47:657.
9. Williamson JF: Monte-Carlo and Analytic Calculation of Absorbed Dose Near CS-137 Intracavitary Sources. *Int J Radiat Oncol Biol Phys.* 1988;15:227.
10. Williamson JF: The Sievert integral revisited: Evaluation and extension to I-125, Yb-169, and Ir-192 brachytherapy sources. *Int J Radiat Oncol Biol Phys.* 1996;36:1239.
11. Popescu CC, Wise J, Sowards K, et al: Dosimetric characteristics of the Pharma Seed (TM) model BT-125-I source. *Med Phys.* 2000;27:2174.
12. Nath R, Meigooni AS, Muench P, Melillo A: Anisotropy functions for Pd-103, I-125, and Ir-192 interstitial brachytherapy sources. *Med Phys.* 1993;20:1465.
13. Nath R, Meigooni AS, Meli JA: Dosimetry on transverse axes of I-125 and Ir-192 interstitial brachytherapy sources. *Med Phys.* 1993;20:1569.
14. Meigooni AS, Yoe-Sein MM, Al Otoom AY, Sowards KT: Determination of the dosimetric characteristics of InterSource (125) Iodine brachytherapy source. *Appl Radiat Isot.* 2002;56:589.
15. Meigooni AS, Sowards K, Soldano M: Dosimetric characteristics of the InterSource (103) palladium brachytherapy source. *Med Physics.* 2000;27:1093.
16. Meigooni AS, Nath R: A comparison of radial dose functions for PD-103, I-125, SM-145, AM-241, YB-169, IR-192, and CS-137 brachytherapy sources. *Int J Radiat Oncol Biol Phys.* 1992; 22:1125.
17. Meigooni AS, Kleiman MT, Johnson JL, et al: Dosimetric characteristics of a new high-intensity Ir-192 source for remote afterloading. *Med Phys.* 1997;24:2008.
18. Meigooni AS, Johnson JL, Kleiman MT, et al: Dosimetric characteristics of a new HDR source. *Radiology.* 1996;201:1235.
19. Meigooni AS, Gearheart DM, Sowards K: Experimental determination of dosimetric characteristics of best (R) I-125 brachytherapy source. *Med Phys.* 2000;27:2168.
20. Meigooni AS, Bharucha Z, Yoe-Sein M, Sowards K: Dosimetric characteristics of the best (R) double-wall Pd-103 brachytherapy source. *Med Phys.* 2001;28:2568.
21. Meigooni AS, Meli JA, Nath R: Influence of the variation of energy-spectra with depth in the dosimetry of Ir-192 using LIF TLD. *Phys Med Biol.* 1988;33:1159.
22. Pradhan AS, Quast U: In-phantom response of LiF TLD-100 for dosimetry of Ir-192 HDR source. *Med Phys.* 2000;27:1025.
23. Kirov AS, Williamson JF, Meigooni AS, Zhu Y: TLD, diode and Monte Carlo dosimetry of an Ir-192 source for high dose-rate brachytherapy. *Phys Med Biol.* 1995;40:2015.
24. Watanabe Y, Roy J, Harrington PJ, Anderson LL: Experimental and Monte Carlo dosimetry of the Henschke applicator for high dose-rate Ir-192 remote afterloading. *Med Phys.* 1998;25:736.
25. Karaiskos P, Angelopoulos A, Sakelliou L, et al: Monte Carlo and TLD dosimetry of an Ir-192 high dose-rate brachytherapy source. *Med Phys.* 1998;25:1975.
26. Anctil JC, Clark BG, Arsenault CJ: Experimental determination of dosimetry functions of Ir-192 sources. *Med Phys.* 1998;25:2279.
27. Patel NS, Chiu-Tsao ST, Williamson JF, et al: Thermoluminescent dosimetry of the Symmetra TM I-125 model I25.S06 interstitial brachytherapy seed. *Med Phys.* 2001;28:1761.
28. Gearheart DM, Drogin A, Sowards K, et al: Dosimetric characteristics of a new I-125 brachytherapy source. *Med Phys.* 2000;27:2278.
29. Duggan DM, Johnson BL: Dosimetry of the I-Plant Model 3500 iodine-125 brachytherapy source. *Med Phys.* 2001;28:661.
30. Reniers B, Vynckier S, Scalliet P: Dosimetric study of the new InterSource (125) iodine seed. *Med Phys.* 2001;28:2285.
31. Nath R, Yue N: Dosimetric characterization of a newly designed encapsulated interstitial brachytherapy source of iodine-125-model LS-1 Brachyseed (TM). *Appl Radiat Isot.* 2001;55:813.
32. Meigooni AS, Yoe-Sein MM, Al Otoom AY, Sowards KT: Determination of the dosimetric characteristics of InterSource (125) Iodine brachytherapy source. *Appl Radiat Isot.* 2002;56:589.
33. Wallace RE: Model 3500 I-125 brachytherapy source dosimetric characterization. *Appl Radiat Isot.* 2002;56:581.
34. Anagnostopoulos G, Baltas D, Karaiskos P, et al: Thermoluminescent dosimetry of the select Seed I-125 interstitial brachytherapy seed. *Med Phys.* 2002;29:709.
35. Wallace RE, Fan JJ: Report on the dosimetry of a new design (125)Iodine brachytherapy source. *Med Phys.* 1999;26:1925.
36. Popescu CC, Wise J, Sowards K, et al: Dosimetric characteristics of the Pharma Seed (TM) model BT-125-I source. *Med Phys.* 2000; 27:2174.
37. Meigooni AS, Gearheart DM, Sowards K: Experimental determination of dosimetric characteristics of Best (R) I-125 brachytherapy source. *Med Phys.* 2000;27:2168.
38. Wallace RE, Fan JJ: Dosimetric characterization of a new design (103)palladium brachytherapy source. *Med Phys.* 1999;26:2465.
39. Nath R, Yue N, Shahnazi K, Bongiorni PJ: Measurement of dose-rate constant for Pd-103 seeds with air kerma strength calibration based upon a primary national standard. *Med Phys.* 2000;27:655.
40. Sloboda RS, Wang RQ: Combined experimental and Monte Carlo verification of Cs-137 brachytherapy plans for vaginal applicators. *Phys Med Biol.* 1998;43:3495.
41. Perera H, Williamson JF, Monthofer SP, et al: Rapid 2-dimensional dose measurement in brachytherapy using plastic scintillator sheet—Linearity, signal-to-noise ratio, and energy response characteristics. *Int J Radiat Oncol Biol Phys.* 1992;23:1059.
42. Li ZF, Palta JR, Fan JJ: Monte Carlo calculations and experimental measurements of dosimetry parameters of a new Pd-103 source. *Med Phys.* 2000;27:1108.
43. Li ZF, Fan JJ, Palta JR: Experimental measurements of dosimetric parameters on the transverse axis of a new I-125 source. *Med Phys.* 2000;27:1275.
44. Dale RG: Some theoretical derivations relating to the tissue dosimetry of brachytherapy nuclides, with particular reference to I-125. *Med Phys.* 1983;10:176.
45. Williamson JF, Dempsey JF, Kirov AS, et al: Plastic scintillator response to low-energy photons. *Phys Med Biol.* 1999;44:857.
46. Kirov AS, Shrinivas S, Hurlbut C, et al: New water equivalent liquid scintillation solutions for 3D dosimetry. *Med Phys.* 2000;27:1156.
47. Kirov AS, Hurlbut C, Dempsey JF, et al: Towards two-dimensional brachytherapy dosimetry using plastic scintillator: New highly efficient water equivalent plastic scintillator materials. *Med Phys.* 1999;26:1515.

48. Kirov AS, Binns WR, Dempsey JF, et al: Towards two-dimensional brachytherapy dosimetry using plastic scintillator: Localization of the scintillation process. *Nucl Instr Meth Phys Research Section A-Accel Spectrom Detect Assoc Equip.* 2000;439:178.

49. Fluhs D, Heintz M, Indenkampen F, et al: Direct reading measurement of absorbed dose with plastic scintillators—The general concept and applications to ophthalmic plaque dosimetry. *Med Phys.* 1996;23:427.

50. Quast U, Fluhs D, Heintz M, et al: Tissue equivalent plastic scintillator probes: Fast, precise Ir-192 afterloading dosimetry. *Radiother Oncol.* 31[suppl 1];22:1994. Abstract.

51. Niroomand-Rad A, Blackwell CR, Coursey BM, et al: Radiochromic film dosimetry: Recommendations of AAPM Radiation Therapy Committee Task Group 55. *Med Phys.* 1998;25:2093.

52. Monroe JI, Dempsey JF, Dorton JA, et al: Experimental validation of dose calculation algorithms for the GliaSite (TM) RTS, a novel I-125 liquid-filled balloon brachytherapy applicator. *Med Phys.* 2001;28:73.

53. Chan GH, Prestwich WV: Dosimetric properties of the new I-125 BrachySeed (TM) model LS-1 source. *Med Phys.* 2002; 29:190.

54. Skwarchuk MW, Ochran TG, Komaki R, et al: The use of radiochromic film to measure dose distributions resulting from high dose rate (192)Iridium single catheter treatments. *Int J Radiat Oncol Biol Phys.* 1996;34:173.

55. Pai S, Reinstein LE, Gluckman G, et al: The use of improved radiochromic film for in vivo quality assurance of high dose rate brachytherapy. *Med Phys.* 1998;25:1217.

56. Dempsey JF, Low DA, Mutic S, et al: Validation of a precision radiochromic film dosimetry system for quantitative two-dimensional imaging of acute exposure dose distributions. *Med Phys.* 2000;27:2462.

57. Muench PJ, Meigooni AS, Nath R, McLaughlin WL: Photon energy-dependence of the sensitivity of radiochromic film and comparison with silver-halide film and LIF TLDS used for brachytherapy dosimetry. *Med Phys.* 1991;18:769.

58. McLaughlin WL, Soares CG, Sayeg JA, et al: The use of a radiochromic detector for the determination of stereotaxic radiosurgery dose characteristics. *Med Phys.* 1994;21:379.

59. Chiutsao ST, Delazerda A, Lin J, Kim JH: High-sensitivity gafchromic film dosimetry for I-125 seed. *Med Phys.* 1994;21:651.

60. Tolli H, Johansson KA: Absorbed dose determination at short distance from Co-60 and Ir-192 brachytherapy sources. *Phys Med Biol.* 1998;43:3183.

61. Dunderstadt JJ, Martin WR: *Transport theory.* New York; London: Wiley; 1979.

62. Berger MJ: Energy deposition in water by photons from point isotropic sources 1051. *J Nucl Med.* 1968;suppl-25.

63. Loevinger R: Absorbed dose from interstitial and intracavitary sources. In Simon N, ed. *Afterloading in Radiotherapy.* Rockville, Md: Bureau of Radiological Health, US Department of Health, Education and Welfare Publication No. (FDA) 72-8024, BRH/DMRE 72-4., 1972.

64. Kahn H: *Applications of Monte Carlo.* 19 April 1954, rev. 27 April 1956 ed. Santa Monica, Calif: Rand Corp; 1956.

65. Messel H, Crawford DF: *Electron—Photon Shower Distribution Function Tables for Lead, Copper, and Air Absorbers,* 1st ed. Oxford: Pergamon Press; 1970.

66. Zaider M, Brenner DJ, Wilson WE: The applications of track calculations to radiobiology 1. Monte-Carlo simulation of proton tracks. *Radiat Res.* 1983;95:231.

67. Paretzke HG, Turner JE, Hamm RN, et al: Spatial distributions of inelastic events produced by electrons in gaseous and liquid water. *Radiat Res.* 1991;127:121.

68. Hamm RN, Turner JE, Wright HA, Ritchie RH: Calculated ionization distributions in small volumes in liquid water irradiated by protons. *Radiat Res.* 1984;97:16.

69. Berger MJ, Seltzer SM: Calculation of energy and charge deposition and of the electron flux in a water medium bombarded with 20-MEV electrons 1050. *Ann NY Acad Sci.* 1969;161:8.

70. Briesmeister JF: A general Monte Carlo N-Particle transport code, version 4A. Los Alamos National Laboratory. LA-12625. 1993.

71. Ford RL, Nelson WR: The EGS code system: Computer programs for the Monte Carlo simulation of electromagnetic showers (version 3). 210. 1978. Stanford, Calif, Stanford Linear Accelerator Center.

72. Chibani O: Simulation du transport des particules (photons, electrons et poasitrons) — Le systeme GEPTS, Thesis No.1303. 1994. Paul Sabatier University, Toulouse, France. Thesis/Dissertation.

73. Weinberg AM, Wigner EP: *The Physical Theory of Neutron Chain Reactors.*. Chicago: University of Chicago Press; 1958: 1958.

74. Williamson JF: Comparison of measured and calculated dose-rates in water near I-125 and IR-192 seeds. *Med Phys.* 1991; 18:776.

75. DeMarco JJ, Hugo G, Solberg TD: Dosimetric parameters for three low-energy brachytherapy sources using the Monte Carlo N-Particle code. *Med Phys.* 2002;29:662.

76. Wuu CS, Zaider M: A calculation of the relative biological effectiveness of 125I and 103Pd brachytherapy sources using the concept of proximity function. *Medical Physics.* 1998; 25:2186.

77. Wuu CS, Kliauga P, Zaider M, Amols HI: Microdosimetric evaluation of relative biological effectiveness for 103Pd, 125I, 241Am, and 192Ir brachytherapy sources. *Int J Radiat Oncol Biol Phys.* 1996;36:689.

78. Dale RG: A Montecarlo derivation of parameters for use in the tissue dosimetry of medium and low-energy nuclides. *Br J Radiol.* 1982;55:748.

79. Burns GS, Raeside DE: Monte-Carlo estimates of specific absorbed fractions for an I-125 point-source in water. *Med Phys.* 1983;10:197.

80. Williamson JF, Morin RL, Khan FM: Monte-Carlo evaluation of the sievert integral for brachytherapy dosimetry. *Phys Med Biol.* 1983;28:1021.

81. Williamson JF: Monte-Carlo evaluation of specific dose constants in water for I-125 seeds. *Med Phys.* 1988;15:686.

82. Sanchez-Reyes A, Tello JJ, Guix B, Salvat F: Monte Carlo calculation of the dose distributions of two Ru-106 eye applicators. *Radiother Oncol.* 1998;49:191.

83. Rivard MJ: Monte Carlo calculations of AAPM Task Group Report No. 43 dosimetry parameters for the MED3631-A/(MI)-I-125 source. *Med Phys.* 2001;28:629.

84. Bohm TD, Pearson DW, Das RK: Measurements and Monte Carlo calculations to determine the absolute detector response of radiochromic film for brachytherapy dosimetry. *Med Phys.* 2001; 28:142.

85. Wierzbicki JG, Rivard MJ, Waid DS, Arterbery VE: Calculated dosimetric parameters of the IoGold I-125 source model 3631-A. *Med Phys.* 1998;25:2197.

86. Berger MJ: Distribution of absorbed dose around point sources of electrons and beta particles in water and other media. *J Nucl Med.* 1971;suppl-23.

87. Clairand I, Ricard M, Gouriou J, et al: DOSE3D: EGS4 Monte Carlo code-based software for internal radionuclide dosimetry. *J Nucl Med.* 1999;40:1517.

88. Furhang EE, Chui CS, Sgouros G: A Monte Carlo approach to patient-specific dosimetry. *Med Phys.* 1996;23:1523.

89. Furhang EE, Chui CS, Kolbert KS, et al: Implementation of a Monte Carlo dosimetry method for patient-specific internal emitter therapy. *Med Phys.* 1997;24:1163.

90. Kellerer AM: Considerations on the random traversal of convex bodies and solutions for general cylinders. *Radiat Res.* 1971; 47:359.

91. Kellerer AM: Chord-length distributions and related quantities for spheroids 1065. *Radiat Res.* 1984;98:425.

92. Loevinger R, Budinger TF, Watson EE, Society of Nuclear Medicine (Medical Internal Radiation Dose Committee: *MIRD primer for absorbed dose calculations.* New York: Society of Nuclear Medicine; 1988.

93. Katagiri M, Hikoji M, Kitaichi M, et al: Effective doses and organ doses per unit fluence calculated for monoenergetic 0.1 Mev to 100 MeV electrons by the MIRD-5 phantom. *Radiat Protect Dosim.* 2000;90:393.

94. Bardies M, Myers MJ: Computational methods in radionuclide dosimetry. *Phys Med Biol.* 1996;41:1941.

95. Bardies M, Pihet P: Dosimetry and microdosimetry of targeted radiotherapy. *Curr Pharm Des.* 2000;6:1469.

96. Toohey RE, Stabin MG, Watson EE: The AAPM/RSNA physics tutorial for residents—Internal radiation dosimetry: Principles and applications. *Radiographics.* 2000;20:533.

97. Zanzonico PB: Internal radionuclide radiation dosimetry: A review of basic concepts and recent developments. *J Nucl Med.* 2000;41:297.

98. Siegel JA, Thomas SR, Stubbs JB, et al: MIRD pamphlet no. 16: Techniques for quantitative radiopharmaceutical biodistribution data acquisition and analysis for use in human radiation dose estimates. *J Nucl Med.* 1999;40:37S.

99. Watson EE, Stabin MG, Siegel JA: MIRD formulation. *Med Phys.* 1993;20:511.

100. Humm JL, Roeske JC, Fisher DR, Chen GTY: Microdosimetric Concepts in Radioimmunotherapy. *Med Phys.* 1993;20:535.

101. Leichner PK, Kwok CS: Tumor dosimetry in radioimmunotherapy—Methods of calculation for beta-particles. *Med Phys.* 1993;20:529.

102. Pan ZY, Wolf W: Computer package for the calculation of the radiation-dose to patients, based on the MIRD approach. *J Nucl Med.* 1985;26:318.

103. Bateman J, Rossi HH: RBE studies with monoenergetic neutrons. A. Opacification studies. NYO-2740-6. *NYO Reports.* 1969;235.

104. Bateman JL, Johnson HA, Bond VP, Rossi HH: The dependence of RBE on the energy of fast neutrons for spermatogonia depletion in mice. *Radiat Res.* 1968;35:86.

105. Bateman JL, Rossi HH, Kellerer AM, et al: Dose-dependence of fast neutron RBE for lens opacification in mice. *Radiat Res.* 1972;51:381.

106. Bond VP, Meinhold CB, Rossi HH: Low-dose RBE and Q for x-ray compared to gamma-ray radiations. *Health Phys.* 1978;34:433.

107. Hall EJ, Kellerer AM: The biophysical properties of 3.9-GeV nitrogen ions. 3. OER and RBE determinations using Vicia seedlings. *Radiat Res.* 1973;55:422.

108. Hall EJ, Novak JK, Kellerer AM, et al: RBE as a function of neutron energy. I. Experimental observations. *Radiat Res.* 1975;64:245.

109. Kellerer AM, Hall EJ, Rossi HH, Teedla P: RBE as a function of neutron energy. II. Statistical analysis. *Radiat Res.* 1976;65:172.

110. Kellerer AM, Rossi HH: RBE and the primary mechanism of radiation action. *Radiat Res.* 1971;47:15.

111. Kellerer AM, Rossi HH: Dependence of RBE on neutron dose. *Br J Radiol.* 1972;45:626.

112. Wolf C, Lafuma J, Masse R, et al: Neutron RBE for induction of tumors with high lethality in Sprague-Dawley rats. *Radiat Res.* 2000;154:412.

113. Ling CC, Li WX, Anderson LL: The relative biological effectiveness of I-125 and Pd-103. *Int J Radiat Oncol Biol Phys.* 1995; 32:373.

114. Nath R, Meigooni AS, Melillo A: Some treatment planning considerations for Pd-103 and I-125 permanent interstitial implants. *Int J Radiat Oncol Biol Phys.* 1992;22:1131.

115. Zellmer DL, Gillin MT, Wilson JF: Microdosimetric single event spectra of yb-169 compared with commonly used brachytherapy sources and teletherapy beams. *Int J Radiat Oncol Biol Phys.* 1992;23:627.

116. Zellmer DL, Shadley JD, Gillin MT: Comparisons of measured biological response and predictions from microdosimetric data applicable to brachytherapy. *Radiat Protect Dosim.* 1994;52:395.

117. Kellerer AM, Chmelevsky D: Concepts of microdosimetry. I. Quantities. *Radiat Environ Biophys.* 1975;12:61.

118. Kellerer AM, Chmelevsky D: Concepts of microdosimetry II. Probability distributions of the microdosimetric variables. *Radiat Environ Biophys.* 1975;12:205.

119. Kellerer AM, Chmelevsky D: Concepts of microdosimetry. III. Mean values of the microdosimetric distributions. *Radiat Environ Biophys.* 1975;12:321.

120. Rossi HH, Zaider M: *Microdosimetry and Its Applications.* Berlin/Heidelberg: Springer-Verlag; 1996.

121. International Commission on Radiation Units and Measurements: *Microdosimetry 32.* Bethesda, Md: ICRU, 1983.

122. Zaider M, Rossi HH: On the application of microdosimetry to radiobiology. *Radiat Res.* 1988;113:15.

123. Cauchy A: Memoire sur la rectification des courbes et la quadrature des surface courbes. *Qevres completes.* Paris: Gauthier Villard; 1908.

124. Kellerer AM, Rossi HH: Generalized Formulation of Dual Radiation Action. *Radiat Res.* 1978;75:471.

125. Zaider M: There is no mechanistic basis for the use of the linear-quadratic expression in cellular survival analysis. *Med Phys.* 1998; 25:791.

126. Rossi HH: The radiobiological significance of spatial and temporal distribution of energy absorbed from ionizing radiations. [Review] [36 refs]. *Basic Life Sci.* 1991;58:325.

127. Rossi HH: The role of microdosimetry in radiobiology. *Radiat Environ Biophys.* 1979;17:29.

128. Rossi HH: Interpretation of biological response in terms of microdosimetry. *Ann NY Acad Sci.* 1969;161:260.

129. Lea DE, Catcheside DG: The mechanism of the induction by radiation of chromosome aberrations in tradescantia. *J Genetic.* 1942;44:216.

130. Zaider M, Dicello J: RBEOER: A Fortran program for the computation of RBEs, OERs, survival ratios and the effects of fractionation using the theory of dual radiation action. Los Alamos Scientific Laboratory Report LA-7196-MS, 1-19. 1978.

131. Sur RK, Levin CV, Donde B, et al: Prospective randomized trial of HDR brachytherapy as a sole modality in palliation of advanced esophageal carcinoma—An International Atomic Energy Agency Study. *Int J Radiat Oncol Biol Phys.* 2002;53:127.

132. Nag S, Tippin D, Ruymann FB: Intraoperative high-dose-rate brachytherapy for the treatment of pediatric tumors: The Ohio State University experience. *Int J Radiat Oncol Biol Phys.* 2001; 51:729.

133. Nag S, Shasha D, Janjan N, et al: The American Brachytherapy Society recommendations for brachytherapy of soft tissue sarcomas. *Int J Radiat Oncol Biol Phys.* 2001;49:1033.

134. Nag S, Erickson B, Parikh S, et al: The American brachytherapy society recommendations for high-dose-rate brachytherapy for carcinoma of the endometrium. *Int J Radiat Oncol Biol Phys.* 2000;48:779.

135. Blasko JC, Mate T, Sylvester JE, et al: Brachytherapy for carcinoma of the prostate: Techniques, patient selection, and clinical outcomes. *Semin Radiat Oncol.* 2002;12:81.

136. Kucera H, Mock U, Knocke TH, et al: Radiotherapy alone for invasive vaginal cancer: Outcome with intracavitary high dose rate brachytherapy versus conventional low dose rate brachytherapy. *Acta Obstetricia et Gynecologica Scandinavica.* 2001;80:355.

137. Leung TW, Wong VYW, Kwan KH, et al: High dose rate brachytherapy for early stage oral tongue cancer. *Head Neck—J Sci Special Head Neck.* 2002;24:274.

138. Lu JJ, Bains YS, Abdel-Wahab M, et al: High-dose-rate remote afterloading intracavitary brachytherapy for the treatment of extrahepatic biliary duct carcinoma. *Cancer J.* 2002;8:74.

139. Suh JH, Barnett GH: Brachytherapy for brain tumor. *Hematol Oncol Clin North Am.* 1999;13:635.

140. Guix B, Finestres F, Tello JI, et al: Treatment of skin carcinomas of the face by high-dose-rate brachytherapy and custom-made surface molds. *Int J Radiat Oncol Biol Phys.* 2000;47:95.

141. Baglan KL, Martinez AA, Frazier RC, et al: The use of high-dose-rate brachytherapy alone after lumpectomy in patients with early-stage breast cancer treated with breast-conserving therapy. *Int J Radiat Oncol Biol Phys.* 2001;50:1003.

142. Anderson LL, Nath R., Olch AJ, et al: American Endocurietherapy Society recommendations for dose specifications in brachytherapy. *Endocurietherapy Hyperthem Oncol.* 1991;7:1.

143. Anderson LL, Hoffman MR, Harrington PJ, Starkschall G: Atlas generation for intraoperative high dose rate brachytherapy. *J Brachyther Int.* 1997;13:333.

144. Chiu-Tsao S-T: I-125 Episcleral ete plaque for treatment of intra-ocular malignancies. In Williamson JF, Thomadsen BR, Nath R, eds. *Brachytherapy Physics, AAPM Summer School 1994.* Madison, Wisc: American Association of Physicists in Medicine; 1994:451.

145. International Commission on Radiological Units and Measurements: *Dose and volume specification for reporting intracavitary therapy in gynecology 113.* Bethesda, Md.: ICRU; 1985.

146. Fung AY, Alektiar KM, Silvern DA, Zaider M: Treatment-plan optimization for soft-tissue sarcoma brachytherapy using a genetic algorithm. *Int J Radiat Oncol Biol Phys.* 2000;47:1385.

147. Amols HI, Rosen II: A 3-film technique for reconstruction of radioactive seed implants. *Med Phys.* 1981;8:210.

148. Rosen II, Khan KM, Lane RG, Kelsey CA: The effect of geometric errors in the reconstruction of IR-192 seed implants. *Med Phys.* 1982;9:220.

149. Biggs PJ, Kelley DM: Geometric reconstruction of seed implants using a 3-film technique. *Med Phys.* 1983;10:701.

150. Rosenthal MS, Math R: An automatic seed identification technique for interstitial implants using 3 isocentric radiographs. *Med Phys.* 1983;10:475.

151. Siddon RL, Chin LM: 2-film brachytherapy reconstruction algorithm. *Med Phys.* 1985;12:77.

152. Todor DA, Cohen GN, Amols HI, Zaider M: Operator-free, film-based 3D seed reconstruction in brachytherapy. *Phys Med Biol.* 2002;47:2031.

153. Tubic D, Zaccarin A, Pouliot J, Beaulieu L: Automated seed detection and three-dimensional reconstruction. I. Seed localization from fluoroscopic images or radiographs. *Med Phys.* 2001; 28:2265.

154. Tubic D, Zaccarin A, Beaulieu L, Pouliot J: Automated seed detection and three-dimensional reconstruction. II. Reconstruction of permanent prostate implants using simulated annealing. *Med Phys.* 2001;28:2272.

155. Meli JA: Source localization. In Williamson JF, Thomadsen BR, Nath R, eds. *AAPM Summer School 1994.* Madison, Wisc: Medical Physics Publishing Company; 1995:236.

156. *Radium Dosage: The Manchester System,* 2nd ed. Baltimore: Williams & Wilkins; 1967.

157. Anderson L: Spacing nomograph for interstitial implant of I-125 seeds. *Med Phys.* 1976;3:48.

158. Anderson LL, Moni JV, Harrison LB: A nomograph for permanent implants of Pd-103 seeds. *Int J Radiat Oncol Biol Phys.* 1993;27:129.

159. Cohen GN, Amols HI, Zelefsky MJ, Zaider M: The Anderson nomograms for permanent interstitial prostate implants: A briefing for practitioners. *Int J Radiat Oncol Biol Phys.* 2002;53:504.

160. Hilaris BS, Nori D, Anderson LL: *An Atlas of Brachytherapy.* New York: Macmillan; 1988.

161. Pierquin B, Wilson JF, Chassagne D: *Modern Brachytherapy.* New York: Masson; 1987.

162. Pierquin B, Marinello G: *A Practical Manual of Brachytherapy 9.* Madison, Wis: Medical Physics Pub; 1997.

163. Pierquin B: *Brachytherapy.* St. Louis: WH Green; 1978.

164. Gillin MT, Albano KS, Erikson B: Classical systems II for planar and volume temporary interstitial implants: The Paris system and other systems. In Williamson JF, Thomadsen BR, Nath R, eds. *Brachytherapy Physics, AAPM Summer School 1994.* Madison, Wisc: American Association of Physicists in Medicine; 1995:324.

165. Kneschaurek P, Wehrmann R, Hugo C, et al: Die Flabmethode zur intraoperativen Bestrahlung. *Strahlentherapie und Onkologie.* 1995;171:61.

166. Sloboda RS: Optimization of brachytherapy dose distribution by simulated annealing. *Med Physics.* 1992;19:964.

167. Pouliot J, Tremblay D, Roy J, Filice S: Optimization of permanent I-125 prostate implants using fast simulated annealing. *Int J Radiat Oncol Biol Phys.* 1996;36:711.

168. Silvern DA: Automated OR prostate brachytherapy treatment planning using genetic optimization. 1998. Columbia University in the City of New York. Thesis/Dissertation.

169. Yu Y, Schell MC: A genetic algorithm for the optimization of prostate implants. *Med Phys.* 1996;23:2085.

170. Gallagher RJ, Lee EK: Mixed integer programming optimization models for brachytherapy treatment planning. *Proc AMIA Annual Fall Symposium.* 1997;278.

171. Lee EK, Gallagher RJ, Silvern D, et al: Treatment planning for brachytherapy: An integer programming model, two computational approaches and experiments with permanent prostate implant planning. *Phys Med Biol.* 1999;44:145.

172. Zaider M, Zelefsky MJ, Lee EK, et al: Treatment planning for prostate implants using magnetic-resonance spectroscopy imaging. *Int J Radiat Oncol Biol Phys.* 2000;47:1085.

173. Chambers L: *Practical Handbook of Genetic Algorithms.* Boca Raton, Fla: CRC Press; 1995.

174. Grefenstette JJ, American Association for Artificial Intelligence, Bolt BaNi, Naval Research Laboratory (U.S.): *Genetic Algorithms and Their Applications: Proceedings of the Second International Conference on Genetic Algorithms, July 28-31, 1987 at the Massachusetts Institute of Technology, Cambridge, Mass.* Hillsdale, NJ: Erlbaum Associates; 1987.

175. Man KF, Tang KS, Kwong S: *Genetic Algorithms Concepts and Designs.* London: Springer; 1999.

176. Zalzala AMS, Fleming PJ: *Genetic Algorithms in Engineering Systems.* London: Institution of Electrical Engineers; 1997.

177. Kirkpatrick S, Gelatt CD, Vecchi MP: Optimization by simulated annealing. *Science.* 1983;220:671.

178. Press WH: *Numerical Recipes in FORTRAN: The Art of Scientific Computing,* 2nd ed. Cambridge, England: Cambridge University Press; 1992.

179. Metropolis NA, Rosenbluth A, Rosenbluth M, et al: Equation of state calculations by fast computing machines. *J Chem Phys.* 1953;21:1087.

180. International Commission on Radiation Units and Measurements: *Determination of Absorbed Dose in a Patient Irradiated by Beams of X or Gamma Rays in Radiotherapy Procedures 20.* Washington, DC: International Commission on Radiation Units and Measurements; 1976.

181. Schulz RJ: Further improvements in close distributions are unlikely to affect cure rates. *Med Phys.* 1999;26:1007.

182. Wefer AE, Hricak H, Vigneron DB, et al: Sextant localization of prostate cancer: Comparison of sextant biopsy, magnetic resonance imaging and magnetic resonance spectroscopic imaging with step section histology. *J Urol.* 2000;164:400.

183. Kurhanewicz J, Vigneron DB, Nelson SJ, et al: Citrate as an in-vivo marker to discriminate prostate-cancer from benign prostatic hyperplasia and normal prostate peripheral zone—Detection via localized proton spectroscopy. *Urology.* 1995;45:459.

184. Kurhanewicz J, Vigneron DB, Nelson SJ: Three-dimensional magnetic resonance spectroscopic imaging of brain and prostate cancer. *Neoplasia.* 2000;2:166.

185. Kurhanewicz J, Vigneron DB, Males RG, et al: The prostate: MR imaging and spectroscopy—Present and future. *Radiol Clin North Am.* 2000;38:115.

186. Scheidler J, Hricak H, Vigneron DB, et al: Prostate cancer: Localization with three-dimensional proton MR spectroscopic imaging—Clinicopathologic study. *Radiology.* 1999;213:473.

187. International Commission on Radiation Units and Measurements: *Radiation Quantities and Units.* Washington, DC: International Commission on Radiation Units and Measurements; 1980.

188. American Association of Physicists in Medicine. Specification of brachytherapy source strength. Task Group No. 32. Report 21. 1987. New York, American Institute of Physics.

189. Kliauga P, Dvorak R: Microdosimetric measurements of ionization by monoenergetic photons 1199. *Radiat Res.* 1978;73:1.

190. Comité Français pour le Mésure des Rayonnements Ionisants. Recommendations pour la Détermination des Doses Absorbées en Curiethérapie. CFMRI No.1. 1983. Paris, CFMRI.

191. Burlin TE: A general theory of cavity ionization. *Br J Radiol.* 1966;39:727.

Instruments and Techniques in Brachytherapy

12

Kaled M. Alektiar, MD and Michael J. Zelefsky, MD

The word brachytherapy means treatment with radioactive sources placed at a short ("brachy" is Greek for "short") distance from the body. The history of brachytherapy dates back to the late 19th century when radium was discovered in 1898 by Marie and Pierre Curie, and soon after that the use of radium in the treatment of cancer began. In 1917 the first report on radium therapy in bladder and prostate cancer was published by Janeway and colleagues[1] from Memorial Sloan-Kettering Cancer Center (MSKCC).

The treatment of cancer with brachytherapy continued to flourish in the early part of the 20th century; however, by the 1950s its use became increasingly confined to gynecologic applications due to the following events: (1) major technologic development of x-ray machines capable of producing a wide range of high energy photons and electrons, (2) concern about radiation exposure, and (3) the drive to achieve a homogeneous dose distribution throughout the treated volume.

The concept of afterloading was first introduced into clinical practice by Henschke[2] in the 1960s, which allowed the rapid placement of radiation sources into nonradioactive channels that had first been positioned into the tumor. This ingenious technique, coupled with the introduction of man-made isotopes with a wide range of energies, led to an increase in the use of brachytherapy alone or more commonly in combination with external beam radiotherapy (EBRT).

The introduction of three-dimensional (3D) conformal, and more recently, intensity-modulated radiation therapy (IMRT), treatment planning in EBRT has led to a resurgence in the interest of brachytherapy as a form of conformal radiotherapy. This is largely due to the intrinsic property of brachytherapy that allows maximal tumor dose while minimizing the dose to the surrounding normal tissue, a concept that continues to be the main goal of radiotherapy. This could be enhanced even more by using high-dose-rate (HDR) remote afterloading treatment with its different optimization schemes.

GENERAL PRINCIPLES

Brachytherapy procedures are categorized as using implants that are temporary or as using those that are permanent. Both types are discussed in this chapter.

Temporary Implants

Temporary implants fall into four categories: (1) interstitial implants that are placed directly within the tumor bed; (2) intracavitary implants, where an applicator is placed into body cavities such as the uterus or the rectum; (3) intraluminal implants, in which an afterloading catheter is placed inside a body viscera such as the esophagus or the bronchus; and (4) intraoperative implants, in which the sources are placed into a surface applicator that is in direct contact with the tumor bed.

INTERSTITIAL

Iridium-192 (^{192}Ir) is the most commonly used isotope for temporary interstitial implants that can be done free hand or stabilized by a template.

Free Hand

The instruments needed for free hand temporary implants include: (1) nylon afterloading catheters 50 cm long with a thin leader portion; (2) nylon afterloading catheters 50 cm long with a sealed end; (3) straight stainless steel needles, 17 gauge and 15 cm long; (4) curved stainless steel needles, 15 and 20 cm long; (5) a 15 cm stainless steel ruler; (6) metal buttons, which prevent the plastic afterloading catheters from slipping (a silk suture is threaded through each of the two holes at the button and through the skin; when crimped, the metal button prevents the radioactive sources from slipping as well; and (7) plastic hemispheric buttons that separate the skin from the metal buttons to prevent electron scatter from the metal buttons once the catheters are loaded (Fig. 12-1).

These instruments should be wrapped in a package and gas sterilized. Autoclaving could damage the plastic afterloading catheters. The catheters have either dummy sources at 1 cm intervals (Fig. 12-2) or a wire that provides stability and prevents kinking, especially in loop implants. The catheters with dummy sources come in different colors to assist in their identification when multiple catheters are used.

TECHNIQUES

SEALED END TECHNIQUE. This method is used to implant tumors or tumor beds that are accessible from one side only, like tumors in the thoracic or abdominal cavities.

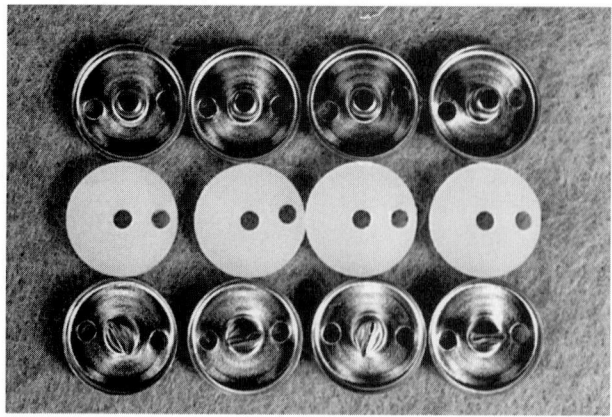

Figure 12–1. Plastic and metal buttons used in securing the sources inside the afterloading catheters. *Upper row* shows uncrimped metal buttons, *center row* shows plastic buttons, and *lower row* shows metal buttons with the tubular portion crimped.

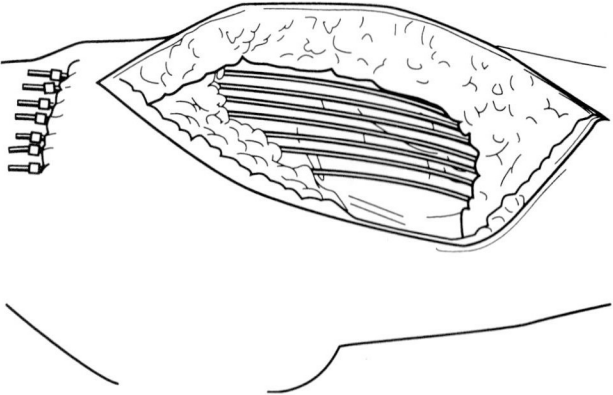

Figure 12–3. Sealed-end technique. Illustration of afterloading catheters with distal ends embedded inside the tumor bed. The proximal ends are sutured to the skin via buttons.

Another indication for this method is when it is desirable to decrease the number of entrance and exit points of the catheters as in soft tissue sarcomas (Fig. 12-3).[3,4]

The first step in this procedure is to insert a straight or curved stainless steel needle through the skin and into the tumor or tumor bed (Fig. 12-4). The second step is to thread the sealed end of the afterloading catheter through the needle and push it until it emerges from the tip of the needle. The third step is to hold the sealed end of the catheter and at the same time pull the needle out. In the fourth step, the catheter is advanced as much as desired to cover the tumor or tumor bed with enough margin. Then chromic catgut sutures are used to stabilize the catheters in the tumor bed. This process is repeated until an adequate number of catheters is used.

In planar implants, the catheters are usually placed parallel and 1 cm apart. In multi-planar implants, the catheters are usually spaced 1.2 to 2 cm apart with 1.5 to 2 cm between planes. A nomogram designed by Anderson et al.[5] can be used to determine the exact spacing between catheters in planar implants.

The plastic hemispheric and metal buttons are slid over the part of the catheter that is outside the skin and the metal buttons are crimped and sutured to the skin to prevent catheter slippage. The free ends of the catheters are folded and kept together inside a tightened Penrose drain.

THROUGH AND THROUGH TECHNIQUE. This technique is used when both sides of the tumor are accessible, as in tumors in the breast,[6,7] lip,[8] skin, and neck nodes.[9,10] The first step is to insert the needle through the skin into the tumor or tumor bed and then to exit through the skin again on the opposite side of the tumor. It is desirable to mark the entrance and exit points of each needle inserted on the skin so that the catheters will be placed parallel to each other. The second step is to thread the thin end of the catheter through the needle until it exits from the tip of the needle. In the third step, the thin end of the catheter and tip of the needle are pulled so that the wider portion of the plastic catheter is following the needle. Now the catheter has an entrance and exit point through the skin and each of these ends is stabilized in place by

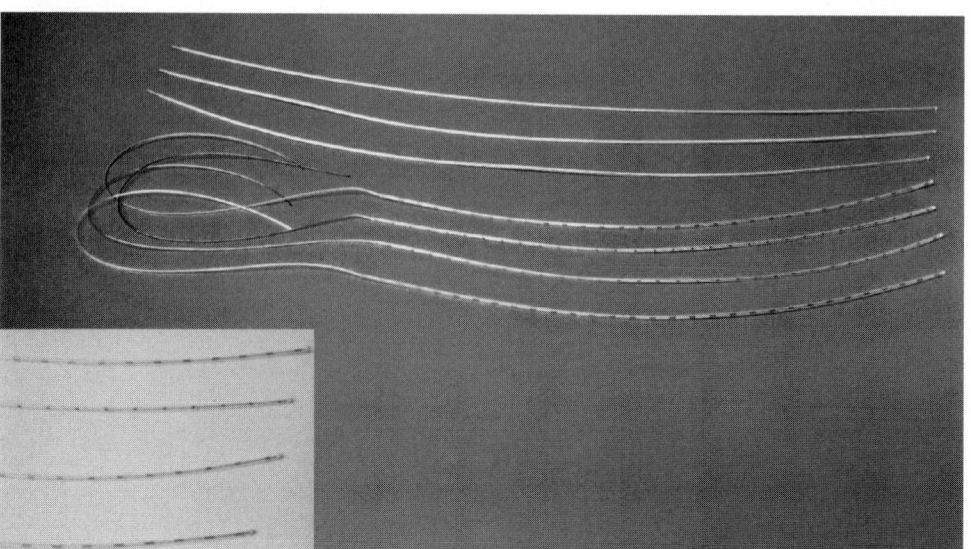

Figure 12–2. Top three catheters with wires and bottom four catheters with dummy sources. *Insert* shows a magnified view of the different sizes of the dummy sources.

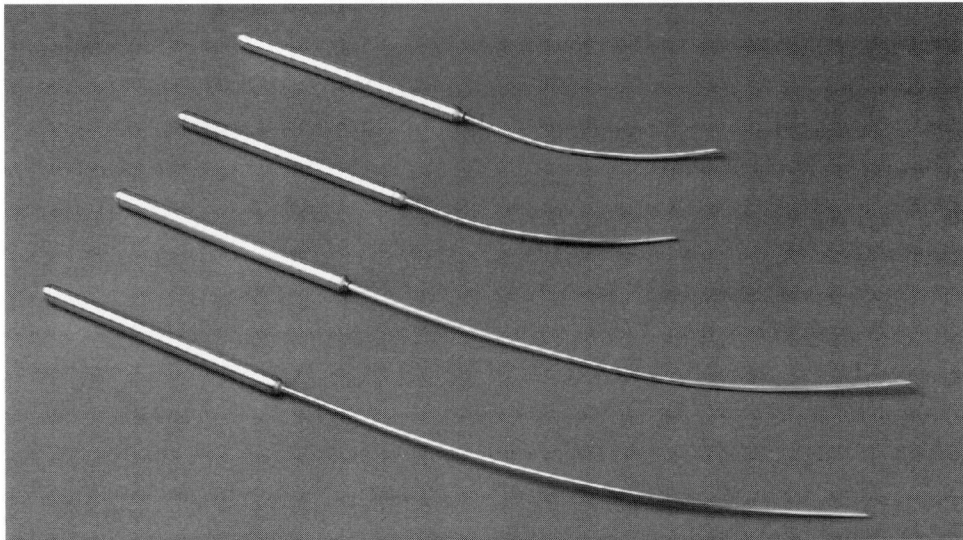

Figure 12–4. Short curved trocars (*top*) and long curved trocars (*bottom*).

plastic hemispheric and metal buttons that are crimped and sutured to the skin (Fig. 12-5). The ends of plastic catheters are cut off with at least 4 cm extending beyond the metal buttons.

LOOP TECHNIQUE. This technique is mainly used in the treatment of cancer of the oral cavity[11,12] or oropharynx.[13] A good example of the loop technique is in the base of tongue (Fig. 12-6). It involves the percutaneous introduction of a curved trocar by means of submental approach through the base of tongue. The catheter is threaded through the trocar and looped back through an adjacent trocar, creating a loop in the base of tongue. Both ends exit the skin of the neck. An array of loops is created to encompass the target volume plus about a 1 to 1.5 cm margin. The spacing between each end of the loop is 1 cm and between each plane is 1 to 1.5 cm.

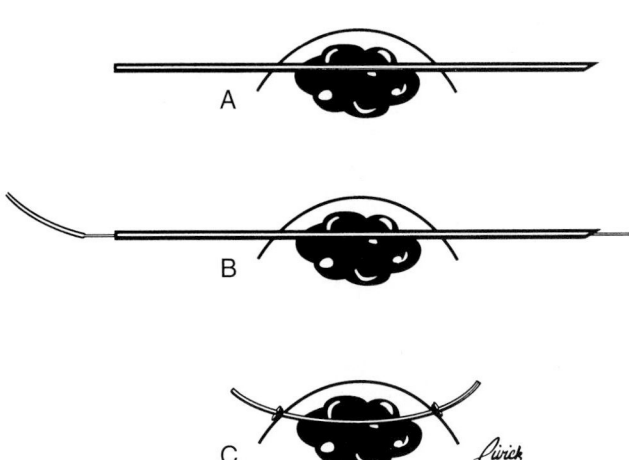

Figure 12–5. Through-and-through technique. The needle passes through the tumor bed, penetrating the skin surfaces on entrance and exit (**A**). The leader of an afterloading catheter is threaded through the stainless steel needle (**B**). The catheter is then pulled through the implant area and secured on each end (**C**).

TREATMENT PLANNING AND DELIVERY

The procedures used in the treatment planning of temporary implants are as important as those used in external beam radiotherapy planning.

The planning of a temporary implant starts either at or before the implant procedure itself, where tumor volume or tumor bed measurements are obtained and spacing between catheters is determined. A single-plane implant is usually sufficient for tumors less than 1.5 cm thick or for tumor bed implants (Fig. 12-7). A two-plane implant is recommended for tumors thicker than 1.5 cm but less than 2.5 cm with spacing at 1.2 to 2 cm between catheters and 1.5 to 2 cm between planes. A volume implant is recommended for larger tumors.

The next step is source localization, which determines the relationship between the sources themselves and surrounding structures. This localization process is best done on a simulator from which two or more films can be obtained at arbitrary isocentric angles. The afterloading catheters are usually 50 cm long. This excess length is not needed in most cases; therefore, they need to be cut, leaving a stump 3 to 4 cm long with a beveled edge. The films are obtained with dummy sources at 1 cm intervals that are already inside the afterloading catheters, or if wires are used, they should be replaced with dummy sources at this time. These localization films should not only demonstrate the target volume but also reference points at the surrounding normal structure. For example, in the case of soft tissue sarcoma of the thigh in a young man, this would include skin, neurovascular bundle, and testicles.

Computerized treatment plans are an integral part of modern brachytherapy, and they should be obtained in all cases. For temporary implants, the treatment time is determined by dividing the prescribed dose by a treatment dose rate selected from appropriately generated isodose-rate contours. Planar implants are mainly used as an adjunct to surgical excision, and therefore the thickness of tissue that requires irradiation is rather small. In practice it is assumed that 1 cm treatment region thickness is

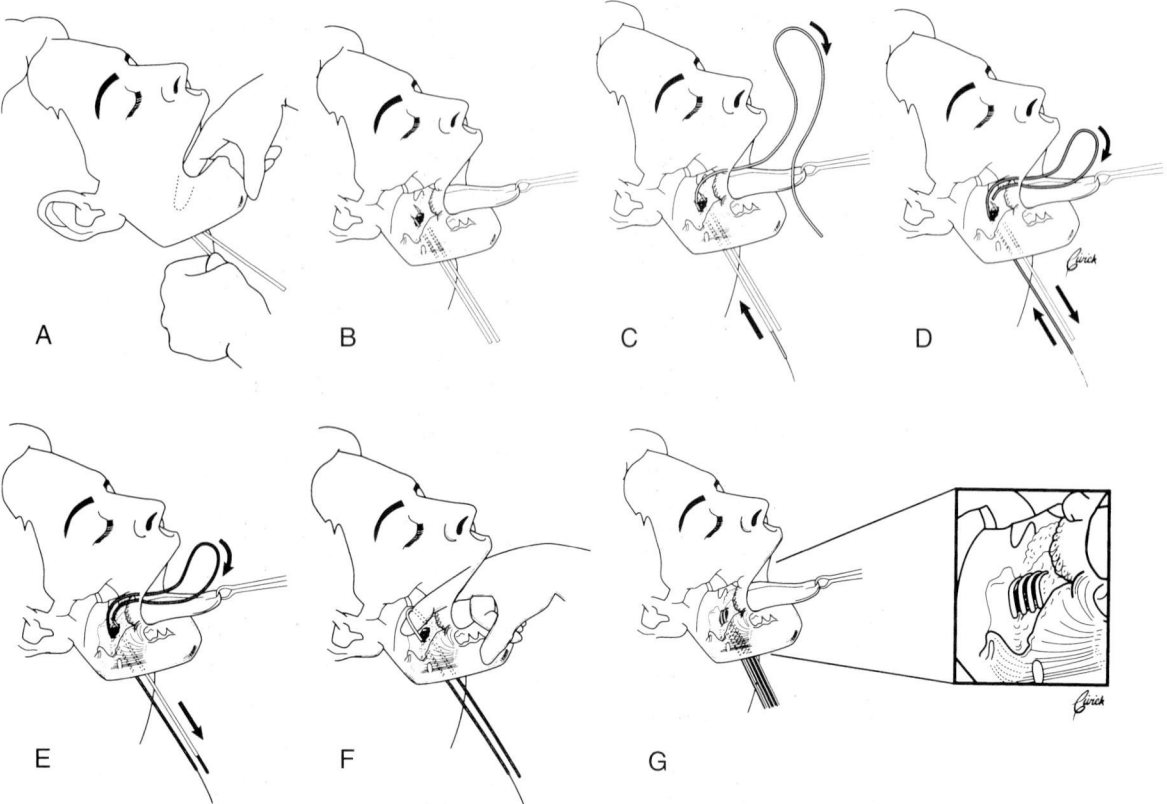

Figure 12–6. Loop technique. The stainless steel needles are inserted into the submental area with one hand until they exit through the base of tongue, guided by the index finger of the other hand (**A**). Two stainless steel needles are shown exiting through the base of tongue (**B**). The blind end of the afterloading catheter is first inserted through the submental end of one of the needles until it exits through the mouth (**C**). The blind end is then reversed and threaded through the oral end of the other needle (**D**). A full loop is created when the blind end exits through the submental end of the second needle (**E**). The stainless steel needles are removed, and the loop is pulled loosely against the surface of the base of tongue (**F**), allowing room for post-insertion edema. Two looped afterloading catheters in position (**G**), four loops cover half of the base of tongue (*inset*).

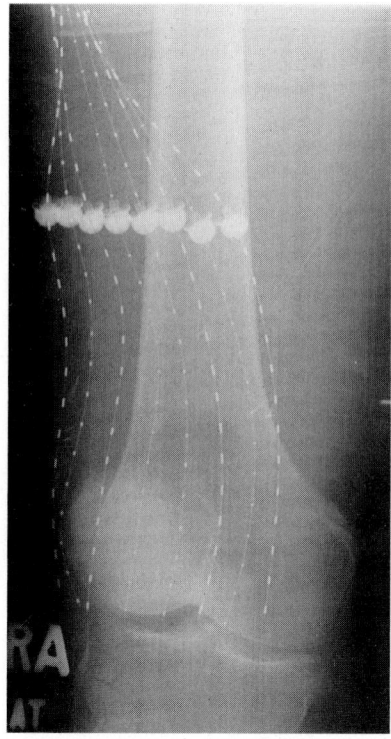

Figure 12–7. X-ray of a single-plane implant.

adequate for potential microscopic disease. At MSKCC the implant dose is prescribed to the median peripheral dose rate (MPDR) line. The MPDR is obtained from several computer planes throughout the target volume, and in each plane the first isodose rate line that is continuous (i.e., without gaps) is selected. Then the lowest isodose rate line among all the planes is chosen. This is referred to as the MPDR. For example, in a planar implant of soft tissue sarcoma, four transverse cuts were obtained. In the first cut, the 10 Gy/day line was the first line that covered all seeds continuously, in the second cut it was 9 Gy/day, the third 10 Gy/day, and the fourth 10 Gy/day. The MPDR will be 9 Gy/day (Fig. 12-8). If the planar implant is performed properly, the range of MPDR should be 8 to 12 Gy/day and its thickness close to 1 cm. At MSKCC a special form is used to determine the MPDR, the duration of an implant, and the total dose of radiation to adjacent structure (Fig. 12-9). If the total dose of the implant in the previous example is 45 Gy, then the duration of the implant will be 45 Gy divided by 9 Gy/day equal to 5 days.

The computerized planning of volume implants is evolving due to the advances in tumor imaging and the ability to reconstruct the tumor/tumor bed volume in three dimensions. Ideally, the dose should be prescribed to the dose rate line that encompasses the target volume in a similar fashion to choosing an isodose line for prostate cancer using 3D treatment planning (Fig. 12-10). If the

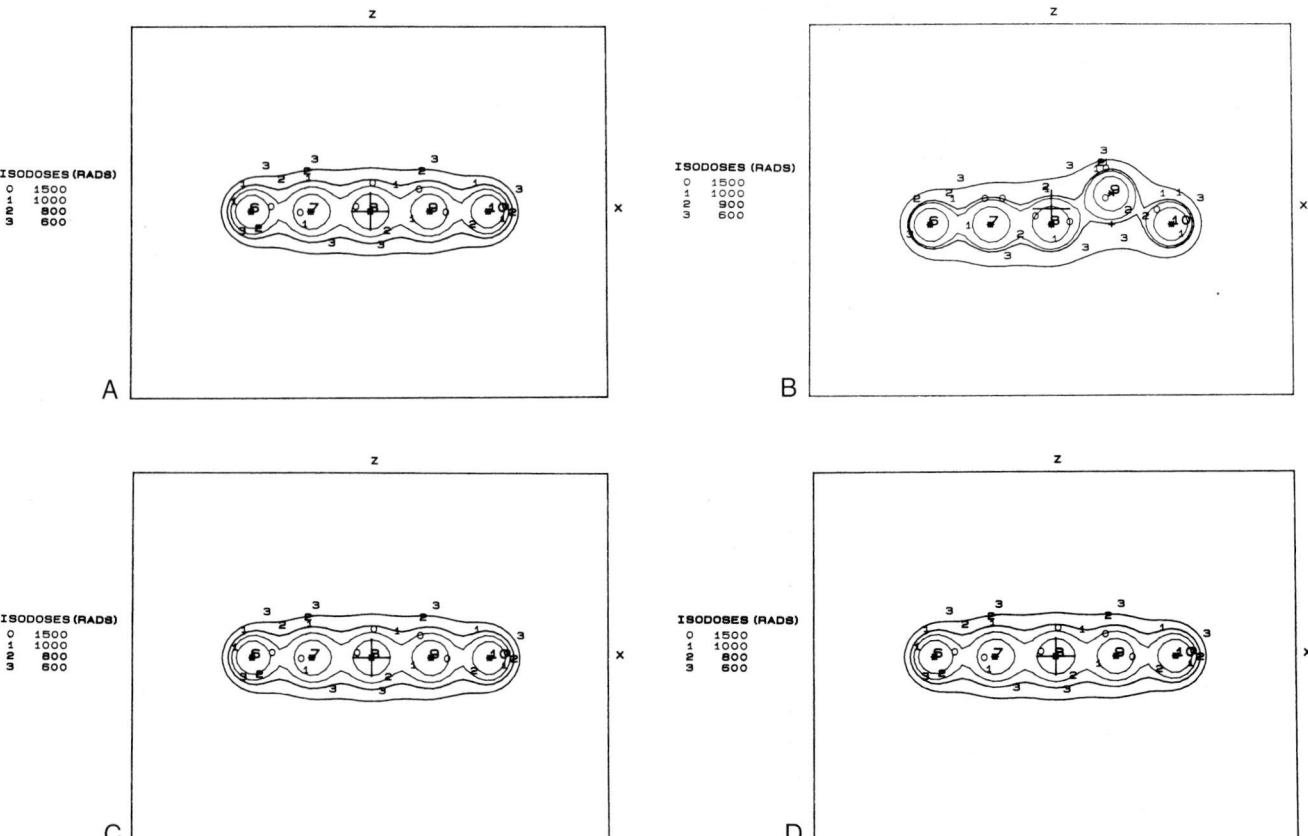

Figure 12–8. Determining the median peripheral dose rate (MPDR) line from a set of isodose plans. In **A, C,** and **D,** the first isodose rate line that is continuous is the 1000 Gy/day line, but in **B,** it is 900 cGy/day. Therefore, the MPDR is 900 cGy/day.

implant was performed without the use of 3D imaging, at least a target projection should be drawn on orthogonal simulation films. The dose is then prescribed to the isodose-rate contour in a similar fashion as planar implantation.

Before loading any patient, it is essential to notify the nursing staff to allow sufficient time to take care of the patient's immediate needs before loading. The patient should be informed of the whole procedure, including how to identify a missing ribbon and restriction on movement outside the room and on visitation. Also, patients need to be reassured that while they are loaded, they will be cared for by nursing staff and doctors. ^{192}Ir is available in two forms, either as plastic ribbons or as wire. The latter is rarely used in the United States, although very common in Europe. The ^{192}Ir in plastic ribbons is commercially available (Best Industries, Inc., Springfield, Va.). The ribbons contain several cylinders of stainless steel ^{192}Ir seeds, each measuring about 3 mm in length and 0.5 mm in diameter. Each ribbon can be customized to have from 1 to 18 seeds at standard 1 cm spacing.

The loading of the ^{192}Ir is performed in the patient's room behind a bedside shield (Fig. 12-11). A systematic approach to loading will significantly decrease the exposure to personnel. The simulation films with each catheter numbered and the number of seeds per ribbon clearly identified should be at the bedside. The crimped tubular portion of the metal buttons should be uncrimped using a long hemostat and dummy sources or wires pulled out. The patency of the catheters should be checked with a wire to identify any kinks that would otherwise obstruct the advancement of the ribbons.

The ^{192}Ir ribbons are stored within a lead shield container (Fig. 12-12) with a numbered tag on each end corresponding with the appropriate catheter number. At least two persons are needed to load a patient: one person to remove each ribbon from the lead container and verbally identify its number and the other person (radiation oncologist) to insert the ribbon in the corresponding catheter. The person who is loading should stand behind the bedside lead shield and hold each ribbon with a long forceps (at least 20 cm long) from the tip that contains the radioactive seeds (Fig. 12-13). The other hand should hold on to the beveled end of the afterloading catheter to guide the ribbon through it. Having a beveled end will facilitate this process significantly.

The tubular portion of the metal buttons should be crimped, and every ribbon should be manually checked to make sure it will not slide out of the catheter. Using a marking pen, a line should be drawn on each side of overlap between the ribbon and the catheter. This will assist in identifying any slippage of the ^{192}Ir ribbons later. These procedures can be done quickly with minimum exposure compared with the exposure that someone might receive if a ribbon fell out due to inadequate crimping.

After this is accomplished, the exposure rate should be measured at the surface of the patient near the implant and at 1 meter using an ionization type survey meter (Fig. 12-14). These numbers should be written on the yellow radiation precaution tags and posted on the room's door and patient's hospital chart. If the exposure rate is greater than 2 mrem/hour at 1 meter, bedside lead shielding should be used (which is the case in all ^{192}Ir implants). It

Patient's Name:_____   Medical Record Number: _____

TEMPORARY IMPLANTS

EVALUATION OF DOSIMETRY AND DETERMINATION OF THE TIME OF
IMPLANTATION

(FILE IN RT FOLDER)

1. Obtain the inner continuous curve around plane of implant for each of the
    standard cuts.

    1. _____ cGy/day   6. _____ cGy/day
    2. _____ cGy/day   7. _____ cGy/day
    3. _____ cGy/day   8. _____ cGy/day
    4. _____ cGy/day   9. _____ cGy/day
    5. _____ cGy/day   10. _____ cGy/day

2. Obtain from the above the median isodose rate curve, which will be called the
    MPDR (Median Peripheral Dose Rate): _____ cGy/day.

3. Correlate all isodose curves with the location of the tumor in the x-ray films.
    Determine whether the tumor is covered properly by the MPDR. If yes, proceed
    to step #4. If not, go back to steps 1 - 2 and obtain the next lower curve, which
    will be the new MPDR: _____ cGy/day.

4. Decide the median peripheral dose (MPD): _____ cGy/day.

5. Divide the MPD in cGy by the MPDR in cGy/day to determine the duration of
    implantation as _____ days. Multiply this figure by 24 hours and derive the
    implantation time as _____ days and _____ hours.

6. Mark on the x-ray film points of interest (e.g., skin, spinal cord, rectum, etc.) for
    which separate dose determinations should be made.

Point of Interest	Maximum Dose Rate	Total Dose
_____	_____ cGy/day	_____ cGy
_____	_____ cGy/day	_____ cGy
_____	_____ cGy/day	_____ cGy

    Radioactive sources inserted: Date _____ Time_____
    Radioactive sources inserted: Date _____ Time_____

    Date: _____   Signature: _____

Figure 12–9. Temporary implant evaluation form.

is also preferable to use a corner room in order to decrease
exposure to adjoining rooms.

A note should be written by the radiation oncologist
describing the loading procedure and stating the date and
time of the loading and the planned unloading, the total
dose, the number of ^{192}Ir ribbons, the total activity, and
activity per seed. The name and the beeper number of the
person who can be reached if there is any concern about
the radioactive source position should be clearly identified
to the nursing staff.

While the patient is loaded, he or she should be visited
by the radiation oncologist twice a day including weekends,
and the number and the positions of the ^{192}Ir ribbons and
catheters should be checked in addition to the patient's
progress. The time of the visits should also be noted in
the patient chart.

The unloading procedure should be systematic and
quick to decrease exposure. The equipment needed for
this procedure is similar to that needed for loading
i.e., a pair of long forceps, hemostat and scissors (see
Fig. 12-13). The unloading is done behind a bedside lead
shield. First the metal buttons should be uncrimped, then
each ribbon pulled out of its corresponding catheter and
handed to the other person in the room who has the ^{192}Ir
lead shield container to store them.

After all ribbons are removed and accounted for, the
attention is directed to the afterloading catheters. First
the metal button's silk sutures are removed, and then the
plastic catheters should be removed gently. In loop and
through-and-through type implants, one side of the
catheter is pulled out gently and cut, and then the catheter
is pulled from the other side to prevent having any part
of the catheter outside the skin pulled back through the
wound in the removal process. If there are any bleeding
points, they can be easily controlled with pressure. After

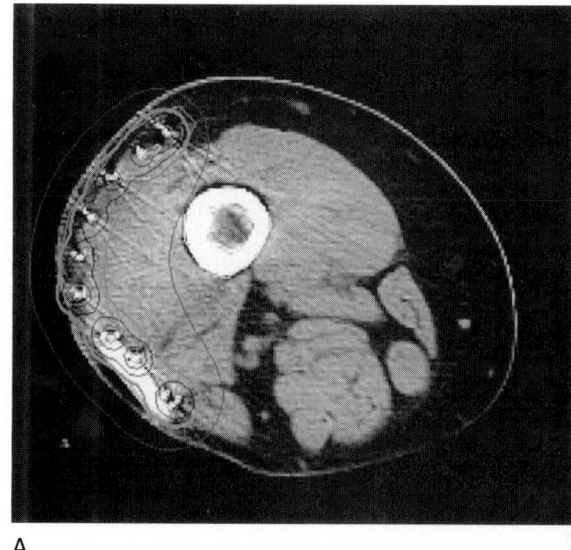

A

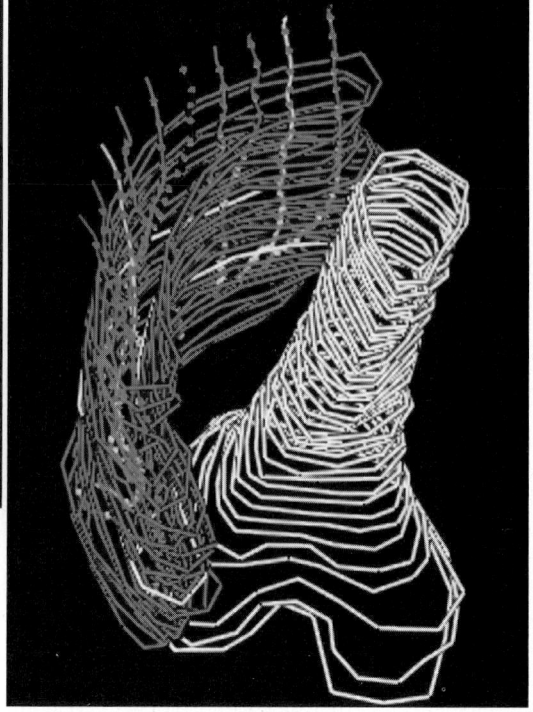

B

Figure 12–10. Computed tomography–based planning of an interstitial
implant. **A,** Transverse view outlining the dose distribution in relationship
to the target volume and adjacent normal structures (bone). **B,** Beam's-eye
view of the catheters, target, and bone. See also Color Figure 12-10.

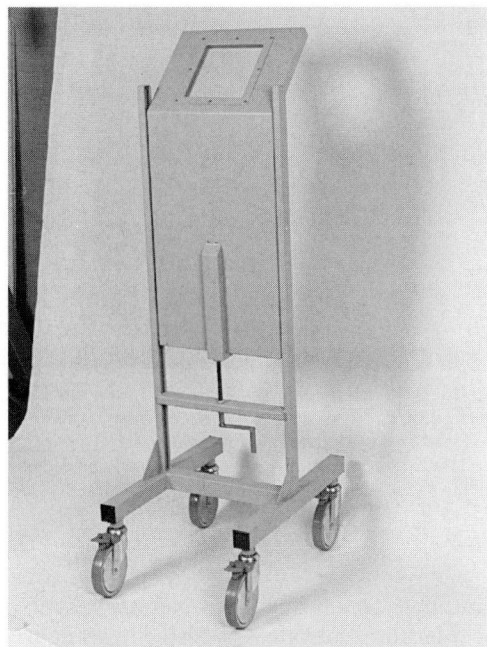

Figure 12–11. Adjustable, rolling bedside shield with leaded glass window. (Courtesy of Radiation Products Design, Inc., 5218 Barthel Industrial Drive, Albertville, NM 55301-9766.)

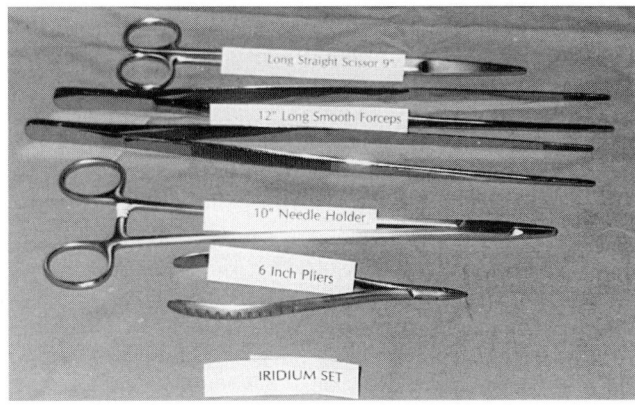

Figure 12–13. Iridium set. These instruments are used for the loading and unloading of iridium-192.

the catheters are pulled, they should be individually checked to make sure there are no missing pieces that could have been left behind inadvertently.

The patient and the room should be monitored for radioactivity to assure that all seeds are accounted for. At this point, all radiation precaution tags should be removed. A note should be written in the patient's chart describing the procedure, uploading time, total dose delivered, and full accounting of all implanted seeds. If a patient has a draining tube, it is advisable to leave it in place throughout the treatment and remove it after the unloading in order to preserve the geometry of the implant.

For most temporary interstitial implants, ^{192}Ir is the most commonly used isotope; however, high activity iodine-125 (^{125}I) (10 to 40 mCi) does have a distinct advantage over ^{192}Ir due to its lower energy (27 to 35 Kev). This low energy enables the surrounding tissue to attenuate more effectively the gamma rays, which in turn minimize the radiation dose to surrounding normal tissue.[14] For example, high activity ^{125}I soft tissue sarcoma implants in young patients decreases the dose delivered to the gonads, thyroid, and breast, as shown in Table 12-1. The other advantage is the minimal radiation protection required for hospital personnel and family members. The implant procedure for ^{125}I is identical to ^{192}Ir except that the afterloading catheters need to have a larger diameter to accommodate the ^{125}I ribbons, which are thicker than ^{192}Ir ribbons.

All that the patient must do when visitors or medical personnel enter the room is cover the implanted region with a lead-impregnated rubber piece. The disadvantages of high-activity temporary ^{125}I seeds are their cost and the complexity of physics planning. High-activity ^{125}I is also used in eye plaques[15] (Fig. 12-15) and brain implants.[16]

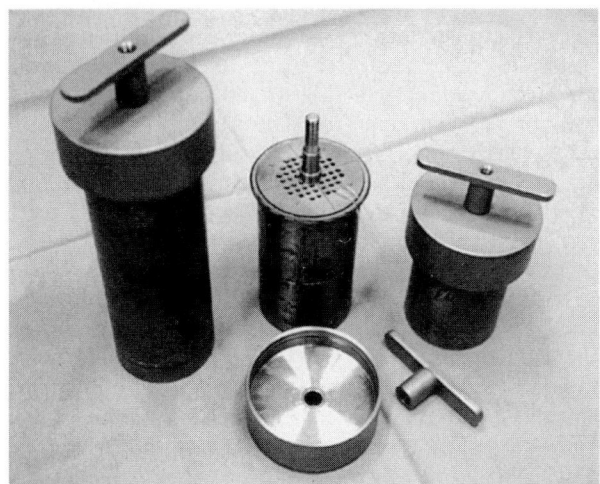

Figure 12–12. Container used for transporting the iridium-192 sources. The sources are placed inside the lead pig shown at center, then placed inside either of the other two lead pigs for additional protection. (Courtesy of Radiation Products Design, Inc., Albertville, NM.)

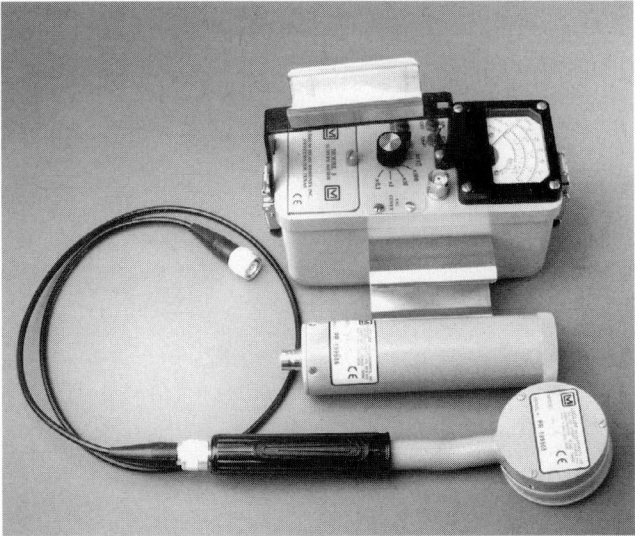

Figure 12–14. Dual function survey meter. It could be used as a Geiger counter to detect any lost radioactive sources or ionization type meter to measure exposure.

Table 12–1 Comparisons of ^{192}Ir and High Activity ^{125}I Treatment of a 17-Year-Old Patient with Desmoid Right Posterior Thigh

	^{192}Ir	^{125}I
Target dose	Homogeneous	Homogeneous
Skin average, Gy/d	262 (60 cm²)	68 (60 cm²)
Skin max, Gy/d	422	210
Right ovary, Gy/d	151	17
Left ovary, Gy/d	43	1
Breasts, Gy/d	11	0
Thyroid, Gy/d	8	0

Data from Harrison, Zelefsky, Armstrong, et al: Brachytherapy and function preservation in the localized management of soft tissue sarcomas of the extremity. *Semin Radiat Oncol.* 1993;3:260.

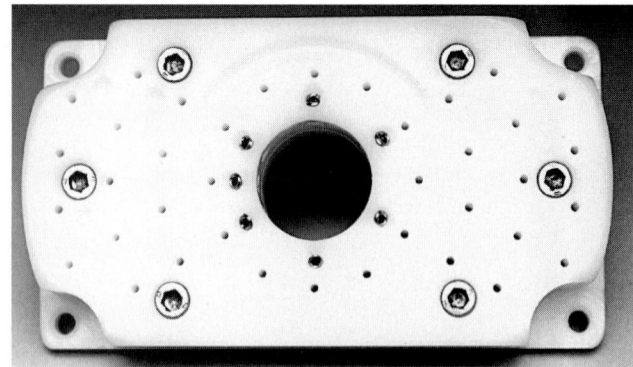

Figure 12–16. Syed-Neblett gynecologic template. The two lucite plates are joined by six machine screws that tighten to grasp as many as 38 stainless steel afterloading needles. An additional six needles fit into the grooves of a 2 cm diameter vaginal cylinder that is placed in the central opening of the template. (Courtesy of Best Industries, Inc., Springfield, Va.)

Template

Proper maintenance of accurate radioactive source position during the treatment is an integral part of interstitial brachytherapy. This is not a problem when implanting an extremity or base of tongue with plastic catheters; however, it could be a problem when implanting a prostate, vagina, female urethra, or rectum. In these situations, it is preferable to use stainless steel needles instead of plastic catheters and to secure the needle position by a stabilizer or template.

These templates are commercially available or can be custom made. The basic components of most of these templates include: (1) a set of hollow stainless steel needles, (2) a rectal or vaginal obturator with peripheral grooves to accommodate needles and a central bore to accommodate a tandem, if desired, and (3) a set of two identical plates made of acrylic plastic or silicone material, superimposed and held together by screws so that the needles are locked in place.

The two most commonly used templates are the Syed-Neblett and the Universal Martinez template. Our

discussion here is on the Syed-Neblett template. The Universal Martinez template is discussed in detail in Chapter 48, Cancer of the Uterine Cervix. There are different types of Syed templates for different sites, and by far, the most commonly used is the gynecologic template. Others include rectal, prostate, and female urethra templates.

The gynecologic template is mainly used for cervical and vaginal cancer. It consists of two lucite plates (Fig. 12-16) with a central large opening to place a 2 cm diameter vaginal obturator and 38 small peripheral holes in concentric circles or arcs to accommodate 38 stainless steel hollow needles. An additional six needles could be placed around the vaginal obturator in specially designed grooves. This brings the total number of needles that could be used up to 44. These needles are arranged in concentric circles or arcs with 1 cm distance between adjacent needles, and this arrangement could cover an area of 4 × 10 cm in a "butterfly" distribution. The 17-gauge needles supplied with the template are 15 and 20 cm long, but shorter needles (11 cm) are also available to treat shallow regions. The vaginal obturator has a central opening for placement of vaginal or uterine tandem. The two plates are joined by six screws that tighten to grasp the stainless steel needles. A larger version of this template could accommodate 10 additional needles, which enables implanting a 6 × 10 cm area. These additional needles are usually placed anteriorly and posteriorly, thus forming a third complete circle. In practice these needles are rarely loaded because of the high dose of radiation to the bladder and rectum. Currently, there is a Syed gynecologic template made of a single rubber plate without metal screws and rigid plastic needles, which allows for computed tomography (CT)-based treatment planning (Fig. 12-17). The gynecologic template is indicated in the treatment of (1) cervical cancer,[17] including early-stage disease if the cervical canal is obliterated due to tumor, fibrosis, or prior surgery (carcinoma of cervical stump); locally advanced cervical cancer, stage III A, B; and recurrent cervical cancer after surgery; and (3) vaginal cancer.[18]

The rectal template is similar to the gynecologic template, but instead of a butterfly distribution, it has three

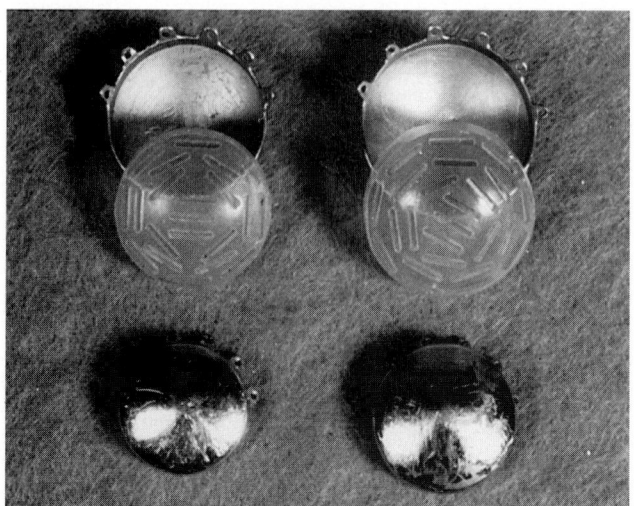

Figure 12–15. Eye plaques. Four sizes are shown, with gold outer shell and silicone insert, which holds the radioactive seeds in place.

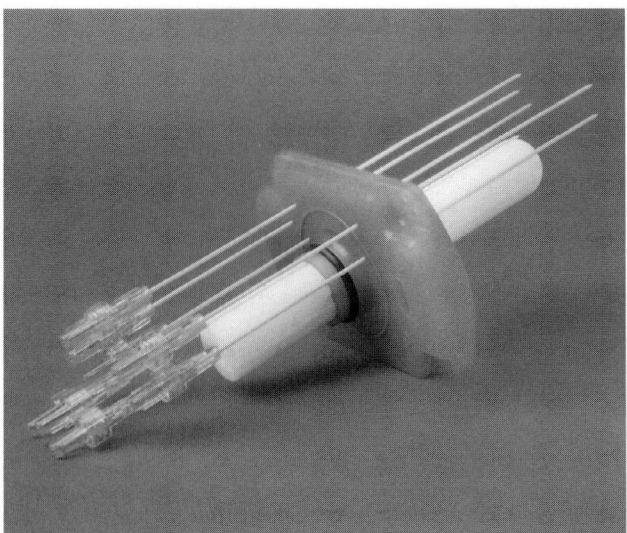

Figure 12–17. Computed tomography–compatible Syed template. The template comprises a single-plate rubber. The needles are made of hard plastic. No metals are used to secure the template and needles.

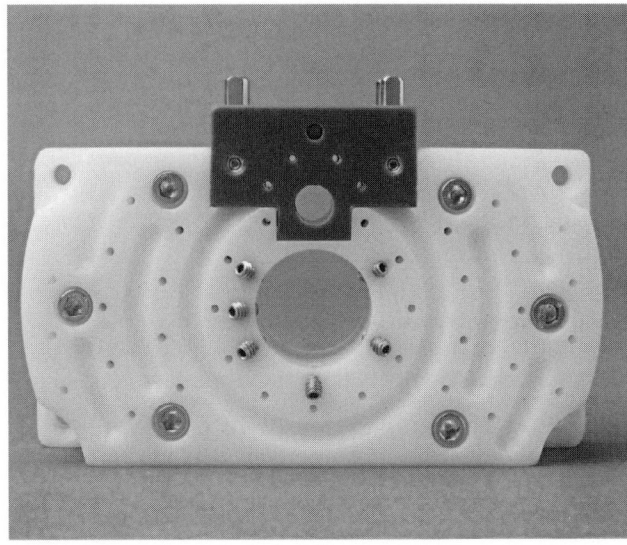

Figure 12–19. Urethral template. Similar to Syed gynecologic template with the addition of an apparatus to accommodate a Foley catheter and surrounding needles.

concentric circles that accommodate up to 36 needles (Fig. 12-18). A rectal tube could be passed through a central hole in the template.

The prostate template has two concentric circles—the inner one contains 6 holes and the outer one 12 holes. Up to 18 needles can be inserted transperineally through the prostate and seminal vesicles with the tip of the needles about 1 cm above the bladder neck.

The urethral template has two concentric circles with a total of 17 needles. This template is a single plate with a central hole for a Foley catheter (Fig. 12-19). It is useful in the treatment of distal urethral tumors in females. Our discussion is limited to gynecologic templates.

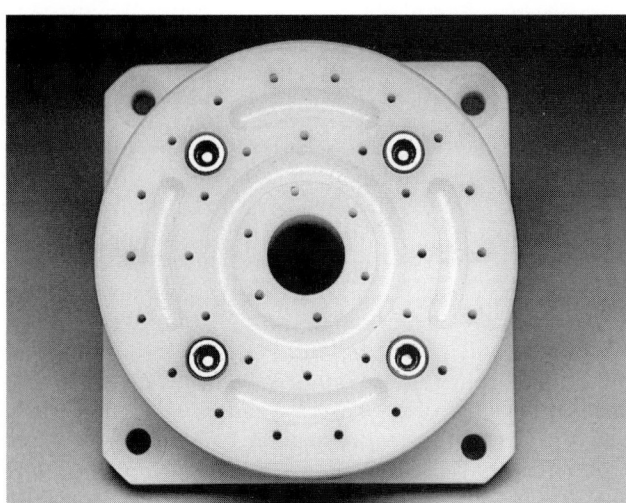

Figure 12–18. Syed-Neblett rectal template. The two lucite plates are joined by four machine screws that tighten to grasp as many as 36 stainless steel afterloading needles. (Courtesy of Best Industries, Inc., Springfield, Va.)

TECHNIQUES

Template insertion is done in the operating room under general anesthesia. A bimanual pelvic examination is done to determine the extent of cervical or vaginal cancer. The vagina and perineum are prepped in the usual manner with Betadine solution, and the patient is draped. Gold or silver marker seeds are inserted into the anterior and posterior cervical lips with an MD Anderson marker applicator (Fig. 12-20). Marker seeds should also be inserted into the vaginal wall to identify the lower border of any vaginal involvement. If a uterine tandem is used, the endometrial canal needs to be sounded and the measurement recorded. This is followed by dilation of the cervical canal by a Hegar or Haynes dilator. Then a Foley catheter is inserted in the bladder with the balloon filled with 7 mL of contrast mixed with saline. The bladder is not drained so that any inadvertent puncture will be identified by urine leakage from the hollow needles.

The instruments needed for this template include: (1) gynecologic template; (2) 2 cm diameter vaginal obturator; (3) Allen wrenches and six screws to tighten the two plates; (4) screws to fix the obturator to the template; (5) 17-gauge stainless steel needles, 15 cm and 20 cm in length; (6) sharp stylets for needle insertion; (7) straight vaginal or uterine tandem; (8) afterloading plastic catheters with dummy sources; (9) rubber needle caps to secure the ^{192}Ir ribbons inside the needles; and (10) a ruler. With the new CT-compatible Syed-Neblett template (see Fig. 12-17), there is no need for the screws or Allen wrench.

A guide needle is inserted into the deepest portion of the tumor to determine the depth of the implanted volume. This depth is established from imaging (CT or magnetic resonance imaging) as well as examination under anesthesia. The position of the needle is checked by vaginal and rectal examinations. The vaginal obturator with the tandem in the central hole is inserted until it is pushed against the cervical os.

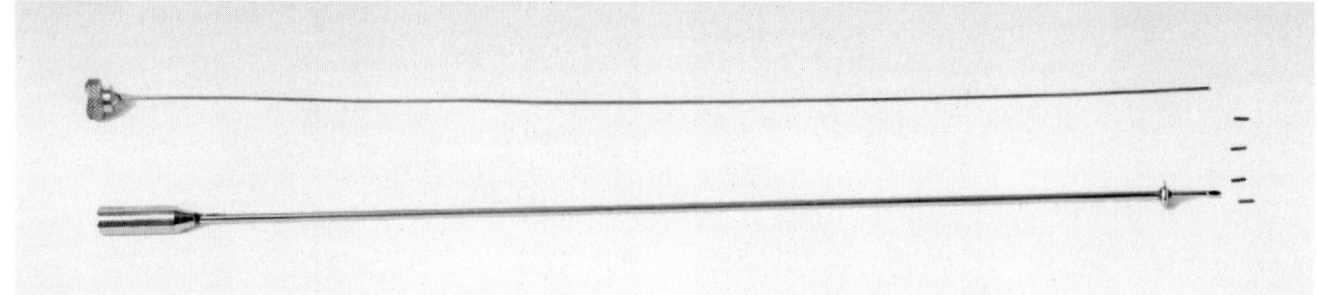

Figure 12–20. Cervical marker with silver seeds.

The Syed template is then inserted over the obturator and the guide needle. If no tandem is going to be used, needles are inserted through the obturator's grooves. Then an appropriate number of needles to cover the tumor volume is inserted through the template. The needles should be placed to a depth so that their distal tips line up with the tip of the guide needle.

It is important to ensure that the needles did not penetrate into the rectum or bladder by verifying the position of every needle on vaginal and rectal examination, as well as by checking for any urine leakage through the needles or deflation of the Foley catheter balloon.

The needles should not be pushed more than 3 to 4 cm beyond the level of the external os. The use of laparoscopy at the time of insertion, especially in those who had prior hysterectomy, decreases the possibility of the needles entering the peritoneal cavity.[19] In addition, the use of transrectal ultrasound during the insertion of the needles might be very helpful in providing real-time visualization of the target volume and adjacent normal structures.[20]

The needles are fixed by tightening the screws on the template and the obturator with an Allen wrench. The four corners of the template are sutured to the perineum. The space between the perineum and the template should be fitted with gauze to prevent necrosis of the vulva or thigh. A rectal tube is inserted in the rectum at this time to accommodate the dummy sources that must be placed in the rectum for dose calculation at the time of simulation.

TREATMENT PLANNING AND DELIVERY

After the patient recovers from anesthesia, she needs to be transferred to the simulator to have localization films taken. Dummy sources should be placed into the needles, rectum, and the tandem (if used). It is advisable not to load all the needles at once because it will make it difficult to visualize all the dummy sources. After an orthogonal pair of films are taken, the patient is returned to her room.

A significant part of the planning is done before the surgical insertion to determine the tumor volume and its relationship to the cervical lips and pelvic side wall. This relationship will determine the depth to which the guide needle must be inserted and the position of the most lateral needles to be used, respectively. Preplanning also includes determining the number of ^{192}Ir ribbons needed, number of seeds per ribbon, and the differential source strength

loading, facilitating the appropriate number of ^{192}Ir ribbons to be ordered. This includes extra ribbons to account for potential changes based on the postinsertion planning.

After localization films are taken, a computerized plan is created to determine the optimal implant dosimetry. *This step is extremely important because early experience with this template led to high complication rates.* However, certain guidelines were proposed by Syed et al.[21] to reduce those complications, including:

1. If the intrauterine tandem is used, none of the central six source guides should be loaded. If there is no central bulky tumor, do not use the anterior three and posterior three guides in the second diameter of the Syed-Neblett applicator to reduce the dose to the rectum and bladder.
2. If the central six guides are implanted as well as the tandem, then only four seeds of ^{192}Ir per guide should be loaded.
3. The activity of the ^{192}Ir sources should be in the range of 0.25 to 0.35 mgRaeq per seed to avoid exceeding 80 cGy/hour to point A.
4. Differential unloading of tandem and central guides, or higher activity sources (0.4 mgRaeq per seed) in the lateral guides, should be used to achieve higher doses to point B, pelvic wall, and lymph nodes while sparing the rectum and bladder.
5. To prevent slipping of the tandem into the vagina, the tandem is fixed at the conclusion of the procedure rather than at the start.

The dose is prescribed to an isodose-rate contour in a similar fashion to MPDR in planar implant. The dose to the rectum, vagina, and bladder should be taken into consideration when choosing the isodose-rate contour. Using MPDR for dose prescription of a volume implant relies on the assumptions that the needles cover all the tumor volume; therefore, if the MPDR covers all the needles, it will cover the tumor. The dose should be prescribed to the tumor volume visualized on CT or MRI imaging. The use of CT-based planning[21,22] helps tremendously in permitting more accurate, anatomically based dosimetric analysis (Fig. 12-21). Currently, inverse planning for gynecologic interstitial implants is being investigated to try to simulate IMRT planning.[23]

The loading is done in the patient's room from behind a lead shield. After inserting the ^{192}Ir ribbons into the hollow guides, the needles are covered with the plastic caps

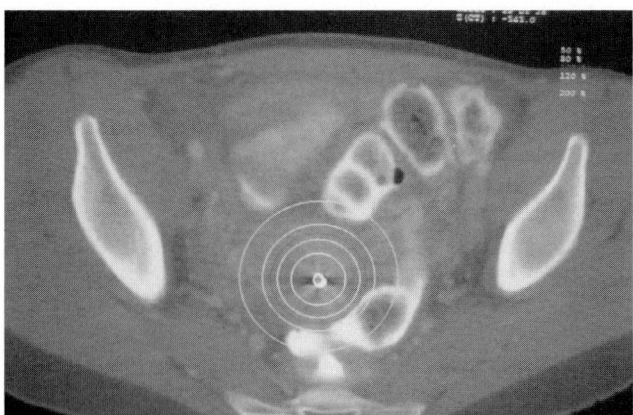

Figure 12–21. Computed tomography–based planning for a Syed gynecologic implant.

to prevent slippage. It is important to ensure that while inserting a ^{192}Ir ribbon, the position of the adjacent ribbons is not altered. If the tandem is to be loaded, three sources of cesium-137 (^{137}Cs) in combinations of 15 + 10 + 5 or 10 + 5 + 5 are used. The patient should be on bed rest and on pain and antidiarrheal medications. The number and position of the ribbons should be checked twice a day, and the patient should also be examined for signs of bleeding, infection, or acute abdomen.

After the appropriate dose has been delivered, the radioactive sources are removed, sutures are cut, and the whole template is removed in one continuous motion. An analgesic needs to be given to the patient before removal of the template. If there is bleeding from needle exit points in the perineum, pressure should be applied. This will stop the oozing in most cases. The room needs to be surveyed to detect any residual radioactivity.

The debate on whether the Syed template provides better dose distribution than conventional tandem and ovoids for patients with intact cervix is still ongoing. Hsu et al. compared the dosimetry of both using a hypothetical computer model. They found better coverage in the parametrial regions, but underdosage in the central cervical regions with the interstitial system. The sparing of the adjacent normal organs was better with the interstitial system due to more rapid dose drop-off outside the treated volume with the interstitial system.[24]

INTRACAVITARY

Intracavitary applicators are primarily used to treat gynecologic malignancies. Medically inoperable rectal cancer could also be treated with intracavitary brachytherapy with or without EBRT.

Intravaginal Applicators

The use of intravaginal HDR brachytherapy in the treatment of endometrial cancer was pioneered by Henschke at MSKCC in the mid-1960s.[2] The usefulness and safety of this technique has been demonstrated.[25,26] Intravaginal brachytherapy is also indicated in the postoperative radiation treatment of cervical cancers and the definitive treatment of early superficial vaginal cancers.[27] At MSKCC,

the most common vaginal applicator is a cylinder connected to a ^{192}Ir HDR remote afterloader.

TECHNIQUE

Our discussion is limited to postoperative HDR brachytherapy in endometrial cancer. The procedure is done on an outpatient basis without anesthesia or sedation. The patient is placed in the lithotomy position on a gynecologic examination table and a pelvic examination is performed. The largest diameter cylinder that the vagina can accommodate is chosen and the length of the vagina is measured. The cylinder should be inserted with its dome against the vaginal cuff, and one finger should be placed at the introitus, then the cylinder is pulled out and the distance between the tip of the cylinder and the tip of the measuring finger is measured. The target volume is usually one half to two thirds the measured vaginal length.

TREATMENT PLANNING AND DELIVERY

Cylinder diameters range from 2 to 5 cm (Fig. 12-22). The dose is usually prescribed to a 0.5 cm depth from the surface of the cylinder, and with the use of ^{192}Ir HDR, the dose distribution can be optimized in such a way that the dose will taper down as it gets closer to the introitus and, at the same time, improve the depth dose distribution by lowering the dose to the vaginal surface relative to that at 0.5 cm (Fig. 12-23). When intravaginal HDR brachytherapy is used alone, the dose is usually 7 Gy per fraction × 3 with 2 week intervals between fractions. If EBRT is used as well, the dose per fraction should be decreased to 5 Gy.[28] The standard cylinder has only one central channel, which might lead to anisotropy near the dome region, especially if dose optimization was not used. This could represent a problem if there is a positive margin or gross disease at the vaginal vault. A modified cylinder with a central channel, as well as peripheral channels, could overcome this limitation.[29]

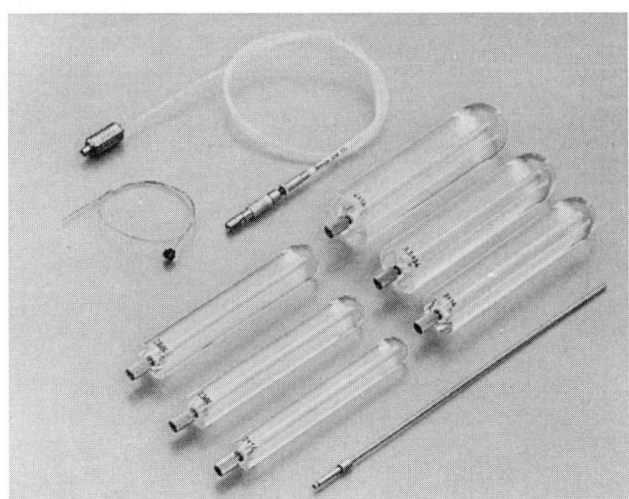

Figure 12–22. High-dose-rate vaginal cylinder set. Different diameter cylinders are shown, along with transport tube, dummy source, and central source tube. (Courtesy of Gamma-Med, Frank Barker Association Inc., Pequannock, NJ.)

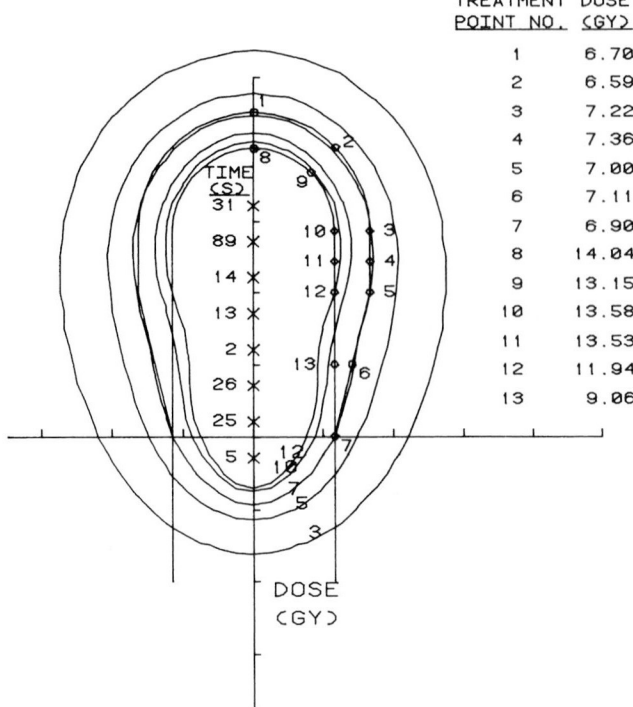

TREATMENT POINT NO.	DOSE (GY)
1	6.70
2	6.59
3	7.22
4	7.36
5	7.00
6	7.11
7	6.90
8	14.04
9	13.15
10	13.58
11	13.53
12	11.94
13	9.06

Figure 12–23. Least-squares optimized dwell times to produce doses as close as possible to 7.0 Gy at target points 1 through 7 and as uniform as possible among points 8 through 12 for 2.3 cm diameter vaginal applicators. (From Anderson LL: Physical optimization of afterloading techniques. *Strahlentherapie.* 1985;161:264.)

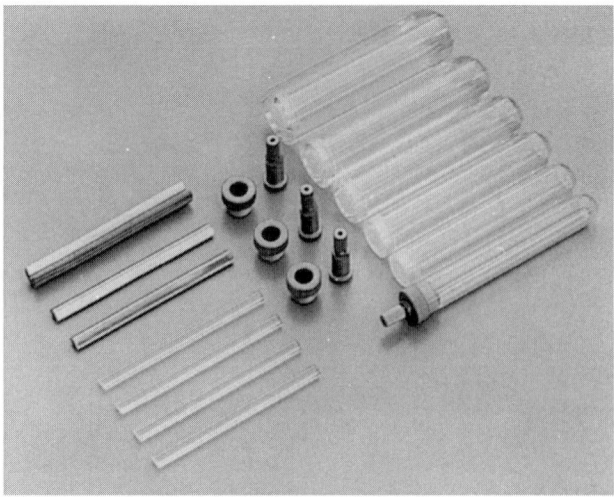

Figure 12–24. Shielded vaginal cylinder set. Various tungsten shields can be arranged to shield the treatment diameter in increments of 90 degrees. (Courtesy of Gamma-Med, Frank Barker Association Inc., Pequannock, NJ.)

Other institutions use different types of low-dose-rate (LDR) vaginal applicators, including vaginal colpostats, domed cylinders, and the MIRALVA applicator, which incorporates two ovoid sources and central tandem colpostats.[30] The isotope used in those cylinders is ^{137}Cs. The disadvantage of the domed cylinder is again anisotropy, which can be corrected by using a high intensity ^{137}Cs source (which is shorter than regular sources) at the tip next to the vaginal vault; or by using the T-shaped source arrangement in which the source next to the vault is perpendicular to the long axis of the vagina. Some vaginal cylinders are provided with added lead shielding (Fig. 12-24) to protect the rectum, bladder, or selected parts of the vagina (Fig. 12-25).

The choice of the applicator (cylinder vs. colpostat) should be patient and institution dependent.[31] Kim et al. compared the dosimetry of a cylinder applicator to that of a vaginal colpostat. The dose distribution, for the most part, was similar. However, with the colpostat system, cold spots could easily occur depending on the amount of packing and the magnitude of separation between the two colpostats.[32] Since the cylinder applicator is easier to insert and does not require packing, it is our applicator of choice.

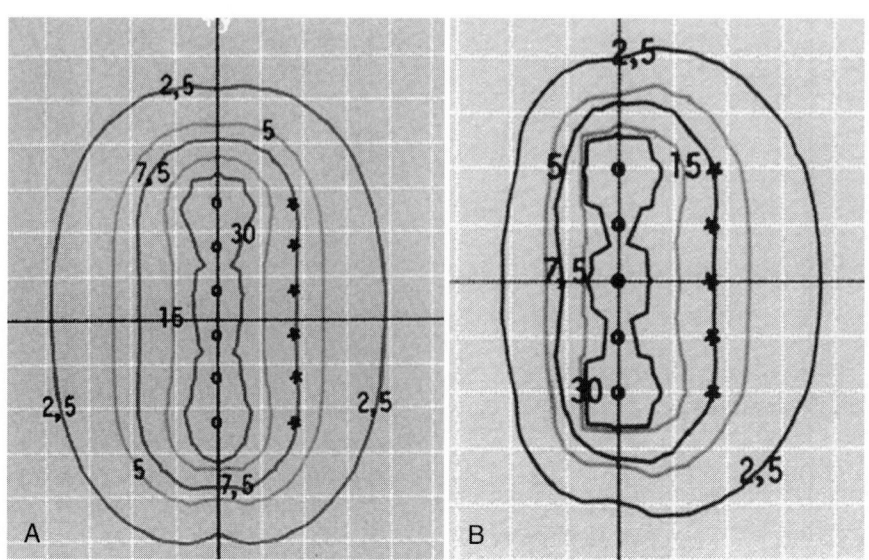

Figure 12–25. Isodose distribution for vaginal cylinder. Unshielded (**A**) and partial shielding (**B**) on the left side only. (Courtesy of Gamma-Med, Frank Barker Association Inc., Pequannock, NJ.)

Cervical Applicators

The two most commonly used applicators in the United States are the Henschke and Fletcher applicators. The Fletcher applicator is described later in Chapter 48 (Cancer of the Uterine Cervix). The Henschke applicator was the first afterloading applicator, representing a significant milestone in the history of modern brachytherapy.

This applicator consists of a uterine tandem and two ovoids attached to each other by an adjustable pivot yoke that prevents rotation of the tandem. The tandem is available in three different curvatures to accommodate for different uterine positions. Each ovoid is available in three different diameters. The smallest is 2 cm and is provided with anterior and posterior tungsten inserts for partial shielding of the bladder and rectum. Hemispheric nylon caps could be placed over the 2 cm ovoid to increase its diameter to 2.5 or 3 cm (Fig. 12-26).

Henschke applicators can be autoclaved or gas sterilized, and each set should contain three tandems, two ovoids (2 cm diameter), two pairs of plastic hemispheric nylon caps (2.5 and 3 cm diameters), uterine sound, ruler, and a cervical flange.

TECHNIQUE

The insertion of the Henschke applicator is done under general anesthesia. Bimanual pelvic examination is done by the radiation oncologist and the gynecologist to determine the extent of the disease and the position of the cervix and the uterus. A Foley catheter is inserted and the 10 mL balloon is inflated using a radiopaque agent. A marker applicator (see Fig. 12-20) is used to implant seeds into the anterior and posterior cervical lips and the lower extent of any vaginal involvement. A pair of retractors is used to visualize the external cervical os, and a uterine sound is inserted into the uterine cavity to measure its length. To prevent inward displacement of the cervix and uterus during sounding and dilation, a tenaculum is used (Fig. 12-27).

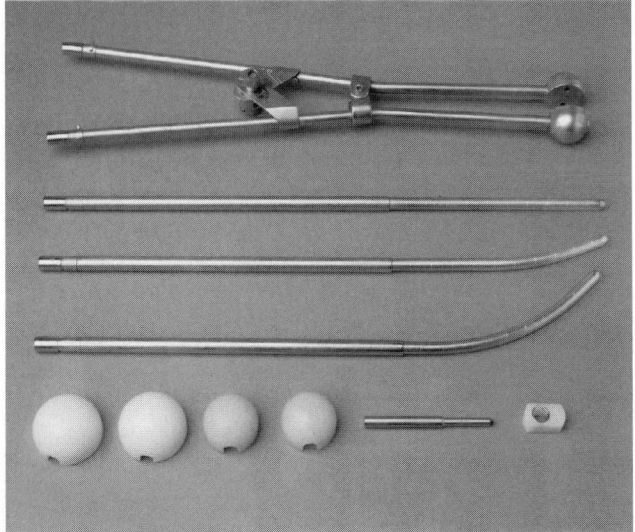

Figure 12–26. Henschke applicator set. *Top*: ovoids; *middle*: straight, semi-curved, and curved tandems; *bottom*: two 3 cm ovoid cups, two 2.5 cm cups, Allen wrench, and a flange or a stopper.

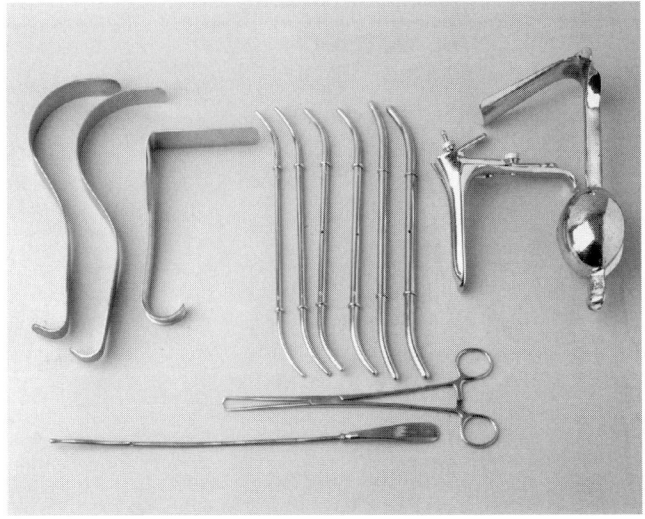

Figure 12–27. *Left*: vaginal retractors; *middle*: dilators; *right*: speculum and weighted speculum; *bottom*: tenaculum and a uterine sound.

After measuring the uterine length, Hegar or Hanks uterine dilators are used, starting with the smallest diameter and increasing to 8 mm, the diameter of the tandem. During dilation, the inserted dilator length should be equal to the measured uterine length in order to prevent perforation. Depending on uterus position, one of three curved tandems is selected and the cervical flange is tightened in place, corresponding to the length of the uterine cavity.

After inserting the tandem, the two ovoids are inserted into the lateral vaginal fornices. The size of the ovoids used should be the largest that the upper vagina can accommodate. The most commonly used size is 2.5 cm. Henschke ovoids in general conform easily to a narrow vagina; therefore, there is no need to use a minicolpostat. The two ovoids are separated as much as possible without causing a downward displacement. The tandem should be equidistant from the two ovoids and in the same horizontal plane that bisects the two ovoids.

All three components of the applicator are now connected and fastened to prevent any dislocation or rotation. Packing is done with 22-inch gauze soaked in Betadine and held with forceps in such a way that the gauze only comes in direct contact with the vaginal mucosa to avoid inadvertent laceration. During the packing, the tenaculum must be removed, but a suture placed into the cervical lip might be used as a substitute for counter retraction. This is a very important aspect of the packing because it prevents the inward displacement of the cervix away from the ovoids. The packing process starts between the posterior wall of the vagina and the ovoids, and then the same process is repeated anteriorly. This process should be alternated until the whole vagina is packed. At no time should the gauze make a complete loop around the tandem and ovoids because that complicates the unpacking process. The adequacy of posterior packing should be checked by rectal examination.

The applicator is secured in place using 0-silk suture sewn through the labia majora above the applicator. A rectal tube is inserted into the rectum and secured in

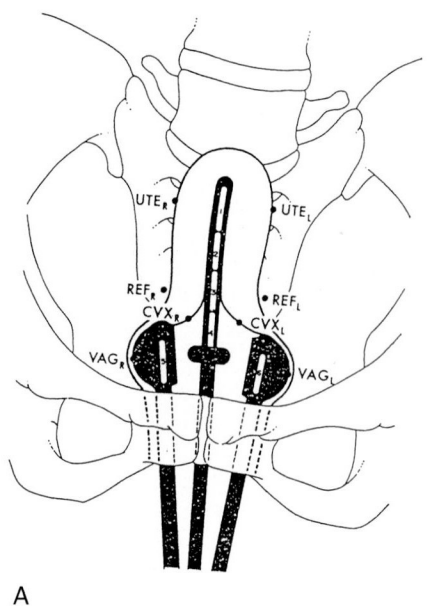

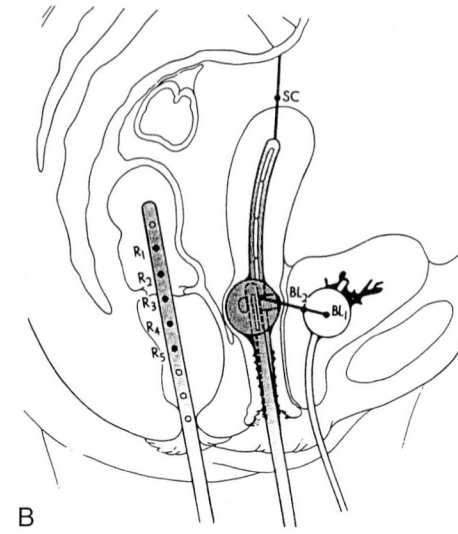

A

B

Figure 12–28. Treatment points (**A**) and tolerance points (**B**) used to optimize loading of a Henschke applicator by the least-squares method. (**A** from Rosenstein LM: A simple computerized program for optimization of source loading in cervical intracavitary applicators. *Br J Radiol.* 1977;50:119; **B** from Anderson LL: Physical optimization of afterloading techniques. *Strahlentherapie.* 1985;161:264.)

place using tape. Postoperative orders should include a low residue diet, and bed rest with instructions about allowed movements in the bed and elevation, as well as pain and antidiarrheal medications. After the patient recovers from anesthesia, she is taken to the simulator and a pair of orthogonal films are taken with dummy sources in the tandem, the two ovoids, and the rectal tube.

TREATMENT PLANNING AND DELIVERY

At MSKCC, the dosimetry planning is computerized and optimized based on an algorithm proposed by Rosenstein et al.[33] This algorithm uses dose criterion points including (1) target points representing the cervix, the uterus, the vagina, and the reference points (point A) and (2) tolerance points representing the rectum, bladder,

and sigmoid colon (Fig. 12-28). With this optimization, the tolerance points are those for which the target dose is stated as an upper limit. Table 12-2 gives the doses achieved at the criterion points relative to the target or tolerance doses specified, together with the weighing factor used for each point's contribution to the sum of squares.[34] It is essential to mention that the Henschke avoids are shielded as in Fletcher ovoids in order to decrease the dose to the bladder and rectum.[35,36]

One of the biggest shortcomings of intracavitary brachytherapy in cervical cancer has been the lack of correlation between prescription points and the target volume. But recently there has been significant interest in trying to implement 3D imaging of the cervical applicators.[37-39] Trying to integrate positron emission tomography–guided 3D imaging is also being investigated in cervical cancer.[40] These advances in imaging and planning will have a major impact on the way brachytherapy is prescribed in cervical cancer (Fig. 12-29). With the use of

Table 12–2 Example Case: Doses Achieved Relative to Specified Target and Tolerance Dose with Low-Dose-Rate Remote Afterloader

Point (%)	Weight	Desired Dose (Gy)	Achieved Dose (%)
Reference (avg)	—	30	100
Cervix (avg)	1.0	58.5	97
Vagina (avg)	1.0	30	103
Uterus 1 (avg)	1.0	25.5	92
Uterus 2 (avg)	1.0	30	101
Uterus 3 (avg)	1.0	30	103
Rectum 1	4.0	<10.5	95
Rectum 2	4.0	<10.5	101
Rectum 3	4.0	<10.5	103
Rectum 4	4.0	<10.5	101
Rectum 5	4.0	<10.5	95
Sigmoid colon	1.0	<10.5	82
Bladder, center	1.0	<13.5	98
Bladder, surface	0.0	<24	94

Data from Anderson LL: Plan optimization and dose evaluation in brachytherapy. *Semin Radiat Oncol.* 1993;3:290.

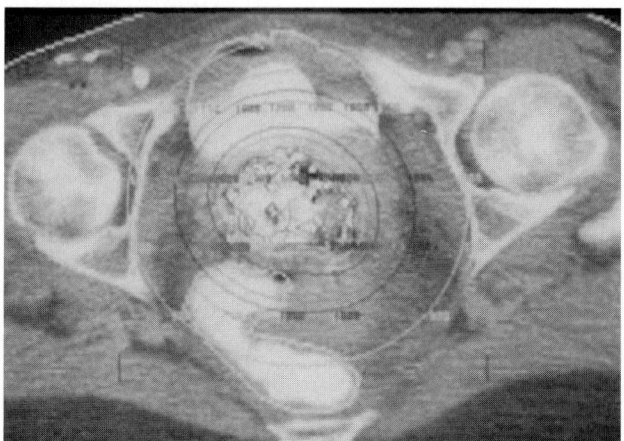

Figure 12–29. A cross-section of computed tomography–based planning of a cervical intracavitary applicator.

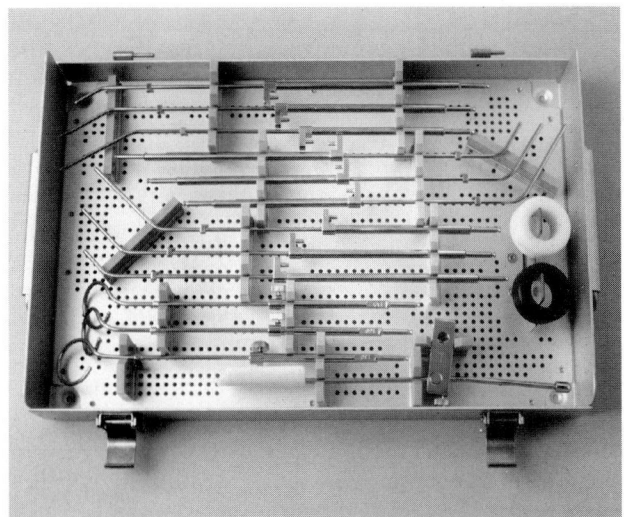

Figure 12–30. A set of computed tomography–compatible high-dose-rate cervical applicators.

CT/MRI-compatible applicators, the quality of imaging will be significantly enhanced, thus further facilitating accurate anatomically based planning (Fig. 12-30).

After the dose is prescribed, the patient is loaded in her room either manually or, more commonly, by a remote afterloader that allows complete radiation protection to medical personnel and visitors. While hospitalized, the patient should be examined daily for any signs of bleeding, acute abdomen, or infection.

When the treatment is finished, the applicator is disconnected from the remote afterloader. The 0-silk sutures are cut and packing is gently removed. Finally, the ovoid spreading is released and the applicator is rotated 45 degrees and gently removed. The clinician should look for any mucosal laceration or excessive bleeding. The room should be surveyed to detect any radioactivity.

Our discussion so far has focused on LDR ^{137}Cs, but there has been a surge in the use of pulsed LDR and HDR brachytherapy, which are discussed in Chapter 13, High Dose Rate Brachytherapy.[41,42]

Uterine Applicators

Since the use of preoperative radiation therapy in the management of uterine cancer has declined, fewer institutions are using the Heyman or Simon capsules.[43] The latter is an afterloading technique that uses thin ^{137}Cs sources connected to a steel wire that would be loaded after the packing is finished. In patients who have a medically inoperable uterine cancer, the Fletcher-Suit-Delclos applicator with one or two tandems (depending on uterus size) could be used in addition to two ovoids in the management of this subset of patients with uterine cancer. In a study by Rouanet et al.,[44] 250 patients with endometrial cancer were treated with radiation alone using a Fletcher-Suit-Delclos applicator with one or two tandems (depending on uterine size) and two ovoids followed by EBRT. The total combined dose to point A ranged from 75 Gy to 85 Gy. The 5-year disease-specific survival was 76.5%. HDR intracavitary brachytherapy,

either alone or combined with external beam radiation, could also be used to definitively treat uterine cancer.[45]

INTRALUMINAL BRACHYTHERAPY

Intraluminal brachytherapy is a form of brachytherapy in which the afterloading catheters are inserted directly into the lumen of a viscera instead of into an applicator as in intracavitary brachytherapy. This method of treatment has gained significant popularity since the introduction of HDR brachytherapy, especially in lung cancer.[46-50] LDR is still being used but to a lesser extent due to the significant advantages of HDR with regard to exposure, hospitalization, and dose optimization.

High-Dose-Rate Intraluminal Brachytherapy

Esophageal cancer is used as an example of this treatment method.[51] Intraluminal brachytherapy could be used as a boost following external beam radiation in patients with potentially curable disease, or alone in patients with recurrent tumor.

TECHNIQUE

The esophageal lumen should be open enough to accommodate the intraluminal catheter further and without extensive periesophageal extension.

The procedure is done on an outpatient basis using a nasogastric tube (10 or 12 Fr) or a special afterloading tube (4 mm in diameter) that has a radiopaque marker at its distal end. If a nasogastric tube is used, there is no need for sedation or local anesthesia. The applicator is slowly advanced into the esophagus while the patient is being asked to swallow, and typically it is placed at least 3 cm beyond the distal edge of the tumor.

TREATMENT PLANNING AND DELIVERY

The length of the esophagus that needs to be treated is defined as the longest tumor measurement on pretreatment barium swallow, CT scan, or endoscopy plus 1 cm margin proximally and distally. The dose is prescribed at 1 cm depth from the source train at midposition of the active treatment length. Treatment is given once a week × 3 to 5 Gy per fraction, with the first HDR brachytherapy fraction given after 2 weeks of EBRT completion.

A Radiation Therapy Oncology Group phase I/II trial evaluating concurrent EBRT and chemotherapy followed by intraluminal brachytherapy showed a high rate of fistulae (12%) in patients treated with this regimen.[52] Patients with recurrent disease could be treated with 5 Gy per fraction × 3 at 1 week intervals. Unlike with definitive treatment, the palliative effects of HDR intraluminal brachytherapy have been encouraging.[53,54]

Low-Dose-Rate Intraluminal Brachytherapy

Biliary tract cancer is used as an example of this technique. In patients with unresectable or incompletely resected tumors, it is suggested that brachytherapy plus EBRT with or without chemotherapy might be a valid approach.[55]

TECHNIQUE

Intraluminal brachytherapy can be administered to patients along an existing drainage tube or by percutaneous transhepatic cannulation.

LDR ^{192}Ir is the most widely used isotope. The procedure is usually done with the assistance of an interventional radiologist. An afterloading catheter with dummy sources inside is inserted along the percutaneous drain under fluoroscopic guidance. In order to identify the tumor volume, a transhepatic cholangiogram is performed either through the T tube in patients who underwent surgical biliary bypass or percutaneously in those who did not. The distal end of the afterloading catheter should be passed to a point well beyond the cholangiographically demonstrated stenosis and the proximal end should be fixed to the skin using the plastic hemispherical spacer and the stainless steel button.

TREATMENT PLANNING AND DELIVERY

Next, localization films of the afterloading catheter with the dummy sources inside are taken (Fig. 12-31). The treatment length is determined by the tumor volume on cholangiogram plus 2 cm margin both proximally and distally. This wide margin is needed due to the tendency of cholangiocarcinoma to have submucosal extension; however, the anastomosis site between the bile duct and the small intestine (surgical bypass) should be excluded from a high dose of radiation.

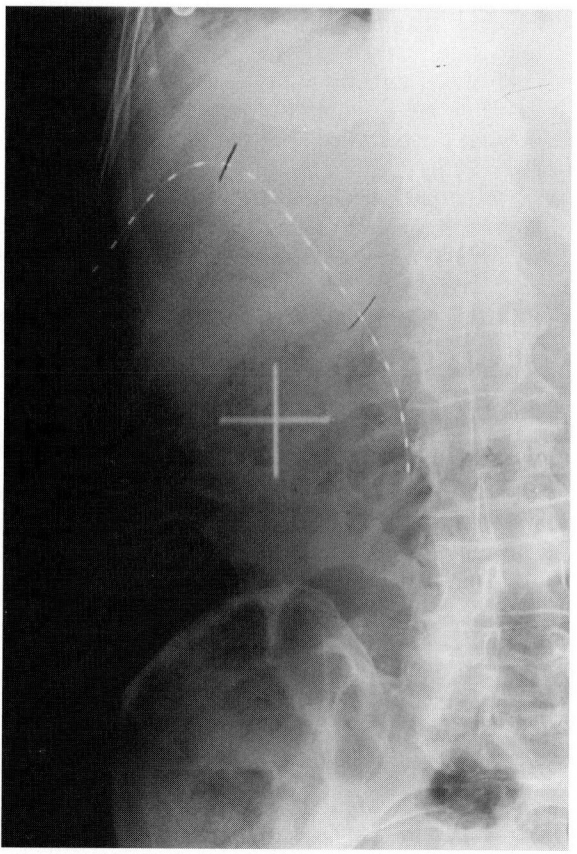

Figure 12–31. Simulation film of intraluminal biliary tract implant showing dummy seeds positioned at the distal end of the catheter. Markings indicate the active length to be used in the treatment.

The usual dose of the intraluminal brachytherapy boost is 20 to 30 Gy prescribed to a 1 cm distance from the source. This treatment is usually given after 45 to 50.4 Gy EBRT. The loading of the ^{192}Ir is done in the patient's room and is usually left in place for 2 to 3 days. During hospitalization, special care must be taken to maintain the potency of the biliary tract to prevent obstructive cholangitis. When the desired dose is delivered, ^{192}Ir seeds are unloaded and the patient and room are surveyed, followed by removal of the plastic catheters.

HIGH-DOSE-RATE INTRAOPERATIVE BRACHYTHERAPY

Intraoperative radiation allows the clinician to directly visualize the tumor bed area and to displace the surrounding normal tissue from the radiation field. For these reasons, it is possible to deliver a high dose of radiation to the tumor while minimizing the dose to the surrounding organs.[56]

Electrons generated by a linear accelerator have been used to deliver this type of radiation; however, this technique is obviously very expensive due to shielding requirements and cost. Its applications are limited due to the difficulty of getting the field of radiation to conform to different anatomic sites.

The introduction of HDR brachytherapy as an alternative to electrons may popularize the use of intraoperative radiation because it is relatively cheap and has the potential for use in any body part. A specially designed intraoperative HAM (Harrison, Anderson, and Mick) catheter applicator is placed in the tumor bed area and is connected to the ^{192}Ir HDR remote afterloader (Fig. 12-32). The HAM applicator is pliable and conforms to surface curvature as shown in Figure 12-33. The other advantage of this technique is the ability to treat a large volume with a precise matching.

At MSKCC, HDR intraoperative brachytherapy has been used in the treatment of rectal cancer,[57-59] retroperitoneal sarcomas,[60] gynecologic cancers,[61] and pediatric tumors.[62] The treatment is given in 1 fraction with a dose that ranges from 12 to 17.5 Gy and is prescribed to a depth of 1 cm from the source.

Permanent Implants

Unlike temporary implants, permanent implants are not afterloaded. Therefore, manual instruments are an essential component in handling the radioactive sources during the entire implant procedure. The instruments needed depend on the type of the implant; a Mick applicator is used for volume implants, and if a tumor bed is implanted, a seed in a carrier is used.

INSTRUMENTS

Mick Applicator

This applicator is commercially available (Mick Medical Instruments, Inc., Bronx, NY), allowing precise and quick placement of radioactive seeds in the tumor through previously inserted needles.

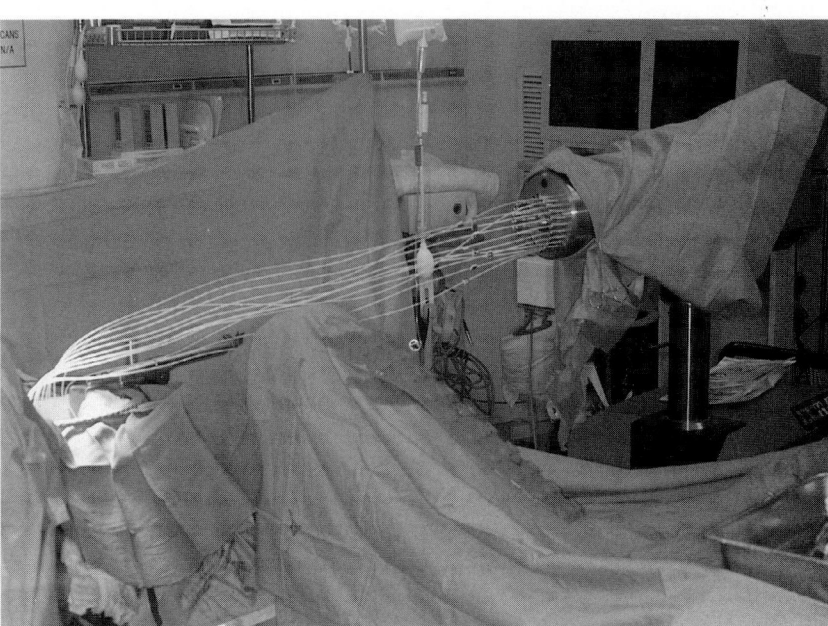

Figure 12–32. Harrison, Anderson, and Mick (HAM) applicator being connected to high-dose-rate treatment machine via transport tubes.

The instrument includes a magazine for handling the radioactive seeds and a stainless steel tray that contains 17-gauge stainless steel needles, the applicator itself, and a stainless steel ruler (Fig. 12-34). Each magazine has a cartridge inside, which is loaded with stacked-up radioactive sources. The magazine in turn has a head plunger, which is inserted into a corresponding slot on the cartridge and turned clockwise until it stops. This arrangement allows the release of one seed at a time into the applicator. A special magazine holder that has five holes to hold five magazines is available. Attached to the holder is a tag that records the number of magazines, number of seeds per magazine, and the activity per seed on the day of the implant. The stainless steel needles have a standard length of 15 cm, but some models accommodate shorter (10 cm) or longer (20 cm) needles. The applicator itself has a needle receptor that holds the needle firmly in place. To detach the needle from the applicator, two buttons located on each side of the receptor must be pushed simultaneously. This feature prevents inadvertent detachment of the needles. Another receptor accommodates the magazine and a stylet that guides each individual seed after it has been released from the magazine through the needle and into the tumor. The other function of the stylet is seed release, whereby every time the stylet is pulled back beyond the magazine receptor, a seed is released. The stainless steel tray with all its contents as well as the magazines are sterilized by autoclaving just before use.

Iodine-125 Seeds in Carriers (Suture Seeds)

In planar implant, the tissue being implanted is not firm enough to support loose seeds as with volume implants. In these cases, a mesh tube of Vicryl absorbable suture material is used with ^{125}I seeds embedded in it (Fig. 12-35). Each suture has ten ^{125}I seeds spaced 1 cm from center to center, and at one end the suture is connected to a half-circle taper point surgical needle. The suture is housed in a stainless steel ring that provides complete shielding. Each ring should have a tag stating the activity per seed on the day of the implant.

TECHNIQUES, TREATMENT PLANNING, AND DELIVERY

Permanent implants are done for the most part under general anesthesia, and the technique and treatment planning depend on the type of implant performed.

Volume Implants

Even though most of the work on ^{125}I volume implants is on prostate cancer,[63-65] this technique could be used virtually in any solid organ of the body. These implants are done using the Mick applicator. The cornerstone of the permanent implant is the accurate determination of the tumor volume, because unlike temporary implants, once

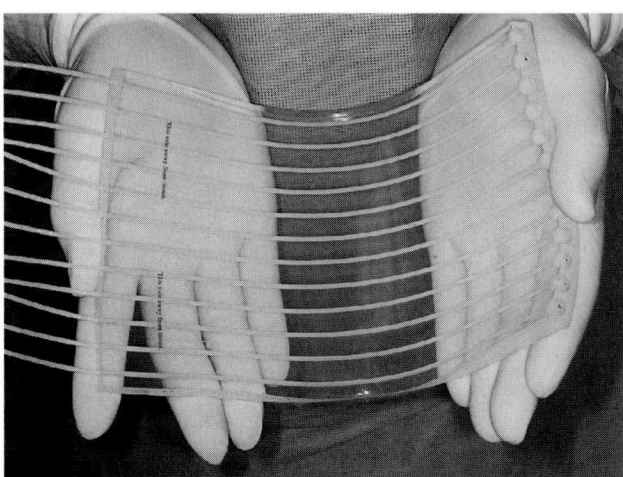

Figure 12–33. Hand-held Harrison, Anderson, and Mick (HAM) applicator to indicate the degree of its flexibility and conformity to curvature. The HAM applicator is made of a slab of tissue-equivalent material.

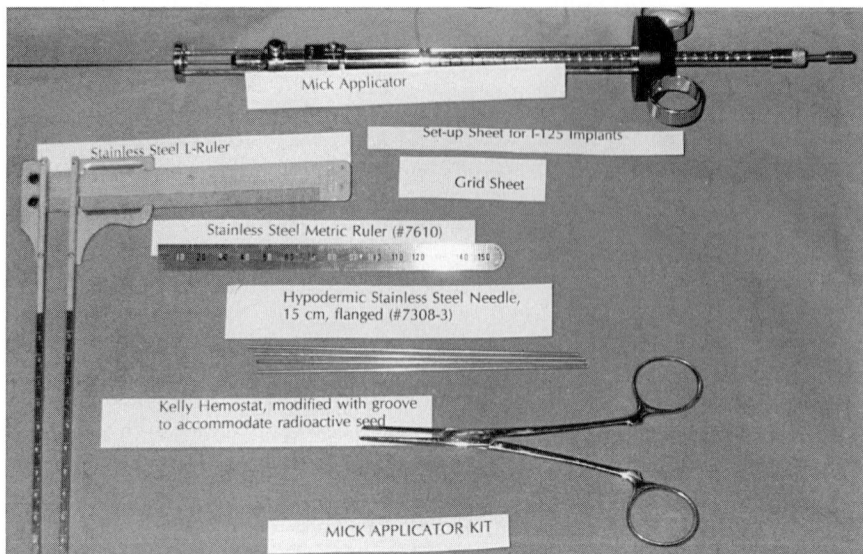

Figure 12–34. Mick applicator kit.

the seeds are implanted, there is nothing that can be done to modify or optimize the dose distribution.

The tumor volume dimensions are determined from imaging (e.g., CT, MRI) or during surgery. The most difficult dimension to measure intraoperatively is the depth, and the best approach is to insert a 15-cm long needle through the maximum thickness of the tumor and subtract the protruding length of the needle from its total length of 15 cm.

Based on the average of three dimensions of the tumor volume, a nomogram published by Anderson[66] determines the total number of ^{125}I seeds and the spacing between needles (Fig. 12-36). Other factors that must be used in the nomogram, in addition to the average dimension, include the seed strength in mCi at the day of the implant and the selected spacing between ^{125}I seeds. This

spacing (preferably 1 cm) is determined in such a way that the maximum number of seeds may be inserted through one needle. To determine the number of seeds from the nomogram, a straight line is drawn that starts with the average dimension value located on the far left column of the nomogram. This point is then connected to another point on the "seed strength" column. The line created is then extended until it intersects with the "number of seeds" column. To determine the spacing between needles, two additional straight lines need to be drawn. The first line starts at the same point where the previous line ended on the "number of seeds" column and connects with a point on the second average dimension column (middle of the nomogram). This line is extended until it reaches the tie line. The second line starts at the same point where the first line ended on the tie line and connects with a point on the spacing along needle column (the value is usually 1 cm). This second line is extended until it reaches the "spacing between needles" column.

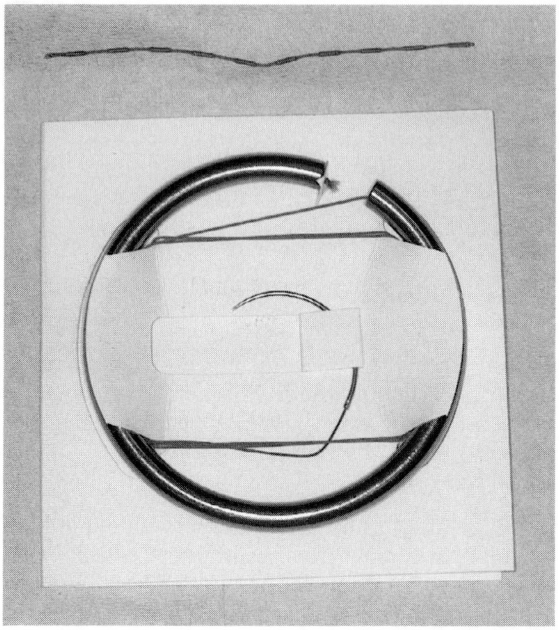

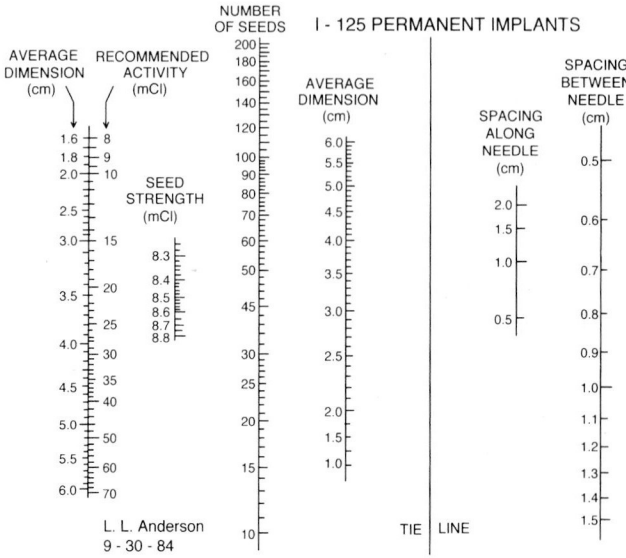

Figure 12–35. ^{125}I seeds in carrier. The metal ring is used to house the seeds before use.

Figure 12–36. A nomogram for ^{125}I volume implants.

The number of sources per needle is determined from the average depth of the implant and the spacing between seeds in each needle. The total number of needles required for a volume implant is determined by dividing the total number of seeds by the number of seeds per needle.

Next, the predetermined number of 17-gauge needles are inserted into the tumor one at a time and parallel to one another. After all needles are inserted, the Mick applicator is connected one needle at a time and the radioactive seeds are inserted through the needle at the selected spacing. When the predetermined number of seeds per needle is reached, the needle is pulled out and the process is repeated for each remaining needle (Fig. 12-37). A record should be kept of the total number of seeds used, activity per seed, and seed spacing along the needle. Throughout the procedure, attention should be paid to any loose seeds that may have fallen around the implanted area.

At the end of the implant procedure, a full accounting of all seeds should be done and any free seeds should be collected in a small lead container with a tag showing the number of seeds, the activity, and the date. A Geiger counter should be used to detect any loose seeds that may have been left behind inadvertently in the Mick applicator, its accessories, and all drained fluids, sheaths, equipment, and so on. After all this is finished, a note is written in the patient's chart describing the procedure and stating the total number of seeds implanted, the activity per seed, and the time of implant. Postoperative localization films are taken to determine the dose and dose distribution. Although these two factors may not be modified once a permanent implant has been done, their evaluation is an important quality assurance measure and enables the radiation oncologist to compare his or her data with that from other institutions.

The traditional method of dose calculation and distribution has been the matched peripheral dose (MPD), which is defined as the dose for which the contour volume is equal to the volume of an ellipsoid having the same dimensions as the measured dimension of the tumor volume. This definition assumes that both the target volume and the volume isodose contour are similar in shape, which is not the case in many volume implants. This discrepancy leads the MPD to overestimate the MPD (the dose that covers 100% of the target) and not to take into consideration any geographic miss (Fig. 12-38).

There have been significant strides in the planning of prostate implants over the past decade.[67-70] At MSKCC, we have developed and successfully implemented an intraoperative conformal optimization and planning system for ultrasound-based prostate implants.[71,72] At the time of implant, patients are placed in the extended lithotomy position and a urinary catheter is inserted. An ultrasound probe is positioned in the rectum, and the prostate and normal anatomy are identified. Needles are inserted through the perineal template at the periphery of the prostate. The prostate is subsequently scanned from apex to base, and these 0.5 cm images are transferred to the treatment planning system using a PC-based video capture system. On the computer monitor, the prostate contours as well as the urethra are digitized on each axial image. Needle positions are identified on each image, and their coordinates are incorporated into a genetic algorithm optimization program. This sophisticated optimization system incorporates acceptable dose ranges allowed within the target as well as dose constraints for the rectal wall and urethra.

After the optimization program identifies the optimal seed-loading pattern and the dose calculations are completed, isodose displays are superimposed on each transverse ultrasound image and carefully evaluated. Dose volume histograms for the target volume, rectum, and urethra are also carefully assessed. If portions of the target volume are found to be underdosed or higher urethral doses on selected images are observed, appropriate adjustments are made with the deletion of a seed or insertion of new needle positions, and revised isodose distributions are immediately generated. The entire planning

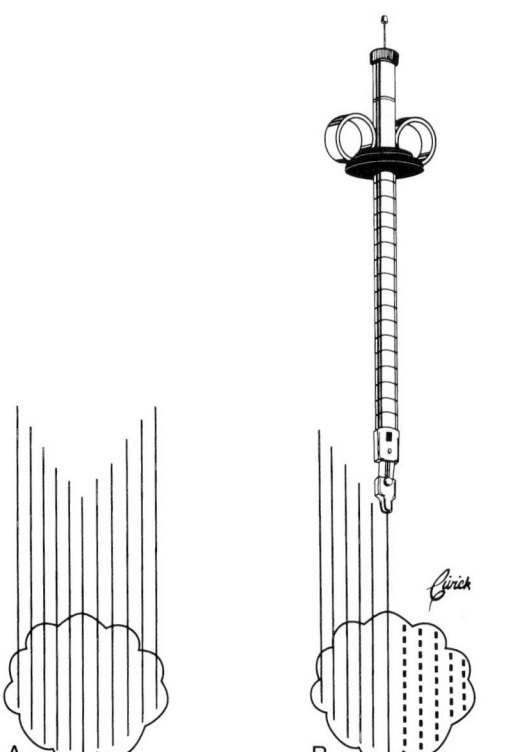

Figure 12–37. Volume implants technique. **A**, Diagram of needles placed with desired spacing within the tumor. **B**, Insertion of ^{125}I seeds into the tumor using the Mick applicator.

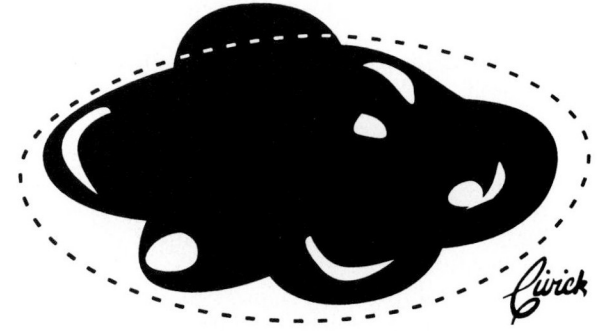

Figure 12–38. Matched peripheral dose (MPD). This illustration demonstrates the shortcoming of the MPD method. The *dotted line* represents the MPD, and the *black volume* is the tumor. Note that the dotted line underestimates the tumor volume in certain areas, causing a geographic miss, and overestimates it in others.

process, from the contouring of images to the generation of the seed loading patterns, requires approximately 10 minutes. Seeds are then loaded with a standard applicator.

Planar Implant

In planar implants ^{125}I is used in the form of suture seeds, which could be sewn into the tissue directly or using a Dexon mesh. This latter approach is used when there is inadequate tissue to support the suture seeds or there is a critical structure in the target area. Planar implants are used in the treatment of lung cancer if there is a concern about the margin of resection,[73] neck node,[9,10] and rectal cancer,[74] to name a few.

The implant procedures are identical for both types except that the suture seeds are first sewn onto the Dexon mesh instead of the tumor bed. First, the target area length and width are measured. Then a modified planar implant nomogram is used to determine the total number of ^{125}I seeds and the spacing between seeds' rows that would deliver 160 Gy MPD. As in volume implants, localization films are taken postoperatively.

APPLICATION TO ANATOMIC SITES

Only sites that are not extensively covered elsewhere in this textbook are discussed here.

Skull Base Tumors

Permanent interstitial implants alone or in combination with EBRT could be used to re-irradiate recurrent tumors or treat primary tumors after subtotal resection, respectively. This technique of radiation allows the delivery of high doses of radiation to very inaccessible areas.[75,76] With the advances in stereotactic radiosurgery, however, the indication for this technique has diminished.

TECHNIQUE
SELECTION. Patients with primary tumor, status post-subtotal resection, or recurrent tumor after EBRT are selected. The tumor could be of any histologic type (e.g., meningioma, chordoma, invasive pituitary adenoma, sarcoma). In order for the implant to be successful, the tumor mass needs to be localized rather than diffuse.

ISOTOPES. Permanent low activity (0.4 to 0.5 mCi) ^{125}I seeds are used.

PROCEDURES. The procedure is done under general anesthesia, usually at the time of surgery when there is gross residual disease left. The tumor volume is determined from preoperative CT and MRI and, more importantly, intraoperatively.

Surgical exploration is essential in determining the extent of the tumor as well as providing access for source placement. ^{125}I sources are inserted into the tumor mass either with a Mick applicator or Vicryl suture seeds. In thin lesions and where there is no adequate tissue to support the suture seeds, a biologic adhesive is used to glue the seeds to the tumor bed.

Following the implant, orthogonal pair localization films and CT scans are taken to calculate the dose and verify the position of the sources in relation to the tumor mass. The dose is prescribed in terms of MPD like other permanent implants; however, if 3D imaging of the implanted tumor is available, the dose could be prescribed in terms of minimal peripheral dose.

Nasopharynx

External beam radiotherapy is the main treatment for primary nasopharyngeal cancer. Brachytherapy is used primarily in patients who have developed local recurrence after high doses of external beam radiation.[77-79] But some advocate its use also for locally advanced disease.[80]

TECHNIQUE
SELECTION. All patients with recurrent nasopharyngeal malignancies are potential candidates for brachytherapy. Patients with intracranial extension are not suitable for brachytherapy due to the rapid falloff of dose with increased distance of the tumor from the source.

ISOTOPES. High activity ^{125}I or ^{192}Ir is generally used for intracavitary brachytherapy, whereas ^{125}I seeds have been commonly used for permanent interstitial brachytherapy.

PROCEDURES. The nasopharynx is a small yet anatomically complex area composed of superior, posterior, lateral, anterior, and inferior surfaces. Discussions of brachytherapy techniques have generally not regarded the anatomic variation in these sites. Different techniques are needed for each site in order to achieve both an optimal distribution of dose to the tumor and as low a dose as possible to the surrounding normal tissue.[81]

1. Permanent implants: For lesions located in the superior and posterior wall of the nasopharynx, permanent implants can be done with the help of a surgical exposure or via the nasal or oral cavity.[82-84] Permanent implants are appropriate when accurate determination of the tumor volume can be made based on findings from physical examination and CT scan or MRI. Individual ^{125}I seeds of desired activity are used. These seeds are implanted with either a single-seed applicator or a Mick applicator. Following the implant with ^{125}I seeds, orthogonal films of the nasopharynx are taken and isodose curves are generated. The dose delivered depends on the dose already received from external beam irradiation. For patients with recurrent disease, we have generally delivered 45 to 50 Gy via external beam, plus ^{125}I implants for 160 Gy MPD.
2. Temporary implants: For diffuse lesions or those involving a lateral wall or posterior nasal cavity, permanent implants with seeds are very difficult. Also, the tendency of tumors in this area to extend laterally toward the lateral retropharyngeal space makes the dosimetry of a permanent implant suboptimal. However, this area is suited for a temporary implant.

A custom-designed nasopharyngeal applicator can be contoured to bend toward the side of the nasopharynx that requires brachytherapy. The patient has a CT scan done with the applicator and dummy sources in place. With this information, the implant can be appropriately planned. A hole is drilled in the applicator at a specific angle, designed so that an iridium ribbon placed through the applicator would exit with a specific orientation to the main axis of the applicator, which houses a second ribbon. In this manner, two ^{192}Ir ribbons are placed in the applicator to cover the target volume. It is clear that appropriate doses of radiation can be delivered to the lateral nasopharynx with relative sparing of the uninvolved normal tissues. The same is true of the posterior nasal cavity, which was also involved in this particular patient, as seen on the CT scan.

Appropriately sized endotracheal tubes are usually required. Through the tubes, the desired isotope can be inserted into the nasopharynx, whether it be ^{137}Cs or ^{192}Ir or high activity ^{125}I. Alternatively, special applicators can be made with synthetic materials. After the insertion of the intracavitary applicator, orthogonal x-rays are taken and computerized treatment planning is done to determine the isodose-rate contour to which the dose of radiation will be prescribed. The typical dose of an intracavitary boost is usually 15 to 20 Gy.

Nasopharyngeal implants are usually very well tolerated. Other than minimum bleeding after interstitial implantation of ^{125}I seeds, there are no other notable problems. The patient can be observed for 24 hours in the hospital and discharged if there is no bleeding. For intracavitary implantation, no particular acute or post-insertion problems have been reported. The patients are followed with periodic physical examinations and MRI or CT scans.

Lip

Malignant lip tumors are most commonly squamous cell cancer.

TECHNIQUE
SELECTION. Early lesions (T1 and small T2) can be treated by interstitial implant alone or in combination with EBRT.[85,86]

ISOTOPES. Temporary interstitial implants can be done with either iridium or iodine.

PROCEDURES. After infiltration of local anesthesia, 14-gauge angiocatheters are placed through the lesion with approximately 1 cm spacing in a single plane. The target volume includes the tumor volume plus 0.5 to 1 cm margins. Localization films are taken, and computer dosimetry is done.

In cases in which implant alone is used, doses in the 60 Gy range are usually adequate. When implant is combined with external radiation, the lip receives 50 to 54 Gy and the involved neck, 60 Gy.

Uninvolved neck sites are treated to 50 Gy, then 2 weeks later, the implant delivers an additional 20 to 30 Gy in 2 to 3 days. While the implant is loaded, it is recommended that the patient wear a radiation-shield prosthesis to protect the gingiva, oral tongue, floor of mouth, and mandible, if possible.

Oral Tongue

Early tongue cancers are successfully managed by either surgery or radiotherapy. When radiation therapy is given, numerous authors[11,12,87,88] have shown that treatment outcome is superior when all or part of the dose is delivered via an interstitial implant.

By far the largest experience in the literature is from Decroix et al.[89] from the Curie Institute in Paris. These authors reported on 602 patients with T1, T2, or T3 squamous cell cancers of the oral tongue. The majority (312 patients) had implant alone, with 148 patients having external beam plus implant, 69 patients having implant and surgery, 67 patients having external beam alone, and only 6 patients having surgery alone. T1 and T2 tumors were most often managed with an implant alone, delivering 70 Gy in 6 to 9 days. Larger T2 and most T3 lesions received external radiation, with the more responsive tumors being boosted with implant and the less responsive ones boosted with external beam. Local control was obtained in 86% for T1, 80% for T2, and 68% for T3 tumors. This compares quite favorably with the primary surgical data from MSKCC,[90] indicating local control of 85% for T1, 77% for T2, and 50% for T tumors.

TECHNIQUE
SELECTION. Implant alone is preferred for T1 lesions. For T2 lesions, either implant alone or implant with external beam can be used. For these patients, management of the primary site must be integrated with management of the neck. For N0 patients, combining external beam with implant allows for the delivery of elective neck irradiation simultaneous with irradiation to the tongue, followed by implant boost to the tongue. For N+ patients, in whom the neck is treated with surgery and radiation, external beam is given to the neck and tongue, followed by implant to the tongue and a neck dissection a few weeks later.

ISOTOPES. LDR ^{192}Ir or high activity ^{125}I can be used.

PROCEDURES. There are a number of techniques for implanting the oral tongue, but the loop technique is the most favorable. Trocars are introduced via a submental approach and are looped over the tongue mucosa. The target volume includes the tumor volume plus 1 cm margin around it. Care is taken to keep the catheters as far from the mandible as possible. The catheters are loaded after localization films are taken and computed dosimetry is performed. When implant alone is used, a total dose of 60 to 70 Gy is given.

For lesions treated with external beam and implant, the external radiation is done first. The dose to the primary and upper neck is approximately 50 Gy. Two to three weeks later, an implant is done, as described, with the boost dose being 20 to 25 Gy. As opposed to the situation with base of tongue implants, a tracheostomy is not required for an oral tongue implant. The patient needs to wear a tongue prosthesis to protect the palate through the implant duration.

A small subset of patients have an excision of a small tongue lesion but have very close or positive margins. Clearly, in this situation, the major treatment goal is to control the disease with minimum loss of tongue. Ange et al.[91] have described the use of implant alone after excision that leaves close or positive margins, with all 23 patients in their series achieving local control.

Floor of Mouth

As in oral tongue cancer, when radiation is used, it is preferable for at least a portion of the treatment to be delivered via an implant.[92] If the lesion abuts or is tethered to the periosteum of the mandible, it is probably better to treat the tumor with surgery in order to avoid the placement of radioactive sources against the mandible. Placement of sources in this location can lead to osteonecrosis.

TECHNIQUE
SELECTION. As is the case with tongue cancer, early lesions can be treated with implant alone; however, for T1N0 and T2N0 tumors, combined external beam plus implant is used.

ISOTOPES. The isotopes used are similar to those used for the oral tongue treatment.

PROCEDURES. The loop technique is preferred. The target volume includes the tumor volume plus 1 cm margin. When implant is used alone, the dose of radiation is 60 to 70 Gy. When combined with external beam radiotherapy, the dose is 20 to 25 Gy for the implant and 50 to 54 Gy for the external beam. Care should be taken to keep the implant as far from the mandible as possible.

Buccal Mucosa

Carcinoma of the buccal mucosa is a relatively rare tumor in the United States, accounting for only 4% of all oral cancers.

TECHNIQUE
SELECTION. Small lesions (T1 and early T2) can be managed by surgery or by an interstitial implant alone. Moderately advanced lesions can be resected or treated with external beam radiation, with implant as a boost.

ISOTOPES. The isotopes used are similar to those used for the oral tongue treatment.

PROCEDURES. Small lesions (<1 cm thickness) can be treated with a single-plane implant. Eighteen-gauge angiocatheters are placed through the skin anteriorly and through the lesion and exit skin posteriorly. The catheters are then fixed in place with small metal buttons. Orthogonal x-rays are taken for localization of the catheters and dosimetric calculations. Iridium seeds in

nylon ribbons are then placed in the catheters. The target volume includes the tumor volume plus 1 cm margin. A planned dose of 60 to 70 Gy is given over 6 days if the implant is used alone. When the implant is combined with external beam radiotherapy, the dose is 20 to 25 Gy. A lead obturator is used to shield the normal mucosa from excessive radiation.

Neck Nodes

The two main modalities used in the management of metastatic neck nodes from head and neck squamous cell cancer are surgery and/or external beam radiotherapy. However, in the subgroup of patients in whom the lymph nodes are attached to the carotid the local control with any of those two modalities is very poor.[9] At Stanford a treatment approach that includes combination of gross surgical resection of the tumor without sacrifice of the carotid artery, along with ^{125}I permanent implant at the time of surgery and external beam radiotherapy if it was not used before, have yielded a 79% control rate in the implanted volume.[10] Unfortunately, most of those patients developed distant metastasis.

TECHNIQUE
SELECTION. Patients who are suitable for implants are those with advanced neck disease that adheres to the carotid artery and in whom a gross resection alone will leave a positive or unsure margin. Patients with subcutaneous metastasis or bilateral neck disease are not good candidates.

ISOTOPES. Permanent ^{125}I seeds are used in most centers. Temporary ^{192}Ir or high activity ^{125}I could be used instead; however, the dose of radiation to the surrounding normal tissue is higher with the latter, especially considering that many of those patients have already received prior radiation.

PROCEDURES. Permanent ^{125}I implants are best done at the time of surgery, after the neck mass has been resected. Suture seeds can be sewn directly into the tumor bed as shown in Figure 12-39, or through a Dexon mesh in a single-planar implant that covers the tumor bed. If there is any gross residual disease left, a volume implant can be done using a Mick applicator. To decrease wound complication and potentially carotid artery exposure, a 1 to 2 cm thick tissue layer should be placed between the seeds and the skin. Postoperatively, localization films are taken and the dose is calculated from the implant.

Rectal Cancer

Primary radiation therapy is not the treatment of choice for rectal cancer; however, intracavitary HDR brachytherapy[93,94] or interstitial brachytherapy[95] in addition to EBRT could have a role in the management of this disease in medically inoperable patients. Intraoperative HDR brachytherapy[57,58] or permanent ^{125}I implants[74] have a significant role in the management of patients

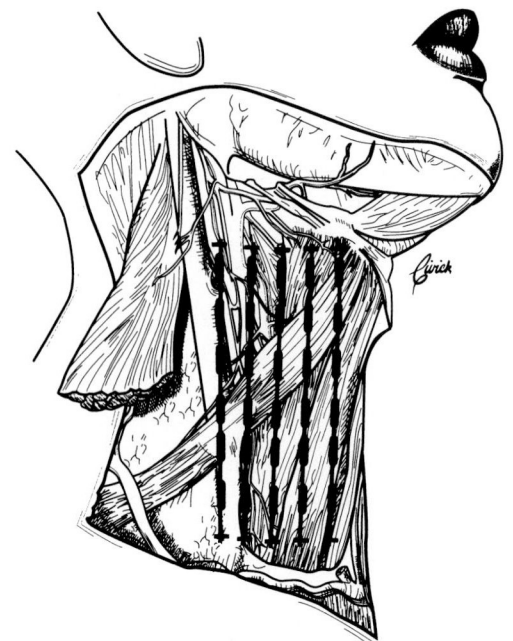

Figure 12–39. Planar ^{125}I implant in the neck using seeds in the carrier, which are directly embedded into the tumor bed.

with recurrent or initially unresectable rectal cancer in whom brachytherapy is used as an adjuvant treatment to resection after preoperative EBRT and chemotherapy. In patients with recurrent tumor and prior EBRT, only brachytherapy is used.

TECHNIQUE
SELECTION. In medically inoperable patients, brachytherapy is used 2 to 3 weeks following a course of EBRT to the pelvis with or without chemotherapy. Intracavitary HDR brachytherapy in this setting is simpler and more convenient than interstitial brachytherapy, especially in medically inoperable patients who may not tolerate general anesthesia very well. It also does not require the strict selection criteria of the Papillon technique (i.e., lesion size, grade, tumor configuration, location).[96] However, if the tumor mass does not respond to EBRT and is deeply penetrating, then a multiplane interstitial implant would be preferable. Transrectal ultrasound could be of significant assistance in this regard.

In patients who present with unresectable tumor, EBRT and chemotherapy are first given. Then, in 4 to 6 weeks, patients undergo surgery and either ^{125}I permanent implant or intraoperative HDR brachytherapy is used as a boost. The main advantage of HDR intraoperative radiation therapy over ^{125}I permanent implant is the ability to displace or shield adjacent bowel, uninvolved ureters, and other radiosensitive structure. At present, most patients at MSKCC with unresectable rectal cancer are enrolled in a phase I/II prospective trial using preoperative EBRT to 50.4 Gy plus chemotherapy. In 6 weeks the patient undergoes resection and HDR intraoperative radiation therapy boost to 15 Gy if there is a positive or uncertain margin.

ISOTOPES. For intracavitary brachytherapy, HDR ^{192}Ir is used. In temporary interstitial implant LDR ^{192}Ir is used, and for permanent implant, ^{125}I is used.

PROCEDURES
INTRACAVITARY HIGH-DOSE-RATE BRACHYTHERAPY. This procedure is done on an outpatient basis under topical anesthesia. The tumor volume is defined from rectal examination, sigmoidoscopy, barium enema, ultrasound, or MRI. The target volume includes the tumor volume plus 1 to 2 cm margin proximally and distally depending on the size and location of the tumor. Complication rates increase if the treatment length exceeds 7 cm or the anal sphincter is included in the target volume.[93]

The treatment is usually given with a 2 cm diameter cylinder with a dose of 3 Gy per fraction × 3 at 1-week intervals. The dose is prescribed to 0.5 cm depth from the surface of the cylinder. The most commonly used cylinder is the one with a 180-degree lead shield to protect the rest of the rectal circumference from high doses of radiation (Fig. 12-40).

TEMPORARY INTERSTITIAL IMPLANT. This procedure is performed under general or epidural anesthesia after the patient's bowel has been prepped with the proper combination of antibiotic similar to the one used for rectal surgery.

Single- or multiplane implant is used depending on the extent of the tumor, which should be determined from examination under anesthesia and sigmoidoscopy. Straight trocars are inserted through the perianal skin, then afterloading catheters with dummy sources are threaded through. At the time of trocar insertion, one double-gloved finger should be placed in the rectum to avoid entrance into the rectal lumen. The catheters should be placed parallel and 0.5 cm away from the rectal mucosa.

In a single-plane implant, catheters should be placed 1 cm apart, and 1.2 to 2 cm in multiplane implant with 1.5 to 2 cm between planes uniformly throughout the

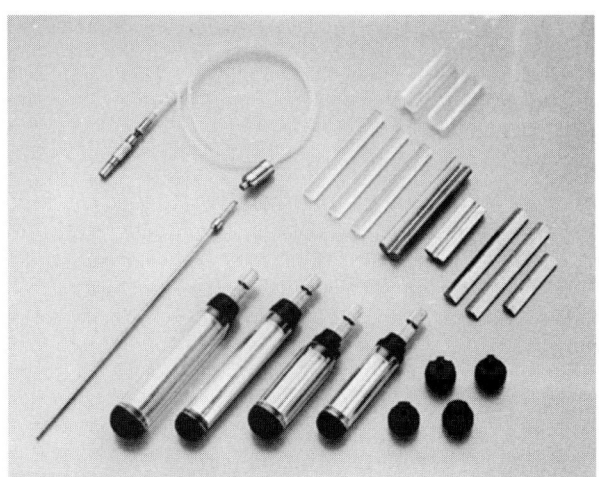

Figure 12–40. Shielded rectal cylinder set. Various lead shields can be arranged to shield the treatment diameter in increments of 90 degrees. The transport tube and central source tube are also shown. (Courtesy of Gamma-Med, Frank Barker Association Inc., Pequannock, NJ.)

tumor volume. A Syed template would be useful in this setting. To reduce the dose of radiation to the rest of the rectal wall, a custom-made plug is inserted to distend the rectal lumen.

Following the implant, the patient should be placed on diphenoxylate hydrochloride (Lomotil) and a low-residue diet. Occasionally, a diverting colostomy might be needed to prevent obstruction. This may represent a limitation for this technique, because those patients requiring colostomy for the large part are medically inoperable. Orthogonal pair films are taken postoperatively to determine the target volume; the dose of ^{192}Ir boost is usually 25 to 30 Gy depending on the dose of EBRT.

PERMANENT ^{125}I IMPLANT. A planar or volume implant is used, depending on the extent of residual disease after resection. If the patient has a positive or unsure margin, then a suture seed planar implant with or without a Dexon mesh is used. If there is a gross residual disease, a volume implant is performed using a Mick applicator.

It is *very* important that the surgeon and radiation oncologist work together to identify the area or volume that needs to be implanted and to assure that all possible measures are taken to keep the small bowel out of the target area. For example, a portion of the omentum could be mobilized and placed over the implanted area to increase the distance between the ^{125}I seeds and the bowel.

INTRAOPERATIVE HIGH-DOSE-RATE BRACHYTHERAPY. After the patient undergoes the resection, the surgeon and radiation oncologist identify and measure the area of positive or unsure margin. A retractor is used to displace adjacent organs, and lead shield discs of different diameters are used to shield any other organ or structure that is not involved and that could not be displaced.

After measuring the tumor bed dimensions, an appropriately sized intraoperative applicator is selected. Once the position of this applicator has been secured by packing and the position confirmed by fluoroscopy, the applicator catheters will be attached to the cables of the HDR remote afterloader. A dose of 12–17.5 Gy is given to the tumor bed in a single fraction at a depth of 1 cm from the source.

When there is gross residual disease, an interstitial ^{125}I permanent implant will be used in addition to the intraoperative boost. After this has been completed, the catheters are disconnected from the applicator, all packing gauzes and shielding discs are accounted for, and the applicator is removed as well as the retractor. Finally, the surgeon closes the patient and completes the procedure.

The use of brachytherapy in the management of anal cancer has declined due to the risk of necrosis and the high number of local and lymph node failures reported.[97]

Cancer of the Female Urethra

Primary carcinoma of the female urethra is exceedingly rare. The most common location is near the meatus, and the most common histology is squamous cell carcinoma.

Interstitial brachytherapy has been used in the management of this disease, and most data have demonstrated that in well-selected cases, this treatment modality provides

good results.[98,99] A study by Foens et al.[100] has shown a superior local regional control with combined EBRT and brachytherapy compared with one modality alone.

TECHNIQUE
SELECTION. Ideal candidates for interstitial implants are those with tumor less than 4 cm, involving the distal urethra, low grade, T1N0M0 (tumor invading subepithelial connective tissue) and early T1N0M0 (invading periurethral muscles). In patients with advanced T2, T 3, T4 or N+ disease, the result with any single treatment modality is poor.

ISOTOPES. The isotope used is LDR ^{192}Ir.

PROCEDURES. The implant is done under general anesthesia with the patient in the lithotomy position. The extent of the tumor should be determined from CT or MRI, examination under anesthesia, and cystourethroscopy to rule out bladder base invasion.

The Memorial Hospital urethral applicator (see Fig. 12-19) or the Syed template could be used. A 28-gauge Foley catheter with a 30 mL capacity balloon and a stainless steel tube inside is inserted into the bladder. The Foley balloon is inflated with a radiopaque agent and pulled back against the bladder neck. This arrangement of the catheter not only provides drainage but also stabilization of the implant. Two plexiglass templates with a central hole to accommodate the Foley catheter and six peripheral holes for needles are used. These holes are arranged in a circle of 1 cm radius, and the distance between the holes is also 1 cm. The first template is passed through the Foley catheter to the urethral meatus and is fixed in that position by a thumb screw. Six 17-gauge, sealed-tip, stainless steel needles are inserted through the peripheral holes of both templates.

The target volume includes the tumor plus a 1 to 2 cm margin. Postoperatively, orthogonal pair localization films are taken. The dose is usually 60 Gy when implant is used alone or 20 to 30 Gy when combined with EBRT (45 Gy).

CANCER OF THE PENIS

Squamous cell carcinoma of the penis is uncommon, representing about 1% of male cancers. Therefore, experience in the treatment of this disease with brachytherapy or EBRT is scarce.[101,102] Gerbaulet et al.[103] reported an 82% local control in 109 patients treated with ^{192}Ir implant alone.

TECHNIQUE
SELECTION. Tumors smaller than 4 cm and with an invasion of the corpora cavernosa of less than 1 cm are suitable for treatment.

ISOTOPES. The isotope used is LDR ^{192}Ir.

PROCEDURES. It is preferable to proceed first with circumcision. After healing is complete, the interstitial implant is done. This procedure is done under general anesthesia or epidural anesthesia. The implant technique used by Gerhaulet at the Institute Gustave-Roussy in France is as follows: Needles are inserted through the lesion parallel, 1 cm apart, and perpendicular to the long axis of the penis. A single-plane implant is usually used. Preperforated plexiglass templates are placed on the lateral surface of the penis on each side to stabilize the needles. The target volume includes the tumor plus a 1.5 to 2 cm margin in all directions. Postoperatively, orthogonal pair localization films are taken, and the patient is loaded with ^{192}Ir after the edema has subsided. The dose is 60 to 65 Gy.

REFERENCES

1. Janeway HH, Barringer BS, Failla G: *Radiation Therapy in Cancer at the Memorial Hospital New York.* Paul B Hoeber; New York: 1917.
2. Henschke UK, Hilaris BS, Maran GD: Remote afterloading with intracavitary applicators. *Radiology.* 1964;83:344.
3. Harrison LB, Franzese F, Gaynor JJ, et al: Long-term results of a prospective randomized trial of adjuvant brachytherapy in the management of completely resected soft tissue sarcomas of the extremity and superficial trunk. *Int J Radiat Oncol Biol Phys.* 1993;27:259.
4. Alektiar KM, Leung D, Zelefsky MJ, et al: Adjuvant brachytherapy for primary high-grade soft tissue sarcoma of the extremity. *Ann Surg Oncol.* 2002;9:48.
5. Anderson LL, Hilaris BS, Wagner LK: A nomograph for planar implant planning. *Endocurie Hypertherm Oncol.* 1985;1:9.
6. Vicini F, Baglan K, Kestin L, et al: The emerging role of brachytherapy in the management of patients with breast cancer. *Semin Radiat Oncol.* 2002;12:31.
7. Kuske RR: Breast brachytherapy. *Hematol Oncol Clin North Am.* 1999;13:543.
8. Beauvois S, Hoffstetter S, Peiffert D, et al: Brachytherapy for lower lip epidermoid cancer: tumoral and treatment factors influencing recurrences and complications. *Radiother Oncol.* 1994;33:195.
9. Kennedy JT, Krause CJ, Loevy S: The importance of tumor attachment to the carotid artery. *Arch Otolaryngol.* 1977;103:70.
10. Paryani SB, Goffinet DR, Fee WE, et al: Iodine 125 suture implants in the management of advanced tumors in the neck attached to the carotid artery. *J Clin Oncol.* 1985;3:809.
11. Inoue T, Yoshida K, et al: Phase III trial of high- vs. low-dose-rate interstitial radiotherapy for early mobile tongue cancer. *Int J Radiat Oncol Biol Phys.* 2001;51:171.
12. Fujita M, Hirokawa Y, Kashiwado K, et al: Interstitial brachytherapy for stage I and II squamous cell carcinoma of the oral tongue: Factors influencing local control and soft tissue complications. *Int J Radiat Oncol Biol Phys.* 1999;44:767.
13. Harrison LB, Lee HJ, Pfister DG, et al: Long term results of primary radiotherapy with/without neck dissection for squamous cell cancer of the base of tongue. *Head Neck.* 1998;20:668.
14. Harrison LB, Zelefsky MJ, Armstrong JG, et al: Brachytherapy and function preservation in the localized management of soft tissue sarcomas of the extremity. *Semin Radiat Oncol.* 1993;3:260.
15. Shields CL, Shields JA, Cater J, et al: Plaque radiotherapy for uveal melanoma: Long-term visual outcome in 1106 consecutive patients. *Arch Ophthalmol.* 2000;118:1219.
16. Gutin PH, Prados MD, Phillips TL, et al: External irradiation followed by an interstitial high activity iodine-125 implant "boost" in the initial treatment of malignant gliomas: NCOG study 6G-82-2. *Int J Radiat Oncol Biol Phys.* 1991;21:5601.
17. Syed AM, Puthawala AA, Abdelaziz NN, et al: Long-term results of low-dose-rate interstitial-intracavitary brachytherapy in the treatment of carcinoma of the cervix. *Int J Radiat Oncol Biol Phys.* 2002;54:67.
18. Tewari KS, Cappuccini F, Puthawala AA, et al: Primary invasive carcinoma of the vagina: Treatment with interstitial brachytherapy. *Cancer.* 2001;91:758.
19. Choi JC, Ingenito AC, Nanda RK, et al: Potential decreased morbidity of interstitial brachytherapy for gynecologic malignancies using laparoscopy: A pilot study. *Gynecol Oncol.* 1999;73:210.
20. Stock RG, Chan K, Terk M, et al: A new technique for performing Syed-Neblett template interstitial implants for gynecologic malignancies using transrectal-ultrasound guidance. *Int J Radiat Oncol Biol Phys.* 1997;37:819.
21. Erickson B, Albano K, Gillin M: CT-guided interstitial implantation of gynecologic malignancies. *Int J Radiat Oncol Biol Phys.* 1996;36:699.
22. Eisbruch A, Johnston CM, Martel MK, et al: Customized gynecologic interstitial implants: CT-based planning, dose evaluation, and optimization aided by laparotomy. *Int J Radiat Oncol Biol Phys.* 1998;40:1087.
23. Lessard E, Hsu IC, Pouliot J: Inverse planning for interstitial gynecologic template brachytherapy: Truly anatomy-based planning. *Int J Radiat Oncol Biol Phys.* 2002;54:1243.
24. Hsu IC, Speight J, Hai J, et al: A comparison between tandem and ovoids and interstitial gynecologic template brachytherapy dosimetry using a hypothetical computer model. *Int J Radiat Oncol Biol Phys.* 2002;52:538.
25. Alektiar KM, McKee A, Venkatraman E, et al: Intravaginal high-dose-rate brachytherapy for Stage IB (FIGO Grade 1, 2) endometrial cancer. *Int J Radiat Oncol Biol Phys.* 2002;57:707.
26. Horowitz NS, Peters WA III, Smith MR, et al: Adjuvant high dose rate vaginal brachytherapy as treatment of stage I and II endometrial carcinoma. *Obstet Gynecol.* 2002;99:235.
27. Ogino I, Kitamura T, Okajima H, Matsubara S: High-dose-rate intracavitary brachytherapy in the management of cervical and vaginal intraepithelial neoplasia. *Int J Radiat Oncol Biol Phys.* 1998;40:881.
28. Reisinger S, Nori D, Lewis JL: Postoperative intravaginal radiation therapy as an adjunct to external irradiation in high-risk endometrial adenocarcinoma: An evaluation of two different dose schedules. *Endocurie Hypertherm Oncol.* 1991;7:35.
29. Demanes DJ, Rege S, Rodriquez RR, et al: The use and advantages of a multichannel vaginal cylinder in high-dose-rate brachytherapy. *Int J Radiat Oncol Biol Phys.* 1999;44:211.
30. Perez CA, Slessinger E, Grigsby PW: Design of an afterloading vaginal applicator (MIRALVA). *Int J Radiat Oncol Biol Phys.* 1990;18:1503.
31. Nag S, Erickson B, Parikh S, et al: The American Brachytherapy Society recommendations for high-dose-rate brachytherapy for carcinoma of the endometrium. *Int J Radiat Oncol Biol Phys.* 2000;48:779.
32. Kim RY, Pareek P, Duan J, et al: Postoperative intravaginal brachytherapy for endometrial cancer: Dosimetric analysis of vaginal colpostats and cylinder applicators. *Brachytherapy.* 2002;1:138.
33. Rosenstein LM: A simple computer program for optimization of source loading in cervical intracavitary applicators. *Br J Radiol.* 1977;50:119.
34. Anderson LL: Plan optimization and dose evaluation in brachytherapy. *Semin Radiat Oncol.* 1993;3:290.
35. Mohan R, Ding IY, Toraskar J, et al: Computation of radiation dose distributions for shielded cervical applicators. *Int J Radiat Oncol Biol Phys.* 1984;11:823.
36. Mohan R, Ding IY, Martel MK, et al: Measurements of radiation dose distributions for shielded cervical applicators. *Int J Radiat Oncol Biol Phys.* 1984;11:861.
37. Weeks KJ, Montana GS: Three-dimensional applicator system for carcinoma of the uterine cervix. *Int J Radiat Oncol Biol Phys.* 1997;37:455.
38. Fellner C, Potter R, Knocke TH, Wambersie A: Comparison of radiography- and computed tomography-based treatment planning in cervix cancer in brachytherapy with specific attention to some quality assurance aspects. *Radiother Oncol.* 2001;58:53.
39. Lerma FA, Williamson JF: Accurate localization of intracavitary brachytherapy applicators from 3D CT imaging studies. *Med Phys.* 2002;29:325.
40. Mutic S, Grigsby PW, Low DA, et al: PET-guided three-dimensional treatment planning of intracavitary gynecologic implants. *Int J Radiat Oncol Biol Phys.* 2002;52:1104.
41. Nag S, Chao C, Erickson B, et al: The American Brachytherapy Society recommendations for low-dose-rate brachytherapy for carcinoma of the cervix. *Int J Radiat Oncol Biol Phys.* 2002;52:33.
42. Nag S, Erickson B, Thomadsen B, et al: The American Brachytherapy Society recommendations for high-dose-rate brachytherapy for carcinoma of the cervix. *Int J Radiat Oncol Biol Phys.* 2000;48:201.

43. Fishman DA, Roberts KB, Chambers JT, et al: Radiation therapy as exclusive treatment for medically inoperable patients with stage I and II endometrioid carcinoma with endometrium. *Gynecol Oncol.* 1996;61:189.

44. Rouanet P, Dubois JB, Gely S, et al: Exclusive radiation therapy in endometrial carcinoma. *Int J Radiat Oncol Biol Phys.* 1993; 26:223.

45. Nguyen TV, Petereit DG: High-dose-rate brachytherapy for medically inoperable stage I endometrial cancer. *Gynecol Oncol.* 1998;71:196.

46. Yao MS, Koh WJ: Endobronchial brachytherapy. *Chest Surg Clin N Am.* 2001;11:813.

47. Kelly JF, Delclos ME, Morice RC, et al: High-dose-rate endobronchial brachytherapy effectively palliates symptoms due to airway tumors: The 10-year M. D. Anderson cancer center experience. *Int J Radiat Oncol Biol Phys.* 2000;48:697.

48. Stout R, Barber P, Burt P, et al: Clinical and quality of life outcomes in the first United Kingdom randomized trial of endobronchial brachytherapy (intraluminal radiotherapy) vs. external beam radiotherapy in the palliative treatment of inoperable non-small cell lung cancer. *Radiother Oncol.* 2000;56:323.

49. Langendijk H, de Jong J, Tjwa M, et al: External irradiation versus external irradiation plus endobronchial brachytherapy in inoperable non-small cell lung cancer: A prospective randomized study. *Radiother Oncol.* 2001;58:257.

50. Lagerwaard FJ, Murrer LH, de Pan C, et al: Mucosal dose prescription in endobronchial brachytherapy: A study based on CT-dosimetry. *Int J Radiat Oncol Biol Phys.* 2000;46:1051.

51. Gaspar LE, Nag S, Herskovic A, et al: American Brachytherapy Society (ABS) consensus guidelines for brachytherapy of esophageal cancer. Clinical Research Committee, American Brachytherapy Society, Philadelphia. *Int J Radiat Oncol Biol Phys.* 1997;38:127.

52. Gaspar LE, Winter K, Kocha WI, et al: A phase I/II study of external beam radiation, brachytherapy, and concurrent chemotherapy for patients with localized carcinoma of the esophagus (Radiation Therapy Oncology Group Study 9207): final report. *Cancer.* 2000; 88:988.

53. Sur RK, Levin CV, Donde B, et al: Prospective randomized trial of HDR brachytherapy as a sole modality in palliation of advanced esophageal carcinoma—An International Atomic Energy Agency study. *Int J Radiat Oncol Biol Phys.* 2002;53:127.

54. Spencer GM, Thorpe SM, Blackman GM, et al: Laser augmented by brachytherapy versus laser alone in the palliation of adenocarcinoma of the oesophagus and cardia: A randomized study. *Gut.* 2002;50:224.

55. Morganti AG, Trodella L, Valentini V, et al: Combined modality treatment in unresectable extrahepatic biliary carcinoma. *Int J Radiat Oncol Biol Phys.* 2000;46:913.

56. Hu KS, Enker WE, Harrison LB: High-dose-rate intraoperative irradiation: Current status and future directions. *Semin Radiat Oncol.* 2002;12:62.

57. Harrison LB, Minsky BD, Enker WE, et al: High dose rate intraoperative radiation therapy (HDR-IORT) as part of the management strategy for locally advanced primary and recurrent rectal cancer. *Int J Radiat Oncol Biol Phys.* 1998;42:325.

58. Alektiar KM, Zelefsky MJ, Paty PB, et al: High-dose-rate intraoperative brachytherapy for recurrent colorectal cancer. *Int J Radiat Oncol Biol Phys.* 2000;48:219.

59. Shoup M, Guillem JG, Alektiar KM, et al: Predictors of survival in recurrent rectal cancer after resection and intraoperative radiotherapy. *Dis Colon Rectum.* 2002;45:585.

60. Alektiar KM, Hu K, Anderson L, et al: High-dose-rate intraoperative radiation therapy (HDR-IORT) for retroperitoneal sarcomas. *Int J Radiat Oncol Biol Phys.* 2000;47:157.

61. Gemignani ML, Alektiar KM, Leitao M, et al: Radical surgical resection and high-dose-rate intraoperative radiation therapy (HDR-IORT) in patients with recurrent gynecologic cancers. *Int J Radiat Oncol Biol Phys.* 2001;50:687.

62. Goodman KA, Wolden SL, La Quaglia MP, et al: Intraoperative high-dose rate brachytherapy for pediatric solid tumors: A 10-year experience. *Brachytherapy.* 2003;2(3):139.

63. Merrick GS, Wallner KE, Butler WM: Permanent interstitial brachytherapy for the management of carcinoma of the prostate gland. *J Urol.* 2003;169:1643.

64. Grimm PD, Blasko JC, Sylvester JE, et al: 10-year biochemical (prostate-specific antigen) control of prostate cancer with ^{125}I brachytherapy. *Int J Radiat Oncol Biol Phys.* 2001;51:31.

65. Zelefsky MJ, Wallner KE, Ling CC, et al: Comparison of the 5-year outcome and morbidity of three-dimensional conformal radiotherapy versus transperineal permanent iodine-125 implantation for early-stage prostatic cancer. *J Clin Oncol.* 1999;17:517.

66. Anderson LL: A spacing nomograph for interstitial implants of 125-I seeds. *Med Phys.* 1976;3:48.

67. Nag S, Beyer D, Friedland J, et al: American Brachytherapy Society (ABS) recommendations for transperineal permanent brachytherapy of prostate cancer. *Int J Radiat Oncol Biol Phys.* 1999;44:789.

68. Nag S, Bice W, DeWyngaert K, et al: The American Brachytherapy Society recommendations for permanent prostate brachytherapy postimplant dosimetric analysis. *Int J Radiat Oncol Biol Phys.* 2000;46:221.

69. Nag S, Ellis RJ, Merrick GS, et al: American Brachytherapy Society recommendations for reporting morbidity after prostate brachytherapy. *Int J Radiat Oncol Biol Phys.* 2002;54:462.

70. Nag S, Ciezki JP, Cormack R, et al: Intraoperative planning and evaluation of permanent prostate brachytherapy: Report of the American Brachytherapy Society. *Int J Radiat Oncol Biol Phys.* 2001;51:1422.

71. Zelefsky MJ, Yamada Y, Cohen G, et al: Postimplantation dosimetric analysis of permanent transperineal prostate implantation: Improved dose distributions with an intraoperative computer-optimized conformal planning technique. *Int J Radiat Oncol Biol Phys.* 2000;48:601.

72. Zelefsky MJ, Yamada Y, Marion C, et al: Improved conformality and decreased toxicity with intraoperative computer-optimized transperineal ultrasound-guided prostate brachytherapy. *Int J Radiat Oncol Biol Phys.* 2003;55:956.

73. Hilaris BS: Lung brachytherapy. An overview and current indications. *Chest Surg Clin N Am.* 1994;4:45.

74. Minsky BD, Cohen AM, Enker WE, et al: Radiation therapy for unresectable rectal cancer. *Int J Radiat Oncol Biol Phys.* 1991;2l:1283.

75. Kumar PP, Patil AA: Interstitial brachytherapy for skull base tumors. *Neurosurg Clin N Am.* 2000;11:639.

76. Gutin PH, Leibel SA, Crumley RL, et al: Brachytherapy of recurrent tumors of the skull base and spine with interstitially implanted Iodine-125 sources. *Neurosurgery.* 1987;20:930.

77. Mazeron JJ, Noel G, Simon JM: Head and neck brachytherapy. *Semin Radiat Oncol.* 2002;12:95.

78. Law SC, Lam WK, Ng MF, et al: Reirradiation of nasopharyngeal carcinoma with intracavitary mold brachytherapy: an effective means of local salvage. *Int J Radiat Oncol Biol Phys.* 2002;54:1095.

79. Wang CC, Busse J, Gitterman M: A simple afterloading applicator for intracavitary irradiation of carcinoma of the nasopharynx. *Radiology.* 1975;115:737.

80. Levendag PC, Lagerwaard FJ, de Pan C, et al: High-dose, high-precision treatment options for boosting cancer of the nasopharynx. *Radiother Oncol.* 2002;63:67.

81. Harrison LB, Nori D, Hilaris BS, et al: Nasopharynx. In: *Interstitial Brachytherapy by the Interstitial Collaborative Working Group.* New York: Raven Press Ltd; 1990:95.

82. Harrison LB, Sessions RB, Fass DE, et al: Nasopharyngeal brachytherapy with access via a transpalatal flap. *Am J Surg.* 1992; 164:173.

83. Vikram B, Hilaris B: Transnasal permanent interstitial implantation of carcinoma of the nasopharynx. *Int J Radiat Oncol Biol Phys.* 1984;10:153.

84. Harrison LB, Weissberg JB: A technique for interstitial nasopharyngeal brachytherapy. *Int J Radiat Oncol Biol Phys.* 1987;13:451.

85. de Visscher JG, Grond AJ, Botke G, van der Waal I: Results of radiotherapy for squamous cell carcinoma of the vermilion border of the lower lip. A retrospective analysis of 108 patients. *Radiother Oncol.* 1996;39:9.

86. Beauvois S, Hoffstetter S, Peiffert D, et al: Brachytherapy for lower lip epidermoid cancer: Tumoral and treatment factors influencing recurrences and complications. *Radiother Oncol.* 1994;33:195.

87. Mendenhall W, Van Ase W, Bova F, et al: Analysis of time-dose factors in squamous cell carcinoma of the oral tongue and floor of mouth treated with radiation therapy alone. *Int J Radiat Oncol Biol Phys.* 1981;7:1005.

88. Chu A, Fletcher G: Incidence and causes of failure to control by irradiation the primary lesions in squamous cell carcinomas of the anterior two-thirds of the tongue and floor of mouth. *Am J Roent.* 1973;117:502.

89. Decroix Y, Ghossein N: Experience of the Curie Institute in treatment of cancer of the mobile tongue. I. Treatment policies and results. *Cancer.* 1981;47:496.

90. Spiro R, Stong E: Epidermoid carcinoma of the mobile tongue treatment by partial glossectomy alone. *Am J Surg.* 1971;122:707.

91. Ange D, Lindberg R, Guillamondegui O: Management of squamous cell carcinoma of the oral tongue and floor of mouth after excisional biopsy. *Radiology.* 1975;116:143.

92. Marsiglia H, Haie-Meder C, Sasso G, et al: Brachytherapy for T1-T2 floor-of-the-mouth cancers: The Gustave-Roussy Institute experience. *Int J Radiat Oncol Biol Phys.* 2002;52:1257.

93. Kaufman N, Nori D, Shank, B, et al: Remote afterloading intraluminal brachytherapy in the treatment of rectal, rectosigmoid, and anal cancer: A feasibility study. *Int J Radiat Oncol Biol Phys.* 1989;17:663.

94. Vuong T, Belliveau PJ, Michel RP, et al: Conformal preoperative endorectal brachytherapy treatment for locally advanced rectal cancer: Early results of a phase I/II study. *Dis Colon Rectum.* 2002;45:1486.

95. Syed AM, Puthawala A, Neblett D, et al: Primary treatment of carcinoma of the lower rectum and anal canal by a combination of external irradiation and interstitial implant. *Radiology.* 1978;128:199.

96. Papillon J: Rectal and anal cancers. Conservative treatment by irradiation—An alternative to rectal surgery. Berlin, Heidelberg, New York: Springer-Verlag; 1982:66.

97. Papillon J, Montbarbon JF: Epidermoid carcinoma of the anal canal. *Dis Colon Rectum.* 1987;30:324.

98. Garden AS, Zagars GK, Delclos L: Primary carcinoma of the female urethra. Results of radiation therapy. *Cancer.* 1993; 71:3102.

99. Milosevic MF, Warde PR, Banerjee D, et al: Urethral carcinoma in women: Results of treatment with primary radiotherapy. *Radiother Oncol.* 2000;56:29.

100. Foens CS, Hussey DH, Stables JJ, et al: A comparison of the roles of surgery and radiation therapy in the management of carcinoma of the female urethra. *Int J Radiat Oncol Biol Phys.* 1991;21:961.

101. Soria JC, Fizazi K, Piron D, et al: Squamous cell carcinoma of the penis: Multivariate analysis of prognostic factors and natural history in monocentric study with a conservative policy. *Ann Oncol.* 1997;8:1089.

102. Crook J, Grimard L, Tsihlias J, et al: Interstitial brachytherapy for penile cancer: An alternative to amputation. *J Urol.* 2002; 167:506.

103. Gerbaulet A, Lambin P: Radiation therapy of cancer of the penis. *Urol Clin North Am.* 1992;19:325.

High Dose Rate Brachytherapy

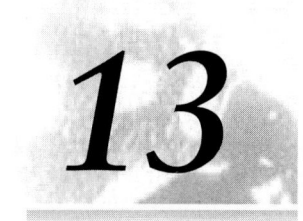

Andre Abitbol, MD, Subir Nag, MD,

I-Chow Joe Hsu, MD, Jean Pouiliot, PhD,

Alan A. Lewin, MD, and Colin G. Orton, PhD

The miniaturization of a high-activity radiation source and the development of a computerized remote-controlled delivery system has led to the advent of a new brachytherapy modality: high dose rate (HDR) brachytherapy. The dose rate usually delivered by a commercially available HDR brachytherapy apparatus is 100 to 300 Gy per hour and is higher than the International Commission on Radiation Units and Measurements (ICRU) Report No. 38 definition.[1] Distinct from low dose rate (LDR) brachytherapy, this modality represents a radical departure from traditional brachytherapy. Long accustomed to LDR regimens that allow repair of sublethal injury during the treatment time (typically 48 to 120 hours), the radiation oncologist must adjust the time-dose-fractionation regimen to compensate for the potential loss of the therapeutic ratio inherent with HDR brachytherapy. Appropriately, the development of good radiobiologic models now permits the use of rational regimens that are radiobiologically sound and, at the same time, clinically useful. Moreover, the American Brachytherapy Society (ABS) has published a number of articles on the recommended use of HDR brachytherapy for a number of sites.[2-10] Although these published guidelines are based primarily on nonrandomized trials, they do represent a consensus opinion of experts in the ABS. The use of HDR brachytherapy will necessitate the development of new brachytherapy systems and apparatuses. For example, a dedicated HDR suite with appropriate shielding may be necessary for high-volume practices and may add considerable cost. The delivery system may require different applicators and dosimetric considerations. Establishing a good quality assurance program for an HDR brachytherapy program requires close collaboration with the medical physicist and radiation therapists. The necessity for prompt dosimetry and rapid delivery of treatment (typically minutes) increases the chance for error in dosimetric calculations. The experience with HDR brachytherapy in the United States is increasing rapidly but well-established clinical protocols are still lacking.

Notwithstanding these considerations, HDR brachytherapy has many clinical advantages. Treatment can be delivered expeditiously on an outpatient basis and, if required, can be integrated with a course of external beam radiation therapy (EBRT). This modality increases the patient's comfort and reduces the risk of acute complications by obviating the need for hospitalization, prolonged bed rest, and, frequently, general anesthesia associated with low dose rate brachytherapy. The miniaturization of the radiation source and the applicator allows a more facile application, enhances accessibility to tumor sites, and increases the potential for dose optimization. The near infinite dose variation within each delivery step (*dwell times*) and the multiplicity of delivery channels allow greater dose conformity to the tumor and dose reduction to normal surrounding organs. However, this greater flexibility of dose variation with HDR brachytherapy does not replace the bad geometry of a poorly placed application. The resultant effects may be suboptimal dosimetry and clinical outcome (as cautioned by Nag and Samsami).[11] The use of a remote-controlled system eliminates radiation exposure to staff. Moreover, the use of brachytherapy can be extended to clinical situations not readily managed with LDR brachytherapy (intraoperative situations, pediatric tumors, and critically ill patients).

DOSE OPTIMIZATION FOR HIGH DOSE RATE BRACHYTHERAPY

Significant technological improvements have been made in imaging devices, and better quality images are obtained. More details of the anatomy can be seen, sharper organ boundaries can be delimited, and with the development of functional imaging,[12] it is often possible to see tumors within organs. In parallel to modern imaging modalities, computer speed and capacity have experienced exponential growth. Visually impressive planning programs are available off the shelf and can be used to calculate dose distributions within minutes.

The use of a programmable remote afterloading unit to move a single radioactive source (^{192}Ir) along many catheters represents a flexible system that can generate a wide variety of dose distributions from a given implant simply by adjusting the length of time (dwell time) that the source dwells at any location within a catheter (dwell position). This flexibility allows the full benefit of the recent three-dimensional planning system based on computed tomography (CT) or magnetic resonance imaging (MRI).

Dose distribution can be manually obtained by adjusting relative dwell time values until an acceptable solution is found, the computer being used only to calculate the dose distribution once the plan has been decided by the dosimetrist. This approach, or combination of it with standard optimization algorithms such as geometrical or dose point optimization, requires time and skill. An important distinction must be made between a planning system where doses are optimized based on anatomic structures versus a geometrically optimized planning system where the doses are optimized based on location of the active dwells. The use of an anatomy-based optimization is the final step toward a truly anatomy-based conformal dose planning.

Inverse Planning Dose Optimization

Few algorithms that specifically use the anatomy (target and organs at risk, as well) to guide the optimization have been developed. Tumor shape and the relative positions between the organs at risk and the tumors and the intent of the clinicians all contribute to define the objectives and dose constraints of the optimization engine. One approach is to obtain an optimized plan for each set of constraints and present all the possible solutions to the planner. Then, the planner can use his or her experience or a decision-making tool to select the solution that provides the best fit for the clinical goals.[13] Alternatively, one can combine the conflicting constraints as a weighted sum.[14-16] This way, coverage, conformity, and uniformity of the dose distribution must be balanced for all volumes of interest, targets, and organs at risk alike. Weight factors or importance factors are used to prioritize the dose constraints. This approach, called inverse planning, has been successfully developed and implemented at the University of California at San Francisco (UCSF).[17-18]

Since inverse treatment planning begins with the description of the desired dose distribution, it represents a change of paradigm in the planning process. It can be understood as an expert system that combines a user-to-computer translator to gather the anatomic dose constraints of the clinician, and as an optimization engine that finds the best solution to fulfill the constraints. Clinical target volumes (CTV) and critical organs (CO) are contoured on each slice of the scan used for CT- or MRI-based planning. Dwell source positions are automatically determined based on CTV and CO. Dwell times are automatically optimized. The algorithm accepts multiple CTV and CO, each with their own dose prescription or constraint, using dose constraint potentials (DCPs). These DCPs convert the dose delivered to a dose control point i to a penalty value W_i. The farther the dose at point i is from the prescribed dose range, the larger the penalty value W_i. If the dose at point i is exactly inside the prescribed dose range, the penalty value W_i is null. This conversion is defined by the following relations where the parameters D_{min}, S_{min}, D_{max}, and S_{max} are, respectively, the minimum dose constraint, the slope of the minimum dose constraint, the maximum dose constraint, and the slope of the maximum dose constraint.

$$S_{min}(D_{min} - D_i) \quad \text{if } D_i < D_{min}$$

$$W_i = \begin{cases} S_{max}(D_i - D_{max}) & \text{if } D_i < D_{max} \\ 0 & \text{if } D_{min} \leq D_i \leq D_{max} \end{cases}$$

The two slopes of these DCPs correspond to two penalty factors: one on the minimum dose (S_{min}), the other on the maximum dose (S_{max}). These penalty factors force the dose to drop and remain inside the acceptable range between the minimum (D_{min}) and the maximum (D_{max}) doses prescribed by the clinician. With these penalty factors, the importance of one clinical criterion over the other can be adjusted. Finally, the sum of the penalty values W_i over m dose control points. Finally, the penalty values W_i are summed over m dose control points to obtain the global penalty E_n for the dose delivery on the given volume n:

$$E_n = \Sigma_i (W_i/m)$$

For example, for a usual prostate case, the sum could be performed on two target volumes (the prostate and a dominant intraprostatic lesion defined with magnetic resonance spectroscopy [MRS]) and three organs-at-risk volumes (urethra, bladder, and rectum). The objective function value E(k) of the dwell time distribution of iteration k is given by the sum of the global penalty of each volume.

$$E(k) = \Sigma_n (E_n(k))$$

The value E(k) is used to compare a given dwell time distribution k relative to the next k+1. The closer to the clinical objective, the smaller is the objective function value. Since this function can be adapted to the clinician's prescription owing to the dose constraint potentials, it is called the *adaptable objective function*.

The minimization of the adaptable objective function requires an optimization technique that allows for wider sampling and hill climbing to escape from a local minimum. This is due to the fact that the cost function E(k) is mathematically nonlinear and therefore presents multiple minimums. Simulated annealing (SA), first introduced by Kirkpatrick,[19] and other related algorithms (Fast SA, Very Fast SA) are optimization techniques that can process cost functions with arbitrary boundary conditions with the statistical guarantee of finding an optimal solution. Equally important, SA class algorithms are easily coded compared to other nonlinear optimization algorithms. It has been shown that the fast simulated annealing algorithm can be used to govern an optimization process to automatically and rapidly produce a plan for prostate permanent implant[15,20] treatments, as well as for afterloading HDR prostate treatments.[2]

The inverse planning tool was used for dose planning of more than 200 patients[17-18,21-22] with anatomic sites including prostate, gynecologic (vaginal cylinders, tandem-ovoids, and interstitial templates), rectum, sarcomas, base of tongue, and nasopharynx. In prostate treatment the urethra can be considered as a second target as it requires the full dose, but also protection from high dose spots. One can also include other critical organs such as the bulb of the penis[23] and specifically protect the neurovascular bundles or boost a dominant intraprostatic lesion. The concept of prescribing at a given point no longer applies for inverse planning; the prescription is global. The approach of inverse planning allows the increase of the number of organs at risk with specific dose constraints without adding to the complexity of the problem. In the case of the treatment of prostate, for instance, the dose received by the bulb of the penis can be significantly reduced by including it as an additional organ at risk. It was shown that on average, the volume of the bulb receiving 75% of the prescribed dose is reduced by 80% for a small penalty of 2% on the target coverage.[24]

Clinical Implementation

The clinical implementation of the inverse planning algorithm results in a workload shift; more emphasis is placed on contouring the anatomy, while little time (if any) is spent adjusting the dose distribution following optimization. Zero time is needed for dwell position determination and dwell time adjustment, as these tasks are automatic and completely transparent to the user.

Since CT or MRI contours of the CTV and CO are used not only to define the anatomy, but also to constrain the dose distribution, they provide the clinician with added flexibility and control to shape the dose distribution. The availability of inverse planning tools allows the planning of complex dose distributions that were not considered before. New organs at risk, not taken into account before, such as the bulb of the penis[23] or the neurovascular bundles, will become an integral part of the dose constraints.

As we move from the two-dimensional brachytherapy planning system to the new three-dimensional era, the necessity of an inverse planning algorithm becomes clear. With hundreds of active dwell positions, irregularly shaped volumes, multiple target and organ volumes, and multiple organ sensitivities, the chance of finding dwell times that would optimally satisfy all the requirements manually becomes more and more remote. Armed with the next generation brachytherapy planning system, systematic evaluation of partial organ tolerance on a finer scale will become possible. This understanding of partial organ tolerance will be the key to the next generation of brachytherapy.

RADIOBIOLOGY OF HIGH DOSE RATE BRACHYTHERAPY

Repair of Sublethal Damage

The major radiobiologic difference between LDR and HDR brachytherapy relates to repair of sublethal damage. This is vitally important because it is the differences in repair between tumor and late-responding normal tissue cells that make radiotherapy a viable way to treat cancer. These differences in repair cause the shapes of survival curves to differ, as illustrated in Figure 13-1. Survival curves for some tumor cells tend to be flatter (more linear) and have a greater initial negative slope than those for late-reacting normal tissue cells.[25] Inasmuch as survival curves for late-reacting normal tissue cells are "curvier," these curves have a larger shoulder at low doses and therefore greater potential for repair of sublethal damage. A fractionated course of

radiotherapy capitalizes on this concept. Using multiple fractions of radiation, each of small size, allows more repair of the normal tissue compared with that of some cancer cells. There is essentially a "window of opportunity" whereby treatment at dose/fraction below the crossover point of the two survival curves in Figure 13-1 results in more killing of tumor than normal tissue cells, and this is the reason we fractionate. It should be noted that this crossover point will be highly tumor- and normal tissue-specific, which is why the optimal dose/fraction is not the same for all clinical situations.

Because repair takes time, with typical half-times for repair on the order of 1 hour,[26-30] it is generally agreed that at least 6 hours should be allowed between fractions if this repair advantage of fractionation is to be fully realized. Alternatively, irradiating continuously at LDR allows sufficient time *during* the treatment for repair to occur. Then the major radiobiologic difference between HDR and LDR is that the repair advantage with HDR is realized by using many low-dose fractions separated by enough time for most repairs to occur *between* fractions, whereas, with LDR, the repair advantage is realized by using a dose rate low enough to allow repair during the irradiation. Replacing LDR with HDR necessitates the simulation of the dose-rate effect of LDR by the fractionation effect of HDR. This is illustrated by the cell survival curves shown in Figure 13-2.[31] The *dashed line* represents the single-dose survival curve at high dose rate (too high to allow any repair during the irradiation). With continuous LDR irradiation, the curve (*dotted line*) moves to the right (*more survival*) due to increased repair, and straightens out, since most repairable damage will be repaired, leaving only irreparable damage, which varies linearly with dose.[32] This is the so-called *dose-rate effect*.[32] Selecting the HDR dose/fraction that generates a fractionated survival curve that falls exactly along this continuous irradiation line achieves equivalency between the HDR and LDR regimens. This is shown by the d_{eq} Gy/fraction *"wavy" line* in Figure 13-2. The "waviness" of this survival curve is a result of the repetitive shoulder

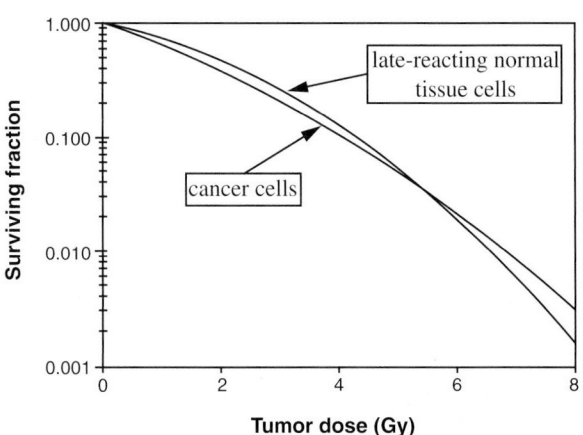

Figure 13–1. Survival curves for late-reacting normal tissue cells tend to be more curved and have a shallower initial slope (i.e., a more pronounced "shoulder") compared with those for cancer cells. In terms of the linear-quadratic (L-Q) model, this means that the a/b ratio is lower for late-reacting normal tissues than for tumors.

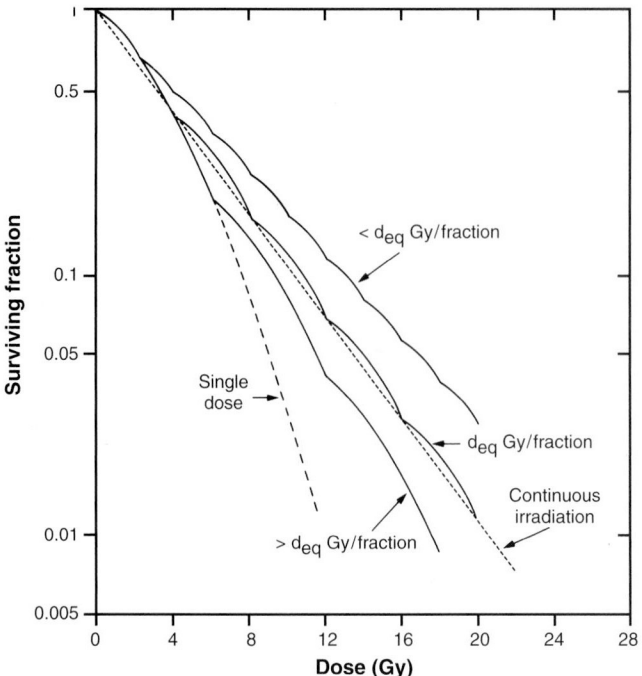

Figure 13–2. Hypothetical cell-surviving fraction curves illustrating the effect of changing the dose per fraction for high dose rate (HDR). At dose per fraction d_{eq} the survival curve for HDR treatment is equivalent to a continuous course of LDR therapy for the L-Q model parameters assumed. For dose per fraction greater than d_{eq}, there is decreased cell survival, and with less than d_{eq} there is increased survival. (From Orton CG: High and low dose rate remote afterloading: A critical comparison. In Sauer R, ed. *International Radiation Therapy Techniques—Brachytherapy.* Berlin: Springer-Verlag; 1991:53).

for each fraction, which represents repair between successive fractions. Treating at a low dose/fraction ($<d_{eq}$ Gy/fraction) will result in more repair and hence a shallower survival curve, as shown by the *upper curve in* Figure 13-2. Conversely, treating at a higher dose/fraction ($>d_{eq}$ Gy/fraction) causes the survival curve to become steeper.

Although Figure 13-2 illustrates how survival curves for HDR and LDR can be similar, it does not address the important effect of the differences in shapes of the survival curves of cancer and late-responding normal tissue cells shown in Figure 13-1. Complete equivalence of HDR and LDR regimens requires that the HDR and LDR survival curves be coincident for both tumor and normal tissue cells. Although not obvious from Figure 13-2, it can be shown that it is theoretically possible to find a value of d_{eq} for which this will occur.[27] Demonstrating this requires the use of a mathematical model that represents the shapes of these survival curves. Dale[28] did just this using the linear-quadratic model for cell survival.

THE LINEAR QUADRATIC MODEL

The L-Q equation for cell surviving fraction, *S*, is:

$$\ln S = -N(\alpha d + G\beta d^2)$$

where *d* is the dose/fraction (of HDR or LDR), *N* is the number of fractions, α and β are parameters that define the "curviness" of the survival curves, and *G* is a function that accounts for the repair that occurs during and between fractions.[28,33,34] Clearly, *G* depends on dose rate, dose/fraction, time between fractions, and the rate of repair. Dale[28] published equations to account for changes in all these variables.

Using Dale's equations, it has been shown that HDR surviving fractions can exactly match those with LDR for both cancer and normal tissue cells, with a reasonable number of HDR fractions, if it is assumed that tumor cells repair faster that normal cells.[35] For example, if the half-times for repair are assumed to be 0.5 hour for tumor and 1.5 hours for late-reacting normal tissue cells,[26,27,29,30] a course of 60 Gy at LDR can be matched by a 7-fraction HDR regimen at 6 Gy/fraction, using representative L-Q model α and β parameters. This is illustrated in Figure 13-3.

Note that in Figures 13-1 and 13-3 it has been assumed that the dose to normal tissues is the same as the

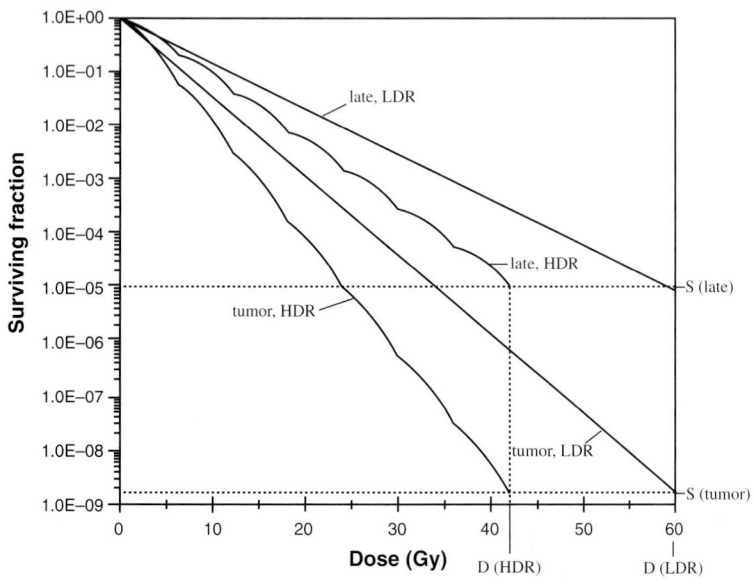

Figure 13–3. Hypothetical survival curves illustrating how a course of high dose rate therapy in 7 fractions, each of 6 Gy, can be equivalent as far as late-reacting normal tissues and tumor are concerned to a low dose rate regimen of 60 Gy in 72 hours.

tumor dose. However, a major advantage of brachytherapy is that this is a highly conformal type of radiotherapy, so the important physical advantage of brachytherapy has been neglected. This can be accounted for in L-Q model calculations by the use of the "geometrical sparing factor."[36]

GEOMETRICAL SPARING FACTOR

Since brachytherapy dose distributions are significantly inhomogeneous, it is not readily obvious how to compare tumor and normal tissue doses. One way to do this is to reduce these dose distributions to "effective" doses, where the "effective dose" is that which, if delivered uniformly to the tumor or normal tissue, exhibits the same local control or risk of injury, respectively, as the inhomogeneous distribution it depicts.[34] Then the geometrical sparing factor (f) can be defined as:

$$f = \frac{\text{effective dose to normal tissues}}{\text{effective dose to tumor}}$$

which, for brachytherapy, should normally be less than unity.

This can have a profound effect on the comparison of tumor and normal tissue cell survival curves, as illustrated in Figure 13-4, in which the tumor curve and the late-responding normal tissue curve for $f = 1$ (*dashed*) are the same as the two curves shown in Figure 13-1, although taken out to higher doses.

If, as illustrated, the dose axis represents the tumor dose, and a modest geometrical sparing factor of 0.8 is assumed, the normal tissue curve shifts 20% to the right and the crossover point moves all the way out to about 8 Gy. The "window of opportunity" now opens considerably, giving a much wider range of doses over which the repair advantage of normal tissues can be exploited. For example, using the L-Q model, one can show that with $f = 0.8$, the number of HDR fractions required to be equivalent to LDR (shown in Fig. 13-3) reduces from 7 to 6, and with $f = 0.6$, this number reduces to only 4. Hence,

a modest improvement in geometrical dose sparing makes use of an HDR program practical.[36,37] It has even been demonstrated that geometrical sparing, combined with slow repair of late-reacting normal tissue cells similar to that observed with the continuous hyperfractionated accelerated radiotherapy (CHART) experience,[38] could make HDR superior to LDR.[39]

With this radiobiologic model, the resultant calculations provide only a fair representation of the highly complex biological changes that occur in tissues exposed to a course of brachytherapy. For example, reoxygenation, repopulation, and the inverse dose-rate effect have been neglected. Nevertheless, analysis of results of several decades of experience with tens of thousands of patients treated for cervical cancer shows that replacing LDR with an HDR regimen that has four to seven fractions[40] is feasible, and affirms the concordance of theory and clinical practice.

In summary, radiobiologic modeling shows that it is possible to replace LDR brachytherapy with HDR without a decrease in the probability of tumor control or an increased risk of complications. The number of fractions necessary to achieve equivalency between HDR and LDR regimens is multifactorial and depends on the radiobiologic properties of the irradiated tissues (e.g., the relative half-times of repair of tumor and normal-tissue cells) and the physical "geometrical sparing" of the normal tissues. Commonly used HDR regimes with four to seven fractions seem to satisfy these requirements.

CLINICAL USES OF HIGH DOSE RATE BRACHYTHERAPY

High dose rate brachytherapy has been used in various sites. Its predominant use has been in the treatment of lung, cervical, and endometrial cancers and, to a lesser extent, in esophageal, biliary, rectal, brain, head and neck, soft tissue sarcomas, and skin.[41] High dose rate brachytherapy is increasingly being incorporated as a component of prostate cancer and as a solitary radiotherapeutic treatment of breast cancer. Its use in the lung is dealt with in some detail to illustrate the general technique of HDR brachytherapy, and its use in other locations is discussed less fully.

CARCINOMA OF THE CERVIX

Role of High Dose Rate Brachytherapy

High dose rate brachytherapy in the treatment of carcinoma of the cervix is increasingly accepted as an alternative to low dose rate brachytherapy. Major cooperative group trials in the United States allow substitution of HDR for LDR protocols. The National Institute of Health Consensus Conference on Carcinoma of the Cervix also allowed a similar substitution.[42] Although the role of HDR brachytherapy has been more established in certain European and Asian countries, there is increasing adoption of this modality in the United States. Establishing an HDR brachytherapy program for carcinoma of the cervix requires a significant commitment

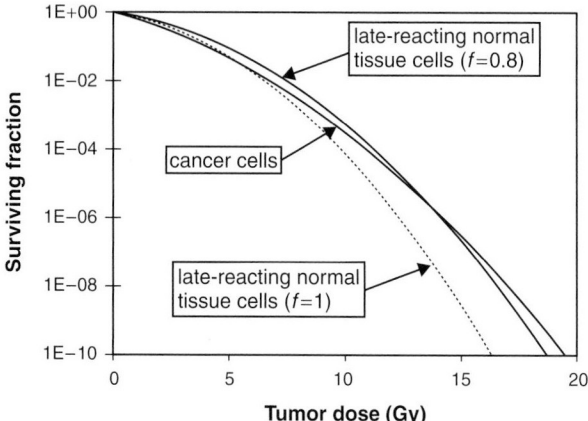

Figure 13–4. Effect of geometrical sparing of normal tissues on the crossover point for tumor and normal tissue survival curves. With the L-Q model parameters used here, the crossover point moves from about 5 Gy when the geometrical sparing factor (f) = 1 (see Fig. 13-1), out to about 13 Gy when $f = 0.8$.

of resources and time.[43] Despite a large published database, there is no established optimal dose fractionation regimen and technique.[44] There is increasing radiobiologic modeling available to guide the radiation oncologist in establishing an HDR brachytherapy program.[45] The advantages of HDR brachytherapy (discussed earlier in this chapter) account for its greater acceptability in the United States. Its patient care advantages include outpatient therapy and the avoidance of prolonged bed rest (with its attendant discomfort and risk of deep vein thrombosis, cardiac decompensation, and pulmonary atelectasis).[46] Additionally, the avoidance of cervical dilation because of miniaturization of the radiation source and streamlining of the applicator reduces the need for general anesthesia. Physical advantages include potentially greater dose sparing of the rectum and bladder by temporary retraction (*geometrical sparing factor*) and dose optimization. Moreover, the rapid delivery of treatment minimizes the risk of applicator displacement within the patient. It is generally more facile to integrate, earlier in the treatment course, the brachytherapy component with EBRT.[47] These advantages must be contrasted with the greater number of treatments required (typically five or six applications) and the increased "labor intensiveness."

High Dose Rate Brachytherapy System

An HDR brachytherapy system comprises three components: a miniaturized radiation source, a dose fractionation regimen, and an HDR uterovaginal applicator.

DOSE FRACTIONATION

Although the initial dose fractionation schedules used in the United States and worldwide vary considerably, there has been a momentum toward standardization of dose per fraction and number of fractions and interfraction time intervals.[48] The most commonly used regimens use fraction sizes between 5 and 7 Gy in 4 to 6 fractions, given on a weekly basis.[49-51] The brachytherapy has usually been given concurrently or after EBRT. When patients with cancer of the cervix are treated with LDR brachytherapy, the intracavitary application is typically

performed after the EBRT component to the pelvis. When an HDR technique is used, EBRT (in combination with concurrent chemotherapy) and brachytherapy may be integrated earlier, typically after 2 weeks (20 Gy) of EBRT. A typical treatment scenario is henceforth described. Using an initial four-field box technique delivering 19.8 Gy (1.8 Gy per fraction), EBRT (with concurrent chemotherapy) is then continued 4 days per week (2.0 Gy per fraction) for nonbulky stages I and II (<4 cm primary) using an anterior-posterior–posterior-anterior (AP–PA) technique with a midline block to a total dose of 45.8 Gy (Table 13-1). For bulky lesions (stages IB and II ≥4 cm or stages IIIA and B and stage IVA), EBRT continues 4 days weekly (1.8 Gy per fraction) to a baseline dose of 45.0 to 50.4 Gy (Table 13-3).[49] This is followed by supplemental doses to the involved parametria/sidewalls to a total dose of 54.0 to 59.4 Gy with special attention given to avoiding additional small bowel irradiation. Anatomic distortion by the tumor may technically preclude the insertion of a tandem at 19.80 Gy. EBRT therefore continues to 39.60 Gy (four-field box technique) and tandem insertion is reattempted. Six weekly HDR uterovaginal applications, each delivering 6.0 Gy to point A, are performed (not concurrently with EBRT) for both bulky and nonbulky categories following 19.80 Gy EBRT, or alternatively, 4 to 5 HDR applications, each delivering 6.0 Gy to point A following 39.60 Gy. The midline blocking is designed to block the approximate 6 Gy isodose line. The relative simplicity of this regimen allows for the same fraction size and interfraction time interval for nearly all cases. The only variable is the number of fractions, which depends on the integration of HDR brachytherapy and EBRT. The earlier integration of HDR in the radiotherapeutic management readily allows for the total duration of the treatment program to be shorter than 55 days. Extended duration of radiation therapy (external and brachytherapy) for cervical carcinoma beyond 55 days is adversely associated with a lesser control rate and survival.[51] Moreover, the earlier integration (Table 13-2) of HDR brachytherapy provides an enhanced ability to concentrate dose delivery to the primary tumor and to reduce symptoms such as bleeding. The potential disadvantage of earlier integration of HDR brachytherapy is the reduced dose to

Table 13–1   Radiotherapeutic Schemas for Carcinoma of the Cervix: Low Bulk (Stage I/II <4 cm)

Treatment	Week 1	Week 2	Week 3	Week 4	Week 5	Week 6	Week 7	Week 8
EBRT (Gy): (cumulative)*	9	18	25.2	32.4	39.6	46.8	50.4–54	—
Midline Bladder/Rectal Shielding*	—	—	+	+	+	+	+	
HDRB (Gy), Point A	—	—	6	6	6	6	6	6‡
Bladder/Rectal† (Gy)(Cumulative)	9	18	24.3	28.8	33.3	37.8	42.3	46.8 (or 49.8 Gy‡)

*Bladder and rectum shielded after 19.8 Gy EBRT.
†Bladder and rectal doses are typically limited to 75% of point A for each HDRB application.
‡Based on tumor response, a 7th HDRB application is optional during week 8 of therapy. The 6th and 7th application fraction size may be reduced to 5 Gy each to point A.
EBRT, external beam radiation therapy; HDRB, high dose rate brachytherapy.

Table 13–2   Radiotherapeutic Schema for Bulky Carcinoma of the Cervix: Stage I/II ≥ 4 cm or Stage III/IVA (Early Integration of HDRB)

Treatment	Week 1	Week 2	Week 3	Week 4	Week 5	Week 6	Week 7	Week 8
EBRT (Gy): (cumulative)	9	18	25.2	32.4	39.6	46.8	54	59.4
HDRB (Gy), point A	—	—	6*†	6*†	6*†	6*†	6*†	6*†
			(or 5‡)	(or 5‡)	(or 5‡)	(or 5‡)	(or 5‡)	(or 5‡)
Midline rectal/bladder shielding§	—	—	*	*	*	†	†	†
	—	—	—	—	—	‡	‡	‡
Bladder/rectal¶ (Gy)(cumulative)	9	18	24.3*	28.8*	33.3*	37.8*	42.3*	46.8*
			(or 29.7†	(or 41.4†	(or 53.1†	(or 57.6†	(or 62.1†	(or 61.9‡)
			or 28.8‡)	or 39.7‡)	or 50.7‡)	or 54.4‡)	or 58.2‡)	

†If bladder or rectal shield is used after 39.6 Gy when using 6 Gy to point A per HDR application, omit the sixth 6-Gy HDR application to keep total rectal/bladder dose (EBRT + HDRB) to <62 Gy.

‡Alternatively, 6 HDR applications may be performed (after midline shielding of the rectum/bladder at 39.6 Gy) and each HDR application fraction size is reduced to 5.0 Gy to point A to keep total rectal/bladder dose (EBRT + HDRB) to <62 Gy.

§Bladder and rectum may be shielded after 19.8 Gy EBRT (*) or after 39.6 Gy EBRT (††).

¶Bladder and rectal dose are limited to 75% of point A for each HDR brachytherapy application.

EBRT, external beam radiation therapy; HDRB, high dose rate brachytherapy.

the periphery of the tumor in bulky barrel-shaped tumors (when combined simultaneously with the use of a midline bar to shield the bladder and rectum). A minor variation from the regimen described earlier for bulky tumors allows for the early integration of HDR brachytherapy (at 19.8 Gy) using a fraction size of 6 Gy and omission of the midline bar until a dose of EBRT 39.6 Gy is reached while continuing the 4-field box technique (except during the weekly brachytherapy day). This strategy allows for a greater and more facile integration of the brachytherapy and EBRT components while emphasizing the dose concentration in the bulky primary site. At this point, AP–PA techniques of EBRT are used to boost the involved pelvic sidewalls/parametria as described earlier. This regimen may allow for a reduction of planned number of HDR applications by one and allows for the shortening of the treatment duration. Alternatively, 6 weekly HDR applications of 5 Gy each delivered to point A may be substituted. This allows completion of the treatment program in 8 weeks and keeps the total rectal/bladder dose (EBRT + HDR brachytherapy) to less than 62 Gy. Hence, earlier integration of HDR brachytherapy is almost always possible using these strategies. These schemas are depicted in Table 13-1.

The ABS has recommended a number of therapeutic schemas for the integration of EBRT and HDR brachytherapy.[51] Following 19.8 Gy (1.8 Gy/fraction) EBRT for nonbulky tumors, fraction sizes of 7.5 Gy, 6.5 Gy, and 6.0 Gy are used for 6, 7, or 8 fractions, respectively. Following 45 Gy (1.8 Gy/fraction) EBRT for nonbulky tumors, fraction sizes 6.0 and 5.3 Gy are used in 5 and 6 fractions, respectively. For bulky tumors, the ABS suggests fraction sizes 6.5 Gy and 5.8 Gy for 5 and 6 applications, respectively, following 45 Gy (1.8 Gy/fraction) EBRT. Alternatively, fraction size 7.0 Gy, 6.0 Gy, and 5.3 Gy are used for 4, 5, and 6 applications, respectively, following 50.4 Gy EBRT. In order to deliver the treatment program (EBRT, HDR, chemotherapy) within the 55 days recommended duration, the ABS allows a variation of performing two applications per

Table 13–3   Radiotherapeutic Schemas for Bulky Carcinoma of the Cervix: Stage I/II ≥4 cm or Stage III/IVA (Delayed Integration of HDRB*)

Treatment	Week 1	Week 2	Week 3	Week 4	Week 5	Week 6	Week 7	Week 8
EBRT (Gy): (cumulative)	9	18	27	36	43.2	50.4	57.6	59.4
Midline Bladder/Rectal Shielding*	—	—	—	—	+	+	+	+
HDRB (Gy), Point A	—	—	—	—	6	6	6	6 (or 5 × 2)‡
Bladder/Rectal† (Gy)(cumulative)	9	18	27	36	44.1	48.6	53.1	57.6 (or 60.5 Gy)‡

*Bladder and rectum are shielded after 39.6 Gy EBRT.

†Rectal and bladder dose limited to 75% of point A dose for each HDRB application.

‡A 5th additional HDRB application is optional, but is recommended, and may be preferentially done during week 8 of therapy. In that situation, reduce the HDRB dose per fraction for the 4th and 5th applications (performed during week 8) to 5 Gy each to keep total bladder/rectal dose (EBRT + HDRB) to <62 Gy.

EBRT, external beam radiation therapy; HDRB, high dose rate brachytherapy.

week following integration of HDR brachytherapy after 45 or 50 Gy EBRT.

UTEROVAGINAL APPLICATOR

Applicator Description

Several uterovaginal applicators and one prototype composed of three interconnected components are commercially available: tandem, colpostat such as a ring ovoid, and a rectal retractor (depicted in Fig. 13-5). The tandem is available with three angulations and three lengths (2, 4, and 6 cm). The thin caliber of the tandem approximates the diameter of a typical uterine sound. The ring ovoid is available in three diameters (26, 30, and 34 mm), each with its own plastic cap (3 to 4 mm thick) and corresponding angulation to match the tandem (30, 45, and 60 degrees). Because this is a fixed-geometry system, the ring ovoid is connected to the tandem in the patient at the time of insertion, thereby ensuring that the tandem is situated at the epicenter of the ring. Hence, anterior or posterior displacement of the ring ovoid is prevented. Other systems use a separate tandem with a pair of culpostats attached to it. Lastly, a rectal retractor with built-in metal markers is introduced in the vagina and connected to the applicator. The metal markers readily identify the posterior vaginal mucosa on radiographic films and facilitate dose calculation for the rectum (Fig. 13-6).

Applicator Placement

The applicator is inserted under intravenous sedation either in an operating room suite or in a dedicated procedure suite with available pulse oximetry and

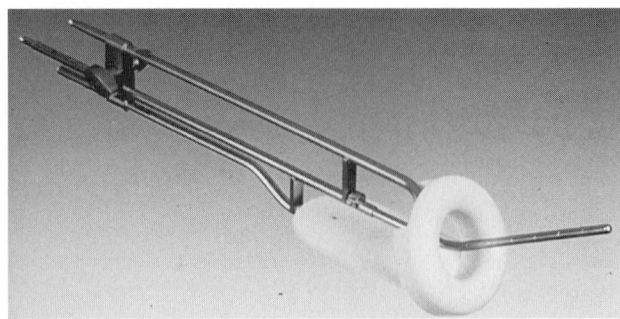

Figure 13–5. Uterovaginal high dose rate ring applicator. (Courtesy of Nucletron Corporation).

electrocardiographic and respiratory monitoring by certified anesthetic personnel. The miniature size of the radiation source and the use of a slim tandem (typically of the same caliber as a uterine sound) allows for the intrauterine placement without cervical canal dilation. This obviates the need for general anesthesia or spinal anesthesia. It is highly recommended to verify the accuracy of the placement intraoperatively under ultrasound guidance. Inserting sufficient sterile saline solution in the urinary bladder (typically 150 to 200 mL) enhances the resolution of the image. Sagittal and axial images are performed intraoperatively to ensure there is no fundal penetration or creation of false tracts inside the uterine wall. Gently wiggling the tandem during the imaging procedure helps to discern the tandem within the uterine cavity. The tip of the tandem should be situated within 1.0 to 1.5 cm of the fundal serosa in the normal-sized uterus (<8 cm uterine cavity length using a 6-cm length

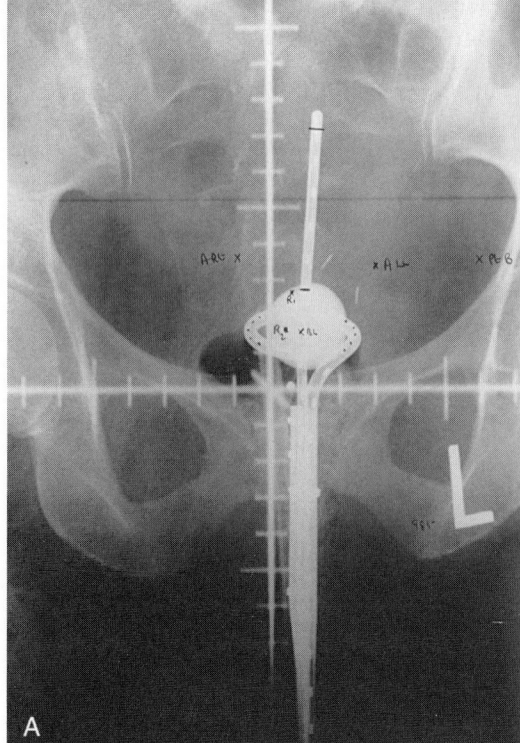

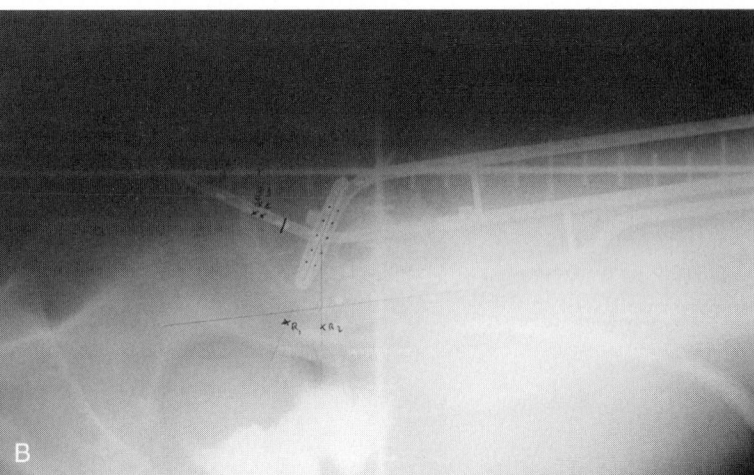

Figure 13–6. Anterior-posterior (**A**) and lateral (**B**) orthogonal radiographs of uterovaginal application.

tandem). In large size uteri, the distance between the tip of the tandem and the fundal serosa may be farther in the initial application, but may decrease as the uterus size decreases with further external irradiation with chemotherapy and HDR brachytherapy. The application placement is completed with the placement of the vaginal ovoid (typically the largest size that is acceptable by the anatomy) and bladder and rectal retraction. Retractors or vaginal packing or both are used for the purpose of retraction. The application may be secured by means of an external immobilizing device and may be adjusted in its anterior or posterior orientation to avoid excessive anteflexion or retroflexion of the uterus. Generally, the application is centered in the midline. The external immobilizing device assures greater geometrical reproducibility between subsequent applications. Moreover, some centers elect to retract caudally the applicator and uterus by clasping the cervix and connecting the clasp to the external immobilizing device, thereby reducing the potential radiation exposure of the rectosigmoid colon, small bowel, and bladder.

DOSE PRESCRIPTION POINTS

Dose prescription is to point *A*, which is defined as 2 cm cephalad along the axis of the tandem and 2 cm laterally from the epicenter of the ring ovoid plus an allowance of 5 mm for the plastic cap covering. Bladder and rectal computerized dose calculations are illustrated in Figure 13-7. The specifications of bladder and rectal dose calculations are given in ICRU Report No. 38[52] and are illustrated in Figure 13-8. The rectal and bladder maximal dose allowance per application is 75% of point *A*. Newer MRI- and CT-compatible uterovaginal applicators are now commercially available. They may allow for image-based dose distributions and potential integration of EBRT and brachytherapy dosimetry to arrive at composite dose distributions.

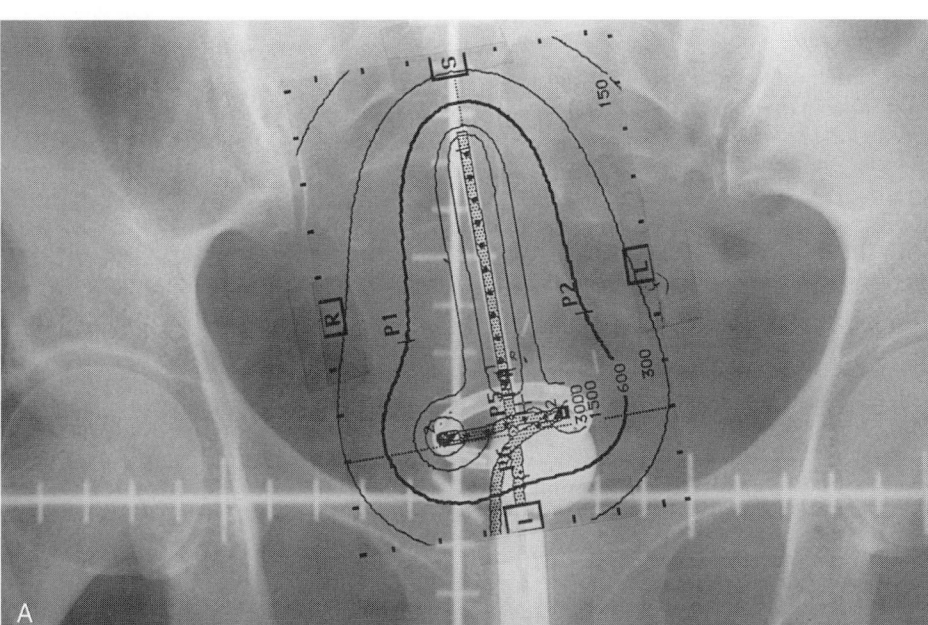

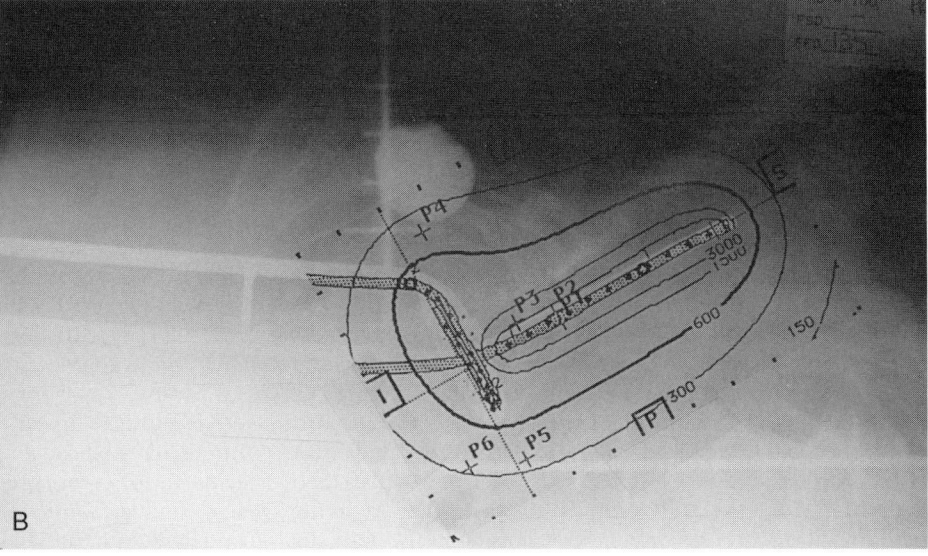

Figure 13–7. Anterior-posterior (**A**) and lateral (**B**) isodose distributions of uterovaginal application.

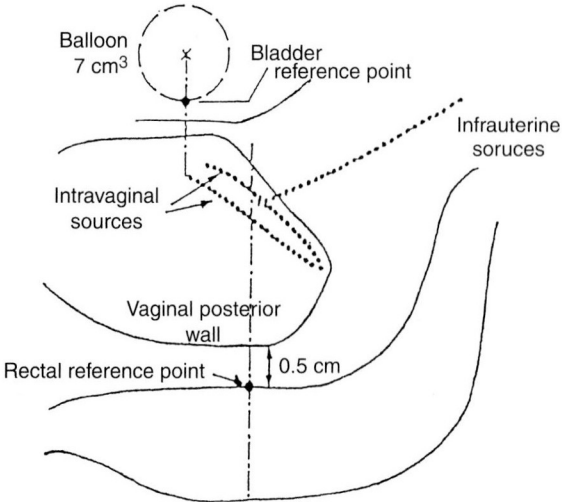

Figure 13–8. Illustration of bladder and rectal dose specifications from the International Commission on Radiation Units and Measurements Report No. 38.

RESULTS

The paucity of controlled randomized trials comparing LDR and HDR brachytherapy in carcinoma of the cervix makes analysis of these studies difficult. Unfortunately, most of the published reports have been nonrandomized studies. The earlier studies using HDR brachytherapy showed good local control and survival rates compared with those obtained with LDR; however, some increased late small bowel complications were noted initially when HDR brachytherapy dose used exceeded 9 Gy per fraction.[53] Modifications of the treatment regimens using lower doses per HDR fraction (< 8 Gy to point A) and a greater number of fractions resulted in equivalent control rates comparable to that of LDR without an increase in toxicity.[53-59] A reasonable number of fractions of HDR applications could balance the need for avoidance of toxicity while maintaining a clinically practical treatment program.

The results of two meta-analyses comparing LDR and HDR brachytherapy series have generally confirmed the equivalency of both modalities in terms of control rate and toxicity.[60,61] In a comparison of the published results of HDR brachytherapy regimens (in treating 4283 patients) with the results of LDR (in treating 5100 patients), Orton[60] showed overall 5-year survival rates of 61.2% and 55.5% for HDR and LDR, respectively. Notwithstanding the constraints of comparing populations of patients treated in various centers with different regimens of HDR and LDR in a nonrandomized fashion, Orton concluded that the evidence suggests the results of HDR are at least not inferior to those achieved by LDR brachytherapy. The incidence of severe complications with HDR was 3.5% compared with 7.7% with LDR.[61] Fu and Phillips confirmed similar conclusions in their large analysis.[44] There have been two randomized studies comparing the use of HDR with the use of LDR brachytherapy in carcinoma of the cervix.[62,63] Shigematsu and colleagues[62] reported on 143 patients treated with HDR brachytherapy compared with 106 patients treated with LDR for stages IIB and III disease. Although the randomization process was compromised (some patients randomized to LDR were actually treated with HDR because of limited LDR availability), there was no difference in survival between LDR- and HDR-treated patients. Superior local control was found for the HDR treatment arm compared with the LDR arm.

A randomized study of LDR versus HDR brachytherapy from a single institution has been reported from India.[63] With more than 482 patients, the authors demonstrated no difference in local control, survival, and severe complications between the two treatment modalities. However, there was a statistical difference in rectal complication, with a 20% rate in the LDR group and only a 6% rate in the HDR group. Although a large, well-controlled, randomized study has not been done in the United States, the available literature, controlled and uncontrolled, documents the feasibility of HDR brachytherapy and suggests the equivalency of local control, survival, and complication rates.

COST EFFECTIVENESS

The cost effectiveness of HDR in comparison with that of LDR is complex and controversial. It also depends on the patient load.[64] HDR equipment is more expensive than LDR equipment, unless remote afterloading is used; then it is similar. The cost of constructing a shielded HDR room can be considerable. A resource utilization study comparing costs of LDR with those of HDR brachytherapy reported by Bastin and colleagues[65] revealed that LDR brachytherapy was 244% more expensive than HDR brachytherapy, primarily because of hospital and operating room expenses. Potential cost savings with HDR brachytherapy may be of importance in the present climate of health care cost containment in the United States.

CARCINOMA OF THE ENDOMETRIUM

Adjuvant Radiation Therapy

High dose rate brachytherapy (either as a sole modality or in addition to EBRT) is commonly used to treat the vaginal cuff after hysterectomy in patients with intermediate to high risk for vaginal recurrence. Indications may include high-grade adenocarcinoma histology, clear cell carcinoma or serous papillary carcinoma histology, deep myometrial invasion, and extrauterine (including lymph node metastases) or cervical spread. The role of EBRT in endometrial carcinoma following hysterectomy in stage I disease remains controversial. A survival advantage was not demonstrated in a multicenter randomized trial by Creutzberg et al.[66] This study included patients with adenocarcinoma, adenosquamous, papillary serous, and clear cell carcinoma histologies. Fédération International de Gynécologie et d' Obstétrique (FIGO) grade I with deep myometrial (>50%) invasion, grade II with any myometrial invasion, and grade III with superficial myometrial (<50%) invasion were eligible. The survival advantage of postoperative EBRT appears to be limited to the subpopulation of higher risk stage 1 disease with grade III histology with deep myometrial invasion,[67] and this group was not eligible. While the options of EBRT alone, vaginal brachytherapy alone, or a combination of both exist for stage I disease, the ultimate choice requires clinical judgment regarding the risk of locoregional recurrence, morbidity, costs of adjuvant therapy, and potential for salvage of patients with vaginal recurrences. If the clinical endpoint is a survival advantage, the more intense radiotherapeutic regimens appear to benefit mostly the more aggressive stage I or greater uterine tumors.[67] However, a locoregional recurrence rate of 18% was found in the control group without EBRT. These patients were older than age 60 and had either deep myometrial invasion greater than 50% with grade I to II or superficial myometrial invasion less than 50% with grade III. This contrasted to a locoregional recurrence of 5% with EBRT and was problematic to the authors.[66] There is no demonstrated advantage to adding vaginal brachytherapy following EBRT in early-stage endometrial carcinoma. Conversely, most locoregional recurrences occur in the vagina and may be prevented effectively with vaginal brachytherapy alone. However, the combination of EBRT and vaginal brachytherapy is certainly indicated in the setting of vaginal recurrence and is effective as a salvage therapy, with 69% 3-year survival.[66] Additionally, brachytherapy can be used for primary treatment in inoperable endometrial carcinoma.

TECHNIQUE OF VAGINAL BRACHYTHERAPY

If pelvic EBRT is given, the dose is usually about 40 to 45 Gy in 20 to 25 treatments, respectively. Brachytherapy is usually performed by a single-line source placed centrally in a vaginal cylinder. The largest diameter of a cylinder that comfortably fits the vagina is used. Vaginal diameters of 2 cm or less are to be avoided because of the decreased depth dose incumbent with a small source to vaginal surface distance. A vaginal cylinder with a diameter of 3 cm or greater is preferable. The superior portion of the vagina (3 to 5 cm) is usually treated in most cases, although in certain centers a longer length may be preferable in clear cell or serous histologies.[68-73]

A linear source such as Iridium 192, as used in a vaginal cylinder, may pose the potential for dose inhomogeneity at the vaginal apex due to source anisotropy. The actual clinical importance of dose anisotropy is not well defined. Certain centers prefer to use an ovoid or circular ring placed at the vaginal apex to circumvent this potential problem.[74]

BRACHYTHERAPY DOSE

The dose prescription point is either defined at the vaginal surface or at 0.5 cm from the surface of the vaginal cylinder. In either case, both doses (vaginal surface and 0.5 cm depth) are recorded as recommended by the ABS.[74] It is not recommended to use 1.0 cm from the surface applicator as a prescription dose point. The dose per fraction has varied from 4.5 to 16 Gy, and the number of fractions has varied from 2 to 7.[68-73] The interval between fractions is usually 1 to 2 weeks, but more commonly once weekly. When a lower dose of about 5 Gy per fraction is chosen, a larger number of fractions is used (3 or 4) or EBRT is added, or both. The consensus report also advises the use of dose optimization for the cylinder or an angle source delivery system to be introduced to ensure uniform dose at depth and eliminate the potential dose reduction at the vaginal apex due to source anisotropy.[74]

A commonly used regimen combining EBRT and HDR brachytherapy is the following: 45 Gy in 25 fractions of EBRT (four-field box technique); 2 to 3 fractions of HDR spaced 1 week apart delivering 5.5 Gy and 4.0 Gy each, respectively, prescribed at 0.5 cm depth are administered at the completion of EBRT. Some centers prefer to deliver 3.5 Gy at a depth of 0.5 cm or 5 Gy at the vaginal surface twice weekly for 3 applications. This allows for completion of the treatment program combining EBRT and vaginal brachytherapy within 7 weeks. A tabular summary of the treatment parameters combining EBRT and vaginal brachytherapy in the adjuvant setting is given in Table 13-4 and Table 13-5 for prescription point depth 0.5 cm and vaginal surface, respectively. Although a regimen for vaginal HDR brachytherapy alone is not well established, a dose of 21 Gy (at 0.5 cm depth) given in 3 treatments spaced 1 to 2 weeks apart is used in some centers. The ABS has made recommendations for both prescription points (0.5 cm depth, vaginal surface). Tables 13-6 and 13-7 provide a tabular summary of the recommendations. Some centers prefer to deliver vaginal brachythereapy twice weekly and include a therapeutic schema.

RESULTS

The 5-year survival results vary from 72% to 97%, depending on the usual prognostic parameters such as stage, grade, and depth of myometrial invasion.[68-72] The severe late complication rate (grade III or IV) is usually less than 1% and depends on the dose per fraction employed.[68-72] Generally, doses per fraction of more than 7 Gy should be avoided (especially if EBRT is added). The incidence of vaginal shortening also depends very

Table 13–4   Endometrial Carcinoma: Postoperative Combined External Radiation Therapy (EBRT) and Vaginal High Dose Rate Brachytherapy Regimens (Dose Prescription Point @ 0.5 cm depth)

EBRT (Gy)/5 weeks (1.8 Gy/Rx)	Vaginal HDR dose (Gy)	Vaginal Dose Prescription Point (depth: cm)	HDR Fractions, *n*	Interfraction HDR Interval (days)
45	5.5*	0.5	2	7
45	4.0*	0.5	3	7
45	3.5	0.5	3	3-4

*Recommended by the American Brachytherapy Society. From Nag S, Erickson B, Parikh S, et al: The American Brachytherapy Society Recommendations for HDR Brachytherapy for Carcinoma of the Endometrium. *Int J Radiat Oncol Biol Phys.* 2000;48:779.

Table 13–5 Endometrial Carcinoma: Postoperative Combined External Beam Radiation Therapy (EBRT) and Vaginal High Dose Rate (HDR) Brachytherapy Regimens (Dose Prescription Point @ Vaginal Surface)

EBRT (Gy)/5 weeks (1.8 Gy/Rx)	Vaginal HDR dose (Gy)	Vaginal Dose Prescription Point (depth: cm)	HDR Fractions, n	Interfraction HDR Interval (days)
45	8.0*	0.0	2	7
45	6.0*	0.0	3	7
45	5.0	0.0	3	3-4

*Recommended by the American Brachytherapy Society. From Nag S, Erickson B, Parikh S, et al: The American Brachytherapy Society Recommendations for HDR Brachytherapy for Carcinoma of the Endometrium. *Int J Radiat Oncol Biol Phys.* 2000;48:779.

much on the dose per fraction; it was as high as 70% when 9 Gy per fraction was used at a 1-cm depth and reduced to 31% when the dose was reduced to 4.5 Gy per fraction.[73] Other factors implicated in an increased risk of morbidity include the use of a small (2-cm) diameter vaginal cylinder, the addition of pelvic EBRT, and treatment dose prescription beyond 0.5 cm.[68]

INOPERABLE ENDOMETRIAL CARCINOMA

Indications

Some patients with adenocarcinoma of the endometrium are not candidates for surgery because of severe co-morbid medical problems (obesity, cardiovascular disease, diabetes mellitus, and hypertension). This subset is treated by radiation therapy. A combination of EBRT and brachytherapy or brachytherapy alone is used depending on the size of the uterine cavity, histologic grade, and other risk factors for lymph node involvement. The previously mentioned conditions that preclude these patients from surgery also place them at added risk for anesthesia and prolonged bed rest. In particular, when LDR brachytherapy is used, the incidence of thromboembolic events and cardiac decompensation may be significant.[46]

Technique

Various applicators may be used.[70,75] The simplest involves the introduction of a tandem and colpostat, but this has the limitation of not irradiating the uterine surface homogeneously. Some authors have used a curved tandem, turning it to the left and right in alternate insertions. A Y-shaped applicator, comprising two abutting tandems, is easy to use and irradiates the fundus more

evenly by allowing the tip of each tandem to lodge in each cornu (Fig. 13-9). Other possibilities include insertion of modified Heyman capsules or multiple catheters.[75] The dose is commonly specified at 2.0 cm caudally from the fundus (at the midline) and 2 cm laterally. To ensure a more homogeneous dose to the entire myometrium and dose optimization, a preplanning magnetic resonance image of the uterus and intraoperative ultrasonography (as described earlier for carcinoma of the cervix) are useful.

Dose Schedules

The dose per fraction has ranged from 5 to 12 Gy, and 4 to 6 fractions are commonly used.[69,70,75-82] The dose or the dose per fraction is reduced if EBRT can be added. The current optimal regimen remains undefined. A useful treatment regimen guideline is provided by the ABS regarding using HDR brachytherapy alone or combined with EBRT.[74] A summary of the treatment parameters in tabular form is presented in Table 13-8.

Clinical Results

Rotte[70] compared his results using LDR and HDR brachytherapy regimens (historic controls) alone and found no difference in survival, stage for stage. Interestingly, he noted a decreased rate of thromboembolic events from 7.5% to 0% when switching from an LDR to an HDR regimen. The toxicity is higher when patients are treated with a high dose per fraction and ranges around 7%.[78,81-83]

The 5-year survival rate for stage I is 70% to 80% and is slightly lower than the rate expected with surgery.

Table 13–6 Endometrial Carcinoma: Postoperative Vaginal High Dose Rate Brachytherapy Regimens: Dose Prescription Point @ 0.5 cm Depth (without External Beam Radiation Therapy [EBRT]

EBRT	Vaginal HDR dose (Gy)	Vaginal Dose Prescription Point (depth: cm)	HDR Fractions, n	Interfraction HDR Interval (days)
0	7.0*	0.5	3	7-14
0	5.5*	0.5	4	7
0	4.7*	0.5	5	7
0	3.5	0.5	6	3-4

*Recommended by the American Brachytherapy Society. From Nag S, Erickson B, Parikh S, et al: The American Brachytherapy Society Recommendations for HDR Brachytherapy for Carcinoma of the Endometrium. *Int J Radiat Oncol Biol Phys.* 2000;48:779.

Table 13–7   Endometrial Carcinoma: Postoperative Vaginal High Dose Rate [HDR] Brachytherapy Regimens: Dose Prescription Point @ Vaginal Surface (without External Beam Radiation Therapy [EBRT])

EBRT	Vaginal HDR dose (Gy)	Vaginal Dose Prescription Point (depth: cm)	HDR Fractions, *n*	Interfraction HDR Interval (days)
0	10.5*	0.0	3	7-14
0	8.8*	0.0	4	7
0	7.5*	0.0	5	7
0	5.0	0.0	6	3-4

*Recommended by the American Brachytherapy Society. From Nag S, Erickson B, Parikh S, et al: The American Brachytherapy Society Recommendations for HDR Brachytherapy for Carcinoma of the Endometrium. *Int J Radiat Oncol Biol Phys.* 2000;48:779.

TREATMENT OF VAGINAL RECURRENCES

The radiotherapeutic treatment of vaginal recurrences following definitive surgical therapy for endometrial carcinoma has generally achieved modest results.[84] The salvage rate for isolated vaginal recurrences is 40% to 80%.[85-87] The treatment consists of combined EBRT and vaginal brachytherapy. Vaginal brachytherapy is integrated at the completion of EBRT (45 Gy in 5 weeks) and should be used selectively for residual masses less than 0.5 cm in thickness. Alternative techniques of interstitial therapy may be more suitable for bulkier vaginal recurrences following EBRT or for previously irradiated (with EBRT) patients. A tabular list of ABS treatment guidelines[74] using HDR brachytherapy is presented in Table 13-9.

LUNG CANCER

Because of the high prevalence of lung cancer and the easy accessibility of endobronchial disease (by flexible bronchoscope), the lung is a common site of HDR brachytherapy.

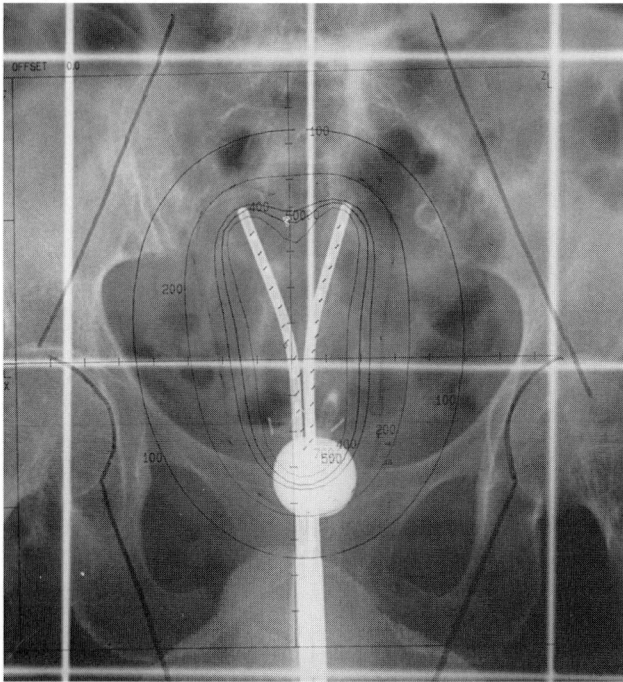

Figure 13–9. Y-shaped applicator for irradiating carcinoma of the endometrium.

The advent of HDR brachytherapy popularized the use of endobronchial brachytherapy. The treatment can be given by means of flexible bronchoscopy over a short time period (a few minutes) on an outpatient basis with the use of local anesthetic and mild sedation, as opposed to a prolonged and uncomfortable treatment by LDR.

Indications for High Dose Rate Endobronchial Brachytherapy

Goals and indications for HDR endobronchial brachytherapy are:

1. Palliation of endobronchial disease recurrent after significant pretreatment with EBRT in non–small-cell lung cancer. Patients with severe pulmonary compromise due to underlying chronic obstructive lung disease precluding the use of EBRT may be candidates for endobronchial HDR brachytherapy for palliation of bronchial symptoms. In either scenario, these patients typically have significant acute or subacute dyspnea, severe cough, hemoptysis, or clinical signs of obstructive pneumonitis (e.g., fever, malaise associated with leukocytosis) in addition to the symptomatology mentioned earlier.
2. Palliation of endobronchial disease from metastatic cancers.
3. Boosting of EBRT for primary lung cancers: HDR endobronchial brachytherapy may likewise be used in the initial management of patients treated with external irradiation and chemotherapy. This allows

Table 13–8   Primary Inoperable Endometrial Carcinoma: Treatment Guidelines*

EBRT (1.8 Gy/Rx)	Dose of HDR Fraction†	HDR fractions, *n*	HDR Interfraction Interval (weeks)
45	8.5	2	1
45	6.3	3	1
45	5.2	4	1
0	8.5	4	1
0	7.3	5	1
0	6.4	6	1
0	5.7	7	1

*Recommended by the ABS. From Nag S, Erickson B, Parikh S, et al: The American Brachytherapy Society Recommendations for HDR Brachytherapy for Carcinoma of the Endometrium. *Int J Radiat Oncol Biol Phys.* 2000;48:779.
†Dose prescribed at 2 cm from the midpoint of the intrauterine source.

Table 13–9   Endometrial Carcinoma: Vaginal Recurrences: Radiotherapeutic Guidelines (External Beam Radiation Therapy [EBRT] and Vaginal High Dose Rate [HDR] Brachytherapy)*

EBRT (1.8 Gy/Rx)	HDR Fraction Size	HDR Fractions, *n*	Dose Prescription Point	HDR Interfraction Interval
45	7.0	3	0.5 cm depth	1
45	6.0	4	0.5 cm depth	1
45	6.0	5	Vaginal surface	1
45	7.0	4	Vaginal surface	1

*Recommended by the American Brachytherapy Society. From Nag S, Erickson B, Parikh S, et al: The American Brachytherapy Society Recommendations for HDR Brachytherapy for Carcinoma of the Endometrium. *Int J Radiat Oncol Biol Phys.* 2000;48:779.

for rapid resolution of bronchial symptoms in patients treated with curative or palliative intent. It is important to recognize that the limited penetration of dose of endobronchial HDRB requires the careful selection of patients with predominant bronchial symptomatology. Bulky extrinsic peribronchial disease beyond 1.5 to 2 cm from the source catheter will not be significantly impacted by HDR endobronchial brachytherapy. Although the role of HDR endobronchial brachytherapy is primarily palliative, its routine use as a boost for EBRT or as an adjunct to surgery has not been established in patients treated for cure and awaits further clinical trials.[88-92] However, selective use of HDR endobronchial brachytherapy in combination with EBRT to achieve a more rapid palliation of obstructive pneumonitis, high-grade airway obstructive lesions, or hemoptysis is a reasonable option.

Technique

Close cooperation among individual team members (pulmonologist, radiation oncologist, radiation physicist, nursing staff, endoscopy staff, and radiation therapists) is essential. Although the procedures (bronchoscopy, fluoroscopy, localization films, and HDR treatment) are ideally performed in a dedicated HDR brachytherapy suite, minimal patient movement may also be achieved by performing the catheter placement and localization films in close proximity to the treatment room, that is, using simulator and linear accelerator rooms if the institution lacks a dedicated HDR suite.

Bronchoscopy

Standard fiberoptic bronchoscopy techniques are used to evaluate the airway and locate the involved site. The use of a 6-French catheter requires the brush channel of the bronchoscope to have a minimum diameter of 2.2 mm. Centers using 5-French catheters may use bronchoscopes with a brush channel diameter of 2 mm.

Connecting the bronchoscope to a video camera system allows all participants to monitor the bronchoscopic findings and is highly recommended. If the monitor system is not available, the bronchoscope can be connected to a teaching head to allow the radiation oncologist to visualize the lesion. It is extremely important to visualize the relationship of the proximal

and distal (if possible) extent of the tumor to fixed structures such as the tracheal carina and to note the distances involved and visualize them fluoroscopically, if possible. This permits radiographic localization of the lesion on treatment-planning films.

Catheter Placement

Although both 5- and 6-French catheters are commercially available, it is preferable to select the 6-French catheter since this allows the HDR source to more easily negotiate tight curves. Confirmation of the proper length and size of catheter should be done before beginning the procedure. Commercially available catheters come in 100- or 150-cm lengths. Since the computer software is programmed automatically for a length of 100 cm, appropriate changes in the formatting of the program are necessary when a 150-cm-long catheter is used. The catheter is placed through the brush channel of the bronchoscope and is negotiated under fluoroscopy control to a location distal to the obstruction and, if possible, lodged in one of the smaller bronchi. Placement of the catheter past a high-grade obstructive endobronchial lesion requires meticulous care to reduce the likelihood of bleeding. Additional catheters are inserted if more than one bronchus requires treatment. To ease the withdrawal of the bronchoscope after catheter placement, a 150-cm-long metal wire is inserted into the afterloading catheter to add rigidity and prevent kinking. The pulmonologist then slowly withdraws the bronchoscope under fluoroscopy while at the same time pushing ("pull-push technique") the afterloading catheter in to prevent catheter displacement. The catheter is then securely taped to the nose, its position marked in ink to alert the radiation oncologist of possible displacement, and the catheter is labeled to identify the index bronchus targeted for treatment. The external length of the catheter from the tip of the nostril is noted, as an added precaution. When multiple catheters are used, the procedure is repeated, and each catheter is labeled with adhesive tape marked with a number and site (e.g., bronchus).

Localization X-Ray Films

Localization x-ray films, with radiopaque dummy wires in the catheters, should be obtained with an orthogonal technique, the three-film method, or special localization jigs.[93] The location of the lesion and the target length are marked on the x-ray films to determine the length to be irradiated and the proximal/distal dwell positions.

Treatment Planning

The radiation oncologist advises the physicist or dosimetrist of the treatment parameters including dose, prescription point, length, location, and number of catheters to be irradiated. The dose has been prescribed at various points from 0.5 to 2.0 cm. Although there is no consensus regarding a dose prescription point, 1.0 cm from the source is commonly used.[94,95] The length to be irradiated usually includes the endobronchial tumor and a 1.0- to 2.0-cm margin, both proximally and distally, which typically represents a 5- to 7-cm bronchial segment. Figure 13-10 provides an illustrative case using two catheters. Some centers, such as Ohio State University, use an abbreviated, preplanned dosimetry based on precalculated plans for 3-, 5-, 7-, and 10-cm lengths of irradiated bronchial segments. The prescribed dose of 5 or 7.5 Gy at 1 cm from the source using equal times is used for single catheter placements with minimal curvature. This simplified dosimetry shortens considerably the waiting time between catheter placement and actual treatment delivery.[96] For the use of multiple catheter placements, the use of individualized image-based planning is mandated.

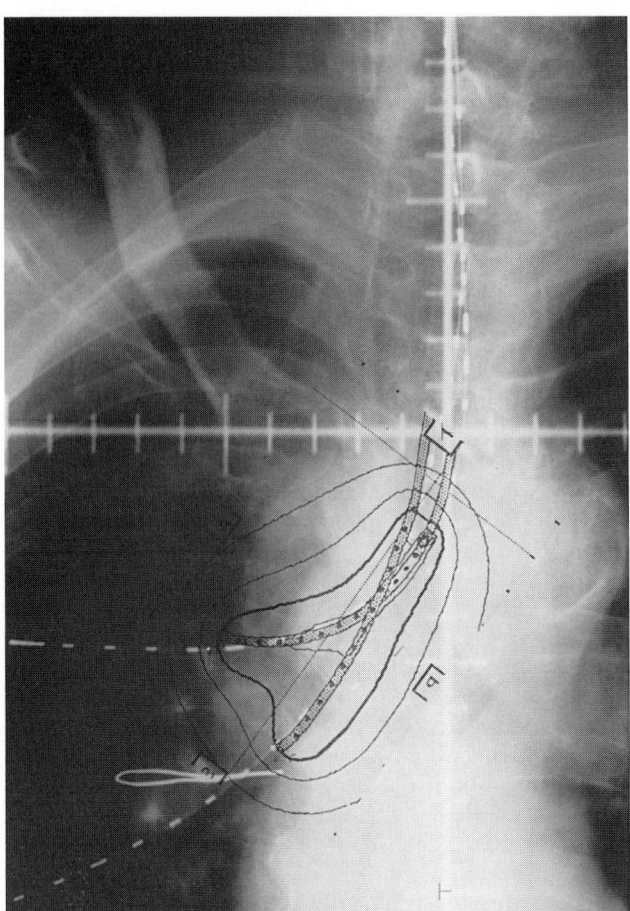

Figure 13–10. Two-catheter endobronchial application with superimposed dose distribution (posterior-anterior radiograph).

Brachytherapy Treatment

Confirmation of the patency of the catheter and completion of quality assurance checks are performed. The patient then undergoes treatment under constant video and audio monitoring. The catheter is disconnected from the patient after treatment, and, as an important precautionary measure, both the catheter and the patient are surveyed for any residual radioactivity before the catheter is discarded.

Dose and Fractionation

Although various dose schedules have been used ranging from 15 Gy in 1 fraction to 20 Gy divided into 5 fractions, the most commonly used interval between fractions is 1 week and the fraction size is typically between 5 Gy (repeated 3 or 4 times) and 10 Gy (repeated twice).[95] The ABS recommends several regimens including 7.5 Gy weekly for 3 weeks or 2 fractions of 10 Gy each or 4 fractions of 6 Gy each in all cases prescribed at 1.0 cm when the use of HDR brachytherapy is a solitary modality for palliation (Table 13-10).[97] There are no convincing data to suggest clinical superiority of any singular regimen. Radiobiologic modeling, likewise based on the linear quadratic model, also suggests equivalency.[96] The ABS recommends an HDR dose of three 5 Gy fractions (weekly) or two 7.5 Gy fractions (weekly) as a boost to EBRT (60 Gy in 30 fractions or 45 Gy in 15 fractions) (Table 13-11).[97] The prescription point is defined as 1.0 cm from the central axis of the catheter. In the rare case of endobronchial brachytherapy used as a sole treatment modality in previously unirradiated patients, HDR doses of five 5 Gy fractions or three 7.5 Gy fractions are advised by the ABS.[97] See Table 13-10 for a summary of the treatment parameters used in an HDR brachytherapy program for definitive and palliative situations.

Clinical Results

BENEFITS

The clinical results obtained by a number of institutions indicate subjective improvement rates of 50% to 100% and bronchoscopic objective response rates of 59% to 100%.[98-107] There is an inherent difficulty in analyzing the reasons for the variability of end results because of

Table 13–10   Palliative High Dose Rate Endobronchial Brachytherapy Schema*

Prescription Point	Fraction Size (Gy)	Fractions, n	Interfraction Interval (weeks)	External Radiation Therapy (Gy)†
1 cm	6.0	3	1	0
1 cm	7.5	2	1	0
1 cm	10	2	1	0

*Recommended by American Brachytherapy Society. From Nag S, Kelly JF, Horton JL, et al: The American Brachytherapy Society recommendations for HDR brachytherapy for carcinoma of the lung. *Oncology.* 2001;15:371.
†Patients have been previously irradiated to full doses of external beam radiation therapy or are not candidates for this therapy.

Table 13–11   High Dose Rate Endobronchial Brachytherapy Boost Schema*

Prescription Point	Fraction Size (Gy)	Fractions, n	Interfraction Interval (weeks)	External Radiation Therapy†
1 cm	5.0	3	1	60 Gy (30 Rx) or 45 Gy (15 Rx)
1 cm	7.5	2	1	60 Gy (30 Rx) or 45 Gy (15 Rx)

*Recommended by American Brachytherapy Society. From Nag S, Kelly JF, Horton JL, et al: The American Brachytherapy Society recommendations for HDR brachytherapy for carcinoma of the lung. *Oncology.* 2001;15:371.
†Patients have been previously irradiated to full doses of external beam radiation therapy or are not candidates for this therapy.

different study designs: the inhomogeneous groups of patients; treatment of advanced tumors; the use of additional treatments (including lasers, EBRT, prior therapy); and the variety of dose and fractionation schedules used.

Select patients with predominantly endobronchial disease who are candidates for EBRT with chemotherapy may receive an endobronchial boost using HDR brachytherapy in order to achieve rapid improvement of severe bronchial symptoms or obstructive pneumonitis or both.[98,101,108-110] An uncommon clinical scenario is the patient with an occult endobronchial or tracheal lesion who can be treated with endobronchial HDR brachytherapy alone or in combination with EBRT. Encouraging results have been published in a small series of patients indicating cause-specific survival between 78% and 100%.[111-114] A report of endobronchial HDR brachytherapy as a sole treatment modality for early-stage disease in medically inoperable patients by Marsiglia et al. indicates a survival of rate of 78%. The median follow-up was 2 years among this series of 34 patients. The regimen used was 30 Gy in 6 fractions of 5 Gy each once weekly.[115] Endobronchial HDR brachytherapy may be used for minimal bulk residual disease after surgical resection. Macha et al. have reported on 19 patients treated with 5 Gy fractions (total 20 Gy) with favorable results.[103]

COMPLICATIONS

Radiation bronchitis and stenosis are occasionally seen after HDR endobronchial brachytherapy.[116] Since the dose is typically prescribed at 1 cm from the radiation source, narrower airways (i.e., distal) may be expected to receive higher bronchial mucosa doses. Other contributing factors such as tumor destruction of the bronchial wall remain unclear. Radiation bronchitis can vary from grade I (mild mucosal inflammation), which invariably occurs, to grade IV. Grade IV is characterized by significant fibrosis that results in circumferential narrowing, requiring dilation or stent placement. Speiser and Spratling[116] reported an overall incidence of 29%, 22%, 20%, and 29%, respectively, for grades I through IV radiation bronchitis.

The serious complication of fatal hemoptysis may result from soft tissue destruction caused by the high dose of radiation delivered to the area of the pulmonary artery, or the failure of treatment to control tumor with resultant progression of disease.[117] Significant risk factors for the development of fatal hemoptysis may include a heavy pretreatment dose of external beam irradiation, multiple courses of endobronchial brachytherapy, a left

upper lobe bronchial location, or long irradiated bronchial segments.[118,119] Reports of the incidence of fatal hemoptysis vary considerably in range—zero to 50%, with a median value of 8%.[120]

CANCER OF THE ESOPHAGUS

Indications

The development of a successful combined modality regimen (concurrent radiation and chemotherapy)[121] has renewed interest in improving local control of esophageal cancer. Despite the use of EBRT and concurrent chemotherapy, local failures occur in 30% to 40% of cases. HDR brachytherapy has been used either alone or in combination with EBRT, both for palliation and for potential cure as a boost treatment following EBRT. The palliative role of HDR brachytherapy alone is well established, but the role of HDR brachytherapy boost therapy following curative therapy with EBRT and concurrent chemotherapy remains to be defined. A multi-institutional Radiation Therapy Oncology Group (RTOG) phase I/II study of external irradiation, brachytherapy, and concurrent cisplatin and 5-fluorouracil obtained a 12% incidence of fistulization leading to 3 deaths among the 49 entered patients.[122] The median survival in this series was 11 months, and the final local persistence or recurrence was 63%. Follow-up assessment of swallowing function in this study among surviving patients revealed that 92% of patients were able to swallow at least liquids at some point after therapy.[123] These sobering results have raised the issue that previous trials reporting positive results did not integrate concurrent chemotherapy, which is the current standard of care.

Technique

The treatment is usually given via a nasogastric tube or a special esophageal applicator. Figure 13-11 provides an example of such an application. The largest possible diameter applicator that can be easily inserted should be used to minimize the dose to the mucosa relative to the dose at depth. However, the standardization of applicator diameter has not been established.[124] The site to be irradiated can be confirmed by fluoroscopy or endoscopy. Usually, the area involved by tumor with the margin of 2 cm cephalad and 2 cm caudad is treated.

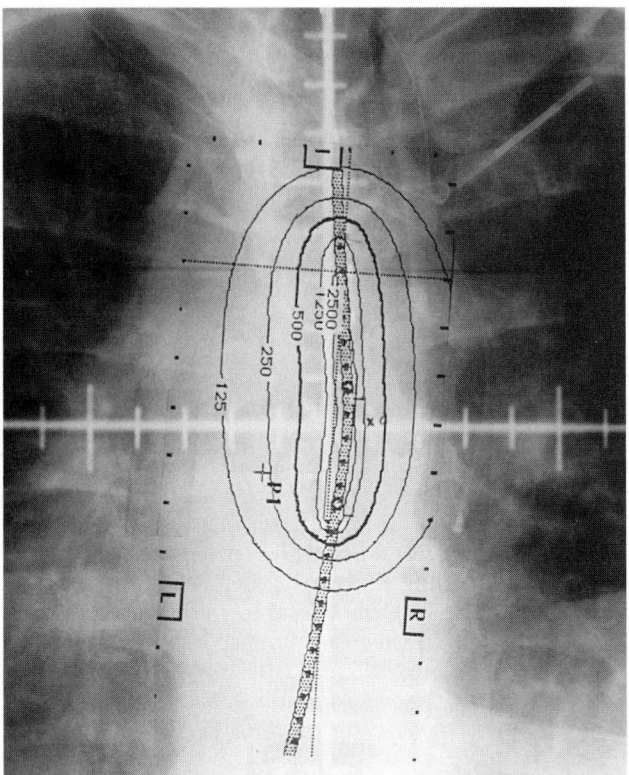

Figure 13–11. Applicator for intraluminal brachytherapy for carcinoma of the esophagus.

Dose

The dose is generally prescribed at 1 cm. Doses of 5 to 15 Gy per fraction have been given for 1 to 4 fractions before, concurrent with, or after EBRT. The advantage of giving brachytherapy after EBRT is to allow shrinkage of the tumor to deliver a more uniform dose to the residual tumor. The advantage of giving the brachytherapy initially is to have rapid relief of the major symptom, dysphagia. The ABS currently recommends an HDR dose regimen of fractions of 10 Gy each prescribed at 1 cm from the source. An esophageal applicator with an external diameter of 6 to 10 mm should be used. EBRT delivering 50 Gy in 5 weeks and concurrent chemotherapy should precede the dose.[125] Hence, the brachytherapy component is delayed until radiation therapy and chemotherapy are completed.

Clinical Results

Controlled clinical trials (randomized and historical) have evaluated HDR brachytherapy primarily as a palliative modality. Although the following trials attest to the efficacy of HDR brachytherapy (either alone or in combination with external irradiation) in the palliation of dysphagia, these trials may not be germane in the current era of concurrent EBRT and chemotherapy. EBRT combined with brachytherapy gave survival results of 78%, 31%, and 17% at 1, 3, and 5 years, respectively, compared with 56%, 19%, and 10% for 1-, 3-, and 5-year survivals obtained by EBRT alone, as reported by Yin and colleagues.[126,127] The improvements were

statistically significant for the 1- and 3-year survival rate, but not for the 5-year survival rate. In another randomized trial examining palliation of dysphagia, Sur et al. found that the group receiving EBRT alone (35 Gy in 15 treatments) had a 12-month survival of 16% compared with a 69% 12-month survival in the group receiving 35 Gy EBRT followed by 12 Gy in 2 fractions of HDR brachytherapy.[128] There was an improvement in the relief of dysphagia with the addition of HDR brachytherapy at 3 months (82% vs. 24%), and at 6 months (84% vs. 13%). Flores and colleagues[129] reported significant improvement of performance status, swallowing ability, weight, and pain control with intracavitary irradiation. Of 171 patients, 33% were still alive at 1 year, 26% at 2 years, and 19% at 3 years after therapy. Rowland and Pagliero[130] obtained significant relief of dysphagia at 6 weeks in 70% of the squamous cell carcinoma patients treated. However, only about 10% survived symptom-free at 1 year, which may have been due to the advanced nature of the disease. Hishikawa and colleagues,[131] in a nonrandomized trial, showed a better survival of patients treated with EBRT plus HDR brachytherapy compared with those treated by EBRT alone (28% compared with 4% 2-year survival). The local control rate was also higher (63% vs. 20%). The validity of the results of these studies in the current era of combined external irradiation and concurrent chemotherapy has been raised.[122] Since most of the trials did not incorporate concurrent chemotherapy and radiation therapy,[121] these results may no longer be applicable in curative treatment in light of the RTOG study combining EBRT and concurrent chemotherapy and brachytherapy.[122] Based on this trial, HDR brachytherapy trials are currently not being planned in the RTOG and extreme caution is encouraged in the use of external irradiation, concurrent chemotherapy, and brachytherapy.

CARCINOMA OF THE PROSTATE

The transrectal ultrasound-guided implant technique is the backbone of modern prostate brachytherapy. Whether it is permanent or temporary, HDR or LDR, each type of modern prostate brachytherapy uses a similar technique of transperineal insertion of seed-bearing needles or afterloading catheters. This is based on the original technique described by Holm in 1983.[132] Using ultrasound guidance, a real-time image of the implant volume can be seen and the position of each implant needle adjusted to ensure accurate placement. This method led to improvements in the quality of prostate brachytherapy and resurgence of interest in the technique. In most HDR implants, afterloading catheters are typically secured in position using a perineal template. The location of the catheters is determined using ultrasounds, orthogonal x-ray or a CT scan.[133-135] Each catheter's position is then transferred into a computer, and by using the treatment planning software, the optimal loading is determined. Single or multiple fractions can be delivered via the same afterloading catheter using the remote afterloader during outpatient sessions or short hospital stays.

There are many reasons why HDR brachytherapy may be useful in the delivery of conformal radiotherapy to the prostate. Modern HDR brachytherapy can be optimized based on the actual catheter position using computer algorithms. This allows a more homogeneous dose within the implant volume and better coverage of the target volume.[136] Recent advances in treatment planning may provide further refinement of dosimetry by using inverse planning algorithms.[137,138] Hsu et al. compared the dosimetry data generated from three-dimensional conformal EBRT with HDR brachytherapy and showed significantly less rectal and bladder volume irradiated using HDR brachytherapy boost compared with conformal EBRT.[139] An example of implant dosimetry is given in Figures 13-12 and 13-13. Besides the dosimetric advantages, there are other practical advantages of HDR brachytherapy compared with traditional LDR brachytherapy. Since the HDR treatment is delivered within a few minutes, similar to EBRT, and is always carried out in the shielded environment of the HDR treatment room, the patient does not need to be isolated between treatments and can stay in an unshielded room with other patients. There is no radiation exposure to hospital personnel or to the patient's family members. Since an HDR implant is a closed system, there is no risk of seed migration. The effect of postimplant edema can be accounted for by performing a dose calculation soon after the implant. Finally, by treating multiple patients with a single radioactive source, there is the potential for cost saving compared to permanent seed implant boost (see Fig. 13-13).

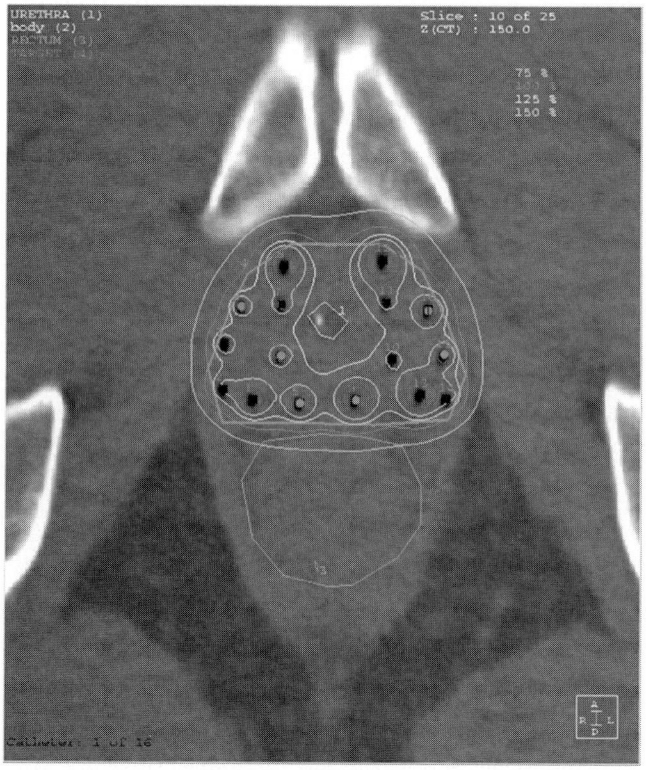

Radiobiology of HDR Prostate Brachytherapy

Clinical gain has been predicted and reported using alternative fractionation schemes in radiotherapy.[140,141] The linear-quadratic model represents the basis for estimating the clinical effects of alternative fractionation schemes. In this model, the response of tissue to altered fractionation is determined by the tissue's alpha-beta ratio. Brenner et al. estimated the alpha-beta ratio for prostate carcinoma based on mature clinical data and showed that prostate cancer has a low alpha-beta ratio of 1.5 Gy.[142] Several studies have supported this finding.[143-145] If this is indeed the case, then prostate cancer's alpha-beta ratio is significantly lower than the alpha-beta ratio of dose-limiting structures around the prostate (3 to 5 Gy). This suggests there is a potential gain for treating prostate cancer using hypofractionated radiotherapy.[146-148] Hsu et al. calculated this potential biological dose gain based on the linear quadratic model and comparison of HDR dosimetry with conformal EBRT.[139] They showed a potential increase of 7% to 64% in the biologic dose delivered to the prostate without an increase in the biologic dose delivered to the rectum using HDR boost. It is clear from this study that if the radiobiologic hypothesis is correct, hypofractionation radiotherapy may indeed be a more effective form of radiotherapy for prostate cancer and may have fewer side effects.

Figure 13–12. A three-dimensional brachytherapy planning system is an important part of modern brachytherapy. Critical organs such as the urethra, rectum, and bladder are contoured during the treatment planning process; in this way, the dose delivered to the critical organs can be accurately controlled. See also Color Figure 13-12.

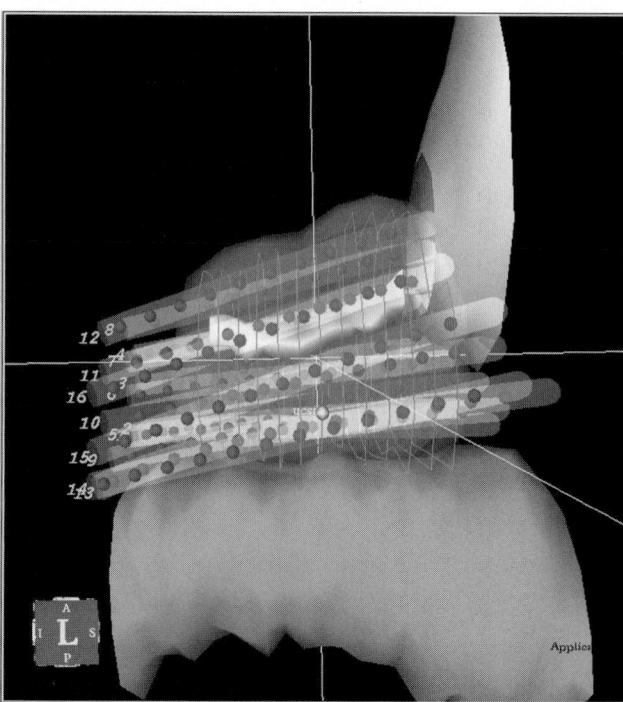

Figure 13–13. Very conformal dose distribution can be delivered to the prostate using modern brachytherapy treatment system. A steep dose falloff outside of the implant volume decreases the dose and volume of radiated normal structures. See also Color Figure 13-13.

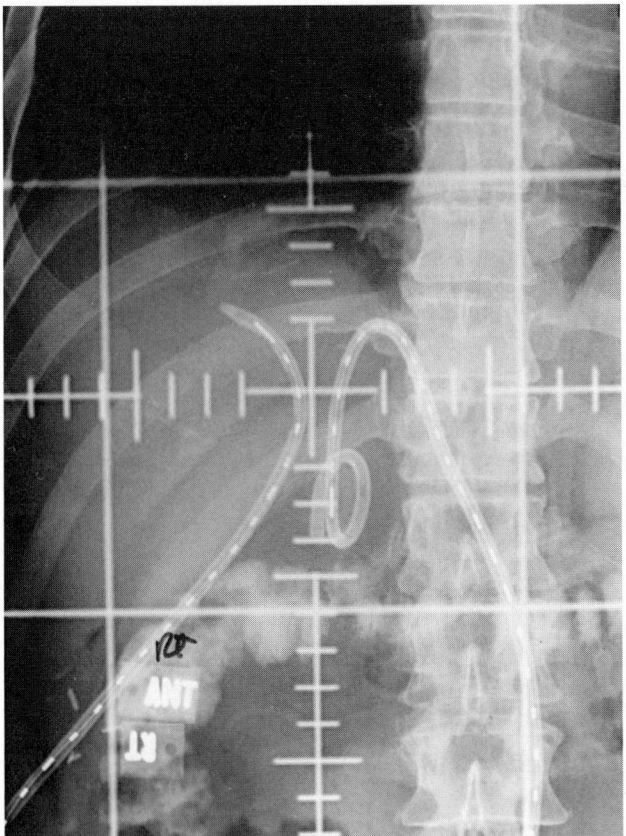

Figure 13–14. Anterior-posterior simulation film of stents with high dose rate catheters and dummy strands for biliary application.

Dose and Clinical Results

The dose per fraction delivered is variable, but about 5 Gy per fraction at a distance of 1 cm from the source is commonly used for 3 to 4 fractions (15 to 20 Gy in 3 to 4 weeks) to boost 45 Gy EBRT. An HDR dose escalation phase I/II study for patients with unresectable or partially resectable disease at the University of Miami used an HDR fraction size 7 Gy at 1 cm depth following external beam irradiation (45 Gy/standard fractionation).[168] The treatment protocol increased the number of HDR fractions from 1 to 3 weekly (total external plus brachytherapy 52 Gy, 59 Gy, 66 Gy, respectively). The corresponding median survivals of the 3 sequential dose groups were 9, 12.2, and 20.3 months, respectively. This did not reach statistical significance, but the complete or partial response rate was significantly improved statistically (25% for total dose of 52 Gy vs. 80% for doses 59 and 66 Gy). One of 18 patients in this series experienced a grade III toxicity.

HEAD AND NECK CANCERS

Indications

Brachytherapy, especially using manually afterloaded ^{192}Ir, has been widely used in the head and neck area. HDR brachytherapy may be used in select cases as an outpatient procedure and to permit optimization.[169-174] These reports used HDR brachytherapy with or without external beam irradiation. A tabular summary is in Table 13-14. For patients treated with HDR alone, however, these advantages are offset by the need for multiple fractions, especially since critical structures in the head and neck area (e.g., spinal cord, brain, mandible) may be intolerant of a high dose per fraction. Lau et al. have cautioned about the loss of the therapeutic ratio with 6.5 Gy twice daily.[170] Lau reported a 53% control rate among 25 patients with predominantly T1 and T2 lesions and recommended LDR brachytherapy.[170] Alternatively, comparing HDR and LDR brachytherapy for T1-2N0M0 oral tongue cancer patients, Inoue reported in a randomized trial of 29 patients 2-year local control of 100% and 86%, respectively.[171] Inoue used 60 Gy in 10 fractions over 6 days for the HDR regimen. Inoue suggests equivalency between HDR and LDR regimens. The nasopharynx is a site within the head and neck area that is easily accessible by an intracavitary HDR applicator.[175,176] Moreover, thin residual tumors (<10 mm) following EBRT and chemotherapy may be more suitable candidates.[169] In Rotterdam, doses of 18 Gy in 6 fractions are delivered by a special nasopharynx applicator to boost 60 to 70 Gy of EBRT.[176] The authors reported a 5-year local relapse-free survival rate of 96% for T1-2 cancers versus 57% for T4 cancers. Currently, there are limited data regarding HDR brachytherapy with or without EBRT for salvage therapy of locally recurrent nasopharyngeal carcinoma following definitive EBRT.

Table 13–14   High Dose Rate Brachytherapy for Head and Neck Cancer

Reference	EBRT Dose (Gy)	Fraction Size (Gy)	Fractions, n	Equivalent Dose* (Gy)	Patients, n	Local Control, %
Dixit et al[169]	0	3	20	65	3	N/A
Lau et al[170]	0	6.5	7	63	27	53
Inoue et al[171]	0	6	10	80	14	100
Donath et al[172]	0	4.5-5	10	54-63	13	90
Leung et al[173]	0	5.5-6	10	71-80	13	100
Yu et al[174]	50	2.7	6	67	12	79
Dixit et al[169]	40-48	3	7	63-71	18	80

*Equivalent dose for tumor effects @ 2 Gy/day using linear quadratic model with an α/β ratio of 10.[28,34,39]

Dose

The use of HDR brachytherapy catheters incorporated in removable dental molds allows repeated fractionated outpatient brachytherapy for palate or sinus sites in a highly reproducible manner without requiring repeated catheter insertion into the tumor.[177] Doses of about 15 to 20 Gy in 3 to 5 fractions can be delivered in this manner to boost 45 to 50 Gy EBRT.

The use of HDR interstitial brachytherapy in the head and neck region in accessible sites (e.g., cheek, lip, tongue) as boost therapy following EBRT may be considered in lieu of LDR brachytherapy and may obviate the need for hospitalization. Typically, treatment schedules of 3 to 4 Gy per HDR fraction twice daily 6 hours apart for 4 to 5 fractions are used following 45 to 50 Gy EBRT.[178]

Intraoperative HDR Brachytherapy

Another innovative approach is the use of intraoperative HDR brachytherapy. This permits normal tissues to be retracted or shielded during brachytherapy. The catheters are removed immediately after the single dose of radiation, hence minimizing inconvenience and permitting the use of brachytherapy in difficult-to-reach areas such as the base of skull.[179,180] Doses of 7.5 to 15.0 Gy are given if an external beam of 45 to 50 Gy is added. In recurrent tumors in which no further EBRT can be given, the single intraoperative dose is 15 to 20 Gy. Intraoperative HDR brachytherapy can access many sites in the head and neck area that are difficult to treat or are inaccessible by either LDR removable brachytherapy or electron beam intraoperative radiation therapy.[180] It has been used extensively in IORT of rectal cancer.

SOFT TISSUE SARCOMAS

Indication

The role of EBRT following wide local resection of soft tissue sarcoma is well established. Irradiation of large volumes of normal tissues has at times been associated with significant soft tissue fibrosis. There is increasing interest in using HDR brachytherapy either alone as a substitute for EBRT or as a boost therapy in combination with EBRT, with the hope of reducing treatment-related morbidity. There is a limited database regarding the use of HDR brachytherapy.

Technique and Dose

A perioperative technique for soft tissue sarcomas uses HDR brachytherapy catheters implanted along the tumor bed after gross excision of tumor. The area implanted includes the tumor bed and a 2- to 5-cm margin proximally and distally. Optimized treatment planning can be used to deliver a more homogeneous dose. Doses

equivalent to 60 Gy LDR (40 to 50 Gy) are given in 12 to 15 fractions if the HDR is given alone.[181,182] If EBRT (45 to 50 Gy) is added, the brachytherapy dose is limited to 18 to 25 Gy in 4 to 7 fractions.[182] It is important to delay the start of this brachytherapy for at least 1 week to allow well-established wound healing. Caution should be exercised in the use of HDR brachytherapy over neurovascular bundles since the tolerance of nerves may be a limiting factor.

Remote HDR brachytherapy has some theoretical advantages over manually afterloaded LDR brachytherapy (e.g., ability for optimization, elimination of radiation exposure hazard). However, there is little experience in the use of HDR brachytherapy in soft tissue sarcomas, and HDR brachytherapy remains investigational.[181-187] The ABS has summarized its recommendations for the use of HDR brachytherapy in patients with adult soft tissue sarcomas.[188]

PEDIATRIC TUMORS

LDR brachytherapy has been used in children to reduce the adverse effects of EBRT.[189-191] However, LDR brachytherapy is difficult to perform in young children and infants because of the need for prolonged sedation; immobilization; and close, frequent monitoring. HDR brachytherapy is currently undergoing trials at Ohio State University and Columbus Children's Hospital in an effort to reduce radiation exposure to personnel and permit brachytherapy in infants.[192-194] The minimum peripheral dose is 36 Gy in 12 fractions prescribed at 0.5 cm (3 Gy per treatment given twice a day, 6 hours apart).[188,193] Therapeutic guidelines for the use of HDR brachytherapy following EBRT are not available. Although the long-term morbidity of HDR brachytherapy in young children is not fully known, one may expect it to preserve organ functions similar to the experience with LDR brachytherapy.[189] The use of HDR brachytherapy should be restricted to select pediatric tumors in controlled clinical trials until long-term data are available.

BREAST CARCINOMA

Boost Therapy

INDICATION

The use of brachytherapy as a boost following EBRT or as a partial breast irradiation strategy in lieu of EBRT in breast conservation therapy (BCT) has generated increasing attention. A large randomized trial from the European Organization for Research and Treatment of Cancer has demonstrated the benefit of boost therapy in improving local control in patients with breast cancer with negative margins.[195] The practical preference of most radiation oncologists to use electron beam as a boost technique must be balanced by its limitation in certain scenarios. Large breasts, deep-seated tumors, or both may hamper the use of electron beam. Moreover, positive or close margins or unknown margin status may indicate a greater risk of subclinical tumor burden and may require higher doses of radiation. A more focused technique using breast brachytherapy as a boost technique may facilitate delivery of radiation as opposed to that delivered with EBRT.[196]

TECHNIQUE

The success of breast brachytherapy is predicated by the need to precisely define the CTV (discussed earlier in this chapter). The ABS has published guidelines to assist in the accuracy of the treatment.[197] A 2-cm margin around the lumpectomy cavity is recommended unless limited by the chest wall or skin. A practical way of defining the cavity is the intraoperative placement of clips at the periphery of the cavity to assist in the localization of the implanted volume and to guarantee adequacy of dosimetry coverage. A newer technique of cavity outlining using injection of biologically inert contrast in the cavity under ultrasound guidance as proposed by Kuske may also facilitate accurate placement of catheters when under real-time fluoroscopic or mammographic guidance.[196] A minimum of two brachytherapy planes is required for most implants unless limited by the thinness of breast tissue (<2 cm). Assurance of correct spacing between needles (in the same plane) or planes of needles is necessary. The ABS recommends adequate treatment planning to assure dose homogeneity within the CTV and criteria to judge quality.

DOSE

The optimal dose schedule for HDR boost therapy remains undefined. The ABS recommends a dose equivalency of 10 to 20 Gy LDR.[96]

PARTIAL BREAST IRRADIATION

Indication

Breast conservation therapy (BCT) has traditionally combined limited breast tissue resection and EBRT directed to the entire breast. Most breast recurrences are anatomically situated in close proximity to the lumpectomy site. The need for whole breast irradiation must be counterbalanced by the potential long-term risk of increased sequelae and the long treatment duration of EBRT. An abbreviated course of partial breast irradiation (PBI) would increase the logistical availability of BCT to more women and may achieve a more facile integration of chemotherapy. Careful selection of patients for PBI is critical to achieve success. Patients with multicentric disease, inadequate excision, extensive intraductal component, and infiltrating lobular carcinoma are not recommended to have PBI.[196]

Technique and Dose

The technique is outlined earlier. Strict therapeutic guidelines as outlined in RTOG protocol No. 95-17 and at the William Beaumont Hospital[198-201] are essential. A high quality assurance program including the use of dose volume histogram must be an integral part of the treatment program.[202] The RTOG phase I/II trial of partial breast irradiation has demonstrated on a group-wide basis a high adequate coverage of the CTV in 97% of the patients treated. The RTOG used HDR doses of 3.4 Gy in 10 fractions over 5 days. The RTOG is planning a phase III randomized trial between EBRT whole breast and PBI. The ABS is recommending a HDR dose of 34 Gy in 10 fractions .[197]

Clinical Results

An earlier, large randomized trial of PBI at the Christie Hospital analyzed 708 patients, comparing 40 Gy whole breast EBRT (6 MeV) in 15 fractions to 40 to 42.5 Gy partial breast in 8 fractions of 10 MeV electrons. Researchers were limited by the lack of adequate margin assessment.[203,204] The 7-year local failure rates were 11% and 20% for whole breast and partial breast irradiation, respectively. The poor results among the PBI patients were ascribed primarily to failures among the infiltrating lobular histology patients. The local 7-year recurrence rates were 8% and 34% for lobular histology and 11% and 15% for ductal histology for whole breast versus partial breast irradiation. The difference is due to a significant difference of failure outside of the index quadrant in the lobular histology patients. North American trials (phase I/II) of PBI from the Ochsner Clinic, William Beaumont Hospital, and the RTOG have accrued 50, 174, and 100 patients, respectively.[200,205,206] The Ochsner study has a single breast recurrence (2%) with a median follow-up of 75 months. The William Beaumont trial study with a median follow-up of 36 months has no breast recurrence. Matched pair analyses of the Ochsner and William Beaumont studies confirm the equivalent rates of local control between whole breast irradiation and PBI groups.[200,206] The William Beaumont Hospital series has evolved from an LDR to an HDR program and currently uses 34 Gy in 10 fractions over 5 days. A phase III randomized trial comparing PBI to whole breast irradiation is recommended to determine the long-term efficacy of PBI.[196]

INTRAOPERATIVE HIGH DOSE RATE BRACHYTHERAPY

Indications

Maximum surgical debulking allows the residual micro- or macroscopic component to be amenable to intraoperative and perioperative brachytherapy techniques.[207-209] Intraoperative HDR brachytherapy has much promise because normal tissues can be displaced or partially shielded during the irradiation. Unfortunately, because of the limited availability of a shielded operating room, only a few centers have reported using intraoperative HDR brachytherapy.[209-212] Intraoperative HDR brachytherapy may have certain technical advantages over electron beam intraoperative therapy, particularly in steeply sloped surfaces, narrow cavity spaces, and in certain highly angulated directions inaccessible to the electron beam.

Technique

The surgery is performed in a shielded operating room with remote anesthesia and a video monitoring system. Maximal surgical debulking is attempted whenever possible. The tumor bed is irradiated using special intraoperative applicators incorporated with HDR catheters, parallel and 1 cm apart. The use of a fixed-geometry applicator with an array of 1-cm–spaced catheters allows the patient to be treated without delay using preplanned dosimetry for the selected applicator. Normal tissues are either retracted away from the high-dose area or shielded. Doses of 10 to 20 Gy are usually given as a single fraction over 10 to 60 minutes. A 2 to 4 cm displacement of tissue typically results in an 80% to 93% dose reduction, whereas 1 to 5 mm of lead shielding reduces the normal tissue dose by 20% to 80%, respectively.[209]

SKIN

Indications

Little interest has developed over the use of brachytherapy for skin cancers. Most basal cell and squamous cell carcinomas addressed radiotherapeutically are treated with orthovoltage or EBRT. Yet the availability of orthovoltage equipment has decreased in most radiation oncology departments. The ready availability of EBRT has supplanted orthovoltage therapy. EBRT presents certain constraints, however. These include an initial decrement of dose at the skin surface (necessitating bolus equivalent material), greater bone dose absorption underneath skin (than soft tissue) and dose decrement at the periphery of the field in highly sloped surfaces. Since most skin cancers are superficial (i.e., <3 mm), 6 MeV electrons are typically used. A comparison of dose distribution of 6 MeV electrons (with 0.5-cm bolus) compared to the Freiburg (*registered name*) applicator (for HDR) for treatment of a skin cancer of the hand is presented in tabular form (Table 13-15). Dose distributions in Table 13-15 indicate a superior dose profile for HDR (compared to electron beam) with less dose delivered to the subcutaneous tissues and deeper tissues (e.g., bone, joints, tendons, lacrimal gland). The Freiburg applicator offers certain practical advances in the use of brachytherapy: (1) malleability and ease of adaptability to various skin contours including sloped surfaces; (2) variability of

sizes; (3) no need for bolus. We are selectively using a regimen of 4 Gy at 2 mm depth twice weekly for 9-10 treatments (total 36-40 Gy). For deeper tumors and larger size lesions necessitating photon or electron therapy, we use a boost dose of HDR (4 Gy twice weekly for 3 to 4 fractions) following 50 Gy external beam standard fractionation with resultant flattening of the mass to less than 5-mm thickness.

The disadvantage of the Freiburg HDR applications are the labor intensiveness, with a typical time of 1 to 2 hours for treatment setup verification on the simulator, and repeat dosimetry if necessary. These disadvantages may be balanced by the fewer number of treatment fractions used in view of the enhanced dose distribution.

FUTURE TRENDS IN HIGH DOSE RATE BRACHYTHERAPY

It is expected that the use of HDR brachytherapy will greatly expand over the next decade and that refinements will occur primarily in the integration of imaging (CT, MRI, intraoperative ultrasonography) and optimization of dose distribution. It is anticipated that better tumor localization and normal tissue definition will help to optimize dose distribution to the tumor and reduce normal tissue exposure.

The ability to readily integrate HDR brachytherapy and EBRT will result in increasing use of HDR brachytherapy in investigational protocols. Dose constraints of brachytherapy generally require that it follow maximal cytoreductive EBRT. However, with HDR it is increasingly possible to integrate brachytherapy earlier in the treatment course and emphasize the brachytherapy component.

Collaborative efforts among various institutions are needed to standardize the methodology and dose fractionation of HDR brachytherapy. The recognition of a need for consensus development has spurred the creation of the Clinical Research Committee of the ABS. This committee has already published consensus guidelines. Further efforts are urgently required to form consensus opinions and standardization in HDR brachytherapy. The development of well-controlled randomized trials addressing issues of efficacy, toxicity, quality of life, and costs versus benefits will ultimately define the role of HDR brachytherapy in the therapeutic armamentarium.

Table 13–15 Comparison of Electrons and High Dose Rate (HDR) Freiburg Flap Application DRB for the Treatment of Skin Cancer

Depth, cm	6 MeV Electron (0.5 c Bolus), % Dose	HDR Normalized @ 0.2 cm Depth, % Dose
0.0	88	105-110
0.5	98	85
1.0	98	65
1.5	78	55
2.0	36	30

REFERENCES

1. International Commission on Radiation Units and Measurements: *ICRU Report 38: Dose and Volume Specification for Reporting Intracavitary Therapy in Gynecology*. Bethesda, Md.: International Commission on Radiation Units and Measurements; 1985.
2. Nag S, Abitbol A, Anderson LL, et al. Consensus guidelines for high dose rate remote brachytherapy (HDR) in cervical, endometrial, and endobronchial tumors. *Int J Radiat Oncol Biol Phys*. 1993;27:1241.
3. Nag S, Dobelbower R, Glasgow G, et al: Inter-society standards for brachytherapy: A joint report from AAPM, ABS, ACMP, and ACRO. *Int J Radiat Oncol Biol Phys*. (Submitted, 2001).

4. Nag S, Erickson B, Parikh S, et al: The American Brachytherapy Society recommendations for HDR brachytherapy for carcinoma of the endometrium. *Int J Radiat Oncol Biol Phys.* 2000;48:779.

5. Nag S, Kelly JF, Horton JL, et al: The American Brachytherapy Society recommendations for HDR brachytherapy for carcinoma of the lung. *Oncology.* 2001;15:371.

6. Nag S, Kuske RR, Vicini F, et al: The American Brachytherapy Society recommendations for brachytherapy for carcinoma of the breast. *Oncology.* 2001;15:195.

7. Nag S, Orton C, Petereit D, et al: The American Brachytherapy Society recommendations for HDR brachytherapy of the cervix. *Int J Radiat Oncol Biol Phys.* 2000;48:201.

8. Nag S, Shasha D, Janjan N, et al: The American Brachytherapy Society recommendations for brachytherapy of soft tissue sarcomas. *Int J Radiat Oncol Biol Phys.* 2001;49:1033.

9. Nag S, Vikram B, Demanes JD, et al: The American Brachytherapy Society recommendations for HDR brachytherapy for head and neck carcinoma. *Int J Radiat Oncol Biol Phys.* 2001;50:1190.

10. Rodriguez R, Nag S, Mate T, et al: High dose rate brachytherapy for prostate cancer: Assessment of current clinical practice and recommendations of The American Brachytherapy Society. *J. Brachyther Int.* 2001;17:265.

11. Nag S, Samsami N: Pitfalls of inappropriate optimization. *J Brachyther Int.* 2000;16:187.

12. Kurhanewicz J, Vigneron B, Nelson S: Three-dimensional magnetic resonance spectroscopic imaging of brain and prostate cancer. *Neoplasia.* 2000;2:166.

13. Lahanas M, Baltas D, Zambouglou N: Anatomy-based three-dimensional dose optimization in brachytherapy using multiple objective genetic algorithm. *Med Phys.* 1999;26:9.

14. Lessard E, Pouliot J: Anatomy-based dose optimization for HDR-brachytherapy of the prostate using fast simulated annealing algorithm. *Med Phys.* 2001;28:773.

15. Pouliot J, Tremblay D, Roy J, Filice S: Optimization of permanent ^{125}I prostate implants using fast simulated annealing. *Int J Radiat Oncol Biol Phys.* 1996;36:711.

16. Kneschaurek P, Schiessl W, Wehrmann R: Volume-based dose optimization in brachytherapy. *Int J Radiat Oncol Biol Phys.* 1999;45:811.

17. Hsu I-C, Lessard E, Weinberg V, Pouliot J: Comparison of inverse planning and geometrical optimization for prostate high dose rate brachytherapy. Presented at the 23rd American Brachytherapy Society Meeting, Orlando, Fla. May 24, 2002.

18. Pouliot J, Charra-Brunaud C, Kim YB, et al: Inverse planning for HDR brachytherapy: Clinical implementation. Presented at the 23rd American Brachytherapy Society Meeting, Orlando, Fla. May 24, 2002.

19. Kirkpatrick S, Gelatt CD, Vecchi PM: Optimization by simulated annealing. *Science.* 1983;220:671.

20. Pouliot J, Taschereau R, Coté C, et al: Dosimetric aspects of permanent radioactive implants for the treatment of prostate. *Physics in Canada.* 1999;55:61.

21. Lachance B, B-Nadeau D, Lessard E, et al: Early clinical experience with anatomy-based inverse planning dose optimization for HDR boost of the prostate. *Int J Radiat Oncol Biol Phys.* 2002;54:1.

22. Lessard E, Hsu I-C, Pouliot J: Inverse planning for interstitial gynecological template brachytherapy: Truly anatomy based planning. *Int J Radiat Oncol Biol Phys.* 2002;54:5.

23. Fisch BM, Pickett B, Weinberg V, Roach M, III: Dose of radiation received by the bulb of the penis correlates with risk of impotence after three-dimensional conformal radiotherapy for prostate cancer. *UROL.* 2001;57.

24. Lessard E, Hsu I-C, Fish B, Pouliot J: Inverse planning ability to protect the bulb of the penis and other organs at risk in HDR-brachytherapy of the prostate. *Med Phys.* 2002;29:6.

25. Hall EJ: *Radiobiology for the Radiologist.* 5th ed. Philadelphia: Lippincott Williams & Wilkins; 2000:401.

26. Brenner DJ, Hall EJ: Conditions for the equivalence of continuous to pulsed low dose rate brachytherapy. *Int J Radiat Oncol Biol Phys.* 1991;20:181.

27. Brenner DJ, Hall EJ: Fractionated high dose rate versus low dose rate regimens for intracavitary brachytherapy of the cervix. *Br J Radiol.* 1991;64:133.

28. Dale RG: The application of the linear-quadratic dose-effect equation to fractionated and protracted radiotherapy. *Br J Radiol.* 1985;58:515.

29. Fowler JF: Why shorter half-times for repair lead to greater damage in pulsed brachytherapy. *Int J Radiat Oncol Biol Phys.* 1993;26:353.

30. Thames HD: Effect-independent measurements of tissue responses to fractionated irradiation. *Int J Radiat Biol Phys.* 1984;45:l.

31. Orton CG: High and low dose rate remote afterloading: A critical comparison. In Sauer R, ed. *International Radiation Therapy Techniques—Brachytherapy.* Berlin: Springer-Verlag; 1991:53.

32. Hall EJ: *Radiobiology for the Radiologist.* 5th ed. Philadelphia: Lippincott Williams & Wilkins; 2000:74.

33. Barendsen GW: Dose fractionation, dose rate and iso-effect relationships for normal tissue responses. *Int J Radiat Oncol Biol Phys.* 1982;8:1981.

34. Orton CG: Recent developments in time-dose modelling. *Australas Phys Eng Sci Med.* 1991;14:57.

35. Dale RG: What minimum number of fractions is required with high dose-rate remote afterloading? *Br J Radiol.* 1987;60:301.

36. Dale RG: The use of small fraction numbers in high dose-rate gynecological afterloading: Some radiobiological considerations. *Br J Radiol.* 1990;63:290.

37. Stitt J, Fowler J, Thomadsen B, et al: High dose rate intracavitary brachytherapy for carcinoma of the cervix: The Madison system: 1. Clinical and radiobiological considerations. *Int J Radiat Oncol Biol Phys.* 1992;24:335.

38. Bentzen SM, Saunders MI, Dische S: Repair half-times estimated from the observations of treatment-related morbidity after CHART or conventional radiotherapy in head and neck cancer. *Radiotherapy Oncol.* 1999;53:219.

39. Orton, CG: High-dose-rate brachytherapy may be radiobiologically superior to low dose rate due to slow repair of late-responding normal tissue cells. *Int J Radiat Oncol Biol Phys.* 2001;49:183.

40. Orton CG, Seyedsadr M, Somnay A: Comparison of high and low dose rate remote afterloading for cervix cancer and the importance of fractionation. *Int J Radiat Oncol Biol Phys.* 1991;21:1425.

41. Nag S, Owen J, Pajak T, et al: Survey of brachytherapy practice in the U.S.; A report of the Clinical Research Committee of The American Endocurietherapy Society. *Int J Radiat Oncol Biol Phys.* 1995;31:103.

42. Consensus Statement: National Institutes of Health Consensus Development Conference Statement on Cervical Cancer. *Gynecol Oncol.* 1997;66:351.

43. Houdek P: Design and implementation of a program for high dose rate brachytherapy. In Nag S, ed. *High Dose Rate Brachytherapy: A Textbook.* Armonk, N.Y.: Futura Publishing; 1994:27.

44. Fu K, Phillips T: High-dose-rate versus low-dose-rate intracavitary brachytherapy for carcinoma of the cervix. *Int J Radiat Oncol Biol Phys.* 1990;19:791.

45. Ling CC, Sahoo N, Leibel S, et al: High dose rate gynecological applications—Radiobiological considerations based on the alpha-beta model. *Radiother Oncol.* 1993;8:118.

46. Dusenbery K, Carson L, Potish R: Perioperative morbidity and mortality of gynecologic brachytherapy. *Cancer.* 1991;67:2786.

47. Abitbol A, Stitt J, Schwade J, Lewin A: High dose rate brachytherapy for carcinoma of the cervix. In Nag S, ed. *High Dose Rate Brachytherapy: A Textbook.* Armonk, N.Y.: Futura Publishing; 1994:373.

48. Nag S, Abitbol A, Anderson LL, et al: Consensus guidelines for high dose rate remote brachytherapy (HDR) in cervical, endometrial, and endobronchial tumors. *Int J Radiat Oncol Biol Phys.* 1993;27:1241.

49. Abitbol A, Wolfson A, Lewin A, et al: Management of stage I-B, II-A, and II-B carcinoma of the cervix: Results of an institutional clinical trial. *Am J Clin Oncol.* 1996;19:223.

50. Nag S, Young D, Orton C, *Int J Radiat Oncol Biol Phys*: Survey of the brachytherapy practice for carcinoma of the cervix: A report of the Clinical Research Committee of the American Brachytherapy Society. *Gynecol Oncol.* 1999;73:111-118.

51. Nag S, Orton C, Petereit D, et al: The American Brachytherapy Society Recommendations for HDR Brachytherapy of the Cervix. *Int J Radiat Oncol Biol Phys.* 2000;48:201.

52. ICRU: *Dose and Volume Specification for Reporting Intracavitary Brachytherapy for Gynecology. Report No. 38.* Bethesda, Md: International Commission on Radiation Units and Measurements; 1985.

53. Joslin CA: The cathetron as part of the radical management of cervix cancer. *Br J Radiol.* 1980;17:11.

54. Rotte K: A randomized clinical trial comparing a high dose-rate with a conventional dose-rate afterloading machine (the Cathetron). *Int J Radiat Oncol Biol Phys.* 1983;9:931.

55. Arai T, Morita S, Kutsutani Y, et al: Relationships between total iso-effect dose and number of fractions for the treatment of uterine cervical carcinoma by high dose-rate intracavitary irradiation. *Br J Radiol.* 1980;17:89.

56. Sato S, Yajima A, Suzuki M: Therapeutic results using high-dose-rate intracavitary irradiation in cases of cervical cancer. *Gynecol Oncol.* 1984;19:143.

57. Arai T, Nakano T, Morita S, et al: High-dose-rate remote afterloading intracavitary radiation therapy for cancer of the uterine cervix: A 20-year experience. *Cancer.* 1992;69:175.

58. Akine Y, Arimoto H, Ogino T, et al: High-dose-rate intracavitary irradiation in the treatment of carcinoma of the uterine cervix: Early experience with 84 patients. *Int J Radiat Oncol Biol Phys.* 1988;14:893.

59. Chen M-S, Lin F-J, Hong C-H, et al: High-dose-rate afterloading technique in the radiation treatment of uterine cervical cancer: 399 cases and 9 years experience in Taiwan. *Int J Radiat Oncol Biol Phys.* 1991;20:915.

60. Orton CG: High dose rate versus low dose rate brachytherapy for gynecological cancer. *Semin Radiat Oncol.* 1993;3:232.

61. Orton CG, Seyedsadr M, Somnay A: Comparison of high and low dose rate remote afterloading for cervix cancer and the importance of fractionation. *Int J Radiat Oncol Biol Phys.* 1991;21:1425.

62. Shigematsu Y, Nishiyama K, Masaki N, et al: Treatment of carcinoma of the uterine cervix remotely controlled afterloading intracavitary radiotherapy with high-dose rate: A comparative study with a low-dose rate system. *Int J Radiat Oncol Biol Phys.* 1983;9:351.

63. Patel FD, Sharma SC, Pritam SN, et al: Low dose rate versus high dose rate brachytherapy in the treatment of carcinoma of the uterine cervix: A clinical trial. *Int J Radiat Oncol Biol Phys.* 1993;28:335.

64. Jones GW, Lukka H: HDR versus LDR brachytherapy for squamous cell carcinoma of the cervix. An economic analysis. In Mould RF, ed. *International Brachytherapy.* Veenendaal, The Netherlands: Nucletron; 1992:516.

65. Bastin K, Buchler D, Stitt J, et al: Comparative cost analysis of high dose rate versus low dose rate brachytherapy for gynecological cancer. *Am J Clin Oncol.* 1993;16:256.

66. Creutzberg CL, van Putten WLJ, Koper PCM, et al: Surgery and postoperative radiotherapy versus surgery alone for patients with stage-1 endometrial carcinoma: Multicentre randomised trial. *Lancet.* 2000;355:1404.

67. Aalders J, Abeler V, Kolstad P, et al: Postoperative external irradiation and prognostic parameters in stage I endometrial carcinoma: Clinical and histopathologic study of 540 patients. *Obstet Gynecol.* 1980;56:419.

68. Mandell LM, Nori D, Anderson LL, Hilaris BS: Postoperative vaginal radiation in endometrial cancer using a remote afterloading technique. *Int J Radiat Oncol Biol Phys.* 1985;11:473.

69. Stitt JA: High-dose-rate intracavitary brachytherapy for gynecologic malignancies. *Oncology.* 1992;6:59.

70. Rotte K: Technique and results of HDR afterloading in cancer of the endometrium. In Martinez AA, Orton CG, Mould RF, eds. *Brachytherapy HDR and LDR.* Columbia, Md: Nucletron; 1990:68.

71. Peschel RE, Healey G, Smith RJ: High dose rate remote afterloading for endometrial cancer. *Endo Hyper Oncol.* 1989;5:209.

72. Lybert MLM, van Putten WLJ, Ribot JG, et al: Endometrial carcinoma: High dose rate brachytherapy in combination with external irradiation—A multivariate analysis of relapses. *Radiother Oncol.* 1989;16:245.

73. Sorbe BG, Smeds AC: Postoperative vaginal irradiation with high dose rate afterloading technique in endometrial carcinoma stage I. *Int J Radiat Oncol Biol Phys.* 1990;18:305.

74. Nag S, Erickson B, Parikh S, et al: The American Brachytherapy Society recommendations for HDR brachytherapy for carcinoma of the endometrium. *Int J Radiat Oncol Biol Phys.* 2000;48:779.

75. Rippa P, Seppo K, Kauppila MD: Comparison of Heyman packing and Cathetron afterloading methods in the treatment of endometrial cancer. *Br J Radiol.* 1985;58:437.

76. Stitt JA: Dose specification for inoperable endometrial carcinoma: The Madison system. *Activity/Int Selectron Brachyther J.* 1991;5:32.

77. Kucera H, Weghaupt K: Treatment of inoperable endometrial carcinoma with intracavitary high dose rate iridium irradiation. *Strahlenther Onkol.* 1986;9:508.

78. Taina E: High versus low dose rate intracavitary radiotherapy in the treatment of carcinoma of the uterus. *Acta Obstet Gynecol Scand.* 1981;103:1.

79. Snelling MD, Hambert HE: The treatment of carcinoma of the cervix and endometrium using the Cathetron at the Middlesex Hospital. *Clin Radiol.* 1979;30:253.

80. Sipila P, Kauppila A: Intracavitary irradiation of endometrial carcinoma using a high intensity Co-60 afterloading method. *Acta Oncol.* 1989;28:601.

81. Sorbe B, Frankendal B: Intracavitary irradiation of endometrial carcinoma stage I by a high dose rate afterloading technique. *Gynecol Oncol.* 1989;33:135.

82. Sorbe B, Kjelligren O, Stenson S: Prognosis of endometrial carcinoma stage I in two Swedish regions: A study with special regard to the effects of intracavitary irradiation with high dose rate afterloading technique. *Acta Oncol.* 1990;29:29.

83. Nori D, Stitt JA, Pao L: The role of high dose rate brachytherapy in carcinoma of the endometrium. In Nag S, ed. *High Dose Rate Brachytherapy: A Textbook.* Armonk, N.Y.: Futura Publishing; 1994:385.

84. Chadha M: Gynecologic brachytherapy-II: Intravaginal brachytherapy for carcinoma of the endometrium. *Semin Radiat Oncol.* 2002;12:53.

85. Poulsen MG, Roberts SJ: The salvage of recurrent endometrial carcinoma in the vagina and pelvis. *Int J Radiat Oncol Biol Phys.* 1988;15:809.

86. Sears JD, Greven KM, Hoen HM, et al: Prognostic factors and treatment outcome for patients with locally recurrent endometrial cancer. *Cancer.* 1994;74:1303.

87. Mandell LR, Nori D, Hilaris B: Recurrent stage I endometrial carcinoma: Results of treatment and prognostic factors. *Int J Radiat Oncol Biol Phys.* 1985;6:1103.

88. Reddi RP, Marbach JC: HDR remote afterloading brachytherapy of carcinoma of the lung. *Selectron Brachyther J.* 1992;6:21.

89. Mehta MP, Speiser BL, Macha HN: High dose rate brachytherapy for lung cancer. In Nag S, ed. *High Dose Rate Brachytherapy: A Textbook.* Armonk, N.Y.: Futura Publishing; 1994:237.

90. Aygun C, Weiner S, Scariato A, et al: Treatment of non–small cell lung cancer with external beam radiotherapy and high dose rate brachytherapy. *Int J Radiat Oncol Biol Phys.* 1992;23:127.

91. Bastin KT, Mehta MP, Kinsella TJ: Thoracic volume radiation sparing following endobronchial brachytherapy: A quantitative analysis. *Int J Radiat Oncol Biol Phys.* 1993;25:703.

92. Sutedja T, Zoetmulder F, Zandwijk N: High dose rate brachytherapy improves resectability in squamous cell lung cancer. *Chest.* 1992;102:308.

93. Loeffler EL: Quality control in brachytherapy. In Rotte K and Kiffer J, eds. *Changes in Brachytherapy, Quality Control in Brachytherapy.* Nuremberg, Germany: DE Wacholz KG; 1989.

94. Speiser BL: High dose-rate endobronchial brachytherapy: Whither goest thou? *Int J Radiat Oncol Biol Phys.* 1992;23:250.

95. Speiser BL, Spratling L: Remote afterloading brachytherapy for the local control of endobronchial carcinoma. *Int J Radiat Oncol Biol Phys.* 1993;25:579.

96. Nag S, Gupta N: A simple method of obtaining equivalent doses for use in HDR brachytherapy. *Int J Radiat Oncol Biol Phys.* 2000;46:507.

97. Nag S, Kelly JF, Horton JL, et al: The American Brachytherapy Society recommendations for HDR brachytherapy for carcinoma of the lung. *Oncology.* 2001;15:371.

98. Aygun C, Weiner S, Scariato A, et al: Treatment of non–small cell lung cancer with external beam radiotherapy and high dose rate brachytherapy. *Int J Radiat Oncol Biol Phys.* 1992;23:127.

99. Bedwinek J, Petty A, Bruton C, et al: The use of high dose rate endobronchial brachytherapy to palliate symptomatic endobronchial recurrence of previously irradiated bronchogenic carcinoma. *Int J Radiat Oncol Biol Phys.* 1992;22:23.

100. Burt PA, O'Driscoll BR, Notley HM, et al: Intraluminal irradiation for the palliation of lung cancer with high dose rate microselectron. *Thorax.* 1990;45:765.

101. Chang LFL, Horvath J, Peyton W: High dose rate afterloading intraluminal brachytherapy in malignant airway obstruction of lung cancer. *Int J Radiat Oncol Biol Phys.* 1994;28:589.

102. Delclos ME, Komaki R, Garden A, et al: High dose rate remote afterloading endobronchial brachytherapy for recurrent endobronchial lesions. *Radiology*. 1996;281:279.

103. Macha HN, Wahlers B, Reichle C, et al: Endobronchial radiation therapy for obstructing malignancies: Ten years' experience with iridium-192 high-dose radiation brachytherapy afterloading technique in 365 patients. *Lung*. 1995;173:271.

104. Miller JI, Jr, Phillips TW: Neodymium:YAG laser and brachytherapy in the management of inoperable bronchogenic carcinoma. *Ann Thorac Surg*. 1990;50:190.

105. Speiser B, Spratling L. Intermediate dose rate remote afterloading brachytherapy for intraluminal control of bronchogenic carcinoma. *Int J Radiat Oncol Biol Phys*. 1990;18:1443.

106. Stout R, Barber PV, Burt PA, et al: Intraluminal brachytherapy in bronchial carcinoma. *Br J Radiol*. 1990;63:16 [abstract].

107. Sutedja G, Baris G, Schaake-Koning C, et al: High dose rate brachytherapy in patients with local recurrence after radiotherapy of non–small cell lung cancer. *Int J Radiat Oncol Biol Phys*. 1992;24:551.

108. Cotter GW, Craig L, Ellingwood KE, et al: Inoperable endobronchial obstructing lung cancer treated with combined endobronchial and external beam irradiation: A dosimetric analysis. *Int J Radiat Oncol Biol Phys*. 1993;27:531.

109. Huber RM, Fischer R, Hautmann H, et al: Does additional brachytherapy improve the effect of external irradiation? A prospective, randomized study in central lung tumors. *Int J Radiat Oncol Biol Phys*. 1997;38:533.

110. Reddi RP, Marbach JC: HDR remote afterloading brachytherapy of carcinoma of the lung. *Selectron Brachyther J*. 1992;6:21.

111. Perol M, Caliandro R, Pommier P, et al: Curative irradiation of limited endobronchial carcinomas with high-dose-rate brachytherapy. Results of a pilot study. *Chest*. 1997;111:1417.

112. Saito M, Yokoyama A, Kurita Y, et al: Treatment of roentgenographically occult endobronchial with external beam radiotherapy and intraluminal low dose rate brachytherapy: second report. *Int J Radiat Oncol Biol Phys*. 2000;47:673.

113. Sutedja G, Baris G, van Zandwijk N: High dose rate brachytherapy has a curative potential in patients with intraluminal squamous cell lung cancer. *Respiration*. 1994;61:167.

114. Tredaniel J, Hennequin C, Zalcman G, et al: Prolonged survival after high dose rate endobronchial radiation for malignant airway obstruction. *Chest*. 1994;105:767.

115. Marsiglia H, Baldeyrou P, Lartigau E, et al: High-dose-rate brachytherapy as a sole modality for early-stage endobronchial carcinoma. *Int J Radiat Oncol Biol Phys*. 2000;47:665.

116. Speiser BL, Spartling L: Radiation bronchitis and stenosis secondary to high dose rate endobronchial irradiation. *Int J Radiat Oncol Biol Phys*. 1993;25:589.

117. Speiser B, Spratling L: Fatal hemoptysis: Complication or failure of treatment. *Int J Radiat Oncol Biol Phys*. 1993;25:925 [Letter].

118. Bedwinek J, Petty A, Bruton C, et al: The use of high dose rate endobronchial brachytherapy to palliate symptomatic endobronchial recurrence of previously irradiated bronchogenic carcinoma. *Int J Radiat Oncol Biol Phys*. 1991;22:23.

119. Khanavkar B, Stern P, Alberti W, et al: Complications associated with brachytherapy alone or with laser in lung cancer. *Chest*. 1991;99:1062.

120. Mehta MP, Speiser BL, Macha HN: High dose rate brachytherapy for lung cancer. In Nag S, ed. *High Dose Rate Brachytherapy: A Textbook*. Armonk, N.Y.: Futura Publishing; 1994:237.

121. Herskovic A, Martz K, Al-Sarraf A, et al: Combined chemotherapy and radiotherapy compared with radiotherapy alone in patients with cancer of the esophagus. *N Engl J Med*. 1992;326:1593.

122. Gasper LE, Winter K, Kocha WI, et al: A phase I/II study of external beam radiation, brachytherapy, and concurrent chemotherapy for patients with localized carcinoma of the esophagus (Radiation Therapy Oncology Group Study 9207). *Cancer*. 2000;88:988.

123. Gasper LE, Winter K, Kocha WI, et al: Swallowing function and weight change observed in a phase I/II study of external-beam radiation, brachytherapy and concurrent chemotherapy in localized cancer of the esophagus (RTOG 9207). *Cancer: Sci Ameri J*. 2001;7:388.

124. Gaspar L: Radiation therapy for esophageal cancer: Improving the therapeutic ratio. *Semin Oncol*. 1994;4:192.

125. Gaspar LE, Nag S, Herskovic A, et al: American Brachytherapy Society (ABS) Consensus Guidelines for Brachytherapy of Esophageal Cancer. *Int J Radiat Oncol Biol Phys*. 1997;38:127.

126. Zhao R-F, Zhang PH, Wang HG, et al: Combination of external irradiation and intracavitary cesium-37 radiotherapy for esophageal carcinoma. *Chin J Radiat Oncol Phys Biol*. 1990;2:85.

127. Flores AD, Rowland CG, Yin W-B: High-dose rate brachytherapy of carcinoma of the esophagus. In Nag S, ed. *High Dose Rate Brachytherapy: A Textbook*. Armonk, N.Y.: Futura Publishing; 1994:275.

128. Sur RK, Kochar R, Negi PS, Gupta BD: High dose rate intraluminal brachytherapy in palliation of esophageal carcinoma. *Endocuriether Hypertherm Oncol Int J*. 1994;10:25.

129. Flores A, Nelems B, Evans K, et al: The impact of new radiotherapy modalities on the surgical management of cancer of the esophagus and cardia. *Int J Radiat Oncol Biol Phys*. 1989;17:937.

130. Rowland CG, Pagliero KM: Intracavitary irradiation in palliation of carcinoma of the esophagus and cardia. *Lancet*. 1985;2:981.

131. Hishikawa Y, Kamikonya N, Tanaka S, et al: Radiotherapy or esophageal carcinoma: Role of high dose rate intracavitary irradiation. *Radiother Oncol*. 1987;9:13.

132. Holm H, Juul N, Pedersen J, et al: Transperineal iodine-125 seed implantation in prostate cancer guided by transrectal ultrasonography. *J Urol*. 1983;130:283.

133. Demanes J, Rodriguez RR, Altieri GA: High dose rate prostate brachytherapy: The California Endocurietherapy (CET) Method. *Radiother Oncol*. 2000;57:289.

134. Edmundson G, Rizzo N, Teahan M, et al: Concurrent Treatment Planning for Outpatient High Dose Rate Prostate Template Implants. *Int J Radiat Oncol Biol Phys*. 1993;27:1215.

135. Mate TP, Gottesman JE, Hatton J, et al: High dose-rate afterloading 192Iridium prostate brachytherapy: Feasibility report. *Int J Radiat Oncol Biol Phys*. 1998;41:525.

136. Kolkman-Deurloo IKK, Visser AG, Niël CGJH, et al: Optimization of interstitial volume implants. *Radiother Oncol*. 1994;31:229.

137. Lessard E, Pouliot J: Inverse planning anatomy-based dose optimization for HDR-brachytherapy of the prostate using fast simulated annealing algorithm and dedicated objective function. *Med Phys*. 2001;28:773.

138. Taschereau R, Roy J, Pouliot J: Monte Carlo simulations of prostate implants to improve dosimetry and compare planning methods. *Med Phys*. 1999;26:1952.

139. Hsu I-C, Pickett B, Shinohara K, et al: Normal tissue dosimetric comparison between HDR prostate implant boost and conformal external beam radiotherapy boost: Potential for dose escalation. *Int J Radiat Oncol Biol Phys*. 2000;46:851.

140. Fu KK, Pajak TF, Trotti A, et al: A Radiation Therapy Oncology Group (RTOG) phase III randomized study to compare hyperfractionation and two variants of accelerated fractionation to standard fractionation radiotherapy for head and neck squamous cell carcinomas: First report of RTOG 9003 [see comments]. *Int J Radiat Oncol Biol Phys*. 2000;48:7.

141. Horiot JC, Bontemps P, van den Bogaert W, et al: Accelerated fractionation (AF) compared to conventional fractionation (CF) improves loco-regional control in the radiotherapy of advanced head and neck cancers: Results of the EORTC 22851 randomized trial [see comments]. *Radiother Oncol*. 1997;44:111.

142. Brenner D, Hall E: Fractionation and protraction for radiotherapy of prostate carcinoma. *Int J Radiat Oncol Biol Phys*. 1999; 43:1095.

143. King CR, Fowler JF: A simple analytic derivation suggests that prostate cancer alpha/beta ratio is low. [Comment In: *Int J Radiat Oncol Biol Phys*. 2001;51:1 UI: 21407940]. *Int J Radiat Oncol Biol Phys*. 2001;51:213.

144. Fowler J, Chappell R, Ritter M: Is alpha/beta for prostate tumors really low? *Int J Radiat Oncol Biol Phys*. 2001;50:1021.

145. Brenner D, Martinez AA, Edmundson G, et al: Direct evidence that prostate tumors show high sensitivity to fractionation (low a/b ratio), similar to late-responding normal tissue. *Int J Radiat Oncol Biol Phys*. 2002;52:6.

146. D'Souza WD, Thames HD: Is the alpha/beta ratio for prostate cancer low? [Comment on: *Int J Radiat Oncol Biol Phys.* 2001;51:213 UI: 21407968]. *Int J Radiat Oncol Biol Phys.* 2001;51:1.

147. Duchesne GM, Peters LJ: What is the alpha/beta ratio for prostate cancer? Rationale for hypofractionated high-dose-rate brachytherapy [editorial]. *Int J Radiat Oncol Biol Phys.* 1999;44:747.

148. Fowler JF, Chappell RJ, Ritter MA: The prospects for new treatments for prostate cancer. *Int J Radiat Oncol Biol Phys.* 2002;52:3.

149. Borghede G, Hedelin H, Holmäng S, et al: Irradiation of localized prostatic carcinoma with a combination of high dose rate iridium-192 brachytherapy and external beam radiotherapy with three target definitions and dose levels inside the prostate gland. *Radiother Oncol.* 1997;44:245.

150. Borghede G, Hedelin H, Holmäng S, et al: Combined treatment with temporary short-term high dose rate iridium-192 brachytherapy and external beam radiotherapy for irradiation of localized prostatic carcinoma. *Radiother Oncol.* 1997;44:237.

151. Dinges S, Deger S, Koswig S, et al: High-dose rate interstitial with external beam irradiation for localized prostate cancer—Results of a prospective trial. *Radiother Oncol.* 1998;48:197.

152. Dinges S, Loening SA, Budach V: [Combined iridium 192 afterloading therapy of prostate carcinoma]. *Schweizerische Rundschau für Medizin Praxis.* 1997;86:1908.

153. Kestin LL, Martinez AA, Stromberg JS, et al: Matched-pair analysis of conformal high-dose-rate brachytherapy boost versus external-beam radiation therapy alone for locally advanced prostate cancer. *J Clin Oncol.* 2000;18:2869.

154. Martinez A, Gonzalez J, Stromberg J, et al: Conformal prostate brachytherapy: Initial experience of a phase I/II dose-escalating trial. *Int J Radiat Oncol Biol Phys.* 1995;33:1019.

155. Martinez AA, Kestin LL, Stromberg JS, et al: Interim report of image-guided conformal high-dose-rate brachytherapy for patients with unfavorable prostate cancer: The William Beaumont phase II dose-escalating trial. *Int J Radiat Oncol Biol Phys.* 2000;47:343.

156. Martinez AA, Pataki I, Edmundson G, et al: Phase II prospective study of the use of conformal high-dose-rate brachytherapy as monotherapy for the treatment of favorable stage prostate cancer: A feasibility report. *Int J Radiat Oncol Biol Phys.* 2001;49:61.

157. Kovács G, Galalae R, Loch T, et al: Prostate preservation by combined external beam and HDR brachytherapy in nodal negative prostate cancer. *Strahlenther Onkol.* 1999;175:87.

158. Kovacs G, Wirth B, Bertermann H, et al: Prostate preservation by combined external beam and HDR brachytherapy at nodal negative prostate cancer patients—An intermediate analysis after ten years experience. *Int J Radiat Oncol Biol Phys.* 1996;36:198.

159. Stromberg JS, Martinez AA, Horwitz EM, et al: Conformal high dose rate iridium-192 boost brachytherapy in locally advanced prostate cancer: Superior prostate-specific antigen response compared with external beam treatment [see comments]. *Cancer J Scientific Amer.* 1997;3:346.

160. Galalae RM, Kovacs G, Schultze J, et al: Long-term outcome after elective irradiation of the pelvic lymphatics and local dose escalation using high-dose-rate brachytherapy for locally advanced prostate cancer. *Int J Radiat Oncol Biol Phys.* 2002;52:81.

161. Stromberg J, Martinez A, Gonzalez J, et al: Ultrasound-guided high dose rate conformal brachytherapy boost in prostate cancer: Treatment description and preliminary results of a phase I/II clinical trial. *Int J Radiat Oncol Biol Phys.* 1995;33:161.

162. Rodriguez RR, Nag S, Mate TP, et al: American Brachytherapy Society recommendatuions for high dose rate brachytherapy for prostate cancer. *J Brachyther.* 2002;17:265-282.

163. Yoshioka Y, Nose T, Yoshida K, et al: High-dose-rate interstitial brachytherapy as a monotherapy for localized prostate cancer: Treatment description and preliminary results of a phase I/II clinical trial. *Int J Radiat Oncol Biol Phys.* 2000;48:675.

164. Nag S, Tai DL, Gold RE: Biliary tract neoplasms: A simple management technique. *South Med J.* 1984;77:593.

165. Herskovic A, Heaston D, Engler MJ, et al: Irradiation of biliary carcinoma. *Radiology.* 1981;139:219.

166. Haffty BG, Mate TP, Greenwood LH, et al: Malignant biliary obstruction: Intracavitary treatment with a high-dose-rate remote afterloading device. *Radiology.* 1987;164:574.

167. Urban MS, Siegel JH, Pavlou W, et al: Treatment of malignant biliary obstruction with a high-dose rate remote afterloading device using a 10F nasobiliary tube. *Gastrointest Endosc.* 1990;36:292.

168. Lu JJ, Bains YS, Abdel-Wahab M, et al: High-dose-rate remote afterloading intracavitary brachytherapy for the treatment of extrahepatic biliary duct carcinoma. *Cancer: Sci Ameri J.* 2002;8:74.

169. Dixit S, Baboo HA, Rakesh V, et al: Interstitial high dose rate brachytherapy in head and neck cancers: Preliminary results. *J Brachyther Int.* 1997;13:363.

170. Lau HY, Hay JH, Flores AD, et al: Seven fractions of twice daily high dose-rate brachytherapy for node-negative carcinoma of the mobile tongue results in loss of therapeutic ratio. *Radiother Oncol.* 1996;39:15.

171. Inoue T, Yamazaki H, et al: Phase III trial of high and low dose rate interstitial radiotherapy for early oral tongue cancer. *Int J Radiat Oncol Biol Phys.* 1996;36:1201.

172. Donath D, Vuong T, Shnouda G, et al: The potential uses of high-dose-rate brachytherapy in patients with head and neck cancer. *Eur Arch Otorhinolaryngol.* 1995;252:321.

173. Leung TW, Wong VYW, Wong CM, et al: Technical hints for high dose rate interstitial tongue brachytherapy. *Clin Oncol.* 1998;10:231.

174. Yu L, Vikram B, Chadha M, et al: High dose rate interstitial brachytherapy in patients with cancers of the head and neck. *Endocurietherapy/Hyperthermia Oncol.* 1996;12:1.

175. Mazeron JJ, Noel G, Simon JM: Head and neck brachytherapy. *Semin Radiat Oncol.* 2002;12:95.

176. Levendeg PC, Peters R, Meeuwis CA, et al: A new applicator design for endocavitary brachytherapy of nasopharynx. *Radiother Oncol.* 1997;45:95.

177. Jolly DE, Nag S: Technique for construction of dental molds for high-dose-rate remote brachytherapy. *Spec Care Dent.* 1992;12(5):219-334.

178. Nag S, Vikram B, Demanes JD, et al: The American Brachytherapy Society recommendations for HDR brachytherapy for head and neck carcinoma. *Int J Radiat Oncol Biol Phys.* 2001;50:1190.

179. Nag S, Dixit S, Mountain R, Schuller D: Intraoperative high dose rate brachytherapy of head and neck cancer. *Radiother Oncol.* 1994;31:S30.

180. Nag S, Schuller D, Pak V, et al: Pilot study of intraoperative high dose rate brachytherapy for head and neck cancer. *Radiother Oncol.* 1996;41:125.

181. Alekhteyar KM, Porter AT, Ryan C, et al: Preliminary results of hyperfractionated high dose rate brachytherapy in soft-tissue sarcoma. *Endocuriether Hypertherm Oncol Int J.* 1993;9:56 [abstract].

182. Donath D, Clark C, Kaufmann MD, et al: Postoperative adjuvant high dose rate brachytherapy in the treatment of poor-prognosis soft-tissue sarcoma. *Endocuriether Hypertherm Oncol Int J.* 1993;9:48 [abstract].

183. Nag S, Porter AT, Donath D: The role of high dose rate brachytherapy in the management of adult soft tissue sarcomas. In Nag S, ed. *High Dose Rate Brachytherapy: A Textbook.* Armonk, N.Y.: Futura Publishing; 1994:393.

184. Chuba R, Ben-Josef EB, Porter AT, et al: Adjuvant brachytherapy for primary and recurrent soft tissue sarcoma at WSU. *Radiother Oncol.* 1996;39:S4 [abstract].

185. Crownover RL, Marks KE, Zehr RJ: Initial results with high dose rate brachytherapy for soft-tissue sarcomas. *Sarcoma.* 1997;1:196.

186. Koizumi M, Inoue T, Yamazaki H, et al: Perioperative fractionated high-dose rate brachytherapy for malignant bone and soft tissue tumors. *Int J Radiat Oncol Biol Phys.* 1999;43:989.

187. Yoshida K, Inoue T, Kuizumi M, et al: Perioperative high dose rate brachytherapy for bone and soft tissue tumors. *Nippon Acta Radiologica (Tokyo).* 1996;41:1635.

188. Nag S, Shasha D, Janjan N, et al: The American Brachytherapy Society recommendations for brachytherapy of soft tissue sarcomas. *Int J Radiat Oncol Biol Phys.* 2001;49:1033.

189. Flamant F, Gerbaulet A, Nihoul-Fekete C, et al: Long-term sequelae of conservative treatment by surgery, brachytherapy and chemotherapy for vulval and vaginal rhabdomyosarcoma in children. *J Clin Oncol.* 1990;8:1847.

190. Fontanesi J, Kun L, Pao W, et al: Brachytherapy as primary or "boost" irradiation in 18 children with solid tumors. *Endocuriether Hypertherm Oncol Int J.* 1991;7:195.

191. Gerbaulet AP, Esche BA, Hail CM, et al: Conservative treatment for lower gynecological tract malignancies in children and adolescents: The Institut Gustave-Roussy experience. *Int J Radiat Oncol Biol Phys.* 1989;16:655.

192. Nag S, Grecula JC, Ruymann F: Aggressive chemotherapy, organ preserving surgery, and high dose rate remote brachytherapy in the treatment of rhabdomyosarcoma in infants and young children. *Cancer.* 1993;72:2769.

193. Nag S, Fernandes PS, Martínez-Monge R, Ruymann FB: Use of brachytherapy to preserve function in children with soft-tissue sarcomas. *Oncology.* 1999;13:361.

194. Nag S, Olson T, Ruymann F, et al: High dose rate brachytherapy in childhood sarcomas: A local control strategy preserving bone growth and function. *Med Ped Oncol.* 1995;25:463.

195. Bartelink H, Horiot JC, Poortmans P, et al: Recurrence rates after treatment of breast cancer with standard radiotherapy with or without additional radiation. *N Engl J Med.* 2001;345:1378.

196. Vicini F, Baglan K, Kestin L, et al: The emerging role of brachytherapy in the management of patients with breast cancer. *Semin Radiat Oncol.* 2002;12:31.

197. Nag S, Kuske RR, Vicini F, et al: The American Brachytherapy Society recommendations for carcinoma of the breast. *Oncology.* 2001;15:195.

198. Kuske RR, Bolton JS, McKinnon WMP, et al: 5-year results of a prospective phase II trial of wide-volume brachytherapy as the sole method of breast irradiation in $T_{is}, T_1, T_2, N_{0-1}$ breast cancer. *Proc of 40th Annual ASTRO Meeting.* 1998;113:181.

199. Kuske RR, Bolton JS, Wilinzick RM, et al: Brachytherapy as the sole method of breast irradiation in TIS, T1, T2N0-1 breast cancer. *Int J Radiat Oncol Biol Phys.* 1994;30:245.

200. Vicini FA, Baglan KL, Kestin LL, et al: Accelerated treatment of breast cancer. *J Clin Oncol.* 2001;19:1993.

201. Kestin LL, Jaffray DA, Edmundson GK, et al: Improving the dosimetric coverage of interstitial high-dose-rate breast implants. *Int J Radiat Oncol Biol Phys.* 2000;46:35.

202. Vicini FA, Kestin JS, Kuske RR, et al: Dose-volume analysis for quality assurance of interstitial brachytherapy for breast cancer. *Int J Radiat Oncol Biol Phys.* 1999;45:803.

203. Ribeiro GG, Magee B, Swindell R, et al: The Christie Hospital breast conservation trial: An update at 8 years from inception. *Clin Oncol (R Coll Radiol).* 1993;5:278.

204. Magee B, Swindell R, Harris M, et al: Prognostic factors for breast recurrence after conservative breast surgery and radiotherapy: Results from a randomized trial. *Radiother Oncol.* 1996;39:223.

205. Kuske RR, Bolton JS, McKinnon WMP, et al: 5-year results of a prospective trial of wide-volume brachytherapy as the sole method of breast irradiation in TIS, T1, T2, N0-1 breast cancer. *Int J Radiat Oncol Biol Phys.* 1998;42:181.

206. King TA, Bolton JS, Kuske RR, et al: Long-term results of wide-field brachytherapy as the sole method of radiation therapy after segmental mastectomy for TIS,1,2) breast cancer. *Am J Surg.* 2000;180:299.

207. Nag S, Tippin D, Ruymann FB: Intraoperative high-dose-rate brachytherapy for the treatment of pediatric soft tissue sarcomas. *Int J Radiat Oncol Biol Phys.* 2000;51:729-735.

208. Nori D, Williams H: Intraoperative brachytherapy: Rationale and future directions. In Mould RF, ed. *International Brachytherapy Programme & Abstracts, 7th International Brachytherapy Working Conference.* Baltimore, Md., 6-8 September, 1992. Veenendaal, The Netherlands: Nucletron International; 1992:132.

209. Nag S, Orton C: Development of intraoperative high dose rate brachytherapy for treatment of resected tumor beds in anesthetized patients. *Endocuriether Hypertherm Oncol Int J.* 1993;9:187.

210. Dritschilo A, Harter KW, Thomas D, et al: Intraoperative radiation therapy of hepatic metastases: Technical aspects and report of a pilot study. *Int J Radiat Oncol Biol Phys.* 1988;14:1007.

211. Lukas P, Kneschaurek P, Ries G, et al: A new modality for intra-operative radiotherapy using a high dose rate afterloading unit. In *Proceedings of Sixth International High Dose Rate Remote Afterloading Conference, Budapest, Hungary, May 2-4, 1991.* South China, Maine: Health Service Consultants; 1991:62.

212. Abitbol A, Lewin A, Brown W, et al: Video-assisted thoracoscopic limited resection and high-dose-rate brachytherapy of non–small cell carcinoma of the lung: Rationale and technical considerations. In Brown WT, ed. *Atlas of Video-Assisted Thoracic Surgery.* Philadelphia: WB Saunders; 1994:236.

Total Body Irradiation

Brenda Shank, MD, PhD, FACR

14

RATIONALE

Purposes of Total Body Irradiation

Total body irradiation (TBI) and other large-field variations, such as total lymphoid irradiation (TLI) and total abdominal irradiation (TAI), have played an important role in preparative cytoreductive regimens for bone marrow transplantation (BMT). There are three main purposes of TBI: immunosuppression (lymphocyte cell kill) to allow engraftment of donor marrow; eradication of malignant cells (leukemias, lymphomas, and some solid tumors); and eradication of cell populations with genetic disorders (e.g., Fanconi's anemia, thalassemia major).

Advantages of Total Body Irradiation Compared with Chemotherapy

There are many theoretical advantages of TBI as a systemic agent when compared with chemotherapy: (1) there is no sparing of "sanctuary" sites such as the testes; (2) the dose delivered is fairly homogeneous and independent of blood supply; (3) there is no cross-resistance with other agents; (4) since no detoxification or excretion of a chemical agent is necessary, there is no alteration of dose if these mechanisms are impaired; and (5) the dose distribution within the body may be tailored by either blocking normal tissues that are more sensitive or "boosting" areas at greater risk of recurrence.

Because of the toxicity of the high TBI doses that would be required to immunosuppress adequately for consistent donor marrow engraftment, and to eradicate malignancies sufficiently to obtain cures, TBI has been combined with chemotherapeutic agents. Most commonly in leukemias, cyclophosphamide (Cy) has been used, with the most frequently used schedule being 60 mg/kg per day for 2 days, either before or after TBI. Etoposide (VP-16) has also been frequently used, either instead of Cy or in addition to Cy.

More recently, TBI has been used in nonmyeloablative doses (1 to 2 Gy) along with immunotherapy (donor lymphocyte infusions [DLI]) to achieve marrow chimeras and even sustained remissions in some leukemia patients after autologous grafting.

Current Cytoreductive Therapy Usage

From data published by the International Bone Marrow Transplant Registry (IBMTR), the majority of allogeneic marrow transplants (73%) are performed for leukemia.[1] Other malignancies make up 10% and aplastic anemia, 8%, with the remainder for genetic disorders and immune deficiencies. TBI has been a major component of most regimens for leukemia, although many centers have been investigating the use of alternative chemotherapy-only regimens with some success. Because of the continued widespread use of TBI for the leukemias, however, the use of this modality for the leukemias is emphasized in this chapter. Also included are some of the important results in other diseases. Examples of TBI usage are listed in Table 14-1.

Table 14–1 Diseases in Which Total Body Irradiation or Other Large Fields Are Used for Marrow Transplantation

Malignant

Leukemias
    Acute lymphoblastic leukemia*
    Acute myeloid leukemia*
    Chronic myeloid leukemia*
    Hairy cell leukemia
Lymphomas or other myeloproliferative diseases
    Non-Hodgkin's lymphoma*
    Refractory Hodgkin's disease (no or minimal prior irradiation)
    Myelodysplasia
    Multiple myeloma
Pediatric solid tumors
    Neuroblastoma
    Ewing's sarcoma
Adult solid tumors
    Small cell carcinoma of lung
    Testicular carcinoma

Non-Malignant

Immune disorders
    Aplastic anemia (total lymphoid irradiation)
Genetic disorders
    Osteopetrosis
    Wiskott-Aldrich syndrome
    Thrombocytopenia-absent radii syndrome
    Fanconi's anemia (total abdominal irradiation)

*Most common.

In addition, the indications for the use of TAI and TLI are covered. These fields are often adequate when only immunosuppression is needed, as for aplastic anemia, or when only nodal areas need to be treated, as in refractory Hodgkin's disease without marrow involvement.

Many investigators have been looking at alternative regimens containing only chemotherapy for cytoreduction, to avoid the toxicities attributed to TBI.[2] Although various regimens have been tried, the most common alternative in patients with leukemia has been the use of busulfan (Bu), in various doses, to replace TBI.[3] However, other toxicities are associated with such regimens, such as seizures,[4] a high incidence (19%) of veno-occlusive disease (VOD) compared with TBI/Cy (1%),[5] and a high incidence (30%) of hemorrhagic cystitis compared with TBI/Cy (14%).[5] The incidence of fatal interstitial pneumonitis (IP), however, appears to be low compared with that from TBI/Cy (5% vs. 32%) in patients who had received prior thoracic irradiation to doses greater than 20 Gy.[6] Growth in children given Bu/Cy was found to be no better than that in children who received TBI/Cy in a study from Johns Hopkins.[7]

Nonrandomized data collected by IBMTR suggest very little difference between these two types of regimens in disease-free survival in any of the leukemias.[2] An analysis of 123 patients in the Japanese Bone Marrow Transplant Registry indicated a decreased relapse rate (16% vs. 37%) and improved overall survival (77% vs. 51%) with TBI-containing regimens (mostly TBI/Cy) compared with chemotherapy-only regimens (mostly Bu/Cy).[8]

Several randomized studies have compared Bu/Cy with TBI-containing regimens (Table 14-2).[9-19] In a French multi-institutional study (Group d'Études de la Greffe de Moelle Osseuse [GEGMO]),[9] there was an advantage to the TBI/Cy regimen over Bu/Cy in acute myeloid leukemia (AML) patients in first remission, in terms of relapse rate, overall and disease-free survival, and mortality. A long-term follow-up of four randomized studies for myeloid leukemia, which included this GEGMO study, still demonstrated a 10% lower survival rate after Bu/Cy compared with TBI/Cy, but the difference was not statistically significant.[20] A randomized study of TBI/Cy versus Bu/Cy for autologous purged marrow transplants in AML patients demonstrated that for all endpoints (relapse, relapse-free survival, overall survival, and incidence of VOD), TBI/Cy was equivalent to or better than Bu/Cy, although with only 35 patients randomized, none of these reached statistical significance.[21]

Table 14-2 Randomized Studies Comparing Total Body Irradiation–Containing Regimens with Busulfan–Cyclophosphamide for Conventional Allogeneic Bone Marrow Transplantation

Disease/Stage	Regimen	Patients, n	Time of Analysis, yr	Disease-Free Survival, %	Actuarial Overall Survival, %	Actuarial Relapse, %	Reference
AML-1st (GEGMO)	TBI/Cy	50	2	72 ($P < 0.01$)	75 ($P < 0.02$)	14 ($P < 0.04$)	Blaise et al.[9]
	Bu/Cy	51	2	47	51	34	
CML-CP (Seattle)	TBI/Cy	66	3	—	80 (NS)	13 (NS)	Clift et al.[10,11,12]
	Bu/Cy	68	3	—	78	11	
Acute leukemia >1st and CML >1st CP (SWOG)	TBI/VP16	61	3	25	52*/11† (NS)*/(NS)†	—	Blume et al.[13]
	Bu/Cy	61	3	28	37*/24†	—	
CML-CP (GEGMO)	TBI/Cy	56	2	— (NS)	— (NS)	11‡, 31§ ($P = 0.04$)	Cosset et al.[14]; Devergie et al.[15]
	Bu/Cy	66	2	—	—	4	
CML-CP (Berlin)	TBI/Cy	16	2	—	63 ($P = 0.24$)	—	Schwerdtfeger et al.[16]
	Bu/Cy	16	2	—	81	—	
CML-CP (Baltimore)	TBI/Cy	18	1.7	56 (NS)	56 (NS)	0	Miller et al.[17]
	Bu/Cy	19	1.7	52	52	0	
Acute leukemia/CML Early disease	TBI/Cy	61	7	66 (NS)	67 (NS)	27 (NS)	Ringden et al.[18,19]
	Bu/Cy	59	7	68	72	21	
Late disease (Nordic BMTG)	TBI/Cy	18	7	49 ($P = 0.09$)	49 ($P = 0.05$)	36 (NS)	
	Bu/Cy	29	7	17	17	50	

*"Good-risk" patients.
†"Bad-risk" patients.
‡Single-dose TBI (11%).
§Fractionated TBI (31%).
AML, acute myeloid leukemia; BMTG, Bone Marrow Transplant Group; Bu, busulfan; CML, chronic myeloid leukemia; CP, chronic phase; Cy, cyclophosphamide; GEGMO, Croup d'Etude de la Greffe de Moelle Osseuse; NS, not statistically significant; SWOG, Southwest Oncology Group; TBI, total body irradiation; VP-16, etoposide; 1st, first remission.

When these randomized patients were analyzed in combination with 40 nonrandomized AML patients, there was a statistically significant improvement in disease-free survival at 2 years (*P* = 0.04) in the TBI/Cy subset of patients who were in second or later remission (38% vs. 7%).[22]

In chronic myeloid leukemia (CML), TBI-containing regimens appear to be equivalent to Bu/Cy in five randomized studies[10-17] in terms of disease-free and overall survival; however, in the GEGMO study,[14,15] TBI/Cy showed a trend toward a better engraftment rate (*P* = 0.06), and the relapse rate was higher (*P* = 0.04) in the TBI/Cy arms (11% for single-dose TBI and 31% for fractionated TBI) when compared with the Bu/Cy arm (4%), although this was not reflected in either disease-free survival or overall survival rates. It should be noted that the SWOG study[13] also included acute leukemia patients in greater than first remission as well as CML patients in greater than first chronic phase. The Nordic study,[18,19] however, favored TBI/Cy over Bu/Cy in advanced disease patients, with highly significant differences out to 7 years in both overall and disease-free survival rates.

Many other chemotherapeutical agents have been used with or without TBI for cytoreduction before transplant. Most frequently used have been etoposide (VP-16)[23] or cytosine arabinoside (AraC).[24] Further discussion of these agents follows in the section regarding the interaction with chemotherapy under "Biological Principles"; these agents and others have been reviewed in detail elsewhere.[2,25]

BIOLOGIC PRINCIPLES

In Vitro Data

NORMAL LYMPHOCYTES

Immunosuppression, the clinical manifestation of reduced lymphocyte numbers or activity, is one of the important functions of TBI. Cell culture studies, supported by studies of lymphocyte survival in vivo, demonstrate either no or a very small shoulder on the cell survival curve, indicating minimal repair.[26,27] The slope of the survival curve has varied in different studies, but there has been a trend toward a lesser radiosensitivity for T lymphocytes compared with B lymphocytes.

Lymphocyte survival in patients undergoing TBI appears similar to the in vitro data; one study of the decrease in absolute lymphocyte concentration during the course of a hyperfractionated TBI regimen showed no shoulder to the survival curve and an *effective* D_0 of about 3.8 Gy, where *effective* D_0 was defined as the fractionated dose required by a given regimen to reduce the cell population to 37% in the straight line portion of the survival curve.[28]

LEUKEMIC CELLS

Leukemic cells have also been considered to demonstrate either no shoulder or a minimal shoulder on the cell survival curve. Since many investigators have studied survival in various leukemic cells, there are now sufficient data to indicate the following: (1) the shoulder and slope of survival curves vary widely for different cell types and for different cell lines from the same type of leukemia;[29,30] (2) some cell lines show no repair at all, whereas others exhibit definite repair;[30-32] and (3) most human hematopoietic cell lines studied have survival curves that fit the linear quadratic (LQ) model of cell survival.[30,32]

When survival was studied in a human acute lymphoblastic leukemia (ALL) cell line (Reh), using a common TBI hyperfractionation regimen (1.25 Gy/fraction, three fractions per day), the resulting survival curve could be readily explained by complete repair between fractions and minimal regrowth between fractions.[32] The single-dose survival curve in this cell system fit the LQ model, with a continuously downward curving shape.

Animal Data

IMMUNOSUPPRESSION

In marrow transplantation, the degree of immunosuppression is reflected clinically in the success of engraftment of donor marrow. It was shown in dogs that the rate of engraftment increases with increasing doses of irradiation.[33,34] Furthermore, single-dose irradiation was more immunosuppressive in dogs than fractionated irradiation, for the same total dose.[34] Other studies in mice, rats, and monkeys also show that, with fractionated irradiation, higher total doses are necessary for engraftment with single-dose irradiation.[35,36]

In one murine study,[37] both low-dose-rate, single-dose TBI (0.05 Gy/minute) and fractionated TBI required higher total doses for engraftment compared with high-dose-rate, single-dose TBI (1 Gy/minute); increasing the interval between fractions from 6 to 24 hours required an additional dose increase. In another murine study, low-dose-rate, single-dose TBI (0.04 Gy/minute) to 7.5 Gy total dose was equivalent to a hyperfractionated TBI schedule of 1.25 Gy three times a day to the same total dose, in terms of the effect on the hemopoietic system.[38] No significant repopulation between fractions was seen with the fractionated course.

A murine study across various degrees of genetic disparity between donor and host demonstrated that engraftment depends critically on the TBI dose; the required TBI dose increased with greater genetic disparity.[39] Although one might expect that donor T cells might suppress host marrow and, therefore, enhance engraftment, another murine study showed that the addition of an increasing number of donor T cells did not affect the TBI dose required to achieve equivalent erythroid engraftment.[40]

LEUKEMIA

One important question has been the issue of sequencing of TBI with Cy; traditionally in marrow transplantation regimens, Cy was given before TBI, but in the last decade, many centers changed to delivering TBI first, with the advantage of better tolerance of the many fractions of TBI in fractionated regimens, especially when the patient was in the standing position. A murine study suggested that there is a greater antileukemic effect of Cy followed by TBI, compared with the reverse order.[41] This study was done by transferring the spleens from leukemic mice treated with either regimen to nonleukemic mice and monitoring the development of leukemia and survival in the recipient mice.

LUNG TOXICITY

Radiobiological studies in animals and humans have shown that increasing the number of fractions, for a given total dose, contributes greatly to decreasing the incidence of IP.[42,43] As a corollary, increasing the number of fractions allows one to increase the total dose for the same biological effect. In a murine study, the $LD_{50/30}$ (lethal dose for 50% of the animals in 30 days) due to IP was increased by 21% with an increase from one to six fractions, with a dose rate of 0.25 Gy/minute.[42] With a lower dose rate (0.08 Gy/minute), the increase in $LD_{50/30}$ with the increased number of fractions was less (14%), but still evident.

Graft-versus-host disease (GVHD) also plays a significant role in the development of IP. In the previously cited murine study that looked at the issue of engraftment as a function of the addition of varying amounts of donor T lymphocytes, it was found that the increasing numbers of T cells significantly increased the risk of pulmonary toxicity.[40]

Sequencing studies in mice have shown that there is less lung damage when Cy is given 12 to 24 hours after TBI compared with 24 to 48 hours before TBI.[44,45] In contrast, a different murine study showed a high incidence of early deaths when the majority of irradiation was given before chemotherapy.[46]

Schedule Optimization (Theoretical)

In 1979 and 1980, Peters and his associates[47,48] suggested that the use of fractionated TBI would be better than single-dose TBI; this suggestion was based on basic radiobiologic knowledge of hematopoietic and normal tissue effects. Various clinical studies have shown that a fractionated regimen, either daily fractionation or multiple fractions per day, decreased toxicity in a number of organs. Since then, many investigators have attempted to use available data to model the effects of TBI and to optimize its schedule.

Vriesendorp[35,49] took the approach of calculating the surviving fraction of cells, which determines tissue damage and organ function, for various fractionation schemes of TBI, using the multihit, multitarget model of cell survival. His calculated results show the impressive sparing of lung and intestines that could be expected with increasingly fractionated TBI regimens. The immune system survival results had suggested that immunosuppression with these highly fractionated regimens would be poor; however, the calculated results for the immune system were in error. When corrected and expanded to include some of the high-total-dose regimens (15 Gy) used today, it was found that immunosuppression is predicted to be excellent with these high total doses, and normal tissues continue to be spared.[50]

Vitale and his colleagues[51] performed calculations on the effectiveness of various dose rates and fractionation schemes for lung and leukemia relative to their own regimen of 9.9 Gy in three fractions at a dose rate of 0.05 Gy/minute. They found a greater dose rate effect in lung than in leukemic cells, but this became insignificant in the more highly fractionated schemes such as 15 Gy in 12 fractions. At any dose rate, the antileukemic effect relative to lung was greatest with this highly fractionated regimen (which allowed the greatest total dose to be given).

O'Donoghue and colleagues[52] compared schedules that were isoeffective for lung damage, using a mathematical model for leukemic cell kill that considered leukemic cell doubling time. They concluded that "accelerated hyperfractionation" schedules were optimal. With a minimum of 6 hours between fractions for maximal repair, two fractions per day was considered to be most practical. With the additional constraint of no treatments on weekends, they concluded that the optimal schedule for rapidly dividing cells (doubling time of 2 to 4 days) would be 10 fractions of 1.37 Gy per fraction in 5 days. For longer doubling times, a smaller dose per fraction would be optimal. Their recommendation for a practical schedule is 1.3 to 1.5 Gy per fraction for 10 fractions in 5 days. No randomized trial has been done to compare this scheme with others, but data at Mount Sinai Medical Center suggest that immunosuppression at 1.5 Gy per fraction as suggested is equivalent to that for the three fractions per day regimen (1.25 Gy/fraction) used extensively at Memorial Sloan-Kettering Cancer Center (MSKCC) to the same total dose (15 Gy); in CML patients, excellent clinical results have been achieved with no untoward toxicity.[53,54]

In another publication,[55] O'Donoghue also suggested that single-dose, low-dose-rate TBI could potentially be radiobiologically equivalent to fractionated TBI, but this would require unduly long treatment times (about 24 hours), which would be very impractical for most centers today.

Interaction with Chemotherapy

AGENTS USED

The principle chemotherapeutic agents that have been used with TBI are Cy, VP-16, and AraC. With Cy, toxicities of greatest concern have been IP and hemorrhagic cystitis. In the literature, either Cy alone[56,57] or AraC alone[24,58] can cause IP; it has been difficult to separate the contribution of Cy or AraC to IP when used in combination with TBI, especially when so many other factors contribute to this complication. IP is considered further in the section on toxicity. Sequencing of Cy with TBI has been a major question. Several studies have addressed this issue; these are discussed in the next section. Neither VP-16 nor AraC are as effective as Cy in immunosuppressive ability.[59]

The agent VP-16 has been increasingly used in regimens for ALL. Major toxicities in combination with TBI have not appeared to be a problem. AraC, on the other hand, has been implicated in an increased risk of renal toxicity, which had been seen rarely in transplant patients when Cy was the only chemotherapeutic agent used.

SEQUENCING

Traditionally, TBI had been given after Cy, but when institutions began fractionating irradiation, it was found to be more convenient for the patient and the department to give TBI before Cy, so that the patient experienced less nausea and vomiting during TBI, especially when the patient was in the standing position as in the treatment protocol developed at MSKCC. It was noted that there was improved acute tolerance of TBI when this was done, although no randomized studies have addressed this issue. Animal studies (see the previous section on leukemia) have suggested potential advantages for either alternative;[41,60] clinical results have not suggested any advantage for either in terms of relapse or survival, but no randomized studies have been done.

Physiologic Considerations

ORTHOSTATIC HYPOTENSION

Occasionally, patients have experienced syncope during the course of TBI in the standing position; most often, this has been attributable to the administration of a phenothiazine, which can cause orthostatic hypotension. Use of nonphenothiazine antiemetics usually ameliorates this problem. Occasionally, especially in patients with aplastic anemia, syncope may be caused by brain hypoxia resulting from a combination of anemia and hypotension in the standing position. Transfusion with packed red cells usually eliminates this problem.

NAUSEA AND VOMITING

The most common acute side effects observed, regardless of regimen used, have been nausea and vomiting. These have been noted to be less intense with fractionated regimens compared with single-dose regimens,[61] but they have persisted. One report indicated that emesis was universal after one fraction of 1.2 Gy in a hyperfractionated regimen and showed that there was a statistically significant diminution over the 4 days of that regimen.[62]

Many agents other than phenothiazines, such as metoclopramide and dexamethasone, have been used in attempts to control emesis. Several studies have attested to the antiemetic efficacy of ondansetron and granisetron, 5-hydroxytryptamine subtype 3 (5-HT$_3$) antagonists, for TBI.[63,64] A randomized, double-blind, placebo-controlled trial of ondansetron during fractionated TBI showed that ondansetron was superior to placebo for both number of emetic episodes ($P = 0.005$) and the time to the onset of emesis ($P = 0.003$) when given prophylactically 1.5 hours before each fraction of TBI.[65] Another double-blind, placebo-controlled trial during single-dose TBI also showed a statistically significant reduction in emetic

events with a single 8 mg dose of ondansetron at the initiation of TBI.[66]

PHYSICAL PRINCIPLES

Reproducibility

To ensure reproducibility from one fraction to another and consistency throughout the course of one fraction, patient position and immobilization must be considered. Various patient positions were described by Shank.[67] In brief, patients today are either treated standing up with anterior and posterior fields, or lying supine or prone or both with anterior and posterior fields, lateral fields, or a combination of both. When the patient is lying down, the patient is comfortable and motion during relatively short fractions (10 to 15 minutes) is minimal. When the patient is standing for that long, however, some type of immobilization is necessary.

Many centers have developed some form of TBI stand to help support and immobilize the patient.[68-71] An example of such a stand developed at MSKCC is shown in Figure 14-1.[50,69] It incorporates a bicycle seat and hand grips for greater patient security, as well as devices to control movement of the thorax region and to support lung shields and port film holders. This stand increased the accuracy and reproducibility of lung shield placement.

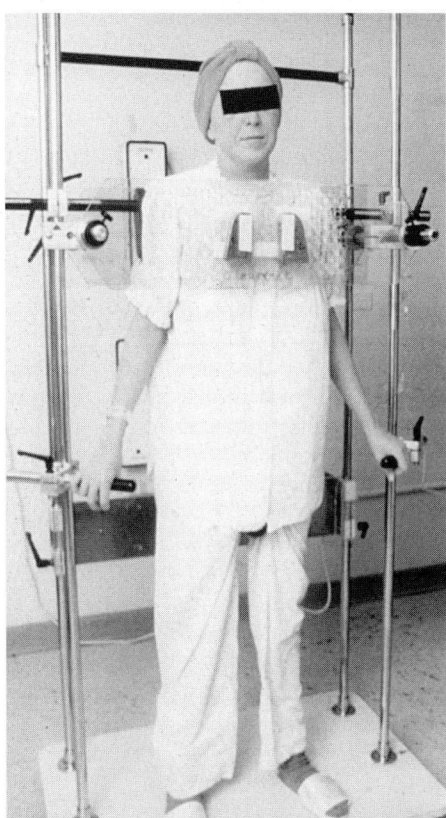

Figure 14–1. Patient with lung shields in place on a total body irradiation stand designed at Memorial Sloan-Kettering Cancer Center.

Another device described in the literature is a plaster vest that also supports lung shields.[72]

Homogeneity

It is assumed, in patients with leukemia, that leukemic cells may be dispersed anywhere throughout the body, including within the skin. Most centers in the United States have used energies that range from that of ^{60}Co (1.25 MV) to 10 MV with a linear accelerator; these, of course, have a dose buildup region upon entering tissue, which could potentially result in underdosing the skin. Even higher energies, up to 25 MV, have also been used, especially in Europe, but these would appear to have little advantage.

When energies greater than that of ^{60}Co are used for TBI, it is necessary to introduce a screen made of a tissue-equivalent material between the beam and the patient to maintain dose homogeneity.[67] This screen allows adequate buildup of dose in the skin to prevent underdosage. As an example, with 6 MV photons, a screen made of 1 cm Lexan results in a surface dose (at 1 mm) of about 95% relative to the prescribed dose at the midline from that single beam. Of course, the final dose to the surface depends on the dose from the opposing beam as well.

At some institutions, compensators have also been used at the neck, feet, and other areas to increase homogeneity, especially when beams of 10 MV or greater have been used.[67] TBI dose variability within the patient of ±5% is considered excellent, but ±10% is considered acceptable.

Dose Rate

When TBI is given in a single dose to a total dose of 10 Gy, it is necessary to use a low dose rate (≤0.05 Gy/minute) to decrease the probability of IP.[73,74] When higher dose rates are used, it is necessary to decrease the total dose given,[75,76] although this may contribute to a higher relapse rate as noted in one study when 5 Gy total dose was used at a dose rate of 0.4 to 0.9 Gy/minute.[76] For fractionated TBI schedules, the dose rate becomes less important, although in a mouse study, there was still a dose-rate effect for fraction sizes of 2 Gy per fraction or more.[77] When fraction sizes of 1.5 Gy or less are used, dose rates usually range from 0.05 to 0.18 Gy/minute.

At the large distances used to ensure that the entire unflexed body is in the beam with some margin around the patient, the dose rate is usually in the desired range. For infants, who may be treated supine and prone, on a mat on the floor (closer to the head of the machine compared with adults), it may be desirable to reduce the dose rate by means of lead beam attenuators.

Blocking

Many centers use lung shields during TBI. Most use partially attenuating shields (1 half-value layer [HVL]) throughout the course of treatment,[78] but at least one institution has used thick blocks (7 HVL) for one treatment out of the TBI course with none the remainder of the time.[79] Some institutions have attempted to shield the lungs with the patient's arms, by treating the patient laterally. However, as the position is difficult to reproduce, and it is difficult to assess the dosimetry, this method is not recommended.

It is relatively easy to simulate treatment with the patient in the standing position (Fig. 14-2). Films are taken in both the anterior and the posterior position with a wire marker on the skin as a reference point. After the blocks are designed on the anterior film, a final reference point may be determined both anteriorly and posteriorly for a tattoo to guide block placement during the course of treatment: midway between the blocks at a level corresponding to the superior edge of the blocks. The same blocks, carefully labeled *right* and *left*, may be used both anteriorly and, when reversed, posteriorly for treatment.

One institution has used partial-transmission liver shielding to decrease the incidence of VOD and has also used renal shielding (70% transmission) to minimize renal dysfunction in the setting of cytoreduction that includes both AraC and Cy.[80] Late renal dysfunction (at 18 months) is significantly less with the use of these blocks.[81] Long-term results with respect to relapse and survival are not yet available.

With leukemias, the lenses should not be shielded because of the possible eye or orbital involvement with disease. With some diseases, it is possible to use eye shielding. For example, in aplastic anemia, when the

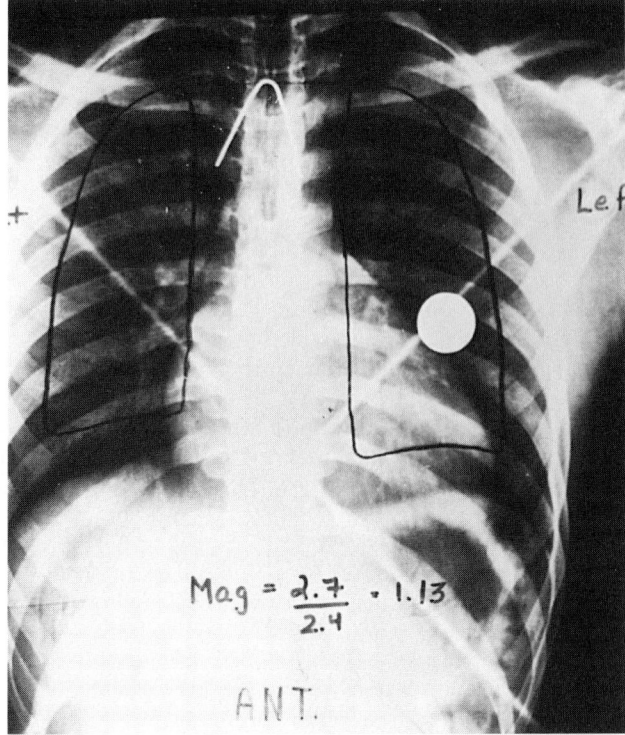

Figure 14–2. Example of simulation for lung blocks. The patient is in the standing position with a wire marker on the skin as a reference point and a quarter on the skin to aid in the calculation of magnification.

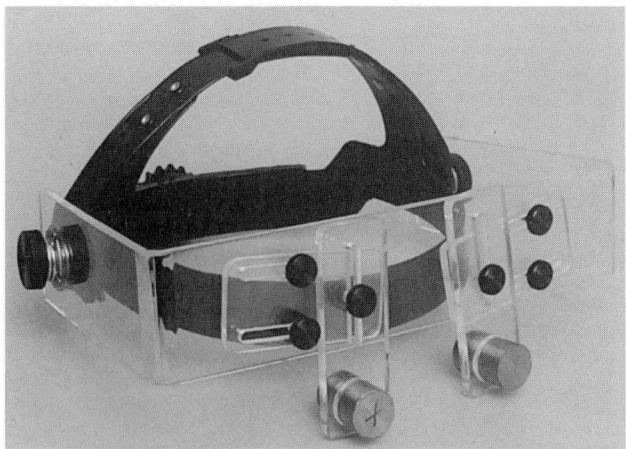

Figure 14–3. Example of eye shields that may be used for reduction of the lens dose in patients without malignant disease who require total body irradiation for immunosuppression.

donor is unrelated, intensive cytoreduction is necessary for engraftment, but there are no malignant cells to be concerned about. When TBI is part of such a cytoreductive regimen, adjustable eye shields can be used, as was done at MSKCC in a protocol for aplastic anemia patients (Fig. 14-3).[82] Of course, if intensive cytoreduction is not necessary, TLI or TAI may be used and the eyes are outside the field.

"Boosting"

When lung blocks were initiated, it was felt that it was necessary to supplement the dose to marrow-containing ribs in the area of the lung blocks to ensure that an adequate dose was given to all potential sites of leukemia.[78] When this is done, careful treatment planning using CT scans through the area beneath the lung blocks is necessary (Fig. 14-4) so that the appropriate energy of electrons and thickness of bolus are used. Guidelines used were to aim for 90% of the electron dose at the inner chest wall and less than 10% of the dose at midplane in the core of the lungs.

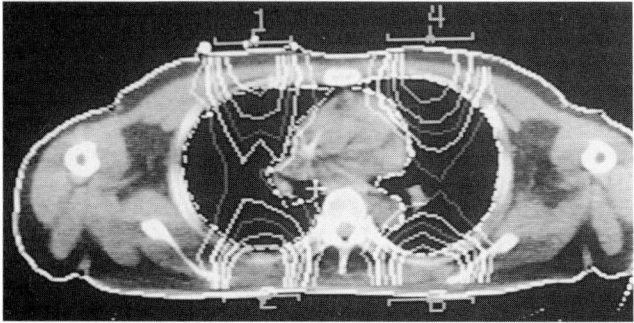

Figure 14–4. Example of electron boost planning for the chest wall after the use of lung blocks. The 90% isodose is at the inner chest wall; no more than 10% of the dose is delivered to the core of the lungs. See also Color Figure 14-4.

Dutreix and colleagues[83] calculated that blocking lungs was theoretically equivalent to merely lowering the total body dose by a small percentage. On that basis, the Institut Gustave-Roussy did not add an electron boost to lungs. They reported no difference in relapse rate in their patients compared with other centers where lung boosts were given.[84] As a result, several centers have eliminated this step.

In the Seattle experience, 25% of the boys who survived more than 5 months after transplantation developed primary testicular relapse.[85] After noting a high relapse rate in the testes in the MSKCC patients with leukemia (4/28 males), Shank and colleagues[86] added a 4-Gy testes boost with electrons to all their leukemia TBI protocols. This was usually given in one fraction unless prior testicular irradiation had been given. With prior testicular treatment, this dose was split into two fractions in 2 days, or not given at all if that treatment were within 1 to 2 months of the transplantation. No further relapses occurred in more than 300 male patients after this added boost.

Splenic irradiation before TBI is a logical boost treatment in patients with CML, especially when the spleen is enlarged, since it frequently harbors a large leukemic cell burden. In a European study, there was a trend toward an improved survival in CML patients who received splenic irradiation compared with those who did not.[87] Radiobiological[88] and clinical studies[89] support this concept. In a prospective randomized study, however, no significant survival advantage was seen when splenic irradiation was given up to 14 days before BMT in 239 patients with chronic-phase CML, but follow-up was quite short.[90] In an update, one subset of patients did benefit with splenic irradiation.[91] Patients who did not receive T-depleted BMT and had blood basophil levels less than 3% before transplantation had a relapse rate at 8 years of 8% with splenic irradiation compared with 30% without it ($P < 0.05$). If splenic irradiation is done, a liver/spleen radionuclide scan is very useful to carefully plan this treatment (Fig. 14-5).

In some diseases such as the lymphomas, it is desirable to boost sites of residual gross disease or other areas at particular risk since failures of transplantation are most often in sites of initial involvement. For example, boost treatments to total doses of 12 to 20 Gy have been added to TBI regimens in areas of gross residual disease, such as the mediastinum.[92] Locoregional irradiation as a "boost" to initial or residual disease sites is often added to high-dose chemotherapy-only regimens with evidence of improved local control, freedom from relapse, and survival in nonrandomized studies of both Hodgkin's disease[93-95] and non-Hodgkin's lymphomas.[96-98]

A novel type of supplemental treatment that may be thought of as a hematopoietic boost is the use of antibody radionuclide conjugates, such as I-131-labeled anti-CD45 antibody.[99,100] This antibody, which is found on nearly all hematopoietic cells except mature red cells and platelets, is also found on 85% to 90% of acute leukemia cells. Substantially greater doses of radiation can be delivered to hematopoietic tissues compared with liver, lung, or kidney, with toxicity that is not appreciably greater than that with TBI/Cy alone.

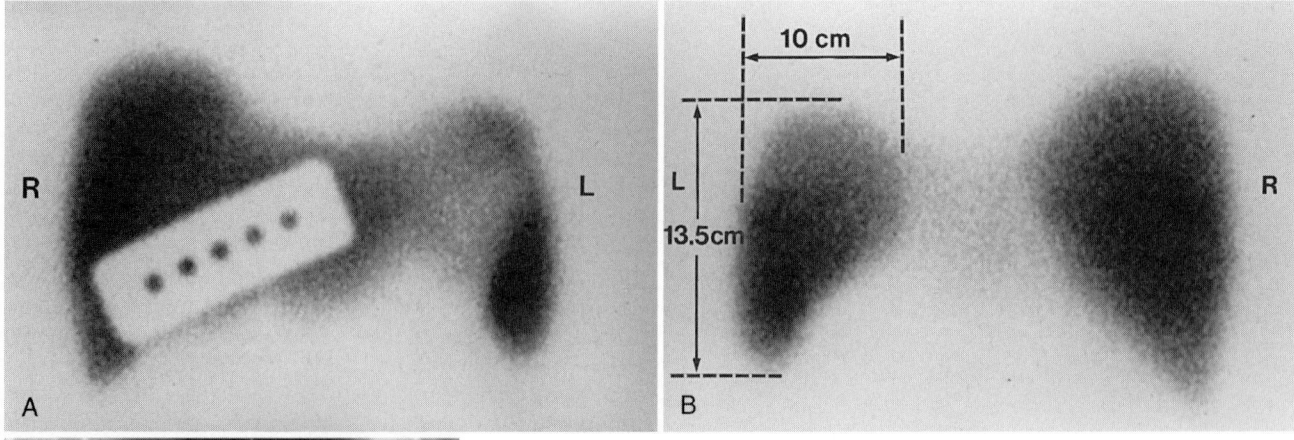

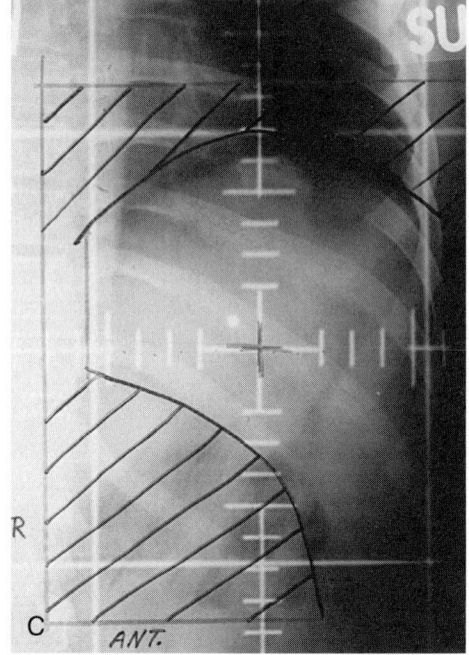

Figure 14–5. Planning for spleen irradiation. **A,** Anterior liver-spleen scan with radioactive markers 2 cm apart for magnification. **B,** Posterior liver-spleen scan for spleen length and width measurements, corrected by magnification. **C,** Spleen field simulation with size and shape obtained from scans described in parts **A** and **B**.

Special Dosimetry

Special considerations contribute to the dose distribution in the patient when TBI is used. For example, with a patient in the standing position at one end of a room at a large distance from the source, the gantry may be somewhat angled in a way that increases the distance from the source to the feet compared with the distance from the source to the vertex, resulting in a lesser dose to the feet than to the vertex. There is a large amount of internal scatter from within the patient, and there is scatter from the wall behind the patient and even from the TBI stand itself. With any given setup at an institution, it is important to make careful measurements of the dose at various sites, including behind lung blocks, on many patients, to understand the dose distribution for that system. At the low dose rates encountered, ion chambers are usually the best means of measuring the doses. For extensive discussions of dosimetry and dose calibration, see the publications of Briot and colleagues[101] and Van Dyk and colleagues.[102,103]

RESULTS OF CLINICAL STUDIES

Immunosuppression

ENGRAFTMENT

With conventional matched sibling allografts, nonengraftment is rare (1% to 2%);[104,105] engraftment, as measured by a white cell count greater than 500/mm³, is noted from 1.5 to 3 weeks from the day of BMT (median: 17 days).[28] In human leukocyte antigen (HLA)-nonidentical transplants from related nonsibling donors, graft failure was found to be a function of the degree of donor incompatibility.[105]

When donor marrow has been T-cell–depleted as a means of preventing GVHD, graft failures have been reportedly more frequent. Single-dose TBI (7.5 to 10 Gy) has been shown to be more effective in preventing rejection than fractionated TBI to a relatively low total dose of 10 to 12 Gy.[1,106-108] Many reports have indicated that either higher total doses of fractionated TBI[109-112] (Fig. 14-6) or the addition of TLI to TBI[106,113-116]

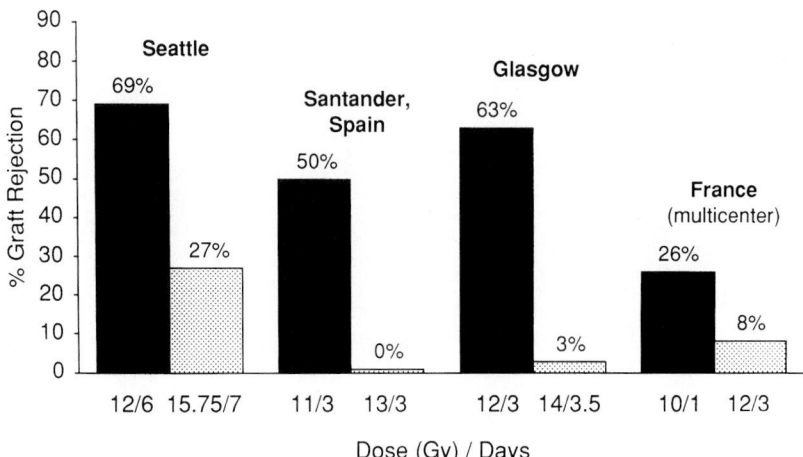

Figure 14–6. Graft rejection in patients with a T-cell–depleted bone marrow transplant as a function of the total dose of total body irradiation used in nonrandomized comparisons of different fractionation schemes from four centers (see references 109-112).

(Fig. 14-7) may prevent graft rejection in a large proportion of patients receiving T-cell–depleted marrow, although this improvement has not always been found with either increased TBI dose[98,99] or the addition of TLI.[100] In the analysis of T-cell–depleted marrow, this improvement has not always been found with either increased TBI dose[117,118] or the addition of TLI.[119] In the analysis of T-cell–depleted transplants reported by the IBMTR,[1] higher total doses ($\geq$11 Gy) and higher dose rates ($\geq$0.14 Gy/minute) were associated with significantly fewer rejections. Single fraction low-dose TBI (1 to 2 Gy) has been used as immunosuppressive therapy prior to hematopoietic cell transplantation and allogeneic donor lymphocyte infusion.[120,121] Donor chimerism, often unstable, has been achieved, as have sustained complete remissions in some patients, but GVHD has been a problem. However, the feasibility and potential of such an approach has been established.

APLASTIC ANEMIA

In severe aplastic anemia, large-field irradiation is useful only to prevent rejection since there are no malignant cells to eradicate. To prevent rejection, Cy alone is insufficient, so cytoreductive regimens have usually included either TBI or TLI to enhance engraftment, either as a single dose[122,123] or fractionated.[82] The advantage of using TLI for immunosuppression is that normal tissues outside of the field can be spared, namely brain and eye, kidneys, lungs, and much of the small bowel. Shank and colleagues[82] have determined that, for a one-log peripheral blood lymphocyte decrease, TBI to 6 Gy is equivalent to TLI to 10 Gy, when fractionated as done at MSKCC: TBI in 2 Gy daily fractions and TLI given in 1 Gy fractions, three fractions per day.

In patients with aplastic anemia who receive T-cell–depleted marrow transplants, no rejection and no GVHD was seen when the TLI dose was increased to 18 Gy with twice-daily fractions, although follow-up was short.[115,116] TAI has also been used for severe aplastic anemia and, more commonly, for Fanconi's anemia.[124,125] These fields do not spare small bowel and kidneys, but they do spare brain, eyes, and lung and are easy to administer in small children, since the block arrangement is less complicated. Some regimens do not use any irradiation, such as that of the Seattle group, which uses only Cy and antithymocyte globulin.[126]

Long-term survival in severe aplastic anemia is generally in the range of 65% to 75%, but GVHD has generally remained a problem.[127] Survival at 5 years for Fanconi's anemia patients who have been transplanted is similar.[128] The most serious long-term complication encountered with the anemias has been second malignancies; this is discussed in the later section on toxicity.

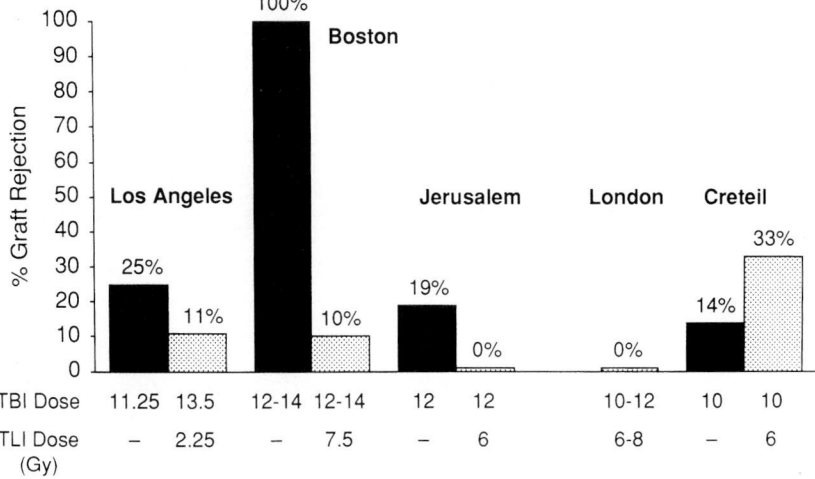

Figure 14–7. Graft rejection in patients with a T-cell–depleted bone marrow transplant with and without the addition of total lymphoid irradiation (TLI); all comparisons within institutions are nonrandomized (see references 106, 113-116, 119).

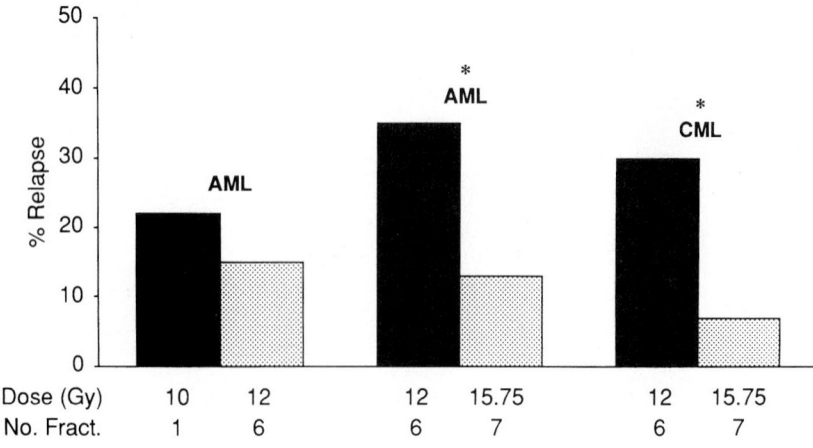

Figure 14–8. Leukemic relapse as a function of the total dose of total body irradiation in the three randomized studies from Seattle comparing different fractionation schemes for patients receiving conventional transplants (see references 129-134). Asterisk indicates statistically significant findings. AML, acute myeloid leukemia; CML, chronic myeloid leukemia.

Eradication of Malignancy

Leukemic relapse is a reflection of the efficacy of leukemic cell kill, which is dependent upon many factors in addition to the cytoreductive transplant regimen; these factors include the leukemic cell burden, pretransplant chemotherapy, drug resistance, and graft-versus-leukemia effect.

Several studies have examined the influence of total TBI dose, dose rate, and fractionation on leukemic relapse. Three randomized studies in Seattle compared schedules.[129-134] These studies (Fig. 14-8) showed that the higher doses, which can be achieved with fractionation, decrease the relapse rate as might be expected radiobiologically. In the CML study, survival was initially lower in the high-dose group because of an increased early mortality, but at 5 years, there is no statistically significant difference in survival.[129,132] In the first AML study comparing single-dose

TBI with fractionated daily TBI, survival was significantly better with fractionated TBI.[130,133] In the second study, which compared two daily fractionation schemes, no difference in survival was seen.[131,134]

Dose escalation has been attempted to levels above 15 Gy for TBI.[135,136] One study achieved a maximum tolerated dose of 16 Gy in 2-Gy fractions given twice a day 6 hours apart.[135] Another study used 50% lung transmission blocks with electron chest wall boosts in those areas, and kidney shielding to a maximum dose of 16 Gy. In nine patients receiving autologous peripheral blood stem cells, with three patients each at 16 Gy, 18 Gy, and 20 Gy (2 Gy per fraction twice daily), toxicity was moderate with four patients achieving complete remissions, and one remaining disease-free at 5 years post-transplant.[136]

Results from nonrandomized studies with regard to relapse rate are quite variable (Fig. 14-9), with only the

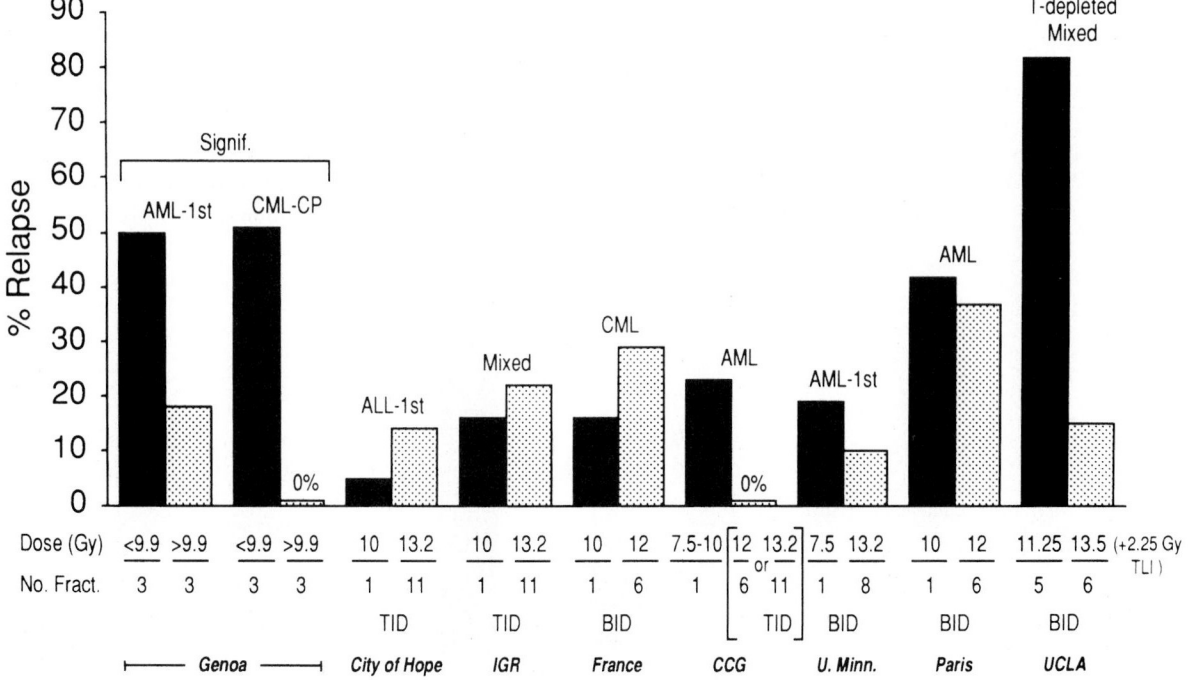

Figure 14–9. Leukemic relapse as a function of total dose of total body irradiation in nonrandomized studies from many centers using different fractionation schemes (see references 84,106,137-139,147-151). With the exception of the last study, all patients received conventional transplants. ALL, acute lymphoblastic leukemia; AML, acute myeloid leukemia; CML, chronic myeloid leukemia; CP, chronic phase; TLI, total lymphoid irradiation; 1st, first remission.

study from Genoa (see first two sets of bar graphs in Fig. 14-9) showing a significant difference in relapse rate.[137-139] In that study, patients with CML and AML were treated with a nominal dose of 9.9 Gy given in three fractions of 3.3 Gy each. Actual doses calculated retrospectively, however, were found to differ considerably. The difference in relapse between patients who received greater than 9.9 Gy compared with patients who received less than 9.9 Gy translated into a highly significant difference in survival (74% at 8 years compared with only 38%, respectively). The total dose was the most significant factor affecting relapse; dose rate was of only borderline significance.

ACUTE LYMPHOBLASTIC LEUKEMIA

Comparative studies (Table 14-3) between allogeneic BMT and maintenance chemotherapy for ALL have shown decreased relapse rates and improved disease-free survival in the BMT arm of the studies,[140-143] but this is not always statistically significant. The success of transplant depends upon remission status. In children with ALL in second remission, the relapse rate at 5 years is only 13% and disease-free survival is 64%.[144]

The Seattle group compared two fractionated dose schedules in a nonrandomized study: 2.25 Gy daily for 7 days to 15.75 Gy total dose (26 patients), and 1.2 Gy three times daily for 4 days to 14.4 Gy total dose (23 patients).[145] The group receiving the 15.75 Gy total dose had a lower relapse rate and better disease-free survival at 3 years, but these differences were not statistically significant.

Allogeneic transplant, when a matched donor is available, has the advantage over autologous transplant, based on the available data (see Table 14-3). A study from Rome has demonstrated a significantly better disease-free survival and lower relapse rate for allogeneic BMT compared with autologous BMT,[146] whereas others show a significantly lower relapse rate, but no difference in disease-free survival[142] or a trend toward a higher disease-free survival rate with allogeneic transplants.[152-154] For patients who do not have matched donors for an allogeneic transplant, however, an autologous BMT is possible using marrow obtained in remission, then purged of leukemic cells by chemotherapeutic or immunologic methods.[142,146,152-154] An advantage of autologous BMT over chemotherapy alone has not been conclusively demonstrated, but the data in Table 14-3 suggest an improved disease-free survival with autologous BMT; the major disadvantage is a high relapse rate, which suggests either that the graft-versus-leukemia effect is important or that purging is insufficient. Long-term disease-free survival is in the range of 25% to 30%, with the best results in patients in first remission.

ACUTE MYELOID LEUKEMIA

In AML, a large number of studies have shown an improved disease-free survival rate with BMT compared with continued chemotherapy (Table 14-4).[156-162] Not much difference has been observed between allogeneic and autologous BMT,[157,160,163,164] with disease-free survival for either being about 50%. Long-term leukemia-free survival from IBMTR data is 51% for patients in first remission, 31% in second or greater remission, and 21% in relapse.[1] In an analysis from MSKCC, children with AML had a 0% relapse rate when transplanted in first remission and 13% in second remission, and disease-free survival was about 70% for either first or second remission.[144] These low relapse rates were attributed to the high total TBI dose (13.2 to 14.4 Gy) used with their hyperfractionated regimen, the addition of a 4 Gy testes boost, and the sequencing of Cy after TBI.

Two randomized scheduling trials for AML in first remission have been done in Seattle.[130,131,133,134] First, single dose TBI was compared with daily fractionation[130,133] (six fractions of 2 Gy each for a total dose of 12 Gy). Event-free survival was significantly better with the daily fractionation scheme, primarily due to decreased early mortality (Fig. 14-10). When this same fractionation scheme was compared with another daily fractionation scheme (seven fractions of 2.25 Gy each for a total dose

Table 14–3   Percentage Disease-Free Survival of Acute Lymphoblastic Leukemia Patients According to Postinduction Treatment

| Study | Population | Disease-Free Survival, % | | | Time of Analysis, yr | Reference |
		Allo BMT	Auto BMT	Chemo		
Seattle	C, CR2 or >	34	—	0	4	Johnson and Thomas[155]
London	C, CR2	35	—	20	5	Chessells et al.[140]
CCG	C, CR2	39* 60†	—	19	3	Harris et al.[141]
Rome	C + A, CR1	52	29	—	3	Arcese et al.[146]
Italy	C, CR1	57	50	—	2.5	Uderzo et al.[154]
Newcastle	A, CR1	30	30	12	3	Proctor et al.[142]
France	C + A, CR1	71	40	—	4	Blaise et al.[152]
Minneapolis	C, CR2	27	20	—	4	Kersey et al.[153]
Zagreb	A, CR1	52	—	24	3	Mrsic et al.[143]

*Cyclophosphamide and total body irradiation.
†High-dose cytosine arabinoside and total body irradiation.

A, adults; Allo, allogeneic; Auto, autologous; BMT, bone marrow transplantaion; C, children; Chemo, chemotherapy; CR1, first remission; CR2, second remission.

Table 14–4   Percentage Disease-Free Survival of Acute Myeloid Leukemia Patients According to Postinduction Treatment

Study	Population	Disease-Free Survival, %			Time of Analysis, yr	Reference
		Allo BMT	*Auto BMT*	*Chemo*		
UCLA	Adults	40*	—	27*	4	Champlin et al.[165]
Seattle/SWOG	Adults	48	—	26	4	Applebaum et al.[158]
Royal Marsden	Children + adults	64	—	29	3	Powles et al.[159]
CCG	Children	47	—	34	8	Nesbit et al.[166]
CCG†	Children	55	51	—	3	Woods et al.[167]
IBMTR-German AML Coop. Group	Adults	54	—	40		Gale et al.[156]
Paris (SHIP)	Children	83	—	52	3	Schalson et al.[168]
EORTC	Adults	54	49	30	4	Zittoun et al.[157]
ECOG	Adults	42	54	—	3	Cassileth et al.[163]
MD Anderson	Adults	36‡	—	19‡	3	Zander et al.[169]
AML-80	Children	43	—	31	6	Dahl et al.[170]
Netherlands	Adults	51	35	—	3	Lowenberg et al.[164]
Bordeaux (BGMT)	Adults	66	41	16	2.5	Reiffers et al.[160]
Lyon	Adults	41	—	27	7	Archimbaud et al.[161]
Spain	Adults	70	—	10	3	Conde et al.[162]
	Adults <45 yr	70	—	17	3	

*Overall survival.
†Included patients with myelodysplastic syndrome.
‡Crude overall survival.
Allo, allogeneic; AML, acute myeloid leukemia; Auto, autologous; BMT, bone marrow transplantation; Chemo, chemotherapy; IBMTR, International Bone Marrow Transplant Registry.

of 15.75 Gy) in a second trial, there was no difference in relapse-free survival (both ≈55% at 6 years).[131,134] Although the relapse rate was less with the regimen with the higher total dose of 15.75 Gy, mortality was also greater.

The Seattle group has also analyzed its nonrandomized experience with the two daily fractionation schemes described previously for patients in untreated first

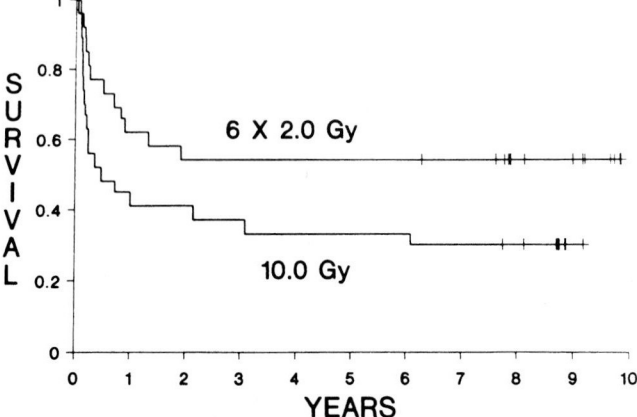

Figure 14–10. Event-free survival of patients with acute myelocytic leukemia in first remission who were randomized on the Seattle study to either single-dose total body irradiation (10 Gy) or fractionated TBI (6 × 2 Gy) after 60 mg/kg per day cyclophosphamide × 2 days, before allogeneic bone marrow transplantation from an HLA-identical sibling. (From Thomas, ED: Total body irradiation regimens for marrow grafting. *Int J Radiat Oncol Biol Phys.* 19:1285, 1990.)

relapse.[134] GVHD prophylaxis was methotrexate and cyclosporine for all 19 patients in the 12 Gy total dose regimen and for 22 patients in the 15.75 Gy total dose regimen. Methotrexate only was used for GVHD prophylaxis in 30 patients in the 15.75 Gy regimen. Although nonrelapse mortality was 50% in the first year in the group that received 15.75 Gy followed by methotrexate only, disease-free survival was best in this group (≈27% at 7 years) because of the relatively low probability of relapse (<30%).

CHRONIC MYELOID LEUKEMIA

Many studies have shown that CML patients have a better survival rate when transplanted in the first chronic phase. Long-term disease-free survival for patients in first chronic phase who have been transplanted with unmanipulated marrow from a matched sibling donor is about 60% to 70%.[132,171,172] With T-cell depletion of donor marrow, there is an increased risk of relapse, resulting in a lower disease-free survival rate.[173] In either group, with or without T-cell depletion, patients who develop chronic GVHD have less risk of relapse, demonstrating a graft-versus-leukemia effect.

In the same patients in the Genoa study described at the beginning of this section on the eradication of malignancy, a later analysis looked at the presence of mixed chimerism, that is, the presence of host marrow cells as well as donor cells.[174] It was found that the patients who did not have mixed chimerism were the patients who had received the higher mean TBI dose (>9.9 Gy); these patients were more likely to remain in remission.

LYMPHOMAS

Non-Hodgkin's Lymphomas

The first marrow transplants in patients with non-Hodgkin's lymphoma were done on those in relapse; the surprising success in some of these otherwise hopeless patients encouraged others to perform BMT earlier in the course of intermediate or high-grade non-Hodgkin's lymphoma. It was shown that aggressive cytoreduction (TBI/Cy) followed by autologous BMT as early treatment was highly successful in patients with the poor prognostic features of high serum lactic dehydrogenase, bulky mediastinal or abdominal disease, or both.[92,175,176] At 5 years, 79% of patients were alive and free of disease in the group who underwent autologous BMT after induction chemotherapy, compared with only 31% in the group of patients who elected to wait and undergo BMT only at failure of chemotherapy.

From data gathered by the European Bone Marrow Transplant Group (EBMTG), patients who have relapsed but responded to chemotherapy, achieving a complete or partial response, may achieve a 40% progression-free survival at 5 years after an autologous BMT.[177] With a more aggressive cytoreductive regimen (TBI/VP-16/Cy), even patients with relapsed and resistant disease may be successfully treated (57% disease-free survival at a median follow-up of >42 months).[178-180]

Some patients may not be considered good candidates for an autologous BMT, because of severe marrow dysfunction or the presence of lymphoma in the marrow, but may have a matched donor for an allogeneic BMT. Although GVHD and regimen-related toxicity is higher than with an autologous BMT, the relapse rate is low, perhaps as a result of a "graft-versus-lymphoma" effect. A case-control study by the EBMTG demonstrated that there was no difference in progression-free survival, even though there was a statistically significant greater relapse rate in the autologous group (48% vs. 24%).[181]

The role of BMT in low-grade non-Hodgkin's lymphoma is as yet undefined.[182] The indolent course of most of these patients makes it difficult to justify the risks of early mortality from BMT, and makes investigational studies difficult to assess, since results will be meaningful only after a decade.

There is a long history (since 1923) of reports documenting excellent symptomatic and objective responses in patients with highly radiosensitive tumors (lymphomas and leukemias) treated with low-dose TBI without BMT. The most rewarding responses were in the indolent non-Hodgkin's lymphomas and in chronic lymphocytic leukemia. Typical regimens in the more recent era (1975 on) have consisted of 10 to 15 cGy per fraction, two to three fractions per week, to a total dose of 150 to 200 cGy. Although as many as 80% to 85% of lymphoma patients achieved a complete response,[183,184] few studies followed patients for a long term, and hematopoietic toxicity has been severe in some studies. Results of randomized comparisons of TBI versus chemotherapy for chronic lymphocytic leukemia have been mixed, with two studies favoring TBI[185,186] and one favoring chemotherapy (chlorambucil and prednisone).[187] But in all these studies, follow-up was short. In another study with both chronic

lymphocytic leukemia and indolent lymphoma patients, TBI and chemotherapy with the same agents were equivalent.[188] One long-term study demonstrated a recurrence-free survival of 19% at 10 years after TBI for advanced-stage, low-grade non-Hodgkin's lymphoma. This excellent survival without any maintenance therapy suggested that low-dose TBI should be first-line therapy in this group of patients.[189]

Hodgkin's Disease

Patients with refractory or relapsed *Hodgkin's disease* may be salvaged by BMT also. In patients who had not had prior irradiation, a group at MSKCC found disease-free survival to be 65% at 20+ months follow-up using a regimen involving "boost" irradiation to any areas of gross disease, followed by TLI/VP-16/Cy and autologous BMT.[190,191] In Seattle, various regimens were used over a period of 21 years for such patients; more than half of the regimens did not use irradiation, and the rest incorporated TBI.[192] These investigators concluded that (1) BMT should be performed early after relapse and (2) HLA-matched sibling marrow resulted in a lower relapse rate compared with autologous marrow.

Patients who have received prior irradiation usually are not eligible for either a TLI- or TBI-containing preparative regimen. At Stanford, a nonrandomized comparison of patients receiving an autologous BMT after either chemotherapy (bis-chloroethyl-nitrosourea [BCNU]), or TBI/VP-16/Cy indicated no difference at 4 years in relapse, overall survival, or event-free survival between the two regimens, although the populations differed with respect to prior therapy.[193]

TOXICITY

Acute Side Effects

The most obvious acute side effects are nausea and vomiting, which tend to occur a few hours after the first fraction of fractionated irradiation, and have been noted to decrease with time over a course of hyperfractionated irradiation. The successful use of ondansetron or granisetron to control this has been described in the section on physiologic considerations.

Other acute side effects frequently encountered include oral mucositis, diarrhea, and parotiditis. These, along with nausea and vomiting, have been shown to be less with hyperfractionated (twice-daily) irradiation compared with single-dose irradiation in a French study that randomized dose rates but not the fractionation.[194,195] The dose rate per se had no obvious effect on acute side effects for either fractionation. Another study showed that no parotiditis occurred with fractionated TBI (12 Gy in six fractions) compared with a 40% incidence with single-dose TBI (10 Gy).[196]

The major factor responsible for the transient xerostomia associated with BMT is probably TBI.[197] Some patients develop severe dental caries without fluoride prophylaxis; therefore, dental assessment and fluoride prophylaxis are recommended for all TBI patients. Prophylactic acyclovir, which is effective against herpes simplex virus, has been found effective in decreasing the severity of mucositis.[198] One agent, pentoxifylline, was thought initially in clinical observations to decrease mucositis and other later toxicities of acute GVHD, VOD, and renal insufficiency; however, in a randomized controlled trial, it was found to be of no benefit.[199] Fatigue is universal over the course of TBI, with any fractionation scheme. Some patients will develop skin erythema and, later, even hyperpigmentation.

Late Toxicities

REGIMEN-RELATED TOXICITY

The term *regimen-related toxicity* refers to all toxicities related to the preparative (cytoreductive) regimen[200] and should be distinguished from transplant-related morbidity, which can refer to other toxicities related to transplantation, such as from prophylactic medications, pancytopenia, or GVHD. An empirical grading system for eight individual organs has been devised by the Seattle group.[201] When all regimen-related toxicities were grouped together, one study[200] showed that the only major factor that increased the risk in allogeneic transplant patients was higher TBI dose, when two regimens with daily fractionation were compared (12 Gy in six fractions of 2 Gy vs. 15.75 Gy in seven fractions of 2.25 Gy). Although the higher dose was administered more commonly to relapsed patients and patients who received mismatched grafts, the TBI dose was still the only high-risk factor for allogeneic transplant patients that emerged in a multivariate analysis. An allogeneic BMT per se increased the risk for regimen-related toxicity when compared with an autologous transplant.

GRAFT-VERSUS-HOST DISEASE

The immune response of donor T lymphocytes against host normal tissues in spite of apparent histocompatibility between donor and host, that is, GVHD, can be a significant contributor to organ toxicity. Acute GVHD is a distinctive syndrome consisting, to variable degrees, of dermatitis, hepatitis, and enteritis, appearing within 100 days of allogeneic transplant.

Acute GVHD may be staged (+1 to +4) at each organ site by severity, based on (1) the intensity of the skin rash and percentage of body surface area involved, (2) the extent of bilirubin elevation for liver involvement, and (3) the severity of diarrhea for the gastrointestinal tract.[202] An overall grade of GVHD from zero (none) to IV (life-threatening), which predicts the clinical course, is then assigned based on the staging at each organ site. IP, as discussed later, is related to the severity of acute GVHD. The histopathology has been well described in the literature.[203]

Chronic GVHD, which is considered to develop more than 100 days after allogeneic transplantation, tends to result in more widespread organ involvement (skin, liver, lung, eye, and gastrointestinal tract) and behaves more like an autoimmune process.

Many agents have been used for the prevention of acute GVHD, such as methotrexate alone,[204] cyclosporine alone,[205] combined methotrexate and cyclosporine,[205] or a regimen of methotrexate, antithymocyte globulin, and prednisone.[204] The latter regimen decreased the incidence of GVHD when compared in a randomized study to methotrexate alone.[204] Methotrexate combined with cyclosporine was superior to cyclosporine alone in another randomized study, demonstrating an advantage in survival as well as in GVHD reduction.[205]

Other approaches to reducing GVHD include the use of polyvalent intravenous immunoglobulin,[206] and donor marrow T-lymphocyte depletion.[207,208] Although the latter technique can be highly successful in eliminating GVHD, problems encountered include graft failure and, in patients with CML, a higher incidence of relapse, presumably due to the loss of a graft-versus-leukemia capability during the T-lymphocyte depletion process.

INTERSTITIAL PNEUMONITIS

One of the major contributors to mortality after BMT has been IP, with a minimum incidence of about 20% even in patients who have not received TBI as part of their cytoreductive regimen.[79] IP has usually been fatal in approximately two thirds of patients who develop it,[78,79] although there now may be somewhat fewer fatalities with the advent of a useful treatment (combined ganciclovir and immunoglobulin[209,210]) for IP caused by one of the organisms most frequently responsible, cytomegalovirus.

Complicating any analysis of IP and its risk factors is the use of varying definitions of IP in the literature. Some investigators consider only idiopathic IP, while others consider all IP, including that of known infectious cause. The time frame also varies, with some considering only IP that develops in 100 or fewer days, while others may consider any IP, even as remote as 1 to 2 years after BMT. It is advisable to consider all IP, but to define the causes, since the cytoreductive regimen could potentially play a role in IP of any cause, even infectious.

In spite of the difficulties cited, some factors that put patients at risk for developing IP have been identified. Factors that may increase the risk of IP may be divided into patient-related factors over which we have little or no control, such as older patient age, increased body weight,[211] 1.5 m² or greater body surface area,[212] male sex,[213] and a diagnosis of CML compared with other leukemias.[201,214] GVHD, over which we only have partial control, has been shown in many studies to increase the risk of IP.[212-218] The use of T-cell–depleted transplants, which minimizes the incidence and severity of GVHD, results in a very low incidence of IP.[61,117,219-221]

The immediate cause of IP can often be diagnosed as an infectious agent, such as cytomegalovirus or *Pneumocystis carinii*. Patients who are seropositive for cytomegalovirus, or who develop cytomegalovirus viruria or viremia, are at increased risk for cytomegalovirus IP.[210]

Factors related to the transplant procedure that influence IP are the cytoreductive regimen, including Cy[56,57] and TBI, and agents used after BMT for GVHD prophylaxis, such as methotrexate.[222] In a nonrandomized retrospective comparison of TBI/Cy and Bu/Cy, patients who had the TBI/Cy preparation for BMT had a greater decrease in carbon monoxide diffusion than patients who had Bu/Cy.[213]

TBI techniques may be altered in various ways to minimize IP. Fractionation has been found to be extremely important. There is a lower incidence of IP and fewer fatalities from IP when TBI is fractionated than when single-dose TBI is used, even though the total dose with the fractionated regimen is higher. This was found in a large number of nonrandomized studies,[79,84,86,147-150,218,223,224] as well as the randomized study from Seattle (Fig. 14-11).[130] The only exception was in the low-dose-rate arm of a study that randomized patients to high and low dose rates; in that low-dose-rate arm, there was no significant difference between single-dose or hyperfractionated TBI.[194]

Lung shields can reduce the dose to a large percentage of the lung and, theoretically, reduce IP as a result. Some of the decrease in IP in the fractionation studies seen in Figure 14-11 may be attributable to the concomitant use of lung blocks when TBI was fractionated, as in the study from MSKCC.[86] In the study from the Institut Gustave-Roussy, however, lung shields were used in both single-dose and fractionated TBI, and the beneficial effect of fractionation in reducing IP was still observed.[84] In a study from Croatia, using the same TBI regimen with and without lung blocks, IP was 8% with lung shielding compared with 27% without such shields.[225]

Investigators from Glasgow studied the effects of different TBI regimens, which incorporated lung shielding, on pulmonary function at various times after BMT.[226] The regimens were single-dose TBI to 9.5 Gy with a lung dose of 8 Gy, and fractionated regimens, which varied from 12 to 14.4 Gy in six to eight fractions with lung doses between 11 and 13.5 Gy. Impairment of lung function was seen in all instances after BMT, especially with

respect to gas exchange; these gradually improved to normal, as is also seen in a Milan study of pulmonary function tests.[227] There was significantly less marked impairment in patients who had undergone the fractionated regimens compared with single-dose TBI, in spite of the lesser total lung dose received with single-dose TBI. In addition, they noted that patients who had the single-dose regimen had a slower and less complete recovery of gas exchange.

Reducing the total lung dose in a single-dose (10 Gy) regimen does not appear to be the answer to reducing IP. When this was attempted in a study that randomized patients between total lung doses of 6 and 8 Gy.[228] IP was essentially the same (23% vs. 28%, respectively), and relapse was significantly higher in the 6 Gy group.

Dose rate is important with single-dose TBI, with very low-dose rates (0.025 Gy/min) resulting in a low incidence of IP (10%) and fatal IP (5%), but treatment times are extremely lengthy to achieve this (i.e., 7 hours).[229] One study using a high instantaneous dose rate (0.21 to 0.235 Gy/min) reported a very high IP incidence (8 of 11 patients), which was fatal in half of the patients.[223] Two studies suggest that with fractionated TBI, dose rate is of little importance, which is the result expected if the dose per fraction is within the shoulder of the cell survival curve or if the dose per fraction is below the flexion point for the tissue of interest. Clearly small fractions or very low dose rates spare the lung from the component of IP that is due to direct radiation effect on the lung.[194,215]

Prior pulmonary irradiation is also a consideration in the development of lung toxicity. The carbon monoxide transfer coefficient dropped to a significantly greater extent after BMT in patients who had received prior pulmonary irradiation.[216] In another study, in which

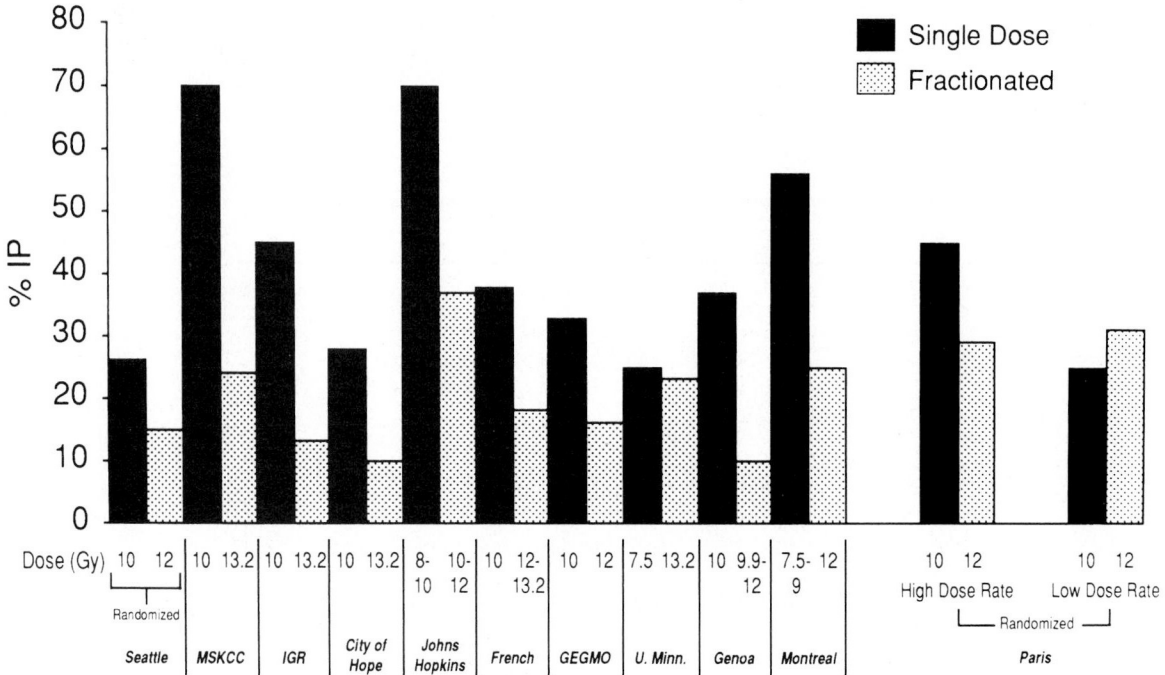

Figure 14–11. Comparison of the incidence of interstitial pneumonitis (IP) for single-dose and fractionated regimens from many institutions; all studies were nonrandomized with the exception of the first, from Seattle, and the last, which randomized to different dose rates, but not fractionation schemes (see references 79, 84, 86, 130, 147-149, 194, 218, 223, 224).

lymphoma patients were treated with high-dose therapy and autologous BMT, an acute respiratory failure thought secondary to pulmonary alveolar hemorrhage occurred in 26% of patients and was associated with the use of thoracic radiation for malignant disease just before BMT.[230] In another study in patients who received TBI, prior bleomycin treatment was found to significantly enhance lung toxicity.[213]

CATARACTS

With single-dose TBI, it has been found that the incidence of cataract development is very high (Table 14-5), 80% to 100% when patients are followed 8 to 10 years.[231-237] As many as 59% of these patients required surgery for this condition.[232]

The incidence of cataract development is considerably less (5% to 30%) when TBI is fractionated,[148,231-233,235, 237-241] with only about 20% requiring surgery[231,232,236] (see Table 14-5). One exception is a study with rapid fractionation (10.5 to 12 Gy in only 1.5 to 3 days), in which 63% of patients developed cataracts.[242] Other factors that contribute to the development of cataracts include the use of steroids,[231,239] high-dose-rate TBI,[238] the use of non–T-cell-depleted grafts,[236] prior cranial irradiation,[243,244] and the development of GVHD.[231]

HEPATIC DYSFUNCTION

Many hepatic disorders may occur after BMT: GVHD; chronic hepatitis; infections (viral, fungal, bacterial); drug reactions; leukemic infiltrates; and, a potentially fatal complication, VOD of the liver, which has risen in incidence as cytoreductive regimens have become more intense. VOD is manifested histologically by partial or complete occlusion of terminal hepatic venules by reticulin fibers, associated with sinusoidal dilatation and congestion, hepatocyte atrophy, and loss in zone 3 of the acinus.[245-247] When VOD is fatal, massive centrilobular hemorrhage is seen.[247] Clinically, the disease is defined by the triad of hepatomegaly, weight gain, and jaundice.[248]

Chemotherapy and TBI are considered the principle causes of VOD, but the etiology of the disease is undoubtedly multifactorial. With respect to TBI, a higher total dose (>12 Gy compared with 12 Gy) played a role in one study.[249] Fractionation has usually resulted in a lower incidence of VOD when results of single-dose (10 Gy) TBI have been compared with those of fractionated TBI (12 to 14 Gy),[84,133,148,250-252] but a few exceptions have been noted.[194,196,253] In single-dose regimens, the dose rate has been important, with minimal VOD with dose rates 0.07 Gy/minute or less compared with an incidence as high as 50% with dose rates of 0.18 to 1.20 Gy/minute.[246] A randomized study of dose rate, in both single-dose and fractionated TBI, did not show a difference in VOD.[194]

There is a significantly higher incidence of chronic hepatitis in patients who have an abnormal alanine aminotransferase level prior to BMT, but survival is unaffected.[254]

RENAL DYSFUNCTION

Renal changes have been noted in some studies after BMT.[255-260] Characteristics include: (1) increased serum creatinine and decreased creatinine clearance, (2) increased blood urea nitrogen, (3) a decreased glomerular filtration rate, (4) anemia, (5) hypertension without obvious cause, (6) peripheral edema, and (7) elevated lactic dehydrogenase.[255,260] The pathological appearance includes extreme subendothelial widening of glomerular basement membranes, endothelial cell dropout, arteriolar intimal thickening, and atrophic tubules.[255]

Analyses have suggested various risk factors that contribute to this morbidity. The combination of AraC plus Cy has been suggested in one study.[255] In another, a stepwise regression analysis suggested contributions from TBI, the use of cyclosporine for GVHD prophylaxis, and the use of the antifungal agent amphotericin B.[257] Renal dysfunction was strongly correlated with total TBI dose and dose per fraction in two studies.[258,259]

Table 14–5   Incidence of Cataract Development After Bone Marrow Transplantation

Study	TBI		None, %	References
	Single-Dose, %	*Fractionated, %*		
Seattle	85 (59% need surgery)	19 (20% need surgery)	19	Sanders[235]
		50 (>12 Gy; 33% need surgery)		Benyunes et al.[232]
		34 (≤12 Gy; 22% need surgery)		
Cardiff	83	0	—	Livesey et al.[233]
Stockholm	100 (10 Gy)	—	0	Calissendorff et al.[234]
	0 (8 Gy + eyeshield)			
England	—	63 (rapid fractionation)	9	Bray et al.[242]
Minneapolis	27 (3 yr) [NS]	12 (3 yr)	—	Kim et al.[148]
Paris	11 (low dose rate)	2 (low dose rate)	—	Ozsahin et al.[238]
	24 (high dose rate)	10 (high dose rate)	—	
London	100 (9 yr; non–T-cell-depleted)	—	—	Hamon et al.[236]
	72 (9 yr; T-cell depleted)	—	—	
Baltimore	—	18 (with steroids)	12	Dunn et al.[239]
	—	4 (without steroids)	—	
Helsinki	100	0	—	Lappi et al.[240]

ENDOCRINE DYSFUNCTION

Many abnormalities in endocrine function have been noted after BMT, manifested, for example, as hypothyroidism, growth deficits, impaired sexual development, and infertility. Decreased morbidity has generally been noted with fractionated TBI compared with single-dose TBI. An excellent review of this subject by Sanders and her colleagues from Seattle[261] has been published.

Thyroid function has been shown to be altered more frequently with transplant regimens containing TBI.[262] In several studies a much higher incidence of compensated hypothyroidism as well as overt hypothyroidism was found in children who had received single-dose TBI (10 Gy) compared with fractionated TBI (12 to 15.75 Gy over 4 to 7 days).[235,261,263,264]

Gonadal function is depressed in the majority of patients who receive single-dose TBI but appears to be less frequently affected in patients who receive fractionated TBI,[264] as measured by basal and stimulated luteinizing hormone levels and follicle-stimulating hormone levels. With single-dose TBI, menarche and the development of secondary sexual characteristics are significantly delayed, but with fractionated TBI, about 50% of the patients experience normal pubertal development.[237] Although most women develop primary gonadal failure, a few have recovered, and pregnancies have been reported from several institutions.[237,261,263,265,266] The first report of a successful full-term pregnancy with an embryo from donated oocytes in a woman who had undergone an allogeneic BMT appeared in 1994.[267]

GROWTH RETARDATION

Two factors can contribute to growth retardation of children who receive TBI: depressed growth hormone and a direct radiation effect on bone growth. Growth hormone deficiency is found in about 40% to 55% of children who have received TBI, but if they have had prior cranial irradiation, this incidence climbs to as high as 90%.[237] Less growth retardation occurs with fractionated TBI compared to single-dose TBI.[268-270]

ALTERATION IN COGNITIVE FUNCTION

Few studies have looked at cognitive function after marrow transplantation. A case report described somnolence syndrome 8 weeks after irradiation in an adult with AML who underwent cytoreduction with Cy and a rapid TBI course (2.2 Gy twice daily for 3 days to a total dose of 13.2 Gy).[271] A study in children showed no significant changes in IQ or in an adaptive behavior scale.[272] Hyperfractionated TBI resulted in no alterations in cognitive testing in a study of 58 patients.[273]

One study of patients who received TBI demonstrated an increasing cognitive dysfunction with increasing TBI dose, by both univariate and multivariate analysis.[274] Another study by the same group has shown that 75% of adults with malignant disease (primarily leukemia) who are candidates for marrow transplantation had a cognitive impairment before the transplant procedure, when tested for 11 functional indices.[275] Most common was a memory impairment. Prior history of cranial irradiation was the variable most strongly associated with impaired function, but there were also trends associating impairment with high-dose AraC, as well as central nervous system disease treated with intrathecal chemotherapy. Children with ALL who have more than one course of cranial irradiation also have increasing toxicity, with greater decrements in IQ and achievement.[276]

SECONDARY MALIGNANCIES

An association between irradiation for BMT and the development of secondary malignancies (SMs) is controversial. A report from Paris implicated total abdominal irradiation, which was used in preparation for BMT for severe aplastic anemia and Fanconi's anemia, in an unusually high incidence of SM at 8 years (22% ± 11% SE).[277] In contrast, there was only a 1.4% incidence at 10 years when aplastic anemia patients in Seattle were prepared with chemotherapy only.[126] It should be noted that there is an association of squamous cell carcinoma with Fanconi's anemia, even without irradiation.[278] Another analysis from Seattle with 2246 patients (320 with aplastic anemia and 1926 with hematologic malignancies) cited a 1.4% incidence of SM and implicated TBI as well as antithymocyte globulin as risk factors for GVHD.[279] An analysis of European BMT data that compared immunosuppression with BMT for aplastic anemia showed that patients who were immunosuppressed had a similar incidence of SM (0.9%) compared to those who had a BMT (0.8%).[280] In the patients who developed solid tumors in the BMT group, there was a relative risk of 20.7 for irradiation. Surprisingly, all 15 patients who developed solid tumors were male.

In contrast to these studies, other investigators suggest no association with irradiation.[281,282] In a registry study of 9880 patients, the distribution of the 127 SMs seen was similar to that in other organ transplant patients not given irradiation, only immunosuppression.[281]

CURRENT CLINICAL INDICATIONS AND FUTURE DIRECTIONS

Leukemias

In *AML*, BMT is usually done in first remission, especially with poor risk factors, or in early relapse. Poor risk factors include (1) certain chromosomal rearrangements, such as trisomy 8, t(6;9), t(9;22), or abnormalities of chromosomes 5, 7, or 11; (2) prior myelodysplasia; (3) secondary AML; (4) acute megakaryocytic leukemia; and (5) refractoriness to initial induction.[283] Allogeneic transplants are usually done if there is a suitable matched donor (see Table 14-4), but if there is not, an autologous BMT may be done with marrow purged of residual leukemic cells.

In *ALL*, since there is a reasonable long-term cure rate with standard multiagent chemotherapy, BMT is usually reserved for patients who are refractory or who relapse.

Exceptions are made for patients who are considered poor risk, such as those with certain chromosome abnormalities, for example, t(9;22), the Philadelphia chromosome; t(8;14); or t(4;11).[283]

Patients with *CML* usually undergo transplantation in chronic phase, since long-term disease-free survival is considerably better when they are transplanted early in the course of their disease.

In all of the leukemias, the major challenges continue to be the reduction of early morbidity and GVHD without compromising leukemic cell kill. Innovative techniques of radiolabeled antibodies appear promising, and newer supportive care measures are continually being developed. Low-dose nonmyeloablative TBI with donor lymphocyte infusion holds promise, providing that the high rate of severe GVHD can be reduced.

Myelodysplasias

Myelodysplastic syndromes may be quite successfully treated with allogeneic BMT. A report from Seattle, summing up their experience with BMT after TBI/Cy in 93 patients with greater than 5% blasts in their marrow or peripheral blood, demonstrates a disease-free survival rate at 4 years of 41% overall.[284] In particular, patients who were younger than 40 years old and were not defined as having excess blasts had no relapses and had a 4-year disease-free survival of 62%. As a result, BMT was recommended early in the course of disease, before any progression.

Lymphomas

Non-Hodgkin's lymphoma patients may receive an autologous BMT after cytoreduction with chemotherapy only or with a TBI-containing regimen. In general, appropriate patients are those who are refractory, relapsed, or at high risk. Results are better in high-risk patients when they undergo transplantation "up-front," rather than after relapsing.[92] High-risk patients include those with bulky mediastinal or any abdominal disease or those with a high lactate dehydrogenase level or both. The role of purging for these patients is unclear.

Hodgkin's disease patients who are refractory or relapsed patients may be eligible for autologous BMT.[285-287] If they have only had chemotherapy previously, they may receive irradiation as part of their cytoreduction procedure. More than half of these patients may be salvaged by such a regimen, as demonstrated in the patients treated at MSKCC with a TLI-containing protocol.[95,191] Patients with certain poor-risk features may be treated with a BMT also. A group from Genoa has considered patients at poor risk when they are older than age 40 or have a high lactic dehydrogenase level, anemia, bulky mediastinal disease, or extranodal disease.[285] Using a chemotherapy-only regimen, this group has achieved an 87% disease-free survival rate at 3 years, which compares favorably with their historical control patients with similar poor risk factors, who have a 33% disease-free survival rate without autologous BMT.

Multiple Myeloma

Several promising regimens have been reported in the literature for autologous BMT in multiple myeloma patients who have a large tumor burden; many contain melphalan ± TBI, and others have multiple chemotherapeutic agents and TBI. The value of purging in this disease is unclear. In a recent study from France, which used multiagent chemotherapy and TBI, a 40% event-free survival rate was reported.[288] This was a relatively young group of patients with a median age of 44. A group from Milan is achieving a survival benefit in a high-risk group defined by a high labeling index of the tumor.[289]

Anemias

Severe aplastic anemia has already been considered in some detail in the earlier section "Results of Clinical Studies." Patients who have been heavily transfused require sufficiently aggressive treatment to allow engraftment since they have been sensitized to allografts by their transfusions. TLI, which spares many sensitive structures, along with Cy, is theoretically ideal for this purpose, provided a sufficiently high dose is given. Although the optimal dose is not defined, our prior studies suggest that somewhere in the range of 900 cGy may be recommended.[82]

Pediatric Malignancies

Although some initial transplant studies for Ewing's sarcoma and neuroblastoma suggested that TBI may have a role in BMT for pediatric malignancies, there appears to be little enthusiasm today for TBI-containing regimens for children with solid tumors. In neuroblastoma, overall survival at 2 years with a TBI-containing transplant regimen was better than that for comparable patients previously treated by the same group (39% vs. 12%).[290] However, it was clear that current intensive regimens were still inadequate.

Genetic Disorders

Many patients with genetic disorders have successfully received allogeneic transplants after preparation with regimens containing TBI. Examples of diseases treated include Wiskott-Aldrich syndrome,[291] thalassemia major,[292] and infantile malignant osteopetrosis.[293] Total TBI doses may be kept low (4 to 7 Gy), minimizing any effects on bone growth and endocrine function in these children.

REFERENCES

1. Bortin MM, Horowitz MM, Rimm AA: Progress report from the international bone marrow transplant registry. *Bone Marrow Transplant.* 1992;10:113.
2. Copelan EA, Deeg HJ: Conditioning for allogeneic marrow transplantation in patients with lymphohematopoietic malignancies

without the use of total body irradiation [Review]. *Blood.* 1992; 80:1648.

3. Tutschka PJ, Copelan EA, Kapoor N: Replacing total body irradiation with busulfan as conditioning of patients with leukemia for allogeneic marrow transplantation. *Transplant Proc.* 1989;21:2952.

4. DeLaCamara R, Tomas JF, Figuera A, et al: High dose busulfan and seizures. *Bone Marrow Transplant.* 1991;7:363.

5. Morgan M, Dodds A, Atkinson K, et al: The toxicity of busulphan and cyclophosphamide as the preparative regimen for bone marrow transplantation. *Br J Haematol.* 1991;77:529.

6. Van der Jagt RHC, Appelbaum FR, Petersen FB, et al: Busulfan and cyclophosphamide as a preparative regimen for bone marrow transplantation in patients with prior chest radiotherapy. *Bone Marrow Transplant.* 1991;8:211.

7. Wingard JR, Plotnick LP, Freemer CS, et al: Growth in children after bone marrow transplantation: Busulfan plus cyclophosphamide versus cyclophosphamide plus total body irradiation. *Blood.* 1992;79:1068.

8. Inoue T, Ikeda H, Yamazaki H, et al: Role of total body irradiation as based on the comparison of preparation regimens for allogeneic bone marrow transplantation for acute leukemia in first complete remission. *Strahlenther Onkol.* 1993;169:250.

9. Blaise D, Maraninchi D, Archimbaud E, et al: Allogeneic bone marrow transplantation for acute myeloid leukemia in first remission: A randomized trial of a busulfan-Cytoxan versus Cytoxan-total body irradiation as preparative regimen: A report from the Groupe d'Etudes de la Greffe de Moelle Osseuse. *Blood.* 1993;79:2578.

10. Clift RA, Buckner CD, Thomas ED, et al: Marrow transplantation for chronic myeloid leukemia: A randomized study comparing cyclophosphamide and total body irradiation with busulfan and cyclophosphamide. *Blood.* 1994;84:2036.

11. Clift RA, Storb R: Marrow transplantation for CML: The Seattle experience. *Bone Marrow Transplant.* 1996;17(suppl 3):S1.

12. Clift RT, Radich J, Appelbaum FR, et al: Long-term follow-up of a randomized study comparing cyclophosphamide and total body irradiation with busulfan and cyclophosphamide for patients receiving allogeneic marrow transplants during chronic phase of chronic myeloid leukemia. *Blood.* 1999;94:3960.

13. Blume KG, Kopecky KJ, Henslee-Downey JP, et al: A prospective randomized comparison of total body irradiation-etoposide versus busulfan-cyclophosphamide as preparatory regimens for bone marrow transplantation in patients with leukemia who were not in first remission. *Blood.* 1993;81:2187.

14. Cosset JM, Devergie A, Blaise D, et al: Busulfan-Cytoxan (BuCy) versus Cytoxan-total body irradiation (CyTBI) as conditioning regimen before allogeneic bone marrow graft; results of two French randomized trials for chronic myeloid leukemia (CML) and acute myeloid leukemia (AML). *Int Congress Radiat Oncol.* 1993:363. Abstract.

15. Devergie A, Blaise D, Attal M, et al: Allogeneic bone marrow transplantation for chronic myeloid leukemia in first chronic phase: a randomized trial of busulfan-Cytoxan versus Cytoxan-total body irradiation as preparative regimen: a report from the French Society of Bone Marrow Graft (SFGM). *Blood.* 1995;85:2263.

16. Schwerdtfeger R, Kirsch A, Sonntag S, et al: Allogeneic bone marrow transplantation in chronic myeloid leukemia—What is the best conditioning regimen? *Bone Marrow Transplant.* 1993;12(suppl 2):13.

17. Miller G, Wagner JE, Vogelsang GB, et al: A randomized trial of busulfan-cyclophosphamide (Bu-Cy) versus cyclophosphamide-total body irradiation (Cy-TBI) as preparative regimen for patients with chronic myelogenous leukemia (CML). *Blood.* 1991;78 (suppl 1):291a. Abstract.

18. Ringden O, Ruutu T, Remberger M, et al: A randomized trial comparing busulfan with total body irradiation as conditioning in allogeneic marrow transplant recipients with leukemia: A report from the Nordic Bone Marrow Transplant Group. *Blood.* 1994;83:2723.

19. Ringden O, Remberger M, Ruutu T, et al: Increased risk of chronic graft-versus-host disease, obstructive bronchiolitis, and alopecia with busulfan versus total body irradiation: Long-term results of a randomized trial in allogeneic marrow recipients with leukemia. *Blood.* 1999;93:2196.

20. Socie G, Clift RA, Blaise D, et al: Busulfan plus cyclophosphamide compared with total-body irradiation plus cyclophosphamide before marrow transplantation for myeloid leukemia: Long-term follow-up of 4 randomized studies. *Blood.* 2001;98:3569.

21. Dusenbery KE, Daniels KA, McClure JS, et al: Randomized comparison of cyclophosphamide-total body irradiation vs. busulfan-cyclophosphamide conditioning in autologous bone marrow transplantation for acute myeloid leukemia. *Int J Radiat Oncol Biol Phys.* 1995;31:119.

22. Dusenbery KE, Steinbuch M, McGlave PB, et al: Autologous bone marrow transplantation in acute myeloid leukemia: The University of Minnesota experience. *Int J Radiat Oncol Biol Phys.* 1996; 36:335.

23. Blume KG, Forman SJ: High-dose etoposide (VP-16)-containing preparatory regimens in allogeneic and autologous bone marrow transplantation for hematologic malignancies. *Semin Oncol.* 1992;19:63.

24. Weyman C, Graham-Pole J, Emerson S, et al: Use of cytosine arabinoside and total body irradiation as conditioning for allogeneic marrow transplantation in patients with acute lymphoblastic leukemia: A multicenter survey. *Bone Marrow Transplant.* 1993;11:43.

25. Copelan EA: Conditioning regimens for allogeneic bone marrow transplantation. *Blood Rev.* 1992;6:234.

26. Kwan DK, Norman A: Radiosensitivity of human lymphocytes and thymocytes. *Radiat Res.* 1977;69:143.

27. Szcylik C, Wiktor-Jedrzejczak W: The effects of x-irradiation in vitro on subpopulations of human lymphocytes. *Int J Radiat Biol.* 1981;39:253.

28. Shank B, Andreeff M, Li D: Cell survival kinetics in peripheral blood and bone marrow during total body irradiation for marrow transplantation. *Int J Radiat Oncol Biol Phys.* 1983;9:1613.

29. Weichselbaum RR, Greenberger JS, Schmidt A, et al: In vitro radiosensitivity of human leukemia cell lines. *Radiology.* 1981; 139:485.

30. Lehnert S, Rybka WB, Suissa S, et al: Radiation response of haematopoietic cell lines of human origin. *Int J Radiat Biol.* 1986; 49:423.

31. Rhee JG, Song CW, Kim TH, et al: Effect of fractionation and rate of radiation dose on human leukemic cells, HL-60. *Radiat Res.* 1985;101:519.

32. Shank B: Hyperfractionation (T.I.D.) vs. single dose irradiation in human acute lymphocytic leukemia cells: Application to TBI for marrow transplantation. *Radiother Oncol.* 1993;27:30.

33. Vriesendorp HM, Johnson PM, Fey TA, et al: Optimal dose of total body irradiation for allogeneic bone marrow transplantation. *Transplant Proc.* 1985;17:517.

34. Storb R, Raff RF, Appelbaum FR, et al: Comparison of fractionated to single-dose total body irradiation in conditioning canine littermates for DLA-identical marrow grafts. *Blood.* 1989;74:1139.

35. Vriesendorp HM: Radiobiological speculations on therapeutic total body irradiation. *Crit Rev Oncol Hematol.* 1990;10:211.

36. Down JD, Tarbell NJ, Thames HD, et al: Syngeneic and allogeneic bone marrow engraftment after total body irradiation: Dependence on dose, dose rate, and fractionation. *Blood.* 1991;77:661.

37. Van Os R, Thames HD, Konings AWT, et al: Radiation dose-fractionation and dose-rate relationships for long-term repopulating hemopoietic stem cells in a murine bone marrow transplant model. *Radiat Res.* 1993;136:118.

38. Girinski T, Socie G, Cosset JM, et al: Similar effects on murine haemopoietic compartment of low dose rate single dose and high dose rate fractionated total body irradiation. Preliminary results after a unique dose of 750 cGy. *Br J Radiol.* 1990;61:797.

39. Van Os R, Konings AWT, Down JD: Radiation dose as a factor in host preparation for bone marrow transplantation across different genetic barriers. *Int J Radiat Biol.* 1992;61:501.

40. Down JD, Mauch P, Warhol M, et al: The effect of donor T lymphocytes and total-body irradiation on hemopoietic engraftment and pulmonary toxicity following experimental allogeneic bone marrow transplantation. *Transplant.* 1992;54:802.

41. Loewenthal E, Weiss L, Samuel S, et al: Optimization of conditioning therapy for leukemia prior to BMT. I. Optimal synergism between cyclophosphamide and total body irradiation for eradication of murine B cell leukemia (BCL1). *Bone Marrow Transplant.* 1993;12:109.

42. Evans RG: Radiobiological considerations in magna-field irradiation. *Int J Radiat Oncol Biol Phys.* 1983;9:1907.

43. Wara WM, Phillips TL, Margolis LW, et al: Radiation pneumonitis: A new approach to the derivation of time-dose factors. *Cancer.* 1973;32:547.

44. Yan R, Peters LJ, Travis EL: Cyclophosphamide 24 hours before or after total body irradiation: Effects on lung and bone marrow. *Radiother Oncol.* 1991;21:149.

45. Collis CH, Steel GG: Lung damage in mice from cyclophosphamide and thoracic irradiation: The effect of timing. *Int J Radiat Oncol Biol Phys.* 1983;9:685.

46. Okunewick JP, Kociban DL, Young CK, et al: Effect of radiation and drug order in preparatory regimens for bone marrow transplantation. In: Proceedings of the 36th Annual Meeting of the Radiation Research Society; April, 1988; Philadelphia. Abstract, p 157.

47. Peters LJ, Withers HR, Cundiff JH, et al: Radiobiological considerations in the use of total-body irradiation for bone-marrow transplantation. *Radiology.* 1979;131:243.

48. Peters L: Discussion: The radiobiological bases of TBI. *Int J Radiat Oncol Biol Phys.* 1980;6:785.

49. Vriesendorp HM: Prediction of effects of therapeutic total body irradiation in man. *Radiother Oncol.* 1990;1(suppl):37.

50. Shank B, Hoppe RT: Radiotherapeutic principles of hematopoietic cell transplantation. In Blume KG, Forman SJ, Appelbaum FR, eds: *Thomas' Hematopoietic Cell Transplantation, 3rd ed.* Boston: Blackwell Scientific, 2003:178.

51. Vitale V, Scarpati D, Frassoni F, et al: Total body irradiation: Single dose, fractions, dose rate. *Bone Marrow Transplant.* 1989; 4(suppl 1):233.

52. O'Donoghue JA, Wheldon TE, Gregor A: The implications of *in-vitro* radiation-survival curves for the optimal scheduling of total-body irradiation with bone marrow rescue in the treatment of leukemia. *Br J Radiol.* 1987;60:279.

53. Fruchtman S, Scigliano E, Isola L, et al: Hyperfractionated total body irradiation (HF-TBI) and whole allogeneic marrow grafts: An intensive, safe, and highly efficacious approach to the cure of leukemia. *Blood.* 1995;86(suppl 1):945a. Abstract.

54. Singh H, Isola L, Richards S, et al: Higher dose total body irradiation with allogeneic BMT for CML-CP results in fewer relapses. *Blood.* 2000;96:358b. Abstract.

55. O'Donoghue JA: Fractionated versus low dose-rate total body irradiation. Radiobiological considerations in the selection of regimes. *Radiother Oncol.* 1986;7:241.

56. Mark GJ, Lehimgar-Zadeh A, Ragsdale BD: Cyclophosphamide pneumonitis. *Thorax* 1978;33:89.

57. Spector JI, Zimbler H, Ross JS: Early-onset cyclophosphamide-induced interstitial pneumonitis. *JAMA.* 1979;242:2852.

58. Andersson BS, Luna MA, Yee C, et al: Fatal pulmonary failure complicating high-dose cytosine arabinoside therapy in acute leukemia. *Cancer.* 1990;65:1079.

59. Gassmann W, Uharek L, Wottge H-U, et al: Comparison of cyclophosphamide, cytarabine, and etoposide as immunosuppressive agents before allogeneic bone marrow transplantation. *Blood.* 1988;72:1574.

60. Blackett NM, Aguado M: The enhancement of haemopoietic stem cell recovery in irradiated mice by prior treatment with cyclophosphamide. *Cell Tissue Kinet.* 1979;12:291.

61. Shank B, O'Reilly RJ, Cunningham I, et al: Total body irradiation for bone marrow transplantation: The Memorial Sloan-Kettering Cancer Center experience. *Radiother Oncol.* 1990;1(suppl):68.

62. Spitzer TR, Deeg HJ, Torrisi J, et al: Total body irradiation (TBI) induced emesis is universal after small dose fractions (120 cGy) and is not cumulative dose related. *Proc Am Soc Clin Oncol.* 1990; 9:14. Abstract.

63. Hewitt M, Cornish J, Pamphilou D, et al: Effective emetic control during conditioning of children for bone marrow transplantation using ondansetron, a 5-HT3 antagonist. *Bone Marrow Transplant.* 1991;7:431.

64. Spitzer TR, Friedman CJ, Bushnell W, et al: Double-blind, randomized, parallel-group study on the efficacy and safety of oral granisetron and oral ondansetron in the prophylaxis of nausea and vomiting in patients receiving hyperfractionated total body irradiation. *Bone Marrow Transplant.* 2000;26:203.

65. Spitzer TR, Bryson JC, Cirenza E, et al: Randomized double-blind, placebo-controlled evaluation of oral ondansetron in the prevention of nausea and vomiting associated with fractionated total-body irradiation. *J Clin Oncol.* 1994;12:2432.

66. Tiley C, Powles R, Catalano J, et al: Results of a double blind placebo controlled study of ondansetron as an antiemetic during total body irradiation in patients undergoing bone marrow transplantation. *Leuk Lymphoma.* 1992;7:317.

67. Shank B: Techniques of magna-field irradiation. *Int J Radiat Oncol Biol Phys.* 1983;9:1925.

68. Glasgow GP, Wang S, Stanton J: A total body irradiation stand for bone marrow transplant patients. *Int J Radiat Oncol Biol Phys.* 1989;16:875.

69. Kutcher GJ, Bonfiglio P, Shank B, et al: Combined photon and electron technique for total body irradiation. *European Society for Therapeutic Radiology and Oncology.* 1988;31. Abstract.

70. Miralbell R, Rouzaud M, Grob E, et al: Can a total body irradiation technique be fast and reproducible? *Int J Radiat Oncol Biol Phys.* 1994;29:1167.

71. Gerbi BJ, Dusenbery KE: Design specifications for a treatment stand used for total body photon irradiation. *European Society for Therapeutic Radiology and Oncology.* 1988;31. Abstract.

72. Breneman JC, Elson HR, Little R, et al: A technique for delivery of total body irradiation for bone marrow transplantation in adults and adolescents. *Int J Radiat Oncol Biol Phys.* 1990;18:1233.

73. Bortin MM: Pathogenesis of interstitial pneumonitis following allogeneic bone marrow transplantation for acute leukemia. In Gale RP, ed. *Recent Advances in Bone Marrow Transplantation.* New York: Alan R Liss; 1983:445.

74. Fryer CJH, Fitzpatrick PJ, Rider WD, et al: Radiation pneumonitis: Experience following a large single dose of radiation. *Int J Radiat Oncol Biol Phys.* 1978;4:931.

75. Kim TH, Kersey JH, Sewchand W, et al: Total body irradiation with a high-dose-rate linear accelerator for bone-marrow transplantation in aplastic anemia and neoplastic disease. *Radiology.* 1977;122:523.

76. Fyles GM, Messner HA, Lockwood G, et al: Long-term results of bone marrow transplantation for patients with AML, ALL, and CML prepared with single dose total body irradiation of 500 cGy delivered with a high dose rate. *Bone Marrow Transplant.* 1991; 8:453.

77. Tarbell NJ, Amato DA, Down JD, et al: Fractionation and dose rate effects in mice: A model for bone marrow transplantation in man. *Int J Radiat Oncol Biol Phys.* 1987;13:1065.

78. Shank B, Hopfan S, Kim JH, et al: Hyperfractionated total body irradiation for bone marrow transplantation: I. Early results in leukemia patients. *Int J Radiat Oncol Biol Phys.* 1981;7:1109.

79. Pino y Torres JL, Bross DS, Lam W-C, et al: Risk factors in interstitial pneumonitis following allogenic bone marrow transplantation. *Int J Radiat Oncol Biol Phys.* 1982;8:1301.

80. Lawton CA, Barber-Derus SW, Murray KJ, et al: Technical modifications in hyperfractionated total body irradiation for T-lymphocyte deplete bone marrow transplant. *Int J Radiat Oncol Biol Phys.* 1989;17:319.

81. Lawton CA, Barber-Derus SW, Murray KJ, et al: Influence of renal shielding on the incidence of late renal dysfunction associated with T-lymphocyte deplete bone marrow transplantation in adult patients. *Int J Radiat Oncol Biol Phys.* 1992;23:681.

82. Shank B, Brochstein JA, Castro-Malaspina H, et al: Immunosuppression prior to marrow transplantation for sensitized aplastic anemia patients: Comparison of TLI with TBI. *Int J Radiat Oncol Biol Phys.* 1988;14:1133.

83. Dutreix J, Janoray P, Bridier A, et al: Biologic and anatomic problems of lung shielding in whole-body irradiation. *J Natl Cancer Inst.* 1986;76:1333.

84. Cosset JM, Baume D, Pico JL, et al: Single dose versus hyperfractionated total body irradiation before allogeneic bone marrow transplantation: A non-randomized comparative study of 54 patients at the Institut Gustave-Roussy. *Radiother Oncol.* 1989; 15:151.

85. Sanders JE, Flournoy N, Thomas ED, et al: Marrow transplant experience in children with acute lymphoblastic leukemia: An analysis of factors associated with survival, relapse, and graft-versus-host disease. *Med Pediatr Oncol.* 1985;13:165.

86. Shank B, Chu FCH, Dinsmore R, et al: Hyperfractionated total body irradiation for bone marrow transplantation. Results in seventy leukemia patients with allogeneic transplants. *Int J Radiat Oncol Biol Phys.* 1983;9:1607.

87. Gratwohl A, Gluckman E, Goldman J, et al: Effect of splenectomy before bone marrow transplantation on survival in chronic granulocytic leukemia. *Lancet.* 1985;2:1290.

88. Barrett AJ, Longhurst P, Humble JG, et al: Effect of splenic irradiation on circulating colony-forming cells in chronic granulocytic leukemia. *Br Med J.* 1977;1:1259.

89. Ravalese J III, Madoc-Jones H, Ling M, et al: Splenic irradiation prior to high dose chemotherapy and allogeneic bone marrow transplantation for chronic myelogenous leukemia. *Int J Radiat Oncol Biol Phys.* 1993;27:312 Abstract.

90. Gratwohl A, Hermans J, Biezen AV, et al: No advantage for patients who receive splenic irradiation before bone marrow transplantation for chronic myeloid leukemia. *Bone Marrow Transpl.* 1992;10:147.

91. Gratwohl A, Hermans J, Biezen AV, et al: Splenic irradiation before bone marrow transplantation for chronic myeloid leukemia. *Br J Haematol.* 1996;95:494.

92. Chadha M, Shank B, Fuks Z, et al: Improved survival of poor prognosis diffuse histiocytic (large cell) lymphoma managed with sequential induction chemotherapy, "boost" radiation therapy, and autologous bone marrow transplantation. *Int J Radiat Oncol Biol Phys.* 1988;14:407.

93. Mundt AJ, Sibley G, Williams S, et al: Patterns of failure following high-dose chemotherapy and autologous bone marrow transplantation with involved field radiotherapy for relapsed/ refractory Hodgkin's disease. *Int J Radiat Oncol Biol Phys.* 1995; 33:261.

94. Poen JP, Hoppe RT, Horning SJ: High-dose therapy and autologous bone marrow transplantation for relapsed/refractory Hodgkin's disease: The impact of involved field radiotherapy on patterns of failure and survival. *Int J Radiat Oncol Biol Phys.* 1996;36:3.

95. Moskowitz CH, Nimer SD, Zelenetz AD, et al: A 2-step comprehensive high-dose chemoradiotherapy second-line program for relapsed and refractory Hodgkin disease: Analysis by intent to treat and development of a prognostic model. *Blood.* 2001; 97:616.

96. Mundt AJ, Williams SF, Hallahan D: High dose chemotherapy and stem cell rescue for aggressive non-Hodgkin's lymphoma: Pattern of failure and implications for involved-field radiotherapy. *Int J Radiat Oncol Biol Phys.* 1997;39:617.

97. Fouillard L, Laporte JP, Labopin M, et al: Autologous stem-cell transplantation for non-Hodgkin's lymphomas: The role of graft purging and radiotherapy posttransplantation. Results of a retrospective analysis on 120 patients autografted in a single institution. *J Clin Oncol.* 1998;16:2803.

98. Philip T, Guglielmi C, Hagenbeek A, et al: Autologous bone marrow transplantation as compared with salvage chemotherapy in relapses of chemotherapy-sensitive non-Hodgkin's lymphoma. *N Engl J Med.* 1995;333:1540.

99. Matthews DC, Appelbaum FR, Eary JE, et al: Phase I study of (131)I-anti-CD45 antibody + cyclophosphamide and total body irradiation for advanced leukemia and myelodysplastic syndrome. *Blood.* 1999;94:1237.

100. Matthews DC, Appelbaum FR, Eary JF, et al: Development of a marrow transplant regimen for acute leukemia using targeted hematopoietic irradiation delivered by 131I-labeled anti-CD45 antibody, combined with cyclophosphamide and total body irradiation. *Blood.* 1995;85:1122.

101. Briot E, Dutreix A, Bridier A: Dosimetry for total body irradiation. *Radiother Oncol Suppl.* 1990;1:16.

102. Van Dyk J: Dosimetry for total body irradiation. *Radiother Oncol.* 1987;9:107.

103. Van Dyk J, Galvin JM, Glasgow GP, Podgorsak EB: *The Physical Aspects of Total and Half Body Photon Irradiation.* AAPM Report No. 17. New York: American Institute of Physics; 1986.

104. Storb R, Appelbaum F, Schuening F, et al: Bone marrow transplantation and massive total body irradiation. In Ricks RC, Fry SA, eds. *The Basis for Radiation Accident Preparedness: II. Clinical Experience and Follow-up Since 1979.* New York: Elsevier; 1990:109.

105. Anasetti C, Amos D, Beatty PG, et al: Effect of HLA compatibility on engraftment of bone marrow transplants in patients with leukemia or lymphoma. *N Engl J Med.* 1989;320:197.

106. Champlin R, Ho WG, Mitsuyasu R, et al: Graft failure and leukemia relapse following T-lymphocyte depleted bone marrow transplantation; effect of intensification of immunosuppressive conditioning. *Transplant Proc.* 1987;19:2616.

107. Guyotat D, Dutou L, Ehrsam A, et al: Graft rejection after T-cell depleted marrow transplantation: Role of fractionated irradiation. *Br J Haematol.* 1987;65:499.

108. Patterson J, Prentice HG, Brenner MK, et al: Graft rejection following HLA matched T-lymphocyte depleted bone marrow transplantation. *Br J Haematol.* 1986;63:221.

109. Burnett AK, Robertson AG, Hann IM, et al: In vitro T-depletion of allogeneic bone marrow: Prevention of rejection in HLA-matched transplants by increased TBI. *Bone Marrow Transplant.* 1986;1(suppl 1):121.

110. Racadot E, Herve P, Beaujean F, et al: Prevention of graft-versus-host disease in HLA-matched bone marrow transplantation for malignant diseases: Multicentric study of 62 patients using 3-pan-T monoclonal antibodies and rabbit complement. *J Clin Oncol.* 1987;5:426.

111. Iriondo A, Hermosa V, Richard C, et al: Graft rejection following T lymphocyte depleted bone marrow transplantation with two different TBI regimens. *Br J Haematol.* 1987;65:246.

112. Martin PH, Hansen JA, Torok-Storb B, et al: Graft failure in patients receiving T cell-depleted HLA-identical allogeneic marrow transplants. *Bone Marrow Transplant.* 1988;3:445.

113. Soiffer RJ, Mauch P, Tarbell NJ, et al: Total body irradiation to prevent graft rejection in recipients of HLA non-identical T cell-depleted allogeneic marrow. *Bone Marrow Transplant.* 1991;7:23.

114. James ND, Apperley JF, Kam KC, et al: Total lymphoid irradiation preceding bone marrow transplantation for chronic myeloid leukemia. *Clin Radiol.* 1989;40:195.

115. Slavin S, Or R, Naparstek E, et al: New approaches for the prevention of rejection and graft-versus-host disease in clinical bone marrow transplantation. *Israel J Med Sci.* 1986;22:264.

116. Slavin S, Or R, Weshler Z, et al: The use of total lymphoid irradiation for abrogation of host resistance to T-cell depleted marrow allografts. *Bone Marrow Transplant.* 1986;1(suppl 1):98.

117. Kernan NA, Bordignon C, Heller G, et al: Graft failure after T-cell-depleted human leukocyte antigen identical marrow transplants for leukemia: I. Analysis of risk factors and results of secondary transplants. *Blood.* 1989;74:2227.

118. Poynton CH, MacDonald D, Byrom NA, et al: Rejection after T cell depletion of donor bone marrow. *Bone Marrow Transplant.* 1987;2(suppl 1):153.

119. Ganem G, Kuentz M, Beaujean F, et al: Additional total lymphoid irradiation (TLI) in preventing graft failure of T cell depleted bone marrow transplantation (BMT) from HLA identical siblings: Results of a prospective randomized study. *Bone Marrow Transplant.* 1987;2(suppl 1):156.

120. McSweeney PA, Niederwieser D, Shizuru JA, et al: Hematopoietic cell transplantation in older patients with hematologic malignancies: Replacing high-dose cytotoxic therapy with graft-versus-tumor effects. *Blood.* 2001;97:3390.

121. Ballen KK, Becker PS, Emmons RV, et al: Low-dose total body irradiation followed by allogeneic lymphocyte infusion may induce remission in patients with refractory hematologic malignancy. *Blood.* 2002;100:442.

122. Ramsay NKC, Kim TH, McGlave P, et al: Bone marrow transplantation for severe aplastic anemia following preparation with cyclophosphamide and total lymphoid irradiation. In Young NS, Levine AS, Humphries RK, eds. *Aplastic Anemia: Stem Cell Biology and Advances in Treatment.* New York: Alan R Liss; 1984:315.

123. Kim TH, Kersey JH, Khan FM, et al: Single dose total lymphoid irradiation combined with cyclophosphamide as immunosuppression for human marrow transplantation in aplastic anemia. *Int J Radiat Oncol Biol Phys.* 1979;5:993.

124. Vitale V, Barra S, Corvo R, et al: The role of thoraco-abdominal irradiation before marrow transplantation. *Bone Marrow Transplant.* 1991;7(suppl 3):35.

125. Gluckman E: Radiosensitivity in Fanconi anemia: Application to the conditioning for bone marrow transplantation. *Radiother Oncol.* 1990;18(suppl 1):88.

126. Witherspoon RP, Storb R, Pepe M, et al: Cumulative incidence of secondary solid malignant tumors in aplastic anemia. *Blood.* 1992;79:289.

127. Storb R: Allogeneic marrow transplantation in patients with severe aplastic anemia. *Transplant Rev.* 1993;3:33.

128. Flowers MED, Doney KC, Storb R, et al: Marrow transplantation for Fanconi anemia with or without leukemic transformation: An update of the Seattle experience. *Bone Marrow Transplant.* 1992;9:167.

129. Thomas ED: Total body irradiation regimens for marrow grafting. *Int J Radiat Oncol Biol Phys.* 1990;19:1285.

130. Thomas ED, Clift RA, Hersman J, et al: Marrow transplantation for acute nonlymphoblastic leukemia in first remission using fractionated or single-dose irradiation. *Int J Radiat Oncol Biol Phys.* 1982;8:817.

131. Clift RA, Buckner CD, Appelbaum FR, et al: Allogeneic marrow transplantation in patients with acute myeloid leukemia in first remission: A randomized trial of two irradiation regimens. *Blood.* 1990;76:1867.

132. Clift RA, Buckner CD, Appelbaum FR, et al: Allogeneic marrow transplantation in patients with chronic myeloid leukemia in the chronic phase: A randomized trial of two irradiation regimens. *Blood.* 1991;77:1660.

133. Deeg HJ, Sullivan KM, Buckner CD, et al: Marrow transplantation for acute non lymphoblastic leukemia in first remission: Toxicity and long-term follow-up of patients conditioned with single dose or fractionated total body irradiation. *Bone Marrow Transplant.* 1986;1:151.

134. Clift R, Buckner CD, Bianco J, et al: Marrow transplantation in patients with acute myeloid leukemia. *Leukemia.* 1992; 6 (suppl 2):104.

135. Peterson FB, Deeg HJ, Buckner CD, et al: Marrow transplantation following escalating doses of fractionated total body irradiation and cyclophosphamide. A phase I trial. *Int J Radiat Oncol Biol Phys.* 1992;23:1027.

136. McAfee SL, Powell SN, Colby C, Spitzer TR: Dose-escalated total body irradiation and autologous stem cell transplantation for refractory hematologic malignancy. *Int J Radiat Oncol Biol Phys.* 2002;53:151.

137. Frassoni F, Scarpati D, Bacigalupo A, et al: The effect of total body irradiation dose and chronic graft-versus-host disease on leukemic relapse after allogeneic bone marrow transplantation. *Br J Haematol.* 1989;73:211.

138. Scarpati D, Frassoni F, Vitale V, et al: Total body irradiation in acute myeloid leukemia and chronic myelogenous leukemia: Influence of dose and dose-rate on leukemia relapse. *Int J Radiat Oncol Biol Phys.* 1989;17:547.

139. Frassoni F: Eradication of leukemic marrow and prevention of leukemia relapse with total body irradiation and bone marrow transplantation. *Med Oncol Tumor Pharmacother.* 1991; 8:189.

140. Chessells JM, Rogers DW, Leiper AD, et al: Bone-marrow transplantation has a limited role in prolonging second marrow remission in childhood lymphoblastic leukemia. *Lancet.* 1986; 1:1239.

141. Harris R, Feig S, Coccia P, et al: ALL in second remission: A CCSG study comparing intensive maintenance chemotherapy to bone marrow transplantation. *Proc Am Soc Clin Oncol.* 1987; 6:163. Abstract.

142. Proctor SJ, Hamilton PJ, Taylor P, et al: A comparative study of combination chemotherapy versus marrow transplant in first remission in adult acute lymphoblastic leukemia. *Br J Haematol.* 1988;69:35.

143. Mrsic M, Nemet D, Labar B, et al: Chemotherapy versus allogeneic bone marrow transplantation in adults with acute lymphoblastic leukemia. *Transplant Proc.* 1993;25:1268.

144. Brochstein JA, Kernan NA, Groshen S, et al: Allogeneic bone marrow transplantation after hyperfractionated total-body irradiation and cyclophosphamide in children with acute leukemia. *N Engl J Med.* 1987;317:1618.

145. Buckner CD, Doney K, Sanders J, et al: Marrow transplantation for patients with acute lymphoblastic leukemia: The Seattle experience. *Leukemia.* 1992;6(suppl 2):193.

146. Arcese W, Meloni G, Giona F, et al: Idarubicin plus ARA-C followed by allogeneic or autologous bone marrow transplantation in advanced acute lymphoblastic leukemia. *Bone Marrow Transplant.* 1991;7(suppl 2):38.

147. Socie G, Devergie A, Girinsky T, et al: Influence of the fractionation of total body irradiation on complications and relapse rate for chronic myelogenous leukemia. *Int J Radiat Oncol Biol Phys.* 1991;20:397.

148. Kim TH, McGlave PB, Ramsay N, et al: Comparison of two total body irradiation regimens in allogeneic bone marrow transplantation for acute non-lymphoblastic leukemia in first remission. *Int J Radiat Oncol Biol Phys.* 1990;19:889.

149. Blume KG, Forman SJ, Snyder DS, et al: Allogeneic bone marrow transplantation for acute lymphoblastic leukemia during first complete remission. *Transplant.* 1987;43:389.

150. Devergie A, Reiffers J, Vernant JP, et al: Long-term follow-up after bone marrow transplantation for chronic myelogenous leukemia: Factors associated with relapse. *Bone Marrow Transplant.* 1990;5:379.

151. Feig SA, Nesbit ME, Buckley J, et al: Bone marrow transplantation for acute non-lymphocytic leukemia. A report from the Children's Cancer Study Group of sixty-seven children transplanted in first remission. *Bone Marrow Transplant.* 1987;2:365.

152. Blaise D, Gaspard MH, Stoppa MA, et al: Allogeneic or autologous bone marrow transplantation for acute lymphoblastic leukemia in first complete remission. *Bone Marrow Transplant.* 1990;5:7.

153. Kersey JH, Weisdorf D, Nesbit ME, et al: Comparison of autologous and allogeneic bone marrow transplantation for treatment of high-risk refractory acute lymphoblastic leukemia. *N Engl J Med.* 1987;317:461.

154. Uderzo C, Coleselli P, Messina C, et al: Allogeneic BMT versus autologous BMT in childhood acute lymphoblastic leukemia (ALL): An Italian cooperative study of vincristine (VCR), R-TBI and cyclophosphamide. *Bone Marrow Transplant.* 1991; 7(suppl 2):132.

155. Johnson FL, Thomas ED: Treatment of relapsed acute lymphoblastic leukemia in childhood. *N Engl J Med.* 1984; 310:263. Letter.

156. Gale RP, Buchner T, Horowitz MM, et al: Chemotherapy versus bone marrow transplants for adults with acute myelogenous leukemia (AML) in first remission. *Blood.* 1993;82:168a. Abstract.

157. Zittoun R, Mandelli F, Willemze R, et al: Prospective phase III study of autologous bone marrow transplantation (ABMT) v short intensive chemotherapy (IC) v allogeneic bone marrow transplantation (allo-BMT) during first complete remission (CR) of acute myelogenous leukemia (AML). *Blood.* 1993;82:85a. Abstract.

158. Appelbaum FR, Fisher LD, Thomas ED: Chemotherapy v. marrow transplantation for adults with acute nonlymphocytic leukemia: A 5-year follow-up. *Blood.* 1988;72:179.

159. Powles RL, Morgenstern G, Clink HM, et al: The place of bone-marrow transplantation in acute myelogenous leukemia. *Lancet.* 1980;1:1047.

160. Reiffers J, Gaspard MH, Maraninchi D, et al: Allogeneic bone marrow transplantation versus chemotherapy in first-remission acute myeloid leukemia. *J Clin Oncol.* 1989;7:979. Letter.

161. Archimbaud E, Thomas X, Michallet M, et al: Prospective genetically randomized comparison between intensive postinduction chemotherapy and bone marrow transplantation in adults with newly diagnosed acute myeloid leukemia. *J Clin Oncol.* 1994;12:262.

162. Conde E, Iriondo A, Rayon C, et al: Allogeneic bone marrow transplantation versus intensification chemotherapy for acute myelogenous leukemia in first remission: A prospective controlled trial. *Br J Haematol.* 1988;68:219.

163. Cassileth PA, Andersen J, Lazarus HM, et al: Autologous bone marrow transplant in acute myeloid leukemia in first remission. *J Clin Oncol.* 1993;11:314.

164. Lowenberg B, Verdonck LJ, Dekker AW, et al: Autologous bone marrow transplantation in acute myeloid leukemia in first remission: Results of a Dutch prospective study. *J Clin Oncol.* 1990;8:287.

165. Champlin RE, Ho WG, Gale RP, et al: Treatment of acute myelogenous leukemia. A prospective controlled trial of bone marrow transplantation versus consolidation chemotherapy. *Ann Intern Med.* 1985;102:285.

166. Nesbit ME Jr, Buckley JD, Feig SA, et al: Chemotherapy for induction of remission of childhood acute myeloid leukemia followed by marrow transplantation or multiagent chemotherapy: a report from the Children's Cancer Group. *J Clin Oncol.* 1994;12:127.

167. Woods WG, Kobrinsky N, Buckley J, et al: Intensively timed induction therapy followed by autologous or allogeneic bone marrow transplantation for children with acute myeloid leukemia or myelodysplastic syndrome: A Children's Cancer Group pilot study. *J Clin Oncol.* 1993;11:1448.

168. Schalson G, Michel G, Landman-Parker J, et al: Allogeneic bone marrow transplantation (BMT) is the most effective treatment for acute myeloblastic leukemia in childhood. *Blood*. 1993;82:169a. Abstract.

169. Zander AR, Keating M, Dicke K, et al: A comparison of marrow transplantation with chemotherapy for adults with acute leukemia of poor prognosis in first complete remission. *J Clin Oncol*. 1988;6:1548.

170. Dahl GV, Kalwinsky DK, Mirro J Jr, et al: Allogeneic bone marrow transplantation in a program of intensive sequential chemotherapy for children and young adults with acute nonlymphoblastic leukemia in first remission. *J Clin Oncol*. 1990;8:295.

171. Gratwohl A, Hermans J, Niederwieser D, et al: Bone marrow transplantation for chronic myeloid leukemia: Long-term results. *Bone Marrow Transplant*. 1993;12:509.

172. Clift RA, Appelbaum FR, Thomas ED: Treatment of chronic myeloid leukemia by marrow transplantation. *Blood*. 1993; 82:1954.

173. Goldman JM, Gale RP, Horowitz MM, et al: Bone marrow transplantation for chronic myelogenous leukemia in chronic phase. *Ann Intern Med*. 1988;108:806.

174. Frassoni F, Strada P, Sessarego M, et al: Mixed chimerism after allogeneic marrow transplantation for leukemia: Correlation with dose of total body irradiation and graft-versus-host disease. *Bone Marrow Transplant*. 1990;5:235.

175. Gulati SC, Shank B, Black P, et al: Autologous bone marrow transplantation for patients with poor-prognosis lymphoma. *J Clin Oncol*. 1988;6:1303.

176. Freedman AS, Takvorian T, Neuberg D, et al: Autologous bone marrow transplantation in poor-prognosis intermediate-grade and high-grade B-cell non-Hodgkin's lymphoma in first remission: A pilot study. *J Clin Oncol*. 1993;11:931.

177. Goldstone AH: High-dose therapy for the treatment of non-Hodgkin's lymphoma. In Armitage JO, Antman KH, eds. *High-Dose Cancer Therapy: Pharmacology, Hematopoietins, Stem Cells*. Baltimore: Williams & Wilkins; 1992:662.

178. Gulati S, Acaba L, Yahalom J, et al: Autologous bone marrow transplantation for acute myelogenous leukemia using 4-hydroperoxycyclophosphamide and VP-16 purged bone marrow. *Bone Marrow Transplant*. 1992;10:129.

179. Shepherd JD, Barnett MJ, Connors JM, et al: Allogeneic bone marrow transplantation for poor-prognosis non-Hodgkin's lymphoma. *Bone Marrow Transplant*. 1993;12:591.

180. Gulati S, Yahalom J, Acaba L, et al: Treatment of patients with relapsed and resistant non-Hodgkin's lymphoma using total body irradiation, etoposide, and cyclophosphamide and autologous bone marrow transplantation. *J Clin Oncol*. 1992;10:936.

181. Chopra R, Goldstone AH, Pearce R, et al: Autologous versus allogeneic bone marrow transplantation for non-Hodgkin's lymphoma: a case-controlled analysis of the European Bone Marrow Transplant Group Registry data. *J Clin Oncol*. 1992;10:1690.

182. Stewart FM: Indications and relative indications for stem cell transplantation in non-Hodgkin's lymphoma. *Leukemia*. 1993;7:1091.

183. Chaffey JT, Hellman S, Rosenthal DS, et al: Total-body irradiation in the treatment of lymphocytic lymphoma. *Cancer Treat Rep*. 1977;61:1149.

184. Qasim MM: Total body irradiation as a primary therapy in non-Hodgkin lymphoma. *Clin Radiol*. 1979;30:287.

185. Johnson RE, Ruhl U: Treatment of chronic lymphocytic leukemia with emphasis on total body irradiation. *Int J Radiat Oncol Biol Phys*. 1976;1:387.

186. Kempin S, Shank B: Radiation in chronic lymphocytic leukemia. In Gale RP, Rai KR, eds. *Chronic Lymphocytic Leukemia: Recent Progress and Future Direction*. New York: Alan R Liss; 1987:337.

187. Rubin P, Bennett JM, Begg C, et al: The comparison of total body irradiation vs chlorambucil and prednisone for remission induction of active chronic lymphocytic leukemia: An ECOG study: Part I: Total body irradiation-response and toxicity. *Int J Radiat Oncol Biol Phys*. 1981;7:1623.

188. Jacobs P, King HS: A randomized prospective comparison of chemotherapy to total body irradiation as initial treatment for the indolent lymphoproliferative diseases. *Blood*. 1987;69:1642.

189. Lybeert MLM, Meerwaldt JH, Deneve W: Long-term results of low dose total body irradiation for advanced non-Hodgkin's lymphoma. *Int J Radiat Oncol Biol Phys*. 1987;13:1167.

190. Yahalom J, Gulati S, Shank B, et al: Total lymphoid irradiation, high-dose chemotherapy and autologous bone marrow transplantation for chemotherapy-resistant Hodgkin's disease. *Int J Radiat Oncol Biol Phys*. 1989;17:915.

191. Yahalom J, Gulati SC, Toia M, et al: Accelerated hyperfractionated total-lymphoid irradiation, high-dose chemotherapy, and autologous bone marrow transplantation for refractory and relapsing patients with Hodgkin's disease. *J Clin Oncol*. 1993; 11:1062.

192. Anderson JE, Litzow MR, Appelbaum FR, et al: Allogeneic, syngeneic, and autologous marrow transplantation for Hodgkin's disease: The 21-year Seattle experience. *J Clin Oncol*. 1993; 11:2342.

193. Horning SJ, Negrin RS, Chao NJ, et al: Autologous stem cell transplant for recurrent or refractory Hodgkin's disease: Comparative results of total body irradiation (TBI) and chemotherapy-only high dose regimens. *Blood*. 1993;82:445a. Abstract.

194. Ozsahin M, Pene F, Touboul E, et al: Total-body irradiation before bone marrow transplantation; results of two randomized instantaneous dose rates in 157 patients. *Cancer*. 1992;69:2853.

195. Belkacemi Y, Pene F, Touboul E, et al: Total-body irradiation before bone marrow transplantation for acute leukemia in first or second complete remission. Results and prognostic factors in 326 consecutive patients. *Strahlenther Onkol*. 1998;174:92.

196. Valls A, Granena A, Carreras E, et al: Total body irradiation in bone marrow transplantation. Fractionated vs single dose. Acute toxicity and preliminary results. *Bull Cancer*. 1989;76:797.

197. Jones LR, Toth BB, Keene HJ: Effects of total body irradiation on salivary gland function and caries-associated oral microflora in bone marrow transplant patients. *Oral Surg Oral Med Oral Pathol*. 1992;73:670.

198. Shepp DH, Dandliker PS, Flournoy N, et al: Sequential intravenous and twice-daily oral acyclovir for extended prophylaxis of Herpes simplex virus infection in marrow transplant patients. *Transplant*. 1987;43:654.

199. Clift RA, Bianco JA, Appelbaum FR, et al: A randomized controlled trial of pentoxifylline for the prevention of regimen-related toxicities in patients undergoing allogeneic marrow transplantation. *Blood*. 1993;82:2025.

200. Bearman SI, Appelbaum FR, Buckner CD, et al: Regimen-related toxicity in patients undergoing bone marrow transplantation. *J Clin Oncol*. 1988;6:1562.

201. Petersen FB, Bearman SI: Preparative regimens and their toxicity. In Forman SJ, Blume KG, Thomas ED, eds. *Bone Marrow Transplantation*. Boston: Blackwell Scientific; 1994:79.

202. Glucksberg H, Storb R, Fefer A, et al: Clinical manifestations of graft-versus-host disease in human recipients of marrow from HL-A-matched sibling donors. *Transplantation*. 1974;18:295.

203. Slavin RE, Santos GW: The graft versus host reaction in man after bone marrow transplantation: Pathology, pathogenesis, clinical features, and implication. *Clin Immunol Immunobiol*. 1973;1:472.

204. Ramsay NKC, Kersey JH, Robison LL, et al: A randomized study of the prevention of acute graft-versus-host disease. *N Engl J Med*. 1982;306:392.

205. Storb R, Deeg HJ, Whitehead J, et al: Methotrexate and cyclosporine compared with cyclosporine alone for prophylaxis of acute graft versus host disease after marrow transplantation for leukemia. *N Engl J Med*. 1986;314:729.

206. Sullivan KM, Kopecky KJ, Buckner CD, et al: Intravenous IgG to prevent graft-versus-host disease after bone marrow transplantation. *N Engl J Med*. 1990;323:705. Letter.

207. Reisner Y, Kapoor N, Kirkpatrick D, et al: Transplantation for acute leukaemia with HLA-A and B non-identical parental marrow cells fractionated with soybean agglutinin and sheep red blood cells. *Lancet*. 1981;2:327.

208. Kernan NA: T-cell depletion for prevention of graft-versus-host disease. In Forman SJ, Blume KG, Thomas ED, eds. *Bone Marrow Transplantation*. Boston: Blackwell Scientific; 1994:124.

209. Emanuel D, Cunningham I, Jules-Elysee K, et al: Cytomegalovirus pneumonia after bone marrow transplantation successfully treated with the combination of ganciclovir and high-dose intravenous immune globulin. *Ann Intern Med*. 1988;109:777.

210. Enright H, Haake R, Weisdorf D, et al: Cytomegalovirus pneumonia after bone marrow transplantation: Risk factors and response to therapy. *Transplantation*. 1993;55:1339.

211. Ozsahin M, Schwartz LH, Pene F, et al: Is body weight a risk factor of interstitial pneumonitis after bone marrow transplantation? *Bone Marrow Transplant.* 1992;10:97. Correspondence.

212. Ozsahin M, Belkacemi Y, Touboul E, et al: The influence of body surface on interstitial pneumonitis following bone marrow transplantation. *Int Congress Radiat Oncol.* 1993;546. Abstract.

213. Hartsell WF, Ghalie R, Rubin D, et al: Pulmonary complications of bone marrow transplantation (BMT): A comparison of total body irradiation and cyclophosphamide (TBI-Cy) to busulfan and cyclophosphamide (Bu-Cy). *Int J Radiat Oncol Biol Phys.* 1993;27(suppl 1):186. Abstract.

214. Granena A, Carreras E, Rozman C, et al: Interstitial pneumonitis after BMT: 15 years experience in a single institution. *Bone Marrow Transplant.* 1993;11:453.

215. Gogna NK, Morgan G, Downs K, et al: Lung dose rate and interstitial pneumonitis in total body irradiation for bone marrow transplantation. *Australas Radiol.* 1992;36:317.

216. Badier M, Guillot C, Delpierre S, et al: Pulmonary function changes 100 days and one year after bone marrow transplantation. *Bone Marrow Transplant.* 1993;12:457.

217. Wingard JR, Mellits ED, Sostrin MB, et al: Interstitial pneumonitis after allogeneic bone marrow transplantation: Nine-year experience at a single institution. *Medicine.* 1988;67:175.

218. Sutton L, Kuentz M, Cordonnier C, et al: Allogeneic bone marrow transplantation for adult acute lymphoblastic leukemia in first complete remission: Factors predictive of transplant-related mortality and influence of total body irradiation modalities. *Bone Marrow Transplant.* 1993;12:583.

219. Latini P, Aristei C, Aversa F, et al: Lung damage following bone marrow transplantation after hyperfractionated total body irradiation. *Radiother Oncol.* 1991;22:127.

220. Latini P, Aristei C, Aversa F, et al: Interstitial pneumonitis after hyperfractionated total body irradiation in HLA-matched T-depleted bone marrow transplantation. *Int J Radiat Oncol Biol Phys.* 1992;23:401.

221. Ho VT, Weller E, Lee SJ, et al: Prognostic factors for early severe pulmonary complications after hematopoietic stem cell transplantation. *Biol Blood Marrow Transplant.* 2001;7:223.

222. Ginsberg SJ, Comis RL: The pulmonary toxicity of antineoplastic agents. *Semin Oncol.* 1982;9:34.

223. Kim TH, Rybka WB, Lehnert S, et al: Interstitial pneumonitis following total body irradiation for bone marrow transplantation using two different dose rates. *Int J Radiat Oncol Biol Phys.* 1985;11:1285.

224. Bacigalupo A, van Lint MT, Frassoni F, et al: Late complications of allogeneic bone marrow transplantation. *Med Oncol Tumor Pharmacother.* 1991;8:261.

225. Labar B, Bogdanic V, Nemet D, et al: Total body irradiation with or without lung shielding for allogeneic bone marrow transplantation. *Bone Marrow Transplant.* 1992;9:343.

226. Tait RC, Burnett AK, Robertson AG, et al: Subclinical pulmonary function defects following autologous and allogeneic bone marrow transplantation: relationship to total body irradiation and graft-versus-host disease. *Int J Radiat Oncol Biol Phys.* 1991;20:1219.

227. Gandola L, Siena S, Bregni M, et al: Prospective evaluation of pulmonary function in cancer patients treated with total body irradiation, high-dose melphalan, and autologous hematopoietic stem cell transplantation. *Int J Radiat Oncol Biol Phys.* 1990;19:743.

228. Girinsky T, Socie G, Ammarguellat H, et al: Consequences of two different doses to the lungs during a single dose of total body irradiation: Results of a randomized study on 85 patients. *Int J Radiat Oncol Biol Phys.* 1994;30:821.

229. Barrett A, Depledge MH, Powles RL: Interstitial pneumonitis following bone marrow transplantation after low dose rate total body irradiation. *Int J Radiat Oncol Biol Phys.* 1983;9:1029.

230. Jules-Elysee K, Stover DE, Yahalom J, et al: Pulmonary complications in lymphoma patients treated with high-dose therapy and autologous bone marrow transplantation. *Am Rev Resp Dis.* 1992;146:485.

231. Deeg HJ, Flournoy N, Sullivan KM, et al: Cataracts after total body irradiation and marrow transplantation: A sparing effect of dose fractionation. *Int J Radiat Oncol Biol Phys.* 1984; 10:957.

232. Benyunes MC, Sullivan KM, Deeg HJ, et al: Cataracts after bone marrow transplantation: Long-term follow-up of adults treated with fractionated total body irradiation. *Int J Radiat Oncol Biol Phys.* 1995;32:661.

233. Livesey SJ, Holmes JA, Whittaker JA: Ocular complications of bone marrow transplantation. *Eye.* 1989;3:271.

234. Calissendorff B, Bolme P, el Azazi M: The development of cataract in children as a late side-effect of bone marrow transplantation. *Bone Marrow Transplant.* 1991;7:427.

235. Sanders JE: Late effects in children receiving total body irradiation for bone marrow transplantation. *Radiother Oncol Suppl.* 1990;1:82.

236. Hamon MD, Gale RP, MacDonald ID, et al: Incidence of cataracts after single fraction total body irradiation: The role of steroids and graft versus host disease. *Bone Marrow Transplant.* 1993;12:233.

237. Deeg HJ: Delayed complications of marrow transplantation. *Marrow Transpl Rev.* 1992;2:10.

238. Ozsahin M, Belkacemi Y, Pene F, et al: Total-body irradiation and cataract incidence: A randomized comparison of two instantaneous dose rates. *Int J Radiat Oncol Biol Phys.* 1993;28:343.

239. Dunn JP, Jabs DA, Wingard J, et al: Bone marrow transplantation and cataract development. *Arch Ophthalmol.* 1993;111:1367.

240. Lappi M, Rajantie J, Uusitalo RJ: Irradiation cataract in children after bone marrow transplantation. *Graefes Arch Clin Exp Ophthalmol.* 1990;228:218.

241. Belkacemi Y, Labopin M, Vernant JP, et al: Cataracts after total body irradiation and bone marrow transplantation in patients with acute leukemia in complete remission: A study of the European Group for Blood and Bone Marrow Transplantation. *Int J Radiat Oncol Biol Phys.* 1998;41:659.

242. Bray LC, Carey PJ, Proctor SJ, et al: Ocular complications of bone marrow transplantation. *Br J Ophthalmol.* 1991;75:611.

243. Fife K, Milan S, Westbrook K, et al: Risk factors for requiring cataract surgery following total body irradiation. *Radiother Oncol.* 1994;33:93.

244. Zierhut D, Lohr F, Schraube P, et al: Cataract incidence after total-body irradiation. *Int J Radiat Oncol Biol Phys.* 2000;46:131.

245. Sloane JP, Norton J: The pathology of bone marrow transplantation. *Histopathology.* 1993;22:201.

246. Shulman HM, Hinterberger W: Hepatic veno-occlusive disease-liver toxicity syndrome after bone marrow transplantation. *Bone Marrow Transplant.* 1992;10:197.

247. Carreras E, Granena A, Rozman C: Hepatic veno-occlusive disease after bone marrow transplant. *Blood Rev.* 1993;7:43.

248. McDonald GB: Venoocclusive disease of the liver following marrow transplantation. *Marrow Transplant Rev.* 1993;3:50.

249. McDonald GB, Hinds MS, Fisher LD, et al: Veno-occlusive disease of the liver and multiorgan failure after bone marrow transplantation: a cohort study of 355 patients. *Ann Intern Med.* 1993;118:255.

250. McDonald GB, Sharma P, Matthews DE, et al: Venocclusive disease of the liver after bone marrow transplantation: Diagnosis, incidence, and predisposing factors. *Hepatology.* 1984;4:116.

251. Resbeut M, Cowen D, Blaise D, et al: Fractionated or single-dose total body irradiation in 171 acute myeloblastic leukemias in first complete remission: Is there a best choice? *Int J Radiat Oncol Biol Phys.* 1995;31:509.

252. Girinsky T, Benhamou E, Bourhis J-H, et al: Prospective randomized comparison of single-dose versus hyperfractionated total-body irradiation in patients with hematologic malignancies. *J Clin Oncol.* 2000;18:981.

253. Belkacemi Y, Ozsahin M, Rio B, et al: Is veno-occlusive disease incidence influenced by the total-body irradiation technique? *Semin Oncol.* 1995;171:694.

254. Locasciulli A, Bacigalupo A, Alberti A, et al: Predictability before transplant of hepatic complications following allogeneic bone marrow transplantation. *Transplantation.* 1989;48:68.

255. Lawton CA, Cohen EP, Barber-Derus SW, et al: Late renal dysfunction in adult survivors of bone marrow transplantation. *Cancer.* 1991;67:2795.

256. Tarbell NJ, Guinan EC, Niemeyer C, et al: Late onset of renal dysfunction in survivors of bone marrow transplantation. *Int J Radiat Oncol Biol Phys.* 1988;15:99.

257. Van Why SK, Friedman AL, Wei LJ, et al: Renal insufficiency after bone marrow transplantation in children. *Bone Marrow Transplant.* 1991;7:383.

258. Rhoades JL, Lawson CA, Cohen EP, et al: Incidence of bone marrow transplant nephropathy (BMT-Np) after twice-daily hyperfractionated total body irradiation. *Cancer J Sci Am.* 1997; 3:116. Abstract.

259. Miralbell R, Bieri S, Mermillod B, et al: Renal toxicity after allogeneic bone marrow transplantation: The combined effects of total-body irradiation and graft-versus-host disease. *J Clin Oncol.* 1996;14:579.

260. Bergstein J, Andreoli SP, Provisor AJ, et al: Radiation nephritis following total-body irradiation and cyclophosphamide in preparation for bone marrow transplantation. *Transplantation.* 1986;41:63.

261. Sanders JE, Long-term Follow-up Team: Endocrine problems in children after bone marrow transplant for hematologic malignancies. *Bone Marrow Transplant.* 1991;8(suppl 1):2.

262. Carlson K, Lonnerholm G, Smedmyr B, et al: Thyroid function after autologous bone marrow transplantation. *Bone Marrow Transplant.* 1992;10:123.

263. Sanders JE, Seattle Marrow Transplant Team: The impact of marrow transplant preparative regimens on subsequent growth and development. *Semin Hematol.* 1991;28:244.

264. Thomas BC, Stanhope R, Plowman PN, et al: Endocrine function following single fraction and fractionated total body irradiation for bone marrow transplantation in childhood. *Acta Endocrinol.* 1993;128:508.

265. Samuelsson A, Fuchs T, Simonsson B, et al: Successful pregnancy in a 28-year-old patient autografted for acute lymphoblastic leukemia following myeloablative treatment including total body irradiation. *Bone Marrow Transplant.* 1993;12:659.

266. Giri N, Vowels MR, Barr AL, et al: Successful pregnancy after total body irradiation and bone marrow transplantation for acute leukemia. *Bone Marrow Transplant.* 1992;10:93.

267. Rio B, Letur-Konirsch H, Ajchenbaum-Cymbalista F, et al: Full-term pregnancy with embryos from donated oocytes in a 36-year-old woman allografted for chronic myeloid leukemia. *Bone Marrow Transplant.* 1994;13:487.

268. Hovi L, Saarinen UM, Siimes MA: Growth failure in children after total body irradiation preparative for bone marrow transplantation. *Bone Marrow Transplant.* 1991;8(suppl 1):10.

269. Brauner R, Fontoura M, Zucker JM, et al: Growth and growth hormone secretion after bone marrow transplantation. *Arch Dis Childhood.* 1993;68:458.

270. Cohen A, Rovelli A, Bakker B, et al: Final height of patients who underwent bone marrow transplantation for hematological disorders during childhood: A study by the Working Party for Late Effects-EBMT. *Blood.* 1999;93:4109.

271. Goldberg SL, Tefferi A, Rummans TA, et al: Post-irradiation somnolence syndrome in an adult patient following allogeneic bone marrow transplantation. *Bone Marrow Transplant.* 1992;9:499.

272. Kramer JH, Crittenden MR, Halberg FE, et al: A prospective study of cognitive functioning following low-dose cranial radiation for bone marrow transplantation. *Pediatrics.* 1992;90:447.

273. Wenz F, Steinvorth S, Lohr F, et al: Prospective evaluation of delayed central nervous system (CNS) toxicity of hyperfractionated total body irradiation (TBI). *Int J Radiat Oncol Biol Phys.* 2000;48:1497.

274. Andrykowski MA, Altmaier EM, Barnett RL, et al: Cognitive dysfunction in adult survivors of allogeneic marrow transplantation: Relationship to dose of total body irradiation. *Bone Marrow Transplant.* 1990;6:269.

275. Andrykowski MA, Schmitt FA, Gregg ME, et al: Neuropsychologic impairment in adult bone marrow transplant candidates. *Cancer.* 1992;70:2288.

276. Mulhern RK, Ochs J, Fairclough D, et al: Intellectual and academic achievement status after CNS relapse: A retrospective analysis of 40 children treated for acute lymphoblastic leukemia. *J Clin Oncol.* 1987;5:933.

277. Socie G, Henry-Amar M, Cosset JM, et al: Increased incidence of solid malignant tumors after bone marrow transplantation for severe aplastic anemia. *Blood.* 1991;78:277.

278. Reed K, Ravikumar TS, Gifford RRM, et al: The association of Fanconi's anemia and squamous cell carcinoma. *Cancer.* 1983; 52:926.

279. Sullivan KM, Mori M, Sanders J, et al: Late complications of allogeneic and autologous marrow transplantation. *Bone Marrow Transplant.* 1992;10:127.

280. Socie G, Henry-Amar M, Bacigalupo A, et al: Malignancies occurring after the treatment for aplastic anemia: A survey on 1680 patients conducted by the European Group for Bone Marrow Transplantation (EBMT)—Severe Aplastic Anemia Working Party. *Blood.* 1992;80:169a. Abstract.

281. Kolb HJ, Guenther W, Duell T, et al: Cancer after bone marrow transplantation. *Bone Marrow Transplant.* 1992;10:135.

282. Neglia J, Shapiro R, Haake R, et al: Second neoplasms following bone marrow transplantation (BMT). *Blood.* 1992;80:169a. Abstract.

283. Jones RJ, Santos GW: Bone marrow transplantation in acute leukemia. *Marrow Transplant Rev.* 1991;1:39.

284. Anderson JE, Appelbaum FR, Fisher LD, et al: Allogeneic bone marrow transplantation for 93 patients with myelodysplastic syndrome. *Blood.* 1993;82:677.

285. Carella AM, Carlier P, Congiu A, et al: Autologous bone marrow transplantation as adjuvant treatment for high-risk Hodgkin's disease in first complete remission after MOPP/ABVD protocol. *Bone Marrow Transplant.* 1991;8:99.

286. Rapoport AP, Meisenberg B, Sarkodee-Adoo C, et al: Autotransplantation for advanced lymphoma and Hodgkin's disease followed by post-transplant rituxan/GM-CSF or radiotherapy and consolidation chemotherapy. *Bone Marrow Transplant.* 2002;29:303.

287. Ferme C, Mounier N, Divine M, et al: Intensive salvage therapy with high-dose chemotherapy for patients with advanced Hodgkin's disease in relapse or failure after initial chemotherapy: Results of the Groupe d'Etudes des Lymphomes de l'Adulte H89 Trial. *J Clin Oncol.* 2002;20:467.

288. Fermand J-P, Chevret S, Ravaud P, et al: High-dose chemoradiotherapy and autologous blood stem cell transplantation in multiple myeloma: Results of a phase II trial involving 63 patients. *Blood.* 1993;82:2005.

289. Gandola L, Caracciolo D, Stern A, et al: High-dose sequential chemoradiotherapy, a widely applicable regimen, confers survival benefit to patients with high-risk multiple myeloma. *J Clin Oncol.* 1994;12:503.

290. Philip T, Bernard JL, Zucker JM, et al: High-dose chemoradiotherapy with bone marrow transplantation as consolidation treatment in neuroblastoma: An unselected group of stage IV patients over 1 year of age. *J Clin Oncol.* 1987;5:266.

291. Rimm IJ, Rappeport JM: Bone marrow transplantation for the Wiskott-Aldrich syndrome: Long-term follow-up. *Transplantation.* 1990;50:617.

292. Brochstein JA, Kirkpatrick D, Giardina PJ, et al: Bone marrow transplantation in two multiply transfused patients with thalassaemia major. *Br J Haematol.* 1986;63:445.

293. Coccia PF, Krivit W, Cervenka J, et al: Successful bone-marrow transplantation for infantile malignant osteopetrosis. *N Engl J Med.* 1980;302:701.

Intraoperative Radiation Therapy

15

Harvey B. Wolkov, MD, Theodore L. Phillips, MD, and Christopher Biggs, MD

RATIONALE

Radiation therapy's principal role in cancer management is the control of local-regional disease. For most types of cancer, the ability of radiation therapy to control local disease increases with the ability to deliver higher doses of radiation to a tumor volume. Not infrequently, the total radiation dose that can be safely delivered to a tumor volume is limited by the tolerance of adjacent normal structures. Despite the use of computed tomography (CT)–assisted three-dimensional treatment planning and intensity-modulated radiation therapy (IMRT), which allow more precise definition of treatment volumes, the dose-limiting toxicity of regional normal tissues remains a limitation of high-dose external beam radiation therapy (EBRT).

Intraoperative radiation therapy (IORT) is a technique that allows the delivery of a large single dose of electron or orthovoltage radiation, *at the time of surgery,* to a tumor or tumor bed. Direct visualization of the tumor volume allows greater accuracy in determining areas at potential risk of spread and allows sensitive adjacent normal tissues to be moved or shielded from the path of the radiation beam. This allows a larger dose of radiation to be delivered safely and provides an improved therapeutic ratio of local control to complications.

Advantages of IORT include:

1. Exclusion of dose-limiting structures from the radiation beam.
2. Reduction or in some cases elimination of postoperative external beam dose.
3. Immediate and accurate targeting of "at risk" margins of resection.
4. Hypofractionation and higher log cell kill in the treatment of radioresistant tumors.
5. Extending the margin of resection beyond anatomically removable boundaries.
6. Treatment of previously irradiated recurrent tumors, eliminating or reducing dose to structures that have reached their dose tolerance.
7. Elimination of time between surgery and EBRT, resulting in treatment when the tumor cell burden is lowest.

Interstitial implants and brachytherapy molds have also been used as intraoperative boost techniques. Beam IORT has certain advantages, however, including (1) the ability to treat large volumes, (2) a homogeneous dose distribution, (3) the potential to limit tumor seeding, and (4) avoidance of trauma to normal tissues associated with interstitial implantation. Disadvantages of beam IORT include inability to treat under the abdominal wall or chest wall and the complete surface of cavities.

HISTORICAL OVERVIEW

Intraoperative radiation therapy dates back to the early 1900s, when Beck[1] and Finsterer[2] independently used this technique for the treatment of advanced gastrointestinal malignancies. In the 1930s, Eloesser,[3] using 200 kV(p) x-rays at Stanford Medical Center, reported the safe treatment of six patients with advanced gastric and rectal tumors. The early interest in IORT waned with the advent in the 1950s of megavoltage equipment that allowed larger doses of radiation to be delivered to deep-seated cancers without the necessity of surgical exposure.

In Japan, the deleterious side effects of high-dose radiation therapy to the intestines and kidneys in the management of gastric carcinoma resulted in a resurgence of interest in IORT. In the 1960s, the pioneering work by Abe, at the University of Kyoto, with electron beam IORT spurred significant interest in this technique. By 1981 there were 27 institutions in Japan participating in prospective clinical trials evaluating IORT.

In 1976, based on successful clinical studies in Japan, Goldson and his colleagues at Howard University Hospital reintroduced IORT with electron beams in the United States. Once the technical feasibility of this procedure was established, other academic institutions began clinical investigations. These included the Massachusetts General Hospital (MGH), National Cancer Institute (NCI), Mayo Clinic, and the New England Deaconess Hospital. In 1983, IORT was first introduced in the nonuniversity or private hospital setting at the Radiation Oncology Center in Sacramento, Calif. Ever since there has been wide dissemination of the technique throughout the United States. Throughout Europe and Asia, clinical programs that have added to the understanding of the potential of this modality have been developed.

BIOLOGICAL PRINCIPLES

The main biological advantage of IORT is the ability to remove normal tissue from the path of the radiation beam, thereby decreasing normal tissue toxicity. Several potential biologic disadvantages exist for single-dose versus fractionated radiation. These include the possible limitations of the cellular processes of repair, repopulation, redistribution, and reoxygenation. By combining fractionated EBRT and IORT, one can minimize the theoretical disadvantages.

Early normal tissue tolerance data necessary for the development of IORT were generated from clinical and laboratory studies performed by Abe and associates[4-6] at the University of Kyoto. Abe and Arakawa[7] subjected dogs to laparotomy and single-dose IORT and noted that the major retroperitoneal blood vessels tolerated significant doses of radiation without significant acute toxicity, whereas treatment to the intestine could result in perforation and obstruction. During the last two decades, a large series of laboratory studies independently performed at the NCI and Colorado State University (CSU) using a canine animal model better defined the acute and late radiation effects on normal tissues in the abdomen, pelvis, retroperitoneum, and thorax. Investigators at the NCI examined the effect of delivering single intraoperative electron doses of 20 to 50 Gy to the abdominal aorta and vena cava.[8,9] These studies demonstrated that the major blood vessels maintained their structural integrity with single IORT doses as high as 50 Gy. Radiation doses greater than 30 Gy were associated with histopathological changes of subintimal and medial fibrosis with loss of the elastic elements in the walls of the aorta and vena cava within 1 year after IORT. Investigators at CSU defined tissue tolerance with ED_{50} values, which estimate the dose at which 50% of animals will develop complications from IORT in the presence or absence of preoperative or postoperative EBRT. Gillette and colleagues,[10] using the radiographic endpoint of aortic narrowing on x-ray films, demonstrated an ED_{50} of 38 Gy for IORT alone and 31 Gy for conventional fractionated EBRT combined with IORT with follow-up of 5 years. Gillette and colleagues[10,11] noted the development of large thrombi and aneurysms at 4 to 5 years after 30 Gy of IORT alone and 50 Gy of EBRT combined with 20 Gy of IORT. These investigators noted an ED_{50} of 29.2 Gy for thrombus formation at 5 years and 23.5 Gy when combined with 50 Gy of EBRT.

Large-animal studies confirmed Abe's clinical finding that hollow viscera are very sensitive to IORT. Incidental inclusion of the intestines within the IORT field resulted in perforation in several animal trials at the NCI.[8,9] Doses of 20 Gy to the small bowel resulted in mucosal ulceration and atrophy with subsequent fibrosis of the muscularis. IORT delivered to the intestine resulted in obstruction after 20 to 30 Gy and perforation after 45 Gy. Investigators at CSU delivered IORT doses of 12.5 to 40 Gy to the intestines followed by 50 Gy of EBRT and noted the development of mucosal atrophy and ulceration at doses of 17.5 and 32.5 Gy, respectively.[12] In defunctionalized (surgically bypassed) small bowel, structural integrity was maintained with IORT doses up to 45 Gy. Duodenal bypass should be considered if a portion of the duodenal wall must be included in the IORT field.

Tolerance of the liver and bile duct to IORT has been studied in rabbit and dog models. Todoroki[13] demonstrated in the rabbit model that both biliary fibrosis and hepatic parenchymal atrophy developed with single IORT doses greater than 30 Gy. Sindelar and colleagues,[14] using a dog model, noted fibrosis and stenosis of the extrahepatic biliary tree at dose levels greater than 20 Gy.

The short-term tissue tolerance of the pancreas to IORT was investigated in the canine model by Heijmans and colleagues.[15] These investigators reported doses up to 25 Gy to be well tolerated with no change in endocrine function at 1-year follow-up. IORT doses of 35 Gy produced a significant reduction in serum insulin levels and glucose clearance rates without the overt development of diabetes.

The genitourinary tract has also proved to be sensitive to relatively low doses of IORT. Investigations at the NCI demonstrated parenchymal atrophy and necrosis of the kidney at doses of greater than 20 Gy.[9] Investigators at CSU delivered 15 Gy to canine kidneys followed by wedge cortex biopsies every 4 weeks and noted a biphasic drop in tubular epithelial cells.[16] The tubular epithelial cell volume decreased to 15% of the original volume by 24 weeks with an accompanying increase in glomerular and interstitial vascular fibrosis. Irradiation of the ureter using a single dose greater than 30 Gy resulted in fibrosis and progressive obstruction.[9] McChesney-Gillette and colleagues[16] noted an ED_{50} of 32.5 Gy for radiographic evidence of hydroureter at 5 years. When 50 Gy preceded IORT, the ED_{50} for radiographic abnormalities was 29 Gy. Shaw and colleagues[17] reported 50% obstruction with hydronephrosis after dose levels of 10 Gy and 70% obstruction after doses of 15 to 20 Gy. The bladder is relatively tolerant of IORT. Using a canine model, the bladder wall has been demonstrated to maintain its structural integrity up to 50 Gy; however, the ureteral orifice has been found to develop progressive inflammation and fibrosis and sporadic occlusion at dose levels greater than 25 Gy.[18,19] Matsumoto and colleagues[20] reported transient ureterovesical junction obstruction in 3 of 36 patients who received 25 to 30 Gy intraoperatively followed by 30 to 40 Gy of EBRT to the ureteral orifice. An additional patient developed progressive hydronephrosis requiring urinary diversion 12 years after treatment.[16]

Radiation injury to peripheral nerves is a potential dose-limiting toxicity in the treatment of pelvic and retroperitoneal tumors. Early clinical observations revealed the development of pain with evidence of sensory or motor changes in the distribution of irradiated nerves within 6 to 9 months after IORT.[21] Shaw and colleagues[17] observed neuropathy at IORT doses of 15 Gy, a lower dose than that previously reported in the canine model.[22] Histologic changes to irradiated nerves include increased endoneural, perineural, and epineural fibrous connective

Table 15-1 Normal Tissue Tolerance to Intraoperative Radiation Therapy Doses

Organ or Tissue	Maximum Tolerable Dose, Gy	Effects
Large blood vessels (arota and vena cava)	50	Fibrosis (>30 Gy) Aneurysms and thrombosis (>30 Gy IORT or 50 Gy EBRT + 20 Gy IORT)
Kidney	10	Atrophy, fibrosis (<20 Gy)
Ureter	20	Fibrosis, stenosis (20 Gy)
Bile duct	20	Fibrosis, stenosis (20 Gy)
Esophagus (full thickness)	20	Ulceration, stricture ($\geq$20 Gy)
Small intestine	20	Ulceration, fibrosis, stenosis ($\geq$20 Gy); obstruction, perforation ($\geq$30 Gy)
Colon	45	Fibrosis, stenosis, ulceration ($\geq$45 Gy); perforation (>50 Gy)
Nerve	30	Neuropathy, fiber loss (>15 Gy); paralysis (>40 Gy)
Bone	38	50% empty lacunae (>38.6 Gy IORT or >32 Gy IORT + 50 Gy EBRT)

EBRT, external beam radiation therapy; IORT, intraoperative radiation therapy.

tissue with a corresponding decreased number of axons and myelin. Necrosis and thickening of the media of small arteries and arterioles can also be demonstrated. At high IORT doses, total disruption of vessels and areas of hemorrhage and telangiectasis around nerve bundles can be seen.[22,23] LeCouteur and colleagues[24] were unable to demonstrate significant abnormalities in peripheral nerves with EBRT doses up to 80 Gy. However, significant histopathological abnormalities were demonstrated with IORT doses greater than 15 Gy. The ED_{50} for vessel disruption and hemorrhage was 19.5 Gy with IORT only and 18.7 Gy when combined with EBRT. These studies demonstrate the importance of shielding spinal roots and peripheral nerves if possible when these structures are included in an IORT field. Investigators at CSU[25] delivered concomitant IORT and intraoperative hyperthermia to dogs and noted a higher incidence of peripheral neuropathy with a shorter latency to development compared with dogs that received IORT alone.

The long-term tolerance of thoracic structures has been investigated in the laboratory setting.[26-28] Minor histologic changes are noted at IORT doses of 20 Gy; however, doses greater than 30 Gy to full-thickness esophagus are associated with chronic inflammation and occasionally severe focal mucosal ulceration. If only a portion of the circumference of the esophagus is treated in an IORT field, doses up to 40 Gy are tolerated. The atrium of the heart demonstrates obliterative endarteritis of the microvasculature with late fibrosis of the myocardium with IORT doses above 20 Gy.[26]

Powers and colleagues[29] examined the late effects of experimentally delivered IORT to the lumbar–para-aortic area of dogs, with long-term follow-up at 5 years after 15 to 55 Gy of IORT alone, 10 to 47.5 Gy of IORT combined with 50 Gy of EBRT, or 60 to 80 Gy of EBRT alone. These investigators noted an ED_{50} of 28.5 Gy for empty bone lacunae at 5 years and 14.4 Gy when combined with 50 Gy of EBRT. An incidental finding of concern was the development of osteosarcoma 4 to 5 years after treatment in 21% of dogs that had received 25 Gy of IORT, with or without EBRT. No bone tumors could be demonstrated in dogs receiving EBRT alone at doses of 50 to 80 Gy. Malignant tumor induction was also described within the IORT field in 7 of 148 dogs treated at the NCI with a median latency period of 40 months.[30]

The tolerance of surgically manipulated tissues has also been studied with the canine model. Arterial anastomoses have been demonstrated to heal after doses of 45 Gy; however, fibrosis leading to occlusion has been noted at that dose. Johnstone and colleagues[31] noted frequent late vascular graft occlusion with IORT doses greater than 25 Gy. Intestinal suture lines have been shown to heal after doses up to 45 Gy. Bile duct fibrosis and stenosis may develop after doses of greater than 20 Gy, and biliary-enteric anastomoses have failed to heal at dose ranges of 20 to 45 Gy.[32] The various tissue tolerances with or without prior surgery are summarized in Tables 15-1 and 15-2.

PHYSICAL PRINCIPLES

Intraoperative radiation therapy is a technique that allows an improved dose distribution to a tumor volume while sparing contiguous normal tissues. The most common radiation modality used to date for IORT is the megavoltage electron beam, although there are facilities using orthovoltage x-rays for this purpose. The main disadvantage of orthovoltage x-rays is their poor penetration through tissue, which results in greater heterogeneity of dose within a given tumor volume. Another disadvantage is the concern over doses delivered to structures deep to the tumor as well as long-term bone complications secondary to the increased bone absorption of orthovoltage x-rays.

Modified linear accelerators are the most common type of equipment used for generating an IORT electron beam. EBRT provides good dose homogeneity with rapid falloff of dose beyond the treatment volume. Linear

Table 15-2 Surgically Manipulated Tolerance Intraoperative Radiation Therapy Doses

Tissue	Maximum Tolerable Dose, Gy	Effects
Aortic anastomosis	45	Fibrosis, stenosis (>20 Gy)
Intestinal anastomosis	5	Fibrosis, stenosis (>20 Gy)
Biliary anastomosis	20	Suture line disruption (20 Gy)
Bronchial stump	40	Mild fibrosis (40 Gy)

accelerators generally provide electron energies from 6 to 21 MeV. The upper energy limit is determined by the following considerations: (1) the largest tumor depth to be treated, (2) the depth (e.g., depth of the maximal dose, d_{max}; 90% isodose, d_{90}; or 80% isodose, d_{80}) at which treatment will be prescribed, and (3) the variation in central axis depth-doses for flat versus beveled treatment cones or applicators. Our experience indicates that energies above 12 MeV are rarely required. Linear accelerators are generally found in a radiation oncology department; however, several facilities have "dedicated" units that are located in an existing operating suite. These dedicated facilities make IORT more readily applicable, but the cost is substantial.[33]

In most institutions, conventional linear accelerators are modified to deliver electron beam IORT. Modifications include the accelerator patient support assembly that must be equipped with a purely mechanical braking system that replaces the normal motorized controls. This ensures against unplanned motion of the assembly during treatment. An IORT collimation or applicator system is necessary; this consists of a main frame adaptor that attaches to the head of the linear accelerator; a double set of clear acrylic (Lucite) or aluminum applicators that attach to the main frame; and a video-assisted viewing system for observing the actual treatment (Figs. 15-1 to 15-3). The applicators in use at most centers are generally circular and range from 4 to approximately 10 cm. In addition to circular cones, rectangular and elliptical cones have been constructed. The applicators are available with unbeveled or beveled ends of 15 and 30 degrees that aid in treating sloping surfaces such as the pelvic side wall. An additional set of applicators is useful for field planning in the operating room. In addition, they prevent normal tissue, such as bowel, from slipping into the treatment field. To reduce leakage through the side of the acrylic cones, a stainless steel collar can be used. Additional modifications can include a side-mounted right-angled periscope inserted into the main frame adaptor that allows an illuminated "beam's

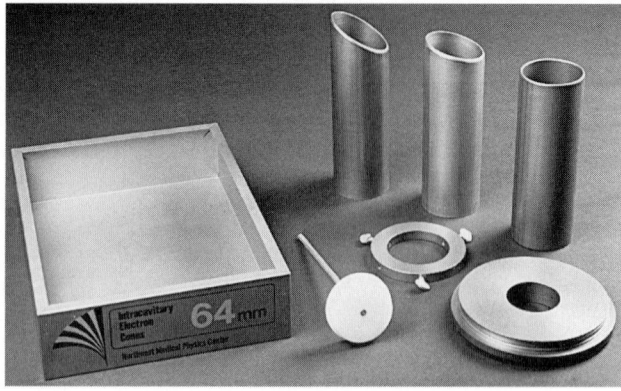

Figure 15–2. The Jones cone system, components of a 6.4-cm diameter aluminum cone set including three cones, an alignment rod, a clamping ring, and an aperture plate. (From Jones D, Taylor E, Travaglini J, et al: A noncontracting intraoperative electron cone apparatus. *Int J Radiat Oncol Biol Phys.* 1989;16:1643.)

eye view" of the tumor volume before the delivery of IORT, and a small hole in the transparent applicator that allows blood to be suctioned. This ensures that blood does not accumulate over the tumor bed and interfere with proper dose delivery.

Other specialized equipment necessary for IORT can include a separate patient anesthesia monitoring system

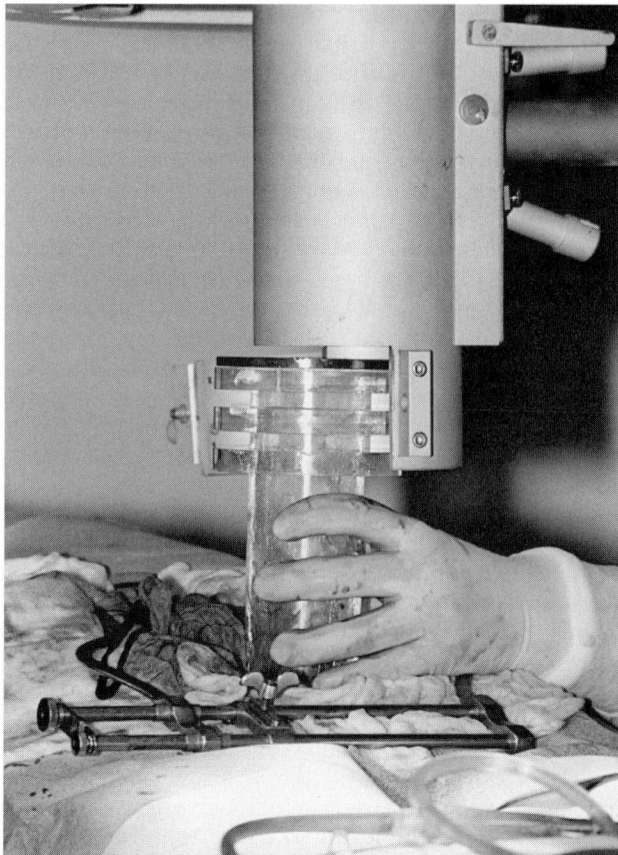

Figure 15–3. Docking of applicator to adaptor attached to linear accelerator. (From Wolkov H, Chenery S, Asche D, et al: Practical and technical considerations in establishing an intraoperative radiation therapy program in the community practice. *Radiology.* 1988;168:255.)

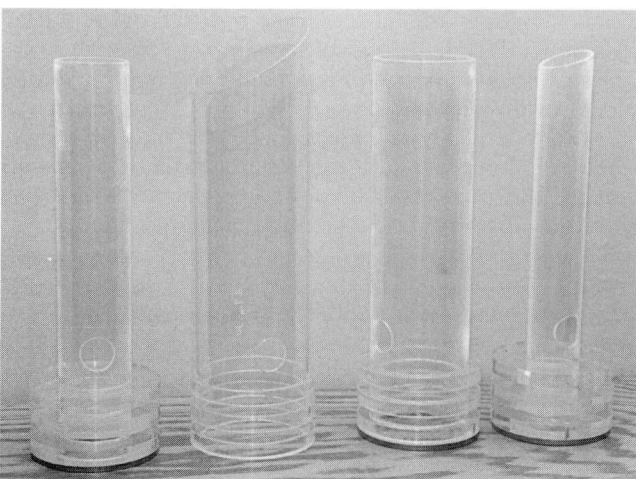

Figure 15–1. Transparent applicators of various diameters and beveled ends used for intraoperative radiation therapy. (From Jones D, Taylor E, Travaglini J, et al: A noncontracting intraoperative electron cone apparatus. *Int J Radiat Oncol Biol Phys.* 1989;16:1643.)

consisting of a close-up video camera and monitor in addition to the standard patient-monitoring system used in most treatment facilities. Since the IORT suite must be able to function as an operating room, equipment such as operating room lights, armbands, IV poles, lithotomy stirrups, and other standard equipment should be available. When a patient is transported from the operating room to the radiation oncology facility, a portable anesthesia unit and electrocardiographic monitoring equipment are necessary.

Physics equipment, which is necessary in addition to the standard tools used to calibrate the reference electron beam sizes, includes a thin window pancake ionization chamber for the measurement of IORT output factors and surface doses, and film densitometry equipment for isodose curve determination. A two-dimensional automatic isodose plotter is helpful in view of the large number of films that must be scanned to obtain a complete record of all applicators, bevels, and beam energies.

In the past 5 years portable linear accelerators that may be moved from one OR to another have been developed. Some of these require no added shielding in the OR. They contain a backstop to absorb bremsstrahlung emitted from the patient.

TECHNIQUE

A multidisciplinary team composed of the radiation oncologist; the surgeon with oncologic expertise; the anesthesiologist; and the support staff, which include operating room nurses, radiation therapists, and physics staff, is required for IORT.

Techniques for IORT vary among institutions depending on the location of the IORT treatment machine and the type of supporting equipment used. A typical technique is described to illustrate the general approach to delivering IORT.

The radiation oncologist consults on any potential candidate for IORT preoperatively and obtains consent. Once a diagnosis of malignancy has been established and surgical resection has been completed, but before anastomoses are performed, the surgeon and radiation oncologist determine areas of residual disease or areas at high risk for disease recurrence. For unresectable disease, information from computed tomography (CT) or magnetic resonance imaging (MRI), correlated with operative findings possibly including intraoperative ultrasonography, is used to determine the tumor thickness and the energy of the beam required. In general gross unresectable disease is poorly controlled by IORT and is rarely treated today. A sterilized treatment cone of appropriate size and shape (i.e., bevel angle) that best encompasses the target volume and treatment site is selected and the depth of treatment is determined. This information is relayed to the physicist who is present at the treatment site so that the appropriate electron energy can be calibrated.

Before patient transport, incisions are temporarily closed with a running continuous suture or clamps and the wound is covered with a sterile adhesive dressing. The patient is placed on a Surgilift stretcher and transported to the radiation oncology department while under portable anesthesia. The patient is then transferred to the treatment couch and reprepared and redraped. After involved personnel are regowned and regloved, the incision is reopened by the surgeon and the treatment applicator cone is verified, placed on the treatment volume, and "docked" to the radiation therapy machine. This involves maneuvering the treatment table underneath the accelerator head and adjusting the gantry angle of the linear accelerator to provide alignment between the treatment cone and the accelerator head. The correct placement of the treatment cone is confirmed by viewing the treatment field using the illuminated periscope to ensure that there has not been slippage of normal tissues inside the treatment cone and that blood has not accumulated. The IORT team exits the treatment room, and the irradiation is delivered while the patient and anesthesia equipment are monitored. Transportation of the patient is avoided with dedicated OR facilities and portable linear accelerators.

Generally, a dose of between 10 and 20 Gy is delivered, depending on the area and volume of potential close or positive margin. The energy of electrons is selected on the basis of the thickness of the tumor bed. After the actual delivery of the IORT is completed, which takes approximately 3 minutes, the position of the treatment applicator is checked to ensure that there has been no movement of the applicator. The cone is then undocked from the accelerator and removed from the patient. This procedure is repeated if another field is to be treated. Generally, clips are later placed around the irradiated volume so that it can be visualized radiographically later, at the time of a subsequent external beam treatment simulation.

After the IORT procedure, the wound is closed and the anesthetized patient is returned to the operating room if transport was required. Once wound healing has taken place, approximately 4 to 6 weeks after IORT, a postoperative course of EBRT may be given.

More recently there have been several intraoperative machines manufactured, designed specifically for use in unshielded operating rooms. Several use orthovoltage energy x-rays. There is also an X-band linear accelerator that delivers intraoperative electrons. The design of this machine allows for use of electrons ranging from 4 MeV to 12 MeV. Its portability allows the machine to be used in multiple operating rooms, even between different hospitals. Careful dosimetry and positioning of the machine make its use in most operating rooms feasible.

SPECIAL DOSIMETRY

Before the clinical use of an IORT system, extensive characterization of the beam parameters must be determined and documented. It is necessary to independently measure the following parameters for each applicator, bevel, and electron energy: (1) central axis data, including the depth of the maximal dose (d_{max}), percentage depth-dose (% DD), surface dose, and bremsstrahlung effect; (2) applicator parameters such as output factors, source-to-surface distance correction factors, leakage laterally from the applicator and photon collimator setting;

(3) dose distribution data including isodose curves, beam flatness, and penumbra; and (4) shielding data. Although extensive IORT physics data have been described in the literature,[34-37] these data are strongly dependent on the type of accelerator, photon collimator setting, and IORT applicator system being used. It is therefore not possible to rely on measurements from other centers.

The study and comparison of dose distribution for beveled and unbeveled applicators reveal significant differences. The isodose remains relatively parallel to the surface in oblique incidence,[38] but the shape near the beam edge is strongly influenced by the bevel angle. The radiation oncologist must be aware of the difference in depth of penetration and shape of the 90% isodose curve that occurs when a beveled applicator is used. It is very important to have sample isodose distributions for beveled and unbeveled applicators available to the clinician at the time of treatment planning.

Another important clinical parameter is the width of the 90% isodose, W_{90}, which is normally less than the applicator diameter. This is important, since underdosage of peripheral areas of the tumor occurs if too small an applicator diameter is chosen for a given target volume. Only for high-energy electron beams does W_{90} approach the actual diameter of the applicator. A margin of 0.5 cm around the tumor volume could be required for unbeveled applicators, whereas a margin in excess of 1.0 cm may be required for the small-diameter beveled applicators.

Another clinically significant feature of the isodose curves is the presence of "hot spots" near the surface at the circumference of the field. These are produced by electrons scattered from the sides of the applicator into the beam. The location and magnitude of the hot spots depend on beam energy, adjustable photon collimator opening, applicator bevel, and applicator size. Surface dose may not be as high as the maximum dose and full isodose curves are needed for each applicator to determine if bolus is required.

When large areas are treated, field matching is of critical importance. Because electron beam isodose curves diverge with depth, if matching of fields is done at the surface of the treatment volume, hot spots will be created at depths where isodose curves overlap. Matching fields at depth result in cold spots at the surface of the treatment volume. Several methods described in the literature provide guidelines for optimally matching flat rectangular fields.[36,39,40] These solutions include the use of small gaps or the use of bolus, or both, to shift the isodose curves. Nonrectangular and beveled applicators present a significantly more complex problem. The dose to normal tissues encompassed by the treatment cone can be mitigated by the insertion of lead sheets. The central axis dose can be decreased to under 10% if a sufficient thickness of lead is used; these generally range from 2.4 mm for 6 MeV electron beams to 7.1 mm for 18 MeV beams.[31] When lead shields are used, backscatter occurs and must be considered in the dose calculations. Backscatter off the lead shield can be decreased by placing 1 cm of wet gauze between the lead and the surrounding tissue. A task force of the American Association of Physicists in Medicine recently published recommendations for the delivery and

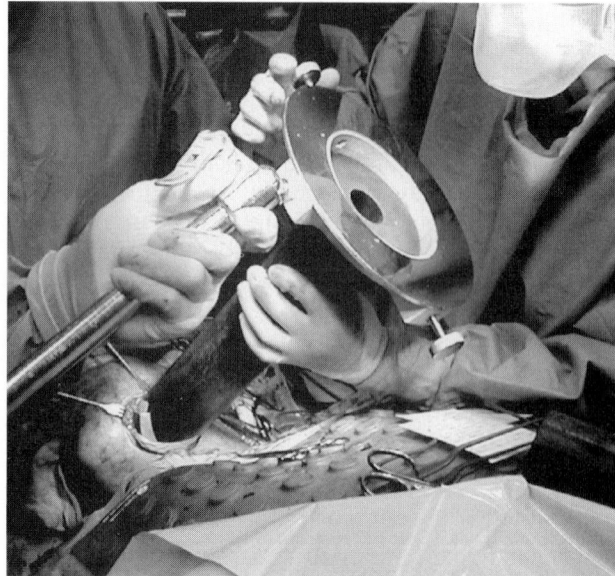

Figure 15–4. Applicator from the portable intraoperative radiation therapy Mobetron system being placed into the wound and attached to the docking ring and the support assembly. Note the polished surface of the ring used for laser alignment. Photos by the authors at the University of California, San Francisco.

documentation of the IORT procedure and an outline of a quality assurance reporting procedure[41] (Figs. 15-4 to 15-6).

TREATMENT RESULTS

Colorectal Carcinoma

Locally advanced or recurrent colorectal tumors present a particularly difficult problem for the surgeon and radiation oncologist. Local tumor invasion into adjacent

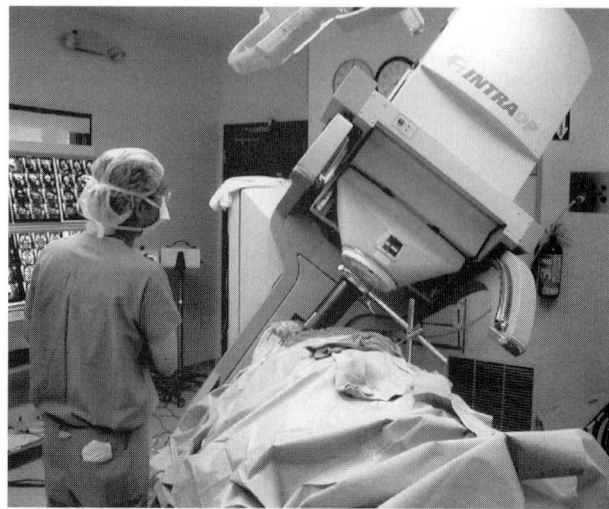

Figure 15–5. Mobile linear accelerator docking with the table-mounted applicator using a no-touch system with laser alignment. The alignment lights can be seen on the screen on the lower part of the accelerator. Photos by the authors at the University of California, San Francisco.

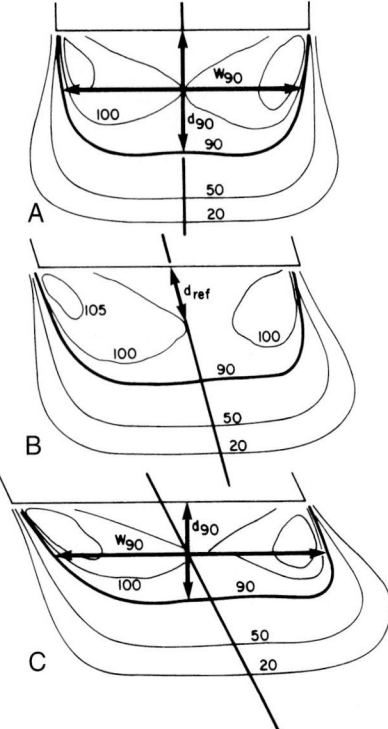

Figure 15–6. Isodose distributions for an 8.8 cm cone at 15 MeV, showing the effect of applicator bevel on the distribution of the relative dose. **A,** Unbeveled. **B,** 15-degree bevel. **C,** 30-degree bevel. The depth of the 90% isodose, d_{90}, measured perpendicular to the surface and the width of the same isodose, W_{90}, as illustrated in *parts A* and *C*, show how these parameters delineate the volume of tissue receiving 90% of the prescribed dose (prescribed to 100%). Distal narrowing of the volume is seen in all three examples as well as the symmetry in the volume resulting from the applicator bevel. d_{ref}, reference dose. (From Wolkov H, Chenery S, Asche D, et al: Practical and technical considerations in establishing an intraoperative radiation therapy program in the community practice. *Radiology.* 1988;168:255.)

pelvic structures such as the sacrum or pelvic side wall often preclude the surgeon from performing an adequate surgical resection. A limited number of approaches have been attempted to address this problem. Preoperative radiation or chemoradiotherapy in the primary setting have offered increased resectability and reasonable local control rates. For example, in several preoperative radiation therapy trials, 40% to 75% of patients have been able to be resected with curative intent. However, local recurrence rates remained in the 35% to 45% range.[42-44]

Attempts at using EBRT alone have shown local failure rates of approximately 90% and 5-year survival rates under 10%.[45,46] Surgery in combination with EBRT appears to be superior to radiation alone. Shield and colleagues[47] reported a 70% local failure rate with gross residual disease despite doses of 60 Gy to the operative bed. Ghossein and colleagues[48] noted the instance of local failure and survival for patients treated with microscopic disease to be 16% and 84%, respectively, whereas patients with gross disease had figures of 50% and 39%, respectively.

Several groups have investigated the ability of IORT to improve the outcome of surgery, with or without EBRT and chemotherapy. At Mayo Clinic and MGH, IORT

was used as a boost with 45 to 55 Gy EBRT in patients presenting with colorectal lesions that were unresectable, had residual disease postoperatively, or had locally recurrent disease. The dose was prescribed to the 90% isodose line at both institutions. Microscopical residual disease was treated to 10 to 12.5 Gy; gross residual disease 2 cm in diameter or less received 16 Gy; and gross disease 2 cm or greater received 17.5 to 20 Gy. Local control rates at Mayo Clinic and MGH were excellent when IORT was combined with EBRT and surgical resection. Investigators at Mayo Clinic reported on 69 patients who received IORT for advanced primary and recurrent colorectal carcinoma.[49] They demonstrate IORT in field recurrences in zero of 20 (0%) primary cases and 5 of 50 (10%) of the recurrent cases. The regional local failure rate, defined as recurrence within the external beam field, was 4 of 20 (20%) in primary cases and 16 of 50 (32%) in patients with recurrent disease. In a historical comparison, local failure was documented in 13 of 17 (76%) patients treated with EBRT alone versus 4 of 20 (20%) patients treated with the addition of IORT.[49] Survival at 3 years was 50% in the IORT group versus 24% for surgery and EBRT alone.

The MGH experience has been extensively reviewed.[50-54] Willett and colleagues[53] reported 5-year actuarial local control and disease-free survival rates of 88% and 53%, respectively, in 20 patients after complete resection for primary locally advanced rectal and rectosigmoid carcinoma. In 22 patients with residual disease after attempted surgical extirpation, the 5-year actuarial local control rate was 60% and the disease-free survival rate was 47%. Rates of local control and disease-free survival were found to correlate with the extent of residual disease. In the setting of macroscopic residual disease, the 5-year actuarial local control rate was 50% and the disease-free survival rate was 17%. For patients who had microscopic residual disease, these figures were 69% and 47%, respectively.

In the recurrent setting results are less encouraging. Willett and colleagues[54] reported that the 5-year actuarial local control and disease-free survival rates in 30 patients who underwent preoperative EBRT and surgical resection with IORT were 26% and 19%, respectively. In patients who underwent complete resection, the determinate local control and disease-free survival rates were 62% and 54%, respectively. Of 17 patients who underwent partial resection, these figures were 18% and 6%, respectively.

The Radiation Therapy Oncology Group (RTOG) conducted a phase I/II study in advanced unresectable or recurrent carcinoma of the rectum. Lanciano and colleagues[56] reported the 2-year actuarial local control rate within the IORT field and external beam field to be 65% and 38%, respectively. Local control and survival rates were dependent on the amount of residual disease before IORT. The actuarial local control and survival rates at 2 years were 77% and 88%, respectively, in the setting of no gross residual disease but decreased to 10% and 48%, respectively, in the presence of gross residual disease. The success of pelvic control was found to be a function of primary unresectability versus recurrent disease status. Pelvic control at 2 years decreased from

83% in the primary unresectable group to 28% in the recurrent or residual group.

The RTOG initiated a phase III trial for locally recurrent colorectal carcinoma to evaluate the effectiveness of IORT with and without the hypoxic radiosensitizer etanidazole (SR-2508). Due to poor patient accrual, this study was not completed successfully.

More recently, several series have focused attention on the use of chemotherapy, in particular 5-FU in combination with IORT as multimodality therapy. Promising preliminary results are suggesting that the use of IORT in a multimodality setting may provide improved local control and survival. These data also suggest a new focus for randomized trials with the concomitant or adjuvant use of chemotherapy with IORT.

At the Mayo Clinic 123 patients were treated for recurrent previously unirradiated rectal cancers. All received EBRT, with or without 5-FU. They show an 84% actuarial local control rate, with an overall survival (OS) of 24% (negative surgical margins) and 18% (gross residual) at 5 years, with a 54% distant metastasis rate. Later, in a series of 61 patients with locally advanced disease, they retrospectively demonstrate a 95% local control rate (negative margins) and find a statistically significant difference between preoperative versus postoperative EBRT + 5-FU. The distant metastasis rate remains at 50%, however.[58,59] They specifically reviewed a series of 51 patients, all of whom had recurrent, locally advanced rectal cancer, and who had also received previous external beam radiotherapy. With 20 of them receiving 5-FU, they achieved a 72% 2-year actuarial in field control rate, with a 2-year survival of 48% and a 5-year survival of 12%. Again, the distant metastasis rate was 50%. Reirradiation with EBRT showed a trend toward improved outcome.[60]

The University of Texas at Houston treated 43 patients with locally advanced, previously unirradiated recurrent tumors with preoperative EBRT and chemotherapy (5-FU with or without CDDP). At 26 months Lowy and colleagues show a 74% local control rate, with a 58% 5-year actuarial survival.[61]

At the Harvard Joint Center, 40 patients treated for positive margins at resection all received preoperative EBRT, with 30 receiving 5-FU. The local control rates for initial and recurrent disease were 73% and 27%, respectively.[62]

With a median follow-up of 17.5 months, Memorial Sloan-Kettering Cancer Center showed a 2-year actuarial local control rate of 81% for primary disease, and 63% for recurrent. Patients received preoperative 5-FU, leukovorin, and EBRT, and achieved a disease-free survival of 69% and 47% for primary and recurrent disease, respectively.[62] Their series using intra-operative high dose rate brachytherapy (IOHDR) did not appear to be as successful, with 74 locally recurrent patients, 29 of whom received external beam radiotherapy (EBRT) and 33 of whom received 5-FU. With a median follow-up of 22 months, the 5-year actuarial local control rate was 39%, with an OS of 23%. Margin status and the addition of EBRT were predictive of survival.[64] A more recent review of 111 patients who received IORT as part of their therapy showed that a 67% local control rate was achieved at 23 months, with a distant metastasis rate of 45%.[65]

Table 15–3 Radiation Therapy Oncology Group Phase I/II Rectal Cancer*

	2-Yr Local Control, %	2-Yr Survival (Actuarial), %
Within IORT field	65	—
Within EBRT field	38	—
Gross total resection	77	88
Gross residual	10	48

*From Lanciano R, Calkins A, Wolkov H, et al: A study of intraoperative radiotherapy in advanced unresectable carcinoma of the rectum: A Radiation Therapy Oncology Group (RTOG) study. *J Surg Oncol.* 1993;53:20.
EBRT, external beam radiation therapy; IORT, intraoperative radiation therapy.

MGH treated 73 recurrent or unresectable rectal cancers with intra-operative electron radiotherapy (IOERT) and 5-FU. Disease-specific survival and local control were significantly better in the patients who received 5-FU as part of their adjuvant therapy.[66] They later report on recurrent rectal patients who received preoperative EBRT with IORT and show a local control rate of 35% with 5-year OS of 27%. In this later series the use of chemotherapy did not significantly predict clinical outcome.[67]

In Japan, a series of 78 patients treated with IORT for recurrent locally unresectable rectal cancers was compared to 248 stage-matched patients who received surgery alone. Survival, disease-free survival, and local recurrence were significantly more favorable in patients who received IORT. Local control rates were 97% and 88% with and without the use of IORT. Although this is a retrospective analysis, it is suggestive of a potential survival benefit to the use of IORT in recurrent rectal cancer patients, and points to the need for randomized data confirming the use of this therapy.[68]

Several conclusions can be drawn from these series (Tables 15-3 to 15-5):

1. Local control is reasonably attained with the use of IORT and chemotherapy.
2. Margin negative status and attempt at curative resection predicts a more favorable outcome.
3. The use of EBRT pre- or postoperatively may improve local control and survival.
4. Distant metastasis rates of about 50% continue to affect survival, and attention to distant disease will

Table 15–4 Massachusetts General Hospital Experience with IORT and Rectal Cancer

Extent of Resection	Primary		Recurrent	
	5-Yr Local Control, %	5-Yr DFS, %	5-Yr Local Control, %	5-Yr DFS, %
Complete	88	53	62	54
Partial	60	32	18	6
Micro +	69	47	—	—
Micro −	50	17	—	—
Unresectable	—	—	0	0

DFS, disease-free survival; IORT, intraoperative radiation therapy.

Table 15–5   Intraoperative Radiation Therapy and Chemotherapy in Rectal Cancer

Institution	Disease Status	Chemotherapy	Local Control, %	Survival, %	Metastases, %
Mayo Clinic	Recurrent	5-FU	84	24 – margins	54
				18 + margins	
Mayo Clinic	Locally advanced	5-FU	95		50
Mayo Clinic	Recurrent prev. unirradiated	5-FU	72 (2 yr)	12 (5 yr)	50
Univ. Texas	Locally advanced	5-FU +/– CDDP	74	58 (5 yr)	—
Joint Center	Positive margins	5-FU	73 (primary)	—	—
			27 (recurrent)		
Memorial Sloan-Kettering	Locally advanced	5-FU Leucovorin	—	69 primary (DFS)	—
				47 recurrent (DFS)	

DFS, disease-free survival.

increase the importance of IORT and the role of local control.

5. Prospective trials are needed to assess the roles of additional EBRT (pre- or postoperatively), chemotherapy, and IORT in recurrent rectal cancer.

Pancreatic Carcinoma

Pancreatic cancer continues to pose a difficult problem for surgeons and radiation oncologists alike. Surgical management continues to be the mainstay of treatment for curative intent; however, the vast majority of patients present with unresectable disease. Resection alone produces disappointing results.[69] Despite combination therapy, the local-regional failure rate remains high, and therefore suggests that local therapy may aid in disease-free survival.[70,71] Because dose intensification in the peripancreatic area is severely limited by local tolerance, IORT may provide an ideal opportunity to remove sensitive structures such as duodenum and stomach from the path of the radiation. IORT has been used either alone[72-75] or in combination with EBRT with or without chemotherapy.[76-81]

In the absence of EBRT, IORT alone appears ineffective.[75,77] Abe and colleagues[67] showed equivalent survival for surgery ± IORT. Abe and colleagues[70] used a combination of EBRT and IORT with an improved median survival of 12 months. Several investigators have also combined moderate doses of IORT (15 to 20 Gy) with 40 to 50 Gy of EBRT and have reported improved survival.[74,75,78,79] In a multivariate analysis, Shibamoto and colleagues[82] at the University of Kyoto suggest that low disease burden was associated with better survival in patients with unresectable pancreatic cancers treated with EBRT and IORT compared to EBRT alone. Many reports have not shown a survival benefit when IORT is added to EBRT.[77-86]

Promising results combining postoperative radiotherapy with chemotherapy for resected tumors suggest that IORT would be best used in a combined modality setting.[62,87]

Analysis of RTOG 85-05 examined IORT with postoperative EBRT and 5-FU chemotherapy for locally advanced pancreatic carcinoma.[80] Patients received 20 Gy IORT with postoperative EBRT to 50.4 Gy in combination with 5-FU. Median survival was 9 months. Median survival was very similar to the results obtained in the series using EBRT and 5-FU without IORT. The local control rate could not be evaluated adequately. An update demonstrated 6% survival at 24 months.[88]

The Mayo Clinic demonstrated an advantage in local control in patients who were treated with a combination of EBRT and IORT versus IORT alone (actuarial local control rate at 2 years was 66% vs. 20%).[81,89] However, improved local control did not translate into a survival advantage. Sequencing of treatment was altered so that EBRT (50 to 54 Gy with or without 5-FU chemotherapy) was delivered preoperatively. With this program, 27% of their patients did not receive IORT because of documented abdominal disease progression at the time of restaging at 2 to 2.5 months after completion of preoperative EBRT. This approach did not result in a decrease in the incidence of abdominal disease. However, there was a trend toward improved actuarial local control at 1 year (86% vs. 65%) in this highly selected patient population.

Two prospective randomized clinical trials have been performed at NCI.[90,91] The first evaluated the use of IORT (20 Gy) versus postoperative EBRT (45 Gy) for resectable tumors. When operative deaths were excluded from the analysis, preliminary results suggested an improvement in the disease-free interval in patients treated with IORT (18.4 vs. 12 months). Survival was improved but not statistically significant. Local control was significantly improved with the use of IORT, with 80% local control at 12 months, whereas the control group uniformly failed locally within 12 months. The second prospective, randomized trial examined unresectable stage III or IV tumors. Randomization was between biliary and gastric bypass and 60 Gy of postoperative EBRT delivered in a split-course fashion (20 Gy over 2 weeks × 3) with 5-FU versus gastric and biliary bypass IORT (25 Gy) and 50 Gy of postoperative EBRT with 5-FU.

In addition, intraoperative radiation therapy has been found to be of great palliative benefit, with approximately 70% to 95% of patients experiencing significant pain reduction after the IORT procedure.[74,75,92,93]

In a phase I/II trial at Kyoto University in Japan, a radiosensitizer, KU-2285 (a nitroimidazole derivative) was given before IORT in 30 patients with unresectable, unresected, or macroscopical residual tumors, 23 of which were pancreatic. Eleven patients without evidence of distant spread of disease treated with KU-2285 plus IORT and EBRT had a median survival time of 11 months and a local control rate of 50% at 1 year. This compared well with a survival of 8 months and local control of 28% for 22 matched historical patients.[94] They further reviewed a series of 138 patients receiving pancreaticoduodenectomy with and without IORT. The median IORT dose was 25 Gy. The median survival was 17 versus 11 months in those patients receiving IORT plus EBRT who had negative surgical margins, although this was not statistically significant. Those with positive margins had a difference in survival with borderline significance. Interestingly, patients who received intra-arterial or intraportal chemotherapy had a significantly better survival, although this represented a small fraction of the patients reviewed.[95]

At Pennsylvania Hospital, 105 unresectable or locally advanced patients were treated with either IOERT or intraoperative I[125] seed implantation, with age- and disease-matched controls receiving only EBRT. The complication rate was significantly lower in the EBRT versus I[125] groups. The actuarial local control rate for the IOERT group was 70% at 2 years, with an actuarial survival of 18 months. All patients received multimodality therapy, including EBRT and chemotherapy.[96]

MD Anderson performed a prospective, preoperative treatment protocol that enrolled patients with resectable localized pancreatic head cancer. This consisted of preoperative 5-FU and 30 Gy EBRT in 10 fractions. After restaging, 20 of 35 enrolled patients went on to pancreaticoduodenectomy with IOERT. The 3-year survival was 23% for this group with a median follow-up of 37 months. This is a promising approach, with excellent results, albeit in a group of highly selected patients.[97]

At the Catholic University Hospital in Rome, 46 patients with cancers of the pancreatic head underwent resection. Twenty-six patients also received intraoperative radiotherapy with postoperative EBRT. Overall 5-year survival and local control were 13% and 48.6%, respectively, with a median survival of 10 months for the surgery-alone group and 14.3 in the combined modality arm ($P = .06$). Adjuvant radiotherapy was an independent prognostic factor for survival ($P < .01$) and local control ($P = .03$) on multivariate analysis.[98]

At the San Raffaele H. Scientific Institute in Milan, 127 patients were taken to surgery with IORT. These were compared with 76 patients treated with surgery alone. In the 49 patients with local disease, IORT improved local control and OS when compared to surgery alone. Multivariate analysis, controlling for age, grade, margin status, chemotherapy, and EBRT, showed a significant improvement in outcome for patients who received IORT. In patients with locally advanced tumors, IORT affected local control but not survival. This series is the first to show an improvement in OS with the use of IORT in pancreatic cancer when matched to untreated patients, and points to the particular need for a randomized study using IORT in pancreatic cancer.[99]

These data suggest that IORT is helpful in improvement of local control, but its impact on OS remains uncertain. In conjunction with chemotherapy, either systemically or intrahepatically, IORT may yet show an improvement in survival as control of distant disease improves, and the importance of local control increases. The role of hypoxic or radiosensitizers in conjunction with IORT is also quite promising, and may afford a further advantage to the use of this modality in both resectable and locally advanced pancreatic cancer.

Gastric Carcinoma

Despite recent advances in the local management of gastric carcinoma, local control continues to be a problem. In the Minnesota reoperation series, after curative resection, 23% of patients had local-regional failure as the only component of failure.[100] Papachristou and Fortner[101] demonstrated an incidence of 25% local-regional recurrence irrespective of stage. A recent intergroup trial showed an advantage to combined modality therapy, although local failure in the combined arm was 19% (vs. 29% in the surgery-alone arm).[114]

The Japanese experience in the management of gastric carcinoma has been reviewed.[74,102-104] Nonrandomized clinical trials have been performed comparing survival rates of patients undergoing surgery versus surgery with IORT. Patients received doses ranging from 28 Gy for microscopic disease to 35 Gy for macroscopical disease. For patients with tumors confined to the gastric wall, 5-year survival rates were not significantly different for IORT versus resection alone. However, for patients with regional lymph node involvement, gastric wall penetration, or extragastric extension of tumor, there was a significant increase in the 5-year actuarial survival rates for patients who underwent IORT (Table 15-6).

There have been two randomized trials involving IORT in the management of gastric carcinoma. The NCI conducted a small, prospective, randomized trial of IORT for patients with gastric carcinoma[105,106] in which it compared conventional therapy consisting of gastrectomy and postoperative EBRT versus gastrectomy plus 20 Gy of IORT to the tumor bed. The patient population primarily had advanced disease. Forty-one patients were entered into the study intraoperatively, with 16 patients randomly assigned to receive 20 Gy of IORT plus misonidazole before irradiation and 25 patients randomly assigned to receive conventional therapy. The study failed to demonstrate any difference between the IORT group and the control group with respect to survival or recurrence rates; however, a difference was noted in the pattern of recurrence. Local-regional disease failures occurred in 7 of 16 (44%) patients in the IORT-treated group and in 23 of 25 (92%) patients treated with conventional treatment. Of 23 patients in whom disease recurred after they received conventional therapy, all (100%) experienced local-regional failures, with 20 recurrences noted in the gastric bed (87%). Of 10 patients in the IORT group with recurrences, 7 (70%) had local-regional failures, with 5 (50%) recurrences in the gastric bed. Although the numbers were small, the

Table 15–6   Results of Intraoperative Radiation Therapy in Carcinoma of the Pancreas

Study	Design	Disease Status	Survival	Local Control, %
RTOG 85-05	Postoperative EBRT + IORT + 5-FU	Locally advanced	9 mo	—
Mayo Clinic	EBRT + IORT	Resectable	—	66
	IORT			20
NCI	EBRT	Resectable	12 mo	0
	IORT		18.4 mo	80
Kyoto Univ.	IORT + EBRT + KU-2285	Unresectable or	11 mo	50 (1 yr)
	Matched controls	Gross residual	8 mo	28 (1 yr)
Pennsylvania Hospital	EBRT + IORT + Chemo	Unresectable	18 mo	70 (2 yr)
MD Anderson	Prospective preoperative EBRT, 5-FU, then IORT	Resectable	38% (3 yr)	—

EBRT, external beam radiation therapy; IORT, intraoperative radiation therapy; NCI, National Cancer Institute; RTOG, Radiation Therapy Oncology Group.

authors concluded that IORT and EBRT were equivalent with respect to disease control and survival after complete resection of locally advanced gastric carcinoma.

A randomized trial[107] from Beijing was conducted involving 200 patients, mostly with stage III or IV disease randomly assigned to receive surgery alone or surgery plus IORT. A dose of 25 to 40 Gy was delivered to the operative bed and regional lymphatics using 8 to 10 MeV electrons. A survival advantage was demonstrated at 8 years in patients with stage III disease treated with IORT compared with those who received surgery alone (51.4% vs. 22.1%).

Extrahepatic Biliary Carcinoma

Because of the high local recurrence rates with biliary carcinoma, IORT would seem to provide an ideal opportunity for improvement of local disease. Surgical resection with definitive irradiation is associated with local recurrence rates of up to 80%.[108,109] IORT for unresectable EHBD lesions has been reported in studies from Japan and the United States. The Japanese experience consists of 59 patients treated at 12 institutions with a single IORT dose of 25 to 40 Gy.[110,111] The mean survival time in this series was 10.2 months, similar to results obtained with EBRT. Todoroki and colleagues[112] delivered IORT doses of 25 to 30 Gy to 11 patients after preoperative EBRT for advanced biliary carcinoma and noted recanalization of the bile duct in 8 patients. Survival was 63% at 1 year.

The RTOG conducted a small phase I/II trial of EBRT with IORT in the treatment of EHBD cancer. Of eight patients who completed protocol treatment, including IORT, only one patient was alive without evidence of disease with a median follow-up of 10.5 months. The local in-field recurrence or persistent disease was documented in only one of eight patients (12.5%).[113]

Soft Tissue Sarcoma

Retroperitoneal sarcoma has a high local recurrence rate, and postoperative EBRT has been shown to improve local control.[115,116] Despite the use of this modality,

however, normal tissue tolerance precludes the use of high dose EBRT in abdominal or retroperitoneal sites.

The MGH experience includes 12 patients treated preoperatively with EBRT followed by surgical resection and IORT doses of 15 to 20 Gy.[117] Local control was 75% overall and 90% in patients treated for microscopical disease. Dubois and associates[118] demonstrated local control of 87% in completely resected soft tissue sarcomas with IORT doses of 10.0 to 25 Gy.

A randomized trial of IORT in patients with retroperitoneal sarcoma was performed by the NCI.[119] Randomization consisted of resection followed by IORT (20 Gy), followed by 40 to 45 Gy of postoperative EBRT versus surgical resection, followed by 50 to 55 Gy of postoperative EBRT. The number of local-regional recurrences was significantly lower in the IORT group (6 of 15) versus the control group (16 of 20). There was no significant difference in median survival between the two groups. Significantly fewer bowel complications were also noted in the IORT group, but radiation-related peripheral neuropathy was more frequent.

At the Cape Cod Hospital, 37 patients with primary or recurrent retroperitoneal sarcoma were treated with a preoperative course of external beam radiotherapy. This was followed by attempted resection and IOERT to 10 to 20 Gy. Of the 37 patients, 20 went on to receive IOERT and were compared to 17 patients without the IOERT. For the group who underwent gross total resection, OS and local control were 74% and 83%, respectively. The group without IOERT had OS and local control rates of 30% and 61%. This uncontrolled study is at least suggestive that aggressive local therapy using IORT may affect survival.[120]

At the University of Heidelberg, all patients treated with radiotherapy for soft tissue sarcoma were reviewed. Intraoperative radiotherapy was used in various sites, including limb, trunk, and retroperitoneum. External beam radiotherapy was used when possible. IORT was used in 92/251 patients (37%). For the grossly resected patients, multivariate analysis identified grade ($P < 0.001$), age (older than 55 years), and retroperitoneal site ($P < 0.004$) as independently associated with recurrence-free survival. IORT was associated with a decreased relative risk of death or recurrence ($P < 0.02$).[121]

At the Mayo Clinic, 87 patients with primary or recurrent sarcomas were treated with IOERT to the retroperitoneum or other sites. Seventy-two patients had a gross total resection. IOERT doses ranged from 8.75 to 30 Gy (median 15). In addition all tumors received EBRT. All patients were followed prospectively for outcome and toxicity evaluation. The overall estimated 5-year survival was 47%. Patients with tumors greater than 10 cm had a significantly poorer outcome. There was a 77% local control rate (seven in-field recurrences), with 56% of patients having recurrence of some kind.[122]

Most investigation into IORT for sarcoma suggests a local control advantage. As is a common theme in IORT investigation regardless of site, the more complete the resection, the better the prognosis. As better modalities for distant disease emerge, the importance of local control and, therefore, IORT in the management of sarcoma will increase (Table 15-7).

Gynecological Cancer

There are several small series on the use of IORT in recurrent or advanced gynecologic malignancies. Goldson and colleagues[123] used IORT for patients with cervical cancer in early trials. The para-aortic nodes or pelvic side walls, or both, were treated with IORT with and without EBRT in 19 patients. Eleven patients had positive para-aortic nodes. Median survival was 17 months in 11 patients with positive para-aortic nodes and 33 months in the 8 patients with negative nodes.

The University of Navarre, Spain, treated 27 patients with IORT of which 19 had recurrent disease. At 12 months, local control was 63%.[124] Peripheral neuropathy without motor dysfunction developed in five patients after IORT. Monge and associates[125] reviewed their results of IORT in the management of 26 recurrent gynecologic malignancies. For patients who had previously received EBRT the local control rate was 33%. However, local control was 77% in previously unirradiated tumors. The 4-year survival was 7% and 33%, respectively, indicating that IORT may be in previously unirradiated patients.

The Mayo Clinic reviewed IORT in a series of 21 patients, 19 with recurrent disease and 2 with locally advanced primary gynecologic malignancies. Actuarial local control at 5 years was 71% (80% for microscopic

residual and 61% for gross residual). Local control within the IORT field was 80% (90% for microscopic and 68% for gross). Actuarial disease-free survival was 40% at 5 years overall, and was 70% in patients with microscopic disease. Grade III or higher toxicity was attributable to IORT in 29% of patients.[126]

The French Cooperative IORT Group reports a retrospective multicenter study of IORT in the management of recurrent carcinoma of the cervix.[127] Seventy patients with pelvic recurrence were treated with 18 to 19 Gy intraoperatively with a mixture of adjuvant EBRT and chemotherapy. OS rates at 1, 2, and 3 years were 47%, 17%, and 8%, respectively. Survival differences were not statistically significant in any of the treatment groups. The overall local control rate was 21%, notwithstanding more than half (37/67) of patients receiving only a partial resection.

At Memorial Sloan-Kettering, recurrent gynecological tumors were treated with radical resection and HDR-IORT. Seventeen patients underwent treatment, with local recurrences from cervical, uterine, and vaginal cancers. All had received previous EBRT. The 3-year actuarial local control rate was 67%, 83% for those with gross total resection. Only 25% local control was achieved, however, in patients with gross local residual.[128]

At the University of Navarra, 67 patients with recurrent or high risk cervical cancer were treated with IOERT as part of their therapeutical regimen. Previously unirradiated patients underwent concurrent EBRT and chemotherapy to a dose of 45 Gy (with CDDP and 5-FU). The 10-year local in-field control rate was 69.4% (92.8% for initial and 46.4% for recurrent disease). Involved lymph nodes and subtotal resection were predictive for poor outcome (Table 15-8).[129]

Bladder

Matsumoto and colleagues[130,131] treated 117 patients with IORT and EBRT for bladder cancer. Patients received 30 Gy IORT with 4 to 6 MeV electrons followed by 30 to 40 Gy of postoperative EBRT. The 3-, 5-, and 10-year survival rates were 91.0%, 85.2%, and 68% for patients with T1 lesions, and 78.3%, 64.3%, and 41.16% for patients with T2 lesions, respectively.

Table 15–7   Local Control and Survival with Intraoperative Radiation Therapy for Sarcoma

Experience	Local Control, %	Survival, %
MGH	75 (90 microscopical dz)	—
Dubois	87	—
NCI (RP only)	80 vs. 60	No difference
Cape Cod Hospital (RP only)	74 vs. 30	83 vs. 61
Mayo Clinic	77 (3.5 yr)	47

MGH, Massachusetts General Hospital; NCI, National Cancer Institute; RP, retroperitoneal.

Table 15–8   Local Control in Advanced and Recurrent Gynecological Tumors

Institution	Disease Characteristics	Local Control, %
University Navarre	Recurrent/Primary advanced IORT + 5-FU/CDDP	46.4 (recurrent) 92.8 (primary)
University Navarre	Recurrent/Primary advanced	63
Mayo Clinic	Recurrent/Primary advanced	71 (3 yr actuarial) 80 (in-field)
Memorial Sloan-Kettering	Recurrent	67 (overall) 83 (GTR)

CDDP, cisplatin; GTR, ; IORT, intraoperative radiotherapy.

Normal bladder function was preserved in 95% of patients treated with IORT. This report suggests that IORT plus EBRT is associated with low recurrence rates and good bladder function after therapy in patients with early-stage bladder carcinoma.

A series of advanced (T3) tumors was treated with 15 Gy IORT and adjuvant preoperative chemoradiotherapy.[132] Patients received a radical cystectomy. At 23 months, local control was achieved in 13 of 17 patients without residual disease in the bladder specimen. Three of six patients with residual tumor in the bladder developed recurrent disease. Distant failure occurred first in all instances of recurrence.

At the Centre Hospitalier, Lyon, IOERT was used in conjunction with transurethral resection, EBRT, and concomitant chemotherapy for bladder-preserving treatment of infiltrating bladder cancer. Twenty-seven patients underwent transurethral resection, followed by 48 Gy EBRT (2 Gy/fraction) with concurrent cisplatin. This was followed by cystoscopy and cystotomy with IOERT to 15 Gy. At least half of the patients also received MTX, vinblastine, and CDDP. The OS at 5 years was 53%, and the cystectomy-free survival rate was 48.1%. Five patients recurred locally, 2 in regional nodes and 10 distantly. With three cases of mucosal necrosis managed well medically, this unique prospective trial demonstrates a promising coordination of IOERT, EBRT, and chemotherapy to achieve excellent local control and survival with modest morbidity.[133]

Head and Neck

Intraoperative radiotherapy has been used in several series for both primary and recurrent head and neck cancer. In most settings the use of IORT is associated with either high risk or previously irradiated patients, and most series report a high rate of gross residual disease. Despite this, local control rates (if margin status is taken into consideration) are reasonable. There are no prospective series, and therefore results can be difficult to compare.

The Methodist Hospital of Indiana[134] treated 28 patients between 1982 and 1984 with advanced or recurrent squamous cell carcinoma. OS at 1 year was 67%. The local in-field control rate for close margins was 87%; microscopically positive margins, 75%; and for gross residual disease, 0%. Margin status was significant in predicting local failure. In a later series of 47 patients, all of whom received previous radiotherapy, median survival was 29 months with a 2-year actuarial local control rate of 61.5%. These results are remarkable given that 41 patients had microscopically positive margins, and 6 had gross residual disease.[135]

In a larger series, Freeman et al. treated 104 patients with mixed histology. Most cases represented recurrent, previously irradiated disease. Average IORT dose was 15 to 20 Gy. Local control with a minimum of 2 years follow-up was 40%. Interestingly, this series included autopsy findings in 25 local recurrences, 22 of which had recurrence outside the IORT field edge. Squamous histology showed local control rates of 44% for microscopically positive margins, 30% for close margins, and 43% for gross residual disease. Salivary gland tumors had similar results.[136] Skull-based lesions of mixed histology, reported separately, were treated with 15 to 20 Gy IORT. Fifty-six percent of the patients were treated for recurrence, with 79% having received previous EBRT. Local control was 64% at 12 months. Control rates were 86% for microscopically positive, 54% for close, and 50% for gross margins. These are two of a few trials that fail to show a difference in local control by margin status.[137]

Toita et al. reported on 25 patients with IORT for advanced or recurrent cases with doses ranging from 10 to 30 Gy. The in-field control rate was 54.1% with a 2-year OS of 45%. The OS for cases with close margins was 70%; microscopical residual, 33%; and gross residual, 0%. Margin status significantly predicted local control: 81.8% for close, 54.5% for microscopically positive, and 0% for grossly positive margins.[138] UCSF described 44 patients treated with IOEBRT from 1991 to 1995. Thirty-six (78%) were recurrent, and 10 (22%) were primary high-risk cases. Histology was mixed. Twenty-five resections had microscopically positive margins, and 20 had close or negative margins. One patient had gross residual disease. The 2-year actuarial in-field control rate was 61.7%. There were 19 total relapses, 14 of which were locoregional, and 6 of which were in-field (3 of these had simultaneous separate regional failure). Four patients recurred as distant metastasis only. Interestingly, of the 17 patients in this retrospective cohort who had postoperative radiotherapy, none had an in-field failure.[139,140]

The Technical University in Aachen, Germany has used IORT in the palliative treatment of unresectable tumors. They report on 95 patients, 71% of whom had gross residual disease at surgery. Only 11 patients had microscopically negative margins. Local control was 17% in patients with gross residual disease, and 64% in those with negative margins.[141] Separately, 84 previously irradiated patients were treated with IORT, with a median survival of 6.8 months, and a median time to recurrence of 3.7 months. Local recurrence rates were 51/62 in gross, 7/12 in microscopically positive, and 6/12 in microscopically negative margins. Of the 84 patients, 62 were left with gross disease at surgery. This work suggests that gross residual disease is not adequately treated with IORT alone.[142] This is further borne out by a similar series of subtotally resected patients at the University of Navarra in Spain, where local failure was 71.4% for gross residual disease, and 57.1% for a macroscopic resection.[143]

Ohio State University has used IORT in primary high risk disease and for recurrence. In a series of 40 previously unirradiated cases, doses of 10 to 15 Gy were delivered for a local control rate of 70% at 16 months. For those receiving or not receiving postoperative EBRT, the local control rates were 79% and 50%, respectively. Twenty-four month OS was 88% versus 33% for completing or not completing postoperative external beam therapy. This series differs from most in that, with definitive intent, 35/40 patients had negative margins on frozen section.[144] In recurrent, previously irradiated patients, the results were not as promising. Thirty-eight previously irradiated patients had a 66% in-field recurrence rate, with 6-month, 1-year, and 2-year in-field control rates of 41%, 19%, and 13%, respectively, and a median survival of 7 months. Seven patients had metastases at recurrence, and 92% had close or positive margins, with none of the patients receiving EBRT postoperatively (Table 15-9).[145]

Miscellaneous Sites

Intraoperative radiation therapy has been evaluated in the management of intracranial tumors[146-149] and various thoracic malignancies.[150-153] These studies suggest IORT may be feasible in these sites, but the series are small, and the results must be interpreted with caution.

In the pediatric population, IORT has been performed in patients with Wilms' tumor,[154-156] neuroblastoma,[156-158] Ewing's sarcoma,[156,159] and osteosarcoma.[160,161] Although these series are encouraging, organized cooperative group trials have not been performed. However, the Children's Cancer Study Group will be undertaking a pilot study in the near future to evaluate the role of IORT in pediatric malignancies (P. Schomberg, personal communication).

TOXICITY

Complications associated with IORT appear to be very acceptable. Noyes and colleagues[162] reviewed the surgical complications associated with IORT in three phase II prospective studies from the RTOG. The three intra-abdominal disease sites included advanced malignancies of the stomach, pancreas, and rectum. IORT was delivered in 129 patients, and 98 patients underwent palliative surgical procedures only. There was no morbidity associated with the patient transport process, delivery of anesthesia, or IORT procedure itself. There was no statistical difference in surgical mortality between the IORT (2.3%) and the non-IORT (1.2%) groups. Major complications occurred at each treatment site that mirrored the complication rate in the surgical literature

for the management of gastric, rectal, and pancreatic cancers. For gastric carcinoma, a higher incidence of pancreatitis was noted in patients whose pancreatic resection margin was included in the IORT field. In patients treated on the pancreatic protocol, there appeared to be a higher rate of infection in the IORT-treated group; however, this was within the reported range of wound infections for pancreatic surgery without IORT. Major operative hemorrhage was a common complication reported during the resection of recurrent rectal carcinomas in both the IORT and the non-IORT group. This study confirmed reports from other investigators[163-166] that suggested there is no significant difference in surgical complication rates between patients treated with IORT and those treated without IORT.

The toxicity of IORT-related treatment has correlated well with laboratory observations. Ureteral and bile duct stenosis and fibrosis have been observed clinically when these structures have been included in the IORT field.[13,50] Upper gastrointestinal hemorrhage has been observed in the treatment of unresectable pancreatic carcinoma; the hemorrhage is thought to be due to ulceration of the C-loop of the duodenum, which is included in the IORT field.

Several investigators have reported IORT-related neuropathy or pelvic pain, or both, when treating tumors in various sites, including retroperitoneal sarcoma, extremity sarcoma, gynecological malignancies, and locally advanced rectal cancer. Shaw and colleagues[17] reported the development of unilateral pain, numbness, weakness, or a combination of symptoms in the lower extremities of 32% of patients treated with IORT, surgery, and EBRT for various pelvic tumors. Investigators at Mayo Clinic[47] and the University of Navarre, Spain,[167] independently reported a 32% incidence of neuropathy in patients treated for rectal carcinoma with surgery, IORT, and EBRT. Both institutions reported the resolution of pain in 42% of cases. The development of IORT-induced neuropathy appears related to (1) recurrent disease treated with prior surgery or EBRT, or both; (2) overlap of matching IORT fields; (3) the total IORT dose; and (4) the volume irradiated. Other complications of IORT have infrequently been reported and are well documented in the literature.[92,119,124,163,167,168]

Table 15–9 Results of Head and Neck Treatment with Intraoperative Radiotherapy

Study	Patient Characteristics	Local Control, %	Survival, %
Methodist Hospital of Indiana	Advanced primary or recurrent previously unirradiated	Close margins, 87 Micro + margins, 75 Gross residual, 0	67 (1 yr)
Methodist Hospital of Indiana Freeman et al	Recurrent, previously irradiated Recurrent, most previously irradiated	61.5 40 (overall) 88 (in IORT field)	29 mo (median) —
Toita et al	Advanced or recurrent +/− EBRT	54	70 (close margins) 33 (micro + margins) 0 (gross residual)
UCSF	Advanced or recurrent +/− EBRT	61.7 (1 yr)	—
Ohio State University	Advanced or recurrent previously unirradiated	79 (+ postop XRT) 50 (− postop XRT)	88 (+ postop XRT) 33 (− postop XRT)
Ohio State University	Advanced or recurrent previously irradiated	34 (no postop XRT)	7 mo (median)

EBRT, external beam radiation therapy; IORT, intraoperative radiation therapy; XRT, radiation therapy.

CLINICAL INDICATIONS AND FUTURE PROSPECTS

On the basis of clinical trials performed in the United States and abroad, general conclusions can be made regarding the current status of IORT. Clinical studies suggest an improvement in local control and possibly survival in patients who have locally advanced gastric carcinoma with evidence of nodal involvement or extragastric extension. Currently it is the standard of care at several institutions throughout Japan to deliver IORT to all patients with locally advanced gastric cancer. In the United States, IORT is still considered investigational in these patients. For advanced primary colorectal carcinomas, there also appears to be improved local control and a trend toward improved survival in patients with recurrent or locally advanced primary colorectal carcinoma, providing that gross resection can be performed.

The role of IORT in the management of pancreatic carcinoma is largely palliative in nature. In patients who have undergone an aggressive surgical resection, there appears to be improved local control, but most series do not support a survival benefit.

Patients with retroperitoneal sarcoma demonstrate improved local tumor control and decreased chronic intestinal complications with a combined IORT-EBRT approach. There does not appear to be a survival advantage with IORT over EBRT alone. Further evaluation of IORT combined with preoperative versus postoperative EBRT with and without aggressive chemotherapy appears justified for locally advanced primary and recurrent retroperitoneal sarcomas.

Intraoperative radiation therapy is a developing technology whose role in the management of other tumor sites, such as lung, esophagus, bladder, prostate, brain, and of the pediatric malignancies remains to be defined. IORT has been shown to be feasible and associated with acceptable morbidity. It appears to improve local control and functions as an effective boosting technique when combined with maximal surgical resection and EBRT with or without chemotherapy in most treatment sites.[169]

It is anticipated that further technological improvements, such as improved collimation systems, can be expected in the future. Currently under development are sophisticated mobile electron beam accelerators that may allow IORT to be shared among several operating rooms, thereby decreasing the costs associated with the modification of existing surgical suites.[170]

Improving the biological effectiveness of IORT will involve the study of radiation dose modifiers such as hypoxic cell sensitizers. Although the early experience with the hypoxic sensitizer misonidazole in the treatment of pancreatic carcinoma was disappointing, Tepper and colleagues[171] demonstrated the feasibility of this approach. Currently under investigation are new-generation sensitizing agents, such as etanidazole, which appear promising.[55]

Prospective clinical trials are crucial to further define the role of IORT. Participation in organized clinical trials will allow patient access to consensus-based treatment programs that can be monitored closely to provide sound quality assurance. Local-regional intensification programs involving IORT, EBRT, surgery, and innovative chemotherapy regimens will require further investigation. In an era of cost consciousness, an accurate assessment of the relative cost efficacy of IORT may be necessary to ensure a future for this emerging treatment technique.[56]

REFERENCES

1. Beck C: External roentgen treatment of internal structures eventration treatment. *NY Med J.* 1909;89:621.
2. Finsterer H: Zur Therapie inoperable Magen und Dormkorzinome mit freilegung und nachfolgender Rontgenbestrahlung. *Strahlentherapie.* 1915;6:205.
3. Eloesser L: The treatment of some abdominal cancers by irradiation through the open abdomen combined with cautery excision. *Ann Surg.* 1937;106:645.
4. Abe M, Takahashi M: Intraoperative radiotherapy: The Japanese experience. *Int J Radiat Oncol Biol Phys.* 1981;7:863.
5. Abe M, Takahashi M, Ono K, et al: Japan gastric trials in intraoperative radiotherapy. *Int J Radiat Oncol Biol Phys.* 1988;15:1431.
6. Abe M, Takahashi M, Yabumoto E, et al: Clinical experiences with intraoperative radiotherapy of locally advanced cancers. *Cancer.* 1980;45:40.
7. Abe M, Arakawa M: Fundamental studies on surgical irradiation. Histological and hematological changes following irradiation during laparotomy in dogs. *Jpn Soc Cancer Ther.* 1967;2:271.
8. Sindelar WF, Kinsella T, Tepper J, et al: Experimental and clinical studies with intraoperative radiotherapy. *Surg Gynecol Obstet.* 1983;157:205.
9. Sindelar WF, Tepper J, Travis E, et al: Tolerance of retroperitoneal structures to intraoperative radiation. *Ann Surg.* 1982;196:601.
10. Gillette EL, Powers BE, McChesney SL, et al: Response of aorta and bronchial arteries to experimental intraoperative irradiation. *Int J Radiat Oncol Biol Phys.* 1989;17:1247.
11. Gillette EL, Powers BE, McChesney SL, et al: Aortic wall injury following intraoperative irradiation. *Int J Radiat Oncol Biol Phys.* 1988;15:1401.
12. Ahmadu-Suka F, Gillette EL, Withrow SJ, et al: Pathologic response of the pancreas and duodenum to experimental intraoperative radiation. *Int J Radiat Oncol Biol Phys.* 1988;14:1197.
13. Todoroki T: The late effects of single massive irradiation with electrons of the liver hilum in rabbits. *Jpn J Gastroenterol Surg.* 1978;11:169.
14. Sindelar WF, Tepper J, Travis EL: Tolerance of bile duct to intraoperative irradiation. *Surgery.* 1982;92:533.
15. Heijmans HJ, Mehta DM, Kleibeuker JH, et al: Intraoperative irradiation of the canine pancreas: Short term effects. *Radiother Oncol.* 1993;29:347.
16. McChesney-Gillette SL, Gillette EL, Powers BE, et al: Ureteral injury following experimental intraoperative irradiation. *Int J Radiat Oncol Biol Phys.* 1989;17:791.
17. Shaw EG, Gunderson LL, Martin JK, et al: Peripheral nerves and ureteral tolerance to intraoperative radiation therapy: Clinical and dose-response analysis. *Radiother Oncol.* 1990;18:247.
18. Kinsella TJ, Sindelar WF, DeLuca AM, et al: Tolerance of the canine bladder to intraoperative radiotherapy: An experimental study. *Int J Radiat Oncol Biol Phys.* 1988;14:939.
19. DeLuca AM, Johnstone PA, Ollayos CW, et al: Tolerance of the bladder to intraoperative radiation in a canine model: A five year follow-up. *Int J Radiat Oncol Biol Phys.* 1994;30:339.
20. Matsumoto K, Kakizoe T, Shuichi M, et al: Clinical evaluation of intraoperative radiotherapy for carcinoma of the urinary bladder. *Cancer.* 1981;47:509.
21. Kinsella TJ, Sindelar WF, DeLuca AM: Tolerance of peripheral nerve to intraoperative radiotherapy (IORT): Clinical and experimental studies. *Int J Radiat Oncol Biol Phys.* 1985;11:1941.
22. Kinsella TJ, Sindelar WF, Lack E, et al: Preliminary results of a randomized study of adjuvant radiation therapy in resectable adult retroperitoneal sarcomas. *J Clin Oncol.* 1988;6:18.
23. Kinsella TJ, DeLuca AM, Barnes M, et al: Threshold dose for peripheral nerve injury following intraoperative radiotherapy (IORT)

in a large animal model. *Int J Radiat Oncol Biol Phys.* 1991; 20:697.

24. LeCouteur RA, Gillette EL, Powers BE, et al: Peripheral neuropathies following experimental intraoperative radiation therapy (IORT). *Int J Radiat Oncol Biol Phys.* 1989;17:583.

25. Vujaskovic Z, Gillette SM, Powers B, et al: Effects of intraoperative irradiation and intraoperative hyperthermia on canine sciatic nerve: Neurologic and electrophysiologic study. *Int J Radiat Oncol Biol Phys.* 1996;34:125.

26. Barnes M, Pass H, DeLuca A, et al: Response of the mediastinal and thoracic viscera of the dog to intraoperative radiation therapy (IORT). *Int J Radiat Oncol Biol Phys.* 1987;13:371.

27. Tochner ZA, Pass HI, Sindelar WF, et al: Long term tolerance of thoracic organs to intraoperative radiotherapy. *Int J Radiat Oncol Biol Phys.* 1992;22:65.

28. Sindelar WF, Hoekstra JH, Kinsella TJ, et al: Response of canine esophagus to intraoperative electron beam radiotherapy. *Int J Radiat Oncol Biol Phys.* 1988;15:663.

29. Powers BE, Gillette EL, McChesney SL, et al: Bone necrosis and tumor induction following experimental intraoperative irradiation. *Int J Radiat Oncol Biol Phys.* 1989;7:559.

30. Barnes M, Dupray P, DeLuca A, et al: Tumor induction following intraoperative radiotherapy: Late results of the National Cancer Institute canine trials. *Int J Radiat Oncol Biol Phys.* 1990;19:651.

31. Johnstone PAS, Sprague M, DeLuca AM, et al: Effects of intraoperative radiotherapy on vascular grafts in a canine model. *Int J Radiat Oncol Biol Phys.* 1994;29:1015.

32. Tepper JE, Sindelar WF, Travis EL: Tolerance of canine anastomosis to intraoperative radiation therapy. *Int J Radiat Oncol Biol Phys.* 1983;9:987.

33. Wolkov HB: The economics of intraoperative radiation therapy. In Abe M, Dobelbower RR, eds. *Intraoperative Radiation Therapy.* Boca Raton, Fla: CRC Press; 1989:393.

34. Biggs PJ, Epp ER, Ling CC, et al: Dosimetric field shaping and other considerations for intraoperative electron therapy. *Int J Radiat Oncol Biol Phys.* 1981;7:875.

35. McCullough EC, Anderson JA: The dosimetric properties of an applicator system for intraoperative electron beam therapy utilizing a Clinac-18 accelerator. *Med Phys.* 1982;9:261.

36. Fraas BA, Miller RW, Kinsella TJ, et al: Intraoperative radiation therapy at the National Cancer Institute: Technical innovations and dosimetry. *Int J Radiat Oncol Biol Phys.* 1985;11:1299.

37. Wolkov HB, Chenery SG, Asche DR, et al: Practical and technical considerations in establishing an intraoperative radiation therapy program in the community practice. *Radiology.* 1988;168:255.

38. Almond PR: Radiation physics of electron beams. In Du V, Tapley N, eds. *Clinical Applications of the Electron Beam.* New York: John Wiley; 1976:64.

39. Shaw EG, Blackwell CR, McCullough EC, et al: Resident Essay Award: Matching intraoperative electron beam fields: Dosimetry and clinical considerations. *Int J Radiat Oncol Biol Phys.* 1987;13:1303.

40. Bagne F: Adjacent fields of high energy x-rays and electrons: Flat surfaces. *Phys Med Biol.* 1978;23:1186.

41. Palta JR, Biggs PJ, Hazle JD, et al: Intraoperative electron beam radiation therapy: Technique, dosimetry, and dose specification: Report of task force 48 of the radiation therapy committee, American Association of Physicists in Medicine. *Int J Radiat Oncol Biol Phys.* 1995;33:725.

42. Stevens KR, Allen CV, Fletcher WS: Preoperative radiotherapy for adenocarcinoma of the rectosigmoid. *Cancer.* 1976;37:2866.

43. Emani B, Pilepich M, Willett C, et al: Management of unresectable colorectal carcinoma (preoperative radiotherapy and surgery). *Int J Radiat Oncol Biol Phys.* 1982;8:1295.

44. Dosoretz DE, Gunderson LL, Hoskins B, et al: Preoperative irradiation for localized carcinoma of the rectum and rectosigmoid: Patterns of failure, survival and future treatment strategies. *Cancer.* 1983;52:814.

45. Cummings BJ, Rider WD, Harwood AR, et al: External beam radiation therapy for adenocarcinoma of the rectum. *Dis Colon Rectum.* 1983;26:30.

46. Wang CC, Schultz MD: The role of radiation therapy in the management of the sigmoid, rectosigmoid, and rectum. *Radiology.* 1976;79:1.

47. Shield SE, Mortenson JA, Gunderson LL, et al: Long term survival in patterns of failure after post operative radiation therapy for subtotally resected rectal adenocarcinoma. *Int J Radiat Oncol Biol Phys.* 1989;16:459.

48. Ghossein NA, Samala EC, Alpert S, et al: Elective post operative radiotherapy after incomplete resection of colorectal cancer. *Dis Colon Rectum.* 1981;24:252.

49. Gunderson LL, Mortenson JA, Kvols LK, et al: Indications for and results of intraoperative irradiation for locally advanced colorectal cancer. In Vaeth JM, Meyer JL, eds. *The Role of High Energy Electrons in the Treatment of Cancer. Frontiers of Radiation Therapy and Oncology.* Vol 25. Basel, Switzerland: S Karger; 1991:284.

50. Gunderson LL, Cohen AM, Dosoretz DE, et al: Residual, unresectable, or recurrent colorectal cancer: External beam irradiation and intraoperative electron beam boost ± resection. *Int J Radiat Oncol Biol Phys.* 1983;9:1597.

51. Tepper JE, Cohen A, Orlow E, et al: Intraoperative irradiation of rectal cancer. In Abe M, Dobelbower R, eds. *Intraoperative Radiation Therapy.* Boca Raton, Fla: CRC Press; 1989:279.

52. Gunderson LL, Martin JK, Beart RW, et al: External beam and intraoperative electron irradiation for locally advanced colorectal cancer. *Ann Surg.* 1988;27:52.

53. Willett CG, Shellito PC, Tepper JE, et al: Intraoperative electron beam radiation therapy for primary locally advanced rectal and rectosigmoid carcinoma. *J Clin Oncol.* 1991;9:843.

54. Willett CG, Shellito PC, Tepper JE, et al: Intraoperative electron beam radiation therapy for recurrent locally advanced rectal or rectosigmoid carcinoma. *Cancer.* 1991;67:1504.

55. Halberg FE, Cosmatis D, Gunderson LL, et al: RTOG #89-06: A phase I study to evaluate intraoperative radiation therapy and the hypoxic cell sensitizer etanidazole in locally advanced malignancies. *Int J Radiat Oncol Biol Phys.* 1994;28:201.

56. Wolkov HB: The economics of intraoperative radiation therapy. In Dobelbower RR, Abe M, eds. *Intraoperative Radiation Therapy.* Boca Raton, Fla: CRC Press; 1989:393.

57. Lanciano R, Calkins A, Wolkov H, et al: A study of intraoperative radiotherapy in advanced unresectable carcinoma of the rectum: A Radiation Therapy Oncology Group (RTOG) study. *J Surg Oncol.* 1993;53:20.

58. Gunderson LL, Nelson H, Martenson JA, et al: Intraoperative electron and external beam irradiation with or without 5-fluorouracil and maximum surgical resection for previously unirradiated, locally recurrent colorectal cancer. *Dis Colon Rectum.* 1996;39: 1379.

59. Gunderson LL, Nelson H, Martenson JA, et al: Locally advanced primary colorectal cancer: Intraoperative electron and external beam irradiation ± 5-FU. *Int J Radiat Oncol Biol Phys.* 1997; 37:601.

60. Haddock MG, Gunderson LL, Nelson H, et al: Intraoperative irradiation for locally recurrent colorectal cancer in previously irradiated patients. *Int J Radiat Oncol Biol Phys.* 2001;49:1267.

61. Lowy AM, Rich TA, Skibber JM, et al: Preoperative infusional chemoradiation, selective intraoperative radiation, and resection for locally advanced pelvic recurrence of colorectal adenocarcinoma. *Ann Surg.* 1996;223:177.

62. Kim HK, Jessup JM, Beard CJ, et al: Locally advanced rectal carcinoma: Pelvic control and morbidity following preoperative radiation therapy, resection, and intraoperative radiation therapy. *Int J Radiat Oncol Biol Phys.* 1997;38:777.

63. Harrison LB, Minsky BD, Enker WE, et al: High dose rate intraoperative radiation therapy (HDR-IORT) as part of the management strategy for locally advanced primary and recurrent rectal cancer. *Int J Radiat Oncol Biol Phys.* 1998;42:325.

64. Alektiar KM, Zelefsky MJ, Paty PB, et al: High-dose-rate intraoperative brachytherapy for recurrent colorectal cancer. *Int J Radiat Oncol Biol Phys.* 2000;48:219.

65. Shoup M, Guillem JG, Alektiar KM, et al: Predictors of survival in recurrent rectal cancer after resection and intraoperative radiotherapy. *Dis Colon Rectum.* 2002;45:585.

66. Nakfoor BM, Willett CG, Shellito PC, et al: The impact of 5-fluorouracil and intraoperative electron beam radiation therapy on the outcome of patients with locally advanced primary rectal and rectosigmoid cancer. *Ann Surg.* 1998;228:194.

67. Lindel K, Willett CG, Shellito PC, et al: Intraoperative radiation therapy for locally advanced recurrent rectal or rectosigmoid cancer. *Radiother Oncol.* 2001;58:83.

68. Sadahiro S, Suzuki T, Ishikawa K, et al: Intraoperative radiation therapy for curatively resected rectal cancer. *Dis Colon Rectum.* 2001;44:1689.

69. Tepper JE, Nordi GL, Suite HD: Carcinoma of the pancreas: Review of the MGH experience from 1963-1975. *Cancer.* 1975;37:1519.

70. Gastrointestinal Tumor Study Group: Comparative therapeutic trial of radiation with or without chemotherapy in pancreatic carcinoma. *Int J Radiat Oncol Biol Phys.* 1979;5:1643.

71. Whittington R, Solin L, Mohiuddin M, et al: Multimodality therapy of localized unresectable pancreatic adenocarcinoma. *Cancer.* 1984;54:1991.

72. Abe M, Takahashi M: Intraoperative radiotherapy: The Japanese experience. *Int J Radiat Oncol Biol Phys.* 1981;5:863.

73. Abe M, Takahashi M, Yabumoto E, et al: Clinical experience with intraoperative radiation therapy of locally advanced cancers. *Cancer.* 1980;45:40.

74. Abe M, Shibamoto Y, Takahashi M, et al: Intraoperative radiation therapy for carcinomas of the stomach and the pancreas. *Ann Radiol.* 1989;32:482.

75. Kawamura M, Kataoka M, Fujii T, et al: Electron beam intraoperative radiation therapy (EBIORT) for localized pancreatic carcinoma. *Int J Radiat Oncol Biol Phys.* 1992;23:751.

76. Gunderson LL, Martin JK, Earle JD, et al: Intraoperative and external beam irradiation ± resection: Mayo pilot experience. *Mayo Clin Proc.* 1984;59:691.

77. Gunderson LL, Martin JK, Kvols LK, et al: Intraoperative and external beam irradiation ± 5-FU for locally advanced pancreatic cancer. *Int J Radiat Oncol Biol Phys.* 1987;13:319.

78. Shipley WU, Wood WC, Tepper JF, et al: Intraoperative electron beam irradiation for patients with unresectable pancreatic cancer. *Ann Surg.* 1984;200:289.

79. Wood W, Shipley WU, Gunderson LL, et al: Intraoperative irradiation for unresectable pancreatic carcinoma. *Cancer.* 1982;49:1272.

80. Tepper JE, Noyes D, Krall JM, et al: Intraoperative radiation therapy of pancreatic cancer: A report of RTOG 85-05. *Int J Radiat Oncol Biol Phys.* 1991;21:1145.

81. Garton GR, Gunderson LL, Nagorney DM, et al: High dose preoperative external beam and intraoperative radiotherapy for locally advanced pancreatic carcinoma. *Int J Radiat Oncol Biol Phys.* 1993;27:1153.

82. Shibamoto Y, Manabe T, Ohshio G, et al: High dose intraoperative radiotherapy for unresectable pancreatic cancer. *Int J Radiat Oncol Biol Phys.* 1996;34:57.

83. Dobelbower RR, Howard JM, Bagne F, et al: Treatment of cancer of the pancreas by precision high dose rate (PHD) external beam and intraoperative electron beam therapy (IOEBT). *Int J Radiat Oncol Biol Phys.* 1989;16:205.

84. Rich TA: Radiation therapy for pancreatic cancer: Eleven years experience at the JCRT. *Int J Radiat Oncol Biol Phys.* 1985;1:759.

85. Tuckson WB, Goldson AL, Ashereyeri E, et al: Intraoperative radiotherapy for patients with carcinoma of the pancreas. The Howard University Hospital Experience 1978-1986. *Ann Surg.* 1988;207:648.

86. Shibamoto Y, Manube T, Baba N, et al: High dose, external beam and intraoperative radiotherapy in the treatment of resectable and unresectable pancreatic carcinoma. *Int J Radiat Oncol Biol Phys.* 1990;19:605.

87. Gastrointestinal Tumor Study Group: Therapy of locally unresectable pancreatic carcinoma: A randomized comparison of high dose (6000 rads) radiation alone, moderate dose radiation (4000 rads + 5 fluorouracil) and high dose radiation + 5 fluorouracil. *Cancer.* 1981;48:1705.

88. The Radiation Therapy Oncology Group and the American College of Radiology: *RTOG Report.* Vol 17. July 1993.

89. Roldan GE, Gunderson LL, Nagorney DM, et al: External beam versus intraoperative and external beam irradiation for locally advanced pancreatic cancer. *Cancer.* 1988;61:1110.

90. Sindelar WF, Kinsella WT: Randomized trial of intraoperative radiotherapy in unresectable carcinoma of the pancreas. *Int J Radiat Oncol Biol Phys.* 1986;12(suppl 1):148. Abstract.

91. Sindelar WF, Kinsella WT: Randomized trial of intraoperative radiotherapy in resected carcinoma of the pancreas. *Int J Radiat Oncol Biol Phys.* 1986;12(suppl):148. Abstract.

92. Calvo FA, Azinovic I, Zornoza G, et al: Pancreatic cancer. In Calvo FA, Santos M, Brady LW, eds. *Intraoperative Radiotherapy: Clinical Experiences and Results.* Berlin: Springer-Verlag; 1992:57.

93. Dobelbower RR, Konski AA, Merrick HW, et al: Intraoperative electron beam radiation therapy (IOEBRT) for carcinoma of the exocrine pancreas. *Int J Radiat Oncol Biol Phys.* 1991;20:113.

94. Shibamoto Y, Ohshio G, Hosotani R, et al: A phase I/II study of a hypoxic cell radiosensitizer KU-2285 in combination with intraoperative radiotherapy. *Br J Cancer.* 1997;76:1474.

95. Kokubo M, Nishimura Y, Shibamoto Y, et al: Analysis of the clinical benefit of intraoperative radiotherapy in patients undergoing macroscopically curative resection for pancreatic cancer. *Int J Radiat Oncol Biol Phys.* 2000;48:1081.

96. Schuricht AL, Spitz F, Barbot D, et al: Intraoperative radiotherapy in the combined-modality management of pancreatic cancer. *Am Surg.* 1998;64:1043.

97. Pisters PW, Abbruzzese JL, Janjan NA, et al: Rapid-fractionation preoperative chemoradiation, pancreaticoduodenectomy, and intraoperative radiation therapy for resectable pancreatic adenocarcinoma. *J Clin Oncol.* 1998;16:3843.

98. Alfieri S, Morganti AG, Di Giorgio A, et al: Improved survival and local control after intraoperative radiation therapy and postoperative radiotherapy: A multivariate analysis of 46 patients undergoing surgery for pancreatic head cancer. *Arch Surg.* 2001;136:343.

99. Reni M, Panucci MG, Ferreri AJ, et al: Effect on local control and survival of electron beam intraoperative irradiation for resectable pancreatic adenocarcinoma. *Int J Radiat Oncol Biol Phys.* 2001;50:651.

100. Gunderson LL, Sosin H: Adenocarcinoma of the stomach: Areas of failure in a reoperation series (second or symptomatic look): Clinicopathologic correlation and implications for adjuvant therapy. *Int J Radiat Oncol Biol Phys.* 1982;8:1.

101. Papachristou DN, Fortner JG: Local recurrence of gastric adenocarcinoma after gastrectomy. *J Surg Oncol.* 1981;18:47.

102. Abe M: Intraoperative radiation therapy for gastrointestinal malignancy. In De Cosse JJ, Sherlock P, eds. *Clinical Management of Gastrointestinal Cancer.* New York: Martinus Nijhoff; 1984:327.

103. Takahashi M, Abe M: Intraoperative radiotherapy for carcinoma of the stomach. *Eur J Surg Oncol.* 1986;12:247.

104. Abe M, Takahashi M, Ono K, et al: Japan gastric trials in intraoperative radiation therapy. *Int J Radiat Oncol Biol Phys.* 1988;15:1431.

105. Sindelar WF, Kinsella TJ, Tepper JE, et al: Randomized trial of intraoperative radiotherapy in carcinoma of the stomach. *Am J Surg.* 1993;165:178.

106. Sindelar WF, Kinsella TJ: Randomized trial of intraoperative radiotherapy in locally advanced gastric cancer. *Proc Am Soc Clin Oncol.* 1987;6:91.

107. Jiang Y, Lu J, Chen G: Intraoperative radiotherapy for gastric cancer. *Strahlenther Onkol.* 1992;168:477.

108. Kopelson G, Galdabini S, Warshaw A, et al: Patterns of failure after curative surgery for extrahepatic biliary carcinoma: Implications for adjuvant therapy. *Int J Radiat Oncol Biol Phys.* 1981;11:413.

109. Buskirk SJ, Gunderson LL, May GR: Analysis of failure following curative irradiation of gallbladder and extrahepatic duct carcinoma. *Int J Radiat Oncol Biol Phys.* 1984;10:2013.

110. Abe M: History of intraoperative radiation therapy. In Abe M, Dobelbower RR, eds. *Intraoperative Radiation Therapy.* Boca Raton, Fla.: CRC Press; 1989:1.

111. Abe M, Takahashi M, Yabumoto E, et al: Clinical experiences with intraoperative radiotherapy of locally advanced cancers. *Cancer.* 1980;45:40.

112. Todoroki T, Iwasaki Y, Okamura T, et al: Intraoperative radiotherapy for advanced carcinoma of the biliary system. *Cancer.* 1980;46:2179.

113. Wolkov HB, Graves G, Wen M, et al: Intraoperative radiation therapy of extrahepatic biliary carcinoma: A report of RTOG 8506. *Am J Clin Oncol.* 1992;15:323.

114. Macdonald JS, Smalley SR, Benedetti J, et al: Chemoradiotherapy after surgery compared with surgery alone for adenocarcinoma of the stomach or gastroesophageal junction. *N Engl J Med.* 2001;345:725.

115. Tepper JE, Suit HD, Wood WC, et al: Radiation therapy of retroperitoneal soft tissue sarcomas. *Int J Radiat Oncol Biol Phys.* 1984;10:825.

116. Harrison LB, Gutierrez E, Fischer JJ: Retroperitoneal sarcomas. The Yale experience and a review of the literature. *J Surg Oncol.* 1986;32:159.

117. Willett CG, Suit HD, Tepper JE, et al: Intraoperative electron beam radiation therapy for retroperitoneal soft tissue sarcoma. *Cancer.* 1991;68:278.

118. Dubois JB, Debrigode C, Hay M, et al: Intraoperative radiotherapy in the soft tissues. *Radiother Oncol.* 1995;34:160.

119. Sindelar WF, Kinsella TJ, Chen PW, et al: Intraoperative radiotherapy in retroperitoneal sarcomas. Final results of a prospective randomized, clinical trial. *Arch Surg.* 1993;128:402.

120. Gieschen HL, Spiro IJ, Suit HD, et al: Long-term results of intraoperative electron beam radiotherapy for primary and recurrent retroperitoneal soft tissue sarcoma. *Int J Radiat Oncol Biol Phys.* 2001;50:127.

121. Lehnert T, Schwarzbach M, Willeke F, et al: Intraoperative radiotherapy for primary and locally recurrent soft tissue sarcoma: morbidity and long-term prognosis. *Eur J Surg Oncol.* 2000; 26(suppl A):S21.

122. Petersen IA, Haddock MG, Donohue JH, et al: Use of intraoperative electron beam radiotherapy in the management of retroperitoneal soft tissue sarcomas. *Int J Radiat Oncol Biol Phys.* 2002;52:469.

123. Goldson AL, Delgado G, Ashayeri, et al: Intraoperative electron beam radiation therapy for gynecological malignancies. In Dobelbower RR, Abe M, eds. *Intraoperative Radiation Therapy.* Boca Raton, Fla: CRC Press; 1989:247.

124. Calvo FA, Ortiz de Urbina D, DeLa Fuente F, et al: Gynecologic cancer. In Calvo FA, Santos M, Brady LW, eds. *Intraoperative Radiotherapy: Clinical Experiences and Results.* Berlin: Springer-Verlag; 1992:79.

125. Monge RM, Jurado M, Azinovic I, et al: Intraoperative radiotherapy in recurrent gynecological cancer. *Radiother Oncol.* 1993;28:127.

126. Garton GR, Gunderson LL, Webb MJ, et al: Intraoperative radiation therapy in gynecologic cancer: The Mayo Clinic experience. *Gynecol Oncol.* 1993;48:328.

127. Maché MA, Gerard SP, Dubois JB, et al: Intraoperative radiation therapy in recurrent carcinoma of the uterine cervix: Report of the French Intraoperative Group on 70 patients. *Int J Radiat Oncol Biol Phys.* 1996;34:21.

128. Gemignani ML, Alektiar KM, Leitao M, et al: Radical surgical resection and high-dose intraoperative radiation therapy (HDR-IORT) in patients with recurrent gynecologic cancers. *Int J Radiat Oncol Biol Phys.* 2001;50:687.

129. Martinez-Monge R, Jurado M, Aristu JJ, et al: Intraoperative electron beam radiotherapy during radical surgery for locally advanced and recurrent cervical cancer. *Gynecol Oncol.* 2001;82:538.

130. Matsumoto L, Kakizoe T, Mikuriya S, et al: Clinical evaluation of intraoperative radiotherapy for carcinoma of the urinary bladder. *Cancer.* 1981;47:509.

131. Matsumoto K: Intraoperative radiation therapy for bladder cancer. In Dobelbower RR, Abe M, eds. *Intraoperative Radiation Therapy.* Boca Raton, Fla: CRC Press; 1989:217.

132. Calvo FA, Abuchaibe O, Aristu J: Bladder cancer. In Calvo FA, Santos M, Brady LW, eds. *Intraoperative Radiotherapy: Clinical Experiences and Results.* Berlin: Springer-Verlag; 1992:73.

133. Rostom YA, Chapet O, Russo SM, et al: Intra-operative electron radiotherapy as a conservative treatment for infiltrating bladder cancer. *Eur J Cancer.* 2000;36:1781.

134. Garrett P, Pugh N, Ross D, et al: Intraoperative radiation therapy for advanced or recurrent head and neck cancer. *Int J Radiat Oncol Biol Phys.* 1987;13:785.

135. Rate WR, Garrett P, Hamaker R, et al: Intraoperative radiation therapy for recurrent head and neck cancer. *Cancer.* 1991; 67:2738.

136. Freeman SB, Hamaker RC, Singer MI, et al: Intraoperative radiotherapy of head and neck cancer. *Arch Otolaryngol Head Neck Surg.* 1990;116:165.

137. Freeman SB, Hamaker RC, Singer MI, et al: Intraoperative radiotherapy of skull base cancer. *Laryngoscope.* 1991;101:507.

138. Toita T, Nakano M, Takizawa Y, et al: Intraoperative radiation therapy (IORT) for head and neck cancer. *Int J Radiat Oncol Biol Phys.* 1994;30:1219.

139. Ling SM, Roach M III, Fu KK, et al: Local control after the use of adjuvant electron beam intraoperative radiotherapy in patients with high-risk head and neck cancer: The UCSF experience. *Cancer J Sci Am.* 1996;2:321.

140. Coleman CW, Roach M III, Ling SM, et al: Adjuvant electron-beam IORT in high-risk head and neck cancer patients. *Front Radiat Ther Oncol.* 1997;31:105.

141. Spaeth J, Andreopoulos D, Unger T, et al: Intra-operative radiotherapy—5 years of experience in the palliative treatment of recurrent and advanced head and neck cancers. *Oncology.* 1997;54:208.

142. Schleicher UM, Phonias C, Spaeth J, et al: Intraoperative radiotherapy for pre-irradiated head and neck cancer. *Radiother Oncol.* 2001;58:77.

143. Martinez-Monge R, Azinovic I, Alcalde J, et al: IORT in the management of locally advanced or recurrent head and neck cancer. *Front Radiat Ther Oncol.* 1997;31:122.

144. Nag S, Schuller D, Pak V, et al: IORT using electron beam or HDR brachytherapy for previously unirradiated head and neck cancers. *Front Radiat Ther Oncol.* 1997;31:112.

145. Nag S, Schuller DE, Martinez-Monge R, et al: Intraoperative electron beam radiotherapy for previously irradiated advanced head and neck malignancies. *Int J Radiat Oncol Biol Phys.* 1998;42:1085.

146. Goldson AL, Streeter OE, Ashayeri E, et al: Intraoperative radiotherapy for intracranial malignancies: A pilot study. *Cancer.* 1984;54:2807.

147. Matsutani M: Intraoperative radiation therapy for malignant brain tumors. In Dobelbower RR, Abe M, eds. *Intraoperative Radiation Therapy.* Boca Raton, Fla: CRC Press; 1989:137.

148. Saki N, Yamada H, Andoh T, et al: Intraoperative radiation therapy of malignant glioma. *Neurol Med Chir (Tokyo).* 1991;31:702.

149. Matsutani M, Nakamura O: Intraoperative radiation therapy (IORT) for cerebral glioblastoma. In Abe M, Takahashi M, eds. *Intraoperative Radiation Therapy. Proceedings of the Third International Symposium on Intraoperative Radiation Therapy.* Elmsford, NY: Pergamon Press; 1991:147.

150. Calvo FA, Santos M, Ortiz de Urbina D, et al: Intraoperative radiotherapy in thoracic tumors. In Vaeth JM, Meyer JL, eds. *The Role of High Energy Electrons with Treatment of Cancer. Frontiers of Radiation Therapy and Oncology.* Vol 25. Basel, Switzerland: S Karger; 1991:307.

151. Dubois JB, Gu SD, Hay MH, et al: Intra-operative radiation therapy (IORT) in non-small cell lung carcinomas (NSCLC). In Abe M, Takahashi M, eds. *Intraoperative Radiation Therapy. Proceedings of the Third International Symposium on Intraoperative Radiation Therapy.* Elmsford, NY: Pergamon Press; 1991:177.

152. Ogata T, Matsuura K, Kure M, et al: Combined surgery and intraoperative radiation therapy (IORT) for thoracic esophageal cancer. In Abe M, Takahashi M, eds. *Intraoperative Radiation Therapy. Proceedings of the Third International Symposium on Intraoperative Radiation Therapy.* Elmsford, NY: Pergamon Press; 1991:183.

153. Arimoto T, Takamura A, Tomita M, et al: Intraoperative radiotherapy for esophageal carcinoma-significance of IORT dose for the incidence of fatal tracheal complication. *Int J Radiat Oncol Biol Phys.* 1993;27:1063.

154. Halberg FE, Harrison MR, Salvatierra O Jr, et al: Intraoperative radiation therapy for Wilms' tumor in situ or ex vivo. *Cancer.* 1991;67:2839.

155. Ohnuma N, Takahashi H, Tanable M, et al: Multimodality therapy combined with intraoperative radiation therapy for malignant abdominal tumor in children. In Abe M, Takahashi M, eds. *Intraoperative Radiation Therapy. Proceedings of the Third International Symposium on Intraoperative Radiation Therapy.* Elmsford, NY: Pergamon Press; 1991:345.

156. Haase GM, Meagher DP, McNeely LK, et al: Electron beam intraoperative radiation therapy for pediatric neoplasms. *Cancer.* 1994;74:740.

157. Matsuura K, Ogata T, Sugimoto T, et al: Intraoperative radiation therapy (IORT) for advanced abdominal neuroblastoma. In

Abe M, Takahashi M, eds. *Intraoperative Radiation Therapy. Proceedings of the Third International Symposium on Intraoperative Radiation Therapy.* Elmsford, NY: Pergamon Press; 1991:350.

158. Masaki H, Saeki M, Tsuchida Y, et al: Intraoperative radiation therapy for advanced neuroblastoma. In Abe M, Takahashi M, eds. *Intraoperative Radiation Therapy. Proceedings of the Third International Symposium on Intraoperative Radiation Therapy.* Elmsford, NY: Pergamon Press; 1991:352.

159. Calvo FA, Abuchaibe O, Villas C: Ewing's sarcoma. In Calvo FA, Santos M, Brady LW, eds. *Intraoperative Radiotherapy: Clinical Experiences and Results.* Berlin: Springer-Verlag; 1992:99.

160. Calvo FA, Azinovic I, Amillo S, et al: Osteosarcoma. In Calvo FA, Santos M, Brady LW, eds. *Intraoperative Radiotherapy: Clinical Experiences and Results.* Berlin: Springer-Verlag; 1992:99.

161. Sasai K, Shibamoto Y, Takahashi M, et al: Intraoperative radiation therapy for osteosarcoma: Its technique. In Abe M, Takahashi M, eds. *Intraoperative Radiation Therapy. Proceedings of the Third International Symposium on Intraoperative Radiation Therapy.* Elmsford, NY: Pergamon Press; 1991:378.

162. Noyes RD, Weiss SM, Krall JM, et al: Surgical complications of intraoperative radiation therapy: The Radiation Therapy Oncology Group experience. *J Surg Oncol.* 1992;50:209.

163. Tepper JE, Gunderson LL, Orlow E, et al: Complications of intraoperative radiation therapy. *Int J Radiat Oncol Biol Phys.* 1984;10:1831.

164. Gunderson LL, Shipley WU, Suit HD, et al: Intraoperative irradiation: A pilot study combining external beam photons with "boost" dose intraoperative electrons. *Cancer.* 1982;49:2259.

165. Avizonis VN, Sause WT, Noyes RD: Morbidity and mortality associated with intraoperative radiotherapy. *J Surg Oncol.* 1989; 41:241.

166. Cromack DT, Maher MM, Hoekstra H, et al: Are complications in intraoperative radiation therapy more frequent than in conventional treatment? *Arch Surg.* 1989;124:229.

167. Calvo FA, Azinovic I, Pardo F, et al: Colorectal cancer. In Calvo FA, Santos M, Brady LW, eds. *Intraoperative Radiotherapy: Clinical Experiences and Results.* Berlin: Springer-Verlag; 1992:99.

168. Wolkov HB: Intraoperative electron beam therapy in the community environment. In Vaeth JM, Meyer JL, eds. *The Role of High Energy Electrons in the Treatment of Cancer. Frontiers of Radiation Therapy and Oncology.* Vol 25. Basel, Switzerland: S Karger; 1991:322.

169. Pelton J, Lanciano R, Hoffmann J: The influence of surgical margins on advanced cancer treated with intraoperative radiation therapy and surgical resection. *J Surg Oncol.* 1993;53:30.

170. Meurk ML, Schonberg RG, Haynes G, et al: The development of a small, economic mobile unit for intraoperative electron beam therapy. *Am J Clin Oncol.* 1993;16:459.

171. Tepper JE, Shipley WA, Warshaw A, et al: The role of misonidazole combined with intraoperative radiation therapy in the treatment of pancreatic carcinoma. *J Clin Oncol.* 1987;5:579.

Imaging

Head and Neck

16

Nancy J. Fischbein, MD, and Nancy Lee, MD

Advances in imaging have revolutionized the diagnosis and treatment of neoplasms of the head and neck. In this chapter we will first review basic principles and applications of computed tomography (CT), magnetic resonance imaging (MRI), and positron emission tomography (PET). We will then review the normal imaging anatomy of the head and neck and discuss the imaging appearance of common pathologies.

DIAGNOSTIC IMAGING TECHNIQUES

Computed Tomography

CT makes use of ionizing radiation to generate cross-sectional images based on differences in x-ray attenuation of various tissues. Modern scanners are typically helical, meaning that x-ray source rotation and patient translation occur simultaneously, resulting in the acquisition of a "volume" of data that is then partitioned and reconstructed into individual slices.[1] Helical scanning allows for rapid data acquisition to diminish artifacts related to motion (breathing, swallowing, gross patient motion). The rapid data acquisition also allows for more and thinner slices to be obtained, which facilitates diagnosis by decreasing partial volume averaging effects. It also allows for improved quality of multiplanar reconstructions. The most recent advance in CT imaging has been the introduction of the so-called "multislice" scanners.[2,3] Multislice scanners have a variable number of parallel arcs of detectors that are capable of simultaneously acquiring volumes of data. The increased speed that results from multislice sampling can be traded for improved longitudinal resolution, increased volume of coverage, or improved signal to noise.

CT of the head and neck should be performed with thin sections, usually ≤3 mm, in the axial plane. Direct coronal imaging or coronal reformations (Fig. 16-1) may be useful in some situations. Additional angled views can also be useful in specific situations (e.g., to throw artifacts related to dental amalgam off of vital structures). Unless one is primarily interested in bony structures, CT of the head and neck is usually performed following injection of iodinated contrast material. The opacification of vessels helps to separate them from other structures such as lymph nodes and also helps to delineate pathology. Iodinated contrast material carries a small risk of minor or significant allergic reaction and a risk of nephrotoxicity in patients who already have some degree of renal dysfunction or are at risk of this (e.g., diabetics).

CT is useful in the very ill or uncooperative patient in whom MR imaging is compromised by patient motion. CT is also useful in patients for whom MR is contraindicated by the presence of ferromagnetic aneurysm clips or other such devices. CT easily demonstrates differences in attenuation among air, bone, fat, and soft tissue, but is far less sensitive to subtle differences in tissue composition than is MR. In the head and neck, while CT is excellent for imaging the larynx and most cervical nodal groups, MR generally provides more information about the extent of primary tumors and better information about skull base involvement, perineural spread of disease, and intracranial extension. CT is also useful for assessing bone destruction and may be useful for planning reconstructive surgeries.

Magnetic Resonance

MR exploits differences in tissue relaxation characteristics and spin density to produce an image that is exquisitely sensitive to soft tissue contrast.[4,5] Depending on the parameters that one selects, variable tissue characteristics and contrast will be produced. Multiple different types of sequences in multiple planes are generally necessary to fully characterize lesions of the head and neck. Slice thickness should be no more than 5 mm, and a gadolinium-based contrast agent is generally used to enhance detection of pathology and improve tissue characterization and differential diagnosis. In some circumstances, thinner sections covering a smaller anatomic area may be necessary for more precise diagnosis.

In the head and neck, we typically obtain the following imaging sequences:

- Sagittal, axial, and coronal T1-weighted images
- Axial fast spin-echo T2-weighted images with fat saturation
- Axial and coronal post-gadolinium T1-weighted images with fat saturation

Additional planes may be useful in some circumstances (e.g., coronal fast spin-echo T2-weighted images with fat saturation for paranasal sinus pathology). Additional sequences such as MR angiography (MRA) may

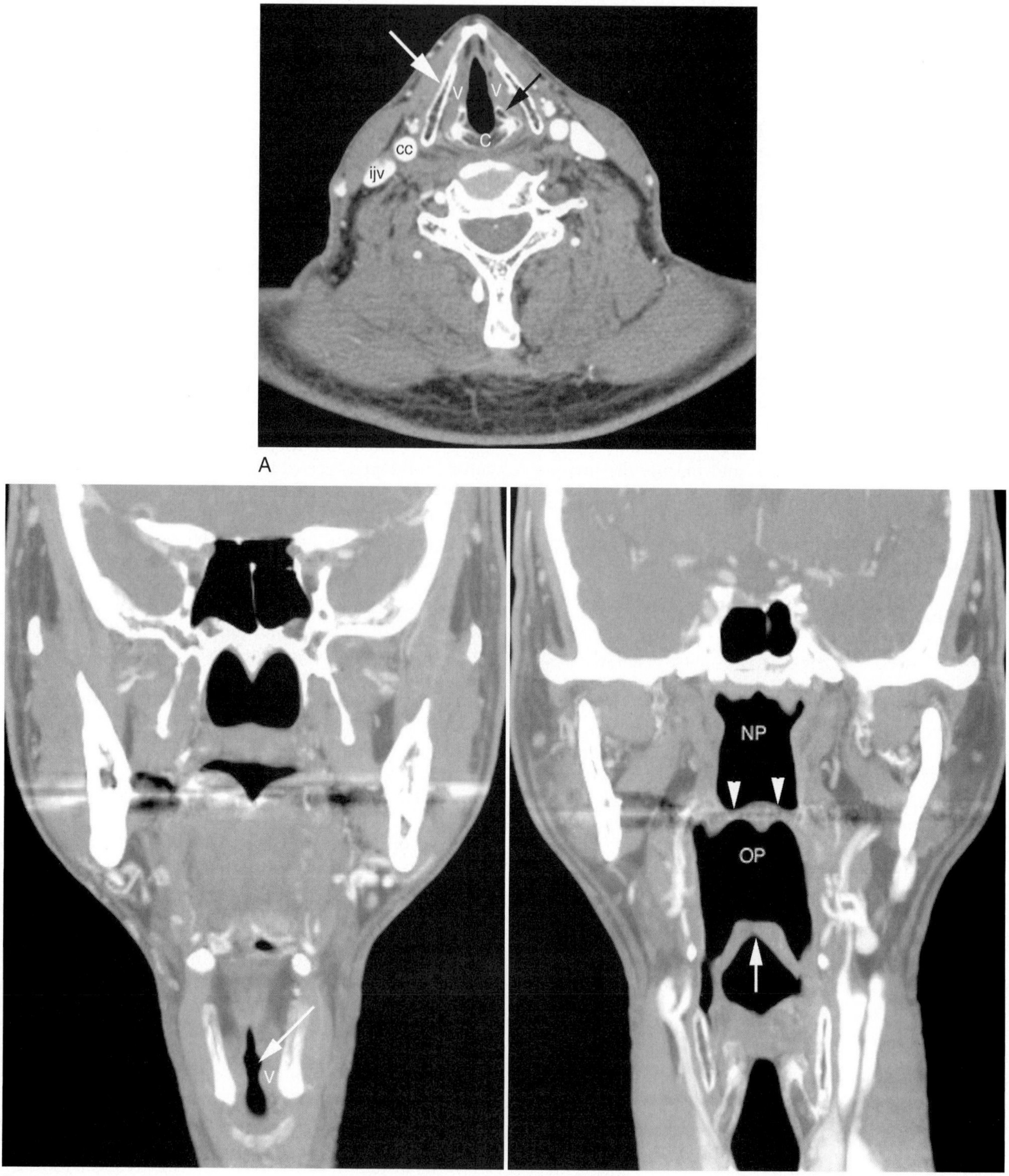

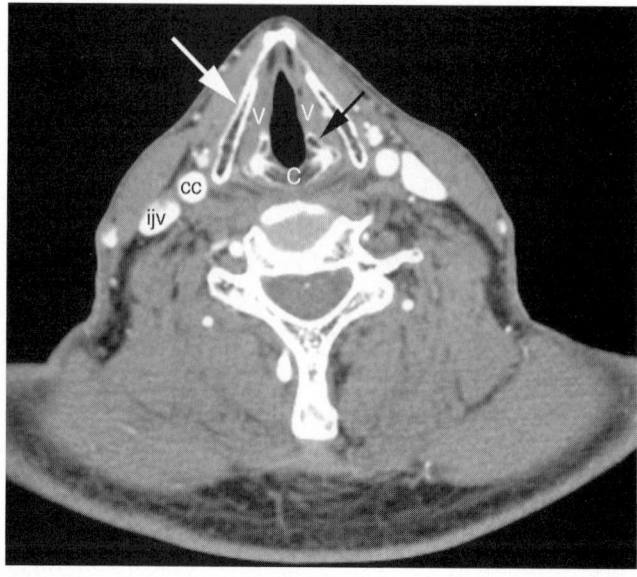

A

B

C

Figure 16–1. **A,** Axial 2.5-mm-thick slice from a contrast-enhanced computed tomography (CT) scan of the neck. Note the excellent depiction of the normal larynx, with the true vocal cords (*V*), cricoid cartilage (*C*), arytenoid cartilage (*black arrow*), and thyroid cartilage (*white arrow*) indicated. Also shown are the common carotid artery (*cc*) and internal jugular vein (*ijv*). **B,** Coronal reformation of the axial CT data demonstrates the true vocal cord (*V*) and laryngeal ventricle (*arrow*). **C,** A more posterior coronal reformation demonstrates the epiglottis (*white arrow*), oropharyngeal airway (*OP*), soft palate (*arrowheads*), and nasopharyngeal airway (*NP*).

be useful in certain circumstances (e.g., paragangliomas) but are not necessary for evaluation of most neoplasms of the head and neck. Modalities in widespread use in the brain (magnetic resonance spectroscopy, diffusion-weighted imaging, functional MRI) have not yet found a place in routine head and neck imaging.

On a T1-weighted image, fat is bright and fluid (such as cerebrospinal fluid) is relatively dark. Muscle and most pathologies are of intermediate signal intensity. The large amount of fat in the head and neck provides intrinsic tissue contrast, which makes the T1-weighted image very sensitive to infiltrative processes that obliterate tissue planes or that replace marrow fat (Fig. 16-2A). Some hemorrhagic or proteinaceous lesions may result in intrinsic T1-shortening such that they appear bright on a T1-weighted image. On a T2-weighted image, fluid is very bright and most pathologies are relatively bright, while muscle is quite dark. The fast spin-echo technique is useful in limiting artifacts related to motion and magnetic susceptibility as compared with a conventional spin-echo T2-weighted image. Since fat remains bright on a fast spin-echo image, however, fat saturation should ideally be applied. In the nasal cavity and paranasal sinuses, T2-weighted images are particularly useful in distinguishing neoplastic masses from polyps, thickened mucosa, and retained secretions (Fig. 16-2B). Gadolinium is useful for demonstrating pathology and tailoring a differential diagnosis based on enhancement characteristics. Postgadolinium imaging is also useful in assessing perineural spread of tumor, cavernous sinus invasion, and meningeal infiltration (Figs. 16-2C and 16-2D). Fat saturation should ideally be applied on a postgadolinium image; otherwise, the contrast between an enhancing lesion and surrounding fat may actually be reduced as compared with the pregadolinium image. As low-field scanners often do not have fat saturation available, high-field (1.5 T) imaging is generally preferred for patients with head and neck cancer. If a patient is severely claustrophobic, sedation may be necessary to accomplish the scan.

As mentioned earlier, in most cases MRI is preferred to CT because of its superior soft tissue contrast and increased sensitivity to processes such as perineural spread of tumor. In the acutely ill or uncooperative patient, or the patient with an absolute contraindication to MRI, good-quality CT can be useful. It is important for the clinician to be aware of MRI safety considerations and relative and absolute contraindications to MRI.[6,7]

Positron Emission Tomography

PET offers information regarding tissue metabolism rather than simply demonstrating anatomy. The most common radiopharmaceutical in use for cancer imaging at present is ^{18}F-fluorodeoxyglucose (FDG). This is taken up into tissues in proportion to the glycolytic rate, which is generally increased in neoplastic processes. FDG does accumulate in some normal structures to a variable degree (sublingual glands, lymphoid tissue of Waldeyer's ring),[8] and one needs to be aware of the appearance of a normal FDG PET scan (Fig. 16-3).

Focal, asymmetrical uptake becomes a concern for a tumor, but is nonspecific as FDG is also concentrated in areas of inflammation. Situations where FDG PET scanning is particularly helpful include the search for an unknown primary lesion in a patient presenting with metastatic neck disease (Fig. 16-4), the assessment of residual or recurrent disease following primary therapy, and the search for synchronous or metachronous primary lesions or distant metastases.[9,10] FDG PET can also be useful for staging the neck. However, there may be a significant number of false-negative studies in patients with clinically N0 necks, as small tumor deposits (on the order of 1 to 4 mm) may not be detectable on FDG PET scan, but will be found if a neck dissection is performed.

IMAGING THE HEAD AND NECK

The anatomy of the head and neck is extremely complex. To facilitate communication and differential diagnosis, the supra- and infrahyoid neck are usually discussed as a series of spaces.[11-13] We will be discussing primarily the pharyngeal mucosal space, from which squamous cell carcinomas (SCCs), lymphomas, and numerous minor salivary gland tumors may arise. In this discussion we will refer to the traditional divisions of this space into the nasopharynx, oropharynx, oral cavity, and hypopharynx. The larynx, located in the infrahyoid visceral space, will also be discussed. The deeper spaces of the head and neck may become involved by deep extension of primarily mucosal lesions or may be the site of origin of soft-tissue sarcomas and other nonsquamous neoplasms.

Spatial Anatomy of the Head and Neck

The spaces of the suprahyoid neck are defined by the three layers of the deep cervical fascia (the superficial, middle, and deep layers). The spaces so defined include the pharyngeal mucosal space, parapharyngeal space, masticator space, parotid space, carotid space, retropharyngeal space, and perivertebral space. These spaces and their critical contents are demonstrated in Figure 16-5. In a discussion of head and neck cancer, however, which is largely represented by SCC of the mucosa of the upper aerodigestive tract, we will discuss lesions arising in the nasopharynx, oropharynx, oral cavity, hypopharynx, and larynx. The infrahyoid neck has traditionally been taught from the point of view of surgical triangles, but can also be described as a series of spaces, which facilitates understanding and interpretation of cross-sectional imaging modalities such as CT and MRI. The spaces of the infrahyoid neck are also defined by the three layers of the deep cervical fascia and include the superficial space (external to the superficial layer of the deep cervical fascia); visceral space (including the thyroid gland, larynx, and esophagus); carotid space; retropharyngeal space; and prevertebral space. These spaces and their critical contents are demonstrated in Figure 16-6.

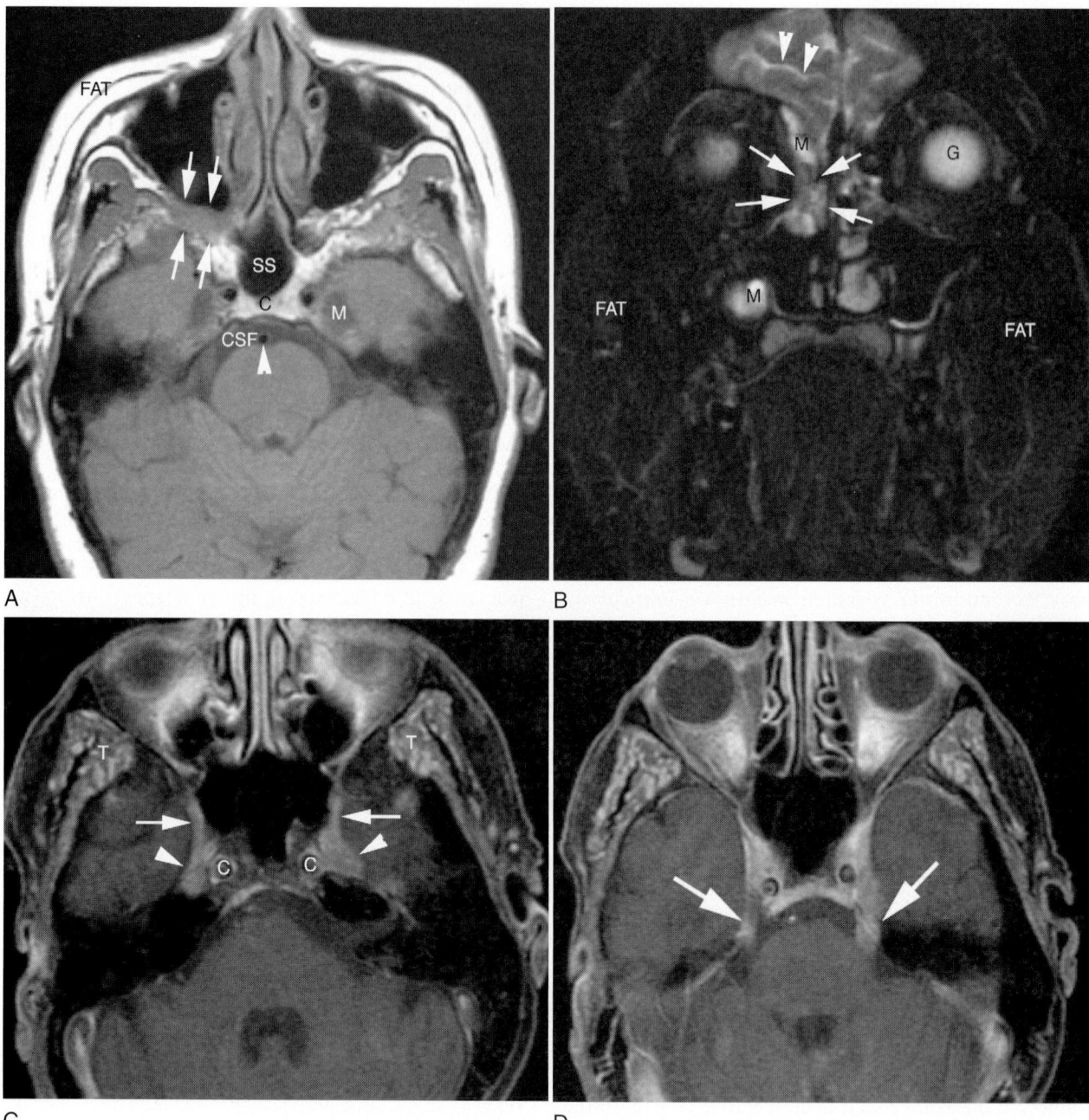

Figure 16–2. A, An axial T1-weighted image is shown. Note that fat (as seen in the subcutaneous region, *FAT,* and also in the marrow of the *clivus, C,*) is extremely bright, while fluid (as seen in cerebrospinal fluid in the prepontine cistern (*CSF*) and Meckel's cave (*M*) is dark. Soft tissue such as muscle and brain parenchyma are intermediate in signal intensity, while air (as in the sphenoid sinus, *SS*) is black. The white arrowhead indicates the flow void of the basilar artery. White arrows indicate nasopharyngeal carcinoma infiltrating the fat of the right *pterygopalatine fossa,* which appears expanded and of lower signal intensity than the normal mostly fatty space on the left. **B,** A coronal fast spin-echo T2-weighted image with fat saturation is shown. Note that the signal from subcutaneous fat (*FAT*) is completely suppressed. Fluid appears bright, as seen with CSF in a cerebral sulcus (*arrowheads*) and the vitreous humor within the ocular globe (*G*). Mucoid material (*M*) within the maxillary, frontal, and ethmoid sinuses is extremely bright. In contrast, a highly cellular inverting papilloma (*white arrows*) is of intermediate signal intensity and shows clearly in contrast to thickened mucosa and sinonasal secretions. **C,** A postgadolinium axial T1-weighted image with fat saturation is shown. Subcutaneous fat appears dark because its signal has been suppressed. Gadolinium administration can be confirmed by looking at the sinonasal mucosa, which enhances brightly post-gadolinium. Orbital fat appears bright because of local failure of fat saturation due to inhomogeneity of the local magnetic field due to the proximity and morphology of the maxillary sinus. Abnormal enhancement is seen along foramen rotundum (*white arrows*) and in the cavernous sinuses (*white arrowheads*) due to lymphomatous infiltration of the trigeminal nerves. Increased enhancement of the temporalis muscles bilaterally (*T*) is related to denervation change from involvement of V3. **D,** A slightly more superior postgadolinium axial T1-weighted image with fat saturation demonstrates abnormal thickening and enhancement of the cisternal segments of the trigeminal nerves bilaterally, also due to lymphomatous infiltration.

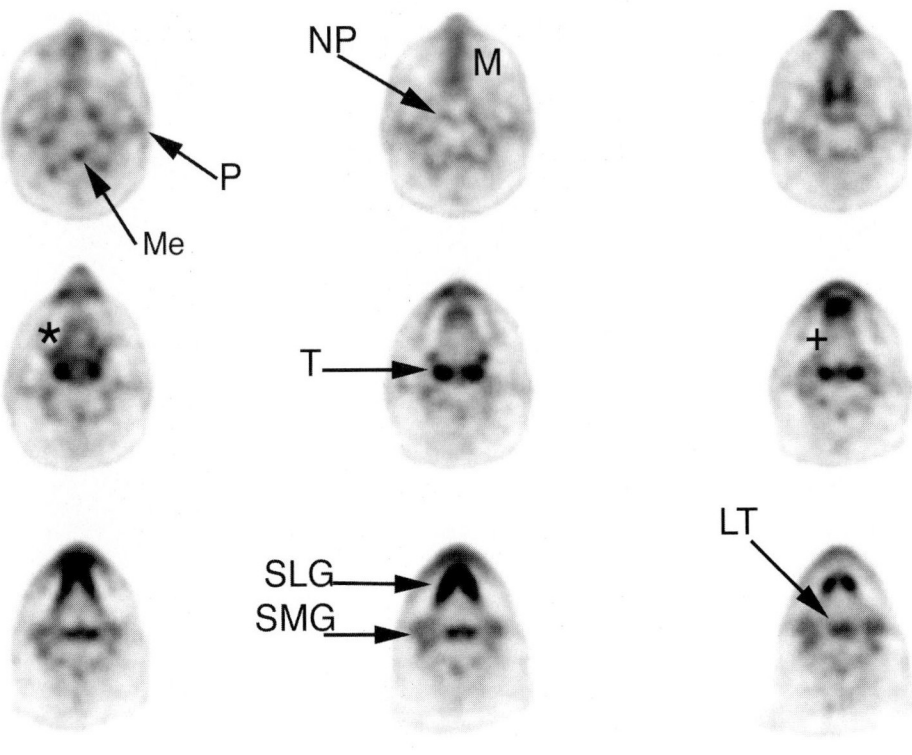

Figure 16–3. Normal ^{18}F-fluorodeoxyglucose positron emission tomography scan. Areas of greatest activity include the palatine tonsils (*T*), lingual tonsils (*LT*), and sublingual glands (*SLG*). The medulla (*Me*) also shows significant activity. Intermediate activity is seen in the parotid glands (*P*), submandibular glands (*SMG*), and nasopharynx (*NP*). Bone, air, and fat are photopenic, as is seen in the maxillary sinus (*M*), maxilla (***), and mandible (+).

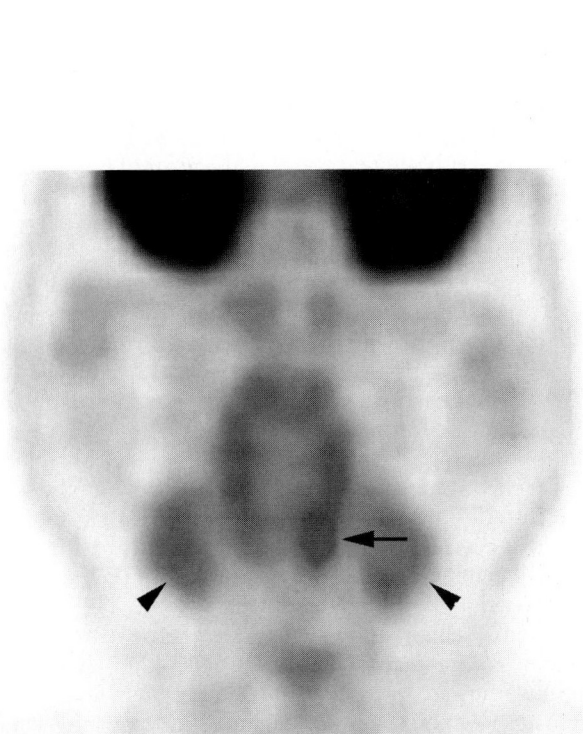

Figure 16–4. ^{18}F-fluorodeoxyglucose positron emission tomography scan in a patient who presented with metastatic cervical lymphadenopathy, fine-needle aspiration positive for squamous cell carcinoma (SCC). Routine head and neck examination was unremarkable. The scan in the coronal plane demonstrates asymmetrical activity in the lower pole of the left tonsil (*arrow*). Focused clinical evaluation revealed slight firmness in the lower pole of the tonsil, and a biopsy was positive for SCC. Arrowheads indicate the submandibular glands.

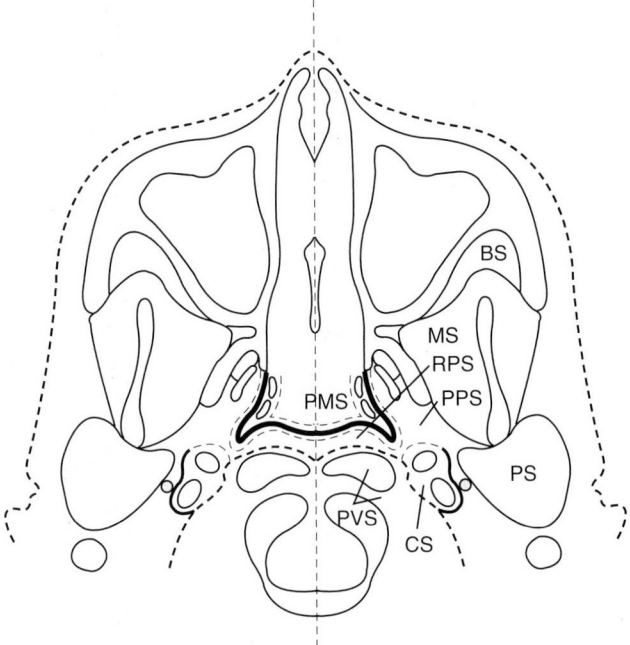

Figure 16–5. Diagram of the spatial anatomy of the suprahyoid neck at the mid-nasopharyngeal level. The spaces are defined by the three layers of the deep cervical fascia: superficial layer (*solid line*), middle layer (*dotted line*), and deep layer (*dashed line*). In addition, the pharyngobasilar fascia, which connects the superior constrictor muscle to the skull base, is shown as a dark curvilinear line superficial to the middle layer of the deep cervical fascia. The spaces include the pharyngeal mucosal space (*PMS*), retropharyngeal space (*RPS*), parapharyngeal space (*PPS*), carotid space (*CS*), parotid space (*PS*), masticator space (*MS*), and perivertebral space (*PVS*). The buccal space (*BS*) is not a true fascia-defined compartment. (Modified from Harnsberger HR: CT and MRI of masses of the deep face. *Curr Probl Diagn Radiol.* 1987;16:141. Used with permission.)

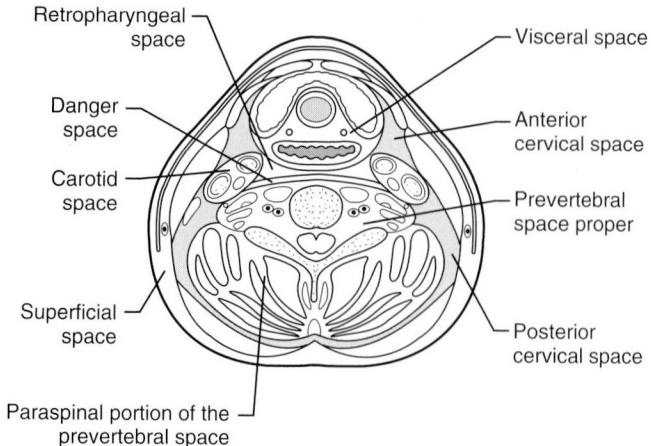

Figure 16–6. Diagram of the spatial anatomy of the infrahyoid neck at the mid-thyroid level. The spaces are again defined by the three layers of the deep cervical fascia. The superficial layer encircles the neck completely, splitting to encircle the sternocleidomastoid and trapezius muscles. External to this layer is the superficial space of the infrahyoid neck. The middle layer encircles and defines the visceral space, which includes the trachea, esophagus, and thyroid gland. The deep layer of fascia defines the perivertebral space, which includes the prevertebral space proper and the paraspinal portion of the prevertebral space. The carotid space is defined by contributions from all three fascial layers. The posterior cervical space is largely fat-filled and contains multiple lymph nodes. (Modified from Smoker WR, Harnsberger HR: Differential diagnosis of head and neck lesions based on their space of origin. 2. The infrahyoid portion of the neck. *AJR Am J Roentgenol.* 1991;157:155. Used with permission.)

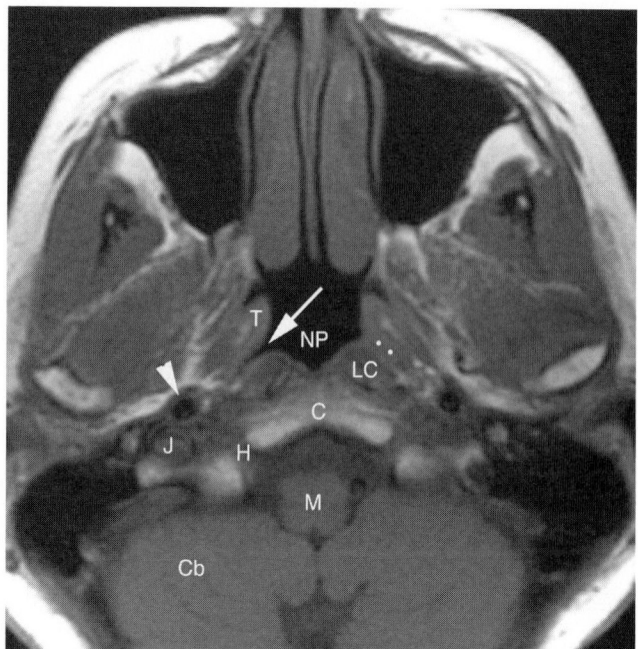

Figure 16–7. Axial T1-weighted image of the normal nasopharynx. Nasopharyngeal airway (*NP*), *longus colli* muscle (*LC*), clivus (*C*), *torus tubarius* (*T*), hypoglossal canal (*H*), internal jugular vein (*J*), internal carotid artery (*white arrowhead*), medulla (*M*), and cerebellum (*Cb*) are indicated. The straight white arrow indicates air in the right lateral pharyngeal recess (*Rosenmüller's fossa*); on the left, the mucosal surfaces of the *fossa* are coapted (*white dots*).

Nasopharynx

NORMAL ANATOMY

The nasopharynx is bounded anteriorly by the posterior nasal cavity at the level of the choana; posterosuperiorly by the lower clivus, upper cervical spine, and prevertebral muscles; and inferiorly by the palate. Its contents include mucosa, lymphoid tissue (adenoids), pharyngeal constrictor muscles, the levator palatini muscle, and the torus tubarius (the projecting posterior lip of the pharyngeal opening of the Eustachian tube). Because of the location of the pharyngeal opening of the Eustachian tube, nasopharyngeal masses may obstruct the tube, causing dysfunction and serous otitis. The so-called *Rosenmüller's fossa* represents the uppermost aspect of the lateral recess of the nasopharynx and is a common site of origin of nasopharyngeal cancers. The normal nasopharynx is shown in Figure 16-7.

PATHOLOGY

Nasopharyngeal carcinoma (NPC) is the most common malignant lesion of the nasopharynx. NPC may be small and confined to *Rosenmüller's fossa* or large with extension to the skull base, intracranial structures, and deep spaces of the head and neck.[14] Lymphadenopathy is often a prominent feature of even early NPC, and the imaging appearance of normal and pathologic lymph nodes

is discussed later. Nasopharyngeal carcinomas most commonly metastasize to retropharyngeal, level II, and level V nodes. Note that the classification of lymph nodes based on anatomic "levels" is discussed later in the Lymph Nodes section.

Contralateral retropharyngeal, level II, and level V nodes are also at significant risk because of rich bilateral lymphatic drainage. NPC generally presents as an asymmetric, infiltrative mass that is intermediate in signal intensity on both T1- and T2-weighted images, and shows homogeneous enhancement post-gadolinium (Fig. 16-8). Small lesions are typically limited by the surrounding pharyngobasilar fascia; once this barrier is breached, the tumor may directly invade the skull base, usually at the level of the petroclival fissure and foramen lacerum. Skull base involvement is best detected on T1-weighted images, which show loss of the normal bright signal of marrow fat (Fig. 16-9). The sinus of Morgagni, which allows passage of the cartilaginous portion of the Eustachian tube and the levator veli palatini muscle, is a natural defect that may allow extension of NPC laterally into the parapharyngeal space and carotid space. A tumor may then involve V3 and extend intracranially via the foramen ovale. Cavernous sinus extension and perineural spread of disease (usually along V3) are often best demonstrated on post-gadolinium T1-weighted images with fat saturation (Fig. 16-10).

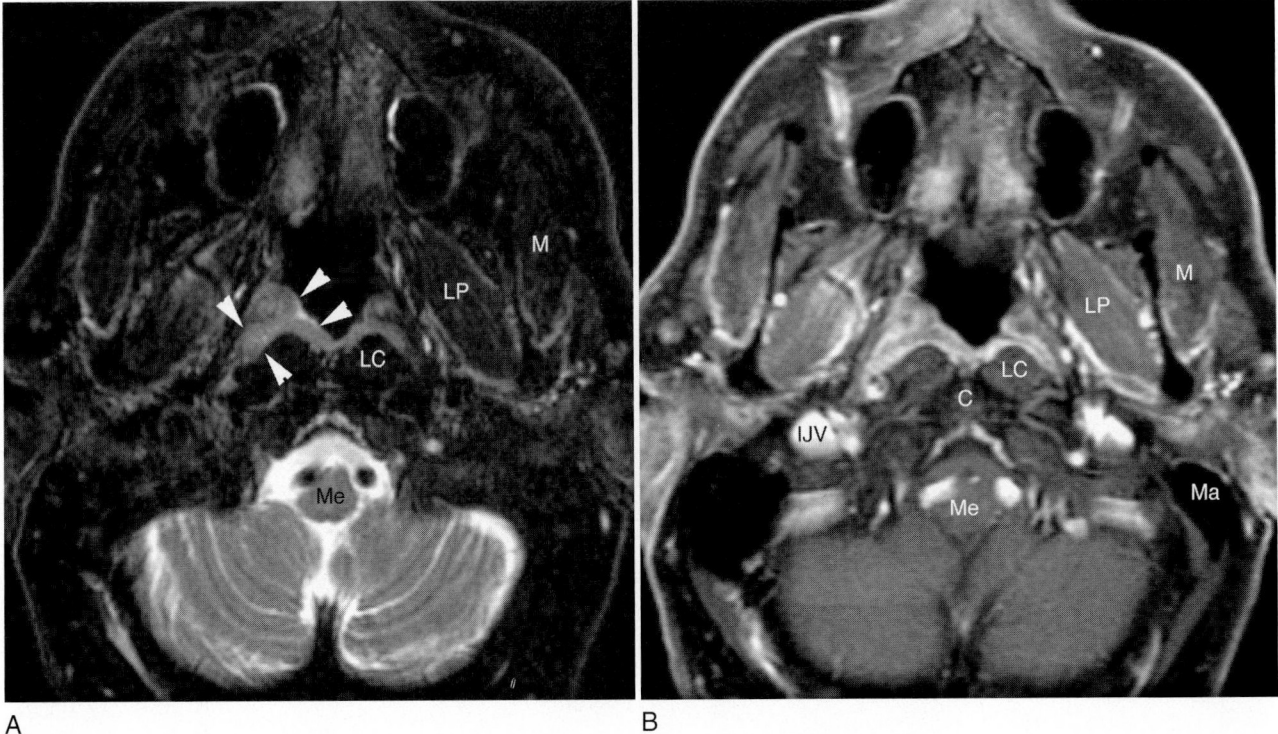

A   B

Figure 16–8. A, Axial fast spin-echo T2-weighted image through the nasopharynx in a patient who presented with a neck mass (not shown). The right *Rosenmüller's fossa* is expanded by an intermediate-signal intensity soft tissue mass that also infiltrates along the mucosa overlying the *torus tubarius* and toward the midline (*arrowheads*). Biopsy-proven nasopharyngeal carcinoma. Also indicated are the *longus colli* (*LC*), lateral pterygoid (*LP*), and masseter (*M*) muscles, and medulla (*Me*). **B,** Axial postgadolinium T1-weighted image with fat saturation shows moderate homogeneous enhancement of the mass. Also labeled are the *clivus* (*C*), internal jugular vein (*IJV*), and mastoid (*Ma*).

Oropharynx

NORMAL ANATOMY

The oropharynx is bounded anteriorly by the circumvallate papillae of the tongue and the anterior tonsillar pillars, which separate the oropharynx from the oral cavity.[15] Posteriorly it is bounded by the pharyngeal constrictor muscles and superiorly by the soft palate. Inferiorly it is separated from the larynx by the epiglottis and glossoepiglottic fold and from the hypopharynx by the pharyngoepiglottic fold. Its contents include the tongue base, palatine tonsils, soft palate, and oropharyngeal mucosa and constrictor muscles from the level of the palate to the hyoid bone. The normal oropharynx is shown in Figure 16-11.

PATHOLOGY

SCC accounts for most tumors of the oropharynx, followed by lymphoma, minor salivary gland lesions, and mesenchymal tumors.[16] The appearance of SCC varies somewhat with the specific subsite involved, and the tumor may be variably exophytic or deeply infiltrative. Tumors of the *tonsillar fossa* may be occult when small and may present with cervical nodal disease. Tonsil cancers most commonly metastasize to level II lymph nodes. Larger tumors of the *tonsillar fossa* may

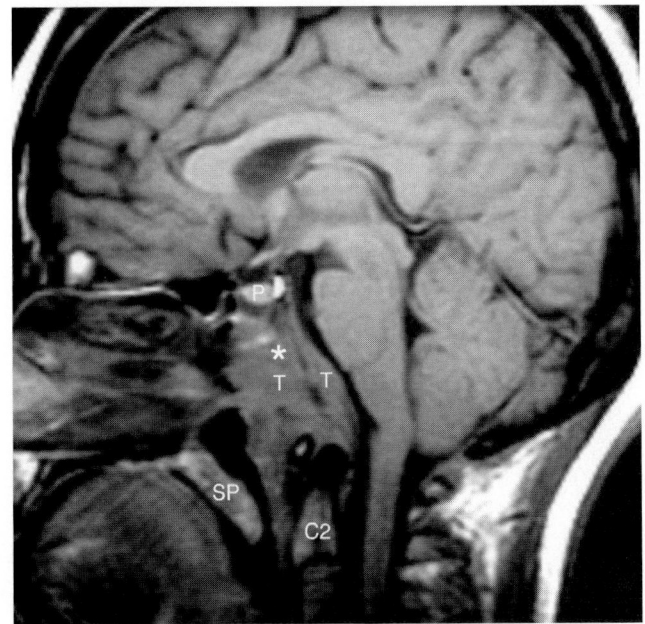

Figure 16–9. Sagittal T1-weighted image in a patient with nasopharyngeal carcinoma shows loss of the normal high-signal intensity in the *clivus* (***) and replacement by infiltrative tumor. The tumor (*T*) is also seen in the nasopharynx and involving the retro-clival dura. The clival involvement may be easily missed on a CT scan. Also shown are the pituitary gland (*P*), C2 vertebral body (*C2*), and the soft palate (*SP*).

Text continued on page 382

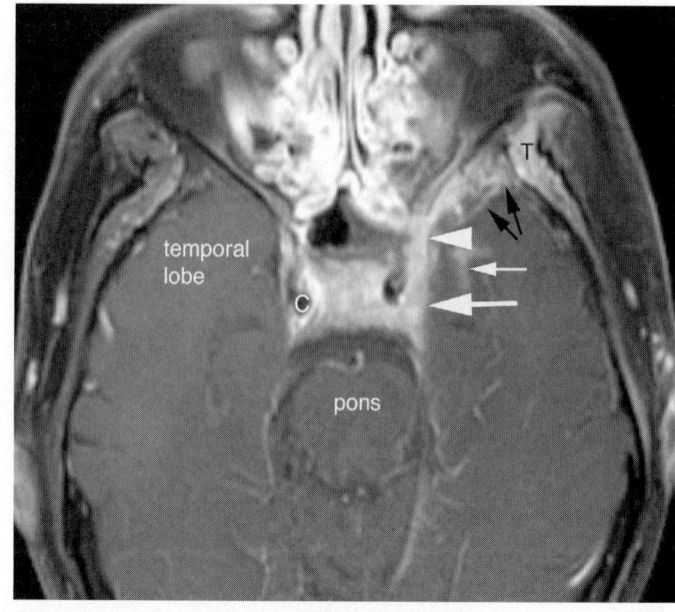

A

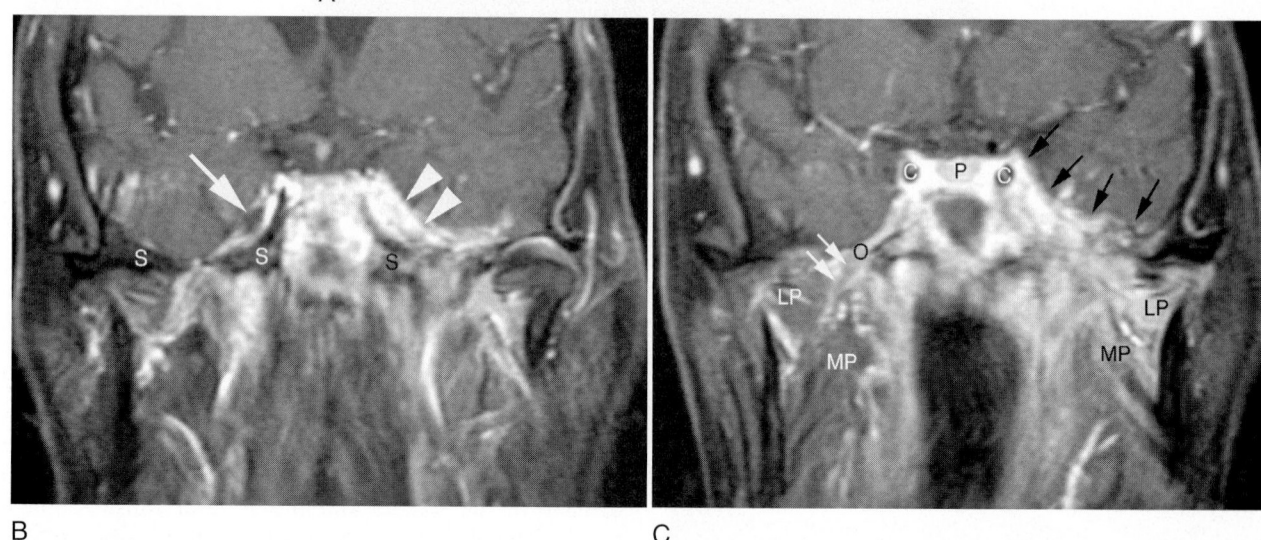

B   C

Figure 16–10. A, Axial post gadolinium T1-weighted image with fat saturation in a patient with recurrent nasopharyngeal carcinoma and left trigeminal nerve motor and sensory symptoms demonstrates intracranial extension of tumor to the left cavernous sinus (*large white arrow*) and also involvement of the left foramen rotundum (*white arrowhead*). There is abnormal enhancement and filtration of the dura of the left middle cranial fossa (*small black arrows*), as well as of the greater wing of the sphenoid. Denervation change with asymmetrical enhancement is seen in the left temporalis muscle (*T*). A small focus of brain parenchymal enhancement (*small white arrow*) is due to radiation necrosis from prior therapy. Also indicated are the right cavernous carotid artery (*C*), the pons, and the temporal lobe. **B,** Coronal post-gadolinium T1-weighted image with fat saturation in the same patient demonstrates fluid signal intensity in the normal right Meckel's cave (*white arrow*), as well as normal suppressed marrow fat in the right greater wing of the sphenoid (*white S*). On the synptomatic left side, Meckel's cave (*white arrowheads*) is expanded and the expected fluid has been replaced by infiltrative tumor. Abnormal signal intensity is seen in the tumor-involved sphenoid wing (*black S*). **C,** A slightly more anterior coronal post gadolinium T1-weighted image with fat saturation shows normal foramen ovale (*O*) and V3 (*white arrows*) on the right, as well as normal intermediate signal intensity of the medial (*MP*) and latteral (*LP*) pterygoid muscles. On the left, tumor has invaded laterlly through the pharyngobasilar fascia ans has extended intracranially along V3, with abnormal enhancing soft tissue seen in the left cavernous sinus, Meckel's cave, and dura (*black arrows*). Infiltrating tumor has obscured normal anatomy, and it is difficult to separate V3 from the surrounding tumor-infiltrated soft tissues. The cavernous cartoid arteries are indicated (*C*). Denervation change is present in the muscles of mastication due to tumor invasion of V3, and this manifests as abnormal enhancement of the left medial and lateral pterygoid muscles (*MP, LP*) as compared with the right.

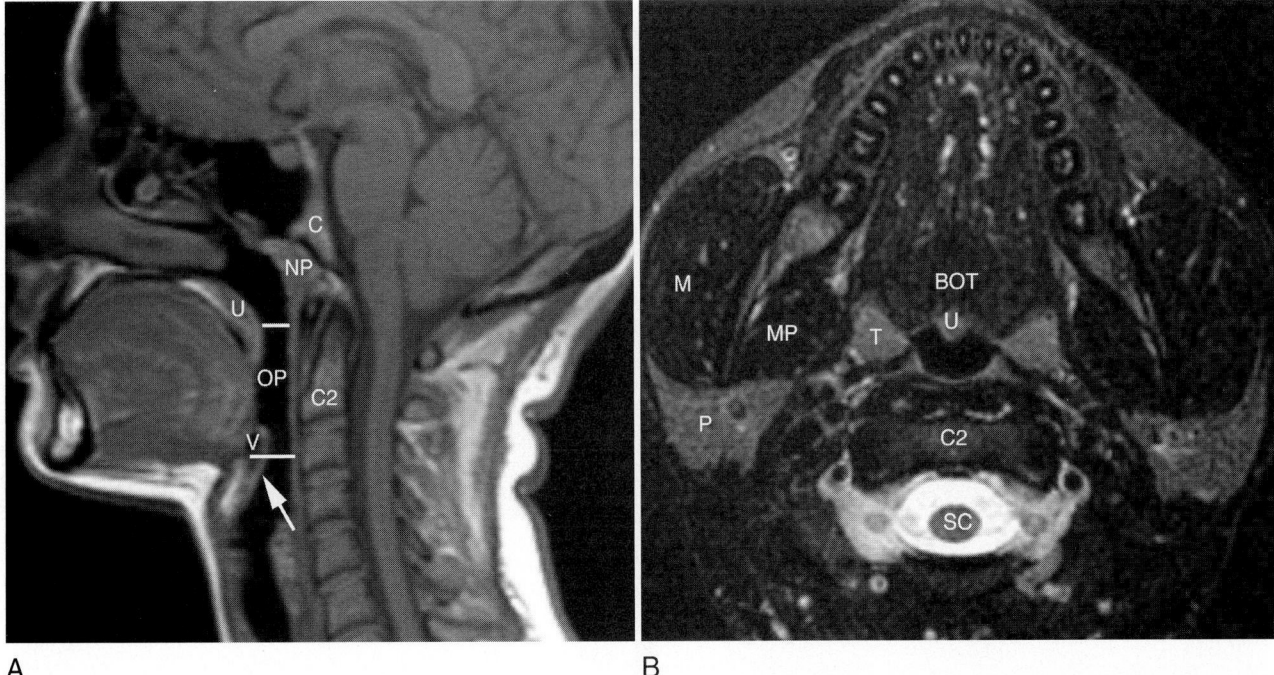

A   B

Figure 16–11. A, Sagittal T1-weighted image shows the oropharynx (*OP*) extending from the soft palate (*U*) superiorly to the level of the bottom of the vallecula (*V*) inferiorly. Also shown are the normal nasopharyngeal soft tissues (*NP*), the *clivus* (*C*), the C2 vertebral body, and the epiglottis (*white arrow*). **B,** Axial fast spin-echo T2-weighted image with fat saturation of the normal oropharynx shows the uvula (*U*), base of tongue (*BOT*), and palatine tonsils (*T*). Also shown are the spinal cord (*SC*), C2 vertebral body, medial pterygoid (*MP*) and masseter (*M*) muscles, and the parotid gland (*C*).

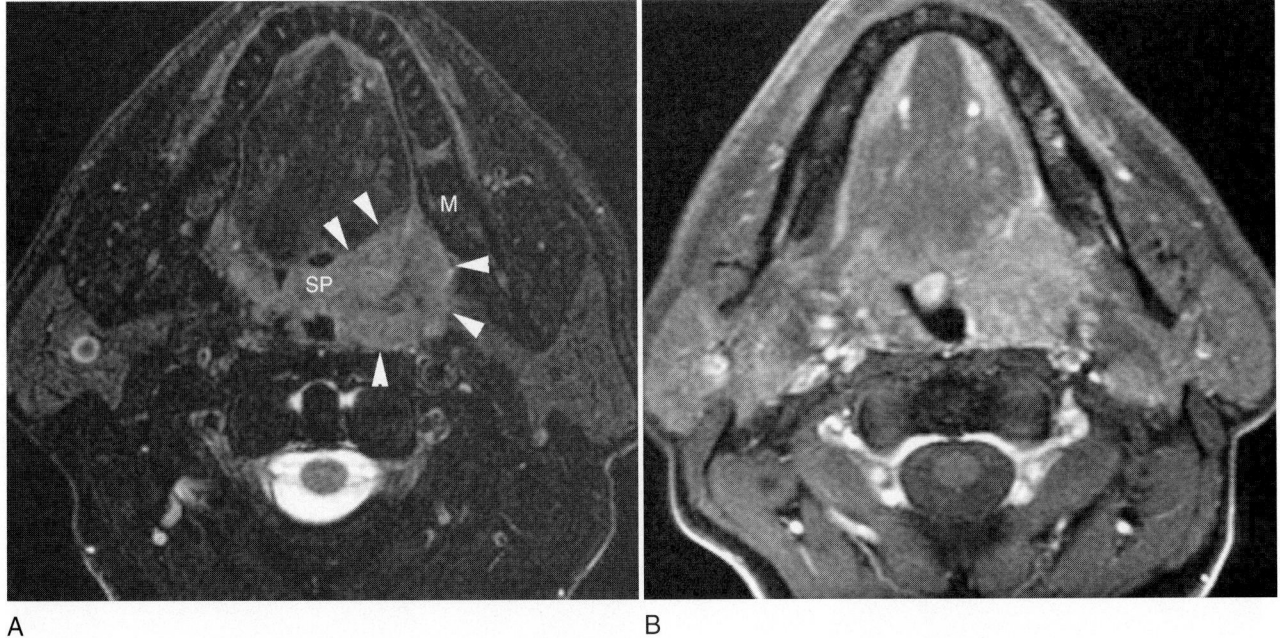

A   B

Figure 16–12. A, Axial fast spin-echo T2-weighted image with fat saturation in a patient with squamous cell carcinoma demonstrates a large mass in the left tonsillar *fossa* (*arrowheads*), extending into the soft palate (*SP*). The mass abuts but does not invade the mandible (*M*) and the base of tongue. **B,** Post-gadolinium, the mass demonstrates moderate homogeneous enhancement.

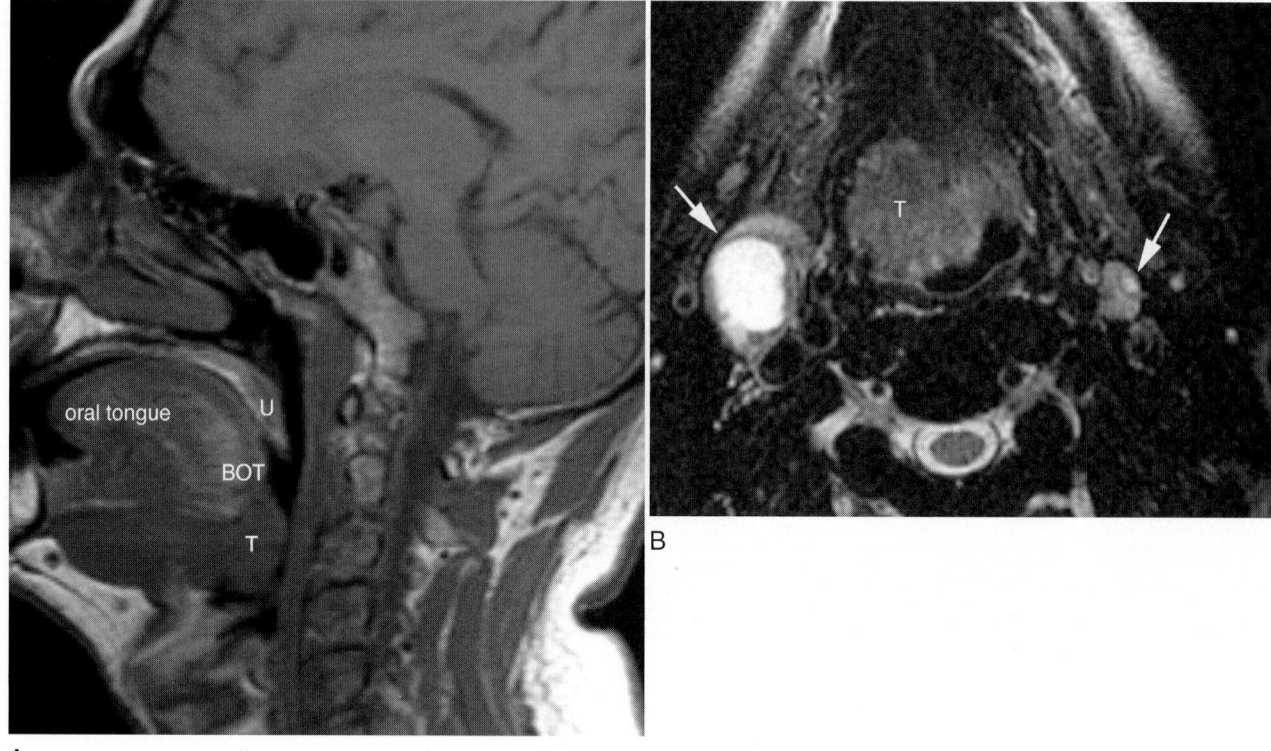

Figure 16–13. A, Sagittal T1-weighted image shows an exophytic soft tissue mass (*T*) arising from the base of tongue (*BOT*) in this patient with squamous cell carcinoma of the base of the tongue. The uvula is shown above (*U*). No significant invasion into the oral tongue or floor of mouth is noted in this largely exophytic lesion. **B,** Axial FSE T2-weighted image with fat saturation demonstrates the intermediate signal intensity primary mass lesion (*T*), as well as bilateral heterogeneous, level IIA metastatic lymph nodes (*arrows*).

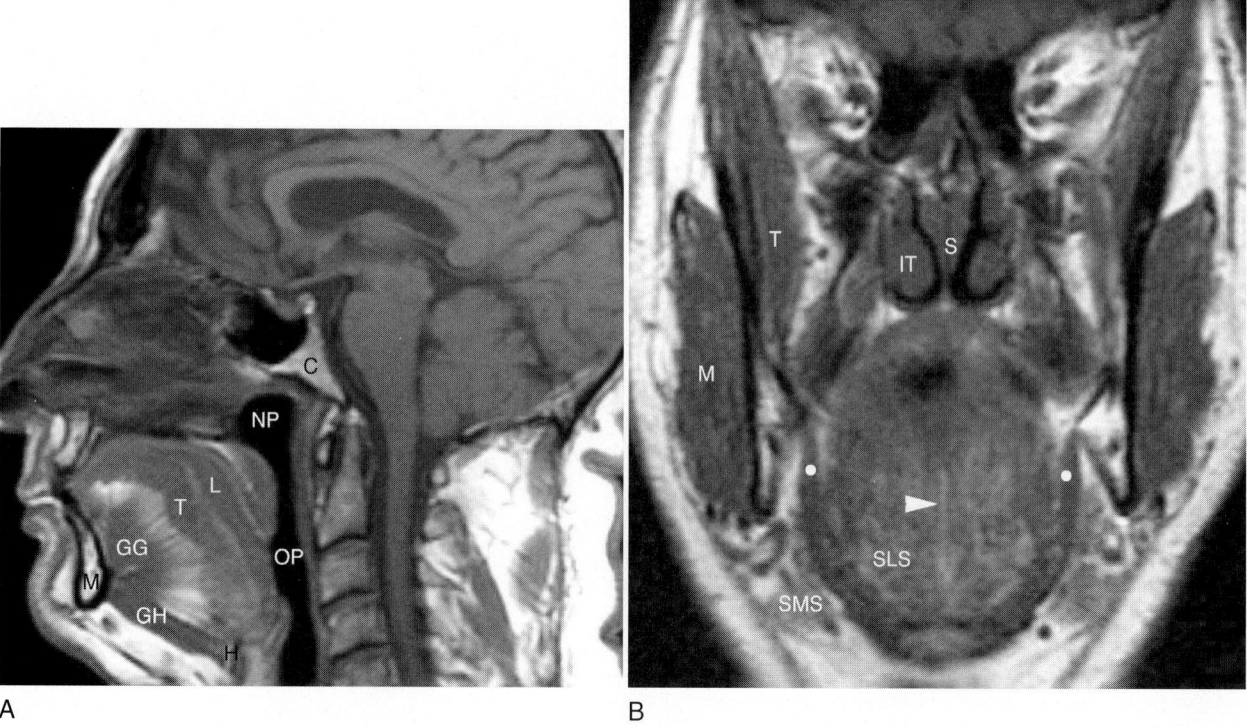

Figure 16–14. A, Sagittal T1-weighted image of the oral cavity. Well seen are the longitudinal (*L*) and transverse (*T*) muscle fibers of the tongue, as well as the genioglossus (*GG*) and geniohyoid (*GH*) muscles. Also indicated are the genu of the mandible (*M*), the hyoid bone (*H*), the nasopharyngeal (*NP*) and oropharyngeal (*OP*) airways, and the normal *clivus* (*C*) showing fatty-signal intensity in the clival marrow. **B,** Coronal T1-weighted image of the oral cavity shows the mylohyoid muscle (•), forming the U-shaped muscular floor of the mouth and separating the sublingual space above (*SLS*) from the submandibular space below (*SMS*). The midline fatty lingual septum is indicated by the white arrowhead. Also shown are the masseter (*M*) and *temporalis* (*T*) muscles, the inferior turbinate (*IT*), and the nasal septum (*S*).

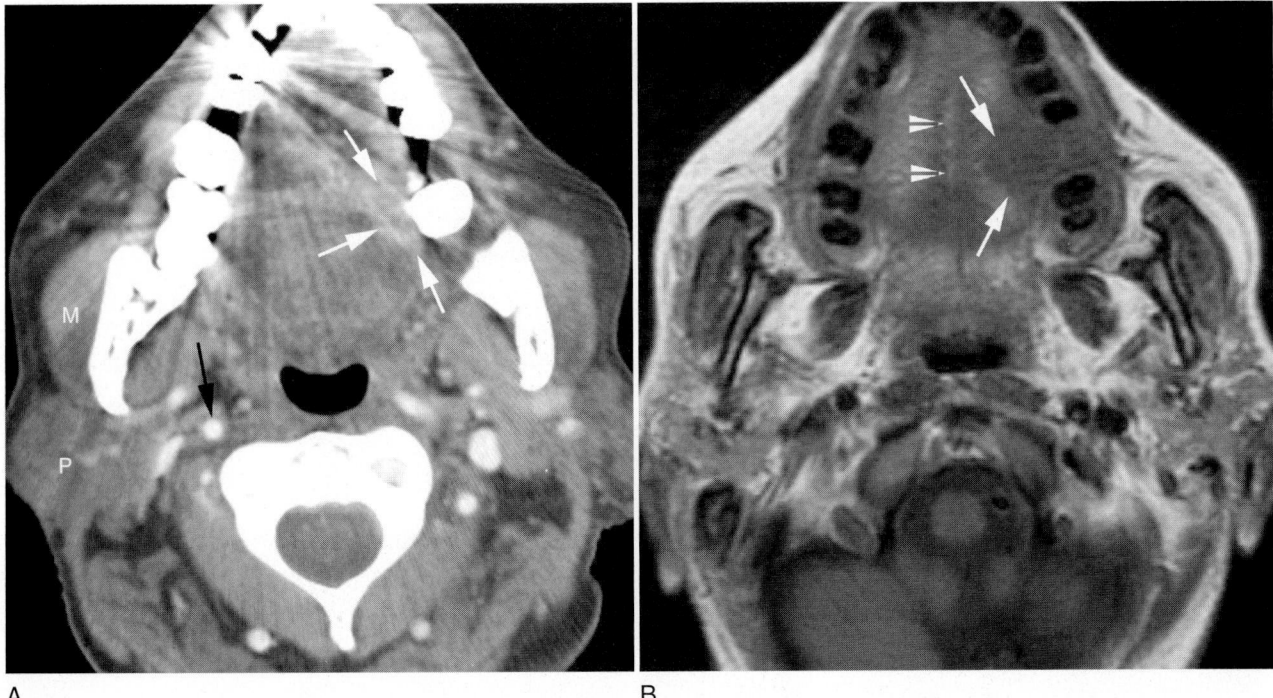

A   B

Figure 16–15. A, Contrast-enhanced CT scan in a patient with an ulcerative lesion of the left lateral tongue is significantly limited by dental artifact but does show a subtle mass in the left oral tongue (*white arrows*). Also indicated are the masseter muscle (*M*), parotid gland (*P*), and right internal carotid artery (*black arrow*). **B,** Axial T1-weighted magnetic resonance image in the same patient nicely demonstrates an infiltrative mass (*arrow*) in the left hemitongue that does not extend to the midline lingual septum (*arrowheads*). A biopsy confirmed squamous cell carcinoma.

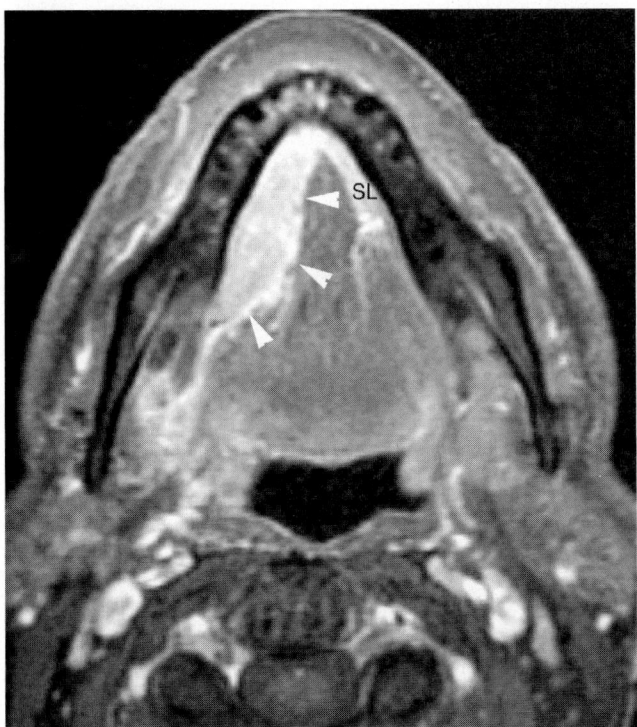

Figure 16–16. Axial post-gadolinium T1-weighted image with fat saturation in a patient with squamous cell carcinoma of the floor of the mouth. The lesion has extended into and extensively infiltrates the right sublingual gland/space (*arrowheads*). The normal left sublingual gland is shown for comparison (*SL*).

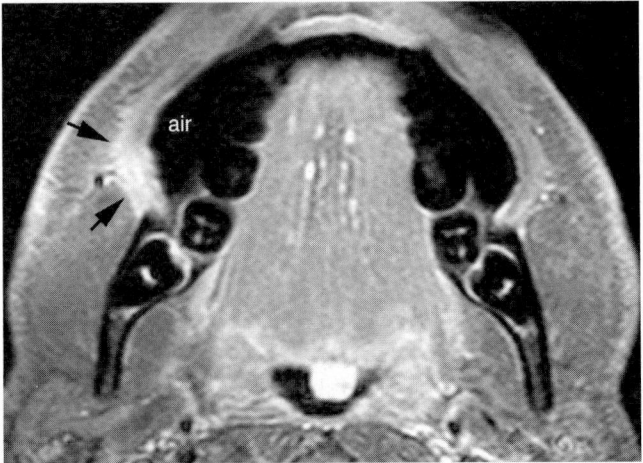

Figure 16–17. Axial post-gadolinium T1-weighted image in a patient with buccal carcinoma, performed using the puffed cheek technique. Note the air between the buccal mucosa and the mandible. The right sided carcinoma (*black arrows*), which infiltrates the underlying buccinator muscle, is well seen as compared with the normal left side.

spread anteriorly or posteriorly to involve the tonsillar pillars or anteriorly to invade the tongue. They may extend deeply to invade the constrictor muscles and then gain access to the parapharyngeal space and skull base. Tumors of the base of the tongue, when small, may be difficult to separate from normal lingual tonsillar tissue. Malignancy of the tongue base is usually asymmetrical, crossing midline only when large. Patterns of spread include posterolaterally to the tonsillar pillar and pharyngeal wall, submucosally into the supraglottic larynx, or anteriorly into the floor of the mouth. Nodal metastases are common with base of tongue tumors, with level II nodes most commonly involved, followed by level III nodes. Contralateral level II nodes are also commonly involved. The imaging features of lymphomas and minor salivary tumors are similar to SCC, and clinical examination and tissue sampling are necessary to make a specific diagnosis in most cases. Representative *tonsillar fossa* and base of tongue lesions are shown in Figures 16-12 and 16-13.

Oral Cavity

NORMAL ANATOMY

The oral cavity is anterior to the oropharynx and separated from it by the circumvallate papillae; soft palate; and anterior tonsillar pillars, which make up its posterior

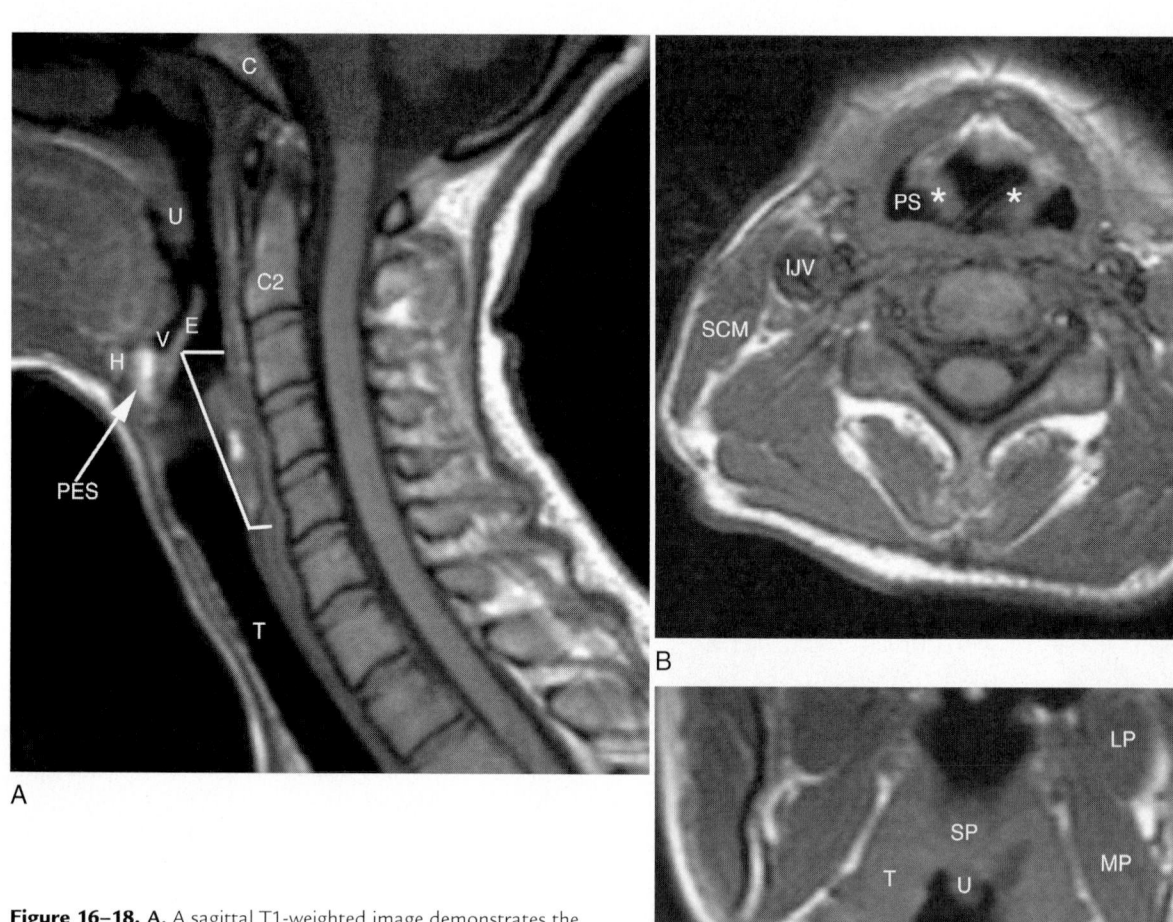

Figure 16–18. **A,** A sagittal T1-weighted image demonstrates the superior to inferior extent of the hypopharynx (*white lines*), from the bottom of the vallecula (*V*) to the bottom of the cricoid cartilage. Also shown are the *clivus* (*C*), uvula (*U*), C2 vertebral body (*C2*), epiglottis (*E*), hyoid bone (*H*), trachea (*T*), and fat in the pre-epiglottic space (*PES*). **B,** Axial T1-weighted image demonstrates the normal aryepiglottic folds (***) and pyriform sinus (*PS*), as well as the sternocleidomastoid muscle (*SCM*) and internal jugular vein (*IJV*). **C,** Coronal T1-weighted image demonstrates the epiglottis (*E*) and pyriform sinuses (*PS*). Also shown are the soft palate (*SP*) and uvula (*U*), the palatine tonsil (*T*), the medial (*MP*) and lateral pterygoid (*LP*) muscles, the masseter muscle (*M*), and the submandibular gland (*SMG*).

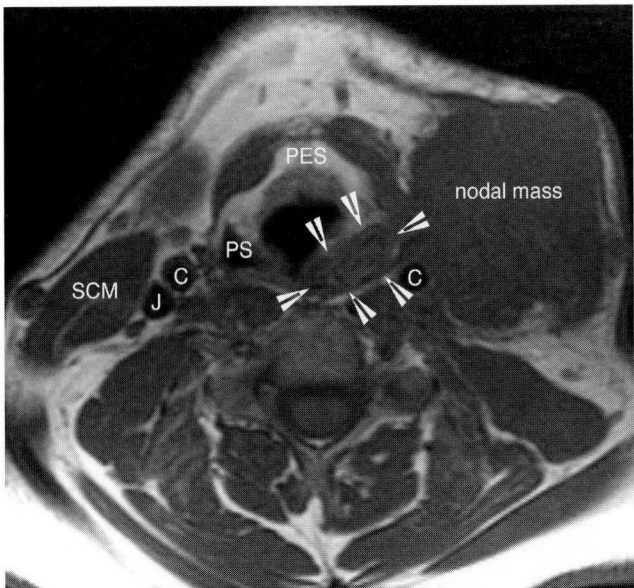

Figure 16–19. Axial T1-weighted image in a patient who presented with a large nodal mass due to metastatic squamous cell carcinoma demonstrates a relatively small primary tumor in the left pyriform sinus (*arrowheads*). The normal right pyriform sinus (*PS*) is shown for comparison. Also shown are the common carotid arteries (*C*), the right internal jugular vein (*J*) (*note that the left IJV is severely compressed or occluded by mass effect and is not visible*), fat in the pre-epiglottic space (*PES*), and the sternocleidomastoid muscle (*SCM*).

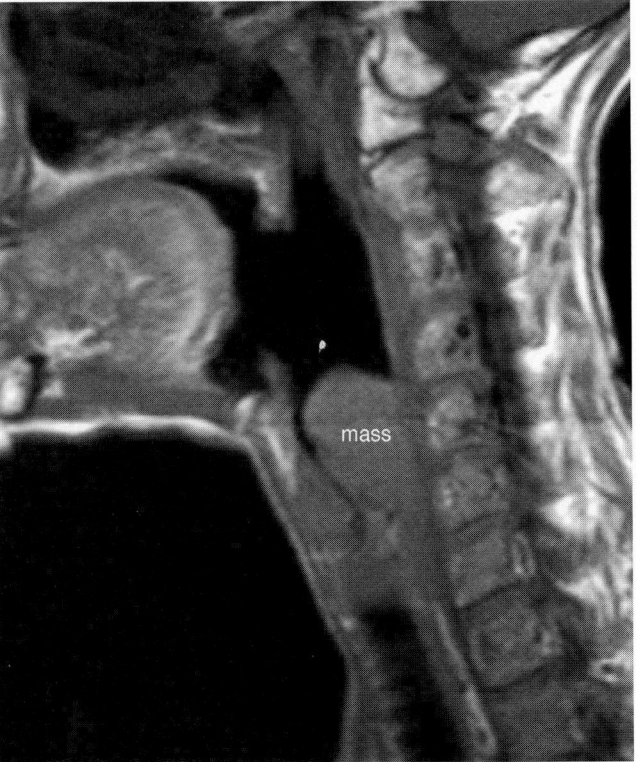

Figure 16–21. Sagittal T1-weighted image demonstrates a large hypopharyngeal mass, extending exophytically from the posterior pharyngeal wall. The inferior extent of the lesion is not clear from imaging alone.

boundary.[17] The oral cavity is bounded superiorly by the hard palate, laterally by the cheek, and inferiorly by the mylohyoid muscle. In addition to the mucosal area of the oral cavity (the dominant structure of which is the oral

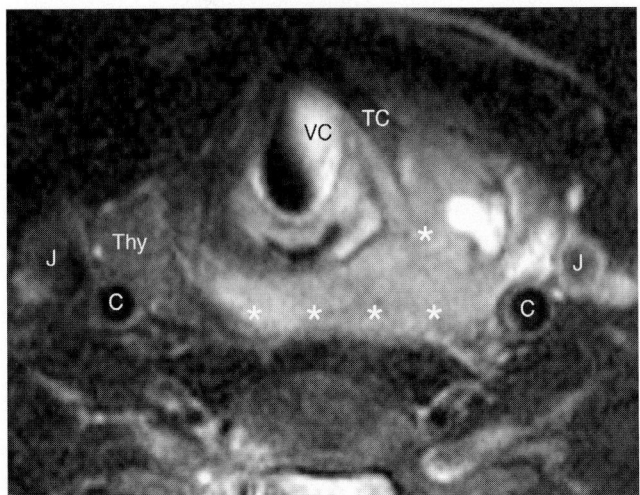

Figure 16–20. Axial fast spin-echo T2-weighted image with fat saturation from a patient with a large hypopharyngeal mass (*asterisks*) that involved the postcricoid region and extended into the cervical esophagus, invaded the thyroid gland (the normal right thyroid, is shown for comparison), eroded the left thyroid cartilage (*TC*), and infiltrated the cricoid cartilage. Tumor also extends through the cricothyroid joint, and the left vocal cord (*VC*) is enlarged and edematous due to denervation change. The common carotid arteries (*C*) and internal jugular veins (*J*) are indicated.

tongue), the mylohyoid muscle cleaves the lower oral cavity into the sublingual and submandibular spaces (Fig. 16-14). The sublingual space is frequently invaded by tumors of the floor of the mouth. The submandibular space is most commonly involved by inflammatory processes or metastases to level I lymph nodes. Direct extension to the submandibular space by SCC of the oral cavity is uncommon.

PATHOLOGY

All surfaces of the oral cavity are covered by mucosa, so there are many potential sites of origin of SCC. In addition, numerous minor salivary glands are distributed subepithelially throughout the oral cavity and can give rise to benign or malignant salivary tumors. SCC of the oral tongue, floor of the mouth, and gingivobuccal surfaces is well assessed by clinical examination. In cases of small or superficial lesions, imaging may be normal even though direct inspection clearly demonstrates a neoplasm. CT and MRI are most useful for assessing deep extension of malignant processes, involvement of critical structures such as the neurovascular bundle, and the presence of associated pathologic lymphadenopathy. They are also useful for presurgic and radiotherapy planning. Representative cases are illustrated in Figures 16-15 and 16-16. Because mucosal surfaces are usually coapted during scanning, which limits sensitivity

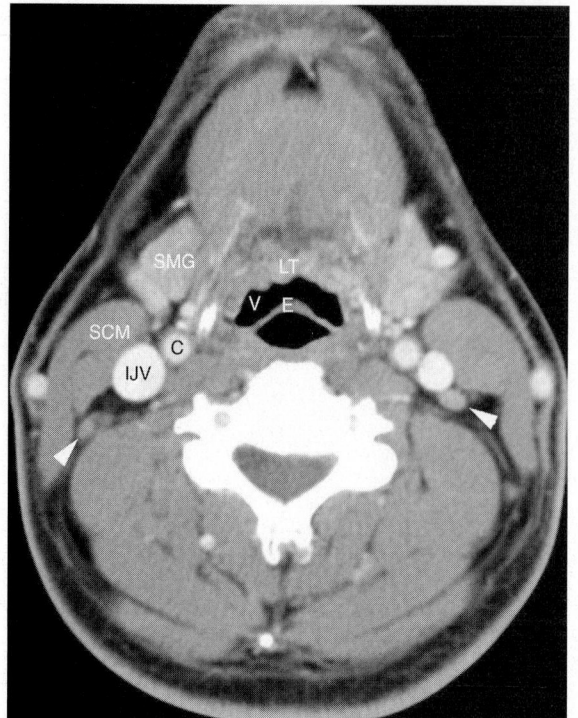

Figure 16–22. A series of axial contrast-enhanced computed tomography scans through the larynx, from cephalad to caudad. **A,** Indicated are the free edge of the epiglottis (*E*), the vallecula (*V*), lingual tonsillar tissue (*LT*) at the base of the tongue, submandibular gland (*SMG*), sternocleidomastoid muscle (*SCM*), common carotid artery (*C*), and internal jugular vein (*IJV*). The white arrowheads indicate normal level II lymph nodes. **B,** Image through the high supraglottic level shows the pyriform sinus (*PS*) and aryepiglottic fold (*white arrowhead*), as well as fat in the pre-epiglottic space (*PES*) and the superior cornu of the thyroid cartilage (*black arrowhead*). The strap muscles (*SM*) are indicated. **C,** Image through the low supraglottic level shows the thyroid notch (*N*), the false vocal cords (*white arrowheads*), and the fat-filled paralaryngeal space (*P*). Ossified segments of the thyroid cartilage are indicated (*black arrowheads*). **D,** Image through the glottic level shows the true vocal cord (*VC*), the thin anterior commissure (*white arrowhead*), and the arytenoid (*A*) and cricoid (*C*) cartilages. The calcified but not ossified thyroid lamina is indicated (*black arrowheads*), as is the top of the thyroid gland (*T*). **E,** Image through the subglottic larynx shows the cricoid cartilage (*C*), the inferior cornua of the thyroid cartilage (*black arrowheads*), and the cricothyroid membrane (*white arrowheads*). The cricopharyngeus muscle/proximal cervical esophagus is also indicated (*CPM/CE*). The "x" indicates the expected position of the right recurrent laryngeal nerve, which runs in the tracheoesophageal groove and at this level is immediately adjacent to the cricothyroid joint.

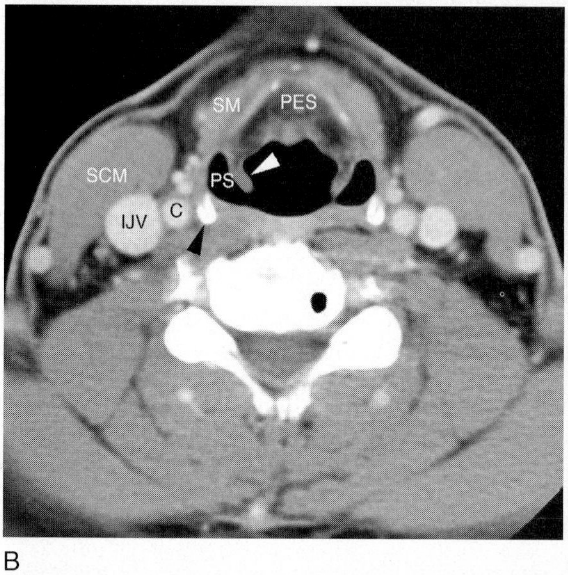

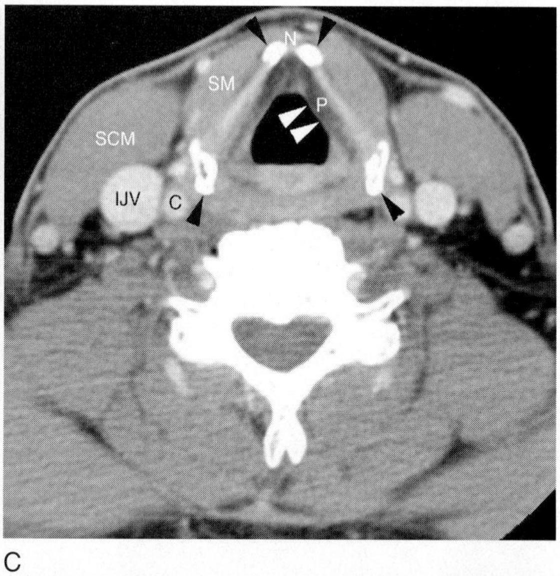

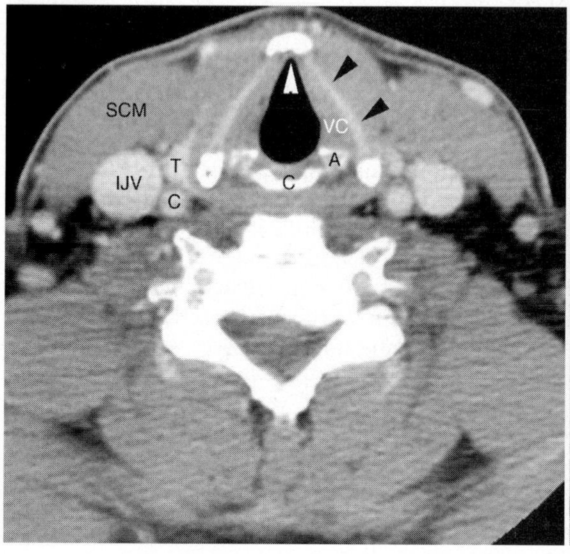

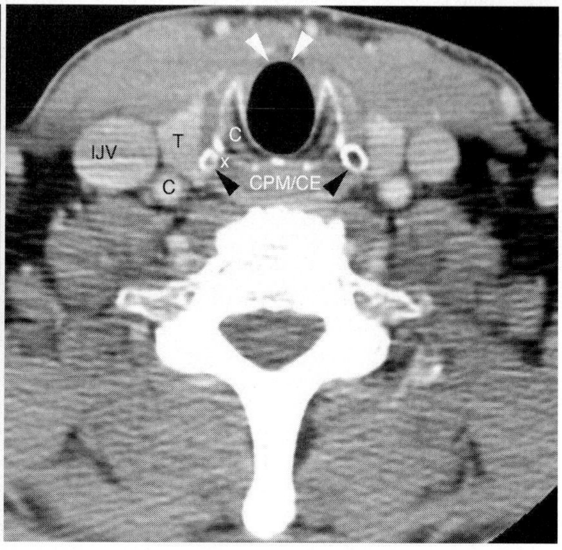

for small lesions and subtle deep invasion, it may be useful to have the patient perform a "puffed cheek" maneuver[18] to improve the assessment of oral cavity cancers, especially those of the buccal mucosa (Fig. 16-17). Cancers of the oral tongue most commonly metastasize to ipsilateral level II lymph nodes, followed by level I nodes, while cancers of the floor of the mouth most commonly metastasize to level I nodes followed by level II nodes.

Hypopharynx

NORMAL ANATOMY

The hypopharynx extends from the level of the hyoid bone and *valleculae* to the cricopharyngeus (or inferior margin of the cricoid cartilage on imaging studies). Its three major anatomic subsites include the pyriform sinus, postcricoid area, and posterior pharyngeal wall. The pyriform sinus is shaped like an inverted pyramid, with its apex at the level of the cricoarytenoid joint. The postcricoid area extends from the level of the arytenoid cartilages to the inferior border of the cricoid cartilage and is the anterior wall of the lower pharynx. The posterior hypopharyngeal wall extends from the level of the vallecula to the level of the cricoarytenoid joints (Fig. 16-18).

PATHOLOGY

The contents of the hypopharynx are the extensive squamous mucosal surfaces, minor salivary glands, and inferior pharyngeal constrictor muscles. SCC is the most common cause of hypopharyngeal pathology.[19] The pyriform sinus is the hypopharyngeal subsite most commonly involved with SCC (Fig. 16-19). SCC arising in this location tends to invade the soft tissues of the neck early and is frequently accompanied by pathologic lymphadenopathy. Ipsilateral metastatic nodes are common in both levels II and III. The extensive submucosal growth of hypopharyngeal tumors and invasion of adjacent organs are often not apparent on clinical examination, but are readily detected on cross-sectional imaging (Fig. 16-20). The sagittal plane is particularly useful in assessing the superoinferior extent of lesions of the posterior pharyngeal wall (Fig. 16-21), but the exact boundary of inferior extension into the cervical esophagus is often difficult to define by imaging and must be assessed endoscopically.

Larynx

NORMAL ANATOMY

The larynx is an anatomically complex region that consists of a mucosal surface draped over a supporting cartilaginous skeleton made up of the cricoid, thyroid, and

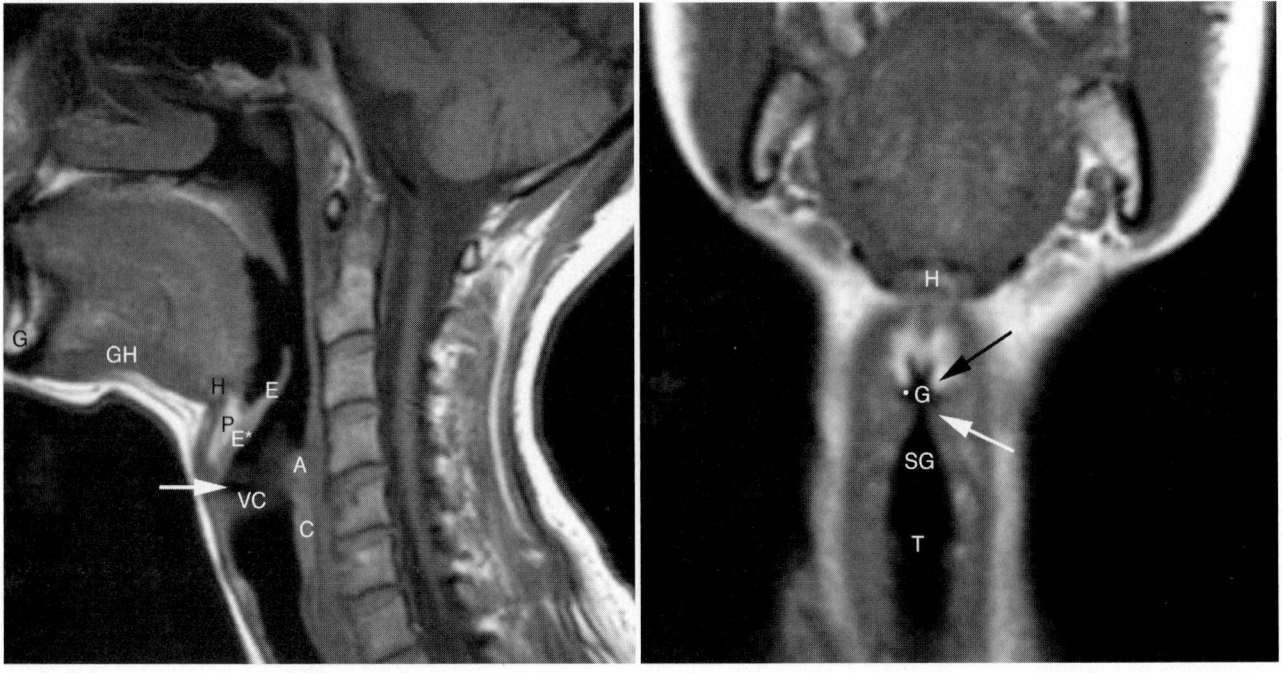

A   B

Figure 16–23. A, Sagittal T1-weighted image through the normal larynx. The free margin (*E*) and fixed portion (*E**) of the epiglottis are shown, as is the fat-filled pre-epiglottic space (*P*), the laryngeal ventricle (*white arrow*), the true vocal cord (*VC*), and the arytenoid (*A*) and cricoid (*C*) cartilages. The hyoid bone (*H*), genu of the mandible (*G*), and geniohyoid muscle (*GH*) are also shown. The supraglottis extends from the tip of the epiglottis above to the laryngeal ventricles below, the glottis includes the true vocal cords and the anterior and posterior commissures, and the subglottis extends from the undersurface of the true cords to the inferior surface of the cricoid cartilage. **B,** Coronal T1-weighted image through the normal larynx. The glottic level (*G*), laryngeal ventricle (•), subglottis (*SG*), body of the hyoid bone (*H*) and trachea (*T*) are indicated. The white arrow traverses the vocalis muscle and points to the edge of the true vocal cord, while the black arrow traverses the paralaryngeal fat and points to the false vocal cord.

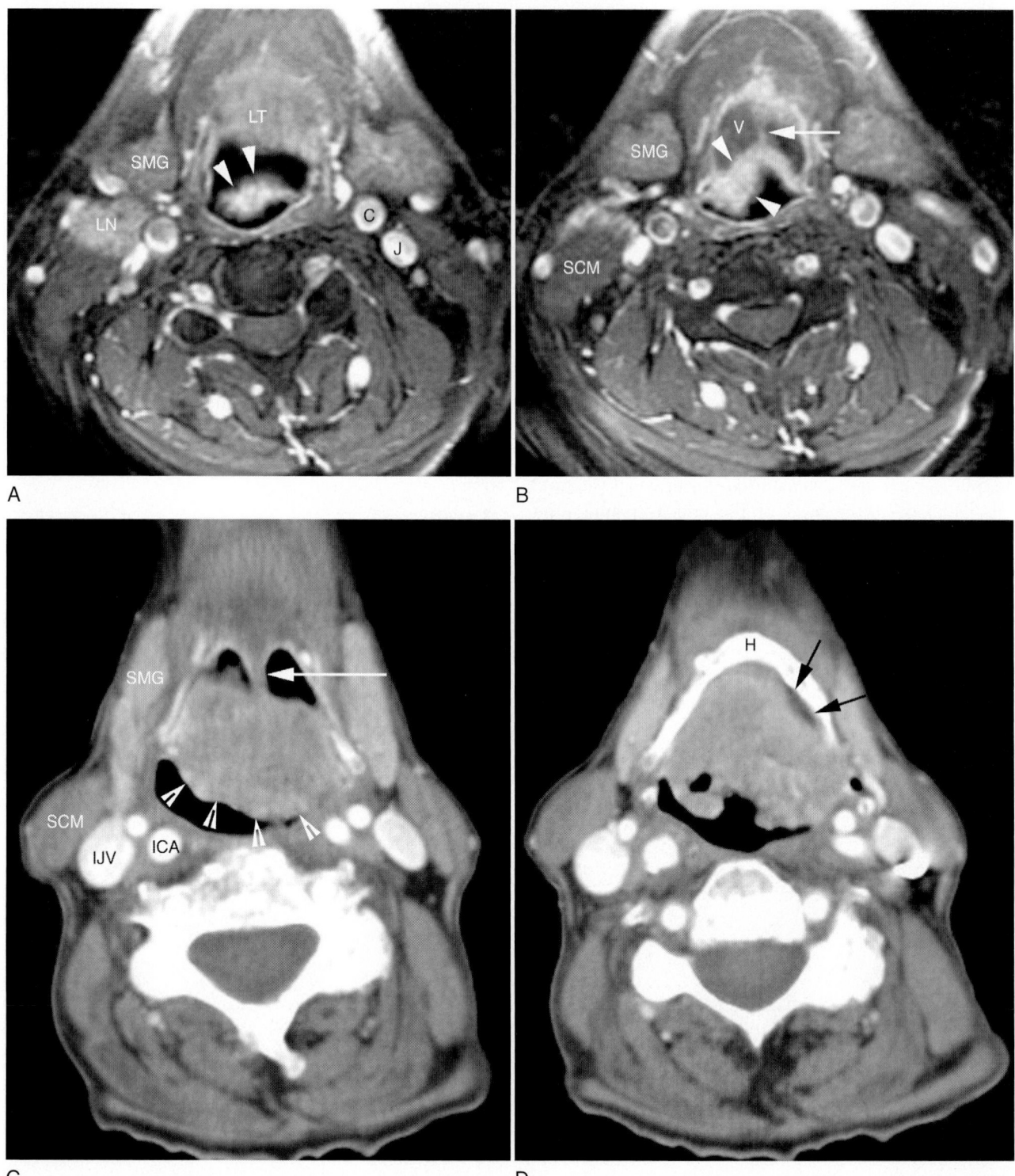

Figure 16–24. A and **B,** Axial post-gadolinium T1-weighted images with fat saturation in a patient with a small supraglottic cancer who presented with a neck mass and mild dysphagia. Indicated are the primary tumor, which infiltrates and thickens the free margin of the epiglottis (*white arrowheads*), as well as the metastatic level IIa lymph nodes (*LN*). Also shown are the lingual tonsils (*LT*), the glossoepiglottic fold (*white arrow*), the submandibular gland (*SMG*) and the sternocleidomastoid muscle (*SCM*). **C** and **D,** Axial images from a postcontrast CT scan in a patient with a massive supraglottic cancer who presented with dysphagia, odynophagia, and cachexia. Indicated is the primary tumor (*white arrowheads*), which infiltrates and thickens the epiglottis and aryepiglottic folds. There is extensive infiltration of the pre-epiglottic fat, with a tumor abutting the posterior aspect of the hyoid bone (*H*) and only a thin sliver of preserved hypodense preepiglottic fat seen on the left (*black arrows*).

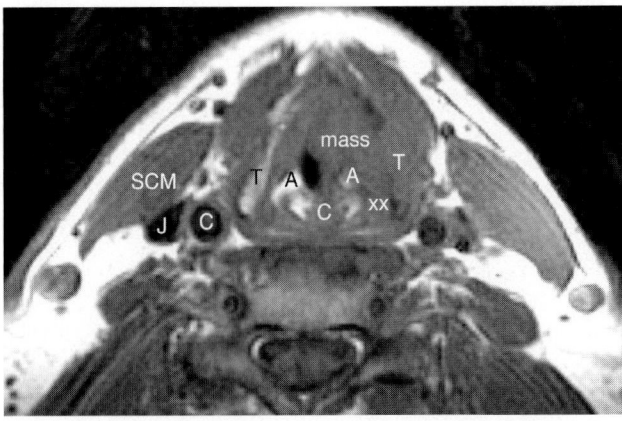

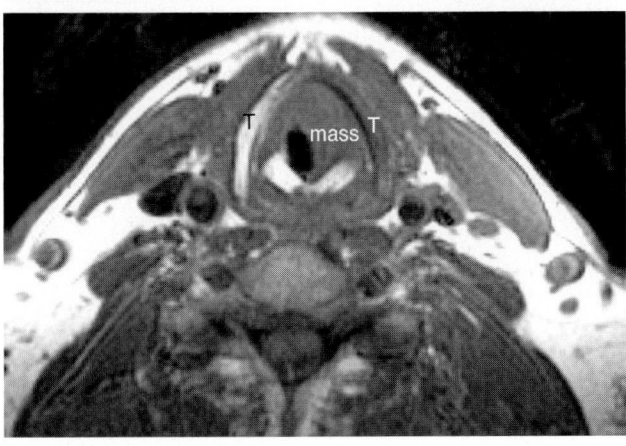

Figure 16–25. Axial T1-weighted images in a patient with squamous cell carcinoma of the glottic larynx. **A,** A large mass infiltrates the left true vocal cord and involves the anterior commissure. The left thyroid (*T*) and arytenoid (*A*) cartilages have abnormal signal intensity and are infiltrated by the tumor, while the right thyroid and arytenoid cartilages are ossified and have normal fatty signal intensity. The mass markedly widens the left cricothyroid joint (*xx*). **B,** A more inferior image at the undersurface true card level shows the extension of the tumor submucosally in the left true vocal cord and anterior commissure, with extension across midline to involve the right true vocal cord. Involvement of the left thyroid cartilage (*T*) is clear.

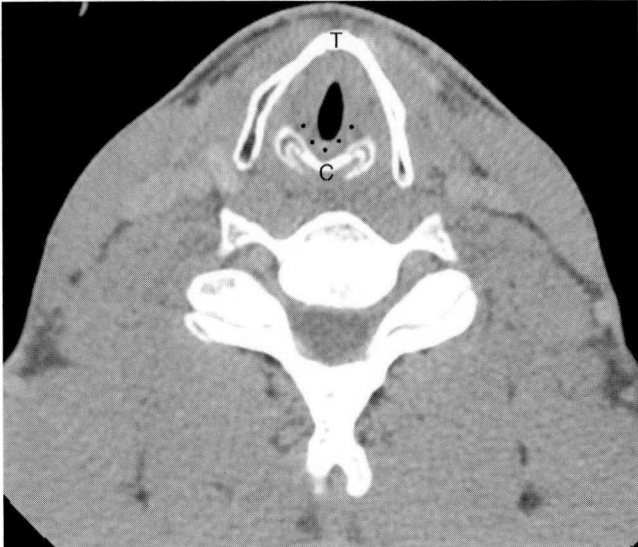

Figure 16–26. Axial computed tomography scan in a patient with adenoid cystic carcinoma of the trachea and subglottis demonstrates abnormal soft tissue thickening (*black dots*) anterior to the cricoid cartilage (*C*). Normally the air column should appear to directly contact the anterior surface of the cricoid, as in Figure 16-22**E**. The thyroid cartilage is also indicated (*T*).

arytenoid cartilages.[20] Structures that are part of the larynx include the epiglottis, aryepiglottic folds, and true and false vocal cords. Between the mucosal surfaces and the cartilaginous skeleton lie the predominantly fat-filled pre-epiglottic and paraglottic spaces. The endolarynx is usually divided into three segments (Figs. 16-22 and 16-23). The supraglottis extends from the tip of the epiglottis above to the laryngeal ventricles below and includes the epiglottis, aryepiglottic folds, pre-epiglottic space, false vocal cords, arytenoid cartilages, and the paraglottic (paralaryngeal) space. The glottis includes the true vocal cords and both the anterior and posterior commissures. On a normal axial CT scan or magnetic resonance image, less than 1 mm of tissue should be discernible at the level of the commissures. The subglottic area extends from the undersurface of the true vocal cords above to the inferior surface of the cricoid cartilage. As the mucosal surface of the subglottic area is closely applied to

the cricoid cartilage, any tissue seen on the airway side of the subglottic larynx should be viewed with suspicion. The site of origin of SCC within the larynx also dictates the likelihood of accompanying metastatic nodal involvement. The supraglottic larynx has a rich network of draining lymphatics and therefore a propensity toward metastatic nodal disease, while the glottic and subglottic larynx are far less likely to develop nodal metastases. Ipsilateral level II and III metastatic nodes are present in 50% to 70% of supraglottic cancers, while contralateral level II and III nodes are seen in 10% to 20% of cases.[21,22] Glottic cancers have a lower incidence of ipsilateral and a far lower incidence of contralateral nodal metastases.

The larynx is a site where CT may be superior to MRI for assessing the extent of a primary tumor. Though MRI has superior soft tissue contrast and superior sensitivity for cartilage invasion, it is often severely limited by breathing, coughing, and swallowing motion. Spiral and multislice CT scanners allow the rapid acquisition of images, often in a single breath hold, and facilitate high-quality multiplanar reformations.

PATHOLOGY

The vast majority of laryngeal neoplasms are SCCs. These tumors are usually well assessed by laryngoscopy, but imaging is useful for the assessment of submucosal and deep extension. The imaging of each laryngeal subsite raises certain unique issues. Supraglottic lesions (Fig. 16-24) tend to be large at the time of diagnosis because there is no hoarseness until the true vocal cord is involved, and nodal metastases are common at presentation. Anterior supraglottic lesions (those involving the epiglottis) spread

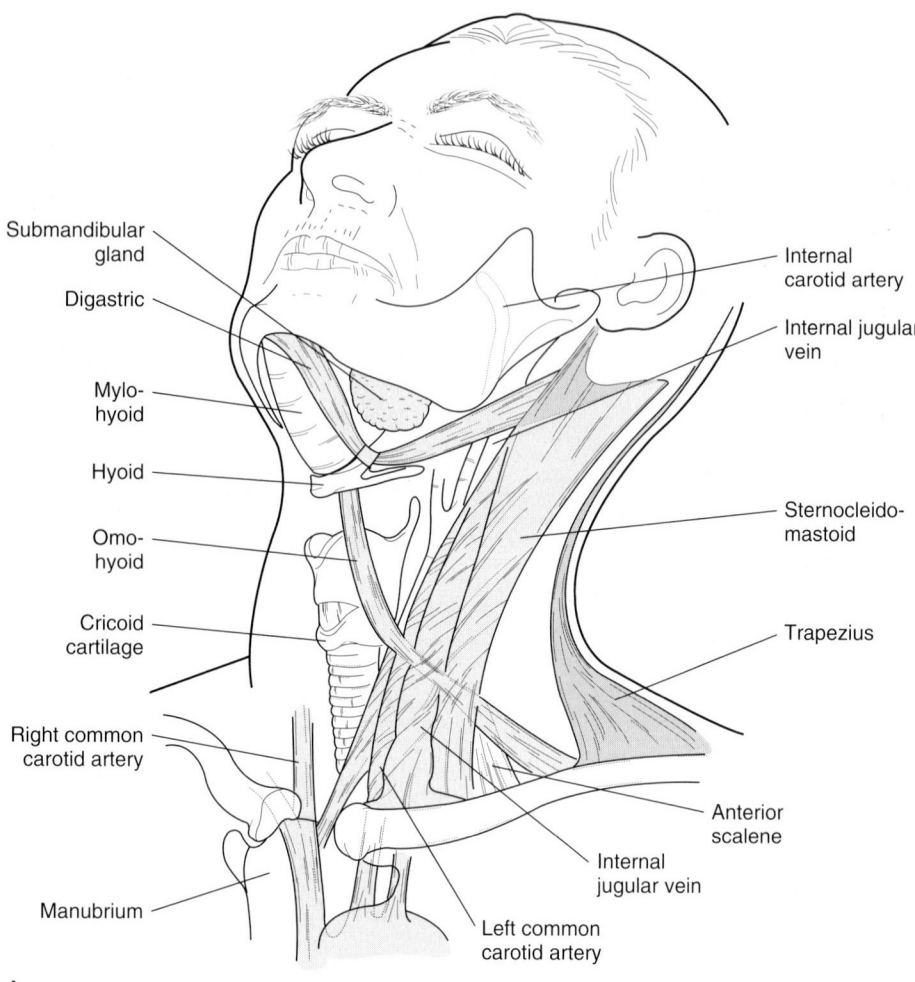

Submandibular
gland

Digastric

Mylo-
hyoid

Hyoid

Omo-
hyoid

Cricoid
cartilage

Right common
carotid artery

Manubrium

Internal
carotid artery

Internal jugular
vein

Sternocleido-
mastoid

Trapezius

Anterior
scalene

Internal
jugular vein

Left common
carotid artery

A

Figure 16–27. A, Line drawing of neck from left anterior view demonstrates anatomy relevant to nodal classification.

Continued

initially into the pre-epiglottic space, and later may access the tongue base above and the paraglottic space below. The pre-epiglottic space is optimally viewed on a sagittal T1-weighted image, which is very sensitive to infiltration of the normally bright pre-epiglottic fat by intermediate signal intensity tumor. Posterolateral supraglottic cancers (aryepiglottic fold, false vocal cord, laryngeal ventricle) may grow exophytically off the aryepiglottic folds or spread submucosally into the paraglottic space from the false cords and ventricle. Glottic SCCs often present early with voice change and/or hoarseness, and T1 lesions are often not visible on cross-sectional imaging studies. More advanced lesions are imaged to assess paraglottic and subglottic extension, as well as cartilage involvement (Fig. 16-25). Particular attention should be paid to the anterior and posterior commissures, which require thin-section technique. The subglottis is relatively easy to assess, as the area below the undersurface of the true cord has no normal

tissue between the mucosal surface and the cricoid cartilage, so any soft tissue thickening is pathologic (Fig. 16-26).

The laryngeal cartilages normally calcify with age, and eventually ossify. Assessing involvement of the laryngeal cartilages by tumor is an important part of the radiologic evaluation of SCC of the larynx.[23] CT can be used to assess asymmetric sclerosis and gross destruction, while MR is better suited to assess replacement of normal tissue by an infiltrating tumor. Both modalities are limited by their inability to separate tumor involvement from reactive changes, and the only sure indicators of neoplastic involvement are gross cartilage destruction or the presence of a tumor on both sides of the cartilaginous structure. Multiple studies have demonstrated that the radiologic ability to conclusively demonstrate cartilage involvement by tumor (except with gross destruction or tumor on both sides of the cartilage) is limited.

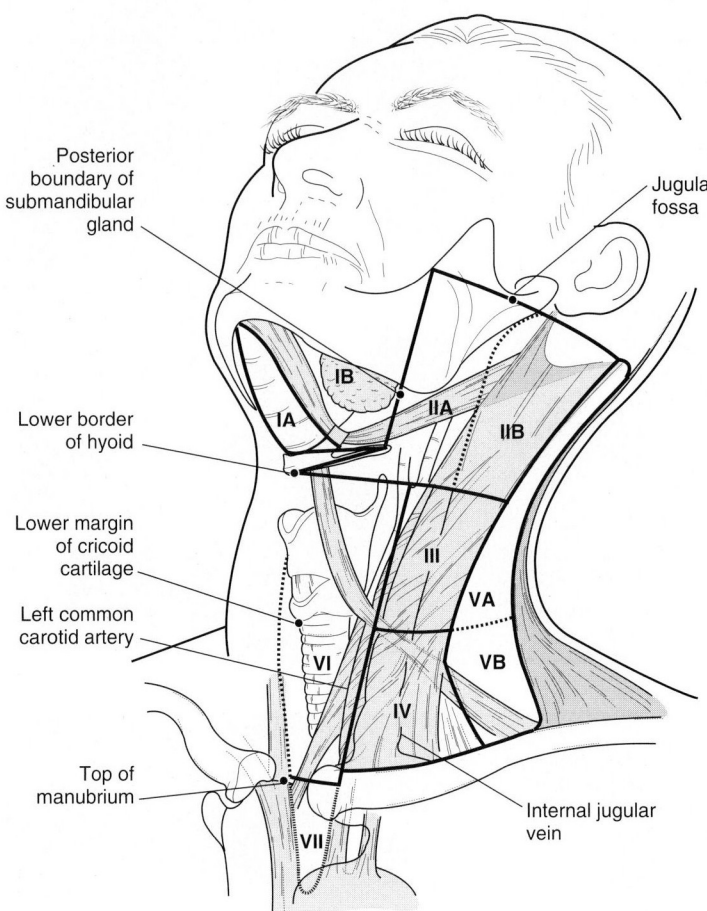

Figure 16–27. cont'd B, Nodal classification levels are indicated with regard to anatomic landmarks. Note that the posterior margin of the submandibular gland separates levels I and II, while the separation of levels II and III from level V is the posterior edge of the sternocleidomastoid muscle. The posterior edge of the internal jugular vein separates level IIA and IIB nodes. (Reprinted with permission from Som PM, Curtin HD, Mancuso AA: An imaging-based classification for the cervical nodes designed as an adjunct to recent clinically based nodal classifications. *Arch Otolaryngol Head Neck Surg.* 1999;125:388.)

B

Table 16–1   Summary of Imaging-Based Nodal Classification

Nodes	Boundaries	Subcategories
Level I	Above hyoid bone, below mylohyoid muscle, anterior to back of SMG	IA: between medial margins of anterior bellies of digastric muscles IB: posterolateral to level IA
Level II	From skull base to lower body of hyoid bone, posterior to back of SMG and anterior to back of SCM	IIA: anterior, lateral, medial, or posterior to IJV; and inseparable from IJV (if posterior to IJV) IIB: posterior to IJV with a fat plane separating nodes and vein
Level III	From lower body of hyoid to lower cricoid cartilage arch, anterior to back of SCM	
Level IV	From lower cricoid arch to level of clavicle, anterior to line connecting back of SCM and posterolateral margin of ASM, lateral to CAs	
Level V	Posterior to back of SCM from skull base to clavicle. Below cricoid arch, posterior to line connecting back of SCM and posterolateral margin of ASM.	VA: from skull base to bottom of cricoid arch, posterior to SCM VB: from cricoid arch to clavicle, posterior to line connecting back of SCM and posterolateral margin of ASM
Level VI	Between CAs from level of lower body of hyoid bone to top of manubrium	
Level VII	Between CAs below level of top of manubrium, caudal to level of innominate vein	

ASM, anterior scalene muscle; CA, carotid artery; IJV, internal jugular vein; SMG, submandibular gland; SCM, sternocleidomastoid muscle.
N. B. The supraclavicular and retropharyngeal nodes are not part of this numbered classification scheme. The retropharyngeal lymph nodes are defined as being within 2 cm of the skull base and medial to the internal carotid arteries, while the supraclavicular nodes are defined as at or caudal to the level of the clavicle as seen on each axial scan, lateral to the carotid artery on each side of the neck, and above and medial to the ribs.
Summarized from Som PM, Curtin HD, Mancuso AA: Imaging-based nodal classification for evaluation of neck metastatic adenopathy. *AJR Am J Roentgenol.* 2000;174:837.

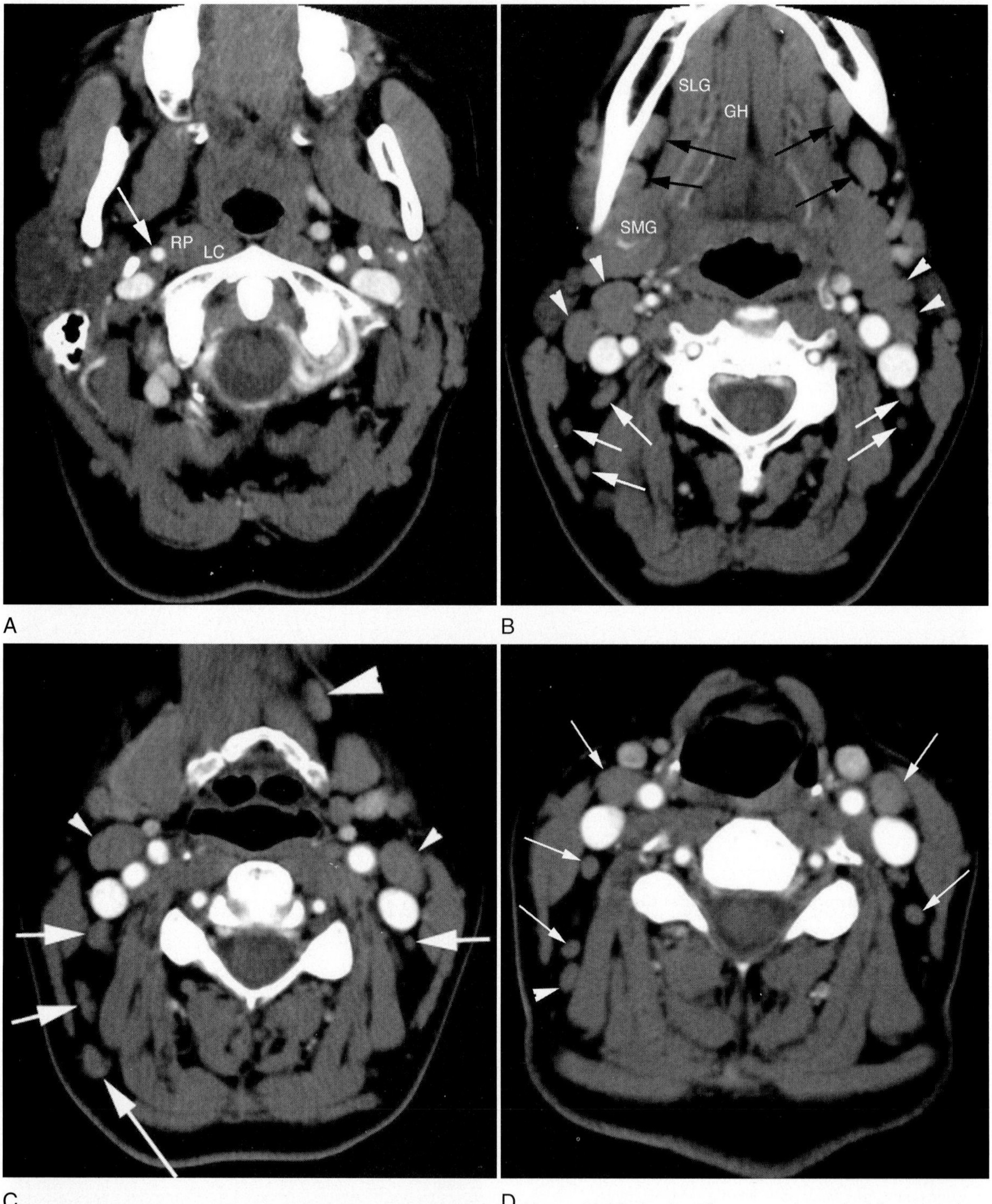

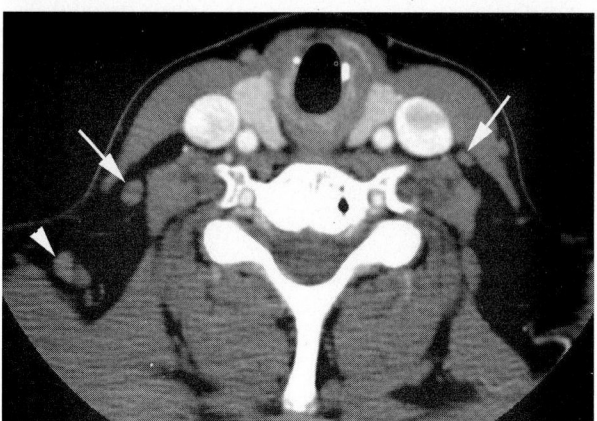

A

B

C

D

Figure 16–28. A series of contrast-enhanced axial computed tomography images in a patient with lymphoma demonstrates the imaging-based nodal classification. **A,** A retropharyngeal (*RP*) node is seen within 2 cm of the skull base, anterolateral to the longus colli muscle (*LC*) and medial to the internal carotid artery (*white arrow*). **B,** A scan through the suprahyoid neck shows level IB (*black arrows*), level IIA (*white arrowheads*), and level IIB (*white arrows*) lymph nodes. Also shown are the submandibular (*SMG*) and sublingual glands (*SLG*), and the geniohyoid muscle (*GH*). **C,** A scan at the level of the hyoid bone shows a level IA node (*large white arrowhead*), level IIA (*small white arrowheads*) and IIB (*short white arrows*) nodes, and a level VA node (*long white arrow*). **D,** A scan of the infrahyoid neck above the level of the cricoid cartilage demonstrates multiple level III lymph nodes (*white arrows*). A level VA node (*white arrowhead*) is also seen. Note that this node would be transected by a line through the back of the sternocleidomastoid muscle; when a lymph node is transected by a line that defines the level, the side of the line on which the bulk of the node lies is the level in which the node should be classified. **E,** A scan below the level of the cricoid cartilage shows level IV nodes (*white arrows*) and a level VB node (*white arrowhead*).

E

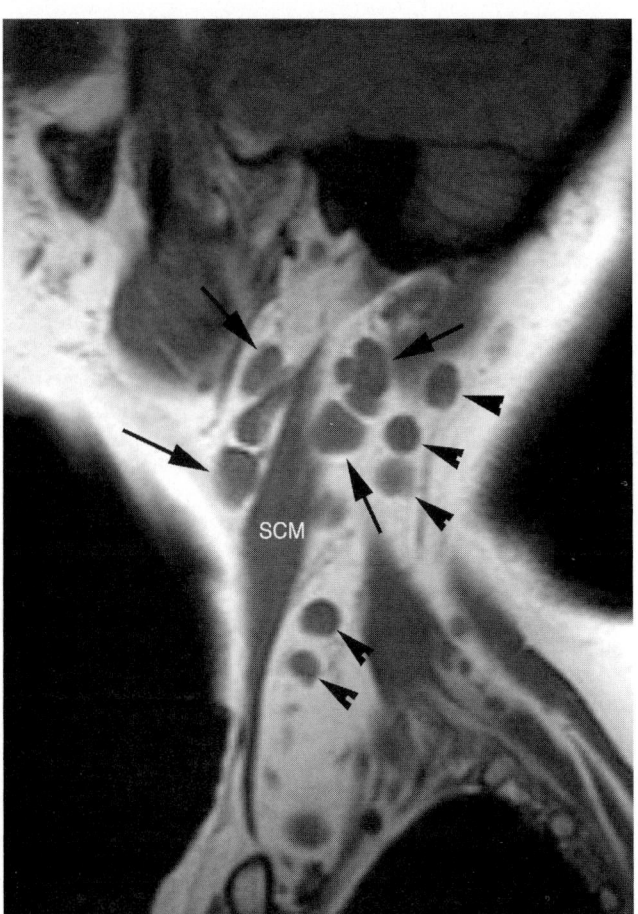

A

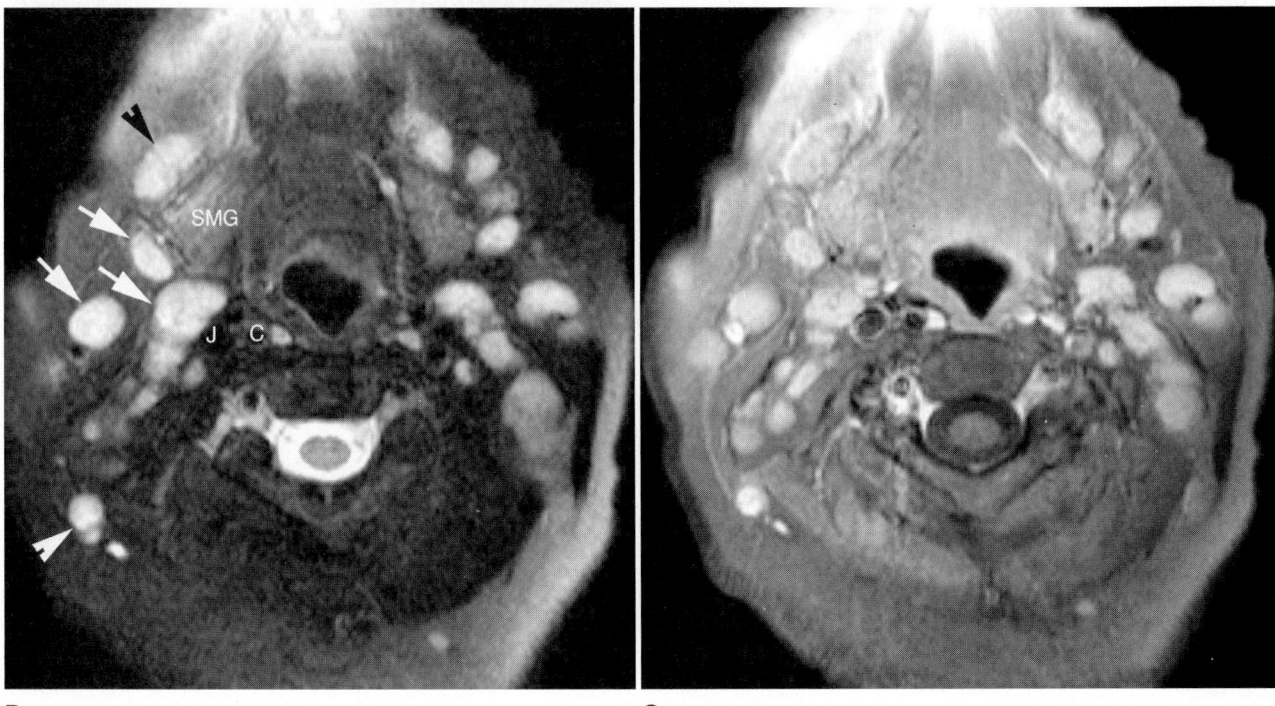

B   C

Figure 16–29. Magnetic resonance images from a patient with multiple reactive lymph nodes. **A,** Sagittal T1-weighted image shows multiple smooth, round or ovoid, homogeneous level II (*black arrows*) and level V (*black arrowheads*) nodes. Note that high-level V nodes can be difficult to distinguish from level IIB nodes, and this often must be assessed in multiple planes. **B,** Fast spin-echo T2-weighted image just above the hyoid bone shows level IB (*black arrowhead*), IIA and B (*white arrows*), and VA (*white arrowhead*) nodes. **C,** Post-gadolinium, the nodes show moderate, homogeneous contrast enhancement.

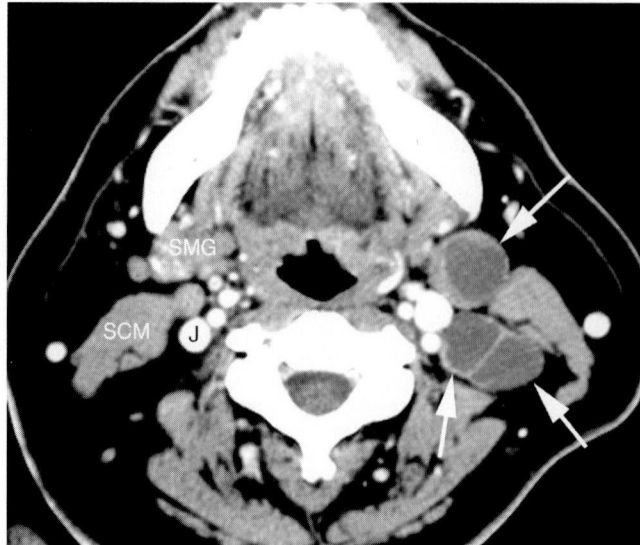

Figure 16–30. Axial contrast-enhanced computed tomography scan of the suprahyoid neck in a patient with metastatic nodal disease (*arrows*) from a tonsil primary. The tumor-involved nodes show extensive necrosis or cystic degeneration or both, as evidenced by central nonenhancement and a thin peripheral rim of enhancing tissue. These nodes are all located in level IIA, as even the more posterior nodes are inseparable from the internal jugular vein.

Lymph Nodes

Assessment of the cervical lymph nodes for metastatic involvement is an important issue in the evaluation of the patient with head and neck cancer. Lymph nodes are seen on all cross-sectional studies of the head and neck. Lymph nodes have historically been described using anatomy-based terminology (e.g., jugulodigastric, spinal accessory), but have more recently been described using nodal "levels" that group nodes on the basis of clinical and pathophysiologic information (Fig. 16-27). These nodal levels have been translated to cross-sectional imaging,[24,25] and this imaging-based classification is summarized in Table 16-1 and illustrated in Figure 16-28. On imaging studies, normal nodes are usually less than 10 mm in short axis diameter. They show intermediate density on CT scans and on MRI show homogeneous intermediate signal intensity on T1-weighted images, mild hyperintensity on T2-weighted images, and homogeneous enhancement post-gadolinium (Fig. 16-29). Metastatic deposits may lead to nodal enlargement, but more importantly to nodal heterogeneity. Areas of cystic degeneration, keratin pools, or frank necrosis result in nodal heterogeneity (notably a focal lack of enhancement on postgadolinium T1-weighted images) that is considered to represent neoplastic involvement in a patient who has head and neck cancer (Fig. 16-30; also as shown in Fig. 16-13*B*). Pathologic nodes may also show extracapsular spread of the tumor, manifest as irregular margination and invasion of adjacent fat or other structures. Of particular interest is extension of nodal disease to involve the carotid artery. The imaging assessment of carotid invasion is difficult. In general a

carotid artery that is contacted by tumor over 270 degrees or more of its circumference is likely invaded, but actual adventitial involvement may need to be assessed intraoperatively.

The particular difficulty in the assessment of nodal involvement by head and neck cancer is the fact that a normal-sized, nonnecrotic node is not necessarily normal since small foci of tumors may not be appreciable by standard CT and MRI methods. Ultrasound-guided fine-needle aspiration (FNA) can improve sensitivity and specificity,[26] but has not found wide acceptance in the United States. FDG PET can offer an additional assessment of nodal involvement, but it is also relatively insensitive to small metastatic foci.[27,28] Furthermore, even a grossly enlarged (but homogeneous) node may be reactive rather than tumor-involved. Choosing a "cut-off" size for calling a node normal or tumor-involved represents a tradeoff between sensitivity and specificity, and leads to probabilities rather than definite answers.[29,30] It is certainly useful to assess the cervical lymph nodes using CT or MRI since clinically occult nodal disease will be detected in some cases, and suspected involvement confirmed in others, but the neck must be managed based on clinical predictors of nodal metastasis that are suggested by the site and size of the primary tumor.[21] Further advances in "functional" nodal imaging using alternative PET tracers, super-paramagnetic iron oxide particles,[31] and sentinel node imaging[32] will likely alter nodal assessment in coming years.

Post-Treatment Imaging

The assessment of the post-therapeutic head and neck cancer patient is complicated by tissue distortion from prior surgery and flap reconstruction,[33] as well as radiation effects on the tissues. These changes may make it difficult to detect recurrent neoplasm or new primary or nodal sites of disease. This difficulty can be somewhat alleviated by obtaining a good baseline scan 6 to 8 weeks following completion of therapy to establish a standard for future comparison (Fig. 16-31). Things to assess on the post-treatment scan include the expected changes based on the patient's therapy, the presence of a new or enlarging mass, perineural spread of disease, denervation changes in muscle, skull base or cavernous sinus involvement or both, and metastatic disease. It is also important to recognize the normal striated appearance of the muscular component of a musculocutaneous flap as compared with the nonstriated and mass-like appearance of recurrent cancer (Fig. 16-32). FDG PET can also be helpful in the assessment of a residual or recurrent tumor, as it is not compromised by tissue distortion.[34,35] FDG PET does, however, suffer from nonspecificity and its inability to conclusively distinguish inflammation from a tumor.

The effects of radiation will be seen on all tissues within the radiation port (Fig. 16-33).[36] Reactive changes within the skin and subcutaneous tissues will be seen, with skin thickening and reticulation of the subcutaneous and deep investing fat. The pharyngeal mucosa shows

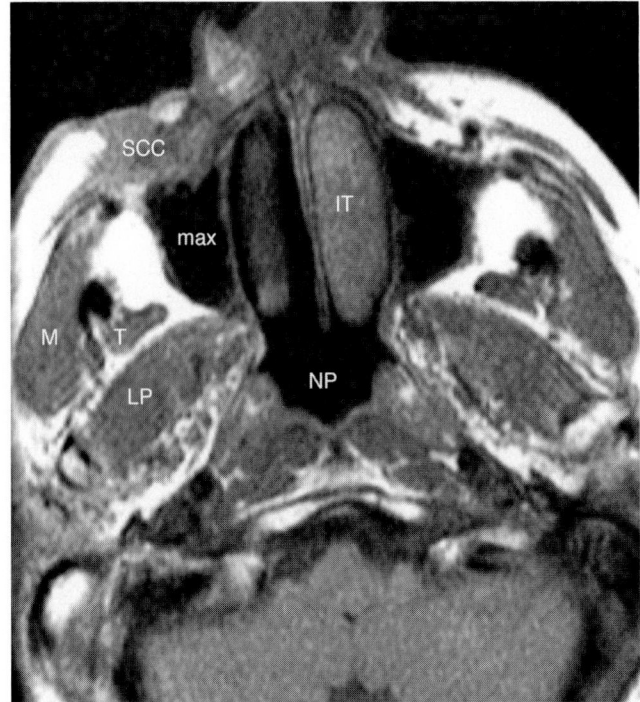

A

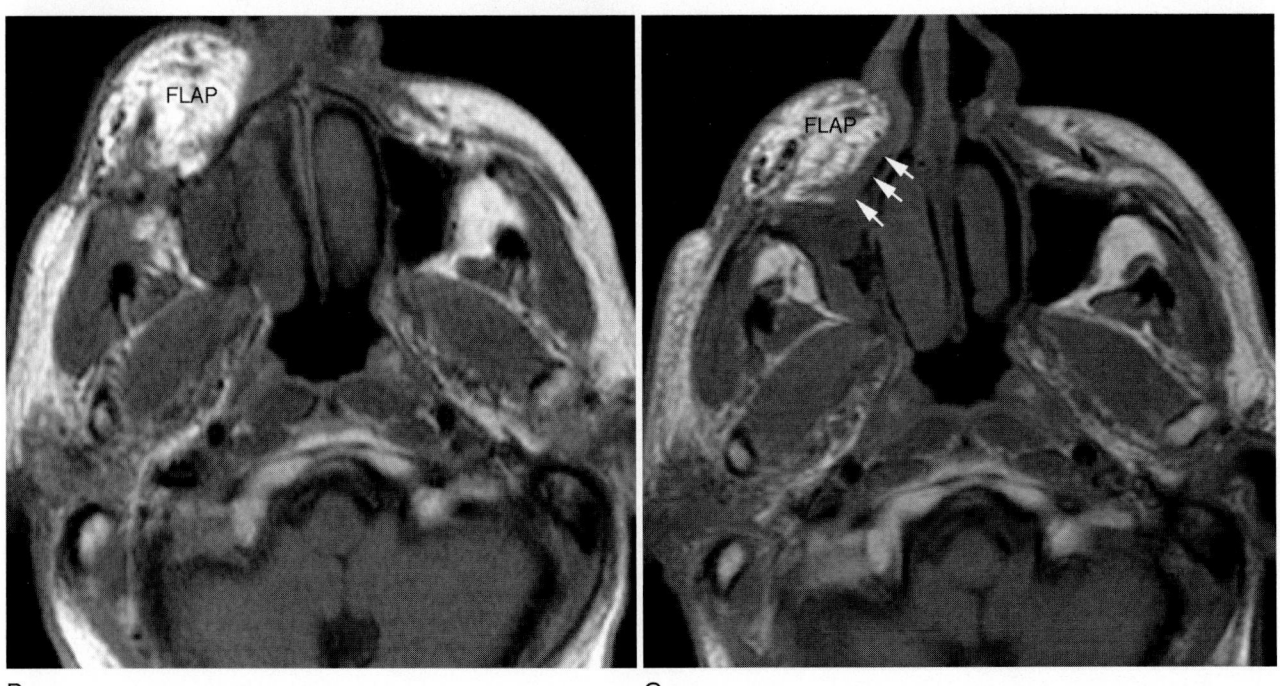

B   C

Figure 16–31. A, Preoperative axial T1-weighted image of a patient with squamous cell carcinoma of the right cheek s/p-status post multiple local dermatological procedures demonstrates a soft tissue mass (*SCC*) that is infiltrating from the skin to the anterior wall of the maxillary sinus (*max*). Also shown are the inferior turbinate (*IT*); nasopharyngeal airway (*NP*); and masseter (*M*), *temporalis* (*T*), and lateral pterygoid (*LP*) muscles. **B,** Baseline axial T1-weighted image following surgical resection, placement of radial forearm free flap, and external beam radiation therapy. **C,** A follow-up scan 3 months later demonstrates new soft tissue along the deep margin of the flap (*arrows*). Clinically the patient was asymptomatic with no new findings on physical examination. A biopsy confirmed recurrent squamous cell carcinoma.

increased enhancement, and there may be pooling of secretions dependently in the pharynx due to decreased motility and difficulty swallowing. The epiglottis and aryepiglottic folds are often dramatically and diffusely thickened. Edema in the retropharyngeal space and carotid sheath may be seen, as well as edema tracking generally along fascial planes. These changes may gradually improve over time, though in some patients they will persist for many years following completion of therapy.

Salivary glands may show increased enhancement compared to normal, and they may gradually atrophy over time. Finally, the marrow of the skull base and cervical spine may show marked fatty infiltration due to conversion of red to yellow marrow.

Radiation may also have more focal effects on tissues that received particularly high doses of radiation, leading to focal areas of tissue necrosis. This can be particularly problematic with regard to bony or cartilaginous

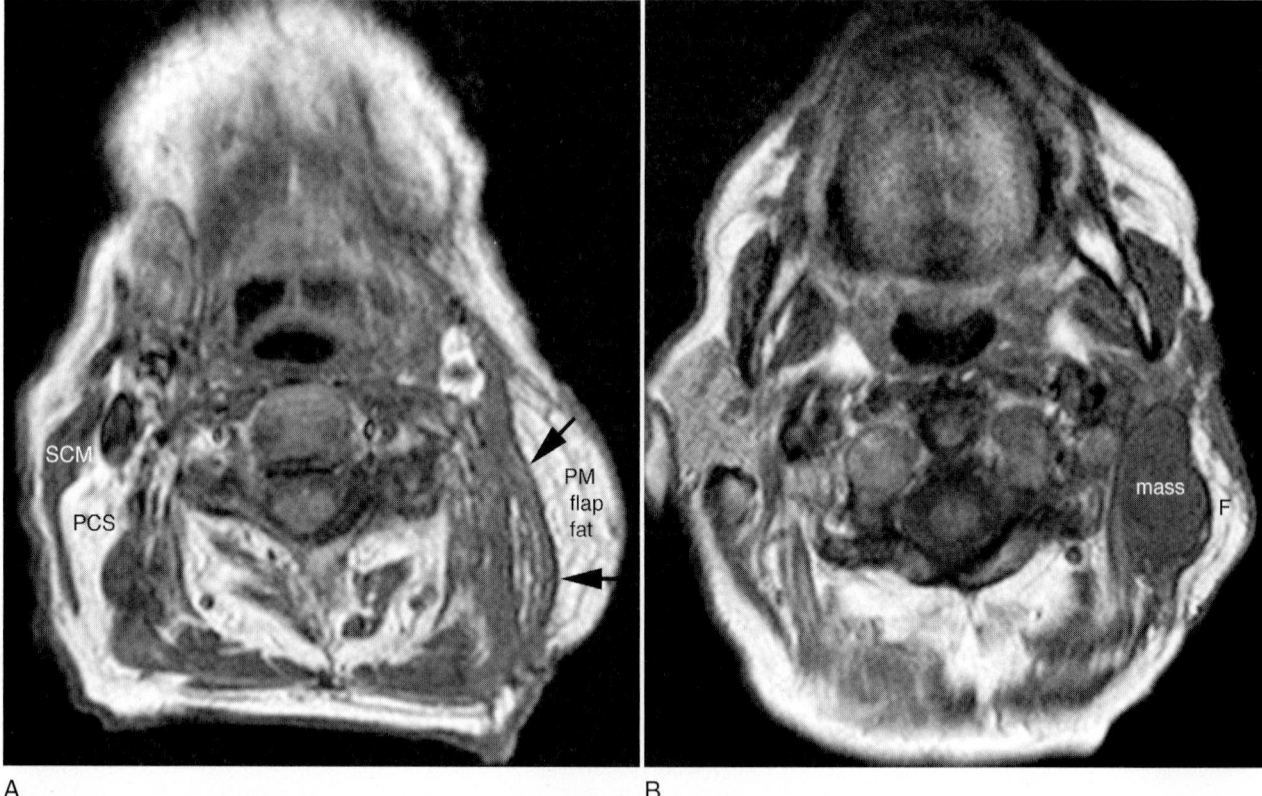

Figure 16–32. A, Axial T1-weighted image of a patient who has undergone left radical neck dissection and reconstruction with a pectoralis major myocutaneous flap. The fatty component of the flap is indicated *(PM flap fat)*, as is the muscular component *(black arrows)*, which demonstrates a striated architecture. Indicated on the contralateral side are the sternocleidomastoid muscle *(SCM)* and the fat-filled posterior cervical space *(PCS)*. **B,** More superiorly, at the top of the flap *(F)*, a more homogeneous, rounded area of soft tissue signal intensity is present. This represents a recurrent tumor and should not be confused with the muscular component of the flap.

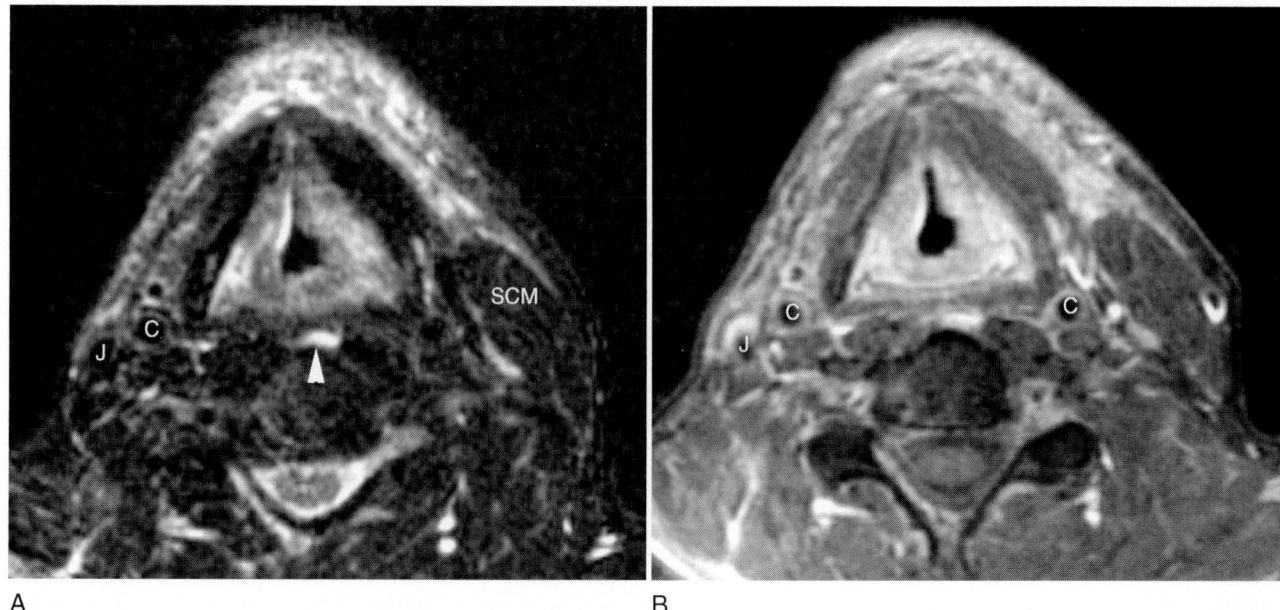

Figure 16–33. A, Axial fast spin-echo T2-weighted image with fat saturation in a patient who has undergone right modified radical neck dissection and external beam radiation therapy for metastatic squamous cell carcinoma. Generalized edema of the skin and subcutaneous fat is seen, as is diffuse thickening of the glottic soft tissues and retropharyngeal edema *(arrowhead)*. **B,** A post-gadolinium T1-weighted image with fat saturation in the same patient demonstrates diffuse gadolinium enhancement of the superficial soft tissues of the neck and the glottis.

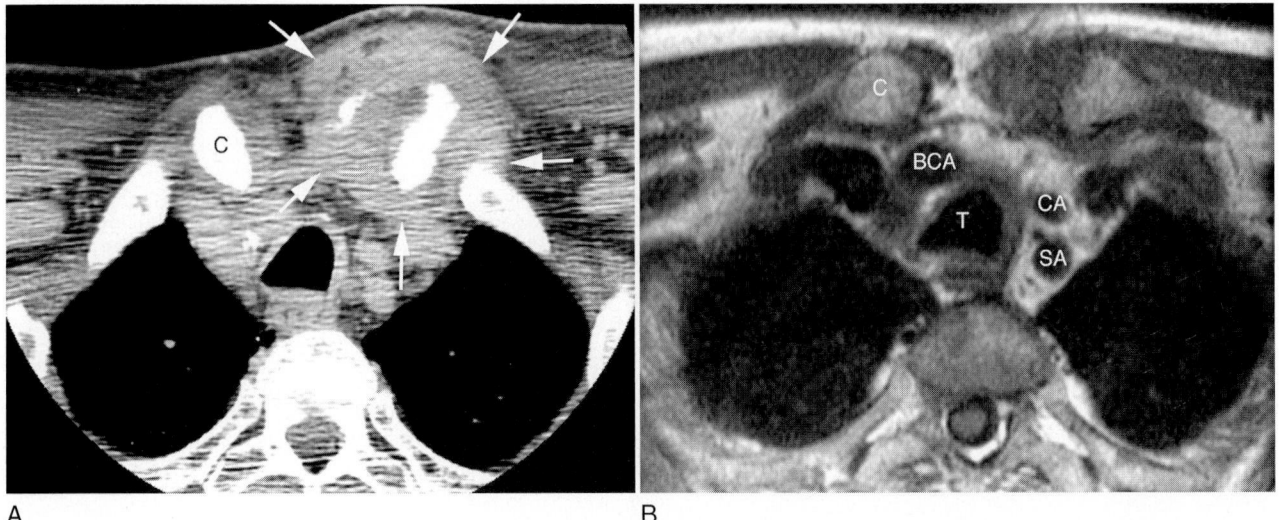

Figure 16–34. A, A computed tomography scan of the neck in a patient with a history of prior surgery and radiation for laryngeal cancer demonstrates a large mass (*arrows*) around the left clavicular head. The normal right clavicular head (*C*) is shown for comparison. Multiple fine-needle aspirations demonstrated only reactive cells, and the patient was treated with a long course of antibiotics for presumed osteoradionecrosis of the clavicle. **B,** A follow-up T1-weighted magnetic resonance image 6 months later shows near-complete regression of the soft tissue mass. Shown are the clavicular head (*C*), trachea (*T*), brachiocephalic artery (*BCA*), left common carotid artery (*CA*), and subclavian artery (*SA*).

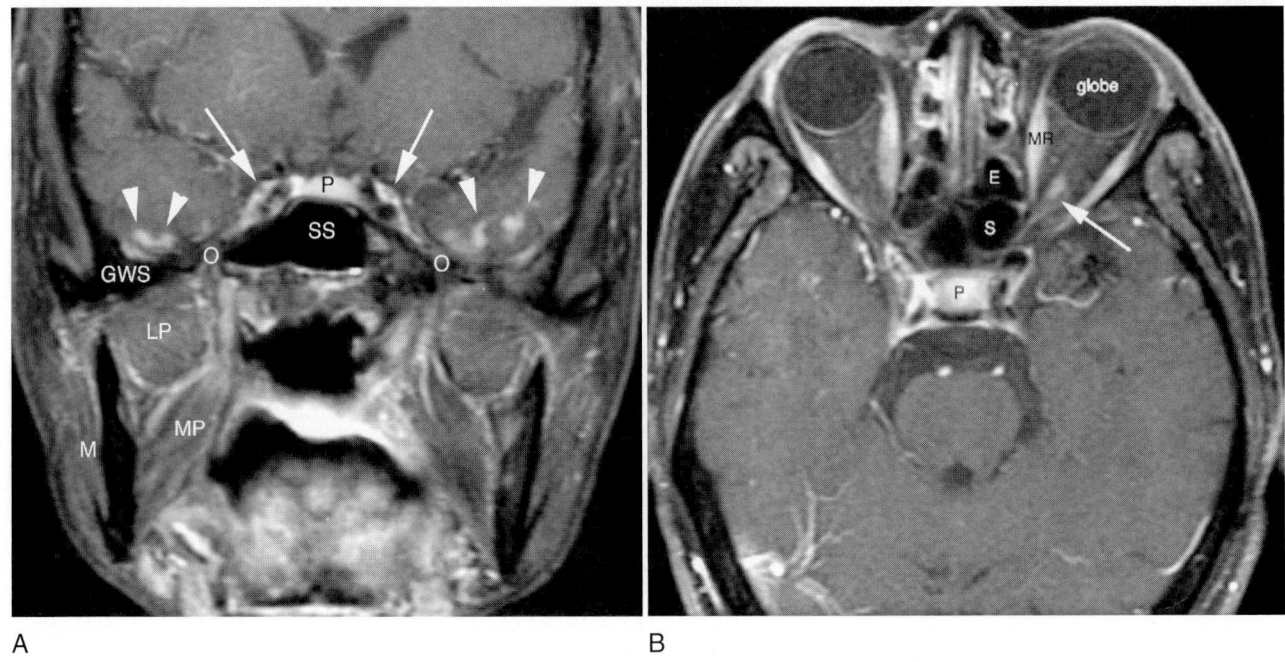

Figure 16–35. A, Coronal postgadolinium T1-weighted image with fat saturation in a patient who has undergone prior high-dose radiation therapy for nasopharyngeal carcinoma. Areas of irregular enhancement in the inferior temporal lobes bilaterally (*arrowheads*) are consistent with radiation necrosis. Also shown are the cavernous sinuses (*white arrows*); pituitary gland (*P*); sphenoid sinus (*SS*); foramen ovale (*O*); and the lateral pterygoid (*LP*), medial pterygoid (*MP*), and masseter (*M*) muscles. The greater wing of the sphernoid bone (*GWS*), which forms the floor of the middle cranial fossa is also indicated. **B,** Axial postgadolinium T1-weighted image with fat saturation in the same patient, who complained of visual loss in his left eye. Abnormal enhancement of the left optic nerve is seen (*white arrow*), presumably due to radiation-induced optic neuritis. Also shown are the ocular globe, medial rectus muscle (*MR*), ethmoid (*E*) and sphenoid (*S*) sinuses, and pituitary gland (*P*).

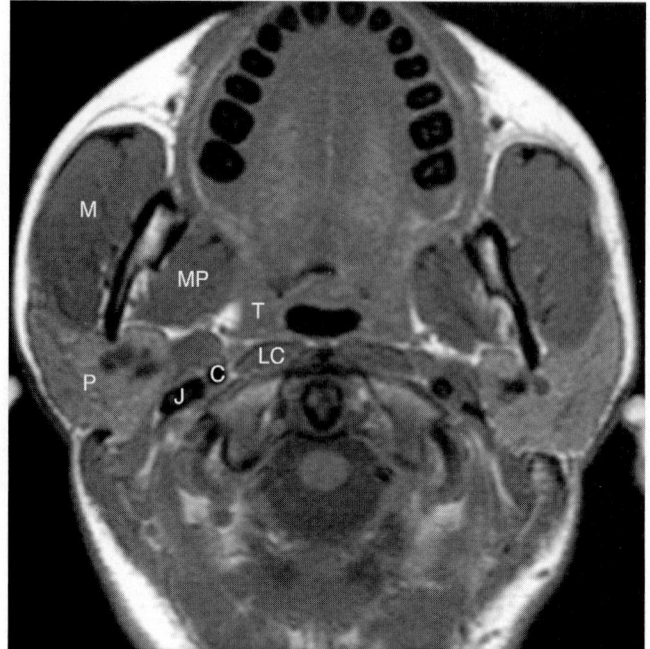

A

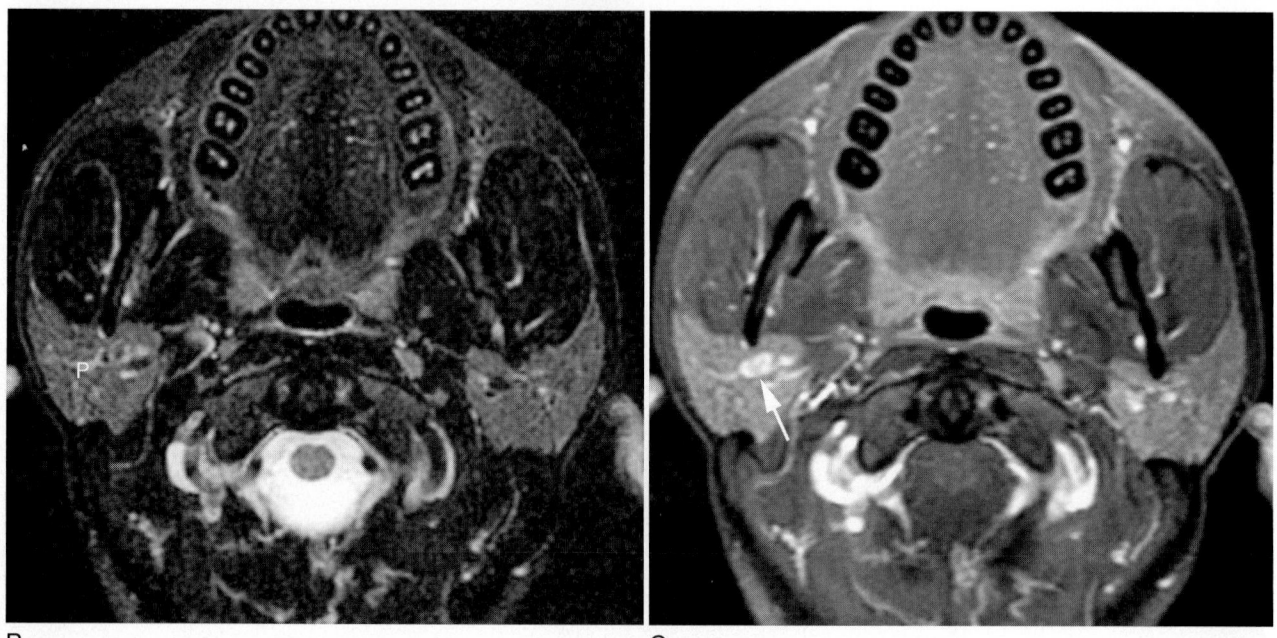

B   C

Figure 16–36. Magnetic resonance appearance of the normal parotid gland. **A,** Axial T1-weighted image shows the normal parotid gland (*P*), with signal intensity greater than muscle but less than fat. No visible plane separates the superficial from the deep lobe, and the facial nerve cannot be identified as it traverses the gland. Also shown are the masseter (*M*) and medial pterygoid (*MP*) muscles, tonsil (*T*), longus colli (*LC*) muscle, internal carotid artery (*C*), and internal jugular vein (*J*). **B,** Axial fast spin-echo T2-weighted image with fat saturation shows the parotid gland (*P*) is mildly hyperintense compared with muscle. **C,** Post-gadolinium, the gland demonstrates mild homogeneous enhancement. The retromandibular vein (*arrow*) is seen within the gland.

structures and may lead to osteoradionecrosis (Fig. 16-34) or chondronecrosis. This is particularly problematic in the larynx and also at the skull base, notably in the patient who has undergone high-dose radiation therapy for the treatment of nasopharyngeal carcinoma. Patients treated with high-dose radiation for nasopharyngeal carcinoma may develop necrosis of the temporal lobes and also radiation-induced optic neuropathy or other cranial neuropathies (Fig. 16-35). These complications should be reduced with the use of more conformal methods of treatment.

Salivary Glands

The major salivary glands include the paired parotid, submandibular, and sublingual glands.[37] The bulk of the parotid gland lies posterior to the masseter muscle, below and anterior to the external auditory canal and mastoid tip. The remainder of the gland extends medially through the stylomandibular notch. The division of the gland into "superficial" and "deep" lobes is artificial in that there is no anatomical cleavage plane between them, but the plane of the facial nerve is used as

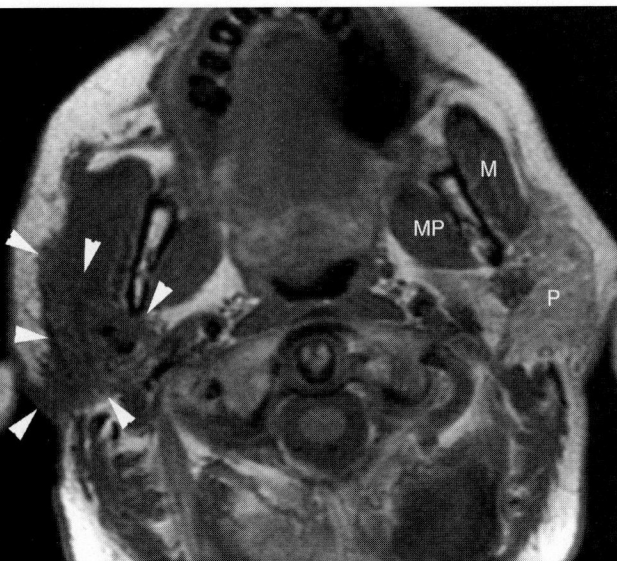

Figure 16–37. An axial T1-weighted image in an elderly male demonstrates diffuse infiltration of the right parotid gland with abnormal soft tissue (*arrows*) that extends to the skin surface and is poorly marginated from the right masseter muscle. Surgical resection confirmed high-grade salivary duct carcinoma that was found to infiltrate the skin, subdermal lymphatics, and masseter muscle. Also shown for comparison is the normal left parotid gland (*P*), as well as the masseter (*M*) and medial pterygoid (*MP*) muscles.

parotid gland has a high adipose content and is relatively bright on a T1-weighted image, while it is relatively low-signal intensity on T2-weighted images and shows mild homogeneous enhancement postgadolinium (Fig. 16-36). Tumors of the parotid gland are particularly well seen on T1-weighted images as the normal fatty parenchyma is replaced by infiltrative or mass-like soft tissue (Fig. 16-37). Low-grade malignancies have imaging characteristics identical to benign salivary tumors, and tissue sampling is needed to make the distinction. Higher-grade neoplasms often have irregular, infiltrative margins. In addition, parotid malignancies may extend centrally along the facial nerve, and the facial nerve needs to be carefully assessed in patients with parotid malignancy (Fig. 16-38).

The submandibular gland lies in the submandibular space, below the plane of the mylohyoid muscle but wrapping around its dorsal free edge. It does not have a significant adipose component and is therefore of intermediate soft-tissue signal intensity on MRI rather than having a fatty signal intensity like the parotid gland. Submandibular gland malignancies may appear relatively well circumscribed (Fig. 16-39) or may have infiltrative margins. Neoplasms of the floor of the mouth may obstruct the submandibular duct (Wharton's duct) and lead to ductal dilatation or glandular inflammation or both (Fig. 16-40).

The sublingual gland lies in the floor of the mouth, in the sublingual space, just superior to the mylohyoid muscle. The gland is usually intermediate in signal intensity on T1-weighted images and moderately bright on T2-weighted images. On CT, the normal sublingual space is relatively hypodense due to the fluid content of the gland and ducts and the normal fat that is present in the sublingual space. The sublingual space is frequently involved by inferior extension of tongue and

an internal reference. The facial nerve cannot be directly visualized within the parotid gland or routine imaging studies. Normal structures that can be seen within the parotid gland include the retromandibular vein and as many as three to five normal lymph nodes. The adult

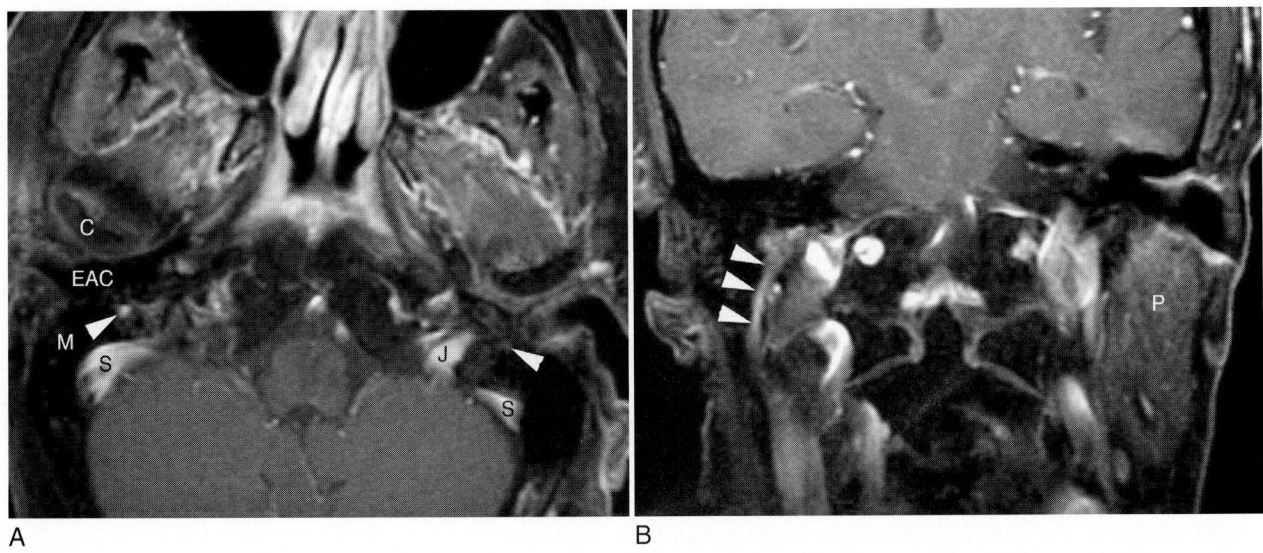

Figure 16–38. A patient with a history of prior right parotidectomy for carcinoma ex pleomorphic adenoma presents with a new facial nerve palsy. **A,** Axial post-gadolinium T1-weighted image with fat saturation shows asymmetrical enlargement and enhancement of the right descending mastoid segment of the facial nerve (*white arrowhead*) as compared with the left. Also shown are the external auditory canal (*EAC*), mandibular condyle (*C*), mastoid air cells (*M*), sigmoid sinus (*S*), and internal jugular vein (*J*). **B,** Coronal post-gadolinium T1-weighted image with fat saturation shows absence of the right parotid gland (the left gland is indicated, *P*) and diffuse enlargement and enhancement of the descending mastoid segment of the right facial nerve (*arrowheads*). Perineural spread of the tumor was confirmed surgically.

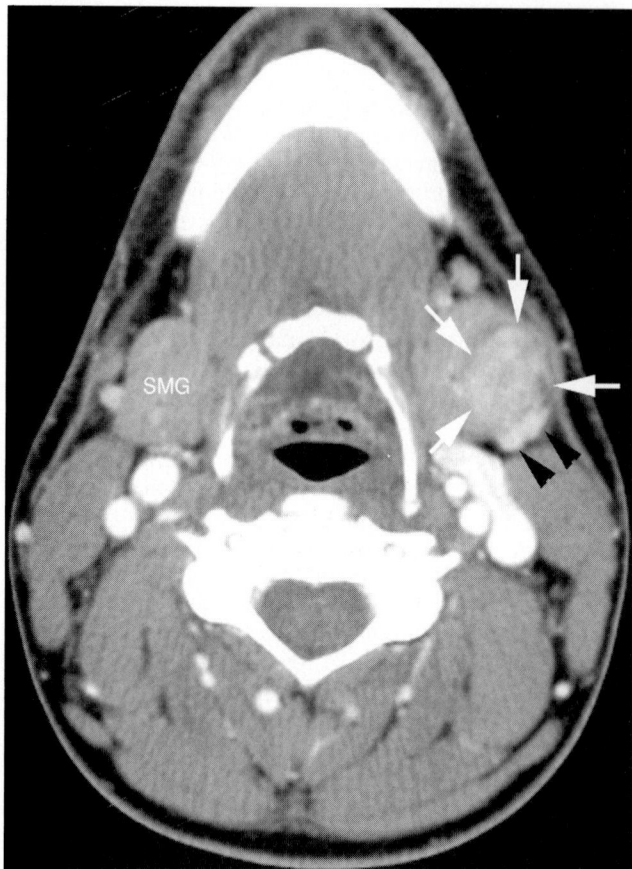

Figure 16–39. Axial contrast-enhanced computed tomography scan in a 36-year-old man presenting with a mass in the submandibular region demonstrates a fairly well-circumscribed mildly enhancing mass (*white arrows*) in the left submandibular gland. The facial vein (*black arrowheads*) is displaced posteriorly. Fine-needle aspiration demonstrated a low-grade mucoepidermoid carcinoma. Also indicated is the contralateral normal submandibular gland (*SMG*).

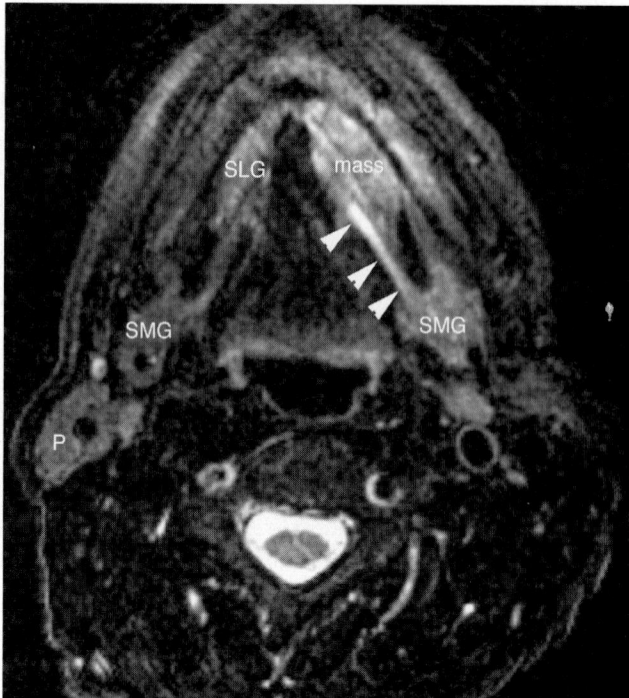

Figure 16–40. Axial fast spin-echo T2-weighted image with fat saturation in a patient with squamous cell carcinoma of the left floor of mouth (*mass*). The mass caused obstruction and dilation of the submandibular duct (*arrowheads*). The left submandibular gland (*SMG*) appears mildly hyperintense compared with the right, presumably due to obstruction and inflammation. The right sublingual gland (*SLG*) and parotid gland (*P*) are also shown.

floor-of-mouth SCCs, or by minor salivary gland tumors, a situation which is usually well assessed with coronal plane MRI or CT imaging (Fig. 16-41).

Nasal Cavity/Paranasal Sinuses

The nasal cavity and paranasal sinuses are connected by multiple ostia. A mass lesion may obstruct drainage from one of the sinuses, and a patient will present with (often unilateral) sinusitis. As many patients with sinonasal symptoms undergo limited coronal CT screening, it is important to review these films with an eye to detecting an underlying mass lesion or areas of aggressive bone destruction or soft tissue infiltration in order not to overlook a more significant pathology than just inflammatory mucosal disease. In addition, the nasal cavity and paranasal sinuses are intimately related to important adjacent structures (orbit, cribriform plate, pterygopalatine fossa, sella turcica, clivus), and these areas need to be carefully assessed for tumor extension in a patient with a sinonasal malignancy. Once a tumor has accessed the

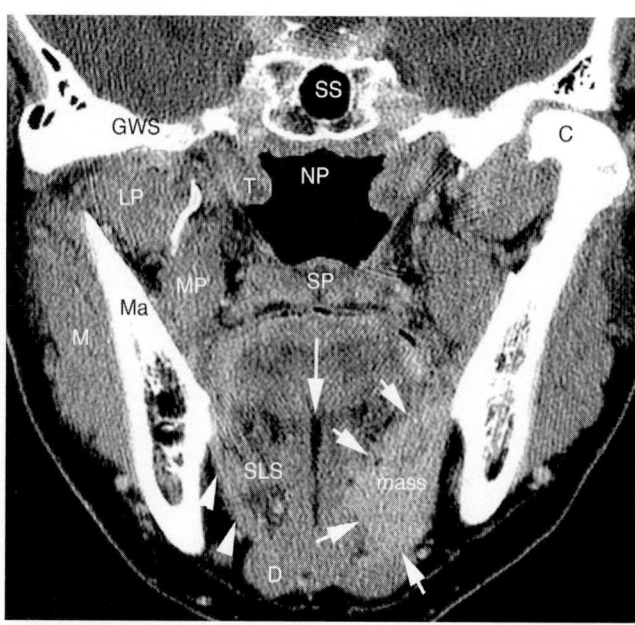

Figure 16–41. Coronal contrast-enhanced computed tomography scan in a patient with adenoid cystic carcinoma of the left sublingual gland (*mass, short white arrows*). The normal mixed fat density right sublingual space is shown (*SLS*), as is the mylohyoid muscle (*white arrowheads*). The midline fatty lingual septum is also indicated (*long white arrow*). The scan also demonstrates the mandibular ramus (*Ma*), greater wing of the sphenoid (*GWS*), mandibular condyle (*C*), and sphenoid sinus (*SS*). The nasopharyngeal airway (*NP*), torus tubarius (*T*), and soft palate (*SP*) are shown, as are the masseter (*M*), medial pterygoid (*MP*), and lateral pterygoid (*LP*) muscles.

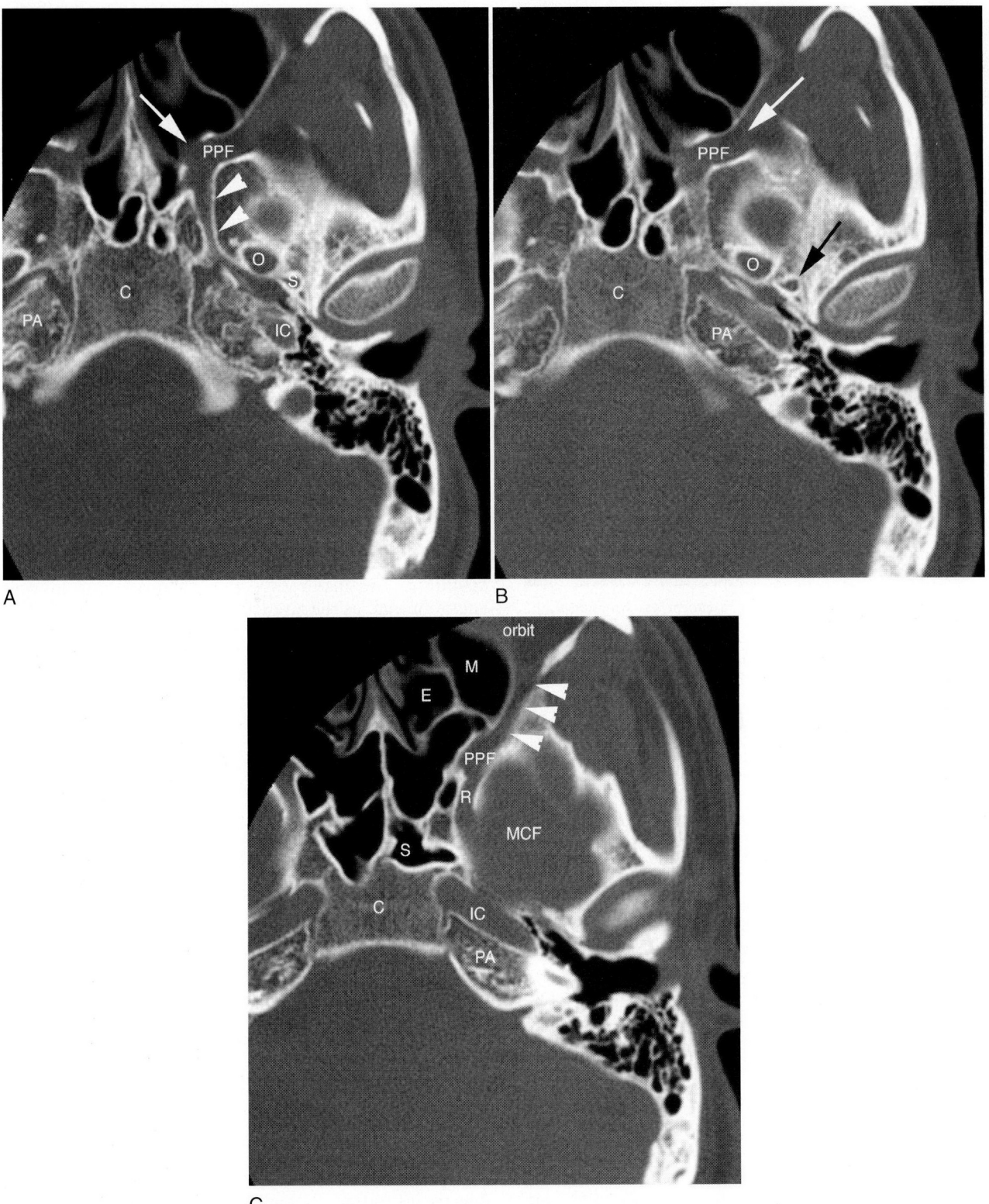

Figure 16–42. Axial computed tomography images in bone window from inferior to superior illustrate the anatomy and interconnections of the *pterygopalatine fossa*. **A,** A relatively inferior image shows the *pterygopalatine fossa* (PPF), which connects medially with the nasal cavity via the sphenopalatine foramen (*white arrow*) and posteriorly with the *foramen lacerum* via the vidian canal (*double white arrowheads*). Also shown are the *foramen ovale* (O, which transmits V3, the third division of the trigeminal nerve), *foramen spinosum* (S, which transmits the middle meningeal artery), the carotid canal (IC), the *clivus* (C), and the petrous apex (PA). **B,** A slightly more superior section also demonstrates the lateral communication of the PPF with the infratemporal fossa (*parapharyngeal and masticator spaces*) via the pterygomaxillary fissue (*white arrow*). *Foramen spinosum* is indicated here by the black arrow. **C,** A more superior section shows an additional posterior communication of the PPF, which connects to the middle cranial fossa (MCF) via foramen rotundum (R), which transmits V2, the second division of the trigeminal nerve. At this level the PPF connects to the orbit anteriorly via the inferior orbital fissure (*arrowheads*). Also shown are the sphenoid (S), ethmoid (E), and maxillary sinuses (M).

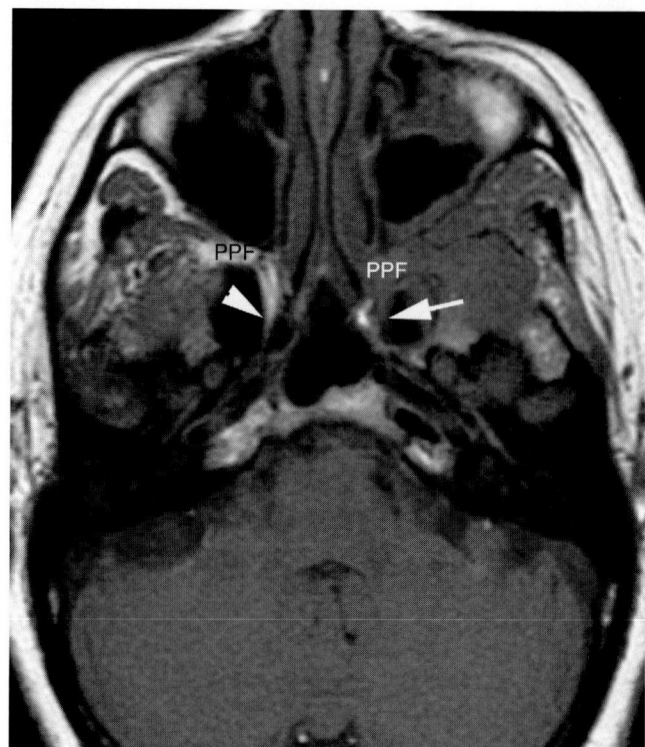

Figure 16–43. Axial T1-weighted image in a patient with lymphoma shows normal fat in the right pterygopalatine fossa (*PPF, black letters*) and some fat in the right vidian canal (*white arrowhead*). On the left, the PPF is expanded and the fat is infiltrated with abnormal soft tissue, which also extends posteriorly in the vidian canal (*white arrow*) and laterally into the infratemporal fossa.

pterygopalatine fossa, it can spread throughout the head and neck, as well as intracranially, due to the multiple interconnections of this space (Fig. 16-42). Because the normal pterygopalatine fossa contains only fat and a few small neural and vascular structures, pregadolinium T1-weighted images should be carefully scrutinized for replacement of the normal high-signal intensity fat by abnormal intermediate-signal intensity soft tissue (Fig. 16-43). The retroantral fat should also be scrutinized in a patient with a maxillary sinus malignancy, as should the nasal septum and hard palate in a patient with a nasal cavity malignancy.

MRI and CT imaging are often complementary in the assessment of the patient with a sinonasal malignancy, though MRI generally yields more information.[38,39] CT is useful for assessing bone erosion and for certain aspects of surgical planning, but MRI provides far more detailed information about the extent of the tumor. Of note, on CT it is often difficult to separate the soft-tissue density of a tumor from the opacification of adjacent sinuses due to obstruction with resultant mucosal inflammation and accumulation of secretions. MRI facilitates the distinction of tumor versus mucosal edema and secretions. On T1-weighted images, edematous mucosa and trapped secretions may be isointense to the tumor or may show areas of intrinsic T1 shortening (high signal)

related to inspissation and elevated protein content (Fig. 16-44*A*). On T2-weighted images, sinonasal neoplasms are usually of intermediate signal intensity. Edematous mucosa, on the other hand, typically has very high signal intensity, and trapped secretions may be very bright if relatively fluid or very dark if very desiccated and inspissated (Fig. 16-44*B*). Post-gadolinium, sinonasal tumors typically show moderate homogeneous enhancement, while inflamed and edematous mucosa shows marked enhancement and trapped secretions show no enhancement. A coronal fast spin echo (FSE) T2-weighted image is often particularly helpful in distinguishing a tumor from adjacent mucosal disease (Fig. 16-45).

The sinonasal cavities are commonly involved by SCC, lymphoma, and minor salivary gland tumors. Any of these lesions may cause aggressive bone destruction and infiltration and invasion of adjacent soft tissue structures, making a preoperative specific diagnosis impossible by imaging alone. In addition, esthesioneuroblastoma is an important consideration for tumors that arise high in the nasal vault, while mucosal melanomas are also seen with some frequency. The preoperative distinction among these lesions is generally not possible with imaging alone, and tissue sampling is required for definitive diagnosis. The major exception to this is the juvenile angiofibroma, as the large and numerous flow voids in a nasal cavity lesion in an adolescent male are pathognomonic for this diagnosis (Fig. 16-46). Certain other imaging features can occasionally be helpful in the preoperative differential diagnosis, as mucosal melanomas may show areas of increased signal intensity on pregadolinium T1-weighted images due to hemorrhage or melanin content or both (Fig. 16-47),[40] while esthesioneuroblastoma may demonstrate peripheral intracranial cysts (Fig. 16-48).[41]

Thyroid Gland

NORMAL ANATOMY

The thyroid gland lies within the visceral space of the infrahyoid neck, wrapping around the upper trachea. It usually consists of a right and a left lobe, connected across the midline by the thyroid isthmus. In at least 50% of patients, a pyramidal lobe may be seen extending superiorly from the isthmus along the course of the thyroglossal duct in the neck. The thyroid gland is highly vascular and is divided by multiple fibrous *septae*.

The normal thyroid gland is intrinsically dense on CT due to its iodine content and enhances intensely and homogeneously following administration of iodinated contrast (Fig. 16-49). In a patient suspected of having or known to have thyroid carcinoma, administration of iodinated contrast should be avoided if the patient is to undergo radioiodine imaging or therapy, since the iodine from the contrast material will saturate the gland. These patients are usually best assessed by MRI, which provides exquisite detail of the extent of disease while avoiding the administration of an iodine-based contrast

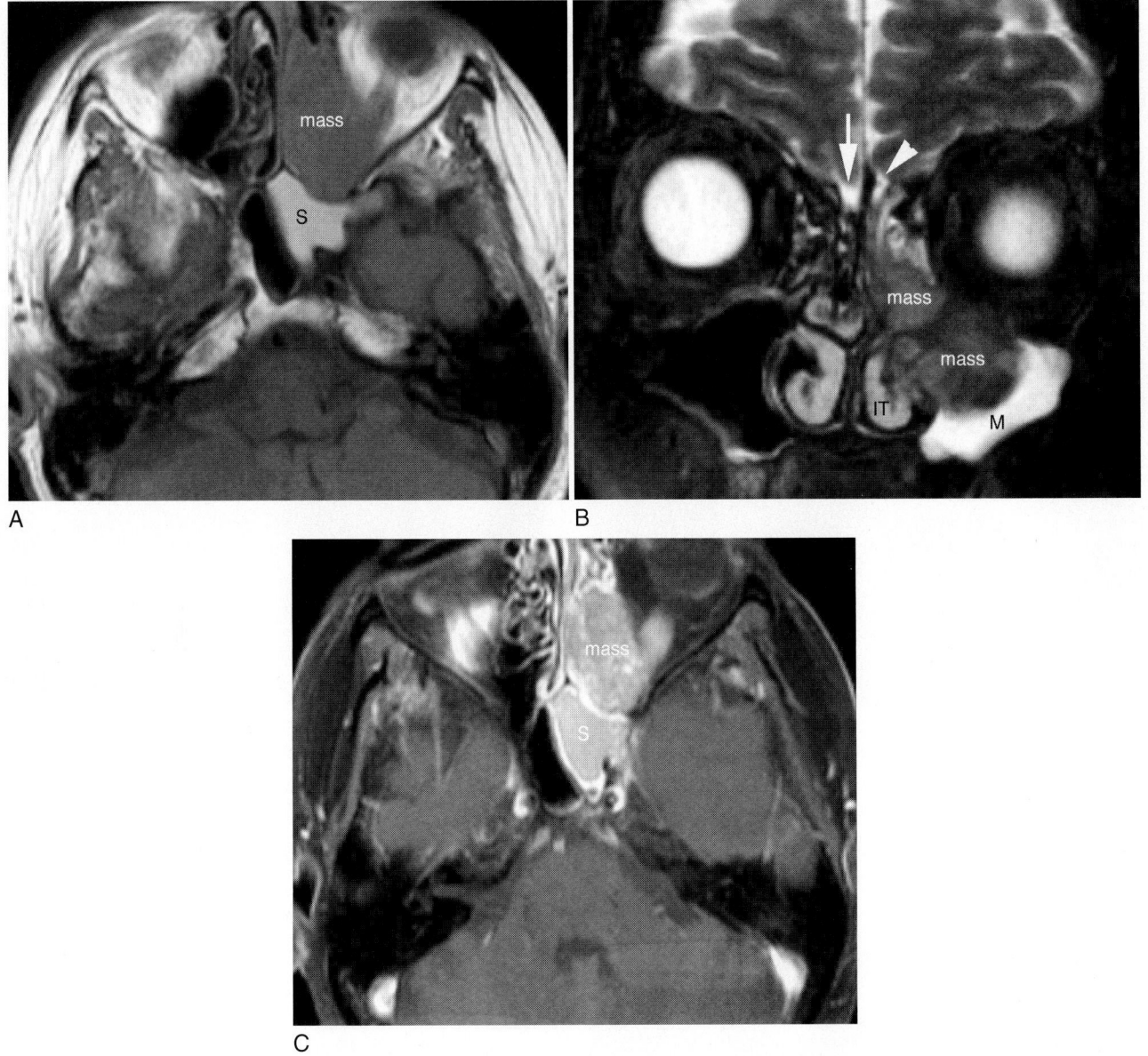

Figure 16–44. Images from a patient with squamous cell carcinoma of the left ethmoid sinus and nasal cavity. **A,** Axial T1-weighted image shows the tumor (*mass*) is intermediate-signal intensity. Trapped secretions within the left sphenoid sinus (*S*) are bright due to inspissation and elevated protein content. **B,** Coronal fast spin-echo T2-weighted image shows the tumor is of intermediate signal intensity (*mass*) and easily distinguished from inflammatory mucosal edema and secretions in the obstructed left maxillary sinus (*M*). The tumor involves the inferior turbinate (*IT*). With tumors of the ethmoid sinus or upper nasal cavity, the cribriform plate with tumors of the ethmoid roof must be closely scrutinized for any evidence of intracranial extension. The cerebrospinal fluid (CSF) space below the right gyrus rectus and above the right cribriform plate (*white arrow*) is larger than the CSF space on the left (*white arrowhead*), suggesting possible skull base transgression by tumor and attenuation of the subarachnoid space because of extradural or dural involvement by tumor. **C,** On a post-gadolinium T1-weighted image with fat saturation, the tumor is seen to enhance with moderate intensity and homogeneity. The material in the sphenoid is somewhat more difficult to distinguish from a tumor, demonstrating the use of pregadolinium T1-weighted imaging when dealing with lesions of the paranasal sinuses, and of the the head and neck in general.

agent. On MRI, the normal thyroid gland is of homogeneous intermediate signal intensity on T1- and T2-weighted images and shows intense and homogeneous enhancement post-gadolinium.[42]

PATHOLOGY

Unlike other tumors of the head and neck, which are primarily assessed by CT and MRI, thyroid pathology is often initially addressed by ultrasound (US) and nuclear medicine studies using radiolabeled iodine. Cross-sectional imaging with CT or MRI is used secondarily to evaluate the deep tissue extent of a mass that is to be surgically removed, or for the assessment of nodal metastases or chest disease. In many cases a thyroid lesion is picked up incidentally on a cross-sectional imaging study ordered for another purpose, but most of these lesions prove to be colloid cysts or adenomas rather than thyroid malignancies.

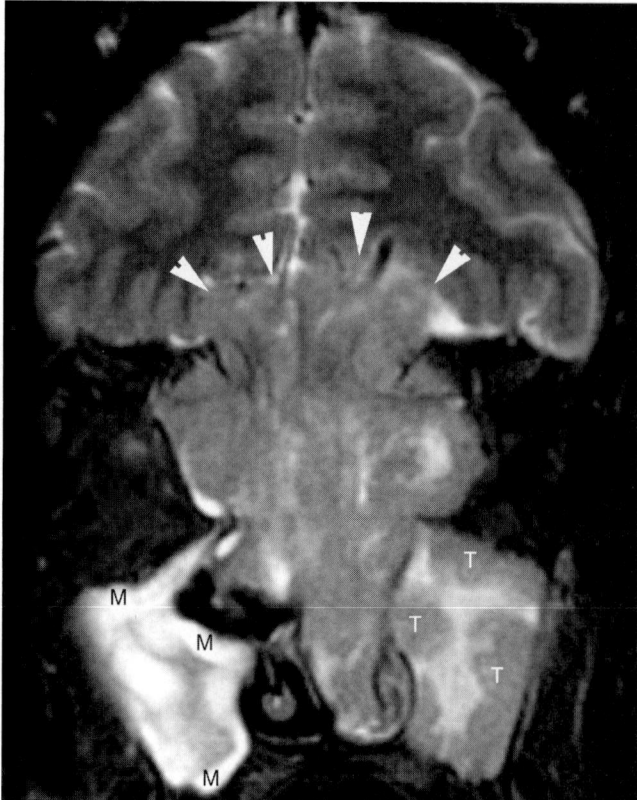

Figure 16–45. Coronal fast spin-echo T2-weighted image with fat saturation in a young man with a sinonasal undifferentiated carcinoma (SNUC). A large mass fills the nasal cavity and ethmoid sinuses, extends into the orbits bilaterally, and also has a large intracranial component (*arrowheads*). In addition, the tumor can be seen spreading submucosally in the left maxillary (*T*), as distinct from high-signal intensity secretions located more centrally in the left maxillary sinus. By comparison, the left maxillary sinus shows edematous mucosa (*M*), with heterogeneous trapped secretions more centrally.

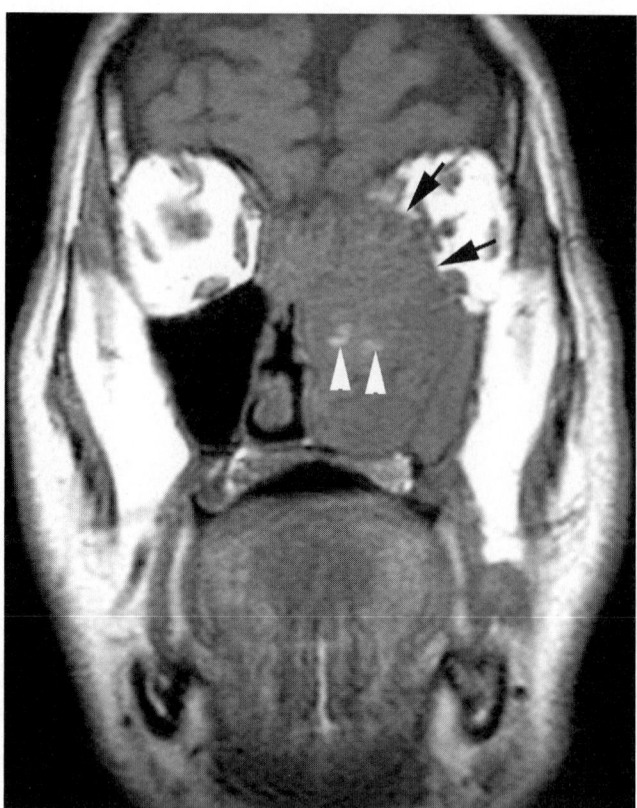

Figure 16–47. Coronal T1-weighted image in an elderly male with unilateral nasal obstruction and epistaxis demonstrates a large, intermediate-signal intensity mass filling the left nasal cavity and left ethmoid sinus, as well as extending into the left maxillary sinus and anterior cranial fossa. There is also extension into the left orbit (*black arrows*). Small foci of intrinsic high-signal intensity are present (*white arrowheads*), consistent with foci of hemorrhage or melanin or both in this patient with melanotic sinonasal melanoma.

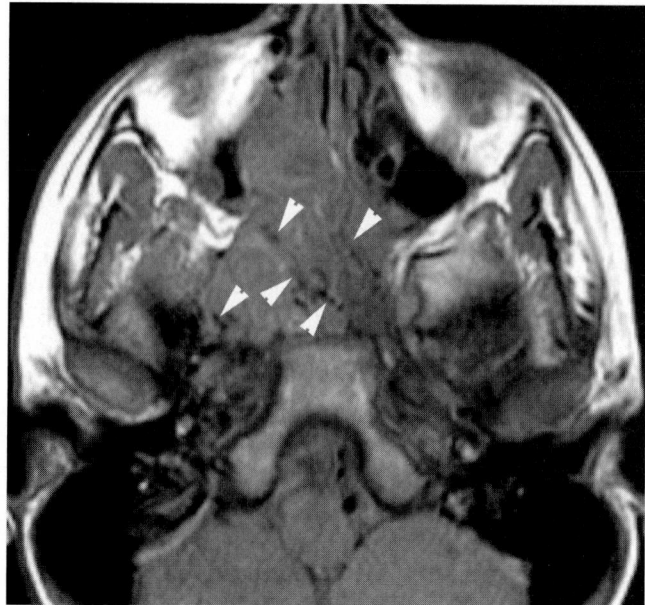

Figure 16–46. Axial T1-weighted image in a teenage male presenting with nasal obstruction and epistaxis demonstrates a large mass extensively involving the sinonasal cavity and remodeling the right skull base. Multiple areas of intralesional serpiginous hypointensity (*arrowheads*) are consistent with flow voids and in this clinical setting are diagnostic of juvenile angiofibroma.

A thyroid malignancy may simulate a benign process on cross-sectional imaging, and tissue sampling is usually necessary for definitive diagnosis. Both papillary and follicular carcinomas of the thyroid may present as well-circumscribed lesions that have variable enhancement characteristics on CT or MRI. Cyst formation may result in well-circumscribed areas of fluid density or intensity, and calcifications may be seen as well. On US, neoplasms are typically hypoechoic, and on radioiodine studies they are seen as cold nodules. If a lesion is allowed to grow unchecked, invasion into adjacent structures will be seen, and possibly airway compromise (Fig. 16-50). In addition, cervical nodal metastatic disease may be evident. On MRI, the presence of intrinsic T1 shortening in lymph nodes is highly suspicious for metastatic thyroid cancer (Fig. 16-51) due to either the thyroglobulin content or the propensity of these nodes to undergo hemorrhage. On CT, nodes involved with metastatic thyroid cancer may appear cystic.

More aggressive thyroid cancers, notably anaplastic thyroid cancer, have a high propensity to invade adjacent structures early in their course. Encasement of the carotid arteries, airway invasion, and vertebral column invasion are common, as are nodal and distant metastases.

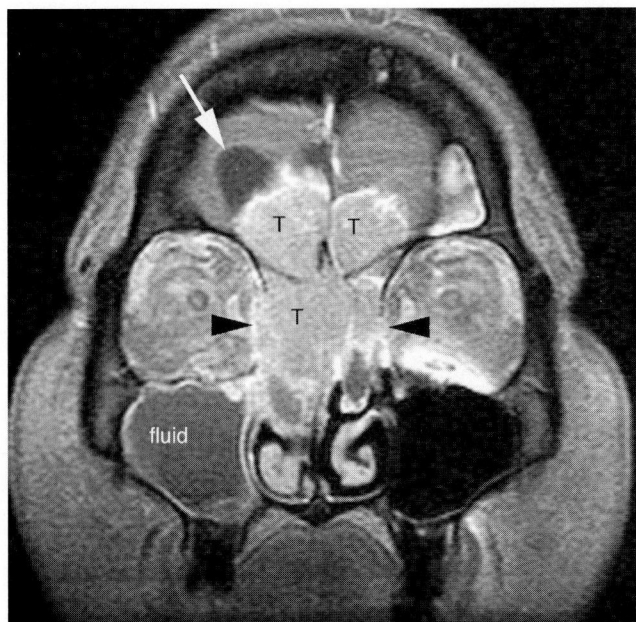

Figure 16–48. Coronal post-gadolinium T1-weighted image with fat saturation in a 45-year-old woman with headache and epistaxis demonstrates a large tumor (*T*) centered in the upper nasal vault, but with extension into both orbits (*black arrowheads*) and significant intracranial extension. A peripheral intracranial cyst is present (*white arrow*), and these cysts have been noted in association with esthesioneuroblastoma, which was the pathologically confirmed diagnosis in this case. The tumor obstructs the *ostium* of the right maxillary sinus and has resulted in fluid accumulation (fluid) in the sinus.

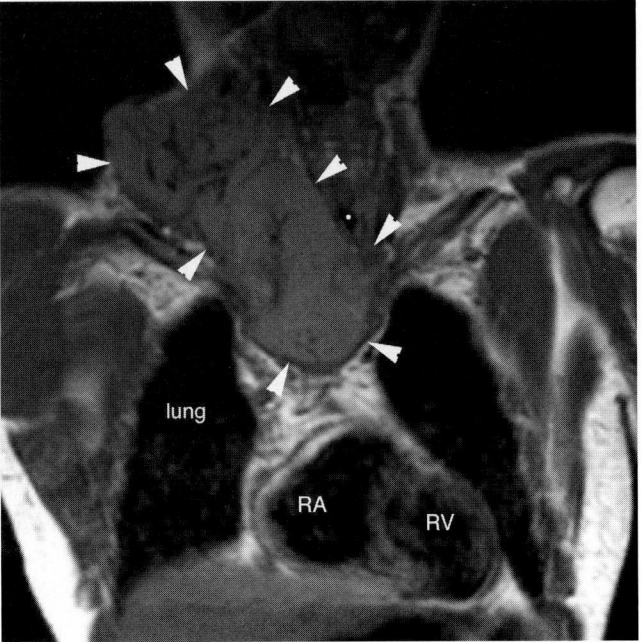

Figure 16–50. Coronal T1-weighted image in a young man presenting with a neck mass and stridor demonstrates a huge soft tissue mass (*arrowheads*) involving the right lower neck, compressing the trachea (*white dot*) and extending into the superior mediastinum. The mass is highly vascular, as evidenced by multiple serpiginous hypointense structures that represent flow voids. The lung, right atrium (*RA*), and right ventricle (*RV*) are shown. Tissue sampling confirmed follicular carcinoma of the thyroid.

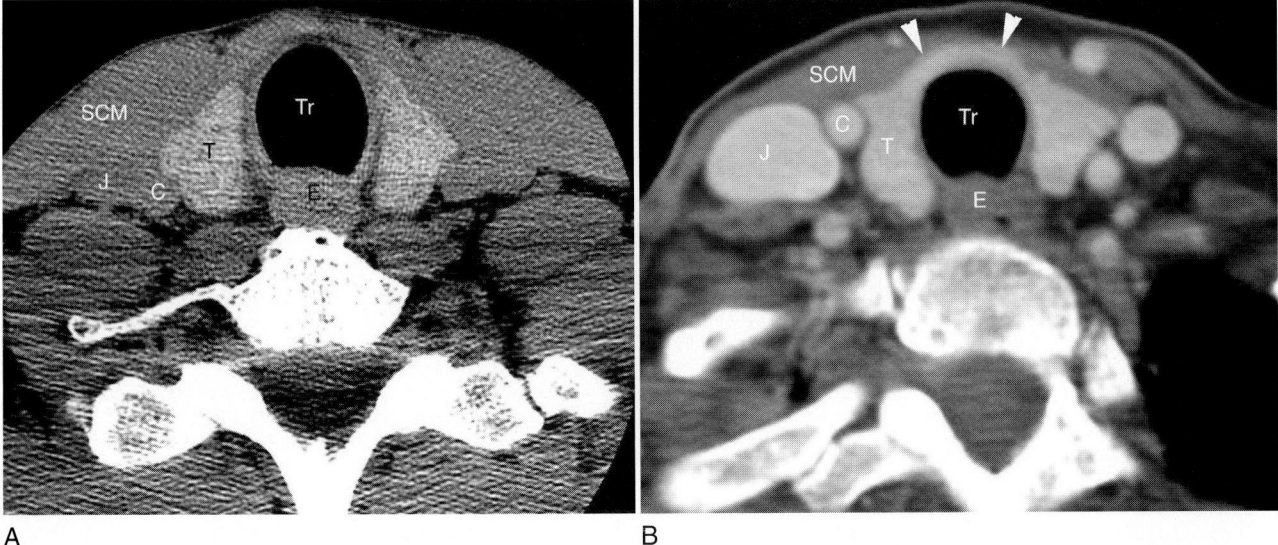

A   B

Figure 16–49. A, Axial noncontrast computed tomography demonstrates the intrinsic high density of the normal thyroid gland (*T*). Also shown are the trachea (*Tr*), esophagus (*E*), sternocleidomastoid muscle (*SCM*), common carotid artery (*C*), and internal jugular vein (*J*). The scan also demonstrates the difficulty of distinguishing vessels from other structures on noncontrast examination. **B,** Axial contrast-enhanced computed tomography scan through the lower neck shows homogeneous enhancement of the thyroid gland. The narrow thyroid isthmus (*arrowheads*) is seen connecting the right and left lobes of the thyroid.

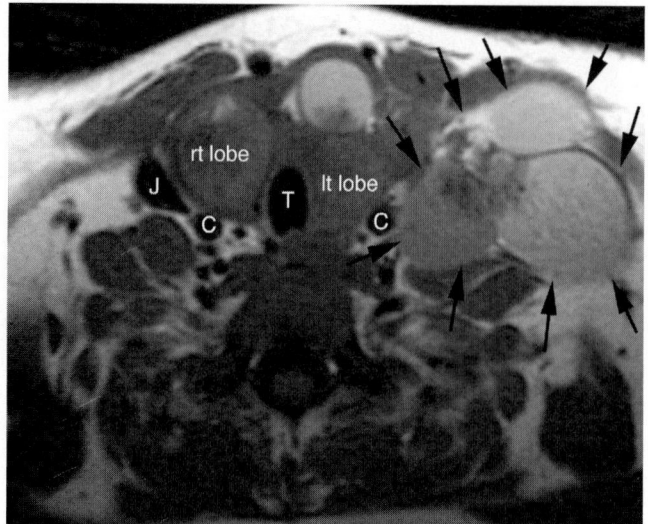

A

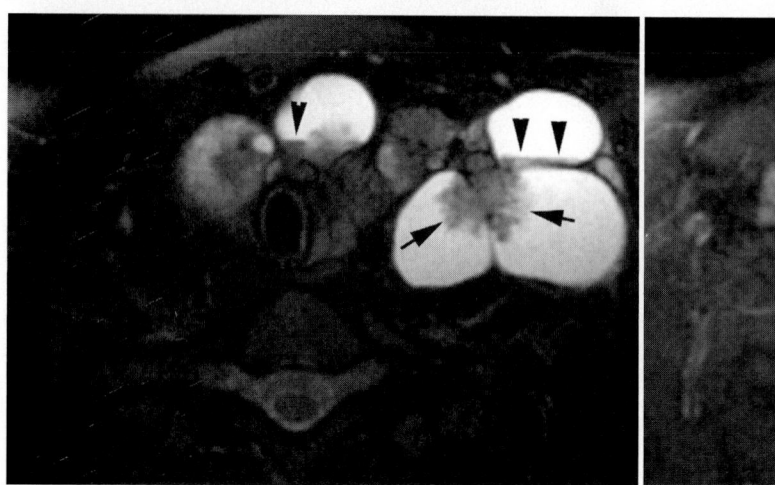

B

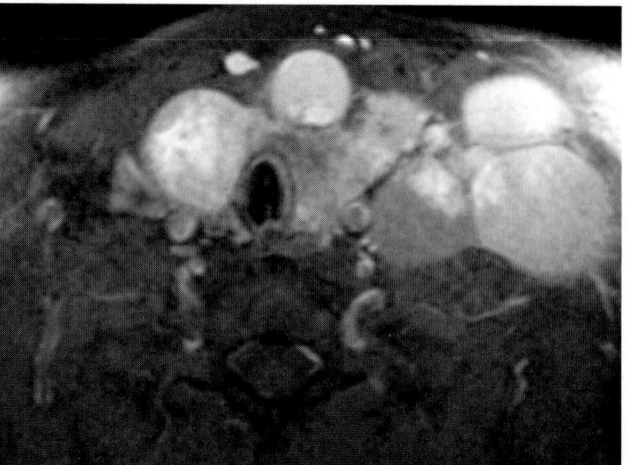

C

Figure 16–51. Magnetic resonance images of the neck in a young woman who has neglected a long-standing, progressively enlarging neck mass. **A,** Axial T1-weighted image demonstrates enlargement and heterogeneity of the right and left lobes of the thyroid. The trachea (*T*), common carotid arteries (*C*), and right internal jugular vein (*J*) are shown for orientation. Also demonstrated is a large, heterogeneous, mostly hyperintense mass (*black arrows*) consistent with a metastatic nodal mass. The High signal intensity of the nodes on a pre-gadolinium 71-weighted image is highly suggestive of metastatic thyroid cancer. **B,** Axial fast spin-echo T2-weighted image with fat saturation demonstrates papillary frond-like solid elements of the tumor (*black arrows*) as well as fluid-fluid levels (*black arrowheads*) consistent with hemorrhage into partly cystic lymph nodes. **C,** Post-gadolinium T1-weighted image with fat saturation shows heterogeneous enhancement of the solid areas of the tumor. Tissue sampling diagnosed papillary carcinoma of the thyroid.

Other thyroid malignancies include medullary carcinoma, lymphoma, and metastatic disease. The imaging features are generally nonspecific and tissue sampling and correlation with clinical history are necessary to make an accurate diagnosis.

REFERENCES

1. Brink JA, Heiken JP, Wang G, et al: Helical CT: Principles and technical considerations. *Radiographics.* 1994;14:887.
2. Rydberg J, Buckwalter KA, Caldemeyer KS, et al: Multisection CT: Scanning techniques and clinical applications. *Radiographics.* 2000;20:1787.
3. Lewis MA: Multislice CT: Opportunities and challenges. *Br J Radiol.* 2001;74:779.
4. Hendrick RE: The AAPM/RSNA physics tutorial for residents. Basic physics of MR imaging: An introduction. *Radiographics.* 1994;14:829.
5. Plewes DB: The AAPM/RSNA physics tutorial for residents. Contrast mechanisms in spin-echo MR imaging. *Radiographics.* 1994;14:1389.
6. Price RR: The AAPM/RSNA physics tutorial for residents. MR imaging safety considerations. Radiological Society of North America. *Radiographics.* 1999;19:1641.
7. Kanal E, Borgstede JP, Barkovich AJ, et al: American College of Radiology White Paper on MR Safety. *AJR Am J Roentgenol.* 2002;178:1335.
8. Jabour BA, Choi Y, Hoh CK, et al: Extracranial head and neck: PET imaging with 2-[F-18]fluoro-2-deoxy-D-glucose and MR imaging correlation. *Radiology.* 1993;186:27.
9. Rege S, Maass A, Chaiken L, et al: Use of positron emission tomography with fluorodeoxyglucose in patients with extracranial head and neck cancers. *Cancer.* 1994;73:3047.
10. McGuirt WF, Greven K, Williams D III, et al: PET scanning in head and neck oncology: A review. *Head Neck.* 1998;20:208.
11. Harnsberger HR: CT and MRI of masses of the deep face. *Curr Probl Diagn Radiol.* 1987; 16:141.
12. Harnsberger HR, Osborn AG: Differential diagnosis of head and neck lesions based on their space of origin. 1. The suprahyoid part of the neck. *AJR Am J Roentgenol.* 1991;157:147.
13. Smoker WR, Harnsberger HR: Differential diagnosis of head and neck lesions based on their space of origin. 2. The infrahyoid portion of the neck. *AJR Am J Roentgenol.* 1991;157:155.
14. Ng SH, Chong VF, Ko SF, Mukherji SK: Magnetic resonance imaging of nasopharyngeal carcinoma. *Top Magn Reson Imaging.* 1999;10:290.

15. Hermans R, Lenz M: Imaging of the oropharynx and oral cavity. Part I: Normal anatomy. *Eur Radiol.* 1996;6:362.

16. Lenz M, Hermans R: Imaging of the oropharynx and oral cavity. Part II: Pathology. *Eur Radiol.* 1996;6:536.

17. Laine FJ, Smoker WR: Oral cavity: Anatomy and pathology. *Semin Ultrasound CT MR.* 1995;16:527.

18. Weissman JL, Carrau RL: "Puffed-cheek" CT improves evaluation of the oral cavity. *AJNR Am J Neuroradiol.* 2001;22:741.

19. Pameijer FA, Mukherji SK, Balm AJ, van der Laan BF: Imaging of squamous cell carcinoma of the hypopharynx. *Semin Ultrasound CT MR.* 1998;19:476.

20. Becker M: Larynx and hypopharynx. *Radiol Clin North Am.* 1998;36:891.

21. Lindberg R: Distribution of cervical lymph node metastases from squamous cell carcinoma of the upper respiratory and digestive tracts. *Cancer.* 1972;29:1446.

22. Shah J: Patterns of cervical lymph node metastases from squamous cell carcinomas of the upper aerodigestive tract. *Am J Surg.* 1990;160:405.

23. Becker M: Neoplastic invasion of laryngeal cartilage: Radiologic diagnosis and therapeutic implications. *Eur J Radiol.* 2000;33:216.

24. Som PM, Curtin HD, Mancuso AA: An imaging-based classification for the cervical nodes designed as an adjunct to recent clinically based nodal classifications. *Arch Otolaryngol Head Neck Surg.* 1999;125:388.

25. Som PM, Curtin HD, Mancuso AA: Imaging-based nodal classification for evaluation of neck metastatic adenopathy. *AJR Am J Roentgenol.* 2000;174:837.

26. van den Brekel MW, Castelijns JA, Stel HV, et al: Modern imaging techniques and ultrasound-guided aspiration cytology for the assessment of neck node metastases: A prospective comparative study. *Eur Arch Otorhinolaryngol.* 1993;250:11.

27. Stoeckli SJ, Steinert H, Pfaltz M, Schmid S: Is there a role for positron emission tomography with 18F-fluorodeoxyglucose in the initial staging of nodal negative oral and oropharyngeal squamous cell carcinoma? *Head Neck.* 2002;24:345.

28. Adams S, Baum RP, Stuckensen T, et al: Prospective comparison of 18F-FDG PET with conventional imaging modalities (CT, MRI, US) in lymph node staging of head and neck cancer. *Eur J Nucl Med.* 1998;25:1255.

29. van den Brekel MW: Lymph node metastases: CT and MRI. *Eur J Radiol.* 2000;33:230.

30. Curtin HD, Ishwaran H, Mancuso AA, et al: Comparison of CT and MR imaging in staging of neck metastases. *Radiology.* 1998;207:123.

31. Anzai Y, Prince MR: Iron oxide-enhanced MR lymphography: The evaluation of cervical lymph node metastases in head and neck cancer. *J Magn Reson Imaging.* 1997;7:75.

32. von Buchwald C, Bilde A, Shoaib T, Ross G: Sentinel node biopsy: The technique and the feasibility in head and neck cancer. *ORL J Otorhinolaryngol Relat Spec.* 2002;64:268.

33. Hudgins PA, Burson JG, Gussack GS, Grist WJ: CT and MR appearance of recurrent malignant head and neck neoplasms after resection and flap reconstruction. *AJNR Am J Neuroradiol.* 1994;15:1689.

34. Anzai Y, Carroll WR, Quint DJ, et al: Recurrence of head and neck cancer after surgery or irradiation: Prospective comparison of 2-deoxy-2-[F-18]fluoro-D-glucose PET and MR imaging diagnoses. *Radiology.* 1996;200:135.

35. Fischbein NJ, AAssar OS, Caputo GR, et al: Clinical utility of positron emission tomography with 18F-fluorodeoxyglucose in detecting residual/recurrent squamous cell carcinoma of the head and neck. *AJNR Am J Neuroradiol.* 1998;19:1189.

36. Mukherji SK, Mancuso AA, Kotzur IM, et al: Radiologic appearance of the irradiated larynx. Part I. Expected changes. *Radiology.* 1994;193:141.

37. Weissman JL: Imaging of the salivary glands. *Semin Ultrasound CT MR.* 1995;16:546.

38. Weissman JL, Tabor EK, Curtin HD: Magnetic resonance imaging of the paranasal sinuses. *Top Magn Reson Imaging.* 1990;2:27.

39. Hasso AN, Lambert D: Magnetic resonance imaging of the paranasal sinuses and nasal cavities. *Top Magn Reson Imaging.* 1994;6:209.

40. Yousem DM, Li C, Montone KT, et al: Primary malignant melanoma of the sinonasal cavity: MR imaging evaluation. *Radiographics.* 1996;16:1101.

41. Som PM, Lidov M, Brandwein M, et al: Sinonasal esthesioneuroblastoma with intracranial extension: Marginal tumor cysts as a diagnostic MR finding. *AJNR Am J Neuroradiol.* 1994;15:1259.

42. Loevner LA: Imaging of the thyroid gland. *Semin Ultrasound CT MR.* 1996;17:539.

Thorax

17

Dmitry Bolkhovets, MD, Kenneth E. Rosenzweig, MD, and Michelle S. Ginsberg, MD

Accurate diagnosis is one of many important aspects of treatment planning. With the rapidly progressing radiologic imaging technologies and the increased computing power of imaging equipment, abnormal findings can be localized with increasing accuracy. The location of an abnormality can be pinpointed with increasing precision. However, accurate radiologic diagnosis depends on both anatomic knowledge and understanding of the disease processes.

Imaging has an invaluable role in every stage of patient care. When the patient presents for initial diagnosis, identification of the disease and accurate staging is of utmost importance. Following treatment, assessment of response and complications are often followed radiologically. Finally, imaging plays a central role in the post-treatment monitoring for early detection of disease recurrence. At any of these stages, imaging may also be to direct image-guided biopsies.

IMAGING MODALITIES

While all existing imaging modalities have found application in the diagnosis of diseases of the chest, the chest radiograph—the oldest technique—remains the most commonly ordered initial radiologic study.[1] In addition to conventional screen-film techniques, digital radiography, which captures images directly in computer format, is becoming more prevalent. Cross-sectional imaging such as computed tomography (CT) or magnetic resonance imaging (MRI) often is the next step in the diagnostic workup. CT is the second most commonly used thoracic imaging technique offering the most comprehensive examination of the mediastinum, lung parenchyma, pleura, and chest wall. The advent of helical CT in the 1990s allowed for faster scanning and volume acquisition of data with re-formation options and three-dimensional reconstruction capabilities. Helical CT was made possible by the development of *slip-ring technology*, which allows the tube and detector to rotate around a continuously moving table on which a patient lies. Thus, the tube and detector acquire data in a corkscrew, or helical, path. The next generation of scanners, the *multidetector-row CT (MDCT)* scanners, took the helical technology one step further by simultaneously acquiring data through multiple detectors. In addition to further decreasing scanning time, multidetector technology reduces or even completely eliminates the mismatch between longitudinal (axial) and transverse resolution, which further improves three-dimensional reconstruction capabilities. MDCT decreases motion artifact and improves the quality of images, particularly in a patient in distress or an uncooperative pediatric patient. Faster scanning also allows the entire examination to be performed during optimal contrast enhancement of the cardiovascular system. For example, faster imaging using an MDCT scanner allows CT angiography for evaluation of pulmonary embolism and vascular abnormalities. Three-dimensional reconstruction allows anatomic examination of the airway and virtual bronchoscopy.[1]

MRI is based on the magnetic properties of the proton (the nucleus of the hydrogen atom). MRI contrast depends on several factors including the difference in the behavior of protons in different tissues in response to magnetization as well as proton density. MRI provides soft tissue contrast resolution superior to that of CT.[2] MRI contrast agents, most of which are based on gadolinium, are widely used with a safety record superior to that of iodinated contrast agents used in CT scanning.[2]

MRI offers the advantages of excellent soft tissue contrast, multiplanar capability, intrinsic flow sensitivity, and lack of ionizing radiation.[2] In clinical applications, MRI of the thorax is reserved for (1) specific problematic cases where mediastinal, chest wall, vertebral body, or vascular invasion needs to be further assessed after a CT of the chest has been performed, or (2) evaluating the mediastinum of patients for whom the administration of iodinated contrast material is contraindicated. The multiplanar capability of MRI aids in the evaluation of chest wall and pleural abnormalities, particularly in the apical regions.[3] CT and MRI may play complementary roles in evaluating chest wall disorders such as mesenchymal tumors, primary and secondary malignancies, inflammatory conditions, and infectious disease. CT more readily demonstrates soft tissue calcification and bone destruction whereas MRI better delineates the extent of invasive tumors, soft tissue involvement, and infiltration of bone marrow as well as vascular involvement. The ability of MRI to evaluate the lung parenchyma is limited by artifact from multiple air–soft tissue interfaces, cardiac and respiratory motion, and poor signal-to-noise ratio.[2]

In addition to imaging based on depiction of anatomic and morphologic structures, functional imaging is widely used in thoracic imaging. ^{18}F-fluorodeoxyglucose (FDG) is a D-glucose analog that is most commonly used in positron emission tomography (PET) imaging of the thorax. The fluorine incorporated in the FDG undergoes decay with emission of a positron that after an annihilation reaction with an electron produces two photons that can be detected by a camera. Because malignant tissues have high rates of metabolism, they disproportionately accumulate FDG. Increased glucose metabolism by malignant cells may allow physiologic differentiation between benign and malignant abnormalities. As inflammatory lesions also can demonstrate increased uptake of FDG, differentiation between malignancy and inflammatory lesions may be difficult. At the same time, some malignant lesions such as bronchioloalveolar carcinoma may not demonstrate uptake on PET scan. Quantification of FDG uptake by a lesion may assist in this differentiation as well as affect prognosis. The standardized uptake value (SUV) is a widely used semi-quantitative method for measuring FDG uptake.[5-7]

FDG PET is used in examination and staging of lung cancer, differentiating benign from malignant solitary pulmonary nodules, and in diagnosis and assessment of treatment response of lymphoma.[1,8] In the staging of lung cancer, FDG PET is useful in evaluating local disease, lymph node involvement, and distant metastatic sites. The accuracy of FDG PET in demonstrating intrathoracic metastatic nodal disease is greater than that of CT or MRI. Whole-body PET is useful in detection of unsuspected extrathoracic metastases. Conventional imaging often does not allow differentiation of tumor from post-treatment scarring. Increased FDG uptake at the sites of residual radiographic abnormalities may suggest persistent or recurrent tumor.[8] In addition to its role in the staging of lung cancer, whole-body PET scanning is used in the diagnosis and staging of many other neoplasms including malignant melanoma, lymphoma, colorectal cancer, and head and neck tumors. Combining the PET scan with its sensitivity to detect lesions with a CT scan's high special resolution may increase the diagnostic accuracy of both modalities.[9,10] Recently, an integrated PET/CT scanner (fusion scanner) was developed. The fusion scanner combines a high-resolution, high-sensitivity PET scanner with a fast multidetector CT scanner. In addition to precise matching of PET and CT images, combining the two devices in one unit allows use of the CT data to measure the differences in the absorption of the PET emission by different parts of the patient's body (*attenuation correction*).[10] Faster scanning may reduce the artifact created by patient movement and respiration.[9]

ANATOMY OF THE THORAX

The major components of the thorax are the lungs and mediastinum, which are surrounded by the chest wall. Any structure in the thorax can give rise to a malignant neoplasm or become involved in a metastatic process.

Lungs

The right lung is larger than the left lung and consists of three lobes. The left lung has only two lobes. In the right lung, the major fissure runs obliquely and separates the lower lobe from the upper and middle lobes. In addition, the minor fissure that runs horizontally separates the upper and middle lobes. Only the major fissure is found in the left lung. It runs obliquely, separating the upper and lower lobes. The lobes are further subdivided into segments. Ten segments are found in the right lung, whereas only eight segments are found in the smaller, left lung.[11]

Pleura

The lungs are enveloped by the pleura, which consists of the visceral and parietal layers. The potential space between the layers can fill with fluid (exudate, transudate, blood), resulting in an effusion. Pneumothorax results when air accumulates in the pleural space.

Mediastinum

The mediastinum is commonly divided into anterior, middle, and posterior compartments based on the lateral chest radiograph. A line drawn along the back of the heart and front of the trachea divides the anterior and middle mediastinum, whereas the line connecting a point on each thoracic vertebra about a centimeter behind its anterior margin separates the middle and posterior compartments (Fig. 17-1).[12,13] Neoplasms usually arise from normal structures contained in each compartment. The anterior mediastinum contains the thymus, fat, and lymph nodes, and the most common neoplasms found in that area are thymoma, lymphoma, and germ cell tumors. Thyroid abnormalities that extend from the neck into the mediastinum are most commonly found in the anterior mediastinum but may also extend to the middle and posterior mediastinum, as well. The middle mediastinum contains the heart, pericardium, great vessels, trachea, bronchi, esophagus, and lymph nodes. Esophageal tumors, tracheal tumors, and lymph nodes are typically located in this compartment. The posterior mediastinum contains autonomic nerves, vessels, and lymph nodes. Neurogenic tumors and lymphadenopathy usually present in this location.[13,14] Besides primary and secondary tumors of these compartments, other vascular and developmental lesions can occur, but they are beyond the scope of this chapter.

Chest Wall

The chest wall consists of the ribs, sternum, intercostal muscles, nerves, blood vessels, skin, and subcutaneous tissues. These structures can give rise to a malignant lesion or become a site of metastatic involvement.

DISEASES OF THE THORAX

A great variety of pathologic processes occur in the thorax: both neoplastic (benign or malignant) and non-neoplastic, which range from congenital anomalies to infectious,

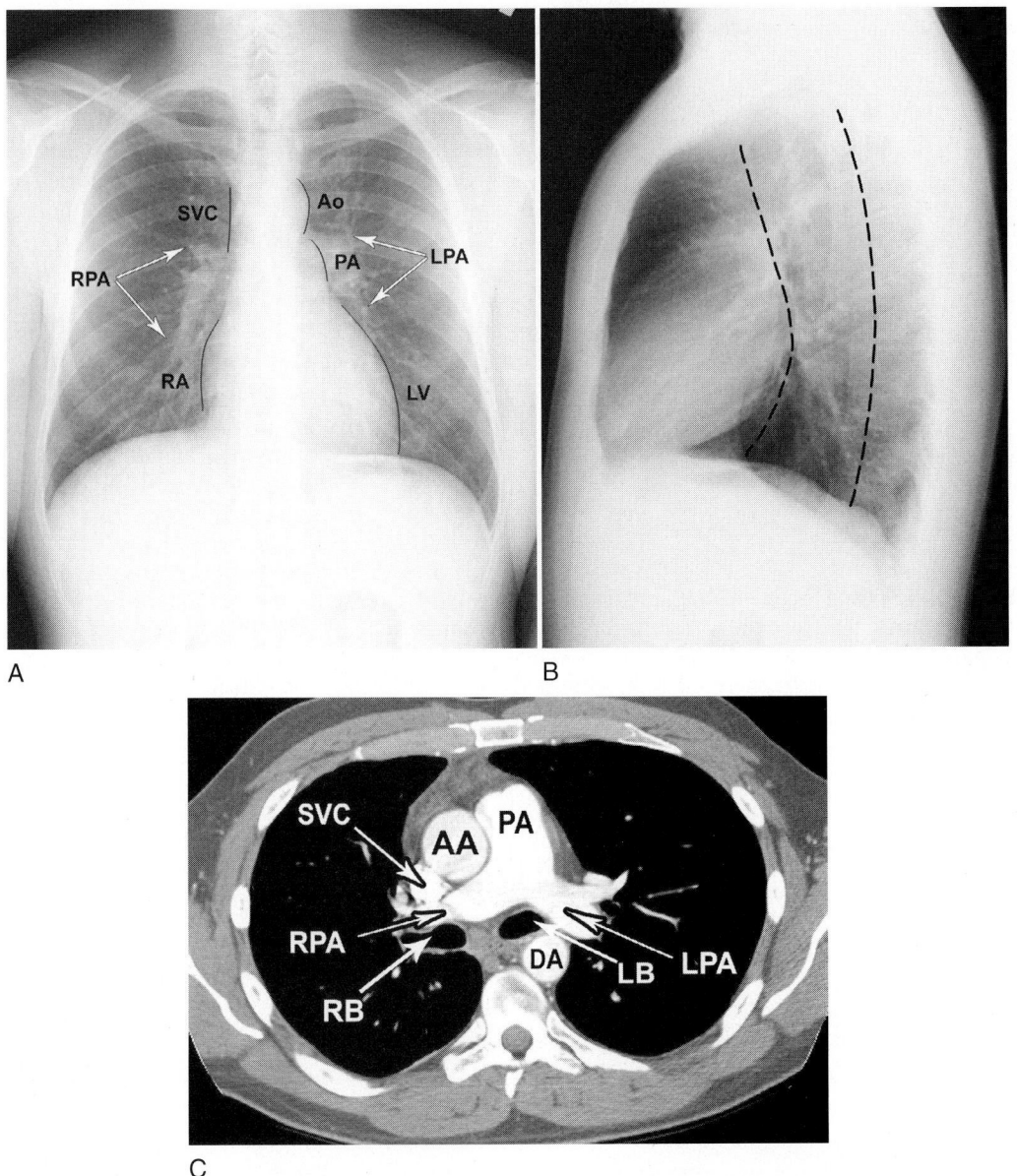

Figure 17–1. A, B: Normal posterior-anterior (PA) and lateral radiographs. **A**, Ao—aortic arch segment; SVC—superior vena cava; PA—main pulmonary artery segment; RPA—right pulmonary artery; LPA—left pulmonary artery; RA—right atrium; LV—left ventricle. **B**, Division of the mediastinum into anterior, middle, and posterior compartments. **C**, Axial computed tomography image at the level of carina: AA—ascending aorta; PA—main pulmonary artery; SVC—superior vena cava; RPA—right pulmonary artery; LPA—left pulmonary artery; RB—right main bronchus; LB—left main bronchus; DA—descending aorta.

inflammatory, and post-traumatic conditions. The scope of this discussion is limited only to the most common malignant neoplasms in the lungs, pleura, mediastinum, and chest wall that are usually amenable to radiation therapy. This treatment modality itself causes reactive changes in normal tissues; radiologic manifestations of such response are discussed at the end of this section.

Lung Malignancies

In 2003, there were an estimated 171,900 new cases of lung cancer in the United States: 91,800 in men and 80,100 in women. About 157,200 of these people will die

from the disease. Lung cancer is the leading cause of cancer death in both men and women, accounting for 31% of all cancer deaths in men and 25% of all cancer deaths in women. Smoking is responsible for at least 30% of all cancer deaths and 87% of all lung cancers; compared to nonsmokers, lung cancer mortality rates are 22 times higher for male and 12 times higher for female smokers. In addition, an estimated 3000 nonsmoking adults die each year from lung cancer caused by second-hand smoking.[15]

Histologically, the most common subtypes of lung cancer, in order of decreasing frequency, include adeno, squamous cell, small cell, and large cell carcinoma. Adenocarcinomas are further subdivided into several

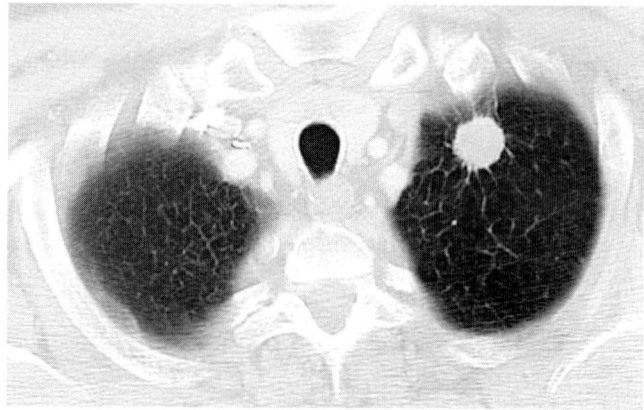

Figure 17–2. Two-centimeter nodule in the left upper lobe (adenocarcinoma at surgery).

histologic subtypes, including bronchioloalveolar carcinoma. There are major differences in therapeutic approaches to patients with small cell lung carcinoma and the other types of lung cancer; therefore, all primary lung malignancies are usually divided into non–small cell and small cell categories.[16,17]

NON–SMALL CELL LUNG CANCER

The most common cell types of lung cancer have a certain, typical radiographic presentation. It should be noted, however, that there is significant overlap between radiographic appearances of lung cancer. In addition, the relative frequency of different categories of this disease, as well as "typical" radiographic findings, have been changing in the past few decades.[18]

ADENOCARCINOMA

Adenocarcinoma is the most common cell type of bronchogenic carcinoma and accounts for approximately half of all cases. It typically presents as a small (often <3 cm), peripheral, round or oval solitary pulmonary nodule. It is commonly smoothly marginated, but spiculated margins can also occur (Figs. 17-2 to 17-4).[17] Calcifications are rare but are occasionally seen on CT scans. Central lesions have a higher frequency of hilar and mediastinal metastases at presentation.[17] Distant metastases are frequently present at the time of diagnosis. Peripheral tumors may directly invade the pleura and grow circumferentially around the lung, mimicking diffuse malignant mesothelioma.[19] Central tumors may directly invade mediastinal structures or extend via the pulmonary veins to invade the left atrium.

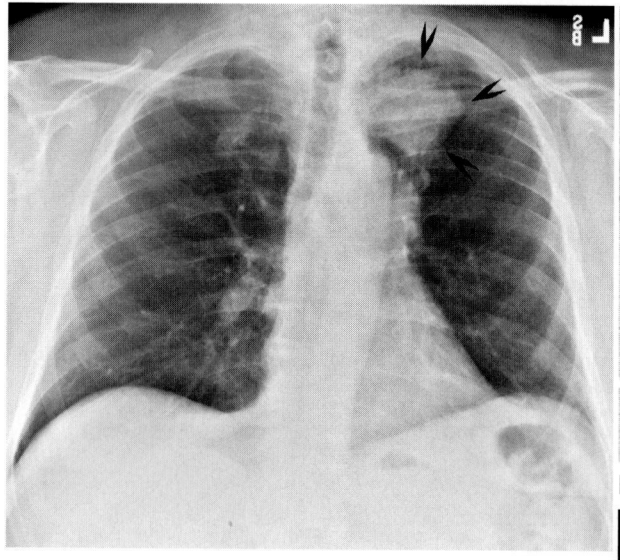

A

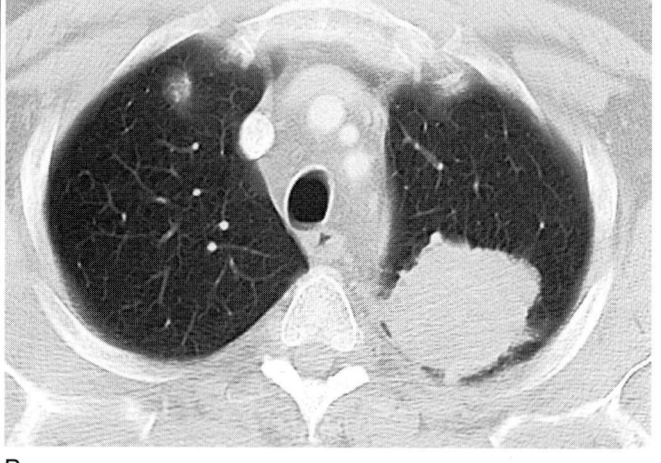

B

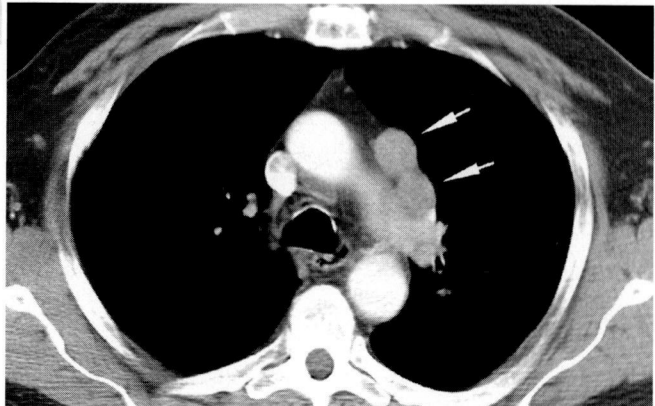

C

Figure 17–3. A, Adenocarcinoma presenting as a left upper lobe mass on PA radiograph (*arrowheads*). **B,** Same patient: CT scan. **C,** Same patient: CT scan demonstrates associated para-aortic lymphadenopathy (*arrows*).

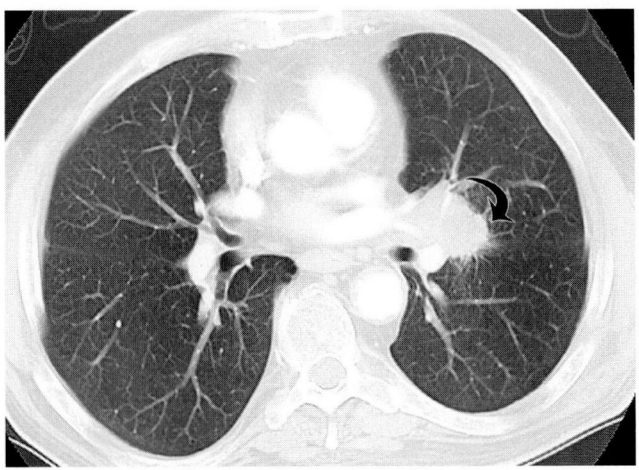

Figure 17–4. Centrally located spiculated mass directly invading the mediastinum, suggesting adenocarcinoma.

BRONCHIOLOALVEOLAR CARCINOMA

Bronchioloalveolar carcinoma, a subtype of adenocarcinoma, commonly presents as a well-circumscribed, peripherally located solitary nodule.[17,20] CT scan may reveal surrounding ground glass opacity. Cavitation is an infrequent finding in adenocarcinoma.[21] Bronchioloalveolar carcinoma can present as multifocal disease; several patterns have been described. It may present as multiple well-defined nodules of varying size involving one or both lungs. Another pattern of presentation can be focal, poorly defined or scattered lung opacities that may coalesce, causing opacification of a lobe or rarely the entire lung, and resemble pneumonia. Reticulonodular opacities similar in appearance to interstitial lung disease have been described (Fig. 17-5).[17,21] High-resolution CT may demonstrate air attenuation and pseudocavitation within the nodules corresponding to small bronchi and cystic spaces.[17,22] Unusual radiographic appearances include lobar atelectasis and expansile consolidation without air bronchograms.[17,23,24]

SQUAMOUS CELL CARCINOMA

Squamous cell carcinoma is a slow-growing malignancy with late metastasis predominantly to the liver, adrenal glands, kidneys, and bones.[17] Its typical presentation is described as a central endobronchial obstructing lesion with associated atelectasis or postobstructive pneumonia (Figs. 17-6 to 17-7). In addition, mucoid impaction or bronchiectasis may occur.[17] With increasing frequency,[18] these tumors present as a solitary peripheral nodule with or without cavitation.[25] When the tumor cavitates, the inner wall is typically thick and irregular and, if secondarily infected, may develop an air-fluid level (Fig. 17-8).[26] Extensive necrosis, however, may result in a thin-walled cavity. Squamous cell carcinoma is the most common histologic type found in Pancoast or superior sulcus tumors.[17]

LARGE CELL CARCINOMA

The majority of large cell carcinomas present as a large (average size >4 cm) peripheral mass with poorly defined margins. Cavitation and calcification of the tumor may

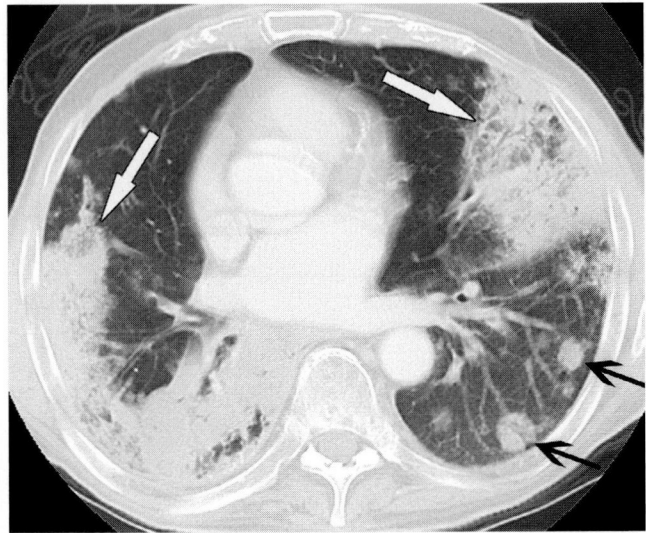

A

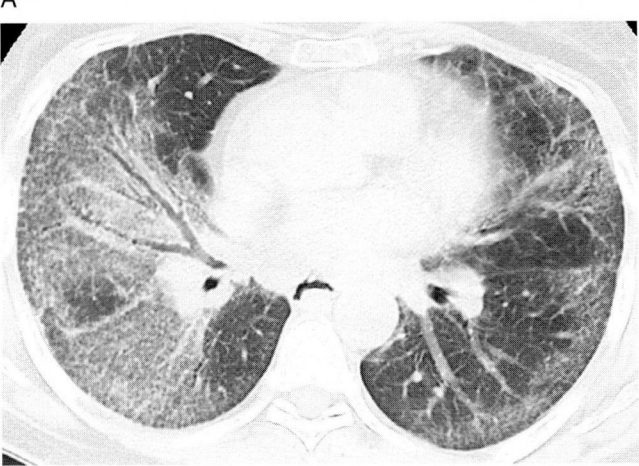

B

Figure 17–5. Bronchioloalveolar carcinoma. **A,** Both discrete nodules and dense consolidations are seen in this patient. **B,** Diffuse ground-glass opacities.

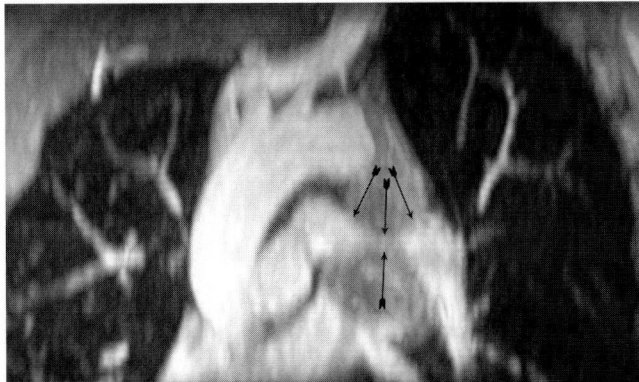

Figure 17–6. Gadolinium-enhanced coronal magnetic resonance image shows a central lesion encasing the left pulmonary artery (*arrows*). This patient with squamous cell carcinoma required pulmonectomy.

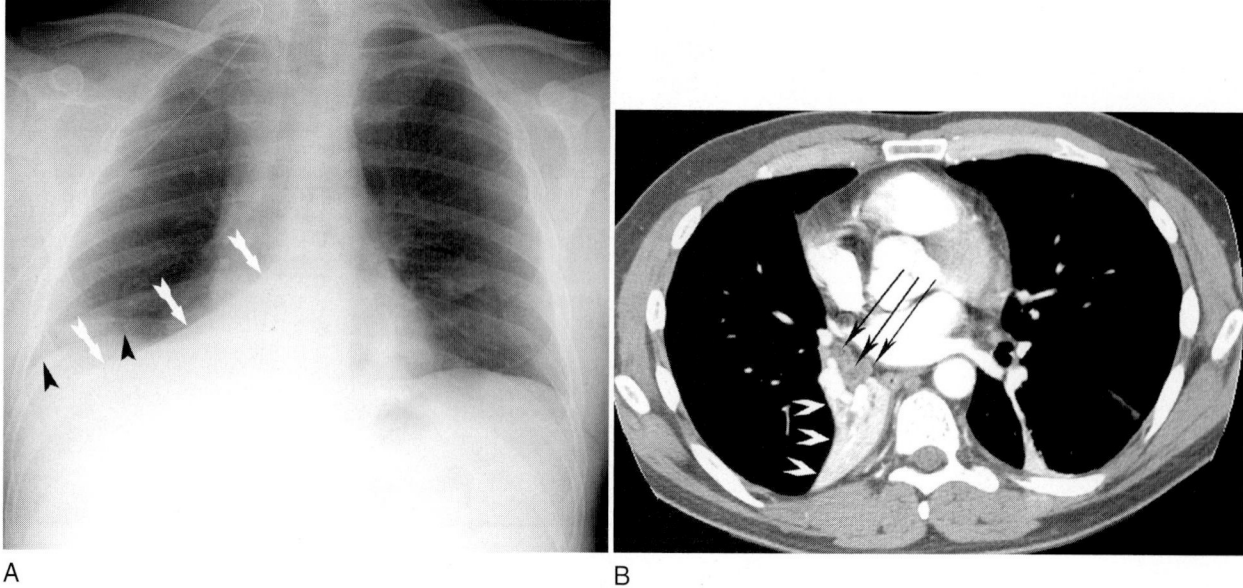

Figure 17–7. Right lower lobe collapse. Endobronchial lesions are among a number of causes of lung collapse due to obstruction. Among other numerous causes of lung lobar collapse, enlarged lymph nodes, a foreign body, and mediastinal mass are common. **A,** Volume loss in the right hemithorax with elevated hemidiaphragm (*arrowheads*), inferior and medial displacement of the minor fissure with a dense opacity representing the collapsed right lower lobe (*arrows*). **B,** CT of the same patient shows bronchial obstruction by low-density mucus (*arrows*) and a completely collapsed right lower lobe (*arrowheads*).

occur. These tumors grow rapidly and metastasize early via lymphatic and hematogenous routes, often presenting with hilar or mediastinal adenopathy.[17] Giant cell carcinoma is a subtype with multiple giant cells and a more aggressive behavior and poorer prognosis.

A variant of large cell carcinoma is large cell neuroendocrine carcinoma (LCNEC), or intermediate cell neuroendocrine carcinoma. It has a poorer prognosis than classic large cell carcinoma.[27] The ability to express neuroendocrine markers also places LCNEC into a broad category of neuroendocrine tumors of the lung, including

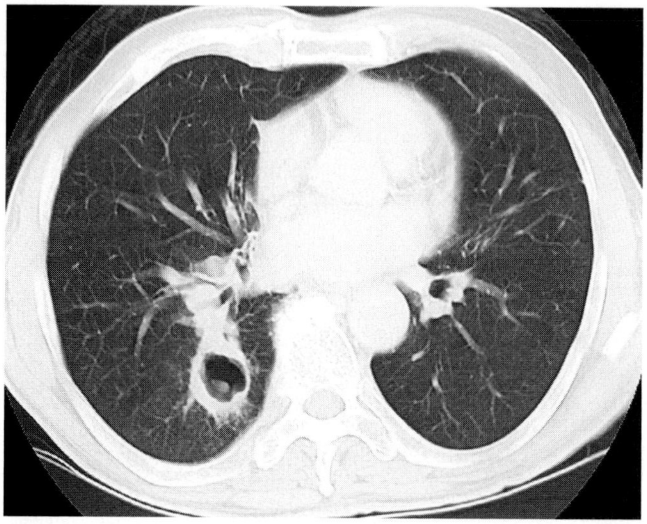

Figure 17–8. Thick-walled cavity—a frequent appearance of squamous cell carcinoma of the lung.

atypical carcinoid, typical carcinoid, and small cell lung carcinoma.[27,28]

MULTIPLE LUNG PRIMARY TUMORS

Multiple lung carcinomas are present in less than 1% of all lung cancers. Synchronous lesions are defined as the simultaneous presence of tumors that are physically distinct and separate, and can have different histology. If the histology is the same, however, the tumors should be present in different segments or lobes of the lung and originate from carcinoma in situ. No carcinoma in lymphatics or extrapulmonary metastases should be present at the time of diagnosis. Simultaneous lesions not meeting these criteria most likely represent metastases.[29] Metachronous lesions are defined as a second primary cancer appearing after a time interval in a patient considered cured of the initial cancer. Metachronous lesions comprise at least two thirds of multiple pulmonary neoplasms, and on average are recognized 4 to 5 years after the first primary. Up to one third of patients surviving resection for lung cancer may develop a second primary tumor.[30] These lesions are regarded as metachronous primary tumors rather than metastases if they show unique histologic features. If histology is the same, then in order to meet the criteria for a metachronous lesion, the cancer-free interval should be at least 2 years and the tumor must originate from carcinoma in situ or in a different lobe or lung. There should be no carcinoma in lymphatics common to both the old and the new lesions, and no extrapulmonary metastasis should exist at the time of diagnosis.[29] Squamous cell cancer is the most common histologic type of multiple carcinomas; adenocarcinoma, however, is currently the most common cell type. The reason for this trend is unknown, but the change in contents of cigarettes and filters that now contain more nitrates and less nicotine is suspected.[31,32]

STAGING

Accurate preoperative staging in patients with non–small cell lung cancer is important for selecting those patients with localized disease who are likely to benefit from surgical resection.[33,34] Cure rates and survival for non–small cell lung cancer are predicted by staging.[35] The TNM staging system of the American Joint Committee on Cancer is the most widely accepted and used classification system for preoperative and postoperative staging. Mediastinal lymph nodes are involved with disease in approximately one quarter of newly diagnosed lung cancer patients.[33,36] The evaluation of these lymph nodes is the primary goal of intrathoracic staging of non–small cell lung cancer. The current noninvasive imaging techniques evaluate lymph nodes based on either size (CT) or metabolism (PET).[37] Conventional cross-sectional imaging techniques provide excellent anatomic information used in staging, but they have limitations differentiating benign and malignant lymph nodes based on size criteria. CT of the chest remains the most widely accepted imaging modality for evaluation of the primary tumor (the *T* classification); nodal metastases (the *N* classification); and distant metastases, especially the adrenal glands (the *M* classification).[16] Even though not absolutely essential, intravenous contrast is usually administered when a CT scan of the chest is performed for staging. Intravenous contrast helps distinguish between normal vascular structures and lymph nodes and aids in evaluation of the degree of mediastinal invasion.[35] CT alone, however, often cannot accurately differentiate between benign lymph node enlargement and metastasis, and its accuracy for mediastinal staging has not improved over the past decade despite improvement in resolution.[33] For example, normal-sized lymph nodes may contain metastases, while enlarged lymph nodes may have benign underlying etiology. The most commonly used criterion is a short axis diameter equal to or greater than 1 cm, even though up to 40% of lymph nodes identified as abnormal using this method can be benign. CT scanning, however, provides an extra benefit of guidance when selective biopsy is required.[35] PET can be useful in suggesting metastatic involvement of lymph nodes, but it can be falsely positive in a number of inflammatory and infectious conditions. In addition, very small lesions, typically less than 1 to 1.2 cm, can be beyond the detection ability of PET. Current evidence indicates that PET is more sensitive and specific for evaluation of mediastinal lymph nodes.[33,38,39] In addition, PET may be superior to CT in more accurately predicting long-term survival in non–small cell lung cancer patients.[40] The recently developed fusion scanners that combine CT and PET may provide an optimal and cost-effective method for lung cancer staging. This technology, however, still needs to be evaluated in clinical trials.[33] The role of MRI currently remains limited to evaluation of superior sulcus tumors, brachial plexus, and vertebral invasion. Intravenous contrast may improve the accuracy of MRI in detection of abnormal

mediastinal lymph nodes.[35] MRI's accuracy for anatomic imaging of mediastinal lymph nodes is comparable with that of CT and exceeds the accuracy of CT in evaluating hilar lymph nodes.[41] CT often combined with PET currently remains the study of choice for mediastinal staging of non–small cell lung cancer.[35,41]

METASTASES FROM LUNG CANCER

Extrathoracic metastases are found in almost half of the newly diagnosed lung cancer patients.[33,36] The adrenal glands are one of the most common sites of metastases from lung cancer. At the time of presentation, 5% to 10% of patients with lung cancer have adrenal metastases (Fig. 17-9). Metastases to the liver, brain, and skeletal system are also common.[33,35] The more unusual sites of metastases include the kidneys, pancreas, and small bowel. Serosal and mesenteric implants may become quite large and invade and perforate the adjacent bowel.

When a clinician suspects distant metastases (e.g., neurologic symptoms, abdominal or flank pain, pathologic fractures, or abnormal serum liver enzyme levels,[33] the preferred workup includes CT or MRI scan with contrast of the brain and ^{99m}Tc bone scan. Inclusions of the adrenals and partial imaging of the liver on the chest CT scan are currently routine. When an adrenal lesion is greater than 3 cm in size, it likely represents a metastasis and warrants further workup with CT, MRI, or sometimes percutaneous biopsy.[33] A liver lesion in an asymptomatic patient is relatively unlikely to represent a metastasis, with most incidentally discovered lesions being cysts or hemangiomas. When clinically indicated, evaluation with contrast-enhanced CT or MRI scan or occasionally percutaneous biopsy is performed.[35] Distant metastases can still be missed due to the limited area of coverage by each technique. PET has reportedly overcome some of the limitations of other staging techniques and is gaining more widespread use as it is becoming readily available at many institutions. There is evidence

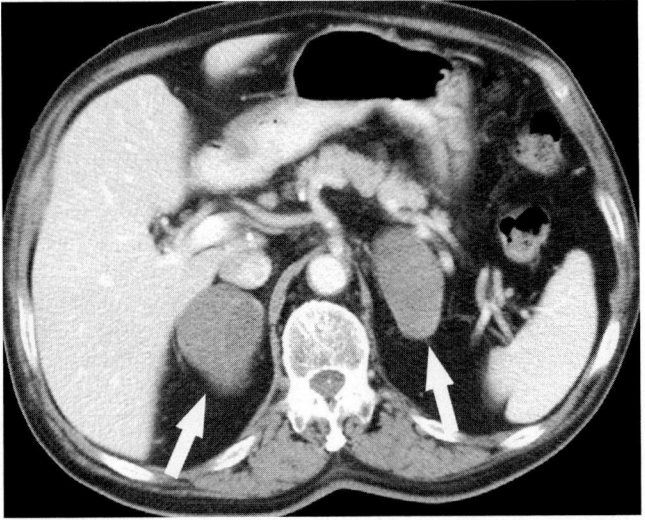

Figure 17–9. Bilateral adrenal masses consistent with metastases from large cell carcinoma of the lung.

that a whole-body PET scan can detect an additional 10% to 20% of distant metastases.[33,35,42] MRI of the brain is more sensitive than CT and detects smaller lesions in greater numbers but does not identify more patients with metastatic cancer or affect survival. Bone scan is a sensitive test in detecting bone metastases, but it has a relatively high false-positive rate. Unless evidence for metastatic disease is overwhelming, an abnormal bone scan may not be conclusive even with the addition of skeletal MRI, and tissue confirmation of a metastatic lesion may be required.[35]

INVASIVE STAGING

Noninvasive staging methods cannot provide tissue diagnosis that is often required for the evaluation of tumor resectability.[37] Histologic evaluation of mediastinal lymph nodes is currently considered essential for accurate staging, but techniques such as bronchoscopy and mediastinoscopy also have limitations and, like any invasive procedures, are associated with morbidity.

Invasive techniques include needle biopsy such as transbronchial needle aspiration, transthoracic needle aspiration, or endoscopic ultrasound-guided needle aspiration, as well as open surgical biopsy performed by mediastinoscopy.[37] To achieve consistent and reproducible classification of the mediastinal lymph nodes, the following schema that describes 14 nodal stations has been adopted by the American Joint Committee on Cancer and other organizations.[16]

Small Cell Lung Cancer

Small cell lung cancer (SCLC) is a rapidly proliferating, biologically aggressive form of lung cancer that has a short survival without treatment.[44] These tumors probably arise from neuroendocrine cells, that contain neurosecretory granules, and may secrete peptide hormones.[17] SCLC is associated with tobacco use.[45]

The typical presentation of this disease is a centrally located tumor, frequently associated with mediastinal extension and often extensive encasement of mediastinal structures, as well as compression of the tracheobronchial tree. Rarely, SCLC may present as a peripheral tumor that is often associated with hilar adenopathy and atelectasis. The peripheral tumor itself may not be visible on radiographic studies, and extensive extrathoracic metastases to the liver, bone marrow, adrenal glands, and the brain may be the initial presentation.[17] Rarer presentations of the disease also include a solitary lesion within the lung parenchyma that may mimic the appearance of non–small cell cancer. The appearance of SCLC may overlap with a more unusual presentation of non–small cell lung cancer that can manifest as a central mass with a similar metastatic pattern. A pleural effusion may be present, and when malignant, it affects the staging and patient's outcome.[46]

A two-stage classification developed by the Veterans Administration Lung Cancer Study Group is widely accepted for staging of SCLC. When the entire tumor is confined to the thorax and can be included in a single radiation therapy port, the disease is defined as limited stage. Most patients, however, present with extensive disease involving distant metastases and noncontiguous metastases to the contralateral lung, which requires systemic treatment.[17,44,45]

Imaging modalities currently used in initial staging of SCLC are CT of the chest and upper abdomen including the entire liver and adrenal glands, a bone scan, and CT or MRI examination of the brain. PET may offer additional benefit in staging and restaging of SCLC, but its use is still under investigation.

Metastatic Lung Lesions

The lung is one of the most common sites for metastases that are found at autopsy.[47] Breast, colon, kidneys, and uterus, as well as head and neck cancers, are the common malignancies with pulmonary metastases.[48] Many other less common malignant neoplasms are known to frequently metastasize to the lung, including choriocarcinoma, osteosarcoma, testicular tumors, melanoma, Ewing's sarcoma, and thyroid carcinoma. CT is the modality of choice for detection of pulmonary metastases. It typically demonstrates multiple peripherally located round nodules of various sizes indicative of the hematogenous route of spread (Fig. 17-10) or diffuse thickening of the interstitium, which represents lymphangitic carcinomatosis.[49] While the finding of multiple pulmonary nodules carries a significant chance of the diagnosis of metastases,[50] not all pulmonary metastatic lesions have this typical appearance; several atypical findings have been described. These atypical appearances include cavitation, calcification, and hemorrhage around the metastatic nodule.[47,51]

A persistent lung lesion seen after chemotherapy that demonstrates no change or an initial decrease in size followed by no change may represent a "sterilized metastases." At histology no viable tumor is identified and only necrosis or fibrosis, or both, are seen. It is, however,

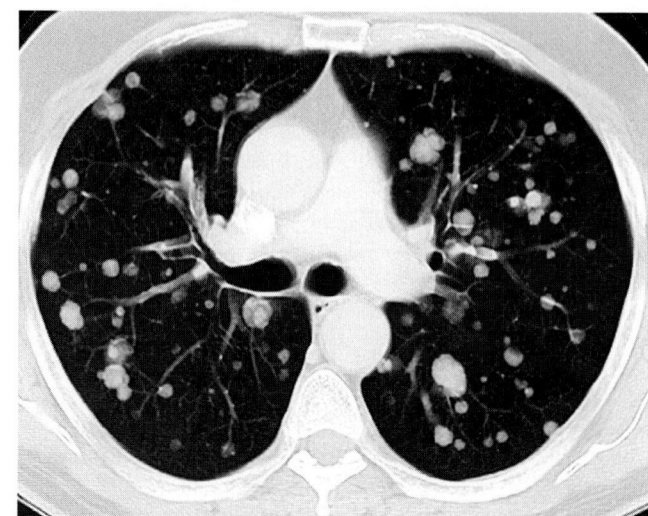

Figure 17–10. Multiple nodules of varying sizes—a typical appearance of hematogenous pulmonary metastases.

difficult to radiologically exclude active disease. These lesions are most commonly seen in treated metastases from testicular cancer, choriocarcinoma, thyroid cancer, sarcoma, and breast cancer.

Unusual Tumors

While the great majority of primary lung malignancies fall into the category of adenocarcinoma, squamous cell carcinoma, large cell undifferentiated carcinomas and small cell carcinoma, a number of benign and malignant lesions of mesenchymal, epithelial, lymphoreticular, and vascular origin have been described. These lesions are rare and represent less than 1% of all lung neoplasms.[52]

Lung Cancer Screening

Screening of a high-risk population (primarily cigarette smokers) for lung cancer using a low-dose helical CT has gained popularity in recent years. CT is superior to plain film radiograph in the detection of small lung nodules, which may represent early-stage lung cancer. Its usefulness, however, remains controversial, since decrease in mortality associated with earlier detection has not been proven. In addition, it has not been determined whether an increase in the number of tumors detected at an early stage represents a true stage shift or just a statistic bias. A large number of false-positive results may also lead to unnecessary workup with associated patient morbidity. More clinical trials aimed at resolving the controversies that surround lung cancer screening programs are currently under way.[53,54]

MEDIASTINAL MASSES

The organs and structures of the mediastinum are composed of a multitude of tissues that can give rise to both benign and malignant neoplasms. Significant differences exist between adults and children in incidence of mediastinal lesions. Primary thymic neoplasms, thyroid masses, and lymphomas are the most frequently encountered mediastinal neoplasms in adults, whereas in pediatric patients neurogenic tumors, germ cell neoplasms, and foregut cysts are most common, representing 80% of mediastinal tumors in that population.[55,56] Overall, two thirds of mediastinal masses are benign. Most patients with mediastinal masses are asymptomatic, and 83% of asymptomatic mediastinal masses are benign. In contrast, in patients with symptoms caused by a mediastinal mass, the diagnosis of malignancy is made in 57% of cases.[55] On cross-sectional imaging, invasion and obstruction of adjacent structures are suggestive of malignancy.[55]

Thymoma

Thymoma is a rare tumor, but it is the most frequent lesion in the mediastinum and the most common primary tumor of the thymus. Most thymomas present in adults

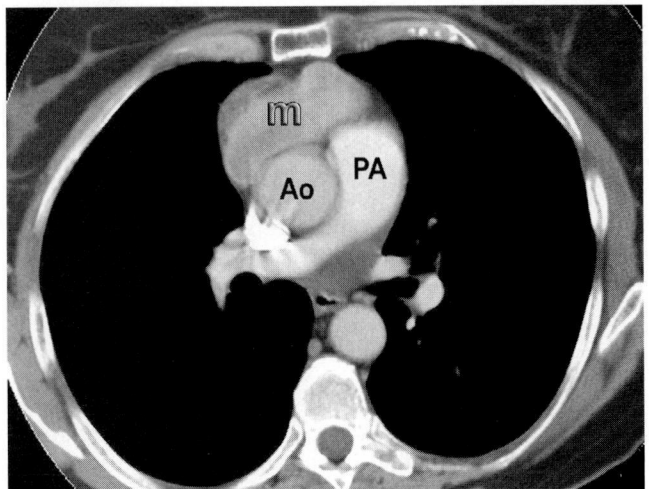

Figure 17–11. Thymoma: anterior mediastinal mass with smooth borders. Ao—ascending aorta; PA—main pulmonary artery; m—anterior mediastinal mass.

in the fifth and sixth decades of life. The majority of these tumors are found in the anterior mediastinum (Fig. 17-11), but occasionally they are encountered in the neck and posterior mediastinum. A number of classifications of thymomas exist based on histologic type and the ability to invade adjacent structures.[57] Noninvasive thymomas are usually seen on CT as well-defined oval, rounded, or lobulated masses that can be partially or completely surrounded by fat. MRI demonstrates a homogenous mass with well-defined margins that is isointense with skeletal muscle on T1-weighted images and demonstrates high signal intensity on T2-weighted images. Homogeneous enhancement is typically seen upon administration of intravenous contrast, but cystic or hemorrhagic areas that do not enhance can be present occasionally. Invasive thymomas have ill-defined margins and a heterogeneous appearance with septations and intratumoral loculations seen especially well on T2-weighted images. Calcifications are occasionally seen in noninvasive thymomas; invasive thymomas rarely calcify.[58,59] Thymomas are followed in frequency of incidence by neurogenic tumors and benign cysts, together representing 60% of mediastinal masses in all patients.

Germ Cell Tumor

Germ cell tumor is a neoplasm that takes origin from rests of primitive germ cells that normally migrate from the yolk sac to the urogenital ridge during early embryogenesis. Germ cell tumors commonly occur in the gonads, but the anterosuperior mediastinum is the most common site of extragonadal germ cell tumors in adults.

The majority of mediastinal germ cell tumors are benign with mature teratoma as the most common histologic type. It is a slow-growing tumor that typically occurs in young patients and is frequently an incidental finding on chest radiographs of asymptomatic patients. It usually presents as a sharply demarcated rounded or lobulated mass that may occasionally contain teeth, skeletal parts, or fat-fluid levels. Mature teratoma typically includes all three germinal layers, whereas another benign neoplasm, dermoid cyst, contains only elements derived from the ectodermal layer. On imaging studies, benign germ cell tumors present as a heterogeneous, predominately cystic mass with solid components, well defined margins, and often calcification.

Seminoma is a malignant neoplasm and the second most common mediastinal germ cell tumor that commonly occurs in men in the third or fourth decade of life. Histologically it is identical to the neoplasm that occurs in the testes. It may cause superior vena cava syndrome and metastasize to bone, lungs, liver, and thoracic lymph nodes. Mediastinal seminomas are usually sensitive to radiation and chemotherapy. Less common malignant histologic types include nonseminomatous neoplasms such as teratoma with embryonal cell carcinoma (teratocarcinoma), endodermal sinus tumor, choriocarcinoma, and embryonal cell carcinoma.

Malignant germ cell tumors grow rapidly and invade adjacent mediastinal structures. Unlike their benign counterparts, they usually have an imaging appearance of heterogeneous solid masses with irregular margins that only rarely show calcification (Fig. 17-12). CT and MRI play a complementary role in evaluating calcification and invasion of the chest wall and adjacent mediastinal structures.[13,60]

Lymphoma

Lymphoid neoplasms comprise a number of conditions that are classified based on morphology, immunophenotype, genetic and clinical features.[61] These neoplasms are commonly placed into two major categories: non-Hodgkin's and Hodgkin's lymphoma. Hodgkin's disease is a discrete type of lymphoma, whereas the non-Hodgkin's lymphoma category includes a heterogeneous group of diseases that differ in histopathologic types as well as clinical manifestations.[62] Non-Hodgkin's lymphoma accounts for 4% of all cancer cases in adults in this country. The incidence of Hodgkin's disease is almost eight times lower than the incidence of non-Hodgkin's lymphoma. People infected with HIV and organ transplant recipients are at higher risk of developing the disease.[15]

Non-Hodgkin's and Hodgkin's lymphomas differ not only in their histologic characteristics, but also in demographics and clinical behavior. Thoracic involvement at presentation is more common in Hodgkin's disease than in non-Hodgkin's lymphoma.[62]

Hodgkin's Lymphoma

Hodgkin's disease virtually always begins in lymph nodes and predictably spreads from one lymph node group to another with radiographic evidence of intrathoracic disease seen in two thirds of patients at the time of presentation. The mediastinal lymphadenopathy most frequently involves anterior mediastinal and paratracheal lymph nodes followed by subcarinal, superior diaphragmatic, paraesophageal, and internal mammary groups. Extensive mediastinal lymphadenopathy can cause obstruction of the superior vena cava or compress the esophagus and major airways (Fig. 17-13).

When lung parenchymal involvement occurs, it is almost always associated with hilar or mediastinal lymphadenopathy. The most frequent pattern of lung parenchymal disease in Hodgkin's lymphoma is multiple pulmonary nodules. The second pattern is reticular; it is thought to be caused by obstruction of lymphatic or venous drainage by enlarged hilar and mediastinal lymph nodes and presents with septal lines. Finally, Hodgkin's lymphoma may present as lobar or segmental consolidation with air bronchograms indistinguishable from pneumonia. Pleural effusions may develop and are usually a consequence of lymphatic or venous obstruction.[62]

Non-Hodgkin's Lymphoma

This condition usually presents at a more advanced stage than Hodgkin's disease. Superior mediastinal lymphadenopathy is less frequently found. Lung parenchymal involvement of non-Hodgkin's lymphoma is much less common at presentation and is found in less than 5% of patients, but unlike Hodgkin's disease, it may be isolated (Fig. 17-14). All three radiologic patterns of lung parenchymal involvement found in Hodgkin's disease— pulmonary nodules, reticular pattern, and consolidation with air bronchograms—can be seen in non-Hodgkin's lymphoma as well. Pleural effusions also occur and are usually associated with mediastinal lymphadenopathy.[62]

PLEURAL TUMORS

Among various pleural tumors, metastatic disease represents the most common neoplasm.[63] Primary pleural neoplasms are less common than invasion of the pleura by a secondary malignancy such as bronchogenic carcinoma, breast cancer, lymphoma, and ovarian or gastric

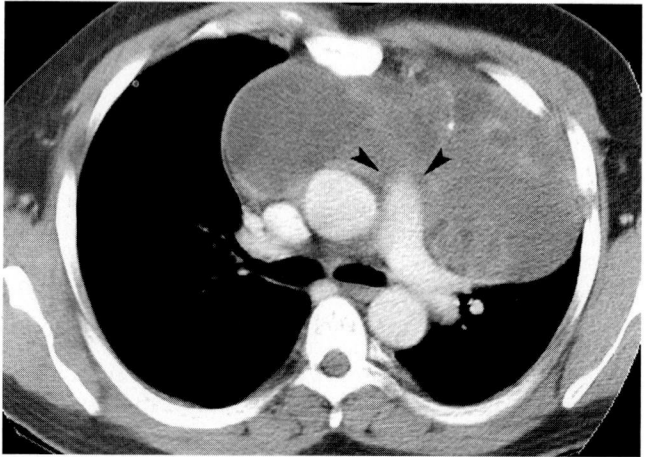

Figure 17–12. Nonseminomatous germ cell tumor: large heterogeneous anterior mediastinal mass encasing the great vessels. *Arrowheads* point to encasement of main pulmonary artery.

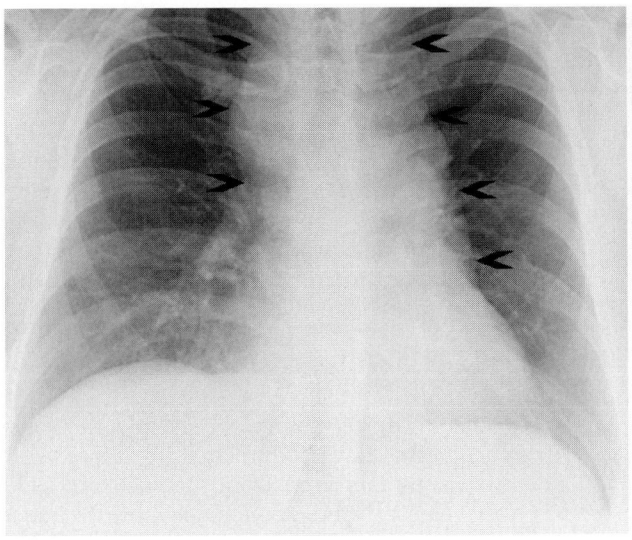
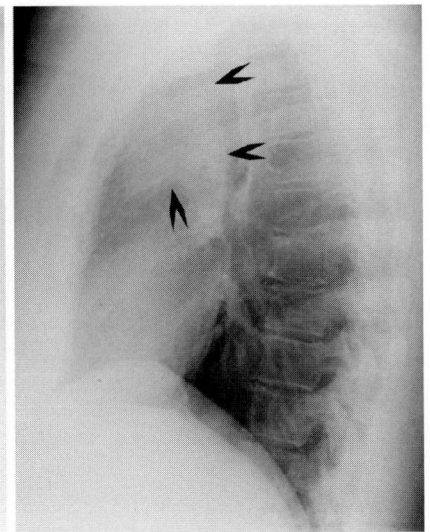

A

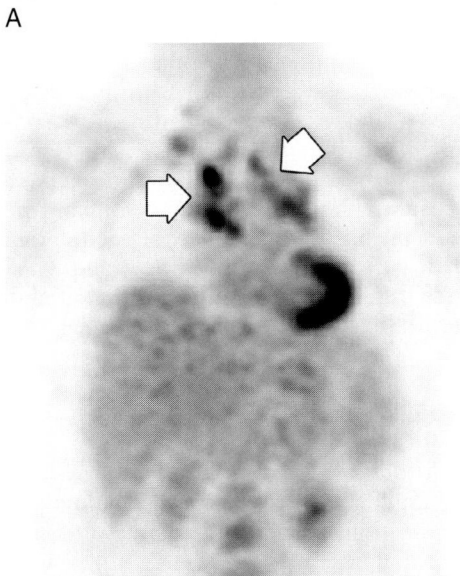

B

Figure 17–13. Non-Hodgkin's lymphoma. **A**, PA and lateral radiographs show enlargement of the mediastinal contour and the corresponding soft tissue mass in the superior retrosternal space due to lymphadenopathy. **B**, ¹⁸F-fluorodeoxyglucose positron emission tomography (FDG-PET) coronal image demonstrates increased metabolic activity in the corresponding mediastinal lymph nodes.

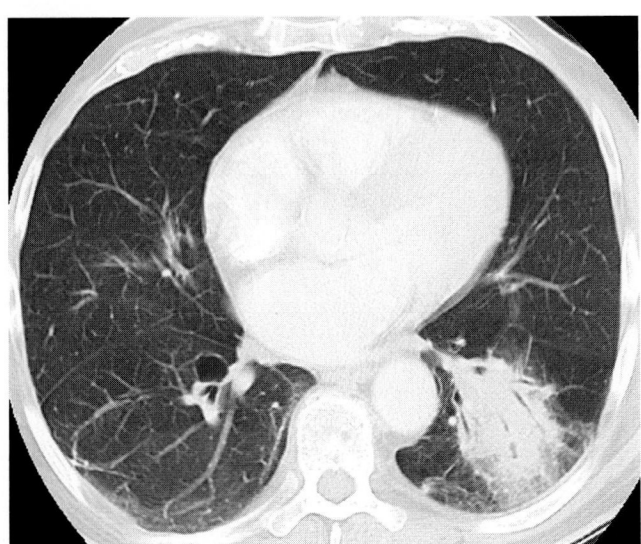

Figure 17–14. Primary lymphoma of the lung presenting as a dense consolidation with air bronchograms.

carcinoma.[63,64] Primary pleural neoplasms are most commonly mesothelioma and less commonly localized fibrous tumor and pleural liposarcoma.[64]

Mesothelioma

Mesothelioma of the pleura is a rare, aggressive, and usually fatal malignant neoplasm that in 80% of cases reported in the Western World affects individuals occupationally exposed to asbestos through various industries.[65-67] Mesothelioma appears to have a complex etiology in which environmental carcinogens (asbestos and erionite), ionizing radiation, viruses, and genetic factors act alone or in concert to cause malignancy.[67,68] Between 2000 and 3000 new cases are expected to be diagnosed annually in the United States. The tumor affects both visceral and parietal pleura. Its natural history involves aggressive local growth with encasement and invasion of the lung, vital mediastinal structures, and the chest wall.[65,66]

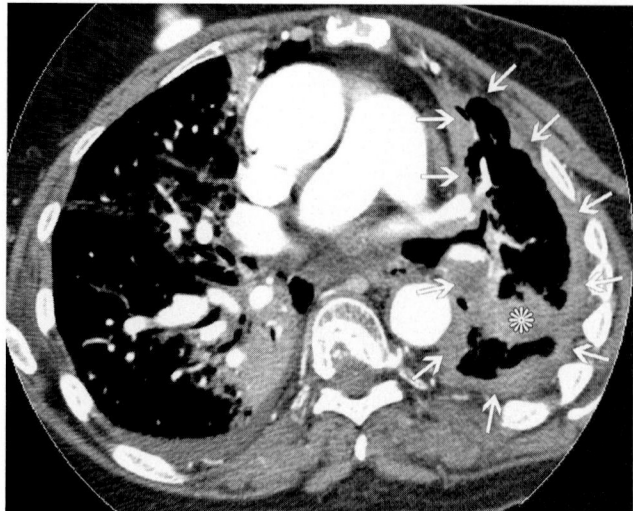

Figure 17–15. Mesothelioma: circumferential left pleural mass extending into the major fissure (*asterisk*) and encasing the lung (*arrows*).

Difficulties in diagnosis, staging, and treatment set this disease apart from other malignancies.[66] The pathologic diagnosis of mesothelioma is difficult because it may mimic metastatic adenocarcinoma[65] and may have a variable radiologic presentation.[65]

Chest radiographs, CT, MRI, and FDG PET scanning are commonly used in the diagnosis and staging of malignant mesothelioma. The most common radiographic findings on CT include pleural thickening, including thickening of the pleural surfaces of the interlobar fissures, and pleural effusions (Fig. 17-15). Contraction of the involved hemithorax is frequently present.[69] Mediastinal shift as well as disease beyond the parietal pleura, chest wall, mediastinum, lymph nodes, and diaphragm can also be seen.[69]

When pleural thickening is present, the main differential diagnosis in addition to mesothelioma includes pleural thickening due to benign causes (empyema, infections, fibrothorax, and idiopathic exudates) and adenocarcinoma involving the pleura.[70] Mediastinal pleural involvement, circumferential pleural thickening, nodularity, irregularity of pleural contour, and infiltration of the chest wall or diaphragm, or both, are most suggestive of a malignant disease both on CT and MRI, whereas pleural calcification on CT is suggestive of a benign cause.[70,71]

Localized Tumor of the Pleura

Solitary fibrous tumor of the pleura is a nonepithelial neoplasm that is unrelated to asbestos exposure.[72,73] These tumors arise from mesenchymal cells underlying the pleura[74] and arise much more frequently from the visceral than the parietal or mediastinal pleura. The tumor may have benign or malignant histologic features, but these do not always predict the clinical behavior of the tumor. In most cases, the tumor appears pedunculated[74] and has the appearance of a circumscribed, spheric or ovoid, noncalcified lesion arising along the pleural surface[63] (Fig. 17-16). Fibrous tumors of the pleura are characterized by low signal intensity on all MRI sequences, which is explained by high collagen content within the tumors' stroma and which might help include this in the preoperative differential diagnosis of a pleural-based mass.[75]

CHEST WALL MASSES

A multitude of disorders affect the chest wall, including congenital and infectious abnormalities, inflammatory and infectious conditions, and soft-tissue and bone tumors. Tumors may arise from any tissue found in the

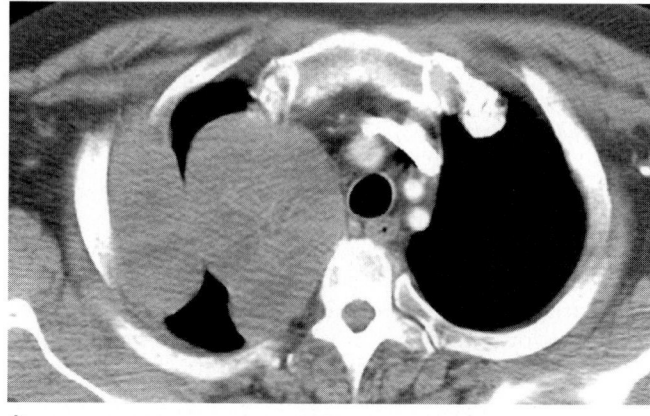

A

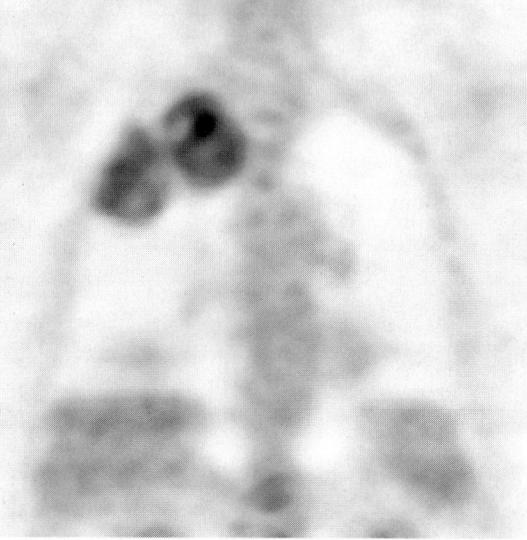

B

Figure 17–16. Malignant fibrous tumor of the pleura. **A,** CT scan demonstrating a large bilobed right pleural mass. **B,** Increased metabolic activity seen on FDG PET coronal image.

chest wall: muscles, bone, cartilage, fat, fibrous connective tissue, nerves, breast tissue, blood, and lymphatic vessels. As masses expand into the lung, they usually displace the pleura and produce an obtuse angle with the chest wall on radiographs, CT scans, and MR images. When rib changes are detected, a mass can be reliably diagnosed as extrapleural.[76]

RADIATION CHANGES

Cancers in the chest treated with radiation are lung, breast, esophageal, and mediastinal tumors, most commonly lymphoma, and head and neck tumors.[77,78] Radiation therapy is used for cure, and palliation, either alone or in combination with surgery or chemotherapy.[77]

Radiation-induced thoracic injuries are classified as lung injuries, mediastinal injuries, cardiovascular injuries, and chest wall injuries, and their appearance varies with the angle of the beam and shape of the radiation portal. The severity or radiation damage to the lung is determined by technical factors (total dose, dose rate and fractionation, portals and beam arrangement) as well as patient factors such as preexisting lung condition and functional capacity of the irradiated portion of the lung. Chemotherapeutic agents potentate the effect of radiation injury, whereas steroids may alleviate the manifestations of radiation pneumonitis.[78] Most manifestations of radiation-induced injury are subclinical, and the patients remain asymptomatic. The radiation-induced lung disease is usually, but not always, confined to the radiation volume.[77,78]

Radiation-induced lung disease occurs in two clinical stages: (1) the early stage, which usually occurs in the first 4 to 12 weeks, is characterized by radiation-induced pneumonitis and (2) the late stage, which represents radiation fibrosis. The evolution of the fibrosis extends over a period of 6 to 24 months and usually remains stable after 2 years (Fig. 17-17).[78] CT is a sensitive and accurate method of evaluation of radiation-induced lung disease. Libshitz and Shuman described four patterns of findings in irradiated lung. The first two patterns are believed to reflect the acute exudative stage of radiation-induced injury. The first pattern is represented by ground-glass opacity or homogeneous consolidation, and the second involves patchy consolidation in the lung that does not conform to the shape of the portal. The third pattern, presumed to correspond to an organizing or proliferative phase of radiation-induced pneumonitis, is described as discrete consolidation that conforms to the shape of the portal but does not outline it uniformly. Finally, the fourth pattern that corresponds to the chronic fibrotic phase has the appearance of solid consolidation that conforms to the irradiated areas of the lung (Fig. 17-18).[13,78,79] The usual findings of fibrosis are volume loss, architectural distortion, bronchiectasis, and pleural thickening. These bronchiectatic changes become stable 9 to 12 months after the completion of radiation therapy. Filling in of these bronchiectatic bronchi at a later stage may serve as an indicator of locally recurrent bronchogenic carcinoma.[80]

More uncommon complications of radiation treatment to the lung include pulmonary necrosis, and bronchiolitis

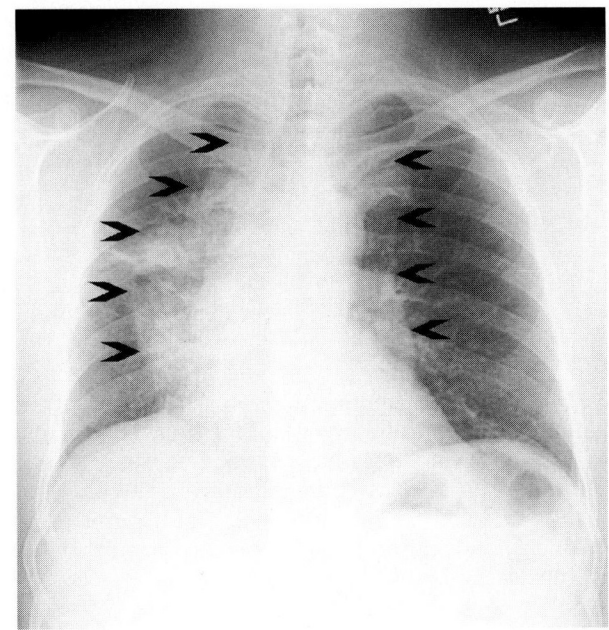

Figure 17–17. Postradiation changes: bilateral paramediastinal consolidation with sharply defined borders (*arrowheads*) corresponding to the radiation port.

obliterans with organizing pneumonia. In addition, spontaneous pneumothorax, mesothelioma, and lung cancer have been described as complications of radiation therapy.[77]

Radiation effects are not limited to the lungs. In the mediastinum, radiation effects include thymic cysts, calcified lymph nodes, and injuries to the esophagus. Cardiovascular complications have also been described; their onset is usually late and gradual. These injuries include premature coronary artery stenosis, calcifications of the ascending aorta, pericardial disease, valvular injuries, and conduction abnormalities. Breast cancer risk

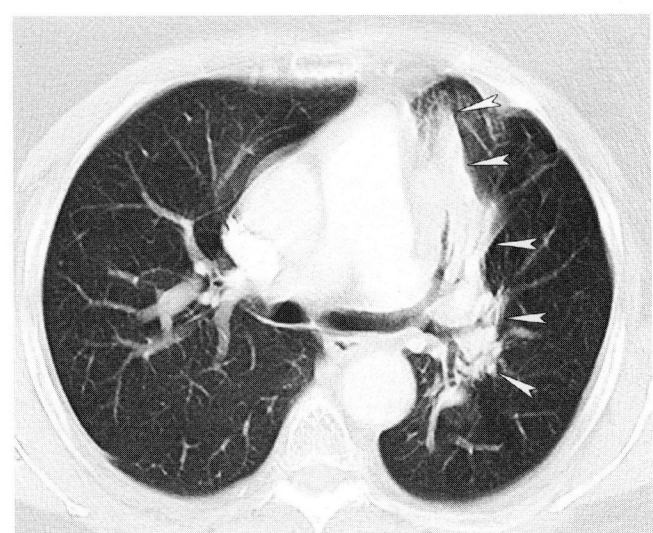

Figure 17–18. Postradiation changes: left paramediastinal lung consolidation with sharp borders that conforms to the radiation port.

is increased in women who receive thoracic irradiation before the age of 30. Chest wall complications are also well-recognized albeit infrequent. They include radiation-induced sarcomas, osteochondromas, and rib or clavicle fractures.[77]

CONCLUSION

Imaging is a vital part in the initial diagnosis and staging, monitoring of treatment response and complications, and follow-up for recurrence of malignancies of the thorax. Radiologic technology has advanced rapidly with the advent of rapid acquisition multislice CT, MRI, and PET scanning. In the future we can look forward to many applications of three-dimensional imaging, refinements in noninvasive CT and MRI angiography, as well as functional and molecular imaging. The rapid acquisition of data and digital transmission of images will further facilitate the access to studies by clinicians.

REFERENCES

1. Frush DP, Donnelly LF, Chotas HG: Contemporary pediatric thoracic imaging. *AJR Am J Roentgenol.* 2000;175:841.
2. Lufkin RB: *The MRI Manual, 2nd ed.* St. Louis: Mosby; 1998: xiii, 466.
3. Knisely BL, Broderick LS, Kuhlman JE: MR imaging of the pleura and chest wall. *Magn Reson Imaging Clin N Am.* 2000;8:125.
4. Kuhlman JE, Bouchardy L, Fishman EK, Zerhouni EA: CT and MR imaging evaluation of chest wall disorders. *Radiographics.* 1994;14:571.
5. Pandit N, Gonen M, Krug L, Larson SM: Prognostic value of [(18)F]FDG-PET imaging in small cell lung cancer. *Eur J Nucl Med Mol Imaging.* 2003;30:78.
6. Vansteenkiste JF, Stroobants SG, Dupont PJ, et al: Prognostic importance of the standardized uptake value on (18)F-fluoro-2-deoxy-glucose-positron emission tomography scan in non–small-cell lung cancer: An analysis of 125 cases. Leuven Lung Cancer Group. *J Clin Oncol.* 1999;17:3201.
7. Jeong HJ, Min JJ, Park JM, et al: Determination of the prognostic value of [(18)F]fluorodeoxyglucose uptake by using positron emission tomography in patients with non–small cell lung cancer. *Nucl Med Commun.* 2002;23:865.
8. Erasmus JJ, McAdams HP, Patz EF Jr, et al: Thoracic FDG PET: State of the art. *Radiographics.* 1998;18:5.
9. Townsend DW, Beyer T: A combined PET/CT scanner: The path to true image fusion. *Br J Radiol.* 2002;75 Spec No:S24.
10. Steinert HC, von Schulthess GK: Initial clinical experience using a new integrated in-line PET/CT system. *Br J Radiol.* 2002;75 Spec No:S36.
11. Pearson FG: *Thoracic Surgery, 2nd ed.* New York: Churchill Livingstone; 2002:xxv, 1942.
12. Felson B: *Chest Roentgenology.* Philadelphia: WB Saunders; 1973:viii, 574.
13. McLoud TC: *Thoracic Radiology.* St. Louis: Mosby; 1998: xvi, 541.
14. Kawashima A, Fishman EK, Kuhlman JE, Nixon MS: CT of posterior mediastinal masses. *Radiographics.* 1991;11:1045.
15. American Cancer Society: *Cancer Facts & Figures.* Atlanta: The Society; 2003:v.
16. The American Thoracic Society and The European Respiratory Society: Pretreatment evaluation of non–small-cell lung cancer. *Am J Respir Crit Care Med.* 1997;156:320.
17. Patz EF Jr: Imaging bronchogenic carcinoma. *Chest.* 2000;117:90S.
18. Quinn D, Gianlupi A, Broste S: The changing radiographic presentation of bronchogenic carcinoma with reference to cell types. *Chest.* 1996;110:1474.

19. Rosado-de-Christenson ML, Templeton PA, Moran CA: Bronchogenic carcinoma: Radiologic-pathologic correlation. *Radiographics.* 1994;14:429; quiz 447.
20. Epstein DM: Bronchioloalveolar carcinoma. *Semin Roentgenol.* 1990;25:105.
21. Berkmen YM: The many faces of bronchiolo-alveolar carcinoma. *Semin Roentgenol.* 1977;12:207.
22. Adler B, Padley S, Miller RR, Muller NL: High-resolution CT of bronchioloalveolar carcinoma. *AJR Am J Roentgenol.* 1992; 159:275.
23. Weisbrod GL, Towers MJ, Chamberlain DW, et al: Thin-walled cystic lesions in bronchioalveolar carcinoma. *Radiology.* 1992;185:401.
24. Huang D, Weisbrod GL, Chamberlain DW: Unusual radiologic presentations of bronchioloalveolar carcinoma. *Can Assoc Radiol J.* 1986;37:94.
25. Haque AK: Pathology of carcinoma of lung: An update on current concepts. *J Thorac Imaging.* 1991;7:9.
26. Hartman TE, Tazelaar HD, Swensen SJ, Muller NL: Cigarette smoking: CT and pathologic findings of associated pulmonary diseases. *Radiographics.* 1997;17:377.
27. Iyoda A, Hiroshima K, Toyozaki T, et al: Clinical characterization of pulmonary large cell neuroendocrine carcinoma and large cell carcinoma with neuroendocrine morphology. *Cancer.* 2001; 91:1992.
28. Carretta A, Ceresoli GL, Arrigoni G, et al: Diagnostic and therapeutic management of neuroendocrine lung tumors: A clinical study of 44 cases. *Lung Cancer.* 2000;29:217.
29. Martini N, Melamed MR: Multiple primary lung cancers. *J Thorac Cardiovasc Surg.* 1975;70:606.
30. Bower SL, Choplin RH, Muss HB: Multiple primary bronchogenic carcinomas of the lung. *AJR Am J Roentgenol.* 1983;140:253.
31. Lee PN: Lung cancer and type of cigarette smoked. *Inhal Toxicol.* 2001;13:951.
32. Hoffmann D, Djordjevic MV, Hoffmann I: The changing cigarette. *Prev Med.* 1997;26:427.
33. Toloza EM, Harpole L, McCrory DC: Noninvasive staging of non–small cell lung cancer: A review of the current evidence. *Chest.* 2003;123:137S.
34. Miller JD, Gorenstein LA, Patterson GA: Staging: The key to rational management of lung cancer. *Ann Thorac Surg.* 1992; 53:170.
35. Silvestri GA, Tanoue LT, Margolis ML, et al: The noninvasive staging of non–small cell lung cancer: The guidelines. *Chest.* 2003; 123:147S.
36. Jemal A, Thomas A, Murray T, Thun M: Cancer statistics, 2002. *CA Cancer J Clin.* 2002;52:23.
37. Toloza EM, Harpole L, Detterbeck F, McCrory DC: Invasive staging of non–small cell lung cancer: A review of the current evidence. *Chest.* 2003;123:157S.
38. Dwamena BA, Sonnad SS, Angobaldo JO, Wahl RL: Metastases from non–small cell lung cancer: Mediastinal staging in the 1990s—Meta-analytic comparison of PET and CT. *Radiology.* 1999;213:530.
39. von Haag DW, Follette DM, Roberts PF, et al: Advantages of positron emission tomography over computed tomography in mediastinal staging of non–small cell lung cancer. *J Surg Res.* 2002;103:160.
40. Dunagan D, Chin R Jr, McCain T, et al: Staging by positron emission tomography predicts survival in patients with non–small cell lung cancer. *Chest.* 2001;119:333.
41. Boiselle PM: MR imaging of thoracic lymph nodes. A comparison of computed tomography and positron emission tomography. *Magn Reson Imaging Clin N Am.* 2000;8:33.
42. Saunders CA, Dussek JE, O'Doherty MJ, Maisey MN: Evaluation of fluorine-18-fluorodeoxyglucose whole body positron emission tomography imaging in the staging of lung cancer. *Ann Thorac Surg.* 1999;67:790.
43. Mountain CF, Dresler CM: Regional lymph node classification for lung cancer staging. *Chest.* 1997;1718.
44. Niell HB: Extensive stage small cell lung cancer. *Curr Treat Options Oncol.* 2001;2:71.
45. Simon GR, Wagner H: Small cell lung cancer. *Chest.* 2003; 123:259S.
46. Komaki R, Chasen MH, Travis WD, et al: Oncodiagnosis panel: 1999. Cancer of the lung: Oncodiagnosis. *Radiographics.* 2001;21:1573.

47. Quint LE, Park CH, Iannettoni MD: Solitary pulmonary nodules in patients with extrapulmonary neoplasms. *Radiology.* 2000; 217:257.

48. Ginsberg MS, Griff SK, Go BD, et al: Pulmonary nodules resected at video-assisted thoracoscopic surgery: Etiology in 426 patients. *Radiology.* 1999;213:277.

49. Seo JB, Im JG, Goo JM, et al: Atypical pulmonary metastases: Spectrum of radiologic findings. *Radiographics.* 2001;21:403.

50. Gross BH, Glazer GM, Bookstein FL: Multiple pulmonary nodules detected by computed tomography: Diagnostic implications. *J Comput Assist Tomogr.* 1985;9:880.

51. Ginsberg MS, Panicek DM: Subcentimeter pulmonary nodules detected in patients with sarcoma. *Sarcoma.* 2000;4:63.

52. Gimenez A, Franquet T, Prats R, et al: Unusual primary lung tumors: A radiologic-pathologic overview. *Radiographics.* 2002;22:601.

53. Swensen SJ, Jett JR, Hartman TE, et al: Lung cancer screening with CT: Mayo Clinic experience. *Radiology.* 2003;226:756.

54. Henschke CI, McCauley DI, Yankelevitz DF, et al: Early lung cancer action project: Overall design and findings from baseline screening. *Lancet.* 1999;354:99.

55. Laurent F, Latrabe V, Lecesne R, et al: Mediastinal masses: Diagnostic approach. *Eur Radiol.* 1998;8:1148.

56. Azarow KS, Pearl RH, Zurcher R, et al: Primary mediastinal masses. A comparison of adult and pediatric populations. *J Thorac Cardiovasc Surg.* 1993;106:67.

57. Santana L, Givica A, Camacho C: Best cases from the AFIP: Thymoma. *Radiographics.* 2002;22 Spec No:S95-S102.

58. Santana L, Givica A, Camacho C: Best cases from the AFIP: Thymoma. *Radiographics.* 2002;22:S95.

59. Sakai F, Sone S, Kiyono K, et al. MR imaging of thymoma: Radiologic-pathologic correlation. *Am J Roentgenol.* 1992; 158:751.

60. Drevelegas A, Palladas P, Scordalaki A: Mediastinal germ cell tumors: A radiologic-pathologic review. *Eur Radiol.* 2001; 11:1925.

61. Harris NL, Jaffe ES, Diebold J, et al: World Health Organization classification of neoplastic diseases of the hematopoietic and lymphoid tissues: Report of the Clinical Advisory Committee meeting—Airlie House, Va, November 1997. *J Clin Oncol.* 1999;17:3835.

62. Au V, Leung AN: Radiologic manifestations of lymphoma in the thorax. *AJR Am J Roentgenol.* 1997;168:93.

63. Dynes MC, White EM, Fry WA, Ghahremani GG: Imaging manifestations of pleural tumors. *Radiographics.* 1992;12:1191.

64. Bonomo L, Feragalli B, Sacco R, et al: Malignant pleural disease. *Eur J Radiol.* 2000;34:98.

65. Miller BH, Rosado-de-Christenson ML, Mason AC, et al: From the archives of the AFIP. Malignant pleural mesothelioma: Radiologic-pathologic correlation. *Radiographics.* 1996;16:613.

66. Zellos LS, Sugarbaker DJ: Diffuse malignant mesothelioma of the pleural space and its management. *Oncology (Huntingt).* 2002; 16:907; discussions 916, 919, 925.

67. Carbone M, Kratzke RA, Testa JR: The pathogenesis of mesothelioma. *Semin Oncol.* 2002;29:2.

68. Heineman EF, Bernstein L, Stark AD, Spirtas R: Mesothelioma, asbestos, and reported history of cancer in first-degree relatives. *Cancer.* 1996;77:549.

69. Kawashima A, Libshitz HI: Malignant pleural mesothelioma: CT manifestations in 50 cases. *AJR Am J Roentgenol.* 1990; 155:965.

70. Statement on malignant mesothelioma in the United Kingdom. *Thorax.* 2001;56:250.

71. Hierholzer J, Luo L, Bittner RC, et al: MRI and CT in the differential diagnosis of pleural disease. *Chest.* 2000;118:604.

72. Rusch VW: Diagnosis and treatment of pleural mesothelioma. *Semin Surg Oncol.* 1990;6:279.

73. Briselli M, Mark EJ, Dickersin GR: Solitary fibrous tumors of the pleura: Eight new cases and review of 360 cases in the literature. *Cancer.* 1981;47:2678.

74. de Perrot M: Fibrous tumors of the pleura. *Curr Treat Options Oncol.* 2000;1:293.

75. Ferretti GR, Chiles C, Cox JE, et al: Localized benign fibrous tumors of the pleura: MR appearance. *J Comput Assist Tomogr.* 1997;21:115.

76. Jeung MY, Gangi A, Gasser B, et al: Imaging of chest wall disorders. *Radiographics.* 1999;19:617.

77. Mesurolle B, Qanadli SD, Merad M, et al: Unusual radiologic findings in the thorax after radiation therapy. *Radiographics.* 2000;20:67.

78. Park KJ, Chung JY, Chun MS, Suh JH: Radiation-induced lung disease and the impact of radiation methods on imaging features. *Radiographics.* 2000;20:83.

79. Libshitz HI, Shuman LS: Radiation-induced pulmonary change: CT findings. *J Comput Assist Tomogr.* 1984;8:15.

80. Libshitz HI, Sheppard DG: Filling in of radiation therapy-induced bronchiectatic change: A reliable sign of locally recurrent lung cancer. *Radiology.* 1999;210:25.

18

Abdomen

Bilal Hameed, MD, and Fergus V. Coakley, MD

Imaging of intra-abdominal malignancy has steadily evolved in recent decades. Current radiologic modalities allow for the accurate detection, characterization, and staging of many tumors. Contrast-enhanced computed tomography (CT) is the workhorse of oncologic abdominal imaging, with supplementation by ultrasound (US) and magnetic resonance (MR) imaging in select situations. Targeted biopsy can be performed under US or CT guidance, although US guidance is preferred if the lesion is clearly visible sonographically. MR-guided biopsy is available only in a few centers and is not part of routine practice. Positron emission tomography (PET) shows great promise in the staging of intra-abdominal malignancy, although PET lacks the spatial resolution for accurate anatomical localization before surgery. Combined PET/CT scanners are beginning to enter clinical practice, and may provide the optimal combination of anatomic and metabolic imaging for the detection and localization of malignant disease sites. In this chapter, we review basic principles and applications of abdominal CT because CT is the cornerstone of modern abdominal imaging. We then review the normal relevant imaging anatomy and the standard radiologic approach to cholangiocarcinoma, gallbladder carcinoma, pancreatic carcinoma, retroperitoneal lymphadenopathy, and gastric carcinoma. These sites and diseases have been chosen for specific discussion because of their pertinence to radiation oncology.

COMPUTED TOMOGRAPHY TECHNOLOGY AND TERMINOLOGY

Three distinct generations of CT technology are currently in use. In order of historical development and scanner speed, they are conventional CT, spiral (or helical) CT, and multi-slice (or multi-detector) CT. Rapid scanning is a desirable feature in abdominal CT for two reasons. First, unlike the brain, the abdomen moves with respiration, and imaging during a single breath hold removes the risk of respiratory misregistration (i.e., structures missed between slices because successive breath holds are not identical). Furthermore, in uncooperative patients, rapid scanning helps reduce image degradation by motion artifact. Second, many applications in abdominal imaging are affected by the time images are acquired relative to the bolus of intravenous contrast medium, and accurate diagnosis may require imaging precisely timed to one or more phases of enhancement. Sir Godfrey Hounsfield

invented CT in 1972, with initial clinical installations in 1974. The first CT scanner developed by Hounsfield in his laboratory at EMI required several hours to acquire the data for a single slice and took several days to reconstruct the corresponding image. Data acquisition and image reconstruction became progressively faster during the 1970s and 1980s, although the speed of the scanners remained limited by the need for "stop-start" slice-by-slice acquisition. That is, in conventional CT, an axial slice is generated by rotating an x-ray tube and detector array in a 360-degree circle around the patient. After a 360-degree rotation, the rotating gantry reverses direction to prevent disruption of the tethered cables that transfer the data from the detector array to the computer. Such sequential slice acquisition limits the speed of conventional CT, prevents volumetric data acquisition, results in slice misregistration, and limits temporal resolution such that multi-phase volumetric scanning is not possible. The development of spiral (or helical) CT in the late 1980s signified a technological breakthrough. In spiral CT, data is carried from the rotating gantry to the computer by slip rings, which allows for continuous x-ray tube rotation and data transfer. Scanning can be performed while the patient is moved slowly but continuously through the gantry. The ability to continuously scan allows for "non-stop" volumetric data acquisition. Data is gathered on a three-dimensional volume in a spiral fashion. Images are reconstructed from the data volume. Physical and clinical performance studies of spiral CT were first reported at the 1989 Radiological Society of North America meeting.[1] The first commercially available spiral CT scanner was released in 1990 (Somatom Plus, Siemens Medical Systems, Malvern, Pa.).[2]

Spiral CT was an important technological advance, but many limitations and compromises remained. The rotational speed of the x-ray tube was generally 1 rotation per second, and clinical results suggested that a pitch (ratio of longitudinal distance moved by the tabletop during one x-ray tube rotation to beam collimation) greater than 2 was undesirable. As a result, either large volumes could be covered, or thin sections acquired, but not both. The Elscint CT Twin scanner employed a dual array of two side-by-side detector rows, and represented an early version of multi-slice technology.[3] However, while this scanner was an improvement over single detector spiral CT in terms of coverage,[4] substantial limitations persisted. It was not until 1998 that a scanner with four detector rows became commercially available (Lightspeed,

General Electric Medical Systems, Waukesha, Wisc.). Modern multi-slice CT using four or more detector rows essentially abolishes the remaining obstacles to rapid isotropic (i.e., equal resolution in all three dimensions) volumetric imaging by using multiple side-by-side detectors simultaneously. The most recent scanners use up to 16 detector rows. Such multi-slice CT systems can collect multiple slices of data in about 350 milliseconds and reconstruct a 512 × 512 matrix image from millions of data points in less than a second. An entire body cavity (brain, chest, or abdomen) can be scanned in 5 to 10 seconds using the most advanced multi-slice CT systems. Faster imaging with modern scanners is due not only to multiple detector rows, but also to increased x-ray tube rotational speed. Many commercial scanners are now capable of a complete rotation in 0.5 second or less. Multi-slice CT has been a major advance in several areas of abdominal imaging, particularly those requiring imaging in multiple phases of enhancement after intravenous contrast medium administration (Fig. 18-1) and rapid near-isotropic volumetric acquisition, such as CT angiography (Fig. 18-2). The ability to acquire scans of the abdomen

during multiple phases of enhancement is particularly helpful when both arteriographic and parenchymal phases of enhancement are required for complete evaluation. For example, the arteriographic phase is critical for the assessment of arterial encasement in pancreatic cancer, but parenchymal enhancement phases are required for demonstration of the primary tumor and detection of hepatic metastases.

A potential source of confusion that arises with respect to multi-slice CT is the definition of pitch. Pitch can be defined in one of two ways: (1) as the ratio of longitudinal distance moved by the tabletop during one x-ray tube rotation to beam collimation or (2) the ratio of longitudinal distance moved by the tabletop during one x-ray tube rotation to slice thickness. In single-detector spiral CT, these two definitions are the same, since the slice thickness is the beam collimation. In multi-slice CT, the collimated beam is split into several slices, and therefore the definitions of pitch are different. For example, a four-channel multi-slice scanner acquiring 2.5 mm thick slices (beam collimation of 10 mm) at a tabletop speed of 15 mm per 1 second x-ray tube rotation could be defined as having

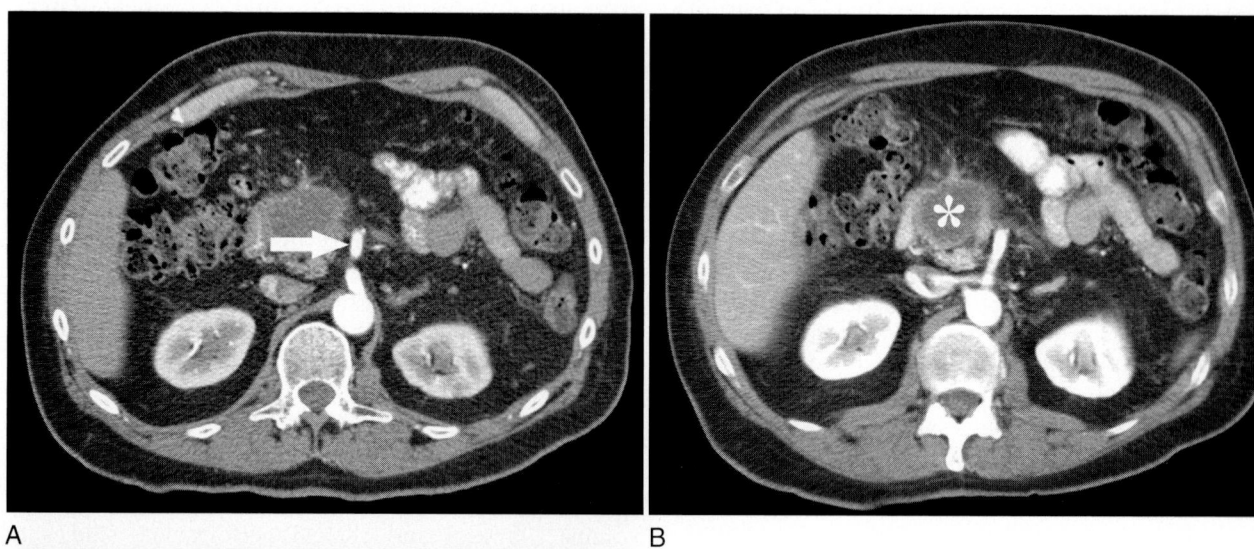

A
B

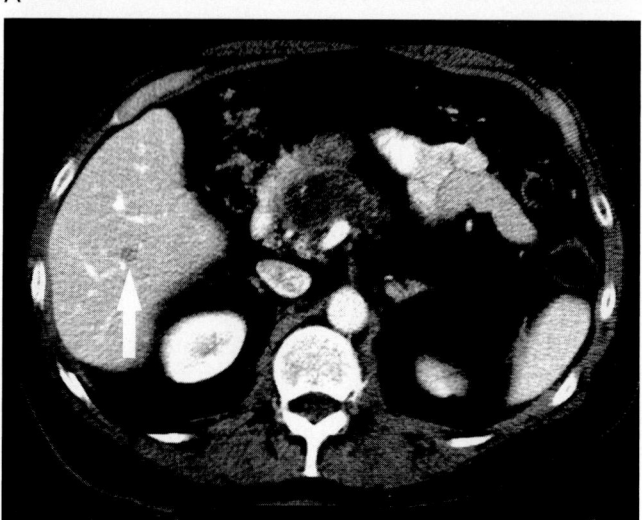

C

Figure 18–1. The ability to obtain multiple sequential images in different phases of enhancement is a major advantage of multi-slice computed tomography (CT), since different parameters are optimally evaluated in different phases of enhancement. **A,** Multi-slice CT performed during the arteriographic phase of enhancement in a 67-year-old patient with pancreatic cancer. The superior mesenteric artery (*arrow*) is well opacified, and is not encased by tumor. **B,** Image obtained in a slightly later phase of enhancement shows a greater degree of parenchymal enhancement. The tumor (*asterisk*) is well seen and is predominantly hypovascular. **C,** Image obtained in the portal venous stage of enhancement and displayed at a liver window shows a small hypodense lesion (*arrow*) in the liver, which may be a metastasis.

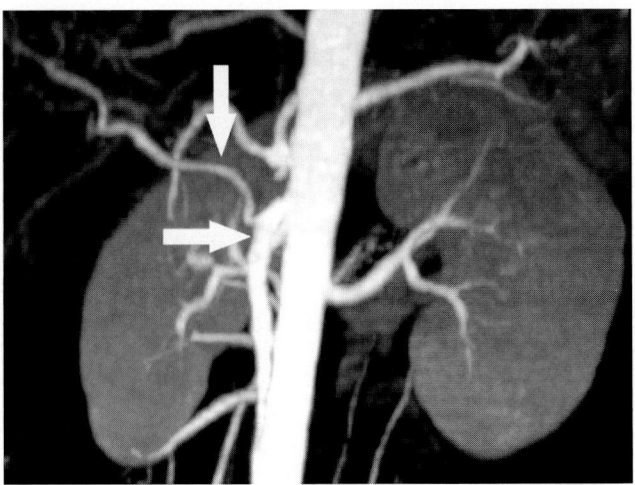

Figure 18–2. Computed tomography (CT) arteriogram in a 26-year-old patient being evaluated as a potential living related right hepatic lobe donor. An aberrant right hepatic artery (*vertical arrow*) is seen arising from the superior mesenteric artery (*horizontal arrow*). With the advent of multi-slice CT, noninvasive arteriography can be performed routinely and with near-isotropic resolution (i.e., equal spatial resolution in all three planes), and the era of diagnostic catheter angiography is coming to an end.

a pitch of 6 (longitudinal distance moved by the tabletop during one x-ray tube rotation/slice thickness = 15/2.5 = 6) or 1.5 (longitudinal distance moved by the tabletop during one x-ray tube rotation/beam collimation = 15/10 = 1.5). There is no current consensus on which definition is preferable. While most manufacturers use the ratio of longitudinal distance moved by the tabletop during one x-ray tube rotation to slice thickness, there are arguments related to basic science and calculation of radiation dose that suggest the alternative definition is more appropriate. In any event, it is important to clarify which definition of pitch is being used when describing CT protocols and parameters for multi-slice scanners.

One of the unfortunate consequences of the increased ability to obtain multi-phase imaging has been a corresponding increase in confusion with respect to the proper terminology for these studies.[5] It has reasonably been suggested that the term *phase* should not be applied to non-contrast images.[6] It also seems reasonable to use the term *arteriographic phase* for early arterial images in which contrast is primarily within the arteries, and the term *parenchymal arterial phase* for the subsequent period of early tissue enhancement when hypervascular masses are most prominent. Later periods of image acquisition can be referred to as *portal venous* or *delayed*, as appropriate. Until a universal terminology is established, it is probably best to avoid unclear terms such as *dual* or *triple* phase studies, and instead describe the specific phases acquired.

CHOLANGIOCARCINOMA

Normal Anatomy

Bile is collected from the hepatocytes by a system of small intrahepatic ducts that drain from the liver through the right and left hepatic ducts. The right and left hepatic ducts join together shortly after leaving the liver in the porta hepatis. This confluence forms the common hepatic duct. The common hepatic duct joins with the cystic duct from the gallbladder to form the common bile duct. The common bile duct lies lateral to the common hepatic artery and anterior to the portal vein. The distal one third of the common bile duct passes though the pancreatic head to terminate at the ampulla of Vater. US and CT have limited ability to distinguish the entry-point of the cystic duct, and therefore the term *common duct* is frequently used in radiologic parlance to refer to both the common hepatic duct and common bile duct in combination. The regional lymph nodes for the biliary system are the pericholedochal, hilar, peripancreatic (pancreatic head group only), periduodenal, periportal, celiac, and superior mesenteric nodes.

Pathology

Cholangiocarcinomas are adenocarcinomas of the biliary ductal epithelium, and account for more than 90% of bile duct malignancies. Based on location, cholangiocarcinomas are divided into intrahepatic, proximal extrahepatic (i.e., perihilar), and distal extrahepatic. Perihilar cholangiocarcinomas, also known as Klatskin's tumors, originate at the confluence of the right and left hepatic ducts and are the most common.[7] Distal extrahepatic cholangiocarcinomas, originating from the common duct between the upper border of the pancreas and the ampulla of Vater, are the second most common. Intrahepatic cholangiocarcinomas are the least common. Cholangiocarcinomas are infiltrative tumors, and typically invade and occlude adjacent structures such as the bile ducts, portal veins, and hepatic arteries. As a result, cholangiocarcinomas are often locally advanced before clinical presentation with features of biliary obstruction such as painless jaundice, pruritus, dark urine, and pale stools. Regional extension occurs into the liver, and lymph nodes of the celiac and pancreaticoduodenal chains. Distant metastases may appear in the peritoneum, thoracic lymph nodes, and surgical or drain incisions. Intrahepatic cholangiocarcinomas may involve hepatoduodenal ligament, para-aortic, retro pancreatic, or common hepatic artery nodes. In addition, perihilar and left intrahepatic cholangiocarcinomas may spread along the left gastric nodes adjacent to the lesser curvature of the stomach.[8]

Imaging of Cholangiocarcinoma

INTRODUCTION

The traditional standard of reference for the diagnosis and staging of cholangiocarcinoma has been the combination of conventional cholangiography and angiography.[9] Modern cross-sectional imaging has largely replaced the need for these invasive tests, both with respect to diagnosis and staging. The diagnosis of cholangiocarcinoma should be suspected when US, CT, or MRI demonstrate dilated intrahepatic ducts with nondilated extrahepatic ducts in a patient with painless jaundice. Because of the infiltrative nature of cholangiocarcinoma, the primary tumor may or may not be seen, and visualization of a mass is not required to suggest the diagnosis. Potential differential diagnoses in this setting include postsurgical stricture (either iatrogenic bile duct injury or biliary enteric anastomotic stricture) or malignant masquerade (other hepatic masses, such as metastases, very rarely result in biliary dilation). Postsurgical strictures will usually be evident from the clinical history. Malignant masquerade is a rare non-neoplastic fibrous proliferation that occurs at the hilum of the liver and clinically and radiologically mimics perihilar cholangiocarcinoma.[10] In a series of 94 patients with suspected obstructive malignancy at the hilum, 8 were found to have malignant masquerade at pathologic analysis.[10] The eight patients ranged in age from 37 to 66 years, and all presented with obstructive jaundice. One later developed cholangiographic changes of sclerosing cholangitis, and it may be that malignant masquerade represents a localized mass-like form of sclerosing cholangitis.[11]

CONVENTIONAL CHOLANGIOGRAPHY

Conventional cholangiography can be performed by endoscopic retrograde cholangiopancreatography (ERCP), or percutaneous transhepatic cholangiography (PTC). ERCP has the advantages of excluding ampullary pathology by direct endoscopic evaluation and allowing for simultaneous tissue sampling. Palliative endobiliary stenting can also be performed at the same sitting. ERCP is usually favored over PTC, but the latter may be appropriate when attempts at ERCP have been unsuccessful. PTC may allow access in proximal lesions with obstruction of both right and left hepatic ducts. Tissue may be obtained for cytologic analysis and drainage performed. The typical appearance of a cholangiocarcinoma at conventional cholangiography is of a tight irregular stricture of variable length associated with marked dilation of the proximal biliary tract (Fig. 18-3).

ULTRASOUND

US is frequently the initial investigation requested in patients with suspected biliary obstruction. Klatskin tumors classically manifest at US as segmental dilation and nonunion of the right and left hepatic ducts in the porta hepatis (Fig. 18-4). The papillary and nodular ductal variants of cholangiocarcinoma are relatively easy to see at US; papillary tumors form polypoid intraluminal masses, while nodular cholangiocarcinoma manifests as a discrete smooth mass with associated mural thickening.[12] Smaller or infiltrative tumors may be missed, although experienced operators can demonstrate high sensitivity. In a retrospective study of 49 patients with pathologically proved cholangiocarcinoma, US demonstrated the tumor in 47 (96%) cases, a mass was demonstrated in 44, and focal or diffuse thickening of the bile duct wall in 3.[13] In a study of 39 patients with Klatskin tumors undergoing preoperative US,[14] ductal masses were detected in 34 patients (87%). Masses were isoechoic in 22 (65%), hypoechoic in 7 (21%), and hyperechoic in 5 (15%). Morphologic tumor patterns included nodular

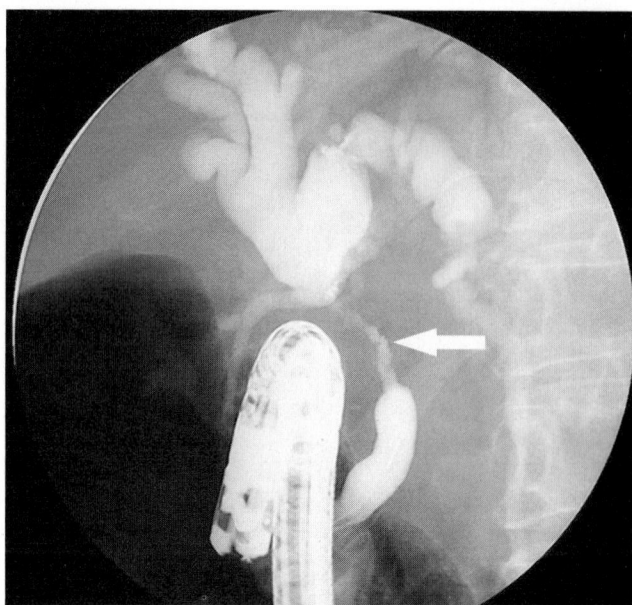

Figure 18–3. ERCP in a 64-year-old woman with cholangiocarcinoma. A tight irregular stricture (*arrow*) is seen in the mid- to upper common duct and is associated with moderate to marked dilation of the intrahepatic biliary system.

mural thickening (n = 19; 56%), irregular infiltration (n = 9; 26%), and intraductal polypoid masses (n = 6; 18%). Vascular involvement is an important determinant of irresectability, and portal vein involvement can be assessed with an accuracy of up to 91% by Doppler US.[15] In a study of 22 patients with hilar cholangiocarcinoma, vascular involvement was evaluated by Doppler US and arteriography, using operative findings as the standard of reference. Vascular patency or involvement was correctly determined by Doppler US in 19 patients (86%), compared to 18 by arteriography (82%).[16]

COMPUTED TOMOGRAPHY

Depending on referral practices, CT may be the first investigation requested in patients with painless jaundice.

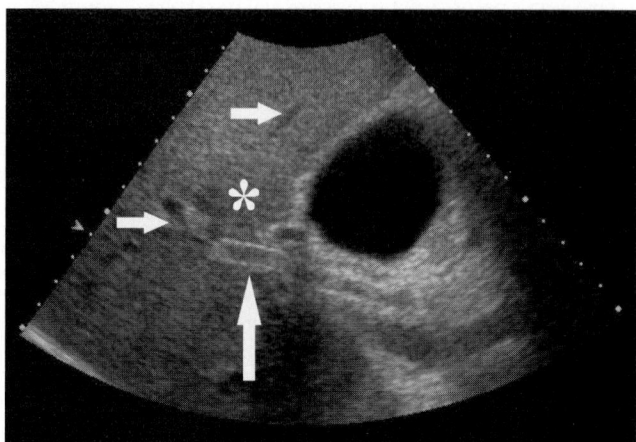

Figure 18–4. Ultrasound in a 56-year-old man with cholangiocarcinoma. A subtle mass (*asterisk*) is seen in the central liver. Dilated bile ducts (*horizontal arrows*) are visible at the periphery of the mass. A plastic endobiliary stent (*vertical arrow*) traversing the tumor is also visible.

The CT findings in Klatskin tumors resemble those seen at US, namely segmental dilatation and nonunion of the right and left hepatic ducts in the porta hepatis (Fig. 18-5). The reported frequency with which a primary tumor mass is seen varies from 40% to 91%.[17-20] Delayed enhancement is a relatively recently described finding that has been reported in 36% to 74% of cases (Fig. 18-6).[19,20] In one study, 3 of 47 cholangiocarcinomas were seen only on delayed images.[20] The optimal time for acquisition of delayed images is 10 to 20 minutes after contrast media injection.[19] Lobar atrophy is a nonspecific but useful ancillary feature of cholangiocarcinoma that may be better appreciated at CT than US. Lobar atrophy usually indicates both biliary and portal venous obstruction in that lobe. Another advantage of CT is the ability to detect metastases, such as nodal or peritoneal deposits. Adenopathy in cholangiocarcinoma arising secondary to primary sclerosing cholangitis should be interpreted with caution, since nodal enlargement in this context may be reactive or metastatic. Occasionally, CT may suggest the diagnosis of peripheral intrahepatic cholangiocarcinoma when a patient with vague or nonspecific symptoms is found to have a hypodense hepatic mass with peripheral enhancement, biliary dilation, and delayed enhancement.[21]

MAGNETIC RESONANCE IMAGING

MRI findings in cholangiocarcinoma resemble those seen at CT, isolated intrahepatic biliary dilatation with or without a visible mass (Fig. 18-7). While MRI is frequently reserved for patients with contraindications to contrast-enhanced CT, such as elevated creatinine or contrast allergy, the modality has several attractive imaging characteristics that may assist in tumor evaluation. MR cholangiography provides similar information to conventional cholangiography, and may obviate the need for invasive biliary imaging.[22] MR angiography can be used to assess vascular involvement and may replace catheter angiography for vascular evaluation. In a study of 27 preoperative

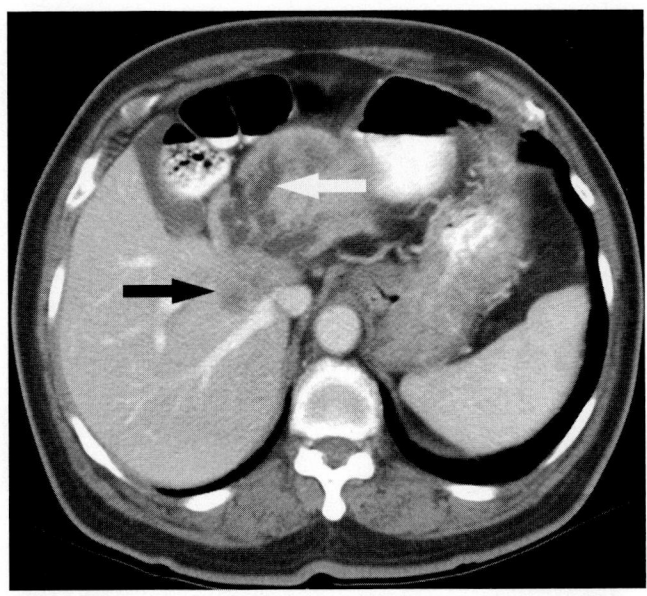

Figure 18–5. Contrast-enhanced CT in a 72-year-old man with cholangiocarcinoma. A hypodense mass (*black arrow*) is present in the central liver, with associated marked biliary dilation (*white arrow*) in the left hepatic lobe. The left lobe is also atrophic.

patients with Klatskin tumors, evaluation of vascular involvement by MRI and US were compared with intraoperative findings.[23] Encasement, thrombosis, occlusion, and nonvisualization were considered to be evidence of vascular involvement. Twelve of 16 involved veins were detected at MRI compared to 13 of 16 at US. There was one false-positive diagnosis of inferior vena cava involvement at both MR imaging and US. These results suggest that MRI and US provide comparable results for assessment of hepatic vein involvement by tumor. Central hypointensity on T2-weighted images appears to be a characteristic finding in intrahepatic cholangiocarcinoma (Fig. 18-8) and reflects severe fibrosis.[24]

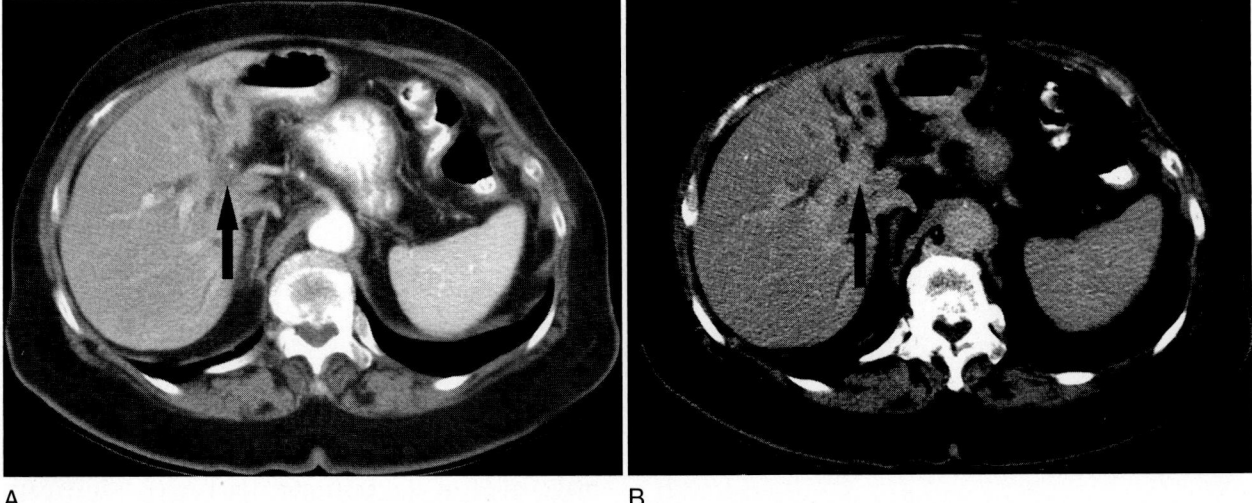

A   B

Figure 18–6. A relatively recently recognized characteristic of cholangiocarcinoma is that the tumor often demonstrates delayed enhancement, and some cholangiocarcinomas may only be seen several minutes after administration of intravenous contrast. **A,** Contrast-enhanced computed tomography (CT) in a 63-year-old woman with cholangiocarcinoma. The tumor (*arrow*) is hypovascular during the portal venous phase of enhancement. **B,** CT obtained 10 minutes after the administration of intravenous contrast. The tumor (*arrow*) is now slightly hypervascular with respect to the adjacent hepatic parenchyma.

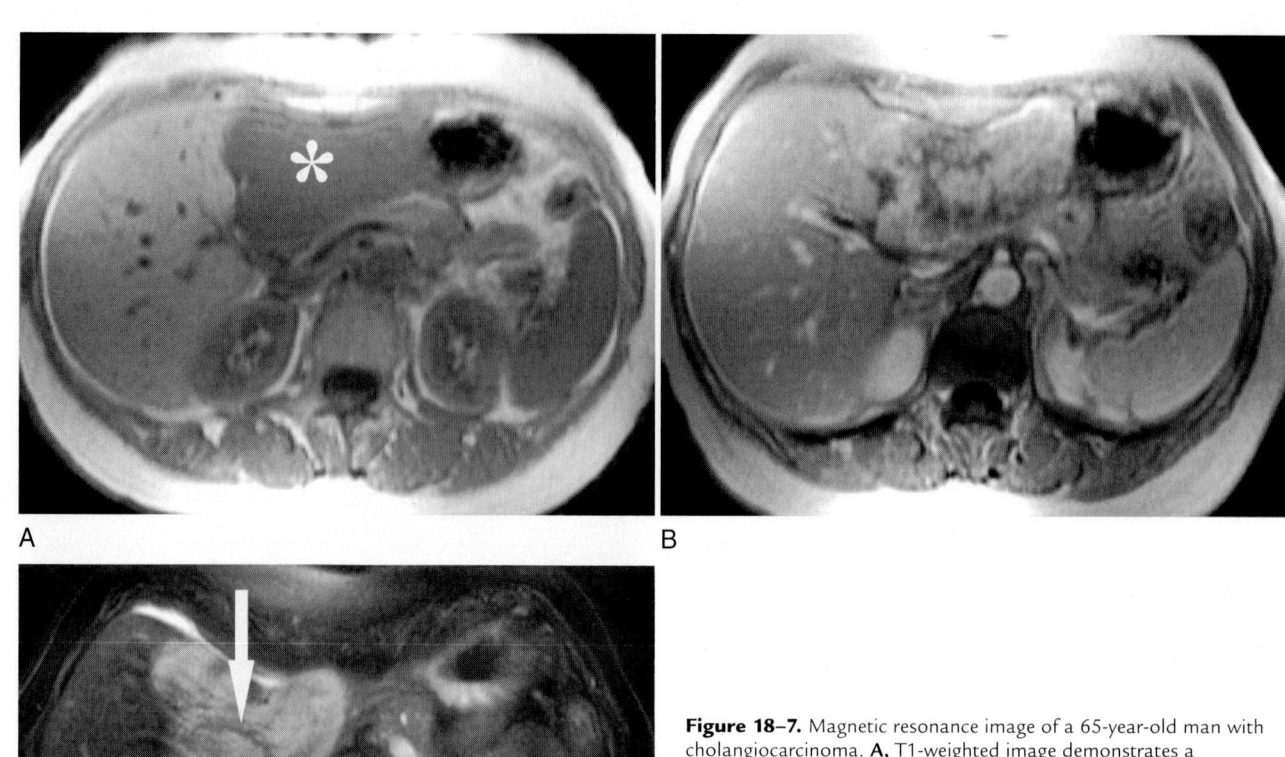

A

B

C

Figure 18–7. Magnetic resonance image of a 65-year-old man with cholangiocarcinoma. **A,** T1-weighted image demonstrates a hypointense mass (*asterisk*) replacing much of the left hepatic lobe. **B,** After the administration of intravenous gadolinium, the mass demonstrates heterogeneous enhancement. **C,** T2-weighted image shows a linear region of central hypointensity (*arrow*) within the mass.

POSITRON EMISSION TOMOGRAPHY

Early results suggest PET scanning may have a role to play in the evaluation of cholangiocarcinoma,[25] since it may detect cholangiocarcinoma tumors as small as 1 cm diameter and can simultaneously detect distant metastases. In a study of 54 patients, 26 with cholangiocarcinoma and 28 with no disease or benign disease, true-positive PET scans were obtained in 24 of 26 cholangiocarcinoma patients with only two false-positive results (sensitivity of 92% and specificity of 93%). Regional or hepatoduodenal lymph node metastases were detected with PET in only 2 of 15 cases, whereas distant metastases (peritoneal carcinomatosis, pulmonary metastases) were diagnosed in 7 of 10 cases.[26]

GALLBLADDER CARCINOMA

Anatomy

The gallbladder lies in the gallbladder fossa on the inferior surface of the liver. Both the gallbladder fossa and the middle hepatic vein lie in the plane that divides the liver into right and left lobes. The gallbladder is divided anatomically into fundus, body (corpus), infundibulum, and neck. The infundibulum connects the body to the cystic duct and is a frequent site of stone impaction (Hartmann's pouch). The cystic duct carries bile from the gallbladder and joins the common hepatic duct, to form the common bile duct. The arterial supply of the gallbladder is from the cystic artery, which is usually a branch of the right hepatic artery. Venous drainage is predominantly through the cystic vein to the portal vein, but also through small veins that empty directly into the liver. The regional lymph nodes for the gallbladder are the pericholedochal, hilar, peripancreatic (pancreatic head group only), periduodenal, periportal, celiac, and superior mesenteric nodes.

Pathology

Gallbladder carcinoma is the most common primary hepatobiliary malignancy and the fifth most common malignancy of the gastrointestinal tract. Most patients are elderly women.[27] Approximately 80% of gallbladder carcinomas occur in the fundus or body. The most common presenting symptom is abdominal pain (83%), followed by nausea and vomiting (45%).[28] Involvement

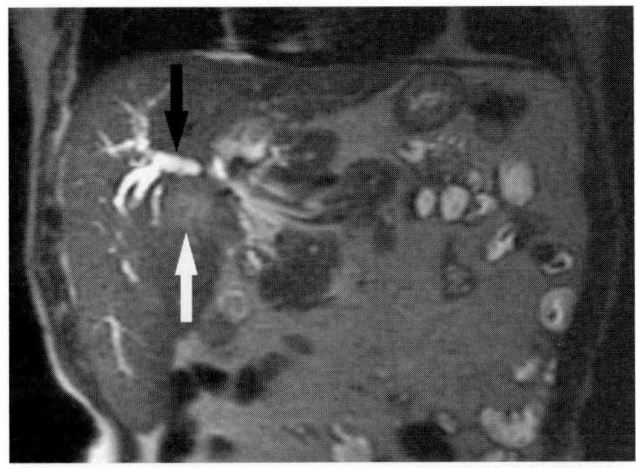

A

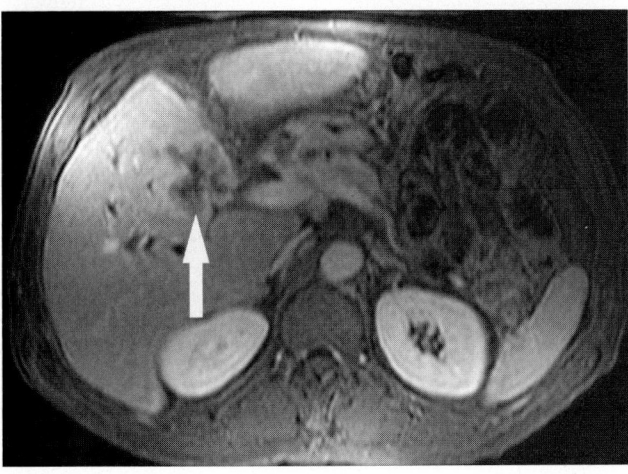

B

Figure 18–8. Magnetic resonance image of a 55-year-old woman with cholangiocarcinoma. **A,** T2-weighted coronal image shows moderately dilated intrahepatic bile ducts (*black arrow*) to the level of an ill-defined mass (*white arrow*) in the central liver. **B,** The mass (*arrow*) is well seen on this T1-weighted image after the administration of intravenous gadolinium.

of the liver, either by direct invasion or hematogenous metastases, is frequently present at diagnosis. Nodal metastases usually develop in the cystic duct, common bile duct, porta hepatis, and pancreaticoduodenal node chains. The para-aortic nodes may ultimately be involved. Intraperitoneal seeding may also occur.

Imaging of Gallbladder Carcinoma

INTRODUCTION

Gallbladder carcinoma is usually advanced at the time of diagnosis, and early-stage tumors are rarely encountered.[29] As a result, imaging findings are usually relatively obvious and can be well assessed by US, CT, or MRI. Radiologic findings include focal or diffuse thickening of the gallbladder wall (49%), a solid mass replacing the gallbladder in the gallbladder fossa (37%), or an intraluminal mass in the gallbladder (14%). Associated findings include invasion of adjacent structures such as the

liver (67%), coexistent gallstones (64%), biliary duct dilation (38%), coexistent porcelain gallbladder (4%), and distant metastases outside the liver (3%).[30] While gallbladder cancer may manifest as an intraluminal mass at imaging, it should be remembered that gallbladder polyps may be found in up to 2.5% of asymptomatic patients[31] and that most small non-calculous gallbladder filling defects are benign. In a study of 143 polyps, gallbladder polyps less than 1.5 cm in diameter removed by laparoscopic cholecystectomy, the final diagnoses were cholesterol polyp (74%), adenoma (11%), adenomyomatosis (7%), adenocarcinoma (4%), and hyperplastic or inflammatory polyp (4%).[32] Historical reports have suggested the risk of gallbladder carcinoma in patients with a porcelain gallbladder is between 12% and 61%,[33] and such numbers are frequently quoted in clinical practice. Two recent series of 10,741 and 25,900 cholecystectomy specimens from UCLA and Massachusetts General Hospital, respectively, have suggested the true risk is 0% to 7%.[33,34]

ULTRASOUND

Sonographic findings of gallbladder carcinoma include variable degrees of gallbladder wall thickening and irregularity (Fig. 18-9). Gallbladder wall thickening can also be seen with chronic cholecystitis and adenomyomatosis, but the wall thickening of these inflammatory and hyperplastic conditions is usually more diffuse than the relatively focal changes typical of gallbladder carcinoma. With more advanced disease, US may demonstrate a necrotic mass, direct hepatic invasion, biliary dilation, or hepatic metastases. Ultrasound is of limited use in the evaluation of nodal, peritoneal, or more distant metastases. Occasionally tumefactive sludge may mimic an intraluminal mass, but mobility on changes in patient position and absence of flow on Doppler insonation help in the correct identification of sludge.[35] Endoscopic US has been used in some centers to study gallbladder carcinoma, and early results suggest this modality may be helpful in assessing the depth of wall invasion.[36] Loss of the normal multiple-layer pattern of the gallbladder wall has been reported as the most specific finding at endoscopic US in the diagnosis of gallbladder carcinoma.[37]

COMPUTED TOMOGRAPHY

CT is helpful in both the diagnosis and staging of gallbladder carcinoma because it can detect gallbladder masses, wall thickening, and hepatic invasion (Fig. 18-10). Spiral CT has an accuracy of 83% to 86% in the local staging of gallbladder carcinoma.[38] The reported sensitivity for the detection of nodal metastases was more limited, ranging from 36% to 47%. CT has reasonably high positive predictive values for the detection of hepatic invasion of less than 2 cm (77%), hepatic invasion of more than 2 cm (100%), involvement of the common duct (90%), or invasion of the pancreas (100%).[39]

MAGNETIC RESONANCE IMAGING

MRI findings in gallbladder carcinoma resemble those seen at CT (Fig. 18-11). MRI and MR cholangiopancreatography

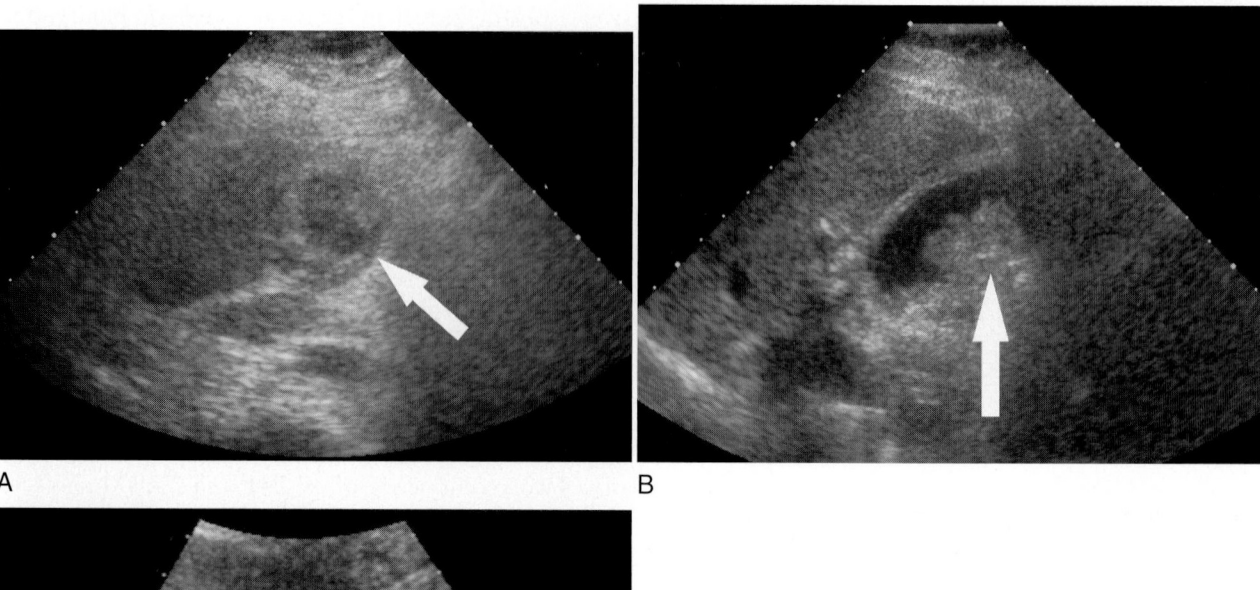

A

B

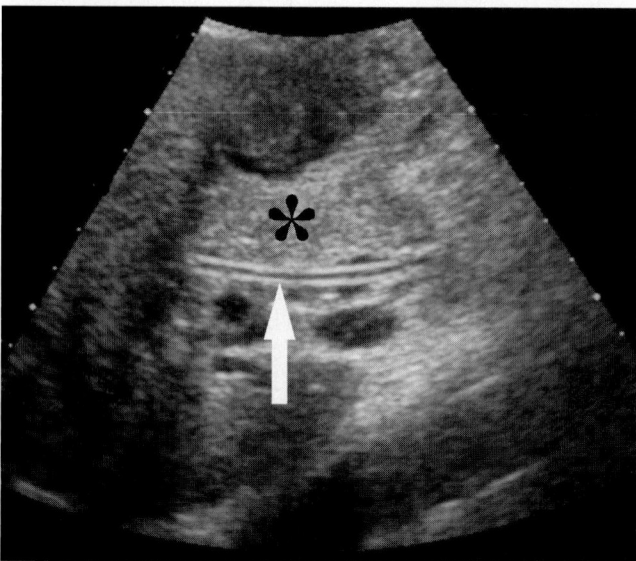

C

Figure 18–9. Gallbladder cancer has three main gross morphologic patterns, as illustrated in these three different cases. **A,** Ultrasound (US) of the gallbladder in an 80-year-old woman shows irregular circumferential wall thickening (*arrow*). **B,** US of the gallbladder in a 75-year-old woman shows an irregular polypoid mass (*arrow*) extending into the lumen. **C,** US of the gallbladder in an 87-year-old woman shows complete replacement of the gallbladder by a large irregular mass (*asterisk*). The mass has infiltrated the adjacent common duct, which contains a plastic endobiliary stent (*arrow*).

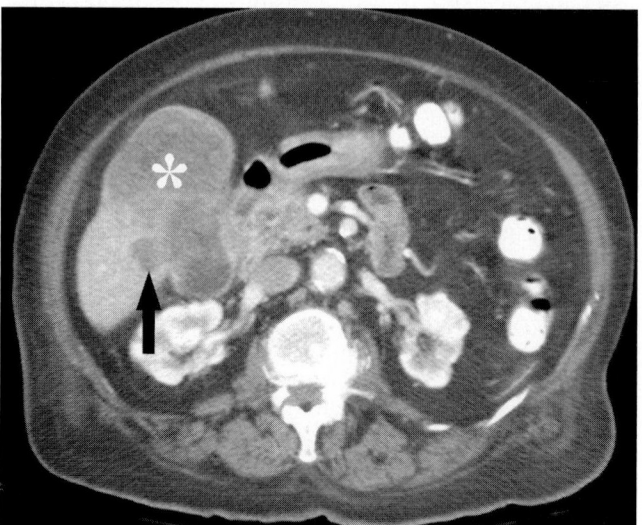

Figure 18–10. Contrast-enhanced CT of the gallbladder in a 74-year-old man. The gallbladder is almost completely replaced by a large cancer (*asterisk*) that is also invading the adjacent liver (*arrow*).

can provide information relevant to preoperative staging of gallbladder carcinoma. Gallbladder carcinoma manifested at MR imaging as focal gallbladder wall thickening with an eccentric mass in 76% of cases. The most common types of regional spread demonstrated are direct hepatic invasion (91%), lymphadenopathy (76%), and biliary tract invasion (62%). Sensitivity for direct hepatic invasion is reported as 100%, and sensitivity for lymph node metastasis as 92%.[40]

PANCREATIC CARCINOMA

Anatomy

The pancreas is an exocrine and endocrine gland, situated transversely in the retroperitoneum, at the level of the L1 and L2 vertebrae. The head lies within the duodenal sweep, while the body and tail extend to the gastric border of the spleen. While several systems for describing the anatomic subdivisions of the pancreas have been

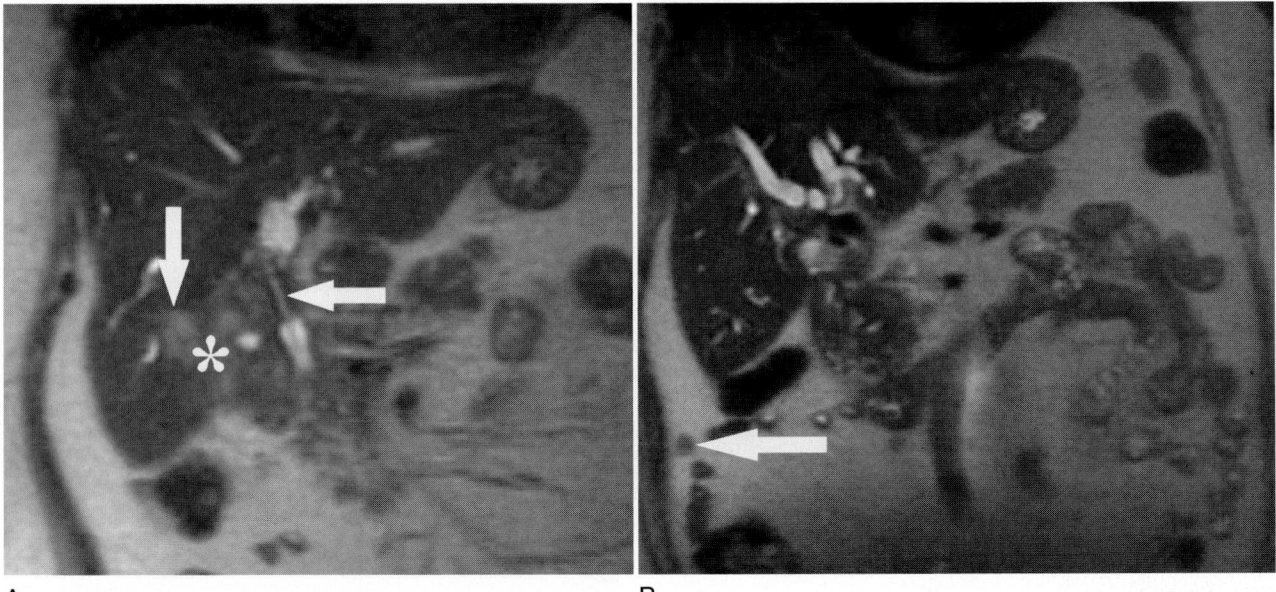

Figure 18–11. Magnetic resonance image of an 85-year-old woman with gallbladder carcinoma. **A,** T2-weighted coronal image demonstrates a mass (*asterisk*) of intermediate intensity replacing the gallbladder and invading the liver (*vertical arrow*). The mass also encases the adjacent common duct, which contains a stent (*horizontal arrow*). **B,** A contiguous T2-weighted coronal image demonstrates a small peritoneal implant (*arrow*) adjacent to the hepatic flexure. Peritoneal spread of biliary malignancy is not unusual, and should be specifically sought out.

proposed, the TNM classification is straightforward and divides the pancreas into head, body, and tail.[41] According to this classification, the head lies to the right of the left border superior mesenteric vein, the body lies between the left border of the aorta and the left border of the superior mesenteric vein, and the tail lies to the left of the left border of the aorta (Fig. 18-12). The pancreatic head lies posterior to the stomach and transverse colon and anterior to the inferior vena cava. The common bile duct courses through the pancreatic head to the ampulla of Vater. The pancreatic body lies anterior to the superior mesenteric vessels. The pancreatic tail extends laterally to abut the spleen and splenic flexure of the colon and lies anterior to the left kidney. The blood supply of the pancreas is derived from the pancreaticoduodenal branches of the gastroduodenal and superior mesenteric arteries and from direct branches of the splenic artery. Pancreatic venous drainage is through the portal system to the liver. The pancreas has an extensive system of lymphatic drainage, primarily to superior and inferior pancreatico-duodenal, porta hepatis, and supra pancreatic nodes, but also to para-aortic nodes.

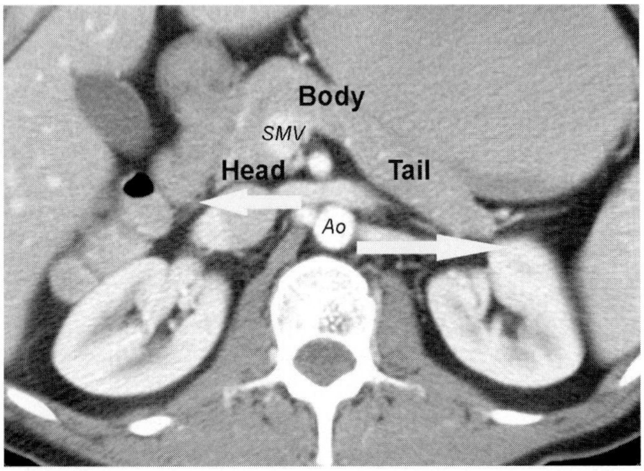

Pathology

Most pancreatic cancers are adenocarcinomas arising from the pancreatic ductal epithelium. Pancreatic adeno-carcinoma is often far advanced by the time symptoms occur. Approximately 75% of all pancreatic carcinomas occur within the head or body of the pancreas. Pancreatic cancer typically spreads first to regional lymph nodes, then to the liver, and finally to more distant sites such as the lungs. Regional nodes of the pancreas include supraperipancreatic nodes above the head and body, infrapancreatic nodes below the head and body, periceliac nodes, anterior and posterior pancreaticoduo-denal nodes, pyloric nodes, peribiliary nodes, and proxi-mal mesenteric nodes. Nodal involvement is seen in approximately 73% of patients undergoing surgical resection, and lowers the 5-year survival from 26% to 5%.[42] Unfortunately, both CT and PET are of very limited accuracy in the evaluation of regional adenopathy in pancreatic cancer.[43,44] Carcinoma of the head of the pancreas typically compresses the common bile duct and pancreatic duct and causes biliary and pancreatic ductal dilation. Peritoneal involvement is more common with carcinoma of the body and tail than with carcinoma of the head, presumably because such tumors are less likely to cause obstructive jaundice and therefore present in a more advanced stage.

Figure 18–12. The pancreas may be divided into the head, body, and tail. The heads lies to the right of the left border of the superior mesenteric vein (SMV). The tail lies to the left of the left border of the aorta (Ao). The body lies between the head and tail.

Imaging of Pancreatic Carcinoma

INTRODUCTION

Imaging modalities for pancreatic carcinoma include transabdominal US, endoscopic US, CT, MRI, PET, and conventional cholangiography.[45] Apart from distant metastases, involvement of the major vessels is the most important parameter for determining resectability in patients with pancreatic adenocarcinoma. Two problems commonly arise in imaging pancreatic carcinoma across all these modalities. First, pancreatic carcinoma is often infiltrative and the tumor may be poorly defined and difficult to appreciate. Even quite large tumors can be of similar appearance to the adjacent pancreatic parenchyma and difficult to visualize. Such tumors may be diagnosed predominantly through the indirect findings of pancreatic or biliary dilation (Fig. 18-13). Second, pancreatic carcinoma may be difficult to distinguish from focal chronic pancreatitis.

ULTRASOUND

Transabdominal US is of limited use in the diagnosis of pancreatic carcinoma because of suboptimal acoustic contrast and variable obscuration of the pancreas by overlying bowel. US may be helpful in the initial workup of patients, since it can distinguish obstructive from nonobstructive jaundice and thus guide further investigations. Endoscopic US is an evolving modality that shows great promise in the diagnosis and staging of pancreatic carcinoma. Endoscopic US remains the most sensitive and specific method to identify pancreatic masses. Early results suggest endoscopic US is more accurate than CT for staging pancreatic malignancy, including the evaluation of vascular invasion and local resectability. In a study of 151 patients with pancreatic carcinoma, the overall accuracy for T and N staging was 85% and 72% for endoscopic US compared to only 30% and 55% for CT, respectively. The ability to accurately predict vascular invasion was 93% for endoscopic US compared to 62% for CT. Endoscopic US was 93% accurate for predicting local resectability versus 60% for CT.[46] In a study of 21 patients with pancreatic carcinoma, endoscopic US demonstrated an accuracy of 81% in the assessment of vascular involvement compared to 38% for selective venous angiography.[47] Endoscopic US can also be combined with targeted fine-needle aspiration biopsy, and has shown a sensitivity of 93% and a specificity of 100% in establishing the correct diagnosis when employed in patients with pancreatic masses in whom prior biopsies have been nondiagnostic.[48]

COMPUTED TOMOGRAPHY

CT is the most frequently used modality for the evaluation of pancreatic carcinoma. CT-guided biopsy can be performed to provide a tissue diagnosis. The primary finding on contrast-enhanced CT is a focal hypodense mass (Fig. 18-14). The sensitivity of spiral CT for the detection of pancreatic carcinoma is between 89% and 97%.[49] The overall accuracy of spiral CT in the determination of resectability has been reported as 77%.[49] In a study of 80 evaluable major vessels in 25 patients, tumor contact

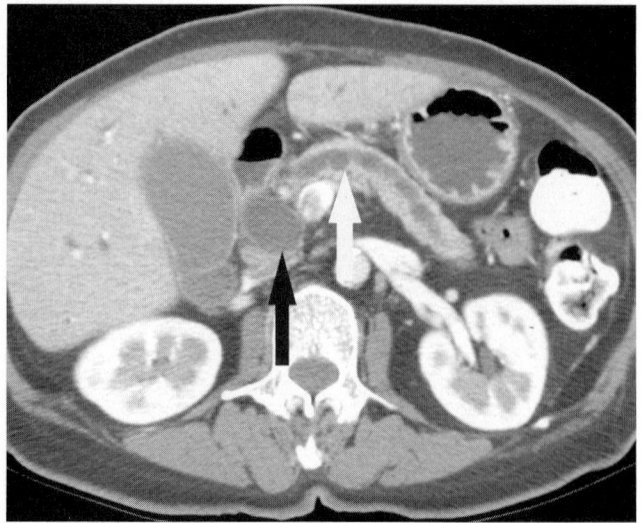

A

B

Figure 18–13. Computed tomography (CT) is the primary modality used to evaluate patients with suspected pancreatic cancer, but tumors may be infiltrative, Isodense, and difficult to directly visualize. **A,** Contrast-enhanced CT section in a 56-year-old man with painless jaundice and weight loss shows dilation of the pancreatic duct (*white arrow*) with atrophy of the surrounding pancreas. These findings are indirect signs that strongly suggest the presence of a malignant obstruction. **B,** CT section at a more inferior level, where the pancreatic and common bile ducts are no longer dilated, shows the pancreatic head (*arrow*). No definite mass can be seen. At surgery, a 3 cm pancreatic carcinoma was found in the pancreatic head.

with more than 50% of the vessel circumference demonstrated a sensitivity of 84% and specificity of 98% in the diagnosis of vascular invasion (Fig. 18-15).[50] The development of spiral CT has allowed imaging of pancreatic carcinoma in several different phases of enhancement, and each may provide useful information. Arteriographic images are helpful in the evaluation of arterial encasement by pancreatic carcinoma.[51] With respect to tumor detection, some studies have suggested tumor to background contrast is greater in the late arterial phase (scan delay of 40 to 70 seconds, sometimes called the pancreatic phase) than in the standard portal venous phase,[52,53] although other studies have suggested late

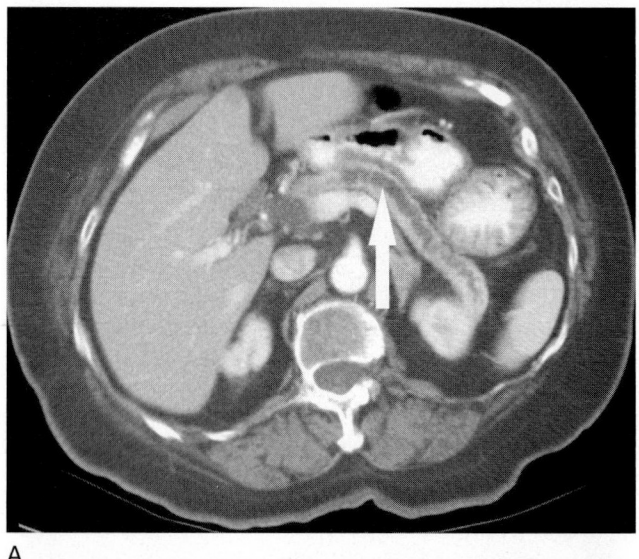

A

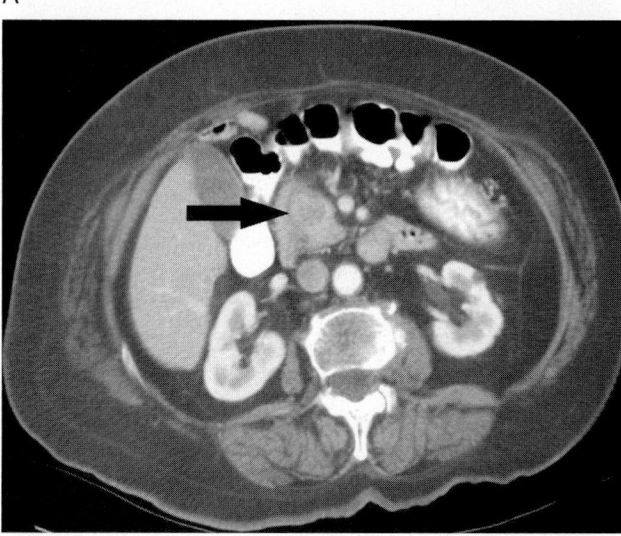

B

Figure 18–14. Contrast-enhanced computed tomography in a 64-year-old woman with pancreatic carcinoma. **A,** Section through the pancreas demonstrates marked ductal dilation (*arrow*) and atrophy of the surrounding gland. **B,** Section at a more inferior level shows the malignant mass (*arrow*) in the pancreatic head.

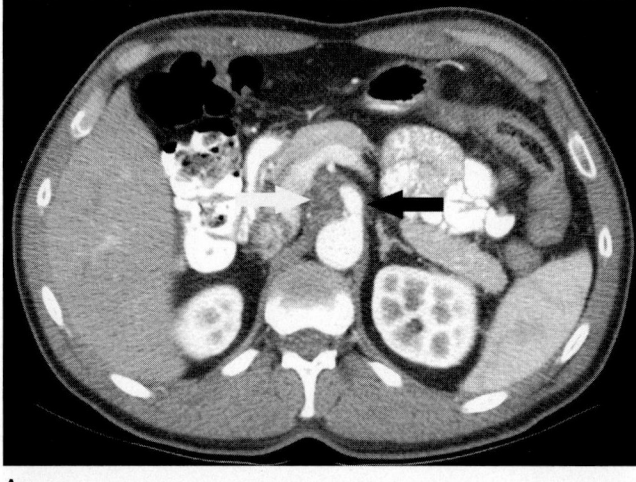

A

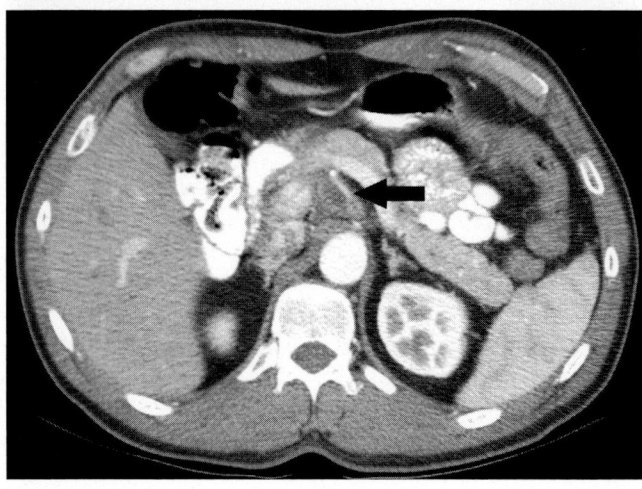

B

Figure 18–15. Contrast-enhanced computed tomography in a 58-year-old man with pancreatic carcinoma. **A,** Section through the origin of the celiac artery (*black arrow*) shows infiltrative tumor (*white arrow*) surrounding the vessel. Tumor contact with more than 50% of the circumference of the vessel is strongly predictive of vascular invasion and irresectability. **B,** Section at a more inferior level showing the celiac artery (*black arrow*) is both narrowed and encased by tumor.

arterial phase images do not improve pancreatic tumor detection when compared to standard portal venous phase images.[54,55] Accordingly, baseline studies for pancreatic carcinoma can reasonably be protocoled to include three phases: early arterial (arterial encasement), late arterial (tumor detection), and portal venous (hepatic evaluation).

CONVENTIONAL CHOLANGIOGRAPHY

After CT, ERCP is perhaps the second commonest investigation performed in patients with suspected pancreatic carcinoma (Fig. 18-16). Brush cytology and forceps biopsy can be used to provide a tissue diagnosis. Endobiliary stents can also be inserted at the time of ERCP, although this may not always be appropriate in patients who are surgical candidates; two separate studies of periampullary tumors and proximal cholangiocarcinoma

have shown that preoperative endobiliary stenting is associated with increased bacterial contamination of the biliary system, wound and intra-abdominal complications, and postoperative infections.[56,57] The principal disadvantage of conventional cholangiography, such as ERCP or percutaneous transhepatic cholangiography, is that these invasive procedures have a major complication rate on the order of 3%. Such complications include sepsis, bleeding, bile leak, and death.[58,59]

MAGNETIC RESONANCE IMAGING

MRI is used mainly as a problem-solving modality in patients with suspected pancreatic carcinoma, typically in patients with an equivocal CT scan or with contraindications to iodinated contrast such as contrast allergy, or elevated creatinine. However, the ability of MRI to simultaneously image the pancreatic parenchyma and

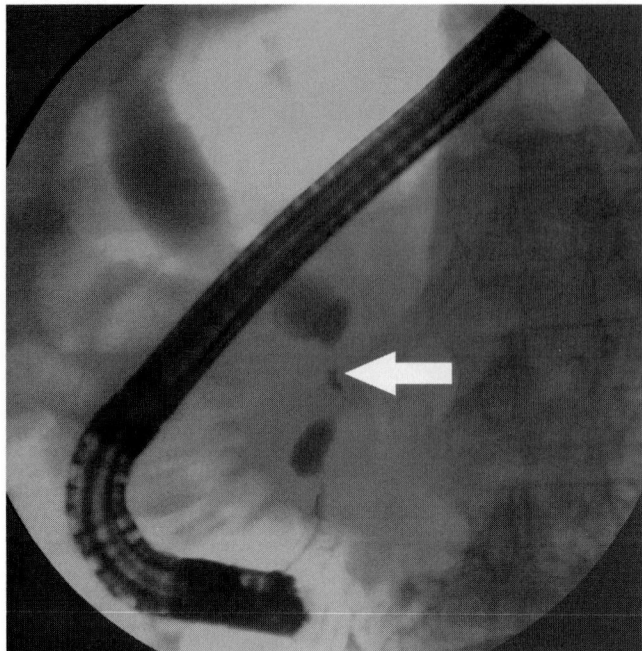

Figure 18–16. Endoscopic retrograde cholangiopancreatography in a 69-year-old man with pancreatic carcinoma. A tight irregular stricture (*arrow*) is seen in the distal common bile duct, with marked biliary dilation above the stricture.

vasculature with gadolinium enhancement and the pancreaticobiliary system with MRCP provides an attractive combined assessment that may be superior to more traditional methods (Fig. 18-17).[60-62] For example, in a study of 124 patients with suspected pancreatic carcinoma where the standard of reference was biopsy or 1 year of clinical follow-up, the sensitivity and specificity of MRCP for the diagnosis of pancreatic cancer was 84% and 97%, respectively, compared to a sensitivity and specificity of 70% and 94% for ERCP.[60] Another study concluded that mangafodipir trisodium-enhanced MR imaging was as accurate as contrast-enhanced spiral CT for the detection and staging of pancreatic

cancer, but offered improved detection of small pancreatic masses and of liver metastases.[61] In a study of 33 patients with suspected pancreatic carcinoma, MRI was significantly better in the assessment of resectability than spiral CT.[62]

POSITRON EMISSION TOMOGRAPHY

Initial studies suggest PET scanning may be helpful in the diagnosis of pancreatic carcinoma, detection of distant metastases, and evaluation of recurrent disease. In a study comparing PET and CT for tumor diagnosis in 73 patients with suspected pancreatic malignancy, PET had higher sensitivity (93% versus 80%) and specificity (93% versus 74%).[63] In another study of 65 patients with suspected pancreatic carcinoma, PET again demonstrated higher sensitivity and specificity than CT in the diagnosis of pancreatic carcinoma (92% and 85% vs. 65% and 61%).[64]

RETROPERITONEAL LYMPHADENOPATHY

Anatomy

The retroperitoneal space is bounded by the posterior parietal peritoneum anteriorly and the lumbar spine posteriorly. The retroperitoneal space contains the kidneys, adrenal glands, pancreas, nerve roots, lymph nodes, abdominal aorta, and inferior vena cava. The retroperitoneal (or lumbar) lymph nodes are the regional lymph nodes for the organs of the retroperitoneal space, and also for the testes, ovaries, fallopian tubes, and uterus (which are embryologically derived from the retroperitoneum). The retroperitoneal nodes are divided by the aorta and inferior vena cava into three groups: those lying to the left of the aorta (left para-aortic or left lumbar group), those lying between the aorta and inferior vena cava (inter-aortocaval or intermediate lumbar group), and those lying to the right of the inferior vena cava (right para-caval or right lumbar group).

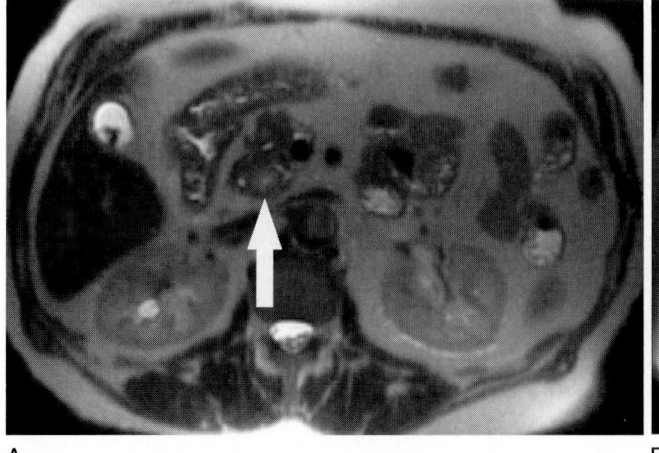
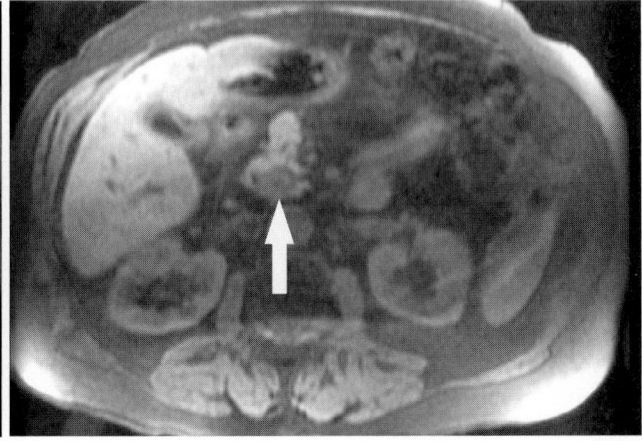

A   B

Figure 18–17. Magnetic resonance images of a 75-year-old man with pancreatic carcinoma. **A,** T2-weighted axial section shows a mildly hyperintense mass (*arrow*) in the pancreatic head. **B,** T1-weighted axial image after the administration of intravenous gadolinium demonstrates the mass (*arrow*) to be mildly hypointense.

Pathology

Virtually any malignancy can spread to the retroperitoneal nodes, particularly when widely disseminated. Tumors that commonly involve the retroperitoneal nodes include malignancies of the gastrointestinal tract, pancreas, kidney, and genitourinary system. The latter includes tumors of the testes, ovaries, and prostate. It is also common for lymphoma to involve the retroperitoneal nodes. In men presenting with a retroperitoneal nodal mass, where biopsy demonstrates a germ cell histology, careful evaluation of the testes is important because the retroperitoneal adenopathy may represent a primary extragonadal germ cell tumor, or metastatic disease from a testicular primary. Testicular US in a patient with retroperitoneal germ cell tumor may demonstrate a typical primary testicular cancer (i.e., ovoid hypoechoic mass), or a dense echogenic focus. Such lesions are usually primary germ cell malignancies, often seminomas.[65] Occasionally no tumor is found within such a hypoechoic mass, and these are regarded as regressed primary tumors.[66] Echogenic foci are thought to represent "scars" or "burnt-out" tumors.[67]

Imaging of Retroperitoneal Adenopathy

INTRODUCTION

Retroperitoneal adenopathy can be defined as an abnormal increase in the number or size of retroperitoneal nodes. This is a clinically useful operational definition, but includes an element of subjectivity as to what constitutes "abnormal." As a result, retroperitoneal adenopathy is often defined in imaging studies as the presence of nodes with a short axis diameter of 1 cm or more. While this definition has the advantage of objectivity, it does not really reflect daily practice. It should be noted that both definitions are based on nodal size, with the implicit assumption that nodal size reflects pathology. This assumption is of limited validity; normal-sized nodes can contain microscopic metastases and enlarged nodes may be reactive and not cancer-containing. Ideally, imaging evaluation would use a parameter that reflects node content rather than node size. Lymphangiography and PET are two modalities that at least partially reflect node content, though neither is routinely used for retroperitoneal nodal assessment, and CT and MRI remain the primary modalities in common usage. Because of poor acoustic contrast and variable obscuration by overlying bowel gas, US is of limited use in evaluation of the retroperitoneum, though large nodal masses may sometimes be visible.

Computed Tomography

Normal retroperitoneal lymph nodes are either invisible or appear on CT as small round or oval densities less than 1 cm in diameter (Fig. 18-18). Abnormal nodes are also seen as soft tissue densities, but of greater size and number. Adenopathy can occasionally be confluent or calcified. The accuracy of CT evaluation of retroperitoneal

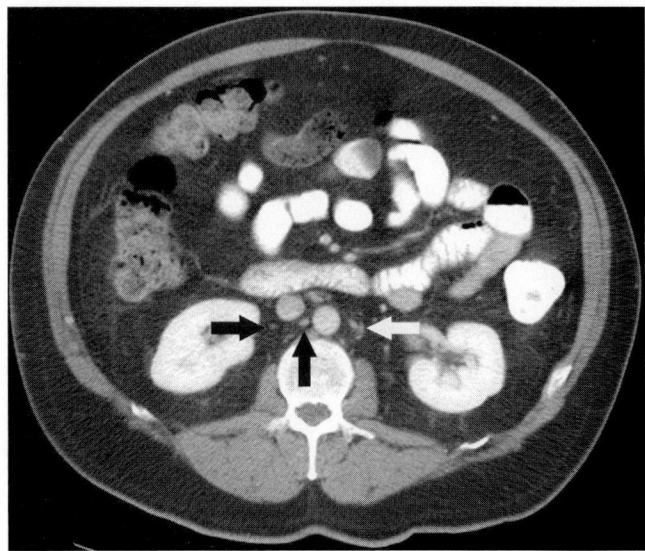

Figure 18–18. Contrast-enhanced computed tomography in a 42-year-old man illustrating normal retroperitoneal nodes. The nodal chains include left para-aortic (*white arrow*), inter-aortocaval (*vertical black arrow*), and right para-caval (*horizontal black arrow*) groups.

nodes is partially disease specific, and this will be illustrated by describing nodal assessment in testicular, endometrial, ovarian, and renal cancers. Right-side testicular cancer typically spreads to inter-aortocaval or paracaval nodes at the level of the entry of the right renal vein into the inferior vena cava (Fig. 18-19). Left-sided testicular cancers typically spread to left para-aortic nodes at the level of the entry of the left renal vein into the inferior vena cava (Fig. 18-20). These nodal sites should be carefully scrutinized in patients with testicular cancer. A study of 70 patients with newly diagnosed clinical stage 1 testicular nonseminomatous germ cell cancer, undergoing preoperative CT, showed that a short axis size threshold of 1 cm had a sensitivity of 37% and a specificity of 100% in the diagnosis of nodal metastases.

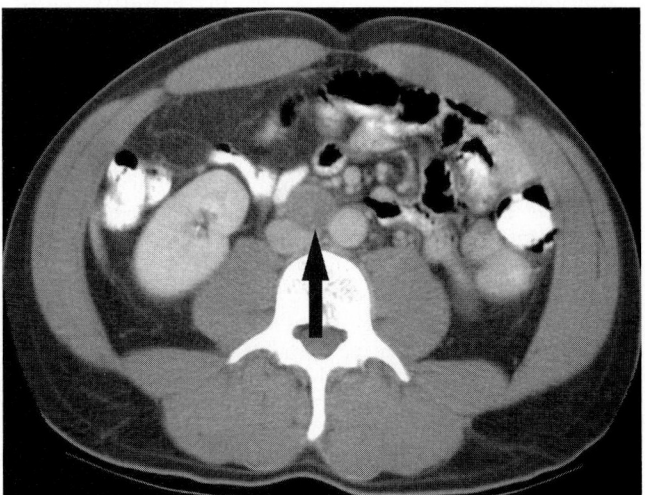

Figure 18–19. Contrast-enhanced computed tomography in a 42-year-old man with a right-sided testicular cancer. An anterior inter-aortocaval nodal metastasis (*arrow*) is visible.

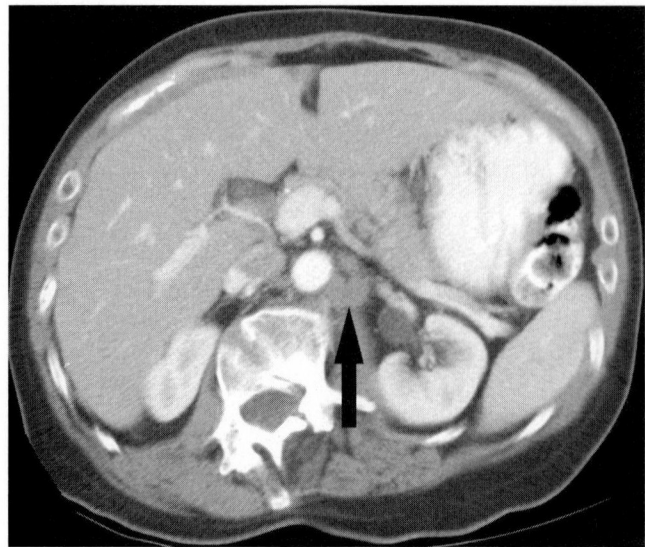

Figure 18–20. Contrast-enhanced computed tomography in a 27-year-old man with a left-sided testicular cancer. A left para-aortic nodal metastasis (*arrow*) is visible.

Progressively lower size thresholds demonstrated greater sensitivity but lower specificity, so that a 4 mm threshold had a sensitivity of 93% and a specificity of 58%. The same study also showed that nodes lying anterior to the center of the aorta were more likely to be metastatic than nodes of similar size lying more posteriorly.[68] The incidence of para-aortic nodal metastases in patients with clinical stages IA, IB, II, and III endometrial carcinoma is 2.5%, 8.5%, 15.7%, and 33.3%, respectively.[69] Deep myometrial invasion, cervical involvement, and lymphovascular space invasion also significantly increase the likelihood of nodal metastases. In a study of 56 women with endometrial carcinoma who had preoperative CT scans and lymph node sampling, the sensitivity and specificity of CT for detecting nodal metastases were 57% and 92%, respectively.[70] This study used a short axis diameter of at least 1.5 cm to define adenopathy. Ovarian cancer can spread to pelvic and retroperitoneal nodes. In a study of 71 patients undergoing preoperative CT or MRI, the incidence of nodal metastases at surgery was 28% (20/71).[71] CT showed a sensitivity of 50% and a specificity of 95% in the diagnosis of nodal metastases, using a 1 cm short axis diameter threshold. The evaluation of retroperitoneal adenopathy in renal cell carcinoma illustrates the importance of clinical context, because nodal enlargement in this setting is often reactive rather than metastatic. In a study of 163 patients undergoing preoperative CT and using a short axis threshold of 1 cm to define adenopathy,[72] lymphadenopathy was found in 43 patients, only 18 of whom had nodal metastases at surgery (positive predictive value of 43%). No adenopathy was detected in 120 patients, 5 of whom had metastases at surgery (negative predictive value of 96%).

MAGNETIC RESONANCE IMAGING

MRI is rarely employed as the primary imaging modality for assessment of retroperitoneal adenopathy since CT, even without intravenous contrast, is usually adequate. In general, the same size criteria are used at MRI as are used at CT, although a recent study suggests different size criteria may be appropriate.[73] In a group of testicular cancer patients without metastases undergoing surveillance imaging, the 95th percentile for maximum short axis diameter of retroperitoneal nodes at various locations ranged from 3 to 5 mm.

POSITRON EMISSION TOMOGRAPHY

PET (Fig. 18-21) allows detection of small malignant nodes not identified or not meeting size criteria for malignancy by CT, or when lack of retroperitoneal fat or postsurgical change makes it difficult to identify retroperitoneal nodes with CT.[74] PET scanning is also gaining importance in diagnosing and staging of cervical cancer. In a study comparing PET and CT in 101 consecutive patients with carcinoma of the cervix treated by chemotherapy and radiotherapy as clinically indicated and followed for a median of 15.4 months, baseline CT and PET showed retroperitoneal adenopathy in 7 and 21 patients, respectively. The 2-year progression-free survival, based solely on retroperitoneal adenopathy, was 64% in patients negative by both modalities, 14% in patients positive by both modalities, and 18% in patients negative on CT but positive on PET. Multivariate analysis demonstrated that the most significant prognostic

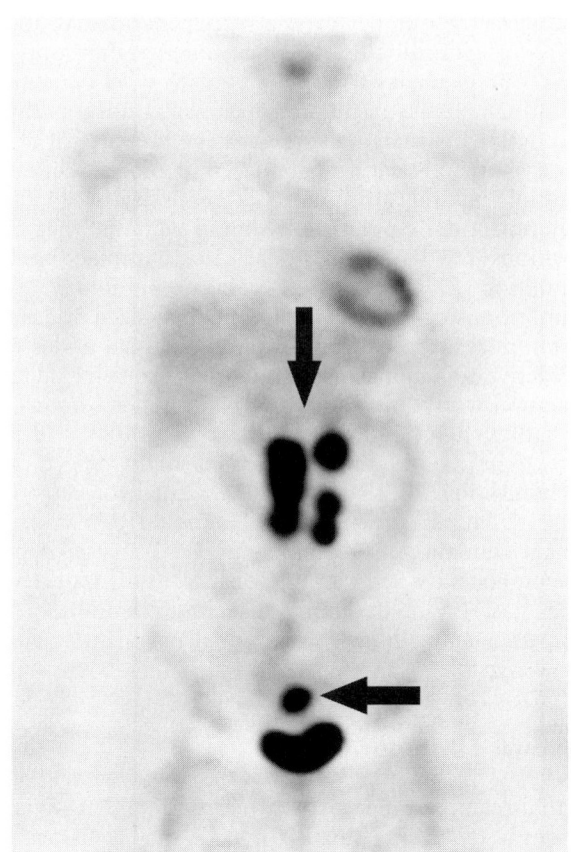

Figure 18–21. Positron emission tomography scan in a 51-year-old woman with endometrial cancer and retroperitoneal nodal metastases. The primary tumor (*horizontal arrow*) is seen above the bladder, and the nodal metastases (*vertical arrow*) are seen in the retroperitoneum.

factor for progression-free survival was the absence of positive retroperitoneal nodes on PET. These results suggest PET detects abnormal lymph nodes more often than CT, and that PET findings are a better predictor of outcome.[75]

LYMPHANGIOGRAPHY

Lymphangiography (Fig. 18-22) has largely fallen into disuse. Because it is an invasive and technically challenging procedure, few practicing radiologists have the necessary training to perform or interpret lymphangiograms, and the available data do not suggest any incremental clinical benefit. Even when lymphangiography was available, it was largely confined to a few specialist centers and reserved for evaluation of testicular and cervical cancer. A recent meta-analysis reviewed the performance of lymphangiography, CT, and MRI in nodal assessment in cervical cancer. The three modalities had similar accuracy, and the authors concluded that as CT and MRI are less invasive than lymphangiography and also assess local tumor extent, they should be considered the preferred adjuncts to clinical evaluation of invasive cervical cancer.[76] In a study comparing CT and lymphangiography in 50 patients with intra-abdominal metastatic testicular cancer, CT was more effective than lymphangiography. CT showed metastatic disease in 21 patients compared to 7 for lymphangiography. In the detection of relapse, lymphangiography showed nodal enlargement in 4 of 8 cases compared to 8 of 8 for CT.[77]

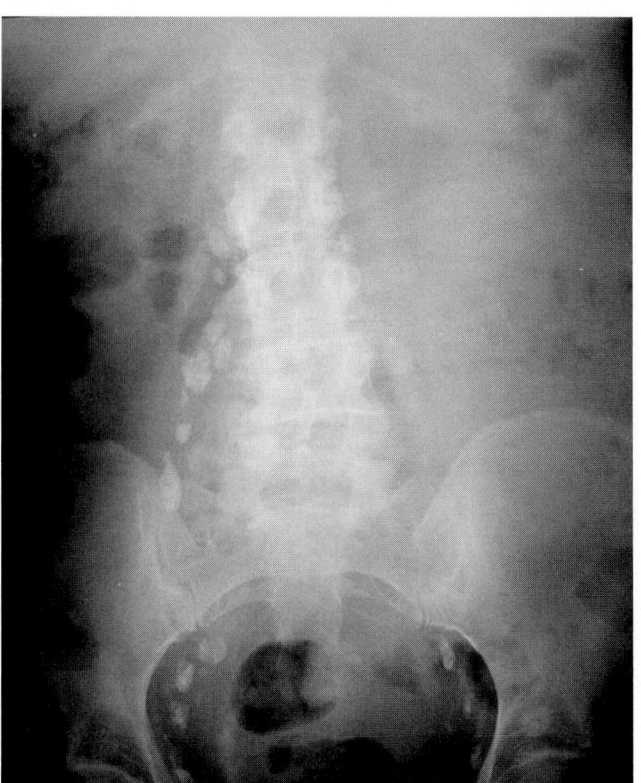

Figure 18–22. Lymphangiogram in a 24-year-old man with testicular cancer. Normal lymph nodes are opacified by contrast, which is injected into small lymphatics on the dorsum of the feet. The study is invasive, technically challenging, and now rarely performed.

GASTRIC CANCER

Anatomy

The stomach lies in the left upper quadrant and is divided into fundus, body, and antrum. The gastroesophageal junction (cardia) and gastroduodenal junction are protected by the lower esophageal sphincter and pyloric sphincter, respectively. The shorter right border of the stomach forms the lesser curvature and the longer left border forms the greater curvature. The stomach wall is made up of five layers: mucosal, submucosal, muscular, subserosal, and serosal. The stomach is in contact with the esophagus, duodenum, diaphragm, liver, spleen, anterior abdominal wall, transverse colon, mesocolon, left adrenal gland, left kidney, pancreas, greater omentum, and small bowel loops, and any of these structures may be involved by extension of gastric carcinoma. The arterial blood supply to the stomach is from the celiac trunk, through the left and right gastric, short gastric, and left and right gastroepiploic arteries. Venous drainage parallels the arterial supply, but enters the portal vein to the liver. Lymphatic drainage generally follows the blood supply to the stomach, and local nodes are located at the cardia, along the greater and lesser curvatures, and near the pylorus. Regional nodes lie along the left gastric, common hepatic, splenic, and celiac arteries. Involvement of hepatoduodenal, portal, mesenteric, and retroperitoneal is classified as distant metastases.[78]

Pathology

Adenocarcinoma of the stomach constitutes between 90% and 95% of all gastric malignancies. Nearly all the carcinomas arise from the mucus-secreting cells of the gastric crypts. Gastric cancers are more common on the lesser curvature. Most lesions are ulcerative and require differentiation from benign gastric ulcers. Findings that suggest malignancy are heaped-up ulcer margins and a diameter greater than 2 cm. Gastric cancer spreads by direct extension to the nearby structures, by lymphatics to locoregional and distant nodes, and hematogenously to the liver and systemic sites such as the lungs and bones. Eponymous sites of distant nodal involvement include the left supraclavicular (Virchows) nodes and left axillary (Irish) nodes. Peritoneal spread is also common, and eponymous sites of peritoneal involvement include the ovary (Krukenberg's tumor) and anterior rectal wall (rectal shelf of Blummer).

Imaging of Gastric Carcinoma

INTRODUCTION

Gastroscopy is the standard of reference for the diagnosis of gastric carcinoma, with a reported accuracy of more than 95%. Endoscopic US may be helpful to supplement endoscopy. CT and MRI are useful for detection of metastases in advanced disease. The double contrast upper-gastrointestinal examination with air and barium has been largely replaced by gastroscopy, but may still be useful in select cases in order to direct endoscopy to areas of the stomach that require particular scrutiny. Even in Japan, where double contrast upper-gastrointestinal examinations are still frequently performed as a first line investigation, approximately 26% (7 of 27) of gastric cancers may be completely occult radiographically.[79]

ENDOSCOPIC ULTRASOUND

Endoscopic US provides high spatial resolution images of the gastric wall, allowing visualization of all five layers, and also allows for evaluation of perigastric nodes. In a study of 119 patients with gastric cancer undergoing preoperative endoscopic US, the modality demonstrated an accuracy of 70% and 65% in the prediction of depth of tumor invasion and nodal involvement, respectively.[80] In another study, the overall accuracy, sensitivity, and specificity of endoscopic US in the diagnosis of lymph nodal metastases was reported as 79%, 79%, and 80%, respectively.[81]

COMPUTED TOMOGRAPHY

CT is of limited value in the primary diagnosis of gastric cancer (Fig. 18-23). In the preoperative staging of gastric carcinoma, the criteria to be assessed with CT includes extension of the tumor along the wall and adjacent areas, lymph node metastases, and distant metastases.[82] The use of water as a negative contrast agent to produce gastric distention by water may assist tumor visualization and assessment. In a study of 71 patients with gastric cancer undergoing thin section spiral CT, the sensitivity for early stage tumors was only 26% (12 of 46), although all 29 advanced tumors were seen.[83] The overall T-staging was correct in only 66% (27 of 41). CT is more commonly used for detection of metastatic disease. In a study of 56 patients with node-positive gastric cancer undergoing spiral CT, the sensitivity, specificity, and accuracy in the detection of liver metastases were 89%, 98%, and 96%,

respectively.[84] However, peritoneal dissemination was not detected in 15 of 56 patients (27%), and stage IV disease was not correctly diagnosed in 18 of 40 patients (45%).

Magnetic Resonance Imaging

MRI is rarely used to evaluate gastric carcinoma, and only a few studies have been reported. While the high tissue contrast and multi-planar capability of MRI are potentially attractive features for imaging gastric pathology, no convincing advantage has been shown for MRI over CT. In a study of 30 patients with gastric carcinoma undergoing preoperative MRI and CT, MRI and CT were of similar accuracy in T staging (73% and 67%, respectively). Accuracy for nodal staging was also similar for MRI and CT (55% and 59%, respectively).[85]

REFERENCES

1. Kalender WA, Seissler W, Vock P: Single-breath-hold spiral volumetric CT by continuous patient translation and scanner rotation. *Radiology.* 1989;173:414.
2. Kalender WA: Technical foundations of spiral CT. *Semin Ultrasound CT MR.* 1994;15:81.
3. Liang Y, Kruger RA: Dual-slice spiral versus single-slice helical scanning: Comparison of the physical performance of two computed tomography scanners. *Med Phys.* 1996;23:205.
4. Coakley FV, Cohen MD, Waters DJ, et al: The detection of pulmonary metastases with pathological correlation in a canine model: Effect of breathing on the accuracy of spiral CT. *AJR Am J Roentgenol.* 1997;169:1615.
5. Catalano O: Proper terminology for multiple-phase helical CT of the liver. *AJR Am J Roentgenol.* 2001;176:547. Letter.
6. Dodd GD: AJR proper terminology for multiple-phase helical CT of the liver. *AJR Am J Roentgenol.* 2001;176:547. Reply.
7. Klatskin G: Adenocarcinoma of the hepatic duct at its bifurcation within the porta hepatis: An unusual tumor with distinctive clinical and pathological features. *Am J Med.* 1965;38:241.
8. Tsuji T, Hiraoka T, Kanemitsu K, et al: Lymphatic spreading pattern of intrahepatic cholangiocarcinoma. *Surgery.* 2001;129:401.
9. Yeo CJ, Pitt HA, Cameron JL: Department of Surgery, Johns Hopkins University, Baltimore, Md. Cholangiocarcinoma. *Surg Clin North Am.* 1990;70:1429.
10. Hadjis NS, Collier NA, Blumgart LH: Malignant masquerade at the hilum of the liver. *Br J Surg.* 1985;72:659.
11. Goematis B, Giannopoulos A, Papachristou DN, et al: Sclerosing cholangitis of the bifurcation of the common hepatic duct. *Mt Sinai J Med.* 1982;49:38.
12. Bloom CM, Langer B, Wilson SR: Role of US in the detection, characterization, and staging of cholangiocarcinoma. *Radiographics.* 1999;19:1199.
13. Robledo R, Muro A, Prieto ML: Extrahepatic bile duct carcinoma: US characteristics and accuracy in demonstration of tumors. *Radiology.* 1996;198:869.
14. Hann LE, Greatrex KV, Bach AM: Cholangiocarcinoma at the hepatic hilus: Sonographic findings. *AJR Am J Roentgenol.* 1997;168:985.
15. Smits NJ, Reeders JW: Imaging and staging of biliopancreatic malignancy: Role of ultrasound. *Ann Oncol.* 1999;10(Suppl 4):20.
16. Looser C, Stain SC, Baer HU, et al: Staging of hilar cholangiocarcinoma by ultrasound and duplex sonography: A comparison with angiography and operative findings. *Br J Radiol.* 1992;65:871.
17. Sans N, Fajadet P, Galy-Fourcade D, et al: Is capsular retraction a specific CT sign of malignant liver tumor? *Eur Radiol.* 1999;9:1543.
18. Feydy A, Vilgrain V, Denys A, et al: Helical CT assessment in hilar cholangiocarcinoma: Correlation with surgical and pathologic findings. *AJR Am J Roentgenol.* 1999;172:73.

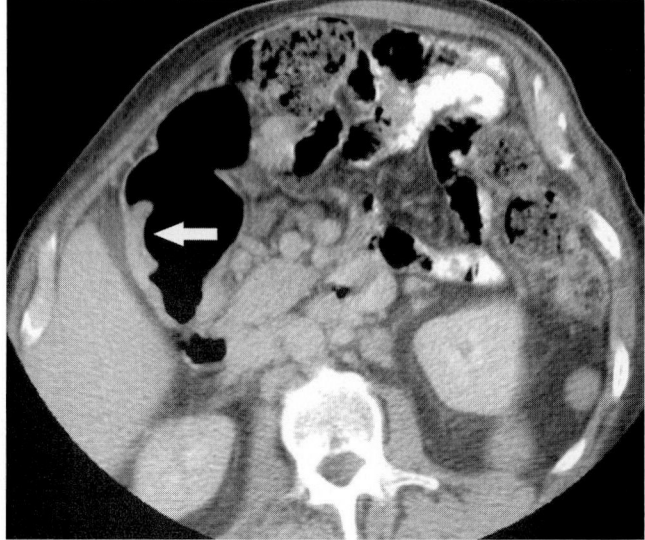

Figure 18–23. Contrast-enhanced computed tomography in a 77-year-old man with gastric cancer. The tumor is seen as an elevated ulcerated mass (*arrow*).

19. Keogan MT, Seabourn JT, Paulson EK, et al: Contrast-enhanced CT of intrahepatic and hilar cholangiocarcinoma: Delay time for optimal imaging. *AJR Am J Roentgenol.* 169:1493.

20. Lacomis JM, Baron RL, Oliver JH III, et al: Cholangiocarcinoma: Delayed CT contrast enhancement patterns. *Radiology.* 1997;203:98.

21. Valls C, Guma A, Puig I, et al: Intrahepatic peripheral cholangiocarcinoma: CT evaluation. *Abdom Imaging.* 2000;25:490.

22. Schwartz LH, Coakley FV, Sun Y, et al: Neoplastic pancreaticobiliary duct obstruction: Evaluation with breath hold MR cholangiopancreatography. *AJR Am J Roentgenol.* 1998;170:1491.

23. Hann LE, Schwartz LH, Panicek DM, et al: Tumor involvement in hepatic veins: Comparison of MR imaging and US for preoperative assessment. *Radiology.* 1998;206:651.

24. Maetani Y, Itoh K, Watanabe C, et al: MR imaging of intrahepatic cholangiocarcinoma with pathologic correlation. *AJR Am J Roentgenol.* 2001;176:1499.

25. Torok N, Gores GJ: Cholangiocarcinoma. *Semin Gastrointest Dis.* 2001;12:125.

26. Kluge R, Schmidt F, Caca K, et al: Positron emission tomography with [(18)F]fluoro-2-deoxy-D-glucose for diagnosis and staging of bile duct cancer. *Hepatology.* 2001;33:1029.

27. Nardi M, D'Amico G, Basti M, et al: Cancer of the gallbladder. *Minerva Chir.* 1997;52:583.

28. Cunningham CC, Zibari GB, Johnston LW: Primary carcinoma of the gall bladder: A review of our experience. *J La State Med Soc.* 2002;154:196.

29. Levy AD, Murakata LA, Rohrmann CA Jr: Gallbladder carcinoma: Radiologic-pathologic correlation. *Radiographics.* 2001;21:295.

30. Rooholamini SA, Tehrani NS, Razavi MK, et al: Imaging of gallbladder carcinoma. *Radiographics.* 1994;14:291.

31. Moriguchi H, Tazawa J, Hayashi Y, et al: Natural history of polypoid lesions in the gallbladder. *Gut.* 1996;39:860.

32. Huang CS, Lien HH, Jeng JW, et al: Role of laparoscopic cholecystectomy in the management of polypoid lesions of the gallbladder. *Surg Laparosc Endosc Percutan Tech.* 2001;11:242.

33. Stephen AE, Berger DL: Carcinoma in the porcelain gallbladder: A relationship revisited. *Surgery.* 2001;129:699.

34. Towfigh S, McFadden DW, Cortina GR, et al: Porcelain gallbladder is not associated with gallbladder carcinoma. *Am Surg.* 2001;67:7.

35. Ueno N, Tomiyama T, Tano S, et al: Diagnosis of gallbladder carcinoma with color Doppler ultrasonography. *Am J Gastroenterol.* 1996;91:1647.

36. Fujita N, Noda Y, Kobayashi G, et al: Diagnosis of the depth of invasion of gallbladder carcinoma by EUS. *Gastrointest Endosc.* 1999;50:659.

37. Mizuguchi M, Kudo S, Fukahori T, et al: Endoscopic ultrasonography for demonstrating loss of multiple-layer pattern of the thickened gallbladder wall in the preoperative diagnosis of gallbladder cancer. *Eur Radiol.* 1997;7:1323.

38. Yoshimitsu K, Honda H, Shinozaki K, et al: Helical CT of the local spread of carcinoma of the gallbladder: Evaluation according to the TNM system in patients who underwent surgical resection. *AJR Am J Roentgenol.* 2002;179:423.

39. Ohtani T, Shirai Y, Tsukada K, et al: Spread of gallbladder carcinoma: CT evaluation with pathologic correlation. *Abdom Imaging.* 1996;21:195.

40. Schwartz LH, Black J, Fong Y, et al: Gallbladder carcinoma: Findings at MR imaging with MR cholangiopancreatography. *J Comput Assist Tomogr.* 2002;26:405.

41. TNM Atlas: *Illustrated Guide to the TNM/pTNM-Classification of Malignant Tumors.* 3rd ed. Heidelberg, Germany: Springer-Verlag; 1989.

42. Gebhardt C, Meyer W, Reichel M, et al: Prognostic factors in the operative treatment of ductal pancreatic carcinoma. *Langenbecks Arch Surg.* 2000;385:14.

43. Zeman RK, Cooper C, Zeiberg AS, et al: TNM staging of pancreatic carcinoma using helical CT. *AJR Am J Roentgenol.* 1997;169:459.

44. Valinas R, Barrier A, Montravers F, et al: [18 F-fluorodeoxyglucose positron emission tomography for characterization and initial staging of pancreatic tumors]. *Gastroenterol Clin Biol.* 2002;26:888.

45. Del Frate C, Zanardi R, Mortele K, et al: Advances in imaging for pancreatic disease. *Curr Gastroenterol Rep.* 2002;4:140.

46. Gress FG, Hawes RH, Savides TJ, et al: Role of EUS in the preoperative staging of pancreatic cancer: A large single-center experience. *Gastrointest Endosc.* 1999;50:786.

47. Ahmad NA, Kochman ML, Lewis JD, et al: Endosonography is superior to angiography in the preoperative assessment of vascular involvement among patients with pancreatic carcinoma. *J Clin Gastroenterol.* 2001;32:54.

48. Wiersema MJ: Accuracy of endoscopic ultrasound in diagnosing and staging pancreatic carcinoma. *Pancreatology.* 2001;1:625.

49. Valls C, Andía E, Sanchez A, et al: Dual-phase helical CT of pancreatic adenocarcinoma assessment of resectability before surgery. *AJR Am J Roentgenol.* 2002;178:821.

50. Lu DSK, Reber HA, Krasny RM, et al: Local staging of pancreatic cancer: Criteria for unresectability of major vessels as revealed by pancreatic-phase, thin-section helical CT. *AJR Am J Roentgenol.* 1997;168:1439.

51. Raptopoulos V, Steer ML, Sheiman RG, et al: The use of helical CT and CT angiography to predict vascular involvement from pancreatic cancer: Correlation with findings at surgery. *AJR Am J Roentgenol.* 1997;168:971.

52. Lu DS, Vedantham S, Krasny RM, et al: Two-phase helical CT for pancreatic tumors: Pancreatic versus hepatic phase enhancement of tumor, pancreas, and vascular structures. *Radiology.* 1996;199:697.

53. O'Malley ME, Boland GW, Saez M, et al: Pancreatic-phase versus portal vein-phase helical CT of the pancreas: Optimal temporal window for evaluation of pancreatic adenocarcinoma. *AJR Am J Roentgenol.* 1999;172:605.

54. Graf O, Boland GW, Warshaw AL, et al: Arterial versus portal venous helical CT for revealing pancreatic adenocarcinoma: Conspicuity of tumor and critical vascular anatomy. *AJR Am J Roentgenol.* 1997;169:119.

55. Keogan MT, McDermott VG, Paulson EK, et al: Pancreatic malignancy: Effect of dual-phase helical CT in tumor detection and vascular opacification. *Radiology.* 1997;205:513.

56. Hochwald SN, Harrison LE, Blumgart LH, et al: A preoperative biliary stent is associated with increased complications after pancreaticoduodenectomy. *Arch Surg.* 1998;133:149.

57. Hochwald SN, Burke EC, Jarnagin WR, et al: Association of preoperative biliary stenting with increased postoperative infectious complications in proximal cholangiocarcinoma. *Arch Surg.* 1999;134:261.

58. Bilbao MK, Dotter CT, Lee TG, et al: Complications of retrograde cholangiography (ERCP): A study of 10,000 cases. *Gastroenterology.* 1976;70:314.

59. Harbin WP, Meuller P, Ferrucci JT: Transhepatic cholangiography: Complications and use pattern of the fine-needle technique. *Radiology.* 1980;135:15.

60. Adamek HE, Albert J: Pancreatography and endoscopic retrograde cholangiopancreatography: A prospective controlled study. *Lancet.* 2000;356:190.

61. Schima W, Függer R, Schober E, et al: Diagnosis and staging of pancreatic cancer: Comparison of mangafodipir trisodium-enhanced MR imaging and contrast-enhanced helical hydro-CT. *AJR Am J Roentgenol.* 2002;179:717.

62. Sheridan MB, Ward J, Guthrie JA, et al: Dynamic contrast-enhanced MR imaging and dual-phase helical CT in the preoperative assessment of suspected pancreatic cancer: A comparative study with receiver operating characteristic analysis. *AJR Am J Roentgenol.* 1999;173:583.

63. Stollfuss JC, Glatting G, Friess H, et al: 2-(fluorine-18)-fluoro-2-deoxy-D-glucose PET in detection of pancreatic cancer: Value of quantitative image interpretation. *Radiology.* 1995;195:339.

64. Delbeke D, Rose DM, Chapman WC, et al: Optimal interpretation of FDG PET in the diagnosis, staging and management of pancreatic cancer. *J Nucl Med.* 1999;40:1784.

65. Glazer HS, Lee JKT, Melson GL, et al: Sonographic detection of occult testicular neoplasms. *AJR Am J Roentgenol.* 1991;138:673.

66. Gross GW, Rohner TJ, Lombard JS, et al: Metastatic seminoma with regression of testicular primary: Ultrasonographic detection. *J Urol.* 1986;136:1086.

67. Imaging of retroperitoneal adenopathy. In Hricak H, Hamm B, Kim B: *Imaging of the Scrotum: Textbook and Atlas.* New York: Raven Press; 1995:49.

68. Hilton S, Herr HW, Teitcher JB, et al: CT detection of retroperitoneal lymph node metastases in patients with clinical stage I testicular nonseminomatous germ cell cancer: Assessment of size and distribution criteria. *AJR Am J Roentgenol.* 1997;169:521.

69. Hirahatake K, Hareyama H, Sakuragi N, et al: A clinical and pathologic study on para-aortic lymph node metastasis in endometrial carcinoma. *J Surg Oncol.* 1997;65:82.

70. Connor JP, Andrews JI, Anderson B, et al: Computed tomography in endometrial carcinoma. *Obstet Gynecol.* 2000;95:692.

71. Forstner R, Hricak H, Occhipinti KA, et al: Ovarian cancer: Staging with CT and MR imaging. *Radiology.* 1995;197:619.

72. Studer UE, Scherz S, Scheidegger J, et al: Enlargement of regional lymph nodes in renal cell carcinoma is often not due to metastases. *J Urol.* 1990;144:243.

73. Grubnic S, Vinnicombe SJ, Norman AR, et al: MR evaluation of normal retroperitoneal and pelvic lymph nodes. *Clin Radiol.* 2002;57:193.

74. Vesselle HJ, Miraldi FD: FDG PET of the retroperitoneum: Normal anatomy, variants, pathologic conditions, and strategies to avoid diagnostic pitfalls. *Radiographics.* 1998;18:805.

75. Grigsby PW, Siegel BA, Dehdashti F: Lymph node staging by positron emission tomography in patients with carcinoma of the cervix. *J Clin Oncol.* 2001;19:3745.

76. Scheidler J, Hricak H, Yu KK, et al: Radiological evaluation of lymph node metastases in patients with cervical cancer. A meta-analysis. *JAMA.* 1997;278:1096.

77. Williams MP, Husband JE: Computed tomography scanning and post-lymphangiogram radiography in the follow-up of patients with metastatic testicular cancer. *Clin Radiol.* 1989;40:47.

78. Fleming ID, Cooper JS, Henson DE, et al., eds: *Manual for Staging of Cancer. American Joint Committee on Cancer.* 5th ed. Philadelphia: JB Lippincott; 1997.

79. Shindoh N, Nakagawa T, Ozaki Y, et al: Overlooked gastric carcinoma: Pitfalls in upper gastrointestinal radiology. *Radiology.* 2000;217:409.

80. Wang JY, Hsieh JS, Huang YS, et al: Endoscopic ultrasonography for preoperative locoregional staging and assessment of resectability in gastric cancer. *Clin Imaging.* 1998;22:355.

81. Chen CH, Yang CC, Yeh YH: Preoperative staging of gastric cancer by endoscopic ultrasound: The prognostic usefulness of ascites detected by endoscopic ultrasound. *J Clin Gastroenterol.* 2002;35:321.

82. Angelelli G, Ianora AA, Scardapane A, et al: Role of computerized tomography in the staging of gastrointestinal neoplasms. *Semin Surg Oncol.* 2001;20:109.

83. Fukuya T, Honda H, Kaneko K, et al: Efficacy of helical CT in T-staging of gastric cancer. *J Comput Assist Tomogr.* 1997; 21:73.

84. Adachi Y, Sakino I, Matsumata T, et al: Preoperative assessment of advanced gastric carcinoma using computed tomography. *Am J Gastroenterol.* 1997;92:872.

85. Sohn KM, Lee JM, Lee SY, et al: Comparing MR imaging and CT in the staging of gastric carcinoma. *AJR Am J Roentgenol.* 2000;174:1551.

19

Pelvis

Oguz Akin, MD, and Hedvig Hricak, MD

Radiotherapy has always been image-based, but the precision of the "image" has evolved. Historically, the images were two-dimensional x-ray projections. The availability of three-dimensional (3D) anatomical data, first provided by computed tomography (CT), dramatically improved anatomic display, and with the advances of treatment planning, started "image-based" 3D conformal radiation therapy (3D-CRT). Within the past decade, an advanced form of 3D-CRT, intensity-modulated radiotherapy (IMRT), has led to further improvement in the dose distribution conformality using computer-optimized intensity modulation. IMRT, however, requires high precision in tumor localization for dose escalation and mandates that medical imaging enlarges its scope from morphology to information about metabolism and function. The spatial and temporal resolution of anatomic images has reached new heights, resulting in detection of smaller lesions and routine clinical use of positron emission tomography (PET), and magnetic resonance spectroscopic imaging allows noninvasive biologic imaging of cancer. These advances have tremendous potential for improved cancer care through the increased sensitivity in tumor detection, more accurate staging, and treatment follow-up. All of these advances, however, necessitate continuous improvement in our knowledge of advantages and limitations of modern imaging. This chapter focuses on clinically relevant, applied anatomy and provides an overview of pelvic oncologic imaging.

PELVIC ANATOMY

The pelvis is an osseous ring supported by musculature and connective tissue and contains reproductive organs, the lower urinary tract, parts of the small bowel, rectosigmoid colon, the related blood vessels, nerves, and lymphatics. Figure 19-1 *(A–H)* illustrates the normal pelvic anatomy seen on axial CT images.

An imaginary oblique line passing from the sacral promontory to the superior aspect of the symphysis pubis divides the pelvis into the false or *greater* pelvis superiorly and the true or *lesser* pelvis inferiorly. The false pelvis is related with the abdominal cavity anteriorly and superiorly and contains most of the small bowel, parts of the colon, and the common iliac vessels. The true pelvis contains some small bowel, the rectum, the urinary bladder, and the reproductive organs. Levator ani muscles define the inferior border of the lesser pelvis and separate

it from the perineum. The pelvic inlet is the superior opening of the lesser pelvis, while the pelvic outlet is the inferior opening.[1]

In terms of pathways of disease dissemination, dividing the pelvis into intraperitoneal and extraperitoneal compartments is of more significance than the anatomic division of true and false pelvis.

The peritoneal reflections within the pelvis form several important recesses that are important in treatment planning since these recesses may harbor fluid collections or metastases. The rectovesical space is the most caudal portion of the peritoneal cavity and is formed by the peritoneal reflection between the rectum and the urinary bladder. In males, the layers of peritoneum lining the rectovesical space are fused inferiorly to form Denonvilliers' fascia, which lies between the prostate and the rectum. However, in females, the rectovesical space is divided by the indentation of the uterus into a vesicouterine recess anteriorly and a rectouterine cul-de-sac (pouch of Douglas) posteriorly. In females, the inferior portion of the peritoneum lining the rectouterine recess is fused and forms the rectovaginal septum. The pararectal fossae are lateral extensions of the rectovesical space. Indentation of the urinary bladder to the pelvic peritoneum causes formation of the supravesical space cranially and paravesical spaces laterally on each side.[1]

The prevesical space, also known as the *space of Retzius*, is the largest extraperitoneal recess in the pelvis and lies between the anterior abdominal wall anteriorly and the umbilicovesical fascia posteriorly. It extends cranially to the level of the umbilicus and its caudal boundary is formed by the puboprostatic ligament in the male and the pubovesical ligament in the female. The prevesical space is laterally related with the paravesical connective tissue. The perivesical space, which is bounded by the umbilicovesical fascia, contains the urinary bladder, obliterated umbilical arteries, and urachus running from the apex of the bladder to the umbilicus.[1]

The perineum is a diamond-shaped space located inferior to the pelvic floor muscles. The boundaries of perineum are the symphysis pubis and the arcuate pubic ligament anteriorly; the inferior pubic ramus, ischial ramus, and ischial tuberosity laterally; and the coccyx posteriorly. The superficial transversus perinei muscle divides the perineum into two triangles: urogenital triangle anteriorly and anal triangle posteriorly. The urogenital triangle contains external urogenital organs and the anal triangle contains the anus.[1]

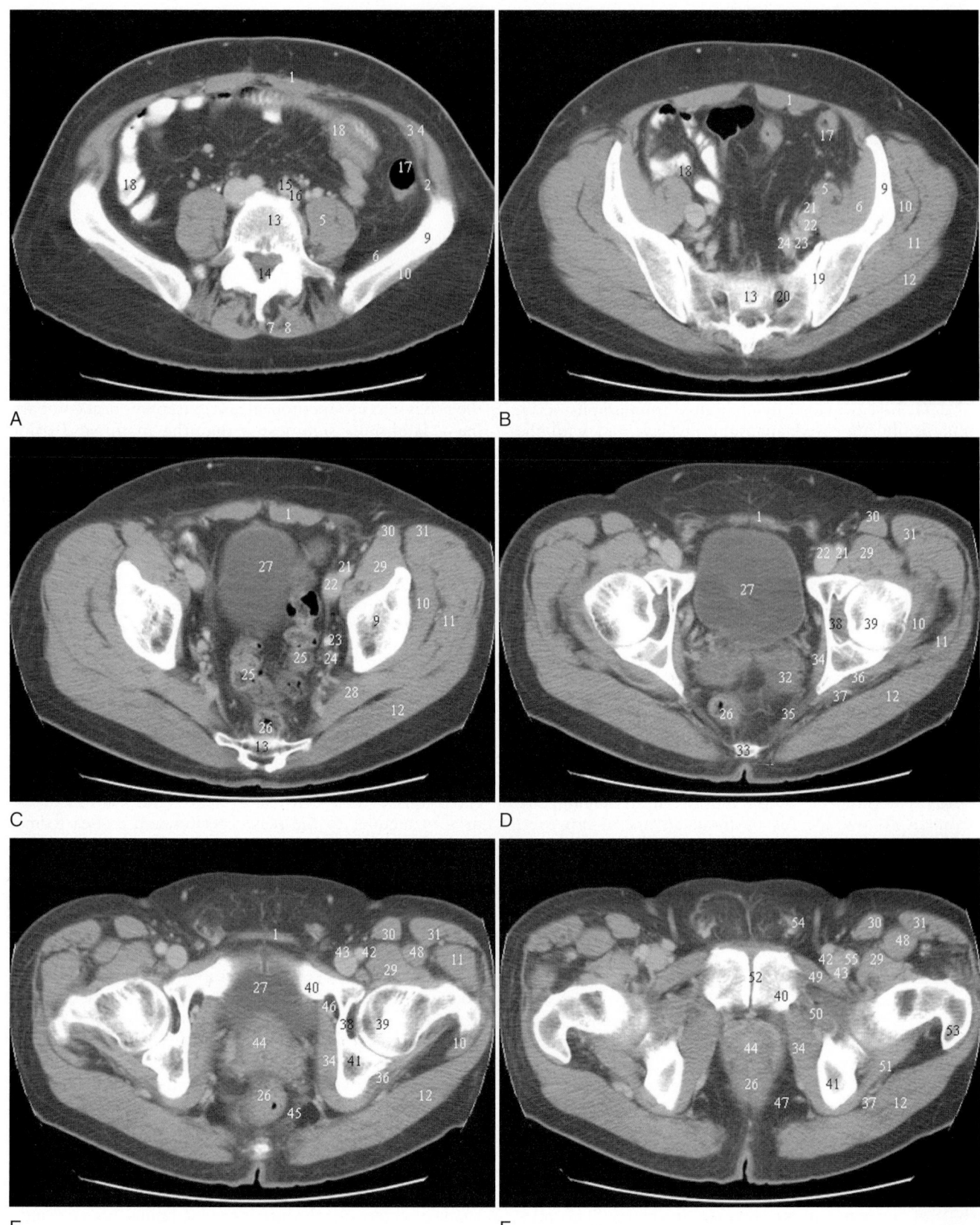

Figure 19–1. Axial contrast-enhanced computed tomography images depicting normal pelvic anatomy (**A–H**). 1. Rectus abdominis muscle; 2. Transverse abdominis muscle; 3. Internal oblique muscle; 4. External oblique muscle; 5. Psoas muscle; 6. Iliacus muscle; 7. Transversospinal muscle; 8. Erector spinae muscle; 9. Iliac bone; 10. Gluteus minimus muscle; 11. Gluteus medius muscle; 12. Gluteus maximus muscle; 13. Sacrum; 14. Spinal canal; 15. Common iliac artery; 16. Common iliac vein; 17. Descending colon; 18. Small bowel; 19. Sacroiliac joint; 20. Sacral foramen; 21. External iliac artery; 22. External iliac vein; 23. Internal iliac artery; 24. Internal iliac vein; 25. Sigmoid colon; 26. Rectum; 27. Urinary bladder; 28. Piriformis muscle; 29. Iliopsoas muscle;

continued

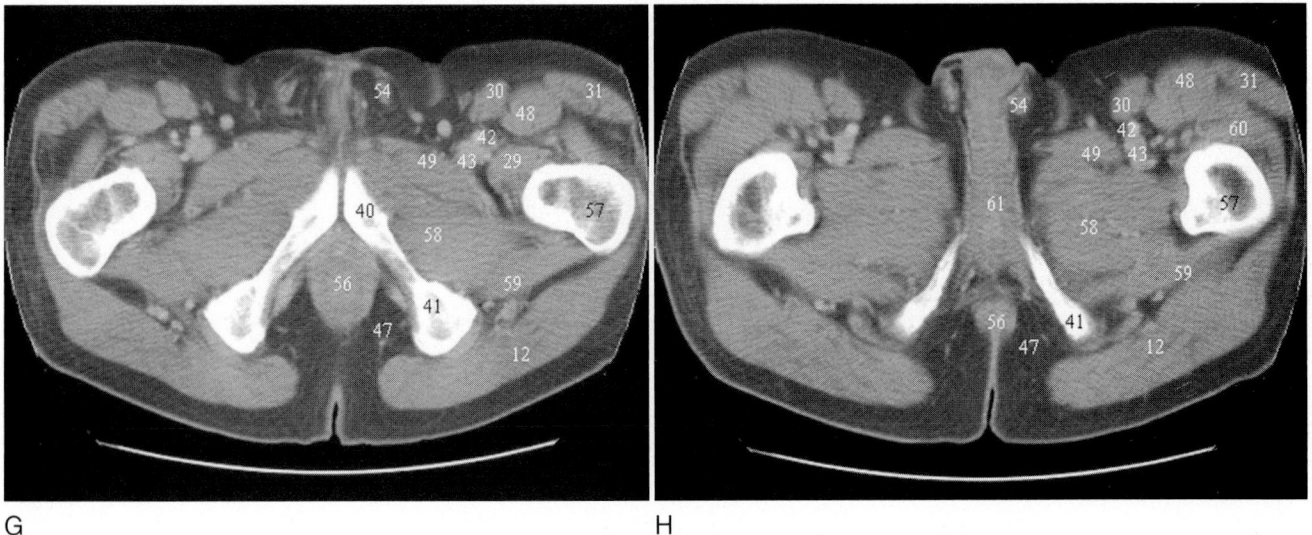

G   H

Figure 19–1. cont'd, 30. Sartorius muscle; 31. Tensor fascia latae muscle; 32. Seminal vesicle; 33. Coccyx; 34. Obturator internus muscle; 35. Coccygeus muscle; 36. Gemellus superior muscle; 37. Sciatic nerve and vessels; 38. Acetabular fossa; 39. Femoral head; 40. Pubis; 41. Ischium; 42. Femoral artery; 43. Femoral vein; 44. Prostate; 45. Levator ani muscle; 46. Obturator fossa; 47. Ischiorectal fossa; 48. Rectus femoris muscle; 49. Pectineus muscle; 50. Obturator externus muscle; 51. Gemellus inferior muscle; 52. Symphysis pubis; 53. Greater trochanter; 54. Spermatic cord; 55. Deep femoral artery; 56. Anal canal; 57. Femur; 58. Adductor muscles; 59. Quadratus femoris muscle; 60. Vastus muscles; 61. Penis.

Blood Vessels

The common iliac bifurcation is located approximately at the level of the third to fourth lumbar vertebra. The common iliac arteries run anterior to the common iliac veins. The common iliac arteries are divided into internal and external iliac arteries at the level of the fifth lumbar to first sacral vertebra. Two branches of external iliac artery that can be identified on imaging are the inferior epigastric artery and the deep circumflex iliac artery. The internal iliac arteries course posteroinferiorly and at the lower margin of the sacroiliac joints divide into anterior and posterior trunks.[1]

Pelvic Lymph Nodes

Lymphatics from pelvic organs drain to pelvic nodal chains bilaterally and to the retroperitoneum. Familiarity with the lymphatic drainage pathways is of great importance for staging pelvic tumors. Figure 19-2 (A–D) illustrates pelvic lymph node groups on axial CT images.

The most peripheral lymph nodes draining the pelvis are the inguinal nodes (see Fig. 19-2D). The inguinal lymph nodes are divided into superficial and deep groups. The superficial inguinal nodes drain the anus, the perianal skin, and the round ligament of the uterus. The lymph from the gluteal region and the anterior abdominal wall below the level of the umbilicus also drain to lateral nodes in this group. The medial group of superficial lymph nodes receives lymphatics from the perineal genitalia. The lower group of superficial inguinal lymph nodes receives superficial lymphatics from the lower extremity. The deep inguinal lymph nodes are located on the medial side of the femoral vein. They receive efferents from the deep lymphatics of the lower extremity, a small number of efferents from the superficial inguinal nodes, and lymphatic drainage from the glans penis or clitoris. The superficial and deep inguinal nodes drain to the external iliac lymph nodes.[1]

The external iliac lymph nodes accompany the external iliac vessels and are divided into medial, posterior, and lateral groups (see Fig. 19-2B and C). The medial group of the external iliac lymph nodes drains the urinary bladder, prostate, membranous part of the urethra, cervix, and upper part of the vagina. The posterior group receives lymphatics from the internal iliac nodes via the obturator lymph nodes. The lateral group drains lymph from the superficial and deep inguinal nodes. The external iliac lymph nodes drain to the posterior and lateral common iliac nodes.[1]

The internal iliac nodes accompany the internal iliac vessels and drain lymph from all of the pelvic viscera such as the body of the uterus, prostate gland, upper part of the vagina, seminal vesicles, vas deferens, lower part of the ureters, and bladder (see Fig. 19-2B). They also receive lymphatic drainage from the deeper parts of the perineum, the buttock muscles, and the posterior aspect of the thigh. They send efferents to the external iliac and common iliac chains. The sacral lymph nodes, which drain directly into lumbar lymphatics, and the anatomic obturator lymph nodes, which are occasionally present in the obturator canal, are members of the internal iliac group.[1]

The common iliac lymph nodes accompany the common iliac vessels and are divided into lateral, medial, and posterior groups (see Fig. 19-2A). The lateral group directly drains the external iliac lymph nodes. The posterior group receives efferents from both the internal and external iliac lymph nodes. The medial common iliac

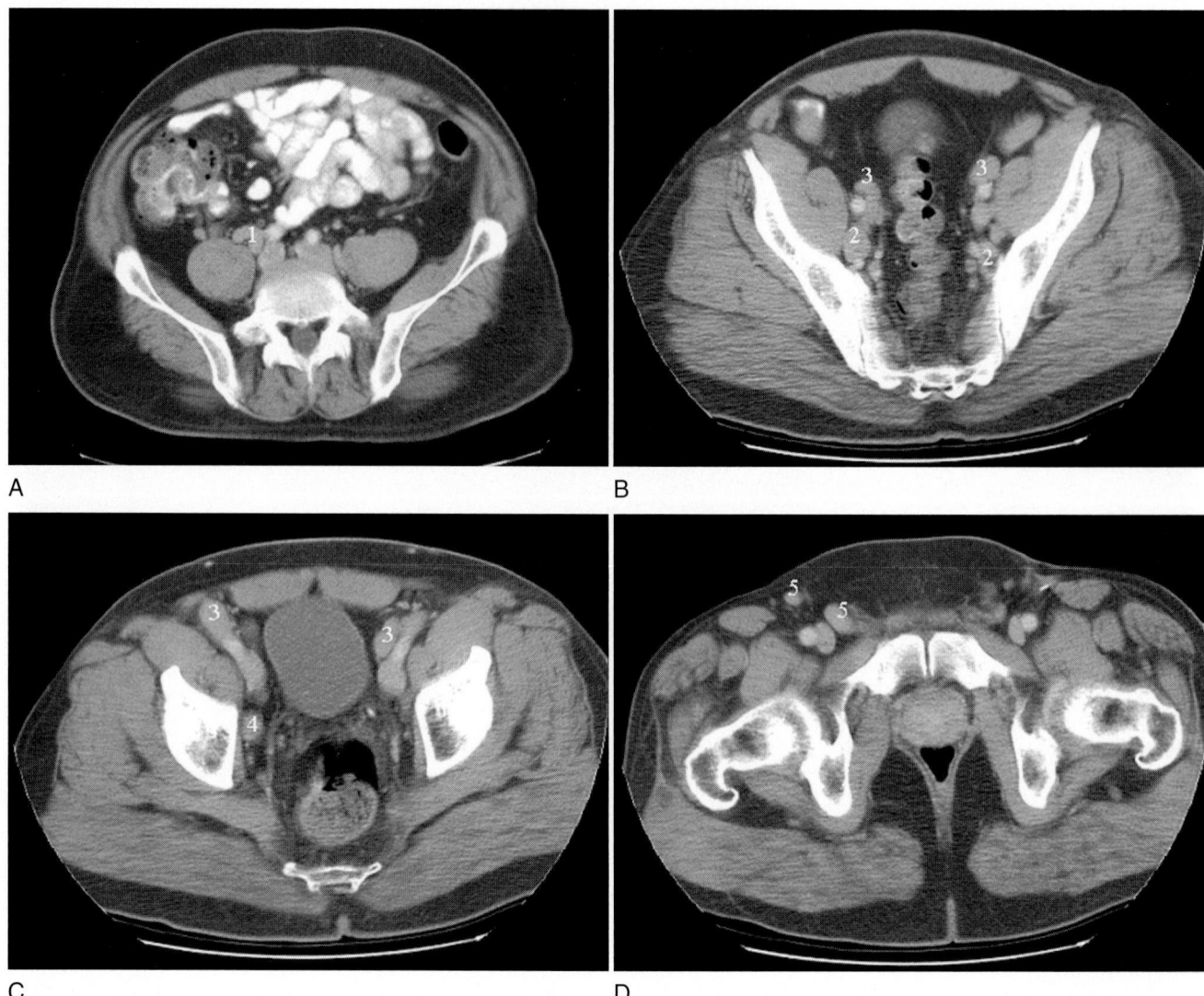

Figure 19–2. A–D, Axial contrast-enhanced computed tomography images depicting pelvic lymphadenopathy. 1. Common iliac lymphadenopathy; 2. Internal iliac lymphadenopathy; 3. External iliac lymphadenopathy; 4. Obturator lymphadenopathy; 5. Inguinal lymphadenopathy.

group receives lymph from the internal iliac nodes. The common iliac nodes drain into the left and right lateral aortic nodal chains, which are part of the lumbar nodes.[1]

The lumbar lymph nodes are divided into right lateral aortic, left lateral aortic, and preaortic lymph node groups. The right lateral aortic chain includes paracaval and retrocaval lymph nodes. The preaortic chain also includes precaval lymph nodes.[1]

Bones and Muscles

The pelvic skeleton is composed of two paired, innominate bones; the sacrum; and the coccyx. The innominate bones are formed by three separate bones: ilium, ischium, and pubis. The acetabulum, which is a socket for the head of the femur, is formed by the fusion of these three bones on each side laterally. The two innominate bones unite anteriorly at the symphysis pubis and posteriorly at the sacrum.[1]

The psoas muscles originate from the vertebral bodies and transverse processes of the 12th thoracic to 4th lumbar vertebrae. At the level of the first sacral vertebra, psoas muscle unites with the iliacus muscle, which originates from the upper two thirds of the iliac fossa and sacral ala. Then, iliopsoas muscle inserts on the lesser trochanter of the femur.[1]

The levator ani and coccygeus muscles are the main muscles of the pelvic diaphragm. The levator ani muscle originates from the pubis, ischium, and the fascia of the obturator internus muscle and inserts on the coccyx and the anococcygeal raphe. The coccygeus muscle arises from the ischial spine and attaches to the coccyx posterior to the levator ani. The other pelvic floor muscles are the deep and superficial transversalis perinei muscles, the ischiocavernosus and bulbocavernosus muscles, and the external anal sphincter muscle.[1]

The obturator internus muscle arising from the anterolateral wall of the true pelvis and the piriformis muscle arising from the lateral aspect of the sacrum insert on the greater trochanter of the femur and form part of the pelvis sidewall.[1]

Uterus and Cervix

The uterus is located posterior to the urinary bladder and anterior to the rectum (Fig. 19-3A–D). In women of reproductive age, the uterus is normally 6 to 9 cm in length. The uterine volume varies with the menstrual cycle and is greatest during the secretory phase.[2]

On T2-weighted magnetic resonance images, three distinct uterine layers can be differentiated: the endometrium, junctional zone, and myometrium. The endometrium is of high signal intensity on T2-weighted images and occupies the central portion of the uterus.

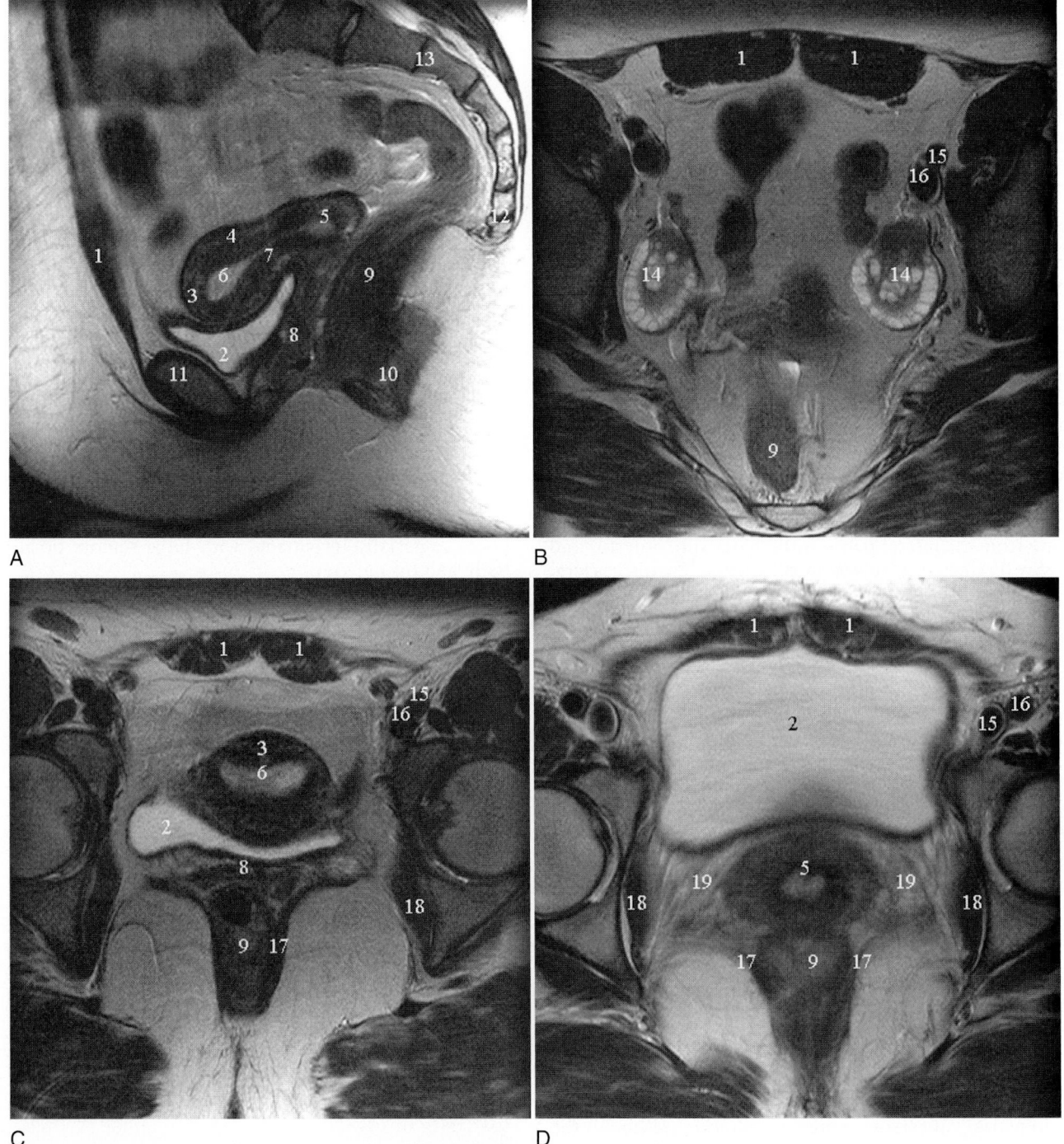

Figure 19–3. Magnetic resonance imaging anatomy of normal uterus and ovaries. Sagittal (**A**) and axial (**B–D**) T2-weighted images. 1. Rectus abdominis muscle; 2. Urinary bladder; 3. Fundus uterus; 4. Corpus uterus; 5. Cervix; 6. Endometrium; 7. Junctional zone; 8. Vagina; 9. Rectum; 10. Anal canal; 11. Pubis; 12. Coccyx; 13. Sacrum; 14. Ovary; 15. External iliac artery; 16. External iliac vein; 17. Levator ani muscle; 18. Internal obturator muscle; 19. Parametrium.

The myometrium, which is of medium signal intensity on T2-weighted images, is separated from the endometrium by a low-signal-intensity region called the *junctional zone*. There is no histological equivalent to the junctional zone. It just represents inner myometrium, which has lower water content than the outer myometrium (see Fig. 19-3A, C).[2,3]

In premenarchal females, the endometrium is either very thin or absent, and the junctional zone is indistinct. The myometrium has lower signal intensity than in postmenarchal females. In postmenopausal women, the zonal anatomy is again indistinct, the endometrium is less than 3 mm thick, and the myometrium is of lower signal intensity compared with that of premenopausal females.[2]

The parametrium is a cellular connective tissue contiguous with the bare areas of the uterus that are not covered by the peritoneum. The parametrium is found adjacent to the lateral margins of the uterus, where the peritoneum reflects to form the broad ligaments and anteriorly between the uterus and the bladder beneath the peritoneal reflection of the vesicouterine pouch. Parametrial tissue contains ureters, blood vessels, and lymphatics (see Fig. 19-3D).[2,4,5]

The broad ligaments of the uterus are formed by the reflections of the peritoneum as it passes over the fallopian tubes and enclose the fallopian tubes, round ligaments, uterine vessels, and ovarian ligaments. The round ligaments originate at the lateral angles of the uterus and pass through the inguinal canal to insert the labia majora. The suspensory ligaments of the uterus are the vesicouterine, cardinal, and uterosacral ligaments. The vesicouterine ligaments are located between the cervix and the urinary bladder base. The cardinal ligaments originate from the lateral pelvic wall, divide into anterior and posterior slips, and surround the cervix. The uterosacral ligaments pass between the cervix and sacrum and encircle the rectum. The uterine suspensory ligaments are clinically significant because they form local pathways for tumor spread, particularly in cervical carcinoma.[2]

The cervix is the inferior portion of the uterus (see Fig. 19-3A, D). On T2-weighted magnetic resonance images, the cervix demonstrates a high-signal-intensity inner area with a surrounding low-signal-intensity stroma. The inner zone represents epithelium and mucus. The stroma of the cervix, which has a high concentration of elastic fibrous tissue within its inner portion, demonstrates low signal intensity on T2-weighted images. Smooth muscle strands predominate toward the periphery of the cervix, resulting in an area of medium signal intensity similar to that of myometrium.[2,4,5]

ENDOMETRIAL CANCER

Endometrial carcinoma is the fourth most common cancer in females and the most common invasive gynecologic malignancy in the United States.[6] Up to 90% of endometrial cancers are adenocarcinomas. Although the exact etiology of endometrial cancer is still unknown, two distinct mechanisms may play a role in its origin: (1) unopposed estrogen stimulation, causing endometrial hyperplasia, which then progresses to carcinoma; and (2) spontaneous carcinoma arising from atrophic or inert endometrium.[7]

The most important prognostic factors in endometrial cancer include the histologic grade of the tumor, the stage of the tumor, depth of myometrial invasion, and the lymph node status.[8] Because of the inability of clinical staging to assess the depth of myometrial invasion or the presence of lymphadenopathy, the International Federation of Gynecology and Obstetrics (FIGO) revised the staging of endometrial cancer to incorporate surgical findings. Surgical staging, however, is not suitable for elderly and obese patients and those with additional medical problems that make them poor candidates for surgery. Noninvasive cross sectional imaging is particularly helpful in such cases to depict the depth of myometrial invasion, tumor extent, and presence of lymphadenopathy. Pretreatment imaging improves patient care by impacting the type and extent of surgery or radiation treatment or both.[3]

Ultrasound is a simple technique that can depict endometrial tumors (Fig. 19-4). The use of transabdominal ultrasonography in staging of endometrial cancer is not advocated. However, transvaginal ultrasonography is helpful in the evaluation of myometrial invasion, with accuracy rates varying between 68% and 99%.[3] Myometrial invasion is suggested when the tumor disrupts the subendometrial halo and extends asymmetrically into myometrium.[9] The limitations of ultrasound include: (1) poor soft tissue contrast resolution, which hampers delineation between tumor, adjacent myometrium, and coexisting pathology such as uterine leiomyomas; (2) a relatively small field of view, which precludes assessment the cervix, parametrium, and the lymph nodes, especially in patients with large tumors or large body habitus or both.[3]

CT is widely used for the preoperative evaluation of endometrial carcinoma to assess the extent of disease

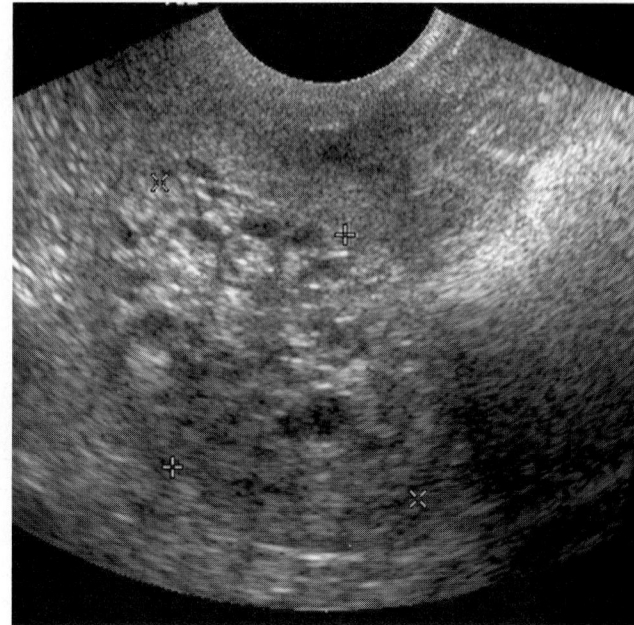

Figure 19–4. Transvaginal ultrasound depicts large heterogeneous mass containing cystic areas within the endometrial cavity.

and lymph node status.[3] The accuracy of preoperative staging with conventional CT for endometrial cancer varies between 84% and 88%.[10,11] However, even by using helical computed tomography, magnetic resonance imaging (MRI) was reported to be more sensitive and specific than CT for preoperative staging of endometrial cancer.[12]

At present, magnetic resonance is the most accurate imaging modality for the pretreatment evaluation of endometrial cancer. The reported staging accuracy of MRI for endometrial cancer is between 83% and 92%.[13-15] A suggested MRI protocol includes orthogonal T2-weighted, transverse T1-weighted, and sagittal, dynamic, contrast-enhanced, T1-weighted sequences.[3] This protocol is optimal for detection of primary tumor, myometrial and cervical involvement, local spread, and lymphadenopathy.[3]

Endometrial tumors are isointense to myometrium on T1-weighted sequences and demonstrate a variable appearance on T2-weighted sequences (Fig. 19-5). Following dynamic administration of contrast, they enhance less than the normal myometrium, which is more marked on early phases.[3] Stage 0 (carcinoma in situ) tumors appear as normal or widened endometrium. Stage I endometrial cancers are confined to uterine corpus. In stage IA, the tumor is limited to endometrium and may demonstrate normal or diffuse or focal abnormal signal intensity with smooth endometrial-myometrial interface. Stage IB tumors penetrate into myometrium less than 50% with partial or full-thickness disruption of the junctional zone and irregular endometrial-myometrial interface. In stage IC, the tumor extends into myometrium more than 50%; however, the outer stripe of myometrium is intact. Stage II endometrial cancers extend beyond the uterine corpus into the cervix. In stage IIA, the internal os and endocervical canal are widened; however, low-signal-intensity, fibrous cervical stroma is intact. In stage IIB, fibrocervical stroma is disrupted. Stage III endometrial cancers extend beyond the uterus but not to the true pelvis. In stage IIIA, outer myometrium is irregular and disrupted. The ovaries may be involved by direct extension or as metastases. Parametrial involvement is seen as disruption of the serosa and direct tumor extension into parametrial fat. Stage IIIB tumors involve the upper vagina, which is seen as disruption of the low-signal-intensity vaginal wall. In stage IIIC disease, there is lymph node involvement, which can be diagnosed when the short axis of lymph nodes exceeds 1 cm. Unfortunately, metastatic and hyperplastic lymphadenopathy cannot be distinguished based on signal intensity characteristics. Stage IV tumors extend beyond the true pelvis. In stage IVA there is disruption of tissue planes with loss of low-signal-intensity wall of bladder, rectum, or both, indicating invasion of these organs. In stage IVB, there is distant organ metastasis.[3]

CERVICAL CANCER

Cervical carcinoma is the sixth most common solid malignant neoplasm in women in the United States.[6] Cervical cancer occurs more commonly in young women with low socioeconomic status. Risk factors include early age at first intercourse, several sexual partners, nulliparity, smoking, and a history of sexually transmitted diseases. There is strong evidence that the human papilloma virus is a main cause of cervical cancer. Cervical cancer arises at the squamocolumnar junction. The two main histologic

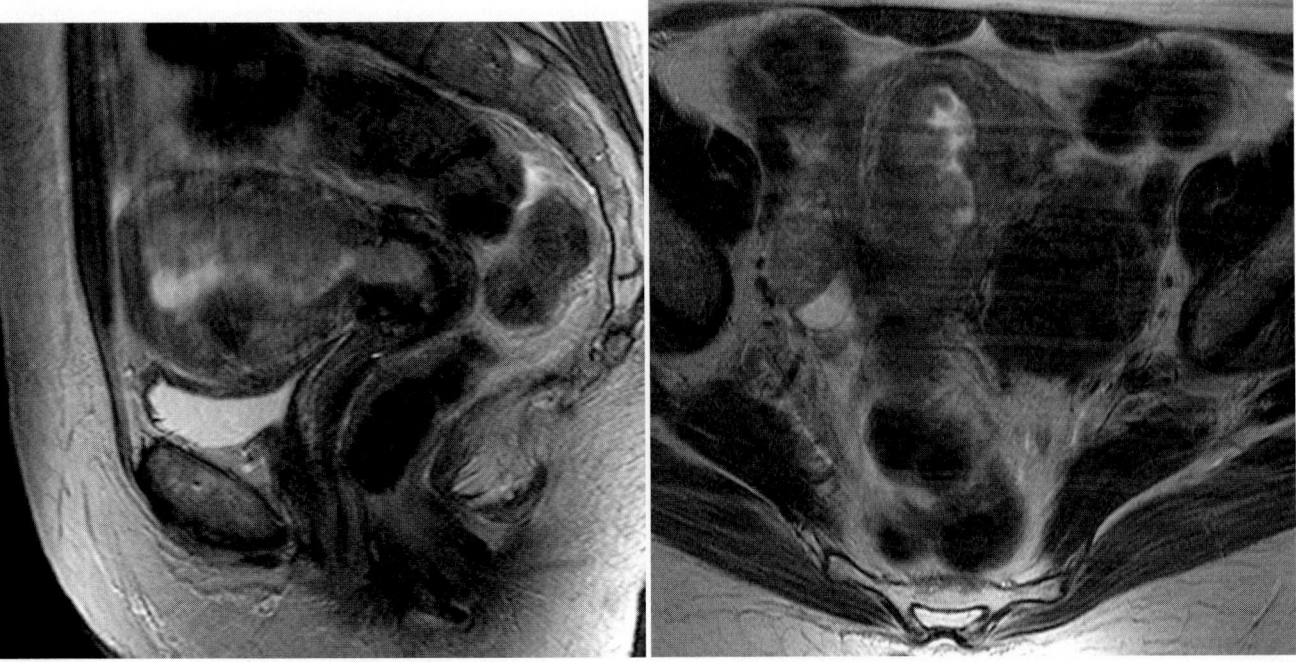

A   B

Figure 19–5. Sagittal (**A**) and axial (**B**) T2-weighted magnetic resonance images depict endometrial cancer. Note that the low-signal intensity junctional zone is disrupted, indicating myometrial invasion.

types are: squamous cell carcinoma, which accounts for the 80% to 90% of cases, and adenocarcinoma, which has a worse prognosis. Tumor prognostic factors include the histologic grade of the tumor, the location of the tumor (exocervix versus endocervix), tumor volume, depth of stromal invasion, adjacent organ invasion, and lymph node status.[4]

The FIGO staging system includes findings obtained from physical examination, examination under anesthesia, cystoscopy, rectosigmoidoscopy, barium enema, biopsy, intravenous pyelography, and chest radiography. There is a discrepancy between clinical staging and intraoperative or pathologic findings in 20% to 35% of cases depending on the stage of the tumor.[4,16-18] In addition, lymph node metastases and extension into adjacent organs are difficult to detect clinically.

The diagnosis of cervical cancer is made by cytology or biopsy. Imaging is warranted when tumor diameter is greater than 2 cm, the clinical examination to determine tumor size is difficult, or when the tumor is primarily endocervical in location. The role of imaging in the pretreatment evaluation of cervical cancer is to define the extent of tumor to decide suitable treatment modality.

Ultrasound has a low diagnostic value in cervical cancer staging. Patient's habitus, lack of soft tissue contrast, and operator dependence are limitations of ultrasound in the staging of pelvic malignancies.[4] CT cannot differentiate normal cervical tissue from tumor and is therefore also limited to evaluate tumor size and stromal invasion[4] (Fig. 19-6). CT was found to be 65% accurate in the staging of cervical carcinoma compared with 90% accuracy of MRI. In evaluating lymph node metastasis, both modalities were alike with an accuracy of 86%.[19] MRI is accepted as the most accurate imaging modality in the staging of cervical cancer and provides important

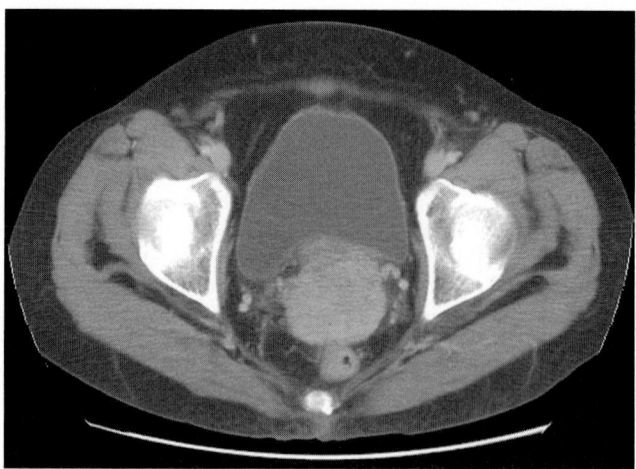

Figure 19–6. Contrast-enhanced axial computed tomography image demonstrates large cervical mass.

information in selecting patients for surgery or radiation therapy.

Cervical cancer appears as a relatively high-signal-intensity mass within low-signal-intensity cervical stroma on T2-weighted sequences (Fig. 19-7). The contrast enhancement of cervical cancer varies considerably. Since contrast enhancement makes the tumor isointense with the surrounding cervical and parametrial tissue on T1-weighted images, it does not increase the ability of MRI in tumor depiction and stromal or parametrial invasion.[20-24] Contrast enhancement may help in the evaluation of tumor extension into the pelvic wall or adjacent organs.[24]

Stage 0 (carcinoma in situ) tumors are not visible on MRI. Stage I tumors are confined to the cervix. Depending

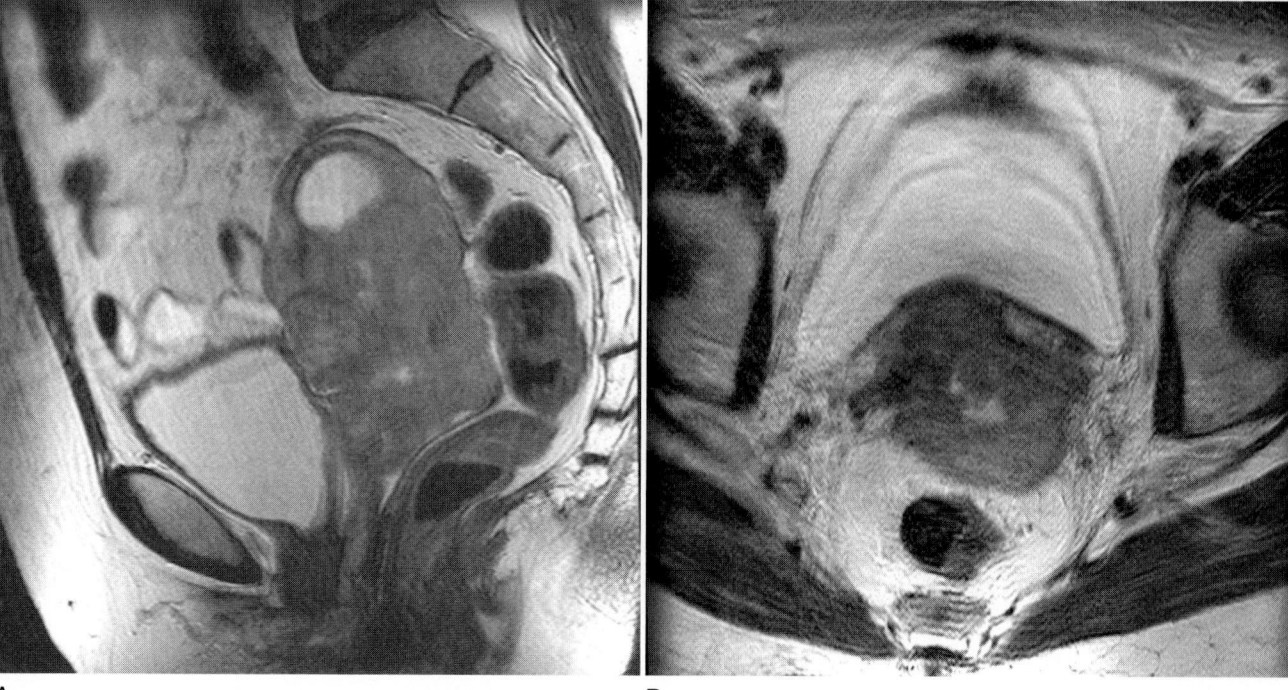

A   B

Figure 19–7. Sagittal (**A**) and axial (**B**) T2-weighted magnetic resonance images demonstrate a large cervical mass growing into the uterus.

on the size of the lesion, these tumors can be detected by their high signal intensity within a low-signal-intensity cervical ring on T2-weighted images. The depth of stromal invasion can be determined easily. Preservation of a low-signal-intensity cervical stripe is a good indicator for the exclusion of parametrial invasion. Complete disruption of the cervical ring, indicating full-thickness stromal involvement, may hamper exclusion of parametrial involvement. Stage II tumors extend beyond the cervix. In stage IIA tumors, less than two thirds of the upper vagina is involved, which is seen as loss of normal low signal intensity and thickening of the vagina. The tumor is classified as stage IIB when there is parametrial invasion. The tumor extends directly through low-signal-intensity cervical stroma into the parametrium. Stage IIIA tumors extend into the lower third of the vagina, which is indicated by loss of low signal intensity and thickening of the lower part of the vagina. In stage IIIB tumors, there is pelvic side wall invasion, and hydronephrosis can be seen if there is ureteral involvement. Stage IV tumors invade the bladder or rectum, which is indicated by the loss of normal low signal intensity and thickening of the walls of these adjacent structures.[20-24]

Signal intensity characteristics are not helpful in differentiating between malignant and hyperplastic lymph nodes. MRI has a sensitivity of 62%, a specificity of 98%, and an accuracy of 93% in detecting metastatic lymphadenopathy in cervical cancer if the upper limit of normal lymph nodes is accepted as 1 cm in the short axis.[25] MRI and CT are not significantly different in the detection of metastatic lymphadenopathy in cervical cancer.[26]

VAGINA AND VULVA

The vagina is a fibromuscular tube extending between the uterus and the vestibule, the cleft between the labia minora. The vulva consists of mons pubis, labia majora, labia minor, clitoris, vestibular bulb, vestibular glands, and the vestibule of the vagina.

On cross-sectional images, the vagina is located between the bladder and urethra anteriorly and rectum and anal canal posteriorly (see Fig. 19-3A). The upper vagina is attached to the uterine cervix near the external os and forms anterior and posterior fornices. The posterior vaginal fornix is deeper than the anterior fornix.[2,27]

Cancer of the Vagina

Most of the primary vaginal malignancies are squamous cell carcinomas. Adenocarcinomas are only 5% to 10% of primary vaginal malignancies. Clear cell adenocarcinoma of the vagina is a subtype of adenocarcinoma associated with maternal ingestion of diethylstilbestrol during pregnancy. Vaginal melanomas and vaginal sarcomas are other rare primary vaginal malignancies. In children younger than age 6, the most common primary vaginal malignancy is embryonal rhabdomyosarcoma (sarcoma botryoides). Metastases to the vagina are more common than the primary tumors and usually occur by direct extension from adjacent organs such as the endometrium, cervix, rectum, or bladder.[27]

The most important prognostic factors in vaginal malignancies are tumor stage and tumor size. Staging of vaginal cancer according to FIGO includes clinical examination, chest x-ray, complete blood count, and biochemical profile. Often cystoscopy, sigmoidoscopy, barium enema, and intravenous pyelography are also included in FIGO staging.[27]

Cross-sectional imaging has been increasingly used in the evaluation of patients with vaginal cancers. Ultrasound is limited in the evaluation of the cervix and vagina. Both ultrasound and CT have low soft tissue contrast and are therefore not good enough in depicting early vaginal cancer. CT is useful in the evaluation of advanced disease and in the assessment of lymph node status. MRI has excellent soft tissue resolution and is therefore very useful in evaluating the tumor size, location, and extent of disease.[27]

On T2-weighted magnetic resonance images, vaginal carcinomas appear as intermediate– to high–signal-intensity masses. When the tumor is confined to the vaginal wall (stage I), the normal low-signal-intensity vaginal wall is intact on T2-weighted sequences. Stage II lesions invade paravaginal tissues but do not extend to the pelvic side wall. On T2-weighted sequences, the interface between fat and tumor is not well defined and there is medium to high signal intensity similar to tumor intensity within paravaginal tissues. In stage III tumors there is increased signal intensity within pelvic floor muscles on T2-weighted images, indicating extension into the pelvic wall. Stage IVA tumors invade the bladder or rectum or extend beyond the true pelvis. Direct tumor extension into the bladder or rectum can be seen as disruption of soft tissue planes and increased signal intensity within the bladder or rectal wall.[27]

Cancer of the Vulva

Vulvar cancer is a rare malignancy occurring most commonly in women older than age 60. The most common histologic type is squamous cell carcinoma. The other vulvar cancers consist of melanoma, Bartholin gland cancer, Paget's disease, sarcomas, basal cell carcinoma, and adenocarcinoma.[27]

Prognosis of vulvar carcinoma depends on tumor size, depth of tumor invasion, and lymph node metastases. CT is useful in the evaluation of advanced disease and lymph node status. MRI is superior to both ultrasound and CT in evaluating local extension of the tumor.[27]

Stage I vulvar cancers are less than 2 cm in size and can be seen as high-signal-intensity lesions on T2-weighted sequences. Stage II tumors are larger than 2 cm but confined to the vulva. In stage III tumors, there is invasion of the lower urethra with or without involvement of the vagina and anus. A high–signal-intensity mass extending into these structures can be seen on T2-weighted magnetic resonance images. In stage IVA, tumor extension to the upper urethra, bladder, rectal mucosa, or pelvic bones can be seen as areas of intermediate– to high–signal-intensity within these structures.[27]

OVARIES

The ovaries lie in the lateral pelvic sidewall recesses called ovarian fossae, between the obliterated umbilical artery anteriorly and the internal iliac artery and the ureter posteriorly (see Fig. 19-3*B*).[28]

The size and appearance of the ovary vary with age. At birth the ovary measures $1.5 \times 0.5 \times 0.3$ cm and is situated within the false pelvis. During adolescence the ovaries enlarge to reach adult size and move to the true pelvis. In the adult, the ovary measures approximately $3 \times 1.5 \times 1$ cm and weighs 2 to 8 grams. After menopause, the ovary becomes atrophic, measuring less than 2 cm in diameter and weighing only 1 to 2 grams.[28]

The ovarian suspensory ligament extends from the lateral pelvic wall to the tubal aspect of the ovary and contains the ovarian artery and vein. The tubo-ovarian ligament originates from the lateral uterine angle and attaches to the uterine aspect of the ovary.[28]

The ovarian arteries originate directly from the aorta. A small ovarian branch of the uterine artery supplies the ovary in addition to the ovarian artery. The ovarian veins drain to the inferior vena cava on the right side and to the left renal vein on the left side.[28]

Ovarian Cancer

Ovarian cancer is the fifth most common cause of cancer-related deaths in women and the most common cause of death from gynecologic malignancy.[6] Approximately 90% of ovarian cancers are of epithelial origin, with subtypes such as serous, mucinous, endometrioid, clear cell, and undifferentiated. Nonepithelial cancers of the ovary include malignant granulosa cell tumor, dysgerminoma, immature teratoma, endodermal sinus tumor, and metastases.[29,30]

The FIGO staging system of ovarian cancer reflects the three primary mechanisms of ovarian cancer spread: local, peritoneal, and lymphatic. Stage I ovarian cancer refers to tumor confined to one or both ovaries. Stage II indicates ovarian cancer with peritoneal metastases confined to the true pelvis. Stage III refers to ovarian cancer with extrapelvic peritoneal metastases or nodal disease. Stage IIIA indicates that there are microscopic implants. Stage IIIB refers to implants smaller than 2 cm and Stage IIIC indicates that the implants are larger than 2 cm. Stage IV consists of ovarian cancer with distant metastases such as malignant pleural effusion and intrahepatic metastases. The management of ovarian cancer is closely related to stage. The standard of care for FIGO stage I, II, IIIA, and IIIB ovarian cancer is an exploratory staging laparotomy. The standard of care for resectable FIGO stage IIIC ovarian cancer is primary surgical cytoreduction (i.e., debulking) followed by adjuvant chemotherapy. Optimal debulking refers to the reduction of all tumor sites to a maximal diameter of less than 1 cm. The management of FIGO stage IV disease is primary chemo-cytoreduction. Considering different management options, the importance of imaging is in the distinction among FIGO stages IIIA, IIIB, and stage IIIC disease. Furthermore, in the category of FIGO stage IIIC disease,

the importance of imaging is in the detection of nonresectable disease. Important for patient management is also the assignment of FIGO stage IV disease. There are two potential pitfalls in assigning FIGO stage IV disease. On imaging, the presence of pleural effusion can be benign or malignant. The findings of pleural thickening or nodularity in addition to the presence of pleural effusion indicate the malignant nature of effusion. In the absence of those findings, thoracentesis is essential. The other important distinction is to differentiate liver surface implants (peritoneal spread and therefore stage III disease) from true intraparenchymal metastases (as a result of hematogenous spread and therefore stage IV disease).[29,31]

In patients with an adnexal mass, ultrasound is very accurate in the assessment of tumor location (e.g., differentiation of uterine from adnexal masses), as well as distinguishing between a benign and malignant adnexal lesion (Fig. 19-8). Doppler ultrasound findings are also very helpful in addition to morphologic features of the mass depicted on gray-scale ultrasound.[32,33] If ultrasound findings are inconclusive, MRI is recommended for further evaluation.[34] The use of contrast media in MRI allows a better characterization of solid nodules within a cystic lesion or presence of necrosis within a solid lesion. In the characterization of adnexal masses, MRI also demonstrates a high inter- and intraobserver agreement.[35,36] CT is not commonly used in the characterization of an adnexal mass. Characterization of an adnexal mass on CT relies on the depiction of morphologic features such as enhancing mural nodularity or heterogeneity and necrosis within the solid lesion (Fig. 19-9). Presence of ancillary findings such as ascites and peritoneal carcinomatosis are strong indicators of a malignant adnexal mass by ultrasound, CT, or MRI.

Ovarian cancer can spread by local continuity to the opposite ovary; uterus; and adjacent structures such as the sigmoid colon, urinary bladder, and pelvic sidewall. Imaging criteria for rectosigmoid and urinary bladder invasion include focal obliteration of the fat plane between the tumor and these organs.

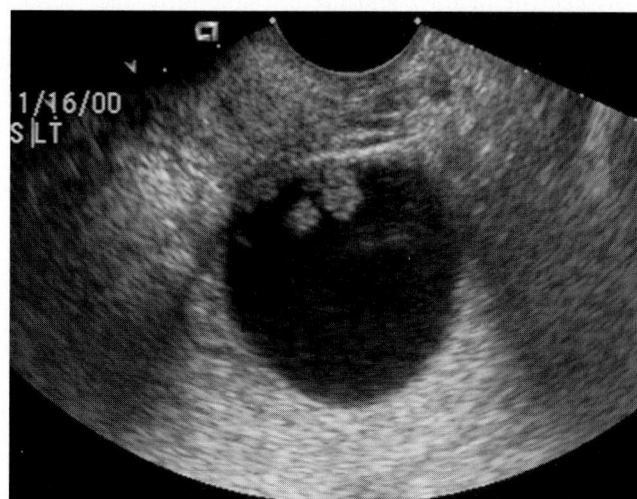

Figure 19–8. Ovarian serous adenocarcinoma. Transvaginal ultrasound depicts a cystic ovarian mass with nodular solid components.

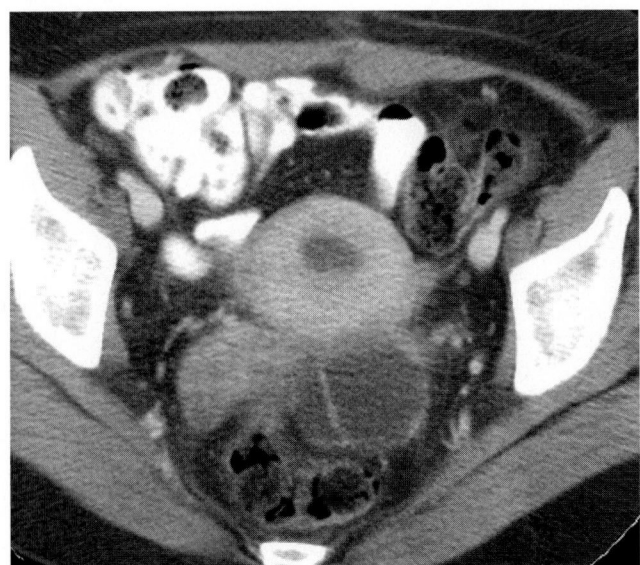

Figure 19–9. Contrast-enhanced axial computed tomography reveals a left ovarian cystic mass with thick nodular wall.

Peritoneal spread is the most common route of ovarian cancer spread. Peritoneal nodules are commonly seen in the pouch of Douglas, right paracolic gutter, right subphrenic space, and left paracolic gutter. Peritoneal metastases appear as nodular or plaque-like enhancing soft tissue masses of varying sizes. Ascites in a patient with ovarian cancer usually indicates its malignant nature. Ascitic fluid often outlines small peritoneal implants, facilitating their detection.

Ovarian cancer can also spread to lymph nodes. Most commonly, nodal disease is seen along the aortocaval and paraortic retroperitoneal sites. Second, nodal spread along the broad ligament can reach the internal iliac, obturator, and external iliac vessels. Third, lymph node involvement can occur via the round ligament to the external iliac and inguinal nodes. Superior diaphragmatic lymphadenopathy is considered as distant nodal disease and indicates advanced ovarian cancer.

Hematogeneous spread from ovarian cancer commonly occurs to sites such as the liver, lung, pleura, adrenal gland, and spleen. Bone and brain metastases are rare.

PROSTATE AND SEMINAL VESICLES

The normal adult prostate measures approximately $4 \times 3 \times 3$ cm, and weighs 15 to 20 grams. It is shaped like an inverted pyramid and surrounds the prostatic urethra (Fig. 19-10A–D).[37,38]

The prostate is histologically composed of glandular and nonglandular elements. The prostatic urethra and the anterior fibromuscular stroma are the major nonglandular components. The glandular portion of the prostate consists of inner and outer components, both of which are divided into two. The inner prostate consists of periurethral glandular tissue and the transitional zone and the outer prostate consists of the central and peripheral zones.[37,38]

The prostatic urethra is divided into proximal and distal parts by the verumontanum, which lies midway between the prostatic apex and the bladder neck. The proximal half of the prostatic urethra is surrounded by a cuff of smooth muscle known as the *preprostatic sphincter*, which prevents the passage of major ducts into the proximal part of the prostatic urethra.[37,38]

The periurethral glands and the transitional and central zones are related exclusively to the proximal prostatic urethra. The peripheral zone surrounds all three components as well as the distal prostatic urethra. The ducts of the peripheral zone drain exclusively to the distal prostatic urethra.[37,38]

The zonal description of prostate anatomy is clinicopathologically more significant than the older lobar nomenclature. First, the zones are clearly defined on histologic sections. In addition, prostatic pathologies have a zonal distribution. Prostatic adenocarcinomas arise 70% in the peripheral zone, 20% in the transitional zone, and 10% in the central zone. On the contrary, nodules of benign prostatic hyperplasia arise either in the transitional zone or the submucosal periurethral glands of the proximal urethra. Prostatitis is a disease of the glandular prostate, with a predilection for the peripheral zone.[37-39]

From an imaging viewpoint, the glandular prostate is arbitrarily divided into two components: peripheral zone and the central gland. The term "central gland" refers collectively to the periurethral, transitional, and central zones. In young men the central gland comprises mainly the central zone, while in older men with benign prostatic hyperplasia, the central gland comprises mainly the transitional zone.[37-39]

The true or anatomic capsule of the prostate is a 2-to 3-mm thick fibromuscular tissue layer surrounding the prostate. The anatomic capsule should not be confused with the surgical or pseudo-capsule, which develops around the central gland in the aging hyperplastic prostate.[37,38]

Anteriorly, the prostate is separated from the symphysis pubis and the pubic bones by vessels and connective tissue. The puboprostatic ligaments run from the prostatomembranous junction to the pubic bones. Posteriorly, the prostate is separated from the rectum by areolar tissue and Denonvilliers' fascia. Posterosuperiorly, the seminal vesicles lie between the bladder base and rectum. Laterally, the prostate is surrounded by the periprostatic venous plexus and the muscles of the pelvic floor. The lateral venous plexus, arteries, and nerves collectively comprise the neurovascular bundles, which pass craniocaudally along the posterolateral aspect of the prostate. The neurovascular bundles pierce the capsule; therefore, extracapsular extension of tumor occurs preferentially along them. Inferiorly, the apex of the prostate abuts the genitourinary membrane. The urethra exits the prostate to enter the genitourinary membrane and becomes the membranous urethra. The genitourinary membrane is suspended between the inferior pubic rami just below the symphysis pubis.[37,38]

The seminal vesicles are paired accessory glands located superior to the prostate gland, posterior to the urinary bladder, and anterior to the rectum. Each seminal vesicle consists of a single tube coiled upon itself. In its medial portion, the tube is constricted and forms an excretory duct. The excretory duct of the seminal vesicle and the ductus deferens join to form an ejaculatory

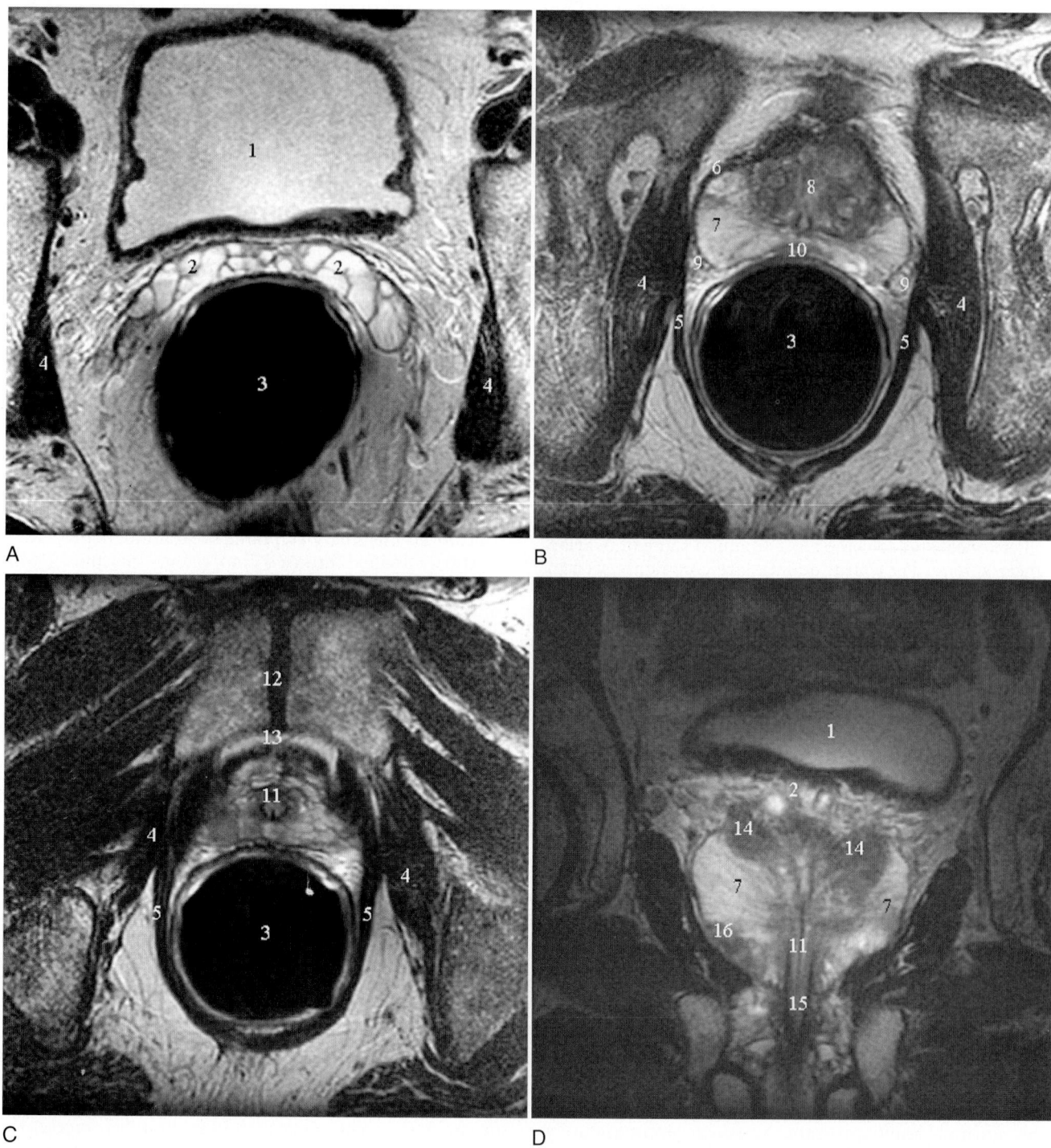

Figure 19–10. Magnetic resonance imaging anatomy of prostate. Axial (**A–C**) and coronal (**D**) T2-weighted images. 1. Urinary bladder; 2. Seminal vesicles; 3. Rectum; 4. Obturator internus muscle; 5. Levator ani muscle; 6. Prostatic capsule; 7. Peripheral zone; 8. Transitional zone; 9. Neurovascular bundle; 10. Denonvilliers' fascia; 11. Prostatic urethra; 12. Symphysis pubis; 13. Retropubic space; 14. Central zone; 15. Membranous urethra; 16. Tumor.

duct. The ejaculatory ducts pass obliquely within the prostate gland and at the verumontanum join to the prostatic urethra (see Fig. 19-10A).[38,40]

Prostate Cancer

Prostate cancer is the most common cancer seen in men and the second most common cause of cancer-related deaths after lung cancer. About 189,000 new cases of prostate cancer are expected among men in the United States. However, more than 80 percent of these estimated new cases are diagnosed at local and regional stages with nearly 100 percent 5-year relative survival rates.[6] Autopsy studies showed that 30% to 46% of men older than age 50 have microscopic prostate cancer, but less than 20% of men develop clinically overt prostate cancer in their lifetime.[41,42] Unlike other aggressive cancers, prostate cancer has less predictable behavior. Prognostic factors include the size, histologic grade, and stage of the tumor.

Prostate cancer is suspected due to an abnormal digital rectal examination or elevated serum prostate-specific antigen (PSA), which are recommended in yearly checkups for men older than age 50. Diagnosis of prostate cancer is made by histopathologic examination of tissue specimens obtained from the prostate, which also allows estimation of tumor grade. Imaging findings have no role in the early detection and diagnosis of prostate cancer but provide valuable information in staging the disease. Another role of imaging is guidance for biopsy.[39]

Transrectal ultrasound provides high-resolution images of the prostate gland because a high-frequency (5 to 7.5 MHz) probe can be placed close to the prostate. Ultrasound also allows examination of the prostate in multiple planes and provides very accurate measurements of the prostate gland. The other major use of transrectal ultrasound is guidance for biopsy.[39] Only prostate cancers located in the peripheral zone can be reliably detected by ultrasound. Prostate cancer is usually seen as a hypoechoic area relative to the peripheral zone (Fig. 19-11). However, up to 40% of prostate cancers are isoechoic, hampering their detection with ultrasound.[43,44] The finding of a hypoechoic area within the peripheral zone is not specific for prostate carcinoma and can also be seen in benign processes such as prostatitis.[39,44] Distortion of the normal internal anatomy of the prostate is another important sign that may help in detection of prostate carcinoma, especially in advanced cases.[44]

CT, even with contrast enhancement, lacks the soft tissue resolution for the detection of prostate cancer within a normal prostate. Additionally, CT has no advantages over ultrasound in guidance for biopsy.[39] However, CT is very useful in the detection of distant metastases and lymph nodes.[39]

MRI provides the best quality of images demonstrating normal zonal anatomy of the prostate.[39] On T2-weighted magnetic resonance images, prostate cancer is seen most commonly as a low–signal-intensity area within the high–signal-intensity normal peripheral zone. The detection of prostate cancer on MRI, like transrectal ultrasound, is reliable only in tumors located in the peripheral zone. Even in the peripheral zone, postbiopsy changes, prostatitis, dystrophic changes, changes secondary to radiation, or hormonal ablation therapy can be seen as low–signal-intensity areas mimicking tumor.[39] It has been shown that MRI should be performed at least 3 weeks after biopsy to prevent under- or over-staging of tumor extent on MRI. The role of MRI in evaluating prostate cancer is mainly to demonstrate extracapsular and seminal vesicle invasion (Fig. 19-12). MRI findings of extracapsular extension include: irregular bulge of the prostate margin; contour deformity with step-off or angulated margin; overt disruption of the capsule with direct tumor extension; obliteration of recto-prostatic angle; and asymmetry of neurovascular bundles. Seminal vesicle invasion is diagnosed when contiguous low–signal-intensity tumor extension into and around seminal vesicles is demonstrated, or when a tumor extension along the ejaculatory duct results in nonvisualization of the ejaculatory duct, decreased signal intensity of seminal vesicles, and loss of the seminal vesicle wall on T2-weighted images.[45,46]

Magnetic resonance spectroscopy is a new technique used in prostate imaging that provides metabolic information by detection of cellular metabolites: citrate, creatine, and choline. In tumor localization, combined use of MRI and magnetic resonance spectroscopy provides the highest specificity (91%) among noninvasive methods. Combined use of magnetic resonance spectroscopy also improves detection of extracapsular extension.[47-49]

The Tumor Node Metastasis (TNM) staging classification is widely used for staging prostate cancer and can be applied to imaging. T1 prostate cancers are nonpalpable tumors that are discovered incidentally during transurethral resection of the prostate or because of an elevated PSA. T2 tumors represent clinically localized palpable cancers. The tumor is classified as stage T3 if it spreads beyond the prostatic capsule. T4 tumors represent cancers invading adjacent structures such as the bladder, rectum, or pelvic side wall. The N classification denotes the presence or absence of lymphatic involvement, and the M classification indicates distant metastasis.

The primary goal of local staging is to differentiate patients with tumors confined to the prostate (T1 and 2) from patients with tumors that have extracapsular or seminal vesicle invasion (T3). Patients with organ-confined disease can be treated with surgery or radiation therapy. However, patients with extracapsular extension are not surgical candidates and are treated with radiation, hormonal, or combination therapy. Accurate preoperative surgical planning aims to decrease the rate of positive surgical margins while maximizing erectile potency rates. Similarly, radiation treatment aims to deliver a specific dose of radiation to a defined volume of tumor while minimizing radiation exposure to surrounding tissues.

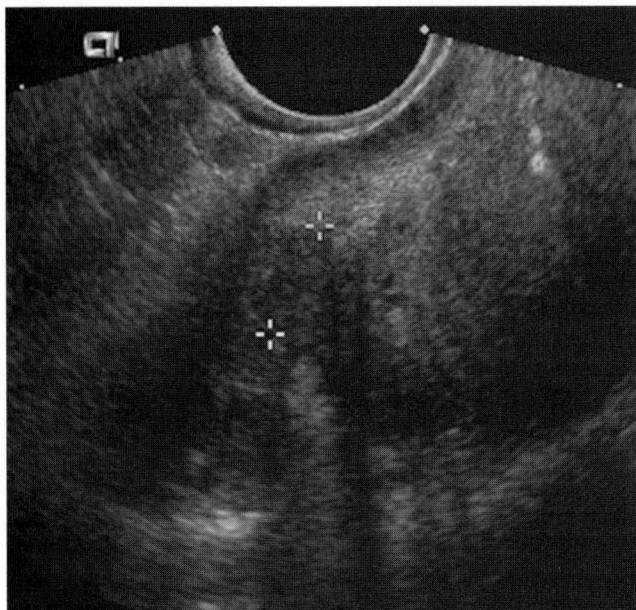

Figure 19–11. Transrectal ultrasound of prostate depicts hypoechoic tumor within the peripheral zone.

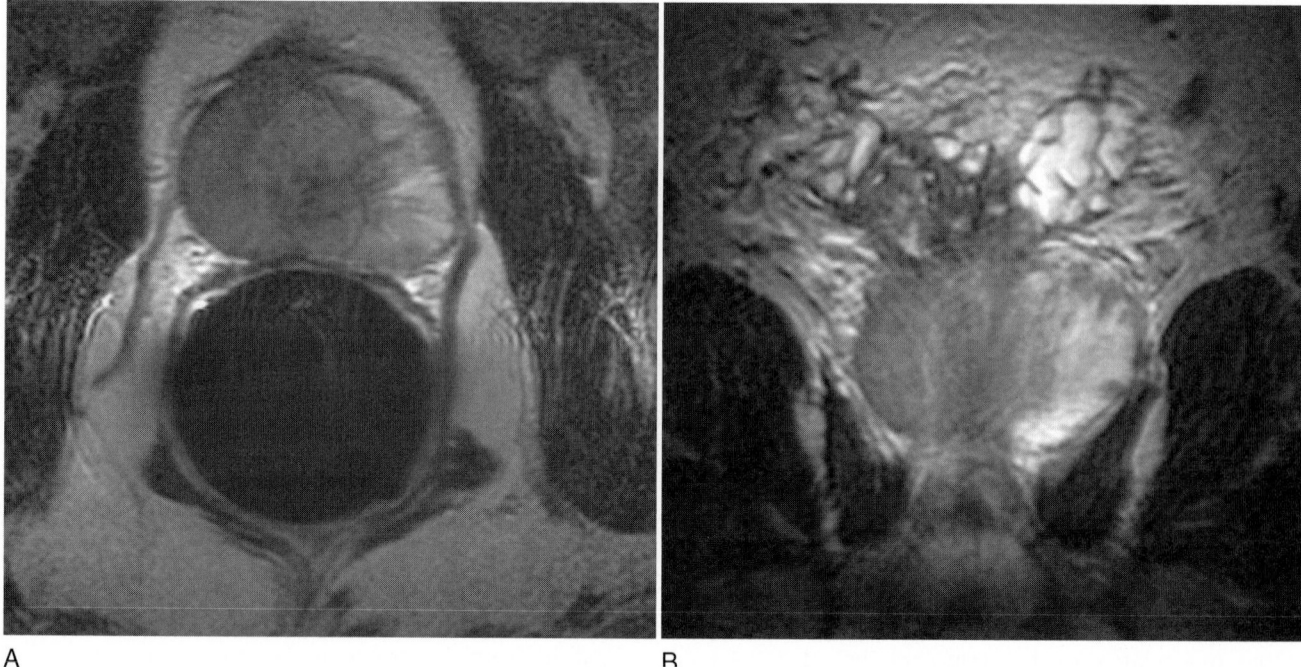

A B

Figure 19–12. Axial (**A**) and coronal (**B**) T2-weighted magnetic resonance images of the prostate reveal large tumor involving the right side of prostate. Tumor invades seminal vesicles (**B**).

Clinical staging, although inexpensive and simple, is not accurate enough to make treatment decisions. Therefore, imaging plays an important role in the staging of prostate cancer. Among the currently available imaging techniques, MRI is the most accurate method for local staging.[39] MRI is cost-effective, especially for patients who have an intermediate risk for having extracapsular extension and recurrent cancer defined by clinical prognostic factors such as digital rectal examination (stages T1 and 2), preoperative PSA (10 to 20 ng/mL), and biopsy Gleason score (5 to 7).[39]

TESTES

The testes are located within the scrotum. The scrotal septum divides the scrotal sac into two compartments. The normal adult testis measures 4 to 5 cm long, 2 to 3 cm wide, and 2 to 3 cm in anteroposterior diameter. The weight of the testis is 15 to 25 grams. The appendix of the testis, which is a müllerian duct remnant, is located at the upper pole of the testis.[50]

An outpouching of peritoneum called *tunica vaginalis* envelops each testis anterolaterally. At the posterolateral bare area of the testis is the epididymis. The *tunica albuginea* is a dense fibrous connective tissue capsule covering the testis itself. Along the posterior aspect of the testis, tunica albuginea invaginates into testis and forms mediastinum testis. Septae from mediastinum testis divide the testis into pyramidal lobules. Convoluted seminiferous tubules within the lobules of the testis straighten to form *rete testis* in the region of the mediastinum testis. The efferent ductules run from the rete testis to the duct of epididymis. The *ductus deferens (vas deferens)* is a continuation of the duct of epididymis. The

ductus deferens is about 30 cm long and extends to the ejaculatory duct. The ductus deferens, testicular vessels, and lymphatics are surrounded by a connective tissue fascia called spermatic cord. Each layer of the anterior abdominal wall musculature and parts of the cremasteric muscle contribute to form spermatic cord.[50]

The testicular arteries arise from the aorta or renal artery. The veins of the testis converge at the mediastinum testis and form pampiniform plexus.[50]

Testicular Tumors

Testicular tumors are rare, constituting only 1% of all malignant neoplasms in men, but are the most common malignancy occurring in young men and adolescents.[6,51] They can be classified into germ cell tumors, arising from spermatogenic cells, and non–germ cell tumors, deriving from the sex cords (Sertoli cells) and stroma (Leydig cells). Germ cell tumors constitute 95% of testicular neoplasms and are almost uniformly malignant. However, non–germ cell primary tumors of the testis are malignant in only 10% of cases. The secondary tumors of the testis include tumors such as lymphoma, leukemia, and metastases.[51]

Testicular tumors most commonly present with painless scrotal enlargement or as an incidental testicular nodule. Pain is an uncommon presenting symptom, reported by approximately 10% of patients. In some cases, testicular neoplasia may initially be misdiagnosed as orchitis. Testicular tumors sometimes may undergo regression, necrosis, and scarring (so-called burned-out germ cell tumors); therefore, some patients may have normal or small testes at presentation. Some patients, especially those who have an aggressive histologic tumor type, may present with metastases. A small group of patients with hormonally active tumors present with endocrine abnormalities, most commonly gynecomastia.[50,51]

Ultrasonography performed with high frequency transducers is the most commonly used primary imaging modality for the initial workup and evaluation of a scrotal mass, as well as in the staging of a known testicular tumor (Fig. 19-13). It has been shown to be almost 100% sensitive in the detection of scrotal masses. Intratesticular versus extratesticular pathologic conditions can be differentiated with 98% to 100% sensitivity.[52,53] The normal testis demonstrates a homogeneous echotexture. The covering tunica albuginea is generally not seen as a separate structure; except in mediastinum testis, where it can be seen as an echogenic line invaginating into the testis. The epididymis is isoechoic or slightly hyperechoic compared with the testis.

Ultrasound is very helpful in the localization of the scrotal mass, whether intratesticular or extratesticular. Further morphologic characterization of the lesion such as cystic or solid is also possible. Solid intratesticular masses are frequently malignant. Testicular tumors are usually hypoechoic compared with the surrounding testicular parenchyma. Some tumors can be heterogeneous, containing calcifications or cystic areas. Color Doppler ultrasound may be helpful to identify an isoechoic mass or differentiate a complex cystic lesion from a solid mass.[51]

MRI can be a useful problem-solving tool in the rare cases in which ultrasound is inconclusive.[54] The normal testis demonstrates a homogeneous, intermediate signal intensity on T1-weighted images and high signal intensity on T2-weighted images. The tunica albuginea appears as a thin low–signal-intensity line surrounding the testis on both T1-weighted and T2-weighted images. The epididymis is isointense or slightly hypointense relative to the testis on T1-weighted images and hypointense on T2-weighted images.[50,51]

Testicular tumors often demonstrate homogeneous medium signal intensity similar to normal testis on T1-weighted images and decreased signal intensity within high signal intensity of normal testis on T2-weighted images. Homogeneous or heterogeneous high–signal-intensity tumors or tumors with similar signal intensity to testis can also be seen.[50] MRI is very sensitive in depicting the tumors; however, specificity as to tumor type is low.

PENIS

The penis is composed of two lateral corpora cavernosa and the ventral and medial corpus spongiosum. The posterior portions of the corpora cavernosa called the *crura* and the expanded posterior end of corpus spongiosum called the *bulb of penis* form the radix penis located in the perineum. The major portions of the corpora cavernosa and the corpus spongiosum are found within the shaft of the penis. At its distal end, the corpus spongiosum expands to form the glans penis. The tunica albuginea, which is composed of fibrous tissue, covers all three corpora. Buck's fascia is a fibrous envelope that separates the corpora cavernosa from the corpus spongiosum. The suspensory ligaments of the penis blend with Buck's fascia and extend to the symphysis pubis.[55]

Penile Carcinoma

Carcinoma of the penis is a rare disease. Most penile cancers are squamous cell carcinomas. Penile carcinoma's etiology is unclear, but it is seldom seen in circumcised men and it is related to the presence of foreskin, irritant effects of smegma, and poor hygiene. Treatment depends on the degree of involvement and ranges from partial penile amputation to total penectomy.[55]

MRI is a useful tool to evaluate penile tumors that appear iso- to hypointense on T1-weighted images and hypointense on T2-weighted images compared with the surrounding corporeal body. MRI is especially useful when the tumor extends into the radix penis, which is difficult to evaluate clinically. Depiction of tumor extension into the bulb of penis or across the urogenital diaphragm is important in determining treatment options, which include radiation or surgery.[55]

URINARY BLADDER AND URETHRA

The urinary bladder is extraperitoneal and located behind the symphysis pubis. In the male, the bladder base is related to the base of the prostate gland, seminal vesicles, and ductus deferens. In the female, the bladder base is related to the cervix, vagina, periurethral muscles, and urethra. In infants, the internal sphincter of the urinary bladder neck lies above the symphysis pubis and the upper border of the full urinary bladder rises to the level of the first sacral vertebra. In adults, the urinary bladder neck is located at the level of the symphysis pubis, and the full urinary bladder reaches the level of the second or third sacral vertebra.[56]

The male urethra is about 18 to 20 cm long and is divided into three segments: prostatic, membranous, and penile urethra. The penile urethra is also divided into

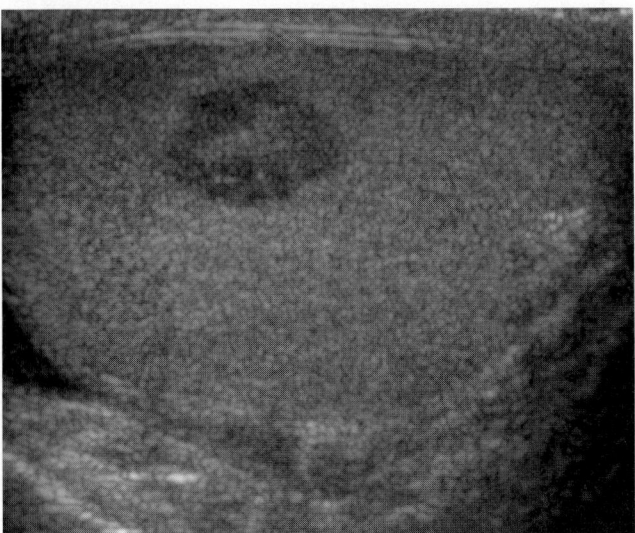

Figure 19–13. Scrotal ultrasound reveals heterogeneous hypoechoic mass in testis.

bulbar and anterior portions. The prostatic urethra is the 3 to 4 cm portion surrounded by the prostate gland. The membranous urethra is 1 cm long, extending from the apex of the prostate to the bulb of penis passing through the urogenital diaphragm. The wall of the membranous urethra consists of an inner layer of smooth muscle bundles and an outer, thicker layer of striated muscle fibers called the *external sphincter*. The penile urethra is 15 cm long and is located within the corpus spongiosum.[37,55]

The female urethra is 4 cm long and extends from the internal urethral orifice of the bladder to the external urethral orifice just anterior to the vaginal opening. The female urethra is divided into three portions: the upper, middle, and lower thirds. The upper third is composed mainly of an external muscular coat, which is continuous with the bladder neck. The middle third of the urethra is surrounded by an outer layer of circular striated muscle and inner layer of smooth muscle in submucosa. The lower third of the female urethra is almost entirely of fibrous tissue.[56]

Bladder Cancer

Bladder carcinoma is the most common malignancy of the urinary tract. It occurs more commonly in males than females.[6] Most bladder cancers are of epithelial origin and up to 90% are transitional cell carcinomas. Squamous cell carcinomas (5% to 10%) and adenocarcinomas (2%) are the other types of epithelial bladder cancers. Squamous cell carcinomas are associated with chronic inflammatory diseases of the urinary bladder.[56]

The prognosis of urinary bladder cancer depends on histologic type, pattern of tumor growth, and anatomic extent of disease at the time of diagnosis. Most patients present with superficial disease, for which transurethral resection and multiple cystoscopic biopsies are sufficient for diagnosis, staging, and definitive therapy. Staging with cross-sectional imaging is necessary when deeply invasive tumors are detected (Figs. 19–14 and 19–15). Evaluation of bladder cancer consists of determining the site, number and growth pattern of the tumors, depth of muscular and perivesical invasion, and lymph node status.

On cross-sectional imaging, it is difficult to differentiate tumors that are confined to the mucosa and submucosa (stage T1) from tumors superficially invading the muscle wall (stage T2). Deep muscle invasion (stage T3a) is diagnosed when there is interruption of the urinary bladder wall. Perivesical fat invasion (stage T3b) can be diagnosed when there is infiltration in the perivesical fat. However, inflammatory changes can mimic tumor invasion into perivesical fat and may cause over-staging. Direct invasion of adjacent organs (stage T4) can also be easily seen on CT or MRI. Detection of lymph node metastasis depends on demonstration of enlarged regional lymph nodes. However, metastatic lymph nodes cannot be differentiated from hyperplastic ones.

Different numbers of staging accuracies for bladder carcinoma were reported with CT (40% to 92%) and with MRI (50% to 96%). Dynamic contrast-enhanced MRI provides increased tumor detection and staging accuracy for superficial lesions. Limitations of both MRI and CT include their inabilities to depict small tumor growth

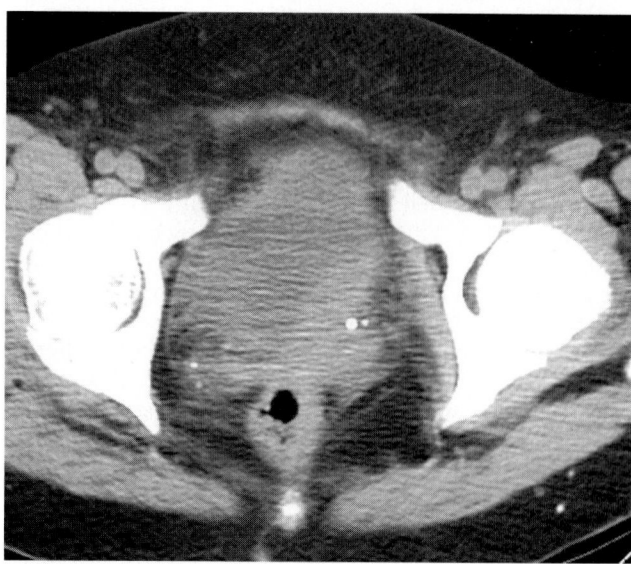

Figure 19–14. Contrast-enhanced axial computed tomography image reveals bladder cancer causing thickening of the left posterolateral wall.

into the muscle layer of the bladder wall or differentiate between tumor and inflammatory changes.[57–63]

RECTUM AND SIGMOID COLON

The sigmoid colon is usually located in the true pelvis. It is an intraperitoneal organ. The rectosigmoid junction is located approximately at the level of the third segment of the sacrum. The rectosigmoid junction forms an acute angle and is fixed by the mesentery. The rectum is the terminal portion of the colon and ends at the anus.

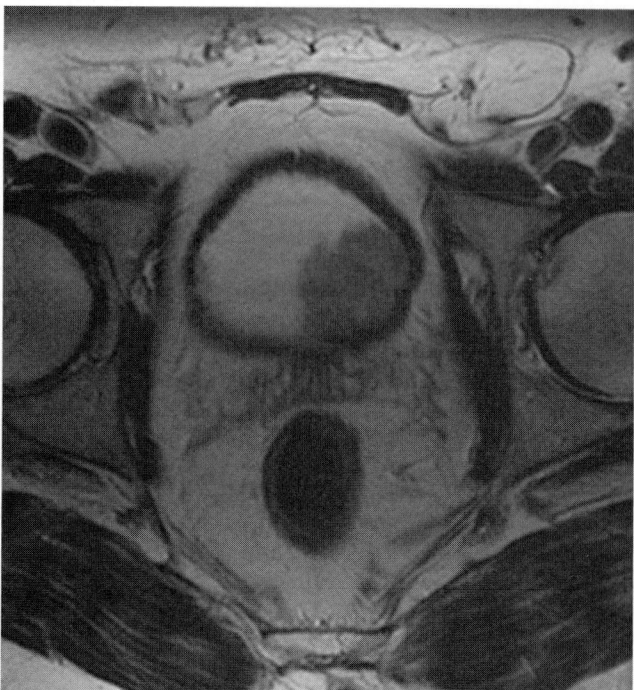

Figure 19–15. Axial T2-weighted magnetic resonance image depicts bladder cancer on left posterolateral wall. Note that the normal low signal intensity of bladder wall is preserved, excluding tumor invasion.

Anatomically, the rectum comprises a 10- to 12-cm long rectum proper and a 2.5- to 3-cm long anal canal. The upper portion of the rectum is totally covered by peritoneum. The dorsal part of the rectum is not covered by the peritoneum. The anterior and lateral aspects of the rectum are also covered by peritoneum to the level of the fifth sacral or first coccygeal vertebra. The peritoneal reflection anteriorly creates the rectovesical fossa in the male and the rectouterine fossa (pouch of Douglas) in the female. The lateral peritoneal recesses form the pararectal spaces. The ischiorectal fossae are located laterally to the rectum and bounded laterally by the obturator internus muscle and the levator ani muscle.[64]

The anal canal is the external aperture of the colon and terminates at the anus. The levator ani muscle attaches laterally to the anal canal and acts as an accessory sphincter. It consists of three parts: the iliococcygeus muscle, the pubococcygeus muscle, and the puborectalis muscle. The puborectalis muscle is also known as the sphincter muscle of the rectum. Two sphincters surround the anal canal. The internal anal sphincter is a 2- to 3-mm thick ring, formed by the thickening of circular fibers of the muscularis propria. The external anal sphincter is elliptical in shape with three concentric layers of striated muscle fibers: deep, superficial, and subcutaneous parts.[64]

Rectal Cancer

Colorectal carcinoma is the most common cancer of the gastrointestinal tract, and the second most common cause of cancer-related death in the United States.[6] The most common histologic type of sigmoid and rectal cancer is adenocarcinoma. The standard surgical management for rectal carcinoma was once abdominoperineal resection and formation of permanent colostomy. However, new surgical techniques such as low-anterior resection with anal sphincter sparing and local excision, have become more popular for well-differentiated, early-stage tumors. Accurate preoperative staging of rectal cancer determines the choice of surgical approach and the need for adjuvant radio- or chemotherapy. In addition, the degree of tumor invasion through the layers of the rectal wall and the patient's nodal status are very important features that determine the risk of local tumor recurrence.[65,66] For these reasons, correct preoperative local staging of rectal cancer is essential.

Transrectal ultrasound and MRI are commonly used for assessing tumor penetration through the rectal wall layers and nodal status. Unlike CT, both transrectal ultrasound and MRI can distinguish the layers of the rectal wall and allow depiction of tumor growth through these layers. According to the TNM staging system, a stage T1 tumor is limited to the mucosa and submucosa and does not extend to the muscularis propria. Stage T2 refers to tumors that partially involve the muscularis propria. A stage T3 tumor totally disrupts the muscular layer and extends into the perirectal fat. When invasion is present in adjacent organs or structures, the tumor is identified as stage T4 (Fig. 19-16).

For the local staging of rectal cancer, the reported accuracy of transrectal ultrasound ranges between 70% and 81%, and that for MRI between 71% and 91%. Most understaging errors occur due to the inability to detect microscopic or minimal invasion with both methods. Regarding overstaging, inflammatory changes in perirectal fat mimicking tumor invasion are reported to be the most frequent cause.[67-74]

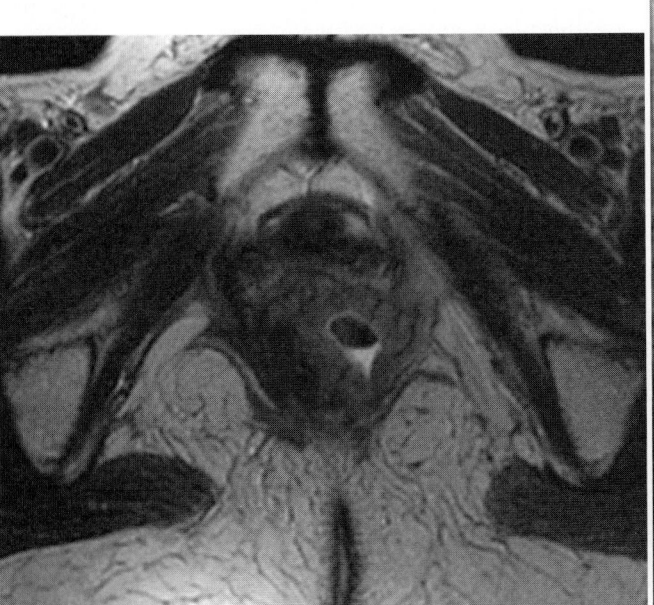
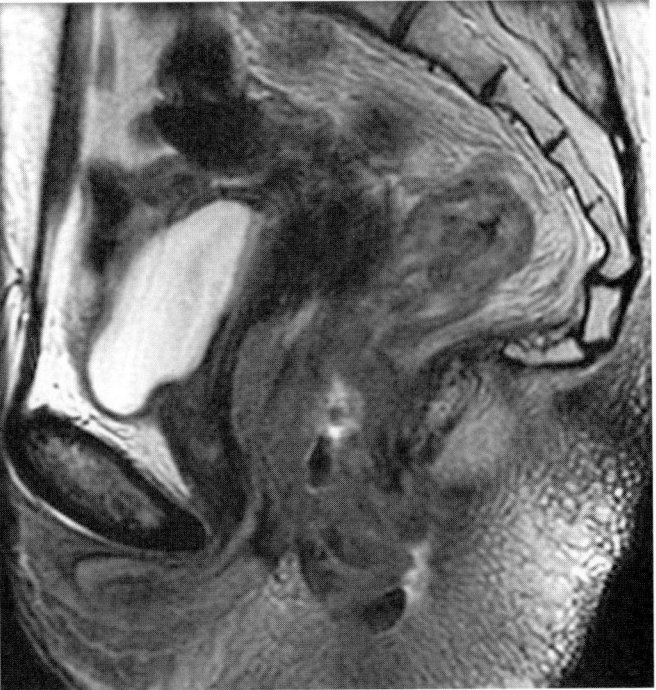

A   B

Figure 19–16. Axial (**A**) and sagittal (**B**) T2-weighted magnetic resonance images reveal rectal cancer causing thickening in rectal wall and invading vagina.

REFERENCES

1. Carrington B, Hricak H: Anatomy of the pelvis. In Hricak H, Carrington BM, eds. *MRI of the Pelvis. A Text Atlas*. London: Martin Dunitz Ltd; 1991:43.
2. Carrington B, Hricak H: The uterus and vagina. In Hricak H, Carrington BM, eds. *MRI of the Pelvis. A Text Atlas*. London: Martin Dunitz Ltd; 1991:93.
3. Ascher SM, Reinhold C. Imaging of cancer of the endometrium. *Radiol Clin North Am*. 2002;40:563.
4. Scheidler J, Heuck AF: Imaging of cancer of the cervix. *Radiol Clin North Am*. 2002;40:577.
5. Nicolet V, Carignan L, Bourdon F, Prosmanne O: MR imaging of cervical carcinoma: A practical staging approach. *Radiographics*. 2000;20:1539.
6. Jemal A, Thomas A, Murray T, et al: Cancer statistics, 2002. *CA Cancer J Clin*. 2002;52:23.
7. Barakat RR, Grigsby PW, Zaino SP: Corpus epithelial tumors. In Hoskins WJ, Perez CA, Young RC, eds. *Principles and Practice of Gynecologic Oncology*. Philadelphia: Lippincott Williams & Wilkins; 2000:919.
8. Boronow RC, Morrow CP, Creaseman WT, et al: Surgical staging in endometrial carcinoma: Clinical-pathologic findings of a prospective study. *Obstet Gynecol*. 1984;63:825.
9. Gordon AN, Fleischer AC, Dudley BS, et al: Preoperative assessment myometrial invasion of endometrial adenocarcinoma by sonography (US) and magnetic resonance imaging (MRI). *Gynecol Oncol*. 1989;34:175.
10. Balfe DM, Van Dyke J, Lee JK, et al: Computed tomography in malignant endometrial neoplasms. *J Comput Assist Tomogr*. 1983; 7:677.
11. Walsh JW, Goplerud DR: Computed tomography of primary, persistent and recurrent endometrial malignancy. *AJR Am J Roentgenol*. 1982;139:1149.
12. Hardesty L, Sumkin JH, Hakim C, et al: The ability of helical CT to pre-operatively stage endometrial carcinoma. *AJR Am J Roentgenol*. 2001;176:603.
13. Hirano Y, Kubo K, Hirai Y, et al: Preliminary experience with gadolinium-enhanced dynamic MR imaging for uterine neoplasms. *Radiographics*. 1992;12:243.
14. Hricak H, Rubinstein LV, Gherman GM, et al: MR imaging evaluation of endometrial carcinoma: Results of an NCI cooperative study. *Radiology*. 1991;179:829.
15. Lien HH, Blomlie V, Trope C, et al: Cancer of the endometrium: Value of MR imaging in determining depth of invasion into the myometrium. *AJR Am J Roentgenol*. 1991;157:1221.
16. Chung CK, Nahhas WA, Zaino R, et al: Histologic grade and lymph node metastasis in squamous call carcinoma of the cervix. *Gynecol Oncol*. 1981;12:348.
17. Cobby M, Browning J, Jones A, et al: Magnetic resonance imaging, computed tomography and endosonography in the local staging of carcinoma of the cervix. *Br J Radiol*. 1990;63:673.
18. Kim SH, Choi BI, Lee HP, et al: Uterine cervical carcinoma: Comparison of CT and MR findings. *Radiology*. 1990;175:45.
19. Subak LL, Hricak H, Powell CB, et al: Cervical carcinoma: Computed tomography and magnetic resonance imaging for preoperative staging. *Obstet Gynecol*. 1995;86:43.
20. Lien HH, Blomlie V, Kjorstad K, et al: Clinical stage I carcinoma of the cervix: Value of MRI in determining degree of invasiveness. *AJR Am J Roentgenol*. 1991;156:1191.
21. Sironi S, Belloni C, Taccagni GL, et al: Carcinoma of the cervix: Value of MRI in detecting parametrial involvement. *AJR Am J Roentgenol*. 1991;156:753.
22. Togashi K, Nishimura K, Sagoh T, et al: Carcinoma of the cervix: Staging with MRI. *Radiology*. 1989;171:245.
23. Hricak H, Lacey CG, Sandles LG, et al: Invasive cervical carcinoma: Comparison of MRI and surgical findings. *Radiology*. 1988;166:623.
24. Hricak H, Hamm B, Semelka RC, et al: Carcinoma of the uterus: Use of gadopentetate dimeglumine in MRI. *Radiology*. 1991;181:95.
25. Kim SH, Kim SC, Choi BI, et al: Uterine cervical carcinoma: Evaluation of pelvic lymph node metastasis with MRI. *Radiology*. 1994;190:807.
26. Scheidler J, Hricak H, Yu KK, et al: Radiological evaluation of lymph node metastases in patients with cervical cancer: A meta-analysis. *JAMA*. 1997;278:1096.
27. Chang SD: Imaging of the vagina and vulva. *Radiol Clin North Am*. 2002;40:637.
28. Carrington B: The adnexae. In Hricak H, Carrington BM, eds. *MRI of the Pelvis. A Text Atlas*. London: Martin Dunitz Ltd; 1991:185.
29. Coakley FV: Staging ovarian cancer: Role of imaging. *Radiol Clin North Am*. 2002;40:609.
30. Koonings PP, Campbell K, Mishell DR, et al: Relative frequency of primary ovarian neoplasms: A 10-year review. *Obstet Gynecol*. 1989;74:921.
31. Boente MP, Chi DS, Hoskins WJ: The role of surgery in the management of ovarian cancer: Primary and interval cytoreductive surgery. *Semin Oncol*. 1998;25:326.
32. Cohen LS, Escobar PF, Scharm C, et al: Three-dimensional power Doppler ultrasound improves the diagnostic accuracy for ovarian cancer prediction. *Gynecol Oncol*. 2001;82:40.
33. Kinkel K, Hricak H, Lu Y, et al: US characterization of ovarian masses: A meta-analysis. *Radiology*. 2000;217:803.
34. Rieber A, Nussle K, Stohr I, et al: Preoperative diagnosis of ovarian tumors with MR imaging: Comparison with transvaginal sonography, positron emission tomography, and histological findings. *AJR Am J Roentgenol*. 2001;177:123.
35. Hricak H, Chen M, Coakley FV, et al: Complex adnexal masses: Detection and characterization with MR imaging-multivariate analysis. *Radiology*. 2000;214:39.
36. Stevens SK, Hricak H, Stern JL: Ovarian lesions: Detection and characterization with gadolinium-enhanced MR imaging at 1.5 T. *Radiology*. 1991;181:481.
37. Hricak H: The prostate gland. In Hricak H, Carrington BM, eds. *MRI of the Pelvis. A Text Atlas*. London: Martin Dunitz Ltd; 1991:249.
38. Coakley FV, Hricak H: Radiologic anatomy of the prostate gland: A clinical approach. *Radiol Clin North Am*. 2000;38:15.
39. Yu KK, Hricak H: Imaging prostate cancer. *Radiol Clin North Am*. 2000;38:59.
40. Hricak H: The seminal vesicles. In Hricak H, Carrington BM, eds. *MRI of the Pelvis. A Text Atlas*. London: Martin Dunitz Ltd; 1991:313.
41. Kabalin JN, McNeal JE, Price HM, et al: Unsuspected adenocarcinoma of the prostate in patients undergoing cystoprostatectomy for other causes: Incidence, histology and morphometric observations. *J Urol*. 1989;141:1091.
42. Quinlan DM, Partin AW, Walsh PC: Can aggressive prostatic carcinomas be identified and can their natural history be altered by treatment? *Urology*. 1995;46:77.
43. Shinohara K, Wheeler TM, Scardino PT: The appearance of prostate cancer on transrectal ultrasonography: Correlation of imaging and pathological examinations. *J Urol*. 1989;142:76.
44. Shinohara K, Scardino PT, Carter SS, et al: Pathologic basis of the sonographic appearance of the normal and malignant prostate. *Urol Clin North Am*. 1989;16:675.
45. Schnall MD, Imai Y, Tomaszewski J, et al: Prostate cancer: Local staging with endorectal surface coil MR imaging. *Radiology*. 1991; 178:797.
46. Yu KK, Hricak H, Alagappan R, et al: Detection of extracapsular extension of prostate carcinoma with endorectal and phased-array coil MR imaging: Multivariate feature analysis. *Radiology*. 1997; 202:697.
47. Scheidler J, Hricak H, Vigneron DB, et al: Prostate cancer: Localization with three-dimensional proton MR spectroscopic imaging—Clinicopathologic study. *Radiology*. 1999;213:473.
48. Wefer AE, Hricak H, Vigneron DB, et al: Sextant localization of prostate cancer: Comparison of sextant biopsy, magnetic resonance imaging and magnetic resonance spectroscopic imaging with step-section histology. *J Urol*. 2000;164:400.
49. Yu KK, Scheidler J, Hricak H, et al: Prostate cancer: Prediction of extracapsular extension with endorectal MR imaging and three-dimensional proton MR spectroscopic imaging. *Radiology*. 1999;212:481.
50. Hricak H: The testis. In Hricak H, Carrington BM, eds. *MRI of the Pelvis. A Text Atlas*. London: Martin Dunitz Ltd; 1991:343.
51. Ulbright TM, Amin MB, Young RH: *Tumors of the Testis, Adnexa, Spermatic Cord, and Scrotum. Atlas of Tumor Pathology, Fasc 25, Ser 3*. Washington, DC: Armed Forces Institute of Pathology; 1999:1.
52. Schwerk WB, Schwerk WN, Rodeck G: Testicular tumors: Prospective analysis of real-time US patterns and abdominal staging. *Radiology*. 1987;164:369.

53. Rifkin MD, Kurtz AB, Pasto ME, Goldberg BB: Diagnostic capabilities of high-resolution scrotal ultrasonography: Prospective evaluation. *J Ultrasound Med.* 1985;4:13.

54. Serra AD, Hricak H, Coakley FV, et al: Inconclusive clinical and ultrasound evaluation of the scrotum: Impact of magnetic resonance imaging on patient management and cost. *Urology.* 1998;51:1018.

55. Hricak H: The penis and male urethra. In Hricak H, Carrington BM, eds. *MRI of the Pelvis. A Text Atlas.* London: Martin Dunitz Ltd; 1991:383.

56. Hricak H: The bladder and female urethra. In Hricak H, Carrington BM, eds. *MRI of the Pelvis. A Text Atlas.* London: Martin Dunitz Ltd; 1991:417.

57. Husband JE, Olliff JF, Williams MP, et al: Bladder cancer: Staging with CT and MR imaging. *Radiology.* 1989;173:435.

58. Tanimoto A, Yuasa Y, Imai Y, et al: Bladder tumor staging: Comparison of conventional and gadolinium-enhanced dynamic MR imaging and CT. *Radiology.* 1992;185:741.

59. Persad R, Kabala J, Gillatt D, et al: Magnetic resonance imaging in the staging of bladder cancer. *Br J Urol.* 1993;71:566.

60. Barentsz JO, Ruijs SH, Strijk SP: The role of MR imaging in carcinoma of the urinary bladder. *AJR Am J Roentgenol.* 1993; 160:937.

61. Kim B, Semelka RC, Ascher SM, et al: Bladder tumor staging: Comparison of contrast-enhanced CT, T1- and T2-weighted MR imaging, dynamic gadolinium-enhanced imaging, and late gadolinium-enhanced imaging. *Radiology.* 1994;193:239.

62. Barentsz JO, Jager GJ, Witjes JA, et al: Primary staging of urinary bladder carcinoma: The role of MRI and a comparison with CT. *Eur Radiol.* 1996;6:129.

63. Narumi Y, Kumatani T, Sawai Y, et al: The bladder and bladder tumors: Imaging with three-dimensional display of helical CT data. *AJR Am J Roentgenol.* 1996;167:1134.

64. Hricak H: The rectum and sigmoid colon. In Hricak H, Carrington BM, eds. *MRI of the Pelvis. A Text Atlas.* London: Martin Dunitz Ltd; 1991:463.

65. Fazio VW, Tjandra JJ: Primary therapy of carcinoma of the large bowel. *World J Surg.* 1991;15:568.

66. Izbicki JR, Blochle C: Colorectal carcinoma: Impact of staging on surgical treatment. *Endoscopy.* 1993;25:117.

67. Gualdi GF, Casciani E, Guadalaxara A, et al: Local staging of rectal cancer with transrectal ultrasound and endorectal magnetic resonance imaging. Comparison with histologic findings. *Dis Colon Rectum.* 2000;43:338.

68. Zagoria RJ, Schlarb CA, Ott DJ, et al: Assessment of rectal tumor infiltration utilizing endorectal MR imaging and comparison with endoscopic rectal sonography. *J Surg Oncol.* 1997;64:312.

69. Kim NK, Kim MJ, Yun SH, et al: Comparative study of transrectal ultrasonography, pelvic computerized tomography, and magnetic resonance imaging in preoperative staging of rectal cancer. *Dis Colon Rectum.* 1999;42:770.

70. Chan TW, Kressel HY, Milestone B, et al: Rectal carcinoma: Staging at MR imaging with endorectal surface coil. *Radiology.* 1991;181:461.

71. Indinnimeo M, Grasso RF, Cicchini C, et al: Endorectal magnetic resonance imaging in the preoperative staging of rectal tumors. *Int Surg.* 1996;81:419.

72. Schnall MD, Furth EE, Rosato EF, et al: Rectal tumor stage: Correlation of endorectal MR imaging and pathologic findings. *Radiology.* 1994;190:709.

73. Blomqvist L, Holm T, Rubio C, et al: Rectal tumours—MR imaging with endorectal and/or phased-array coils, and histopathological staging on giant sections. *Acta Radiol.* 1997;38:437.

74. Maldjian C, Smith R, Kilger A, et al: Endorectal surface coil MR imaging as a staging technique for rectal carcinoma: A comparison study to rectal endosonography. *Abdom Imaging.* 2000;25:75.

Clinical Radiation Oncology

Primary and Metastatic Brain Tumors in Adults

20

Ashwatha Narayana, MD and *Steven A. Leibel, MD*

Primary brain and central nervous system tumors accounted for an estimated incidence of 18,300 new cases diagnosed in the year 2003 in the United States.[1] They will account for approximately 13,100 deaths in the same year. There is an early peak of 2 to 3 per 100,000 in the annual age-specific incidence of primary brain tumors in children up to the age of 4 years. A decline occurs between 15 and 24 years, followed by a steady rise, reaching a plateau of 21 per 100,000 between 75 and 79 years of age.[2] Several histopathologically different tumors arise in the brain, reflecting the diversity of phenotypically distinct cells within the central nervous system (CNS) that have a capacity for neoplastic transformation.[3] Malignant gliomas are considered first in this chapter. Many of the principles of brain tumor management are discussed in this section. Tumors that are most common in children but also seen in adult patients are reviewed in Chapter 53, Pediatric Central Nervous System Tumors, and only briefly presented here. The chapter closes with a discussion on the management of metastatic brain tumors.

ANAPLASTIC ASTROCYTOMA AND GLIOBLASTOMA MULTIFORME

Epidemiology

Malignant gliomas make up 35% to 45% of primary brain tumors, and of these, nearly 85% are glioblastoma multiforme.[3] The incidence of anaplastic astrocytoma peaks in children younger than 10 years of age and then remains constant in each subsequent decade of life. In contrast, glioblastoma multiforme is uncommon before the age of 20 years, whereas the rate of occurrence increases dramatically after the age of 40.[3] The incidence of malignant gliomas has increased at least twofold among the elderly over the past 2 decades.[4]

Current knowledge of the molecular biology and genetics of astrocytic neoplasms has been well summarized.[5] Two genetic pathways, a progression pathway and a de novo pathway, that lead to glioblastoma multiforme development have been proposed (Fig. 20–1).[6] It is hypothesized that *p53* gene mutations represent an early genetic event in astrocytoma development. This change alone is insufficient to produce progression to a more advanced histologic grade. Loss of heterozygosity (LOH) for chromosome 17p is associated with transition to grade 2 tumors. Malignant progression to anaplastic astrocytoma is associated with LOH for chromosomes 9p (*CDKN2* [cyclin-dependent kinase] [*p16/MTS1*] gene), 13q, or 19q and *CDK4* gene amplification. Subsequent LOH on chromosome 10 and amplification of the epidermal growth factor receptor *(EGF-R)* and murine double minute 2 *(mdm-2)* genes characterize further progression to glioblastoma multiforme.

A second, *p53*-independent, pathway may lead more directly to glioblastoma multiforme development.[6] This pathway is associated with normal *p53* and with LOH for chromosomes 9p, 10, and 17p and amplification of the *EGF-R* and perhaps the *CDK4* gene. Consistent genetic abnormalities have not been demonstrated for 25% to 50% of adult astrocytomas, and

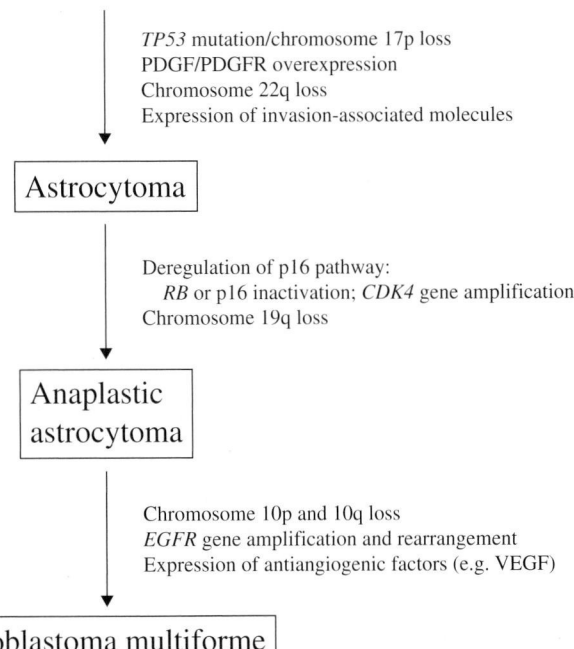

TP53 mutation/chromosome 17p loss
PDGF/PDGFR overexpression
Chromosome 22q loss
Expression of invasion-associated molecules

Astrocytoma

Deregulation of p16 pathway:
   RB or p16 inactivation; *CDK4* gene amplification
Chromosome 19q loss

Anaplastic astrocytoma

Chromosome 10p and 10q loss
EGFR gene amplification and rearrangement
Expression of antiangiogenic factors (e.g. VEGF)

Giloblastoma multiforme

Figure 20–1. Molecular alterations characteristic of different stages of astrocytoma progression. PDGF = platelet-derived growth factor; R = receptor; VEGF = vascular endothelial growth factor.

alterations of presently unknown genes may be responsible for the genesis and progression of these tumors.

Several hereditary syndromes are associated with an increased risk of brain tumors including neurofibromatosis-1 (chromosome involved: *17q12-17q22*) and neurofibromatosis-2 *(22q)*, tuberous sclerosis *(9q32-34 or 11q)*, Li-Fraumeni syndrome *(17p[p53])*, nevoid basal cell carcinoma syndrome *(9q31 or 1q22)*, familial polyposis *(5q)*, Turcot syndrome *(5q)*, Gardner syndrome *(5q)*, and von Hippel-Lindau disease *(3p13-14.3 and 3p25-26)*. With the exception of Turcot syndrome, all are inherited in an autosomal dominant pattern.[7] In addition to the association between hereditary syndromes and brain tumors, certain families of brain tumor patients have aggregations of brain tumors and extraneural malignancies. Germ-line *p53* mutations have been frequently identified in glioma patients with multifocal lesions, a different second primary malignancy, and a family history of cancer.

Although some environmental factors have been linked with brain tumor development, they do not appear to be responsible for most brain tumors.[8] Apart from a predisposing genetic syndrome that is present in less than 5% of patients with brain tumors, the only other firmly established cause is ionizing radiation.[9] Radiation-induced gliomas have been reported, and 25% of such cases have arisen in children with acute lymphoblastic leukemia who received prophylactic cranial irradiation and chemotherapy.

Anatomy

The brain is divided into supratentorial and infratentorial compartments by the tentorium cerebelli. The supratentorial compartment includes the cerebral hemispheres and the sellar, pineal, and diencephalon regions, whereas the infratentorial compartment includes the midbrain, pons, medulla, and cerebellum. The cerebral hemispheres are connected by the corpus callosum and are divided into the frontal, parietal, occipital, and temporal lobes. The frontal lobes are concerned with behavior organization, planning and association, and speech; the parietal lobes with motor, sensory, and complex intellectual functions; the occipital lobes with vision; and the temporal lobes with behavior, memory, speech, emotion, and auditory-visual pathways.[10]

The brain is housed within the bony calvarium, made up of the frontal, ethmoid, parietal, sphenoid, temporal, and occipital bones. The posterior margin of the lesser wings of the sphenoid marks the anterior aspect of the lateral cerebral (Sylvian) fissure, the junction of the frontal and temporal lobes of the brain. The base of the skull can be approximated on the surface of the patient by a line, called the orbitomeatal or Reid's base line, which extends from the infraorbital rim to the external auditory meatus.[11]

Most malignant gliomas arise in the cerebral hemispheres, and the lobar distribution is directly related to the amount of white matter present in each region. Among 1578 patients with supratentorial malignant gliomas entered into Radiation Therapy Oncology Group (RTOG) trials, 44% were located in the frontal, 30% in the temporal, and 22% in the parietal lobes, whereas 4% arose at other sites.[12]

Pathology

Central nervous system tumors are generally classified as follows: (1) gliomas, (2) neuronal/glioneuronal neoplasms, (3) embryonal neoplasms, (4) meningeal neoplasms, and (5) miscellaneous nonglial neoplasms (Table 20-1). Reliance on a pathological classification of brain tumors is a requisite for treatment. Indeed, histopathology is more important than anatomic staging in determining the clinical behavior and prognosis of these tumors. Tumor classification is based on histologic evidence of differentiation; however, expression of histologic features may vary widely within tumors of a given type, particularly diffuse gliomas. This regional heterogeneity makes interpretation of small biopsy samples difficult; this is especially true of astrocytomas. Unfortunately, these difficulties can have significant implications on the diagnosis and grading of these tumors.

Astrocytic gliomas, which are the most common primary brain tumors, arise from astrocytes, the supporting cells of the brain and spinal cord. The cytoplasmic processes that extend from the astrocytes contain a characteristic filamentous protein, glial fibrillary acidic protein (GFAP), which provides an immunohistochemical marker for these tumors.[13] The characteristic histopathological features of anaplastic astrocytomas include moderate hypercellularity, moderate cellular and nuclear pleomorphism, variable mitotic activity, and microvascular proliferation (Fig. 20-2). The presence of tumor necrosis is the hallmark that distinguishes anaplastic astrocytoma from glioblastoma multiforme (Fig. 20-3).

Neuropathologists have not uniformly agreed on a single classification system for astrocytic gliomas. As shown in Table 20-2, several schemes that define three or four grades of malignancy are used in clinical practice.[14-18] The World Health Organization (WHO) system,[16] which divides astrocytic tumors into four grades, from grade 1, corresponding to pilocytic astrocytomas to grade IV, corresponding to the glioblastoma multiforme, is used more often.

Astrocytic gliomas with similar histopathologic features may vary in their clinical behavior. Objective indicators of tumor proliferative potential, including bromodeoxyuridine (BrdU) and Ki-67 labeling indices, have been used to better predict prognosis. Cellular incorporation of BrdU is a marker of the DNA synthesis phase of the cell cycle, whereas antibodies to Ki-67 label an antigen that is present in all phases of the cell cycle except G_0. A shortcoming of BrdU is that it must be introduced by intravenous administration before surgery, and Ki-67 can be examined only on frozen tissue sections. Another antibody to the Ki-67 antigen, MIB-1, can be studied in paraffin tissue sections, making labeling index studies for prognostication more generally available.[13]

Table 20–1   Histopathology of Brain Tumors

Major Classification	Variants	WHO Grades
Glioma		
Astrocytic: circumscribed	Pilocytic astrocytoma	I
	Subependymal giant cell astrocytoma (SEGA)	I
	Pleomorphic xanthoastrocytoma (PXA)	II
Astrocytic: diffuse	Astrocytoma	II
	Anaplastic astrocytoma	III
	Glioblastoma multiforme	IV
Oligodendroglial	Oligodendroglioma	II
	Anaplastic oligodendroglioma	III
Mixed gliomas	Oligoastrocytoma	II
	Anaplastic oligoastrocytoma	III
Ependymal	Subependymoma	I
	Myxopapillary ependymoma	I
	Ependymoma	II
	Anaplastic ependymoma*	III
Choroid plexus	Choroid plexus papilloma	I
	Choroid plexus carcinoma*	III
Cranial & Peripheral Nerve Tumors	Schwannoma	I
Neuronal & Glioneuronal Tumors	Gangliocytoma/ganglioglioma	I–III
	Desmoplastic infantile ganglioma (DIG)	I
	Dysplastic cerebellar gangliocytoma	I
	Central neurocytoma	I
	Dysembryoplastic neuroepithelial tumor	I
	Paraganglioma	I
Pineal Parenchymal Tumors (PPT)	Pineocytoma	II
	PPT with intermediate differentiation	III
	Pineoblastoma	IV
Embryonal Tumors	Medulloepithelioma*	IV
	Primitive neuroectodermal tumor (PNET),* including medulloblastoma and variants*	IV
	Atypical teratoid/rhabdoid tumor (AT/RT)	IV
	Cerebral neuroblastoma/ganglioneuroblastoma	IV
	Ependymoblastoma*	IV
	Olfactory neuroblastoma (esthesioneuroblastoma)	IV
Meningeal Tumors	Meningioma	I
	Atypical meningioma	II
	Anaplastic (malignant) meningioma	III
Germ Cell Tumors	Hemangiopericytoma†	II–III
	Germinoma	NA
	Mature teratoma	NA
	Nongerminomatous germ cell tumors	NA
Tumors of the Sellar Region	Craniopharyngioma: adamantinomatous	I
	Craniopharyngioma: papillary	I
Hemopoietic Neoplasms	Primary CNS lymphoma (PCNSL)	NA
	Secondary lymphoma/leukemia	NA
	Histiocytic tumors and histiocytoses	NA
Secondary Tumors/Metastases	Carcinomas and sarcomas	NA

WHO, World Health Organization; NA, not applicable.
*Indicates those tumors with a tendency to disseminate throughout the CNS.
†Origin of hemangiopericytoma is uncertain.

Clinical Presentation

The presenting symptoms and signs of brain tumors are divided into those associated with a mass effect and increased intracranial pressure and those that are focal. The most common presenting symptom is headache, and approximately 20% of patients with supratentorial tumors present with seizures. Alterations in personality, mood, mental capacity, and concentration are frequently seen early in the clinical course.[3] The focal neurologic symptoms and signs observed with supratentorial brain tumors are summarized in Table 20-3.

Routes of Spread

Malignant gliomas form as an expansile mass that conforms to the barriers of the cortical convolutions, deep nuclear structures, and adjacent myelinated nerve fibers.[19,20] Microscopic examination typically shows a

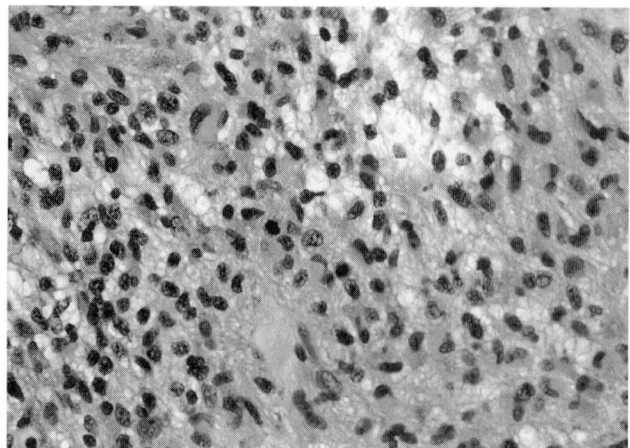

Figure 20–2. Anaplastic astrocytoma showing hypercellularity and pleomorphic nuclei. Tumor necrosis is absent. (Hematoxylin and eosin; original magnification ×250.)

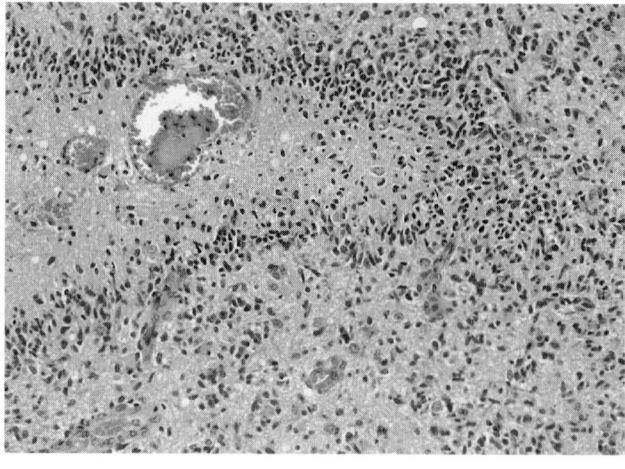

Figure 20–3. Glioblastoma multiforme with the hallmark features of necrosis with peripheral pseudopalisading of neoplastic nuclei. (Hematoxylin and eosin; original magnification ×100.)

gradient of infiltrating tumor cells that decreases with the distance from the periphery of the mass. As they enlarge, malignant gliomas extend directly into adjacent lobes, infiltrate throughout the ipsilateral cerebral hemisphere, and disseminate along anatomically defined nerve fiber pathways. In some cases individual cells, facilitated by the accompanying edema, may infiltrate for long distances from the main tumor mass. Multicentric gliomas are found in less than 5% of patients.[21] Dissemination by seeding through the cerebrospinal fluid pathways occurs in approximately 10% of cases but is usually a late event, often appearing at a time when its effects are inconsequential compared with those of the recurrent primary tumor mass. Metastases rarely arise outside the CNS.

Diagnostic Studies

Computed tomography (CT) and magnetic resonance imaging (MRI) play an indispensable role in the management of brain tumors. CT is almost universally available and, with contrast enhancement, is a reliable screening and diagnostic method for suspected supratentorial brain

tumor lesions. MRI is now more frequently used in patients with malignant brain tumors and has become the screening procedure of choice for diagnosing and localizing tumors in the brainstem, posterior fossa, and spinal cord and for defining the extent of low-grade gliomas. MRI is superior to CT for detecting and localizing brain tumors because MRI produces images in any plane and offers high resolution and contrast without being compromised by bone artifact.[22] On the other hand, CT can better image calcification found in some low-grade gliomas and can distinguish an acute bleed.

On noncontrast CT studies, gliomas may be hypodense, isodense, or hyperintense with the surrounding brain, or they may be calcified.[22] A considerable mass effect may be present. Although the majority of malignant gliomas enhance with iodinated contrast media, as many as 30% of anaplastic astrocytomas present as nonenhancing lesions. Tumor enhancement appears in an irregular ringlike configuration that surrounds a central low-attenuation area of necrosis or cyst formation. Peripheral to the enhancing zone, there is a nonenhancing low-attenuation region of brain edema. The perimeter of the enhancing lesion does not define the true tumor

Table 20–2   Grading Systems for Astrocytic Gliomas

Kernohan (Svien et al.*)	Ringertz† (Burger et al[15])	WHO (Kleihues et al.[16])	St. Anne-Mayo (Daumas-Duport et al.[17])	UCSF (Davis[18])
Astrocytoma grade 1	Astrocytoma	Pilocytic astrocytoma grade 1	Astrocytoma grade 1	Mildly anaplastic astrocytoma
Astrocytoma grade 2	Anaplastic astrocytoma	Astrocytoma grade 2	Astrocytoma grade 2	Moderately anaplastic astrocytoma
		Anaplastic astrocytoma grade 3	Astrocytoma grade 3	Highly anaplastic astrocytoma
Astrocytoma grade 3 Astrocytoma grade 4	Glioblastoma multiforme	Glioblastoma multiforme grade 4	Astrocytoma grade 4	Glioblastoma multiforme

*From Svien HJ, Mabon RF, Kernohan JW: Astrocytomas. *Proc Staff Mayo Clin.* 1949;24:54.
†From Ringertz N: "Grading" of gliomas. *Acta Pathol Microbiol Scand.* 1950;27:51.
WHO, World Health Organization; UCSF, University of California, San Francisco.
Modified from Bruner JM: Neuropathology of malignant gliomas. *Semin Oncol.* 1994;21:126.

Table 20–3   Focal Neurologic Symptoms and Signs Associated with Supratentorial Tumors

Anatomic Region	Symptoms or Signs or Both
Frontal lobe	Personality change
	Slowing of contralateral hand movements
	Contralateral spastic hemiplegia
	Mood elevation
	Difficulty in adapting to new situations
	Loss of initiative
	Dysphagia ± lip, tongue, and hand movement
	Apraxia (if dominant lobe involved)
Bifrontal involvement	Bilateral hemiparesis
	Spastic bulbar palsy
	Impairment of intellect
	Lability of mood
	Dementia
	Primitive grasp, suck, and snout reflexes
Temporal lobe	Impairment of recent memory
	Homonymous quadrantanopsia
	Auditory hallucinations
	Aggressive behavior
Nondominant lobe	Minor perceptual problems
	Spatial disorientation
Dominant lobe	Dysnomia
	Impaired perception of verbal commands
	Fluent Wernicke-like aphasia
Parietal lobe	Mild hemiparesis
	Mild to severe sensory loss
	Homonymous hemianopia
	Visual inattention
Nondominant lobe	Perceptual abnormalities
	Anosognosia
	Apraxia for self-dressing
Dominant lobe	Alexia
	Dysgraphia
	Other forms of apraxia
Occipital lobe	Contralateral homonymous hemianopia
	Visual aberrations
Bilateral occipital involvement	Cortical blindness
	Herniation syndromes
Thalamus or basal ganglia or both	Contralateral sensory abnormalities
	Intermittent contralateral paresthesias
	Neuropathic pain syndrome
	Contralateral intention tremor
	Hemiballistic-like movement disorder
	Hydrocephalus due to trapping of lateral horn of ventricle

Modified from Levin VA, Gutin PH, Leibel S: Neoplasms of the central nervous system. In DeVita VT Jr, Hellman S, Rosenberg SA, eds. *Cancer Principles and Practice of Oncology.* 4th ed. Philadelphia: JB Lippincott; 1993:1679.

size; tumor cells may extend well beyond the region of enhancement into areas of brain that otherwise appear normal.

Typically, T2-weighted MRI abnormalities extend beyond the corresponding CT boundaries of contrast enhancement and low attenuation. In both low-grade and malignant gliomas, parenchymal infiltration by isolated tumor cells may be present in regions of T2-weighted abnormality that appear normal on CT. Tumor may even be found in normal-appearing brain adjacent to the T2-weighted abnormality. Malignant gliomas display significant enhancement with gadolinium-labeled diethylenetriamine pentaacetic acid (gadolinium), forming ringlike configurations comparable to those seen on CT (Fig. 20-4). As with CT, tumor tissue may extend beyond the enhancing lesion. Thus, MRI does not define the peripheral extent of tumor involvement better than CT.[23] The use of flare sequence (T2 image with fluid suppression) may help to better define the true extent of the disease by suppressing the cerebrospinal fluid signal from the tumor induced edema.

Imaging studies are performed after surgical resection to determine the presence of residual tumor and to provide a baseline for subsequent treatment. Enhancement resulting from surgical trauma may be indistinguishable from residual tumor even after a complete surgical resection. Postsurgical enhancement develops as early as the fifth postoperative day, peaks after 2 weeks, and may persist for months. Therefore, imaging should be performed within the first 96 hours after surgery.[24]

Corticosteroids, which act to reestablish the blood-brain barrier (BBB), have a profound impact on the area of enhancement, and diminution in the area of enhancement may be due to corticosteroids alone. To determine a radiographic response to therapy, patients should be on the same or a lower dose of corticosteroids than the dose at the time of the pretreatment scan.[25]

Positron emission tomography (PET) is an imaging method that uses a positron-emitting radioisotope-labeled biologic tracer to provide metabolic data about the tumor and surrounding normal brain.[26] The use of the fluorinated glucose analog (^{18}F)-2-fluoro-2-deoxyglucose (^{18}FDG) as an imaging agent is based on the observation that malignant cells use glucose at a greater rate than normal tissue. ^{18}FDG uptake directly correlates with the degree of malignancy (i.e., low-grade gliomas tend to have ^{18}FDG uptake that is the same as or less than cerebral white matter), whereas malignant gliomas take up the same or more ^{18}FDG than does gray matter. ^{18}FDG-PET is also used to identify tumor recurrence, differentiate between radiation-induced brain necrosis and recurrent high-grade gliomas, discriminate residual tumor from postoperative enhancement seen on MRI and CT, and localize brain tumor biopsy sites.[26]

Single photon emission computed tomography (SPECT) with thallium-201 (^{201}Tl) is another imaging approach used in brain tumor management. Actively dividing tumors preferentially take up thallium through the adenosine triphosphate cell membrane pump, permitting tumor to be distinguished from surrounding normal brain.[27] Like ^{18}FDG-PET, ^{201}Tl-SPECT is a noninvasive method of tumor grading as well as a means for measuring response to treatment, identifying recurrent tumors, differentiating recurrent tumor from radiation necrosis, and localizing stereotactic biopsy sites.

Magnetic resonance spectroscopy (MRS) is an evolving technique that allows the in vivo collection and measurement of chemical information from a selected volume of brain tissue.[28] By developing the techniques that suppress the dominant water proton signal, one can study the components that are normally overwhelmed by the body's water protons. In human brain, the four main

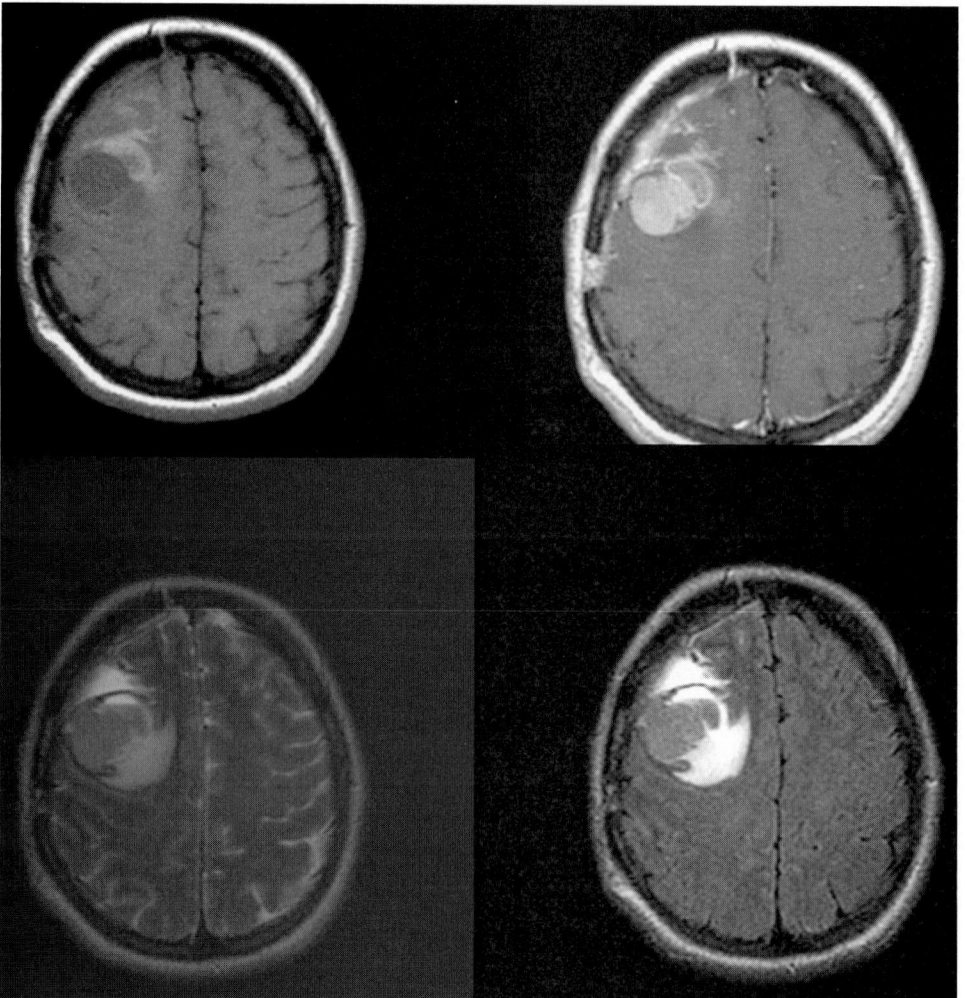

Figure 20–4. Axial magnetic resonance image of high-grade astrocytoma of right frontal lobe with T1- weighted images without and with contrast, flare sequence, and T2-weighted image, clockwise from upper left corner.

components seen are N-acetylaspartate (NAA), creatine (CR), choline (CHO), and lactate (LAC). While NAA is found in the normal nerve cells, choline serves as a marker of cellular integrity and cellularity. Creatine is a marker for cellular energy, while lactate is seen when there is significant anaerobic metabolism. The MRS of a patient with a malignant glioma is shown in Figure 20-5. Generally, a tumor exhibits increased choline, decreased NAA, and decreased creatine levels. On the other hand, necrotic tissue would show increased levels of lactate and decreased levels of all the other metabolites. The possible uses of MRS in brain tumors include the in vivo differentiation of tumors,[29] differentiation between tumor recurrence and necrosis following stereotactic radiosurgery (SRS) procedure,[28] and in target delineation for dose escalation.[30] Poor-quality spectroscopy due to presence of clips, radioactive seeds, clotted blood, and skull bone within the measured volume may make it very difficult to interpret findings. Possible solutions include acquisition of better technical data with multi-voxel images, serial follow-up information, and better interpretation that may make this technique more useful in the coming years.

Staging

There is no accepted staging system for gliomas. The American Joint Committee on Cancer (AJCC) had proposed a staging scheme for primary brain tumors based on T and M (dissemination within and rarely outside the CNS) as well as G for tumor grade. Because this system was not generally adapted to clinical use, it was removed from the 1997 AJCC staging manual.

Prognostic Factors

A major contribution of the cooperative group brain tumor studies has been the identification of pretreatment characteristics that affect the outcome in patients with malignant gliomas. A nonparametric recursive partitioning technique was applied to an analysis of 1578 patients accrued to three successive RTOG trials.[31] Age, histologic appearance, KPS, mental status, duration of symptoms, neurologic functional class, extent of surgery, and radiation dose were identified as significant partitioning

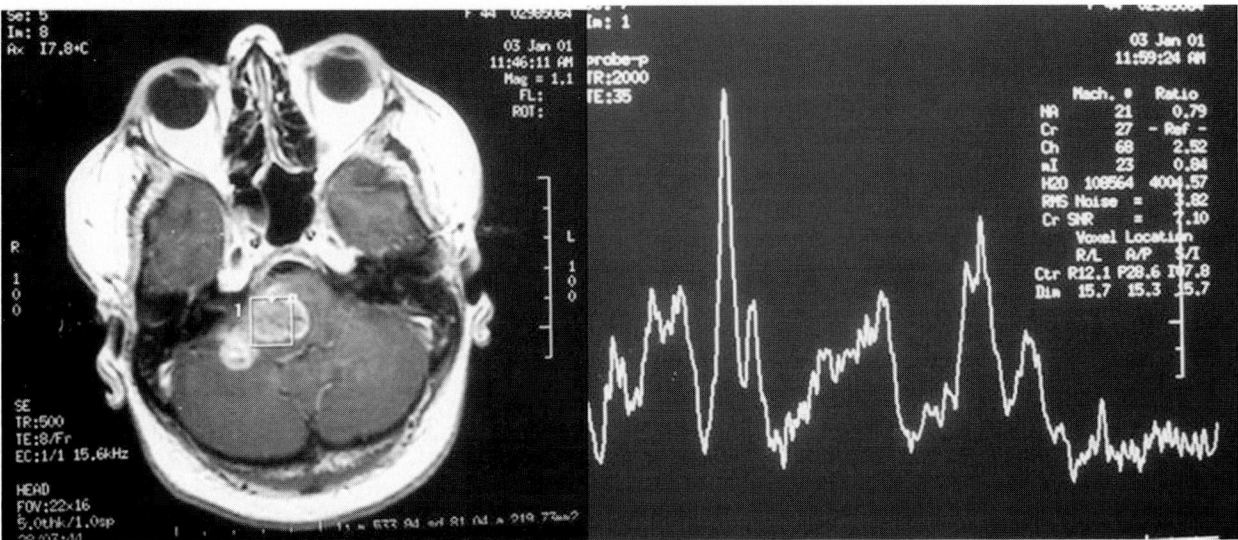

Figure 20–5. Single voxel spectroscopy on a patient with high-grade brainstem glioma.

covariates. As shown in Table 20-4, six patient classes were defined with median survival times ranging from 4.6 to 58.6 months and 2-year survival rates of 4% to 76%. These classes were used to define favorable (classes I and II, 12% of the patients evaluated), intermediate (classes III and IV, 43%), and poor (classes V and VI, 45%) prognosis subgroups. This information is important for interpreting correctly the results of studies comparing different treatment regimens and for assessing the potential of new therapeutic methodologies.

Standard Therapeutic Approaches

SURGERY

The combination of surgery, radiation therapy, and chemotherapy represents the standard approach to the treatment of malignant gliomas. Generally, surgery is performed through an open craniotomy. The goals of surgery are to provide a histologic diagnosis, alleviate intracranial hypertension and focal neurologic deficits due to a mass effect, and permit rapid corticosteroid dose tapering.[32] Furthermore, a large tumor mass left in the brain can serve as a nidus for cerebral edema after radiation therapy. The influence of surgical resection in malignant gliomas has been controversial. The aim of palliation of symptoms was always clear, but the survival advantage was debated. However, the evidence suggests that patients with more complete resections, designed to minimize the volume of residual tumor, live longer and have an improved functional status compared with those who undergo a biopsy or partial resection only. An analysis of the RTOG database of 645 patients with malignant gliomas revealed a median survival of 11.3 months with total resection, 10.4 months with sub-total resection, and 6.6 months with biopsy alone.[12] However, tumor size was not found to be a predictor of survival. Advances in neurosurgery, including diagnostic ultrasound, lasers, ultrasonic tissue aspirators, cortical mapping, functional imaging, and computer-assisted stereotactic laser techniques, have improved the ability of neurosurgeons to radically remove intracranial tumors.[33]

A closed needle biopsy, using CT- or MRI-coupled stereotactic techniques, may be indicated in many clinical

Table 20–4   Patient Classes for Malignant Gliomas According to Recursive Partitioning Analysis of Prognostic Factors

Class	Characteristic	Median Survival, mo	2-Yr Survival, %
I	AAF, age <50 yr, normal mental status	58.6	76
II	AAF, age ≥50 yr, KPS 70-100, >3 mo time to first symptom	37.4	68
III	AAF, age <50 yr, abnormal mental status or GBM, age <50 yr, KPS 90-100	17.9	35
IV	GBM, age <50 yr, KPS <90 or AAF, age ≥50 yr, ≤3 mo time from first symptom or GBM, KPS 70-100, ≥ partial resection, "work" neurologic functional status	11.1	15
V	GBM, age ≥50 yr, KPS 70-100, ≥ partial resection, "home" or "hospital" neurologic functional status or GBM, age ≥50 yr, KPS 70-100, biopsy only, received >54.4 Gy or age ≥50 yr, KPS <70, normal mental status	8.9	6
VI	GBM, age ≥50 yr, KPS 70-100, biopsy only, received ≤54.5 Gy or age ≥50 yr, KPS <70, abnormal mental status	4.6	4

AAF, Astrocytoma with atypical or anaplastic features; GBM, glioblastoma multiforme; KPS, Karnofsky performance status.
Data from Curran WJ Jr, Scott CB, Horton J, et al: Recursive partitioning analysis of prognostic factors in three Radiation Therapy Oncology Group malignant glioma trials. *J Natl Cancer Inst.* 1993;85:704.

settings. A biopsy is preferred for tumors located in functionally important or inaccessible areas of the brain. In addition, surgical resection is not practical for patients with significant tumor infiltration across the midline and around the ventricular system or for those with diffuse, nonfocal lesions.[34]

RADIATION THERAPY

Randomized trials conducted by the Brain Tumor Cooperative Group (BTCG) and the Scandinavian Glioblastoma Study Group (SGSG) provided seminal evidence that external beam irradiation favorably affects the outcome of malignant gliomas. BTCG trials 6901 and 7201 demonstrated a significant survival advantage for irradiated patients who received 50 to 60 Gy to the whole brain (in single daily fractions of 1.7-2.0 Gy, 5 days per week) either alone or with chemotherapy compared with those treated with either resection and supportive care only ($P = 0.001$) or with chemotherapy alone ($P < 0.01$).[35,36] The median survival of patients receiving 60 Gy was 2.3 times longer than that observed for nonirradiated patients. Nearly 30% of irradiated patients in the SGSG trial maintained a full or partial working capacity, whereas the nonirradiated patients progressively deteriorated, and none regained their original performance level.[37] Randomized trials of postoperative radiation therapy in gliomas is shown in Table 20-5. These studies were so convincing that virtually all patients with malignant gliomas receive some mode of radiation therapy.

CHEMOTHERAPY

Adjuvant chemotherapy is also part of the standard therapeutic regimen for malignant gliomas. The addition of chemotherapy to radiation therapy improves the 1-year survival by 10% and the 2-year survival by 8.6%.[38] The nitrosoureas, especially carmustine (bis-chloroethylnitrosourea, BCNU), are the most active single agents, and no other drug or drug combination has been found to be more effective against these tumors.[39] An exception is the combination of procarbazine, lomustine (CCNU), and vincristine (PCV), which was shown in a subset analysis of a Northern California Oncology Group (NCOG) randomized trial to be more effective than BCNU for highly anaplastic astrocytomas.[40] However, a subsequent retrospective analysis of the RTOG database did not confirm the benefit of PCV in anaplastic astrocytomas.[41] A recently reported Medical Research Council (MRC) phase III trial of 674 patients using 60 Gy ± PCV chemotherapy showed no difference is median survival (9.5 vs. 10 months).[42] Also, no benefit of chemotherapeutic agents such as Tirapazamine, Topotecan, Taxol, B-IFN, and Thalidomide was noted when used with standard radiation in RTOG phase II trials.[43]

Temozolomide is an alkylating agent that has shown promise in both gliomas and brain metastases. It is a derivative of dacarbazine and an inactive prodrug that undergoes hydrolysis to active metabolite 5-(3-methyl triazen-1-yl) imiadazole-4-carboxamide (MTIC) when absorbed and results in methylation of guanine at O6 and n7 positions at the DNA. It has several advantages over conventional chemotherapy agents. These include oral administration, rapid absorption, 100% bioavailability, ability to cross the BBB, its linear pharmacokinetics, and minimal delayed myelosuppression. A large multicenter phase II trial in recurrent gliomas refractory to PCV chemotherapy treated with Temozolomide showed 35% response rate and 6 month progression-free survival (PFS) of 46% and was subsequently FDA approved for relapsed anaplastic astrocytoma (AA).[44] A randomized phase II international trial comparing Temozolomide to procarbazine in 225 recurrent glioblastoma multiforme patients showed improved disease-free survival (21% vs. 8%) and overall survival (OS) (7.3 vs. 5.8 months).[45] Better quality of life in all seven quality of life domains tested was noted. Another phase II trial of 60 Gy with 75 mg/M^2 per day of Temozolomide followed by 6 cycles of 200 mg/M^2 × 5 days/month in 64 patients showed an impressive 16-month median OS and a 2-year OS of 31%.[46] Based on these data, there is an ongoing

Table 20–5   Randomized Trials of Postoperative Trials in High-Grade Gliomas

Study (Ref.)	Study Group	Radiation Dose Gy/n fractions	Patients Randomized (analyzed), n	Median Survival (wk)	Overall Survival P Value
Shapiro et al, 1976[65]	CT	—	16 (16)	30	NR
	RT+CT	60	17 (17)	44.5	Not significant
Andersen, 1978*	Surgery alone	—	57 (57)	15	<0.005
	RT	45/25	51 (51)	23	Survival at 6 mo
Walker et al, 1978[35d]	Surgery alone	—	42 (31)	14[c]	0.001
	RT	50-60/25-35	93 (68)	36[c]	
Walker et al, 1980[36d]	CT	—	111 (111)	31	0.003
	RT	60/30-35	118 (118)	37	
Kristiansen et al, 1981[37]	Surgery alone	—	38 (38)	23	NR
	RT±CT	45/25	80 (80)	47	Significant
Sandberg-Wollheim et al, 1991†	CT	—	87 (87)	42	0.028
	RT+CT	58/27	84 (84)	62	

*From Anderson AP: Postoperative irradiation of glioblastomaas. Results in a randomized series. *Acta Radiol Oncol.* 1978;17:475
†From Sandberg-Wallheim M, Mahlstrom P. Stromblad LG, et al: A randomized study of chemotherapy with procarbazine, vincristine and lomustine with and without radiation therapy for astrocytoma grades 3 and/or 4. *Cancer.* 1991;68:22.
From Laperriere N, Zuraw L, Cairncross G, et al: Radiotherapy for newly diagnosed malignant glioma in adults: A systematic review. *Radiother Oncol.* 2002;64:259.

European Organization for Research and Treatment of Cancer (EORTC) phase III trial comparing Temozolomide and CCNU as an adjuvant chemotherapy agent in malignant gliomas.

Several new agents including antiepidermal growth factors and antiangiogenic agents, as well as novel techniques of drug delivery, are under investigation.[47]

Techniques of Radiotherapy

Most malignant gliomas are unifocal at the time of initial presentation, and after treatment the majority recur at or within 1 to 2 cm of their original location.[48] Thus, limited treatment portals are used for malignant gliomas. Intracranial metastases that appear after partial brain irradiation do not affect the ultimate outcome because they are nearly always accompanied by relapse at the primary tumor site. Whole-brain radiation therapy (WBRT) is commonly recommended for patients with multifocal tumors, but even for these lesions, relapses occur most frequently in the sites of known disease.[49]

The conventional dose schedule is 59.4 to 60 Gy, given in single daily fractions of 1.8 to 2.0 Gy, 5 days per week. With this scheme, approximately 25% of patients with glioblastoma multiforme and 50% of those with anaplastic astrocytoma exhibit a significant radiographic response. Rapid fractionation schemes (such as 30 to 36 Gy in 10 to 12 fractions of 3.0 Gy each) may be appropriate for some elderly or poor-performance-status patients with glioblastoma multiforme who have relatively short survival expectancies.

The gross target volume (GTV) represents a three-dimensional reconstruction of the location of the tumor, determined by merging data from contrast-enhanced CT scans and MRI studies. The integration of MRI into CT-based treatment planning provides complementary information for accurately defining the tumor volume. When MRI- and CT-derived tumor volumes were compared, MRI clearly defined larger volumes. However, CT scans also defined abnormalities that were not always perceptible with MRI. Only 43% of the composite CT-MRI volume was apparent on both studies; 37% of the composite volume was only evident on MRI, and 21% was apparent only on CT.[50]

Little agreement exists as to the definition of the clinical target volume (CTV) or the planning target volume (PTV). A shrinking field approach is used in RTOG trials. The initial PTV (PTV1) encompasses the enhancing lesion (GTV) and edema (CTV) with a 2 cm margin. After 46 Gy of a conventionally fractionated treatment course, the PTV (PTV2) is reduced to include only the enhancing lesion with a 2.5 cm margin. Using the extent of edema to define the PTV has some limitations. The identification of peritumoral edema is subjective, and its volume may vary with corticosteroid dosage.[25] An analysis of the patterns of failure using the RTOG-defined PTVs demonstrated that nearly all relapses occurred within the reduced PTV2 at the site of the enhancing tumor.[51] Based on these data, we define the CTV by adding a margin of approximately 2.5 cm around the T1 contrast or a 1.5 cm margin around the flare sequence

enhancement series. The PTV is determined by adding an additional 0.5 cm margin to the CTV to account for treatment uncertainties.

Patients are fixed in a custom-designed immobilization device and treated in the supine or prone position, depending on tumor location. When conventional treatment-planning techniques are used, 90-degree orthogonal simulator radiographs are obtained. Outlines of the GTV and PTV are drawn on a contour of the head, taken through the central plane defined by the proposed treatment portals. Although treatments are commonly planned from CT or MRI images or both, MRI data can be acquired in axial, coronal, and sagittal planes without compromise of spatial or contrast detail. These images can be readily superimposed on simulator films to localize the tumor more accurately for portal design. The contour is digitally transferred to a treatment-planning computer, radiation beams are defined, and isodose distributions are generated. The PTV should be encompassed in its entirety while minimizing the dose to contralateral brain tissue and other critical structures.

Field arrangements and beam energy are selected after consideration of the location of the tumor within the brain and the geometry of the PTV. Lateral opposed fields are used only when extensive bilateral tumor involvement is present. This technique is suboptimal for most lesions because a substantial volume of normal brain tissue will be irradiated to the same dose as the tumor. Lateral and vertex (or angled vertex) fields in a wedge-pair arrangement are typically used for lateral lesions, and a three-field approach or wedge-arc rotation is used for more midline tumors.

Three-dimensional conformal radiation therapy (3D-CRT) is ideally suited for the treatment of brain tumors. Three-dimensional treatment plans are designed directly from CT (and MRI) image data sets, and the target volume and surrounding normal tissues are displayed using the beam's eye view technique. The use of multiple 3D-planned nonaxial coplanar and noncoplanar fields can often reduce the volume of normal brain tissue treated to high doses. This approach may allow higher than traditional doses to be safely administered to select patients. Interstitial brachytherapy and radiosurgery are also being used to augment the dose from conventional radiation therapy. Radiosurgery is discussed in Chapter 25.

Intensity-modulated radiation therapy (IMRT) is an advanced form of 3D-CRT that uses inverse planning and computer-controlled radiation dose deposition. This advantage of precision delivery of radiation enables dose escalation and sparing of normal tissues. The brain IMRT treatment planning consists of immobilization using an aquaplast face mask. A CT simulation with IV contrast is performed with the acquisition of 3-mm size thickness images. The previously obtained MRI data is superimposed on the CT images using a fusion program. GTV, CTV, and PTV are defined as in a 3D-CRT plan. All normal structures are outlined in three dimensions. User-defined constraints including maximum and minimum dose constraints both for the PTV and the normal structures are prescribed. As in 3D-CRT, noncoplanar beams would be used. The plan consists of an intensity profile that is created for each beam. The profiles are

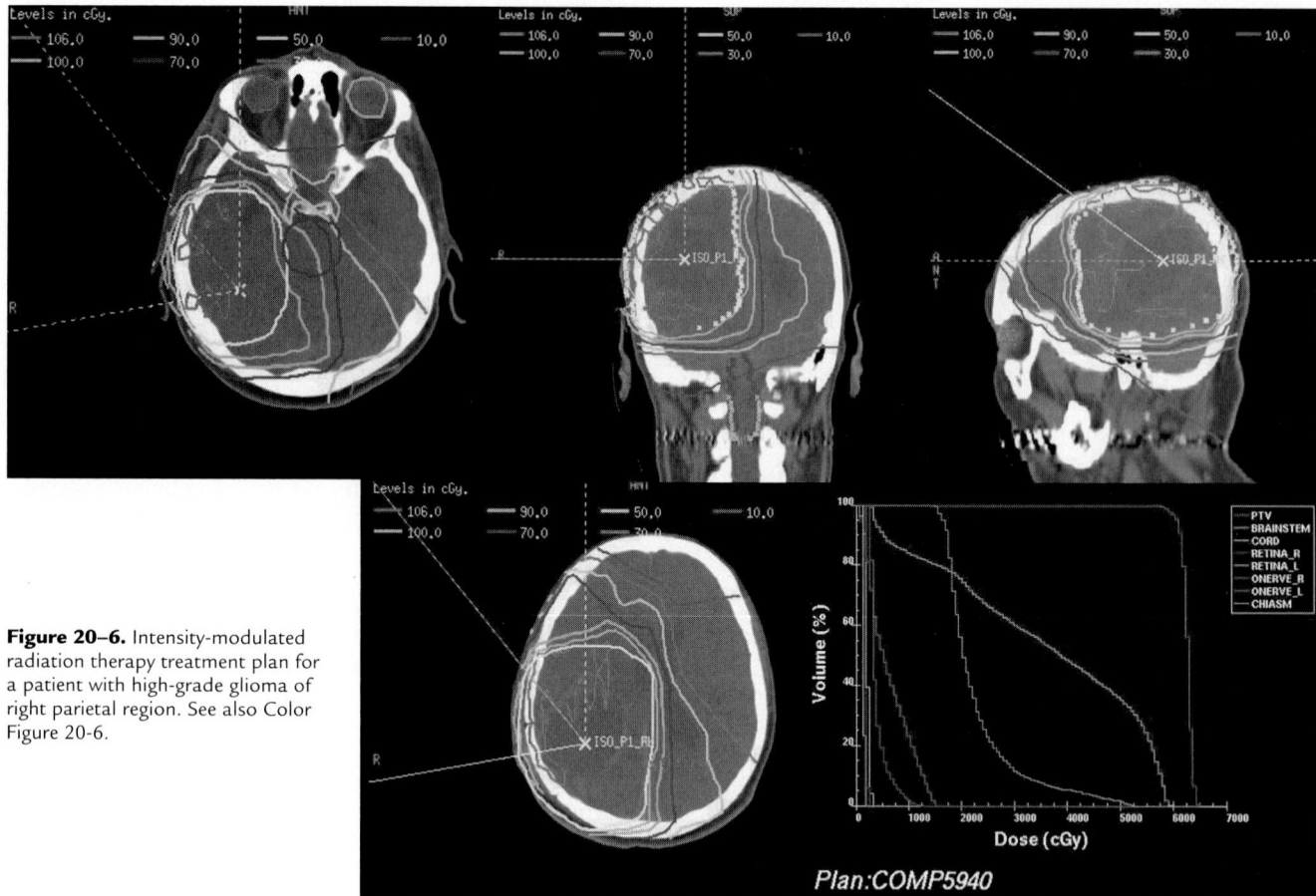

Figure 20–6. Intensity-modulated radiation therapy treatment plan for a patient with high-grade glioma of right parietal region. See also Color Figure 20-6.

translated to leaf motion of the dynamic multi-leaf collimator using a leaf sequencer algorithm (Fig. 20-6). We have seen that the use of IMRT decreases the dose to critical structures such as optic chiasm and brainstem when compared to the 3D conformal plan.[52] There is evidence that use of IMRT decreases the dose to the cochlea in children with medulloblastoma when used for the posterior fossa boost.[53] The use of IMRT for dose escalation in brain tumors is presently being explored.[54]

Normal Tissue Reactions

Several adverse neurologic reactions may be observed in patients receiving cranial irradiation. They are classified into acute reactions, early-delayed reactions, and late-delayed injuries. With daily fractions of 1.8 to 2.0 Gy, the acute reaction most often presents as mild headache and nausea, beginning within a few hours after the first treatment and becoming progressively less severe with each succeeding fraction.[55] The pathogenesis is thought to be increased cerebral edema caused by radiation-induced permeability changes in the BBB. Corticosteroids may prevent or relieve most symptoms. Thus, if symptoms of increased intracranial pressure are present, patients undergoing cranial irradiation should be protected with corticosteroids (e.g., dexamethasone, 8 to 16 mg per 24 hours), administered for at least 48 to 72 hours before beginning treatment.

The early-delayed reaction (also called *radiation encephalopathy*) is characterized by transient, self-limited neurologic deterioration, somnolence, or focal encephalopathy.[56] Early-delayed encephalopathy occurs in 15% to 40% of patients with primary or metastatic brain tumors. This reaction, which begins within 1 to 12 weeks after the completion of radiation therapy, usually peaks by 8 weeks after treatment and resolves spontaneously within the subsequent 4 months. Patients complain of headache, lethargy, and an exacerbation of their neurologic symptoms. At times, corticosteroid therapy and intensive medical support may be required. Declines in long-term memory within 1 to 2 months after irradiation, followed by recovery 4 to 8 months later, have also been observed.

The early-delayed reaction is thought to result from transient demyelination, resulting from damage to proliferating oligodendrocytes, and temporary changes in the BBB. CT and MRI studies during this period may show apparent tumor enlargement, increased tumor enhancement, and edema, and in some cases new enhancement may appear. These changes appear to relate to intralesional reactions, indicative of tumor response, or localized perilesional edema and demyelination, or both. It is important to recognize that the appearance of new findings during the early post-treatment interval does not always indicate that the tumor has recurred or that a change in therapy is warranted.

Late-delayed radiation injuries vary in their appearance and severity from asymptomatic white matter changes to cerebral atrophy, hemorrhagic vascular telangiectasia, neurobehavioral impairment, pituitary-hypothalamic dysfunction, and potentially fatal necrosis. Rarely, therapeutic irradiation can cause an occlusive arterial cerebrovasculopathy[106] or secondary neoplasia.

Approximately 3% to 9% of patients irradiated for brain tumors develop clinically detectable focal radiation necrosis.[58] Radiation necrosis may appear as early as 3 months but usually develops within 1 to 2 years after treatment is completed.[102] The breakdown of white matter may induce marked edema and marked mass effect. The symptoms of focal necrosis frequently recapitulate those of the tumor, leading the clinician to suspect recurrence. MRI may show a contrast-enhancing mass with extensive white matter alterations on T_2-weighted images. Histopathologic findings are generally limited to the white matter and include focal coagulation necrosis and demyelination. Endothelial cell atypia and a unique form of fibrinoid necrosis of small arterial vessels are characteristic features that suggest the underlying pathophysiology.

Because neither the symptoms nor the radiographic findings clearly distinguish tumor from necrosis, the clinical diagnosis of radiation necrosis may be difficult to confirm. [18]FDG-PET, ^{201}Tl-SPECT, and MRS studies may help to differentiate necrosis from recurrent tumor. However, many patients have a mixture of necrosis and tumor. Thus, a biopsy may be required to confirm the diagnosis, especially when the injury occurs at or near the tumor site.

Corticosteroids may improve or stabilize the neurologic symptoms associated with the effects of radiation injury. Surgical resection is frequently beneficial to patients with favorably situated focal necrotic lesions who deteriorate neurologically and become steroid-dependent.[59] There is some evidence that anticoagulation may lead to clinical improvement when surgery is not feasible.

Radiation necrosis is uncommon at doses below 60 Gy with conventionally fractionated irradiation.[60] The probability of necrosis increases with larger daily fraction sizes (2.2 to 2.5 Gy). For patients treated with hyperfractionated irradiation (twice-daily fractions of 1.2 Gy), the incidence of necrosis increased from 4.6% for 64.8 Gy to 19.2% for 81.6 Gy. Individual host factors, including the use of chemotherapy, may alter sensitivity and increase the risk of injury.

Diffuse white matter injury develops in at least 40% of patients irradiated for intracranial neoplasms.[61] The T2-weighted magnetic resonance images reveal hyperintensity of the periventricular white matter. Cerebral cortical atrophy occurs in 17% to 50% of patients treated for brain tumors. Enlarged cerebral sulci and ventricular dilatation are seen on neuroimaging studies. The abnormalities that accompany white matter change and cerebral atrophy are discernible within the first year after irradiation and persist or progress thereafter. They tend to be more severe with larger treatment volumes, higher doses, older age, longer intervals after irradiation, and chemotherapy. Clinical features range from mild lassitude or personality change to incapacitating dementia. Some patients with cerebral atrophy may also develop gait abnormalities and urinary incontinence suggestive of the syndrome of normal pressure hydrocephalus. Many patients with radiographic changes have no symptoms, but in those who do, the degree of impairment correlates approximately with the severity of the MRI appearance.

Decreased levels of intellectual function have been observed in adults after cranial irradiation. Certain cognitive functions, such as memory, may be more susceptible to decline than others.[62] Impairment is most pronounced in those who have had chemotherapy and WBRT. Intellectual decline is first discernible within 4 to 6 months after treatment and becomes more pronounced by 2 to 3 years of follow-up. Memory loss may prevent patients from returning to their premorbid occupation. However, an analysis found that 60% of long-term survivors irradiated for gliomas were employed at occupations comparable to those they had held before treatment. Patients treated with partial brain irradiation tended to have a higher Karnofsky performance status (KPS), superior memory function, and a better employment history compared with those who received WBRT.[63]

Neuropsychologic testing of patients treated for various brain tumors who failed to retain their premorbid social or occupational levels of function demonstrated that newly learned tasks requiring attention and immediate problem-solving ability were performed poorly. In contrast, tests that evaluated long-term memory and overlearned material were generally consistent with premorbid levels.[64] IQ testing alone is a less sensitive indicator of changes in cognitive function in adults. Prompt neuropsychologic intervention when necessary and early return to work after treatment may lead to improvement in or recovery of cognitive function.

Outcome

The median survival times using conventional radiotherapy alone or with chemotherapy consistently range from 9 to 14 months.[38] The median survival for patients with glioblastoma multiforme is 10 to 12 months, whereas the 3-year survival rate is only 6% to 8%.[28] The median survival for patients with anaplastic astrocytoma is 36 months, and the 3-year survival rate is approximately 50%.

VOLUME OF RADIATION. In the BTCG 8001 trial, patients were randomized to receive either 60-Gy WBRT or 43-Gy WBRT with 17.2-Gy boost. No difference in survival or recurrence was noted.[65] In a Japanese trial patients were randomized to 40-Gy WBRT with 18-Gy boost or 56-Gy local field radiation alone.[66] Again, the 2-year survival was no different in this study (43% vs. 39%), indicating that large volume irradiation is unnecessary in high-grade gliomas.

DOSE OF RADIATION. Radiation dose is another important consideration. In an MRC phase III trial, 444 patients were randomized to either 45 Gy in 20 fractions or 60 Gy in 30 fractions (1:2 randomization). A benefit of 60 Gy was seen in terms of 1-year survival (29% vs. 39%) and the median survival (9 vs. 11 months).[67] In the

RTOG phase III trial, patients received either 60 Gy WBRT or 60 Gy WBRT with a 10-Gy boost. There was no benefit with the boost in terms of the median survival (9.3 vs. 8.2 months).[68] Researchers at the University of Michigan reported dose escalation to 80 Gy and 90 Gy with 3D-CRT and showed no difference in patterns of relapse or survival, indicating the absence of benefit with dose escalation beyond 60 Gy in malignant gliomas.[69,70]

RADIATION SENSITIZERS. Multiple randomized trials conducted by RTOG, BTSG, and others have failed to show any survival benefit with Misonidazole or other agents when compared with radiotherapy alone.[71,72] Difluoromethylornithine (DFMO), an inhibitor of polyamine synthesis, has not shown any benefit in a phase III clinical trial.[73] RSR-13, a synthetic allosteric modifier of hemoglobin, showed a median survival of 12.3 months when used along with 60 Gy in a phase II study and is being presently tested in a phase III trial.[74]

Two halogenated pyrimidine analogs, bromodeoxyuridine (BUdR) and iododeoxyuridine (IUdR), have been tested and in randomized trials have failed to show any benefit. NCOG data had shown a median survival of 252 weeks with BUdR with concomitant radiation and chemotherapy in anaplastic astrocytoma compared to 82 weeks without BUdR.[75] However, an RTOG trial of 60 Gy in 30 fractions combined with PCV chemotherapy with or without BUdR in 189 patients of anaplastic astrocytoma had to be prematurely closed due to lack of benefit (1-year survival—68% vs. 82%) and higher toxicity.[76]

ALTERED FRACTIONATION. Again, multiple randomized trials conducted by the RTOG, the EORTC, and others have failed to show any survival benefit with hyperfractionation when compared with conventional RT alone.[71,77] Similarly, several trials using different accelerated fractionation regimens have been reported, and none have shown a survival benefit over conventional irradiation. An EORTC trial involving 60 Gy given in either conventional fractionation or with 3 fractions of 2 Gy given in a single day, 4 hours apart, in 340 patients showed no difference in survival or any increased toxicity.[78] Doses of 64 and 70.4 Gy in 1.6-Gy twice-daily fractions with BCNU tested in RTOG trial showed no benefit.[79] Shortening the treatment time has again failed to show any improvement.[80] A Johns Hopkins trial of 30 Gy in 10 fractions followed by 2 weeks rest and then another 21 Gy in 7 fractions to reduced fields in 219 patients showed a survival similar to RTOG recursive partitioning analysis (RPA) groups I to VI patients.[81]

BRACHYTHERAPY. An earlier BTSG trial that randomized malignant glioma patients to 60 Gy radiation ± I-125 seed implant to 50 Gy showed a survival benefit with the addition of brachytherapy (median survival—13 vs. 16 months).[82] However, these data are questionable since the information was presented as an abstract only and never published. Similarly, an NCOG phase II trial had shown median survival of 38 months in anaplastic astrocytoma and 20 months in glioblastomas.[83] However, a randomized trial done at Princess Margaret Hospital that randomized patients to 50 Gy external beam radiation with or without temporary I-125 seed implant to 60 Gy did not show any survival benefit (median survival—13.2 vs. 13.8 months).[84]

STEREOTACTIC RADIOSURGERY. Several retrospective trials had indicated a possible survival advantage with the addition of an SRS boost to high-grade gliomas.[85-88] The RTOG conducted a randomized trial of conventional radiotherapy to 60 Gy and BCNU alone or preceded by a radiosurgery boost to 15 to 24 Gy in patients with glioblastoma multiforme measuring 4 cm or less.[89] However, the results were disappointing. The median survival (14 vs. 13.7 months), 2-year survival (22% vs. 18%), and 3-year survival (16% vs. 8%) were similar with or without the boost. There was no improvement in any RPA class. No increased toxicities were seen with the addition of the SRS boost. Failures were still predominantly local (>90%).

CHEMOTHERAPY. No chemotherapeutic regimen tested by the BTCG[71] and by the RTOG (with the Eastern Cooperative Oncology Group [ECOG])[90] has offered an advantage over BCNU alone. In contrast, a reanalysis of a randomized trial by the NCOG (6G-61) found that both time to progression ($P = 0.025$) and survival ($P = 0.021$) were improved in patients with highly anaplastic astrocytomas who received PCV, compared with those who received BCNU. A difference was not observed for glioblastoma multiforme.[40] However, a retrospective analysis of the RTOG database did not confirm the benefit of PCV in anaplastic astrocytomas.[41]

Some of the newer biologic agents being presently explored in high-grade gliomas include tyrosine kinase inhibitors,[47] matrix metalloproteinase inhibitors,[91] and antitenascin antibodies.[92]

LOW-GRADE ASTROCYTOMA

Incidence

Low-grade astrocytomas make up 5% to 15% of adult primary brain tumors and 67% of low-grade gliomas, the remainder of low-grade gliomas being mixed oligoastrocytomas (19%) and oligodendrogliomas (13%).[93] Unlike the incidence of their malignant counterparts, the incidence of low-grade astrocytomas decreases with increasing age. They are most common between the ages of 20 and 40 years and rarely occur after the age of 50.

Anatomy

Low-grade astrocytomas in adults typically involve the cerebral hemispheres. Among 995 cases of supratentorial astrocytomas culled from the literature, 42% were located in the frontal lobes, 37% in the temporal, 5% in the parietal, and 10% in more than one lobe, whereas 6% presented at other sites.[93]

Pathology

Astrocytomas are well-differentiated tumors that display increased cellularity compared with normal brain tissue and have mild to moderate nuclear pleomorphism (Fig. 20-7). Microcysts are frequently present, a feature that distinguishes astrocytomas from reactive gliosis.[13] The majority of low-grade astrocytomas are classified as grade 2 in the WHO system and grades 1 and 2 in the St. Anne-Mayo scheme. Pilocytic astrocytomas are classified as grade 1 in the WHO system (see Table 20-2).

The various astrocytoma subtypes, including the fibrillary, protoplastic, gemistocytic, and pilocytic forms, are distinguished by their intracytoplasmic fibrillary processes, demonstrated by staining for GFAP. Fibrillary astrocytomas, the most common subtype, and protoplasmic astrocytomas have been referred to as "ordinary astrocytomas"[93] and share a similar prognosis. Over time, at least 50% of these tumors transform into more anaplastic lesions. Gemistocytic astrocytomas are composed of large, plump astrocytes with abundant eosinophilic cytoplasm. Because gemistocytes commonly transform into highly anaplastic cells, they behave in an aggressive fashion and should be treated as anaplastic gliomas.

Pilocytic astrocytomas typically occur in the first 2 decades of life but also arise in adults. They are composed of fusiform cells with unusually long wavy processes. Endothelial proliferation may be present but does not signify malignancy.[94] Pilocytic astrocytomas have a long natural history and rarely dedifferentiate into tumors with more malignant histologic appearances.

Although low-grade astrocytomas are often similar in their histologic appearance, their biologic behavior may vary considerably. By labeling cells undergoing DNA

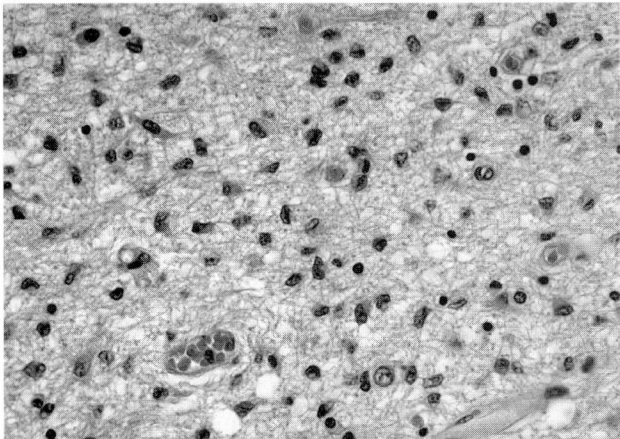

Figure 20–7. Low-grade astrocytoma showing mildly increased cellularity with uniform cells and nuclei. (Hematoxylin and eosin, original magnification ×250.)

synthesis in situ with BrdU, one can determine the percentage of S-phase cells or the BrdU labeling index (LI). In one study, 85% of patients exhibiting a low growth rate with an LI of less than 0.7% survived 3 years. The 3-year survival of patients with an LI of 0.7% to 2.2% was 65%, whereas only 25% of those with an LI of more than 2.2% survived.[95] These data suggest that patients with a high LI should be considered for more aggressive treatment programs.

Clinical Presentation

About two-thirds of adult patients with low-grade astrocytomas present with seizures but are otherwise neurologically intact.[93] Others exhibit a slowly progressive neurologic syndrome consisting of headache, vomiting, motor deficit, visual or sensory loss, language disturbance, or personality change. Symptoms may be present for months or years before a diagnosis is made. Seizures are associated with a better survival, whereas the presence of functional deficits predicts a poorer outcome.

Routes of Spread

Pilocytic astrocytomas are well circumscribed and grow by expansion, whereas the nonpilocytic tumors diffusely infiltrate adjacent tissues in a pattern similar to that of malignant gliomas. One variant, called gliomatosis cerebri, found in the second and third decade of life, may involve considerable areas of the cerebral hemispheres, cerebellum, and brainstem. The widespread nature of this lesion has been regarded as evidence for multifocal astrocytic neoplastic transformation.

Diagnostic Studies

Pilocytic astrocytomas appear on CT as discrete, enhancing lesions. The classic appearance is a large cyst with an enhancing mural nodule. Ordinary astrocytomas appear as diffuse, poorly defined, low-density, nonenhancing lesions.[22] Approximately 40% of ordinary astrocytomas enhance, and calcification is found in 10% of cases.[49,145] MRI typically shows low-signal intensity changes on T1-weighted images, high-signal intensity on T2, and an absence of enhancement (Fig. 20-8). Tumor volumes defined by T2-weighted MRI are larger than those defined by low attenuation on CT (representing tumor plus edema).

Grouping

Bauman and associates have proposed a grouping system for predicting the survival for patients with low-grade gliomas using RPH based on a database of 401 patients.[96] Age, KPS, and presence or absence of contrast enhancement were used as prognostic indicators. Group I

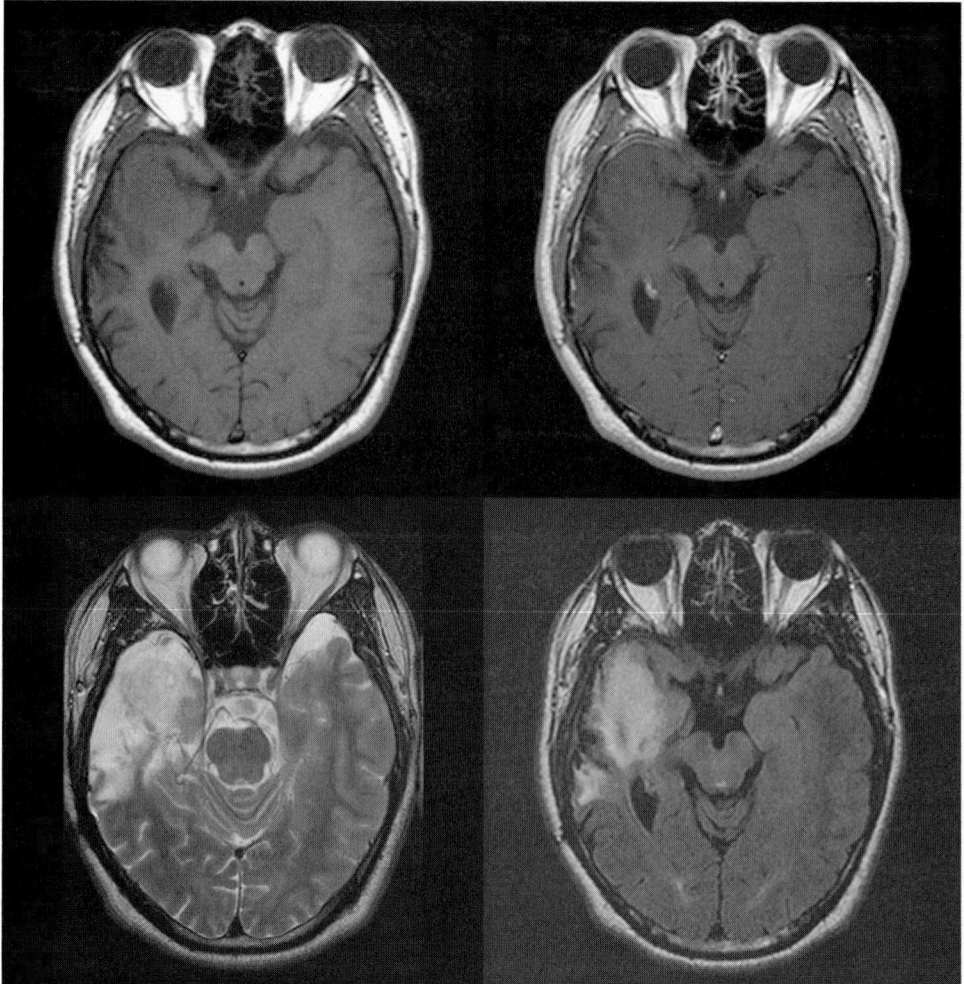

Figure 20–8. Axial magnetic resonance image of low-grade astrocytoma of right temporal lobe with T1- weighted images without and with contrast, flare sequence, and T2-weighted image, clockwise from upper left corner.

(KPS <70 and age older than 40) had the worst median survival of 12 months. Group II (KPS >70, age older than 40, and contrast enhancement present) had a median survival of 46 months. Group III (KPS >70, age older than 40, and contrast enhancement absent or KPS <70 and age younger than 40) had a median survival of 87 months. Group IV (KPS >70, age 18 to 40) had the best median survival of 128 months.

Standard Therapeutic Approaches

The outcome of patients diagnosed and treated in the CT–MRI era is notably better than that reported in the past when the conditions of diagnosis were different than they are now. Median survival times in recent series range from 7.2 to 12.9 years,[145-149] as compared with 5 years or less in older series, raising concerns over the value of the older literature in making treatment decisions today.[97] The improved outcomes appear to be related to the early diagnosis of neurologically intact patients who exhibit only seizures at the time of diagnosis. These factors have been the source of controversy regarding the optimal management of low-grade

astrocytomas, and a number of different therapeutic approaches have been recommended.[98]

SURGERY

The goals of surgery are to establish a tissue diagnosis, to remove as much tumor as possible without increasing the neurologic deficit, and to remove an epileptogenic focus if present.[98] Pilocytic astrocytomas are relatively well circumscribed, and 60% to 80% are amenable to total removal. Long-term survival approaches 100% after complete surgical resection.[99] After partial resection, survival rates range from 80% to 90% at 5 years, 70% to 80% at 10 years, and 50% to 60% at 20 years. The 10- to 20-year survival after biopsy alone varies from 40% to 50%.

Resection of the more common diffuse astrocytomas is limited by the lack of clear demarcation between the infiltrating tumor and normal brain tissue. Newer surgical techniques make the attempted resection safer, more complete, and more likely to control seizures. Most series show an improvement in time to progression and survival with more extensive surgery.[100,101,102] In one series, 80% of adult patients with completely resected tumors survived 5 years, compared with 50% for subtotal resection and 45% for biopsy.[100] Others, however, have not shown a correlation between the extent of resection and prognosis.[103,104]

The earlier diagnosis of patients with low-grade astrocytomas has raised questions regarding the timing of therapeutic intervention. There is general agreement that large symptomatic and progressive tumors should be treated at diagnosis, and a complete surgical resection should be attempted. A diagnostic biopsy should be performed on patients with deep or unresectable symptomatic tumors. Patients with small, asymptomatic (other than medically controlled seizures), apparently indolent tumors may be considered for close observation. Surgical intervention is offered should the tumor change its radiographic appearance or cause new symptoms or medically uncontrollable seizures.

Alternatively, more aggressive local treatment in the form of surgery alone or surgery and postoperative irradiation can be offered. Arguments for performing immediate surgery are to confirm the diagnosis and to identify patients with nonenhancing anaplastic tumors. Complete resection of smaller tumors may improve survival,[105] obviate the need for irradiation, and decrease the risk of malignant transformation, the most common cause of death from low-grade astrocytomas.

RADIATION THERAPY

Patient selection, the dose, and the timing of postoperative irradiation are controversial issues. Postoperative irradiation is not indicated for completely resected pilocytic astrocytomas.[103] There are insufficient data relative to the role of radiation therapy for incompletely resected tumors. Therefore, after subtotal resection or biopsy, the following may be recommended: immediate irradiation or close follow-up, deferring treatment until there is disease progression.

Opinions differ regarding the need for postoperative irradiation for completely resected ordinary astrocytomas. The 5-year recurrence-free survival rates of patients with supratentorial astrocytomas or mixed oligoastrocytomas who undergo total or radical subtotal tumor resection range from 52% to 95%.[103,104] The outcome in adult patients after total resection has been found in some series to be similar to that of patients undergoing less extensive surgery.[103] Thus, in adults postoperative irradiation has been recommended after complete resection by some, whereas others suggest that radiotherapy be withheld until recurrence.[103,105]

Most retrospective reviews suggest that postoperative irradiation is beneficial for incompletely resected nonpilocytic astrocytomas. A major question concerns whether radiotherapy should be given immediately after surgery or be delayed until recurrence or progression. Patients with intractable seizures or with large, progressive, symptomatic, unresectable or incompletely resected tumors should be considered for radiotherapy. Immediate postoperative irradiation has been recommended for patients older than 40 years who appear to benefit most from this treatment approach.[98,100,103] Postoperative irradiation is commonly deferred in patients with well-controlled seizures who present with otherwise asymptomatic tumors. Proponents of this approach argue that with CT and MRI, the disease is diagnosed earlier in its natural history than in the past and that it is unclear whether early irradiation provides an outcome advantage over delayed irradiation, whether irradiation can delay or prevent tumor dedifferentiation, or whether it even alters the prognosis.[102,106] Of 525 patients with biopsy-proven astrocytomas reported in the literature from the CT era, 423 (80%) received immediate postoperative radiotherapy, whereas 98 (19%) were not irradiated, and 4 (1%) had deferred treatment for malignant tumor transformation.[101] Thus, the safety of deferring postoperative radiotherapy cannot be gleaned from the retrospective data.

A randomized trial of early versus delayed radiotherapy in adult patients was conducted by the EORTC.[107] In this trial, 311 patients with low-grade gliomas were randomized to no immediate therapy or 54 Gy postoperative radiation. In this study, biopsy alone was the surgical procedure in 40% of the patients; the histology was oligodendroglioma in 25% of the patients. With a median follow-up of 5 years, the 5-year disease free survival was better with immediate postoperative radiation (37% vs. 44%). However, the 5-year OS was the same (63% vs. 66%), indicating that deferring the postoperative therapy is an option for selected group of patients.

CHEMOTHERAPY

Chemotherapy has little established role in adult low-grade astrocytomas. In a Southwest Oncology Group (SWOG) trial, patients with incompletely excised tumors were randomly assigned to receive radiotherapy alone or with CCNU. The median survival of all patients was 4.45 years with no difference between the two treatment arms.[101] Levin and colleagues[108] treated 22 adult patients with contrast-enhancing astrocytomas with radiotherapy and BrdU followed by 1 year of PCV chemotherapy. The estimated 6-year survival was 79%, comparing favorably with the outcome for enhancing low-grade gliomas reported by others. Levin has recommended neoadjuvant procarbazine and CCNU followed by radiotherapy in adults younger than age 45 years with infiltrating astrocytomas. There is an RTOG trial that allows observation alone for completely resected low-grade gliomas in patients younger than 40 years and randomizes subtotally resected young patients and older patients after any kind of resection to postoperative radiation to 54 Gy with or without PCV chemotherapy for six cycles. This study has just completed the accrual and the results are awaited.

Techniques of Radiotherapy

Limited radiation fields are used for the treatment of low-grade astrocytomas. The PTV encompasses the T2-weighted MRI-defined GTV with a 2-cm margin of normal brain. In general, contrast administration is not helpful since enhancement is either weak or absent altogether. Nearly all recurrences occur at the original primary tumor site. Three-dimensionally designed complex treatment plans with multiple fields are used whenever appropriate to limit the high-dose volume and to minimize the risk of long-term radiation sequelae. Doses of 50.4 to 54 Gy in daily fractions of 1.8 to 2.0 Gy, five fractions per week, are usually recommended.

Outcome

Representative survival rates for adults with low-grade astrocytomas are summarized in Table 20-6. Note that for irradiated patients treated since 1975, 5-year survival rates range from 50% to 79% and 10-year rates range from 30% to 67%. In one series, the 5-year survival for nonirradiated patients was 65%. In that report, 35% of patients were treated with surgery alone and 65% received postoperative irradiation.[100] Unfortunately, no information is given regarding the criteria used to select patients for a particular treatment program. Young age,

good performance status, complete resection, pilocytic histologic appearance, and low proliferative potential are favorable prognostic features.

The optimal dose of radiation remains unclear. In a randomized trial conducted by the EORTC involving 379 patients, no survival difference was observed when 45 Gy was compared with 59.4 Gy. With a median follow-up of 6 years, the 5-year disease-free survival (47% vs. 50%) and the 5-year OS were the same (58% vs. 59%).[109] In this study, biopsy alone was the surgery done in 45% of the patients; the histology was oligodendroglioma in 25% of the patients. In another combined NCCTG, RTOG, and ECOG study, patients were randomized to receive 50.4 Gy in 28 fractions or 64.8 Gy in 36 fractions. With a median follow-up of 6.3 years, the 5-year disease-free survival (44% vs. 40%) and the 5-year OS were again the same (72% vs. 64%), indicating that lower doses of RT are probably as effective as higher doses of radiation for low-grade gliomas.[110]

Table 20–6   Outcome in Adults with Low-Grade Astrocytoma Treated with Surgery Alone or Surgery and Radiotherapy

Reference	Dates of Study	Cases, *n*	Treatment	Survival Rate, %	
				5-Yr	10-Yr
Leibel et al*	1942-1967	78	S	23	15
			S + RT	35	24
Fezakas[†]	1958-1974	41	S	22	—
			S + RT	48	18
Garcia et al[‡]	1950-1979	80	S	21	10
			S + RT	50	25
Medbery et al[§]	1960-1986	50	S + RT	45	32
			≥50 Gy	55	45
			<50 Gy	22	13
Shaw et al[¶]	1960-1982	121	S	32	11
			S + RT ≥53 Gy	68	39
			S + RT <53 Gy	47	21
Whitton & Bloom[104]	1960-1985	60	S + RT	36	26
Shibamoto et al[¶]	1965-1989	71	S + RT	54 (age >30)	33
North et al**	1975-1984	52	S + RT	53 (age 20-50)	—
				32 (age >50)	—
McCormack et al[††]	1977-1988	53	S + RT	64	48
Philippon et al[100]	1978-1987	179	S	65	—
			S + RT	55	—
Eyre et al[101]	1980-1985	54	S + RT	50	30
Van Glabbeke et al[‡‡]	1985-1991	391	S + RT 45 Gy	58	—
			S + RT 59.4 Gy	59	—
Stalpers et al[§§]	1980-1991	164	S + RT	79	67

*From Leibel SA, Sheline GE, Wara WM, et al: The role of radiation therapy in the treatment of astrocytomas. *Cancer.* 1975;35:1551.
[†]From Fazekas JT: Treatment of grades I and II brain astrocytomas: The role of radiotherapy. *Int J Radiat Oncol Biol Phys.* 1977;2:661.
[‡]From Garcia DM, Fulling KH, Marks JE: the value of radiation therapy in addition to surgery for astrocytomas of the adult cerebrum. *Cancer.* 1985;55:919.
[§]From Medbery CA III, Straus KL, Steinberg SM, et al: Low-grade astrocytomas: Treatment results and prognostic variables. *Int J Radiat Oncol Biol Phys.* 1988;15:837.
[¶]From Shaw EG, Daumas-Duport C, Scheithauer BW, et al: Radiation therapy in the management of low-grade supratentorial astrocytomas. *J Neurosurg.* 1989;70:853.
[¶]From Shibamoto Y, Kitakabu Y, Takahashi M, et al: Supratentorial low grade astrocytoma. Correlation of CT findings with effect of radiotherapy and prognostic variables. *Cancer.* 1993;72:190.
**From North CA, North RB, Epstein JA, et al: Low-grade cerebral astrocytomas. Survival and quality of life after radiation therapy. *Cancer.* 1990;66:6.
[††]From McCormack BM, Miller DC, Budzilovich GN, et al: Treatment and survival of low-grade astrocytoma in adults—1977-1988. *Neurosurgery.* 1992;31:636.
[‡‡]From Van Glabbeke M, Karim ABMF, Hamers H, et al: No improvement in survival by increased radiation dose given postoperatively to patients with low-grade brain tumors: An EORTC randomized phase II study. *Proc ASCO.* 1995;14:145. Abstract.
[§§]From Stalpers L, Bauman G, Sneed P, et al: Radiotherapy of grade II gliomas. *Eur J Cancer.* 1995;31A(suppl 5):S57. Abstract.
S, surgery alone; S + RT, surgery and postoperative irradiation; —, data not available.

OLIGODENDROGLIOMA

Incidence

Oligodendrogliomas, which comprise less than 5% of adult primary brain tumors, occur most commonly between the ages of 25 and 49 years.[98] Losses of genetic information from chromosomes 1p (75%) and 19q (81%) are commonly seen in oligodendroglioma specimens, whereas losses on 17p (19%) and *p53* gene mutations are notably less frequent, suggesting that early events in their oncogenesis are distinct from those associated with astrocytic tumors. On the other hand, anaplastic oligodendrogliomas show additional allelic losses involving chromosomes 9 and 10 and in some cases *EGF-R* gene amplification in a pattern similar to that of anaplastic astrocytomas, indicating a common progression pathway.[111]

Anatomy

More than 80% of oligodendrogliomas arise in the white matter of the cerebral hemispheres, most commonly in the frontal, temporal, and parietal lobes.[98] Approximately 15% are found in the third or lateral ventricles, and the remainder arise in the posterior fossa.

Pathology

Oligodendrogliomas are composed of small, uniform cells with round central nuclei and distinct cytoplasmic borders. Formalin fixation causes a perinuclear halo that produces a "fried egg" or "honeycomb" appearance. The cells lack fibrillary cytoplasmic processes. A rich, vascular network, called "chicken-wire" vessels, divides the tumor into discrete lobules. Calcification is a frequent feature (Fig. 20-9).[13] Anaplastic oligodendrogliomas, which represent only 3.5% of malignant gliomas,[174] may

evolve from low-grade oligodendrogliomas or arise de novo. They have recognizable oligodendroglial components but also exhibit features of anaplasia, including nuclear pleomorphism, vascular endothelial proliferation, mitoses, and necrosis.[112]

A two-tiered system, low-grade and anaplastic, is used to grade oligodendrogliomas.[112] Patients with grades 1 or 2 tumors have a median survival of 9.8 years and 5- and 10-year survival rates of 73% and 49%, respectively, whereas those with grade 3 or 4 tumors have a median survival of 4.6 years and 5- and 10-year survival rates of 45% and 26%.[113]

Many oligodendrogliomas are admixed with astrocytoma or ependymoma components. The presence of 10% to 25% of the minor component is required to make the diagnosis of a mixed oligoastrocytoma.[93] The median survival for patients with low-grade mixed oligoastrocytomas is 7 years and the 5- and 10-year survival rates are 63% and 33%, respectively.[13] Most oligoastrocytomas and 50% to 75% of oligodendrogliomas recur as anaplastic astrocytomas or glioblastoma multiforme.

Clinical Presentation

Oligodendrogliomas present in a fashion similar to that of hemispheral astrocytomas. However, two features distinguish them from astrocytomas: the antecedent history, averaging 7 to 8 years, tends to be longer, and seizures are more common, occurring in 70% to 90% of patients by the time of diagnosis.[3] Headache, altered mental status, papilledema, and focal neurologic deficits are also common at presentation.

Patterns of Spread

Oligodendrogliomas grow in a diffuse infiltrative pattern. They may invade the cerebral cortex or expand centrally into the deep midline structures. Ventricular extension accounts for a 5% to 10% incidence of spread through the cerebrospinal fluid pathways. Metastases may occur to the spinal cord and rarely to extracranial sites.[114]

Diagnostic Studies

A provisional diagnosis may be made by CT or MRI. Oligodendrogliomas are typically hypodense or isodense, poorly defined, and nonenhancing on CT. Calcification is present in 60% of cases, and peritumoral edema is minimal. They are of low signal intensity on T1-weighted MRI and hyperintense on T2-weighted studies except for regions of signal void that correspond to fragments of calcium (Fig. 20-10).[22] Some aggressive low-grade oligodendrogliomas enhance on CT and MRI.[98] Anaplastic oligodendrogliomas and mixed gliomas more often enhance and may contain hemorrhagic and necrotic areas. Although these tumors do rarely spread through the cerebrospinal fluid, cytological and spinal MRI studies are not obtained unless clinically warranted.

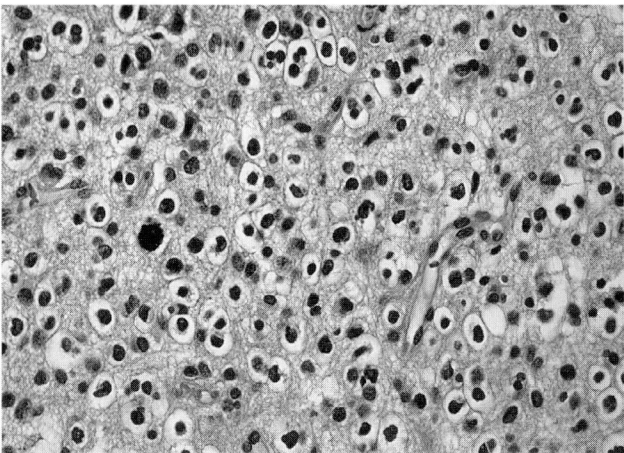

Figure 20–9. Low-grade oligodendroglioma showing uniform cells with clear cytoplasm and fragments of calcification. (Hematoxylin and eosin, original magnification ×250.)

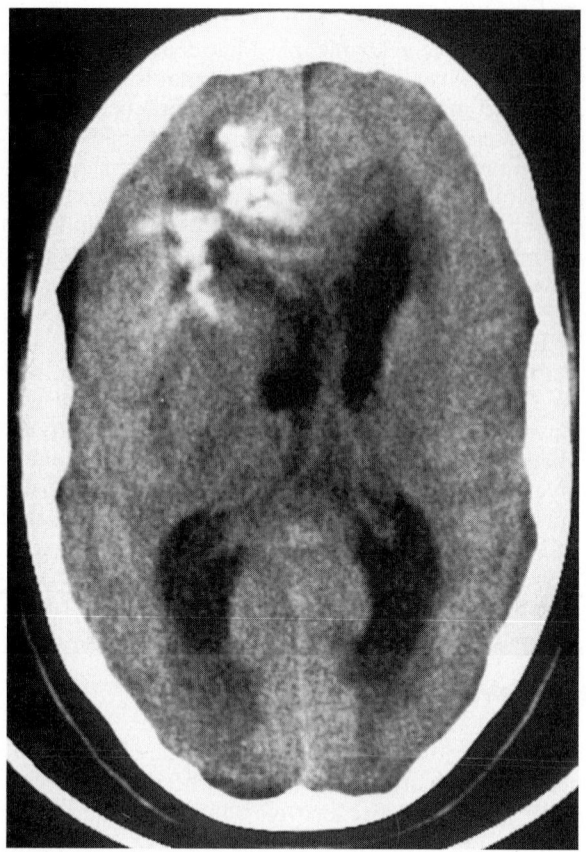

Figure 20–10. Axial computed tomographic image of low-grade oligodendroglioma with poorly defined, nonenhancing mass and marked calcification.

Standard Therapeutic Approaches

SURGERY

Surgery is required for histologic confirmation. The principles of surgical resection are similar to those for cerebral astrocytomas, with gross total removal being the goal when this is consistent with good neurologic outcome. The margins of oligodendrogliomas can appear to be more distinct than those of astrocytomas but generally they are infiltrative, and surgical cure is unlikely.[3] The extent of resection[104,105] and postoperative tumor volume[105] have been shown to affect survival in some series but not in others.[115] As in the case of low-grade astrocytomas, some small asymptomatic (except for controlled seizures) tumors can be observed, delaying surgical intervention until there is disease progression. However, if feasible, large, symptomatic, or progressive tumors should be resected.[98]

RADIATION THERAPY

Conclusions regarding the value of radiotherapy are contradictory, and the lack of randomized trials precludes the statement of firm recommendations. The infrequent occurrence of oligodendrogliomas and their variable and often long natural history make it difficult to evaluate the effect of radiotherapy on these tumors. Certain histologic features affect the prognosis,[116] and it is likely that many retrospective studies contain patients with both differentiated and anaplastic oligodendrogliomas.

Patients with completely resected low-grade oligodendrogliomas can be observed, deferring radiotherapy until the time of recurrence. Large, symptomatic unresectable or incompletely resected tumors should receive postoperative irradiation.[98] On the other hand, certain small asymptomatic (except for controlled seizures) tumors may be observed after subtotal resection, delaying radiotherapeutic intervention until there is tumor progression. Patients with pure or mixed anaplastic oligodendrogliomas should routinely receive postoperative irradiation.

CHEMOTHERAPY

Anaplastic oligodendrogliomas are chemosensitive tumors. PCV used in standard and higher-dose regimens (intensive PCV) produces response rates of 75% or more in newly diagnosed anaplastic oligodendrogliomas, anaplastic oligoastrocytomas, and oligodendrogliomas, and rates of 68% or more in recurrent tumors.[117,118] To test the efficacy of chemotherapy in newly diagnosed pure and mixed anaplastic oligodendrogliomas, the RTOG, ECOG, NCCTG, and SWOG have conducted a trial comparing radiotherapy alone with neoadjuvant intensive PCV chemotherapy (four 6-week cycles) followed by radiotherapy. The study has met the target accrual and the results are awaited. The RTOG has just opened another phase II trial of preradiotherapy temozolomide chemotherapy for six cycles to delay radiotherapy (59.4 Gy) in partial responders or to even withhold it in complete responders in pure or mixed anaplastic oligodendroglioma patients.

Radiation Therapy Techniques

The PTV for radiotherapy encompasses the MRI-defined GTV with a 2-cm margin. A dose of 54 Gy in daily 1.8-Gy fractions is used. Patients with pure and mixed anaplastic oligodendrogliomas receive 59.4 to 60 Gy in daily fractions of 1.8 to 2.0 Gy using an approach similar to that used for malignant gliomas.

Outcome

Outcome data from representative series are shown in Table 20-7. Five-year survival rates for irradiated patients range from 36% to 83% and 10-year rates vary from 8% to 56%. In contrast, 5-year survival rates for nonirradiated tumors range from 25% to 74% and 10-year rates vary from 12% to 59%. Marked changes in neuroimaging and the quality of surgery, radiation therapy, and patient management occurred over the long time intervals spanned by these studies. Age, completeness of resection, performance status, and histopathologic features affect the prognosis.[113,119,120,121]

For incompletely resected oligodendrogliomas, several studies suggest a benefit for postoperative irradiation during the first 5 years after treatment, but this effect

Table 20–7   Outcome of Surgery Alone or Surgery and Radiotherapy for Oligodendroglioma

Reference	Dates of Study	Cases, *n*	Treatment	Survival Rate, %	
				5-Yr.	10-Yr.
Reedy et al*	1950-1980	48	S	67	46†
			S + RT	63	51†
Lindegaard et al[119]	1952-1977	170	S	36	8
			S + RT		
Bullard et al[121]	1940-1983	71	S	48‡	17‡
			S + RT	60‡	15‡
Wallner et al§	1940-1983	25	S	55‡	18
			S + RT ≥45 Gy	78‡	56
Shaw et al¶	1960-1982	19	S—GTR	74	59
		8	S—STR	25	25
		26	S + RT <50 Gy	39	20
		29	S + RT ≥50 Gy	62	31
Nijjar et al	1958-1984	68	S + RT	66	30
Gannett et al[120]	1956-1984	63	S	51	36
			S + RT	83	46
Sun et al[115]	1961-1985	46	S	31	16
			S + RT	57	43
Shimizu et al¶	1957-1990	31	S	25	—
			S + RT	74	—

*From Reedy DP, Bay JW, Hahn JF: role of radiation therapy in the treatment of cerebral oligodendroglioma: An analysis of 57 cases and a literature review. *Neurosurgery.* 1983;13:499.
†8-year survival.
‡Data estimated from graphs.
§From Wallner KR, Gonzales M, Sheline GE: Treatment of oligodendrogliomas with or without postoperative irradiation. *J Neurosurg.* 1988;68:684.
¶From Shaw EG, Scheithauer BW, O'Fallon JR, et al: Oligodendrogliomas: The Mayo Clinic experience. *J Neurosurg.* 1992;76:428.
¶From Shimizu KY, Tran LM, Mark RJ, Selch: Management of oligodendrogliomas. *Radiology.* 1993;186:569.
GTR, gross total resection; S, surgery alone; S + RT, surgery and postoperative irradiation; STR, subtotal resection; —, data not available.

diminishes over time. Lindegaard and colleagues[119] reported that radiotherapy prolonged the median survival of patients with incompletely resected tumors but did not influence the overall cure rate. Gannett and associates[120] found a significant improvement in survival with postoperative irradiation. Irradiated patients had 5- and 10-year survival rates of 83% and 46%, respectively, compared with 51% and 36% for those treated with surgery alone ($P = 0.032$). Patients in each treatment group were equally distributed with respect to prognostic factors. On the other hand, Bullard and colleagues[121] found no outcome improvement with the addition of radiotherapy, although the percentage of patients surviving in the irradiated group was consistently higher than in the nonirradiated group during the first 5 years after treatment.

Winger and colleagues[122] reported median survival times of 1.1 years for mixed anaplastic oligoastrocytomas and 5.3 years for anaplastic oligodendrogliomas treated with radiotherapy and chemotherapy. In contrast, Shaw and associates[113] found that patients with high-grade mixed oligoastrocytomas and high-grade oligodendrogliomas had similar outcomes with median survival times and 5- and 10-year survival rates of 4.3 years, 45% and 23%, respectively, for high-grade oligoastrocytomas and 4.6 years, 45% and 26%, for high-grade oligodendrogliomas.

Cairncross et al.[117] have noted that a subset of oligodendrogliomas is very responsive to chemotherapy. Those patients who had tumors with deletion of 1p

chromosome had a 100% response rate and a median survival of more than 10 years.[117] This group has also noted that 1p deletion predicted a longer progression-free survival after radiotherapy compared to patients who did not have the deletion (55 vs. 6.2 months).[118]

PRIMARY CENTRAL NERVOUS SYSTEM LYMPHOMA

Epidemiology

Until the 1980s, primary CNS lymphomas represented less than 2% of intracranial neoplasms.[123] However, during the last 2 decades, there has been a threefold to more than 10-fold increase in incidence.[124] Although this partly reflects the higher prevalence of acquired immuno-deficiency states (especially acquired immunodeficiency syndrome [AIDS]), the incidence is also increasing within the apparently immunocompetent general population. The peak incidence in human immunodeficiency virus (HIV)-negative patients is in the fifth to seventh decades of life with a 3:2 to 2:1 male-to-female ratio. In contrast, immunocompromised patients are frequently diagnosed in the third and fourth decades, and nearly all are male.[193] The molecular genetics and pathogenesis of primary CNS lymphoma have not been elucidated. Epstein-Barr virus (EBV) genome-protein expression is present in two-thirds of HIV-related primary CNS lymphomas but in only 15% of immunocompetent patients, suggesting that

EBV does not play an essential role in the pathogenesis of primary CNS lymphoma in immunocompetent patients and that HIV-related and HIV-negative primary CNS lymphoma may represent pathogenetically distinct entities.[124]

Anatomy and Routes of Spread

Central nervous system lymphomas most frequently arise in the supratentorial paraventricular region of the brain but also occur in the cerebellum and brainstem. Rarely, they present only in the leptomeninges or spinal cord.[125] Multifocal tumors are present at diagnosis in 25% to 50% of immunocompetent patients and in 60% to 80% of AIDS patients. CNS lymphomas tend to infiltrate extensively along the corpus callosum and other deep white matter tracts. They frequently traverse the ependyma to involve the ventricular surface or spread peripherally into the overlying leptomeninges. Cytologic examination of cerebrospinal fluid reveals malignant or suspicious cells in up to two-thirds of immunocompetent patients and in nearly all AIDS patients. Ocular lymphoma is found in association with primary CNS lymphoma in about 20% of patients at diagnosis.[198] Lymphoma can also begin within the globe. Of patients presenting with ocular lymphoma, 50% to 80% will subsequently develop CNS lymphoma within a median of 9 months.[126]

Pathology

Histologic examination shows perivascular cuffs and sheets of lymphoid tumor cells infiltrating brain tissue with expansion of the Virchow-Robin spaces. The neoplastic cells are similar to those of non-Hodgkin's lymphoma arising in extranodal sites. They are predominantly of B-cell origin, the majority being high-grade large cell or small noncleaved cell lymphomas, with large cell immunoblastic the most common subtype. Intermediate-grade lymphomas are less common, and low-grade subtypes and T-cell lymphomas are rare.[124]

Clinical Presentation

Presenting symptoms include focal neurologic deficits, seizures, neuropsychiatric disturbance, headache, lethargy, and confusion.[127] Neck or back pain and symptoms or signs of myelopathy may indicate parenchymal spinal cord involvement, whereas blurred vision or floaters suggest ocular lymphoma.

Diagnostic Studies

The diagnostic evaluation begins with a cranial MRI. Single or multiple densely and uniformly contrast-enhancing lesions in the paraventricular regions, basal ganglia, thalamus, or corpus callosum are characteristic findings (Fig. 20-11). Irregular ring enhancement may be present on imaging studies in AIDS-related primary CNS lymphoma, making it difficult to distinguish lymphoma from toxoplasmosis and other opportunistic infections.[3]

Cerebrospinal fluid cytologic examination and an ophthalmologic evaluation that includes a slit-lamp examination are also performed. A spinal MRI is obtained only if parenchymal spinal cord involvement is suspected.[125] Because systemic involvement at the time of diagnosis (or relapse) is extremely rare, extensive testing for occult systemic lymphoma is not warranted. However, CNS metastases are common in AIDS patients with systemic non-Hodgkin's lymphoma. Thus, a systemic staging evaluation is recommended for AIDS patients with a suspected primary CNS lymphoma.

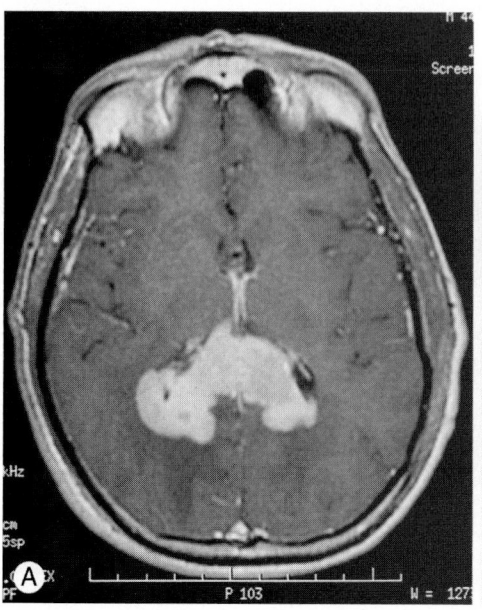
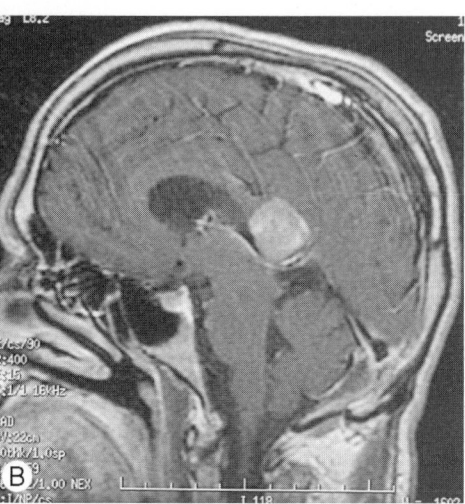

Figure 20–11. A, Axial and **B,** sagittal T1-weighted magnetic resonance images of primary nervous system lymphoma showing a contrast-enhancing lesion at the splenium of the corpus callosum.

Standard Therapeutic Approaches

SURGERY

The role of surgery is to establish a tissue diagnosis, and this is best obtained by stereotactic biopsy. Because of the multifocal nature of this tumor, extensive resections produce little survival benefit and increase the risk of postoperative deficits.[125] Large single hemispheric lesions may be surgically reduced when intracranial pressure cannot be medically controlled.

CORTICOSTEROIDS

Primary CNS lymphomas respond dramatically to corticosteroid therapy. At least 90% of patients improve clinically, whereas 40% of lesions shrink considerably and 10% disappear on CT and MRI. Tumor biopsy after corticosteroid therapy may be problematic due to the disappearance of a target for biopsy and may yield nondiagnostic tissue. Thus, when the diagnosis of primary CNS lymphoma is suspected, corticosteroids should be withheld, if possible, until a tissue diagnosis has been obtained.[125]

RADIATION THERAPY

WBRT with corticosteroids has been the standard treatment for primary CNS lymphoma. Recommended doses range from 40 to 55 Gy, often with a 10- to 20-Gy boost to the tumor bed using conventional fractionation schedules. The RTOG examined the efficacy of high-dose radiotherapy in a prospective study (trial 8315).[128] Patients with non–AIDS primary CNS lymphoma were treated with WBRT to 40 Gy plus an additional 20-Gy boost to the tumor. The median survival from the start of radiotherapy was only 11.6 months, and the 1- and 2-year survival rates were 48% and 28%, respectively. Because relapse within the boost volume occurs as frequently as outside the volume,[129] patients at Memorial Sloan-Kettering Cancer Center (MSKCC) receive 45 Gy to the whole brain without a supplemental boost. For patients with primary leptomeningeal lymphoma, the craniospinal axis is treated to 39.6 Gy, and areas of grossly identifiable tumor are given an additional 5.4 to 10.8 Gy.

When ocular lymphoma is present at the time of diagnosis of cerebral lymphoma, the eyes are treated to 36 Gy concurrently with the brain. A similar dose is used if an ocular recurrence develops in a patient who has had previous cranial irradiation.[125] Radiotherapy improves visual acuity in up to 75% of patients with symptomatic ocular lymphoma, unless extensive retinal damage has already occurred.[200] The treatment of isolated ocular lymphoma is controversial. Although some advocate treatment with ocular and WBRT, it is our policy to administer only ocular radiotherapy because of the potential toxicity of WBRT.

CHEMOTHERAPY

Several reports have documented improved survival when chemotherapy is added to radiation therapy.[125,129,130] Lipophilic agents, such as methotrexate and cytarabine, are used most frequently. Chemotherapy is given before radiotherapy, both to assess response and to reduce the risk of late neurotoxicity. The outcome is better with high-dose methotrexate-based regimens, often combined with intrathecal chemotherapy. In contrast, the efficacy of standard systemic non-Hodgkin's lymphoma regimens has been less encouraging, perhaps due to the limited penetration of many of the agents through the intact BBB.[125]

DeAngelis and colleagues[129] at MSKCC gave oral dexamethasone, high-dose intravenous methotrexate (1 g/m^2 weekly for two doses) with leucovorin rescue plus intra-Ommaya methotrexate (six doses of 12 mg each, twice weekly) followed by WBRT. Subsequently, high-dose intravenous cytarabine (two daily doses of 3 g/m^2 each separated by 24 hours) was administered. Complete response rates were 64% after preirradiation chemotherapy and 87% after all treatment. The median survival was 42.5 months. The median time to progression was 41 months for patients treated with chemotherapy and radiotherapy, compared with 10 months for a group of patients treated with radiotherapy alone ($P = 0.003$).

Of concern in the MSKCC trial was the observation of dementia and ataxia among 27% of patients over the age of 50 years who achieved a complete response. These findings were not seen in younger patients.[125] This has led to the policy of deferring radiotherapy in select older patients who respond to chemotherapy until the time of disease progression. Others are exploring regimens in which radiotherapy is withheld until recurrence to avoid radiation-induced neurotoxicity. Neuwelt and associates[131] used the technique of osmotic BBB disruption with intra-arterial mannitol followed by intra-arterial high-dose methotrexate (2.5 g) with leucovorin rescue in combination with systemic cyclophosphamide, procarbazine, and dexamethasone. Among 16 evaluable patients treated with this approach, 81% had a complete response and 19% a partial response. Ten patients subsequently relapsed and nine received radiation therapy. The median survival was 44.5 months. Six of seven nonirradiated complete responders retained good cognitive function.

Outcome

Historically, survival times from the onset of symptoms to death with no treatment or surgical resection alone ranged from 0.9 to 4.6 months.[124] Representative outcome results from the RTOG and single institutional trials are shown in Table 20-8. The median survival for radiotherapy alone varies from 12 to 20 months, and only 3% to 4% of patients survive for 5 years.[125] Median survival times for treatment programs that include high-dose methotrexate-based chemotherapy range from 33 to 42 months. Age younger than 60 and good performance status are favorable prognostic indicators. The treatment and outcome of AIDS-related primary CNS lymphoma are detailed in Chapter 67, HIV-related malignancies.

Table 20–8 Outcome in Patients with Primary Central Nervous System Lymphoma

Reference	Patients, *n*	Radiotherapy Regimen, Gy	Chemotherapy Regimen	Median, mo	Survival % 1-Yr	Survival % 2-Yr
Nelson et al[128]	41	40 WB + 20 boost	None	11.6	48	28
Schultz et al*	51	41.4 WB + 18 boost	CTX, DOX, VCR, DEX	12.8	58	40
O'Neill et al†	46	50.4 WB	CTX, DOX, VCR, PRED, HD-ara-C	11.3	43	29
DeAngelis et al[129]	31	40 WB + 14.4 boost	HD- and IO-MTX, HD-ara-C	42.5	80	75
Glass et al[130]	13	30 WB	HD-MTX	33	75	55
Neuwelt et al[131]	16	50 WB (9 patients at relapse)	IA mannitol, IA-MTX, CTX, PROCARB, DEX	44.5	75	70

*From Schultz C, Scott C, Wasserman T, et al: Pre-irradiation chemotherapy (CTX) with Cytoxan, Adriamycin, vincristine, and Decadron (CHOD) for primary central nervous system lymphomas (PCNSL): Initial report of Radiation Therapy Oncology Group (RTOG) protocol 86-06. *Proc Am Soc Clin Oncol.* 1994;13:174. Abstract.
†From O'Neill BP, O'Fallon JR, Earle JD, et al: Primary central nervous system non-Hodgkin's lymphoma: Survival advantages with combined initial therapy? *Int J Radiat Oncol Biol Phys.* 1995;33:663.
ara-C, cytarabine; CTX, cyclophosphamide; DEX, dexamethasone; DOX, doxorubicin; HD, high-dose; IA, intra-arterial; IO, intra-Ommaya; MTX, methotrexate; PRED, prednisone; PROCARB, procarbazine; VCR, vincristine; WB, whole brain.

RTOG and SWOG together have conducted a phase II trial in which HIV-negative patients received methotrexate, procarbazine, vincristine, and intra-Ommaya methotrexate over 10 weeks followed by WBRT to 45 Gy in 25 fractions of 1.8 Gy. Three weeks later, two cycles of high-dose cytarabine were given. Grade III or higher hematologic toxicities were noted in two-thirds of the patients. In an interim analysis, complete response to therapy was noted in 45 of the 78 evaluable patients on the study. The overall and the progression-free survival times were 3.3 and 1.5 years, respectively. However, 15% of the patients experienced severe delayed neurologic toxicity.[132]

UNCOMMON ADULT PRIMARY BRAIN TUMORS

Brainstem Glioma

Brainstem gliomas account for less than 2% of brain tumors in adults.[133] In a series of brainstem gliomas including patients of all ages, adults constitute about one third of those reported. The outcome of adults treated for brainstem gliomas is summarized in Table 20-9. Shrieve and associates[133] reported 41 pediatric and 19 adult patients who received 66 to 78 Gy with a hyperfractionation schedule of 1.0 Gy twice daily. The median survival time

Table 20–9 Outcome in Adults with Brainstem Glioma

Reference	Dates of Study	Patients, *n*	Dose, Gy	Median, mo	Survival % 1-Yr	Survival % 2-Yr	Survival % 5-Y
Kim et al*	1960-1975	30	50-60	15	55	40	30
Grigsby et al†	1950-1983	19 (pons)	49.8 (median)	33	84	68	47
		31 (thalamus)		14	68	35	21
Shibamoto et al‡	1962-1987	27	57-65	15	—	—	23
Shrieve et al[133]	1984-1990	19	66-78	44	68	53	—
	1973-1986	11	(HPFx) 16-59	8	36	18	—
Prados et al[134]	1987-1991	42	72-78 (HPFx)	16	—	—	—

*From Kim TH, Chin HW, Pollan S, et al: Radiotherapy of brain stem tumors. *Int J Radiat Oncol Biol Phys.* 1980;6:51.
†From Grigsby PW, Thomas PR, Schwartz HG, Fineberg BB: Multivariate analysis of prognostic factors in pediatric and adult thalamic and brainstem tumors. *Int Radiat Oncol Biol Phys.* 1989;16:649.
‡From Shibamoto Y, Takahashi M, Dokoh S, et al: Radiation therapy for brain stem tumor with special reference to CT feature and prognosis correlations. *Int J Radiat Oncol Biol Phys.* 1989;17:71.
HPFx, hyperfractionation schedule, 1.0 Gy twice daily; —, data not available.

and 1- and 2-year survival rates for children were 16 months and 63% and 32%, respectively, compared with 44 months and 68% and 53% for adults ($P = 0.43$). Prognostic covariates identified in children were not significant in their adult population. The 2-year survival for patients with thalamic and midbrain tumors (40%) was similar to that of patients with tumors arising in the pons or medulla (57%, $P = 0.67$). Furthermore, the 2-year survival (54%) of patients with diffuse tumors was the same as that of patients with focal tumors (50%). Compared with patients treated with conventional fractionation, there was a trend toward an improvement in outcome with hyperfractionation ($P = 0.08$). In an update of that series, the median survival of 42 adult patients was 16 months, and the median time to progression was 11.4 months. There was no benefit to increasing the dose above 72 Gy.[134] Similarly, in a randomized trial done by the Pediatric Oncology Group (POG), there was no benefit of hyperfractionated irradiation to 70.2 Gy compared to 54 Gy conventional fractionation.[135] Chemotherapy has not shown any benefit in the management of brainstem gliomas. In fact, a detrimental effect of combining cisplatinum with radiation has been noted in childhood brainstem gliomas.[136] As a result, radiotherapy alone by conventional fractionation to 54 Gy in symptomatic or large brainstem lesions is recommended.

Ependymoma

Ependymomas represent about 5% of all intracranial gliomas.[137] Although they are most common in children, approximately one-third occur in adults. The incidence peaks at 5 years and again at 34 years of age. Between 30% and 40% of ependymomas arise in the supratentorial brain, and 40% to 60% of tumors in this location occur in adults. The remaining 60% to 70% of ependymomas arise in the infratentorial brain, and 25% of these occur in adults.

Although the correlation between survival and histopathologic grade is controversial, histopathologic grade is a useful predictor of outcome.[138] Ependymomas are separated into low-grade and high-grade lesions (ependymoma and anaplastic ependymoma in the WHO classification). The 5-year survival for low-grade tumors ranges from 60% to 80%, whereas it varies from 10% to 47% for high-grade tumors. Supratentorial ependymomas generally have poorer prognoses than their infratentorial counterparts due to a greater proportion of lesions that are high grade[139] and the tendency for larger volumes of residual disease to be present after surgical resection.[140]

Most ependymomas cannot be completely excised because of their location and growth characteristics.[140] Postoperative irradiation improves local tumor control and survival and is an accepted part of the standard treatment for these tumors. Although most ependymomas are slow-growing, circumscribed tumors that seldom spread, others are more aggressive and may disseminate throughout the cerebrospinal fluid pathways. The frequency of tumor seeding, the identification of patients who are at high risk for dissemination, and the volume of

the CNS to treat are controversial topics. A literature review found that local relapse had the greatest impact on the development of spinal seeding, regardless of tumor grade or site.[141] The incidence of spinal dissemination was 3.3% in locally controlled patients and 9.5% in those with uncontrolled primary tumors ($P < 0.05$). The risk of seeding was not affected by prophylactic spinal irradiation.[142]

Treatment volumes recommended for low-grade supratentorial ependymomas vary from generous local fields to fields encompassing the whole brain. For low-grade infratentorial tumors they include local fields, the whole brain with cervical spine extension, and craniospinal axis irradiation.[138] The outcome with partial-brain irradiation appears to be comparable with that of whole-brain or craniospinal axis irradiation. Thus, low-grade supratentorial ependymomas are treated using a PTV of 2 cm beyond the MRI-defined lesion to a dose of 54 Gy. Patients with low-grade infratentorial ependymomas are treated in a similar fashion. The dose is modified if there is extension below the foramen magnum. The craniospinal axis is treated to 36 Gy when the spinal fluid contains malignant cells or when there is radiographic evidence of seeding.

Many authors recommend inclusion of the entire craniospinal axis in the treatment of anaplastic supratentorial and posterior fossa ependymomas, although some use WBRT with an additional boost for high-grade supratentorial lesions located away from the ventricular system.[143] However, despite the apparent superiority of craniospinal irradiation in some series, improvements in imaging, the finding that spinal seeding is uncommon in the absence of local relapse, and the identification of similar patterns of failure in patients treated with local fields or to the craniospinal axis have led some investigators to question the routine use of craniospinal, WBRT, or even entire posterior fossa.[141] Currently, at MSKCC we treat high-grade ependymomas with local fields using a PTV of 2 to 3 cm beyond the MRI-defined lesion to a dose of 59.4 Gy. The value of chemotherapy in adults with ependymomas and anaplastic ependymomas is not well defined.[3]

The outcome of adult patients with ependymoma is summarized in Table 20-10. Shaw and colleagues[144] and Vanuytsel and associates[141] found no differences between the outcomes in children and those in adults. In contrast, some series report better survival in adults,[145] whereas others have observed a better outcome in children.[139] Four of the six adult patients reported by Chin and colleagues[139] had high-grade supratentorial tumors, accounting for the poorer outcomes observed in adults in their series. In German prospective trials HIT 88/89 and 91 in anaplastic ependymomas, the only significant prognostic factor was the extent of resection. The irradiation volume did not influence the overall three-year survival of 75%.[146]

Medulloblastoma

About 30% of patients with medulloblastoma are 16 years of age or older (median 22 to 28 years) when first diagnosed.[147] In adults, medulloblastomas more

Table 20–10   Outcome in Adults with Ependymoma

Reference	Dates of Study	Patients, *n* (age, yr)	Tumor Dose, Gy	Survival, % 5-Yr	10-Yr
Chin et al[139]	1962-1974	6 (>16)	34.5-60	17	—
		10 (≤16)		50	—
Salazar et al*	1959-1979	21 (>12)	43-60	19	19
		30 (≤12)		47	47
Garrett & Simpson†	1958-1980	13 (≥18)	—	83	—
		37 (<18)		29	—
Read[145]	1956-1980	32 (>15) sup	42.5-50	40	40
		inf 21 (≤15)		65	65
				15	15
				28	28
Shaw et al[144]	1963-1983	15 (>18)	35-61	73	60
		18 (≤18)		51	51
Vanuytsel et al‡	1952-1988	35 (≥16)	24-59.2	57	48
		58 (<16)		48	39

*From Salazar OM, Castro-Vita H, Van Houtte P, et al: Improved survival in cases of intracranial ependymoma after radiation therapy: Late report and recommendations. *J Neurosurg.* 1983;59:652.
†From Garrett PG, Simpson WJK: Ependymomas: Results of radiation treatment. *Int J Radiat Oncol Biol Phys.* 1983;9:1121.
‡From Vanuytsel LJ, Bessell EM, Ashely SE, et al: Long-term results of a policy of surgery and radiotherapy. *Int J Radiat Oncol Biol Phys.* 1992;23:313.
—, data not available; sup, supratentorial; inf, infratentorial.

frequently arise laterally in the cerebellar hemispheres or cerebellopontine angle (38% to 67%) than in children (7% to 9%). Thus, adults commonly present with lateral cerebellar dysfunction. The desmoplastic histopathological variant of medulloblastoma is more common in adults (25% to 47%) than in children (13% to 18%).[148] On microscopic examination, thick bundles of collagen are found to divide the tumor into follicular nests of anaplastic cells. These changes have been thought to result from extension of the tumor to the leptomeninges, which incites a proliferation of fibrous connective tissue. However, the finding of LOH at chromosome 9q with this histologic subtype suggests that desmoplastic medulloblastomas may be pathogenetically distinct from their classic counterparts.[149] Approximately 30% of adults have disease outside the primary site,[147] similar to the rates reported in the pediatric literature.

Radiotherapy to the entire craniospinal axis is essential. The dose to the craniospinal axis is 36 Gy in daily fractions of 1.8 Gy. A boost of 18 Gy is given to the posterior fossa to bring the total to 54 Gy. At MSKCC we have used a 3D-conformal approach to deliver the posterior fossa boost and to give an additional 5.4 Gy in three fractions (total 59.4 Gy) to the primary site.

The role of chemotherapy in adult medulloblastomas is not well defined. Combinations of vincristine and CCNU,[148] procarbazine and hydroxyurea,[147] and other nitrosourea-based regimens[148] have been used. Prados and colleagues[229] found an improvement in survival (P = 0.03) and time to progression (P = 0.05) with adjuvant nitrosourea-based chemotherapy, and they recommend that chemotherapy be given to poor-risk patients. A retrospective study of 47 patients from Royal Marsden Hospital indicated a better 5-year survival of 76% with a combination of radiation therapy and chemotherapy compared with 37% with radiotherapy alone.[148] However, the patients who received chemotherapy also had higher poterior fossa dose, earlier spinal radiation and more total resection which could have contributed to the better survival.

The outcome in adults with medulloblastoma is summarized in Table 20-11. Five-year survival rates range from 46% to 81%, and 10-year rates vary from 38% to 55%, comparable with the rates reported in children.[149-150] Prados and colleagues[147] divided patients into good-risk and poor-risk groups. The criteria for the poor-risk category were disease beyond the primary site and less than a 75% tumor resection. The 5-year disease-free survival rates for good- and poor-risk adult patients were 58% and 32% (P = 0.05), respectively, similar to the rates reported for good-risk and poor-risk children (59% and 26%).[150]

Frost and associates[151] found on univariate analysis that M classification (P = 0.0005), functional status at the time of radiotherapy (P = 0.005), and the presence or absence of hydrocephalus preoperatively (P = 0.02) had a significant impact on disease-free survival, whereas subtotal tumor removal (P = 0.04) was the only covariate that affected posterior fossa relapse. The T classification has less prognostic value in adults than in children,[151] and tumor location and desmoplastic histologic appearance do not affect the prognosis.[148] A recent histologic analysis of a large series of 181 medulloblastoma patients revealed a lower labeling index and higher apoptotic index in adults, indicating a biologic difference between the two age groups, thus potentially raising the question of less aggressive therapy for adult medulloblastoma.[152]

Table 20–11   Outcome in Adults with Medulloblastoma

Reference	Dates of Study	Patients, n	Median Age (range), yr	Survival, % 5-Yr	Survival, % 10-Yr
Kopelson et al*	1962-1969	17	24 (16-41)	46	46
Hughes†	1960-1981	15	23.5 (16-46)	63	38
Haie et al‡	1961-1982	20	26.5 (16-47)	78	55
Skolyszewski et al§	1974-1980	13	22.4 (16-52)	62	—
Bloom et al[148]	1952-1981	47	24 (16-54)	54	40
Frost et al[151]	1955-1988	48	25 (16-48)	62	41
Prados et al[147]	1975-1991	47	28 (16-56)	60 Good risk: 81 Poor risk: 54	—

*From Kopelson G, Linggood RM, Kleinman GM: Medulloblastoma in adults: Improved survival with supervoltage radiation therapy. *Cancer.* 1982;49:1334.
†From Hughes PG: Cerebellar medulloblastoma in adults. *J Neurosurg.* 1984;60:994.
‡From Haie C, Schlienger M, Contans JP, et al: Results of radiation treatment of medulloblastoma in adults. *Int J Radiat Oncol Biol Phys.* 1985;11:2051.
§From Skolyszewski J, Glinski B: Results of postoperative irradiation of medulloblastoma in adults. *Int J Radiat Oncol Biol Phys.* 1989;16:479.
—, data not available.

BRAIN METASTASES

Epidemiology

Metastases to the brain occur in as many as 30% of patients with systemic cancer and represent the most common type of intracranial tumor.[153] Brain metastases exert a profound effect on the quality and length of survival, and despite the best current management, they represent the direct cause of death in one-third to one-half of affected patients.[55] Although brain metastases can arise from any primary cancer, certain tumors such as melanoma and carcinomas of the lung (especially small cell and adenocarcinoma), breast, and colorectum have a propensity to metastasize to the brain.[154] About one-half of patients present with only a single lesion, and an additional 20% have only two. Most brain metastases, particularly those that arise from primary sites other than the lung, occur at a late stage when metastatic dissemination is present elsewhere in the body.

Anatomy

Brain metastases arise from hematogenous spread to the white matter of the watershed area of the brain at the junction of the gray and white matter. Most metastatic tumors distribute themselves between the supratentorial and infratentorial compartments in proportion to the relative weight and blood supply of these structures (i.e., 85% in the cerebral hemispheres, 10% to 15% in the cerebellum, and 1% to 3% in the brain stem).[154] Certain metastatic tumors, particularly small cell lung cancer and tumors arising in the prostate, uterus, or gastrointestinal tract, have a predilection to the cerebellum.

Most brain metastases grow as spherical, well-demarcated, solid masses that displace rather than destroy adjacent tissue. They may be surrounded by minimal to extensive edema. Some rapidly growing metastases undergo central necrosis or cystic change, and others, especially those from melanoma, choriocarcinoma, and testicular carcinoma, may be hemorrhagic. *Carcinomatous encephalitis* is a clinical syndrome caused by widespread invasion of the cerebral cortex by small or microscopic foci of tumor that may or may not be seen on imaging studies.[155]

Pathology

The microscopic appearance of a brain metastasis resembles the primary tumor from which it arises. Thus, in patients with an unknown primary cancer, extirpation of the metastasis with microscopic examination often provides an important clue as to the original site of the primary tumor.[55]

Clinical Presentation

The most common presenting signs and symptoms are summarized in Table 20-12. They usually begin insidiously and evolve over a period of days or a few weeks. The spread of edema through the white matter frequently determines the speed of onset and progression of signs and symptoms.[94] Hemorrhage into a tumor may cause a more sudden onset or acute worsening of symptoms.[155]

Diagnostic Studies

Gadolinium-enhanced MRI is the best diagnostic test for brain metastases.[55] MRI can detect small lesions not seen on CT, particularly in the cerebellum and brainstem. The T2-weighted image reveals an area or areas of hyperintensity in the white matter, encompassing both the tumor and surrounding edema.

Although the clinical history combined with the results of MRI establish the diagnosis of brain metastasis with reasonable certainty, a definitive diagnosis of metastatic

Table 20–12   Presenting Symptoms and Signs in 363 Patients with Brain Metastases

Symptoms	%*	Signs	%*
Headache	49	Impaired cognitive function	58
Focal weakness	30	Hemiparesis	59
			27
			31
Mental disturbances	32	Mild–moderate	27
Gait ataxia	21	Severe	31
Seizures	18	Hemisensory loss	21
Focal motor	4	Papilledema	20
Generalized	7	Gait ataxia	19
Other focal	7	Aphasia	18
Speech difficulty	12	Visual field cut	7
Visual disturbance	6	Limb ataxia	6
Sensory disturbance	6	Depressed level of consciousness	4
Limb ataxia	6		

*Patients may present with more than one symptom or sign.
From Posner JB: *Neurologic Complications of Cancer.* Philadelphia: FA Davis; 1995:37, 77, 311.

brain tumor cannot be made on scan results alone. Even a typical radiographically defined lesion may prove to be a primary tumor, an abscess, or another lesion.[153] A known systemic cancer increases the likelihood of brain metastases, and multiple lesions make the diagnosis even more likely. However, if doubt exists, a biopsy is required to establish the correct diagnosis.

Grouping

Although no generally accepted grouping system exists for brain metastases, one was proposed by investigators from the RTOG based on a RPA of prognostic factors.[156] Three groups were defined by KPS (<70 vs. ≥70), age (younger than 65 vs. 65 or older), status of the primary tumor (controlled vs. uncontrolled), and extent of metastases (brain only vs. brain and other sites). The definition and corresponding survival for each group are shown in Table 20-13. The application of this scheme is important

Table 20–13.   Proposed Staging System for Brain Metastases Based on Recursive Partitioning Analysis of Prognostic Factors

Stage	Characteristics	Median Survival, mo
I	KPS ≥70, primary controlled, age <65 y, metastases to brain only	7.1
II	KPS ≥70, primary uncontrolled	4.2
	KPS ≥70, primary controlled, age ≥65 y	
	KPS ≥70, primary controlled, age <65 y, metastases to brain and other sites	
III	KPS <70	2.3

KPS, Karnofsky performance status.
Data from Gaspar L, Scott C, Rotman M, et al: Recursive partitioning analysis (RPA) of prognostic factors in three Radiation Therapy Oncology Group (RTOG) brain metastases trials. *Int J Radiat Oncol Biol Phys.* 1997;37:745.

to ensure that new treatment techniques for brain metastases are tested in homogeneous patient groups.

Standard Treatment Approaches

Because the majority of patients with metastatic brain lesions have or will soon develop widely disseminated disease, treatment is dictated by the need to achieve immediate short-term palliation and the desire for durable symptom-free remission. With early diagnosis and vigorous treatment, many of the symptoms associated with brain metastases can be reversed, often returning the patients to a useful life, at least temporarily. The median survival of patients with symptomatic brain metastases is approximately 1 month without treatment and 2 months with corticosteroid administration. Survival is longer and the quality of life better if brain metastases are treated.[55]

CORTICOSTEROIDS

Corticosteroids rapidly ameliorate many symptoms of brain metastasis and should be used at the onset for all symptomatic patients. Symptomatic but stable patients can begin with approximately 16 mg of dexamethasone (or equivalent) daily in two to four divided doses. Patients who are receiving WBRT should receive steroids for at least 48 hours before treatment. Steroid tapering may begin during week 2 of radiotherapy. For patients receiving 16 mg of dexamethasone, the drug should be tapered by 2 to 4 mg every fifth day. If the patient develops symptoms of either brain tumor or steroid withdrawal, the dosage is increased to the next level for 4 to 8 days before the taper is started again. If symptoms return after drug withdrawal, the full dexamethasone regimen is restarted.[55] An alternative approach is to begin at 16 mg per day for 4 days followed by 8 mg for 4 days and 4 mg per day until the completion of treatment.

SURGERY

Surgery is used to establish the diagnosis of metastatic brain disease when it is uncertain and as a treatment for single metastases. When the brain metastasis is resectable with a minimal risk of neurologic injury, surgical extirpation may provide local tumor control and immediate relief of neurologic signs and symptoms due to a mass effect.[154] Patients with a single accessible lesion, controlled or absent extracranial disease, a KPS of at least 70, age younger than 60, and a life expectancy of at least 2 months are most likely to benefit from surgery.[153] Such patients live longer, have fewer recurrences of cancer in the brain, and enjoy a better quality of life compared with those treated by radiotherapy alone. After tumor removal, steroids can usually be discontinued, whereas it is more difficult to discontinue steroids after radiotherapy because residual tumor often remains as a nidus for continuing brain edema. Based on accepted selection criteria, only 9% of patients seen at MSKCC were ideal candidates for surgical extirpation.[157] Rates of complete resection vary from 70% to 79%, whereas the operative mortality is 1% to 7%, and 5% to 22% of patients develop worsening of neurologic deficits.[55] The outcome after surgery varies with the primary tumor type. Renal cell, lung, and breast carcinomas carry a better prognosis (median survival 11 to 12 months), whereas melanoma and colorectal cancers have a worse outcome (6.5 to 8 months).[154]

Although surgery is usually not the approach of choice for patients with multiple metastases, the presence of multiple brain metastases does not always constitute a contraindication to surgery. A patient with two accessible lesions that cannot be controlled by radiotherapy or chemotherapy (not lymphoma and leukemia, small cell lung cancer, or germ cell tumor) may be treated surgically.[158] Furthermore, patients with a large metastatic lesion causing uncontrollable neurologic symptoms may be candidates for resection, even if multiple brain metastases are present, before irradiation of the smaller lesions.

Approximately 5% to 20% of patients with brain metastases present with an unknown primary tumor.[158] Most metastases arise from lung or renal cell carcinoma and melanoma. When a patient without known cancer presents with brain metastases, a search for the primary tumor should ensue before treatment of the metastatic brain disease is begun. If no other lesion is found and if the brain lesion is single and surgically accessible, extirpation is indicated to establish the diagnosis and for therapy. If multiple lesions are present or if a single lesion is surgically inaccessible, a stereotactical needle biopsy is warranted.

WHOLE-BRAIN RADIATION THERAPY

Radiotherapy is the appropriate treatment for most patients with brain metastases, including those with multiple lesions and those with single metastases who are not candidates for surgery. The standard approach is to treat the whole brain to 30 Gy in 10 daily fractions of 3 Gy each over 2 weeks.[159] The advantages of WBRT include simple clinical setup, its ease of delivery as an outpatient, its low cost, its minimal disruption of quality of life, and its good palliation as a single modality. Depending on the symptom, the response rate varies from 70% to 90%. Overall, neurologic function is improved in 50% of patients. Functional improvement is dependent on the degree of neurologic impairment at the time of treatment. Approximately two-thirds of patients with severe neurologic dysfunction improve, whereas one-third of those with moderate dysfunction improve to normal or near normal. The median time to improvement is 1 to 2 weeks in patients with severe dysfunction and 3 weeks for those with moderate impairment. The durability of response is problematic, as the median time to progression is only 2 to 3 months. Overall, 75% to 80% of remaining life is spent in an improved or stable neurologic state.[160]

RTOG has tried five schedules of fractionation varying from 20 Gy in a week to 40 Gy in 4 weeks in three randomized trials. All the regimens were similar in improvement in neurologic function (50%), duration of improvement (9 to 12 weeks), time to progression (10 weeks), survival (15 to 18 weeks), or the quality of palliation.[160] Another RTOG trial that compared accelerated fractionation (54.4 Gy in twice-daily 1.6-Gy fractions) with conventional irradiation (30 Gy in daily 3-Gy fractions) was negative.[161] Neither concomitant misonidazole[162] nor BrdU[163] has improved the outcome. Rapid dose schedules such as 10 Gy in one fraction or 15 Gy in two fractions yield a shorter duration of improvement, a lower response rate, and earlier relapse.[164] Furthermore, high-dose fractions often lead to severe acute side effects and in some cases cerebral herniation and death. A minority of patients, perhaps only 10% to 20%, who have been treated with 30 Gy in 10 fractions to the whole brain and who survive for longer than 1 year develop radiation-induced dementia. In a series by DeAngelis et al.,[165] 12 patients treated with WBRT to a dose of 25 to 39 Gy in 3 to 6Gy/fx ± surgery developed late toxicity. These patients had no evidence of disease by CT or at the time of surgery performed for a variety of reasons. All of these patients had severe dementia, ataxia, and incontinence 5 to 36 months (median—14 months) after therapy. CT scan revealed evidence of cortical atrophy, ventricular dilatation, and hypodensity of white matter. Thus, for patients who have favorable characteristics and are expected to have a good prognosis (such as RTOG class I), a protracted treatment course with daily fractions of 1.8 to 2 Gy to a total of 45 to 50 Gy is recommended.

Most series report no survival differences by tumor type. Studies from MSKCC indicate that patients harboring metastases from breast and lung carcinoma are likely to respond to radiotherapy both clinically and by scan, and those who respond are unlikely to die of their metastatic brain tumor. Patients with melanoma, colon cancer, and renal cancer are less likely to have a radiographic response even when there is a clinical response and they are more likely to die of their metastatic brain tumor than of systemic disease.[157] However, occasional responses by these patients to irradiation, documented by CT or MRI, make treatment of all patients desirable.

The outcome of two randomized trials comparing surgery and radiotherapy with whole brain radiotherapy alone is summarized in Table 20-14. In the study by Patchell and associates,[153] the recurrence rate was 20% in the surgery group and 52% in the radiation-only group (P < 0.02), and the median time to recurrence was more than 59 weeks for combined treatment and 21 weeks for radiation alone (P < 0.0001). The median duration of functional independence, defined as KPS greater than or equal to 70, was 38 weeks for combined treatment and 8 weeks for radiation alone (P < 0.005). Noordijk and colleagues found that the median survival of patients with inactive extracranial disease was 12 months for combined treatment and 7 months for radiotherapy alone (P = 0.02).[166] In contrast, there was no benefit from combined treatment in patients with active extracranial disease or in those older than 60 years of age (median survival 5 months in both groups).

WBRT is generally recommended after surgical resection of metastatic tumors. There is good evidence suggesting that postoperative irradiation decreases relapse both at the site of surgical removal and elsewhere in the brain.[167] Patchell et al. randomized 95 patients with

Table 20–14   Outcome of Randomized Trials Comparing Surgery and Radiotherapy with Radiotherapy Alone for Patients with a Solitary Brain Metastasis

Reference	Date of Study	Patients, n	Dose Fractionation Scheme, Gy/fx, n	Survival Median, mo	Survival 1-Yr, %
Patchell et al[153]	1985-1988	48	36/12	3.5*	5
			36/12 + surgery	9*	45
Noordijk et al[166]	1985-1991	66	40/10†	6‡	24
			40/10 + surgery	10‡	48

*Difference significant, $P < 0.01$.
†Treament given in twice-daily fractions of 2 Gy.
‡Difference significant, $P = 0.04$
fx, fractions; —, data not available.

solitary metastasis to surgery with or without 50.4-Gy WBRT. They noted a benefit of WBRT in terms of decreased recurrence at the site of original disease—10% versus 46%; recurrence at other sites in brain—14% versus 37%; recurrence anywhere in the brain—18% versus 70%; and death due to neurologic causes—14% versus 44%. However, the OS (48 weeks) and functionally independent survival (36 weeks) were the same in both arms.[167] Hence, a protracted radiotherapy course should be considered in favorable-prognosis patients because shorter treatment courses do not appear to prevent recurrence and may increase toxicity.

Patients who initially respond to irradiation and subsequently relapse may be candidates for reirradiation. A dose of 19.8 to 25.2 Gy in 1.8-Gy fractions is used. Although the response rate (40%) is lower than after initial irradiation, some patients do benefit from another course of treatment. Patients who have had a good clinical and radiographic response to radiotherapy and who survive 6 months after the initial treatment are the best candidates for reirradiation.

STEREOTACTIC RADIOSURGERY

SRS is an excellent alternative to surgical extirpation of solitary and multiple brain metastases (see Chapter 25, Radiosurgery). The rationale for SRS in brain metastases

includes the pseudo-spherical shape of the lesion that makes it an ideal target, the site at gray-white matter junction, which is a relatively non-eloquent location, thus permitting the delivery of single large doses; increased use of MRI where most lesions are detected while still relatively small (<3cm); the pseudocapsule of the lesions, which allows tight margins; and the hypothesis that better local control may improve the survival in these patients.

Several reports support the use of radiosurgery in the initial treatment of patients with one or two favorable brain metastases or in those who relapse after whole-brain irradiation. Table 20-15 shows data from the 10 largest SRS series, which consistently show a freedom from progression of around 90% and a median survival of 9 months.[169-178] These survival results are comparable to those observed for surgical resection. There has never been a randomized trial comparing SRS with surgical resection. Multi-institutional retrospective data of SRS for solitary metastasis that come closest to addressing this issue was reported by Auchter et al.[178] A total of 122 patients with solitary brain metastasis were treated to a 37.5-Gy median dose WBRT with SRS boost to 15 to 24 Gy. With a 123-week follow-up, the local control was 86%. The infield recurrence rate was 14% and the intracranial recurrence outside SRS volume was 22%. The median overall and functionally independent

Table 20–15   Ten Large Series with Stereotactic Radiosurgery

Institution	Patients	Lesion	Dose (Gy)	Volume (cc)	FFP (median), %	MST (mo)
Moriarty[176]	353	643	15	2.5	88	10.5
Goodman[173]	258	682	18.5	1.7	82	9.1
Kihlstrom[175]	236	311	20	NR	91	7
Gerosa[172]	225	343	21	5.7	88	9.2
Joseph[174]	190	431	20	2.8	86	7.8
Pirzkall[177]	160	235	27	4.5	94	7.0
Flickinger[170]	157	229	16	3.0	89	10
Fukuoka[171]	130	215	25	5.5	96	8
Chen[169]	122	163	17	2.7	86	12
Auchter[178]	120	189	26	5.3	94	7.4

FFP, freedom from progression; MST, median survival time; NR, not reported.

survival rates were 56 and 44 weeks, respectively, indicating that the SRS is at least equivalent, if not superior to, surgical resection.

Many randomized trials have tried to address the benefit of SRS when given in addition to WBRT. Kondziolka et al. reported a small randomized trial of 27 patients with 2 to 4 metastases to WBRT ± SRS. The median time to local failure was 6 versus 36 months and the median survival was significantly better with the addition of SRS boost (7.5 vs. 11 months).[179] The local failure decreased from 100% to 8% at 1 year with SRS. In the recently completed RTOG 9508 trial, 333 patients with 1 to 3 metastases were randomized to 37.5-Gy WBRT with or without SRS boost.[180] A survival benefit was noted in RPA class I, solitary metastasis, and non–small cell lung cancer patients. Local control at 1 year was 71% with WBRT compared with 82% with the addition of SRS boost. Improved KPS was also noted with the addition of SRS boost (27% vs. 43%) at 6 months.

There is a suggestion that treatment outcome may not be compromised by omitting immediate whole-brain irradiation in patients treated with SRS for limited brain metastasis. Retrospective data by Sneed on 105 patients, 62 of whom were treated with SRS alone, showed an OS of 11-month and 1-year freedom from progression of 75%.[181] Although the brain FFP was lower (28% vs. 69%) with the omission of upfront WBRT, with salvage it was the same (62% vs. 73%), indicating that it could be an option for patients with 1 to 2 metastases. Similar results have been reported from the University of Pittsburgh, the Cleveland Clinic, and the University of Heidelberg.[177,182,183] A word of caution comes from Regine et al., who noted that 70% of patients were symptomatic at the time of recurrence and 60% had neurological deficits. Regine et al. recommended that adjuvant WBRT should be considered a mainstay of treatment in brain metastases.[184]

At MSKCC, we would recommend SRS only for 1 to 2 metastases with WBRT reserved for tumor recurrence or for new brain tumors when the patients have poor performance status and progressive systemic disease. We would repeat SRS for good performance status patients. For those with 3 to 4 metastases, we would recommend WBRT together with SRS boost. WBRT alone would be recommended for patients with progressive systemic disease, poor performance status, and four or more lesions. However, SRS boost may be considered for RPA class I/II patients with four or fewer residual lesions.

Chemotherapy

Brain metastases from breast, small cell and non–small cell lung cancer, and melanoma have been treated with chemotherapy, and various regimens have been used.[185] Response rates of 45% to 55% for metastases arising from carcinoma of the breast, 28% for melanoma, and 30% for small cell and non–small cell lung cancer have been reported. Chemotherapy can be considered in select

patients who progress locally after whole-brain irradiation.[55] Temozolomide has shown promise in the management of brain metastases. In a recently reported phase II trial of 30 Gy WBRT with 6- to 9-Gy boost along with 60 mg/M^2 per day of temozolomide, followed by 6 cycles of the drug at 150 mg/M^2 in 20 patients, 15% showed a complete response, 40% showed a partial response, and 25% had stable disease.[186] In another recently reported phase III trial of WBRT of 30 Gy given in 10 fractions with or without the drug at a dose of 75 mg/M^2 concurrently and then six additional cycles in 134 patients revealed an improved OS (5.6 vs. 7.9 months) and time to treatment progression (6 vs. 7.5 months).[187] The role of temozolomide and SRS alone with salvage therapy, when necessary, needs to be tested in a prospective trial.

CONCLUSION

Over the past decades there have been significant strides in imaging, neurologic techniques, radiation delivery systems, and recognition of prognostic factors in the management of adult brain tumors. Unfortunately, the treatment results have not changed significantly.

It is unlikely that the results of conventional treatment with surgery, radiation, and chemotherapy will dramatically improve the outcome. A better understanding of molecular events in the development of brain tumors has resulted in the use of targeted biologic agents in clinical trials presently under way. Quality of life issues in the management of brain tumors must be recognized. Therapy has to be customized because selective patients benefit from aggressive treatment. Also, there is a need to reduce the toxicities of therapy. Therefore, participation in properly conducted experimental studies remains the best option for patients with brain tumors.

ACKNOWLEDGMENTS

The authors gratefully acknowledge the assistance of Dr. Marc Rosenblum of the Memorial Sloan-Kettering Cancer Center for contributing the pathology photomicrographs used in this chapter and Eve S. Ferdman for carefully reviewing and editing this work.

REFERENCES

1. Jemal A, Murray T, Samuela A, et al: Cancer statistics, 2003. *CA Cancer J Clin.* 2003;53:5.
2. Greig NH, Reis LG, Yancik R, et al: Increasing annual incidence of primary malignant tumors in the elderly. *J Natl Cancer Inst.* 1990;82:1621.
3. Levin VA, Gutin PH, Leibel S: Neoplasms of the central nervous system. In DeVita VT Jr, Hellman S, Rosenberg SA, eds. *Cancer Principles and Practice of Oncology,* 5th ed. Philadelphia: JB Lippincott; 1997:2022.
4. Desmeules M, Mikkelsen T, Mao Y: Increasing incidence of primary malignant brain tumors: Influence of diagnostic models. *J Natl Cancer Inst.* 1992;84:442.
5. Wong AJ, Zoltick PW, Moscatello DK: The molecular biology and molecular genetics of astrocytic neoplasms. *Semin Oncol.* 1994;21:139.

6. van Meyel DJ, Ramsay DA, Casson AG, et al: p53 mutation, expression, and DNA ploidy in evolving gliomas: Evidence of two pathways of progression. *J Natl Cancer Inst.* 1994;86:1011.

7. Bondy M, Wiencke J, Wrensch M, et al: Genetics of primary brain tumors: A review. *J Neurooncol.* 1994;18:69.

8. Savitz DZ, Ahlbom A: Epidemiologic evidence on cancer in relation to residential and occupational exposures. In Carpenter DO, ed. *Biologic Effects of Electric and Magnetic Fields.* New York: Academic Press; 1994:233.

9. Bernstein M, Laperriere N: Radiation-induced tumors of the nervous system. In Gutin PH, Leibel SA, Sheline GE, eds. *Radiation Injury to the Nervous System.* New York: Raven Press; 1991:455.

10. Kornblith PL, Walker MD, Cassidy JR: Neoplasms of the central nervous system. In DeVita VT Jr., Hellman S, Rosenberg SA, eds. *Cancer Principles and Practice of Oncology.* 2nd ed. Philadelphia: JB Lippincott; 1985:1437.

11. Meschan I: *An Atlas of Anatomy Basic to Radiology.* Philadelphia: WB Saunders; 1975:209.

12. Simpson JR, Horton J, Scott C, et al: Influence of location and extent of surgical resection on survival of patients with glioblastoma multiforme: Results of three consecutive Radiation Therapy Oncology Group (RTOG) clinical trials. *Int J Radiat Oncol Biol Phys.* 1993;26:239.

13. Brumer JM: Neuropathology of malignant gliomas. *Semin Oncol.* 1994;21:126.

14. Rinertz N: "Grading" of gliomas. *Acta Pathol Microbol Scand.* 1950;27:51.

15. Burger PC, Vogel FS, Green SB, et al: Glioblastoma multiforme and anaplastic astrocytoma. Pathologic criteria and prognostic implications. *Cancer.* 1985;56:1106.

16. Kleihues P, Burger PC, Scheithauer BW: *Histological Typing of Tumours of the Central Nervous System.* 2nd ed. Berlin: Springer-Verlag; 1993;11.

17. Daumas-Duport C, Scheithauer B, O'Fallon J, et al: Grading of astrocytomas: A simple and reproducible method. *Cancer.* 1988; 62:2152.

18. Davis RL: Grading of gliomas. In Fields, WS, ed. *Primary Brain Tumors. A Review of Histologic Classification.* New York: Springer-Verlag; 1989:150.

19. Burger PC: Classification, grading and patterns of spread of malignant gliomas. In Apuzzo MLJ, ed. Malignant Cerebral Gliomas. Park Ridge, Ill: American Association of Neurological Surgeons; 1990:3.

20. Coons SW, Johnson PC: Histopathology of astrocytomas: Grading, patterns of spread, and correlation with modern imaging modalities. *Semin Radiat Oncol.* 1991;1:2.21.

21. Barnard RO, Geddes JF: The incidence of multifocal cerebral gliomas. A histologic study of large hemisphere sections. *Cancer.* 1987;60:1519.

22. Byrne TN: Imaging of gliomas. *Semin Oncol.* 1994;21:162.

23. Earnest F IV, Kelly PJ, Scheithauer BW, et al: Cerebral astrocytomas: Histopathologic correlation of MR and CT-contrast enhancement with stereotaxic biopsy. *Radiology.* 1988;166:823.

24. Cairncross JG, Pexman JH, Rathbone MP, et al: Postoperative contrast enhancement in patients with brain tumor. *Ann Neurol.* 1985; 17:570.

25. Cairncross JG, Macdonald DR, Pexman JHW, et al: Steroid-induced CT changes in patients with recurrent malignant glioma. *Neurology.* 1988;38:724.

26. American Academy of Neurology: Therapeutics and technology assessment: Positron emission tomography. *Neurology.* 1991; 41:163.

27. Lorberboym M, Baram J, Feibel M, et al: A prospective evaluation of thallium-201 single photon emission computerized tomography for brain tumor burden. *Int J Radiat Oncol Biol Phys.* 1995; 32:249.

28. Chamberlain MC, Murovic JA, Levin VA: Absence of contrast enhancement on CT brain scans of patients with supratentorial malignant gliomas. *Neurology.* 1988;38:1371.

29. De Stefano N, Caramanos Z, Preul MC, et al: In vivo differentiation of astrocytic brain tumors and isolated demyelinating lesions of the type seen in multiple sclerosis using ^{1}H magnetic resonance spectroscopic imaging. *Ann Neurol.* 1998; 44:273.

30. Pirzkall A, McKnight TR, Graves EE, et al: MR-spectroscopy guided target delineation for high-grade gliomas. *Int J Radiat Oncol Biol Phys.* 2001;50:915.

31. Curran WJ Jr, Scott CB, Horton J, et al: Does extent of surgery influence outcome for astrocytoma with atypical or anaplastic foci (AAF)? A report from three Radiation Therapy Oncology Group (RTOG) clinical trials. *Int J Radiat Oncol Biol Phys.* 1993;26:239.

32. Berger MS: Malignant astrocytomas: Surgical aspects. *Semin Oncol.* 1994;21:172.

33. Kelly PJ: Stereotactic resection and its limitations in glial neoplasms. *Stereotact Funct Neurosurg.* 1992;59:84.

34. Lunsford LD, Coffey RJ: Stereotactic surgery in the diagnosis and treatment of malignant intracranial gliomas. In Apuzzo MLJ, ed. *Malignant Cerebral Gliomas.* Park Ridge, Ill: American Association of Neurological Surgeons;1990:115.

35. Walker MD, Alexander E Jr, Hunt WE, et al: Evaluation of BCNU and/or radiotherapy in the treatment of anaplastic gliomas. *J Neurosurg.* 1978;49:333.

36. Walker MD, Green SB, Byar DP, et al: Randomized comparisons of radiotherapy and nitrosoureas for the treatment of malignant glioma after surgery. *N Engl J Med.* 1980;303:1323.

37. Kristiansen K, Hagen S, Kollevold T, et al: Combined modality therapy of operated astrocytomas grade III and IV. Confirmation of the value of postoperative irradiation and lack of potentiation of bleomycin on survival time: A prospective multicenter trial of the Scandinavian Glioblastoma Study Group. *Cancer.* 1981;47:649.

38. Fine HA, Dear KGB, Loeffler JS, et al: Meta-analysis of radiation therapy with and without adjuvant chemotherapy for malignant gliomas in adults. *Cancer.* 1993;71:2585.

39. Lesser GJ, Grossman S: The chemotherapy of high-grade astrocytomas. *Semin Oncol.* 1994;21:220.

40. Levin VA, Silver P, Hannigan J, et al: Superiority of post radiotherapy adjuvant chemotherapy with CCNU, procarbazine and vincristine (PCV) over BCNU for anaplastic gliomas: NCOG 6G61 final report. *Int J Radiat Oncol Biol Phys.* 1990;18:321.

41. Prados MD, Scott C, Curran WJ Jr, et al: Procarbazine, lomustine, and vincristine (PCV) chemotherapy for anaplastic astrocytoma: A retrospective review of radiation therapy oncology group protocols comparing survival with carmustine or PCV adjuvant chemotherapy. *J Clin Oncol.* 1999;17:3389.

42. Medical Research Council Brain Tumor Working Party. Randomized trial of procarbazine, lomustine, and vincristine in the adjuvant treatment of high grade astrocytoma: A medical research council trial. *J Clin Oncol.* 2001;19;509.

43. Seifenheld WF, Mehta MP, Del Rowe J, et al: Five years of glioblastoma (GBM) phase II trials at the radiation therapy oncology group (RTOG). *Proceedings of ASCO.* 2002;21:71a.

44. Macdonald DR: Temozolomide for recurrent high-grade glioma. *Semin Oncol.* 2001;28(4 suppl 13):3.

45. Yung WK, Albright RE, Olsen J, et al: A phase II study of temozolomide vs. procarbazine in patients with glioblastoma multiforme at first relapse. *Br J Cancer.* 2000;83:588.

46. Stupp R, Dietrich PY, Ostermann Kraljevic SO, et al: Promising survival for patients with newly diagnosed glioblastoma multiforme treated with concomitant radiation plus temozolomide followed by adjuvant temozolomide. *J Clin Oncol.* 2002;20:1375.

47. Ambrad AA, Stea B, Martinez J, et al: ZD1839 ("Iressa") an EGFT tyrosine kinase inhibitor radiosensitizes glioblastoma multiforme by inhibition of a cell survival pathway. *Int J Radiat Oncol Biol Phys.* 2002;54(suppl):95. Abstract.

48. Hochberg PH, Pruitt A: Assumptions in the radiotherapy of glioblastomas. *Neurology.* 1980;30:907.

49. Wallner KE: Radiation therapy treatment planning for malignant astrocytomas. *Semin Radiat Oncol.* 1991;1:17.

50. Thornton AF Jr, Sandler HM, Ten Haken RK, et al: The clinical utility of magnetic resonance imaging in 3-dimensional treatment planning of brain neoplasms. *Int J Radiat Oncol Biol Phys.* 1992;24:767.

51. Nelson DF, Curran WJ Jr., Scott C, et al: Hyperfractionated radiation therapy and bis-chlorethyl nitrosourea in the treatment of malignant glioma—Possible advantage observed at 72 Gy on 1.2 Gy b.i.d. fractions: Report of the Radiation Therapy Oncology Group protocol 8302. *Int J Radiat Oncol Biol Phys.* 1993;25:193.

52. Hunt MA, Zelefsky MJ, Wolden S, et al: Treatment planning and delivery of intensity-modulated radiation therapy for primary nasopharynx cancer. *Int J Radiat Oncol Biol Phys.* 2001;49:623.

53. Huang E, Teh BS, Strother DR, et al: Intensity-modulated radiation therapy for pediatric medulloblastoma: Early report on the reduction of ototoxicity. *Int J Radiat Oncol Biol Phys.* 2002;52:599.

54. Shaw EG, Stieber V, Tatter S, et al: A Phase I dose escalating study of intensity modulated radiation therapy (IMRT) for the treatment of glioblastoma multiforme (GBM). *Int J Radiat Oncol Biol Phys.* 2002;54:206. Abstract.

55. Posner JB: *Neurologic Complications of Cancer.* Philadelphia: FA Davis; 1995:37,77,311.

56. Leibel SA, Sheline GE: Tolerance of the central and peripheral nervous system in therapeutic irradiation. In Lett JT, Altman KI, eds. *Advances in Radiation Biology.* New York: Academic Press; 1987:257.

57. Sheline GE, Wara WM, Smith V: Therapeutic irradiation and brain injury. *Int J Radiat Oncol Biol Phys.* 1980;6:1215.

58. Soffietti R, Sciolla R, Giordana MT, et al: Delayed adverse effects after irradiation of gliomas: Clinicopathological analysis. *J Neuroncol.* 1985;3:187.

59. Gutin PH: Treatment of radiation necrosis of the brain. In Gutin PH, Leibel SA, Sheline GE, eds. *Radiation Injury to the Nervous System.* New York: Raven Press; 1991:271.

60. Marks JE, Baglan RJ, Prassad SC, et al: Cerebral radionecrosis: Incidence and risk in relation to dose time, fractionation and volume. *Int J Radiat Oncol Biol Phys.* 1981;7:243.

61. Curran WJ, Hecht-Leavitt C, Schut L, et al: Magnetic resonance imaging of cranial radiation lesions. *Int J Radiat Oncol Biol Phys.* 1987;13:1093.

62. Roman DD, Sperduto PW: Neuropsychological effects of cranial radiation: Current knowledge and future directions. *Int J Radiat Oncol Biol Phys.* 1995;31:983.

63. Kleinberg L, Wallner K, Malkin MG: Good performance status of long-term disease-free survivors of intracranial gliomas. *Int J Radiat Oncol Biol Phys.* 1993;26:129.

64. Hochberg FH, Slotnick B: Neuropsychologic impairment in astrocytoma survivors. *Neurology.* 1980;30:172.

65. Shapiro WR, Young DF: Treatment of malignant glioma. A controlled study of chemotherapy and irradiation. *Arch Neurol.* 1976;33:494.

66. Kita M, Okawa T, Tanka M, et al: Radiotherapy of malignant glioma-prospective randomized clinical study of whole brain vs. local irradiation [in Japanese]. *Gan No Rinsho.* 1989;35:1289.

67. Bleehen NM, Stenning SP: A Medical Research Council trial of two radiotherapy doses in the treatment of grades 3 and 4 astrocytoma. The Medical Research Council Brain Tumor Working Party. *Br J Cancer.* 1991;64:769.

68. Nelson DF, Diener-West M, Horton J, et al: Combined modality approach to treatment of malignant gliomas—Re-evaluation of RTOG 7401/ECOG 1374 with long-term follow-up: A joint study of the Radiation Therapy Oncology Group and the Eastern Cooperative Oncology Group. *NCI Monogr.* 1988;6:279.

69. Lee SW, Fraass BA, Marsh LH, et al: Patterns of failure following high-dose 3-D conformal radiotherapy for high-grade astrocytomas: A quantitative dosimetric study. *Int J Radiat Oncol Biol Phys.* 1999;43:79.

70. Chan JL, Lee SW, Fraass BA, et al: Survival and failure pattern of high-grade gliomas after three-dimensional conformal radiotherapy. *J Clin Oncol.* 2002;20:1635.

71. Deutsch M, Green SB, Strike TA, et al: Results of a randomized trial comparing BCNU plus radiotherapy, streptozotocin plus radiotherapy, BCNU plus hyperfractionated radiotherapy, and BCNU following misonidazole plus radiotherapy in the postoperative treatment of malignant glioma. *Int J Radiat Oncol Biol Phys.* 1989;16:1389.

72. Nelson DF, Diener-West M, Weinstein AS, et al: A randomized comparison of misonidazole sensitized radiotherapy plus BCNU and radiotherapy plus BCNU for treatment of malignant glioma after surgery: Final report of an RTOG study. *Int J Radiat Oncol Biol Phys.* 1986;12:1793.

73. Prados MD, Wara WM, Sneed PK, et al: Phase III trial of accelerated hyperfractionation with or without difluromethylornithine (DFMO) versus standard fractionated radiotherapy with or without DFMO for newly diagnosed patients with glioblastoma multiforme. *Int J Radiat Oncol Biol Phys.* 2001;49:71.

74. Kleinberg L, Grossman SA, Carson K, et al: Survival of patients with newly diagnosed glioblastoma multiforme treated with RSR13 and radiotherapy: Results of a phase II new approaches to brain tumor therapy CNS Consortium Safety and Efficacy Study. *J Clin Oncol.* 2002;20:3149.

75. Phillips TL, Levin VA, Ahn DK, et al: Evaluation of bromodeoxyuridine in glioblastoma multiforme: A Northern California Cancer Center phase II study. *Int J Radiat Oncol Biol Phys.* 1991;21:709.

76. Prados MD, Scott C, Sandler H, et al: A Phase 3 randomized study of radiotherapy plus procarbazine, CCNU, and vincristine (PCV) with or without BUdR for the treatment of anaplastic astrocytoma: A preliminary report of RTOG 9404. *Int J Radiat Oncol Biol Phys.* 1999;45:1109.

77. Curran WJ, Scott CB, Yunk WKA, et al: No survival benefit of hyperfractionated radiotherapy (RT) to 72 Gy & carmustine versus standard RT & carmustine for malignant glioma patients. Preliminary results of RTOG 90-06. *Proc Am Soc Clin Oncol.* 1996;15:154. Abstract.

78. Horiot JC, van den Bogaert W, Ang KK, et al: European Organization for Research on Treatment of Clinical Trials using radiotherapy with multiple fractions per day. A 1978-1987 survey. *Front Radiat Ther Oncol.* 1988;22:149.

79. Coughlin C, Scott C, Langer C, et al: Phase II, two-arm RTOG trial (94-11) of bischloroethyl-nitrosourea plus accelerated hyperfractionated radiotherapy (64.0 or 70.4 Gy) based on tumor volume (> 20 or < 20 cm(2), respectively) in the treatment of newly-diagnosed radiosurgery-ineligible glioblastoma multiforme patients. *Int J Radiat Oncol Biol Phys.* 2000;48:1351.

80. Brada M, Sharpe G, Rajan B, et al: Modifying radical radiotherapy in high grade gliomas: Shortening the treatment time through acceleration. *Int J Radiat Oncol Biol Phys.* 1999;43:287.

81. Kleinberg L, Grossman SA, Piantadosi S, et al: The effects of sequential versus concurrent chemotherapy and radiotherapy on survival and toxicity in patients with newly diagnosed high-grade astrocytoma. *Int J Radiat Oncol Biol Phys.* 1999;44:535.

82. Green SB, Shapiro WR, Burger PC, et al: A randomized trial of interstitial radiotherapy (RT) for newly diagnosed malignant glioma: Brain Tumor Cooperative Group (BTCG) trial 8701. *Proc Am Soc Clin Oncol.* 1994;13:174. Abstract.

83. Prados MD, Gutin PH, Phillips TL, et al: Highly anaplastic astrocytoma: A review of 357 patients treated between 1977 and 1989. *Int J Radiat Oncol Biol Phys.* 1992;23:3.

84. Laperriere NJ, Leung PM, McKenzie S, et al: Randomized study of brachytherapy in the initial management of patients with malignant astrocytoma. *Int J Radiat Oncol Biol Phys.* 1998;41:1005.

85. Kondziolka D, Flickinger JC, Bissonette DJ, et al: Survival benefit of stereotactic radiosurgery for patients with malignant glial neoplasms. *Neurosurgery.* 1997;41:776.

86. McDermott MW, Sneed PK, Chang SM, et al: Results of radiosurgery for recurrent gliomas. In Kondziolka D, ed. *Radiosurgery 1995.* Vol 1. Basel, Switzerland: Karger; 1996:107.

87. Nwokedi EC, DiBiase SJ, Jabbour S, et al: Gamma knife stereotactic radiosurgery for patients with glioblastoma multiforme. *Neurosurgery.* 2002;50:41.

88. Sarkaria JN, Mehta MP, Loeffler JS, et al: Radiosurgery in the initial management of malignant gliomas; survival comparison with the RTOG recursive partitioning analysis. *Int J Radiat Oncol Biol Phys.* 1995;32:931.

89. Souhami L, Scott C, Brachman D, et al: Randomized prospective comparison of stereotactic radiosurgery (SRS) followed by conventional radiotherapy (RT) with BCNU to RT with BCNU alone for selected patients with supratentorial glioblastoma multiforme (GBM): Report of RTOG 93-05 protocol. *Int J Radiat Oncol Biol Phys.* 2002;54:94. Abstract.

90. Chang CH, Horton J, Schoenfeld D, et al: Comparision of postoperative radiotherapy and combined postoperative radiotherapy and chemotherapy in the multidisciplinary management of malignant gliomas. A joint Radiation Therapy Oncology Group and Eastern Cooperative Oncology Group study. *Cancer.* 1983;52:997.

91. Groves MD, Puduvalli VK, Hess KR, et al: Phase II trial of temozolomide plus the matrix metalloproteinase inhibitor, marimastat, in recurrent and progressive glioblastoma multiforme. *J Clin Oncol.* 2002;20:1383.

92. *Reardon DA, Akabani G, Coleman RE, et al: Phase II trial of murine (131)I-labeled antitenascin monoclonal antibody 81C6 administered into surgically created resection cavities of patients with newly diagnosed malignant gliomas. *J Clin Oncol.* 2002; 20:1389.

93. Shaw EG, Scheithauer BW, O'Fallon JR: Management of supratentorial low-grade gliomas. *Semin Radiat Oncol.* 1991;1:123.

94. Laperriere N, Zuraw L, Cairncross G, et al: Radiotherapy for newly diagnosed malignant glioma in adults: A systematic review. *Radiother Oncol.* 2002;64:259.

95. Hoshino T, Ahn D, Prados MD, et al: Prognostic significance of the proliferative potential of intracranial gliomas measured by bromodeoxyuridine labeling. *Int J Cancer.* 1993;53:550.

96. Bauman G, Lote K, Larson D, et al: Pretreatment factors predict overall survival for patients with low-grade glioma: A recursive partitioning analysis. *Int J Radiat Oncol Biol Phys.* 1999;45:923.

97. Vertosick FT Jr, Selker RG, Arena VC: Survival of patients with well-differentiated astrocytomas diagnosed in the era of computed tomography. *Neurosurgery.* 1991;28:496.

98. MacDonald DR: Low grade gliomas, mixed gliomas, and oligodendrogliomas. *Semin Oncol.* 1994;21:236.

99. Forsyth PA, Shaw EG, Scheithauer BW, et al: Supratentorial pilocytic astrocytomas. A clinicopathologic, prognostic and flow cytometric study of 51 patients. *Cancer.* 1993;72:1335.

100. Philippon JH, Clemenceau SH, Fauchon FH, et al: Supratentorial low-grade astrocytoma in adults. *Neurosurgery.* 1993;32:554.

101. Eyre HJ, Crowley JJ, Townsend JJ, et al: A randomized trial of radiotherapy versus radiotherapy plus CCNU for incompletely resected low-grade gliomas: A Southwest Oncology Group study. *J Neurosurg.* 1993;78:909.

102. Shapiro WR: Low-grade gliomas: When to treat? *Ann Neurol.* 1993;2;31:437. Editorial.

103. Shaw EG, Daumas-Duport C, Scheithauer BW, et al: Radiation therapy in the management of low-grade supertentorial astrocytomas. *J Neurosurg.* 1989;70:783.

104. Whitton AC, Bloom HJ: Low-grade glioma of the cerebral hemispheres in adults: A retrospective analysis of 88 cases. *Int J Radiat Oncol Biol Phys.* 1990;18:783.

105. Berger MS, Deliganis AV, Dobbins J, et al: The effect of extent of resection on recurrence in patients with low-grade cerebral hemisphere gliomas. *Cancer.* 1994;74:1784.

106. Cairncross JG, Laperriere NJ: Low-grade glioma: To treat or not to treat? *Arch Neurol.* 1989;46:1238.

107. Karim AB, Afra D, Cornu P: Randomized trial on the efficacy of radiotherapy for central low-grade glioma in the adult: EORTC Study 22845 with the MRC Study BR04: An interim analysis. *Int J Radiat Oncol Biol Phys.* 2002;52:316.

108. Levin VA, Prados MR, Wara WM, et al: Radiation therapy and bromodeoxyuridine chemotherapy followed by procarbazine, lomustine, and vincristine for the treatment of anaplastic gliomas. *Int J Radiat Oncol Biol Phys.* 1995; 32:75.

109. Karim AB, Maat B, Hatlevoll R, et al: A randomized trial on dose response in radiation therapy of low-grade glioma: European Organization for Research and Treatment of Cancer (EORTC) Study 22844. *Int J Radiat Oncol Biol Phys.* 1996;36:549.

110. Shaw E, Arusell R, Scheithauer B, et al: Prospective randomized trial of low- versus high-dose radiation therapy in adults with supratentorial low-grade glioma: Initial report of a North Central Group/Eastern Cooperative Oncology Group Study. *J Clin Oncol.* 2002;20:2267.

111. Reifenberger J, Reifenberger G, Liu L, et al: Molecular genetic analysis of oligodendroglial tumors show preferential allelic deletions on 19q and 1p. *Am J Pathol.* 1994;145:1175.

112. Buger PC, Rawling C, Cox ED, et al: Clinicopathologic correlations in the oligodendroglioma. *Cancer.* 1987;59:1345.

113. Shaw EG, Scheithauer BW, O'Fallon JR: Astrocytomas (A), oligoastrocytomas (OA), and oligodendrogliomas (O): A comparative survival study. *Neurology.* 1992;42(suppl 3):342. Abstract.

114. Harsh GR IV, Wilson CB: Neuroepithelial tumors of the adult brain. In Youmans JR, ed. *Neurological Surgery.* 3rd ed. Philadelphia: WB Saunders; 1990:3040.

115. Sun ZM, Genka S, Shitara N, et al: Factors possibly influencing the prognosis of oligodendroglioma. *Neurosurgery.* 1992;76:428.

116. Ludwig CL, Smith MT, Godfrey AD, et al: A clinicopathological study of 323 patients with oligodendrogliomas. *Ann Neurol.* 1986;19:15.

117. Cairncross JG, Ueki K, Zlatescu MC, et al: Specific genetic predictors of chemotherapeutic response and survival in patients with anaplastic oligodendrogliomas. *J Natl Cancer Inst.* 1998; 90:1473.

118. Bauman GS, Ino Y, Ueki K, et al: Allelic loss of chromosome 1p and radiotherapy plus chemotherapy in patients with oligodendrogliomas. *Int J Radiat Oncol Biol Phys.* 2000;48:825.

119. Lindegaard K-F, Mark SJ, Eide GE, et al: Statistical analysis of clinicopathological features, radiotherapy, and survival in 170 cases of oligodendroglioma. *J Neurosurg.* 1987;67:224.

120. Gannett DE, Wisbeck WM, Silbergeld DL, et al: The role of postoperative irradiation in the treatment of oligodendroglioma. *Int J Radiat Oncol Biol Phys.* 1994;30:567.

121. Bullard DE, Rawling CE III, Phillips B, et al: Oligodendroglioma. An analysis of the value of radiation therapy. *Cancer.* 1987; 60:2179.

122. Winger MJ, MacDonald DR, Cairncross JG: Supratentorial anaplastic gliomas in adults: The prognostic importance of extent of resection and prior low-grade glioma. *J Neurosurg.* 1989;71:487.

123. Zimmerman HN: Malignant lymphomas of the central nervous system. *Acta Neuropathol.* (Berlin). 1975;6(suppl):69.

124. Jellinger KA, Paulus W: Primary central nervous system lymphomas—New pathological developments. *J Neurooncol.* 1995;24:33.

125. DeAngelis LM: Current management of primary central nervous system lymphoma. *Oncology.* 1995;9:63.

126. Peterson K, Gordon KB, Heinenmann MH, et al: The clinical spectrum of ocular lymphoma. *Cancer.* 1993;72:843.

127. Tomlinson PH, Kurtin PJ, Suman VJ, et al: Primary intracerebral lymphomas: A clinicopathological study. *J Neurosurg.* 1985; 82:558.

128. Nelson DF, Martz KL, Bonner H, et al: Non-Hodgkin's lymphoma of the brain: Can high dose, large volume radiation therapy improve survival? Report on a prospective by the Radiation Therapy Oncology Group (RTOG): RTOG 8315. *Int J Radiat Oncol Biol Phys.* 1992;23:9.

129. DeAngelis LM, Yahalom J, Thaler HT, et al: Combined modality therapy for primary CNS lymphoma. *J Clin Oncol.* 1992;10:635.

130. Glass J, Gruber ML, Cher L, et al: Preirradiation methotrexate chemotherapy of primary central nervous system lymphoma: long-term outcome. *J Neurosurg.* 1994;81:188.

131. Neuwelt EA, Goldman DL, Dahlborg SA, et al: Primary CNS lymphoma treated with osmotic blood-brain barrier disruption: Prolonged survival and preservation of cognitive function. *J Clin Oncol.* 1991;9:1580.

132. DeAngelis LM, Seiferheld W, Schold SC, et al: Combination chemotherapy and radiotherapy for primary central nervous system lymphoma: Radiation Therapy Oncology Group Study 93-10. *J Clin Oncol.* 2002;20:4643.

133. Shrieve DC, Wara WM, Edwards MS, et al: Hyperfractionated radiation therapy for gliomas of the brainstem in children and in adults. *Int J Radiat Oncol Biol Phys.* 1992;24:599.

134. Prados MD, Wara WM, Edwards MS, et al: The treatment of brain stem and thalamic gliomas with 78 Gy of hyperfractionated radiation therapy. *Int J Radiat Oncol Biol Phys.* 1995; 32:85.

135. Mandell LR, Kadota R, Freeman C, et al: There is no role for hyperfractionated radiotherapy in the management of children with newly diagnosed diffuse intrinsic brainstem tumors: Results of a Pediatric Oncology Group phase III trial comparing convention vs. hyperfractionated radiotherapy. *Int J Rad Oncol Biol Phys.* 1999;43:959.

136. Freeman CR, Kepner J, Kun LE, et al: A detrimental effect of a combined chemotherapy-radiotherapy approach in children with diffuse intrinsic brain stem gliomas? *Int J Radiat Oncol Biol Phys.* 2000;47:561.

137. Kricheff II, Becker M, Schneck SA, et al: Intracranial ependymomas. A study of survival in 65 cases treated by surgery and irradiation. *Am J Roentgenol.* 1964;91:167.

138. Leibel SA, Sheline GE: Radiation therapy for neoplasms of the brain. *J Neurosurg.* 1987;66:1.

139. Chin HW, Maruyama Y, Markesbery W, et al: Intracranial ependymoma: Results of radiation therapy at the University of Kentucky. *Cancer.* 1982;49:2276.

140. Marks JE, Adler SI: A comparative study of ependymomas by site of origin. *Int J Radiat Oncol Biol Phys.* 1982;8:37.

141. Paulino AC: The local field in infratentorial ependymoma: Does the entire posterior fossa need to be treated? *Int J Rad Oncol Biol Phys.* 2001;49:757.

142. Vanuytsel L, Brada M: The role of prophylactic spinal irradiation in localized intracranial ependymoma. *Int J Radiat Oncol Biol Phys.* 1991;21:825.

143. Goldwein JW, Leahy JM, Packer RJ, et al: Improved survival in cases of intracranial ependymoma after radiation therapy: Late report and recommendations. *J Neurosurg.* 1983;59:652.

144. Shaw EG, Evans RG, Scheithauer BW, et al: Postoperative radiotherapy of intracranial ependymoma in pediatric and adult patients. *Int J Radiat Oncol Phys.* 1987;13:1457.

145. Read G: The treatment of ependymoma of the brain and spinal canal by radiotherapy: A report of 79 cases. *Clin Radiol.* 1984; 35:163.

146. Abacioglu U, Uzel O, Sengoz M, et al: Medulloblastoma in adults: Treatment results and prognostic factors. *Int J Radiat Oncol Biol Phys.* 2002;54:855.

147. Prados MD, Warnick RE, Wara WM, et al: Medulloblastoma in adults. *Int J Radiat Oncol Biol Phys.* 1994;32:1145.

148. Bloom HJG, Bessell EM: Medulloblastoma in adults: A review of 47 patients treated between 1952 and 1981. *Int J Radiat Oncol Biol Phys.* 1990;18:763.

149. Schofield D, West DC, Anthony DC, et al: Correlation of loss of heterozygosity at chromosome 9q with histological subtype in medulloblastomas. *Am J Pathol.* 1995;146:472.

150. Evans AE, Jenkin RD, Sposto R, et al: The treatment of medulloblastoma. Results of a prospective randomized trial of radiation therapy with and without CCNU, vincristine, and prednisone. *J Neurosurg.* 1990;72:572.

151. Frost PJ, Laperriere HJ, Wong CS, et al: Medulloblastoma in adults. *Int J Radiat Oncol Biol Phys.* 1995;32:951.

152. Sarkar C, Pramanik P, Karak AK, et al: Are childhood and adult medulloblastomas different? A comparative study of clinico-pathological features, proliferation index and apoptotic index. *J Neurooncol.* 2002;59:49.

153. Patchell RA, Tibbs PA, Walsh JW, et al: A randomized trial of surgery in the treatment of single metastases to the brain. *N Engl J Med.* 1990; 322:494.

154. Delattre JY, Krol G, Tahler HT, et al: Distribution of brain metastases. *Arch Neurol.* 1988;45:741.

155. Maiuri F, D'Andrea F, Gallicchio B, et al: Intracranial hemorrhages in metastatic brain tumors. *J Neurosurg Sci.* 1985;29:37.

156. Gaspar L, Scott C, Rotman M, et al: Recursive portioning analysis (RPA) of prognostic factors in three Radiation Therapy Oncology Group (RTOG) brain metastases trials. *Int J Radiat Oncol Biol Phys.* 1997;37:745.

157. Cairncross JG, Kim J-H, Posner JB: Radiation therapy for brain metastases. *Ann Neurol.* 1980;7:529.

158. Moser R, Johnson M: Surgical management of brain metastases: How aggressive should we be? *Oncology.* 1989;3:123.

159. Coia LR: The role of radiation therapy in the treatment of brain metastases. *Int J Radiat Oncol Biol Phys.* 1992;23:229.

160. Borgelt B, Gelbert R, Kramer S, et al: The palliation of brain metastases: Final results of the first two studies of the Radiation Therapy Oncology Group. *Int J Radiat Oncol Biol Phys.* 1980;6:1.

161. Murray KJ, Scott C, Greenberg HM, et al: A randomized phase III study of accelerated hyperfractionation versus standard in patients with unresected brain metastases: A report of the Radiation Therapy Oncology Group (RTOG) 9104. *Int J Radiat Oncol Biol Phys.* 1997;39:571.

162. Komarnicky LT, Phillips TL, Martz K, et al: A randomized phase III protocol for the evaluation of misonidazole combined with radiation in the treatment of patients with brain metastases (RTOG-7916). *Int J Radiat Oncol Biol Phys.* 1991;20:53.

163. Phillips TL, Scott CB, Leibel SA, et al: Results of a randomized comparison of radiotherapy and bromodeoxyuridine with radiotherapy alone for brain metastases; report of RTOG trial 89-05. *Int J Radiat Oncol Biol Phys.* 1995;33:339.

164. Borgelt B, Gerber R, Larson M, et al: Ultra-rapid high dose irradiation scheduled for the palliation of brain metastases: Final results of the first two studies of the Radiation Therapy Oncology Group. *Int J Radiat Oncol Biol Phys.* 1981;7:1633.

165. DeAngelis LM, Delattre JY, Posner JB: Radiation-induced dementia in patients cured of brain metastases. *Neurology.* 1989;39:789.

166. Noordijk EM, Vecht CJ, Haaxma-Reiche H: The choice of treatment of single brain metastasis should be based on extracranial tumor activity and age. *Int J Radiat Oncol Biol Phys.* 1994;29:711.

167. Patchell RA, Tibbs PA, Regine WF, et al: Postoperative radiotherapy in the treatment of single metastases to the brain: A randomized trial. *JAMA.* 1998;280:1485.

168. Cooper JS, Steinfeld AD, Lerch IA: Cerebral metastases: Value of reirradiation in selected patients. *Radiology.* 1990;174:883.

169. Chen JC, Petrovich Z, O'Day S, et al: Stereotactic radiosurgery in the treatment of metastatic disease to the brain. *Neurosurgery.* 2000;47:268.

170. Flickinger JC, Lunsford LD, Somaza S, et al: Radiosurgery: Its role in brain metastasis management. *Neurosurg Clin North Am.* 1996;7:497.

171. Fukuoka S, Seo Y, Takanashi M: Radiosurgery of brain metastases with the Gamma Knife. *Stereotact Funct Neurosurg.* 1996;66:193.

172. Gerosa M, Nicholato A, Severi F, et al: Gamma Knife radiosurgery for intracranial metastases: From local tumor control to increased survival. *Stereotact Funct Neurosurg.* 1996;66:184.

173. Goodman KA, Sneed PK, McDermott MW, et al: Relationship between pattern of enhancement and local control of brain metastases after radiosurgery. *Int J Radiat Oncol Biol Phys.* 2001; 50:139.

174. Joseph J, Adler JR, Cox RS: Linear accelerator-based sterotactic radiosurgery for brain metastases: The influence of number of lesions on survival. *Clin Oncol.* 1996;14:1085.

175. Kihlstrom L, Karlsson B, Lindquist C: Gamma knife surgery for cerebral metastases: Implications for survival based on 16 years experience. *Stereotact Funct Neurosurg.* 1993;61:45.

176. Moriarty TM, Loeffler JS, Black PM: Long term follow-up of patients treated with sterotactic radiosurgery for single or multiple brain metastases. In Kondziolka D, ed: *Radiosurgery 1996.* Vol 1. Basel, Switzerland: Karger: 1996:83.

177. Pirzkall A, Debus J, Lohr F, et al: Radiosurgery alone or in combination with whole brain radiotherapy for brain metastases. *J Clin Oncol.* 1998;16:3563.

178. Auchter RM, Lamond JP, Alexander E., et al: A multiinstitutional outcome and prognostic factor analysis of radiosurgery for resectable single brain metastasis. *Int J Radiat Oncol Biol Phys.* 1996;35:27.

179. Kondziolka D, Patel A, Lunsford LD, et al: Stereotactic radiosurgery plus whole brain radiotherapy versus radiotherapy alone for patients with multiple brain metastases. *Int J Radiat Oncol Biol Phys.* 1999;45:427.

180. Sperduto PW, Scott C, Andrews D, et al: Stereotactic radiosurgery with whole brain radiation therapy improves survival to patients with brain metastases: Report of Radiation Therapy Oncology Group III 95-08 study. *Int J Radiat Oncol Biol Phys.* 2002;54:3. Abstract.

181. Sneed PK, Lamborn KR, Forstner JM, et al: Radiosurgery for brain metastases: is whole brain radiotherapy necessary? *Int J Radiat Oncol Biol Phys.* 1999;43:549.

182. Flickinger JC, Kondziolka D, Lunsford LD, et al: A multi-institutional experience with sterotactic radiosurgery for solitary brain metastases. *Int J Radiat Oncol Biol Phys.* 1994;28:797.

183. Chidel MA, Suh JH, Reddy CA, et al: Application of recursive partitioning analysis and evaluation of the use of whole brain radiation among patients treated with stereotactic radiosurgery for newly diagnosed brain metastases. *Int J Radiat Oncol Biol Phys.* 2000;47:993.

184. Regine WF, Huhn JL, Patchell RA, et al: Risk of symptomatic brain tumor recurrence and neurologic deficit after radiosurgery alone in patients with newly diagnosed brain metastases: results and implications. *Int J Radiat Oncol Biol Phys.* 2002;52:333.

185. Hoang-Xuan K, Delattre J-Y: Treatment of brain metastases. In Hildebrand J, ed: *Management in Neuro-Oncology.* European School of Oncology Monographs. Berlin: Springer-Verlag; 1992:23.

186. Dardougas C, Milladou A, Skarleas C: Concomitant temozolomide (TMZ) and radiotherapy (RT) followed by adjuvant with temozolomide in patients with brain metastases from solid tumors. *Proc Am Soc Clin Oncol.* 2001;20:75b. Abstract 2048.

187. Antonadou D, Coliarakis N, Paraskevaidis M, et al: Whole brain radiotherapy alone or in combination with temozolomide for brain metastases. A phase III study. *Int J Radiat Oncol Biol Phys.* 2002;54(2 suppl):93.

Meningeal Tumors

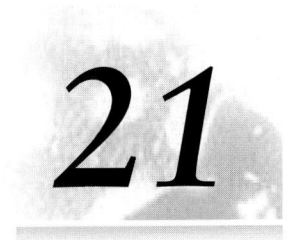

Brian J. Goldsmith, MD

EPIDEMIOLOGY

Meningiomas make up approximately 20% of all primary intracranial tumors.[1,2] Reported incidence rates are between 1 and 5 per 100,000,[2-10] with the range of values perhaps reflecting differences in study design and population exposure to etiologic risk factors. The Central Brain Tumor Registry of the United States estimates approximately 8600 new cases of meningioma in the United States in 2002.[2] Most meningiomas are grossly unifocal. In computed tomography (CT) era series, multiple synchronous lesions are seen in 40% or fewer of cases,[11-16] with the majority of authors reporting multiplicity rates of between 5% and 9%.[12-15] Intracranial sites for meningioma are listed in order of incidence in Table 21-1. Metastases are extremely rare.[17,18] The female/male ratio is approximately 2:1 for all meningiomas,[1,7,8] and 1:1 for anaplastic meningiomas.[19] The incidence of benign meningioma increases with age, with a peak in the seventh decade of life. The incidence of anaplastic meningioma rises to a plateau in the third decade, where it remains relatively constant thereafter.[19] Patients with benign and anaplastic meningioma present at a mean age of 58 ± 15 years (standard error of the mean), and 57 ±

14 years, respectively.[19] In the pediatric population, meningiomas are less common, constituting 1% to 4% of all intracranial tumors. There is no female preponderance as seen with adult meningiomas, and there is a common (24%) association with neurofibromatosis.[20,21]

Factors considered for possible causal relationship with meningioma have included ionizing radiation, trauma, viral infection, and sex hormones,[22-27] and of these only ionizing radiation has been clearly identified as an etiologic agent. In addition, associations between meningioma and type 2 neurofibromatosis, and between meningioma and breast cancer, have been recognized.

Ionizing Radiation

Several case reports have identified intracranial meningioma in patients with a history of previous scalp irradiation for tinea capitis,[28-30] suggesting an etiologic role. From 1910 to 1959, an estimated 20,000 children in the United States and 200,000 worldwide received such treatments.[31] Ron and associates[32] compared the incidence of meningioma in a cohort of 10,834 children treated with ionizing radiation in Israel for tinea capitis with that of a nonirradiated control group. With an estimated 1.5 Gy delivered to the brain surface, the relative risk (RR) was 9.5 times that of the control group (95% confidence interval [CI], 3.5 to 25.7). The mean interval between irradiation and diagnosis with meningioma was 20 years. Rubinstein and associates[33] retrospectively analyzed 201 patients with intracranial meningioma, 43 of whom had received childhood radiation for tinea capitis, and identified several distinctive clinical and histological features in the irradiated subgroup. A statistically significant ($P < 0.001$) difference in location was seen favoring falx cerebri, parasagittal, or convexity regions in the irradiated group, corresponding to the site of scalp treatment. Presentation with seizures was more common in the irradiated group ($P < 0.005$), perhaps reflecting the predominantly supratentorial location of the tumors. Histologically, the radiation-associated meningiomas (RAM) had a significantly higher incidence of (1) high cellularity, (2) pleomorphic nuclei, and (3) numerous giant cells ($P < 0.001$). Following resection, recurrence

Table 21–1   Intracranial Sites of Meningioma

Site	Incidence, %
Cerebral convexity	34
Parasagittal	22
Sphenoid ridge	17
Lateral ventricle	5
Cerebellar convexity	5
Tentorium	4
Tuberculum sellae/parasellar	3
Olfactory groove	3
Intraorbital	2
Cerebellopontine angle	2
Foramen magnum	1
Clivus	1
Other	1

Data from Rohringer M, Sutherland GR, Louw DF, et al: Incidence and clinicopathologic features of meningioma. *J Neurosurg.* 1989;71:665.

rates were 25% versus 11% ($P < 0.05$) in the RAM and non-RAM groups, respectively.[33] In a recent comparison between 16 RAM and 17 non-RAM tumors, Rienstein et al.[34] found no significant differences in the number of genetic changes and the extent and frequency of chromosomes 1 and 22 losses, suggesting similar molecular pathways for tumorigenesis, regardless of radiation exposure (see Type 2 Neurofibromatosis and Chromosome 22 later).

Trauma

Head trauma, hypothesized by some to promote tumorigenesis during the increased mitotic activity of the reparative process, has not been convincingly shown to cause meningioma. In a recent multicenter study of 330 meningioma cases matched to 1132 controls, Preston-Martin and colleagues[27] found no statistically significant relationship between trauma and meningioma—results that refute the authors'[25,26,35] earlier observations in Los Angeles County. No increased incidence of meningioma was found in a Mayo Clinic review of 3587 residents of Olmstead County who sustained head trauma between 1935 and 1974 associated with loss of consciousness, amnesia, or skull fracture,[36] and a case-control study from Schlehofer and colleagues[37] actually found a history of head trauma protective, with an RR of 0.5.

Viral Infection

Viral antigen and DNA have been found in meningioma by several investigators.[38,39] It has been hypothesized that infection with papovavirus may promote meningioma by causing the loss of a tumor suppressor gene on chromosome 22.[40,41] However, the etiologic role of viral infection has not yet been examined epidemiologically.

Sex Hormones

Several clinical findings suggest a possible biologic role of female sex hormones in the etiology and regulation of growth of meningiomas: (1) the incidence in women is twice that of men[1,7,8]; (2) the RR of developing meningioma after breast cancer diagnosis is significantly elevated (1.75; 95% CI, 1.08 to 2.68)[42]; (3) the RR of developing breast cancer between the ages of 50 and 64 after meningioma diagnosis is significantly elevated (1.92; 95% CI, 1.02 to 3.29)[42]; (4) there is a reported relationship between pregnancy and increased rate of progression of symptoms in patients with meningioma[43]; and (5) approximately three quarters of meningiomas are progesterone receptor positive.[44-49] However, epidemiologic evidence to date is limited, conflicting, and does not confirm a causal relation between sex hormones and meningioma. Schlehofer and coworkers[50] found no relation between parity and incidence of meningioma, but found a reduced risk associated with a premenopausal bilateral oophorectomy, and Ryan and coworkers[23] showed no relation between risk of meningioma and

parity or history of hysterectomy. A recent phase III trial evaluating the antiprogestin mifepristone (RU486) for the treatment of unresectable meningioma showed no response (unpublished data, presented at the 2001 meeting of the American Society for Clinical Oncology). Future epidemiologic studies are needed to carefully examine the relation between incidence of meningioma and parity, number of pregnancies, number of births, age at menarche, age at menopause, history of hysterectomy, and oral contraceptive and postmenopausal estrogen use.

Type 2 Neurofibromatosis and Chromosome 22

Losses on 22q are the most frequent genomic alterations observed in meningioma.[51,52] Type 2 neurofibromatosis (bilateral acoustic neurofibromatosis, NF2), characterized cytogenetically by loss of the *NF2* gene from 22q12, is associated with an increased incidence of meningioma.[53] Based on the most common chromosomal aberrations identified in the various grades of meningioma, a model for progression has been proposed by Weber et al.[51] that initiates the clonal expansion from normal meningeal cells to benign World Health Organization (WHO) grade I meningioma with loss on 22q. The model continues with cumulative genetic alterations on other chromosomes in higher grade tumors (loss on 1p, 6q, 10, 14q, 18q, and gain on 1q, 9q, 12q, 15q, 17q, and 20 in atypical WHO grade II; followed by loss on 9p and amplification on 17q in anaplastic WHO grade III).

Breast Cancer

Both the risk of developing meningioma in patients who have had breast cancer and the risk of developing breast cancer in patients who have had meningioma are higher than in the general population.[42] The association may be explained by a hormonal effect or possibly by a shared chromosome 22 abnormality.[54,55]

PATHOLOGY

Meningiomas are thought to arise from arachnoidal cap cells that are found on the outer surface of the arachnoidal membrane between the dura and pia mater. Cells of the arachnoidal membrane uniquely display both mesenchymal and epithelial characteristics, capable of fibro-lipo-chondro-osteoblastic differentiation as well as of well-formed desmosomal connections between tumor cells and other structural and histochemical features usually attributed to epithelial neoplasms. Though the extent meningioma literature is largely based on similar legacy classification systems, most neuro-oncology communities have now adopted the 2000 WHO system[56] to optimize uniformity of communication among institutions. This new system endeavors to predict the likelihood of recurrence and aggressive behavior, primarily on the basis of histologic subtype and grade.

Conventional histologic subtypes, including *meningothelial, fibrous, transitional, psammomatous, angiomatous, microcystic, secretory, lymphoplasmacyterich,* and *metaplastic,* have no apparent prognostic importance.[56] In contrast, four rare variants (each constituting <1% of all meningiomas) have characteristically aggressive behavior:

Clear Cell, composed of sheets of clear, glycogen-rich, polygonal cells forming only a few vague whorls; often with extensive stromal and perivascular hyalinization; frequently deceptively benign appearance with few mitotic figures.[57]

Chordoid, mimic chordoma with lobular, low-power architecture and production of stroma mucosubstances, but with scant reactivity for chordoma-typical epithelial membrane antigen, cytokeratin, and S-100.[58]

Rhabdoid, usually seen in association with conventional histologic subtypes, with increasing prominence with each recurrence; characterized by sheets of loosely cohesive cells with eccentric nuclei and hyaline paranuclear inclusions.[59]

Papillary, seen both as the predominant morphology and in association with one of the conventional histologic subtypes; characterized by a striking papillary pattern with foci of necrosis, numerous mitotic figures, and local invasiveness.[60]

Since the 1993 revision of the WHO classification system,[58] characteristically aggressive hemangiopericytomas and hemangioblastomas have been deemed nonmeningothelial in origin and are no longer classified as meningiomas.

The 2000 WHO grading scheme is based largely on the work of Perry et al.[61]:

Grade I (benign): lacking criteria for grades II (atypical) or III (anaplastic).

Grade II (atypical): Either of the following criteria:

1. High mitotic index (e.g., four or more mitoses per 10 high power fields or 2.5 or more per mm^2)
2. Presence of at least three of the following features:

Hypercellularity
Small cell formation with high nucleus:cytoplasm ratio
Prominent nucleoli
Sheeting architecture
Foci of necrosis

Grade III (anaplastic): Either of the following criteria:
1. Excessive mitotic activity (e.g., 20 or more mitoses per 10 high power fields or 12.5 or more per mm^2)
2. Focal or diffuse loss of meningothelial differentiation at the light microscope level resulting in sarcoma, carcinoma, or melanoma-like appearance

Examples of the different histopathologic types are shown in Figure 21-1. The WHO system does *not* treat brain invasion as a de facto criterion of malignancy and suggests appending the phrase "with brain invasion" to the diagnosis. In contradistinction, Perry et al. recommend classifying otherwise benign-appearing meningiomas with brain invasion as grade II, based on their prognostic similarity.[61] Clear cell and chordoid histologic subtypes

are assigned grade II, and rhabdoid and papillary histologic subtypes are assigned grade III classification, even in the absence of the criteria described previously.

Proliferation indices based on MIB-1 labeling of Ki-67 nuclear protein or PC10 labeling of proliferating cell nuclear antigen (PCNA) are powerful adjuncts that offer additional prognostic information. High indices reflect increased proliferative activity and recurrence potential.[62-67] However, inter-institutional and inter-observer variation presently preclude cutoff levels to distinguish between grades. The 2000 WHO system recommends that a phrase such as "with high proliferative activity" be added to pathology reports if indices are conspicuously higher than expected for the histopathologic grade.

At the time of this chapter's preparation, the 2000 WHO grading scheme has not yet been examined for prognostic use in new radiotherapy studies. However, meningioma grade, as defined by similar legacy systems,[58,68,69] has been established of clear prognostic importance, with atypia and anaplasia associated with more frequent and earlier recurrence.[68-71] For example, postradiotherapy 5-year progression-free survival (PFS) rates of 94% versus 78% for 1993 WHO grade I versus grade II ($P = 0.02$),[70] 95% versus 0% for 1993 WHO grade I versus grade II/III ($P < 0.01$),[71] and 89% versus 49% for University of California San Francisco (UCSF) system benign versus malignant ($P = 0.001$)[68] have been reported.

CLINICAL PRESENTATION AND DIAGNOSTIC EVALUATION

In practice, the radiation oncologist's relationship with the meningioma patient usually begins in the postoperative setting, after a thorough diagnostic evaluation, optimal resection, and confirmation of histologic diagnosis has been undertaken by the neurosurgeon. Evaluation begins with a detailed history and physical examination. Presenting complaints and physical findings, listed in order of frequency, are found in Tables 21-2 and 21-3, respectively. Patients with visual complaints should be evaluated with formal visual field and acuity testing before surgery or radiation therapy. Patients with hearing loss should be tested with formal audiometry.

Pediatric patients with convexity or parasagittal meningiomas often present with seizures, focal deficits, or signs of increased intracranial pressure (ICP), and those with intraventricular lesions typically present with elevated ICP, hemiparesis, and hemianopia. In addition to these typical presenting signs and symptoms, increasing head circumference as a first sign of meningioma is also seen in children.[72]

Adult patients with spinal meningioma most often present with pain (72%), which usually antedates other symptoms by months to years, followed by sensory loss and weakness, followed by bowel and bladder dysfunction.[73] Children with spinal meningioma, unlike adults, most often present with extremity weakness (57%), followed by back pain, bowel and bladder dysfunction, and extremity pain. In children, back and extremity pain may be expressed as increased irritability.[74]

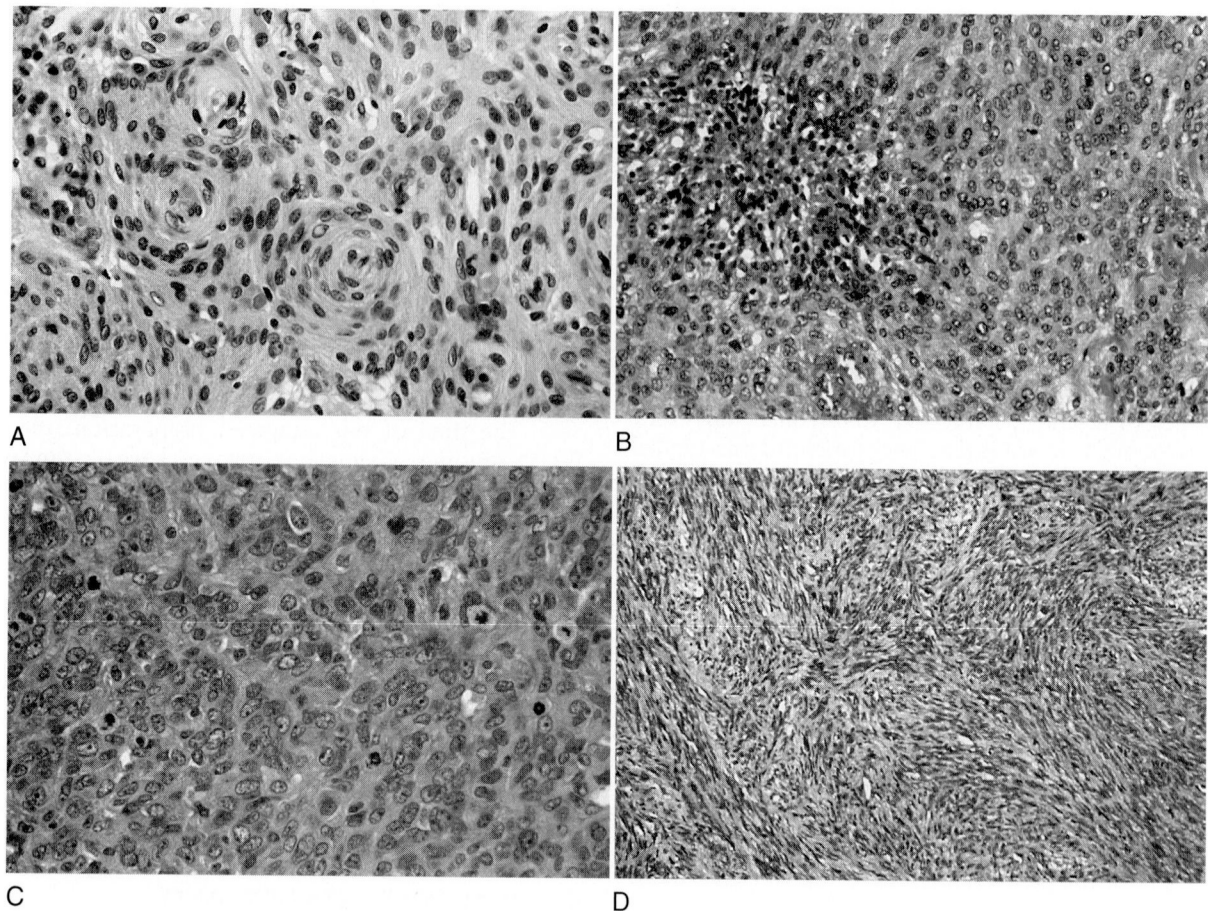

Figure 21–1. A (upper left), Grade I (benign) meningioma. This example exhibits meningothelial whorls and intranuclear pseudoinclusions. There is no mitotic activity. **B (upper right),** Grade II (atypical) meningioma. Focal necrosis (upper left) and isolated mitoses characterize this example. **C (lower left),** Grade III (anaplastic) meningioma. A high mitotic rate and loss of differentiated meningothelial features are evident in this lesion. **D (lower right),** Grade III meningioma. shown here is a fibrosarcoma-like histologic presentation. See also Color Figure 21–1A-D.

CT or magnetic resonance imaging (MRI) with contrast yields information regarding tumor size, location, potential resectability, and proximity to critical neurologic structures. Meningiomas are generally well circumscribed and smooth in contour. Most are homogeneously high density on unenhanced CT scans, 25% to 33% are isodense, about 1% are hypodense, and a few demonstrate mixed attenuation. The majority demonstrate moderate to intense homogeneous enhancement following administration of a contrast agent, with the degree of enhancement dependent on tumor vascularity and extracellular accumulation of the contrast material. Peritumoral edema is seen in 60% of cases, and associated bony changes (destruction or hyperostosis) in 15% to 20%.[75] The degree

Table 21–2 Presenting Complaints

Complaints	Incidence, %
Headache	37
Personality change/confusion	22
Paresis	19
Generalized seizures	19
Visual impairment	16
Focal seizures	15
Ataxia	15
Aphasia	10
Decreasing level of consciousness	7
Paresthesia	6
Diplopia	3
Vertigo	1
Decreased hearing	1

Data from Rohringer M, Sutherland GR, Louw DF, et al: Incidence and clinicopathologic features of meningioma. *J Neurosurg.* 1989;71:665.

Table 21–3 Physical Findings

Finding	Incidence, %
Paresis	30
Non-focal exam	26
Memory deficit	15
Cranial nerve deficit other than CN II	12
Visual field deficit	10
Paresthesia	9
Aphasia	9
Papilledema	8
Decreased visual acuity	6
Altered level of consciousness	5
Nystagmus	3
Decreased hearing	2

Data from Rohringer M, Sutherland GR, Louw DF, et al: Incidence and clinicopathologic features of meningioma. *J Neurosurg.* 1989;71:665.

of preoperative peritumoral edema seen on CT has been reported to correlate positively with the probability of brain invasion.[76]

On magnetic resonance images, meningiomas are typically isointense with gray matter on both T_1- and T_2-weighted images, and intensely enhanced when contrast is used. A radiographic feature that is suggestive of, but not specific for, meningioma is linear meningeal thickening and enhancement adjacent to a peripherally located cranial mass—the so-called "dural tail sign."[75,77] This has been reported in 60% of meningiomas, but has also been seen in chloroma, lymphoma, and sarcoidosis. In the case of meningioma, the enhancement of the dural tail usually represents reactive changes and does not necessarily indicate neoplastic involvement.[78] Collagen-rich fibrous and densely cellular transitional meningiomas are relatively low in tumor water content with resultant typical T_2-weighted hypointensity (seen in 90% of cases). The sparse stroma and high water tumor content of transitional meningiomas and the dilated blood vessels of angiomatous meningiomas render them typically hyperintense on T_2-weighted images (seen in 66% of cases). Although these variations allow for good differentiation between fibrous/transitional and meningothelial/angiomatous histologic findings, further separation between fibrous and transitional, or meningothelial and angiomatous is not possible by T_2 criteria. Although several authors have reported that MRI cannot reliably predict tumor histology,[75,79,80] a report by Kaplan and associates[81] found that the correct conventional histologic subtype could be predicted 96% of the time with a combination of T_2 criteria and adjunctive imaging features, including mass effect, peritumoral edema, and intratumoral cyst formation. Preoperative distinction between conventional subtypes with similar recurrence potential is largely academic, however, since the use of MRI in predicting the relevant, rare, aggressive variants or tumor grade, or both, has not been established.[75,79,80] On magnetic resonance images, intratumoral inhomogeneities are often seen associated with calcifications, central necrosis, pseudocysts, and vascular spaces. Intratumoral hemorrhage is unusual. Displacement of the gray-white interface, peritumoral edema, and adjacent encephalomalacic changes are better seen with MRI than CT, whereas osseous changes and calcification are better seen with CT than MRI.[75,82]

STANDARD THERAPEUTIC APPROACHES

Meningiomas are well managed with total excision, if achievable with acceptable morbidity, resulting in an expected 5-, 10-, and 15-year overall survival (OS) of approximately 85%, 75%, and 70%, and a 5-, 10-, and 15-year PFS of 90%, 80%, and 67%, respectively.[83-87] However, about one in three meningiomas are not fully resectable[85] because of tumor location, size, and proximity to adjacent critical central nervous system CNS and vascular structures. In the skull base, total resection is accomplished about half the time[85,88] and its likelihood correlates inversely with preoperative factors including prior irradiation, vessel encasement, multiple fossa involvement,

and cranial nerve palsies.[88] Subtotal resection alone is inadequate therapy, with inferior 5-, 10-, and 15-year PFS rates of approximately 60%, 45%, and 10%[85,89-93] and cause-specific survival (CSS) rates of 80%, 66%, and 50%,[87] respectively.

Radiotherapy after subtotal resection has been shown to significantly improve both PFS[70,87,89-91] and CSS,[87] with low morbidity.[68-70,90,91,94,95] Adjuvant irradiation, rather than observation, is considered by many[68,87,90,96,97] to be the standard of care for subtotally resected meningiomas.

Patients who are not surgical candidates should be considered for radiotherapy alone, which has been shown to have both palliative efficacy and long-term PFS in the majority of cases.[69,87,94,98,99]

Optimal salvage therapy for unirradiated patients is irradiation, either after re-resection or alone for the inoperable recurrent lesion.[90-92,100]

Radiotherapy experience with pediatric meningiomas is limited and its role is unclear.[20,101] Treatment must be on an individualized and carefully selected basis because of the greater potential for morbidity in the developing child.[102]

Preoperative embolization of highly vascular meningiomas, in selected patients, safely achieves intraoperative hemostasis and facilitates surgical resection,[103-105] and has replaced preoperative radiotherapy in this role.

TECHNIQUES OF CONFORMAL RADIATION THERAPY

Optimal radiation therapy requires meticulous attention to tumor volume as delineated by the neurosurgeon's description, as well as CT and MRI findings. MRI is generally superior to CT, with its exquisite resolution, absence of bone artifact, intense tumor contrast enhancement, and coronal and sagittal viewing advantages. Khoo et al.[82] have compared MRI and CT for radiotherapy treatment planning. They observed that MRI-defined meningioma volumes are larger but not inclusive of CT-defined volumes, suggesting complementary spatial information and a role for composite CT/MRI volumes. Both preoperative and postoperative studies should be used in treatment planning when available. In cases where conformal radiotherapy will be employed without surgery, the planning tumor volume (PTV) consists of the entire gross tumor volume (GTV) plus a margin of 1 cm along dural surfaces for benign WHO grade I lesions, and at least 2 cm for atypical WHO grade II and anaplastic WHO grade III lesions. For infiltrative tumors, a rim of adjacent brain parenchyma should be included. Tighter margins (e.g., 2 mm) for low grade meningiomas[70] are feasible with fractionated stereotactic radiotherapy (see Innovative Therapies later).

In the postoperative setting, the GTV for benign meningioma is the postoperative remnant. For atypical and anaplastic lesions, treatment planning is based on the entire preoperative GTV. The conformal radiotherapy PTV consists of the GTV plus a margin of 1 cm along dural surfaces for benign WHO grade I lesions, and at least 2 cm for atypical WHO grade II and anaplastic WHO grade III lesions.

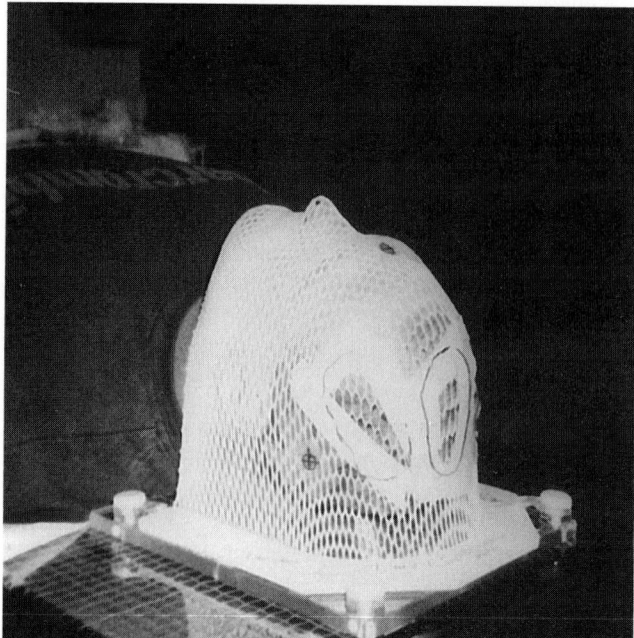

Figure 21–2. Radiotherapy immobilization system.

Excellent precision is achieved by use of an immobilization system, consisting of a head support, a thermoplastic mask that is molded to the patient's head, and a frame that locks the mask and head in a reproducible position (Fig. 21-2). CT and MRI-assisted computerized treatment planning should be used. Treatment-planning scans should be obtained with the patient in the treatment position, wearing the immobilization device with radiopaque fiducials. The use of such careful tumor localization and immobilization techniques has been shown to have greater prognostic importance than tumor size or radiotherapy dose, and has been associated with a 5-year PFS, which is significantly better (98% vs. 77%, P = 0.002) than that achieved without such techniques.[68]

Optic nerve sheath meningiomas require precision conformal therapy, such as described by Eng and colleagues.[106] The patient is positioned supine with the head rotated laterally, so that the affected optic nerve is approximately perpendicular to the horizontal plane. The appropriate angle of lateral head rotation can be estimated from diagnostic CT scans. In the series from Eng's group, this value ranged from 15 to 27 degrees. Neck flexion should establish an imaginary vertical line on the lateral simulation film from the center of the orbit to a point just superior to the pituitary sella. In this position, the patient's head is immobilized with a head support, thermoplastic mask, and locking frame as just described. The treatment-planning CT scan is then obtained with the patient in this position, wearing the immobilization mask. Three small half-beam blocked fields are set up isocentrically with axes lying in the horizontal plane (Fig. 21-3). Treatment table rotation is used to produce a vertex field and two superior-lateral fields. The superior-lateral fields are angled to avoid the contralateral eye and optic nerve. The beams are split perpendicular to the vertical axis and the anterior half is blocked in order to prevent anterior divergence toward the globe.

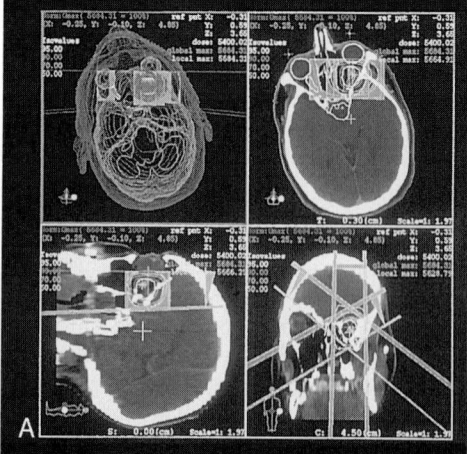

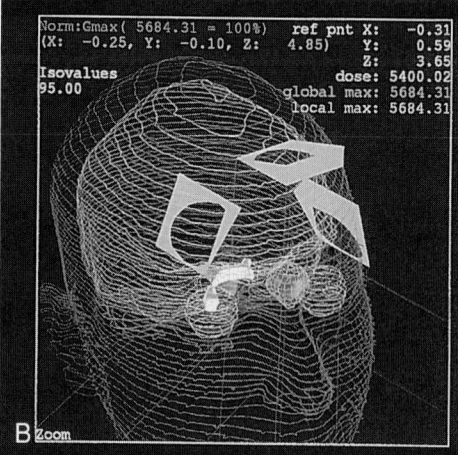

Figure 21–3. Precision conformal therapy technique for optic nerve sheath meningioma, beams, and beam splitter orientation. (Courtesy of Tzvetan Tzvetanov, MS, and Computerized Medical Systems, Inc.)

Differential field weighting is used to optimize the isodose distribution, and the prescribed isodose volume (with 5% or less heterogeneity) should encompass the gross tumor with appropriate margin, based on tumor grade, as described earlier (Fig. 21-4).

For other intracranial sites, multiple static fields or rotational arcs should be selected to minimize dose to the uninvolved CNS tissues. Lateralized lesions are best treated with a wedged-pair technique. Lesions near the midline (particularly parasellar and medial sphenoid lesions) should be approached with either arcs (in a manner similar to that used for the treatment of pituitary adenoma) or three fields (laterals and vertex) (Fig. 21-5). Opposed lateral fields should be avoided in practically all cases to prevent unnecessarily irradiating lateral CNS structures such as the temporal lobes. Careful conformal technique should limit inhomogeneity of dose to less than 10%, and ideally less than 5%. No portion of the optic nerve or chiasm should receive more than 100% of the prescribed dose, and at 1.8 Gy per fraction, its total dose should be kept at or below 54 Gy.[107] A dose of 54 Gy at 1.8 Gy per fraction, 5 days a week, is generally given to benign (WHO grade I) meningiomas, and for atypical and anaplastic (WHO grade II and III) lesions the dose is increased to 59.4 Gy. Dose recommendations are not

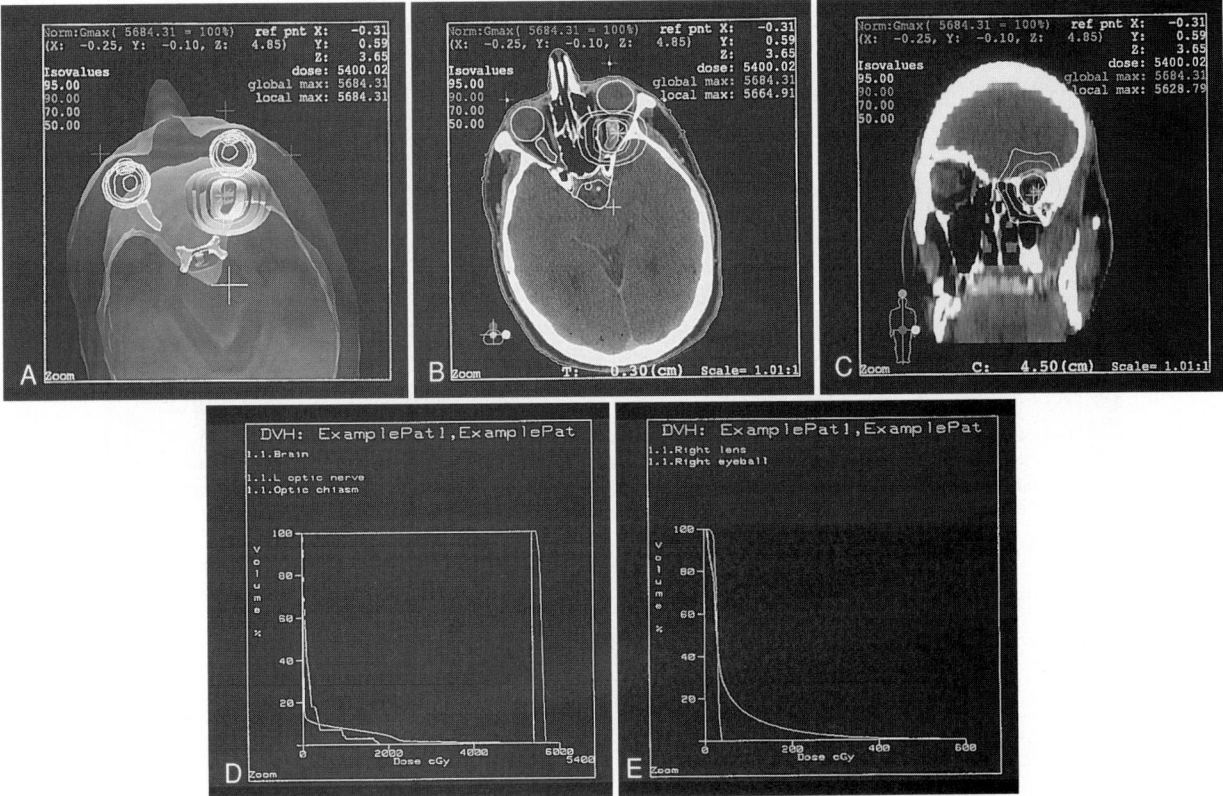

Figure 21–4. Precision conformal therapy technique for optic nerve sheath meningioma, example of 3D isodose plan (A–C), and dose volume histograms (D–E). See also Color Figure 21–4. (Courtesy of Tzvetan Tzvetanov, MS, and Computerized Medical Systems, Inc.)

based upon dose-response analysis, since all large studies have failed to demonstrate a positive correlation on multivariate analysis—likely the result of treatment within a rather narrow dose range (50 to 60 Gy) in most reports. Of note, one exception is the Massachusetts General Hospital (MGH) series,[108] which reported superior local control for atypical and anaplastic tumors treated to doses greater than or equal to 60 cobalt Gy equivalent (*P* = 0.025 and 0.002, respectively, albeit based on only 15 and 13 cases). The selection of 54 Gy for benign (WHO grade I) meningiomas is based on its proven efficacy and low probability of associated complications (see Outcome and Recommendations and Critical Normal Tissues later). Conversely, 59.4 Gy for atypical and anaplastic (WHO grades II and III) lesions is recommended because such tumors are associated with a significantly inferior local control and outcome, and this represents the maximum tolerable conventionally fractionated conformal radiotherapy dose for CNS lesions. Anaplastic lesions may be considered for radiosurgery boost following external beam radiotherapy, if the tumor volume is small.

CRITICAL NORMAL TISSUES: RADIATION INJURY

Common acute toxicities of irradiation for meningioma are, in general, mild and include fatigue, skin erythema, and varying degrees of in-field alopecia (which may be transient or permanent). If the external auditory canal and middle ear are within the irradiated field, an external otitis and serous otitis media are common. Less often seen are acute transient symptoms suggestive of increased intracranial pressure (headache, nausea, vomiting) and exacerbation of preradiation therapy neurologic deficits.[109] Late effects (Table 21-4) are dependent on the region irradiated. Chronic otitis[91] and decreased hearing[70,91,94] have been reported after irradiation of the ear. Retinopathy[68,94,110] and optic neuropathy[68,70,91,107,108,111-113] have been reported following irradiation of the globe and the anterior visual pathway, respectively. Cerebral necrosis[68,69,91,95,108,113] and focal neurologic deficits suggestive of late brain injury have been seen, particularly after doses greater than 60 Gy and dose per fraction greater than 1.8 to 2.0 Gy and with opposed lateral field arrangement.[108,109] Hypopituitarism manifested by hyposecretion of growth hormone, luteinizing hormone, follicle-stimulating hormone, corticotropin, and thyrotropin (in their order of radiosensitivity) is expected after irradiation of the hypothalamic-pituitary axis region and has been reported after radiation therapy for meningioma.[111] Mechanisms of injury and time-dose analyses for radiation injury to the visual apparatus,[107,109,110,112,114] brain,[109,115] and pituitary gland[109,116] are available to the interested reader.

Goldsmith and coworkers[68] reported a crude 3.6% (5 of 140 patients) incidence of radiation complications (see Table 21-4). One of the two patients with cerebral necrosis recovered after decompressive craniotomy and the second died of bronchopneumonia secondary to chronic brain syndrome. As a consequence of the recognition of

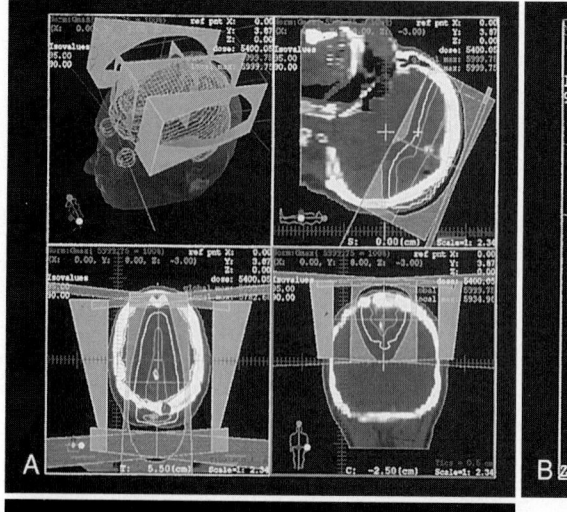
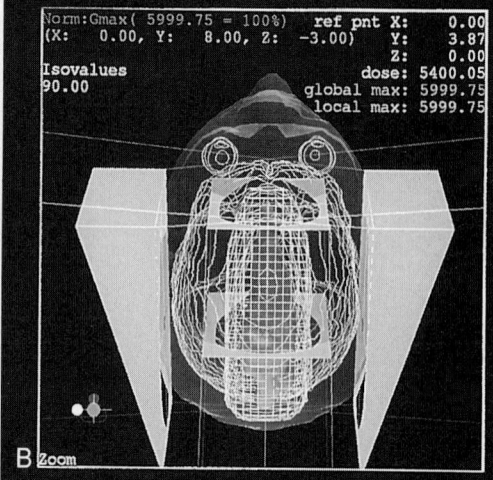
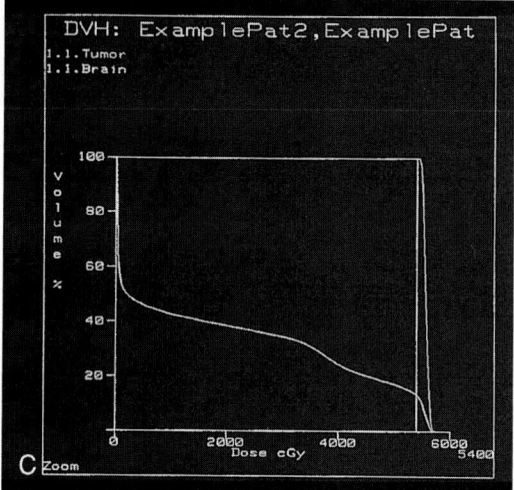

Figure 21–5. Example of three-field 3D isodose plan (A and B) and dose volume histogram (C) for a falx meningioma. See also Color Figure 21–5. (Courtesy of Tzvetan Tzvetanov, MS, and Computerized Medical Systems, Inc.)

these complications and a subsequent analysis of optic neuropathy risk,[107] UCSF has established an institutional policy to avoid using high-dose opposed lateral technique for irradiation of the CNS and to avoid exceeding a maximum dose of 54 Gy to the optic nerve whenever possible.

Glaholm and coworkers[69] reported a crude 2% (4 of 186 patients) incidence of late radiation complications (see Table 21-4). All four patients were treated before 1980, when all fields were generally not treated daily, resulting in higher dose per fraction to the surrounding brain. Of note, in two patients initially irradiated for benign and six for "aggressive benign" meningiomas, the disease recurred with frankly anaplastic meningioma. This transformation to a less differentiated histologic finding, however, is not considered a radiation complication, as it has been reported in 14% to 26% of patients managed with surgery alone.[117]

It is important to emphasize that many of the reported cases of radiotherapy complications are from a treatment era when opposed lateral fields were commonly employed. This technique often unnecessarily irradiated uninvolved CNS tissues, and has been abandoned in practice by most radiation oncologists. The future incidence of complications is expected to decline substantially as modern treatment planning techniques become uniformly applied.

OUTCOME AND RECOMMENDATIONS

Preoperative

Experience with preoperative radiation therapy as a means of achieving intraoperative hemostasis and improving resectability for highly vascular tumors is limited,[100,118,119] and its efficacy has not been clearly established. On the other hand, preoperative embolization experience in this setting has been extensive and favorable.[103-105] Therefore, preoperative radiation therapy should be reserved only for patients with highly vascular meningiomas *and* contraindications for embolization.

Postoperative

Although postoperative radiotherapy for subtotally resected meningioma has never been evaluated in a randomized trial, large institutional retrospective analyses (Table 21-5) from the UCSF and the Royal Marsden Hospital (RMH), as well as several other studies,[71, 87,91,94,98,113,120,121] strongly support its role following subtotal resection.

The UCSF experience with postoperative radiotherapy has been reported and updated.[68,89,100] Barbaro and

Table 21–4   Radiation Toxicity Data

Reference	Crude Rate	Complication	Dose$_{Rx}$, Gy	Dose$_{max}$, Gy
Goldsmith et al.[68]	5/140	Retinopathy	54	27
		Retinopathy	49.23	37
		Optic neuropathy	54	56.7
		Cerebral necrosis	60	66.67
		Cerebral necrosis	55.8	56.7
Glaholm et al.[69]	4/186	Memory deficit	NR	NR
		Memory deficit	NR	NR
		Memory deficit	NR	NR
		Paraplegia	NR	NR
Miralbell et al.[91]	6/36	Chronic otitis	48.7	NR
		Hearing deficit	48.7	NR
		Hearing deficit	52	NR
		Memory deficit	69.6	NR
		Hypogonadism	55.8	NR
		Cerebral necrosis*	71.6†	NR
Forbes and Goldberg[94]	4/31	Retinopathy	NR	NR
		Hearing deficit	NR	NR
		Hearing deficit	NR	NR
		Hearing deficit	NR	NR
Taylor et al.[90]	0/23	None detected	—	—
Yamashita et al.[95]	3/7	CNS necrosis‡	60	NR
		CNS necrosis§	79.8	NR
		Neurologic decline§	60	NR

CNS, central nervous system; Dose$_{max}$, maximum dose delivered to injured structure; Dose$_{Rx}$, prescribed dose; NR, not reported.
*Large recurrent invasive tumor treated with mixed beam photons/protons.
†Dose in cobalt-Gy-equivalent.
‡Recurrent tumor irradiated after three previous operations.
§Recurrent malignant meningioma.

colleagues[89] reported UCSF's 1968-1978 pre-CT, megavoltage (MV) era results. After a mean follow-up period of 78 months, crude recurrence rates were 60% after subtotal resection versus 32% after subtotal resection plus radiation therapy. Five-year actuarial freedom from recurrence was 59% after subtotal resection versus 77% after subtotal resection plus radiation therapy. Median time to recurrence was 66 and 125 months, respectively (P < 0.05). Irradiated patients had more favorable outcomes than the nonirradiated, despite having more surgically unfavorable[85] skull base sites in the irradiated cohort.

Goldsmith et al.[68] have since updated the UCSF subtotal resection plus radiation therapy experience with a review of 140 patients (117 benign, 23 malignant) treated between 1967 and 1990. Patients received a median dose of 54 Gy, conventionally fractionated, via arcs or 2- or 3-field static fields. From 1967 to 1980, tumor volume was defined by the surgeon's description of tumor site and extent. From 1981 to 1990, the volume was based on both radiographic data from CT, MRI, or both and the surgeon's description. In general, benign tumor PTV included the postoperative tumor remnant plus a 1 to 2 cm margin of adjacent tissue. Malignant tumor (as defined by pre-1994 UCSF grading system) PTVs included the preoperative tumor volume plus a 1 to 3 cm margin. Five-year PFS was 89% and 48% for benign and malignant meningiomas, respectively (P = 0.001), and 10-year PFS for benign meningioma was 77%. No malignant tumor was followed for as long as 10 years. Local control of orbital, parasellar, and posterior fossa tumors, notoriously difficult to completely resect and therefore associated with higher recurrence rates in the surgical literature,[85] did not differ significantly from all other sites. For benign meningiomas, multivariate analysis revealed that improved PFS was not associated with tumor size or increasing minimum tumor dose but *was* associated with younger age (P = 0.01) and treatment after 1980 with innovative technologies (P = 0.002). Five-year PFS for patients treated after 1980 (when CT or MRI imaging was used for treatment planning) was 98%, as compared with 77% for patients treated before 1980. No statistically significant parameter predictive of improved outcome was identified for malignant meningioma.

Glaholm and colleagues[69] have reported the treatment of 186 patients between 1963 and 1983 at the RMH. Histologic grade information as defined by the RMH legacy system was available in 171 cases: 117 tumors were benign, 28 were "aggressive benign," 9 were malignant, and 17 were classified as "meningioma" (not otherwise specified). Twenty-three patients were treated after gross total resection because of uncertainty regarding the completeness of the resection or aggressive or malignant histology. Eighty-two were treated after subtotal resection with minimal macroscopic residuum. Forty-six had bulky residual disease. All patients were treated with megavoltage

Table 21–5   Treatment Data for Postoperative Radiation Therapy versus Surgery Alone

Reference	Patients Treated, n		Dose, Gy	Actuarial 5-Year Local Control Rate, %				Actuarial 10-Year Local Control Rate, %			
				Benign		Anaplastic		Benign		Anaplastic	
	STR	STR + RT		STR	STR + RT	STR	STR + RT	STR	STR + RT	STR	STR + RT
Barbaro et al.[89]	30	54	52.53 (mean)	59	77	—	—	0	52	—	—
Goldsmith et al.[68]	—	140	54 (median)	—	89	—	48	—	77	—	—
Glaholm et al.[69]	—	186	50–55	—	84	—	35	—	74	—	—
Nutting et al.[122]	—	82	55–60	—	92	—	—	—	87	—	—
Condra et al.[87]	55	17	53.3 (median)	52	87	—	—	40	82	—	—
Miralbell et al.[91]	79	36	NR	59	88	—	—	—	—	—	—
Connel et al.[123]		54	54 (median)	—	76	—	—	—	—	—	—

NR, not reported; STR, subtotal resection or biopsy alone, STR + RT, subtotal resection or biopsy plus radiation therapy; —, data not available.

radiation therapy (cobalt, 6 or 8 MV). PTV encompassed the preoperative tumor volume plus a 2 to 4 cm margin. Patients were treated daily to 50 to 55 Gy over 6 to 6.5 weeks. The amount of residual disease was not a significant prognostic factor for PFS: 5-, 10-, and 15-year PFS were 78%, 67%, and 56% in patients with minimum residuum versus 81%, 68%, and 61% in those with bulky residuum, respectively. Paradoxically, the worst results were seen with patients irradiated after gross total resection, with a 10-year PFS of 40%. This finding was attributed to high risk prognostic factors that were typical in this group of patients. Both malignant and "aggressive benign" histologies were associated with poor outcome following postoperative radiotherapy, with 5-year PFS of 35%, 44%, and 84% for malignant, "aggressive benign," and benign tumors, respectively. Karnofsky performance scores (KPS) greater than 50 were associated with superior CSS: 5-, 10-, and 15-year CSS were 83%, 70%, and 63% for patients with KPS greater than 50, compared with 49%, 44%, and 35% for KPS less than or equal to 50, respectively. Younger patients did better, with 5- and 10-year CSS of 84% and 73% for age younger than 60, compared with 59% and 42% for age 60 or older. On multivariate analysis, only tumor grade (benign vs. aggressive benign vs. malignant), extent of surgery (gross total resection vs. subtotal resection), and KPS were independent prognostic factors. Timing of radiotherapy (primary vs. salvage) did not influence survival.

Nutting et al.[122] have subsequently updated the RMH experience (1962-1992) with an analysis limited to 82 benign skull base meningiomas. Sixty-two patients were irradiated primarily after macroscopic excision ($n = 9$), subtotal resection ($n = 45$), biopsy ($n = 6$), undetermined surgery ($n = 2$). Twenty received radiotherapy after recurrence and a second operation: partial resection ($n = 10$) and biopsy ($n = 10$). All patients were treated with three fields using a 6 or 8 MV linear accelerator, and received 55 to 60 Gy in 33 fractions to the preoperative tumor volume plus 2 to 3 cm margin. Before 1973, tumor volumes were defined on the basis of surgical information. Subsequently, volumes were CT- or MRI-based. Five- and 10-year PFS were 92% and 83%, respectively. Age, gender, KPS, tumor site, extent of surgery, treatment era, use of CT or MRI diagnostic imaging, and primary versus recurrent tumor were evaluated for prognostic significance. Only tumor site was significant on univariate and multivariate analysis, with sphenoid ridge tumors having a 10-year PFS (69%) inferior to parasellar (90%) and other sites (100%). Sphenoid ridge tumors had a fivefold increased risk of progression, compared with other sites. The authors hypothesized that this difference might be the consequence of relatively larger tumors presenting at the sphenoid ridge, though they did not perform a size analysis, and size has not been convincingly demonstrated elsewhere[68,123] as a risk factor for treatment failure. Modern treatment era therapy (1970 and after vs. pre-1970) had a nonstatistically significant beneficial impact on both PFS and OS.

Condra and colleagues[87] have described 17 patients managed with postoperative adjuvant radiotherapy at the University of Florida between 1964 and 1992 after subtotal resection for benign meningioma. All were treated with conventionally fractionated megavoltage irradiation to 50 to 70 Gy (median 53.3 Gy). The PTV encompassed the tumor bed with a 2 cm margin. Five-, 10-, and 15-year PFS rates were 87%, 87%, and 87%, equivalent to total resection and significantly better ($P = 0.0001$) than subtotal resection-alone during the same period (5-, 10-, and 15-year PFS rates of 52%, 40%, and 30%). Fifteen-year CSS after total resection, subtotal resection plus radiation therapy, and subtotal resection alone were 88%, 86%, and 51% respectively ($P = 0.0003$), reflecting that many subtotal resection-alone patients were not successfully salvaged.

Miralbell et al.[91] described 17 patients with benign meningioma irradiated at the MGH after subtotal resection between 1968 and 1986 with either megavoltage photons alone or in combination with 160 MV protons. Eight-year PFS was 88%, superior to the 48% subtotal resection-alone PFS during the same period ($P = 0.057$) despite the fact that there were more high-grade lesions in the irradiated group than the nonirradiated group. Neither sex, age, pathology score, pathologic grade, extent of surgery, dose, nor radiation therapy technique (photons vs. photons/protons) were significant predictors of outcome on univariate analysis, albeit the sample size for this analysis was small. Wenkel and colleagues[113] subsequently updated the MGH experience with a review of 46 patients irradiated with combined photons and 160 MV protons after subtotal resection, biopsy, or recurrence for benign meningioma between 1981 and 1996. Five- and 10-year PFS were 100% and 88%, respectively. No dose response was observed.

Connell and colleagues[123] reported on 54 patients with benign meningioma irradiated at the University of Chicago after subtotal resection between 1984 and 1995. All were treated with megavoltage irradiation, conventionally fractionated to 45 to 60 Gy (median 54 Gy). The PTV encompassed the residual tumor with a 2 cm margin. Study methodology was flawed by clinical classification of tumor progression when follow-up scans were not available. Five-year PFS was incongruously poor (76%) for exclusively CT-era treatment and the median time to progression was surprisingly short (14 months). Both of these findings were attributed in accompanying editorials to probable misclassification of radiation-induced cerebral edema as tumor progression. Residual tumor size (expressed as greatest dimension, determined from radiology reports, scans, and tumor reconstructions from treatment ports), sex, age, site, histologic subtype, primary versus recurrent, dose, and biopsy versus partial resection were all evaluated for prognostic significance in PFS and CSS. No factor but postoperative residual tumor size was statistically significant, though this finding has also been called into question by the study's inexact means of determining size and classifying progression.

Milosevic and colleagues[124] have reported the Princess Margaret Hospital experience with adjuvant radiotherapy for atypical and anaplastic meningioma. "Atypical," in this case, was defined as the presence of mitoses, nuclear atypia, or necrosis. Between 1966 and 1990, 59 patients were irradiated: 24 primarily, 35 after at least one recurrence. Extent of most recent surgery before radiation was gross total in 17, subtotal resection in 35, biopsy in 3, and none or unknown in 4. All patients received megavoltage radiation. The PTV included the tumor as described by the neurosurgeon (before 1976) or CT/MRI (after 1975), plus 3 to 4 cm margin. Median dose was 50 Gy in 25 fractions. The 5-year CSS and OS were 34% and 26%, respectively. Nonstatistically significant improvement in CSS was seen in patients whose tumors were primarily irradiated (44% vs. 28% for those irradiated for salvage), atypical (51% vs. 27 for anaplastic), and totally excised (47% vs. 28% for subtotally excised). Statistically significant improvement in CSS was observed in younger patients (50% in those younger than age 59 vs. 0% for older patients), patients treated in the CT era (38% vs. 0% for pre-CT era), and those treated to a dose of 50 Gy or higher (42% vs. 0% for less than 50 Gy). On multivariate analysis, age, CT era, and radiation dose remained independently prognostic.

In summary, postoperative adjuvant radiotherapy has been clearly established as superior to subtotal resection alone for benign meningioma, with a 40% to 50% improvement in 10-year PFS[87,89-91] and 20% improvement in CSS.[87] These results approach those obtained in patients managed with total excision. After subtotal resection, observation alone unnecessarily subjects the patient to an increased risk of recurrence with a concomitant risk of requiring a second craniotomy. Moreover, when irradiation is delayed until the time of recurrence, the efficacy of therapy may be jeopardized if the meningioma should undergo malignant transformation to a more aggressive tumor[63,117] or develop increasing tumor burden with compromised performance status and likelihood of salvage.

Radiation Therapy Alone for Unresectable Tumors

Patients deemed unresectable because of technical considerations or medical condition are candidates for radiotherapy alone, which has been shown by several investigators to be associated with substantial palliative benefit in terms of improved or stabilized neurologic status, and durable PFS in the majority of cases. Maire and colleagues[99] have described the Hôpital Saint-André experience with radiotherapy alone for 44 inoperable or unresectable patients. Between 1981 and 1993, all patients were irradiated with 6 to 9 MV photons to a PTV that encompassed the GTV plus 1 to 1.5 cm margin via 3 to 4 isocentric portals. Median dose was 52 Gy at 1.8 Gy per fraction. After a median follow-up of 40 months, the crude PFS rate was 41/44. When reported in combination with 51 patients treated for other indications (subtotal resection, salvage after recurrence, and total resection with unfavorable histology), overall neurologic performance improved in 72%.

Glaholm et al.[69] reported the treatment of 32 unresectable patients at RMH with megavoltage radiation alone between 1963 and 1983. PTV encompassed the GTV plus a 2 to 4 cm margin. Patients were treated daily to 50 to 55 Gy over 6 to 6.5 weeks. PFS at 5, 10, and 15 years was 53%, 47%, and 47%. Neurologic performance improved in 38%.

Forbes and Goldberg[94] described 19 patients who were treated after biopsy only or no exploration. Patients were treated with 4 or 8 MV photons, conventionally fractionated, to a mean dose of 52.8 Gy (range 37.2 to 60). After a median follow-up of 45 months, 4-year PFS was 64%.

Pourel and coworkers[71] recently reviewed the Centre Alexis Vautrin experience, including nine patients managed with conventionally fractionated conformal radiotherapy alone between 1978 and 1997. After a median follow-up of 45 months, 5-year actuarial PFS was 80%.

Carella et al.[98] reported on 11 patients treated between 1964 and 1980 with RT alone without pathologic confirmation. Patients were treated with either cobalt or 4 MV photons, most receiving 55 to 60 Gy over 6 to 6.5 weeks. After a follow-up of 3 to 6 years, crude survival rate was 100%, nine patients experienced neurologic improvement, two remained stable, and none had neurologic deterioration.

Condra and colleagues[87] described seven inoperable or unresectable patients irradiated between 1964 and 1992 to 50 to 55 Gy. Crude 5-year PFS and CSS was 6/7.

Radiation Therapy after Recurrence

Salvage therapy for unirradiated patients with recurrent, progressive disease should include irradiation, either as an adjuvant to re-resection or alone for the inoperable/unresectable recurrent lesion. In this setting, PFS with the addition of RT is superior to that seen with surgery alone for salvage (Table 21-6).[90-92,100]

Wara and associates[100] reported the results of 16 patients treated from 1942 to 1972 with irradiation at the time of recurrence (with or without reoperation). Between 1942 and 1950, patients were treated with orthovoltage to a total dose of 30 to 40 Gy. After 1950, irradiation was megavoltage quality, with a total dose of 45 to 55 Gy given in daily increments of 1.8 Gy over about 5.5 weeks. The crude salvage rate was 50% (8 of 16), which was superior to the 37% (10 of 27) salvage rate seen in patients managed with reoperation alone at the same institution during the same period.

Taylor et al.[90] reported on 10 patients treated between 1973 and 1985 for recurrent benign meningioma. All received megavoltage irradiation, conventionally fractionated, to a total dose of 50 to 63 Gy. The treatment

Table 21–6 Salvage Radiation Therapy Data

	Patients, n			Salvage Rate	
Reference	Surg*	RT†	Endpoints	Surg*	RT†
Wara et al.[100]	27	16	Crude LC	10/27	8/16
Taylor et al.[90]	15	10	10 yr LC	30%	89%‡
Miralbell et al.[91]	18	16	8 yr LC	11%	78%§
Kokubo et al.[125]		20	5 yr PFS		41%
Pourel et al.[71]		14	5 yr PFS		73%

LC, local control.
*Treated with surgical salvage only.
†Treated with salvage radiation therapy with or without re-resection.
‡Statistically significant difference: *P* = 0.01.
§Statistically significant difference: *P* = 0.001.

volume encompassed the tumor bed with a 2 to 4 cm margin. The 10-year actuarial local control rate was 89%, which was significantly better (P = 0.01) than the 30% local control rate seen in patients managed without adjuvant radiation therapy at the same institution during the same period. Although the local control rate following radiation therapy for salvage (89%) compared favorably with that seen with immediate postoperative radiation therapy (82%, see earlier discussion under Postoperative), the authors emphasized that withholding radiation therapy initially after subtotal resection was associated with an inferior determinant survival, and that their excellent salvage results should not be interpreted as a justification for not irradiating meningiomas initially after subtotal resection.

Miralbell and colleagues[91] reported 19 patients treated at MGH after recurrence between 1968 and 1986 with either megavoltage photons alone or in combination with 160 megavolt protons. Eight-year PFS was 78%, which was superior to the 11% PFS seen in patients managed with surgery alone at the same institution during the same period, (P = 0.001).

Kokubo et al.[125] reported 20 patients treated at Kyoto University after recurrence between 1964 and 1998 with megavoltage photons. Block margins were 1 to 2 cm from the GTV, and doses ranged from 50 to 61.2 Gy, conventionally fractionated. Five patients were treated in the pre-CT era. Thirteen, four, and three patients had 1, 2, and 3 previous operations, respectively. Ten tumors were histologically benign, four were atypical, and six were anaplastic. Five-year PFS was 41% (benign) and 30% (atypical and anaplastic).

Pourel et al.[71] described 14 patients treated after first recurrence with conventionally fractionated conformal radiotherapy between 1978 and 1997. After a median follow-up of 35 months, 5-year actuarial PFS was 73%.

Optic Nerve Sheath Meningioma

Several investigators have reported very encouraging preliminary results with irradiation for meningiomas arising from the optic nerve sheath.[126-128] Smith and colleagues[129] first reported their experience with five patients treated between 1975 and 1980. Four of the five patients experienced improvement in visual acuity, fields, or color perception 2 to 10 months after irradiation. Improvement was temporary in only one case (with acuity declining at 3 years), and no patients demonstrated definite tumor progression after a follow-up of 3 to 48 months.

Kennerdell and colleagues[130] subsequently reported six patients irradiated to a total dose of approximately 55 Gy in 28 to 32 fractions. All had progressive loss of visual acuity or fields before radiation therapy, and all experienced improved visual acuity and fields after therapy, which was maintained throughout the period of follow-up (30 to 84 months). None had marked tumor shrinkage or progression. In the same series, 18 patients were managed with observation alone, and 10 had surgery only. Nine of the 18 observed patients had an initial visual acuity of 20/40 or better, and none of these 9 patients maintained this level of acuity for longer than 5 years. Only 2 of

10 patients managed with surgery alone had ultimate visual acuity better than detection of hand motion. Based on this data, several authors[109,130-132] have recommended an individualized treatment strategy as follows:

Observation of patients with good visual acuity at 6 month intervals with annual CT or MRI evaluation,
Irradiation if visual acuity declines below 20/40 or if the visual field is further constricted during the period of observation,
Observation for patients who present with no light perception and a tumor confined to the orbit,
Total excision of the tumor and nerve if the meningioma is large and markedly displacing the globe or progressing intracranially.

The experience at UCSF with irradiation of optic nerve sheath meningiomas has been very favorable, with the majority of patients experiencing resolution of visual field deficits within a few months of completing external beam radiotherapy (personal communication, D.A. Larson). As a result, observation is not encouraged at this institution, and all patients are offered radiotherapy using the technique described by Eng and associates.[106]

Spinal Meningioma

The optimal treatment of spinal meningioma is total excision. A large series from the Cleveland Clinic[73] reported only one recurrence among 80 patients managed with complete tumor removal. Subtotal resection in their experience was unusual (7% of all spinal meningioma cases), and disease recurred in only two of seven such cases, at 13 and 16 years. The authors concluded that unlike intracranial meningiomas, subtotally resected spinal meningiomas often pursue an indolent course. No radiation oncology literature has addressed the role of radiation therapy in such patients, so treatment recommendations are lacking. The UCSF policy is to treat subtotally resected spinal meningiomas with a total dose of 50.4 to 54 Gy, since in general it is felt that the potential complications of recurrence or further surgery outweigh the risks of radiation therapy.

Meningioma in the Pediatric Population

Pediatric skull base meningiomas are rare, and their treatment with irradiation is even more rare. Most pediatric patients are managed with surgery alone, resulting in an overall 20-year survival rate of 62%.[21] As a consequence, there is little radiotherapy literature addressing this topic, and there are no established treatment recommendations.[20,101] Leibel et al.[101] reported three patients with intracranial lesions irradiated after subtotal resection. The first, with a convexity malignant meningioma, had a minimal response to 50 Gy with concurrent cytoxan chemotherapy, and died 4 months later of uncontrolled disease. The second, also with a convexity malignant meningioma, received 32 Gy after a partial resection, followed by complete excision 6 months later, but this patient died due to postoperative complications. The third, with a benign transitional meningioma of the posterior fossa, was treated to 50.4 Gy and recurred 4 years later. This was again subtotally resected, and the patient was followed for an additional 9 years without progression. Irradiation for recurrence was also reported in three cases by Leibel et al.[101] All three patients had benign meningiomas that had recurred after subtotal resection. The first was treated to 50.6 Gy and was free of recurrence at 6 years. The second was treated to 52.88 Gy followed 6 months later by total excision, and was free of disease 9 years later. The third received 50 Gy, but died of uncontrolled disease 3 months later. The unimpressive results and small number of patients make interpretation of this data difficult. The authors concluded that when the tumor location and potential neurologic sequelae of recurrence and salvage surgery permit, radiotherapy may be withheld. Reasonable indications for radiotherapy (to a dose of 50 to 54 Gy) would include: (1) malignant histology, (2) incompletely resected benign meningioma at a site where the potential complications of recurrence or further surgery outweigh the risks of radiotherapy, and (3) progressive unresectable disease.

Innovative Therapies

STEREOTACTIC RADIOSURGERY

Radiosurgery (RS) is emerging as an effective and low-morbidity treatment option for patients with small-to-medium sized tumors (generally ≤3 cm) in sites that can be treated without exceeding tolerance dose constraints of nearby critical structures. Kondziolka and coworkers[133] reported the treatment of 99 patients with benign meningioma, between 1987 and 1992, at the University of Pittsburgh. Forty-three percent were treated primarily, and 57% had at least one prior surgery. Patients received a single-fraction median tumor margin dose of 16 Gy (range 9 to 25 Gy). Median maximal tumor dose was 32 Gy (range 18 to 50 Gy). The individual dose chosen depended on tumor volume, surgical history, irradiation history, neurologic status, tumor location, and the radiosensitivity of nearby critical structures. Although the analysis was undertaken 5 to 10 years after all the treatments were delivered, 32% of the patients were followed with imaging less than or equal to 4 years, and 14% for less than or equal to 2 years. The observed local control rate was 95%. Three patients (actuarial rate 5% between 31 and 120 months) experienced delayed neurologic sequelae consistent with radiation injury including: visual acuity deterioration (at 6 months, recovered), hemianopsia (at 31 months, permanent), hemiparesis (at 12 months, recovered), and abducens nerve palsy (at 18 months, recovered) in the same patient; worsened preexisting oculomotor palsy (at 3 months, permanent); and hemianopsia (at 30 months, permanent). Since restricting optic chiasm dose to below 8 Gy and conforming the RS plan with more sophisticated planning software, no subsequent patients developed delayed visual complications.

Stafford et al.[97] reviewed the Mayo Clinic experience of RS for 190 patients with meningioma. Forty-one percent were treated primarily, and 59% had at least one prior surgery. One hundred sixty-eight patients had benign tumors, and 13 and 9 had atypical and anaplastic grades, respectively. The median number of isocenters was 9 (range 1 to 21). Most tumors (93%) were prescribed to the 50% isodose line, and the median prescription isodose volume was 8.2 cm³. Median dose at the tumor margin was 16 Gy (range 12 to 36 Gy). Generally dose at the tumor margin was 20, 18, and 16 Gy for tumor volumes of less than 4.2, 4.2 to 14.1, and more than 14.1 cm³. After a median follow-up of 39 months, actuarial 5-year PFS was 89%. Five-year PFS rates for benign, atypical, and anaplastic grades were 93%, 68%, and 0%, respectively (P < 0.0001). Twenty-four patients (13%) had treatment-related complications, including 15 new or worsened cranial neuropathies.

Villavicencio et al.[134] described the treatment of 56 patients with skull base meningiomas (53 benign, 3 atypical) between 1988 and 1994. All tumors measured less than 5 cm in diameter and were situated more than 5 mm from the optic chiasm. Seventy-five percent of the lesions measured 3 cm or less. Nineteen patients were treated without prior surgery, and 36 had at least one prior surgical procedure. Seven had been previously irradiated to 40 to 60 Gy (4 for the same tumor, 2 for other tumors). All patients were treated with a dedicated stereotactic 6 MV linear accelerator. Mean single fraction dose to the tumor margin was 15 Gy (range 9 to 18.5 Gy). After a median follow-up of 26 months, actuarial PFS was 95%. Two of three recurrences were marginal. None of the atypical meningiomas had recurred. Five patients (9%) had long-term complications, one of whom developed optic neuropathy with complete loss of vision in the left eye 6 months after receiving 10 Gy to the left aspect of the optic chiasm.

Presently, the lack of effective primary therapies for anaplastic meningiomas and salvage therapies for recurrent meningiomas after radiation therapy failure argue in favor of RS as an appropriate, reasonably safe, and effective treatment option for these selected cases, either as primary therapy or as a boost following conventionally fractionated radiation therapy. However, for benign meningiomas that have not failed conventional radiotherapy, there are a few arguments against the routine use of RS: (1) the lack of long-term RS efficacy data, and (2) the potential for late radiation injury to normal CNS structures, particularly cranial nerves. Cranial neuropathy, which is uncommon after radiation therapy using modern treatment techniques, is a salient risk more commonly reported in the RS literature. A compelling radiobiologic rationale for fractionated radiotherapy of meningioma is avoidance of late-responding tissue injury. Considering the good to excellent results achieved with conventionally fractionated conformal radiation therapy for subtotally resected and unresectable or inoperable benign meningiomas, the use of RS in this setting should be considered investigational.

FRACTIONATED STEREOTACTIC RADIOTHERAPY

Fractionated stereotactic radiotherapy combines the precision of stereotactic positioning with the radiobiologic advantage of fractionation. Debus et al.[70] reported the

University of Heidelberg's experience treating 189 patients between 1985 and 1998 with a PTV of CTV plus 2 mm, using mask immobilization attached to a stereotactic frame. Three to five noncoplanar isocentric fields were employed, and a (mean) dose of 56.8 Gy was prescribed to the isocenter with the 90% isodose line encompassing the PTV. Eighty-two patients had 1993 WHO grade I tumors, 8 were grade II, 39 were benign according to the university's legacy grading system, and 59 were treated without tissue diagnosis. All had macroscopic disease targets: 59 unresected tumors, 50 after subtotal resection, 3 after biopsy, and 77 after recurrence. After a median follow-up of 35 months, 5-year PFS was 94% and 78% for benign and atypical tumors ($P = 0.02$), with no marginal failures. Pretreatment neurologic deficits improved in 45% and worsened in 7% of patients. Grade 3 toxicity (reduced vision, trigeminal neuropathy, and hypopituitarism) was seen in 2%.

INTENSITY-MODULATED RADIOTHERAPY

Inverse planning and intensity modulation offer more variables that can be manipulated to achieve target goals of coverage, conformality, and homogeneity, while meeting critical normal tissue constraints. The complex—and often concave—shape of meningiomas and their frequent proximity to dose-limiting structures make them suitable candidates for intensity-modulated radiotherapy (IMRT) dose distribution optimization evaluation. Pirzkall et al.[135] have compared conformal and IMRT isodose plan qualities for four patients with challenging, complex-shaped meningiomas of the following sites: clivus, frontobasal/ethmoid, sphenoid/retro-orbital, and cavernous sinus. Conformal PTV doses had to be limited to 52 Gy to not exceed critical structure dose limits (54 Gy to optic chiasm and optic nerve, 36 Gy to lacrimal gland, and 54 Gy to brainstem). In contrast, IMRT techniques yielded superior target coverage and conformality with equivalent dose homogeneity, and took less time to plan. Dose plan quality differences between IMRT and conformal radiotherapy are sensitive to tumor shape and proximity to dose-limiting structures, and are therefore expected to be less compelling for convex shaped and non–skull base tumors. Given the absence of strong evidence for dose-response within the range commonly employed for meningioma, it also remains to be seen whether the dose distribution advantages of IMRT will prove clinically relevant. Escalating target dose while maintaining acceptable normal tissue complication probabilities may have a role in the management of atypical and anaplastic meningioma.

BRACHYTHERAPY

Pioneering work with ^{125}I brachytherapy has been reported in the management of meningioma[136-140] for the primary therapy of unresectable lesions, inoperable patients, and anaplastic lesions, and salvage therapy following surgical or radiation therapy failure, or both, with promising results. Gutin and associates[140] reported the treatment of eight patients between 1981 and 1986, six of whom had anaplastic histology. Most had undergone multiple surgical resections for recurrent tumor. Two

were treated primarily with a combination of external beam radiation therapy and brachytherapy, and six had failed after previous external irradiation. After all accessible and safely resectable tumor was removed, the volume considered at risk for failure was implanted with ^{125}I sources, with either microsurgical or stereotactic technique. Primarily treated patients received 50 Gy via external radiation therapy followed by 50 Gy via brachytherapy. Patients treated for recurrence received 80 to 150 Gy (in addition to their previous external irradiation to 50 to 60 Gy). Two patients who had tumors that were not fully accessible experienced recurrence outside the implanted volume and died of uncontrolled disease, one at 8 and one at 9 months. A third patient experienced recurrence at 28 months, and the remaining five patients were stable without evidence of recurrence at 2 to 54 months follow-up (mean 30 months). In general, the treatment was well tolerated with only one of eight patients experiencing neurologic deficits attributable to radiation necrosis.

Vuorinen et al.[141] permanently implanted I-125 seeds into 44 meningiomas using stereotactic technique and 3-D dose planning, administering between 100 and 150 Gy to the GTV margin. After a median follow-up of 19 months, 1- and 2-year actuarial CSS were 78% and 62%, respectively. Preoperative cranial nerve III, V, or VI signs were present in 17 patients and subsided in 8. Cranial nerve V deficits developed or increased in 9 of the 25 patients with parasellar-clival meningiomas.

The lack of effective primary therapies for anaplastic meningiomas and salvage therapies for recurrent meningiomas after radiation therapy failure argue in favor of ^{125}I brachytherapy as an appropriate, safe, and effective treatment option in these cases. However, in light of good to excellent results seen after conventionally fractionated radiation therapy for subtotally resected and unresectable or inoperable meningiomas, and the lack of long-term brachytherapy data, the use of ^{125}I in these patients should be considered investigational and not recommended for routine clinical application.

HIGH LINEAR ENERGY TRANSFER IRRADIATION

Meningiomas abutting the spinal cord and brainstem that are not fully resectable pose a treatment planning challenge because of the need to deliver a therapeutic tumor dose that approaches or exceeds the tolerance of adjacent critical neurologic tissues. High linear energy transfer (LET) particle radiation, like radiosurgery, has the advantage of excellent dose localization (i.e., high tumor dose with an extremely steep dose gradient at the target border and little radiation to adjacent structures). High LET particle treatment has been employed in the management of various tumors (including meningioma) adjacent to the spinal cord and brainstem at the University of California Lawrence Berkeley Laboratory.[142,143] Results have been encouraging, with a local control rate of 62% at a median 20 months follow-up, and the incidence of serious complications is acceptable at 13%.

Experience with mixed photon and proton irradiation of benign intracranial meningioma has been reported by Wenkel et al.[113] Between 1981 and 1996, 46 patients were treated at the MGH and Harvard Cyclotron Laboratory (HCL). Median GTV dose was 59 cobalt gray equivalent (CGE), with a range of 53.1 to 74.1 CGE. Typically, 48 CGE was administered with protons at 1.92 CGE per fraction, with the balance via 4 or 10 MV photons at 1.8 Gy per fraction. Seventeen patients were treated shortly after subtotal resection (*n* = 9) or biopsy (*n* = 8); twenty-nine patients were treated after recurrence. After a median follow-up of 53 months, 5- and 10-year OS was 93% and 77%, respectively. Five- and 10-year PFS was 100% and 88%, respectively. No dose response for local control was observed. The maximum dose constraints for critical normal tissues were lowered during the period of this study (e.g., optic chiasm and nerve ≤62 CGE before 1996, ≤56.4 CGE between 1996 and 1997, and ≤54 CGE thereafter). Eight patients (17%) developed one or more grade 3 or 4 long-term neurologic toxicities. Four of four patients with optic neuropathy received optic structure doses in excess of 54 Gy. No ophthalmologic toxicity was seen in patients treated with current dose constraints. MGH and Loma Linda University are now conducting a prospective randomized dose searching trial for benign meningioma, comparing 55.8 CGE with 63 CGE.

Hug et al.[108] reported the contemporary MGH-HCL 1993 WHO grades II and III meningioma series, with patients treated with either photons alone (*n* = 15) or mixed photons and protons (*n* = 16). Between 1973 and 1995, 31 patients were treated for atypical (*n* = 15) or anaplastic (*n* = 16) disease. In general, the PTV included the GTV plus 1 cm, with a cone down to GTV only after 50 to 54 Gy. Mean PTV doses were 62 Gy/CGE (range 50 to 68 Gy/CGE) and 58 Gy/CGE (range 40 to 72 Gy/CGE) for atypical and anaplastic grades, respectively. Five- and 8-year PFS was 38% and 19% for atypical grade, and 52% and 17% for anaplastic grade (*P* = NS). Dose greater than or equal to 60 Gy/CGE was independently associated with superior PFS for both atypical and anaplastic grades: 5- and 8-year atypical meningioma PFS 90% and 45% for high dose versus 0% and 0% for low dose, *P* = 0.025; 5- and 8-year anaplastic meningioma PFS 100% and 33% for high dose versus 0% and 0% for low dose, *P* = 0.0006. Although statistically significant, these results need to be interpreted with caution because so few patients were studied. Three of thirty-one patients (9%) experienced late complications: two cerebral necroses (after 59 Gy and 72 CGE) and one optic neuropathy (dose to optic nerve ≤60 CGE). High LET therapy, along with fractionated stereotactic and IMRT, may play an important future role in dose escalation for grades II and III meningioma.

HORMONAL THERAPY

Although several investigators reported encouraging preliminary results with salvage hormonal therapy for unresectable meningioma,[144-146] subsequent trials have been disappointing. The Southwest Oncology Group studied the anti-estrogen tamoxifen[146] in 21 patients with unresectable meningioma. All patients received tamoxifen 40 mg per m^2 twice a day for 4 days, then 10 mg twice a day thereafter until progression. Of 19 evaluable patients, 1 (5%) achieved an MRI documented partial response,

2 had a minor response of short duration (4 and 20 months), 6 (32%) remained stable for a median of 31 months, and 10 (53%) progressed. The Southwest Oncology Group and Eastern Cooperative Oncology Group subsequently conducted a phase III placebo-controlled trial evaluating the anti-progestin mifepristone (RU486) for the treatment of unresectable nonanaplastic meningioma. One hundred ninety-three patients were enrolled, and at 2 years 80 patients per arm were evaluable. No significant difference in response was seen (unpublished data, presented at the 2001 meeting of the American Society for Clinical Oncology).

RADIOGRAPHIC FOLLOW-UP RECOMMENDATIONS

At UCSF, post-treatment scans (CT or MRI) are obtained annually for non–optic nerve sheath WHO grade I, and twice-a-year for grade I optic nerve sheath, grade II and III lesions, largely based on and corresponding to the mean tumor volume doubling times reported by Jaaskelainen.[147] Such careful follow-up is warranted because the potential for salvage is substantial (see earlier discussion under Innovative Therapies).

ACKNOWLEDGMENTS

I am deeply indebted to and most appreciative of the efforts of Tzvetan Tzvetanov, MS, and Computerized Medical Systems, Inc., for their assistance in the preparation of the chapter's three-dimensional treatment planning and dose volume histogram figures.

REFERENCES

1. Longstreth WT Jr, Dennis LK, McGuire VM, et al: Epidemiology of intracranial meningioma. *Cancer*. 1993;72:639.
2. Surawicz TS, McCarthy BJ, Kupelian V, et al: Descriptive epidemiology of primary brain and CNS tumors: Results from the Central Brain Tumor Registry of the United States, 1990-1994. *Neurooncol*. 1999;1:14.
3. Preston-Martin S: Descriptive epidemiology of primary tumors of the brain, cranial nerves and cranial meninges in Los Angeles County. *Neuroepidemiology*. 1989;8:283.
4. Sutherland GR, Florell R, Louw D, et al: Epidemiology of primary intracranial neoplasms in Manitoba, Canada. *Can J Neurol Sci*. 1987;14:586.
5. Kurland LT, Schoenberg BS, Annegers JF, et al: The incidence of primary intracranial neoplasms in Rochester, Minnesota, 1935-1977. *Ann N Y Acad Sci*. 1982;381:6.
6. Sankila R, Kallio M, Jaaskelainen J, et al: Long-term survival of 1986 patients with intracranial meningioma diagnosed from 1953 to 1984 in Finland. Comparison of the observed and expected survival rates in a population-based series. *Cancer*. 1992;70:1568.
7. Helseth A, Mork SJ, Johansen A, et al: Neoplasms of the central nervous system in Norway. IV. A population-based epidemiological study of meningiomas. *Apmis*. 1989;97:646.
8. Staneczek W, Janisch W: Epidemiologic data on meningiomas in East Germany 1961-1986: incidence, localization, age and sex distribution. *Clin Neuropathol*. 1992;11:135.
9. Sant M, Crosignani P, Bordo BM, et al: Incidence and survival of brain tumors: A population-based study. *Tumori*. 1988;74:243.
10. Lovaste MG, Ferrari G, Rossi G: Epidemiology of primary intracranial neoplasms. Experiment in the Province of Trento, (Italy), 1977-1984. *Neuroepidemiology*. 1986;5:220.

11. Andrioli GC, Rigobello L, Iob I, et al: Multiple meningiomas. *Neurochirurgia (Stuttg)*. 1981;24:67.

12. Butti G, Assietti R, Casalone R, et al: Multiple meningiomas: A clinical, surgical, and cytogenetic analysis. *Surg Neurol*. 1989;31:255.

13. Domenicucci M, Santoro A, D'Osvaldo DH, et al: Multiple intracranial meningiomas. *J Neurosurg*. 1989;70:41.

14. Locatelli D, Bottoni A, Uggetti C, et al: Multiple meningiomas evaluated by computed tomography. *Neurochirurgia (Stuttg)*. 1987;30:8.

15. Lusins JO, Nakagawa H: Multiple meningiomas evaluated by computed tomography. *Neurosurgery*. 1981;9:137.

16. Borovich B, Doron Y, Braun J, et al: The incidence of multiple meningiomas—Do solitary meningiomas exist? *Acta Neurochir (Wien)*. 1988;90:15.

17. Shuangshoti S, Hongsaprabhas C, Netsky MG: Metastasizing meningioma. *Cancer*. 1970;26:832.

18. Batsakis JG: Pathology consultation. Extracranial meningiomas. *Ann Otol Rhinol Laryngol*. 1984;93:282.

19. Rohringer M, Sutherland GR, Louw DF, et al: Incidence and clinicopathological features of meningioma. *J Neurosurg*. 1989;71:665.

20. Shah MV, Haines SJ: Pediatric skull, skull base, and meningeal tumors. *Neurosurg Clin N Am*. 1992;3:893.

21. Deen HG Jr, Scheithauer BW, Ebersold MJ: Clinical and pathological study of meningiomas of the first two decades of life. *J Neurosurg*. 1982;56:317.

22. Choi NW, Schuman LM, Gullen WH: Epidemiology of primary central nervous system neoplasms. II. Case-control study. *Am J Epidemiol*. 1970;91:467.

23. Ryan P, Lee MW, North B, et al: Risk factors for tumors of the brain and meninges: Results from the Adelaide Adult Brain Tumor Study. *Int J Cancer*. 1992;51:20.

24. Mills PK, Preston-Martin S, Annegers JF, et al: Risk factors for tumors of the brain and cranial meninges in Seventh-Day Adventists. *Neuroepidemiology*. 1989;8:266.

25. Preston-Martin S, Mack W, Henderson BE: Risk factors for gliomas and meningiomas in males in Los Angeles County. *Cancer Res*. 1989;49:6137.

26. Preston-Martin S, Paganini-Hill A, Henderson BE, et al: Case-control study of intracranial meningiomas in women in Los Angeles County, California. *J Natl Cancer Inst*. 1980;65:67.

27. Preston-Martin S, Pogoda JM, Schlehofer B, et al: An international case-control study of adult glioma and meningioma: the role of head trauma. *Int J Epidemiol*. 1998;27:579.

28. Munk J, Peyser E, Gruszkiewicz J: Radiation induced intracranial meningiomas. *Clin Radiol*. 1969;20:90.

29. Beller AJ, Feinsod M, Sahar A: The possible relationship between small dose irradiation to the scalp and intracranial meningiomas. *Neurochirurgia (Stuttg)*. 1972;15:135.

30. Modan B, Baidatz D, Mart H, et al: Radiation-induced head and neck tumors. *Lancet*. 1974;1:277.

31. Shore RE, Albert RE, Pasternack BS: Follow-up study of patients treated by x-ray epilation for tinea capitis: Resurvey of post-treatment illness and mortality experience. *Arch Environ Health*. 1976;31:21.

32. Ron E, Modan B, Boice JD Jr, et al: Tumors of the brain and nervous system after radiotherapy in childhood. *N Engl J Med*. 1988;319:1033.

33. Rubinstein AB, Shalit MN, Cohen ML, et al: Radiation-induced cerebral meningioma: A recognizable entity. *J Neurosurg*. 1984;61:966.

34. Rienstein S, Loven D, Israeli O, et al: Comparative genomic hybridization analysis of radiation-associated and sporadic meningiomas. *Cancer Genet Cytogenet*. 2001;131:135.

35. Preston-Martin S, Yu MC, Henderson BE, et al: Risk factors for meningiomas in men in Los Angeles County. *J Natl Cancer Inst*. 1983;70:863.

36. Annegers JF, Laws ER Jr, Kurland LT, et al: Head trauma and subsequent brain tumors. *Neurosurgery*. 1979;4:203.

37. Schlehofer B, Blettner M, Becker N, et al: Medical risk factors and the development of brain tumors. *Cancer*. 1992;69:2541.

38. Martini F, Iaccheri L, Lazzarin L, et al: SV40 early region and large T antigen in human brain tumors, peripheral blood cells, and sperm fluids from healthy individuals. *Cancer Res*. 1996;56:4820.

39. Ibelgaufts H, Jones KW, Maitland N, et al: Adenovirus-related RNA sequences in human neurogenic tumors. *Acta Neuropathol (Berl)*. 1982;56:113.

40. Zang KD, May G, Fischer H: Expression of SV 40-related T-antigen in cell cultures of human meningiomas. *Naturwissenschaften*. 1979;66:59.

41. Weiss AF, Portmann R, Fischer H, et al: Simian virus 40-related antigens in three human meningiomas with defined chromosome loss. *Proc Natl Acad Sci U S A*. 1975;72:609.

42. Helseth A, Mork SJ, Glattre E: Neoplasms of the central nervous system in Norway. V. Meningioma and cancer of other sites. An analysis of the occurrence of multiple primary neoplasms in meningioma patients in Norway from 1955 through 1986. *Apmis*. 1989;97:738.

43. Goldberg M, Rappaport ZH: Neurosurgical, obstetric and endocrine aspects of meningioma during pregnancy. *Isr J Med Sci*. 1987;23:825.

44. Grunberg SM, Weiss MH, Spitz IM, et al: Treatment of unresectable meningiomas with the antiprogesterone agent mifepristone. *J Neurosurg*. 1991;74:861.

45. Poisson M, Pertuiset BF, Hauw JJ, et al: Steroid hormone receptors in human meningiomas, gliomas and brain metastases. *J Neuro Oncol*. 1983;1:179.

46. Schnegg JF, Gomez F, LeMarchand-Beraud T, et al: Presence of sex steroid hormone receptors in meningioma tissue. *Surg Neurol*. 1981;15:415.

47. Magdelenat H, Pertuiset BF, Poisson M, et al: Progestin and oestrogen receptors in meningiomas. Biochemical characterization, clinical and pathological correlations in 42 cases. *Acta Neurochir (Wien)*. 1982;64:199.

48. Yu ZY, Wrange O, Haglund B, et al: Estrogen and progestin receptors in intracranial meningiomas. *J Steroid Biochem*. 1982;16:451.

49. Blankenstein MA, Blaauw G, Lamberts SW: Progestin and estrogen receptors in human meningioma. *Clin Neuropharmacol*. 1984;7:363.

50. Schlehofer B, Blettner M, Wahrendorf J: Association between brain tumors and menopausal status. *J Natl Cancer Inst*. 1992;84:1346.

51. Weber RG, Bostrom J, Wolter M, et al: Analysis of genomic alterations in benign, atypical, and anaplastic meningiomas: Toward a genetic model of meningioma progression. *Proc Natl Acad Sci U S A*. 1997;94:14719.

52. Zang KD: Meningioma: A cytogenetic model of a complex benign human tumor, including data on 394 karyotyped cases. *Cytogenet Cell Genet*. 2001;93:207.

53. Collins VP, Nordenskjold M, Dumanski JP: The molecular genetics of meningiomas. *Brain Pathol*. 1990;1:19.

54. Larsson C, Bystian C, Skoog L: Chromosomal mutations in human breast carcinoma. *Genes Chromosomes Cancer*. 1990;2:181.

55. Iida A, Kurose K, Isobe R: Mapping of a new target region of allelic loss to a 2-cM interval at 22q13.1 in primary breast cancer. *Genes Chromosomes Cancer*. 1998;21:108.

56. Kleihues P, Louis DN, Scheithauer BW, et al: The WHO classification of tumors of the nervous system. *J Neuropathol Exp Neurol*. 2002;61:215.

57. Zorludemir S, Scheithauer BW, Hirose T, et al: Clear cell meningioma. A clinicopathologic study of a potentially aggressive variant of meningioma. *Am J Surg Pathol*. 1995;19:493.

58. Kleihues P, Burger PC, Scheithauer BW: The new WHO classification of brain tumors. *Brain Pathol*. 1993;3:255.

59. Perry A, Scheithauer BW, Stafford SL, et al: "Rhabdoid" meningioma: An aggressive variant. *Am J Surg Pathol*. 1998;22:1482.

60. Ludwin SK, Rubinstein LJ, Russell DS: Papillary meningioma: A malignant variant of meningioma. *Cancer*. 1975;36:1363.

61. Perry A, Scheithauer BW, Stafford SL, et al: "Malignancy" in meningiomas: A clinicopathologic study of 116 patients, with grading implications. *Cancer*. 1999;85:2046.

62. Fukui M, Iwaki T, Sawa H, et al: Proliferative activity of meningiomas as evaluated by bromodeoxyuridine uptake examination. *Acta Neurochir (Wien)*. 1986;81:135.

63. Shibuya M, Hoshino T, Ito S, et al: Meningiomas: Clinical implications of a high proliferative potential determined by bromodeoxyuridine labeling. *Neurosurgery*. 1992;30:494.

64. Spaar FW, Ahyai A, Blech M: DNA-fluorescence-cytometry and prognosis (grading) of meningiomas—A study of 104 surgically removed tumors. *Neurosurg Rev*. 1987;10:35.

65. Cobb MA, Husain M, Andersen BJ, et al: Significance of proliferating cell nuclear antigen in predicting recurrence of intracranial meningioma. *J Neurosurg*. 1996;84:85.

66. Takeuchi H, Kubota T, Kabuto M, et al: Prediction of recurrence in histologically benign meningiomas: proliferating cell nuclear antigen and Ki-67 immunohistochemical study. *Surg Neurol.* 1997;48:501.

67. Colvett KT, Hsu DW, Su M, et al: High PCNA index in meningiomas resistant to radiation therapy. *Int J Radiat Oncol Biol Phys.* 1997;38:463.

68. Goldsmith BJ, Wara WM, Wilson CB, et al: Postoperative irradiation for subtotally resected meningiomas. A retrospective analysis of 140 patients treated from 1967 to 1990. *J Neurosurg.* 1994; 80:195.

69. Glaholm J, Bloom HJ, Crow JH: The role of radiotherapy in the management of intracranial meningiomas: The Royal Marsden Hospital experience with 186 patients. *Int J Radiat Oncol Biol Phys.* 1990;18:755.

70. Debus J, Wuendrich M, Pirzkall A, et al: High efficacy of fractionated stereotactic radiotherapy of large base-of-skull meningiomas: long-term results. *J Clin Oncol.* 2001;19:3547.

71. Pourel N, Auque J, Bracard S, et al: Efficacy of external fractionated radiation therapy in the treatment of meningiomas: a 20-year experience. *Radiother Oncol.* 2001;61:65.

72. Herz DA, Shapiro K, Shulman K: Intracranial meningiomas of infancy, childhood and adolescence. Review of the literature and addition of 9 case reports. *Childs Brain.* 1980;7:43.

73. Levy WJ Jr, Bay J, Dohn D: Spinal cord meningioma. *J Neurosurg.* 1982;57:804.

74. Murovic J, Sundaresan N: Pediatric spinal axis tumors. *Neurosurg Clin N Am.* 1992;3:947.

75. Sheporaitis LA, Osborn AG, Smirniotopoulos JG, et al: Intracranial meningioma. *AJNR Am J Neuroradiol.* 1992;13:29.

76. Mantle RE, Lach B, Delgado MR, et al: Predicting the probability of meningioma recurrence based on the quantity of peritumoral brain edema on computerized tomography scanning. *J Neurosurg.* 1999;91:375.

77. Tien RD, Yang PJ, Chu PK: "Dural tail sign": A specific MR sign for meningioma? *J Comput Assist Tomogr.* 1991;15:64.

78. Tokumaru A, O'Uchi T, Eguchi T, et al: Prominent meningeal enhancement adjacent to meningioma on Gd-DTPA-enhanced MR images: histopathologic correlation. *Radiology.* 1990; 175:431.

79. Elster AD, Challa VR, Gilbert TH, et al: Meningiomas: MR and histopathologic features. *Radiology.* 1989;170:857.

80. Demaerel P, Wilms G, Lammens M, et al: Intracranial meningiomas: correlation between MR imaging and histology in fifty patients. *J Comput Assist Tomogr.* 1991;15:45.

81. Kaplan RD, Coons S, Drayer BP, et al: MR characteristics of meningioma subtypes at 1.5 tesla. *J Comput Assist Tomogr.* 1992;16:366.

82. Khoo VS, Adams EJ, Saran F, et al: A comparison of clinical target volumes determined by CT and MRI for the radiotherapy planning of base of skull meningiomas. *Int J Radiat Oncol Biol Phys.* 2000;46:1309.

83. Adegbite AB, Khan MI, Paine KW, et al: The recurrence of intracranial meningiomas after surgical treatment. *J Neurosurg.* 1983;58:51.

84. Marks SM, Whitwell HL, Lye RH: Recurrence of meningiomas after operation. *Surg Neurol.* 1986;25:436.

85. Mirimanoff RO, Dosoretz DE, Linggood RM, et al: Meningioma: Analysis of recurrence and progression following neurosurgical resection. *J Neurosurg.* 1985;62:18.

86. Jaaskelainen J: Seemingly complete removal of histologically benign intracranial meningioma: Late recurrence rate and factors predicting recurrence in 657 patients. A multivariate analysis. *Surg Neurol.* 1986;26:461.

87. Condra KS, Buatti JM, Mendenhall WM, et al: Benign meningiomas: Primary treatment selection affects survival. *Int J Radiat Oncol Biol Phys.* 1997;39:427.

88. Levine ZT, Buchanan RI, Sekhar LN, et al: Proposed grading system to predict the extent of resection and outcomes for cranial base meningiomas. *Neurosurgery.* 1999;45:221.

89. Barbaro NM, Gutin PH, Wilson CB, et al: Radiation therapy in the treatment of partially resected meningiomas. *Neurosurgery.* 1987;20:525.

90. Taylor BW Jr, Marcus RB Jr, Friedman WA, et al: The meningioma controversy: Postoperative radiation therapy. *Int J Radiat Oncol Biol Phys.* 1988;15:299.

91. Miralbell R, Linggood RM, de la Monte S, et al: The role of radiotherapy in the treatment of subtotally resected benign meningiomas. *J Neuro Oncol.* 1992;13:157.

92. Stafford SL, Perry A, Suman VJ, et al: Primarily resected meningiomas: outcome and prognostic factors in 581 Mayo Clinic patients, 1978 through 1988. *Mayo Clin Proc.* 1998;73:936.

93. Mathiesen T, Lindquist C, Kihlstrom L, et al: Recurrence of cranial base meningiomas. *Neurosurgery.* 1996;39:2.

94. Forbes AR, Goldberg ID: Radiation therapy in the treatment of meningioma: The Joint Center for Radiation Therapy experience 1970 to 1982. *J Clin Oncol.* 1984;2:1139.

95. Yamashita J, Handa H, Iwaki K, et al: Recurrence of intracranial meningiomas, with special reference to radiotherapy. *Surg Neurol.* 1980;14:33.

96. Black PM, Villavicencio AT, Rhouddou C, et al: Aggressive surgery and focal radiation in the management of meningiomas of the skull base: preservation of function with maintenance of local control. *Acta Neurochir (Wien).* 2001;143:555.

97. Stafford SL, Pollock BE, Foote RL, et al: Meningioma radiosurgery: Tumor control, outcomes, and complications among 190 consecutive patients. *Neurosurgery.* 2001;49:1029.

98. Carella RJ, Ransohoff J, Newall J: Role of radiation therapy in the management of meningioma. *Neurosurgery.* 1982;10:332.

99. Maire JP, Caudry M, Guerin J, et al: Fractionated radiation therapy in the treatment of intracranial meningiomas: Local control, functional efficacy, and tolerance in 91 patients. *Int J Radiat Oncol Biol Phys.* 1995;33:315.

100. Wara WM, Sheline GE, Newman H, et al: Radiation therapy of meningiomas. *Am J Roentgenol Radium Ther Nucl Med.* 1975;123:453.

101. Leibel SA, Wara WM, Sheline GE, et al: The treatment of meningiomas in childhood. *Cancer.* 1976;37:2709.

102. Kennedy JD, Haines SJ: Review of skull base surgery approaches: With special reference to pediatric patients. *J Neuro Oncol.* 1994;20:291.

103. Manelfe C, Lasjaunias P, Ruscalleda J: Preoperative embolization of intracranial meningiomas. *AJNR Am J Neuroradiol.* 1986; 7:963.

104. Nelson PK, Setton A, Choi IS, et al: Current status of interventional neuroradiology in the management of meningiomas. *Neurosurg Clin N Am.* 1994;5:235.

105. Oka H, Kurata A, Kawano N, et al: Preoperative superselective embolization of skull-base meningiomas: Indications and limitations. *J Neuro Oncol.* 1998;40:67.

106. Eng TY, Albright NW, Kuwahara G, et al: Precision radiation therapy for optic nerve sheath meningiomas. *Int J Radiat Oncol Biol Phys.* 1992;22:1093.

107. Goldsmith BJ, Rosenthal SA, Wara WM, et al: Optic neuropathy after irradiation of meningioma. *Radiology.* 1992;185:71.

108. Hug EB, Devries A, Thornton AF, et al: Management of atypical and malignant meningiomas: role of high-dose, 3D-conformal radiation therapy. *J Neuro Oncol.* 2000;48:151.

109. Capo H, Kupersmith MJ: Efficacy and complications of radiotherapy of anterior visual pathway tumors. *Neurol Clin.* 1991;9:179.

110. Parsons JT, Bova FJ, Fitzgerald CR, et al: Radiation retinopathy after external-beam irradiation: Analysis of time-dose factors. *Int J Radiat Oncol Biol Phys.* 1994;30:765.

111. al-Mefty O, Kersh JE, Routh A, et al: The long-term side effects of radiation therapy for benign brain tumors in adults. *J Neurosurg.* 1990;73:502.

112. Parsons JT, Bova FJ, Fitzgerald CR, et al: Radiation optic neuropathy after megavoltage external-beam irradiation: Analysis of time-dose factors. *Int J Radiat Oncol Biol Phys.* 1994; 30:755.

113. Wenkel E, Thornton AF, Finkelstein D, et al: Benign meningioma: Partially resected, biopsied, and recurrent intracranial tumors treated with combined proton and photon radiotherapy. *Int J Radiat Oncol Biol Phys.* 2000;48:1363.

114. Parsons JT, Bova FJ, Fitzgerald CR: Tolerance of the visual apparatus to conventional therapeutic irradiation. In Sheline GE, ed. *Radiation Injury to the Nervous System.* New York: Raven Press; 1991:283.

115. Leibel SA, Sheline GE: Tolerance of the brain and spinal cord to conventional irradiation. In Sheline GE, ed. *Radiation Injury to the Nervous System.* New York: Raven Press; 1991:239.

116. Littley MD, Shalet SM, Bearswell CG: Radiation and the hypothalamic-pituitary axis. In Sheline GE, ed. *Radiation Injury to the Nervous System.* New York: Raven Press; 1991:303.

117. Jaaskelainen J, Haltia M, Servo A: Atypical and anaplastic meningiomas: Radiology, surgery, radiotherapy, and outcome. *Surg Neurol.* 1986;25:233.

118. Fukui M, Kitamura K, Nakagaki H, et al: Irradiated meningiomas: A clinical evaluation. *Acta Neurochir (Wien).* 1980;54:33.

119. Fukui M, Kitamura K, Ohgami S, et al: Radiosensitivity of meningioma—Analysis of five cases of highly vascular meningioma treated by preoperative irradiation. *Acta Neurochir (Wien).* 1977;36:47.

120. Solan MJ, Kramer S: The role of radiation therapy in the management of intracranial meningiomas. *Int J Radiat Oncol Biol Phys.* 1985;11:675.

121. Petty AM, Kun LE, Meyer GA: Radiation therapy for incompletely resected meningiomas. *J Neurosurg.* 1985;62:502.

122. Nutting C, Brada M, Brazil L, et al: Radiotherapy in the treatment of benign meningioma of the skull base. *J Neurosurg.* 1999;90:823.

123. Connell PP, Macdonald RL, Mansur DB, et al: Tumor size predicts control of benign meningiomas treated with radiotherapy. *Neurosurgery.* 1999;44:1194.

124. Milosevic MF, Frost PJ, Laperriere NJ, et al: Radiotherapy for atypical or malignant intracranial meningioma. *Int J Radiat Oncol Biol Phys.* 1996;34:817.

125. Kokubo M, Shibamoto Y, Takahashi JA, et al: Efficacy of conventional radiotherapy for recurrent meningioma. *J Neuro Oncol.* 2000;48:51.

126. Moyer PD, Golnik KC, Breneman J: Treatment of optic nerve sheath meningioma with three-dimensional conformal radiation. *Am J Ophthalmol.* 2000;129:694.

127. Fineman MS, Augsburger JJ: A new approach to an old problem. *Surv Ophthalmol.* 1999;43:519.

128. Lee AG, Woo SY, Miller NR, et al: Improvement in visual function in an eye with a presumed optic nerve sheath meningioma after treatment with three-dimensional conformal radiation therapy. *J Neuro Ophthalmol.* 1996;16:247.

129. Smith JL, Vuksanovic MM, Yates BM, et al: Radiation therapy for primary optic nerve meningiomas. *J Clin Neuro Ophthalmol.* 1981;1:85.

130. Kennerdell JS, Maroon JC, Malton M, et al: The management of optic nerve sheath meningiomas. *Am J Ophthalmol.* 1988;106:450.

131. Dutton JJ: Optic nerve sheath meningiomas. *Surv Ophthalmol.* 1992;37:167.

132. Ito M, Ishizawa A, Miyaoka M, et al: Intraorbital meningiomas. Surgical management and role of radiation therapy. *Surg Neurol.* 1988;29:448.

133. Kondziolka D, Levy EI, Niranjan A, et al: Long-term outcomes after meningioma radiosurgery: Physician and patient perspectives. *J Neurosurg.* 1999;91:44.

134. Villavicencio AT, Black PM, Shrieve DC, et al: Linac radiosurgery for skull base meningiomas. *Acta Neurochir (Wien).* 2001;143:1141.

135. Pirzkall A, Carol M, Lohr F, et al: Comparison of intensity-modulated radiotherapy with conventional conformal radiotherapy for complex-shaped tumors. *Int J Radiat Oncol Biol Phys.* 2000;48:1371.

136. Kumar PP, Good RR, Patil AA, et al: Permanent high-activity iodine-125 in the management of petroclival meningiomas: Case reports. *Neurosurgery.* 1989;25:436.

137. Kumar PP, Patil AA, Leibrock LG, et al: Brachytherapy: A viable alternative in the management of basal meningiomas. *Neurosurgery.* 1991;29:676.

138. Kumar PP, Patil AA, Syh HW, et al: Role of brachytherapy in the management of the skull base meningioma. Treatment of skull base meningiomas. *Cancer.* 1993;71:3726.

139. Kumar PP, Patil AA, Leibrock LG, et al: Continuous low dose rate brachytherapy with high activity iodine-125 seeds in the management of meningiomas. *Int J Radiat Oncol Biol Phys.* 1993;25:325.

140. Gutin PH, Leibel SA, Hosobuchi Y, et al: Brachytherapy of recurrent tumors of the skull base and spine with iodine-125 sources. *Neurosurgery.* 1987;20:938.

141. Vuorinen V, Heikkonen J, Brander A, et al: Interstitial radiotherapy of 25 parasellar/clival meningiomas and 19 meningiomas in the elderly. Analysis of short-term tolerance and responses. *Acta Neurochir (Wien).* 1996;138:495.

142. Castro JR, Collier JM, Petti PL, et al: Charged particle radiotherapy for lesions encircling the brain stem or spinal cord. *Int J Radiat Oncol Biol Phys.* 1989;17:477.

143. Saunders WM, Chen GT, Austin-Seymour M, et al: Precision, high dose radiotherapy. II. Helium ion treatment of tumors adjacent to critical central nervous system structures. *Int J Radiat Oncol Biol Phys.* 1985;11:1339.

144. Grunberg SM: The role of progesterone receptors in meningioma. *Cancer Treat Res.* 1991;58:127.

145. Lamberts SW, Tanghe HL, Avezaat CJ, et al: Mifepristone (RU 486) treatment of meningiomas. *J Neurol Neurosurg Psychiatry.* 1992;55:486.

146. Goodwin JW, Crowley J, Eyre HJ, et al: A phase II evaluation of tamoxifen in unresectable or refractory meningiomas: A Southwest Oncology Group study. *J Neuro Oncol.* 1993;15:75.

147. Jaaskelainen J, Haltia M, Laasonen E, et al: The growth rate of intracranial meningiomas and its relation to histology. An analysis of 43 patients. *Surg Neurol.* 1985;24:165.

22

Skull Base Tumors: Chemodectomas— Nonchromaffin Paragangliomas

Mary Austin-Seymour, MD and Daniel R. Reed, DO

Paraganglia are collections of neuroepithelial cells that probably have their origin in the neural crest.[1] Tumors that may develop from paraganglia are most commonly found in the temporal bone or cervical region. These low-grade malignancies are called *paragangliomas*. Paragangliomas are classified as chromaffin and nonchromaffin, depending on whether the tumor produces catecholamines and therefore reacts with chromic acid.[2] Most tumors of extra-adrenal paraganglionic tissue do not have a positive chromaffin reaction and are therefore called nonchromaffin paragangliomas. The proper term for such tumors is *nonchromaffin paragangliomas*, preceded by the site of origin.

Chemodectoma is a term also used to describe nonchromaffin paragangliomas. This term was introduced initially to describe carotid body tumors that originate from cells with chemoreceptor function.[3] It was derived from the Greek words *chemia* (infusion), *decesthai* (receive), and *oma* (tumor). Much of the literature uses the term chemodectoma to describe all nonchromaffin paragangliomas, and this discussion also considers chemodectomas to be synonymous with nonchromaffin paragangliomas. The term *glomus body tumor* is also used to describe these tumors.

EPIDEMIOLOGY AND GENETICS

Most series have a marked female predominance in the nonfamilial form of this tumor.[4,5] Most patients are middle-aged, although patients with a family history may present at a younger age. Some series report an increased incidence of carotid body tumors at high altitudes.[6] A few tumors may have endocrine activity and cause symptoms of pheochromocytomas or carcinoid apudomas.[7] The incidence of metastasis is about 10% or less.[8,9]

The familial occurrence of nonchromaffin paragangliomas was first noted in 1933.[10] Familial tumors account for about 10% of all cases.[2] Familial tumors are much more likely to be multicentric and bilateral than sporadic tumors. In one series, multicentricity was noted in 55% of familial cases.[5] Familial paragangliomas appear to follow an autosomal dominant transmission, with variable penetrance and expressivity.[2,11,12] Genetic analysis has identified three different genetic types of paraganglioma: paraganglioma 1 (*PGL1*) 11q23, paraganglioma 2 (*PGL2*) 11q13, and paraganglioma 3 (*PGL3*).[13-15] These genes include *PGL1* succinate-ubiquinone-oxidoreductase subunit D (SDHD) and *PGL3* succinate-ubiquinone-oxidoreductase subunit C (SCHC).

ANATOMY

The most common location of paragangliomas is the carotid body; these account for 60% to 70% of all head and neck cases.[2] The carotid body is located adjacent to the bifurcation of the common carotid artery. The next most common location is the temporal bone. The distribution and number of paraganglia within the temporal bone vary among individuals. The most common location is along the superior bulb of the internal jugular vein (glomus jugulare). The next most common locations are along the tympanic branch of cranial nerve IX (glomus tympanicum) and the auricular branch of cranial nerve X. These temporal bone paraganglia are located in close relationship to cranial nerves IX to XI. About 20% of the temporal bone paraganglia are in the tympanic canaliculus. Other head and neck locations for paraganglia include the region of the ciliary nerve in the orbit, vagus nerve, and larynx.

PATHOLOGY

Nonchromaffin paragangliomas are hypervascular tumors that are histologically benign in appearance. They resemble normal paraganglia and have nests of round or polygonal epithelioid cells surrounded by an elaborate vasculature.[16] The relative amounts of epithelioid and vascular tissue may vary. Figure 22-1 shows a typical paraganglioma. As described earlier, the chromaffin reaction used to identify catecholamines is almost always negative for the paragangliomas under discussion. This reaction is not sensitive enough to identify the small amounts of catecholamines in these paragangliomas.

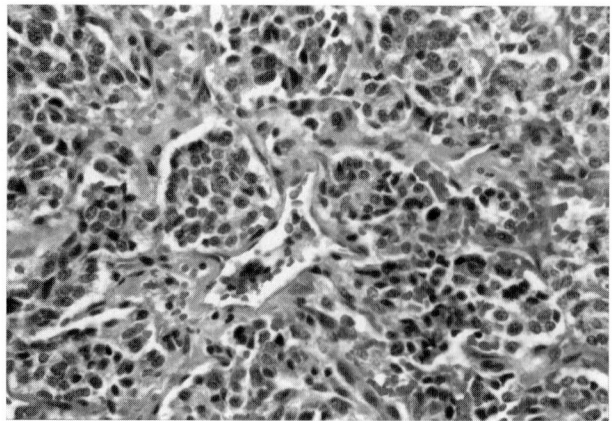

Figure 22–1. The microscopic appearance of a typical paraganglioma.

A formaldehyde-induced fluorescence technique is a more sensitive method to identify the catecholamines. This technique requires fresh or frozen tissue.[16] Another more specific diagnostic technique is the use of immuno-histochemical staining for neuron-specific enolase.[16] One study showed the presence of aneuploidy in 37% of para-gangliomas.[17] This is evidence for the neoplastic nature of these lesions.

CLINICAL PRESENTATION

Paragangliomas of the carotid body usually present as an asymptomatic mass located at the bifurcation of the common carotid artery.[18] Often, this has been present for several years. More advanced disease may present with palsies of cranial nerves IX, X, and XII; pain; dysphagia due to extension into the parapharyngeal space; or carotid sinus syndrome. Paragangliomas in the temporal bone present insidiously, and the symptoms vary with the site of the paraganglioma within the temporal bone. Lesions in the region of the jugular bulb present with headaches and cranial nerve deficits of IX to XI. These tumors may cause extensive bone destruction and, with extension of the tumor to the posterior cranial fossa, deficits of cranial nerves V to XII may develop. Lesions in the region of the middle ear present with progressive conductive hearing loss and pulsatile tinnitus.[19] Vertigo may also be present.

ROUTES OF SPREAD

The predominant pattern of spread of paragangliomas is local. Lymph node and distant metastases are rare.[20] Carotid body paragangliomas expand as they grow and displace the internal and external carotid arteries. As described, temporal bone paragangliomas can erode and destroy the temporal bone as well as involve the posterior cranial fossa. Medially, they may extend to the internal auditory canal and involve cranial nerves VII and VIII. Laterally, they may grow through the tympanic membrane and appear as masses in the external auditory canal.

DIAGNOSTIC STUDIES

The initial diagnostic study for all patients suspected of having a paraganglioma is a computed tomography (CT) scan. Since these tumors are hypervascular, there is intense enhancement with contrast administration. Large tumors may have areas of low attenuation, which represent hemorrhage and necrosis.[21] Usually these lesions have smooth contours. Figure 22-2 shows the typical CT appearance of a carotid paraganglioma. Paragangliomas greater than 2 cm have a characteristic appearance on magnetic resonance imaging (MRI) of both hyperintensity and hypointensity on both T1- and T2-weighted images.[22] Serpentine or channel-like areas of signal void, which represent the vascular flow voids of the dominant vessels of the tumor, can be seen. Figure 22-3 shows an MRI of a paraganglioma. The use of contrast with MRI may enhance the specificity of the image.[23,24] Angiography is used to evaluate patients preoperatively and to confirm the diagnosis when the CT scan is equivocal. Figure 22-4 shows a typical angiogram with intense vascularity of the paraganglioma and splaying of the internal and external carotid arteries. The combination of a characteristic angiogram and typical CT/MRI findings is considered equivalent to a biopsy. If there are questionable features of the imaging studies, biopsy may be necessary.

The paragangliomas of the temporal bone have additional imaging requirements. The CT evaluation of the temporal bone is extremely important. Typically the bone windows in the region of the tumor reveal irregular demineralization or destruction of bone.[22] Figure 22-5 shows bone destruction from a paraganglioma. Paragangliomas tend to grow along preexisting pathways in the temporal bone such as fissures, vascular channels, and foramina. Recent work has explored the role of contrast-enhanced MRI in the diagnosis of these lesions. A characteristic dip in the enhancement of the sigmoid sinus and jugular

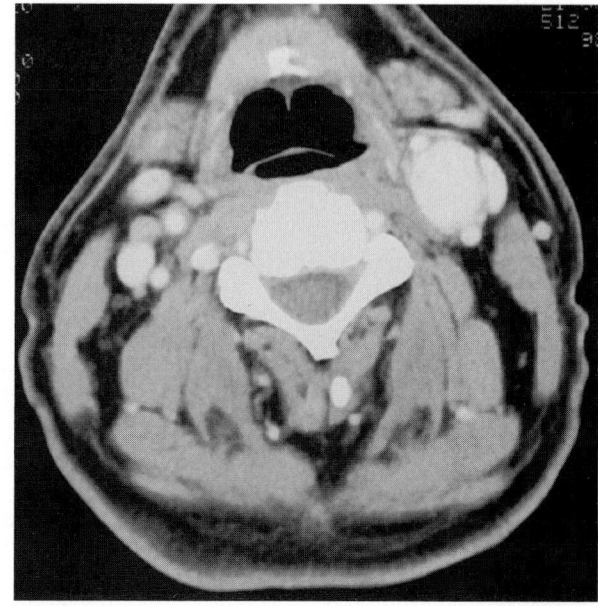

Figure 22–2. Computed tomographic scan of a carotid paraganglioma shows intense enhancement of the tumor.

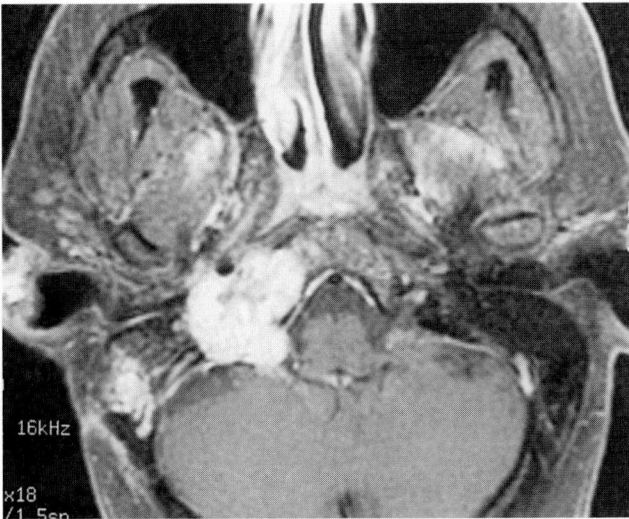

Figure 22–3. Magnetic resonance imaging scan of temporal bone paraganglioma shows areas of both hyperintensity and hypointensity and extension into the posterior fossa.

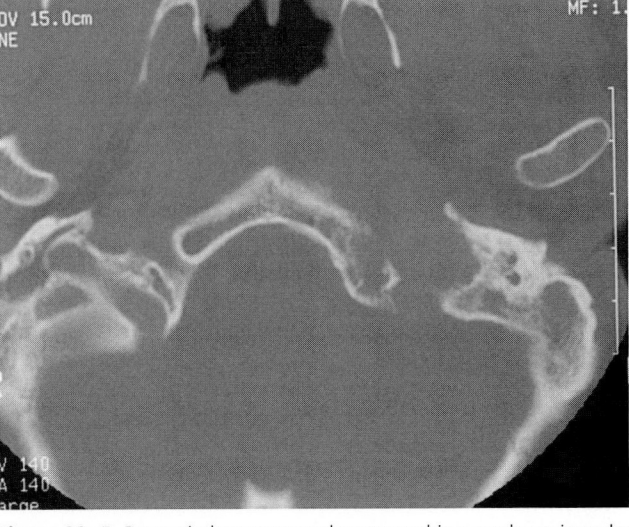

Figure 22–5. Bone window computed tomographic scan shows irregular destruction of bone by a paraganglioma.

bulb has been described.[25] Small paragangliomas of the temporal bone may require angiography for diagnosis. Figure 22-6 shows the typical angiographic appearance of a moderate-sized temporal bone paraganglioma. Angiography may also be done for larger lesions as part of preoperative therapeutic embolization.

Patients with a positive family history require a more extensive radiographic evaluation because of the possibility of bilateral tumors. These patients should have bilateral carotid angiography and consideration should be given to *m*-iodobenzylguanidine scintigraphy.[26]

STAGING

There is no generally accepted staging system for paragangliomas. Lesions are considered to be early when they are small without cranial nerve palsies and with little or no bone destruction. Advanced tumors have significant bone destruction or cranial nerve palsies.

STANDARD THERAPEUTIC APPROACHES

The primary treatment for paragangliomas is radiation or surgery. Occasionally, patients are treated with radiation after subtotal surgical removal. The selection of

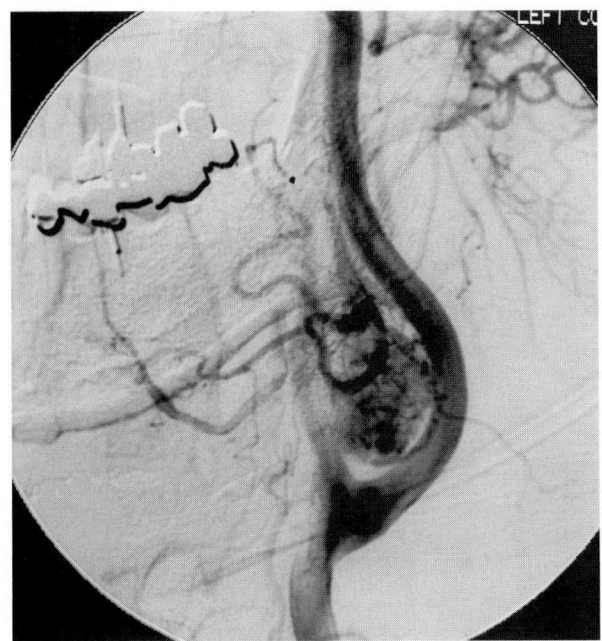

Figure 22–4. Angiogram of a carotid paraganglioma shows the intense vascularity of the tumor and splaying of the internal and external carotid arteries.

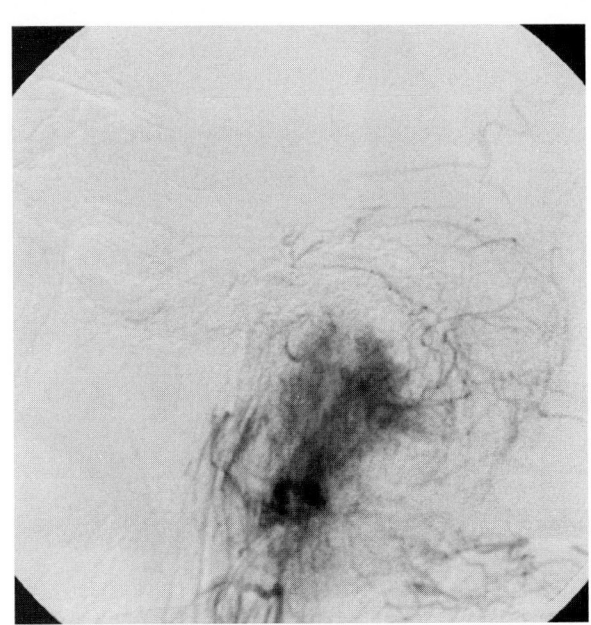

Figure 22–6. Angiogram of a moderate-sized temporal bone paraganglioma shows intense vascularity.

treatment for a given patient is determined by many factors, including the location of the lesion, the likely complications of surgical removal or radiation treatment, prior treatment (if any), and the general condition of the patient. One notable feature of radiation treatment is that most patients continue to have a radiographic or palpable abnormality after treatment.[27] The usual course after treatment is slow regression of the mass. The long-term effectiveness of treatment is judged by lack of progression of the mass and permanent improvement in clinical signs and symptoms.

Most carotid body paragangliomas are amenable to surgical removal. Resection of large tumors may be associated with a risk of vascular or neurologic complications. Preoperative embolization of tumors decreases the likelihood of intraoperative hemorrhage. Large tumors that would require ligation or reconstruction of the carotid arteries should be considered for radiation treatment, as should fixed or unresectable tumors. Because most carotid body paragangliomas are treated surgically, less data exists on the results of radiation treatment for paragangliomas in this region compared with the temporal bone. The limited amount of data suggests that the long-term control (83% to 88%) is similar to the results reported for irradiated temporal bone tumors.[28,29]

Because of the location of paraganglioma in the temporal bone, many of these tumors are treated with radiation alone. Surgery for most tumors in the temporal bone may be complicated by new cranial nerve deficits.[30-33] Radiation treatments are effective for these tumors (88% to 100% control rate) with a low risk of complications and improvements in clinical symptoms.[30,34-36] For these reasons, most temporal bone paragangliomas are initially treated with irradiation. Surgical treatment is used for early tumors of the middle ear and possibly of the jugular foramen, and for the few patients whose tumors progress after irradiation.

SIMULATION AND TREATMENT PLANNING

The radiation treatment for paragangliomas consists of localized treatment to an adequate volume. All available diagnostic information should be used in determining the gross tumor volume (GTV). As discussed in the section on diagnostic imaging, CT, MRI, and angiograms all have a role in determining the nature and extent of a paraganglioma. The clinical target volume (CTV) is the GTV plus a margin for microscopic tumor extension. Since lymph node spread is rare for paragangliomas, the CTV only needs to account for microscopic extent in the region of the GTV. The target volume to be treated is the planning target volume (PTV). The PTV takes into account intrafractional and interfractional variations. The treatment of this volume ensures that the CTV receives the prescribed dose. Although the temporal bone paragangliomas do not move with physiologic processes, one should account for the factors of daily setup variation and patient motion during treatment.

Most paragangliomas are well treated using wedge-pair techniques. The usual orientation of the fields is in the anterior-posterior plane. For lesions in the temporal bone, exit through the opposite eye must be avoided. This can be accomplished by careful selection of the angles or by positioning the patient in a hyperextended position with the chin up. Another alternative is a superior-inferior orientation of the wedge pair. All of these patients benefit from immobilization of the head. Three-dimensional treatment planning is essential for the treatment of large lesions and is also useful for small to moderate-sized lesions as well.

Simulation films for a typical treatment of a temporal bone paraganglioma are shown in Figures 22-7 and 22-8. The patient was immobilized in a thermoplastic face

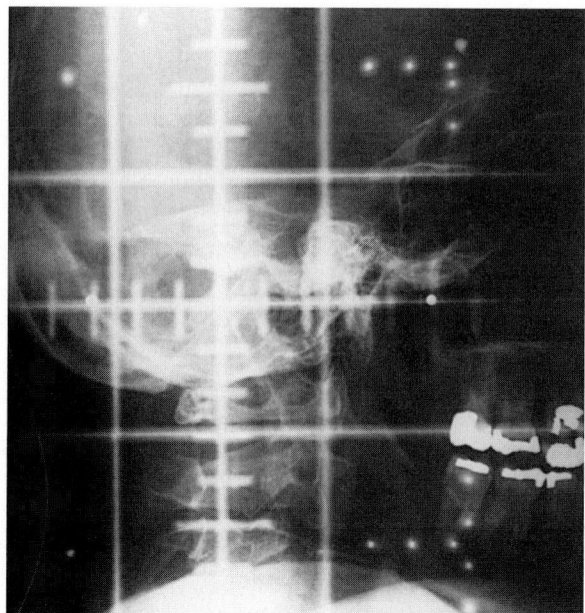

Figure 22–7. This patient had a temporal bone paraganglioma recurrent after surgery. The right anterior oblique simulation film is an example of a typical treatment field.

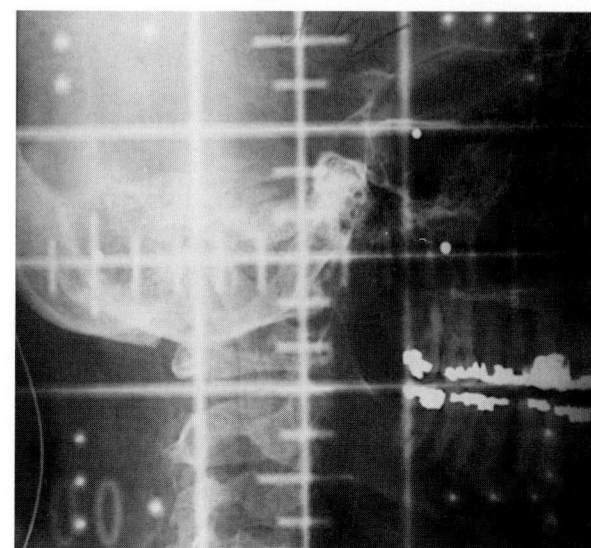

Figure 22–8. The right posterior oblique simulation film shows that the angle was chosen to avoid exit through the left eye.

mask and underwent three-dimensional treatment planning. A treatment planning CT scan was done with the patient in the mask on a flat couch. The CTV was drawn on each CT image by the treating clinician. A margin to account for interfractional and intrafractional variations was added to create the PTV. In addition, the critical normal structures, including both globes and the brainstem, were drawn on each CT image. Beam's eye view (BEV) techniques were used to determine the optimal angles of the right anterior and posterior oblique fields. Figure 22-9 shows the BEV for the right posterior oblique field. At the time of simulation, the position of the isocenter in the patient was verified using anterior-posterior and lateral BEVs generated by the treatment planning program. In addition, the simulation films were checked against the BEVs for the oblique fields. The dose distribution was optimized using appropriate field margins for penumbra and wedges so that the PTV was homogeneously treated (Fig. 22-10).

A prescribed dose of 45 to 50 Gy in daily fractions of 1.8 to 2 Gy is generally used. A review by Kim and associates[34] demonstrated a high recurrence rate (22%) in patients treated with doses of less than 40 Gy in 4 weeks. Doses to the brainstem and spinal cord should be within tolerance with good treatment planning. Intensity-modulated radiotherapy, fractionated stereotactic radiotherapy, and stereotactic radiosurgery (SRS) are additional possible treatment modalities. Currently, SRS is being used with increasing frequency.

STEREOTACTIC RADIOSURGERY

Stereotactic radiosurgery is an emerging treatment modality for paragangliomas of the skull base. The primary advantages are decreased radiation exposure to normal surrounding tissues and a dramatically shortened length of therapy. Stereotactic radiosurgery is performed by two main techniques: the Leksell Gamma Knife Unit and LINAC (linear accelerator)-based treatment. Both delivery systems are used successfully in the treatment of paragangliomas.[37-42] These techniques use stereotaxic frame-based target localization, using axial, coronal, and sagittal imaging for three-dimensional planning, with submillimeter accuracy. Imaging techniques of CT, MRI, and angiography are used in conjunction to increase the accuracy of tumor localization.[43] Figures 22-11A–C demonstrate the excellent coverage of the target by the 50% isodose surface. The prescribed or margin dose range in reported series range from a mean of 15 Gy to 19.4 Gy (Table 22-1).[37-42]

Small paragangliomas of the temporal bone can be considered for treatment with SRS. However, the results for SRS at this time have a fairly short median follow-up time for a tumor that may have late failures. In addition, the PTV must not be too narrow in order to minimize the risk of marginal recurrences.

TREATMENT TOXICITY

In 1990 Springate and Weichselbaum[30] published a review of reports in the literature for temporal bone paragangliomas treated with external beam radiotherapy. They analyzed complications and determined that serious complications were rare (2% to 3%). The complications consisted of bone necrosis (1.7%) and brain necrosis/abscess (0.84%). A single second malignancy (fibrosarcoma) was reported. In a single institution report on the long-term results for radiation treatment of temporal bone tumors, the complication rate was low, as well.[44] There were no instances of brain or bone necrosis, but facial nerve palsies developed in two patients who received high doses (64 Gy and 66 Gy).

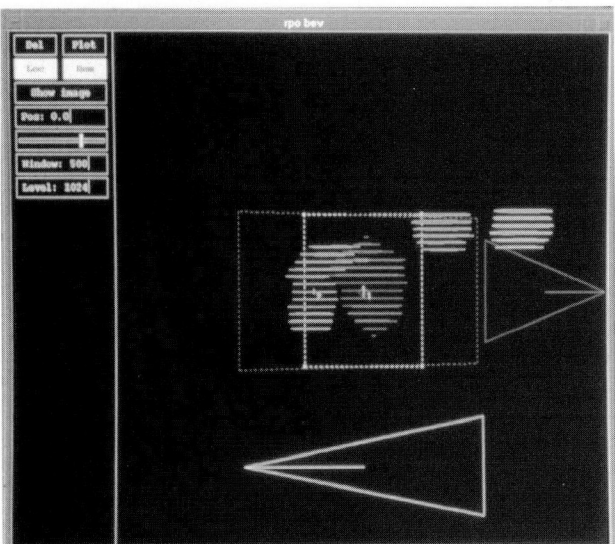

Figure 22–9. Beam's eye view of the right posterior oblique field shows the planning target volume, brainstem, and globes. Note that the left eye is excluded. See also Color Figure 22-9.

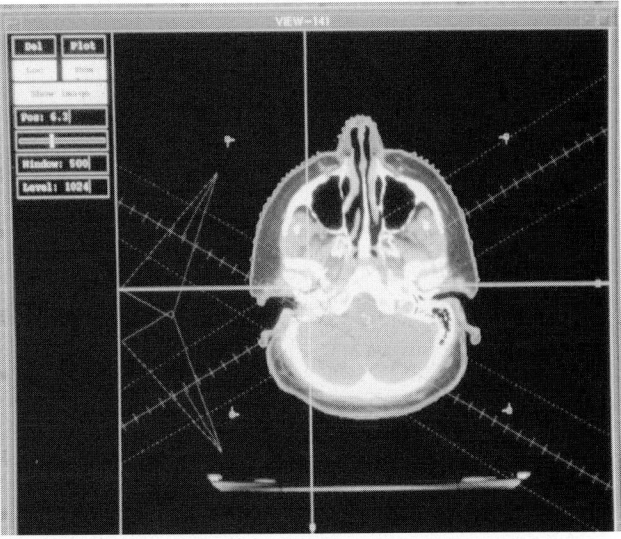

Figure 22–10. Dose distribution for treatment of a recurrent temporal bone paraglioma. The 100% isodose line corresponds to 5040 cGy. The planning target volume and the 95% isodose line are also shown. See also Color Figure 22-10.

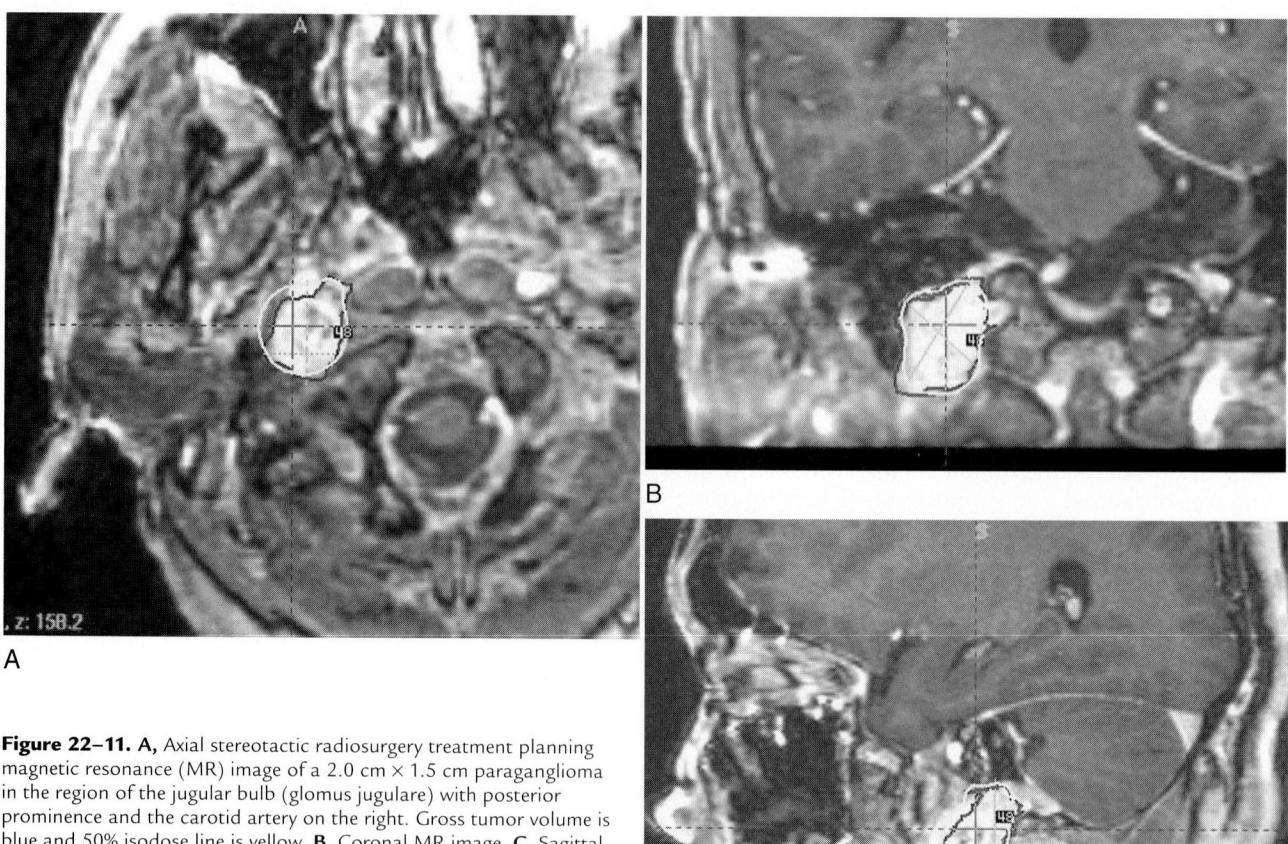

Figure 22–11. A, Axial stereotactic radiosurgery treatment planning magnetic resonance (MR) image of a 2.0 cm × 1.5 cm paraganglioma in the region of the jugular bulb (glomus jugulare) with posterior prominence and the carotid artery on the right. Gross tumor volume is blue and 50% isodose line is yellow. **B,** Coronal MR image. **C,** Sagittal MR image. (Courtesy of James G. Douglas, MD, MS.) See also Color Figure 22-11.

Table 22–1   Stereotactic Radiosurgery of Paragangliomas: Dosing and Target Size

References	Patients, *n*	Margin Dose	Max. Dose	Prescribe Isodose	Volume
Liscak et al[37]	14	19.4 Gy (10–25)	37.4 Gy		5.5 cm³ (0.7–11.3)
Liscak et al[38]	66	16.5 Gy (10–30)	32 Gy (20–60)		5.7 cm³ (0.5–27)
Eustacchio et al[39]	13	13.5 Gy (12–20)		50% (30–50%)	6.4 cm³ (4.6–13.7)
Jordan et al[40]	8	16.3 Gy (12–20)	33 Gy (22–46.5)		9.81 cm³ (4.29–17.25)
Foote et al[41]	25	15.0 Gy (12–18)		50%	10.4 cm³ (1.2–29.3)
Feigenberg et al[42]	5	15.0 Gy (12.5–15)		80% (2), 70% (3)	10.84 cm³ (4.9–18.4)

Table 22–2   Local Control of Chemodectomas Treated with Fractionated Radiation

Reference	Dose, Gy	Local Control*	Follow-up, yr
Powell et al[44]	35–66	39/46	9 (median)
Wang et al[45]	29–67.5	12/15	5–33
Hinerman et al[46]	37.7–60	40/43	11.1 (median)
Konefal et al[47]	46–55	20/22	10.5 (mean)
Cummings et al[48]	35/3 wk	42/45	10 (median)
Sharma et al[49]	40–50	33/40	13 (mean)

*Number of patients with local control out of total number studied.

Table 22–3   Stereotactic Radiosurgery of Paragangliomas: Outcome

		Radiographic Size		Symptom		
Reference	Follow-up, mo	*Reduction*	*Stable*	*Progression*	*Improvement*	*Progression*
Liscak et al[37]	20.5 (6–42)	29% (4/14)	71% (10/14)	0%	43% (6/14)	21% (3/14)
Liscak et al[38]	24 (3–70)	37% (19/52)	54% (28/52)	0%	29% (15/52)	6% (3/52)
Eustacchio et al[39]	37.6 (5–68)	31% (4/13)	46% (6/13)	7% (1/13)	38% (5/13)	0%
Jordan et al[40]	27 (7–102)	50% (4/8)	38% (3/8)	0%	50% (4/8)	13% (1/8)
Foote et al[41]	35 (10–113)	68% (17/25)	32% (8/25)	0%	60% (15/25)	4% (1/25)
Feigenberg et al[42]	27 (14–50)	60% (3/5)	0%	40% (2/5)	40% (2/5)	40% (2/5)

OUTCOME

Successful radiation treatment of paragangliomas with conventional external beam irradiation results in symptomatic improvement and long-term absence of tumor progression. As discussed earlier, patients often have a persistent radiographic abnormality after treatment. Springate and Weichselbaum[30] comprehensively reviewed the results of treatment for temporal bone paragangliomas in articles published between 1965 and 1988. The patients had been treated between 1932 and 1983. The control rate was 93%, with a low incidence of complications.

Long-term results were reported by Powell and coworkers[44] in 84 patients. Radiation therapy alone was used in 46 patients with temporal bone tumors. Seven of these patients experienced recurrences. The 10-year actuarial control rate is 90% and the 25-year actuarial local control rate is 73%. Improvement in pain was seen in virtually all patients, and cranial nerve palsies improved in 20% of the patients. Similar 10-year results have been reported in many series and are summarized in Table 22-2.[44-49]

Several published series between 1998 and 2002 demonstrate effective local control and symptom improvement in patients treated with stereotactic radiosurgery (Table 22-3).[37-42] Local control or tumor reduction is achieved in 60% to 100% of treated patients, and symptomatic improvement is reported in 29% to 60% of patients. Radiologic tumor progression was observed in only 3 of 131 patients.[39,42] Progression of symptoms, or new symptoms, including tinnitus, hearing loss, facial nerve dysfunction, and vertigo have been reported in 4% to 40% of patients.

REFERENCES

1. Lawson W: The neuroendocrine nature of the glomus cells: An experimental, ultrastructural, and histochemical tissue culture study. *Laryngoscope.* 1980;90:120.
2. Sobol SM, Dailey JC: Familial multiple cervical paragangliomas: Report of a kindred and review of the literature. *Otolaryngol Head Neck Surg.* 1990;102:382.
3. Mulligan RM: Chemodectoma in the dog. *Am J Pathol.* 1950;26:681.
4. Parry DM, Frederick PL, Strong LC, et al: Carotid body tumors in humans: Genetics and epidemiology. *J Natl Cancer Inst.* 1982;68:573.
5. van der Mey AGL, Furns JHM, Brons EN, et al: Does intervention improve the natural course of glomus tumors? A series of 108 patients seen in a 32 year period. *Ann Otol Rhinol Laryngol.* 1992;101:635.
6. Saladana MJ, Salem LE, Travezan R: High altitude hypoxia and chemodectomas. *Hum Pathol.* 1973;4:251.
7. Farrior JB III, Hyams VJ, Benke RH, et al: Carcinoid apudoma arising in a glomus jugulare tumor: Review of endocrine activity in glomus jugulare tumors. *Laryngoscope.* 1980;90:110.
8. Zbaran P, Lehmann W: Carotid body paraganglioma with metastases. *Laryngoscope.* 1985;95:450.
9. Hodge KM, Beyers RM, Peters LJ: Paragangliomas of the head and neck. *Arch Otolaryngol.* 1988;114:872.
10. Chase WH: Familial and bilateral tumors of the carotid body. *J Pathol Bacteriol.* 1993;36:1.
11. Tran LP, Velanovich V, Kaufmann CR: Familial multiple glomus tumors: Report of a pedigree and literature review. *Ann Plast Surg.* 1994;32:89.
12. van Barrs F, Cremers C, van den Borek P, et al: Genetic aspect of nonchromaffin paraganglioma. *Hum Genet.* 1982;60:305.
13. Heutink P, van der Mey AG, Sandkuijl LA, et al: A gene subject to genomic imprinting and responsible for hereditary paragangliomas maps to chromosome 11q23-qter. *Hum Mol Genet.* 1992;1:7.
14. Mariman EC, van Beersum SE, Cremers CW, et al: Analysis of a second family with hereditary non-chromaffin paragangliomas locates the underlying gene at the proximal region of chromosome 11q. *Hum Genet.* 1993;91:357.
15. Niemann S, Muller U: Mutations in SDHC cause autosomal dominant paraganglioma, type 3. *Nat Genet.* 2000;26:268.
16. Enzinger FAA, Weiss SW: *Soft Tissue Tumors,* 3rd ed. St. Louis: Mosby Year-Book; 1993:969.
17. van der Mey AGL, Cornelisse CJ, Hermans J, et al: DNA flow cytometry of hereditary and sporadic paragangliomas (glomus tumors). *Br J Cancer.* 1991;63:298.
18. Krupski WC, Effeney DJ, Ehrenfeld WK, et al: Cervical chemodectoma. Technical considerations and management options. *Am J Surg.* 1982;144:215.
19. Alford BR, Guilford FR: A comprehensive study of tumor of glomus jugulare. *Brain.* 1953;76:576.
20. Lee JH, Barich F, Karnell LH, et al: National Cancer Data Base report on malignant paragangliomas of the head and neck. *Cancer.* 2002;94:730.
21. Som PM, Bergeron RT: *Head and Neck Imaging,* 2nd ed. St. Louis: Mosby Year-Book;1994:480.
22. Som PM, Bergeron RT: *Head and Neck Imaging,* 2nd ed. St. Louis: Mosby Year-Book; 1991:1073.
23. Vogl T, Bürning R, Schedel H, et al: Paragangliomas of the jugular bulb and carotid body: MR imaging with short sequences and Gd-DTPA enhancement. *AJR.* 1989;153:587.
24. Phelps PD, Cheesman AD: Imaging jugulotympanic glomus tumors. *Arch Otolaryngol Head Neck Surg.* 1990;116:940.
25. Vogl TJ, Mack MG, Juergens M, et al: Skull base tumors: Gadodiamide injection—enhanced MR imaging—Drop-out effect in the early enhancement pattern of paragangliomas versus different tumors. *Radiology.* 1993;188:339.

26. van der Mey AGL, Maaswinkel-Mooy PD, Cornelisse CJ, et al: Genomic imprinting in hereditary glomus tumors: Evidence for new genetic theory. *Lancet.* 1989;60:1291.

27. Mukherji SK, Kasper ME, Tart RP, et al: Irradiated paragangliomas of the head and neck: CT and MR appearance. *Am J Neuroradiol.* 1994;15:357.

28. Guedea F, Mendenhall WM, Parsons JT, et al: Radiotherapy for chemodectoma of the carotid body and ganglion nodosum. *Head Neck.* 1991;13:509.

29. Verniers DA, Keus RB, Schouwenburg PF, et al: Radiation therapy, an important mode of treatment for head and neck chemodectomas. *Eur J Cancer.* 1992;28A:1028.

30. Springate SC, Weichselbaum RR: Radiation or surgery for chemodectoma of the temporal bone: A review of local control and complications. *Head Neck.* 1990;12:303.

31. Green JD, Brackman DE, Nguyen CD, et al: Surgical management of previously untreated glomus jugulare tumors. *Laryngoscope.* 1994;104:917.

32. Watkins LD, Mendoza N, Cheesman AD, Smon L: Glomus jugulare tumors: A review of 61 cases. *Acta Neurochir.* 1994; 130:66.

33. Patel SJ, Sekhar LN, Cass SP, Hirsch BE: Combined approaches for resection of glomus jugulare tumors: A review of 12 cases. *J Neurosurg.* 1994;80:1026.

34. Kim J-A, Elkon D, Lim M-L, et al: Optimum dose of radiotherapy for chemodectomas of the middle ear. *Int J Radiat Oncol Biol Phys.* 1980;6:815.

35. Larner JM, Hahn SS, Spaulding CA, Constable WC: Glomus jugulare tumors. Long-term control by radiation therapy. *Cancer.* 1992;69:1813.

36. Schild SE, Foote RL, Buskirk SJ, et al: Results of radiotherapy for chemodectomas. *Mayo Clin Proc.* 1992;67:537.

37. Liscak R, Vladyka V, Simonova G, et al: Leksell gamma knife radiosurgery of the tumor glomus jugulare and tympanicum. *Stereotact Funct Neurosurg.* 1998;70(suppl 1):152.

38. Liscak R, Vladyka V, Wowra B, et al: Gamma Knife radiosurgery of the glomus jugulare tumour—Early multicentre experience. *Acta Neurochir (Wien).* 1999;141:1141.

39. Eustacchio S, Leber K, Trummer M, et al: Gamma knife radiosurgery for glomus jugulare tumours. *Acta Neurochir (Wien).* 1999;141:811.

40. Jordan JA, Roland PS, McManus C, et al: Stereotactic radiosurgery for glomus jugulare tumors. *Laryngoscope.* 2000;110:35.

41. Foote RL, Pollock BE, Gorman DA, et al: Glomus jugulare tumor: Tumor control and complications after stereotactic radiosurgery. *Head Neck.* 2002;24:332; discussion 338.

42. Feigenberg SJ, Mendenhall WM, Hinerman RW, et al: Radiosurgery for paraganglioma of the temporal bone. *Head Neck.* 2002;24:384.

43. Phillips MH, Stelzer KJ, Griffin TW, et al: Stereotactic radiosurgery: A review and comparison of methods. *J Clin Oncol.* 1994; 12:1085.

44. Powell S, Peters N, Harmer C: Chemodectoma of the head and neck: Results of treatment in 84 patients. *Int J Radiat Oncol Biol Phys.* 1992;22:919.

45. Wang M-L, Hussey DH, Doornbos JF, et al: Chemodectoma of the temporal bone: A comparison of surgical and radiotherapeutic results. *Int J Radiat Oncol Biol Phys.* 1988;14:643.

46. Hinerman RW, Mendenhall WM, Amdur RJ, et al: Definitive radiotherapy in the management of chemodectomas arising in the temporal bone, carotid body, and glomus vagale. *Head Neck.* 2001:May;363.

47. Konefal JB, Pilepich MV, Spector GJ: Radiation therapy in the treatment of chemodectomas. *Laryngoscope.* 1987;97:1331.

48. Cummings BJ, Beale FA, Garrett PG, et al: The treatment of glomus tumors in the temporal bone by megavoltage radiation. *Cancer.* 1984;53:2635.

49. Sharma PD, Johnson AP, Whitton AC: Radiotherapy for jugulotympanic paragangliomas (glomus jugulare tumors). *J Laryngol Oncol.* 1984;98:621.

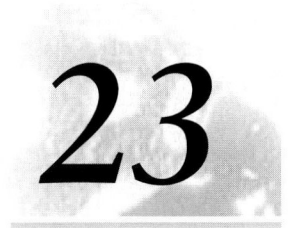

Skull Base Tumors: Chordomas and Chondrosarcomas

John E. Munzenrider, MD, Judy Adams, CMD,
and Norbert J. Liebsch, MD, PhD

ANATOMY, PATHOLOGY, AND INCIDENCE OF SKULL BASE TUMORS

The skull base can be divided into anterior, middle, and posterior regions, corresponding to the anterior, middle, and posterior fossae of the cranium. The undersurfaces of the frontal, temporal, parietal, and occipital lobes of the brain and that of the cerebellum occupy these fossae. The cranial nerves, brainstem, and cerebral blood vessels traverse the skull base through specific, named foramina. This anatomically complex, bony, protective structure is composed of six separate bones: the temporal, frontal, parietal, sphenoid, occipital, and zygomatic bones.

Skull base and cervical spine tumors are estimated to represent between 3% and 11% of primary bone tumors, which have an estimated annual incidence in the United States of 84 in 100,000. Histologically, osteosarcoma and chondrosarcoma are the most common primary bone tumors, although benign and malignant neoplasms of any histologic type can occur at these sites. Osteosarcoma not infrequently involves the maxilla or the mandible but is seen relatively infrequently at the skull base. Chordoma, a rare tumor thought to originate in rests of the embryonal notochord, always occurs in the midline, with 35% to 40% occurring in the skull base. Some benign tumors, such as pituitary adenomas, acoustic neuromas, benign meningiomas, and craniopharyngiomas, as well as atypical and malignant meningiomas and advanced epithelial tumors involving the paranasal sinuses and nasopharynx can also be seen in the skull base.[1,2]

Accurate pathologic diagnosis is essential, since treatment, patterns of spread, and prognosis can be quite different for tumors of the various cell types. The cartilaginous tumors offer a particular challenge to the pathologist. Of 255 patients reviewed at the Massachusetts General Hospital (MGH), 40% of patients referred with a diagnosis of chordoma were rediagnosed as having chondrosarcomas, resulting in an almost equal proportion of each tumor type being included in that series: 125 chordomas and 130 chondrosarcomas.[3]

Chordomas are characterized by lobules of cohesive polygonal and rounded cells arranged in nests and cords, embedded in a flocculent myxoid ground substance. The cytoplasm may be granular, eosinophilic, or, less frequently, clear. The hallmark of the chordoma is the presence of so-called *psysaliferous cells*, containing numerous intracytoplasmic vacuoles, which may indent the nucleus. Nuclear pleomorphism can be seen, although the nuclei are more commonly uniformly round. Mitotic counts vary, necrosis is infrequent, and vascular invasion is rare. The chondroid variant of chordoma contains a mixture of the typical chordoma pattern and cartilaginous features. These chondrosarcomatous-appearing areas are characterized by small cells arranged in lacunae, which lack cytoplasmic vacuolation, embedded in a hyaline matrix.[3] Special immunohistochemical stains may be helpful in classifying these tumors.[4]

Skull base tumors can be discovered on imaging studies performed to evaluate specific symptoms, such as headaches, gait disturbance, hearing loss, nasal or eustachian tube obstruction, visual loss, or ocular dysmotility. The diagnosis can also present as an incidental finding on studies done following trauma. In 97 patients with skull base tumors (49 low-grade chondrosarcomas, and 48 chordomas), the most common symptoms at presentation were headache (in 67% of chordoma patients and 49% of chondrosarcoma patients) and intermittent diplopia (in 75% of chordoma patients and 78% of chondrosarcoma patients). Decreased visual acuity or hearing, facial numbness or weakness, tinnitus, dysphagia, and dysarthria were also present initially in those patients.[5]

Regardless of presenting symptoms or histologic classification, patients with skull base tumors present a formidable management problem. Total resection is usually not possible due to involvement of adjacent critical normal structures, such as the optic nerves, optic chiasm, cranial nerves, major blood vessels, and brain and brainstem. The adjacency of these structures may also limit the radiation dose that can be delivered safely. This is less of a problem with tumors such as benign meningiomas, schwannomas, giant cell tumors, pituitary adenomas, and craniopharyngiomas, for which relatively lower doses (54 to 60 Gy) are generally prescribed. However, epithelial and sarcomatous tumors require much higher radiation doses (68 to 76 Gy) to achieve local control. When tumors requiring higher doses are adjacent to multiple dose-limiting normal structures, the radiation modalities and techniques that can best localize the dose delivered to the defined target are especially attractive.

Fractionated particle beam therapy has been shown to offer a significant advantage for patients with cartilaginous tumors of the skull base.[6,7] The Harvard Cyclotron's fixed horizontal 160 MeV proton beam has maximum penetration in tissue of 16.0 cm. This energy is particularly well suited for treating skull base tumors. The majority of skull base tumor patients treated with fractionated proton beam therapy have had chordomas and low-grade chondrosarcomas. The remainder of this chapter discusses techniques developed for such patients, results of that treatment, and a currently operative protocol in that patient population.

PROTON THERAPY AT THE HARVARD CYCLOTRON LABORATORY

In 1973, what has proved to be a most durable collaboration between the MGH Radiation Oncology Department (formerly Radiation Medicine Service) and the Harvard Cyclotron Laboratory (HCL) commenced, with the express purpose of studying human tumor and normal tissue responses to fractionated proton beam radiotherapy.[8] This program complemented a single-fraction proton stereotactic radiosurgery program, dating to 1961,[9,10] that currently involves collaboration between the MGH radiation oncology and neurosurgery departments. The improved dose localization properties of high-energy protons relative to high-energy x-rays make such beams of particular interest for clinical radiotherapy: the dose delivered to a defined target (tumor, vascular anomaly, or other structure) can usually be increased without a corresponding increase in the dose to adjacent dose-limiting normal tissues. Normal tissue beyond the target volume receives additional and superfluous radiation dose from an exponentially decreasing x-ray beam, but none from a proton beam, as shown in Figure 23-1.

The positively charged protons have very favorable physical characteristics for clinical radiotherapy, most importantly, a finite range in tissue as a function of their energy. Any reduction in the volume of non-target tissue included in the high-dose region is primarily due to the absence of dose beyond the end of range of the proton beam. There can also be a lower dose in the entrance region of each beam as well. This ability to achieve reduced dose in both the exit and entrance path of the proton beam remains the predominant factor in developing superior treatment plans with charged particle beams, relative to those that can be achieved with supervoltage x-rays. Proton dose distributions that conform in three dimensions to the defined target volume can best be realized by use of computerized three-dimensional (3D) treatment planning programs. Since protons are low LET (linear energy transfer) particles, they do not have any significant biologic advantage over conventional supervoltage x-rays.[11]

The Harvard Cyclotron's fixed horizontal 160 MeV proton beam has maximum penetration in tissue of 16 cm. This energy is particularly well suited for intracranial, paracranial, and cervical spine tumors in general, and for

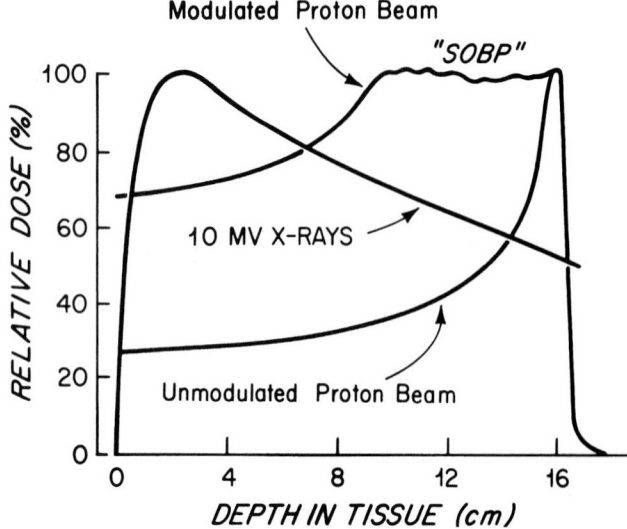

Figure 23–1. Central axis depth dose for 160 MeV mono-energetic and a modulated ("spread out") proton beam, shown with the depth dose curve for a 10 MV linear accelerator beam. Note that dose falls to 0 at approximately 16 cm depth with the proton beam, while the dose from the x-ray beam continues to decrease exponentially off the scale.

skull base tumors in particular. The majority of skull base tumor patients treated with protons have had chordomas and low-grade chondrosarcomas; fractionated particle beam therapy has been shown to offer a significant advantage for patients with these tumors.[6,7] Techniques developed for these patients have been successfully applied to other tumors arising at the skull base, including benign, atypical, and malignant meningiomas, soft tissue and bone sarcomas,[12] and advanced epithelial tumors involving the paranasal sinuses and nasopharynx.

Initial Patient Evaluation

Patients who did not have their primary surgery at MGH are reviewed at the MGH-Massachusetts Eye and Ear Infirmary (MEEI) Skull Base Center Rounds, with consultation from neurosurgeons, otologists, skull base surgeons, pathologists, and neuroradiologists, to obtain optimal understanding of the current patient status and to assess whether additional surgery might facilitate treatment. The primary goal of any additional surgery that might be recommended is to reduce or eliminate tumor bulk, so as to achieve better geometry between the tumor and the dose-constraining normal tissues. Such improved tumor–normal tissue geometry may allow a more optimal dose distribution to the residual tumor to be achieved, with maximal sparing of adjacent dose-limiting normal tissues. Occipital-cervical spine fusion may also be recommended for patients thought to be orthopedically unstable, due to bone destruction by tumor. Endocrine, auditory, and ophthalmologic status is formally assessed before initiation of treatment in patients expected to receive significant radiation dose to the hypothalamic-pituitary axis, the middle ear, and the optic nerves and chiasm, respectively.

Three-Dimensional Treatment Planning

Tissue inhomogeneity, such as air cavities or bone, result in much greater dose perturbations with charged particles than with x-rays. Because of varying amounts of muscle, bone, and air at the skull base, it is critical to accurately quantitate the tissue density along the beam path, so that precise compensation for inhomogeneities can be incorporated into the treatment plan.[13-15] It is also crucial that the patient be precisely aligned to the compensator during treatment, so that dose delivered to the target will be distributed as planned. Techniques for patient immobilization, treatment planning, aperture and compensator specification and fabrication, and treatment techniques used for proton beam therapy at the Harvard Cyclotron Laboratory are subsequently described.

Patients are immobilized in the treatment position[16,17] with various combinations of an individualized mouthpiece, a thermoplastic face mask, and a body mold. A treatment planning computed tomographic (CT) scan is performed on the immobilized patient using contiguous slices of 1 to 3 mm thickness throughout the tumor region. The CT scan data set is transferred to the treatment planning computer, and contours outlining the targets and critical normal tissues throughout the treatment volume are manually drawn on the computer monitor on serial CT sections. Usually, two target volumes are drawn for each patient, with the smaller defining the macroscopic tumor demonstrated on imaging studies, and the larger adding an appropriate margin to allow for microscopic extension not detectable on the imaging studies. Targets are determined from operative notes, consultation with the operating surgeon, and from preoperative and postoperative imaging studies, specifically CT and magnetic resonance imaging (MRI) scans. Optic nerves and chiasm, middle ear, brainstem and spinal cord, and the temporal lobes are also defined on the planning scan. Target volumes generally do not overlap with normal tissues, so as to make an explicit statement regarding tumor location relative to that of dose-limiting normal tissues.

The *beam's-eye view* feature of the interactive treatment planning program is employed to define treatment apertures that encompass the defined target from multiple angles, while minimizing dose to defined normal tissues.[18] Treatment plans are developed to deliver the prescribed dose, while limiting the dose delivered to the optic nerves and chiasm and to the brainstem and spinal cord surface and center to the defined tolerance levels. A dose gradient will exist in cases in which the target abuts or displaces any of these normal structures. The target abutting the structure receives the constraining dose for that structure, with the dose rapidly increasing to the prescribed level in the rest of the tumor volume. Dose contour at depth is shaped with portal-specific compensators. Both apertures and compensators are specified by the treatment planning system to a computer-controlled milling machine and are individually fabricated for each field from brass and tissue-equivalent plastic, respectively. Each separate portal requires an aperture-compensator set, with as many portals being employed as are necessary to obtain optimal target coverage while minimizing the dose to normal tissue. An average of seven separate proton portals and two to three x-ray portals are used for the treatment of most skull base tumors.

Three-dimensional dose distributions throughout the entire volume of interest are reviewed before plan implementation, so that unexpected dose variations can be corrected before actual treatment.

Dose and Fractionation

The prescribed tumor dose varies with histology. Generally, lower doses, ranging from 54 to 63 CGyEq (CGyEq [cobalt gray equivalent] = proton Gy $\times$ RBE [relative biologic effectiveness] 1.1)[8] are given to benign tumors, such as acoustic neuromas, benign meningiomas, and craniopharyngiomas. For more "radioresistant" tumors, target doses ranging from 66.6 to 79.2 CGyEq have been prescribed to the macroscopic tumor volume, while the larger volume thought to potentially contain microscopic tumor only is prescribed a lower dose, on the order of 50 to 54 CGyEq. The Cyclotron has generally been available only 4 days per week, with the fifth day reserved for the stereotactic radiosurgery program. Early in the program, patients received four fractions of 2.1 CGyEq per week. Since normal tissue tolerance is related to dose per fraction, the daily increment was changed to 1.8 CGyEq, with patients getting four proton and one x-ray treatment per week. In a few cases, all treatment was given with protons, daily for 3 days, and twice daily on the fourth day. In such cases, the interfraction interval was 7 hours or more. The use of x-rays can also achieve some skin sparing, since the entrance dose from the proton beam increases as the proton beam is modulated (spread out), as shown in Figure 23-1.

Treatment Techniques and Documentation

Patients are treated in the same immobilization device used for the treatment planning scan. Patient position is verified radiographically before each treatment. Setup accuracy and reproducibility is $\pm$ 1 to 2 mm.[16,17]

The primary and secondary targets (T1 and T2) and the brainstem, optic nerves, and chiasm of a patient with a clival chordoma are shown in Figure 23-2A. 3D dose distributions are calculated and can be displayed on the monitor as traditional isodose lines (see Fig. 23-2A) or as a color wash display (Fig. 23-2B). Figure 23-2C shows an application of the *patch technique*, which is used to contour the dose around the brainstem by treating a portion of the target with, in this example, a left posterior oblique (LPO) portal and the remainder with a right lateral portal. Tumor extension toward the right side anterior to the brainstem, which is inadequately covered by the LPO portal, is treated by the right lateral portal, with dose delivered by that portal stopping (ranging out) in the target that has already been treated by the LPO portal. Alternatively, the range of the right lateral portal could be increased, and the LPO used to treat only that portion of the target extending posterior to the posterior margin of the right lateral portal. Small *hot spots* are created with this technique in that portion of the target

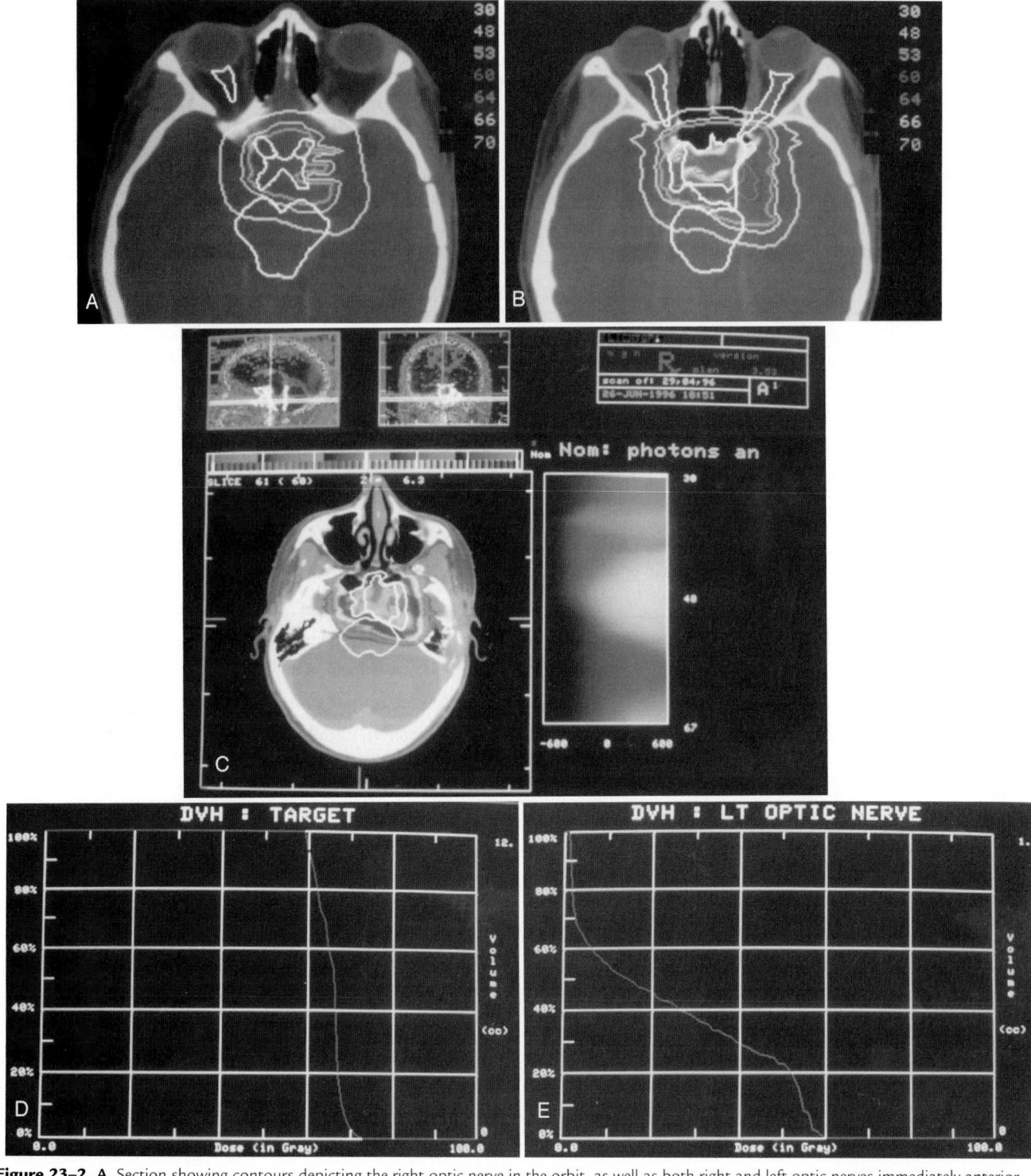

Figure 23–2. A, Section showing contours depicting the right optic nerve in the orbit, as well as both right and left optic nerves immediately anterior to the optic chiasm, which are also shown. Brainstem is also drawn. Dose distribution is shown in isodose lines. The entire chiasm and proximal optic nerves receive at least 53 Gy, but 60 Gy is not received by any structures at this level. **B,** A CT section 6 mm inferior to that shown in 2A shows both optic nerves, as well as both primary (smaller) and secondary (larger) target volumes, which include the entire sellar contents. Brainstem is also contoured. The posterior portion of the target volume receives a dose less than or equal to 60 Gy, while the anterior portion of the target volume receives a dose gradient from 60 to 53 Gy. **C,** At a level of 2.4 cm inferior to the chiasm, smaller and larger volumes both receive a uniform dose, as shown by the magenta color. A dose gradient exists across the brainstem from approximately 30 Gy (blue) up to 64 Gy (red-magenta transition at the edge of the brainstem). **D** and **E,** The dose volume histograms for the primary target (macroscopic disease) *(D)* and the left optic nerve *(E)*. Note that virtually all the target receives greater than 60 CGyEq, but the prescribed dose of 66.6 CGyEq is achieved in only 40% to 50% of the target. None of the left optic nerve receives greater than 60 CGyEq. See also Color Figure 23-2.

Neuropsychologic effects were evaluated by a battery of standard psychologic instruments designed to examine specific cognitive function. Thirty-eight patients were studied at specified intervals following initial evaluation and treatment. Median prescribed tumor dose was 68.4 CGyEq (range, 66.6 to 72 CGyEq); some portion of the brain adjacent to the defined target volume received the prescribed dose. Seventeen patients were restudied 48 months or more after treatment. No adverse effects on cognitive function were demonstrated. Performance on tests of verbal and nonverbal learning and memory, simultaneous attention and concentration, and language and visuospatial processing either remained stable or improved slightly over time, possibly as a result of repetition of the tests. Statistically significant slowing of motor speed and reaction time was shown for the group as a whole. Self-reported assessments of mood and psychiatric symptoms showed progressive improvement in anxiety, depression, and self-perceived cognitive efficiency. Fatigue levels remained stable over the course of observation. It appeared that over the first 12 to 18 months after treatment, the patients either improved or stabilized from an emotional standpoint, while some degree of motor slowing was appearing during that same time frame.[27]

Treatment techniques have been modified to try to decrease the frequency of brain injury. A minimum of two portals are usually treated each day, to decrease the daily dose increment delivered to non–target tissues in the entrance region. A greater number and variety of beam directions are also being employed, including not only direct lateral portals but both simple and compound angles of approach for posterior, oblique, or superior portals.

VISION

Neurovisual changes following treatment have been described.[28] More recently, visual function was evaluated in 274 patients with minimum follow-up of 12 months. Prescribed tumor doses ranged from 61 to 76 CGyEq, with the dose to the optic nerves and chiasm constrained at less than or equal to 60 CGyEq; one optic nerve was allowed to receive up to 64 CGyEq if abutted by tumor, and vision in the contralateral eye was good. Optic neuropathy occurred in 12 patients (4.4%): 1 had unilateral hemianopia only, whereas 9 patients developed unilateral and 2 patients developed bilateral blindness (grades 2, 3, and 4, respectively). Visual injury became apparent between 7 and 40 months after treatment; median time to injury was 12 months. Dose distributions and dose-volume histograms for the 12 patients with neuropathy and for a matched control group of 24 patients without toxicity were reviewed. In the injured patients, maximum dose to the optic structures ranged from 50.21 to 69.6 CGyEq, with median dose being 59.43 CGyEq. Various parameters were examined for prognostic value, including minimum, mean, and maximum dose to optic structures; the volume receiving 50, 55, and 60 CGyEq; the presence or absence of diabetes and hypertension; the number of surgical procedures; and distance between the optic structures and the superior extension of the tumor. The separation between the optic structures and the superior extension of the tumor was the only parameter found to be significantly related to the development of optic neuropathy.[29] Treatment plans incorporating the patch technique are now carefully scrutinized before implementation, to assess dose to the optic structures and to determine that optimal beam angles and portal separation have been chosen.

HEARING

The relationship between dose to auditory pathways and audiologic outcome has been assessed in 33 patients. All had had a normal baseline audiogram, had received at least 15 CGyEq to the ipsilateral auditory structures, were free of recurrent tumor near those structures, and had had a follow-up audiogram. Significant hearing loss was documented on audiogram in 15 patients, occurring at 2, 3, 4, and 5 years in 3, 1, 10, and 1 patient, respectively. Four individual structures were outlined on the treatment planning scan in each ear of each patient: the cochlea, its nucleus, the eighth nerve, and the middle ear. The dose that had been delivered to each of the 264 outlined structures (eight structures per patient in 33 patients) was determined. No patient receiving less than or equal to 59 CGyEq to the cochlea or auditory nerve developed hearing loss, whereas almost two thirds of those receiving greater than or equal to 60 CGyEq to either structure manifested significant loss. Progression to severe hearing loss was usually quite rapid after onset.[30]

CRANIAL NEUROPATHY

Twenty-seven patients were evaluated for cranial neuropathies following high-dose irradiation given for chordoma (14), chondrosarcoma (11), acoustic neuroma (1), and meningioma (1). With mean follow-up of 74 months (range, 40 to 110 months), clinically evident cranial nerve dysfunction that had developed following treatment and could not be attributed to tumor progression was seen in 17 nerves in 15 patients. Cranial nerves and their related nuclei were drawn on the planning scan used for the treatment, and the dose that had been delivered to each of the 594 outlined structures (22 structures per patient in 27 patients) was determined. The actual dose delivered to the nerve was found to predict the likelihood of injury, which increased from an estimated probability of 1% at 60 CGyEq (0.5% to 3%, 95% confidence limits) to 5% at 70 CGyEq (64 to 81 CGyEq, 95% confidence limits), as shown in Figure 23-5. The slope of the dose-response curve at 50% was 3.2 (2.2 to 5.4, 95% confidence limits). There was no significant relation between the latency period for appearance of nerve dysfunction and the dose delivered to the nerve or its nucleus.[19] The dose delivered to the optic structures is constrained, as noted earlier, but no constraints are employed for the other cranial nerves. The doses to cochlea and the eighth nerve, however, are kept as low as possible.

ENDOCRINOPATHY

Neuroendocrine changes following treatment have been described.[31] More recently, endocrine function was evaluated before and after treatment in 79 skull base

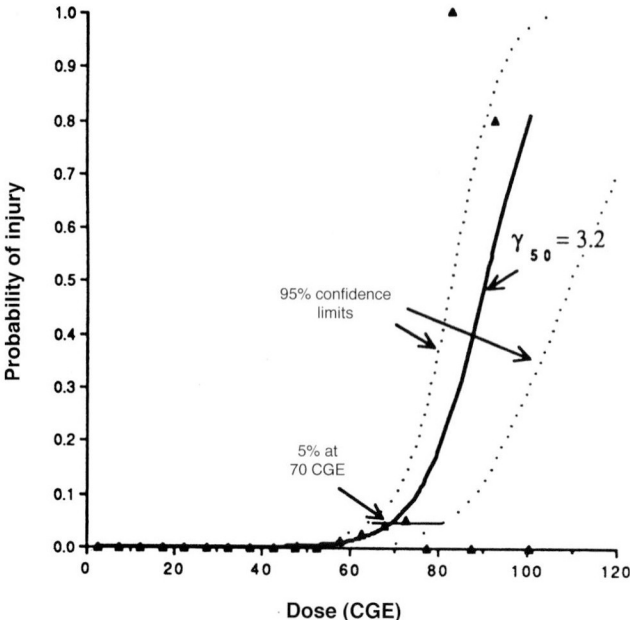

Figure 23–5. Probability of cranial nerve injury as function of dose. Data points are shown by triangles, while the solid line represents the logistic regression of complication probability. The slope of the dose response curve at 50% is indicated by gamma. The 95% confidence limits indicate the probable range of dose at which a given complication rate could be seen. (Reprinted from Urie MU, Fullerton B, Tatsuzaki H, et al: A dose response analysis of injury to cranial nerves and/or nuclei following proton beam radiation therapy. *Int J Radiat Oncol Biol Phys.* 1992;23:27, with permission from Elsevier.)

sarcoma patients who received greater than or equal to 40 CGyEq to the pituitary gland. Median prescribed tumor dose was 68.4 CGyEq, ranging from 48.6 to 75.6 CGyEq. The pituitary gland and a portion of the hypothalamus received the same dose as the tumor in centrally placed upper clival lesions. Relatively lower pituitary doses would generally have been received by chondrosarcoma patients with tumors arising laterally in the temporal bone, and by patients with either histologic type confined to the lower clivus. Endocrinopathy appeared after treatment in 32 of the 79 patients (40%). Growth hormone level was deficient in only 2 patients (3%), but deficiencies in luteinizing hormone, prolactin, thyroid-stimulating hormone, and cortisone were detected in 12 to 18 patients (15% to 23%). Probability of surviving free of endocrinopathy at 5 years was 72% (L. Renard et al., 1997).

Endocrinopathy has developed as late as 8 to 10 years after treatment. Patients whose pituitary-hypothalamic axis will receive greater than or equal to 40 CGyEq are strongly advised to have lifelong endocrine surveillance, since undiagnosed and untreated hormone deficiencies can be disabling and potentially fatal. Most of these hormonal deficiencies are readily replaced with oral hormonal supplementation, although males require transdermal or injected replacement therapy. Secondary amenorrhea is not uncommon; of the women so affected, at least two have delivered healthy full-term infants following pituitary stimulation. Male fertility appears to have been less severely impaired than female fertility.

DISCUSSION

Locally progressive disease and ultimate death usually result within a few years of diagnosis in most patients with skull base sarcomas who are treated with conventional postoperative radiotherapy.[32] The local control and survival rates achieved with the techniques described both in this paper and at Lawrence Berkeley Laboratory (LBL)[7] are markedly superior to results previously reported for skull base chordomas and chondrosarcomas. These improved results can be attributed to the higher doses delivered, primarily because of the improved dose-localization characteristics of the particle beam employed (protons in these patients, helium ions at LBL), and the availability of computerized 3D treatment planning. Whether equally favorable results can be accomplished with single fraction stereotactic radiosurgery or with conformal intensity modulated x-ray therapy remains to be demonstrated.

Complication rates, although higher than desired, may be acceptable, particularly when weighed against the major morbidity and ultimately fatal outcome in patients with uncontrolled tumor growth. Tumor recurrence and treatment-related morbidity can appear at various times after treatment, requiring ongoing surveillance of tumor size and configuration and neurologic, visual, auditory, and endocrine status. This aids in recognizing and treating tumor recurrences, extensions, metastasis, or complications as expeditiously as possible.

In 1985, MGH and LBL collaborated to initiate a randomized prospective clinical trial. Local tumor control and normal tissue effects were to be prospectively assessed in patients with skull base and cervical spine chordomas and chondrosarcomas randomly assigned to receive doses of either 66.6 or 72 CGyEq, given predominantly with protons or with helium ions. The trial was initially coordinated through the National Cancer Institute-sponsored Radiation Therapy Oncology Group (RTOG), and later through the Proton Radiation Oncology Group (PROG). Loma Linda University Medical Center[33] subsequently joined PROG, while treatment with helium ions was terminated at LBL. As the trial progressed, it became apparent that there were two separate groups in this population, in terms of the risk of both local failure and survival. Treatment failures were significantly more likely in female patients with skull base chordoma, and in patients of either sex with cervical spine tumors of either histologic type. Lower-risk patients (males with skull base chordomas and all patients with skull base chondrosarcomas) had a significantly better treatment outcome than did higher-risk patients (females with skull base chordomas and all patients with cervical spine tumors). Because of these differences, the protocol was modified in May 1993. Lower-risk patients continue to be randomized between the original dose levels (66.6 vs. 72 CGyEq), using the normal tissue dose constraints defined earlier. Higher-risk patients (females with skull base chordomas and all patients with cervical spine tumors of either histologic type) were to be randomized between 72 and 79.2 CGyEq. Dose constraints for the patients in the 72 CGyEq arm remained unchanged, but were increased by 5% for patients randomized to the 79.2 CGyEq arm.

Through June 1997, 292 patients were randomized, 239 at MGH-HCL, 24 at UCSF-LBL, and 29 at Loma Linda University Medical Center.

The observed gender difference was recently discussed in detail.[34] The reason for the apparently worse prognosis for females with skull base nonchondroid chordomas is unknown. Preliminary analysis of our data has not demonstrated a relationship between post-treatment endocrinopathy and a worse treatment outcome in females with nonchondroid chordomas, suggesting that physiologic or radiation-induced endocrine changes in women after treatment are not responsible for the difference; a more detailed analysis of this aspect of the problem is needed. We are currently studying the prognostic significance of the presence or absence of hormone receptors (estrogen and progesterone) in the tumor.

Both tumor volume[3,35] and minimum tumor dose[35] are significant prognostic factors for local failure. At least in some patients, tumor volume can be reduced by additional surgery before treatment. Surgical reduction of tumor bulk may create a better tumor–normal tissue configuration and allow a higher dose to be delivered to the tumor than would have been possible had the patient been treated with the presenting geometrically unfavorable tumor–normal tissue relationship. As discussed earlier, the majority of local recurrences take place in lower dose regions where the tumor abuts or displaces a dose-constraining normal tissue.[20] A recent analysis has quantified the magnitude of this dose deficiency in the patients receiving prescribed doses ranging from 66.6 to 75.6 CGyEq. A higher proportion of the prescribed dose was delivered to a greater percentage of the target volume in patients prescribed to receive lower doses, while mean dose was greater in patients prescribed to receive higher doses. There was little variation in minimum dose, regardless of dose prescribed, since the same normal tissue dose constraints were applied for all patients. The apparent dose difference between the two arms in the randomized trial, 5.4 CGyEq, was reached on average in 30% to 40% of the target.[36] This emphasizes that every effort should be made to minimize dose inhomogeneity in the target due to dose constraints imposed by the proximity of the optic nerves, optic chiasm, and brainstem, and to increase the minimum dose to the defined target, since minimum dose has been shown to be significantly related to local control.[35]

Surgery for locally recurrent tumor is recommended only if significant or near-total tumor resection can be anticipated, or for a reasonable expectation of relief by such surgery from distressing symptoms or disability from progressive tumor growth. Some patients have received stereotactic radiosurgery for tumor progression, but a clear-cut benefit from such treatment has not consistently been demonstrated. No systemic treatment has been of value in patients with recurrent disease. Local radiation has been palliative to patients with progressive tumor outside the original high-dose treatment area (e.g., drop metastasis, cerebellar involvement, bone metastasis).

Fractionated proton treatment can be given to patients with histologies requiring generally lower doses than those used for the chordomas and chondrosarcomas. However, more treatment options for such patients with fractionated conformal x-ray therapy are available. Proton beam techniques do offer the potential for decreasing normal tissue doses, which may be particularly important when treating pediatric patients.[23, 37-39]

In summary, 3D-planned high-dose radiation therapy delivered with combined proton and supervoltage x-ray techniques following surgical removal of as much tumor as possible appears to represent the best management policy currently available for patients with skull base chordomas and chondrosarcomas and tumors of other histologic types that require a high radiation dose to achieve local control. This potentially hazardous treatment is expensive, time-consuming, and demanding, both for patients and for those involved in their care. Nonetheless, it offers patients with such tumors a major advancement in outcome, relative to that expected with conventional supervoltage x-ray techniques.[32,40]

ACKNOWLEDGMENTS

This work was supported by Grant CA 21239 from the National Cancer Institute, Department of Health and Human Services. Editorial assistance from Tina Hennessey and assistance with follow-up by Susan Dean, Pat McManus, Ena Chang, Juergen Debus, and June Kim are gratefully acknowledged.

REFERENCES

1. Dahlin DC: *Bone Tumors*, 2nd ed. Springfield, Ill: Charles C Thomas; 1967.
2. Netherlands Committee on Bone Tumors: *Radiologic Atlas of Bone Tumors*, vol 1. Baltimore: Williams & Wilkins; 1966.
3. O'Connell JX, Renard LG, Liebsch NJ, et al: Base of skull chordoma: A correlative study of histologic and clinical features of 62 cases. *Cancer.* 1994;74:2261.
4. Rosenberg AE, Brown GA, Bhan AK, Lee JM: Chondroid chordoma: A variant of chordoma—A morphological and immuno-histochemical study. *Am J Clin Pathol.* 1994;101:36.
5. Volpe NJ, Liebsch NJ, Munzenrider JE, Lessell S: Neuro-ophthalmologic findings in chordoma and chondrosarcoma of the skull base. *Am J Ophthalmol.* 1993;115:97.
6. Austin-Seymour M, Munzenrider J, Goitein M, et al: Fractionated proton radiation therapy of chordoma and low grade chondrosarcoma of the base of skull. *J Neurosurg.* 1989;70:13.
7. Castro JR, Linstadt DE, Bahary JP, et al: Experience in charged particle irradiation of tumors of the skull base: 1977-1992. *Int J Radiat Oncol Biol Phys.* 1994;29:647.
8. Suit HD: Potential for improving survival rates for the cancer patient by increasing the efficacy of treatment of the primary lesion [American Society of Therapeutic Radiology Presidential Address October 1981]. *Cancer.* 1982;50:1227.
9. Kjellberg RN, Shintani A, Frantz AG, et al: Proton beam therapy in acromegaly. *N Engl J Med.* 1968;278:689.
10. Kjellberg RN, Hanamura T, Davis KR, et al: Bragg-Peak proton beam therapy for arteriovenous malformations of the brain. *N Engl J Med.* 1983;309:269.
11. Urano M, Verhey LJ, Goitein M, et al: Relative biological effectiveness of modulated proton beams in various murine tissues. *Int J Radiat Oncol Biol Phys.* 1984;10:509.
12. Hug EB, Fitzek MM, Liebsch NJ, Munzenrider JE: Locally challenging osteo- and chondrogenic tumors of the axial skeleton: Results of combined proton and photon radiation therapy using three-dimensional treatment planning. *Int J Radiat Oncol Biol Phys.* 1995;31:467.
13. Goitein M, Abrams M: Multi-dimensional treatment planning: 1. Delineation of anatomy. *Int J Radiat Oncol Biol Phys.* 1983;9:777.

14. Goitein M: Compensation for inhomogeneities in charged particle radiotherapy using computed tomography. *Int J Radiat Oncol Biol Phys.* 1978;4:499.

15. Urie M, Goitein M, Wagner M: Compensating for heterogeneities in proton radiation therapy. *Phys Med Biol.* 1983;29:553.

16. Verhey LJ, Munzenrider JE, Goitein M, et al: Precise positioning of patients for radiation therapy. *Int J Radiat Oncol Biol Phys.* 1982;8:289.

17. Rosenthal SJ, Urie MM, Thornton A: Advances in head and neck immobilization for radiotherapy [abstract]. *Med Phys.* 1993;20:868.

18. Goitein M, Abrams M, Rowell D, Pollari H, Wiles J: Multi-dimensional treatment planning: II. Beam's eye-view, back projection and projection through CT sections. *Int J Radiat Oncol Biol Phys.* 1983;9:789.

19. Urie MU, Fullerton B, Tatsuzaki H, et al: A dose response analysis of injury to cranial nerves and/or nuclei following proton beam radiation therapy. *Int J Radiat Oncol Biol Phys.* 1992;23:27.

20. Austin JP, Urie MM, Cardenosa G, Munzenrider JE: Probable causes of recurrence in patients with chordoma and chondrosarcoma of the base of skull and cervical spine. *Int J Radiat Oncol Biol Phys.* 1993;25:439.

21. Oot RF, Melville GE, New PF, et al: The role of MR and CT in evaluating clival chordomas and chondrosarcomas. *Am J Roentgenol.* 1988;151:567.

22. Munzenrider JE, Hug EB, McManus P, et al: Skull base chordomas: Treatment outcome and prognostic factors in adult patients following conformal treatment with 3D planning and high dose fractionated combined proton and photon radiation therapy [abstract]. *Int J Radiat Oncol Biol Phys.* 1995;32:209.

23. Benk V, Liebsch NJ, Munzenrider JE, et al: Base of skull and cervical spine chordomas in children treated by high-dose irradiation. *Int J Radiat Oncol Biol Phys.* 1995;31:577.

24. Fagundes MA, Hug EB, Liebsch NJ, et al: Radiation therapy for chordomas of the base of skull and cervical spine: Patterns of failure and outcome after relapse. *Int J Radiat Oncol Biol Phys.* 1995;33:579.

25. Debus J, Hug EB, Munzenrider JE, et al: Brainstem tolerance to conformal radiotherapy of skull base tumors. *Int J Radiat Oncol Biol Phys.* 1997;39:976.

26. Santoni R, Finkelstein DM, Liebsch NJ, et al: Temporal lobe damage following surgery and high dose photon and proton irradiation in 96 patients affected by chordomas and chondrosarcomas of the base of skull. *Int J Radiat Oncol Biol Phys.* In press.

27. Glosser G, McManus P, Munzenrider JE, et al: Neuropsychological function in adults after high dose fractionated radiation therapy of skull base tumors. *Int J Radiat Oncol Biol Phys.* 1997;38:231.

28. Habrand JL, Austin-Seymour M, Birnbaum S, et al: Neurovisual outcome following proton radiation therapy. *Int J Radiat Oncol Biol Phys.* 1989;16:1601.

29. Kim J, Hug EB, Liebsch NJ, et al: Tolerance of optic nerve to high dose fractionation proton and x-ray therapy [abstract]. *Int J Radiat Oncol Biol Phys.* 1997;39:272.

30. Schoenthaler R, Fullerton B, Maas A, et al: Relationship between dose to auditory pathways and audiological outcomes in skull base tumor patients receiving high-dose proton/photon radiotherapy. Proceedings of the 38th Annual ASTRO meeting. *Int J Radiat Oncol Biol Phys.* 1996;36(1):291.

31. Slater JD, Austin-Seymour M, Munzenrider J, et al: Endocrine function following high dose proton therapy for tumors of the upper clivus. *Int J Radiat Oncol Biol Phys.* 1988;15:607.

32. Catton C, O'Sullivan B, Bell R, et al: Chordoma: Long-term follow-up after radical photon irradiation. *Radiother Oncol.* 1996;41:67.

33. Slater JM, Archambeau JO, Miller DW, et al: The proton treatment centre at Loma Linda University Medical Center: Rationale for and description of its development. *Int J Radiat Oncol Biol Phys.* 1992;22:383.

34. Halperin EC: Why is female sex an independent predictor of shortened overall survival after proton/photon radiation therapy for skull base chordomas? *Int J Radiat Oncol Biol Phys.* 1997;38:225.

35. Terahara A, Hug EB, Liebsch NJ, et al: Analysis of the relationship between tumor dose inhomogeneity and local control in patients with skull base chordoma [abstract]. *Int J Radiat Oncol Biol Phys.* 1996;36:369.

36. Hanssens P, Urie M, Niemierko A, et al: Tumor doses inhomogeneity: Possible implications for radiation dose escalation studies. Submitted for publication.

37. Archambeau JO, Slater JD, Slater JM, et al: Role for proton beam irradiation in treatment of pediatric CNS malignancies. *Int J Radiat Oncol Biol Phys.* 1992;22:287.

38. Wambersie A, Gregoire V, Brucher JM: Potential clinical gain of proton (and heavy ion) beams for brain tumors in children. *Int J Radiat Oncol Biol Phys.* 1992;22:275.

39. Miralbell R, Lomax A, Bortfeld T, et al: Potential role of proton therapy in the treatment of pediatric medulloblastoma/primitive neuroectodermal tumors: Reduction of the supratentorial target volume. *Int J Radiat Oncol Biol Phys.* 1997;38:477.

40. Hug EB, Munzenrider JE: Charged particle therapy for base of skull tumors: Past accomplishments and future challenges. *Int J Radiat Oncol Biol Phys.* 1994;29:911.

Pituitary Tumors

24

David Huang, MD and Francine E. Halberg, MD

The role of radiotherapy in the management of pituitary tumors has become more clearly defined with the adoption of pituitary microsurgery and the development of high-resolution magnetic resonance imaging (MRI) and sensitive hormone assays. The management of pituitary tumors requires a multidisciplinary team, including representatives from endocrinology, neurosurgery, neuroradiology, laboratory medicine, neuro-ophthalmology, and radiation oncology.

The goals of pituitary adenoma therapy are to remove or destroy the tumor, control hypersecretion, and restore lost function without producing hypopituitarism or injury to surrounding normal tissue. Because surgical resection accomplishes these goals most rapidly, with prompt decompression of mass effects and improvement in pituitary function, it is generally the treatment of first choice. Postoperative radiation therapy is indicated in the setting of persistent hypersecretion or incomplete resection or documented recurrence. Primary radiotherapy is an excellent alternative in patients who are medically inoperable or who refuse surgery.

EPIDEMIOLOGY

Pituitary tumors constitute approximately 10% of all intracranial neoplasms. Up to 22% of apparently normal pituitary glands have been found to contain pituitary adenomas at autopsy.[1] Most are therefore asymptomatic. The incidence of macroadenomas appears to be equal between the sexes.[2,3] However, clinical manifestations from microadenomas appear more frequently in women than in men. Seventy percent of these tumors present between the ages of 30 and 50 years old. Only 3% to 7% occur under the age of 20 years. The epidemiology of pituitary adenomas is not well understood. There is evidence that endocrine-inactive pituitary adenomas are the result of a monoclonal expansion of a genetically aberrant cell.[4] The concept of one cell–one hormone has been disproven. Pituitary adenomas either produce in vivo, or have the capacity to produce, functional anterior pituitary hormones, imperfect or uncoupled portions of those hormones, and other products.[5] In general, pituitary adenomas have low proliferative activity[5,6] and mitoses are generally rare. A monoclonal antibody, Ki-67, evaluates growth fraction; kinetic analysis found that all adenomas contained proliferating cells with a growth fraction from 0.1% to 3.7%.[7] Low values were present in patients with endocrine-inactive adenomas, slightly higher values in acromegalic patients, and a broad spectrum of values from 0.1% to 3.7% in patients with prolactinomas and Cushing's disease. Tumors that were frankly invasive have higher Ki-67 values than noninvasive adenomas.[8]

Cytologic characteristics that are typically used to assess growth in malignancy, including hypercellularity; variations in nuclear size, shape, and chromatin content; presence of multinucleated cells; and so on, are unreliable in pituitary tumors. Pituitary tumors cannot be classified as benign or malignant on the basis of pathologic criteria. Local invasion of bone and soft tissue is common with benign adenomas, and cellular pleomorphism does not correspond with clinical malignancy.

Pituitary neoplasms can be best understood in the context of their surrounding normal anatomy and the physiology of the pituitary gland.

ANATOMY

Anatomically, the pituitary gland is a midline structure resting in the sella turcica, a cavity of the sphenoid bone (Fig. 24-1). This cavity is so named due to its shape, which resembles a Turkish saddle. The pituitary gland is bordered by the sphenoid sinuses inferiorly. The diaphragm sella, an extension of the dura, separates the pituitary from the neural structures above it, the most relevant being the optic chiasm. The posterior border of the sella is formed by the dorsum sellae, a thin bony structure with two prominences, the posterior clinoids, at the superior-lateral margins. The corresponding anterior wall of the sella contains a superior prominence known as the tuberculum sellae with two lateral projections, the anterior clinoids. Lateral to the sella are the cavernous sinuses, which include the internal carotid arteries and the second, third, fourth, and sixth cranial nerves. Normal sella dimensions are approximately 15 mm anterior-posterior and 12 mm superior-inferior. Tumors of the pituitary may compress the remainder of the pituitary gland and may expand the sella. They may erode the walls and extend laterally into the cavernous sinuses. Superiorly they may affect the optic chiasm and hypothalamus and inferiorly, the sphenoid sinus. Tumors arising in the pituitary gland, if unchecked, can ultimately extend into the temporal lobe, third ventricle, and posterior fossa.

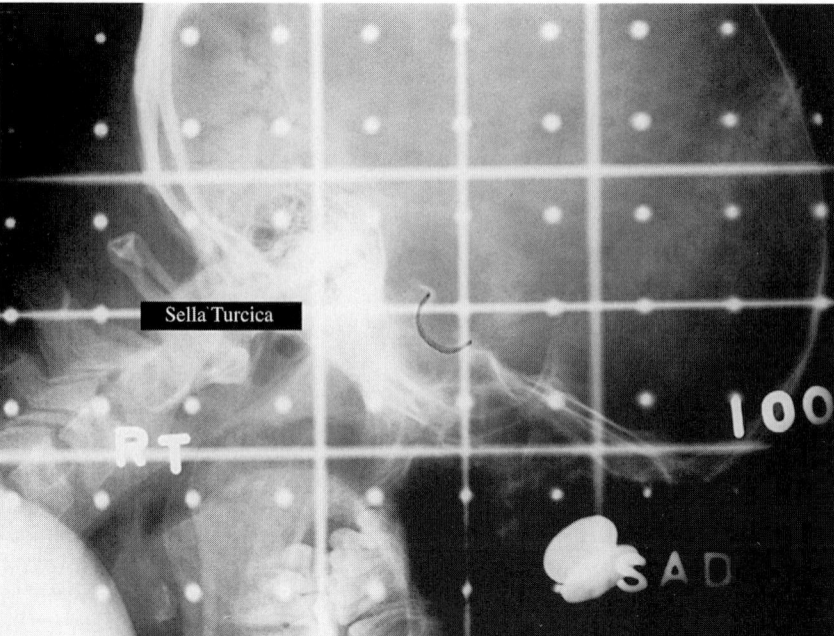

Figure 24–1. Lateral simulation radiograph with label denoting the sella turcica and a lead marker on the contralateral eye.

The pituitary gland is essentially composed of two lobes, the anterior and the posterior. A stalk made up of neural and vascular elements connects the pituitary to the hypothalamus. The anterior lobe of the pituitary arises from Rathke's pouch, an evagination of ectodermal tissue from the roof of the oral cavity. These cells migrate up to surround the anterior aspect of the posterior lobe and stalk. The anterior lobe is involved in the synthesis and release of a number of polypeptides and hormones. Hormonal release from the anterior pituitary is regulated by a feedback mechanism of target gland hormones. Pituitary tumors arise from the anterior lobe.

The posterior lobe and stalk arise from a down-pocketing of the third ventricle floor. The posterior lobe contains terminal axons from neurons in the supraoptic and paraventricular nuclei of the hypothalamus. Secretory granules synthesized in the hypothalamic nuclei are transported down the stalk to the posterior lobe, where they are released as pituitary hormones. Posterior pituitary hormones are oxytocin and vasopressin. Pituitary tumors do not arise in the posterior lobe.

PATHOLOGY

Light microscopy demonstrates normal-appearing pituitary cells but with loss of acinar stromal pattern. Pituitary adenomas are classified as endocrine-active or endocrine-inactive (Table 24-1). Using immunohistochemical and electron microscopic techniques, endocrine-active adenomas can be classified on the basis of the hormones produced: growth hormone (GH), prolactin, mixed GH-prolactin, corticotropic cell, acidophilic stem cell, thyrotropic cell, and gonadotropic cell. The majority (about 70%) of pituitary tumors produce one or two hormones that are detectably elevated in blood and are associated with well-defined clinical syndromes. Silent corticotropic adenomas contain immunoreactive adrenocorticotropic hormone but are not associated with signs of hypercortisolemia. Endocrine-inactive tumors are predominantly of two cell types: null cell and oncocytomas, which produce no hormone. Hormonally inactive glycoprotein-producing adenomas make up the remainder of the endocrine-inactive tumors. Pituitary carcinomas are exceedingly rare, with only 36 cases reported in the past century.

CLINICAL PRESENTATION

The most common presentations of pituitary tumors are endocrine abnormalities. These abnormalities may be a manifestation of hypersecretion in endocrine-active tumors or hyposecretion secondary to compression of the pituitary gland or hypothalamic stalk. Hypothyroidism, adrenal insufficiency, or growth deficiency may result from compression. Table 24-2 summarizes the more common endocrine abnormalities associated with hypersecretion.

Pituitary adenomas vary greatly in size. Most such endocrine-active tumors are microadenomas, which are defined as adenomas with diameters less than 10 mm.[9]

Table 24–1 Morphologic Classification of Pituitary Adenomas

Prolactin cell
Growth hormone cell
Mixed: growth hormone cell–prolactin cell
Acidophilic stem cell
Thyrotropic cell
Gonadotropic cell
Corticotropic cell
Undifferentiated cell:
    Nononcocytic (mixed cell)
    Oncocytic (oncocytoma)

Table 24–2 Clinical Syndromes Associated with Endocrine-Active Pituitary Adenomas

Hormone Produced	Clinical Syndrome
Prolactin	Amenorrhea, galactorrhea
	Impotence in men
Growth hormone	Gigantism and acromegaly
Corticotropin	Cushing's disease, Nelson's syndrome after adrenalectomy
Thyroid-stimulating hormone (rare)	Hyperthyroidism

Conversely, macroadenomas measure 10 mm or greater. Macroadenomas occur more frequently than microadenomas in females. However, microadenomas occur equally in males and females. Overall they tend to have a long natural history, and subtle symptoms and signs of tumors may not be recognized. Pituitary tumors may present with mass effect. Approximately 20% of patients present with headache. Tumors extending superiorly may cause visual loss, usually visual field defects, either bitemporal hemianopia or, less commonly, superior temporal defects. Tumors may extend laterally and cause ophthalmoplegia from cranial nerve involvement.

DIAGNOSTIC EVALUATION

A history and physical examination may demonstrate clinical syndromes of hormonal imbalance, ophthalmologic deficits, or neurologic effects from a pituitary adenoma. The diagnosis of an endocrine-active pituitary tumor is based on selected radioimmunoassays for hormone levels (Table 24-3).[10] The diagnostic neuroimaging procedure of choice is magnetic resonance imaging (MRI). Gadolinium enhancement should be used for microadenomas (diameter <10 mm).[11,12] Figure 24-2 shows a pituitary adenoma before surgery. With respect to defining a tumor volume for treatment planning, the diagnostic MRI and, if obtained, high-resolution computed tomography (CT) scan are essential. However, head position for treatment is different than head position for diagnostic imaging studies; therefore, a CT scan with the head in treatment position is usually obtained during simulation for treatment planning (see Simulation section).

Neuro-opthalmologic examination with baseline formal visual field testing is indicated in individuals with visual symptoms or tumor encroaching on the optic apparatus. This may be repeated later in follow-up to assess change.

STAGING

Hardy and Vizini[13] developed a staging system based on the symmetry and integrity of the floor of the sella. Wilson[14] at the University of California at San Francisco (UCSF) modified Hardy's classification, incorporating the prognostic value of local growth characteristics and size (Table 24-4). These staging systems have gained partial acceptance, predominately by neurosurgeons.

Table 24–3 Pituitary Tumor Diagnostic Evaluation

General

History
Physical examination, including careful neurologic examination

Endocrine Evaluation

Pituitary hormone levels: serum prolactin, fasting growth hormone
Growth hormone dynamics (including glucose suppression, insulin tolerance, thyrotrophin-releasing hormone stimulation)
Serum ACTH, urine 17-ØH corticosteroids and free-cortisol, response to dexamethasone suppression
Gonadal function: follicle-stimulating hormone, luteinizing hormone, plasma estradiol, testosterone
Thyroid function: thyroxine, tri-iodothyroxine, thyroid-stimulating hormone

Radiologic Studies

Magnetic resonance imaging, thin section with contrast
Skull films

Special Tests

Neuro-ophthalmologic examination, visual field testing

Other

Complete blood count, serum chemistries, urinalysis
Chest x-ray
Skeletal survey in acromegaly
Selective bilateral simultaneous venous sampling of ACTH from inferior petrosal sinuses (in Cushing's disease with negative neuroimaging)

ACTH, adrenocorticotropic hormone.

STANDARD THERAPEUTIC APPROACHES

The role of radiation therapy depends on whether the lesion is surgically resectable and, postoperatively, how effectively the resection has controlled any mass effects and hypersecretion (when present).[15]

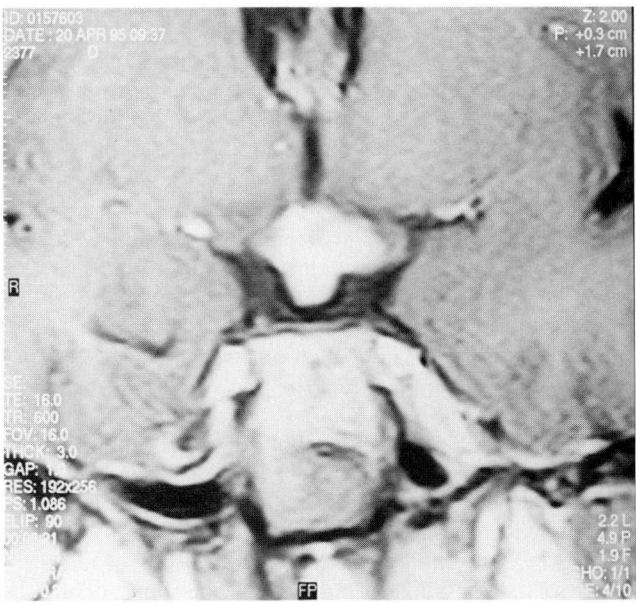

Figure 24–2. Coronal magnetic resonance imaging scan showing a pituitary adenoma.

Table 24–4 Staging of Pituitary Adenomas: Anatomic Classification of Pituitary Adenomas, Radiographic and Operative

Relationship of Adenoma to Sella & Sphenoid Sinuses (Grade)

Floor of sella intact
I.   Sella normal or focally expanded, tumor <10 mm
II. Sella enlarged, tumor ≥10 mm
Sphenoid
III. Localized perforation of sellar floor
IV. Diffuse destruction of sellar floor
Distant spread
V.   Spread via cerebrospinal fluid or blood-borne

Extrasellar Extension (Stage)

Suprasellar extension
0: None
A: Occupying cistern
B: Recesses of third ventricle obliterated
C: Third ventricle grossly displaced
Parasellar extension
D: Intracranial (intradural), anterior, middle, or posterior fossa
E: Into or beneath cavernous sinus (extradural)

Surgery

The trans-sphenoidal approach is the preferred surgical technique for almost all pituitary adenomas, regardless of size, because it is safer and better tolerated than the alternative frontal craniotomy approach.[13] With larger tumors, the trans-sphenoidal approach is feasible as suprasellar extension drops into the sella with progressive resection. Contraindications to the trans-sphenoidal approach are minimal or disproportionately little enlargement of the sella relative to a large suprasellar mass, extrasellar extension into the middle fossa with the volume of the extrasellar mass being greater than the intrasellar volume, unusually fibrous tumors that cannot be removed trans-sphenoidally (a situation noted at the time of trans-sphenoidal procedure), and, lastly, the rare situation in which an unrelated intracranial pathology may complicate the trans-sphenoidal approach (e.g., a parasellar aneurysm).

For patients with pituitary microadenomas, trans-sphenoidal resection alone is the treatment of choice.[16,17] The initial treatment for prolactin-secreting microadenomas should be trans-sphenoidal resection or medical management with bromocriptine. The management of the rare and aggressive thyroid-stimulating hormone (TSH) adenoma is not well defined. For larger pituitary adenomas, trans-sphenoidal surgery is also the initial treatment of choice, as mass effects can be decompressed quickly, endocrine-hypersecretion decreased or eliminated, and existing pituitary function retained or improved most rapidly. Surgical decompression also helps predict which patients will need adjuvant therapy.

The transcranial approach is uncommonly used except in cases of intracranial extension or if the trans-sphenoidal approach is limited by the anatomy (insufficient pneumatization of the sphenoid sinus or a small sella.)

Medical Management

The medical management of pituitary adenomas, particularly prolactin-secreting adenomas, is assuming an increasingly important role.[10] Bromocriptine has been recommended as initial therapy for patients with prolactin-secreting macroadenomas.[18] Bromocriptine is a dopamine receptor agonist and a prolactin inhibitor. It has been used to induce tumor regression of macroadenomas. For larger adenomas, this therapy has usually preceded either trans-sphenoidal resection or radiation therapy. Bromocriptine does not produce a permanent reduction in prolactin levels and does not eliminate the risk of tumor growth during pregnancy; nonetheless, long-term bromocriptine is an option for managing hyperprolactinemia. The appropriate duration of therapy is still an open question.

In Cushing's disease, drugs that inhibit adrenocortical secretion are often used as adjuvant therapy after surgery or radiation therapy.[19] Ketoconazole inhibits the cytochrome P450 enzymes needed for adrenal steroid biosynthesis. Metyrapone, an 11 β-hydroxylase inhibitor in conjunction with aminoglutethimide, which blocks the conversion of cholesterol to pregnenolone, are used in combination to control hypercortisolism in patients before surgery or after therapy while awaiting response to treatment. Mitotane is an adrenocortical cytotoxic agent, which both alone and together with pituitary irradiation has previously been recommended in the management of patients with Cushing's disease. Mitotane, however, has a number of side effects and is limited by delayed response.

Somatostatin-analogues such as octreotide have been evaluated in the management of GH-secreting and thyrotropin-producing pituitary tumors, where they may be the drug of first choice if tumor resection is not possible.[20,21] These drugs are used while awaiting the radiation therapy effect to take place. However, they are not a good long-term alternative as yet, since three-times-daily subcutaneous administration is required. Other drugs, such as newer long-acting dopamine agonists, are under investigation.

Radiation Therapy

The role of radiation therapy has decreased markedly as techniques for diagnosing smaller endocrine-active adenomas have improved and particularly as the trans-sphenoidal resection of adenomas has been widely adopted. Postoperative radiation therapy is used to eradicate any significant remaining tumor, prevent regrowth, and further decrease persistently elevated circulating hormone levels.[22,23] For medically inoperable patients or those who refuse surgery, conventional radiation therapy, either alone or in conjunction with medical treatment, is recommended.[24]

Comparison of results of primary radiation therapy with those of surgical resection is difficult. Patients receiving radiation therapy often have larger or invasive tumors or are elderly. The series involving radiation therapy tend to be older, and CT or MRI scanning were often not used, so the tumor burden may have been large. Nonetheless, progression after primary radiation therapy is infrequent in large, primary radiotherapy series. Overall, radiation therapy controls tumor growth in more than 90% of patients with endocrine-inactive, prolactin-secreting, and GH-secreting pituitary adenomas.[22,24,25] It is less effective in controlling endocrine-hypersecretion, and decreases in circulating hormone levels may take months to years to achieve (see Outcomes section).

SIMULATION

At the time of treatment planning for radiotherapy, the patient is positioned supine. The head and neck are flexed and positioned in a rigid tilted head holder as shown in Figure 24-3. The patient's chin is tucked down, and the angle of elevation of the head and neck off of the treatment couch is adjusted such that the plane of rotation of the radiation beam will be across the upper forehead or frontal region, posterior to the eyes. The head is typically held at a 45-degree angle. Tilting-head baseplate immobilization systems are commercially available. The head holder set-up can also be easily constructed out of the styrofoam used for block fabrication. A section of the styrofoam is cut in a 45-degree angle, such that a Timo B standard head holder can be inserted into it. At UCSF, we use a 10-cm styrofoam thickness (rather than the standard 8 cm). This styrofoam piece, containing the Timo B, is then inserted into a standard head immobilization system (e.g., Aquaplast, Uniframe). The patient's head is positioned, then Aquaplast is used to rigidly hold the position and attach the patient's head to the immobilization system holder. This essentially prevents motion during simulation and treatment. It also fits into a CT scanner (see Fig. 24-3).

Typically, 5.0 × 5.0 cm fields are set up, centered on the sella. Lateral and coronal simulation radiographs are taken with a lead marker on the contralateral eyelid (Fig. 24-4 and see Fig. 24-1). The central axis is indicated by two small marks placed bilaterally and one midline on the mask. A treatment planning CT scan is then obtained, with a therapist or dosimetrist, ensuring that cuts are obtained through the central axis and at 5 mm intervals through the treatment volume defined at simulation.

If sophisticated treatment planning equipment is not available (or as an additional backup), a contour is taken through the plane of rotation of the radiation beam, with marks showing the isocenter. The isocenter is marked on the patient or mask bilaterally and in the midline. After simulation, the contour is traced onto paper and the target volume is drawn, referenced to the isocenter. The contour is then entered into the treatment planning system.

RADIATION TREATMENT PLAN

A great deal of progress has been made in radiation therapy technique and treatment planning for pituitary tumors. However, the basic principles remain the same: to deliver a curative dose to the pituitary tumor while minimizing the dose delivered to adjacent normal structures. The treatment planning system used for designing pituitary treatment fields must allow for precise calculations of dose delivered to critical, immediately adjacent normal tissues, which include the optic chiasm and optic nerves, temporal lobes, brain stem, and hypothalamus. It must also be able to calculate the dose to the remainder

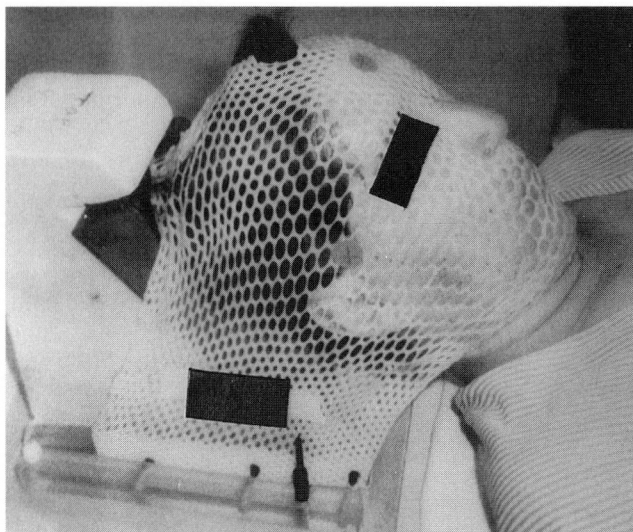

Figure 24–3. Lateral view of patient positioned with head immobilized in a tilted head holder. Note the styrofoam cut out at a 45-degree angle, supporting a standard Timo B head holder, attached to the table with a standard head immobilization system. Note also the central axis marks midline and laterally.

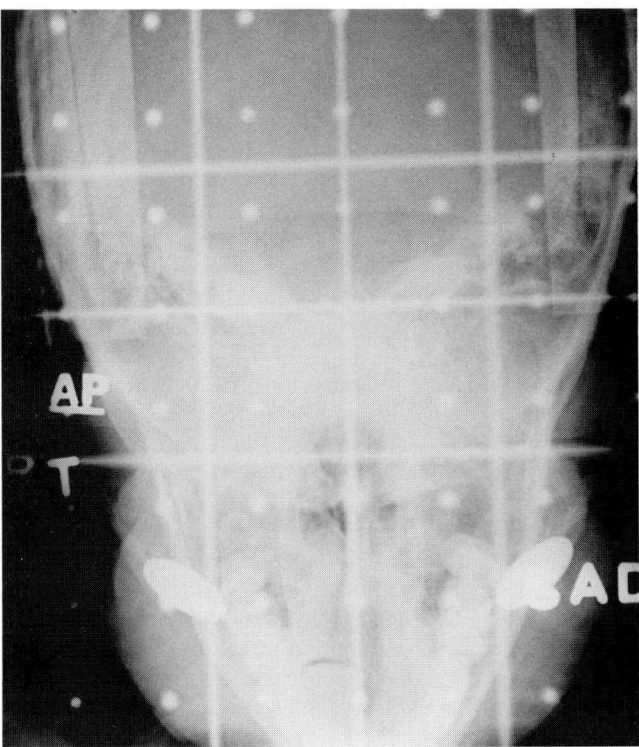

Figure 24–4. Coronal stimulation radiograph. (See Fig. 24-1 for lateral simulation radiograph.)

of the brain and assess the dose to the eyes and thyroid so that these structures can be eliminated from the field or receive the minimal possible dose.

In choosing the target volume, clinical, radiologic, and surgical findings must be incorporated. Both preoperative and postoperative high-resolution MRI scans are particularly helpful. As pituitary tumors are generally slow growing, the postoperative MRI should be obtained approximately 6 weeks after surgery, so that postsurgical changes have begun to resolve. Treatment planning systems that can integrate MRI studies into the planning process and thus allow for the most accurate treatment fields are now available. For most adenomas, the tumor volume defined on the original and postoperative diagnostic MRI scans, and hopefully well visualized on the treatment planning CT scan, plus a 1.5 to 2 cm margin, is generally used. This usually results in the aforementioned 5-cm treatment field. With larger, invasive tumors, particularly those with significant suprasellar, lateral, sphenoidal, or other intracranial involvement, or in situations in which the tumor volume cannot be well defined, planning of the target volume must take these considerations into account and will generally lead to a slightly larger margin around the known tumor volume.

Pituitary tumors should be treated with high-energy photon beams since they penetrate deeply and the tumors are centrally located. When this method is used with an 18 MeV accelerator, hair loss does not occur, which represents a significant benefit, as these patients are fully functional and do not have a malignancy. The most common techniques for treating pituitary adenomas include the bicoronal wedged arc technique (described later) and three-field plans with opposed lateral fields and a vertex field. Opposed lateral fields alone give too high a dose to the temporal lobes. For all but the very largest tumors, the dose distribution from the bicoronal arc technique appears to be superior to three-field or two-field techniques, with a lower dose to normal brain. This technique is also applicable to other small midline brain tumors, including craniopharyngiomas and gliomas of the third or fourth ventricle.

For most pituitary tumors, the target volume is relatively easily encompassed with a rotational technique. Bilateral 110-degree arc rotations are employed, with a 30-degree wedge, which is reversed for the second arc. Visually, the linear accelerator delivers the radiation beam as it rotates from the level of the ears superiorly to midline, forming a 110-degree arc. The wedge filter, which moves along with the beam, compensates well for skull nonuniformity and the use of a partial arc. The contralateral arc is then treated after the wedge position is reversed (Fig. 24-5).

Although the majority of patients can be treated with the bicoronal arc technique, each patient's tumor size and, to a lesser extent, skull shape varies, and thus each plan must be individualized. In general, generous margins around the tumor volume are not employed. The field size is chosen to enclose the target volume in the 95% isodose line, with dose decreasing rapidly outside of this volume. Thus, the highest dose point is within the pituitary tumor and does not exceed 5% above that prescribed for the target volume.

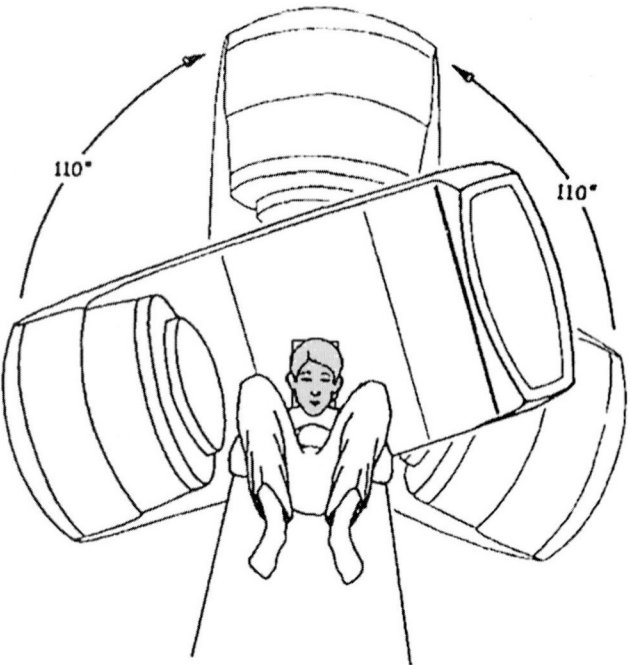

Figure 24–5. Schematic of bilateral arc rotations on a high-energy linear accelerator.

For eccentrically located tumors, the axis of rotation, thickness of the wedge, or length of the arc may vary from that just described. For very large pituitary tumors, the target volume may be best encompassed with a conformal plan that employs multiple intersecting beams, each with individualized blocking and wedges. Such a set-up often requires couch rotation, gantry, and collimator angles to be combined for the best dose distribution. Figure 24-6 shows an isodose distribution for a 5-cm diameter tumor volume (indicated by dotted circle delineating target volume). Bicoronal 110-degree arcs with moving 30-degree wedges are used on an 18 MeV accelerator. The dose-volume-histogram (DVH) for this plan, showing normal tissues and tumor dose volumes using the bicoronal arc technique, is shown in Figure 24-7. The arc technique provides excellent sparing of normal brain tissue. Nine percent of brain volume receives greater than 50% dose in the arc technique, compared with 17% of brain volume when the corresponding three-field technique is used. The arc technique also provides greater sparing of the brain stem than the three-field technique. The two techniques yield comparable high-dose regions (in both cases, 8% of the brain volume receives more than 60% of the dose) and tumor coverage.

Although intensity-modulated radiotherapy (IMRT) has been used by some to treat pituitary tumors, we do not currently advocate its use in this region. IMRT often involves inhomogeneities that may cause hotspots to occur within the critical structures adjacent to the tumor target. Such excessive dose may significantly contribute to risk of toxicity, and in the setting of generally benign disease, the increased risk of damage to vision is unacceptable. IMRT offers no advantage over three-dimensional conformal radiotherapy in the treatment of such tumors.

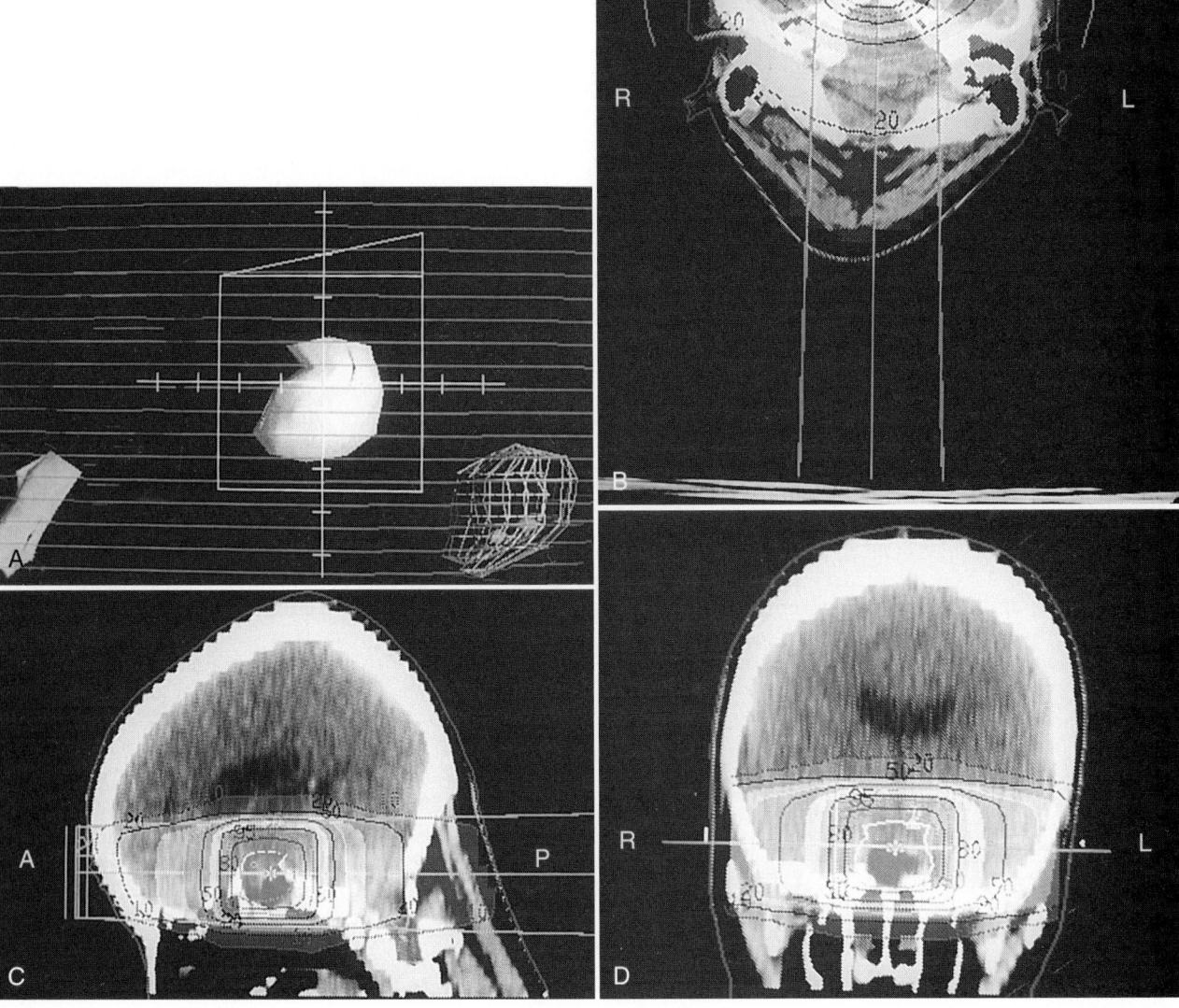

Figure 24–6. Isodose curves for a 5 cm diameter tumor volume: 18 MeV, bicoronal 110-degree arcs with moving 30-degree wedge filters. **A,** Lateral beam's-eye-view display showing the relationship of the target volume to the eyes and brainstem. **B,** Axial plane; **C,** sagittal plane; **D,** coronal plane. See also Color Figure 24-6.

DOSE

Data from retrospective analyses of pituitary tumor control rates, as well as analyses of complications, have defined the recommended radiation dose and fractionation. Older series established a dose that provides good tumor response with a low risk of complications. Doses less than 40 Gy have been reported to result in poor tumor control. Doses greater than 50.4 Gy or daily doses above 2 Gy are associated with higher complication rates with no proven increase in tumor control. The older series, however, predominantly used clinical assessment.

This is no longer valid in the era of functional bioassays and high-resolution MRI scanning. Nor have complication rates been reassessed in the era of more sophisticated treatment planning. The most common side effect from pituitary radiotherapy remains hypopituitarism. This is a dose-related phenomenon and it would be worth exploring whether there are certain clinical situations in which lower doses could be used. For example, Littley and coworkers[26,27] described equal reductions in circulating hormone levels in patients with acromegaly and hyperprolactinemia using regimens of 20 Gy in 8 fractions over 11 days versus 35 to 40 Gy in 15 fractions over 21 days.

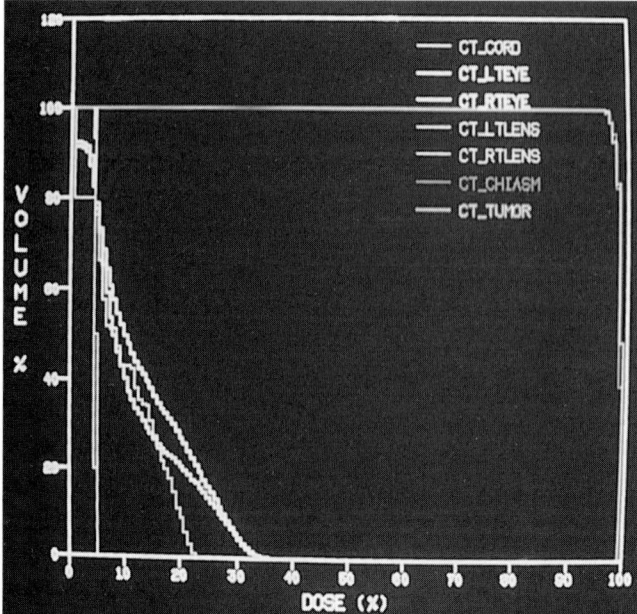

Figure 24–7. Dose volume histogram for bicoronal arc technique in the pituitary gland. The top 100% line is the tumor dose. Other normal structure doses are also shown. See also Color Figure 24-7.

There may be no significant improvement of the local control rate by increasing total irradiation doses between 48 and 60 Gy.[28] More dose-response information with long-term follow-up is clearly needed to better define dose requirements in the modern era. Based on available data, we continue to recommend daily fractions of 1.8 Gy to a total dose of 45 Gy. For adrenocorticotropic hormone (ACTH)- and TSH-secreting tumors we usually treat to a slightly higher dose, 50.4 Gy. Dose is prescribed to the 95% isodose volume. It should be noted that there are very few, if any, associated acute symptoms or side effects with the bicoronal arc, high-energy photon technique. Most patients can carry on their normal activities, including full-time work, while under treatment.

CRITICAL NORMAL TISSUES, COMPLICATIONS OF RADIOTHERAPY

The most common late complication of pituitary radiotherapy is hypopituitarism. Fortunately, other significant complications are rare with modern radiotherapeutic techniques. Possible other late complications include vision loss, carcinogenesis, cerebral infarction, and brain necrosis.

Hypopituitarism

The rate of hypopituitarism increases with time and may only be detected years after radiotherapy. The reported incidence varies greatly. Combining data from numerous series, at least half of the patients will develop at least one anterior pituitary hormone deficit within 5 years of receiving radiotherapy. The radiation target volume will include the entire pituitary and stalk and a significant portion of the hypothalamus in virtually all patients. Even with 1.8 Gy per day fractions, 5 days per week, to a total dose of 45 Gy, the development of hormone deficiencies is common. Equally common is a slight increase in prolactin levels after radiotherapy, attributed to hypothalamic and pituitary stalk dysfunction both from preexisting mass effect in certain tumors and from radiation-induced damage to hypothalamic prolactininhibitory centers.

In patients who develop hormonal deficiencies, the first is usually GH deficiency. In the past this has not been treated. However, there is increasing evidence that persistent GH deficiency in adults may decrease longevity, resulting from adverse changes in lipid and carbohydrate metabolism, cardiac function, renal function, and psychological well-being. The next anterior pituitary hormones lost are generally the gonadotropes, and finally either thyrotropins or adrenocorticotropins. The hypothalamus, rather than the anterior pituitary gland, may be responsible for these deficiencies,[29,30] as deficiencies have been noted in hypothalamic hormone-releasing factors. Patients with GH-secreting tumors are predisposed to hypopituitarism, presumably on the basis of small vessel disease. Radiation therapy does not cause diabetes insipidus.

It is clear that surgery alone carries a lower risk of hypopituitarism than radiotherapy. Radiotherapy alone has a lower risk of hypopituitarism than when surgery and radiation are combined.

In summary, hypothalamic-pituitary dysfunction following external beam irradiation is common, and patients must be observed indefinitely for this possibility. Deficiencies may be noted within several months of radiation therapy, although commonly these deficiencies take years to manifest themselves. Patients need to be tested at least yearly. With improved radioimmunoassays and physiological tests of endocrine function, hypopituitarism should be detected earlier and treated more rigorously than in the past. Despite the fact that endocrinologic deficiencies can be corrected with medical management, the risk of hypopituitarism continues to be the main disadvantage of radiotherapy.

Vision Loss

Loss of vision after pituitary radiation therapy has been reported predominantly from older series in which larger dose fraction sizes were used. In fact, a recent literature review evaluated 471 patients with non–GH-secreting pituitary adenomas treated with radiation therapy and found vision loss in only 7 patients (1.5%). In each case, larger fraction sizes than are currently recommended were used.[31] The same study reported results of pituitary radiotherapy for acromegaly/GH-secreting pituitary adenomas. Of 1000 cases, 23 patients had vision loss (2.3%). Only 2 patients (0.2%) were treated at fractions of 1.8 Gy per day. Therefore, the potential for loss of vision should not be viewed as a contraindication to radiation therapy, as the risk is much less than 1% with modern equipment, techniques, and dose fractionation schedules. In fact, radiation therapy has been documented to improve tumor-related visual field and visual acuity deficits in the majority of patients and to stabilize visual deficits in the remainder of patients.[31]

Carcinogenesis

Radiation-induced carcinogenesis is extremely rare. A review of 334 patients with pituitary adenomas treated with postoperative radiotherapy who were followed for 3760 person years after surgery found 5 patients with probable radiation-induced tumors.[32] These tumors were of a different type than the previous tumor and therefore not a recurrence; they occurred within the previously irradiated volume; and there was a latent period of at least several years between completion of initial therapy and the appearance of the second tumor. Tumors in this series appeared from 6 to 21 years after treatment. The risk of developing a second tumor was placed at 1.3% at 10 years and 1.9% at 20 years. The relative risk of developing a second brain tumor was 9.38% compared to the normal population. However, the risk of second malignancy in patients treated for pituitary adenomas without radiation therapy is not known. A literature review in the same paper found 57 possible radiation-induced tumors: 18 gliomas, 27 sarcomas, and 12 meningiomas with latencies of approximately 7, 9, and 13 years, respectively.[32]

In summary, the risk of developing a second brain tumor after pituitary radiation therapy is small. However, as patients generally have a long life expectancy after pituitary tumor irradiation, it is important for clinicians and patients to understand the risk.

Radiation Necrosis

Radiation necrosis is also an exceedingly rare complication of pituitary radiotherapy. In fact, most reports of radiation-induced brain necrosis were in patients treated with large fractions, multiple courses of radiotherapy, or in the days of orthovoltage irradiation. Sheline and coworkers[33] reviewed approximately 5000 patients treated with radiation therapy for pituitary adenomas; 20 cases of radiation necrosis were found. They defined the Neuret as a unit of biological effect and calculated the incidence of radiation-induced brain necrosis in patients receiving less than 1000 Neurets to be on the order of 0.04%. Doses of 45 to 50.4 Gy in 1.8 Gy fractions are equivalent to 860 to 910 Neurets. Thus, radiation necrosis is not expected with these doses, particularly in the era of high energy linear accelerators and modern treatment techniques.

Previous reports have suggested that patients with acromegaly were predisposed to radiation-induced brain injury. A review of more than 1000 acromegalic patients treated with radiation therapy revealed only 2 cases of radiation necrosis (0.2%).[33]

Changes seen on MRI or CT scan or both have been reported in some patients receiving radiation therapy for pituitary adenomas, but these findings were not clinically significant.[34] Positron emission tomography scans have not demonstrated any evidence of altered blood flow or oxygen consumption in similarly irradiated patients.[35] Radiation-induced brain necrosis should not be considered a contraindication to radiation therapy.

Cerebral Infarction

The risk of radiation-induced cerebral infarction is also very low. Several reports suggest radiation-induced intracranial arterial occlusion in patients with pituitary tumors who received 50 to 60 Gy.[36] Hirata and coworkers[37] reviewed previously reported cases and were unable to relate this complication to radiation dose. Radiation-induced cerebrovascular accidents would be expected to increase with increasing dose. Flickinger and coworkers[38] reported that 7 patients of 156 who had received radiation therapy for pituitary adenomas developed a cerebral infarction. Multivariate analysis documented that the risk of a cerebrovascular accident was related to patient age but not to dose. The evidence that radiation therapy for pituitary adenomas causes stroke is weak, and the number of irradiated patients who subsequently developed a stroke is small.

In view of the large numbers of patients who have been treated with radiation, it is evident that aside from hypopituitarism, other complications from pituitary radiation therapy, including vision loss, carcinogenesis, brain necrosis, and cerebral infarction are indeed rare problems.

BRACHYTHERAPY

Brachytherapy has a limited role, if any, in the management of pituitary tumors. Radioactive sources deliver very high doses to highly restricted volumes. Prescription doses may range from 500 to 1500 Gy. These volumes must be small to avoid complications. With implant techniques, the dose distribution throughout the adenoma or pituitary gland is also highly variable. In one report, only 51% of patients were free of complications after implantation of ^{90}Y or ^{198}Au radioactive sources.[39] However, Sandler and colleagues[40] reported long-term follow-up of Cushing's disease treated with interstitial irradiation. Brachytherapy must be limited to small, essentially intrasellar tumor volumes. This is precisely the situation in which trans-sphenoidal adenomectomy is most successful. We therefore recommend trans-sphenoidal resection as the treatment of choice for microadenomas and small intrasellar pituitary adenomas.

RADIOSURGERY

Radiosurgery (RS) delivers a very high dose of radiation to a very small volume, producing a lesion similar to surgical ablation. Good response rates and low complication rates have been reported. Histological response has been shown to also be more intensive with RS than with fractionated radiotherapy.[42] Multiple series of RS using linear accelerator as well as Gamma Knife techniques for pituitary adenomas show excellent results in both a definitive as well as an adjuvant setting.[43,44]

Early on, Kjellberg reported on GH and ACTH secreting pituitary adenomas treated with primary proton beam RS.[45] At their 5-year follow-up, 80% of patients with ACTH tumors and 50% of GH tumors had normalized hormone levels. However, hypopituitarism requiring hormonal replacement occurred in half the patients. Stereotactic RS does appear to provide a more rapid hormonal response than conventional RT, although there does not appear to be a difference in the long run.[44]

Linear accelerator-based RS has been reported by several institutions for treatment of pituitary adenomas. Yoon reported excellent control (20 of 21 patients who received such treatment for pituitary macroadenomas).[46] Doses ranged from 10 to 27 Gy, with limitation of dose to the optic pathways of 6 Gy. Mitsumori et al. showed a high rate of disease control, demonstrating a tumor control rate of 100% for stereotactic RS versus 85% for external beam radiotherapy at 3 years.[47] However, there was a higher incidence of toxicity, predominantly damage to the temporal lobe, associated with this form of RS (20%) when compared with external beam radiotherapy (0%). Leber also reported a high tumor control rate with linear accelerator-based RS as well as an increased risk of documentable optic neuropathy.[48]

Gamma Knife RS has also been used. Initially, high doses of up to 100 Gy were used, but doses have been significantly reduced.[49] Reports of control have been promising[50,51] with minimal risk of toxicity. Izawa reports a 91% rate of overall tumor growth control (in both functional and nonfunctional lesions), as well as an 80% rate of decreased hormonal production in secreting adenomas using a mean marginal dose of 20.5 Gy.[52] Zhang et al. reported excellent growth hormone level normalization with a rate of 96% at 3 years, as well as a radiographic response rate of 92% at 3 years after Gamma Knife RS was used as primary therapy for patients with acromegaly.[53] Mean marginal dose was 31.3 Gy in this series. Ikeda et al. reported 82% and 100% cure rates for patients receiving RS for postsurgical residual tumors with and without cavernous sinus involvement, respectively.[54] RS for the treatment of ACTH has also been successful. Pollock reported an 82% tumor growth control for these lesions.[55] Median marginal dose used was 20 Gy.

Such high-dose-per-fraction RS may subject patients to a higher risk of toxicity to the sensitive adjacent structures. Acute or chronic cranial neuropathy may result. Care must be taken to limit dose delivered to the optic chiasm and optic nerves to avoid damage to vision. Tishler et al. reported on the development of optic neuropathy after RS in 24% of patients receiving greater than 8 Gy per fraction to the optic pathway versus 0% in those receiving less than 8 Gy.[56] Ove et al. also demonstrate the safety of a single 8-Gy dose to these structures.[57] Fortunately, the other surrounding neurovascular structures in the cavernous sinus region are less radiosensitive and may tolerate the ablative doses of RS more easily.[58] With careful use, RS may be more capable of avoiding radiation-induced injury to the surrounding structures. It may be useful in the cavernous sinus region as long as there is separation between it and the optic pathway.

Our current recommendation at UCSF is to limit the dose to 8 Gy in a single fraction to the optic structures. With stable immobilization, accurate imaging, and precise planning systems, safe delivery of such treatment is possible. This is accomplished with our Gamma Knife if there is a separation of at least 3 mm between the tumor target and the optic nerves or chiasm.

Stereotactic charged-particle RS has a much longer history. At the University of California at Berkeley, 475 patients with pituitary tumors were treated with charged-particle radiotherapy, with excellent control of both tumor growth and hormone secretion. Hypopituitarism developed in approximately one-third of patients, with cranial nerve injury in 1% of patients.[41] The proton beam facility at Harvard Medical School has reported similar results.[59]

RS is more often used for recurrent disease rather than as primary or adjuvant therapy. It may not be appropriate as there may be disease left unaddressed by this focal treatment in the adjuvant setting. Most commonly, RS is used in the setting of recurrent tumor in the cavernous sinus out of the range for surgical intervention.

OUTCOME

Results of radiation therapy for pituitary tumors from a number of institutions have recently been updated. Results are presented in terms of disease-free and progression-free survival, and local control for each pituitary tumor cell type. Prognostic factors that may affect results from radiation therapy are not well defined. Patient age, gender, and performance status; whether or not tumor is confined to sella; and presence of visual deficits have not been found to affect survival or be of prognostic significance.[60,61] There is conflicting information on whether surgery before radiation therapy improves 10-year disease-free survival.

If a recurrence develops after adequate dose radiation therapy, it would be noted within 10 years. Grigsby et al. suggests that there is a low but persistent risk of failure in patients receiving postoperative radiation therapy for pituitary adenomas beyond that time.[62] This appears to be a dose-response phenomenon, as patients who experienced a recurrence had received a significantly lower mean dose than patients who did not (37.9 Gy vs. 46.2 Gy). This led McCollough and coworkers[63] to review all reports on patients treated with a dose of 45 Gy or greater with modern equipment and techniques, who did not receive medical therapy, and in whom there was a known time to recurrence after radiation therapy. Twenty-six patients in six publications were identified. All 26 failures occurred before 10 years after radiotherapy. Therefore, it is important to look at recent results of radiation therapy with dose and length of follow-up in mind.

Acromegaly

For many years, external beam radiotherapy alone was used to treat patients with acromegaly. The UCSF data and a review of the literature reveal that radiotherapy was successful in controlling mass effect associated with larger GH-secreting adenomas. The efficacy of radiation therapy in these older series was based predominantly on clinical responses. Current criteria for cure have been defined as basal GH levels less than 5 ng/mL, glucose-suppressed GH levels less than 2 ng/mL, and normalization of serum somatomedin-C levels.[64] Insulin-like growth factor I (IGF-I) levels may also be affected, although normalization is not common after radiotherapy.[65] Newer radiotherapy series report basal hormone levels but may not include all of the aforementioned criteria. Unfortunately, GH levels tend to fall slowly after radiation therapy, with only half of patients normalizing by 2 to 5 years after primary radiotherapy. By 10 years, 70% to 90% of patients have normalized. Longer series reveal that GH levels continue to fall past 15 years of follow-up.[64] Reduction to normal GH levels occurs sooner in patients with pretreatment GH levels of less than 100 ng/mL. Importantly, reversal of many signs and symptoms of acromegaly may be noted before normalization of GH levels.

Table 24-5 summarizes recent series with long follow-up.[50,62,65-67] Patients were treated either with surgery followed by radiation therapy or with radiation therapy alone. Failure of surgery to control GH levels in patients with pituitary adenomas was not associated with a poor response to radiotherapy. Since acromegaly and elevated GH levels can cause crippling orthopedic and cosmetic deformities and are associated with an increased risk of mortality from metabolic effects, initial surgery is recommended to provide the most rapid reduction in basal GH levels. GH levels normalize after surgery in 60% to 90% of patients, depending on preoperative GH level. Patients in whom postoperative GH levels are less than 5 ng/mL have an excellent prognosis. Patients with persistently elevated GH levels after surgery require additional therapy. We recommend conformal external beam radiotherapy, 45 Gy in 1.8 Gy fractions. Since the effects of radiation therapy may take months to years, bromocriptine or newer medical approaches may be used as additional therapy while full response to pituitary irradiation is pending. Reduction of GH levels with bromocriptine is not as consistent as reduction of prolactin levels in prolactinomas. Treatment recommendations are the same for patients with delayed recurrence of GH hypersecretion after surgery and the occasional patient who is a poor operative candidate.

Prolactinoma

Prolactin-secreting pituitary adenomas are the most common type of pituitary adenoma. They cause amenorrhea, galactorrhea, and infertility in women. Men tend to present with local mass effect (e.g., headache, visual deficits, significant hypopituitarism) and a history of decreased libido and impotence. Both sexes may ultimately develop osteopenia. The diagnosis of a prolactinoma requires a serum level of greater than 200 ng/mL in women and greater than 100 ng/mL in men or clear radiographic evidence of an intrasellar tumor. Normal serum prolactin values should be less than 25 ng/mL. Mild hyperprolactinemia in the range of 25 to 150 ng/mL may result from any lesion that compresses the pituitary stalk or otherwise prevents delivery of prolactin-inhibiting factor from the hypothalamus, or from a prolactinoma. Levels above 1000 ng/mL have been associated with invasive prolactinomas.

Surgery, radiotherapy, bromocriptine, or virtually all combinations of these therapies have been advocated in the treatment of prolactinoma. Clinical series are not easily compared. The probability of cure decreases with the magnitude of the pretreatment prolactin level. It is important to remember that mildly elevated prolactin levels (25 to 150 ng/mL) after radiotherapy may be due to hypothalamic damage. In fact, mild prolactin elevation is also often seen after radiotherapy for non–prolactin-producing adenomas. Most treatment recommendations include dopamine-agonist therapy as the initial management of choice for prolactinomas. Long-term use of bromocriptine in patients with microprolactinomas is generally accepted, as bromocriptine therapy does not lead to a permanent reduction in prolactin levels or adenoma size after cessation of the drug. Microadenomas at UCSF are resected in patients with a desire for pregnancy, in male patients, and in patients who have prolactin levels or MRI studies that indicate growth on bromocriptine, or patients who prefer a surgical approach.

Table 24–5   Acromegaly: Results of Treatment

Reference	Patients, n	Treatment	Results Endpoint	Finding, % (y)
Eastman et al[66]	87	S + RT or RT	GH <5 ng/mL	30 (5)
				53 (10)
				77 (15)
				89 (20)
Grigsby et al[60]	12	S + RT	Disease-free survival	76 (10)
Grigsby et al[62]	22	RT	Disease-free survival	69 (10)
Abosch et al[68]	193	S	GH <5 ng/mL	76% (immediate)
	119	S	GH <2.5 ng/mL	93% (10)
Ludecke et al[67]	30	RT	GH <10	88% (5)

GH, growth hormone; RT, radiotherapy; S, surgery; y, years of follow-up.

There are concerns that bromocriptine may not prevent the risk of tumor expansion during pregnancy. Initially, treatment with bromocriptine suppression of prolactinomas followed by radiation therapy just before attempts at pregnancy was suggested, such that the probability of gonadotropin deficiencies secondary to surgical resection or late radiation therapy effects would be minimized.[68] Other investigators recommend surgery before attempts at pregnancy, or just bromocriptine.[69] Transsphenoidal resection of most macroadenomas is recommended. However, long-term cure of hyperprolactinemia after surgery for macroadenomas occurs rarely, generally in patients with tumors smaller than 2 cm. Bromocriptine may be used before surgery to reduce tumor volume. Persistent hyperprolactinemia after surgery is managed with bromocriptine. Irradiation is reserved for patients who cannot tolerate bromocriptine or have progression on treatment, generally 45 Gy in 1.8 Gy fractions.

Several series evaluated radiotherapy alone or following surgery and found that serum prolactin levels decrease after radiotherapy in virtually all patients.[27,61,68,70-74] Normalization of prolactin levels, however, occurs in only about 50% of patients, with an additional 20% to 30% of patients having levels just above normal (Table 24-6).

Mixed Adenomas

Mixed adenomas are generally prolactin- and GH-secreting adenomas. Any patient with elevated GH levels should be treated with initial trans-sphenoidal adenomectomy. Criteria for postoperative radiotherapy are the same as those for GH-secreting and prolactin-secreting adenomas.

Adrenocorticotropic Hormone-Secreting Adenomas

Hypersecretion of ACTH by a pituitary adenoma causes Cushing's disease. Most patients present with signs of hypercortisolemia, which occur early; therefore, most patients have microadenomas at the time of diagnosis. The diagnosis is based on sustained hypercortisolism and a loss of circadian variation in urinary 17-OH corticosteroids and free-cortisol. A diagnosis is established with documentation of nonsuppressability of hypercortisolemia by low-dose dexamethasone and less than 50% suppressability with high-dose dexamethasone in the setting of normal or only slightly elevated plasma ACTH levels. Low or undetectable ACTH levels, on the other hand, suggest Cushing's syndrome, which is caused by an adrenal neoplasm. Extremely high ACTH levels suggest an ectopic ACTH-producing tumor. Because these pituitary tumors are small, MRI does not always document them. If a high-quality MRI scan does not document an adenoma and the radiologist has expertise, bilateral simultaneous selective venous sampling of ACTH from the inferior petrosal sinuses is done to identify a diagnostic 2:1 ACTH gradient from the sinuses to peripheral blood.[17]

Patients with Cushing's disease often have a number of associated medical problems, such as hypertension, diabetes, electrolyte imbalances, hypothyroidism, and immunosuppression. These problems resolve rapidly once ACTH hypersecretion is normalized. Therefore, surgery is the initial treatment of choice, as normalization of cortisol levels may take months to years after radiotherapy. The presence of extrasellar extension worsens the prognosis after surgery. Patients with pituitary hyperplasia rather than a discrete pituitary adenoma are also felt to be at higher risk for recurrence following pituitary surgery. In the UCSF experience, however, such patients are rare.

Radiation therapy is indicated for patients who have residual adenoma tissue after trans-sphenoidal surgery.[75] Disease can recur as late as 8 years after surgery, whereas late recurrence after radiation therapy is not common with conventional doses. With radiation therapy, however, interim medical therapy may be necessary while waiting for ACTH levels to decrease. Radiation therapy is also indicated in the rare patient who is an extremely high surgical risk. Table 24-7 summarizes recent radiotherapy results.[61,75-77] The definition of "cure" or "remission" varies from series to series and includes normalization of hormone levels and lack of clinical manifestations and radiologic evidence of tumor, as well as more sophisticated endocrinologic evaluation with 24-hour urinary-free cortisol and dexamethasone-suppression tests. Approximately 50% to 70% of patients are reported to

Table 24–6   Prolactinoma: Results of Treatment

Reference	Patients, n	Treatment	Results	
			Endpoint	Finding, % (y)
Littley et al[26]	58	S + RT or RT	Normal prolactin	50 (10)
Tsagarakis et al[69]	36	RT	Normal prolactin	50 (2–13)
Grigsby et al[74]	17	RT	Disease-free: normal prolactin or clinically	82 (10)
Grigsby et al[73]	28	S + RT	Disease-free: normal prolactin or clinically	93 (10)
Johnston et al[72]	14	S + RT or RT	Normal prolactin	43 (9)
Rush et al[70]	10	RT	Normal prolactin	70 (3–8)
Clarke et al[75]	14	S + RT or RT	Normal prolactin	71 (7.5)
Hughes et al[61]	19	S + RT	Normal prolactin	62 (5)
	6	RT	Normal prolactin	50 (5)

RT, radiotherapy; S, surgery; y, years of follow-up.

Table 24–7   Cushing's Disease: Results of Treatment

			Results	
Reference	Patients, *n*	Treatment	*Endpoint*	*Finding,% (y)*
Hughes et al[61]	40	RT	Disease-free	59 (10)
Howlett et al[77]	21	RT	Remission	57 (9.5)
Howlett et al[77]	9	RT*	Remission	56 (3)
Vicente et al[76]	14	RT*	Remission	61 (1)
			Remission	70 (2)
Littley et al[78]	24	RT	Tumor Control/Remission	33% (7.7)

RT, radiotherapy; y, years of follow-up.
*Radiotherapy after surgical failure.

achieve remission after radiotherapy. Detailed endocrinologic evaluation years after radiotherapy has shown that most patients do not obtain normal plasma cortisone levels with dynamic testing, although these patients are clinically in remission.

Treatment recommendations for children with Cushing's disease are essentially the same as for adults. Children may be more sensitive to pituitary radiotherapy, if indicated. Cure rates are reported to be about 80%, with a more rapid decrease in cortisone levels after radiotherapy.

We recommend 50.4 Gy in 1.8 Gy fractions for patients with ACTH-secreting adenomas, favoring a slightly higher dose, as the control rates may be lower for ACTH-secreting adenomas treated with 45 Gy.

NELSON'S SYNDROME

Nelson's syndrome is a result of ACTH hypersecretion by a pituitary adenoma that occurs in approximately 20% to 40% of patients treated with bilateral adrenalectomy for Cushing's syndrome. It may be brought on by an absence of the negative feedback loop of cortisol on the hypothalamus, leading to chronic overstimulation of the pituitary gland by ACTH-releasing factor. The loss of cortisol inhibition allows the pituitary to secrete vast amounts of ACTH and may promote rapid growth of the adenoma. Cutaneous melanocytes are also stimulated by the high ACTH levels. The development of hyperpigmentation in a patient known to have undergone adrenalectomy is diagnostic of Nelson's syndrome; however, the diagnostic tests used for Cushing's disease are also required in this setting.

Nelson's syndrome pituitary tumors are usually large and aggressive and respond poorly to therapy. Trans-sphenoidal surgery offers the best hope of disease control. Because these tumors usually have extrasellar extension, however, surgical cure is achieved in less than 30% of patients. If ACTH levels remain elevated, radiotherapy and medical therapy are indicated. A dose of 45 Gy is recommended. Approximately half of the small number of patients with Nelson's syndrome reported in the literature have been documented to benefit from radiation therapy with progressive depigmentation, shrinkage of the tumor, and decreasing ACTH levels.[76] As bilateral adrenalectomy is now rarely performed, the incidence of Nelson's disease has decreased dramatically.

Endocrine-Inactive Pituitary Adenomas

Endocrine-inactive adenomas, sometimes referred to as nonfunctioning pituitary adenomas and formerly classified as chromophobe adenomas, constitute approximately 25% of pituitary tumors. Sensitive radioimmunoassays demonstrate that approximately 50% of these tumors produce a hormone that is generally inactive. Therefore, these tumors usually present with symptoms from mass effects. Mild hyperprolactinemia may be present from compression of the pituitary stalk. In addition to the assessment of pituitary hormone function and an MRI scan, a determination of pituitary glycoprotein hormone subunits should be performed.

Treatment recommendations for endocrine-inactive adenomas vary. If an endocrine-inactive tumor is documented in a completely asymptomatic patient with normal pituitary function, the majority of authorities feel that these patients should simply be followed with serial MRI scans. Symptomatic patients with endocrine-inactive adenomas should undergo trans-sphenoidal resection. This leads to rapid decompression of the optic chiasm and can avert pituitary insufficiency in most patients. In patients with pituitary insufficiency, trans-sphenoidal surgery may improve function. Response is assessed clinically and with MRI scans. In certain cases, the inactive alpha or beta glycoprotein subunits produced by some nonfunctional pituitary tumors can also serve as markers.

Indications for postoperative radiation therapy are controversial. Some authors feel that surgery alone is sufficient in the case of near-gross total removal.[78] At UCSF we recommend postoperative radiotherapy for tumors that are frankly invasive and incompletely resected and for very large tumors that are likely to be at least microscopically invasive. Table 24-8 summarizes recent results of radiotherapy for nonfunctional adenomas, with approximately 90% control.[60,62,78-81] We recommend 45 Gy in 1.8 Gy fractions. RS for residual disease is selectively recommended.

Thyroid-Stimulating-Hormone-Secreting Tumors

Thyroid-stimulating-hormone-secreting pituitary tumors are very rare. They are diagnosed on the basis of elevated TSH levels and MRI documentation of a pituitary tumor.

Table 24–8   Nonfunctional Pituitary Adenomas: Results of Treatment

Reference	Patients, n	Treatment	Results Endpoint	Finding, % (y)
Flickinger et al[79]	112	S + RT	Progression-free survival or RT	89 (10)
Grigsby et al[62]	81	S + RT	Disease-free survival	89.9 (10)
Grigsby et al[60]	19	RT	Disease-free survival	79.6 (10)
Tsang et al[80]	128	S + RT	Progression-free survival	91 (10)
Brada et al[81]	199	S + RT	Progression-free survival	98 (10)
	31	RT	Progression-free survival	95 (10)
McCord et al[82]	98	S + RT	Progression-free survival	95 (10)
	23	RT	Progression-free survival	95 (10)

RT, radiotherapy; S, surgery; y, years of follow-up.

They are generally large and locally aggressive. Surgery is recommended as initial therapy[82]; however, tumor regrowth and persistent hypersecretion are common after surgery alone, and these tumors tend to have an aggressive history. Therefore, postoperative radiation therapy is recommended.

There is little information on the efficacy of radiation therapy in this setting. Because of the worse natural history of these tumors, we recommend a slightly higher tumor dose, 50.4 Gy in 1.8 Gy fractions.

REIRRADIATION OF PITUITARY ADENOMA

Although excellent control rates are achieved following moderate-dose radiotherapy to pituitary adenomas, patients occasionally develop a recurrence in the previously irradiated field. Because of concerns about optic chiasm and surrounding brain radiotolerance, reirradiation has generally been avoided. Schoenthaler and associates[83] reported on 15 patients with pituitary adenomas that recurred at a median of 9 years after radiotherapy (with a median initial radiation dose of 48.8 Gy), who then received a second course of radiation (median 42.0 Gy). Median follow-up after irradiation was 10 years. Local control was maintained in 80% of patients; all patients developed hypopituitarism; two patients developed temporal lobe injury; and no visual complications were noted. Similar data have been reported by Flickinger and associates[84]; therefore, reirradiation could be considered if there is a long interval from first radiotherapy to recurrence and other therapeutic modalities to treat the recurrence have been unsuccessful. Stereotactic RS has also been used in this setting; however, data are very limited.

FOLLOW-UP

Patients treated with radiation therapy for their pituitary adenoma need to be followed for life. They need serial endocrinologic evaluation by an endocrinologist to monitor for and correct hypopituitarism secondary to radiation therapy. Formal ophthalmologic follow-up is indicated for patients who present with visual deficits. Patients also need

to be followed for response to treatment, with serial hormone determinations and yearly MRI scanning. These tests will typically demonstrate reduction in tumor size or an empty sella within several years following completion of radiation therapy. One can also see remineralization of the sella and a decrease in the size of the pituitary fossa after radiotherapy.

REFERENCES

1. Kernohan JW, Sayre GP: Tumors of the pituitary gland and infundibulum. *Atlas of Tumor Pathology.* Washington, D.C.: Armed Forces Institute of Pathology; 1956; Section X, Fascicle 36.
2. Annegers JF, Coulam CB, Abbour CF, et al: Pituitary adenomas in Olmsted County, Minnesota, 1935-1977. *Mayo Clin Proc.* 1978;53:641.
3. Faglia G: Epidemiology and pathogenesis of pituitary adenomas. *Acta Endocrinol.* 129:1, 1993.
4. Alexander JM, Biller BM, Bikkal H, et al: Clinically nonfunctioning pituitary tumors are monoclonal in origin. *J Clin Invest.* 1990;86:336.
5. Scheithauer BW, Horvath E, Kovacs K, et al: Plurihormonal pituitary adenomas. *Semin Diagn Pathol.* 1986;3:69.
6. Landolt AM, Shibata T, Kleihues P: Growth rate of human pituitary adenomas. *J Neurosurg.* 1987;67:803.
7. Nagashima T, Murovic, JA, Hoshino T, et al: The proliferative potential of human pituitary tumors in situ. *J Neurosurg.* 1986;64:588.
8. Knosp E, Kitz K, Perneczky A: Proliferation activity in pituitary adenomas: Measurement by monoclonal antibody Ki-67. *Neurosurgery.* 1989;25:927.
9. Hardy J: Transsphenoidal surgery of hypersecretion in pituitary tumors. In Kohler PO, Ross PT (eds.) Diagnosis and Treatment of Pituitary Tumors. New York, Elsevier, 1973:179.
10. Aron DC, Tyrell JB, Wilson CB: Pituitary tumors: Current concepts in diagnosis and management. *West J Med.* 1995;162:340.
11. Newton DR, Dillon WP, Norman D, et al: Gd-DTPA-enhanced MR imaging of pituitary adenomas. *Am J Neuroradiol.* 1989;10:949.
12. Miki Y, Matsuo M, Nishizawa S, et al: Pituitary adenomas and normal pituitary tissue: Enhancement patterns on gadopentetate-enhanced MR-imaging. *Radiology.* 1990;177:35.
13. Hardy J, Vezina JL: Trans-sphenoidal neurosurgery of intracranial neoplasm. In Thompson RA, Green JR, eds. *Advances in Neurology: Neoplasia in the Nervous System.* Vol 15. New York: Raven Press; 1976:261.
14. Wilson CB: Surgical management of endocrine-active pituitary adenomas. In *Oncology of the Nervous System.* Walker, MD, ed. (series volume in *Cancer Treatment and Research,* WL, McGuire, ed.) Boston: Martinus Nijhoff; 1983:117.
15. Halberg FE, Sheline GE: Radiotherapy of pituitary tumors. *Endocrin Metab Clin.* 1987;16:667.

16. Ross DA, Wilson CB: Results of transsphenoidal microsurgery for growth hormone-secreting pituitary adenoma in a series of 214 patients. *J Neurosurg.* 1988;68:854.

17. Wilson CB: Pituitary neoplasms. In Holland JF, Frei E III, eds. *Cancer Medicine.* Philadelphia: Lea & Febiger; 1993:1131.

18. Bevan JS, Webster J, Burke CW, Scanlon MF: Dopamine agonists and pituitary tumor shrinkage. *Endocr Rev.* 1992;13:220.

19. Atkinson AB: The treatment of Cushing's syndrome. *Clin Endocrinol (Oxf).* 1991;34:507.

20. Lamberts SWJ, Reubi JC, Krenning EP: Somatostatin analogs in the treatment of acromegaly. *Endocrin Metab Clin North Am.* 1992;21:737.

21. Chanson P, Weintraub BD, Harris AG: Octreotide therapy for thyroid-stimulating hormone-secreting pituitary adenomas: A follow-up of 52 patients. *Ann Intern Med.* 1992;119:236.

22. Fisher BJ, Gaspar LE, Noone B: Giant pituitary adenomas: Role of radiotherapy. *Int J Radiat Oncol Biol Phys.* 1993;25:667.

23. Woollons AC, Hunn MK, Rajapakse YR, et al: Non-functioning pituitary adenomas: Indications for postoperative radiotherapy. *Clin Endocrinol (Oxf).* 2000;53:713.

24. Sheline GE, Tyrrell B: Pituitary adenomas. *Radiation Oncology Annual.* New York: Raven Press; 1983:1.

25. Zierhut D, Flentje M, Adolph J, et al: External radiotherapy of pituitary adenomas. *Int J Radiat Oncol Biol Phys.* 1995;33:307.

26. Littley MD, Shalet SM, Swindell R, et al: Low-dose pituitary irradiation for acromegaly. *Clin Endocrinol (Oxf).* 1990;32:261.

27. Littley MD, Shalet SM, Reid H, et al: The effect of external pituitary irradiation on elevated serum prolactin levels in patients with pituitary macroadenomas. *Q J Med.* 1991;81:985.

28. Isobe K, Ohta M, Yasuda S, et al: Postoperative radiation therapy for pituitary adenoma. *J Neuro Oncol.* 2000;48:135.

29. Lustig RH, Schriock EA, Kaplan SL, et al: Effect of growth hormone-releasing factor on growth hormone release in children with radiation-induced growth hormone deficiency. *Pediatrics.* 1985;76:274.

30. Littley MD, Shalet SM, Beardwell CG, et al: Hypopituitarism following external radiotherapy for pituitary tumors in adults. *Q J Med.* 1989;70:145.

31. Rush SC, Kupersmith MJ, Lerch I, et al: Neuro-ophthalmological assessment of vision before and after radiation therapy alone for pituitary macroadenomas. *J Neurosurg.* 1990;72:594.

32. Brada M, Ford D, Ashley S, et al: Risk of second brain tumor after conservative surgery and radiotherapy for pituitary adenoma. *Br Med J.* 1992;304:1343.

33. Sheline GE, Wara WM, Smith V: Therapeutic irradiation and brain injury. *Int J Radiat Oncol Biol Phys.* 1980;6:1215.

34. Al-Mefty O, Kersh JE, Routh A, et al: The long-term side effects of radiation therapy for benign brain tumors in adults. *J Neurosurg.* 1990;73:502.

35. Beaney RP, Gibbs JS, Brooks DJ, et al: Absence of irradiation induced ischaemic temporal lobe damage in patients with pituitary tumors. *J Neuro Oncol.* 1987;5:129.

36. Hashimoto N, Handa H, Yamashita J, et al: Long-term follow-up of large or invasive pituitary adenomas. *Surg Neurol.* 1986;25:49.

37. Hirata Y, Matsukado Y, Mihara Y, et al: Occlusion of the internal carotid artery after radiation therapy for the chiasmal lesion. *Acta Neurochir (Wien).* 1985;74:141.

38. Flickinger JC, Nelson PB, Taylor FH, et al: Incidence of cerebral infarction after radiotherapy for pituitary adenoma. *Cancer.* 1989;63:2404.

39. Fraser R, Doyle GF, Joplin CW, et al: The assessment of endocrine effect and the effectiveness of ablative pituitary treatment by ^{90}Y and ^{198}Au implantation. In Kohler PO, Ross GT, eds. *Pituitary Tumors.* New York: Elsevier; 1973:35.

40. Sandler LM, Richards NT, Carr DH, et al: Long-term follow-up of patients with Cushing's disease treated by interstitial irradiation. *J Clin Endocrinol Metab.* 1989;65:441.

41. Levy RP, Fabrikant JI, Frankel KA, et al: Progress in heavy particle radiotherapy. *Gan To Kagaku Ryoho.* 1994;21:929.

42. Nishioka H, Hirano A, Haraoka J, Nakajima N: Histological changes in the pituitary gland and adenomas following radiotherapy. *Neuropathology.* 2002;22:19.

43. Kjellberg RN, Kliman B: Bragg peak proton treatment for pituitary-related conditions. *Proc R Soc Med.* 1974;67:32.

44. Alexander E, Loeffler J: Clinical experience with Linac radiosurgery. In Gildenberg P, Tasker R, eds: Textbook of Stereotactic and Functional Neurosurgery. New York, McGraw-Hill, 1998, p. 745.

45. Kjellberg RN, Kliman B, Swisher B, et al: Proton beam therapy of Cushing's disease and Nelson's syndrome. In Black PM, ed. *Secretory Tumors of Pituitary Gland.* New York: Raven Press, 1984:191.

46. Yoon S, Suh T, Jang H, et al: Clinical results of 24 pituitary macroadenomas with linac-based stereotactic radiosurgery. *Int J Radiat Oncol Biol Phys.* 1998;41:849.

47. Mitsumori M, Shrieve DC, Alexander E III, et al: Initial clinical results of Linac-based stereotactic radiosurgery and stereotactic radiotherapy for pituitary adenomas. *Int J Radiat Oncol Biol Phys.* 1998;42:573.

48. Leber KA, Bergloff J, Pendl G: Dose-response tolerance of the visual pathways and cranial nerves of the cavernous sinus to stereotactic radiosurgery. *J Neurosurg.* 1998;88:43.

49. Degerblad M, Rahn T, Bergstrand G, et al: Long-term results of stereotactic radiosurgery to the pituitary gland in Cushing's disease. *Acta Endocrinol Copenhagen.* 1986;112:310.

50. Pan L, Zhang N, Wang E, et al: Pituitary adenomas: The effect of gamma knife radiosurgery on tumor growth and endocrinopathies. *Stereotact Funct Neurosurg.* 1998;70:119.

51. Lim YJ, Leem W, Kim TS, et al: Four years' experience in the treatment of pituitary adenomas with gamma knife radiosurgery. *Stereotact Funct Neurosurg.* 1998;70:95.

52. Izawa M, Hayashi M, Nakaya K, et al: Gamma knife radiosurgery for pituitary adenomas. *J Neurosurg.* 2000;93s:19.

53. Zhang N, Pan L, Wang EM, et al: Radiosurgery for growth hormone-producing pituitary adenomas. *J Neurosurg.* 2000;93s:6.

54. Ikeda H, Jokura H, Yoshimoto T: Transsphenoidal surgery and adjuvant gamma knife treatment for growth hormone-secreting pituitary adenoma. *J Neurosurg.* 2001;95:285.

55. Pollock B, Young W. Stereotactic radiosurgery for patients with ACTH-producing pituitary adenomas after prior adenalectomy. *Int J Radiat Oncol Biol Phys.* 2002;54:839.

56. Tishler RB, Loeffler JS, Lunsford D, et al: Tolerance of cranial nerves of the cavernous sinus to radiosurgery. *Int J Radiat Oncol Biol Phys.* 1993;27:215.

57. Ove R, Kelman D, Amin PP, Chin LS: Preservation of visual fields after peri-sellar gamma-knife radiosurgery. *Int J Cancer.* 2000;90:343.

58. Jackson IM, Noren G: Role of gamma knife radiosurgery in acromegaly. *Pituitary.* 1999;2:71.

59. Suit H, Urie M: Proton beams in radiation therapy. *J Natl Cancer Inst.* 1992;84:155.

60. Grigsby PW, Simpson JR, Stokes S, et al: Results of surgery and irradiation or irradiation alone for pituitary adenomas. *J Neuro Oncol.* 1988;6:129.

61. Hughes MN, Llamas KJ, Yelland ME, et al: Pituitary adenomas: Long-term results for radiotherapy alone and post-operative radiotherapy. *Int J Radiat Oncol Biol Phys.* 1993;27:1035.

62. Grigsby PW, Simpson JR, Fineberg B: Late regrowth of pituitary adenomas after irradiation and/or surgery. Hazard function analysis. *Cancer.* 1989;63:1308.

63. McCollough WM, Marcus RBJ, Rhoton ALJ, et al: Long-term follow-up of radiotherapy for pituitary adenoma: The absence of late recurrence after greater than or equal to 4500 cGy. *Int J Radiat Oncol Biol Phys.* 1991;21:607.

64. Melmed S: Acromegaly. *N Engl J Med.* 1990;322:966.

65. Barkan AL, Halasz I, Dornfeld KJ: Pituitary irradiation is ineffective in normalizing plasma insulin-like growth factor I in patients with acromegaly. *J Clin Endocrinol Metab.* 1997;82:3187.

66. Eastman RC, Gorden P, Glatstein E, et al: Radiation therapy of acromegaly. *Endocrinol Metab Clin North Am.* 1992;21:693.

67. Ludecke DK, Lutz BS, Niedwork G: The choice of treatment after incomplete adenomectomy in acromegaly: Proton versus high-voltage radiation. *Acta Neurochir (Wien).* 1989;96:32.

68. Abosch A, Tyrrell JB, Lamborn KR, et al: Transsphenoidal microsurgery for growth hormone-secreting pituitary adenomas: initial outcome and long-term results. *J Clin Endocrinol Metab.* 1998;83:3411.

69. Tsagarakis S, Grossman A, Plowman PN, et al: Megavoltage pituitary irradiation in the management of prolactinomas: Long-term follow-up. *Clin Endocrinol (Oxf).* 1991;34:399.

70. Molitch ME: Pregnancy and the hyperprolactinemic woman. *N Engl J Med.* 1985;312:1364.

71. Rush SC, Newall J: Pituitary adenoma: The efficacy of radiotherapy as the sole treatment. *Int J Radiat Oncol Biol Phys.* 1989;17:165.

72. Johnston DG, Hall K, Kendall TP, et al: The long-term effects of megavoltage radiotherapy as sole or combined therapy for large prolactinomas: Studies with high definition computerized tomography. *Clin Endocrinol (Oxf)*. 1986;24:675.

73. Grigsby PW, Simpson JR, Emami BN, et al: Prognostic factors and results of surgery and postoperative irradiation in the management of pituitary adenomas. *Int J Radiat Oncol Biol Phys*. 1989;16:1411.

74. Grigsby PW, Stokes S, Marks JE, et al: Prognostic factors and results of radiotherapy alone in the management of pituitary adenomas. *Int J Radiat Oncol Biol Phys*. 1988;15:1103.

75. Clarke SD, Woo SY, Butler EB, et al: Treatment of secretory pituitary adenomas with radiation therapy. *Radiology*. 1993;188:759.

76. Vicente A, Estrada J, dela Cuerda C, et al: Results of external pituitary irradiation after unsuccessful transsphenoidal surgery in Cushing's disease. *Acta Endocrinol (Copenh)*. 1991;125:470.

77. Howlett TA, Plowman PN, Wass JAH, et al: Megavoltage pituitary irradiation in the management of Cushing's disease and Nelson's syndrome: Long-term follow-up. *Clin Endocrinol*. 1989;31:309.

78. Littley MD, Shalet SM, Beardwell CG, et al: Long-term follow-up of low-dose external pituitary irradiation for Cushing's disease. *Clin Endocrinol (Oxf)*. 1990;33:445.

79. Flickinger JC, Nelson PB, Martinez AJ, et al: Radiotherapy of nonfunctional adenomas of the pituitary gland. Results with long-term follow-up. *Cancer*. 1989;63:2409.

80. Tsang RW, Brierly JD, Panzarella T, et al: Radiation therapy for pituitary adenoma: Treatment outcome and prognostic factors. *Int J Radiat Oncol Biol Phys*. 1994;30:557.

81. Brada M, Rajan B, Traish D, et al: The long-term efficacy of conservative surgery and radiotherapy in the control of pituitary adenomas. *Clin Endocrinol*. 1993;38:571.

82. McCord MW, Buatti JM, Fennel EM, et al: Radiotherapy for pituitary adenoma: Long-term outcome and sequelae. *Int J Radiat Oncol Biol Phys*. 1998;39:437.

83. Mindermann T, Wilson CB: Thyrotropin-secreting pituitary adenomas. *Neurosurg*. 1993;79:521.

84. Schoenthaler R, Albright NW, Wara WM, et al: Re-irradiation of pituitary adenoma. *Int J Radiat Oncol Biol Phys*. 1992;24:307.

85. Flickinger JC, Deutsch M, Lunsford LD: Repeat megavoltage irradiation of pituitary and suprasellar tumors. *Int J Radiat Oncol Biol Phys*. 1989;17:171.

Radiosurgery

Dennis C. Shrieve, MD, PhD, David A. Larson, MD, PhD, and Jay S. Loeffler, MD

25

Stereotactic radiosurgery (SRS) is the delivery of a single high dose of ionizing radiation to an intracranial target defined using stereotactic imaging. Several different delivery techniques result in a dose distribution that is highly conformal to the target. Dose fall-off outside the target is precipitous and therefore only the target and immediately surrounding normal tissue are included in the high-dose region. SRS was developed by Swedish neurosurgeon Lars Leksel of the Karolinska Institute in Stockholm, initially for treatment of functional disorders.[1] After more than 30 years of development, radiosurgery has entered the mainstream of medical care. Since the 1960s, more than 200,000 patients have been treated with some form of radiosurgery, most within the past 5 years. Radiosurgery is now practiced at more than 200 facilities in the United States.

In North America, patients who undergo radiosurgery are usually selected, treated, and followed by a dedicated multidisciplinary radiosurgery team of experts including radiation oncologists, neurosurgeons, physicists, nurses, and technologists; the same radiosurgery team provides quality assurance. This multidisciplinary approach to therapy has received support from the radiosurgery task forces of societies representing both neurosurgery and radiation oncology.[2-4]

TECHNIQUES

STEREOTAXIS. The term stereotactic (from the Greek *stereo* + *taxis*, ordered in three dimensions) refers to techniques in which intracranial targets are localized precisely in three-dimensional space for introduction of a probe for biopsy or for delivery of localized radiotherapy. The basis for construction of the stereotactic space is the rigid application of a head frame to the patient's skull. Stereotactic imaging is then performed with a localizer fitted over the patient's head and attached to the frame. Fiducial markers in the localizer box define x, y, and z coordinates for any location in the defined space above the frame and appear on each image obtained. Imaging may be done with either computed tomography (CT) or magnetic resonance imaging (MRI) technology or both with "fusion" of the two imaging modalities (Fig. 25-1).

SRS DELIVERY SYSTEMS. At present, radiosurgery is performed by using one of three forms of high-energy radiation. The radiosurgery technology most commonly available around the world uses high-energy x-rays generated from a clinical linear accelerator, or "linac." Gamma-ray radiosurgery with the Gamma Knife (AB Elekta, Stockholm), although not yet as widely available as linac radiosurgery, has been increasing in usage at numerous centers and has been used to treat more patients than other radiosurgery technologies. Radiosurgery with charged particles (e.g., protons or heavy ions) produced by a cyclotron or synchrotron is the technology least frequently used, but may be most suitable for large target volumes. Any radiosurgery treatment-planning system should provide rapid, three-dimensional visualization of the target and isodose distribution superimposed on CT scans, magnetic resonance images, and angiograms.

Gamma Knife

More than 150 Gamma Knife units are now located around the world, including more than 70 in the United States. As of the year 2003, more than 200,000 patients had been treated with this technology. The Gamma Knife unit consists of a central core containing 201 cobalt 60 (^{60}Co) sources surrounded by two hemispheric, cast-iron shields and a steel entrance door (Fig. 25-2). The sources are situated in individual beam channels in the central core directed convergently toward a single target point (isocenter) at the hollow center of the radiation unit (see Fig. 25-2). Collimation of the beams is provided by a collimator helmet, which is attached to the treatment table and contains 201 collimators projecting to 4, 8, 14, or 18 mm diameter at the isocenter (see Fig. 25-2).

After stereotactic frame placement and imaging, treatment planning consists of selection of a number of individual "shots" or radiation doses to small volumes within the target, each with a unique isocenter coordinate. Treatment plans are evaluated and optimized using dose-volume histograms (DVH). Once treatment planning is completed, the patient lies on the treatment table which is adjusted so that the patient's head, fixed within the stereotactic frame, is moved into the collimator helmet (Fig. 25-3). The frame is oriented within the helmet in the x, y, and z

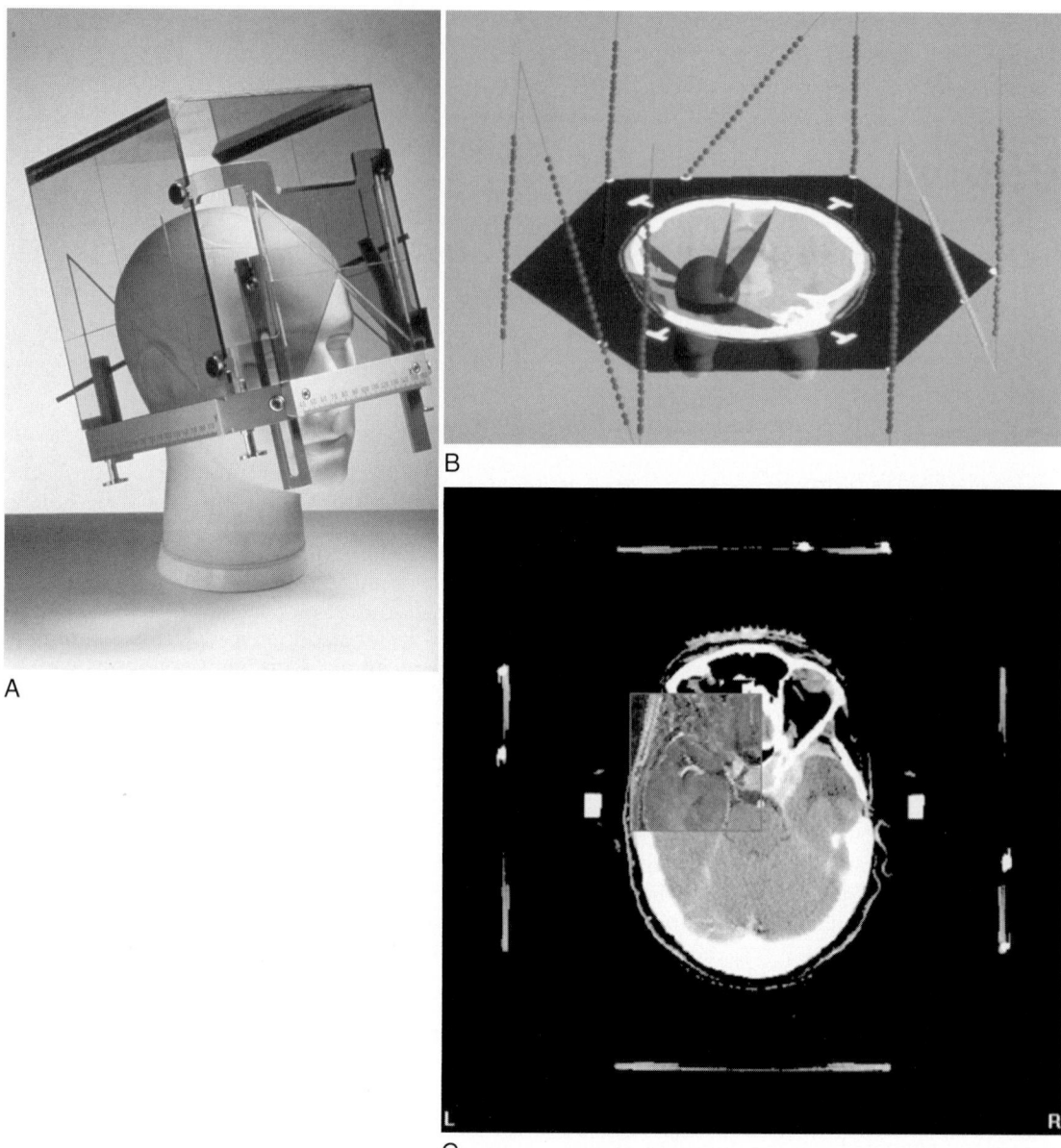

Figure 25–1. A, Leksell stereotactic frame with magnetic resonance (MR)-compatible localizer. Note "N"-shaped fiducial markers on localizer and scale on frame for patient positioning during treatment. **B,** Computer rendering of computed tomography (CT) slice depicting stereotactic space defined by "N"-shaped fiducials from linac radiosurgery planning system. Note projection of collimator (red) and paths of arcs for delivery of treatment (blue). **C,** Stereotactic CT of patient with left cavernous sinus meningioma with overlying "fused" MR (blue box). Note excellent fusion of images and fiducials, indicating they are level within stereotactic space. See also Color Figure 25-1.

directions so that the radiation beams will align with the target site according to the treatment plan. Several different isocenters may be treated in sequence during the treatment session in order to make the isodose surface conform closely to any irregular three-dimensional target contour (Fig. 25-4). It takes about 10 to 15 minutes to place the patient in position and treat each isocenter. Because ^{60}Co has a half-life of 5 years, treatment times must be progressively increased.

Figures 25-5 through 25-7 represent examples of Gamma Knife plans for ateriovenous malformation (AVM), metastatic disease, and a benign acoustic schwannoma, respectively. In each, the dose was prescribed at the 50% isodose line (yellow), which was required to conform tightly to the target configuration

(red or blue). The 25% isodose line (green) is also shown. The crosses represent projections of isocenter locations onto the MR image plane.

Linear Accelerator

Linear accelerator, or linac, radiosurgery is widely available, in part because existing linacs may be modified for radiosurgery with relatively little expense. It is likely that more than 30,000 patients have been treated with linac radiosurgery. Although many treatment centers use a linac unit that has been modified for radiosurgical use, dedicated stereotactic linac units that are specially designed and have excellent mechanical accuracy are now available.

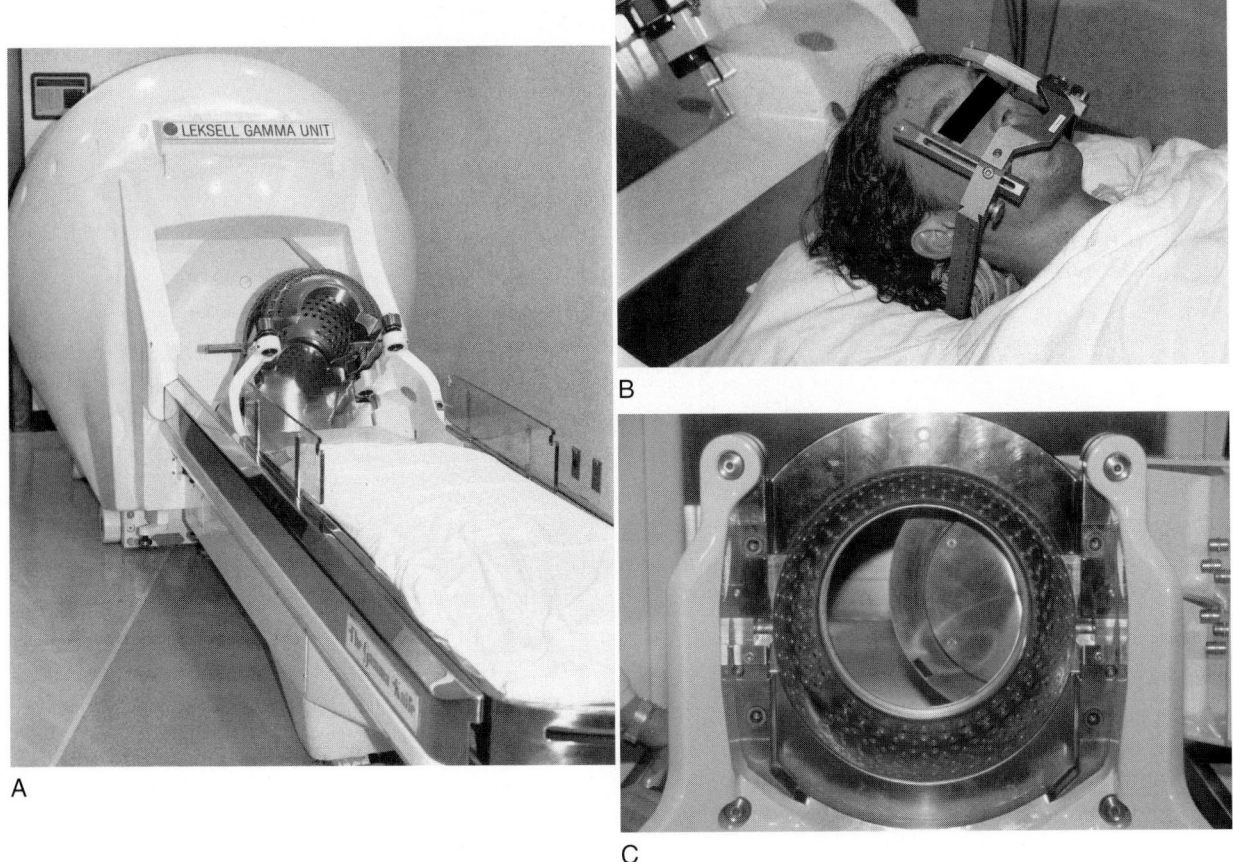

Figure 25–2. A, Schematic of Gamma Knife unit showing patient in treatment position, source and beams directed to isocenter through primary and secondary collimators. **B,** Leksell Gamma Knife unit with patient in helmet ready to enter into treatment position. **C,** Closeup of Gamma Knife helmet. The 8 designates this helmet as having collimators projecting to 8 mm at the isocenter.

"Home-grown" linac planning systems are now being replaced by commercially available systems that are approved by the U.S. Food and Drug Administration for this purpose.

Like the Gamma Knife, linacs have a defined isocenter at the intersection of the axis of rotation of the gantry and the treatment couch and the central axis of the

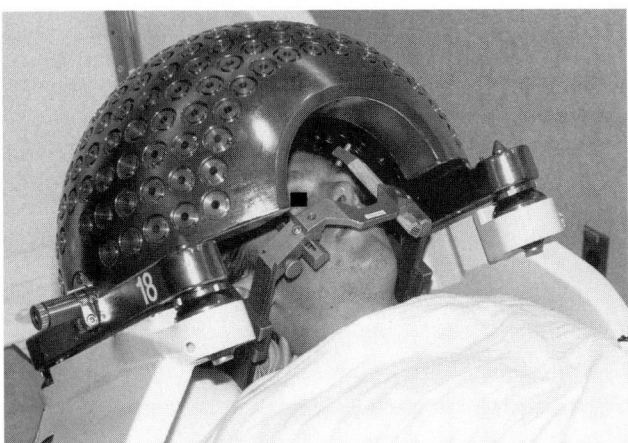

Figure 25–3. A patient positioned in a Gamma Knife helmet before entry into the Gamma Knife core.

photon beam (Fig. 25-8). Targets may be treated with single or multiple isocenter plans. Initial linac systems used special circular collimators of diameters from 5–60 mm to reduce the penumbra of the beam and the radiation dose to normal tissues. However, the use of circular collimators greatly limits the potential for isodose shaping, especially when using single isocenter plans. Excellent conformity is now possible using micro multileaf collimation and either multiple fixed fields or dynamic arc radiosurgery. In the latter, the field shape is constantly changing to conform to the beam's eye view outline of the target volume (Fig. 25-9). This treatment strategy has been shown to produce isodose distributions with conformity indices as good as those reported for multiple isocenter Gamma Knife plans.[5]

Further improvement in conformity of linac radiosurgery plans is obtained using intensity-modulated delivery methods. Coupled with inverse treatment planning systems, avoidance of normal structures adjacent to the target volume is also possible. Clearly the future of linac-based stereotactic radiotherapy and radiosurgery lies in the ability to produce conformal treatment plans entirely covering a target while using intensity modulation to avoid adjacent critical structures.[6] Such treatment may often be delivered through a single isocenter and with prescription to the greater than 80% isodose line, thereby reducing dose inhomogeneity within the target.

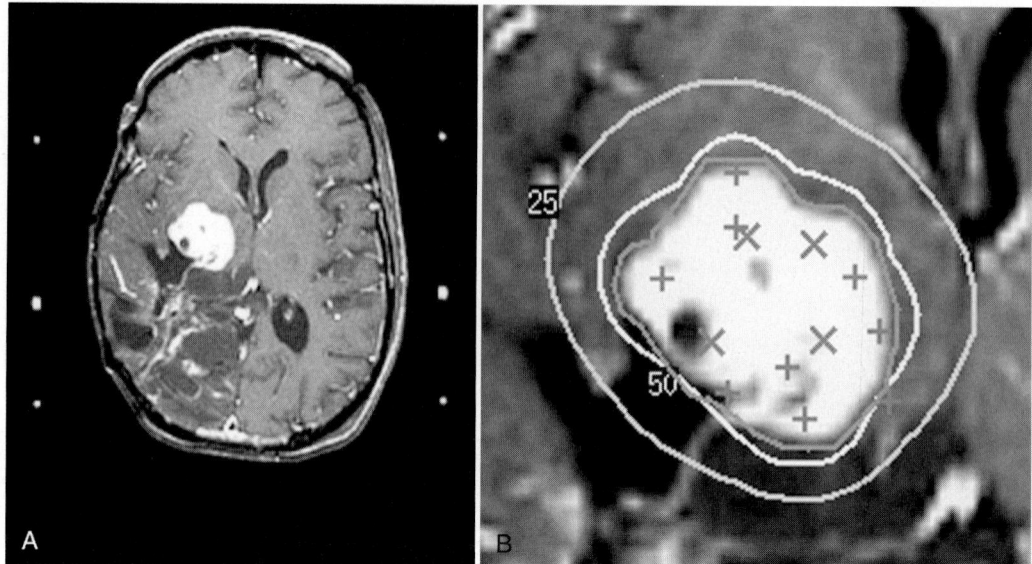

Figure 25–4. A, Magnetic resonance image of right parietal glioblastoma in a 39-year-old man with focal recurrence 15 years following diagnosis and treatment with 60 Gy external beam, chemotherapy, and brachytherapy boost. **B,** 13 isocenters were used to obtain conformity of 50% isodose line to tumor volume. Three different collimator helmets were employed (18 mm × 3, 14 mm × 7, 8 mm × 3). The target volume was 20.2 mL and a dose of 11 Gy was prescribed to the 50% isodose line representing the target periphery. See also Color Figure 25-4B.

To align the patient's head with respect to the linac beam, some groups have the patient lie on the treatment couch with the head supported and positioned on a separate, floor-mounted, stereotactic fixture, whereas others use only the treatment couch together with the standard alignment lasers associated with linac technology. Many groups recommend that target positioning be verified radiographically before each individual treatment. With most systems, patients are treated while they lie supine, although some systems require that the patient be in a sitting position. In most cases, beam-entrance patterns trace a series of noncoplanar arcs on the scalp, one arc for each of several positions to which the table is turned.[7]

Particle-Beam Irradiation

Charged particle-beam radiosurgery has been used predominantly in North America and the Soviet Union over the past 40 years, during which more than 6000 patients have been treated, some receiving therapy in as many as 4 fractions rather than 1.[8] In contrast to x-ray or Gamma Knife techniques, which require a large number of convergent radiation beams to produce a highly focal dose distribution, charged-particle beams produced by cyclotrons or synchrotrons produce a highly focal dose distribution with only a few beams because of the Bragg ionization peak produced by each individual beam. The width of the Bragg peak and its depth in relation to the scalp are adjusted to match the target's dimensions and depth in brain. Patients usually are treated with two to six stationary, intersecting beams, each with its own irregularly shaped collimator that conforms to the contour of the target. To ensure an acceptable three-dimensional dose distribution, compensators may be interposed in the beams to compensate for skull curvature and tissue inhomogeneities. As in linac or Gamma Knife radiosurgery, the three-dimensional dose distribution produced by a few intersecting particle beams falls off rapidly with distance from the target periphery, but it can be made more homogeneous within the target.

RADIOBIOLOGICAL EFFECT

Usually, radiosurgery delivers little or no clinically important radiation dose beyond the target volume, in part because of the steep dose gradient at the target's margins and in part because the minimum target isodose contour (usually 50% to 80%) conforms closely to the three-dimensional configuration of the target. Therefore, radiosurgery doses are high and inhomogeneous. The biological effectiveness of radiation depends on the total dose of radiation, the dose per fraction, and the type of tissue irradiated. For late responding tissues, like normal central nervous system or vasculature, there is a strong dependence on dose per fraction. With radiosurgery, total dose and dose per fraction are high and variations in both according to isodose distributions produce sharply changing biological effects. Within the target periphery, dose inhomogeneity (sharply rising dose from target margin to isocenter) has a disproportionate radiobiological effect and may substantially elevate the potential for a cure or complication. Beyond the target's perimeter, the radiobiological effect declines rapidly due to decreasing dose and dose per fraction, a characteristic that may spare normal tissue but that may permit the survival of potential infiltrative disease just outside the radiologically apparent target.[9]

Intracranial Target Lesions

Intracranial targets for radiosurgery fall into one of four categories based on two criteria: (1) whether the target tissue's

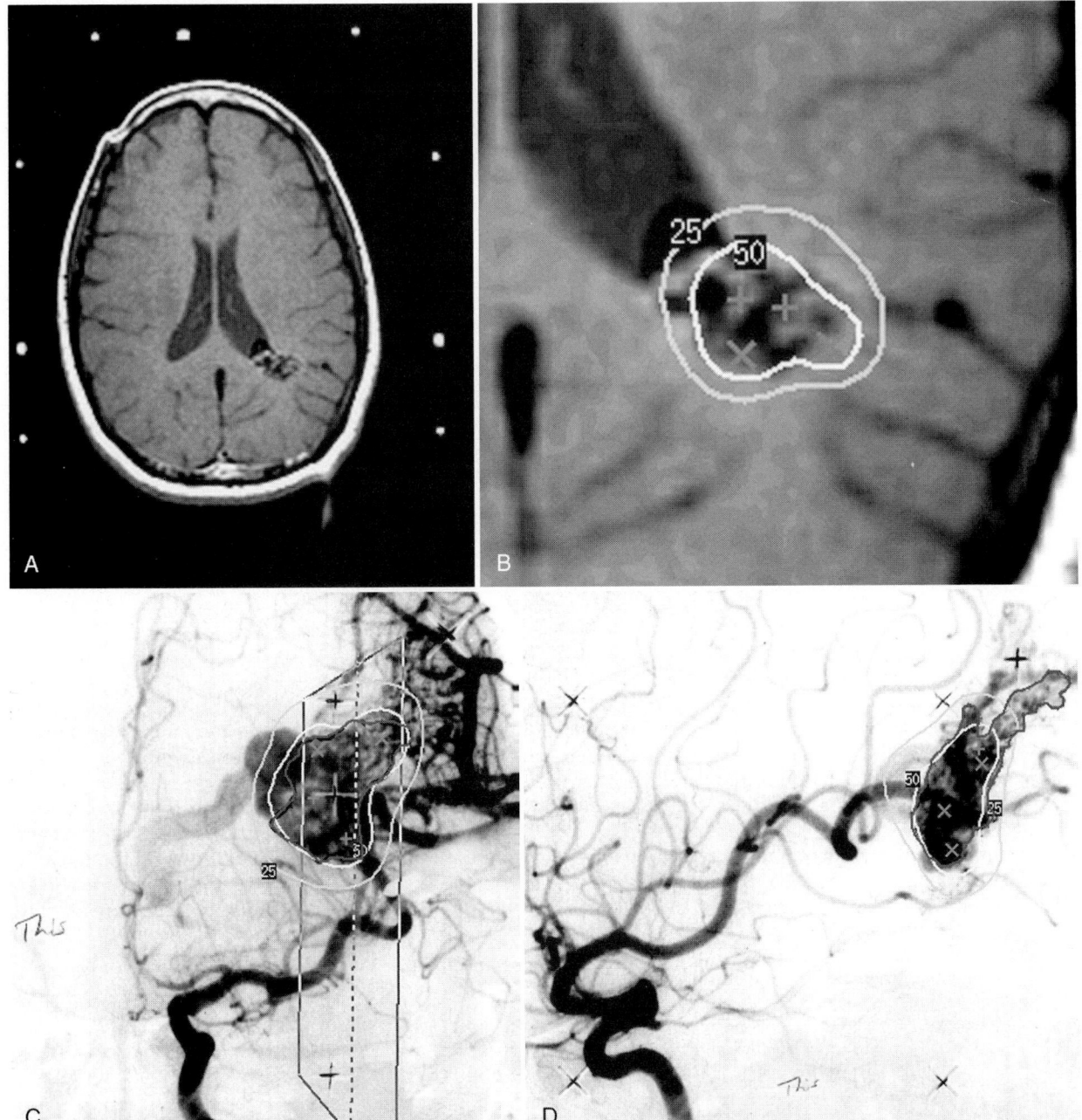

Figure 25–5. A, Magnetic resonance image of a 41-year-old woman with left parietal arteriovenous malformation (AVM). **B**, Four isocenters were used (14 mm x 1, 8 mm x 3) and 18.5 Gy was delivered to the 50% isodose line. **C** and **D**, Angiographic orthogonal views of the AVM with isodose distribution superimposed on anteroposterior [**C**] and sagittal (**D**) angiograms. See also Color Figure 25-5B–D.

radiobiological response to radiosurgery is early or late; and (2) whether the target volume contains any normal tissue.[9]

- Category A: Target volumes containing an AVM are late responding in both normal and abnormal tissue because the target volume contains some normal brain.
- Category B: Target volumes containing a benign tumor, such as meningioma, pituitary adenoma, and acoustic neuroma, are also late responding and show a marked radiobiological effect, but predominantly in abnormal tissue, because the target contains no normal tissue.
- Category C: Target volumes containing a low-grade glial tumor also contain some normal brain, but show a

more substantial effect in late-responding normal tissue than in early-responding tumor tissue. Radiosurgery is recommended for these tumors only occasionally.
- Category D: Target volumes containing a metastasis show an early response and a moderately large effect, but predominantly in early-responding abnormal tissue because the target volume contains no normal tissue. Glioblastomas may be considered to be in category D, although they may contain a small amount of normal tissue.

For small targets in categories A and B, it is to be anticipated that the ratio of patients cured to those with

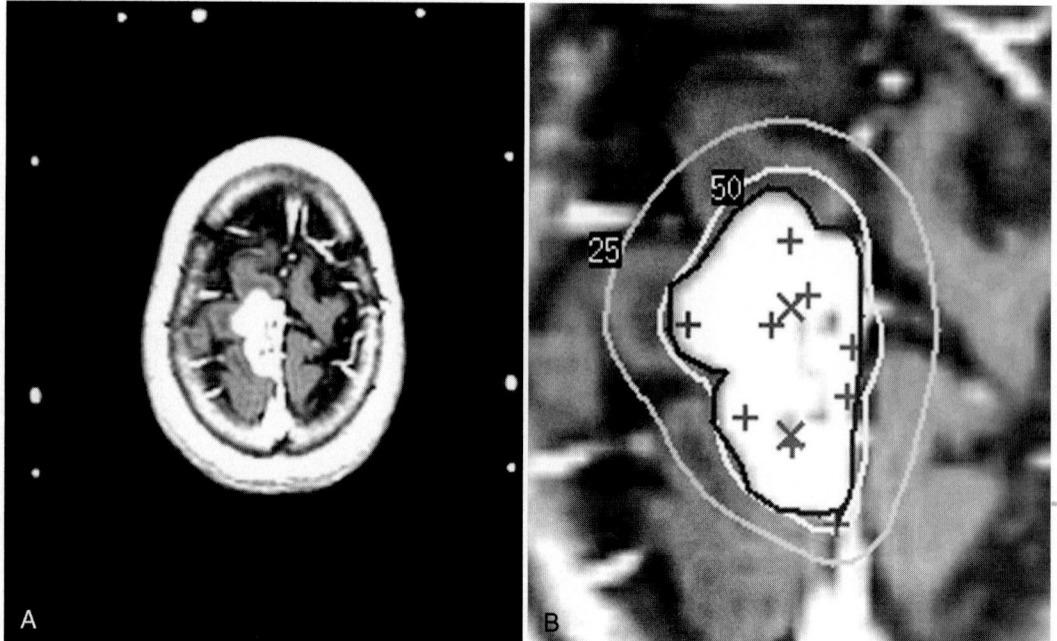

Figure 25–6. A, Magnetic resonance image of a dural-based mass at the right superior frontoparietal convexity, immediately adjacent to the falx. The patient was a 65-year-old man who had been previously diagnosed with adenocarcinoma of the colon. **B,** 11 isocenters (18 mm × 2, 14 mm × 5, 8 mm × 4) were used to cover the 13 mL target volume with the 50% isodose line. The clinician prescribed 16 Gy. See also Color Figure 25-6B.

complications (therapeutic ratio) will bear little relation to the fractionation scheme used, whether single or multiple. For AVMs (category A), clinical data on fractionated treatments to a dose sufficient to test this prediction are not available. The clinical data available so far on radiosurgery for meningioma (category B) are not dissimilar to the best reported results of fractionated radiation therapy planned with CT or MR imaging.[10-12] For metastases (category D), it might be thought that fractionated

treatments would be preferable to single-fraction treatments because hypoxic tumor cells might reoxygenate and become more radiosensitive between fractions. The therapeutic ratio appears to be better with radiosurgery for metastatic lesions than with fractionated treatment, although a valid comparison is not possible because no studies have used sufficiently high fractionated doses. Why fractionation is not more important for these targets is not entirely understood, although the explanation may

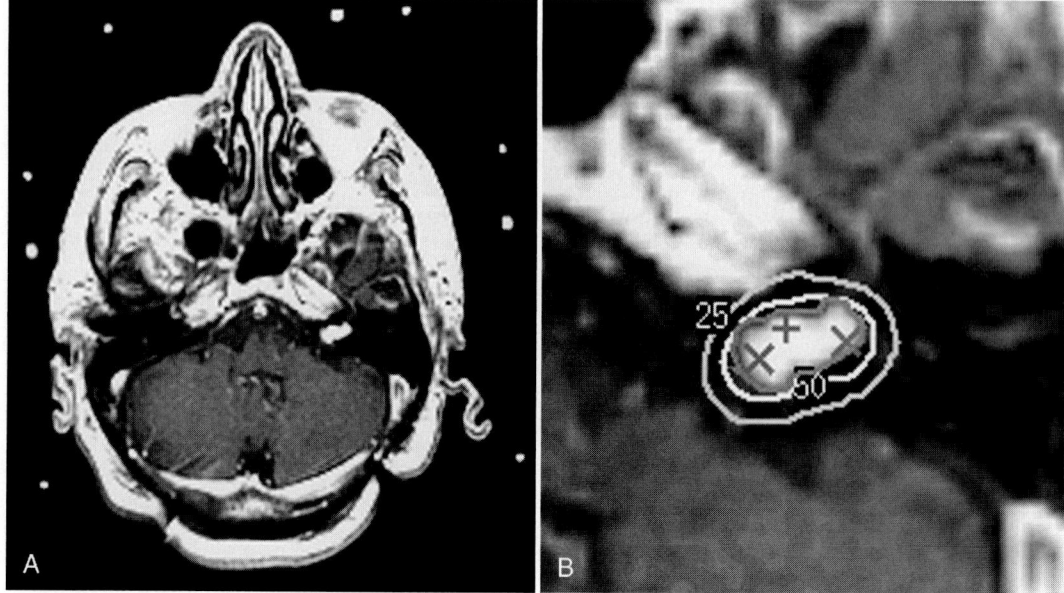

Figure 25–7. A, Magnetic resonance image (MRI) of a left acoustic neuroma in a 72-year-old man who had developed sudden onset of left sensorineural hearing loss 2 years earlier. MRI showed a small acoustic neuroma and the patient was observed. His hearing deteriorated, however, and a repeat scan at 2 years showed tumor progression. **B,** The Gamma Knife isodose plan. The patient received 14 Gy at the target periphery, delivered with three isocenters (8 mm × 3). The target volume was 0.4 cm². See also Color Figure 25-7B.

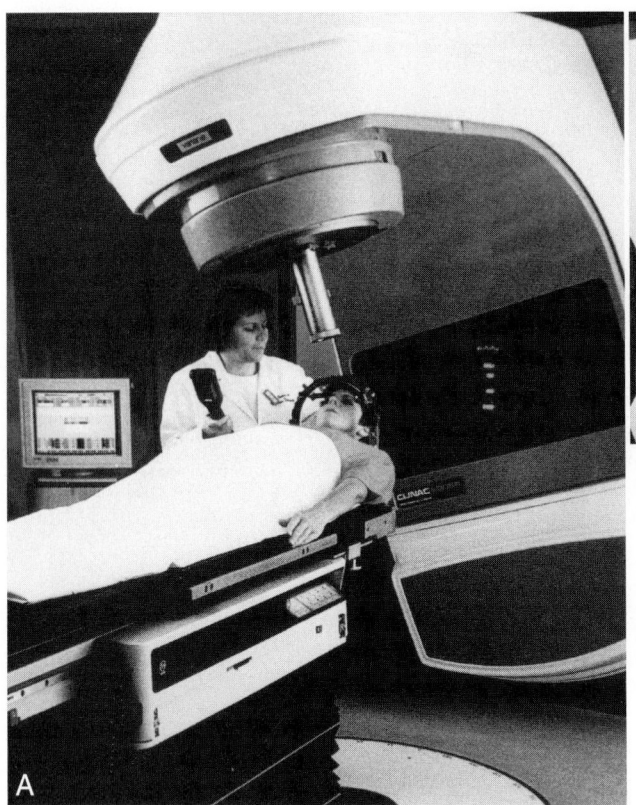

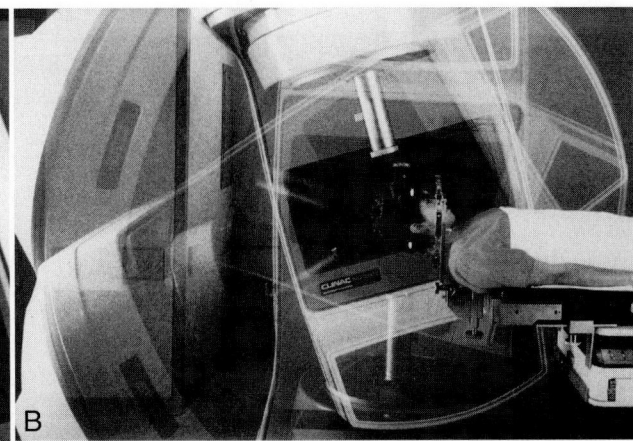

Figure 25–8. A, Schematic of linear accelerator demonstrating patient position for radiosurgery on table extension. Also note rotation of table and gantry about isocenter. **B**, Multiple exposures showing the arcing motion of the linac gantry and collimator during radiosurgery.

relate to the treatment volume. Usually, for small targets, a single fraction does not produce enough damage to normal tissue to have clinical consequences. In any case, most patients with lesions in category C and many in category D, except those with recurrent tumors, undergo fractionated irradiation as part of their therapy.

Radiation Dose

In all radiosurgery techniques, the volume of normal brain tissue beyond the target that receives a moderate to high dose of radiation increases approximately as the cube of the average diameter of the target volume. As complications of irradiation affecting normal tissue may correlate with the volume of normal tissue receiving a dose of a specified magnitude, at least to some extent, isoeffect dose levels may be expected to follow a power law, by which a log-log plot of isoeffective dose versus target diameter approximates a straight line with negative slope. The *empirical* power law dose-diameter isoeffect curve developed by Kjellberg and colleagues[13] for proton radiosurgery is thought to correspond to a 1% risk for radiation necrosis of human brain tissue. The *theoretical* integrated logistic model dose-diameter curve developed by Flickinger14—obtained from a mathematical model that predicts the relationship of dose to volume for a 3% risk for radiation necrosis—closely resembles Kjellberg's 1% curve, for both Gamma Knife and linac radiosurgery. In each case, a log-log plot of isoeffective dose versus diameter approximates a straight line with negative slope. Although insufficient clinical data are available to confirm

the level or slope of these curves, no doubt several variables, in addition to dose and volume, influence the probability of radiation damage. Still, Flickinger's model can be helpful in comparing treatment plans to determine, for each particular patient, which plan has the least potential to cause complications (Fig. 25-10).

With the possible exception of AVMs (see following), there are no good dose response data for SRS. Most centers base doses on tumor volume and any restriction based on adjacent normal structures such as optic chiasm. RTOG 9005 determined the maximum tolerated dose (MTD) of SRS in previously irradiated patients being treated for recurrence.[15] Dose escalation was performed with stratification of patients into 3 categories based on maximum tumor diameter: less than 20 mm, 21-30 mm, and 31-40 mm. As expected, patients with smaller tumors tolerated higher doses. For the group with tumors less than 20 mm, 24 Gy was established as safe. Further dose escalation in this group was not possible due to lack of patient accrual at the 27 Gy level (presumably due to reluctance of clinicians to treat patients at this dose.) MTDs of 18 Gy and 15 Gy were established for patients with tumors 21-30 mm and greater than 30 mm in diameter, respectively.

While these results are extremely valuable and may serve as guidelines, several factors should be kept in mind when choosing SRS dose.[16] First, patients in RTOG 9005 were previously irradiated patients. Patients receiving SRS as a boost to whole-brain radiotherapy (WBRT), for example, for metastatic disease, may neither require nor tolerate the doses established as MTD in the protocol. Some clinicians decrease doses by approximately

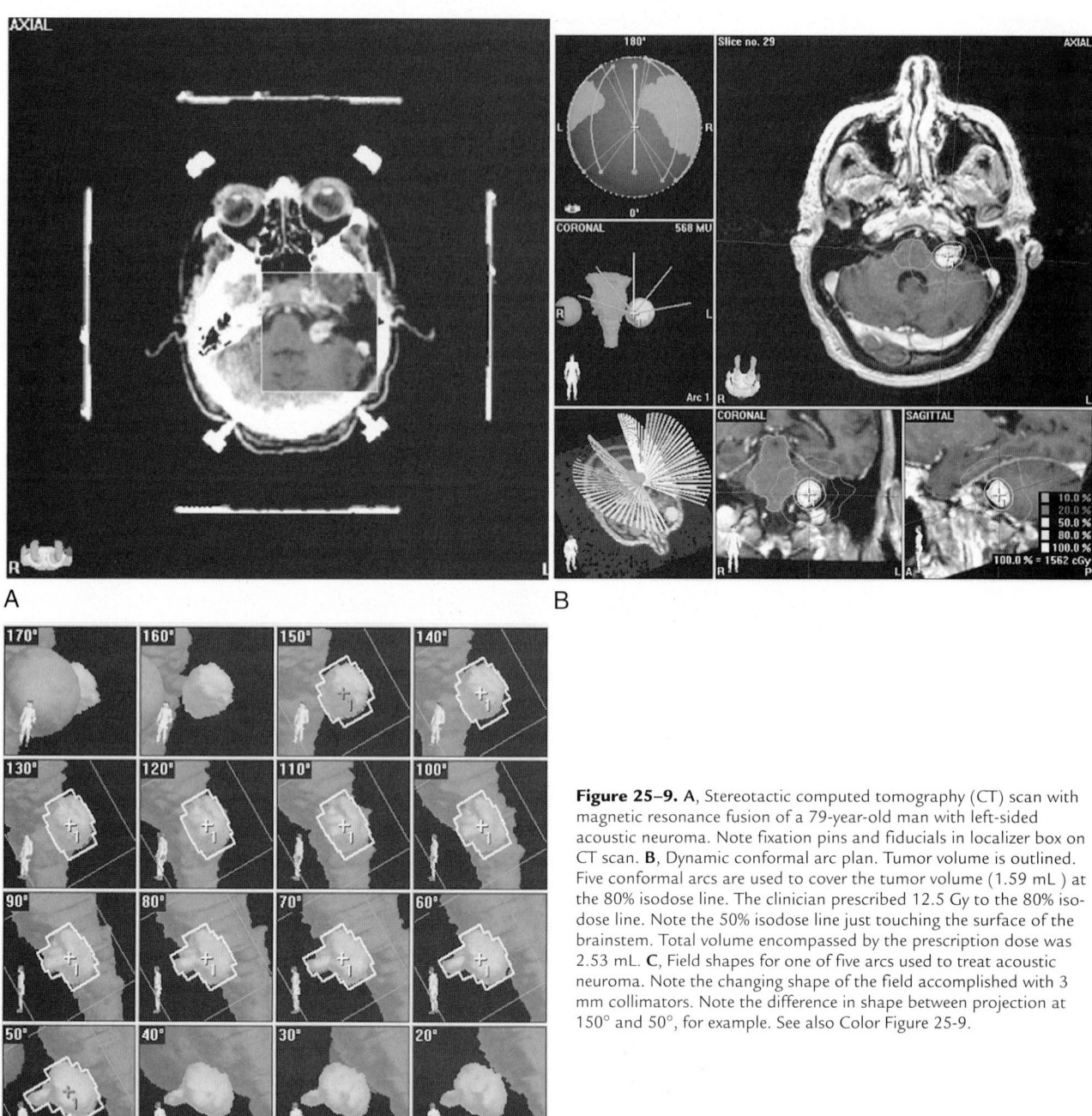

Figure 25–9. A, Stereotactic computed tomography (CT) scan with magnetic resonance fusion of a 79-year-old man with left-sided acoustic neuroma. Note fixation pins and fiducials in localizer box on CT scan. **B,** Dynamic conformal arc plan. Tumor volume is outlined. Five conformal arcs are used to cover the tumor volume (1.59 mL) at the 80% isodose line. The clinician prescribed 12.5 Gy to the 80% isodose line. Note the 50% isodose line just touching the surface of the brainstem. Total volume encompassed by the prescription dose was 2.53 mL. **C,** Field shapes for one of five arcs used to treat acoustic neuroma. Note the changing shape of the field accomplished with 3 mm collimators. Note the difference in shape between projection at 150° and 50°, for example. See also Color Figure 25-9.

10% when treating as a boost compared to treatment with SRS alone. Other special circumstances may also apply. For example, it is clear that acoustic neuroma is well treated with doses far below the RTOG MTDs and that these doses would result in unnecessary toxicity (see later).

As complications of radiosurgical treatment have been documented more thoroughly, there has been a general reduction in dose levels prescribed. Central to the practice of radiosurgery are four general principles: (1) slowly proliferating tissues may not manifest a response for months or years after treatment; (2) a slow response does not necessarily indicate that the lesion is radiation resistant; (3) the latent interval can be decreased by increasing the dose delivered; and (4) response often reflects proliferative activity rather than intrinsic radiation sensitivity.[17] Radiosurgical targets that are slowly proliferative include AVMs and benign tumors (meningioma, pituitary adenoma, and acoustic neuroma). Those lesions and other slowly growing tumors usually do not require a radiation dose that unduly risks damage to normal tissue in order to produce a rapid response or tumor necrosis.

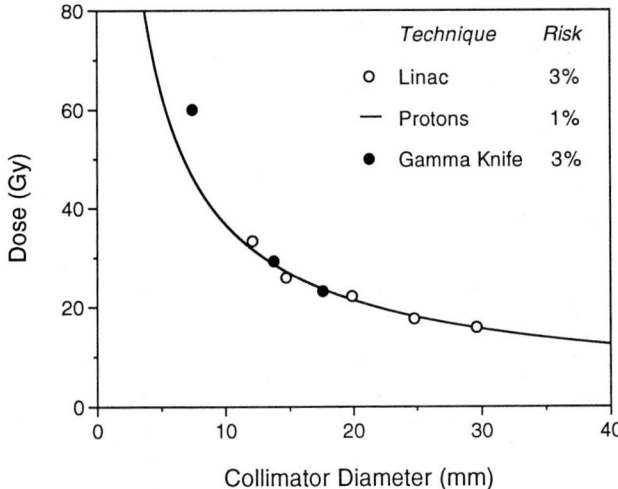

Figure 25–10. Plot of isoeffective dose versus target diameter. The *solid line* represents the empirical power law dose-diameter isoeffect curve developed by Kjellberg [Kjellberg, 1983 #1726] for proton radiosurgery, thought to correspond to a 1% risk for radiation necrosis of human brain tissue. The *open* (linac) and *closed* (Gamma Knife) *circles* represent individual calculation points corresponding to a 3% risk for radiation necrosis, based on the theoretic integrated logistic model developed by Flickinger [Flickinger, 1989 #517]. A log-log plot of these data and the solid line would approximate a straight line with negative slope.

RESULTS OF RADIOSURGICAL TREATMENT

Arteriovenous Malformations

The natural history of AVMs represents a potentially life-threatening intracranial process, as is evident from the retrospective study of 160 patients with untreated AVMs (mean follow-up, 23.7 years) in which Ondra and associates[18] found an annual rate of spontaneous hemorrhage of 3.9% and annual morbidity and mortality rates of 2.4% and 1.0%, respectively. It appears that AVMs are cured, with no further risk of hemorrhage, when total microsurgical resection or total radiosurgical obliteration can be angiographically demonstrated.[19] Because there seems to be a persistent risk of hemorrhage during the latent interval following radiosurgery, complete microsurgical excision of the AVM is the preferred therapy whenever it can be accomplished safely. When this is not possible, radiosurgery can obliterate both superficial AVMs and deep-seated, relatively inaccessible AVMs, with low morbidity and mortality rates and minimal hospitalization (Table 25-1). Radiosurgery induces a progressive thickening of the vascular wall and luminal thrombosis, which takes months to years to complete. In most series, the obliteration rates at 2 years after radiosurgical treatment of small AVMs are higher (90% to 100%) than those for larger AVMs (50% to 70%).[20-24] This is due to the higher minimum doses delivered to smaller AVMs.[25] Minimum doses of 13 and 25 Gy are associated with in-field obliteration rates of 50% and 98%, respectively.[26]

The rate of permanent residual neurologic injury after radiosurgery for AVM is 3% to 4%.[24,27-29] In about one-third of patients, follow-up magnetic resonance images show transient increased T_2 signal changes surrounding the target that develop about 6 to 18 months after radiosurgery and resolve a year or so thereafter. These changes are highly dependent on the location and size of the target.[30] About one-third of patients who develop these T_2 signal changes also have transient neurologic symptoms.

Benign Tumors

For most benign intracranial tumors, fractionated radiation therapy has been the preferred treatment, and it produces few significant complications, especially when performed with three-dimensional planning and delivery. Whether fractionated radiation therapy or radiosurgery is performed, it is *not* necessary to cause significant tumor necrosis or to obtain a complete radiographic response. Rather, the goal is to halt the tumor's growth permanently and, in the case of a hormonally active pituitary tumor, to halt abnormal hormone production permanently, as well. For most benign tumors, neither fractionated radiotherapy or SRS is likely to rapidly decompress mass effect from tumor.

Benign tumors commonly treated by radiosurgery are acoustic neuromas, meningiomas, and pituitary adenomas releasing somatotropin or adrenocorticotropin (Table 25-2). Clinical observations on the radiosurgery

Table 25–1   Results of Radiosurgery for Arteriovenous Malformations

Reference	Technique	Minimum Dose, Gy	AVMs Treated, n	Angiographic Obliteration	
				Rate, %	Time, y
Columbo et al[24]	Linac	19-40	67	75	2
Fabrikant et al[20] and Levy et al[23]	Particle	11.5-45	48	92	3
Forster[22]	Gamma Knife	25	96	59	2
Friedman and Bova[24]	Linac	10-25	21	81	2
Lindquist and Steiner[27] and Steiner et al[28]	Gamma Knife	10-30	573	82	2
Lunsford et al[29]	Gamma Knife	18-25	46	80	2

Adapted from Loeffler JS, Flickinger JC, Shrieve DC, and Larson DA: Radiosurgery for the treatment of intracranial lesions. In DeVita VT, Helman S, Rosenberg SA, eds. *Important Advances in Oncology.* Philadelphia: JB Lippincott; 1995:141.

Table 25–2   Results of Radiosurgery for Benign Tumors

Tumor	Reference	Technique	Minimum Dose, Gy	Tumors Treated, n	Local Control, %	Follow-Up, y
Acoustic neurinoma	Kondziolka et al[36]	Gamma Knife	12-20	162	98	5-10 actuarial
	Mendenhall et al[37]	Linac	10-22.5	32	100	
	Noren et al[38]	Gamma Knife	10-35	227	85	2.25 mean 4.5 median
Meningioma	Loeffler et al[43]	Linac	10-20	97	96	2 actuarial
	Engenhart et al[44]	Linac	10-50	17	100	
	Kondziolka et al[12]	Gamma Knife	10-25	97	95	3 median 4 actuarial
Acromegaly	Kjellberg and Abe[46] and Kjellberg[47]	Particle	30-150	581	88*	20 actuarial
	Levy et al[23]	Particle	30-50	318	95*	10 actuarial
Cushing's disease	Kjellberg and Abe[46] and Kjellberg[47]	Particle	30-150	180	63*	3.7 median
	Levy et al[23]	Particle	50-150	82		
	Sheehan et al[33]	Linac	3.6-30	44		

*Normalization of hormone levels.

Adapted from Loeffler JS, Flickinger JC, Shrieve DC, and Larson DA: Radiosurgery for the treatment of intracranial lesions. In DeVita VT, Helman S, Rosenberg SA, eds. *Important Advances in Oncology*. Philadelphia: JB Lippincott; 1995:141.

of these lesions have provided fundamental information about the tolerance to single-fraction treatment on the part of the pituitary gland, the cranial nerves of the cavernous sinus, and the mesial temporal lobes.[31-35]

ACOUSTIC NEUROMA. The role of radiosurgery for acoustic neuroma as an alternative to microsurgery is a topic of lively debate. The radiosurgical progression-free survival rate with acoustic neuromas has been reported to be greater than 85%.[36-38] The early use of high doses in the range of 20 Gy at the tumor margin resulted in high rates of transient cranial nerve V and VII neuropathies. There was also hearing loss in approximately half of patients with useful hearing at the time of SRS. Due to these toxicities and the high rate of tumor control, doses have decreased over the past 10 years (see Table 25-2). Flickinger et al reported a 98% control rate in more than 100 patients treated with the gamma knife to less than or equal to 13 Gy.[39] In the same group of patients there was no reported facial weakness and a 91% hearing preservation rate. Similar results have been obtained by other institutions,[40] and marginal doses in the range of 12–13 Gy have become standard.

Fractionated stereotactic radiotherapy, or staged radiosurgery, has been used to treat acoustic neuromas with very similar results as those reported for SRS. Tumor control rates are greater than 90% for treatment regimens of 50–54 Gy in standard fractions or 20–35 Gy in fractions of 4–5 Gy. Virtually no incidence of cranial neuropathy has occurred and there has been excellent preservation of hearing.[41,42]

MENINGIOMA. Based on findings available to date, radiosurgery appears to be safe and effective in producing a durable arrest of growth of small, inoperable, recurrent, or residual meningiomas. In a series of 97 patients with meningiomas reviewed by Loeffler and associates,[43] 67%

of patients were treated for recurrence after their first operation (see Table 25-2). Although the 2-year actuarial freedom from progression rate was 96%, 14 patients had complications, including cranial neuropathies in 5 patients and malignant edema in 5; 2 of those patients required reoperation. The complication rates were significantly higher for the larger or deep-seated tumors. The investigators concluded that fractionated radiation therapy may be preferable for this subset of lesions. Engenhart and colleagues[44] similarly showed excellent control rates (82%) but a high complication rate (42%) among patients who were treated radiosurgically for large meningiomas. Kondziolka and colleagues[12] showed excellent 2-year control rates (96%) and a low complication rate (6%) among patients treated with radiosurgery for small meningiomas. While these studies indicate that radiosurgery holds promise for the treatment of small meningiomas, patients must accrue in trials and be followed for several more years before its efficacy in comparison with surgery and radiation therapy[10] can be judged definitively. Larger meningiomas (>3 cm) may be more safely treated with fractionated conformal radiotherapy.

PITUITARY ADENOMA. Pituitary adenomas have been treated with radiosurgery for about 40 years, especially with particle accelerators. Long-term follow-up has shown excellent local control rates of 85% to 95%. Data suggests that SRS will produce a more rapid correction of abnormalities due to hormonally active tumors compared with fractionated radiotherapy (median time to correction 8.5 versus 18 months).[45] Sheehan et al reported on 43 patients treated with Gamma Knife SRS for Cushing's disease.[33] 63% of patients achieved normal or below normal urinary free-cortisol levels at a median time of 12.1 months following SRS. Complication due to SRS for pituitary tumors is a rare occurrence. Of more than 1300 patients represented in Table 25-2 who were treated with radiosurgery for pituitary adenomas, 0.3% developed subsequent blindness, 0.7% subsequent visual field cuts, and 0.9% subsequent oculomotor deficits. Particles have been used to treat pituitary tumors for more than 40 years. Radiosurgery has been shown to normalize increased hormone levels in a majority of patients.[23,46,47]

At this stage of experience with radiosurgery, a comparison with radiation therapy in the management of benign intracranial tumors[17] permits the following conclusions: (1) radiosurgery may provide a more rapid radiographic and hormonal response than fractionated radiation therapy but there are no data to suggest that control rates differ; and (2) acute effects (e.g., edema) and subacute effects (e.g., cranial neuropathies) are more common with radiosurgery than with radiation therapy, especially in cases of the larger and deep-seated lesions. There continues to be increasing interest in fractionated stereotactic radiotherapy to take full advantage of the conformity of stereotactic techniques while taking advantage of the well-known normal tissue-sparing properties of fractionated radiation.

Brain Metastases

The median survival for patients with symptomatic metastases to the brain is about 1 month if they remain untreated and about 3 to 6 months if they undergo conventional WBRT, irrespective of the fractionation scheme used. As compared with patients receiving only WBRT, those treated with surgery and radiation therapy for solitary brain metastases have a significantly longer survival (40 weeks versus 15 weeks, P <0.01) and improved quality of life, and significantly fewer patients have recurrence at the initial metastatic site (20% versus 52%, P <0.02).[48] Systemic chemotherapy has not been shown to influence the outcome to any great extent. When patients with extracranial metastases are considered for promising therapies with biological response modifiers, those with brain metastases are usually excluded. Therapies aimed at control of intracranial metastases are therefore of great potential value.

Because of their biological and physical characteristics, metastatic lesions would seem to be optimally suited for radiosurgery. They are usually relatively small (<30 mm) when diagnosed, and they are often nearly spheric and radiographically distinct. They are minimally invasive and displace normal brain parenchyma circumferentially beyond the target volume, reducing the risk of radiation injury to normal tissue. Although surgery for metastases has certain advantages in that it provides immediate resolution of mass effect, provides diagnostic information if needed, and entails no risk of radiation necrosis, radiosurgery has the substantial advantage that the entire extent of disease can usually be encompassed within the treatment volume because treatment is linked directly to three-dimensional visualization of the tumor. Moreover, radiosurgery avoids the risks of hemorrhage, infection, and tumor seeding, and, as it requires minimal hospitalization, the costs of therapy are less than those of surgery.[49] Local control can be expected in 73% to 98% of patients treated with radiosurgery (Table 25-3).[50-55] The results of radiosurgical treatment for single brain metastases appear to be at least equivalent to those of surgery (Table 25-4).[50,56,57]

In a multicenter study reported by investigators from several Gamma Knife facilities,[53] 116 patients were treated with Gamma Knife radiosurgery for single brain metastases (mean minimal dose, 17.5 Gy). Local control of tumor was achieved in 99 patients (85%). Among all patients, the 2-year actuarial tumor control rate was 67% ± 8%, with a plateau in the curve at 18 months. These findings suggest that, for most patients treated, the local control rates are durable. Multivariate analysis showed that the patients who experienced better local control were those who underwent whole-brain irradiation in addition to radiosurgery and, paradoxically, those with lesions of histologies known to be resistant to fractionated radiation therapy (melanoma and renal cell carcinoma)—a finding also reported by others.[58] Median survival from the time of radiosurgery was 11 months, and patients with breast cancer had the best survival rates.

In a series of 421 metastatic lesions in 248 patients who were treated at one center over a 7-year period,[50] the control rates for lesions with radiation-resistant histological findings were statistically equal to those of other lesions. Multivariate analysis showed only two factors that were predictive of enhanced local control: a supratentorial versus infratentorial site (RR, 2.3; P = 0.009) and treatment of primary tumor versus recurrent tumor (RR, 4.6; P = 0.035). The median survival for the entire group was 9.4 months from the time of radiosurgery. In multivariate analysis, the absence of systemic disease (RR, 4.4; P = <0.001) and age younger than 60 years

Table 25–3   Results of Radiosurgery for Brain Metastases

Reference	Technique	Patients Treated, n	Lesions Treated, n	Dose, Gy*	Local Control, %	Median Follow-Up, mo
Alexander et al[50]	Linac	248	421	15.0	89	26.0
Engenhart et al[51]	Linac	71	124	17.0	94	7.0
Fuller et al[52]	Linac	27	47	24.6	88	5.0
Flickinger et al[53]	Gamma Knife	116	116	17.5	85	9.0
Kihlstrom et al[54]	Gamma Knife	300	200	29.0	94	—
Mehta et al[55]	Linac	40	58	18.3	73	6.5

*Median dose to tumor periphery.

Adapted from Loeffler JS, Flickinger JC, Shrieve DC, and Larson DA: Radiosurgery for the treatment of intracranial lesions. In Devita VT, Helman S, Rosenberg SA, eds. *Important Advances in Oncology*. Philadelphia: JB Lippincott; 1995:141.

Table 25–4 **Comparison of Radiosurgical and Surgical Treatment for Patients with a Single Brain Metastasis**

Reference	Patients, *n*	Treatment	Median Survival, wk	Median KPS >70, wk	Local Failure, %	Neurologic Deaths, %
Alexander et al[50]	147	Radiosurgery*	49	36	11	18
Mehta[56]	19	Radiosurgery*	40	36	11	17
Patchell et al[48]	25	Surgery + RT	40	38	20	29

*Patients in these studies fit the eligibility criteria used in the study by Patchell et al.[48]
KPS, Karnofsky performance status; RT, radiation therapy.
Adapted from Loeffler JS, Flickinger JC, Shrieve DC, and Larson DA: Radiosurgery for the treatment of intracranial lesions. In DeVita VT, Helman S, Rosenberg SA, eds. *Important Advances in Oncology.* Philadelphia: JB Lippincott; 1995:141.

(RR, 1.6; *P* = 0.002) were factors associated with longer survival. Seven percent of patients required surgery for the development of symptomatic mass effect from 1 to 22 months after radiosurgery.

In a single institution randomized prospective trial Kondziolka et al.[59] examined the relative efficacy of WBRT (30 Gy in 12 fractions) alone compared to the same WBRT plus SRS. Patients with two to four brain metastases with known histology were eligible. Twenty-seven patients were accrued before stopping rules were met. Local failure at 1 year was 100% for WBRT alone versus 8% with the addition of SRS. There was no significant difference in overall survival between the groups.

RTOG 9508 has also studied the benefit of WBRT (37.5 Gy in 15 fractions) compared to WBRT plus a boost with SRS in patients with 1, 2, or 3 brain metastases.[60] At 1 year the local control rates were 82% and 71% for WBRT+SRS and WBRT alone (*P* = 0.01), respectively. There was no statistical difference in the rate of grade 3 or 4 toxicities between the groups. For patients with single metastases, a significant survival benefit was demonstrated for the addition of SRS (6.5 versus 4.9 months). Similar significant survival advantages of 1.6-2 months were demonstrated for patients in RTOG RPA Class I,[61] patients under 50 years of age, and those with non–small-cell lung cancer, regardless of the number of metastases. Karnofsky performance status (KPS) score was improved or stable at 3 months in 50% versus 33% in SRS-treated patients versus those receiving WBRT alone (*P* = 0.02), respectively and at 6 months in 43% versus 27% (*P* = 0.03), respectively. However, at the time of the initial report, this difference had not reached statistical significance (*P* = 0.107).

Within the range of doses commonly used for radiosurgery, there appears to be no clear-cut dose-response relationship, and the range of doses used does not appear to correlate with outcome. Most radiosurgical teams prefer to use a lower dose for larger lesions in order to minimize the risk of complications. Therefore, the response rate can be expected to correlate with target size. Among reported series, complete response was achieved in 78% of patients with lesions with tumor volumes less than 2 cm^3 and in 50% of those with tumor volumes 10 cm^3 or greater, and subsequent progression occurred in only 4% of complete responders versus 20% of partial responders.[55] In another series,[50] tumor volume greater than 3 cm^3 was significantly associated with higher rates of local failure in univariate analysis, although in multivariate analysis the association was not significant (*P* = 0.06).

It may be that whole-brain irradiation administered concomitantly with radiosurgery improves the outcome of treatment for patients with brain metastases. Fuller and associates[52] reported significantly improved local control within the radiosurgical target region or elsewhere in the brain for patients undergoing radiosurgery plus whole-brain irradiation as compared with those who received only radiosurgery, although there was no significant difference in survival rates for the two groups. Similarly, Flickinger and associates[53] showed that significantly fewer patients receiving whole-brain irradiation plus radiosurgery had recurrence at the radiosurgical target site.

In order to avoid the often debilitating toxicity of WBRT in long-term survivors, many groups may omit WBRT and use SRS alone in selected circumstances. Sneed et al. retrospectively reviewed the outcome of 62 patients treated with SRS alone versus 43 patients treated with SRS plus WBRT for single or multiple brain metastases.[62] Patients receiving SRS alone were at significantly greater risk for developing new brain metastases (69% versus 28%, *P* = 0.03) at 1 year. Salvage therapy in these patients was either repeat SRS or WBRT. Overall 74% of the SRS-alone group were spared WBRT. There was no difference in overall survival between the groups. In general, most patients who undergo radiosurgery for lesions metastatic to the brain experience clinical improvement and reduced steroid requirements, and only 11% to 25% eventually die of neurologic causes.[52,55]

Glioblastoma Multiforme

Although surgical resection followed by irradiation and chemotherapy lengthens the survival of patients who have glioblastoma multiforme, most patients die as a result of persistence or local recurrence of their tumor.[63] For highly selected patients with small glioblastomas—a minority of the patients affected with this lesion—a highly conformal brachytherapy boost has improved survival following conventional fractionated radiation therapy.[64-66] Because conformal dose distributions of radiosurgery and brachytherapy are similar, it has been proposed that radiosurgery may provide an effective therapeutic boost and may have a similar potential for improving survival (Table 25-5). In fact, many clinicians now offer radiosurgery as an alternative to brachytherapy. Radiosurgery, which is noninvasive, is attractive both from the patient's standpoint as well as from that of health care providers.

Guidelines for selecting patients who may benefit from radiosurgery appear to be similar to those for selecting patients for brachytherapy. Larson and colleagues[67] performed a multivariate analysis of 189 patients with malig-

Table 25–5   Stereotactic Irradiation Boost Therapy for Primary and Recurrent Glioblastoma Multiforme

Tumor Type	Reference	Boost Technique	Dose, Gy*	Patients, n	Median Survival, mo	ReoperationRate, %
Primary	Shrieve et al[69]	Radiosurgery	12.0	78	19.9	50
Primary	Mehta et al[68]	Radiosurgery	12.0	50	11.0	10
Primary	Green et al[66]	Brachytherapy†	50.0	56	18.0	64
Primary	Scharfen et al[64]	Brachytherapy†	52.9	106	22.0	38
Primary	Wen et al[65]	Brachytherapy†	60.0	66	12.0	50
Recurrent	Shrieve et al[75]	Radiosurgery	13.0	86	10.2	22
Recurrent	Shrieve et al[75]	Brachytherapy†	50.0	32	11.5	44
Recurrent	Scharfen et al[64]	Brachytherapy†	52.9	66	12.0	38

*Median dose to tumor periphery.
†With iodine 125.
Adapted from Loeffler JS, Flickinger JC, Shrieve DC, and Larson DA: Radiosurgery for the treatment of intracranial lesions. In DeVita VT, Helman S, Rosenberg SA, eds. Important advances in Oncology. Philadelphia: JB Lippincott; 1995:141.

nant glioma treated with the Gamma Knife. These investigators explored a broad spectrum of criteria for patient selection and treatment. The main endpoints of their study were survival and complications, and the analysis was designed to determine factors that were associated with better or worse outcomes. Multivariate analysis selected five variables significantly associated with decreased survival: higher pathologic tumor grade, older age of the patient, lower KPS score, larger tumor volume, and bifocal versus unifocal tumor. It is likely that variations in published reports regarding survival rates after radiosurgery or brachytherapy for malignant glioma can be attributed, in part, to substantial differences in patient populations with respect to these five variables. Patients with unfavorable constellations of these variables are unlikely to benefit from radiosurgery. In the absence of a randomized trial, however, the relative roles of radiosurgery and brachytherapy remain unknown.

Acute complications were reported in 0% of patients reported by Mehta and colleagues,[68] as compared with 9% reported by Larson and colleagues,[67] and 12% reported by Shrieve and colleagues.[69] Chronic problems or reoperations or both were reported in 22% of the patients reported by Shrieve and colleagues[69] who had reoperation for necrotic tumor, and 13% of patients reported by Mehta and colleagues[68] who had clinically significant necrosis. Because some patients may not survive long enough to experience chronic complications, the actuarial risk of chronic complications may be substantially higher than that given by these crude percentages, although Larson and colleagues[67] found chronic complications in only 17% of patients evaluated at least 1 year after radiosurgery who had a constellation of problems. Most authors report a high rate of chronic corticosteroid dependency among long-term survivors. Approximately half the patients evaluated at any interval after radiosurgery may expect to have a stable or improved KPS score, as compared with the initial KPS score, whereas 10% to 25% of patients may experience a decrease of greater than 20 points in their KPS score.[67]

Most formal institutional protocols for radiosurgical treatment of glioblastoma require that patients meet the following criteria: a KPS score of at least 70; a unifocal, well-demarcated tumor that enhances, with administration of contrast material, on CT or MR imaging; and a target dimension no greater than 3–4 cm. In addition, patients with primary tumors must undergo conventional external-beam irradiation to approximately 60 Gy in 30–33 fractions. Current data do not show a clear-cut dose-response relationship within the narrow range of radiation doses used.

Shrieve et al.[69] published results on 78 patients with GBM treated with surgery followed by standard external-beam irradiation plus an SRS boost to the residual tumor or tumor bed. Median survival was 19.9 months for all patients. Patients younger than 40 had a median survival of 48.6 months. Comparison of the outcome by RTOG prognostic class[70] suggested an improvement over historic controls in all three classes included (Table 25-6).

RTOG Protocol 93-05 randomized patients with primary GBM to standard postoperative treatment with RT (60 Gy) and BCNU chemotherapy versus SRS followed by the standard treatment.[71] Eligible patients had GBM less than 4 cm in maximum diameter and KPS score greater than 60. SRS dose of 15-24 Gy according to RTOG 90-05[72] size criteria was used. A total of 204 patients were randomized and 186 analyzed. With a median follow-up time of 44 months, median survival was 14.1 months for patients not receiving upfront SRS compared with 13.7 months for patients who received upfront SRS. The median survival of patients in this trial of approximately 14 months is better than that found in most studies.[73] All patients in the study were treated at institutions with SRS capability. The relative good outcome in these patients may be related to the selection criteria for SRS.

SUMMARY

Radiosurgical facilities are now being established in community hospitals, and the number of patients treated radiosurgically is increasing every year. The number of cooperative group trials of radiosurgical applications is also increasing, and changes in practice patterns are occurring. Lower radiation doses are now prescribed for tumors with a benign histology and for vascular lesions, and a greater proportion of lesions originally considered unsuited to radiosurgery, such as malignant tumors, are being treated radiosurgically. Radiosurgery is also being incorporated into staged treatment protocols, together with embolization, surgery, and radiation therapy; and it is being used as immediate adjuvant therapy to prevent recurrence, in preference to observation followed by treatment at recurrence.[74]

Table 25–6 Summary of Patient Survival Time by RTOG Prognostic Class*

| | Current Study (radiosurgery boost) | | | | | RTOG Protocol (no radiosurgery) | | | | | |
| | Survival Time | | | | | Survival Time | | | | | |
RTOG Class	No. of Patients	Median (mos)	1 yr (%)	2 yrs (%)	3 yrs (%)	No. of Patients	Median (mos)	1 yr (%)	2 yrs (%)	3 yrs (%)	Difference[†]
III	27	29.5	93	58	48	175	17.9	66[‡]	35	22[‡]	11.6
IV	29	19.2	86	23	18	457	11.1	45[‡]	15	8[‡]	8.1
V	22	18.2	86	23	5	395	8.9	31[‡]	6	2[‡]	9.3

*Classes based on Curran et al.[70]
[†]Differences in median survival time in months between SRS-treated patients and patients from the same RTOG class who were not treated with SRS.
[‡]Figures were extrapolated by the authors from survival curves published by Curran et al.

Also resulting from such work are certain generalizations that define radiosurgery. It has been established that the larger the target volume, the less the dose that can be delivered safely[72] and the lower the probability of achieving control or obliteration of the target lesion. It is known that the development of symptomatic radiation necrosis is related to the dose, volume, site, and histology of the target lesion, and that cranial nerves II and VIII are particularly vulnerable to damage by radiation. Radiosurgery is especially damaging, also, to late-responding tissue, such as abnormal blood vessels, which accounts for the high overall response to radiosurgical treatment of vascular tumors and AVMs. Tentatively, certain conclusions seem justified:

- Based on clinical results and complication rates, the different radiosurgery techniques appear to be equally effective.
- Radiosurgery produces a large radiobiological effect within the target volume.
- For the majority of benign intracranial targets, radiosurgery provides control while causing only mild to moderate toxicity; that toxicity should be reduced with developing techniques that entail more elaborate three-dimensional planning and lower radiation doses or fractionation.
- For AVMs, radiosurgery is particularly effective; retrospective data demonstrate low toxicity and high efficacy and indicate that obliteration rates and the time to obliteration of the lesion are dose-dependent and inversely related to volume.
- For small metastatic brain tumors, irrespective of histology, radiosurgery is highly effective and produces few complications; clinical data suggest that it is an excellent alternative to surgery for neurologically intact patients, but its role for patients with multiple lesions has not been established.
- For glioblastoma, radiosurgery appears to have efficacy and toxicity resembling that of brachytherapy.

REFERENCES

1. Leksell L: The stereotaxic method and radiosurgery of the brain. *Acta Chir Scand*. 1951;102:316.
2. Larson DA, Bova F, Eisert D, et al: Current radiosurgery practices: Results of an ASTRO survey. *Int J Radiat Oncol Biol Phys*. 1994;28:523.
3. Larson DA, Bova F, Eisert D: Consensus statement on stereotactic radiosurgery and quality improvement. *Int J Radiat Oncol Biol Phys*. 1994;28:527.
4. Lunsford LD, Alexander E, III, Chapman P: Consensus statement on stereotactic radiosurgery. *Neurosurg*. 1994;34:193.
5. Shrieve DC, Watson GA, Jensen RL, et al: Conformity of LINAC-Based SRS Utilizing Dynamic Arcs with MMLC. *Int J Radiat Oncol Biol Phys*. 2001;51:126.
6. Nakamura JL, Pirzkall M, Carol M, et al: Comparison of intensity modulated radiosurgery to gamma knife for challenging skull base lesions. *Int J Radiat Oncol Biol Phys*. 2001;51:125.
7. Kooy HM: Linear accelerators in stereotactic radiosurgery. In Alexander E, III, Loeffler JS, Lunsford LD, eds. *Stereotactic Radiosurgery*. New York: McGraw-Hill; 1993:67.
8. Levy RP, Fabrikant JI, Frankel KA, et al: Charged particle radiosurgery of the brain. *Neurosurg Clin N Am*. 1990;1:955.
9. Larson DA, Flickinger JC, Loeffler JS: The radiobiology of radiosurgery. *Int J Radiation Oncology Biol Phys*. 1993;25:557.
10. Goldsmith BJ, Wara WM, Wilson CB, et al: Postoperative irradiation of subtotally resected meningiomas. *J Neurosurg*. 1994;80:195.
11. Hakim R, Alexander E, III, Loeffler JS, et al: Results of linear accelerator-based radiosurgery for intracranial meningiomas. *Neurosurg*. 1998;42:446.
12. Kondziolka D, Lunsford LD, Coffey RJ, Flickinger JC: Stereotactic radiosurgery of meningiomas. *Journal of Neurosurgery*. 1991;74:552.
13. Kjellberg RN, Hanamura T, Davis KR, et al: Bragg-peak proton-beam therapy for arteriovenous malformations of the brain. *N Engl J Med*. 1983;309:269.
14. Flickinger JC: An integrated formula for prediction of complications from radiosurgery. *Int J Radiation Oncology Biol Phys*. 1989;17:879.
15. Shaw E, Scott C, Souhami L, et al: Single dose radiosurgical treatment of recurrent previously irradiated primary brain tumors and brain metastases: Final report of RTOG protocol 90-05. *Int J Radiat Oncol Biol Phys*. 2000;47:291.
16. Flickinger JC, Kondziolka D, Lunsford LD: Dose selection in stereotactic radiosurgery. *Neurosurg Clin N Am*. 1999;10:271.
17. Larson DA, Flickinger JC, Loeffler JS: Stereotactic radiosurgery: Techniques and results. In DeVita VT, Hellman S, Rosenberg SA, eds. *Cancer: Principles and Practice of Oncology Updates*. Philadelphia: Lippincott; 1993:1.
18. Ondra SL, Troupp H, George ED, Schwab K: The natural history of symptomatic arteriovenous malformations of the brain: A 24-year follow-up assessment. *Journal of Neurosurgery*. 1990;73:387.
19. Stein BM, Sisti MB, Kader A: Microsurgery and radiosurgery in small AVMs. *J Neurosurg*. 1993;79:795.
20. Fabrikant JI, Levy RP, Steinberg GK, et al: Charged particle radiosurgery for intracranial arteriovenous malformations. *Neurosurg Clin N Am*. 1992;3:99.
21. Colombo F, Benedetti A, Pozza F, et al: Linear accelerator radiosurgery of cerebral arteriovenous malformations. *Neurosurgery*. 1989;24:833.
22. Forster DE: The Sheffield "Gamma Knife" experience: Results in arteriovenous malformation radiosurgery in 507 patients. In Lunsford LD, ed. *Stereotactic Radiosurgery Update*. New York: Elsevier; 1992:113.
23. Levy RP, Fabrikant JI, Lyman JT, et al: Clinical results of stereotactic heavy-charged particle radiosurgery of pituitary gland. In

Steiner L, Lindquist C, Forster D, et al, eds. *Radiosurgery: Baseline and Trends*. New York: Raven Press; 1992:149.

24. Friedman WA, Bova FJ: Linear accelerator radiosurgery for arteriovenous malformations. *Journal of Neurosurgery*. 1992;77:832.

25. Loeffler JS, Alexander E, Siddon RL, et al: Stereotactic radiosurgery for intracranial arteriovenous malformations using a standard linear accelerator. *Int J Radiation Oncology Biol Phys*. 1989;17:673.

26. Flickinger JC, Pollack BE, Kondziolka D, Lunsford LD: A dose-response analysis of arteriovenous malformation obliteration after radiosurgery. *Int J Radiat Oncol Biol Phys*. 1996;36:873.

27. Lindquist C, Steiner L: Stereotactic radiosurgical treatment of arteriovenous malformations of the brain. In Lunsford LD, ed. *Modern Stereotactic Neurosurgery*. Boston: Martinus Nijhoff; 1988:491.

28. Steiner L, Lindquist C, Adler JR, et al: Clinical outcome of radiosurgery for cerebral arteriovenous malformations. *Journal of Neurosurgery*. 1992;77:1.

29. Lunsford LD, Kondziolka D, Flickinger JC, et al: Stereotactic radiosurgery for arteriovenous malformations. *J Neurosurg*. 1991;75:517.

30. Flickinger JC, Lunsford LD, Kondziolka D, et al: An analysis of neurodiagnostic imaging changes following Gamma Knife radiosurgery for arteriovenous malformations. *Int J Radiat Oncol Biol Phys*. 1992;23:19.

31. Mehta MP, Kinsella TJ: Cavernous sinus cranial neuropathies: Is there a dose-response relationship following radiosurgery? *Int J Radiat Oncol Biol Phys*. 1993;27:477.

32. Morita A, Coffey RJ, Foote RL, et al: Risk of injury to cranial nerves after gamma knife radiosurgery for skull base meningiomas: Experience in 88 patients. *J Neurosurg*. 1999;90:42.

33. Sheehan JM, Vance ML, Sheehan JP, et al: Radiosurgery for Cushing's disease after failed transsphenoidal surgery. *J Neurosurg*. 2000;93:738.

34. Tishler RB, Loeffler JS, Lunsford LD, et al: Tolerance of cranial nerves of the cavernous sinus to radiosurgery. *Int J Radiation Oncology Biol Phys*. 1993;27:215.

35. Leber KA, Bergloff J, Pendl G: Dose-response tolerance of the visual pathways and cranial nerves of the cavernous sinus to stereotactic radiosurgery. *J Neurosurg*. 1998;88:43.

36. Kondziolka D, Lunsford LD, McLaughlin MR, Flickinger JC: Long-term outcomes after radiosurgery for acoustic neuromas. *N Engl J Med*. 1998;339:1426.

37. Mendenhall WM, Friedman WA, Bova FJ: Linear accelerator-based stereotactic radiosurgery for acoustic schwannomas. *Int J Radiation Oncology Biol Phys*. 1994;28:803.

38. Noren G, Greitz D, Hirsch A, et al: Gamma Knife radiosurgery in acoustic neurinoma. In Steiner L, Lindquist C, Forster D, et al, eds. *Radiosurgery: Baseline and Trends*. New York: Raven Press; 1992:141.

39. Flickinger JC, Kondziolka D, Niranjan A, Lunsford LD: Results of acoustic neuroma radiosurgery: An analysis of 5 years' experience using current methods. *J Neurosurg*. 2001;94:1.

40. Miller RC, Foote RL, Coffey RJ, et al: Decrease in cranial nerve complications after radiosurgery for acoustic neuromas: Prospective study of dose and volume. *Int J Radiat Oncol Biol Phys*. 1999;43:305.

41. Varlotto JM, Shrieve DC, Alexander E, III, et al: Fractionated stereotactic radiotherapy for the treatment of acoustic neuromas: Preliminary results. *Int J Radiat Oncol Biol Phys*. 1996;36:141.

42. Williams JA: Fractionated stereotactic radiosurgery for treatment of acoustic neuromas. *Stereotactic and Functional Neurosurg*. 1999;73:45.

43. Loeffler JS, Flickinger JC, Shrieve DC, Larson DA: Radiosurgery for the treatment of intracranial lesions. In DeVita VT, Hellman S, Rosenberg SA, eds. *Important Advances in Oncology*. Philadelphia: JB Lippincott; 1995:141.

44. Engenhart R, Kimmig BN, Hover K, et al: Stereotactic single high dose radiation therapy of benign intracranial meningiomas. *Int J Radiation Oncology Biol Phys*. 1990;19:1021.

45. Mitsumori M, Shrieve DC, Alexander E, III, et al: Initial clinical results of Linac-based stereotactic radiosurgery and stereotactic radiotherapy for pituitary adenoma. *Int J Radiat Oncol Biol Phys*. 1998;42:573.

46. Kjellberg RN, Abe M: Stereotactic Bragg peak proton beam therapy. In Lunsford LD, ed. Modern Stereotacitc Neurosurgery. Boston: Martinus Nijhoff; 1988:463.

47. Kjellberg RN: Proton beam (PB) therapy of pituitary tumors. Paper presented at: International Stereotactic Radiosurgery Symposium; June 19-21, 1991; Pittsburgh.

48. Patchell, RA, Tibbs PA, Walsh JW, et al: A randomized trial of surgery in the treatment of single metastases to the brain. *N Engl J Med*. 1990;322:494.

49. Noyes WR, Auchter RM, Craig B, et al: Cost analysis of radiosurgery versus resection for single brain metastases. In Kondziolka D, ed. *Radiosurgery 1995*. Basel, Switzerland: Karger; 1995:172.

50. Alexander E, III, Moriarity T, Davis R, et al: Stereotactic radiosurgery for definitive, noninvasive treatment of brain metastases. *J Nat Can Inst*. 1995;87:34.

51. Engenhart R, Kimmig B, Hover K, et al: Long-term follow-up for brain metastases treated with single high dose radiation. *Cancer*, 1993;71:1353.

52. Fuller BG, Kaplan ID, Adler J, et al: Stereotactic radiosurgery for brain metastases: The importance of adjuvant whole brain irradiation. *Int J Radiat Oncology Biol Phys*. 1992;23:413.

53. Flickinger JC, Kondziolka D, Lunsford LD, et al: A multi-institutional experience with stereotactic radiosurgery for solitary brain metastasis. *Int J Radiat Oncology Biol Phys*. 1994;28:797.

54. Kihlstrom L, Karlsson B, Lindquist C: Stereotactic radiosurgery for single and multiple cerebral metastases. *Acta Neurochir (Wien)*. 1993;122:158.

55. Mehta MP, Rozental JM, Levin AB, et al: Defining the role of radiosurgery in the management of brain metastases. *Int J Radiat Oncol Biol Phys*. 1992;24:619.

56. Mehta MP. Radiosurgery for brain metastases. In DeSalles AAF, Goetsch SJ, eds. *Stereotactic Surgery and Radiosurgery*. Madison: Medical Physics Publishers; 1993:353.

57. Patchell RA, Cirrincione C, Thaler HT, et al: Single brain metastases: Surgery plus radiation or radiation alone. *Neurology*. 1986;36:447.

58. Loeffler JS, Alexander E, III: Radiosurgery for the treatment of intracranial metastases. In Alexander E, III, Loeffler JS, Lunsford LD, eds. *Stereotactic Radiosurgery*. New York: McGraw-Hill; 1993:197.

59. Kondziolka D, Patel A, Lunsford LD, et al: Stereotactic radiosurgery plus whole brain radiotherapy versus radiotherapy alone for patients with multiple brain metastases. *Int J Radiat Oncol Biol Phys*. 1999;45:427.

60. Sperduto PW, Scott C, Andrews D, Schell M, et al: Stereotactic radiosurgery with whole brain radiation therapy improves survival in patients with brain metastases: Report of Radiation Therapy Oncology Group (RTOG) Phase III Trial 9508. *Int J Radiat Oncol Biol Phys*. 2002; 54 (Suppl):3.

61. Gaspar LE, Scott C, Rotman M, Asbell S, et al: Recursive partitioning analysis (RPA) of prognostic factors in three Radiation Therapy Oncology Group (RTOG) brain metastases trials. *Int J Radiat Oncol Biol Phys*. 1997;37:754.

62. Sneed PK, Lamborn KR, Forstner JM, et al: Radiosurgery for brain metastases: Is whole brain radiotherapy necessary? *Int J Radiat Oncol Biol Phys*. 1999;43:549.

63. Leibel SA, Scott CB, Loeffler JS: Contemporary approaches to the treatment of malignant gliomas with radiation therapy. *Seminars in Oncology*. 1994;21:198.

64. Scharfen CO, Sneed PK, Wara WM, et al: High activity iodine-125 interstitial implant for gliomas. *Int J Radiat Oncology Biol Phys*. 1992;24:583.

65. Wen PY, Alexander E, Black PM, et al: Long-term results of stereotactic brachytherapy used in the initial treatment of patients with glioblastomas. *Cancer*. 1994;73:3029.

66. Green SB, Shapiro WR, Burger PC, et al: A randomized trial of interstitial radiotherapy (RT) for newly diagnosed glioma: Brain Tumor Cooperative Group (BTCG) trial 8701. Paper presented at: 30th Annual Meeting of the American Society of Clinical Oncology; May 14-17, 1994, Dallas, Tx.

67. Larson DA, Gutin PH, McDermott MW, et al: Multicenter trial update: Glioma. Paper presented at: 6th Annual Leksell Gamma Knife Society Meeting; May 1994, Kyoto.

68. Mehta MP, Masciopinto J, Baskin K, et al: Glioblastoma treated with external beam radiotherapy and stereotactic radiosurgery boost. *Int J Radiat Oncol Biol Phys*. 1993;27:152.

69. Shrieve DC, Alexander EI, Black PM, et al: Treatment of patients with primary glioblastoma multiforme with standard postoperative radiotherapy and radiosurgical boost: Prognostic factors and long-term outcome. *J Neurosurg*. 1999;90:72.

70. Curran WJJ, Scott CB, Horton J, et al: Recursive partitioning analysis of prognostic factors in three Radiation Therapy Oncology Group Malignant Glioma Trials. *J Natl Cancer Inst.* 1993;85:704.

71. Souhami L, Scott C, Brachman D, et al: Randomized prospective comparison of stereotactic radiosurgery (SRS) followed by conventional radiotherapy (RT) with BCNU to RT with BCNU alone for selected patients with supratentorial glioblastoma multiforme (GBM): Report of RTOG 93-05 protocol. *Int J Radiat Oncol Biol Phys.* 2002; 54 (Suppl):94.

72. Shaw E, Scott C, Souhami L, et al: Radiosurgery for the treatment of previously irradiated recurrent primary brain tumors and brain metastases: Initial report of Radiation Therapy Oncology Group Protocol 90-05. *Int J Radiat Oncol Biol Phys.* 1996;34:647.

73. Seiferheld WF, Mehta MP, Del Rowe J, et al: Five years of glioblastoma multiforme (GBM) phase II trials at the RTOG. Paper presented at: Thirty-eighth Annual Meeting of the American Society for Clinical Oncology, 2002; Orlando, Fla.

74. Lunsford LD: Contemporary management of meningiomas: Radiation therapy as an adjuvant and radiosurgery as an alternative to surgical removal? *J Neurosurg.* 1994;80:187.

75. Shrieve DC, Alexander E, III, Wen Py et al: Comparison of stereotactic radiosurgery and brachytherapy in the treatment of recurrent glioblastoma multiforme. *J Neruosurg.* 1995;36:275.

Spinal Cord Tumors

David E. Linstadt, MD

26

PRIMARY TUMORS INVOLVING THE SPINAL CORD

Epidemiology and Genetics

Primary tumors involving the spinal cord are uncommon[1] and tend to occur in young patients. In adults, they are outnumbered by primary brain tumors at a ratio of roughly 20:1; for children, a ratio of 5:1 is reported by most centers. Tumors arising from the spinal canal and vertebrae show a more heterogeneous age distribution. The rarity of primary spinal tumors makes it difficult to establish a clear-cut association with specific cytogenetic abnormalities. Some investigators have found an association between spinal and brain ependymomas and the loss of sequences in chromosome arm 22q, suggesting the presence of one or more ependymoma tumor supressor genes in this location.[2-4] Pediatric ependymomas and astrocytomas have been associated with loss of chromosome arm 17p.[3,4] Some myxopapillary and papillary ependymomas have been associated with bcl-2 oncoprotein expression.[5] Other ependymomas have been associated with mutations in the MEN1 gene and loss of heterozygosity in the chromosome arm 11q region.[6]

Prior exposure to therapeutic irradiation probably increases the risk for developing spinal canal meningiomas, soft tissue sarcomas, vertebral body sarcomas, and possibly spinal cord gliomas, although the magnitude of this risk is unclear. Neurofibromatosis is strongly associated with an increased incidence of spinal canal neurofibrosarcoma and has been associated with intracranial and spinal cord ependymoma, as well.[2] This latter association may be indirect, with the actual cause being the loss of a separate ependymoma tumor supressor gene located near the *NF2* gene.[3]

Anatomy

The spinal cord extends from the level of the foramen magnum to the L1-L2 vertebral level in most adults. Below the termination of the cord, the spinal canal contains the lumbar cistern, an enlargement of the subarachnoid space that surrounds the cauda equina. The spinal subarachnoid space terminates inferiorly at the S2-S3 level and does not extend laterally beyond the spinal canal. The subarachnoid space limits the volume at risk for harboring metastases borne by the cerebrospinal fluid (CSF). Below S2-S3, the spinal canal forms an extradural space, which continues inferiorly into the coccyx.

The cord proper lies within the spinal canal, with the dura intimately applied to the bony and ligamentous structures forming the periphery of the canal. In addition to the cord, the spinal canal includes the subarachnoid space, vessels, nerve roots, and meninges. The spinal canal is encased by the elements of the vertebrae and intervertebral ligaments, with the vertebral bodies located anteriorly; the pedicles, lamina, and transverse processes laterally; and the spinous processes posteriorly.

Tumors involving the spinal cord have often been classified by their anatomic relationship relative to the dura. The majority of extradural lesions are metastatic. Intradural, extramedullary tumors are roughly evenly divided between primary and metastatic tumors, while intradural, intramedullary tumors are most often primary gliomas.

Approximately 10% of all primary tumors involving the cord arise from the vertebrae, 65% from the spinal canal, and 25% from the cord proper. For purposes of treatment, it is useful to group primary tumors based on whether they arise from the cord, spinal canal, or vertebrae (Table 26-1). This system helps to predict whether radical surgery is feasible. It also suggests whether the normal spinal cord must be included within the high-dose irradiation volume or could instead be partially excluded from treatment with the use of sophisticated irradiation techniques.

Table 26–1   Common Primary Tumor Types Involving the Spinal Cord

Location	Histologic Types
Vertebral body (excluding myeloma/plasmacytoma)	Osteogenic sarcoma
	Chondrosarcoma
	Chordoma
Spinal canal	Neurofibrosarcoma
	Malignant schwannoma (neurilemoma)
	Meningioma
Spinal cord/cauda equina	Astrocytoma
	Ependymoma
	Oligodendroglioma

Pathology

The histology of spinal tumors correlates strongly with location. Primary tumors of bone (osteogenic sarcoma, chondrosarcoma, and chordoma) comprise most primary vertebral tumors aside from myeloma or plasmacytoma. Chordomas in particular are concentrated in sacral locations. Soft tissue sarcomas (particularly nerve sheath tumors such as malignant schwannoma or neurofibrosarcoma) and meningiomas comprise most spinal canal tumors. Astrocytomas and ependymomas account for the majority of primary cord tumors, with oligodendrogliomas occurring rarely. Other histologies such as vertebral body hemangiomas, lipomas, and arteriovenous malformations (AVMs) are occasionally encountered. Cauda equina ependymomas account for 60% of all spinal ependymomas and are generally included with intramedullary ependymomas when radiotherapy results are reported. Although spinal ependymomas (cord and cauda) outnumber astrocytomas two to one, intramedullary tumors are almost evenly divided between ependymomas and astrocytomas.

Grade is an important consideration for several tumor types. Low-grade spinal canal sarcomas appear to be at low risk for both local and distant recurrence if completely resected. High-grade, malignant meningiomas are probably at higher risk for recurrence than the more typical benign meningiomas. The importance of grade is uncertain for ependymomas, as some series have identified grade as a significant prognostic factor,[7-9] and others have not.[10] The overall risk of subsequent intracranial failure for low-grade spinal ependymomas is low, on the order of 7%.[11] However, this value is probably higher for histologically malignant ependymomas.[12,13] Myxopapillary ependymomas reportedly have a particularly favorable prognosis.[9]

Grade is clearly the most important factor influencing outcome for spinal astrocytomas.[14,15] Although prolonged survival is generally the rule for patients with low-grade astrocytomas, malignant astrocytomas such as glioblastoma multiforme (GBM) and highly anaplastic (Grade 3) astrocytoma (HAA) are aggressive tumors characterized by rapid local recurrence following treatment, craniospinal axis dissemination, and short survival.[13-17] The pilocytic astrocytoma subtype reportedly has a better prognosis than the diffuse fibrillary astrocytoma subtype.[18]

Clinical Presentation

Patients with primary spinal tumors generally present with local or distal neurological symptoms produced by spinal cord dysfunction. Local symptoms often include focal pain, segmental or nerve root weakness, and sensory deficits corresponding to a dermatomal distribution. These symptoms and signs usually correspond closely to the level of the lesion within the cord. Distal symptoms are produced by involvement of the cord's long tracts, creating paresis, sensory deficits, and autonomic dysfunction diffusely below the level of the cord lesion. Depending on the location of the lesion, long tract signs may be relatively lateralized (e.g., the Brown-Sécquard

syndrome). Since the cord is substantially shorter than the spine in adults, an intrinsic cord lesion is generally located anatomically a few vertebral bodies above the clinical cord level (e.g., a T8 cord segment astrocytoma may lie at the level of the T6 vertebral body).

Routes of Spread

Primary cord tumors, particularly high-grade ependymomas and malignant astrocytomas, can spread via the subarachnoid CSF throughout the craniospinal axis. Low-grade astrocytomas and ependymomas generally remain localized. Primary tumors arising from the spinal canal and vertebrae occasionally spread hematogeneously, with the lungs being the most frequent metastatic site. Lymphatic metastases are rarely encountered with any primary spinal tumor.

Diagnostic and Staging Studies

The workup for primary cord tumors is chiefly radiographical. Magnetic resonance imaging (MRI) with gadolinium for contrast is the imaging study of choice.[19] Standard or metrizamide-enhanced computed tomographic (CT) myelography is indicated for patients unable to undergo MRI (e.g., pacemaker-dependent patients). Intramedullary tumors usually extend for multiple segments of cord, and sagittal MRI is particularly useful for delineating the rostral and caudal extent of tumor. Imaging of the entire craniospinal axis is required for all ependymomas since spinal axis metastases develop in 5% to 15% of intracranial ependymomas.[20] These spinal "drop metastases" can produce the initial symptoms of a disseminated, primary intracranial ependymoma.

The entire neuraxis should also be imaged for cord HAAs and GBMs. Low-grade spinal astrocytomas and oligodendrogliomas do not require imaging of the entire craniospinal axis. CT scanning of the chest to rule out pulmonary metastases should be performed for vertebral osteogenic sarcomas and chondrosarcomas, as well as for spinal canal neurofibrosarcomas. Other tests such as angiography may be of limited use for AVMs or meningiomas. CSF cytology may be informative, but its use in determining treatment or influencing outcome is controversial. No chemical markers appear to be clinically useful in the diagnosis or follow-up of spinal tumors. The role of the bromodeoxyuridine (BrdU) and Ki-67 labeling indices as prognostic indicators for spinal ependymomas is under investigation.[21,22] An elevated cyclin D1 labeling index, high MIB-1 proliferation index, and *p53* immunolabeling might be indicative of high grade in ependymomas, although a correlation with clinical outcome is unclear.[5,23]

Staging System

Presently there is no commonly accepted TNM-type staging system for primary cord tumors. Primary vertebral body tumors and spinal canal tumors should be staged using the American Joint Committee on Cancer

(AJCC) staging systems for bone and soft tissues, respectively.[24]

Standard Therapeutic Approaches

Surgical exploration combining maximal resection (preferably en bloc) with minimal risk of iatrogenic injury is the preferred initial treatment procedure. In addition to decompressing the cord, essential histologic information is obtained. There is no role for preoperative irradiation or irradiation without a prior attempt at histologic diagnosis. As many as 4% of radiographically diagnosed "cord gliomas" have proven to be benign upon pathologic examination, with infarcts, demyelinating processes, amyloidosis, and sarcoidosis comprising some of the disease processes which mimic gliomas.[25]

The anatomic location and histology of the tumor have important implications for treatment. Complete resection of primary vertebral body tumors is infrequent; the radiation oncologist must generally deal with residual macroscopic tumor requiring radiation doses greatly exceeding normal spinal cord tolerance. Charged particle beams are generally employed in this setting. Completely resected, low-grade spinal canal sarcomas and meningiomas generally do not require postoperative irradiation. Subtotally resected meningiomas may be managed with observation, conventional megavoltage irradiation, or charged particle beams. Charged particle beams are preferred to irradiate subtotally resected or high-grade sarcomas of the spinal canal.

The extent of resection is variable for primary cord gliomas. Using modern microsurgical techniques with intraoperative monitoring, complete resection of low-grade gliomas has become more common, and outcome has been successful without the use of adjuvant radiotherapy.[26,27] Postoperative megavoltage irradiation provides favorable long-term results following subtotal resection. Craniospinal irradiation is employed in the management of malignant as well as benign, multifocal ependymomas.

The favorable location of ependymomas of the cauda equina usually permits complete resection. Intramedullary ependymomas frequently have tissue planes separating the tumor and cord that facilitate complete resection, as well. Low-grade astrocytomas and oligodendrogliomas are infiltrative and generally lack tissue planes separating the tumor from normal cord. Aggressive resection in this situation can result in substantial neurologic injury, so subtotal resection or biopsy is often performed. However, aggressive resection has been performed successfully in some expert hands.[28] If frozen sections suggest HAA or GBM, resection is usually abandoned after biopsy is performed.

The treatment approach for primary spinal canal and vertebral tumors differs from that for primary cord tumors because a small distance (often on the order of millimeters) physically separates the tumor from the cord. This distance often allows aggressive surgery without an unacceptably high risk of cord injury.

Chemotherapy is not indicated in the management of low-grade cord gliomas, although concurrent treatment with carmustine (bis-chloroethyl-nitrosourea [BCNU]) might be useful with HAAs or GBMs. Osteogenic sarcomas arising from the vertebrae should be treated with aggressive chemotherapy, as performed in other osseous sites. The role of adjuvant chemotherapy for other soft tissue and bone sarcomas is less clear, but in view of the high risk of systemic recurrence, might be considered for high-grade lesions. Adjuvant chemotherapy with procarbazine, lomustine (chloroethyl-cyclohexyl-nitrosourea [CCNU]), and vincristine (PCV) may be considered for malignant (but not benign) meningiomas.

Role of Radiation Therapy

The radiation oncologist faces four basic clinical situations when evaluating a patient with a primary cord glioma:

1. Completely resected, localized, low-grade glioma
2. Subtotally resected, localized, low-grade glioma
3. High-grade astrocytoma (GBM, HAA)
4. Malignant ependymoma and benign, multifocal ependymoma

The radiotherapeutic approach is different for each situation (Table 26-2). Postoperative irradiation is not

Table 26–2   Radiotherapeutic Management of Primary Spinal Tumors

Type	Treatment and Total Radiation Dose (Gy)*
Low-grade glioma,† complete resection	Observation
Low-grade glioma,† subtotal resection	Focal field XRT,‡ 50.4
High-grade (malignant) glioma (HAA, GBM)	Focal field XRT, 54
Malignant ependymoma and benign multifocal ependymoma	Craniospinal XRT to 45, then 9 focal boost to gross tumor sites (54 total)
Meningioma, completely resected	Observation
Meningioma, subtotally resected	Observation vs. focal field XRT, 50.4-54, or Charged particle beams,§ 52-54 Eq
Spinal canal sarcomas and vertebral body chondrosarcomas, chordomas, osteogenic sarcomas	Charged particle beams,§ 60-72 Eq

*Total dose prescribed using standard (1.8 Gy) once-daily fractions with megavoltage photons unless otherwise specified.
†Includes astrocytoma, ependymoma, and oligodendroglioma.
‡XRT = megavoltage photon irradiation
§Protons or helium ions

indicated for completely resected low-grade gliomas.[26,29,30] Incompletely resected low-grade astrocytomas and ependymomas are generally treated with postoperative focal irradiation. High-grade (malignant) astrocytomas are palliatively irradiated with focal fields. Malignant ependymoma and multifocal, benign ependymomas are treated with curative-intent, craniospinal irradiation.

Completely resected spinal canal meningiomas require no additional therapy, since the risk of recurrence is only on the order of 6%.[31] However, subtotally resected meningiomas have a higher risk of local recurrence, making postoperative irradiation a reasonable consideration.

Nerve sheath sarcomas are approached in a similar manner: Postoperative irradiation is generally withheld if the tumor has been completely resected. Particle beam irradiation is given if macroscopic tumor remains. Incompletely removed vertebral chondrosarcomas and chordomas are likewise irradiated with charged particles (see Table 26-2). Osteogenic sarcomas are treated with a combination of chemotherapy, surgery, and postoperative particle beam irradiation if complete resection is not achieved.

Simulation

The approach to radiation treatment planning for spinal tumors will undergo a tremendous change in the next few years as intensity-modulated radiation therapy (IMRT) becomes more widely available. When possible, IMRT should be used to treat spinal tumors with curative intent, due to the advantages obtained by reducing the acute toxicity caused by irradiation of nearby gastrointestinal structures, as well as reducing the risk of long-term radiation injury to radiosensitive organs such as the lung, kidney, and liver. Where IMRT is unavailable, though, more conventional treatment techniques are employed, beginning with a formal simulation before the start of irradiation. Low-grade cord gliomas are treated with megavoltage photon fields encompassing the radiographically apparent lesion with a 3 to 5 cm margin of normal spinal cord (or brainstem for high cervical lesions) both rostrally and caudally. Preoperative sagittal MRI is the most useful study for determining the size and location of the portals. Field width rarely needs to exceed 7 to 8 cm, since only the cord requires irradiation in this setting. Sophisticated immobilization devices are rarely needed, although thermoplastic face masks are useful for tumors located in the cervical spine. A typical clinical setup for a patient with a thoracic cord glioma is shown in Figure 26-1.

Whether to include an associated syrinx (a dilated, fluid-filled intramedullary cavity) in the treatment volume is controversial. At times, the syrinx is formed by local mass effect resulting in obstruction of the central canal of the spinal cord; in this situation, the syrinx is not part of the neoplastic process, but instead represents a reaction of normal tissue to the nearby tumor bulk. At other times, the tumor itself may be forming a cystic cavity or syrinx, and the syrinx must be regarded as a part of the malignant process. Clinically distinguishing these situations from one another is often difficult. In general,

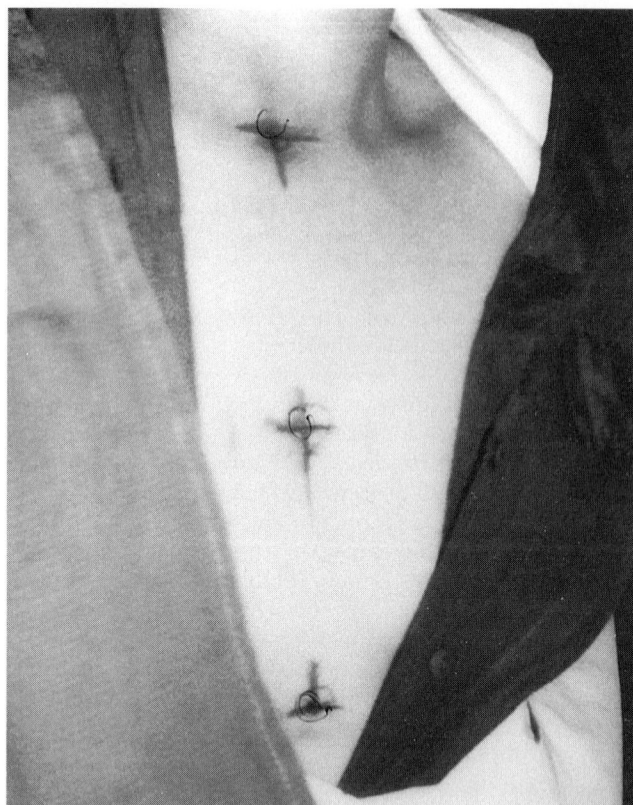

Figure 26–1. Clinical setup showing cephalad and caudal field borders for a localized low-grade thoracic spinal cord glioma.

a small syrinx is included in the treatment volume. A syrinx extending for virtually the entire length of the cord, associated with a histologically low-grade tumor, generally would not be completely encompassed by the treatment fields.

Tumors in the upper cervical spine are generally treated with opposed lateral fields to avoid unnecessary irradiation of the aerodigestive mucosa. Tumors located more caudally are often treated with differentially weighted anterior-posterior–posterior-anterior (AP-PA) fields using compensators. Use of beam-split abutting opposed lateral and AP-PA fields to treat tumors at the cervicothoracic junction is discouraged; the risk of overdosing the normal cord and underdosing the tumor owing to setup variation or error far outweighs any advantage in reducing acute morbidity. When the use of such abutting fields is unavoidable, the use of a matching beam-split technique using independent jaws is required. The match line should be shifted 1 cm after every 10 Gy to minimize the risk of inadvertent overlap. A medulloblastoma-type "gap" technique should only be used when treating the craniospinal axis, and the gap should never be located over a site of macroscopic disease.

Wedged pair, posterior, oblique fields offer the theoretical advantage of decreased morbidity by minimizing exit dose in any given location; however, the planning and setup are technically more difficult, and scrupulous verification is necessary to ensure adequate coverage during treatment. Care must also be taken with this technique to ensure that the kidneys, liver, or substantial portions of the lungs are not irradiated beyond tolerance. The use of three-dimensional (3D) conformal treatment planning with dose-volume histograms has greatly improved the reliability and safety of this technique (Fig. 26-2).

Caudal ependymomas have historically been treated with generous fields extended inferiorly to encompass the entire thecal sac and laterally as far as the sacroiliac joints to encompass the sacral nerve roots. The justification for extended fields has been to comprehensively irradiate the subarachnoid space, which many incorrectly believe extends laterally along the sacral nerve roots. However, the subarachnoid space terminates inferiorly at the S2-S3 level and does not extend laterally beyond the confines of the spinal canal. Enlarging the fields laterally beyond the bony canal is thus inconsistent with the physical location of the subarachnoid space and only serves to unnecessarily irradiate a larger volume of normal tissue. Similarly, CSF-borne metastases from the cauda would be expected to spread from the primary tumor in a cephalad direction as well as caudally. It is logically inconsistent to extend fields caudally well beyond the termination

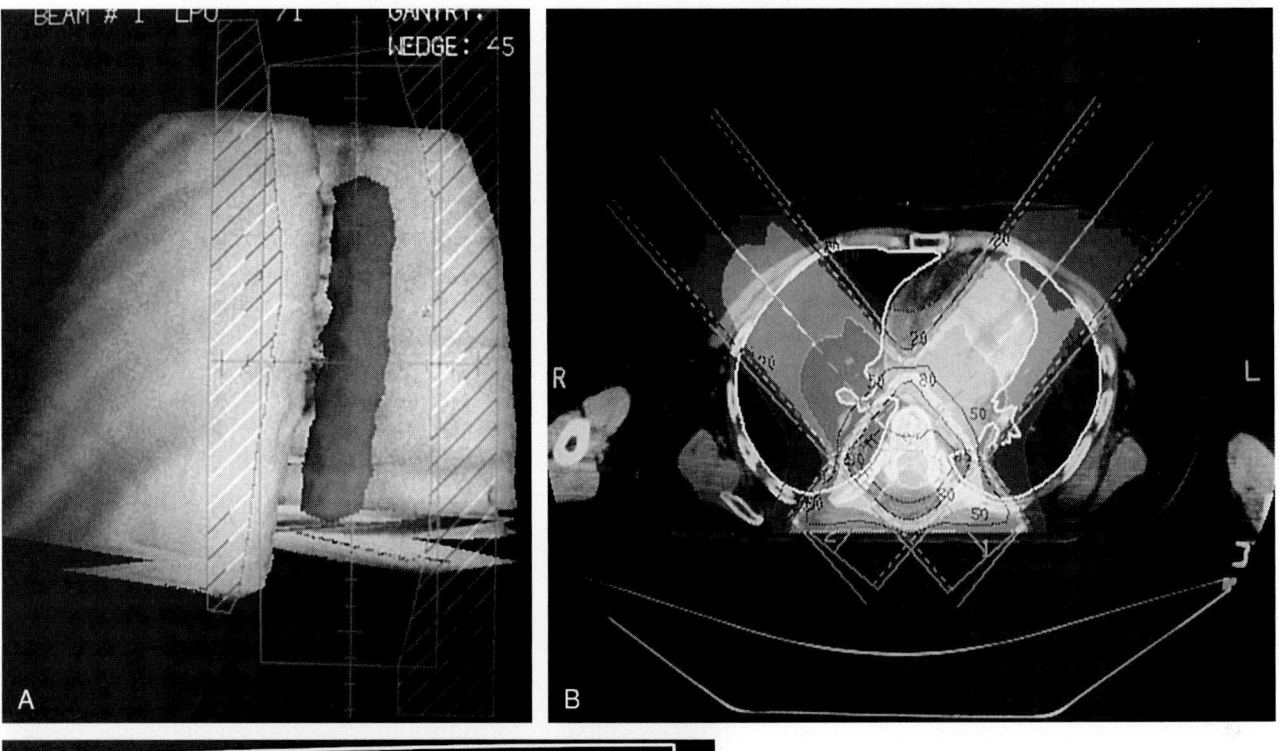

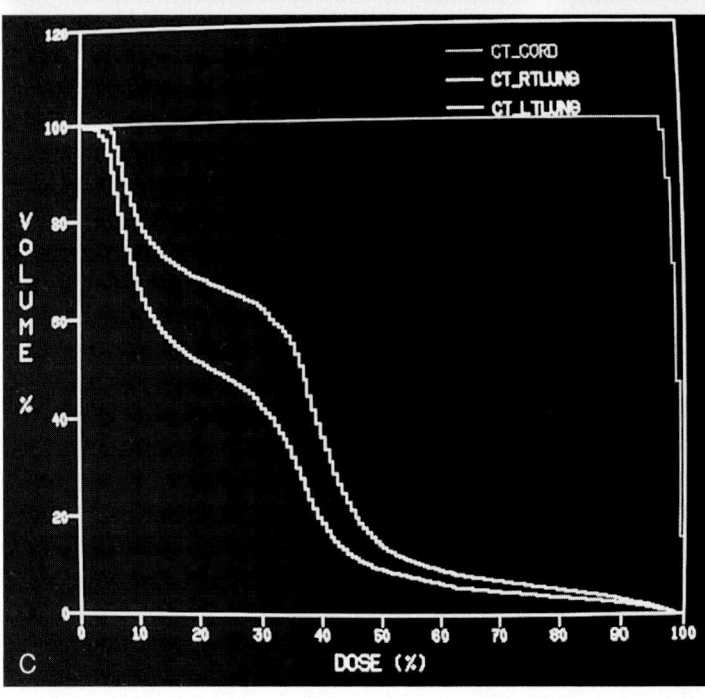

Figure 26-2. A, Beam's eye view achieved using three-dimensional conformal reconstruction of a thoracic cord glioma target volume and adjacent lungs with a posterior oblique wedged-pair irradiation technique. Custom low melting point alloy blocking is designed using the beam's eye view of the target volume. **B,** Transverse section showing dosimetry from the treatment plan developed using the target volume derived from **A**. Note the substantial portion of lung included in the beam's exit path at this level. **C,** Dose-volume histogram derived from the treatment plan shown in **B** using dosimetry information for the entire treatment volume. Virtually the entire target volume receives 100% of the total dose of 50.4 Gy at 1.8 Gy per fraction. Despite the impressive amount of lung included in the exit beam shown in **B,** the histogram shows that only 10% to 15% of each lung atually receives more than 25 Gy (50% of the total dose) under this plan. Nonetheless, 40% of the left lung and 60% of the right lung receives a dose greater than 15 Gy (30% of the total dose). See also Color Figure 26-2.

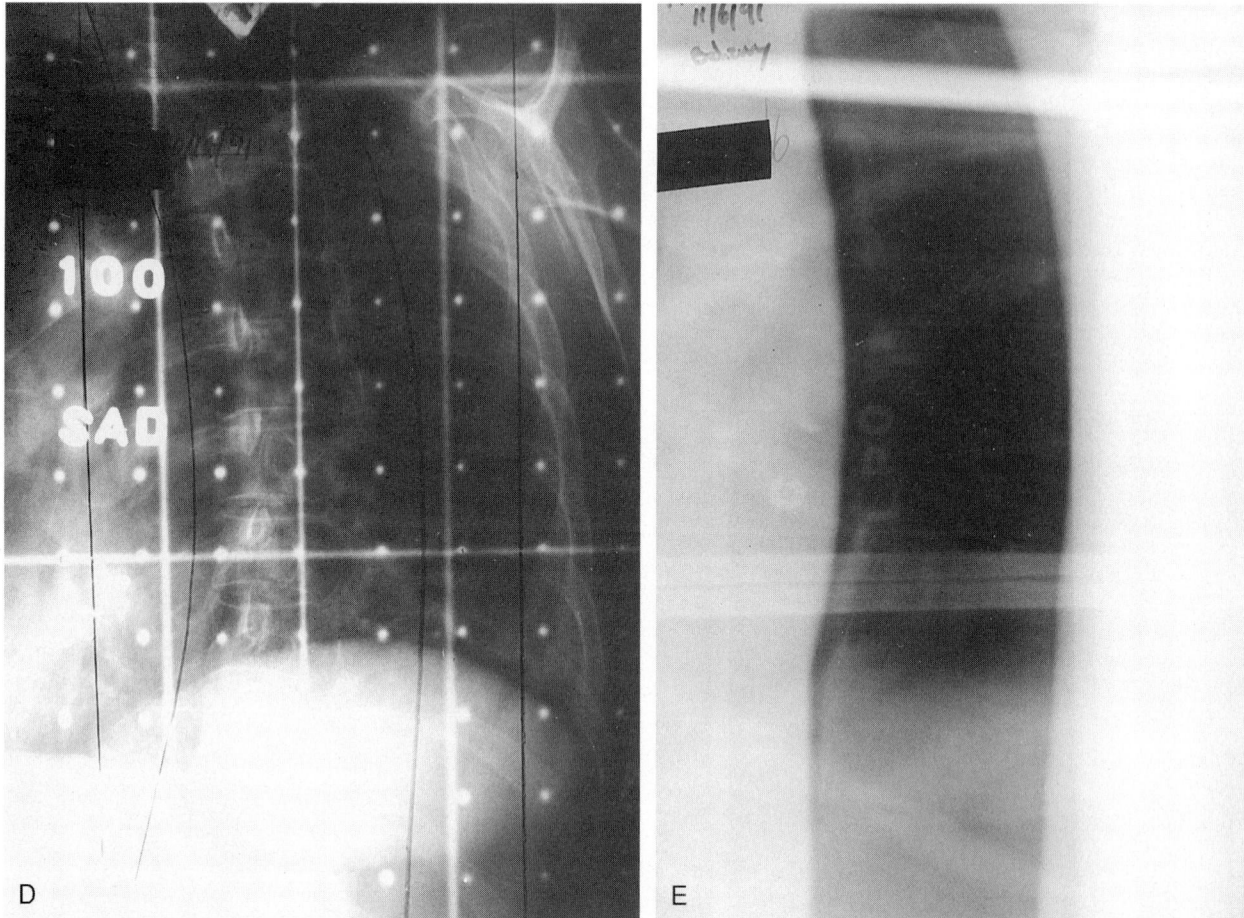

Figure 26–2. (*cont'd*) **D,** Verification simulator film taken with the beam's eye view geometry based on the treatment plan developed in **A, B,** and **C. E,** Port film taken during treatment on the linear accelerator using the treatment field shown in **D** confirms the accuracy of the daily patient setup.

of the subarachnoid space, while arbitrarily stopping fields only a few vertebral bodies cephalad to the primary tumor, where no similar barrier to spread exists.

It is worth noting that a series from Iowa with small numbers of cauda ependymomas found that adjuvant thecal sac irradiation was beneficial when "piecemeal" rather than "en bloc" resection was performed.[32] However, several other series found no advantage to the use of traditional extended fields over focal fields.[8,33] Following an uncomplicated resection, the use of fields extended inferiorly and laterally to encompass the entire sacrum appear unnecessary from both a clinical and theoretic standpoint.

Craniospinal axis irradiation using a medulloblastoma-type technique is advised for malignant ependymomas, as well as for multifocal, benign ependymomas. Care should be taken to ensure that the matchline does not cut through macroscopic disease, and that the matchline is moved 1 to 2 cm every 10 Gy to minimize inadvertent setup overlap causing overdosage of the normal cord. Focal boost fields with 3 to 5 cm craniocaudal margins should be applied to macroscopic disease sites after the entire neuraxis is treated. Prophylactic craniospinal irradiation is not advised for GBMs or HAAs despite their propensity for CSF dissemination. Since local failure is

inevitable, the increased morbidity of neuraxis irradiation to control microscopic, asymptomatic disease is inappropriate. Focal fields encompassing the symptomatic, macroscopic disease with a 3 to 5 cm margin are used instead.

Spinal canal meningiomas are treated with focal fields encompassing the preoperative tumor volume with a 3 to 5 cm margin in cephalocaudal dimension, usually using megavoltage beams. Spinal canal sarcomas as well as sarcomas of bone generally require extremely high doses of radiation, far exceeding the tolerance of the normal cord, for local control to be achieved. Charged particle beams are generally required in this setting to avoid irradiating the normal cord while adequately encompassing the tumor, which is generally located only a few millimeters away. A technical description of such treatment techniques is available in Chapter 69, Particle Radiation Therapy.

Radiation Treatment Plan

Preoperative sagittal MRI and operative findings are the most useful studies defining the volume to be irradiated. When 3D conformal treatment planning is unavailable, contours should be taken at several levels, particularly in the lumbosacral region, to ensure homogeneity of dose throughout the length of the field. 3D conformal planning using CT scanning with magnetic resonance fusion is generally employed when charged particle beam therapy is undertaken for spinal canal and vertebral body primary tumors.

Low-grade astrocytomas and benign ependymomas are treated with daily fractions of 1.8 Gy to a total dose of 50.4 Gy over 5.5 weeks.

Malignant ependymomas and benign multifocal ependymomas are treated with 18 Gy fractions. The entire craniospinal axis is treated to a dose of 45 Gy, followed by a boost to macroscopic disease sites to 50.4 to 54 Gy total.

Malignant astrocytomas (HAA, GBM) are treated palliatively with focal fields using 1.8 Gy fractions to a total dose of 54 Gy.

Unless observation is chosen, subtotally resected spinal canal meningiomas may be irradiated in one of two ways: either 1.8 Gy daily fractions to a total dose of 50.4 to 54 Gy, or with twice-a-day fractions of 1 Gy (minimum 5- to 6-hour interfraction interval) to 54 Gy. (The hyperfractionated approach has the theoretical advantage of minimizing the risk of radiation injury to the normal spinal cord and has been used safely when incidentally irradiating the cervical cord during treatment for brainstem gliomas.[34]) Since the risk of long-term local recurrence for subtotally resected intracranial meningiomas is less than 10% when the minimum tumor dose is 52 Gy or greater,[35] a reasonable approach is to use a plan in which the maximum dose in the treatment volume is 54 Gy, with a minimum dose to the meningioma of 52 Gy.

Experience with soft tissue and bone sarcomas from extremity sites suggests that doses in the range of 60 to 66 Gy are required to eradicate microscopic disease. Still higher doses are required to control macroscopic disease. These doses clearly exceed cord tolerance, so conventional x-ray therapy cannot be used safely in this situation. The physical dose-distribution advantages of charged particle beams can be exploited here. These beams have extremely sharp lateral penumbras as well as Bragg peak behavior that allow accurate placement of the beam within a few millimeters of the spinal cord, without actually including the cord in the high-dose volume. With mixtures of photons, protons (and in the past, helium and neon ions), radiation doses in the range of 65 to 72 GyEq can be delivered to the tumor, while the dose to the cord is limited to less than 45 GyEq. Primary vertebral chordomas, chondrosarcomas, and osteogenic sarcomas are treated similarly. Patients with these types of tumors should be referred to the few national centers (e.g., Harvard, Loma Linda) with particle beam capabilities.

Brachytherapy

There is no established role for brachytherapy in the management of primary cord gliomas. Temporary ^{192}Ir and permanent ^{125}I implants have been used rarely to manage paraspinal sarcomas, occasionally with concurrent placement of a gold foil shield separating the seeds from the cord. Outcome has been poor in situations in which resection of the tumor has required opening of the dura.[36] Currently, brachytherapy plays little role in the management of most primary tumors involving the spinal cord.

Critical Normal Tissues (Radiation Myelitis)

The spinal cord and cauda equina are the critical dose-limiting structures in the treatment of primary tumors involving the spinal cord. The cauda equina, consisting of peripheral nerve, is probably more resistant to radiation injury than the cord. Myelopathy was observed to be much more frequent when intrathecal [198]Au was used alone or in addition to external beam treatment[20,37]; this form of therapy is now obsolete.

It has been postulated that the risk of cord injury depends on the location and length of cord irradiated, but no contemporary data exist to support this widely held notion. Older reports in the literature suggested that the thoracic cord was more sensitive to radiation injury than the cervical cord.[38] During the period when this information was gathered, it was common to treat with only one field per day. Since most fields involving the cervical cord were opposed laterals, the dose delivered daily to the cervical cord was the prescribed mid-plane dose. The thoracic cord, on the other hand, was usually irradiated with AP-PA opposed fields, and the radiation dose it received on "PA days" was substantially higher than the mid-plane dose. Since fraction size dominates as a risk factor for radiation cord injury, the radiobiologic dose received by the cord under the "one-field-a-day" approach was much greater than the prescribed mid-plane dose. Thus, the reputed anatomic variability in cord sensitivity appears to be a radiobiologic artifact created by an obsolete treatment technique.[39] Unlike the brain, where a relationship apparently exists between the volume irradiated and the subsequent risk of radiation injury, the length of cord irradiated appears to have little impact on the risk of radiation injury.[40,41]

The radiation tolerance of the *normal* spinal cord using once-daily fractions of 1.8 to 2 Gy has been traditionally listed as 45[42] to 50 Gy.[38,43] The 45 Gy value reportedly entails a 5% risk of myelitis at 5 years (TD$_{5/5}$), which seems a gross overestimate. A University of Florida review of head and neck cancer patients whose cervical cords were incidentally irradiated found a 0.4% incidence of radiation myelitis with total doses between 45.01 and 50 Gy (2 of 471), compared with a 0% incidence with 40.01 to 45 Gy (0 of 514 patients), and 0% incidence (0 of 75 patients) with doses of more than 50 Gy.[44] A 6% incidence of cervical myelitis was reported in 72 head and neck cancer patients whose cords were treated with at least 55 Gy.[45] In that series, the minimum follow-up was 2 years, radiation fraction sizes ranged from 1.5 to 2 Gy, and 26 patients received total doses in excess of 60 Gy. Based partly on these data, contemporary experts have suggested that the TD$_{5/5}$ for human spinal cord is actually on the order of 57 to 61 Gy, and the $TD_{5/50}$ is in the range of 68 to 73 Gy.[40,41,46,47] The spinal cord is particularly vulnerable to injury when larger fraction sizes are used; the Medical Research Council Lung Cancer Working Party reported on radiation myelopathy developing in 1048 lung cancer patients undergoing thoracic irradiation with palliative intent.[48] No radiation myelitis developed using 3 Gy × 10 fractions (30 Gy total); but myelitis developed in 2.5% of patients receiving 3 Gy × 13 fractions (39 Gy total).

Although it seems logical to assume that cord injured by growing tumor and surgical trauma would be more sensitive to radiation injury than incidentally irradiated normal spinal cord, many series suggest that cord involved by tumor may be safely irradiated to standard tolerance levels. In the Massachusetts General Hospital (MGH) series, 26 patients with various histologic conditions were postoperatively irradiated to the equivalent of 40 to 50 Gy with standard fractionation and none developed radiation myelopathy.[49] Likewise, none of 29 Medical College of Virginia spinal cord ependymoma and astrocytoma patients treated with doses between 45 and 55 Gy developed radiation-related neurologic deficits.[50] In the series from the University of California at San Francisco (UCSF), 39 patients with primary cord and cauda tumors received total doses ranging between 45 and 54.7 Gy and only one case of radiation myelitis developed.[13] Higher total radiation doses have been well tolerated; four ependymoma patients were treated at the Mayo Clinic to doses of 55 Gy and greater without complications.[12]

Outcome

Treating primary spinal tumors with postoperative irradiation is generally successful in terms of survival, less so in terms of local control, and difficult to evaluate in terms of long-term neurologic outcome. Survival of patients with low-grade spinal gliomas is substantially better than that achieved with histologically similar intracranial gliomas, probably because salvage of locally recurrent tumors with additional surgery is often effective.

The exact degree of neurologic impairment caused by irradiation is difficult to determine because injury due to direct tumor growth as well as surgical trauma must be taken into account. As a general rule, it seems that a majority of patients either improve neurologically or stabilize with irradiation.[51]

Spinal ependymoma patients do well, with 5- and 10-year survival rates in the 70% to 100% range (Table 26-3). Unfortunately, local recurrence ultimately develops in roughly one third of irradiated patients. Delayed local failures are far from rare; most series include several late recurrences developing more than 5 or 10 years after initial treatment, indicating the need for long-term follow-up. The majority of recurrences develop within the irradiated volume.

A Mallinckrodt series of 37 patients with primary "cord tumors" found a statistically significant dose-response relationship: Survival was 23% for those receiving less than 40 Gy total dose, compared with 83% for those with total doses of 40 Gy or greater.[37] This analysis combined ependymomas, astrocytomas, unbiopsied tumors, and lymphoma together. When ependymomas have been analyzed exclusively, no series has found a statistically significant dose-response relationship in the 40 to 54 Gy range.[11-13,20,32,33,52] In the Mayo Clinic series, 4 patients were irradiated to total doses of 55 Gy or greater, with one in-field failure still noted at this dose level.[12] The UCSF series included 9 ependymoma patients treated with doses between 45 and 50.4 Gy and another 9 with doses between 50.4 and 52.9 Gy. The local recurrence rate was 33% in both dose ranges.[13] Presently, there are no convincing data that demonstrate improved outcome with total doses above 50.4 Gy.

Results for low-grade spinal astrocytomas are similar to those achieved with ependymomas, with long-term survival in the 60% to 90% range, but a relatively high incidence of local recurrence (Table 26-4). Most failures develop within 2 to 3 years of treatment. Low-grade astrocytomas tend to fail locally, although craniospinal axis metastases are occasionally encountered.[11,13] Like ependymomas, there is no evidence for a dose-response relationship to suggest improved local control or survival with total doses exceeding 50.4 Gy.[11,13]

Table 26–3 Spinal Ependymomas: Reported Results with Postoperative Irradiation

Author	Patients, n	Actuarial Survival (%)		LFR (%)*
		5 yr	10 yr	
Garcia[37]	8 (cord)	60	60	38
	10 (cauda)	100	70	10
Shaw et al[12]	22	95	95	32
Whitaker et al[7]	43	69	62	—
Waldron et al[8]	59	83	75	19
Linstadt et al[13]	18	93	93	33
Schild et al[9]	35	97	93	—
McLaughlin et al[23]	9	100	100	None
Abdel-Wahab et al[52]	—	94	68	—
Hulshof et al[86]	34	—	91	25

*Crude incidence, not actuarial risk.
LFR, local failure rate; not reported.

Table 26–4   Spinal Astrocytomas: Reported Results with Postoperative Irradiation

| Author | Patients, *n* | Actuarial Survival (%) | | LFR (%)* |
		5 yr	10 yr	
Garcia[37]	14	60	50	50
Koppelson et al[11]	9	89	89	22
Linstadt et al[13]	12	91	91	33
Huddart et al[87]	27	59	52	59
Hulshof et al[86]	12	—	43	—
Jyothirmayi et al[51]	15	79	—	—
Abdel-Wahab et al[52]	—	64	54	—
McLaughlin et al[10]	8	—	—	1
Minehan et al[18]	79	—	50%	—
pilocytic	43	—	81%	—
diffuse fibrillary	25	—	15%	—

*Crude incidence, not actuarial risk.
LFR, local failure rate; not reported.

Postoperative irradiation for malignant astrocytomas provides palliation, but long-term results are dismal. Extremely rapid local recurrence, CSF dissemination, and short survival times are the rule, regardless of the total dose of radiation used (Table 26–5).

Published results regarding irradiation of subtotally resected spinal meningiomas are virtually nonexistent. However, extrapolation from the experience with intracranial meningiomas potentially supports the use of postoperative irradiation in this setting.

Spinal canal sarcomas respond favorably to charged particle irradiation. Castro and coworkers[53,54] at Lawrence Berkeley Laboratory (LBL) treated 14 patients with neurofibrosarcoma and other soft tissue sarcoma histologies whose tumors abutted or encircled the spinal cord. All had macroscopic residual tumor when irradiated. With a mix of photons and helium and neon ions, a median dose of 65 GyEq was delivered to the tumor, but the cord dose was generally limited to less than 45 GyEq. The 4-year actuarial local control rate was 56%, and the 4-year actuarial survival rate was 77%. There was 1 case of radiation myelitis in a patient whose cord dose reached 55 GyEq.

The experience with primary tumors arising from the vertebral bodies is similar. Twenty-four LBL patients were irradiated with particles for spinal chordoma and chondrosarcoma.[54] Mean doses were 72 GyEq (chondrosarcoma) and 65 GyEq (chordoma); gross tumor was present at the time of irradiation in 92% of cases. The 3-year actuarial local control rate for chondrosarcoma was 83%; the 3-year survival rate was 69%. Corresponding values for chordoma were 33% local control and 48% survival. There were no neurologic complications. Fourteen patients with sacral chordomas did particularly well, with a 5-year actuarial survival rate of 85% and a 55% local control rate.[55] Similar results have been reported with the use of protons at MGH.[56] The 5-year survival rate for proton treatment of cervical chondrosarcomas and chordomas using doses of 56.8 to 80 GyEq was 58%; as with the LBL series, better outcome was seen with chondrosarcomas than with chordomas.[57] Investigators in Hannover, Germany also reported a benefit from high-dose (60 to 70 Gy) postoperative radiotherapy after subtotal resection of spinal chordoma, although results were best when en bloc resection could be performed.[58]

Experience with vertebral osteogenic sarcomas is limited. Five such patients were treated at LBL; local control was achieved in two without treatment-related complications.[54] Fifteen osteogenic sarcoma patients treated at MGH with mixed protons and photons achieved a 5-year local control rate of 59%, and a 5-year overall survival rate of 44%.[59]

Table 26–5   High-Grade Spinal Astrocytomas (Including Highly Anaplastic Astrocytomas and Glioblastoma Multiforme): Reported Results with Postoperative Irradiation

Author	Patients, *n*	Survival (%)	Median Survival
Koppelson and Linggood[14]	5	0	2 years
Linstadt et al[13]	3	0	6 months
Cohen et al[17]	19	21*	6 months
Jyothirmayi et al[51]	6	0	10 months
McLaughlin et al[10]	4	0	—

*Unclear if any long-term survivors exist.

Treatment of Recurrent Spinal Cord Gliomas

Only minimal information is available regarding management of recurrent, previously irradiated cord and cauda tumors, and what does exist is largely anecdotal. Many patients suffer devastating neurologic impairment from recurrent disease and do not benefit from heroic attempts at salvage. More localized recurrences in patients with reasonable neurologic and performance status should be managed aggressively, since prolonged survival is often achieved.

Surgery is the mainstay of salvage treatment. Low-grade tumors can be treated with reexcision including cordectomy, if necessary. These tumors appear to be particularly appropriate candidates for radical resection. In the experience at New York University, 29 patients (26 of whom had recurrent intramedullary tumors, with 18 previously irradiated) underwent attempted radical resection.[17] Complete resection was obtained in 14, with "99% removal" in another 7. Although all three patients with malignant astrocytomas died from neuraxis dissemination, only one local recurrence was reported for low-grade tumors. Follow-up was short (range, 6 to 36 months) so long-term local control and survival rates are unknown. Lower extremity neurologic function appeared satisfactory, with stabilization or improvement in 72% of patients. However, patients unable to stand or walk preoperatively did not improve. Long-term disease-free survival following recurrence has also been reported following total removal or cordectomy in both the Mayo Clinic and UCSF series.[12,13]

Reirradiation has been attempted sporadically. Both experimental and clinical data suggest that the spinal cord and lung, unlike the heart and kidney, partially recover from subclinical radiation injury, suggesting that reirradiation of the cord might therefore be safely attempted.[60] In the UCSF series, 16 patients with spinal cord tumors suffered local failure. Four underwent repeat subtotal resection and reirradiation. No patients with multifocal or high-grade disease benefitted from retreatment. Two others with low-grade recurrences survived several years with high Karnofsky Performance Status values (≥80) following reirradiation. Both had initially undergone subtotal resections (one localized low-grade astrocytoma, one localized low-grade ependymoma) followed by 50.4 Gy to focal fields. After developing in-field recurrence and undergoing repeat subtotal resection, both patients were reirradiated with focal fields with 1 Gy fractions given twice daily to doses of 30 and 27 Gy. The cumulative doses were 77 Gy to the cauda equina for the ependymoma and 80 Gy to the cervical cord for the astrocytoma. No long-term radiation injuries developed.

SPINAL CORD COMPRESSION FROM METASTATIC DISEASE

Natural History

Epidural spinal metastases develop in 5% of patients with systemic cancer at some time during their illness, causing 20,000 cases of cord and cauda compression annually.[61] Primary carcinomas originating from the breast, lung, and prostate account for about half of all cases of cord compression. Other histologic types (including lymphoma, renal cell carcinoma, myeloma, melanoma, gastrointestinal carcinomas, gynecologic carcinomas, and sarcomas) account for the remainder.

Cord compression is most commonly caused by local progression of a vertebral body or neural arch osseous metastasis, which ultimately grows into the spinal canal. Less commonly, paraspinal metastases extend through vertebral foramina to involve the cord. The majority of lesions (85%) are located anterior to the cord, and often multiple epidural metastases exist simultaneously.

Ninety percent of patients have been diagnosed with cancer before they develop cord compression. Depending on histology, cord compression can develop soon after diagnosis (e.g., lung cancer: average 6 months) or with a prolonged interval between diagnosis and compression (e.g., breast cancer: average 4 years). Cord compression has been reported to develop as late as 19 years after initial diagnosis of the primary tumor.

Symptoms

Pain is the most common initial symptom (present in 90% to 95% of patients) and can be either local or radicular in nature. It usually precedes all other symptoms by several weeks to months. *Weakness* is rarely the first symptom (2%) but is common at diagnosis (75%). *Sensory loss* is present in 50% of patients at diagnosis, but is rarely the initial symptom. *Autonomic dysfunction* is usually a late manifestation associated with an unfavorable prognosis, but is present in upwards of 50% of patients at the time of diagnosis.

Workup

History, physical, and a high index of suspicion are essential for making the diagnosis of cord compression. All patients with back pain and a history of cancer should be evaluated for possible spinal cord compression. One prospective series of cancer patients suggested that the likelihood of cord compression was approximately 30% when any one of the following risk factors was present: back pain, abnormal neurologic examination, or evidence of vertebral metastases on plain x-rays.[62] When two factors were present, the probability of cord compression was 60% to 70%; when all three features were present, the likelihood of cord compression was more than 90%.

Imaging

MRI with gadolinium is the radiographic study of choice to evaluate possible malignant spinal cord compression (SCC). Patients unable to undergo MRI should be evaluated by metrizamide-enhanced CT myelography. In addition to the clinical area of interest, the study should evaluate the entire spine to determine the complete extent of the lesion and to detect possible synchronous lesions located elsewhere along the spinal axis. One retrospective series reported that multiple levels of cord compression existed in 39% of patients with apparently clinically localized SCC, and that more than two thirds of patients with multiple levels of SCC had more than one spinal region involved.[63]

Diagnostic Approach

The following approach is suggested to evaluate the cancer patient with new back pain: If the neurologic examination is *abnormal*, a screening saggital MRI of the entire spine is performed. If the neurologic examination is *normal*, a screening saggital MRI of the entire spine is still performed.

When the saggital screening MRI detects epidural disease, a full MRI of the affected area is performed. This approach results in more rapid performance of the definitive study compared with the old approach of first performing plain films ± bone scans, followed by MRI when radiographic or scintigraphic abnormalities were noted.[64] It also results in a less expensive MRI examination if no epidural disease is detected and has proven to be cost-effective compared with the traditional approach.[64] This approach might be criticized as excessively "high-tech," and it probably detects far more cases of painful bony metastases than actual cord compression. Nonetheless, the patient's long term functional status is clearly superior when a painful bony metastasis is irradiated early on, rather than later when neurologic deficits from cord compression have developed.

A widespread belief held among radiation oncologists is that referral for radiation treatment of SCC occurs most frequently on Fridays, generally late in the afternoon. The validity of this belief is supported by a retrospective study of 443 SCC patients from The Netherlands, which showed that 30% of such referrals came on Friday, 12% on Monday, 17% on Tuesday, 15% on Wednesday, 20% on Thursday, 5% on Saturday, and 1% on Sunday ($p < .002$).[65]

Treatment

Management options vary among irradiation, neurosurgical decompression with or without postoperative irradiation, and chemotherapy. Currently, irradiation and corticosteroids are the mainstay of treatment.[61]

STEROIDS

Glucocorticoid therapy (dexamethasone) is generally started immediately upon diagnosis; the initial dose is controversial. Extremely high dexamethasone doses (100 mg intravenous bolus upon diagnosis followed by 24 mg orally qid for 3 days, then tapered) did not influence neurologic outcome in two prospective studies, but appeared to hasten pain relief.[66,67] At UCSF, 10 mg of dexamethasone is given intravenously, followed by 4 to 6 mg orally or intravenously every 6 hours. The

dexamethasone dose is gradually tapered once the initial high-dose radiation fractions are completed.

Some investigators have suggested that steroids may be safely omitted for favorable patients with SCC undergoing irradiation (those presenting without neurologic deficits or radiculopathy symptoms only, and no massive vertebral involvement). One prospective phase II trial from Italy contained 20 such patients; all were ambulatory at the end of treatment, and median survival was 14 months.[68] Conversely, a randomized trial of high-dose dexamethasone (96 mg × 4 days, then tapered) versus no steroid was performed in 57 irradiated SCC patients in Denmark. The corticosteroid treatment resulted in superior outcome with respect to ambulation rates 6 months after treatment (59% for the steroid group versus 33% for the group not receiving steroids.)[69] However, there was no difference between groups with respect to median survival.

SURGERY

The traditional approach, decompressive laminectomy, offers poor exposure for the majority of tumors that arise from anterior bony structures. A successful outcome (defined as ambulation after treatment) is achieved in about 30% of patients. Historically, complications have been high, with 10% surgical mortality, 10% significant morbidity, and 10% of patients experiencing further neurologic deterioration.[70] More recently, selective surgery with vertebral body resection and stabilization has been performed for anterior tumors.[71] This approach appears to have substantially improved results with approximately 80% to 90% of patients ambulatory postoperation, although mortality and serious morbidity rates remain in the 5% to 15% range. Currently there are several clear indications for proceeding with surgical intervention:

1. Diagnosis unknown or doubtful for malignancy.
2. Instability of spine or bony compression of the cord.
3. Previous x-ray therapy (XRT) at site of compression precludes irradiation.
4. Neurologic status deteriorates during XRT. (This approach of radiation followed by surgery has been associated with a much higher rate of wound complications.[72])

IRRADIATION

Treatment of cord compression with either irradiation alone or postoperative irradiation appears to achieve better results than decompressive laminectomy alone. A large retrospective review from Memorial Sloan-Kettering Cancer Center (MSKCC) examined results with radiation alone (170 patients) and surgery plus postoperative XRT (65 patients).[73] There was no significant difference in outcome between the two treatment groups, with 46% of patients ambulatory following treatment in the surgery plus XRT group versus 49% in the XRT-alone group. Conversely, a retrospective study from Australia found the combination of surgery followed by irradiation (38 patients) to be superior to either surgery alone (19 patients) or radiotherapy alone (37 patients).[74]

A prospective, randomized trial from the University of California at Los Angeles compared irradiation alone with decompressive laminectomy and postoperative XRT. The study was small (16 patients received surgery plus XRT; 13 received XRT alone), but found no difference between treatment arms with respect to pain relief, improved ambulation, or improved sphincter function.[75] Another small, randomized, prospective trial from the MD Anderson Center compared radiotherapy alone versus surgical decompression plus irradiation and found no difference in outcome.[76] It is important to note that there are no data comparing irradiation alone with selective anterolateral-approach surgery, and this new procedure (perhaps combined with postoperative XRT) might prove to be superior to XRT alone.

Dogma states that XRT should commence within 30 minutes to 2 hours once the diagnosis of SCC has been made. There do not appear to be any objective scientific data that document the benefit of starting irradiation within this time interval, although rapid intervention seems prudent. With the proper use of steroids, a delay of several hours before irradiation may be acceptable. Each case must be managed individually; a patient who is ambulatory or paraparetic has a roughly 40% to 80% chance of remaining ambulatory with treatment, indicating the need for immediate XRT. On the other hand, paralyzed patients have only a remote chance of regaining ambulation. A "more than 2-hour delay" before starting XRT seems particularly unlikely to substantially affect outcome for paralyzed patients.

The standard radiation portal encompasses the site of the cord compression with a 5-cm craniocaudal margin (two vertebral bodies above and below the gross disease). In the high cervical spine, opposed lateral fields are generally appropriate. In the thoracic spine, PA-only fields are often used with the dose specified at a depth of 6 cm; differentially weighted AP-PA fields can also be used if desired. In the lumbar region, AP-PA opposed fields are most often used because the greater depth of cord and cauda (often 8 to 10 cm) makes the entry dose excessively high for single PA fields and because of variability of cord and cauda depth at different locations within the field. Since the metastasis usually originates from the anterior vertebral body, an adequate dose to the whole vertebra should be delivered.

Radiation doses are usually given once daily with initially large fractions (3 to 5 Gy) and then decreased in size after 3 to 4 doses and taken to total doses in the 20 to 40 Gy range. The UCSF treatment policy has been to deliver 4 Gy daily × three fractions, followed by 2 Gy × 12 (total dose 36 Gy in 15 fractions given over 3 weeks). This regimen appears to be well tolerated and achieves satisfactory outcome. Alternative schemes such as 4 Gy × 5, 3 Gy × 10 or (for selected patients with highly favorable long-term prognosis) 2 Gy × 20 are reasonable. An Italian series reported that a short course scheme of a single 8-Gy fraction followed by a second 8-Gy fraction given 1 week later was comparable in outcome to a more protracted regimen using daily fractions of 5 Gy × 3, 4 days of rest, and then 3 Gy × 5 (30 Gy total).[77]

CHEMOTHERAPY

Cytotoxic chemotherapy has been suggested as an alternative to irradiation or surgery for some highly chemosensitive tumors (e.g., lymphoma, Ewing's sarcoma, germ cell tumors, and neuroblastoma). Most reports are anecdotal. The efficacy of chemotherapy has not been prospectively compared with radiation or surgery but might be appropriate where radiation-related bone growth retardation is an overriding concern, or in situations in which neither XRT nor surgery is feasible.

Prognostic Factors

The most important factor influencing functional outcome is the extent of neurologic impairment when treatment begins.[78,79] In the MSKCC series of patients treated with XRT alone, 79% of patients who were ambulatory at the start of irradiation remained so at the end of treatment.[73] In contrast, only 45% of paraparetic patients became ambulatory, and only 3% of paralyzed patients later walked. Results were similar for the patients treated with both surgery and postoperative XRT (64%, 45%, and 10% post-treatment ambulation rates, respectively).

The Rigshospitalet in Copenhagen reported similar post-treatment ambulation rates in 345 patients treated with laminectomy, radiation, or both.[80] Of initially ambulatory patients, 79% remained ambulatory, compared with 21% of paraparetic patients. There did appear to be a better outcome for *paralyzed* patients treated with laminectomy plus XRT (13% post-treatment ambulation rate) versus XRT alone (4%).

One retrospective review has suggested a better outcome with laminectomy plus XRT than with XRT alone for *paraparetic* patients.[81] In that series, post-treatment ambulation rates were 64% for XRT alone, but 82% with combined therapy. No series has suggested a better outcome for *ambulatory patients* treated with combined surgery plus XRT compared with XRT alone.

Somewhat counterintuitively (given the usual rush to initiate XRT as soon as possible), a longer time interval between the onset of motor deficits and the initiation of radiotherapy appears to result in better functional outcome. A retrospective review of 96 SCC patients from Hannover, Germany found that 89% of patients showed improved motor function with irradiation when their motor symptoms had been present for 14 days or longer before the start of radiotherapy; only 2% deteriorated.[82] In contrast, only 12% of patients improved when their motor symptoms had been present for less than 14 days before the start of radiation, and 49% deteriorated despite treatment. The effect was particularly pronounced when motor symptoms had been present for less than 48 hours before the start of irradiation: Only 6% of such patients experienced improved motor function from treatment while 65% deteriorated. A followup prospective, observational study of 98 patients from the same investigators confirmed these findings.[83] In that series the post-treatment ambulation rates were 86% for patients whose symptoms developed more than 14 days before the start of irradiation, 55% for symptoms developing 8 to 14 days before treatment, and 35% for those whose symptoms developed 1 to 7 days before treatment.

However, they do strongly indicate that the intrinsic biology of the tumor causing the SCC is the major factor influencing functional outcome,[83] and the slower the development of motor deficits, the better. Consequently, while the perceived need to initiate radiotherapy emergently may benefit all those involved psychologically, it may not provide any meaningful improvement in the patient's long-term functional outcome.

Survival

Survival correlates best with ambulatory status at the end of treatment.[84] In a series of 56 breast cancer patients irradiated for cord compression, the 1-year actuarial survival rate was 66% for patients who were ambulatory at the end of irradiation versus 10% for nonambulatory patients.[85] For irradiated patients with SCC caused by prostate cancer, median survival for post-treatment walking patients was 10 months, compared with 2 months for nonwalking patients.[77]

REFERENCES

1. Michalski J, Garcia D. Spinal Canal: In Perez C, Brady L, eds. *Principles and Practice of Radiation Oncology.* 3rd ed. Philadelphia: Lippincott-Raven; 1998:851.
2. von Haken MS, White EC, Daneshvar-Shyesther L, et al: Molecular genetic analysis of chromosome arm 17p and chromosome arm 22q DNA sequences in sporadic pediatric ependymomas. *Genes Chromosomes Cancer.* 1996;17:37.
3. Hulsebos TJ, Oskam NT, Bijleveld EH, et al: Evidence for an ependymoma tumour suppressor gene in chromosome region 22pter-22q11.2. *Br J Cancer.* 1999;81:1150.
4. Huang B, Starostik P, Kuhl J, et al: Loss of heterozygosity on chromosome 22 in human ependymomas. *Acta Neuropathol (Berl).* 2002;103:415.
5. Rushing EJ, Brown DF, Hladik CL, et al: Correlation of bcl-2, p53, and MIB-1 expression with ependymoma grade and subtype. *Mod Pathol.* 1998;11:464.
6. Lamszus K, Lachenmayer L, Heinemann U, et al: Molecular genetic alterations on chromosomes 11 and 22 in ependymomas. *Int J Cancer.* 2001;91:803.
7. Whitaker SJ, Bessell EM, Ashley SE, et al: Postoperative radiotherapy in the management of spinal cord ependymoma. *J Neurosurg.* 1991;74:720.
8. Waldron JN, Laperriere NJ, Jaakkimainen L, et al: Spinal cord ependymomas: A retrospective analysis of 59 cases. *Int J Radiat Oncol Biol Phys.* 1993;27:223.
9. Schild SE, Nisi K, Scheithauer BW, et al: The results of radiotherapy for ependymomas: The Mayo Clinic experience. *Int J Radiat Oncol Biol Phys.* 1998;42:953.
10. McLaughlin MP, Buatti JM, Marcus RB, Jr., et al: Outcome after radiotherapy of primary spinal cord glial tumors. *Radiat Oncol Investig.* 1998;6:276.
11. Kopelson G, Linggood RM, Kleinman GM, et al: Management of intramedullary spinal cord tumors. *Radiology.* 1980;135:473.
12. Shaw EG, Evans RG, Scheithauer BW, et al: Radiotherapeutic management of adult intraspinal ependymomas. *Int J Radiat Oncol Biol Phys.* 1986;12:323.
13. Linstadt DE, Wara WM, Leibel SA, et al: Postoperative radiotherapy of primary spinal cord tumors. *Int J Radiat Oncol Biol Phys.* 1989;16:1397.
14. Kopelson G, Linggood RM: Intramedullary spinal cord astrocytoma versus glioblastoma: The prognostic importance of histologic grade. *Cancer.* 1982;50:732.
15. Rodrigues GB, Waldron JN, Wong CS, et al: A retrospective analysis of 52 cases of spinal cord glioma managed with radiation therapy. *Int J Radiat Oncol Biol Phys.* 2000;48:837.
16. Cooper P, Epstein F: Radical resection of intramedullary spinal cord tumors in adults. Recent experience in 29 patients. *J Neurosurg.* 1985;63:492.
17. Cohen A, Wisoff J, Allen J, et al: Malignant astrocytomas of the spinal cord. *J Neurosurg.* 1989;70:50.
18. Minehan KJ, Shaw EG, Scheithauer BW, et al: Spinal cord astrocytoma: Pathological and treatment considerations. *J Neurosurg.* 1995;83:590.
19. Wara W, Linstadt D, Larson D: Management of primary brain stem gliomas and spinal cord gliomas. *Semin Radiat Oncol.* 1991;1:50.
20. Marks JE, Adler SJ: A comparative study of ependymomas by site of origin. *Int J Radiat Oncol Biol Phys.* 1982;8:37.
21. Asai A, Hoshino T, Edwards M, et al: Predicting the recurrence of ependymomas from the bromodeoxyuridine labeling index. *Childs Nerv Syst.* 1992;8:273.
22. Schroder R, Ploner C, Ernestus RI: The growth potential of ependymomas with varying grades of malignancy measured by the Ki-67 labeling index and mitotic index. *Neurosurg Rev.* 1993;16:145.
23. McLaughlin MP, Marcus RB, Jr., Buatti JM, et al: Ependymoma: Results, prognostic factors and treatment recommendations. *Int J Radiat Oncol Biol Phys.* 1998;40:845.
24. AJCC: Bone and soft tissue sarcoma. In Greene FL, Page DL, Fleming I, et al, eds. *AJCC Cancer Staging Manual.* 6th ed. New York: Springer; 2002:185.
25. Lee M, Epstein FJ, Rezai AR, et al: Nonneoplastic intramedullary spinal cord lesions mimicking tumors. *Neurosurgery.* 1998;43:788.
26. Lee TT, Gromelski EB, Green BA: Surgical treatment of spinal ependymoma and post-operative radiotherapy. *Acta Neurochir (Wien).* 1998;140:309.
27. Chang C, McCormick P, Stein B, et al: *Radical Treatment of Primary Intramedullary Spinal Cord Tumors.* Kyoto, Japan: International Congress of Radiation Oncology; 1993:95.
28. Epstein F, Epstein N: Surgical treatment of spinal cord astrocytomas of childhood. A series of 19 patients. *J Neurosurg.* 1982;57:685.
29. Constantini S, Miller D, Allen J, et al: Radical excision of intramedullary spinal cord tumors: Surgical morbidity and long-term follow-up evaluation in 164 children and young adults. *J Neurosurg.* 2000;93:183.
30. Goh K, Velasquez L, Epstein F: Pediatric intramedullary spinal cord tumors: Is surgery alone enough? *Pediatr Neurosurg.* 1997;27:34.
31. Solero CL, Fornari M, Giombini S, et al: Spinal meningiomas: Review of 174 operated cases. *Neurosurgery.* 1989;25:153.
32. Wen BC, Hussey DH, Hitchon PW, et al: The role of radiation therapy in the management of ependymomas of the spinal cord. *Int J Radiat Oncol Biol Phys.* 1991;20:781.
33. Lodin K, Dattoli M, Milcu M: *Radiation Therapy for Adult Spinal Cord Ependymomas: The Case for Limited Volume Treatment.* Scottsdale, Ariz.: Proceedings from the 72nd Annual American Radium Society Meeting, April 21–25, 1990; 1990:5.
34. Linstadt DE, Edwards MS, Prados M, et al: Hyperfractionated irradiation for adults with brainstem gliomas. *Int J Radiat Oncol Biol Phys.* 1991;20:757.
35. Goldsmith B, Wara W, Wilson C, et al: Post-operative external beam irradiation for sub-totally resected meningioma. *Int J Radiat Oncol Biol Phys.* 1992;24:126.
36. Armstrong J, Fass D, Bains M, et al: Paraspinal tumors: Techniques and results of brachytherapy. *Int J Radiat Oncol Biol Phys.* 1991;20:787.
37. Garcia D: Primary spinal cord tumors treated with surgery and postoperative irradiation. *Int J Radiat Oncol Biol Phys.* 1985;11:1933.
38. Wara WM, Phillips TL, Sheline GE, et al: Radiation tolerance of the spinal cord. *Cancer.* 1975;35:1558.
39. Schultheiss TE: Spinal cord radiation "tolerance": Doctrine versus data. *Int J Radiat Oncol Biol Phys.* 1990;19:219.

40. Levin V, Leibel S, Gutin P: Neoplasms of the central nervous system. In Devita V, Hellman S, Rosenberg S, eds. *Cancer Principles and Practice of Oncology.* 6th ed. Philadelphia: Lippincott Williams & Wilkins; 2001:2117.

41. Schultheiss TE, Kun LE, Ang KK, et al: Radiation response of the central nervous system. *Int J Radiat Oncol Biol Phys.* 1995; 31:1093.

42. Rubin P, Cooper R, Phillips T: In Rubin P, Cooper R, Phillips T, eds. *Radiation Biology and Radiation Pathology Syllabus.* Chicago: American College of Radiology; 1975.

43. Phillips TL, Buschke F: Radiation tolerance of the thoracic spinal cord. *Am J Roentgenol Radium Ther Nucl Med.* 1969;105:659.

44. Marcus R, Million R: The incidence of myelitis after irradiation of the cervical spinal cord. *Int J Radiat Oncol Biol Phys.* 1990;19:3.

45. Jeremic B, Djuric L, Mijatovic L: Incidence of radiation myelitis of the cervical spinal cord at doses of 5500 cGy or greater. *Cancer.* 1991;68:2138.

46. Kim YH, Fayos JV: Radiation tolerance of the cervical spinal cord. *Radiology.* 1981;139:473.

47. van der Kogel AJ: Retreatment tolerance of the spinal cord. *Int J Radiat Oncol Biol Phys.* 1993;26:715.

48. Macbeth FR, Wheldon TE, Girling DJ, et al: Radiation myelopathy: Estimates of risk in 1048 patients in three randomized trials of palliative radiotherapy for non–small cell lung cancer. The Medical Research Council Lung Cancer Working Party. *Clin Oncol (R Coll Radiol).* 1996;8:176.

49. Kopelson G: Radiation tolerance of the spinal cord previously damaged by tumor and operation: Long term neurological improvement and time-dose-volume relationships after irradiation of intraspinal gliomas. *Int J Radiat Oncol Biol Phys.* 1982;8:925.

50. Chun H, Schmidt-Ullrich R, Wolfson A, et al: External beam radiotherapy for primary spinal cord tumors. *J Neurooncol.* 1990; 9:211.

51. Jyothirmayi R, Madhavan J, Nair MK, et al: Conservative surgery and radiotherapy in the treatment of spinal cord astrocytoma. *J Neurooncol.* 1997;33:205.

52. Abdel-Wahab M, Corn B, Wolfson A, et al: Prognostic factors and survival in patients with spinal cord gliomas after radiation therapy. *Am J Clin Oncol.* 1999;22:344.

53. Castro J, Collier J, Petti P, et al: Charged particle radiotherapy for lesions encircling the brain stem or spinal cord. *Int J Radiat Oncol Biol Phys.* 1989;17:477.

54. Nowakowski VA, Castro JR, Petti PL, et al: Charged particle radiotherapy of paraspinal tumors. *Int J Radiat Oncol Biol Phys.* 1992; 22:295.

55. Schoenthaler R, Castro JR, Petti PL, et al: Charged particle irradiation of sacral chordomas. *Int J Radiat Oncol Biol Phys.* 1993; 26:291.

56. Austin-Seymour M, Munzenrider J, Goitein M, et al: Progress in low-LET heavy particle therapy: Intracranial and paracranial tumors and uveal melanomas. *Radiat Res Suppl.* 1985;8:S219.

57. Munzenrider J: Proton therapy with the Harvard cyclotron. *Int Cong Ser.* 1994;1077:83.

58. Klekamp J, Samii M: Spinal chordomas—Results of treatment over a 17-year period. *Acta Neurochir (Wien).* 1996;138:514.

59. Hug EB, Fitzek MM, Liebsch NJ, et al: Locally challenging osteo- and chondrogenic tumors of the axial skeleton: Results of combined proton and photon radiation therapy using three-dimensional treatment planning. *Int J Radiat Oncol Biol Phys.* 1995;31:467.

60. Neider C, Milas L, Ang K: Tissue tolerance to reirradiation. *Semin Radiat Oncol.* 2000;10:200.

61. Byrne T: Spinal cord compression from epidural metastases. *N Engl J Med.* 1992;327:614.

62. Rodichok LD, Harper GR, Ruckdeschel JC, et al: Early diagnosis of spinal epidural metastases. *Am J Med.* 1981;70:1181.

63. Cook A, Lau T, Tomlinson M, et al: Magnetic resonance imaging of the whole spine in suspected malignant spinal cord compression: impact on management. *Clin Oncol (R Coll Radiol).* 1998;10:39.

64. Ruckdeschel J, Patterson S, Cuthbertson D, et al: Rapid, cost-effective diagnosis of spinal cord compression due to cancer. *Cancer Control.* 1995;2:320.

65. Poortmans P, Vulto A, Raaijmakers E: Always on a Friday? Time pattern of referral for spinal cord compression. *Acta Oncol.* 2001;40:88.

66. Greenberg H, Kim J, Posner J: Epidural spinal cord compression from metastatic tumor: Results with a new treatment protocol. *Ann Neurol.* 1980;8:361.

67. Vecht CJ, Haaxma-Reiche H, van Putten WL, et al: Initial bolus of conventional versus high-dose dexamethasone in metastatic spinal cord compression. *Neurology.* 1989;39:1255.

68. Maranzano E, Latini P, Beneventi S, et al: Radiotherapy without steroids in selected metastatic spinal cord compression patients. A phase II trial. *Am J Clin Oncol.* 1996;19:179.

69. Sorensen S, Helweg-Larsen S, Mouridsen H, et al: Effect of high-dose dexamethasone in carcinomatous metastatic spinal cord compression treated with radiotherapy: A randomised trial. *Eur J Cancer.* 1994;30A:22.

70. Black P: Spinal metastasis: Current status and recommended guidelines for management. *Neurosurgery.* 1979;5:726.

71. Sundaresan N, Digiacinto GV, Hughes JE, et al: Treatment of neoplastic spinal cord compression: Results of a prospective study. *Neurosurgery.* 1991;29:645.

72. Ghogawala Z, Mansfield F, Borges L: Spinal radiation before surgical decompression adversely affects outcomes of surgery for symptomatic metastatic spinal cord compression. *Spine.* 2001; 26:818.

73. Gilbert R, Kim J, Posner J: Epidural spinal cord compression from metastatic tumor: Diagnosis and treatment. *Ann Neurol.* 1978;3:40.

74. Milcross C, Davies M, Fisher R, et al: The efficacy of treatment for malignant epidural spinal cord compression. *Australas Radiol.* 1997;41:137.

75. Young RF, Post EM, King GA: Treatment of spinal epidural metastases. Randomized prospective comparison of laminectomy and radiotherapy. *J Neurosurg.* 1980;53:741.

76. Payne R, Gaughan E, Chou C, et al: A randomized trial of radiation therapy alone versus best decompressive surgery plus radiaton for single site spinal cord compression: Interim analysis. *Proc Annu Meet Am Soc Clin Oncol.* 1997;16:A275 (Abstract).

77. Maranzano E, Latini P, Beneventi S, et al: Comparison of two different radiotherapy schedules for spinal cord compression in prostate cancer. *Tumori.* 1998;84:472.

78. Kim RY, Spencer SA, Meredith RF, et al: Extradural spinal cord compression: Analysis of factors determining functional prognosis—Prospective study. *Radiology.* 1990;176:279.

79. Turner S, Marosszeky B, Timms I, et al: Malignant spinal cord compression: A prospective evaluation. *Int J Radiat Oncol Biol Phys.* 1993;26:141.

80. Sorensen S, Borgesen SE, Rohde K, et al: Metastatic epidural spinal cord compression. Results of treatment and survival. *Cancer.* 1990;65:1502.

81. Landmann C, Hunig R, Gratzl O: The role of laminectomy in the combined treatment of metastatic spinal cord compression. *Int J Radiat Oncol Biol Phys.* 1992;24:627.

82. Rades D, Blach M, Nerreter V, et al: Metastatic spinal cord compression. Influence of time between onset of motoric deficits and start of irradiation on therapeutic effect. *Strahlenther Onkol.* 1999;175:378.

83. Rades D, Heidenreich F, Karstens J: Final results of a prospective study of the prognostic value of the time to develop motor deficits before irradiation in metastatic spinal cord compression. *Int J Radiat Oncol Biol Phys.* 2002;53:975.

84. Kovner F, Spigel S, Rider I, et al: Radiation therapy of metastatic spinal cord compression. Multidisciplinary team diagnosis and treatment. *J Neurooncol.* 1999;42:85.

85. Maranzano E, Latini P, Checcaglini F, et al: Radiation therapy of spinal cord compression caused by breast cancer: Report of a prospective trial. *Int J Radiat Oncol Biol Phys.* 1992;24:301.

86. Hulshof MC, Menten J, Dito JJ, et al: Treatment results in primary intraspinal gliomas. *Radiother Oncol.* 1993;29:294.

87. Huddart R, Traish D, Ashley S, et al: Management of spinal astrocytoma with conservative surgery and radiotherapy. *Br J Neurosurg.* 1993;7:473.

Cancer of the Nasopharynx

Nancy Lee, MD and Karen K. Fu, MD

27

EPIDEMIOLOGY

Nasopharyngeal carcinoma is uncommon in most parts of the world. The incidence is highest among Southern Chinese, particularly those originating from Kwantung Province, followed by Chinese mixed populations of Southeast Asia, and Eskimos.[1,2] It is of intermediate incidence in North Africa and in the Philippines and it is rare among whites and Japanese. The age-adjusted incidence rate (per 100,000 population per year) ranges from 28.8 in Hong Kong to 17.2 in Eskimos, Indians, and Aleuts in Alaska; 16.8 in Singapore; 4.6 in the Philippines; 2.8 in Algeria; and 0.6 in the United States and Japan.[3,4] The peak incidence occurs in the fourth and fifth decade of life, and the male/female ratio is 2:1 to 3:1.

ETIOLOGY

The etiology of nasopharyngeal carcinoma is most likely multifactorial. Current epidemiological and experimental data suggest at least three major etiological factors: 1) viral, 2) genetic, and 3) environmental.

Epstein-Barr virus (EBV) has long been associated with nasopharyngeal carcinoma. Antibody titers to EBV have been found to be elevated in nasopharyngeal carcinoma patients regardless of their ethnic and geographic origin. The EBV genome has been demonstrated by nucleic acid hybridization in biopsies from nasopharyngeal carcinoma. Recent studies showed that EBV nuclear antigen (EBNA-1) was expressed in nearly all cases and that latent membrane protein (LMP1) was expressed in approximately two thirds of cases of EBV-positive nasopharyngeal carcinomas.[5] Using real-time polymerase chain reaction (PCR) technology, Lo et al.[6] were able to detect circulating EBV DNA in 96% of nasopharyngeal carcinoma patients in Hong Kong. The plasma EBV DNA levels correlated with the disease stage. Recently, LMP1 has also been shown to increase the production of vascular endothelial growth factor (VEGF).[7] LMP1-induced VEGF production is mediated in part by cyclooxygenase-2 (COX-2), which is overexpressed in tumors.

The high incidence of nasopharyngeal carcinoma among Southern Chinese and Southeast Asian populations of Southern Chinese descent suggests a genetically determined susceptibility. Highly significant differences in histocompatibility human leukocyte antigen (HLA) patterns have been found between Chinese nasopharyngeal carcinoma patients and control subjects. There is a significant increase of HLA-A2 and HLA-B-SIN2 in Chinese patients.[8] However, the high-risk HLA pattern is not present in all nasopharyngeal carcinoma patients and such a pattern is present in some individuals with no nasopharyngeal carcinoma.

The decreased incidence of nasopharyngeal carcinoma in successive generations of Chinese born in America[9] suggests a role for environmental factors in the etiology of this disease. Various environmental factors such as poor ventilation, occupational exposures to smoke or dusts and diet or both have been implicated. The ingestion of salted fish during early childhood has been suggested as the most important environmental factor among the Southern Chinese with nasopharyngeal carcinoma.[2,10,11] Dimethylnitrosamine, a carcinogen found in salted fish, has been shown to induce carcinoma in the upper respiratory tract of rats.[10]

ANATOMY

The nasopharynx is a roughly cuboidal open chamber located below the base of skull and behind the nasal cavity. It measures 4.0 to 5.5 cm in its widest transverse diameter, 2.5 to 3.5 cm in its anterior-posterior diameter, and approximately 4.0 cm in height.

Anteriorly, the nasopharynx is in continuity with the nasal cavity through the posterior choanae, which are separated by the nasal septum. The posterior wall lies at the level of the first two cervical vertebrae and is continuous with the roof. The roof is formed by the basisphenoid, basiocciput, and the anterior arch of the atlas. The lymphoid tissue in this area forms the pharyngeal tonsil (adenoids) (Fig. 27-1). Each of the lateral walls contains the eustachian tube orifice, which is surrounded by the torus tubarius (Fig. 27-1), a prominence in the cartilaginous portion of the tube. Behind the torus tubarius is a recess called Rosenmüller's fossa (Figs. 27-1 and 27-2). The lateral walls, including Rosenmüller's fossa, are the most common sites of origin of nasopharyngeal carcinoma. The floor of the nasopharynx consists of the upper surface of the soft palate and communicates with the oropharynx via the pharyngeal isthmus. The isthmus is bounded by the uvula anteriorly, the palatopharyngeal arches laterally, and the posterior pharyngeal wall posteriorly.

The posterior wall of the nasopharynx is made up of four anatomic layers: the mucous membrane of the

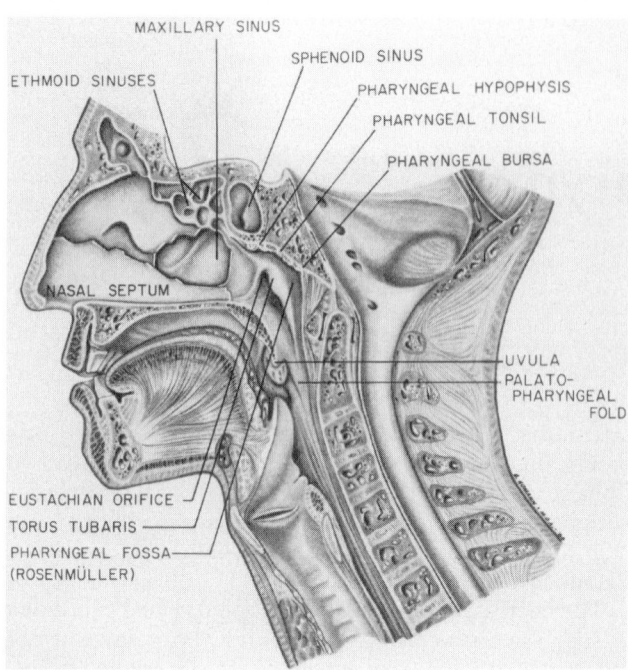

Figure 27–1. Mid-sagittal section of the head showing the nasopharynx and related structures. (From MacComb WS, Fletcher GH: *Cancer of the Head and Neck*. Baltimore: Williams & Wilkins; 1967:154.)

pharynx; the pharyngeal aponeurosis; the superior constrictor muscle of the pharynx; and the buccopharyngeal fascia, which is loosely connected with the adjacent prevertebral fascia. The muscular wall of the nasopharynx is incomplete. In the upper nasopharynx, the lateral walls consist of only two layers: the mucous membrane and the pharyngeal aponeurosis. This area of muscular deficiency is called the sinus of Morgagni, through which the cartilaginous part of the eustachian tube enters the pharyngeal wall along with the levator veli palatini muscle.

The pharyngeal fascia of the posterior and lateral walls of the nasopharynx is attached to the pharyngeal tubercle on the basiocciput just in front of the foramen magnum. It extends laterally on each side to the ridge on the undersurface of the petrous pyramid, just in front of the carotid canal and anteriorly to the apex of the petrous portion of the temporal bone, and then to the posterior border of the medial pterygoid plate. This fascia is continuous with the fibrous tissue occupying the foramen lacerum, which is separated from the middle cranial fossa only by fibrocartilaginous tissue. Five other foramina are adjacent to the wall of the nasopharynx: the foramen ovale, the foramen spongiosum, the carotid canal, the jugular foramen, and the hypoglossal canal (Fig. 27-3). The foramen lacerum and the foramen ovale constitute the *petrosphenoidal crossway*, providing an easy pathway into the cranium, and are in close anatomic relationship to the cavernous sinus and hence the II, III, IV, and VI cranial nerves, the trigeminal ganglion of the fifth nerve and its branches.

Anterior to the eustachian tube, the lateral wall of the nasopharynx is in close relation with the maxillopharyngeal space, which is limited laterally by the ascending

ramus of the mandible. In this space is the mandibular nerve descending from the foramen ovale. Posterior to the eustachian tube, Rosenmüller's fossa is in close relationship with the lateral pharyngeal or retroparotidian space. The lateral pharyngeal or retroparotidian space is limited anteriorly by the parotid gland and the styloid process and its muscles; posteriorly by the transverse process of the first cervical vertebra; and laterally by the sternocleidomastoid muscle. It contains the lateral pharyngeal nodes, including the lateral retropharyngeal node of Rouvière; the internal carotid artery; the internal jugular vein; and the glossopharyngeal, vagus, spinal accessory, and hypoglossal nerves, as well as the cervical sympathetic nerves as they emerge from the base of skull (Fig. 27-4).

Blood supply to the nasopharynx is provided by one direct and two indirect branches of the external carotid artery. They are: (1) the ascending pharyngeal artery and two branches of the maxillary artery; (2) the artery of the pterygoid canal (vidian artery); and (3) the sphenopalatine artery. Venous drainage is via the pharyngeal plexus, which communicates with the pterygoid plexus above and drains into the internal jugular vein below. The pharyngeal plexus also communicates with the veins of the orbit through the inferior ophthalmic vein. Nerve supply to the nasopharynx is primarily derived from branches of the glossopharyngeal (IX), the vagus (X), and the sympathetic nerves, although the maxillary (V_2) branch of the trigeminal (V) nerve supplies the sensory innervation of the anterior portion of the roof and floor of the nasopharynx and the motor innervation of the tensor veli palatini.

LYMPHATIC DRAINAGE

The nasopharynx has a rich lymphatic plexus, particularly in the roof and in the posterior and lateral walls. The lymphatics from the nasopharynx have three major pathways (Fig. 27-5):

1. One path is through the lateral pharyngeal wall to the lateral pharyngeal (parapharyngeal) nodes in the lateral pharyngeal or retroparotid space. The uppermost of this group of nodes is the lateral retropharyngeal node of Rouvière (see Fig. 27-5).
2. From these lateral pharyngeal nodes, efferent channels pass to the jugular chain, especially to the jugulodigastric (subdigastric) nodes. Some lymphatic channels may bypass the lateral pharyngeal wall and drain directly to the jugulodigastric node.
3. Another path is by direct channel to the deep nodes of the posterior triangle, the spinal accessory nodes. The uppermost node of this chain lies beneath the sternocleidomastoid muscle at the tip of the mastoid process.

From these primary groups of nodes, further extensions proceed down the jugular chain to the mid and lower jugular nodes and down the spinal chain to the mid and lower posterior cervical nodes in the posterior triangle. Lymphatic channels crossing the midline account for contralateral or bilateral involvement. Rarely, carcinoma

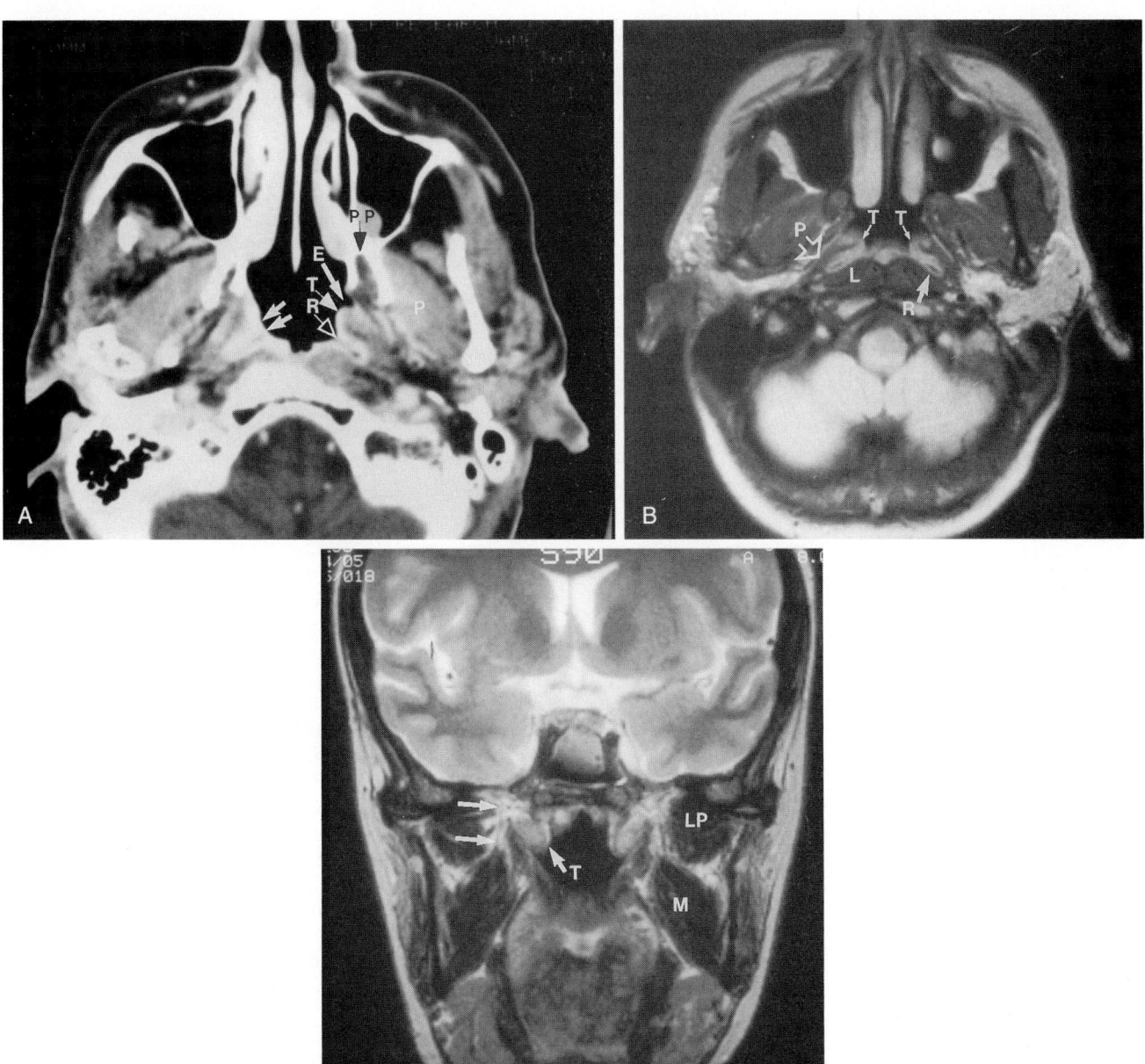

Figure 27–2. Normal computed tomography (CT) and magnetic resonance imaging (MRI) images of the nasopharynx. **A,** Axial postcontrast CT scan obtained through the midnasopharynx. Just posterior to the medial pterygoid plate (*PP*) is a small recess representing the orifice of the eustachian tube (*E*). Posterior to this and separating the fossa of Rosenmüller (*R*) from the eustachian orifice is a protuberance that extends in the nasopharyngeal airway, the torus tubarius (*T*). Lateral to the pterygoid plates is the lateral pterygoid muscle (*P*). Note the normal asymmetry of the fossa of Rosenmüller (*double white arrows*), which can occasionally simulate early carcinoma. Also of importance is the symmetrical parapharyngeal space, which contains branches of the internal maxillary artery and small veins of the pterygoid plexus. The parapharyngeal space separates the deep lobe of the parotid gland from the soft tissues of the nasopharynx and serves as a landmark for deep invasion from carcinoma of the nasopharynx. **B,** Axial "proton density"–weighted MRI scan through the nasopharynx showing soft tissue contrast achieved with MRI scanning in this region. Note the higher-signal-intensity mucosal adenoidal tissue, which is easily separated from the underlying musculature of the deep pharyngeal soft tissues. Also note the musculature of the masticator space, including the masseter muscle, deep head of the temporalis muscle, lateral and medial pterygoid muscles, as well as the tensor veli and levator veli palatini muscles. Note the symmetric convex appearance of the longest capitis muscles (*L*) positioned directly behind the mucosa of the nasopharynx and Rosenmüller's fossa (*R*). Posterior and lateral to the torus tubarius (*T*) is the parapharyngeal space (*P*), containing fat and separating the deep structures from the deep lobe of the parotid gland. **C,** Coronal T2-weighted MRI scan showing the intimate relationship of the superior recess of the nasopharynx to the skull base, the torus tubarius (*T*), the levator veli palatini muscle (*double arrows*), the medial pterygoid muscle (*M*), the lateral pterygoid (*LP*) muscle, the mandible, and the masseter muscle. Positioned in the midline are the tongue and soft palate.

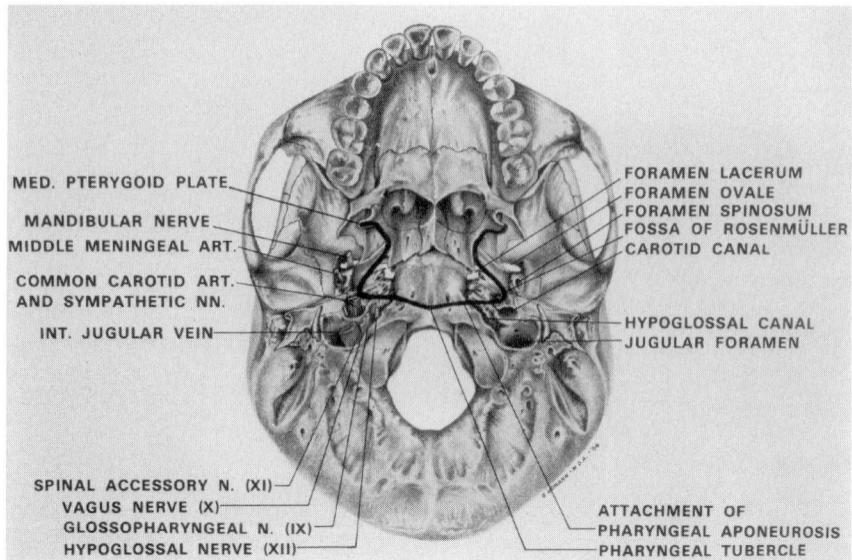

Figure 27–3. Basal view of the skull showing the bony attachments of the nasopharyngeal wall. The bony foramina of the base of the skull are shown on the right and the structures occupying these foramina appear on the left. (From MacComb WS, Fletcher GH: *Cancer of the Head and Neck.* Baltimore: Williams & Wilkins; 1967:155.)

of the nasopharynx may spread to the submaxillary and submental nodes. Spread to the parotid nodes can occur via the lymphatics of the eustachian tube.

PATHOLOGY

The majority of malignant nasopharyngeal tumors (80% to 99%) arise from the epithelium and should be considered as variants of squamous cell carcinoma. According to the World Health Organization (WHO),

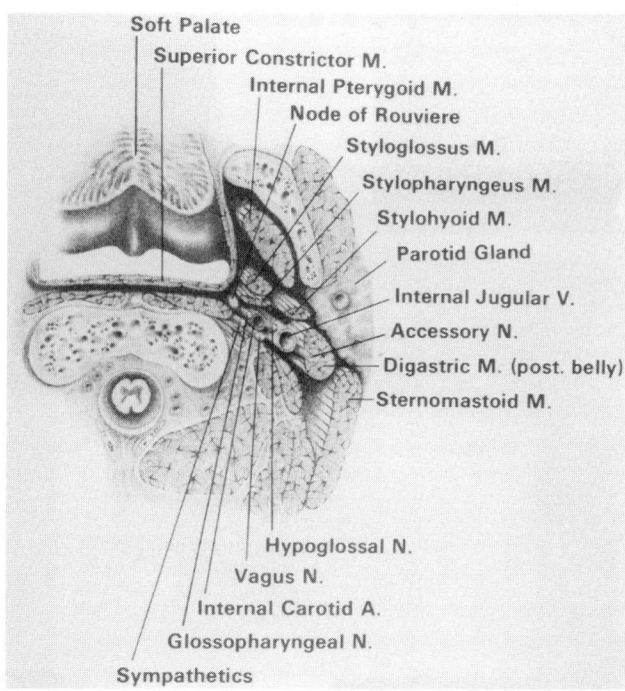

Figure 27–4. Poststyloid portion of the lateral pharyngeal space and its contents. (From MacComb WS, Fletcher GH: *Cancer of the Head and Neck.* Baltimore: Williams & Wilkins; 1967:157.)

carcinomas of the nasopharynx are classified into three histological types: (1) squamous cell carcinoma, (2) nonkeratinizing carcinoma, and (3) undifferentiated carcinoma.[12] The histological distinctions among these three types are by no means sharp. Some lesions share intermediate features and some are histological hybrids. The term *lymphoepithelial carcinoma* or *lymphoepithelioma* is used to describe nonkeratinizing and undifferentiated nasopharyngeal carcinomas in which numerous lymphocytes are found among the tumor cells.

The distribution of WHO histopathologic types varies with geography. In North America, about 20% of nasopharyngeal carcinomas are type 1, 10% type 2, and 70% type 3.[13] In Hong Kong, about 3% are type 1, 9% type 2, and 88% type 3.[14] In addition, nasopharyngeal histology also correlates with race and national origin.[15] WHO type 1 comprised 75% of the U.S. nasopharyngeal carcinoma cases and were found most often in U.S.-born, nonHispanic whites. WHO types 2 and 3 comprised the remaining 25% and were more common in Asians. Asians had the highest proportion of WHO types 2 and 3.

Malignant lymphoma in the nasopharynx is less common. Other malignant tumors such as adenocarcinoma, plasmacytoma, melanoma, and sarcomas are relatively uncommon.

CLINICAL PRESENTATION

A neck mass is the most frequent presenting symptom and sign in carcinoma of the nasopharynx.[16] The next most common symptoms are epistaxis, decreased hearing, nasal obstruction, pain, and cranial nerve deficits.

Cervical lymphadenopathy is present in 87% of patients.[17] Typically, a mass is visible in the upper posterior neck and palpable beneath the superior aspect of the sternocleidomastoid muscle at the tip of the mastoid. This is due to metastasis in the parapharyngeal or superior posterior cervical nodes of the spinal accessory chain or both. Bilateral cervical lymph node metastases occur

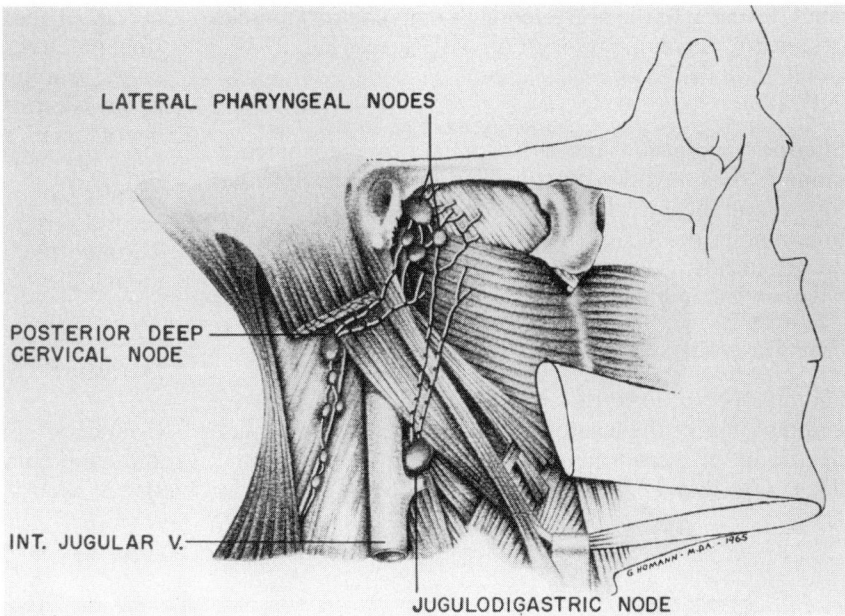

Figure 27–5. Major lymphatic drainage of the nasopharynx. (From MacComb WS, Fletcher GH: *Cancer of the Head and Neck.* Baltimore: Williams & Wilkins; 1967:158.)

LATERAL PHARYNGEAL NODES

POSTERIOR DEEP CERVICAL NODE

INT. JUGULAR V.

JUGULODIGASTRIC NODE

in about 50% of cases. The most frequently involved nodes are the upper posterior cervical, parapharyngeal, and jugulodigastric nodes. The midjugular and midposterior cervical nodes are the next most commonly involved, followed by the lower jugular and supraclavicular nodes. The submental nodes and occipital nodes may become involved in the presence of massive cervical lymphadenopathy. Rarely, patients may present with metastatic preauricular nodes.

Nasal twang in speech occurs as a consequence of nasal obstruction, loss of nasopharyngeal resonance, and mechanical interference with normal movement of the soft palate. Nasal discharge, epistaxis, and coughing up of blood-tinged sputum from postnasal drip are symptoms due to local tumor effect.

Impaired hearing of the conductive type, usually unilateral with or without tinnitus and serous otitis media, occurs as a result of obstruction of the eustachian tube orifice by the primary tumor.

Cranial nerve deficits can result from direct extension intracranially with compression of the II to VI cranial nerves (the petrosphenoidal syndrome of Jacod) or from lateral retropharyngeal lymph node metastases in the retroparotid space with involvement of the IX to XII cranial nerves and the cervical sympathetic nerve (the syndrome of the retroparotid space of Villaret). The petrosphenoidal syndrome is characterized by unilateral neuralgia of the trigeminal (V) type, unilateral ptosis (III), complete ophthalmoplegia (III, IV, and V) and amaurosis (II). The syndrome of retroparotid space is characterized by difficulty in swallowing (IX and X); perversion of taste in the posterior third of the tongue (IX); hyperesthesias, hypoesthesias, or anesthesias of the mucous membrane of the soft palate, pharynx, and larynx; respiratory and salivary problems (X); hemiparesis of the soft palate; paralysis and atrophy of the trapezius and sternocleidomastoid muscles (XI); and unilateral paralysis and atrophy of the tongue (XII). This may be accompanied or preceded by Horner's syndrome due to compression of the cervical sympathetic nerve. The cranial nerves V and

VI are most frequently involved while cranial nerves I, VII, and VIII are rarely involved.

Pain results from the compression of the trigeminal nerve or its branches and from invasion of the bones of the skull. Facial pain and occipital and temporal headaches are most common. Pain in lifting the head and extending the neck can occur as a consequence of posterior invasion of the prevertebral muscles.

Sore throat occurs secondary to tumor extension into the oropharyngeal wall. Trismus results from invasion of the pterygoid muscles or involvement of the motor branches of the fifth nerve. Proptosis occurs with posterior orbital invasion.

Distant metastasis at presentation is detected in about 3% of cases.[18] The bones, lungs, and liver are the most common distant metastatic sites.

ROUTES OF SPREAD

Local Extension

ANTERIOR

Anteriorly, direct extension into the nasal cavity is common. Invasion into the lateral wall of the nasal cavity may lead to destruction of the pterygoid plates. Invasion of the posterior ethmoid and maxillary sinuses is less common. Orbital invasion can occur in advanced disease.

SUPERIOR AND POSTERIOR

Superiorly and posteriorly, the tumor can directly invade the base of the skull, the sphenoid sinus, and the clivus. The foramen lacerum, located directly above Rosenmüller's fossa, is a weak spot in the base of the skull, through which the tumor can gain access into the cavernous sinus and the middle cranial fossa and invade cranial nerves II to VI. Tumor may also invade through the foramen ovale into the middle cranial fossa, the petrous part of the temporal bone, and the cavernous sinus. Invasion of the prevertebral (longus capitus) muscles posteriorly is commonly seen on MRI scans (Fig. 27-6).

INFERIOR

Inferiorly, extension into the oropharynx is not uncommon. It may involve the tonsillar pillars, the tonsillar fossae, and the lateral and posterior oropharyngeal walls. Invasion of the C1 vertebra posteriorly and inferiorly occurs in advanced disease. Direct invasion of the soft palate is uncommon.

LATERAL

Lateral spread into the lateral parapharyngeal space and invasion of the levator and tensor veli palatini muscles occur early and are commonly seen on MRI scans (Figs. 27-6 and 27-7). Invasion of the pterygoid muscles

occurs in more advanced disease. Direct tumor extension or lateral retropharyngeal lymph node metastasis in the parapharyngeal space can lead to compression or invasion of cranial nerve XII as it exits through the hypoglossal canal, cranial nerves IX to XI as they emerge from the jugular foramen and the cervical sympathetic nerves. Compression or direct invasion of the internal carotid artery can also occur in advanced disease. Through the eustachian tube, tumor can directly invade the middle ear.

Lymphatic Spread

Lymphatic spread to the ipsilateral nodes is common and is present in 85% to 90% of cases.[17] Bilateral spread occurs in about 50% of cases. Metastasis to the

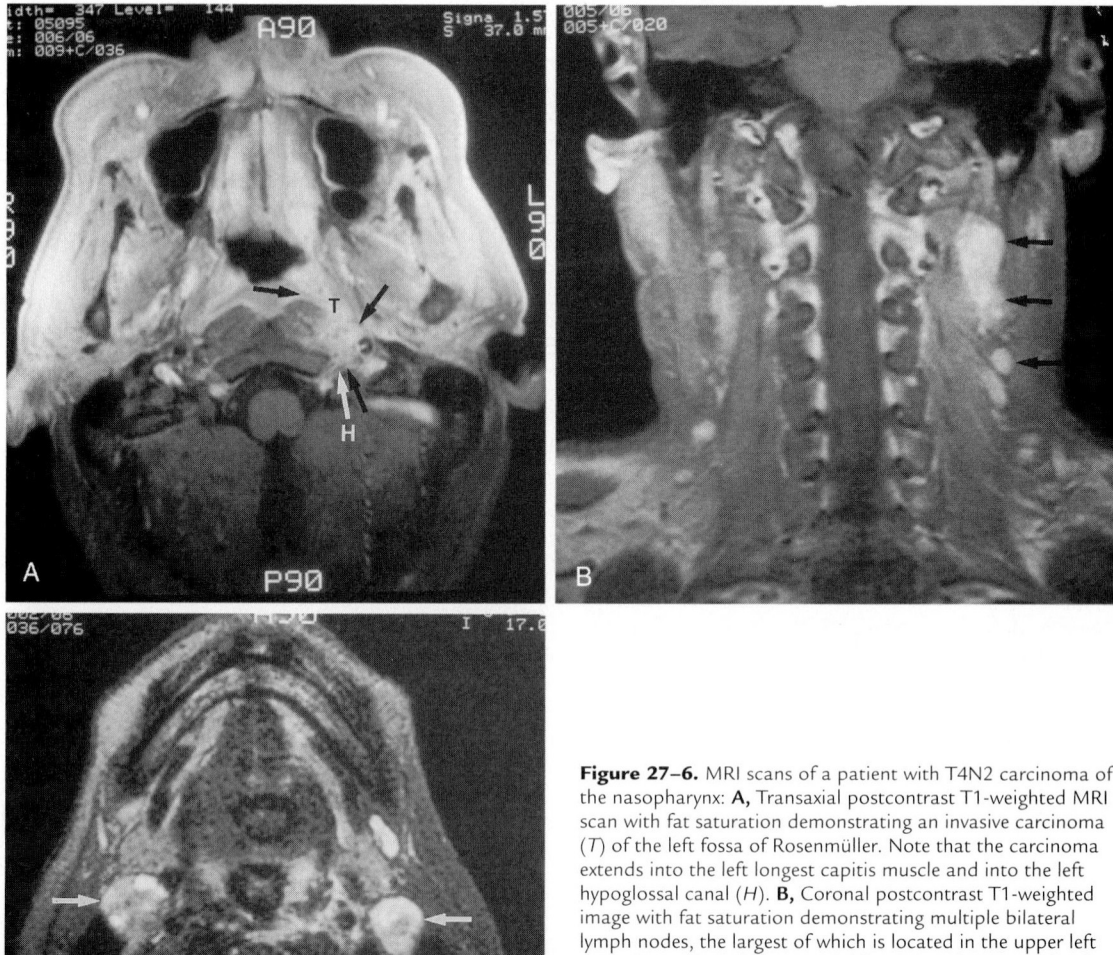

Figure 27–6. MRI scans of a patient with T4N2 carcinoma of the nasopharynx: **A,** Transaxial postcontrast T1-weighted MRI scan with fat saturation demonstrating an invasive carcinoma (*T*) of the left fossa of Rosenmüller. Note that the carcinoma extends into the left longest capitis muscle and into the left hypoglossal canal (*H*). **B,** Coronal postcontrast T1-weighted image with fat saturation demonstrating multiple bilateral lymph nodes, the largest of which is located in the upper left posterior cervical chain. **C,** Axial fast-spin-echo T2-weighted MRI scan through the neck demonstrating bilateral enlarged, inhomogeneous lymphadenopathy. Note the foci of high signal intensity within the lymph nodes, indicating malignant invasion (*arrows*).

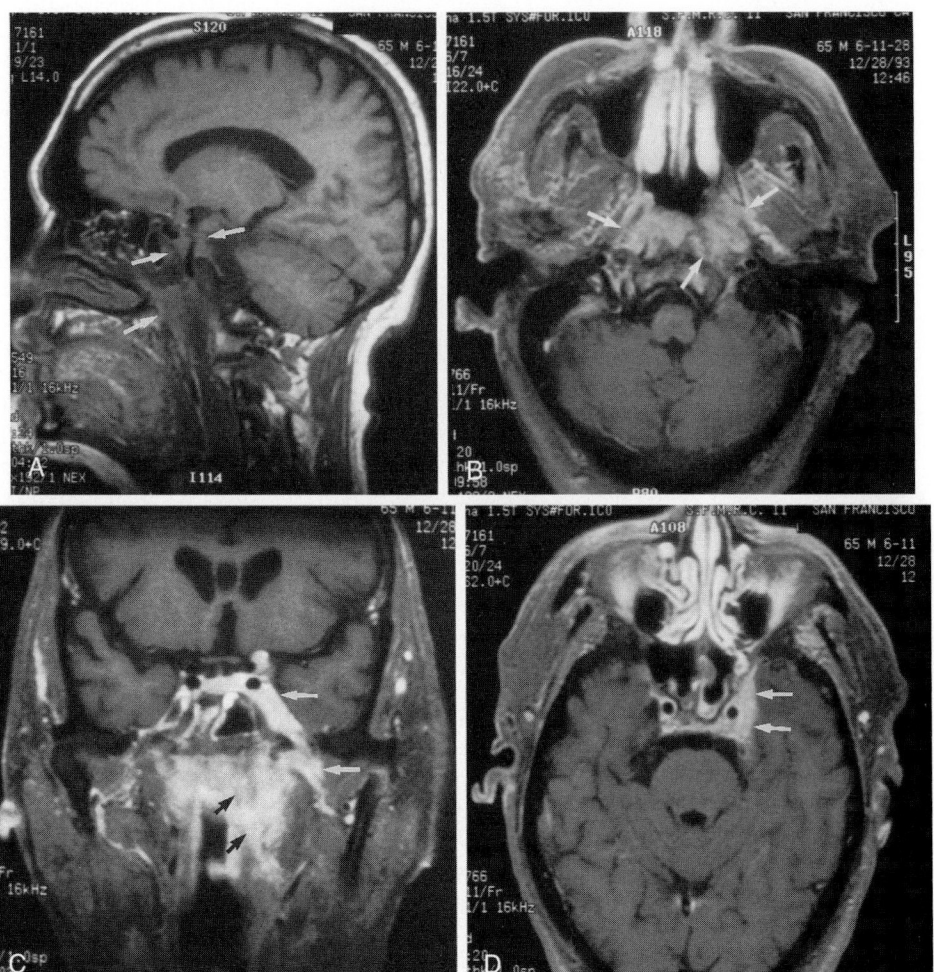

Figure 27–7. MRI scans of a patient with T4, N0 carcinoma of the nasopharynx. **A,** Sagittal T1-weighted MRI scan demonstrates abnormal soft tissue (*arrows*) in the region of the left cavernous sinus extending from the upper nasopharynx. **B,** Axial post-contrast T1-weighted image following fat saturation demonstrating an invasive carcinoma that extends across midline to involve both Rosenmüller's fossae (*arrows*). **C,** Coronal T1-weighted postcontrast MRI scan demonstrating the invasive carcinoma of the nasopharynx (*black arrows*) with extension through the foramen ovale along the course of the third division of the fifth cranial nerve into the cavernous sinus (*white arrows*). **D,** Axial postcontrast T1-weighted image through the cavernous sinus demonstrating an enhancing tumor that has expanded the left cavernous sinus (*arrows*) as it courses along the third division of the fifth cranial nerve.

contralateral nodes only is uncommon. The distribution of clinically palpable nodes at diagnosis is shown in Fig. 27-8. Spread to the lateral and posterior retropharyngeal lymph nodes occurs early and is frequently seen on MRI or CT scans, although the nodes are not palpable (Fig. 27-9). Metastasis to the jugulodigastric and superior posterior cervical nodes is also common. From these first echelon nodes, further metastasis to the midjugular and posterior cervical, lower jugular, and posterior cervical

and supraclavicular nodes can occur. Occasionally, spread to the submental and occipital nodes occurs as a result of lymphatic obstruction due to extensive cervical lymphadenopathy. Metastasis to the mediastinal lymph nodes may occur when supraclavicular lymphadenopathy is present. Distant lymph node metastasis is often reported in autopsy series.

Hematogeneous Spread

Distant metastasis is present in 3% of the cases at diagnosis and may occur in 18% to 50% or more of cases during the course of the disease.[18-23] An 80% incidence rate has been reported in a small autopsy series.[24] The incidence of distant metastasis is highest in patients with advanced neck node metastasis,[19,25-27] particularly in the low neck.[28,29] Bone is the most common distant metastatic site followed by the lungs and liver.

DIAGNOSTIC AND STAGING STUDIES

Diagnosis of nasopharyngeal carcinoma is established by biopsy of a primary tumor in the nasopharynx, which usually can be done under local anesthesia in the

Nasopharynx

N0	N1	N2A	N2B	N3A	N3B	N1-N3 / Total
22	18	16	23	8	82	147 / 169 = 87%

Figure 27–8. Distribution of clinically palpable cervical lymph nodes at diagnosis. (From Fletcher GH: *Textbook of Radiotherapy*, 3rd ed. Philadelphia: Lea & Febiger; 1980:260.)

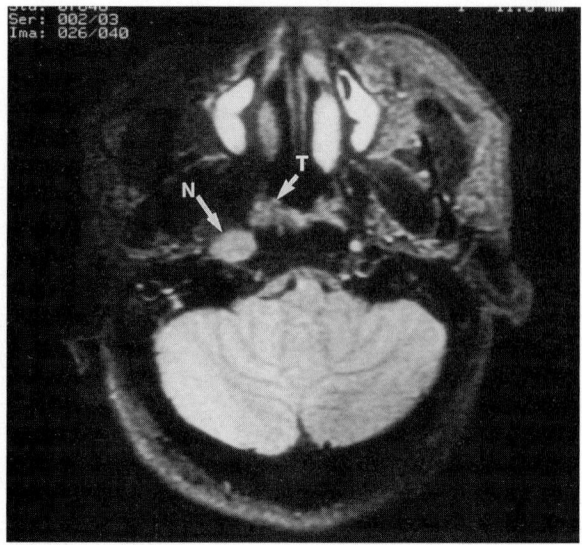

Figure 27–9. Axial T2-weighted MRI scan through the midnasopharynx showing the presence of a metastatic right lateral retropharyngeal lymph node (*N*). Note its location lateral and posterior to the tumor (*T*) in the right fossa of Rosenmüller.

outpatient clinic. Biopsy with direct visualization under general anesthesia may be necessary to obtain a positive tissue diagnosis when the tumor is not visible or when the patient cannot cooperate. Not infrequently the tumor is submucosal and not visible. In cases suspicious for a nasopharyngeal primary tumor, but without a visible tumor, random biopsies should be taken from the most commonly involved sites: Rosenmüller's fossa on each of the lateral walls and the superior posterior wall of the nasopharynx. Fine needle aspiration of a neck mass may establish the presence of metastatic nasopharyngeal carcinoma in cervical lymph nodes. This may precede biopsy of the nasopharynx when the primary tumor is not clinically detectable.

The following pretreatment diagnostic evaluations are recommended:

1. Complete history and physical examination;
2. MRI or CT scans of the nasopharynx, paranasal sinuses, base of the skull, nasal cavity, and the neck;
3. Posterior-anterior and lateral chest x-ray;
4. Complete blood count, urinalysis, and liver function tests;
5. EBV-specific serologic tests: IgA anti-viral capsule antigen (VCA) titers;
6. Bone scan in patients with advanced locoregional disease, symptoms suggestive of bone metastasis, or an elevated serum alkaline phosphatase;
7. CT scan of the abdomen in patients with abnormal liver function tests or clinical suspicion of liver metastasis;
8. CT scan of the chest when the chest x-ray is abnormal or there is clinical suspicion of lung metastasis;
9. Pretreatment dental evaluation and initiation of dental prophylaxis.

The nasopharynx is best visualized with a fiberoptic endoscope. However, when the nasal cavity is completely obstructed due to tumor extension, the tumor may be visualized through indirect mirror examination or with a flexible fiberoptic endoscope. Complete physical examination should include careful palpation of the neck, cranial nerve examination, percussion and auscultation of the chest, palpation of the abdomen for possible liver involvement, and percussion of the spine and bones for possible bone metastasis.

Both MRI and CT scans are useful in diagnostic imaging of the nasopharynx, as well as in radiotherapy treatment planning. However, MRI is the imaging technique of choice in the staging evaluation of nasopharyngeal carcinoma.[30-32] Since the current T classification system requires a search for tumor invasion into the soft tissue, such as parapharyngeal space, and bony structures, MRI may be necessary for proper staging since CT has limitations in accurately defining the tumor extent in these regions.[33] MRI is capable of multiplanar display of tumor extent and is superior to CT scans in delineating muscle, other soft tissue involvement, and evaluating the skull base (Figs. 27-6, 27-7, and 27-10).[33-35] In post-treatment follow-up examinations, it has the ability to differentiate radiation fibrosis from persistent or recurrent tumor based on T2-weighted signal intensities and with gadolinium enhancement and fat suppression.[36] MRI and CT scans can also detect lymph node metastasis that may not be evident on clinical examination[37] (see Fig. 27-9). CT scan is superior to MRI in the detection of early bone invasion.[32,34] CT scan with bone windows is useful to demonstrate the extent of invasion of the base of the skull or cervical vertebrae, although MRI is preferable. The major limitation of CT is its poor tissue differentiation, which may be problematic in the evaluation of patients after radiotherapy.[35]

The close association between EBV and nasopharyngeal carcinoma, regardless of geographical and ethnic background, has provided a tumor marker for the diagnosis of this disease. Both immunoglobulin A (IgA) anti-VCA and IgG anti-early antigen (EA) antibodies are sensitive for the diagnosis of nasopharyngeal carcinoma, although IgA anti-VCA is more specific.[13] Elevated IgA antibody titers have been reported in more than 90% of untreated patients with nasopharyngeal carcinoma from Hong Kong, East Africa, and California.[38-40] Positive IgA anti-VCA and IgG anti-EA serologies are primarily associated with WHO type 2 and type 3 nasopharyngeal carcinoma. Elevated IgA anti-VCA antibody titers were detected in 82%, and IgG anti-EA antibody titers were detected in 86% of patients with nonkeratinizing carcinoma and undifferentiated carcinomas, but in only 16% and 35%, respectively, of patients with squamous cell carcinomas in a North American study.[13] Elevated serum IgA anti-VCA antibodies may be demonstrated in patients months before the onset of symptoms and may serve as a screening test in high-risk patients.[41,42]

STAGING CLASSIFICATION

Various staging systems have been formulated for nasopharyngeal carcinoma.[10,43-49] The most widely used systems in the English literature are the American Joint Committee on Cancer (AJCC), Union International Centre Cancer (UICC), and Ho systems. The latest versions of the AJCC

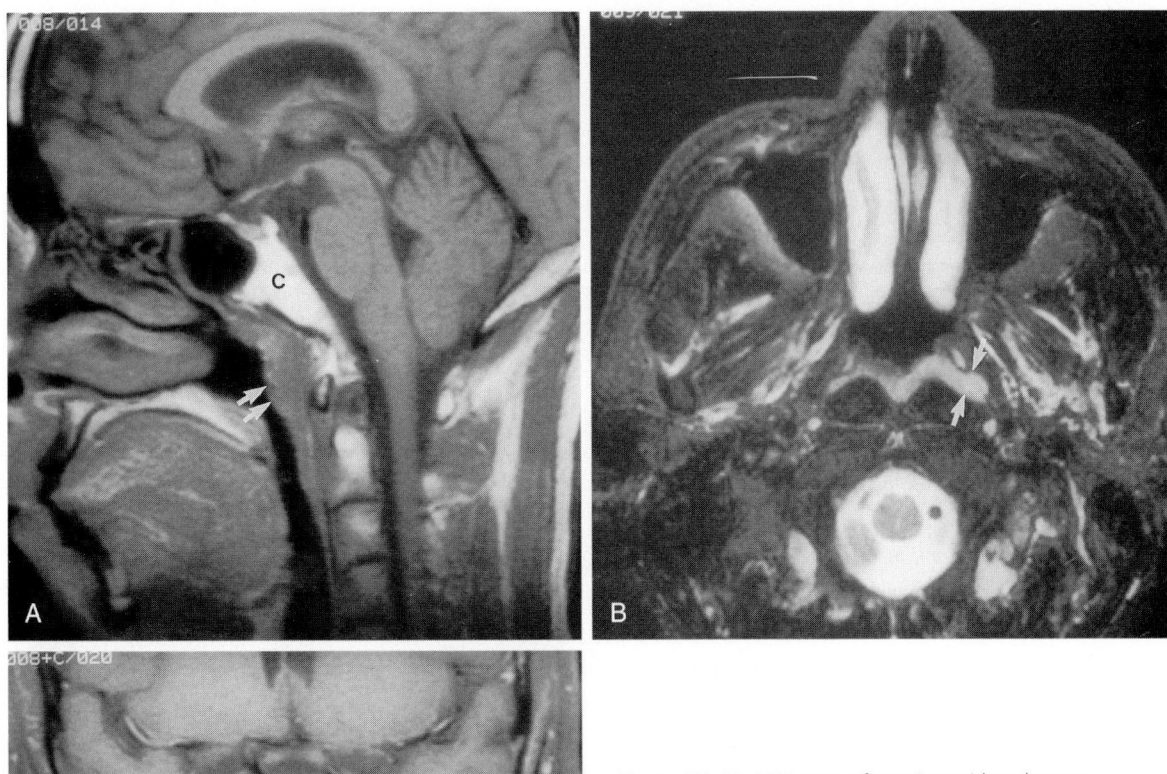

Figure 27–10. MRI scans of a patient with early stage carcinoma of the nasopharynx. **A,** Sagittal T1-weighted MRI scan. A soft tissue mass can be visualized in the upper nasopharynx (*arrows*). Note the soft tissue mass does not invade the normal high-signal-intensity marrow of the clivus (C). **B,** Axial T2-weighted MRI scan. Expansion of the left fossa of Rosenmüller by a high-signal-intensity mass can be identified (*arrows*). While normal asymmetry of the adenoidal tissue may be seen, it will not result in mass effect as is seen here. This is the earliest appearance of nasopharyngeal carcinoma confined to the mucosa of the nasopharynx. **C,** Coronal T1-weighted MRI scan following contrast administration. The mass within the left upper recess of the nasopharynx (*arrow*) is visualized. However, it has little in the way of signal intensity difference from surrounding normal mucosa. There is no invasion of the skull base or the cavernous sinus.

and UICC (2002) systems are virtually identical. Table 27-1 shows the AJCC and Ho systems currently in use. Each system has its limitations. In the AJCC and UICC systems, the designation of T1 or T2, which is based on the extent of involvement within the nasopharynx, is not meaningful and carries no prognostic significance.[47,50] In the latest version of the AJCC (2002) staging system with regard to T2 lesions, it is divided into *with* or *without* parapharyngeal involvement, which has prognostic significance.[50a] Those with parapharyngeal space involvement are at higher risk for local and regional recurrence, as well as a high rate of distant metastases.[51] Cranial nerve involvement has been shown to carry a worse prognosis than base of the skull involvement[27,28,46,52]; however, both are included in the T4 classification in the AJCC and the UICC systems and the T3 in Ho's system. With respect to N-stage classification, the Ho system, which is based on the level or location of neck node involvement, appears to be superior to the AJCC and

the UICC system, which are based on size, number, and laterality of the lymph nodes involved.[28,47,53] Because of these limitations, modifications of both Ho's and AJCC classification have been proposed and are shown in Table 27-1.[43,53] The adequacy of these new modified staging classifications will require further clinical confirmation. Retrospective comparison of the 1997 or the 2002 AJCC with the 1988 AJCC classification in patients staged with CT or MRI scans suggest a more even stage distribution and better correlation with prognosis with the 1997 or the 2002 AJCC classification.[54]

STANDARD THERAPEUTIC APPROACHES

Because of the anatomic location and the propensity for early bilateral lymph node metastases and involvement of the lateral retropharyngeal node of Rouvière,

Table 27–1 **Classification of Nasopharyngeal Carcinoma**

Stage-Classification	Ho (1978)		AJCC 2002			
T stage	T1	Tumor confined to the nasopharynx (space behind the choanal orifices and nasal septum and above the posterior margin of the soft palate in the resting position).	T1	Tumor confined to the nasopharynx		
	T2	Tumor extended to the nasal fossa, oropharynx, or adjacent muscles or nerves below the base of the skull	T2	Tumor extends to soft tissue of oropharynx or nasal fossa or both 2a Without parapharyngeal extension 2b With parapharyngeal extension		
	T3	Tumor extended beyond T2 limits: T3a Bone involvement below the base of the skull. (Floor of the sphenoid sinus is included in this category.) T3b Involvement of the base of the skull. T3c Involvement of the cranial nerve(s). T3d Involvement of the orbits, laryngopharynx (hypopharynx), or infratemporal fossa.	T3 T4	Tumor invades bony structures or paranasal sinuses or both Tumor with intracranial extension and/or involvement of cranial nerves, infratemporal fossa, hypopharynx, or orbit		
N stage	N0	None palpable.	NX	Regional lymph nodes cannot be assessed		
	N1	Node(s) wholly in the upper cervical level bounded below by the skin crease extending laterally and backward from or just below the thyroid notch (laryngeal eminence).	N0 N1	No regional lymph node metastases Unilateral metastasis in lymph node(s), ≤6 cm in greatest dimension, above the supraclavicular fossa		
	N2	Node(s) palpable between the crease and the supraclavicular fossa, the upper limit being a line joining the upper margin of the sternal end of the clavicle and the apex of an angle formed by the lateral surface of the neck and the superior margin of the trapezius.	N2 N3	Bilateral metastasis in lymph node(s), ≤6 cm in greatest dimension, above the supraclavicular fossa Metastasis in lymph nodes 3a >6 cm in dimension 3b Extension to the supraclavicular fossa		
	N3	Node(s) palpable in the supraclavicular fossa and/or skin involvement in the form of carcinoma en cuirasse or satellite nodules above the clavicles.				
M stage	M0	No hematogeneous metastases.	MX	Distant metastases cannot be assessed		
	M1	Hematogeneous metastases present, and/or lymph nodal metastases below the clavicle.	M0 M1	No distant metastases Distant metastases		
Stage	I	T1, N0	0	T1s,	N0,	M0
	II	T2 and/or N1	I	T1,	N0,	M0
	III	T3 and/or N2	IIA	T2a,	N0,	M0
	IV	N3 (any T)	IIB	T1,	N1,	M0
	V	M1		T2,	N1,	M0
				T2a,	N1,	M0
				T2b,	N0,	M0
				T2b,	N1,	M0
			III	T1,	N2,	M0
				T2a,	N2,	M0
				T2b,	N2,	M0
				T3,	N0,	M0
				T3,	N1,	M0
				T3,	N2,	M0
			IVA	T4,	N0,	M0
				T4,	N1,	M0
				T4,	N2,	M0
			IVB	Any T,	N3,	M0
			IVC	Any T,	any N,	M1

AJCC, American Joint Committee on Cancer.
From Greene FL, Page DL, Fleming ID, et al, eds: *AJCC Cancer Staging Manual,* 6th ed. New York: Springer; 2002.

which usually is unresectable surgically, nasopharyngeal carcinoma is primarily managed with radiotherapy. Cervical lymph node metastases from nasopharyngeal carcinoma, even when they are bulky, are very radioresponsive and curable locoregionally. Radiotherapy, consisting of external beam irradiation or brachytherapy or both, is also the mainstay of treatment for locally recurrent disease. In patients with distant metastasis, radiotherapy can offer significant palliation.

Although surgery is not used in the treatment of the primary tumor, radical neck dissection is the treatment of choice for resectable neck disease that is persistent or recurrent after radiotherapy.[55,56] Surgery has also been used to salvage select patients with locally recurrent disease.[57-60] Chemotherapy has been used as induction or neoadjuvant therapy before radiotherapy, as a radiosensitizer during radiotherapy, or as an adjuvant after radiotherapy in the treatment of advanced nasopharyngeal carcinoma.[61-64,65,66] Thus far, prospective randomized trials comparing neoadjuvant or adjuvant chemotherapy combined with radiotherapy to radiotherapy alone have not shown a survival benefit.[67-69] A phase III trial by the Head and Neck Intergroup in the United States compared radiotherapy alone to radiotherapy plus concurrent and adjuvant chemotherapy for stage III and IV disease.[70] Chemotherapy consisted of cisplatin 100 mg/m^2 every 3 weeks during radiotherapy and cisplatin 80 mg/m^2 plus 5-fluorouracil (5-FU) infusion 1000 mg/m^2/day, 4 days every 4 weeks after the completion of radiotherapy. Radiotherapy was delivered at 1.8 to 2 Gy per fraction per day, 5 days a week, to a total dose of 70 Gy. An update of the Intergroup trial[71] showed that at 5 years, the overall survival was 37% versus 67% ($P < 0.001$) and progression-free survival was 29% versus 58% in favor of the combined modality arm ($P < 0.001$). Significant differences were found in the overall survival and progression-free survival between the histological types for all patients treated. The overall survival was 37% for WHO I, 55% for WHO II, and 60% for WHO III ($P < 0.001$).

Chemotherapy alone or combined with reirradiation is also used in the palliation of recurrent or metastatic disease. Complete response rates of 15% to 44% have been achieved with combination chemotherapy in recurrent or metastatic nasopharyngeal carcinoma,[62,64,67,72]

although long-term disease control and survival are uncommon.

INTENSITY-MODULATED RADIATION THERAPY

Intensity-modulated radiation therapy (IMRT) is replacing conventional radiotherapy in the treatment of nasopharyngeal carcinoma in an increasing number of institutions in the United States. With this technique, the intensity of the radiation beams can be modulated so that a high dose can be delivered to the tumor with an improved target volume coverage while significantly reducing the dose to the surrounding normal tissues.[73-76]

At the University of California, San Francisco (UCSF), we have been using IMRT in the treatment of nasopharyngeal carcinoma since 1995. The following describes the evolution of our techniques in the treatment planning and delivery of IMRT for nasopharyngeal carcinoma.

Simulation and Treatment Planning Computed Tomography Procedures

The patient's head position should be hyperextended at the initial simulation so that there is adequate separation between the primary and retropharyngeal lymph nodes and the upper neck nodes.[77] The tip of the uvula and the base of the occiput should be on a plane parallel to the beam axis (Fig. 27-11). The head and neck, and in some cases the shoulders, are immobilized using a thermoplastic mask with the neck supported on a Timo (S-type, MED-TEC)[76,78] (Fig. 27-12). A pair of orthogonal radiographs is taken for isocenter localization at the initial simulation. The isocenter on the initial simulation film is placed at the anticipated treatment isocenter. Treatment

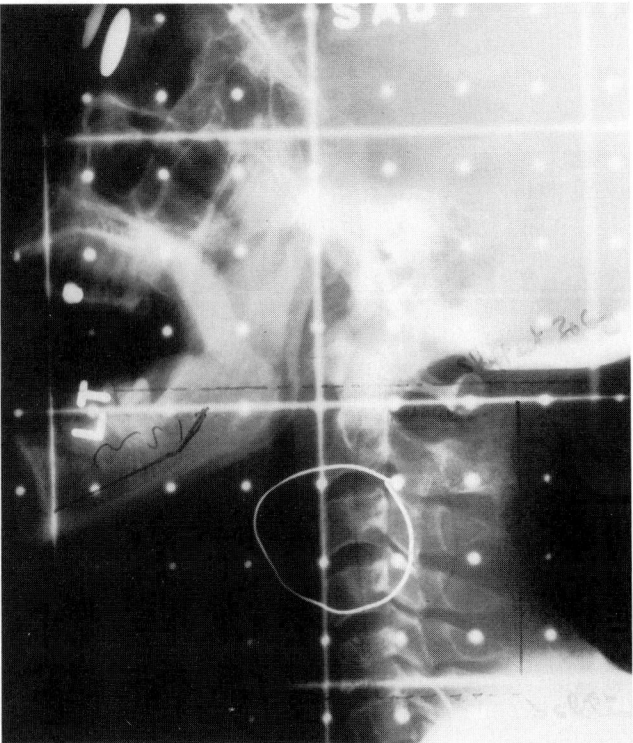

Figure 27–11. Initial simulation film of the lateral nasopharynx. (From Sultanem K, Shu HK, Xia P, et al: Three-dimensional intensity-modulated radiotherapy in the treatment of nasopharyngeal carcinoma: The University of California–San Francisco Experience. *Int J Radiat Oncol Biol Phys.* 2001;48:713.)

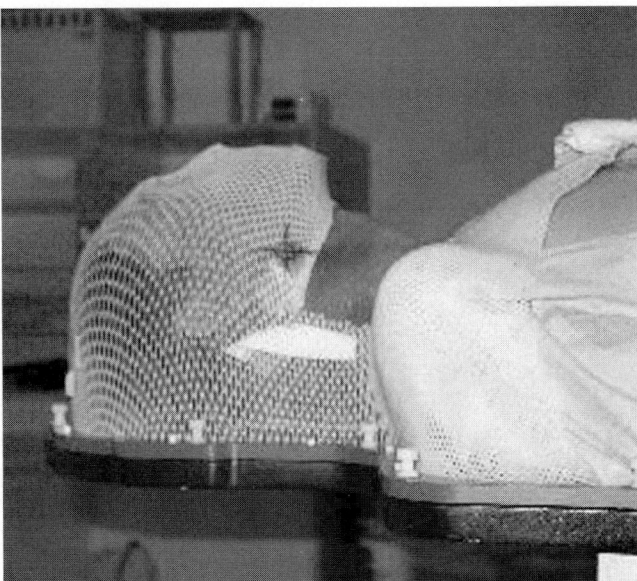

Figure 27–12. Head, neck, and shoulder immobilization using a thermoplastic mask with the neck supported on a Timo (S-type, MED-TEC).

planning CT scans are then obtained. In the region that contains the primary gross tumor volume (GTV), CT scan slice thickness should be 3 mm or less. The regions above and below the primary tumor target volume may be scanned with slice thickness of 5 mm.

Treatment Volume

The treatment volume should encompass the GTV as well as regions of microscopic disease and potential spread or the clinical target volume (CTV). The GTV is determined by clinical examination as well as MRI and CT scans. All patients should have a pretreatment MRI scan for precise target volume delineation unless medically contraindicated. Whenever possible, fusion of the diagnostic MRI images and the treatment planning CT images should be performed to accurately delineate the GTV and the surrounding critical normal structures. For disease clinically confined to the nasopharynx, the GTV should include the primary tumor in the nasopharynx, retropharyngeal lymphadenopathy, and all gross nodal disease.

The CTV is defined as the GTV plus areas containing potential microscopic disease. This volume should include at least the entire nasopharynx; retropharyngeal lymph nodal regions; clivus; skull base; pterygoid fossae; parapharyngeal space; inferior sphenoid sinus; posterior third of the nasal cavity; and posterior third of the maxillary sinuses.

The CTV should also include the following lymph nodal groups that are at high risk of potential microscopic spread of disease: bilateral upper deep jugular (junctional, parapharyngeal), submandibular, subdigastric (jugulodigastric), midjugular, posterior cervical, and retropharyngeal lymph nodes, and "circumferential margin to account for patient motion and set-up errors should be added." Bilateral lower neck and supraclavicular nodes, which are at a lower risk for microscopic spread, are also included in the CTV. Alternatively, a separate low anterior neck field (anterior-posterior) can be used to match the IMRT fields.

The lymph node groups at risk are outlined on the treatment planning CT scans according to image-based nodal classification.[79-82]

The surrounding critical normal structures, including the brainstem, spinal cord, optic nerves, chiasm, parotid glands, pituitary, temporomandibular (TM) joints, middle and inner ears, and skin should also be outlined on the treatment planning CT scans.

Treatment Planning and Delivery

Various treatment planning systems are available commercially. At the UCSF Medical Center, three different treatment planning software systems have been used for IMRT: a modification of the CT-based forward planning system developed at the University of Michigan (U-M Plan),[83] forward planning system by the ADAC-Pinnacle Corporation, and two inverse treatment-planning systems developed by the NOMOS Corporation (i.e., the Peacock and Corvus planning systems).[84,85] Treatment is delivered using linear accelerators equipped with a computer-controlled auto-sequence multi-leaf collimator (MLC) system (Siemens Medical Systems, Concord, Calif.), a multivane dynamic MLC (MIMiC), or a dynamic MLC system (Varian Oncology Systems, Palo Alto, Calif.). Examples of a 10-field forward plan, an inverse Peacock plan delivered using the mimic collimator, and an inverse Corvus plan delivered using MLC are shown in Figures 27-13 through 27-15.

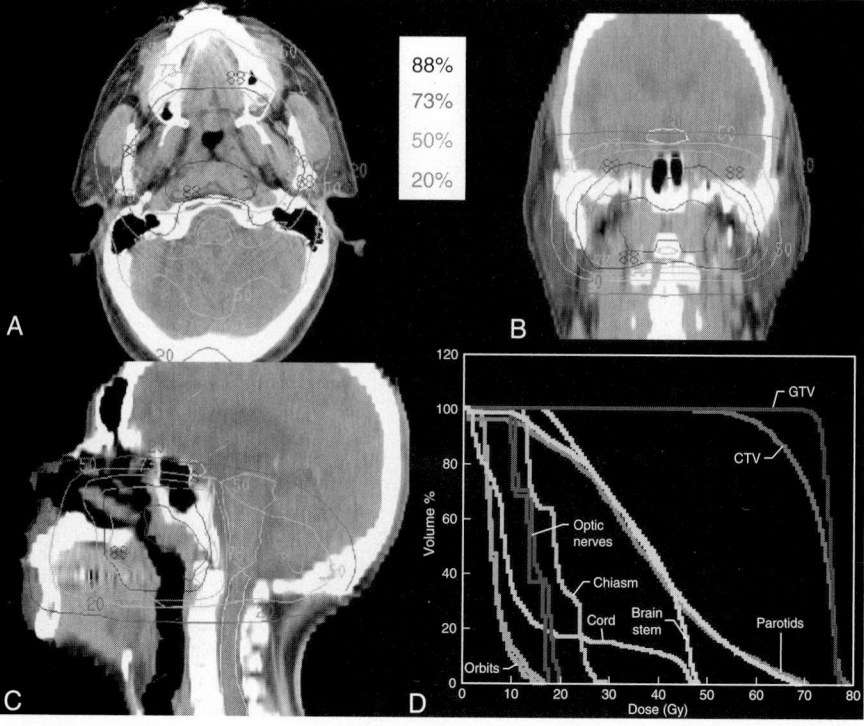

Figure 27–13. Isodose curves of a 10-field forward intensity-modulated radiotherapy plan for a patient with T1N1 carcinoma of the nasopharynx displayed on the axial (**A**), coronal (**B**), and sagittal (**C**) planes through the centroid of the primary tumor and the Dose Volume Histogram (**D**) for the relevant structures. (From Lee N, Xia P, Quivey JM, et al: Intensity-Modulated Radiotherapy in the Treatment of Nasopharyngeal Carcinoma: An Update of the UCSF Experience. *Int J Radiat Oncol Biol Phys.* 2002;53:15.). See also Color Figure 27-13.

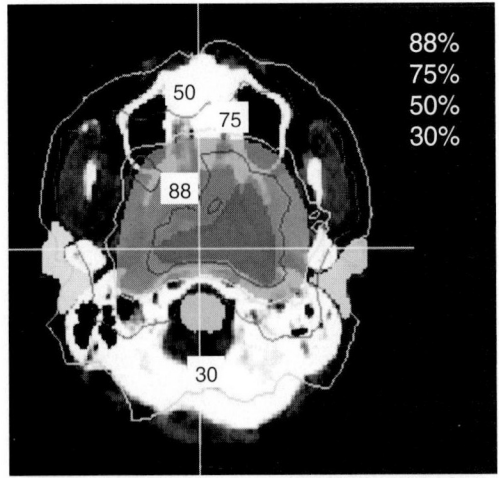

A

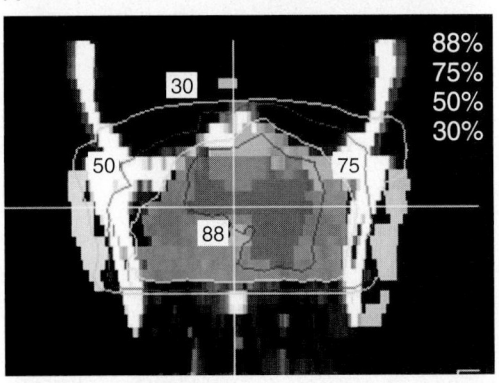

B

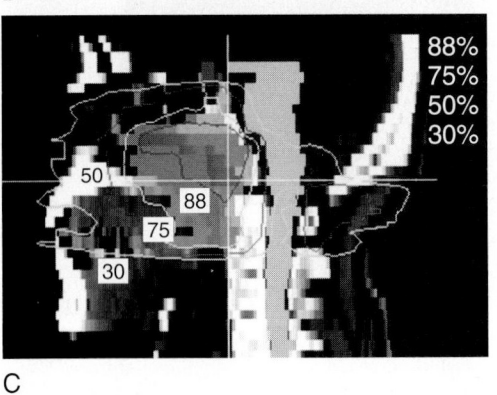

C

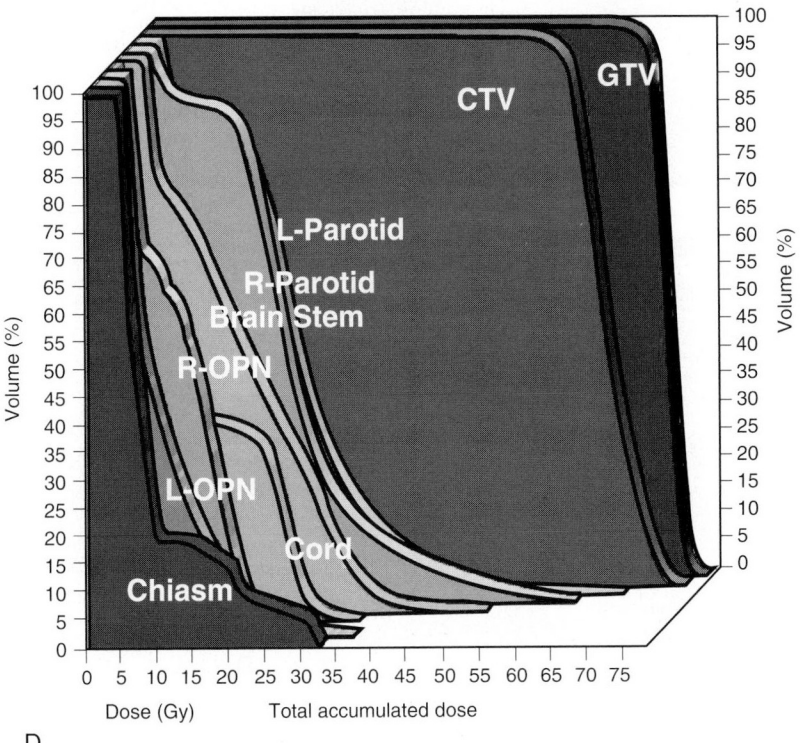

D

Figure 27–14. Isodose curves of an inverse IMRT plan delivered using multivane dynamic multi-leaf collimator (MIMiC) for a patient with T4N1 carcinoma of the nasopharynx displayed on the axial (**A**), coronal (**B**), and sagittal (**C**) planes through the centroid of the primary tumor and the Dose Volume Histogram for the relevant structures (**D**). The gross tumor volume is shown in red and the clinical target volume is shown in orange. (From Lee N, Xia P, Quivey JM, et al: Intensity-modulated radiotherapy in the treatment of nasopharyngeal carcinoma: An update of the UCSF Experience. *Int J Radiat Oncol Biol Phys.* 2002;53:16.) See also Color Figure 27-14.

Since 1995, several different radiotherapy techniques and IMRT methods have evolved at UCSF. In our initial experience, the primary tumor was treated with IMRT and the neck was treated with conventional radiotherapy.[77] The upper neck above the vocal cords was irradiated with opposed-lateral fields. The lower neck and the supraclavicular fossae were treated with a single anterior field. The IMRT field was matched with the opposed-lateral neck field with a split-beam technique. The opposed-lateral neck field was also matched to the lower neck and supraclavicular field with a split-beam technique.

More recently, a second technique treated the primary and the upper neck above the vocal cords with IMRT and the lower neck and the supraclavicular fossae with an anterior field. These two fields were matched with a split-beam technique. The dose uncertainties at the match lines led us to our third technique, in which we used an extended-field IMRT (EF-IMRT) that treated the primary tumor along with all the regional lymph nodes

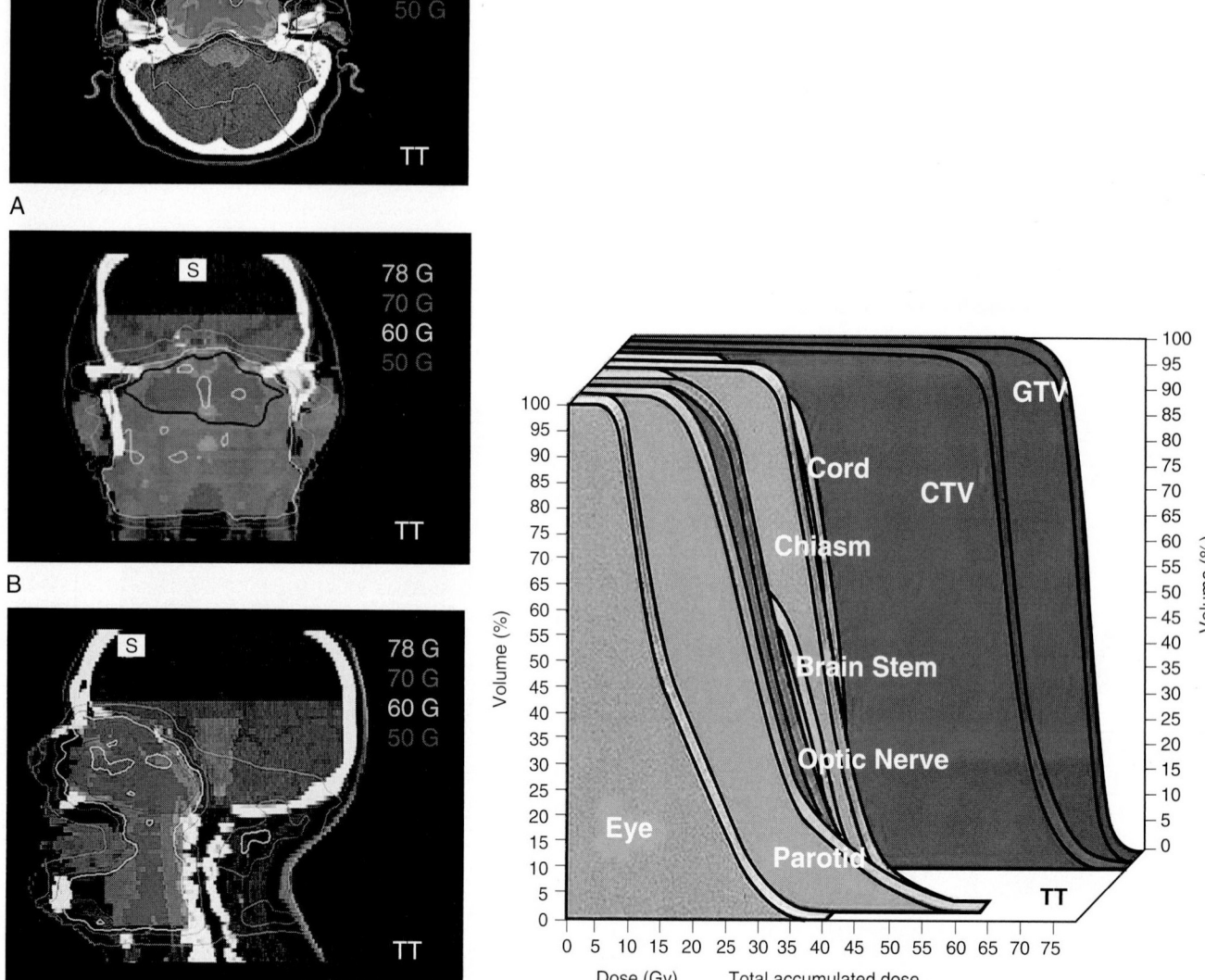

Figure 27–15. Isodose curves of an inverse IMRT plan using nine coplanar gantry angles delivered with conventional MLC for a patient with T3N0 carcinoma of the nasopharynx displayed on the (**A**) axial, (**B**) coronal, and (**C**) sagittal planes through the centroid of the primary tumor and the Dose Volume Histogram for the relevant structures (**D**). The GTV is shown in red and the CTV is shown in magenta. (From Lee N, Xia P, Fischbein N, et al: Intensity-modulated radiotherapy for head and neck cancer: The UCSF Experience focusing on target. *Int J Radiat Oncol Biol Phys.* 2003;57(1):49-60.) See also Color Figure 27-15.

including the supraclavicular nodes. However, due to the extended field size, application of this EF-IMRT technique may be limited by the field size constraints of the available linear accelerators.

Beam Energy

Megavoltage beams, 6 MV or greater x-rays, are used for the irradiation of the primary tumor. The neck is irradiated with a combination of 6 MV x-rays and 9 MeV electrons. X-rays with energy greater than 6 MV should

not be used for the irradiation of the cervical lymph nodes.

Dose and Fractionation

The prescribed dose is 70 Gy to the GTV and positive neck nodes, 59.4 Gy to the high risk CTV, and 50 to 54 Gy to the low risk clinically negative neck. The prescribed dose fractionation is 1.8 Gy/fraction per day, 5 days per week to the CTV to a total dose of 59.4 Gy to the high-risk CTV and 50.4 Gy to the low-risk CTV.

The GTV receives a higher dose per fraction on a daily basis and is typically 2.12 Gy/fraction per day.

Dose volume histograms are generated for all target volumes and critical normal structures. Guidelines for the dose constraints to normal tissues follow:

Brainstem and optic nerves	54 Gy or less than or equal to 60 Gy to 1% of the volume
Spinal cord	45 Gy or less than or equal to 50 Gy to 1% of the volume
Mandible	70 Gy or less than or equal to 75 Gy to 1 mL of the volume
Temporal lobes	60 Gy or less than or equal to 65 Gy to 1% of the volume
Parotid glands	Mean dose of less than or equal to 26 Gy to at least one parotid gland whenever possible.

These dose constraints include all scattered and transmitted doses. The critical normal structure constraints are the most important treatment planning priorities, followed by the tumor target volume prescription goals, and then the planning goals for the salivary glands.

BRACHYTHERAPY

Brachytherapy with intracavitary insertions[86-94] or interstitial implants[95-98] has been used as a boost treatment of T1 to T3 carcinoma of the nasopharynx after external beam irradiation or in the treatment of recurrent disease, either alone or in combination with external beam irradiation. Because of the rapid falloff of dose with an increase in the distance from the radioactive source, brachytherapy is not suitable for treatment of tumors with intracranial extension.

Various applicators and techniques have been used for the delivery of intracavitary brachytherapy for carcinoma of the nasopharynx.[88-91,92,99] In the past, intracavitary brachytherapy was delivered using low-dose-rate techniques. More recently, remote afterloading, fractionated high-dose-rate techniques on an outpatient basis are more commonly used. Since 1997 at UCSF, we have been using a remote afterloading intracavitary brachytherapy

technique with the Rotterdam Nasopharynx Applicator described by Dr. Peter C. Levendag.[99,100]

In a modification of the technique described by Levendag et al.,[100] the mucosa of the nasal cavity and the nasopharynx is first sprayed with a decongestant (0.05% oxymetazoline hydrochloride) and anesthetized with 5% cocaine hydrochloride applied topically with cotton Q-tips. The soft palate is anesthetized with Cetacaine (benzocaine, tetracaine hydrochloride, butamben, and benzalkonium chloride) spray. Two 5 French pediatric feeding tubes with an outer diameter of 1.65 mm and an inner diameter of 1.09 mm, respectively, are then introduced into the nasopharynx and withdrawn through the mouth to serve as guide tubes for the Rotterdam Nasopharynx Applicator. The applicator is then guided intraorally over the pediatric feeding tubes into the nasopharynx and the nasal cavity by pulling the nasal portion of the pediatric feeding tubes. Placement of the applicator into the nasopharynx is facilitated by gentle pushing of the oral portion of the pediatric feeding tubes intraorally with a pair of forceps. After the applicator is positioned in the nasopharynx and the nasal cavity, the pediatric feeding tubes are withdrawn, and the applicator is secured in place with a plastic clamp placed over the external portion of the applicator outside the nose (Fig. 27-16). Dummy iridium-192 sources in afterloading catheters are then inserted into each of the tubes of the applicator. After lead markers are placed on the contralateral outer canthus and tragus, a pair of orthogonal anterior-posterior and lateral localization x-ray films with the dummy sources in place are obtained (Fig. 27-17). The points of interest, including the nasopharynx, base of skull, node of Rouvière, pituitary, optic chiasm, spinal cord, and the palate points, are marked on the localization films.[101] Treatment planning and optimization is then performed with a computer software program (Plato brachytherapy afterloading planning system from Nucletron Corp., Netherlands). A dose of 5 to 6 Gy in two fractions, 5 to 6 hours apart, is prescribed at the isodose curve that passes through the nasopharynx points as a boost treatment for T1 to T2 lesions after 65 Gy of external beam radiotherapy. The dose for reirradiation of recurrent tumors depends on the

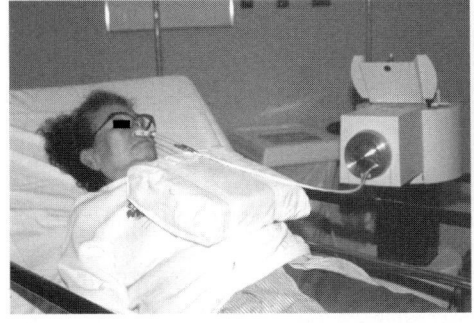
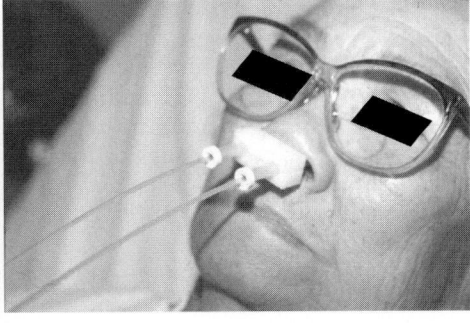

A   B

Figure 27–16. A, A patient with the Rotterdam nasopharynx applicator in place. The afterloading catheters are connected to a remote-controlled high-dose-rate afterloading machine (microSelectron HDR, Nucletron-Oldeft Nucletron). **B,** Close-up view of the Rotterdam nasopharynx applicator secured in place with a plastic clamp placed over the external portion of the applicator just outside the nose.

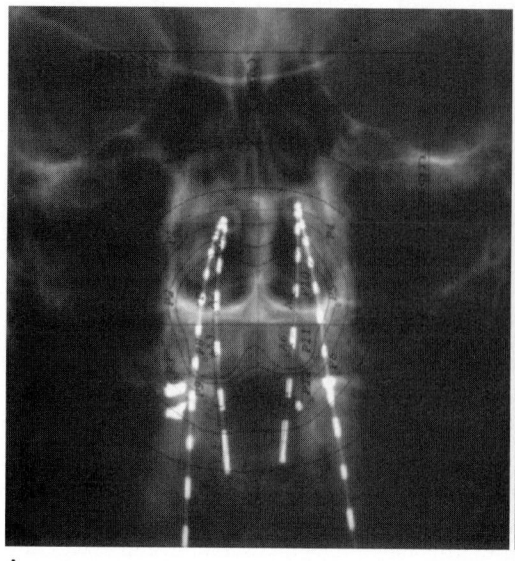 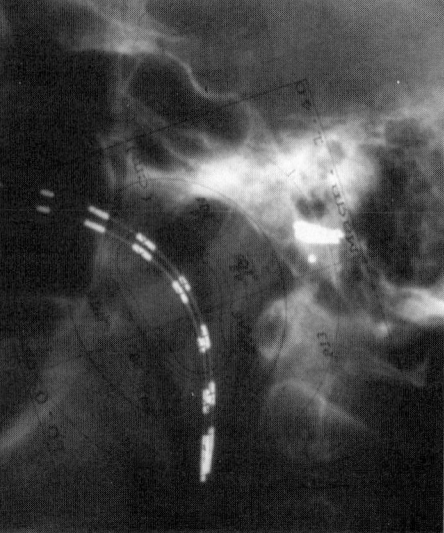

A   B

Figure 27–17. A, Lateral and **B,** anterior-posterior localization films of an intracavitary brachytherapy boost using the Rotterdam Nasopharynx Applicator with the dummy sources inserted.

previous dose of external beam radiotherapy. After treatment planning, afterloading catheters are then inserted into the applicator and connected to a remote-controlled high-dose-rate afterloading machine (microSelectron HDR, Nucletron-Oldeft Nucletron) for treatment delivery. Upon completion of treatments, the nose clamp and the afterloading catheters are removed. Two 5 French pediatric feeding tubes are reinserted into the applicator and the applicator is withdrawn through the mouth by pushing it into the nose while gently pulling on the feeding tubes exiting the mouth.

Several approaches have been used for permanent interstitial implantation of carcinoma of the nasopharynx at different institutions. They include the transnasal approach[95] and the transoral approach[96] for lesions in the middle and low posterior wall; implantation of iodine-125 seeds through a transpalatal flap for lesions in the superior or high posterior wall; and the split-palate approach with gold-198 seeds.[102]

COMPLICATIONS

In the past, because of the large treatment volume and high dose required for nasopharyngeal carcinoma in most patients, various complications occurred after conventional radiotherapy.[103] The overall complication rate ranged from 31% to 66%.[21,27,103,104] Severe complication rates of 6% to 15% and fatal complication rates of 1% to 3% have been reported.[21,27,103,104] The complication rates are increased with concurrent chemotherapy[105] or coexisting medical conditions such as diabetes or hypertension. However, using modern three-dimensional conformal radiotherapy techniques including IMRT, these complication rates should decrease.[74,75,77]

Xerostomia was by far the most common sequela with conventional radiotherapy. Most patients experience some degree of dry mouth permanently. However, with IMRT, most patients recover their salivary gland function more rapidly and completely.[74,75,77] Dental problems, a consequence of decreased saliva and altered

salivary consistency, occurred in 4% to 17% of patients treated with conventional radiotherapy.[21,104] Dental prophylaxis with topical fluorides and good dental care before, during, and after radiotherapy can reduce the incidence of dental caries.

Chronic otitis media occurred in 3% to 18% and hearing loss in 6% to 8% of the patients.[21,29,104] The incidence of hearing impairment was related to the dose to the inner ear and was significantly higher in patients who received more than 50 Gy to the cochlea.[106]

Trismus occurred as a result of fibrosis and contraction of pterygoid muscles or fibrosis of the temporomandibular joint in 5% to 10% of patients.[21,29,104] Mandible exercise may prevent progression of the trismus and surgical intervention may be necessary occasionally to relieve severe trismus.

Severe neck fibrosis usually resulted from the use of a large dose per fraction[29] and neck irradiation using anterior-posterior opposed fields,[21] especially when compensators were not used. The use of doses less than or equal to 2 Gy/fraction and the use of a combination of photon and electron beam for treatment of posterior cervical nodes should reduce the incidence of this complication.

Soft tissue or bone necrosis or both have been described in 5% to 16 %[21,27,104] and brain necrosis in 2% to 3% of patients.[27,29]

Cranial nerve dysfunction, usually affecting cranial nerves IX to XII, and in particular the twelfth nerve, may result from soft tissue fibrosis along the course of the nerves and entrapment in the lateral retroparotid space. The incidence is approximately 1% to 6%.[21,27,29,104]

Transverse radiation myelitis has been reported in 1% to 4% of patients.[21,29,104,107] Improvement in tumor localization and treatment planning with the aid of CT and MRI scans and careful treatment techniques should prevent this devastating treatment complication.

Because a portion of the orbit and sometimes the eye, especially in patients with advanced disease, is usually included in the treatment volume, optic nerve injury and radiation retinopathy with impairment of vision can occur in patients after radiotherapy for nasopharyngeal

Table 27–2   Carcinoma of the Nasopharynx: Control of the Primary Tumor According to 1992 AJCC T-Stage After Conventional Radiotherapy

| First Author | Stage % (Patients, *n*) | | | |
	T1	T2	T3	T4
Hoppe (1976)	87 (38)	94 (16)	68 (19)	44 (9)
Mesic (1981)	97 (34)	84 (102)	73 (45)	71 (70)
Chu (1984)	76 (25)	79 (14)	37 (19)	55 (22)
Vikram (1985)		74 (47)	100 (3)	63 (57)
Wang (1990)	76 (17)	54 (23)	34 (11)	42 (10)
	67* (14)	84* (30)	78* (12)	52* (12)
Perez (1992)	85† (21)	75† (33)	67† (26)	40† (63)
Bailet (1992)	64 (28)		61 (71)	

*Twice daily accelerated fractionation treatment.
†10-year actuarial rate.

carcinoma when using conventional techniques.[21,108,109] Retinopathy has occurred after a dose of less than 50 Gy.[108,109] Optic nerve injury can occur after 50 Gy, and the incidence increases with increase of fraction size.[108] Limiting the fraction size to less than or equal to 2 Gy/fraction per day and a dose of 45 Gy or less to the retina and 54 Gy or less to the optic nerve should prevent this complication.

Hypothalamic-pituitary or thyroid dysfunction or both can occur in 1% to 6% of long-term survivors.[29,104,110-113] The true incidence of endocrine dysfunction following radiotherapy of nasopharyngeal carcinoma may be higher as most patients have not been routinely evaluated for endocrine function during follow-up examinations. Since most of these endocrine dysfunctions can be corrected medically, periodic evaluation of the hypothalamic, pituitary, and thyroid function may be indicated in the follow-up examination of patients after radiotherapy for nasopharyngeal carcinoma.

Carotid stenosis has been reported in patients who undergo irradiation of the head and neck region. Interval from radiotherapy was a significant independent predictor for severe carotid stenosis. Some have recommended a routine duplex ultrasound screening test in these patients.[114]

RESULTS OF TREATMENT

The local-regional control rates by radiotherapy in select series are shown in Tables 27-2 and 27-3.

Control of the primary lesion using conventional radiotherapy varied with the T classification (see Table 27-2), ranging from 67% to 97% for T1 lesions, 54% to 94% for T2 lesions, 34% to 78% for T3 lesions, and 40% to 71% for T4 lesions.[20,21,27,104,115-117] Local control rate increased with increase in dose[20,27,104,116,118] and field size.[20,21] Interruption of treatment for 3 weeks or longer adversely affected local control.[116] Boost treatment with intracavitary brachytherapy[89] and the use of twice-daily split-course accelerated fractionation improved local control.[119] Nonkeratinizing squamous cell carcinoma and undifferentiated carcinoma had better local control than keratinizing squamous cell carcinoma in T2 to T3 lesions but not in T1 or T4 lesions.[27] Control of cervical lymph node metastasis from carcinoma of the nasopharynx by conventional radiotherapy is excellent even with extensive disease in the neck (see Table 27-3). The control rate of cervical lymph node metastasis ranged from 82% to 100% for N0, 86% to 92% for N1, and 78% to 89% for N2 to N3 disease.[21,27,104]

Five-year survival rates ranged from 36% to 58% (Table 27-4).[20,21,104,115,117,120] The 5-year survival rate correlated with the T-stage, as well as with the N-stage (Tables 27-5 and 27-6), being 60% to 76% for T1, 48% to 68% for T2, 27% to 55% for T3, and 0% to 29% for T4 lesions[21,117]; 42% to 78% for N0, 27% to 70% for N1, and 32% to 52% for N2 to N3 disease. The prognosis is poor when nodes in the lower neck or the supraclavicular fossa or both are involved.

Table 27–3   Carcinoma of the Nasopharynx: Control of Cervical Lymph Node Metastases According to 1992 AJCC N-Stage* After Conventional Radiotherapy

| First Author | Stage, % (Patients, *n*) | | | |
	N0	N1	N2	N3
Hoppe (1976)	96 (24)	92 (25)	87 (15)	89 (18)
Mesic (1981)	100 (35)	90 (30)	88 (59)	82 (114)
Perez (1992)	82* (48)	86* (23)	78* (72)	

*Ten-year actuarial rate.

Table 27–4   Carcinoma of the Nasopharynx: 5-Year Survival After Conventional Radiotherapy (1992 AJCC Staging System)*

First Author	Patients, *n*	5-Yr Survival, %
Hoppe (1976)	82	57 (actuarial)
Mesic (1981)	251	52 (actuarial disease-free)
Chu (1985)	80	36 (actuarial)
Vikram (1984)	107	56 (actuarial)*
Wang (1990)	185	43 (absolute)
Bailet (1992)	103	58 (actuarial)

*Estimated from survival curve.

Table 27–5   Carcinoma of the Nasopharynx: 5-Year Survival After Conventional Radiotherapy According to 1992 AJCC T-Stage*

| First Author | 5-Yr Survival, % (Patients, *n*) | | | |
	T1	*T2*	*T3*	*T4*
Hoppe (1976)	76* (38)	68* (16)	55* (19)	0* (9)
Wang (1990)	60 (52)	48 (58)	27 (33)	29 (42)

*Actuarial disease-free survival.
AJCC, American Joint Committee on Cancer.

With IMRT, excellent local and regional control was achieved in 97% and 98% of the patients treated at UCSF, respectively (Figs. 27-18 and 27-19).[77] However, distant metastases remained high; the distant metastases-free rate was 66% at 4 years (Fig. 27-20). The overall survival was 88% (Fig. 27-21). Similar to the UCSF experience, preliminary results from the Memorial Sloan-Kettering Cancer Center based on 38 patients with a median follow-up of 22 months also showed an excellent 2-year local-regional control rate of 97%. The 2-year freedom-from-distant-metastases rate was 79%, which was not significantly different from their non-IMRT experience.[121]

In addition to stage, several other factors may influence prognosis: histologic type, age, sex, EBV-specific IgA antibody titer, serum EBV DNA levels, tumor angiogenesis, HLA antigen pattern, and cell-mediated immune status. Lymphoepitheliomas and undifferentiated carcinomas have been reported to be more radiosensitive and associated with better prognosis than squamous cell carcinoma in some series.[20,25,104,117,122-124]

Younger patients appear to have better 5-year survival rates than older patients.[10,20,27,125] In Ho's series, the difference in 5-year survival between patients younger than 40 years of age and those 40 years or older was statistically significant (57.8% vs. 43.4%, *P* = 0.001).[10] In a retrospective review of 119 patients younger than 30 years of age from the Children's Cancer Study Group,[126] the overall 5-year survival and relapse-free survival rates from diagnosis were 51% and 36%, respectively, and were not significantly different from other series of adult patients.

Better prognosis for females than males has been shown in some series, although the difference is not statistically significant in most series.[10,20,21,115,125]

Table 27–6   Carcinoma of the Nasopharynx: 5-Year Survival After Conventional Radiotherapy According to 1992 AJCC N-Stage*

| First Author | 5-Yr Survival, % (Patients, *n*) | | | |
	N0	*N1*	*N2*	*N3*
Hoppe (1976)	78* (24)	70* (25)	42* (15)	39* (18)
Chu (1984)	42† (25)	27† (11)	52† (19)	27† (25)
Wang (1990)	60‡ (67)	42‡ (19)	32‡ (99)	

*Actuarial disease-free survival.
†Actuarial survival.
‡Absolute survival.

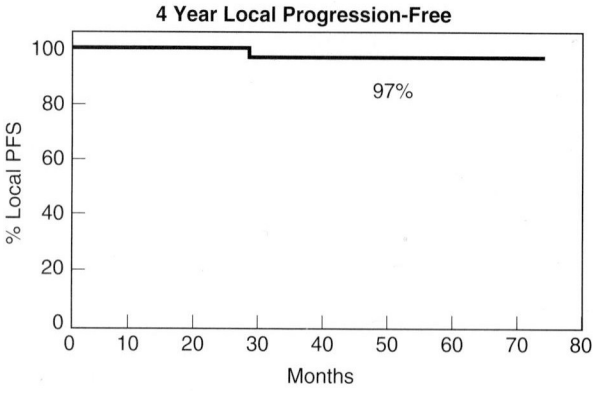

Figure 27–18. Kaplan-Meier estimate of local progression-free probability. (From Lee N, Xia P, Quivey JM, et al: Intensity-modulated radiotherapy in the treatment of nasopharyngeal carcinoma: An update of the UCSF Experience. *Int J Radiat Oncol Biol Phys.* 2002;53:17.)

EBV antibody titer following treatment may be a significant prognostic factor.[127-129] In a multicenter follow-up study, increasing titers of IgA anti-EA antibodies in patients in apparent clinical remission 1 year after radiotherapy were highly significant for prediction of relapse.[127] In another study from Taiwan, 72% to 100% of the patients who developed recurrent nasopharyngeal carcinoma demonstrated elevated IgA, as well as IgG, anti-VCA antibody titers 1 year after radiotherapy, although during the first year following radiotherapy, some decrease and fluctuation of seropositive rates were observed in both the cured and recurrent patients.[129] However, in one North American study, sequential measurements of various EBV antibody titers was not useful in post-treatment monitoring of patients.[130] Recently circulating EBV DNA concentration has been shown to be an independent prognostic indicator.[131]

A pilot study at UCSF showed that tumor angiogenesis (measured with microvessel density) and c-erB2 expression were significant prognostic factors for nasopharyngeal carcinoma.[132] This has not been confirmed by other studies to date. With further development of the microarray technology, additional tumor markers may be identified to be of prognostic significance in the future.

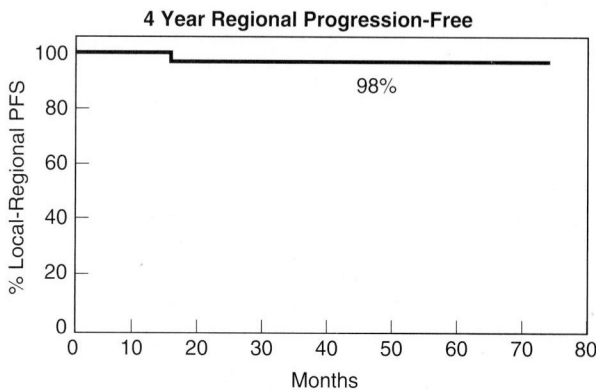

Figure 27–19. Kaplan-Meier estimate of regional progression-free probability. (From Lee N, Xia P, Quivey JM, et al: Intensity-modulated radiotherapy in the treatment of nasopharyngeal carcinoma: An update of the UCSF Experience. *Int J Radiat Oncol Biol Phys.* 2002;53:18.)

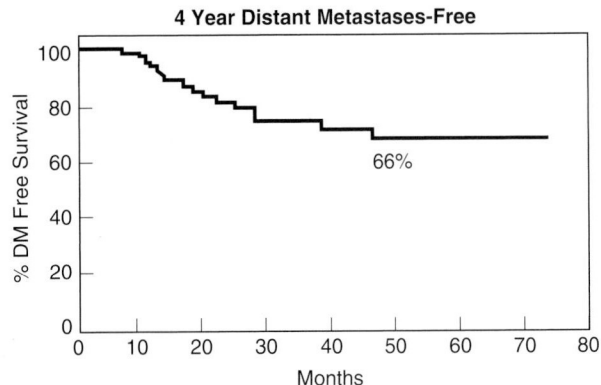

Figure 27–20. Kaplan-Meier estimate of distant-metastasis-free probability. (From Lee N, Xia P, Quivey JM, et al: Intensity-modulated radiotherapy in the treatment of nasopharyngeal carcinoma: An update of the UCSF Experience. *Int J Radiat Oncol Biol Phys.* 2002;53:18.)

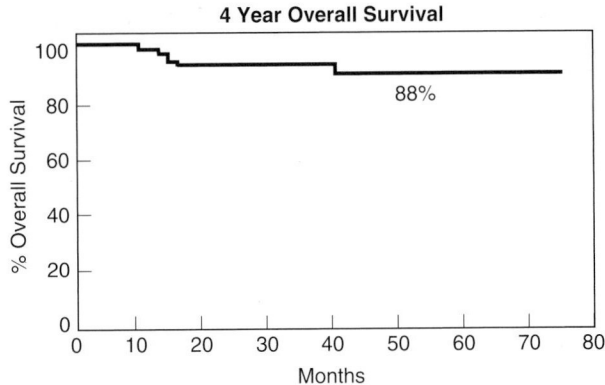

Figure 27–21. Kaplan-Meier estimate of overall survival. (From Lee N, Xia P, Quivey JM, et al: Intensity-modulated radiotherapy in the treatment of nasopharyngeal carcinoma: An update of the UCSF Experience. *Int J Radiat Oncol Biol Phys.* 2002;53:18.)

REIRRADIATION OF RECURRENT CARCINOMA

Significant palliation and occasional long-term survival can be achieved without excessive risk in patients with recurrent nasopharyngeal carcinoma.[60,88,91,93,98,102,120,133-135] Various radiation therapy modalities, including external beam irradiation, intracavitary brachytherapy, interstitial implantation, particle beam radiotherapy, and stereotactic radiosurgery have been used.[60,88,91,93,96,98,120,133-138] The treatment technique and the dose of reirradiation depend on the extent of disease at recurrence and the dose of previous radiotherapy. Superficial recurrent disease limited to the nasopharynx may be treated with intracavitary brachytherapy or interstitial implant alone, or combined with hyperfractionated external beam radiotherapy with or without concurrent chemotherapy. Currently at UCSF, recurrent nasopharyngeal carcinoma is treated with IMRT delivering a dose of 60 Gy at 1.44 Gy/fraction, twice-daily, 6 hours apart, 5 days per week concurrent cisplatin chemotherapy to the GTV while the CTV receives a dose of 50 Gy at 1.2 Gy/fraction, twice-daily. Alternatively once-a-day fractionation using IMRT to 60 Gy can be used if a desirable plan is achieved, concurrent with chemotherapy. High-dose brachytherapy can be considered in patients with residual disease limited to the nasopharynx after external beam radiotherapy.

Particle beam radiotherapy has a more favorable physical dose distribution than conventional photon irradiation, and heavily charged particle irradiation may have additional biological advantages. Using heavily charged particle irradiation, a local control rate of 45% and a 5-year survival of 31% was achieved in a small series of patients with recurrent disease involving the base of the skull with or without cranial nerve deficits.[136]

Results of reirradiation of select patients with recurrent nasopharyngeal carcinoma are shown in Table 27-7. The 5-year actuarial survival rate ranged from 20% to 45%.[60,88,91,93,120,134,135] However, long-term local control, which depends on the extent of recurrent disease, was possible in only 14% to 60% of the patients retreated. Survival after retreatment appears to correlate with the time of recurrence after initial radiotherapy,[88,93,134] extent of recurrent disease, and dose of reirradiation.[88,91,135] Five-year actuarial survival was 13% in patients whose disease recurred 2 years or less after initial radiotherapy and 66% in those with recurrence more than 2 years after initial treatment.[88] Five-year actuarial survival was 38% for stage T1 to T2 and 15% for stage T3 to T4 disease at recurrence.[88] It was 45% with doses greater than or equal to 60 Gy and 0% with doses less than 60 Gy, although most of the patients who received lower doses had more advanced recurrent disease.[88]

Following reirradiation, severe complications occurred in 4% to 48% of the patients (see Table 27-7). The

Table 27–7   Results of Retreatment of Recurrent Carcinoma of the Nasopharynx

First Author	Patients, n	Local Control, %	5-Yr Survival, %	Severe Complications, %
Hwang (1998)	74	49	37	23
Yan (1983)	162	14	23	34[†]
Vikram (1986)	15	61*	55*	20
Wang (1987)	51	—	45[‡]	4
Pryzant (1992)	53	35	21	15
Wei (1993)	34	63	33	20

*2-year actuarial.
[†]29 of 85 patients who survived 5 years.
[‡]In patients who received ≥60 Gy.

incidence of severe complications of reirradiation increased with the increase of total cumulative dose of external beam irradiation; it was 4% with doses less than or equal to 100 Gy and 39% with doses greater than 100 Gy.[91] Late normal tissue complications of reirradiation should decrease with the use of hyperfractionation and three-dimensional conformal radiotherapy techniques including IMRT and particle beam radiotherapy.

REFERENCES

1. Tai THP MR: Analytical epidemiology: Risk factors for nasopharyngeal carcinoma. *Curr Opin Oncol.* 2001;8:156.
2. Tai THP MR: Descriptive epidemiology of nasopharyngeal cancer. *Curr Opin Oncol.* 2001;8:114.
3. Parkin DM, Muir CS, Whelan SL, et al: Cancer incidence in five continents. *Epidemiology.* In Parkin DM, Muir CS, Whelan SL, eds. Lyon, France: IARC Scientific Publications: 1992;182.
4. Lanier A, Bender T, Talbot M, et al: Nasopharyngeal carcinoma in Alaskan Eskimos, Indians, and Aleuts: A review of cases and study of Epstein-Barr virus, HLA, and environmental risk factors. *Cancer.* 1980;46:2100.
5. Liebowitz D: Nasopharyngeal carcinoma: The Epstein-Barr virus association. *Semin Oncol.* 1994;21:376.
6. Lo YMD, Chan LYS, Lo KW, et al: Quantitative analysis of cell-free Epstein-Barr virus DNA in plasma of patients with nasopharyngeal carcinoma. *Cancer Res.* 1999;59:1188.
7. Murono S, Inoue H, Tanabe T, Joab I, et al: Induction of cyclooxygenase-2 by Epstein-Barr virus. Latent membrane protein 1 is involved in vascular endothelial growth factor production in nasopharyngeal carcinoma cells. *Proc Nat'l Acad Sci.* 2001;98:6905.
8. Simons MJ, Wee GB, Goh EH, et al: Immunogenetic aspects of nasopharyngeal carcinoma. IV. Increased risk in Chinese of nasopharyngeal carcinoma associated with a Chinese-related HLA profile (A2, Singapore 2). *J Natl Cancer Inst.* 1976;57:977.
9. Buell P: The effect of migration on the risk of nasopharyngeal cancer among Chinese. *Cancer Res.* 1974;34:1189.
10. Ho JH: An epidemiologic and clinical study of nasopharyngeal carcinoma. *Int J Radiat Oncol Biol Phys.* 1978;4:182.
11. Yu MC: Diet and nasopharyngeal carcinoma. *Prog Clin Biol Res.* 1990;346:93.
12. International histological classification of tumors: Histological typing of upper respiratory tract tumors. *World Health Organization.* 1978;19:32.
13. Neel HBI: Nasopharyngeal carcinoma: Diagnosis, staging, and management. *Oncology.* 1992;6:87.
14. McGuire LJ, Lee JC: The histopathologic diagnosis of nasopharyngeal carcinoma. *Ear Nose Throat J.* 1990;69:229.
15. Marks JE, Phillips JL, Menck HR: The national cancer data base report on the relationship of race and national origin to the histology of nasopharyngeal carcinoma. *Cancer.* 1998;83:582.
16. Skinner DW, Van-Hasselt CA, Tsao SY: Nasopharyngeal carcinoma: Modes of presentation. *Ann Otol Rhinol Laryngol.* 1991;100:544.
17. Lindberg RD: Distribution of cervical lymph node metastases from squamous cell carcinoma of the upper respiratory and digestive tracts. *Cancer.* 1972;29:1446.
18. Ahmad A, Stefani S: Distant metastases of nasopharyngeal carcinoma: A study of 256 male patients. *J Surg Oncol.* 1986;33:194.
19. Bedwinek JM, Perez CA, Keys DJ: Analysis of failures after definitive irradiation for epidermoid carcinoma of the nasopharynx. *Cancer.* 1980;45:2725.
20. Chu AM, Flynn MB, Achino E, et al: Irradiation of nasopharyngeal carcinoma: Correlations with treatment factors and stage. *Int J Radiat Oncol Biol Phys.* 1984;10:2241.
21. Hoppe RT, Goffinet DR, Bagshaw MA: Carcinoma of the nasopharynx: Eighteen years' experience with megavoltage radiation therapy. *Cancer.* 1976;37:2605.
22. McNeese MD, Fletcher GH: Retreatment of recurrent nasopharyngeal carcinoma. *Radiology.* 1981;138:191.
23. Moench HC, Phillips TL: Carcinoma of the nasopharynx: Review of 146 patients with emphasis on radiation dose and time factors. *Am J Surg.* 1972;124:515.
24. Lynn TC, Huang SC, Tu SM: Treatment of nasopharyngeal carcinoma. *Excerpta Med Int Congr Ser.* 1982;571:408.
25. Frezza G, Barbieri E, et al: Patterns of failure in nasopharyngeal cancer treated with megavoltage irradiation. *Radiother Oncol.* 1986;5:287.
26. Johansen LV, Mestre M, Overgaard J: Carcinoma of the nasopharynx: Analysis of treatment results in 167 consecutively admitted patients. *Head Neck.* 1992;14:200.
27. Perez CA, Devinen VR, Marcial-Vega V, et al: Carcinoma of the nasopharynx: Factors affecting prognosis. *Int J Radiat Oncol Biol Phys.* 1992;23:271.
28. Teo P, Shiu W, Leung SF, et al: Prognostic factors in nasopharyngeal carcinoma investigated by computer tomography—An analysis of 659 patients. *Radiother Oncol.* 1992;23:79.
29. Lee AW, Law SC, Ng SH, et al: Retrospective analysis of nasopharyngeal carcinoma treated during 1976-1985: Late complications following megavoltage irradiation. *Br J Radiol.* 1992;65:918.
30. Poon PY, Fau-Tsang VH, Tsang VH, Fau-Munk PL, Munk PL: Tumour extent and T stage of nasopharyngeal carcinoma: A comparison of. *Can Assoc Radiol J.* 2000;51:287, quiz 286.
31. Lanzieri CF, Bangert B: Magnetic resonance imaging of the nasopharynx. *Top Magn Reson Imaging.* 1990;2:39.
32. Mancuso AA, Harnsberger HR, Dillon WP: Nasopharynx, parapharyngeal space, skull base, cranial nerves V and IX-XII, and sympathomimetics. In Grayson TH, Eckhart C, eds. *Workbook for MRI and CT of the Head and Neck.* Baltimore: Williams & Wilkins; 1989;123.
33. Sievers KW, Greess H, Baum U, et al: Paranasal sinuses and nasopharynx CT and MRI. *Eur J Radiol.* 2000;33:185.
34. Dillon WP, Harnsberger HR: The impact of radiologic imaging on staging of cancer of the head and neck. *Semin Oncol.* 1991;18:64.
35. Glazer HS, Niemeyer JH, Balfe DM, et al: Neck neoplasms: MR imaging. Part II. Post treatment evaluation. *Radiology.* 1986;160:349.
36. Gong QY, Zheng GL, Zhu HY: MRI differentiation of recurrent nasopharyngeal carcinoma from postradiation fibrosis. *Comput Med Imaging Graph.* 1991;15:423.
37. Som PM: Detection of metastasis in cervical lymph nodes: CT and MR criteria and differential diagnosis. *AJR Am J Roentgenol.* 1992;158:961.
38. Henle G, Henle W: Epstein-Barr virus-specific IgA serum antibodies as an outstanding feature of nasopharyngeal carcinoma. *Int J Cancer.* 1976;17:1.
39. Wara WM, Wara DW, Phillips TL, et al: Elevated IGA in carcinoma of the nasopharynx. *Cancer.* 1975;35:1313.
40. Ho HC, Ng MH, Kwan HC, et al: Epstein-Barr-virus-specific IgA and IgG serum antibodies in nasopharyngeal carcinoma. *Br J Cancer.* 1976;34:655.
41. Zeng Y: Seroepidemiological studies on nasopharyngeal carcinoma in China. *Adv Cancer Res.* 1985;44:121.
42. Zong YS, Shan JS, Ng MH, et al: Immunoglobulin A against viral capsid antigen of Epstein-Barr virus and indirect mirror examination of the nasopharynx in the detection of asymptomatic nasopharyngeal carcinoma. *Cancer.* 1992;69:3.
43. AJCC: Pharynx. In Beahrs OH, Henson DE, Hulter RVP, Kennedy BJ, et al, eds. *Manual for Staging of Cancer.* Philadelphia: JB Lippincott Company; 1992:31.
44. Clinical S: Recommendation, Nasopharyngeal Carcinoma: Etiology and Control. In De-The G, Ito Y, eds. *International Agency for Research on Cancer.* Lyon, France: Scientific Publications No. 20; 1978:594.
45. Huang SC: Nasopharyngeal cancer: A review of 1605 patients treated radically with cobalt 60. *Int J Radiat Oncol Biol Phys.* 1980;6:401.
46. Huang SC, Lui LT, Lynn TC: Nasopharyngeal cancer: Study III. A review of 1206 patients treated with combined modalities. *Int J Radiat Oncol Biol Phys.* 1985;11:1789.
47. Neel HBI, Taylor WF: New staging system for nasopharyngeal carcinoma. Long-term outcome. *Arch Otolaryngol Head Neck Surg.* 1989;115:1293.
48. Teo PM, Tsao Sy, Ho JH, et al: A proposed modification of the Ho stage-classification for nasopharyngeal carcinoma. *Radiother Oncol.* 1991;21:11.

49. UICC: Pharynx. In Spiessl B, et al, eds. *TNM Atlas*. Berlin: Springer-Verlag; 1992:20.

50. Sham JS, Wei WI, Nicholls J, et al: Extent of nasopharyngeal carcinoma involvement inside the nasopharynx. Lack of prognostic value on local control. *Cancer*. 1992;69:854.

50a. Greene FL, Page DL, Fleming ID, et al: eds. AJCC Cancer Staging Manual, 6th ed. New York, Springer; 2002.

51. Xiao GL, Gao L, Xu GZ: Prognostic influence of parapharyngeal space involvement in nasopharyngeal carcinoma. *Int J Radiat Oncol Biol Phys*. 2002;52:957.

52. Sham JS, Cheung YK, Chay D, et al: Cranial nerve involvement and base of the skull erosion in nasopharyngeal carcinoma. *Cancer*. 1991;68:422.

53. Teo PM, Leung SF, Yu P, et al: A comparison of Ho's, International Union Against Cancer, and American Joint Committee stage classifications for nasopharyngeal carcinoma. *Cancer*. 1991; 67:434.

54. Ozyar E, Yildiz F, Akyol FH, Atahan IL: Comparison of AJCC 1988 and 1997 classifications for nasopharyngeal carcinoma. *Int J Radiat Oncol Biol Phys*. 1999;44:1079.

55. Yen KL, Hsu LP, Sheen TS, et al: Salvage neck dissection for cervical recurrence of nasopharyngeal carcinoma. *Arch Otolaryngol Head Neck Surg*. 1997;123:725.

56. Wei WI, Ho WK, Cheng AC, et al: Management of extensive cervical nodal metastasis in nasopharyngeal carcinoma after radiotherapy: A clinicopathological study. *Arch Otolaryngol Head Neck Surg*. 2001;127:1457.

57. Fee WE Jr, Roberson JB, Gioffinet DR, et al: Long-term survival after surgical resection for recurrent nasopharyngeal cancer after radiotherapy failure. *Arch Otolaryngol Head Neck Surg*. 2002; 128:280.

58. Tu GY, Hu YH, Xu GZ, et al: Salvage surgery for nasopharyngeal carcinoma. *Arch Otolaryngol Head Neck Surg*. 1988;114:328.

59. WI W: Salvage surgery for recurrent primary nasopharyngeal carcinoma. *Crit Rev Oncol Hematol*. 2000;33:91.

60. Wei WW, Ho CM, Lan KH, et al: Surgical resection for nasopharynx cancer. In Johnson JT, Didolkar MS, eds. *Head and Neck Cancer*. Hong Kong: Elsevier Science; 1993:465.

61. Al-Sarraf M, Reddy MS: Nasopharyngeal carcinoma. *Curr Treat Options Oncol*. 2002;3:21.

62. Cvitkovic E, Bachouchi M, Armand JP: Nasopharyngeal carcinoma. Biology, natural history, and therapeutic implications. *Hematol Oncol Clin North Am*. 1991;5:821.

63. Dimery IW, Hong WK: Overview of combined modality therapies for head and neck cancer. *J Natl Cancer Inst*. 1993;85:95.

64. Fandi A, Altun M, Azli N, et al: Nasopharyngeal cancer: Epidemiology, staging, and treatment. *Semin Oncol*. 1994;21:382.

65. Ali H, Al-Sarraf M: Chemotherapy in advanced nasopharyngeal cancer. *Oncology*. 2000;14:1223.

66. Huncharek M, Kupelnick B: Combined chemoradiation versus radiation therapy alone in locally advanced nasopharyngeal carcinoma. *Am J Clin Oncol*. 2002;25:219.

67. Orecchia R, Airoldi M, Sola B, et al: Results of chemotherapy plus external reirradiation in the treatment of locally advanced recurrences of nasopharyngeal carcinoma. *Eur J Cancer B Oral Oncol*. 1992;28b:109.

68. Hareyama M, Sakata K, Shirato H, et al: A prospective, randomized trial comparing neoadjuvant chemotherapy with radiotherapy alone in patients with advanced nasopharyngeal carcinoma. *Cancer*. 2002;94:2217.

69. Ma J, Mai HQ, Hong MH, et al: Results of a prospective randomized trial comparing neoadjuvant chemotherapy plus radiotherapy with radiotherapy alone in patients with locoregionally advanced nasopharyngeal carcinoma. *J Clin Oncol*. 2001; 19:1350.

70. Al-Sarraf M, LeBlanc M, et al: Chemoradiotherapy versus radiotherapy in patients with advanced nasopharyngeal cancer: phase III randomized intergroup study 0099. *J Clin Oncol*. 1998; 16:1310.

71. Al-Sarraf M, LeBlanc M, Giri PG, et al: Superiority of 5-year survival with chemoradiotherapy vs. radiotherapy in patients with locally advanced nasopharyngeal cancer. Intergroup 0099 Phase III study: Final report. *Proc Am Soc Clin Oncol*. 2001;20:227a.

72. Choo R, Tannock I: Chemotherapy for recurrent or metastatic carcinoma of the nasopharynx. A review of the Princess Margaret Hospital experience. *Cancer*. 1991;68:2120.

73. Nutting C, Dearnaley DP, Webb S: Intensity-modulated radiation therapy; a clinical review. *Br J of Radiol*. 2000;73:439.

74. Eisbruch A, Martel MK: Parotid gland sparing in patients undergoing bilateral head and neck irradiation; techniques and early results. *Int J Radiat Oncol Biol Phys*. 1996;36:469.

75. Eisbruch A, Ten Haken RK, Kim HM: Dose, volume, and function relationship in parotid salivary glands following conformal, and intensity-modulated irradiation of head and neck cancer. *Int J Radiat Oncol Biol Phys*. 1999;45:577.

76. Xia P, Fu KK, Wong GW: Comparison of treatment plans involving intensity-modulated radiotherapy for nasopharyngeal carcinoma. *Int J Radiat Oncol Biol Phys*. 2000;48:329.

77. Lee N, Xia P, Quivey JM: Intensity-modulated radiotherapy in the treatment of nasopharyngeal carcinoma: An update of the UCSF experience. *Int J Radiat Oncol Biol Phys*. 2002;53:12.

78. Thornto AF, Thornto AF, Jr., Ten Harken RK, Gerhadsson A: Three-dimensional motion analysis of an improved head immobilization system for simulation, CT, MRI, and PET imaging. *Radiother Oncol*. 1991;20:224.

79. Som P, Curtin HD, Mancusco AA: Imaging-based nodal classification for evaluation of neck metastatic adenopathy. *AJR Am J Roentgenol*. 2000;174:837.

80. Nowak PJCM, Wijers OB, Lagerwaard FJ: A three-dimensional CT-based target definition for elective irradiation of the neck. *Int J Radiat Oncol Biol Phys*. 1999;45:33.

81. Gregoire V, Coche E, Cosnard G, et al: Selection and delineation of lymph node target volumes in head and neck conformal radiotherapy. Proposal for standardizing terminology and procedure based on the surgical experience. *Radiother Oncol*. 2000; 56:135.

82. Martinez-Monge R, Fernandes PS, Gupta N, et al: Cross-sectional nodal atlas: A tool for the definition of clinical target volumes in three-dimensional radiation therapy planning. *Radiology*. 1999; 211:815.

83. Lichter AS, Sandler HM, Robertson JM: Clinical experience with three dimensional treatment planning. *Semin Radiat Oncol*. 1992;2:257.

84. Carol MP: Integrated 3D conformal multivane intensity-modulated delivery system for radiotherapy. In Hounsell AR, Williams PC, eds. *XIth International Conference on the Use of Computers in Radiation Therapy*. Vol. 172. Manchester, United Kingdom: Christie Hospital, NHS Trust; 1994.

85. Carol MP, Peacock C: A system for planning and rotational delivery of intensity modulated fields. *Int J Radiat Oncol Biol Phys*. 1995;6:56.

86. Levendag PC, Schmitz PI, Jansen PP, et al: Fractionated high-dose-rate brachytherapy in primary carcinoma of the nasopharynx. *J Clin Oncol*. 1998;16:2213.

87. Levendag PC, Lagerwaard FJ, Noever I, et al: Role of endocavitary brachytherapy with or without chemotherapy in cancer of the nasopharynx. *Int J Radiat Oncol Biol Phys*. 2002;52:755.

88. Wang CC: Re-irradiation of recurrent nasopharyngeal carcinoma—Treatment techniques and results. *Int J Radiat Oncol Biol Phys*. 1987;13:953.

89. Wang CC: Improved local control of nasopharyngeal carcinoma after intracavitary brachytherapy boost. *Am J Clin Oncol*. 1991;14:5.

90. Zhang YW, Liu TF, Fi CX: Intracavitary radiation treatment of nasopharyngeal carcinoma by the high dose rate afterloading technique. *Int J Radiat Oncol Biol Phys*. 1989;16:315.

91. Pryzant RM, Wendt CD, Delclos L, et al: Re-treatment of nasopharyngeal carcinoma in 53 patients. *Int J Radiat Oncol Biol Phys*. 1992;22:941.

92. Teo P, Tsao SY, Leung SF: Afterloading intracavitary radiation treatment of nasopharyngeal carcinoma. Description of a technique and preliminary treatment results. *Acta Oncol*. 1989; 28:525.

93. Hwang JM, Fuk K, Phillips TL: Results and prognostic factors in the retreatment of locally recurrent nasopharyngeal carcinoma. *Int J Radiat Oncol Biol Phys*. 1998;41:1099.

94. Lee N, Hoffman R, Phillips TL, et al: Managing nasopharyngeal carcinoma with intracavitary brachytherapy—One institution's 45 year experience. *J Brachytherapy*. 2002;1:74.

95. Vikram B, Mishra S: Permanent iodine-125 (I-125) boost implants after external radiation therapy in nasopharyngeal cancer. *Int J Radiat Oncol Biol Phys*. 1994;28:699.

96. Harrison LB, Sessions RB, Fass DE, et al: Nasopharyngeal brachytherapy with access via a transpalatal flap. *Am J Surg.* 1992;164:173.

97. Choy D, Sham JS, Wei WI, et al: Transpalatal insertion of radioactive gold grain for the treatment of persistent and recurrent nasopharyngeal carcinoma. *Int J Radiat Oncol Biol Phys.* 1993; 25:505.

98. Syed AM, Puthawala AA, Damore SJ, et al: Brachytherapy for primary and recurrent nasopharyngeal carcinoma: 20 years' experience at Long Beach Memorial. *Int J Radiat Oncol Biol Phys.* 2000;47(5):1311.

99. Levendag PC, Peters R, Meeuwis CA, et al: A new applicator design for endocavitary brachytherapy of cancer in the nasopharynx. *Radiother Oncol.* 1997;45:95.

100. Levendag PC, Lagerwaard FJ, Noever I, et al: High Dose Rate Brachytherapy for Cancer of the Head and Neck. In Nag S, ed. *High Dose Rate Brachytherapy: A Textbook.* Armonk, NY: Futura Publishing Company; 1994:237.

101. Levendag PC, Peters R, Meeuwis CA: A new applicator design for endocavitary brachytherapy of cancer in the nasopharynx. *Radiother Oncol.* 1997;45:95.

102. Kwong DL, Wei Wi, Cheng AC, et al: Long term results of radioactive gold grain implantation for the treatment of persistent and recurrent nasopharyngeal carcinoma. *Cancer.* 2001;91:1105.

103. Lee AW, Law SC, Foo W, et al: Retrospective analysis of patients with nasopharyngeal carcinoma treated during 1976–1985: Survival after local recurrence (see comments). *Int J Radiat Oncol Biol Phys.* 1993;26:773.

104. Mesic JB, Fletcher GH, Goepfert H: Megavoltage irradiation of epithelial tumors of the nasopharynx. *Int J Radiat Oncol Biol Phys.* 1981;7:447.

105. Peters LJ, Harrison ML, Dimery IW, et al: Acute and late toxicity associated with sequential treatment of carcinoma of the nasopharynx. *Int J Radiat Oncol Biol Phys.* 1988;14:623.

106. Grau C, Moller K, Overgaard M, et al: Sensori-neural hearing loss in patients treated with irradiation for nasopharyngeal carcinoma. *Int J Radiat Oncol Biol Phys.* 1991;21:723.

107. Tokars RP, Griem ML: Carcinoma of the nasopharynx and optimization of radiotherapeutic management for tumor control and spinal cord injury. *Int J Radiat Oncol Biol Phys.* 1979; 5:1741.

108. Parsons JT, Fitzgerald CR, Hood CI: The effects of irradiation on the eye and optic nerve. *Int J Radiat Oncol Biol Phys.* 1983; 9:609.

109. Wara WM, Irvine AR, Neger RE: Radiation retinopathy. *Int J Radiat Oncol Biol Phys.* 1979;5:81.

110. de-Schryuver A, Ljunggren JG, Baryd I: Pituitary function in long term survival after radiation therapy of nasopharyngeal tumors. *Acta Radiol Ther.* 1973;12:497.

111. Lam KS, Ho JH, Lee AW, et al: Symptomatic hypothalamic-pituitary dysfunction in nasopharyngeal carcinoma patients following radiation therapy: A retrospective study. *Int J Radiat Oncol Biol Phys.* 1987;13:1343.

112. Rosenthal MB, Goldfine ID: Primary and secondary hypothyroidism in nasopharyngeal carcinoma. *JAMA.* 197;236:1591.

113. Samaan NA, Vieto R, Schultz PN: Hypothalamic, pituitary and thyroid dysfunction after radiotherapy to the head and neck. *Int J Radiat Oncol Biol Phys.* 1982;8:1857.

114. Cheng SW, Ting AC, Lam LK, Wei Wi: Carotid stenosis after radiotherapy for nasopharyngeal carcinoma. *Arch Otolaryngol Head Neck Surg.* 2000;126:517.

115. Bailet JW, Mark RJ, Abemayor E, et al: Nasopharyngeal carcinoma: Treatment results with primary radiation therapy. *Laryngoscope.* 1992;102:965.

116. Vikram B, Mishra UB, Strong EW, et al: Patterns of failure in carcinoma of the nasopharynx: I. Failure at the primary site. *Int J Radiat Oncol Biol Phys.* 1985;11:1455.

117. Wang CC: Carcinoma of the nasopharynx. In Wang CC, ed. *Radiation Therapy for Head and Neck Neoplasms: Indications, Techniques, and Results.* Chicago: Year Book Medical Publishers; 1990:261.

118. Vikram B, Strong EW, Manolatos S, et al: Improved survival in carcinoma of the nasopharynx. *Head Neck Surg.* 1984;2:123.

119. Wang CC: Accelerated hyperfractionation radiation therapy for carcinoma of the nasopharynx. Techniques and results. *Cancer.* 1989;63:2461.

120. Vikram V: Permanent iodine-125 implants for recurrent carcinoma of the nasopharynx: Early results. *Endocurie Hyperth Oncol.* 1986;2:83.

121. Wolden S, Pfister D, Zelefsky M, et al: Intensity modulated radiation therapy improves locoregional control for nasopharyngeal carcinoma. *Proceedings of ASCO.* 2002;21:240a.

122. Cammoun M, Ellouz R, Behi J, et al: Histological types of nasopharyngeal carcinoma in an intermediate risk area. *IARC Sci Publ.* 1978;20:13.

123. Hoppe RT, Williams J, Warnke R, et al: Carcinoma of the nasopharynx—The significance of histology. *Int J Radiat Oncol Biol Phys.* 1978;4:199.

124. Shanmugaratnam K: Histopathology of nasopharyngeal carcinoma: Correlations with epidemiology, survival rates and other biological characteristics. *Cancer.* 1979;44:1029.

125. Hsu MM, Huang SC, Lynn TC, et al: The survival of patients with nasopharyngeal carcinoma. *Otolaryngol Head Neck Surg.* 1982;90:289.

126. Jenkin RD, Anderson JR, Jereb B, et al: Nasopharyngeal carcinoma—A retrospective review of patients less than thirty years of age: A report of Children's Cancer Study Group. *Cancer.* 1981; 47:360.

127. de-Vathaire F, Sancho-Giarnier H, De-The H, et al: Prognostic value of EBV markers in the clinical management of nasopharyngeal carcinoma (NPC): A multicenter follow-up study. *Int J Cancer.* 1988;42:176.

128. Henle W, Ho JH, Henle G, et al: Nasopharyngeal carcinoma: Significance of changes in Epstein-Barr virus-related antibody patterns following therapy. *Int J Cancer.* 1977;20:663.

129. Lynn TC, Tu SM, Kawamura A, Jr: Long-term follow-up of IgG and IgA antibodies against viral capsid antigens of Epstein-Barr virus in nasopharyngeal carcinoma. *J Laryngol Otol.* 1985; 99:567.

130. Neel HBI, Taylor WF: Epstein-Barr virus-related antibody. Changes in titers after therapy for nasopharyngeal carcinoma. *Arch Otolaryngol Head Neck Surg.* 1990;116:1287.

131. Lo YMD, Chan ATC, Chan LYS, et al: Molecular prognostication of nasopharyngeal carcinoma by quantitative analysis of circulating Epstein-Barr virus DNA. *Cancer Res.* 2000;60:6878.

132. Roychowdhury DF, Tseng A, Fu KK, et al: New prognostic factors in nasopharyngeal carcinoma. *Cancer.* 1996;77:1419.

133. Hwang HN: Nasopharyngeal carcinoma in the People's Republic of China: Incidence, treatment, and survival rates. *Radiology.* 1983;149:305.

134. Yan JH, Hu YH, Gu XZ: Radiation therapy of recurrent nasopharyngeal carcinoma. Report on 219 patients. *Acta Radiol (Oncol).* 1983;22:23.

135. Lee AW, Foo W, Law SC, et al: Reirradiation for recurrent nasopharyngeal carcinoma: Factors affecting the therapeutic ratio and ways for improvement. *Int J Radiat Oncol Biol Phys.* 1997;38:43.

136. Feehan PE, Castro JR, Phillips TL, et al: Recurrent locally advanced nasopharyngeal carcinoma treated with heavy charged particle irradiation. *Int J Radiat Oncol Biol Phys.* 1992;23:881.

137. Kondziolka D, Lunsford LD, Choi KN, et al: Stereotactic radiosurgery for squamous cell carcinoma of the nasopharynx. Locally advanced paranasal sinus and nasopharynx tumors treated with hyperfractionated radiation and concomitant infusion cisplatin. *Laryngoscope.* 1991;67:2748.

138. Chua DT, Shan JS, Hung KN, et al: Stereotactic radiosurgery as a salvage treatment for locally persistent and recurrent nasopharyngeal carcinoma. *Head Neck.* 1999;21:620.

Cancer of the Oropharynx

Kenneth S. Hu, MD, Louis B. Harrison, MD,
Bruce Culliney, MD, Adam Dicker, MD, PhD, and
Roy B. Sessions, MD

Tumors of the oropharynx comprise approximately 5000 new cases each year in the United States.[1] Patients with a history of tobacco or alcohol use are at increased risk for these tumors. Such a history can also be associated with other metachronous or synchronous tumors of the aerodigestive tract. The prognosis for oropharyngeal carcinoma depends on the location of the primary tumor and the stage at presentation. The most important cause of death is locoregional recurrence, which, if it occurs, usually manifests itself within 2 years. Patients who survive are at risk for developing a second or third primary cancer in the upper aerodigestive tract or in the lower respiratory tract. The treatment strategies are numerous for these patients, and advances in organ preservation with attention to quality of life (QOL) will be among the major issues for oncologists in the next decade.

ANATOMY OF THE OROPHARYNX

The pharynx is divided into the nasopharynx, oropharynx, and hypopharynx (Fig. 28-1). The oropharynx is located between the soft palate superiorly and the hyoid bone inferiorly. It is continuous with the oral cavity anteriorly and communicates with the nasopharynx above and the supraglottic larynx and hypopharynx below. Within the oropharynx are four different sites: soft palate, tonsillar region (fossa and pillars), base of tongue, and posterior and lateral pharyngeal wall between the nasopharynx and the pharyngoepiglottic fold (Fig. 28-2).

Soft Palate

The soft palate includes the uvula and incompletely separates the oral cavity and oropharynx from the nasopharynx. It is continuous laterally with the tonsillar pillars and attaches anteriorly to the hard palate. It forms both the roof of the oropharynx and the floor of the nasopharynx. The soft palate demarcates the oral cavity from the oropharynx as well as the oropharynx from the nasopharynx. Tumors arising from the oropharyngeal surface are far more common than are those arising from the nasopharyngeal surface.

Tonsillar Region

The palatine (or faucial) tonsils, located posteriorly on the lateral wall of the oropharynx, are almond-shaped structures of largely lymphoid tissue embedded in a fibrous capsule. The tonsillar fossa, which encases the palatine tonsil, is bounded by an anterior and posterior portion, commonly called the "pillars." The tonsillar pillars contain the palatoglossus and palatopharyngeus muscles, respectively, and converge superiorly to join with the soft palate. The inferior portion of the fossa is the glossopalatine sulcus.

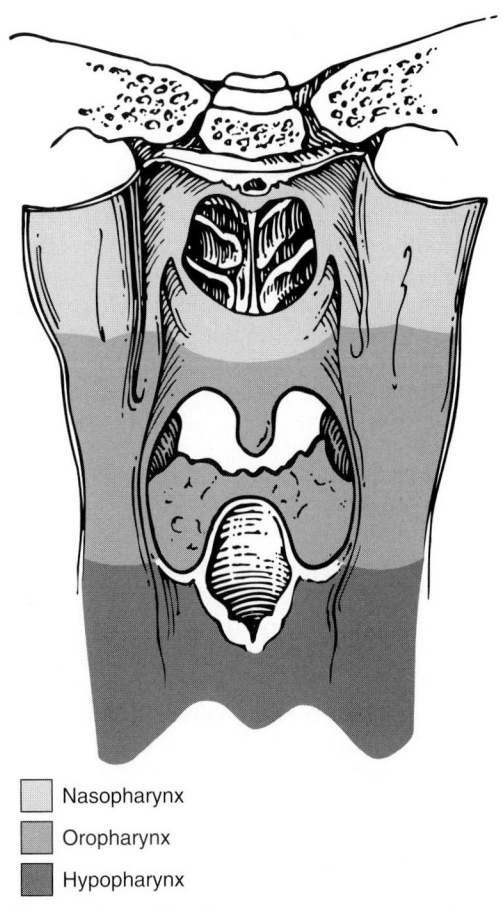

Nasopharynx

Oropharynx

Hypopharynx

Figure 28–1. Regions of the pharynx.

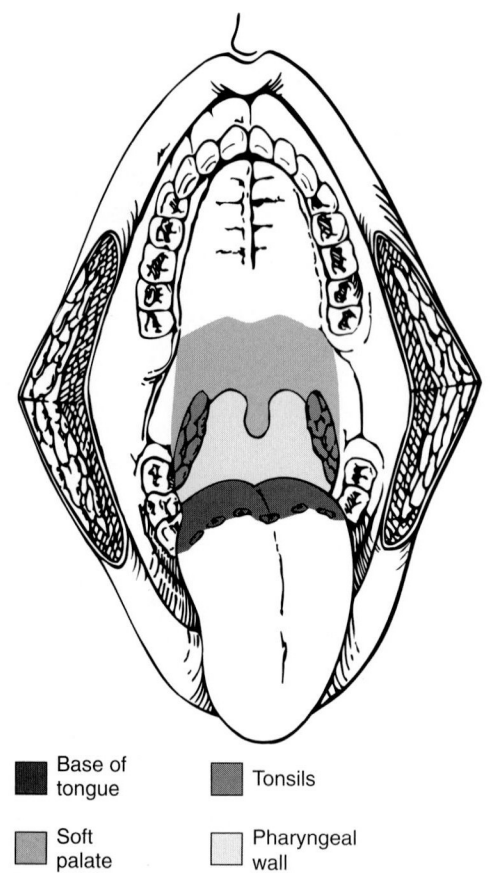

■ Base of tongue

■ Soft palate

■ Tonsils

□ Pharyngeal wall

Figure 28–2. Topographic surface anatomy of the oropharynx; view from oral cavity.

Base of Tongue

The base of tongue is defined as the tissue that extends inferiorly from the circumvallate papilla to the vallecula (base of the epiglottis) and encompasses the pharyngoepiglottic and glossoepiglottic folds. Laterally, it extends to the glossopalatine sulcus. The tongue musculature is composed of the genioglossus, styloglossus, palatoglossus, and hypoglossus muscles. The blood supply is identical to that of the oral tongue, and innervation is via the hypoglossal nerve.

Pharyngeal Wall

The posterior pharyngeal wall starts at the inferior aspect of the nasopharynx in the region of the soft palate and extends to the level of the epiglottis inferiorly. It comprises the posterolateral surfaces of the oropharynx. The pharyngeal constrictor muscles constitute the framework of the pharyngeal wall. The wall is related to the second and third cervical vertebrae and contains the mucosa, submucosa, pharyngobasilar fascia, underlying superior constrictor muscle, and buccopharyngeal fascia. The lateral aspect of the pharyngeal wall is continuous with the pharyngoepiglottic fold and continues into the lateral aspect of the piriform sinus. Nerve supply is from cranial nerves IX and X. The pharyngeal wall is rich in

lymphatics with primary drainage to the retropharyngeal nodes and levels II and III.

Lymphatics of the Oropharynx

The lymphatic drainage of the neck was described in a classic paper by Rouviere[2] in 1938 and has been refined by others.[3,4] The lymph node groups are described by clinical levels I to V as depicted in Figure 28-3.

The primary drainage of the oropharynx is to the jugulodigastric (level II) nodes located in the upper deep jugular chain. The tonsillar region, pharyngeal portion of the soft palate, lateral and posterior oropharyngeal walls, and base of tongue are also drained by the retropharyngeal and parapharyngeal nodes. These nodes are located in the retropharyngeal and parapharyngeal space that is closely related to cranial nerves IX through XII, the internal jugular vein, and the internal carotid artery at the base of skull. The parapharyngeal lymph nodes are also known as the junctional nodes, owing to the junction of the spinal accessory (level V) and upper internal jugular lymphatic chains.

The probability of lymphatic metastasis is related to size and location of the primary tumor within the oropharynx. The order of progression of lymph node metastases usually proceeds superiorly, from the high cervical first-echelon nodes (level II) inferiorly to the midcervical and lower cervical nodes (levels III and IV). Skip metastasis can occur in which a particular lymph node level is bypassed, but this is very unusual. Candela et al.,[5] from 1965 to 1986, evaluated 333 previously untreated patients with primary squamous cell carcinoma (SCC) of the oropharynx or hypopharynx to ascertain the prevalence of neck node metastases by neck level. The patients underwent classic radical neck dissections. Isolated skip metastases outside of level II, III, or IV occurred in only one patient (0.3%). Otherwise, level I or V involvement was always associated with nodal metastases at other levels.[5]

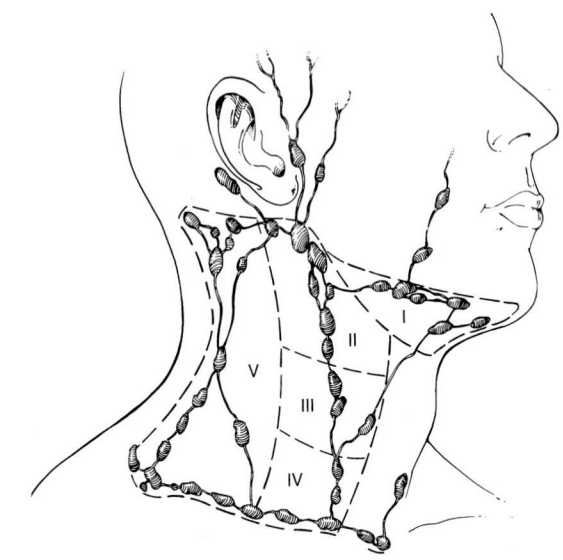

Figure 28–3. Anatomic lymph node levels of the neck.

Table 28–1   Percentage Incidence of Cervical Lymph Node Metastasis as Determined by Clinical Examination

	N0	N1	N2
Oropharyngeal wall			
T1	75	0	25
T2	70	10	20
T3	33	23	45
T4	24	24	52
Soft palate			
T1	92	0	8
T2	64	12	25
T3	35	26	39
T4	33	11	56
Tonsillar fossa			
T1	30	41	30
T2	33	14	54
T3	30	18	52
T4	11	13	77
Base of tongue			
T1	30	15	55
T2	29	15	57
T3	26	23	52
T4	16	9	76

Adapted from Lindberg R: Distribution of cervical lymph node metastases from squamous cell carcinoma of the upper respiratory and digestive tracts. *Cancer.* 1972;29:1446.

Tumors located in the midline (base of tongue, soft palate, and posterior pharyngeal wall) exhibit a higher propensity for bilateral lymphadenopathy. The probability of cervical node metastases, as demonstrated by clinical examination of the soft palate, tonsillar fossa, base of tongue, and oropharyngeal wall, is shown in Table 28-1.[6]

PATHOLOGY

More than 90% of tumors of the oropharynx are SCCs, the remainder being malignant melanomas, minor salivary gland tumors, sarcomas, plasmacytomas, lymphomas, and other rare tumors.[7] Benign and malignant tumors that can be found in the oropharynx are listed in Table 28-2. Metastases to the oropharynx do occur.[8-11] Lymphoepithelioma is more common in the tonsillar region and base of tongue. The distinction between lymphoepithelioma and SCC is important, with the former likely to be particularly radiosensitive.[12] Non-Hodgkin's lymphoma is seen in approximately 5% of tonsillar malignancies and is rarely encountered in the base of tongue.

CLINICAL PRESENTATION AND PATTERNS OF SPREAD

Patients with primary tumors of the oropharynx frequently are asymptomatic until their primary tumors reach a significant size or metastasize to a lymph node in the neck. The usual complaints are that of vague discomfort, irritation, or a mass in the neck. The manifestation of symptoms depends on the location of the primary

Table 28–2   Differential Diagnosis of an Oropharyngeal Mass

Malignant
  Squamous cell carcinoma
  Minor salivary gland tumor
  Lymphoma
  Sarcoma
  Melanoma
  Plasmacytoma
  Other
Benign
  Papilloma
  Retention cyst
  Fibroma
  Lipoma
  Hemangioma
  Lymphangioma
  Neuroma
  Other

tumor within the oropharynx. Some tumors are visualized easily and frequently are found by dentists and clinicians (e.g., tonsil), whereas others are not visualized as easily. The most common complaint is of pain, which can be attributed either to deep infiltration of tumor or to referred pain. The following sections list some of the possible clinical scenarios based on the site of the primary tumor within the oropharynx.

Soft Palate

Tumors of the soft palate are almost exclusively found on the anterior surface (the oropharynx portion as opposed to the nasopharynx portion) (Fig. 28-4). In a study of 359 male U.S. military veterans diagnosed with 424 cancers of the oral cavity and oropharynx, tobacco smoking was found to be more strongly associated with soft-palate lesions than with lesions in more anterior sites.[13] Tumors can extend to involve the tonsillar pillars and the base of

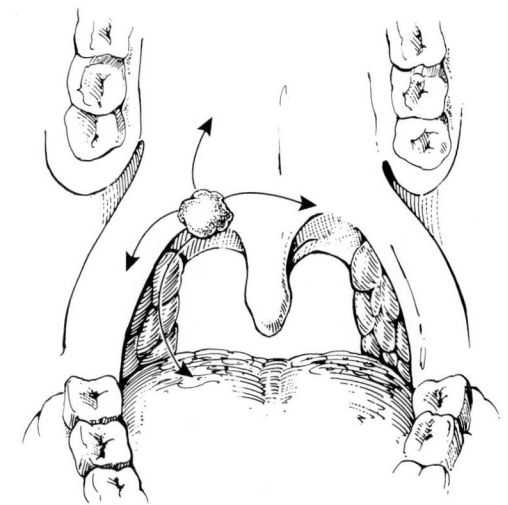

Figure 28–4. Patterns of tumor spread in soft palate.

tongue. Occasionally, these lesions may extend laterally and superiorly as far as the nasopharynx. Involvement of the palatine nerve can result in tumor tracking along this pathway, with extension into the cranium. Lymphatic involvement is primarily to level II. Lesions of the midline and uvula can result in bilateral nodal metastases more frequently than lateralized lesions.

Tonsil

The most common location for a primary tumor of the oropharynx is the anterior tonsillar pillar and tonsil. Common presenting symptoms are ipsilateral referred otalgia, discomfort, poorly fitting dentures, or a sensation of a lump or foreign body in the throat. Lesions involving the anterior tonsillar pillar can appear as areas of dysplasia, inflammation, or a superficial spreading or exophytic lesion. Frequently, these lesions become endophytic, ulcerate, and can spread laterally to the buccal mucosa and directly to the retromolar trigone (Fig. 28-5). Inferior extension to the base of tongue is common. Perez et al.[14] reported that of 218 patients presenting with SCC of the tonsillar region, the soft palate was involved in 131 (60%) and extension to the base of tongue occurred in 120 (55%). Superior extension can involve the soft and hard palate. Medial extension can involve the oral tongue. The close proximity of the anterior tonsillar pillar to the mandible places the periosteum and bone at risk in advanced cases. Posterior extension with destruction of the tonsillar pillars can involve the pterygoid muscles, with subsequent trismus and pain. The lymphatic drainage is primarily to level II but can involve level I and the retropharyngeal and parapharyngeal nodes.

Tumors of the tonsillar fossa (in contrast to those of the tonsillar pillar) are either exophytic or ulcerative and present in more advanced stages than do tumors of the

pillars or soft palate. Approximately 75% of patients will present with stage III or IV disease, for which the patterns of extension are similar to those of the tonsillar pillar. In addition, lateral extension can involve the parapharyngeal space toward the base of skull, causing neurological signs and symptoms. Tumors of the posterior tonsillar pillar can extend inferiorly and involve the pharyngoepiglottic fold and the posterior aspect of the thyroid cartilage. These lesions also more frequently involve the level V nodes due to extension to the spinal accessory chain group.

The probability of clinical lymph node involvement is greater with tumors of the tonsillar fossa, especially contralateral involvement in contrast to that of the tonsillar pillar. The lymphatic drainage depends on the location of the primary tumor. Lindberg[6] described nodal metastases in 76% of patients with tonsillar fossa tumors. The most common nodal group was level II. Contralateral lymph nodes were detected in 11% of patients. In contrast, tumors of the anterior tonsillar pillar or retromolar trigone region have an incidence of ipsilateral lymph node metastases of 45%, level II being the most common nodal-bearing region. Contralateral adenopathy occurred in only 5% of patients.

Base of Tongue

SCC of the base of tongue is highly insidious. The base of tongue is almost devoid of pain fibers, and frequently these tumors are asymptomatic until they have progressed significantly. Many who present with a neck node are found, on examination, to have a base-of-tongue lesion. Visualization of this area on physical examination is difficult; therefore, a lesion is often missed.[15] Patients may experience the sensation of a mass or discomfort in the throat, with bleeding and pain at later stages. Patients also might experience difficulty in swallowing or speaking. Occasionally, referred otalgia is the first symptom. If the size of the primary tumor increases such that it involves the pterygoid muscles, trismus can result.

Extension anteriorly can involve the oral tongue, superior and lateral extension can involve the tonsil, and inferior extension can involve the vallecula, epiglottis, and pre-epiglottic space (Fig. 28-6). Locally advanced base-of-tongue tumors can infiltrate the deep muscle and cause fixation.

Lymph node metastasis is common due to the rich lymphatic drainage of the base of tongue. The most common first-echelon nodal region is level II, though involvement of levels III and IV also is seen. Approximately 70% or more of patients will present with ipsilateral metastases, and 10% to 20% will present with bilateral nodal metastases.

Pharyngeal Wall

Tumors of the pharyngeal wall region generally are diagnosed in an advanced stage due to the silent location in which they develop. Symptoms include pain, bleeding, and a mass in the neck. Disease involvement can extend

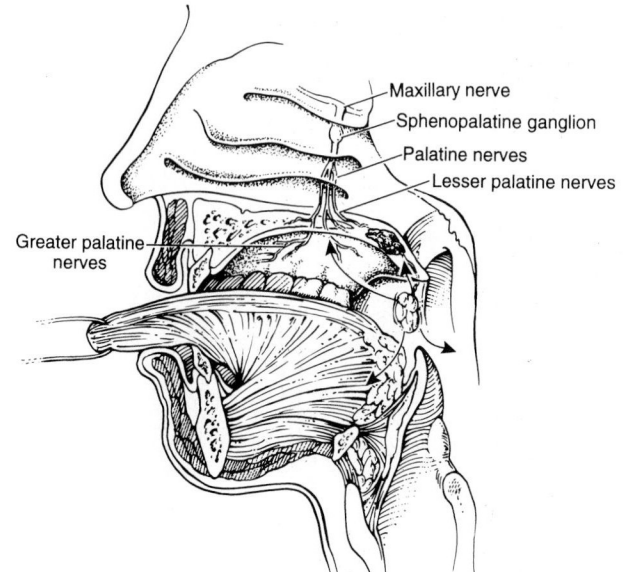

Figure 28–5. Patterns of spread of tonsillar carcinoma.

Maxillary nerve
Sphenopalatine ganglion
Palatine nerves
Lesser palatine nerves
Greater palatine nerves

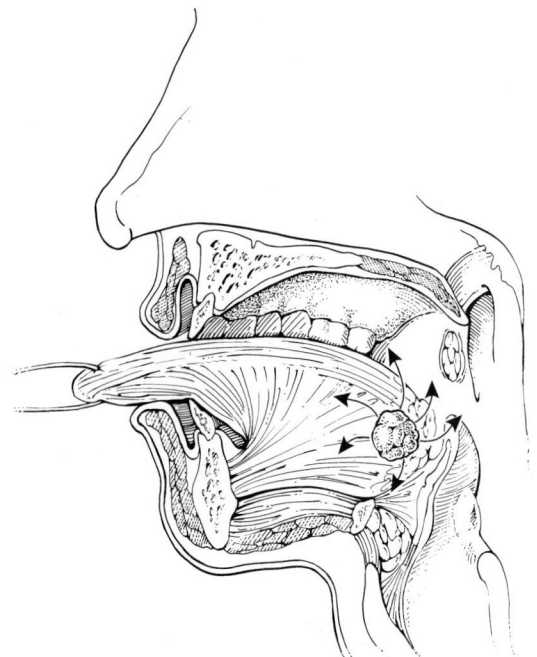

Figure 28–6. Patterns of spread of base-of-tongue cancer.

to the nasopharynx superiorly, the prevertebral fascia posteriorly, and piriform sinuses and hypopharyngeal wall inferiorly. Clinically palpable cervical lymph node metastases are present in 25% of patients with T1 lesions, 30% with T2 lesions, 66% with T3 lesions, and more than 75% with T4 disease. Because most

pharyngeal wall tumors extend past the midline, bilateral cervical metastases are common. Retropharyngeal lymph nodes are at particular risk for involvement and should be addressed.

Referred Otalgia

Referred otalgia can be one of the first symptoms that a patient experiences with a mass in the oropharynx. The pathway for this referred pain is mediated by cranial nerves IX and X. The pathophysiology for otalgia depends on the site of pain (Fig. 28-7).

DIAGNOSTIC EVALUATION

History

The history should be part of a comprehensive evaluation of any patient with head and neck cancer. Patients usually present with pain and dysphagia and, occasionally, referred otalgia. If the history strongly reveals tobacco and alcohol use, efforts should be made to determine whether the patient is an alcoholic and continues to smoke. Alcoholic smokers are at risk for other chronic diseases of the heart, lung, peripheral vascular system, and liver, and may present with signs of malnutrition. Before instituting any therapeutic modality, patients should cease alcohol and tobacco use. It may be necessary to guide the patient toward cessation programs. Clearly, those who discontinue smoking will better tolerate treatment and obtain a better result.[16]

Figure 28–7. Neural pathways of referred otalgia. For pain sensed in the front of the helix and tragus, the skin of the anterior wall of the external auditory canal, the tympanic membrane, and the temple, pain is referred via the *auriculotemporal nerve*, which joins the lingual nerve, where the two become the mandibular nerve and enter the foramen ovale. The sensation of deep ear pain is via the *tympanic nerve (Jacobson's)*, which joins the *glossopharyngeal nerve (cranial nerve [CN] IX)* as the two traverse the jugular foramen. These general somatic afferent fibers innervate the base of tongue, inner surface of the tympanic membrane, and upper pharynx. Pain sensation in the back of the pinna, the posterior wall of the external auditory canal, and the external surface of the tympanic membrane is via the *auricular nerve (Arnold's)*, which joins the superior *laryngeal nerve (CN X)*, which in turn innervates the larynx, pharynx, and epiglottis as it traverses the jugular foramen.

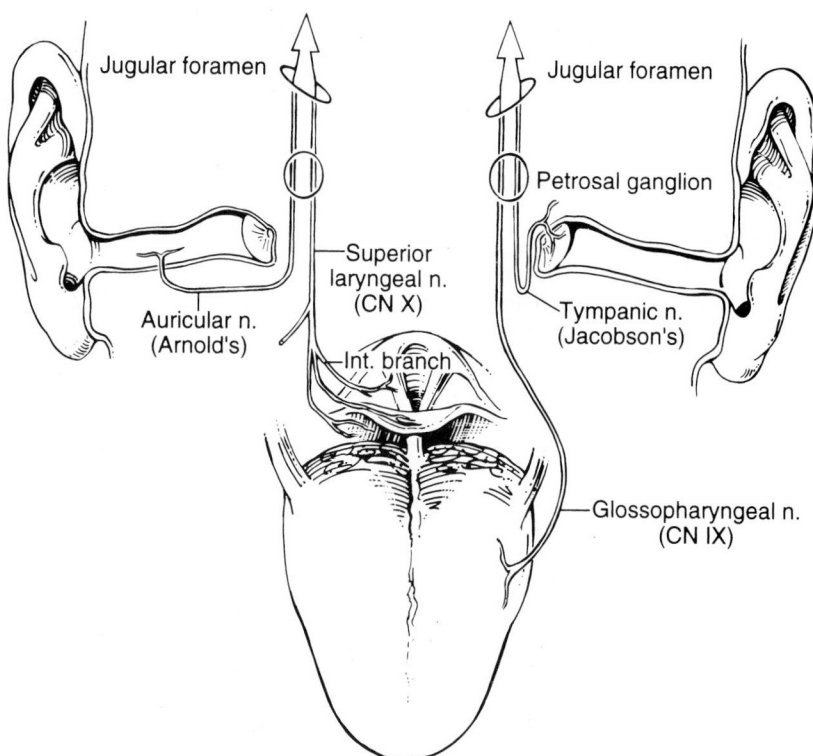

Physical Examination

Specific aspects of the physical examination should include evaluation of the lesion (exophytic or infiltrative), tongue mobility, and palatal motion. Fixation of the tongue will result in incomplete protrusion or deviation of the tongue to the side of tumor involvement. In patients with a smoking and drinking history, three sites have a greater propensity for developing carcinoma than do others in the oral cavity and oropharynx: floor of mouth, ventrolateral tongue, and lingual aspect of the retromolar trigone and the anterior tonsillar pillar.[17,18]

For tumors of the tonsil or lateral pharyngeal wall, the examiner should test for anesthesia in the distribution of the ipsilateral mental nerve (V3). Any abnormality might suggest involvement of the inferior alveolar nerve in its pathway as it courses through the mandible or the base of skull and may direct the appropriate imaging study.[12] The tonsil is adjacent to the ascending ramus of the mandible, and posterolateral to the tonsil is the parapharyngeal space. Tumors may extend into this area and be palpable in the neck on bimanual palpation. Owing to the relationship of the anterior tonsil (palatoglossus muscle) and the base of tongue, tonsillar cancers frequently extend into this region.

After completion of the direct visual examination, indirect mirror examination followed by indirect fiber-optic nasopharyngoscopy is performed. We photograph or extensively diagram the physical findings in every patient. This often includes a videotape. Such records are an excellent means of documenting the physical findings and of comparing future examination results to the initial presentation; they also serve as a teaching tool.

At the conclusion of the examination of the oral cavity and oropharynx, bimanual palpation of the floor of mouth, mandible, and base of tongue should be performed. In select cases, an examination under anesthesia is recommended to obtain information that is not completely accessible during an office examination.

Initial Workup and Radiographic Evaluation

In addition to a history and physical examination, a complete blood cell count, screening profile, and chest roentgenogram are recommended. Biopsy of a suspicious lesion is necessary to confirm the diagnosis.[19] A more detailed metastatic workup is indicated only when strong clinical or laboratory suspicion of metastatic disease exists.

Staging

The current staging criteria for tumors of the oropharynx, as defined by the American Joint Committee on Cancer,[20] is listed in Table 28-3. This is a clinical staging system, not a pathological staging system. If radiographical information reveals a discrepancy from clinical examination, this should be noted (e.g., clinical—cT2, N2b, radiographic—rN2c). Current staging allows the

Table 28–3 Classification of Oropharyngeal Cancer

Primary tumor (T)	
T1	Tumor ≤2 cm in greatest dimension
T2	Tumor >2 cm but not >4 cm in greatest dimension
T3	Tumor >4 cm in greatest dimension
T4a	Tumor invades deep/extrinsic muscles of tongue, medial pterygoid, larynx, hard palate, or mandible
T4b	Tumor invades lateral pterygoid muscle, pterygoid plates, lateral nasopharynx, or skull base or encases carotid artery
Regional lymph nodes (N)	
N0	No regional lymph node metastasis
N1	Metastasis in a single ipsilateral node, ≤3 cm in greatest dimension
N2a	Metastasis in a single ipsilateral node, >3 cm but <6 cm
N2b	Metastasis in multiple ipsilateral nodes, >3 cm but <6 cm
N2c	Metastasis in bilateral or contralateral lymph nodes, none >6 cm
N3	Metastasis in a lymph node >6 cm
Distant metastasis (M)	
M0	No distant metastasis present
M1	Distant metastasis present
Stage	
Stage I	T1, N0, M0
Stage II	T2, N0, M0
Stage III	T3, N0, M0 or T1-3, N1, M0
Stage IVa	T4a, N0-2, M0 or T1-3, N2, M0
IVb	T4b, any N, M0 or any T, N3, M0
IVc	Any T, any N, M1

Greene FL, Page DL, Fleming ID, et al (eds): *AJCC Cancer Staging Manual*, 6/E, New York: Springer 2002.

radiographical findings to factor into the staging designation.

Dental Evaluation and Prophylaxis

Treatment of the oropharynx by external beam radiation therapy (EBRT) can result in a number of temporary and permanent effects on the oral cavity and oropharynx. Among these are mucositis, xerostomia, and infections. Dentulous patients are at increased risk for dental caries due to the reduction in salivary flow, pH, and proliferation of bacteria believed to be responsible for caries. A complete dental evaluation should be performed before any therapy is undertaken. This includes panorex even in edentulous patients (to rule out retained dental elements), identification of nonrestorable teeth for pretreatment extraction, construction of dental trays for fluoride rinse and protection against scatter radiation from metal fillings, as well as education about long-term oral hygiene.

STANDARD THERAPEUTIC APPROACHES

Treatment decisions depend on both the ability of a particular modality to control the primary tumor and on the state of the neck and its associated morbidity. In general, early-stage disease can be treated by either radiation therapy (RT) or surgery, whereas more advanced lesions are often treated by combinations of these methods. RT is chosen more often than surgery for most early lesions because the cure rates are high and the functional outcome is better. Generally, chemotherapy is reserved for patients with advanced disease or for certain organ-sparing protocols. In the following sections, outcomes are reported by subsite of the oropharynx. The results from altered fractionation and chemoradiation trials are then summarized with regard to oropharyngeal tumors.

Soft Palate

SELECTION OF THERAPEUTIC MODALITY

Early Disease

For early-stage lesions of the soft palate, either surgical resection or RT has provided excellent local control. Most patients are treated with RT because the results are excellent and the functional result is probably better. Also, because many lesions are near the midline, radiation treatment of the primary site and both sides of the neck is easy. In general, more morbidity ensues with surgical therapy to these same areas, especially if postoperative radiation becomes necessary.

Advanced Disease

Patients with advanced soft-palate disease usually receive combined surgery and postoperative RT. The use of RT alone has been reported, and the results for advanced-stage lesions are suboptimal.[21] However, increasing evidence demonstrates that concurrent chemoradiation improves locoregional control and survival compared to radiation alone and is therefore gaining wider acceptance as an alternative treatment option for advanced oropharynx cancers.[22-24]

Tonsillar Region

SELECTION OF THERAPEUTIC MODALITY

Early Disease

Early lesions in the tonsillar region can be treated by RT or surgery. The use of RT as the definitive treatment for tumors of the tonsillar fossa is appropriate for T1, T2, and T3 (exophytic) tumors. Radiation is generally preferred because the results are excellent, and the functional outcome is better. Treatment entails portals that include the primary site and ipsilateral neck, including the retropharyngeal nodes. Care is taken to avoid irradiating the contralateral parotid gland to reduce the incidence of xerostomia. For those patients treated surgically, either a transoral or mandibulotomy approach is generally used for the primary site. When better exposure is required, a combined lip-splitting incision with an anterior midline or lateral mandibulotomy is used. If there is superficial extension to the periosteum of the mandible, a partial mandibulectomy may be performed. For clinically negative neck nodes, a modified supraomohyoid neck dissection, as a staging procedure, is often performed. If nodes are positive, postoperative radiation is added.

Advanced Disease

Patients with stage III and IV tonsillar disease can be managed in several ways. For infiltrative or endophytic T3 or T4 lesions, either surgery combined with postoperative RT or an organ-preserving approach involving chemotherapy should be used. Definitive radiation with the addition of a neck dissection for node-positive patients is often used if the primary site is early stage. However, for locally advanced lesions, combined-modality treatment consisting of surgery followed by RT is traditionally recommended; however, based on recent trials, chemoradiation and planned neck dissection in those with advanced neck disease should be considered.[22-24] Surgery for advanced disease generally entails a segmental mandibulectomy.

Base of Tongue

SELECTION OF THERAPEUTIC MODALITY

Early Disease

Early-stage base-of-tongue disease is successfully treated with either surgery or definitive RT. The results are equivalent for local control and survival. The morbidity of a surgical procedure must be weighed against the morbidity of RT. In the overwhelming majority of cases, RT is selected because it provides a better functional result and quality-of-life outcome.

Surgical Therapy

Select patients with small base-of-tongue lesions and negative neck nodes can be managed with primary resection and elective neck dissection. A significant percentage will be found to harbor positive microscopic nodes, thereby necessitating postoperative RT. Therefore, for purposes of maximizing functional outcome and using only one modality, primary RT is the preferred strategy. Surgery generally is reserved for patients who cannot receive RT or for those with particularly endophytic, locally advanced lesions that are difficult to control with RT alone.

In contrast, patients with nodal metastases routinely will undergo a surgical procedure in the neck if the primary tumor is being treated by radiation alone. Preferably, the neck dissection is performed at the completion of RT. If the primary tumor is being managed surgically, surgery followed by RT is preferred. In our practice, patients generally undergo a combination of EBRT and a brachytherapy (BT) implant (discussed later). In this setting, the implant and neck dissection are carried out during the same anesthetic period, approximately 3 weeks after the EBRT. Andersen et al.[25] have shown that preservation of the spinal accessory nerve in a modified neck dissection in patients with clinically evident nodal metastases was not associated with increased risk of treatment failure in the dissected neck.

Base-of-tongue tumors may be resected transorally or via a mandibulotomy and transhyoid pharyngotomy. The transoral approach is indicated only for small, well-circumscribed lesions that are located superficially. The mandibulotomy technique allows superior access and is frequently combined with a graft.[26] Frequently, when a patient has evidence of bone invasion or close encroachment of tumor to bone, a mandibulectomy is performed. The use of a flap or plate with this procedure depends on the age of the patient, amount of tissue resected, and anticipated functional or cosmetic outcome.

Patients with advanced tumors usually require a major or total glossectomy. In addition, some patients may require a total glossectomy due to local extension of their tumor. The need for laryngeal resection (either subtotal supraglottic resection or total laryngectomy) depends on the extent of disease and the risk of aspiration. In most patients in whom a laryngectomy is deemed necessary for base-of-tongue cancer, the indication is for prevention of chronic aspiration, not for oncological purposes.

Postoperatively, patients will spend a great deal of time learning to swallow and avoiding aspiration. If the dysfunction is significant, the patient may require placement of a percutaneous endoscopic gastrostomy (PEG), which can be performed at the time of surgery.[27] A prosthesis may have to be constructed to aid speech and swallowing. Speech rehabilitation is started as soon as possible while the patient is still in the hospital.

Advanced Disease

Major resection has traditionally been recommended in patients with advanced base-of-tongue disease. This often entails a total laryngectomy as well as a bone or tongue resection followed by postoperative RT. Although significant advances have been made for the laryngectomy, a significant rehabilitation process ensues for all patients, and some never regain the ability to communicate orally. In an effort to improve QOL, other approaches such as the combined use of chemotherapy and RT for organ preservation are now considered appropriate treatment options. RT alone (with the addition of neck dissection for patients with palpable nodes at presentation) is also used for certain moderately advanced lesions. Most patients, even those with advanced disease, can be offered nonsurgical options that provide local control equivalent to that achieved surgically and better QOL. Primary surgery is not common in most centers, including our own.

Pharyngeal Wall

SELECTION OF THERAPEUTIC MODALITY

Early Disease

Early lesions of the pharyngeal wall can be treated by RT or surgery. RT is generally preferred because the results are good to excellent and confer less functional impairment than is likely after surgery. Treatment portals are the primary site and bilateral neck, including the retropharyngeal nodes. For those treated surgically, a transhyoid approach or anterior pharyngotomy is generally used for the primary site. A bilateral modified neck dissection is often performed. If nodes are positive, postoperative RT is added.

Advanced Disease

Most locally advanced lesions are best approached with combined-modality treatment consisting of surgery followed by RT or an organ-preservation strategy. A number of different surgical approaches can be used, among them a circumferential pharyngectomy, pharyngoesophagectomy, pharyngolaryngectomy, or pharyngolaryngoesophagectomy.[28] When primary repair is impossible, a number of reconstructive options are available: pectoralis major myocutaneous flap, free revascularized radial forearm flap, transposed stomach,[29] or free revascularized jejunum.[30] Due to the high incidence of retropharyngeal and cervical lymph node involvement, postoperative RT is recommended.

SIMULATION

Radiation Techniques

For optimal treatment planning, a thorough review of the diagnostic films, endoscopic findings, and description of the examination under anesthesia is a prerequisite to determine the target volume.

In general, oropharyngeal cancer patients are treated with a three-field technique that uses isocentrically opposed lateral fields matched to a lower anterior neck field. Either 4-MV or 6-MV energies or ^{60}Co is used. Patients are generally treated in the supine position, with the neck maximally extended on a well-fitting headrest. To facilitate neck extension, we use a headrest and cloth straps placed around the patient's wrists and attached by Velcro to a wooden board by the patient's feet. This aids in pulling the shoulders inferiorly to maximize exposure of the head and neck. A shoulder pull-down device must be used for lesions extending inferiorly into the larynx or hypopharynx such that the shoulders are out of the lateral portals. In such cases, the patient should be reminded not to swallow during treatment or while the simulation films are taken. Contour at the level of the vocal cords and tissue compensators are chosen to homogenize the dose to the larynx.

A bite block is used to facilitate immobilization and reduce the amount of normal tissue situated in the treatment field. For base-of-tongue tumors, the bite block keeps the primary tumor within the field, whereas for a soft-palate tumor it helps to reduce the amount of tongue that would be unnecessarily treated. It may be customized by molding 2.4-mm Aquaplast around a tongue depressor blade and inserting it into the patient's mouth while the patient is in the desired treatment position. The bite block must be placed as far posteriorly as possible to ensure that it functions properly. If dental fluoride trays are to be worn during treatment, they should be in place during the simulation. The setup is performed under radiographic guidance. Additional neck or shoulder immobilization may be considered particularly if three-dimensional (3D) or intensity-modulated radiation therapy (IMRT) techiques are used.

The spinal cord must be blocked at the junction of the lateral portals and low anterior neck field to prevent overdosage. This may be positioned in the posterior-inferior aspect of the portal field or the superior central portion of the low anterior neck field, depending on where the tumor volume is located and if the larynx can be shielded. In the first phase of treatment, we typically treat to a dose of 45 Gy, then come down off cord by splitting the initial field along the middle of the vertebral body into an anterior photon field and posterior electron strip.

Treatment planning computed tomographic (CT) scans to define tumor, the clinical target volume (CTV), and the planning target volume (PTV) are obtained if 3D therapy or IMRT is to be delivered. CT scans with 3-mm slices should be obtained in the region containing target volume while images of those areas below or above the target should be acquired with 5-mm thick cuts. In accordance with International Commission on Radiation Units (ICRU) Report #50, the gross tumor volume is all gross disease determined by clinical examination, the CTV is defined as the gross tumor volume plus areas containing potential microscopic disease. Typically, this is a margin of 1 to 2 cm with a minimum of 5 mm. The PTV has an additional margin on the CTV to compensate for treatment setup error and internal organ motion. The minimum additional margin of 5 mm is needed.

Lymph nodes at risk in patients with oropharyngeal lesion include: (1) submental (Level Ia) if the submandibular lymph nodes or floor of mouth is involved; and (2) submandibular (Level Ib), especially for base of tongue, tonsil cancers, or patients with involvement of the upper jugular nodes. Upper, middle, and lower jugular lymph nodes, supraclavicular lymph nodes (Levels II to IV), and retropharyngeal/parapharyngeal nodes are treated bilaterally in nearly all cases except if unilateral irradiation of a tonsil lesion is considered (see Fig. 28-3). Posterior cervical lymph nodes (level V) must be included if jugular nodal metastases exist.

Soft Palate

The CTV should include the primary site and involved lymph nodes with elective treatment of potential occult disease in the ipsilateral jugular, supraclavicular, and retropharyngeal nodes as well as the contralateral neck nodes for midline lesions using opposed lateral portals and a low anterior neck field matched above the larynx. Figure 28-8 demonstrates a typical field.

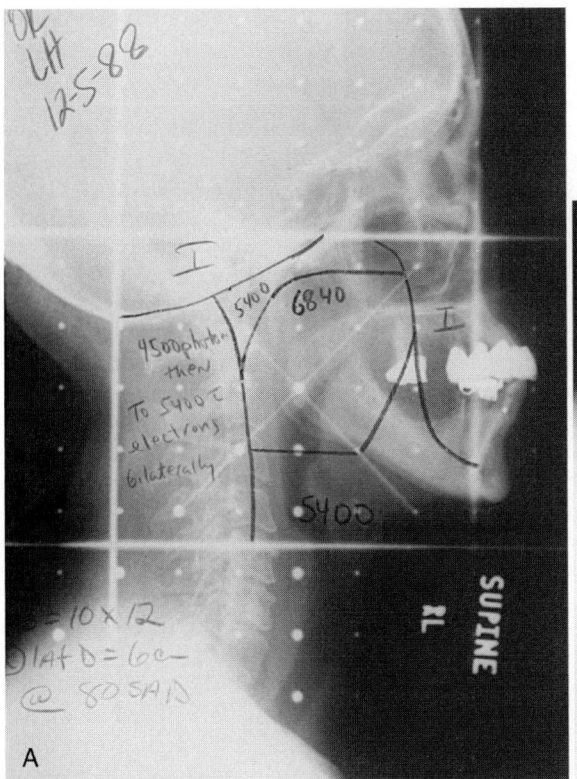
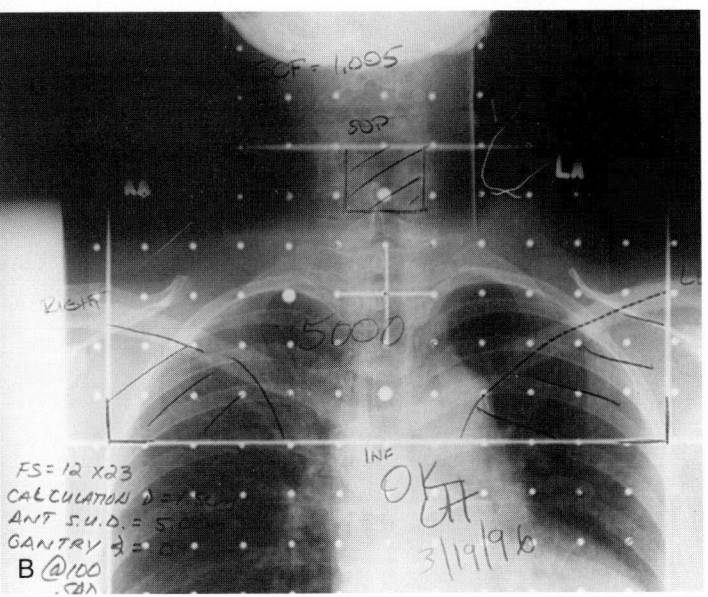

Figure 28–8. Simulation films of patient with early-stage cancer of the soft palate. This patient was treated with external-beam radiation therapy to the primary site and both sides of the neck. Opposed lateral portals **(A)** were used in conjunction with a low anterior neck field **(B).** The primary site and low neck regions received 45 Gy, after which a spinal cord block was placed. Then the primary site and upper neck regions, including the retropharyngeal nodes, were treated to 54 Gy. The final dose to the primary site was 68.4 Gy. Fraction size is 1.8 Gy per day. The lower neck is treated with an anterior portal to 50 Gy over 5 weeks. The posterior neck regions are boosted with electrons to protect the spinal cord to 54 Gy. The spinal cord is protected at the junction of the lateral and low anterior fields by a midline block in the low neck field. The block also protects the larynx. On setup, the field junction is placed above the thyroid notch, but below the hyoid bone.

Tonsil

Lesions that cross the midline, involve the tongue base, or involve N2 or more advanced neck disease should be treated with bilateral opposed portals and a low neck field that protects the larynx and spinal cord at the field junction.

For lateralized lesions of the tonsil and soft palate, radiation is given via a wedged pair that incorporates the primary site and the ipsilateral neck. The upper neck is treated in the same portals as is the primary site; the low neck is treated with a single anteroposterior field, with the larynx and the spinal cord protected at the field junction. In general, most T1 to T2 lesions in patients with an N0 or N1 neck can be treated with ipsilateral fields (Fig. 28-9). At the time of simulation, a bite block is used and all scars are marked with wire. A CT scan is performed to assist in treatment planning for lesions treated unilaterally. For patients who will receive bilateral radiation, a planning CT scan is generally not required.

The CTV of the ipsilateral treatment should include the primary lesion as well as the ipsilateral jugular vein and retropharyngeal/supraclavicular lymph nodes. Attention should be given to outline the contralateral salivary gland so that it may be avoided during treatment planning. If disease extends to the base of tongue, then EBRT alone is not as effective as EBRT plus implant to the tongue.[31] In this case, full-dose EBRT is delivered, followed by an interstitial ^{192}Ir implant as a boost to the tongue portion of the target.

Base of Tongue

Primary RT is the preferred definitive treatment for most tumors of the base of tongue. It is the sole primary therapy for most T1, T2, and many T3 (exophytic) tumors. For infiltrative or endophytic T3 or T4 lesions, either surgery combined with postoperative RT or an organ preservation approach using RT and chemotherapy should be used. The target volume of the parallel opposed fields should include the base of tongue and margin that will incorporate a portion of the oral tongue, vallecula, pharyngeal walls, and suprahyoid epiglottis, and the superior portion of the preepiglottic space. Due to the high probability of lymph node metastasis, these portals include the bilateral regional and retropharyngeal lymph node groups. This is true, too, in the case of the patient with a clinically "negative neck."

Our preferred strategy entails EBRT followed by an interstitial ^{192}Ir implant as a boost to the base of tongue. (See Brachytherapy section later.) We believe that this offers the most consistent, excellent local control and best functional results compared with either EBRT alone or to primary surgery.

Pharyngeal Wall

Definitive radiation with the addition of a neck dissection for node-positive patients can be considered in patients with T1-2 tumors. For pharyngeal wall tumors, radiation treatment planning is more complicated due to the close proximity of the spinal cord to the primary lesion and involved pharyngeal lymph nodes, both of which may extend posterolaterally around the anterior portion of the vertebral body. Therefore, particular attention must be given to the posterior edge of the off-cord treatment field. A number of strategies have been suggested to overcome this problem.[32] First, the sharpest beam edge must be used to avoid underdosing the posterior aspect of the tumor. This is accomplished by the use of a 6-MV or 4-MV beam and a split beam technique, which blocks the posterior field, thereby eliminating posterior divergence. Second, custom cerrobend blocks should be used to define the posterior border. Third, the posterior border should be placed at the most anterior aspect of the spinal cord. Finally, frequent portal films throughout treatment are necessary to ensure proper setup and spinal cord protection.

Another method of addressing pharyngeal wall tumors that wrap around the spine has been described by Grimard et al.,[33] who use an asymmetric arc technique consisting of two posterior arcs with closure of one jaw beyond the central axis. Each arc delivers the total dose to each ipsilateral side, whereas the median region of the U-shaped volume is treated by the summation of both arcs. Alternatively, conformal planning with 3D therapy or IMRT may be considered.

Dose and Fractionation

PRIMARY SITE

In general for T1-2 lesions involving the soft palate, tonsil, pharyngeal wall, and T1 lesions of the tongue base, doses of 66 to 70 Gy 6½ to 7 weeks with conventional fractionation (1.8 to 2.0 Gy/fraction) are recommended for definitive radiotherapy. However, for T3-4 oropharyngeal and T2 base-of-tongue cancers, several studies have demonstrated better locoregional control when either accelerated or hyperfractionated regimens are compared to conventional fractionation.[34-40] Thus, the dose may range from 70 to 81.6 Gy, depending on the radiation regimen chosen. We favor a delayed, accelerated, hyperfractionated schedule in which a concomitant boost is delivered as a second daily dose to the final conedown field during weeks 5 and 6 of radiation. The dose given is 1.6 Gy after an interfraction interval of 6 hours after 1.8 Gy is delivered to the A.M. field. A total of 16 Gy is delivered with the concomitant boost in addition to 54 Gy given in the A.M. for a total 70 Gy/6 weeks.

For locally advanced lesions treated, the addition of concurrent chemotherapy to either conventional or altered fractionated radiation has been beneficial compared to radiation alone.[22-24,41] We have combined our delayed, accelerated, hyperfractionated schedule with concurrent cis-platinum (100 mg/m^2 weeks 1 and 4 of radiation) to treat head and neck cancer including oropharyngeal lesions that are unresectable[42] or require organ preservation.[43]

For patients undergoing BT implant boost, the primary site is treated to a dose of 54 Gy in 30 fractions

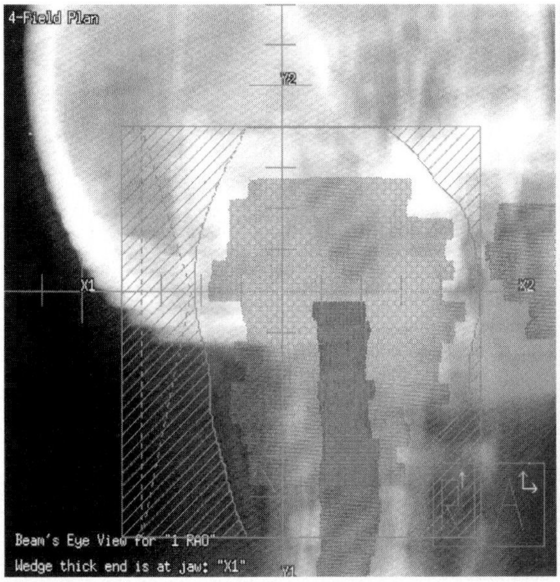

A

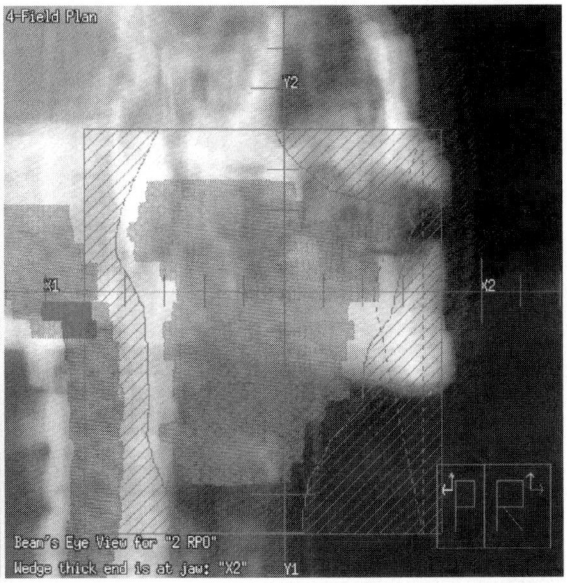

B

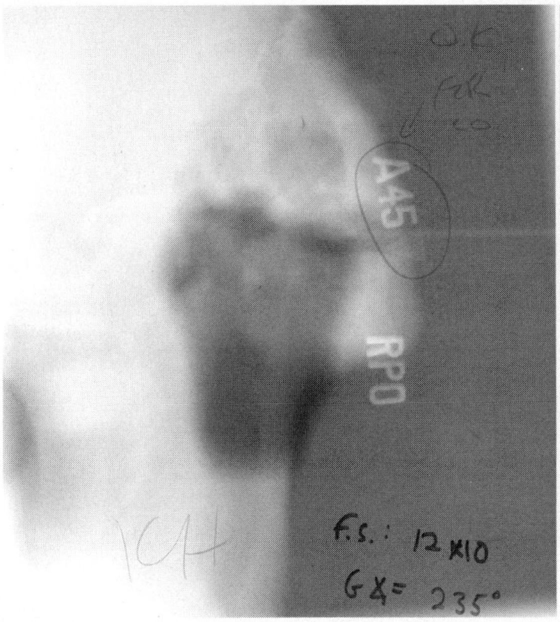

Beam's Eye View for "1 RAO"
Wedge thick end is at jaw: "X1"

Beam's Eye View for "2 RPO"
Wedge thick end is at jaw: "X2"

4-Field Plan

4-Field Plan

C

A45

RPO

f.s.: 12×10
G∢= 235°

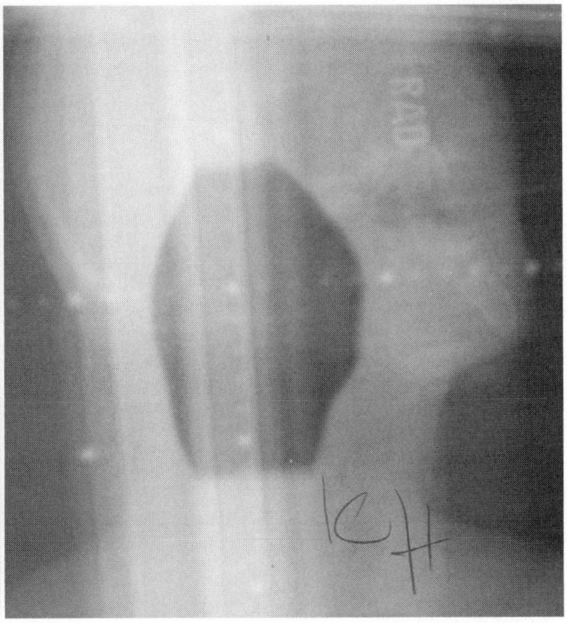

D

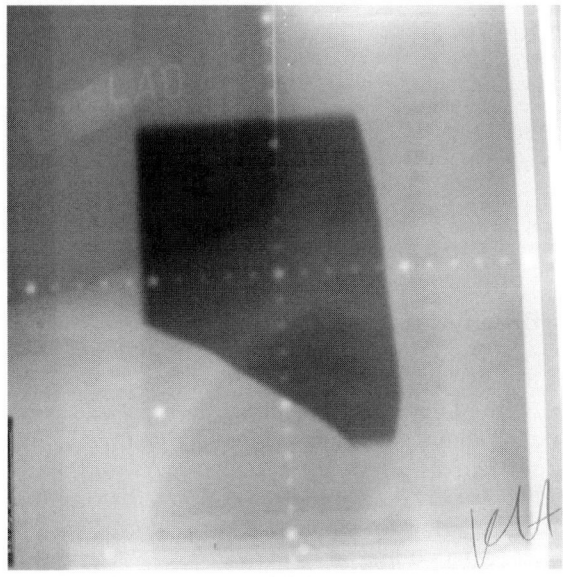

E

Figure 28–9. Simulation of an early-stage tonsil cancer with a wedge-pair technique and localization films of a tonsil cancer implant. The patient is a 43-year-old HIV-positive female who presented with a T2N0 right tonsillar carcinoma and was treated with an ipsilateral wedge-pair technique to cover the primary site. These fields were matched with an angled oblique field to treat the ipsilateral neck electively. The primary site received 70 Gy in 2-Gy fractions while the low anterior neck received 50 Gy in 2-Gy fractions. Fifteen months later, the patient presented with a metachronous left tonsillar squamous cell carcinoma with involved cervical lymph node. She underwent tonsillectomy and neck dissection. Margins were positive and multiple lymph nodes were involved. She was subsequently treated with a brachytherapy boost to the tonsillar site and wedge-pair technique to treat the contralateral neck and primary site. The brachytherapy boost was needed to treat the primary site for the positive margin as a full course of external beam radiation could not be given without exceeding normal tissue tolerance. **A–E,** 3D-planned wedge-pair fields treating the initial primary lesion involving the right tonsil matched above the larynx to an ipsilateral low neck field.

Continued

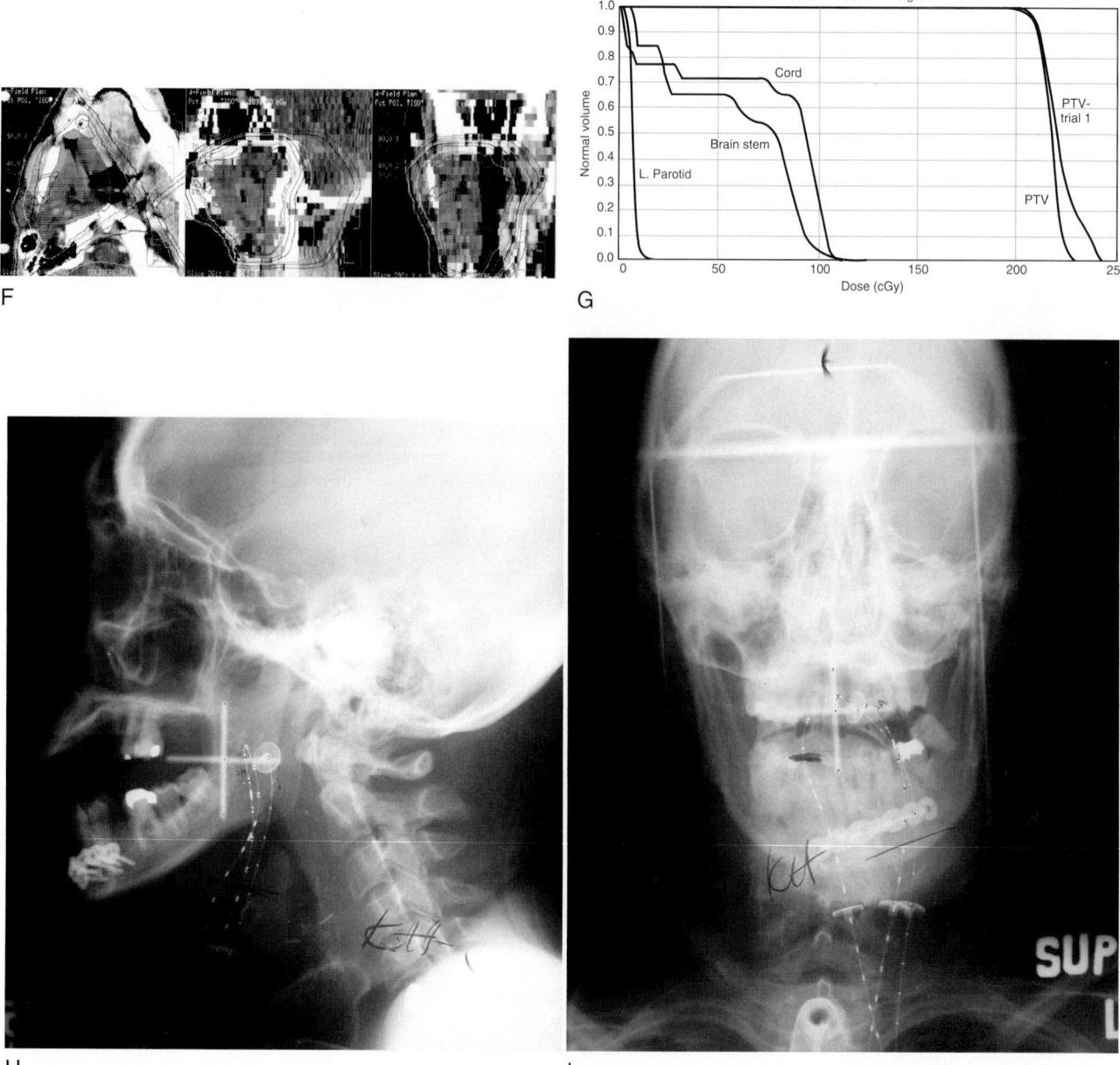

Figure 28–9 cont'd. F, Dose to the contralateral parotid gland was limited to less than 5% of the total dose to the ipsilateral lesion. **G,** Dose-volume histogram analysis showing dose delivered to tumor and within normal limits of critical normal tissues including spinal cord and contralateral parotid. **H–I,** Radiographs illustrating placement of a temporary interstitial Ir-192 brachytherapy implant into the left tonsillar fossa. This area was supplemented with external beam radiation to the primary site and left neck. See also Color Figure 28–9A, B, and F.

(1.8 Gy per fraction). At that point, photons are used to treat the tongue and the anterior upper neck to 54 Gy, and electrons are used to treat the posterior neck to 54 Gy. We generally boost the area of palpable nodes with an additional 6 Gy with electrons, bringing the total to 60 Gy.

NECK

For clinically negative neck nodes, all patients receive 50 to 54 Gy in 5 to 6 weeks. For clinically positive lymph nodes, this should be followed by either an additional boost to therapeutic doses to the neck or by neck dissection.[44] For patients with palpable nodes, our preference is

to perform neck dissection after boosting involved lymph nodes to a preoperative dose of 60 Gy.[45]

Brachytherapy

Brachytherapy, usually in combination with external beam radiotherapy, is commonly applied to oropharyngeal carcinomas, particularly the base-of-tongue and velotonsillar areas. Pharyngeal wall tumors may be implanted, but due to their remote location, often require surgical intervention for optimal exposure. Our preference is to use afterloading ^{192}Ir radioisotope for temporary interstitial implants or I-125 for permanent implants.[80-83]

However, remote after-loading using high activity ^{192}Ir, delivered high dose rate (HDR) or pulsed dose rate (PDR), has gained favor in some institutions due primarily to the reduction in personnel exposure as well as dose optimization planning.

A typical case involving a base of tongue lesion is illustrated in Figure 28-10. In an effort to reduce the implant volume and treat all disease at the primary site and neck simultaneously, the patient begins first with external beam radiotherapy. When a neck dissection is planned, the implantation and dissection are performed during the same anesthetic period. A BT boost to the tongue base (20 to 30 Gy) is performed approximately 3 weeks after EBRT (50 to 54 Gy). The implant consists of ^{192}Ir afterloading catheters placed with a looping technique,[46,47] which involves the percutaneous introduction of curved trocars by means of a submental approach through the base of tongue. The catheter is threaded through the trocar and looped back through an adjacent trocar, creating a loop in the tongue. For patients with disease extension toward the pharyngoepiglottic fold, lateral loops are added to encompass this region.[46] Both ends exit the skin of the neck. An array of loop is fashioned to encompass the target volume plus a 1.0- to 1.5-cm margin. The spacing between each end of the loop is 1 cm and between each plane is 1.0 to 1.5 cm. As a safety precaution, a temporary tracheostomy is performed in patients immediately before the implantation. A temporary nasogastric feeding tube is placed at the completion of the procedure.

Localization films are taken as the patient can tolerate. The location of dummy seeds in the catheters are digitized into a treatment planning system. Seed ribbons are customized to provide coverage without severe hot spots. Patients are loaded several days after the procedure, after the majority of the swelling has subsided and patients are able to suction themselves and perform tracheostomy care. Efforts are made to protect the palate by use of a customized shield that is under patient control.

CRITICAL NORMAL TISSUE

Dose-limiting Tissues

The dose-limiting tissues include spinal cord, mandible, and mucosa.

Effects of Treatment on Normal Tissue

The major sequelae of RT can be divided into acute and chronic side effects. These depend on total dose, fraction size, fractionation, prior or concomitant therapy (i.e., surgery or chemotherapy), and target volume. The potential acute effects on the oral cavity and pharynx after approximately 1 week of RT include mucositis, sore throat, loss of taste, and xerostomia (if any of the major salivary glands are in the treatment portal). The decrease in saliva changes the microflora in the mouth and can dramatically increase the number of dental caries in the patient. Fluoride gel treatments are effective in reducing

the subsequent incidence of dental caries. Approximately 5% of patients develop sialadenitis within 24 hours of the first irradiation treatment, and this resolves within 24 to 48 hours. The skin experiences erythema, peeling, and tanning. If the capacity of the basal cell layer to repopulate the epidermis is overwhelmed, the result is moist desquamation. Likewise, epilation of hair-bearing areas with accompanying loss of sweat and sebaceous gland function occurs.

The late effects after definitive RT can include xerostomia, dental caries, altered sense of taste, lymphedema, hypothyroidism, epilation, trismus, cervical fibrosis, atrophy of the mucosa and skin, as well as soft-tissue and bone ulceration/necrosis. In the latter process, radiation is believed to exert an avascular effect on tissues and epithelia that are thinner and more susceptible to injury. The process usually starts with ulceration of soft tissues, which can progress to bone exposure. If bone is then injured, bone necrosis or osteoradionecrosis can result. Treatment is frustrating and difficult. For minor bone exposures, conservative measures are used, débridement being performed when indicated. For refractory cases, hyperbaric oxygen treatment has been advocated. Factors that can influence osteoradionecrosis include elective dental extraction after RT and treatment of tumors near bone.[48,49] In the modern era, osteonecrosis should be an uncommon event (<5%).[50]

The use of BT implants can also contribute to osteoradionecrosis. Harrison[51] pointed out that the patients who developed complications usually received the BT implant as the initial mode of therapy and the entire tumor bed was implanted. When EBRT was used for initial treatment, the boost was administered to the smaller volume of residual disease and the incidence of soft-tissue ulceration and osteoradionecrosis was reduced greatly. Technique also plays a role, the nonlooping technique being associated with a higher reported injury rate than the looping technique.[51,52]

PROGNOSTIC FACTORS

Commonly reported prognostic factors for locoregional control, disease-free or overall survival. Include T classification, N-status, gender, and performance status.[53,54] Multiple studies have investigated various radiographic parameters and molecular markers as potential predictive factors in patients treated definitely for oropharynx cancers. In contrast to cancers involving the larynx,[55] hypopharynx,[56] and nasopharynx,[57] pretreatment CT-determined primary tumor volume is not predictive for local control after definitive radiotherapy alone using conventional[58] or altered fractionated radiation.[59] This outcome is likely due to the fact that size is already incorporated as part of the T-staging for oropharynx but not in older staging systems for the other sites. Encouraging results from single institution studies have reported that a high intratumoral microvessel density predicts for poorer local control and worse overall survival after definitive radiation of oropharynx carcinoma[60] and that a high Ki-67 labeling index is associated with local relapse[61] and shorter mean time to relapse[62] after definitive resection

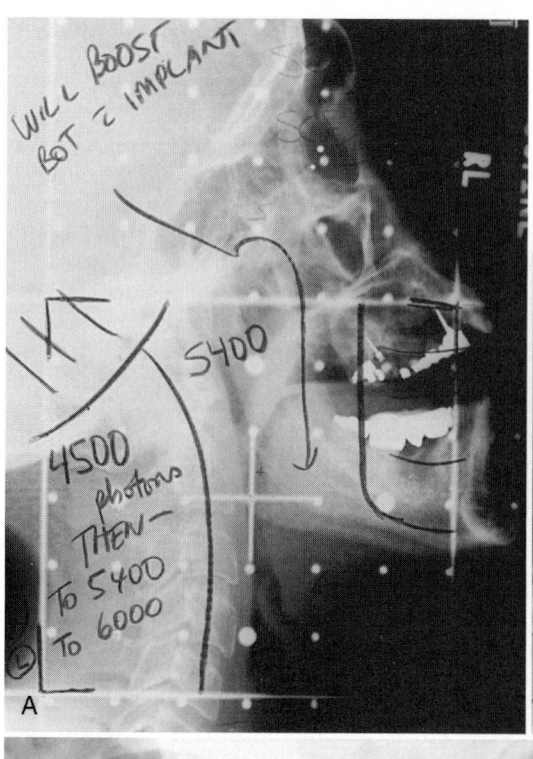

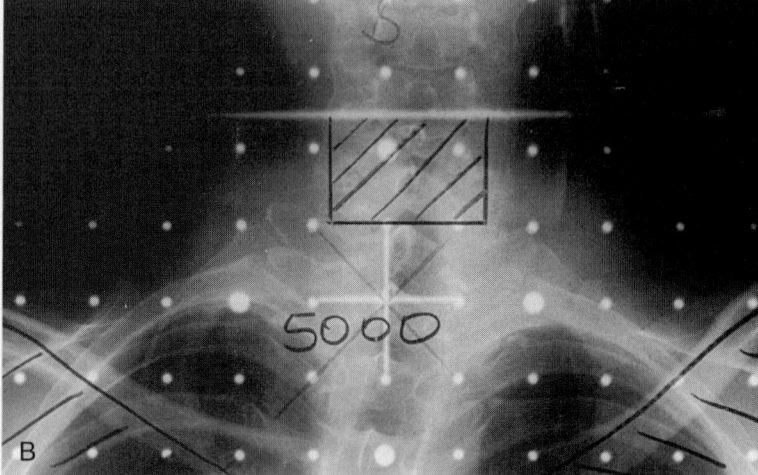

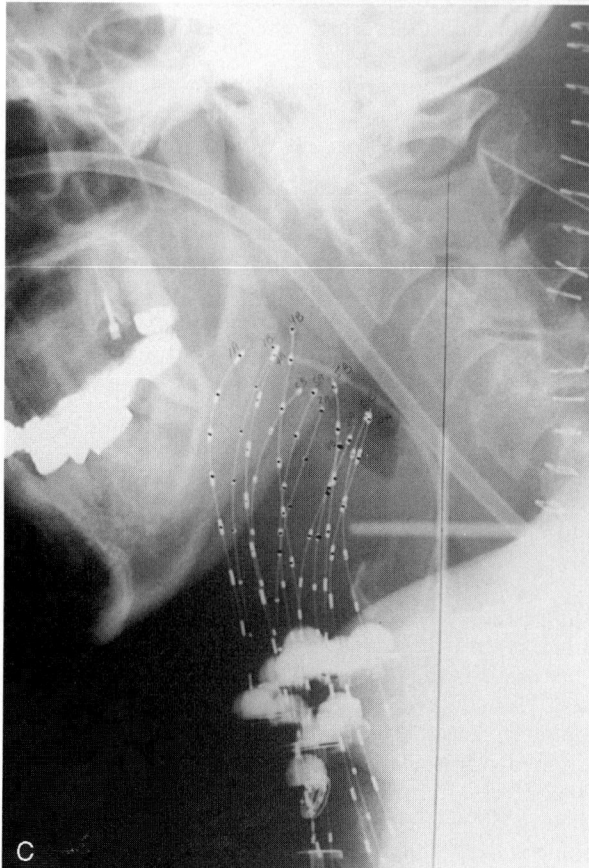

Figure 28–10. A patient with a T2N2 squamous cancer of the left side of the base of tongue. The treatment plan consisted of initial external-beam radiation therapy to the primary site and the entire neck bilaterally. This was followed by a left radical neck dissection and an implant, both done with the same anesthesia. **A,** The simulation film shows the primary site outlined and the neck node with wire around it. A bite block is in place. A total of 45 Gy was given to the primary site and both upper necks, after which a spinal cord block was placed. The primary and upper neck was then treated with 54 Gy. Fraction size was 1.8 Gy/day. After that, the bed of the lymph node in the left neck was boosted on the right and to 5940 on the left. **B,** The low neck was treated with a single anterior field to 50 Gy/5 weeks. A midline block protects the spinal cord at the field junction. **C,** Approximately 3 weeks after the external radiation was completed, the patient was taken to the operating room and a left radical neck dissection and an Ir-192 implant were done. The figure shows the catheters looped through the base of the tongue by the submental approach. Also visible are the skin staples from the neck surgery. The implant delivered an additional 28 Gy. The neck specimen was histologically negative. The patient had no evidence of disease at 6 years. He had a soft tissue ulcer in the tongue that healed with conservative management.

and postoperative radiation. Overexpression of PCNA (an estimate of growth fraction),[62,63] Vascular Endothelial Growth Factor (VEGF), or thrombospondin-1 (both markers of angiogenesis) have shown no predictive value in oropharynx patients treated with either definitive radiotherapy or combined surgery and radiation.[60,62,63] P53 overexpression studies have yielded conflicting results

regarding its prognostic value for this tumor site.[60-62] Hypoxia as detected by Eppendorf measurement of cervical lymph nodes involved with head and neck cancer has been associated with worse radiation[64-66] or chemoradiation response[67] of the involved lymph node. Anemia has also been associated with poor outcome after radiation[54,68] and its correction may improve outcome.[69] Overexpression of a hypoxia-induced transcription factor, hif-1-α (hypoxia-inducible factor one-alpha), was shown in one study of 98 patients who had oropharyngeal cancers correlated with likelihood of complete response at the primary and nodal sites after radiation treatment. It also correlated with local failure-free, disease-free, and overall survival on multivariate analysis.[70] These markers remain to be validated in larger, multi-institutional trials.

OUTCOMES

Soft Palate

EARLY DISEASE

Definitive External Beam Radiotherapy

Two major series examine the use of EBRT alone or in conjunction with planned neck dissection. Amdur et al.[21] analyzed 75 patients with SCC of the soft palate, uvula, or both. Patients received between 60 and 70 Gy. The ultimate local control rates after surgical salvage of irradiation failures for T1 through T4 lesions were 100%, 84%, 45%, and 25%, respectively. Overall, 13% of patients treated with continuous-course irradiation experienced irradiation-related bone or soft-tissue complications. Weber et al.[71] reviewed the experience at the University of Texas MD Anderson Hospital. Treatment to the primary site consisted of RT for 150 patients, surgery alone for 28 patients, and combined therapy for 10 patients. Local control rates for T1 through T4 lesions were 91%, 77%, 77%, and 35%, respectively. Local control was obtained in 88% of patients with N0 necks and in 77% of patients with nodal involvement. In addition, these investigators found that patients with tumor extension to the tongue base, midline tumors, or tumors that extended across the palatine arch had inferior survival compared with those who did not exhibit those features ($P < .05$).[71]

Combined External Beam Radiotherapy and Brachytherapy Implant

The use of a BT implant for small soft-palate lesions has been reported extensively by French investigators. Esche et al.[72] described 43 patients with carcinoma of the soft palate and uvula who were treated by interstitial implant and EBRT. Patients received 50 Gy external irradiation to the oropharynx and neck, followed by 20 to 35 Gy by a low dose rate (0.4 Gy to 1 Gy/hour) interstitial ^{192}Ir implant. This therapy yielded a local control of 92%, with no local failures in 34 T1 primary tumors. One serious complication was seen. Overall actuarial survival was 60% at 3 years and 37% at 5 years, but cause-specific survivals were 81% and 64%. The leading cause of death was other aerodigestive cancers, with an actuarial rate of occurrence of 10% per year after treatment of a soft-palate cancer.

Mazeron et al.[73] reported on a subset of patients with early-stage tumors who received EBRT to the primary tumor and neck nodes to a dose of 45 Gy, followed by 30 Gy delivered by a ^{192}Ir implant to the primary tumor. Local control was 85% for soft-palate tumors. Regional control was 97% for patients with N0 disease and 88%

for patients with N1 through N3 disease. Soft-tissue ulceration occurred in 17 patients, all of whom healed spontaneously.

Pernot et al.[74] reported on 277 patients with velo-tonsillar cancer (oropharyngeal cancer excluding base of tongue and valleculae) who were treated by BT either alone (14 patients) or combined with external beam irradiation (263 patients) using an afterloading ^{192}Ir technique. Thirty-five percent of the patients had soft-palate lesions. Of the patients treated for early lesions in the soft palate, the local control rates for T1-2,N0 and T1-2,N1-3 were 90% and 86%, respectively. No local recurrence was detected after 3 years.

External Beam Radiation Therapy versus External Beam Radiation Therapy + Brachytherapy

The need for an implant was analyzed retrospectively by Mazeron et al.,[44] who reported T1 and T2 carcinomas of the soft palate and uvula treated definitively by EBRT alone (16 patients), ^{192}Ir implant alone (14 patients), or a combination of the two methods (29 patients). Two techniques of implantation were used: the guide-gutter technique (33 patients) and the plastic-tube technique (10 patients). Local failure was 25% after EBRT alone, 0% after ^{192}Ir implant alone, and 18% after combined therapy. No local failures were seen with the plastic-tube technique compared with 15% for guide gutters. Only two nodal failures were observed (3%). Crude 5-year disease-free survival was 33%. Severe complications were limited to one incident of osteonecrosis, one soft-tissue necrosis, and one case of partial palatal incompetence. Xerostomia was reduced when implantation was used for part or all of the treatment. This is not conclusive proof that an implant is required, and these results may be difficult to duplicate without the requisite expertise in brachytherapy. Clearly, patient selection factors are important in these results.

Fractionated High-Dose Rate or Pulsed-Dose Rate Brachytherapy

In an effort to minimize occupational radiation exposure and decrease the patient isolation period while minimizing normal tissue complications, Levendag reported an initial experience combining EBRT with high-dose (HDR—1 Gy/minutes) or pulsed-dose rate (PDR) BT in 38 patients—19 soft palate tumors (14 T1-2) and 19 tonsillar cancers.[75] Twice-a-day fractions of 3.0 to 5.4 Gy HDR to a dose of 15 to 27 Gy or 4×2 Gy–8×1 Gy/day of PDR to a dose of 20 to 28 Gy were delivered within 1 to 2 weeks after completion of EBRT (46 to 50 Gy, median cumulative dose of 66 Gy). At a mean follow-up of 2.6 years, 87% of soft palate tumors were locally controlled. The incidence of grade 3 mucositis or ulceration was no different between patients treated with PDR versus HDR and similar to those reported after low dose-rate brachytherapy.

Clearly, RT is very effective for patients with early disease (Fig. 28-11), but is suboptimal for patients with advanced disease. The need for a BT implant has not been proven. However, there are anecdotal comments related to improved salivary function in those patients who received an implant, due to the decreased external-beam

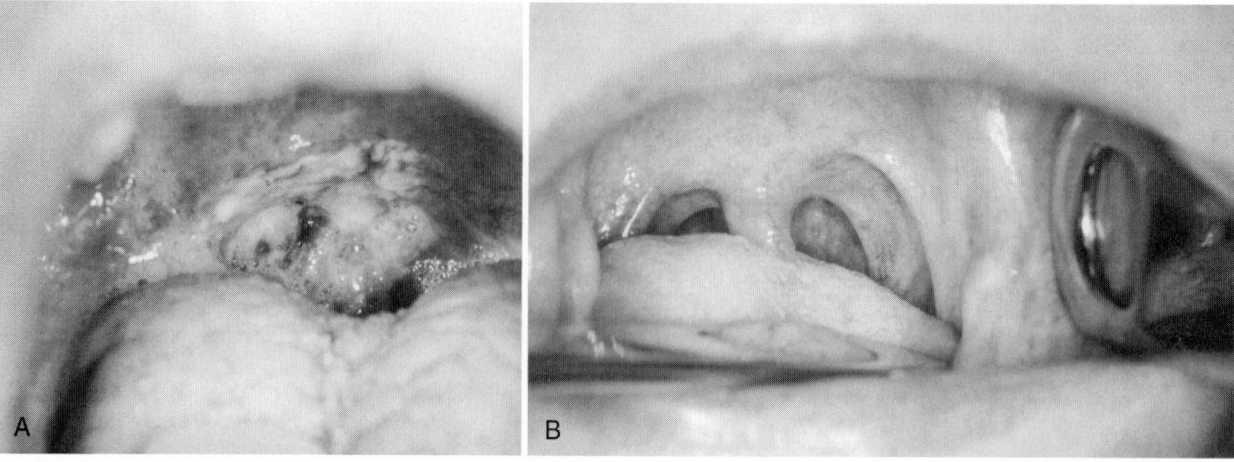

Figure 28–11. Results after treatment of a patient with a T2N0 squamous cell cancer of the soft palate, before **(A)** and after **(B)** radiation therapy. This patient was treated with external-beam radiation therapy to the primary site and both sides of the neck. Opposed lateral portals were used in conjunction with a low anterior neck field. Then the primary site and upper neck regions, including the retropharyngeal nodes, were treated to 54 Gy. The final dose to the primary site was 68.4 Gy. Fraction size is 1.8 Gy per day. The lower neck is treated with an anterior portal to 50 Gy over 5 weeks. The posterior neck regions are boosted with electrons to protect the spinal cord to 54 Gy. The patient currently has no evidence of disease. See also Color Figure 28–11.

dose to the major salivary glands. Patient selection is important, and a radiation oncologist with experience in palatal implants must perform the therapy.

ADVANCED DISEASE

Most advanced soft-palate tumors should be treated with combined surgery and postoperative RT. RT alone has been reported to offer suboptimal results.[21]

RECURRENT DISEASE AND SALVAGE

The treatment strategy for recurrence relates to tumor resectability. In those patients who have resectable disease, surgery should precede RT. If prior RT was undertaken, then "adjuvant" BT to the tumor bed may be considered if there are concerns about the margins of resection.

Patients who have previously received "full-tolerance" RT and who later develop either a second primary tumor or recurrence can be salvaged with a BT implant. Maulard et al.[76] reported on 28 patients with prior irradiation of the oropharynx who underwent salvage BT for an SCC of the tonsil or soft palate. The patients had no evidence of regional metastatic disease. Salvage BT consisted of two split-course implantations performed 1 month apart, delivering 35 and 30 Gy, respectively. Fifteen patients (54%) were disease-free before the second implant, and 23 (82%) were clinically disease-free at the end of treatment. Five local failures have been observed, without any influence of the tumor size, the topographic site of the tumor, or the histology. Of the four patients in whom EBRT had failed previously, three were disease-free after salvage brachytherapy. The overall local control rate was 68%, with a mean follow-up of 41 months. Soft-tissue necrosis was observed in four cases and, in all patients, the interval between previous RT and salvage treatment was short (mean, 7 months).

BT implant is a reasonable option for salvage therapy in patients with recurrent and second cancers occurring in the oropharynx. However, as with any retreatment

situation, the complication rate will be higher than it is with primary therapy.

Tonsil

EARLY DISEASE

Surgery Alone

The use of surgery as the sole treatment for early tonsillar disease is not reported frequently. However, excellent local control rates ranging from 80% to 90% have been reported.[30,53,77] When there is extension to the lateral pharyngeal wall or base of tongue, local recurrence approaches 33% and 47%, respectively.[78-80] The degree to which local control can be obtained depends on the extension of disease outside the tonsillar fossa.

External Beam Radiation Therapy Alone

There are no definitive randomized studies comparing surgery versus EBRT. However, no obvious differences between these modalities in locoregional control or absolute survival can be determined based on the reported literature.[77,81-92] If local control is maintained in patients by EBRT alone, the greatest risk to these patients is the development of future aerodigestive malignancies.[51] In general, the results using conventionally fractionated EBRT alone (1.8 to 2.0 Gy/dose over 6.5 to 7 weeks to doses of 65 to 70 Gy) are excellent for early-stage tumors (Table 28-4).[53,85-87,93]

Mendenhall updated the University of Florida experience where definitive radiation to the primary site is the institutional policy for treatment of 400 tonsillar cancers over a 23-year period with a minimum of 2-year follow-up.[81] Patients were treated with continuous course conventionally fractionated radiation (n = 160, median total dose 66 Gy) or using hyperfractionation (n = 240, median total dose 77 Gy). Only 18 patients received

Table 28–4   Tonsillar Carcinoma: Local Control and Survival with External-Beam Radiation Therapy with or without Brachytherapy Implant

Study and Institution	Patients, n	Median Follow-up, mo	T3–4, %	Local Control, %				Local Control, %				5-year Survival, %	
				T1	T2	T3	T4	N0	N1	N2	N3	DFS	Overall
Remmler et al.[78] MD Anderson	112	50	63	100	89	68	24	95	95	95	95	48	85
Wong et al.[86] MD Anderson	150	36	50	94	79	59	50	100	100	100	68	—	—
Bataini et al.[85] Institut Curie	698	60	72	89	84	63	43	ns	ns	ns	ns	ns	ns
Pernot et al.*[84] Centre Alexis	277	36	36	89	86	69	—	ns	ns	ns	ns	62	ns
Mazeron et al.*[73] Henri Mondor	165	60	0	100	94	—	—	ns	ns	ns	ns	71	53

*With implant.
DFS, disease-free survival; ns, not significant.

chemotherapy, 147 underwent planned neck dissection, and 107 underwent an interstitial BT boost. Five-year rates of local control were: T1 ($n = 56$), 83%, T2 ($n = 150$), 81%, T3 ($n = 126$), 74%, and T4 ($n = 68$), 60%. Of the 83 local recurrences, 36 underwent salvage therapy and 17 were successfully salvaged. The ultimate local control rates were T1, 92%, T2, 89%, T3, 77%, and T4, 65%. Five-year disease-specific survivals by 1998 American Joint Committee on Cancer stage were: I, 100%, II, 86%, III, 82%, IVa, 63%, and IVb, 22%. Absolute overall survival at 5 years was: I, 51%, II, 60%, III, 57%, IVa, 47%, and IVb, 14%. No severe acute radiation-related complications were reported; however, 5% (19/400) developed severe late complications including osteoradionecrosis requiring mandibulectomy ($n = 8$), dysphagia requiring gastrostomy ($n = 6$), bone exposure necessitating debridement and hyperbaric treatment ($n = 3$), orocutaneous fistula ($n = 1$), and fatal aspiration pneumonia ($n = 1$).

Remmler et al.[78] reported on 160 patients, the majority of whom received EBRT as the sole therapy. Primary tumor control rates were 100% for T1 lesions, 89% for T2, 68% for T3, and 24% for T4. In addition, radiation therapeutic control of cervical metastases in patients was excellent (95%). When a planned neck dissection was performed 5 weeks after RT, the control of cancer in the neck was 100%. The incidence of distant metastases was 10% and was unaffected by the selection of therapy. The 2- and 5-year determinate survival figures for 112 patients treated with RT alone were 67% and 48%, respectively, whereas 31 patients treated with RT followed by neck dissection achieved a 5-year survival rate of 48% (Table 28-5).

Lower doses or split-course radiation results in poorer locoregional control.[54] Using RT alone, Bataini et al.[85] reported that in tumors arising from the glossopalatine sulcus, characterized by involvement of the tongue, inferior local control is achieved as compared with similar therapy for tumors arising from other sites within the tonsillar region.

Ipsilateral External Beam Radiation Therapy

For patients with T1 and T2 lesions, treatment of the ipsilateral neck alone is usually possible without having to irradiate the contralateral neck, which minimizes irradiation to the contralateral salivary gland and reduces the incidence of xerostomia (Fig. 28-12). Eisbruch demonstrated that patients treated unilaterally report less

Table 28–5   Base-of-Tongue Carcinoma: Local Control and Survival with External-Beam Radiation Therapy Alone

Study and Institution	Patients, n	Median Follow-up, yrs	T3–4, %	Local Control, %				Local Control, %				5-year Overall Survival, %			
				T1	T2	T3	T4	N0	N1	N2	N3	T1	T2	T3	T4
Jaulerry et al[145] Institut Curie	166	5	58	96	57	45	23	86	79	58	61	49	29	23	16
Spanos et al[144] MD Anderson Cancer Center	174	10*	54	91	71	78	52	NS	NS	NS	NS	100	58	38	20
Foote[146] University of Florida	84	8	54	89	88	77	36†	NS	NS	NS	NS	100	86	56	36†
Houssett[47] Hospital Necker	54	8	0	78	47	—	—	4	9	—	40	17	17	—	—

*Extrapolated.
†Average of stages IVa and IVb.
ns, not significant.

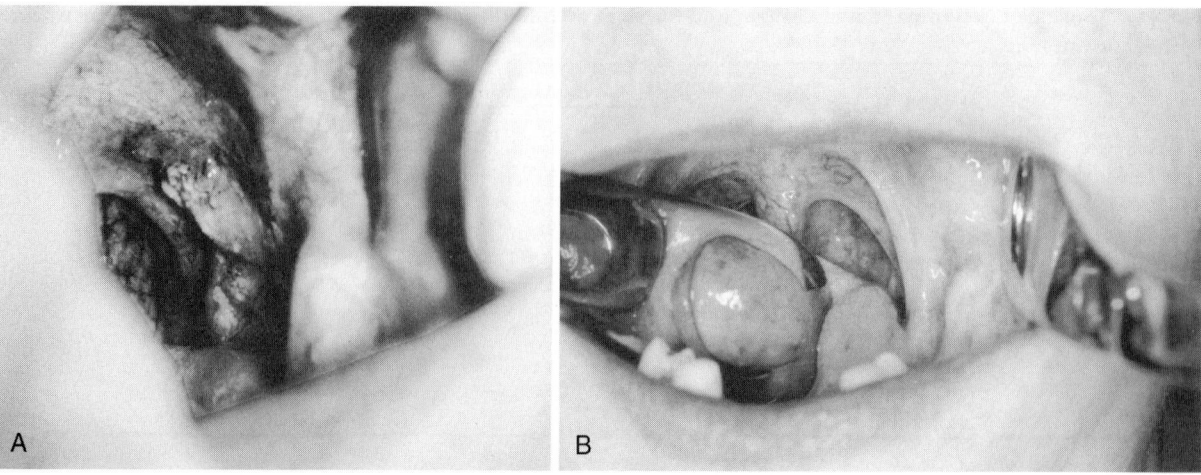

Figure 28–12. A patient with a T2N0 squamous cell cancer of the tonsil, before **(A)** and after **(B)** radiation therapy. The patient was treated with external beam radiation therapy to the primary site and ipsilateral neck using an ipsilateral wedge-pair beam arrangement in conjunction with an ipsilateral low anterior neck field. The final dose to the primary site was 70.2 Gy. Fraction size was 1.8 Gy/day. The lower neck was treated with an anterior portal to 50 Gy over 5 weeks. See also Color Figure 28–12.

xerostomia and better *QOL* compared to those treated with intensity-modulated radiotherapy delivery of bilateral radiation with contralateral parotid sparing.[94] However, careful patient selection is required to minimize the risk of contralateral neck failure. Two major series have documented excellent outcomes using ipsilateral neck EBRT.

O'Sullivan reported the results of 228 tonsillar carcinomas treated with ipsilateral radiotherapy over a 20-year period at Princess Margaret Hospital.[95] Eligible patients typically had T1 or T2 tumors (191 T1-2, 30 T3, 7 T4) with N0 (133 N0, 35 N1, 27 N2-3) disease. During this period, only 16 patients were treated surgically. Radiation was typically delivered with wedged-pair Cobalt beams and an ipsilateral low anterior neck field delivering 50 Gy in 4 weeks (90% isodose line) to the primary volume. At a median follow-up of 5.7 years, the 3-year local control rate was 77%, regional control 80%, and cause-specific survival 76%. Contralateral neck failure occurred in 3% (8/228). All patients with T1 lesions or N0 neck status had 100% contralateral neck control. Patients with a 10% or greater risk of contralateral neck failure included those with T3 lesions, lesions involving the medial one third of the soft hemipalate, tumors invading the middle third of the ipsilateral base of tongue, and N1 disease.

Jackson reported an 18-year experience of 178 patients receiving ipsilateral treatment using limited fields for tonsillar cancers.[96] Patients presented primarily with T1-2 (117/178—66%) and N0 (101/178—57%) disease, but 29% (52/178) had T3 tumors and 30% had N1 disease, with 63% presenting with stage III/IV disease. Sixty Gy/25 fxns (50 to 66 Gy) was delivered to gross tumor volume with a 1-cm margin and first echelon lymph nodes using 2 or 3 wedged fields. The length of follow-up was not stated. The rate of locoregional control and contralateral neck recurrence by stage following ipsilateral radiotherapy were: I (*n* = 23)—91%, 0%; II (*n* = 43)—74%, 2%; III (*n* = 82)—51%, 4%; IV (*n* = 30)—53%, 0%. Patients with N0 (*n* = 101) or N1

(*n* = 54) disease had contralateral failure rates of 0% and 4%, respectively. None of the 23 patients with N2-3 disease had contralateral failure; however, the determinate risk for contralateral failure may have been obscured by the 52% incidence of ipsilateral failure. The authors were unable to relate the risk of contralateral neck failure according to the degree of tumor extension along the glossopalatine fold due to the retrospective nature of the study. The overall rate of local control was 75% (T1-2, 84% and T3,4, 58%) and overall survival was 56%.

External Beam Radiation Therapy and Brachytherapy

The goal of implantation when combined with EBRT is to improve local control of the tumor while preserving salivary function and lessening muscular fibrosis.

Pernot et al.[74] reported on 277 patients, 101 of whom had advanced disease (T3). The 5-year local control, disease-specific survival, and overall survival rates by T classification (T1, T2, T3) were as follows: local control, 89%, 86%, and 69%, respectively; disease-specific survival, 78%, 62%, and 46%, respectively; and overall survival, 62%, 53%, and 43%, respectively. No local recurrence was detected after 3 years. In a later update of 361 cases, the 5-year outcomes of patients with tonsil, posterior pillar, or soft palate cancers (group A) were compared to those involving the anterior pillar and glossopharyngeal sulcus (group B).[84] Local control was better in group A patients compared to those in group B as follows: T1, 94% versus 75%, T2, 93% versus 67%, and T3, 71% versus 51%, respectively. Disease-specific and overall survival was also better in group A as follows: T1: 88%, 65% versus 55%, 48%; T2: 78%, 63% versus 43%, 38%; and T3: 53%, 49% versus 27%, 27%, respectively. Multivariate analysis revealed that a treatment interval of fewer than 20 days between EBRT and BT and an overall treatment time of fewer than 55 days yielded better outcomes. Complications in this patient population appeared to be related to a total dose greater than 80 Gy, dose rate greater than 0.7 Gy/hour, treated surface area greater than 12 cm², treatment volume greater than 30 mL, and absence of leaded protection.[97]

External Beam Radiation Therapy versus External Beam Radiation Therapy and Brachytherapy

Mazeron et al.[98] reported on 165 T1-2 SCCs of the faucial arch. Because of institutional policy changes, these authors could compare patients who received EBRT alone with those with EBRT and implantation. Those who received an implant were first treated by EBRT to the tumor site and neck areas (45 Gy in 25 fractions over 5 weeks) and then received a 30-Gy low-dose rate iridium implant. For patients with clinically positive nodes, either additional 25- to 30-Gy electron-beam irradiation to the nodes or neck dissection was added. Both local control (77% vs. 94% at 5 years; P < .01) and disease-free survival (56% vs. 71%; P = .03) were improved for the implant group. No randomized study has shown whether this combined approach is superior to EBRT alone. Nonetheless, even advocates of the use of EBRT alone agree that the addition of an implant can improve local control when disease extends into the tongue.[31]

High-Dose Rate Brachytherapy

High-dose rate BT (HDR-BT) as boost treatment with external beam radiation has been reported in 2 small series to offer excellent local control for early-stage tonsil, base of tongue, and soft palate tumors with local control of 83% to 87%, but lower with T3-4 tumors (42% to 47%).[31,58] Fractionated HDR-BT using BID treatments of 1.2 to 3.0 Gy fractions was combined with EBRT to total cumulative doses of 66 to 72 Gy. Successful surgical salvage was 50% to 60% among those who failed locally with no obvious increase in surgical complications such as fistula or flap necrosis. Rates of serious complications (primarily soft tissue ulcer and mandibular osteoradionecrosis) were reported in 10% to 16% and similar to those reported by low-dose-rate BT reports.

ADVANCED DISEASE

The management of patients with advanced tonsillar lesions is more complex and controversial. Some argue for RT alone, reserving surgery for salvage.[100,101] Others advocate surgery and postoperative RT.[102,103] Definitive chemoradiation also represents a treatment option to be considered in eligible patients.

Surgery and Post-operative Radiation

Traditionally, combined modality therapy is recommended in patients with advanced disease. Surgery frequently results in close or positive margins and multiple positive neck nodes. Two reports highlight the importance of postoperative adjuvant RT in advanced cases. The first, by Zelefsky et al.,[103] reported the long-term treatment results for advanced oropharyngeal carcinomas treated with surgery and postoperative RT at the Memorial Sloan-Kettering Cancer Center. Twenty patients with SCC of the tonsillar fossa were treated with surgery plus RT. The 7-year actuarial local control rate for tonsillar fossa lesions was 83%. Local control was

achieved in 94% of patients with T3 lesions and in 75% of patients with T4 lesions. Among patients with positive or close margins who received postoperative doses of 60 Gy or more, the long-term control rate was 93%. At 7 years, the overall survival for all patients was 52%, and the disease-free survival was 64%. The actuarial incidence of neck failure was 18%. For all patients, the likelihood of having distant metastasis at 7 years was 30%.

The second study, by Foote et al., evaluated 72 patients who had surgery either with or without postoperative adjuvant RT for advanced disease.[77] These investigators noted that the main pattern of treatment failure was above the clavicles. This occurred in 39% of patients treated with surgery alone compared with 31% of patients undergoing surgery and postoperative adjuvant RT (despite the more advanced neck disease of the surgery and RT group) and was significantly related (P = .002) to the overall clinical tumor, node, metastasis (TNM) stage. Five-year overall survival rates for patients with clinical stage III and IV disease who were treated with surgery and postoperative adjuvant RT were 100% and 78%, compared with 56% and 43%, respectively.

When such results are compared to similar staged patients treated with either surgery or radiation alone, others have reported inferior locoregional control,[104] disease-free survival,[82] and overall survival.[102] In contrast, Spiro and Spiro[105] reviewed 162 patients with carcinoma of the tonsillar fossa treated between 1969 and 1983 with radiotherapy alone or combined modality therapy. Combined surgery and RT were used in 29% of patients with stage II disease, 40% of patients with stage III disease, and 67% of patients with stage IV disease. The 3-year determinate local control rates were 89%, 83%, 58%, and 49% for stages I through IV, respectively. The overall 2-year crude survival is 58%. No survival benefit was seen in advanced-stage disease, but this might reflect a selection bias against combined-modality treatment compared to those receiving radiotherapy alone.

A number of retrospective reports have examined preoperative RT (45 to 50 Gy over 5 weeks) versus definitive RT or neck dissection.[90,91,106] No advantage to preoperative RT was seen. Thus preoperative RT for resectable lesions for which surgery is planned is no longer used as a strategy for the primary site. Patients with early-stage primary lesions but advanced neck disease are often treated with definitive RT to the primary with preoperative radiation to the neck followed by planned neck dissection.

External Beam Radiation Therapy and Brachytherapy

The use of a combination of external megavoltage irradiation and interstitial ^{192}Ir implants for T3 lesions has been reported by Puthawala et al.[107] Local control of disease in patients with T3 and T4 lesions was 79%, compared with 95% for T1-2 lesions. Treatment-related complications such as soft-tissue necrosis or osteoradionecrosis occurred in 6% of patients in the primary group and 23% in the recurrent group. No significant functional or aesthetic impairments were reported.

Pernot reported on 277 velotonsillar lesions discussed earlier in this section. For patients with T3 lesions treated with EBRT plus brachtherapy, local control, disease-free survival, and overall survival were 69%, 46%, and 43%, respectively.

A number of investigators have reported that patients with tumor that extends to the tongue have an inferior outcome compared with patients with no tongue extension. However, when an implant is used, this difference is negated. In the retrospective report of Leborgne et al.,[108] local relapse was 64% and the 3-year disease-free survival rate was 23% in 39 patients with tongue extension who were treated with EBRT alone, as compared with 40% and 60%, respectively, for patients treated with EBRT plus BT. Local relapse in patients with no tongue extension treated with EBRT alone was 33%.

RECURRENT DISEASE AND SALVAGE

Surgical salvage of recurrent disease after RT has a greater chance of success for tumors of the anterior tonsillar pillar than for those in the tonsillar fossa. Gehanno et al.[80] reported on salvage surgery for 50 patients with tumors of the tonsillar region. The actuarial survival rates at 3 and 5 years after salvage surgery were 38% and 24%, respectively. Compared with primary surgery, a higher postoperative mortality (8% vs. 1.4%) was also seen. Tumor extension that required resection into the tongue base was a negative prognostic factor; survival declined dramatically in such cases.

Peiffert et al.[109] reported on using BT salvage (60 Gy) in 73 patients who presented with velotonsillar SCC in a previously irradiated area. The 5-year actuarial local control rates for T1N0 and T2N0 disease were 80% and 67%, respectively. The regional relapse rate was 10% in both groups. Grade 2 complications occurred in 13% of patients, and these were related to neither the volume treated nor to the dose rate. No grade 3 or 4 complications occurred. The 5-year specific survival rate is 64%. Of note, 42% of the patients in this series died from another carcinoma.

Puthawala et al.,[107] using implantation alone, obtained a 75% local control rate in patients with recurrent

disease, with a 2-year absolute disease-free survival rate of 42%. Treatment-related complications such as soft-tissue necrosis or osteoradionecrosis occurred in 23% of these patients who had received previous RT.

Base of Tongue

EARLY DISEASE

Surgery Alone versus Radiotherapy

Surgical results for early base-of-tongue tumors reflect relatively high local control rates—from 75% to 85%.[110, 111] Primary EBRT, alone or followed by a planned neck dissection, also has a high local control rate of approximately 80% to 90% for T1 to T2 lesions and 70% to 85% for T3 tumors (Table 28-6). Survival for radiotherapy is similar to that after surgery, but with a lower risk of severe complications than surgery.[112] Of interest, tumor growth patterns were predictive of the response to RT (see Table 28-6). The primary control rate at 2 years for patients with exophytic tumors was 84%, as opposed to 58% for patients with ulcerative or infiltrative tumors ($P = .04$).

External Beam Radiation Therapy and Brachytherapy

Data from numerous authors have shown that the local control for early-stage tumors is in the range of 80% to 100% when treated with combined EBRT and BT implantation. Pernot reported a 5-year local control of 93% and 72% for T1 ($n = 14$) and T2 ($n = 27$), respectively, base-of-tongue tumors treated with a combined EBRT and BT approach. Corresponding 5-year disease-specific survivals were 76% and 62%, respectively.[84]

Housset et al.[47] have evaluated a comparison among surgery plus postoperative RT, EBRT plus implantation, and EBRT alone for a series of patients with T1 to T2 base-of-tongue lesions. This series is unique in that it attempts to address the issue of which management strategy is optimal. Demographical and oncological

Table 28–6 Base-of-Tongue Carcinoma: Local Control and Survival with External-Beam Radiation Therapy and Brachytherapy Implant Boosts

Study and Institution	Patients, n	Median Follow-up, mo	T3–4, %	Local Control, %				Local Control, %				5-year Survival, %	
				T1	T2	T3	T4	N0	N1	N2	N3	DFS	Overall
Remmler et al.[78]	112	50	63	100	89	68	24	95	95	95	95	48	85
Harrison et al.[114-115] MSKCC	36	22	31	100	100	80	100	100	100	100	100	ns	85
Housset et al.[47] University of Paris	29	96	All T1–T2	100	80	—	—	94	100	—	94	ns	52
Puthwala et al.[116] Long Beach	70	60	74	100	88	75	67	84*	81	78	50	67	35
Goffinet et al.[147] Stanford University	14	32	50	71†	—	—	—	ns	ns	ns	ns	76	ns

DFS, disease-free survival; MSKCC, Memorial Sloan-Kettering Cancer Center; ns, not significant.
*Without salvage.
†Not broken down.

characteristics of the patients were well balanced except that, among the EBRT-alone group, there was a significantly greater number of patients with exophytic (more favorable) lesions. Despite this imbalance, the patients who received EBRT alone suffered approximately twice the local failure rate than the other two groups (40% vs. 20%). This study suggests that EBRT plus implantation is certainly oncologically equivalent to surgery plus postoperative RT and that EBRT alone is inferior.

ADVANCED DISEASE

Advanced base-of-tongue tumors are poorly controlled with one treatment modality. The natural history of advanced tumors of the base of tongue can be gleaned from Dupont et al.,[113] who reported on 34 patients with advanced SCC of the base of tongue (20 with T3 and 14 with T4 lesions) treated by surgical resection. These patients underwent an operative procedure as the sole definitive form of treatment. Twenty-eight patients (82%) presented with clinically positive cervical nodal metastases. The local control at 2 years was 27% ($n = 9$) and the overall survival was 20% ($n = 7$). Of note, 44% of patients ($n = 15$) required laryngectomy as part of the primary surgical treatment and 15% ($n = 5$) required laryngectomy due to chronic aspiration, resulting in a total of 59% of patients who required total laryngectomy. Of the 19 patients who had a unilateral neck dissection, failure in the neck was experienced by 53% (70% contralateral, 30% ipsilateral).

Information regarding definitive EBRT for carcinomas of the base of tongue spans at least 5 decades. Data are typically from single institutions and do not take into account developments in diagnostic radiology and radiation oncology. For advanced tumors, definitive RT produced a local control rate of approximately 50%, as compared with 75% to 90% for surgery and postoperative RT.[110]

External Beam Radiation Therapy and Brachytherapy

The series reported by Harrison et al.[52] involves mainly patients with stage III and IV disease who were treated with EBRT plus implantation and neck dissection. Patients who would have required laryngectomy had they undergone primary surgery received neoadjuvant chemotherapy followed by EBRT and implantation as part of a larynx preservation study. Sixty-eight patients were managed by this approach between 1981 and 1995. The range of follow-up was 1 to 151 months, with a median follow-up of 36 months. In this series, the actuarial local control rate at both 5 and 10 years was 88%; regional control was 96% at both 5 and 10 years; distant metastasis-free survival rates were 91% and 76%, respectively; disease-free survival rates were 80% and 67%, respectively; and overall survival rates were 86% and 52%, respectively. After EBRT, 78% of dissected necks were pathologically negative. With surgical salvage, the local control rate was 94%.[51-52,114-115] Almost identical results have been reported by Goffinet[46] from Stanford University and Puthawala et al.[116] A dose-response effect

appears to occur, with higher local control being associated with doses of at least 75 Gy.[117]

In the authors' opinion, the treatment of choice for patients with SCC of the base of tongue is definitive RT, including a BT implant. The overwhelming majority of patients present with stage III or IV disease. In general, treatment consists of 50 to 54 Gy with EBRT and a 20- to 30-Gy boost to the base of tongue via a ^{192}Ir implant using afterloading catheters. Necks are managed with elective radiation alone in the N0 group or with radiation plus neck dissection in the group with palpable neck node metastases. The data make clear that most patients' disease will be controlled with this strategy. We believe that this approach should be considered the treatment of choice whenever feasible. For those few advanced-stage patients who cannot be managed with an organ-preserving approach, surgery followed by RT is generally used.

Surgery and Post-operative Adjuvant Radiotherapy

Recognizing that advanced carcinomas treated surgically will need postoperative RT, Zelefsky et al.[103] reported the long-term treatment results for base-of-tongue and tonsillar fossa carcinomas treated at the Memorial Sloan-Kettering Cancer Center. Between 1973 and 1986, 51 patients were treated with surgery plus RT. Indications included advanced disease (stage T3 or T4, 66%); close or positive margins (64%), and multiple positive neck nodes (84%). The 7-year actuarial local control rate is impressive: 81% for carcinomas of the base of tongue. Local control was achieved in 94% and 75% of patients with T3 and T4 lesions, respectively. For patients with positive or close margins who received postoperative doses of 60 Gy or more, the long-term control rate was 93%. The authors also examined the influence of treatment interruptions. The actuarial control rate among patients who required a treatment break was 64%, in contrast to those who did not require interruption of their treatment, in whom the actuarial control rate was 93% ($P = .05$). At 7 years, the overall survival for all patients was 52%, and the disease-free survival was 64%. For all patients, the likelihood of having distant metastasis at 7 years was 30%.

RECURRENT DISEASE AND SALVAGE

The approach to the patient with recurrent base-of-tongue disease depends on the initial therapy the patient received. The use of surgery alone as the salvage procedure in cases of base-of-tongue cancer treated previously with RT was reported by Pradhan et al.[104] In approximately one third of the patients, local control was achieved for at least 1 year. Thirty-five patients required a total glossectomy, 26 of whom did not undergo removal of the larynx. Only 13 patients were alive more than 3 years after salvage.

Others have used ^{192}Ir afterloading techniques in patients who received full-tolerance radiation (with or without previous surgery). Langlois et al.[105] reported on 123 patients treated for recurrence or new cancer of the tongue or oropharynx arising in previously irradiated tissues. The actuarial local control rate was 67% at 2 years and 59% at 5 years. Local control of the tumor was reasonable in most of these patients, though the actuarial survival was only 48% at 2 years and 24% at 5 years. The complication rate was slightly higher; 28 patients developed mucosal necrosis.

Mazeron et al.[106] had similar results: Actuarial local control was 72% at 2 years and 69% at 5 years. Although local control of the tumor was achieved in the majority of these patients, only 14% remained alive at 5 years. The best results were achieved in patients with lesions of the faucial arch and posterior pharyngeal wall; local control was achieved in 100% of these patients. Patients with lesions of the base of tongue and of the glossotonsillar sulcus had suboptimal results; local control was achieved in only 61%.

Due to the high complication rates, Housset et al.[107] compared two techniques of iridium implantation for salvage. Patients received either single-course implants, delivering 60 Gy, or split-course implants with a source shift, the goal being to decrease treatment complications. The first and second course of the split-course implants delivered 35 and 30 Gy, respectively, at a 1-month interval. The active lines of the second implant were placed parallel to and between the lines of the first implant. This shift in the source position resulted in a more uniform dose within the treated volume, with a 60% reduction in the high-dose sleeves. The overall local failure rate was 45.5% (25 of 55). The difference between the local failure rate after single-course implants (52%) and after split-course implants (37.5%) was not statistically significant. The only complication noted in the 40 patients in whom immediate local control was achieved after either implantation technique was mucosal necrosis. Of note, the split-course implants were associated with a two-and-a-half-fold decrease in the incidence of necrosis: 43% (9 of 21) in the single-course group and 16% (3 of 19) in the split-course group ($P = .05$).

Pharyngeal Wall

Surgery Alone

The use of surgical resection alone for pharyngeal wall tumors has been reported by Guillamondegui et al.[108] Twenty-eight percent of patients had recurrent tumors above the clavicles. Salvage in the form of RT or surgery was successful in less than one third of those patients. Patients with positive retropharyngeal nodes had an increased rate of distant metastases (22%) compared with those who did not have positive nodes (15%).

Radiation Therapy

Fein et al.,[32] from the University of Florida, retrospectively compared the effect of the use of once-daily to twice-daily fractionation on local control in 99 patients with carcinomas of the hypopharyngeal or oropharyngeal wall or both. The local control rates for patients treated with once-daily versus twice-daily fractionation were, for T1 lesions, 100% versus 100%; for T2 lesions, 67% versus 92%; for T3 lesions, 43% versus 80%; and

for T4 lesions, 17% versus 50%. These investigators also examined their former technique (posterior border placed at middle of the vertebral body when the portals were reduced off the spinal cord) compared with their current, modified technique (posterior border placed at posterior edge of the vertebral body). The local control rates were, for T1 lesions, 100% each; for T2 lesions, 57% versus 100%; for T3 lesions, 46% versus 73%; and for T4 lesions, 29% versus 75%.[32]

Meoz-Mendez et al.[109] reported on 164 patients treated at the MD Anderson Cancer Center for carcinomas of the hypopharynx and pharyngeal walls. Local control rates for T1 through T4 lesions were 71%, 73%, 61%, and 37%, respectively. For patients with T3 and T4 tumors, the combination of surgery and RT was superior to RT alone (75% local control vs. 51%).

Surgery and Radiation Therapy

Marks et al.[110] retrospectively compared the results of treatment in 51 patients after low-dose (25 to 30 Gy) preoperative RT and surgery to the results in those who had definitive RT. No difference was found in local control or survival (17%); however, the surgery plus RT group experienced a significant number of complications (fistula, 31%; carotid rupture, 14%; operative mortality, 14%). The same authors updated their experience with a group consisting of 89 patients.[118] These patients were treated with high doses of radiation (50 to 72 Gy) either for preoperative intent or for definitive therapy. Treatment outcome, survival, and tumor and nodal control were better for the RT-plus-surgery group than for the RT-alone group. The patterns of relapse differed for the two groups, with low-dose preoperative irradiation and surgery offering greater control of the primary tumor and high-dose irradiation achieving better control of nodal disease. To draw any conclusions from this article is difficult, as the reported study spanned almost 20 years, during which time many technological advances were made in radiation oncology, anesthesia, and surgery.

Spiro et al.[28] reviewed a 12-year experience with 295 patients treated for SCC of the pharynx at the Memorial Sloan-Kettering Cancer Center. Of these patients, 78 had lesions in the posterior wall. Surgery was the definitive therapy for the primary tumor in 73%. A second group of 21 patients with more extensive tumors required a laryngectomy and complex reconstruction, often with postoperative RT, and five had lesions that were implanted after access was provided by a mandibulotomy. The cumulative 5-year survival for the entire group was 32% and ranged from 44% in those with favorable lesions to 15% in those with extensive tumors. The overall complication rate was 50%. For the group that received an implant, local control was excellent.

The use of a BT implant (either ^{192}Ir or ^{125}I) and EBRT was reported by Son and Kacinski[119] for a small group of patients. The local control rate was 86% and actuarial survival was 82% at 5 years. These results are impressive but must be confirmed. In general, results in patients with extensive lesions still leave much to be desired, despite radical surgery and aggressive RT, and creative BT techniques warrant further investigation.

ROLE OF ALTERED FRACTIONATED RADIATION AND CHEMOTHERAPY IN ORGAN

Preservation Therapy of Advanced Oropharyngeal Carcinoma

Patients with advanced tumors of the oropharynx who require extensive surgery with or without total laryngectomy have typically experienced suboptimal results. Due to the size and location of these tumors, primary surgery can have a significant impact on the functional, psychological, and cosmetic consequences for these patients. The previous standard for organ preservation was established by the Veterans Affairs Laryngeal Cancer Study Trial[120,121] in which induction chemotherapy plus conventionally fractionated EBRT (which allowed preservation of the larynx in 66%) produced survival rates equivalent to those undergoing total laryngectomy with postoperative EBRT. However, recent studies and meta-analyses have demonstrated that a concurrent chemoradiation appears superior to the Veterans Affairs regimen or to EBRT alone and have brought into question the benefit of induction chemotherapy.[42-44,122-127] Forastiere's preliminary results of Radiation Therapy Oncology Group-91-11 demonstrated that in patients with larynx cancer requiring total laryngectomy and randomized to (A) conventional fractionated EBRT (70 Gy/7 weeks) alone, (B) the Veterans Affairs Regimen, or (C) concurrent cisplatin (CDDP) (100 mg/m^2 weeks 1, 4, and 7) with conventional fractionated EBRT (70 Gy/7 wks), those in arm C had superior laryngectomy-free survival compared to the other arms.[123] Numerous trials restricted to oropharynx cancers have demonstrated similar findings.

Concurrent Chemotherapy with Conventionally Fractionated Radiation

Calais reported a landmark French intergroup (GORTEC) phase III randomized trial designed to test whether adding concurrent chemotherapy to conventionally fractionated radiotherapy improves outcome compared to conventionally fractionated radiotherapy alone for patients with advanced-stage oropharynx carcinoma.[42-44] The 226 patients with stage III (32%) and IV (68%) carcinoma were randomized to 70 Gy/7 weeks or 70 Gy with 3 cycles of concurrent carboplatin (70 mg/m^2/ × 4 days)/5-fluorouracil (600 mg/m^2/ × 4 days) (weeks 1, 4, and 7). The arms were balanced with regard to stage, sex, tumor site, performance status, age, and histology. Acute toxicities were increased in the concurrent arm, including grade 3 or 4 mucositis (71% vs. 39%, P = .005), dermatitis (67% vs. 59%, P = .02), and need for feeding tube (36% vs. 15%, P = .02) compared to the control arm. However, the incidence of treatment-related mortality (1% [1/109] vs. 0%), overall treatment duration (52 vs. 50 days, respectively), and treatment interruption greater than 3 days (19% vs. 16%, respectively) were similar. Severe cervical fibrosis was increased in the combined modality treatment group (12% vs. 3%, P = .08, respectively) but the overall rate of severe chronic toxicity was 14% versus 9%, respectively. At a median follow-up of 35 months, patients in the combined modality arm had a higher 3-year locoregional control (66% vs. 42%, P = .03), disease-free survival (42% vs. 20%, P = .04), and overall survival (51% vs. 31%, P = .02), but no difference in rate of distant metastases (11% vs. 11%, respectively). The approximately 20% improvement in survival and locoregional control argues for the addition of concurrent chemotherapy in patients with advanced oropharynx cancer treated with definitive radiation. However, the optimal chemoradiotherapy regimen with regard to fractionation scheme and chemotherapy agents remains to be defined.

Altered Fractionated Radiation

Withers analyzed outcomes from nine centers using widely different dose-fractionation radiation regimens treating a total of 676 tonsil carcinomas (range of total dose 50 to 72 Gy, dose per fraction 1.8 to 3.3 Gy, and overall treatment time 3 to 8 weeks).[128] Total dose and treatment duration were significant treatment parameters affecting local control, but dose per fraction was not important. The data were most consistent with the model of delayed accelerated tumor repopulation occurring 30 days after the beginning of treatment with a compensatory dose of 0.73 Gy per day of treatment prolongation. Thus shortening treatment duration to minimize accelerated repopulation or increasing total dose without adding to late complications have become important areas of investigation. Attempts to improve locoregional control with altered fractionation have seemed promising in single-institution studies.[34-38,81,88]

Based on such evidence, the Radiation Therapy Oncology Group conducted a landmark trial (RTOG-90-03) comparing the leading U.S. altered fractionated regimens for multiple head and neck cancer sites, including oropharynx cancers (60%).[39] The 1073 patients with primarily advanced squamous cell cancers of the head and neck were randomized to 4 arms: (A) conventional fractionation (CF) 2 Gy daily, 5 days a week to 70 Gy over 7 weeks; (B) split-course accelerated fractionation (S-AF) with 1.6 Gy twice daily to 67.2 Gy over 6 weeks with an intentional 2-week break after 38.4 Gy and an interfraction interval of 6 hours; (C) delayed concomitant boost (DCB) with daily morning 1.8-Gy treatments and 1.5-Gy afternoon concomitant boost for the last 12 days of treatment with a 6-hour interfraction interval and a total dose of 72 Gy over 6 weeks; and (D) pure hyperfractionation (HF) with 1.2 Gy twice daily with an interfraction interval of 6 hours to a dose of 81.6 Gy/7 weeks. Eligible sites included oropharynx, oral cavity, hypopharyx, and supraglottic larynx with stage III/IV disease or stage II if hypopharynx or base of tongue was the tumor origin. In a preliminary analysis with a median follow-up of 23 months for all analyzable patients, the DCB and HF arms had significantly better 2-year locoregional control compared to CF (54.5% vs. 54.4% vs. 46%, respectively, P = .05 DCB vs. CF and P = .045 HF vs. CF) and trends toward improved disease-free survival (39.3% vs. 37.6% vs. 31.7%, respectively, P = .054 DCB vs. CF and P = .067 DCB vs. CF) were seen in the both the DCB radiation arm and hyperfractionation arms compared to conventional fractionation. Overall survival was no different. Acute grade 3-4 toxicity was increased compared to CF (59% vs. 55% vs. 35%, respectively). Chronic grade 3-4 toxicity was increased at 3 months for the delayed concomitant boost arm (37% vs. 27%), but was not different by 6 to 24 months compared to the control arm. There was no difference in chronic grade 3-4 toxicity in the hyperfractionated arm (28% vs. 27%) compared to CF.

Horiot reported results of the EORTC 22791 randomized trial comparing a hyperfractionation regimen of 1.15 Gy twice daily (4 to 6 hours between fractions) to 80.5 Gy over 7 weeks versus CF of 1.8 to 2.0 Gy to 70 Gy over 7 to 8 wks in the treatment of 356 patients with T2-3N0-1 oropharyngeal cancers excluding the base of tongue.[40] With a mean follow-up of about 4 years, hyperfractionation improved 5-year actuarial local regional control compared to conventional fractionation (59% vs. 40%, respectively, P = 0.02) with a trend toward improved survival (38% vs. 29%, respectively, P = 0.08). T3 tumors benefited from hyperfractionation, but not T2 lesions. More severe acute mucositis occurred in the hyperfractionation, but did not increase the incidence of treatment interruption. The incidence of grade 2 or 3 late effects was no different between the two arms.

Combining Chemotherapy with Altered Fractionated Radiation

As both the addition of concurrent chemotherapy and altered fractionated radiation have been shown independently to improve outcome for head and neck cancer patients, the present challenge is to find the optimal chemoradiation regimens that offer high rates of locoregional control, are not unduly morbid, offer maximal preservation of organ function and may be integrated with new biological agents.[39,42-44,123] Multiple phase II and randomized studies have reported possible regimens. The benefit of induction chemotherapy remains to be defined.

Phase II Studies

Our group published the results of a phase II trial treating 82 patients with unresectable head and neck cancer using the DCB radiation technique (70 Gy/6 weeks, twice daily RT last 2 weeks) with concurrent CDDP (100 mg/m^2) given every 3 weeks for 2 cycles.[42] Adjuvant chemotherapy was given in 68%. Although 40% had initial skull base invasion, the response rate was 94% with 60% complete responses. Oropharynx cancers comprised 23% (12/82) of all tumors treated. For all patients at a minimal follow-up of 3 years, the 3-year local control, overall survival, and distant-metastasis-free survival was 58%, 36%, and 58%, respectively. Seventy percent of patients with base of skull invasion were locally controlled. The treatment was reasonably well tolerated. The 3-year local control for oropharynx cancers was 64%. All patients experienced grade 3 acute mucositis, usually during the concomitant boost phase. Twenty-four percent required a treatment break, the majority requiring less than 1 week. Two deaths due to sepsis occurred during treatment. Severe chronic toxicity occurred in three patients with one osteoradionecrosis, one frontal lobe necrosis, and one case of lung toxicity secondary to adjuvant chemotherapy. Given the especially poor prognosis of this group,

the local control was good and survival better than expected with such an aggressive chemoradiation program.

A modified version of DCB radiation was reported by Bieri in which a planned total dose of 69.6 Gy was shortened to a total of 5.5 weeks, and one third received primarily concurrent CDDP-based chemotherapy.[129] Among the 55 patients with oropharynx carcinoma (76% stage III/IV), locoregional control at 3 years was 69.5% at a median follow-up of 32 months. Eighty-two percent experienced grade 3 or 4 mucositis. Patients receiving chemotherapy had greater rates of grade 3 dysphagia (68% vs. 25%, P = .003) and hospitalization (37% vs. 14%, P = .08) and greater need for a nasogastric tube (68% vs. 22%, P = .001). Late Radiation Therapy Oncology Group grade 3/4 complications occurred in 12%, consisting of laryngeal edema, mucosal necrosis, and mandibular osteoradionecrosis.

A phase II study using induction chemotherapy followed by concurrent chemoradiation was reported by Vokes' group.[130] Sixty-one patients with advanced oropharyngeal carcinomas (97% IV, 82% T3-4, and 85% N2-3) were treated with 3 cycles of CDDP (100 mg/m^2), 5FU (640 mg/m^2 per day × 5 days), leucovorin (300 to 600 mg/m^2 per day × 6 days), and IFN-alpha (2 MU/m^2 per day × 6 days) for 3 cycles. Then they proceeded to concurrent chemoradiotherapy if at least a near-complete response was obtained. This consisted of split courses of weekly concurrent hydroxyurea (2000 mg/day × 5 days) and 5FU (800 mg/m^2 × 5 days) with 9 to 10 Gy/5 days given every other week to a total dose of 68 to 75 Gy for gross disease. Neck dissections (n = 35) were performed for N2/3 disease. After induction chemotherapy, 65% obtained a complete response and 34% a partial response. Sixteen patients underwent resection of the primary tumor (11 organ sparing and 13 after induction chemotherapy). At a median follow-up of 39 months (68 months among survivors), locoregional control was 70%, distant-metastases-free survival 89%, disease-free survival 64%, and overall survival 51%. Locoregional control was 100% in patients with T1-2 (n = 11) or N0 (n = 1), 81% for T3 (n = 16), 53% for T4 (n = 34), and 67% to 69% N1-3 (n = 60). No difference was noted in local control among those undergoing surgery of the primary site versus those treated with chemoradiation alone (5-year LC 66% vs. 72%). Regional control was obtained in 98%. An update with 93 patients showed similar results.[131] Acute toxicity was substantial with severe or life-threatening mucositis in 57% and leukopenia in 65% during the induction phase, while 81% had grade 3 or 4 mucositis during the concurrent chemoradiation. The authors concluded that the treatment sequence of induction chemotherapy followed by concurrent chemoradiation and optional organ-preservation surgery is promising, but that less toxic regimens must be identified.[124]

Bensadoun reported on 54 unresectable oropharynx and hypopharynx carcinoma patients treated with concomitant hyperfractionated radiation (75.6 to 80.4 Gy) and 3 cycles of 5FU/CDDP (750 mg/m^2 per day or 750 mg/day × 5 days and 100 mg/m^2, respectively, on weeks 1, 4, 7).[132] The regimen was acutely toxic (4% mortality from treatment-related septicemia, 86% grade 3/4 mucositis by cycle 2 of chemotherapy, grade 3 or

4 neutropenia in 43% by cycle 2), but no patient required a treatment break greater than 4 days due to mucositis. No grade greater than 3 late toxicities were reported; grade 2 xerostomia was reported in 70%, and grade 2 cervical fibrosis in 45%. At a median follow-up of 16 months, locoregional control was 67% at 6 months and disease-specific survival 72% at 2 years. Other chemoradiation regimens for oropharyngeal carcinomas with encouraging locoregional control rates but short-term follow-up or small patient numbers include those using concurrent weekly paclitaxel (30 to 50 mg/m² per week)[133] and induction chemotherapy with preoperative concurrent chemoradiation followed by organ-preserving surgery.[134]

Randomized Trials of Altered Fractionation with or without Chemotherapy

Concurrent chemotherapy with hyperfractionated radiation was explored by Brizel in a phase III randomized trial.[41] The 116 patients with advanced head and neck cancer were randomized to hyperfractionated radiation alone treated with 1.25 Gy twice a day (6-hour interfraction interval) 5 days a week to 75 Gy over a 6-week period versus a concurrent chemoradiation arm consisting of 5FU/CDDP given on weeks 1 and 6 of split-course hyperfractionated radiation. In contrast to the control arm, an intentional 1-week treatment break was required in the experimental arm and the total dose was slightly lower (70 Gy). Both groups received 2 adjuvant courses of 5FU/CDDP after completion of radiation. At a median follow-up of 41 months, the chemoradiation showed improved locoregional (70% vs. 44%, $P = 0.01$) and a trend toward improved 3-year overall survival (55% vs. 34%, $P = 0.07$), and relapse-free survival (61% vs. 41%, $P = 0.08$). However, patients in the chemoradiation arm developed more acute toxicity including the requirement for more feeding tubes (44% vs. 29%) and worse hematalogic suppression. Three-quarters of patients in both arms experienced confluent mucositis. Chronic toxicity was no different with about a 10% incidence of necrosis of the skin or bone in both arms. The trial has been criticized, not only for the added toxicity, but because of the imbalance in the proportion of advanced neck disease (44% vs. 63%, in the RT vs. CT/RT arms, respectively) treated in the concurrent chemoradiation, which may have accounted for the difference in locoregional control.

Jeremic reported a phase III randomized study testing whether daily low-dose CDDP improved outcome for patients undergoing hyperfractionation radiation compared to those treated with the same hyperfractionated radiation alone in locally advanced head and neck squamous cell cancers (37% were oropharynx).[135] The 130 patients with stage III or IV disease were randomized to 1.1 Gy twice a day to 77 Gy/7 weeks alone or with CDDP 6 mg/m² per day. At a median follow-up of 79 months, the investigational arm showed improved locoregional control (50% vs. 36% at 5 years, $P = .041$), progression-free survival (46% vs. 25% at 5 years, $P = .0068$), and overall survival (46% vs. 25% at 5 years, $P = .0075$) as well as fewer distant metastases (14% vs. 43% at 5 years,

$P = .0013$). The latter result was unexpected and raised the possibility that concurrent daily CDDP may affect the incidence of distant metastases by a direct systemic effect or secondarily through improved locoregional control. Daily concurrent chemotherapy was well tolerated with neither an increase in acute grade 3 mucositis and esophagitis nor in late skin, bone, or salivary gland severe effects.

A German multicenter randomized trial tested whether the combination of hyperfractionated accelerated radiation (69.6 Gy/5 1/2 weeks) with carboplatin (70 mg/m²)/5FU (600 mg/m² per day × 5 days) on weeks 1 and 5 of RT improved outcome compared to the same radiation regimen alone.[136] Two-hundred forty patients with stage III (4%)/IV (96%) oropharyngeal ($n = 178$) and hypopharynx ($n = 62$) tumors were entered in a 2 × 2 study randomizing patients to receive radiation with or without chemotherapy and then again to receive G-CSF or not. G-CSF was administered to determine its effect on mucositis. Treatment was tolerable in both study arms with higher mucosal and hematological toxicity in the CT/RT arm, but no difference in duration of treatment (41 vs. 42 days) or total radiation dose delivered (68.5 Gy vs. 69.9 Gy) in the CT/RT versus RT arms, respectively. Response rates at 6 weeks after treatment were similar: 92% (CR = 40%) after CT/RT and 88% (CR = 34%) after RT alone. At a median follow-up of 22 months, the 1- and 2-year rates of locoregional control were 69% and 51% after CT/RT compared to 58% and 45% after RT ($P = 0.14$). On subset analysis, patients with oropharyngeal carcinomas had 1-year improved survival with local control after chemoradiation (60% vs. 40%, $P = 0.01$) and a trend toward improved locoregional control (70% vs. 58%, 1-year and 51% vs. 42% 2-year, $P = .07$) compared to RT alone. Patients in the CT/RT had increased grade 3 and 4 toxicities including mucositis (68% vs. 52%, $P = .01$), vomiting (8% vs. 2%, $P = .02$) and hematological toxicity (neutropenia—18% vs. 0%) with similar rates of dermatitis (30% vs. 28%). Patients receiving CT/RT had more swallowing problems and continuous need for feeding tubes (51% vs. 25%, $P = .02$). Interestingly, patients receiving G-CSF had reduced locoregional control (55% vs. 38%, $P = .0072$) and decreased mucositis ($P = .06$). This raises the issue of possible tumor radioprotection and certainly deserves further evaluation.

Altered Fractionated Radiation versus Chemoradiation

The GORTEC group conducted a randomized trial for 109 unresectable SCCs of the head and neck to receive accelerated radiation (62 to 64 Gy/3 weeks) or moderately accelerated radiation (62 to 64 Gy/5 weeks) with CDDP (100 mg/m² day 1, 16, and 32) and 5FU (1 gm/m² days 1 through 5 and 31 through 35).[137] In the concurrent CT/RT arm 2 additional cycles of 5FU/CDDP were given 4 and 7 weeks after local treatment. Most patients had T4 and N3 status (90%, mean nodal diameter 8 cm) and the most frequent site was the oropharynx. The patients were well balanced with respect to age, performance status, tumor site, and stage. The trial was stopped early due to increased treatment-related deaths in the

CT/RT arm. At preliminary report, no statistical difference in locoregional control, event-free, or overall survival could be detected between the two arms.

Conclusion

In summary, these trials raise the question of which radiation regimen is optimal for the various subsets of head and neck cancer patients (unresectable vs. resectable, organ preservation in patients with cancers of the larynx/ hypopharynx vs. oropharynx, and so on) and whether the addition of concurrent chemotherapy with accelerated radiation outweighs its concomitant intensification of acute and chronic toxicities. The best chemoradiation regimen that maximizes *QOL* remains to be defined and must be evaluated in the context of possible integration with novel targeted-biological therapies.

QUALITY OF LIFE

Much interest has been expressed in patient *QOL* since the start of this decade. Oncologists are recognizing that a cured patient who is disabled as a result of treatment is not the same as a patient who requires significant intervention by the health care system or dependence on society for social services. Measures of *QOL*, although still evolving, are now important parts of research protocols. We currently use a number of tools to study this process. One such tool is the Memorial Symptom Assessment Scale (MSAS), a comprehensive symptom measure that records (1) prevalence of 32 physical and psychological symptoms commonly experienced by cancer patients, (2) symptom characteristics, and (3) measures of symptom distress.[138] Another such tool is the Functional Assessment of Cancer Therapy (FACT), a multidimensional

33 item *QOL* instrument. A study in a mixed cancer population ($n = 545$) demonstrated the internal consistency and validity of the total and subscale scores for various domains of well-being.[139] Each score is calculated as the sum of the responses given to specific groups of questions relating to physical, emotional, social, and functional well-being.

A third *QOL* evaluation tool is the head and neck performance status scale (PSS). This interviewer-rated scale yields separate scores reflecting a patient's ability to eat in public, comprehensibility of speech, and normalcy of diet. The scale has been validated and used in prior surveys of patients with base-of-tongue cancer. Each score corresponds to a description of the functional capability that attends it. The higher the score, the better the function. A score of 100 indicates normal function and is the best possible score.[140]

Harrison et al.[141] retrospectively examined patients with SCC of the base of tongue who were treated with primary RT or primary surgery, comparing the *QOL* and functional outcome. Patients had been treated primarily by RT or surgery depending on the philosophy of their primary clinician. Primary RT consisted of 45 to 54 Gy EBRT followed by a ^{192}Ir implant that delivered an additional 2000 to 3000 Gy over 2 to 3 days. In those with involved lymph nodes, a neck dissection was performed at the same time as the implantation. Primary surgery consisted of resection of the base-of-tongue lesion, neck dissection, and postoperative RT. Both groups had similar local control (80% to 90%). A subjective PSS for head and neck cancer patients was used to assess the QOL in these patients (0 to 100, where 0 = worst function and 100 = normal function), measuring the patient's ability to eat in public, comprehensibility of speech, and normalcy of diet (Fig. 28-13).[139] Patients treated with RT had consistently better performance status and *QOL* scores. This

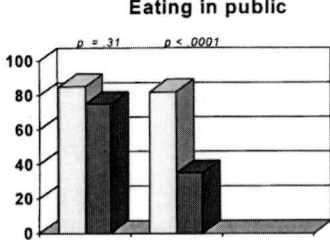

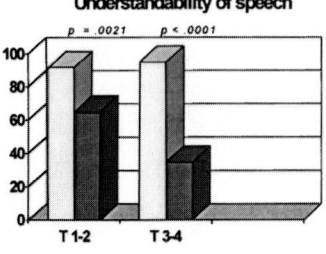

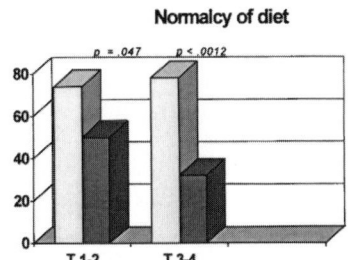

Figure 28–13. Performance status scales for normalcy of diet, eating in public, and comprehensibility of speech after treatment for squamous cell cancer of the base of tongue: a comparison of primary radiation therapy and primary surgery. (Performance status scale for head and neck patients adapted from Puthawala AA, Syed AM, Gates TC: Iridium-192 implants in the treatment of tonsillar region malignancies. *Arch Otolaryngol.* 1985;111:812.)

was true for those with early (T1 to T2) as well as more advanced (T3 to T4) disease. In addition, comparison of scores for early and advanced disease treated by primary RT revealed no difference in all three functional categories for T1 to T2 as compared with T3 to T4 disease ($P = .84$), showing that QOL scores remain high for all stages. For surgery, functional status deteriorated significantly when comparing T1 to T2 and T3 to T4 lesions ($P = .0014$), consistent with the fact that larger tumors require more extensive operations. The investigators' results show that RT provides a better performance status than surgery for base-of-tongue cancer, whether the patient exhibits early or advanced disease. Functional scores remained high for all T stages treated with irradiation but deteriorated with more advanced T stages for patients treated surgically.[141]

In addition to QOL issues, Harrison et al.[141-143] examined the long-term socioeconomic outcomes for patients with cancer of the base of tongue who were treated with an organ preservation approach. At the time of follow-up (median, 5 years), patients' annual incomes were similar to those at the time of presentation (89% exceeding $20,000; 52% exceeding $60,000). Of those working full-time, 72% were still in full-time work, and 83% of those working part-time were in part-time work.

QOL has recently been recognized as an issue of paramount importance in the decision analysis for managing patients with head and neck cancer, and confirmatory studies that use objective criteria are needed to compare in more detail the various treatment modalities for oropharyngeal cancers. Clearly, QOL issues must factor strongly into the decision-making process and selection of the appropriate management strategy.

REFERENCES

1. Wingo PA, Tong T, Bolden S: Cancer statistics, 1996. *CA Cancer J Clin.* 1996;46:5.
2. Rouviere H: *Anatomy of the Human Lymphatic System.* Ann Arbor, Mich.: Edwards Brothers; 1938.
3. Fisch UP: Cervical lymphography in cases of laryngopharyngeal carcinoma. *J Laryngol Otol.* 1964;78:715.
4. Haagensen CD et al: *The Lymphatics in Cancer.* Philadelphia: Saunders; 1972.
5. Candela FC, Kothari K, Shah JP: Patterns of cervical node metastases from squamous carcinoma of the oropharynx and hypopharynx. *Head Neck.* 1990;12:197.
6. Lindberg R: Distribution of cervical lymph node metastases from squamous cell carcinoma of the upper respiratory and digestive tracts. *Cancer.* 1972;29:1446.
7. Crawford BE, Callihan MD, Corio RL, et al: Oral pathology. *Otolaryngol Clin N Am.* 1979;12:29.
8. Low WK, Sng I, Balakrishnan A: Palatine tonsillar metastasis from carcinoma of the colon. *J Laryngol Otol.* 1994;108:449.
9. Mochimatsu I, Tsukuda M, Furukawa S, Sawaki S: Tumors metastasizing to the head and neck—A report of seven cases [Review]. *J Laryngol Otol.* 1993;107:1171.
10. Tesei F, Farneti G, Cavicchi O, et al: A case of Merkel-cell carcinoma metastatic to the tonsil. *J Laryngol Otol.* 1992; 106:1100.
11. Asami K, Yokoi H, Hattori T, et al: Metastatic gall bladder carcinoma of the palatine tonsil [Review]. *J Laryngol Otol.* 1989; 103:211.
12. Johnson J: Oropharynx. In Gluckman JL, Gullane P, Johnson J, eds. *Practical Approach to Head and Neck Tumors.* New York: Raven Press; 1995:91.
13. Boffetta P, Mashberg A, Winkelmann R, Garfinkel L: Carcinogenic effect of tobacco smoking and alcohol drinking on anatomic sites of the oral cavity and oropharynx. *Int J Cancer.* 1992;52:530.
14. Perez CA, Purdy JA, Breaux SR, et al: Carcinoma of the tonsillar fossa: A nonrandomized comparison of preoperative radiation and surgery or irradiation alone: Long-term results. *Cancer.* 1982; 50:2314.
15. Shugar MA, Nosal P, Gavron JP: Technique for routine screening for carcinoma of the base of tongue. *J Am Dent Assoc.* 1982; 104:646.
16. Brownian GP, Wong G, Hodson I, et al: Influence of cigarette smoking on the efficacy of radiation therapy in head and neck cancer [see comments]. *N Engl J Med.* 1993;328:159.
17. Mashberg A, Meyers H: Anatomical site and size of 222 early asymptomatic oral squamous cell carcinomas: A continuing prospective study of oral cancer: II. *Cancer.* 1976;37:2149.
18. Mashberg A, Samit AM: Early diagnosis of asymptomatic oral and oropharyngeal squamous cancers. *CA Cancer J Clin.* 1995;45:328.
19. Shaha AR, Shah JP: Biopsy techniques in head and neck. *Surg Oncol Clin N Am.* 1995;4:15.
20. American Joint Committee on Cancer: *Manual for Staging of Cancer.* 6th ed. New York: Springer-Verlag; 2002.
21. Amdur RJ, Mendenhall WM, Parsons JT, et al: Carcinoma of the soft palate treated with irradiation: Analysis of results and complications. *Radiother Oncol.* 1987;9:185.
22. Calais G, Alfonsi M, Bardet, E: Randomized trial of radiation therapy versus concomitant chemotherapy and radiation therapy for advanced-stage oropharynx carcinoma. *J Natl Cancer Inst.* 1999;91:2081.
23. Calais G, Alfonsi M, Bardet E: [Stage III and IV cancers of the oropharynx: Results of a randomized study of GORTEC comparing radiotherapy alone with concomitant chemotherapy]. *Bull Cancer.* 2000;87(Spec No):48.
24. Calais G, Alfonsi M, Bardet E: Radiation (RT) alone versus RT with concomitant chemotherapy (CT) in stages III and IV oropharynx carcinoma. Final results of the 94-01 GORTEC randomized study. *Int J Radiat Oncol Biol Phys.* 2001;51:1.
25. Andersen PE, Shah JP, Cambronero E, Spiro RH: The role of comprehensive neck dissection with preservation of the spinal accessory nerve in the clinically positive neck. *Am J Surg.* 1994; 168:499.
26. Spiro RH, Gerold FP, Strong EW: Mandibular "swing" approach for oral and oropharyngeal tumors. *Head Neck Surg.* 1981;3:371.
27. Shike M, Bemer YN, Gerdes H, et al: Percutaneous endoscopic gastrostomy and jejunostomy for long-term feeding in patients with cancer of the head and neck. *Otolaryngol Head Neck Surg.* 1989; 101:549.
28. Spiro RH, Kelly J, Vega AL, et al: Squamous carcinoma of the posterior pharyngeal wall. *Am J Surg.* 1990;160:420.
29. Spiro RH, Bains MS, Shah JP, Strong EW: Gastric transposition for head and neck cancer: A critical update. *Am J Surg.* 1991;162:348.
30. Michiwaki Y, Schmelzeisen R, Hacki T, Michi K: Functional effects of a free jejunum flap used for reconstruction in the oropharyngeal region. *J Craniomaxillofac Surg.* 1993;21:153.
31. Million RR: Squamous cell carcinoma of the head and neck: Combined therapy: Surgery and post-operative irradiation. *Int J Radiat Oncol Biol Phys.* 1979;5:2161.
32. Fein DA, Mendenhall WM, Parsons JT, et al: Pharyngeal wall carcinoma treated with radiotherapy: Impact of treatment technique and fractionation. *Int J Radiat Oncol Biol Phys.* 1993;26:751.
33. Grimard L, Szanto J, Girard A, et al: Asymmetric arc technique for posterior pharyngeal wall and retropharyngeal space tumors. *Int J Radiat Oncol Biol Phys.* 1995;31:611.
34. Ang KK, Peters LJ, Weber RS, et al: Concomitant boost radiotherapy schedules in the treatment of carcinoma of the oropharynx and nasopharynx. *Int J Radiat Oncol Biol Phys.* 1990;19:1339.
35. Wang CC: Local control of oropharyngeal carcinoma after two accelerated hyperfractionation radiation therapy schemes. *Int J Radiat Oncol Biol Phys.* 1988;14:1143.
36. Ang KK: Altered fractionation trials in head and neck cancer. *Semin Radiat Oncol.* 1998;8:230.
37. Cummings BJ: Benefits of accelerated hyperfractionation for head and neck cancer. *Acta Oncol.* 1999;38:131.
38. Million RR, Parsons JT, Cassisi NJ: Twice-a-day irradiation technique for squamous cell carcinomas of the head and neck. *Cancer.* 1985;55(suppl):2096.

39. Fu KK, Pajak T, Trotti A: A Radiation Therapy Oncology Group (RTOG) phase III randomized study to compare hyperfractionation and two variants of accelerated fractionation to standard fractionation radiotherapy for head and neck squamous cell carcinomas: First report of RTOG 9003. *Int J Radiat Oncol Biol Phys.* 2000;48:7.

40. Horiot JC, LeFur R, Nguyen T: Hyperfractionation versus conventional fractionation in oropharyngeal carcinoma: Final analysis of a randomized trial of the EORTC cooperative group of radiotherapy. *Radiother Oncol.* 1992;25:231.

41. Brizel DM, Albers ME, Fisher SR, et al: Hyperfractionated irradiation with or without concurrent chemotherapy for locally advanced head and neck cancer. *N Engl J Med.* 1998;338:1798.

42. Harrison LB, Raben A, Pfister D: A prospective phase II trial of concomitant chemotherapy and radiotherapy with delayed accelerated fractionation in unresectable tumors of the head and neck. *Head Neck.* 1998;20:497.

43. Hu KH, Nwokedi E, Harrison LB, et al: Delayed accelerated hyperfractionated radiation with concurrent CDDP without induction chemotherapy for organ preservation therapy of stage III/IV head and neck cancer, Abs # 844, European Society of Therapeutic Radiation Oncology, Prague 2002.

44. Har-El G, Shaha A, Chaudry R, et al: Carcinoma of the uvula and midline soft palate: Indication for neck treatment. *Head Neck.* 1991;14:99.

45. Lee HJ, Zelefsky MJ, Harrison LB, et al: Long-term regional control after radiation therapy and neck dissection for base of tongue carcinoma. *Int J Radiat Oncol Biol Phys.* 1997;38:995.

46. Goffinet DR, Fee WE Jr, Wells J, et al: ^{192}Ir pharyngoepiglottic fold interstitial implants. The key to successful treatment of base tongue carcinoma by radiation therapy. *Cancer.* 1985;55:941.

47. Housset M, Baillet F, Dessard-Diana B, et al: A retrospective study of three treatment techniques for T1-T2 base of tongue lesions: Surgery plus postoperative radiation, external radiation plus interstitial implantation and external radiation alone. *Int J Radiat Oncol Biol Phys.* 1987;13:511.

48. Spanos WJ Jr, Shukovsky LJ, Fletcher GH: Time, dose, and tumor volume relationships in irradiation of squamous cell carcinomas of the base of the tongue. *Cancer.* 1976;37:2591.

49. Bedwinek JM, Shukovsky LJ, Fletcher GH, Daley TE: Osteonecrosis in patients treated with definitive radiotherapy for squamous cell carcinomas of the oral cavity and naso- and oropharynx. *Radiology.* 1976;119:665.

50. Parsons JT, Million RR, Cassisi NJ: Carcinoma of the base of the tongue: Results of radical irradiation with surgery reserved for irradiation failure. *Laryngoscope.* 1982;92:689.

51. Harrison LB, Sessions RB, Strong EW, et al: Brachytherapy as part of the definitive management of squamous cancer of the base of tongue. *Int J Radiat Oncol Biol Phys.* 1989;17:1309.

52. Harrison LB, Zelefsky MJ, Sessions RB, et al: Base-of-tongue cancer treated with external beam irradiation plus brachytherapy: Oncologic and functional outcome. *Radiology.* 1992;184:267.

53. Perez CA, Patel M, Chao K: Carcinoma of the tonsillar fossa: Prognostic factors and long-term therapy outcome. *Int J Radiat Oncol Biol Phys.* 1998;42:1077.

54. Johansen LV, Grau C, Overgaard J: Squamous cell carcinoma of the oropharynx—An analysis of treatment results in 289 consecutive patients. *Acta Oncol.* 2000;39:985.

55. Pameijer FA, Mancuso A, Mendenhall W: Can pretreatment computed tomography predict local control in T3 squamous cell carcinoma of the glottic larynx treated with definitive radiotherapy? *Int J Radiat Oncol Biol Phys.* 1997;37:1011.

56. Pameijer FA, Mancuso A, Mandenhall W: Evaluation of pretreatment computed tomography as a predictor of local control in T1/T2 pyriform sinus carcinoma treated with definitive radiotherapy. *Head Neck.* 1998;20:159.

57. Chua DT, Shan J, Kwong D: Volumetric analysis of tumor extent in nasopharyngeal carcinoma and correlation with treatment outcome. *Int J Radiat Oncol Biol Phys.* 1997;39:711.

58. Hermans R, Op de Beeck K: The relation of CT-determined tumor parameters and local and regional outcome of tonsillar cancer after definitive radiation treatment. *Int J Radiat Oncol Biol Phys.* 2001;50:37.

59. Nathu RM, Mancuso A, Zhu T: The impact of primary tumor volume on local control for oropharyngeal squamous cell carcinoma treated with radiotherapy. *Head Neck.* 2000;22:1.

60. Aebersold DM, Beer K, Laissue J: Intratumoral microvessel density predicts local treatment failure of radically irradiated squamous cell cancer of the oropharynx. *Int J Radiat Oncol Biol Phys.* 2000;48:17.

61. Grabenbauer GG, Muhlfriedel G, Rodel F: Squamous cell carcinoma of the oropharynx: Ki-67 and p53 can identify patients at high risk for local recurrence after surgery and postoperative radiotherapy. *Int J Radiat Oncol Biol Phys.* 2000;48:1041.

62. Sittel C, Eckel H, Damm M: Ki-67 (MIB1), p53, and Lewis-X (LeuM1) as prognostic factors of recurrence in T1 and T2 laryngeal carcinoma. *Laryngoscope.* 2000;110:1012.

63. Jaskulski D, deRiel J, Mercer W: Inhibition of cellular proliferation by antisense oligodeoxynucleotides to PCNA cyclin. *Science.* 1988;240:1544.

64. Nordsmark M, Overgaard M, Overgaard J: Pretreatment oxygenation predicts radiation response in advanced squamous cell carcinoma treated by radiation therapy. *Radiother Oncol.* 1996;41:31.

65. Nordsmark M, Overgaard J: A confirmatory prognostic study on oxygenation status and loco-regional control in advanced head and neck squamous cell carcinoma treated by radiation therapy. *Radiother Oncol.* 2000;57:39.

66. Brizel DM, Sibley G, Prosnitz L: Tumor hypoxia adversely affects the prognosis of carcinoma of the head and neck. *Int J Radiat Oncol Biol Phys.* 1997;38:285.

67. Vanselow B, Eble M, Rudat V: Oxygenation of advanced head and neck cancer: Prognostic marker for the response to primary radiochemotherapy. *Otolaryngol Head Neck Surg.* 2000;122:856.

68. Overgaard J, Hansen H, Overgaard M: A randomized double-blind phase III study of nimorazole as a hypoxic radiosensitizer of primary radiotherapy in supraglottic larynx and pharynx carcinoma. Results of the Danish Head and Neck Cancer Study (DAHANCA) Protocol 5-85. *Radiother Oncol.* 1998;46:135.

69. Glaser CM, Millesi W, Komek G: Impact of hemoglobin level and use of recombinant erythropoietin on efficacy of preoperative chemoradiation therapy for squamous cell carcinoma of the oral cavity and oropharynx. *Int J Radiat Oncol Biol Phys.* 2001;50:705.

70. Aebersold DM, Burri P, Beer K: Expression of hypoxia-inducible factor-1 alpha: A novel predictive and prognostic parameter in the radiotherapy of oropharyngeal cancer. *Cancer Res.* 2001;61:2911.

71. Weber RS, Peters LJ, Wolf P, Guillamondegui O: Squamous cell carcinoma of the soft palate, uvula, and anterior faucial pillar. *Otolaryngol Head Neck Surg.* 1988;99:16.

72. Esche BA, Haie CM, Gerbaulet AP, et al: Interstitial and external radiotherapy in carcinoma of the soft palate and uvula. *Int J Radiat Oncol Biol Phys.* 1988;15:619.

73. Mazeron JJ, Crook J, Martin M, et al: Iridium 192 implantation of squamous cell carcinomas of the oropharynx [Review]. *Am J Otolaryngol.* 1989;10:317.

74. Pernot M, Malissard L, Taghian A, et al: Velotonsillar squamous cell carcinoma: 277 cases treated by combined external irradiation and brachytherapy-results according to extension, localization, and dose rate. *Int J Radiat Oncol Biol Phys.* 1992;23:715.

75. Levendag PC, Schmitz P, Jansen P: Fractionated high-dose-rate and pulsed-dose-rate brachytherapy: First clinical experience in squamous cell carcinoma of the tonsillar fossa and soft palate. *Int J Radiat Oncol Biol Phys.* 1997;38:497.

76. Maulard C, Housset M, Delanian S, et al: Salvage split course brachytherapy for tonsil and soft palate carcinoma: Treatment techniques and results. *Laryngoscope.* 1994;104:359.

77. Foote RL, Schild S, Thompson W: Tonsil cancer. Patterns of failure after surgery alone and surgery combined with postoperative radiation therapy. *Cancer.* 1994;73:2638.

78. Remmler D, Medina JE, Byers RM, et al: Treatment of choice for squamous carcinoma of the tonsillar fossa. *Head Neck Surg.* 1985;7:206.

79. Weichert KA, Aron B, Maltz R, Shumrick D: Carcinoma of the tonsil: treatment by a planned combination of radiation and surgery. *Int J Radiat Oncol Biol Phys.* 1976;1:505.

80. Gehanno P, Depondt J, Guedon C, et al: Primary and salvage surgery for cancer of the tonsillar region: A retrospective study of 120 patients [see comments]. *Head Neck.* 1993;15:185.

81. Mendenhall WM, Amdur RJ, Stringer SP, et al: Radiation therapy for squamous cell carcinoma of the tonsillar region: A preferred alternative to surgery? *J Clin Oncol.* 2000;18:2219.

82. Hicks WL Jr, Kurialcose M, Loree T: Surgery versus radiation therapy as single-modality treatment of tonsillar fossa carcinoma: The Roswell Park Cancer Institute experience (1971-1991). *Laryngoscope.* 1998;108:1014.

83. Mizono GS, Diaz RF, Fu KK, Boles R: Carcinoma of the tonsillar region. *Laryngoscope.* 1986;96:240.

84. Pernot M, Hoffstetter S, Peiffert D: Role of interstitial brachytherapy in oral and oropharyngeal carcinoma: Reflection of a series of 1344 patients treated at the time of initial presentation. *Otolaryngol Head Neck Surg.* 1996;115:519.

85. Bataini JP, Asselain B, Jaulerry C, et al: A multivariate primary tumour control analysis in 465 patients treated by radical radiotherapy for cancer of the tonsillar region: Clinical and treatment parameters as prognostic factors [see comments]. *Radiother Oncol.* 1989;14:265.

86. Wong CS, Ang K, Fletcher G: Definitive radiotherapy for squamous cell carcinoma of the tonsillar fossa. *Int J Radiat Oncol Biol Phys.* 1989;16:657.

87. Amornmarn R, Prempree T, Jaiwatana J: Radiation management of carcinoma of the tonsillar region. *Cancer.* 1984;54:1293.

88. Gwozdz JT, Morrison W, Garden A: Concomitant boost radiotherapy for squamous carcinoma of the tonsillar fossa. *Int J Radiat Oncol Biol Phys.* 1997;39:127.

89. Gluckman JL, Black RJ, and Crissman, JD: Cancer of the oropharynx. *Otolaryngol Clin North Am.* 1985;18:451.

90. Givens CD Jr, Johns ME, Cantrell RW: Carcinoma of the tonsil. Analysis of 162 cases. *Arch Otolaryngol.* 1981;107:730.

91. Rabuzzi DD, Mickler A, Clutler D: Treatment results of combined high-dose preoperative radiotherapy and surgery for oropharyngeal cancer. *Laryngoscope.* 1982;92(9 Pt 1):989.

92. Garrett PG, Beale F, Cumminges B: Carcinoma of the tonsil: The effect of dose-time-volume factors on local control. *Int J Radiat Oncol Biol Phys.* 1985;11:703.

93. Shukovsky LJ, Fletcher GH: Time-dose and tumor volume relationships in the irradiation of squamous cell carcinoma of the tonsillar fossa. *Radiology.* 1973;107:621.

94. Eisbruch A, Kim H, Terrel J: Xerostomia and its predictors following parotid-sparing irradiation of head-and-neck cancer. *Int J Radiat Oncol Biol Phys.* 2001;50:695.

95. O'Sullivan B, Warde P, Grice B: The benefits and pitfalls of ipsilateral radiotherapy in carcinoma of the tonsillar region. *Int J Radiat Oncol Biol Phys.* 2001;51:332.

96. Jackson SM, Hay J, Flores A: Cancer of the tonsil: The results of ipsilateral radiation treatment. *Radiother Oncol.* 1999;51:123.

97. Pernot M, Luporsi E, Hoffstetter S, et al: Complications following definitive irradiation for cancers of the oral cavity and the oropharynx (in a series of 1134 patients). *Int J Radiat Oncol Biol Phys.* 1997;37:577.

98. Mazeron JJ, Belkacemi Y, Simon JM, et al: Place of iridium 192 implantation in definitive irradiation of faucial arch squamous cell carcinomas. *Int J Radiat Oncol Biol Phys.* 993; 27:251.

99. Rudoltz MS, Perkin R, Luthmann R: High-dose-rate brachytherapy for primary carcinomas of the oral cavity and oropharynx. *Laryngoscope.* 1999;109:1967.

100. Mendenhall WM, Parsons JT, Cassisi NJ, Million RR: Squamous cell carcinoma of the tonsillar area treated with radical irradiation. *Radiother Oncol.* 1987;10:23.

101. Kaplan R, Million RR, Cassisi NJ: Carcinoma of the tonsil: results of radical irradiation with surgery reserved for radiation failure. *Laryngoscope.* 1977;87:600.

102. Dasmahapatra KS, Mohit-Tabatabai MA, Rush BF Jr, et al: Cancer of the tonsil. Improved survival with combination therapy. *Cancer.* 1986;57:451.

103. Zelefsky MJ, Harrison LB, Armstrong JG: Long-term treatment results of postoperative radiation therapy for advanced stage oropharyngeal carcinoma. *Cancer.* 1992;70:2388.

104. Perez CA, Carmichael T, Deviveni VR, et al: Carcinoma of the tonsillar fossa: A nonrandomized comparison of irradiation alone or combined with surgery: Long-term results. *Head Neck.* 1991; 13:282.

105. Spiro JD, Spiro RH: Carcinoma of the tonsillar fossa. An update. *Arch Otolaryngol Head Neck Surg.* 1989;115:1186.

106. Quenelle DJ, Crissman JD, Shumrick DA: Tonsil carcinoma—Treatment results. *Laryngoscope.* 1979;89:1842.

107. Puthawala AA, Syed AM, Gates TC: Iridium-192 implants in the treatment of tonsillar region malignancies. *Arch Otolaryngol.* 1985;111:812.

108. Leborgne JH, Leborgne F, Barlocci LA, Ortega B: The place of brachytherapy in the treatment of carcinoma of the tonsil with lingual extension. *Int J Radiat Oncol Biol Phys.* 1986; 12:1787.

109. Peiffert D, Pernot M, Malissard L, et al: Salvage irradiation by brachytherapy of velotonsillar squamous cell carcinoma in a previously irradiated field: Results in 73 cases [see comments]. *Int J Radiat Oncol Biol Phys.* 1994;29:681.

110. Weber RS, Gidley P, Morrison WH, et al: Treatment selection for carcinoma of the base of the tongue. *Am J Surg.* 1990;160:415.

111. Foote RL, Olsen KD, Davis DL, et al: Base of tongue carcinoma: Patterns of failure and predictors of recurrence after surgery alone. *Head Neck.* 1993;15:300.

112. Hinerman RW, Parsons JT, Mendenhall WM, et al: External beam irradiation alone or combined with neck dissection for base of tongue carcinoma: An alternative to primary surgery. *Laryngoscope.* 1994;104:1466.

113. Dupont JB, Guillamondegui OM, Jesse RH: Surgical treatment of advanced carcinomas of the base of the tongue. *Am J Surg.* 1978; 136:501.

114. Harrison LB, Lee H, Kraus DH, et al: Long term results of primary radiation therapy for squamous cancer of the base of tongue. *Radiother Oncol.* 1996;39:S6(abst).

115. Harrison LB, Kraus DH, Zelefsky MJ, et al: Long term results of primary radiation therapy for squamous cell cancer of the base of tongue. *Proc Int Mtg Head Neck Cancer.* 1996;71(abst).

116. Puthawala AA, Syed AM, Eads DL, et al: Limited external beam and interstitial ^{192}iridium irradiation in the treatment of carcinoma of the base of the tongue: A ten year experience. *Int J Radiat Oncol Biol Phys.* 1988;14:839.

117. Crook J, Mazeron JJ, Marinello G, et al: Combined external irradiation and interstitial implantation for T1 and T2 epidermoid carcinomas of base of tongue: The Creteil experience (1971-1981). *Int J Radiat Oncol Biol Phys.* 1988;15:105.

118. Kramer S, Gelber RD, Snow JB, et al: Combined radiation therapy and surgery in the management of advanced head and neck cancer: Final report of study 73-03 of the Radiation Therapy Oncology Group. *Head Neck Surg.* 1987;10:19.

119. Son YH, Kacinski BM: Therapeutic concepts of brachytherapy/megavoltage in sequence for pharyngeal wall cancers. Results of integrated dose therapy. *Cancer.* 1987;59:1268.

120. The Department of Veterans Affairs Laryngeal Cancer Study Group. Induction chemotherapy plus radiation compared with surgery plus radiation in patients with advanced laryngeal cancer. *N Engl J Med.* 1991;324:1685.

121. Spaulding MB, Fischer SG, Wolf GT: The Department of Veterans Affairs Cooperative Laryngeal Cancer Study Group. Tumor response, toxicity, and survival after neoadjuvant organ-preserving chemotherapy for advanced laryngeal carcinoma. *J Clin Oncol.* 1994;12:1592.

122. Domenge C, Hill C, Lefebvre J: Randomized trial of neoadjuvant chemotherapy in oropharyngeal carcinoma. French Groupe d'Etude des Tumeurs de la Tete et du Cou (GETTEC). *Br J Cancer.* 2000;83:1594.

123. Forastiere AA, Berley B, Maor M: Phase III trial to preserve the larynx: Induction chemotherapy and radiotherapy versus concomitant chemoradiotherapy versus radiotherapy alone, Intergroup Trial R91-11. *Proc ASCO, 2001.* 2001;20:2a.

124. Pignon JP, Bourhis J: Meta-analysis of chemotherapy in head and neck cancer: Individual patient data vs literature data. *Br J Cancer.* 1995;72:1062.

125. Pignon JP, Bourhis J, Domenge C: Chemotherapy added to locoregional treatment for head and neck squamous-cell carcinoma: Three meta-analyses of updated individual data. MACH-NC Collaborative Group. Meta-Analysis of Chemotherapy on Head and Neck Cancer. *Lancet.* 2000;355:949.

126. El-Sayed S, Nelson N: Adjuvant and adjunctive chemotherapy in the management of squamous cell carcinoma of the head and neck region. A meta-analysis of prospective and randomized trials. *J Clin Oncol.* 1996;14:838.

127. Munro AJ: An overview of randomised controlled trials of adjuvant chemotherapy in head and neck cancer. *Br J Cancer.* 1995;71:83.

128. Withers HR, Peters L, Taylor J: Local control of carcinoma of the tonsil by radiation therapy: An analysis of patterns of fractionation in nine institutions. *Int J Radiat Oncol Biol Phys.* 1995;33:549.

129. Bieri S, Allal A, Dulgueror P: Concomitant boost radiotherapy in oropharynx carcinomas. *Acta Oncol.* 1998;37:687.

130. Vokes EE, Kies M, Haraf D: Induction chemotherapy followed by concomitant chemoradiotherapy for advanced head and neck cancer: Impact on the natural history of the disease. *J Clin Oncol.* 1995;13:876.

131. Kies MS, Haraf D, Athanasiadis I: Induction chemotherapy followed by concurrent chemoradiation for advanced head and neck cancer: Improved disease control and survival. *J Clin Oncol.* 1998;16:2715.

132. Bensadoun RJ, Etienne M, Chassonville D: Concomitant b.i.d. radiotherapy and chemotherapy with cisplatin and 5-fluorouracil in unresectable squamous-cell carcinoma of the pharynx: Clinical and pharmacological data of a French multicenter phase II study. *Int J Radiat Oncol Biol Phys.* 1998;42:237.

133. Machtay M, Rosenthal D, Algazy K: Pilot study of organ preservation multimodality therapy for locally advanced resectable oropharyngeal carcinoma. *Am J Clin Oncol.* 2000;23:509.

134. Giralt JL, Gonzalez J, del Campo J: Preoperative induction chemotherapy followed by concurrent chemoradiotherapy in advanced carcinoma of the oral cavity and oropharynx. *Cancer.* 2000;89:939.

135. Jeremic B, Shibamoto Y, Milicic B: Hyperfractionated radiation therapy with or without concurrent low-dose daily cisplatin in locally advanced squamous cell carcinoma of the head and neck: A prospective randomized trial. *J Clin Oncol.* 2000;18:1458.

136. Staar S, Rudat V, Stuetzer H: Intensified hyperfractionated accelerated radiotherapy limits the additional benefit of simultaneous chemotherapy—Results of a multicentric randomized German trial in advanced head-and-neck cancer. *Int J Radiat Oncol Biol Phys.* 2001;50:1161.

137. Bourhis J, Lapeyre M, Tortochaux J, et al: Preliminary results of the GORTEC 96-01 randomized trial, comparing very accelerated radiotherapy versus concomitant radiochemotherapy for locally inoperable head and neck squamous cell carcinoma. *Proc of ASCO Abs 905,* Vol 21, 2002.

138. Portenoy RK, Thaler HT, Kornblith AB, et al: The Memorial Symptom Assessment Scale: An instrument for the evaluation of symptom prevalence, characteristics and distress. *Eur J Cancer.* 1994;30A:1326.

139. Cella DF, Tulsky DS, Gray G, et al: The Functional Assessment of Cancer Therapy scale: Development and validation of the general measure. *J Clin Oncol.* 1993;11:570.

140. List MA, Ritter-Sterr C, Lansky SB: A performance status scale for head and neck cancer patients. *Cancer.* 1990;66:564.

141. Harrison LB, Zelefsky MJ, Armstrong JG, et al: Performance status after treatment for squamous cell cancer of the base of tongue—a comparison of primary radiation therapy versus primary surgery. *Int J Radiat Oncol Biol Phys.* 1994;30:953.

142. Harrison LB, Zelefsky MJ, Pfister D, et al: Detailed quality of life assessment in patients treated with primary radiotherapy for squamous cell cancer of the base of the tongue. *Head Neck.* 1997;19:169.

143. Harrison LB, Zelefsky MJ, Pfister D, et al: Detailed quality of life assessment on long term survivors of primary radiation therapy for cancer of the base of tongue. *Head Neck.* 1997;19:169.

144. Spanos WJ Jr, Shukovsky LJ, Fletcher GH: Time, dose, and tumor volume relationships in irradiation of squamous cell carcinomas of the base of the tongue. *Cancer.* 1976;37:2591.

145. Jaulerry C, Rodriguez J, Brunin F, et al: Results of radiation therapy in carcinoma of the base of the tongue. The Curie Institute experience with about 166 cases. *Cancer.* 1991;67:1532.

146. Foote RL, Parsons JT, Mendenhall WM, et al: Is interstitial implantation essential for successful radiotherapeutic treatment of base of tongue carcinoma? *Int J Radiat Oncol Biol Phys.* 1990; 18:1293.

147. Goffinet DR, Fee WE Jr, Wells J, et al: Iridium-192 pharyngoepiglottic fold interstitial implants. The key to successful treatment of base of tongue carcinoma by radiation therapy. *Cancer.* 1985;55:941.

Cancer of the Oral Cavity

29

Nancy Lee, MD and Theodore L. Phillips, MD

EPIDEMIOLOGY AND GENETICS

Approximately 19,400 cases of oral cavity cancer are seen in the United States each year, with 5200 deaths.[1] It is more commonly seen among males than females with an approximate ratio of 3:2.[2] It is predominantly a disease of middle-aged men with a history of exposure to various carcinogenic chemicals, including tobacco smoke and alcohol. There is a clear dose-response relationship between the amount and duration of tobacco smoke exposure and the incidence of oral cavity cancer. In countries such as India, where smokeless tobacco (snuff) is popular, oral cancer is also common, although the risk is lower than for smoking (relative risk, 4.2 vs. 10 to 15). The use of betel nuts is also related to oral cancer, particularly buccal mucosal cancer.[3] Alcohol appears to act as a co-carcinogen and has a topical effect in that mucosal areas directly exposed to alcohol have a higher incidence of oral cancer.[4] Recently, for reasons unclear, there is an increasing trend in tongue cancer in young Americans who never had any exposure to tobacco or alcohol.[5]

Genetic abnormalities such as those seen with Fanconi's syndrome, ataxia telangiectasia, and xeroderma pigmentosum are associated with higher risk, as is human immunodeficiency virus (HIV) infection. Dietary deficiency can cause a higher incidence, as in vitamin A deficiency. A diet high in fruits and vegetables and antioxidants appears to reduce the risk. Human papillomavirus types 6, 11, 16, and 18 have been associated with head and neck cancer.

The spectrum of molecular changes seen in oral cancer varies by country of origin.[6] Mutations of *p53* are common in oral cancers in patients from countries with European populations; for example, 47% of Europeans with oral cancer show mutated *p53*, whereas in patients from India and Southeast Asia, only 7% show mutations. Patients from these areas have tumors with abnormal *ras* genes, which include mutations, loss of heterozygosity (H-*ras*), and amplification (K-*ras* and N-*ras*). Loss of *Rb* gene function may be necessary in combination with *p53* mutation for oncogenesis. It has been widely observed that oral cancers express transforming growth factor-alpha (TGF-α) and epidermal growth factor receptor (EGFR), which may trigger the autocrine growth pathway.[7]

ANATOMY

The oral cavity extends from the skin–vermilion junction of the lips to the junction of the hard and soft palate above, and to the line of circumvallate papillae below, and is divided into the following specific areas (Figs. 29-1 through 29-3).

LIPS. The lip begins at the junction of the vermilion border with the skin and includes only the vermilion surface, or that portion of the lip that comes into contact with the opposing lip. It is divided into an upper lip and a lower lip joined at the commissures of the mouth.

ORAL TONGUE (ANTERIOR TWO THIRDS OF THE TONGUE). The oral tongue is the freely mobile portion of the tongue that extends anteriorly from the line of circumvallate papillae to the undersurface of the tongue at the junction of the floor of the mouth. It is composed of four areas: the tip, the lateral borders, the dorsum, and the undersurface (nonvillous surface of the tongue).

FLOOR OF THE MOUTH. This is a semilunar space over the mylohyoid and hyoglossus muscles, extending from the inner surface of the lower alveolar ridge to the under surface of the tongue. Its posterior boundary is the base

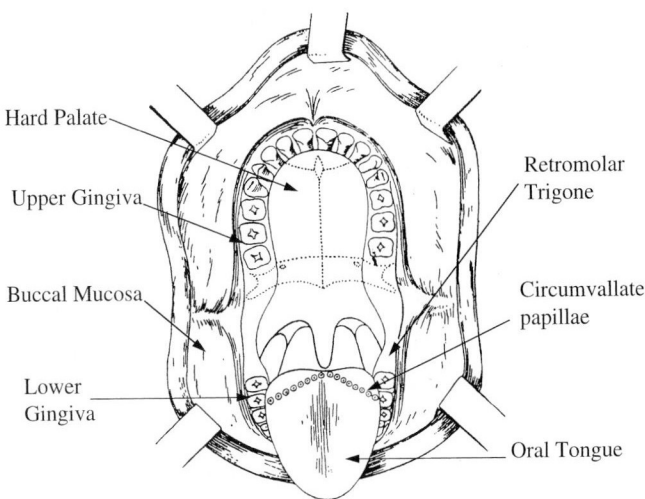

Figure 29–1. Anterior view of oral cavity with structures labeled.

631

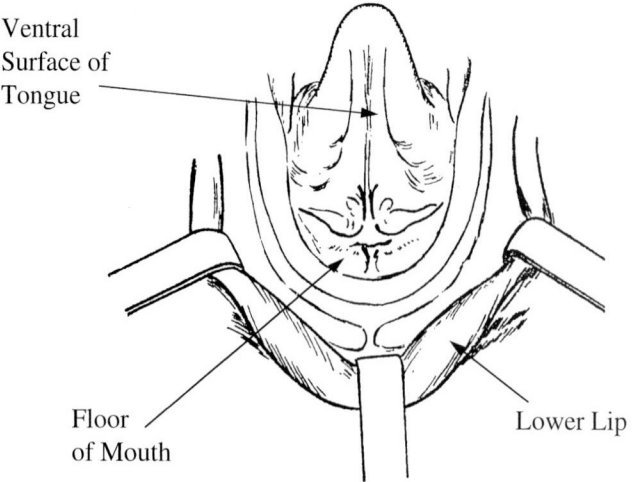

Figure 29–2. View of ventral surface of tongue and floor of mouth.

of the anterior pillar of the tonsil. It is divided into two sides by the frenulum of the tongue and contains the ostia of the submaxillary and sublingual salivary glands.

BUCCAL MUCOSA. This includes all the membrane lining of the inner surface of the cheeks and lips, from the line of contact of the opposing lips to the line of attachment of mucosa of the alveolar ridge (upper and lower) and pterygomandibular raphe.

UPPER GINGIVA. The upper gingiva is the upper ridge of the alveolar process of the maxilla and its covering mucosa, which extends from the line of attachment of mucosa in the upper gingival buccal gutter to the junction of the hard palate. Its posterior margin is the upper end of the pterygo-palatine arch.

LOWER GINGIVA. This ridge includes the alveolar process of the mandible and its covering mucosa, which extends from the line of attachment of mucosa in the buccal gutter to the line of free mucosa of the floor of the

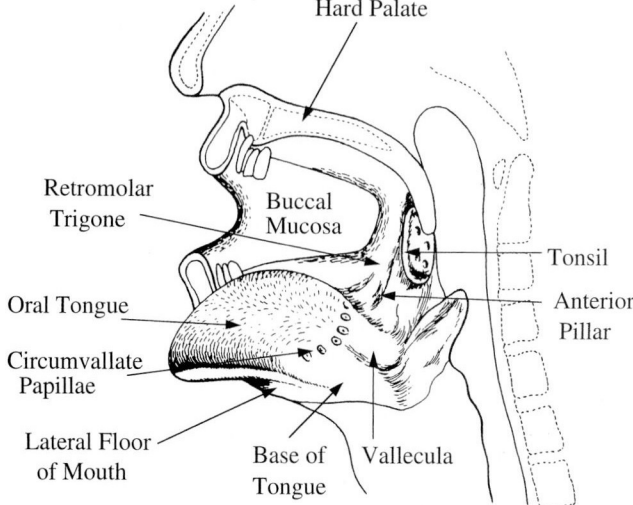

Figure 29–3. Lateral view of oral cavity.

mouth. Posteriorly, it extends to the ascending ramus of the mandible.

RETROMOLAR TRIGONE (RETROMOLAR GINGIVA). This is the attached mucosa overlying the ascending ramus of the mandible from the level of the posterior surface of the last molar tooth to the apex superiorly, adjacent to the tuberosity of the maxilla.

HARD PALATE. This is the semilunar area between the upper alveolar ridge and the mucous membrane covering the palatine process of the maxillary palatine bones. It extends from the inner surface of the superior alveolar ridge to the posterior edge of the palatine bone.

PATHOLOGY

Squamous cell carcinoma is the dominant tumor in the oral cavity and accounts for 95% of the cases. The majority of squamous cancers are moderately differentiated. Tumor grade has little prognostic value. Second in incidence are the various tumors of minor salivary origin, including adenoid cystic carcinoma, mucoepidermoid carcinoma, and adenocarcinoma. Sarcomas can arise in the oral submucosal tissues and from the bones. Ameloblastomas are benign but locally invasive tumors that arise in the mandible or maxilla.

STAGING AND GROUPING SYSTEM

The preferred clinical staging is the American Joint Committee on Cancer (AJCC) system 6th ed.[8] (Table 29-1). T4 lesions have been divided into T4a (resectable disease) versus T4b (unresectable disease).

DIAGNOSTIC AND STAGING STUDIES

The evaluation of the patient with oral cancer begins with a careful oral examination and biopsy of the lesion. The delineation of the gross extent is sometimes aided by toluidine blue staining. Bone invasion should be evaluated by Panorex dental radiographs for the mandible and by computed tomography (CT) scans with bone windows for maxillary and deeper mandibular invasion. The extent of lymph node involvement in the neck is determined by physical examination and a magnetic resonance imaging (MRI) scan. MRI appears superior to CT for determination of local invasion of soft tissues. The best initial staging study is MRI, with CT used for problem cases in which bone invasion may be present.

GENERAL THERAPEUTIC APPROACHES

Surgery Alone

Surgical resection of the primary lesion, either with the laser or by intraoral conventional resection, is the treatment of choice for many T1 lesions of the lip, tongue, and

Table 29–1   Classification of Oral Cavity Cancer

Primary Tumor (T)

TX	Primary tumor cannot be assessed
T0	No evidence of primary tumor
Tis	Carcinoma in situ
T1	Tumor ≤2 cm in greatest dimension
T2	Tumor >2 cm but not >4 cm in greatest dimension
T3	Tumor >4 cm in greatest dimension
T4	(lip) Tumor invades adjacent structures (e.g., through cortical bone, tongue, skin of neck)
T4	(oral cavity)
	T4a—Tumor invades adjacent structures (e.g., through cortical bone, into deep [extrinsic] muscle of the tongue [genioglossus, hyoglossus, palatoglossus, and styloglossus]
	T4b—Tumor invades masticator space, pterygoid plates, or skull base, or encases internal carotid artery, or both

Regional Lymph Nodes (N)

NX	Regional lymph nodes cannot be assessed
N0	No regional lymph node metastases
N1	Metastases in a single ipsilateral lymph node, ≤3 cm in greatest dimension
N2	Metastasis in a single ipsilateral lymph node, >3 cm but not >6 cm in greatest dimension, or in multiple ipsilateral lymph nodes, none >6 cm in greatest dimension, or in bilateral or contralateral lymph nodes, none >6 cm in greatest dimension
N2a	Metastasis in a single ipsilateral lymph node >3 cm but not >6 cm in greatest dimension
N2b	Metastasis in multiple ipsilateral lymph nodes, none >6 cm in greatest dimension
N2c	Metastasis in bilateral or contralateral lymph nodes, none >6 cm in greatest dimension
N3	Metastasis in a lymph node >6 cm in greatest dimension

Distant Metastases (M)

MX	Distant metastasis cannot be assessed
M0	No distant metastasis
M1	Distant metastasis

Stage Grouping

Stage 0	T1s	N0	M0
Stage I	T1	N0	M0
Stage II	T2	N0	M0
Stage III	T3	N0	M0
	T1	N1	M0
	T2	N1	M0
	T3	N1	M0
Stage IVA	T4a	N0	M0
	T4a	N1	M0
	T1	N2	M0
	T2	N2	M0
	T3	N2	M0
	T4a	N2	M0
Stage IVB	T4b	Any N	M0
	Any T	N3	M0
Stage IVC	Any T	Any N	M1

From Greene FL, Page DL, Fleming ID, et al, eds: *AJCC Cancer Staging Manual, 6th ed.* New York: Springer; 2002.

floor of the mouth. This is often accompanied by a neck dissection, either supra-omohyoid or comprehensive. Some early T2 tumors may also be treated by surgery alone, but a neck dissection must be added.

Radiotherapy Alone

Tumors classified as T1 and select cases of early T2 can be treated with radiation alone. Lesions of the lip and floor of the mouth can be treated by external beam radiotherapy or brachytherapy or both. Oral tongue lesions do not respond well to external beam radiotherapy; therefore, surgery is probably the better treatment modality with brachytherapy or peroral cone plus external beam as alternatives.

Combined Radiotherapy and Surgery

For locally advanced carcinomas, radiotherapy combined with surgery achieves the most optimal results. Combination therapy is indicated when the primary lesions are large, deeply infiltrative, or necrotic; when there is bone invasion or deep muscle infiltration; when cervical lymph node metastases are present; when there is invasion of the soft tissues in the neck; and when there is known residual disease beyond the margins of resection. Even T1 lesions may require postoperative treatment if tumor invasion is deep, even in the presence of negative margin. It is strongly recommended that the radiation oncologist review all slides with the pathologist to determine whether adjuvant radiotherapy is indicated.

The selection of patients and the planning of the combined treatment should be done jointly by the radiation oncologist and the head-and-neck surgeon.

Combined Chemotherapy and Radiotherapy

Chemotherapy has been combined with radiotherapy in the management of patients with unresectable oral cavity cancer with the goals of increasing local control and survival as well as decreasing distant metastases. The chemotherapeutic agents most commonly used include cisplatin, Taxol, fluorouracil (5-FU), methotrexate, and bleomycin. Except for one randomized study reported by Lo and colleagues, which showed increased survival in patients with oral cavity lesions receiving 5-FU concurrently with radiotherapy as compared with patients receiving radiotherapy alone,[9] there has been no definitive evidence for improved local control or survival in oral cancer when single-agent chemotherapy is combined with radiotherapy. Enhanced radiation mucositis has been commonly observed with concurrent drug and radiation administration, especially when 5-FU is given concurrently with radiation.

Postoperative Radiotherapy

The aims of postoperative radiotherapy are (1) to prevent local recurrence when there is known residual gross or microscopical disease after surgery, (2) to prevent recurrence in the neck when there are large or multiple lymph node metastases and tumor invasion of the soft tissues in the neck, and (3) to control occult disease in the cervical lymph nodes that were not resected surgically.[10]

When radiotherapy is given postoperatively, usually a dose of 63-66.6 Gy is delivered in 1.8 Gy daily fractions, five fractions a week, to the primary site and involved neck areas. Clinically or pathologically uninvolved neck areas receive 54 Gy.[11] It is generally believed that tumor cells trapped in the surgical scars are less well oxygenated and therefore more radioresistant, and that higher radiation doses are required to eradicate them than are required preoperatively. However, this belief has not been adequately tested. Apparent differences in doses required preoperatively and postoperatively may be due to proliferation of tumor cells in the postoperative period before radiotherapy starts. The volume that is irradiated should include the entire surgical bed and the entire neck. Postoperative radiotherapy can be started as soon as wound healing is complete, usually within 2 to 3 weeks after surgery.

SIMULATION

To assure daily reproducibility of treatment setups, the patient is placed in the supine position with the head on a Timo or other head-holding device. The involved lymph nodes, commissures of the lips, and any scars in postoperative patients are outlined with thin solder wire. The head is then immobilized in the neutral position with a face mask. Either the vacuum-forming technique or thermoplastic techniques are satisfactory and superior to bite blocks. For patients with short necks, the shoulders should be lowered by the patient's pulling on a tensioning device looped under the feet. If a three-dimensional (3D) plan is to be generated, orthogonal films for the superior (oral cavity) volume are taken and the supraclavicular-neck field is simulated. CT scans are then taken in the treatment position with the mask in place. If a 3D plan is not used, opposing portals are simulated. A 3D plan should be used for any but simple opposed-lateral fields. Details of simulation for specific sites are given in the following sections.

GENERAL TECHNIQUES OF RADIOTHERAPY AND TREATMENT PLANS

Megavoltage External Beam Radiotherapy

Megavoltage external beam radiotherapy in combination with surgery or interstitial brachytherapy is the most frequently used radiotherapy technique in the treatment of carcinoma of the oral cavity. Megavoltage beams with an energy range between 4 and 6 MV having a maximum dose at about 1 to 1.5 cm below the skin surface are most suitable. When higher energy beams (>4 MV) are used, bolus material may be necessary to bring the maximum dose closer to the skin surface to adequately treat superficial lymph nodes and surgical scars.

The treatment volume encompassing the primary tumor with adequate margins and cervical lymph nodes of concern is outlined on the treatment simulation films or the skin or both. Metallic wires or gold seeds or silver clips placed in the tumor periphery are helpful in localizing the tumor volume on the simulation films. Normal tissues that are in the field but need not be irradiated are shielded with individual, tailor-made lead blocks mounted on the treatment field template on a tray. Alternately, multi-leaf collimator shaping can be employed. Examples are shown in Figures 29-4 through 29-6 for treatment of an advanced carcinoma of the tongue. Weekly port films are obtained with the patient on the treatment machine to verify the actual volume irradiated. Treatment planning is then done using a 3D planning computer. After the treatment volumes have been established and verified, the isocenter of the treatment volume may be tattooed on the skin so that ink markings outlining the treatment field are not necessary.

Tissue-compensating filters made of copper alloy are used with opposing portals when the variation of the separation is greater than 3 cm. All fields are treated daily. The usual dose fractionation is 1.8 to 2 Gy per day, five daily treatments per week for definitive cases and 1.8 to 2 Gy per fraction for postoperative cases. The total

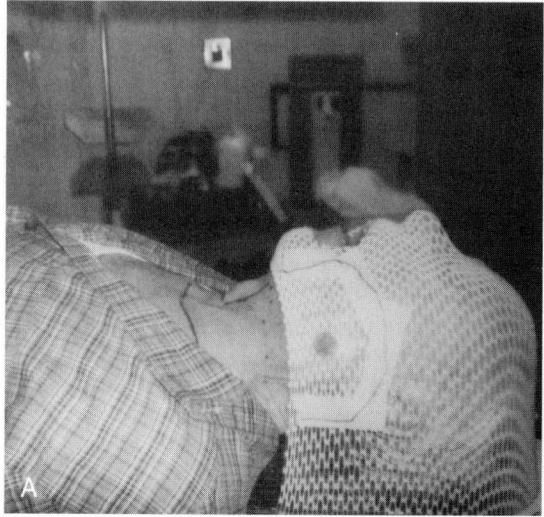 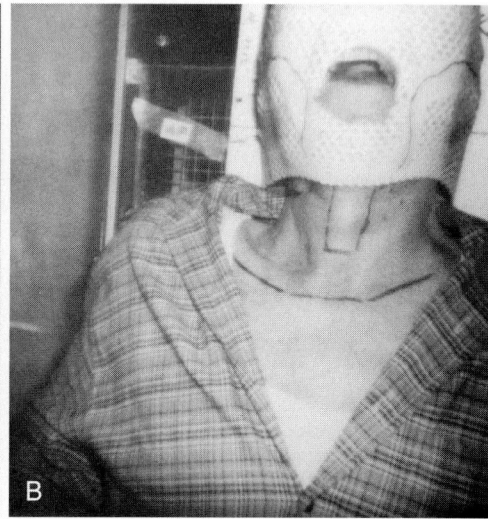

Figure 29–4. A, Lateral view of patient in mask showing lateral and anterior low neck fields for treating oral tongue cancer. **B,** Anterior supraclavicular portal.

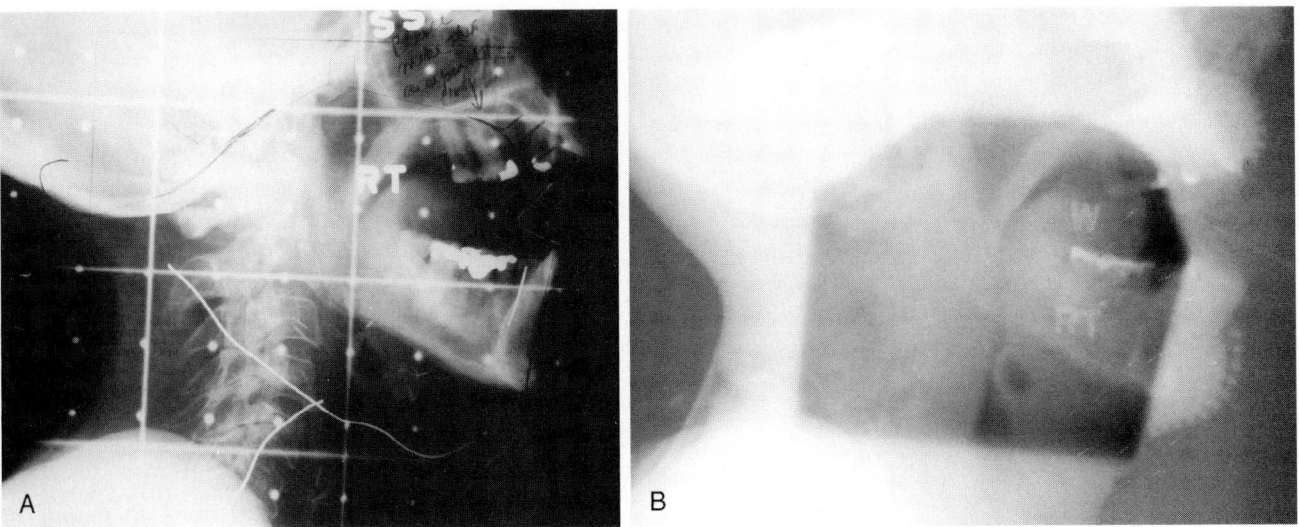

Figure 29–5. A, Simulation film of lateral port for tongue carcinoma. **B,** Portal film of lateral port.

dose depends on the extent of the disease and whether external beam radiotherapy is used alone or in combination with interstitial radiotherapy or surgery. When definitive external beam alone is used, the total dose is usually in the range of 70 to 74 Gy. The spinal cord is shielded after 44 Gy and the treatment fields are further reduced to 54 to 60 Gy so that only a limited volume containing the gross disease is irradiated with a higher dose.

PERORAL CONE RADIOTHERAPY

Intraoral cone radiotherapy using 100 to 250 kVP x-rays or 6 MeV electron beams is suitable for the treatment of select small lesions, less than 3 cm in diameter, in the floor of the mouth. For the proper administration of this

radiotherapy modality, it is necessary that adequate coverage of the lesion is achieved with the intraoral cone and that patient immobilization be maintained during treatment. The use of a special immobilizing chair that locks the patient and applicator in a rigid unit is advised for orthovoltage treatment, as shown in Figure 29-7. The analysis by Phillips[12] on the time-dose relationships in peroral radiotherapy for oral cancer suggested that surface doses between 55 Gy in 18 days and 60 Gy in 26 days will result in good control rates with acceptable risk of soft tissue or bone necrosis. Wang[13] has described a technique for using peroral cones with electron beams (Fig. 29-8).

The advantages of peroral radiotherapy over interstitial radiotherapy or external beam radiotherapy in properly selected patients are as follows: (1) only a small volume is irradiated, therefore salivary gland function is

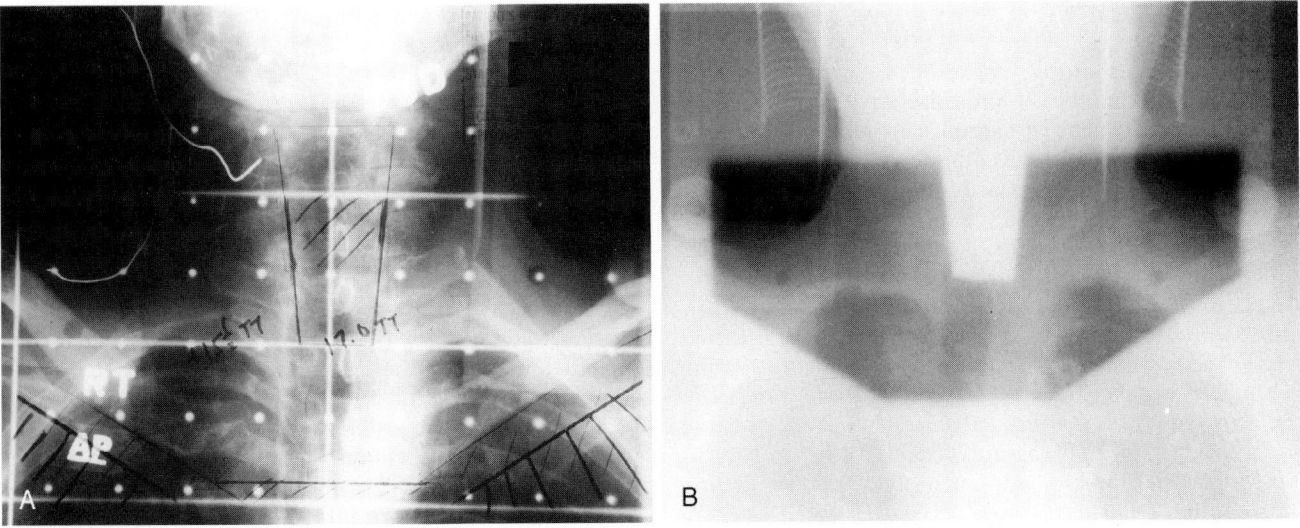

Figure 29–6. A, Simulation film of anterior port for supraclavicular and low neck treatment. **B,** Portal film of anterior port.

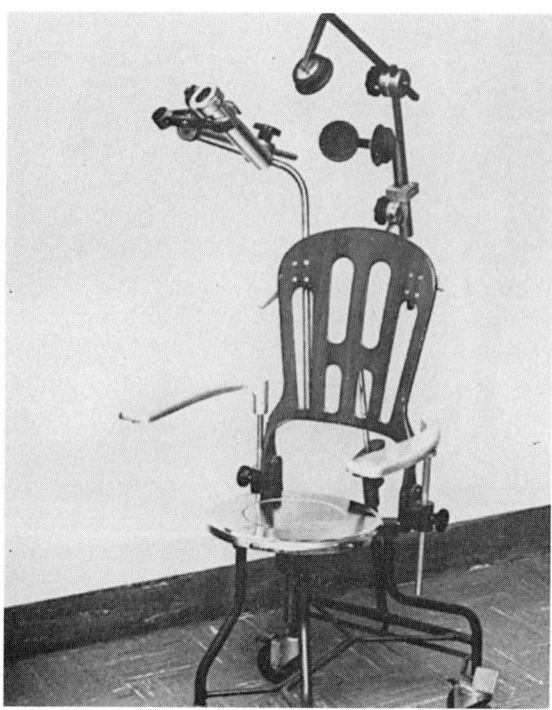

Figure 29–7. Peroral cone for orthovoltage with treatment chair. (From Phillips TL: Peroral roentgen therapy. *Radiology.* 1968;90:525.)

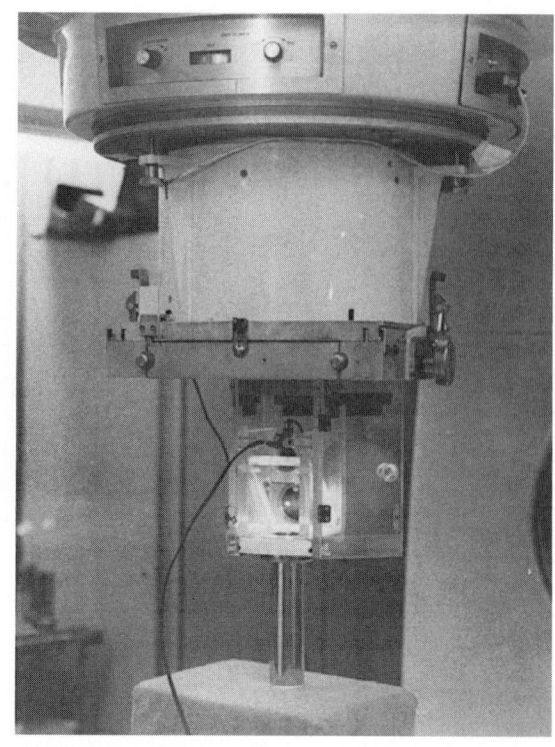

Figure 29–8. Electron beam peroral cone set up at Massachusetts General Hospital. (From Wang CC: Technical and radiotherapeutic considerations of intra-oral cone electron beam radiation therapy for head and neck cancer. *Semin Radiat Oncol.* 1992;2:171.)

preserved and late dental problems avoided; (2) no hospitalization or anesthetics are necessary; (3) the risk of bone necrosis is minimal.

Peroral radiotherapy can also be used in combination with external beam radiotherapy to deliver a boost dose to lesions that are marginally encompassed by an intraoral cone. The boost should be given before the external beam treatment and is usually 21 to 27 Gy in 3 Gy fractions.

BRACHYTHERAPY

Interstitial radiotherapy, either alone or in combination with external beam radiotherapy, is for selected cases in the treatment of carcinoma of the oral tongue, floor of the mouth, and buccal mucosa.[14-16] The radioactive isotopes used in the past in interstitial radiotherapy of oral carcinomas included radium-226, cesium-137, gold-198, and tantalum-182. Iridium 192 used in the form of pins (epingles), wires, or seeds preloaded in a plastic ribbon have the advantage of being suitable for afterloading techniques. At the University of California, San Francisco (UCSF), we prefer to use afterloading techniques with iridium 192 for temporary interstitial implants of oral cavity lesions whenever possible. Iodine 125 may be substituted and is the isotope of choice for permanent implants. The use of remote afterloading of iridium sources with high dose rate (HDR) is replacing the use of hand-loaded seeds in ribbons in many institutions. These techniques minimize

exposure to personnel and allow optimization of dose distribution.[17]

When the tumor thickness is 1 cm or less, a single-plane implant is adequate. When the tumor thickness is greater than 1 cm, then a double-plane implant or volume implant is necessary to deliver a relatively uniform dose to the tumor volume. The Patterson-Parker or Quimby[18,19] tables are often used for treatment planning; however, dosimetry is best done by a computer using localization films of the actual implant.

When interstitial radiotherapy is used alone, for patients who present with early-staged T1 to T2N0 disease, the usual implant dose is 60 to 70 Gy delivered over a period of 6 to 7 days.[20,21] For oral tongue lesions, if a combination of external beam radiotherapy and interstitial implant is considered, several series have reported on the importance of adequate interstitial implant dose. The total implant dose is correlated with local control. Those patients who received an external beam dose less than 40 Gy along with a higher brachytherapy dose achieved higher local control rates than those who received a lower brachytherapy dose.[22-24] If the patients have neck disease, surgery ± postoperative radiotherapy is recommended over radiotherapy alone.

No adjustment of total dose is made when the dose rate of the minimum tumor dose is between 30 and 60 cGy per hour.[25] Examples of a single-plane iridium implant and a volume iridium implant and the isodose distributions are shown in Figures 29-9 and 29-10.

Surface mold radiotherapy can be used as a primary treatment for select initial or recurrent superficial lesions

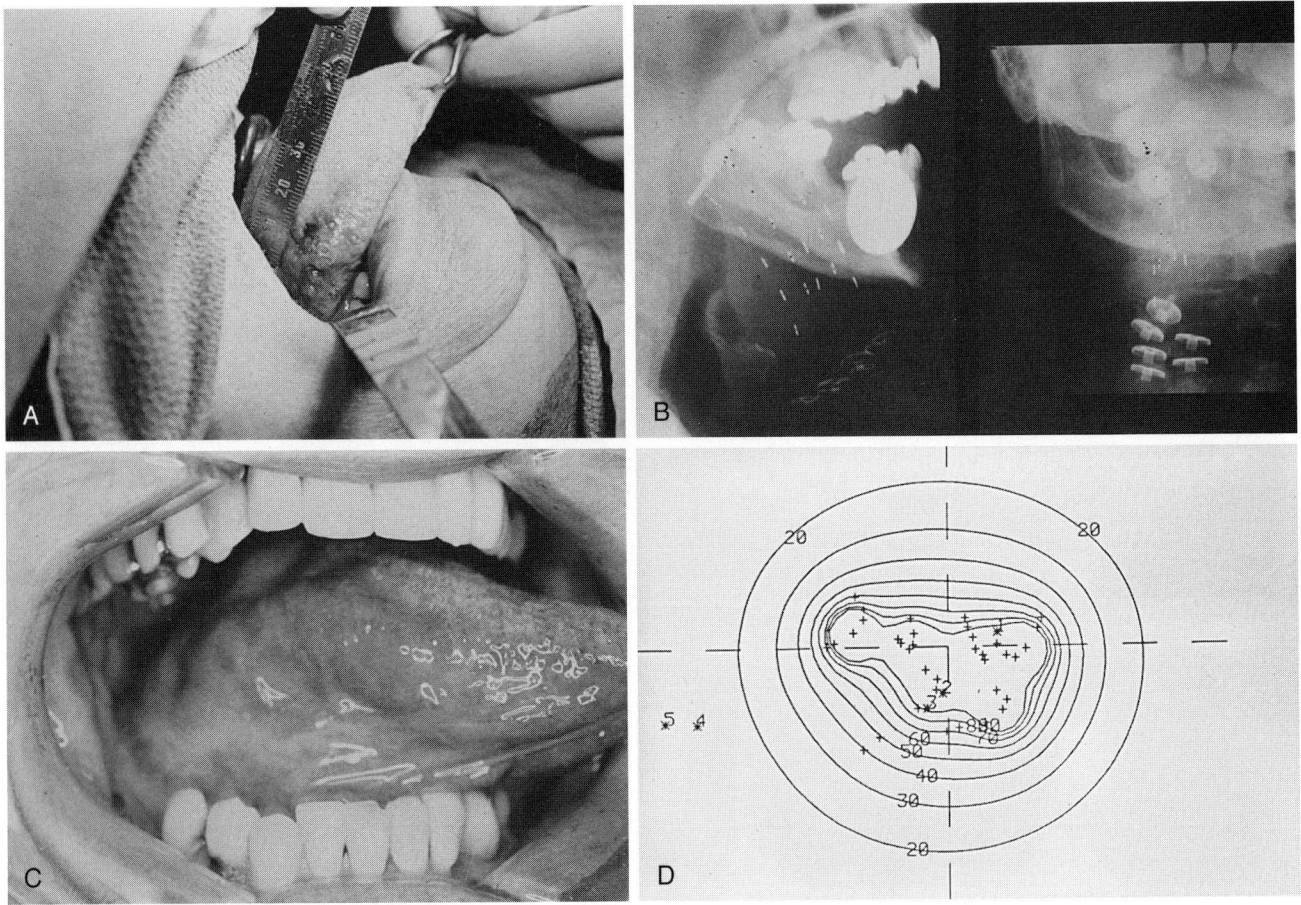

Figure 29–9. A, Carcinoma of the right oral tongue before brachytherapy. **B,** Double-plane implant for T2 squamous cell cancer of oral tongue—lateral and anterior-posterior radiographs. **C,** Appearance of tongue 1 year after implant. Note normal saliva and intact teeth. **D,** Isodose plot of the double-plane implant.

of the hard palate, lower gingiva, and floor of the mouth. An impression is usually made of the surface to be irradiated and a mold in the form of a partial dental plate is made of dental plaster. After distribution of radioactive isotopes has been outlined, iridium seeds or wires or tubes for HDR treatment can be inserted into the predrilled holes or grooves in the mold and sealed with dental plaster. Treatment can be carried out on an outpatient basis with the patient wearing the surface mold several hours a day, or the patient can be admitted into the hospital and wear the surface mold for most of the day except mealtimes. HDR remote afterloading with fractionated delivery may be used with surface molds. Surface mold radiotherapy is not adequate for lesions greater than 1 cm in depth.

CARCINOMA OF THE LIP

Clinical Presentation

Second to the skin, carcinoma of the lip is the most common cancer of the head and neck. In the United States, lip cancer accounts for 12.7 per 100,000 annually.[26] It is rare among blacks and Asians. It accounts for approximately 25% of all carcinomas of the oral cavity. Approximately 90% of the carcinomas of the lip arise

from the lower lip. Most frequently, it affects elderly men in the sixth and seventh decades of life. The incidence rates are generally stable or falling among males worldwide but rising among many female populations. Chronic exposure to sunlight appears to be a predisposing factor for the development of carcinoma of the lip. Carcinoma of the lip occurs most frequently in light-complected, fair-skinned persons who work outdoors.[27] Other possible etiologic factors are tobacco smoking and viruses.

The majority of carcinomas of the lower lip are moderately to well differentiated squamous cell carcinomas. Basal cell carcinomas make up the majority of upper lip lesions.[28] Basal cell carcinomas arising from the skin that invade the lips secondarily should be considered carcinomas of the skin.

Carcinoma of the lower lip frequently appears as a thickening of the mucous membrane initially. Later, desquamation and ulceration that does not heal may develop. There may be a history of long-standing keratosis or leukoplakia.[29]

Routes of Spread

Carcinoma of the lip tends to be localized. It usually spreads by direct invasion of the surrounding soft tissue,

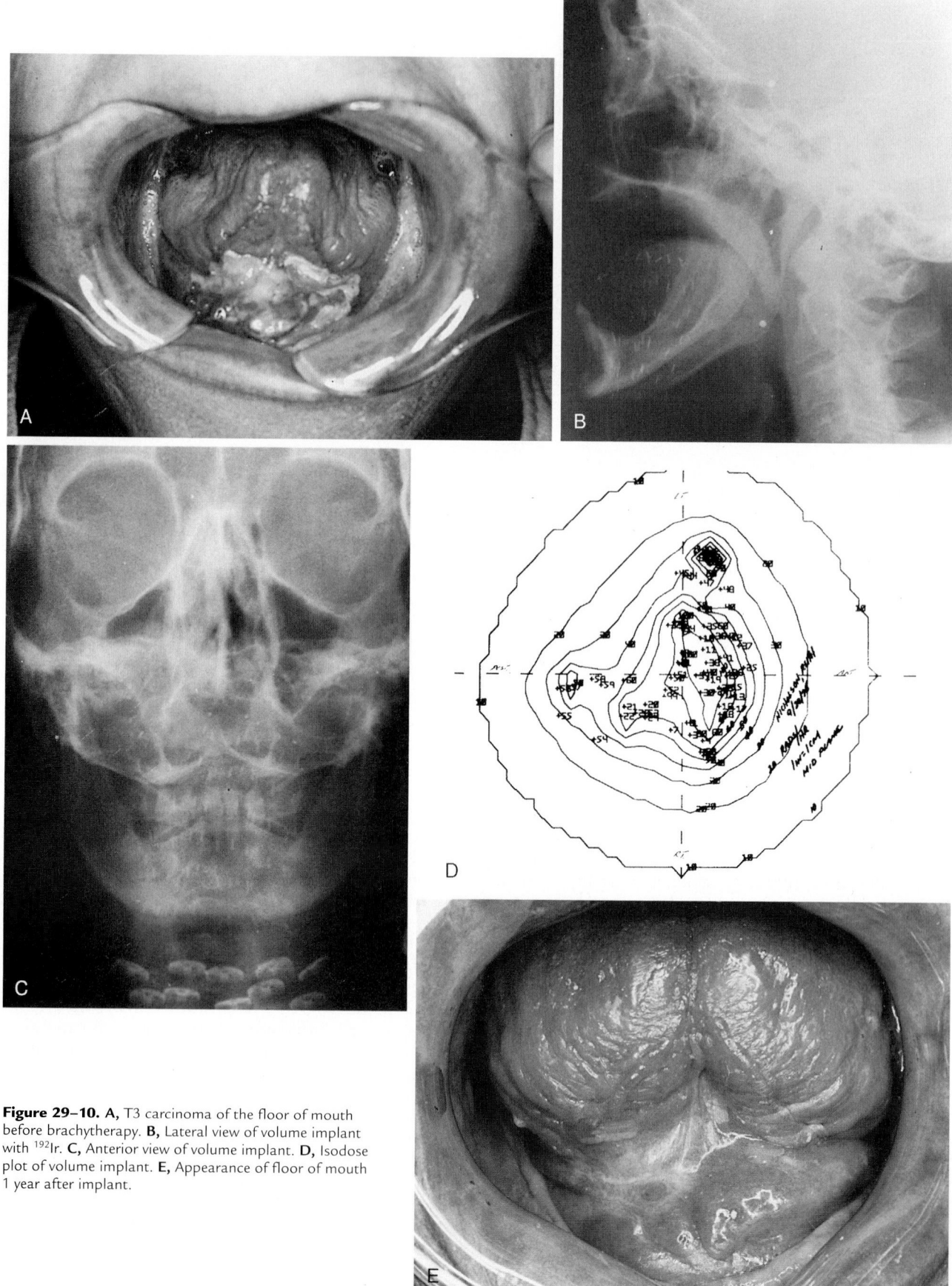

Figure 29–10. A, T3 carcinoma of the floor of mouth before brachytherapy. **B,** Lateral view of volume implant with ¹⁹²Ir. **C,** Anterior view of volume implant. **D,** Isodose plot of volume implant. **E,** Appearance of floor of mouth 1 year after implant.

skin, and bone and infrequently metastasizes to regional lymph nodes.[30] The incidence of lymph node metastasis varies with the extent of the primary lesion. The average incidence of regional lymph node metastasis is about 3% to 8% on presentation, and approximately an equal proportion of patients develop cervical lymph node metastasis subsequent to treatment of the primary lesion. There is rare incidence of perineural spread, often into the mandibular canal.[31]

Lymph node metastasis from carcinoma of the lower lip most frequently involves the ipsilateral prevascular submandibular nodes. Carcinoma arising near the midline of the lower lip usually metastasizes to the submental nodes. Carcinoma at or near the commissure may metastasize rarely to the facial nodes within the substance of the cheek. Carcinoma of the upper lip may metastasize directly to the upper cervical, preauricular, or submandibular nodes. However, contralateral metastases are infrequent. Distant metastasis from carcinoma of the lip is extremely rare.

Treatment Approach

Carcinoma of the lip can be treated successfully with either radiotherapy or surgery.[32] The choice of treatment depends on the extent of disease, the functional and cosmetic results of the treatment, expediency, the patient's age, and the available treatment personnel and facilities.[33] Radiotherapy is usually indicated for moderately large (≥3 cm) infiltrative lesions that would otherwise require a complicated plastic surgery with less satisfactory cosmetic and functional results. Radiation is also indicated for tumors involving the commissure because surgical excision of the commissure would not yield satisfactory cosmetic and functional results.[34] Elderly patients who are at high risk for complications of general anesthesia or who have persistent or recurrent disease after surgery should be considered for radiotherapy. Radiotherapy is also administered postoperatively when the surgical margin is inadequate and there is invasion of the soft tissues of the neck by the cervical lymph node metastasis, and in combination with surgery for advanced resectable disease. Surgery is usually preferred for small lesions, young patients, very advanced disease with bone invasion, cervical lymph node metastasis, and recurrent disease after radiotherapy.

Radiotherapy modalities commonly used for carcinoma of the lip include external beam radiotherapy with orthovoltage x-rays or electron beam[35] and interstitial implants with radium or iridium.[16] The "sandwich" technique has also been used in some centers; however, fractionated external beam radiotherapy usually yields more satisfactory cosmetic results, especially for moderately advanced disease. When interstitial radiotherapy is used, a dose of 60 to 70 Gy in 6 to 8 days is usually adequate.

When external beam radiotherapy is used, a lead cut-out is usually made to outline the treatment volume. A lead shield can be inserted between the inner surface of the lip and the gingiva to prevent irradiation of the intraoral structures. The treatment volume should include the lesion with adequate margins. Leukoplakic changes on the lip adjacent to the lesion should also be included in the treatment volume. For small superficial tumors, a single field with 100 to 150 kV x-rays is sufficient. For deeper, more advanced tumors, 200 to 250 kV x-rays or electrons are usually used. The optimal dose-fractionation schedule depends on the volume of irradiation. For small lesions (≤2 cm in diameter), a dose of 45 Gy to 50 Gy in 15 fractions over 3 weeks is usually adequate, with good cosmetic results. For larger lesions, more protracted treatments with 50 to 70 Gy in 4 to 7 weeks are often used. The base of the skull should be adequately covered in cases with perineural involvement (Fig. 29-11). The neck is usually not irradiated unless cervical lymph node metastasis is present. Acute moist skin and mucous membrane reactions are managed with frequent cleansing and saline soaks. Topical antibiotics are rarely used unless there is infection.

Treatment Outcome

Results of radiotherapy in select series of patients treated with radiotherapy for carcinoma of the lip are shown in Table 29-2.[34,36-38] Control of the primary lesion can be achieved with external beam irradiation or interstitial implants in the majority of patients. Those with recurrent disease after radiotherapy or cervical lymph node metastasis are usually treated surgically. Death due to uncontrolled carcinoma of the lip is uncommon (<10% in most series). The local control rate by interstitial implant is comparable to that achieved with external irradiation, although for larger lesions, better cosmetic results are obtained with protracted external beam radiotherapy.

CARCINOMA OF THE ORAL TONGUE

Clinical Presentation

Second to carcinoma of the lip, carcinoma of the oral tongue is the most common carcinoma of the oral cavity. It is more common in males than in females. The peak incidence occurs in the fifth through seventh decades of life. It is often associated with poor oral hygiene, alcoholism, and heavy tobacco smoking. In the past, it has been associated with syphilis. There also has been an association with Plummer-Vinson syndrome in Sweden, and chewing betel nuts mixed with slaked lime and tobacco in India.

Carcinoma of the oral tongue most frequently arises from the lateral border of the tongue, especially the posterior portions of the oral tongue. Grossly, it may be exophytic, papillary, or infiltrative, with superficial ulcerations. The majority of carcinomas of the oral tongue are moderately to well differentiated squamous cell carcinomas. Areas of leukoplakia and carcinoma in situ associated with invasive carcinoma are not uncommon.

Carcinoma of the oral tongue commonly presents as a growth or ulcer with or without local pain. When the disease becomes more advanced, the patient may complain of pain in the ear on the same side of the lesion,

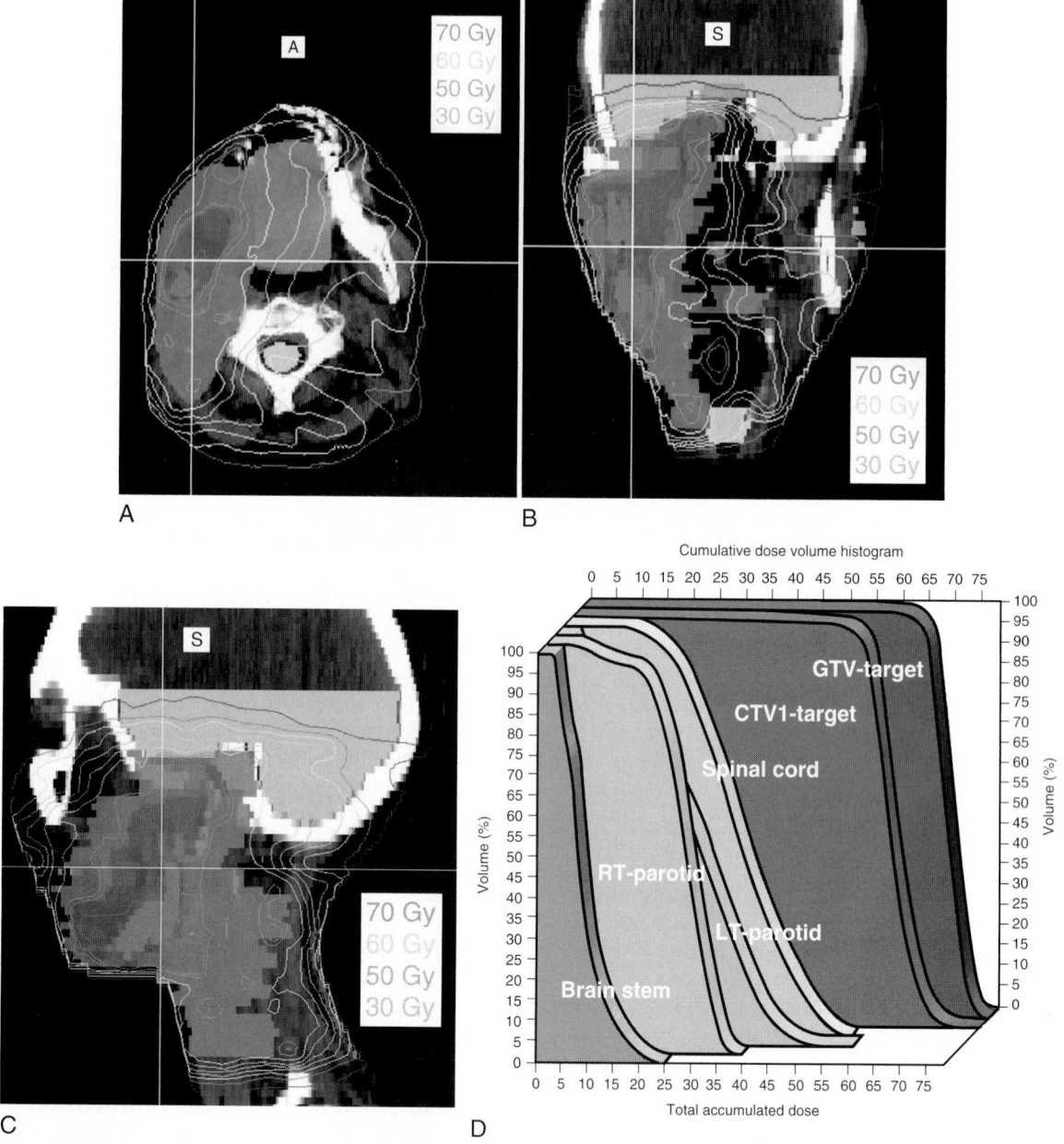

Figure 29–11. Isodose curves of an inverse intensity-modulated radiotherapy plan using seven coplanar gantry angles delivered with conventional multi-leaf collimator for a patient with recurrent carcinoma of the lip with perineural invasion displayed on the axial (**A**), coronal (**B**), and sagittal (**C**) planes through the centroid of the primary tumor and the Dose Volume Histogram for the relevant structures (**D**). The gross tumor volume is shown in red and the clinical target volume (including a margin for set-up errors) is shown in magenta. See also Color Figure 29-11.

Table 29–2   Results of Radiotherapy of Carcinoma of the Lip

Institution (Y, Follow-up)	Patients, n	Stage	Local Control Rate, %	Disease-Free Survival	Overall Survival
USC/UCLA (1987, 20 y)[36]	108	T1	98.9		
		T2	76.5		
		T3	100		
PMH (1993, 5 y)[37]	117	T1	96		
		T2-T3	94		
Netherlands (1996, 10 y)[34]	89	T1	98.9		
	17	T2	76.5		
	2	T3	100		
Italy (1998, 5 y)[38]	57	T1-3	94	81	76

owing to involvement of the lingual nerve, hypersalivation, and dysphagia. When there is extreme involvement of the tongue or fixation of the tongue, swallowing and speech may become difficult. Patients usually die of uncontrolled local disease with hemorrhage, inanition, aspiration, or other complications.

Routes of Spread

Carcinoma of the oral tongue usually spreads by direct invasion into the floor of the mouth, anterior tonsillar pillar, base of tongue, and mandible. Approximately 30% to 40% of the patients have cervical lymph node metastasis on presentation. The thickness as well as the T stage of the tongue lesion is directly correlated with the incidence of lymph nodal involvement.[21,39] The subdigastric nodes are most frequently involved. The submandibular and midjugular lymph nodes are less commonly involved, and the submental, lower jugular, and posterior cervical nodes are rarely involved. Distant metastasis is seldom detected before death. Lungs, liver, and bones are the most common distant metastatic sites. Approximately 19% of patients develop a second malignant tumor. The majority of the second cancers are in the upper respiratory-digestive tract. The distribution of lymph nodes reported by Lindberg[40] is shown in Figure 29-12.

Treatment Approach

Surgery followed by radiotherapy, for both the primary as well as the bilateral necks is the preferred treatment modality for carcinoma of the oral tongue. Invasive pattern T1 and T2, T3 or T4 lesions, bone invasion, multiple cervical lymph node metastases, close or positive margins, lymphovascular, or perineural invasion are indications for postoperative radiotherapy. Attempts to spare the parotid glands can be made to reduce xerostomia (Fig. 29-13). With the excellent functional outcome of the reconstructed oral tongue after hemiglossectomy,[41,43] definitive radiotherapy with or without chemotherapy is reserved for selected cases (i.e., if the patient is medically

inoperable or if the lesion is unresectable). It must include brachytherapy to be effective.

Surgery is indicated for small lesions (<1 cm) located on the dorsum, the tip, or the lateral border of the tongue that can be excised without resulting in dysfunction, especially in young patients. Certain carcinomas of the tongue arising from syphilitic glossitis, lesions that are edematous and deeply infiltrative, lesions that have invaded the mandible, lesions that have invaded the glossopalatine sulcus, and advanced lesions with multiple lymph node metastases are best managed with combined radiotherapy and surgery. Surgery is also preferred in elderly patients who tolerate partial glossectomy better than radiotherapy and in whom preservation of speech is not important. Although recurrence in the primary lesion after radiotherapy is very seldom salvaged by surgery, metastatic cervical lymph node metastasis that develops after the primary lesion has been controlled with radiotherapy can be successfully managed by surgery in the majority of patients.

When external irradiation is used in combination with interstitial implants in selected cases of carcinoma of the oral tongue, usually 40 Gy are delivered in 2 Gy fractions, five daily fractions per week, before the implant. The implant should deliver at least 40 Gy. Although the primary lesion may shrink after the external irradiation, the treatment volume for the interstitial implant is usually determined before any treatment is initiated. The treatment volume for external irradiation should include the primary lesion as well as the regional lymph nodal areas. The lymph node areas are treated to 54 to 60 Gy. When lymph nodes are clinically involved, neck dissection should be considered instead of radiotherapy as it offers better local control. In this clinical scenario, the preference is surgery followed by postoperative radiotherapy when indicated.

Interstitial implant is an integral part of radiotherapy for carcinoma of the oral tongue if definitive radiotherapy is the primary treatment approach.[44] The implant dose is directly correlated with local control.[22-24] External radiotherapy alone is not recommended as it is rarely successful. Early superficial lesions can be controlled with a single-plane interstitial implant or peroral radiotherapy alone. For lesions greater than 1 cm in thickness, double-plane or volume implants in combination with external irradiation are usually used. Brachytherapy has also been used in the postoperative setting for T1-2N0 squamous cell carcinomas of the oral tongue and the floor of mouth with close or positive margins. The recommended dose is 60 Gy.[45,46] High rates of locoregional control, close to 90%, with low risk of chronic sequelae have been reported.[45,46]

The most important step in treatment planning for interstitial implants is the determination of the treatment volume. Sometimes the true extent of the tumor cannot be adequately determined without anesthesia because of pain. With the patient under general anesthesia, it is not uncommon to find a tumor more extensive than anticipated. For this reason, it is always a good idea to bring a surplus of needles to the operating room when radium needles are used.

For interstitial implants of carcinoma of the tongue and floor of the mouth, dose rates in the range of 30 to

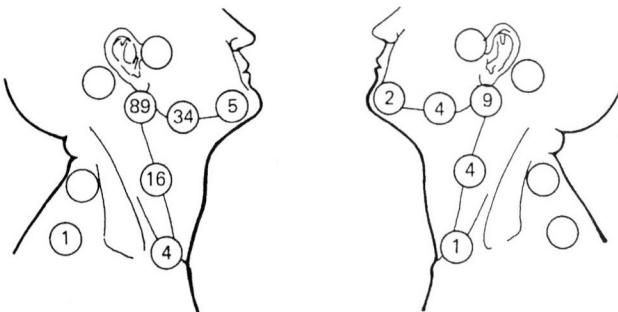

Figure 29–12. Distribution of 105 lymph nodes in 302 patients for oral tongue. (From Lindberg RD: Distribution of cervical lymph node metastases from squamous cell carcinoma of the upper respiratory and digestive tracts. *Cancer.* 1972;29:1446.)

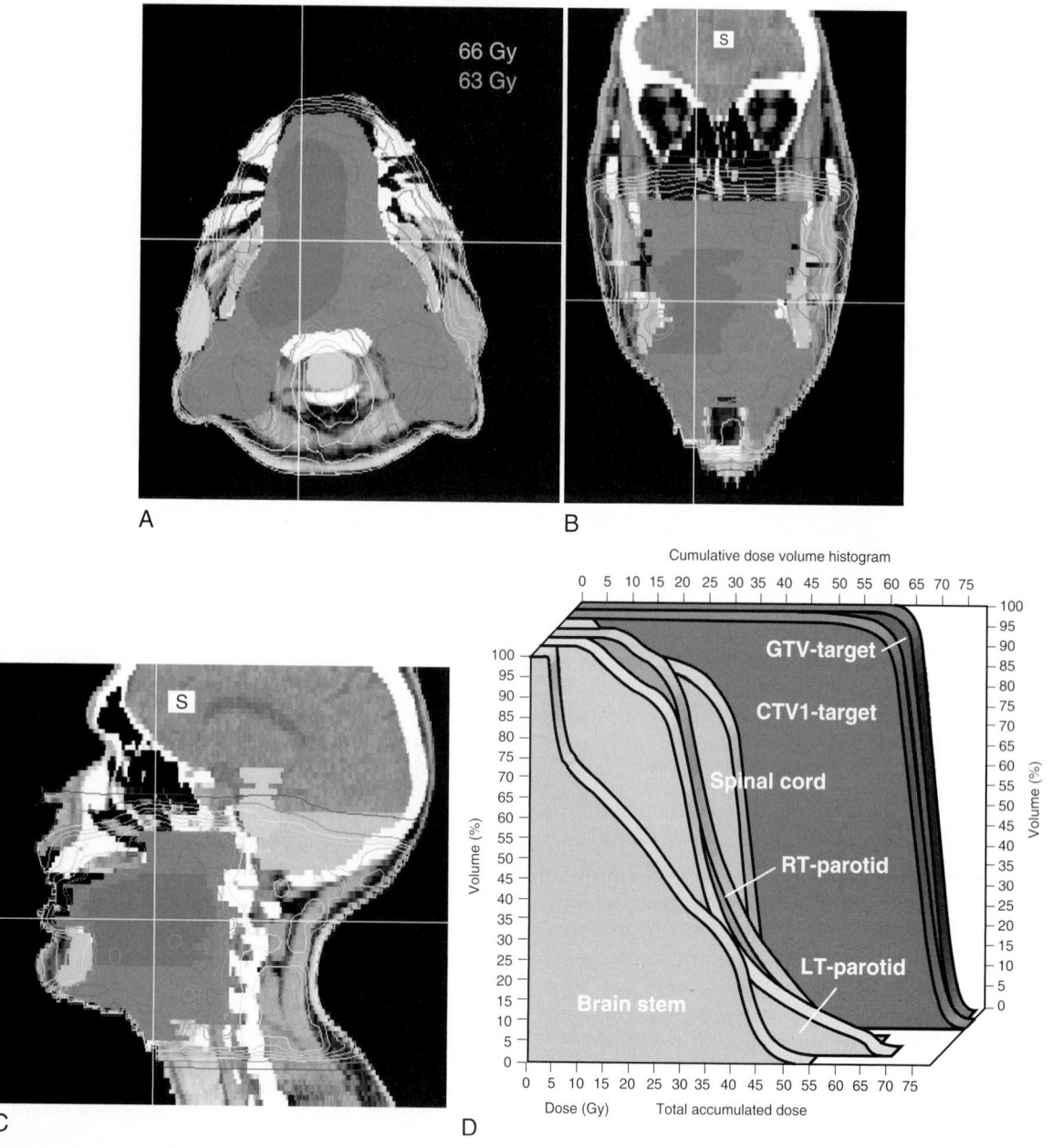

Figure 29–13. Isodose curves of an inverse intensity-modulated radiotherapy plan using seven coplanar gantry angles delivered with conventional multi-leaf collimator for a patient receiving post-operative radiotherapy for a T2N2b carcinoma of the oral tongue displayed on the axial (**A**), coronal (**B**), and sagittal (**C**) planes through the centroid of the primary tumor and the Dose Volume Histogram for the relevant structures (**D**). The gross tumor volume is shown in red and the clinical target volume (including a margin for set-up errors) is shown in magenta. A low neck/supraclavicular field is matched to the IMRT plan. See also Color Figure 29-13.

100 cGy per hour for the minimum tumor dose have been commonly used when low dose rate (LDR) brachytherapy is the treatment approach. Although some authors[18,47] recommend adjustments of the total dose according to the dose rate, we agree with Pierquin and coworkers[48] that for dose rates between 30 and 100 cGy per hour, no adjustment of total dose is indicated. Overcorrection of dose for reduced overall treatment time may lead to a high incidence of local recurrence.[49,50]

Although patients are usually able to speak and swallow with the implant in place, it is good practice to maintain adequate hydration with intravenous fluids

unless the patient's oral fluid intake is adequate. A liquid to semisolid diet is well tolerated during the implant period. We have used antibiotics routinely during the implant and for 1 week after the implant for oral cavity lesions. Patients are also encouraged to irrigate the mouth with salt and baking soda solutions or half-strength peroxide solutions during and after the implant. Analgesics are prescribed whenever necessary. The peak reaction of mucous membranes usually does not occur until several days to 1 week after the implant.

Localization films of the implant are usually taken on the day of the procedure. Computer dosimetry provides detailed information on the dose distribution within the implant volume. The dose distribution in several parallel planes intersecting the tumor volume should be obtained. An isodose curve that encompasses the entire tumor volume on all the planes that intersect the volume should be used to calculate the minimum tumor dose. Sometimes part of the implant may be removed during the course of treatment when there is a volume of overdosage within the implant. The optimal minimum tumor doses for local control vary with the size of the primary lesions. For T1 and select small T2 lesions, implant alone is used with a dose of 60 to 70 Gy. For larger T2 lesions, a total dose between 75 to 80 Gy is delivered by using both intestitial implant and external beam radiotherapy. The incidence of soft tissue and bone necrosis depends on the total dose as well as on tumor volume but is independent of the dose rate.[51] It is important to separate the ribbons from the mandible by the use of dental rolls sutured in place.

Currently at UCSF, high dose rate (HDR) fractionated interstitial brachytherapy is the preferred treatment approach for patients undergoing implantation. A phase III trial of high and low dose interstitial radiotherapy for early oral tongue cancer showed that HDR can be an alternative to LDR with the advantage of eliminating exposure to the medical staff.[17] If not using HDR, an afterloading technique using iridium seeds is preferable because of the reduced radiation exposure to the medical and paramedical personnel. The afterloading technique also allows more time for optimal placement of needles, since no radiation exposure occurs during the procedure.

Treatment Outcome

Radiotherapy results for carcinoma of the oral tongue are given in Table 29-3.[24,52-55] Most of the patients in the series reported by Wendt and associates[54] and Mazeron and associates[53] did not have cervical lymph node metastasis at the time of treatment, whereas 50% of the patients in the series reported by Fletcher[56] presented with cervical lymph node metastasis. The incidence of occult metastasis in early-staged squamous cell carcinoma of the oral tongue is between 20% and 48%.[57]

Because interstitial radiotherapy is an integral part of radiotherapy in patients receiving radiotherapy alone for carcinoma of the oral tongue, a small area of the mandible usually receives a dose in excess of 75 Gy. The incidence of osteonecrosis was 19% in the series reported by Delclos and coworkers.[58] Most of the necrosis healed with conservative management, although 35% of the bone necrosis in that series required surgical treatment. Another series reported a 38% complication rate, such as erosive ulcerations and bone exposure, in patients who received brachytherapy for stage I and II disease.[59] The patients who also received external beam radiotherapy in addition to brachytherapy had higher complications than those treated with brachytherapy alone.

Survival after radiotherapy for carcinoma of the oral tongue is directly related to the stage of disease. In a series of 204 patients treated between 1940 and 1971, reported by Fu and associates,[51] the overall 5-year actuarial survival was 32% and determinate survival was 47% for all stages. The prognosis for patients who had cervical lymph node metastasis on presentation and persistent or recurrent disease at 3 months after treatment was significantly poorer than the prognosis for patients who had no cervical lymph node metastasis on presentation and those who were free of disease at 3 months after treatment. A recent series of 370 stages T1 and T2 cases reported by Shibuya and associates showed that the 5-year primary tumor control was 85% for superficial lesions, 70% for exophytic lesions, and 45% for infiltrative lesions. The 5-year overall survivals for stages T1, T2a, and T2b were 84%, 78%, and 72%, respectively. (T2a lesions are lesions >2 cm but ≤3 cm, and T2b lesions are lesions >3 cm but ≤4 cm.)[59]

CARCINOMA OF THE FLOOR OF THE MOUTH

Clinical Presentation

Carcinoma of the floor of the mouth accounts for approximately 15% of all carcinomas of the oral cavity. Similar to carcinoma of the oral tongue, carcinoma of

Table 29–3 Results of Radiotherapy of Carcinoma of the Oral Tongue

Institution (Yr, Follow-up)	Patients, n	Stage	Local Control, %	Treatment
Univ. of FL (1994, 2 yr)[52]	18	T1	79	EBRT + IMP
	48	T2	72	
France (1990, 5 yr)[53]	70	T1N0	87	IMP only
	83	T2N0	92	
MDA (1990, 5 yr)[54]	18	T1	81	Mostly IMP alone
	85	T2	70	
MGH (1989, 5 yr)[55]	56	T1	80	EBRT and IOC or
	86	T2	64	IMP
UCSF (1976, 5 yr)[25]	12	T1	83	EBRT + IMP
	38	T2	74	
	8	T3	38	

EBRT, external beam radiation therapy; IMP, interstitial implant; IOR, intraoral cone.

the floor of the mouth is often associated with tobacco smoking, heavy alcohol consumption, and poor oral hygiene. It is more common in males than in females. The male-to-female ratio is approximately 2.5:1. Most of the patients are between 50 and 70 years old, with a peak incidence between 55 and 65 years.

The majority of the carcinomas of the floor of the mouth are moderately to well differentiated squamous cell carcinomas. Clinically, they usually present as a growth or an ulcer, most often on one or the other side of the midline. Invasion of the tongue is common, and sometimes it may be difficult to distinguish whether a primary growth is arising from the floor of the mouth or from the oral tongue. The frenulum is frequently involved. With more advanced lesions, patients may complain of otalgia from referred pain, hypersalivation, difficulties in speech, and bleeding. A significant number of patients with carcinoma of the floor of the mouth develop a second primary cancer. In the series reported by Fu and Lichter,[51] 55 of 153 (36%) of the patients had a second primary cancer. The majority of the second primary sites are in the upper aerodigestive tracts.

Routes of Spread

Carcinomas of the floor of the mouth usually spread by direct invasion into the tongue, the lower alveolar ridge, the mandible, and the submandibular glands. Approximately 30% of the patients have cervical lymph node metastasis on presentation. The submandibular lymph nodes are most frequently involved. Metastasis to subdigastric nodes, midjugular nodes, and submantle nodes are less frequent. The incidence of lymph node metastasis is directly proportional to the stage of the primary lesion; 9% for T1 lesions, 25% for T2 lesions, and 68% for T3 and T4 lesions (Fig. 29-14). Similarly, 20% of the patients without initial lymph node metastasis subsequently develop cervical lymph node metastasis. Distant metastasis occurs in approximately 9% of the patients. Lungs, liver, bone, and mediastinal lymph nodes are the most common sites of distant metastasis.

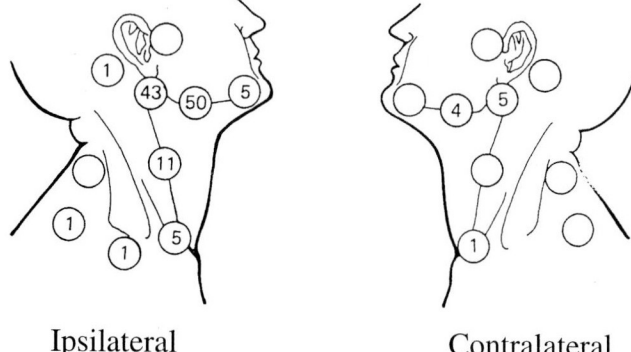

Ipsilateral   Contralateral

Figure 29–14. Distribution of 79/258 positive lymph nodes in floor of mouth. (From Lindberg RD: Distribution of cervical lymph node metastases from squamous cell carcinoma of the upper respiratory and digestive tracts. *Cancer.* 1972;29:1446.)

Treatment Approach

Radiotherapy or surgery is a treatment option for early-staged disease. A combination of surgery followed by postoperative radiotherapy is recommended for operable stage III and IV disease, especially when there is invasion of the mandible and the presence of large or multiple cervical lymph node metastases or extensive involvement of the musculature of the tongue. For advanced, inoperable stage III and IV disease, a combination of chemotherapy and radiotherapy should be considered. Surgery is used in the treatment of recurrent disease after radiotherapy.

Radiotherapy modalities for carcinoma of the floor of the mouth consist of external beam irradiation, peroral cone irradiation, and interstitial implants. Interstitial implants alone or peroral cone irradiation may be used for superficial or exophytic T1 lesions. For most carcinomas of the floor of the mouth without bone invasion, we recommend external beam irradiation with 50 to 54 Gy delivered at 2 Gy per fraction, five fractions per week, to the primary lesion with adequate margins and the upper neck, including the submandibular and subdigastric nodes, followed by a boost to the primary lesion with 20 Gy using interstitial implant, peroral cone irradiation, or external beam irradiation. The lower neck is routinely irradiated when cervical lymph node metastasis is present. For advanced, unresectable lesions not amenable to implant, patients can be treated with external beam radiotherapy using accelerated hyperfractionation with a concomitant boost technique. The boost portion of treatment encompasses any visible tumor plus a margin, and we prefer using three-dimensional conformal radiotherapy (Fig. 29-15).

Similar interstitial radiotherapy techniques for carcinoma of the oral tongue are used for carcinoma for the floor of the mouth, as shown in Figure 29-10. The iridium seeds in nylon ribbons are afterloaded into nylon tubes extending from the skin of the submental region to the floor of the mouth. The nylon tubes are pulled in behind stainless steel needles, which are then removed. For large lesions, the catheters are usually placed with the use of needles inserted through the submental skin to the dorsum of the tongue, to deliver an adequate dose throughout the tumor volume. If the tubes terminate in the floor of the mouth, the iridium ribbons must protrude at least 1 cm or have double-strength seeds at the tip. Alternately, longer dwell times can be used with HDR. A recent report from Japan indicated that HDR can achieve high control rates for carcinoma of the floor of mouth and the advantage of HDR versus LDR was the elimination of radiation exposure for the medical staff.[60] The recommended HDR dose was 6000 cGy.

Treatment Outcome

Bone and soft tissue necrosis develops in approximately 13% to 21% of the patients,[58,61,62] usually within 2 years after treatment. Most of the necroses heal with conservative management, although some patients require hemimandibulectomy. The results of radiotherapy of carcinoma of the floor of the mouth, as reported

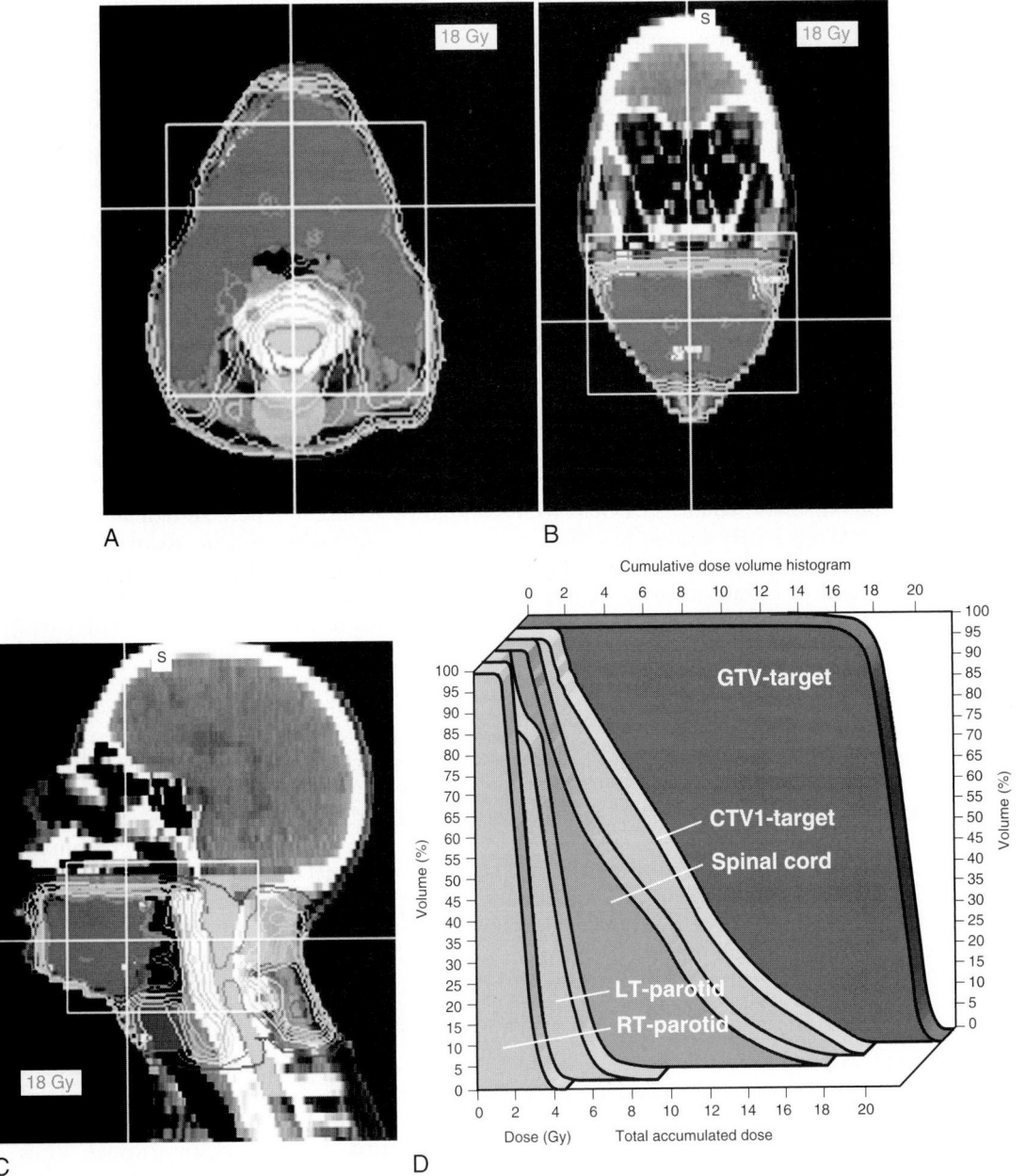

Figure 29–15. Isodose curves of an inverse intensity-modulated radiotherapy plan using seven coplanar gantry angles delivered with conventional multi-leaf collimator of a *boost plan* to the gross tumor volume (GTV) with a margin for a patient with T4N1 carcinoma of the floor of mouth displayed on the axial (**A**), coronal (**B**), and sagittal (**C**) planes through the centroid of the primary tumor and the DVH for the relevant structures (**D**). The GTV is shown in red and the clinical target volume (including a margin for set-up errors) is shown in magenta. See also Color Figure 29-15.

in several recent series, are given in Table 29-4.[45,60,62] Most patients were treated with a combination of external irradiation and interstitial implants. Some early lesions were treated with interstitial implants or external irradiation alone. The control of the primary lesion is directly proportionate to the stage of the disease. Control of the cervical lymph node metastasis is also related to the N staging. Approximately two thirds of cases of N1 disease (lesion <3 cm in diameter) can be controlled with radiation alone or in combination with surgery.

Table 29–4   Carcinoma of the Floor of the Mouth and Local Control

Institution (Yr, Follow-up)	Stage	Patients, *n*	Local Control, %
Japan (1998, 5 yr)[63]	T1-T3	41	94
France (2002, 5 yr)[62]	T1	79	93
	T2	81	88
France (1991, 5 yr)[48]	T1	84	97
	T2	100	72
	T3	17	51

Following treatment, the most common site of failure is the site of the primary lesion, with or without simultaneous failure in the cervical lymph nodes. Approximately 80% of the recurrences appear within 2 years following treatment. Failure in the cervical lymph nodes alone or in distant metastasis alone is rare.

A recent series of 160 patients from France showed that brachytherapy alone offers excellent local control of 89% for T1 and T2 lesions with a 5-year survival of 76%.[62] In spite of the good local control rate of carcinoma of the floor of the mouth, actuarial survival of these patients is poor, owing to a significant number of deaths from intercurrent disease or a second primary cancer. In the series of 153 patients with carcinoma of the floor of the mouth reported by Fu and Lichter,[51] the 5-year actuarial and determinate survival rates were 35% and 60%, respectively, for the entire group of patients. Data from Washington University showed that in a retrospective study of 280 patients treated with surgery or radiation, the overall 5-year disease-specific survival was 56%.[63] Recurrence at the primary site (41%) was the most common site of failure followed by neck recurrence of 19%. Metastasis occurred in 30%. Twenty percent of the patients had second primaries and 53% died of their second primary disease.

CARCINOMA OF THE BUCCAL MUCOSA

Clinical Presentation

After carcinoma of the lip, oral tongue, floor of the mouth, and lower gum, carcinoma of the buccal mucosa is the fifth most common carcinoma of the oral cavity. Squamous cell carcinoma of the buccal mucosa comprises approximately 10% of all oral cancers in the United States and Western Europe. It is the most common carcinoma of the oral cavity in India, Malaysia, and Taiwan. It usually occurs in the sixth and seventh decades of life and is more prevalent in males than in females. Tobacco and betel nut chewing appear to play an important role in the etiology of these tumors.[64]

Carcinomas of the buccal mucosa often occur in association with preexisting leukoplakia and tend to have multiple primary sites and recurrence. Excision of the oral leukoplakia may reduce the subsequent development of carcinoma.[65] They usually arise in the area adjacent to the lower molars along the occlusal line of the teeth. Clinically, there are three distinct types: exophytic, ulcerative, and verrucous. The patient may present with pain or bleeding, trismus, or cervical lymphadenopathy. In advanced stages, the tumor may destroy the entire cheek and invade the adjacent bones and the neck. Infection is common and mastication becomes difficult. Death usually occurs as a result of poor nutrition and general debilitation.[66,67]

Routes of Spread

Carcinomas of the buccal mucosa frequently spread by direct invasion into the gingivobuccal sulcus, the upper and lower alveolar ridges, the hard palate, the maxilla, and the mandible. Lymph node metastasis occurs in approximately 9% to 31% of the patients during the course of the disease.[66,67] The submandibular lymph nodes are most frequently involved; involvement of the upper cervical and the parotid lymph nodes is less common. The risk of subclinical disease is 16%.[68] Distant metastases are rare, as patients often die of uncontrolled local disease before distant metastases are manifested clinically.

Treatment Approach

Radiotherapy alone can be considered in small lesions involving the commissure or in the mid cheek without sulcus invasion. Otherwise, surgery followed by postoperative radiotherapy is the recommended treatment modality for all buccal mucosa carcinomas, including T1 lesions. A recent report stated that T-classification and negative margins are not adequate predictors of local control and even early buccal tumors could benefit from adjuvant therapy to enhance local control.[69] In another series, local recurrence occurred in all patients with stage I and II disease treated with wide local excision.[70] In cases that are inoperable, radiotherapy in combination with chemotherapy can be used. Surgery is also considered in patients who recur after radiotherapy as salvage. One series reported a 5-year actuarial disease-free survival after surgical salvage of 59.7%.[71]

When the tumor has invaded the buccogingival sulcus, the gingiva, or bones, a combination of surgery (i.e., composite resection) and post-operative radiotherapy is typically used. Marginal or segmental mandibulectomy or partial maxillectomy should be performed when tumor invasion to the nearby bony structures is clinically suspected. 3D conformal therapy should be done from the beginning of the treatment to spare the contralateral parotid. Because the buccal mucosa lesions are lateralized, treatment of the contralateral buccal mucosa is not necessary. The details of such a 3D plan are shown in Figures 29-16 and 29-17.

Interstitial implants with iridium wires or seeds in nylon ribbons can be considered for treatment of early, small lesions that have not invaded the buccogingival sulcus, the gingiva, or bone. Usually a minimum tumor dose of 60 to 70 Gy in 5 to 8 days is delivered through a single-plane or double-plane implant on the thickness of the lesion.

Treatment Outcome

Reports of the select retrospective studies of carcinoma of the buccal mucosa can be found in Table 29-5.[70,72-76] A recent prospective, randomized trial from India examined the role of postoperative radiotherapy in stages III and IV carcinoma of the buccal mucosa. The 3-year actuarial disease-free survival was 68% versus 38%, with and without postoperative radiotherapy. The 3-year actuarial overall survival was 94% versus 84%, respectively.

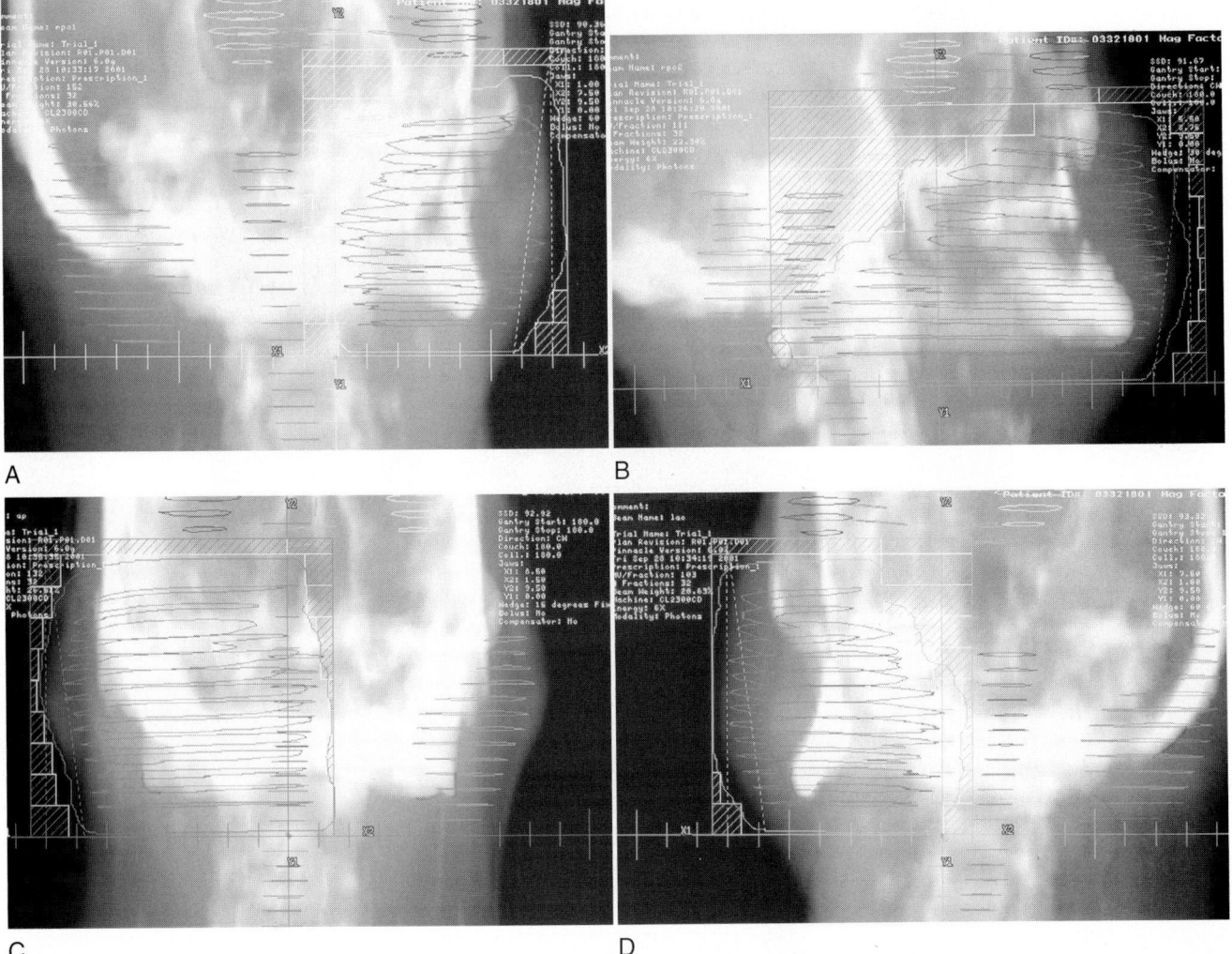

Figure 29–16. 3-D reconstructed radiographs of a patient who required post-operative radiotherapy for buccal mucosa cancer. The neck was treated with conventional techniques.

Surgery can be used to salvage patients that failed radical radiotherapy. One series reported an overall 5-year actuarial disease-free survival after salvage surgery to be 59.7%. At recurrence, T stage and whether there is skin infiltration were the factors that significantly influenced disease-free survival.[71]

CARCINOMA OF THE UPPER GINGIVA

Clinical Presentation

Carcinomas of the upper gingiva are much less common than those of the lower gingiva. They frequently invade the maxillary antrum and are often difficult to differentiate from a primary carcinoma arising from the floor of the maxillary sinus. They usually affect men in the fifth and sixth decades of life.

Carcinomas of the upper gingiva usually arise in the region of the molar and premolar teeth. They often appear as papillary growths. The majority of cases are well differentiated squamous cell carcinomas.

Patients usually present with a history of ill-fitting dentures, ulceration around the teeth that fails to heal, or bleeding. Trismus is present in advanced cases.

Routes of Spread

Carcinomas of the upper gingiva usually spread by direct invasion into the maxillary sinus or the upper gingivobuccal sulcus. Lymph node metastasis most frequently involves the submandibular lymph nodes. The subdigastric and upper cervical nodes are less frequently involved. At diagnosis, 18% to 52% of patients have positive lymph nodes.

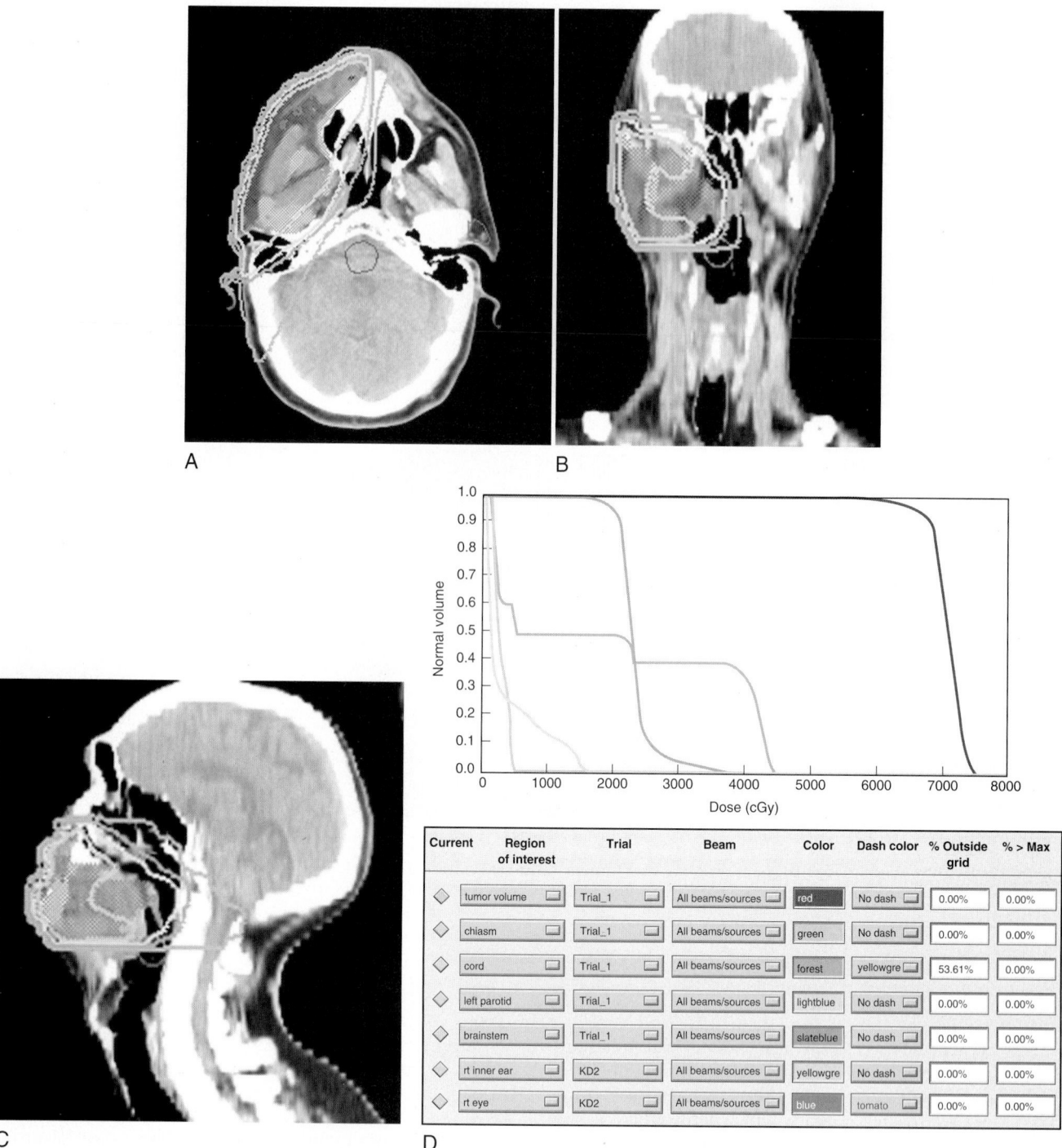

Figure 29–17. **A,** 3D treatment plan for buccal mucosal cancer, axial plane. **B,** 3D plan, coronal plane. **C,** 3D plan, sagittal view. **D,** Dose-volume histogram. See also Color Figure 29-17.

Treatment Approach

Because of early bone involvement and the risk of bone exposure after the tumor is irradiated, surgery is the treatment of choice for carcinomas of the upper gingiva.

Except for early superficial lesions, most tumors of the hard palate and upper gingiva are treated with surgery. Postoperative radiotherapy is added in high-risk patients. For definitive radiotherapy, the patient is treated with opposed-lateral fields or wedge pairs to 70 Gy. In the postoperative setting, doses of 63 to 66 Gy are delivered. A balloon filled with water can be used to compensate for postsurgical tissue defects. Postoperative radiotherapy usually begins 2 to 3 weeks after surgery.

Table 29–5   Carcinoma of the Buccal Mucosa

Institution (Yr, Follow-up)	Patients, n	LR, %	LRR, %	DSS, %	OS, %
UCLA (1999, 5 yr)[73]	27	26			60
Rotterdam (1988, 5 yr)[75]	49		45		52
India (1989, 2 yr)[74]	185	37			
Mayo Clinic (1999, 5 yr)[70]	31	80			52
Taiwan (1997, 3 yr)[72]	57		39	62	55
France (1995, 5 yr)[76]	42		43	74	48

LR, local recurrence; LRR, local regional recurrence; DSS, disease-specific survival; OS, overall survival.

Treatment Outcome

In the review of the Memorial Sloan-Kettering Cancer Center experience, of 61 patients with upper gingival tumor treated mostly with surgery, the 5-year survival rate was 51% (31/61). Clinical stage was the only predicator of survival.[77] In another series of 82 patients from Japan, the 5-year local control rate was 61% with a 5-year actuarial survival of 45%.[78]

CARCINOMA OF THE LOWER GINGIVA

Clinical Presentation

Carcinoma of the lower gingiva accounts for about 12% of carcinomas of the oral cavity. It usually occurs at an advanced age and is rare in persons younger than age 40. Males are affected more frequently than females.

Carcinomas of the lower gingiva usually arise in the region of the molar teeth. They can be ulcerative, exophytic, or verrucous in their gross appearance. They can be multicentric in origin. Leukoplakia is frequently present. The majority of carcinomas of the lower gingiva are well differentiated or moderately well differentiated squamous cell carcinomas.

Patients with carcinoma of the lower gingiva not infrequently present with a history of ill-fitting dentures or bleeding upon mastication. The dentist is frequently consulted first. A history of tooth extraction and surgical incision of a suspected abscess is not uncommon. Otalgia can occur because of secondary infection. Trismus and pain can result from bone invasion.

Routes of Spread

Tumor spreads mainly through the occlusal ridge alone or in combination with penetration of the buccal or lingual plates in edentulous patients.[79,80] Lymph node metastasis is present in 13% to 24% of patients with carcinoma of the lower gingiva. The submandibular lymph nodes are most frequently involved. Involvement of the subdigastric and upper cervical nodes is less common. Direct invasion of the mandible may be present in 50% of the patients on initial examination. The actual extent of bone involvement may exceed that shown on radiographs.

Treatment Approach

Because of frequent bone involvement and lymph node metastasis, surgery has been the primary treatment modality in the management of carcinoma of the lower gingiva. Early superficial lesions can be expeditiously treated by a simple excision or marginal resection with skin graft. In patients with more advanced disease, postoperative radiotherapy can reduce the incidence of local recurrence. Clear margins should be achieved as inadequate margins result in a high rate of local recurrence. One series showed that the 5-year local control rate in the presence of positive margins was 49% versus 100% with negative margins and survival was 11% versus 91%.[81] In addition, patients with advanced T stage, radiologic or histologic evidence of mandibular invasion, tumors involving the symphyseal region, and decreased tumor differentiation have high propensity for regional metastases. Therefore, elective treatment of the neck should be considered.[82] One series reported that larger tumor size is more important than mandibular invasion in predicting local control—larger tumors that have a higher propensity for local recurrence require a more extensive surgical resection.[83]

Early superficial lesions, less than 2 cm in diameter, can be adequately treated with 60 Gy using electrons in 3 to 4 weeks using a peroral cone. Orthovoltage should not be used over bone. For more advanced unresectable disease, an external beam irradiation with 70 Gy in 2 Gy fractions may be used in selected cases in combination with chemotherapy. Oblique- or right-angle, wedged-pair field arrangements can be used to spare the contralateral salivary glands.

Treatment Outcome

Local control of carcinomas of the lower gingiva treated with radiotherapy alone was achieved in 71.5% (5/7) of T1 lesions, 70% (7/10) of T2 lesions, 59% (10/17) of T3 lesions, and 29% (4/14) of T4 lesions in the series reported by Fletcher.[68] The 5-year survival rate of 108 patients treated between 1947 and 1960 at the M.D. Anderson Hospital was 46%.[68] Most series report excellent local control with surgery followed by postoperative radiotherapy when indicated. Results from select series are shown in Table 29-6.[81,84]

CARCINOMA OF THE RETROMOLAR TRIGONE

Clinical Presentation

Carcinomas of the retromolar trigone are rare. Indirect extension into the anterior tonsillar pillar or the buccal mucosa occurs early. Frequently, they are indistinguishable from carcinomas arising from the anterior tonsillar pillar.

Table 29–6   Carcinoma of the Lower Gingiva

Institution (Yr, Follow-up)	Patient, *n*	LC, %	LRC, %	DSS, %	OS, %
MDACC (1996, 2 yr)[82]	61		95	61	
Japan (2002, 5 yr)[81]	50	85		73	50

LC, local control; LRC, local regional control; DSS, disease-specific survival; OS, overall survival.

They are usually moderately differentiated squamous cell carcinomas.

Routes of Spread

Carcinomas of the retromolar trigone frequently metastasize to the subdigastric lymph nodes. The submandibular and upper cervical lymph nodes are affected less often. The incidence on diagnosis is about 30%.

Treatment Approach

These lesions are treated in a highly selected manner similar to that of tonsillar pillar tumors. T1 and early T2 tumors are treated with megavoltage external beam irradiation. However, surgical resection is the preferred modality. More advanced tumors require surgery and postoperative radiotherapy (Fig. 29-18).

Selected early lesions of the retromolar trigone can be treated with external beam irradiation alone using mixed electrons and photons with single lateral fields or parallel opposing fields with 2:1 loading favoring the diseased side. Usually a dose of 66 to 74 Gy in 2 Gy fractions is administered. Prophylactic treatment of the neck is essential as lesions located in the retromolar trigone have a high propensity for metastases in the neck. When there is bone involvement, surgery and postoperative irradiation are used. A recent report showed that surgery in combination with radiotherapy offered the better locoregional control and disease-free survival than radiotherapy alone.[85]

Treatment Outcome

M.D. Anderson Hospital reported results of 159 patients with squamous cell carcinoma of the anterior faucial pillar and retromolar trigone region treated with radiation.[86] Local control with radiation alone for T1 lesions was 71% (12/17); for T2 lesions, 70% (51/81); for T3 lesions, 76% (19/25); and three of five T4 lesions were controlled. Most of the failures were treated with surgery, and the ultimate control rate was 100% for T1, 94% for T2, and 92% for T3. The overall N0 neck failure rate was 11%. The authors recommend elective treatment of subdigastric and upper jugular nodes to the level of the hyoid. The 5-year determinate survival rate in the series was 83%. See Table 29-7 for select results of treatment for carcinoma of the retromolar trigone.[85,87]

CARCINOMA OF THE HARD PALATE

Clinical Presentation

Primary malignancies of the hard palate are rare. In one series of 5000 cases of oral cancer, only 25 (0.5%) had squamous cell carcinoma of the hard palate.[88] In another study, squamous cell carcinoma accounted for 3% of all oral cancers.[89] Patients complain of ill-fitting

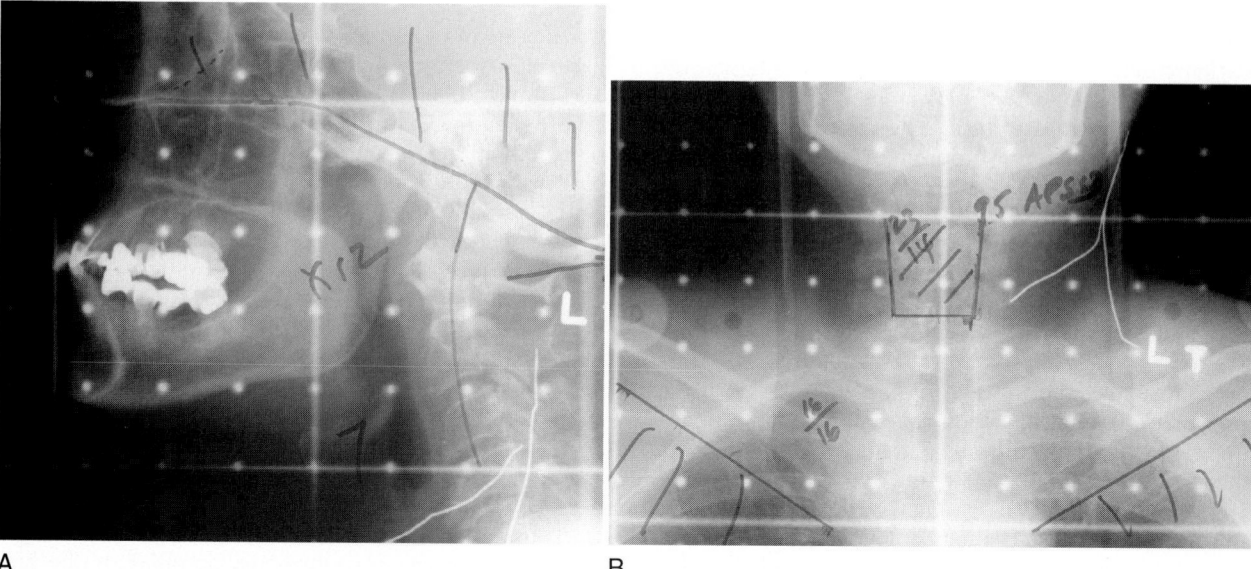

A   B

Figure 29–18. A, Simulation film of a patient with cancer of the retromolar trigone, lateral view. **B,** Simulation film of the low neck and supraclavicular fossae.

Table 29–7   Carcinoma of the Retromolar Trigone

Institution (Yr, Follow-up)	Patients, n	LRC, %	DSS, %	OS, %
Washington Univ. (2001, 5 yr)[85]	65	74	68	22
MDACC (1984, 5 yr)[87]	110	83		26

LRC, local regional control; DSS, disease-specific survival; OS, overall survival.

dentures, pain, intermittent bleeding, or a sore that does not heal.

Routes of Spread

The majority of hard palate lesions originate in the minor salivary glands. Adenoid cystic types spread hematogeneously to lungs and bone and along the second branch, V2, of the fifth cranial nerve to the base of the skull. Lymph node spread is present in less than 10% of patients.

Treatment Approach

Carcinomas of the hard palate are primarily treated with surgical resection. For high-grade mucoepidermoid tumors and for adenoid cystic tumors, postoperative irradiation is indicated (Fig. 29-19). Very superficial lesions of the hard palate can be treated with surface molds.

Except for early superficial lesions, most tumors of the hard palate and upper gingiva are treated with surgery. Postoperative radiotherapy is added in high-risk patients. For definitive radiotherapy, the patient is treated with opposed-lateral fields or wedge pairs to 66 to 74 Gy in 2 Gy fractions. In the postoperative setting, doses of 63 to 66 Gy using 1.8 Gy per fraction are administered.

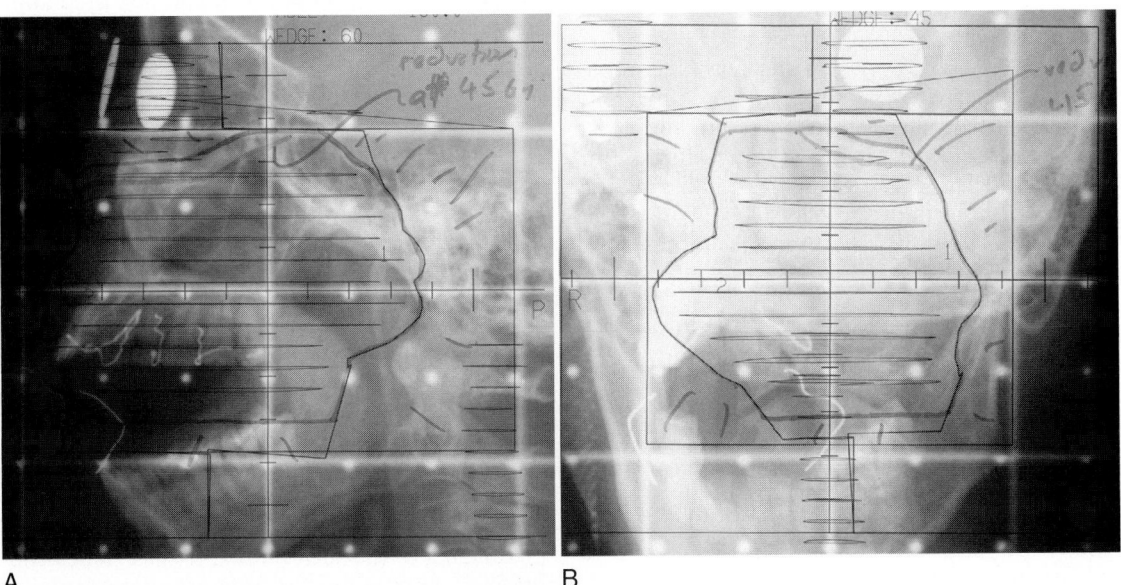

A   B   C

Figure 29–19. A-C, 3D treatment reconstructed radiographs of a patient with hard palate adenoid cystic carcinoma, who required postoperative radiotherapy.

A prosthesis (i.e., obturator) can be placed over the postsurgical defect during radiotherapy. Alternatively, a balloon filled with water can be used to compensate for postsurgical tissue defects. Postoperative radiotherapy usually begins 2 to 3 weeks after surgery.

Treatment Outcome

Owing to the rarity of this disease, limited information is available. Evans and Shah[90] reported their 15-year experience from the Memorial Sloan-Kettering Cancer Center. For stage I squamous cell carcinoma of the hard palate, the 5-year disease-free survival rate was 75% (6/8); all patients were treated with surgery alone. For stage II disease, 46% (6/13) were disease free at 5 years; postoperative radiotherapy was added in one patient. In stage III disease, the 5-year disease-free survival rate was 40% (4/10); one patient in the group received postoperative radiotherapy. In stage IV patients, 8% (1/12) of patients treated with surgery alone, 25% (1/4) of those treated with radiotherapy alone, and none (0/2) of those treated with the combined modality were disease free at 5 years. In another series of patients with squamous cell carcinoma of the hard palate, from the University of Virginia, select early-stage lesions were equally effectively treated by radiotherapy as surgery during the supervoltage era.[91] Patients with a clear margin after surgical resection had improved local control.[91] See Table 29-8 for select results of carcinoma of the hard palate.[91-93]

CRITICAL NORMAL TISSUES

Acute and Late Effects

Acute changes occur in the oral mucosa, the salivary glands, and the taste buds during irradiation. Unless the parotid glands are shielded, xerostomia occurs after a few weeks. For most oral cancers, most of the parotids can be shielded to prevent this complication. Acute mucositis cannot be avoided. For the definitive treatment of lesions with radiotherapy, the goal is to achieve mucositis that is either patchy (grade 2) or confluent (grade 3). Simple erythema (grade 1) usually means that the protraction of the treatment is too long and tumor proliferation during radiotherapy will be too great. Excellent oral care is required, as detailed in the next section, to avoid grade 4 reactions, which require hospitalization. Nutritional support is also required, as discussed later.

Late effects are seen as bone necrosis in the mandible and the maxilla, which occurs after breakdown of the mucosa and exposure of the bone with ensuing osteomyelitis.[94,95] The teeth must be maintained in good repair to avoid extractions, which can lead to infection. Soft tissue necrosis is frequently seen after both brachytherapy and peroral cone treatment. It is painful but usually heals without surgery. Necrotic mandible often must be resected.

DENTAL AND ORAL CARE

Proper dental care is essential in the management of patients with head and neck cancer. After radiotherapy, there is increased susceptibility to infection and development of dental caries. This is due to the decreased amount and pH of the saliva, diminished vascular supply, reduced number of osteoblasts and osteoclasts, altered normal metabolism of bone, and impaired ability to heal in response to physical, chemical, and biological injuries after head and neck irradiation. As a result, osteoradionecrosis develops in patients following head and neck irradiation, especially if proper preradiotherapy dental care was not done. The mandible is most commonly involved and the maxilla is rarely affected. The risk of osteonecrosis is directly related to the radiation dose to the bone. The incidence and severity of dental decays and osteonecrosis can be minimized with proper dental care and hygiene before, during, and after head and neck irradiation.

Before radiotherapy begins, the teeth and soft tissues of the oral cavity are carefully examined, pertinent radiographs are obtained, and the findings are recorded. We do not recommend routine extraction of all teeth included in the irradiated volume. The only teeth removed are those that are unsalvageable, likely to require extraction shortly after irradiation, or potentially damaging to the surrounding tissues. When tooth extraction is done before or after irradiation, the underlying alveolar bone must be smoothed to allow primary closure of the gingival tissues. Antibiotics are used routinely as a prophylaxis against infection. All patients are given dental prophylaxis with cleansing of their teeth and instructed on oral hygiene. Mouth irrigation with 1% sodium fluoride solution is started during radiotherapy and continued permanently after radiotherapy to minimize radiation caries.

During radiotherapy, patients are encouraged to irrigate the mouth with a salt and baking soda solution (1/2 to 1 teaspoon of salt and 1/2 to 1 teaspoon of baking soda in 1 quart of warm water) three to four times daily. Moniliasis is a common complication during irradiation of the head and neck. This can be effectively controlled with systemic antifungal agents. Once the patient has been placed on an agent, it is important to maintain its use until the completion of radiotherapy. Otherwise, moniliasis usually recurs if treatment is discontinued during the course of radiotherapy.

Table 29–8   Carcinoma of the Hard Palate

Institution (Yr, Follow-up)	Patients, *n*	LC, %	DSS, %	OS, %
United Kingdom (2001, 5 yr)[92]	26	69		55
Univ. of Virginia (1980, 5 yr)[91]	66			72
Washington Univ. (1993, 10 yr)[93]	13	92	77	34

LC, local control; DSS, disease-specific survival; OS, overall survival.

After radiotherapy, the patients are continued on a good oral hygiene program and topical fluoride applications (mouth rinses) as well as a fluoride-containing dentifrice. Caries are filled and there are no unusual contraindications for endodontic procedures. Extractions are performed whenever necessary and antibiotics are routinely used to minimize the risk of infection. When osteonecrosis develops, it is usually managed conservatively with topical or systemic antibiotics and analgesics initially. Good oral hygiene is imperative. Loose spicules of bone above the gingival crest are gently removed. Healing may take place over a period of several months. Partial mandibulectomy is performed only if conservative management fails and the patient continues to have persistent pain, infection, or trismus.

Nutrition

Maintenance of good nutrition is important for patients with head and neck cancer. Most patients receiving radiation therapy to the head and neck area do experience some eating problems during the treatment. This is due, in part, to the side effects of radiation therapy such as the loss of sense of taste, decreased saliva, and inflammation of the mucous membranes, resulting in soreness of the mouth and dysphagia. The postponement of dentures to avoid irritation of the mucous membranes in edentulous patients makes mastication difficult. The psychological impact, mental stress, discomfort, and pain associated with the disease may also contribute to a decreased appetite and food intake. Patients who have undergone head and neck surgery may experience difficulties in chewing and swallowing because of the loss of their normal tissues and because of injury to the nerves necessary for these functions. It is important to inform the patient and his or her family of the treatment side effects and the potential problems of eating that may arise and to emphasize the importance of good nutrition during and after treatment. The assistance of a dietitian experienced in working with cancer patients can be very helpful in providing guidance for a well-balanced diet. Modification of the consistency and texture of the food may be necessary. Small, frequent meals of soft to semiliquid foods may be better tolerated. Dietary modifications are best worked out on an individual basis, tailored to the patient's usual eating habits, cultural practices, and religious beliefs. Psychological and social support and the cooperation of the patient's family may be essential in providing adequate dietary intake.

Dietary supplements such as instant breakfast, Sustagen, Ensure, or other homemade substitutes are soothing to the mucosa and easy to swallow and provide a substantial amount of calories as well as essential vitamins.

In patients with severe pain and dysphagia or problems of mastication or excessive weight loss, tube feeding may be necessary. The aim of a dietary program during head and neck irradiation is to provide adequate nutrition and prevent weight loss. Percutaneous gastrostomy tube placement may be required for patients who lose more than 10% of their body weight.

REFERENCES

1. Jemal A, Murray T, Samuels A, et al: Cancer Statistics, 2003. *CA Cancer J Clin.* 2003;53:5.
2. Funk GF, Karnell LH, Robinson RA, et al: Presentation, treatment, and outcome of oral cavity cancer: a national cancer data base report. *Head Neck.* 2002;24:165.
3. Chen YK, Huang HC, Lin LM, et al: Primary oral squamous cell carcinoma: An analysis of 703 cases in southern Taiwan. *Oral Oncol.* 1999;35:173.
4. Johnson NW, Warnakulasurity S, Tavassoli M: Hereditary and environmental risk factors: clinical and laboratory risk matters for head and neck, especially oral cancer and pre-cancer. *Eur J Cancer.* 1996;56:5.
5. Schantz S, Yu GP: Head and Neck Cancer Incidence Trends in Young Americans, 1993-1997, with a Special Analysis for Tongue Cancer. *Arch Otolaryngol Head Neck Surg.* 2002;128:268.
6. Paterson IC, Everson JW, Prime SS: Molecular changes in oral cancer may reflect aetiology and ethnic origin. *Eur J Cancer.* 1996;Part B:150.
7. Wong DT: TGF-alpha and oral carcinogenesis. *Eur J Cancer.* 1993;29B:3.
8. American Joint Committee on Cancer Lip and Oral Cavity. In Fleming ID, Henson DE, et al., eds. *AJCC Cancer Staging Manual,* 6th ed. Philadelphia: Lippincott; 2002.
9. Lo TCM, Wiley AL, Ansfield FJ: Combined radiation therapy and 5 fluorouracil for advanced squamous cell carcinoma of the oral cavity and oropharynx: A randomized study. *Am J Roentgenol.* 1976;126:229.
10. Parsons JT, Mendenhall WM, Stringer SP, et al: An analysis of factors influencing the outcome of postoperative irradiation for squamous cell carcinoma of the oral cavity. *Int J Radiat Oncol Biol Phys.* 1997;39:137.
11. Peters LJ, Goepfert H, Ang KK, et al: Evaluation of the dose for postoperative radiation therapy of head and neck cancer: first report of a prospective randomized trial. *Int J Radiat Oncol Biol Phys.* 1993;26:3.
12. Phillips TL: Peroral roentgen therapy. *Radiology.* 1968;90:525.
13. Wang CC: Technical and radiotherapeutic considerations of intra-oral cone electron beam radiation therapy for head and neck cancer. *Semin Radiat Oncol.* 1992;2:171.
14. Goffinet DR: Brachytherapy for head and neck cancer. *Semin Radiat Oncol.* 1993;3:250.
15. Shaha D, Harrison LB, Chiu-Tsao ST: The role of brachytherapy in head and neck cancer. *Semin Radiat Oncol.* 1998;8:270.
16. Harrison LB: Applications of brachytherapy in head and neck cancer. *Semin Surg Oncol.* 1997;13:177.
17. Inoue T, Teshima T, Murayama S, et al: Phase III trial of high and low dose rate interstitial radiotherapy for early oral tongue cancer. *Int J Radiat Oncol Biol Phys.* 1996;36:1201.
18. Quimby EH: Dosage table for linear radium sources. *Radiology.* 1944;43:572.
19. Johns HE, Cunningham JR: *The Physics of Radiology,* 4th ed. Springfield, Ill: Charles C. Thomas; 1983.
20. Leung TW, Wong V, Wong CM, et al: High dose rate brachytherapy for carcinoma of the oral tongue. *Int J Radiat Oncol Biol Phys.* 1997;39:1113.
21. Matsuura K, Hirokawa Y, Fujita M, et al: Treatment results of stage I and II oral tongue cancer with interstitial brachytherapy: maximum tumor thickness is prognostic of nodal metastasis. *Int J Radiat Oncol Biol Phys.* 1998;40:535.
22. Mendenhall WM, Van Cise WS, Bova FJ, Million RR: Analysis of time-dose factors in squamous cell carcinoma of the oral tongue and floor of mouth treated with radiation therapy alone. *Int J Radiat Oncol Biol Phys.* 1981;7:1005.
23. Chu A, Fletcher G: Incidence and causes of failures to control by irradiation of the primary lesions in squamous cell carcinomas of the anterior two-thirds of the tongue and floor of mouth. *Am J Roentgenol.* 1973;117:502.
24. Fu KK, Ray JW, Chan EK, Phillips TL: External and interstitial radiation therapy of carcinoma of the oral tongue, a review of 32 years' experience. *Am J Roentgenol.* 1976;126:107.
25. Fu KK, Chan EK, Phillips TL, Ray JW: Time, dose and volume factors in interstitial radium implants of carcinoma of the oral tongue. *Radiology.* 1976;119:209.

26. Moore S, Johnson N, Pierce A, Wilson D: The epidemiology of lip cancer: A review of global incidence and aetiology. *Oral Dis.* 1999;5:185.

27. Pogoda JM, Preston-Martin S: Solar radiation, lip protection, and lip cancer risk in Los Angeles County women (California, United States). *Cancer Causes Control.* 1996;7:458.

28. Huynh N, Vaness MJ: Basal cell carcinoma of the lip treated with radiotherapy. *Australas J Dermatol.* 2002;43:15.

29. MacKay EN, Sellers AH: A statistical review of carcinoma of the lip. *Can Med Assoc J.* 1964;90:670.

30. Cross JE, Guralnick E, Daland EM: Carcinoma of the lip: A review of 563 case records of carcinoma of the lip at Pondville Hospital. *Surg Gynecol Obstet.* 1948;81:153.

31. Byers RM, O'Brien J, Waxler J: The therapeutic and prognostic implications of nerve invasion in cancer of the lower lip. *Int J Radiat Oncol Biol Phys.* 1978;4:215.

32. Stranc MF, Fogel M, Dische S: Comparison of lip function: surgery vs RT. *Br J Plast Surg.* 1987;40:598.

33. de Visscher JG, Grond AJ, et al: Surgical treatment of squamous cell carcinoma of the lower lip: evaluation of long-term results and prognostic factors–A retrospective analysis of 184 patients. *J Oral Maxillofac Surg.* 1998;56:814.

34. de Visscher JGAM, Grond AJK, Botke G, van der Wall I: Results of radiotherapy for squamous cell carcinoma of the vermilion border of the lower lip. A retrospective analysis of 108 patients. *Radiother Oncol.* 1996;39:9.

35. Sykes AJ, Allan E, Irwin C: Squamous cell carcinoma of the lip: the role of electron treatment. *Clin Oncol (R Coll Radiol).* 1996;8:384.

36. Petrovich A, Parker RG, Luxton G, et al: Carcinoma of the lip and selected sites of the head and neck skin. A clinical study of 896 patients. *Radiother Oncol.* 1987;8:11.

37. Cerezo L, Liu FF, Tsang R, Payne D: Squamous cell carcinoma of the lip: Analysis of the Princess Margaret Hospital experience. *Radiother Oncol.* 1993;28:142.

38. Tombolini V, Bonanni A, Valeriani M, et al: Brachytherapy for squamous cell carcinoma of the lip. The experience of the Institute of Radiology of the University of Rome La Sapienza. *Tumori.* 1998;84:478.

39. Yamazaki H, Inoue T, Teshima T, et al: Tongue cancer treated with brachytherapy: Is thickness of tongue cancer a prognostic factor for regional control? *Anticancer Res.* 1998;18:1261.

40. Lindberg RD: Distribution of cervical lymph nodes metastases from squamous cell carcinoma of the upper respiratory and digestive tracts. *Cancer.* 1972;29:1446.

41. Lyos AT, Evans GRD, Perez D: Tongue reconstruction: Outcomes with the rectus abdominis flap. *Plast Reconstr Surg.* 1999;103:442.

42. Yokoo S, Komori T, Umeda M: Functional reconstruction of mobile tongue and suprahyoid muscles after resection of cancer of the tongue. *Br J Oral Max Surg.* 2001;39:252.

43. Salibian AH, Allison GR, Armstrong WB: Functional hemitongue reconstruction with the microvascular ulnar forearm flap. *Reconstr Surg.* 1999;104:654.

44. Fujita M, Hirokawa Y, Kashiwado K, et al: Interstitial brachytherapy for stage I and II squamous cell carcinoma of the oral tongue: Factors influencing local control and soft tissue complications. *Int J Radiat Oncol Biol Phys.* 1999;44:767.

45. Lapeyre M, Hoffstelter S, Peiffert D, et al: Postoperative brachytherapy alone for T1-2N0 squamous cell carcinomas of the oral tongue and floor of mouth with close or positive margins. *Int J Radiat Oncol Biol Phys.* 2000;48:37.

46. Chao KS, Emani B, Akhileswaran R, et al: The impact of surgical margin status and use of an interstitial implant on T1,T2 oral tongue cancers after surgery. *Int J Radiat Oncol Biol Phys.* 1996;36:1039.

47. Paterson R: *The Treatment of Malignant Disease by Radiotherapy,* 2nd ed. Baltimore: Williams & Wilkins; 1963:210.

48. Mazeron JJ, Simon JH, LePechoux C, et al: Effect of dose rate on local control and complications in definite irradiation of T1-2 squamous cell carcinomas of mobile tongue and floor of the mouth with interstitial Iridium-192. *Radiother Oncol.* 1991;21(1):39.

49. Burgers JM, Awwad HK, van Der Laarse R: Relation between local cure and dose-time-volume factors in interstitial implants. *Int J Radiat Oncol Biol Phys.* 1985;11:715.

50. Awwad HK, Burgers JM, Marcuse HR: The influence of tumor dose specification on the early clinical results of interstitial radium tongue implant. *Radiology.* 1974;110:177.

51. Fu KK, Lichter A: Carcinoma of the floor of mouth: An analysis of treatment results and sites and causes of failures. *Int J Radiat Oncol Biol Phys.* 1976;1:829.

52. Fein DA, Mendendall WM, Parson JT, et al: Carcinoma of the oral tongue: A comparison of results and complications of treatment with radiotherapy and/or surgery. *Head Neck.* 1994;16:358.

53. Mazeron JJ, Crook JM, Benck V, et al: Iridium 192 implantation of T1 and T2 carcinomas of the mobile tongue. *Int J Radiat Oncol Biol Phys.* 1990;19:1369.

54. Wendt CD, Peters LJ, Delclos L, et al: Primary radiotherapy in the treatment of stage I and II oral tongue cancers: Importance of the proportion of therapy delivered with interstitial therapy. *Int J Radiat Oncol Biol Phys.* 1990;18:1287.

55. Wang CC, Kelly J, August M, Donoff B: Early carcinoma of the oral cavity: A conservative approach with radiation therapy. *J Oral Maxillofac Surg.* 1995;53:687.

56. Fletcher GH: Elective irradiation of subclinical disease in cancers of the head and neck. *Cancer.* 1972;29:1450.

57. Haddadin KJ, Soutar DS, Oliver RJ, et al: Improved survival for patients for clinically T1/T2, N0 tongue tumors undergoing a prophylactic neck dissection. *Head Neck.* 1999;21:517.

58. Delclos L, Lindberg RD, Fletcher GH: Squamous cell carcinoma of the oral tongue and floor of mouth: Evaluation of interstitial radium therapy. *Am J Roentgenol.* 1976;126:223.

59. Shibuya H, Hoshina M, Takeda M, et al: Brachytherapy for stage I and II tongue cancer: An analysis of past cases focusing on control and complications. *Int J Radiat Oncol Biol Phys.* 1993;26:51.

60. Inoue T, Yamazaki H: High dose rate versus low dose rate interstitial radiotherapy for carcinoma of the floor of mouth. *Int J Radiat Oncol Biol Phys.* 1998;41:53.

61. Grimard L, Mazeron JJ, Pierquin B: Curietherapy versus external irradiation combined with curietherapy in stage II squamous cell carcinomas of the floor of the mouth. *Endocurie Hypertherm Oncol.* 1990;7:97.

62. Marsiglia H, Haie-Meder C, Sasso G, et al: Brachytherapy for T1-2 floor-of-the-mouth cancers: The Gustave-Roussy Institute experience. *Int J Radiat Oncol Biol Phys.* 2002;52:1257.

63. Sessions DG, Specter GJ, Lenox J, et al: Analysis of treatment results for floor-of-mouth cancer. *Laryngoscope.* 2000;110:1764.

64. Lampe I: Radiation therapy of cancer of the buccal mucosa and lower gingiva. *Am J Roentgenol.* 1955;73:628.

65. Saito T, Suguira C, Hirai A, et al: Development of squamous cell carcinoma from pre-existent oral leukoplakia: With respect to treatment modality. *Int J Oral Maxillofac Surg.* 2001;30:49.

66. Conley J, Sadoyama JA: Squamous cell carcinoma of the buccal mucosa: A review of 90 cases. *Arch Otolaryngol.* 1973;97:330.

67. Bloom ND, Spiro RH: Carcinoma of the cheek mucosa: A retrospective analysis. *Am J Surg.* 1980;140:556.

68. MacComb WS, Fletcher GH, Healey JE Jr: *Cancer of the Head and Neck.* Baltimore: Williams & Wilkins; 1967:110.

69. Sieczka E, Datta R, Singh A, et al: Cancer of the buccal mucosa: are margins and T-stage accurate predictors of local control? *Am J Otolaryngol.* 2001;22:395.

70. Strome SE, To W, Strawderman M, et al: Squamous cell carcinoma of the buccal mucosa. *Otolaryngol Head Neck Surg.* 1999;120:375.

71. Cherian T, Sebastian P, Ahamed MI, et al: Evaluation of salvage surgery in heavily irradiated cancer of the buccal mucosa. *Cancer.* 1991;68:295.

72. Fang FM, Leung SW, Huang CC, et al: Combined-modality therapy for squamous carcinoma of the buccal mucosa: treatment results and prognostic factors. *Head Neck.* 1997;19:506.

73. Chhetri DK, Rawnsley JD, Calcaterra TC: Carcinoma of the Buccal Mucosa. *Otolaryngol Head Neck Surg.* 2000;123:566.

74. Chaudhary AJ, Pande SC, Sharma V, et al: Radiotherapy of carcinoma of the buccal mucosa. *Semin Surg Oncol.* 1989;5:322.

75. Pop L, Eijkenboom WMH, De Boer MF, et al: Evaluation of treatment results of squamous cell carcinoma of the buccal mucosa. *Int J Radiat Oncol Biol Phys.* 1989;16:483.

76. Lapeyre M, Peiffert D, Malissard L, et al: An original technique of brachytherapy in the treatment of epidermoid carcinomas of the buccal mucosa. *Int J Radiat Oncol Biol Phys.* 1995;33:447.

77. Soo KC, Spiro RH, King W, et al: Squamous carcinoma of the gums. *Am J Surg.* 1988;156:281.

78. Shibuya H, Horiuchi I, Suzuki S, et al: Oral carcinoma of the upper jaw. Results of radiation treatment. *Acta Radiol Oncol.* 1984; 23:331.

79. Hong SX, Cha IH, Lee EW, Kim J: Mandibular invasion of lower gingival carcinoma in the molar region: its clinical implications on the surgical management. *Int J Oral Maxillofac Surg.* 2001;30:130.

80. McGregor AD, MacDonald G: Routes of entry of squamous cell carcinoma to the mandible. *Head Neck Surgery.* 1988;10:294.

81. Shingaki S, Nomura T, Masahito T, et al: Squamous cell carcinomas of the mandibular alveolus: Analysis of prognostic factors. *Oncology.* 2002;62:17.

82. Eicher SA, Overholt SM, El-nagger AK, et al: Lower gingival carcinoma. *Arch Otolaryngol Head Neck Surg.* 1996;122:634.

83. Overholt SM, Eicher SA, Wolf P, Weber RS: Prognostic factors affecting outcome in lower gingival carcinoma. *Laryngoscope.* 1996;106:1335.

84. Byers RM, Newman R, Russell N, Yue A: Results of treatment for squamous carcinoma of the lower gum. *Cancer.* 1981;47:2236.

85. Huang CJ, Chao KS, Tsai J, et al: Cancer of retromolar trigone: Long-term radiation therapy outcome. *Head Neck.* 2001;23:758.

86. Lo K, Fletcher GH, Byers R, et al: Results of irradiation in the squamous cell carcinomas of the anterior faucial pillar-retromolar trigone. *Int J Radiat Oncol Biol Phys.* 1987;13:969.

87. Byers RM, Anderson B, Schwarz EA, et al: Treatment of squamous carcinoma of the retromolar trigone. *AM J Clin Oncol.* 1984; 7:647.

88. New GB, Hallberg OE: The end results of the treatment of malignant tumors of the palate. *Surg Gynecol Obstet.* 1941; 73:520.

89. Chierici G, Silverman S, Forsythe B: A tumor registry study of oral squamous carcinoma. *J Oral Med.* 1968;53:91.

90. Evans JF, Shan J: Epidermoid carcinoma of the palate. *Am J Surg.* 1981;142:451.

91. Chung CK, Johns ME, Cantrell RW, Constable MB: Radiotherapy in the management of primary malignancies of the hard palate. *Laryngoscope.* 1980;90:576.

92. Yorozu A, Sykes AJ, Slevin NJ: Carcinoma of the hard palate treated with radiotherapy: A retrospective review of 31 cases. *Oral Oncol.* 2001;37:493.

93. Kovalic JJ, Simpson JR: Carcinoma of the hard palate. *J Otolaryngol.* 1993;22:118.

94. Vanderpuye V, Goldson A: Osteoradionecrosis of the mandible. *J Natl Med Assoc.* 2000;92:579.

95. Fujita M, Hirokawa Y, Kashiwado K, et al: An analysis of mandibular bone complications in radiotherapy for T1 and T2 carcinoma of the oral tongue. *Int J Radiat Oncol Biol Phys.* 1996;34:333.

Cancer of the Hypopharynx

30

Michael J. Zelefsky, MD

EPIDEMIOLOGY

Approximately 2500 cases of hypopharyngeal cancer are diagnosed in the United States each year, 75% to 80% of which arise in the pyriform sinuses, while 15% to 20% originate from the posterior pharyngeal wall. Postcricoid cancers constitute about 5% of cases. The male-to-female ratio ranges from 5:1 to 7:1 for pyriform sinus cancer and 3:1 to 4:1 for pharyngeal wall cancer.[1,2] Postcricoid cancers occur predominantly in women. The age-specific incidence rate for white males increases from the 40- to 44-year old group (0.4/100,000) to the 65- to 69-year-old group (9.6/100,000) and then subsequently declines (4.3/100,000) for the 85-year-old group.[2] Among African-American males, the incidence continues to increase with age (up to 15.8/100,000 in the 85-year-old group).[2] In general, the prognoses for hypopharyngeal tumors are notoriously poor because of the following associated factors: extensive local-regional spread of disease through the submucosal route, abundant lymphatic drainage of the region with a greater propensity for distant metastatic spread; clinical presentation at an advanced stage; frequent association with nutritional depletion; concurrent medical problems conferred by tobacco and alcohol abuse; and occurrence in patients with a predisposition for the development of second malignancies (secondary to mucosal field cancerization).

ETIOLOGY

Tobacco and alcohol use are clearly associated with the development of hypopharyngeal cancer.[3-5] While tobacco alone is known to be carcinogenic, the role of alcohol in the etiology of hypopharyngeal cancer has been underappreciated. A prevailing opinion is that alcohol potentiates carcinogenesis in tobacco-exposed mucosa.[6] However, evidence points to an independent role for alcohol.[4,7,8] The data suggest a synergistic interaction between tobacco and alcohol with regard to the risk of inducing hypopharyngeal cancer, particularly for people with heavy alcohol consumption.[4,8]

Among cigarette smokers, the use of unfiltered cigarettes or black tobacco (with higher concentrations of carcinogenic N-nitrosamines) increases the risk of cancer.[4] For a similar reason, smoking marijuana (with its high tar burden and aromatic hydrocarbon content) appears to confer even greater risk.[6] Moist snuff (smokeless

tobacco) consumption also exposes the pharynx to carcinogens.[9,10] The latter is noteworthy in that snuff consumption increased by 38% in the United States between 1981 and 1993.[11] A growing prevalence of snuff dipping among young males has been suggested as a reason for this increase.[11]

Dietary factors predisposing to the development of hypopharyngeal cancer may include a diet low in carotenoids[3,6] and iron-deficiency anemia. This anemia has been associated with postcricoid cancers in women in Scandinavia and Great Britain and usually occurs in this setting along with dysphagia (from hypopharyngeal webs) and atrophy of the oral mucosa (manifested by loss of tongue papillae). The triad of iron-deficiency anemia, dysphagia, and glossitis is known as the Plummer-Vinson syndrome in Scandinavia and the Paterson-Brown Kelly syndrome in Great Britain.

Genetic susceptibility of the host influences the likelihood of cancer development.[3] DNA repair capability, which can be indirectly measured by assessment of chromosomal breakage induced by in vitro exposure to bleomycin,[12] was demonstrated in a case-control study to be a strong predictor of the risk of upper aerodigestive tract cancer.[13] A positive family history of cancer of the respiratory or upper digestive tract among first-degree relatives (especially siblings) also has been associated with an increased risk of head and neck cancer.[14]

GENETICS AND CYTOGENETICS

Genetic abnormalities that appear to be causally linked to the etiology of head and neck cancer are point mutations in the *p53* gene[15] and *bcl*-2 overexpression. In the case of *bcl*-2, the protein encoded by the *bcl*-2 gene is overexpressed in head and neck cancers among heavy smokers.[16] This is hypothesized to result from the chromosomal translocation t(14;18)(q32;q21), which juxtaposes the *bcl*-2 proto-oncogene with the immunoglobulin heavy-chain gene,[17] a juxtaposition that occurs in 85% of non-Hodgkin's follicular lymphomas.[18] It is further hypothesized that carcinogens from cigarette smoke act upon the *bcl*-2 site and increase the rate of the t(14;18) translocation.[16,17]

Other oncogenes may be involved in the pathogenesis of head and neck cancer; these include *p16* (CDKN2), PRAD1 (cyclin D1), EMS1, the epidermal growth factor (EGF) receptor gene, *erb*-B-2 (*neu*), *myc*, and *ras*.[6,15,19-22]

Particular oncogenes are expected to act at distinct points along a multistep pathway in a manner analogous to the colorectal model demonstrated by Vogelstein and associates.[22,23]

As a vector of proto-oncogenes, human papillomavirus infection may also contribute to the etiology of hypopharyngeal cancer.[24] Integration of its DNA into the host genome could affect gene expression or regulation. One study has associated detection of human papillomavirus DNA in laryngeal and hypopharyngeal tumor specimens with both decreased disease-specific survival and decreased local-regional control.[24]

ANATOMY

The hypopharynx (the inferior portion of the pharynx) is subdivided into three sites: the pyriform sinuses (the paired recesses lateral to the larynx), the posterior pharyngeal wall, and the postcricoid region. The hypopharynx functions to guide food into the esophagus, and away from the larynx, during normal swallowing. The hypopharynx extends from the level of the hyoid bone to the inferior edge of the cricoid cartilage, corresponding to the C4 through C6 vertebral bodies. It envelops the larynx, as shown in Figure 30-1. The oropharynx lies above, the cervical esophagus below, the larynx anteriorly and medially, and the retropharyngeal space posteriorly.

The bilateral pyriform sinuses (laryngopharyngeal sulci) lie just distal to the glossopharyngeal sulci of the oropharynx. The pharyngoepiglottic fold demarcates each pyriform sinus from the oropharynx (Fig. 30-2). Underlying and inferior to this fold is the pharyngoepiglottic muscle, which constitutes the anterior wall of the pyriform fossa. The medial wall is composed of the mucosal surface overlying the aryepiglottic muscle (lateral to the aryepiglottic fold), as well as the surface lateral to the arytenoid cartilage. Lateral boundaries are the thyrohyoid membrane (upper portion) and thyroid cartilage (lower portion). Inferiorly, the sinus tapers to an apex, the level of which varies among individuals but usually is no lower than the lower border of the cricoid cartilage. The apex is composed of loose, expansile connective tissue. Posteriorly, the pyriform sinus opens to the remainder of the hypopharyngeal lumen.

The postcricoid area is the caudally sloping mucosal surface that overlies the posterior lamina of the cricoid cartilage (see Fig. 30-2). The posterior surfaces of the arytenoid cartilages form the superior boundary of this region. The posterior cricoarytenoid muscles lie immediately underneath the mucosa. Inferiorly, the postcricoid area is continuous with the cervical esophagus.

The posterior pharyngeal wall is continuous with the lateral walls of the two pyriform sinuses (see Fig. 30-1). The wall itself, from the inner to outer aspect, is composed of the following: mucosal lining, submucosa, fibrous layer (pharyngobasilar fascia), muscular layer, and a deeper layer of fascia (visceral fascia). The muscular layer is composed mainly of the inferior constrictor muscle, with contributions from the distal portion of the middle constrictor muscle superiorly, and the cricopharyngeal muscle inferiorly. Behind the posterior pharyngeal wall, loose connective tissue forms a potential space (the retropharyngeal space) between this wall and the prevertebral fascia. Posterolaterally lie the carotid spaces, which contain the neurovascular bundles; these are intimately associated with the deep cervical lymph nodes and vessels.

Sensory nerve supply to the hypopharynx is provided through both the internal branch of the superior laryngeal nerve and the recurrent laryngeal nerve. Motor supply is predominantly via the recurrent laryngeal nerve. Both are branches of the vagus nerve (cranial nerve X). The internal branch of the superior laryngeal nerve runs submucosally along the anterolateral wall of the pyriform sinus and exits the laryngeal framework superolaterally through an opening in the thyrohyoid membrane. This branch eventually joins the vagus nerve, which synapses with the auricular nerve of Arnold at the jugular ganglion; this pathway allows for referred otalgia (see section on clinical presentation). Branches of the recurrent laryngeal nerve course submucosally through both the postcricoid region and the pyriform fossa.

LYMPHATIC DRAINAGE

A rich lymphatic network drains the hypopharynx. One pathway of ductal drainage is via the ascending route taken by the internal branch of the superior laryngeal nerve (see previous discussion). Together with this nerve, lymph vessels as well as the superior laryngeal artery and vein traverse an opening in the lateral aspect of the thyrohyoid membrane. Lymph then drains predominantly into the level II (upper jugular) and level III (midjugular)

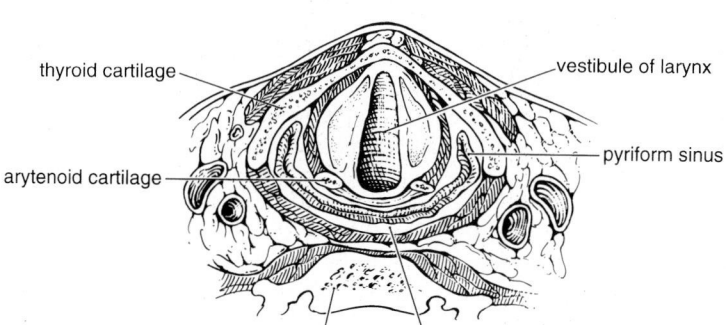

thyroid cartilage

vestibule of larynx

pyriform sinus

arytenoid cartilage

C5 vertebral body

posterior pharyngeal wall

Figure 30–1. Axial view of the hypopharynx.

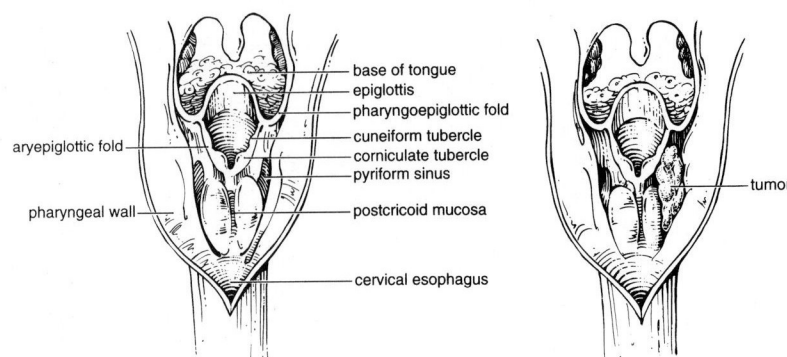

Figure 30–2. Posterior view of the hypopharynx.

nodal groups. Another pathway is via the paratracheal nodes, which lie posterior to the thyroid gland in the tracheoesophageal grooves. These then drain into the level IV (lower jugular) group as well as into the anterior mediastinal nodes.

The retropharyngeal lymph nodes can also be accessed from the hypopharynx. These nodes are located high in the retropharyngeal space and are divided into a medial group and a lateral group (Fig. 30-3). (The latter are also called the nodes of Rouvière.) Both groups are above the level of the hyoid bone. Below the hyoid, the retropharyngeal space contains fat only. Yet, as there are no fascial barriers within this space, once tumor penetrates it, neoplastic cells can migrate freely throughout. Cephalad spread results in nodal involvement. Caudal dissemination allows disease to access the mediastinum, with which the retropharyngeal space is contiguous. This space thus becomes an additional vertical pathway through which tumor cells may travel.

PATHOLOGY

Squamous cell carcinomas constitute more than 95% of carcinomas of the hypopharynx. Among pyriform sinus carcinomas, approximately one third have been found to be nonkeratinizing and 40% poorly differentiated in one large series.[25] The same report noted the tumor growth pattern at the periphery of biopsy specimens to be infiltrating in 80% and pushing in 20%.[25] Trends toward increased local-regional relapse were found for keratinizing (vs. nonkeratinizing) tumors and for those with infiltrating (vs. pushing) margins.[25]

This information has greater relevance in light of reports from the Department of Veterans Affairs Cooperative Laryngeal Cancer Study Group that demonstrate that the histologic growth pattern of the tumor (for cancer of the larynx) is a significant predictor of both complete tumor response to neoadjuvant chemotherapy[26] and disease-free survival.[27] Cancers with blunt, thick invading cords of tumor responded less frequently—and were associated with a poorer disease-free survival rate—than those with thin, irregular infiltrating cords. The latter pattern is thought to reflect rapidly growing tumor with a high proliferative rate.[26]

The basaloid variant of squamous cell carcinoma occasionally arises in the hypopharynx.[28] Its prognostic significance is uncertain. Other rare tumors of the hypopharynx include minor salivary gland tumors, sarcomas of various types (fibrosarcomas, liposarcomas, synovial cell sarcomas, and malignant fibrous histiocytomas), and lymphomas.

CLINICAL PRESENTATION

Symptoms

The most common presenting symptoms of cancer of the hypopharynx are sore throat, odynophagia, and a neck mass. A neck mass may be the sole presenting symptom in up to 25% of cases.[29,30] Dysphagia and weight loss frequently occur with locally advanced disease and can occur in early stages. Airway obstruction requiring emergency tracheostomy occurs in 5% to 10% of cases. Other symptoms may include otalgia, neck pain, hoarseness, foreign body sensation and mucus retention in the throat, aspiration, and hemoptysis.

Otalgia occurs as a referred pain from a mass lesion in the hypopharynx pressing on or invading the internal branch of the superior laryngeal nerve. This nerve eventually joins the auricular nerve of Arnold at the jugular foramen, which supplies sensory innervation to the posterior aspect of auricle and posterior and inferior aspects of the external auditory canal. Referred otalgia through this pathway is a dull, aching pain of the external ear.

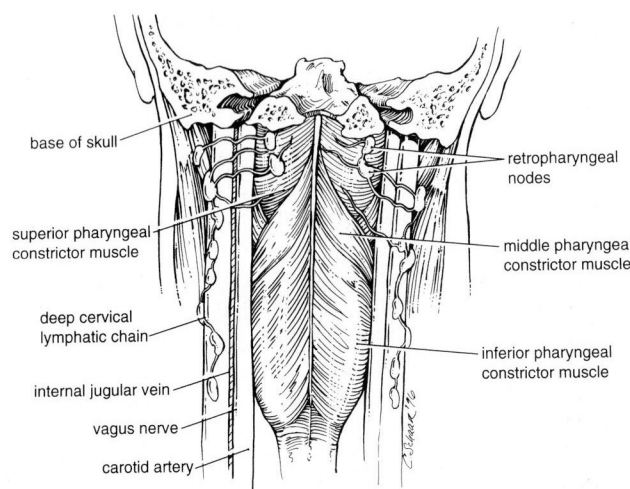

Figure 30–3. Schematic posterior view of the retropharyngeal lymph nodes.

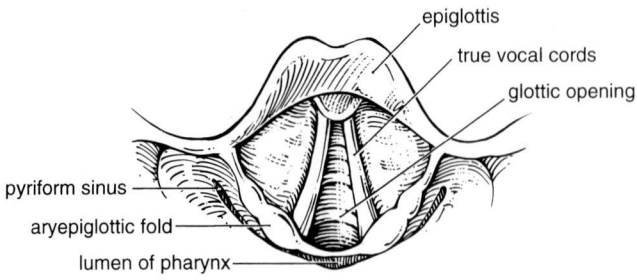

Figure 30–4. Endoscopic view of normal larynx and hypopharynx.

The hallmark of postcricoid carcinoma is dysphagia, which is a presenting symptom in more than 90% of cases.[31-33] Among posterior wall cancers, dysphagia heralds the disease in 45% to 90% of patients.[30,34-36] Cachexia is thus not a rare finding in patients with cancer of the hypopharynx. Other comorbidities may include malnutrition due to alcohol abuse, alcohol-induced liver disease, and chronic obstructive pulmonary disease.

Physical Examination

Indirect mirror and direct endoscopic examination of the laryngopharynx are mandatory for evaluation of disease. Schematic endoscopic views of the normal and diseased hypopharynx are shown in Figures 30-4 and 30-5. Pooling of secretions and arytenoid edema may be prominent findings, especially with tumors of the pyriform apex and postcricoid region. It is not unusual for these findings to obscure visualization of the primary lesion itself. Tumors of the upper (membranous) portion of the pyriform sinus tend to be locally infiltrating, exophytic lesions, while those of the lower (cartilaginous) portion tend to be widely infiltrating, ulcerative lesions. Lesions arising from the cartilaginous portions of the hypopharynx have been associated with a poorer prognosis compared with lesions from the membranous portion of the pyriform region,[37-39] and so it is important to note from which portion the tumor arises. It is also important to differentiate a lesion of the medial wall of the pyriform fossa from a lesion arising from the aryepiglottic fold proper, as the latter carries a better prognosis.[40] Posterior wall tumors can present as submucosal bulges with or without ulceration.

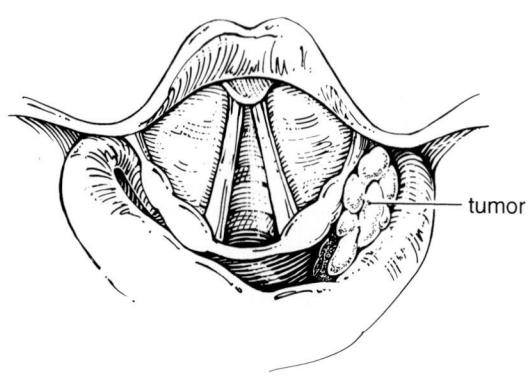

Figure 30–5. Endoscopic view of bulky, exophytic T1 pyriform sinus cancer.

Side-to-side manipulation of the thyroid cartilage is helpful in determining posterior extent of disease. Postcricoid and posterior wall tumors can either displace the thyroid cartilage and larynx anteriorly, or, in deeply invasive disease, fix these structures to the prevertebral fascia. Either scenario results in loss of the crepitation (or thyroid click) that is usually produced when the superior horns of the thyroid cartilage are dragged medially against and across the anterior aspect of the vertebral column. Tenderness of the thyroid cartilage itself suggests cartilaginous invasion by tumor.

The neck should be examined with attention to the location, size, and mobility of any palpable lymph nodes.

ROUTES OF DISEASE SPREAD

Local

Noteworthy routes of local spread include submucosal extension of disease, not infrequently associated with skip metastases and intervening normal-appearing mucosa.[41] Such spread allows for both vertical and horizontal migration of the tumor. Medial extension results in involvement of endolaryngeal structures. The primary tumor can also extend directly into the soft tissues of the neck through the thyrohyoid membrane, through the thyroid cartilage, or around the posterior border of the thyroid ala. In the latter two instances, the thyroid gland may also be invaded. Tumors arising in the pyriform apex often invade the thyroid cartilage.[42]

Nodal

For pyriform sinus cancers, palpable lymph nodes can be found at presentation in 70% to 75% of patients.[43-46] Bilateral or contralateral nodes are present in 10% to 14%.[43,45,47] Neck dissection increases the yield of node positivity by exposing occult disease. Upon dissection, up to 40% to 50% of patients with clinically N0 necks can be found to harbor nodal metastases.[48,49]

Posterior wall tumors present with palpable nodes in 40% to 60% of cases.[36,50-53] The incidence of bilaterality ranges from 10% to 35%,[50,51,53] depending on the location of the primary tumor in the medial-to-lateral dimension. The incidence is higher with more medially located tumors, due to submucosal anastomoses of lymphatic capillaries. Occult metastases have been found in 54% to 66% of N0 patients upon neck dissection.[30,54] Between 30% and 40% of patients have retropharyngeal lymph nodes involved with tumor.[50,55,56]

Postcricoid cancers present with palpable nodes in 33% to 45% of patients.[31-33,57-59] Bilateral or contralateral nodes are present in 8% to 18%.[32,59] Among patients with T4 tumors, 50% have clinically apparent nodal disease, and 33% have bilateral involvement.[33] Occult metastases may frequently be present in paratracheal lymph nodes or the thyroid gland (which is also true for tumors originating in the adjacent apex of the pyriform sinus).[54,60-63] Such subclinical disease must be taken into account when the treatment is planned.[64-67]

Distant

Of patients with hypopharyngeal cancer, 20% to 30% develop clinically overt distant metastases within 2 years, despite treatment. The autopsy incidence of distant metastases among 108 patients treated in the modern era at a single institution was found to be 60%; however, only 13% of these patients had pathologic local-regional control of disease.[68] Autopsy studies reporting on heterogeneous cases of head and neck cancer have shown a 19% to 42% incidence of distant metastases among patients who have no evidence of local-regional disease at postmortem examination.[69] This suggests the presence of micrometastatic spread of disease at the time of initial diagnosis. Results from a Radiation Therapy Oncology Group (RTOG) analysis of the effect of local-regional control on distant metastatic dissemination for 237 cancers of the hypopharynx support this hypothesis: local-regional control of disease at 6 months was associated with a slight reduction in the incidence of distant metastases at 0.5 to 2.5 years from 43% to 40% (P = 0.054).[70]

The most common metastatic sites, in decreasing order, are lung, mediastinal nodes, liver, and bone.[68]

DIAGNOSTIC AND STAGING STUDIES

Routine staging studies should include a chest x-ray, blood tests to evaluate liver function, and a computed tomographic (CT) scan of the head and neck. The CT scan should be done before biopsy of the tumor to avoid imaging postbiopsy edema, which obscures radiologic definition of tumor extent.[71] The CT scan is useful for precise delineation of tumor extent, with particular reference to the following: visualizing inferior extent of tumor (for which fiberoptic endoscopy alone is often inadequate); detecting invasion of the laryngeal framework and extralaryngeal/extrapharyngeal spread into the soft tissues of the neck; detecting submucosal spread toward the midline via the paraglottic space (anteromedial to the pyriform sinus); and detecting posterior spread into the

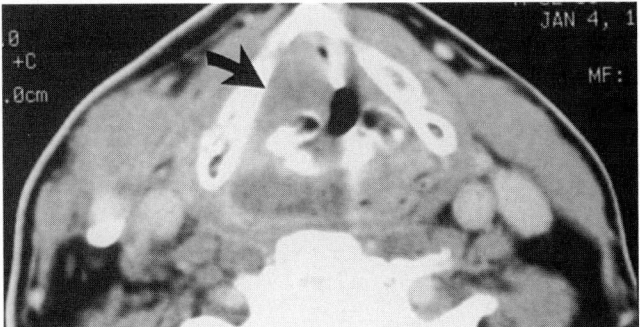

Figure 30–7. Pyriform sinus cancer extending into paraglottic space. Endoscopically, mass effect upon the laryngeal vestibule was apparent.

retropharyngeal space (Figs. 30-6, 30-7, and 30-8).[72] It is also useful for disclosing clinically occult metastatic lymphadenopathy, particularly positive retropharyngeal nodes, contralateral nodes, and extracapsular extension of disease.

Magnetic resonance imaging (MRI) is an important adjunctive study in two situations: (1) for determining whether cartilage invasion is present,[73] and (2) for determining the extent of paraglottic space invasion.[74] These are pertinent issues when conservation laryngopharyngeal surgery is being considered, because cartilage invasion and extensive paraglottic space invasion are contraindications to such surgery.

Helical (spiral) computed tomography provides a rapid and practical means for three-dimensional (3D) imaging of the upper airway.[75] It can be used to produce a 3D airway cast—similar to a laryngogram done in years past (but not requiring instillation of foreign material). In demonstrating tumor mass effect upon adjacent airway structures clearly, the 3D laryngogram provides a complementary view of tumor extent.

Biopsy of the primary lesion should be performed under general anesthesia. Due to the risk of synchronous primary malignancies amid vulnerable mucosa, bronchoscopy and esophagoscopy should also be done at this time.[76,77] Open biopsy of a neck mass to obtain a tissue diagnosis should be avoided, as this contaminates the neck oncologically.

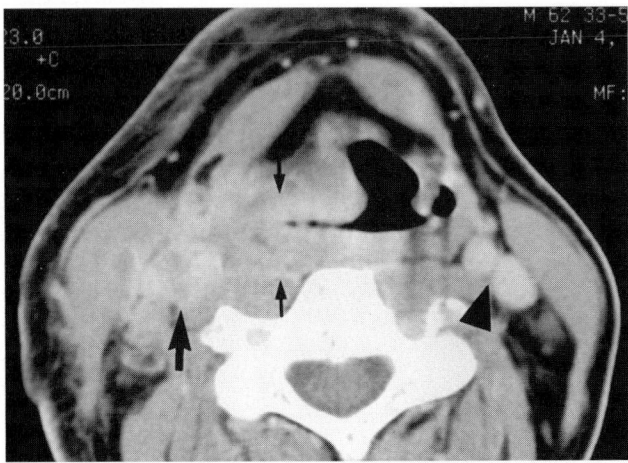

Figure 30–6. T4 pyriform sinus cancer extending into soft tissues of neck. *Thin arrows* indicate primary lesion. *Thick arrow* indicates lymphadenopathy with fixation to carotid vessels. *Arrowhead* indicates normal carotid vessels on the left.

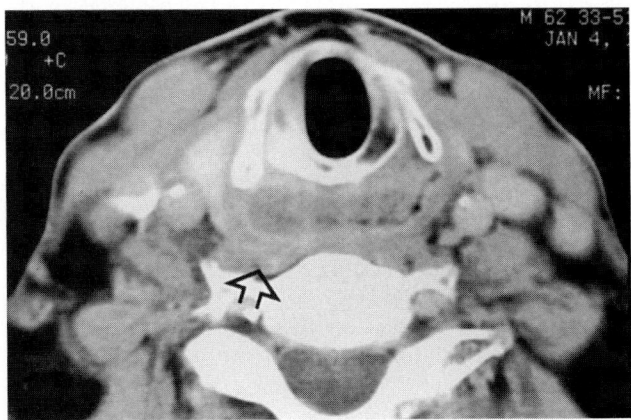

Figure 30–8. Pyriform sinus cancer with retropharyngeal space involvement *(arrow)*.

STAGING

The 2002 American Joint Committee on Cancer (AJCC) staging[78] for all hypopharyngeal cancers is given in Table 30-1. Stage Note that the staging for T2 lesions maintains the size parameter as well the proviso that there is no fixation of the hemilarynx. Stage T4a includes invasion of the thyroid gland, cricoid and thyroid cartilage hyoid bone, or esophagus. Stage T4b includes invasion of the prevertebral fascia, encasement of the carotid artery, or invasion of the mediastinal structures.

STANDARD THERAPEUTIC APPROACHES

Pyriform Sinus: Early-Stage (T1–T2) Disease

Either a primary conservative surgical approach or primary radiation therapy is a suitable treatment option for early-stage pyriform sinus cancer. Features allowing for conservative therapy are the following: all T1 tumors as well as T2 exophytic tumors of the upper or membranous portion of the pyriform sinus, lack of extension to the apex, lack of disease extension to the arytenoids, intact vocal cord mobility, uncompromised airway, and nonfixed neck nodes.[38,39,79-90] Tumors originating in or extending to the apex frequently invade the thyroid cartilage, which often necessitates its removal in surgical management of disease respecting oncologic principles.[42] Furthermore, in obtaining clear surgical margins on apical disease, the cricoid cartilage often must be sacrificed, necessitating permanent tracheostomy. In addition, patients require adequate pulmonary function to undergo a conservative hypopharyngeal surgery.

Early-stage favorable disease is not commonly encountered. In each of three separate series of more than 400 patients, T1 and T2 tumors (endophytic included) with nonfixed nodes constituted 12% to 16% of the cases; categorizing disease by the additional features listed previously would further winnow the number of patients actually presenting with favorable disease.[40,84,85,89] Earlier detection of hypopharyngeal cancer, however, may increase the fraction of patients who are eligible for a larynx-conserving approach.

Conservative surgery consists of partial laryngopharyngectomy and ipsilateral modified radical neck dissection (or bilateral for N2c disease).[82,89,91-95] In the setting of an N0 or N1 neck, a lateral neck dissection (involving removal of level II, III, and IV nodes) may be performed instead. Partial laryngopharyngectomy removes the upper portion of the pyriform sinus and adjacent marginal laryngeal structures (false cords, epiglottis, and possibly the ipsilateral arytenoid cartilage). In the setting of positive margins, multiple positive lymph nodes, or extracapsular extension of disease, surgery is followed by postoperative radiotherapy to maximize locoregional control of disease.[45,47,49,60,96-98]

When primary radiation therapy is decided upon, a planned neck dissection may follow radiotherapy, approximately 3 to 4 weeks after completion of radiotherapy. This approach may be performed if any single lymph node is greater than 2 or 3 cm or if multiple positive lymph nodes are present on initial clinical examination,

Table 30–1 Classification of Hypopharyngeal Cancers

Primary Tumor (T)

TX	Primary tumor cannot be assessed
T0	No evidence of primary tumor
Tis	Carcinoma in situ

Hypopharynx

T1	Tumor limited to one subsite of hypopharynx and ≤2 cm in greatest dimension
T2	Tumor involves more than one subsite of hypopharynx or an adjacent site, or measures >2 cm but not >4 cm in greatest diameter without fixation of hemilarynx
T3	Tumor measures >4 cm in greatest dimension or with fixation of hemilarynx
T4a	Tumor invades thyroid/cricoid cartilage, hyoid bone, thyroid gland, esophagus, or central compartment soft tissue*
T4b	Tumor invades prevertebral fascia, encases carotid artery, or involves mediastinal structures

*Note: Central compartment soft tissue includes prelaryngeal strap muscles and subcutaneous fat.

Hypopharynx

NX	Regional lymph nodes cannot be assessed
N0	No regional lymph node metastasis
N1	Metastasis in a single ipsilateral lymph node, ≤3 cm in greatest dimension
N2	Metastasis in a single ipsilateral lymph node, >3 cm but not >6 cm in greatest dimension, or in multiple ipsilateral lymph nodes, none >6 cm in greatest dimension
N2a	Metastasis in a single ipsilateral lymph node >3 cm but not >6 cm in greatest dimension
N2b	Metastasis in multiple ipsilateral lymph nodes, none >6 cm in greatest dimension
N2c	Metastasis in bilateral or contralateral lymph nodes, none >6 cm in greatest dimension
N3	Metastasis in a lymph node >6 cm in greatest dimension

Distant Metastasis (M)

MX	Distant metastasis cannot be assessed
M0	No distant metastasis
M1	Distant metastasis

Stage Grouping: Oropharynx and Hypopharynx

Stage 0	Tis	N0	M0
Stage I	T1	N0	M0
Stage II	T2	N0	M0
Stage III	T3	N0	M0
	T1	N1	M0
	T2	N1	M0
	T3	N1	M0
Stage IV	T4a	N0	M0
	T4a	N1	M0
	T1	N2	M0
	T2	N2	M0
	T3	N2	M0
	T4a	N2	M0
Stage IVB	T4b	Any N	M0
	Any T	N3	M0
Stage IVC	Any T	Any N	M1

From Greene FL, Page DL, Fleming ID, et al, eds: AJCC Cancer Staging Manual, 6th ed. New York: Springer; 2002.

unless there has been early complete regression of neck disease.[39,40,81,88,99,100]

Amdur et al.[101] reported on 101 patients treated at the University of Florida with radiotherapy alone with or without a planned neck dissection. The 5-year actuarial local control rates for T1 and T2 tumors were 90% and 80%, respectively. After surgical salvage, the ultimate local control was 95% and 91%, respectively. One univariate analysis apical involvement for T1 tumors was associated with an inferior local control compared to patients with no apical involvement (1/3—33% vs. 14/14—100%).

While the local-regional control and survival outcomes are similar for conservative surgery and radiotherapy (Tables 30-2 and 30-3),[81,83,102,103] primary radiation therapy may be the preferable treatment option secondary to its associated superior functional outcomes involving speech and swallowing. Nevertheless, there is an increased risk of swallowing dysfunction after radiotherapy for early-stage lesions. In the University of Florida series (101) 6% of patients experienced difficulty swallowing, requiring a permanent gastrostomy tube after radiotherapy alone. Although as noted there are potential significant complications after radiotherapy alone, the risk of severe toxicity and significant dysfunction is more prevalent after conservation surgery. Furthermore, the risk of chronic aspiration secondary to pharyngolaryngeal dyssynergia (due to sacrifice of the superior laryngeal nerve) after conservation surgery is less often observed after definitive radiotherapy.[82,93,94,104,105]

Pyriform Sinus: Locally Advanced (T3–T4) Resectable Disease

Standard management for unfavorable, resectable disease (i.e., disease not meeting criteria specified previously, though still resectable) consists of the following: total laryngectomy and partial pharyngectomy combined with neck dissection; either primary closure or pharyngeal reconstruction—the latter with a myocutaneous flap, gastric pull-up, or microvascular free tissue transfer (in a one-stage procedure); and postoperative radiation therapy. Beyond the locally invasive features of the primary tumor, the resectability of a tumor is also determined by a surgeon's aggressiveness and skill, as well as the extent of the patient's willingness to accept postoperative complications and longer-term impairment of speech and swallowing. Tumor fixation to the cervical spine or a massive T4 tumor always confers unresectability, as does bulky cervical lymphadenopathy fixed to the neurovascular bundle.

Postoperative radiation therapy is preferred to preoperative irradiation. A randomized trial by the RTOG, RTOG 73-03, has been the definitive study of this sequencing issue.[106,107] Postoperative irradiation was associated with significantly improved local-regional control for all anatomic subsites combined. Among hypopharyngeal cases only, actuarial local-regional control and survival at 4 years were 61% and 28%, respectively, for the postoperative group, compared with 50% and 18% for the preoperative group. While other studies

have suggested an increased perioperative complication rate in patients with hypopharyngeal cancer in particular who are treated with preoperative irradiation,[29,86,108,109] this relationship was not confirmed in RTOG 73-03.

For stage III and IV disease, surgery in combination with postoperative radiation therapy results in better localregional control rates (and possibly survivorship) than surgery alone. Retrospective data supporting this conclusion are outlined in Tables 30-4 and 30-5. The only randomized trial that compared surgery alone with surgery plus postoperative radiation therapy in the management of locally advanced head and neck cancer, including pharyngeal carcinomas, did not adequately address the question.[110] The case mixture was heterogeneous, the sample size small, and the distribution of prognostic factors between groups unequal despite randomization.[111] Furthermore, the total dose of radiation administered (50 Gy) was too low to eradicate microscopic disease in an operative bed.

Because distant metastases remain a common reason for treatment failure despite adequate local-regional control of disease,[70,85,111,112] systemic therapy is an important consideration in the management of patients with stage III or IV disease. In randomized trials involving heterogeneous cases of advanced head and neck cancers, induction chemotherapy has been shown to affect the incidence of distant metastases.[113-115] Adjuvant chemotherapy both after definitive local-regional therapy (as maintenance chemotherapy)[116,117] and concurrent with local therapy (in the sequence surgery-chemotherapy-radiation therapy)[118] may also reduce the rate of distant failure. Similarly, chemotherapy as part of a larynx-preserving treatment approach may result in decreased failure below the clavicles, as it has been shown in the management of advanced laryngeal cancer.[119]

Larynx-conserving treatment regimens in which aggressive surgery is avoided have been reported.[120-136] Early results from a randomized trial led by the European Organization for Research in Cancer Therapy comparing induction chemotherapy (three cycles of cisplatin and 5-fluorouracil) and radiotherapy with primary surgery and postoperative radiotherapy suggested that larynx preservation might be a viable strategy in managing hypopharyngeal cancer, as survival was not compromised.[120] At 3 years, the crude survival rates were 53% and 56% for the chemotherapy-radiotherapy approach and surgery plus postoperative radiotherapy, respectively, and 28% of patients in the chemotherapy-radiotherapy arm were free of disease, with an intact, functioning larynx. Follow-up data from this trial confirm these positive results: Survival rates in the two arms remained equivalent, while in the experimental arm, local progression-free survival with a functional larynx was achieved in 35% of patients at 5 years.[121]

Recently, investigators from the University Hospital Center in St. Etienne, France reported the outcome of patients with pyriform sinus cancers treated with various hyperfractionated radiotherapy and concomitant chemotherapy treatment schedules.[122] In one group of 24 patients, carboplatin (days 1 to 16 and 16 to 27) was given in conjunction with hyperfractionated radiotherapy (1.6 Gy twice daily) to a total dose 67.2 Gy. In a second

Table 30–2   Carcinoma of the Pyriform Sinus: Results of Radiation Therapy Alone, with Curative Intent

Institution (Year)	Patients, n	Local-regional Control, %	3-Year NED Survival, %*	5-year NED Survival, %*
Institut Curie[†] (1982):				
Overall[40]	434	47[§§]	26**	19**
T1-2N0[40,167]	33	70[§§]	42**	34**
T1-2N1-3[40,167]	57	47[§§]	34**	21**
T1-2N2-3[40,168]	36	42[§§]	22**	15**
T3N0-1[40,168]	71		46–50**	
T4N0-1[40,168]	124		28–29**	
T3-4N0-1[40]	195	53[§§]	33**	24**
T3-4N2-3[40,168]	149	35[§§]	13**	9**
M.D. Anderson (1982)[84]	48	79[§§]	48[‡]*	
U. of Michigan (1984):				
Lateral epilarynx/upper pyriform sinus[38]	93	43[§§]		45**
Lower pyriform sinus[38,169]	61	31[§§]		26**
Stage III	21			57**
Stage IV	38			15**
Ctr. Paul Lamarque[†] (1986):[89]				
Overall	209	25[§§]		5**
T1-2N0	24	75[§§]		
T1-2N1-3	37	41[§§]		
T1-2N1-2b	19	68[§§]		
T1-2N2c-3	18	11[§§]		
T3-4N0	29	31[§§]		
T3-4N2c-3	95	4[§§]		
Inst. Gustave-Roussy (1987):[85]				
T1-2N0-1,[¶] membranous pyriform sinus	31		65**	40**
Mass. General (1990):[90]				
Overall Conventional RT	127	44[††]	21**	
T1-T2		68[§§]		
T3-T4		20[§§]		
T1-2N0	11		73**	
T1-2N1	9		56**	
T1-2N2-3	7		14**	
T3N0-1	33		27**	
T4N0-1	11		9**	
T3-4N0-1	44		23**	
T3-4N2-3	56		5**	
T1-4N0-1, membranous pyriform sinus	31		55**	
T1-4N0-1, cartilaginous pyriform sinus	33		18**	
Mass. General (1990):[90]				
T1-T4, hyperfractionated radiation therapy	54	61[§§]		
T1-T2	31	82[§§]		
T3-T4	23	33[§§]		
French Head and Neck Study Group (1991) [166]:				
T1-2 with palpable nodes	60		32**	18**
U. of Florida[‡‡] (1993):[39]				
Favorable T1-2 overall	73	79[§§]		43**
T1-2N0	15	90[§§]		62**
T1-2N1	13	54[§§]		45**
T1-2N2-3	31	65[§§]		32**
T2, conventional RT	23	65[§§]		
T2, hyperfractionated RT	16	94[§§]		
M.D. Anderson (1995)[170] hyperfractionated radiation	39	85[§§]		

NED, no evidence of disease.

*Actuarial, unless otherwise noted.

[†]Lymph node staging converted from the following non-AJCC lymph node staging used in this report: N1, ipsilateral palpable, mobile, nodes; N2, bilateral or contralateral palpable, mobile nodes; N3, any fixed node.

[‡]At 2 years.

[§]Local control only.

[¶]N1 nodes less than 2 cm only.

**Crude data, for all numbers in this column for this institution.

[††]Actuarial local control at 5 years, for all numbers in this column for this institution.

[‡‡]A planned neck dissection followed radiation in 19 cases.

[§§]Actuarial local control only at 2 years.

Table 30–3   Carcinoma of the Pyriform Sinus: Results of Conservative Surgery (Partial Laryngopharyngectomy and Neck Dissection) and Pre- or Postoperative Radiation Therapy

Institution (Year)	Patients, n	Local-regional Control, %	3-Year NED Survival, %*	5-year NED Survival, %*
Washington U.† (1981):[94]				
T1-T4	80	77¶	46	39‡‡
M.D. Anderson‡ (1981):[104]				
T2-T4§	19	32¶		
Ctr Paul Lamarque** (1986):[89]				
T1-T2 overall	73	43¶		
T1-T2N1-2b	13	69¶		37††
French Head and Neck Study Group (1991):[166]				
T1-T2 with palpable nodes	39		32	18‡‡
Hospital Laënnec‡‡ (1993):[93]				
Favorable T2§§	34	94		

NED, no evidence of disease.
*Actuarial.
†Preoperative radiotherapy, 3000 cGy in 3 weeks, given by ipsilateral portal only, with dose prescribed to midplane.
‡15 patients received postoperative radiotherapy, 4 preoperative radiotherapy.
§16% T2, 74% T3, 10% T4; overall 60% had pathologically involved neck nodes.
¶Minimum follow-up of 18 months.
**An unspecified number of patients underwent total laryngopharyngectomy.
††Overall actuarial survival.
‡‡Preoperative chemotherapy, various regimens, given in 91% of patients; postoperative radiotherapy, 4500–7000 cGy over 6–10 weeks, for 91% of patients.
§§62% clinically node-negative, 41% pathologically node-negative.

group of 22 patients, carboplatin and 5-FU were given with a delayed concomitant boost approach. For these latter patients, 1.8 Gy single daily fraction was delivered for the first 2 weeks followed by 1.5 Gy twice daily for the next 3 weeks to a dose of 63 Gy. The 2-year local control and larynx preservation rates for the first and second groups were 67% and 55%, respectively. In both treatment groups, unplanned hospitalizations due to treatment-related toxicity occurred in 63% and 86%, respectively. No differences in survival outcomes were observed.

Pyriform Sinus: Unfavorable, Unresectable Disease

Concomitant chemotherapy and radiation therapy is rapidly becoming the standard management for locally advanced, unresectable head and neck cancer, including hypopharyngeal cancer.[136] Randomized trials involving heterogeneous groups of unresectable, epithelial head and neck cancers have demonstrated the survival benefit of this approach as compared with induction chemotherapy with radiotherapy, as well as the use of hyperfractionated radiotherapy regimens without chemotherapy.[137,138] The chemotherapeutic agent most commonly used in the concomitant setting is cisplatin, as it is associated with high response rates, while it often exacerbates the mucositis caused by radiotherapy.[139-141] In most series mucositis is observed in approximately 70% to 80% of treated patients and pretreatment placement of a percutaneous gastrostomy is recommended. Chemotherapy typically is given at the start of weeks 1 and 4 of a radiotherapy treatment schedule (see "Techniques of Radiotherapy" later in this chapter for further discussion).[139,140,142]

Alternative approaches to the management of unresectable hypopharyngeal cancer include radiation therapy alone, radiation therapy followed by chemotherapy, or chemotherapy alone. The selection of a treatment approach largely depends on the medical condition of the patient, which indicates the level of aggressiveness with which control and cure of disease may be pursued.

Fixed cervical lymph nodes associated with an otherwise resectable primary tumor constitute a separate category of unresectable disease. In this situation, preoperative radiotherapy with or without concomitant chemotherapy may be used for downsizing of neck nodes in an attempt to make neck surgery possible. The usual dose administered is approximately 50 Gy in conventional fractionation to the primary lesion and with a boost to the primary lesion to 70 Gy to 72 Gy depending upon the tumor response at this site. The region of gross neck disease can be boosted to 60 Gy. Neck surgery follows 4 to 8 weeks later if the mass in the neck becomes resectable (i.e., regresses off the neurovascular bundle). Another situation in which preoperative radiotherapy should be considered is when emergency tracheostomy has been performed through obstructing tumor. Because of tumor spillage beyond the usual surgical confines of disease associated with this procedure, radiation therapy should be started as soon as possible.[143]

Carcinoma of the Posterior Pharyngeal Wall

Surgical resection of posterior pharyngeal wall tumors often leaves microscopical disease at the resection margins, due to the difficulty of obtaining a deep margin at the prevertebral fascia, and to a high incidence of submucosal

Table 30–4   Carcinoma of the Pyriform Sinus: Results of Surgery Alone

Institution (Year)	Patients, n	Local-regional Control, %	3-Year NED Survival, %*	5-year NED Survival, %*
Osaka U. (1973)[81]	31[†††]		37[‡‡]	33[‖‖]
MSKCC (1976):[48]				
Overall	301[§††]		44[‖§]	25[‖‖]
Stage I	28[§††]			43[‖‖]
Stage II	75[§††]			38[‖‖]
Stage III	165[§††]			19[‖‖]
Stage IV	33[§††]			9[‖‖]
Mayo Clinic (1976):[29,172]	82[¶‡†]			
Stage I-II	31[§‖†]	71[¶¶]		
Stage II	24[§‖†]		81[§§]	
Stage III-IV	50[§‖†]	58[¶¶]	52[§§]	45[‖‖]
Roswell Park (1977):[173,174]				
Overall	67[#‡‡]	31[¶¶]		25[‖‖]
T1-2N0	6[@††]			67[‖‖]
T1-2N1	27[†††]			19[‖‖]
T3-4N0-1	34[@††]			23[‖‖]
Yale (1977)[175]	25[**†]		24[‖]	
U. of Iowa (1977)[176]	19[†††]	63[¶¶]	47[‖]	47[‖‖]
M. D. Anderson (1982)[84]	203[‡‡‡]	61[¶¶]	40[§§]	25[‖‖]
U. of Virginia (1983)[177]	22[‡‡‡]	39[¶¶]	32[‖§]	
UCSF (1984)[178]	21[##‡]	86[¶¶]	62[@@]	48[@@]
Rocky Mountain Cancer Data System*** (1987)[171]				
Overall	118[†††]		59[@@]	41[@@]
Stage I-II	32[†††]		75[@]	48[@]
Stage III-IV	86[†††]		54[@]	39[@]
Medical College of Virginia (1994)[111]	65[†††]	43[¶¶]	24[¶¶]	20[@]

MSKCC, Memorial Sloan-Kettering Cancer Center; NED, no evidence of disease.

*Actuarial, unless noted otherwise.

†Nearly all patients had locally advanced disease.

‡Overall determinate survival.

§78% treated with surgery alone; 59% of all patients had pyriform sinus primary tumors; 35% and 6% had posterior pharyngeal wall and postcricoid primaries, respectively.

‖Crude NED survival, for all numbers in this column for this institution.

¶Included in this group are an unspecified number of pharyngeal wall and postcricoid primary tumors; among all 162 patients treated with various modalities, 72% had pyriform sinus primary tumors, while 23% and 5% had pharyngeal wall and postcricoid primary tumors, respectively.

#Does not include 14 patients (d>) some of whom were treated by surgery alone (d>) who died from unrelated causes within 3 years of treatment.

@2 patients with T1N0 disease and 2 with T3N1 disease received immediate postoperative irradiation for microscopically positive margins.

**21 of 25 patients had T3 or T4 primary tumors.

††16 of 19 patients had stage III disease.

‡‡90% of patients had T3 or T4 primary tumors, and 52% had N2 or N3 nodal disease.

§§Actuarial NED survival at 2 years.

‖‖Overall actuarial survival.

¶¶Determinate calculation.

##18 of 21 patients had stage III or IV disease.

@@Overall crude survival, for all numbers in this column from the same report.

***Data collected from a wide geographic area, representing a cross-sectional view of treatment for hypopharyngeal cancer from 1973 to 1983 and also reflecting inherent selection biases; the large majority of cases were pyriform sinus cancers.

†††76% of patients had stage III or IV disease; 77% of cancers originated in the pyriform sinus, 23% at other hypopharyngeal subsites or unspecified.

spread of disease longitudinally.[61] Consequently, when surgery is performed as primary therapy, postoperative radiation therapy is usually indicated.[144] Occasionally, selected patients may undergo larynx-conserving surgery alone as the only therapy for management of disease.[35,36,145-147] Data from series reporting on surgery alone for pharyngeal wall cancer are outlined in Table 30-6.

Other investigators advocate that definitive radiation therapy with or without concomitant chemotherapy be the standard management for posterior pharyngeal wall tumors, since the outcomes do not appear to be markedly different from those of surgery alone (Table 30-7), and the morbidity of a major operation can be spared.[90,148]

When disease is unresectable, strong consideration should be given to concomitant chemotherapy and radiotherapy for patients having a good performance status (see section on unresectable pyriform sinus cancer).

Postcricoid Carcinoma

As with posterior pharyngeal wall tumors, inadequate margins of resection are a common problem in the surgical management of this rare cancer. Extensive resections are required not only to encompass potential areas of "skip" metastases resulting from submucosal migration

Table 30–5 Carcinoma of the Pyriform Sinus: Results of Surgery and Postoperative Radiation Therapy

Institution (Year)	Patients, n	Local-regional Control, %	3-Year NED Survival, %*	5-year NED Survival, %*
M.D. Anderson (1979)[179]				
T3-4N2-3	47‡‡	81‡‡	23†	
M.D. Anderson (1982)[84]	125‡‡	89‡‡	50§	40‖
Inst. Gustave-Roussy (1983)[96]	34¶‡	78#	50‖	
Ctr. Paul Lamarque** (1986):[89]				
Overall	154‡‡	36‡‡		33‖†
T1-2N0	0‡‡			
T1-2N1-3	54‡‡	43‡‡		
T1-2N1-2b	13‡‡	69‡‡		
T1-2N2c-3	41‡‡	34‡‡		
T3-4N0	22‡‡	68‡‡		
T3-4N2c-3	40‡‡	28‡‡		
Inst. Gustave-Roussy (1987)[85]	199‡‡	82‡‡	48††	33††
U. of Hong Kong/Queen Mary Hospital (1993)[112]				
Overall	109‡‡	61#		35‖†
Stage I	9‡‡			74‖†
Stage II	17‡‡			63‖†
Stage III	42‡‡			32‖†
Stage IV	41‡‡			14‖†
Free University Hospital, Amsterdam (1994)[180]	32§§	84‡‡	41‖‖	22‖
Medical College of Virginia (1994)[111]	45¶¶	86‡‡	55‖‖	45††

NED, no evidence of disease.

*Actuarial, unless noted otherwise.

†Crude NED survival 2 years.

‡86% of patients had T3 or T4 primary tumors, and 58% had N2 or N3 nodal disease.

§Actuarial NED survival at 2 years.

‖Overall actuarial survival, for all numbers in this column for this institution.

¶Unspecified hypopharyngeal tumors; most patients with T3 or T4 primary tumors, and half with N2c or N3 disease.

#Regional control at 2 years.

**Lymph node staging here converted from the following non-AJCC lymph node staging used in this report: N1, ipsilateral palpable, mobile, nodes; N2, bilateral or contralateral palpable, mobile, nodes; N3, any fixed node.

††Crude overall survival.

‡‡76% had tumors originating in the pyriform sinus, 17% in the postcricoid region, and 7% at the posterior pharyngeal wall.

§§All with T3 or T4 disease.

‖‖Overall actuarial survival at 2 years.

¶¶96% of patients had stage III or IV disease; 93% of cancers originated in the pyriform sinus, 7% at the posterior wall.

of tumor cells, but also to encompass potential regional spread of disease to paratracheal lymph nodes.[62] For these very reasons, postoperative radiotherapy is also indicated—unless primary radiation therapy is given instead. Results of treatment of postcricoid carcinoma are shown in Table 30-8. Definitive irradiation appears to confer a survival outcome similar to that of primary surgery. This latter approach, especially for bulky tumors, should be used in conjunction with concomitant chemotherapy.

TECHNIQUES OF RADIOTHERAPY

Pretreatment Dental Consultation

Dental consultation before simulation is necessary so that the patient's dental status can be evaluated and steps can be taken to minimize the potentially deleterious impact of planned radiotherapy on oral health. These steps include removal of teeth affected by caries and placement of the patient on a regimen of daily fluoride application.

Pretreatment Nutritional Assessment

For patients with a marginal nutritional status, consideration should be given to having them undergo a percutaneous endoscopic gastrostomy before irradiation to ensure optimal nutrition during treatment.

Patient Immobilization

The patient is in the supine position for simulation and treatment. The neck should be maximally extended on a headrest that fits the patient well, with the chin positioned superiorly. This position serves to maximally displace the oral cavity and mandible from the planned treatment field. The shoulders should be displaced inferiorly as much as possible to maximize the utility of lateral portals in treatment delivery. Inferior displacement of the shoulders can be accomplished by the patient's pulling on two ends of a strap wrapped around a footboard. Immobilization for optimal reproducibility of the setup position is achieved through the use of a custom-made mask made of thermoplastic material (e.g., Aquaplast). A bite block can be placed in the oral cavity,

Table 30–6 Carcinoma of the Posterior Pharyngeal Wall of the Hypopharynx (± Pharyngeal Wall Tumors of the Oropharynx): Results of Surgery Alone

Institution (Year)	Patients, n	Local-regional Control, %	3-Year NED Survival, %	5-Year NED Survival, %
M.D. Anderson (1967)[56]	39*	44	44	
MSKCC (1967)[30]	73†			22
Osaka U. (1973)[81]	13		36	22
M.D. Anderson (1978)[50]				
Overall	94†	72	41‡	
T1	5	80	60	
T2	22	86	64	
T3	32	75	41	
T4	35	60	26	
MSKCC (1990)[36]	78†§	59¶	39**	32††

MSKCC, Memorial Sloan-Kettering Cancer Center.
*Includes patients with tumors of oropharyngeal walls; excludes patients living with less than 3-year follow-up.
†Includes patients with tumors of oropharyngeal walls.
‡2-year NED survival, for all numbers in this column for this institution.
§Primary surgery in 57 patients, primary radiotherapy in 21; 32 of 57 surgical patients had conservation surgery alone, while 21 had radical surgery and postoperative irradiation.
¶Local control only; neck failure occurred in 21% of all patients.
**Determinate 2-year NED survival.
††Overall actuarial survival.

which can also function to remind the patient that he or she should not swallow during the actual treatment, so that the larynx does not move during treatment. This device should be made of a tissue-equivalent material.

Simulation

The most commonly used technique for treatment of pyriform sinus, posterior pharyngeal wall, and postcricoid cancers involves the use of opposed lateral photon fields (Fig. 30-9), a low anterior neck (LAN) photon field (Fig. 30-10), and posterior cervical electron fields. General guidelines for the design of these portals are listed in Table 30-9. The gross tumor volume, clinical target volume, and planning target volume are defined in Table 30-10. Topical anatomic features, such as palpable lymphadenopathy and the anterior surface of the neck (and stoma, if postlaryngopharyngectomy), should be outlined on the skin with radiopaque wire so that these structures can be visualized on simulation films.

The lateral photon portals should encompass as much of the clinical target volume as possible without having the entrance beam (as determined by the light field on the skin) go through the shoulder. A contour is obtained at the level of the vocal cords, and tissue compensators are chosen (on the basis of a two-dimensional plan) to homogenize the dose in the region of the larynx. The spinal cord must be blocked at the junction of the lateral portals and low anterior neck field to prevent overdosage of the cord. In treating hypopharyngeal cancers, this cord block should be placed at the posterior-inferior aspect of both lateral

portals (rather than at the midline of the LAN portal) so that tumor is not shielded from the radiation beam.

Special attention must be given to placement of the posterior border of the off-cord portal for tumors involving the posterior pharyngeal wall, as well as for tumors associated with bulky retropharyngeal lymphadenopathy. As tumor or lymphadenopathy may extend posterolaterally around the anterior aspect of the vertebral column to make for a horseshoe-shaped target volume, optimal inclusion of the clinical target volume within the cone-down field requires that the posterior edge of the field be placed as far posterior as possible without including the spinal cord. This can be achieved by placing the central axis of the cone-down field at the posterior aspect of the vertebral bodies and using a split-beam technique—where the posterior half of the beam is blocked and posterior divergence of the beam is thus avoided.[148] Photons of 6 MV should be used for this cone-down field, as the field edge will be sharp, while beam constriction associated with higher energies can be avoided.[148,149] Alternatively, conformal radiation therapy—either using an isocentric rotational technique with multileaf collimation[150] or a static five-field technique[151]—may effectively address the problem of a horseshoe-shaped target volume (Fig. 30-11).

Patients with short necks or those unable to displace their shoulders inferiorly pose a separate treatment planning challenge: Their shoulders lie within the same transverse plane as the inferior aspect of the gross tumor volume, preventing the use of the standard opposed lateral fields. One solution to this problem involves the use of lateral fields that are angled inferiorly to obtain better inferior coverage of the gross tumor volume and clinical target volume, and elimination of the standard LAN field.[152,153] Inferior angulation is done by rotating the foot of the treatment table 10 to 20 degrees away from the gantry. Alternating use of no wedges and 15-degree wedges in these treatment fields allows for requisite homogeneity in the dose distribution. A 3D dose distribution for this technique is shown in Figure 30-12. (For comparison, a 3D dose distribution for a standard three-field technique is shown in Figure 30-13.) A customized tissue compensator based on a 3D treatment plan could provide for optimal dose homogeneity.[153]

Tumors with extension of disease into the cervical esophagus require the use of multiple fields in a complicated treatment plan similar to a thyroid plan; this involves at least one set of wedged anterior oblique fields. An example of such a treatment plan is shown in Figure 30-14.

When the upper mediastinum has radiographically evident lymphadenopathy or is deemed to be at significant risk for harboring occult disease, it should be treated in addition to the low anterior neck portal (Fig. 30-15). The depth of the mediastinal lymph nodes should be determined in the anterior-to-posterior dimension on a CT scan. Adequate dose delivery to these lymph nodes may require the use of parallel opposed anteroposterior and posteroanterior fields rather than just an extended LAN field prescribed to a greater depth. When an antero-posterior-posteroanterior arrangement is used, a cumulative dose of only 45 Gy (rather than 50 Gy) is prescribed

Table 30–7   Carcinoma of the Posterior Pharyngeal Wall of the Hypopharynx (± Pharyngeal Wall Tumors of the Oropharynx): Results of Radiation Therapy Alone

Institution (Year)	Patients, n	Local-regional Control, %	3-Year NED Survival, %	5-Year NED Survival, %
MSKCC (1967)[30]	41*		17	
Mass. General (1971)[181]	37	51†	25	17
Emory U. (1971)[145]	18		11‡	
U. of Toronto (1971)[182]	18	33		
Osaka U. (1973)[81]	9		38	33
M.D. Anderson (1978)[51]				
Overall	164*	60§	14?	
T1	11	91		
T2	45	73		
T3	62	61		
T4	46	37		
Washington U. (1978)[52]	13*		17¶	
Inst. Gustave-Roussy (1978)[183]	122#	32§	24@	3
U. of Virginia (1981)[34]	24**	57††	46	25
U. of Liverpool (1982)[35]	17			0
U. of Michigan (1984)[38]	45	47		30‡‡
Washington U. (1985)[184]	34*	24	26§§	6‡‡
Yale‖ (1987)[163]	14*	86	82¶¶	82¶¶
Mass. General (1990)[90]				
Conventional fractionation:				
Overall	61		30	
T1	11	89	64	
T2	21	29	22	
T3	23	42	29	
T4	6	20	0	
Hyperfractionation:				
T1	3	100		
T2	18	70		
T3	10	39		
T4	2	100		
U. of Florida (1993)[148]				
Overall	75			
T1	5	100		
T2	24	76		
T3	36	51		
T4	10	25		
Stage I	4##			50‡‡
Stage II	22			36
Stage III	24			26
Stage IVA	24			28
Stage IVB	25			5
Centro di Riferimento Oncologico (1995)[146]	32@@	53		0

MSKCC, Memorial Sloan-Kettering Cancer Center; NED, no evidence of disease.
*Includes patients with tumors of oropharyngeal walls.
†Local control only.
‡2-year NED survival, for all numbers in this column for this institution.
§Local control only at 1 year, for all numbers in this column for this institution.
‖Crude overall survival at minimum follow-up of 1 year.
¶3-year overall actuarial survival.
#83% of patients had T3 or T4 lesions, 80% of tumors were ulcerated, and 42% of patients had N3 disease.
@Greater than 1 year overall survival.
**About 50% of patients were N0.
††Local control only for those patients receiving at least 6000 cGy.
‡‡Overall actuarial survival, for all numbers in this column for this institution.
§§Crude overall survival at 2 years.
‖Treatment involves brachytherapy with ^{192}Ir or ^{125}I followed by external beam irradiation.
¶¶Actuarial NED survival.
##Data analyzed by stage also includes 25 patients with pharyngeal wall tumors of the oropharynx.
@@Group of patients with adverse prognostic features.

Table 30–8   Postcricoid Carcinoma: Results of Treatment

Institution (Year)	Patients, n	Local-regional Control, %	3-Year Survival, %	5-Year Survival, %
Natl. Ctr. for Radiotherapy, Sheffield (1971)[31]				
Radiation:	103			8
<5 cm	33			18
>5 cm	70			3
U. of Toronto (1971)[182]				
Surgery	4			25
Radiation	15			7
Holt Radium Inst. (1971)[182]				
Radiation:	39			
<5 cm, neg. nodes		36		
>5 cm, neg. nodes		9		
Osaka U. (1973)[81]				
Radiation	17		37	31
Surgery	8		20	20
U. of Liverpool (1978)[32]				
Radiation	28*			22
Surgery	29†			31
Holt Radium Inst. (1986)[33]				
Radiation	102			22
St. James Hospital (1986)[185]				
Surgery	30		20	16
Helsinki U. (1990)[186]				
Radiation	35		22	16
Mass. General (1990)[90]				
Radiation	17		18‡	
U. of Liverpool (1995)[67]				
Radiation	50	48¶		25
T1-T2 subset				49
Surgery	67§	69¶		18
T1-T2 subset				44

*Nearly all T1N0 or small T2N0.
†More advanced disease than in those treated with radiation alone; treated with pharyngolaryngectomy and deltopectoral skin flap.
‡2-year NED survival.
§Patients treated with surgery tended to be in better physical condition and tended to have more advanced disease than those treated by irradiation.
¶P = 0.039.

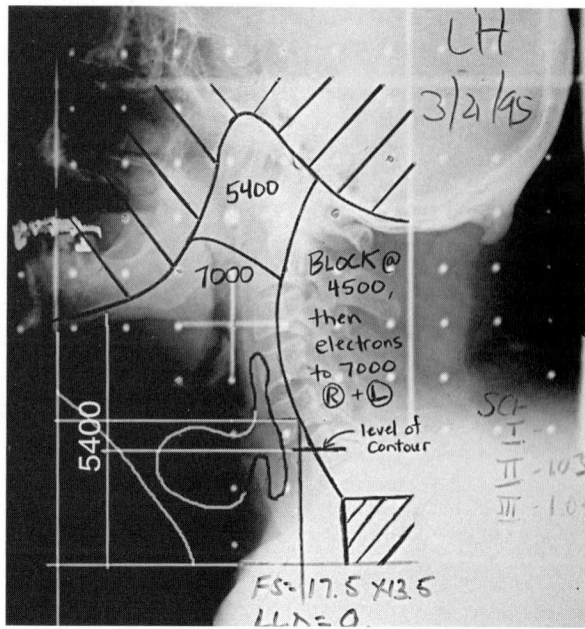

Figure 30–9. Typical lateral photon portals, cone-down fields, and doses for hypopharyngeal cancer. Level of contour is indicated. *Horizontal white line* above level of contour and *vertical dark line* posterior to thyroid cartilage delineate the region encompassed by tissue compensators. Anterior *curved white line* delineates the skin surface at the anterior neck. A strip of the superior and anterior neck is blocked after 54 Gy, as indicated by the *vertical white line* inside the anterior border of the treatment portal.

to protect the spinal cord. Any additional dose, if desired, must be delivered by a set of off-cord (oblique or lateral) fields; this necessitates the formulation of a two-dimensional treatment plan with isodose distributions at the outset of the treatment course for evaluation of the maximal spinal cord dose.

In the postoperative setting, the tracheal stoma should be irradiated. This is recommended because of the significant risk of recurrence at this site secondary to occult paratracheal lymphadenopathy or microscopic disease in the parastomal soft tissues. The stoma could be treated in the lateral, upper neck fields but is usually treated in the LAN field because of its low position. In the latter instance, if 6 MV photons are used, a bolus should be used at the stoma to bring the skin dose close to 100% of the prescription dose.

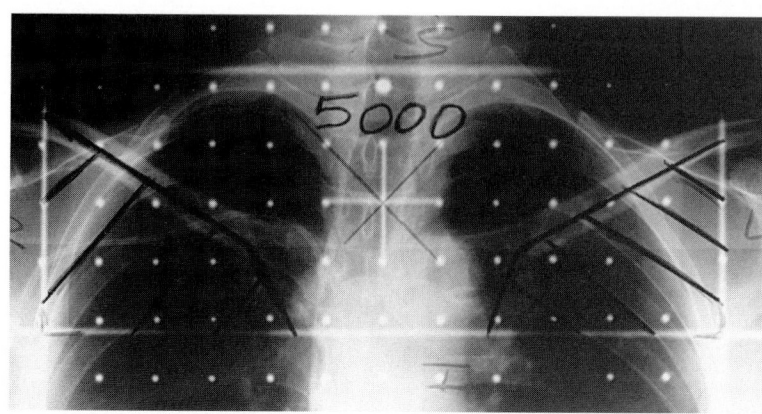

Figure 30–10. Typical low anterior neck portal.

Table 30–9   Guidelines to Design of Treatment Portals for Radiotherapy of Hypopharyngeal Cancer

Opposed Lateral Photon Fields
Additional shaping:

Superior border:	1.5 cm above the top of C1 to include the retropharyngeal and junctional nodes
Inferior border:	As low as possible without entrance beam going through the shoulder (as determined by the lightfield on the skin); this border should be at least 2 cm below inferior edge of the cricoid cartilage to include the apex of the pyriform sinus
Anterior border:	1.0 to 1.5 cm beyond the skin surface to include thyroid cartilage in its entirety, and anterior soft tissues (for a posterior pharyngeal wall primary tumor, this border may be placed just posterior to the skin surface to exclude a small strip of anterior skin)
Posterior border:	Up to 4500 cGy—just beyond the posterior spinous process of C2 to include level V lymph nodes
	After 4500 cGy—curved border along middle of vertebral bodies of cervical spine; if tumor extends to or arises from the posterior pharyngeal wall, the posterior border should be placed at posterior edge of vertebral bodies using a split beam technique with 6MV photons (see text)
Additional shaping:	With Cerrobend blocks to exclude spinal cord at posteroinferior aspect of field, as well as oral cavity, a portion of the mandible, and cerebellum
	Cone-down field 2:
	After 5400 cGy to exclude regions of neck only at risk for having microscopic disease (additional Cerrobend blocking added to superior aspect of field to exclude region of retropharyngeal nodes; occasionally thin strips of blocking are also added to anterior and inferior aspects of field)

Low Anterior Neck Field

Superior border:	Matched on skin to inferior border of opposed lateral fields; the spinal cord at the junction of fields is blocked in the upper fields
Inferior border:	With low risk of mediastinal disease—below heads of clavicles, with blocking inferior to inferior aspect of clavicles
	With high risk of mediastinal disease—5 cm below head of clavicles, with lateral blocking extended inferiorly so that mediastinal portion of field is about 8 cm wide
Lateral borders:	Positioned to exclude lateral 1/3 of clavicles

Posterior Electron Strips

Matched on skin to off-cord photon fields

Dose and Fractionation for Postoperative Radiotherapy

When postoperative radiotherapy is administered, a cumulative dose of 63 Gy is delivered to the primary tumor bed after a field reduction off the spinal cord at 45 Gy and a second field reduction to exclude low-risk regions of the neck after 54 Gy. The dose is divided in daily fractions of 1.8 Gy each. Dose is prescribed to the isocenter (at the midplane along the central axis) for these lateral photon fields. The posterior neck is boosted with appositional electron fields to 54 Gy if that side of

the neck had been uninvolved by lymphadenopathy on anterior neck dissection, or 63 Gy if involved. The electron energy is selected on the basis of the thickness of soft tissue between the skin and vertebral column or the depth of the lymph nodes on a CT or MRI scan. The LAN is treated to a cumulative dose of 50 Gy, divided in daily fractions of 2 Gy each. Dose is prescribed to d_{max} below

Table 30–10   Tumor and Target Volume Definitions in the Radiotherapy of Hypopharyngeal Cancer

Gross Tumor Volume (GTV)

Gross visible, palpable, or demonstrable extent of primary tumor and metastatic lymphadenopathy

Clinical Target Volume (CTV)

GTV and regions of potential microscopic disease (includes upper, middle, and lower jugular lymph nodes, spinal accessory lymph nodes, junctional and retropharyngeal lymph nodes, retropharyngeal space, thyroid and cricoid cartilages, pre-epiglottic and paraglottic spaces, paratracheal lymph nodes, parastomal soft tissues if stoma is present, supraclavicular lymph nodes, and occasionally upper mediastinal lymph nodes)

Planning Target Volume (PTV)

GTV plus margin (1.5 cm margin for standard three-field technique) to compensate for patient movement and inaccuracies in beam and patient set-up

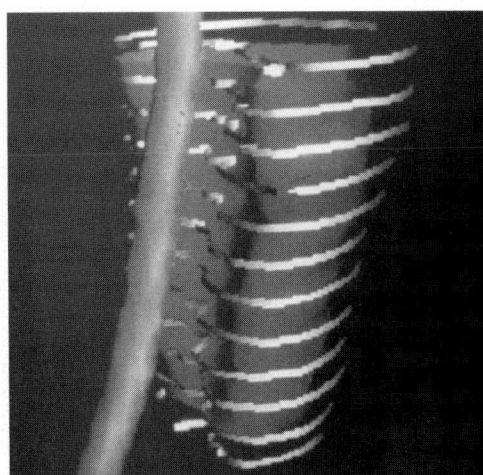

Figure 30–11. Three-dimensional view of a horseshoe-shaped target volume and the spinal cord for a treatment plan using an isocentric rotational technique with multileaf collimation. (From Esik O, Burkelbach J, Boesecke R, et al: Three-dimensional photon radiotherapy planning for laryngeal and hypopharyngeal cancers: 2. Conformation treatment planning using a multileaf collimator. *Radiother Oncol.* 1991;20:238. With kind permission from Elsevier Science Ireland Ltd., Bay 15K, Shannon Industrial Estate, Co. Clare, Ireland.)

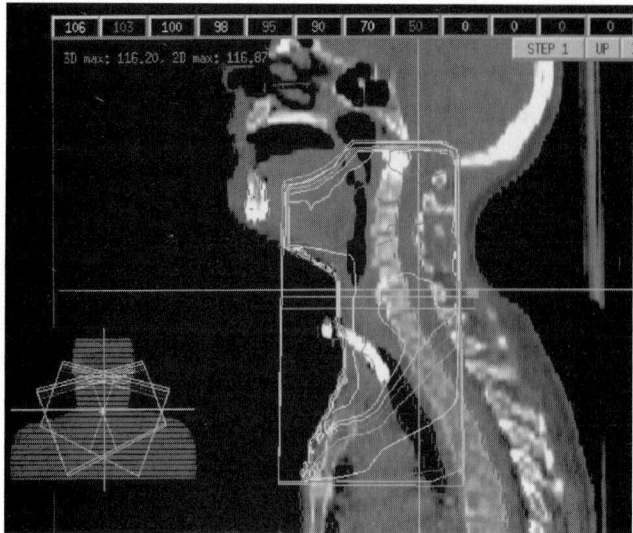

Figure 30–12. Three-dimensional dose distribution for inferiorly angled, lateral fields in the treatment of hypopharyngeal cancer. (Courtesy of Scott L. Sailer, MD.)

a point on the skin along the course of the lower jugular (level IV) lymph node chain. The stoma is often boosted with electrons to 60 Gy.

In the setting of positive margins or gross residual disease after surgery, the cumulative dose to the final cone-down field can be increased to 66.6 to 70.2 Gy.

Postoperative radiotherapy after gastric pull-up reconstruction of the alimentary tract, or after microvascular free tissue transfer of a jejunal segment, presents an interesting issue: Can the transposed stomach or grafted jejunum tolerate a standard postoperative dose of 63 Gy? Available evidence indicates that this dose appears to be safe, at least after gastric transposition.[154,155] In a series of 120 patients at Memorial Sloan-Kettering Cancer Center (MSKCC), late bleeding manifested by persistently low

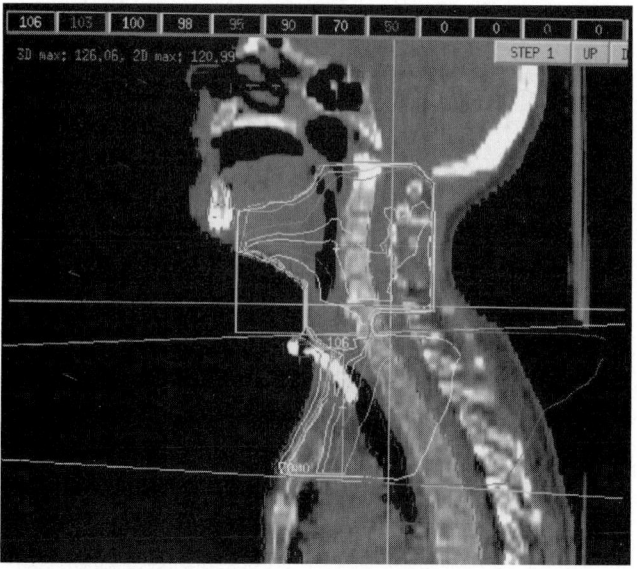

Figure 30–13. Three-dimensional dose distribution for the standard three-field technique fields in the treatment of hypopharyngeal cancer. (Courtesy of Scott L. Sailer, MD.)

hemoglobin concentrations with endoscopic evidence of gastritis was found in only four patients, while one additional patient required surgical intervention to control hemorrhage.[155] After free jejunal interposition, a mean dose of 56 Gy resulted in no radiation-related complications in a series of 20 patients.[156] Nevertheless, caution should be exercised in such clinical situations treating to standard doses due to the lower dose threshold tolerance of jejunal or gastric mucosa.

Dose and Fractionation for Primary Radiotherapy, and Integration of Chemotherapy

The treatment policy at MSKCC for the nonsurgical management of hypopharyngeal carcinomas involves concomitant cisplatin chemotherapy and radiotherapy employing a delayed concomitant boost technique during the last 2 weeks of a 6-week treatment course. Induction chemotherapy with cisplatin and 5-fluorouracil can be given as well for tumors considered resectable, as done in the randomized trial of the Department of Veterans Affairs Laryngeal Cancer Study Group.[119] The only exception to this treatment policy is for T1 tumors and, occasionally, select exophytic T2 tumors: These are treated with radiation therapy alone, conventionally fractionated at 1.8 to 2 Gy per day, to a total dose ranging from 66 to 72 cGy—the higher doses reserved for bulkier tumors.

If induction chemotherapy is given, it consists of two to three cycles of cisplatin (100 mg/m², bolus IV infusion, given on days 1, 22, and 43) and 5-fluorouracil (1000 mg/m², continuous IV infusion, given on days 1 to 5, 22 to 26, and 43 to 47). Concomitant chemotherapy involves the administration of cisplatin (100 mg/m², bolus IV infusion) on days 1 and 22 of the radiotherapy schedule (or days 64 and 85 of the overall treatment schedule when induction chemotherapy is given).

At our institution, radiotherapy using a concomitant boost involves the delivery of a second daily fraction to the final cone-down field during weeks 5 and 6 of irradiation.[157-159] The dose given with this fraction is 1.6 Gy per day. It is delivered in the afternoon, at least 5 hours after the regular daily fraction of 1.8 Gy. A total of 16 Gy is delivered with these boost fractions. When this is added to the 54 Gy delivered over 6 weeks with the regular daily fractions, the cumulative dose is 70 Gy.

The rationale for this fractionation scheme is threefold: (1) It shortens the overall treatment time of irradiation to increase dose intensity; (2) It concentrates dose delivery during that portion of the radiotherapy schedule when tumor clonogen repopulation accelerates, in order to negate this effect; and (3) it limits twice-a-day irradiation to only a portion of the treatment schedule to minimize the acute toxicity of such fractionation, where it is temporally separated from concomitant chemotherapy administration.[160-162]

Another accepted fractionation schedule used commonly at other institutions is that of hyperfractionated radiotherapy for the entire treatment course. Cumulative doses of 74.4 to 76.8 Gy are typically prescribed, divided in

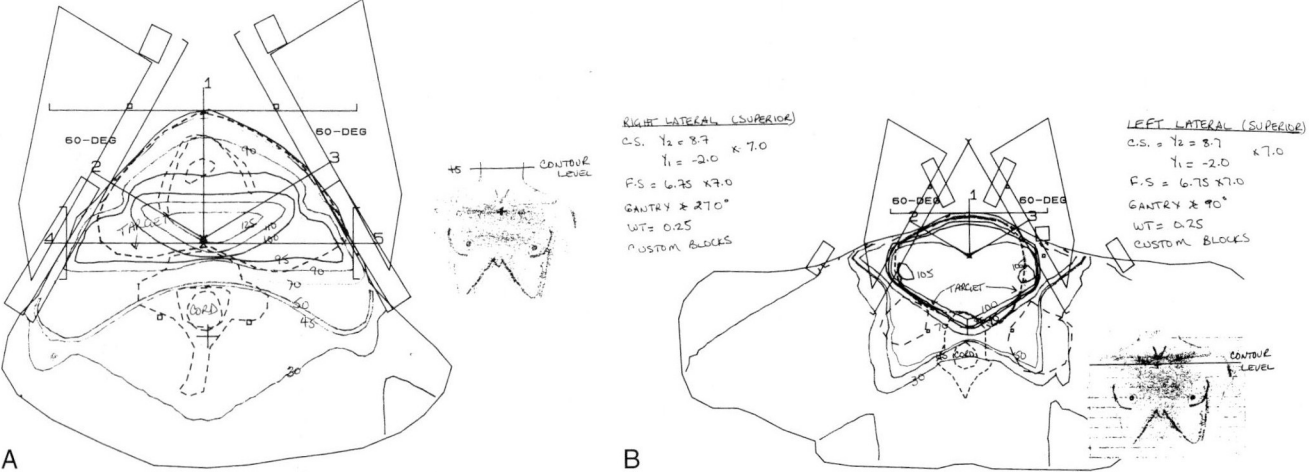

Figure 30–14. A and B, Treatment plan for the "boost" portion of treatment for a patient with hypopharyngeal cancer extending into cervical esophagus. A treatment-planning CT scan was obtained, and isodose distributions are shown at the two levels indicated.

twice-daily fractions of 1.2 Gy each. Hyperfractionated radiotherapy administered in this manner usually precludes the possibility of concomitant chemotherapy due to the attendant acute toxicity of mucositis.

BRACHYTHERAPY

Brachytherapy is rarely done for hypopharyngeal cancers. Two techniques have been published.[163,164]

CRITICAL NORMAL TISSUES

Acute Effects

The major dose-limiting toxicity of radiotherapy for hypopharyngeal cancer is mucositis. This is accompanied by symptoms of sore throat, dysphagia, and hoarseness.

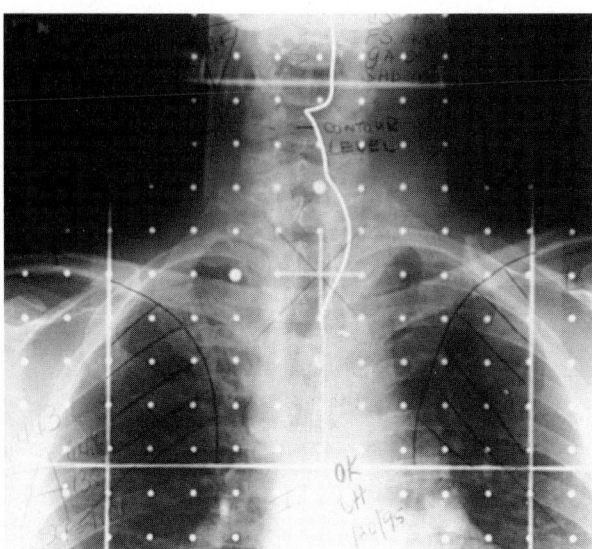

Figure 30–15. Extended low anterior neck field to include the upper mediastinum.

Xerostomia and dysgeusia invariably occur with the standard doses administered. As all of these symptoms can lead to significant weight loss, the patient's nutritional status should be closely monitored by the radiation oncologist. Enteral hyperalimentation with percutaneous endoscopic gastrostomy-tube feeding often is necessary. To ensure adequate nutrition, this tube may be placed before initiation of radiotherapy. The increasing severity of these reactions with greater volumes of tissue irradiated establishes the basis for, and importance of, a shrinking field technique.

Laryngeal edema is usually induced by radiotherapy, and this may persist for up to 6 months after completion of treatment. It often is limited to the arytenoids. Biopsy to rule out persistent or recurrent disease should be done only if careful follow-up reveals progressive edema that is unresponsive to conservative measures. One should also have a strong index of suspicion for the presence of tumor, as biopsy is associated with the risk of laryngeal necrosis.[88]

Late Effects

Late laryngeal chondronecrosis in the preserved larynx or soft tissue necrosis of the pharyngeal wall occurs in 2% to 4% of patients.[40,51,53,84,86,87] Severe laryngeal edema requiring tracheostomy occurs in 1% to 6% of patients.[40,51,53,86,87] Permanent gastrostomy for inability to swallow becomes necessary for 2% to 7% of patients treated with radiotherapy alone,[40,53,86,87] and up to 16% of patients treated with surgery and postoperative irradiation.[84,165] Subcutaneous fibrosis of the soft tissues of the neck occurs in up to 11% of patients.[84]

The treatment-related mortality rate of radiation therapy alone is 1% to 3%.[40,53,84] The figure rises to 5% to 6% when surgical salvage of severe complications is attempted.[51,86] This surgical mortality is usually due to wound breakdown, pharyngocutaneous fistula, or hemorrhage from carotid artery rupture. Mortality from irradiation alone is usually secondary to cachexia after pharyngeal/esophageal stricture (or inability to swallow),

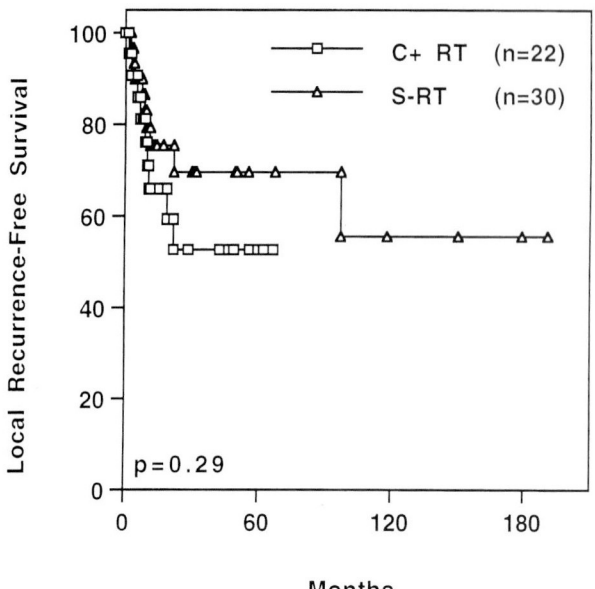

Figure 30–16. Actuarial local control using larynx-preserving therapy *(C + RT)* as compared with surgery and postoperative radiotherapy *(S-RT)* at MSKCC.

aspiration pneumonia, asphyxia due to laryngeal edema, or carotid blow-out.[40,84,106]

OUTCOME

Outcomes of treatment for large series of patients are listed in Tables 30-2 through 30-8. Data on locoregional control, 3-year survival, and 5-year survival have been collated from the published reports indicated. Between 90% and 95% of all recurrences occur within 2 years of treatment. Actuarial data from MSKCC comparing a

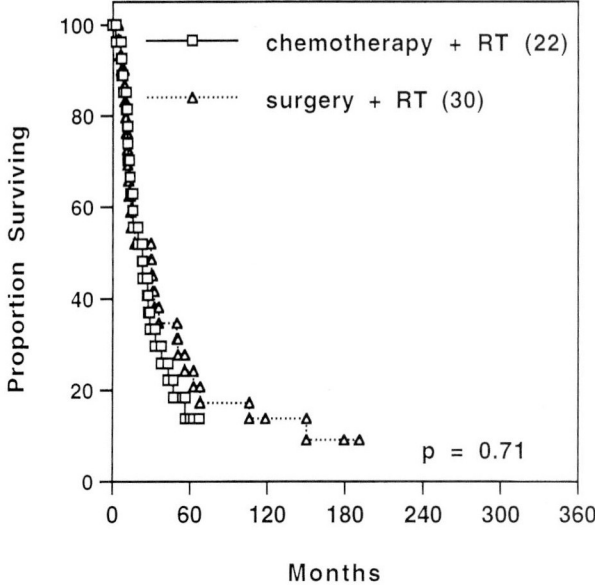

Figure 30–17. Actuarial survival using larynx-preserving therapy *(chemotherapy + RT)* as compared with surgery and postoperative radiotherapy *(surgery + RT)* at MSKCC.

larynx-preservation treatment approach with standard therapy (surgery and postoperative irradiation) for advanced hypopharyngeal cancer are shown in Figures 30-16 and 30-17.

REFERENCES

1. Marks JE, Spector JG: Hypopharynx. In Perez CA, Brady LW, eds. *Principles and Practice of Radiation Oncology,* 2nd ed. Philadelphia: JB Lippincott; 1992:725.
2. Murthy AK, Galinsky D, Hendrickson FR: Hypopharynx. In Laramore GE, ed. *Radiation Therapy in Head and Neck Cancer.* Berlin: Springer-Verlag; 1989:107.
3. Spitz MR: Epidemiology and risk factors for head and neck cancer. *Semin Oncol.* 1994;21:281.
4. Tuyns AJ, Esteve J, Raymond L, et al: Cancer of the larynx/ hypopharynx, tobacco and alcohol. *Int J Cancer.* 1988;41:483.
5. Spitz MR, Fueger JJ, Goepfert H, et al: Squamous cell carcinoma of the aerodigestive tract: A case comparison analysis. *Cancer.* 1988;61:203.
6. Wolf GT, Lippman SM, Laramore GE, et al: Head and neck cancer. In Holland JF, Frei E III, Bast RC Jr., et al, eds. *Cancer Medicine,* 3rd ed. Philadelphia: Lea & Febiger; 1993:1211.
7. Blot WJ, McLaughlin JK, Winn DM, et al: Smoking and drinking in relation to oral and pharyngeal cancer. *Cancer Res.* 1989;48:3282.
8. Day JL, Blot WJ, Austin DF, et al: Racial differences in risk of oral and pharyngeal cancer: Alcohol, tobacco, and other determinants. *J Natl Cancer Inst.* 1993;85:465.
9. Winn DM, Blot WJ, Shy CM, et al: Snuff dipping and oral cancer among women in the southern United States. *N Engl J Med.* 1981;304:745.
10. Mattson ME, Winn DM: Smokeless tobacco: Association with increased cancer risk. *NCI Monogr.* 1989;8:13.
11. Hoffman D, Djordjevic MV, Fan J, et al: Five leading U.S. commercial brands of moist snuff in 1994: Assessment of carcinogenic N-nitrosamines. *J Natl Cancer Inst.* 1995;87:1862.
12. Hsu TC, Johnston DA, Cherry LM, et al: Sensitivity to genotoxic effects of bleomycin in humans: Possible relationship to environmental carcinogenesis. *Int J Cancer.* 1989;43:403.
13. Spitz MR, Fueger JJ, Beddingfield NA, et al: Chromosome sensitivity to bleomycin-induced mutagenesis: An independent risk factor for upper aerodigestive tract cancers. *Cancer Res.* 1989;49:4626.
14. Copper MP, Jovanovic A, Nauta JJP, et al: Role of genetic factors in the etiology of squamous cell carcinoma of the head and neck. *Arch Otolaryngol Head Neck Surg.* 1995;121:157.
15. Sidransky D: Molecular genetics of head and neck cancer. *Curr Opin Oncol.* 1995;7:229.
16. Gallo O, Bianchi S, Porfirio B: *Bcl-2* overexpression and smoking history in head and neck cancer. *J Natl Cancer Inst.* 1995;87:1024.
17. Bell DA, Liu Y, Cortopassi GA: Occurrence of *bcl-2* oncogene translocation with increased frequency in the peripheral blood of heavy smokers. *J Natl Cancer Inst.* 1995;87:223.
18. Yunis JJ, Oken MM, Kaplan ME, et al: Distinctive chromosomal abnormalities in histologic subtypes of non-Hodgkins lymphoma. *N Engl J Med.* 1982;307:1231.
19. Frank JL, Bur ME, Garb JL, et al: *p53* tumor suppressor oncogene expression in squamous cell carcinoma of the hypopharynx. *Cancer.* 1994;73:181.
20. Frank JL, Garb JL, Banson BB, et al: Epidermal growth factor receptor expression in squamous cell carcinoma of the hypopharynx. *Surg Oncol.* 1993;2:161.
21. Issing WJ, Wustrow TP, Heppt WJ: Oncogenes related to head and neck cancer. *Anticancer Res.* 1993;13:2541.
22. Brachman DG: Molecular biology of head and neck cancer. *Semin Oncol.* 1994;21:320.
23. Vogelstein B, Fearon ER, Hamilton SR, et al: Genetic alterations during colorectal tumor development. *N Engl J Med.* 1988; 319:525.
24. Clayman GL, Stewart MG, Weber RS, et al: Human papillomavirus in laryngeal and hypopharyngeal carcinomas. *Arch Otolaryngol Head Neck Surg.* 1994;120:743.

25. Martin SA, Marks JE, Lee JY, et al: Carcinoma of the pyriform sinus: Predictors of TNM relapse and survival. *Cancer.* 1980;46:1974.

26. Spaulding MB, Fischer SG, Wolf GT, et al: Tumor response, toxicity, and survival after neoadjuvant organ-preserving chemotherapy for advanced laryngeal cancer. *J Clin Oncol.* 1994;12:1592.

27. Truelson JM, Fischer SG, Beals TE, et al: DNA content and histologic growth pattern correlate with prognosis in patients with advanced squamous cell carcinoma of the larynx. *Cancer.* 1992;70:56.

28. Banks ER, Frierson HF Jr, Mills SE, et al: Basaloid squamous cell carcinoma of the head and neck: A clinicopathologic and immuno-histochemical study of 40 cases. *Am J Surg Pathol.* 1992;16:939.

29. Carpenter RJ III, DeSanto LW, Devine KD, et al: Cancer of the hypopharynx: Analysis of treatment and results in 162 patients. *Arch Otolaryngol.* 1976;102:716.

30. Cunningham MP, Catlin D: Cancer of the pharyngeal wall. *Cancer.* 1967;20:1859.

31. Kalavathi N: Factors influencing cure in the radiotherapy of post cricoid carcinoma. *Clin Radiol.* 1970;21:248.

32. Stell PM, Carden EA, Hibbert J, et al: Post-cricoid carcinoma. *Clin Oncol.* 1978;4:215.

33. Farrington WT, Weighill JS, Jones PH: Post-cricoid carcinoma: A ten-year retrospective study. *J Laryngol Otol.* 1986;100:79.

34. Talton BM, Elkon D, Kim J, et al: Cancer of the posterior hypo-pharyngeal wall. *Int J Radiat Oncol Biol Phys.* 1981;7:597.

35. Raine CH, Stell PM, Dalby J: Squamous cell carcinomas of the posterior wall of the hypopharynx. *J Laryngol Otol.* 1982;96:997.

36. Spiro RH, Kelly J, Vega AL, et al: Squamous carcinoma of the posterior pharyngeal wall. *Am J Surg.* 1990;160:420.

37. Marks JE: The endolarynx and hypopharynx. In Moss WT, Cox JD, eds. *Radiation Oncology,* 6th ed. St. Louis: Mosby; 1989:232.

38. Ahmad K, Fayos JV: Role of radiation therapy in carcinoma of the hypopharynx. *Acta Radiol Oncol.* 1984;23(Fasc 1):21.

39. Mendenhall WM, Parsons JT, Stringer SP, et al: Radiotherapy alone or combined with neck dissection for T1-T2 carcinoma of the pyriform sinus: An alternative to conservation surgery. *Int J Radiat Oncol Biol Phys.* 1993;27:1017.

40. Bataini P, Brugere J, Bernier J, et al: Results of radical radiothera-peutic treatment of carcinoma of the pyriform sinus: Experience of the Institut Curie. *Int J Radiat Oncol Biol Phys.* 1982;8:1277.

41. Harrison D: Pathology of hypopharyngeal cancer in relation to surgical management. *J Laryngol Otol.* 1970;84:349.

42. Kirchner JA: Pyriform sinus cancer: A clinical and laboratory study. *Ann Otol Rhinol Laryngol.* 1975;84:793.

43. Lindberg R: Distribution of cervical lymph nodes from squamous cell carcinoma of upper respiratory and digestive tracts. *Cancer.* 1972;29:1446.

44. Horwitz SD, Caldarelli DD, Hendrickson FR: Treatment of carcinoma of the hypopharynx. *Head Neck Surg.* 1979;2:107.

45. Bataini JP, Bernier J, Brugere J, et al: Natural history of neck disease in patients with squamous cell carcinoma of oropharynx and pharyngolarynx. *Radiother Oncol.* 1985;3:245.

46. Lefebvre JL, Castelain B, De La Torre JC, et al: Lymph node invasion in hypopharynx and lateral epilarynx carcinoma: A prognostic factor. *Head Neck Surg.* 1987;10:14.

47. Marks JE, Devineni VR, Harvey J, et al: The risk of contralateral lymphatic metastases for cancers of the larynx and pharynx. *Am J Otolaryngol.* 1992;13:34.

48. Shah JP, Shaha AR, Spiro RH, et al: Carcinoma of the hypo-pharynx. *Am J Surg.* 1976;132:439.

49. Marks JE, Breaux S, Smith PG, et al: The need for elective irradia-tion of occult lymphatic metastases from cancers of the larynx and pyriform sinus. *Head Neck Surg.* 1985;8:3.

50. Guillamondegui OM, Meoz R, Jesse RH: Surgical treatment of squamous cell carcinoma of the pharyngeal walls. *Am J Surg.* 1978;136:474.

51. Meoz-Mendez RT, Fletcher GH, Guillamondegui OM, et al: Analysis of the results of irradiation in the treatment of squamous cell carcinomas of the pharyngeal walls. *Int J Radiat Oncol Biol Phys.* 1978;4:579.

52. Marks JE, Freeman RB, Lee F, et al: Pharyngeal wall cancer: An analysis of treatment results, complications, and patterns of failure. *Int J Radiat Oncol Biol Phys.* 1978;4:587.

53. Mendenhall WM, Parsons JT, Mancuso AA, et al: Squamous cell carcinoma of the pharyngeal wall treated with irradiation. *Radiother Oncol.* 1988;11:205.

54. Ogura JH, Biller HF, Wette R: Elective neck dissection for pharyn-geal and laryngeal cancers: An evaluation. *Ann Otol Rhinol Laryngol.* 1971;80:646.

55. Ballantyne AJ: Significance of retropharyngeal nodes in cancer of the head and neck. *Am J Surg.* 1964;108:500.

56. Ballantyne AJ: Principles of surgical management of cancer of the pharyngeal walls. *Cancer.* 1967;20:664.

57. Dalley VM: Cancer of the laryngopharynx. *J Laryngol.* 1968;82:407.

58. McCrea RS, Dickie WA: Carcinoma of the hypopharynx and cervical esophagus: A review of sixty-one cases. *J Laryngol.* 1968;82:421.

59. Willatt DJ, Jackson SR, McCormick MS, et al: Vocal cord paralysis and tumor length in staging postcricoid cancer. *Eur J Surg Oncol.* 1987;13:131.

60. Biller H, Davis W, Ogura J: Delayed contralateral cervical metastasis with laryngeal and laryngopharyngeal cancers. *Laryngoscope.* 1971;81:1499.

61. Harrison DFN: Surgical management of cancer of the hypopharynx and cervical oesophagus. *Br J Surg.* 1969;56:95.

62. Harrison DFN: Role of surgery in the management of postcricoid and cervical esophageal neoplasms. *Ann Otol.* 1972;81:465.

63. Harrison DFN: Thyroid gland in the management of laryngo-pharyngeal cancer. *Arch Otolaryngol.* 1973;97:301.

64. Harris HH, Butler E: Surgical limits in cancer. *Arch Otolaryngol.* 1968;87:64.

65. Harrison DFN: Resection of the manubrium. *Br J Surg.* 1977;64:374.

66. Weber RS, Marvel J, Smith P, et al: Paratracheal lymph node dissection for carcinoma of the larynx, hypopharynx, and cervical esophagus. *Otolaryngol Head Neck Surg.* 1993;108:11.

67. Jones AS, McRae RD, Phillips DE, et al: The treatment of node neg-ative squamous cell carcinoma of the postcricoid region. *J Laryngol Otol.* 1995;109:114.

68. Kotwall C, Sako K, Razack MS, et al: Metastatic patterns in squa-mous cell cancer of the head and neck. *Am J Surg.* 1987;154:439.

69. Zbären P, Lehmann W: Frequency and sites of distant metastases in head and neck squamous cell carcinoma. *Arch Otolaryngol Head Neck Surg.* 1987;113:762.

70. Leibel SA, Scott CB, Mohiuddin M, et al: The effect of local-regional control on distant metastatic dissemination in carcinoma of the head and neck: Results of an analysis from the RTOG head and neck database. *Int J Radiat Oncol Biol Phys.* 1991;21:550.

71. Silverman PM, Bossen EH, Fisher SR, et al: Carcinoma of the larynx and hypopharynx: Computed tomographic-histopathologic correlations. *Radiology.* 1984;151:697.

72. Million RR, Cassisi NJ, Mancuso AA: Hypopharynx: Pharyngeal walls, pyriform sinus, postcricoid pharynx. In Million RR, Cassisi NJ, eds. *Management of Head and Neck Cancer: A Multidisciplinary Approach,* 2nd ed. Philadelphia: JB Lippincott; 1994:505.

73. Castelijns JA, Gerritsen GJ, Kaiser MC, et al: Invasion of laryngeal cartilage by cancer: Comparison of CT and MR imaging. *Radiology.* 1987;166:199.

74. Wenig BL, Ziffra KL, Mafee MF, et al: MR imaging of squamous cell carcinoma of the larynx and hypopharynx. *Otolaryngol Clin North Am.* 1995;28:609.

75. Silverman PM, Zeiberg AS, Sessions RB, et al: Three-dimensional imaging of the hypopharynx and larynx by means of helical (spiral) computed tomography: Comparison of radiologic and otolaryngologic evaluation. *Ann Otol Rhinol Laryngol.* 1995;104:425.

76. McGuirt WF, Matthews B, Koufman JA: Multiple simultaneous tumors in patients with head and neck cancer: A prospective, sequential panendoscopic study. *Cancer.* 1982;50:1195.

77. McGuirt WF: Panendoscopy as a screening examination for simultaneous primary tumors in head and neck cancers: A prospective sequential study and review of the literature. *Lancet.* 1982;92:569.

78. American Joint Committee on Cancer: Pharynx (including base of tongue, soft palate and uvula). In *AJCC Cancer Staging Manual,* 6th ed. New York: Springer-Verlag; 2002:33.

79. Baclesse F: Roentgentherapy in cancer of the hypopharynx. *JAMA.* 1949;140:525.

80. Baclesse F: Classification topographique des cancer de l'hypopharynx. In Baclesse F, ed. *Tumeurs Malignes du Pharynx et du Larynx.* Paris: Masson & Co; 1960:283.

81. Inoue T, Shigematsu Y, Sato T: Treatment of carcinoma of the hypopharynx. *Cancer*. 1973;31:649.

82. Freeman RB, Marks JE, Ogura JH: Voice preservation in treatment of carcinoma of the pyriform sinus. *Laryngoscope*. 1979;89:1855.

83. Million RR, Cassisi NJ: Radical irradiation for carcinoma of the pyriform sinus. *Laryngoscope*. 1981;91:439.

84. El Badawi SA, Goepfert H, Fletcher GH, et al: Squamous cell carcinoma of the pyriform sinus. *Laryngoscope*. 1982; 92:357.

85. Vandenbrouck C, Eschwege F, De la Rochefordiere A, et al: Squamous cell carcinoma of the pyriform sinus: Retrospective study of 351 cases treated at the Institut Gustave-Roussy. *Head Neck Surg*. 1987;10:4.

86. Mendenhall WM, Parsons JT, Devine JW, et al: Squamous cell carcinoma of the pyriform sinus treated with surgery and/or radiotherapy. *Head Neck Surg*. 1987;10:88.

87. Mendenhall WM, Parsons JT, Cassisi NJ, et al: Squamous cell carcinoma of the pyriform sinus treated with radical radiation therapy. *Radiother Oncol*. 1987;9:201.

88. Fu KK: The endolarynx and hypopharynx. In Cox JD, ed. *Moss Radiation Oncology: Rationale, Technique, Results*, 7th ed. St. Louis: Mosby; 1994:214.

89. Dubois JB, Guerrier B, Di Ruggiero JM, et al: Cancer of the piriform sinus: Treatment by radiation therapy alone and with surgery. *Radiology*. 1986;160:831.

90. Wang CC: Carcinoma of the hypopharynx. In Wang CC: *Radiation Therapy for Head and Neck Neoplasms: Indications, Techniques, and Results*, 2nd ed. Chicago: Year Book Medical Publishers; 1990:207.

91. Ogura JH, Jurema AA, Watson RK: Partial laryngopharyngectomy and neck dissection for pyriform sinus cancer. *Laryngoscope*. 1960;70:1399.

92. Ogura JH, Marks ME, Freeman RB: Results of conservation surgery for cancers of the supraglottis and pyriform sinus. *Laryngoscope*. 1980;90:591.

93. Laccourreye O, Merite-Drancy A, Brasnu D, et al: Supracricoid hemilaryngopharyngectomy in selected pyriform sinus carcinoma staged as T2. *Laryngoscope*. 1993;103:1373.

94. Marks JE, Kurnik B, Powers WE, et al: Carcinoma of the pyriform sinus: An analysis of treatment results and patterns of failure. *Cancer*. 1978;41:1008.

95. Krespi YP, Sisson GA: Voice preservation in pyriform sinus carcinoma by hemicricolaryngopharyngectomy. *Ann Otol Rhinol Laryngol*. 1984;93:306.

96. Arriagada R, Eschwege F, Cachin Y, et al: The value of combining radiotherapy with surgery in the treatment of hypopharyngeal and laryngeal cancers. *Cancer*. 1983;51:1819.

97. Fletcher GH: Place of irradiation in the management of head and neck cancer. *Semin Oncol*. 1977;4:375.

98. Mendenhall WM, Parsons JT, Springer SP, et al: Squamous cell carcinoma of the head and neck treated with irradiation: Management of the neck. *Semin Radiat Oncol*. 1992;2:163.

99. Jesse RH, Lindberg RD: The efficacy of combining radiation therapy with a surgical procedure in patients with cervical metastasis from squamous carcinoma of the oropharynx and hypopharynx. *Cancer*. 1975;35:1163.

100. Mendenhall WM, Million RR, Cassisi NJ: Squamous cell carcinoma of the head and neck treated with radiation therapy: The role of neck dissection for clinically positive neck nodes. *Int J Radiat Oncol Biol Phys*. 1986;12:733.

101. Amdur RJ, Mendenhall WM, Stringer SP, et al: Organ preservation with radiotherapy for T1-T2 carcinoma of the pyriform sinus. *Head and Neck*. 2001;23:353.

102. Harrison LB, Zelefsky MJ, Armstrong JG, et al: Performance status after treatment for squamous cell cancer of the base of tongue: A comparison of primary radiation therapy versus surgery. *Int J Radiat Oncol Biol Phys*. 1994;30:953.

103. Million RR: Carcinomas of the larynx and hypopharynx: Curative treatment with preservation of laryngeal function. *Front Radiat Ther Oncol*. 1993;27:31.

104. Goepfert H, Lindberg RD, Jesse RH: Combined laryngeal conservation surgery and irradiation: Can we expand the indications for conservation therapy? *Otolaryngol Head Neck Surg*. 1981;89:974.

105. Sheed DP, Scatliff JA, Kirchner JA: A cineradiographic study of postresectional alterations in oral pharyngeal physiology. *Surg Gynecol Obstet*. 1960;110:69.

106. Kramer S, Gelber RD, Snow JB, et al: Combined radiation therapy and surgery in the management of advanced head and neck cancer: Final report of study 73-03 of the Radiation Therapy Oncology Group. *Head Neck Surg*. 1987;10:19.

107. Tupchong L, Scott CB, Blitzer PH, et al: Randomized study of preoperative versus postoperative radiation therapy in advanced head and neck carcinoma: Long-term follow-up of RTOG study 73-03. *Int J Radiat Oncol Biol Phys*. 1991;20:21.

108. Vandenbrouck C, Sancho H, Le Fur R, et al: Results of a randomized clinical trial of preoperative irradiation versus postoperative in treatment of tumors of the hypopharynx. *Cancer*. 1977;39:1445.

109. Hamby L, McGrath PC, Luce EA, et al: Optimizing primary treatment for advanced laryngeal and pyriform sinus carcinoma. *Am J Surg*. 1992;164:629.

110. Kokal WA, Neifeld JP, Eisert D, et al: Postoperative radiation as adjuvant treatment for carcinoma of the oral cavity, larynx, and pharynx: Preliminary report of a prospective randomized trial. *J Surg Oncol*. 1988;38:71.

111. Frank JL, Garb JL, Kay S, et al: Postoperative radiotherapy improves survival in squamous cell carcinoma of the hypopharynx. *Am J Surg*. 1994;168:476.

112. Ho CM, Lam KH, Wei WI, et al: Squamous cell carcinoma of the hypopharynx: Analysis of treatment results. *Head Neck*. 1993; 15:405.

113. Schuller DE, Metch B, Stein DW, et al: Preoperative chemotherapy in advanced resectable head and neck cancer: Final report of the Southwest Oncology Group. *Laryngoscope*. 1988;98:1205.

114. Schuller DE, Stein DW, Metch B: Analysis of treatment failure patterns: A Southwest Oncology Group study. *Arch Otolaryngol Head Neck Surg*. 1989;115:834.

115. Paccagnella A, Orlando A, Marchiori C, et al: Phase III trial of initial chemotherapy in stage III or IV head and neck cancers: A study by the Gruppo di Studio sui Tumori della Testa e del Collo. *J Natl Cancer Inst*. 1994;86:265.

116. Head and Neck Contracts Program: Adjuvant chemotherapy for advanced head and neck squamous carcinoma: Final report of the Head and Neck Contracts Program. *Cancer*. 1987;60:301.

117. Jacobs C, Makuch R: Efficacy of adjuvant chemotherapy for patients with resectable head and neck cancer: A subset analysis of the Head and Neck Contracts Program. *J Clin Oncol*. 1990; 8:838.

118. Laramore GE, Scott CB, Al-Sarraf M, et al: Adjuvant chemotherapy for resectable squamous cell carcinomas of the head and neck: Report on Intergroup Study 0034. *Int J Radiat Oncol Biol Phys*. 1992;23:705.

119. The Department of Veterans Affairs Laryngeal Cancer Study Group: Induction chemotherapy plus radiation compared with surgery plus radiation in patients with advanced laryngeal cancer. *N Engl J Med*. 1991;324:1685.

120. Lefebvre JL, Sahmoud T: Larynx preservation in hypopharynx squamous cell carcinoma: Preliminary results of a randomized study (EORTC 24891). *J Clin Oncol*. 1994;13:283.

121. Lefebvre JL, Chevalier D, Luboinski B, et al: Larynx preservation in pyriform sinus cancer: Preliminary results of a European Organization for Research and Treatment of Cancer phase III trial. *J Natl Cancer Inst*. 1996;88:890.

122. Prades JM, Schmitt TM, Timoshenko AP, et al. Concomitant chemoradiotherapy in pyriform sinus cancer. *Arch Otolaryngol Head Neck Surg*. 2002;128:384.

123. Zelefsky MJ, Kraus DH, Pfister DG, et al: Combined chemotherapy and radiotherapy versus surgery and postoperative radiotherapy for advanced hypopharynx cancer. *Head Neck*. 1996;18:405.

124. Kraus DH, Pfister DG, Harrison LB, et al: Larynx preservation with combined chemotherapy and radiation therapy in advanced hypopharynx cancer. *Otolaryngol Head Neck Surg*. 1994; 111:31.

125. Pfister DG, Strong E, Harrison L, et al: Larynx preservation with combined chemotherapy and radiation therapy in advanced but resectable head and neck cancer. *J Clin Oncol*. 1991;9:850.

126. Clayman GL, Weber RS, Guillamondegui O, et al: Laryngeal preservation for advanced laryngeal and hypopharyngeal cancers. *Arch Otolaryngol Head Neck Surg*. 1995;121:219.

127. Shirinian MH, Weber RS, Lippman SM, et al: Laryngeal preservation by induction chemotherapy plus radiotherapy in locally advanced head and neck cancer: The M.D. Anderson Cancer Center experience. *Head Neck*. 1994;16:39.

128. Jacobs C, Goffinet DR, Goffinet L, et al: Chemotherapy as a substitute for surgery in the treatment of advanced resectable head and neck cancer. *Cancer*. 1987;60:1178.

129. Vikram B, Bosl G, Pfister D, et al: New strategies for avoiding total laryngectomy in patients with head and neck cancer. *NCI Monogr*. 1988;6:361.

130. Vikram B, Malamud S, Gold J, et al: Chemotherapy rapidly alternating with accelerated radiotherapy for advanced carcinomas of the hypopharynx and upper esophagus: A feasibility study. *Head Neck*. 1991;13:415.

131. Karp DD, Vaughan CW, Carter R, et al: Larynx preservation using induction chemotherapy plus radiation therapy as an alternative to laryngectomy in advanced head and neck cancer: A long-term follow-up report. *Am J Clin Oncol*. 1991;14:273.

132. Taylor SG, Murthy AK, Vannetzel J-M, et al: Randomized comparison of neoadjuvant cisplatin and fluorouracil infusion followed by radiation versus concomitant treatment in advanced head and neck cancer. *J Clin Oncol*. 1994;12:385.

133. Urba SG, Forastiere AA, Wolf GT, et al: Intensive induction chemotherapy and radiation for organ preservation in patients with advanced resectable head and neck carcinoma. *J Clin Oncol*. 1994;12:946.

134. Leyvraz S, Pasche P, Bauer J, et al: Rapidly alternating chemotherapy and hyperfractionated radiotherapy in the management of locally advanced head and neck carcinoma: Four-year results of a phase I/II study. *J Clin Oncol*. 1994;12:1876.

135. Koch WM, Lee DJ, Eisele DW, et al: Chemoradiotherapy for organ preservation in oral and pharyngeal carcinoma. *Arch Otolaryngol Head Neck Surg*. 1995;121:974.

136. Vokes EE, Weichselbaum RR: Measurable impact: Multimodality therapy of head and neck cancer. *Int J Radiat Oncol Biol Phys*. 1993;27:481.

137. Adelstein DJ, Li Y, Adams GL, et al: An intergroup phase III comparison of standard radiation therapy and two schedules of concurrent chemoradiotherapy in patients with unresectable squamous cell head and neck cancer. *J Clin Oncol*. 2003;21:92.

138. Brizel DM, Albers ME, Fisher SR, et al: Hyperfractionated irradiation with or without concurrent chemotherapy for locally advanced head and neck cancer. *N Engl J Med*. 1998; 338:1798.

139. Al-Sarraf M, Pajak TF, Marcial VA, et al: Concurrent radiotherapy and chemotherapy with cisplatin in inoperable squamous cell carcinoma of the head and neck. *Cancer*. 1987;59:259.

140. Marcial VA, Pajak TF, Mohiuddin M, et al: Concomitant cisplatin chemotherapy and radiotherapy in advanced mucosal squamous cell carcinoma of the head and neck: Long-term results of the Radiation Therapy Oncology Group study 81-17. *Cancer*. 1990;66:1861.

141. Coughlin CT, Richmond RC: Biologic and clinical developments of cisplatin combined with radiation: Concepts, utility, projections for new trials, and the emergence of carboplatin. *Semin Oncol*. 1989;16:31.

142. Harrison LB, Pfister DG, Fass DE, et al: Concomitant chemotherapy-radiation therapy followed by hyperfractionated radiation therapy for advanced unresectable head and neck cancer. *Int J Radiat Oncol Biol Phys*. 1991;21:703.

143. Parsons JT: Time-dose-volume relations in radiation therapy. In Million RR, Cassisi NJ, eds. *Management of Head and Neck Cancer: A Multidisciplinary Approach*, 2nd ed. Philadelphia: JB Lippincott; 1994:203.

144. Amdur RJ, Parsons JT, Mendenhall WM, et al: Postoperative irradiation for squamous cell carcinoma of the head and neck: An analysis of treatment results and complications. *Int J Radiat Oncol Biol Phys*. 1989;16:25.

145. Wilkens SA: Carcinoma of the posterior pharyngeal wall. *Am J Surg*. 1971;122:477.

146. Barzan L, Barra S, Franchin G, et al: Squamous cell carcinoma of the posterior pharyngeal wall: Characteristics compared with the lateral wall. *J Laryngol Otol*. 1995;109:120.

147. McNeill R: Surgical management of carcinoma of the posterior pharyngeal wall. *Head Neck Surg*. 1981;3:389.

148. Fein DA, Mendenhall WM, Parsons JT, et al: Pharyngeal wall carcinoma treated with radiotherapy: Impact of treatment technique and fractionation. *Int J Radiat Oncol Biol Phys*. 1993;26:751.

149. Laughlin JS, Mohan R, Kutcher GJ: Choice of optimum megavoltage for accelerators for photon beam treatment. *Int J Radiat Oncol Biol Phys*. 1986;12:1551.

150. Esik O, Burkelbach J, Boesecke R, et al: Three-dimensional photon radiotherapy planning for laryngeal and hypopharyngeal cancers: 2. Conformation treatment planning using a multileaf collimator. *Radiother Oncol*. 1991;20:238.

151. van Mierlo IJM, Levendag PC, Eijkenboom WMH, et al: Radiation therapy for cancer of the pyriform sinus: A failure analysis. *Am J Clin Oncol*. 1995;18:502.

152. Andrew JW, Eapen L, Kulkarni NS: Homogeneous irradiation of the short-necked laryngeal cancer patient. *Int J Radiat Oncol Biol Phys*. 1984;10:549.

153. Sailer SL, Sherouse GW, Chaney EL, et al: A comparison of postoperative techniques for carcinomas of the larynx and hypopharynx using 3-D dose distributions. *Int J Radiat Oncol Biol Phys*. 1991;21:767.

154. Devineni VR, Hayden R, Fredrickson J, et al: Tolerance of gastric mucosal flap to postoperative irradiation. *Laryngoscope*. 1991;101:462.

155. Spiro RH, Bains MS, Shah JP, et al: Gastric transposition for head and neck cancer: A critical update. *Am J Surg*. 1991;162:348.

156. Petruzzelli GJ, Johnson JT, Myers EN, et al: The effect of postoperative radiation therapy on pharyngoesophageal reconstruction with free jejunal interposition. *Arch Otolaryngol Head Neck Surg*. 1991;117:1265.

157. Knee R, Fields RS, Peters LJ: Concomitant boost radiotherapy for advanced squamous cell carcinoma of the head and neck. *Radiother Oncol*. 1985;4:1.

158. Ang KK, Peters LJ, Weber RS, et al: Concomitant boost radiotherapy schedules in the treatment of carcinoma of the oropharynx and nasopharynx. *Int J Radiat Oncol Biol Phys*. 1990;19:1339.

159. Schmidt-Ullrich RK, Johnson CR, Wazer DE, et al: Accelerated superfractionated irradiation for advanced carcinoma of the head and neck: Concomitant boost technique. *Int J Radiat Oncol Biol Phys*. 1991;21:563.

160. Withers HR: Biological basis for altered fractionation schemes. *Cancer*. 1985;55:2086.

161. Peters LJ, Ang KK: The role of altered fractionation in head and neck cancers. *Semin Radiat Oncol*. 1992;2:180.

162. Dische S: Radiotherapy: New fractionation schemes. *Semin Oncol*. 1994;21:304.

163. Son YH, Kacinski BM: Therapeutic concepts of brachytherapy/megavoltage in sequence for pharyngeal wall cancers. *Cancer*. 1987;59:1268.

164. Son YH, Skomro-Dicker C: Crossing and looping methods in radical interstitial therapy for lateral and posterior oro-/hypopharyngeal tumors. *Int J Radiat Oncol Biol Phys*. 1983;9:401.

165. Lee NK, Goepfert H, Wendt CD: Supraglottic laryngectomy for intermediate-stage cancer: U.T. M.D. Anderson Cancer Center experience with combined therapy. *Laryngoscope*. 1990;100:831.

166. French Head and Neck Study Group: Early pharyngolaryngeal carcinomas with palpable nodes. *Am J Surg*. 1991;162:377.

167. Bataini JP, Brugere J, Jaulerry C, et al: Radiation treatment of lateral epilaryngeal cancer. *Am J Clin Oncol*. 1984;7:641.

168. Bataini JP: Head and neck cancer and the radiation oncologist. *Radiother Oncol*. 1991;21:1.

169. Ahmad K, Fayos JV: High-dose radiation therapy in carcinoma of the pyriform sinus. *Cancer*. 1984;53:2091.

170. Garden AS, Morrison WH, Ang KK, et al: Hyperfractionated radiation in the treatment of squamous cell carcinomas of the head and neck: A comparison of two fractionation schedules. *Int J Radiat Oncol Biol Phys*. 1995;31:493.

171. Pingree TF, Davis RK, Reichman O, et al: Treatment of hypopharyngeal carcinoma: A 10-year review of 1,362 cases. *Laryngoscope*. 1987;97:901.

172. Carpenter RJ, DeSanto LW: Carcinoma of the hypopharynx. *Surg Clin North Am*. 1977;57:723.

173. Razack MS, Sako K, Marchetta FC, et al: Carcinoma of the hypopharynx: Success and failure. *Am J Surg*. 1977;134:489.

174. Razack MS, Sako K, Kalnins I: Squamous cell carcinoma of the pyriform sinus. *Head Neck Surg*. 1978;1:31.

175. Kirchner JA, Owen JR: Five hundred cancers of the larynx and pyriform sinus: Results of treatment by radiation and surgery. *Laryngoscope*. 1977;87:1288.

176. Eisbach KJ, Krause CJ: Carcinoma of the pyriform sinus: A comparison of treatment modalities. *Laryngoscope*. 1977; 87:1904.

177. Driscoll WG, Nagorsky MJ, Cantrell RW, et al: Carcinoma of the pyriform sinus: Analysis of 102 cases. *Laryngoscope*. 1983;93:556.

178. Yates A, Crumley RL: Surgical treatment of pyriform sinus cancer: A retrospective study. *Laryngoscope*. 1984;94:1586.

179. Byers RM, Krueger WW, Saxton J: Use of surgery and postoperative radiation in the treatment of advanced squamous cell carcinoma of the pyriform sinus. *Am J Surg*. 1979; 138:597.

180. Slotman BJ, Kralendonk JH, Snow GB, et al: Surgery and postoperative radiotherapy and radiotherapy alone in T3-T4 cancers of the pyriform sinus. *Acta Oncol*. 1994;33:55.

181. Wang CC: Radiotherapeutic management of carcinoma of the posterior pharyngeal wall. *Cancer*. 1971;27:894.

182. Bryce D: The conventional surgical management of carcinoma of the hypopharynx. *J Laryngol Otol*. 1971;85:1221.

183. Pene F, Avedian V, Eschwege F, et al: A retrospective study of 131 cases of carcinoma of the posterior pharyngeal wall. *Cancer*. 1978;42:2490.

184. Marks JE, Smith PG, Sessions DG: Pharyngeal wall cancer: A reappraisal after comparison of treatment methods. *Arch Otolaryngol*. 1985;111:79.

185. Hennessy TPJ, O'Connell R: Carcinoma of the hypopharynx, esophagus and cardia. *Surg Gyn Obstet*. 1986;162:243.

186. Kajanti M, Mantyla M: Carcinoma of the hypopharynx: A retrospective analysis of the treatment results over a 25-year period. *Acta Oncol*. 1990;29(Fasc 7):903.

Cancer of the Larynx

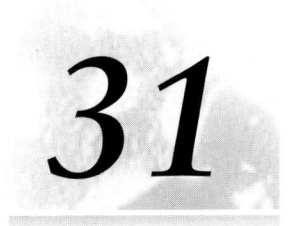

Nancy Lee, MD   and   Theodore L. Phillips, MD

EPIDEMIOLOGY, ETIOLOGY, AND GENETICS

Tumors of the larynx constitute about 2% of all cancers and are the most common cancers of the upper aerodigestive tract. The ratio of glottic to supraglottic carcinomas is about 3:1.

Patients with a history of smoking are at high risk for these cancers. The use of black tobacco carries a higher risk than the use of blond tobacco. People who employ their voices extensively in their work also appear to be at higher risk. The role of alcohol is less clear for glottic cancer but has been implicated in supraglottic cancer. The tumors can begin as dysplasia, progress to in situ lesions, and finally progress to invasive lesions.

Mutation of the *p53* gene is common and is seen in 47% of the patients who are cigarette smokers but in only 14% of those who are nonsmokers. Fifty-five percent of the tumors among drinkers and 20% among nondrinkers had *p53* mutations.[1] Changes in *p53* and proliferating cell nuclear antigen expression may be associated with human papillomavirus infection and could play a role in the carcinogenesis of laryngeal cancer.[2,3] In addition, coexpression of three genes, namely, *bax*, *bcl-2*, and *p53*, plays a critical role in the apoptotic mechanisms of laryngeal carcinoma.[4]

Some have advocated that the overexpression of *p53* is associated with tumor bulk and poor local control in T1 glottic cancer,[5] while others have found that *p53* status is not a marker for prognosis and clinical outcome in laryngeal carcinoma.[6] Low levels of cyclin D1 have been suggested to correlate with radioresistance in early-stage larynx carcinoma.[7]

ANATOMIC CONSIDERATIONS

Anatomically, the larynx is contiguous with the lower portion of the pharynx above and is connected with the trachea below. It extends from the tip of the epiglottis at the level of the lower border of the C3 vertebra to the lower border of the cricoid cartilage at the level of the C6 vertebra. The larynx is subdivided into three anatomical regions: the supraglottis, glottis, and subglottis regions (Fig. 31-1). The supraglottis includes the epiglottis, aryepiglottic folds, arytenoids, and false cords (ventricular bands). The glottis consists of the true vocal cords and the anterior and posterior commissures (the mucosa between the arytenoids). The lower boundary of

the glottis is a horizontal plane 1 cm below the apex of the ventricle or 5 mm below the free margin of the vocal cords. The subglottis extends from the lower boundary of the glottis to the inferior margin of the cricoid cartilage. The appearance of the larynx as seen in the indirect mirror examination is shown in Figure 31-2. The cartilaginous framework of the larynx is important in diagnostic radiology and in evaluating simulation and port films. The relationship of the various cartilages to surface anatomy is shown in Figure 31-3. The thyroid, cricoid, and most of the arytenoid cartilages are composed of hyaline cartilage, which begins to ossify at about 20 years of age. The epiglottis, the corniculate and cuneiform cartilages, and the apex and vocal process of the arytenoids are made up of elastic cartilage, which does not ossify and therefore is not radiopaque.

The anterior limits of the larynx consist of the lingual surface of the suprahyoid epiglottis, the thyrohyoid membrane, the anterior commissure, and the anterior wall of the subglottic region, which is composed of the thyroid cartilage, the cricothyroid membrane, and the anterior arch of the cricoid cartilage (see Fig. 31-3B). It is important to note that the anterior commissure is usually within 1 cm of the skin surface. The posterior and lateral limits include the aryepiglottic folds, the arytenoids, the interarytenoid space, and the posterior surface of the

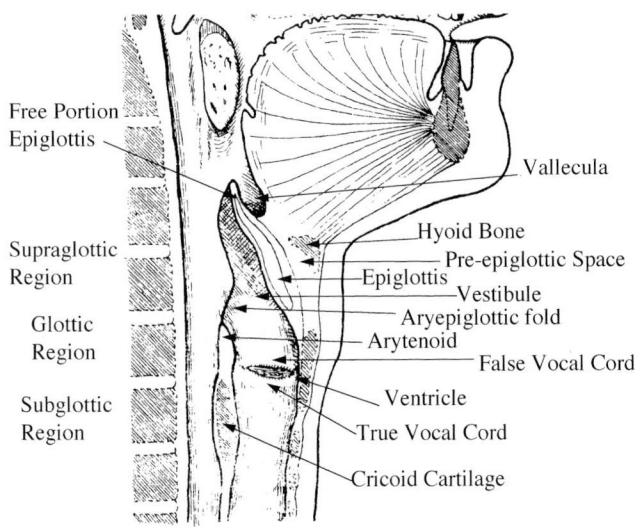

Figure 31–1. Anatomic regions and structures of the larynx.

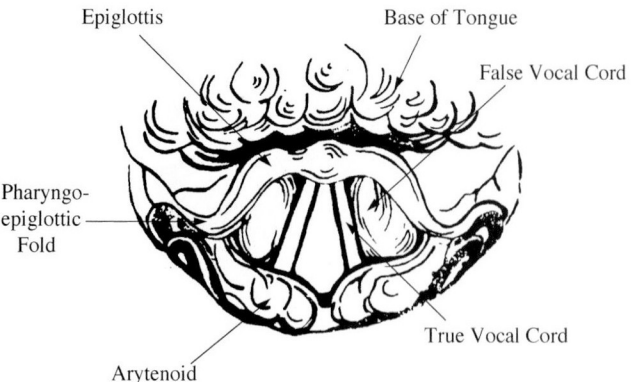

Figure 31–2. Structures of the larynx as seen by indirect mirror examination.

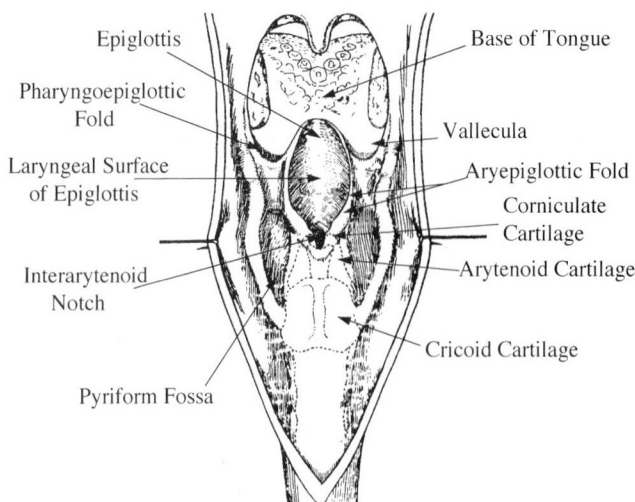

Figure 31–4. Structures of the larynx as seen from behind.

subglottic space formed by the mucous membrane covering the cricoid cartilage. The superolateral limits consist of the tip and the lateral borders of the epiglottis. The inferior limit is the inferior edge of the cricoid cartilage (Fig. 31-4). The anatomy of the larynx can also be appreciated on computed tomography (CT) scans. The key structures are seen in Figure 31-5.

LYMPHATIC DRAINAGE

The supraglottis has a rich lymphatic network. The lymphatic channels from the supraglottis pass through the thyrohyoid membrane and drain into the subdigastric (jugulodigastric), midjugular (jugulocarotid), and lower jugular (jugulo-omohyoid) nodes of the jugular chain. The distribution of positive lymph nodes as determined by Lindberg[8] is shown in Figure 31-6.

The lymphatic network is less developed in the subglottis. Lymphatic channels from the subglottic area unite to form three lymphatic pedicles, one anterior and two posterolateral. The anterior channels pass through the cricothyroid membrane and drain into the mid- and lower jugular nodes or terminate in the prelaryngeal node

(Delphian node), from which lymphatics drain into the pretracheal and supraclavicular nodes. The posterolateral lymphatic channels pass through cricotracheal membrane and terminate in the highest paratracheal nodes.

The true vocal cords are devoid of lymphatic capillaries. Lymphatic spread from glottic cancer occurs when there is tumor extension into the supraglottis or the subglottis.

PATHOLOGY

At least 95% of all malignant neoplasms of the larynx are squamous cell carcinoma or one of its variants. Carcinomas arising from the true vocal cords are usually well differentiated or moderately well differentiated. Carcinomas of the supraglottis and subglottis are less differentiated than those of the vocal cords. Carcinoma in situ occurs in the vocal cords but is rare in the supraglottis.

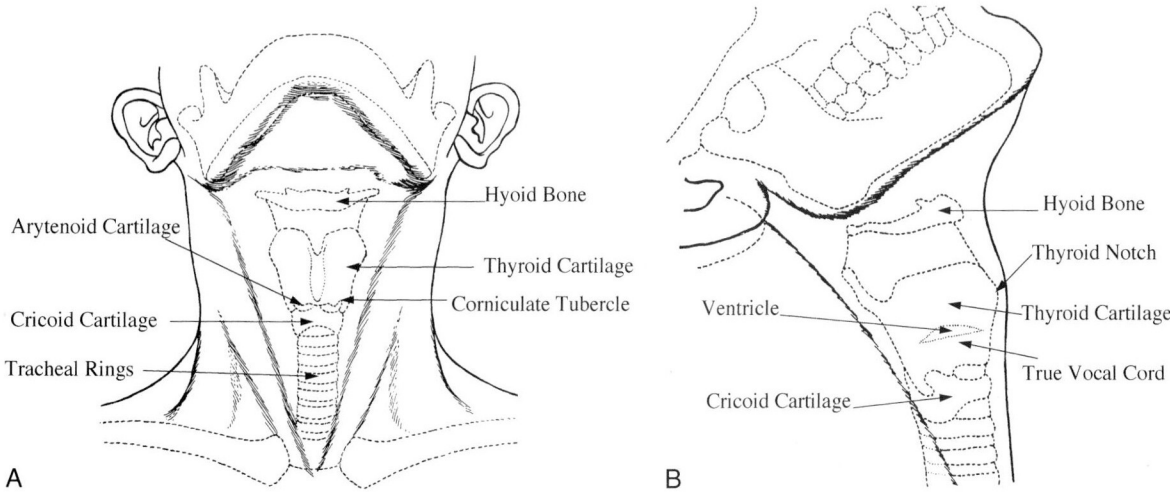

Figure 31–3. **A,** Anterior view of surface anatomy with cartilages shown. **B,** Lateral view of surface anatomy with cartilages shown.

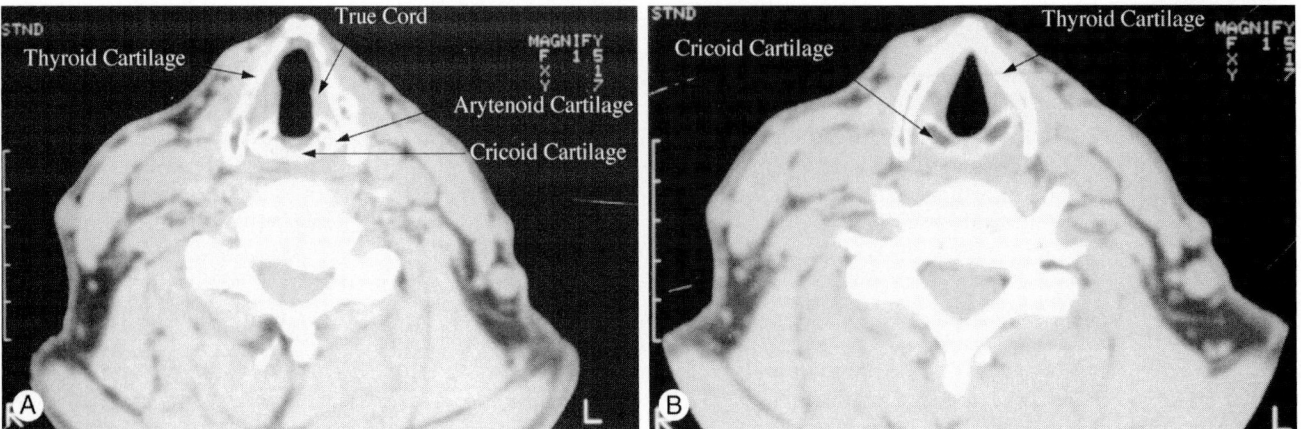

Figure 31–5. Structures of the larynx as seen on computed tomography scans at the level of true vocal cords (**A**) and subglottis (**B**).

Verrucous carcinoma is an uncommon but distinct variety of squamous cell carcinoma. It accounts for 1% to 2% of the carcinomas of the vocal cord. It is a bulky, exophytic, papillomatous, low-grade squamous cell carcinoma. Typically it has a heavily keratinized surface and a blunt, well-demarcated, invasive, deep margin, often with a broad base. Bona fide cases of verrucous carcinoma do not metastasize. The phenomenon of anaplastic transformation of verrucous carcinoma following radiotherapy (RT) remains controversial.[9,10]

Other rare tumors of the larynx include malignant minor salivary gland tumors, small cell carcinoma, lymphoma, plasmacytoma, chemodectoma, carcinoid, pseudosarcoma, soft-tissue sarcoma, chondrosarcoma, osteosarcoma, and malignant melanoma.

CLINICAL PRESENTATION

Sore throat and odynophagia are the most common presenting symptoms of carcinoma of the supraglottis. The patient may experience a foreign body sensation and difficulty in swallowing. Unilateral otalgia occurs as referred pain by way of the vagus nerve and the auricular nerve of Arnold. A change in voice occurs when an exophytic mass touches the vocal cords. Hoarseness is seldom an initial symptom and occurs with invasion of the vocal cords. Hemoptysis is uncommon. Because of the high incidence of lymph node metastasis, a neck mass may be the first sign of carcinoma of the supraglottis. Weight loss, dyspnea, foul breath, and aspiration occur with advanced disease.

Hoarseness is the most common presenting symptom of early vocal cord cancer. Sore throat, otalgia, localized pain owing to cartilage invasion, and dyspnea are symptoms of advanced disease.

Carcinoma of the subglottis is rare. It is relatively asymptomatic in the early stage. The most common presenting symptom is dyspnea, which occurs as a result of narrowed airway owing to tumor growth. Hoarseness, odynophagia, and hemoptysis are less common.

ROUTES OF SPREAD

Lymphatic

The incidence of lymph node metastasis from carcinoma of the supraglottis at the time of diagnosis is 55%, with 16% being bilateral.[8] The subdigastric and midjugular nodes are most commonly involved. The lower jugular nodes are less commonly involved, and the posterior cervical and supraclavicular lymph nodes are occasionally involved. The incidence of lymph node metastasis increases with the T stage and when there is extension into the base of the tongue and hypopharynx. The incidence of histologically positive lymph nodes in elective neck dissections for carcinoma of the larynx is 37%.[11] The incidence of subsequent lymph node metastasis in initially N0 necks following treatment is 14%.[12]

For carcinoma of the vocal cords, the incidence of lymph node metastasis at diagnosis is low: approximately 0% to 2% for T1, 3% to 7% for T2, 15% to 20% for T3, and 20% to 30% for T4 lesions.[13-16] The pattern of lymph node metastasis depends on the site of involvement and follows that of the supraglottis or subglottis. However, the incidence of lymph node metastasis from primary vocal cord carcinomas with supraglottic or subglottic involvement is not as high as the incidence of

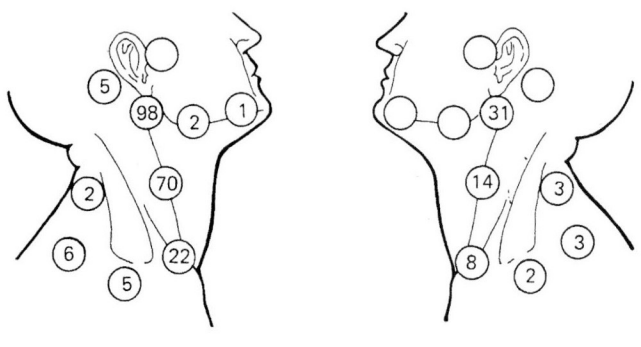

Ipsilateral   Contralateral

Figure 31–6. Distribution of lymph node metastases from carcinoma of the supraglottic larynx. (From Lindberg RD, et al: Distribution of cervical lymph node metastases from squamous cell carcinoma of the upper respiratory and digestive tracts. *Cancer.* 1992;29:1446, 1450.)

node involvement in primary supraglottic or subglottic carcinomas.

The incidence of lymph node metastasis from carcinoma of the subglottis varies from 20% to 50%.[17,18] The prelaryngeal (Delphian), lower jugular, pretracheal, paratracheal, and upper mediastinal lymph nodes are most commonly involved. The midjugular and supraclavicular lymph nodes are less commonly involved.

Distant Metastasis

The incidence of distant metastasis is approximately 13% to 19% for carcinoma of the supraglottic larynx.[12,19] The lung is the most common distant metastatic site. Bone, mediastinal lymph node, and liver metastases are less common.

DIAGNOSTIC EVALUATION

A careful history and physical examination are mandatory in the evaluation of a patient with carcinoma of the larynx. A flexible fiberoptic endoscope or rigid endoscope (Hopkin's rod) is particularly helpful in the examination of a patient whose larynx is not well visualized with indirect mirror examination. These devices allow excellent visualization of the infrahyoid epiglottis and anterior commissures, which may be difficult to see with indirect laryngoscopy. In addition to determining the tumor extent, it is essential to assess the mobility of the vocal cords. Such endoscopes may be attached to a photographic device, allowing documentation of the tumor size and location.

The neck is carefully palpated to determine the presence, size, and location of lymph node metastasis. Localized tenderness or a mass over the thyroid cartilage is suggestive of thyroid cartilage invasion. Loss of thyrovertebral crackle is a sign of postcricoid extension.

Routine laboratory tests include a chest radiograph, complete blood count, and liver function tests. The hemoglobin level may have prognostic value in patients irradiated for carcinoma of the larynx.[20,21] If the liver function tests or serum alkaline phosphatase is abnormal, further studies such as liver and bone scans may be indicated.

Both CT scan with contrast enhancement and magnetic resonance imaging (MRI) with and without contrast are useful in the diagnostic imaging of laryngeal cancer. These studies are preferably performed before biopsy of the tumor, as postbiopsy edema may cause overestimation of tumor extent. The relative usefulness of CT scan versus MRI remains controversial, but it is our experience that MRI is more useful in delineating the soft-tissue extent of the primary tumor, and CT is better for evaluating early bone invasion. They are equal in detecting lymph node involvement.

Both CT and MRI scans are useful in determining pre-epiglottic and periglottic space invasion, subglottic and extralaryngeal extension, and cartilage invasion. CT scans are also useful in the detection of subclinical lymph node metastasis. With CT scans, correct T-classification is possible in 70% to 80% of cases, and N stage in about 80%.[22] The limitations of CT include the subtle evaluation of tumor-induced cartilage and bone defects and the detection of superficial tumors.

Compared with CT, the multiplanar capability of MRI provides superior definition of anatomy and tumor extent.[23] MRI appears to be more effective in detecting cartilage invasion.[24] MRI is as effective as CT in defining lymph node metastasis and extension into the carotid sheath. The disadvantages of MRI are longer scanning time and motion artifact.[22]

Pulmonary function tests are performed in patients being considered for supraglottic laryngectomy or partial laryngopharyngectomy.

Direct laryngoscopy with biopsy of the tumor is the most valuable and essential step in the diagnosis and staging of carcinoma of the larynx. It is usually combined with bronchoscopy and esophagoscopy to rule out multiple tumors.

STAGING

The TNM staging system of the 2002 American Joint Committee on Cancer for carcinoma of the larynx is shown in Table 31-1.[25] Primary tumor (T) classification is based on the extent of involvement within the larynx, extralaryngeal extension, cartilage invasion, and mobility of the vocal cords. T4 lesions have been divided into T4a, which is resectable, and T4b, which is unresectable, leading to the division of stage IV into IVA and IVB. Regional lymph node (N) classification is based on size and number, as well as on ipsilateral, bilateral, or contralateral lymph node involvement.

GENERAL THERAPEUTIC APPROACHES AND THE ROLE OF RADIATION THERAPY

The treatment objective for carcinoma of the larynx is to obtain the best cure rate with the optimal preservation of organ function.[26-30] RT or surgery alone has been the primary treatment modality for select cases of early carcinoma of the larynx. RT is delivered primarily with external beam irradiation. Surgical procedures include endoscopic stripping, laser excision, laryngofissure, cordectomy, hemilaryngectomy, or vertical partial laryngectomy for early glottic carcinoma and supraglottic laryngectomy for early supraglottic carcinoma. Total laryngectomy is necessary in the surgical treatment of advanced carcinoma of the larynx.

Recently, concurrent chemotherapy combined with RT has been used in the treatment of advanced operable laryngeal cancer (excluding T4 lesions) with organ preservation in many patients and with no compromise of survival.[31] Although randomized trials for advanced, mostly inoperable head and neck cancer including carcinoma of the larynx have shown increased local-regional control with concurrent RT and single-agent chemotherapy (i.e., 5-fluorouracil, cisplatin, bleomycin, mitomycin C, and methotrexate) most trials showed no significant improvement in survival.[32-36]

Selection of a treatment modality for an individual patient depends on a number of factors: site and extent

Table 31–1 Classification of Laryngeal Cancer

Primary Tumor (T)

TX	Primary tumor cannot be assessed
T0	No evidence of primary tumor
Tis	Carcinoma in situ

Supraglottis

T1	Tumor limited to one subsite of supraglottis, with normal vocal cord mobility
T2	Tumor invades mucosa of more than one adjacent subsite of supraglottis or glottis or region outside the supraglottis (e.g., mucosa of base of tongue, vallecula, medial wall of pyriform sinus) without fixation of the larynx
T3	Tumor limited to larynx with vocal cord fixation and/or invades any of the following: postcricoid area or preepiglottic tissues
T4	Tumor invades through thyroid cartilage and/or extends to soft tissues of the neck, thyroid, and/or esophagus.
T4a	Tumor invades through the thyroid cartilage and/or invades tissues beyond the larynx (e.g., trachea, soft tissues of neck including deep extrinsic muscle of the tongue, strap muscles, thyroid, or esophagus).
T4b	Tumor invades prevertebral space, encases carotid artery, or invades mediastinal structures.

Glottis

T1	Tumor limited to vocal cord(s) (may involve anterior or posterior commissures), with normal mobility
T1a	Tumor limited to one vocal cord
T1b	Tumor involves both vocal cords
T2	Tumor extends to supraglottis and/or subglottis, and/or with impaired vocal cord mobility
T3	Tumor limited to the larynx, with vocal cord fixation
T4	Tumor invades through thyroid cartilage and/or to other tissues beyond the larynx (e.g., trachea, soft tissues of neck, including thyroid, pharynx)
T4a	Tumor invades through the thyroid cartilage and/or invades tissues beyond the larynx (e.g., trachea, soft tissues of neck including deep extrinsic muscle of the tongue, strap muscles, thyroid, or esophagus).
T4b	Tumor invades prevertebral space, encases carotid artery, or invades mediastinal structures.

Subglottis

T1	Tumor limited to the subglottis
T2	Tumor extends to vocal cord(s), with normal or impaired mobility
T3	Tumor limited to larynx, with vocal cord fixation
T4	Tumor invades through cricoid or thyroid cartilage and/or extends to other tissues beyond the larynx (e.g., trachea, soft tissues of neck, including thyroid, esophagus)

T4a	Tumor invades cricoid or thyroid cartilage and/or invades tissues beyond the larynx (e.g., trachea, soft tissues of neck including deep extrinsic muscle of the tongue, strap muscles, thyroid, or esophagus).
T4b	Tumor invades prevertebral space, encases carotid artery, or invades mediastinal structures.

Regional Lymph Nodes (N)

NX	Regional lymph nodes cannot be assessed
N0	No regional lymph node metastasis
N1	Metastasis in a single ipsilateral lymph node, 3 cm or less in greatest dimension
N2	Metastasis in a single ipsilateral lymph node, more than 3 cm but not more than 6 cm in greatest dimension, or in multiple ipsilateral lymph nodes, none more than 6 cm in greatest dimension, or in bilateral or contralateral lymph nodes, none more than 6 cm greatest dimension
N2a	Metastasis in a single ipsilateral lymph node more than 3 cm but not more than 6 cm in greatest dimension
N2b	Metastasis in multiple ipsilateral lymph nodes, none more than 6 cm in greatest dimension
N2c	Metastasis in bilateral or contralateral lymph nodes, none more than 6 cm in greatest dimension
N3	Metastasis in a lymph node more than 6 cm in greatest dimension

Distant Metastasis (M)

MX	Distant metastasis cannot be assessed
M0	No distant metastasis
M1	Distant metastasis

Stage Grouping

Stage 0	Tis	N0	M0
Stage I	T1	N0	M0
Stage II	T2	N0	M0
Stage III	T3	N0	M0
	T1	N1	M0
	T2	N1	M0
	T3	N1	M0
Stage IVA	T4a	N0	M0
	T4a	N1	M0
	T1	N2	M0
	T2	N2	M0
	T3	N2	M0
	T4a	N2	M0
Stage IVB	T4b	Any N	M0
	Any T	N3	M0
Stage IVC	Any T	Any N	M1

From Greene FL, Page DL, Fleming ID, et al, eds: *AJCC Cancer Staging Manual.* 6th ed. New York: Springer; 2002:41.

of disease involvement, vocal cord mobility, cartilage invasion, tumor growth characteristics, histology, general medical condition of the patient, occupation, patient compliance for close follow-up examinations, patient preference, sex of the patient, cost, and availability of surgical or radiation oncology expertise.

Early lesions of the vocal cords can be treated successfully with either surgery or RT; however, the voice quality is better after RT. Advanced lesions with fixed vocal cords owing to extensive cartilage invasion are best

managed with surgery with postoperative RT.[37] Exophytic lesions are more responsive to RT than are infiltrative lesions. RT alone or concurrent with chemotherapy may be the preferred treatment for poorly differentiated carcinoma. Conservation surgery may be the preferred treatment for early verrucous carcinoma of the vocal cord. Patients with medical contraindications for general anesthesia or patients who refuse surgery are treated with RT. Patients with poor pulmonary function who are not suitable for supraglottic laryngectomy or partial laryngopharyngectomy are treated with RT. RT may be the preferred initial treatment in patients whose occupation requires intact voice function. Patients who are not reliable for close follow-up examinations may require aggressive treatment from the start. Of note, the prognosis of females irradiated for laryngeal cancer is usually better than that of males.

Carcinoma of the Supraglottis

Early (T1N0) superficial exophytic lesions can be treated with RT or supraglottic laryngectomy, with excellent local control and preservation of voice.[38] For intermediate-size, infiltrative lesions with or without extensive cervical lymph node metastasis (N2 or N3) that can be removed with conservation surgery, supraglottic laryngectomy with or without radical neck dissection combined with postoperative RT offers the best functional and therapeutic results.[39-41]

Supraglottic laryngectomy is contraindicated when there is arytenoid fixation, bilateral arytenoid involvement, involvement of the apex of the pyriform sinus, invasion of the thyroid or cricoid cartilage, involvement of the postcricoid region, impaired vocal cord mobility, extension into the glottic area, and extensive involvement of the base of the tongue. Elderly patients or those with chronic lung disease may not tolerate supraglottic laryngectomy because of postoperative difficulty swallowing and consequent complications of aspiration.

RT is the preferred initial treatment for superficial exophytic lesions (T1,T2N0), with surgery reserved for RT failures. RT is also the preferred treatment for poorly differentiated early carcinoma of the supraglottis. Moderately advanced supraglottic carcinoma with vocal cord involvement and extensive neck disease (T2N2-3) can be treated with RT with or without a radical neck dissection, with preservation of voice. Other than early T1N0 lesions, an altered fractionated schedule—either hyperfractionation or accelerated fractionation using a concomitant boost technique—is recommended.

The role of postradiotherapy neck dissection in patients who have a complete response after definitive RT is controversial. A single institution's experience of 121 patients with node-positive supraglottic carcinoma who underwent definitive RT and achieved a complete response locoregionally 4 to 6 weeks after treatment resulted in very few isolated neck recurrences. Therefore, postradiotherapy neck dissection is not routinely recommended.[42]

For advanced operable carcinoma of the supraglottis (T3-4N0-3), surgery combined with RT offers the best local-regional control rate.[37] In most centers, when RT is combined with surgery for carcinoma of the larynx, it is usually given postoperatively. In a randomized trial by the Radiation Therapy Oncology Group (RTOG) comparing preoperative and postoperative RT for carcinoma of the larynx, local-regional control was significantly better with postoperative RT, although the difference in survival was not significant.[43]

Although total laryngectomy combined with postoperative RT has been used in the treatment of advanced operable carcinoma of the larynx, a randomized trial by the Department of Veterans Affairs, Laryngeal Cancer Study Group has shown that induction chemo-therapy with three cycles of cisplatin and 5-fluorouracil infusion and definitive RT can be effective in preserving the larynx in 62% of patients with advanced laryngeal cancer without compromising overall survival.[44] The RTOG[31] conducted a larynx preservation trial, randomizing patients to induction chemotherapy (modeled after the Veterans Affairs trial) and RT versus concomitant chemoradiotherapy (cisplatin given on days 1, 22, 43) versus RT alone. This trial showed that for 547 patients with stage III and IV potentially resectable cancer of the supraglottic and glottic larynx, treated to 70 Gy in 2 Gy/fractions, the 2-year local-regional control rates were 78% for the concurrent arm, 61% for the induction arm, and 56% for the RT-alone arm. Time to laryngectomy was significantly increased with concurrent chemoradiotherapy. This result is so far only published in abstract form.

Select patients with advanced supraglottic carcinoma, patients who are medically unsuitable for surgery, and patients with inoperable disease are treated with RT, preferably with chemotherapy. Females with exophytic T3-4N0 or N1 lesions may be treated initially with RT alone. For moderately advanced and advanced supraglottic carcinoma treated with RT alone, retrospective comparisons suggest a higher local-regional control rate with hyperfractionated or accelerated hyperfractionated RT.[45-47] A phase III RTOG randomized trial showed that hyperfractionation and accelerated fractionation with concomitant boost are more efficacious than standard fractionation for locally advanced head and neck cancer in terms of local control and disease-free survival.[48] Stage II to IV supraglottic larynx carcinoma was included in this study, however, primary glottic laryngeal cases were not included. In addition, a phase II trial conducted by the RTOG tested whether two cycles of cisplatin given concurrently with accelerated fractionation with concomitant boost can further improve the local control and disease-free survival rate in locally advanced head and neck cancer patients. Cancer of the larynx was included in this study. Eighty-three percent of the patients had stage IV disease. Toxicity was not significantly enhanced when compared with concurrent chemotherapy and RT using standard fractionation. Preliminary data is encouraging with a 1-year survival rate of 81.3%.[48a]

Carcinoma of the Glottis

CARCINOMA IN SITU. Carcinoma in situ can be treated successfully with endoscopic stripping, laser excision,[49-52] or RT.[16,53-55] Some of these lesions may be understaged owing to an inadequate biopsy. An incidence of 16% to 63% of invasive carcinoma developing in patients treated by conservation surgery[56] has been reported. RT is the initial treatment of choice for recurrent in situ lesions because excellent control and preservation of excellent voice quality can be achieved with minimal morbidity.

EARLY (T1-T2) VOCAL CORD CARCINOMA. RT is the preferred initial treatment, with surgery reserved for salvage of RT failures in most centers. Although similar cure rates can be achieved with hemilaryngectomy or cordectomy for select T1-T2 vocal cord carcinomas, voice quality is usually better after RT than after surgery. If RT fails, salvage surgery is successful in 75% to 85% of the patients in whom surgery is attempted. Conservation surgery with voice preservation may still be possible in select patients with recurrent vocal cord carcinoma after RT.[57,58]

T3 VOCAL CORD CARCINOMA. Fixed vocal cord lesions are indicative of deep muscle or cartilage infiltration. Relatively early fixed vocal cord lesions can be treated initially with RT concurrent with chemotherapy, reserving surgery for salvage.[31] Total laryngectomy is the preferred treatment for more advanced lesions with bilateral vocal cord involvement and compromised airway. Local control rates in select cases of T3 vocal cord carcinoma treated with RT alone are approximately 30% to 60%, and approximately 40% to 50% of the failures are salvaged by surgery. Based on the preliminary RTOG larynx preservation trial, which included T3 tumors, the 2-year local-regional control rate is 78% in patients who received concurrent chemotherapy and radiation therapy versus 56% (*P* < 0.01).

ADVANCED (T4) VOCAL CORD CARCINOMA. Advanced (T4) vocal cord carcinoma is best managed with total laryngectomy and postoperative RT. A neck dissection is usually performed when there are positive lymph nodes. Methods of voice rehabilitation after total laryngectomy and postoperative radiation therapy include tracheoesophageal puncture and artificial larynx.[59] Select lesions with minimal cartilage invasion can be treated initially with RT. RT is also used in patients who have medical contraindications to surgery or who have refused total laryngectomy.

Postoperative RT is indicated when there is tumor at or close to the surgical margins; cartilage invasion; involvement of the soft tissues of the neck; extensive subglottic infiltration; multiple (more than one) lymph node metastases; extracapsular nodal extension; and perineural, lymphatic, or vascular invasion.

VERRUCOUS CARCINOMA. Treatment of verrucous carcinoma of the vocal cords has been controversial. Some regard it as a lesion with limited radioresponsiveness, and anaplastic transformation has been reported to occur after RT.[60] However, others have found that RT and surgery are equally effective and that anaplastic transformation rarely occurs.[10,62] Treatment for this rare lesion should be based on the extent of the disease. Small tumors can be treated by excision or partial laryngectomy. RT is recommended for large tumors that would require total laryngectomy if treated surgically.

Carcinoma of the Subglottis

Primary carcinomas of the subglottis are rare. Most of these lesions are relatively advanced at the time of diagnosis and are managed primarily with surgery followed by postoperative RT. RT alone is used for early lesions and for patients who refuse surgery or have medical contraindications to surgery.[63-65]

SIMULATION

Simulation is performed with the patient in the treatment position: supine with the head hyperextended. The head is immobilized with a face mask. The anterior skin of the neck at the midline is outlined with a strip of radiopaque lead foil tape or wire. Palpable cervical lymphadenopathy is outlined with a radiopaque wire. A lateral radiograph is taken after reviewing the field outline with fluoroscopy. During fluoroscopy, motion of the larynx as a result of swallowing and breathing should be noted. If it exceeds 1 cm, the portals should be lengthened. The central axis is tattooed on both sides of the neck to ensure a reproducible daily setup (Fig. 31-7).

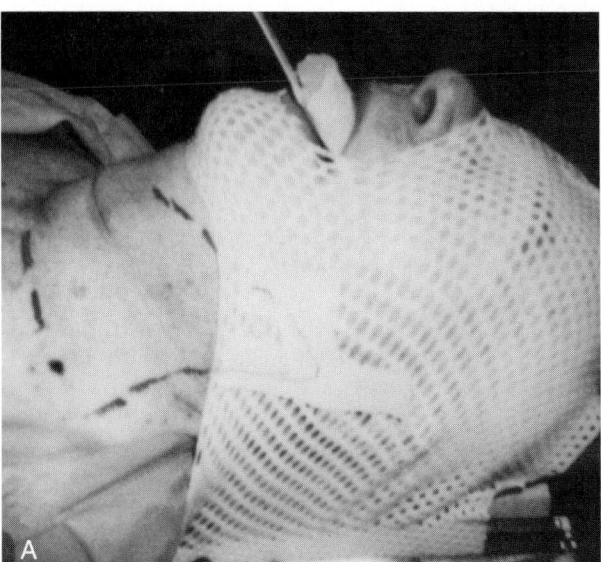
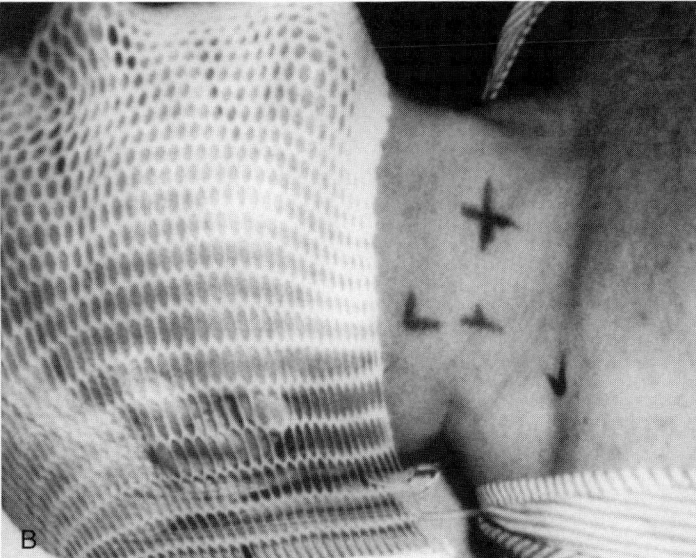

Figure 31–7. Patient in mask in the treatment position for a supraglottic carcinoma (**A**) and glottic cancer (**B**).

All patients should undergo CT treatment planning with 3 mm cuts to accurately define the gross tumor volume unless otherwise contraindicated. This has been reported to correlate with local control.[66-69]

When an anterior low neck field is used, the gantry for the two opposed lateral fields for the upper neck is angled a few degrees so that the lower border of the lateral fields for the upper neck matches the divergence of the upper border of the low neck field on the skin. A lower lateral spinal cord block, 2 cm in height, is placed in the inferior-posterior portion of the lateral upper neck fields to avoid overlap over the spinal cord at depth owing to divergence of the lateral beams. Alternatively, a split-beam technique is used so that the central axes of the beams meet at the junction of the upper and low neck fields and there is no overlap owing to beam divergence. In a patient with a short neck, the shoulders are pulled down with autotraction straps.

RADIOTHERAPY TECHNIQUES

Beam Energy

Linear accelerators with 4 to 6 MV photons or ^{60}Co machines and 6 to 15 MeV electrons for supplemental boosting to the nodes are commonly used. Treatment distance should be at least 80 cm source-to-skin distance (SSD). Because of the skin- and lymph node–sparing effects of higher-energy photons, bolus material is used with photon energies of 6 MV or more. In a study of patients with glottic carcinoma irradiated with 6 MV x-rays, a lower local control rate was noted in patients with gross involvement of the anterior commissure.[70] Other studies have reported inferior local control rates with T1 glottic carcinoma with anterior commissure involvement. This may be the result of technical factors (e.g., the use of wedge filters[71] or understaging of these tumors) as in one series, none of the patients had a pretreatment CT scan.[72]

Treatment Volume and Radiation Field Arrangements

CARCINOMA OF THE SUPRAGLOTTIS. Because of the propensity for lymphatic spread, the treatment volume for carcinoma of the supraglottis should include the primary lesion as well as the regional lymphatics in the neck. Other than T1N0 lesions, accelerated fractionated RT using a concomitant boost technique is recommended. A pair of lateral opposed fields is used to irradiate the primary tumor and the upper cervical lymph nodes with a minimum 2 to 3 cm margin around the tumor and positive lymph nodes (Fig. 31-8). A single anterior low neck field is used to irradiate the low neck. A spinal cord block 2 cm in height is placed in the inferior-posterior portion of the lateral upper neck fields to shield the area of overlap on the spinal cord at the junction for the upper and lower neck fields. The upper border of the lateral fields should adequately cover the upper jugular nodes. The lower border of the lateral fields should encompass the larynx, usually at or below the level of C5. If there is

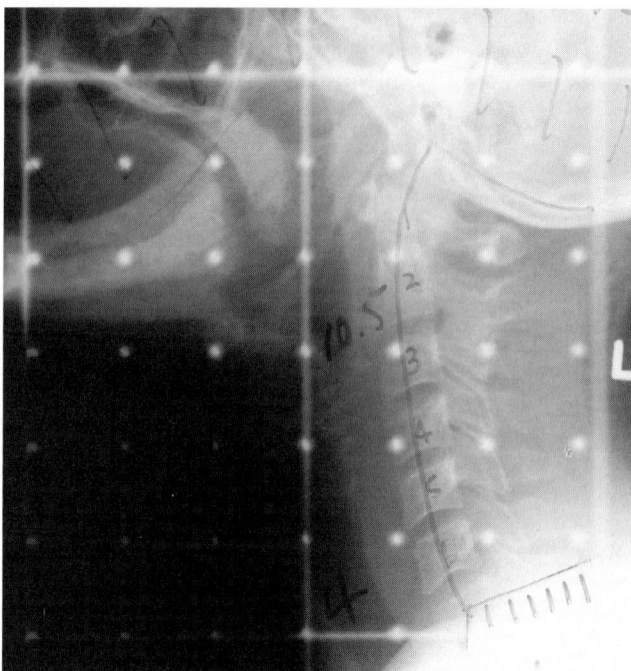

Figure 31–8. Simulation film of a patient with T3N1 carcinoma of the supraglottic larynx.

involvement of the pyriform sinus, lateral or posterior hypopharyngeal wall, or both, the superior border is placed at the base of the skull (above C1) to include the retropharyngeal lymph nodes. The posterior neck should be included in the treatment volume when there are positive lymph nodes in the anterior neck and for T3 and T4 lesions. The spinal cord should be shielded after 45 Gy, and electrons with appropriate energies are used for supplemental boosting to the posterior cervical lymph nodes. The total dose to these opposed-lateral fields is 54 Gy. A second, smaller boost field is delivered concomitantly after 32.4 Gy. The boost fields starts on day 19 of treatment and includes only the primary tumor volume along with any gross nodal disease with at least a 1 to 1.5 cm margin around the initial primary tumor and the positive lymph nodes. The boost fields receive 1.5 Gy per fraction to a total dose of 18 Gy. Figure 31-9 is a three-dimensional CT treatment plan for a patient who presented with T3N0 supraglottic carcinoma.

When there is extensive subglottic involvement or positive lymph nodes in the low neck or supraclavicular fossa, or both, a mediastinal T-field is used for the initial 45 to 50 Gy. The lateral limbs of the T-field should be below the clavicle, and the center portion of the T-field should extend 5 cm below the lower border of the clavicle head to include the upper mediastinum. When there are one or more positive nodes in the posterior low neck, an additional posterior field may be necessary to deliver a supplemental dose to these nodes.

CARCINOMA OF THE GLOTTIS. For T1 and early T2 lesions, two small opposing lateral fields centering on the vocal cords and parallel to the trachea, extending from the upper thyroid notch superiorly to the lower border of

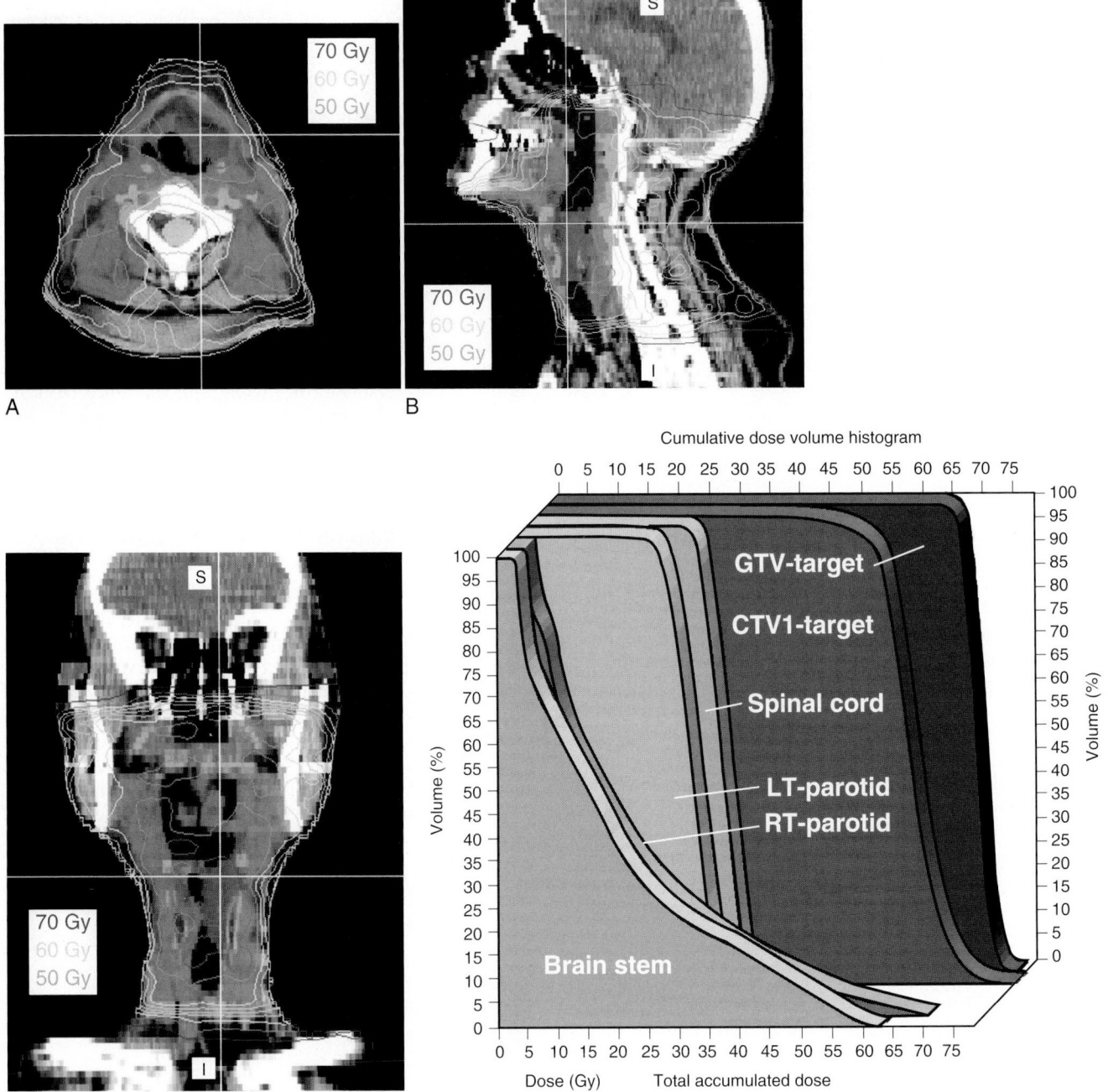

Figure 31–9. Three-dimensional treatment plan for supraglottic larynx cancer. Isodose distribution on the axial plane (**A**), sagittal plane (**B**), and coronal plane (**C**). **D**, Dose-volume histogram. Curves shown for external surface, spinal cord, and tumor as derived from CT scan. See also Color Figure 31-9.

the cricoid (at the lower border of C6) inferiorly, should be used. The anterior border should be 1 cm anterior to the skin surface at the level of the vocal cords. The posterior border of the field should include the anterior portion of the posterior pharyngeal wall. A 5 × 5 cm field is usually sufficient for T1 and early T2 vocal cord carcinomas (see Fig. 31-10). A three-dimensional CT treatment plan for early glottic cancer is depicted in Figure 31-11. Note that all the true and false cords and the upper subglottis are covered by the 95% isodose surface.

The need for elective neck irradiation for T2N0 vocal cord carcinomas is controversial. Wang[15,73] recommended elective irradiation of the subdigastric and midjugular nodes when there is impaired vocal cord mobility. Harwood and colleagues[74] also recommended elective irradiation of at least the first-echelon lymph nodes for all T2 vocal cord carcinomas. However, Mendenhall and associates[75] noted that the risk of occult neck nodes was only 3% when the primary site was controlled and 22% when there was recurrence at the primary site.

They concluded that elective irradiation is not indicated for T2N0 squamous cell carcinoma of the glottis but recommended that a neck dissection be considered in conjunction with the salvage surgery for local recurrence. A similar treatment policy is recommended by Howell-Burke and coworkers.[76] We have not routinely carried out elective neck irradiation when there is minimal extension beyond the vocal cords but have included at least the first-echelon nodes for the initial 45 to 50 Gy when there is extensive supraglottic and infraglottic extension.

For extensive T3 and T4 lesions treated with RT alone, larger lateral fields that include the subdigastric and midjugular nodes and a separate anterior low neck field that includes the lower jugular nodes are used.

CARCINOMA OF THE SUBGLOTTIS. A pair of lateral opposed upper neck fields inferiorly extending at least 2 cm below the primary tumor and superiorly encompassing the upper jugular nodes and an anterior low neck and upper mediastinum T-field are usually used.

Treatment Planning and Dose Fractionation

CARCINOMA OF THE SUPRAGLOTTIS. Tissue-equivalent compensators or wedges, with appropriate angles based on the contours of the neck or CT scan treatment planning, are used to achieve uniform dose distribution within the target volume. For stage I lesions, a dose of 66 to 70 Gy is usually delivered at 2 Gy per fraction to the primary tumor and positive lymph nodes. An additional 2 to 5 Gy may be used to boost large primary tumors and neck nodes using reduced fields. A dose of 50 Gy is delivered to areas at risk for microscopic disease. The dose to the anterior low neck and supraclavicular fossa is calculated at 3 cm depth and to the upper mediastinum at 5 cm depth.

Twice-a-day hyperfractionated RT is recommended for lesions T2 or greater; a total dose of 74.4 to 76.8 Gy at 1.2 Gy/fraction, 2 fractions/day, is delivered to the primary tumor and the upper neck nodes.[45] A minimum daily interfraction interval of 6 hours is recommended to minimize late normal tissue toxicity. The spinal cord is shielded after 45.6 Gy. An alternative technique, described earlier, is to use an accelerated fractionated RT using a concomitant boost technique.[47]

For postoperative RT following total laryngectomy, a total dose of 63 Gy at 1.8 Gy/fraction per day, 5 days/week, is delivered to the tumor bed and the upper neck, with the spinal cord shielded after 45 Gy. An additional 6 to 10 Gy, at 2 Gy per fraction, is delivered through reduced fields to areas of positive margins or gross residual disease. A dose of 50.4 Gy is delivered to the supraclavicular fossa. The tracheal stoma is usually included in the anterior low neck field. It is usually not necessary to place a bolus over the stomal site if ^{60}Co or 4 MV x-rays are used. If higher-energy x-rays are used, bolus of the stomal site is recommended. An additional 10 Gy is delivered through a reduced boost field to the tracheal stoma using 9 to 12 MeV electrons with 0.5 cm bolus. Indications of stoma boost include emergency tracheostomy, subglottic extension, extensive involvement of the soft tissues of the neck, or a surgical scar that crosses over the stoma. Postoperative RT is recommended to begin within 3 to 4 weeks after surgery when the wound is healed.

CARCINOMA OF THE GLOTTIS. For T1-2 carcinoma of the vocal cord, a total dose of 66 to 70 Gy at 2 Gy/fraction per day or 63 to 65.25 Gy at 2.25 Gy/fraction per day, 5 days/week, is commonly used. Lower total doses are used for small tumors, and higher total doses are used for large tumors. A contour of the neck or CT scans of the neck in the treatment volume are used for computerized treatment planning. Open fields, wedged fields (see Figs. 31-10 and 31-11), or mixed open and wedged lateral fields are used, depending on the shape of the neck in the region of the larynx. The objective is to deliver a uniform dose distribution throughout the target volume. For advanced T3 and T4 carcinoma of the glottis and subglottis, the dose fractionation schedule is similar to that for supraglottic carcinomas.

Three-Dimensional Conformal Radiotherapy (Forward-Planned Multi-Segment Technique or Intensity-Modulated Radiotherapy)

Over the past several years, intensity-modulated RT (IMRT) has gained popularity and has proved its value in preserving salivary function in the treatment of head and neck cancer. With this technique, radiation beams can be modulated so that a high dose can be delivered to the tumor target while significantly reducing the dose to the surrounding normal tissues. Please see Chapter 27, Nasopharynx for details of patient setup. Figure 31-12 is an example of an inverse-planned IMRT technique for a patient who presented with T3N1 squamous cell carcinoma of the supraglottic larynx. The patient is a

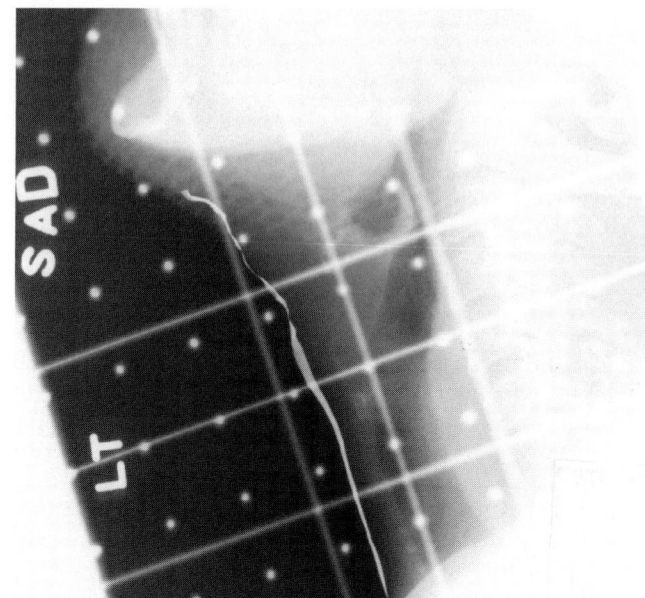

Figure 31–10. Simulation film of patient with T1 or T2 glottic cancer.

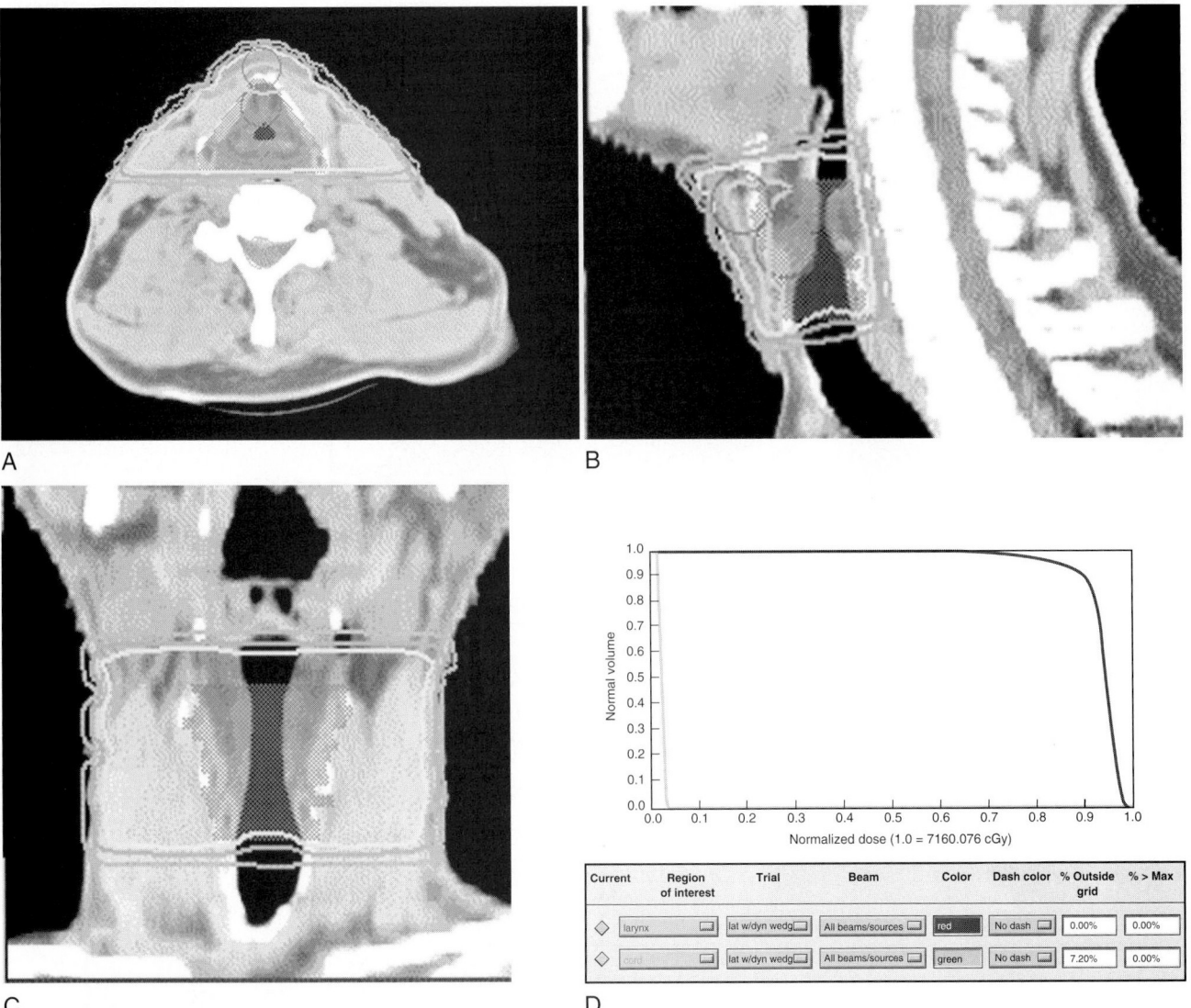

Figure 31–11. Isodose distribution on the axial plane (**A**), sagittal plane (**B**), and coronal plane (**C**). **D**, Dose-volume histogram for the tumor and spinal cord. See also Color Figure 31-11.

psychiatrist who was interested in voice preservation and was concerned about xerostomia. Therefore, we elected to treat him using the Corvus treatment planning system (NOMOS Corporation, Sewickley, Pa). The total treatment time including patient setup was approximately 50 minutes. The patient tolerated treatment well. Although computer-optimized or inverse-planned IMRT is the most ideal IMRT treatment technique, it is not available in every RT clinic and not every patient is a candidate for this method of treatment due to the prolonged treatment time.

At UCSF, we have developed a forward-planned multi-segment technique (FPMS)[77] that achieves a comparable dose distribution to inverse-planned IMRT. Accurate patient setup is essential for this technique. At the first simulation, immobilization is with a head and shoulder mask with the appropriate neck support on a Timo (Uni-Frame System, MED-TEC, Orange City, Iowa). The patient should be supine with the head hyperextended

such that the tip of the uvula and base of skull are parallel to the beam axis (Fig. 31-13). The cervical spinal cord and brainstem should be as straight as possible, parallel to the table. This is very important, especially when using multi-leaf collimators (MLC) to shield the spinal cord and the brainstem. CT scans in serial 3 mm axial slices are obtained for treatment planning. Treatment planning is carried out using the ADAC-Pinnacle Treatment Planning System. The gross tumor volume (GTV) and clinical tumor volume (CTV) as well as surrounding critical normal structures are outlined on the axial CT slices, along with a margin for patient set-up errors. Treatment planning usually takes about 2 to 3 days. Figure 31-14 is an example of an FPMS technique. This patient also presented with a history of T3N1 squamous cell carcinoma of the supraglottic larynx and received concurrent cisplatin chemotherapy with radiation therapy. Because the patient has a short neck and broad shoulders, it was impossible to treat all of his larynx in

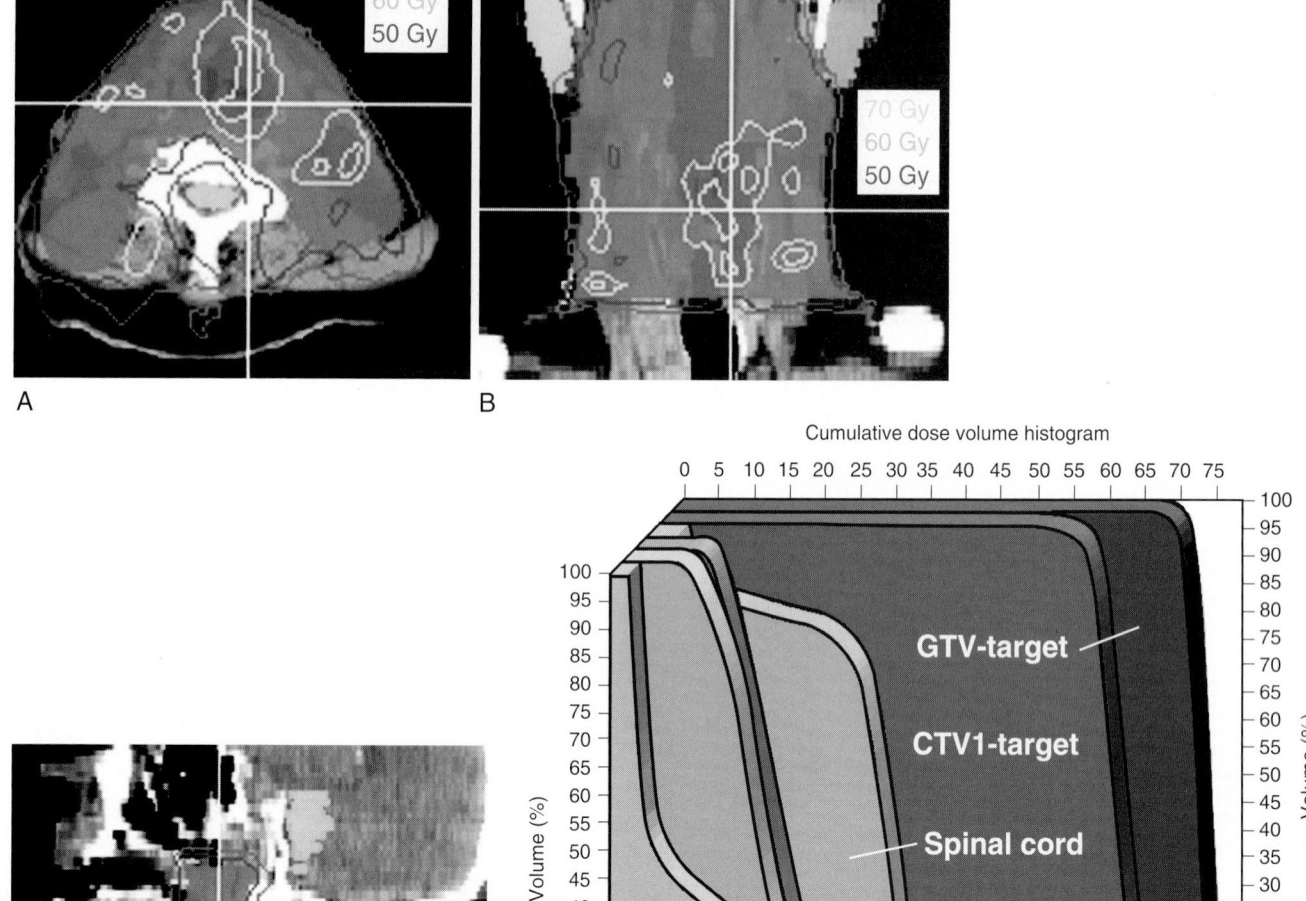

Figure 31–12. Isodose curves of an inverse intensity-modulated radiation therapy plan using seven coplanar gantry angles delivered with conventional multi-leaf collimators for a patient with T3N1 carcinoma of the larynx displayed on the axial (**A**), coronal (**B**), and sagittal (**C**) planes through the centroid of the primary tumor and the dose-volume histogram for the relevant structures (**D**). The gross tumor volume is shown in *red* and the clinical tumor volume (including margin for patient set-up errors) in *magenta*. See also Color Figure 31-12.

the opposed lateral fields without treating his shoulders. The decision was to treat him using IMRT. However, due to his elderly age, he was unable to tolerate the prolonged treatment time associated with inverse-planned IMRT. Therefore, the patient underwent a 13-field FPMS technique.

EFFECTS OF TREATMENT ON NORMAL TISSUES

The acute and late effects of RT or combined RT and surgery for carcinoma of the larynx depend on a number of factors: total dose,[14,78-80] dose per fraction,[14,78,80-82]

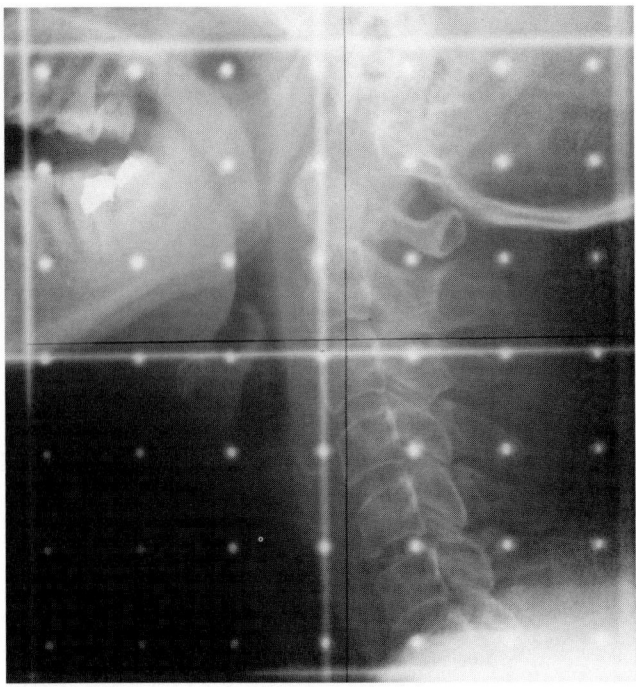

Figure 31–13. Initial simulation film of a lateral view of the larynx. The patient's head is hyperextended and immobilized with a head mask supported on a Timo (Uni-Frame System, MED-TEC, Orange City, Iowa).

treatment volume,[78,80,81,83] overall time,[84] stage of the disease,[14,80,82] sequence of RT and surgery (i.e., pre- vs. postoperative RT),[85,86] surgical technique,[82] and chemotherapy.[87] Daily interfraction interval is also a major determinant of late effects with hyperfractionated RT.[88] Both acute and late normal tissue effects may be exacerbated in the presence of other medical conditions such as diabetes, immune suppression, and collagen vascular disease.

Because of the lack of standardized quantitative criteria for scoring acute and late normal tissue effects of treatment and heterogeneity in treatment techniques among different centers, the incidence and type of complications reported in different series are quite variable and are not directly comparable.

Acute Effects

Acute reactions that occur during fractionated RT for carcinoma of the vocal cords are usually mild. The patient may have an increase of hoarseness, sore throat, dysphagia, patchy mucositis, erythema, and increased pigmentation of the skin in the radiation field. These acute reactions may initially increase and then stabilize toward the latter part of the treatment course. They usually subside completely within 6 to 8 weeks after completion of treatment. In the majority of patients, the voice returns to normal within a few months after treatment.

Acute radiation reactions are more severe during fractionated RT for carcinoma of the supraglottic larynx because of the increased volume of tissues irradiated. In addition to hoarseness and sore throat, change or loss of taste, dry mouth, dysphagia, and weight loss can occur.

The severity of these acute reactions increases with treatment volume.

The acute reactions of twice-daily hyperfractionated or accelerated fractionated RT are usually more severe than those with once-daily conventional fractionated RT.[45,46]

Late Effects

Laryngeal edema of varying degrees may persist after RT for carcinoma of the glottis or supraglottis. In patients irradiated for carcinoma of the glottis, the incidence of mild to moderate laryngeal edema persisting for more than 3 months after RT is about 15.4% to 25%.[78,79,81] The incidence of severe laryngeal edema is about 1.5% to 4.6%.[14,16,76,83,89] The incidence of laryngeal edema increases with greater total dose, field size, dose per fraction, and T stage of the lesion.[14,78,79,81,83,90] In a randomized study to determine the effect of radiation field size on the local control of early glottic carcinomas reported by Inoue and colleagues,[83] 116 patients were treated with a total dose of 60 Gy in 30 fractions over 6 weeks using 4 MV x-rays and wedge filters. Persistent laryngeal edema occurred in 4% of the patients treated with 5×5 cm^2 fields and in 21% of the patients with 6×6 cm^2 fields. The difference was significant, with $P < 0.02$. However, local control rates were similar, being 93% and 95% with a field size of 5×5 cm^2 and 6×6 cm^2, respectively.

Persistent laryngeal edema after RT for carcinoma of the vocal cord often presents a management dilemma to the radiation oncologist and head and neck surgeon. In a series of 247 patients irradiated for carcinoma of the vocal cord, laryngeal edema persisting for more than 3 months following RT developed in 38 patients (15.4%).[79] In 17 (44.7%) of these patients, the laryngeal edema was associated with persistent or recurrent disease, although only 25.4% of the patients with uncontrolled disease had laryngeal edema. Our current policy in the management of patients with persistent laryngeal edema following RT for carcinoma of the vocal cord is to adopt initially conservative measures with voice rest; abstinence from alcohol and cigarettes; and careful, close follow-up examinations, including direct laryngoscopy if necessary. Antibiotics and steroids may be used when there is suspicion of infection or when the edema is severe enough to significantly compromise the airway. If it is mild and stable, if no visible recurrence develops, and especially if it is limited to the arytenoids, no biopsy is attempted because of the risk of inducing laryngeal necrosis. However, if the edema is progressive and unresponsive to conservative measures, and persistent and recurrent disease is strongly suspected, biopsies are carried out to establish the diagnosis. Salvage surgery is performed if biopsies are positive. MRI may be useful in separating edema from tumor.

The risk of late effects in the larynx is strongly dependent on the fraction size.[14,78,81,90] In a series of 208 patients irradiated for T1-T2 carcinomas of the vocal cord reported by Deore and associates,[81] moderate to severe late laryngeal edema developed in 44% of the patients

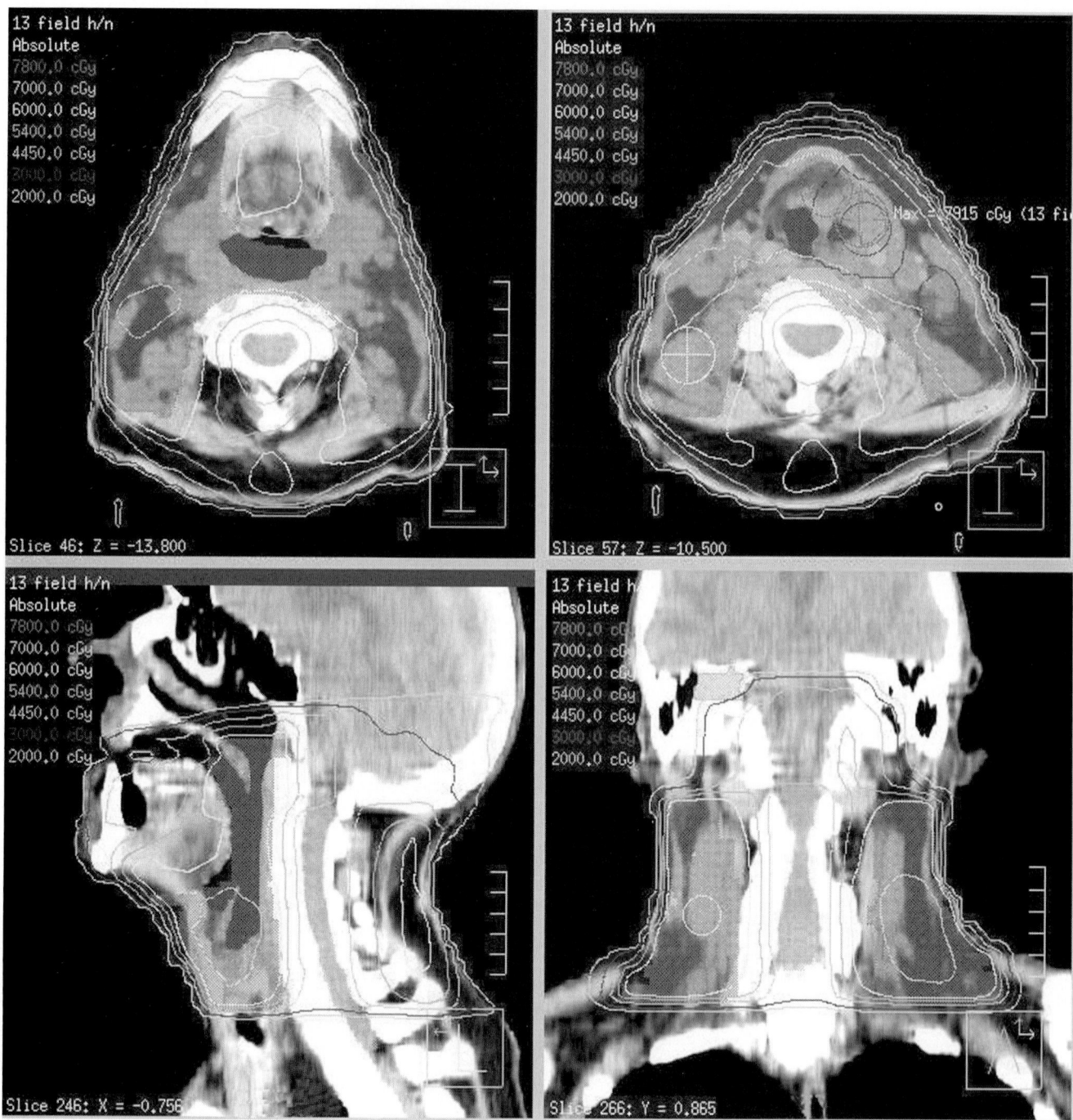

Figure 31–14. Isodose curves of a 13-field forward intensity-modulated radiation therapy plan for a patient with T3N1 carcinoma of the larynx displayed on the axial, coronal, and sagittal planes through the centroid of the primary tumor and the dose-volume histogram for the relevant structures.

who received 50 Gy in 3 weeks at 3.33 Gy/fraction, in 18% of the patients who received 60 Gy in 5 weeks at 2.5 Gy/fraction, and in 17.2% of the patients who received 60.75 Gy in 5.5 weeks at 2.25 Gy/fraction. In a series of 303 patients irradiated for T1 or T2 glottic carcinoma reported by Mendenhall and coworkers,[14] the incidence of moderately severe and severe complications was in 2 of 7 (29%) with 2.25 to 2.55 Gy/fraction and 0 of 14 with 1.75 to 2.24 Gy/fraction when a total dose

of 67 to 70 Gy. It was 0.7% with 2.25 to 2.55 Gy/fraction and 2.2% with 1.75 to 2.24 Gy/fraction for a total dose of 60 to 66 Gy was given.

Late laryngeal necrosis following RT is rare, with a reported incidence of about 0.5% to 1.8% for glottic cancer[17,76,78,89,91] and 1% to 2.5% for supraglottic cancer.[47,92]

In a series of 60 patients with intermediate-stage supraglottic carcinoma who underwent supraglottic

Table 31–2   Carcinoma of the Supraglottis: Local Control with Radiotherapy and Surgical Salvage

Reference	Stage	Patients, n	Initial Local Control, %	Surgical Salvage, n/n*	Ultimate Local Control, %	Larynx Preservation, %
Johansen et al[30]	T1a	74	63			
	T1b	77	63			
	T2	86	62			
	T3	85	45			
	T4	76	42			
Harwood et al[92]	T1N0	87	71			
	T2N0	44	68			
	T3N0	30	56			
	T4N0	94	52			
	T4N1	45	45			
	T4N3	29	41			
Wall et al[95]	T1	38	89			
	T2	132	74			
	T3	50	70			
	T4	28	46			
Hinerman et al[41]	T1	18	100		100	100
	T2	109	85	6/12	91	86
	T3	87	62	16/22	80	68
	T4	21	57	4/4	76	68
Wang[15†]	T1	73	75	5/9	82	
	T2	109	50	9/19	58	
	T3	85	38	10/17	49	
	T4	107	26	3/20	29	

*No. of patients salvaged/no. of patients who underwent salvage.
†Carcinoma of the larynx.

laryngectomy, 50 (83%) underwent postoperative RT.[93] Minor complications occurred in nine patients (14%), including three with vocal cord paralysis, two with dysphagia caused by stricture or esophageal dysmotility, two with fistulas, one with hematoma, and one with wound infection. Significant complications occurred in another nine patients (14%). Seven patients (11%) required gastrostomy for prolonged inability to maintain adequate oral intake; one required intravenous hyperalimentation, and one had a tracheostomy. Major complications included two postoperative deaths and three patients

(5%) who underwent total laryngectomy for intractable aspiration.

OUTCOME OF THERAPY

Carcinoma of the Supraglottis

Recent results of primary RT for carcinoma of the supraglottis are shown in Tables 31-2 and 31-3. Initial local control rates are in the range of 63% to 100% for T1,

Table 31–3   Carcinoma of the Supraglottis: Survival After Radiotherapy and Surgical Salvage

Reference	Stage	Patients, n	5-Y Absolute Survival, %	5-Y Cause-Specific
Johansen et al[30]	I	131	60	74
	II	73	53	78
	III	93	47	59
	IV	101	31	39
	All	218	45.0	
Harwood et al[92]	All	410	41*	62*
Hinerman et al[41]	I	17	65	100
	II	74	59	93
	III	79	53	81
	IVA	87	33	50
	IVB	17	6	13

*Actuarial survival.

50% to 85% for T2, 38% to 70% for T3, and 26% to 46% for T4 lesions. Survival rates are lower than local control rates because of deaths from intercurrent diseases and second primaries. The presence of lymphadenopathy, especially with lymph nodes greater than 3 cm in diameter, has an adverse effect on local control as well as survival.[92,94,95] However, in a multivariate analysis by Freeman and colleagues,[96] local control of supraglottic carcinoma depended on T classification and was not influenced by neck stage. Overgaard and associates[22] noted that in patients with supraglottic carcinoma, females with hemoglobin levels above 13g% and males with levels above 14.5g% had a significantly better prognosis than comparable patients with lower hemoglobin levels. Nguyen-Tan et al.[37] also found that hemoglobin levels greater than or equal to 12.5 g/dL during RT were a favorable prognostic factor for local-regional control and overall survival. However, Wall and coworkers[95] noted no correlation between initial hemoglobin level and the probability of primary tumor control.

Hyperfractionated RT[47,97] and split-course accelerated fractionated RT[46] have been used in the treatment of carcinoma of the supraglottis. Retrospective comparisons suggest higher local control rates with twice-daily fractionated RT for T2-T3 carcinoma of the larynx and hypopharynx than historical controls treated with once-daily fractionated RT.[45] A randomized trial by the RTOG (90-03) comparing the relative efficacy of hyperfractionated or accelerated fractionated RT using a concomitant boost technique without a split course with standard fractionation showed improvement in local control and disease-free survival at 2 years in patients who presented with stage II–IV supraglottic laryngeal carcinoma.[48]

For advanced operable lesions, combined surgery with postoperative RT offers improved local control rates compared with the results of either RT or surgery alone.[37] Wang[15] reported a 5-year actuarial NED (no evidence of disease) rate of 93% for T2, 64% for T3, and 48% for T4 lesions. Approximately 80% of these patients had preoperative RT. Lee and colleagues[93] reported a 5-year determinate disease-free survival of

91% in 60 patients (3 with T1, 32 with T2, 21 with T3, and 4 with T4 lesions) selected from a total of 404 patients who underwent supraglottic laryngectomy. Fifty of the patients (83%) received postoperative RT. There were no failures at the primary site, although four patients developed recurrence in the neck. These results compared favorably with those achieved with supraglottic laryngectomy or RT alone for similar lesions.[39,40] Alternatively, properly selected patients can be treated with concurrent chemotherapy and RT in an attempt to preserve the larynx, as discussed earlier.

In the RTOG randomized trial of preoperative versus postoperative RT for advanced head and neck carcinoma, the 5-year local-regional control rate in patients with supraglottic carcinoma was significantly better with postoperative RT than with preoperative RT (77% vs. 53%, $P = 0.007$).[43] However, this did not result in a statistically significant difference in survival.

Carcinoma of the Glottis

The local control rate of carcinoma in situ of the vocal cords is similar to the results with T1 invasive carcinoma. Pene and Fletcher[99] reported on a series of 79 patients with carcinoma in situ and 7 patients with leukoplakia or atypical hyperplasia or both treated with RT. The initial local control rate was 85%. After surgical salvage of the failures, the ultimate local control rate was 99%. A 5-year recurrence-free rate of 83% was reported by Elman and associates[53] in a group of 69 patients with in situ carcinoma of the vocal cords treated with RT. More recently, Spayne and associates[55] reported the Princess Margaret Hospital experience of 67 patients treated with moderate-dose radiation therapy of 51 Gy in 20 daily fractions. With a median follow-up of 6.5 years, the 5-year actuarial local control rate was 98% with only one patient who developed invasive glottic cancer and eventually underwent salvage laryngectomy.

Results of primary RT for T1 and T2 carcinoma of the glottis are shown in Tables 31-4 through 31-7. For T1 lesions, the initial local control rates are in the range of 83% to 95%, and the ultimate local control rates after

Table 31–4   Stage T1 Carcinoma of the Glottis: Local Control with Radiotherapy and Surgical Salvage

Reference	Patients, n	Initial Local Control, %	Surgical Salvage, n/n (%)*	Ultimate Local Control, %	Larynx Preservation, %
Fletcher[§]	332	89	31/36 (86)	98	
Mittal et al[91]	177	83	23/30 (77)	96	90
Amornmarn et al[89]	86	92	6/7 (86)	99	92
Mendenhall et al[106]	291	95	18/18 (58)	98	95
Wang[15†]	723	90	46/59 (78)	97	90
Johansen et al[102]	358	83	40/55 (73)	94	91
Le et al[84]	315	83	41/52 (79)	97	89
Spector et al[27]	104[‡]	89	7/11 (64)	96	89

*No. of patients salvaged/no. of patients who underwent salvage treatment.
[†]Carcinoma of the larynx.
[‡]Patients treated with a mean dose of 66.5 Gy.
[§]Fletcher GH, Treatment of cancer of the Larynx. *Ear Nose Throat J.* 1977;56(3):91–96.

Table 31–5   Stage T2 Carcinoma of the Glottis: Local Control with Radiotherapy and Surgical Salvage

Reference	Patients, n	Initial Local Control, %	Surgical Salvage, n/n (%)*	Ultimate Local Control, %	Larynx Preservation, %
Fletcher[§]	175	74	36/41 (88)	94	
Haugen et al[100]	45	88[†]	2/2 (100)	85	
Amornmarn et al[89]	34	88	2/4 (50)	94	88
Karim et al[103]	156	81	20/25 (80)	95	
Mendenhall et al[106]	146	82	40/49 (82)	96	82
	82	70		96	76
Wang[15‡]	173	69	28/43 (65)	86	71
Howell-Burke et al[76]	114	68	25/34 (74)	94	74
Le et al[84]	83	67	20/27 (74)	92	72

*No. of patients salvaged/no. of patients who underwent salvage treatment.
[†]Actuarial local control.
[‡]Carcinoma of the larynx.
[§]Fletcher GH, Treatment of Cancer of the Larynx. *Ear Nose Throat J.* 1977;56(3):91-96.

surgical salvage of failures are in the range of 94% to 99%. The larynx is preserved in 89% to 95% of the patients irradiated.

For T2 carcinoma of the glottis treated with primary RT, the initial local control rates are in the range of 67% to 88%. After surgical salvage, the ultimate local control rates are in the range of 85% to 96%. The larynx is preserved in 71% to 88% of the patients irradiated. A recent report showed that hyperfractionation compared with standard fractionation improved local control in patients who present with T2N0 glottic lesions.[100] Impaired vocal cord mobility is associated with lower local control rate and survival in some series.[13,73,74,101] Others report similar results, whether the cord mobility is normal or impaired.[76,102,103] Anterior commissure involvement does not worsen local control and survival in most series[14,16,91,104] Subglottic extension, poorly differentiated histopathology, and the male gender have been associated with poorer results in some series.[73,84,89,104,105] Others have noted no significant difference in the results with respect to subglottic extension, gender, or differentiation.[76,91]

Local control rate is also related to total dose and dose per fraction.[16,27,80,106-110] Local control rates are higher with 2 to 2.25 Gy/fraction than with 1.8 Gy/fraction for

a similar total dose.[78] A recent review of T1 and T2 glottic carcinoma treated at the University of California–San Francisco (UCSF) shows that this is true primarily for T2 lesions, although there is a trend for T1 lesions also.[84] Shorter overall time also leads to improved results.[84] A recent publication supports the fact that pretreatment hemoglobin is an independent prognostic factor for local control in patients with T1, T2 carcinoma of the glottis treated with RT. A level below 12 g/dL significantly decreased local control.[111]

The 5-year determinate survival rates, after adjusting for deaths from intercurrent disease or second primaries, range from 94% to 98% for T1 lesions (see Table 31-6) and 78% to 93% for T2 lesions (see Table 31-7).

Advanced carcinomas of the glottis can be treated with surgery or combined surgery and RT. Results of selective stage T3-T4 carcinoma of the glottis treated with primary RT are shown in Table 31-8. The initial local control rates range from 23% to 62%, and the ultimate local control rates after surgical salvage, 37% to 81%. Five-year determinate or cause-specific survival rates range from 57% to 74%. Alternatively, properly selected patients should be considered and treated with a larynx preservation protocol using concurrent chemotherapy and RT, as discussed earlier.

Table 31–6   Stage T1 Carcinoma of the Glottis: Survival After Radiotherapy and Surgical Salvage

Reference	Patients, n	5-Yr Survival, %
Mittal et al[91]	177	97 (determinate)
Amornmarn et al[89]	86	96 (determinate disease-free)
Mendenhall et al[106]	291	80 (absolute) 98 (cause-specific)
Johansen et al[102]	358	94 (determinate)
Le et al[84]	315	84 (actuarial) 97 (cause-specific)
Spector et al[27]	104	83 (actuarial) 95 (disease-specific)

Table 31–7   Stage T2 Carcinoma of the Glottis: Survival After Radiotherapy and Surgical Salvage

Reference	Patients, n	5-Yr Survival, %
Amornmarn et al[890]	34	88 (determinate disease-free)
Karim et al[103]	156	68 (actuarial) 92 (determinate)
Mendenhall et al[106]	228	77 (absolute) 93 (cause-specific)
Howell-Burke et al[76]	114	69 (actuarial) 92 (determinate)
Le et al[84]	83	78 (actuarial)

Table 31–8 Stage T3–4 Carcinoma of the Glottis: Results of Radiotherapy and Surgical Salvage

Reference	Stage	Patients, *n*	Minimum Follow-up, Y	Initial Local Control, %	Ultimate Local Control, %	5-Y Survival, %
Stewart and Jackson[80]	T3	67	10.0	57	69	57 (determinate)
Harwood et al[105]	T3N0	112	3.0	51	77	74 (determinate)
Harwood et al[108]	T4N0	56	3.0	56		65 (determinate)
Woodhouse et al[16]	T3–T4	17	3.5	50	57	
Van den Bogaert et al[104]	T3	33	5.0	23	37	22 (actuarial)
	T4	2				
Mendenhall et al[14]	T3	47	2.0	62	81	58 (absolute)
Wang[15]*	T3	65	3.0	32	57	

*Carcinoma of the larynx.

Carcinoma of the Subglottis

Data on the results of RT for carcinoma of the subglottis are sparse. Vermund[64] in 1970 reported a 5-year survival rate of 36% in 127 patients treated with primary RT and 42% in 58 patients treated with primary surgery from pooled data in the literature. Warde and colleagues[112] reported on a series of 23 patients treated with initial radical RT. Local control was achieved in 16 patients (70%), and the 5-year actuarial and cause-specific survival rates were 26% and 61%, respectively. More recently, the experience at Princess Margaret Hospital showed that local control was achieved with RT alone in 56% of the patients (*n* = 43) with an ultimate local control rate after attempted surgical salvage of 81.4%. The 5-year actuarial local relapse-free rate was 52% with an overall and cause-specific actuarial survival rate of 50.3% and 66.9%, respectively.[65]

REFERENCES

1. Brennan JA, Boyle JO, Koch WM, et al: Association between cigarette smoking and mutation of the p53 gene in squamous cell carcinoma of the head and neck. *N Engl J Med.* 1995;332:712.
2. Jacob SE, Chacko SS, Pillai MR: Cellular manifestations of human papillomavirus infection in laryngeal tissues. *J Surg Oncol.* 2002;79:142.
3. Sourvinus G, Rizos E, Spandidos DA: p53 Codon 72 polymorphism is linked to the development and not the progression of benign and malignant laryngeal carcinoma. *Oral Oncol.* 2001;37:572.
4. Georgiou A, Gomatos IP, Ferekidis E, et al: Prognostic significance of p53, bax, and bcl-2 gene expression in patients with laryngeal carcinoma. *Eur J Surg Oncol.* 2001;27:574.
5. Narayana A, Vaughan AT, Kathuria S, et al: P53 overexpression is associated with bulky tumor and poor local control in T1 glottic cancer. *Int J Radiat Oncol Biol Phys.* 2000;46:21.
6. Pai HH, Rochon L, Clark B, et al: Overexpression of p53 protein does not predict local-regional control or survival in patients with early-stage squamous cell carcinoma of the glottic larynx treated with radiotherapy. *Int J Radiat Oncol Biol Phys.* 1998;41:37.
7. Yoo SS, Carter D, Turner BC, et al: Prognostic significance of cyclin d1 protein levels in early-stage larynx cancer treated with primary radiation. *Int J Cancer.* 2000;90:22.
8. Lindberg RD: Distribution of cervical lymph node metastases from squamous cell carcinoma of the upper respiratory and digestive tracts. *Cancer.* 1972;29:1446.
9. Batsakis JG, Hybels R, Crissman JD, et al: The pathology of head and neck tumors: Verrucous carcinoma, part 15. *Head Neck Surg.* 1982;5:29.
10. O'Sullivan B, Warde P, Keane T, et al: Outcome following radiotherapy in verrucous carcinoma of the larynx. *Int J Radiat Oncol Biol Phys.* 1995;32:611.
11. Shah JP: Patterns of cervical lymph node metastasis from squamous cell carcinoma of the upper aerodigestive tract. *Am J Surg.* 1990; 160:405.
12. Fu KK, Dedo HH, Phillips TL: Results of integrated management of supraglottic carcinoma. *Cancer.* 1977;40:2874.
13. Kaplan MJ, Johns ME, Clark DA, Cantrell RW: Glottic carcinoma: The roles of surgery and irradiation. *Cancer.* 1984;53:2641.
14. Mendenhall WM, Parsons JT, Million RR: T1-2 squamous cell carcinoma of the glottic larynx treated with radiation therapy: Relationship of dose-fractionation factors to local control and complications. *Int J Radiat Oncol Biol Phys.* 1988;15:1267.
15. Wang CC: Carcinoma of the larynx. In Wang CC, ed. *Indications, Techniques and Results.* Chicago: Yearbook Medical Publishers; 1990:223.
16. Woodhouse RJ, Quivey JM, Fu KK, et al: Treatment of carcinoma of the vocal cords: A review of 20 years experience. *Laryngoscope.* 1981;91:1155.
17. Letterman M: Cancer of the larynx. I: Natural history in relation to treatment. *Br J Radiol.* 1971;44:569.
18. McGavran MH, Bauer WC, and Ogura JH: The incidence of cervical lymph node metastasis from epidermoid carcinoma of the larynx and their relationship to certain characteristics of the primary tumor. A study based on the clinical and pathological findings for 96 patients treated by primary en bloc laryngectomy and radical neck dissection. *Cancer.* 1961;14:55.
19. Mendenhall WM, Parsons JT, Stringer SP, et al: Stage T3 squamous cell carcinoma of the glottic larynx: A comparison of laryngectomy and irradiation. *Int J Radiat Oncol Biol Phys.* 1992;23:725.
20. Overgaard J, Hansen HS, Anderson AP, et al: Misonidazole combined with split-course radiotherapy in the treatment of invasive carcinoma of larynx and pharynx: Report from the DAHANCA II study. *Int J Radiat Oncol Biol Phys.* 1989;16:1065.
21. Overgaard J, Hansen HS, Jorgensen K, et al: Primary radiotherapy of larynx and pharynx carcinoma—An analysis of some factors influencing local control and survival. *Int J Radiat Oncol Biol Phys.* 1986;12:515.
22. Bohndorf K: Assessment of laryngeal carcinoma before therapy: Value of computed tomography and magnetic resonance tomography. *Strahlenther Onkol.* 1991;167:239.
23. Jabour BA, Lufkin RB, Hanafee WN: Magnetic resonance imaging of the larynx. *Top Magn Reson Imaging.* 1990;2:60.
24. Castelijns JA, Gerrisen GJ, Kaiser MC, et al: Invasion of laryngeal cartilage by cancer: Comparison of CT and MR imaging. *Radiology.* 1987;166:199.
25. American Joint Committee on Cancer: Larynx. In Fleming ID, Henson DE, et al, eds. *AJCC Cancer Staging Manual.* 6th ed. Philadelphia: Lippincott-Raven; 2002:41.

26. Bron LP, Soldati D, Zouhair A: Treatment of early stage squamous-cell carcinoma of the glottic larynx: Endoscopic surgery or cricothyroidotomy versus radiotherapy. *Head Neck.* 2001;23:823.

27. Spector JG, Sessions DG, Chao KS, et al: Stage I (T1N0M0) squamous cell carcinoma of the laryngeal glottis; therapeutic results and voice preservation. *Head Neck.* 1999;21:707.

28. Verdonck-de Leeuw IM, Keus RB, Hilgers FJ, et al: Consequences of voice impairment in daily life for patients following radiotherapy for early glottic cancer: Voice quality, vocal function, and vocal performance. *Int J Radiat Oncol Biol Phys.* 1999;44:1071.

29. Hocevar-Boltezar I, Zargi M, Honcodeevar-Boltezar I: Voice quality after radiation therapy for early glottic cancer. *Arch Otolaryngol Head Neck Surg.* 2000;126:1097.

30. Johansen LV, Gray C, Overgaard J: Supraglottic carcinoma: Patterns of failure and salvage treatment after curatively intended radiotherapy in 410 consecutive patients. *Int J Radiat Oncol Biol Phys.* 2002;53:948.

31. Forastiere AA, Berkey B, Ridge JA, et al: Phase III trial to preserve the larynx: Induction chemotherapy and radiotherapy versus concomitant chemoradiotherapy versus radiotherapy alone, Intergroup Trial R91-11. *Proc ASCO.* 2001;30:2a.

32. Lo TCM, Wiley AL, Ansfield FJ: Combined radiation therapy and 5-fluorouracil for advanced squamous cell carcinoma of the oral cavity and oropharynx: A randomized study. *AJR Am J Roentgenol.* 1976;126:229.

33. Fu KK, Phillips TL, Silverberg IJ, et al: Combined radiotherapy and chemotherapy with belomycin and methotrexate for advanced inoperable head and neck cancer: Update for a northern California oncology group randomized trial. *J Clin Oncol.* 1987;5:1410.

34. Gupta NK, Pointon CS, Wilkinson PM: A randomized clinical trial to contrast radiotherapy with radiotherapy and methotrexate given synchronously in head and neck cancer. *Clin Radiol.* 1987;38:575.

35. Bachaud JM, Cohen-Jonathan E, Alzieu C, et al: Combined post-operative radiotherapy and weekly cisplatin infusion for locally advanced head and neck carcinoma: Final report of a randomized trial. *Int J Radiat Oncol Biol Phys.* 1996;36:999.

36. Haffty BG, Son YH, Papc R, et al: Chemotherapy as an adjunct to radiation in the treatment of squamous cell carcinoma of the head and neck: Results of the Yale mitomycin randomized trials. *J Clin Oncol.* 1997;15:268.

37. Nguyen-Tan PF, Le QT, Quivey JM, et al: Treatment results and prognostic factors of advanced T3-4 laryngeal carcinoma: The University of California, San Francisco (UCSF) and Stanford University Hospital (SUH) experience. *Int J Radiat Oncol Biol Phys.* 2001;50:1172.

38. Orus C, Leon X, Vega M, et al: Initial treatment of the early stages (I,II) of supraglottic squamous cell carcinoma: Partial laryngectomy versus radiotherapy. *Eur Arch Otorhinolaryngol.* 2000;257:512.

39. Bocca E: Surgical management of supraglottic cancer and its lymph node metastases in a conservative perspective. *Ann Otol Rhinol Laryngol.* 1991;100:261.

40. Robbins KT, Davidson W, Peters LJ, et al: Conservation surgery for T2 and T3 carcinomas of the supraglottic larynx. *Arch Otolaryngol Head Neck Surg.* 1988;114:421.

41. Hinerman RW, Mendenhall WM, Amdur RJ, et al: Carcinoma of the supraglottic larynx: Treatment results with radiotherapy alone or with planned neck dissection. *Head Neck.* 2002;24:456.

42. Chan AW, Ancukiewicz M, Carball N, et al: The role of postradiotherapy neck dissection in supraglottic carcinoma. *Int J Radiat Oncol Biol Phys.* 2001;50:367.

43. Tupchong L, Scott CB, Blitzer PH, et al: Randomized study of pre-operative versus post-operative radiation therapy in advanced head and neck carcinoma: Long-term-follow-up of RTOG study 73-03. *Int J Radiat Oncol Biol Phys.* 1991;20:21.

44. The Department of Veterans Affairs: Induction chemotherapy plus radiation compared with surgery plus radiation in patients with advanced laryngeal cancer. *N Engl J Med.* 1991;324:1685.

45. Parsons JT, Mendenhall WM, Million RR, et al: Twice-a-day irradiation of squamous cell carcinoma of the head and neck. *Semin Radiat Oncol.* 1992;2:29.

46. Wang CC, Efird J, Nakfoor B, Martins P: Local control of T3 carcinoma after accelerated fractionation: A look at the gap. *Int J Radiat Oncol Biol Phys.* 1996;35:349.

47. Garden AS, Morrison WH, Ang KK, Peters LJ: Hyperfractionated radiation in the treatment of squamous cell carcinoma of the head and neck: A comparison of two fractionation schedules. *Int J Radiat Oncol Biol Phys.* 1995;31:493.

48. Fu KK, Phillips TL, Trotti A, et al: A radiation therapy oncology group (RTOG) phase III randomized study to compare hyperfractionation and two variants of accelerated fractionation to standard fractionation radiotherapy for head and neck squamous cell carcinomas: First report of RTOG 9003. *Int J Radiat Oncol Biol Phys.* 2000;48:7.

48a. Ang KK, Harris J, Gorden AS, et al: Concomittant boost radiation and concurrent cisplatin for advanced head and neck carcinomas: preliminary results of a phase II trial of the RTOG (99-14)2002; 54(2) (Suppl 1):71.

49. Bailey B: Management of carcinoma-in-situ and microinvasive carcinoma of the larynx. In Baily B, Biller H, eds. *Surgery of the Larynx.* Philadelphia: WB Saunders; 1985:229.

50. Lillie J, DeSanto L: Transoral surgery of early chordocarcinoma. *Trans Am Acad Ophthalmol Otolaryngol.* 1973;77:92.

51. Maran D, MacKenzie SR: Carcinoma-in-situ of the larynx. *Head Neck Surg.* 1984;7:28.

52. McGuirt WF, Koufman W: Endoscopic laser surgery: An alternative in laryngeal cancer treatment. *Arch Otolaryngol Head Neck Surg.* 1987;113:501.

53. Elman AJ, Goodman M, Wang CC, et al: In-situ carcinoma of the vocal cords. *Cancer.* 1979;43:2422.

54. Hintz B, Kagan A, Nussbaum H, et al: A "watchful waiting" policy for in-situ carcinoma of the vocal cords. *Arch Otolaryngol Head Neck Surg.* 1981;107:746.

55. Spayne JA, Warde P, O'Sullivan B, et al: Carcinoma-in-situ of the glottic larynx: Results of treatment with radiation therapy. *Int J Radiat Oncol Biol Phys.* 2001;49:1235.

56. Miller A, Fisher HR: Clues to the life history carcinoma-in-situ of the larynx. *Laryngoscope.* 1981;81:1475.

57. Shah JP, Loree TR, Kowalski L: Conservation surgery for radiation-failure carcinoma of the glottic larynx. *Head Neck.* 1990; 12:326.

58. Nichols RD, Mickelson SA: Partial laryngectomy after irradiation failure. *Ann Otol Rhinol Laryngol.* 1991;100:176.

59. Mendenhall WM, Morris CG, Stringer SP, et al: Voice rehabilitation after total laryngectomy and postoperative radiation therapy. *J Clin Oncol.* 2002;20:2500.

60. Kraus FT, Perez-Mesa C: Verrucous carcinoma. Clinical and pathologic study of 105 cases involving oral cavity, larynx and genitalia. *Cancer.* 1966;19:26.

61. Sullivan BO, Warde P, Keane T, et al: Outcome following radiotherapy in verrucous carcinoma of the larynx. *Int J Radiat Oncol Biol Phys.* 1995;32:611.

62. Ferlito A: Diagnosis and treatment of verrucous squamous cell carcinoma of the larynx: A critical review. *Am J Otol Rhinol Laryngol.* 1985;94:575.

63. Guedea F, Parsons T, Mendenhall WM, et al: Primary subglottic cancer. *Int J Radiat Oncol Biol Phys.* 1991;21:1607.

64. Vermund H: Role of radiotherapy in cancer of the larynx as related to the TNM system of staging. A review. *Cancer.* 1970;25:485.

65. Paisley S, Warde P, O'Sullivan B: Results of radiotherapy for primary subglottic squamous cell carcinoma. *Int J Radiat Oncol Biol Phys.* 2002;52:1245.

66. Kraas JR, Underhill TE, D'Agostina RB, et al: Quantitative analysis from CT is prognostic for local control of supraglottic carcinoma. *Head Neck.* 2000;5:282.

67. Hermans R, Vanden Bogaert W, Rijnders A, Baert AL: Value of computed tomography as outcome predictor of supraglottic squamous cell carcinoma treated by definitive radiation therapy. *Int J Radiat Oncol Biol Phys.* 1999;44:755.

68. Hermans R, Vanden Bogaert W, Rijnders A, Baert AL: Predicting the local outcome of glottic squamous cell carcinoma after definitive radiation therapy: Value of computed tomography-determined tumour parameters. *Radiother Oncol.* 1999;50:39.

69. Pameijer FA, Hermans R, Mancuso, et al: Pre-and post-radiotherapy computed tomography in laryngeal cancer: Imaging-based prediction of local failure. *Int J Radiat Oncol Biol Phys.* 1999;45:359.

70. Akins Y, Tokita N, Ogino T, et al: Radiotherapy of T1 glottic cancer with 6 MeV x-rays. *Int J Radiat Oncol Biol Phys.* 1991;20:1215.

71. Nozaki M, Furuta M, Murakami Y, et al: Radiation therapy for T1 glottic cancer: Involvement of the anterior commissure. *Anticancer Res.* 2000;20:1121.

72. Maheshwar AA, Gaffney C: Radiotherapy for T1 glottic carcinoma: Impact of anterior commissure involvement. *J Laryngol Otol.* 2001; 115:298.

73. Wang CC: Carcinoma of the larynx. In Wang CC, ed. *Indications, Techniques and Results.* Chicago, London, Boca Raton, Fla, Littletown, Mass: Year Book Medical Publishers; 1990:223.

74. Harwood AR, Beale FA, Cummings BI, et al: T2 glottic cancer: An analysis of dose-time volume factors. *Int J Radiat Oncol Biol Phys.* 1981;7:1501.

75. Mendenhall WM, Parsons JT, Brant TA: Is elective neck treatment indicated for T2N0 squamous cell carcinoma of the glottic larynx? *Radiother Oncol.* 1989;14:199.

76. Howell-Burke D, Peters LJ, Goepfert H, et al: T2 glottic cancer: Recurrence, salvage, and survival after definitive radiotherapy. *Arch Otolaryngol Head Neck Surg.* 1990;116:A30.

77. Lee N, Akazawa C, Akazawa P, et al: Forward-planned treatment techniques using multi-segments for head and neck cancer. (In press).

78. Dinshaw KA, Sharma V, Agarwal JP: Radiation therapy in T1-2 glottic carcinoma: Influence of various treatment parameters on local control/complications. *Int J Radiat Oncol Biol Phys.* 2000; 48:723.

79. Fu KK, Woodhouse RJ, Quivey JM, et al: The significance of laryngeal edema following radiotherapy of carcinoma of the vocal cord. *Cancer.* 1982;49:655.

80. Stewart JG, Jackson AW: The steepness of the dose response curve both for tumor cure and normal tissue injury. *Laryngoscope.* 1975;85:1107.

81. Deore SM, Supe SJ, Sharman V, et al: The predictive role of bioeffect dose models in radiation-induced late effects in glottic cancers. *Int J Radiat Oncol Biol Phys.* 1992;23:281.

82. Taylor JMG, Mendenhall W, Parsons JT, et al: The influence of dose and time on wound complications following post-radiation neck dissection. *Int J Radiat Oncol Biol Phys.* 1992;23:41.

83. Inoue T, Chatani M, Teshima T: Irradiated volume and arytenoid edema after radiotherapy for T1 glottic carcinoma. *Strahlenther Onkol.* 1992;168:23.

84. Le QT, Fu KK, Kroll S, et al: Influence of fraction size, total dose, and overall time on local control of T1-2 glottic carcinoma. *Int J Radiat Oncol Biol Phys.* 1997;39:115.

85. Freeman RB, Marks JE, Ogura JH: Voice preservation in treatment of carcinoma of the pyriform sinus. *Laryngoscope.* 1979;89:1855.

86. Kramer S, Gelber RD, Snow JB: Combined radiation therapy and surgery in the management of advanced head and neck cancer: Final report of study 73-03 of the Radiation Therapy Oncology Group. *Head Neck Surg.* 1987;10:19.

87. Fu KK: Normal tissue effects of combined radiotherapy and chemotherapy for head and neck cancer. *Front Radiat Ther Oncol.* 1979;13:113.

88. Cox JD, Pajack TF, Marcial VA: ASTRO plenary: Interfraction interval is a major determinant of late effects with hyperfractionated radiation therapy of carcinomas of upper respiratory and digestive tracts: Results from Radiation Therapy Oncology Group Protocol 8313. *Int J Radiat Oncol Biol Phys.* 1991;20:1191.

89. Amornmarn R, Prempree T, Viravathana T, et al: A therapeutic approach to early vocal cord carcinoma. *Acta Radiol (ONCOL).* 1985;24:321.

90. Maciejewski B, Taylor JMG, Withers HR: Alpha/beta value and the importance of size of dose per fraction for late complications in the supraglottic larynx. *Radiother Oncol.* 1986;7:323.

91. Mittal B, Rao DV, Marks JE, et al: Role of radiation in the management of early vocal cord carcinoma. *Int J Radiat Oncol Biol Phys.* 1983;9:997.

92. Harwood AR, Beale FA, Cummings BJ, et al: Supraglottic laryngeal carcinoma: An analysis of dose-time-volume factors in 410 patients. *Int J Radiat Oncol Biol Phys.* 1983;9:311.

93. Lee NK, Goepfert H, Wendt CD: Supraglottic laryngectomy for intermediate-stage cancer: UT MD Anderson Cancer Center experience with combined therapy. *Laryngoscope.* 1990;100:831.

94. Issa PY: Cancer of the supraglottic larynx treated by radiotherapy exclusively. *Int J Radiat Oncol Biol Phys.* 1988;15:843.

95. Wall TJ, Peters LJ, Brown BW, et al: Relationship between lymph node status and primary tumor control probability in tumors of the supraglottic larynx. *Int J Radiat Oncol Biol Phys.* 1985; 11:1895.

96. Freeman D, Mendenhall WM, Parsons JT: Does neck stage influence local control probability in squamous cell cancers of the head and neck? *Int J Radiat Oncol Biol Phys.* 1991;21 (suppl 1):138.

97. Parsons JT, Mendenhall WM, Cassisi NJ, et al: Hyperfractionation for head and neck cancer. *Int J Radiat Oncol Biol Phys.* 1988; 14:649.

98. Bocca E: Surgical management of supraglottic cancer and its lymph node metastases in a conservative perspective. *Ann Otol Rhinol Laryngol.* 1991;100:261.

99. Pene F, Fletcher G: Results in irradiation of the in-situ carcinomas of the vocal cords. *Cancer.* 1976;2586.

100. Haugen H, Johansson KA, Mercke C: Hyperfractionated-accelerated conventionally fractionated radiotherapy for early glottic cancer. *Int J Radiat Oncol Biol Phys.* 2002;52:109.

101. Vanden Bogaert W, Rostyn F, van der Schuern E: The significance of extension and impaired mobility in cancer of the vocal cord. *Int J Radiat Oncol Biol Phys.* 1983;9:181.

102. Johansen LV, Overgaard J, Hjelam-Hansen H, et al: *Int J Radiat Oncol Biol Phys.* 1990;18:1307.

103. Karim Kralendonk JH, Yap LY, et al: Heterogeniety of stage II glottic carcinoma and its therapeutic implications. *Int J Radiat Oncol Biol Phys.* 1987;13:313.

104. Vanden Bogaert W, Rostyn F, van der Schuern E: The primary treatment of advanced vocal cord cancer: Laryngectomy or radiotherapy? *Int J Radiat Oncol Biol Phys.* 1983;9:329.

105. Harwood AR, Deboer G, Kazim F: Prognostic factors in T3 glottic cancer. *Cancer.* 1981;47:367.

106. Mendenhall WM, Amdw RJ, Morris CG, et al: T1-T2N0 squamous cell carcinoma of the glottic larynx treated with radiation therapy. *J Clin Oncol.* 2001;19:4029.

107. Parsons JT, Greene BD, Speer TW: Treatment of early and moderately advanced vocal cord carcinoma with 6-MV x-rays. *Int J Radiat Oncol Biol Phys.* 2001;50:953.

108. Harwood AR, Beale FA, Cummings BJ, et al: T4N0M0 glottic cancer: An analysis of dose-time volume factors. *Int J Radiat Oncol Biol Phys.* 1981;7(11):1507.

109. Kim RY, Marks ME, Salter MM: Early-stage glottic cancer: Importance of dose fractionation in radiation therapy. *Radiology.* 1992;182:273.

110. Schwaibold F, Scariato A, Nunno M, et al: The effect of fraction size on control of early glottic cancer. *Int J Radiat Oncol Biol Phys.* 1988;14:451.

111. Warde P, O'Sullivan B, Bristow RG: T1/T2 glottic cancer managed by external beam radiotherapy: The influence of pretreatment hemoglobin on local control. *Int J Radiat Oncol Biol Phys.* 1998;41:347.

112. Warde P, Harwood A, Keane T: Carcinoma of the subglottis. Results of initial radical radiation. *Arch Otolaryngol Head Neck Surg.* 1987;113:1228.

Tumors of the Salivary Glands

32

Lanceford M. Chong, MD, and John G. Armstrong, MD

Malignant salivary gland tumors are uncommon head and neck cancers. They share many characteristics yet also have features that are uniquely attributable to their respective locations and subtypes. The two main categories are major and minor salivary gland tumors. They are presented separately to distinguish the presentations, natural histories, and therapeutic approaches between and within these groups.

MAJOR SALIVARY GLAND TUMORS

Epidemiology

Tumors of the major salivary glands are uncommon and account for approximately 3% to 4% of all head and neck neoplasms. The parotid gland is overwhelmingly the most frequent gland affected. Parotid gland malignancies are much more common than submandibular and sublingual gland cancers by a factor of 10 and 100, respectively.

The ratio of benign to malignant tumors varies by site, and there is an inverse relationship between the size of the salivary gland and its incidence of malignancy: (1) parotid gland: 80% benign (primarily pleomorphic adenomas), 20% malignant. (2) submandibular gland: 50% benign, 50% malignant. (3) sublingual gland: most are malignant. The average age for benign neoplasms is 40 years while that for malignant tumors is 55 years. The incidence is equivalent for men and women.

The etiology of these malignant tumors is unknown. Radiation-induced salivary gland malignancies have been reported in the literature in association with patients who had been irradiated to the head and neck region for benign conditions (e.g., acne, tinea capitis, infected tonsils) and in survivors of the atomic bomb in Hiroshima and Nagasaki. While an association with female breast cancer has been reported, there is a lack of firm epidemiologic data to support this contention. Nutritional deficiency as a possible cause has been reported in the Arctic Inuit peoples who have a diet low in vitamins A and C. Infection has been cited as a possible cause in whites with the Epstein-Barr virus. Other possible epidemiologic causes include alcohol use, hair dye, and a higher education level.

Anatomy

The major salivary glands comprise the parotid, submandibular, and sublingual salivary glands (Fig. 32-1).

Each are paired glands that have different secretory functions: (1) parotid gland—serous; (2) submandibular gland—seromucous; (3) sublingual gland—mucous.

PAROTID GLAND

The parotid glands are the largest of the salivary glands (see Fig. 32-1). These paired glands are surrounded by a discrete capsule and have the following anatomic landmarks: (1) anterior—wraps around the ascending mandibular ramus anterior to the tragus and extends toward the anterior margin of the masseter muscle; (2) posterior—extends from the angle of the mandible under the earlobe toward the mastoid tip; (3) superior—extends to the inferior aspect of the zygoma at the temporomandibular joint level; (4) inferior—extends to the inferior aspect of the angle of the mandible; (5) medial—borders the parapharyngeal-base of skull; (6) lateral—located below the skin of the preauricular cheek–upper neck. The gland is divided into two lobes by the path of the facial nerve, which exits from the stylomastoid foramen (Fig. 32-2): (1) superficial lobe—accounts for 80% of the gland and is located just lateral to the facial nerve; (2) deep lobe—accounts for 20% of the gland and is located medial to the facial nerve and adjacent to the medial aspect of the angle of the mandible and is connected to the superficial lobe by the isthmus (Fig. 32-3). The deep lobe is in close anatomic proximity to the internal carotid artery, the internal jugular vein, the

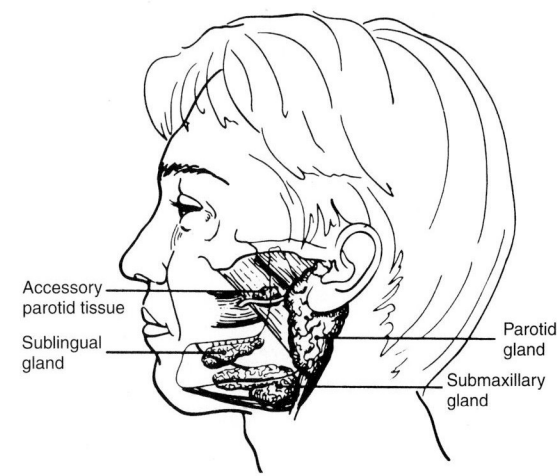

Figure 32–1. The anatomic locations of major salivary glands: parotid, submandibular, sublingual. (From Spiro JD, Spiro RM: Salivary tumors. In Shah J, ed. *Cancer of the Head and Neck*. London: BC Decker; 2001:241.)

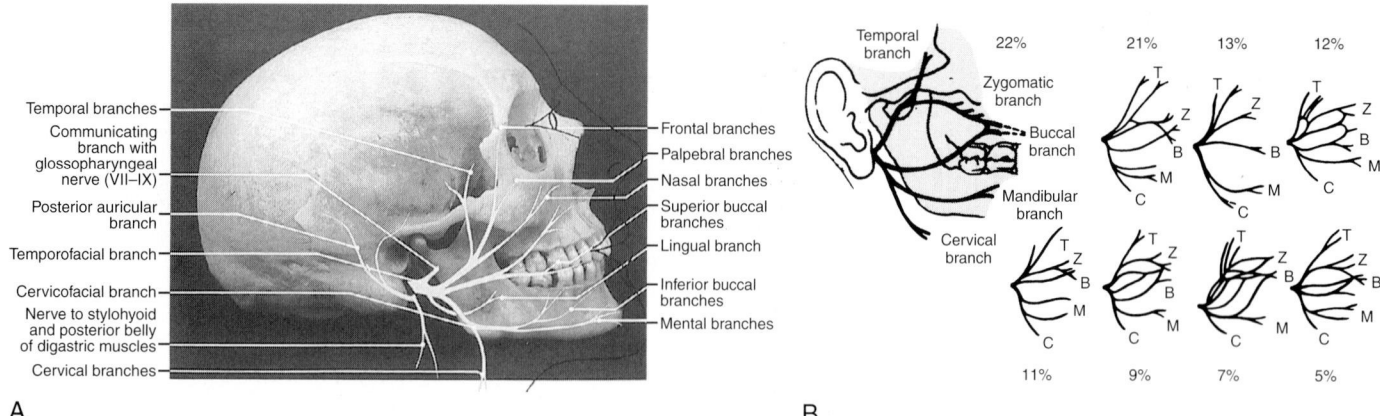

A

B

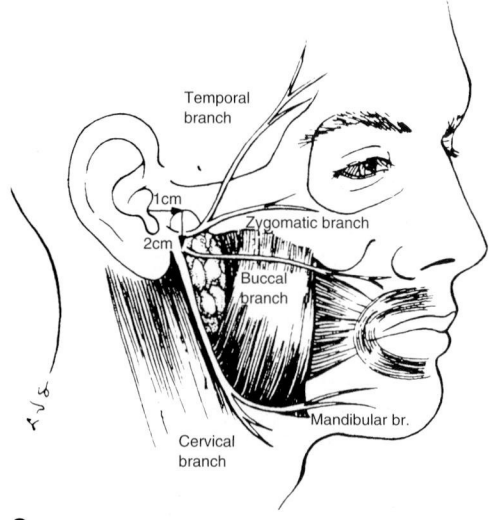

C

Figure 32–2. **A**, Pathway of the facial nerve (CN VII) as it exits the stylomastoid foramen and then branches out into various anatomic regions. **B**, Note the presence of the deep lobe of the parotid gland just medial to the facial nerve. **C**, The facial nerve branches have several distribution variations. (**A** from Leblanc A: *The Cranial Nerves*, 2nd ed. Berlin: Springer-Verlag; 1995:184. **B** from Crumley RL, Kelley TF: Rehabilitation of the patient with tumors of the salivary glands. In Thawley SE, Panje WR, Batsakis JG, et al, eds. *Comprehensive Management of Head and Neck Tumor*. Philadelphia: WB Saunders; 1987:1202, vol. 2. **C** from Som PM, Curtin HD: *Head and Neck Imaging*, 3rd ed. St. Louis: Mosby; 1996:829.)

cervical sympathetic chain, and the cranial nerves IX, X, XI, and XII (Table 32-1).

The parotid gland drains into the oral cavity through Stensen's duct (Fig. 32-4). This duct runs from the upper

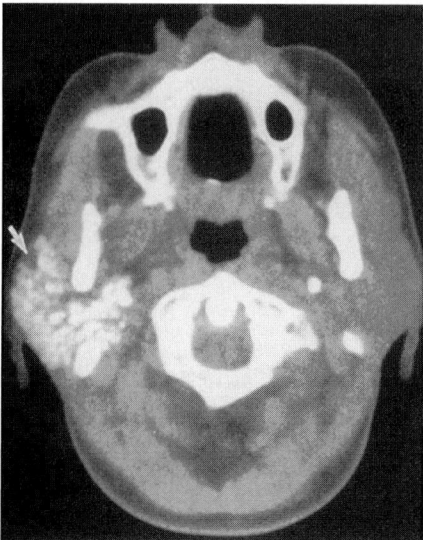

Figure 32–3. Axial view of a noncontrast CT scan of a patient who had previously undergone a right parotid sialogram. Note the superficial lobe, deep lobe, and isthmus of the parotid gland as it wraps around the mandibular ramus. (From Som PM, Curtin HD: *Head and Neck Imaging*, 3rd ed. St. Louis: Mosby; 1996:865.)

anterior third of the parotid gland and exits through the buccal mucosa by the second molar. The lymphatic drainage of the parotid gland progresses in an orderly fashion. Initially, it drains into the periparotid (Fig. 32-5) and intraparotid (Fig. 32-6) nodes that comprise two groups located within the fascia of the gland in two respective locations: between the gland and the superficial fascia and within the parenchyma. It then drains into the submandibular nodes (level I), the upper (level II) and mid (level III) cervical nodes, and sometimes to the retropharyngeal nodes. Drainage to the contralateral nodes is very rare. However, it must be considered if the primary tumor extends across the midline or if there is massive ipsilateral cervical node involvement, which may disrupt the lymphatic pathways and cause spread to the opposite side.

Adjacent to the superficial surface of the parotid gland fascia and anterior to the tragus are the preauricular nodes, which measure less than 3 mm in size and lie within the subcutaneous fat. These lymph nodes receive the lymphatic drainage from the dermis of the upper face, temple of the scalp, eye, nose, and ear. Their involvement is usually associated with skin carcinomas and melanomas in these regions as well as lymphomas. However, primary parotid malignancies do not commonly metastasize to these nodes. Secondary extension into the parotid gland and adjacent facial nerve can sometimes occur. These nodes can then drain into either the inferior parotid nodes (superficial lymph nodes) or into the jugular chain of nodes (level II).

Table 32–1   The Anatomic Relationship of the Major Salivary Glands and Cranial Nerves

Major Salivary Gland	Adjacent Cranial Nerve	Base of Skull Foramen
Parotid		
Superficial/Deep lobes	Facial nerve (CN VII)	Stylomastoid foramen
Deep lobe	Glossopharyngeal nerve (CN IX)	Jugular foramen
	Vagus nerve (CN X)	Jugular foramen
	Accessory nerve (CN XI)	Jugular foramen
	Hypoglossal nerve (CN XII)	Hypoglossal canal
Submandibular	Lingual nerve (CNV3)	Foramen ovale
	Facial nerve (CN VII):	Stylomastoid foramen
	Mandibular/cervical branches	
	Hypoglossal nerve (CN XII)	Hypoglossal canal
Sublingual	Lingual nerve (CN V3)	Foramen ovale

Occasionally, there will be an accessory parotid lobe (Fig. 32-7). This lobe has been reported in 21% of normal adult cadavers.[1] However, in a review of 2261 patients with parotid lesions at Memorial Sloan-Kettering Cancer Center (MSKCC) between 1939 and 1978, only 23 patients (1%) had an accessory parotid gland.[2] Accessory parotid glands are located either cephalad or lateral to the anterior aspect of Stensen's duct and lie over the anterior aspect of the masseter muscle but are separate from the superficial lobe of the parotid gland. Clinically, they are adjacent to Stensen's duct, which is located midway along a line drawn between the tragus of the ear to the lateral upper lip. There can be 1 to 10 tributary ducts from the accessory lobe that will empty into the Stensen's duct. This lobe can be clinically significant in that it may be the primary site of a malignant tumor that presents as an asymptomatic swelling in the mid cheek region.

SUBMANDIBULAR GLAND

The submandibular gland (see Fig. 32-1) is 25% of the size of the parotid gland and measures 3 to 4 cm. These paired glands are surrounded by a capsule and are located in the upper anterior triangle of the neck. They are medial to the proximal half of the mandible (Fig. 32-8). The majority of the gland is over the external surface of the mylohyoid muscle, which forms the muscular floor of mouth in the region between the insertion of the muscle and the mandible and which divides the gland into contiguous superficial and deep portions (Fig. 32-9). The posterior aspect is anterior to but near the lower anterior margin of the parotid gland. The inferior aspect can extend caudad a fair distance and approaches the level of the hyoid bone. Of clinical importance is the fact that the submandibular gland is lateral to and abuts the lingual nerve (cranial nerve V3) and hypoglossal nerve (cranial nerve XII) and is medial to the marginal mandibular and cervical branches of the facial nerve (cranial nerve VII) (see Table 32-1).

The glands drain into the oral cavity through Wharton's duct. This 5 cm duct courses through the niche between the mylohyoid and hypoglossus muscles and emerges in the anterior floor of mouth toward the midline.

The lymphatic drainage of the submandibular glands progresses in an orderly fashion. Initially it drains into the adjacent submandibular nodes (level I) as there are no intraglandular parenchymal nodes. It then drains into the

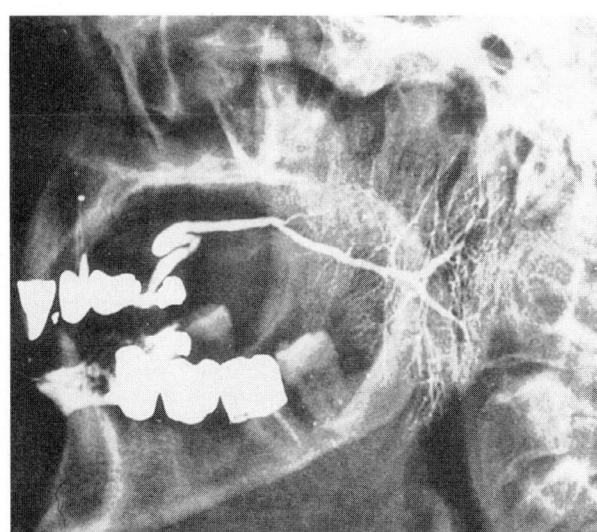

Figure 32–4. Parotid sialogram showing the anatomic location of the gland and Stensen's duct as it exits into the oral cavity by the upper second molar. (From Som PM, Curtin HD: *Head and Neck Imaging*, 3rd ed. St. Louis: Mosby; 1996:836.)

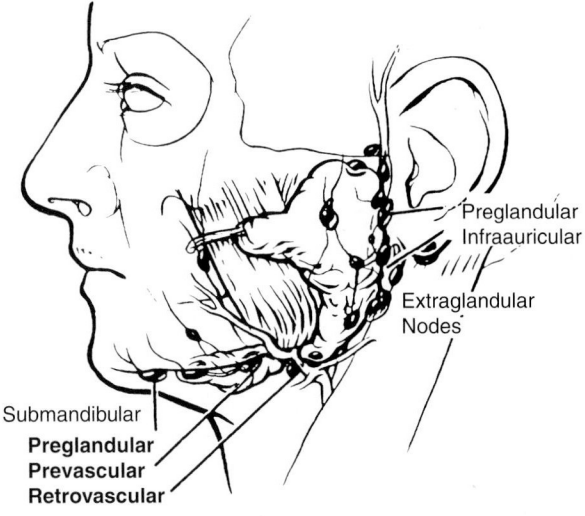

Figure 32–5. Periparotid lymph nodes are located on the surface of the superficial lobe but within the fascia. (From Hoffman H, Funk G, Endres D: Evaluation and surgical treatment of tumors of the salivary glands. In Thawley SE, Panje WR, Batsakis JG, et al, eds. *Comprehensive Management of Head and Neck Tumors*, 1st ed. Philadelphia: WB Saunders; 1987:1112, vol. 2.)

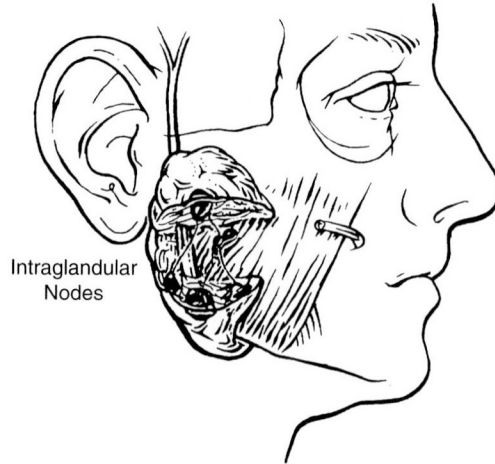

Figure 32–6. Intraparotid nodes are located within the parenchyma of the gland. (From Hoffman H, Funk G, Endres D: Evaluation and surgical treatment of tumors of the salivary glands. In Thawley SE, Panje WR, Batsakis JG, et al, eds. *Comprehensive Management of Head and Neck Tumors.* Philadelphia: WB Saunders; 1987:1112, vol. 2.)

upper (level II) and mid (level III) cervical nodes. Drainage to the contralateral nodes is rare.

SUBLINGUAL GLAND

The paired sublingual salivary glands (see Fig. 32-1) are the smallest of the major salivary glands, 10% the size of parotid glands. These glands do not have a discrete capsule. They are located in the anterior floor of mouth adjacent to the medial aspect of the mandible and occupy a submucosal position. Sublingual salivary glands are adjacent and superior to the mylohyoid muscle in the area of the sublingual depression. They occupy a position just medial to the inner surface of the mandible near the mental symphysis (see Fig. 32-9). It is clinically important to note that the lingual nerve (cranial nerve V3) courses adjacent to the sublingual gland (see Table 32-1).

Primary malignant tumors of the sublingual glands are rare; however, any lesion in this area must be considered malignant until otherwise proven. It may be difficult to clinically rule out a primary squamous cell carcinoma of the anterior floor of mouth in this region.

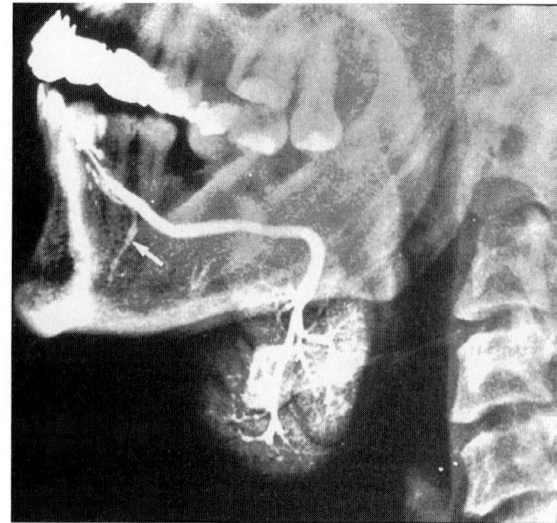

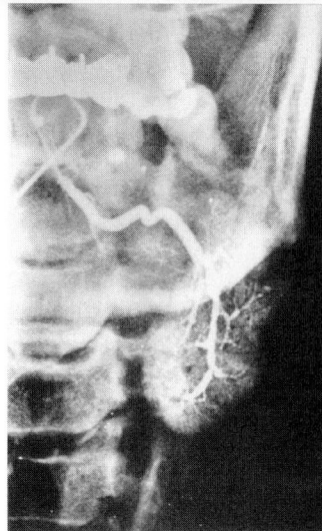

Figure 32–8. A, Lateral sialogram showing the anatomic location of the submandibular gland and Wharton's duct, which drains into the floor of mouth. **B,** Anterior sialogram showing the submandibular gland and the medial pathway of Wharton's duct. (From Som PM, Curtin HD: *Head and Neck Imaging,* 3rd ed. St. Louis: Mosby; 1996:838.)

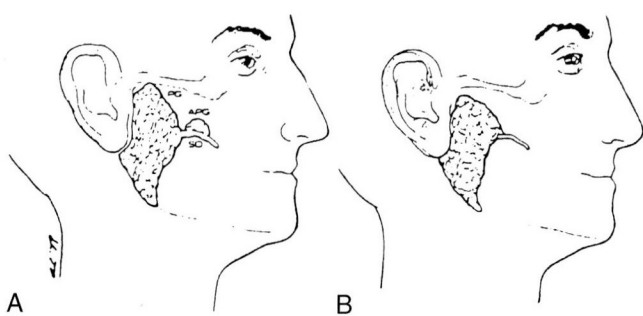

Figure 32–7. A, The accessory parotid lobe is located in the anterior aspect of Stensen's duct. **B,** Normal parotid gland and Stensen's duct. (From Johnson FE, Spiro RH: Tumors arising in accessory parotid tissue. *Am J Surg.* 1979;138:242.)

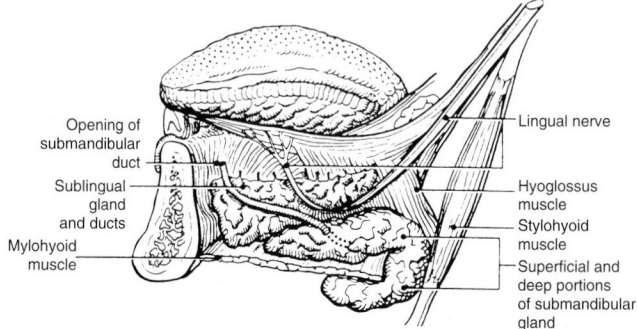

Figure 32–9. Anatomic relationships between the submandibular gland and sublingual gland and the adjacent musculature and cranial nerves. (**A** and **B** from Spiro JD, Spiro RM: Salivary tumors. In Shah J, ed: *Cancer of the Head and Neck.* London: BC Decker; 2001:241.)

These salivary glands drain into the oral cavity via 5 to 15 ducts (Rivinus' ducts) that empty into the sublingual fold of the floor of mouth. Also, these ducts may anastomose to create a larger duct known as Bartholin's duct, which attaches to the submandibular duct.

The lymphatic drainage of the sublingual glands progresses in a predictable, orderly fashion flowing initially to the submental and submandibular nodes and then to the deep jugular nodes.

Pathology

BENIGN TUMORS

BENIGN MIXED TUMORS. Benign mixed tumors are the most common salivary gland tumors. They are referred to as pleomorphic adenomas and may contain glandular elements, connective tissue, cartilage, vascular stroma, and cystic degeneration. They occur at a mean age of 40 years. They are slow growing and can reach huge sizes. By definition, benign tumors do not invade locally; however, enucleation can lead to local recurrence in a significant percentage. With resection of each successive recurrence, the risk of facial nerve damage increases. Frankly malignant mixed tumors also occur and may arise de novo or by evolution from a benign lesion.

PAPILLARY CYSTADENOMA LYMPHOMATOSUM (WARTHIN'S TUMOR). This usually small tumor probably arises from lymphoid elements. It accounts for 5% to 10% of all parotid tumors. It is bilateral in about 10% and occurs predominantly in older men. Recurrence is rare after excision.

BENIGN LYMPHOEPITHELIAL LESIONS (GODWIN'S TUMOR). These lesions account for about 5% of benign tumors and may be an early manifestation of human immunodeficiency infection.

ONCOCYTOMA. This is a benign, slow-growing tumor in the older age group. Occasionally malignant oncocytomas occur.

BASAL CELL ADENOMA. This is a benign tumor that must be distinguished from the unusual occurrence of basal cell cancer of the skin metastatic to intraparotid or periparotid lymph nodes.

MALIGNANT TUMORS

Histopathologic Types

Over the past several years, the World Health Organization has expanded its list of suggested histopathologic typing to include a very comprehensive and varied group of malignant tumors:

Acinic cell carcinoma
Mucoepidermoid carcinoma
Adenoid cystic carcinoma
Polymorphous low-grade adenocarcinoma
Epithelial-myoepithelial carcinoma
Basal cell adenocarcinoma
Sebaceous carcinoma
Papillary cystadenocarcinoma
Mucinous adenocarcinoma
Oncocytic carcinoma
Salivary duct carcinoma
Adenocarcinoma
Myoepithelial carcinoma
Carcinoma in pleomorphic adenoma
Squamous cell carcinoma
Small cell carcinoma
Other carcinomas

The relative incidence of the different histologic types according to gland of origin is detailed in Table 32-2.

MUCOEPIDERMOID CARCINOMA. The majority of these cancers are low-grade cancers that tend to be slow growing, well-circumscribed, and cured by surgery alone. Mucin production may be absent in high-grade tumors, which are invasive and can spread to lymph nodes (Fig. 32-10). Mucoepidermoid carcinoma is the most common cancer of the parotid gland.[3]

ADENOID CYSTIC CARCINOMA. This is the predominant malignant histologic type in submandibular and minor salivary gland tumors.[3] The appearance (Fig. 32-11) can vary from a cribriform pattern (differentiated) to a mixed cribriform pattern and solid features (moderately differentiated) to solid features (undifferentiated). Some authors have observed that the solid variety can have a more malignant behavior. The natural history can be varied, ranging from a matter of months to 20 years or more. The first evidence of recurrence can be 20 years after diagnosis, making it very difficult to ever determine that an individual patient is cured. Lymph node spread is distinctly uncommon (<5%). Adenoid cystic tumors can cause perineural spread, which may track along

Table 32–2   Distribution of Histologic Types of Major Salivary Gland Cancer

Type	Percentage
Parotid (*n* = 1778 cases)	
Mucoepidermoid	32
Adenocarcinoma	16
Malignant mixed	14
Adenoid cystic	11
Acinic	11
Undifferentiated and squamous	16
Submandibular (*n* = 383 cases)	
Adenoid cystic	41
Acinic	17
Mucoepidermoid	12
Malignant mixed	10
Undifferentiated	9
Squamous	9
Adenocarcinoma	2

Data from Memorial Sloan-Kettering Cancer Center.[1]

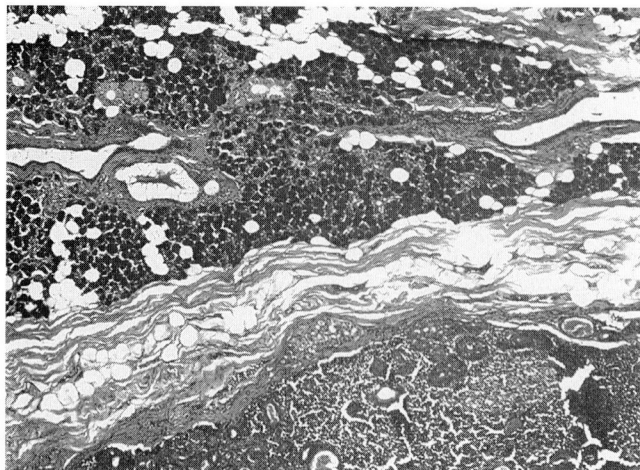

Figure 32–10. Mucoepidermoid carcinoma. There is no classic microscopic appearance as these salivary gland tumors have a wide variation in cellular composition. A predominance of "epidermoid cells" (closely resemble squamous cell carcinomas that form solid areas and nests) or "intermediate cells" (oval cells that contain a small, darkly staining nucleus), or both, is found. See also Color Figure 32-10. (Courtesy of Andrew Huvos, MD, Memorial Sloan-Kettering Cancer Center Department of Pathology.)

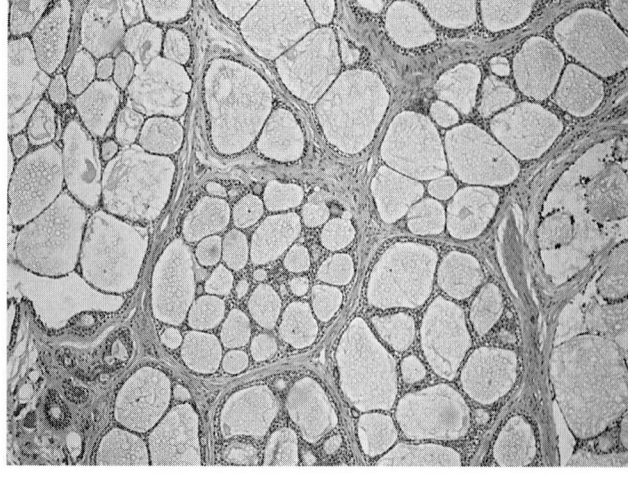

Figure 32–11. Adenoid cystic carcinoma. These are composed of a neoplastic epithelium composed of uniform basaloid cells that contain scant cytoplasm and which are arranged in cords or solid nests. This surrounds a stroma that contains hyaline eosinophilic material or a mucinous myxoid interstitium. See also Color Figure 32-11.

the pathways of the cranial nerves to the base of skull. This is important in planning radiation treatment. Many patients (ultimately up to 40%) will develop pulmonary metastases. As prolonged survival can occur (10 to 20 years) with pulmonary metastases, the primary site must be managed adequately despite the presence of metastatic disease. An example of the management of the primary site in a patient with adenoid cystic cancer and lung metastases is illustrated in Fig. 32-12.

HISTOLOGIC GRADE

The histologic grade or cellular differentiation of the tumor is one of several important factors affecting patient survival. The other indicators include the histologic diagnosis, site, size, degree of fixation, or local extension and facial nerve involvement. Also, regional lymph node and distant metastases are of major importance relating to survival. However, the histologic grade of the tumor is

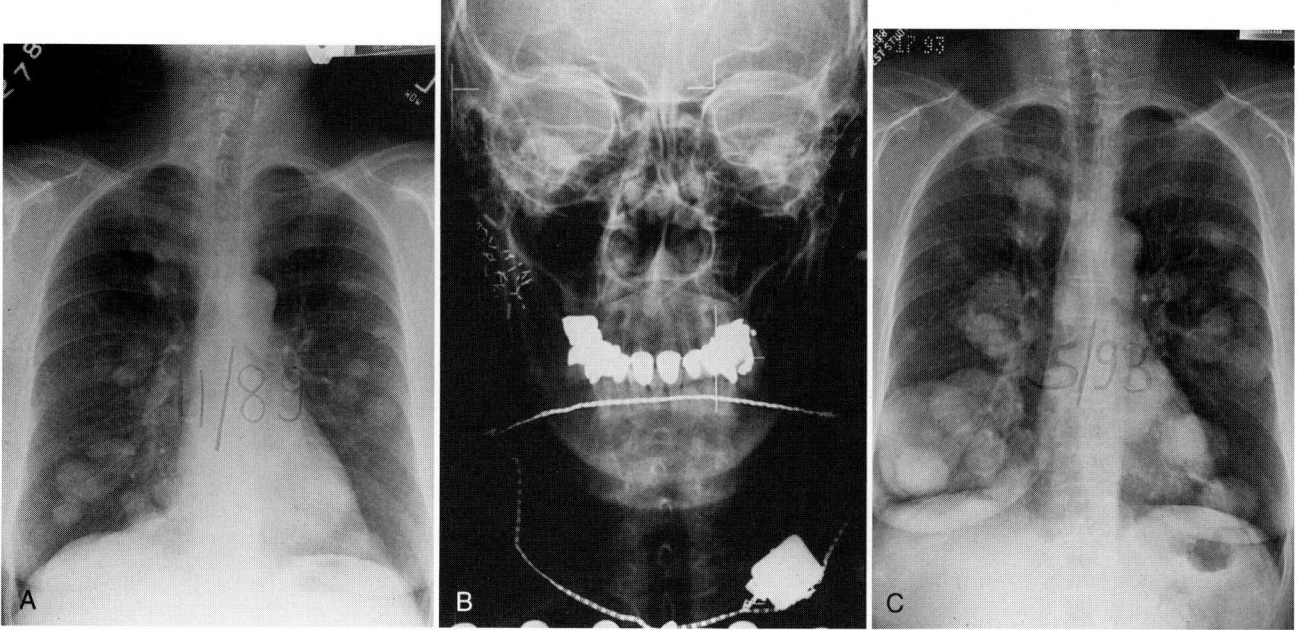

Figure 32–12. **A,** A 52-year-old woman presented in 1989 with adenoid cystic cancer arising in the parotid gland and metastatic to the lungs. The lung radiograph is seen. **B,** The primary tumor was partially resected, with gross disease left behind at the facial nerve. To completely resect the cancer would have necessitated facial nerve sacrifice. Using ^{125}I seeds enmeshed in Vicryl sutures, a dose of 22000 cGy (matched peripheral dose) was delivered. The patient had permanent local control with normal facial nerve function. **C,** A chest radiograph 4 years later shows progression of the metastatic disease. This emphasizes that adenoid cystic clancer patients can live several years despite lung metastases and should therefore have adequate treatment of the primary tumor.

applicable only for adenocarcinoma NOS and mucoepidermoid carcinomas, or when either of these is the malignant component of carcinoma in pleomorphic adenoma. For all of the other subtypes, it is the actual histologic type that defines the grade. For instance, salivary duct carcinoma is high grade while basal cell adenocarcinoma is low grade by definition.

Special Case: Metastatic Disease from Another Primary Site to Involve the Parotid Gland Region

Occasionally, the parotid gland parenchyma or lymph nodes may be the target site of metastatic disease from another primary site. Three pathophysiologic mechanisms explain such occurrences: (1) lymphatic spread; (2) hematogenous dissemination; and (3) direct extension.

Lymphatic spread to the intraglandular and periglandular parotid lymph nodes can occur from primary skin cancers (e.g., squamous cell carcinomas, melanomas) of the scalp, face, and ears. Occasionally there can be lymphatic spread to the parotid nodes from a primary cancer in the palate, tonsil, or nasopharynx.

The majority of hematogenous disseminations are from primary lung cancers. Less frequent other primaries include breast, kidney, and the gastrointestinal tract.

Direct extension of malignant disease to the parotid gland can be seen with adjacent osseous sarcomas or overlying skin lesions.

Patients who develop metastatic disease to the parotid region from another primary site have a grave prognosis with a poor 5-year survival rate.

Clinical Presentation and Evaluation

PAROTID

Primary Site

A thorough history and carefully detailed physical examination are always crucial first steps in the evaluation of patients with a parotid mass. The differential diagnoses of a parotid mass include a malignant tumor as well as several types of benign causes (Table 32-3). Parotid malignancy is usually an asymptomatic mass. However, as the lesion progresses and enlarges, episodic pain occurs in 10% to 20% of cases; subsequently, significant pain can result and become constant. Patients can present with complaints of an inability to move one

Table 32–3 Differential Diagnosis of a Parotid Mass*

1. Metastases to intraparotid nodes
2. Reactive adenopathy
3. Fatty tail of parotid
4. Chronic parotitis
5. Sarcoidosis
6. HIV infection
7. Calculus in duct with obstruction
8. Neoplasms of mandible
9. Cysts (dermoid, bronchial cleft)
10. Prominent transverse process of C1 vertebra
11. Hemangioma, lipoma, lymphangioma

*Other than primary parotid tumors.

side of the face (cranial nerve VII), a shoulder (cranial nerve IX), or one side of the tongue (cranial nerve XII) as the adjacent cranial nerves become involved by the malignant tumor. Clinical presentations can vary according to the histopathology (Table 32-4).

A careful and methodic examination of the patient can provide valuable information regarding the stage of the tumor. The mandibular opening should be measured to rule out trismus due to tumor involvement of the pterygoid plates. Bimanual palpation of the tumor will provide data regarding its dimensions, texture, and mobility. The overlying soft tissues, adjacent mandible, and ipsilateral external auditory canal are sites where tumors can infiltrate and should be carefully evaluated.

The functional status of the adjacent cranial nerves must be documented. This would always include evaluation of the facial nerve (cranial nerve VII), which is involved in 2% to 14% of cases. However, if the deep lobe of the parotid is involved, cranial nerves IX, X, XI, and XII may be affected.

Workup with computed tomography (CT) or magnetic resonance imaging (MRI) can be helpful in selected cases. Slices should cover from above the ears to below the clavicles, thus imaging the base of skull, parotid, retropharyngeal nodes, cervical nodes, and supraclavicular nodes. There are four indications for a pretreatment CT or MRI in parotid gland tumors[4]: (1) deep lobe parotid tumors; (2) neurologically symptomatic tumors; (3) recurrent tumors; and (4) large tumors.

CT and MRI cannot differentiate a benign from a malignant tumor and, thus, are not routinely used for small, mobile, circumscribed lesions. An MRI scan with gadolinium best delineates deep tissue infiltration or perineural extent of the tumor with respect to the facial nerve (cranial VII).

Both benign and malignant salivary tumors may appear well circumscribed on CT or MRI. This may cause one to underestimate the actual extent of infiltration of the cancer.

Although primary and metastatic malignant lesions of the major salivary glands generally show an increased uptake on 2-fluoro-2-deoxy-D-glucose (FDG) positron emission tomography (PET) scans, no large series has evaluated the use of this study in such tumors. Both benign and malignant tumors of the salivary gland show an increase in FDG uptake, and thus one probably would not be able to accurately differentiate between them.

Therefore, at this time, it is not felt that PET scans are helpful in evaluating a primary lesion. However, once a histologic diagnosis has been made establishing a malignancy of the parotid gland, a PET scan may be helpful for evaluation of distant metastasis (personal communication with Heiko Schoder, MD, Department of Nuclear Medicine, MSKCC).

The initial biopsy procedure in a patient suspected of a parotid malignancy can be a fine-needle aspiration (FNA) biopsy. Note that, in general, 80% of parotid masses are benign while 10% are malignant. An FNA biopsy is an accurate diagnostic technique with overall sensitivities of greater than 90% and specificities of greater than 95%.[5-10] If a malignancy is thus diagnosed, one can note if the lesion is a primary parotid lesion or if it is a metastatic lesion to the parotid gland from another

Table 32–4   Summary of Clinical Histologic Presentations in Malignant Tumors of the Salivary Gland

Histology	Incidence	Age Predilection (Decade)	Sex Predilection	Favored Site	Node Metastasis	7th Nerve Involvement	Recurrence	Distant Metastasis	Specific
Acinic cell carcinoma	4	5th	F > M	Parotid	10	3	10–22	Rare	Multifocal, sometimes bilateral
Adenoid cystic carcinoma	2–5	5th–6th	F = M	Minor salivary glands and submaxillary glands	15	26	High*	28	Pain is presenting symptom; long-term survival with distant metastasis not unusual
Mucoepidermoid carcinoma									More patients have low-grade type; half of histology of children in this type
Low grade	17–20	1st–2nd 4th–5th	M > F	None	60	8	17	33	
High grade		6th				High*	75		
Malignant mixed tumor	4	7th	M > F	Parotid and submaxillary glands	33	14	30–40	31	Tumor slow growing; starts sometimes in preexisting pleomorphic adenoma
Squamous cell carcinoma	0.1–3	None	None	Parotids and salivary duct	High*	High*	70	High*	Rapid-growing; nerve palsy a frequent presentation
Adenocarcinoma	2.8	5th–6th	None	Parotid	50	9	67	19	Painless mass usual presentation
Undifferentiated carcinoma	3	7th–8th	F > M	None	50	23	High*	30	May start within preexisting pathology such as mixed cylindroma, or adenocarcinoma

*A high incidence in few cases.

From Shidnia H, Hornback NB: Radiation therapy of tumors of the salivary glands. In Thawley SE, Panje WR, Batsakis JG, Lindberg RD, eds: Comprehensive Management of Head and Neck Tumors, 2nd ed. Philadelphia: WB Saunders; 1999:1185, vol 2.

primary site. In the former situation, appropriate radiographic evaluation and surgical planning can occur and be discussed with the patient. For metastatic lesions to the parotid gland from another primary site, appropriate workup can be initiated to determine the primary site. It should be noted that the routine use of an FNA biopsy in this fashion is controversial as some surgeons feel that it would not change their standard approach, a parotidectomy, and thus would add little to the management of such tumors. Some institutions reserve the FNA biopsy for inoperable or recurrent lesions. However, incisional or excisional biopsies are never performed to establish a tissue diagnosis, as such procedures can increase the likelihood of recurrence, the risk of injury to the facial nerve, and subsequent surgical morbidity (since a wide removal of the biopsy site must then be added to the cancer surgery).

Lymph Nodes

While the overall risk (18%)[11] of lymphatic spread is less common than for mucosal squamous cell carcinomas of the head and neck, it is still essential to carefully evaluate the regional lymph nodes. The influence of tumor histology on the frequency of clinically involved nodes at presentation in 474 previously untreated major salivary gland cancers was reviewed by Armstrong from MSKCC.[12] These data are presented in Table 32-5. The risk of nodal involvement increases with grade and size. However, adenoid cystic cancer, despite often being aggressive histologically and large in size, had only a 2% rate of clinically evident metastases.

Table 32–5   Clinically Involved Nodes at Presentation in Major Salivary Gland Cancers: The Influence of Tumor Histology

Histologic Subtypes	Number (%)
Anaplastic	6/7 (86)
Epidermoid	6/28 (21)
Adenocarcinoma	11/49 (22)
Mucoepidermoid	30/209 (14)
Malignant mixed	11/69 (16)
Acinic	2/55 (2)
Adenoid cystic	1/55 (2)
Oncocytoma	0/2 (0)
TOTAL	67/474 (14)

Data from Armstrong et al.[12]

Table 32–6   Effect of Tumor Histology on Occult Lymph Node Involvement in Major Salivary Gland Cancers

Histologic Subtypes	Number (%)
Epidermoid	9/22 (41)
Adenocarcinoma	7/38 (18)
Mucoepidermoid	26/179 (14)
Acinic	2/53 (4)
Adenoid cystic	2/54 (4)
Anaplastic	1/1
Malignant mixed	0/58
Oncocytoma	0/2
TOTAL	47/407 (12)

Data from Armstrong et al.[12]

In the series reported by Armstrong and associates,[12] overall clinically occult, pathologically positive nodes occurred in 12% (47/407). By univariate analysis, several factors appeared to predict the risk of occult metastases, but multivariate analysis revealed that only size and grade were significant risk factors. Tumors of 4 cm or more had a 20% (32/164) risk of occult metastases, compared with a 4% (9/220) risk for smaller tumors ($P < 0.00001$). High grade tumors (regardless of histologic type) had a 49% (29/59) risk of occult metastases, compared with a 7% (15/221) risk for intermediate or low-grade tumors ($P < 0.00001$). The effect of tumor histology and grade on occult nodal metastases is detailed in Tables 32-6 and 32-7.

It is rare for a low-grade tumor to metastasize to the regional nodes. All high-grade lesions carry a significant risk for nodal metastasis irrespective of the histologic type. High T stage lesions are associated with an increased incidence of nodal metastasis. Submandibular or sublingual primary salivary malignancies have an increased risk for nodal spread compared with parotid salivary malignancies. The histologic type can influence the risk for nodal metastasis as well. Mucoepidermoid carcinoma, squamous cell carcinoma, and undifferentiated carcinoma are associated with a high incidence of nodal metastasis; however, adenoid cystic carcinoma, malignant mixed carcinoma, and acinic cell carcinoma have a low incidence (see Tables 32-5 and 32-6).

The physical examination includes palpation of the preauricular-parotid region (preauricular, intraparotid, and periparotid nodes); submandibular nodes (level I); upper cervical nodes, especially the superior deep jugular nodes and jugulodigastric nodes (level II); and mid cervical nodes (level III). The ipsilateral tonsillar region should be inspected for fullness, which may indicate gross retropharyngeal nodal involvement, particularly when the deep lobe of the parotid is infiltrated by tumor. Any

Table 32–7   Effect of Tumor Grade on Occult Lymph Node Involvement in Major Salivary Gland Cancer

Tumor Grade	Number (%)
Low	2/125 (2)
Intermediate	13/96 (14)
High	29/59 (49)

Data from Armstrong et al.[12]

adenopathy is documented by location, size, number, texture, tenderness, and mobility. The initial radiographic evaluation of the parotid gland may also provide important clinical information regarding the nodal status.

Distant Spread

The most likely site for distant metastasis is the lung, followed by the bones and liver. Adenoid cystic carcinoma, malignant mixed tumor, and mucoepidermoid carcinoma have a risk for distant metastases that ranges from 25% to 35%.[13]

Careful examination of the lungs, percussion of the bones and palpation of the liver should be documented.

A routine chest x-ray should be obtained. Findings that suggest pulmonary metastases are further evaluated with a chest CT scan. Routine bone scans are not indicated unless there is clinical suspicion for osseous metastasis. If a patient is found to have hepatomegaly or elevated liver function tests, or both, an MRI of the liver should be obtained.

SUBMANDIBULAR GLAND

Primary Site

A submandibular salivary gland tumor usually presents as an asymptomatic mass but can be associated with episodic pain in 6% to 7% of cases. However, as the lesion progresses and enlarges, significant pain can develop and become constant. Patients can infrequently present with complaints of decreased sensation in the ipsilateral lower teeth, gums, and lower lip (cranial nerve V3); an inability to move the ipsilateral oral tongue (cranial nerve XII); or facial weakness associated with the marginal mandibular or cervical branch of the facial nerve (cranial VII) as the adjacent cranial nerves become involved with the malignant tumor (14%).

A careful and methodic examination of the patient can provide valuable information regarding the stage of the tumor. Bimanual palpation of the lateral floor of mouth area will provide data regarding tumor dimension, texture, and mobility. The overlying soft tissues and adjacent mandible are sites where tumors can infiltrate and should be carefully evaluated. The functional status of the adjacent cranial nerves must be documented. This includes the marginal mandibular or cervical branch of the facial nerve (cranial nerve VII) or both, the lingual nerve (cranial nerve V_3), or the ipsilateral hypoglossal nerve (cranial nerve XII).

Submandibular gland tumors are seldom imaged since they usually present early and are easily palpated. Note that large primary parotid gland lesions can push down into the submandibular space, thus giving the erroneous clinical impression that there is enlargement of the submandibular gland. If this is suspected in a particular case, one must radiographically evaluate the parotid gland with a CT or MRI. An obstructing calculus within Wharton's duct can cause retrograde pressure and thus result in enlargement of the submandibular gland. Enlargement of upper cervical lymph nodes can displace the submandibular gland, thus forming a "pseudomass."

Based on the particular characteristics of a sub-mandibular tumor, an MRI scan may be indicated to assist in evaluating for deep tissue infiltration or perineural extent of the tumor with respect to the lingual nerve (cranial nerve V$_3$), the hypoglossal nerve (cranial XII), and the marginal mandibular and cervical branches of the facial nerve (cranial nerve VII).

CTs or MRIs cannot generally differentiate between a benign or malignant submandibular mass and thus are not routinely used for small, mobile, circumscribed tumors. However, these studies can determine whether the mass is within the submandibular gland or extrinsic to it (e.g., dermoid, neural lesion, ranula, thyroglossal duct cyst, lymph node). Both benign and malignant salivary tumors may appear well circumscribed on a CT or MRI. This may cause one to underestimate the actual extent of infiltration of the cancer.

Concerns regarding the use of an FDG PET scan are similar to those discussed previously for parotid salivary gland malignancies.

The initial biopsy of a suspicious submandibular salivary gland mass can be an FNA biopsy. Such a procedure is important as only a minority of submandibular masses are primary tumors originating in that gland. Note that, in general, a submandibular gland mass has a 50% chance of being malignant. An FNA biopsy is useful only if it reveals a malignancy. It is important to recognize that the mass may be an enlarged submandibular lymph node (level I), and a careful evaluation of the head and neck for a primary mucosal lesion (e.g., oral cavity, maxillary antrum) must be performed. All suspicious lesions are approached surgically with a submandibular triangle dissection despite a negative FNA biopsy. Incisional or excisional biopsies are never performed to establish a tissue diagnosis, as such procedures increase the probability of recurrence and the risk of surgical morbidity since a wide removal of the biopsy site must be added to the final definitive surgical procedure. The only exception to this rule is when there is a small tumor of the submandibular gland that is surrounded by normal parenchyma—then a simple excision of the submandibular gland may be performed.

Lymph Nodes

Submandibular gland malignancies have an increased risk for nodal metastasis of compared to primary parotid gland lesions (28% vs. 18%, respectively). Otherwise, the general information presented previously for parotid salivary gland malignancies applies to this site.

The physical examination should include palpation of the submandibular nodes (level I), the upper cervical nodes (level II), and the mid cervical nodes (level III). The use of a bimanual palpation technique is particularly helpful in evaluating the submandibular region.

Distant Spread

The information presented previously for parotid gland malignancies is applicable to this site. The most likely region of distant metastasis is to the lung, followed by the bones and liver.

SUBLINGUAL SALIVARY GLAND

Primary Site

A sublingual salivary gland tumor usually presents as an asymptomatic swelling in the anterior floor of mouth. It may be difficult differentiating a primary lesion of the sublingual gland from a primary lesion of the floor of mouth. Up to 15% of patients with such a malignancy can have associated pain. Patients may complain of ipsilateral loss of tongue sensation (cranial nerve V3).

A careful and methodic examination of the patient can provide valuable information regarding the stage of the tumor. Bimanual palpation of the floor of mouth will provide data regarding tumor dimension, texture, and mobility. Because adjacent soft tissues are sites where tumor can infiltrate, they must be carefully evaluated. The functional status of the ipsilateral lingual nerve (cranial nerve V$_3$) must be documented.

Considerations regarding the use of CT, MRI, and FDG PET imaging are similar to those noted previously for submandibular salivary gland tumors.

The initial biopsy procedure of a suspicious sublingual region mass can be an FNA biopsy. Note that, in general, most sublingual salivary gland masses are malignant. Such a procedure is useful only if the biopsy reveals a malignancy. It is important to recognize that the mass may represent a primary minor salivary gland tumor in the anterior floor of mouth. These lesions, despite a negative FNA biopsy, should be resected with a formal cancer procedure. Incisional or excisional biopsies are never performed to establish a tissue diagnosis as such procedures increase the recurrence risk and the risk of surgical morbidity, since a wide removal of the biopsy site must be added to the final definitive cancer surgery.

Lymph Nodes

Sublingual salivary gland malignancies have an increased risk for nodal metastasis compared to parotid gland lesions. Otherwise, the general information presented previously for parotid gland malignancies applies to this site.

The physical examination should include palpation of the submental and submandibular nodes (level I). The use of a bimanual palpation technique is particularly helpful in evaluating this region.

Distant Spread

The information presented previously for parotid salivary gland malignancies applies to this site. The most likely region of distant metastasis is the lung, followed by the bones and liver.

Staging

The American Joint Committee on Cancer (AJCC) has established the staging criteria for major salivary gland tumors.[14] This system is based on an extensive retrospective review of the world's literature.

The AJCC clinical staging is based on two major categories of evaluation: (1) clinical examination findings—size of mass, fixation, extension to adjacent tissues, involvement of adjacent cranial nerves, and (2) radiologic findings.

Periodically, the staging criteria are reviewed and modified in order to better establish a system that reflects contemporary technology and therapeutic interventions. The current AJCC cancer staging criteria (Table 32-8) represents the sixth edition, published in 2002. The following examines the changes from the fifth edition (1997)[15] as it relates to major salivary gland tumors.

I. PRIMARY TUMOR (T) STAGING

The T3 classification was revised to maintain internal consistency of T classification in all head and neck sites. Previously, a T3 tumor represented one that had extra-capsular extension without cranial nerve VII involvement or was more than 4 cm but not more than 6 cm in greatest dimension, or both. The recently revised version defines a T3 tumor as being more than 4 cm or a tumor having extraparenchymal extension, or both.

Previously, a T4 tumor was one that would invade the base of skull, cranial VII, and/or exceeds 6 cm in greatest dimension. The current edition has divided the T4 category into T4a and T4b subclassifications: (1) T4a—tumor that invades the skin, mandible, ear canal, and/or cranial nerve VII; this indicates advanced lesions that are resectable with grossly clear margins. (2) T4b—tumor that invades the base of skull and/or pterygoid plates and/or encases the carotid artery; this classification reflects extension to areas that preclude resection with clear margins.

II. STAGE GROUPING

Major revisions have been made in this area (see Table 32-8).

III. ADDITIONAL DESCRIPTORS:

Residual Tumor (R): (*new category*)

1. RX: Presence of residual tumor cannot be assessed
2. R0: No residual tumor
3. R1: Microscopic tumor
4. R2: Macroscopic tumor

Lymphatic Vessel Invasion (L): (*new category*)

1. LX: Lymphatic vessel invasion cannot be assessed
2. L0: No lymphatic vessel invasion
3. L1: Lymphatic vessel invasion

Venous Invasion (V): (*new category*)

1. VX: Venous invasion cannot be assessed
2. V0: No venous invasion
3. V1: Microscopic venous invasion
4. V2: Macroscopic venous invasion
   "m" suffix: (*new category*)
   Multiple primary tumors in a single site: pT(m) NM
   "y" prefix: (*new category*)
   Classification of T stage during or following initial multimodality therapy: ycTNM or ypTNM
   "r" prefix: (*new category*)
   Notation of a recurrent tumor when staged after a disease-free interval: rTNM

Table 32–8   Classification of Salivary Gland Tumors

Primary Tumor (T)

TX	Primary tumor cannot be assessed
T0	No evidence of primary tumor
T1	Tumor ≤2 cm in greatest dimension without extraparenchymal extension*
T2	Tumor >2 cm but not >4 cm in greatest dimension without extraparenchymal extension*
T3	Tumor >4 cm and/or tumor having extraparenchymal extension*
T4a	Tumor invades skin, mandible, ear canal, and/or facial nerve
T4b	Tumor invades skull base and/or pterygoid plates and/or encases carotid artery

*Note: Extraparenchymal extension is clinical or macroscopic evidence of invasion of soft tissues. Microscopic evidence alone does not constitute extraparenchymal extension for classification purposes.

Regional Lymph Nodes (N)

NX	Regional lymph nodes cannot be assessed
N0	No regional lymph node metastasis
N1	Metastasis in a single ipsilateral lymph node, ≤3 cm in greatest dimension
N2	Metastasis in a single ipsilateral lymph node, >3 cm but not >6 cm in greatest dimension, or in multiple ipsilateral lymph nodes, none >6 cm in greatest dimension, or in bilateral or contralateral lymph nodes, none >6 cm in greatest dimension
N2a	Metastasis in a single ipsilateral lymph node, >3 cm but not >6 cm in greatest dimension
N2b	Metastasis in multiple ipsilateral lymph nodes, none >6 cm in greatest dimension
N2c	Metastasis in bilateral or contralateral lymph nodes, none >6 cm in greatest dimension
N3	Metastasis in a lymph node, >6 cm in greatest dimension

Distant Metastasis (M)

MX	Distant metastasis cannot be assessed
M0	No distant metastasis
M1	Distant metastasis

Stage Grouping

Stage I	T1	N0	M0
Stage II	T2	N0	M0
Stage III	T3	N0	M0
	T1	N1	M0
	T2	N1	M0
	T3	N1	M0
Stage IVA	T4a	N0	M0
	T4a	N1	M0
	T1	N2	M0
	T2	N2	M0
	T3	N2	M0
	T4a	N2	M0
Stage IVB	T4b	Any N	M0
	Any T	N3	M0
Stage IVC	Any T	Any N	M1

From Greene FL, Page DL, Fleming ID, et al, eds: *AJCC Cancer Staging Manual*, 6th ed. New York: Springer; 2002.

"a" prefix: (*new category*)
Stage determined at autopsy: aTNM

Treatment

SURGERY

Surgical resection of the involved major salivary gland is the primary treatment of choice. However, patients must be carefully selected to ensure resectability (see Staging earlier).

PAROTID GLAND

In patients with small lesions located in the tail of the parotid gland, a limited local excision without dissection of the facial (cranial VII) can be considered in highly selected patients. Otherwise, a superficial parotidectomy is the surgical treatment of choice.

For lesions confined to the superficial lobe of the parotid gland, which accounts for around 90% of the cases, the entire superficial lobe is resected in an en bloc fashion (superficial parotidectomy, subtotal parotidectomy, lateral lobe parotidectomy). Generally, an excisional biopsy alone is not done as it would violate the surgical field and is associated with a high recurrence rate. If the tumor is adjacent to the deep lobe, it may be necessary to resect both the superficial lobe and the deep lobe together (total parotidectomy). When the tumor extends to involve the adjacent soft tissues (skin, muscles) or bone, a large en bloc resection of these structures may be required (radical parotidectomy). Stensen's duct is divided and ligated during a typical superficial parotidectomy. Tumor tracking along this duct is rarely seen. The adjacent facial nerve (cranial nerve VII) must be carefully evaluated, and every effort should be made to preserve it. Loss of the facial nerve results in significant disability for the patient. Its innervation of the muscles of facial expression affects mastication, speaking, emotional expression, and socialization. However, in those cases where the facial nerve is enveloped by or adherent to tumor, this would require sacrifice of the nerve. All other situations undergo a dissection and preservation of the facial nerve. Under no circumstance should a piecemeal excision of the parotid tumor be performed in an effort to preserve the facial nerve. In certain instances, it may be possible to preserve part of the uninvolved facial nerve and sacrifice only the branches involved by tumor.

In selected cases where the facial nerve has been sacrificed, it is desirable to perform an immediate cable grafting as long as there are disease-free proximal and distal branches of the facial nerve. Donor nerves include the sensory nerve branches of the cervical plexus or the sural nerves. In cases where the proximal stump of the facial nerve is not available, the hypoglossal nerve (cranial nerve XII) can be anastomosed to the remaining distal portion of the facial nerve. The functional outcome of such nerve grafts are often quite suboptimal, although it usually will allow an improvement in muscle tone. It should be noted that the use of postoperative radiation therapy in these patients is not contraindicated. Radiation can begin at the usual time of 3 to 4 weeks postoperatively with a completely healed incision without any adverse effect on the nerve graft.[16]

With the sacrifice of the facial nerve, closure of the ipsilateral upper eyelid is compromised. This can cause corneal exposure with resultant ulceration, pain, and ultimately blindness. Therefore, it is important to address this functional defect with the placement of a gold weight in the upper eyelid or a tarsorrhaphy in order to protect the eye.

Following a parotidectomy, patients may not uncommonly develop ipsilateral facial sweating and flushing along the distribution of the auriculotemporal nerve during chewing, deglutition, or even when thinking of food. This is known as Frey's syndrome (gustatory sweating) and is due to misdirected regeneration of parasympathetic and sympathetic nerve fibers to the cholinergic receptors of the dermal sweat glands but is generally not a major problem.

For the 10% to 12% of cases involving the deep lobe of the parotid gland, a total parotidectomy is performed. This involves the removal of the entire parotid gland with a cuff of a normal tissue. However, it is difficult to distinguish between the borders of the gland and the adjacent fat, so in reality, the absolute removal of all glandular tissues is nearly impossible. The surgical principles presented earlier for lesions of the superficial lobes still apply to deep lobe lesions.

The overall incidence of occult regional lymph node metastasis is low for parotid gland tumors. Therefore, in general, an elective neck dissection is not performed routinely. However, if the primary lesion is sizable with a high-grade mucoepidermoid carcinoma or squamous cell carcinoma histopathology where there is an increased risk of nodal spread, selective neck dissection is performed.

For patients who present with clinically palpable adenopathy, a therapeutic neck dissection is the procedure of choice. However, if there is limited adenopathy located only in the first echelon nodes, a selective neck dissection can be considered.

SUBMANDIBULAR GLAND

In patients with small lesions of the submandibular salivary gland where the tumor is surrounded by normal parenchyma, a simple excision of the gland is adequate.

For lesions that have extracapsular extension with involvement of the adjacent muscles (digastric, mylohyoid, hypoglossal); nerves (lingual [cranial nerve V_3], hypoglossal [cranial nerve XII], marginal mandibular and cervical branches of the facial nerve [cranial nerve VII]); mandible; sublingual salivary gland; or floor of mouth, an extensive en bloc resection is required. Wharton's duct is divided and ligated. Usually this surgery is performed with a removal of nodal levels I, II, and III (extended supraomohyoid neck dissection).

The general philosophy and therapeutic approach to the lymph nodes are otherwise similar to that previously presented for parotid gland malignant tumors.

SUBLINGUAL GLAND

The anatomic location of the sublingual salivary glands in the floor of mouth bilaterally and their close proximity to the submandibular salivary glands and its Wharton's duct, which empties into the floor of mouth, are important relationships. If the lesion in the sublingual salivary gland is quite localized and small, this can sometimes be surgically resected in an en bloc fashion with a cuff of normal tissue from the floor of mouth without disturbing the drainage of the adjacent submandibular gland through Wharton's duct. More frequently, however, surgical resection of a sublingual salivary gland malignancy would damage Wharton's duct, and thus one would also resect the submandibular salivary gland and perform a type I neck dissection as the operative procedure of choice for these lesions. This approach is similar to that used for the removal of floor of mouth cancers.

RADIATION THERAPY

Indications for Primary Treatment

Medically or surgically unresectable primary or previously unirradiated recurrent malignant salivary gland tumors can be treated with one of the following options: (1) external beam radiation therapy (photons alone, mixed photons and electrons or electrons alone) using conventional or altered fractionation; (2) brachytherapy with or without external beam radiation; or (3) neutron therapy.

EXTERNAL BEAM RADIATION THERAPY

There is no evidence to indicate that unresectable malignant salivary gland tumors do not respond to conventionally fractionated photon radiation therapy. The literature contains reports of partially resected and unresected salivary gland cancers that were successfully treated in this fashion (Table 32-9) and the response rates are similar to those obtained from treating equivalent-sized squamous cell carcinomas of the head and neck.

The use of altered fractionation has been reported with encouraging results. Wang and Goodman[17] from Massachusetts General Hospital treated 14 patients with unresectable malignant parotid carcinomas using accelerated hyperfractionation (1.60 Gy twice a day) photon therapy and various boost techniques to a total dosage of 65 to 70 cGy. The 5-year actuarial local control rate was 82% and the disease-specific survival rate was 55%.

The therapeutic approach of accelerated fractionation external beam photon irradiation with a delayed concomitant boost with concurrent chemotherapy is used at MSKCC. Future studies using this combined modality attack are required. Our experience has shown that a pretreatment evaluation for a percutaneous endoscopic gastrostomy tube for sustenance and close aggressive

Table 32–9   Results of Various Radiation Modalities for Gross Cancer of Salivary Gland Origin

Reference	Site	Stage	Radiation Dose, Gy	Therapy Used	Local Control, % (*n*)
Early-Stage Minor Salivary Cancers					
Fu et al*	Various	NS	50–75	Photon	71 (5/7)
Hioruchi et al†	Various	T1–3	>65	Photon + brachytherapy	73 (8/11)
Ellis et al‡	Various	NS	Range	Photon	86 (6/7)
Weber et al§	Various	NS	Range	Photon	100 (8/8)
Late-Stage and Recurrent Major and Minor Salivary Cancers					
PHOTONS AND BRACHYTHERAPY					
King & Fletcher[19]	Major	Inoperable	50–70	Photon + brachytherapy	63 (10/16)
Armstrong et al‖	Major + Minor	Recurrent	See text		60 (12/20)
Wang & Goodman[17]	Major + Minor	T3–4	65–70	Photon (see text)	100 (10) parotid 78 (15)
Poulsen et al¶	Parotid	Residual**	Wide range	Photon	Minor: 54 (43)
Saroja et al††	Major + Minor	Recurrent Unresectable	18–24	Neutron	Major: 67 (63) Minor: 58 (55)
Catterall & Errington[22]	Major + Minor	Recurrent Unresectable	15.6	Neutron	72 (65)
Laramore et al[21]‡‡	Major + Minor	Recurrent Unresectable	55–70 16.5–22	Photon Neutron	17 (12) 56 (13)

NS, information not stated.

*From Fu K, Leibel S, Levine M, et al: Carcinoma of the major and minor salivary glands: Analysis of treatment results and sites and causes of failures. *Cancer.* 1977;40:2882.

†From Hioruchi J, Shibuya H, Suzuki S, et al: The role of radiotherapy in the management of adenoid cystic carcinoma of the head and neck. *Int J Radiat Oncol Biol Phys.* 1987;13:1135.

‡From Ellis E, Million R, Mendenhall W, et al: The use of radiation therapy in the management of minor salivary gland tumors. *Int J Radiat Oncol Biol Phys.* 1988;15:613.

§From Weber R, Palmer M, El-Naggar A, et al: Minor salivary gland tumors of the lip and buccal mucosa. *Laryngoscope.* 1989;99:6.

‖From Armstrong JG, Harrison LB, Spiro RH, et al: Brachytherapy of malignant tumors of salivary gland origin. *Endocurther Hypertherm Oncol.* 1990;6:19.

¶From Poulsen M, Pratt G, Kynaston B, Tripcony L: Prognostic variables in malignant epithelial tumors of the parotid. *Int J Radiat Oncol Biol Phys.* 1992;23:327.

**Gross residual after surgery.

††From Saroja K, Mansell J, Hendrikson F, et al: An update on malignant salivary gland tumors treated with neutrons at Fermilab. *Int J Radiat Oncol Biol Phys.* 1987;13:1319.

‡‡ Randomized trial.

monitoring of these patients are required due to the prominent acute side effects associated with the resulting mucositis and esophagitis.

BRACHYTHERAPY

For technically implantable lesions, brachytherapy alone or in conjunction with external beam therapy can be used for unresectable malignant parotid tumors. Particularly if the patient was previously treated with radiation therapy and has an unresectable recurrence, brachytherapy alone can be considered as the sole therapeutic modality.

Armstrong et al.[18] reported on 20 patients with recurrent or advanced disease treated with brachytherapy alone using ^{192}Ir or [125]I. Previously, radiation therapy had been administered to 15 of these patients. The implant was to gross disease in 15 of the 20 patients. The actuarial local control rate at 5 years was 60%. Two patients had soft tissue necrosis as a complication and were treated with conservative management. However, two patients with extensive skull base tumors treated with partial surgery and ^{125}I implants for gross residual disease had cerebral abscesses, of which one was fatal.

In unresectable cases with no prior history of radiation, combined external beam and brachytherapy techniques have been employed. King and Fletcher[19] reported on 16 such patients treated in this fashion with 10 (63%) achieving local control.

NEUTRON THERAPY

Neutron therapy is a specialized form of external beam radiation. Its specific therapeutic indication is in cases of unresectable, previously unirradiated primary and recurrent salivary gland malignancies. Only a few institutions in the United States have this modality, including the University of Washington (Seattle) and Wayne State University (Detroit).

Neutrons are a densely ionizing, high linear energy transfer type of particulate radiation that have a limited role in clinical radiation oncology. Fast neutrons are contrasted to photons in the following fashion: (1) the biologic effectiveness of neutrons is much less affected by a hypoxic environment; (2) the lethal effects of neutrons are less dependent on the cell cycle phase compared to photons; (3) the repair of sublethal damage in malignant cells matters less; (4) neutrons are biologically more effective (relative biologic effectiveness [RBE] > 2.6). Also, fast neutrons lack skin sparing and thus can cause a more prominent acute dermal reaction than photons.

Batterman and associates[20] measured the RBE of neutrons to cobalt-60 for human tumors metastatic to lung. RBE was inferred by observation of growth delay. A metastatic adenoid cystic cancer had an RBE of 8 compared with 2.5 to 4 for most other tumors. This observation on limited clinical material prompted an enthusiastic evaluation of the role of neutrons for the treatment of localized salivary cancers.

Neutrons have a high RBE compared with photons. This does not mean, however, that they have a superior therapeutic ratio. Estimates of the exact RBE for salivary cancers are variable and it may simply be that more "radiation effect" was given with the neutron doses than with the photon doses. This may have had two effects—one was the increased local control, and the other was the doubling of severe late effects. In the paper from Laramore and associates,[21] severe late effects were detailed comparing the two treatments. Severe late effects can be assessed by measuring the occurrence of each category of toxicity in each patient. For photons, there were 10 events in 12 categories of toxicity in 12 patients. This represents a 7% occurrence rate (10/144 = 7%). For neutrons, there were 26 events in 12 categories of toxicity in 13 patients, representing a 17% occurrence rate (26/156 = 17%). The outstanding question about neutron therapy is whether equivalent local control could be achieved with photons if the dose of photons were escalated to a point at which the toxicity was equivalent to that of neutron therapy.

The Radiation Therapy Oncology Group (United States) and the Medical Research Council (MRC, England)[21] conducted a major randomized phase III multi-institutional clinical trial of the treatment of 32 patients with unresectable salivary gland tumors with either fast neutrons, photons or electrons, or both. The 10-year likelihood of local control was 56% with neutrons and 17% with photons/electrons. The neutron group had a higher incidence of distant metastasis. The overall survival was not improved with neutrons.

Caterall et al.[22] reported on the MRC cyclotron experience of 65 patients with locally advanced or recurrent malignant salivary gland tumors, 89% of which were stage IV, who were treated with fast neutron radiotherapy. They achieved a 72% local control rate. The 5-year survival rate was 50%. The facial nerve was not damaged by neutron therapy.

INDICATIONS FOR POSTOPERATIVE RADIATION THERAPY

The indications for postoperative radiation therapy include: (1) resectable primary T4 and recurrent tumors; (2) high-grade lesions including adenoid cystic carcinoma; (3) positive or close surgical margins; (4) perineural (including facial nerve)/vascular invasion; (5) concern of the surgeon over the margins or conduct of the procedure (e.g., piecemeal resection, tumor spillage) irrespective of the pathology report; and (6) loco-regional lymph node metastasis.

The use of postoperative radiation therapy has an established and important role in the treatment of major salivary gland tumors. Its employment substantially improves locoregional control in selected cases.

Spiro and colleagues[23] reviewed the experience at MSKCC of 288 patients with parotid malignancies who were primarily treated with surgery (only 12 patients underwent postoperative radiation therapy). Recurrence rates by stage were as follows: (1) stage I: 7%; (2) stage II: 21%; and (3) stage III: 58%.

In comparison, Harrison and colleagues[24] reported on the 5-year actuarial local control rates by T classification of MSKCC patients with major salivary gland malignancies who were treated with surgery and postoperative radiation therapy: (1) T1: 100%; (2) T2: 83%; (3) T3: 80%; (4) T4: 43%. Patients without neck node

Table 32–10   Impact of Postoperative Radiation Therapy on Local Control and Survival in Cancer of Major Salivary Glands

| Reference | Selection | Reason for RT (*n*) | Local Control | | | 5-yr Survival, % |
			Therapy	%	*Follow-up, %*	
King & Fletcher[46]	NS	Positive margins (27)	SX + RT	94	5–20	NS
		Elective (19)				
Guillamondegui et al[45]	NS	Positive margins (15)	SX + RT	86	NS	NS
		Elective (14)				
		No RT (104)	SX	74	5	NS
Tapley*	Parotid	Gross disease (13)	SX + RT	91	NS	NS
		Positive margins (15)				
		Other (5)				
		No RT (54)	SX	70	NS	NS
Fu et al[25]	T1–T3	Positive margins or close (23)	SX + RT	83	NS	NS
		No RT (36)	SX	72	NS	NS
Chung et al†	M0	Positive margins (17)	SX + RT	94	NS	NS
		Perineural				
Fitzpatrick & Theriault‡	TxNx	NS (228)	SX + RT	73	NS	74
		No RT (101)	SX	26	NS	60
Bisset & Fitzpatrick§	Submandibular	NS (54)	SX + RT	69	NS	65
		No RT (30)	SX	30	NS	60
North et al‖	T1–T4	NS (50)	SX + RT	96	NS	76
		No RT (19)	SX	74	NS	60

NS, information not stated; RT, radiation therapy; SX, surgery.

*From Tapley N: Irradiation treatment of malignant tumors of the salivary glands. *Ear Nose Throat J.* 1977;56:110.

†From Chung C, Sagerman R, Ryoo M, et al: The changing role of external beam irradiation in the management of malignant tumors of the major salivary glands. *Radiology.* 1982;145:175.

‡From Fitzpatrick P, Theriault C: Malignant salivary gland tumors. *Int J Radiat Oncol Biol Phys.* 1986;12:1743.

§From Bissett R, Fitzpatrick P: Malignant submandibular gland tumors. *Am J Clin Oncol.* 1988;11:46.

‖From North C, Lee D-J, Piantadosi S, et al: Carcinoma of the major salivary glands treated by surgery or surgery plus postoperative radiotherapy. *Int J Radiat Oncol Biol Phys.* 1990;18:1319.

involvement had an 83% local control rate versus 58% for those with nodal metastasis.

At UCSF, Fu and colleagues[25] reported on 35 patients with minor and major salivary gland carcinomas who had known microscopic disease at or close to the surgical margins following curative surgery. There was a 54% (7/13) recurrence rate in patients who underwent surgery alone compared to a 14% (3/22) rate for those treated with surgery and postoperative radiation therapy.

Various other retrospective reports are reported in the literature detailing the value of adjuvant postoperative radiation therapy (Table 32-10).

The biggest criticism of these studies is that they do not accurately compare the distribution of the many prognostic factors between the surgery-alone patients and the combined-treatment group. These factors include three primary sites; a large number of histologies; and the effect of grade, TNM staging, extent of surgery, margin status, and deep lobe involvement. To control for this large number of variables, Armstrong and associates[26] performed a matched-pair analysis comparing 46 patients treated with surgery and postoperative radiation with 46 prognostically matched patients treated with surgery alone. The large population of patients treated with surgery alone at MSKCC allowed selection (without reference to outcome) of very well matched pairs. This analysis demonstrated that outcome was excellent for stage I and II cancers treated with surgery alone. For patients with T3 and T4 tumors or nodal disease, postoperative radiation therapy significantly improved locoregional control

and survival (Table 32-11). There was a trend toward improved outcome when high-grade tumors were treated with postoperative radiation. Despite the enhancement of local control with radiation, local failures occurred in 51% of stage III and IV tumors, and 37% of high-grade tumors. Harrison and associates[24] reported that local failure was particularly high for T4 tumors, despite the use of surgery and postoperative radiation. This provides a rationale for adjuvant brachytherapy in selected cases. Although the data are limited for adenoid cystic cancer (Table 32-12), most authorities recommend postoperative radiation for all but the smallest tumors.

CLINICAL PREPARATION FOR RADIATION THERAPY

All patients must undergo an initial dental consultation before any radiation therapy. The radiation oncologist

Table 32–11   Postoperative Radiation Therapy: A Matched-Pair Analysis

	Surgery, %	Surgery + Radiation, %
Stage I/II		
5-yr survival	96	82
5-yr local control	91	79
Stage III/IV		
5-yr survival	10	51
5-yr local control	17	51

Data from Armstrong et al.[12]

Table 32–12   Impact of Postoperative Radiation Therapy on Local Control of Adenoid Cystic Cancer

Reference	Surgery, % (n)	Surgery + Radiation, % (n)
Fu et al[25]	30 (10)	90 (10)
Matsuba et al*	24 (19)	60 (36)
Miglianico et al†	44 (38)	78 (43)

*From Matsuba H, Spector G, Thawley SE, et al: Adenoid cystic salivary gland carcinoma: A histopathologic review of treatment failure patterns. *Cancer.* 1986;57:519.
†From Miglianico L, Eschwege F, Marandas P, et al: Cervico-facial adenoid cystic carcinoma: Study of 102 cases. Influence of radiation therapy. *Int J Radiat Oncol Biol Phys.* 1987;13:673.

and dentist must discuss the treatment volume, field arrangements, dosage, and status of the oral cavity. Teeth that are not felt to be salvageable are extracted. Mouth guards are custom made for patients who have significant tooth fillings that will be within the treatment volume so as to decrease the effect of their interaction with radiation associated with focal sites of adjacent mucositis. A lifetime program of fluoride prophylaxis is prescribed. Routine dental evaluations during and after radiation therapy are mandatory.

Baseline thyroid function tests (T3, T4, thyroid-stimulating hormone [TSH]) are obtained before the initiation of radiation and are serially evaluated every 6 months after treatment for up to 5 years. The thyroid gland is a very radiosensitive organ and may show signs of clinical (5%) or chemical (20% to 25%) hypothyroidism in adult patients. Patients who have undergone a hemithyroidectomy can have a risk of as high as 66% of developing a chemical hypothyroidism. If the TSH is increased above the normal range, such patients are started on thyroid hormone replacement therapy irrespective of the T3 and T4 values, which sometimes are within the normal range. Replacement hormonal therapy is continued throughout the life of the patient.

RADIATION ONCOLOGY TREATMENT PLANNING

Simulation

Patients will undergo simulation in a supine position. The head is placed in a holder that will allow hyperextension of the neck. All incisional scars and masses are wired with material appropriate for visualization on regular fluoroscopic simulation films or on the CT scans, depending on which unit is used. A bite block is employed for patients with tumors of the submandibular or sublingual glands; however, it is usually unnecessary for parotid gland tumors. A customized face mask (Fig. 32-13) is created for immobilization and consistency of the head and neck position throughout treatment. A shoulder pull board is employed to bring the shoulder maximally in a caudad direction, particularly when the neck nodes are treated.

At this time, the patient will undergo a fluoroscopically assisted simulation or a CT simulation, depending on whether they will be treated with a two-dimensional or three-dimensional conformal/IMRT treatment plan.[27]

For the patients who undergo a two-dimensional or fluoroscopically assisted simulation, the borders are based on the anatomic structures within the treatment volume

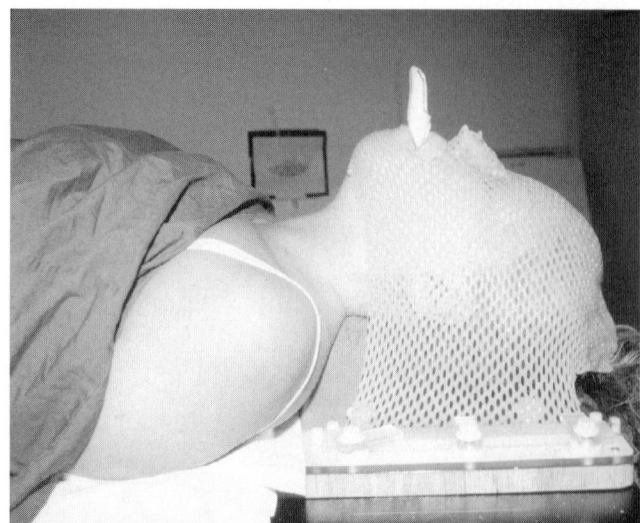

Figure 32–13. Customized face mask and bite block in preparation for CT simulation.

that are peculiar to the salivary gland subsite to be treated. Once the simulation films are evaluated and approved, blocks are drawn on them to shield areas not requiring treatment. Cerrobend blocks are then manufactured.

For the patients who will undergo a CT simulation (Fig. 32-14), the area within the superior and inferior borders of the field, which includes the treatment volume, are scanned using 3 mm slices. No IV contrast is needed. The radiation oncologist then selects the isocenter location on the CT scan, which is then marked on the patient with a permanent tattoo.

COMPUTER TREATMENT PLANNING

The computer data from the CT simulation is downloaded from the CT simulator and transferred to treatment planning computers. The clinical target volume (CTV), which represents the visualized tumor (gross target volume [GTV]) and regions at risk for microscopic disease, such as adjacent tissues or lymph nodes as well as the important adjacent normal structures including the spinal cord, brainstem, optic nerves/chiasm, orbits, cochlea, and the contralateral parotid gland, are contoured. When

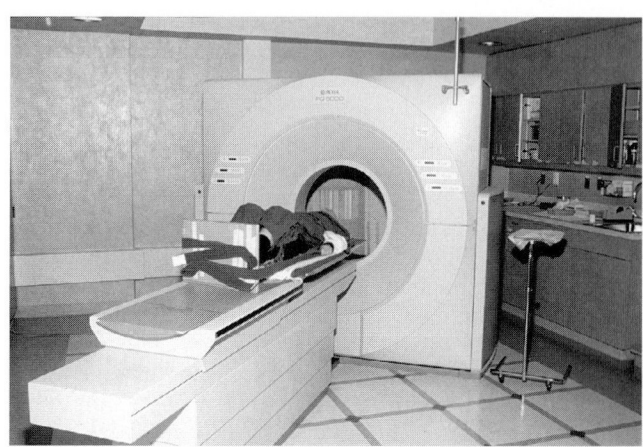

Figure 32–14. CT simulation using head holder, face mask, bite block, and shoulder pull board.

contouring the postoperative surgical bed, the remaining intact contralateral salivary gland is used as an anatomic reference point. A generous margin around the anatomic region of at least 2 cm should be considered in order to cover the entire operative bed with sufficient borders. For patients who have adenoid cystic carcinoma of the salivary gland, the usual approach is to irradiate the pathways of the adjacent cranial nerve up to the base of skull. The detailed and complex pathways of the cranial nerve must be carefully and accurately contoured. LeBlanc[28] has correlated gross anatomic information with associated CT axial images delineating these pathways. The regional lymph node areas will require contouring in specific instances as noted earlier. Several excellent references are available that explore the anatomic region of the respective surgical lymph node group levels (I to VI) with respect to their location on axial CT slices. Nowak et al.[29] correlated

the borders of the surgical levels in the neck (I to VI) with structures seen on a CT scan. They defined the six cervical lymph node regions and noted their respective reproducible landmarks on the CT scan. Wijers et al.[30] presented a more simplified approach for delineating cervical nodal target volume based on CT scans. Chao et al.[31] published guidelines for target volume determination of head and neck lymph nodes. This was based on their analysis of lymph node failure in IMRT-treated patients.

This anatomic data is then used for computer-based complex treatment planning employing the three-dimensional conformal radiation therapy (3DCRT) or intensity-modulated radiation therapy (IMRT) technique, whichever is most appropriate. A thorough discussion between the radiation oncologist and dosimetry staff is held to outline the disease status, treatment goals, areas of concern, and dosage planned. The resulting isodose

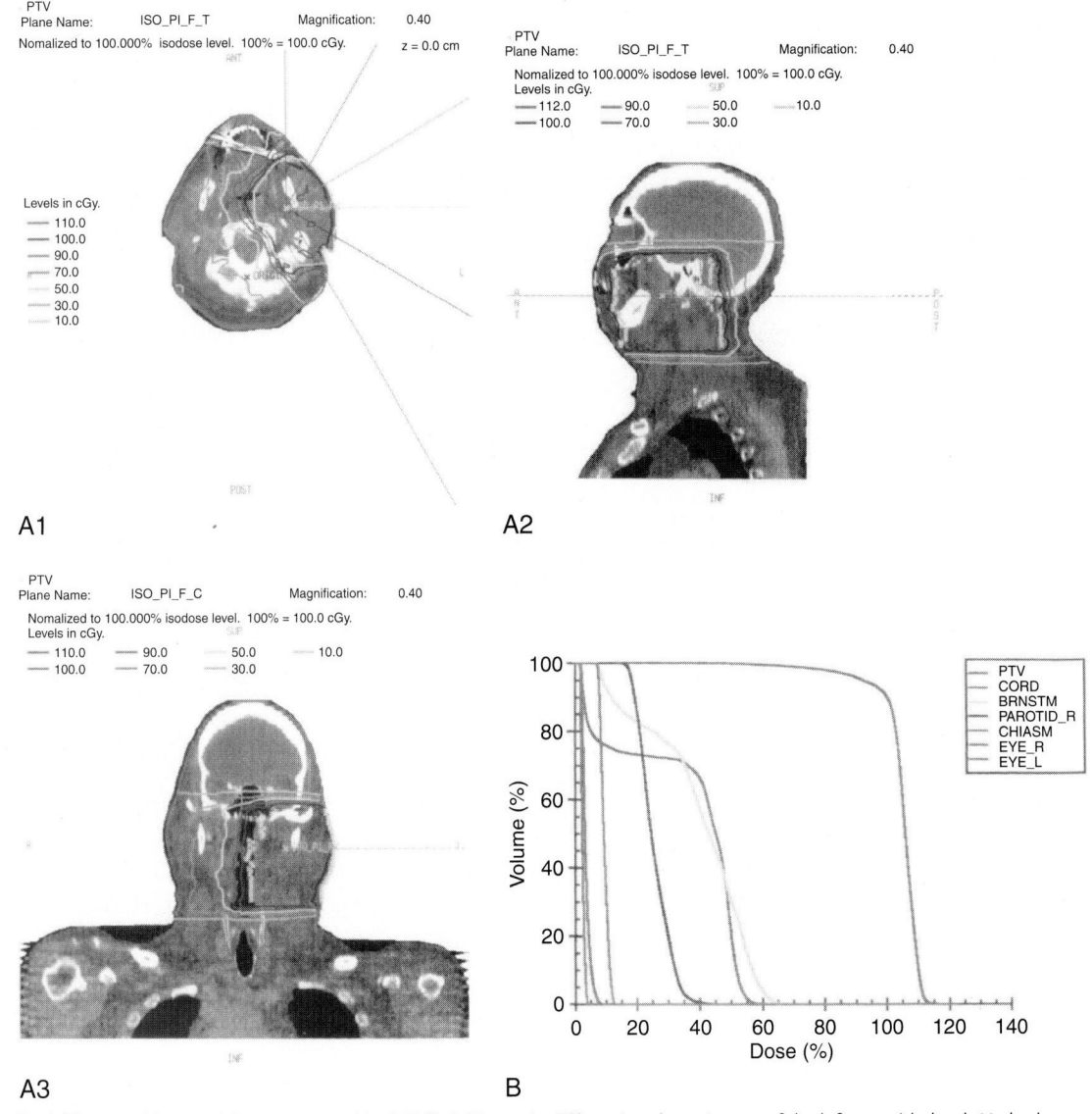

Figure 32–15. A 59-year-old man with an unresectable cT4N2aMO poorly differentiated carcinoma of the left parotid gland. He had progressive severe localized pain in the parotid gland and left facial nerve (CN VII) paralysis. This patient was treated with cisplatin chemotherapy concurrent with accelerated fractionation IMRT-based external beam radiation therapy with a delayed concomitant boost. The left parotid gland and cervical adenopathy were taken to 70 Gy and the left cervical and supraclavicular nodes were taken to 50 to 54 Gy. A complete clinical response was achieved with resolution of all disease on examination and on computed tomography and positron emission tomography scans. **A,** Isodose distributions (A1, axial; A2, sagittal; A3, coronal). **B,** Dose volume histogram. See also Color Figures 32–15A–B.

Continued

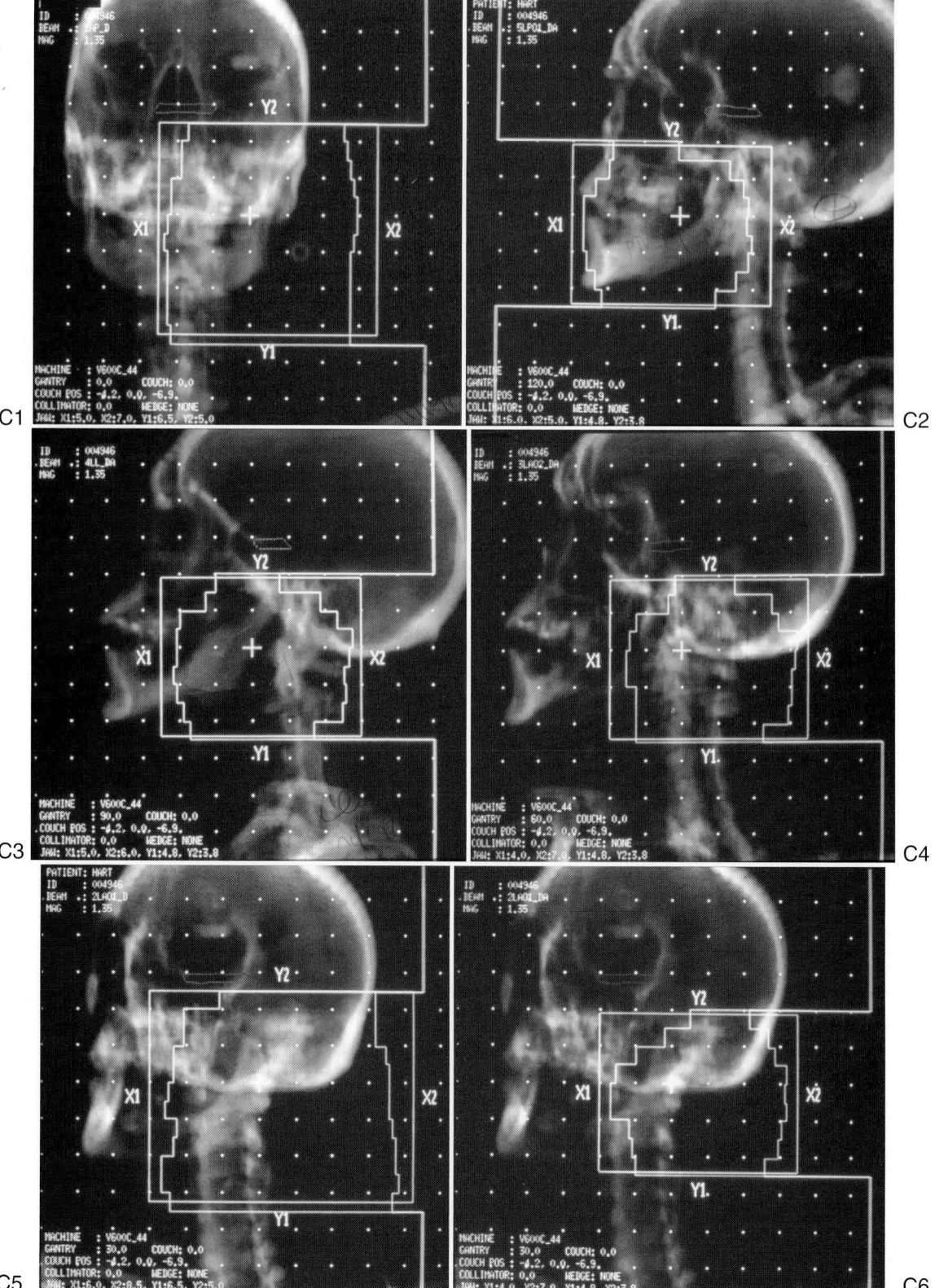

Figure 32–15. *Continued* **C,** Digitally reconstructed radiographs (DRRs).

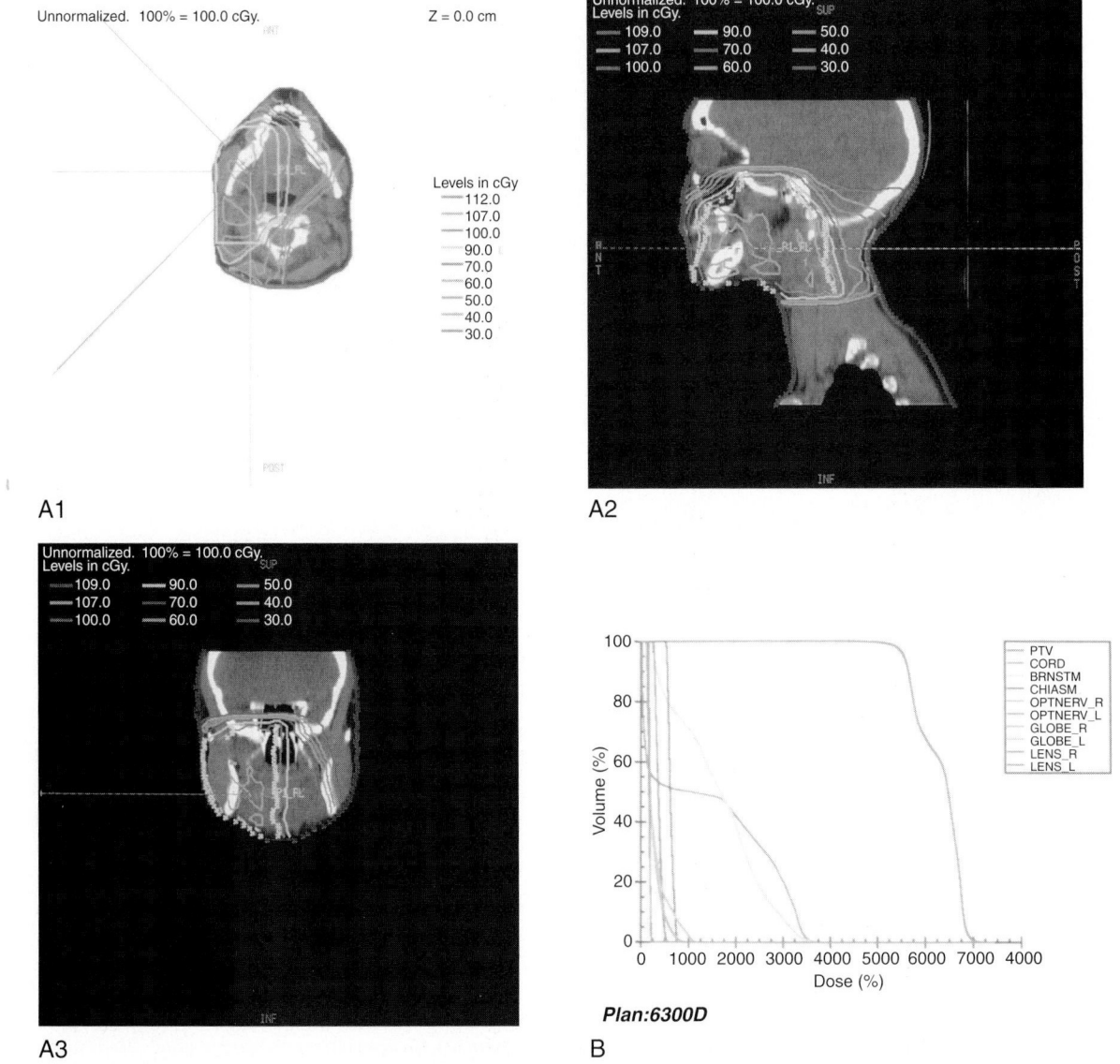

Figure 32–16. A 34-year-old woman with a pT1N0M0 adenoid cystic carcinoma of the right submandibular salivary gland. This patient underwent resection of the gland with pathology findings of positive surgical margins and perineural invasion. Postoperative intensity-modulated radiation therapy–based external beam radiation was administered to a treatment volume consisting of the right submandibular gland area and the pathways of the adjacent lingual nerve (CN V3) and the hypoglossal nerve (CN XII) to the base of skull to a dosage of 54 Gy. The postoperative bed in the submandibular area was then boosted to a total cumulative dosage of 63 Gy. **A,** Isodose distributions (A1, axial; A2, sagittal; A3, coronal). **B,** Dose volume histogram. See also Color Figure 32-16.

curves, dose-volume histograms (DVH) for the tumor area as well as the adjacent critical structures, and the digitally reconstructed radiographs (DRR) are carefully evaluated (See Figs. 32-15 to 32-17).

RADIATION THERAPY TECHNIQUES

Parotid Gland Tumors

PRIMARY SITE. Over the past several decades, multiple techniques have been used for the radiation treatment of parotid gland tumors. These have ranged from very basic to extremely complex plans and are related to the evolution of the therapy units, treatment planning sophistication, and our understanding of normal tissue tolerance.

Radiation therapy approaches include: (1) electrons—lateral en face electron beam (Fig. 32-18); (2) combination of electrons and photons (50% to 80% weighting toward electrons)—lateral en face electron beam and photons using a direct lateral field or a wedge-pair technique; (3) photons—wedge pair using 3DCRT or IMRT approach (Figs. 32-15 to 32-17).

The most frequently used techniques have been with a combination of electrons and photons as a so-called *mixed beam* or photons alone using a wedge pair. Electrons are delivered with a direct lateral en face approach covering the tumor (parotid gland) or tumor bed with a 2 to 3 cm margin.

The general portal margins that would encompass the planning target volume are: (1) superior—top of the zygomatic bone; (2) inferior—hyoid bone–thyroid notch interspace; (3) anterior—2 cm anterior to the upper second molar; (4) posterior—posterior to the mastoid tip;

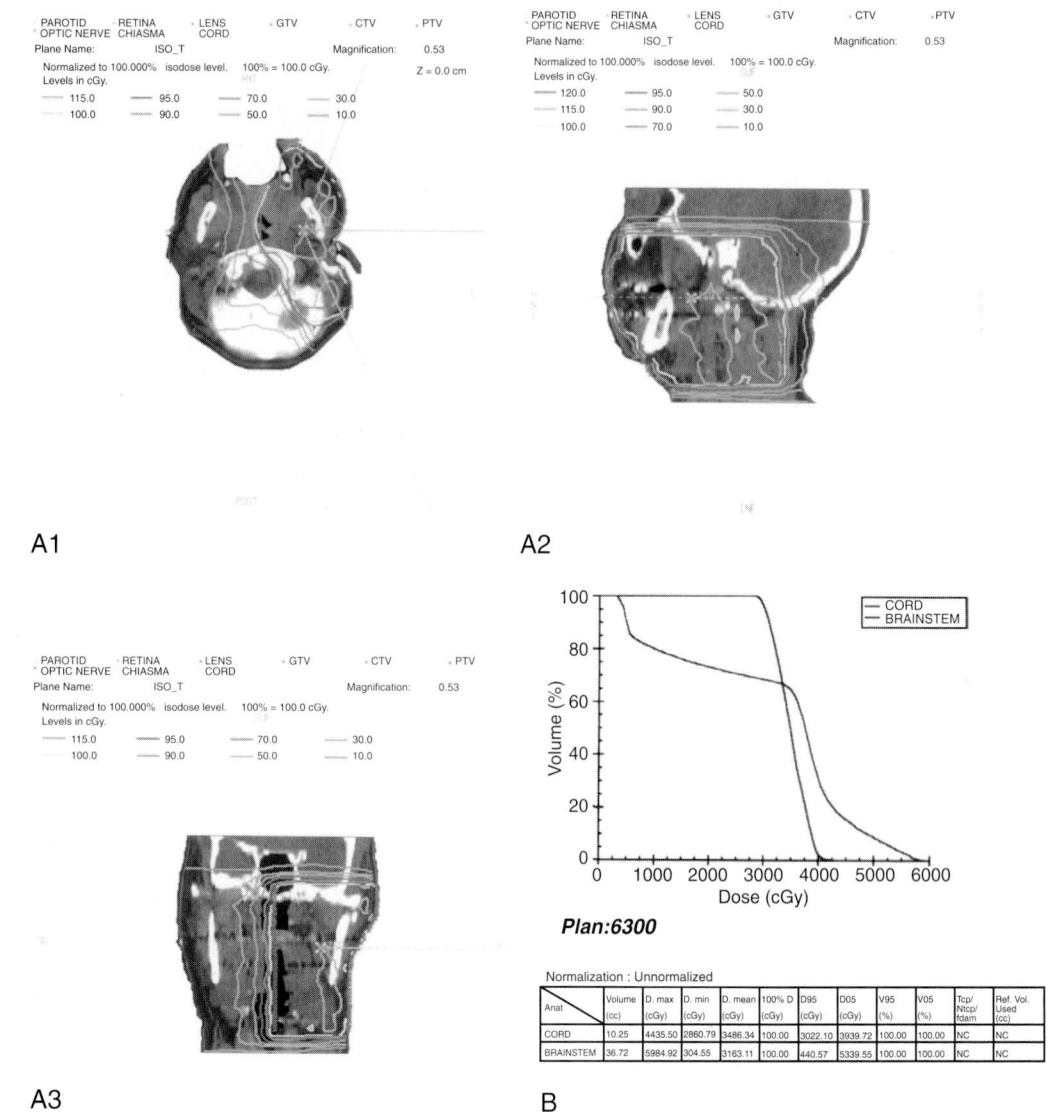

Figure 32–17. A 34-year-old man with a pT4B N0 M0 poorly differentiated mucoepidermoid carcinoma of the left parotid gland (deep lobe) with facial nerve (CN VII) paralysis. This patient underwent a left total parotidectomy with facial nerve sacrifice. A facial nerve graft with a facial sling was performed. The tumor extended superiorly to the left base of skull and had completely encased the facial nerve at the stylomastoid foramen. Pathology evaluation revealed a poorly differentiated mucoepidermoid carcinoma of the left parotid measuring 2.0 cm, which extended into the periparotid soft tissue and skeletal muscle. The carcinoma focally involved the inked resection margin. There was perineural invasion. All 13 lymph nodes were negative for metastatic disease. The patient was felt to be at high risk for local-regional recurrence, and therefore postoperative radiation therapy was adminis-tered to the left parotid gland–left base of skull, left retropharyngeal nodes–left upper cervical nodes using intensity-modulated radiation therapy–based external beam radiation therapy to 63 Gy. The ipsilateral cervical and supraclavicular nodes (off spinal cord) were taken to 50 Gy. **A,** Isodose distributions (A1, axial; A2, sagittal; A3, coronal). **B,** Dose volume histogram. See also Color Figure 32-17.

(5) lateral—2 cm flash of the cheek; (6) medial—2 cm medial from the ipsilateral oropharyngeal area. However, if the accessory parotid gland is involved with tumor, an additional 2 cm margin must be added anteriorly since this is the location of this parotid gland anatomic variation.

The electron portal margins are 1 cm larger than those for photons due to the constriction of the electron isodose curves at depth. The energy of the electron that is chosen depends on the anatomic distance from the skin of the ipsilateral cheek to the oral mucosa and will generally range between 12 and 16 MeV. In some insti-tutions, the ipsilateral external auditory canal, tympanic membrane and middle ear are protected from radiation with the use of a Cerrobend ear plug.

The photon technique using a wedge pair involves an anterior and a posterior oblique ipsilateral attack with wedges (45 and 30 degrees) on a cobalt 60 1.25 MV gamma ray unit or a linear accelerator with 4 to 6 MV x-rays. The basic clinical margin setup is similar to that noted above for electrons but without the added extra 1 cm margin. In order to avoid an exit dose through the contralateral eye, some would use a slight inferior angulation of the beam. Bolus is placed over the scar if clinically indicated.

When a combination of electrons and photons are used, either modality can start first. There is a weighting between 50% and 80% with electrons, but this can also be with the photon component depending on the discretion

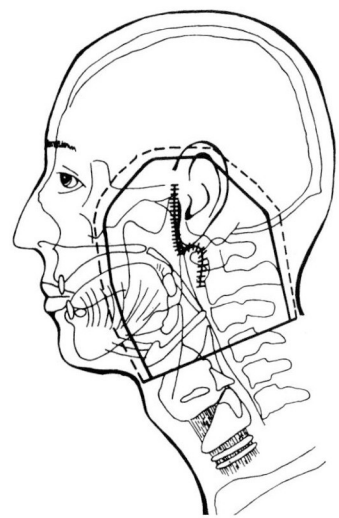

Figure 32–18. Postoperative left lateral electron beam portal for a parotid gland carcinoma. Note that the *dashed line* is 1 cm larger than photon portals due to the constriction of the electron isodose lines at depth. (From Levitt ST, Khan FM, Potish RA, et al, eds. *Levitt and Tapley's Technological Basis of Radiation Therapy: Practical Clinical Applications*, 3rd ed. Philadelphia: Lea & Febiger; 1999:294.)

of the radiation oncologist. By mixing the two different beams, one can decrease the irradiation of the contralateral parotid gland, acute radiation skin reaction, and mucositis.

With the development of CT simulation and sophisticated computer-based treatment planning, the state of the art and the preferred radiation techniques now mandate the use of 3DCRT or IMRT depending on the needs and complexity of the plan. For the majority of cases, 3DCRT using either a two- or three-field approach including wedges is appropriate. However, when the histopathology is adenoid cystic carcinoma, the increased risk of perineural invasion and travel along the pathways of the adjacent cranial nerves (beware of perineural skip lesions) require the treatment volume to include the neural pathways to the base of skull. In such cases, IMRT treatment plans give the best approach.

LYMPH NODES. When there is an indication to treat the regional lymph nodes as presented earlier in the chapter, either electrons (9 MeV) or photons (6MV to 25MV) are employed. Only ipsilateral regional lymph nodes are treated as it is quite rare for there to be involvement of the contralateral cervical nodes, even with multiple ipsilateral cervical nodal involvement. However, if significant bulky nodes are encountered, some would consider the contralateral cervical nodes to be at sufficient risk for metastatic disease and would therefore treat the bilateral neck nodes. Otherwise, the usual approach is to treat the entire ipsilateral cervical and supraclavicular nodes.

With electrons, a direct lateral or en face field is matched to the primary parotid field. Special care must be taken to get the ipsilateral shoulder as far down as possible. This is to allow for the electron cone to be positioned to include the nodes as far down the chain as possible. When multiple cervical lymph nodes are involved, photons should be used to treat the ipsilateral lower cervical nodes as well as the adjacent supraclavicular nodes.

When photons are used, either anteroposterior–posteroanterior (AP/PA) or direct AP fields are used and positioned off the spinal cord. If there is concern regarding the nodal regions in the mid to posterior neck, then the AP/PA approach is employed. These fields are matched with the primary parotid fields, and asymmetric jaws or half beam blocks at the superior margin are used to decrease the overlap of the adjoining field.

RADIATION DOSAGE
PRIMARY TREATMENT

The intact, unresectable parotid gland tumor is considered for neutron therapy. In those patients in whom it is elected instead to undergo photon or electron therapy, or both, an accelerated fractionation with a delayed concomitant boost is used often with concurrent chemotherapy using cisplatin on days 1 and 22. Initially, with phase I, 1.8 Gy is administered per fraction, one fraction per day, 5 days per week for 4 weeks giving a total dosage of 36 Gy. At this point, phase II begins with twice-a-day treatment separated by at least 6 hours. The morning fraction is a continuation of the initial treatment volume and scheme for phase I for the remaining 2 weeks (10 fractions) to a total of 54 Gy. The afternoon fraction is given 6 hours after the morning dose at a fraction size of 1.6 Gy to a cone-down treatment volume that consists of the gross tumor area/primary and adenopathy. This is continued for 2 weeks (10 fractions) to a dosage of 16 Gy. Ultimately, the total cumulative dosage from phase I and II to the gross tumor areas is 70 Gy and to the electively irradiated areas is 54 Gy. The spinal cord dosage is kept to a maximum dosage of 45 Gy.

POSTOPERATIVE TREATMENT TO THE PRIMARY AREA

Postoperative radiation therapy is administered within 6 weeks of surgery or when the incision is completely healed. Extended delays increase the risk for local-regional recurrence of disease and must be avoided if at all possible. A dosage of 1.8 to 2.0 Gy per fraction, 1 fraction per day, 5 days per week is administered to a total cumulative dosage as follows: (1) high-risk areas for microscopic disease in surgically violated regions: 60 Gy (2.0 Gy/fraction) to 63 Gy (1.8 Gy/fraction); (2) small volume of known microscopic disease: 66 Gy; (3) elective irradiation of areas at risk for microscopic disease: 50 Gy (2.0 Gy/fraction) to 54 Gy (1.8 Gy/fraction); and (4) gross residual disease: 70 Gy.

REGIONAL LYMPH NODES

Patients treated by primary radiation therapy are approached with accelerated fractionation radiation therapy with a delayed concomitant boost to 70 Gy, often with concurrent cisplatin chemotherapy, on days 1 and 2 as noted earlier. Any gross adenopathy is included within the primary salivary gland lesion in the afternoon (PM) boost cone-down treatment, which is taken to a total cumulative dosage of 70 Gy. Elective nodal irradiation is administered to 50 Gy (2.0 Gy/fraction) to 54 Gy (1.8 Gy/fraction).

When postoperative radiation therapy is indicated for the ipsilateral regional lymph nodes, a dosage of 50 Gy

(2.0 Gy/fraction) to 54 Gy (1.8 Gy/fraction) is administered. High-risk regions with stage pN2A (>3 cm to <6 cm), stage pN2B (multiple ipsilateral lymph nodes), stage pN3 (>6 cm), extracapsular extension, perineural or perivascular invasion, or a surgical procedure (e.g., excisional or incisional biopsy of a neck node before definitive cancer surgery) are boosted to a total cumulative dosage of 63 Gy.

SUBMANDIBULAR GLAND

Primary Site

The bilaterally paired submandibular salivary glands occupy an anatomic location that is adjacent to the medial rim of the mandible from an area just proximal to the angle of the mandible to the mid aspect of the mandible in the mid to lateral floor of mouth region. The superior extent of the gland is below the mucosa of the lateral floor of mouth region. The inferior extent of the gland approaches the hyoid bone.

The general portal margins that would encompass the planning target volume are: (1) superior—1 cm above the upper border of the tongue; (2) inferior—hyoid bone–thyroid notch interspace; (3) anterior—anterior aspect of the mental symphysis; (4) posterior—base of tongue-jugulodigastric nodal area; (5) lateral—2 cm flash of ipsilateral mandible; (6) medial—midline of tongue.

The radiation therapy techniques for the parotid gland tumors are applicable to this region. Generally, a combination of electrons and photons or photons alone have been used. However, treatment planning with 3DCRT or IMRT for photons represents the best contemporary treatment approach. This will allow a carefully sculpted homogenous dose delivery to the tumor area and good sparing of adjacent structures.

Lymph Nodes

The submandibular salivary glands drain in an orderly fashion to the adjacent submandibular nodes (level I) and then into the upper (level II) and mid (level III) cervical nodes. Contralaterally, lymph node drainage is rare.

The indications for irradiation of the ipsilateral regional lymph nodes are the same as for parotid gland tumors. However, there is up to a 30% incidence of lymph node metastasis in general and some would always include irradiation of the lymph nodes when the primary area is treated.

The treatment volume includes the ipsilateral submandibular, cervical, and supraclavicular nodes. The field arrangements would be similar to those used for parotid gland tumors.

Radiation Dosage

The treatment approaches and dose guidelines for parotid gland tumors are applicable for submandibular gland tumors.

SUBLINGUAL GLAND

Primary Site

In order to treat the sublingual gland region, the general portal margins that would encompass the planning target volume are as follows: (1) superior—1 cm above the upper border of the tongue; (2) inferior—hyoid bone–thyroid notch interspace; (3) anterior—anterior aspect of the mental symphysis; (4) posterior—posterior aspect of the ascending mandibular ramus; (5) lateral—2 cm flash of ipsilateral mandible; (6) medial: 2 cm past midline (however, the entire floor of mouth–submental region will usually require treatment).

Right/left opposed lateral portals are needed to completely encompass this treatment volume, particularly when the regional lymph nodes are included. 3DCRT or IMRT complex treatment planning may be indicated when only the primary tumor area is treated with radiation therapy, as this approach may improve sparing of adjacent structures.

Lymph Nodes

The sentinel nodes are the submental and submandibular nodes. From there, the lymphatic drainage is to the cervical chain and to the supraclavicular nodes in an orderly, predictable fashion. Because of the potential for contralateral lymphatic spread of sublingual gland tumors due to their lateral to mid-line anatomic location, the bilateral nodes must be treated.

The indications for irradiation of the regional lymph nodes are the same as for parotid gland tumors.

Radiation Dosage

The treatment approaches and dose guidelines for parotid gland tumors are applicable for sublingual salivary gland tumors.

Side Effects

CRITICAL NORMAL TISSUES: RADIATION INJURY

Dose-Limiting Tissues

The dose-limiting tissues are the mandible, brain, spinal cord, cochlea eyes, and salivary tissue.

Pathophysiology of Radiation Injury to Salivary Tissue

The normal salivary glands produce about 1 to 1.5 L of saliva daily. The major salivary glands produce 80% of this volume. The parotid glands consist predominantly of serous acini, the submandibular glands contain both mucous and serous acini, and the minor salivary glands are predominantly mucus secretors. During radiation therapy, acute, transient, often painless sialadenitis may occur in the first 24 hours. Significant swelling of the gland within the port is the usual feature. Management is conservative using mild analgesia or anti-inflammatory medication. Serous salivary tissue seems to be more sensitive than mucous tissue, and the saliva becomes reduced in quantity and more ropy, mucous-like, and tenacious. This alteration in character can cause significant symptoms. The magnitude of clinical effect depends largely on the volume of salivary tissue being irradiated, as most clinically useful dose fractionation schedules cause xerosis of any irradiated salivary tissue. Put another way, the only method of sparing salivary function is to avoid irradiating as much salivary tissue as possible.

Permanent xerostomia causes discomfort, alters taste acuity, promotes poor oral hygiene, and accelerates dental decay. The remaining salivary gland tissues are largely obliterated after radiation damage and replaced by collagen. The saliva that is produced is reduced in quantity and has an altered electrolyte content and reduced pH level. The reduced pH favors the growth of bacteria that cause caries and decay. Fluoride supplementation and regular dental hygiene and professional assessment are vital. A home-made mouthwash containing baking soda and salt promotes hygiene and can restore pH toward alkaline values.

Tolerance Doses and Fractionation

Loss of salivary function is usually complete and permanent after doses of 35 Gy in conventional fractionation. Marks and associates[32] noted that only one fifth of patients who received between 40 and 60 Gy had any measurable salivary flow after salivary stimulation. Young patients have better chances of recovery of some salivary function, and the higher the rate of pretreatment salivary flow, the greater the chance of recovery.[33]

ACUTE AND LATE SIDE EFFECTS

Xerostomia

Acute xerostomia will occur for most patients by the third to fourth week of treatment and usually will become more prominent throughout the remaining course of radiation therapy, even with maximum sparing of the contralateral salivary glands, particularly during treatment for parotid gland tumors. With the use of 3DCRT or IMRT, the contralateral and other salivary glands can be spared by limiting the total dosage to 26 Gy, which will allow for a high incidence of substantive salivary recovery in the months following completion of radiation therapy.[27]

TRISMUS

Development of trismus is a potential late effect from radiation therapy, particularly for treatment volumes that include a fair amount of the temporomandibular joint and masseter muscle. If the dosage to this region can be kept to a maximum 50 Gy, this becomes much less of an issue. Diligent daily physical therapy with jaw exercises during treatment and indefinitely thereafter can be quite helpful in limiting and decreasing trismus.

OTITIS MEDIA

When the middle ear–eustachian tube complex is within the entrance or exit beam, the patient can potentially develop otitis media as an acute side effect. This is generally associated with hypoacusis. The patient has the sensation that he or she needs to open his or her mouth and "pop" the ear open, which is similar to the sensation experienced during the takeoff of an airplane. Treatment is with a trial of decongestant initially. If the problem persists, antibiotics can be used. Chronic otitis media may require the placement of a pneumatic tube in the tympanic membrane.

EPILATION

Facial and scalp hair loss will occur within the irradiated volume usually by the fourth to fifth week of treatment. Whether there will be any significant regrowth of hair in the months following completion of treatment depends on the total dosage administered to that area.

DERMAL CHANGES

Depending on the dosage delivered to the skin within the beam entrance or exit sites, there will develop acute radiation dermal changes starting by around weeks 3 to 4 of treatment and will become more prominent as treatment progresses. This will include dryness, hyper-pigmentation, and erythema of varying degrees. These changes will generally fade to a greater or lesser extent depending on the individual patient in the months following completion of treatment. Late effects can sometimes be seen with varying amounts to dermal-soft tissue fibrosis or fullness within the irradiated areas, particularly in regions that have been within the operative field.

DENTAL

Pretreatment dental consultation is essential in every patient. Teeth that are in poor condition and are not felt to have long-term viability need to be extracted before the initiation of radiation therapy. Prophylactic fluoride therapy is initiated and continued during treatment and indefinitely thereafter. Routine dental checkups during and after the course of radiation therapy are essential. Because of the effects on the salivary gland tissues within the radiation portals and the direct effects on the gingiva and arterioles, aggressive dental care is mandatory. The goal is to keep the patient's teeth and gingiva in as good a condition as possible for the long-term and thus prevent the development of osteoradionecrosis, which can occur particularly after extraction of teeth in a heavily irradiated zone.

TASTE

By the third to fourth week of treatment, there generally will be a decrease of taste. In a minority of patients, their taste may take on an extremely salty or sweet character. These side effects will resolve over the months following treatment completion with reasonably good recovery in the majority of patients.

THYROID

The thyroid gland can receive scatter radiation or direct radiation, the latter occurring when the neck nodes are irradiated. Baseline thyroid function tests including a T3, T4, and a TSH are obtained to ensure that the patient's thyroid status is normal at the initiation of treatment. Subsequent to completion of radiation therapy, these thyroid function tests are evaluated every 6 months for up to 5 years. The overall risks of radiation effects on the thyroid are as follows: (1) chemical hypothyroidism—20% to 25%, which increases to 66% in patients who have also undergone a hemithyroidectomy, and (2) clinical hypothyroidism—5%.

MUCOSITIS

Starting around the third to fourth week of treatment, patients will develop progressive acute mucositis to varying degrees with erythema to fibrinous exudates within the irradiated oropharyngeal mucosa. This can be quite symptomatic with pain, particularly with 3DCRT or IMRT treatment plans where hot spots can be problematic. Care issues include good oral hygiene using salt-soda mouthwashes at the outset of treatment and subsequent narcotic analgesics when pain begins. This problem will resolve slowly after completion of radiation therapy. Depending on the severity of the acute mucositis, it may take from 4 to 6 weeks or longer to completely recover, particularly if concomitant chemotherapy has been administered. Some patients note that certain types of foods such as those that are spicy or rather acidic can cause a burning pain within these tissues, sometimes for many months after completion of radiation therapy.

NASAL MUCOSAL CHANGES

Particularly when treating parotid tumors with 3DCRT or IMRT-based radiation therapy, some of the nasal mucosa may be within the beam. In such instances, dryness, congestion, and mild bleeding, particularly when the effected nasal passage is cleaned, can occur acutely during treatment and persist as a chronic effect of treatment.

ORAL CANDIDA

Due to the induction of xerostomia by radiation and the associated changes in the oral pH and flora, some patients may develop oral Candida. This may present with white plaques that may or may not be associated with a bed of erythema. The patient may not have symptoms or have a bad taste or a sore mouth or throat. The radiation oncologist must be on the alert for this development during the weekly status evaluations. Treatment is usually quite effective with topical anti-fungal therapy either as a mouthwash, troche or systemic therapy through pills.

SOFT TISSUE EDEMA

Particularly in areas that had been within the operative field, radiation therapy can be associated with the development of some degree of soft tissue edema. This can occur around the fourth week of treatment but is usually not significant. Late residual soft tissue edema can result but is not generally a cosmetic detriment.

ESOPHAGITIS

When the ipsilateral cervical and supraclavicular nodal areas are treated, there is risk that the patient may develop symptoms of radiation esophagitis. This may occur around the third to fourth week of treatment due to scatter radiation effects on the esophagus, even though treatment techniques used for such nodal radiation would either avoid a direct hit on this organ (e.g., AP/PA off the spinal cord) or limit the amount of radiation (e.g., lateral portal with selected electron energy). Depending on the severity of the symptoms, conservative management may be indicated.

ACUTE PAROTITIS

When a parotid gland is irradiated, an occasional patient will develop acute parotitis within the first 12 hours of the initial fraction. In such cases, an acute inflammatory reaction occurs. The clinical presentation includes area swelling, localized pains, and sometimes a low-grade fever. This is a self-limited problem that will usually resolve spontaneously after several hours. However, we generally prescribe a nonsteroidal anti-inflammatory agent and reassure the patient.

INDUCTION OF MALIGNANCY

This is clearly a potential late complication from radiation therapy that can occur whenever a patient receives such treatment anywhere on the body. The latent period is around 13.3 years. Available data specific to the salivary gland are obtained from atomic bomb survivors and from patients who had received radiation for benign conditions. While the quality of such information is questionable with respect to its use to associate radiation as an etiologic agent for the development of salivary gland malignancies, it is clear that children who received low dose radiation for benign conditions such as thymic enlargement, tinea capitis, or infected tonsils have an increased incidence of such tumors. Mucoepidermoid carcinoma and adenocarcinoma have been reported as the two most common types of malignant salivary gland tumors induced by radiation.[34] In survivors of the atomic bomb, there was a fivefold greater incidence of salivary neoplasia than that expected in a normal population.[35] Besides salivary gland malignancies that could be induced by radiation, the other tissues within the treatment volume also can potentially develop a malignancy such as bone, soft tissue sarcomas, or both; however, the incidence is similarly very rare.

CHEMOTHERAPY

Due to the relatively uncommon incidence and heterogenous nature of salivary gland malignancies, the medical oncology literature in this area is lacking. Generally, chemotherapy is used for the palliative treatment of unresectable recurrent or symptomatic metastatic disease. In some patients with metastases, the disease may behave indolently and be asymptomatic. These patients can function well for a long time, in which case monitoring may be a reasonable option.

Treatment with chemotherapy has response rates between 40% and 50%[36-38] with duration of responses ranging from 5 to 8 months.[39,40]

Active single agents include doxorubicin, cisplatin, paclitaxel, hydroxyurea, bleomycin, and 5-FU. However, single agent therapy has limited activity against malignant salivary gland tumors. The best response rates are associated with combination chemotherapeutic regimens such as cyclophosphamide, doxorubicin, and cisplatin (CAP), for which response rates have been 22% to 100%. Complete response rates of 0% to 40% have been reported for combination chemotherapy.

In selected cases where the primary tumor is unresectable, some patients may be treated with aggressive full course external beam radiation therapy with concomitant chemotherapy. There is no evidence to support the use of chemotherapy in a neoadjuvant or adjuvant role at this time.

Special Cases

ACCESSORY PAROTID GLAND TUMORS

Treatment approaches are similar to those for parotid gland malignancies with surgery as the initial treatment of choice. A standard parotidectomy incision is used with an anterior extension superiorly. Once the lesion is exposed, evaluated and malignancy is confirmed, a wide local excision is performed for localized mobile lesions without extension to the main parotid gland. Such limited surgery alone for these selected lesions is generally curative.

The role for postoperative radiation therapy is similar to that for the main parotid gland.

ADENOID CYSTIC CARCINOMA (CYLINDROMA)

Adenoid cystic carcinoma is a relatively uncommon pathologic subtype comprising approximately 2% to 5% of salivary gland malignancies. It affects male and females equally and is the most common malignant tumor of the minor salivary glands and submandibular.

The initial treatment of choice for adenoid cystic carcinoma is surgical resection. However, it should be noted that this type of malignancy has the propensity not only for perineural spread but also insidious local extension, both of which can make surgery difficult to adequately encompass the potentially involved region. Thus, postoperative radiation therapy is recommended. The routine use of combined surgery and postoperative radiation therapy has been associated with improved local control for both major and minor salivary gland adenoid cystic carcinomas.

There is a 50% incidence of microscopic perineural invasion, particularly of the adjacent cranial nerves. Perineural spread can be associated with skip areas of involvement and therefore one cannot be comfortable with negative neural margins on frozen section. Thus, postoperative radiation therapy of the entire pathway of the adjacent cranial nerve to the base of skull is employed. The resultant base of skull failure from perineural invasion and extension of adenoid cystic carcinoma is associated with significant morbidity and is very difficult to treat effectively. Garden et al[41] found that the base of skull failure was rare whether or not elective radiation was given to the skull base. The policy at MSKCC, however, is to irradiate the adjacent cranial nerve pathway to the base of skull in all of patients who have adenoid cystic carcinoma of the salivary gland (see Fig 32-16).

The overall incidence of regional lymph node metastasis at presentation is 15%. Because the risk for occult nodal metastasis is rare, elective surgical dissection or irradiation is not employed.

Spiro and Huvos reviewed the MSKCC experience of 184 previously untreated patients with adenoid cystic carcinoma of the minor and major salivary glands.[42] Of these, 63% were stage I or II, 43% stage III, and 21% stage IV. Sixty-eight percent were grade 1 (cribriform pattern only), 26% were grade 2 (mixed cribriform pattern and solid features), and only 5% were grade 3 (solid only). All patients were treated with surgery but relatively few received postoperative radiation therapy. The cumulative 10-year survival rate was as follows: (1) stage I/II, 75%; (2) stage III, 43%; and (3) stage IV, 15%. The cause-specific survival at 10 years was 94% for stage I. They arrived at two important conclusions: (1) The clinical stage was the only factor that had significant impact upon survival, and (2) the tumor grade alone was not predictive of survival, regional nodal metastasis, or distant metastasis.

Surgery alone has been associated with a local control rate of 25% to 40%; however, when postoperative radiation therapy is employed, local control rates increase 75% to 80%.

Seventy percent of recurrences from salivary gland malignancies occur generally within the first 2 years of treatment. However, with adenoid cystic carcinomas, most of these local failures occur much later. These patients must be followed closely for many years post treatment.

Adenoidcystic carcinomas can have a natural history of several years even when presenting with metastatic disease. Consideration of controlling the primary tumor is prudent (see Fig. 32-12).

RECURRENT MAJOR SALIVARY GLAND CANCERS

Surgery is the treatment of choice for locally recurrent major salivary gland cancers. To maximize the chances of resectability and control, recurrent lesions must be diagnosed as early as possible. Thus, close follow-up is mandatory for the first 2 to 3 years after the initial treatment.

Unresectable, previously unirradiated, locally recurrent disease can be considered for concurrent chemotherapy and accelerated fractionation external beam radiation therapy if neutron therapy is not a viable option. Brachytherapy can be considered in selected cases.

The role of postoperative radiotherapy in patients with local recurrence who did not receive radiation as part of their initial treatment is not clear. In patients with resected large recurrent tumors and high risk features, postoperative external beam radiation should be considered. Brachytherapy can also be used in selected cases.

Armstrong and associates[43] reviewed the experience at MSKCC of recurrent major salivary gland malignancies in 78 patients who underwent resection of locally confined recurrent major salivary gland cancers. Thirty-eight patients had completely resected tumors, with low- or intermediate-grade histology, without lymph node spread, and the cause-specific survival rate was 83% at 5 years, 70% at 10 years, and 48% at 15 years. Local control for these 38 patients was superior for those with tumors of 3 cm or less compared with those with larger tumors: 80% versus 62% at 5 years, and 73% versus 25% at 10 years (P < 0.05).

The remaining 40 patients had high-risk features (high-grade histology, lymph node metastases, and close or positive margins of resection). Half of the high-risk patients received postoperative radiation therapy and half did not because radiation had been given before the development of local recurrence. Consequently, although local control was enhanced with radiation, this analysis could not determine the role of postoperative radiation. However, the data indicate that surgery alone yielded good local control in patients with small tumors (<3 cm) and no high-risk features, suggesting that postoperative radiation may be unnecessary for these patients if they can be closely followed.

However, another study by Spiro and Spiro at MSKCC reviewed the results of attempted salvage of patients developing locally confined recurrences following initial therapy of their primary tumor. Between 1966 and 1982, 155 patients presented with locally confined new primary carcinomas and were treated surgically with or without radiation therapy.[44] Of the latter group, local failure occurred in 15% (23/155) and only 7 of the 23 were suitable for salvage surgical therapy. All but one of the seven died of their disease, with an actuarial survival rate of only 21% five years after recurrence (Armstrong, unpublished data). In an attempt to explain this discrepancy, it has been postulated that the extent or completeness of therapy administered at the time of the initial diagnosis, before the development of a recurrence, may be an important predictor of the success of management of locally recurrent salivary cancer. The mechanisms of local recurrence following minimal or inadequate initial therapy may differ from the mechanisms of recurrence following aggressive initial therapy. The former may be related to technical factors, whereas the latter may be a manifestation of biologic aggressiveness.

Few other data address the role of postoperative conventional external beam radiotherapy in the management of recurrent tumors of the major salivary glands. Guillamondegui and associates[45] from the MD Anderson Hospital treated 12 patients with surgery or radiotherapy or both for locoregional recurrences. Locoregional control was achieved in 42% (5/12). In contrast, King and Fletcher,[46] from the same institution, reported a crude locoregional control rate of 81% (25/31), with minimum follow-up of 2 years, among patients presenting with postoperative local recurrences treated with radiotherapy. Tu and associates,[47] from the Chinese Academy of Medical Sciences, reported a significant survival advantage with the use of postoperative radiotherapy for recurrent parotid cancers. At 5 years, 89% of the patients (17/19) were alive in the combined-therapy arm compared with 59% (10/17) in the surgery-alone arm.[48] This paper did not compare prognostic factors between the two groups, nor did it detail the patterns of treatment failure. In addition, as the numbers of patients were small, it is difficult to make firm conclusions as to the efficacy of postoperative radiation therapy.

Armstrong and associates reported on 20 patients with recurrent[18] or advanced[12] disease who were treated with ^{192}Ir and ^{125}I brachytherapy as described earlier.[18] Previous radiation therapy had been administered to 15 patients. The implant was to gross disease in 15 of the 20 patients. Actuarial local control was 60% at 5 years. Two patients had soft tissue necrosis as a complication, which was resolved with conservative management. There were two cerebral abscesses, one of which was fatal. Both patients had extensive skull-base tumors treated with partial resection and ^{125}I brachytherapy for gross residual disease.

Brachytherapy can be used in conjunction with resection if the resection margins are close or positive, or in the presence of a T4 tumor. It may also be used as sole treatment of accessible localized recurrent disease previously treated with radiation therapy. Permanent ^{125}I seeds can be implanted directly into the tumor or embedded in Vicryl suture and sewn into tumor beds. The typical matched peripheral dose for ^{125}I implants is 160 Gy. Afterloaded ^{192}Ir can be used as a temporary implant in single or multiple planes for either microscopic residual disease or unresected disease. Typical median peripheral doses are 45 Gy for microscopic disease and 60 Gy for gross disease. A patient with a resectable submandibular cancer with lung metastases who was treated with ^{125}I is illustrated in Figure 32-19.

PLEOMORPHIC ADENOMA (BENIGN MIXED TUMOR)

Pleomorphic adenomas are benign tumors of salivary glands, but they can also occur in lacrimal glands. The pleomorphic adenoma is the most common benign tumor of the parotid glands and accounts for 75% of all parotid epithelial tumors. These adenomas occur rather frequently and generally are found in a relatively young population.

The initial treatment of choice is excision of the tumor with a margin of normal tissue with preservation of the facial nerve. Simple enucleation of the tumor is contraindicated. The likelihood of local recurrence for most patients who undergo uncomplicated surgery is only 1%. The few cases that have local postoperative recurrences can generally be treated again with surgery. However, multiply recurrent tumors will carry up to a 25% risk for further recurrences. With each recurrence, the probability of malignant transformation occurring or facial nerve damage increases.

Pleomorphic adenomas are radioresponsive tumors. In selected cases that are at high risk for local recurrence, the use of postoperative radiation therapy is associated with a cumulative risk of recurrence of 8% at 20 years.[49]

There is an established role for the use of radiation therapy in this benign lesion. The indications for postoperative radiation therapy include: (1) greater than three histologically benign local recurrences, with each recurrence associated with an increasing degree of infiltration; (2) a large lesion (>3 to 5 cm) where surgery is associated with inadequate margins; (3) microscopically positive surgical margins; (4) macroscopic residual disease; and (5) malignant transformation.

The use of postoperative radiation therapy must be based on selective and judicious indications as noted earlier as well as astute clinical judgment. Despite its effectiveness in controlling pleomorphic adenomas, its liberal administration is contraindicated. Because these lesions are benign and are usually found in young patients, the exposure of such patients to the small but definite risk of developing a radiation-induced malignancy as a late complication is unjustified.

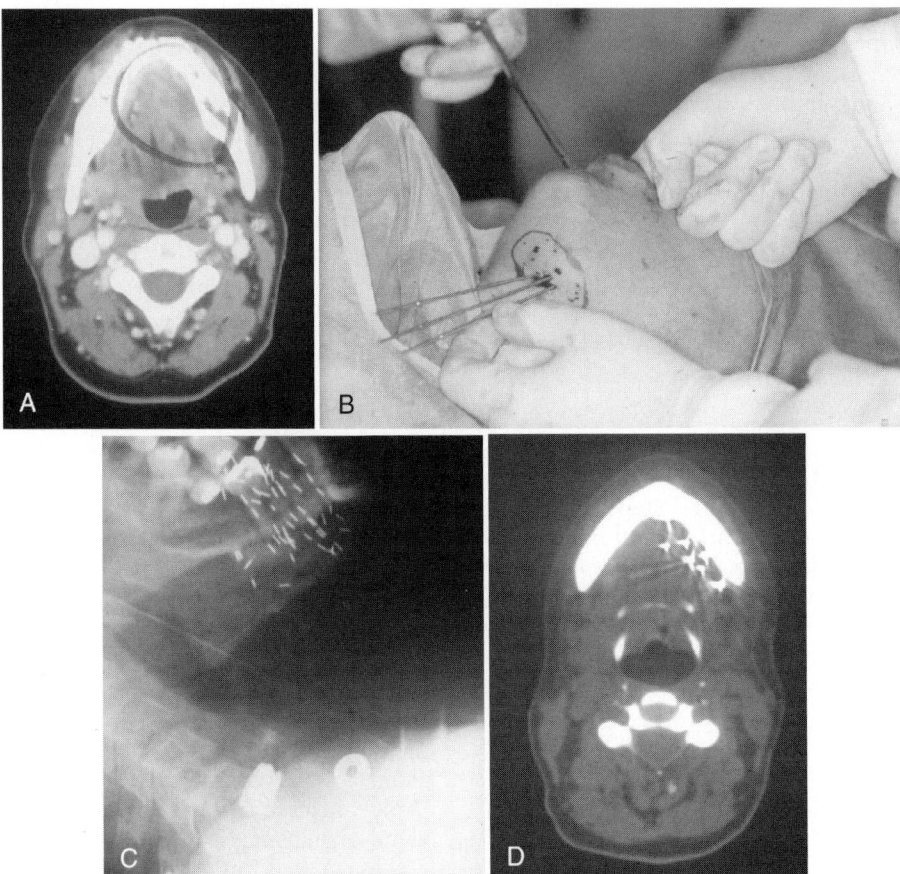

Figure 32–19. An elderly patient with a submandibular malignant mixed tumor. The patient had lung metastases. **A,** Computed tomography (CT) scan showing a left submandibular cancer, which was not resected. **B,** The procedure using Mick afterloading needles to implant ^{125}I seeds into the tumor. One hand is kept in the mouth to guide the needles as they are being implanted. **C,** Localization films with the seeds in place. **D,** A CT scan showing the ^{125}I seeds well localized in the tumor. The matched peripheral dose was 16000 cGy. Local control was achieved for the duration of survival (1 year).

The radiation oncology technical approaches are as presented previously for malignant tumors of the salivary gland. Because this is a benign lesion, there is no attempt to include the regional lymph nodes. However, when malignant transformation is noted in a recurrent lesion, the technique chosen is identical to that for a similar malignant lesion of the salivary gland.

The total cumulative dosage of radiation therapy that is administered for pleomorphic adenomas is 50 to 60 Gy depending on the particular surgical and pathologic characteristics of the case.

MINOR SALIVARY GLAND TUMORS

Epidemiology

While tumors of the major salivary glands are uncommon and account for approximately 3% to 4% of all head and neck cancers, the minor salivary gland tumors are rare. They account for 7% to 10% of all salivary gland tumors.

Minor salivary gland tumors can occur at any age. However, they are rare under the age of 10 years and uncommon before the age of 20 years.

The etiology of malignant minor salivary gland tumors is unknown. The possible causes have been discussed previously for the major salivary gland tumors.

Anatomy

The minor salivary gland tumors involve small, predominantly mucus-secreting glands located beneath the mucosal lining of the upper aerodigestive tract. The highest concentrations of these glands are located in the oral cavity, palate, nasal cavity, and paranasal sinuses. There are approximately 500 to 700 such glands. It should be noted that no minor salivary glands are located in the gingivae or anterior half of the hard palate. Aberrant salivary tissue has been reported in many differing and diverse sites—a lymph node, middle ear, or even the sternoclavicular joint, to name a few.

Pathology

About 50% of minor salivary gland tumors are malignant. The histopathologies include adenoid cystic carcinoma, mucoepidermoid carcinoma, adenocarcinoma, carcinoma in pleomorphic adenoma, acinic cell carcinoma, and oncocytic carcinoma.

In general adenoid cystic carcinoma is the most often encountered malignant minor salivary gland tumor. However, adenocarcinoma is most common in the nasal cavity and paranasal sinuses,[11] while mucoepidermoid carcinoma is highest in the oropharyngeal region, particularly in the base of tongue.[50]

The most frequently encountered benign tumor of the minor salivary glands is the pleomorphic adenoma.

Clinical Presentation and Evaluation

PRIMARY SITE

A thorough history and carefully detailed physical examination are required as the initial steps in evaluating patients with a minor salivary gland mass. The presenting complaint and findings in such tumors varies depending on the site of the lesion in the upper aerodigestive tract. In the oral cavity and oropharynx, there may be a painless swelling in the sub-sites, while in the sinonasal cavities, nasal obstruction may be the presenting symptom.

Palpation and measurement of such a mass, if at all possible, is important. There may be submucosal swelling, which can be ulcerated. Such malignant tumors grow by extensive local infiltration and subsequently will invade the adjacent tissues. Perineural spread is associated with the adenoid cystic carcinoma histopathology, and therefore the adjacent cranial nerves should be examined carefully. These types of malignancies may be clinically indistinguishable from a primary squamous cell carcinoma.

An MRI scan is important in patients with minor salivary gland malignancies, particularly when they arise in the palate, nasal cavity, nasopharynx, and paranasal sinuses. In these regions, the full extent of the disease cannot be fully appreciated by clinical examination alone.

Particularly since there is a 50% risk that minor salivary gland tumors may be malignant, a biopsy is essential. Most of these lesions are accessible and therefore a direct excisional biopsy is performed.

REGIONAL LYMPH NODES

There is an overall 15% risk for cervical lymph node metastasis. This risk, however, is related to the site of origin and the grade of tumor.[11]

The physical examination should include palpation of regional nodes. There may be an increased risk for bilateral or contralateral nodal metastasis, particularly when the primary site is in the oral cavity or oropharynx due to the rich lymphatic pathways in these regions.

DISTANT SPREAD

The ultimate incidence of distant metastasis for minor salivary gland malignancies is 25% overall with an incidence of 50% for adenoid cystic carcinomas. The lung is the site most frequently involved. A staging chest x-ray should be obtained. In cases with abnormalities on this study, a CT scan of the thorax should be performed with contrast for further evaluation. The most common cause of treatment failure for minor salivary gland malignancies is distant metastasis.

The clinical stage of the lesion significantly influences survival. Spiro et al.[51] reviewed the experience at MSKCC and noted the relationship between stage and overall survival at 10 years: (1) stage I, 83%; (2) stage II, 53%; (3) stage III, 35%; (4) stage IV, 24%.

Staging

Minor salivary gland malignancies are staged using the AJCC TNM criteria for squamous cell carcinomas associated with the site of the primary lesion.

Treatment

SURGERY

Surgical resection of malignant minor salivary gland tumors is the primary treatment of choice. However, patients must be carefully selected to ensure resectability. A review of the MSKCC experience by Spiro noted that there were fewer early-stage lesions for the minor salivary gland lesions compared to the major salivary gland malignancies.[11] In fact, almost all of the minor salivary gland malignancies were locally advanced.

The procedure used will depend on the anatomic site of the lesion as well as the tumor size, extent, and grade. For low-grade lesions, a more conservative surgical resection is employed with the goal of achieving negative margins and minimizing extensive surgery with its associated cosmetic and functional impairments. For high-grade lesions, surgery is more aggressive and radical with consideration given to including an ipsilateral neck dissection. The surgical approach will be similar to that used for squamous cell carcinomas of similar stage in that site. This may mean that important functional structures such as the larynx or orbit need to be sacrificed. It is important to note that more radical and extensive surgery does not necessarily translate to further improvement in control of locally advanced tumors. Such procedures, however, are associated with increased morbidity with an adverse impact on the patient's quality of life. Thus, in such cases a less radical surgical approach and the use of planned postoperative radiation therapy can maintain and even improve the chances for control.

The overall incidence of occult regional lymph node metastasis is low for minor salivary gland tumors, especially for adenoid cystic carcinomas. Therefore, in general, an elective neck dissection is not performed routinely. However, if the primary lesion is sizeable with a high-grade mucoepidermoid carcinoma or squamous cell carcinoma histopathology, there is an increased risk of nodal spread, and a selective neck dissection is performed in clinically N0 patients.

For patients who present with clinically palpable adenopathy, a therapeutic neck dissection is performed. However, if there is limited adenopathy in the first echelon nodes, a selective neck dissection can be considered.

RADIATION ONCOLOGY

Indications for Primary Treatment with Radiation Therapy

The medically or surgically unresectable primary or previously unirradiated recurrent malignant minor salivary gland tumors can be approached in a similar fashion with radiation therapy as that previously presented for major salivary gland tumors.

Patients with disease in inaccessible sites or sites where the required surgery would have unacceptable cosmetic or functional results can be treated with radical radiation alone. The techniques are similar to those used for squamous cell cancers in the same location. The radiation doses will be similar to that previously presented for the major salivary gland malignancies. The results of radiation alone for minor salivary cancers are detailed in Table 9. Although relatively small numbers are reported, local control is between 70% and 100%.

Indications for Postoperative Radiation Therapy

Few data are available to support the use of postoperative radiation therapy for minor salivary gland malignancies compared to the data available for such treatment in major salivary gland malignancies. Postoperative external beam radiation therapy has been reported for minor salivary gland malignancies with a local control rate of 75%,[52,53,54,55] compared to 50% reported for surgery alone.[51,52,55] Several series using postoperative radiation therapy for minor salivary gland malignancies are detailed in Table 32-13.

It is hard to make conclusions based on such limited data; however, it would appear that postoperative radiation may improve outcome in selected patients. There is no good hypothesis to explain why postoperative radiation would be effective for selected major salivary gland cancers and ineffective for selected minor salivary gland cancers. Therefore, it is reasonable to recommend postoperative treatment if the resection margins are positive, for T3 to T4 tumors, for node-positive disease, and for high-grade tumors.

The basic pretreatment evaluation and preparation of a patient for the radiation therapy of minor salivary gland malignancies is identical to that presented previously for the major salivary gland tumors.

TREATMENT PLANNING

Simulation

The general approach used for the simulation of major salivary gland tumors is applicable to minor salivary gland malignancies. The technical approach will be similar to that of squamous cell carcinomas of the same anatomic site, size, and extent. Depending on the case, either a fluoroscopically directed simulation or CT simulation will be used. For adenoid cystic carcinomas, in which there is a need to cover the adjacent cranial pathways to the base of skull because of the increased risk for perineural invasion. Therefore, CT simulation will be used in preparation for IMRT treatment planning.

RADIATION THERAPY TECHNIQUE

Primary Site

The specific radiation therapy technical approach will depend on the extent of the primary tumor (lesion size and extension) or the size and anatomic sites of the surgical defect. In general, the approaches that could be considered are similar to the treatment planning and technique options previously presented for the major salivary gland malignancies. However, for minor salivary gland tumors whose primary lesion or surgical bed approaches or crosses the midline and in whom there is a rich lymphatic network with crossover to the contralateral lymph nodes, conventional two-dimensional planning with right/left lateral opposed portals may be the most appropriate approach. In such cases the radiation therapy technique would be similar to that for treatment of squamous cell carcinomas in these respective sites. However, when the histopathology is adenoid cystic carcinoma with its increased risk for perineural invasion and spread to the base of skull, coverage of the entire adjacent cranial nerves to the base of the skull may require a complex treatment plan using an IMRT technique. The goal is to spare the adjacent normal tissues as best as possible from radiation

Table 32–13   Impact of Postoperative Radiation Therapy on Local Control in Cancer of Minor Salivary Glands

Reference	Selection	Reason for RT (*n*)	Local Control	
			Therapy	%
Fu et al[25]	Various sites	Positive margins or close (6)	SX + RT	83
		No RT (16)	SX	75
Ellis et al*	Various sites	Early stage (11)	SX + RT	86
		Late stage (13)	SX + RT	77
Tran et al†	Oral cavity	Positive margin (14)	SX + RT	71
		No RT (10)	SX	50

RT, radiation therapy; SX, surgery.
*From Ellis E, Million R, Mendenhall W, et al: The use of radiation therapy in the management of minor salivary gland tumors. *Int J Radiat Oncol Biol Phys.* 1988;15:613.
†From Tran L, Sidrys J, Sadeghi A, et al: Salivary gland tumors of the oral cavity. *Int J Radiat Oncol Biol Phys.* 1990;18:413.

while still providing an appropriate coverage of the nerve pathways.

Lymph Nodes

There is a 30% incidence of regional lymph node metastasis with minor salivary gland malignancies. The location of the sentinel lymph nodes and their subsequent drainage patterns will depend on the anatomic site of the primary tumor and will be similar to the drainage pattern of squamous cell carcinomas of that region.

In general, the indication for radiation of the regional lymph nodes will be similar to that presented previously for parotid gland malignancies. However, due to the high frequency of a rich lymphatic network with crossover to the contralateral nodes in the oral cavity and oropharyngeal regions, one must consider treating the bilateral neck nodes.

RADIATION DOSAGE

The dosage of radiation therapy required will depend on whether one is dealing with an unresectable primary minor salivary gland malignancy or whether there is high risk for microscopic, macroscopic, or residual gross disease following surgery. The general guidelines presented previously for the major salivary gland malignancies would generally be applicable to the minor salivary gland tumor primary sites and regional lymph nodes, respectively.

Side Effects

The specific side effects associated with radiation therapy for minor salivary gland malignancies will depend on the anatomic site of the primary, whether the regional lymph nodes will need to be included in the field, the cumulative dosage of radiation administered, and the radiation technique employed. In general, the radiation side effects presented previously for the major salivary gland malignancies are applicable to minor salivary gland tumors. However, because of the increased frequency in the use of right/lateral opposed portals, particularly for oral cavity and oropharyngeal lesions, the degree of xerostomia, loss of taste, and mucositis may be more significant.

CHEMOTHERAPY

The use of chemotherapy for minor salivary gland malignancies is based on the data obtained from its application for the major salivary gland tumors and has been presented previously in this chapter.

REFERENCES

1. Frommer J: The human accessory parotid gland: Its incidence, nature and significance. *Oral Surg.* 1977;43:671.
2. Johnson FE, Spiro RH: Tumors arising in accessory parotid tissue. *Am J Surg.* 1979;138:576.
3. Spiro JD, Spiro RH: Salivary tumors. In Shah J, ed. *Cancer of the Head and Neck.* Hamilton, Ontario/London: BC Decker; 2001:240.
4. Eisele DW, Kleinberg LR, O'Malley BB: Management of malignant salivary gland tumors. In Harrison LB, Sessions RB, Hong WK, eds. *Head and Neck Cancer. A Multidisciplinary Approach.* Philadelphia: Lippincott-Raven; 1999:721.
5. O'Dwyer P, Farrar WB, James A: Needle aspiration biopsy of major salivary gland tumors: Its value. *Cancer.* 1986;57:554.
6. Frable MAS, Frable WJ: Fine needle aspiration biopsy of salivary glands. *Laryngoscope.* 1991;101:245.
7. Roland NJ, Caslin AW, Smith PA, et al: Fine needle aspiration cytology of salivary gland lesions reported immediately in a head and neck clinic. *J Laryngol Otol.* 1993;107:1025.
8. Zurrida S, Alasio L, Tradati N, et al: Fine needle aspiration of parotid masses. *Cancer.* 1993;72:2306.
9. Layfield JL, Tan P, Glasgow BJ: Fine needle aspiration of salivary gland lesions. *Arch Pathol Lab Med.* 1987;111:346.
10. Jayaram G, Verma AK, Sood N, et al: Fine needle aspiration cytology of salivary gland lesions. *J Oral Pathol Med.* 1994;23:256.
11. Spiro RH: Salivary neoplasms: Overview of a 35-year experience with 2807 patients. *Head Neck Surg.* 1986;8:177.
12. Armstrong JG, Harrison LG, Spiro RH, et al: The indications for elective treatment of the neck in cancer of the major salivary glands. *Cancer.* 1992;69:615.
13. Wang CC: Tumors of the salivary glands. In Wang CC, ed. *Radiation Therapy for Head and Neck Neoplasms,* 3rd ed. New York: Wiley-Liss; 1997:311.
14. American Joint Committee on Cancer: Major salivary glands (parotid, submandibular, and sublingual). In Greene Fl, Page DL, Fleming ID, et al, eds. *AJCC Cancer Staging Manual,* 6th ed. New York: Springer-Verlag; 2002:69.
15. American Joint Committee on Cancer: Major salivary glands (parotid, submandibular, and sublingual). In Fleming ID, Cooper JS, Henson DE, et al, eds. *AJCC Cancer Staging Manual,* 5th ed. Philadelphia: Lippincott-Raven; 1997:53.
16. McGuitt WF: Effect of radiation therapy on facial nerve cable autografts. *Trans Am Acad Ophthalmol Otolaryngol.* 1976;82:487.
17. Wang CC, Goodman M: Photon irradiation of unresectable carcinomas of salivary glands. *Int J Radiat Oncol Biol Phys.* 1991; 21:569.
18. Armstrong JG, Harrison LB, Spiro RH, et al: Brachytherapy of malignant tumors of salivary gland origin. *Endocurither Hypertherm Oncol.* 1996;6:19.
19. King JJ, Fletcher GH: Malignant tumors of the major salivary glands. *Radiology.* 1971;123:49.
20. Batterman J, Breuer K, Hart G, et al: Observations on pulmonary metastases in patients after single doses and multiple fractions of fast neutrons and cobalt-60 gamma rays. *Eur J Cancer.* 1981; 17:539.
21. Laramore G, Krall J, Griffin T, et al: Neutron versus photon irradiation for unresectable salivary gland tumors: Final report of an RTOG-MRC randomized trial. *Int J Radiat Oncol Biol Phys.* 1993;27:235.
22. Catterall M, Errington RD: The implications of improved treatment of malignant salivary gland tumors by fast neutron radiotherapy. *Int J Radiat Oncol Biol Phys.* 1987;13:1314.
23. Spiro RH, Huvos AG, Strong EW: Cancer of the parotid gland: A clinicopathologic study of 288 primary cases. *Am J Surg.* 1975; 130:457.
24. Harrison LB, Armstrong JG, Spiro RH: Postoperative radiation therapy for major salivary gland malignancies. *J Surg Oncol.* 1990; 45:52.
25. Fu KK, Leibel SA, Levine ML, et al: Carcinoma of the major and minor salivary glands. *Cancer.* 1977;40:2882.
26. Armstrong JG, Harrison LB, Spiro RH, et al: Malignant tumors of major salivary gland origin: A matched pair analysis of the role of combined surgery and postoperative radiation therapy. *Arch Otolaryngol Head Neck Surg.* 1990;116:290.
27. Chong LM, Hunt M: Intensity modulated radiation therapy for head and neck cancer. Fuks Z, Leibel SA, Ling CC, eds. *A practical guide to intensity-modulated radiation therapy.* Madison, Wisc: Medical Physics Publishing; 2003.
28. Leblanc A: *The Cranial Nerves,* 2nd ed. Berlin: Springer-Verlag; 1995.
29. Nowak PJ, Wijers OB, Lagerwaard FJ, et al: A three-dimensional CT-based target definition for elective radiation of the neck. *Int J Radiat Oncol Biol Phys.* 1999;45:33.
30. Wijers OB, Levendag PC, Tan T, et al: A simplified CT-based definition of the lymph node levels in the node negative neck. *Radiother Oncol.* 1999;52:35.

31. Chao KSC, Wippold FJ, et al: Determination and delineation of nodal target volumes for head and neck cancer based on patterns of failure in patients receiving definitive and postoperative IMRT. *Int J Radiat Oncol Biol Phys.* 2002;53:1174.

32. Marks J, Davis CC, Gottsman VL, et al: The effects of radiation on parotid salivary function. *Int J Radiat Oncol Biol Phys.* 1981; 7:1013.

33. Mira J, Wescott W, Starcke E, et al: Some factors influencing salivary function when treating with radiotherapy. *Int J Radiat Oncol Biol Phys.* 1981;7:535.

34. Lawson W, Som ML: Second primary cancer after irradiation of laryngeal cancer. *Ann Otol Rhinol Laryngol.* 1975;84:771.

35. Belsky JL, Takechi N, Yamamoto T, et al: Salivary gland neoplasms following atomic radiation: Additional cases and reanalysis of combined data in a fixed population, 1957–1970. *Cancer.* 1975; 35:555.

36. Dreyfus AI, Clark JR, Fallon BG, et al: Cyclophosphamide, doxorubicin, cisplatin combination chemotherapy for advanced carcinomas of salivary gland origin. *Cancer.* 1987;60:2869.

37. Kaplan MJ, Johns ME, Cantrell RW: Chemotherapy for salivary gland cancer. *Otolaryngol Head Neck Surg.* 1966;95:165.

38. Dimery IW, Legha SS, Shirinian M, et al: Fluorouracil, doxorubicin, cyclophosphamide, and cisplatin combination chemotherapy in advanced or recurrent salivary gland carcinoma. *J Clin Oncol.* 1990;8:1056.

39. Licitra L, Marchini S, Spinazze S, et al: Cisplatin in advanced salivary gland carcinoma. *Cancer.* 1991;68:1874.

40. Creaghan ET, Woods JE, Rubin J, et al: Cisplatin-based chemotherapy for neoplasms arising from salivary glands and contiguous structures in the head and neck. *Cancer.* 1988;62:2313.

41. Garden AS, Weber RS, Morrison WH, et al: The influence of positive margins and nerve invasion in adenoid cystic carcinoma of the head and neck treated with surgery and radiation. *Int J Radiat Oncol Biol Phys.* 1995;32:619.

42. Spiro RH, Huvos AG: Stage means more than grade in adenoid cystic carcinoma. *Am J Surg.* 1992;164:230.

43. Armstrong JG, Harrison LB, Spiro RH, et al: Observation on the natural history and treatment of recurrent major salivary gland cancer. *J Surg Oncol.* 1990;44:138.

44. Spiro R, Spiro J: Cancer of the salivary glands. In Meyers E, Sven J, eds. *Cancer of the Head and Neck*, 2nd ed. London: Churchill Livingstone; 1984:645.

45. Guillamondejui OM, Byers RM, Luna MH, et al: Aggressive surgery in treatment for parotid cancer. The role of adjunctive postoperative radiotherapy. *Am J Roentgenol.* 1975;123:49.

46. King JJ, Fletcher GH: Malignant tumors of the major salivary glands. *Radiology.* 1971;100:381.

47. Tu G-Y, Hu Y, Jiang P, et al: The superiority of combined therapy (surgery and postoperative irradiation) in parotid cancer. *Arch Otolaryngol.* 1982;108:710.

48. Woods J, Weiland L, Chong G, et al: Pathology and surgery of primary tumors of the parotid. *Surg Clin North Am.* 57:565.

49. Dawson AK, Orr JA: Long-term results of local excision and radiotherapy in pleomorphic adenoma of the parotid gland. *Int J Radiat Ncol Biol Phys.* 1985;11:4.

50. DeVries EJ, Johnson JT, Meyers EN, et al: Base of tongue salivary gland tumors. *Head Neck Surg.* 1987;9:329.

51. Spiro RH, Thaler HT, Hicks WF: The importance of clinical staging of minor salivary gland carcinoma. *Am J Surg.* 1991; 162:330.

52. Eapen LJ, Gerig LH, Catton GE, et al: Impact of local radiation in the management of salivary gland carcinomas. *Head Neck Surg.* 1988;10:239.

53. Garden AS, Weber RS, Ang KK, et al: Postoperative radiation therapy for malignant tumors of minor salivary glands. Outcomes and patterns of failure. *Cancer.* 1994;73:2563.

54. Parson JT, Mendenhall WM, Strenger SP, et al: Management of minor salivary gland carcinomas. *Int J Radiat Oncol Biol Phys.* 1996;35:443.

55. Sadeghi A, Tran LM, Mark R, et al: Minor salivary gland tumors of the head and neck: Treatment strategies and prognosis. *Am J Clin Oncol.* 1993;16:3.

Cancer of the Nasal Cavity and Paranasal Sinuses

33

Janice K. Ryu, MD

Malignancies arising from the nasal cavity and paranasal sinuses are relatively rare tumors of the head and neck. They account for only 3% of all upper respiratory tract cancers, with a yearly incidence of 1 per 100,000 people.[1] Because of their rarity, these sites are grouped together in most published reports. It is often difficult to determine the exact site of origin, since most of these tumors present at an advanced stage and extensively involve adjacent sites. Among the tumors arising in this anatomic region, 60% to 90% involve the paranasal sinuses, the majority being in the maxillary antrum. There is a 2:1 male predominance for these tumors.[2,3] Most patients with carcinomas arising in the sinonasal region are older than 40 years of age.[2,4] Esthesioneuroblastoma may occur in much younger patients as well.

Unlike other upper and lower respiratory tract carcinomas, nasal cavity and paranasal sinus cancers have not been associated with cigarette smoking.[5] Chronic sinusitis, although frequently coexistent with malignant tumors in this region, is not a causative agent.[6] However, an increased risk of adenocarcinoma of the nasal cavity and ethmoid sinus has been associated with wood dust exposure.[7-9] Other industrial risk groups include leather tanners[10] and nickel refinery workers (250-fold risk for developing squamous cell carcinoma of the maxillary antrum[11] and >40-fold risk for developing squamous cell carcinoma of the nasal cavity[12]). Thorotrast, a radioactive contrast medium used in the 1960s for radiographic studies of the maxillary sinus, is an established carcinogenic agent for maxillary sinus carcinoma.

CLINICAL PRESENTATION

Early symptoms of nasal cavity and paranasal sinus tumors are vague and mimic sinusitis symptoms; thus the diagnosis of malignancy is often delayed for months. The most common early symptoms of nasal cavity tumors are unilateral nasal obstruction, discharge, and epistaxis. Maxillary antrum cancers do not often exhibit early signs or symptoms. Patients with a maxillary antrum tumor present with complaints of facial pain, numbness, swelling, and nasal obstruction. They may have a facial, intraoral, or intranasal mass, and less frequently proptosis. Patients with tumors of the ethmoid sinus tend to present with ocular problems such as epiphora, proptosis,

diplopia, and eye pain. Primary sphenoidal and frontal sinus tumors are extremely rare. Eye symptoms (diplopia from sixth-nerve palsy) predominate for sphenoidal tumors, and frontal headache and swelling for frontal tumors.

Cervical lymph node metastases on initial presentation are uncommon; most large series report an incidence of less than 10% to 15%. Distant metastases on initial presentation are even less frequent, with a reported incidence of less than 7%.

PATHOLOGY

Most common benign tumors arising in the sinonasal region are inflammatory polyps and benign mixed minor salivary gland tumors. Other tumors are histologically benign but behave in a locally aggressive and destructive manner. These tumors include inverted papillomas and midline granulomas. Inverted papillomas arise from squamous or schneiderian epithelium and most often involve the lateral nasal wall. They may destroy bone and tend to recur if not excised completely. From 10% to 15% of inverted papillomas are associated with malignant squamous degeneration.[13,14] Inverted papillomas are best treated with en bloc resection with medial maxillectomy (recurrence rate <10%).[14,15] Midline granuloma syndrome describes a process of progressive midline facial destruction from various causes including an immunologic or rheumatoid process and lymphomatous proliferation. Often a definitive diagnosis cannot be made on the basis of a biopsy. If the biopsy suggests Wegener's granulomatosis, the treatment consists of systemic steroids or cytotoxic drugs or both. If the biopsy suggests lymphomatosis or reticulosis, the patient should have a systemic workup for lymphoma and be treated with localized radiation if no other disease is found. Midline lethal granuloma is a diagnosis of exclusion and describes progressive, painful destruction of the nasal cavity, paranasal sinuses, and hard palate. Death may eventually result from massive hemorrhage or infection once the base of the skull is eroded. The treatment for this condition is radiation therapy.

The most common malignant histologic type involving the nasal cavity and paranasal sinuses is epithelial in origin with the squamous cell or its variants making up 80% to 85%. Other histologic types are of minor salivary gland origin: adenocarcinoma, adenoid cystic carcinoma, benign mixed, and mucoepidermoid carcinoma. Mucoepidermoid carcinomas are extremely rare in the nasal cavity and paranasal sinuses. On the other hand, roughly 20% of all head and neck adenoid cystic carcinomas arise in this region. Low-grade adenoid cystic carcinomas have a better prognosis than high-grade tumors. Adenocarcinoma of the sinonasal tract can represent a metastasis, most often from kidney, breast, or lung.

Melanoma and olfactory neuroblastoma, also known as esthesioneuroblastoma, are rare epithelial malignancies arising in the nasal cavity. Esthesioneuroblastoma originates from olfactory nerves and is considered a neuroendocrine tumor. It occurs predominantly in young patients between 10 and 20 years old, although a second peak is observed in an older group between the ages of 50 and 60 years.[16-18] Olfactory neuroblastomas have a wide spectrum of clinical behavior. Some are slow growing and tend to be localized, whereas others may be highly aggressive with local destruction and spread as well as distant metastasis. The incidence of cervical nodal involvement is 20%. The most common presenting symptoms are epistaxis, nasal obstruction, and a loss of the sense of smell. Mucosal melanomas are most often found in the nasal cavity and can be primary or metastatic. Overall, less than 1% of melanomas arise from the sinonasal tract. Nasal melanomas can often be amelanotic and may require immunohistochemical and electron microscopic examination for definitive histologic diagnosis. Much more so than the cutaneous melanomas, nasal melanomas have a high incidence of local recurrence,[19,20] and the patient may benefit from postoperative radiation therapy.

Undifferentiated carcinomas have been reported to represent a distinctive, rare, and highly aggressive neoplasm. They are composed of small and medium-sized cells and have to be distinguished from melanoma, lymphoma, olfactory neuroblastoma, rhabdomyosarcoma, neuroendocrine carcinoma, and poorly differentiated squamous cell carcinoma. They present at an advanced stage widely involving the nasal, maxillary, and ethmoid complexes. Orbital and intracranial extension is seen in the majority of cases. Prognosis is extremely poor with 80% to 90% of patients dying within 1 year of extensive local and metastatic disease.[21] The role of systemic chemotherapy as an adjunct to aggressive local therapy needs to be investigated.

Nonepithelial tumors include lymphoma, plasmacytoma, and sarcoma.

PATTERNS OF SPREAD

The nasal cavity and paranasal sinus cancers tend to spread by local extension into adjacent sinuses and bones. To understand the patterns of spread, one must be familiar with the complex anatomy of this region. The nasal cavity and the paranasal sinuses all interconnect with each other via many apertures and often are separated only by thin bony septi, allowing easy invasion of the tumor into adjacent air cavities.

Anatomy

NASAL CAVITY

The coronal and transverse sections of the nasal cavity are illustrated in Figures 33-1 to 33-3. Anteriorly, the nasal cavity begins from the limen nasi, the line of transition from skin to mucous membrane. The nasopharynx is situated directly behind the nasal cavity and communicates with it by the posterior nasal aperture. Inferiorly, the floor is composed of the hard palate. Superiorly, the nasal cavity borders the base of the skull (frontal sinuses, cribriform plate of the ethmoid bone, and ethmoid air cells). The medial walls of the maxillary sinuses define the lateral extent of the nasal cavity. The midline septum divides the nasal cavity into two halves. Three turbinates (or conchae)—superior, middle, and inferior—protrude downward and medially from the lateral wall into the nasal cavity, forming three meatus. The superior turbinate is much smaller than the middle and inferior turbinates and is situated directly in front of the sphenoidal sinus. The nasolacrimal duct drains into the nasal cavity below the inferior turbinate.

The cribriform plate contains the first cranial nerve branches, which distribute their olfactory nerve endings to the upper one third of the septum and superior turbinates. Thus, the cribriform plate serves as an avenue of cancer spread to the anterior cranial fossa from the nasal cavity.

MAXILLARY SINUS

The maxillary sinus (also called the maxillary antrum) is a pyramidal cavity (see Figs. 33-1C, 33-2D, and 33-3A) of approximately 15 cm³ volume ($3.7 \times 2.5 \times 3.0$ cm). The base of the pyramid is composed of the medial wall, which separates the maxillary sinus from the nasal cavity, and the apex is in the zygomatic process. Superiorly, the floor of the orbit forms the roof of the antrum. Anteriorly, the facial wall is located behind the cheek and curves inward into the sinus. Posteriorly, the infratemporal wall borders infratemporal and pterygopalatine fossae. The floor of the maxillary sinus lies inferior to the floor of the nasal cavity, especially in edentulous patients.[22] Secretion from the maxillary sinus is drained into the nasal cavity via openings in the middle meatus. The roots of the second premolar and first two molars penetrate the bony floor of the maxillary sinus.

ETHMOID SINUSES

The ethmoid cells, collectively called a sinus, lie between the nasal cavity and the orbit (see Figs. 33-1B, 33-2C, and 33-3B). The air cells, like a honeycomb, have the thin orbital plate of the frontal bone of the anterior cranial fossa for a roof (fovea ethmoidalis). They are grouped into anterior, middle, and posterior air cells on each side. The anterior cell is closely related to the frontal sinus and connects to the nasal cavity via the middle meatus. The middle ethmoid cell makes a bulge into the lateral wall of the nasal cavity (bulla ethmoidalis) and also communicates with the middle meatus. The posterior ethmoid cells are closely related to the optic canal and nerve and open

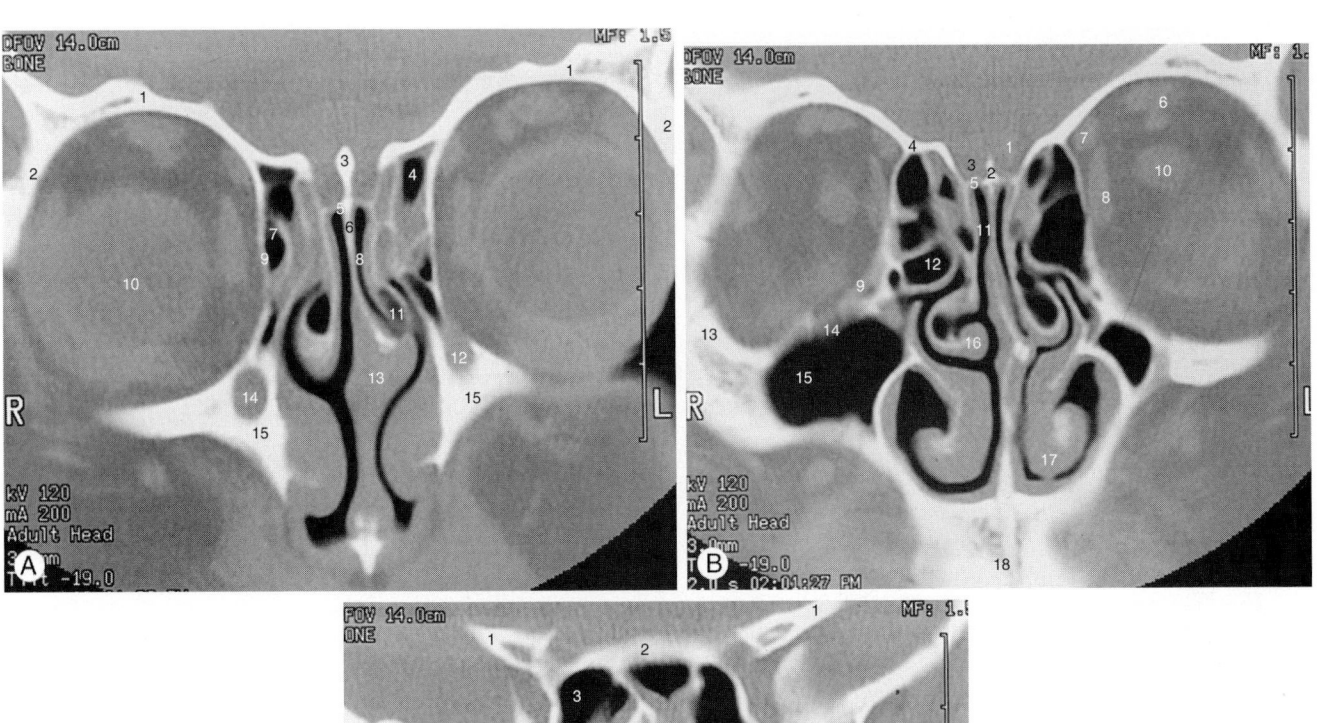

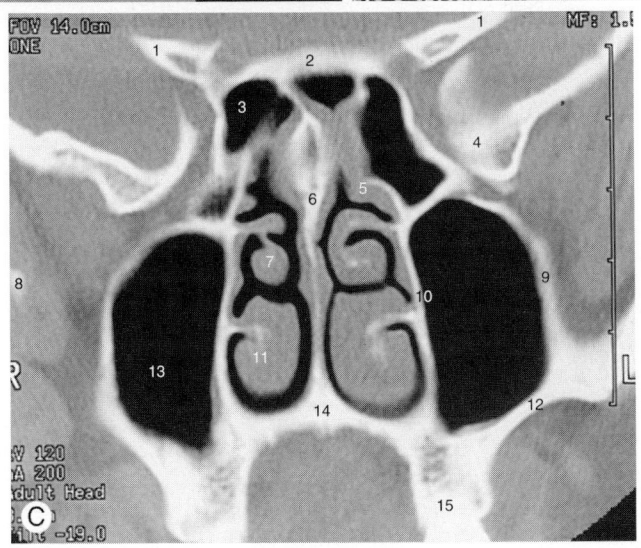

Figure 33–1. Computed tomographic images of the normal anatomy of the paranasal sinuses in the coronal plane (shown in anterior to posterior direction from *part A* to *part C*). **A,** Section through the frontal sinuses, midorbit, anterior ethmoidal sinuses, and nasal cavity. 1, orbital roof; 2, zygomatic process of frontal bone; 3, crista galli; 4, left frontal sinus; 5, cribriform plate; 6, vertical plate of ethmoid bone; 7, anterior ethmoidal air cells; 8, superior extent of nasal cavity; 9, lamina papyracea; 10, right globe; 11, middle turbinate; 12, nasolacrimal duct; 13, nasal septum (bony above, cartilage below); 14, maxillary sinus; 15, maxilla. **B,** Section through the posterior orbit, cribriform plate, middle ethmoidal sinuses, and nasal cavity. 1, anterior cranial fossa; 2, crista galli; 3, olfactory fossa; 4, roof of ethmoidal sinus; 5, cribriform plate; 6, superior rectus muscle; 7, superior oblique muscle; 8, medial rectus muscle; 9, inferior rectus muscle; 10, optic nerve; 11, superior extent of nasal cavity; 12, middle ethmoidal air cells; 13, orbital process of zygoma; 14, infraorbital canal; 15, maxillary sinus; 16, middle turbinate; 17, inferior turbinate; 18, hard palate. **C,** Section through the sphenoidal sinus, maxillary sinus, and the posterior aspect of the nasal cavity. 1, lesser wing of sphenoid; 2, planum sphenoidale; 3, sphenoidal sinus; 4, greater wing of sphenoid; 5, superior turbinate; 6, vomer; 7, middle turbinate; 8, tip of coronoid process; 9, lateral wall of maxillary sinus; 10, medial wall of maxillary sinus; 11, inferior turbinate; 12, inferior wall of maxillary sinus; 13, maxillary antrum; 14, hard palate; 15, alveolar ridge of maxilla.

into the superior meatus. These openings between the nasal cavity and the ethmoid cells are an obvious route of tumor extension. The fragile medial wall of the orbit, formed by the lamina papyracea of the ethmoid bone, is extremely porous and is an easy conduit for tumor spread from the ethmoid sinus into the orbit. The superior portion of the nasal septum separates the right and left ethmoid cells. Most anterior ethmoid air cells extend within 1 cm of the anterior skin surface between the medial canthi. The orbits are conical and the ethmoid sinuses expand posteriorly and inferiorly to form the medial

walls of the orbit. The optic nerves lie at about the same level as the roof of the ethmoid cells.[23] The floor of the orbit rises posteriorly; thus the orbital apex lies superior to the inferior rim of the orbit.

SPHENOIDAL SINUS

The sphenoidal sinus is an air cavity within the body of the sphenoid bone. It is a midline structure located anterior to the clivus, posterior to the superior meatus of the nasal cavity (see Figs. 33-2*B*, 33-2*C*, and 33-3*C*).

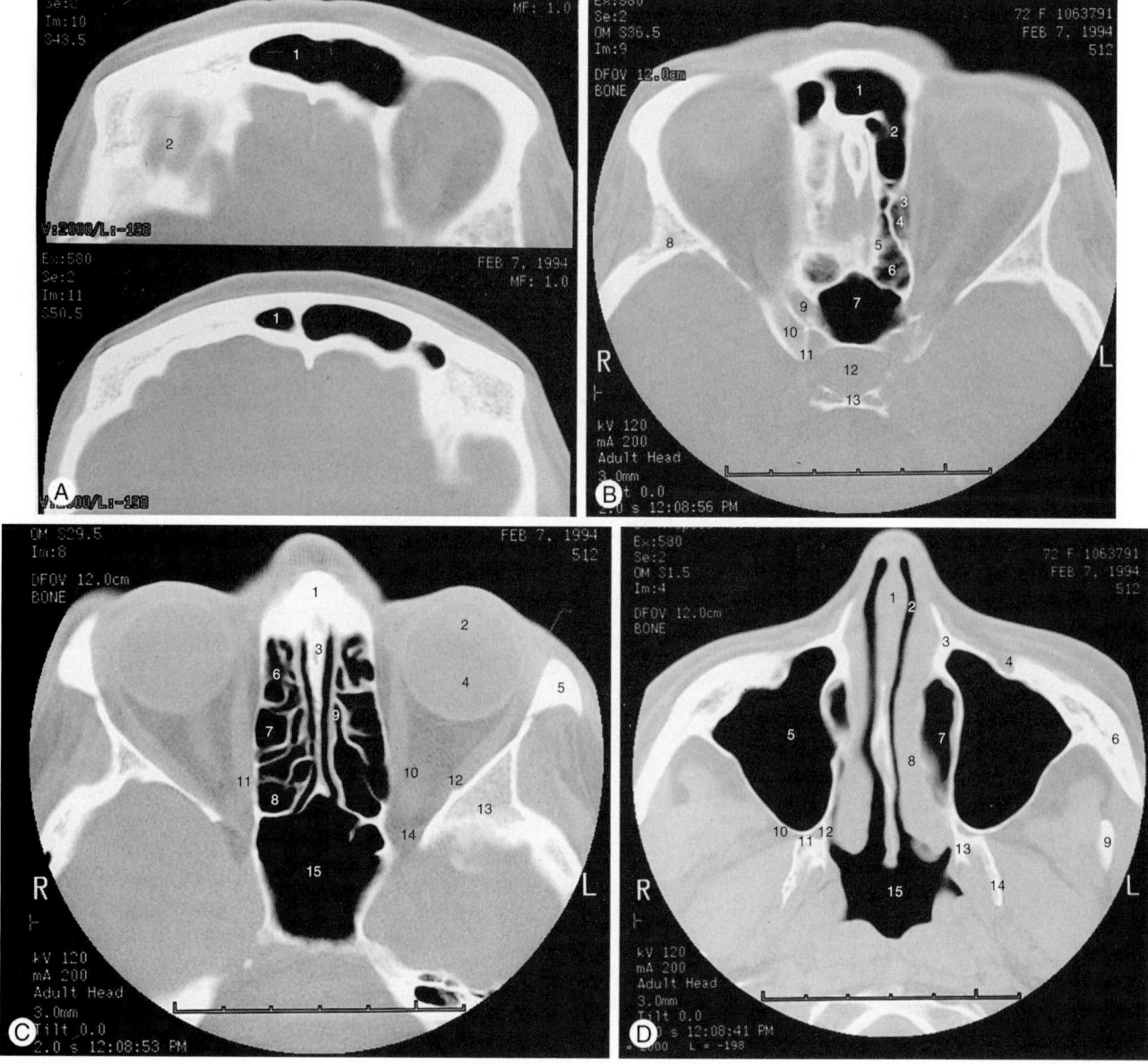

Figure 33–2. Computed tomographic images of normal anatomy of the paranasal sinuses in the transverse plane (shown in superior to inferior direction from *part A* to *part D*). **A,** Sections through the frontal sinuses and roof of the orbit. 1, frontal sinuses; 2, roof of orbit. **B,** Section through the ethmoidal sinus, orbits, and optic chiasm. 1, frontal sinus; 2, anterior ethmoidal air cells; 3, lamina papyracea; 4, middle ethmoidal air cells; 5, cribriform plate; 6, posterior ethmoidal air cells; 7, sphenoidal sinus; 8, greater wing of sphenoid bone; 9, optic canal; 10, squamous portion of temporal bone; 11, anterior clinoid bone; 12, optic chiasm; 13, bony sella. **C,** Sections through the ethmoidal sinus, orbits, and sphenoidal sinus. 1, nasal bone; 2, lens; 3, vertical plate of ethmoid bone; 4, globe; 5, orbital process of zygoma; 6, anterior ethmoidal air cells; 7, middle ethmoidal air cells; 8, posterior ethmoidal air cells; 9, cribriform plate; 10, optic nerve; 11, medial rectus muscle; 12, lateral rectus muscle; 13, greater wing of sphenoid bone; 14, infraorbital fissure; 15, sphenoidal sinus. **D,** Sections through the maxillary antrum, pterygoid plates, and nasopharynx. 1, nasal septum; 2, nasal vestibule; 3, maxilla; 4, infraorbital canal opening; 5, maxillary antrum; 6, zygomatic arch; 7, inferior meatus; 8, inferior turbinate; 9, coronoid process of mandible; 10, perpendicular plate of palatine bone; 11, pterygomaxillary fissure; 12, lower pterygopalatine fossa; 13, medial pterygoid plate; 14, lateral pterygoid plate; 15, nasopharynx.

The cavernous sinuses lie lateral to the sphenoidal sinus with all their vessels (internal carotid artery) and cranial nerves (II, III, IV, V, VI). The pituitary fossa and the optic chiasm lie above and the nasopharynx is located below the sphenoidal sinus. The sphenoidal sinus can be very extensive and may extend laterally between the maxillary nerve and the nerve of the pterygoid canal, inflating the greater wing of the sphenoid bone and pterygoid process.

The sphenoidal sinus opens into the nasal cavity via the sphenoethmoid recess.

FRONTAL SINUS

The pair of frontal sinuses, located within the frontal bone, is irregular in size and shape and often represents an extension of an anterior ethmoid cell (see Figs. 33-1A

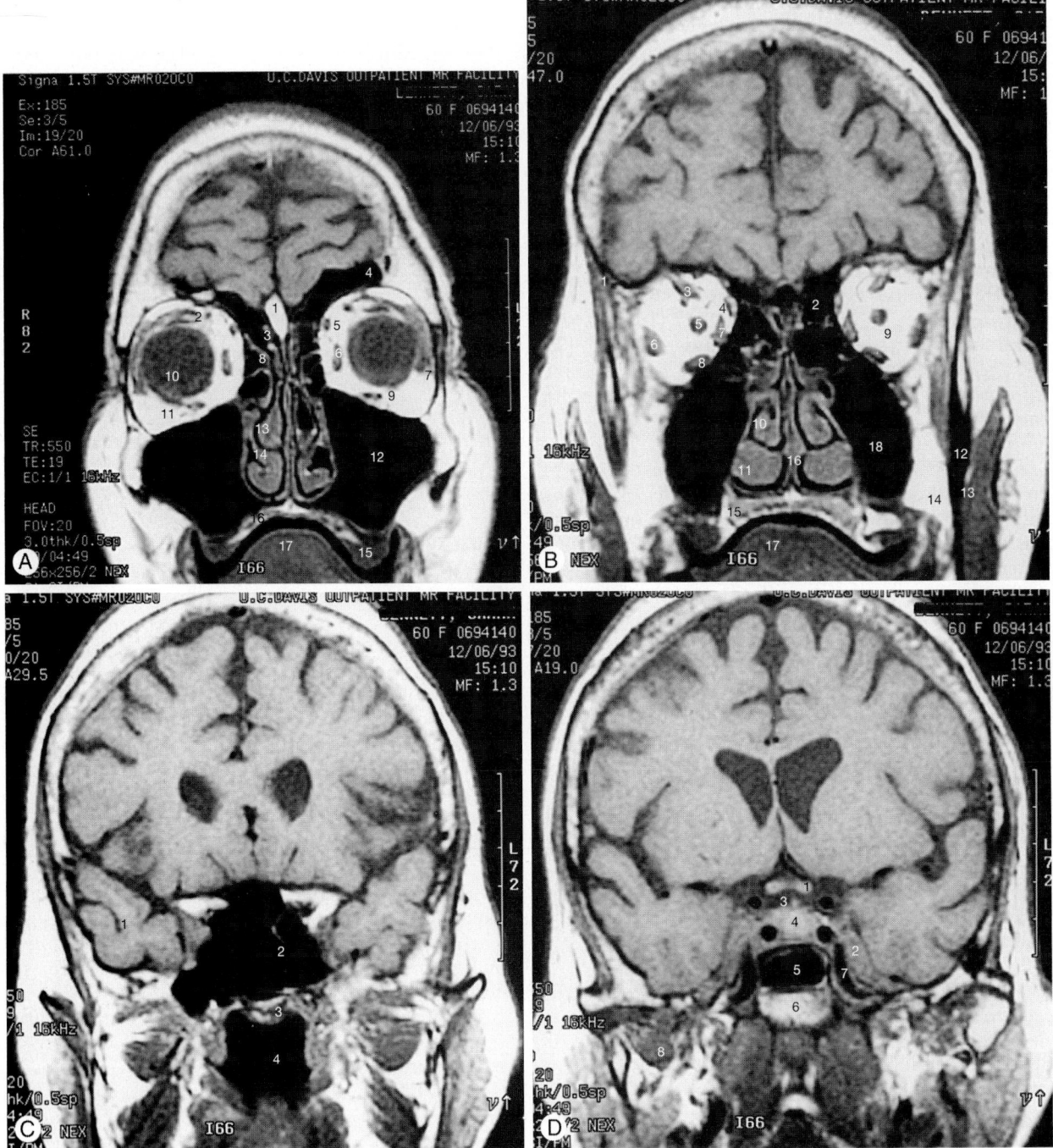

Figure 33–3. Magnetic resonance images of normal anatomy of the paranasal sinuses in the coronal plane (shown in anterior to posterior direction from *part A* to *part D*). **A**, Section through the midglobe, ethmoidal sinus, nasal cavity, and maxillary antrum. 1, crista galli; 2, superior rectus and levator palpebrae superioris muscles; 3, cribriform plate; 4, frontal bone, orbital lamina; 5, superior oblique muscle; 6, medial rectus muscle; 7, lateral rectus muscle; 8, ethmoidal air cells; 9, inferior rectus muscle; 10, globe; 11, periorbital fat; 12, maxillary antrum; 13, middle turbinate; 14, inferior turbinate; 15, maxilla; 16, hard palate; 17, tongue. **B**, Section through posterior orbit, ethmoidal sinus, nasal cavity, and maxillary antrum. 1, temporalis muscle; 2, ethmoidal air cells; 3, superior rectus and levator palpebrae superioris muscles; 4, superior oblique muscle; 5, optic nerve; 6, lateral rectus muscle; 7, medial rectus muscle; 8, inferior rectus muscle; 9, retro-orbital fat; 10, middle turbinate; 11, inferior turbinate; 12, zygomatic bone; 13, masseter muscle; 14, buccal fat pad; 15, hard palate; 16, nasal septum; 17, tongue; 18, maxillary antrum. **C**, Section through the sphenoidal sinus and nasopharynx. 1, temporal lobe; 2, sphenoidal sinus; 3, sphenoid bone; 4, nasopharynx. **D**, Section through the optic chiasm, cavernous sinus, and pituitary gland. 1, optic chiasm; 2, cranial nerve V, maxillary branch (V2); 3, suprasellar cistern; 4, pituitary gland; 5, sphenoidal sinus; 6, clivus; 7, internal carotid artery; 8, lateral pterygoid muscle.

and 33-2A). The sinuses lie above the orbits. The frontal sinus drains into the maxillary sinus via the frontonasal duct.

Local Extension

Nasal cavity carcinomas spread to adjacent sinuses depending on the location of origin: lateral wall tumors destroy the medial maxillary sinus wall and extend into the maxillary antrum, and tumors arising in the middle meatus invade the ethmoid sinus, then the orbit. The sphenoidal sinus and nasopharynx are the next sites of tumor extension in more advanced cases. Esthesioneuroblastomas frequently invade the nasal septum, ethmoid sinuses, orbit, and anterior cranial fossa via the cribriform plate and can involve the frontal brain parenchyma.

Paranasal sinus tumors erode adjacent bone and invade surrounding structures depending on the site of origin in the sinuses. Medial infrastructure lesions of the maxillary sinus invade the nasal cavity early on via the porous medial wall. Lateral infrastructure lesions erode the lateral wall of the antrum and may present as a submucosal mass in the maxillary gingiva. Posterior infrastructure lesions may invade the infratemporal fossa or extend into the pterygopalatine fossa and pterygoid plates. These lesions may invade the orbit by direct superior extension or via extension into the ethmoids.

Suprastructure lesions of the maxillary sinus spread either laterally, invading the malar process of the maxilla and the zygoma, or medially, invading the nasal cavity and ethmoid sinuses. It is not uncommon to encounter a lesion involving the antrum, nasal cavity, and ethmoid sinuses all together, and the site of origin of these tumors may be impossible to determine.

Perineural Spread

The sensory nerve supply of the maxillary, sphenoidal, and ethmoid sinuses; the nasal cavity and palate mucous membrane; the upper teeth and gums; and the adjacent facial skin extending from the lower lid to the upper lip including the nasal vestibule derives from the maxillary branch of the trigeminal nerve (cranial nerve V2). The anterior superior alveolar branch of the infraorbital nerve runs in the facial wall of the maxillary sinus to the upper incisor and canine teeth. The posterior superior alveolar branch (dental nerve) pierces the infratemporal wall and supplies the mucosa of the maxillary antrum. The zygomatic nerve supplies sensory fibers to the lacrimal gland.[24] Involvement of the nerve branches of the maxillary nerve by the tumor often leads to numbness and paresthesias in the skin and mucous membrane of this region.

Perineural extension into the central nervous system is more commonly associated with minor salivary gland tumors, especially with adenoid cystic carcinomas; however, it may occur also with other histologic types, especially in the setting of recurrence after surgery. Commonly involved nerves for perineural spread include

olfactory nerves (from the cribriform plate into the anterior cranial fossa), the infraorbital nerve, and nerves that run through the superior orbital fissure (into the cavernous sinus or middle cranial fossa).[22]

Lymphatic Spread

Lymphatic drainage of the nasal cavity is to the retropharyngeal lymph nodes and the cervical chain. The paranasal sinuses are thought to have sparse capillary lymphatic supply. Thus, the frequency of lymph node involvement is low even in advanced cases unless the tumor involves adjacent areas heavily endowed with lymphatic supply (the nasal cavity, nasopharynx, oral cavity, and skin). About 10% of the patients with nasal cavity or paranasal sinus carcinomas present initially with cervical lymph node metastases and another 10% to 15% develop neck node metastases in follow-up.

DIAGNOSIS AND STAGING

Diagnosis

Physical examination should include inspection and bimanual palpation of the orbit, oral and nasal cavities, and nasopharynx and direct fiberoptic endoscopy. Neurologic examination should emphasize cranial nerve function, since nasal cavity and paranasal sinus tumors are frequently associated with cranial nerve palsies, especially of the trigeminal branches. Cervical lymph nodes are palpated for adenopathy.

Radiologic evaluation is of paramount importance in the diagnosis and staging of nasal cavity and paranasal sinus tumors. Imaging has essentially replaced surgical exploration for staging and tumor mapping in this region. The most useful studies are computed tomography (CT) and magnetic resonance imaging (MRI). CT defines early cortical bone erosion more clearly (Fig. 33-4), whereas MRI better delineates soft tissue. MRI can also differentiate among opacification of the sinuses due to fluid, inflammation, or tumor (Fig. 33-5).[25] CT performs better than MRI in evaluating thin bony structures, such as paranasal sinuses and orbita. MRI may demonstrate subtle perineural spread and involvement of the cranial nerve foramen and canals (Figs. 33-6 and 33-7).[26] MRI is better than CT in evaluating intracranial or leptomeningeal spread. MRI is also more useful in assessing skull base erosion. Sagittal and coronal MRI sections better visualize lesions involving the cribriform plate, basisphenoid, and floor of the middle cranial fossa.[27] Thus, as a single modality, MRI may confer more information than CT.

Pathologic diagnosis is made through a biopsy. Tumors arising from or involving the nasal cavity are amenable to transnasal biopsy. Paranasal sinus tumors are best approached using endoscopic sinus surgery instruments or by an open transcutaneous or transoral procedure. Caldwell-Luc procedures have been used to gain access to the maxillary antrum.

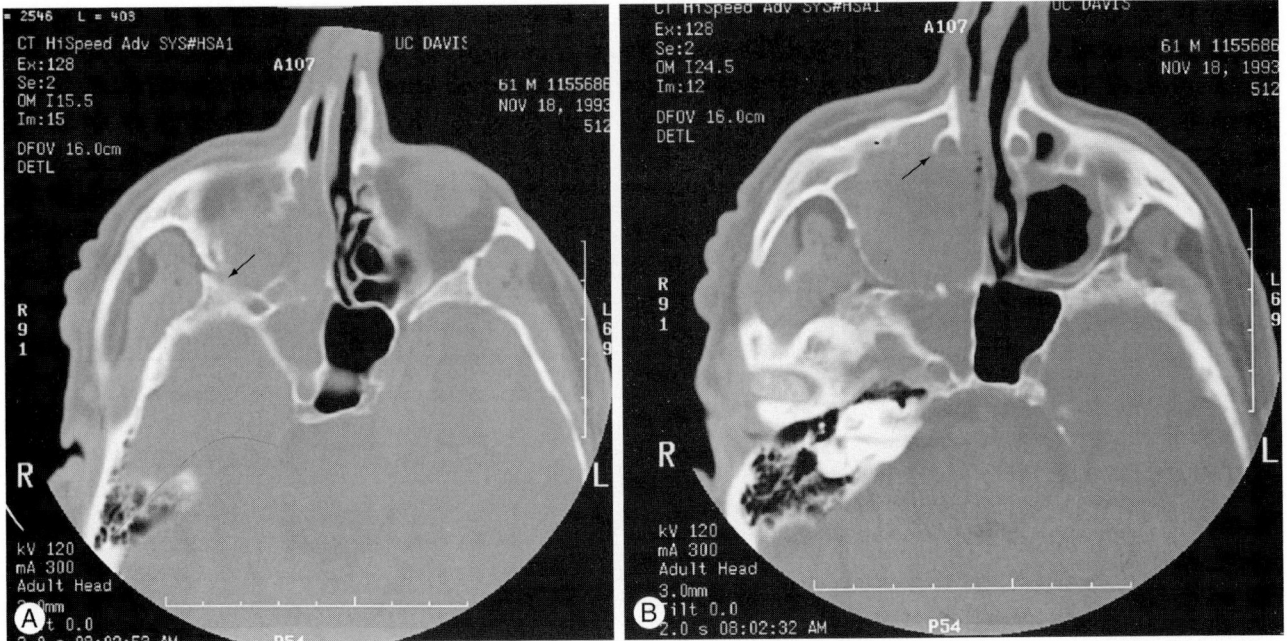

Figure 33–4. Computed tomographic images of a right maxillary antrum carcinoma eroding the medial and lateral walls of the maxillary sinus, extending into the pterygopalatine fossa (**A**, *arrow*) and eroding the lacrimal duct (**B**, *arrow*).

Staging

The staging classification for the epithelial tumors of the nasal cavity and paranasal sinuses has been extensively revised in the sixth edition of the American Joint Committee on Cancer (AJCC) TNM staging system (Table 33-1).[28] In addition to the maxillary sinus, the naso-ethmoid complex has been added as a second site with two regions within the site: the nasal cavity and ethmoid sinuses. The nasal cavity is further divided into four subsites: septum, floor, lateral wall, and vestibule. The ethmoid sinus region is subdivided into two subsites: right and left. For the maxillary sinus, T4 lesions have been divided into T4a (resectable) and T4b

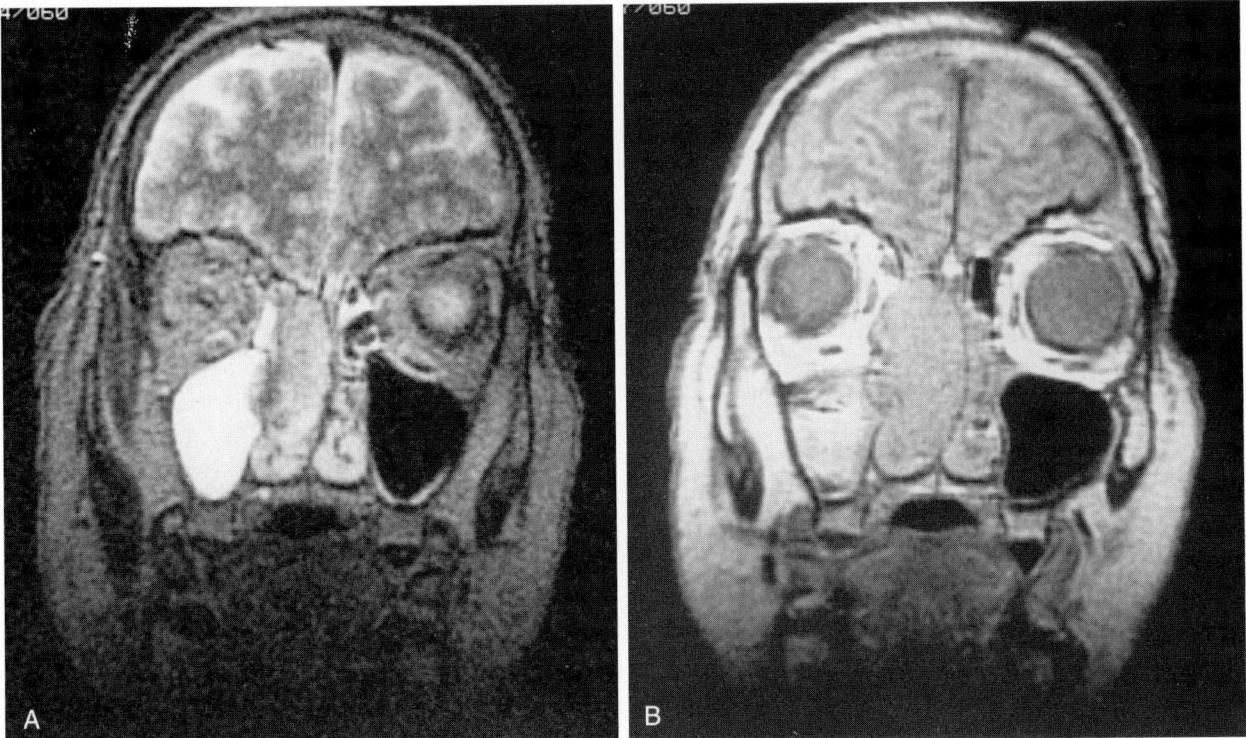

Figure 33–5. Magnetic resonance images of a right nasal cavity carcinoma with possible involvement of the periorbital fat (**A**) and a coexisting fluid-filled maxillary antrum that is uninvolved by the tumor (**B**). MRI is able to distinguish sinusitis and fluid-filled sinus from tumor on a T_2 signal.

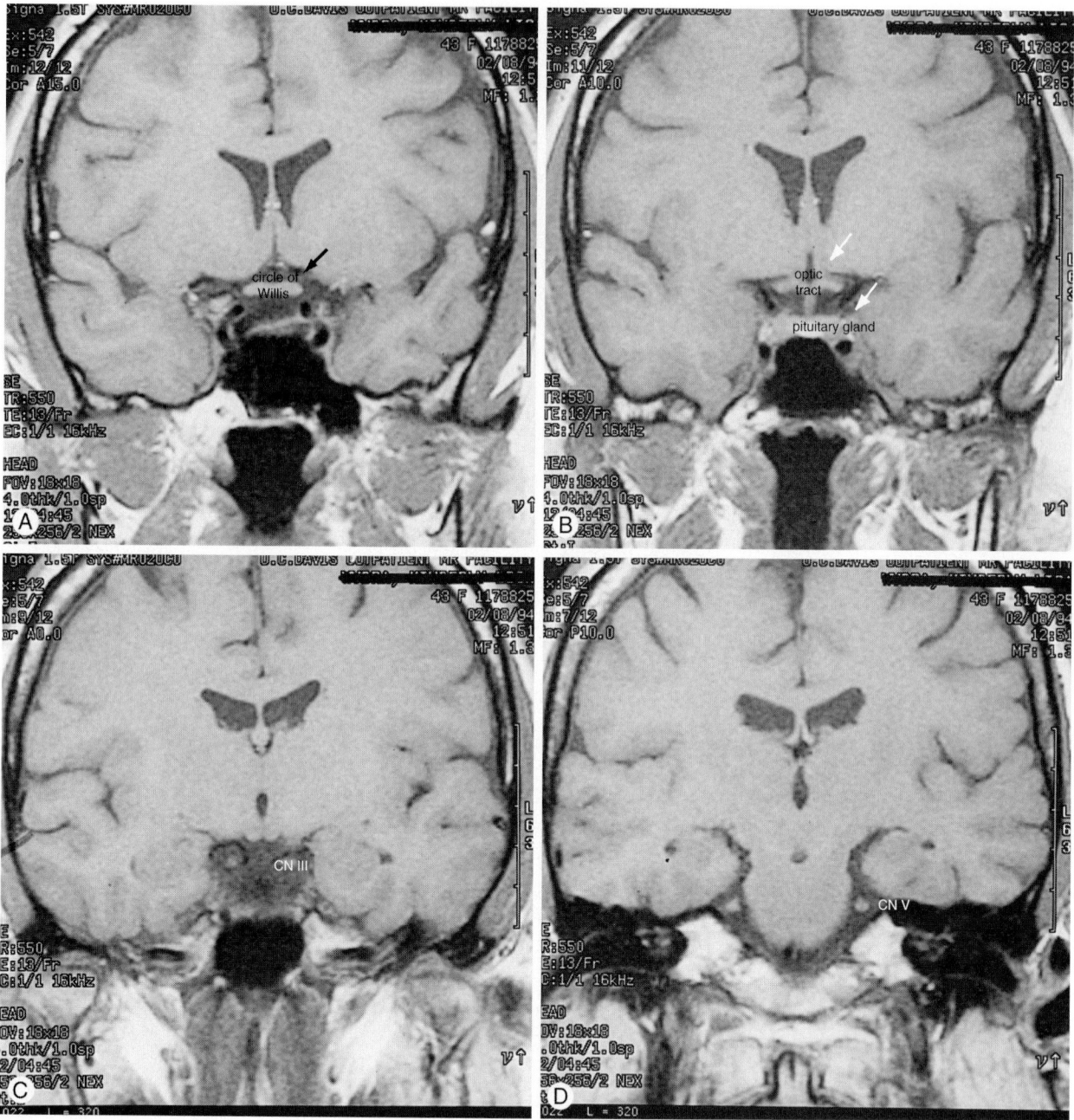

Figure 33–6. Magnetic resonance images of normal cranial nerves in coronal (*A–D*) and transverse (*E–H*) planes. **A,** Optic chiasm and circle of Willis. **B,** Optic chiasm bifurcation and pituitary stalk. **C,** Oculomotor nerve (III). **D,** Trigeminal nerve (V), main trunk.

(unresectable), leading to the division of stage IV into stages IVA, IVB, and IVC. No widely accepted staging classification exists for frontal and sphenoidal tumors, as they are rare.

TREATMENT

Although surgery alone or radiation therapy alone has been used with curative intent in the treatment of select nasal cavity or paranasal sinus carcinomas, most cases warrant combined-modality therapy (Tables 33-2 and 33-3). In recent years, surgery followed by postoperative radiation therapy has been the mainstay of therapy for resectable lesions. Surgery is considered superior to radiation as a single modality for control of small lesions of the nasal septum or those limited to the infrastructure of the maxillary sinus.[3] Although primary radiation therapy has a high cure rate for small squamous carcinomas of the nasal cavity, this approach has a significant chance of optic nerve injury from the high-dose radiation therapy required to achieve a good control rate.[29] Massive tumors with extensive involvement of the nasopharynx, base of skull, sphenoidal sinuses, brain, or optic chiasm are considered unresectable. Some institutions have been studying the efficacy of combined

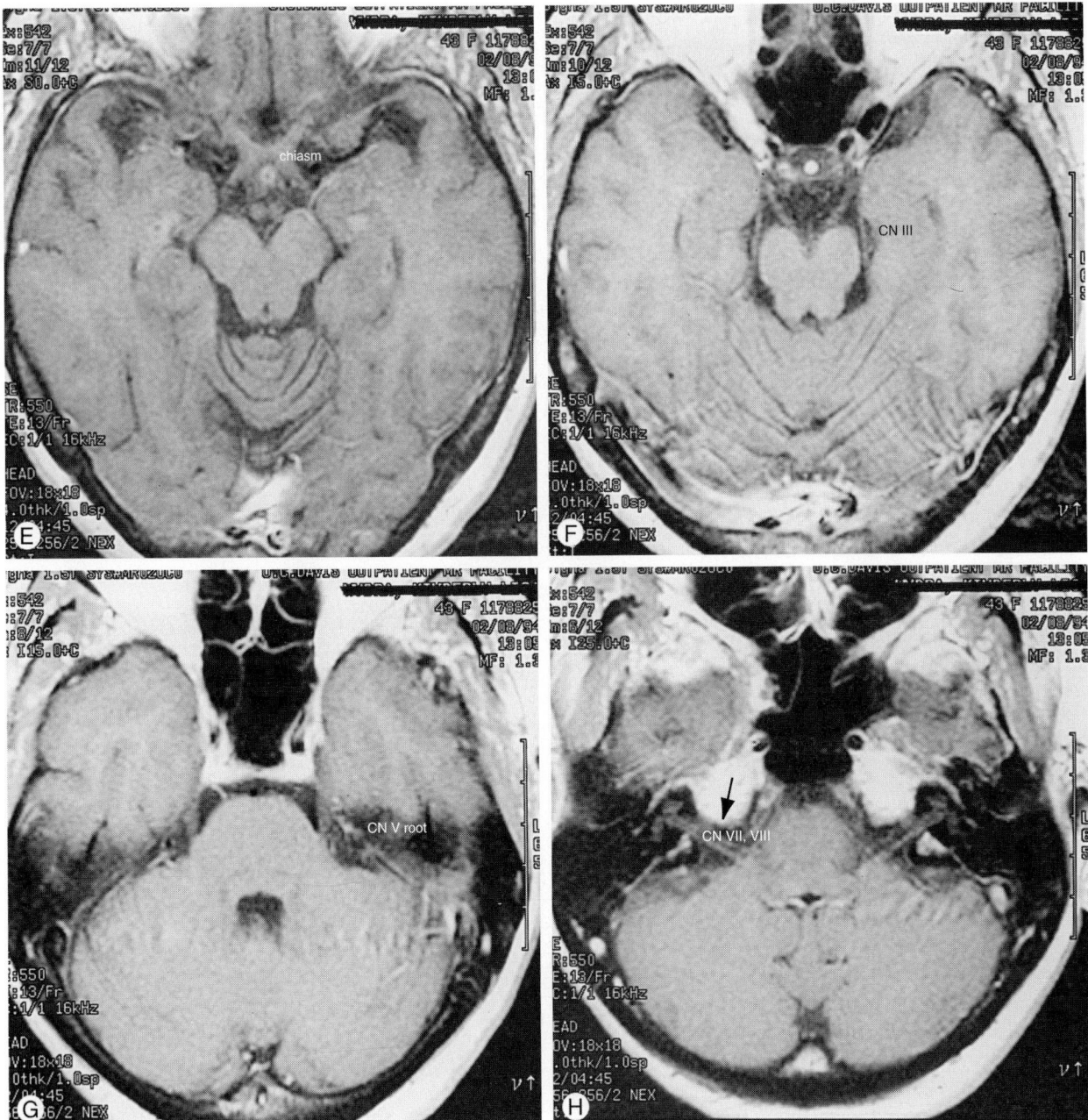

Figure 33–6. cont'd E, Optic chiasm. **F,** Oculomotor nerve (III). **G,** Trigeminal nerve (V). **H,** Facial (VII) and vestibulocochlear (VIII) nerves.

radiation and radiosensitizing chemotherapy for unresectable squamous cell carcinoma of the nasal cavity and paranasal sinuses. Early results of this approach have been promising.[30] If radiation therapy alone is to be used for large lesions, a hyperfractionated regimen may allow the delivery of higher doses than conventional radiation.

Surgery

SURGICAL PROCEDURES

The goal of surgery for nasal cavity and paranasal sinus tumors is to achieve en bloc resection of all involved bone and soft tissue with clear margins while maximizing the cosmetic and functional outcome. The extent and site of the incision depend on the location of the lesion. Limited nasal cavity lesions may be resected with medial maxillectomy. Ethmoid lesions usually require medial maxillectomy and en bloc ethmoidectomy. This is the most common surgical approach for inverted papillomas. The development of a combined craniofacial procedure for lesions involving the inferior surface of the cribriform plate and the roof of the ethmoid bone offers access to the anterior cranial fossa, orbit, and pterygopalatine fossa and allows a rational oncologic resection, dependent on anatomic considerations. In addition, this approach results in excellent cosmesis and improvement

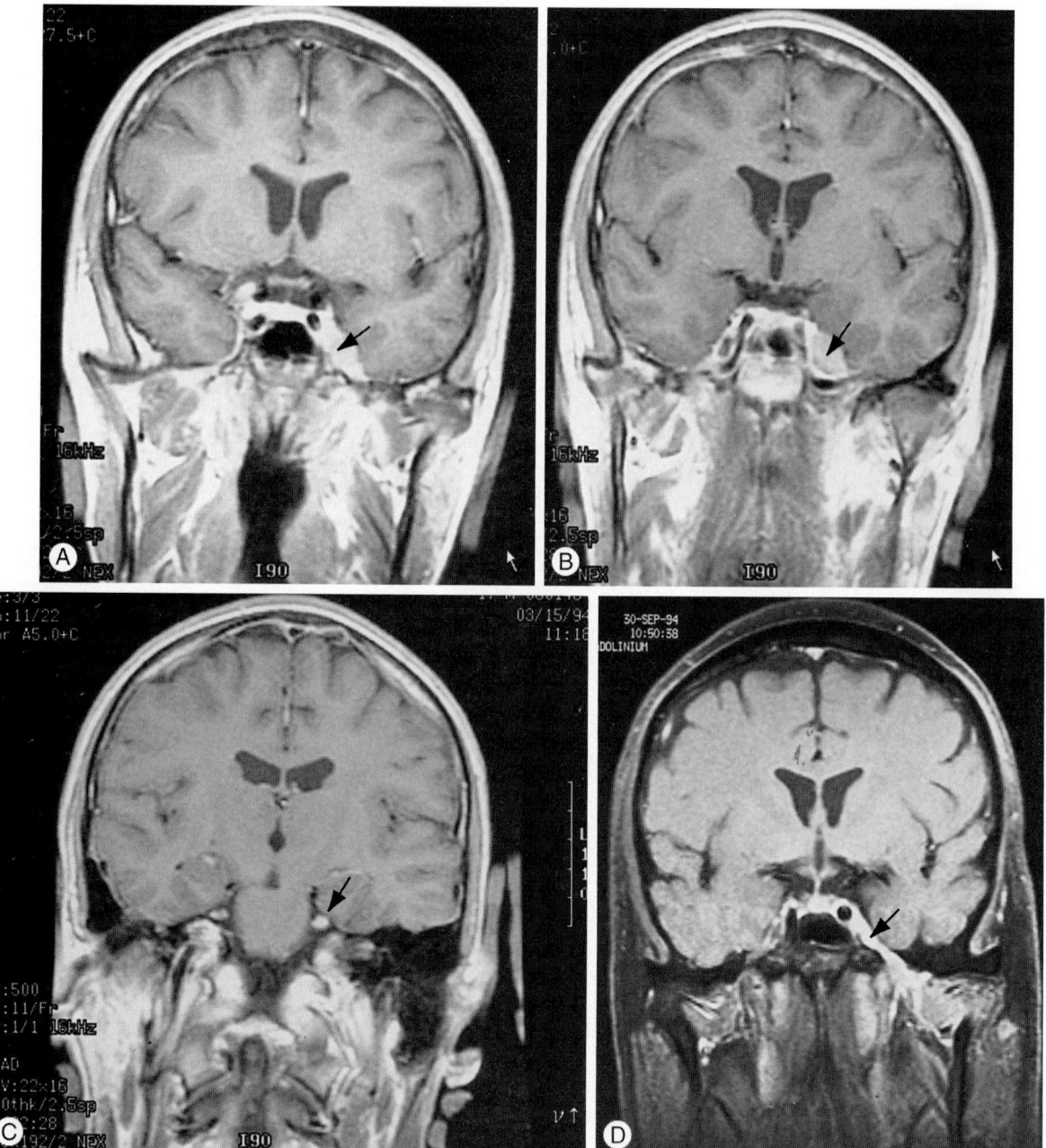

Figure 33–7. Magnetic resonance images of perineural spread in coronal plane involving cavernous sinus, trigeminal nerve and ganglion, and oculomotor nerve. **A,** Left cavernous sinus is expanded by tumor. **B,** Trigeminal ganglion infiltration in Meckel's cavity. **C,** Left trigeminal nerve root enhancement due to perineural spread as it leaves the brainstem. **D,** Enhancement of cavernous sinus by perineural spread along oculomotor nerves.

in the cure of lesions associated with extremely poor prognosis otherwise.[31] The bony defect in the anterior cranial floor is closed with a vascularized pericranial or temporal muscle flap.

Primary surgery for maxillary antral cancers is radical maxillectomy that removes en bloc the entire maxilla and ethmoid sinus via a Weber-Fergusson incision. Patients with tumors limited to the infrastructure do well after surgery alone as long as the margins of resection are adequate. Suprastructure lesions may involve the orbit, necessitating orbital exenteration. Resection of involved periosteum and frozen-section control of adjacent orbital contents with preservation of the eye may be possible in

select lesions with involvement of the periorbita without intraorbital extension. Orbital preservation surgery in select patients with involvement of the bony orbit but not soft tissue does not appear to result in poorer survival or local control than those undergoing exenteration.[32,33] The radical maxillectomy defect is covered with a split-thickness skin graft. As a general rule, the surgical defect should not be obliterated during the initial surgery. An open cavity allows cleansing and direct visual inspection during follow-up.

Base-of-skull surgery has been growing as a discipline of head and neck surgery, addressing the need for more radical resection of extensive tumors involving the

Table 33–1   Classification of Nasal Cavity and Paranasal Sinus Cancers

Primary Tumor (T)

TX	Primary tumor cannot be assessed
T0	No evidence of primary tumor
Tis	Carcinoma in situ

Maxillary Sinus

T1	Tumor limited to maxillary sinus mucosa with no erosion or destruction of bone
T2	Tumor causing bone erosion or destruction including extension into the hard palate and/or middle nasal meatus, except extension to posterior wall of maxillary sinus and pterygoid plates
T3	Tumor invades any of the following: bone of the posterior wall of maxillary sinus, subcutaneous tissues, floor or medial wall of orbit, pterygoid fossa, ethmoid sinuses
T4a	Tumor invades anterior orbital contents, skin of cheek, pterygoid plates, infratemporal fossa, cribriform plate, sphenoid or frontal sinuses
T4b	Tumor invades any of the following: orbital apex, dura, brain, middle cranial fossa, cranial nerves other than maxillary division of trigeminal nerve (V_2), nasopharynx, or clivus

Nasal Cavity and Ethmoid Sinus

T1	Tumor restricted to any one subsite, with or without bony invasion
T2	Tumor invading two subsites in a single region or extending to involve an adjacent region within the nasoethmoidal complex, with or without bony invasion
T3	Tumor extends to invade the medial wall or floor of the orbit, maxillary sinus, palate, or cribriform plate
T4a	Tumor invades any of the following: anterior orbital contents, skin of nose or cheek, minimal extension to anterior cranial fossa, pterygoid plates, sphenoid or frontal sinuses
T4b	Tumor invades any of the following: orbital apex, dura, brain, middle cranial fossa, cranial nerves other than (V_2), nasopharynx, or clivus

Regional Lymph Nodes (N)

NX	Regional lymph nodes cannot be assessed
N0	No regional lymph node metastasis
N1	Metastasis in a single ipsilateral lymph node, 3 cm or less in greatest dimension
N2	Metastasis in a single ipsilateral lymph node, more than 3 cm but not more than 6 cm in greatest dimension, or in bilateral or contralateral lymph nodes, none more than 6 cm in greatest dimension
N2a	Metastasis in a single ipsilateral lymph node, more than 3 cm but not more than 6 cm in greatest dimension
N2b	Metastasis in multiple ipsilateral lymph nodes, none more than 6 cm in greatest dimension
N2c	Metastasis in bilateral or contralateral lymph nodes, none more than 6 cm in greatest dimension
N3	Metastasis in a lymph node, more than 6 cm in greatest dimension

Distant Metastasis (M)

MX	Distant metastasis cannot be assessed
M0	No distant metastasis
M1	Distant metastasis

Stage Grouping

Stage 0	Tis	N0	M0
Stage I	T1	N0	M0
Stage II	T2	N0	M0
Stage III	T3	N0	M0
	T1	N1	M0
	T2	N1	M0
	T3	N1	M0
Stage IVA	T4a	N0	M0
	T4a	N1	M0
	T1	N2	M0
	T2	N2	M0
	T3	N2	M0
	T4a	N2	M0
Stage IVB	T4b	Any N	M0
	Any T	N3	M0
Stage IVC	Any T	Any N	M1

From Greene FL, Page DL, Fleming ID, et al, eds: *AJCC Cancer Staging Manual*, 6th ed. New York: Springer; 2002.

frontal brain, cavernous sinus, sphenoidal sinus, clivus, pterygoid space, and petrous bone. The classic criteria for inoperability include (1) superior extension of the tumor through the dura into the frontal lobes; (2) posterior extension of the tumor beyond the cribriform plate and fovea ethmoidalis to a point where there is excessive traction on the optic chiasm or invasion of the prevertebral fascia or both; (3) involvement of both optic nerves; and (4) lateral extension into the region of the superior orbital fissure and cavernous sinus.[4] In a combined team approach with neurosurgery, many previously unresectable sinonasal tract tumors are successfully resected at some centers. This technique is evolving, and outcomes of such aggressive surgery in those lesions with otherwise dismal prognosis need to be validated.

Table 33–2   Results of Treatment: Combined-Modality Therapy (CMT) of Surgery and Radiation Therapy (RT) Compared with Definitive Radiation

Reference	Study Period	Patients, *n*	Site	Survival Endpoint, Yr	Survival Parameter	Survival Rate, %	
						RT	CMT
Gallagher & Boles[†]	1955–1964	41	Maxillary sinus	5	OS	16	60
Tabb & Barranco[3]	1958–1968	108	Maxillary sinus	5	OS	0	25
Ahmed et al[‡]	1955–1974	56	Maxillary sinus	5	LC*	34	67
Bush & Bagshaw[§]	1956–1974	38	Paranasal sinuses	5	DFS*	23	38
Cheng & Wang[‖]	1960–1970	50	Maxillary sinus	3	DFS	22	58
St. Pierre & Baker[¶]	1964–1975	66	Maxillary sinus	5	OS*	16	58
Amendola et al[**]	1968–1978	39	Maxillary sinus	3	DFS	50	37
Shibuya et al[††]	1953–1982	416	Maxillary sinus	10	OS*	21	34
Shidnia et al[35]	1960–1980	109	Paranasal sinuses	2.5	OS	11	37
Gadeberg et al[‡‡]	1963–1980	80	Paranasal sinuses	5	OS*	10	42
Beale & Garrett[§§]	1964–1979	112	Maxillary sinus	5	OS*	40	51
Flores et al[‖‖]	1970–1978	40	Paranasal sinuses	5	OS	42	74
Isaacs et al[¶¶]	1966–1984	37	Maxillary sinus	2	OS	32	36
Giri et al[66]	1970–1988	37	Maxillary sinus	5	OS*	18	53
Roa et al[***]	1986–1992	39	Paranasal sinuses	3	OS*	32	65

*Reported using an actuarial method.
†From Gallagher TM, Boles R: Symposium: Treatment of malignancies of paranasal sinuses, I. Carcinoma of the maxillary antrum. *Laryngoscope.* 1981;91:133.
‡From Ahmed K, Cordoba RB, Fayos JV: Squamous cell Carcinoma of the maxillary sinus. *Arch Otolaryngol.* 1981;107:48.
§From Bush SE, Bagshaw MA: Carcinoma of the paranasal sinuses. *Cancer.* 1982;50:154.
‖From cheng VST, Wang CC: Carcinomas of the paranasal sinuses: A study of sixty-six cases. *Cancer.* 1977;40:3038.
¶From St. Pierre S, Baker SR: Squamous cell carcinoma of the maxillary sinus: Analysis of 66 cases. *Head Neck Surg.* 1983;5:508.
**From Amendola BE, Eisert D, Hazra TA, et al: Carcinoma of the maxillary antrum: Surgery or radiation therapy? *Int J Radiat Oncol Biol Phys.* 1981;7:743.
††From Shibuya H, Horiuchi JI, Suzuki S, et al: Maxillary sinus carcinoma: Results of radiation therapy. *Int J Radiat Oncol Biol Phys.* 1984;10:1021.
‡‡From Gadeberg CC, Hjelm-Hansen M, Sogaard H, Elbrond O: Malignant tumors of the paranasal sinuses and nasal cavity: A series of 180 patients. *Acta Radiol Oncol.* 1984;23:181.
§§From Beale FA, Garrett PG: Cancer of the paranasal sinuses with particular reference to maxillary sinus cancer. *J Otolaryngol.* 1983;12:377.
‖‖From Flores AD, Anderson DW, Doyle PJ, et al: Paranasal sinus malignancy—A retrospective analysis of treatment methods. *J Otolaryngol.* 1984;13:141.
¶¶From Isaacs JH, Mooney S, Mendenhall WM, Parsons JT: Cancer of the maxillary sinus treated with surgery and/or radiation therapy. *Am Surg.* 1990;56:327.
***From Roa WH, Hazuka MB, Sandler HM, et al: Results of primary and adjuvant CT-based three-dimensional radiotherapy for malignant tumors of the paranasal sinuses. *Int J Radiat Oncol Biol Phys.* 1994;28:857.
DFS, disease-free survival; LC, local control; OS, overall survival.

POSTSURGICAL REHABILITATION

The primary consideration for rehabilitation after radical surgery is function. Preoperative evaluation by a prosthodontist is necessary to obtain dental impressions and to assess the dentition that will remain after surgery. A surgical splint prepared preoperatively is used to fill the defect during the immediate postoperative period. Use of the splint facilitates immediate speech and swallowing. A temporary obturator is then fitted until the cavity completely heals several months later, at which time a permanent obturator can be made.[34]

Table 33–3   Results of Surgery Alone: Maxillary Sinus Cancer

Reference	Study Period	Patients, *n*	5-Yr Survival, %
Gallagher & Boles*	1955–1964	8	50
Tabb & Barranco[3]	1958–1968	19	62
St. Pierre & Baker[†]	1964–1975	10	20

*From Gallagher TM, Boles R: Symposium: Treatment of malignancies of paranasal sinuses, I. Carcinoma of the maxillary antrum. *Laryngoscope.* 1981;91:133.
†From St. Pierre S, Baker SR: Squamous cell carcinoma of the maxillary sinus: Analysis of 66 cases. *Head Neck Surg.* 1983;5:508.

Radiation Therapy

Radiation therapy was more often administered preoperatively in the 1960s and 1970s; however, over the past decade, most centers have been using radiation therapy in the postoperative adjuvant setting after radical surgery for squamous cell carcinomas of the nasal cavity and paranasal sinuses. Although pre- and postoperative radiation may result in similar control rates (Table 33-4), there are definite advantages to surgery before radiation. Preoperative radiation may obscure the initial extent of disease and erroneously lead to a more conservative resection; thus, surgery may not quite encompass the microscopic disease. Preoperative radiation also increases the infection rate and the risk of postoperative wound complications. Radiation therapy in the postoperative setting has the advantage of accurate pathologic review of all structures at risk, and the radiation portals can then be designed to encompass the entire extent of disease with adequate margins. Upfront surgery also allows drainage of infected sinuses before radiation. Postoperative radiation therapy is started 4 to 6 weeks after surgery.

In those patients who are deemed medically inoperable or who refuse radical surgery, primary radiation therapy has been employed with differing success (10%

Table 33–4   Results of Treatment in Maxillary Sinus Tumors: Preoperative and Postoperative Radiation Therapy

Author	Study Period	Patients, *n*	Survival Endpoint, Yr	Survival Rate, %	
				Preop	*Postop*
Jesse*	1952–1961	41	3	45	37
Tabb & Barranco[3]	1958–1968	54	5	32	12
Hu et al[†]	1958–1974	50	5	64	26
Isaacs et al[‡]	1966–1984	11	2	0[§]	80[§]
Korzeniowski et al[∥]	1967–1978	57	5	NA	35
Zaharia et al[¶]	1963–1980	149	5	NA	42

*From Jesse RH: Preoperative versus postoperative radiation in the treatment of squamous carcinoma of the paranasal sinuses. *Am J Surg.* 1965; 110:552. Postop group represents patients treated between 1952 and 1957 and preop group represents those treated between 1958 and 1961.
∥Surgery was incomplete: 35 patients with macroscopic residual and 22 with microscopic residual.
§This series represents small numbers: 6 patients in preoperative group and 5 patients in postoperative group.

to 70% 5-year survival) depending on the stage and extent of the tumor.[35,36]

Minor salivary gland carcinomas are resected first and irradiated postoperatively if the histologic examination reveals a high-grade or adenoid cystic variety, extensive perineural spread, positive or close margins of resection, or extensive primary tumor (T3 or T4). The radiation portals should include neural pathways up to the cranial nerve ganglion at the base of the skull in adenoid cystic carcinomas and high-grade lesions with extensive perineural invasion. There is sparse literature available regarding the outcome of definitive irradiation for unresectable salivary gland tumors of the nasal cavity and paranasal sinuses. The results of definitive conventional photon irradiation of unresectable salivary gland tumors in general were poor (17% local control at 2 years) in at least one randomized trial of photon versus neutron therapy[37]; however, whether neutron therapy offers any advantage over photons is controversial and this controversy is discussed in the preceding chapter on salivary gland tumors.

The neck is treated electively only when the tumor invades the nasopharynx or other lymphatic-rich areas, or is T4 in extent, poorly differentiated, or recurrent. Broader use of elective nodal irradiation is controversial

and is further discussed in "Results of Therapy" later. The neck is irradiated after neck dissection for nodal involvement at presentation according to the usual guidelines for postoperative neck irradiation.

RADIOTHERAPEUTIC TECHNIQUE: EXTERNAL BEAM

It is most advantageous to base the treatment volume on treatment-planning CT with MRI correlation, if available. MRI-derived gross total volumes (GTVs) may be smaller and have less interobserver variation than CT-derived GTVs. CT and MRI are complementary in delineating the GTV.[38] The complex anatomy of this region and the presence of numerous critical, dose-limiting organs such as optic nerves, chiasm, eyes, lacrimal gland, auditory apparatus, pituitary, brainstem, and spinal cord, render tumors of the sinonasal tract ideal candidates for sophisticated treatment planning. Since the introduction of CT-based treatment planning and immobilization devices in the 1980s, improvement in survival rates while reducing the incidence of eye complications has been reported.[39] A three-dimensional (3D) system allows comprehensive visualization of the tumor volume and adjacent normal anatomy through "beam's eye view" displays (Figs. 33-8 and 33-9). Careful definition of the

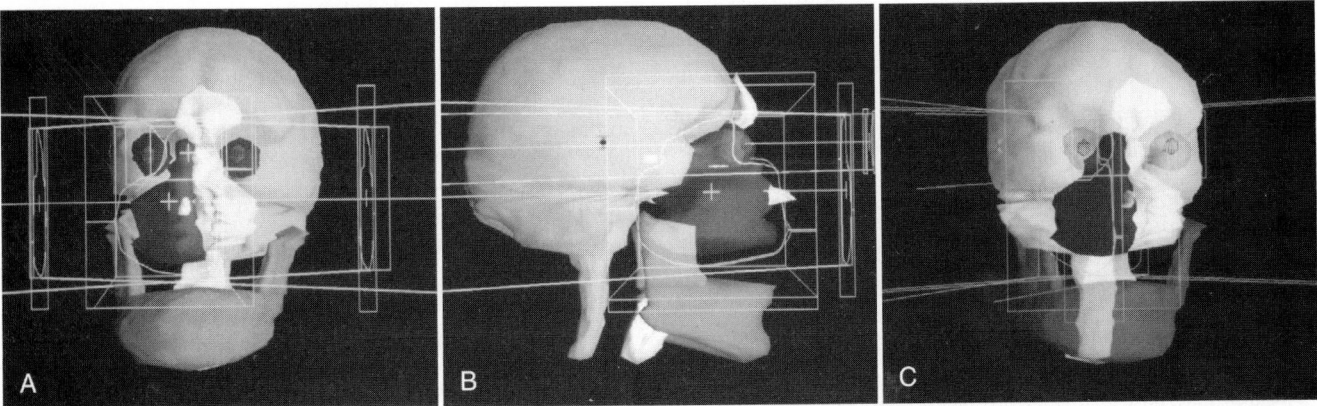

Figure 33–8. Three-dimensional beam's-eye views: four-field technique using opposed lateral portals, and anterior photon and electron portals. **A,** Anterior view. **B,** Lateral view. **C,** Oblique view. See also Color Figure 33-8.

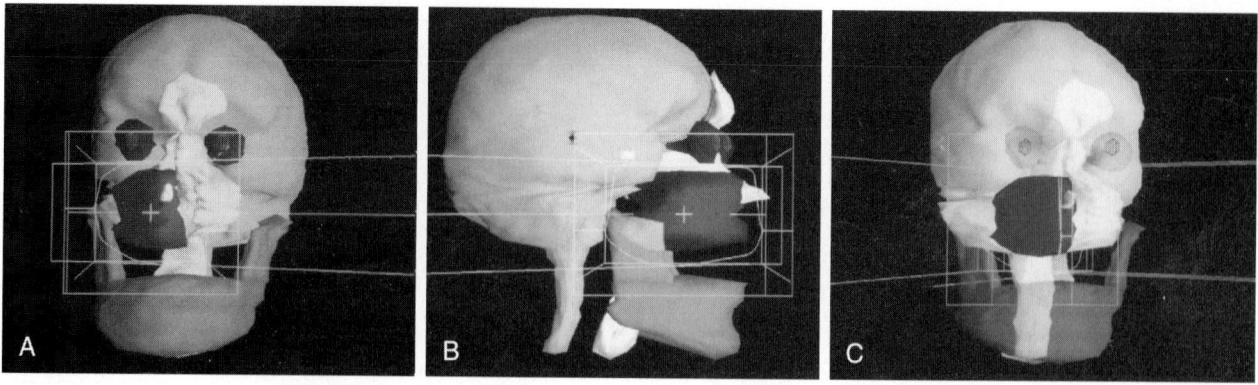

Figure 33–9. Three-dimensional beam's-eye views: wedged-pair portals. **A,** Anterior view. **B,** Lateral view. **C,** Oblique view. See also Color Figure 33-9.

anatomic structures of interest and of the extent of the tumor, together with immobilization devices for precise setup, permits accurate targeting of the tumor. The ability of a 3D system to use nonaxial and noncoplanar fields allows greater flexibility in treatment planning, so that the dose distribution conforms to the tumor volume in 3D space, thus sparing the surrounding normal tissue to a greater extent. Dose-volume histograms (Fig. 33-10) are able to record accurately the doses delivered to differing volumes of adjacent dose-limiting structures. This technology has great potential for improving local control, while decreasing the risk of long-term sequelae of therapy, and allowing dose escalation that has not been possible with conventional two-dimensional treatment-planning systems. Thus, the role of a conformal 3D treatment system will become even more important in the

setting of primary radiation therapy that requires high doses beyond 70 Gy. While 3D conformal plans can provide bilateral sparing of the globe for most patients, it may be more difficult to spare optic nerves, especially on the ipsilateral side, when prescription dose exceeds the normal tissue tolerance doses.

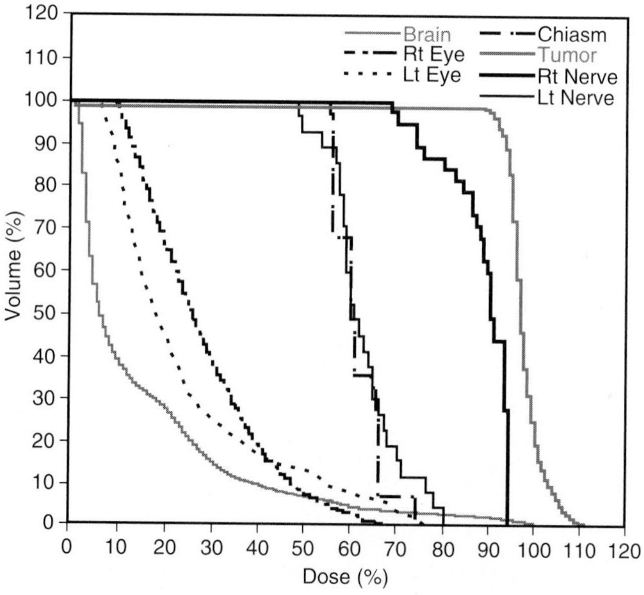

Intensity-modulated radiation therapy (IMRT) using inverse treatment planning systems may render a greater therapeutic ratio for tumors of the paranasal sinuses compared with the more standard forward planning 3D conformal therapy. IMRT can result in better sparing of the optic apparatus, especially in definitive cases where high doses of radiation are necessary for gross tumor eradication. IMRT strategies for paranasal sinus malignancies can be strikingly different in various aspects, such as beam setup; total number of segments; gross, clinical, and planning tumor volume (GTV, CTV, PTV, respectively) dose coverage; and dose statistics for organs at risk (Figs. 33-11 to 33-13).[40]

Among the many advantages of image-based conformal planning in this region is the ability to optimize and show the effects of inhomogeneity corrections for air cavities and dense bone. Conformal planning is especially helpful in the use of anterior electrons, in which the extensive system of air cavities and sloping surfaces present in the paranasal sinuses can significantly distort the isodose curves generated by a nonconformal system, resulting in an overdose to critical structures (i.e., optic nerves and chiasm) and an underdose to the tumor volume.

The radiation therapy of the nasal cavity, ethmoid sinuses, and maxillary sinuses is similar, as the tumor extensively involves two or more sinuses in most cases. A typical target volume in a postoperative setting encompasses both halves of the nasal cavity and ipsilateral maxillary sinus. Ethmoid sinuses and the ipsilateral medial orbital wall are included if the tumor extends superiorly into the ethmoid air cells.

During the initial setup, the patient's head is placed in a neutral supine position (Fig. 33-14). A tongue depressor is placed in the mouth to displace the tongue from the treatment area. In a postoperative setting, the patient wears the obturator for the maxillary defect during the simulation. A CT-compatible thermoplastic

Figure 33–10. Three-dimensional dose-volume histogram. The optic chiasm and the contralateral optic nerve doses are limited to 65% to 70% of the prescribed dose while nearly 80% of the ipsilateral optic nerve receives greater than 90% of the prescribed tumor dose. See also Color Figure 33-10.

Paranasal Sinuses

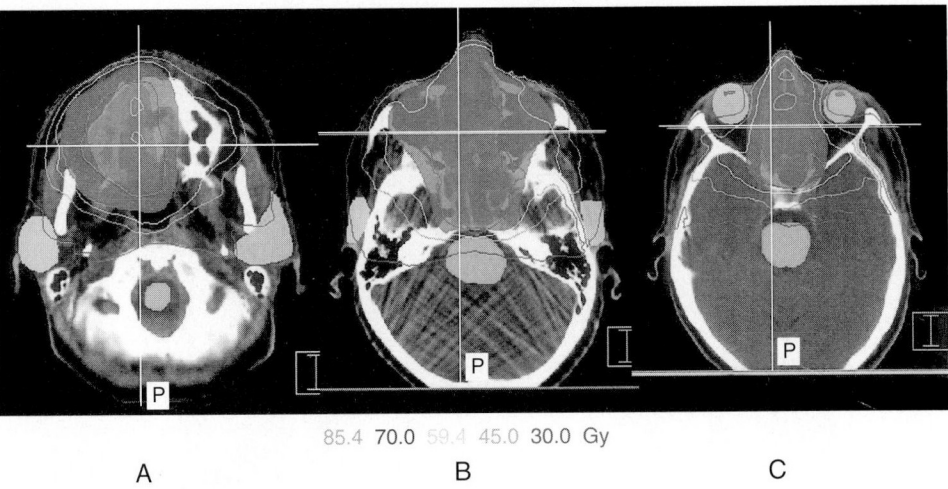

Figure 33–11. Intensity-modulated radiation therapy isodose plans in axial planes (color-wash representations shown here in shades of gray) of a patient with locally advanced (stage T4NxM0) paranasal sinus undifferentiated carcinoma undergoing definitive radiotherapy. The plan was generated on Corvus planning system (Nomos Corp.) using 6 MV photons and MIMic multi-leaf collimator device with six table positions: **A,** At the level of the maxillary sinuses/parotid glands; **B,** at the level of the floor of the orbit/brainstem; **C,** at the level of ethmoid sinuses/mid-orbit. The bilateral eyes are nicely spared (<45 Gy isodose region) as are the brainstem (<45 Gy isodose region) and the parotid glands (<30 Gy isodose region). See also Color Figure 33-11.

85.4 70.0 59.4 45.0 30.0 Gy

A   B   C

Paranasal Sinuses

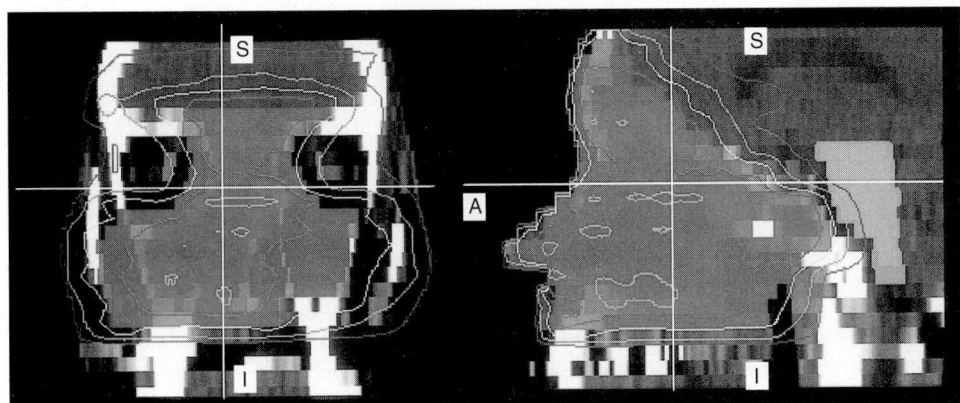

85.4 70.0 59.4 45.0 30.0 Gy

A   B

Figure 33–12. Intensity-modulated radiation therapy isodose plans in sagittal and coronal planes: **A,** coronal view; **B,** sagittal view. See also Color Figure 33-12.

Cumulative dose volume histogram

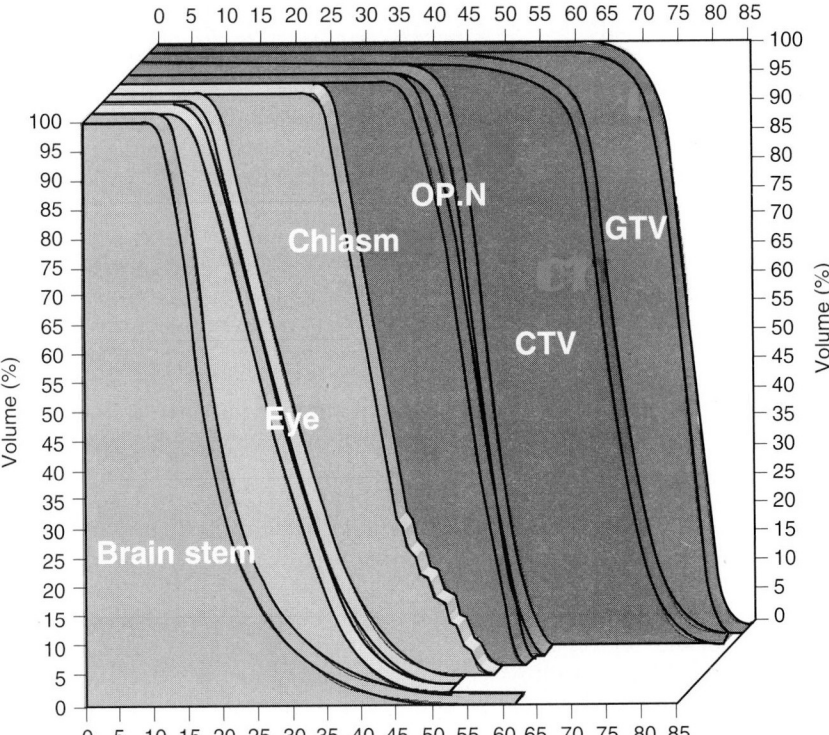

Figure 33–13. Intensity-modulated radiation therapy dose volume histogram. The gross target volume (GTV) receives 70 Gy and the clinical target volume (CTV) receives 59.4 Gy. Less than 10% of the optic chiasm receives greater than 55 Gy. See also Color Figure 33-13.

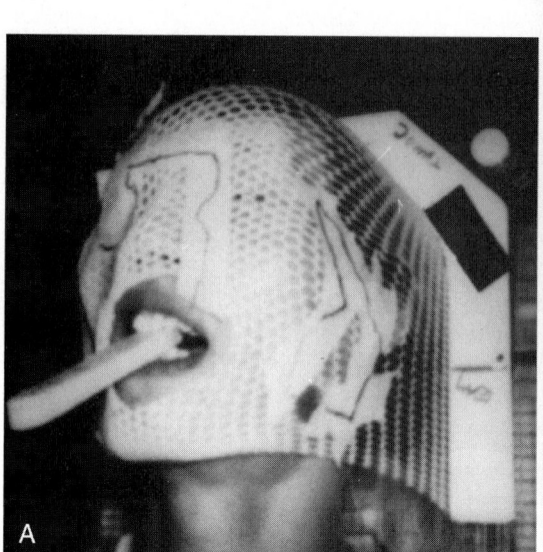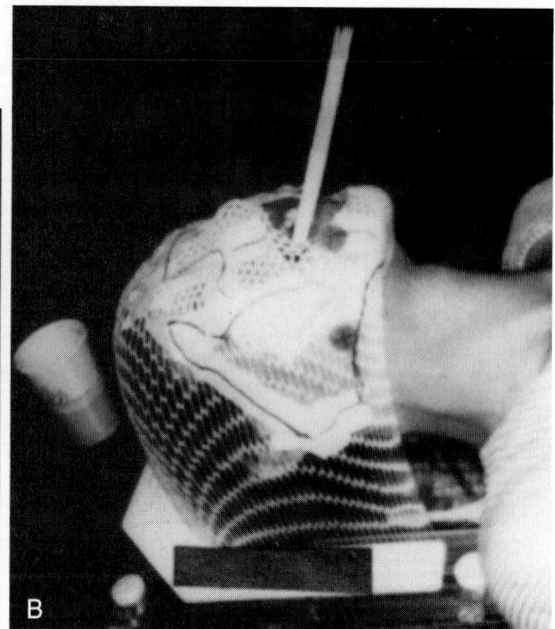

Figure 33–14. A and **B,** Treatment position. The head is placed in a neutral position and immobilized using an Aquaplast mold. A bite block is placed above the oral tongue in the mouth to push the tongue out of the field.

facial mask is made to immobilize the head. An anterior portal is set up with the inferior border splitting the tongue blade (near the commissure of the lips), and the upper border is determined per the superior extension of the tumor. The ipsilateral border should include the entire maxillary sinus and the contralateral border should cover the medial wall of the orbit and medial maxillary wall (just medial to the limbus of the contralateral eye). For massive lesions involving the contralateral maxillary sinus, the lateral border should be extended to include entire contralateral sinuses. The lateral portal is set up with the anterior border flashing the skin of the cheek and the posterior border at the posterior aspect of the clivus, splitting the vertebral bodies. The patient is scanned in the treatment position in the facial mask. For primary radiation therapy of unresectable tumors, CT with intravenous contrast material is recommended to take advantage of the enhancing characteristics of neoplasms. In a postoperative setting, CT without contrast suffices. Thin-cut CT with 3 to 5 mm spacing is recommended through the tumor volume, whereas outside the immediate tumor volume region, 1 cm cuts are obtained from the top of the skull through the mid-neck.

After the tumor volume and normal soft tissue and bony anatomy (e.g., sinuses, skull, base of skull, brain) and critical structures (e.g., eyes, optic nerve, chiasm, brainstem, and spinal cord) are contoured on the CT axial images, beams are placed with a 1.5 to 2 cm margin. The contralateral eye is blocked, and greater than two thirds of the ipsilateral eye[41] are also blocked unless there is intraorbital infiltration by the tumor. Most of these cases would have had orbital exenteration during surgery, and the entire orbital defect is then included in the tumor volume (Fig. 33-15). Compared with a conventional plan, which routinely includes one half to one third of the ipsilateral eye,[22] greater sparing of the ipsilateral eye is

possible without sacrificing tumor control by using a 3D conformal plan (see Fig. 33-10).

In general, four fields, using an anterior and two lateral wedged portals plus an intraorbital electron portal, are used to treat the target volume (Fig. 33-16). Less commonly, three-field techniques (without the anterior electron portal) are used, and for small lesions confined to the ipsilateral maxillary sinus, a wedged pair of anterior and lateral portals is used (Fig. 33-17). With the four-field technique, the eyes are blocked from the anterior and lateral photon portals. The interorbital electron portal makes up the dose to the posterior nasal cavity, ethmoid sinus, and medial orbit. If the three-field technique is used, the anterior border of the lateral portal is placed at the bony canthus and the anterior portal is weighted more heavily (2:1 to 3:1).[22]

The tumor volume is defined as a CT- or MRI-defined gross tumor and by its potential microscopic extension, as well as by the pathologic findings. The target volume includes the tumor volume plus a 1 cm margin so that the tumor volume is included in the 95% isodose line. The computer generates autoblocks with an additional 5 mm margin around the target volume, thus defining the treatment volume. The autoblocks are then edited to ensure sparing of critical structures.

Most commonly, 6 MV photons are used; however, a higher-energy beam may be used in conjunction with low-energy electrons (9 or 12 MeV) in the anterior portals. Lower-energy photons result in a greater dose gradient and a less homogeneous distribution. A typical loading favors the anterior portal by 2:1. The generated isodose curves should reflect the effect of inhomogeneity corrections, although the dose is calculated at the central axis without inhomogeneity corrections (Figs. 33-18 and 33-19). In a postoperative setting, 60 to 63 Gy are prescribed to the target volume at a 1.8 to 2 Gy daily

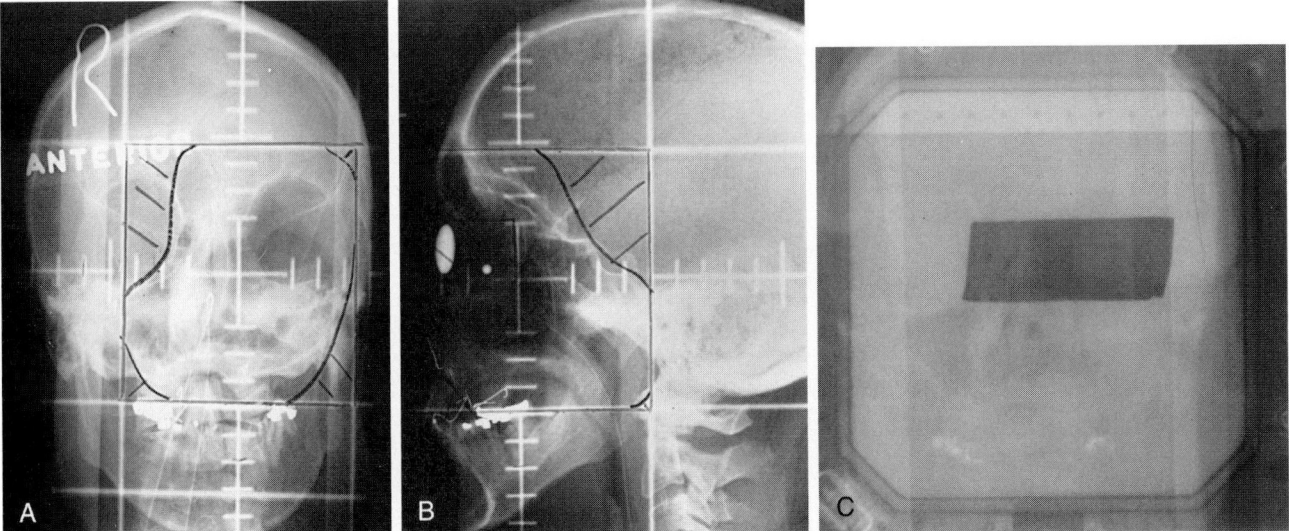

Figure 33–15. Simulation films of a patient undergoing postoperative radiation therapy for a locally advanced paranasal sinus tumor requiring left orbital exenteration. The treatment volume encompasses all the ipsilateral nasal cavity and sinuses including the frontal sinus and orbital bed, contralateral ethmoidal sinus and nasal cavity, and medial maxillary sinus. The patient was treated using a four-field technique that included left and right lateral photon portals, an anterior photon portal, and an electron portal to make up the dose to the left orbital bed, which was blocked from the lateral portals to protect the contralateral eye. **A,** Anterior photon portal including the entire orbital bed. **B,** Lateral photon portal blocking the eye (a dime is placed over the intact eyelid and a canthal marker is placed over the bony canthus). **C,** Anterior electron portal film.

fraction, and an additional cone-down boost may be delivered to the areas of involved margin or gross residual tumor. For unresectable tumors, doses in excess of 70 Gy are recommended. If the tumor involves critical structures or if they cannot be excluded from the high-dose volume by using tight margins, a hyperfractionated regimen (1 to 1.2 Gy twice-daily fractionation) or concurrent delivery of radiosensitizing chemotherapy should be considered. However, it is yet unknown whether optic nerves and chiasm can be differentially spared from the

late effects relative to acute effects on the tissue and tumor by the use of a hyperfractionation scheme.

The dose to the optic nerve and globe should be limited to 50 Gy, and that to the chiasm to 54 Gy. In most cases, the dose delivered to the chiasm can be limited to 70% of the daily prescribed dose. If the tumor extends to the chiasm and the chiasm is included as the primary tumor volume, the dose should be prescribed to 100% isodose line or the isodose line at the chiasm, and great care should be taken to block out the chiasm

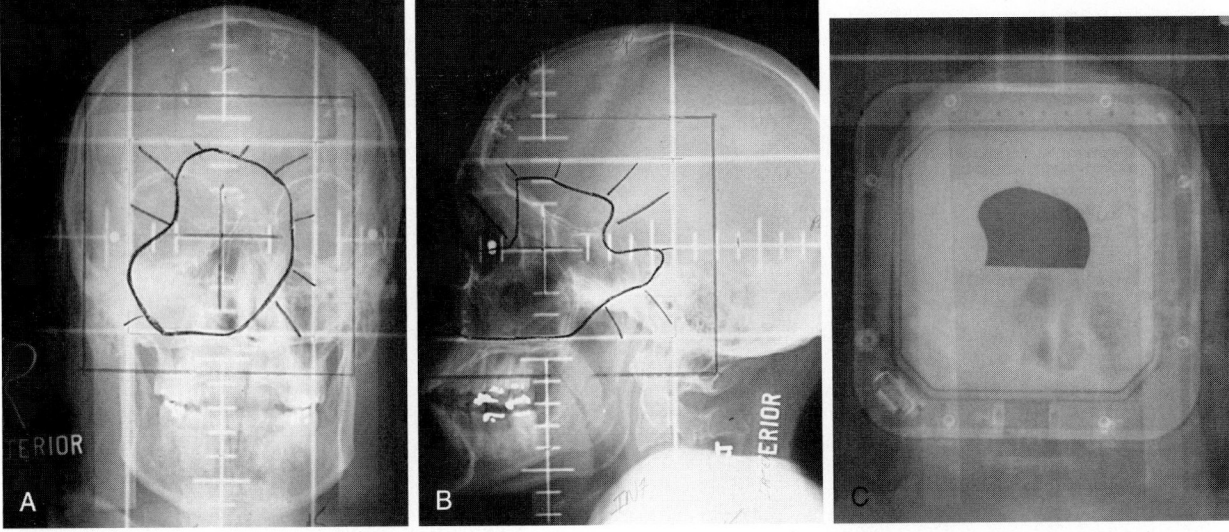

Figure 33–16. Simulation films of a patient undergoing postoperative radiation for undifferentiated carcinoma of the right ethmoidal sinus involving the periorbita and right superior nasal cavity, but not maxillary antrum. The eye was preserved, but the margins of resection were involved in the posterior medial orbital wall. The treatment volume was determined using a treatment-planning CT and includes the ethmoidal sinuses; medial one-half of the ipsilateral orbit, nasal cavity, and maxillary antrum; and medial rim of the contralateral orbit. A four-field technique was used to treat the patient: two lateral portals, an anterior photon portal, and an electron portal. The optic chiasm was blocked from the lateral portals. The eyes were blocked laterally, and the dose was made up using an electron field covering the superior extent of the nasal cavity, the ethmoidal sinus, and the orbits. **A,** Anterior photon portal. **B,** Lateral portals blocking the eyes (canthus markers are placed on the bony canthi). **C,** Anterior electron portal film.

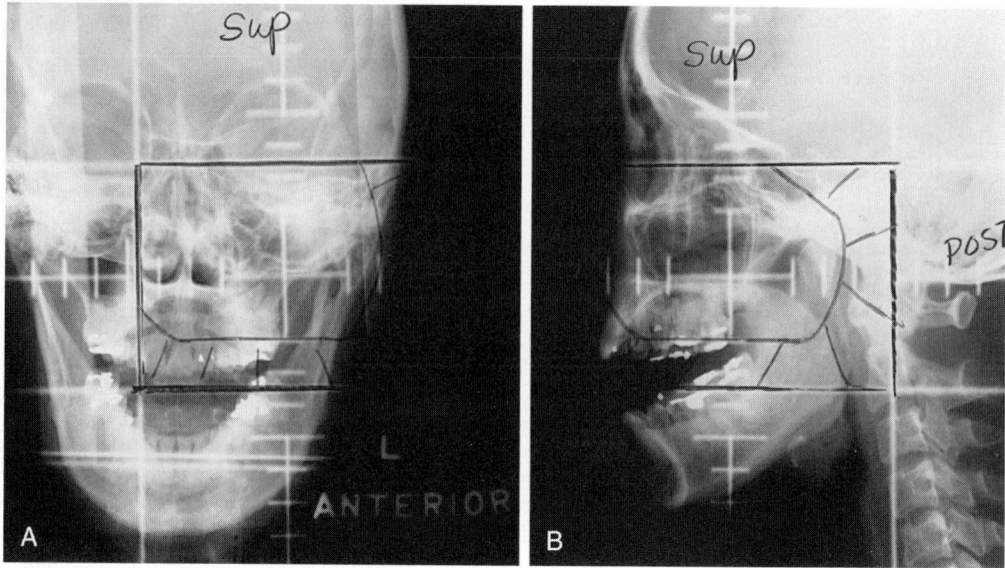

Figure 33–17. Simulation films of wedged-pair setup for a limited lesion involving the maxillary antrum only. The treatment volume includes the ipsilateral maxillary sinus and the nasal cavity. **A,** Anterior portal. **B,** Lateral portal.

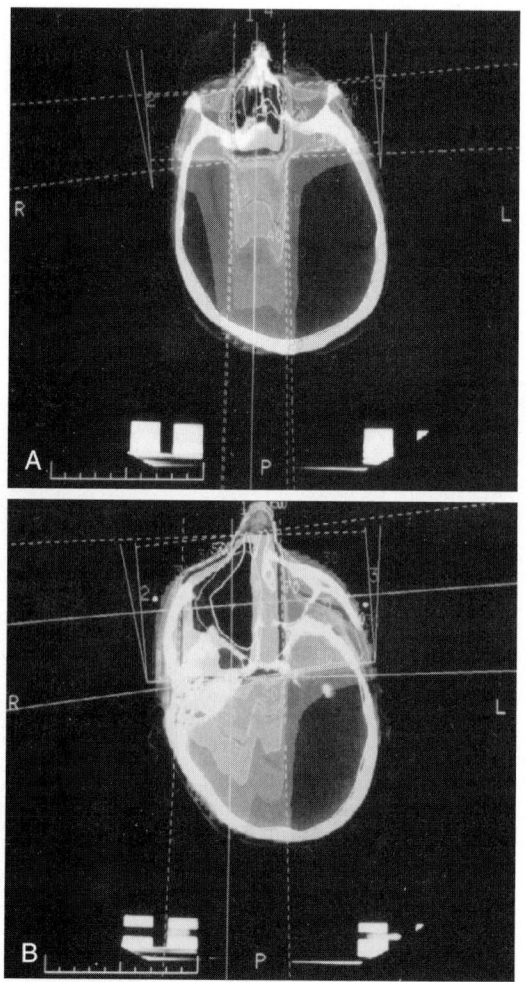

Figure 33–18. Three-dimensional isodose plans (color-wash representations shown here in shades of gray) of a four-field technique. Note the optic chiasm dose at the 60% to 70% region: **A,** At the level of the orbits and chiasm; **B,** at the level of the midantrum. See also Color Figure 33-18.

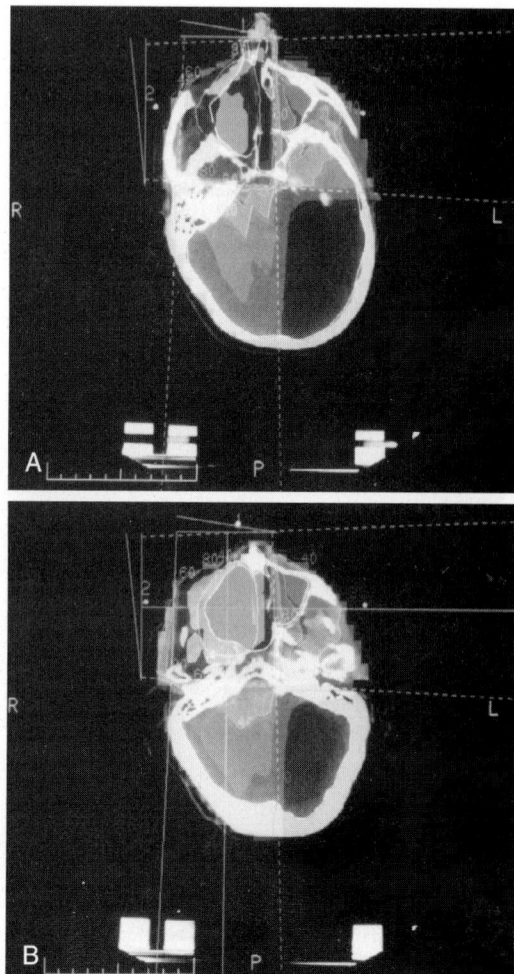

Figure 33–19. Three-dimensional isodose plans (color-wash representations shown here in shades of gray) of a wedged-pair technique: **A,** At the level of the midantrum; **B,** at the level of the lower antrum. See also Color Figure 33-19.

beyond 54 Gy. If there is extensive orbital invasion and the radiation is delivered primarily, the involved eye is encompassed in the anterior volume. All effort should be made to shield the lacrimal gland to avoid painful eye syndrome and to save the contralateral eye. Patients should gaze straight ahead with eyes wide open during treatment so that sparing of the anterior chamber may be attained.

Normal tissue complication probability (NTCP) calculations may be useful in assessing complication risk better than point dose tolerance criteria for the chiasm, optic nerve, and retina.[42] It is important to assess the overall risk of blindness for the patients in addition to the risk for the individual visual pathway structures. Patients should be informed of the risk of radiation-induced damage to the chiasm or eye, or both, and eventual blindness. Preradiation ophthalmologic examination is prudent in all patients undergoing sinus radiation therapy to establish baseline acuity and to detect any preexisting abnormalities.

Tumors arising in the sphenoidal sinus are treated like nasopharynx cancers, through opposed lateral portals using high-energy beams (e.g., 18 MV). A three-field technique may be necessary if there is significant anterior extension. For small lesions of the sphenoidal sinus, a conformal bilateral arc with flying wedges may spare the temporal lobes.

Any tumor at high risk of perineural spread requires generous coverage of the base of the skull.

STEREOTACTIC RADIOSURGERY

More recently there has been an interest in the use of stereotactic radiosurgery for the nasal cavity and paranasal sinus tumors with skull base involvement. Haberman et al.[43] reported their experience at the University of Graz, Austria, treating eight patients who underwent primary surgery and postoperative gamma knife radiosurgery. At 3 years, six patients were alive (all without local recurrence, four without evidence of disease) with no adverse effects. There is a potential for using this technique or a fractionated stereotactic radiotherapy technique as a boost for gross residual disease in addition to conventional image-based radiotherapy in select patients who have small residual tumor volume at the skull base. These new techniques should be investigated further in a prospective trial. Intensity-modulated radiosurgery/radiotherapy using a micro–multi-leaf collimator was compared against forward planning techniques using beam modification by enhanced dynamic wedge.[44] In this report, dose-volume histogram analysis demonstrated that a significant reduction in dose to neighboring critical structures could be achieved through intensity modulation patterns determined from inverse planning, while a marginal change was achieved in the target volume dose uniformity.

INTRACAVITARY BRACHYTHERAPY

The role of intracavitary implants is unclear in the management of nasal cavity and paranasal sinus tumors. External beam radiation therapy is certainly the standard and preferred mode of therapy. Epithelial malignancies in this region tend to be infiltrative and extensively involve adjacent sinuses; thus, generous margins around the tumor bed need to be irradiated for their microscopic extension. Due to the rapid dose falloff of any implant, intracavitary therapy would be limited to surface irradiation only. It may be used in conjunction with external beam therapy as a boost for maxillary antrum tumors. Because of the surface irregularities after radical maxillectomy, the intracavitary mold is custom designed like an obturator, in conjunction with prosthodontic service. The custom mold subsequently has holes drilled to contain catheters for low-dose-rate temporary iridium-192 or cesium-137 or high-dose-rate remote afterloading iridium-192 sources. This technique requires expertise in brachytherapy and mold implantation, and is not recommended for routine use.

Chemotherapy

Although numerous publications have reported a high percentage of good initial responses and some evidence of improved survival with cytotoxic chemotherapy, the efficacy of such therapy as a part of combined treatment for advanced sinonasal carcinoma has yet to be determined in a large clinical trial. The most commonly used regimen has been cisplatin-based.[45,46] Overall response rates ranging from 80% to 90% have been reported in previously untreated patients with paranasal sinus malignancies. Japanese groups reported on the use of intra-arterial 5-fluorouracil chemotherapy as a radiosensitizing agent in an effort to reduce the extent of required surgery.[47,48] Others employed sequential intra-arterial bleomycin and methotrexate followed by preoperative radiation therapy and subsequent radical surgery for advanced maxillary sinus carcinomas with good local control.[49] Lee and colleagues[50] reported an excellent immediate tumor response rate (>90%) using a highly selective intra-arterial infusion of cisplatin-based multiagent induction chemotherapy. More recently, combined radiation therapy and cisplatin-based chemotherapy for radiation sensitization were studied for the definitive management of unresectable base of skull carcinomas with encouraging early results.[30] There is, however, no established role for adjuvant chemotherapy in the management of sinonasal malignancies.

Treatment of Rare Epithelial Tumors

Primary melanomas mostly occur in the nasal cavity and are highly aggressive locally. The main mode of therapy for nasal cavity melanomas is radical surgical excision. Although there is no clear benefit in terms of improved survival for postoperative radiation therapy, postoperative radiation is recommended in most cases of mucosal melanomas. Local failure after surgery alone is much more common in mucosal melanomas compared with cutaneous melanomas because of mucosal melanomas' early lymphovascular invasion and destruction of adjacent structures. Radiation therapy should be delivered for local control in cases of close or involved surgical margins, large lesion size, or recurrence.

Table 33–5 Kadish Staging System for Olfactory Neuroblastoma

Stage A	Tumor confined to the nasal cavity
B	Tumor in nasal cavity that extends to paranasal sinus
C	Tumor that extends to the orbit, base of skull, or cranial cavity or with cervical/distant metastases

Olfactory neuroblastoma is an extremely rare entity arising in the nasal cavity olfactory epithelium. The commonly used Kadish staging system is based on the extent of invasion of adjacent structures (Table 33-5). Prognosis is determined on the basis of stage and resectability. The primary treatment is craniofacial resection. The role of postoperative radiation therapy is controversial. Although some attribute improved local control and survival to aggressive surgical resection via a craniofacial approach combined with radiation therapy,[17,18] others argue that patients treated with surgery alone have better results than with combined surgery and radiation therapy.[51] This may reflect adverse patient selection for the combined-modality therapy. Earlier-stage olfactory neuroblastoma patients enjoy excellent survival with surgery and postoperative radiation therapy: stage A, 96% and stage B, 83% at 5 years.[52] Stage C, however, has a much worse prognosis (53%) because of greater local as well as distant failure. The overall 5-year survival rate is about 50%. Distant metastases develop in 25% to 30% of patients.[53] Chemotherapy has been employed in these advanced cases with limited success.[54-56] A prospective study of 19 patients (4 stage B and 15 stage C) with malignant neuroendocrine tumors of the sinonasal tract conducted at the Massachusetts General Hospital between 1992 and 1998[57] reported an improved outcome for patients with olfactory neuroblastoma and neuroendocrine carcinoma treated with aggressive multimodality therapy. Patients received neoadjuvant cisplatin-etoposide chemotherapy for two cycles and high-dose proton-photon radiotherapy (69.2 cobalt-gray equivalents [CGE] in 1.6 to 1.8 CGE per fraction twice daily in a concomitant boost schedule) with radical surgery reserved for nonresponders. Responders received two more cycles of adjuvant chemotherapy. With the median follow-up of 45 months, 5-year survival and local control rates were 74% and 88%. No radiation-induced visual loss was observed due to the precision delivery of radiation with stereotactic setup and protons; however, four patients developed asymptomatic radiation-induced damage to the frontal or temporal lobe by MRI criteria and two patients showed soft tissue and bone necrosis. Despite sensitivity to platinum-based chemotherapy, patients with high-grade tumors tend to have a more aggressive course than those with lower-grade tumors.[58]

Treatment of Benign and Nonepithelial Tumors

Inverted papillomas are treated with en bloc resection of the medial maxilla with a recurrence rate of less than 10%. Piecemeal or simple excision is associated with an unacceptably high recurrence rate (>50%). Radiation therapy should be considered in patients with incompletely resected lesions, multiple recurrent tumors, and tumors associated with malignancy.

Lethal midline granuloma is a highly destructive process. In the process of ruling out Wegener's granulomatosis, most of the patients with lethal midline granuloma syndrome have failed a trial of systemic steroids. The primary treatment is radiotherapy. All nasal cavity and paranasal sinuses should be included in the treatment portals for the initial 40 Gy, as marginal recurrences have been observed. The final cone-down boost is delivered to the gross areas of destruction at a total dose of 45 to 50 Gy. The local failure rate even at this dose level approaches 30%.[59]

While sinonasal lymphomas are relatively rare in Western countries, in Asian populations they represent the second most frequent group of extranodal lymphomas after gastrointestinal lymphomas. The B-cell phenotype is typically located in the paranasal sinuses and has a slight predominance in Western countries, while the T/NK-cell phenotype is most common in Asian and South American countries and is typically located in the nasal cavity. The T/NK-cell lymphomas have an aggressive, angioinvasive growth pattern that often results in necrosis and bony erosion.[60] Patients with T-lineage disease appear to have a particularly poor outcome.[61] Sinonasal lymphomas tend to present as localized disease (stages I and II) but often relapse in the abdomen. Thus, staging should include endoscopic examination of the gastrointestinal tract. The role of surgery in the management of non-Hodgkin's lymphoma of the paranasal sinuses is limited to biopsy for pathologic diagnosis. Treatment of sinonasal lymphoma depends on the grade and stage of the tumor and follows the general guidelines for the treatment of malignant lymphomas. It may involve local radiation therapy, single-agent or combination anthracycline-based chemotherapy, or combined-modality therapy with chemotherapy followed by consolidated radiation therapy. Aggressive lymphomas involving the base of the skull may require systemic chemotherapy as well as central nervous system prophylaxis.

Nearly one half of head and neck extramedullary plasmacytomas are found in the nasal cavity and paranasal sinuses. These tend to be localized at presentation, although 25% of the cases may also involve cervical lymph nodes. Once multiple myeloma is ruled out, treatment involves local-regional radiation therapy in the dose range of 40 to 45 Gy over 4 to 5 weeks. The local control rate is excellent (>90%), but the ultimate prognosis depends on whether these patients eventually develop systemic myeloma.

Rhabdomyosarcoma is the most commonly found soft tissue sarcoma in the sinonasal tract. These primitive tumors have the morphology of developing striated muscle and constitute one of the "small blue round tumors" of childhood, or peripheral neuroectocrine tumors (PNETs). Eight percent of head and neck rhabdomyosarcomas arise in this region,[62] and they constitute one of the five parameningeal sites of rhabdomyosarcoma (orbit, infratemporal fossa, middle ear, and nasopharynx are the other sites). These are predominantly tumors of the pediatric population and are treated according to the guidelines of the Intergroup Rhabdomyosarcoma Study (IRS). Treatment involves a combined modality including chemotherapy, radiation therapy, and surgery. Unlike rhabdomyosarcomas at other sites, parameningeal rhabdomyosarcomas are less amenable to surgical extirpation; thus, treatment consists predominantly of chemotherapy and local radiotherapy. Hyperfractionated radiotherapy did not result in improvement in a randomized study by IRS-IV. Other soft tissue sarcomas are treated with wide local excision with pre- or postoperative radiation therapy.

Osteosarcoma and chondrosarcoma occur rarely in the nasal cavity and paranasal sinuses. Wide local excision is the primary mode of therapy, although chemotherapy may be used up front to cytoreduce and test in vivo chemosensitivity for osteosarcoma. Radiation therapy has reportedly been used in adjuvant or palliative settings.

COMPLICATIONS OF THERAPY

Katz and colleagues[67] reported a high rate of visual complications for radiation therapy in their series of tumors of the nasal cavity and ethmoid/sphenoid/frontal sinuses. Twenty-one of 78 patients (27%) developed unilateral blindness due to radiation retinopathy or optic neuropathy; however, most of these complications were anticipated because the ipsilateral eye was irradiated to a high dose. Four patients (5%) unexpectedly developed bilateral blindness due to optic nerve injury. All four of these patients received irradiation alone and were treated before 1985. The authors suggest that a combination of surgery and radiation therapy be given in an effort to reduce the total dose needed to achieve local control, and they also suggest improving dose homogeneity within the treatment volume to avoid overdosing the optic nerve.

Late retinal complications of radiation therapy for advanced nasal and paranasal malignancies were retrospectively studied by Takeda et al.[63] Between 1982 and 1996, 43 eyes of 25 patients were exposed to radiotherapy. None of the patients had tumor invasion into the eyes. The patients were followed ophthalmologically for a minimum of 2 years. Radiation retinopathy was observed in seven eyes, with a cumulative incidence of 25% and median interval before the onset of symptoms of 32 months (range 16 to 60). Neovascular glaucoma developed in three eyes, with the cumulative incidence of 7% and median period to the onset of symptoms of 22 months (range 16 to 26). Obstruction of the central retinal artery was observed in one eye. No patients who received less than 50 Gy developed retinal complications. The eyes exposed to greater than 50 Gy with more than 60% retinal area irradiated resulted in a 62% rate of severe retinal complications.

The series of 3D conformal therapy of paranasal sinus malignant tumors reported by Roa and associates[41] revealed more encouraging results with respect to preservation of critical structures. There was only one case of limited optic neuropathy and one case of possible radiation-induced cataract. There was no blindness related to irradiation. Another report of 3D conformal radiotherapy to median PTV doses of 60 Gy for 40 patients with locally advanced paranasal sinuses and nasal cavity tumors suggests an improved visual pathway complication rate. With a median follow-up of 19 months, two patients developed cataracts and one patient developed ipsilateral blindness due to vascular glaucoma.[64]

Neurocognitive effects of therapeutic irradiation for skull base tumors were reported by Meyers et al. from the University of Texas M.D. Anderson Cancer Center.[65] Nineteen patients who received paranasal sinus irradiation at least 20 months and up to 20 years before assessment were given a battery of neuropsychologic tests of cognitive function. Radiation was delivered by a three-field technique with the median dose of 60 Gy (range 50 to 68 Gy). Memory impairment was found in 80% of the patients. One third of the patients manifested difficulty with visual-motor speed, frontal lobe executive functions, and fine motor coordination. Two patients had frank brain necrosis with resultant dementia and blindness, and three had evidence of brain atrophy. Three patients experienced pituitary dysfunction. Neurocognitive symptoms were related to the total dose of radiation delivered, but not to the volume of brain irradiated. Improvement in dose distribution using image-based conformal technique or IMRT should decrease the incidence of these significant late brain injuries.

Other major complications of combined surgery and radiation therapy reported in the past include osteomyelitis or radionecrosis of bone at the base of the skull, or both; meningitis; hemorrhage; and aseptic brain necrosis.[66] With advancement in surgical techniques, antibiotic coverage, and radiotherapeutic techniques, these sometimes fatal complications are seen much less commonly.

RESULTS OF THERAPY

The literature of nasal cavity and paranasal sinus carcinomas is difficult to interpret because of their relatively infrequent incidence and because of the wide variability in surgical and radiotherapeutic techniques employed over the long span of time during which the reported cases were accumulated. Compounding the rarity of these tumors, there are a variety of histologic types of cancers that develop in this anatomic region, all with different biologic behavior. Most reports show overall local control rates from 40% to 60%. Wang[36] reported Massachusetts General Hospital's experience of nasal cavity squamous cell carcinomas from 1960 to 1985 (Table 33-6). Although

Table 33–6 Three-Year Disease-Free Survival after Radiation Therapy Alone or Combined Radiation Therapy and Surgery for Squamous Cell Carcinoma of the Nasal Cavity and Paranasal Sinuses: Massachusetts General Hospital Experience

Site	Survival, n (%)	
	RT Alone	RT and Surgery
Nasal cavity	10 (50)	9 (78)
Maxillary sinus	35 (38)	44 (55)
Ethmoidal sinus	12 (33)	22 (55)

RT, radiotherapy.

the numbers of patients were small, a combination of radiation and surgery appeared to produce better 3-year disease-free survival than radiation alone (78% vs. 50%). He reported similar results in favor of combined surgery and radiation for squamous cell carcinoma of the maxillary and ethmoid sinuses (55% vs. 38%, and 55% vs. 33%, respectively).[36]

Katz and associates[29,67] reported 78 cases of malignant tumors of the nasal cavity (48 patients) and ethmoid/sphenoid/frontal sinuses (30 patients) treated at the University of Florida between 1964 and 1998. These patients were managed with radiation therapy alone (47 patients) or in conjunction with surgery (27 patients). Four patients also received chemotherapy in addition to radiation with or without surgery. The more common histologies included 25 squamous cell carcinomas, 31 minor salivary gland tumors, 14 undifferentiated carcinomas, and 8 esthesioneuroblastomas. The 5-year local control rate for stage I (limited to the site of origin) was 86%; stage II (extension to adjacent sites), 65%; and stage III (destruction of skull base or pterygoid plates, or intracranial extension), 34%. The 5-year actuarial local control rate for patients receiving postoperative irradiation was 79% and for those receiving irradiation alone was 48% ($P = 0.05$). Of the 39 patients who received no elective neck treatment, 33 (85%) did not experience recurrence in the neck compared with 25 (89%) of 28 patients who received elective neck irradiation. They concluded that surgery and postoperative radiation therapy may result in improved local control, absolute survival, and complications when compared with radiation therapy alone. Elective neck irradiation is felt to be unnecessary for patients with early-stage disease.

Lee and Ogura[68] reported on 96 patients with maxillary sinus carcinoma treated at Washington University in St. Louis between 1969 and 1976. A combination of preoperative radiation and surgery produced 5-year overall survival rates of 60%, 45%, 28%, and 38% for T1, T2, T3, and T4 lesions, respectively. None of the 23 patients treated with radiation alone survived 5 years.

A retrospective analysis of 60 cases (46 maxillary antrum and 14 ethmoid sinus) of paranasal sinus cancer treated at Northwestern University between 1970 and 1985 was reported by Sisson and associates.[4] The most common histologic type was squamous cell carcinoma (53%) followed by adenoid cystic carcinoma (17%). The 5-year survival probability for antral and ethmoid cancer was 48% and 68%, respectively. Survival did not differ significantly whether radiation therapy was administered preoperatively or postoperatively (65% vs. 63%, respectively), although there were more advanced (T3 and T4) tumors in the preoperative radiotherapy group. Seven patients with small antral tumors were treated with surgery alone with an 86% 5-year survival rate.

A large retrospective review of 220 patients with nasal cavity and paranasal sinus carcinoma treated at the University of California, Los Angeles, between 1975 and 1994 was reported by Dulguerov et al.[69] With a minimum follow-up of 4 years, the 5-year actuarial survival rate was 63% and the local control rate was 57%. The factors associated with a worse prognosis included squamous or undifferentiated histologies; advancing T

classification; ethmoid location; treatment by radiotherapy alone; and tumor extension to pterygomaxillary fossa, frontal and sphenoid sinuses, cribriform plate, and dura. In multivariate analysis, histology, extension to the pterygomaxillary fossa, and dural invasion remained significant. The authors also performed a systematic review of published articles on patients with malignancies of the nasal and paranasal sinuses during the preceding 40 years and concluded that a progressive improvement in outcome had been made for patients with squamous cell and glandular carcinoma, maxillary and ethmoid sinus primary tumors, and most treatment modalities.

Myers et al[70] reported 5-year and 10-year actuarial disease-specific survival of 52% and 35%, respectively, for patients with paranasal sinus malignancies treated at the University of Texas Southwestern Medical Center between 1980 and 1997. Most patients presented with locally advanced disease (88%) and without nodal involvement (96%) or distant metastasis (96%). About half of the patients presented with squamous cell histology. Sixty-two percent of this study group underwent surgery as part of a multimodality curative treatment plan or alone as curative treatment. Thirteen percent had unresectable local disease and received nonsurgical palliative therapy.

The risk of lymph node metastasis and the controversy surrounding the elective nodal irradiation in patients with maxillary sinus carcinoma was addressed in a report by Le et al.[71] In this retrospective review of 97 patients treated at Stanford University and the University of California, San Francisco between 1959 and 1996, the overall incidence of lymph node involvement at diagnosis was 9%, with the most common sites of nodal involvement at levels 1 and 2. Of 36 patients who had neck irradiation, 25 received elective neck irradiation (ENI) for N0 necks. With the median follow-up of 22 months, the 5- and 10-year actuarial survival rates were 34% and 31%, respectively. Following treatment, the 5-year risk of nodal relapse was 12%. Squamous cell histology was associated with a high incidence of initial nodal involvement and subsequent nodal relapse. Elective nodal irradiation effectively prevented nodal relapse in patients with squamous cell histology. There was no nodal relapse in 13 patients who received ENI while 6 of 26 patients (20%) without ENI relapsed in the neck. Nodal relapse was associated with a high rate of distant metastasis and poorer survival. The authors advocate the use of ENI in patients with T3-T4 squamous cell carcinoma of the maxillary sinus. Results of this study are corroborated by a series reported by Paulino et al.[72] Of 42 patients with squamous cell carcinoma of the maxillary sinus in this series, 9.5% initially presented with cervical lymphadenopathy and 29% later developed recurrence in the neck after undergoing surgical resection of the primary tumor and postoperative irradiation to sinuses without ENI. Greater than a third of the neck recurrence (10.5% of total) represented isolated neck failure. The authors advocate ENI in all stages.

Table 33-7 summarizes several series of results of radiation therapy alone, surgery alone, or combined surgery and radiation for maxillary sinus carcinomas. Overall, it is reasonable to expect 70% to 80% primary-site tumor

Table 33–7   Primary Tumor Control According to T Stage and Treatment Modality for Maxillary Sinus Carcinoma

Reference	Study Period	Treatment Modality	Patients, *n*	Tumor Control, *n/n*			
				T1	T2	T3	T4
Lee & Ogura[68]	1969–1976	RT	35		2/3	0/6	5/35
		CMT	61	5/7	12/11	13/21	12/19
St. Pierre & Baker*†	1964–1975	RT	32	2/4	4/12	1/16	
		Surgery	10	1/1	0/2	0/4	0/3
		CMT	19		1/2	3/5	6/12
Ahmed et al*‡	1955–1974	RT	47		0/1	6/16	9/28
		CMT	9			4/4	2/5

*All squamous cell carcinomas.
†From St. Pierre S, Baker SR: Squamous cell carcinoma of the maxillary sinus: Analysis of 66 cases. *Head Neck Surg.* 1983;5:508.
‡From Ahmed K, Cordoba RB, Fayos JV: Squamous cell carcinoma of the maxillary sinus. *Arch Otolaryngol.* 1981;107:48.
CMT, combined-modality therapy; RT, radiotherapy.

control for early maxillary sinus carcinomas (T1 and T2) and 50% to 60% for more advanced tumors (T3 and T4) after surgery and radiation compared with 50% and 20% to 25%, respectively, after radiation therapy alone. Definitive irradiation of unresectable lesions can achieve 10% to 15% 5-year survival.[30]

The success of therapy for malignant minor salivary gland tumors of the paranasal sinuses and nasal cavity appears to depend on the combination of radiation therapy and surgery and the histologic grade of these tumors.[73] Sixty-six patients, 36 with adenoid cystic carcinoma and 30 with adenocarcinoma, were treated at the University of Texas M.D. Anderson Cancer Center between 1951 and 1980. Most patients were treated with surgery with or without radiation therapy. The local control rates with a minimum follow-up of 2 years were 47% for surgery alone and 76% for planned surgery and irradiation. Patients with high-grade adenoid cystic carcinomas fared significantly worse than those with the low-grade variety. Forty-seven percent of the low-grade patients remained disease free after 5 to 21 years, whereas only 12% of the high-grade group remained disease free between 2 and 3 years after treatment. Although the difference was not as pronounced as in adenoid cystic carcinomas, there was a trend toward better survival among patients with low-grade adenocarcinomas compared with the high-grade group.

In a small retrospective analysis, Naficy et al.[74] reported a 6-year survival rate of 50% for seven patients with adenoid cystic carcinoma of the paranasal sinuses treated by radiation alone, compared with 73% for 10 patients treated by combined surgery and radiation. Overall local control rate was poor at 24%.

Claus et al.[75] reported treatment outcome of 47 patients with adenocarcinoma of the ethmoid sinuses treated with surgery and high-dose postoperative radiation therapy between 1985 and 2001 at the Ghent University Hospital in Belgium. Sixty percent of the cases were locally advanced with T3 and T4 disease. With the median follow-up of 32 months, the 3-year and 5-year disease-free survival rates were 62% and 36%, respectively, and local-regional tumor control rates were 70% and 59%, respectively. Patients presenting with intracranial tumor invasion relapsed within 7 months after the

end of radiotherapy. Radiation-induced dry eye syndrome and optic neuropathy was observed in 7 and 2 patients, respectively, of the 47 cases.

The results of a 3D conformal series of predominantly advanced paranasal sinus malignancies from the University of Michigan compare favorably with older series using conventional planning systems.[41] Between 1986 to 1992, 15 patients were treated with primary radiotherapy to a median prescribed dose of 68.4 Gy for unresectable paranasal sinus malignancies. Postoperative radiation therapy was administered to 24 patients for close margins or microscopic or gross residual disease. The median prescribed doses were 55.8, 59.4, and 67.8 Gy, respectively. With the median follow-up of 4.5 years, the local control at 3 years and actuarial overall survival rate at 4 years for the definitive radiation group were both 32%. The local control rates at 3 and 5 years for the adjuvant group were 75% and 65%, respectively. The actuarial overall survival rates at 3 and 5 years were 65% and 60%, respectively.

Radiation therapy alone has yielded suboptimal results for advanced, resectable nasal cavity and paranasal sinus cancer. Promising results were reported by Harrison and colleagues[30] using concomitant chemotherapy and accelerated radiotherapy in 20 patients with malignant unresectable skull base tumors including 11 T4 paranasal sinus/cavity and 9 T4 nasopharynx cancers. Fifteen had squamous cell carcinoma and five had minor salivary gland histologic types. All patients received accelerated fractionated radiation using a concomitant boost technique to 70 Gy in 6 weeks. Radiotherapy was given once a day at 1.8 Gy per fraction during the first 4 weeks. During the last 2 weeks, the course was accelerated to twice daily with a 1.8 Gy fraction in the morning given to a larger field, and a 1.6 Gy fraction in the afternoon given to a smaller boost field. Cisplatin (100 mg/m²) was given concurrently on days 1 and 22 of radiation. Although the follow-up is relatively short (median follow-up, 11 months), local progression-free survival was 94% at 2 years, and distant metastases-free survival, 57%. The overall survival was 80%. An updated report of this study at minimum follow-up of 3 years demonstrated a continued excellent local control rate of 78% for paranasal sinus tumors.[76] Another report of a prospective trial of multimodality therapy in advanced paranasal sinus carcinoma from the University of Chicago suggests encouraging long-term outcome using neoadjuvant chemotherapy followed by surgery and postoperative concomitant chemoradiotherapy.[77] Fifteen patients with stage III or IV paranasal sinus carcinoma underwent three cycles of cisplatin and 5-fluorouracil (5-FU) induction chemotherapy followed by surgery and postoperative concomitant chemoradiotherapy with hydroxyurea and 5-FU in a week-on/week-off sequence, to a median tumor dose of 60 Gy. Five patients achieved pathologic complete response. The 10-year overall survival, disease-free survival, and local control rates were 56%, 73%, and 79%, respectively.

FUTURE DIRECTION

The presence of gross disease is a major adverse prognostic factor in radiotherapeutic management of nasal cavity and paranasal sinus malignancies. Every effort should be directed to achieve complete resection, leaving only a microscopic residual tumor for postoperative radiation therapy. In massive local tumors, concurrent radiosensitizing chemotherapy and image-based IMRT in conventional or altered fractionation schedules need to be further investigated in hopes of improving the therapeutic ratio. Stereotactic radiosurgery in combination with surgery may provide another therapeutic avenue for select patients with tumors of nasal cavity and paranasal sinuses infiltrating the skull base.

REFERENCES

1. Grant RN, Silverberg E: *Cancer Statistics 1970.* New York: American Cancer Society; 1970:8.
2. Lewis JS, Castro EB: Cancer of the nasal cavity and paranasal sinuses. *J Laryngol Otol.* 1972;86:255.
3. Tabb HG, Barranco SJ: Cancer of the maxillary sinus. *Laryngoscope.* 1971;81:818.
4. Sisson GA, Toriumi DM, Atiyah RA: Paranasal sinus malignancy: A comprehensive update. *Laryngoscope.* 1989;99:143.
5. Preston-Martin S, Henderson BE, Pike MC: Descriptive epidemiology of cancers of the upper respiratory tract in Los Angeles. *Cancer.* 1982;49:2201.
6. Hyams VJ, Batsakis JG, Michaels L: Tumors of the respiratory tract and ear. In Hartmann WH, ed. *Atlas of Tumor Pathology.* Series 2. Washington DC: Armed Forces Institute of Pathology; 1988:58.
7. Acheson ED, Cowdell RH, Hadfield E, et al: Nasal cancer in woodworkers in the furniture industry. *Br Med J.* 1968;2:587.
8. Acheson ED, Pippard EC, Winter PD: Mortality of English furniture makers. *Scand J Work Environ Health.* 1984;10:211.
9. Hernberg S, Westerholm P, Schultz-Larsen, et al: Nasal and sinonasal cancer. Connection with occupational exposures in Denmark, Finland, and Sweden. *Scand J Work Environ Health.* 1983;9:315.
10. Acheson ED, Cowdell RH, Jolles B: Nasal cancer in the Northamptonshire boot and shoe industry. *Br Med J.* 1970;1:385.
11. Enterline PE, March GM: Mortality among workers in a nickel refinery and alloy manufacturing plant in West Virginia. *J Natl Cancer Inst.* 1982;68:925.
12. Torjussen W, Solberg LA, Hgetweit AC: Histopathologic changes of nasal mucosa in nickel workers: A pilot study. *Cancer.* 1979;44:963.
13. Hyams VJ: Papillomas of the nasal cavity and paranasal sinuses. A clinicopathologic study of 315 cases. *Ann Otol Rhinol Laryngol.* 1971;80:192.

14. Myers EN, Fernau JL, Johnson JT, et al: Management of inverted papilloma. *Laryngoscope.* 1990;100:481.
15. Lawson W, LeBenger J, Som P, et al: Inverted papilloma: An analysis of 87 cases. *Laryngoscope.* 1989;99:1117.
16. Kadish S, Goodman M, Wang CC: Olfactory neuroblastoma: A clinical analysis of 17 cases. *Cancer.* 1976;37:1571.
17. Levine PA, McLeon WC, Cantrell RL: Olfactory esthesioneuroblastoma: The University of Virginia experience 1960-1985. *Laryngoscope.* 1990;100:1199.
18. Schwaab G, Micheau C, Pacheco L, et al: Olfactory esthesioneuroma: A report of 40 cases. *Laryngoscope.* 1988;98:872.
19. Batsakis JG, Regezi JA, Solomon AR, et al: The pathology of head and neck tumors: Mucosal melanomas, part 13. *Head Neck Surg.* 1982;4:404.
20. Trapp TK, Fu YS, Calcaterra TC: Melanoma of the nasal and paranasal sinus mucosa. *Arch Otolaryngol Head Neck Surg.* 1987;113:1086.
21. Levine PA, Frierson HF Jr, Stewart FM, et al: Sinonasal undifferentiated carcinoma: A distinctive and highly aggressive neoplasm. *Laryngoscope.* 1987;97:905.
22. Parsons JT, Stringer SP, Mancuso AA, Million RR: Nasal vestibule, nasal cavity, and paranasal sinuses. In Million RR, Cassisi NJ, eds: *Management of Head and Neck Cancer: A Multimodality Approach,* 2nd ed. Philadelphia: JB Lippincott; 1994:551.
23. Bridger MWM, van Norstrand AWP: The nose and paranasal sinuses: Applied surgical anatomy. *J Otolaryngol.* 1978;7 (suppl 6):1.
24. Anderson JE: The cranial nerves. In Anderson JE, ed. *Grant's Atlas of Anatomy,* 7th ed. Baltimore: Williams & Wilkins; 1978: Section 8-6.
25. Som PM, Shapiro MD, Biller HF, et al: Sinonasal tumors and inflammatory tissues: Differentiation with MR imaging. *Radiology.* 1988;167:803.
26. Daniels DL, Pech P, Pojunas KW, et al: Trigeminal nerve: Anatomical correlation with MR imaging. *Radiology.* 1986; 159:577.
27. Virapongse C, Mancuso A, Fitzsimmons J: Value of magnetic resonance imaging in assessing bone destruction in head and neck lesions. *Laryngoscope.* 1986;96:284.
28. Chapter 6: Nasal cavity and paranasal sinuses. In Greene FL, Page DL, Fleming ID, et al, eds: *AJCC Cancer Staging Manual,* 6th ed. New York: Springer; 2002.
29. Parsons JT, Mendenhall WM, Mancusco AA, et al: Malignant tumors of the nasal cavity and ethmoid and sphenoid sinuses. *Int J Radiat Oncol Biol Phys.* 1988;14:11.
30. Harrison LB, Pfister DG, Kraus D, et al: Management of unresectable malignant tumors at the skull base using concomitant chemotherapy and radiotherapy with accelerated fractionation. *Skull Base Surg.* 1994;4:127.
31. Cheesman AD, Lund VJ, Howard DJ: Craniofacial resection for tumors of the nasal cavity and paranasal sinuses. *Head Neck Surg.* 1986;8:429.
32. Imola MJ, Schramm VL Jr: Orbital preservation in surgical management of sinonasal malignancy. *Laryngoscope.* 2002;112:1357.
33. Carrau RL, Segas J, Nuss DW, et al: Squamous cell carcinoma of the sinonasal tract invading the orbit. *Laryngoscope.* 1999; 109:230.
34. Carrau RL, Myers EN, Johnson JT: Paranasal sinus carcinoma—Diagnosis, treatment and prognosis. *Oncology.* 1992;6:43.
35. Shidnia H, Horseback NB, Saghafi N, et al: The role of radiation therapy in treatment of malignant tumors of the paranasal sinuses. *Laryngoscope.* 1984;94:102.
36. Wang CC: Carcinoma of the paranasal sinuses. In Wang CC, ed: *Radiation Therapy for Head and Neck Neoplasms: Indications, Techniques, and Results,* 2nd ed. Littleton, Mass: Year Book Medical; 1990:294.
37. Griffin TW, Pajak TF, Laramore GE, et al: Neutron vs photon irradiation of inoperable salivary gland tumors: Results of an RTOG-MRC cooperative randomized study. *Int J Radiat Oncol Biol Phys.* 1988;15:1085.
38. Rasch C, Keus R, Pameijer FA, et al: The potential impact of CT-MRI matching on tumor volume delineation in advanced head and neck cancer. *Int J Radiat Oncol Biol Phys.* 1997;39:841.
39. Tsujii H, Kamada T, Arimoto T, et al: The role of radiotherapy in the management of maxillary sinus carcinoma. *Cancer.* 1986; 57:2261.

40. Claus F, Mijnheer B, Rasch C, et al: Report of a study of IMRT planning strategies for ethmoid sinus cancer. *Strahlenther Onkol.* 2002;178:572.

41. Roa WH, Hazuka MB, Sandler HM, et al: Results of primary and adjuvant CT-based three-dimensional radiotherapy for malignant tumors of the paranasal sinuses. *Int J Radiat Oncol Biol Phys.* 1994;28:857.

42. Martel MK, Sandler HM, Cornblath WT, et al: Dose-volume complication analysis for visual pathway structures of patients with advanced paranasal sinus tumors. *Int J Radiat Oncol Biol Phys.* 1997;38:273.

43. Habermann W, Zanarotti U, Groell R, et al: Combination of surgery and gamma knife radiosurgery—A therapeutic option for patients with tumors of nasal cavity or paranasal sinuses infiltrating the skull base. *Acta Otorhinolaryngol Ital.* 2002;22:74.

44. Leavitt DD, Watson G, Tobler M, et al: Intensity-modulated radiosurgery/radiotherapy using a micromultileaf collimator. *Med Dosim.* 2001;26:143.

45. LoRusso P, Tapazoglou E, Kish J, et al: Chemotherapy for paranasal sinus carcinoma. *Cancer.* 1988;62:1.

46. Vokes EE, Moran WJ, Mick R, et al: Neoadjuvant and adjuvant methotrexate, cisplatin, and fluorouracil in multimodal therapy of head and neck cancer. *J Clin Oncol.* 1989;7:838.

47. Sakai SM, Hohki A, Fuchihata H, Tanaka Y: Multidisciplinary treatment of maxillary sinus carcinoma. *Cancer.* 1983;52:1360.

48. Sato Y, Morita M, Takahashi HO, et al: Combined surgery, radiotherapy, and regional chemotherapy in carcinoma of the paranasal sinuses. *Cancer.* 1970;25:571.

49. Moseley HS, Thomas LR, Everts EC, et al: Advanced squamous cell carcinoma of the maxillary sinus. *Am J Surg.* 1981;141:522.

50. Lee YY, Dimery IW, Van Tassel P, et al: Superselective intra-arterial chemotherapy of advanced paranasal sinus tumors. *Arch Otolaryngol Head Neck Surg.* 1989;115:503.

51. Biller HF, Lawson W, Sachdev VP, et al: Esthesioneuroblastoma: Surgical treatment without radiation. *Laryngoscope.* 1990;100:1199.

52. Elkon D, Hightower SI, Lim ML, et al: Esthesioneuroblastoma. *Cancer.* 1979;44:1087.

53. Olsen KD, DeSanto LW: Olfactory neuroblastoma: Biologic and clinical behavior. *Arch Otolaryngol.* 1983;109:797.

54. Goldsweig HG, Sundaresan N: Chemotherapy of recurrent esthesioneuroblastoma. Case report and review of the literature. *Am J Clin Oncol.* 1990;13:139.

55. Spaulding CA, Krayak MS, Constable WC, et al: Esthesioneuroblastoma: A comparison of two treatment eras. *Int J Radiat Oncol Biol Phys.* 1988;15:581.

56. Wade PM Jr, Smith RE, Johns ME: Response of esthesioneuroblastoma to chemotherapy: Report of five cases and review of the literature. *Cancer.* 1984;53:1036.

57. Fitzek MM, Thronton AF, Varvares M, et al: Neuroendocrine tumors of the sinonasal tract. Results of a prospective study incorporating chemotherapy, surgery, and combined proton-photon radiotherapy. *Cancer.* 2002;15:2623.

58. McElroy EA Jr, Buckner JC, Lewis JE: Chemotherapy for advanced esthesioneuroblastoma: the Mayo Clinic experience. *Neurosurgery.* 1998;42:1023.

59. Smalley SR, Cupps RE, Anderson JA, et al: Polymorphic reticulosis limited to the upper digestive tract. Natural history and radiotherapeutic considerations. *Int J Radiat Oncol Biol Phys.* 1988;15:581.

60. Vidal RW, Devaney K, Ferlito A, et al: Sinonasal malignant lymphomas: A distinct clinopathological category. *Ann Otol Rhinol Laryngol.* 1999;108:411.

61. Hausdorff J, Davis E, Long G, et al: Non-Hodgkin's lymphomas of the paranasal sinuses: Clinical and pathological features, and response to combined-modality therapy. *Cancer J Sci Am.* 1997; 3:303.

62. Berry MP, Jenkin RDT: Parameningeal rhabdomyosarcoma in the young. *Cancer.* 1981;48:281.

63. Takeda A, Shigematsu N, Suzuki S, et al: Late retinal complications of radiation therapy for nasal and paranasal malignancies: Relationship between irradiated-dose area and severity. *Int J Radiat Oncol Biol Phys.* 1999;44:599.

64. Pommier P, Ginestet C, Sunyach M, et al: Conformal radiotherapy for paranasal sinus and nasal cavity tumors: Three-dimensional treatment planning and preliminary results in 40 patients. *Int J Radiat Oncol Biol Phys.* 2000;48:485.

65. Meyers CA, Geara F, Wong PF, et al: Neurocognitive effects of therapeutic irradiation for skull base tumors. *Int J Radiat Oncol Biol Phys.* 2000;46:51.

66. Giri SPG, Reddy EK, Gemer LS, et al: Management of advanced squamous cell carcinoma of the maxillary sinus. *Cancer.* 1992; 69:657.

67. Katz TS, Mendenhall WM, Morris CG, et al: Malignant tumors of the nasal cavity and paranasal sinuses. *Head and Neck.* 2002;24:821.

68. Lee F, Ogura JH: Maxillary sinus carcinoma. *Laryngoscope.* 1981; 91:133.

69. Dulguerov P, Jacobden MS, Allal AS, et al: Nasal and paranasal sinus carcinoma: are we making progress? A series of 220 patients and a systematic review. *Cancer.* 2001;92(12):3012.

70. Myers LL, Nussenbaum B, Bradford CR, et al: Paranasal sinus malignancies: An 18-year single institution experience. *Laryngoscope.* 2002;112:1964.

71. Le QT, Fu KK, Kaplan MJ, et al: Lymph node metastasis in maxillary sinus carcinoma. *Int J Radiat Oncol Biol Phys.* 2000;46:541.

72. Paulino AC, Fisher SG, Marks JE: Is prophylactic neck irradiation indicated in patients with squamous cell carcinoma of the maxillary sinus? *Int J Radiat Oncol Biol Phys.* 1997;39:283.

73. Goepfert H, Luna MA, Lindberg RD, et al: Malignant salivary gland tumors of the paranasal sinuses and nasal cavity. *Arch Otolaryngol.* 1983;109:662.

74. Naficy S, Disher MJ, Esclamdo RM: Adenoid cystic carcinoma of the paranasal sinuses. *Am J Rhinol.* 1999;14:311.

75. Claus F, Boterberg T, Ost P, et al: Postoperative radiotherapy for adenocarcinoma of the ethmoid sinuses: Treatment results for 47 patients. *Int J Radiat Oncol Biol Phys.* 2002;54:1089.

76. Harrison LB, Raben A, Pfister DG, et al: A prospective phase II trial of concomitant chemotherapy and radiotherapy with delayed accelerated fractionation in unresectable tumors of the head and neck. *Head Neck.* 1998;20:497.

77. Lee MM, Vokes EE, Rosen A, et al: Multimodality therapy in advanced paranasal sinus carcinoma: Superior long-term results. *Cancer J Sci Am.* 1999;5:219.

Cancer of the Thyroid

34

Patrick S. Swift, MD, Steven Larson, MD, and David C. Price, MD

The thyroid gland is unique among the solid organs of the body in its ability to concentrate and use a single element, iodine, in a manner predisposing readily to both diagnostic studies (uptake, scan) and radioisotopic therapy (hyperthyroidism, differentiated carcinoma). Table 34-1 summarizes the relevant radionuclide characteristics of the several isotopes of iodine used in the assessment and management of thyroid disease, as well as their radiation dosimetry.[1] The most common current tracers for the thyroid are ^{123}I for functional uptake and scan, ^{99m}Tc pertechnetate for higher resolution anatomic images of the gland, and ^{131}I for diagnostic thyroid cancer follow-up and therapy. Routine diagnostic studies are now rarely performed with ^{131}I because of the high radiation dose to the thyroid gland and less-than-favorable gamma energy (364 keV) for scintigraphic imaging (see Table 34-1). Because of its short half-life and lack of primary particulate emission, ^{123}I produces only 1% of the radiation exposure to the thyroid gland of an equivalent dose of [131]I. Therefore, it has become the tracer of choice for the majority of diagnostic thyroid studies, particularly when function is an issue (e.g., hyper- or hypothyroidism, "hot" or "cold" nodules). This chapter concentrates on the scintigraphic diagnosis and the radioisotopic and external beam radiotherapy approaches to the management of thyroid cancer.

EPIDEMIOLOGY AND GENETICS

Thyroid cancer is one of the most rapidly increasing cancers in incidence, especially in females. Estimates for new cancer cases in the United States in 2003 were 22,000 total cases, 16,300 female and 5,700 male (F:M ratio = 2.86), representing 1.61% of all new cancer cases[2], with a 5-year relative survival rate during 1992 to 1997 of 95% among white people and 94% among black people.[3] This represents a significant improvement in 5-year survival over the figures of 92% for whites and 88% for blacks in 1974 to 1976, and 83% for whites in 1960 to 1963.[3] Since there is still no effective chemotherapy for most thyroid cancer patients, the majority of this improvement in survival has come from changes in surgical management and the increased use of ^{131}I for therapy. Overall, the incidence of newly diagnosed thyroid cancer ranges from 36 to 60 cases per million population per year, with a mortality rate (1977) of 4 per million in males and 5 per million in females.[4] The incidence is lowest in children, including early teens, but begins to increase in later teens and steadily increases thereafter with each decade until it peaks in the fifth decade of life. In patients with differentiated carcinoma, survival is longer with papillary than with follicular carcinoma and is longer in patients diagnosed in their teens than in patients who develop the disease later in life. The highest recurrence rates occur in the very youngest children and the older adults. In a review of the data on 15,698 patients from the 1993-1997 SEER Program, Gililand et al.[5] noted that the 10-year average survival for patients with papillary carcinoma was 98% and 92% for follicular carcinomas. This represents a mortality rate for follicular carcinoma that is greater than twice that for papillary carcinoma. Medullary carcinoma patients had an 80% 10-year survival rate, while anaplastic cases had only a 13% survival rate.

No single genetic defect is associated with thyroid cancer, with the exception of the well-established chromosome

Table 34–1   Radioactive Isotopes for the Thyroid Gland

Isotope	Half-Life	Mode of Decay	Gamma Energy, keV	Beta Energy, keV	Radiation Exposure, cGy/mCi				
					Thyroid	*Whole Body*	*Red Bone Marrow*	*Ovaries*	*Testes*
[123]I	13.2 hr	EC	159	—	11.8	0.027	0.036	0.041	0.019
[125]I	60.14 d	EC	35	—	888	0.318	0.085	0.026	0.013
[131]I	8.04 d	Beta	364	694	1332	0.333	0.259	0.159	0.100
[99m]Tc	6.02 hr	IT	140	—	0.085	0.013	0.023	0.037	0.010
[201]Tl	3.04 d	EC	73–83*	—	0.925	0.201	0.666	0.444	2.072

*Given as x-rays, not gamma rays.

Beta, beta decay; EC, electron capture; IT, isometric transition.

10 abnormality of the MEN 2 syndromes: MEN 2A (Sipple's syndrome: medullary thyroid cancer, pheochromocytoma, and parathyroid tumors) and MEN 2B (medullary thyroid cancer and pheochromocytoma associated with mucosal neuromas of the tongue and lips and ganglioneuromas of the gastrointestinal tract). Both MEN 2A and MEN 2B are autosomal dominant syndromes. Germline mutations of the *RET* proto-oncogene exist in 95% of patients with hereditary medullary carcinoma of the thyroid.[6] Since the thyroid cell of origin for medullary thyroid cancer (MTC) is the C-cell, arising from the neural crest and responsible for the synthesis of calcitonin rather than thyroid hormones, there is no role for radioiodine in the diagnosis and therapy of MTC.

Some proto-oncogene associations have been recently identified as specific risk factors in the differentiated thyroid cancers, although they are not uniquely etiologic. Activation of the *ras* proto-oncogene family, *K-ras*, *H-ras*, and *N-ras*, has been found in up to 80% of follicular carcinomas and 20% to 60% of papillary and undifferentiated thyroid carcinomas.[7] Other proto-oncogenes such as *PTC* (an aberrant form of the *ret* oncogene), *c-myc*, *N-myc*, *TRK*, *PTEN*, and *c-erbB-2* also have been variously reported in differentiated thyroid carcinomas.[6] Associations between point mutations in the tumor suppressor gene *p53* and undifferentiated thyroid cancer have been identified by Fagin and coworkers.[8] Also, associations between the major histocompatibility complex gene *HLA* alleles *HLA-DR1* and *HLA-DR3* and different thyroid cancers have been described.[9] Familial association has been described in a small number of patients with papillary thyroid carcinoma, but not with follicular.[10] Thus, although some genetic associations are becoming more evident, the process of thyroid carcinogenesis is clearly multifactorial, genetic factors being only one piece of the puzzle.

RADIATION-INDUCED THYROID CANCER

Duffy and Fitzgerald[11] first described an association between childhood radiation exposure to the neck and increased incidence of thyroid carcinoma. Many subsequent publications have confirmed this risk. Maxon and associates[12] showed a linear dose-response relationship that extends up to 10 to 12 Gy, then decreases progressively at higher doses, presumably because higher exposures are more likely to kill the target cell than to cause mutation with continuing cell survival. The risk was expressed as an increase of 5.5 cancers per million persons exposed per cGy per year. Other studies have indicated comparable increases ranging from 1.3 to 8.3 cancers per 1 million people per cGy per year. Modan and associates[13] identified increased risk at thyroid exposures as low as 9 cGy, so there may, in fact, be no lower limit. The latent period from exposure to diagnosis averages around 20 years but can be as short as 10 years and as long as 40 or more years. The majority of the radiation-induced carcinomas are papillary (85%), the remainder being largely follicular with an occasional anaplastic carcinoma. Other head and neck tumors are also increased in incidence in the irradiated population,

as are other forms of thyroid disease (benign nodularity, thyroiditis).

Although most early reports of thyroid radiation carcinogenesis had involved individuals treated with external beam irradiation during childhood for such benign conditions as acne, thymic and tonsillar enlargement, tinea capitis, and so on, subsequent studies also have identified an increased risk of thyroid carcinogenesis following adult thyroid exposure to external radiation, the relative risk being approximately one third that of the risk seen with childhood exposure. On the other hand, none of the many human studies of patients exposed to diagnostic and therapeutic doses of ^{131}I have demonstrated increased risk of thyroid cancer associated with routine medical use of that radioactive isotope. Thyroid carcinogenesis associated with ^{131}I has been demonstrated in animals,[14] and questions remain as to the relative additive risk associated with ^{131}I and other radioactive isotopes of iodine in the increased incidence of thyroid cancer seen in the Hiroshima, Nagasaki, and Marshall Island populations, and most recently in the 1986 Chernobyl reactor accident. The report from the Ukrainian registry on the incidence of thyroid cancer in children of the region before and after the nuclear accident that released an estimated 150 to 200 million Curies of radioactive elements into the atmosphere (more than 450 types of radionuclides) sheds some light on the effect of age at the time of exposure.[15] The greatest increase, a 10-fold increase in incidence, was seen in children under 14 years of age at the time of exposure, whereas a three-fold increase was seen in children aged 15 to 18. Higher incidence rates were seen closer to the most heavily contaminated region. Ninety-three percent of the cases were papillary carcinomas, 3.7% follicular, 2.4% medullary, and 0.35% undifferentiated. The majority of the affected children had received estimated thyroid doses of less than 0.3 Gy (77%), 11% received between 0.3 and 1.0 Gy, and 11% received greater than 1.0 Gy. The incidence rate was noted to rise only 4 years after the event,[16] and is expected to reach a maximum at 15 to 20 years after the disaster.[16] A 20-year collaborative cohort study between Ukraine and the United States is ongoing.[15]

EMBRYOLOGY AND ANATOMY

The normal adult thyroid is a bilobed gland weighing 15 to 20 g. Each lobe measures approximately 4 × 2 × 2 cm. The lobes are usually joined near their lower poles by the thyroid isthmus, crossing the trachea anteriorly just below the cricoid cartilage. In some patients the isthmus is sufficiently substantial to be imageable or even palpable.

Embryologically, each thyroid lobe arises in two parts. The median anlage forms in the floor of the first pharyngeal pouch in the midline at the end of the third week of gestation, descends inferiorly over the next several weeks, and joins in that descent with the lateral anlage arising from the fourth pharyngeal pouch, thus forming the two thyroid lobes. In this descent along the line of the thyroglossal duct, deposits of residual thyroid tissue can be left anywhere from the base of the tongue posteriorly in the midline down the anterior surface of the trachea to the normal thyroid location. This original line of descent can also form a pyramidal lobe arising from the medial aspect of an upper pole, left more often than right. Occasionally in its descent, thyroid tissue may overshoot, extending into the anterior mediastinum. All of these embryologically relevant locations can become a site of primary (or secondary) thyroid neoplasms. Initial thyroid function, in the form of iodine uptake in the developing thyroid tissue, first occurs in the 11th or 12th week of gestation.

Histologically, the thyroid is composed of follicles or acini, each with a basement membrane lined with a single layer of follicular cells responsible for thyroid hormone synthesis. Each follicle has a central space containing thyroglobulin (Tg), the molecule upon which the thyroid hormones are synthesized and stored before release by thyroid-stimulating hormone (TSH) stimulation. A less frequent cell type in the follicular wall is the parafollicular cell, C-cell, or light cell, a cell that derives embryologically from the neural crest tissues in the lateral anlage and is responsible for the synthesis and release of calcitonin.

The thyroid is a highly vascular organ, with a blood flow estimated at 5 mL/g per minute under normal conditions. This may increase as much as 100 times in disease states such as Graves' disease. Each lobe is supplied by a superior thyroid artery to the upper pole and an inferior thyroid artery to the posterior aspect of the lower pole, with a fifth (thyroidea ima) artery sometimes supplying the thyroid in the midline inferiorly. Lymphatic drainage, important with regard to regional tumor spread, is primarily via tracheal lymphatics to a bilateral chain of nodes in the tracheo-esophageal groove. From this initial location, drainage may proceed to other cervical node chains (anterior, posterior triangles). Lymphatic drainage to the superior mediastinum is also common, particularly to nodes associated with the thymus. The Delphian nodes, anterior to the larynx and just above the isthmus, are a frequent site of early tumor metastasis as well. Finally, tumor spread via lymphatics laterally and inferiorly from the thyroid will sometimes reach the supraclavicular nodes. All of these sites of possible lymphatic drainage must be considered in planning external beam radiation therapy of thyroid cancer.

PHYSIOLOGY

The thyroid produces two thyroid hormones, triiodothyronine (T3) and tetraiodothyronine (thyroxine, T4), upon stimulation by TSH from the pituitary gland. These hormones are essential for general control of cellular metabolic activity in all cellular tissues throughout the body. The process of T3 and T4 synthesis involves uptake of iodide from the plasma iodide pool by a 618 amino acid intrinsic membrane glycoprotein, the sodium iodide symporter (NIS).[17] NIS protein is also expressed in other tissues, and so radioiodine used for diagnosis and treatment will also be taken up into these tissues as well, although to a lesser extent than into thyroid. Tissues expressing NIS include salivary glands, gastric mucosa, and lactating

(but **not** nonlactating) mammary gland, as well as about 75% of thyroid cancers. NIS is capable of transporting other anions as well (I–, ClO3–, SCN–, SeCN–, NO3–, Br–, BF4–, IO4–, BrO3–, but perchlorate [ClO4–] is not transported). The mechanism involves cotransport of Na+/I–, in a ratio of 2:1. The interested reader is referred to a recent review of NIS.[18] Once iodine has been transported into the thyroid, there is oxidation of iodide by thyroid peroxidase; iodination of tyrosine bound to Tg with one or two iodine atoms to form monoiodotyrosine (MIT) and diiodotyrosine (DIT); coupling of MIT and DIT to form T3 and T4, also while stored on Tg; and finally, release of T3 and T4 from the thyroid under the control of TSH. All of these normal thyroid metabolic processes also take place in most differentiated thyroid cancers, including responsiveness to TSH, but at a much lower level than in normal thyroid tissue. This fact is the basis for all use of radioiodine in the diagnosis and therapy of differentiated thyroid carcinomas, including the need to do so under maximal TSH stimulation (see later discussion).

PATHOLOGY

As classified by the World Health Organization (WHO),[19] the four broad categories of primary thyroid malignancies include the two differentiated forms, follicular and papillary carcinoma, which arise from the follicular cells; MTC, which arises from the parafollicular or C-cells and which produces and secretes calcitonin rather than T3 and T4; and anaplastic thyroid carcinoma, which is characterized by a lack of differentiated thyroid functional capability. Since the latter two carcinomas do not pick up iodine, there is no role for radioiodine in their diagnosis and therapy. Radioiodine also has no place in the management of the other infrequent malignancies of the thyroid, such as malignant lymphomas and tumor metastases from extrathyroidal primary tumors.

Morphologic characterization that a carcinoma is papillary or follicular is important because these two tumors tend to demonstrate different patterns of metastatic spread, papillary tending to metastasize locally via lymphatics, and follicular more frequently metastasizing hematogenously to lung and bone. In a review of 7845 patients in 13 published series from the literature, Mazzaferri[20] noted that at presentation, nodal metastases were present in 36% of patients with papillary carcinoma and in 17% of those with follicular carcinoma, while distant metastases were present in only 5% of those with papillary but 13% of those with follicular carcinoma. Distant metastases occurred twice as often in the lungs as in the skeleton. These basic differences in tumor spread influence both prognosis and management, with the exception of the appropriateness of radioiodine therapy (which is a function-specific characteristic, not site-specific).

Several variants of papillary carcinoma have been described in addition to the dominant papillary pattern. These include papillary microcarcinoma (<1 cm in diameter); the follicular variant of papillary carcinoma (formerly referred to as mixed papillary-follicular); and the diffuse sclerosing, tall-cell, columnar-cell, and solid variants. The follicular variant of papillary carcinoma should not be confused with follicular carcinoma, as it demonstrates the biologic and prognostic characteristics of papillary rather than follicular. Classification of papillary carcinomas into these variants can be used to better anticipate patient prognosis, as some variants are associated with a good prognosis (papillary microcarcinoma, and the encapsulated, solid, and follicular variants) while the others are associated with a poor prognosis (tall-cell, columnar-cell, and diffuse sclerosing variants).[21] Follicular carcinomas include Hürthle cells to varying degrees, usually a relatively small proportion of the total cellularity. In a few cases there is such an extensive Hürthle cell dominance as to lead to characterization as a Hürthle cell carcinoma, a tumor that is much more aggressive than other follicular cell carcinomas and less likely to concentrate radioiodine well enough to make radioiodine therapy a practical consideration.

Anaplastic carcinoma of the thyroid, although rare, is an extremely aggressive variety of thyroid cancer. It must be carefully distinguished from poorly differentiated medullary carcinoma, lymphoma, and poorly differentiated follicular carcinoma, as each of these has a better prognosis and a different therapeutic approach.[22] The typical presentation of these tumors is a ferociously expanding thyroid mass that quickly extends beyond the capsule of the gland. It has several variants, including spindle cell, squamoid, and giant cell patterns,[23] and has a tendency to occur in elderly female patients.

Numerous studies have identified the prevalence of occult thyroid carcinoma (i.e., papillary microcarcinoma) in routine postmortem examinations in North America to range from a low of 0.49%[24] to a high of 13%,[25] averaging 2.2% in 11 publications in the literature. Comparable studies of thyroid cancer prevalence reported from other countries indicate values ranging as high as 24.2% for Japanese in Hawaii,[26] 28.4% for Japanese in Sendai,[26] and 35.6% in Finland.[27] This observation of the high incidence of (occult) papillary microcarcinoma with little apparent effect on patient survival correlates well with the published experience that small papillary carcinomas less than 1 cm in size have a very low rate of recurrence and thus no impact on mean patient survival no matter what the method of treatment.[28,29] Clearly, a large number of individuals harbor undiscovered (or incidentally discovered) papillary carcinoma, which is quite benign in nature, unlikely to benefit from specific patient management, and not affecting patient survival.

CLINICAL PRESENTATION

Thyroid Nodule

Many thyroid carcinomas present as a palpable nodule first discovered incidentally on routine physical examination. The issue of assessing and managing thyroid nodules is complex and warrants specific discussion.[30,31] Thyroid nodules are a common physical finding. In the Framingham study,[32] solitary palpable thyroid nodules were found in 3% of the population and multiple nodules in an additional 1%. The estimated lifetime risk in that study for development of a palpable thyroid nodule was

estimated to be between 5% and 10%.[33] Their prevalence increases with age. On the other hand, detailed pathologic examination of thyroids at postmortem has demonstrated the prevalence of nodularity to be as high as 50%, one quarter of these being solitary and three quarters multiple.[34] Similarly, high-resolution ultrasonography (7.5 to 10 MHz) has also demonstrated a normal prevalence of multinodularity in the thyroid glands of older patients on the order of 40% to 50%. With abnormal findings this frequent, yet an annual incidence rate of thyroid cancer in the United States that is only 40 per million population per year with a mortality rate one tenth of this,[20] it is a challenge to determine just how aggressively to pursue incidentally discovered thyroid nodules. It is equally difficult to be certain just how aggressive to be in the management of newly diagnosed papillary thyroid carcinoma localized to the thyroid. Nevertheless, there is general agreement that the pathologic diagnosis of thyroid carcinoma requires at minimum surgical removal, customarily total thyroidectomy, and increasing levels of additional management according to various risk factors such as the stage at diagnosis and the progression following initial treatment.

There has been much interest in the past several decades in the assessment of thyroid nodules by radionuclide scintigraphy, mainly because of the unique capability of the thyroid to concentrate iodine and the fact that scintigraphy evolved many years before other imaging modalities such as ultrasonography. In a review of the literature before 1981 (39 publications; including 8177 patients, of whom 5856 went to surgery), Ashcraft and van Herle[35] noted that the probability of cancer in a nodule that is cold with radioiodine was 17%, whereas a warm nodule carried a probability of 9%, and a hot nodule 3%. Note that for hot nodules the probability is the same as that for occult carcinoma in routine postmortem examinations. ^{99m}Tc pertechnetate scintigraphy had a comparable probability of cancer in cold nodules (22%) and warm nodules (13%), but the probability of cancer in a hot nodule was 29%. Others have also noted the higher likelihood of cancer in discrepant nodules that are cold with radioiodine but hot with pertechnetate. Other reported figures for the likelihood of cancer in a solitary nodule that is cold with radioiodine vary widely, from 5%[36] to 29%.[37] On the other hand, the likelihood of cancer in a nodule within a multinodular gland is comparable to the background prevalence of occult thyroid carcinoma, on the order of 1% to 5%. In a patient with a prior history of head-and-neck radiation as a child, however, the likelihood of cancer in a palpable nodule ranges from 20% to 40%, whether the nodule is solitary or multiple. The previous routine use of scintigraphy in evaluating thyroid nodules was based on this ability to characterize thyroid nodules as cold, warm, or hot, and single or multiple, with the corresponding probabilities that they could be thyroid cancer. However, the availability of fine-needle aspiration biopsy (see later discussion) has made scintigraphy largely superfluous and certainly not cost effective, except in the identification of hot thyroid nodules. Similarly, although ultrasonography can identify nodules as small as 1 mm in diameter and can characterize cystic properties of a nodule, such information again does not generally lead to more cost-effective management of the patient.

Fine-needle aspiration biopsy (FNAB) is a relatively accurate and simple, low-risk first step toward pathologic characterization of a thyroid nodule. It is not, however, a true "gold standard," although it is frequently considered as such. Caruso and Mazzaferri,[38] in reviewing 2794 patient FNABs with surgical follow-up, noted that 74% were benign, 4% malignant, 11% indeterminate in morphology, and an additional 11% insufficient for a diagnosis. The sensitivity for malignancy was 91% with a specificity of 57%, a positive predictive value of 47%, and a negative predictive value of 93%. In reviewing 28 published reports of FNAB in the literature before 1981 (11,768 patients, of whom 3736 went to surgery), Ashcraft and van Herle[35] found false-negative and false-positive rates of only 1.6% and 0.9%, respectively. No comment was made on the categories of histologically indeterminate studies, nor on inadequate FNAB samples. Thus, a positive FNAB study is an absolute indication for proceeding to surgery, while a negative FNAB still requires careful consideration of all other relevant contributing factors (age, sex, multinodularity, radiation history, etc.) before a decision about when and whether to repeat the biopsy, or whether to advance to excisional biopsy and lobectomy, can be made. An FNAB diagnosis of *follicular neoplasm* is in a special management category in that the small amount of tissue in a needle biopsy is unlikely to be adequate to properly identify whether the neoplasm has true malignant characteristics, such as vascular invasion. Open biopsy or lobectomy should be considered in such cases.

New efforts to identify RNA fragments or specific tumor- or thyroid-related proteins in FNA material from thyroid nodules or lymph nodes, and potentially peripheral blood, are being examined. The use of reverse transcriptase-polymerase chain reaction analysis (RT-PCR) to identify tumor-specific genes or proteins, such as RET/PTC rearrangements, in FNAs from thyroid nodules or thyroid-specific proteins, such as Tg or thyrotrophin receptors, in FNAs of lymph nodes are showing promise.[39]

Initial Clinical Presentation of Thyroid Cancer

Although frequently found incidentally on routine physical examination, thyroid cancer may present with symptoms and signs of local infiltrative disease, or even distant metastases in lung or skeleton (more frequent with follicular carcinoma). Brain metastases are rare, particularly at diagnosis, but occur in a few percent of patients with advanced disease, as do metastases to the liver or other organs. Locally invasive tumor may be noted by the patient simply as a lump in the neck, but may also involve the recurrent laryngeal nerves with secondary hoarseness, or even directly infiltrate the larynx, pharynx, or esophagus with corresponding symptoms, including hemoptysis. The nodule may be small, rubbery, and mobile on palpation, but more advanced carcinomas may present as a fixed, hard or irregular, nontender thyroid mass, and regional spread may be detectable in the form of an enlarged Delphian node (midline and above the isthmus), or as one or more palpably enlarged cervical or supraclavicular nodes. It is of interest that unilateral cervical lymph node metastases at diagnosis do not adversely affect overall patient survival, as compared with patients with bilateral cervical nodes or with positive mediastinal nodes at diagnosis, in whom the prognosis is progressively worse.[29] In 30% of patients with medullary carcinoma, a prominent symptom will be diarrhea, possibly resulting from the synthesis and release of calcitonin, serotonin, or prostaglandins and generally a sign of more advanced disease with a poor prognosis.

ROUTES OF SPREAD

As previously mentioned, tumor spread can be local, regional, or distant. Local spread is most common with anaplastic, medullary, and papillary carcinoma and is initially intrathyroidal, then through the capsule and into adjacent structures such as paratracheal muscles, trachea, larynx, and esophagus with corresponding symptoms and physical findings. Regional lymphatic spread is commonly to the Delphian node and to nearby unilateral or bilateral cervical nodes, then to the supraclavicular nodes. A parallel or independent path of lymphatic spread is frequently to anterior mediastinal nodes, carrying a poorer prognosis. Hematogenous spread is seen most frequently with follicular carcinoma,[20] most commonly to lung and bone and less frequently to brain, liver, and other organs. More than 45% of anaplastic thyroid cancers will have distant metastases at the time of presentation (lung, bone most common).[22]

DIAGNOSTIC STUDIES

Recommendations regarding optimal approaches to the diagnosis, treatment selection, and the monitoring of treatment response in thyroid cancer are undergoing rapid evolution, due to the availability of recombinant Thyroid Stimulating Hormone (rTSH, thyrogen), sensitive measurements of Tg, and positron emission tomography (PET). The workup of individual patients is determined based on their risk for distant metastases, ability to concentrate radioactive iodine, and in the postablation patient, the presence of Tg in serum.

INITIAL DIAGNOSIS AND TREATMENT OF THE PRIMARY TUMOR. The most important techniques for the diagnosis of thyroid carcinoma are a good physical examination (a small, soft, mobile nodule versus a larger, hard, irregular, fixed nodule with or without palpable evidence of local tissue infiltration, and the presence or absence of enlarged cervical lymph nodes) and a good FNAB. Neither of these modalities is 100% sensitive nor specific, however. As discussed earlier, radionuclide scanning used to play a significant role in the initial work-up of the patient with a thyroid nodule (cold vs. warm or hot nodule), but most clinicians would agree that scintigraphy no longer has a significant role in assessing a newly diagnosed nodule unless hyperthyroidism is also present (hot nodule).[31]

Similarly, ultrasonography, magnetic resonance imaging (MRI), and computed tomography (CT) have been shown to be unreliable in differentiating between benign and malignant nodules. Although each of the latter modalities can be advantageous in detecting bilaterality, local infiltration, and regional nodal involvement, current surgical management generally includes total thyroidectomy and detailed intraoperative assessment for infiltrative and regional nodal involvement, making expensive presurgical imaging redundant.

POSTSURGICAL FOLLOW-UP OF THYROID CANCER. Once the diagnosis of thyroid cancer has been established and treated by total or near-total thyroidectomy, the follow-up and monitoring will be individually tailored to the patient's risk for progression, metastases, and death based on the surgical findings and pathology. All patients with differentiated tumors of papillary, follicular, and Hürthle cell should have an initial ^{131}I diagnostic study performed 2 to 6 months after surgery, and any residual normal thyroid tissue should be ablated. The rationale for this procedure is twofold. If all normal thyroid tissue is removed from the body, then the serum Tg becomes a sensitive and specific tumor marker for recurrence. The second reason for ablation treatment comes from the studies of Mazzaferri, who noted a major benefit from ^{131}I ablation of patients with well-differentiated thyroid cancer.[40] These studies show a clear reduction in risk of recurrence, local and regional metastases, and death. This strategy should be applied in all patients except those at the lowest risk.

A large proportion of the differentiated carcinomas, reportedly 50% to 80% in several published studies, pick up radioactive iodine because of their low-level differentiated function. This iodine uptake is stimulated significantly by TSH. It is essential that all cancer diagnostic scans and therapies be performed at maximal TSH stimulation and maximal dietary iodine depletion. The serum TSH level should be at least above 35 mIU/L (normal: 0.5 to 5.5 mIU/L) and preferably above 50 mIU/L. Dietary iodine content should be restricted to a maximum of 50 µg/day for at least 2 weeks before the study. Such a diet can be obtained from the hospital dietary department or from the literature.[41] The patient must be carefully questioned regarding any recent source of excessive iodine, such as a CT scan with contrast, an intravenous pyelogram or angiographic study; medications such as cold remedies (expectorants), which may be iodine loaded; and so on. Nonionic radiographic contrast media generally require 2 months to clear the system in a patient with normal renal function.

Diagnostic testing for the presence of thyroid cancer that is treatable with ^{131}I may be performed with thyroid withdrawal or using Thyrogen. Recent studies suggest that accuracy for thyroid cancer detection is equivalent.[42]

A standard thyroid withdrawal protocol for thyroid carcinoma ^{131}I scanning is as follows:

1. Six weeks prior to scan, the patient is taken off T4 (Synthroid) and started on T3 (Cytomel) 25 µg twice a day or three times a day. The patient should be questioned in detail about any recent excessive iodine

load (see earlier), and the scan deferred if the patient is believed to be iodine-loaded. Performance of a serum iodine level may help clarify the issue.
2. Two weeks prior to scan, the T3 is discontinued and the patient is started on the stringent low-iodine diet.
3. Four to 5 days prior to scan, blood is drawn for serum TSH and Tg levels.
4. The first day of the study, a pregnancy test is performed if the patient is potentially childbearing, and then 2 to 3 mCi ^{131}I is administered orally. Higher diagnostic doses than this (e.g., 5 to 10 mCi) have been demonstrated to have a partial therapeutic effect on iodine-avid tissue. Thus, if high-dose ^{131}I therapy is needed after the scan, the tumor sites could already be "stunned" from a large (5 to 10 mCi) diagnostic dose, resulting in compromised therapeutic efficacy.
5. At 24 hours, the percentage ^{131}I uptake in the neck is measured with a properly shielded and calibrated thyroid probe, and a single anterior image of the neck is obtained using a scintillation camera with a medium (^{131}I) energy parallel hole collimator.
6. At 72 hours, the neck uptake measurement is repeated, and following intravenous injection of 1 mCi ^{99m}Tc pertechnetate, a repeat anterior neck spot view is obtained as well as complete anterior and posterior whole body scans at both isotope energies. The corresponding ^{99m}Tc images are helpful in identifying the normal structures that pick up iodine and pertechnetate, such as salivary glands, stomach, bowel, and bladder (Fig. 34-1).
7. Additional spot scintiphotos of questionable or suspicious areas can be obtained based on the whole body scan findings.
8. The scan is interpreted in the context of the known TSH level, and a decision is made about the appropriateness and dose of ^{131}I therapy, as discussed further.

For differentiated carcinomas, a properly executed ^{131}I scan is the determinant for consideration of radioisotope therapy. With the rare exception of differentiated tumor patients with a rising serum Tg level and a negative scan, in whom a trial of therapy is a reasonable consideration, no high-dose ^{131}I therapy is given without positive uptake on radioiodine scanning. Such therapy is appropriate even in the absence of any other confirmatory diagnostic imaging test, since residual or recurrent tumor in the thyroid bed or regional nodes may be too small in tumor mass to be detectable by MRI, CT, or ultrasonography. Similarly, diffuse pulmonary micrometastases and small skeletal metastases may also be too small to be detected by other techniques. Demonstration of an elevated serum Tg, particularly with maximum TSH stimulation, is further support for undertaking high-dose ^{131}I therapy in a patient with a positive scan.

Our Thyrogen-stimulated protocol does not require the patient to stop thyroid hormone. Instead, the patient is placed on a low iodine diet, as in step 3, and then receives two daily doses of 0.9 mg Thyrogen intramuscularly, followed by ^{131}I administration at 24 hours after the second dose. Steps 3 through 8 are usually completed as described earlier, and in addition, Tg levels are always obtained at 72 hours after the second dose of Thyrogen.

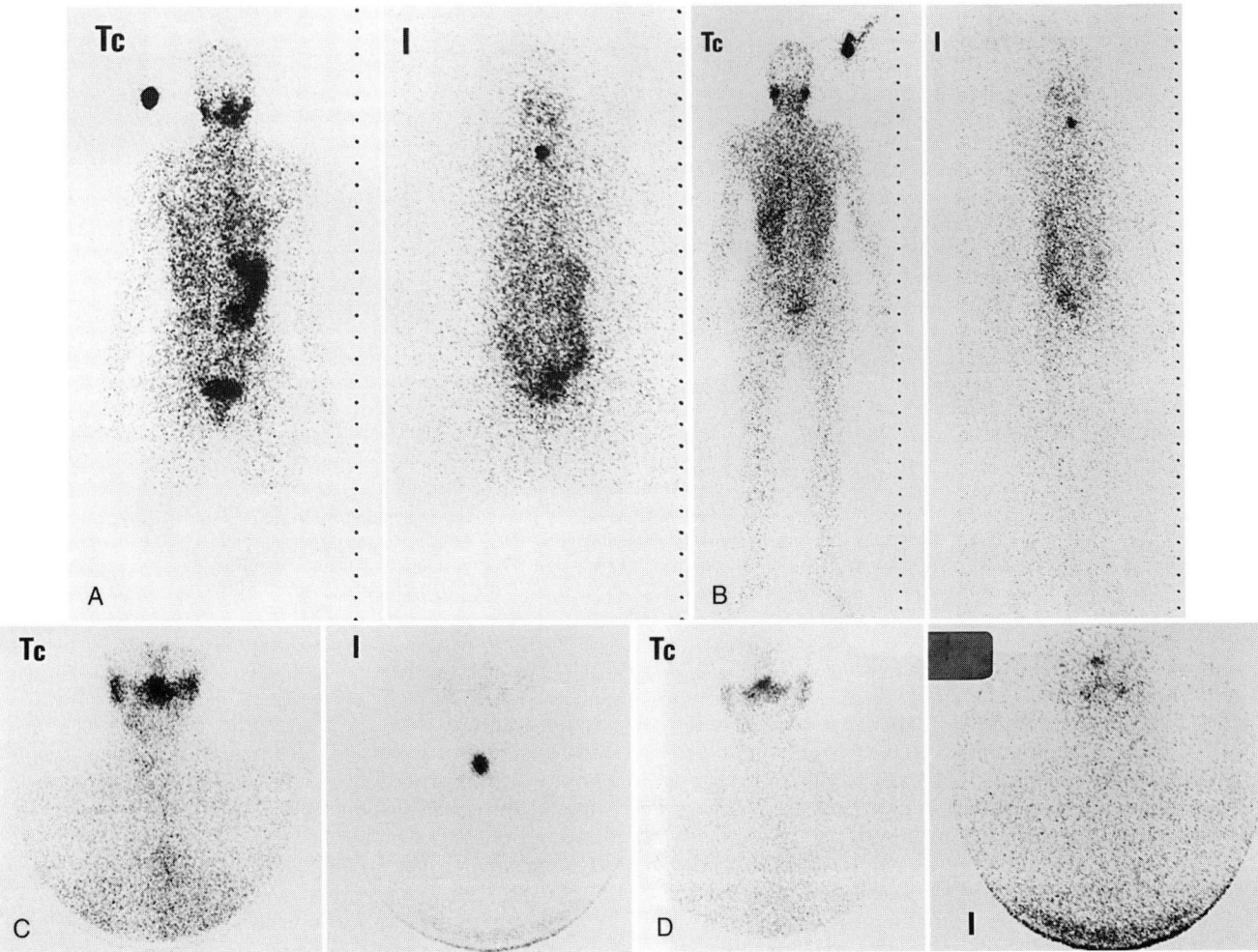

Figure 34–1. The patient is a 24-year-old woman first diagnosed to have papillary carcinoma of the thyroid on biopsy of a 4.5 cm nodule several months previously. The first postsurgical ^{131}I diagnostic scan taken 2 months after total thyroidectomy demonstrates a single focus in the neck seen here on the 72-hour whole-body anterior (**A**) and posterior (**B**) scans as well as spot views of the neck (**C**). Corresponding ^{99m}Tc pertechnetate images are also shown, providing anatomic landmarks. The neck radioiodine uptakes were 0.84% at 24 hours and 0.43% at 72 hours. The patient was treated with 48.2 mCi ^{131}I for ablation of residual thyroid tissue, and a repeat diagnostic ^{131}I study 8 months later (**D**) confirms total ablation of the thyroid remnant.

An increase in Tg to more than 3 to 5 is considered a positive test response, and in the face of a negative ^{131}I dosimetry scan, may be used as a basis for treating the patient, especially those with a high-risk lesion at the time of original surgery (risk factors include age older than 50, evidence of metastases outside the neck, local invasion into surrounding tissues, tumor diameter >5 cm in diameter.

For patients with documented ^{131}I-negative differentiated carcinomas or with medullary or anaplastic carcinoma, ^{131}I therapy is unlikely to be effective. Certainty as to whether the patient's tumor is not iodine-avid will not come until tumor recurrence has been demonstrated by another modality and the tumor site has been shown to be negative with a properly performed radioiodine scan.

Although some interest has been expressed in the use of high-dose (10 to 20 mCi) ^{123}I scanning for the identification of tumor sites, its effectiveness or ineffectiveness has not yet been documented, and the advantage of high tumor-to-background ratios at 72 hours would be lost due to the short (13-hour) half-life of ^{123}I. This inability

to scan at 72 hours could potentially compromise sensitivity for small tumor masses.

Other radiopharmaceuticals have been explored for the assessment of differentiated and undifferentiated non–iodine-avid thyroid cancer. Thallium-201 and ^{99m}Tc sestamibi (*MethoxyIsoButyl Isonitrile*) (MIBI) are nonspecific markers of cellular tissues with good blood flow and have been proven quite effective in identifying sites of persistent, recurrent, and metastatic thyroid cancer.[43] In a review of seven previously published comparative studies, Abdel-Dayem and coworkers[43] noted that ^{201}Tl demonstrated an average sensitivity of approximately 87% for metastatic differentiated thyroid carcinoma, compared with only 44% for ^{131}I scanning, with respective specificities of 95% and 100%.[43] Sensitivity with ^{201}Tl is higher using single photon emission CT (SPECT) (85% vs. 60%),[44] while post-therapy ^{131}I scans demonstrate a considerably higher sensitivity than diagnostic studies (84% vs. 44%) (Fig. 34-2).[45] It is important to perform a whole body scan 5 to 7 days after every patient therapy to fully assess the extent of disease, as well as to document

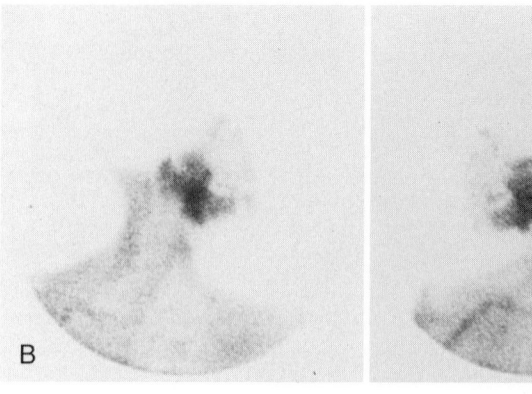

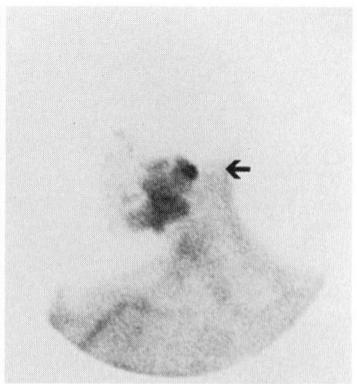

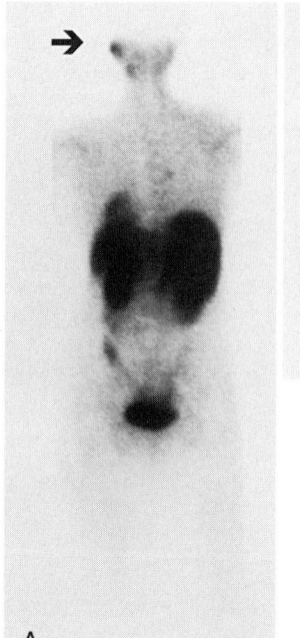

Figure 34–2. Posterior whole body **(A)** and lateral head spot views **(B)** of a ^{99m}Tc-sestamibi scan in a 59-year-old woman first diagnosed to have medullary thyroid carcinoma 19 years previously, treated by total thyroidectomy with bilateral modified radical neck dissection (which demonstrated three positive left cervical nodes). The sestamibi scan was undertaken because of persisting elevation of the serum calcitonin level. The scan demonstrates a single focus at the angle of the left mandible, which was confirmed at surgery to be a tumor-involved lymph node with infiltration into the adjacent parotid gland.

the sites of disease treated by that therapy. Whole-body ^{99m}Tc sestamibi scanning has been used for a much shorter time than ^{201}Tl scanning, but early reports indicate at least an equivalent sensitivity and specificity.[43] There is an advantage to the patient in the use of ^{201}Tl and MIBI imaging in that they appear to be fully effective without requiring the marked hypothyroidism with elevated TSH required for ^{131}I scanning. Further information is still needed on whether sensitivity is truly unaffected by TSH stimulation, and of course a positive scan still requires a subsequent ^{131}I scan to determine if the patient is treatable with ^{131}I.

Both ^{201}Tl and MIBI have been used in medullary (see Fig. 34-2) and anaplastic carcinoma as well as the differentiated carcinomas, with indications that they will be at least equivalently effective. MIBI appears to be particularly useful in Hürthle cell carcinoma, in which ^{131}I uptake is notoriously poor. In a study of 22 such patients with elevated Tg levels, Yen and colleagues[46] found positive ^{131}I scans in 18%, positive ^{201}Tl scans in 68%, and positive MIBI scans in 82%. Again, further published experience is essential. Other tracers that have been explored for thyroid carcinoma imaging, but lack sufficient experience or sensitivity to become standard diagnostic procedures, include pentavalent ^{99m}Tc-DMSA (dimercaptosuccinic acid) and ^{131}I- or ^{123}I-MIBG (metaiodobenzylguanidine) in medullary carcinoma, and recent reports of ^{111}In-Octreotide (a somatostatin analogue) for all thyroid cancers.

Positron emission tomographic scanning with ^{18}F-fluorodeoxyglucose is proving to be an effective imaging modality in selected patients with thyroid cancer.[47,48] At Memorial Sloan-Kettering Cancer Center (MSKCC), PET is performed as a guide to improved staging in patients with elevated Tg and negative ^{131}I diagnostic studies. In addition, most patients with advanced cancers that are metastatic will benefit from PET scanning to improve

staging and to identify potentially treatable lesions in critical locations. FDG PET imaging will also provide prognostic information as well, as lesions with elevated uptake (measured as the standardized uptake value or SUV) have a poorer prognosis[49] (Fig. 34-3) and are unlikely to respond to ^{131}I therapy.[50]

Of the other radiologic techniques available, MRI is proving to be the most useful in the diagnosis and post-thyroidectomy monitoring of all forms of thyroid cancer. Its high resolution is competitive with the best possible ultrasonographic technology (7.5 to 10 MHz) and does not suffer from the limitations of ultrasonography in imaging deeper structures in the neck and retrosternal structures.[51] Where MRI is not available or considered too expensive, ultrasonography of the neck in combination with Tg determination has been shown to be highly sensitive for the detection of local recurrence of differentiated tumors[52] and, in many cases, is the simplest guidance method to assure effective FNAB. Contrast-enhanced MRI can be performed with gadolinium-DTPA, improving sensitivity further and bypassing the adverse feature of CT, which is that it requires a heavily iodinated contrast agent that will interfere with radioiodine diagnostic scanning and ^{131}I therapy. On the other hand, thin-section CT without contrast is the most sensitive technique for demonstrating diffuse pulmonary metastases, with the exception of scintigraphy for those tumors that are iodine-avid.

TUMOR STAGING

Thyroid carcinoma can be staged by the traditional tumor-node-metastasis (TNM) and clinical systems (Tables 34-2 and 34-3). As with other malignancies, prognosis worsens with each increasing stage. Particularly with well-differentiated thyroid carcinomas, age is an

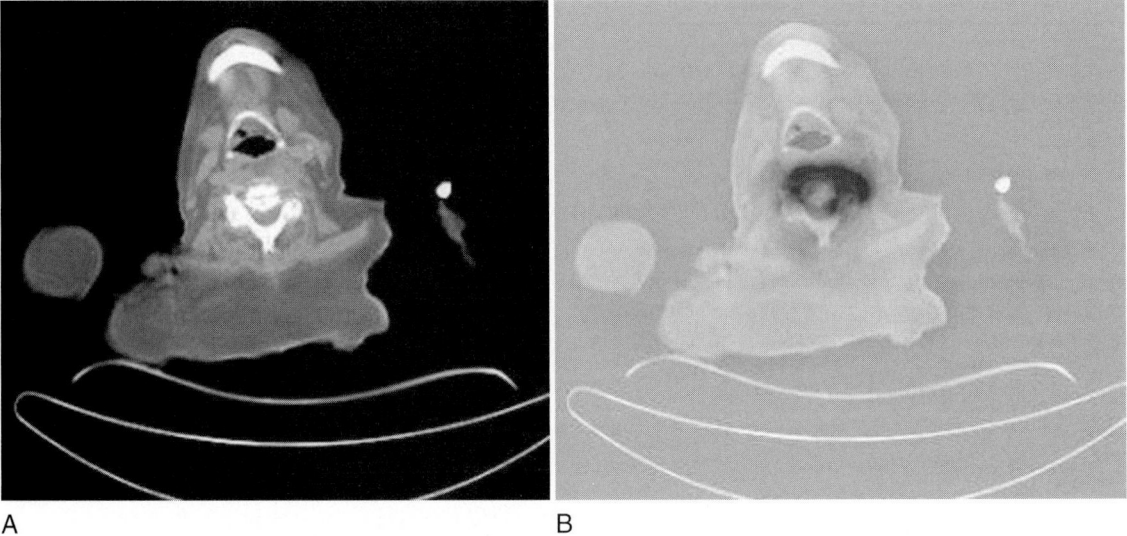

A   B

Figure 34–3. Computed tomography (CT) **(A)** and [18] fluorodeoxy-D-glucose positron emission tomography (PET)/CT **(B)** images of patient with locally advanced thyroid cancer associated with weakness in the left arm. PET/CT shows invasion of tumor into the region of the spinal cord through the left neural foramen of C-5.

additional major factor, with patients older than 45 years of age having a considerably worse prognosis than their younger counterparts.

Other staging systems have been proposed in an attempt to better separate prognostic categories. The European Organization for Research on Treatment of Cancer (EORTC) Prognostic Index, first proposed by Byar and colleagues,[53] assigns numerical values to patient age, patient sex, less-well-differentiated forms of papillary or follicular tumors, anaplastic tumors, local invasion, and single and multiple distant metastases. Based on the derived scores of >109, 84 to 108, 66 to 83, 50 to 65, and <50, the 5-year survival rates in 500 patients were observed to be 5%, 33%, 51%, 80%, and 95%, respectively. This classification has the disadvantage of not including therapy responsiveness among its criteria.

Hay and associates[54] proposed a stratification system termed AGES (*A*ge at diagnosis, *G*rade of tumor, *E*xtent of tumor, and *S*ize of tumor), separating their 860 patients with papillary carcinoma into four groups with 25-year mortalities of 93%, 49%, 7%, and 2%. Their scoring system was subsequently updated to include *M*etastasis, *A*ge at diagnosis, *C*ompleteness of resection, *I*nvasion, and *S*ize (MACIS).[55] A similar system for risk stratification referred to as the AMES score (*A*ge, *M*etastases to distant sites other than lymph nodes, *E*xtent of primary tumor, and *S*ize >5 cm) has been proposed by Cady and Rossi[56] for patients with either papillary or follicular carcinoma. This permitted stratification of their 821 patients into either a high-risk or a low-risk category, the former representing 11% of cases with a 46% 5-year mortality and the latter representing 89% of cases with only a 1.8% 5-year mortality as well as a 5% 5-year recurrence rate. As a result of the AMES stratification, Cady and Rossi recommended only unilateral surgery (subtotal or total lobectomy) with isthmus removal and no radioiodine or thyrosuppressive therapy in the low-risk group. Although helpful in separating patient groups by prognosis, neither the AGES, MACIS, nor AMES systems has come into wide use to date for patient management.

THERAPEUTIC APPROACHES

Initial Surgery

The customary management of all thyroid carcinomas begins with near-total or total thyroidectomy. In our hands, this would include as complete a removal of all thyroid tissue as is possible and detailed examination of regional nodes for macroscopic evidence of spread, with removal of all enlarged nodes. When the tumor is through the thyroid capsule, the surgeon should attempt to remove as much locally infiltrating tissue as possible. If nodes extend retrosternally, the incision should be extended to allow removal of all reachable mediastinal tumor. Although there is some rationale in patients with small (<1 to 1.5 cm) differentiated carcinomas for a more limited surgery (e.g., lobectomy with or without isthmusectomy), standard management in most centers would still be total thyroidectomy. If the primary tumor is so locally extensive and infiltrative that it cannot even be debulked surgically, external beam radiation therapy is the treatment of choice. Even in the presence of distant metastases, total thyroidectomy is important with differentiated tumors because the metastases may be amenable to ^{131}I therapy, and residual thyroid tissue will limit the elevation of TSH achievable before the diagnostic study and therapy. Because of the limited chemotherapy available and the limited effectiveness of external beam therapy in medullary and anaplastic carcinoma, total thyroidectomy and maximum possible tumor removal at initial surgery are particularly important in these patients. In a review of 134 anaplastic thyroid cancer cases managed at the Mayo Clinic from 1949 to 1999, 36% underwent attempts at curative resection, 50% had debulking procedures, and 14% had biopsy only.[22]

Table 34–2 Classification of Thyroid Cancer

Primary Tumor (T)

Note: All categories may be subdivided: (a) solitary tumor,
(b) multifocal tumor (the largest determines the classification.)

TX	Primary tumor cannot be assessed
T0	No evidence of primary tumor
T1	Tumor 2 cm or less in greatest dimension limited to the thyroid
T2	Tumor more than 2 cm but not more than 4 cm in greatest dimension limited to the thyroid
T3	Tumor more than 4 cm in greatest dimension limited to the thyroid or any tumor with minimal extrathyroid extension (e.g., extension to sternothyroid muscle or perithyroid soft tissues)
T4a	Tumor of any size extending beyond the thyroid capsule to invade subcutaneous soft tissues, larynx, trachea, esophagus, or recurrent laryngeal nerve
T4b	Tumor invades prevertebral fascia or encases carotid artery or mediastinal vessels

All anaplastic carcinomas are considered T4 tumors.

T4a	Intrathyroidal anaplastic carcinoma—surgically resectable.
T4b	Extrathyroidal anaplastic carcinoma—surgically unresectable

Regional Lymph Nodes (N)

Regional lymph nodes are the central compartment, lateral cervical, and upper mediastinal lymph nodes.

NX	Regional lymph nodes cannot be assessed
N0	No regional lymph node metastasis
N1	Regional lymph node matastasis
N1a	Metastasis to Level VI (pretracheal, paratracheal, and prelaryngeal/Delphian lymph nodes)
N1b	Metastasis to unilateral, bilateral, or contralateral cervical or superior mediastinal lymph nodes

Distant Metastasis (M)

MX	Distant metastasis cannot be assessed
M0	No distant metastasis
M1	Distant metastasis

Stage Grouping

Separate stage groupings are recommended for papillary or follicular, medullary, and anaplastic (undifferentiated) carcinoma.

Papillary or Follicular
UNDER 45 YEARS

Stage I	Any T	Any N	M0
Stage II	Any T	Any N	M1

Papillary or Follicular
45 YEARS AND OLDER

Stage I	T1	N0	M0
Stage II	T2	N0	M0
Stage III	T3	N0	M0
	T1	N1a	M0
	T2	N1a	M0
	T3	N1a	M0
Stage IVA	T4a	N0	M0
	T4a	N1a	M0
	T1	N1b	M0
	T2	N1b	M0
	T3	N1b	M0
	T4a	N1b	M0
Stage IVB	T4b	Any N	M0
Stage IVC	Any T	Any N	M1

Medullary Carcinoma

Stage I	T1	N0	M0
Stage II	T2	N0	M0
Stage III	T3	N0	M0
	T1	N1a	M0
	T2	N1a	M0
	T3	N1a	M0
Stage IVA	T4a	N0	M0
	T4a	N1a	M0
	T1	N1b	M0
	T2	N1b	M0
	T3	N1b	M0
	T4a	N1b	M0
Stage IVB	T4b	Any N	M0
Stage IVC	Any T	Any N	M1

Anaplastic Carcinoma
All anaplastic carcinomas are considered Stage IV

Stage IVA	T4a	Any N	M0
Stage IVB	T4b	Any N	M0
Stage IVC	Any T	Any N	M1

From Greene FL, Page DL, Fleming ID, et al, eds: *AJCC Cancer Staging Manual,* 6th ed. New York: Springer; 2002.

Radioiodine Therapy

Following total thyroidectomy in patients with differentiated cancers, a baseline whole-body ^{131}I scan is performed 2 to 6 months postoperatively, with full patient preparation as outlined earlier. In patients with a low-risk tumor (no lymphatic spread, no vascular invasion or tumor into or through the capsule, no distant metastases)

Table 34–3 Clinical Classification of Thyroid Cancer

Stage I:	Intrathyroidal
Stage II:	Cervical adenopathy
Stage III:	Locally invasive disease
Stage IV:	Distant metastases

who demonstrate one or several ^{131}I-avid foci only in the thyroid bed in this first scan, treatment should consist of a single dose of oral ^{131}I for ablation of residual thyroid tissue. With small, low-risk tumors, it is much more likely that these foci are residual thyroid and not tumor. Many clinicians treat at this stage with 29.9 mCi ^{131}I by oral capsule, since Nuclear Regulatory Commission (NRC) regulations require that a patient contain less than 30 mCi ^{131}I for discharge from the hospital.[57] However, 29.9 mCi ^{131}I will not fully ablate residual thyroid tissue in all patients. Maxon and coworkers,[58] in reviewing the available literature, noted that a single 30 mCi ^{131}I therapy produced complete ablation of residual thyroid tissue in only 53% of postsurgical patients, while 100 mCi was effective in 86%. Consequently, many practitioners hospitalize the patient and treat with 100 to 150 mCi at the

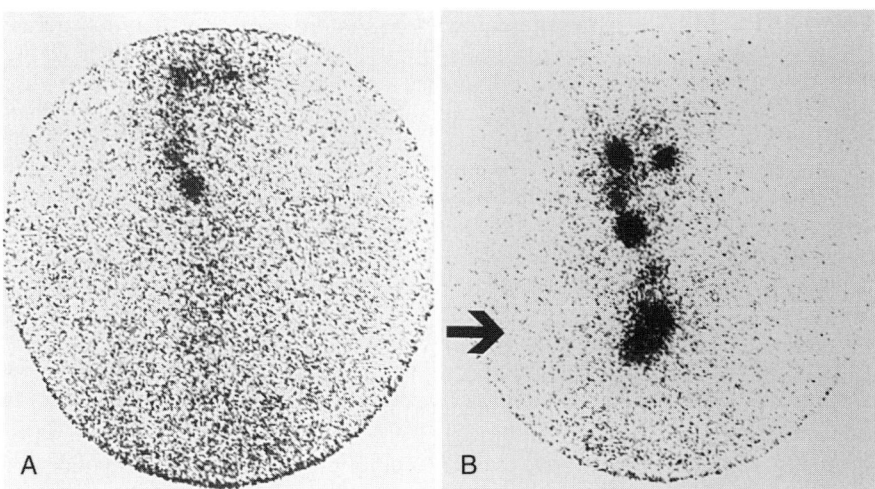

Figure 34–4. The patient is a 17-year-old girl first diagnosed 2 years previously to have an aggressive papillary carcinoma of the thyroid with multiple positive mediastinal lymph nodes. Following her first post-thyroidectomy scan 2 months after surgery, she was treated with 48.1 mCi ^{131}I for two persistent foci in the right thyroid bed, then with an additional 148.1 mCi 1 year later for the same two foci. In a follow-up ^{131}I diagnostic study 1½ years later, the two persisting loci are still seen in the right thyroid bed in the anterior 72-hour spot scintiphotograph **(A)**. The patient was again treated with 197.2 mCi ^{131}I, and the 6-day post-therapy scan **(B)** demonstrates additionally a considerable amount of mediastinal disease *(arrow)* that was not detectable on the 2 mCi diagnostic study. The serum thyroglobulin level at the time of therapy was 193 µg/L with an elevated TSH greater than 150 mIU/L.

outset, achieving 85% to 95% complete ablation. Even in the best surgical hands, 80% or more of total thyroidectomy patients will be found to have a small amount of residual tissue that requires ablative ^{131}I therapy.[58] If the patient was found at surgery to have a high-risk tumor, and particularly if it is known that some of the papillary or follicular neoplasm could not be removed, it is wise to treat the patient in the hospital with 150 mCi ^{131}I, the usual dose for ablation of tumor in the thyroid bed. This is the practice most often followed at MSKCC. We often employ Thyrogen stimulation for this procedure, based on our experience, which has shown it to be equally effective as thyroid withdrawal, as preparation for ablation.[59] The patient should always have a repeat whole-body scan of the therapy dose 5 to 10 days after treatment to evaluate at that higher ^{131}I dose for areas of tumor that were undetected or underestimated in the low-dose diagnostic study (Figs. 34-4 and 34-5).

Approximately 4 to 6 months following the initial ^{131}I ablative therapy, a repeat diagnostic ^{131}I scan is carried out. In the interval, the patient will have been on replacement thyroid hormone. The TSH and Tg also will have been measured at 3 months. If this first post-therapy scan is negative, it is reasonable to repeat it 1 year later, and if still negative, then to follow the patient clinically and with periodic Tg assays. If the first post-therapy scan is positive, but in the same location and with substantially lower radioiodine uptake, and if the patient had a low-risk tumor, a repeat 29.9 mCi ^{131}I therapy would be reasonable, with another scan 6 months later. If that scan is still positive, the patient should then be treated with 150 mCi for persistent/recurrent tumor. On the other hand, if the first post-therapy scan remains positive without reduction in radioiodine uptake, or if there are new foci of uptake, or if the tumor was a high-risk tumor, then the patient should be treated for tumor ablation: 150 mCi for disease in the thyroid bed, and 200 mCi for metastatic disease. This dose schedule (150 or 200 mCi for local/metastatic disease) is used for any reappearance of iodine-avid tumor in the subsequent course of the patient's disease. The basic principle is to continue scanning and treating the patient at 12-month intervals until all detectable tumor has disappeared by ^{131}I scan. Once

that has been achieved, an additional scan is performed 1 to 2 years later, and if this remains negative, the patient can be followed with regular clinical assessments and Tg assays. As discussed in NCRP Report Number 37, with further NRC regulatory detail in Title 10 CFR 20 and

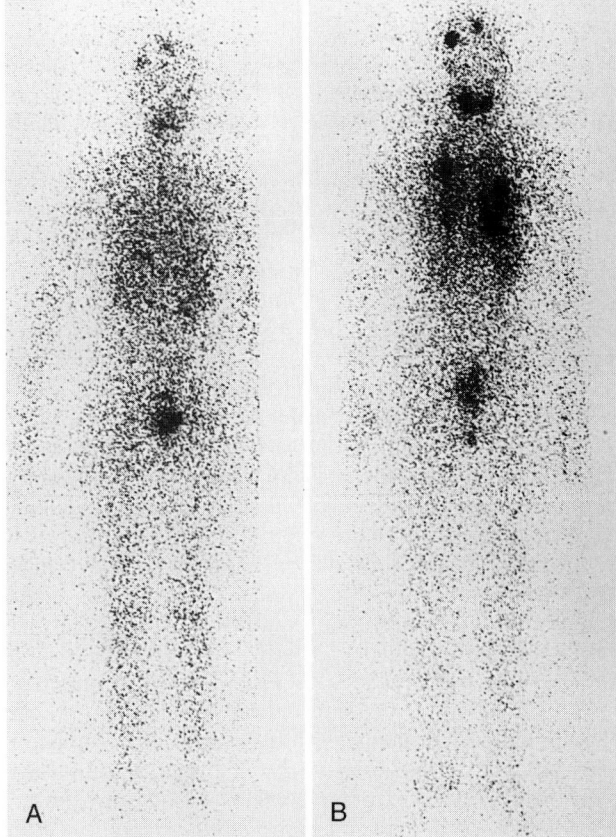

Figure 34–5. **A,** Posterior ^{131}I diagnostic scan in a 55-year-old woman first diagnosed to have papillary thyroid carcinoma 33 years previously. Following total thyroidectomy, she had multiple episodes of tumor recurrence, locally and distantly, with a cumulative ^{131}I dose at this point of almost 800 mCi. Two metastases in the skull are clearly visible, as is some haziness in the lungs. **B,** Seven days following a 196 mCi ^{131}I therapy, the skull metastases are clearly visible, and the lung involvement is much more extensive than was evident on the diagnostic scan.

Title 10 CFR 35.75,[57] patients treated with high doses of ^{131}I are allowed to leave the hospital without restrictions if they contain less than 8 mCi ^{131}I at discharge, and can leave the hospital with certain restrictions with contained doses of 8 to 30 mCi [131]I.

Maxon and coworkers[58] do not recommend the widely used 30/150/200 mCi ^{131}I therapy dose schedule outlined earlier but prefer to individualize dosimetry for each patient. Their goal is to deliver a tissue dose of 300 Gy to residual thyroid tissue in the neck (giving a single-therapy success rate in 81% of the patients, with an average ^{131}I dose of 86.8 mCi) and to deliver a minimum of 85 Gy to tumor-involved lymph nodes (giving complete tumor ablation in 74% of such patients, with an average therapy dose of 156.7 mCi).[58] This dosimetric approach requires quantitative camera scintigraphy at 24, 48, and 72 hours (conjugate views, attenuation correction) and somewhat complex dosimetric calculations, not readily available in many hospitals. It therefore is not practical for most nonacademic hospitals. It also will not be effective for metastatic sites such as lungs and skeleton, where the tissue dosimetry is not calculable. Accurate dosimetry requires a good estimate of tumor or tissue mass, often not achievable with the small amounts of tissue present in many patients with minimal disease, and certainly not achievable with pulmonary or skeletal metastases.

At MSKCC, the practice is to perform dosimetry on patients who are thought to be at high risk for metastases, usually based on criteria such as "AMES," described earlier. Details of the strategy and common protocols are available for review.[59] The goal of therapy is determined by the exposure to normal tissues, and this limits total dose. For example, a maximum of 2 Gy to blood is determined from a combination of whole body counts and the measurement of blood radioactivity clearance. Additional practical limits include maximum doses chosen so that less than 80 mCi is retained at 48 hours in the whole body, if the patient's diagnostic scan has diffuse lung uptake. These doses are determined by methods previously described by Benua et al.[60] to determine maximum tolerated activity (MTA). Typical administered activities range from 250 to 500 mCi for metastatic disease. We believe that the entire sequence of dosimetry is particularly important in patients older than 65 to avoid overtreatment for which altered renal function and prolonged clearance is common.

Hay and colleagues (AGES[54] and MACIS[55] stratification schemes), Cady and Rossi (AMES stratification[56]), McHenry and colleagues,[61] and others have recommended the use of various risk stratification schemes that permit identification of patients with extremely low long-term mortality rates. Based on such risk stratification, they recommend limited surgery such as lobectomy (with a lower incidence of surgical complications) and no adjuvant therapy (radioiodine, T4 suppression) in the low-risk group. At both UCSF and MSKCC, we still follow the management protocol of total thyroidectomy and complete radioiodine ablation because the presence of some thyroid tissue compromises the sensitivity of the serial serum Tg measurements and periodic TSH-stimulated ^{131}I scans in following for recurrence of disease.

An infrequent but clinically challenging decision arises in patients whose scans remain negative but whose serum Tg assays progressively rise. Pacini and associates[62] found that 16 of 17 such patients proved to have scan-positive disease when imaged 5 to 10 days after a 75 to 140 mCi ^{131}I therapy. Similarly, Pineda and associates[63] demonstrated 29 of 35 post-therapy scans to be positive in a group of 17 such patients treated with 150 to 300 mCi ^{131}I after a negative diagnostic scan. In 81% of the patients there was also a post-therapy fall in Tg level. Based on such a high level of response in scan-negative patients with a rising Tg, one therapy is certainly appropriate as a trial, and further therapies are indicated if there is a significant Tg response with or without a positive post-therapy scan. For consideration of such therapy, the patient's Tg level should have risen at least above 5 ng/mL.[63]

Complications of Radioiodine Therapy

Adverse effects from ^{131}I may occur in acute or chronic forms and must be discussed with the patient before obtaining the signed informed consent. The acute symptoms are rarely seen at lower therapy doses (e.g., 30 mCi), but increase in frequency with higher doses ($\geq$150 to 200 mCi). Transient radiation gastritis may cause nausea and vomiting in the first 12 to 48 hours. Since the ^{131}I therapy dose is delivered orally, vomiting in the first 1/2 to 1 hour could result in significant compromise in the therapy. This occurs rarely. Concentration of radioiodine in the salivary glands during the first 24 hours can produce a radiation sialadenitis, with symptoms varying from a mild change in the taste of food to severely inflamed and painful parotid, submaxillary, or submandibular glands. Allweiss and coworkers[64] found that this occurred in 12% of their ^{131}I therapy patients. The acute symptoms can last for several days, and the taste change may persist for weeks or even months. Attention to hydration as well as the use of tart candies or lemons once or twice an hour for the first day helps to minimize or prevent this sialadenitis. Finally, mild symptoms of radiation cystitis can occur if the patient is not encouraged to drink liquids plentifully (1 to 2 cups per hour) and empty the bladder every 2 to 3 hours during the first 24 hours, including throughout the first night. An unsettled bowel or mild diarrhea is an infrequent adverse outcome during the first 1 to 2 days. If the patient has a substantial amount of residual thyroid tissue or tumor tissue picking up the radioiodine very well, this can be a rare cause of regional pain, tenderness, and sometimes tissue swelling in the neck. Transient leukopenia and thrombocytopenia often occur at higher therapeutic ^{131}I doses but are generally mild and not of clinical significance unless the patient already has compromise of marrow function due to prior therapy, or has substantial whole-body retention of the ^{131}I such that the whole blood radiation exposure from a single therapy exceeds 2 to 3 Gy (e.g., in patients with renal failure). Extremely rarely, functioning papillary or follicular metastases may be so extensive that effective high-dose ^{131}I therapy can induce thyrotoxicosis during the first 1 to 2 weeks of tumor lysis, a possibility that can be managed by medications such as propranolol.

The chronic risks associated with high-dose ^{131}I therapy are reproductive, genetic, and carcinogenic. In males, transient oligospermia may occur at lower therapy doses, and permanent oligospermia at higher doses, but in the long-term follow-up of children treated with almost 200 mCi ^{131}I, the incidences of infertility (12%), miscarriages (1.4%), prematurity (8%), and congenital anomalies (1.4%) were found to be the same as in the general population.[65] It is recommended that patients wait at least 6 months after therapy before attempting pregnancy, however. An increase in both leukemia (myelogenous leukemia) and bladder cancer has been described following high-dose ^{131}I therapy, generally with cumulative doses higher than 800 mCi, therapy intervals less than 1 year apart, and single therapy total blood radiation doses greater than 2 Gy.[66] However, the actual relationship of current patterns of therapy to the induction of leukemia, breast cancer, or bladder cancer is not clearcut. In a review of 2753 therapy cases in the literature, Maxon and Smith[66] found only 14 cases (0.5%) of leukemia, so this complication is infrequent and at the lower cumulative therapy doses does not appear to rise above the normal background incidence of leukemia. For example, in one of the few controlled studies in the literature, Hall et al. reported no evidence of increased leukemia incidence in patients treated with an average dose of 125 mCi (4551 MBq). The control group actually had more cases of leukemia than the treated group.[67] However, it would be logical to assume that the frequency does increase with increasing cumulative therapy doses. The incidence of bladder cancer in post-therapy patients is lower than that of leukemia; this complication is seen only at even higher cumulative doses than with leukemia.[68] In a retrospective review of 10,552 Swedish patients treated with an average dose of 13.7 mCi (506 MBq) [131]I and followed for a mean of 15 years, Holm and colleagues[69] found no type of cancer incidence falling outside a 95% confidence interval of the standardized incidence ratio including thyroid, stomach, and bladder cancers and leukemia, although risk for stomach cancer did increase over time ($n = 92$, $P < 0.05$). Finally, late pulmonary fibrosis is a potential concern, but occurs only in patients with diffuse pulmonary metastases and corresponding diffuse pulmonary uptake of the therapy dose (i.e., patients with widespread pulmonary micrometastases). One recommendation in such cases is that individual therapy doses be limited to 75 mCi [131]I.[66]

EXTERNAL BEAM IRRADIATION IN CARCINOMA OF THE THYROID

Indications

Although surgery and radioiodine therapy are the mainstays of intervention for malignancies of the thyroid, there remains a definite group of patients for whom external beam therapy is useful. Historically, the belief that thyroid cancer was radioresistant led to disfavor for this approach. This misconception was based on the fact that the anatomic location of the thyroid and the multiplicity of directions of lymphatic drainage made it very difficult to administer therapeutic doses of external beam irradiation (>55 to 60 Gy) without substantial risk to surrounding normal structures. The thyroid and lymphatics that drain the thyroid lie within a curved bed that lies in the lower neck and upper mediastinum, surrounding the esophagus, vertebral column, and spinal cord. Rouvière[70] and McKormack and Sheline[71] separately identified the lymphatics of concern, which travel down from the thyroid into the upper mediastinum just behind the sternum, as well as upward toward the base of skull in the retropharyngeal chain. Attempts to adequately cover these regions were thwarted by this complexity, resulting in doses less than 45 Gy being delivered to portions of the target area, to respect cord tolerance.[72] Advances in the delivery systems for radiation, especially improved imaging modalities in conjunction with three-dimensional conformal and intensity-modulated treatment planning systems, allow safer delivery of higher doses to the region at risk. The issue of adjuvant radiotherapy for thyroid cancer needs to be readdressed.

Patients who should be considered for adjuvant irradiation in thyroid carcinoma have been well described by Tubiana and associates[72] and O'Connell and associates.[73] They include patients with differentiated thyroid carcinomas who undergo extensive surgery but are found to have microscopic residual disease or are felt to be at high risk of local failure by the experienced surgeon who has carried out the resection[74,75]; patients with gross residual disease after surgery who show little uptake of radioiodine or have substantial bulk of disease remaining after surgery and who are unlikely to take up enough iodine to allow therapeutic doses of radiation; patients with inoperable disease or recurrence after prior radioiodine therapy; and patients with anaplastic lesions that are incompletely resected (who may benefit from combination irradiation and chemotherapy). The presence of nodal involvement by itself is not necessarily an indication for postoperative radiation in the well-differentiated carcinomas.[74,75] Palliative irradiation also plays a role in patients with painful or destructive metastatic sites of disease.[73,76-79]

Technique

Various techniques have been described in the literature, most of which are hampered by the need to reduce the dose to parts of the target volume to keep spinal cord doses below 45 Gy.[73,76-79] Ideally, a technique should be designed that allows the delivery of doses of 55 to 60 Gy to regions known to be microscopically positive, 50 Gy to nodes suspected but unproven, and 65 Gy or greater to macroscopically involved areas in the postoperative or unresectable nonmetastatic cases. Serial cone-down applications would be required to reduce the target volumes as these doses are achieved. The spinal cord dose must be kept at or below the level of 45 to 50 Gy, especially in cases in which concurrent chemotherapy is considered. If chemotherapy is planned concomitantly, then doses should be appropriately reduced. Care must be taken when considering the brachial plexus as well, since doses in excess of 60 Gy may result in plexopathy.

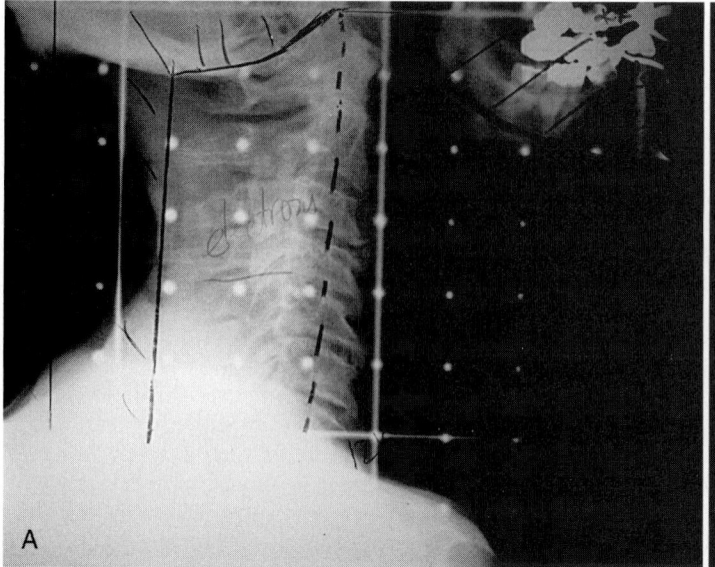

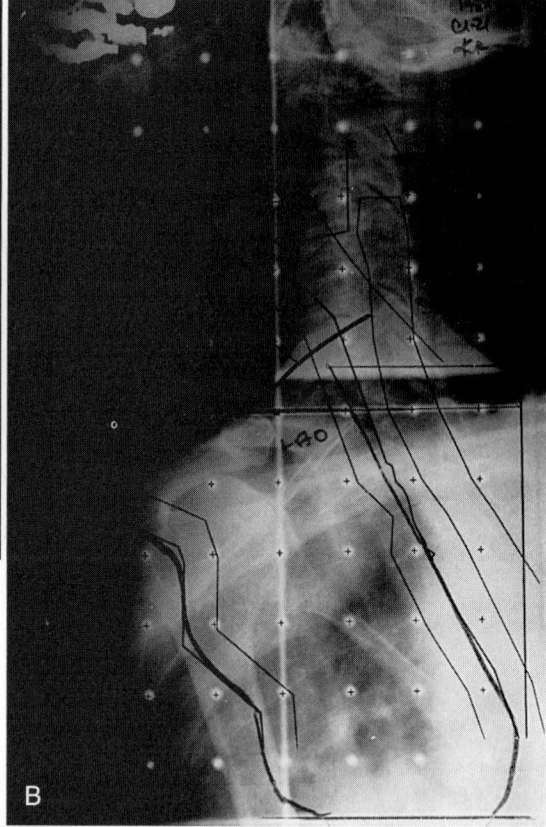

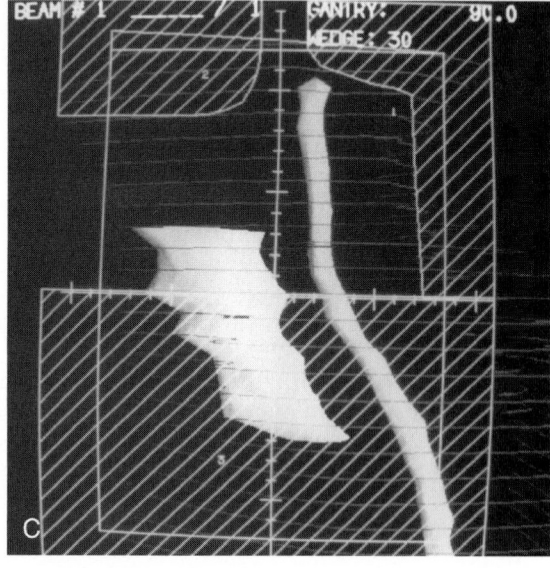

Figure 34–6. A, Lateral simulation film for upper half of field, beam split on the bottom to match the upper border of the lower field. The cord block is drawn in the *dotted line*, to be placed at 45 Gy, with electrons matched on to cover the posterior nodes after 45 Gy. **B,** Oblique simulation film for lower half of field, upper portion, with computed tomographically defined tumor volume, spinal cord, and blocks. See also Color Figure 34–6C.

One such technique is shown in Figures 34-6 and 34-7. CT scanning in the treatment position is carried out, and the target volumes are identified on all slices of the scan. The field is divided into upper and lower sections using independent jaws or beam splitters. The lower portion includes the mediastinum and draining lymphatics and is heavily weighted anteriorly to spare the cord dose from the onset of treatment. The field can be treated initially in an anteroposterior-posteroanterior (AP-PA) fashion, but will need to be switched to a three-field plan after about 30 Gy to allow sufficient remaining cord tolerance to take the area to a dose in excess of 55 Gy. The change should not occur too early, since substantial amounts of lung may be irradiated by the multi-field approach, and an attempt should be made to keep both cord and as much lung tissue as possible below tolerance doses (cord, 45 Gy; lung, 20 Gy). The upper half of the field is treated using a multi-field approach from the outset, or by starting with initial opposed lateral photon fields, followed by an off-cord block at 45 Gy, with electrons added posteriorly for the remainder of the dose. The use of independent jaws with a single isocenter eliminates the need for match-line shifts during therapy if patient immobility is ensured. Alternatively, the central line can be shifted after each 20 Gy to give an improved safety margin, although this becomes quite difficult owing to the location of the thyroid relative to the shoulders.

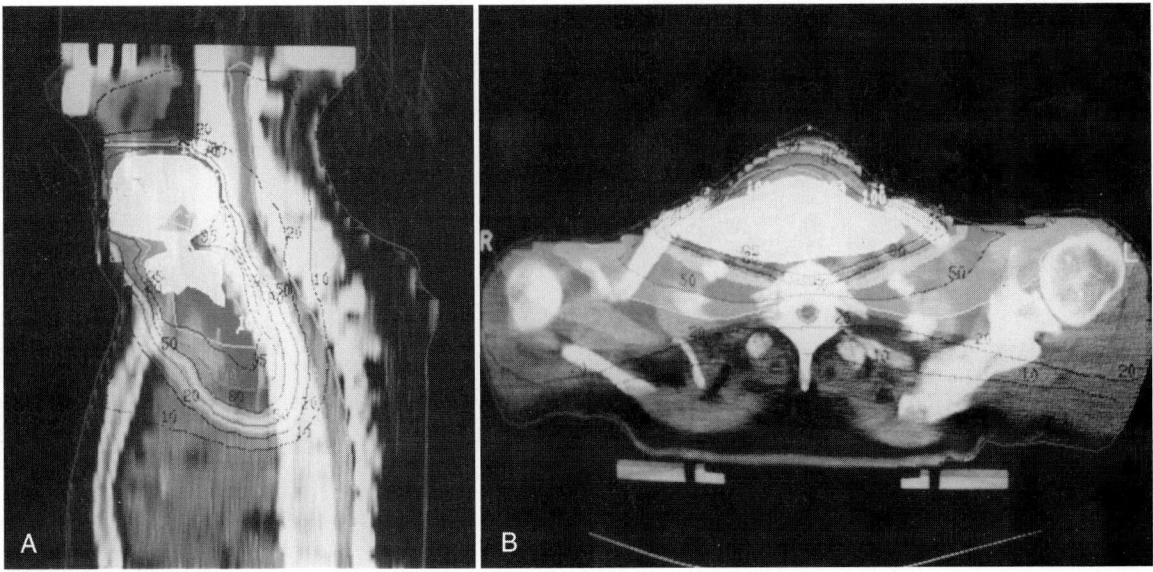

Figure 34–7. A, Sagittal reconstruction of the computed tomography (CT) scan used for treatment planning for the off-cord portion of therapy using the beam split approach, showing superimposed isodose distribution. **B,** Axial slice of CT scan with the superimposed isodose distributions in the lower half of the field for the two-field off-cord boost. See also Color Figure 34–7.

Newer techniques involving intensity-modulated radiation therapy techniques with inverse planning have been described and compared to the older techniques,[80] with a significant improvement in dose distribution. Initial immobilization is critical, as significant respiratory movements can affect the final dose distribution in patients who require coverage of the mediastinal nodes. Definition of the clinical target volume (CTV) will vary depending on the clinical situation. Postoperatively, the CTV will be the initial thyroid bed with or without the regional nodes of interest. The planning target volume (PTV) will include the CTV plus a 0.5 to 1.0 cm margin. In unresectable cases, the PTV will be the gross tumor volume (GTV) plus any clinically relevant nodes. Various plans have been put forth—a nine-field (equispaced around the patient's axis), seven or five fields,[81] and stepping pseudo-arcs[80]—all allowing greater dose delivery to the PTV with reduced dose to the spinal cord when compared to standard three-dimensional treatment plans. IMRT plans may differ significantly in the degree of inhomogeneity seen within the PTV. These inhomogeneities can, however, be used to advantage in what is called a simultaneous integrated boost (SIB)[81]—the delivery of a higher dose per fraction (2 to 2.2 Gy) to the GTV and a lower dose (1.8 Gy) to the remainder of the CTV. By careful identification of organs to be avoided, such as larynx and esophagus in addition to spinal cord, toxicity of therapy may be further reduced in those cases treated with concurrent chemoradiation[80] (Fig. 34-8).

OUTCOME

Differentiated Thyroid Carcinoma

Low-grade papillary and follicular carcinomas of the thyroid are quite benign malignancies with a good prognosis. The combined 25-year survival rate in 1408 patients

(out of a total study group of 1500) at the Mayo Clinic who had papillary carcinoma with no distant metastases at diagnosis or residual tumor post-thyroidectomy was 97%.[82] The 20-year cause-specific survival rate for all 1500 patients with papillary carcinoma was 94.5%, compared with 75.2% in a parallel group of 197 patients with follicular carcinoma. This illustrates the well-established fact that follicular carcinoma is a significantly more aggressive malignancy than papillary carcinoma. In a review of 15 publications involving 9744 patients, Mazzaferri[20] found average 10-year cause-specific survival rates of 88% for papillary and 71% for follicular carcinoma. Many additional factors at diagnosis and in management affect the prognosis.

TUMOR SIZE

In their review of 535 patients with papillary microcarcinoma (previously termed occult papillary carcinoma; tumors <1 cm in diameter) Hay and colleagues[28] found observed survival rates of 90.6% at 10 years and 78.7% at 20 years, but cause-specific survival rates of 99.8% at 10 years, 99.8% at 20 years, and 98.7% at 30 years. This was in spite of multifocality in 20% of patients at diagnosis, as well as bilaterality in 10%, extrathyroidal infiltration in 2%, and positive regional lymph nodes in 32%. Similarly, Mazzaferri,[20] in his review of 1133 patients, noted a 10-year cause-specific survival rate of 99.6% for papillary carcinomas less than 1.5 cm in size at diagnosis, compared with 94.4% for follicular carcinomas. For both histologic types, the mortality rate increases with increasing size above 1.5 cm, with cause-specific 5-year survival rates of 87% and 73%, respectively, for tumors above 4.5 cm.[20] In 1500 patients with papillary carcinoma, Hay[82] found 20-year cause-specific mortality rates of 6% for tumors 2.0 to 3.9 cm, 16% for tumors 4.0 to 6.9 cm, and 50% for tumors 7.0 cm or more in size. Thus, there is little room for augmenting survival by

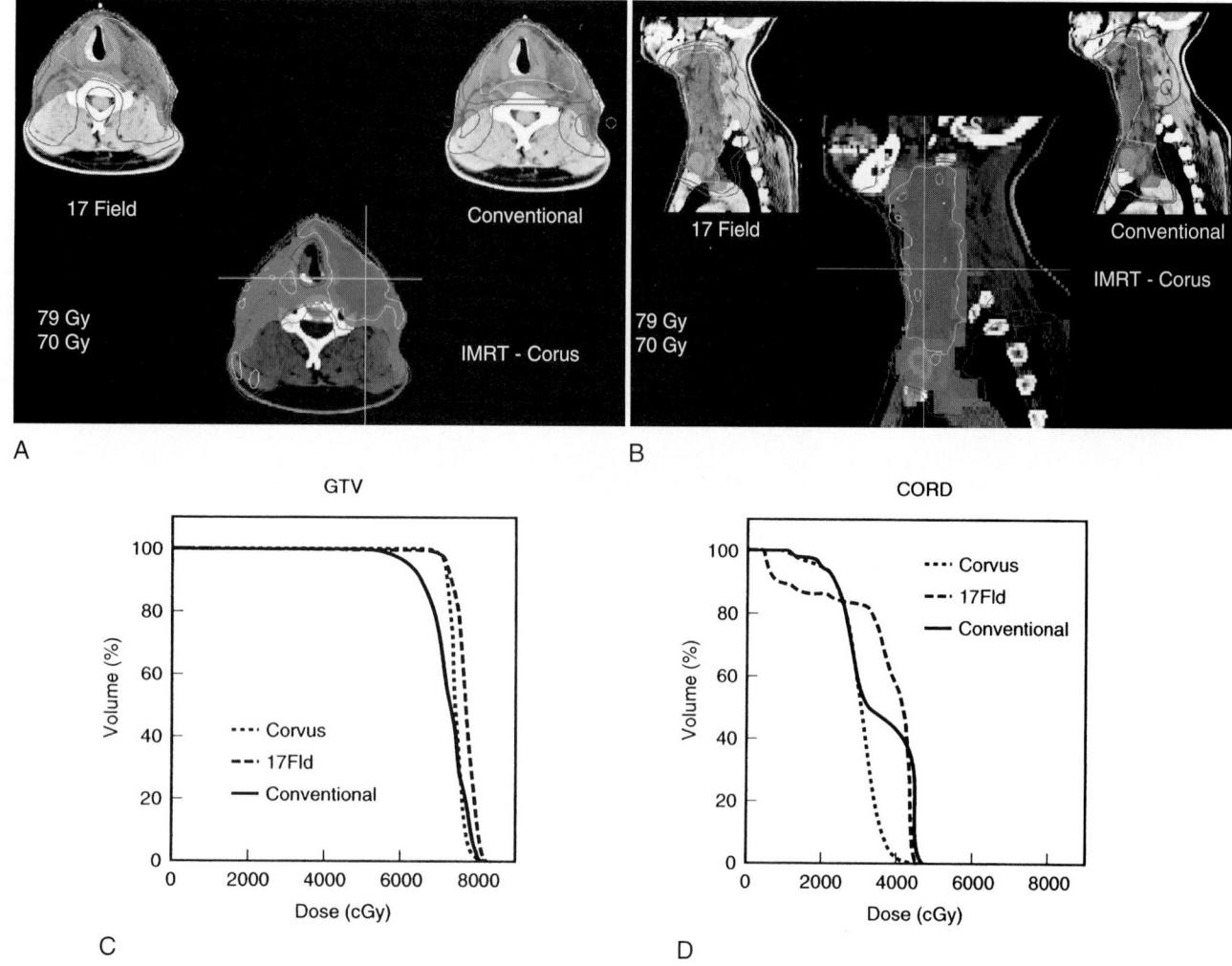

Figure 34–8. A, Axial dose distributions at the level of the larynx in a patient with locally advanced, left-sided anaplastic carcinoma—comparison of standard planning, 17-field three-dimensional treatment plan, and an intensity-modulated radiation therapy plan using the Corvus system. Note the differential dosing allowing laryngeal and cord dose reduction. **B,** Sagittal dose distributions. **C,** Dose-volume histogram comparison for these three plans. **D,** Dose-volume histogram comparison for the spinal cord with these plans. See also Color Figure 34–8.

therapeutic technique in the smaller primary tumors, leading Hay[82] and Mazzaferri,[20,29] along with others, to recommend only near-total thyroidectomy with T$_4$ suppression and no radioiodine therapy in patients with small primary tumors less than 1.5 cm in diameter and no other serious risk factors (e.g., distant metastases, history of childhood irradiation).

AGE AND SEX OF PATIENT

Although thyroid cancer is more common in females by a 2 to 3:1 ratio, mortality is slightly higher in males, although probably not with such significance as to affect management. Hay[82] noted a 20-year cause-specific mortality rate of 4% in women and 9% in men, while Mazzaferri and Jhiang[29] found cause-specific mortalities at 10, 20, and 30 years of 3%, 5%, and 7% in women and 7%, 10%, and 11% in men, respectively. Age also affects patient recurrence and mortality rates. Recurrence rates are highest in patients under 20 years and older than 50 years of age, although mortality rises only in the older population.[29,82] Hay[82] noted a 20-year cause-specific mortality rate for papillary carcinoma of 0.8%, 7%, 20%, and 47% for patients younger than 50 years, 50 to 59 years, 60 to 69 years, and 70 years of age or older at diagnosis. Chow, in a retrospective review of 842 patients with papillary carcinoma, found a 5.4-fold increase in death rate for patients older than 45 years of age.[75] Thus, aggressive management is most important in the older age groups.

EXTENT OF LOCAL AND DISTANT SPREAD

DeGroot and coworkers,[83] in their study of 269 patients with papillary carcinoma, noted that although 21.6% had microscopic capsular invasion, 10.8% had gross capsular invasion, and 46% had multifocal tumor, these local factors did not significantly affect disease-free long-term survival. Similarly, positive cervical adenopathy at diagnosis did not affect disease-free survival in their patient population, although it did slightly increase the incidence of recurrences during the first 10 to 15 years. Hay,[82] on the other hand, found in 1468 papillary carcinoma patients with disease limited to the neck that the 20-year cause-specific mortality rate was 28% in those patients with tumors locally invasive into adjacent soft tissues of the neck, compared with only 1.9% in patients with noninvasive tumors. Mazzaferri and Jhiang[29] reported the 30-year cause-specific survival rate for combined papillary and follicular patients to be 94% if no regional node involvement was present at diagnosis, 90% if there was any regional node involvement, and 78% if there was mediastinal involvement.

The presence at diagnosis of distant metastases is a bad prognostic factor. Hay[82] observed a 69% 10-year cause-specific mortality rate in this group, compared with only 3% in patients with disease confined to the neck. In a review of 13 publications involving 9248 patients with distant metastases at diagnosis, Mazzaferri[20] noted an average 5-year cause-specific mortality rate of 53%. Interestingly, Mazzaferri and Jhiang[29] found that if they excluded the patients with distant metastases at diagnosis in estimating the 30-year cause-specific mortality in their 1355 patients with differentiated carcinoma, the follicular carcinoma mortality rate was only slightly and not significantly higher than that for papillary carcinoma (10% vs. 6%). It is the population of patients with distant metastases, approximately 5% of patients at diagnosis, and an additional 5% to 10% who subsequently develop distant metastases, who represent the most important group for potential benefit from decisions on adjuvant management and the subsequent uses of radioiodine, external beam therapy, and chemotherapy.

STAGE

As previously discussed, several different approaches to staging of thyroid carcinoma exist (e.g., TNM, EORTC, AMES, AGES, MACIS) and all are associated with a worsening prognosis as the tumor stage at diagnosis increases. Such staging can be very helpful in making decisions on how aggressive to be in management.

SURGERY

The extent of initial surgery has been demonstrated to affect both recurrence rate and survival in patients with tumors greater than 1 cm in diameter. DeGroot and associates[83] noted in their papillary carcinoma patients that less extensive initial surgery (lobectomy or bilateral subtotal thyroidectomy) was associated with a statistically significant increase in the rate of recurrence and mortality compared with more extensive surgery (lobectomy plus contralateral subtotal lobectomy or near-total or total thyroidectomy). The addition of a modified or radical neck dissection did not further improve the recurrence rate or survival. Mazzaferri and Jhiang[29] similarly found 30-year recurrence rates of 26% and 40% and mortality rates of 6% and 9% in their stage 2 and 3 papillary and follicular carcinoma patients treated initially with total or near-total thyroidectomy, compared with lesser degrees

of surgery, respectively. Hay[82] in 963 patients with papillary carcinoma staged by his AGES method found that in 866 low-risk patients, the 30-year local recurrence rate was 14% after lobectomy and 4% after bilateral lobar resection, with respective local recurrence rates of 59% and 20% in the 97 high-risk patients. Survival was improved only in the high-risk group, however, and there was no further improvement in survival using total thyroidectomy in comparison with near-total thyroidectomy. In the later MACIS prognostic scoring system of Hay and coworkers[55] applied to 1779 patients with papillary carcinoma, in which completeness of tumor removal at surgery was one factor (but not the extent of thyroidectomy per se), 20-year cause-specific survival rates of 99%, 89%, 56%, and 24% were noted with MACIS scores of less than 6, 6 to 6.99, 7 to 7.99, and more than 8.

DeGroot and colleagues[83] also noted that total thyroidectomy gained no additional survival advantage over near-total thyroidectomy. At the other surgical extreme, Rossi and colleagues[84] reported a 2-year 44% mortality rate in patients with surgically incurable neck disease, and Mazzaferri and Jhiang[29] found in their review of 1355 papillary and follicular patients that tumor invasion of neck structures was associated with a doubling of the mortality rate, and a median survival of only 3.2 years.

In addition to the expectable risks associated with major surgery, such as anesthetic risks, there is risk of hypoparathyroidism (5.9 to 8.4%,[83] 5%[29]) and permanent laryngeal nerve paralysis (1.7%,[83] 2%[29]) associated with total or near-total thyroidectomy. These are risks that will be lower in major academic centers and with highly experienced thyroid surgeons.[29]

The completeness of surgery is an independent prognostic factor. The absence of post-operative residual disease was associated with a reduction in risk of dying of 0.034 compared with those with residual disease in the report by Chow.[75] Tsang, in the review of 382 patients with papillary or follicular carcinoma, found postoperative residual disease to be an independent predictor of cause-specific survival on multivariate analysis.[74] In this report, papillary carcinoma patients with residual disease who received external irradiation showed a significant benefit in both cause-specific survival and loco-regional freedom from relapse, whereas follicular cases failed to show such benefit. Patients with gross postoperative residual disease fared worse than those with microscopic residual in these reports.

RADIOIODINE THERAPY

There are two applications of ^{131}I therapy in the management of differentiated thyroid carcinoma: (1) post-thyroidectomy ablation of residual normal thyroid tissue; and (2) long-term management of patients with regional or distant carcinoma sites, which are iodine-avid and therefore amenable to ^{131}I therapy. Taking the latter use first, it is difficult to assess the effect of radioiodine therapy on outcome in patients with advanced disease because it is invariably the therapy of choice for tumors that are iodine-avid, and no prospective comparative studies have been performed to compare such treatment with matched control subjects managed differently. The closest comparison possible is ^{131}I therapy in advanced-stage patients with iodine-avid metastases versus comparable patients with iodine-nonavid tumors not treated radioisotopically.

Nemec and coworkers[85] noted 10-year survival rates of 70% in patients with pulmonary metastases that concentrated ^{131}I and were so treated, compared with 6% in patients whose pulmonary metastases were not iodine-avid. Reviewing seven published studies involving 806 patients with distant (mainly lung and bone) metastases from differentiated thyroid cancer, Mazzaferri[20] noted that the metastases were iodine-avid in only 54% of the patients and that radioiodine therapy in this group led to a 21% 5- to 10-year mortality rate, compared with a 40% mortality rate in the comparable iodine-nonavid group. There is no dispute regarding the advisability of ^{131}I therapy for persistent or recurrent differentiated thyroid carcinoma in patients whose tumors are iodine-avid.

As with the issue of extent of surgery, however, there is continuing controversy regarding the routine use of ^{131}I for ablation of thyroid remnants after thyroidectomy. Mazzaferri and Jhiang[29] reported that in 1204 patients with papillary or follicular carcinoma in whom initial surgery was complemented with external beam radiotherapy, no medical therapy, thyroid hormone alone, or ^{131}I remnant ablation followed by thyroid hormone maintenance, 30-year recurrence rates were 63%, 40%, 30%, and 15%, and 30-year cause-specific death rates were 32%, 12%, 6%, and 3%, respectively. Almost all of these comparisons were statistically significant, but in fact the baseline risk factors were not equally distributed among the four groups. After further separating groups to almost equalize risk factors, they found that stage 2 and 3 tumor patients treated with ^{131}I still demonstrated a lower 30-year recurrence rate (16% vs. 38%) and cancer mortality rate (3% vs. 9%) than patients who did not receive [131]I. On the other hand, when Hay[82] applied Mazzaferri's criteria for appropriateness of ablative ^{131}I therapy to the relevant 946 patients in his 1500 papillary thyroid carcinoma patient study, the 10-year cause-specific mortality was 2.0% for surgically treated patients and 3.0% for those also treated with ablation. DeGroot and colleagues[83] also noted in their 269 papillary carcinoma patients that "using the Cox model, absence of ablation was not associated with a statistically significant increased risk of death or recurrence," although by X^2 analysis, absence of ablation was associated with increased incidence of deaths in their class I and II patients, and increased risk of recurrence among all patients, among class I and II patients, and among class I and II patients with tumors greater than 1 cm in size. The recommended therapeutic dose of ^{131}I for effective remnant ablation also is somewhat controversial. Johansen and colleagues[86] found that 1073 MBq (29 mCi) and 3700 MBq (100 mCi) were equally effective for remnant ablation (81% vs. 84%). Maxon and colleagues[58] similarly noted 77% complete ablation with approximately 30 mCi therapy, but preferred a delivered dose to the tissue of 300 Gy or greater for maximum effectiveness.

Although this controversy regarding ablation of thyroid remnants remains unresolved, most clinicians would agree that remnant ablation provides advantages in long-term patient follow-up. As a result of having had

total ablation, the patient then begins follow-up with a completely negative ^{131}I diagnostic scan for subsequent comparisons when needed. Also, the absence of any residual thyroid tissue will permit achievement of higher TSH levels for future diagnostic ^{131}I cancer scans, and the baseline and TSH-stimulated Tg levels will be extremely low (e.g., <1 and 4 mcg/L, respectively) so that this, too, will be a more sensitive test for long-term patient monitoring. Complete remnant ablation is widely accepted as standard care.

EXTERNAL BEAM RADIATION

O'Connell and associates[73] reported on a retrospective series of 113 patients with differentiated thyroid cancer treated with external beam radiotherapy at the Royal Marsden Hospital from 1969 to 1991. Of these, 85 had papillary, 24 had follicular, and 4 had Hürthle cell carcinomas. Fifty-three had locally advanced disease and 12 had distant metastases. Radiation was used for the following reasons: 34 had failure to concentrate radioiodine, 21 were poorly differentiated, 24 were inoperable, and 11 were locally recurrent. Tumor doses of 60 Gy were attempted, but the spinal cord was shielded posteriorly after 40 Gy. Seventy-four patients also received [131]I. Of the papillary cases with probable or definite microscopic residual disease after surgery, local failure occurred in 13% (7/53). Complete regression was seen in 41% and partial regression in 22% of patients with macroscopic residual disease. The majority of these patients also received radioiodine, and the combination was well-tolerated.

Chow et al. reported on 842 patients with papillary thyroid carcinoma treated at Queen Elizabeth Hospital in Hong Kong between 1960 and 1997.[75] One hundred five of these patients received external beam radiation in addition to their surgery and radioiodine treatment for locally advanced disease (positive margins, gross residual disease, and pT4). External beam therapy to a median dose of 60 Gy reduced the locoregional relapse risk by two thirds in those with gross residual disease in the neck after surgery.

Tubiana and colleagues[72] reported 66 patients who received prophylactic irradiation after total gross resection of well-differentiated lesions who had multiple nodes involved, upper mediastinal involvement, and invasion of muscles or difficult resections at the time of recurrence. Five- and 15-year relapse-free survival rates of 70% and 53% were seen. In 97 patients irradiated after incomplete resection, these rates were 58% and 39%, but they were only 55% and 7% for 23 initially unresectable patients, 17 of whom were irradiated. In a total of 180 patients who received irradiation for high-risk features, local failure was seen in 25 (14%). The average time from irradiation to local failure was 8.5 years.

Medullary Thyroid Carcinoma

Long-term survival is generally better for hereditary MTC associated with MEN 2A and MEN 2B than for sporadic MTC. In either case, if the tumor is caught early and treated with total thyroidectomy alone while still localized to the thyroid, 10-year cause-specific survival is 95% or greater.[87,88] Extrathyroidal presence of tumor at initial surgery and persistence or recurrence of elevated calcitonin levels post-thyroidectomy are bad prognostic signs associated with significant shortening of survival. If extrathyroidal tumor in the neck can be identified and completely resected upon recurrence, cure rates of 25% to 35% are achievable.[89] Overall 10-year survival rates of 80% with MEN 2A, 55% with sporadic MTC, and less than 50% with MEN 2B have been documented by the German Medullary Thyroid Carcinoma Study Group.[90] Radioiodine ablation of residual thyroid tissue has been shown to have no useful role in the post-thyroidectomy management of MTC.[88]

External beam radiotherapy probably does not have an effect on long-term survival,[91,92] although it can be quite effective in the symptomatic management of extensive regional recurrence or painful bony metastases.[93] The French Federation of Cancer Institutes published a report of 59 patients with medullary carcinoma who underwent surgical resection (total thyroidectomy plus neck dissection) followed by adjuvant radiotherapy to a mean dose of 54 Gy.[94] Eleven patients had residual tumor, and 44 had positive nodes. As this was a retrospective review, there was no unirradiated control arm. Local recurrences occurred in 18 (30%), the majority within the irradiated field. Average survival in this study was 70.5 months.

Various attempts to define effective chemotherapy (e.g., Adriamycin, cisplatin, semustine, and etoposide, alone or in combinations) have been unsuccessful in prolonging survival, with only modest partial remissions on the order of 33% achieved.[87,88,91,92] Symptoms may be treated with somatostatin analogs such as octreotide, which improve the quality, although not the duration, of life.[92]

Anaplastic Thyroid Carcinoma

Anaplastic or undifferentiated thyroid carcinoma is the most aggressive thyroid cancer, with the poorest prognosis and the poorest responsiveness to therapy. There is no role for radioiodine therapy in this malignancy, since lack of differentiation results in failure to concentrate iodine. Radioiodine ablation of thyroid remnants after total thyroidectomy also has no place in the management of these tumors. Many (if not most) anaplastic carcinomas appear to arise from dedifferentiation occurring in well-differentiated tumors. Although this has been reported to be the result of radioiodine or external beam therapy in some patients with differentiated tumors, such radiation-induced dedifferentiation actually occurs quite rarely. Aldinger and associates[95] reported only 10 (4%) patients out of 243 treated with ^{131}I who had progressed from well-differentiated to anaplastic carcinoma, and Tubiana and associates[72] found no cases of dedifferentiation to anaplastic carcinoma among 359 patients previously treated with radioiodine or external beam therapy.

As reviewed by Mazzaferri,[96] median survival from diagnosis in anaplastic carcinoma ranges from 3 to 7 months. Woolner and colleagues,[97] in a study of 119 such patients, found mortalities of 61% at 6 months and 77% at 12 months. Tumor stage (extent of local or distant spread) and patient age appear to be the greatest factors affecting prognosis.[96] Venkatesh and colleagues,[98] in a study of 121 patients, found no significant effect on mean survival provided by extent of surgery (total/subtotal thyroidectomy vs. lobectomy/biopsy resulted in 8.9 vs. 3.3 months, mean survival, $P > 0.1$), radiotherapy (8.5 vs. 5.5 months, $P > 0.2$), chemotherapy (7.3 vs. 5.4 months, $P > 0.2$) or combined chemotherapy and radiotherapy (9.1 vs. 4.8 months, $P > 0.1$). Only limitation of disease to the neck versus distant metastases at diagnosis (8.1 vs. 3.3 months, $P < 0.001$) correlated with prognosis. Several reports of combined surgery, chemotherapy, and fractionated or hyperfractionated radiotherapy have produced only a small number of long-term survivors (up to several years) with a high incidence of therapeutic complications.[95] Since 60% or more of anaplastic carcinoma patients die of locally infiltrative tumor (suffocation),[99] total thyroidectomy with radical neck dissection is important in the initial management of patients with positive regional lymph nodes and without evidence of distant metastases, and external beam radiotherapy may be of additional symptomatic benefit to patients with local tumor recurrence, even though not prolonging survival.

Levendag and colleagues[100] reported on 51 patients who received external beam irradiation after surgery ($n = 15$), biopsy ($n = 8$), or no surgery ($n = 28$). Forty-one percent had metastases at presentation. Twenty-two patients received doses less than 30 Gy, and only 26 received doses greater than 40 Gy. Ninety-four percent died within 1 year, and 32 had local failure as a component of failure, but inadequate doses were used in the majority of patients. In a separate retrospective review of 67 cases from the Netherlands, complete resection was associated with an improved duration of control and survival over incomplete resection (3-year survival 82% vs. 0%), and suggested an improved outcome for those patients treated postoperatively to doses greater than 45 Gy.[101]

Nineteen patients with localized anaplastic giant and spindle cell carcinoma of the thyroid were treated in a prospective study at MSKCC with once-weekly administration of doxorubicin (10 mg/m^2) 1.5 hours before hyperfractionated radiation (1.6 Gy twice a day, with 4-hour intervals between fractions, for 3 days per week to a total dose of 57.6 Gy in 6 weeks).[102] A complete response rate of 84% was seen, with local control maintained in 13 of the 19 (68%). Survival rate at 2 years, however, was only 20%. Treatment was relatively well tolerated, with most patients requiring a 1-week break during therapy secondary to moderate tracheo-esophagitis. In a separate group of 22 patients with well-differentiated papillary, follicular, or mixed carcinomas treated at the same institution with Adriamycin plus once-a-day irradiation to doses of 56 Gy in 5 weeks, a 91% complete response was seen, with 77% local control and a 5-year survival rate of approximately 50%.

Tennvall reported on 55 patients entered into prospective combined modality trials of hyperfractionated radiotherapy, Adriamycin, and surgery for anaplastic thyroid carcinoma.[103] The three trials differed in the dose per fraction (1.0, 1.3, and 1.6 Gy), and the first two trials had split-course radiation (30 Gy preop, 16 Gy postop) as opposed to 46 Gy preop in the third trial. All received concurrent weekly Adriamycin at a dose of 20 mg. Local control was maintained in 60% of the patients, but median survival was short (2 to 4.5 months). Only 16% of patients survived beyond 1 year.

Primary Thyroid Lymphoma

Primary thyroid lymphomas are rare, representing 2% to 5% of non-Hodgkin's extranodal lymphomas.[104] They are commonly associated with preexisting chronic lymphocytic thyroiditis (more than 60% have a history of Hashimoto's thyroiditis),[105] which leads to the development of a mucosa-associated lymphoid tissue tumor (MALToma). These MALTomas can progress to more aggressive lymphomas, such as diffuse large B-cell lymphomas, which comprise the large majority of cases.[105,106] The 5-year overall survival rate in nine published studies reviewed by Mazzaferri and Oertel[104] averaged 59% (368 patients). If the lymphoma is limited to the thyroid at the time of diagnosis, the 5-year survival rate averages 75% to 85%, compared with 35% to 59% if it has extended beyond the gland at diagnosis. Other factors adversely affecting prognosis are high or intermediate tumor grade, age older than 60 years, and goiter duration less than 6 months.

The pathologic subtype of the lymphoma is used to determine the appropriate therapeutic intervention.[105-107] Therefore, adequate tissue for pathologic analysis is critical. In the past, customary therapy was initially surgery for diagnosis, for relief of local compression symptoms, and for tumor debulking, followed by radiotherapy, an approach that achieved a 55% to 70% 5-year survival rate in patients with more advanced disease.[104] More individualized approaches are associated with better outcomes.[106,107] For patients with a diffuse large B-cell lymphoma, appropriate staging is necessary initially. In patients with stage IE or IIE disease, three to four cycles of CHOP chemotherapy, followed by local radiation (mantle or involved field) to a dose of 36 to 42 Gy, resulted in a 10-year failure-free survival of 91%.[107] Those patients with pure, low-grade MALT lymphomas (without evidence of diffuse large cell components) may be appropriately managed with localized therapy alone, such as radiation,[107] avoiding the risks of surgery or chemotherapy.

CONCLUSION

As outlined, the extent of surgery and appropriate use of ^{131}I therapy are the two most important management factors affecting tumor recurrence and patient survival in well-differentiated thyroid carcinoma. In low-risk patients (tumor size <1.5 cm, age younger than 45 years, no distant metastases at diagnosis) the long-term survival rate is greater than 99%, and limited surgery with no adjuvant therapy is appropriate. The bulk of evidence suggests that ^{131}I ablation of residual thyroid tissue provides reduced recurrence and mortality rates, such ablation clearly provides the advantage of being able to follow the patient better with serial Tg assays and TSH-stimulated diagnostic ^{131}I scans. In patients with medullary and anaplastic carcinoma, the completeness of surgical removal of the tumor provides the greatest survival advantage to the patient. In addition, external beam radiotherapy can be important for regionally symptomatic tumor, as it may also be in advanced stages of disseminated differentiated thyroid carcinoma. Radioiodine therapy has no role at all to play in the management of medullary or anaplastic carcinoma, or in other nonfunctional thyroid tumors such as primary thyroid lymphomas. Adjuvant external beam radiation has a limited but significant role in the treatment of patients with residual disease after surgery in differentiated thyroid carcinomas, a palliative role in anaplastic carcinomas and unresectable medullary or differentiated carcinomas, and a curative role in lymphomas.

REFERENCES

1. ICRP: *Radiation Dose to Patients from Radiopharmaceuticals,* ICRP Publication 53. Oxford: Pergamon Press, 1987.
2. Jemal A, Murray T, Samuels A, et al: Cancer statistics, 2003. *CA Cancer J Clin.* 2003;53:5.
3. Wingo PA, Tong T, Bolden S: Cancer statistics 1995. *CA Cancer J Clin.* 1995;45:8.
4. Young JL Jr, Percy CL, Asire AJ, eds: *Surveillance, Epidemiology and End Results: Incidence and Mortality Data, 1973-77.* Washington, DC: National Cancer Institute Publication NIH 81-2330, 1981.
5. Gililland F, Hunt WC, Morris DM, Key CR: Prognostic factors for thyroid carcinoma: A population-based study of 15,698 cases from the SEER Program 1973-1991. *Cancer.* 1997;79:564.
6. Gimm O: Thyroid cancer. *Cancer Letters.* 2001;163:143.
7. Lemoine NR, Mayall ES, Wyllie FS, et al: High frequency of *ras* oncogene activation in all stages of human thyroid tumorigenesis. *Oncogene.* 1989;4:159.
8. Fagin JA, Matsua K, Karmarkar A, et al: High prevalence of mutations of the *p53* gene in poorly differentiated human thyroid carcinomas. *J Clin Invest.* 1993;91:179.
9. Farid NR, Balazs C: Immunogenetics of thyroiditis and thyroid carcinoma. In Farid NR, ed. *Immunogenetics of Endocrine Disorders.* New York: Alan R Liss; 1988:267.
10. Lote K, Andersen K, Nordal E, et al: Familial occurrence of papillary thyroid carcinoma. *Cancer.* 1980;46:1291.
11. Duffy BJ Jr, Fitzgerald PJ: Cancer of the thyroid in children: A report of twenty-eight cases. *J Clin Endocrinol Metab.* 1950;10:1296.
12. Maxon H, Thomas SR, Saenger EL, et al: Ionizing irradiation and the induction of clinically significant disease in the human thyroid gland. *Am J Med.* 1977;63:967.
13. Modan B, Ron E, Werner A: Thyroid cancer following scalp irradiation. *Radiology.* 1977;123:741.
14. Doniach I: Effects including carcinogenesis of ^{131}I and x-rays on the thyroid of experimental animals: A review. *Health Phys.* 1963;9:1357.
15. Tronko M, Bogdanova T, Komissarenko IV, et al: Thyroid carcinoma in children and adolescents in Ukraine after the Chernobyl nuclear accident. *Cancer.* 1999;86:149.
16. Blackburn D, Michel LA, Rosiere A, et al: Occurrence of thyroid papillary carcinoma in young patients: A Chernobyl connection? *J Ped Endocrin Metab.* 2001;14:503.
17. Dai G, Levy O, Carrasco N: Cloning and characterization of the thyroid iodide transporter. *Nature.* 1996;379;458.
18. Dohan O, De La Vieja A, Paroder V, et al: The sodium/iodide symporter (NIS): Characterization, regulation, and medical significance. *Endocr Rev.* 2003;24:48.
19. Hedinger C, Williams ED, Sobin LH: The WHO histological classification of thyroid tumors: A commentary on the second edition. *Cancer.* 1989;63:908.
20. Mazzaferri EL: Thyroid carcinoma: Papillary and follicular. In Mazzaferri EL, Samaan NA, eds. *Endocrine Tumors.* Boston: Blackwell Scientific Publications; 1993:278.

21. Robbins J, Merino MJ, Boice JD Jr, et al: Thyroid cancer: A lethal endocrine neoplasm. *Ann Intern Med.* 1991;115:133.

22. McIver B, Hay ID, et al: Anaplastic thyroid carcinoma: A 50-year experience at a single institution. *Surgery.* 2001;130:1028.

23. Carcingui M, Steeper T, Zampi G, Rosai J: Anaplastic thyroid carcinoma. *Am J Clin Path.* 1985;83:135.

24. Hazard JB, Kaufman N: A survey of thyroid glands obtained at autopsy in a so-called goiter area. *Am J Clin Pathol.* 1952;22:860.

25. Ludwig G, Nishiyama RH: The prevalence of occult papillary carcinoma in 100 consecutive autopsies in an American population. Presented at the 65th Annual Meeting of the International Academy of Pathology; 1976; Boston.

26. Fukunaga FH, Yatani R: Geographic pathology of occult thyroid carcinomas. *Cancer.* 1975;36:1095.

27. Harach HR, Franssila KO, Wasenius V-M: Occult papillary carcinoma of the thyroid. A "normal" finding in Finland. A systematic autopsy study. *Cancer.* 1985;56:531.

28. Hay ID, Grant CS, van Heerden JA, et al: Papillary thyroid microcarcinoma: A study of 535 cases observed in a 50-year period. *Surgery.* 1992;112:1139.

29. Mazzaferri EL, Jhiang SM: Long-term impact of initial surgical and medical therapy on papillary and follicular thyroid cancer. *Am J Med.* 1994;97:418.

30. Mazzaferri EL, de los Santos ET, Rofagha-Keyhani S: Solitary thyroid nodule: Diagnosis and management. *Med Clin North Am.* 1988;72:1177.

31. Mazzaferri EL: Thyroid cancer in thyroid nodules: Finding a needle in a haystack. *Am J Med.* 1992;93:359.

32. Vander JB, Gaston EA, Dawber TR: Significance of solitary nontoxic thyroid nodules. *N Engl J Med.* 1954;251:970.

33. Vander JB, Gaston EA, Dawber TW: The significance of nontoxic thyroid nodules: Final report of a 15 year study of the incidence of thyroid malignancy. *Ann Intern Med.* 1968;69:537.

34. Mortensen JD, Woolner LB, Bennett WA: Gross and microscopic findings in clinically normal thyroid glands. *J Clin Endocrinol Metab.* 1955;15:1270.

35. Ashcraft MW, van Herle AJ: Management of thyroid nodules: II. Scanning techniques, thyroid suppressive therapy, and fine needle aspiration. *Head Neck Surg.* 1981;3:297.

36. Belfiore A, La Rosa GL, La Porta GA, et al: Cancer risk in patients with cold thyroid nodules: Relevance of iodine intake, sex, age, and multinodularity. *Am J Med.* 1992;93:363.

37. Hoffman GL, Thompson NW, Heffron C: The solitary thyroid nodule: A reassessment. *Arch Surg.* 1972;105:379.

38. Caruso D, Mazzaferri EL: Fine needle aspiration biopsy in the management of thyroid nodules. *Endocrinologist.* 1991;1:194.

39. Ringel M: Molecular diagnostic tests in the diagnosis and management of thyroid carcinoma. *Rev Endocr Metab Disord.* 2000; 1:173.

40. Mazzaferri EL, Jhiang SM. Long-term impact of initial surgical and medical therapy on papillary and follicular thyroid cancer. *Am J Med.* 1994;97:418.

41. Lakshmanan M, Schaffer A, Robbins J, et al: A simplified low iodine diet in I-131 scanning and therapy of thyroid cancer. *Clin Nucl Med.* 1988;13:866.

42. Robbins RJ, Tuttle RM, Sharaf RN, et al: Preparation by recombinant human thyrotropin or thyroid hormone withdrawal are comparable for the detection of residual differentiated thyroid carcinoma. *J Clin Endocrinol Metab.* 2001;86:619.

43. Abdel-Dayem HM, Scott AM, Macapinlac HA, et al: Role of ²⁰¹Tl chloride and ⁹⁹ᵐTc sestamibi in tumor imaging. In Freeman LM, ed. *Nuclear Medicine Annual 1994.* New York: Raven Press; 1994:181.

44. Charkes ND, Vitti RA, Brooks K: Thallium-201 SPECT increases detectability of thyroid cancer metastases. *J Nucl Med.* 1990; 31:147.

45. Brendel AJ, Guyot M, Jeandot R, et al: Thallium-201 in the follow-up of differentiated thyroid carcinoma. *J Nucl Med.* 1988; 29:1515.

46. Yen T-C, Lin H-D, Lee C-H, et al: The role of technetium-99m sestamibi whole-body scans in diagnosing metastatic Hürthle cell carcinoma of the thyroid gland after total thyroidectomy: A comparison with iodine-131 and thallium-201 whole-body scans. *Eur J Nucl Med.* 1994;21:980.

47. Blahd WH, Khonsary SA, Brown CV, et al: Thyroid cancer imaging with PET FDG. *J Nucl Med.* 1993;34:12P.

48. Larson SM, Robbins R. Positron emission tomography in thyroid cancer management. *Semin Roentgenol.* 2002;37:169.

49. Wang W, Larson SM, Fazzari M, Tickoo SK, Kolbert K, Sgouros G, Yeung H, Macapinlac H, Rosai J, Robbins RJ. Prognostic value of [18F]fluorodeoxyglucose positron emission tomographic scanning in patients with thyroid cancer. *J Clin Endocrinol Metab.* 2000 Mar;85(3):1107-13.

50. Wang W, Larson SM, Tuttle RM, et al: Resistance of [18f]-fluorodeoxyglucose-avid metastatic thyroid cancer lesions to treatment with high-dose radioactive iodine. *Thyroid.* 2001; 11:1169.

51. Gooding GAW: Sonography of the thyroid and parathyroid. *Radiol Clin N Amer.* 1993;31:967.

52. Franceschi M, Kusic Z, Franceschi D, et al: Thyroglobulin determination, neck ultrasonography and iodine-131 whole-body scintigraphy in differentiated thyroid carcinoma. *J Nucl Med.* 1996;37:446.

53. Byar DP, Green SB, Dor P, et al: A prognostic index for thyroid carcinoma: A study of the EORTC Thyroid Cancer Cooperative Group. *Eur J Cancer.* 1979;15:1033.

54. Hay ID, Grant CS, Taylor WF, et al: Ipsilateral lobectomy versus bilateral lobar resection in papillary thyroid carcinoma: A retrospective analysis of surgical outcome using a novel prognostic scoring system. *Surgery.* 1987;102:1088.

55. Hay ID, Bergstralh EJ, Goellner JR, et al: Predicting outcome in papillary thyroid carcinoma: Development of a reliable prognostic scoring system in a cohort of 1779 patients surgically treated at one institution during 1940 through 1989. *Surgery.* 1993; 114:1050.

56. Cady B, Rossi R: An expanded view of risk-group definition in differentiated thyroid carcinoma. *Surgery.* 1988;104:947.

57. Carey JE, Kumpuris TM, Wrobel MC: Release of patients containing therapeutic dosages of iodine-131 from hospitals. *J Nucl Med Technol.* 1995;23:144.

58. Maxon HR III, Englaro EE, Thomas SR, et al: Radioiodine-131 therapy for well differentiated thyroid cancer: A quantitative radiation dosimetric approach: Outcome and validation in 85 patients. *J Nucl Med.* 1992;33:1132.

59. Robbins RJ, Larson SM, Sinha N, et al: A retrospective review of the effectiveness of recombinant human TSH as a preparation for radioiodine thyroid remnant ablation. *J Nucl Med.* 2002; 43:1482.

60. Benua R, Cicale N, Sonenberg M, Rawson R: The relation of radioiodine dosimetry to results and complications in the treatment of metastatic thyroid cancer. *AJR.* 1962;87:171.

61. McHenry C, Jarosz H, Davis M, et al: Selective postoperative radioactive iodine treatment of thyroid cancer. *Surgery.* 1989; 106:956.

62. Pacini F, Lippi F, Formica N, et al: Therapeutic doses of iodine-131 reveal undiagnosed metastases in thyroid cancer patients with detectable serum thyroglobulin levels. *J Nucl Med.* 1987;28:1888.

63. Pineda JD, Lee T, Ain K, et al: Iodine-131 therapy for thyroid cancer patients with elevated thyroglobulin and negative diagnostic scan. *J Clin Endocrinol Metab.* 1995;80:1488.

64. Allweiss P, Braunstein GD, Katz A, Waxman A: Sialadenitis following I-131 therapy for thyroid carcinoma: Concise communication. *J Nucl Med.* 1984;25:755.

65. Sarkar SD, Beierwaltes WH, Gill SP, Cowley BJ: Subsequent fertility and birth histories of children and adolescents treated with ¹³¹I for thyroid cancer. *J Nucl Med.* 1976;17:460.

66. Maxon H III, Smith HS: Radioiodine-131 in the diagnosis and treatment of metastatic well differentiated thyroid cancer. *Endocrinol Metab Clin North Am.* 1990;19:685.

67. Hall P, Holm LE, Lundell G, et al: Cancer risks in thyroid cancer patients. *Br J Cancer.* 1991;64:159.

68. Edmonds CJ, Smith T: The long-term hazards of the treatment of thyroid cancer with radioiodine. *Br J Radiol.* 1986;59:45.

69. Holm L-E, Hall P, Wiklund K, et al: Cancer risk after iodine-131 therapy for hyperthyroidism. *J Natl Cancer Inst.* 1991;83:1072.

70. Rouvière H: Sur quelques connexions ganglionnaires non encore de©<pi>aacrites des lymphatiques du corps thyroide. *Ann Anat Pathol (Paris).* 1929;6:222.

71. McCormack KR, Sheline GE: Retropharyngeal spread of carcinoma of the thyroid. *Cancer.* 1970;26:1366.

72. Tubiana M, Haddad E, Schlumberger M, et al: External radiotherapy in thyroid cancers. *Cancer.* 1985;55:2062.

73. O'Connell ME, A'Hern RP, Harmer CL: Results of external beam radiotherapy in differentiated thyroid carcinoma: A retrospective study from the Royal Marsden Hospital. *Eur J Cancer.* 1994;6:733.

74. Tsang RW, Brierley JD, et al: The effects of surgery, radioiodine, and external radiation therapy on the clinical outcome of patients with differentiated thyroid carcinoma. *Cancer.* 1998;82:375.

75. Chow SM, Law SC, et al: Papillary thyroid carcinoma: prognostic factors and the role of radioiodine and external radiotherapy. *Int J Radiat Oncol Biol Phys.* 2002;52:784.

76. Tubiana M: External radiotherapy and radionuclide in the treatment of thyroid cancer. *World J Surg.* 1981;5:75.

77. Leeper RD: Thyroid cancer. *Med Clin North Am.* 1985;69:1079.

78. Schlumberger M, Tubiana M, De Vathaire F, et al: Long-term results of treatment of 283 patients with lung and bone metastases from differentiated thyroid carcinoma. *J Clin Endocrinol Metab.* 1986;63:960.

79. Sheline GE, Galante M, Lindsay S: Radiation therapy in the control of persistent thyroid cancer. *Am J Roentgenol Radium Ther Nucl Med.* 1966;97:923.

80. Posner MD, Quivey JM, et al: Dose optimization for the treatment of anaplastic thyroid carcinoma: a comparison of treatment planning techniques. *Int J Radiat Oncol Biol Phys.* 2000;48:475.

81. Nutting CM, Convery DJ, et al: Improvements in target coverage and reduced spinal cord irradiation using intensity-modulated radiotherapy (IMRT) in patients with carcinoma of the thyroid gland. *Radiother Oncol.* 2001;60:173.

82. Hay ID: Papillary thyroid carcinoma. *Endocrinol Metab Clin North Am.* 1990;19:545.

83. DeGroot LJ, Kaplan EL, McCormick M, Straus FH: Natural history, treatment, and course of papillary thyroid carcinoma. *J Clin Endocrinol Metab.* 1990;71:414.

84. Rossi RL, Cady B, Silverman ML, et al: Surgically incurable well-differentiated thyroid carcinoma: Prognostic factors and results of therapy. *Arch Surg.* 1988;123:569.

85. Nemec J, Zamracil V, Pohunkova D, Rohling S: Radioiodine treatment of pulmonary metastases of differentiated thyroid cancer: Results and prognostic factors. *Nuklearmedizin.* 1979;8:86.

86. Johansen K, Woodhouse NJY, Odugbesan O: Comparison of 1073 MBq and 3700 MBq iodine-131 in postoperative ablation of residual thyroid tissue in patients with differentiated thyroid cancer. *J Nucl Med.* 1991;32:252.

87. Grauer A, Raue F, Gagel RF: Changing concepts in the management of hereditary and sporadic medullary thyroid carcinoma. *Endocrinol Metab Clin North Am.* 1990;19:613.

88. Samaan NA, Ordonez NG, Hickey RC: Medullary thyroid carcinoma. In Mazzaferri EL, Samaan NA, eds. *Endocrine Tumors.* Boston: Blackwell Scientific; 1993;334.

89. Tisell L, Hansson G, Jansson S, et al: Reoperation in the treatment of asymptomatic metastasizing medullary thyroid carcinoma. *Surgery.* 1986;99:60.

90. Raue F, Winter J, Spath-Roger M: Register of medullary thyroid carcinoma in Germany. *Henry Ford Hosp Med J.* 1989;37:206.

91. Giuffrida D, Gharib H: Current diagnosis and management of medullary thyroid carcinoma. *Ann Oncol.* 1998;9:695.

92. Vitale G, Caraglia M, et al: Current approaches and perspectives in the therapy of medullary thyroid carcinoma. *Cancer.* 2001; 91:1797.

93. Samaan NA, Schultz PN, Hickey RC: Medullary thyroid carcinoma: Prognosis of familial versus sporadic disease and the role of radiotherapy. *J Clin Endocrinol Metab.* 1988;67:801.

94. Nguyen TD, Chassard JL, Lagarde P, et al: Results of postoperative radiation therapy in medullary carcinoma of the thyroid: A retrospective study by the French Federation of Cancer Institutes-the Radiotherapy Cooperative Group. *Radiother Oncol.* 1992;23:1.

95. Aldinger KA, Samaan NA, Ibanez ML, et al: Anaplastic carcinoma of the thyroid: A review of 84 cases of spindle and giant cell carcinoma of the thyroid. *Cancer.* 1978;41:2267.

96. Mazzaferri EL: Undifferentiated thyroid carcinoma and unusual thyroid malignancies. In Mazzaferri EL, Samaan NA, eds. *Endocrine Tumors.* Boston: Blackwell Scientific; 1993;378.

97. Woolner LB, Beahrs OH, Black BM, et al: Classification and prognosis of thyroid carcinoma: A study of 885 cases observed in a thirty year period. *Am J Surg.* 1961;102:354.

98. Venkatesh YSS, Ordonez NG, Schultz PN, et al: Anaplastic carcinoma of the thyroid: A clinicopathologic study of 121 cases. *Cancer.* 1990;66:321.

99. Tallroth E, Wallin G, Lundell G, et al: Multimodality treatment in anaplastic giant cell thyroid carcinoma. *Cancer.* 1987;60:1428.

100. Levendag PC, De Porre PM, van Putten WL: Anaplastic carcinoma of the thyroid gland treated by radiation therapy. *Int J Radiat Oncol Biol Phys.* 1993;26:125.

101. Pierie JP, Muzikansky A, et al: The effect of surgery and radiotherapy on outcome of anaplastic thyroid carcinoma. *Ann Surg Oncol.* 2002;9:57.

102. Kim JH, Leeper RD: Treatment of locally advanced thyroid carcinoma with combination doxorubicin and radiation therapy. *Cancer.* 1987;60:2372.

103. Tennvall J, Lundell G, et al: Anaplastic thyroid carcinoma: three protocols combining doxorubicin, hyperfractionated radiotherapy and surgery. *Br J Cancer.* 2002;86:1848.

104. Mazzaferri EL, Oertel YC: Primary malignant thyroid lymphoma and related lymphoproliferative disorders. In Mazzaferri EL, Samaan NA, eds. *Endocrine Tumors.* Boston: Blackwell Scientific; 1993;348.

105. Thieblemont C, Mayer A, Dumontet C, et al: Primary lymphoma is a heterogeneous disease. *J Clin Endocrinol Metab.* 2002; 87:105.

106. Belal A, Allam A, Kandil A, et al: Primary thyroid lymphoma. *Am J Clin Oncol.* 2001;24:299.

107. Ha C, Shadle KM, Medeiros LJ, et al: Localized NHL involving the thyroid gland. *Cancer.* 2001;91:629.

Tumors of the Lung, Pleura, and Mediastinum

35

Kenneth E. Rosenzweig, MD and Lee M. Krug, MD

EPIDEMIOLOGY AND ETIOLOGY

Incidence and Mortality

Lung cancer is the leading cause of cancer mortality for men and women, exceeding the combined mortality of breast, ovarian, and cervical cancers combined for women and prostate cancer for men.[1] An estimated 171,900 new cases of lung cancer and 157,200 deaths from lung cancer occurred in 2003.

Smoking and Lung Cancer

The epidemiologic data on smoking and lung cancer fulfill the criteria for causal association, including the consistency of results across studies, the strength of relationship, its specificity, the correct temporal sequence between exposure and disease, and the coherence of the association as evidenced by a dose-response relationship.[2]

It is estimated that cigarette smoking causes 90% of all lung cancers.[3] Multiple genetic alterations of tumor suppressor genes and oncogenes can lead to the pathogenesis of lung cancer. Carcinogens in cigarette smoke are involved in these genetic alterations, mainly through the formation of DNA adducts.[4]

There is a clear dose-response relationship between the risk of lung cancer and the number of cigarettes smoked per day, the degree of inhalation, and the age at initiation of smoking.[5] The relative risk of developing lung cancer decreases as the time from cessation increases.[5]

Occupation and Lung Cancer

Increases in lung cancer risk accompany exposure to carcinogens such as asbestos, radon, bis(chloromethyl) ether, polycyclic aromatic hydrocarbons, chromium, nickel, and inorganic arsenic compounds.[6,7] The association with occupational exposure to these agents appears to be independent of cigarette smoking.

In addition, a number of occupations with high smoking prevalence have increased cancer risk. Women who work as waitresses, cashiers, nurses' aides, and orderlies have smoking prevalences in excess of 40%, as do men who labor as drivers, construction workers, painters, mechanics, and watchmen.[8]

Radon and Lung Cancer

Approximately 10% of lung cancers are thought to be caused by carcinogens other than cigarette smoking. Among nonsmokers, 30% of lung cancer deaths are attributed to radon exposure.[3]

Diet and Lung Cancer

The incidence of lung cancer appears to be inversely related to the intake of many food groups, including dietary carotenoids such as beta carotene and lycopene.[9] The mechanism of this interaction is theorized to be related to scavenging of free radicals or through antioxidative effects.

Chemoprevention of Lung Cancer

The goal of chemoprevention is to use an intervention that can interrupt, arrest, or reverse carcinogenesis.[10] An early, positive trial in the use of chemoprevention demonstrated that the use of 13-cis-retinoic acid led to a decrease of the incidence of second primary cancers (including lung) in patients with treated head and neck cancer.

ANATOMY

Lung

The external anatomy of the lung is dominated by the fissures and the concave cardiac notch on each lung. On both lungs, the oblique fissure extends from the surface of the lung to the hilum and divides the lung into upper and lower lobes, which are connected only by the lobar bronchi and vessels. On the right lung, a horizontal fissure passes from the anterior margin into the oblique fissure to separate the wedge-shaped middle lobe from the upper lobe. This separation is incomplete in most patients. The visceral pleura covering the surface of the lung extends inward to line the depths of the fissures. The trachea divides into a left and right main stem bronchus at the carina. The right main stem bronchus (approximately 4.5 cm long) gives off a right upper lobe bronchus and continues as the bronchus intermedius, which separates into middle and lower lobe bronchi. The left main stem bronchus gives off three branches, but the upper and middle ones are fused before they separate into the upper lobe and lingular lobe. The other branch is the lower lobe bronchus. Each lobar bronchus in turn gives off segmental bronchi totaling 10 segments on each side of the lung.

PATHOGENESIS AND HISTOLOGY

Pathogenesis

There is increasing evidence that lung cancer is derived from a pluripotent stem cell capable of expressing various phenotypes. This epithelial stem cell, in normal histogenesis, differentiates into those cells found in the tracheobronchial tree, including pseudostratified reserved cells, ciliated goblet columnar cells, and neuroendocrine cells as type I and II pneumocytes seen lining the alveoli. Those cells that are capable of division can express hyperplastic, metaplastic, or neoplastic change. Lung cancer may exhibit two or more histologic patterns; the frequency of this occurrence may depend on the number of sections examined. In one study, when at least 10 blocks from each tumor were examined, 45 of the 100 cases showed elements of both squamous cell carcinoma and adenocarcinoma.[11]

SQUAMOUS CELL CARCINOMA

Squamous cell carcinoma arises most frequently in proximal bronchi and is associated with squamous metaplasia and carcinoma in situ. Histologically, the squamous cell tumor is composed of sheets of epithelial cells that may be well or poorly differentiated. Most well-differentiated tumors demonstrate keratin pearl formation. The more poorly differentiated tumors, if determined to be squamous cell carcinomas, have positive keratin staining.

ADENOCARCINOMA

Adenocarcinoma is now the most frequent tumor, accounting for 40% of all lung cancer. Some of this increase is due to better identification of adenocarcinoma, with fewer tumors being classified as undifferentiated large cell tumors. The majority of these tumors are peripheral in origin, arising from surface epithelium or bronchial mucosal glands and can also be seen arising as peripheral scar tumors. Histologically, these tumors form glands and produce mucin. Bronchoalveolar carcinomas arise from type II pneumocytes and grow along alveolar septa, showing little desmoplastic or glandular change. These tumors may present in three different fashions: a solitary peripheral nodule, multifocal disease, or a progressive pneumonic form that appears to spread from lobe to lobe, ultimately encompassing both lungs.

LARGE CELL CARCINOMA

This tumor is the least common of all non–small cell lung (NSCLC) cancers, accounting for approximately 15% of all lung cancers. Using histochemical staining, electron microscopy, and monoclonal antibodies, many tumors previously diagnosed as undifferentiated large cell carcinoma can now be classified more appropriately as poorly differentiated adenocarcinoma or squamous cell carcinoma. For this reason, the incidence of this type of tumor continues to decrease.

IMMUNOHISTOCHEMISTRY

Thyroid transcription factor 1 (TTF-1) is frequently expressed in lung cancers, especially adenocarcinomas and small cell lung cancers. It is helpful in distinguishing lung cancers from other thoracic malignancies.

CLINICAL PRESENTATION

The signs and symptoms manifested by patients suffering from lung cancer depend on the location of the tumor, its locoregional spread, and the effects of metastatic growth. Lung cancer is also associated with paraneoplastic syndromes more frequently than any other tumor. In addition, due to direct effects of locoregional disease, metastases, or general paraneoplastic processes, many patients have anorexia, weight loss, and a decline in performance status at diagnosis. Some patients present with an asymptomatic lesion discovered incidentally on a chest x-ray study.

Routine screening for lung cancer is being investigated once again. In a pilot study of 1000 patients older than age 60 with more than 10 pack-years of smoking, routine screening with low-dose thoracic computed tomography (CT) scans found almost four times as many cancers as chest x-ray alone, and these lesions were six times as likely to be early stage and therefore more curable.[12] Currently, a large national trial is under way to rigorously assess the benefit of screening in this population.

Diagnostic and Staging Procedures

HISTORY AND PHYSICAL EXAMINATION

A detailed history should elicit tobacco use and past exposure to environmental carcinogens, which may suggest a higher probability of lung cancer. Symptoms of metastatic disease in the bone and brain can also be determined. Weight loss of greater than 5% from baseline is one of the most important prognostic indicators in lung cancer treatment. Patients can present with signs and symptoms of paraneoplastic syndromes, more frequently in small cell lung cancer than NSCLCs.

Physical examination of the chest may detect signs of partial or complete obstruction of airways, atelectasis, pneumonia, or pleural effusion. Examination of the neck can reveal evidence of supraclavicular lymphadenopathy, indicative of N3 disease. Lymphadenopathy in the high neck or axilla may represent metastatic disease. Abdominal examination may detect hepatomegaly. Neurologic examination can detect cerebral, base of skull, or spinal cord metastases.

Laboratory studies should include complete blood count, liver function tests, and serum lactate dehydrogenase. Elevated alkaline phosphatase may indicate liver or bone disease. Renal function tests should be performed to assess whether the patient can tolerate intravenous contrast for radiologic examinations and certain types of chemotherapy.

SPUTUM CYTOLOGY

With three sputum samples, up to 80% of central tumors can be diagnosed. The yield is much smaller for peripheral tumors, dropping to less than 20% for peripheral tumors less than 3 cm in diameter.

IMAGING STUDIES

Chest x-ray remains an extremely valuable tool in the diagnosis of lung cancer. However, CT has enormous advantages in its ability to detect lesions that cannot be resolved on chest x-ray. It also plays an important role in staging lung cancer, especially spread to areas of the mediastinum undetected on plain films. Typically, a lymph node is considered normal if it is less than 1 cm in diameter on its short axis. CT may also suggest possible areas of local invasion of the primary tumor to the chest wall, vertebrae, or mediastinal structures. Small pleural effusions or pleural nodules, often undetected on plain films, may be evident on CT. A CT of the chest for lung cancer evaluation should also include part of the upper abdomen, which allows for evaluation of the liver and adrenals for metastatic disease. 18-fluoro-deoxy-glucose positron emission tomography (FDG-PET) scanning can also detect neoplastic activity. Studies have shown CT and PET to be more specific and sensitive than just CT alone.[13] Generally, the sensitivity, specificity, and accuracy of CT scan alone is approximately 70%. CT + PET has an accuracy rate of approximately 90% in single institution studies, although these results may worsen when the technique is studied over multiple institutions. Magnetic resonance imaging (MRI) has not been shown to be more effective than chest CT for lung tumors, but may be helpful in evaluating invasion of the vertebral bodies and the mediastinum.

BRONCHOSCOPY

Using flexible fiberoptic instruments, the proximal tracheobronchial tree can be examined up to the second or third subsegmental subdivision and cytologic or histologic specimens can be obtained. When a visible lesion is identified, the diagnostic yield is well over 90%. Even with no visible lesion, the area of suspicion can be irrigated and lavaged, obtaining cytologic material. Using fiberoptic bronchoscopy and image intensification, peripheral lesions can be reached by cytology brushes, needles, or biopsy forceps, and specimens can be obtained. This is especially effective for lesions greater than 2 cm in diameter. The bronchoscope is also a valuable tool for staging. The site of a primary tumor in a major airway may affect its T-classification, and transbronchoscopic needle aspiration through its airway wall can confirm the presence of a malignancy in mediastinal lymph nodes.

New endobronchial techniques are being developed to detect early lung cancer. Autofluorescence bronchoscopy (AFB) is more sensitive in detecting premalignant and malignant mucosal change as compared to white light bronchoscopy.[14] AFB might also be helpful in detecting dysplastic endobronchial lesions and determination of resection margins. Endobronchial ultrasonography allows detailed imaging of the bronchial wall and peri-bronchial mediastinum and may also add to the evaluation of endobronchial lesions.[14]

MEDIASTINOSCOPY AND MEDIASTINOTOMY

Mediastinoscopy is the most accurate technique to assess superior mediastinal lymph nodes, which are frequently involved in NSCLC. The procedure is simple, safe, and effective in experienced hands. In one large series, the complication rate from cervical mediastinoscopy was 2.3% and the mortality was 0%.[15] In patients suspected of having inoperable disease by virtue of mediastinal involvement as detected by CT scanning, confirmation by mediastinoscopy is indicated. For patients who are potentially operable, it is especially important to sample contralateral mediastinal lymph nodes, to determine if N3 disease is present. Involvement of aorticopulmonary lymph nodes is typically assessed by anterior mediastinotomy (Chamberlain procedure).[16] It is important to remember that these are first-echelon mediastinal lymph nodes for left lung tumors, especially from the left upper lobe, and they may not be sampled when a cervical mediastinoscopy is performed.

THORACOSCOPY

Video-assisted thoracoscopy has been used in the diagnosis and staging of NSCLC. Peripheral nodules can be identified and biopsied or excised using video-assisted techniques, and mediastinal lymph nodes can be sampled for histologic examination. This technique can identify suspected pleural disease and has the ability to accurately assess the status of pleural effusions.

EXTENT OF DISEASE EVALUATION

In 1997, the American Society of Clinical Oncology published guidelines for the workup and treatment of NSCLC. They recommended that in patients without evidence of metastatic disease, a chest x-ray and chest CT are adequate to stage locoregional disease, with biopsy of mediastinal lymph nodes found on CT scan to be greater than 1 cm in shortest transverse diameter. Bone scan and head CAT scan were recommended only when signs or symptoms of disease were present. If a patient is otherwise potentially resectable, a biopsy of a radiographically documented, isolated adrenal or hepatic mass should be performed to rule out metastatic disease.[17]

STAGING OF LUNG CANCER

In 1988, a Tumor Node Metastasis (TNM) staging system that included clinical, surgical, and pathologic assessment was adopted. Using pretreatment minimally invasive techniques only, a significant percentage of patients are clinically understaged compared with the ultimate stage identified by surgical and pathologic staging. The 2002 American Joint Committee on Cancer Staging system is presented in Table 35-1. A diagram of the mediastinal lymph node staging is presented in Figure 35-1. In general, patients being considered for surgical resection are more likely to undergo invasive staging procedures such as mediastinoscopy than patients considered for nonsurgical approaches. Even though pleural and pericardial effusions are technically stage IIIB, they are typically treated in the same fashion as metastatic patients. In our clinical practice, we commonly refer to stage IIIB patients as either "wet" (with an effusion) or "dry" (without an effusion and possibly curable).

PROGNOSTIC FACTORS

Early-Stage (I or II) Non–Small Cell Lung Cancer

The major prognostic determinant for this group is the stage of disease, particularly the size of the tumor and presence or absence of lymph node spread.[18] Sawyer and colleagues reported that in patients with resected N1 disease, positive bronchoscopic findings, smaller tumor size, and a greater number of resected N1 nodes were associated with an improvement in clinical outcome.[19]

Advanced-Stage (III or IV) Non–Small Cell Lung Cancer

Pretreatment stage, performance status, and weight loss are most important.[20] The definitions of weight

---

Table 35–1   Classification of Non–Small Cell Lung Cancer

Primary Tumor (T)

TX	Primary tumor cannot be assessed, or tumor proven by the presence of malignant cells in sputum or bronchial washings but not visualized by imaging or bronchoscopy
T0	No evidence of primary tumor
Tis	Carcinoma in situ
T1	Tumor ≤3 cm in greatest dimension, surrounded by lung or visceral pleura, without bronchoscopic evidence of invasion more proximal than the lobar bronchus (i.e., not in the main bronchus)
T2	Tumor with any of the following features of size or extent: • >3 cm in greatest dimension • Involves main bronchus, ≥2 cm distal to the carina • Invades the visceral pleura • Associated with atelectasis or obstructive pneumonitis that extends to the hilar region but does not involve the entire lung
T3	Tumor of any size that directly invades any of the following: chest wall (including superior sulcus tumors), diaphragm, mediastinal pleura, parietal pericardium; or tumor in the main bronchus <2 cm distal to the carina, but without involvement of the carina; or associated atelectasis or obstructive pneumonitis of the entire lung
T4	Tumor of any size that invades any of the following: mediastinum, heart, great vessels, trachea, esophagus, vertebral body, carina; or separate tumor nodules in the same lobe; or tumor with malignant pleural effusion

Regional Lymph Nodes (N)

NX	Regional lymph nodes cannot be assessed
N0	No regional lymph node metastasis
N1	Metastasis to ipsilateral peribronchial or ipsilateral hilar lymph nodes, or both, and intrapulmonary nodes including involvement by direct extension of the primary tumor
N2	Metastasis to ipsilateral mediastinal or subcarinal lymph nodes, or both
N3	Metastasis to contralateral mediastinal, contralateral hilar, ipsilateral or contralateral scalene, or supraclavicular lymph nodes

Distant Metastasis (M0)

MX	Distant metastasis cannot be assessed
M0	No distant metastasis
M1	Distant metastasis present

Stage Grouping

Occult carcinoma	TX	N0	M0
0	Tis	N0	M0
IA	T1	N0	M0
IB	T2	N0	M0
IIA	T1	N1	M0
IIB	T2	N1	M0
	T3	N0	M0
IIIA	T1	N2	M0
	T2	N2	M0
	T3	N1	M0
	T3	N2	M0
IIIB	Any T	N3	M0
	T4	Any N	M0
IV	Any T	Any N	M1

Residual Tumor

RX	Presence of residual tumor cannot be assessed
R0	No residual tumor
R1	Microscopic residual tumor
R2	Macroscopic residual tumor

From Greene FL, Page DL, Fleming ID, et al, eds: *AJCC Cancer Staging Manual,* 6th ed. New York: Springer, 2002.

loss have varied among researchers, but weight loss of greater than 5% over the past 6 months is frequently used. Serum lactate dehydrogenase, a predictor of survival in small cell lung cancer and other malignancies, also appears to be an independent survival variable. Whether any specific metastatic disease site confers a survival advantage remains controversial. Bone and liver metastases have often been cited as predicting shorter survival. Isolated spleen metastases, though rare, might be associated with a better outcome.[21] The histologic subtype of NSCLC has little influence on survival in advanced disease.

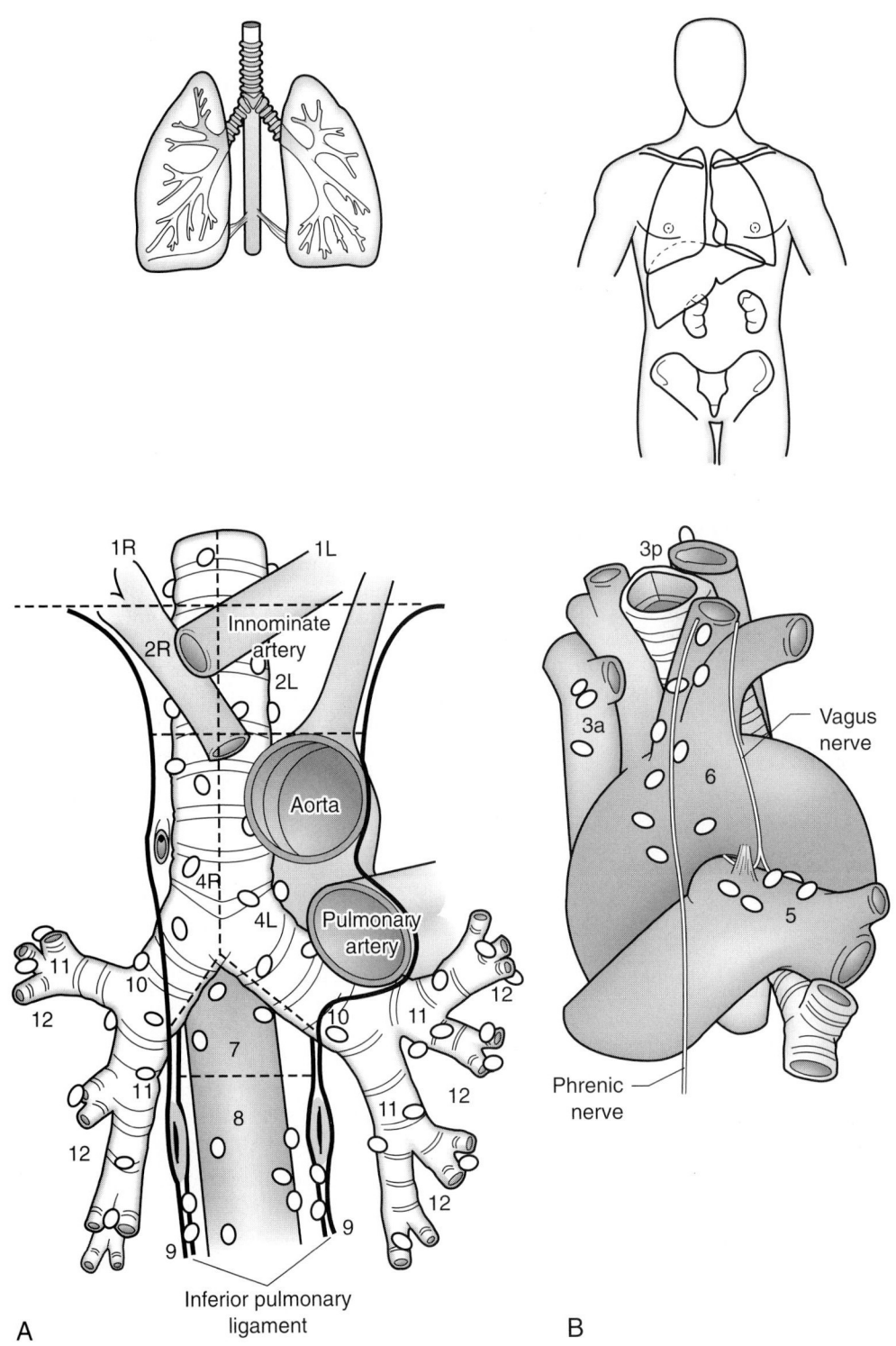

Figure 35–1. Staging of lung cancer.

NON–SMALL CELL LUNG CANCER

Standard Therapeutic Approaches

SELECTION OF THERAPY

Patients with stage I and II disease who are medically fit are treated surgically with very good results. If such patients are medically unfit or refuse surgery, then definitive radiation therapy (RT) offers a potential curative alternative. Selected patients with stage I and II disease are treated with postoperative RT. Chemotherapy is not recommended as standard therapy postoperatively in early-stage disease but is being evaluated.

Stage III disease is a very heterogeneous entity. Practically, it is often easier to consider patients as having either operable, marginally operable, or inoperable tumors. Marginally operable disease consists of tumors that might become operable if they are successfully treated with induction chemotherapy. A typical scenario might be a large central lung tumor that would require pneumonectomy initially, but with tumor shrinkage might be treated with a lobectomy.

There are many reasons that a tumor may be considered unresectable, including: cytologically positive effusions, vertebral body invasion, invasion/encasement of the great vessels, tumor extensively involving the carina or trachea, recurrent laryngeal nerve paralysis, extensive mediastinal lymph node metastases, and N3 disease. A patient may be medically inoperable due to severe coronary artery disease, cor pulmonale, patient refusal, or poor pulmonary function.

The use of neoadjuvant and adjuvant treatment in operable stage III disease is still being determined. There is ample evidence that for many specific situations, the addition of chemotherapy and possibly postoperative RT can improve survival and decrease tumor recurrence.

Stage IV disease is incurable and treatment is palliative. Traditionally this has consisted of palliative chemotherapy, palliative RT, medications, supportive care, and hospice care.

OPERABLE NON–SMALL CELL LUNG CANCER

PATIENT SELECTION

The preoperative assessment of patients considered for surgical treatment of lung cancer includes clinical staging of the disease to assess its resectability, assessment of the cardiopulmonary reserve of the patient to determine whether the intended pulmonary resection is possible, and assessment of the patient with regard to the perioperative risk of the procedure. Traditionally, patients are suitable candidates for pneumonectomy if the ultimate forced expiratory volume in 1 second (FEV 1) is greater that 1.2 L, the patient does not suffer from hypercarbia, and cor pulmonale is not present.[22,23,24] Pulmonary function studies best suited to assess these parameters include spirometry, arterial blood gases, diffusion capacity and, where indicated, ventilation-perfusion scans to estimate the proportions of functioning pulmonary tissue required

to be excised. Patients requiring lobectomy or lesser resections require similar pulmonary function parameters.[25,26] Pulmonary complications increase remarkably when the FEV 1 forced vital capacity (FVC) ratio is below 75% of predicted, indicating significant airway obstruction. FEV 1/FVC ratios of less than 50% of predicted lead to unacceptable postoperative morbidity and mortality.

TECHNIQUE

If complete excision can be obtained by lobectomy, results are equal to those of pneumonectomy.[27] In proximally situated tumors, in which a pneumonectomy may be required for total excision, lung-conserving operations using bronchoplastic procedures to preserve uninvolved lobes (e.g., sleeve lobectomy) have been demonstrated to be feasible, but may have higher local recurrence rates. The role of mediastinal lymphadenectomy as part of the surgical procedure remains hotly debated. Complete mediastinal lymphadenectomy provides the best possible surgical staging by removing all lymph nodes, which can then be analyzed pathologically for metastatic involvement. This can help to identify patents who may require postoperative adjuvant RT. At minimum, for accurate final surgical-pathologic staging, lymph node sampling of all draining areas should be performed at the time of surgical resection. Pneumonectomy should be performed with a mortality of less than 6%, lobectomy less than 3%, and lesser resections 1% or less. These mortality figures are significantly affected by the patient's age, stage of disease, and extent of resection.[28]

Lobectomy has been shown to be superior to more limited surgical resections such as wedge resection or segmentectomy. In a randomized trial conducted by the Lung Cancer Study Group, there was improved local control in patients having the more extensive resection.[29] With the advent of improved imaging and the possible role of screening CT scans, this issue might need to be reexamined. For example, it is probably excessive to remove the entire right lower lobe for a 9 mm squamous cell carcinoma.

RESULTS

Following surgical resection for stage I and II lung cancer, the 5-year survival without recurrence exceeds 50% in stage I and 40% in stage II disease. In completely resected T1N0 tumors, 5-year survival is approximately 80%. Approximately 25% of patients not surviving are tumor free at death, suggesting that surgical resection in early-stage lung cancer renders 80% of patients tumor free.[30]

PATTERNS OF FAILURE FOLLOWING SURGERY

Recognition of prognostic and surgical factors that predict for specific anatomic failure patterns can allow selection of patients for local, systemic, or combined therapy. In general, patients who fail after surgery present with disease outside of the chest 70% of the time, locally 20% of the time, and local and distant simultaneously 10%.[30] Therefore, systemic treatment is most likely to yield benefit postoperatively. Due to the relative chemoresistance of NSCLC, any benefit would likely be modest and would take a large trial to detect. Postoperative treatment is also difficult to tolerate. Unlike breast cancer, where patients recover quickly after modified radical mastectomy or lumpectomy, thoracic surgery, even if done thoracoscopically, requires significant recovery time. It has been shown in many studies that patients are only able to tolerate 60% of the intended treatment after surgery.

Second primary lung cancers occur frequently in all surviving patients at a rate of approximately 1% per year.[31,32]

PREOPERATIVE RADIATION THERAPY

RT may be delivered preoperatively or postoperatively. Theoretically, preoperative induction irradiation may improve resectability of larger tumors, sterilize cells beyond the margins of resection, prevent dissemination by surgical manipulation, and use lower doses of radiation than are required postoperatively when surgical changes induce conditions of hypoxia and relative radioresistance. Compared with postoperative RT, the disadvantages of preoperative RT are that the precise surgical stage may not be known and some patients may be treated unnecessarily, the exact anatomic extent of tumor may not be appreciated, and the risks of postoperative complications are increased.

The initial report of preoperative RT for NSCLC was from Bromley and Szur in 1955. From a large population of patients with early-and intermediate-stage disease, they selected 66 patients who responded to a median of 4700 R and performed resection and lymph node dissection. Complete tumor eradication in the primary tumor and nodes was detected in 47% (29 of 62) of evaluable patients. However, survival was poor with approximately 17% alive at varying follow-up times. This was accounted for in part by the 17% incidence of bronchopleural fistula, which was fatal in all but one patient.[33]

Randomized trials were initiated to answer this question with larger cohorts of patients. The first such major randomized trial was performed by the Veterans Administration. With a minimum follow-up of 4 years in surviving patients, no increase in survival was noted in the pretreatment group. The overall survival rate was 12.5% in the pretreatment arm, compared with 21% in the surgery-alone arm, although this was not statistically significant.[34]

In 1975, the National Cancer Institute published two separate but integrated multi-institutional randomized trials addressing the use of preoperative radiotherapy followed by surgery in both operable and inoperable NSCLC without evidence of preoperative radiotherapy advantage.[35] It is clear from both the nonrandomized and randomized data that preoperative irradiation alone does not improve long-term survival and has no role as a single induction modality in the management of marginally resectable or unresectable stage IIIA or IIIB disease. The use of RT as a single preoperative modality is no longer studied consistently due to the advent of effective chemotherapy agents. Most current trials investigate the use of preoperative concomitant chemoradiotherapy.

POSTOPERATIVE RADIATION THERAPY

The Lung Cancer Study Group (LCSG) investigated the efficacy of postoperative mediastinal irradiation in completely resected stage II and III squamous cell carcinoma of the lung. This trial randomized 210 patients to receive 50 Gy in 25 fractions after surgery versus observation alone. The locoregional failure rate (as first site of failure) was reduced from 41% to 3% with radiotherapy for all node-positive patients. Despite this improvement, the increase in locoregional control with radiotherapy did not translate into a survival benefit for stage II patients because more than two thirds of first failures were distant.[36] Instead of separating patients with N1 and N2 disease, the LCSG combined and analyzed them as a single group.[36] A trend toward improved survival was observed in N2 patients receiving radiotherapy.

The Medical Research Council of the United Kingdom also completed a randomized adjuvant trial in which 308 patients with stage II and III disease were treated with either 40 Gy or no further therapy, although a trend toward improved survival was seen in the N2 subgroup. Again, no overall survival benefit was observed.[37]

The meta-analysis performed by the Medical Research Council confirms these results. They report local recurrences in 276 patients in the surgery-only arms of the trials. There were 195 local recurrences in patients receiving postoperative radiation therapy (PORT). In addition, there was a trend toward improved survival in stage III and N2 patients, although it did not reach significance.[38] Stage I and II patients had decreased survival from PORT, presumably from increased toxicity of treatment without any benefit from the radiation (Figure 35-2).

The meta-analysis has been criticized due to its methodological flaws. The trials studied had variable and unspecified staging, used cobalt-60 or other low energy photons, and had inadequate treatment planning. Also, the interval between surgery and PORT was inconsistent and sometimes not reported.

Machtay and colleagues investigated whether the excess toxicity observed from PORT in the meta-analysis

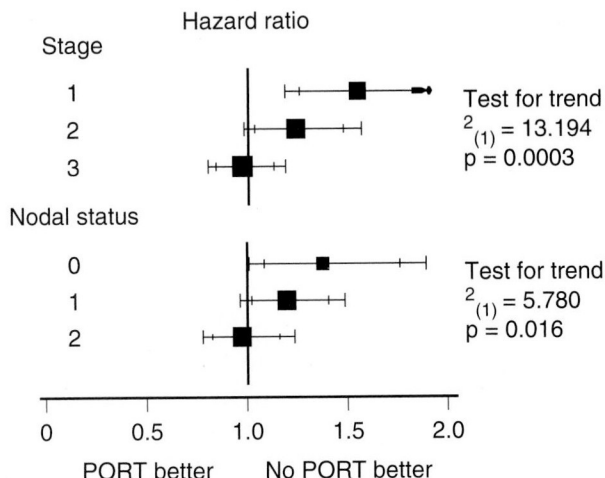

Figure 35-2. Results of the Medical Research Council's Meta-analysis of Postoperative Radiation Therapy. These results show that PORT is of no value to patients with stage I and II disease, but might benefit those with stage III (N2) disease. (From *Lancet.* 1998;352:257.)

was evident in their patient population. They reviewed 202 patients retrospectively who received PORT for stage II and III disease with a median dose of 55 Gy. They found the actuarial rate of death from intercurrent disease was 13.5% compared to an expected rate of 10%. Therefore, there is some toxicity associated from the PORT treatment, but of a lower magnitude than seen in the meta-analysis.

The role of PORT remains controversial. It has not been shown to be beneficial in early-stage disease and should not be recommended in these patients except in the case of suspected residual microscopic or macroscopic disease. It has been shown to improve local control in patients with mediastinal nodal disease, but has no proven survival benefit. There is likely a subgroup of patients, such as those with micrometastatic disease, who will have an improved survival from PORT; however, this patient population has yet to be identified.

Technique of Postoperative Radiation Therapy

Postoperative RT for patients with microscopic residual disease or with resected hilar or mediastinal involvement is planned as follows. The area to be treated is determined by correlating preoperative imaging studies, intraoperative findings, surgical clips, and the pathologic review of the resected specimen. Generally, the objective is to treat the ipsilateral hilum, the mediastinal nodes bilaterally, and the ipsilateral supraclavicular area. Peripheral primary tumors that do not abut the mediastinum or hilum and are not adjacent to the chest wall are usually removed with generous margins. After surgery, their preoperative location is occupied by relocated and uninvolved lung parenchyma, which does not need therapy unless there is clear evidence or strong suspicion of residual disease. The standard postoperative dose is 50.4 Gy in 1.8 Gy fractions

or 50 Gy in 2 Gy fractions. Consequently, the majority of this dose can be given with energy greater than or equal to 6 MV using opposed anterior and lateral fields with appropriate attention to the spinal cord dose. If there is a positive margin, this area is boosted with an additional 10 to 10.8 Gy to bring the total dose to 60 to 61.2 Gy. Half-field wedges can be used to decrease the dose to the spinal cord superiorly where the separation is less than at other levels. One approach is to deliver 41.4 Gy to the target volume with these fields (which will rarely deliver more than 45 Gy to any portion of the spinal cord) and to give the rest of the dose with oblique fields that completely exclude the spinal cord. The use of opposed lateral fields should be discouraged, even for these relatively small doses, due to the excess amount of lung that would be treated. A typical simulation film for PORT is demonstrated in Figure 35-3.

PREOPERATIVE CHEMOTHERAPY

Initial studies using various chemotherapy regimens suggested that preoperative chemotherapy could be administered for selected stage IIIA and a few stage IIIB patients and may be beneficial in this setting.[39,40] Combination chemotherapy with high-dose cisplatin (120 mg/m²), vinca alkaloids, and mitomycin (MVP) was used preoperatively in the stage IIIA patients with clinically apparent ipsilateral mediastinal spread.[41] In a group of 73 patients, the objective major response rate to MVP chemotherapy was 77% with a 10% complete response rate. Overall, 60% of patients underwent complete resections and the median survival was 19 months.[41]

There are multiple trials in which patients undergoing surgical resection were randomized to induction chemotherapy or no treatment.[42,43] The first trial reported by Pass et al. was a small trial that suggested a survival

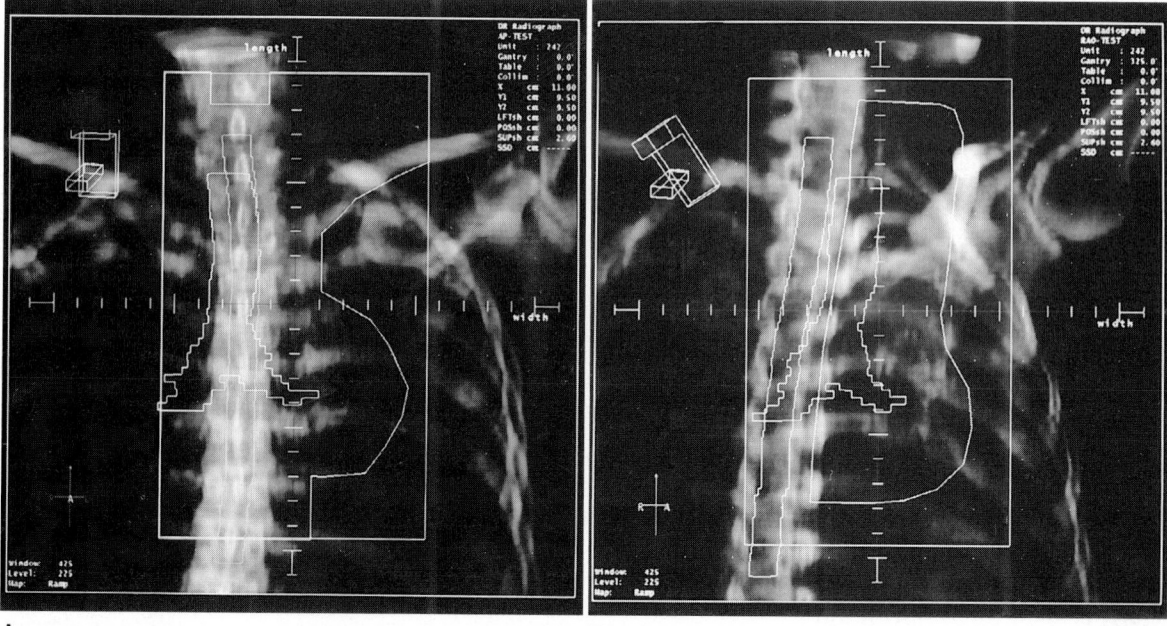

A   B

Figure 35-3. A typical postoperative radiation therapy simulation film. **A,** Anterior field. **B,** Off-cord oblique field. In both films, the carina and the spinal cord are outlined.

Table 35–2   Induction Chemotherapy + Surgery in Stage III NSCLC: Results of Randomized Trials

Investigators	Rx	Patients, *n*	Resect Rate (%)	Med Survival (mo)	5-yr Survival (%)
Pass (1992)	Surgery	14	86	16	12
	CT + Surgery	13	85	29	30
Roth (1994)	Surgery	32	66	11	15
	CT + Surgery	28	61	64	36
Rosell (1994)	Surgery	30	90	8	3
	CT + Surgery	29	85	26	25
Depierre (1999)	Surgery	119	NR	26	28
	CT + Surgery	119		37	39

CT, computed tomography; NR, nonresectable; NSCLC, non–small cell lung cancer.

benefit in patients treated with preoperative cisplatin and etoposide. In 1994, two trials were published, although each closed due to early stopping rules after enrollment of approximately 60 patients. Both trials used induction regimens containing cisplatin and showed a significant increase in survival with chemotherapy and surgery as opposed to surgery alone. The largest trial, from Depierre et al., enrolled 355 patients and treated them with three cycles of induction mitomycin, ifosfamide, and cisplatin and two cycles postoperatively. Median survival improved from 26 months to 37 months but was not statistically significant (Table 35-2).

ADJUVANT CHEMOTHERAPY FOLLOWING COMPLETE RESECTION OF NON–SMALL CELL LUNG CANCER

In 1995, the Non–Small Cell Lung Cancer Collaborative Group published a meta-analysis of 17 trials that contained 4467 patients using adjuvant chemotherapy from 1965 to 1991.[44] This showed decreased survival when alkylating agents were used and no change in survival when 5FU-based regimens were used. However, there was an insignificant ($P = 0.08$) trend toward improved survival by 5% when cisplatin-based chemotherapy was used. Since the publication of the meta-analysis, there have been numerous other trials investigating the role of adjuvant chemotherapy.

The Eastern Cooperative Oncology Group (ECOG) 3590 randomized 488 patients with stage II to IIIA disease after surgery to either RT alone or RT and concurrent cisplatin/etoposide. Five-year survival was 40% and 38%, respectively ($P = NS$).[45]

The International Adjuvant Lung Cancer Trial (IALT) randomized 1867 patients to chemotherapy or no chemotherapy for stage I to III patients following surgical resection. Treatment was determined by the preference of the institution and consisted of cisplatin (80 to 120 mg/m^2) and a second agent that was either etoposide, vinorelbine, vinblastine, or vindesine. Postoperative RT was given at the discretion of the institution. With a median follow-up of 56 months, a significantly improved survival from 40.4% to 44.5% has been shown.[46]

Therefore, the role of adjuvant chemotherapy is still slightly unclear, but it is probably of real benefit. The meta-analysis and the IALT trial certainly suggest that there is a small, significant improvement with the use of postoperative chemotherapy. The ECOG trial was probably too small to detect this. The integration of postoperative chemotherapy and induction chemotherapy has yet to be determined.

PREOPERATIVE CHEMORADIOTHERAPY

The Southwest Oncology Group (SWOG) reported on 126 patients in a phase II trial who received 45 Gy with concurrent cisplatin and etoposide before surgical resection. There was a 59% response rate; 89 patients (71%) underwent resection and 58% had a pathologic complete response or minimal microscopic disease. Despite this, patients with advanced disease (T2-3 N2, T4 N2-3) had only a 12-month median survival. Patients with more limited disease (T1 N2, T4 N0-1) had a 32-month median survival.[47]

SUPERIOR SULCUS TUMORS

The management of superior sulcus tumors (Pancoast tumors) is difficult. RT is an essential component of treatment either as sole therapy, preoperative therapy, postoperative therapy, or as intraoperative brachytherapy.

The use of preoperative RT was pioneered by Paulson.[48] Preoperative doses of 3000 to 3500 R were used to reduce the volume of tumor, thus facilitating complete resection. Operations were performed 1 month after the completion of RT to allow time for pain relief with an accompanying improvement in performance status; resolution of skin changes facilitating good wound healing; and, in some patients, to exclude the emergence of distant metastases, which would make radical local therapy inappropriate. In the initial report of this procedure, five of nine patients followed for more than 1 year were disease free.[49] In a number of series, various preoperative doses of radiation have been used and survival figures range from 20% to 34% at 5 years.

Generally accepted contraindications to surgery in patients with superior sulcus tumors include extensive involvement of the brachial plexus, involvement of the subclavian artery, vertebral bodies, esophagus, mediastinal node metastases, or distant metastases. Figure 35-4 shows a CT scan of a right lung T4 Pancoast tumor. There is gross destruction of the vertebral body and the tumor approximates the spinal cord. The patient was treated with radical RT alone. Patients with unresectable T4 tumors or mediastinal nodal metastases can be treated with radical RT. In general, fields are designed as described in the section on radiation techniques and total doses of 60 Gy or greater are used.

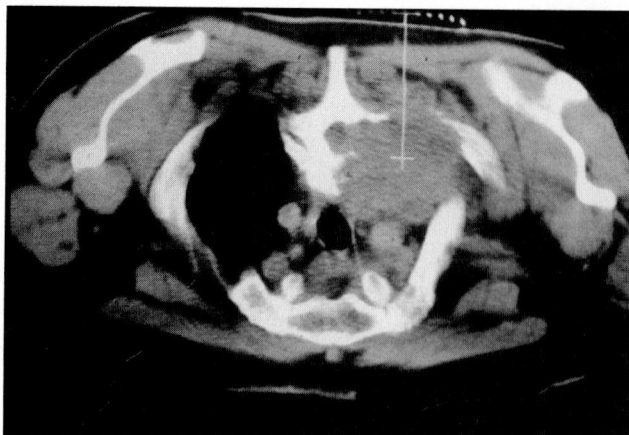

Figure 35–4. Computed tomography scan of a right-lung T4 pancoast tumor. There is gross destruction of the vertebral body and the tumor approximates the spinal cord.

The current standard treatment of superior sulcus tumors generally consists of preoperative chemoradiotherapy to 45 Gy. This is followed 4 weeks later with surgical resection. This regimen was studied in a phase II SWOG protocol that enrolled 111 patients and reported a 65% rate of pathologic complete response or minimal microscopic disease and a 55% two-year survival.[50]

Patients with uncontrolled primary tumors in the superior sulcus often have severe, intractable pain. Therefore, at Memorial Sloan-Kettering Cancer Center (MSKCC), we often offer patients palliative resection of the primary tumor even in the setting of metastatic disease.

Technique for Pancoast Tumors

The basic technique is the same regardless of the setting in which RT is used. The usual technique is to use paired anterior and posterior fields. The dose received by the spinal cord must be calculated superiorly, and must not exceed 110% of the prescription dose. If necessary, a half-field wedge is used as a spinal cord dose-compensator. It is important to use CT scans or MRI scans, or both, to determine field borders. In general, the field encompasses all areas of gross disease with a 2 cm margin. If part of a vertebral body is included in this field, then inclusion of the entire vertebral body should be considered in order to ensure homogenous dose to the vertebral body. A typical simulation film for a patient with a Pancoast tumor is shown in Figure 35-5.

The usual preoperative doses are well within the tolerance of the spinal cord and the fields described here can be used for all of the treatment. If definitive RT alone is used, then the spinal cord dose must be limited to 46 to 48 Gy provided this does not underdose any portion of the tumor. If the tumor approximates the spinal cord, then an absolute maximum of 50 Gy can be given to the spinal cord. It is important to calculate the dose distribution throughout the entire spinal cord to make sure no portion exceeds this maximum. Simple anterior and posterior fields as previously described can be modified to exclude the spinal cord from the latter portion of treatment. Alternatively, paired oblique fields may better cover the target while excluding the spinal cord. When

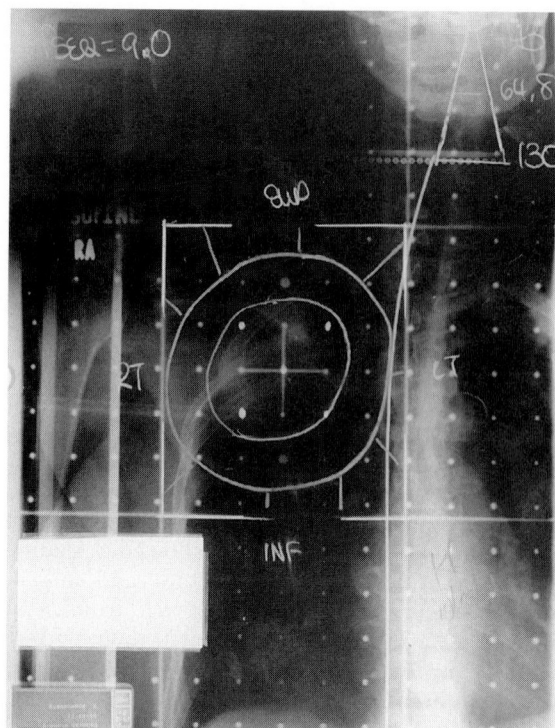

Figure 35–5. Simulation film of a patient with a Pancoast tumor.

RT is used postoperatively, the total dose may be 50 Gy in conventional 1.8 to 2.0 Gy fractions. Consequently, the cord dose must be limited in a similar fashion.

MARGINALLY OPERABLE NON–SMALL CELL LUNG CANCER

There is no standard definition of marginally operable NSCLC. However, the typical clinical situation is a patient with locally advanced disease that might be operable, or require a less morbid surgical procedure, if it responded to induction therapy. Unfortunately, there are no data regarding what percentage of unresectable tumors become resectable with treatment. One major concern is that a patient might receive induction treatment with chemoradiotherapy to 45 Gy and still may be unresectable when the patient is reassessed 1 month after the completion of chemoradiotherapy. In these situations, attempts are made to deliver more radiation to the tumor, but typically only 15 to 20 Gy can be delivered. Therefore, the patient would have been denied the opportunity for definitive treatment.

Intergroup Trial 0139 investigated whether induction chemoradiotherapy to 45 Gy followed by surgical resection was superior to chemoradiotherapy to 61 Gy alone in patients with T1-3 N2 disease. Surgical resection of all tumors were considered technically feasible at the time of registration. Preliminary analysis of 392 eligible patients revealed a lower progression-free survival in patients who received surgery, but overall survival was similar due to the increased treatment-related deaths seen in the surgery arm.[51]

These data suggest that induction chemoradiotherapy followed by surgery will not be of value in patients who are not technically resectable at the time of presentation. The appropriate treatment for these patients is chemotherapy and RT.

INOPERABLE NON–SMALL CELL LUNG CANCER

Radical Radiation Therapy for Inoperable, Early-Stage Non–Small Cell Lung Cancer

Some patients present with surgically resectable disease but have medical contraindications or refuse surgery. For such patients, primary RT offers an alternative and potentially curative approach.[52] The first published experience was from Hilton and Smart of University College Hospital of London, who gave 40 to 55 Gy using orthovoltage equipment to 38 patients.[53] Multiple retrospective series have reported survival rates ranging from 0% to more than 30%.[54-64] A chart of selected series is presented in Table 35-3. Surgery has the highest reported survival rates in stage I and II disease. The results from primary RT are inferior. The observed differences in results between surgery and radiation are due in part to selection bias, because in many instances, patients referred for radiation have worse performance status, are less rigorously staged, and have poor pulmonary function combined with comorbid illnesses.[59] Surgical series reveal that approximately 25% to 50% of clinical stage I patients are upstaged. The rate of occult N1 or N2 disease is as high as 56% if the patient has a positive preoperative bronchoscopy.[64] Therefore, it is important to evaluate cause-specific survival as an endpoint in these studies, since many patients die of intercurrent disease. But even factoring in these biases, RT will always be inferior to aggressive surgery (i.e., lobectomy), since RT is essentially trying to replicate a wedge resection.

More modern series have examined the issues of dose and dose escalation in relation to tumor size, local control, and survival for stage I and II disease. The evidence suggests that radical radiotherapy is an effective treatment primarily for tumors less than 3 cm (T1) when treated to doses of 65 Gy or higher. The highest reported survival was in a series that used the highest median dose, 70.2 Gy.[65] Complete response and local control of larger tumors, however, appears less likely with standard radiation fraction schedules and doses despite availability of modern equipment and CT-based planning.

Elective nodal irradiation of the mediastinum is probably unnecessary for early-stage tumors. The inclusion of large volumes of lung within a radiation port, especially for peripheral T1 and T2 tumors, to prevent regional failure must be balanced against the potential for increased toxicity. The rationale for treating the local tumor volume alone appears justified when the patient's outcome is not negatively impacted if the regional lymph nodes are excluded. The evidence appears to support the use of smaller target volumes to deliver higher doses without compromise of the regional outcome.[57] The regional failure rate is typically less than 10% in reported series where elective nodal areas were not treated.[57,60,65-68] In one series,[61] most patients did receive elective nodal irradiation but still had a failure rate approaching 10%, which suggests that a typical elective dose of 40 Gy is not enough to control occult disease.

Split-course radiation has also been examined for stage I and II NSCLC with mixed results and has generally been discouraged when treating with curative intent.[56,57]

Perhaps the most important issues yet to be elucidated in the treatment of early-stage NSCLC are what dose and fractionation should be used. The need for traditional fractionation of 1.8 to 2 Gy is being challenged. The role of higher doses per fraction, such as 3 to 4 Gy or as high as 10 Gy via stereotactic radiosurgery, are being investigated. 4 Gy per fraction has investigated in a poor performance status population and found to yield adequate control.[69]

Definitive Radiation Therapy for Locally Advanced Non–Small Cell Lung Cancer

RT is the standard therapy for patients with inoperable NSCLC. Essentially, the RT replaces surgery as the definitive treatment. Multiple series have shown that the median and long-term survivals are low when RT alone is used.[70,71] Therefore, there have been investigations as to whether there is any advantage to delivering thoracic radiotherapy in the setting of inoperable disease.

In a multi-institutional cooperative trial, Johnson and associates[72] reported the results of 319 patients with locally advanced, unresectable NSCLC without evidence of distant metastases who were randomized prospectively to one of three arms: chemotherapy alone with vindesine, 3 mg/m^2/wk; standard thoracic irradiation to a dose of 60 Gy in 6 weeks; or combined vindesine and thoracic radiotherapy. Although the overall response rate was superior in the radiotherapy arms (radiotherapy alone, 30%; radiotherapy plus vindesine, 34%; vindesine alone, 10%; $P = 0.001$), the intrathoracic progression rates were similar in the vindesine arm (60%) and in the radiotherapy arm (65%); both median survival and overall

Table 35–3   Selected Studies of Radiation Therapy Alone for Medically Inoperable, Early-Stage, Non–Small Cell Lung Cancer

Study Author	Patients, n	Dose (Gy)	5-yr Survival, %	5-yr Cause-Specific Survival, %	5-yr Local Control, %
Dosoretz	152	60–69	10		
Krol	108	60–65	15	31	25
Kaskowitz	53	63	6	13	0
Sibley	141	55–70	13		
Rosenzweig	32	70.2	33	39	43

survival were also comparable in all three arms. This study has been criticized, however, for the large number of patients in the vindesine-alone arm who received RT and the inadequate number of patients to detect a difference in survival.[73]

A retrospective study from British Columbia that controlled tumor stage and other prognostic factors reported improved survival of 79 days in patients receiving high-dose palliative RT and improved survival of more than 1 year in patients receiving radical RT.[74]

Although it seems clear that thoracic RT offers a survival advantage to patients with disease limited to the thorax, the poor results of these earlier studies led the Radiation Therapy Oncology Group (RTOG) and other groups to investigate methods of improving outcome with radiation alone by initially concentrating on dose intensification with conventional fractionation; the use of altered fractionation; identification of appropriate selection criteria including prognostic factors for the various approaches; the use of innovative treatment planning and technology; and perhaps most importantly, the integration of chemotherapy with RT.

SELECTION OF PATIENTS

Generally accepted eligibility criteria for definitive therapy for lung cancer are based on extent and spread of tumor and the patient's physiologic status. The presence of distant metastases and pleural or pericardial effusions are contraindications. A performance status of 60% or more is preferable, as is adequate pulmonary function. Bleehen and Cox[75] have recommended that the FVC be 45% of predicted, the FEV-1 40% of predicted, single breath diffusing capacity for carbon monoxide corrected for hemoglobin 45% of predicted, and PaO_2 less than or equal to 49 mm Hg. However, these figures should be used as guidelines rather than strict criteria since the use of RT may improve performance status or relieve airway obstruction. In addition, for patients with poor pulmonary function, there is typically no adequate therapeutic option aside from RT, so it is probably still in the patient's best interest to proceed with treatment if he or she is aware of the increased risk of treatment.

RESULTS

Radiation Therapy Alone

The RTOG investigated the effect of various doses of RT on the outcome of 379 patients with locally advanced (T1-3 N0-2) NSCLC.[58] Patients were randomized to receive 40 Gy split-course or 40 Gy, 50 Gy, or 60 Gy continuous-course RT. Median survival was approximately 9 months and 5-year survival was 5%. Between 1 and 3 years, the curves diverged temporarily in favor of 60 Gy, and they subsequently converged. There was no clear effect of dose on survival. However, the in-field failure rate did decrease from 53% to 58% with 40 Gy to 35% with 60 Gy.

Sequential Chemotherapy and Radiation vs. Radiation Alone

Because distant failure is common following RT for locally advanced NSCLC, attempts have been made to improve survival by adding chemotherapy to RT. Combination chemotherapy can produce higher response rates and potentially could be more efficacious in that setting. Initially, most randomized trials were negative, possibly because of failure to select healthier patients and the use of noncisplatin regimens. The Cancer and Leukemia Group B (CALGB) randomized patients with locally advanced NSCLC to receive 60 Gy of thoracic irradiation with ($n = 78$) or without ($n = 77$) induction chemotherapy with vinblastine (five weekly courses of 5 mg/m²) and cisplatin (100 mg/m² twice). The patients were selected by having a performance status of greater than or equal to 80, weight loss of less than or equal to 5%, and hematocrit greater than 30%. Median survival was 14 months with chemotherapy versus 10 months without ($P = 0.006$), and 3-year survival was 23% with chemotherapy versus 11% without.[76] An Intergroup study confirmed in a preliminary manner that this chemotherapy regimen given before 60 Gy of RT improved survival compared to 60 Gy alone.[77] A large randomized study from France tested the value of vindesine, cyclophosphamide, cisplatin, and lomustine added to 65 Gy (split course) of thoracic irradiation. Survival was not increased by the addition of chemotherapy. However, distant metastases were significantly reduced to 45% in the chemotherapy arm ($n = 176$) versus 67% in the RT alone arm ($n = 177$).[78] These data suggest a strong rationale for exploring the combined use of the most effective chemotherapy regimens with more effective thoracic radiation approaches (Table 35-4).

Using a different study design, Kubota and coworkers[79] randomized patients receiving induction chemotherapy to receive ($n = 31$) or not receive ($n = 32$) thoracic irradiation. Thoracic irradiation significantly prolonged the time to progression and increased 2-year survival ($P < 0.05$). This trial shows that even in patients with an excellent response to induction chemotherapy, thoracic RT is still needed to prevent local recurrence.

Table 35-4 **Randomized Trials of Sequential Chemotherapy and Radiation Therapy versus Radiation Therapy Alone**

Study	Patients, n	Chemotherapy	Radiation Therapy Dose (Gy)	5-yr Survival Chemo → RT, %	5-yr Survival RT Alone, %
Dillman (CALGB)	155	Cisplatin/Vinblastine	60	16	6
Sause (RTOG)	490	Cisplatin/Vinblastine	60	8	5
LeChevalier (French)	325	Cisplatin/Vindesine/ CCNU/Cyclophosphamide	65.6	6	3

CALGB, Cancer and Leukemia Group B; CCNU, lomustine; RT, Radiation Therapy; RTOG, Radiation Therapy Oncology Group.

Table 35-5   Randomized Trials of Concurrent Chemotherapy and Radiation Therapy versus Radiation Therapy Alone

Schaake-Konig (EORTC)	Patients, n	2 yr Survival	3 yr Survival	4–5 yr Survival
RT (split) + cDDP 6 mg/m²/d	102	26	16*	NA
RT (split) + cDDP 30 mg/m²/wk	98	19	13	NA
RT (split)			2	NA
Jeremic I	**Patients, n**	**Median Survival (mo)**	**3 yr Survival**	**4–5 yr Survival**
HFx RT (69.6 Gy) + CBDCA/Vp-16 Q wk	52	18	27	21*
HFx RT (69.6 Gy) + CBDCA/Vp-16 Q wk	56	13	16	16
HFx RT	61	8	7	5
Jeremic II	**Patients, n**	**Median Survival (mo)**	**3 yr Survival**	**4–5 yr Survival**
HFx RT + CBDCA/Vp-16 Qd	65	22	NA	23*
HFx RT	66	14	NA	9

*cDDP, cisplatin; CBDCA, carboplatin; Vp-16, etoposide; HFx, hyperfractionation; EORTC, European Organisation for Research and Treatment of Cancer; GLOT, Groupe Lyon-Saint-Etienne d'Oncologie Thoracique.

Concurrent Chemoradiation vs. Radiation Alone

Three major trials have compared concurrent chemo-radiotherapy and radiation alone. The EORTC reported that the addition of cisplatin 6 mg/m² daily to 55 Gy of radiation delivered via a split-course technique was superior to cisplatin 30 mg/m² weekly with the radiation or RT alone. Three-year survival was 16%, 13%, and 2%, respectively.

Jeremic has reported two trials in which carboplatin and etoposide delivered weekly or daily with hyperfractionated RT to 69.6 Gy were superior to the same radiation alone. The results are presented in Table 35-5.

Sequential Chemotherapy and Radiation Therapy vs. Concurrent Chemoradiotherapy

Four trials have compared sequential chemotherapy and radiation and concurrent chemotherapy (Table 35-6). Furuse compared 56 Gy delivered via a split-course technique after induction mitomycin, vinblastine, cisplatin (MVP) chemotherapy to the same regimen delivered concurrently. The 5-year survival increased significantly from 9% to 16%. There was also increased esophagitis.[80]

RTOG 9410 compared: (1) sequential cisplatin/vinblastine chemotherapy and radiation (60 Gy), (2) concurrent cisplatin/vinblastine chemotherapy and 60 Gy, and (3) concurrent cisplatin/oral etoposide with hyperfractionated radiation to 69.6 Gy. At the latest analysis,[81] the concurrent treatment has a significantly improved median survival (14.6 to 17.1 months).

A French trial compared induction cisplatin/vinorelbine followed by 66 Gy with concurrent cisplatin/etoposide/66 Gy followed by cisplatin/vinorelbine. There was no significant difference in survival between the groups.[82]

Finally, a trial from the Czech republic compared 60 Gy or RT delivered either during or after 4 cycles of cisplatin/vinorelbine. They reported a significant increase in survival with the concurrent treatment.[83]

Sequencing of Chemoradiotherapy

The locally advanced multimodality protocol (LAMP)[84] investigated three different schemes of delivering chemoradiotherapy and chemotherapy. All arms used carboplatin and paclitaxel chemotherapy and 66 Gy. In one arm, the chemotherapy and radiation were given sequentially, similar to the CALBG trial. In the second arm, chemotherapy was given initially and then chemoradiotherapy was delivered. In the final arm, chemoradiotherapy was given initially, followed by consolidative chemotherapy with the same agent. Not surprisingly, esophagitis increased dramatically in the arms receiving concurrent chemotherapy. The median survival in the arms with induction chemotherapy was a surprisingly low 11 to 12.5 months. In the arm with early radiation, median survival increased to 16.5 months.

Consolidative Chemotherapy

SWOG 9019[85] used consolidative cisplatin/etoposide after the use of concurrent cisplatin/etoposide/radiation

Table 35–6   Randomized Trials of Sequential Chemotherapy and Radiation Therapy versus Concurrent Chemotherapy and Radiation Therapy

Study	Outcome	Patients, n	Follow-Up	Results (concurrent), %	Results (sequential), %	P value
Furuse	Positive	320	5 yr	16	9	0.04
RTOG	Positive	597	3 yr	26	18	0.038
GLOT	Negative	212	2 yr	35	24	0.55
Czech	Positive	207	2 yr	42	15	0.02

GLOT, Groupe Lyon-Saint-Etienne d'Oncologie Thoracique; RTOG, Radiation Therapy Oncology Group.

in 50 stage IIIB patients. They reported a 3-year survival of 17%. A follow-up study, SWOG 9504, substituted docetaxel as the consolidative agent with an encouraging 3-year survival of 37%.[86] The use of consolidative chemotherapy is being further investigated.

Altered Fractionation Schemes

SPLIT-COURSE RADIATION THERAPY. There are several theoretical advantages to split-course RT. It is postulated that the interval between the courses (usually 2 to 4 weeks) allows for maximal recovery of acute toxicity. Normal cells may repopulate more quickly than cancer cells during the interval and reoxygenation and redistribution of cancer cells may occur, rendering them more radiosensitive during the second course. However, an accelerated repopulation of malignant cells may occur during this interval.[87] In RTOG 73-01, the split-course treatment to 40 Gy had a lower in-field control rate than the continuous treatment.[58] Fowler and colleagues reported a significantly worse outcome in RTOG patients who received a 2 week or more treatment break during their radiation.[88] Split-course treatment is generally out of fashion at this time.

HYPERFRACTIONATED RADIATION THERAPY. Hyperfractionated RT is a method of intensifying radiation effects by delivering smaller dose fractions (e.g., 1.2 Gy per fraction), given more than once per day, increasing the total daily dose to 2.4 Gy or more. Consequently, when given in a continuous course, 5 days per week, the treatment is also described as "accelerated." Theoretically, this approach has a greater effect against cancer cells and keeps chronic side effects at acceptable levels because of the low dose per fraction.

In a randomized phase I/II trial, Cox and coworkers[54] used 69.6 Gy of hyperfractionated RT for locally advanced non–small cell lung cancer and reported a median survival of 13 months in a subgroup of patients with high performance status and minimal weight loss. However, a phase III trial addressing the value of the RTOG-type hyperfractionated radiation scheme compared with standard 60 Gy RT failed to show a survival benefit for hyperfractionation.[78]

HYPERFRACTIONATED ACCELERATED RADIATION THERAPY. Continuous hyperfractionated radiation therapy (CHART) employs many radiobiologic principles in an effort to improve the therapeutic ratio. CHART delivers 54 Gy in three daily doses of 1.5 Gy over 12 continuous days, including weekends. With CHART, treatment is given every day to counteract rapidly proliferating cells. Hyperfractionation with many smaller doses of radiation may reduce long-term toxicity. Accelerating the treatment time from 6 weeks to 2 weeks may also counteract tumor repopulation.

CHART was first examined in a small prospective phase II trial.[89] Some degree of esophageal toxicity was present in all patients. Ten percent of patients developed acute radiation pneumonitis. Two-year survival was 34%.

A phase III randomized study was performed in 13 centers in the United Kingdom. Patients were assigned to either standard radiation of 60 Gy in 30 daily doses of 2 Gy over 6 weeks or CHART. Approximately half of the patients had stage III disease; the remainder had early-stage disease or unknown staging. No other modality of therapy was used. Two-year survival significantly increased from 20% to 29% in the CHART arm. In addition, local control significantly improved from 15% to 23%.[90] Severe esophageal toxicity also increased from 3% to 19%, and acute radiation pneumonitis was 19% in the conventional group and 10% in the CHART arm. However, late pulmonary toxicity and fibrosis requiring treatment at 2 years was present in 16% of living patients who received CHART, as compared to 4% receiving conventional RT. The physical and psychologic symptoms caused by this aggressive regimen have been shown to be tolerable as well.[91]

The use of CHART has been limited by the need to reorganize radiation departments to accommodate the demanding radiation treatment schedule. In addition, patients are hospitalized during their entire course of radiation, which may significantly increase the cost of treatment. Therefore, trials have been conducted using CHART without treatment on weekends (CHARTWELL).[92]

An ECOG trial examined therapy and the feasibility of hyperfractionated accelerated radiation (HART).[93] Twenty-eight patients received 57.6 Gy over 15 days (12 treatment days) in 3 daily fractions of 1.5 Gy, 1.8 Gy, and 1.5 Gy, 4 hours apart. The need to wait 6 hours was avoided by not treating fields containing spinal cord consecutively. They found that this regimen was tolerable, with the main toxicity being esophagitis and moist desquamation of the skin. The HART schedule showed provocative efficacy, with the median survival improving from 13.7 months with 64 Gy in 2 Gy daily fractions compared to 22.2 months with HART.[94]

Three-Dimensional–Conformal Radiation Therapy

Three-dimensional conformal RT (3D-CRT) is a technique whereby precise anatomic data accumulated from high-resolution CT scans are used to build a computerized 3D image of the patient's normal structures and tumor. The optimal radiation beam parameters and orientation are selected by objectively comparing candidate plans using calculations and visual displays. This approach has the potential to maximize the delivery of the prescribed dose to target volumes while reducing exposure to normal structures. An example of a dose distribution obtained with conformational 3D treatment planning is demonstrated in Figure 35-6A. An example of a dose volume histogram generated from a 3D-CRT plan is presented in Figure 35-6C.

Armstrong and associates[95] at MSKCC compared the use of conventional and 3D planning for locally advanced lung cancer and demonstrated that the delivery of high-dose irradiation to the target volume was significantly better with the 3D system. In addition, the 3D system reduced the dose to the lung parenchyma.[95]

At the University of Michigan, patients were treated with doses ranging from 65.1 Gy to 102.9 Gy, depending on the predicted toxicity. They have reported a single case of acute grade 3 pneumonitis and five cases of acute grade 2 pneumonitis.[96] Recently, patients with advanced disease have been receiving neoadjuvant chemotherapy in addition to 3D-CRT. RTOG 9311 also investigated dose

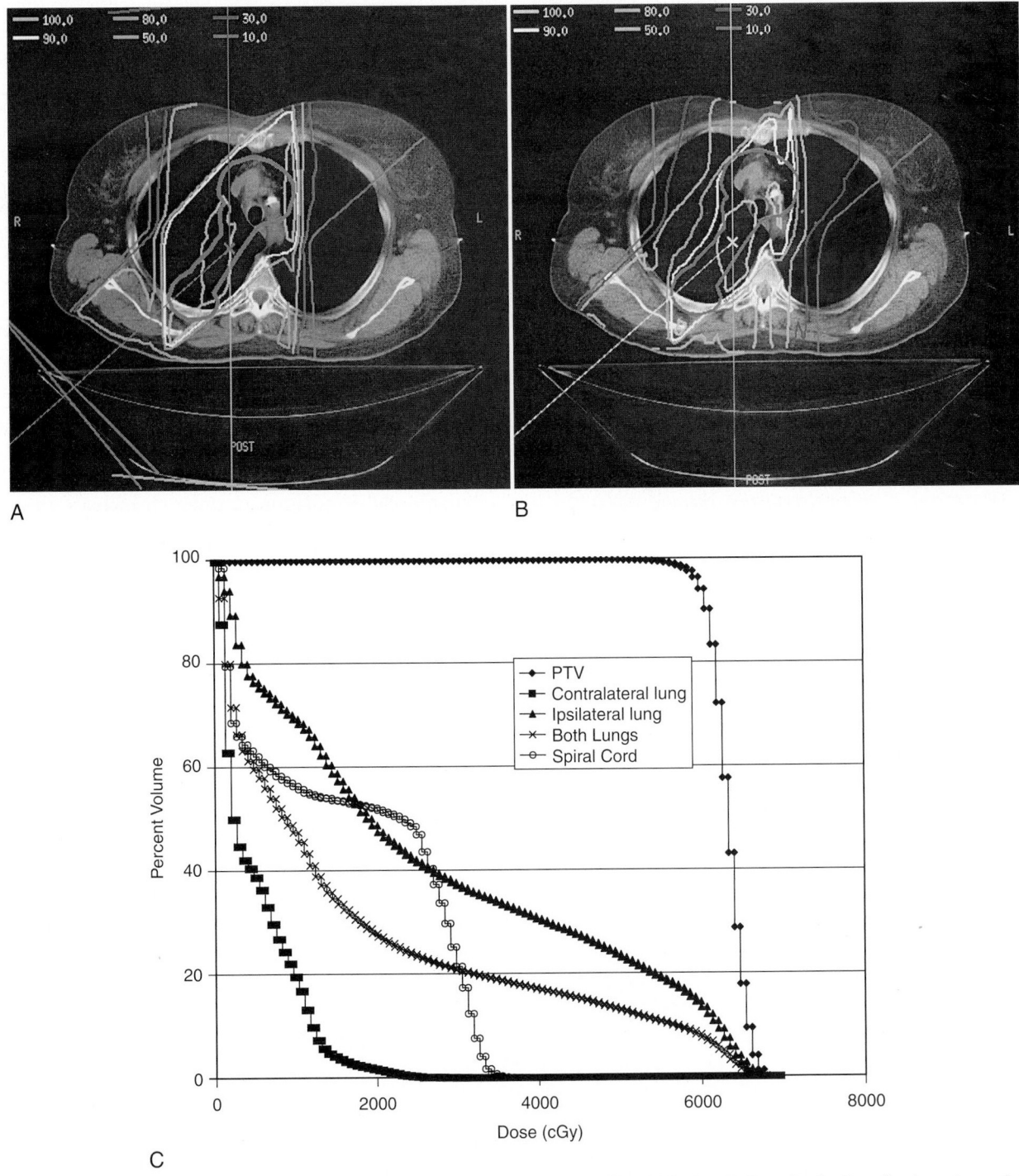

Figure 35–6. A, Dose distribution of a three-dimensional conformal radiation treatment (3D-CRT) plan. **B,** Dose distribution of an intensity-modulated radiation therapy plan. Note how the 90% isodose curve (*yellow*) is more conformal around the PTV (*pink*). **C,** Typical dose volume histogram from a 3D-CRT treatment plan. See also Color Figure 35-6A-B.

escalation using 3D-CRT. They have safely treated tumors to 77.4 Gy if the volume of lung receiving 20 Gy was less than 37% and 90.3 Gy if the volume of lung receiving 20 Gy was less than 25%.[97] MSKCC has demonstrated safe dose escalation to 84 Gy if the normal tissue complication probability was less than 25%.[98]

Technique

The technical objectives of radical RT are to deliver a high dose (≥60 Gy) to gross disease and to keep the dose

to critical normal structures such as the spinal cord and lung parenchyma at or below safe levels.

At simulation, patients are immobilized while supine in custom cradle molds that are used for all phases of planning and therapy. The patient's arms are folded behind the head to allow the use of any oblique treatment angle.

Two-Dimensional Radiation Therapy

For two-dimensional (2D) RT, the usual technique is to initially use paired anterior and posterior fields. The gross tumor and any areas felt to be at risk for tumor recurrence are included in the anterior-posterior/posterior-anterior (AP/PA) fields. The dose to this field is typically 40 Gy and the dose received by the spinal cord must not exceed 110%. If necessary, a half-field wedge can be used as a spinal cord dose-compensator. It is important to use a diagnostic CT scan to determine field borders. In general, the field encompasses all areas of gross disease with a 2 cm margin, the ipsilateral supraclavicular nodes, the sub-carinal nodes, and the contralateral mediastinum. If the subcarinal area is uninvolved, the field's inferior border is two vertebral bodies below the carina. If the carina is clinically involved with tumor, then the inferior border should encompass all the gross disease. A 2-cm margin on the contralateral edge of the vertebral body is sufficient to treat the contralateral mediastinum. For the second part of treatment, only the gross disease is treated to 20 Gy with oblique fields, typically with off-cord oblique fields. Typical 2D simulation films are shown in Figure 35-7.

Three-Dimensional–Conformal Radiation Therapy

When a CT-simulator is used, the CT scan is obtained with 3-mm-thick slices from the larynx to the bottom of the L2 vertebral body. This ensures complete imaging of the thorax and will allow for a high quality digitally reconstructed radiograph. The isocenter is typically placed in the center of the planning target volume (PTV), although any point can be used as long as it is in close approximation to the PTV. Intravenous contrast is typically not used as the contrast may interfere with treatment planning calculations. If contrast is absolutely needed, a second set of CT images can be obtained before the injection of contrast to be used for treatment planning purposes.

If a CT-simulator is not available, a fluoroscopic simulation is performed and anterior and lateral films are taken. The area to be imaged by CT is demarcated on the simulation films and the CT scan is obtained.

Determining the Planning Target Volume

The standard PTV includes the gross tumor and any area that is clinically expected to harbor disease. If elective nodal irradiation is to be used, the ipsilateral hilum, the entire mediastinum, and the ipsilateral supraclavicular area should be included in the volume. A 1- to 2-cm margin is placed around these structures to account for tumor motion and patient setup error.

Elective Nodal Irradiation

As described earlier, standard RT typically involves a dose of 40 Gy to the entire mediastinum, supraclavicular fossa, and ipsilateral hilum, even if there is no evidence of disease in these areas. It has been shown that this elective treatment can significantly add to the morbidity of radiation.[99] Many centers have eliminated elective nodal irradiation in order to increase the dose to the tumor. When RTOG trials were reviewed to estimate the clinical impact of omitting nodal irradiation, they found that when the ipsilateral hilum and mediastinum were incorrectly treated, there was an increased risk of progression.[100] MSKCC reported an elective nodal failure rate of 8% and a local failure rate of 65%,[101] suggesting that until regions of known disease can be better controlled, there is probably no need to treat the whole mediastinum and supraclavicular region electively.

PET Scans

PET scans have been investigated as tools to aid treatment planning. In a detailed study by Mah et al., the

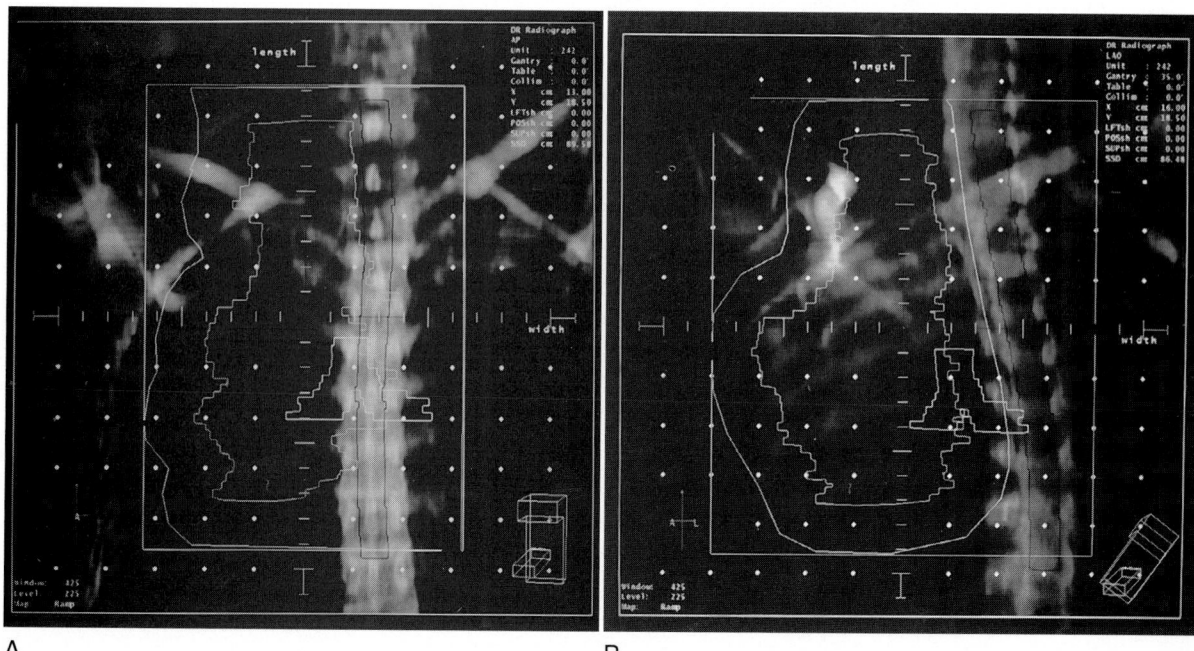

A   B

Figure 35–7. Simulation films of two-dimensional radiation therapy fields. **A,** Shows an anterior field. **B,** Shows an off-cord oblique field. In both films, the gross tumor, carina, and spinal cord are outlined.

treatment volumes of 30 patients were outlined by 3 radiation oncologists using both CT alone and registered CT and PET data.[102] With the addition of PET data, the treatments in 7 of the 30 patients were changed to palliation. In 5 of the remaining 23 patients, PET-positive nodes were detected within 5 cm of the primary tumor as defined by CT alone. The use of PTVs derived with CT alone would have led to geographic miss in 17% to 29% of all patients, as assessed by the combined CT-PET–derived PTVs. Both reduction (24% to 70%) and increase (30% to 76%) in PTV volumes were observed. The range of values quoted here are due to interobserver differences. They also noted that the addition of PET improved contouring consistency among clinicians.

In a prospective treatment planning study, Erdi et al. combined PET images with CT data for 11 NSCLC patients and reported PTV increases for 7 patients, with an average volume increase of 19%. For the other four patients, PTVs decreased by an average of 18%.[103]

Tumor Motion Control

Motion of the tumor and of the lung itself during delivery of each treatment appears to affect the outcome of radiotherapy. Lung tumors have been shown to substantially vary in their position during quiet breathing, causing inaccuracies in treatment delivery.[104-106] Underdosage of the clinical target volume may result if the tumor target moves outside the treatment volume during the administration of radiotherapy. Stevens et al. have reported that lung tumors move during free breathing from 5 to 10 mm and in some cases as much as 4.5 cm.[106] To compensate for this motion, a normal tissue safety margin is typically used to encompass the tumor, which may effectively double the PTV. Thus, approaches have been investigated to reduce the intrafraction organ motion and the volume of lung receiving radiation.

Two distinct techniques have been used to reduce the effects of respiratory motion. The first involves confining radiation delivery to a specified phase in the breathing cycle by gating the linear accelerator while the patient breathes freely. Breathing is monitored with devices that trigger radiation delivery during specific phases of the patient's respiratory cycle.[107] In the second approach, breathing is controlled either voluntarily by the patient or by using an occlusion valve. One example of this approach is active breathing control (ABC), which was developed by Wong et al.[108,109] Another example is the deep inspiration breath hold (DIBH) technique. The DIBH technique involves coaching the patient to the same reproducible deep inspiration level during simulation, radiation treatments, and port film verification. This technique has been shown to increase the theoretical maximum safe dose from 69 Gy to 88 Gy.[110]

TOXICITY OF RADIATION THERAPY TO THE THORAX

Acute side effects begin during the second to third week of conventionally fractionated radiation doses. Dermatitis is rarely severe and can be minimized by avoiding trauma and cosmetics on treated skin. It is treated with aloe vera gel or perfume-free ointments containing petrolatum, mineral oil, mineral wax, and wool wax alcohol (Aquaphor). Esophagitis usually presents as mild to moderate pain on swallowing, which may require a semisolid diet or analgesics (particularly in liquid form). Acute esophagitis generally does not progress to chronic esophagitis, which is rare. Dry, nonproductive cough can be caused by a radiation effect in the trachea or bronchi.

Radiation pneumonitis is the most common significant complication of radical RT and can be fatal in a small percentage of patients. Its incidence is related to dose, fractionation, and volume of lung irradiated. Typically it manifests as fever, dyspnea, tachycardia, and hypoxia. The diffusing capacity may be decreased in the early phase and may be preceded by exercise-induced oxygen desaturation. Radiographs show diffuse inhomogeneous opacification largely confined to the port. If it is symptomatic and other processes have been excluded, it is treated with prednisone (1 mg/kg per day). Prophylaxis against *Pneumocystis carinii* pneumonia with trimethoprim-sulfamethoxazole during prednisone therapy is recommended. It is important to taper steroids very slowly to avoid exacerbations. Patients who have received thoracic radiation and have never exhibited any signs of pneumonitis, and are given high-dose steroids for other reasons, can develop pneumonitis when the steroids are discontinued. Corticosteroids have little impact on radiation damage that has already progressed to fibrosis. There is no indication for the routine use of antibiotics or anticoagulants.

SPECIAL TOPICS IN RADIATION THERAPY FOR NON–SMALL CELL LUNG CANCER

Intraoperative Brachytherapy

The interstitial implantation of radioactive isotopes has been investigated at MSKCC to allow the precise localization of dose in the tumor and spare adjacent normal tissues because of the limited penetration of the low-energy emission. High total tumor dose in the range of 160 Gy is feasible because of the low dose rate (approximately 8 cGy per hour).[111] If there is gross residual disease greater than 1 cm in width, a volume implant is required using hollow needles and the "Mick afterloader" (Mick Radioinstruments, New York). Plaques of residual disease or areas of possible microscopic disease are covered with a planar implant performed either by direct suturing of ^{125}I seeds encapsulated in Vicryl or by evenly spacing of ^{125}I suture seeds in a premeasured Dexon mesh and suturing the mesh directly onto the area at risk. The later technique is well suited to areas such as the major vessels or paraspinal region.[112]

Hilaris[113] reported on 100 patients with stage III non–small cell lung cancer. [125]I implants were performed for unresected or incompletely resected primary tumors and ^{192}Ir implants were used for mediastinal disease. Local control was greater than 70% at 5 years and survival was 22%. Despite these results, intraoperative brachytherapy has not been widely adopted, and although it is theoretically an attractive technique, its superiority to external beam RT alone has not been clearly demonstrated.

Intraluminal Brachytherapy

DEFINITIVE

Huber and colleagues randomized 108 patients to either conventional RT (60 Gy) alone or an endobronchial brachytherapy boost of 4.8 Gy before and after the conventional RT.[114] There was a trend toward improved local control in patients receiving brachytherapy, although it failed to reach significance. There was no difference in overall survival. Criticisms of the trial include that the majority of patient treatment significantly deviated from the protocol. However, it does suggest that endobronchial brachytherapy might play a role in the treatment of primary disease.

PALLIATIVE

The use of high-dose-rate intraluminal brachytherapy is typically performed on an outpatient basis. The treatment catheter is positioned under bronchoscopic guidance and then connected to the remote afterloading machine, which contains a ^{192}Ir source (10 Ci) that travels along the catheter and is programmed to remain at specific locations to deliver a precisely controlled dose over several minutes. In a population of patients that received prior radiation, this approach yielded symptomatic improvement in 75% of patients, and there was a small number of long-term survivors.[115] Similar data were reported by Macha and colleagues,[116] who obtained a response in 79% (44 of 56 patients) receiving 7.5 Gy 1 cm from the source, in four treatments. Radiologic improvement occurred in 88% (22 of 25 patients) with collapse or atelectases, and improvements in FEV 1 and FVC were well documented. Burt and collaborators[117] gave 15 to 20 Gy at 1 cm in one fraction of high-dose-rate intraluminal brachytherapy and reported relief of hemoptysis in 86% (24 of 28), dyspnea in 64% (21 of 33), and cough in 50% (9 of 18) of patients. Unlike other series, they did not use laser therapy before irradiation. Laser treatment provides immediate relief of symptoms, facilitates catheter placement beyond the obstruction, and may increase response rates and duration. Seagren and Harrell[118] reported significantly improved response rates among a population of 36 patients who received laser treatment versus 14 who did not.

Radioprotectants

The radioprotectant amifostine is a sulfhydryl compound. Its metabolites scavenge free radicals that are generated in tissues exposed to radiation.[119] A phase II clinical trial using amifostine with sequential chemotherapy and standard radiation (60 Gy) had no episodes of grade 3 or worse esophagitis or pneumonitis.[120] There was no evidence of tumor protection, either. A randomized prospective trial

from the MD Anderson Cancer Center demonstrated a significant decrease in esophagitis and pneumonitis with twice-weekly use of amifostine with concurrent chemoradiotherapy.[121] However, hypotension was more common in the amifostine arm. RTOG Protocol 98-01 addressed the use of amifostine, and preliminary results reveal that the use of amifostine may not decrease the rate of grade 3 esophagitis.[122] A trial from Singapore showed an insignificant decrease in esophagitis with the use of amifostine in patients receiving concurrent chemoradiotherapy. Antonadou and colleagues reported that in a phase III trial, amifostine reduces the incidence of pneumonitis, lung fibrosis, and esophagitis in radiotherapy patients with lung cancer without compromising antitumor efficacy.[123]

Neutrons

Theoretically, neutron therapy should be useful for large lung tumors that may contain resistant hypoxic components. Schnabel and colleagues[124] randomized 48 patients to receive 18 neutron Gy and compared outcome to 67 controls receiving 54 Gy (photons) and reported no advantage in local control or survival. With increasing follow-up, patients treated with neutrons developed a higher incidence of pneumonitis. The RTOG randomized patients to three arms: 60 Gy photons ($n = 39$), 18 to 20 Gy neutrons ($n = 29$), or combined neutrons and photons ($n = 34$). Median survival was 8, 8, and 7 months, respectively. Severe toxicity rates (mostly pulmonary) were 5%, 31%, and 15%, respectively, confirming the increased risk of therapy with neutrons observed by Schnabel and coworkers.[124] In an attempt to limit this late toxicity, Livingston and collaborators[125] used neutron fields that were smaller and limited to areas of residual disease after induction chemotherapy. The high rates of toxicity were avoided, but high rates of thoracic failure were noted (particularly outside the port).

Prophylactic Cranial Irradiation

The hypothesis that prophylactic cranial irradiation can improve survival is based on the assumption that isolated brain failures occur commonly and lead to death, and that these can be effectively prevented by tolerable doses of radiation. Fifty percent of patients with locally advanced non–small cell lung cancer (LA-NSCLC) will develop central nervous system metastases at some time during the course of their disease. The brain is the first site of relapse in 15% to 30% of these patients.[126]

Four randomized trials of prophylactic cranial irradiation added to chest irradiation (plus or minus chemotherapy) have been reported for patients with locally advanced NSCLC and have not demonstrated improved survival with prophylactic cranial irradiation, although the irradiation did reduce the rate of developing brain metastasis.[126,127-130] Currently, a large RTOG trial is under way to reinvestigate the role of prophylactic cranial irradiation in NSCLC.

New Radiation Therapy Treatment Planning Techniques

Two new radiotherapeutic techniques are now more commonly used in the treatment of NSCLC: intensity-modulated radiation therapy (IMRT) and stereotactic radiosurgery (SRS). Both techniques strive to use advanced radiation treatment planning methods to deliver less radiation dose to the structures at risk (e.g., lung) while treating the tumor to the same dose or an escalated dose.

STEREOTACTIC RADIOSURGERY

Extracranial SRS is currently being investigated in a number of treatment sites as a potential technique to increase dose to the tumor while limiting the normal tissue around the tumor to low doses of radiation. Reports are now being published examining the safety and efficacy of this technique.[131] Whyte and colleagues have reported on 23 patients with tumors between 1 and 5 cm who were treated with this technique at Stanford University.[132] Patients received 15 Gy in a single fraction and this dose was found to be safe and well tolerated. Hof et al. have reported good local control with a short follow-up for patients with stage I NSCLC treated with 19 to 26 Gy of SRS in a single fraction.[133]

INTENSITY-MODULATED RADIATION THERAPY

The advantages of IMRT for NSCLC were demonstrated in a pilot study of six patients previously treated with 3D-CRT who were retrospectively replanned using inverse treatment planning and IMRT.[134] 3D-CRT and IMRT plans were calculated using identical dose volume constraints. Comparisons were made between the maximum dose achievable using the treatment planner's best 3D-CRT plan (typically 3 to 5 wedged fields) and an IMRT plan using the same or similar beam orientations. For all plans, the prescription dose was escalated until the biologic dose constraint for lung was violated. For the six patients, PTV ranged from 229 to 556 cm³, and total lung volumes from 1940 to 3730 cm³. In five of six cases, the prescription dose could be increased with IMRT, on average by 13 Gy. An example of an IMRT plan is presented in Figure 35-6B.

PALLIATION

In view of the poor survival of patients with locally advanced NSCLC and patients with metastatic disease, effective palliation is an important objective. Carroll[135] followed 134 inoperable patients and reported that 64% needed immediate local palliation. Of those with no thoracic symptoms at presentation, half required subsequent local treatment. Thus, a watch-and-wait policy is appropriate for only a minority of patients and it is critical that they be followed carefully to prevent the development of serious local complications of the disease, which may then be less easily palliated. It is important to intervene before superior vena caval obstruction, obstructive pneumonia, or lobar collapse develops. The last two conditions produce a radiographic picture in which tumor and other processes are not easily distinguishable and large radiation fields may be necessary for effective control.

External Beam Radiation Therapy

Various regimens produce a high rate of palliation to some degree, generally sustained for a significant proportion of a patient's survival. Certain symptoms such as hemoptysis of pain are more effectively palliated, while dyspnea, hoarseness, and poor performance status appear to be more refractory. There are no conclusive data proving the palliative superiority of either a more protracted low dose per fraction schedule or a rapid course of large fraction size. The Medical Research Council of Great Britain randomized 369 patients had to either compared 2 fractions of 8.5 Gy 1 week apart (total 17 Gy) versus 30 Gy in 10 fractions versus 27 Gy in 6 fractions. Relief of cough was achieved in approximately 60% and palliation of hemoptysis in approximately 80%, regardless of the treatment regimen. The median duration of palliation was greater than or equal to 50% of survival (median 6 months) for all three treatment approaches.[136]

Distant Metastases

Isolated symptomatic lesions such as bone metastases and spinal cord compression (even if asymptomatic) are managed with palliative courses of radiation (e.g., 30 Gy in 10 fractions). The standard therapy for multiple brain metastases in NSCLC is whole-brain RT. This is accompanied by dexamethasone 4 mg four times daily before and during RT, and anticonvulsants only if seizures occur. The RTOG has studied various dose and fractionation schemes for 1994 patients with brain metastases arising from several primary sites including lung (approximately 50% of patients). The schedules used were 20 Gy in 1 week, 30 Gy in 2 weeks, 30 Gy in 3 weeks, 40 Gy in 3 weeks, and 40 Gy in 4 weeks. The shorter schedules tended to give more rapid relief of neurologic symptoms, but otherwise the schedules had a comparable palliative effect (95% overall), duration of improvement (9 to 13 weeks), and median survival (15 to 18 weeks).[137]

Chemotherapy

Platinum-based palliative chemotherapy has become the standard of care in patients with advanced NSCLC. It has been shown to increase the median survival compared to best supportive care, as well as to improve the quality of life in patients.[138]

ECOG 1594 compared four different platinum-based chemotherapy regimens and found similar results with all four regimens. Response rates ranged from 15% to 21% and 1-year survival ranged from 31% to 36%.[139] Third-generation combination therapies with agents such as gemcitabine, vinorelbine, irinotecan, paclitaxel, and docetaxel with a platinum have been shown to be superior to second-generation combination therapies. Docetaxel has been shown to be superior as a second-line therapy.[140]

New biologic agents attempt to promote tumor growth delay and tumor regression by inhibiting the activation of various receptors. Overexpression of epidermal growth factor receptor (EGFR) in epithelial tumors such as lung cancer has frequently been correlated with poor prognosis, thus stimulating efforts to develop new cancer therapies that target EGFR.[141] The tyrosine kinase inhibitor, gefitinib (Iressa) has been shown to induce tumor regression and was recently approved for use in patients with advanced NSCLC who have failed platinum-based and docetaxel chemotherapies.

SMALL CELL LUNG CANCER

Small cell lung cancer (SCLC) was previously termed *oat cell carcinoma* due to the distinctive small, round shape of the cancer cells. SCLC displays an aggressive growth pattern, a propensity to metastasize, and a remarkable responsiveness to chemotherapy and RT. Although patients can be cured, most die from disease progression due to the rapid development of drug resistance. For this reason, the median survival for patients with metastatic SCLC remains disappointing at 10 months.[142] This is not substantially different from that of patients with NSCLC, a disease much less responsive to chemotherapy. Despite great strides in chemotherapy and radiation, the overall survival rate for patients with SCLC has not changed in the past 20 years.[142]

Pathology

It is rare for SCLC to develop in nonsmokers. Under the microscope, small cell carcinoma appears as small round cells with darkly staining nuclei and scant cytoplasm. In a percentage of cases, a mixed subtype of SCLC and NSCLC is detected. No premalignant histology or molecular marker has been identified for SCLC.

Staging

The staging of SCLC has been simplified to include two stages—limited or extensive—traditionally defined using the Veterans' Administration Lung Study Group criteria.[143] Limited stage disease is confined to one hemithorax and encompassed in a single radiation port. Patients with extensive stage SCLC generally have disease that has spread outside the chest. Common sites of metastasis include the brain, liver, bone, and bone marrow. Patients with involved ipsilateral supraclavicular lymph nodes are generally considered limited stage, while patients with malignant pleural effusions and contralateral supraclavicular lymph node involvement are considered extensive stage.

A thorough work-up is necessary to determine the stage of disease. This may include a bone scan, MRI of the brain, and possibly a bone marrow biopsy. Once a test identifies someone as having extensive disease, the remainder of the workup is superfluous unless it is being done to evaluate a particular symptom. All patients should additionally be screened for electrolyte disturbances. Clinical factors that impact prognosis include stage, performance status, age, gender, and the presence of paraneoplastic syndromes. Several laboratory values have shown significance in predicting poor prognosis, including low serum sodium and high lactate dehydrogenase.[144]

About one third of patients with SCLC present with limited-stage disease. For these patients, long-term survival is a potential, occurring in a small proportion. If cured, these patients require surveillance for second primary malignancies such as NSCLC, particularly if they continue to smoke.[145]

MANAGEMENT OF SMALL CELL LUNG CANCER

Chemotherapy

It was not until chemotherapy trials in the 1970s that survival improved in SCLC from weeks to months. Over the next 20 years, a number of single agents were identified as having significant antitumor activity in SCLC, including cisplatin, carboplatin, cyclophosphamide, doxorubicin, etoposide, ifosfamide, methotrexate, nitrosurea, and vincristine.[142] Several studies have shown that combination therapy is clearly beneficial over single agents, achieving response rates in the range of 80%. The most widely used combinations for SCLC are etoposide plus cisplatin (EP) and cyclophosphamide, doxorubicin, and vincristine (CAV) + etoposide.

Etoposide plus cisplatin has become a standard regimen for front-line therapy of SCLC, in part because it is better tolerated than CAV when given with RT. To avoid the toxicities of cisplatin, namely nausea, vomiting, ototoxicity, and peripheral sensory neuropathy, many oncologists have substituted carboplatin. Carboplatin is easier to administer and does not require aggressive hydration or diuresis. Although nonhematologic toxicities are reduced, however, carboplatin does cause cumulative myelosuppression, anemia, and thrombocytopenia. Several phase II trials have evaluated carboplatin in combination with etoposide for the treatment of SCLC. Response rates are similar to those with cisplatin, ranging from 50% to 63% in patients with extensive disease. The Hellenic Cooperative Oncology Group reported a randomized phase III trial comparing cisplatin with carboplatin.[146] Overall response rates, complete response rates, and median survival did not differ significantly in the two arms.

NEWER AGENTS

A number of other chemotherapeutic drugs that have known activity in NSCLC have also demonstrated activity in SCLC, including paclitaxel, docetaxel, irinotecan, topotecan, gemcitabine, and vinorelbine. For newly diagnosed patients with SCLC, none of these agents has adequate effectiveness as monotherapy; thus, various combinations are under study. Single agents are appropriate in patients treated palliatively for relapse.

Several studies have been conducted to determine whether the addition of paclitaxel to the standard regimens of etoposide and cisplatin or carboplatin improves outcomes. A randomized trial of 133 previously untreated patients with limited or extensive stage disease compared etoposide and cisplatin with etoposide, cisplatin, and paclitaxel.[147] The trial was stopped early after an interim analysis identified eight toxic deaths in the paclitaxel arm versus none in the control arm. The response and survival rates were the same in both arms.

Although permutations of older regimens have been tested, including adding more drugs or escalating doses, little improvement has been made in response or survival over earlier reports of these therapies.[148] At this time, etoposide plus cisplatin or carboplatin is recommended for initial treatment of SCLC.

Thoracic Radiation

SCLC has long been known to be exquisitely sensitive to RT. Early trials used a relatively low dose of RT, presumably because of the rapid response observed. However, establishing whether there was a clear survival advantage to the addition of thoracic RT proved difficult. After 13 randomized trials were performed with conflicting results, a meta-analysis of the data confirmed a small but significant improvement in survival for patients treated with RT.[149] Overall survival at 3 years improved by 5% with younger patients receiving the greatest benefit.

The timing of radiation has been an issue of much controversy. Clearly, toxicity is increased when chemotherapy and radiation are used together. This was evident in two trials using cyclophosphamide-based and doxorubicin-based chemotherapy, showing no difference between concomitant or sequential radiation.[150,151] On the other hand, because of the aggressive nature of SCLC, radiation should theoretically be added early in the treatment to allow the greatest advantage. The National Cancer Institute of Canada compared radiation given concurrently with chemotherapy starting with the second cycle, or radiation given with the final cycle of chemotherapy.[152] Progression-free survival and overall survival were favored in the early radiation treatment arm, although complete remission rates did not differ in the two groups. Severe toxicities were similar in both arms. An overall analysis of several large trials suggests that early radiation results in superior survival.[153]

Twice-daily fractionation has gained attention as a way of potentially improving the results with radiation. Because SCLC is sensitive to radiation even at low doses, administering smaller fractions of radiation more often could theoretically have an antitumor effect while sparing normal tissues. In an Intergroup trial, twice-daily radiation to a dose of 45 Gy (1.5 Gy twice a day) given concomitantly with etoposide and cisplatin resulted in a 5-year survival rate of 23% compared with 16% for daily radiation treatment (1.8 Gy to 45 Gy, $P = 0.04$).[154] The local failure rate was reduced from 52% in the once-daily arm to 36% in the twice-daily arm. Esophagitis did occur more frequently in the twice-daily radiation arm, but this was reversible. This treatment approach has the best results observed in the literature to date and should be attempted in all patients who can tolerate it.

Due to the difficulty and toxicity in delivering twice-daily RT, attempts have been made to replicate the results seen in the Intergroup trial with higher doses of once-daily radiation. Choi et al. reported that 56 to 70 Gy in a once-daily schedule was well tolerated with cycle 4 of etoposide plus cisplatin chemotherapy.[155] A CALGB phase II trial investigated the use of 70 Gy delivered in 2-Gy fractions concurrent with cycle 3 of EP chemotherapy.[156] They found this regimen feasible and reported a median survival of 19.8 months.

In summary, thoracic radiation provides a small survival advantage to patients with limited-stage SCLC. Younger patients receiving radiation concomitantly early in the course of chemotherapy will likely gain the greatest benefit. The local failure rate is still unacceptably high and more advanced techniques or strategies will be needed to improve it.

Surgery

Surgery alone is inadequate therapy for SCLC. In the Medical Research Council study conducted in the 1960s, surgery resulted in a 2-year survival rate of less than 2%.[157] Although a select group of patients may benefit from resection, such as patients with disease confined to the lung (N0, M0)[158] or patients with a mixed histology with NSCLC, surgery is not appropriate for most patients due to the high rate of early metastasis.

RADIATION THERAPY TECHNIQUE FOR SMALL CELL LUNG CANCER

The target volume is determined by correlating imaging studies with bronchoscopic or mediastinoscopy findings. Generally, the objective is to treat all gross disease and to electively treat the ipsilateral hilum, the mediastinal nodes bilaterally, and the ipsilateral supraclavicular area. Such treatment could be accomplished in a manner as described earlier in the section on 2D RT technique. When twice-daily RT is used, the anterior-posterior fields are treated in the morning and afternoon for the first week and only in the morning for the second and third weeks. The off-cord obliques are used for the afternoon treatments in weeks 2 and 3 only. It is important not to decrease the superior-inferior field length for the off-cord treatment. Typical simulation fields are identical to 2D RT fields and are presented in Figure 35-7.

If once-daily RT is used, an anterior-posterior field as described earlier is used for the first course of treatment. Subsequently, off-cord oblique fields to the same tumor volume are used. When higher doses of RT are being used (>60 Gy) it may be appropriate to use 3D-CRT for the second course of treatment. In the CALGB trial discussed earlier, one-half of the patients were treated with 3D-CRT.[156] In these situations, we typically stop the first course of RT at 36 Gy in order to ensure that the cumulative dose to the spinal cord with the 3D plan will be less than 45 Gy.

Prophylactic Cranial Irradiation

The central nervous system is a common place of metastasis for SCLC, occurring in up to 50% of cases in autopsy series.[159] Because the blood-brain barrier provides a sanctuary from the effects of chemotherapy, radiation was studied as a way of decreasing the risk of brain metastases. A meta-analysis of early trials of prophylactic cranial irradiation (PCI) revealed that the benefit was greatest in patients with a complete response to chemotherapy; other patients succumbed to systemic disease.[160] More randomized trials followed evaluating the efficacy of PCI in patients with a complete response, and a subsequent meta-analysis summarized the results.[161] PCI not only decreased the incidence of brain metastasis (relative risk 0.46, $P < 0.001$), but also increased the disease-free survival (relative risk or recurrence or death 0.75, $P < 0.001$) and the overall survival (15% vs. 21% at 3 years). This effect was seen regardless of stage in subgroup analysis, though patients with extensive disease comprised a small percentage. With increasing doses of radiation, the rate of local control improved, but survival was not affected.

The concern for diminished cognitive function after brain irradiation gives many oncologists pause in recommending this treatment, especially in patients with extensive stage disease. The argument holds that the PCI only changes the pattern of relapse, and that radiation can be administered when brain metastases are discovered. However, other factors may contribute to cognitive impairment in these patients, such as chemotherapy effects or subtle paraneoplastic syndromes. In fact, in one randomized trial, neuropsychologic function and the rate of brain CT scan abnormalities did not differ between patients who received or did not receive PCI.[162] Thus, PCI is recommended for patients with a complete response to chemotherapy. Various dose and fractionation regimens have been used and 25 Gy in 10 fractions or 30 Gy in 15 fractions are probably the most commonly delivered.

MESOTHELIOMA

Mesothelioma is a chemoresistant tumor whose epidemiology has been linked with exposure to asbestos. Approximately 2200 people are diagnosed each year in the United States. The median survival is poor, ranging from 4 to 18 months.[163] No single mode of therapy—chemotherapy, radiotherapy, or surgery—has impacted significantly on the survival of these patients. Combined modalities such as surgery followed by adjuvant chemotherapy and radiotherapy have had limited success. Few patients have benefited from this because most patients present with unresectable disease. Thus, there is no standard treatment for mesothelioma.

The 2002 American Joint Committee on Cancer Staging system is presented in Table 35-7.

Surgery

Attempts at local control of the tumor are felt to be a patient's best chance for long-term survival. Two operations have commonly been performed: the extrapleural pneumonectomy (EPP) and the pleurectomy/decortication. The EPP involves en bloc resection of the entire pleura, lung, diaphragm, and ipsilateral half of the pericardium. This operation is associated with a 2-year survival of 30% to 40% and an operative mortality of 5% to 15%. Operative risk appears to be related to patient selection and to the frequency with which the involved thoracic surgeon performs this relatively uncommon procedure. With experience and careful patient selection, the risk of this operation can be reduced to that of a standard pneumonectomy.[164] The second operation, the pleurectomy/decortication, involves resecting all gross tumor without removing the lung. If necessary, the pericardium and the diaphragm are resected and reconstructed. The operative mortality for pleurectomy/decortication is less than that of EPP and is approximately 2%.[165] Although pleurectomy/decortication carries a lower operative risk, it only allows complete resection of tumors in patients who have very early-stage disease with minimal involvement of the visceral pleura. It also limits the dose of adjuvant postoperative RT because the lung is left in place. EPP allows the administration of higher doses of radiation and, therefore, theoretically has a better chance of providing control of local disease.

Chemotherapy

Single-agent chemotherapy has poor activity. No drug has consistently demonstrated a greater than 20% response rate.[166] Combinations of chemotherapeutic agents have been tried in the past with few, if any, improving on the response rates of single agents and without significantly improving survival.

Newer agents such as gemcitabine (a pyrimidine analog) have not been extensively studied in mesothelioma. Gemcitabine alone produced a meager response rate of 7% in one EORTC phase II trial.[167] A phase II study combined gemcitabine, 1000 mg/m^2 on days 1, 8, and 15, with cisplatin 100 mg/m^2 day 1, for patients with advanced mesothelioma.[168] The response rate achieved was 47.6% (10/21 patients with a partial response). No patient achieved a complete response. Several patients had stable disease (9/21 patients). Toxicity was limited to gastrointestinal and hematologic toxicities. There were no treatment-related deaths. Only one patient developed febrile neutropenia. The reported response rate is the highest observed in any trial of advanced mesothelioma. A multicenter Dutch phase II trial used gemcitabine 1250 mg/m^2 days 1 and 8 with cisplatin 80 mg/m^2 on day 8 and reported an 18% response rate.[169]

Recently, a new chemotherapeutic agent, Premetrexed (ALIMTA), a novel antifolate that targets key enzymes in purine and pyrimidine synthesis, was studied in a randomized trial that compared it in combination with cisplatin versus cisplatin alone. This trial demonstrated superiority of Premetrexed/Cisplatin over cisplatin monotherapy with

Table 35–7   New International Mesothelioma Interest Group Staging System for Diffuse MPM

T1	T1a tumor limited to the ipsilateral parietal pleura, including mediastinal and diaphragmatic pleura
	No involvement of the visceral pleura
	T1b tumor involving the ipsilateral parietal pleura, including mediastinal and diaphragmatic pleura
	Scattered foci of tumor also involving the visceral pleura
T2	Tumor involving each of the ipsilateral pleura surfaces (parietal, mediastinal, diaphragmatic, and visceral pleura) with at least one of the following features:
	• involvement of diaphragmatic muscle
	• confluent visceral pleural tumor (including the fissures) or extension to tumor from visceral pleura into the underlying pulmonary parenchyma
T3	Describes locally advanced but potentially resectable tumor
	Tumor involving all of the ipsilateral pleural surfaces (parietal, mediastinal, diaphragmatic, and visceral pleura) with at least one of the following features:
	• involvement of the endothoracic fascia
	• extension into the mediastinal fat
	• solitary, completely resectable focus of tumor extending into the soft tissues of the chest wall
	• nontransmural involvement of the pericardium
T4	Tumor involving all of the ipsilateral pleural surfaces (parietal, mediastinal, diaphragmatic, and visceral) with at least one of the following features:
	• diffuse extension or multifocal masses of tumor in the chest wall, with or without associated rib destruction
	• direct transdiaphragmatic extension of tumor to the peritoneum
	• direct extension of tumor to the contralateral pleura
	• direct extension of tumor to one or more mediastinal organs
	• direct extension of tumor into the spine
	• tumor extending through to the internal surface of the pericardium with or without pericardial effusion, or tumor involving the myocardium

Lymph nodes (N)

NX	Regional lymph nodes cannot be assessed
N0	No regional lymph node metastases
N1	Metastases in the ipsilateral bronchopulmonary or hilar lymph nodes
N2	Metastases in the subcarinal or the ipsilateral mediastinal lymph nodes, including the ipsilateral internal mammary nodes
N3	Metastases in the contralateral mediastinal, contralateral internal mammary, ipsilateral or contralateral supraclavicular lymph nodes

Metastases (M)

MX	Presence of distant metastases cannot be assessed
M0	No distant metastasis
M1	Distant metastasis present

Stage	Description
Stage I	
Ia	T1aN0M0
Ib	T1bN0M0
Stage II	T2N0M0
Stage III	Any T3M0
	Any N1M0
	Any N2M0
Stage IV	Any T4
	Any N3
	Any M1

From International Mesothelioma Interest Group Staging System. Rusch VW: *Chest.* 1995;108:1122.

a response rate of 41% versus 17%, and a median survival of 12.1 months versus 9.3 months, respectively.[170]

Radiation

External beam RT has been ineffective as primary treatment in prolonging survival in mesothelioma patients. It is not possible to administer radiation doses that might be tumoricidal for gross tumor because of the proximity of mesothelioma to structures such as lungs that are radiation intolerant.

To minimize the dose to the lung parenchyma, the standard surgical approach at MSKCC was, for many years, a pleurectomy with intraoperative brachytherapy applied to areas of gross residual disease, followed by external beam RT using photon and electron therapy.[171] Between 1976 and 1988, 164 patients underwent a thoracotomy for mesothelioma, of whom 105 evaluable patients were treated with this combined approach. Brachytherapy was performed in 63% (66/105) of patients and all patients received postoperative external beam RT. The median survival for the entire group was 12.6 months, with 2-year survival of 23%. A favorable subset of patients who had epithelial tumor and complete surgical resection had a median survival of 22.5 months. Radiation pneumonitis occurred in 11% (12/105), and

radiation pericarditis in 7% (8/105) of patients. Local failure or disease progression occurred in 63% (64/105) of patients. This experience highlighted the need for complete resection and the inability to control gross residual tumor by brachytherapy and a moderate dose of external beam RT (median of 4200 cGy).

A prospective trial was completed at MSKCC evaluating the treatment of malignant pleural mesothelioma with hemithoracic RT of 54 Gy.[172] The trial was performed to determine the feasibility, rates of local recurrence, and survival of patients with resectable pleural mesothelioma treated by EPP followed by high-dose hemithoracic RT (54 Gy). Eighty-eight patients were entered on the study. This approach reduced local recurrence, and prolonged survival to a median of 33.8 months for stage I and II tumors. More advanced stages had high risk of early distant relapse and a median survival of 10 months. Adjuvant radiation was well tolerated (grade 0 to 2 fatigue, esophagitis) except for one late esophageal fistula.

TECHNIQUE OF POSTOPERATIVE RADIATION THERAPY

It is ideal to begin hemithoracic radiation within 3 to 6 weeks following EPP, with a total dose of 54 Gy delivered in 30 fractions of 1.8 Gy. Patients can undergo either fluoroscopic or CT simulation. Patients are placed supine with arms akimbo. Customized immobilization is typically not used.

The superior border of the field is the top of T1 at the thoracic inlet, the inferior border at the bottom of L2, and the lateral border flashed skin (Fig. 35-8). If the mediastinal nodes are involved, the medial border should include the mediastinum with the margin extending 1.5 to 2.0 cm beyond the contralateral border of the vertebral bodies. If there is no evidence of mediastinal disease, the medial border should be placed at the contralateral edge of the vertebral body.

A block is placed anteriorly and posteriorly over the abdomen from the start of treatment to shield the stomach and liver from photon irradiation. These blocks typically extend from 1.5 cm from the ipsilateral border of the vertebral bodies to within 2.0 cm to the edge of the chest wall. The blocks cover areas where the diaphragm abutted the abdominal wall, facilitating treatment of this area with electrons. The blocks were not placed where the diaphragm was oblique to the abdominal wall. For left-sided tumors, a block was placed anteriorly over the heart starting at 19.8 Gy. Additional photon blocking was used to exclude the humerus.

Bolus was not routinely placed over the scar or drainage sites, but these sites were included in the radiation field.

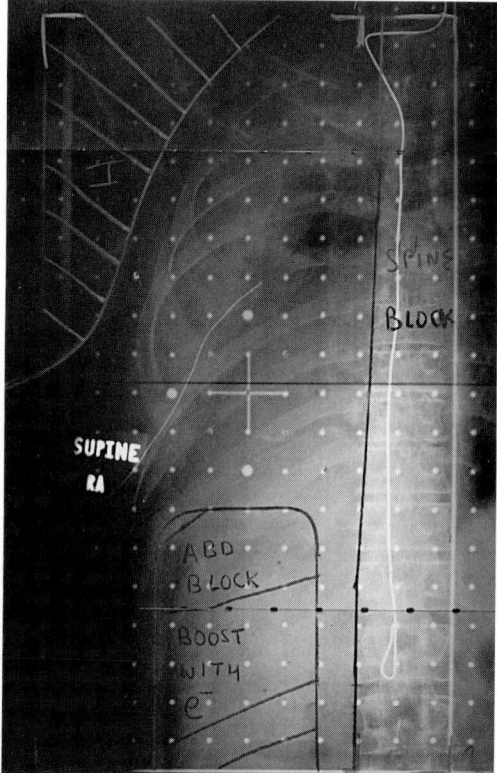

Figure 35–8. Simulation film of right hemithorax following extrapleural pneumonectomy. Field borders are T1 superiorly, L2 inferiorly, the edge of the vertebral body contralaterally, and flashing skin laterally. A block was placed over the abdomen from the start of treatment to shield the stomach and liver from photon irradiation. The blocks covered areas where the diaphragm abutted the abdominal wall, facilitating treatment of this area with electrons. The daily dose of electron irradiation was 153 cGy, as it was assumed there was 15% scatter under the blocks from the photon fields.

At MSKCC, recurrence in the chest wall is rare, even without the use of a scar boost.[173]

Custom lead cut-outs conforming to the blocked areas are used on the photon fields. The blocked abdominal and cardiac regions are treated with electron irradiation. The daily dose of electron irradiation was 1.53 Gy, as there was 15% scatter under the blocks from the photon fields.[174] The dose is normalized to the 90% isodose line and treated with a high enough energy to ensure coverage of the chest wall by the 90% isodose curve.

After 41.4 Gy is delivered, the second phase of the radiation course blocks the spinal cord from the treated field. The final phase typically receives 12.6 Gy in 8 fractions. The superior, inferior, and lateral borders are unchanged from the first phase. The medial border is the ipsilateral edge of the vertebral body, designed to block the spinal cord.

NEOPLASMS OF THE MEDIASTINUM

Anatomy

The boundaries of the mediastinum are the diaphragm inferiorly, the parietal pleura laterally, the sternum at the anterior border, the vertebral column posteriorly, and the thoracic inlet superiorly (Table 35-8). Within the mediastinum are a great number of lymph node drainage areas, and the lymph nodes most likely involved are those immediately adjacent to the tumor. Thus, an anterior mediastinal thymoma might spread on the left to prevascular or level VI lymph nodes as the first echelon of drainage.

TUMORS OF THE THYMUS

Pathology

Several malignant tumors can arise from the thymus, including lymphomas, thymomas, germ cell tumors, carcinoids, and thymic carcinoma. In addition, benign neoplasms also occur. The epithelium of the thymus is the cell of origin of thymomas. Thymomas are composed of bland cells that do not have particular malignant cytologic features. Thymomas, however, can invade surrounding tissues and indeed metastasize within the chest and rarely to other organs.[175] The histologic appearance of localized and invasive tumors tends to be similar

Table 35–8 Anatomical Correlation of Tumor Type Within Mediastinum

Superior	Middle
Lymphoma	Lymphoma
Thyroid	Lung cancer
Thymic tumors	Tumors of heart
Lung cancer	Vascular tumors
Tracheal tumors	
Lymphomas	**Posterior**
Teratomas	Neurogenic tumors
Thymic tumors	Esophageal tumors

except that invasive tumors are not encapsulated or have spread through the capsule. Frequently the distinction between benign and malignant thymomas is a clinical one made by the operating surgeon. If the clinical findings at surgery indicate invasion, the tumor should be treated as a malignant one, even if a subsequent pathology report fails to detect any features of malignancy.

Clinical Presentation

Patients with thymoma are usually between the ages of 40 and 60 years. Thymomas occur rarely in children and tend to be more aggressive. The incidence is approximately equal between the sexes. The etiology of thymoma is unknown. About 30% to 40% of patients diagnosed with thymoma have an anterior mediastinal mass diagnosed or detected on an x-ray film performed for another reason. When symptoms do occur, they result from pressure on surrounding mediastinal structures. Thymomas can present with chest pain, cough, and dyspnea. Of all patients presenting with thymoma, approximately 35% to 50% are associated with myasthenia gravis, 5% with red cell aplasia, and 5% with hypogammaglobulinemia.[175]

About 75% of patients with myasthenia gravis have thymic abnormalities. Of the abnormal thymic glands, 85% have hyperplasia and 15% have thymomas. Removal of the thymus is indicated in all myasthenia gravis patients with tumors. In patients with hyperplasia, thymectomy results in remission of the myasthenia gravis in 35% and improvement in a further 50%.[176]

The main method by which thymoma spreads is by local invasion. Mediastinal lymph nodes may be involved and sometimes pleural metastases occur. These can present in more locally advanced patients and take the form of multiple drop metastases into the pleural space. Alternatively, this can be a presentation at recurrence in a patient whose thorax has previously been opened. Although this presentation implies fairly widespread disease, it is often reasonable to resect such pleural metastases since prolonged survival may result. Patients with thymoma may rarely have metastasis, usually in the setting of advanced local nodal or pleural disease.

Diagnostic and Staging Studies

Because these are anterior mediastinal tumors, they can be clearly seen on a lateral x-ray study. A CT scan allows precise definition of the extent of involvement of the suspected thymoma for staging. A cyst can be differentiated from solid tumors, and pleural and pericardial implants can be identified. An MRI does not have a significant yield beyond that obtained with CT scan. In planning RT (either as sole treatment or postoperatively), the initial diagnostic CT scan is vital. It is important in a postoperative setting to treat the entire area from which the thymoma arose. It must be noted that often a thymoma may have abutted the posterior sternum or anterior chest wall, and this area may be at risk for recurrence if not included in the postoperative radiation fields.

It is important to exclude the possibility that one is dealing with a mediastinal germ cell tumor. Consequently, appropriate serum markers as noted in the section on germ cell tumors should be obtained.

Staging

There is no formal American Joint Committee on Cancer TNM system for staging thymic tumors. A system described by Masaoka and associates[177] is widely used (Table 35-9). Of note, this system classifies pleural or pericardial metastases as stage IVA and lymphatic or hematogenous metastases as stage IVB. At presentation, approximately 40% of patients have the current stage I, 20% stage II, and the remainder stage III.

Standard Therapeutic Approaches

Complete surgical resection is the treatment of choice for thymoma. If the integrity of the capsule of a thymoma is violated, there is a high propensity for local recurrence. Incisional biopsy should be avoided unless the patient is unable to tolerate a resection or has an unresectable tumor. Fine-needle aspiration cytology is an excellent alternative to incisional biopsy. Stage I thymoma can easily be removed with the entire thymus without disturbing the integrity of the capsule. No more than 2% of stage I thymomas develop recurrences, which usually take the form of a localized mediastinal tumor or are caused by pleural, pericardial, or diaphragmatic implants. An aggressive surgical approach is appropriate for stage II and subsets of stage III thymomas. It is important to preserve the phrenic nerves, especially if myasthenia gravis is present. Any involved structures should be resected if technically feasible. This may include lobectomy or pneumonectomy in some instances. A median sternotomy is the usual approach to the anterior mediastinum. Sometimes an alternative approach is chosen if the tumor is predominantly on one side of the thoracic cavity, in which case a thoracotomy may be performed. If an invasive thymoma is documented surgically, it is important that the surgeon place metallic clips to define the margins of resection and identify any postoperative residual disease. RT is usually used postoperatively for stage II and III tumors. Preoperatively, RT may be used to shrink a tumor to render it resectable, and primary RT is indicated for unresectable tumors or for tumors with

Table 35-9 Masaoka Staging System of Thymomas

Stage I	Macroscopically completely encapsulated and microscopically no capsular invasion
Stage II	Macroscopic invasion into surrounding fatty tissue or mediastinal pleura; microscopic invasion into capsule
Stage III	Macroscopic invasion into neighboring organs (pericardium, great vessels, or lung)
Stage IVa	Pleural or pericardial dissemination
Stage IVb	Lymphogenous or hematogenous metastases

From Masaoka A, Monden Y, Nakahara K, Tanioka T: Follow-up study of thymomas with special reference to their clinical stages. *Cancer.* 1981;48:2485.

gross residual disease after surgery. Massive tumors may be treated by induction chemotherapy with resection and postoperative RT. Common regimens include cyclophosphamide, doxorubicin, vincristine, and prednisone (CHOP); cisplatin, doxorubicin, and cyclophosphamide (PAC); and combined cisplatin and etoposide as used in SCLC.

RADIATION TECHNIQUE

The treatment technique is similar to what is used for unresectable NSCLC as described earlier. However, the target volume includes the entire thymus (or bed of resected thymus) and any involved organs. The PTV should include a 1-cm margin around these anatomic structures. For postoperative patients, it is imperative that the preoperative CT scans be available to accurately delineate the tumor bed. In addition, the operative report and pathology report should be scrutinized to determine which areas might have had adherent, invasive disease.

Our approach at MSKCC for postoperative RT is to deliver 45 to 54 Gy in 1.8-Gy fractions 5 days per week. For completely resected stage II patients, we use a dose of 45 Gy. For stage III patients, we typically treat to 50.4 to 54 Gy. For patients with gross residual disease, we try to increase the total dose as high as 60 to 65 Gy depending on the amount of residual tumor and the predicted toxicity from the dose volume histogram.

CHEMOTHERAPY

The use of chemotherapy has not been well studied due to the rarity of this tumor and the fact that most patients are treated with surgical excision.[178] Some investigators have used CHOP chemotherapy and others have used combined etoposide and cisplatin therapy. These treatments result in responses in up to 70% of patients. A regimen of PAC demonstrated a 50% response rate.[179] Currently, the main indication for the use of chemotherapy is as preoperative therapy in an attempt to render a tumor resectable or amenable to radical RT. Chemotherapy is also used for palliation of metastatic disease.

Results of Treatment

INITIAL SERIES

The first reports of megavoltage RT in the treatment of thymoma were by Batata from MSKCC and Marks from South Carolina. Batata reported on 54 patients treated between 1928 and 1972.[180] Patients with invasive thymomas either received surgery alone or surgery plus RT. With surgery alone, none of the 8 patients were disease free at 5 years, while of those receiving surgery plus RT, 6 of 28 were disease free after 5 years. All patients who had incomplete resection and received less than 40 Gy had disease recurrence.

ADJUVANT RADIATION

Curran from Fox Chase reported the results of RT for thymoma.[181] Patients with stage I disease treated with surgery alone had 100% 5-year local control (43 of 43).

Patients treated with gross total resection and RT had a 100% local control (5 of 5). Patients treated with gross total resection without RT had only a 53% local control (13 of 21). Patients treated with subtotal resection and RT had 80% local control (16 of 20), while those treated with subtotal resection without RT had only 50% local control (3 of 6). Curran also provided a meta-analysis of eight previous series with stage II or III patients. Patients with a gross total resection plus RT had local control in 95% (41 of 43), while patients treated with gross total resection without RT had a local control rate of only 72% (52 of 72).

RADIATION FOR GROSS DISEASE

Ciernik and associates[182] from Zurich treated 31 patients with residual macroscopic disease after surgery with 42 to 60 Gy of external beam RT. They noted that epithelial and spindle cell histology and tumors greater than 10 cm had a poor prognosis. Debulking appeared to have no benefit (although it can simplify the technical challenges of radiation planning). Mediastinal control was achieved in 74% (23 of 31 patients). Stage III patients had a 10-year survival of 57% and stage IV patients had 5-year survival of 23% and 10-year survival of 8%. Mornex et al. reported on 90 patients with stage III or IVA thymoma who presented at 10 French cancer centers.[183] They found that with a median dose of 50 Gy, the relapse rate was 14% for patients whose tumor was completely resected and 41% for patients who underwent less extensive surgery.

Malignant Mediastinal Germ Cell Tumors

Malignant mediastinal germ cell tumors account for 5% to 10% of malignant mediastinal tumors and about 2.5% of all mediastinal neoplasms. Males represent approximately 80% of patients developing these tumors.

CLINICAL PRESENTATION

Seminomas are most common in the third decade of life and nonseminomatous germ cell tumors occur in adults from 15 to 35 years of age. These tumors are usually located in the anterior superior mediastinum. Almost one third of patients can present merely by having a routine chest x-ray study performed. As the tumor becomes larger, it can produce substernal pressure and pain radiating to the neck and arms. Superior vena cava obstruction can occur. The more malignant lesions can present with more pain due to local invasion and other symptoms due to local pressure. These tumors have the same histologic appearance as testicular tumors. The histologic distribution is the same with approximately 40% of patients having seminoma and 60% of patients having nonseminomatous germ cell tumors. Approximately 40% of patients with choriocarcinoma develop gynecomastia. Serum beta human chorionic gonadotropin is elevated in about 60% of patients with nonseminomatous germ cell tumors and they have elevated alpha-fetoprotein levels. This often correlates with the presence of embryonic or yolk sac components.[175] It is very important to obtain these serum markers before treatment to assist in diagnoses, to allow monitoring of the response to treatment, and as part of the follow-up of the patients.

PROGNOSTIC FACTORS AND THERAPY

The most important prognostic factor is histologic type. Seminomas are highly curable, whereas nonseminomatous germ cell tumors have a much poorer prognosis. There is little evidence of a role for the routine use of RT for nonseminomatous germ cell tumors. The mainstay of therapy is chemotherapy and surgery. Figure 35-9 shows an MRI of a mediastinal nonseminomatous germ cell tumor. On the other hand, seminomas are traditionally treated with RT either as an adjuvant treatment or sole therapy. The techniques of RT are similar to those described for thymomas. The results of RT for treatment of mediastinal seminoma have been summarized by Emami.[175] Of 78 patients receiving less than 50 Gy, 54 patients were alive and 21 had died of disease. Of 13 patients who received 50 Gy or higher, 12 were alive and only one died of disease. It was difficult in this review to assess the anatomic patterns of failure, but it would appear that higher doses of RT are required than are typically used for seminoma elsewhere in the body. In reviewing the literature, doses in the range of 20 to 60 Gy have been used. Bush and colleagues[184] from Stanford University recommend 40 to 50 Gy in conventional fractionation. They treated 13 patients with definitive megavoltage RT with a follow-up of 5 years. The 10-year

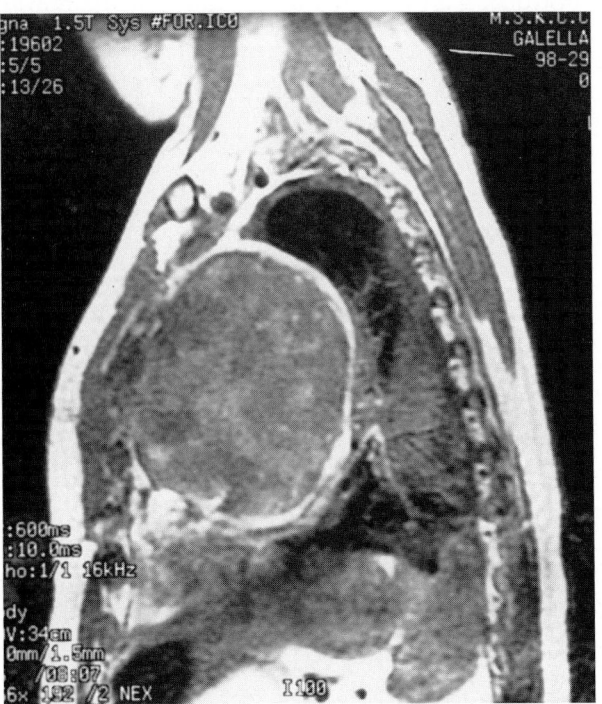

Figure 35–9. This magnetic resonance image (MRI) is from a 54-year old man who presented with substernal discomfort, dysphagia, and elevated serum alpha-fetoprotein. The MRI revealed a massive tumor of the mediastinum with an inhomogeneous appearance. Pathology revealed a yolk sac nonseminomatous germ cell tumor.

survival was 69% and relapse-free survival was 54%. No patients receiving more than 47 Gy to the primary lesion had local or systemic relapse. Although it is not possible to make definitive recommendations regarding doses of RT, it appears reasonable to use approximately 45 Gy to the mediastinal nodal drainage areas and to follow this with a cone-down approach to any gross disease. A cone-down is not necessary if the patient has a resection and RT is being used as adjuvant therapy.

TRACHEAL CANCERS

Pathology

Squamous cell carcinoma of the trachea represents 50% to 60% of all primary tracheal cancers. It is most common in the sixth decade and is often multifocal on presentation with areas of carcinoma in situ and squamous cell metaplasia. It occurs predominantly in the distal third of the trachea. About 60% of cases originate in the posterior or lateral wall. It has the poorest prognosis of all tracheal cancers due to increased frequency of extension to the surrounding structures and mediastinal lymph nodes. At autopsy, metastases can be found in lung, bone, and liver, and local extension to the mediastinum is common. Adenoid-cystic carcinoma (cylindroma) is the second most common tracheal malignancy. It tends to occur in younger patients and is the dominant histology in the upper trachea. The tumor can be indolent with slowly progressive local invasion. Since the tumor arises from the mucus gland in the tracheal wall, the overlying mucosa can be intact. Vertical extension superiorly or inferiorly along the course of the trachea is common. Adenoid-cystic carcinoma tends to metastasize late in the natural history of the disease and about 10% of patients have regional lymph node involvement at the time of surgery. Perineural lymphatic spread can also be observed. Other tumors of the trachea include adenocarcinoma, carcinoid tumors, sarcomas, and direct extension from lung and esophageal cancer. Also, metastases from breast and thyroid cancer can occur.

Clinical Features

The normal trachea has a cross sectional area that is larger than what is usually required for adequate ventilation. Unfortunately, as a result of this, symptoms can present when the disease is rather advanced. These include dyspnea (which can be precipitated by a change in position), cough, wheezing, hemoptysis, and stridor. It is not uncommon for a patient to be incorrectly diagnosed as having asthma. Other symptoms can arise due to mediastinal or secondary spread.

Diagnostic and Staging Studies

A chest x-ray study is not usually helpful, although it may detect gross mediastinal invasion. However, careful examination of the tracheal air column may help to detect a tumor. A CT scan is important to delineate the full extent of luminal tumor and any paratracheal extension. Bronchoscopy should be done in all cases with caution to avoid precipitating airway obstruction. It should be accompanied by esophagoscopy to exclude invasion to the esophagus or invasion by an esophageal cancer into the trachea. There is no recognized staging system for cancer of the trachea.

Management

The treatment of choice for tracheal cancers is resection, if possible. It is very important that an experienced surgeon undertake these very complicated procedures. There is a role for carefully debulking with rigid bronchoscopy and meticulous control of the airway for relief of acute obstruction and patient stabilization before assessing the therapeutic options. Upper tracheal tumors of limited extent may be resected through a cervical collar incision. It is important to position the patient so that the surgeon may extend the approach as it becomes necessary on the basis of operative findings. Tumor of the midtrachea may be approached by an incision including cervical and sternotomy components. A full median sternotomy with a transpericardial approach to the lower trachea and carina may be used. However, a right posterolateral thoracotomy in the fourth interspace provides a better approach to tumors of the lower trachea and most tumors of the carina. The resection rate in the Massachusetts General Hospital series was 74%.[185] It varies according to the type of tumor. Three quarters of adenoid cystic carcinoma were resectable and two thirds of squamous cancers were resected. Factors influencing resectability are excessive linear extent of the tumor, which can leave insufficient trachea for reconstruction. In addition, invasion of critical mediastinal structures and distant metastases preclude resection. The majority of patients in Grillo and Mathieson's series had primary airway reconstruction. A few patients whose tumors involved the upper trachea and approximated the larynx were treated by laryngotracheal resection, with an endostoma being fashioned in the base of the neck or mediastinum.

Postoperative RT is indicated for close of positive margins of resection, lymph node spread, perineural extension, or direct invasion into mediastinal obstructions. Grillo and Mathieson have recommended postoperative RT in almost all resected cases.[185] They suggest that the integrity of the airway anastomosis be established before starting. Intraoperatively, the anastomosis may be protected by oversewing with omentum or intercostal muscle. There are no clear data regarding the optimum dose to use postoperatively. Doses of 50 Gy may be used if the microscopic burden is minimal. However, a dose of up to 60 Gy may be used if the higher postoperative burden is present. If the indication for postoperative RT is a positive margin on the airway itself, then an intraluminal brachytherapy boost may be used to deliver a high dose of radiation to the site of the positive margin. However, if the indication for postoperative RT is extension to other structures, it is unlikely that an intraluminal boost with its very localized dose would significantly cover the entire area at risk.

SIMULATION

Technique is similar to unresectable NSCLC as described earlier. It is important when designing fields for adenoid-cystic carcinoma to be aware of the potential for perineural lymphatic spread along the length of the trachea and to provide wide proximal and distal margins. It may be reasonable to use margins on the order of 4 to 5 cm distally and proximally along the trachea and deliver a dose of 50 Gy , and then reduce the margins to 2 to 3 cm before delivering the final dose. Doses of 60 to 63 Gy should be used, if feasible.

RESULTS OF TREATMENT

Grillo and Mathieson from the Massachusetts General Hospital have reported the largest surgical series.[185] Although actuarial survival was not reported, most patients experienced moderate to long-term survival. Adenoid-cystic histology was distinctly more favorable than squamous cell. No analysis of the role of adjuvant postoperative RT was reported. However, the authors referred most patients for RT, which was delivered with various techniques and doses. They recommend RT after surgery. Chung[186] reported on 20 patients with squamous histology treated with between 45 and 70 Gy, and the median survival was only 5 months. Consequently, when feasible, resection and postoperative RT would appear to be the treatment of choice.

ACKNOWLEDGEMENTS

The authors acknowledge the contributions of Dr. John Armstrong, who prepared this chapter for the previous edition. We would also like to thank Dr. Jana Fox, Dr. Raja Flores, and Ms. Luz Gloder for their help in the preparation of the manuscript, and Dr. Ellen Yorke, Louise Braban, and Laura Happersett for their help in preparation of the figures.

REFERENCES

1. Jemal A, Thomas A, Murray T, Thun M: Cancer statistics, 2002. CA Cancer J Clin. 2002;52:23.
2. Loeb LA, Ernster VL, Warner KE, et al: Smoking and lung cancer: An overview. Cancer Res. 1984;44:5940.
3. Alavanja MC: Biologic damage resulting from exposure to tobacco smoke and from radon: Implication for preventive interventions. Oncogene. 2002;21:7365.
4. Osada H, Takahashi T: Genetic alterations of multiple tumor suppressors and oncogenes in the carcinogenesis and progression of lung cancer. Oncogene. 2002;21:7421.
5. Tyczynski JE, Bray F, Parkin DM: Lung cancer in Europe in 2000: Epidemiology, prevention, and early detection. Lancet Oncol. 2003;4:45.
6. Fraumeni JF Jr: Respiratory carcinogenesis: An epidemiologic appraisal. J Natl Cancer Inst. 1975;55:1039.
7. Fraumeni JF Jr, Blott WJ: Lung and pleura. In Schottenfeld D, Fraumeni JF Jr, eds. Cancer: Epidemiology and Prevention. Philadelphia: WB Saunders; 1982.
8. National Academy of Sciences: Environmental Tobacco Smoke: Measuring Exposure and Assessing Health Effects. Washington, DC: National Academy Press; 1986.
9. Goodman GE: Lung cancer. 1: prevention of lung cancer. Thorax. 2002;57:994.

10. Bertram JS: Rationale and strategies for chemoprevention of cancer in humans. *Cancer Res.* 1987;47:3012

11. Roggli VL, Vollmer RT, Greenberg SD, et al: Lung cancer heterogeneity: A blinded and randomized study of 100 consecutive cases. *Hum Pathol.* 1985;16:569.

12. Henschke CI, McCauley DI, Yankelevitz DF, et al: Early Lung Cancer Action Project: overall design and findings from baseline screening. *Lancet.* 1999;354:99.

13. Vansteenkiste JF, Stroobants SG, De Leyn PR, et al: Lymph node staging in non–small-cell lung cancer with FDG-PET scan: A prospective study on 690 lymph node stations from 68 patients. *J Clin Oncol.* 1998;16:2142.

14. van Zandwijk N: New methods for early diagnosis of lung cancer. *Lung Cancer.* 2002;38:S9.

15. Luke WP, Pearson FG, Todd TR, et al: Prospective evaluation of mediastinoscopy for assessment of carcinoma of the lung. *J Thorac Cardiovasc Surg.* 1986;91:53.

16. McKneal TM, Chamberlain JM: Diagnostic anterior mediastinotomy. *Ann Thorac Surg.* 1966;2:523.

17. Clinical practice guidelines for the treatment of unresectable non–small-cell lung cancer. Adopted on May 16, 1997 by the American Society of Clinical Oncology. *J Clin Oncol.* 1997;15:2996.

18. Mountain CF: A new international staging system for lung cancer. *Chest.* 1986;89(suppl 4):225S.

19. Sawyer TE, Bonner JA, Gould PM, et al: Factors predicting patterns of recurrence after resection of N1 non- small cell lung carcinoma. *Ann Thorac Surg.* 1999;68:1171.

20. Stanley KE: Prognostic factors for survival in patients with inoperable lung cancer. *J Natl Cancer Inst.* 1980;65:25.

21. Downey RJ, Ng KK, Kris MG, et al: A phase II trial of chemotherapy and surgery for non–small cell lung cancer patients with a synchronous solitary metastasis. *Lung Cancer.* 2002;38:193.

22. Reichl J: Assessment of operative risk of pneumonectomy. *Chest.* 1972;62:570.

23. Taube K, Konietzko N: Prediction of postoperative cardiopulmonary function in patients undergoing pneumonectomy. *Thorac Cardiovasc Surg.* 1980;28:348.

24. Putnam JB Jr, Lammermeier DE, Colon R, et al: Predicted pulmonary function and survival after pneumonectomy for primary lung carcinoma. *Ann Thorac Surg.* 1990;49:909.

25. Gass GD, Olsen GN: Preoperative pulmonary function testing to predict postoperative morbidity and mortality. *Chest.* 1986;89:127.

26. Olsen GN, Block AJ, Swenson EW, et al: Pulmonary function evaluation of the lung resection candidate: A prospective study. *Am Rev Respir Dis.* 1975;111:379.

27. Churchill ED, Sweet RH, Sutter L, Scannell JD: The surgical management of carcinoma of the lung. *J Thorac Cardiovasc Surg.* 1950;20:349.

28. Ginsberg RJ, Hill LD, Eagan RT, et al: Modern thirty-day operative mortality for surgical resections in lung cancer. *J Thorac Cardiovasc Surg.* 1983;86:654.

29. Ginsberg RJ, Rubinstein LV: Randomized trial of lobectomy versus limited resection for T1 N0 non-small cell lung cancer. *Ann Thorac Surg.* 1995;60:615.Abstract.

30. Mountain CF, Dresler CM: Regional lymph node classification for lung cancer staging. *Chest.* 1997;111:1718.

31. Feld R, Rubinstein LV, Weisenberger TH: Sites of recurrence in resected stage I non-small-cell lung cancer: A guide for future studies. *J Clin Oncol.* 1984;2:1352.

32. Pairolero PC, Williams DE, Bergstralh EJ, et al: Postsurgical stage I bronchogenic carcinoma: morbid implications of recurrent disease. *Ann Thorac Surg.* 1984;38:331.

33. Bromley L, Szur L: Combined radiotherapy and resection for carcinoma of the bronchus. *Lancet.* 1955;5:937. Abstract.

34. Shields TW, Higgins GA Jr, Lawton R, et al: Preoperative x-ray therapy as an adjuvant in the treatment of bronchogenic carcinoma. *Cancer.* 1982;50:1713.

35. Warram J: Preoperative irradiation of cancer of the lung: Final report of a therapeutic trial. A collaborative study. *Cancer.* 1975;36:914.

36. Effects of postoperative mediastinal radiation on completely resected stage II and stage III epidermoid cancer of the lung. The Lung Cancer Study Group. *N Engl J Med.* 1986;315:1377.

37. Stephens RJ, Girling DJ, Bleehen NM, et al: The role of postoperative radiotherapy in non-small-cell lung cancer: A multicentre randomised trial in patients with pathologically staged T1-2, N1-2, M0 disease. Medical Research Council Lung Cancer Working Party. *Br J Cancer.* PG 1996.

38. Postoperative radiotherapy in non–small-cell lung cancer: Systematic review and meta-analysis of individual patient data from nine randomised controlled trials. PORT Meta-analysis Trialists Group. *Lancet.* 1998;352:257.

39. Takita H, Regal AM, Antkowiak JG, et al: Chemotherapy followed by lung resection in inoperable non-small cell lung carcinomas due to locally far-advanced disease. *Cancer.* 1986;57:630.

40. Raut Y, Huu N, Clavier J, et al: Surgery and chemotherapy. A new method of treatment for squamous cell bronchial carcinoma. *J Thorac Cardiovasc Surg.* 1984;88:754.

41. Martini N, Flehinger BJ, Zaman MB, Beattie EJ Jr: Results of resection in non-oat cell carcinoma of the lung with mediastinal lymph node metastases. *Ann Surg.* 1983;198:386.

42. Pass HI, Pogrebniak HW, Steinberg SM, et al: Randomized trial of neoadjuvant therapy for lung cancer: Interim analysis. *Ann Thorac Surg.* 1992;53:992.

43. Depierre A, Milleron B, Moro-Sibilot D, et al: Preoperative chemotherapy followed by surgery compared with primary surgery in resectable stage I (except T1N0), II, and IIIa non-small- cell lung cancer. *J Clin Oncol.* 2002;20:247.

44. Chemotherapy in non-small cell lung cancer: A meta-analysis using updated data on individual patients from 52 randomised clinical trials. Non-small Cell Lung Cancer Collaborative Group. *BMJ.* 1995;311:899.

45. Keller SM, Adak S, Wagner H, et al: A randomized trial of postoperative adjuvant therapy in patients with completely resected stage II or IIIa non–small-cell lung cancer. *N Engl J Med.* 2000;343:1217.

46. Le Chevalier T: Results of randomized international lung cancer trial (IALT): Cisplatin-based chemotherapy (CT) vs no CT in 1867 patients with resected non-small cell lung cancer. *Proc ASCO.* 2003;22:2. Abstract.

47. Albain KS, Rusch VW, Crowley JJ, et al: Concurrent cisplatin/etoposide plus chest radiotherapy followed by surgery for stages IIIA (N2) and IIIB non–small-cell lung cancer: Mature results of Southwest Oncology Group phase II study 8805. *J Clin Oncol.* 1995;13:1880.

48. Paulson DL: Carcinomas in the superior pulmonary sulcus. *J Thorac Cardiovasc Surg.* 1975;70:1095.

49. Shaw R, Paulson DL, Kee J: Treatment of the superior sulcus tumor by irradiation followed by resection. *Ann Surg.* 1961;154:29.

50. Rusch VW, Giroux DJ, Kraut MJ, et al: Induction chemoradiation and surgical resection for non-small cell lung carcinomas of the superior sulcus: Initial results of Southwest Oncology Group Trial 9416 (Intergroup Trial 0160). *J Thorac Cardiovasc Surg.* 2001;121:472.

51. Albain KS, Scott C, Rusch V, et al: Phase III comparison of concurrent chemotherapy plus radiotherapy (CT/RT) and CT/RT followed by surgical resection for Stage IIIA (pN2) non-small cell lung cancer: Initial results from intergroup trial 0139 (RTOG 93-09). *Proc ASCO.* 2003; 22:621. Abstract.

52. Armstrong JG, Minsky BD: Radiation therapy for medically inoperable stage I and II non- small cell lung cancer. *Cancer Treat Rev.* 1989;16:247.

53. Hilton G: Present position relating to cancer of the lung: Results with radiotherapy alone. *Thorax.* 1960;15:17.

54. Cox JD, Azarnia N, Byhardt RW, et al: A randomized phase I/II trial of hyperfractionated radiation therapy with total doses of 60.0 Gy to 79.2 Gy: Possible survival benefit with greater than or equal to 69.6 Gy in favorable patients with Radiation Therapy Oncology Group stage III non–small-cell lung carcinoma: Report of Radiation Therapy Oncology Group 83-11. *J Clin Oncol.* 1990; 8:1543.

55. Dosoretz DE, Galmarini D, Rubenstein JH, et al: Local control in medically inoperable lung cancer: An analysis of its importance in outcome and factors determining the probability of tumor eradication. *Int J Radiat Oncol Biol Phys.* 1993;27:507.

56. Haffty BG, Goldberg NB, Gerstley J, et al: Results of radical radiation therapy in clinical stage I, technically operable non–small cell lung cancer. *Int J Radiat Oncol Biol Phys.* 1988;15:69.

57. Krol AD, Aussems P, Noordijk EM, et al: Local irradiation alone for peripheral stage I lung cancer: Could we omit the elective regional nodal irradiation? *Int J Radiat Oncol Biol Phys.* 1996; 34:297.

58. Perez CA, Pajak TF, Rubin P: Long-term observations of the patterns of failure in patients with unresectable non-oat cell carcinoma of the lung treated with definitive radiotherapy. *Cancer.* 1987;59:1874.

59. Sandler HM, Curran WJ Jr, Turrisi AT3: The influence of tumor size and pre-treatment staging on outcome following radiation therapy alone for stage I non-small cell lung cancer. *Int J Radiat Oncol Biol Phys.* 1990;19:9.

60. Sibley GS: Radiotherapy for patients with medically inoperable Stage I non–small cell carcinoma: Smaller volumes and higher doses—A review. *Cancer.* 1998;82:433.

61. Kaskowitz L, Graham MV, Emami B, et al: Radiation therapy alone for stage I non-small cell lung cancer. Int J Radiat Oncol Biol Phys. 1993;27:517.

62. Morita K, Fuwa N, Suzuki Y, et al: Radical radiotherapy for medically inoperable non-small cell lung cancer in clinical stage I: A retrospective analysis of 149 patients. *Radiother Oncol.* 1997;42:31.

63. Gauden S, Ramsay J, Tripcony L: The curative treatment by radiotherapy alone of stage I non-small cell carcinoma of the lung. *Chest.* 1995;108:1278.

64. Sawyer TE, Bonner JA, Gould PM, et al: Predictors of subclinical nodal involvement in clinical stages I and II non-small cell lung cancer: Implications in the inoperable and three- dimensional dose-escalation settings. *Int J Radiat Oncol Biol Phys.* 1999;43:965.

65. Rosenzweig K, Dladla N, Schindelheim R, et al: Three-dimensional conformal radiation therapy (3D-CRT) for early stage non–small cell lung cancer. *Clin Lung Cancer.* 2001;3:141.

66. Sibley GS, Jamieson TA, Marks LB, et al: Radiotherapy alone for medically inoperable stage I non-small-cell lung cancer: The Duke experience. *Int J Radiat Oncol Biol Phys.* 1998;40:149.

67. Jeremic B, Shibamoto Y, Acimovic L, Milisavljevic S: Hyperfractionated radiotherapy for clinical stage II non-small cell lung cancer. *Radiother Oncol.* 1999;51:141.

68. Bradley JD, Wahab S, Lockett MA, et al: Elective nodal failures are uncommon in medically inoperable patients with stage I non-small-cell lung carcinoma treated with limited radiotherapy fields. *Int J Radiat Oncol Biol Phys.* 2003;56:342.

69. Slotman BJ, Antonisse IE, Njo KH: Limited field irradiation in early stage (T1-2N0) non-small cell lung cancer. *Radiother Oncol.* 1996;41:41.

70. Dillman RO, Herndon J, Seagren SL, et al: Improved survival in stage III non-small-cell lung cancer: Seven-year follow-up of cancer and leukemia group B (CALGB) 8433 trial [see comments]. *J Natl Cancer Inst.* 1996;88:1210.

71. Sause WT, Scott C, Taylor S, et al: Radiation Therapy Oncology Group (RTOG) 88-08 and Eastern Cooperative Oncology Group (ECOG) 4588: Preliminary results of a phase III trial in regionally advanced, unresectable non-small- cell lung cancer. *J Natl Cancer Inst.* 1995;87:198.

72. Johnson DH, Einhorn LH, Bartolucci A, et al: Thoracic radiotherapy does not prolong survival in patients with locally advanced, unresectable non-small cell lung cancer. *Ann Intern Med.* 1990;113:33.

73. Prosnitz LR: Radiotherapy for lung cancer. *Ann Intern Med.* 1991;114:95.

74. Schaafsma J, Coy P: The effect of radiotherapy on the survival of non-small cell lung cancer patients. *Int J Radiat Oncol Biol Phys.* 1998;41:291.

75. Bleehen NM, Cox JD: Radiotherapy for lung cancer. *Int J Radiat Oncol Biol Phys.* 1985;11:1001.

76. Dillman RO, Seagren SL, Propert KJ, et al: A randomized trial of induction chemotherapy plus high-dose radiation versus radiation alone in stage III non-small-cell lung cancer [see comments]. *N Engl J Med.* 1990;323:940.

77. Sause WT, Scott C, Taylor S, et al: Radiation Therapy Oncology Group (RTOG) 88-08 and Eastern Cooperative Oncology Group (ECOG) 4588: Preliminary results of a phase III trial in regionally advanced, unresectable non-small-cell lung cancer. *J Natl Cancer Inst.* 1995;87:198.

78. Arriagada R, Le Chevalier T, Quoix E, et al: ASTRO (American Society for Therapeutic Radiology and Oncology) plenary: Effect of chemotherapy on locally advanced non–small cell lung carcinoma: A randomized study of 353 patients. GETCB (Groupe d'Etude et Traitement des Cancers Bronchiques), FNCLCC (Federation Nationale des Centres de Lutte contre le Cancer) and the CEBI trialists. *Int J Radiat Oncol Biol Phys.* 1991;20:1183.

79. Kubota K, Furuse K, Kawahara M, et al: Role of radiotherapy in combined modality treatment of locally advanced non-small-cell lung cancer. *J Clin Oncol.* 1994;12:1547.

80. Furuse K, Fukuoka M, Kawahara M, et al: Phase III study of concurrent versus sequential thoracic radiotherapy in combination with mitomycin, vindesine and cisplatin in unresectable stage III non–small-cell lung cancer. *J Clin Oncol.* 1999;17:2692.

81. Curran W, Scott CB, Langer CJ, et al: Long-term benefit is observed in a phase III comparison of sequential vs. concurrent chemo-radiation for patients with unresected stage III nsclc: RTOG 9410. *Proc ASCO.* 2003;22:621.Abstract.

82. Pierre F, Maurice P, Gilles R, et al: A randomized phase III trial of sequential chemo-radiotherapy versus concurrent chemo-radiotherapy in locally advanced non–small cell lung cancer (GLOT-GFPC NPC 95-01 study). *Proc ASCO.* 2001;20:312A. Abstract.

83. Zatloukal PV, Petruzelka L, Zemanova M, et al: Concurrent versus sequential chemoradiotherapy with vinorelbine plus cisplatin in locally advanced non–small cell lung cancer. A randomized Phase II study. *Proc ASCO.* 2002;21:290A. Abstract.

84. Choy H, Curran W, Scott CB, et al: Preliminary report of LAMP: A randomized phase II trial of three chemo-radiation regimens in non–small cell lung cancer. *Proc ASCO.* 2002;21:291A. Abstract.

85. Albain KS, Crowley JJ, Turrisi AT III, et al: Concurrent cisplatin, etoposide, and chest radiotherapy in pathologic stage IIIB non-small-cell lung cancer: A Southwest Oncology Group phase II study, SWOG 9019. *J Clin Oncol.* 2002;20:3454.

86. Gandara DR, Chansky K, Albain KS, et al: Consolidation docetaxel after concurrent chemoradiotherapy in stage IIIB non-small-cell lung cancer: Phase II Southwest Oncology Group Study S9504. *J Clin Oncol.* 2003;21:2004.

87. Withers HR, Taylor JM, Maciejewski B: The hazard of accelerated tumor clonogen repopulation during radiotherapy. *Acta Oncol.* 1988;27:131.

88. Fowler JF, Chappell R: Non–small cell lung tumors repopulate rapidly during radiation therapy. *Int J Radiat Oncol Biol Phys.* 2000;46:516.

89. Saunders MI, Dische S: Continuous, hyperfractionated, accelerated radiotherapy (CHART) in non–small cell carcinoma of the bronchus. *Int J Radiat Oncol Biol Phys.* 1990;19:1211.

90. Saunders M, Dische S, Barrett A, et al: Continuous hyperfractionated accelerated radiotherapy (CHART) versus conventional radiotherapy in non–small-cell lung cancer: A randomised multicentre trial. CHART Steering Committee [see comments]. *Lancet.* 1997;350:161.

91. Bailey AJ, Parmar MK, Stephens RJ: Patient-reported short-term and long-term physical and psychologic symptoms: Results of the continuous hyperfractionated accelerated [correction of acclerated] radiotherapy (CHART) randomized trial in non–small-cell lung cancer. CHART Steering Committee. *J Clin Oncol.* 1998; 16:3082.

92. Saunders MI, Rojas A, Lyn BE, et al: Experience with dose escalation using CHARTWEL (continuous hyperfractionated accelerated radiotherapy weekend less) in non–small-cell lung cancer. *Br J Cancer.* 1998;78:1323.

93. Mehta MP, Tannehill SP, Adak S, et al: Phase II trial of hyperfractionated accelerated radiation therapy for nonresectable non-small-cell lung cancer: Results of Eastern Cooperative Oncology Group 4593. *J Clin Oncol.* 1998;16:3518.

94. Belani CP, Wang W, Johnson DH, et al: Induction chemotherapy followed by standard thoraci radiotherapy vs. hyperfractionated accelerated radiotherapy (HART) for patients with unresectable stage IIIA and IIIB non-small cell lung cancer: Phase III study of ECOG 2597. *Proc ASCO.* 2003;22:622. Abstract.

95. Armstrong J, Burman C, Leibel SA, et al: Conformal three dimensional treatment planning may improve the therapeutic ratio of high dose radiation therapy for lung cancer. *Int J Radiation Oncology Biol Phys.* 1991;21:146.Abstract.

96. Hayman JA, Martel MK, Ten Haken RK, et al: Dose escalation in non–small cell lung cancer (NSCLC) using conformal 3-dimensional radiation therapy (C3DRT): Update of a phase I trial. *Proc ASCO.* 1999;18:459A. Abstract.

97. Graham MV, Winter K, Purdy JA, et al: Preliminary results of a RTOG trial (RTOG 9311), a dose escalation study using 3D conformal radiation therapy in patients with inoperable nonsmall cell lung cancer. *Int J Radiat Oncol Biol Phys.* 2001;51:19. Abstract.

98. Rosenzweig K, Yorke E, Jackson A, et al: Results of a phase I dose escalation trial in inoperable non-small cell lung cancer. *Int J Radiat Oncol Biol Phys.* 2003;59: Abstract.

99. Pu AT, Harrison AS, Robertson JM, et al: The toxicity of elective nodal irradiation in the definitive treatment of non–small cell carcinoma of the lung. *Int J Radiat Oncol Biol Phys.* 1997;39:196. Abstract.

100. Emami B, Scott C, Byhardt R, et al: The value of regional nodal radiotherapy (dose/volume) in the treatment of unresectable non–small cell lung cancer: An RTOG analysis. *Int J Radiat Oncol Biol Phys.* 1996;36:208. Abstract.

101. Rosenzweig KE, Sim S, Mychalczak B, et al: Elective nodal irradiation in the treatment of non–small cell lung cancer with three-dimensional conformal radiation therapy (3D-CRT). *Int J Radiat Oncol Biol Phys.* 2001;49:1229.

102. Mah K, Caldwell CB, Ung YC, et al: The impact of (18)FDG-PET on target and critical organs in CT-based treatment planning of patients with poorly defined non-small-cell lung carcinoma: a prospective study. *Int J Radiat Oncol Biol Phys.* 2002;52:339.

103. Erdi YE, Macapinlac H, Rosenzweig KE, et al: Use of PET to monitor the response of lung cancer to radiation treatment. *Eur J Nucl Med.* 2000;27:861.

104. Ross CS, Hussey DH, Pennington EC, et al: Analysis of movement of intrathoracic neoplasms using ultrafast computerized tomography. *Int J Radiation Oncology Biol Phys.* 1990;18:671.

105. Ekberg L, Holmberg O, Wiltgren L, et al: What margins should be added to the clinical target volume in radiotherapy treatment planning for lung cancer? *Radiother Oncol.* 1998;48:71.

106. Stevens CW, Munden RF, Forster KM, et al: Respiratory-driven lung tumor motion is independent of tumor size, tumor location, and pulmonary function. *Int J Radiat Oncol Biol Phys.* 2001;51:62.

107. Kubo HD, Hill BC: Respiration gated radiotherapy treatment: A technical study. *Phys Med Biol.* 1996;41:83.

108. Wong JW, Sharpe MB, Jaffray DA, et al: The use of active breathing control (ABC) to minimize breathing motion during radiation therapy. *Int J Radiat Oncol Biol Phys.* 1997;39(2 Suppl):164. Abstract.

109. Stromberg JS, Sharpe MB, Kini VR, et al: Active breathing control (ABC) for Hodgkin's desease: Reduction in normal tissue irradiation with deep inspiration and implication for treatment. *Int J Radiat Oncol Biol Phys.* 1998;42(1S):140. Abstract.

110. Rosenzweig KE, Hanley J, Mah D, et al: The deep inspiration breath-hold technique in the treatment of inoperable non-small cell lung cancer. *Int J Radiat Oncol Biol Phys.* 2000;48:81. Abstract.

111. Hilaris BS, Martini N: The current state of intraoperative interstitial brachytherapy in lung cancer. *Int J Radiat Oncol Biol Phys.* 1988;15:1347.

112. Armstrong JG, Fass DE, Bains M, et al: Paraspinal tumors: Techniques and results of brachytherapy. *Int J Radiat Oncol Biol Phys.* 1991;20:787.

113. Hilaris BS, Nori D, Martini N: Intraoperative radiotherapy in stage I and II lung cancer. *Semin Surg Oncol.* 1987;3:22.

114. Huber RM, Fischer R, Hautmann H, et al: Does additional brachytherapy improve the effect of external irradiation? A prospective, randomized study in central lung tumors. *Int J Radiat Oncol Biol Phys.* 1997;38:533.

115. Fass DE, Armstrong JG, Harrison LB, Nori D: Fractionated high dose endobronchial treatment for recurrent lung cancer. *Endocuriether/Hyperthermal Oncol.* 1990;6:211.

116. Macha HN, Koch K, Stadler M, et al: New technique for treating occlusive and stenosing tumours of the trachea and main bronchi: endobronchial irradiation by high dose iridium-192 combined with laser canalisation. *Thorax.* 1987;42:511.

117. Burt PA, O'Driscoll BR, Notley HM, et al: Intraluminal irradiation for the palliation of lung cancer with the high dose rate micro-Selectron. *Thorax.* 1990;45:765.

118. Seagren SL, Harrell J: Prospective trial of palliative high dose rate endobronchial irradiation with or without laser for recurrent non-small cell lung cancer. *Proc ASCO.* 1990;9:224.

119. Smoluk GD, Fahey RC, Calabro-Jones PM, et al: Radioprotection of cells in culture by WR-2721 and derivatives: Form of the drug responsible for protection. *Cancer Res.* 1988;48:3641.

120. Tannehill SP, Mehta MP, Larson M, et al: Effect of amifostine on toxicities associated with sequential chemotherapy and radiation therapy for unresectable non–small-cell lung cancer: Results of a phase II trial. *J Clin Oncol.* 1997;15:2850.

121. Komaki R, Lee JS, Kaplan B, et al: Randomized phase III study of chemoradiation with or without amifostine for patients with favorable performance status inoperable stage II-III non-small cell lung cancer: Preliminary results. *Semin Radiat Oncol.* 2002; 12:46.

122. Movsas B, Scott C, Langer C, et al: Phase III study of amifostine inpatients with locally advanced non–small cell lung cancer receiving chemotherapy and hyperfractionated radiation: RTOG 9801. *Proc ASCO.* 2003;22:636.Abstract.

123. Antonadou D, Pepelassi M, Synodinou M, et al: Prophylactic use of amifostine to prevent radiochemotherapy-induced mucositis and xerostomia in head-and-neck cancer. *Int J Radiat Oncol Biol Phys.* 2002;739.

124. Schnabel K, Vogt-Moykopf I, Berberich W, Abel U: Comparison of neutron and photon irradiation of bronchial carcinoma. *Strahlentherapie.* 1983;159:458.

125. Livingston RB, Griffin BR, Higano CS, et al: Combined treatment with chemotherapy and neutron irradiation for limited non-small-cell lung cancer: A Southwest Oncology Group Study. *J Clin Oncol.* 1987;5:1716.

126. Stuschke M, Eberhardt W, Pottgen C, et al: Prophylactic cranial irradiation in locally advanced non–small-cell lung cancer after multimodality treatment: Long-term follow-up and investigations of late neuropsychologic effects. *J Clin Oncol.* 1999; 17:2700.

127. Cox JD, Stanley K, Petrovich Z, et al: Cranial irradiation in cancer of the lung of all cell types. *JAMA.* 1981;245:469.

128. Umsawadi T, Valdivieso M, Chen T: Role of elective brain irradiation during combined chemoradiotherapy for limited disease non-small cell lung cancer. *J Neurooncol.* 1984;2:253.

129. Mira J, Miller T, Crowley J: Chest irradiation (RT) vs. chest RT + chemotherapy +/– prophylactic brain RT in localized non-small cell lung cancer: A Southwest Oncology Group randomized study. *Int J Radiat Oncol Biol Phys.* 1990;19(Suppl 1):145.

130. Russell AH, Pajak TE, Selim H: Prophylactic cranial irradiation for lung cancer patients at high risk for development of cerebral metastases: Results of a prospective randomized trial conducted by the Radiation Therapy Oncology Group. *Int J Radiat Oncol Biol Phys.* 1991;21:637.

131. Nagata Y, Negoro Y, Aoki T, et al: Clinical outcomes of 3-D conformal hypofractionated single high dose radiotherapy for one or two lung tumors using a stereotactic body frame. *Int J Radiat Oncol Biol Phys.* 2001;51(3 Suppl):352. Abstract.

132. Whyte RI, Crownover R, Murphy MJ, et al: Stereotactic radiosurgery for lung tumors: Preliminary report of a phase I trial. *Ann Thorac Surg.* 2003;75:1097.

133. Hof H, Herfarth KK, Munter M, et al: Stereotactic single-dose radiotherapy of stage I non-small-cell lung cancer (NSCLC). *Int J Radiat Oncol Biol Phys.* 2003;56:335.

134. Yorke E: Advantages of IMRT for dose escalation in radiation therapy for lung cancer. *Med Phys.* 2001;28:1291. Abstract.

135. Carroll M, Morgan SA, Yarnold JR, et al: Prospective evaluation of a watch policy in patients with inoperable non-small cell lung cancer. *Eur J Cancer Clin Oncol.* 1986;22:1353.

136. Inoperable non-small-cell lung cancer (NSCLC): A Medical Research Council randomised trial of palliative radiotherapy with two fractions or ten fractions. Report to the Medical Research Council by its Lung Cancer Working Party. *Br J Cancer.* 1991;63:265.

137. Borgelt B, Gelber R, Larson M, et al: Ultra-rapid high dose irradiation schedules for the palliation of brain metastases: Final results of the first two studies by the Radiation Therapy Oncology Group. *Int J Radiat Oncol Biol Phys.* 1981;7:1633.

138. Billingham LJ, Cullen MH, Woods J, et al: Mitomycin, ifosfamide and cisplatin (MIC) in non–small cell lung cancer (NSCLC): 3. Results of a randomised trial evaluating palliation & quality of life. *Lung Cancer.* 1997;18(Suppl 1):9.

139. Schiller JH, Harrington D, Belani CP, et al: Comparison of four chemotherapy regimens for advanced non-small-cell lung cancer. *N Engl J Med.* 2002;346:92.

140. Shepherd FA, Dancey J, Ramlau R, et al: Prospective randomized trial of docetaxel versus best supportive care in patients with non–small-cell lung cancer previously treated with platinum-based chemotherapy. *J Clin Oncol.* 2000;18:2095.

141. Khalil MY, Grandis JR, Shin DM: Targeting epidermal growth factor receptor: Novel therapeutics in the management of cancer. *Exp Rev Anticancer Ther.* 2003;3:367.

142. Chute JP, Venzon DJ, Hankins L, et al: Outcome of patients with small-cell lung cancer during 20 years of clinical research at the US National Cancer Institute. *Mayo Clin Proc.* 1997;72:901.

143. Zelen M: Keynote address on biostatistics and data retrieval. *Cancer Chemother Rep 3.* 1973;4:31.

144. Yip D, Harper PG: Predictive and prognostic factors in small cell lung cancer: Current status. *Lung Cancer.* 2000;28:173.

145. Tucker MA, Murray N, Shaw EG, et al: Second primary cancers related to smoking and treatment of small-cell lung cancer. Lung Cancer Working Cadre. *J Natl Cancer Inst.* 1997;89:1782.

146. Skarlos DV, Samantas E, Kosmidis P, et al: Randomized comparison of etoposide-cisplatin vs. etoposide-carboplatin and irradiation in small-cell lung cancer. A Hellenic Co-operative Oncology Group study. *Ann Oncol.* 1994;5:601.

147. Mavroudis D, Papadakis E, Veslemes M, et al: A multicenter randomized clinical trial comparing paclitaxel-cisplatin-etoposide versus cisplatin-etoposide as first-line treatment in patients with small-cell lung cancer. *Ann Oncol.* 2001;12:463.

148. Sierocki JS, Hilaris BS, Hopfan S, et al: cis-Dichlorodiammineplatinum(II) and VP-16-213: An active induction regimen for small cell carcinoma of the lung. *Cancer Treat Rep.* 1979; 63:1593.

149. Pignon JP, Arriagada R, Ihde DC, et al: A meta-analysis of thoracic radiotherapy for small-cell lung cancer. *N Engl J Med.* 1992;327:1618.

150. Perry MC, Eaton WL, Propert KJ, et al: Chemotherapy with or without radiation therapy in limited small-cell carcinoma of the lung. *N Engl J Med.* 1987;316:912.

151. Gregor A, Drings P, Burghouts J, et al: Randomized trial of alternating versus sequential radiotherapy/chemotherapy in limited-disease patients with small-cell lung cancer: A European Organization for Research and Treatment of Cancer Lung Cancer Cooperative Group Study. *J Clin Oncol.* 1997;15:2840.

152. Murray N, Coy P, Pater JL, et al: Importance of timing for thoracic irradiation in the combined modality treatment of limited-stage small-cell lung cancer. The National Cancer Institute of Canada Clinical Trials Group. *J Clin Oncol.* 1993;11:336.

153. Murray N, Coldman A: The relationship between thoracic irradiation timing and long-term survival in combined modality therapy of limited stage small cell lung cancer. *Proc ASCO.* 2003; 14:A1099. Abstract.

154. Turrisi AT III, Kim K, Blum R, et al: Twice-daily compared with once-daily thoracic radiotherapy in limited small-cell lung cancer treated concurrently with cisplatin and etoposide. *N Engl J Med.* 1999;340:265.

155. Choi NC, Herndon JE, Rosenman J, et al: Phase I study to determine the maximum-tolerated dose of radiation in standard daily and hyperfractionated-accelerated twice-daily radiation schedules with concurrent chemotherapy for limited-stage small-cell lung cancer. *J Clin Oncol.* 1998;16:3528.

156. Bogart J, Herndon J, Lyss AP, et al: 70 Gy thoracic radiotherapy is feasible concurrent with chemotherapy for limited stage small cell lung cancer: Preliminary analysis of a CALGB phase II trial. *Int J Radiat Oncol Biol Phys.* 2002;54(2 Suppl):103. Abstract.

157. Fox W, Scadding JG: Medical Research Council comparative trial of surgery and radiotherapy for primary treatment of small-celled or oat-celled carcinoma of bronchus. Ten-year follow-up. *Lancet.* 1973;2:63.

158. Shepherd FA, Ginsberg RJ, Patterson GA, et al: A prospective study of adjuvant surgical resection after chemotherapy for limited small cell lung cancer. A University of Toronto Lung Oncology Group study. *J Thorac Cardiovasc Surg.* 1989;97:177.

159. Hirsch FR, Paulson OB, Hansen HH, Vraa-Jensen J: Intracranial metastases in small cell carcinoma of the lung: Correlation of clinical and autopsy findings. *Cancer.* 1982;50:2433.

160. Rosen ST, Makuch RW, Lichter AS, et al: Role of prophylactic cranial irradiation in prevention of central nervous system metastases in small cell lung cancer. Potential benefit restricted to patients with complete response. *Am J Med.* 1983;74:615.

161. Auperin A, Arriagada R, Pignon JP, et al: Prophylactic cranial irradiation for patients with small-cell lung cancer in complete remission. Prophylactic Cranial Irradiation Overview Collaborative Group. *N Engl J Med.* 1999;341:476.

162. Arriagada R, Le Chevalier T, Borie F, et al: Prophylactic cranial irradiation for patients with small-cell lung cancer in complete remission. *J Natl Cancer Inst.* 1995;87:183.

163. Antman KH, Pass HI, Schiff PB: Management of mesothelioma. In DeVita VT, Hellman S, Rosenberg SA, eds. *Cancer: Principles and Practice of Oncology.* New York: Lippincott Williams & Wilkins; 2001:1943.

164. Rusch VW: Indications for pneumonectomy. Extrapleural pneumonectomy. *Chest Surg Clin N Am.* 1999;9:327.

165. McCormack PM, Nagasaki F, Hilaris BS, Martini N: Surgical treatment of pleural mesothelioma. *J Thorac Cardiovasc Surg.* 1982;84:834.

166. Ong ST, Vogelzang NJ: Chemotherapy in malignant pleural mesothelioma. A review. *J Clin Oncol.* 1996;14:1007.

167. van Meerbeeck JP, Baas P, Debruyne C, et al: A phase II study of gemcitabine in patients with malignant pleural mesothelioma. European Organization for Research and Treatment of Cancer Lung Cancer Cooperative Group. *Cancer.* 1999;85:2577.

168. Byrne MJ, Davidson JA, Musk AW, et al: Cisplatin and gemcitabine treatment for malignant mesothelioma: A phase II study. *J Clin Oncol.* 1999;17:25.

169. van Haarst JM, Baas P, Manegold C, et al: Multicentre phase II study of gemcitabine and cisplatin in malignant pleural mesothelioma. *Br J Cancer.* 2002;86:342.

170. Vogelzang NJ, Rusthoven J, Paoletti P, et al: Phase III single-blinded study of premetrexed + cisplatin vs. cisplatin alone in chemonaive patients with malignant pleural mesothelioma. *Proc ASCO.* 2002; 21:2A. Abstract.

171. Hilaris BS, Nori D, Kwong E, et al: Pleurectomy and intraoperative brachytherapy and postoperative radiation in the treatment of malignant pleural mesothelioma. *Int J Radiat Oncol Biol Phys.* 1984;10:325.

172. Rusch VW, Rosenzweig K, Venkatraman E, et al: A phase II trial of surgical resection and adjuvant high-dose hemithoracic radiation for malignant pleural mesothelioma. *J Thorac Cardiovasc Surg.* 2001;122:788.

173. Yajnik S, Rosenzweig K, Mychalczak B, et al: Hemithoracic radiation after extrapleural pneumonectomy for malignant pleural mesothelioma. *Int J Radiat Oncol Biol Phys.* 2003;56:1319.

174. Kutcher GJ, Kestler C, Greenblatt D, et al: Technique for external beam treatment for mesothelioma. *Int J Radiat Oncol Biol Phys.* 1987;13:1747.

175. Graham MV, Emami B: Mediastinum and trachea. In Perez C, Brady LW, eds. *Principles and Practice of Radiation Oncology.* Philadelphia: Lippincott-Raven; 1998:1221.

176. Drachman DB: Myasthenia gravis. *N Engl J Med.* 1994; 330:1797.

177. Masaoka A, Monden Y, Nakahara K, Tanioka T: Follow-up study of thymomas with special reference to their clinical stages. *Cancer.* 1981;48:2485.

178. Thomas CR, Wright CD, Loehrer PJ: Thymoma: State of the art. *J Clin Oncol.* 1999;17:2280.

179. Haniuda M, Miyazawa M, Yoshida K, et al: Is postoperative radiotherapy for thymoma effective? *Ann Surg.* 1996;224:219.

180. Batata MA, Martini N, Huvos AG, et al: Thymomas: Clinicopathologic features, therapy, and prognosis. *Cancer.* 1974;34:389.

181. Curran WJ Jr, Kornstein MJ, Brooks JJ, Turrisi AT III: Invasive thymoma: The role of mediastinal irradiation following complete or incomplete surgical resection. *J Clin Oncol.* 1988;6:1722.

182. Ciernik IF, Meier U, Lutolf UM: Prognostic factors and outcome of incompletely resected invasive thymoma following radiation therapy. *J Clin Oncol.* 1994;12:1484.

183. Mornex F, Resbeut M, Richaud P, et al: Radiotherapy and chemotherapy for invasive thymomas: A multicentric retrospective review of 90 cases. The FNCLCC trialists. Federation Nationale des Centres de Lutte Contre le Cancer. *Int J Radiat Oncol Biol Phys.* 1995;32:651.

184. Bush SE, Martinez A, Bagshaw MA: Primary mediastinal seminoma. *Cancer.* 1981;48:1877.

185. Grillo HC, Mathisen DJ: Primary tracheal tumors: treatment and results. *Ann Thorac Surg.* 1990;49:69.

186. Chung A: Radiotherapy for Primary Carcinoma of the Trachea. *Radiother Oncol.* 1989;14:279.

Cancer of the Esophagus

Bruce D. Minsky, MD

36

EPIDEMIOLOGY, ETIOLOGY, GENETICS, AND CYTOGENETIC ABNORMALITIES

The incidence of esophageal cancer varies by age, sex, and race. Throughout the world, it is a disease of the older population and is rare below the age of 25. The incidence rises steadily with age, reaching a peak in the sixth to seventh decade of life. It varies widely in its incidence according to the country of origin. The highest incidence—more than 100 per 100,000 population—occurs in Linxian, China; the Caspian region of Iran; and the former Soviet Union.

The epidemiology of esophageal cancer has changed during the past decade in that there is an increasing incidence of adenocarcinoma, most commonly occurring at the gastroesophageal (GE) junction.[1]

Squamous Cell Cancer

The National Cancer Institute's Surveillance Epidemiology and End Results (SEER) database reveals that the annual rates per 100,000 population for squamous cell carcinoma decreased 3.4 in 1974-1976 to 2.2 during 1992-1994.[2] In African-American males the incidence is fivefold compared to white males (16.8 vs. 1.0 per 100,000).[3] In most countries, the primary contributing factor is tobacco and alcohol abuse.[4] Diet can have a protective benefit.[5] For example, high intake of raw vegetables and fresh fruit (especially citrus) is associated with a decreased risk.

Adenocarcinoma

In most large referral centers, the incidence of adenocarcinoma of the GE junction represents 60% to 80% of newly diagnosed patients compared with 10% to 15% only 10 years ago.[6] According to data from the SEER database, the incidence of adenocarcinoma in white males doubled from the early 1970s to the late 1980s. In contrast with squamous cell cancer, the male-to-female ratio is 7:1, and there is an increased incidence in whites compared with African Americans. In a Swedish population-based case-control study, Lagergren et al. reported a strong association between symptomatic GE reflux and adenocarcinoma.[7]

Barrett's esophagus is a metaplastic change of the esophageal lining whereby normal squamous epithelium is replaced by columnar epithelium.[8] The pathophysiology, biology, and possible molecular events associated with Barrett's have been extensively reviewed.[9,10] Strong evidence supports the theory that most adenocarcinomas develop from areas of Barrett's esophagus.[11] Anti-reflux medications that relax the lower esophageal sphincter may be a contributing factor. For example, Lagergren et al. reported that patients who used these agents more than 5 years had an increased risk compared to those who never used them.[12] Interestingly, only 10% of patients who have Barrett's develop adenocarcinoma; however, most patients with adenocarcinoma have a history of Barrett's. In fact, most patients with Barrett's will die of other causes.

Although not as prevalent as that reported in patients with squamous cell cancer, tobacco and alcohol abuse also increases the risk of adenocarcinoma.[11] A multicenter case-controlled study identified excess weight (body mass index) as a risk factor.[13] Likewise, a diet high in calories and fat is associated with an increased risk.[14] Although *Helicobacter pylori* is a risk factor for gastric cancer, it does not appear to be associated with adenocarcinoma of the GE junction.[15]

Emerging data suggest that the development of esophagus cancer, similar to many other epithelial-derived carcinomas, is a multistep process that involves a successive activation or deletion of genes and their protein products. This is mediated by regulatory genes.[16-19] For example, *HER-2/neu* expression is associated with advanced disease.[19] Advances in molecular biology techniques have allowed characterization of the genetic changes thought to be responsible for this multistep process.[20,21] In one series microvessel density was a prognostic factor for patients treated with combined modality therapy.[22] Although at this time treatment decisions cannot be made based on molecular markers, their relationship to prognosis is an active area of investigation.

ANATOMY

The esophagus is a hollow viscus lined with primarily keratinized squamous epithelium, which extends from the level of the cricoid cartilage and cricopharyngeus muscle inferiorly to the GE junction. Glandular elements are present and, in the lower 5 to 10 cm, stomach-type glandular epithelium may replace the squamous epithelium (Barrett's esophagus). The lower end of the esophagus is at the squamous columnar junction and the upper end at the cricopharyngeus muscle. The average length is 25 cm.

The esophagus has a rich mucosal and submucosal lymphatic system that is independent of the blood vessels. The submucosal lymphatics may extend long distances, which is why the proximal and distal margins used for radiation treatment planning have traditionally been a minimum of 5 cm. The submucosal plexus drains into the internal jugular, peritracheal, hilar, subcarinal, periesophageal, periaortic, and pericardial lesser curvature lymph nodes, as well as into the left gastric and celiac nodes for lower third lesions.

The esophagus is generally divided into three segments: cervical, thoracic and distal (GE junction). There is no consensus as to the delineation between these segments, and there is overlap among the various definitions.[23] Some definitions use the distance from the incisors (Fig. 36-1), whereas others use anatomic criteria such as the thoracic inlet and carina.

PATHOLOGY

As seen in Table 36-1, various histologic types of tumors arise in the esophagus.[24] The most common are squamous cell and adenocarcinoma. The treatment results discussed in this chapter are limited to these two histologies. Given the increasing incidence of adenocarcinoma of the esophagus compared with squamous cell carcinoma, treatment results must be examined by histology. At present the data

Table 36–1   Classification of Esophageal Cancer

Preinvasive Neoplasia
  Esophageal intraepithelial neoplasia
  Glandular epithelial dysplasia/adenocarcinoma in situ in Barrett's
    mucosa
Invasive Malignant Neoplasia
  Squamous cell carcinoma, NOS
  Basaloid squamous cell carcinoma*
  Squamous cell carcinoma with sarcomatoid features*
  Verrucous squamous cell carcinoma*
  Adenocarcinoma, NOS
  Adenoid cystic carcinoma*
  Mucoepidermoid carcinoma*
  Adenosquamous carcinoma, NOS
  Adenoid cystic carcinoma*
  Mucoepidermoid carcinoma*
  Adenosquamous carcinoma*
  Adenoacanthoma*
  Undifferentiated carcinoma, NOS
  Small cell carcinoma
  Carcinoid tumor
  Malignant melanoma
  Sarcomas
    Leiomyosarcoma
    Fibrosarcoma
    Malignant fibrous histiocytoma
    Osteosarcoma
    Chondrosarcoma
    Synovial sarcoma
    Hemangiopericytoma
    Kaposi's sarcoma
    Rhabdomyosarcoma
    Liposarcoma
    Malignant schwannoma
    Malignant granular cell tumor
    Malignant mesenchymoma
  Choriocarcinoma
  Malignant lymphoma and Hodgkin's disease
  Collision tumors
  Secondary and metastatic tumors
  Unclassified

*Special variants.
NOS, not otherwise specified.

are conflicting, with some series reporting different results by histology and other series reporting no difference. Fortunately, the National Cancer Institute Intergroup randomized trials are now stratified by histology. Until these stratified results are available, the impact of histology cannot be adequately assessed and it is reasonable to treat both histologies similarly.

CLINICAL PRESENTATION

Carcinoma of the esophagus is commonly associated with the symptoms of dysphagia, weight loss, pain, anorexia, and vomiting. The location of the tumor can influence the nature of the symptoms. Dysphagia is by far the most common symptom. The location of the tumor also influences the histologic type. In the upper and middle third, the majority of cancers are squamous cell, whereas in the lower third they are adenocarcinomas.

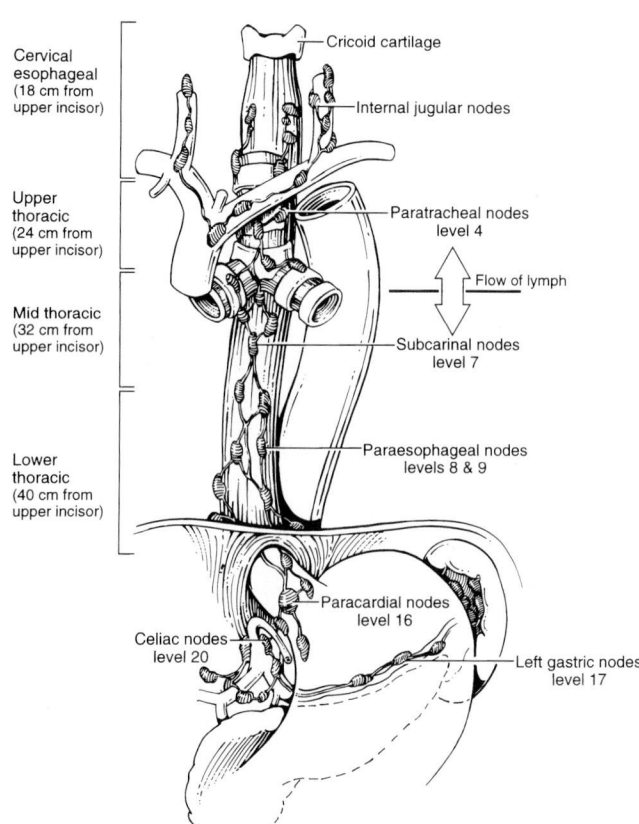

Figure 36-1. Anatomy of the esophagus.

ROUTES OF SPREAD

Esophageal cancer commonly spreads by lymphatics. Since the esophagus is not covered by a serosal lining except for the most distal portion and is in close proximity to many organs and structures, spread by direct extension is also frequent. Lesions of the cervical esophagus may extend to the carotid arteries, pleura, recurrent laryngeal nerves, and trachea. Lesions of the middle third may invade the main stem bronchi, thoracic duct, aortic arch, subclavian artery, intercostal vessels, azygos vein, and right pleura. Tracheoesophageal or broncho-esophageal fistulas are most common in lesions of the middle third and develop in 15% of patients with esophageal cancer. Tumors of the lower third may extend into the pericardium, left pleura, and descending aorta.

Tumors in the upper third metastasize to abdominal nodes in approximately 10% of patients; in the middle third, 25% of tumors metastasize; and in the lower third, 45%. Supraclavicular and infraclavicular nodes are positive 10% of the time with upper-third lesions. Mediastinal nodes are positive in about 50% to 60% of all cases.

The incidence of lymph node involvement increases with T classification. The incidence is also related to the site of the primary tumor in the esophagus. Metastases from the cervical esophagus to the abdominal lymph nodes are unusual, whereas from the upper thoracic esophagus, metastases may occur in greater than 30% of patients. The relative incidence of metastasis is summarized in Figure 36-2.[25] Hematogenous metastases may occur in 25% to 30% of patients at the time of presentation and in as high as 50% of patients at the time of autopsy. The most common sites of metastasis are lung, liver, pleura, bone, kidney, and adrenal gland. Regardless of the anatomic location or histologic subtype, the median survival of patients with distant metastatic disease is 6 to 12 months.

DIAGNOSTIC AND STAGING STUDIES

Diagnosis

The initial diagnosis is often made on endoscopy, which allows observation of the proximal and distal extent of the tumor and biopsy. The barium esophagram will delineate the proximal and distal margins as well as identify a tracheoesophageal fistula. It is helpful for correlation with simulation films. The computed tomography (CT) scan is essential for staging since it can identify extension beyond the esophageal wall and enlarged lymph nodes. Endoscopic ultrasound is highly accurate in determining depth of invasion.[26] CT scan of the chest and abdomen evaluates local extension, nodes, and visceral metastasis. For cervical primaries, a head and neck examination should include lymph nodes as well as all possible mucosal sites of a synchronous primary.

Several studies have examined the effectiveness of 18FDG-positron emission tomography (PET) in the staging of esophageal cancer. Following standard staging for esophageal cancer (including CT scan and endoscopy), undetected metastatic disease was detected by PET in 15% of patients in the series by Flamen et al.[27] and 20% in the series by Downey and associates.[28] There is also a correlation between the intensity of the image seen on PET (defined as SUV-Standardized Uptake Value), and the degree of downstaging following preoperative combined modality therapy.[29] Although it is investigational, PET is highly encouraged.

Staging

The most accurate staging is pathologic.[30] The fifth edition of the American Joint Commission on Cancer (AJCC) and the Union Internationale Contre le Cancer (UICC) TNM staging systems are similar. Although the

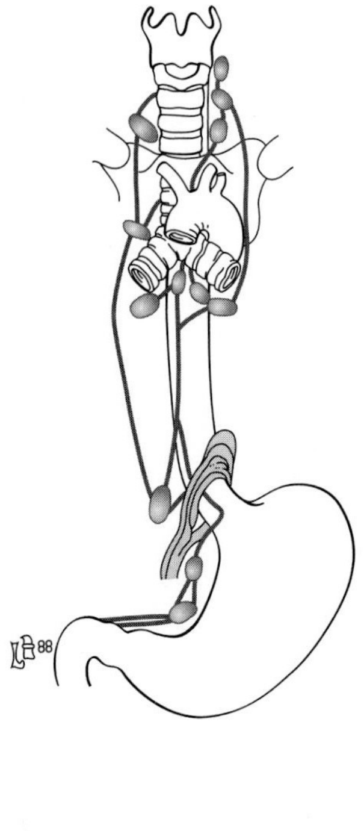

	Primary Site			
	Cervical	Upper Thoracic	Middle Thoracic	Lower Thoracic Cardia
Cervical	14.3	7.9	6.5	5.0
Mediastinal	11.0	85.7	50.1	65.4
Abdominal	2.9	31.8	45.0	92.5

Figure 36-2. Location of the lymph node involvement (%) by esophageal carcinoma is determined by site of primary tumor. (From Sons HU, Borchard F: Cancer of the distal esophagus and cardia. *Ann Surg.* 1986;203:188 and Akiyama H, Tsurumaro M, Kawamura T, et al: Principles of surgical treatment for carcinoma of the esophagus. *Ann Surg.* 1981;194:438.)

length of the primary tumor (> or <5 cm) is prognostic, the AJCC staging system no longer includes length. The sixth edition of the AJCC TNM staging system (Table 36-2)[31] included no major changes from the fifth edition. Additional descriptors in the sixth edition do not affect the stage grouping, but *do* indicate cases needing separate analysis. Similar to the staging system used for gastric and colorectal cancers, the T classification is based on the extension of the primary tumor through the wall.

Since many patients are treated with combined modality therapy alone or preoperatively, clinical staging, although less accurate, may understage patients. This difference in clinical and pathologic staging is why there is commonly a selection bias against the results of nonoperative treatment compared with surgery.

One of the most controversial areas is the delineation between adenocarcinomas of the GE junction and the stomach. These cancers commonly involve both the esophagus and stomach. No standard approach on how to define the organ of origin exists. The most common (and practical) definition is based on where the majority of the tumor is. Whichever organ has the largest percentage of tumor is considered the primary site. Siewert and colleagues have proposed a topographic anatomic classification system to distinguish an adenocarcinoma of the distal esophagus (AEG Type I) from an adenocarcinoma of the gastric cardia (AEG Type II).[32]

STANDARD THERAPEUTIC APPROACHES

There are two general treatment approaches to esophageal cancer: (1) primary treatment (surgical or nonsurgical) or (2) adjuvant treatment (preoperative or postoperative). Primary treatments include surgery alone, radiation therapy alone, and radiation therapy plus chemotherapy (combined modality therapy). Primary therapy can be further subdivided into curative and palliative approaches. Adjuvant therapies include preoperative or postoperative radiation therapy, preoperative chemotherapy, and preoperative combined modality therapy.

There is considerable controversy as to the ideal therapeutic approach. In the 1992-1994 U.S. Patterns of Care Study, treatment approaches included: primary combined modality therapy, 54%; radiation alone, 20%; preoperative combined modality therapy, 13%; postoperative combined modality therapy, 8%; postoperative radiation, 4%; and preoperative radiation, 1%.[33] Various oncology groups have published treatment guidelines; however, there is still no consensus.[34]

TECHNIQUES OF RADIATION THERAPY

Introduction

The design and delivery of radiation therapy for esophageal cancer requires a knowledge of the natural history of the disease, patterns of failure, anatomy, and radiobiologic principles. Furthermore, the use of proper equipment, implementation of methods to decrease

Table 36–2 Classification of Esophageal Carcinomas

Primary Tumor (T)

TX	Primary tumor cannot be assessed
T0	No evidence of primary tumor
Tis	Carcinoma in situ
T1	Tumor invades lamina propria or submucosa
T2	Tumor invades muscularis propria
T3	Tumor invades adventitia
T4	Tumor invades adjacent structures

Regional Lymph Nodes (N)

NX	Regional lymph nodes cannot be assessed
N0	No regional lymph node metastasis
N1	Regional lymph node metastasis

Distant Metastasis (M)

MX	Distant metastasis cannot be assessed
M0	No distant metastasis
M1	Distant metastasis

Tumors of the lower thoracic esophagus:

M1a	Metastasis in celiac lymph nodes
M1b	Other distant metastasis

Tumors of the midthoracic esophagus:

M1a	Not applicable
M1b	Nonregional lymph nodes or other distant metastasis or both

Tumors of the upper thoracic esophagus:

M1a	Metastasis in cervical nodes
M1b	Other distant metastasis

For tumors of midthoracic esophagus use only M1b, since these tumors with metastasis in nonregional lymph nodes and those with metastasis in other distant sites have an equally poor prognosis.

Stage Grouping

0	Tis	N0	M0
I	T1	N0	M0
IIA	T2	N0	M0
	T3	N0	M0
IIB	T1	N1	M0
	T2	N1	M0
III	T3	N1	M0
	T4	Any N	M0
IV	Any T	Any N	M1
IVA	Any T	Any N	M1a
IVB	Any T	Any N	M1b

NOTE: Although additional descriptors do not affect the stage grouping, additional prefixes are used to indicate the need for additional analysis:

Suffix	Reason
m	The presence of multiple primary tumors in a single site, recorded in parentheses: pT(m)NM.
y	When classification is performed during or following initial radiation or chemotherapy or both and is based on the amount of tumor present at the time of the examination, and not an estimate of tumor before therapy: ycTNM or ypTNM.
r	Indicates recurrent tumor: rTNM.
a	Indicates the stage at autopsy: aTNM.

Lymphatic Vessel Invasion (L)

Lx	Cannot be assessed
L0	No lymphatic vessel invasion
L1	Lymphatic vessel invasion present

Venous Invasion (V)

Vx	Cannot be assessed
V0	No venous invasion
V1	Microscopic venous invasion present
V2	Macroscopic venous invasion present

From Greene FL, Page DL, Fleming ID, et al, eds: *AJCC Cancer Staging Manual*, 6th ed. New York: Springer; 2002.

treatment-related toxicity, and a close collaboration with the physics and technology staff is essential.

General Techniques

A number of sensitive organs, depending on the location of the primary tumor, will be in the radiation field. These include, but are not limited to, the spinal cord, lung, heart, intestine, stomach, kidneys, and liver. Minimizing the dose to these structures while delivering an adequate dose to the primary tumor and local-regional lymph nodes is aided by techniques such as patient immobilization, CT-based treatment planning for organ identification and lung correction, and the use of dose-volume histograms.

Although CT can identify adjacent organs and structures, it may be limited in defining the extent of the primary tumor. To assess the consistency of target volume delineation, Tai and colleagues sent sample cases with CT scans to 48 radiation oncologists throughout Canada and asked them to complete questionnaires regarding treatment techniques as well as outline the boost target volumes.[35] There was substantial inconsistency in defining the planning target volume, both in the transverse and longitudinal dimensions. The integration of other imaging modalities in radiation treatment planning such as esophageal ultrasound, PET scan, and magnetic resonance imaging (MRI) are under active investigation.

The standard radiation dose for patients selected for combined modality therapy is 50.4 Gy at 1.8 Gy per fraction.[36] Randomized data from France reveal a higher local control (57% vs. 29%) and 2-year survival rate (37% vs. 23%) with *continuous-course* compared with *split-course* radiation.[37] The radiation field should include the primary tumor with 5-cm superior and inferior margins and 2-cm lateral margins. The primary local-regional lymph nodes should receive the same dose. For cervical (proximal) primary tumors (defined as at or proximal to the carina), the treatment volume includes the bilateral supraclavicular nodes and for GE junction (distal) primaries, the celiac axis nodes must be included.

Some unique features of the AJC staging system have particular relevance to radiation treatment field design. For primary tumors located in the cervical esophagus, supraclavicular lymph nodes are considered nodal (N1) disease and should be included in the radiation field. In contrast, for primary tumors located in the mid or distal esophagus, positive supraclavicular lymph nodes are considered metastatic disease (M1b) and the approach is palliative. For tumors located in the distal esophagus, celiac lymph nodes are also metastatic disease, but are staged as M_{1a} disease and still approached in a potentially curative fashion.

Treatment by Primary Site

From a radiation-treatment-planning viewpoint, tumors at or above the carina are treated as a cervical primary, and the supraclavicular nodes should be included in the radiation field. Tumors below the carina but not extending

to the GE junction are considered mid esophagus and the radiation field does not include the supraclavicular or celiac nodes. Tumors that involve the GE junction are considered distal, and the celiac nodes are included. This simplistic but practical definition is helpful in designing radiation therapy fields.

For cervical primaries, patients are placed supine. Various field designs are possible, and their choice depends on the geometry of the primary tumor in relation to the spinal cord. The ideal design is a three-field technique (two anterior obliques and a posterior). However, since the primary tumor is rarely limited to the midline, the most common approach is anterior-posterior–posterior-anterior (AP–PA) to 39.6 to 41.4 Gy (Fig. 36-3) followed by a left or right opposed oblique pair with photons to 50.4 Gy (Fig. 36-4). Since this technique will exclude the ipsilateral supraclavicular fossa, a separate electron field is added (commonly to a depth of 2 to 3 cm depending on the patient's anatomy), thereby bringing the total dose to 50.4 Gy.

Patients with mid esophageal primaries are placed prone to help exclude the spinal cord from the radiation field. A four-field technique (AP–PA and opposed laterals) is recommended.

For distal (GE junction) primaries, patients are treated supine using the same four-field technique. With a CT simulation, sometimes it is difficult to distinguish a normal stomach from the primary tumor. In this setting, a conventional simulation with barium in addition to a CT simulation may be helpful. The greater curvature of the stomach is commonly used for the anastomosis. Therefore, for patients receiving preoperative treatment, care should be taken to exclude as much of the normal stomach as possible. An example of this technique is seen in Figure 36-5.

In the palliative setting there are various radiation treatment regimens. Since the goal is rapid palliation of

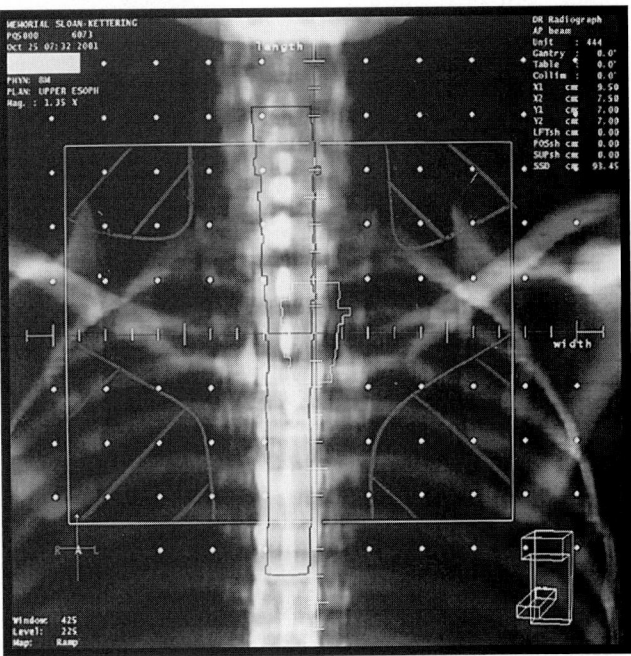

Figure 36-3. An example of the anterior-posterior–posterior-anterior (AP–PA) component for the treatment of a proximal esophageal cancer. See also Color Figure 36-3.

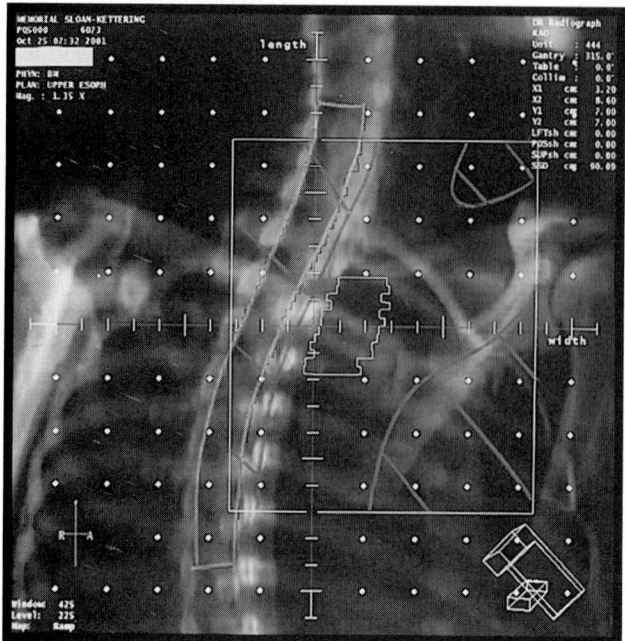

Figure 36-4. An example of the oblique component for the treatment of a proximal esophageal cancer. See also Color Figure 36-4.

symptoms, the most common approach is to treat AP–PA including the primary tumor with 2-cm margins with 10 fractions of 3 Gy/fraction to a total dose of 30 Gy.

CRITICAL NORMAL TISSUES

The most critical normal structures that lie in proximity to the esophagus are the spinal cord, heart, lungs, and kidneys. When radiation is combined with chemotherapy, the radiation fractionation should be 1.8 Gy/day. The spinal cord dose should not exceed 45 Gy. All fields

should be treated daily. Doses to the heart, lungs, and kidneys depend to a large extent on the volume of these organs in the treatment field. Dose-volume histograms are the most effective way to modify treatment techniques to decrease the acute and long-term radiation-related toxicity. Whole-heart irradiation should be limited to 25 to 30 Gy. In the thorax, radiation fields frequently include substantial volumes of lung, especially with oblique or lateral fields. Decreased pulmonary function occurs following irradiation, particularly if large volumes of lung are treated to doses greater than 20 Gy. There is progressive, decreased ventilatory and diffusing capacity as a result of endothelial degeneration and interstitial fibrosis. Fields that include such substantial volumes of lung should be limited to 20 Gy. It is acceptable for small volumes of normal tissue in immediate proximity to the esophagus (excluding the spinal cord) to receive doses as high as 60 Gy. However, since the standard total dose of radiation is 50.4 Gy, this degree of inhomogeneity should be uncommon. Fortunately, even with primaries as distal as the GE junction, there is a limited amount of liver and kidney in the treatment fields.

OUTCOME

Primary Therapy

Primary therapy of esophageal cancer is either surgical or nonsurgical. Although the overall results of these approaches are similar, the patient population selected for treatment with each modality is usually different. For several reasons, this results in a selection bias against nonsurgical therapy. First, patients with poor prognostic features are more commonly selected for treatment with nonsurgical therapy. These features include patients who are not surgical candidates due to medical

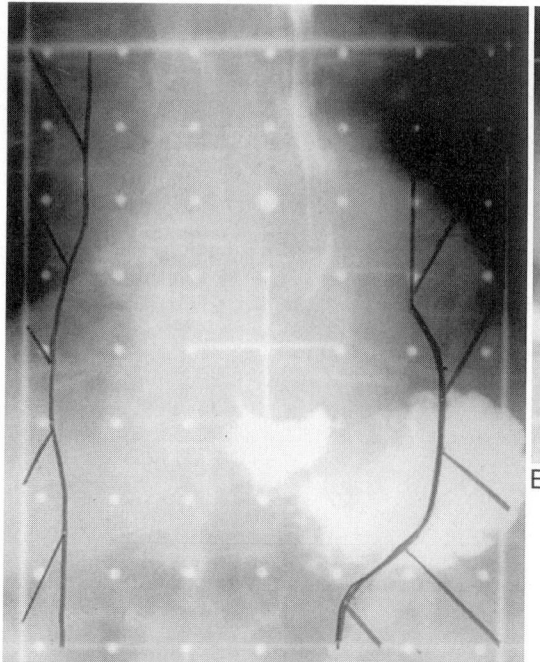

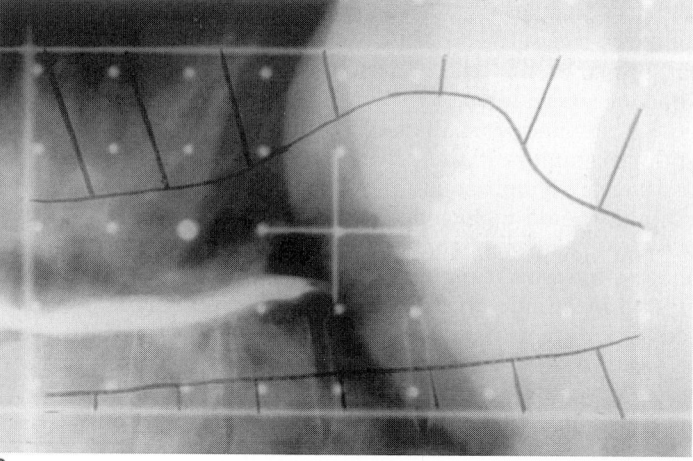

Figure 36-5. An example of a four-field technique for the treatment of a distal esophageal cancer.

contraindications or have primary unresectable or metastatic disease. Second, surgical series report results based on pathologically staged patients whereas nonsurgical series report results based on clinically staged patients. Third, since some patients treated without surgery may be approached in a palliative rather than a curative fashion, the intensity of chemotherapy and the doses and techniques of radiation therapy, in many historic series, were suboptimal.

SURGERY

Surgery is one of two standard therapies for clinically resectable esophageal cancer. Two randomized trials of preoperative chemotherapy (5-FU/cisplatin × 2 cycles) have been performed. The INT 0113 trial revealed no survival advantage.[38] Although the Medical Research Council trial did show a 10% survival advantage, 9% of patients received chemotherapy plus radiation.[39] In the surgical control arm from INT 0113, the median survival was 15 months and the 5-year survival was 20%. Major surgical controversies include the operative approach (transthoracic or Ivor-Lewis esophagectomy vs. transhiatal esophagectomy) and the extent of resection. Due to the high complication rates, the use of a three-field dissection is rarely performed in western countries.[40] Likewise, a minority of surgeons from western countries advocate en bloc resections. Although some phase II trials suggest improved survival with an en bloc resection, this may be due to selection bias since this operation allows more pathologically accurate staging. In a recent series of 111 patients (of which 10% also had preoperative adjuvant therapy), the 5-year survival of the 67 patients with node-positive disease was 26%, which is similar to the surgical control arm of INT 0113.[41]

NONSURGICAL THERAPY

Radiation Therapy Alone

Many historical series have reported results of external beam radiation therapy (EBRT) alone. Most include patients with unfavorable features, such as clinical T_4 disease. Overall, the 5-year survival rate for patients treated with conventional doses of radiation therapy alone is 0% to 10%.[42-44] Shi and colleagues reported a 33% 5-year survival rate with the use of late-course accelerated fractionation to a total dose of 68.4 Gy.[45] However, in the arm of the RTOG 85-01 trial using radiation therapy alone, in which patients received 64 Gy at 2 Gy/day with conventional techniques, all patients were dead of disease by 3 years.[46,47]

There is limited experience using radiation therapy alone for patients with superficial[48] or clinical T_1 disease.[49] The trial by Sykes et al. was limited to 101 patients (90% with squamous cell carcinoma) with tumors less than 5 cm who received 45 to 52.5 Gy in 15 to 16 fractions. The 5-year survival was 20%.[50]

In general, radiation therapy alone should be reserved for palliation or for patients who are medically unable to receive chemotherapy. As discussed later, the results of combined modality therapy are more favorable, making it the standard of care.

Combined Modality Therapy

Six randomized trials have compared radiation therapy alone with combined modality therapy.[46,51-57] Of these trials, five used suboptimal doses of radiation and three used inadequate doses of systemic chemotherapy. The only trial designed to deliver adequate doses of systemic chemotherapy with concurrent radiation therapy was the RTOG 85-01 trial reported by Herskovic et al. (Fig. 36-6).[46,54,57] This Intergroup trial primarily included patients with squamous cell carcinoma. Patients received 4 cycles of 5-FU (1000 mg/m² per 24 hours × 4 days) and Cisplatin (75 mg/m², day 1). Radiation therapy (50 Gy at 2 Gy/day) was given concurrently with day 1 of chemotherapy. Curiously, cycles 3 and 4 of chemotherapy were delivered every 3 weeks (weeks 8 and 11) rather than every 4 weeks (weeks 9 and 13). This intensification may explain, in part, why only 50% of the patients finished all 4 cycles of the chemotherapy. The control arm was radiation therapy alone, albeit a higher dose (64 Gy) than the combined modality therapy arm.

Patients who were randomized to receive combined modality therapy had a significant improvement in both median (14 months vs. 9 months), and 5-year survival (27% vs. 0%, P <0.0001).[54] With a minimum follow-up of 5 years, the 8-year survival was 22%.[57] Histology did not significantly influence the results with 21% of the 107 patients with squamous cell carcinomas alive at 5 years compared with 13% of the 23 patients with adenocarcinoma (P = not significant). The incidence of local failure as the first site of failure (defined as local persistence plus recurrence) was also lower in the combined modality arm (47% vs. 65%). The protocol was closed early due to the positive results. Although African Americans had larger primary tumors, all of which were squamous cell cancers, there was no difference in survival compared with Caucasians.[58]

Based on the positive results from the RTOG 85-01 trial, the conventional nonsurgical treatment for esophageal carcinoma is combined modality therapy.

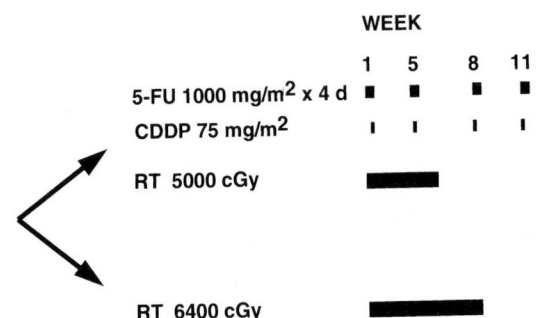

Figure 36-6. Phase III Intergroup trial RTOG 8501 for patients with squamous cell and adenocarcinoma of the esophagus selected for a nonoperative approach.[46,54,57]

Notwithstanding, the local failure rate in the combined modality therapy arm was 47%, indicating room for improvement. Therefore, new approaches such as escalation of the radiation dose were developed in an attempt to improve these results.

Intensification of the Radiation Dose

Two methods have been used to increase the radiation dose to the esophagus: brachytherapy and external beam.

BRACHYTHERAPY. Brachytherapy has been used as primary therapy (usually as a palliative modality)[59-63] as well as a boost following EBRT or combined modality therapy.[59,64-67] It can be delivered by high dose rate or low dose rate.[68] Although there are technical and radiobiologic differences between the two dose rates, there are no clear therapeutic advantages.

Brachytherapy alone is a palliative modality, resulting in a local control rate of 25% to 35% and a median survival of approximately 5 months.[59-62] In the randomized trial from Sur et al., there was no significant difference in local control or survival with high-dose-rate brachytherapy compared with external beam.[60]

A major limitation of brachytherapy is the effective treatment distance. The primary isotope is ^{192}Ir, which is usually prescribed to treat to a distance of 1 cm from the source. Therefore, any portion of the tumor which is greater than 1 cm from the source will receive a suboptimal radiation dose. This limitation has been confirmed by pathologic analysis of treated specimens.[69]

Series that combine brachytherapy with external beam or combined modality therapy report similar results to conventional combined modality therapy. Calais et al. reported a local failure rate of 43% and a 5-year actuarial survival of 18%.[64] Even with the more favorable subset of patients with clinical T1–T2 disease, Yorozu et al. reported a local failure rate of 44% and a 5-year survival of 26%.[70]

In the RTOG 92-07 trial, 75 patients with squamous cell cancers (92%) or adenocarcinomas (8%) of the thoracic esophagus received the RTOG 85-01 combined modality regimen (5-FU/Cisplatin per 50 Gy) followed by a boost during cycle 3 of chemotherapy with either low-dose-rate or high-dose-rate intraluminal brachytherapy.[71] The choice of dose rate was at the investigators' discretion. Due to low accrual, the low-dose-rate option was discontinued and the analysis was limited to patients who received the high-dose-rate treatment. High-dose-rate brachytherapy was delivered in weekly fractions of 5 Gy during weeks 8, 9, and 10. Following the development of several fistulas, the fraction delivered at week 10 was discontinued.

Although the complete response rate was 73%, with a median follow-up of only 11 months, local failure as the first site of failure was 27%. Acute toxicity included 58% grade 3, 26% grade 4, and 8% grade 5 (treatment-related death). The cumulative incidence of fistula was 18%/year and the crude incidence was 14%. Of the six treatment-related fistulas, three were fatal. Given the significant toxicity, this treatment approach should be used with caution.

The American Brachytherapy Society has developed guidelines for esophageal brachytherapy.[72] For example, for patients treated in the curative setting, brachytherapy should be limited to tumors less than or equal to 10 cm with no evidence of distant metastasis. Contraindications include tracheal or bronchial involvement, cervical esophagus location, or stenosis that cannot be bypassed. The applicator should have an external diameter of 6 to 10 cm. If combined modality therapy is used (defined as 5-FU–based chemotherapy plus 45 to 50 Gy), the recommended doses of brachytherapy are 10 Gy in 2 weekly fractions of 5 Gy each for high dose rate and 20 Gy in a single fraction at 4 to 10 Gy/hr for low dose rate. The doses should be prescribed to 1 cm from the source. Lastly, brachytherapy should be delivered after the completion of external beam radiation therapy, not concurrently with chemotherapy.

In summary, in the palliative setting, intraluminal brachytherapy is an effective modality for decreasing symptoms such as dysphagia and bleeding. In patients treated in the curative setting, the addition of brachytherapy does not appear to improve the results compared with radiation therapy or combined modality therapy alone. Therefore, the additional benefit of adding intraluminal brachytherapy to radiation or combined modality therapy, although reasonable, remains unclear.

EXTERNAL BEAM. Based on the tolerability of higher doses of external beam radiation (64.8 Gy) in the Intergroup 0122 trial, this dose was used in the experimental arm of the Intergroup esophageal trial INT 0123 (RTOG 9405).[36] INT 0123 was the follow-up trial to RTOG 8501. In this trial, patients with either squamous cell (85%) or adenocarcinomas (15%) selected for a nonsurgical approach were randomized to a slightly modified RTOG 85-01 combined modality regimen with 50.4 Gy versus the same chemotherapy with 64.8 Gy (Fig. 36-7).

The modifications to the original RTOG 85-01 combined modality therapy arm included: (1) using 1.8 Gy fractions to 50.4 Gy rather than 2 Gy fractions to 50 Gy; (2) treating with 5-cm proximal and distal margins for 50.4 Gy rather than treating the whole esophagus for the first 30 Gy followed by a cone down with 5-cm margins to 50 Gy; (3) cycle 3 of 5-FU/cisplatin did not begin until 4 weeks after completion of radiation therapy rather than 3 weeks; and (4) cycles 3 and 4 of chemotherapy were delivered every 4 weeks rather than every 3 weeks. The trial opened in late 1994 and was closed to accrual in 1999 when an interim analysis revealed it was unlikely that the high dose arm would achieve a superior survival compared with the standard dose arm.

For the 218 eligible patients, there was no significant difference in median survival (13.0 months vs. 18.1 months), 2-year survival (31% vs. 40%), or local/regional failure or local/regional persistence of disease (56% vs. 52%) or both between the high dose and standard dose arms.[36] Although 11 treatment-related deaths occurred in the high dose arm compared with two in the standard dose arm, 7 of the 11 occurred in patients who had received less than or equal to 50.4 Gy.

In addition to increasing the total dose, radiation can be intensified by accelerated doses or hyperfractionation.[45,73,74] Although these approaches are reasonable, most

INT 0123

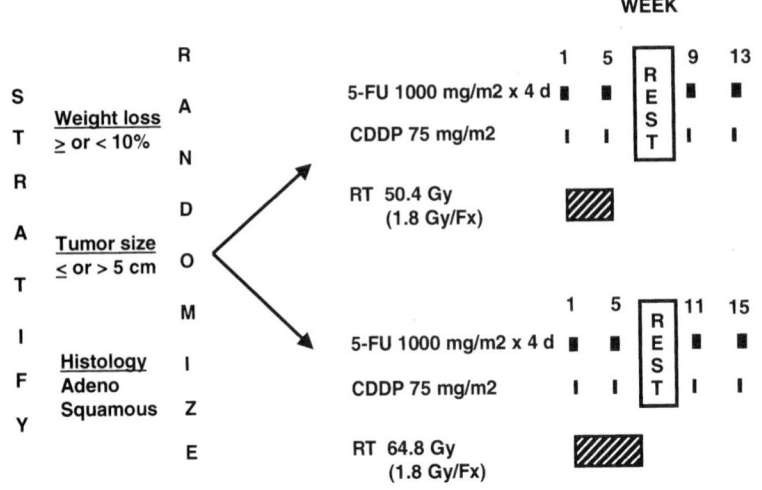

Figure 36-7. Phase III Intergroup trial 0123 (RTOG 94-05) for patients with squamous cell or adenocarcinoma of the esophagus.[36]

series report an increase in acute toxicity without any clear therapeutic benefit. These regimens remain investigational.

In summary, regardless of the technique (brachytherapy or external beam), intensification of the radiation dose beyond 50.4 Gy does not improve the results of combined modality therapy.

Palliation of Dysphagia with Radiation Therapy

Dysphagia is a common problem in patients with esophageal cancer. A major weakness of the series examining palliation is that they are retrospective and most do not use objective criteria to define and assess dysphagia. Some do not report the number of patients presenting with dysphagia or the percentage that are palliated until the time of death. Furthermore, few series carefully examine other variables that may influence the results such as histology, stage, and the location of the primary tumor.

As seen in Table 36-3, a limited number of series have examined the palliative benefits with either radiation alone[52,75-78] or combined modality therapy.[77,79-83] Overall, EBRT alone offers palliation of dysphagia in approximately 70% to 80% of patients.

The most comprehensive and carefully performed analysis of swallowing function in 102 patients receiving combined modality therapy is from Coia et al.[84] Before the start of therapy, 95% of patients had some degree of dysphagia. Within 2 weeks following the start of treatment, 45% had improvement in dysphagia and by the completion of the 6-week therapy, 83% had improvement. Overall, 88% had an improvement in dysphagia. The median time to maximum improvement was 4 weeks (range 1 to 21 weeks) and all but 2 patients could swallow at least soft or solid foods at the time of maximum symptomatic improvement. Even in patients treated in the noncurative setting, 91% had an initial improvement in swallowing and 67% were palliated until the time of their death.

Intraluminal brachytherapy is also an effective albeit more limited method of palliation. It achieves palliation of dysphagia in 40% to 90% of patients.[59-62] As previously discussed, since it is usually prescribed to 1 cm from the source, it may underdose gross disease. There is a selection bias against brachytherapy since it is commonly used for patients who have either failed EBRT or who are medically unable to travel for daily outpatient treatment. Even accounting for these selection biases, given its limited effective range, intraluminal brachytherapy is usually not as successful as EBRT in treating the

Table 36–3 Palliation of Dysphagia from Esophageal Cancer with External Beam Radiation Therapy ± Chemotherapy

Series	Total n	At the End of Treatment	Duration of Palliation
		Palliation of Dysphagia*	
Combined Modality Therapy			
Coia et al[84]	102	88%	67–100% until death
Seitz et al[82]	35	100%[†]	—
Whittington et al[77]	26	—	87% 3-yr actuarial
Algan et al[79]	8	100%	—
Gill et al[80]	71	60%	—
Urba and Turrisi[81]	27	—	59% until death
Izquierdo et al[83]	25	64%	Median 5 mo
Radiation Therapy Alone			
Wara et al[75]	103	89%	6 mo average
Petrovich et al[76]	133	87%	34% ≥6 mo
			18% ≥3 mo
			35% ≤3 mo
Roussel et al[52]	69	70%	
Caspers et al[78]	127	71%	54% until death
Whittington et al[77]	25	—	5% at 9 mo

*See text for the definition and the number of patients presenting with dysphagia.
†Patients had dilation or Nd-YAG laser treatment at the start of therapy.

entire tumor volume. Other modalities such as plastic and metallic stents are available to palliate dysphagia.[85]

Acute and Long-Term Toxicity of Radiation Therapy

The toxicity of radiation therapy is a function of the total dose, technique, and whether the patient has received chemotherapy. During treatment all patients will experience erythema, lethargy, and esophagitis. These begin 2 to 3 weeks after the start of radiation and start to resolve 1 week following the completion of therapy.

The most carefully documented acute radiation-related toxicity data are from the control arm of RTOG 85-01 where patients received radiation therapy alone to a dose of 64 Gy.[46,54] The incidence of acute grade 3 toxicity was 25% and grade 4 toxicity was 3%. There were no treatment-related deaths. The incidence of long-term grade 3+ toxicity was 23% and grade 4+ was 2%.[57] In the control arm of INT 0123 (which was similar to the combined modality therapy arm of RTOG 85-01), the incidence of acute grade 3 toxicity was 43% and grade 4 toxicity was 26%. There were no treatment-related deaths. The incidence of long-term grade 3+ toxicity was 24% and grade 4+ was 13%.[36] As with surgery, radiation therapy can produce esophageal strictures. The incidence of benign stricture (in the absence of local recurrence) is 12%.[84]

The high incidence of fistula reported in the RTOG 92-07 trial of combined modality therapy plus intraluminal brachytherapy (18% actuarial, 14% crude) has not been reported in series using radiation therapy or combined modality therapy without intraluminal brachytherapy. The incidence of other long-term grade 3+ toxicities such as pneumonitis or pericarditis is 5%. If appropriate radiation doses and techniques are used, spinal cord myelitis should not occur.

Treatment-Related Deaths

The incidence of treatment-related death with modern combined modality therapy was only 2% in RTOG 8501[46] and INT 0123 trials.[36] This compares favorably with the 6% reported for the surgery-alone control arm in INT 0113.[38]

Comparison of Radiation and Surgical Therapies

There is one randomized trial addressing the issue of surgical versus nonsurgical therapy. However, the randomization was limited to patients who responded to initial combined modality therapy. The FFCD 9102 trial, reported in abstract form by Bedenne et al., included a total of 445 patients with squamous cell cancer who initially received 2 cycles of 5-FU, cisplatin, and concurrent radiation (either 46 Gy at 2 Gy/day or split-course 15 Gy weeks 1 and 3).[86] The 259 patients who had at least a partial response were then randomized to surgery versus additional combined modality therapy, which included 3 cycles of 5-FU, cisplatin, and concurrent radiation (either 20 Gy at 2 Gy/day or split-course 15 Gy). There was no significant difference in 2-year survival (34% vs. 40%, $P = 0.56$) or median survival (18 months vs. 19 months) in patients who underwent surgery versus additional combined modality therapy.

Nonrandomized comparison of surgical versus nonsurgical therapy from the Intergroup trials reveals that the nonsurgical approaches (RTOG 8501 and INT 0123) offer a survival rate the same if not better than surgery (INT 0113). Although the results are comparable, it is clear that both the nonsurgical and surgical approaches have limited success. Therefore, trials that have combined the two approaches (surgery plus preoperative or postoperative adjuvant therapy) have been developed.

Treatment in the Setting of a Tracheoesophageal Fistula

The presence of a malignant tracheoesophageal fistula is an unfavorable prognostic feature. Although the survival of such patients is limited, they may occasionally survive for a prolonged period. In the historic literature, radiation therapy was considered contraindicated for fear of exacerbating the fistula as the tumor responded. More recently there have been reports to the contrary. In the Mayo Clinic series, 10 patients with a malignant tracheoesophageal fistula received 30 to 66 Gy EBRT and the median survival was 5 months.[87] Of note, none of the patients experienced an increase in the side of the fistula following radiation. In one case report, a patient who developed a fistula while receiving EBRT continued treatment to a total dose of 56.5 Gy. The fistula healed 2 months after completion of radiation.[88] Although the experience is limited, the data suggest that radiation does not necessarily increase the severity of a malignant tracheoesophageal fistula and it may be administered safely. Due to the poor prognosis of this group of patients, it is unclear if radiation improves outcome.

Adjuvant Therapy

ADJUVANT RADIATION THERAPY WITHOUT CHEMOTHERAPY

Preoperative Radiation Therapy

There have been six randomized trials of preoperative radiation therapy for patients with clinically resectable disease.[53,89-93] Overall, preoperative radiation therapy did not increase the resectability rate. The only series to show a significant improvement in survival was from Nygaard and associates; however, their patients also received chemotherapy.[53] A recent meta-analysis from the Oesophageal Cancer Collaborative Group also showed no clear evidence of a survival advantage with preoperative radiation.[94]

Postoperative Radiation Therapy

Despite encouraging nonrandomized reports of postoperative radiation therapy,[95] there have been only two randomized trials limited to patients treated in the adjuvant setting.[96,97] In the series from Teniere et al., there was a significant decrease in local failure in patients with negative nodes.[96] However, neither reported a survival advantage. Although there are no clear data to support it, the only role for postoperative radiation therapy is for patients with positive margins. In this setting, it is reasonable to combine systemic chemotherapy with radiation.

Preoperative Combined Modality Therapy

NONRANDOMIZED TRIALS. In general, the nonrandomized series of preoperative combined modality therapy have used two treatment approaches. Patients either undergo a planned operation or, for various reasons, are selected for an operation. Most trials use 5-FU/cisplatin-based chemotherapy. Recent trials have used taxane-[98-100] or Irinotecan[101]-based chemotherapy. Radiation is delivered either once or twice (BID) daily. In addition to the different treatment schedules, there is also variability of surgical techniques among the trials. The investigators from the University of Michigan use transhiatal esophagectomy whereas most others advocate the Ivor-Lewis approach. The transhiatal esophagectomy is a more conservative approach compared with the more commonly used Ivor-Lewis procedure since the thorax is not entered. There is much debate in the surgical literature as to the relative benefits and risks of these two approaches.

Most of the trials report complete pathologic response rates of approximately 25%.[20] Some report higher rates as well as 3-year survival rates superior to surgery. The 1992-1994 U.S. Patterns of Care survey study reported a significant improvement in survival in patients selected to receive preoperative combined modality therapy compared with combined modality therapy alone.[102] Despite these encouraging results, this approach needs to be confirmed in randomized trials.

RANDOMIZED TRIALS. There have been four randomized trials comparing preoperative combined modality therapy with surgery alone in patients with clinically resectable disease (Table 36-4).[103-105] The series from Le Prise et al. is not included since patients received sequential rather than concurrent chemotherapy plus radiation.[106]

Urba and associates from the University of Michigan randomized 100 patients (75% with adenocarcinoma) to preoperative cisplatin, vinblastine, 5-FU, and concurrent radiation therapy (1.5 Gy BID to 45 Gy), followed on day 42 by a transhiatal esophagectomy versus surgery alone. In the most recent update there was a significant decrease in local recurrence (19% vs. 42%); however, the survival advantage at 3 years (30% vs. 15%) did not reach statistical significance.[105]

In the series from Walsh et al., 113 patients with adenocarcinoma of the mid or distal esophagus (including the cardia) were randomized to two cycles 5-FU/cisplatin plus concurrent pre-operative radiation therapy (2.67 Gy/day to 40 Gy) versus surgery alone.[103] There was a significant improvement in both median survival (16 months vs. 11 months, $P = 0.01$) and 3-year survival (32% vs. 6%, $P = 0.01$). The major criticism of this trial is the high operative mortality rate of 9% and the low 3-year survival (6%) in the surgical control arm.

The third randomized trial of preoperative combined modality therapy was reported by Bosset et al. from the EORTC.[104] A total of 282 patients with clinically resectable squamous cell carcinomas were randomized to preoperative combined modality therapy versus surgery alone. The unconventional preoperative regimen included 3.7 Gy $\times$ 5 followed by a 2-week rest (split course) and another 3.7 Gy/day $\times$ 5. Chemotherapy was limited to low-dose cisplatin 0 to 2 days before (not concurrent with) radiation therapy. Patients who received preoperative combined modality therapy had a significantly greater 3-year disease-free survival (40% vs. 28%) and local disease-free survival rates (relative risk 0.6), but no improvement in median survival (19 months) or overall 3-year survival (36%) compared with surgery alone.

The last trial has been reported in abstract form. The Australasian GI trials group randomized 256 patients (61% with adenocarcinoma) to preoperative cisplatin day 1, followed by 5-FU days 2-5 with concurrent 35 Gy at 2.33 Gy/day versus surgery alone.[107] Comparing preoperative combined modality therapy versus surgery alone, the median overall survival was 22 months versus 19 months ($P = 0.38$). For patients with squamous cell cancer, there was a significant increase in relapse-free survival, but that did not translate into a survival advantage. There was no advantage for adenocarcinomas.

Given the substantial limitations and criticisms of the randomized trials, the Intergroup developed a randomized trial of preoperative combined modality therapy (CALGB C9781). Unfortunately it was closed prematurely due to lack of accrual. Therefore, it is unlikely that

Table 36–4   Randomized Trials of Preoperative Combined Modality Therapy for Esophageal Cancer

				Survival			
Series	n	Histology	Treatment	Pathological Cr (%)	Median (mo)	3-Yr (%)	Local Failure, %
Urba et al[105]	100	75% Adeno	Preop CMT	28	17	30*	19%†
		25% Squamous	Surgery	0	17	15	42%
Walsh et al[103]	113	100% Adeno	Preop CMT	25	16†	32†	—
			Surgery	0	11	6	—
Bosset et al[104]	282	100% Squamous	Preop CMT	26	19	36	—
			Surgery	0	19	36	
Burmeister et al[107]	256	61% Adeno	Preop CMT		22		
			Surgery		19		

*P = not significant
†$P < 0.05$
Adeno, adenocarcinoma; CR, Complete response; Preop CMT, preoperative combined modality therapy; Squamous, squamous cell carcinoma.

the question of the efficacy of preoperative combined modality therapy will ever be clearly answered.

It would be helpful to predict tumors that have a higher likelihood of responding to radiation or combined modality therapy. Correlation with a variety of markers such as p53[108,109] have had variable results. With the further discovery and understanding of various tumor suppressor genes, in the future, these data may be used to help select patients for combined modality therapy.

New Chemotherapeutic Agents

Since 75% to 80% of patients die of metastatic disease, advances in systemic therapies are necessary for further improvement of results. 5-FU has been the most widely used systemic agent in the treatment of esophageal cancer. There are new chemotherapeutic agents in both current practice and development for esophageal cancer. Taxol-based combined modality therapy regimens have shown encouraging results.[98-100,110-112] The RTOG randomized phase II trial E-0113 compares two Taxol-based regimens. Herceptin plus Taxol[113] and oxaliplatin[114] have been combined with radiation therapy. Other agents such as Irinotecan are being used as platforms for new regimens.[115] The development of the ideal regimens and schedules remains an active area of clinical investigation.

New Radiation Treatment Modalities

Although radiation therapy is a critical component in the successful management of esophageal cancers, similar to surgery, intensification has not improved the cure rate. Alternative radiation approaches such as hypoxic cell sensitizers and hyperfractionation have not resulted in a clear survival advantage. Particle irradiation such as helium ions or neutrons have shown increased toxicity with no local control or survival benefit.[116] There is very limited experience with intraoperative radiation as an alternative to external beam radiation.[117] Conformal and intensity modulated radiation therapy are being investigated.[118]

REFERENCES

1. Daly JD, Fry WA, Little AG, et al: Esophageal cancer: Results of an American College of Surgeons Patient Care Evaluation Study. *J Am Coll Surg.* 2000;190:562.
2. Devesa SS, Blot WJ, Fraumeni JF: Changing patterns in the incidence of esophageal and gastric carcinoma in the United States. *Cancer.* 1998;83:2049.
3. Blot WJ, Devesa SS, Kneller RW, et al: Rising incidence of adenocarcinoma of the esophagus and gastric cardia. *JAMA.* 1991;265:1287.
4. Brown LM, Hoover R, Silverman D: Excess incidence of squamous cell esophagus cancer among US black men: Role of social class and other risk factors. *Am J Epidemiol.* 2001;153:114.
5. Launoy G, Milan C, Day NE, et al: Diet and squamous cell cancer of the esophagus: A French multicenter case-control study. *Int J Cancer.* 1998;76:7.
6. Pera M, Pera M: Recent changes in the epidemiology of esophageal cancer. *Surg Oncol.* 2001;10:81.
7. Lagergren J, Bergstrom R, Lindgren A, et al: Symptomatic gastroesophageal reflux as a risk factor for esophageal adenocarcinoma. *N Engl J Med.* 1999;340:825.
8. Spechler SJ, Goyal RK: The columnar-lined esophagus, intestinal metaplasia, and normal Barrets. *Gastroenterology.* 1996;110:614.
9. DeMeester TR: Clinical biology of Barrett's metaplasia, dysplasia to carcinoma sequence. *Surg Oncol.* 2001;10:91.
10. Wijnhoven BP, Tilanus HW, Dinjens WN: Molecular biology of Barrett's adenocarcinoma. *Ann Surg.* 2001;233:322.
11. Gammon MD, Schoenberg JB, Ahsan H: Tobacco, alcohol, and socioeconomic status and adenocarcinoma of the esophagus and gastric cardia. *J Natl Cancer Inst.* 1997;89:1277.
12. Lagergren J, Bergstrom R, Adami HO, et al: Association between medications that relax the lower esophageal sphincter and risk for esophageal cancer. *Ann Int Med.* 2000;133:227.
13. Chow WH, Blot WJ, Vaughan TL: Body mass index and risk of adenocarcinoma of the esophagus and gastric cardia. *J Natl Cancer Inst.* 1998;87:104.
14. Zhang ZF, Kurtz RC, Yu GP, et al: Adenocarcinomas of the esophagus and gastric cardia: The role of diet. *Nutr Cancer.* 1997;27:298.
15. Huang JQ, Subbaramiah S, Chen Y, et al: Meta-analysis of the relationship between *Helicobacter pylori* seropositivity and gastric cancer. *Gastroenterology.* 1998;114:1169.
16. Stein HJ, Feith M: Cancer of the esophagus. In Gospodarowicz M, ed. *Prognostic Factors in Cancer.* New York:Wiley-Liss; 2001:211.
17. Stein HJ, Brucher BLDM, Sendler A, et al: Esophageal cancer: Patient evaluation and pre-treatment staging. *Surg Oncol.* 2001;10:103.
18. Ireland AP, Shibata DK, Chandrasoma P, et al: Clinical significance of *p53* mutations in adenocarcinoma of the esophagus and cardia. *Ann Surg.* 2000;231:179.
19. Ross JS, McKenna BJ: The *HER-2/neu* oncogene in tumors of the gastrointestinal tract. *Cancer Invest.* 2001;19:554.
20. Schrump DS, Altorki N, Forastiere A, Minsky BD: Cancer of the Esophagus. In DeVita VT, Hellman S, Rosenberg SA, eds. *Cancer: Principles and Practice of Oncology.* 6th ed. Philadelphia: Lippincott, Williams & Wilkins; 2001:1051.
21. Reid BJ, Prevo LJ, Galipeau PC, et al: Predictors of progression in Barrett's esophagus II: Baseline 17p (*p53*) loss of heterozygosity identifies a patient subset at increased risk for neoplastic progression. *Am J Gastroenterol.* 2001;96:2839.
22. Hironaka S, Hasebe T, Kamijo T, et al: Biopsy specimen microvessel density is a useful prognostic marker in patients with T2-4M0 esophageal cancer treated with chemoradiotherapy. *Clin Cancer Res.* 2002;8:124.
23. Stein HJ, Sendler A, Fink U, et al: Multidisciplinary approach to esophageal and gastric cancer. *Surg Clin North Am.* 2000;80:659.
24. Begin LR: The pathobiology of *esophageal* cancer. In Roth JA, Ruckdeschel JC, Weisenburger TH, eds. *Thoracic Oncology.* 2nd ed. Philadelphia:WB Saunders; 1995:288.
25. Sons HU, Borchard F: Cancer of the distal esophagus and cardia. *Ann Surg.* 1981;203:188.
26. Kelly S, Harris KM, Berry E, et al: A systematic review of the staging performance of endoscopic ultrasound in gastro-oesophageal carcinoma. *Gut.* 2001;49:534.
27. Flamen P, van Cutsem E, Lerut T, et al: The utility of positron emission tomography with 18F-fluorodeoxyglucose (FDG-PET) to predict the pathologic response and survival of esophageal cancer after preoperative chemoradiation therapy (CRT). *Proc ASCO.* 2001;20:127a [abstract].
28. Downey RJ, Ilson D, Koong H, et al: 18FDG PET measures the pathologic response of esophageal cancer to induction therapy. *Proc ASCO.* 2001;20:127a [abstract].
29. Flamen P, van Cutsem E, Lerut T, et al: Positron emission tomography for assessment of the response to induction radiochemotherapy in locally advanced esophageal cancer. *Ann Oncol.* 2002;13:361.
30. American Joint Committee on Cancer: Esophagus. In Fleming ID, Cooper JS, Henson DE, et al., eds. *AJCC Cancer Staging Manual.* 5th ed. Philadelphia: Lippincott-Raven; 1997:65.
31. American Joint Committee on Cancer: Esophagus. In Greene FL, Page DL, Fleming ID, et al., eds. *AJCC Cancer Staging Manual.* 6th ed. New York: Springer; 2002:91.
32. Siewert JR, Feith M, Werner M, et al: Adenocarcinoma of the esophagogastric junction. Results of surgical therapy based on

anatomic-topographic classification in 1002 consecutive patients. *Ann Surg.* 2000;232:353.

33. Coia LR, Minsky BD, John MJ, et al: The evaluation and treatment of patients receiving radiation therapy for carcinoma of the esophagus. Results of the 1992-1994 Patterns of Care Study. *Cancer.* 1999;85:2499.

34. Coia LR, Minsky BD, John MJ, et al: Patterns of care study decision tree and management guidelines for esophageal cancer. *Radiat Med.* 1998;16:321.

35. Tai P, van Dyk J, Yu E, et al: Variability of target volume delineation in cervical esophageal cancer. *Int J Radiat Oncol Biol Phys.* 1998;42:277.

36. Minsky BD, Pajak T, Ginsberg RJ, et al: INT 0123 (RTOG 94-05) phase III trial of combined modality therapy for esophageal cancer: High dose (64.8 Gy) vs. standard dose (50.4 Gy) radiation therapy. *J Clin Oncol.* 2002;20:1167.

37. Jacob JH, Seitz JF, Langlois C, et al: Definitive concurrent chemoradiation therapy (CRT) in squamous cell carcinoma of the esophagus (SCCE): Preliminary results of a French randomized trial comparing standard vs. split course irradiation (FNCLCC-FFCD 9305). *Proc ASCO.* 1999;18:270a [abstract].

38. Kelsen DP, Ginsberg R, Pajak T, et al: Chemotherapy followed by surgery compared with surgery alone for localized esophageal cancer. *N Engl J Med.* 1998;339:1979.

39. Clark PI: Medical Research Council randomized trial of surgery with or without pre-operative chemotherapy in resectable cancer of the esophagus (MRC Upper GI Tract Cancer Group). *Ann Oncol.* 2000;11:4 [abstract].

40. Nishimaki T, Suzuki T, Suzuki S, et al: Outcomes of extended radical esophagectomy for thoracic esophageal cancer. *J Am Coll Surg.* 1998;186:306.

41. Altorki N, Skinner D: Should en bloc esophagectomy be the standard of care for esophageal carcinoma? *Ann Surg.* 234:581, 2001.

42. De-Ren S: Ten-year follow-up of esophageal cancer treated by radical radiation therapy: Analysis of 869 patients. *Int J Radiat Oncol Biol Phys.* 1989;16:329.

43. Newaishy GA, Read GA, Duncan W, et al: Results of radical radiotherapy of squamous cell carcinoma of the esophagus. *Clin Radiol.* 1982;33:347.

44. Okawa T, Kita M, Tanaka M, et al: Results of radiotherapy for inoperable locally advanced esophageal cancer. *Int J Radiat Oncol Biol Phys.* 1989;17:49.

45. Shi X, Yao W, Liu T: Late course accelerated fractionation in radiotherapy of esophageal carcinoma. *Radiother Oncol.* 1999;51:21.

46. Herskovic A, Martz LK, Al-Sarraf M, et al: Combined chemotherapy and radiotherapy compared with radiotherapy alone in patients with cancer of the esophagus. *N Engl J Med.* 1992;326:1593.

47. Al-Sarraf M, Martz K, Herskovic A, et al: Superiority of chemoradiotherapy (CT-RT) vs radiotherapy (RT) in patients with esophageal cancer. Final report of an Intergroup randomized and confirmed study. Proc ASCO. 1996;15:206 [abstract].

48. Seki K, Karasawa K, Kohno M, et al: The treatment result of definitive radiotherapy for superficial esophageal cancer. *Int J Radiat Oncol Biol Phys.* 2001;51:264 [abstract].

49. Nemoto K, Yamada S, Hareyama M, et al: Radiation therapy for superficial esophageal cancer: A comparison of radiotherapy methods. *Int J Radiat Oncol Biol Phys.* 2001;50:639.

50. Sykes AJ, Burt PA, Slevin NJ, et al: Radical radiotherapy for carcinoma of the esophagus: An effective alternative to surgery. *Radiother Oncol.* 1998;48:15.

51. Araujo CMM, Souhami L, Gil RA, et al: A randomized trial comparing radiation therapy versus concomitant radiation therapy and chemotherapy in carcinoma of the thoracic esophagus. *Cancer.* 1991;67:2258.

52. Roussel A, Jacob JH, Jung GM, et al: Controlled clinical trial for the treatment of patients with inoperable esophageal carcinoma: A study of the EORTC gastrointestinal tract cancer cooperative group. In Schlag P, Hohenberger P, Metzger U, eds. *Recent Results in Cancer Research.* 1st ed. Berlin: Springer-Verlag; 1988:21.

53. Nygaard K, Hagen S, Hansen HS, et al: Pre-operative radiotherapy prolongs survival in operable esophageal carcinoma: A randomized, multicenter study of pre-operative radiotherapy and chemotherapy. The second Scandinavian trial in esophageal cancer. *World J Surg.* 1992;16:1104.

54. Al-Sarraf M, Martz K, Herskovic A, et al: Progress report of combined chemoradiotherapy versus radiotherapy alone in patients

55. Slabber CF, Nel JS, Schoeman L, et al: A randomized study of radiotherapy alone versus radiotherapy plus 5-fluorouracil and platinum in patients with inoperable, locally advanced squamous cell cancer of the esophagus. *Am J Clin Oncol (CCT).* 1998;21:462.

56. Smith TJ, Ryan LM, Douglass HO, et al: Combined chemoradiotherapy vs. radiotherapy alone for early stage squamous cell carcinoma of the esophagus: A study of the Eastern Cooperative Oncology Group. *Int J Radiat Oncol Biol Phys.* 1998;42:269.

57. Cooper JS, Guo MD, Herskovic A, et al: Chemoradiotherapy of locally advanced esophageal cancer. Long-term follow-up of a prospective randomized trial (RTOG 85-01). *JAMA.* 1999;281:1623.

58. Streeter OE, Martz KL, Gaspar LE, et al: Does race influence survival for esophageal cancer patients treated on the radiation and chemotherapy arm of RTOG # 85-01? *Int J Radiat Oncol Biol Phys.* 1999;44:1047.

59. Moni J, Armstrong JG, Minsky BD, et al: High dose rate intraluminal brachytherapy for carcinoma of the esophagus. *Dis Esophag.* 1996;9:123.

60. Sur RK, Singh DP, Sharma SC: Radiation therapy of esophageal cancer: Role of high dose rate brachytherapy. *Int J Radiat Oncol Biol Phys.* 1992;22:1043.

61. Jager J, Langendijk H, Pannebakker M, et al: A single session of intraluminal brachytherapy in palliation of esophageal cancer. *Radiother Oncol.* 1995;37:237.

62. Sur RK, Donde B, Levin VC, et al: Fractionated high dose rate intraluminal brachytherapy in palliation of advanced esophageal cancer. *Int J Radiat Oncol Biol Phys.* 1998;40:447.

63. Maingon P, d'Hombres A, Truc G, et al: High dose rate brachytherapy for superficial cancer of the esophagus. *Int J Radiat Oncol Biol Phys.* 2000;46:71.

64. Calais G, Dorval E, Louisot P, et al: Radiotherapy with high dose rate brachytherapy boost and concomitant chemotherapy for stages IIB and III esophageal carcinoma: Results of a pilot study. *Int J Radiat Oncol Biol Phys.* 1997;38:769.

65. Akagi Y, Hirokawa Y, Kagemoto M, et al: Optimum fractionation for high-dose-rate endoesophageal brachytherapy following external irradiation of early stage esophageal cancer. *Int J Radiat Oncol Biol Phys.* 1999;43:525.

66. Schraube P, Fritz P, Wannenmacher MF: Combined endoluminal and external irradiation of inoperable esophageal carcinoma. *Radiother Oncol.* 1997;44:45.

67. Okawa T, Dokiya T, Nishio M, et al: Multi-institutional randomized trial of external radiotherapy with and without intraluminal brachytherapy for esophageal cancer in Japan. *Int J Radiat Oncol Biol Phys.* 1999;45:623.

68. Caspers RJL, Zwinderman AH, Griffioen G, et al: Combined external beam and low dose rate intraluminal radiotherapy in esophageal cancer. *Radiother Oncol.* 1993;27:7.

69. Sur M, Sur R, Cooper K, et al: Morphologic alterations in esophageal squamous cell carcinoma after preoperative high dose rate intraluminal brachytherapy. *Cancer.* 1996;77:2200.

70. Yorozu A, Dokiya T, Oki Y, et al: Curative radiotherapy with high-dose-rate brachytherapy boost for localized esophageal carcinoma: Dose-effect relationship of brachytherapy with the balloon type applicator system. *Radiother Oncol.* 1999;51:133.

71. Gaspar LE, Qian C, Kocha WI, et al: A phase I/II study of external beam radiation, brachytherapy and concurrent chemotherapy in localized cancer of the esophagus (RTOG 92-07): Preliminary toxicity report. *Int J Radiat Oncol Biol Phys.* 1997;37:593.

72. Gaspar LE, Nag S, Herskovic A, et al: American Brachytherapy Society (ABS) consensus guidelines for brachytherapy of esophageal cancer. *Int J Radiat Oncol Biol Phys.* 1997;38:127.

73. Kim JH, Choi EK, Kim SB, et al: Preoperative hyperfractionated radiotherapy with concurrent chemotherapy in resectable esophageal cancer. *Int J Radiat Oncol Biol Phys.* 2001;50:1.

74. Raoul JL, Le Prise E, Meunier B, et al: Neoadjuvant chemotherapy and hyperfractionated radiotherapy with concurrent low-dose chemotherapy for squamous cell esophageal carcinoma. *Int J Radiat Oncol Biol Phys.* 1998;42:29.

75. Wara WM, Mauch PM, Thomas AN, et al: Palliation for carcinoma of the esophagus. *Radiology.* 1976;121:717.

76. Petrovich Z, Langholz B, Formenti S, et al: Management of carcinoma of the esophagus: The role of radiotherapy. *Am J Clin Oncol (CCT).* 1991;14:80.

77. Whittington R, Coia LR, Haller DG, et al: Adenocarcinoma of the esophagus and esophago-gastric junction: The effects of single and combined modalities on the survival and patterns of failure following treatment. *Int J Radiat Oncol Biol Phys.* 1990;19:593.

78. Caspers RJL, Welvaart K, Verkes RJ, et al: The effect of radiotherapy on dysphagia and survival in patients with esophageal cancer. *Radiother Oncol.* 1988;12:15.

79. Algan O, Coia LR, Keller SM, et al: Management of adenocarcinoma of the esophagus with chemoradiation alone or chemoradiation followed by esophagectomy: Results of sequential nonrandomized phase II studies. *Int J Radiat Oncol Biol Phys.* 1995;32:753.

80. Gill PG, Denham JW, Jamieson GG, et al: Patterns of treatment failure and prognostic factors associated with the treatment of esophageal carcinoma with chemotherapy and radiotherapy either as sole treatment or followed by surgery. *J Clin Oncol.* 1992;10:1037.

81. Urba SG, Turrisi AT: Split-course accelerated radiation therapy combined with carboplatin and 5-fluorouracil for palliation of metastatic or unresectable carcinoma of the esophagus. *Cancer.* 1995;75:435.

82. Seitz JF, Giovannini M, Padaut-Cesana J, et al: Inoperable non-metastatic squamous cell carcinoma of the esophagus managed by concomitant chemotherapy (5-fluorouracil and cisplatin) and radiation therapy. *Cancer.* 1990;66:214.

83. Izquierdo MA, Marcuello E, Gomez de Segura G, et al: Unresectable nonmetastatic squamous cell carcinoma of the esophagus managed by sequential chemotherapy (cisplatin and bleomycin) and radiation therapy. *Cancer.* 1993;71:287.

84. Coia LR, Soffen EM, Schultheiss TE, et al: Swallowing function in patients with esophageal cancer treated with concurrent radiation and chemotherapy. *Cancer.* 1993;71:281.

85. O'Donnell CA, Fullarton GM, Watt E, et al: Randomized clinical trial comparing self-expanding metallic stents with plastic endoprostheses in the palliation of esophageal cancer. *Br J Surg.* 2002;89:985.

86. Bedenne L, Michel P, Bouche O, et al: Randomized phase III trial in locally advanced esophageal cancer: Radiochemotherapy followed by surgery versus radiochemotherapy alone (FFCD 9102). *Proc ASCO.* 2002;21:130a [abstract].

87. Gschossmann JM, Bonner JA, Foote RL, et al: Malignant tracheoesophageal fistula in patients with esophageal cancer. *Cancer.* 1993;72:1513.

88. Arlington A, Bohorquez J: Irradiation of carcinoma of the esophagus containing a tracheoesophageal fistula. *Cancer.* 1993;71:3808.

89. Launois B, Delarue D, Campion JP, et al: Preoperative radiotherapy for carcinoma of the esophagus. *Surg Gynecol Obstet.* 1981;153:690.

90. Arnott SJ, Duncan W, Kerr GR, et al: Low dose preoperative radiotherapy for carcinoma of the esophagus: Results of a randomized clinical trial. *Radiother Oncol.* 1993;24:108.

91. Huang GJ, Gu XZ, Wang LJ, et al: Combined preoperative irradiation and surgery for esophageal carcinoma. In Delarue NC, ed: *International Trends in General Thoracic Surgery.* 1st ed. St. Louis: CV Mosby; 1988:315.

92. Mei W, Xian-Zhi G, Weibo Y, et al: Randomized clinical trial on the combination of preoperative irradiation and surgery in the treatment of esophageal carcinoma: Report on 206 patients. *Int J Radiat Oncol Biol Phys.* 1989;16:325.

93. Gignoux M, Roussel A, Paillot B, et al: The value of preoperative radiotherapy in esophageal cancer: Results of a study of the E.O.R.T.C. *World J Surg.* 1989;11:426.

94. Arnott SJ, Duncan W, Gignoux M, et al: Preoperative radiotherapy in esophageal carcinoma: A meta-analysis using individual patient data (esophageal cancer collaborative group). *Int J Radiat Oncol Biol Phys.* 1998;41:579.

95. Yamamoto M, Yamashita T, Matsubara T, et al: Reevaluation of postoperative radiotherapy for thoracic esophageal carcinoma. *Int J Radiol Oncol Biol Phys.* 1997;37:75.

96. Teniere P, Hay J-M, Fingerhut A, et al: Postoperative radiation therapy does not increase survival after curative resection for squamous cell carcinoma of the middle and lower esophagus as shown by a multicenter controlled trial. *Surg Gynecol Obstet.* 1991;173:123.

97. Fok M, Sham JST, Choy D, et al: Postoperative radiotherapy for carcinoma of the esophagus: A prospective, randomized controlled trial. *Surg.* 1993;113:138.

98. Safran H, Gaissert H, Akerman P, et al: Paclitaxel, cisplatin, and concurrent radiation for esophageal cancer. *Cancer Invest.* 2001;19:1.

99. Ajani JA, Komaki R, Putnam J, et al: A three-step strategy of induction chemotherapy then chemoradiation followed by surgery in patients with potentially resectable carcinoma of the esophagus or gastroesophageal junction. *Cancer.* 2001;92:279.

100. Safran HS, Akerman P, Cioffi W, et al: Paclitaxel and concurrent radiation therapy for locally advanced adenocarcinomas of the pancreas, stomach, and gastroesophageal junction. *Sem Radiat Oncol.* 1999;53:57.

101. Anderson S, Ilson D, Bains M, et al: Phase I trial of cisplatin and escalating dose irinotecan given weekly with concurrent radiation in locally advanced esophageal cancer. *Proc ASCO.* 2001;20:158a [abstract].

102. Coia L, Minsky B, John M, et al: Outcome of patients receiving radiation for cancer of the esophagus: Results of the 1992–1994 patterns of care study. *Proc ASCO.* 1998;17:258a [abstract.

103. Walsh TN, Noonan N, Hollywood D, et al: A comparison of multimodal therapy and surgery for esophageal adenocarcinoma. *N Engl J Med.* 1996;335:462.

104. Bosset JF, Gignoux M, Triboulet JP, et al: Chemoradiotherapy followed by surgery compared with surgery alone in squamous cell cancer of the esophagus. *N Engl J Med.* 1997;337:161.

105. Urba SG, Orringer MB, Turrisi A, et al: Randomized trial of preoperative chemoradiation versus surgery alone in patients with locoregional esophageal cancer. *J Clin Oncol.* 2001;19:305.

106. Le Prise E, Etienne PL, Meunier B, et al: A randomized study of chemotherapy, radiation therapy, and surgery versus surgery for localized squamous cell carcinoma of the esophagus. *Cancer.* 1994;73:1779.

107. Burmeister BH, Smithers BM, Fitzgerald L, et al: A randomized phase III trial of preoperative chemoradiation followed by surgery (CR-S) versus surgery alone (S) for localized resectable cancer of the esophagus. *Proc ASCO.* 2002;21:130a [abstract].

108. Sarbia M, Stahl M, Fink U, et al: Expression of apoptosis-regulating proteins and outcome of esophageal cancer patients treated by combined therapy modalities. *Clin Cancer Res.* 1998;4:2991.

109. Pomp J, Davelaar J, Blom J, et al: Radiotherapy for esophagus carcinoma: The impact of *p53* on treatment outcome. *Radiother Oncol.* 1998;46:179.

110. Kelsen D, Ilson D, Minsky B, Lipton R: Phase I trial of combined modality therapy for localized esophageal cancer: Radiation therapy + concurrent cisplatin and escalating doses of 96 hour infusional paclitaxel. *Proc ASCO.* 1998;17:260a [abstract].

111. Nesbitt J, Ajani JA, Komaki R, et al: Preoperative Taxol-based chemotherapy (CT) followed by chemoradiation therapy (CTRT) in patients (PTS) with potentially resectable esophageal carcinoma (EC). *Proc ASCO.* 1998;17:282a [abstract].

112. Safran H, Gaissert H, Akerman P, et al: Neoadjuvant paclitaxel, cisplatin and radiation for esophageal cancer. *Proc ASCO.* 1998;17:259a [abstract].

113. Safran H, DiPetrillo T, Nadeem A, et al: Neoadjuvant herceptin, paclitaxel, cisplatin, and radiation for adenocarcinoma of esophagus: a phase I study. *Proc ASCO.* 2002;21:141a [abstract].

114. Khushalani KI, Leichman CG, Proulx G, et al: Oxaliplatin in combination with protracted-infusion fluorouracil and radiation: Report of a clinical trial for patients with esophageal cancer. *J Clin Oncol.* 2002;20:2844.

115. Bains MS, Stojadinovic A, Minsky B, et al: A phase II trial of preoperative combined-modality therapy for localized esophageal carcinoma: Initial results. *J Thorac Cardiovasc Surg.* 2002;124:270.

116. Castro JR, Saunders WM, Tobias CA: Treatment of cancer with heavy charged particles. *Int J Radiat Oncol Biol Phys.* 1982;9:465.

117. Hosokawa M, Shirato H, Ohara K, et al: Intraoperative radiation therapy to the upper mediastinum and nerve-sparing three-field lymphadenectomy followed by external beam radiotherapy for patients with thoracic esophageal carcinoma. *Cancer.* 1999;86:6.

118. Nutting CM, Bedford JL, Cosgrove VP, et al: A comparison of conformal and intensity-modulated techniques for esophageal radiotherapy. *Radiother Oncol.* 2001;61:157.

Cancer of the Stomach

Bruce D. Minsky, MD and Raquel T. Wagman, MD

EPIDEMIOLOGY, ETIOLOGY, GENETICS, AND CYTOGENETIC ABNORMALITIES

Epidemiology

Gastric cancer is primarily a disease of older individuals with the median age at diagnosis 65 years (range: 40 to 70 years). The intestinal subtype is seen more commonly in patients older than 40 whereas the diffuse type affects younger patients and has a more aggressive clinical course.[1] Gastric cancer shows a propensity for men both in high- and low-incidence countries.

In a number of studies, the decrease in the incidence of gastric cancer has been attributed to a decrease in the incidence of the intestinal subtype. This trend has been seen in both high- and low-risk populations.[2] In recent years, there has been a decrease in the incidence of gastric cancer arising in the distal portion of the stomach and a concomitant increase in the incidence arising in the proximal portion. Proximal (cardia) gastric cancers tend to be of the diffuse type, which, relative to the intestinal type, is associated with a worse prognosis.[3,4]

Reasons for the improved prognosis reported in Japanese patients with gastric cancer remain unclear, but may include one or more of the following: genetics, early screening, or more extensive surgery.[5,6] Screening programs in Japan identify 50% of newly diagnosed gastric carcinomas as early stage. In contrast, in Great Britain and North America, where formal screening is not performed, the percentage of early gastric cancers is only 10% to 15%.

The incidence of gastric cancer varies widely around the world. The highest death rates are reported in Chile, Costa Rica, Japan, and the former Soviet Union (50, 78, 51, and 53 per 100,000, respectively). In 2003 there were an estimated 22,400 new cases of gastric cancer in the United States, with 13,400 occurring in men and 9000 occurring in women.[7] Approximately 12,100 deaths occurred.

Etiology

Numerous studies have examined the role of various factors that are involved in the development of gastric cancer. These can be broadly grouped into environmental factors, diet, race, and heredity.

DIETARY RISK FACTORS

No single dietary agent has been determined to be the causative factor of gastric cancer. However, in case-controlled studies, gastric cancer appears to be positively correlated with the ingestion of pickled vegetables, salted fish, excessive dietary salt, and smoked meats.[8-10] Fruits and vegetables may have a protective effect.[11,12]

HELICOBACTER PYLORI

Helicobacter pylori is associated with inflammatory conditions in the stomach, in particular chronic atrophic gastritis. Although *H. pylori* by itself cannot cause gastric cancer, a growing body of evidence, including meta-analysis, suggests that it plays an important role in the development of adenocarcinoma of the stomach.[13-16]

GENETIC FACTORS

The genetic basis of gastric cancer and its precursors is being actively investigated. Emerging data suggest that the development of gastric cancer, similar to many other epithelial-derived carcinomas, is a multistep process that involves a successive activation or deletion of genes and their protein products. This is mediated by regulatory genes. Advances in molecular biology techniques have allowed characterization of the genetic changes thought to be responsible for this multistep process.[17]

For example, tumors with high microsatellite instability (MSI) versus low MSI may evolve through different genetic pathways.[18] Another gene important in gastric cancer is CDH1, which encodes E-cadherin, an epithelial cell adhesion molecule. Germline CDH1 mutations have been identified in families with hereditary diffuse gastric cancer in a pattern consistent with autosomal dominant inheritance with incomplete penetrance.[19] HER-2/neu expression is associated with advanced disease.[20]

PREVIOUS RADIATION THERAPY

Limited data suggest that radiation delivered for benign disease may be a risk factor for gastric cancer. In the early 20th century, gastric irradiation was used to suppress gastric acid secretion. Orthovoltage radiation doses ranging from 1500 R to 2000 R in 10 days were used before the development of effective pharmacologic means to treat duodenal ulcers.[21] In a small cohort of patients described by Peters et al., patients who underwent partial gastrectomy and external beam radiation therapy had an increased incidence of gastric cancer.[22] Griem and associates reported on 1831 patients with peptic ulcer disease who were treated with radiation, and compared them to a similar group of medically managed patients over an average of 22 years. Radiation therapy was linked to an increased relative risk (RR) for cancers of the stomach (RR = 2.77, 95% confidence interval), as was partial gastrectomy (RR = 2.60, 95% confidence interval). When surgery was combined with radiation therapy, the risk increased 10-fold.[23] These results were only apparent after extended follow-up.[24]

OTHERS

Various other etiologic agents have been identified such as previous gastric surgery, adenomatous polyps, and chronic atrophic gastritis.[17]

ANATOMY

The stomach is at the first portion of the abdominal diaphragm, also referred to as the cardia. The uppermost portion of the stomach is the fundus or fornix. The major portion of the stomach, the body or corpus, tapers to the pyloric portion. This portion later divides into the pyloric antrum, which narrows into the pyloric canal terminating it, and the pyloric valve, which empties into the first portion of the duodenum. The two borders of the stomach, the concave lesser curvature and the convex greater curvature, both join at the cardia.

Adenocarcinomas of the upper gastrointestinal tract include primaries in both the gastroesophageal (GE) junction and stomach. The treatment of adenocarcinoma of the GE junction is discussed in Chapter 36, Cancer of the Esophagus.

PATHOLOGY

The stomach wall has five layers: mucosal, submucosal, muscular, subserosal, and serosal. The mucosa of the whole stomach is glandular. There are three distinct histologic/anatomic zones: (1) the cardia, which has a small area of predominantly mucus-producing cells; 2) the gastric or fundic glands, which are composed of three cells—mucoid, chief or zymogenic, and parietal; 3) the pyloric glands, which contain mucus-producing cells and associated endocrine cells, which secrete the hormone gastrin into the blood vessels of the lamina propria.

The most common histology (90%) is adenocarcinoma. Subtypes include papillary, tubular, mucinous, signet ring cell, adenosquamous, and squamous cell. Other histologies include sarcoma, carcinoid, small-cell and undifferentiated carcinomas. Lymphomas (mucosa-associated lymphoid tissue, or MALT) and leiomyosarcomas can occur, albeit at a much lower frequency. MALT lymphomas are discussed in Chapter 61, Non-Hodgkin's Lymphoma.

Most gastric carcinomas occur predominantly in the mid-portion of the lesser curvature and the distal stomach. The prognosis of patients with adenocarcinoma of the stomach depends on tumor type, site within the stomach, and the TNM stage. In a review of 5000 cases the distribution of stomach cancers by site were: 50% pyloric; 13% lesser curvature; 10% cardia; and 6% diffuse infiltration of the stomach.

The prognosis of proximal cancers is less favorable than of distal lesions. Borrmann classified stomach cancer into four categories based on the gross morphology. These included type I: polypoid, type II: ulcerative, type III: ulcerating and infiltrating, and type IV: infiltrating. Type IV corresponds to the appearance of linitis plastica, in which infiltration by tumor causes rigidity of the gastric wall. Borrmann types I and II have a more favorable prognosis than Borrmann types III and IV, independent of lymph node involvement.

Numerous classifications based on light microscopy of gastric cancer exist. The World Health Organization classification divides gastric adenocarcinoma into patterns common to carcinomas of other organs and includes well, moderately, or poorly differentiated.

Jarvi and Lauren, based on epidemiologic studies, divided stomach cancers into two main groups: intestinal (expansile) or diffuse (infiltrative). In 1977, Ming proposed a modification of the Jarvi-Lauren classification.[25] He emphasized the growth patterns rather than the tumor's architectural subtypes. The classification divides tumors into two main patterns, expanding and infiltrative, which roughly correspond to the intestinal and diffuse type, respectively. The expanding pattern is more common in his series (67%) and describes tumors that tend to be fungating, whereas the infiltrating tumors tend to be diffuse.

Gastric dysplasia is considered a precursor of gastric adenocarcinoma. Although there is little agreement regarding classification, numerous follow-up studies have correlated biopsy-proven dysphasia with an increased risk of the development of gastric adenocarcinoma.[26]

CLINICAL PRESENTATION

The initial symptoms of gastric cancer are vague and nonspecific. Symptoms generally become evident when tumor involvement has caused significant interference with the lumen or function of the stomach. Patients with proximal lesions may have dysphasia as a presenting symptom. Later, symptoms such as indigestion, post-prandial fullness, and loss of appetite may develop. Hematemesis is not common, but chronic blood loss may occur from an ulcerated lesion. Tumors involving the pylorus in advanced stages generally cause symptoms associated with obstruction. Weight loss and abdominal pain occur in more than half of patients, and one third experience nausea and anorexia.

Routes of Spread

Gastric cancers extend through the gastric wall and into regional lymphatics as well as by direct invasion of adjacent organs (e.g., liver, pancreas, spleen, esophagus, colon, duodenum, gallbladder, or the adjacent mesenteries). Hematogenous spread via the portal vein can involve the liver or the systemic circulation as well as the lungs, bone, and other distant sites. Peritoneal seeding from tumor may involve the gastric serosa through the omentum, parietal peritoneum, ovary (Krukenberg's tumor), and rectal shelf (Blumer). These are signs of advanced carcinomatosis. The degree to which regional lymphatics are involved is determined by the location of the primary lesion in the stomach. Evidence of distant nodal metastases includes the left supraclavicular node (Virchow's node) and left axillary nodes (Irish nodes).

Diagnostic and Staging Studies

The workup for gastric cancer is described in Table 37-1. Although numerous tumor markers have been described in gastric cancer, there is no screening, diagnostic staging, or prognostic tumor marker specific for it. Carcinoembryonic antigen (CEA) is positive in approximately one third of gastric carcinomas and reflects the extent of tumor burden. Postoperative elevated values of CEA are not helpful in predicting recurrence.

Flexible fiberoptic endoscopy with biopsy is more than 90% accurate in diagnosing gastric cancer.[27] The positive yield per biopsy is higher in exophytic tumors than in nonexophytic tumors. In the advanced infiltrating lesion (Borrmann type 4), the diagnosis by biopsy is less accurate. The location of the tumor can affect the diagnostic accuracy. Lesions in the gastric cardia and antrum located behind the *incisura angularis gastris* are particularly difficult from which to obtain a tissue diagnosis. Numerous studies have examined the correlation between radiologic diagnosis, endoscopy, and biopsy. No method alone is usually 100% reliable. The proper combination of radiologic procedures (barium swallow, computed tomography [CT] scan, possibly PET scan) and endoscopy results in the highest number of positive diagnoses. Such information helps the endoscopist direct the biopsy to suspicious areas in which there may not be mucosal abnormalities.

The application of endoscopic ultrasonography (EUS) allows the identification of five gastric wall layers.[28] In staging gastric tumors, EUS diagnoses the depth of penetration of the primary gastric carcinoma with approximately 90% accuracy.[29] EUS can also be used to stage lymph node metastases. However, the accuracy is less compared with the T stage. In one series, EUS had an accuracy of 83%, sensitivity of 54%, and a specificity of 97%. The positive predictive value was 88% and the negative predictive value was 82%.

Table 37–1 Diagnosis and Staging for Gastric Cancer

- History
- Physical examination
- Complete blood count, liver and renal function tests
- CT scan or MRI of the abdomen
- Chest x-ray
- Endoscopy and biopsy
- Upper GI series (*optional*)
- *Optional but recommended*:
    - Endoscopic ultrasound
    - PET scan
    - Laparoscopy

Staging System

In 1988 the American Joint Commission on Cancer (AJCC) and the Union Internationale Contre le Cancer (UICC) shared a joint TNM staging system, based on the fifth edition of the AJCC TNM staging system.[30] The major change from the fifth to the sixth edition is that T2 lesions have been divided into T2a (tumor invades the *muscularis propria*) and T2b (tumor invades the subserosa) (Table 37-2). Additional descriptors do not affect the stage grouping, but do indicate cases needing separate analysis.

As with most other gastrointestinal malignancies, the T classification is based on the extension through the layers of the stomach. Lymph node staging is based on the number of positive regional lymph nodes. Whether a lymph node is staged as nodal (N) or metastatic (M) disease depends on the relationship of the nodes to the primary tumor. In general, regional nodes include those located in the greater and lesser curvatures as well as those in the left gastric, common hepatic, splenic, and celiac arteries. Involvement of other intra-abdominal nodes including hepatoduodenal, retropancreatic, mesenteric, and para-aortic are staged as metastatic disease. Specific regional and distant nodal diseases are listed (see Table 37-2).

Clinical staging can be designated as cTNM and is based on physical examination, radiologic imaging, endoscopy, biopsy, and laboratory findings. Pathologic staging depends on data acquired clinically in addition to surgical and pathologic findings. If there is uncertainty regarding the appropriate T, N, or M staging, the lower (less advanced) category should be used.

STANDARD THERAPEUTIC APPROACHES

Surgery

The primary treatment for local/regional gastric cancer is surgery. An analysis from the U.S. National Cancer Data Base of 50,169 patients treated from 1985 to 1996 who underwent a gastrectomy as a component of their therapy revealed a decrease in overall 5-year survival rate with increasing stage: IA, 78%; IB, 58%; II, 34%; IIIA, 20%; IIIB, 8%; and IV, 7%.[31] In most cases, the determination of resectability for cure or palliation can only be assessed at the time of surgical exploration. The specific surgical procedure is based on the location/extent of the primary tumor and the respective lymph node drainage areas. Laparoscopy can detect disease in the peritoneal cavity and is helpful before a laparotomy.[32]

SUBTOTAL VS. TOTAL GASTRECTOMY

The first randomized prospective trial comparing subtotal with total gastrectomy for distal gastric cancers was reported by Gouzi et al.[33] Both groups had similar morbidity (33%), mortality (1.3% vs. 3.2% respectively), and 5-year survival (48%). Therefore, although elective total gastrectomy can be performed safely, subtotal and total gastrectomy offer equal long-term results in patients

Table 37–2   Classification of Gastric Cancer

Primary Tumor (T)

Tx	Primary tumor cannot be assessed
T0	No evidence of primary tumor
Tis	Carcinoma in situ: intra-epithelial tumor without invasion of the lamina propria
T1	Tumor invades lamina propria or submucosa
T2	Tumor invades muscularis propria or subserosa*
T2a	Tumor invades muscularis propria
T2b	Tumor invades subserosa*
T3	Tumor penetrates serosa (visceral peritoneum) without invasion of adjacent structures[†, ‡]
T4	Tumor invades adjacent structures[†, ‡]

Regional Lymph Nodes (N)[§]

Nx	Regional lymph node(s) cannot be assessed
N0	No regional lymph node metastasis
N1	Metastasis in 1-6 regional lymph nodes
N2	Metastasis in 7-15 regional lymph nodes
N3	Metastasis in >15 regional lymph nodes

Distant Metastasis

Mx	Distant metastasis cannot be assessed
M0	No distant metastasis
M1	Distant metastasis

Stage Grouping

Stage 0	Tis	N0	M0
Stage IA	T1	N0	M0
Stage IB	T1	N1	M0
	T2a/b	N0	M0
Stage II	T1	N2	M0
	T2a/b	N1	M0
	T3	N0	M0
Stage IIIA	T2a/b	N2	M0
	T3	N1	M0
	T4	N0	M0
Stage IIIB	T3	N2	M0
Stage IV	T4	N1-3	M0
	T1-3	N3	M0
	Tany	Nany	M1

*A tumor may penetrate the muscularis propria with extension into the gastrocolic or gastrohepatic ligaments or into the greater or lesser omentum without perforation of the visceral peritoneum covering these structures. In this case, the tumor is classified as T2. If there is perforation of the visceral peritoneum covering the gastric ligaments or the omentum, the tumor should be classified as T3.
[†]The adjacent structures of the stomach include the spleen, transverse colon, liver, diaphragm, pancreas, abdominal wall, adrenal gland, kidney, small intestine, and retroperitoneum.
[‡]Intramural extension to the duodenum or esophagus is classified by the depth of greatest invasion in any of these sites, including the stomach.
[§]A designation of pN0 should be used if all examined lymph nodes are negative, regardless of the total number removed and examined. Regional nodes by the primary tumor site include:
Greater Curvature of Stomach
• Greater curvature
• Greater omental
• Gastroduodenal
• Gastroepiploic, right, or NOS
• Gastroepiploic, left
• Pyloric, including subpyloric and infrapyloric
• Pancreaticoduodenal (anteriorly along first part of the duodenum)
Pancreatic and Splenic Area
• Pancreaticolienal
• Peripancreatic
• Splenic hilum

Continued

Table 37–2   Classification of Gastric Cancer—cont'd

Lesser Curvature of Stomach
• Lesser curvature
• Lesser omental
• Left gastric
• Paracardial; cardial
• Cardioesophageal
• Perigastric, not otherwise specified
• Common hepatic
• Celiac
• Hepatoduodenal
All other lymph nodes are considered distant. They include:
• Retropancreatic
• Para-aortic
• Portal
• Retroperitoneal
• Mesenteric

NOTE: Although additional descriptors do not affect the stage grouping, additional prefixes are used to indicate the need for additional analysis.

Suffix	Reason
m	The presence of multiple primary tumors in a single site, recorded in parentheses: pT(m)NM.
y	When classification is performed during or following initial radiation or chemotherapy or both and is based on the amount of tumor present at the time of the examination, and not an estimate of tumor before therapy: ycTNM or ypTNM.
r	Indicates recurrent tumor: rTNM.
a	Indicates the stage at autopsy: aTNM.

Lymphatic Vessel Invasion (L)

Lx	Cannot be assessed
L0	No lymphatic vessel invasion
L1	Lymphatic vessel invasion present

Venous Invasion (V)

Vx	Cannot be assessed
V0	No venous invasion
V1	Microscopic venous invasion present
V2	Macroscopic venous invasion present

From Greene FL, Page DL, Fleming ID, et al, eds: *AJCC Cancer Staging Manual*, 6th ed. New York: Springer, 2002.

with carcinomas of the distal stomach. Most U.S. surgeons recommend a subtotal gastrectomy providing that both negative margins, and an adequate lymphadenectomy, can be achieved. Proper lymph node staging requires examination of 10 to 15 nodes.[34]

CONVENTIONAL VS. EXTENDED LYMPH NODE DISSECTION

Lymphatic flow in the stomach is complex. Regardless of the location of the primary tumor, numerous nodal groups can be involved from either lymphatic spread occurring in a sequential manner or with metastases to distant lymph nodes without evidence of involvement of perigastric nodes (skipping). In rules established by the Japanese Research Society for Gastric Cancer, the lymph node groups are numbered 1 through 16 and are grouped into four lymph node levels or groups, N1 through N4. The determination of which nodal stations are placed in which nodal groups depends on the location of the primary tumor. By convention, N1 and N2 are considered regional nodes whereas metastasis to N3 and N4 node groups is considered distant metastasis. Most Japanese surgeons recommend an extended dissection. The rationale is that improved local regional control results in improved patient survival. However, the data supporting this hypothesis are controversial. In Japan, there is widespread endoscopic screening, and public health campaigns have resulted in the diagnosis of a larger proportion of early-stage tumors. The cure rates reported by Japanese investigators may be more related to the reduced stage of disease than the more radical surgical approach.[35] Such "stage migration" may be responsible for the improved survival in each stage of the disease.

In Western countries, there is substantial debate regarding how radical the operation should be. Specifically, should the tumor and spleen be resected en bloc, and how many and which lymph nodes should be removed? The extent of the resection is generally subdivided into three categories: D0, D1, and D2. The precise definitions vary, however. In general D0 is a limited operation whereas D1 includes resection of the primary tumor and the primary echelon nodes. The most radical is a D2 resection, which includes dissection of the second echelon nodes as well as an en bloc distal pancreatectomy and splenectomy.

Three randomized trials have addressed the question of the extent of surgery.[36-38] These trials confirm that not only was there no improvement in survival with more radical surgery (D2 vs. D1 vs. D0), but there was a corresponding increase in the incidence of complications. Despite these data, many gastric surgeons advocate a D2 resection and consider a D0 or D1 resection an inadequate cancer operation. The impact of a D2 resection on the results of the INT 0116 trial of postoperative adjuvant combined modality therapy[39] is discussed later in the Outcomes section.

Chemotherapy

Chemotherapy is used in both the adjuvant setting (with or without concurrent radiation therapy) and in the palliative setting for patients with advanced/metastatic disease. Three meta-analyses of the role of postoperative adjuvant 5-FU–based chemotherapy alone reveal conflicting results.[40] Although adjuvant chemotherapy is reasonable, its survival benefit remains unclear. Based on the results of the INT 0116 trial,[39] postoperative combined modality therapy is the standard of care in the adjuvant setting.

Radiation Therapy

Radiation therapy has been used as both an adjuvant treatment as well as a primary treatment modality. In the adjuvant setting it is limited to patients with local/regional disease who have undergone a complete resection with negative margins. Radiation as a primary treatment has been used after an incomplete or noncurative resection. The results are discussed later in the Outcomes section.

TECHNIQUES OF RADIATION THERAPY

The design and delivery of radiation therapy for gastric cancer requires knowledge of the natural history of the disease, patterns of failure, anatomy, and radiobiologic principles. Critical normal tissues that must be considered include the liver, kidneys, small intestine, spinal cord, skin, bone marrow, and the remaining stomach. Furthermore, the use of proper equipment, implementation of methods to decrease treatment-related toxicity, and a close collaboration with the physics and technology staff are essential. General guidelines are offered in Table 37-3.

Radiation technique affects acute and long-term toxicity. For example, in a series by Henning et al., the incidence of grade 4 toxicity with postoperative radiation ± chemotherapy was 14% acute and 5% chronic.[41] The overall incidence of grade 4+ toxicity was lower in the 46 patients treated with greater than or equal to 4 radiation fields (4% crude and 5% 3-year actuarial) compared with the 18 treated with 2 radiation fields (22% crude and 30% 3-year actuarial). These data are consistent with most other abdominal and pelvic malignancies where a multiple-field technique allows a larger volume of small bowel to be excluded from the radiation field when compared with an anterior-posterior–posterior-anterior (AP–PA) technique. However, due to the location of the target volume as well as the proximity of adjacent organs (especially the kidneys and liver), sometimes a multiple-field technique may not always be advantageous. Since the radiation dose for gastric cancer is 45 Gy, the AP–PA technique with high-energy photons may offer, in select cases, the best compromise between decreasing the small bowel volume in the radiation field and limiting the dose to the adjacent organs.

Techniques such as three-dimensional (3-D) treatment planning are helpful to determine if an AP–PA as opposed to a multiple-field technique should be used.[42] Dose volume histograms of the liver and kidneys are obtained. In general, if the dose to a given volume of kidney or liver exceeds its functional tolerance, then a higher dose to that volume is recommended in order to limit the dose to the remaining portion of the organ. For example if 20% of the kidney receives 30 Gy, that 20% will not function. Therefore, delivering 45 Gy to that 20% will not further decrease function, whereas it may allow the delivery of a tolerable dose (<20 Gy) to the remaining 80% of the kidney. With this approach, the largest volume of the organ receives the smallest dose, thereby maintaining function. Exceptions to this approach in the abdomen include the spinal cord and bowel, where the dose may not exceed 50.4 Gy.

Figure 37-1 provides an example of a four-field technique. It must be emphasized that these are *idealized* treatment fields. The borders must be modified based on the location of the primary tumor and the primary nodal drainage. Therefore, the radiation fields will usually be substantially smaller, reflecting this anatomic difference.

CRITICAL NORMAL TISSUES

The biological mechanisms of acute and delayed toxicity, as well as dietary interventions in patients receiving radiation for various malignancies in which the small bowel is in the radiation field, have been previously published.[43-45]

The toxicity (short and long term) in this group of patients is multifactorial and is related to the additive

Table 37–3   Guidelines for Therapy in Gastric Cancer

General Considerations

Target volume: includes the tumor bed, primary lymph nodes, plus an adequate (1.5-2.0 cm) margin.*

The preoperative upper GI series, CT scan, operative findings, and clip placement define the tumor bed and lymph node areas.

The tumor bed includes the maximum preoperative stomach volume. In patients with T3-T4 tumors, it should include the areas of local tumor extension as well as the medial two thirds to three fourths of the left hemidiaphragm.

In the ideal setting, one half to two thirds of the left kidney can be blocked. Likewise, the porta hepatis and retroduodenal lymph nodes can be treated while including only a small portion of the right kidney.

The nodes at risk include the celiac, porta hepatis, subpyloric, gastroduodenal, splenic-suprapancreatic, and retropancreaticoduodenal.

The gastroepiploic nodes are usually removed with the operative specimen.

The porta hepatis nodes are usually covered by a field that extends 2 cm to the right of T11-L1; however, their exact location is best determined from a CT scan.

The celiac axis is located at approximately T12-L1.

In proximal cardia and GE junction primaries, the paraesophageal nodes are at risk. The superior margin of the field should be extended to include 5 cm of the distal esophagus.

Anteroposterior–Posteroanterior (AP–PA) Field

Superior border:	The bottom of T8 or T9 to cover the celiac axis, GE junction, fundus, and the dome of the left hemidiaphragm.
Inferior border:	The bottom of L3 to cover the gastroduodenal nodes and the antrum.
Left border:	Include two thirds to three fourths of the left hemidiaphragm to cover fundus, suprapancreatic nodes, and splenic nodes.
Right border:	Field is 3 to 4 cm lateral to the vertebral bodies to cover the antrum, porta hepatis, and gastroduodenal nodes.

Lateral Field (If Appropriate)

Superior border:	Same as AP–PA field.
Inferior border:	Same as AP–PA field.
Anterior border:	Anterior abdominal wall.
Posterior border:	Include one half to two thirds of the vertebral bodies.

Given the posterior location of fundus, suprapancreatic nodes, and the splenic hilar nodes, lateral fields should be used only if the locations of these structures can be clearly identified and included in the lateral fields.

Blocks

Kidneys:	Blocks are used to spare the kidneys as much as possible and to decrease the amount of small bowel treated both superiorly and anteriorly.
Heart:	Since 5 cm of the distal esophagus are treated with proximal cardia and GE junction primaries, field blocks are needed to limit the dose to the heart. No more than 30% of the heart should receive >40 Gy.
Liver:	No more than 60% of the liver should receive >30 Gy.

*It must be emphasized that these borders are *idealized* and they may require modification based on the preoperative imaging studies, operative findings, clip placement, lymph node involvement, and individual anatomy.
CT, computed tomography; GE, gastroesophageal; GI, gastrointestinal.

risks of multiple operations, radiation therapy, and chemotherapy. Complications of radiation therapy are a function of the volume of the radiation field, overall treatment time, fraction size, radiation energy, total dose, and technique. The most sensitive organs in the radiation field include the stomach, small bowel, spinal cord, liver, and kidneys. Almost all patients will experience acute gastrointestinal and hematologic toxicity with 5% to 10% requiring a treatment break. Gastrointestinal toxicities

include diarrhea, abdominal cramping, nausea, and gastritis. These short-term side effects usually resolve within 1 to 2 weeks following the completion of therapy.

A number of simple radiotherapeutic techniques are available to decrease radiation-related toxicity (Table 37–4). For example, the treatment of all fields each day results in a lower integral dose and more homogeneous dose distribution. The treatment should be designed with the use of computerized radiation dosimetry and be delivered by high-energy linear accelerators, which, by nature of their depth-dose characteristics, deliver a higher dose to the tumor volume while sparing the surrounding normal structures. The fields must be carefully tailored to the primary tumor location and nodal drainage.

OUTCOMES

Rationale for Adjuvant Radiation Therapy

The rationale for adjuvant radiation therapy is based on the patterns of failure following potentially curative surgery (Table 37-5). These failure patterns have been

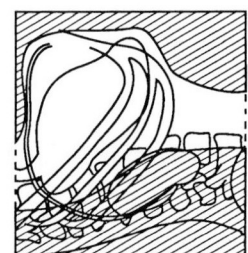

Figure 37–1. Idealized treatment fields for gastric cancer. In this example, a four-field technique is used. These fields should be modified based on the location of the primary tumor and nodal drainage. Therefore, they are usually substantially smaller than they appear in this figure.

Table 37–4   Techniques to Decrease Toxicity

High-energy (≥10-15 MV) linear accelerators.

Treatment 5 days per week and all fields each day.

Port films once per week or more often if clinically indicated.

Computed dosimetry to minimize the hot spots and increase the homogeneity within the target volume.

Three-dimensional treatment planning to generate dose volume histograms for the liver, kidneys, and small intestine.

The ideal field arrangement (AP–PA vs. multiple fields) is the one that (a) delivers the most homogeneous distribution within the target volume while (b) limiting the dose volume to the surrounding organs so as not to exceed the functional tolerance of a given organ. Since the fundus of the stomach usually extends posteriorly, the use of lateral fields commonly increases the dose to the kidneys. Therefore, an AP–PA field arrangement is usually preferred. Occasionally a preoperative upper GI series or CT scan reveals that the stomach is sufficiently anterior to allow the addition of lateral fields.

The spinal cord should be limited to as close to 45 Gy as possible.

If the blood urea nitrogen, creatinine, or both are above normal range, then a renal scan is necessary to determine the relative function of each kidney.

Shaped blocks and, if needed, wedges.

Small bowel contrast for CT scan.

Dose considerations: 45 Gy at 1.8 Gy/d.

AP–PA, anteroposterior–posteroanterior; CT, computed tomography; GI, gastrointestinal.

examined using clinical methods in a series from the Massachusetts General Hospital[46] as well as reoperation methods in a series from the University of Minnesota.[47] The series by Yoo and associates used both clinical and reoperation methods.[48]

The clinical method relies on physical examination, radiologic studies, and, in some patients, operative findings. In contrast, the reoperation method used a planned "second look" operation at least every 6 months. Although this method offers the most accurate appraisal

Table 37–5   Patterns of Failure Following Potentially Curative Surgery in Gastric Cancer Cumulative Incidence of Failure (%)*

Local Failure by TNM Stage	Clinical[46]	Reoperation[47]
T1N0	0	—
T1-2N0	19	—
T3N0	50	—
T4N0	40	—
T1-2 N1-2	24	—
T3N1-2	36	—
T4N1-2	56	—
Failure Site		
Total Local/Regional	38	67
-Gastric Bed	21	54
-Abdominal Scar		5
-Anastomosis	25	26
-Nodes	8	42
Peritoneal Seeding	23	41
-Local		19
-Diffuse		22
Distant	52	22

*Local failure as a component of failure.

of the anatomic distribution of failure, it is no longer used. The failure sites documented in the reoperation series from the University of Minnesota as well as idealized radiation fields covering these failure sites are listed in Figure 37-2.

As seen with other gastrointestinal malignancies, the incidence of local failure increases with increasing penetration of the tumor through the wall of the organ and the presence of lymph node metastasis. Depending on the analytic method used, the incidence of local failure following potentially curative surgery varies from 16% to 23% as the only site of failure and 33% to 67% as a component of failure.[46-48] In the series of 508 patients reported by Yoo et al., the mean time to local failure was 27 months, and, by multivariate analysis, independent factors that predicted a higher incidence of local failure included age older than 50, tumor size greater than 4 cm, proximal location, infiltrative or diffuse type, undifferentiated histology, serosal invasion, and lymph node metastasis.[48] Even in patients in whom a complete (R0) resection is performed, local failure remains a significant clinical problem.

Results of Adjuvant Therapy

POSTOPERATIVE RADIATION THERAPY WITH OR WITHOUT CHEMOTHERAPY

Baeza and colleagues have reported encouraging results from their nonrandomized trials with patients treated in the adjuvant setting (with negative margins).[49] Three

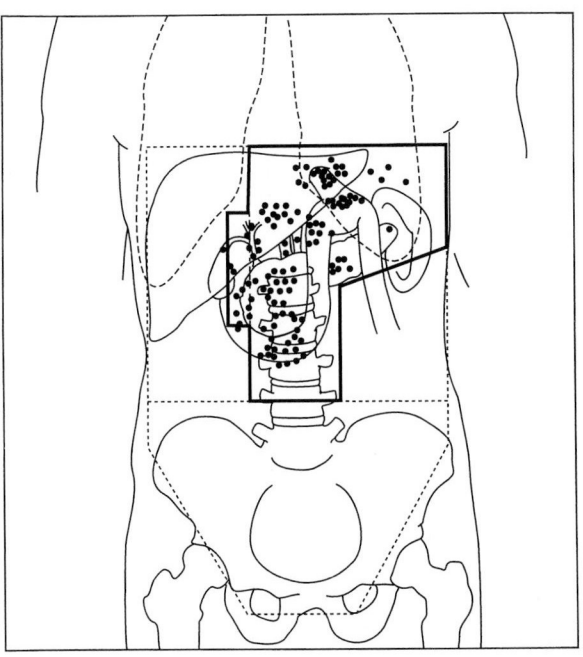

Figure 37–2. Patterns of failure in 82 evaluable patients in the University of Minnesota reoperation series for gastric cancer. The superimposed radiation fields cover the areas of lymph node drainage, gastric remnant, anastomosis, duodenal stump, and gastric bed structures. (Modified from Gunderson LL, Sosin H: Adenocarcinoma of the stomach: Areas of failure in a re-operation series [second or symptomatic look]—Clinicopathologic correlation and implications for adjuvant therapy. *Int J Radiat Oncol Biol Phys.* 1982;8:1.)

randomized trials of postoperative radiation therapy with or without chemotherapy following a complete resection with negative margins have been pereformed. The limited reports by Moertel et al.[50] and Dent and associates[51] did not reveal a clear survival advantage.

The landmark trial is the Intergroup Trial INT 0116 Fig. 37-3).[39] Eligibility included patients with stages IB, II, IIIA, IIIB, and IV nonmetastatic adenocarcinoma of the stomach or gastroesophageal junction. Following a resection with negative margins, patients were randomized to either observation alone or postoperative combined modality therapy consisting of 5 monthly cycles of bolus chemotherapy with 45 Gy concurrent with cycles 2 and 3. During cycles 1, 2, 4, and 5, patients received 5-FU/leucovorin daily × 5 whereas during cycle 2 they received 3 days of 5-FU alone concurrent with the last 3 days of radiation.

A total of 603 patients were registered. Overall, 20% had adenocarcinomas of the GE junction. Pretreatment characteristics were similar in both arms, and most patients had locally advanced disease (69% had T3 or T4 tumors and 85% had positive local/regional nodes). Patients randomized to receive postoperative combined modality therapy had a significant decrease in local failure as the first site of failure (19% vs. 29%) and an increase in median survival (36 months vs. 27 months), 3-year relapse-free survival (48% vs. 31%), and overall survival (50% vs. 41%, $P = 0.005$). The most common acute toxicities were hematologic and gastrointestinal. The incidence of grade 4 toxicity was higher with combined modality therapy (41% vs. 32%). Although 17% could not complete all therapy as planned, there was only one treatment-related death.

In order to minimize radiation-related toxicity, careful pretreatment review of the simulation films was performed. This resulted in the recommendation to the treating radiation oncologist to modify the design or volume of the radiation fields or both in 35% of cases. This illustrates the difficulty in designing gastric adjuvant radiation fields. Smalley and associates have reviewed the gastric anatomy and patterns of failure following surgery, and offer detailed radiation treatment-planning recommendations.[52]

INT 0116 GASTRIC ADJUVANT TRIAL

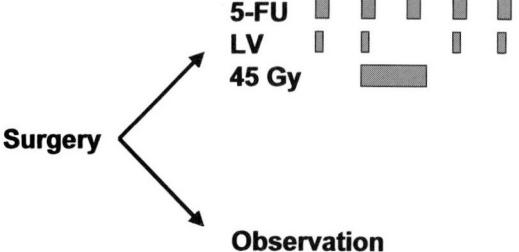

Figure 37–3. Intergroup trial 0116 of adjuvant postoperative combined modality therapy versus observation for patients with T_3 or N_{1-2} disease or both who undergo a complete resection with negative margins.[39] (From Macdonald JS, Smalley SR, Benedetti J, et al: Chemoradiotherapy after surgery compared with surgery alone for adenocarcinoma of the stomach or gastroesophageal junction. *N Engl J Med.* 2001;345:725.)

Some clinicians contend that adjuvant therapy is only a substitute for inferior surgery and is unnecessary if patients undergo a D2 resection. This theory is based on the fact that in the INT 0116 trial, only 10% of patients underwent a D2 resection, while 54% underwent a D0 and 36% underwent a D1 resection. However, data do not support this conclusion. Although the INT 0116 trial was not stratified by the type of resection, there was no significant difference in survival based on the extent of surgery. Furthermore, as previously discussed, the three randomized trials addressing the question of the extent of surgery confirm that there is no improvement in survival with more radical surgery (D2 vs. D1 vs. D0).[36-38] Careful surgical techniques are vital to the successful management of gastric cancer. However, based on the INT 0116 trial, the standard of care for patients with T3 or node-positive disease or both, even following a D2 resection, remains postoperative combined modality therapy.

Most of the trials of combined modality therapy shown in Table 37-6 have not used adequate doses of chemotherapy. In general, patients received 3 to 5 days of bolus 5-FU (350 to 500 mg/m²) during the first and sometimes the last 3 days of radiation therapy. With this schedule, 5-FU is designed as a *radiation sensitizer* rather than as a *systemic therapy*. The European Organization for Research and Treatment of Cancer randomized patients receiving combined modality therapy to short-term 5-FU versus long-term 5-FU and found that those randomized to receive short-plus long-term 5-FU had a median survival of 18 months compared with 10 months for those receiving short-term 5-FU.

Preoperative Radiation Therapy

A randomized trial by Zhang and associates from Beijing revealed a significant improvement in survival with preoperative radiation.[53] A total of 370 patients with adenocarcinoma of the gastric cardia who were younger than 65 years old and, based on endoscopy and CT criteria, had clinically resectable disease, were randomized to preoperative radiation (40 Gy in 20 fractions) followed by surgery 2 to 4 weeks later versus surgery alone. With a median follow-up of 123 to 128 months, there was a significant improvement in survival with preoperative radiation (30% vs. 20%, $P = 0.0094$). Preoperative radiation increased the rate of complete resection with negative margins (80% vs. 62%, $P < 0.001$) without increasing the postoperative morbidity or mortality. The incidence of both local failure (33% vs. 47%) and regional lymph node failure (31% vs. 55%) was also decreased. There was no difference in distant failure (24% vs. 25%). These data suggest that preoperative radiation improves local control and survival. However, randomized trials are needed to confirm the results in Western patients.

Preoperative Combined Modality Therapy

As discussed in Chapter 36, Esophagus, preoperative combined modality therapy achieves a 25% pathologically

Table 37–6   External Beam Radiation Therapy ± Chemotherapy for Gastric Cancer (Select Trials)

Series	% "Curative" Resections	n	Treatment	Survival	Local Failure
Preoperative Randomized Trials					
Zhang et al[53]	83	171	Preop 40 Gy	30% 5-yr I*	33% I*
		199	Surgery	20% 5-yr I	47% I
Postoperative Randomized Trials					
Moertel et al[50]	100	23	Surgery	4% 5-yr I	
	100	39	37.5 Gy + Chemotherapy	23% 5-yr I†	
			Subset Analysis		
		29	(Accepted treatment)	20% 5-yr	39%
		10	(Refused treatment)	30% 5-yr	
		33	Either surgery or refused treatment		54%
Dent et al[51‡]	43	35	20 Gy + Chemotherapy	30% 2-yr	
	48	31	Surgery	40% 2-yr	
			Subset Analysis		
	100	15	20 Gy + Chemotherapy	38% 2-yr	
	100	15	Surgery	60% 2-yr	
INT 0116[39]	100	281	45 Gy + Chemotherapy	50% 3-yr I†	
	100	275	Surgery	41% 3-yr I	
Moertel et al[55]	0	25	35-40 Gy	13 mo (mean) I	
			+ Chemotherapy	I†	
			Surgery	6 mo (mean) I	
Allum et al[76,77]	15	138	Chemotherapy	19% 5-yr	12%
		153	45-50 Gy	12% 5-yr	8% I
		145	Surgery	20% 5-yr	22% I†
Schein et al[78] (GITSG 8274)	0		50 Gy	6% 4-yr I	
	0		50 Gy + Chemotherapy	18% 4-yr I†	
GITSG[79]	0	50	Chemo	11% 3-yr	
	0	45	43.2 Gy + Chemotherapy	7% 3-yr	
Postoperative Nonrandomized Trials					
Safran et al[80]	N/A	27	45-50.5 Gy + Chemotherapy	43% 1-yr	
Henning et al[71]	0	60§	46.8-49.8 Gy median ± IORT	12 Mo median	30% crude 57% 4-Yr actuarial
			± Chemotherapy		
Henning et al[41]	40	63	50.4 Gy median 84% had chemotherapy	17 Mo median	30% crude

†Statistically significant difference.
‡"Division I" only (T1-3N1-2M0).
§Includes 13 patients who received IORT.
N/A, information not available from manuscript; Rx, treatment consisting of combined chemotherapy + radiation.

complete response rate and an 80% to 90% chance of a complete resection and negative margins in patients with adenocarcinoma of the GE junction. Based on these encouraging results, this approach is being used for the treatment of gastric cancer.[54] Although not the standard of care, it is reasonable to treat T2 and lymph-node positive adenocarcinomas involving both the GE junction and stomach with preoperative combined modality therapy. However, if this approach is used, a pretreatment laparoscopy is highly recommended to exclude patients with radiographically undetected peritoneal or liver metastasis or both.[32]

Treatment of Residual and Recurrent Disease

EXTERNAL BEAM RADIATION WITH OR WITHOUT CHEMOTHERAPY

The seminal trial examining the role of postoperative combined modality therapy in gastric cancer was reported by Moertel et al. in 1969.[55] Following laparotomy, patients with advanced gastric cancers were randomized to 30-40 Gy plus 5-FU versus surgery alone delivered as a radiation sensitizer. As seen in Table 37-6, there was a significant improvement in survival with the combination of radiation plus 5-FU.

The remaining randomized trials in Table 37-6 also include patients with unresectable or residual disease or both. It must be emphasized that none of the trials delivered adequate doses of radiation to control residual disease. Following a complete resection with negative margins, 45 Gy is recommended. The dose to adequately treat residual disease is at least 55 to 65 Gy, which, when delivered by external beam, exceeds the tolerance of the stomach and small intestines. The use of intraoperative radiation therapy is an alternative method by which to achieve higher radiation doses, and this approach is discussed later.

Obtaining negative surgical margins is important since, as one would predict, patients who have microscopic or residual disease following surgery have a less favorable outcome than those with negative margins. In a report by Henning et al. of 63 patients treated with postoperative radiation ± 5-FU–based chemotherapy, the median survival for the 25 patients with no residual disease was 19 months versus 17 months for the 28 patients with microscopic residual disease versus 9 months for the 10 patients with gross residual disease ($P = 0.01$).[41] Likewise, there was a corresponding significant decrease in local failure (20% vs. 36% vs. 40%, $P = 0.038$, respectively). The actuarial 4-year survival for the 25 patients treated in the adjuvant setting (no residual disease) was 31%.

Chemotherapeutic agents other than 5-FU are being combined with radiation therapy. Taxanes have both systemic activity as well as radiation-sensitizing properties.[56] Safran and associates have combined Taxol plus concurrent radiation either preoperatively in patients with potentially resectable disease (45 Gy) or as primary therapy in patients with unresectable disease (50.4 Gy).[57] For the 27 patients enrolled in this phase I/II trial, the overall response rate was 56% and the incidence of grade 3+ acute toxicity was 48%. With a median follow-up of 24 months, the 2-year survival was 31%. In patients with adenocarcinoma of the GE junction, Taxol combined with cisplatin and 50.4 Gy is well tolerated.[58,59] Taxol-containing combined modality therapy regimens are being compared in the G-0114 RTOG randomized phase II postoperative gastric adjuvant trial. Irinotecan-based regimens are also in development.[60]

In summary, the randomized data comparing postoperative combined modality therapy with either surgery alone or surgery followed by postoperative chemotherapy in patients with locally unresectable disease are conflicting. Although it is reasonable to treat such patients with combined modality therapy, given the retrospective nature of such series, the use of suboptimal doses of chemotherapy and radiation, and differences in patient selection and prognostic factors, it is difficult to make firm conclusions regarding the relative impact of therapy in this group of patients.

Intraoperative Radiation Therapy

An alternative method of delivering radiation therapy is intraoperative radiation therapy (IORT).[61-67] The theoretical advantage of this approach is the ability to deliver a more intensive dose of radiation to the tumor bed while excluding the surrounding normal tissues from the high-dose field.

The limited randomized trial performed by Sindelar and associates reported that the mean time to local failure was significantly improved in patients who received IORT (21 vs. 8 months).[61] Takahashi and Abe randomized patients based on the day of hospital admission to surgery plus IORT (28 to 35 Gy) versus surgery alone.[62,63] Although there was improved survival with IORT, it was limited to patients with stage III and IV disease.

There are numerous phase I/II trials of IORT + external beam radiation or combined modality therapy.[64,65,68-71] Most include patients with residual disease. Calvo and colleagues reported a 39% 2-year survival.[64] In the series from Coquard and associates, local failure was 25% and the 5-year survival was 47%.[69]

In the phase II RTOG 8504 trial, 27 patients with local/regional-only disease had a 19-month median survival and a 47% 2-year survival. Local failure within the IORT field was 37%.[65] Ogata and colleagues reported a survival of 100% for stage II, 55% for stage III, and 12% for stage IV disease in 58 patients treated with 28 to 30 Gy of a wide field of IORT following a radical gastrectomy.[70]

In the IORT series by Henning et al., the crude incidence of total grade 4 acute toxicity in the 60 patients who received a median of 46.8 Gy ± IORT (91% received 5-FU–based chemotherapy) was 22% and the long-term toxicity was 18%.[71]

The limited data suggest that IORT may be beneficial in select patients with gastric cancer. The optimal method by which to combine it with surgery and external beam radiation has yet to be determined. The use of IORT in gastric cancer, although encouraging, remains investigational.

Palliative Radiation Therapy

In the palliative setting, radiation therapy provides symptomatic relief of symptoms such as bleeding, obstruction, and pain in the majority of patients.[72] Patients with favorable prognostic factors such as a favorable performance status, microscopic as compared with gross residual disease, and who received 5-FU–based chemotherapy tend to have a higher response rate. Overall, the median duration of palliation is 4 to 18 months.[72-74] Rhomberg et al. treated 28 patients (23 with gross unresectable disease and 5 with microscopic residual disease) with a median of 50 Gy plus the radiosensitizer Razoxane.[75] The partial response rate was 89%, local control was 64%, and 96% had rapid pain relief.

CONCLUSIONS

In summary, the incidence of local failure following potentially curative surgery in gastric cancer is substantial. Almost all the series examining the role of postoperative radiation therapy or combined modality therapy in gastric cancer include patients who have microscopic or gross residual disease, thereby making the data difficult to interpret.

Based on the phase III Intergroup trial 0116, the standard adjuvant treatment for a completely resected gastric adenocarcinoma with T3 or node-positive disease or both is postoperative combined modality therapy. It is reasonable to treat patients who have positive margins with the same treatment regimen. Phase I/II trials in progress are examining the use of combining radiation therapy with alternative chemotherapeutic agents such as Taxol and irinotecan.

In the setting of locally unresectable or residual disease, postoperative radiation therapy or combined modality therapy is a reasonable approach, although it is not the standard of care. In those patients selected to receive radiation therapy, it should be combined with adequate doses of chemotherapy. Intraoperative radiation therapy, while promising, remains investigational. In the palliative setting, radiation therapy offers symptomatic relief in the majority of patients. Lastly, careful planning, design, and delivery techniques are central to the successful delivery of radiation therapy with an acceptable rate of complications.

REFERENCES

1. Mecklin JP, Nordling S, Saario I: Carcinoma of the stomach and its heredity in young patients. *Scan J Gastroenterol.* 1988;23:307.
2. Craanen ME, Dekker W, Blok P, et al: Time trends in gastric carcinoma: Changing patterns of type and location. *Am J Gastroenterol.* 1992;87:572.
3. Rhode H, Bauer P, Stutzer H, et al: Proximal compared with distal adenocarcinoma of the stomach: Differences and consequences. German Gastric Cancer TNM Study Group. *Br J Surg.* 1991;78:1242.
4. Munoz N, Connelly R: Time trends of intestinal and diffuse types of gastric cancer in the United States. *Int J Cancer.* 1971; 8:158.
5. Noguchi Y, Yoshikawa T, Tsuburaya A, et al: Is gastric carcinoma different between Japan and the United States? A comparison of patient survival among three institutions. *Cancer.* 2000;89:2237.
6. Theuer CP, Kurosaki T, Ziogas A, et al: Asian patients with gastric carcinoma in the United States exhibit unique clinical features and superior overall and cancer specific survival rates. *Cancer.* 2000;89:1883.
7. Jemal A, Murray T, Samuels A, et al: Cancer Statistics, 2003. *CA Cancer J Clin.* 2003;53:5.
8. Chyou PH, Nomura AM, Hankin JH, et al: A case-cohort study of diet and stomach cancer. *Cancer Res.* 1990;50:7501.
9. Demirer T, Icli F, Uzunalimoglu O, et al: Diet and stomach cancer incidence. A case-control study in Turkey. *Cancer.* 1990;65:2344.
10. Mark SD, Qiao YL, Dawsey SM, et al: Prospective study of selenium levels and incident esophageal and gastric cancer. *J Natl Cancer Inst.* 2000;92:1753.
11. Zhang ZF, Kurtz RC, Yu GP, et al: Adenocarcinomas of the esophagus and gastric cardia: The role of diet. *Nutrit Cancer.* 1997; 27:298.
12. Terry P, Lagergren J, Ye W, et al: Inverse association between intake of cereal fiber and risk of gastric cardia cancer. *Gastroenterology.* 2001;120:387.
13. Eslick GD, Lim LL, Byles JE, et al: Association of *Helicobacter pylori* infection with gastric carcinoma: A meta-analysis. *Am J Gastroenterol.* 1999;94:2373.
14. Huang JQ, Subbaramiah S, Chen Y, et al: Meta-analysis of the relationship between *Helicobacter pylori* seropositivity and gastric cancer. *Gastroenterology.* 1998;114:1169.
15. Castro JR, Saunders WM, Tobias CA: Treatment of cancer with heavy charged particles. *Int J Radiat Oncol Biol Phys.* 1982;9:465.
16. Uemura N, Okamoto S, Yamamoto S, et al: *Helicobacter pylori* and the development of gastric cancer. *N Engl J Med.* 2001;345:784.
17. Schrump DS, Altorki N, Forastiere A, Minsky BD: Cancer of the Esophagus. In DeVita VT, Hellman S, Rosenberg SA, eds. *Cancer: Principles and Practice of Oncology.* 6th ed. Philadelphia: Lippincott, Williams & Wilkins; 2001:1051.
18. Wu CW, Chen GD, Jiang KC, et al: A genome-wide study of microsatellite instability in advanced gastric carcinoma. *Cancer.* 2001;92:92.
19. Chun YS, Lindor NM, Smyrk TC, et al: Germline E-cadherin gene mutations. Is a prophylactic total gastrectomy indicated? *Cancer.* 2001;92:181.
20. Ross JS, McKenna BJ: The *HER-2/neu* oncogene in tumors of the gastrointestinal tract. *Cancer Invest.* 2001;19:554.
21. Carpenter JW, Levin E, Clayman LB, et al: Radiation in the therapy of peptic ulcer. *Am J Roentgen.* 1956;75:374.
22. Peters M, Mackay IR, Buckley D: Occurrence of tumors and effects on longevity after limited x-irradiation in man. *Am J Path.* 1980;101:647.
23. Griem ML, Kleinerman RA, Boice JD, et al: Cancer following radiotherapy for peptic ulcer. *J Natl Cancer Inst.* 1994; 86:842.
24. Griem ML, Justman J, Weiss L: The neoplastic potential of gastric irradiation. IV. Risk estimates. *Am J Clin Oncol (CCT).* 1984;7:675.
25. Ming SC: Gastric carcinoma. A pathobiological classification. *Cancer.* 1977;39:2475.
26. Lansdown M, Quirke P, Dixon MF, et al: High grade dysplasia of the gastric mucosa: A marker for gastric carcinoma. *Gut.* 1990;31:977.
27. Nagao F, Takahashi N: Diagnosis of advanced gastric cancer. *World J Surg.* 1979;3:693.
28. Lambert R, Caletti G, Cho E, et al: International workshop on the clinical impact of endoscopic ultrasound in gastroenterology. *Endoscopy.* 2000;32:549.
29. Lightdale CJ: Diagnosis of esophago-gastric tumors. *Endoscopy.* 1992;24:18.
30. Stomach. In Greene FL, Page DL, Fleming ID, et al., eds. *AJCC Cancer Staging Manual.* 6th ed. New York: Springer; 2002:99.
31. Hundahl SA, Phillips JL, Menck HR: The National Cancer Data Base report on poor survival of U.S. patients treated with gastrectomy. Fifth edition American Joint Committee on Cancer staging, proximal disease and the "different disease" hypothesis. *Cancer.* 2000;88:921.
32. Nord HJ, Brady PG, Lightdale CJ, et al: Diagnostic laparoscopy guidelines for clinical application. *Gastrointest Endosc.* 2001;54:818.
33. Gouzi JL, Huguier M, Fagniez PL, et al: Total versus subtotal gastrectomy for adenocarcinoma of the gastric antrum. A French prospective controlled study. *Ann Surg.* 1989;209:162.
34. Lee HK, Yang HK, Kim WH, et al: Influence of the number of lymph nodes examined on staging of gastric cancer. *Br J Surg.* 2001;88:1408.
35. Otsuji E, Toma A, Kobayashi S, et al: Long-term benefit of extended lymphadenectomy with gastrectomy in distally located early gastric carcinoma. *Am J Surg.* 2000;180:127.
36. Bonenkamp JJ, Hermans J, Sasako M, et al: Extended lymph-node dissection for gastric cancer. *N Engl J Med.* 1999;340:908.
37. Cuschieri A, Weeden S, Fielding J, et al: Patient survival after D1 and D2 resections for gastric cancer: Long-term results of the MRC randomized surgical trial. Surgical Co-operative Group. *Br J Cancer.* 2001;79:1522.

38. Roukos DH, Paraschou P, Lorenz M: Distal gastric cancer and extensive surgery: A new evaluation method based on the study of the status of residual lymph nodes after limited surgery. *Ann Surg Oncol.* 2000;7:719.

39. Macdonald JS, Smalley SR, Benedetti J, et al: Chemoradiotherapy after surgery compared with surgery alone for adenocarcinoma of the stomach or gastroesophageal junction. *N Engl J Med.* 2001;345:725.

40. Gianni L, Panzini I, Tassinari D, et al: Meta-analysis of randomized trials of adjuvant chemotherapy in gastric cancer. *Ann Oncol.* 2001;12:1179.

41. Henning GT, Schild SE, Stafford SL, et al: Results of irradiation or chemoirradiation following resection of gastric adenocarcinoma. *Int J Radiat Oncol Biol Phys.* 2000;46:589.

42. Dicker AP, Minsky BD: Stomach. In Leibel S, Phillips T, eds. *Textbook of Radiation Oncology.* 1st ed. Philadelphia: WB Saunders; 1998:624.

43. Kinsella TJ, Bloomer WD: Tolerance of the intestine to radiation therapy. *Surg Gynecol Obstet.* 1980;151:273.

44. Klimberg VS, Souba WW, Dolson DJ, et al: Prophylactic glutamine protects the intestinal mucosa from radiation injury. *Cancer.* 1990;66:62.

45. Coia L, Myerson R, Tepper JE: Late effects of radiation therapy on the gastrointestinal tract. *Int J Radiat Oncol Biol Phys.* 1995;31:1213.

46. Landry J, Tepper JE, Wood WC, et al: Patterns of failure following curative resection of gastric cancer. *Int J Radiat Oncol Biol Phys.* 1990;19:1357.

47. Gunderson LL, Sosin H: Adenocarcinoma of the stomach: Areas of failure in a reoperation series (second or symptomatic looks). Clinicopathologic correlation and implications for adjuvant therapy. *Int J Radiat Oncol Biol Phys.* 1982;8:1.

48. Yoo CH, Noh SH, Shin DW, et al: Recurrence following curative resection for gastric adenocarcinoma. *Br J Surg.* 2000;87:236.

49. Baeza MR, Giannini O, Rivera R, et al: Adjuvant radiochemotherapy in the treatment of completely resected, locally advanced gastric cancer. *Int J Radiat Oncol Biol Phys.* 2001;50:645.

50. Moertel CG, Childs DS, O'Fallon JR, et al: Combined 5-fluorouracil and radiation therapy as a surgical adjuvant for poor prognosis gastric carcinoma. *J Clin Oncol.* 1984;2:1249.

51. Dent DM, Werner ID, Novis B, et al: Prospective randomized trial of combined oncological therapy for gastric carcinoma. *Cancer.* 1979;44:385.

52. Smalley SR, Gunderson L, Tepper JE, et al: Gastric surgical adjuvant radiotherapy consensus report—rationale and treatment implementation. *Int J Radiat Oncol Biol Phys.* 2002;52:283.

53. Zhang ZX, Gu XZ, Yin WB, et al: Randomized clinical trial on the combination of preoperative irradiation and surgery in the treatment of adenocarcinoma of the gastric cardia (AGC)—Report on 370 patients. *Int J Radiat Oncol Biol Phys.* 1998;42:929.

54. Mansfield PF, Lowy AM, Feig BW, et al: Preoperative chemoradiation for potentially resectable gastric cancer. *Proc ASCO.* 2000; 19:246a [abstract].

55. Moertel CG, Childs DS, Reitemeier RJ, et al: Combined 5-fluorouracil and supervoltage radiation therapy of locally unresectable gastrointestinal carcinoma. *Lancet.* 1969;1:865.

56. Safran HS, Akerman P, Cioffi W, et al: Paclitaxel and concurrent radiation therapy for locally advanced adenocarcinomas of the pancreas, stomach, and gastroesophageal junction. *Sem Radiat Oncol.* 1999;53:57.

57. Safran H, Wanebo H, Hesketh PJ, et al: Paclitaxel and concurrent radiation for gastric cancer. *Int J Radiat Oncol Biol Phys.* 2000;46:889.

58. Kelsen D, Ilson D, Lipton R, et al: A phase I trial of radiation therapy (RT) plus concurrent fixed dose cisplatin (C) with escalating doses of paclitaxel (P) as a 96 hour continuous infusion in patients (PTS) with localized esophageal cancer (EC). *Proc ASCO.* 1999;18:271a [abstract].

59. Enzinger P, Ilson D, Minsky B, et al: Phase I/II neoadjuvant concurrent 96 hour taxol, cisplatin, and radiation therapy: Promising toxicity profile and response in localized esophageal cancer. *Proc ASCO.* 1999;18:271a [abstract].

60. Bains MS, Stojadinovic A, Minsky B, et al: A phase II trial of preoperative combined-modality therapy for localized esophageal carcinoma: initial results. *J Thorac Cardiovasc Surg.* 2002;124:270.

61. Sindelar WF, Kinsella TJ: Randomized trial of resection and intraoperative radiotherapy in locally advanced gastric cancer. *Proc ASCO.* 1987;6:91 [abstract].

62. Abe M: Intraoperative radiation therapy for gastric cancer. In Dobelbower RR, Abe M, eds. *Intraoperative Radiation Therapy.* 1st ed. Boca Raton, FL. CRC Press; 1991:166.

63. Takahashi T, Abe M: Intra-operative radiotherapy for carcinoma of the stomach. *Eur J Surg Oncol.* 1986;12:247.

64. Calvo FA, Aristu JJ, Azinovic I, et al: Intraoperative and external radiotherapy in resected gastric cancer: Updated report of a phase II trial. *Int J Radiat Oncol Biol Phys.* 1992;24:729.

65. Avizonis VN, Buzydolski J, Lanciano R, et al: Treatment of adenocarcinoma of the stomach with resection, intraoperative radiotherapy, and adjuvant external beam radiation: A phase II study from Radiation Therapy Oncology Group 85-04. *Ann Surg Oncol.* 1995;2:295.

66. Chen G, Song S: Evaluation of intraoperative radiotherapy for gastric carcinoma—Analysis of 247 patients. In Abe M, Takahashi M, eds. *Intraoperative Radiotherapy.* New York: Pergamon Press; 1991:190.

67. Kramling HT, Willich N, Denecke H, Grab J: Prospective randomized study on IORT for resectable gastric carcinoma. In Abe M, Takahashi M, eds. *Intraoperative Radiotherapy.* New York: Pergammon Press; 1995:192.

68. Glehen O, Braujard AC, Romestaing P, et al: Intraoperative radiotherapy and external beam radiation therapy in gastric adenocarcinoma with R0-R1 surgical resection. *Eur J Surg Oncol.* 2000;26:S10.

69. Coia LR, Engstrom PF, Paul AR, et al: Long-term results of infusional 5-FU, mitomycin-C, and radiation as primary management of esophageal cancer. *Int J Radiat Oncol Biol Phys.* 1991;20:29.

70. Ogata T, Araki K, Matsuura K, et al: A 10-year experience of intraoperative radiotherapy for gastric carcinoma and a new surgical method of creating a wider irradiation field for cases of total gastrectomy patients. *Int J Radiat Oncol Biol Phys.* 1995;32:341.

71. Henning GT, Schild SE, Stafford SL, et al: Results of irradiation or chemoirradiation for primary unresectable, locally recurrent, or grossly incomplete resection of gastric adenocarcinoma. *Int J Radiat Oncol Biol Phys.* 2000;46:109.

72. Falkson G, Van Eden EB, Sandison AG: A controlled clinical trial of fluorouracil plus imidazole carboxamide dimethyl triazene plus vincristine plus bis-chloroethyl plus radiotherapy in stomach cancer. *Med Pediatr Oncol.* 1976;2:111.

73. Klaassen DJ, MacIntyre JM, Catton GE, et al: Treatment of locally unresectable cancer of the stomach and pancreas: A randomized comparison of 5-fluorouracil alone with radiation plus concurrent and maintenance 5-fluorouracil: An Eastern Cooperative Oncology Group study. *J Clin Oncol.* 1985; 3:373.

74. Mantell BS: Radiotherapy for dysphagia due to gastric carcinoma. *Br J Surg.* 1982;69:69.

75. Rhomberg W, Bohler F, Eiter H, et al: Radiotherapy and razoxane in the palliative treatment of gastric cancer. *Radiat Oncol Invest.* 1996;4:27.

76. Allum W, Hallissey MT, Ward LC, et al: A controlled, prospective randomized trial of adjuvant chemotherapy or radiotherapy in resectable gastric cancer: Interim report. *Br J Cancer.* 1989;60:739.

77. Hallissey MT, Dunn JA, Ward LC, et al: The second British Stomach Cancer Group trial of adjuvant radiotherapy or chemotherapy in resectable gastric cancer: Five-year follow-up. *Lancet.* 1994;343:1309.

78. Schein PS, Smith FP, Woolley PV, et al: Current management of advanced and locally unresectable gastric carcinoma. *Cancer.* 1982;50:2590.

79. Gastrointestinal Tumor Study Group: The concept of locally advanced gastric cancer. Effect of treatment on outcome. *Cancer.* 1990;66:2324.

80. Safran H, Wanebo H, Hesketh PJ, et al: Paclitaxel and concurrent radiation for locally advanced gastric cancer. *Proc ASCO.* 1999;18:273a [abstract].

38

Cancer of the Pancreas

Patricia Lillis-Hearne, MD

EPIDEMIOLOGY, ETIOLOGY, GENETICS AND CYTOGENETIC ABNORMALITIES

Pancreatic cancer is the fifth leading cause of cancer mortality among men and women of all ages; it will strike an estimated 26,300 Americans and caused 28,900 deaths in 2002.[1] A National Cancer Institute (NCI) survey covering 1973 to 1988 showed less than 20% of affected patients survived 1 year and only 3% were alive 5 years after diagnosis.[2,3] Even with the addition of adjuvant radiation and chemotherapy, as well as recent decreases in surgical morbidity, only very modest improvements in survival have been realized. Worldwide, the reported incidence varies considerably. It is unclear whether this represents a true phenomenon or whether it is a reflection of more meticulous reporting patterns in more industrialized countries. In the United States, the incidence of pancreatic cancer is 9 per 100,000 in whites and 15.2/100,000 in blacks with a male-to-female ratio of 1.3:1. Diagnosis is rare before age 45 but rises sharply thereafter.[2] Although the cause of pancreatic cancer is unknown, several environmental factors have been implicated. Smoking, in particular, raises the relative risk 1.5 times.[4] Diets high in meat or fat have also been linked to increased risk, and a diet of fresh fruits and vegetables has been found to be protective.[5] An increased incidence is also found with a prior history of surgery for peptic ulcer disease.[6]

Much controversy was generated in the early 1980s with a report linking pancreatic cancer with coffee consumption,[7] but subsequent prospective studies have failed to confirm this.[8] Both diabetes mellitus[7,9] and chronic pancreatitis[10] are associated with pancreatic cancer, but it is unclear whether this is a cause and effect relationship. Workers employed in manufacturing 2-naphthylamine, benzidine,[11] and gasoline[12] are reported to have a fivefold increased risk. More recently, the study of DNA content, oncogenes, and molecular biology has yielded intriguing data.[13] Molecular histology data has been nicely summarized by Hruban.[14] More and more evidence paints a picture of pancreatic cancer as a disease of acquired and inherited mutations. Tumor suppressor genes regulate cell proliferation and their inactivation can play a profound role in the development of malignancies. There are four specific genes identified as crucial in the development of pancreatic cancer: *p16*, *p53*, *DPC4*, and *BRAC-2*. Oncogenes become active by mutation or amputation. An example is the k-*ras* oncogene, which is often activated in human pancreatic duct carcinomas.[15-19] Data from

Almoguera and colleagues demonstrated that 95% of pancreatic adenocarcinomas contain k-*ras* oncogenes activated by a mutation at codon 12. This mutation is critical to oncogenesis. Shibata and associates noted similar findings in 72% of patients undergoing fine needle aspiration.[16] Kondo and colleagues also found specific mutations of the k-*ras* oncogene at codon 12 in 67% of pure pancreatic juice collected endoscopically in patients with proven pancreatic carcinoma.[20] K-*ras* abnormalities were not detected in healthy controls, patients with chronic pancreatitis, or in three patients with islet cell tumors.[13]

Additionally, mutations can occur in DNA mismatch repair genes. These genes would normally code for proteins that correct errors normally occurring during DNA replication. A summary of genetic abnormalities is provided in Table 38-1. The identification of consistent genetic abnormalities and the observation of higher cancer rates in some families is the genesis of the National Familial Pancreatic Tumor Registry (NFPTR). Familial cases are defined as those in which two or more first-degree relatives are affected. In these individuals the risk extends to second-degree relatives who have a 3.7% chance of developing pancreatic cancer as opposed to .6% in second-degree relatives of sporadic cases.[21]

ANATOMY

The pancreas is an elongated, coarsely lobulated gland lying transversely and retroperitoneally in the posterior abdomen at approximately the L1 to L2 level (Fig. 38-1A). The head lies in the duodenal flexure on the right and the tail extends to the spleen. It is divided into head, uncinate process (considered to be part of the head), neck, body, and tail. Tumors arising to the right of the superior mesenteric vein are considered to be in the head, those

Table 38–1   Genetic Abnormalities in Pancreatic Cancer

Inactivated/ Suppressor Genes	Chromosome	Frequency Seen, %
p53	17p	50–70
p16	9p	95
MKK4	17p	<10
DPC4	18q	50
BRCA2	13q	70

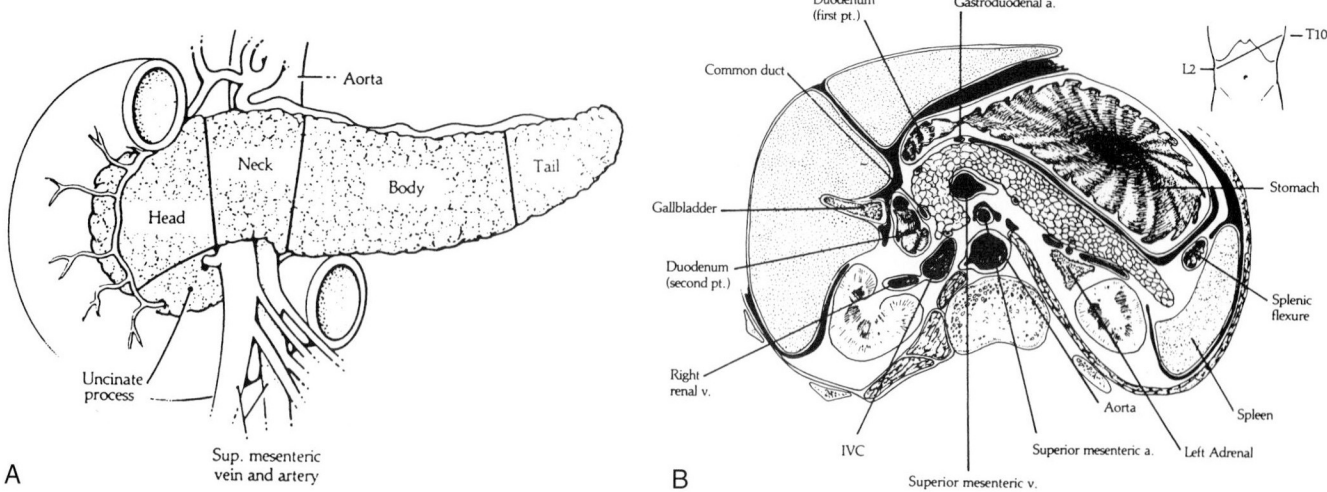

Figure 38–1. A, The five parts of the pancreas in relation to the duodenum and major vessels. The line dividing the body and tail is arbitrary. **B,** Oblique transverse cross section of the upper abdomen along the long axis of the pancreas corresponding approximately to the levels indicated on the inset diagram. In this view relationships of the pancreas to surrounding dose-limiting structures is quite evident. a, artery; IVC, inferior vena cava; pt, part; v, vein.

arising to the left of that vein and left border of the aorta are part of the body, and those arising from the tail are located between the left border of the aorta and the hilum of the spleen. The pancreas is in close contact with surrounding organs including the spleen, stomach, duodenum, jejunum, and kidneys, all of which may all be involved with tumor early on (Fig. 38-1*B*). A rich lymphatic network surrounds the pancreas, including the celiac, superior and inferior pancreaticoduodenal, superior mesenteric, porta hepatis, and pancreaticosplenic nodes (Fig. 38-2*A*). With posterior extension of tumor, the lateral aortic nodes are also at risk. The main venous drainage of the pancreas is via the portal system to the liver. Tumors of the head of the pancreas often cause jaundice due to invasion or compression of the common bile duct.

PATHOLOGY

The most common type of pancreatic cancer is of ductal origin, comprising from 75% to 90% of patients.[22] It is twice as common in the head as in the body or tail. Perineural invasion occurs in approximately 90% of patients, and in more than 85% of patients tumor has extended beyond the organ at the time of diagnosis. The most common extralymphatic sites of involvement are the liver and peritoneum; the lung is the most commonly involved extra-abdominal organ.

Less frequently occurring exocrine tumors such as cystadenocarcinoma or intraductal carcinoma are more common in women and may run a much more indolent course,[23,24] remaining localized for many years and having

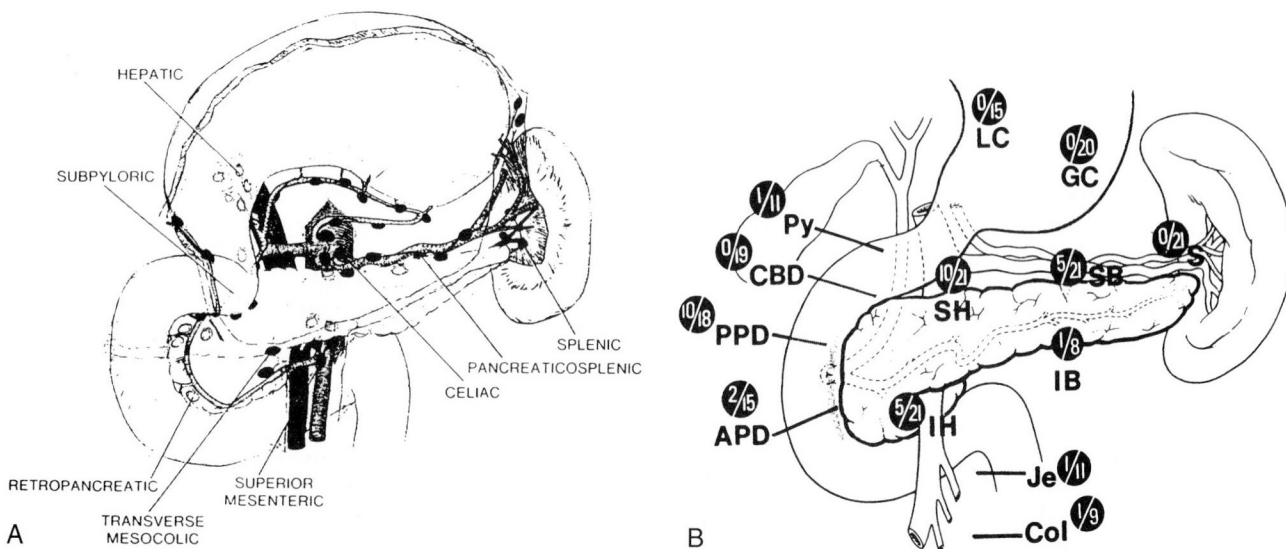

Figure 38–2. A, Lymphatic drainage of the pancreas. Labels indicate representative lymph nodes in the major regional nodal groups. **B,** Lymph node group involvement in 21 patients with duct cancer in the head of the pancreas. APD, anterior pancreaticoduodenal node; CBD, common bile duct; Col, midcolic node; GC, greater curvature; IB, inferior body; IH, inferior head; Je, jejunal node; LC, lesser curvature; PPD, posterior pancreaticoduodenal node; PY, pyloric node; S, splenic node; SB, superior body; SH, superior head. (From Cubilla A, Fortner J, Fitzgerald P: Lymph node involvement in carcinoma of the head of the pancreas. *Cancer.* 1978;41:880. ©1978 American Cancer Society. Reprinted by permission of Wiley-Liss, Inc., a subsidiary of John Wiley & Sons, Inc.)

up to a 50% five-year survival rate.[25] Solid and cystic papillary neoplasms, also known as *Hamoudi tumors*, occur in women in their third decade of life, only rarely metastasize, and have a good prognosis. Acinar cell cancers are rare, associated with fat necrosis and high lipase production, and have a poor prognosis. They may be associated with a clinical picture that includes rash, eosinophilia, and polyarthralgia. Giant cell tumors, which account for only a slight percent of pancreatic cancers, are very large and aggressive and have a very poor survival.[26] Clinical presentation of these less aggressive histologies, however, is indistinguishable from the more aggressive pathologic subtypes.[23] The expression of mucin core protein and mucin carbohydrate appears to correlate with biologic behavior.[27] Several investigators have shown aggressive tumor behavior[28] and particularly poor survival in patients with aneuploid tumors,[29-31] suggesting that ploidy may be an independent prognostic factor.[32] Recent advances in identifying genetic abnormalities in a high percentage of pancreatic cancers can be used to help characterize ambiguous lesions. Cancer metastatic to the pancreas is a relatively uncommon finding. In a series of 2587 consecutive autopsies at the Memorial Sloan-Kettering Cancer Center, 10% of patients were found to have metastases in the pancreas with the most frequent primary sites being breast, lung, or melanoma.[22] The remaining 5% of pancreatic cancers are of endocrine origin and are discussed separately.

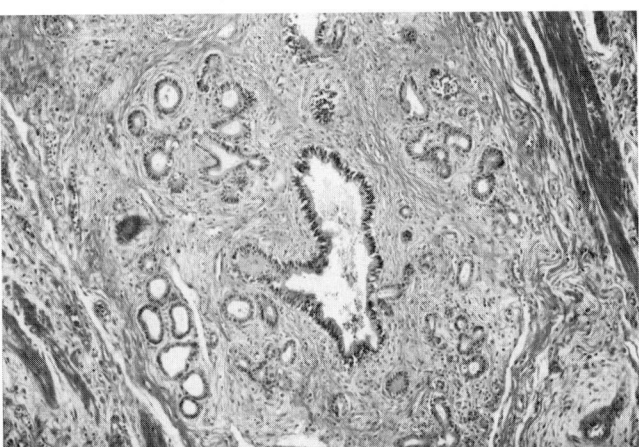

Figure 38–3. Pancreatic adenocarcinoma and dense fibrosis surrounding central pancreatic duct. Hematoxylin and eosin stain; ×16.

may be exceedingly common. A series from Massachusetts General Hospital (MGH) reports a 40% incidence of peritoneal studding in patients clinically felt to be resectable who first underwent laparoscopy before definitive resection.[39] In a patient who has undergone curative therapy, once the therapy fails, local recurrence again dominates the clinical picture.[40,41] In a series of Griffen and associates, only 17% of patients developed disease purely outside the abdominal cavity (Fig. 38-3).

CLINICAL PRESENTATION

More than 80% of patients present with pain, jaundice, or both[33,34]; these symptoms, along with weight loss, constitute a classic triad. Tumors in the body and tail may not cause jaundice or pain until far advanced and thus their prognosis is particularly poor,[35] whereas ampullary cancers have a significantly better prognosis[36] because of earlier clinical presentation. Tumors of the endocrine pancreas may present in a similar fashion but are often recognized due to various clinical syndromes produced by circulating polypeptides elaborated by the tumor.[37] Rarely, presenting symptoms may be diabetes mellitus[9] or acute pancreatitis.[10] Infrequently, patients may present with migratory thrombophlebitis (Trousseau's sign) or with a palpable gallbladder (Courvoisier's sign). Abnormal laboratory tests such as alteration in glucose, amylase, lipase, bilirubin, alkaline phosphatase, lactate dehydrogenase (LDH), or aspartate aminotransferase may all be present but are all also nonspecific.

ROUTES OF SPREAD

Most pancreatic cancers are unresectable at presentation and thus there is sparse literature systematically analyzing patterns of failure. Cubilla and associates[38] reported on the incidence of nodal involvement in completely resected early cancers of the head of the pancreas (Fig. 38-2B), showing that carcinomas in the head tended to spread to multiple nodal groups. In addition to initial spread to regional lymph nodes, early peritoneal seeding

DIAGNOSTIC AND STAGING STUDIES

Preoperative staging of pancreatic cancer to detect resectability is extremely important to avoid unnecessary surgery. Table 38-2 reflects the staging system as revised in January 2003, with the T staging distinguishing between potentially resectable (T3) and unresectable (T4) primary tumors. The stage grouping has also been changed to allow stage III to signify unresectable, locally advanced pancreatic cancer, while stage IV is reserved for patients with metastatic disease. Pancreatic cancer is considered resectable if there is no portal vein or celiac axis involvement and no metastasis evident. Splenic vein involvement does not necessarily preclude resection. Both ultrasound and computed tomography (CT) (Fig. 38-4)

Table 38–2   Evaluation of Pancreatic Mass

History and Physical Laboratory
Complete blood count
Serum chemistries
Lipase/Amylase
Liver functions
Carcinoembryonic antigen
Cancer antigen

Imaging/Diagnosis
Upper gastrointestinal
Computed tomography scan
Ultrasound
ERCP/Biopsy
Arteriogram
Laparoscopy (if no prior surgery)/Biopsy

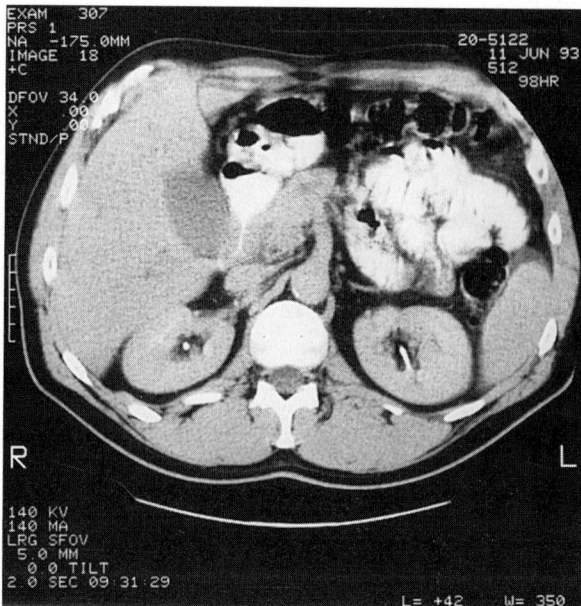

Figure 38–4. Computed tomographic scan showing large pancreatic mass; thin strip of barium indicates near-total duodenal obstruction. This underscores the need to have the treatment field cover the entire duodenal circumference in masses involving the pancreatic head. Note also that a significant volume of the right kidney would be in a field with an anterior-posterior–posterior-anterior arrangement.

can detect pancreatic cancers as small as 2 cm. Both modalities easily detect dilatation of the pancreatic and bile ducts as well as liver metastases.[42] Ultrasound can help distinguish between obstructive and nonobstructive jaundice, but CT is more helpful in providing definition of the tumor and surrounding structures. Magnetic resonance imaging (MRI) at this time offers no advantage over CT.[43,44] However, this is a rapidly changing area of diagnostic radiology, and it is very likely that in the future it may play a larger role in detecting smaller

tumors and vascular involvement. Currently, vascular involvement is most frequently assessed by angiography, though the use of endoscopic ultrasonography (EUS) to assess vessel involvement has been increasing. In skilled hands, EUS images are more sensitive in detecting small tumors (>90%) and in detecting tumor extending into blood vessels. EUS is especially useful in evaluating the portal system. Enlarged lymph nodes are easily seen, though it is not possible to determine whether they are reactive or malignant without a biopsy.[45-48] Percutaneous ultrasound or CT-guided biopsy can safely and easily provide pathologic diagnosis in approximately 90% of cases,[49] but in the case of adenocarcinoma it may cause increased risk of local failure secondary to rapid seeding of tumor.[50] A review from MGH[51] showed a fourfold increased risk of positive peritoneal cytology in patients with prior percutaneous fine needle aspirates. Some institutions thus advocate deferring preoperative biopsy in apparently resectable cases.[52] Older literature suggested a benefit from treating patients already biopsied with low dose (5 to 10 Gy) preopera-tive radiation in an attempt to decrease dissemination of tumor.[53] This is now very rarely done and would not be considered standard of care. Endoscopic retrograde cholangiopancreatography (ERCP) is extremely useful in the differential diagnosis of tumors of the pancreaticobiliary junction (Fig. 38-5). Ampullary and duodenal cancers can be visualized and biopsied during ERCP; pancreatic duct stricture longer than 10 mm, especially if irregular, is more consistent with carcinoma than pancreatitis.[54] Newer, less available imaging methods include nuclear medicine studies using SPECT[55] or radiolabeled antibodies.[56] Supportive serologic evidence of pancreatic cancer includes elevated levels of CA 19-9,[57] elevated levels of carcinoembryonic antigen (CEA), serum elastase, and DU-PAN-2, or low ratio of testosterone to dihydrotestosterone. Unfortunately, no currently available marker is diagnostic or sufficiently sensitive or specific for screening purposes.[58] Following

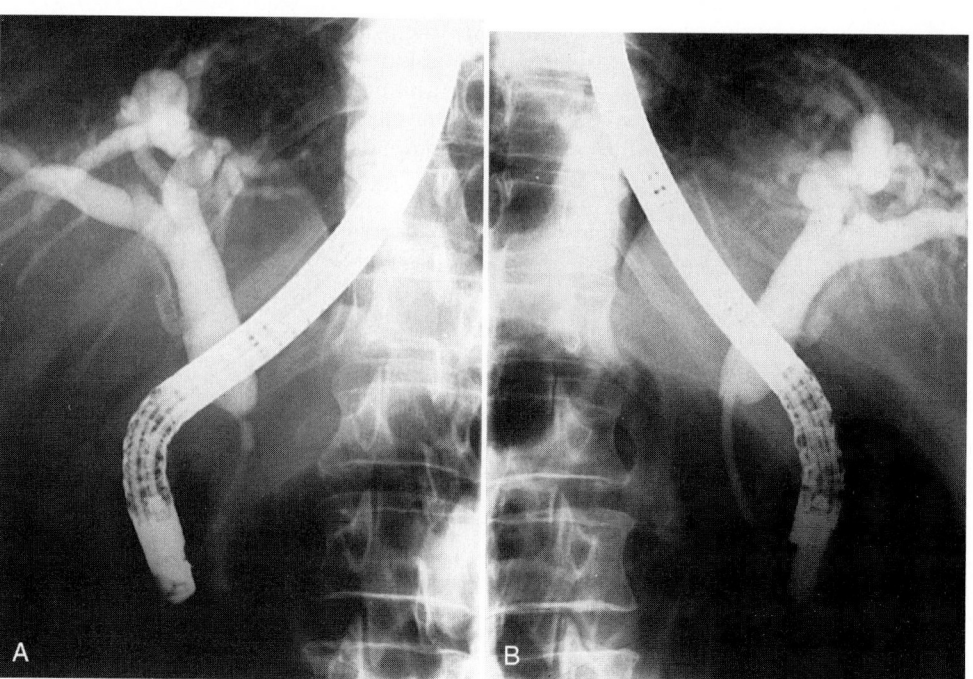

Figure 38–5. Endoscopic retrograde cholangiopancreatography of the same patient shown in Figure 38-4. **A,** Note thin ragged contour of the pancreatic duct—stenosis of the length (see text) is usually indicative of neoplasm. **B,** A stent has successfully been placed in the pancreatic duct to relieve obstructive jaundice.

serial levels of these markers, however, is very useful, and baseline and post-treatment levels of CA 19-9 do correlate with tumor response.[59]

As part of a preoperative staging evaluation, tumors that are apparently localized by ultrasound and dynamic CT are further evaluated by either EUS or angiography since major vascular involvement usually precludes resection. Following this, laparoscopy may be used in patients without prior abdominal surgery to rule out small hepatic or peritoneal metastasis. Investigators at MGH prospectively evaluated 88 patients referred for curative resection using MRI/CT, angiography, and laparoscopy for staging. They identified preoperatively 89% of patients who could not have curative resection. These patients are best spared an operation unless duodenal obstruction is present.[51] Excellent palliation for jaundice can be achieved with endoscopic placement of large stents.[60] Diagnostic workup and TNM staging are outlined in Tables 38-2 and 38-3.

THERAPEUTIC APPROACHES

Options for treating any malignancy include surgery, radiation, and chemotherapy, either singly, sequentially, or in combination. The overall disappointing outcomes in

Table 38–3   Classification of Tumors of the Pancreas

Primary Tumor (T)

TX	Primary tumor cannot be assessed
T0	No evidence of primary tumor
Tis	Carcinoma in situ (This also includes the "PanInIII" classification)
T1	Tumor limited to the pancreas ≤2 cm in greatest dimension
T2	Tumor limited to the pancreas ≥2 cm in greatest dimension
T3	Tumor extends beyond the pancreas, but without involvement of the celiac axis or the superior mesenteric artery
T4	Tumor involves the celiac axis or the superior mesenteric artery (unresectable primary tumor)

Regional Lymph Nodes (N)

NX	Regional lymph nodes cannot be assessed
N0	No regional lymph node metastasis
N1	Regional lymph node metastasis

Distant Metastasis (M)

MX	Distant metastasis cannot be assessed
M0	No distant metastasis
M1	Distant metastasis

Stage Grouping

0	Tis	N0	M0
IA	T1	N0	M0
IB	T2	N0	M0
IIA	T3	N0	M0
IIB	T1	N1	M0
	T2	N1	M0
	T3	N1	M0
III	T4	Any N	M0
IV	Any T	Any N	M1

From Greene FL, Page DL, Fleming ID, et al, eds: *AJCC Cancer Staging Manual*, 6th ed. New York: Springer, 2002.

the treatment of pancreatic cancer have involved all modalities in every order and combination possible. The standard therapeutic approach to pancreatic carcinoma has been surgical and the standard operation for cancers in the pancreatic head has been the pancreaticoduodenectomy or Whipple procedure. During the classic Whipple operation, the gall bladder, distal stomach, and duodenum, the first portion of the jejunum, and the head and portion of the body of the pancreas are resected en bloc. The bile duct is anastomosed to the jejunal remnant, as is the pancreatic remnant. A gastrojejunostomy is then performed along with a vagotomy to prevent upper gastrointestinal hemorrhage, a potentially significant postoperative complication. Total pancreatectomy has been advocated by some as a better operation because it removes more potentially involved tissue and because it avoids a pancreaticojejunal anastomosis, which is the source of significant surgical morbidity and mortality. However, it does result in exocrine insufficiency and brittle diabetes that is difficult to manage,[61] and it confers no survival advantage. Fortner[62] advocates a regional pancreatectomy, which is an en bloc resection of the pancreas and surrounding tissue along with a segment of the mesenteric-portal vein and occasionally major arterial segments. This operation is less frequently performed in the United States because of high operative mortality (8% in Fortner's series) and no clear evidence of survival benefit. Some groups in Japan combine the Whipple procedure with extensive lymph node dissection, claiming better results with no apparent increase in operative mortality.[63] The opposite approach has been taken by several groups in the United States[64,65] that feel there is no compromise of survival when preserving the pylorus in an attempt to avoid postgastrectomy symptoms. In the 1960s and '70s, the pancreaticoduodenectomy was associated with a 20% to 25% in-hospital mortality rate.[66] By the 1980s and '90s, surgical techniques and supportive care improved to the point where this operation now carries only a 1% to 3% mortality rate in major centers.[67] With certainty, the pylorus-preserving pancreaticoduodenectomy improves gastrointestinal function and does not appear to compromise further management. The dramatic improvements in surgical techniques have made it possible to conduct a prospective randomized trial with intraoperative randomization between a standard operation and one with extended retroperitoneal lymph node dissection. This is currently ongoing. What is clear from the surgical literature is that if tumor is knowingly left behind, survival postresection is not much better than after bypass alone.[58] This has led to the question of appropriate surgical management of patients with positive lymph nodes at frozen section. Yeo and colleagues[67] have shown that long-term survival out to 5 years is possible in both lymph node-positive and -negative tumors as long as the patient is otherwise technically suitable for resection. An additional important question answered recently involves determination of the best management of the elderly patient. Sohn and colleagues,[68] as well as Magistrelli and colleagues[69] clearly showed that it is appropriate to perform aggressive surgery in appropriately selected patients into their seventh and eighth decades of life. Several other important points from the surgical literature are worth noting. These involve the importance of both a multidisciplinary approach as well as the importance of an experienced team. The importance of an experienced team is further underscored by series from Robinson et al.[70] and from Sohn et al.[71] at two different institutions, showing the benefit of reoperation at an experienced center: 67% of patients, many deemed unresectable elsewhere, were in fact successfully resected without compromise of their overall outcome. Other series have clearly shown the benefit of decreased in-hospital morbidity and mortality rates as well as survival in those centers with a high volume of cases.[72]

Multiple large series have shown that only 5% to 30% of patients have resectable tumors.[63,73-75] Remaining patients require some form of palliation for pain, duodenal obstruction, or jaundice. Many surgeons feel that a Whipple procedure offers the best palliation,[73,76] while others advocate this procedure only when duodenal obstruction is present.[52] Obstructive jaundice can be relieved percutaneously (albeit with complications up to 35% in some series[58] or with stents that have a >85% success rate and procedure-related mortality of only 1% to 2%.[77] This represents a significant improvement over surgical morbidity. Two randomized trials[78,79] have shown equal survival with both surgical bypass and endoscopic stent placement. In addition to analgesics, percutaneous neurolysis of the celiac ganglion and radiation therapy offer good palliation of pain.

In addition to various surgical approaches, many other avenues have been pursued to improve the outcome for patients with pancreatic cancer. These include not only chemotherapy and pre- and postoperative external beam radiation, but also intraoperative radiation therapy (IORT), brachytherapy with I-125 and Au-198 or Pd-103, and treatment with heavy particles.

Preoperative radiation therapy has been used infrequently. Its goal is improving resectability rates in patients judged to be unresectable. The desire to better tailor the treatment to the patient and to deliver higher radiation doses with concurrent chemotherapy had generally resulted in a shift away from this approach. Renewed interest in neoadjuvant chemotherapy, however, has been awakened with improved outcomes in surgical series.[80,81]

The most common current treatment approach in patients deemed clinically suitable is postoperative radiation with concurrent chemotherapy (Table 38-4). The most commonly used and most effective agent is 5-fluorouracil (5-FU). Retrospective and prospective randomized studies have shown that 5-FU has proven benefit in the adjuvant setting as well as in patients with localized but unresectable tumors. Doses of 5-FU have typically been in the range of 500 mg/m² when given with concurrent radiation. The optimal regimen of chemotherapy has yet to be determined; thus, most clinicians recommend the Gastrointestinal Study Group (GITSG)

Table 38–4 Prospective Randomized Trials of External Beam Radiation Therapy and Chemotherapy

	Reference	Patients, *n*	Median Survival	Local Control, %	2-Yr Survival, %
Resectable					
GITSG*					
Surgery	Kalser & Ellenberg,[83]	22	10.9 mo	—	18
Surgery + EBRT (40 Gy) + 5-FU	GITSG[84]	21	21.0 mo	—	43
Surgery + EBRT (40 Gy) + 5-FU		30	18 mo	—	46
NCI†					
Surgery + EBRT (50 Gy)	Sindelar & Kinsella[122]	16	12 mo	0	
Surgery + IORT (20 Gy)		16	12 mo	80	—
Unresectable					
ECOG					
5-FU	Klaasen et al[147]	44	8.2 mo	32	—
EBRT + 5-FU		47	8.3 mo	32	—
GITSG					
EBRT (60 Gy)	Moertel et al[137]	25	22.9 wk	24	9
EBRT (40 Gy) + 5-FU		83	42.2 wk	26	10
EBRT (60 Gy) + 5-FU		86	40.3 wk	27	10
GITSG					
EBRT (60 Gy) + 5-FU	GITSG‡	73	8.4 mo	58	12
EBRT (60 Gy) + Adriamycin		70	7.5 mo	51	6
GITSG					
EBRT (54 Gy) + 5-FU + SMF	GITSG[82]	22	42 wk	10/22	41 (1-yr)
SMF only		21	32 wk	10/21	19 (1-yr)
MAYO					
EBRT (35–40 Gy)	Moertel et al§	32	6.3 mo	—	—
EBRT (35–40 Gy) + 5-FU		32	10.4 mo	—	—

*Randomized. Registered after closure of surgery-alone arm.
†Stage I control patients received surgery only; all stages received IORT; no patients given chemotherapy.
‡From Gastrointestinal Tumor Study Group: Radiation therapy combined with adriamycin or 5-fluorouracil for the treatment of locally unresectable gastrointestinal pancreatic cancer. *Cancer.* 1985;56:2563.
§From Moertel CG, Childs DS, Reitemeier RJ, et al: Combined 5-fluorouracil and supervoltage radiation therapy of locally unresectable gastrointestinal cancer. *Lancet.* 1969;2:865.
EBRT, external beam radiation therapy; ECOG, Eastern Cooperative Oncology Group; 5-FU, 5-fluorouracil; GITSG, Gastrointestinal Tumor Study Group; IORT, intraoperative radiation therapy; MAYO, Mayo Clinic; NCI, National Cancer Institute; SMF, streptozocin, mitomycin C, 5-fluorouracil.

regimen that demonstrated superiority of chemoradiotherapy over chemotherapy alone.[82] Gemcitabine, a relatively new chemotherapeutic agent, has shown significant promise, but dosing, timing, and sequencing are still under investigation, precluding recommendation of a standard regimen for treatment off protocol.

The major difficulty in treatment of pancreatic cancer is not the radioresistance of the tumor but radiation dose limitations imposed by surrounding normal organs (see Fig. 38-1B) and the frequent presence of distant metastases. Attempts to overcome this problem have included using intraoperative electrons or implantation of the tumor either directly or percutaneously. Obviously, the advantage offered by IORT is precise field localization and the abilities to shield sensitive normal structures and to deliver a relatively high dose quickly. High dose rate brachytherapy has the advantages of reduced radiation exposure to medical personnel and the potential to overcome limitations of attempting to control tumors with a relatively fast doubling time with a low dose rate source.

Discouraging survival statistics, a 50% to 76%[40,41] locoregional failure even after "curative" resection, and the proven survival benefit of adjuvant treatment[83,84] make postoperative radiation with concurrent chemotherapy justifiable in virtually all patients who have had a potentially curative resection of pancreatic cancer. Patients with localized but unresectable cancer can expect doubling of survival with external beam radiation therapy (EBRT) and concurrent 5-FU.[82,85,86] They should be offered treatment unless poor clinical status precludes treatment.

SIMULATION

With the use of multiple fields and high energy photons, doses of up to 60 to 65 Gy can be delivered safely.[87] The addition of chemotherapy requires dose reductions to 50.4 Gy to avoid excessive toxicity.

In patients undergoing an operation, the surgeon should outline the tumor with small vascular clips. If used sparingly, CT artifacts are not significant. Titanium clips produce less interference on CT, but they are often not seen on standard x-ray films. The target volume, which includes the tumor and nodal groups at risk, is further delineated by information obtained on pre- and postoperative CT, preoperative barium studies, ERCP, angiography, ultrasound, and the findings at operation. It is particularly important that the radiation oncologist understand *which surgical procedure was performed* so that this information can be incorporated into treatment planning. Given the overall poor outcome in patients with pancreatic cancer, one may intuitively question the efficacy of prophylactic treatment of nodal groups in patients with gross disease. This issue has never been addressed in a formal or prospective fashion, but findings of long-term survivors as well as demonstrated clinical tolerance of these fields currently supports this practice in any patient treated with curative intent.

The patient is placed in the supine position with arms comfortably on the upper chest or above the head. Renal contrast is given and an initial anterior-posterior (AP) and lateral films are taken to establish the position of the

kidneys. Subsequently oral contrast is given to visualize the stomach and duodenal C-loop, which will localize the position of the head of the pancreas in those patients who have not undergone a Whipple procedure.

Anterior-Posterior–Posterior-Anterior Field: Lateral Borders

For lesions of the head of the pancreas, nodal groups to be treated include the pancreaticoduodenal, suprapancreatic, celiac nodes and those in the porta hepatis. Lesions in the head of the pancreas frequently invade the medial wall of the duodenum, and therefore the entire duodenal loop should be covered for lesions in this location. In the direction of the pancreatic body the treatment volume should extend with a 2 to 3 cm margin beyond gross disease. Care must be taken to keep doses within renal tolerance: often more than 50% of the right kidney is within the field, and thus for lesions of the pancreatic head at least two thirds of the left kidney should be excluded from the anterior-posterior–posterior-anterior (AP–PA) portion of the treatment field. The risk of nodal involvement in this area when the primary tumor is located in the pancreatic head is quite low (see Fig. 38-2B).[38] The risk of renal injury is very low if half of the renal mass receives no more than 18 Gy.[53]

For lesions in the pancreatic body or tail, the target volume includes the tumor with a 2 to 3 cm margin, pancreaticoduodenal, and porta hepatis nodes, lateral suprapancreatic nodes, and nodes of the splenic hilum. It is not necessary to include the whole duodenal loop in the treatment field, and thus most of the right kidney can be spared. Often 50% of the left kidney is in the field when the more lateral nodes are covered (Fig. 38-6).

Anterior-Posterior–Posterior-Anterior Field: Superior and Inferior Borders

Kao and colleagues[88] demonstrated significant variability in the location of the celiac axis and superior mesenteric nodes (Fig 38-7), which emphasizes the need for individualized treatment planning when attempting to cover nodal groups associated with these vessels. For pancreatic head lesions to ensure adequate coverage on the celiac nodes, the superior border should be at the T10/T11 level and the lower border at the L3/L4 level, depending on the preoperative staging studies. Guidelines are identical for lesions of the body and tail, although occasionally the superior margin is higher because of the location of the primary tumor.

Lateral Field Borders

Superior and inferior margins remain the same. Care must be taken to be aware of the location of the kidneys and to take this into account when assigning weighting to the lateral fields. The anterior margin is placed 1.5 to 2 cm beyond gross disease as defined on preoperative CT scan. For the posterior margin, the spinal cord is blocked,

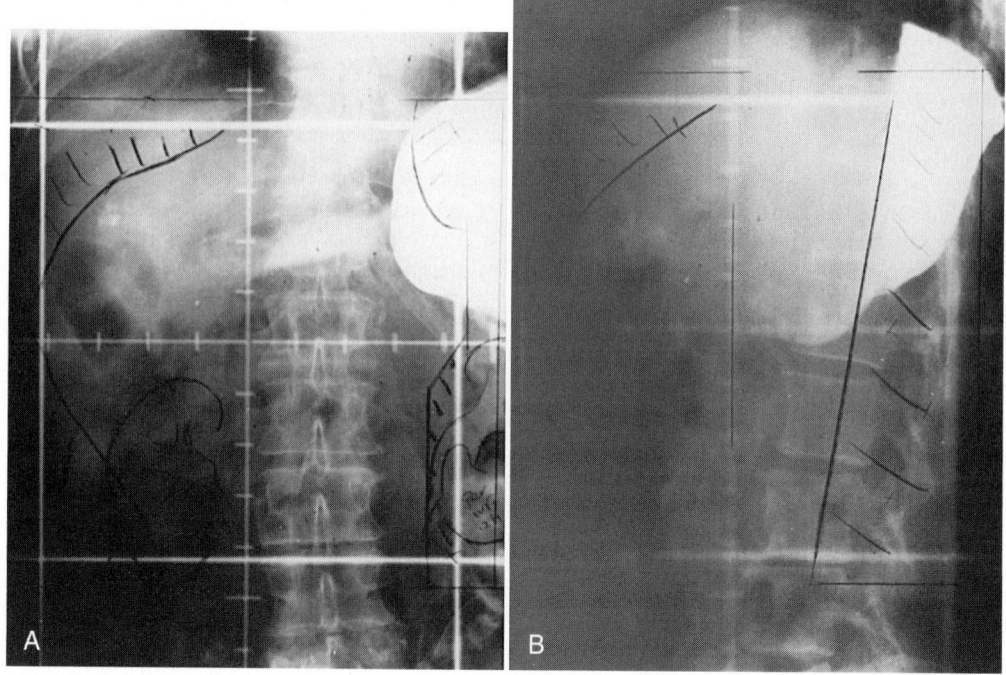

Figure 38–6. A and **B,** Simulation films of the patient shown in Figure 38-4. See text for discussion. Care is taken to include all relevant at-risk regional nodes and to spare as much of one kidney as possible. On the lateral fields, a block should be placed to shield the spinal cord but not block at-risk para-aortic lymph nodes.

but at least 1.5 to 2.0 cm of the anterior portion of the vertebral body is in the field. This is to allow margin on the para-aortic nodes, which are at risk from posterior extension of tumor.

The lateral field contribution is usually limited to 15 to 18 Gy due to inclusion of a large portion of the kidney and liver in the AP–PA fields. If treating to high doses without chemotherapy, field reduction should be made at 50.4 Gy to help diminish the probability of injury to the stomach and small bowel. Otherwise, field reductions should be made at 45 Gy. Boost fields typically dose an additional 9 Gy.

Significantly larger fields encompassing the liver have been studied by some[89] but are not considered to be standard.

New treatment planning software has made possible three-dimensional conformal radiation therapy (3D-CRT) based on CT scanning data (Fig. 38-8). It is possible to determine complete anatomic and dose information for the entire tumor volume and surrounding normal tissues (Fig. 38-9A, B). An approach using tight conformal fields tailored individually to each patient is highly desired when treating aggressively with the newer chemotherapeutic agents that have higher toxicity than 5-FU. Construction of dose-volume histograms shows the volume of normal tissue in the treatment field (Fig. 38-9C). Use of this information to assess the probability of normal tissue complications is under active investigation. The initial simulation is accomplished as described earlier with the patient placed in an immobilization device such as an alpha-cradle. The patient is then CT scanned in the immobilized treatment position on a flat CT tabletop with the CT alignment lasers positioned on the patient's skin marks so that the simulation position can be exactly duplicated. Alternately, a dedicated CT simulator may be used. CT slices are

obtained at 3 to 5 mm intervals. The clinician then outlines the target volume on each CT slice, which includes tumor, areas at risk for microscopic involvement, and an additional 10 mm margin to allow for setup error and patient motion. Other critical organs such as the kidneys and spinal cord are also contoured, and these as well as the target volume and bony landmarks are reconstructed in three dimensions and can be displayed using a beam's eye view (BEV) technique. Beam shaping is then accomplished in this mode, ensuring adequate coverage of the target volume with minimal inclusion of normal tissue. Once the optimal beam arrangement has been determined, the CT image set is used to generate a BEV template at the same magnification as the initial simulation film for each treatment field. Often the isocenter may have been moved during the treatment planning process. At verification the patient is set up again with the initial parameters and changes are then made as determined by the 3D plan. The new BEV template established by the 3D plan is overlaid onto the verification simulation films (obtained for each field). The template can then be used to fabricate custom blocks (Fig. 38-10).

INTRAOPERATIVE RADIATION THERAPY

Preoperative CT is used to do the initial planning with regard to required cone sizes, shapes, and angulations that will be needed. Anticipated electron energy is also determined. Malleable lead shields thick enough to reduce the electron dose by 90% are sterilized. These will be used as secondary collimation to block normal structures within the treatment field. At the time of surgery, maximal exposure of the tumor should be obtained, and the tumor bed should be outlined by surgical metallic

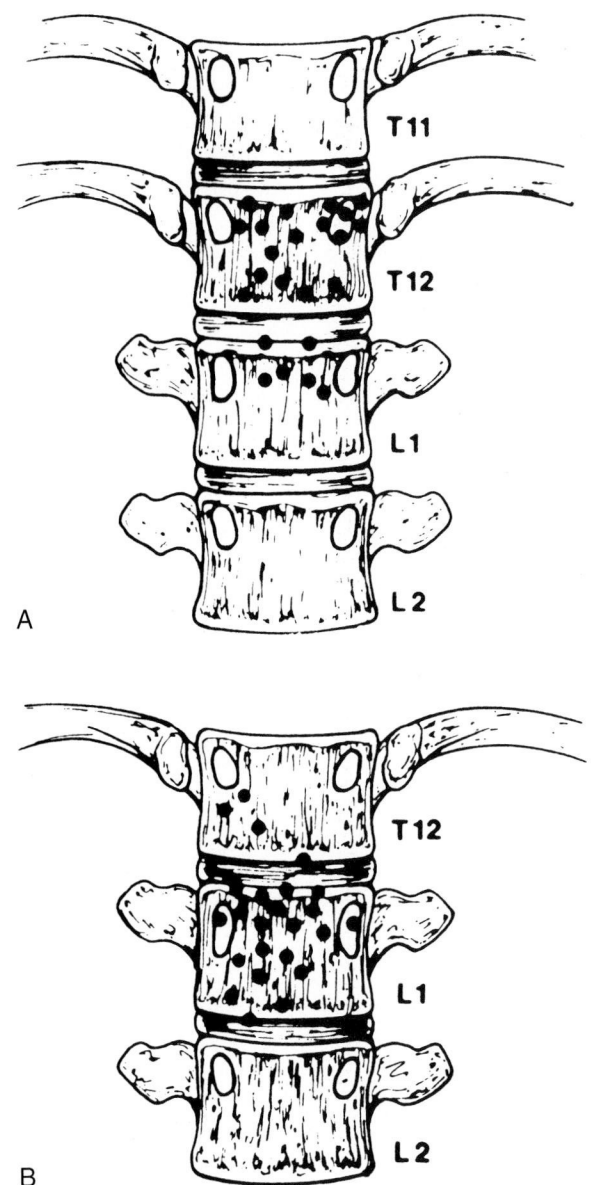

Figure 38–7. Graphic representation of the specific locations of the origin of the celiac axis (**A**) and superior mesenteric arteries (**B**). This underscores the need for individualized treatment planning when covering these nodal groups. (From Kao GD, Whittington R, Coia L: The anatomy of the celiac axis and superior mesenteric artery and its significance in radiation therapy. *Int J Oncol Biol Phys.* 1993;25:131. Reprinted by permission of Elsevier Science, Inc.)

clips. An intraoperative ultrasound supplements the CT information in determining the electron energy to be used. The IORT field should encompass the entire tumor bed as outlined with metallic clips plus a small margin to allow for dose falloff at the field edge. At the same time the cone size should be chosen to spare as much normal tissue as possible. At least two thirds to three-fourths of one functional kidney should be excluded from the field; this can be accomplished with the use of the previously mentioned malleable lead shields. The most common historic dose as well as the current Radiation Therapy Oncology Group recommendation is 15 Gy.

CHEMOTHERAPY

A multitude of published series have shown improved disease-free and overall survival with the addition of 5-FU to radiation. Various doses and schedules have been used; however, no prospective randomized study has clearly shown superiority of one schedule over another. The most commonly used schedule of 5-FU in resected patients has been 500 mg/m^2 intravenous bolus given on the first 3 and last 3 days of radiation. A more intensified 96-hour regimen of 5-FU, 1000 mg/m^2 per 24 hours continuous infusion during the first and fifth weeks of treatment has been shown retrospectively[90] to be superior to bolus 5-FU. A number of studies have also included additional postirradiation adjuvant weekly 5-FU; however, compliance with planned dosing has generally been so haphazard as to preclude any conclusions regarding the true impact of further 5-FU after radiation.[91] Additionally, Gemcitabine and Taxol have been used increasingly. Gemcitabine, both a potent radiosensitizer[92] and cytotoxic agent, has been the focus of intent study since it was shown in a randomized trial to be superior to 5-FU alone.[93] It was also shown to be effective in patients who had previously failed 5-FU.[94] Thus it was an attractive agent to combine with radiotherapy. An early phase II trial with concurrent chemotherapy in non–small cell lung cancer patients was closed due to significant pulmonary toxicity[95] underscoring the laboratory observations of radiation enhancement by a factor of 1.7 to 1.8, even with noncytotoxic concentrations that persisted 24 to 48 hours after exposure. Results are discussed later in the "Outcome" section.

CRITICAL NORMAL TISSUES

Critical normal tissues in a typical field treating pancreatic carcinoma include the liver, small bowel, stomach, and kidney, as well as the pancreas. The pancreas itself is more radioresistant than surrounding organs. This, coupled with overall poor long-term survival, have made reports of radiation injury to the pancreas exceedingly scarce in the literature. Fajardo[96] describes radiation effects to be primarily stromal fibrosis, myointimal proliferation of the arteries, ductal stenosis, and parenchymal atrophy that is similar to the appearance of chronic pancreatitis without the active inflammatory component. Islet cells appear to be more resistant than the exocrine tissue. Autopsy studies in patients treated with helium ions[97] have also shown prominent marked interstitial fibrosis and vascular sclerosis.

OUTCOME

Preoperative Radiation with and without Chemotherapy

Preoperative radiation has been described in several small series in the United States. Pilepich and Miller[98] treated 17 patients preoperatively. Sixteen had been explored and judged to be unresectable based on extension of tumor through the pancreatic capsule. They received 40 to 50 Gy with standard fractionation, and of 11 re-explored

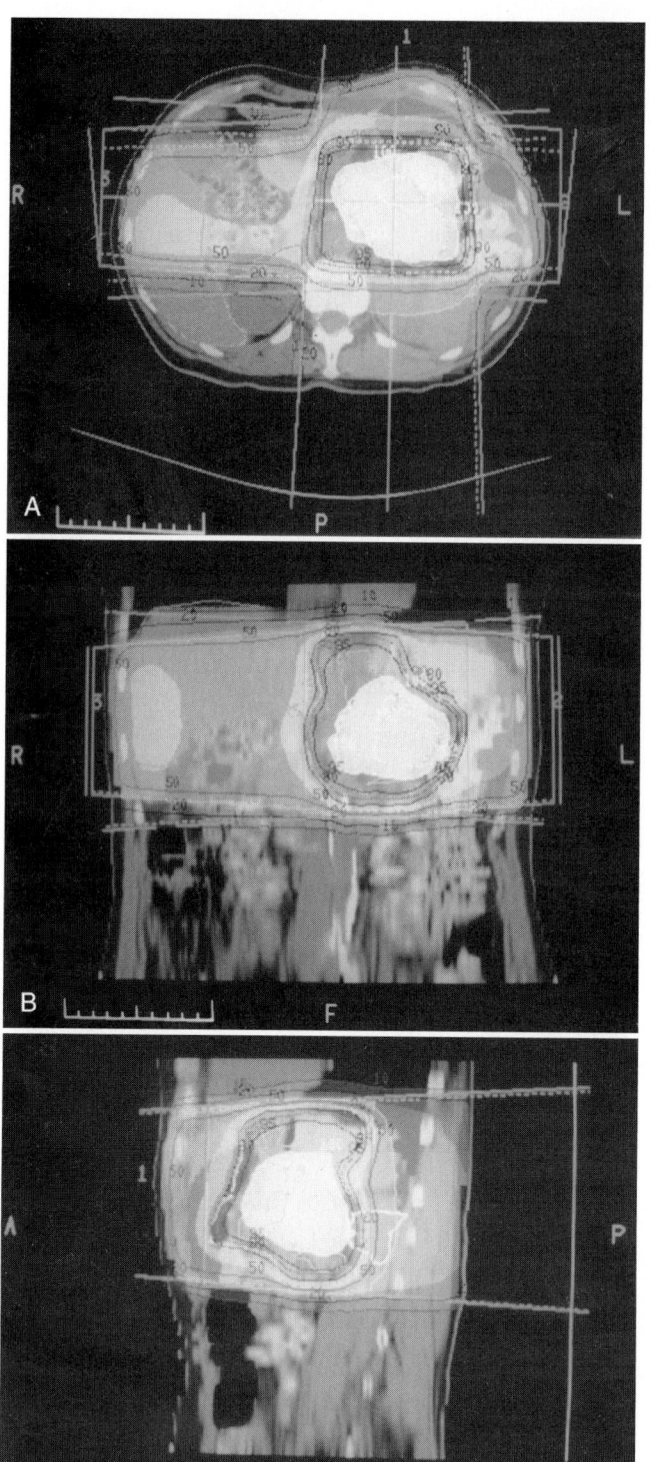

Figure 38–8. Axial (**A**), coronal (**B**), and sagittal (**C**) color-wash isodose distributions of three-field plan with lateral wedges. The tumor bed volume is covered in the 95% isodose line with a hot spot of 104%. The anterior field is weighted 40%, while the laterals have weighting of 30% each. Block margins for this T1N0M0 tumor are 1.0 to 1.5 cm. See also Color Figure 38–8.

patients, 6 were able to undergo radical resection. Two patients remained disease free for 5 years. A second series involved only seven patients,[99] 5 of whom were given 45 Gy preoperatively. There were two 5-year survivors and no clinically detected local recurrence. In Jessup's series[100] of 16 patients, 2 were able to undergo resection after neoadjuvant 5-FU and EBRT and had no evidence of disease at 20 and 22.5 months. In Japan, Ishikawa documented excellent pathologic responses to preoperative

radiation[101] and also noted improved resectability in his series of 22 patients.[102] An added benefit he noted was that no patient developed pancreatic fistulae as compared to a 17% rate of fistulae formation in similar nonirradiated patients who were treated concurrently. For various reasons, neoadjuvant treatment fell out of favor. However, improved surgical outcomes and newer, more effective chemotherapeutic agents have prompted renewed interest with promising early data reported

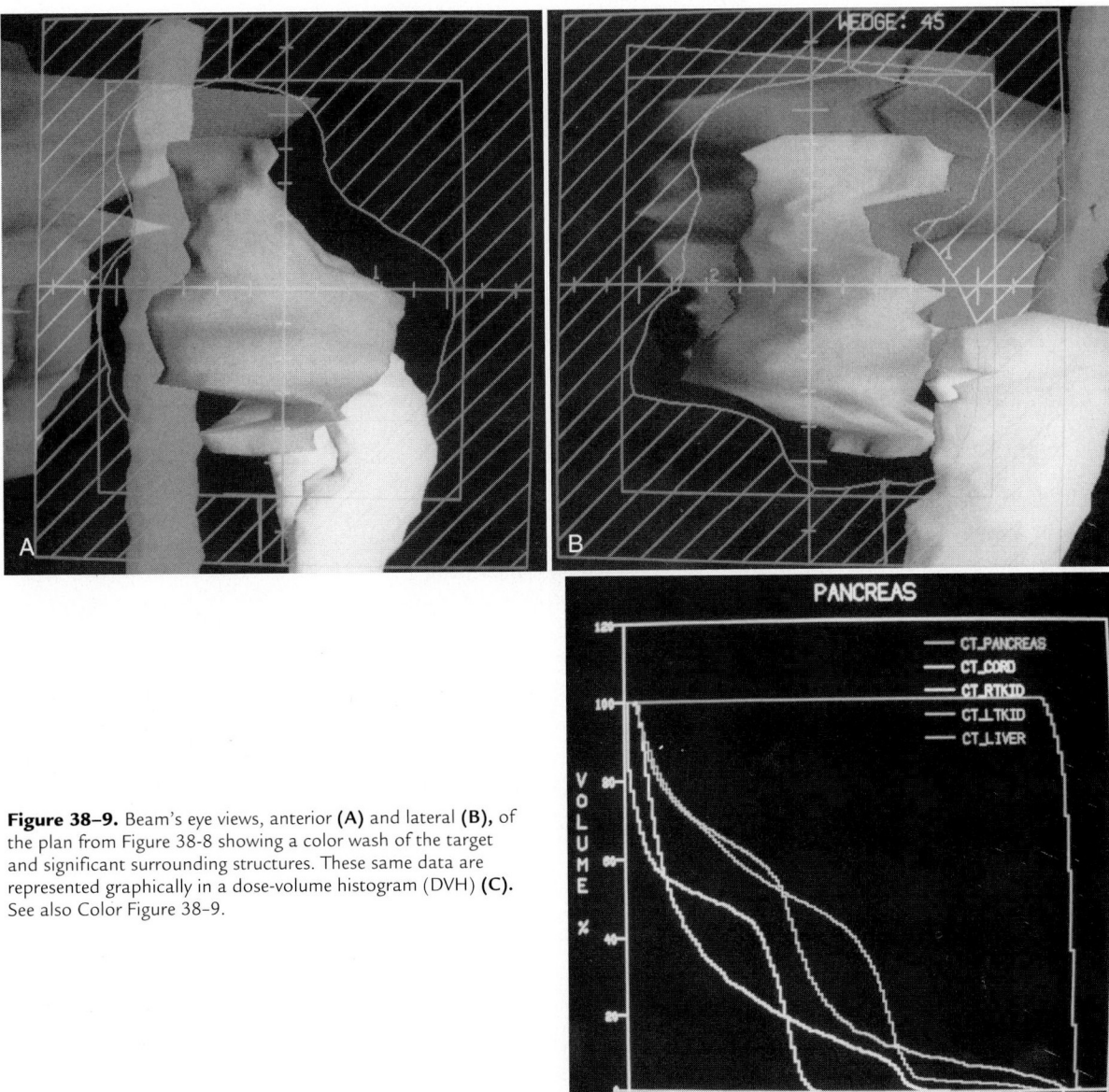

Figure 38–9. Beam's eye views, anterior **(A)** and lateral **(B)**, of the plan from Figure 38-8 showing a color wash of the target and significant surrounding structures. These same data are represented graphically in a dose-volume histogram (DVH) **(C)**. See also Color Figure 38–9.

recently by Gnant at the University of Vienna in Austria.[103]

Chemotherapy Alone

Single agents with a response rate of at least 20% include 5-FU, mitomycin-C, cisplatin,[104,105] ifosfamide,[106] and paclitaxel.[107] Though initial studies showed response rates somewhat less for Gemcitabine, at least one randomized trial showed improved survival compared to 5-FU when used as first-line therapy.[93] Streptozotocin is useful in endocrine tumors and has been incorporated into many regimens, as has doxorubicin (Adriamycin). In combination regimens (fluorouracil, Adriamycin, mitomycin [FAM], streptozocin, mitomycin, fluorouracil [SMF]), response rates as high as 40% have been reported,[82,104] but only 5% are complete responses and median survival has not

exceeded 26 to 32 weeks, which is not much greater than the 24 week mean survival reported for untreated pancreatic cancer.[34,83,105] Various phase I studies have been carried out with the intent of defining an effective and tolerable regimen combining radiation therapy with Gemcitabine.[81,108-111]

For patients with metastatic disease, two controlled trials investigated combination chemotherapy versus best supportive care.[112,113] Mallinson and colleagues[112] noted a significant improvement in survival for patients on the intensive chemotherapy arm versus controls (46 weeks vs. 9 weeks); however, many patients did not have tissue confirmation and these results have never been duplicated. The second trial[113] compared 5-FU and lomustine (CCNU) to best supportive care and found no difference in median survival. Modulation of 5-FU with Leukovorin has not produced improved response rates.[114] Cullinan et al.[115] reported on a trial of three different chemotherapeutic

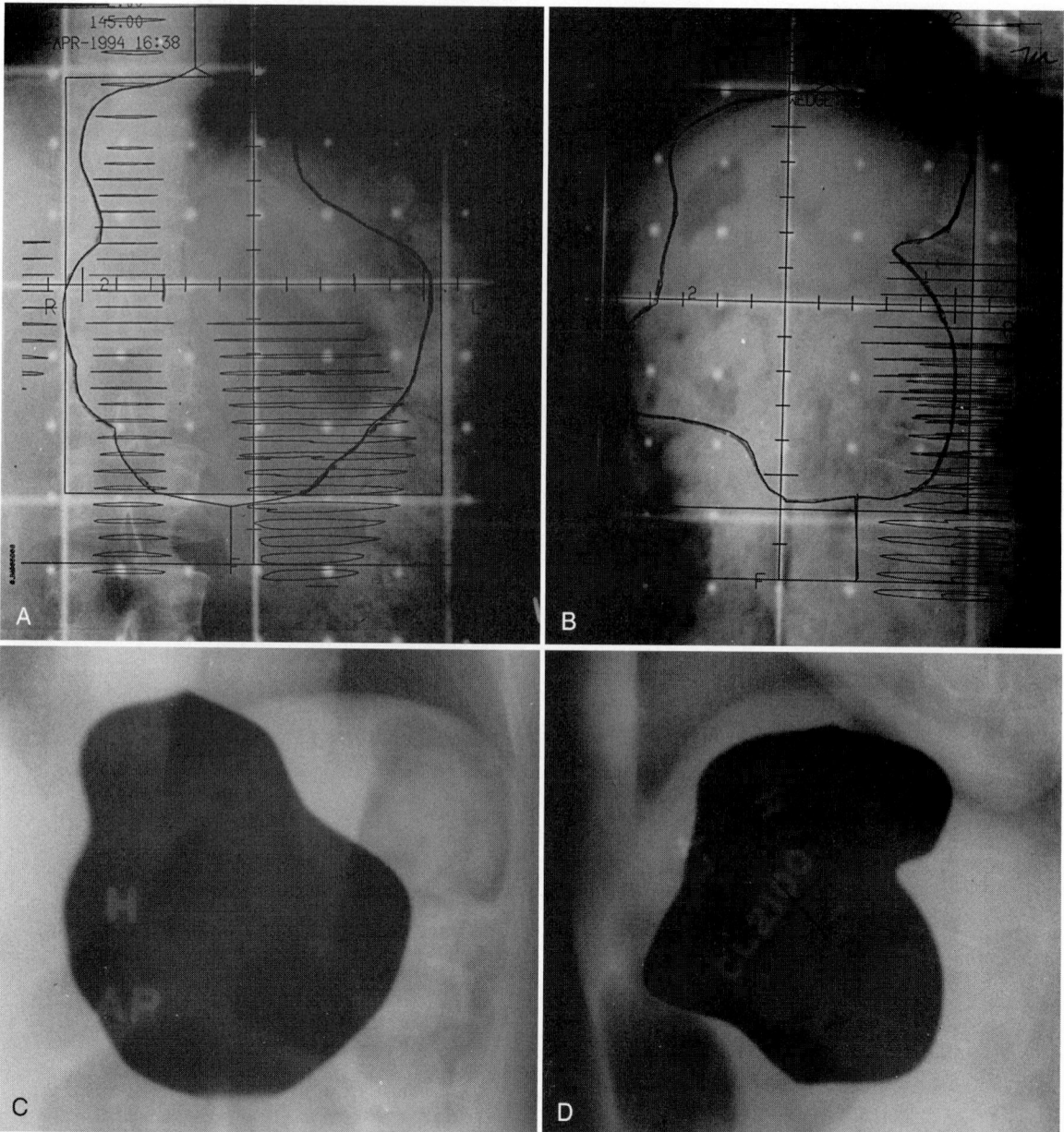

Figure 38–10. Anterior (**A**) and lateral (**B**) simulation and anterior (**C**) and lateral (**D**) port films for the three-dimensional treatment plan shown in Figure 38–8.

regimens for metastatic pancreatic carcinoma, showing all three to be equivalent. In summary, chemotherapy alone has not been shown beneficial for patients with advanced or metastatic disease. These patients are candidates for supportive care with nutrition and analgesics as well as experimental chemotherapy.

In completely resected patients, adjuvant chemotherapy alone may delay recurrence, but no increase in cure rate has been realized.[116] More recent findings of luteinizing hormone–releasing hormone receptors in pancreatic cancers[117] have led to trials with hormonal agents. Results have been mixed and no clear conclusions can be drawn.[118-120] Overall, current data supports the use of chemotherapy only if given in conjunction with radiation therapy or as part of a phase I/II protocol.

Postoperative Radiation with or without Chemotherapy

ADJUVANT THERAPY AFTER CURATIVE RESECTION

In 1974 GITSG undertook a prospective randomized trial giving 40 Gy EBRT and weekly bolus 5-FU versus no adjuvant therapy in potentially curatively resected patients (see Table 38-4).[83] There was a statistically significant improvement in median survival (21 months vs. 11 months) in favor of the irradiated group. Two-year actuarial survival was 43% for the treated group versus 18% for the control group. Subsequently, GITSG closed the observation arm and added an additional 30 patients to the treatment group, again showing the same improved survival.[84] A variety of phase I studies have been carried out with the intent of defining an effective and tolerable regimen combining radiation therapy with Gemcitabine.[108-111,121]

Investigators at the NCI conducted a randomized trial of 32 patients with resected tumors[122] comparing 50 Gy EBRT to 50 Gy EBRT plus a 20 Gy IORT boost. Overall survival was the same in both groups, but the IORT group had increased local control and disease-free survival. Several additional nonrandomized series have shown similar increased survival with adjuvant EBRT.[123-126] Exact criteria for treatment were not always outlined, but presumably these represented patients considered at higher risk for failure compared to those who were not treated. What emerges from various series is that high "T" stage, particularly with pancreatic capsular invasion, positive margins, distal disease, blood vessel invasion, and nodal disease all herald rapid local failure.[65,127-129]

The use of intraoperative electrons to boost the dose to the tumor bed allows high dose delivery to an area at risk while minimizing damage to surrounding radiosensitive tissue (Table 38-5). In the United States IORT has been used primarily for unresectable carcinomas, but in Japan it has been incorporated as part of the treatment for potentially curatively resected lesions. Shibamota et al.[130] reported a mean survival of 14 months in his patients treated with both EBRT and IORT after total resection. Because of small numbers, this trend for improved survival was not statistically significant, but Kawamura[131] subsequently *did* show increased survival in a similar group of 32 patients. This study is difficult to assess since exact details of staging and selection criteria for treatment are not given. Hiraoka et al.[132] treated 14 patients with extended surgery and extended-field IORT with a 5-year survival of 33%. Ozaki et al.[133] reported on 16 patients treated with extended surgery, IORT, and mitomycin; 11 of these were stage III (IUCC) and the group had a 53% survival at 3 years.

TREATMENT FOR LOCALIZED BUT UNRESECTABLE TUMORS

Median survival for localized unresectable cancer of the pancreas treated with bypass alone is 4 to 6 months.[33,34,134-136] EBRT alone does not offer significant improvement.[85,86,137] Hyperfractionated radiation, 1.2 Gy twice daily, was also disappointing though the total dose of 50.4 Gy may have been too low to expect significant benefit.[138] Particle therapy to include pions,[139] neutrons,[140-143] and helium ions[144,145] has been disappointing (Table 38-6). Neutron therapy hoped to take advantage of a higher relative biologic effectiveness (RBE) (2.6 to 3.0) and helium ion therapy was used to take advantage of improved dose localization properties. Even though initial data with helium appeared to be very promising[144] and autopsy studies did confirm tumor kill with minimum effect on adjacent local tissue,[97] a randomized prospective trial comparing helium ions to conventional radiation failed to show a survival benefit in spite of improved local control in the helium arm.[146] The photon arm was split-course and the helium continuous; failures were largely due to distant metastases. EBRT combined with chemotherapy, however, has been shown to confer significant survival advantage over either EBRT or chemotherapy alone (Table 38-7). Although Klaasen et al.[147] found no difference with combined modality treatment,

Table 38–5 Selected Series—Intraoperative Radiation Therapy

	Reference	Patients, *n*	Median Survival, mo	2-Yr Survival, %	Local Failure, %
MGH					
EBRT (45–55 Gy) + IORT (15–20 Gy) ± CT	Shipley et al[164]	29	16.9	30	36
EBRT (45–50 Gy) + IORT (20 Gy) + misonidazole ± CT	Tepper et al[169]	41	12	20	55
MAYO					
EBRT (45–50 Gy) + IORT (17.5–20 Gy) ± CT	Gunderson et al[170]	52	11	8	7
Ohio					
EBRT (19.8–65 Gy) + IORT (12.5–30 Gy) ± CT	Dobelbower et al[134]	26	10.5	—	20
Prospective/Randomized					
Kyoto					
EBRT (50–60 Gy) + IORT (25–33 Gy)	Shibamoto et al[130]	25	6.5	7	—
NCI (unresectable) EBRT (50 Gy) + IORT (25 Gy) + 5-FU	Sindelar & Kinsella[168]	32	8	—	—
RTOG 85-05 EBRT (50.4 Gy) + IORT (20 Gy) + CT*	Tepper et al[165]	51	9	9	—

*Eighteen-month actuarial survival.
CT, computed tomography; EBRT, external beam radiation therapy; IORT, intraoperative radiation therapy; MGH, Massachusetts General Hospital; MAYO, Mayo Clinic; NCI, National Cancer Institute; RTOG, Radiation Therapy Oncology Group.

Table 38–6 Particle Therapy Results in Locally Advanced Pancreatic Cancer

	Reference	Patients, n	Dose	Median Survival, mo	Severe Complications, n/n (%)
Helium					
Lawrence Berkeley Lab					
Nonrandomized (1975–1981*)	Castro et al[145]	94	60 GyE	10	9/94 (9.5)
Prospective, randomized–NCOG	Linstadt et al[146]	21	60–70 GyE	7.8	4/21 (19)
Neutrons					
Fermilab[†]	Cohen et al[141]	77	15–20 Gy	6	36/77 (47)
MDAH-UTMB[‡]	Al-Abdulla et al[140]	15	60 GyE	7	0
Georgetown[§]	Smith et al[143]	19	17–17.5 Gy	6	9/19 (47)

*Several patients received treatment with heavy particles (Ne, C); complications same as in photon group.
[†]Dose in neutrons; RBE not specified.
[‡]13 patients received both photons and neutrons; neutron RBE = 3.1.
[§]Dose in neutrons, RBE = 3.0.
MDAH, M.D. Anderson Hospital; NCOG, Northern California Oncology Group; RBE, relative biologic effectiveness; UTMB, University of Texas Medical Branch (Galveston).

GITSG in a prospective study of 194 patients[137] did find that the addition of 5-FU to EBRT almost doubled the mean survival time (from 5.5 to 10 months) and that at 1 year 40% of the combined modality group was alive versus only 10% of those treated with radiation alone. Other investigators have since duplicated these findings.[85,86] The cooperative groups have also explored the newer chemotherapeutic agents. An Eastern Cooperative Oncology Group trial using protracted infusion 5-FU, Gemcitabine, and external beam radiation therapy (XRT) showed unexpected early toxicity,[148] necessitating early study closure. This underscored earlier studies that suggested that relatively high doses of radiation, large fields including lymph nodes at risk, and Gemcitabine were too toxic. Similar experience of high toxicity suggesting a very narrow therapeutic index with Gemcitabine chemoradiotherapy was demonstrated by researchers at MD Anderson.[149]

An alternate approach investigated at the University of Michigan has consisted of delivering a standard dose of Gemcitabine (1000 mg/m^2) per week along with escalating doses of radiation.[109] Radiation fields were tightly 3D planned, covering only gross tumor volume. Doses ranged from 24 to 42 Gy delivered in 3 weeks with 1.6 to 2.8 Gy

Table 38–7 Selected Series—Brachytherapy

	Reference	Patients, n	Median Survival, mo	Local Control, %	Major Complication, n/n (%)
Memorial Sloan-Kettering					
^{125}I (mean 136.6 Gy) ± EBRT ± CT	Peretz et al[156]	98	7	—	19/98 (19)
Thomas Jefferson					
^{125}I (mean 129 Gy) + EBRT (50–55 Gy) ± CT	Mohiuddin et al[86]	81	12	71	(32)
Massachusetts General					
^{125}I (mean 160 Gy) + EBRT (40–50 Gy) ± CT	Shipley et al[155]	12	11	66	5/12 (42)
Ohio					
^{125}I (mean 140 Gy) + EBRT (48.6–63 Gy) ± CT	Dobelbower et al[151]	12	15	—	5/12 (43)
University of Southern California					
^{125}I (100–150 Gy) + EBRT (30–50 Gy)*	Syed et al[154]	18	14	—	4/18 (22)
Rome					
^{125}I (60–100 Gy) + EBRT (10.5–30 Gy)	Montemaggi et al[153]	7	7	33	3/7 (43)
M.D. Anderson					
^{198}Au[†]	Al-Abdulla et al[140]	25	7	—	6/25 (24)

*Highly selected patients implanted at second laparotomy. If implanted initially, median survival is 10 months.
[†]Twenty-four percent mortality.
CT, computed tomography; EBRT, external beam radiation therapy.

fractions. This study included 37 unresectable or incompletely resected patients, 14 of whom had confirmed or suspected metastatic disease. Median survival of 11.6 months is very promising. More important, patterns of failure suggested that field size reductions did not result in excess failures. Further studies using this approach are planned.

A more aggressive local approach to deliver high doses has been the use of intraoperative brachytherapy (Table 38-8). Direct or percutaneous[150] implantation with I-125, Au-198, or Pd-103 has been reported. Numerous reports using this technique have appeared both in the United States and abroad,[53,85,86,151-154] yielding approximately equal results. Initial reports from MGH in 12 patients treated with bypass, surgery, I-125 implantation and postoperative 40 to 45 Gy showed an 11-month mean survival.[155] Syed[154] reported on 18 patients treated in a similar fashion with a mean survival of 14 months. His patients, however, were highly selected since they were implanted at second laparotomy; those implanted at initial laparotomy had a mean survival of only 10 months. The best survival (mean 15 months) was reported by Dobelbower[151] in his initial series of 12 patients. Long-term follow-up on 81 patients from Thomas Jefferson Medical School[152] showed an excellent local control of 71% but unfortunately no increase in mean survival, which was 12 months for the entire group. Perioperative mortality was 5% and late complications were seen in 32% of patients. The largest series, reported for MSKCC by Peretz, had a total of 98 patients.[156] Mean peripheral dose to the tumor was 136.6 Gy; postoperative complications were high (19/98) and median survival for the whole group was only 7 months.

There are very sparse data on the use of high dose rate brachytherapy. Warszawski[157] developed a technique using CT treatment planning to assure accurate delivery of high doses to the tumor and tolerable dose to surrounding organs. Nine patients were treated with 30 Gy high-activity Ir-192 and subsequent 52 Gy EBRT with concurrent 5-FU/Leukovorin. Results are very preliminary, but all patients had significant pain relief, none had procedure-associated complications, and autopsy in one showed no residual cancer in the treatment field and minimal radiation effects on adjacent small bowel. An alternate means of overcoming the potential drawback of low dose rate I-125 is with the use of Pd-103. With a short half-life of only 17 days, higher total activities can be implanted. The more rapid dose falloff for Pd-103 enhances the sparing effect of brachytherapy on the surrounding normal tissues and the higher dose rate has a theoretical advantage in treating rapidly dividing tumors. Raban et al. reported a small series of patients from MSKCC treated with Pd-103.[158] Median survival was 6.9 months, no different from a similar series of patients treated with I-125. The addition of external beam radiation or chemotherapy did not improve local control or survival. As in other brachytherapy series, palliation of pain was very good with 83% of symptomatic patients reporting durable pain control until the time of death. Complications in this series were felt to be unacceptably high. All in all, the relatively high rate of complications of brachytherapy without demonstrable survival benefit have resulted in a shift toward the use of IORT or high dose conformal radiotherapy when attempting to deliver higher local doses of radiation.

Since Abe's[159] report of the feasibility and safety of the use of intraoperative electrons, many investigators have reported nonrandomized data.[130-133,160-166] Single doses of 15 to 30 Gy are generally given with 15 to 29 Mev electrons. Use of higher doses (up to 50 Gy) have up to a 75% incidence of treatment-related bleeding.[162] IORT alone is no better than bypass surgery[134] with a mean

Table 38–8   Combined-Modality Trials for Locally Advanced and Nonresectable Pancreatic Carcinoma

Reference	Treatment Radiation, Gy	Chemotherapy (mg/m²)	Patients, n	Median Survival, mo
Moertel et al*	35–40	Placebo	32	6.3 (P < 0.05)
	35–40	5-FU (45)†	32	10.4
Moertel et al[137]	60	—	25	5.75 (P < 0.01)
	60	5-FU (500)	31	10
	40	5-FU (500)	28	10.5
GITSG‡	40	5-FU (500)	83	9 (P = 0.19)
	60	5-FU (500)	86	12.25
GITSG‡	60	5-FU (500)	73	9.25
	40	Doxorubicin (15)	70	8.25
GITSG[82]	54	5-FU (500)§ + streptozocin, mitomycin C, 5-FU	22	10.5
	—	Streptozocin, mitomycin C, 5-FU	21	8
Klaasen et al[147] (ECOG)	40	5-FU (600) + 5-FU weekly	47	8.3
	—	5-FU (600 weekly)	44	8.2

*Randomized. Registered after closure of surgery-alone arm.
†Dose is mg/kg.
‡From Gastrointestinal Tumor Study Group: Radiation therapy combined with adriamycin or 5-fluorouracil for the treatment of locally unresectable gastrointestinal pancreatic cancer. *Cancer.* 1985;56:2563.
§5-FU given days 1–3 each 2-week cycle of radiation, then weekly.
ECOG, Eastern Cooperative Oncology Group; 5-FU, 5-fluorouracil; GITSG, Gastrointestinal Tumor Study Group.

survival of around 3.5 months; therefore, treatment is usually given in conjunction with 45 to 50 Gy external beam radiation and 5-FU. Mean survivals in that setting have ranged from 10.5 to 16.5 months.[134,164,167] To ascertain whether this improvement in survival was real or due to selection bias, the NCI and RTOG both undertook randomized trials of IORT. In the NCI trial,[168] patients received 25 Gy IORT with 18 to 22 MeV electrons and postoperative 50 Gy at 1.5 to 1.75 Gy per day compared to controls who received split-course 60 Gy EBRT. Both groups also were given concurrent 5-FU. Treatment-related toxicity was similar in both groups and median survival in each arm was 8 months. Time to disease progression, however, was longer in the IORT group and for the subset of patients with stage III disease (locally infiltrative and involved nodes), time to progression and survival were both prolonged. In RTOG 85-05, patients were given 50.4 Gy EBRT in combination with 5-FU ± 20 Gy IORT. For the 51 fully analyzable patients, the mean survival was only 9 months. This study did confirm the feasibility of using IORT in a multi-institution setting with acceptable morbidity, but it failed to show increased survival benefit of IORT over standard EBRT and 5-FU. The addition of misonidazole, a hypoxic cell sensitizer to IORT,[169] also failed to show any advantage. Though overall survival rates were disappointing, one valuable effect of IORT is the ability to afford significant pain relief; Shipley et al.[164] reported that 50% of his patients had complete pain relief for the duration of their survival. Others have also noted this in up to 90% of their patients.[160,162] IORT unquestionably improves local control: in a series of 159 patients from Mayo,[163] local control at 1 year was 82% for the IORT group versus 48% for standard radiation with 5-FU. Gunderson[170] documented local progression of only 7% in his series of 42 evaluable patients. Peritoneal failure occurred in 26% and distant metastasis in 57%. The majority of distant metastasis occurred in the liver. The vexing problem of local failure in the liver has also been confirmed in two series of curatively resected patients published by Foo[124] and Griffen.[41] In the Mayo series, 36% of patients failed in the liver, and Griffen reports 73% of patients with some component of local failure. To address this problem, Komaki et al.[89] undertook a phase I to II study of 16 patients with either inoperable or locally recurrent disease and gave prophylactic hepatic irradiation. Patients received 61.2 Gy to the tumor along with concurrent 5-FU; during the fourth week the field was expanded to include the liver, which received 23.4 Gy over the remaining 2.5 weeks. Other than temporary elevation of liver enzymes in three fourths of the patients, there were no severe or life-threatening complications. Only two patients demonstrated hepatic metastasis as site of first failure. The RTOG, in a larger setting using the same radiation but more aggressive 5-FU, confirmed that this regimen was tolerable. Their study group consisted of unresectable patients without local metastasis. Hepatic failure as first site of recurrence occurred in 13% and eventually in 32%. Persistent or locally progressive tumor was seen in 73%. The question arising from this series is whether prophylactic hepatic irradiation might be more useful in more favorable patients (i.e., totally resected patients) or whether prophylactic

hepatic irradiation might be combined with a regimen, offering a better chance of local control. To answer this, RTOG 91-02 randomized locally advanced, nonresectable patients to 5-FU, preoperative external beam pancreatic and prophylactic hepatic radiation ± IORT. The main objective was to assess the value of EB-IORT on local control, patterns of failure and overall survival. The outcome of this study has not yet been reported.

Other avenues being explored include newer radiation sensitizers with fewer side effects and the role of radioactively labeled monoclonal antibodies. Misonidazole, an early hypoxic cell radiosensitizer, was disappointing in clinical trials,[169] no doubt in part to limitations in dosing imposed by its main side effect of neurotoxicity. RK-28, a new radiosensitizer, has fewer side effects, is better tolerated systemically, and has been used in preliminary studies directly injected into the tumor just before IORT.[171] Studies are also under way investigating Yttrium-90 conjugated to monoclonal antibodies.[172] Because of the significant problem of distant metastasis, real impact on overall survival awaits the development of accurate and cost-effective screening tests as well as newer systemic agents. Currently the cooperative groups either have open studies or are awaiting maturation of studies incorporating various schedules of radiation, 5-FU, Gemcitabine, or Taxol. In addition, IMRT holds out hope of improvement with its higher dose delivery with less toxicity, but it also still awaits further analysis to assess overall impact.

ENDOCRINE TUMORS

Endocrine tumors comprise approximately 5% of all pancreatic tumors; the enteropancreatic cells are believed to be of neuroectodermal origin and tumors arising from these cells are termed APUDomas (from their ability of **a**mine-**p**recursor **u**ptake and **d**ecarboxylation). These tumors are frequently recognized by the clinical syndromes produced by circulating polypeptides elaborated by malignant cells. Tumors are frequently slow growing with a long natural history.[37] Even with metastasis, survival may be quite long. The primary approach to these tumors is surgical with chemotherapy reserved for unresectable or metastatic disease. There is very sparse anecdotal information on the effects of radiation. The rarity of these tumors has precluded prospective studies of any size. Phan[173] reported on a series of 50 patients, 29 of whom had malignant tumors. Even without adjuvant therapy, 5-year survival was 61%. Status of the surgical margins was of paramount importance. Median survival with negative margins was 71 months vs. 13 months with positive margins.[174-176] Rich[125] reported on three patients, two of whom were treated with IORT achieving good pain palliation. The third patient was able to return to work and lived 61 months from the start of radiation. Gaitan[177] and Keane[178] reported on the use 20 to 25 Gy whole abdominal radiation, suggesting very good results in patients with carcinoid tumors. Patients without the syndrome fared significantly better.[178] Hansen[179] and Torrisi[180] have also reported anecdotal responses to higher doses of radiation in the range of 45 to 50 Gy in patients with other islet cell tumors. Promising data using radionuclide therapy are emerging. Detailed discussions are best found in nuclear medicine textbooks.

REFERENCES

1. Eyre HJ, Gansler T, et al: Cancer statistics, 2002;52:1.
2. National Cancer Institute: *Annual Cancer Statistics Review 1973-1988.* Bethesda, Md: Dept of Health and Human Services, 1991. (NIH Publication no. 91-2789).
3. Gudjonsson B: Cancer of the pancreas: 50 years of surgery. *Cancer.* 1987;60:2284.
4. Farrow DC, Davis S: Risk of pancreatic cancer in relation to medical history and the use of tobacco, alcohol and coffee. *Int J Cancer.* 1990;45:816.
5. Howe GR, Jain M, Miller AB: Dietary factors and the risk of pancreatic cancer: Results of a Canadian population based study. *Int J Cancer.* 1990;45:604.
6. Taylor PR, et al: Induction of pancreatic tumors by longterm duodenogastric reflux. *Gut.* 1989;30:1596.
7. Cuzick J, Babiker AG: Pancreatic cancer, alcohol, diabetes mellitus and gall-bladder disease. *Int J Cancer.* 1989;43:415.
8. Gordis L: Consumption of methylxanthine-containing beverages and pancreatic cancer. *Cancer Letter.* 1990;52:1.
9. Rosa JA, Van Linda BM, Abourizk NN: New onset diabetes mellitus as a harbinger of pancreatic carcinoma. *J Clin Gastroenterol.* 1989;11:211.
10. Lin A, Feller ER: Pancreatic carcinoma as a cause of unexplained pancreatitis: Report of ten cases. *Ann Intern Med.* 1990;113:166.
11. Mancuso TF, el-Attar AA: Cohort study of workers exposed to betanaphthylamine and benzidine. *J Occup Environ Med.* 1967;9:277.
12. Lin RS, Kessler II: A multifactorial model for pancreatic cancer in man. *JAMA.* 1981;245:147.
13. Abrams R, et al: Intensified adjuvant therapy for pancreatic and periampullary adenocarcinoma: Survival and observations regarding patterns of failure, radiotherapy dose and CA 19-9 levels. *Int J Radiat Biol Phys.* 1999;44:1039.
14. Hruban R: Pancreatic Cancer, 1999 Update Symposium. *J Am Coll Surg.* 1998;187:429.
15. Smit VHTB, et al: K-ras codon 12 mutations occur very frequently in pancreatic adenocarcinomas. *Nucleic Acids Res.* 1988;16:7773.
16. Shibata D, et al: Detection of c-K-ras mutations in fine needle aspirates from human pancreatic adenocarcinoma. *Cancer Res.* 1990;130:345.
17. Bos JL: Ras oncogene in human cancer: A review. *Cancer Res.* 1989;49:4682.
18. Gruenewald K, et al: High frequency of Ki-ras codon 12 mutations in pancreatic adenocarcinomas. *Int J Cancer.* 1989;43:1037.
19. Almoguera C, et al: Most human carcinomas of the exocrine pancreas contain mutant c-K-ras genes. *Cell.* 1988;53:549.
20. Kondo H, et al: Detection of point mutations in the K-ras oncogene at Codon 12 in pure pancreatic juice for diagnosis of pancreatic carcinoma. *Cancer.* 1994;73:1589.
21. Hruban RH, et al: Genetics of pancreatic cancer: From genes to families. *Surg Oncol Clin North Am.* 1998;7:1.
22. Cubilla AL, Fitzgerald PJ: Cancer of the exocrine pancreas: The pathologic aspects. *CA Cancer J Clin.* 1985;35:2.
23. Talamini MA, et al: Spectrum of cystic tumors of the pancreas. *Am J Surg.* 1992;163:117.
24. Milchgrub S, et al: Intraductal carcinoma of the pancreas. *Cancer.* 1992;69:651.
25. Abrams R, King D, Wilson J: Objective response of malignant carcinoid to radiation therapy. *Int J Radiat Biol Phys.* 1987;13:869.
26. Wilentz R, Hruban R: Pathology of cancer of the pancreas. *Surg Oncol Clin N Am.* 1998;7:43.
27. Osaka M, et al: Immunohistochemical study of mucin carbohydrates and core proteins in human pancreatic tumors. *Cancer.* 1993;71:2191.
28. Baisch H, Kloeppel G, Reinke B: DNA ploidy and cell cycle analysis in pancreatic and ampullary carcinoma: Flow cytometric study of formalin fixed paraffin embedded tissue. *Virchows Arch.* 1990;417:145.

29. Boettger T, et al: Factors influencing survival after resection for pancreatic cancer. *Cancer.* 1994;73:63.
30. Allison DC, et al: Pancreatic cancer cell DNA content correlates with long term survival after pancreaticoduodenectomy. *Ann Surg.* 1991;214:648.
31. Eskelinen M, et al: Relationship between DNA ploidy and survival in patients with exocrine pancreatic cancer. *Pancreas.* 1991;6:90.
32. Warshaw AL: Implications of malignant-cell DNA content for treatment of patients with pancreatic cancer. *Ann Surg.* 1991;214:645.
33. Kalser MH, Barkin J, MacIntyre MJ: Pancreatic cancer: Assessment of prognosis by clinical presentation. *Cancer.* 1985;56:397.
34. Taskforce, COTP: Staging of cancer of the pancreas. *Cancer.* 1981;47:1631.
35. Nordback IH, et al: Carcinoma of the body and tail of the pancreas. *Am J Surg.* 1992;164:26.
36. Winek T, et al: Prognostic factors for survival after pancreatico-duodenectomy for malignant disease. *Am J Surg.* 1990;159:454.
37. Friesen SR: Tumors of the endocrine pancreas. *N Engl J Med.* 1982;306:580.
38. Cubilla A, Fortner J, Fitzgerald P: Lymph node involvement in carcinoma of the head of the pancreas area. *Cancer.* 1978;41:880.
39. Warshaw AL, Tepper JE, Shipley WU: Laparoscopy in the staging and planning of therapy for pancreatic cancer. *Am J Surg.* 1986;151:76.
40. Tepper JE, Nardi GL, Suit HD: Carcinoma of the pancreas: Review of the MGH experience from 1963-1973: Analysis of surgical failure and implications for radiation therapy. *Cancer.* 1976;37:1519.
41. Griffen JF, et al: Patterns of failure after curative resection of pancreatic carcinoma. *Cancer.* 1990;66:56.
42. Freeney PC, et al: Pancreatic ductal adenocarcinoma: Diagnosis and staging with dynamic CT. *Radiology.* 1988;166:125.
43. Steiner E, et al: Imaging of pancreatic neoplasms: Comparison of MR and CT. *Am J Roentgenol.* 1989;152:487.
44. Warshaw AL, et al: Preoperative staging and assessment of resectability of pancreatic cancer. *Arch Surg.* 1990;125:230.
45. Tio TL, et al: Ampullopancreatic carcinoma: Preoperative TNM classification with endosonography. *Radiology.* 1990;175:455.
46. Snady H, Cooperman A, Siegal J: Endoscopic ultrasonography compared with computed tomography with ERCP in patients with obstructive jaundice or small peripancreatic mass. *Gastrointest Endosc.* 1992;38:27.
47. Palazzo L, et al: Endoscopic ultrasonography in the diagnosis and staging of pancreatic adenocarcinoma: Results of a prospective study with comparison to ultrasonography and CT scan. *Endoscopy.* 1993;25:143.
48. Roesch T, et al: Staging of pancreatic and ampullary carcinoma by endoscopic ultrasonography: Comparison with conventional sonography, computed tomography, and angiography. *Gastroenterology.* 1992;102:188.
49. Ferruci JT, et al: Diagnosis of abdominal malignancy by radiologic fine-needle aspiration biopsy. *Am J Roentgenol.* 1980;134:323.
50. Weiss SM, et al: Rapid intra-abdominal spread of pancreatic cancer. *Arch Surg.* 1985;120:415.
51. Warshaw AL: Implications of peritoneal cytology for staging of early pancreatic cancer. *Am J Surg.* 1991;161:26.
52. Warshaw A, Fernandez-Del Castillo C: Pancreatic carcinoma. *N Engl J Med.* 1992;326:455.
53. Whittington R, et al: Radiotherapy of unresectable pancreatic carcinoma: A six year experience with 104 patients. *Int J Radiat Oncol Biol Phys.* 1981;7:1639.
54. Shemesh E, et al: Role of endoscopic retrograde choloangiopancreatography in differentiating pancreatic cancer coexisting with chronic pancreatitis. *Cancer.* 1990;65:893.
55. Yamamoto K, et al: Human pancreas scintigraphy using Iodine-123-labeled HIPDM and SPECT. *J Nucl Med.* 1990;31:1015.
56. Baum RP: Immunoscintigraphy as a diagnostic tool in pancreatic cancer. *Hepatogastroenterology.* 1990;37:154.
57. Sakahara H, et al: Serum CA 19-9 concentrations and computed tomography findings in patients with pancreatic carcinoma. *Cancer.* 1986;57:1324.
58. Warshaw AL, Swanson RS: Pancreatic cancer in 1988: Possibilities and probabilities. *Ann Surg.* 1988;208:541.
59. Schifeling D, et al: Radiation therapy and 5-Fluorouracil modulated by Leucovorin for adenocarcinoma of the pancreas. *Int J Pancreatol.* 1992;12:239.

60. Speer AG, et al: Randomized trial of endoscopic versus percutaneous stent insertion in malignant obstructive jaundice. *Lancet.* 1987(11 July):57.

61. van Heerden J, et al: Total pancreatectomy for ductal adenocarcinoma of the pancreas. *Am J Surg.* 1981;142:308.

62. Fortner JG: Regional pancreatectomy for cancer of the pancreas, ampulla, and other related sites. *Ann Surg.* 1984;199:418.

63. Funovics JM, et al: Current trends in the management of carcinoma of the pancreatic head. *Hepatogastroenterology.* 1989;36:450.

64. Braasch JW, et al: Pyloric and gastric preserving pancreatic resection. *Ann Surg.* 1986;204:411.

65. Cameron JL, et al: Factors influencing survival after pancreaticoduodenectomy for pancreatic cancer. *Am J Surg.* 1991;161:120.

66. Cameron J, et al: One hundred and forty five consecutive pancreaticoduodenectomies without mortality. *Ann Surg.* 1993;217:430.

67. Yeo C, et al: Pancreaticoduodenectomy for cancer of the head of the pancreas. *Ann Surg.* 1995;221:721.

68. Sohn T, et al: Should pancreaticoduodenectomy be performed in octogenarians? *J Gastrointest Surg.* 1998;2:207.

69. Magisterelli P, et al: Pancreatic resection for periampullary cancer in elderly patients. *Hepatogastroenterology.* 1998;45:242.

70. Robinson E, et al: Reoperative pancreaticoduodenectomy for periampullary carcinoma. *Am J Surg.* 1996;172:432.

71. Sohn T, et al: Reexploration for periampullary carcinoma. Resectability, perioperative results, pathology, and long-term outcome. *Ann Surg.* 1999;229:393.

72. Sosa J, et al: Importance of hospital volume in the overall management of pancreatic cancer. *Ann Surg.* 1998;228:429.

73. Moosa AR: Surgical treatment of pancreatic cancer. *Am J Surg.* 1986;152:503.

74. Connolly MM, et al: Survival in 1001 patients with carcinoma of the pancreas. *Ann Surg.* 1987;206:366.

75. Tsuchiya R, et al: Collective review of small carcinomas of the pancreas. *Ann Surg.* 1986;203:77.

76. Pelligrini C, et al: An analysis of the reduced morbidity and mortality rates after pancreaticoduodenectomy. *Arch Surg.* 1989;124:778.

77. Soehendra N, et al: Malignant jaundice: Results of diagnostic and therapeutic endoscopy. *World J Surg.* 1989;13:171.

78. Smith AC, Dowsett JF, Hatfield ARW: Prospective randomized trial of bypass surgery versus endoscopic stenting in patients with malignant obstructive jaundice. *Gut.* 1989;30:A1513.

79. Anderson JR, et al: Randomized trial of endoscopic endoprosthesis versus operative bypass in malignant obstructive jaundice. *Gut.* 1989;30:1132.

80. Gnant M, et al: Neoadjuvant chemotherapy with Gemcitabine and Docetaxel for locally advanced pancreatic cancer. *Proceed Am Coll Clin Oncol.* 2002;21:149a.

81. Hoffman J, et al: A phase I study of preoperative Gemcitabine with radiation therapy followed by postoperative Gemcitabine in patients with localized resected pancreatic adenocarcinoma. *Proceed Am Coll Clin Oncol.* 1998;17:283a.

82. Group TGS: Treatment of locally unresectable carcinoma of the pancreas: Comparison of combined modality therapy (chemotherapy plus radiotherapy) to chemotherapy alone. *J Natl Cancer Inst.* 1988;80:751.

83. Kalser MH, Ellenberg SS: Pancreatic cancer: Adjuvant combined radiation and chemotherapy following curative resection. *Arch Surg.* 1985;120:899.

84. Group TGTS: Further evidence of effective combined radiation and chemotherapy following curative resection of pancreatic cancer. *Cancer.* 1987;59:2006.

85. Whittington R, et al: Multimodality therapy of localized unresectable pancreatic cancer. *Cancer.* 1984;54:1991.

86. Mohiuddin M, et al: Combined modality treatment of localized unresectable adenocarcinoma of the pancreas. *Int J Radiat Oncol Biol Phys.* 1988;14:79.

87. Dobelbower RR Jr, et al: Precision radiotherapy for cancer of the pancreas: Technique and results. *Int J Radiat Oncol Biol Phys.* 1980;6:1127.

88. Kao GD, Whittington R, Coia L: The anatomy of the celiac axis and superior mesenteric artery and its significance in radiation therapy. *Int J Radiat Oncol Biol Phys.* 1993;25:131.

89. Komaki R, et al: Phase I-II study of prophylactic hepatic irradiation with local irradiation and systemic chemotherapy for adenocarcinoma of the pancreas. *Int J Radiat Oncol Biol Phys.* 1988;15:1447.

90. Bryer M, et al: Adjuvant therapy of resected pancreatic carcinoma. *Proceedings of the 32nd Annual Astro Meeting, 1990;* 19(suppl 1):215.

91. Abrams R, Grochow L: Adjuvant therapy with chemotherapy and radiation therapy in the management of carcinoma of the pancreatic head. *Surg Clin North Am.* 1995;75:925.

92. Lawrence T, et al: Radiosensitization of pancreatic cancer cells by 2′,2′-difluoro-2′-deoxycytidine. *Int J Radiat Biol Physics.* 1996; 34:867.

93. Burris H, et al: Improvements in survival and clinical benefit with Gemcitabine as first line therapy for patients with advanced pancreatic cancer: A randomized trial. *J Clin Oncol.* 1997;15:2403.

94. Rothenberg M, Moore M, Cripps M: A phase II trial of Gemcitabine in patients with 5-FU refractory pancreas cancer. *Ann Oncol.* 1996;7:347.

95. Scalliett P, et al: Gemcitabine with thoracic radiotherapy—A phase II pilot study in chemonaive patients with advanced non–small-cell lung cancer. *Proceed Am Coll Clin Oncol.* 1998; 17:499a.

96. Fajardo L, Berthrong M: Radiation injury in surgical pathology. Part III. Salivary glands, pancreas and skin. *Int J Radiat Oncol Biol Phys.* 1981;5:279.

97. Woodruff KH, et al: Postmortem examination of 22 pancreatic carcinoma patients treated with helium ion irradiation. *Cancer.* 1984;53:420.

98. Pilepich MV, Miller HH: Preoperative irradiation in carcinoma of the pancreas. *Cancer.* 1980;46:1945.

99. Kopelson G: Curative surgery for adenocarcinoma of the pancreas/ampulla of Vater: The role of adjuvant pre or postoperative radiation therapy. *Int J Radiat Oncol Biol Phys.* 1983;9:911.

100. Jessup JM, et al: Neoadjuvant therapy for unresectable pancreatic adenocarcinoma. *Arch Surg.* 1993;128:559.

101. Ishikawa O, et al: Clinical and histological appraisal of preoperative irradiation for adenocarcinoma of the pancreaticoduodenal region. *J Surg Oncol.* 1989;40:143.

102. Ishikawa O, et al: Concomitant benefit of preoperative irradiation in preventing pancreas fistula formation after pancreatoduodenectomy. *Arch Surg.* 1991;126:885.

103. Gnant M, et al: Neoadjuvant chemotherapy with Gemcitabine and Docetaxel for locally advanced pancreatic cancer. *Proceed Am Coll Clin Oncol.* 2002;21:149a.

104. O'Connell MJ: Current status of chemotherapy for advanced pancreatic and gastric carcinoma. *J Clin Oncol.* 1985;3:1032.

105. Arbuck SG: Overview of Chemotherapy for Pancreatic Cancer. *Int J Pancreatol.* 1990;7:209.

106. Loehrer P, et al: Ifosamide: An active drug in the treatment of adenocarcimona of the pancreas. *J Clin Oncol.* 1985;3:367.

107. Safran H, et al: Paclitaxel and concurrent radiation for locally advanced pancreatic and gastric cancer: A phase I study. *J Clin Oncol.* 1997;15:901.

108. Blackstock A, et al: Phase I trial of twice-weekly Gemcitabine and concurrrent radiation in patients with advanced pancreatic cancer. *J Clin Oncol.* 1999;17:2208.

109. McGinn C, et al: Phase I trial of radiation dose escalation with concurrent weekly full dose Gemcitabine in patients with advanced pancreatic cancer. *J Clin Oncol.* 2001;19:4202.

110. Wolff R, et al: Treatment related toxicities with rapid fractionation external beam radiation and concomitant Gemcitabine for locally advanced nonmetastatic adenocarcinoma of the pancreas. *Int J Radiat Biol Phys.* 1998;42:201.

111. Mason K, et al: Maximizing therapeutic gain with Gemcitabine and fractionated radiation. *Int J Radiat Biol Phys.* 1999;44:1125.

112. Mallinson CN, et al: Chemotherapy in pancreatic cancer: Results of a controlled, prospective, randomized multicentered trial. *Br Med J.* 1980;281:1589.

113. Frey C, et al: Randomized study of 5-FU and CCNU in pancreatic cancer. *Cancer.* 1981;47:27.

114. DeCaprio JA, et al: Flourouracil and high dose Leucovorin in previously untreated patients with advanced adenocarcinoma of the pancreas: Results of a phase II trial. *J Clin Oncol.* 1991; 9:2128.

115. Cullinan SA, Moertel CG, Fleming TR: A comparison of three chemotherapeutic regimens in the treatment of advanced pancreatic and gastric carcinoma: Fluorouracil vs Fluorouracil and Doxirubicin vs Fluorouracil, Doxirubicin and Mitomycin. *JAMA.* 1985; 253:2061.

116. Bakkevold KE, et al: Adjuvant combination chemotherapy (AMF) following radical resection of carcinoma of the pancreas and papilla of Vater—Results of a controlled, prospective, randomized multicentre study. *Eur J Cancer.* 1993;29A:698.

117. Friess H: LH-RH receptors in the human pancreas. *Int J Pancreatol.* 1991;10:151.

118. Bakkevold KE, et al: Tamoxifen therapy in unresectable adenocarcinoma of the pancreas and papilla of Vater. *Br J Surg.* 1990; 77:725.

119. Huguier M, et al: Treatment of adenocarcinoma of the pancreas with somatostatin and gonadoliberin (luteinizing hormone-releasing hormone). *Am J Surg.* 1992;164:348.

120. Wong A, Chan A: Survival benefit of Tamoxifen therapy of adenocarcinoma of the pancreas. *Cancer.* 1993;71:2200.

121. Hoffman J, et al: Phase II trial of preoperative radiation therapy and chemotherapy for patients with localized, resectable adenocarcinoma of the pancreas. *J Clin Oncol.* 1998;16:317.

122. Sindelar WF, Kinsella TJ: Randomized trial of intraoperative radiotherapy in resected carcinoma of the pancreas. *Int J Radiat Oncol Biol Phys.* 1986;12:148.

123. Kawamura M, et al: Electron beam intraoperative radiation therapy (EBIORT) for localized pancreatic carcinoma. *Int J Radiat Oncol Biol Phys.* 1992;23:751.

124. Foo ML, Gunderson LL, Nagorney DM: Patterns of failure in grossly resected pancreatic ductal adenocarcinoma treated with adjuvant irradiation ± 5-Fluorouracil. *Int J Radiat Oncol Biol Phys.* 1993;26:483.

125. Rich TA: Radiation therapy for pancreatic cancer: Eleven year experience at the JCRT. *Int J Radiat Oncol Biol Phys.* 1985; 11:759.

126. Whittington R, et al: Adjuvant therapy of resected adenocarcinoma of the pancreas. *Int J Radiat Oncol Biol Phys.* 1991; 21:1137.

127. Bakkevold KE, Kambestad B: Long-term survival following radical and palliative treatment of patients with carcinoma of the pancreas and papilla of Vater—The prognostic factors influencing long-term results. A prospective multicentre study. *Eur J Surg Oncol.* 1993;19:147.

128. Dalton RR, et al: Carcinoma of the body and tail of the pancreas: Is curative resection justified? *Surgery.* 1992;111:489.

129. Nagakawa T, et al: The results and problems of extensive radical surgery for carcinoma of the head of the pancreas. *Jpn J Surg.* 1991;21:262.

130. Shibamoto Y, et al: High dose, external beam and intraoperative radiotherapy in the treatment of resectable and unresectable pancreatic cancer. *Int J Radiat Oncol Biol Phys.* 1990;19:605.

131. Kawamura M, et al: Intraoperative radiation for carcinoma of the pancreas. *Nippon Igaku Hoshasen Gakkai Zasshi.* 1991; 51:1442.

132. Hiraoka T, et al: Combination of intraoperative radiation with resection of cancer of the pancreas. *Int J Pancreatol.* 1990;7:201.

133. Ozaki H, et al: Effectiveness of multimodality treatment for resectable pancreatic cancer. *Int J Pancreatol.* 1990;7:195.

134. Dobelbower RR, et al: Intraoperative electron beam radiation therapy (IOEBRT) for carcinoma of the exocrine pancreas. *Int J Radiat Oncol Biol Phys.* 1991;20:113.

135. Morrow M, Hilaris B, Brennan M: Comparison of conventional surgical resection, radioactive implantation, and bypass procedures for exocrine carcinoma of the pancreas 1975-1980. *Ann Surg.* 1984;199:1.

136. Sarr MG, Cameron JL: Surgical management of unresectable carcinoma of the pancreas. *Surgery.* 1982;91:123.

137. Moertel CG, et al: Therapy of locally unresectable pancreatic carcinoma: Randomized comparison of high dose (6000 Rads) radiation alone, moderate dose radiation (4000 Rads + 5-Fluorouracil), and high dose radiation + 5-Fluorouracil. *Cancer.* 1981;48:1705.

138. Seydel HG, et al: Hyperfractionated radiation and chemotherapy for unresectable localized adenocarcinoma of the pancreas. *Cancer.* 1990;65:1478.

139. Hogstrom KR, et al: Static pion beam treatment planning of deep seated tumors using computerized tomographic scans. *Int J Radiat Oncol Biol Phys.* 1979;5:875.

140. Al-Abdulla, ASM, et al: Experience with fast neutron therapy for unresectable carcinoma of the pancreas. *Int J Radiat Oncol Biol Physics.* 1981;7:165.

141. Cohen L, et al: Response of pancreatic cancer to local irradiation with high energy neutrons. *Cancer.* 1985;56:1235.

142. Kaul R, et al: Pancreatic carcinoma: Results with fast neutron therapy. *Int J Radiat Oncol Biol Phys.* 1981;7:173.

143. Smith FP, et al: Fast neutron irradiation for locally advanced pancreatic cancer. *Int J Radiat Oncol Biol Physics.* 1981;7:1527.

144. Castro JR, et al: Current status of clinical particle radiotherapy at Lawrence Berkeley Laboratory. *Cancer.* 1980;46:633.

145. Castro JR, et al: Clinical problems in radiotherapy of carcinoma of the pancreas. *Am J Clin Oncol.* 1982;5:579.

146. Linstadt D, et al: Comparison of helium-ion radiation therapy and split-course megavoltage irradiation for unresectable adenocarcinoma of the pancreas. Final report of a Northern California Oncology Group Randomized Prospective Clinical Trial. *Radiology.* 1988;168:261.

147. Klaassen DJ, et al: Treatment of locally unresectable cancer of the stomach and pancreas: A randomized comparison of 5-Flourouracil alone with radiation plus concurrent and maintenance 5-Flourouracil—An Eastern Cooperative Oncology Group Study. *J Clin Oncol.* 1985;3:373.

148. Talamonti M, et al: Eastern Cooperative Oncology Group phase I trial of protracted venous infusion fluorouracil plus weekly Gemcitabine with concurrrent radiation therapy in patients with locally advanced pancreas cancer. *J Clin Oncol.* 2000; 18:3384.

149. Crane C, et al: Is the therapeutic index better with Gemcitabine based chemoradiation than chemoradiation in locally advanced pancreatic cancer? *Int J Radiat Biol Phys.* 2002;52:1293.

150. Joyce F, et al: Ultrasonically guided percutaneous implantation of Iodine-I-125 seeds in pancreatic carcinoma. *Int J Radiat Oncol Biol Phys.* 1990;19:1049.

151. Dobelbower RR, et al: I-125 interstitial implant, precision high dose-rate external beam therapy, and 5-FU for unresectable adenocarcinoma of the pancreas and extrahepatic biliary tree. *Cancer.* 1986;58:2185.

152. Mohiuddin M, et al: Long-term results of combined modality treatment with I-125 implantation for carcinoma of the pancreas. *Int J Radiat Oncol Biol Phys.* 1992;23:305.

153. Montemaggi P, et al: Interstitial brachytherapy for pancreatic cancer: Report of seven cases and review of the literature. *Int J Radiat Oncol Biol Phys.* 1991;21:451.

154. Syed AMN, Puthawala AA, Neblett DL: Interstitial Iodine-125 implant in the management of unresectable pancreatic carcinoma. *Cancer.* 1983;52:808.

155. Shipley WU, et al: Iodine-125 implant and external beam irradiation in patients with localized pancreatic carcinoma. A comparative study to surgical resection. *Cancer.* 1980;45:709.

156. Peretz T, et al: Treatment of primary unresectable carcinoma of the pancreas with I-125 implantation. *Int J Radiat Oncol Biol Phys.* 1989;17:931.

157. Warszawski N, et al: Combined isodose curves of high-dose rate interstitial brachytherapy with external beam radiation therapy in pancreatic carcinoma. *Strahlentherapie und Onkologie.* 1992; 168:552.

158. Raben A, et al: Feasibility study of the treatment of primary unresectable carcinoma of the pancreas with 103-Palladium brachytherapy. *Int J Radiat Oncol Biol Phys.* 1996;35:351.

159. Abe M, et al: Clinical experience with intraoperative radiotherapy of locally advanced cancers. *Cancer.* 1980;45:40.

160. Dobelbower RR, et al: Treatment of cancer of the pancreas by precision high dose (PHD) external photon beam and intraoperative electron beam therapy (IOEBT). *Int J Radiat Oncol Biol Phys.* 1989;16:205.

161. Gunderson L, Martin JK, Earle JD: Intraoperative and external beam irradiation with or without resection: Mayo pilot experience. *Mayo Clin Proc.* 1984;59:691.

162. Latz D, Schraube P, Eble MJ: Primare Strahlentherapie des Inoperablen oder Rezidivierten Pankreaskarzinoms-Heidelberger Krankengut von 1982-1992. *Strahlentherapie und Onkologie.* 1993;169:387.

163. Roldan GE, et al: External beam versus intraoperative and external beam irradiation for locally advanced pancreatic cancer. *Cancer.* 1988;61:1110.

164. Shipley WU, et al: Intraoperative electron beam irradiation for patients with unresectable pancreatic carcinoma. *Ann Surg.* 1984;200:289.

165. Tepper J, et al: Intraoperative radiation therapy of pancreatic carcinoma: A report of RTOG 85-05. *Int J Radiat Oncol Biol Phys.* 1991;21:1145.

166. Wood WC, et al: Intraoperative irradiation for unresectable pancreatic carcinoma. *Cancer.* 1982;49:1272.

167. Goldson AL: Intraoperative radiotherapy for pancreatic cancer—Requiem or revival. *Int J Radiat Oncol Biol Phys.* 1991;21:1389.

168. Sindelar WF, Kinsella T: Randomized trial of intraoperative radiotherapy in unresectable carcinoma of the pancreas. *Int J Radiat Oncol Biol Phys.* 1986;12:148.

169. Tepper JE, et al: The role of misonidazole combined with intraoperative radiation therapy in the treatment of pancreatic carcinoma. *J Clin Oncol.* 1987;5:579.

170. Gunderson LL, et al: Intraoperative and external beam irradiation ± 5-FU for locally advanced pancreatic cancer. *Int J Radiat Oncol Biol Phys.* 1987;13:319.

171. Sasai K, et al: Pharmacokinetics of intratumoral RK-28, a new hypoxic radiosensitizer. *Int J Radiat Oncol Biol Phys.* 1992;24:959.

172. Mehta MT, et al: Y-90.B72.3 Against pancreatic cancer: Dosimetric and biologic analysis. *Int J Radiat Oncol Biol Phys.* 1990;19:627.

173. Phan GQ, et al: Pancreaticoduodenectomy for selected periampullary neuroendocrine tumors: Fifty patients. *Surgery.* 1997;122:989.

174. Samloski W, Eyre HJ, Sause W: Evaluation of the response of unresectable carcinoid tumor to radiotherapy. *Int J Radiat Biol Phys.* 1986;12:301.

175. Schupak K, Wallner K: The role of radiation therapy in the treatment of locally unresectable or metastatic carcinoid tumors. *Int J Radiat Biol Phys.* 1991;20:489.

176. Chakravarthy A, Abrams R: Radiation therapy in the management of patients with malignant carcinoid tumor. *Cancer.* 1995;75:1386.

177. Gaitan-Gaitan A, Rider WD, Bush RS: Carcinoid tumor—Cure by irradiation. *Int J Radiat Oncol Biol Phys.* 1975;1:9.

178. Keane TJ, et al: Whole abdominal radiation in the management of gastrointestinal carcinoid tumor. *Int J Radiat Oncol Biol Phys.* 1981;7:1519.

179. Hansen R, Helms J, Winson JF: Nonfunctioning islet cell of the pancreas. *Cancer.* 1988;62:15.

180. Torrisi JR, et al: Radiotherapy in the management of pancreatic islet cell tumors. *Cancer.* 1987;60:1226.

Cancer of the Liver, Bile Duct and Gallbladder

39

Raquel Wagman, MD, and Robin Schoenthaler, MD

RADIATION TOLERANCE

Any discussion about the use of radiation therapy (RT) in the treatment of hepatobiliary malignancies must be prefaced by a description of the radiotolerance of the liver and nearby structures. It is commonly held that there is a low risk of hepatitis if the whole liver receives less than 30 Gy in 3 to 4 weeks, but complication rates rise with whole liver doses exceeding 40 Gy (e.g., liver dysfunction occurs in 75% of patients receiving doses >40 Gy).[1] Fraction size influences the total tolerable dose: Lotze and associates,[2] quoting older literature, state there is a high risk for liver injury if more than 35 Gy is given in 2 Gy fractions and recommend no more than 25 Gy if given in 2.5 Gy fractions, or 21 Gy in 3 Gy fractions. These doses should be attenuated in the presence of certain drugs; Stevens,[1] citing Haddad's work, advocates no more than 20 to 25 Gy to the whole liver with standard fractionation if the patient has received doxorubicin.

With recent studies, a more detailed understanding of partial liver tolerance is emerging. Austin-Seymour and coworkers[3] used integral dose-volume histograms to conclude, "Doses in excess of 30 to 35 GyEq should be limited to 30% or less of the liver when 18 GyEq of whole liver radiation is delivered at 2 GyEq per fraction in addition to primary radiation . . . ." However, this conclusion was based on treatment with charged particles, only 11 patients were studied, and there was only one case of hepatitis. Lawrence and coworkers also used three-dimensional dose-volume histograms in 79 patients, 9 of whom developed radiation hepatitis, to predict the incidence of complications when using 1.5 to 1.65 Gy twice daily with concurrent intra-arterial 5-fluorodeoxyuridine (FUdR). Based on this work, the University of Michigan policy has been to give 66 to 72.6 Gy (with bid fractionation) when less than 33% of the "normal" liver is treated and 48 to 52.8 Gy when 34% to 67% of the liver is radiated ("normal" liver being that not occupied by tumor volume).[4]

Increasing use of intraoperative RT and brachytherapy will result in more sophisticated understanding of bile duct tolerance, as knowledge has thus far been limited by the presence of preexisting ductal injury, the frequency of recurrent or residual disease, and the use of relatively moderate doses of radiation. Kopelson reported asymptomatic biliary fibrosis following external beam doses of 60 Gy, but this has not been a problem clinically (or perhaps is masked by recurrent disease). Both animal and human data seem to show minimal risk to the ducts with single intraoperative RT doses under 20 Gy. Iwasaki and colleagues[5] now keep intraoperative RT doses under 20 Gy because of a high incidence of hepatic artery stenosis, obstruction, and aneurysm after doses of 20 to 30 Gy. Buskirk and associates[6] recommend long-term stent placement as a precaution based on their experience with temporary fibrosis following high brachytherapy doses.

Duodenal and gastric mucosal TD_5 values are reported to be 50 Gy. Virtually all practitioners recommend restriction of dose to these structures to under 55 Gy, and many stay under 50 Gy. The TD_5 and TD_{50} values for kidneys are 23 and 28 Gy, respectively.[7] The same values for spinal cord injury (myelopathy) are 50 and 60 Gy. Table 39-1 provides a summary of these tolerance doses.

HEPATOCELLULAR CARCINOMA

Hepatocellular carcinoma (HCC) is a minor malignancy in the United States (<4/100,000) but a major public health problem (>150/100,000 population) in Africa, China, and areas with high rates of hepatitis B infection (Table 39-2).[8] Multiple conditions have been associated with both animal and human HCC. For humans, the major accepted risk factors include chronic hepatitis B infection, hepatitis C,

Table 39–1 Radiotolerance Summary

Structure	Dose Range
Whole liver	30 Gy (2 Gy/day)
	20–25 Gy with chemotherapy
Partial liver	See text
Bile duct	Single dose <20 Gy
	Fractionated dose: unclear
Hepatic artery	Single dose <20 Gy
	Fractionated dose: unclear
Duodenum and stomach	50–55 Gy (2 Gy/day)
Kidney	<23 Gy (1.8 Gy/day)
Spinal cord	<50 Gy (1.8 Gy/day)

See text for data sources.

Table 39–2 Hepatocellular Carcinoma: International Distribution

Location	Incidence Rate*
Mozambique	113
China	34
Gambia	33
Senegal	26
Burma	26
Philippines	20
Nigeria	15
Korea	14
Brazil	9
Japan	7
Norway	1.8
UK	1.6

*Age-adjusted, in males.
Modified from Muir C, et al: *Cancer Incidence in Five Continents*. IARC Scientific Publications, Vol. V, No. 88. Lyons, France: International Agency for Research in Cancer, 1989.

and cirrhosis, particularly macronodular. In addition, HCC has been linked with genetic hemochromatosis, hereditary tyrosinemia, alpha$_1$-antitrypsin deficiency, aflatoxins, and possibly a promotional relation with alcohol.

The well-known clinical correlation between hepatitis, cirrhosis, and HCC continues to be explored. Tsukuma and associates[9] performed an elegant analysis of an alpha-fetoprotein (AFP) and ultrasonographic screening program of high-risk patients in Japan. They found the cumulative risk of developing HCC at 3 years to be 12.5% among patients with cirrhosis and almost 4% among patients with clinical histories of hepatitis. With the presence of hepatitis C antibody, the risk ratio was 4, and when patients were positive for hepatitis B surface antigen, it was 7. The highest ratio (10.2) was seen among hepatitis patients with cirrhosis and an elevated AFP level.

Work at the molecular level is in its infancy. There is currently no specific oncogene marker for HCC, but Voravud and coworkers[10] have reported that tumors from 12 of 14 HCC patients stained positively for c-*myc*, c-*ras*, and *erbB*-2. In another report, researchers fused HCC cells with activated B cells, producing immunogenic cells that had lost their tumorigenicity.[11] This may have important implications in both the prevention and treatment of HCC and other malignancies.

Anatomy and Physiology

The liver is divided into two lobes and eight subsections. There are no anatomic borders between the subsections and hence no barrier to intrahepatic spread of disease. Lymphatics run between the lobules and usually drain into the liver hilum and cisterna chyle. Drainage along the vena cava occurs approximately 20% of the time.

A unique aspect of liver physiology is the ability to regenerate. This fascinating property, which has implications in malignant transformation as well as in the treatment of liver disease, is just beginning to be understood. A number of molecular regulatory signals are believed to be

involved, including hepatocyte, epidermal, and fibrocyte growth factors, transforming growth factor-α, and possibly the angiotensins.

Pathology

Histologically, early HCCs are generally well differentiated but can eventually show poor differentiation with marked pleomorphism. The only widely agreed upon HCC subcategory is the fibrolamellar type, which tends to occur in younger populations with less preexisting liver disease and is associated with better outcome. The World Health Organization histologic classification[10] recognizes several HCC variants, including childhood, spindle cell, clear cell, combined, carcinosarcoma, and sclerosis; these subcategories are used more, less, or not at all at varying institutions.

Clinical Presentation

The presentation of HCC is often insidious, and clinical symptoms generally herald advanced disease. Unexplained weight loss in cirrhotic patients can be a warning sign. Patients often complain of antecedent malaise, anorexia, and occasionally abdominal pain. Some patients present in florid hepatic failure. Signs include fever of unknown origin, hepatomegaly or a right upper quadrant mass, evidence of portal vein obstruction, bruits, ascites, splenomegaly, or findings attributable to metastatic disease. Screening of high-risk patients with ultrasonography and measurement of AFP levels can help to detect small asymptomatic lesions, although the impact of early detection on survival is still unclear.[13,14]

Routes of Spread

The liver is the site of most disease activity and the primary tumor is often the cause of demise. Locally, there can be spread to vessels, nearby lymph nodes, the stomach, and the diaphragm. Distant sites include bone, lung, peritoneum, and brain.[4]

Diagnostic Studies

The list of imaging studies designed to evaluate local disease is headed by ultrasonography, which, by virtue of its low cost, sensitivity, noninvasive property, and relative simplicity of use, has been effective as both a screening and a diagnostic tool. It is useful in determining the number and size of lesions (lesions as small as 1 cm are detectable),[13] ductal status, and vessel patency. Contrast-enhanced computed tomography (CT) scans have a somewhat higher sensitivity than ultrasonography (94% vs. 81%, per the University of Pittsburgh),[2] but cirrhosis can seriously complicate the picture. CT can sometimes be valuable in evaluating disease beyond the liver, but angiography, particularly angioportography, can be of more help in both the detection of vessel invasion and the identification of variants. Lipiodol-enhanced angiography followed by CT scans a week later can reveal liver lesions as small as 2 mm.[13] Recent data suggest that contrast-enhanced magnetic resonance imaging (MRI) is the most sensitive technique for detecting liver nodules; dynamic hepatic arterial-phase contrast material-enhanced imaging is essential with both CT and MRI for visualization of small hepatic nodules in a background of cirrhosis.[15,16,17,18,19] Intraoperative ultrasonography can be invaluable to the surgeon but generally has minimal relevance to the radiotherapist. Metastatic studies include chest CT and bone scan. Figure 39-1 shows an example of a large hepatoma as seen on CT scan.

The benchmark laboratory study is the serum alpha-fetoprotein (AFP); it is elevated in 70% to 80% of all HCC patients. This rate is lower (≈30%) in the United States and Europe[8] and in patients with fibrolamellar histology. Overall, AFP, when used with a conventional cutoff point of 500 ng/mL, has a sensitivity of 50% and a specificity of 90% in detecting hepatocellular carcinoma in a patient with preexisting liver disease.[20] Higher levels are associated with poorer differentiation and shortened survival times.

A complete laboratory workup includes the AFP assessment, a complete blood count, liver function tests including measurement of the transaminases, alkaline phosphatase and lactate dehydrogenase, prothrombin and partial thromboplastin times (PT/PTT), glucose, cholesterol, albumin, and calcium. Hepatitis B and C serologies should be assessed. Amounts of carcinoembryonic antigen and the glycoprotein CA-19 can be elevated, but this finding is nonspecific. PIVKA-II (des-γ–carboxy prothrombin) assays are obtained at some centers. Table 39-3 provides a general outline of the workup for suspected HCC.

Histologic confirmation of tumor can be obtained through fine-needle aspiration, core biopsy, or open biopsy or resection. Some practitioners also obtain tissue from adjacent liver to determine the extent of coexistent hepatic

Table 39–3   Hepatocellular Carcinoma: Workup

History
   Hepatitis
   Alcohol use
   Environmental exposures
   Transfusions
   Travel
Laboratory Tests
   Alpha-fetoprotein
   Liver function tests
      transaminases
      alkaline phosphatase
      lactate dehydrogenase
      total and direct bilirubin
   Complete blood count (anemia, polycythemia?)
   PT/PTT (prolonged?)
   Glucose (hypoglycemia?)
   Calcium (hypercalcemia?)
   Cholesterol (elevated?)
   Albumin (decreased?)
   Hepatitis B surface antigen
   Hepatitis C antibody
   Carcinoembryonic antigen
   CA19
   PIKVA-II
Imaging Studies
   Ultrasonography
   CT scans with contrast and/or Lipiodol
   Angiography
   Chest x-ray or CT scan
   Bone scan
Histologic or cytologic confirmation

disease. Although these procedures can be technically difficult to perform because of underlying coagulopathies and tumor hypervascularity, in the absence of an elevated AFP, it is generally considered crucial to obtain a tissue diagnosis given the large differential and wide range of treatment options and prognoses. However, for tumors larger than 3 cm, with elevated AFP and clinical and radiographic findings suggesting hepatocellular carcinoma, the false-positive rate for diagnosis of HCC has been shown to be as low as 3%.[21]

The differential diagnosis of liver lesions includes metastasis, cyst, hamartoma, hemangioma, peripheral cholangiocarcinoma, adenoma, focal nodular hyperplasia, hepatoblastoma, melanoma, carcinoid, non-Hodgkin's lymphoma, sarcoma, and several other extremely rare entities.

Staging

Several staging systems have been proposed. Many clinicians categorize tumors as being (1) localized, (2) in liver only but in more than one lobe, or (3) metastatic. The Ugandan system emphasizes both functional (based on liver function test results and presence of cachexia, portal hypertension, ascites) and anatomic (number of lobes) characteristics in the presence or absence of cirrhosis. Okuda and colleagues[16] incorporate tumor size

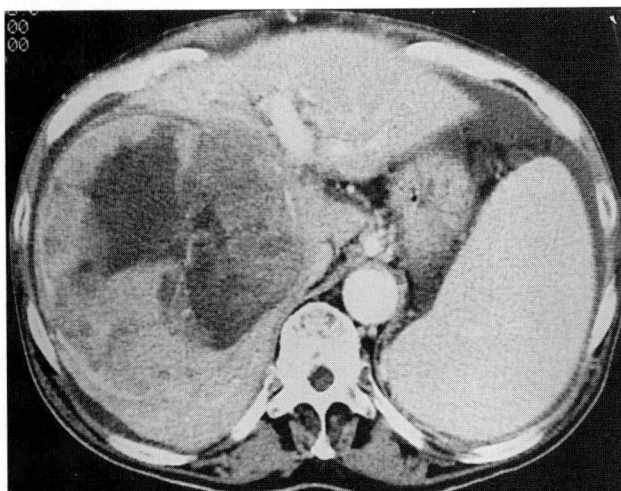

Figure 39–1. Hepatocellular carcinoma as seen on computed tomography scan. (Courtesy of Peter Mueller, MD, Department of Radiology, Massachusetts General Hospital, Boston.)

Table 39–4   Classification of Hepatocellular Carcinoma

Primary Tumor (T)

TX	Primary tumor cannot be assessed
T0	No evidence of primary tumor
T1	Solitary tumor without vascular invasion
T2	Solitary tumor with vascular invasion or multiple tumors, none more than 5 cm
T3	Multiple tumors more than 5 cm or tumor involving a major branch of the portal or hepatic vein(s)
T4	Tumor(s) with direct invasion of adjacent organs other than the gallbladder or with perforation of visceral peritoneum.

Regional Lymph Nodes (N)

NX	Regional lymph nodes cannot be assessed
N0	No regional lymph node metastasis
N1	Regional lymph node metastasis

Distant Metastasis (M)

MX	Distant metastasis cannot be assessed
M0	No distant metastasis
M1	Distant metastasis

Stage Grouping

Stage I	T1	N0	M0
Stage II	T2	N0	M0
Stage IIIA	T3	N0	M0
IIIB	T4	N0	M0
IIIC	Any T	N1	M0
Stage IV	Any T	Any N	M1

From Greene FL, Page DL, Fleming JD, et al, eds. *AJCC Cancer Staging Manual*, 6th ed. New York: Springer; 2002.

(percentage of liver), ascites, and albumin (<3 g/dL) and bilirubin (>3 mg/dL) levels. The TNM system for HCC, as developed by the American Joint Committee on Cancer (AJCC), is presented in Table 39-4.

THERAPEUTIC MODALITIES

Natural History and Prognostic Factors

Hepatocellular carcinoma generally develops insidiously, and many patients present with locally advanced disease, although few have metastatic spread. Outcome and treatment options are complicated by the coexistence of often severe liver disease.

If untreated or untreatable, patients live only a few months. Resectability strongly influences survival time, but only a fraction of patients are surgical candidates. The few surgical studies organized by stage show a sharp stage-related 3-year survival decline (stage I, 50%; stage II, 25%; stages III and IV, 10%[2]), but these rates are still considerably better than results seen in patients treated with any other therapies, as discussed later. In some studies, more than 90% of first failures are in the liver. One autopsy report also showed 57% of patients had disease outside of the liver, one-third in lymph nodes.[22] Overall, however, mortality is generally attributable to tumor-associated

liver failure. Deaths also occur secondary to chronic liver disease, metastatic spread (usually pulmonary), postoperative complications, or as sequelae of treatment.

Surgery

Surgery is currently the only potentially curative treatment modality for HCC patients. The goal is complete gross total resection of tumor with a margin of uninvolved hepatic tissue. Less than 25% of HCC patients are technically and medically surgical candidates.[22,23] Severe cirrhosis is often a contraindication to surgery and can be best evaluated using Child's classification, which uses the severity of encephalopathy and ascites, as well as the absolute values for bilirubin, albumin, and prothrombin time; all Child's C and many Child's B patients are not candidates for surgery. Other limits to curative surgical excision include vascular invasion (particularly the portal or hepatic vein) and multilobe involvement.[24] Contraindications to resection include lymphadenopathy, metastases, prolonged bleeding time, and poor overall medical condition.

Surgical prognostic factors have been identified by several groups. Kemeny and Schneider[22] cite poorer outcomes in patients with lesions greater than 2 cm (vs. 1 cm), elevated bilirubin or alkaline phosphatase levels, profound weight loss (>25%), ascites, and nonfibrolamellar histologies. Dusheiko and colleagues[13] describe a better overall survival in patients with tumors smaller than 2 cm with no extracapsular invasion and histologically negative margins (of >1 cm), and in Child's A patients. Chen and coworkers[24] had improved results in patients with tumors less than 5 cm and without portal vein involvement. The multivariate analysis presented by Ikeda and associates[25] revealed higher recurrence rates after curative resection if there were multiple nodules, high histologic grade, or negative hepatitis C antibody results.

Okuda and associates[16] describe a 3.4% operative mortality rate in Japan, much improved over historical rates because of modern diagnostic, surgical, anesthetic, and postoperative monitoring techniques. Chen and associates[24] had a 4% operative mortality in 120 patients in China, 46% of whom had cirrhosis (none were classified as Child's C). Postoperative morbidity rates have also varied; most modern surveys show severe complication rates of 5% to 10%. These include bleeding, hepatic failure, subphrenic abscess, sepsis, pleural effusion, and bile leakage.[24,25]

Okuda and associates[16] observed a 7-year overall survival rate of 45% in their select group of patients who underwent resection with curative intent. Ikeda and associates[25] reported a 5-year cumulative survival rate of 69% in patients managed very aggressively following recurrence after curative resection. Other surgical survival rates are lower: Chen and associates[24] had a 26% 5-year rate, and rates in the United States are generally under 35%.[26]

Liver transplants have been performed in several institutions internationally. Ringe and Iwatsuki's 1- and 3-year survival rates for liver transplantation were, respectively: stage I, 75% and 75%; stage II, 80% and 60%; stage III, 60% and 40%; and stage IVa, 50% and

15%.[27,28] Almost all deaths were due to hepatic recurrence. These reports include relatively small numbers of carefully selected patients. The 1983 National Institutes of Health Consensus Development Conference emphasized that recurrence is the rule after transplant for HCC but also noted "the procedure may achieve significant palliation."[2] More recently, prolonged survivals have been noted, particularly in patients with small, fibrolamellar lesions without lymph node involvement.

Chemotherapy

The use of chemotherapy has been disappointing. Intravenous (IV) agents, both single and multiple, have an overall response rate of 0% to 20% (average around 15%) with virtually all of these being partial responses. Intra-arterial chemotherapy has a higher response range (15% to 70%, average about 50%)[22] but has not been proven to improve survival. The most commonly used agents include fluorouracil (5-FU) or FUdR, doxorubicin, cisplatin, and mitomycin-C. In some centers, drugs are administered preoperatively in an attempt to increase resectability. Leung et al. found a response rate of 26% in a phase II trial using cisplatin, doxorubicin, 5-FU, and alpha-interferon in 50 patients with unresectable hepatocellular carcinoma. Nine patients underwent surgical resection after achieving a partial response, radiographically and, in four of these patients, histological examination of the resected specimens revealed no viable tumor cells.[29] Other institutions give chemotherapy regionally along with other agents (Gelfoam, microspheres, or the iodized oil Lipiodol). Side effects include varying degrees of transient abdominal pain, fever, nausea, anorexia, and ascites, and sometimes an elevation in liver function test values.[30]

Newer systemic agents are being explored. Hormonal therapy has a theoretical appeal but its efficacy has not yet been borne out by clinical studies of tamoxifen, ketoconazole, and goserelin acetate. Researchers are also evaluating the use of vasoconstrictors, which preferentially constrict portal vein flow. The primary agents under study are the angiotensins, particularly angiotensin II.

Other Modalities

Given the disappointing results with accepted resection methods and classic cytotoxic agents, a number of other modalities have been examined. The hepatic artery is a site of considerable interest, as it is generally the principal supply for the major portion, particularly centrally, of HCC tumors.[22] Quasi-surgical maneuvers include hepatic artery ligation or embolization with Gelfoam, Ivalon sponges, and other such materials. These are contraindicated in the presence of severe cirrhosis, portal vein invasion, or thrombosis.[13] Embolization can have short-lived effects because of recanalization. While some studies suggest an improvement in survival with chemoembolization, randomized trials have failed to confirm this.[22,31,32] Cryosurgery has been attempted in small series. Hyperthermia (generally in conjunction with external

beam radiation therapy) has been used with varying techniques with no impact on survival, but can reduce pain and mass size.[33] Ethanol injections, both percutaneously and intraoperatively, have been used for small primary tumors and for recurrent nodules. Necrosis at the site readily occurs, although hepatic recurrences elsewhere remain the rule. It seems to work best for lesions under 3 cm and is a common technique in Japan.[13] Hot saline has also been used for intralesional injection. A recent report describes no recurrences (with limited follow-up) and pathologic demonstration of no residual tumor in the few patients who underwent post-treatment biopsies.[34] A full list of treatment modalities can be found in Table 39-5.

RADIATION THERAPY

Early on, researchers determined that low doses of anterior-posterior–posterior-anterior (AP-PA) hepatic irradiation were ineffective in controlling gross HCC disease and that higher doses of whole liver irradiation resulted in high rates of radiation hepatitis. Stevens[1] states that 75% of patients treated with 40 Gy or greater to the whole liver will develop liver dysfunction and reports Finney's

Table 39–5   Hepatocellular Carcinoma: Therapeutic Modalities

Surgery
  Curative
    Lesionectomy with margin
    Lobectomy
    Transplant
  Palliative
    Lesionectomy
    Portal vein decompression
    Ductal stent placement
    Repeat resections
    Hepatic artery ligation or embolization
    Chemotherapy pump or reservoir placement

Chemotherapy
  Preoperative, postoperative, or "definitive"
  IA or IV cytotoxins
  +/– Embolization
  +/– Lipiodol
  Hormones

Radioisotopes
  ^{131}I-Antiferritin
  ^{131}I-Lipiodol
  Yttrium-90
  Carcinoembryonic antigen

Radiotherapy
  Historical
  Conformal
  Altered fractionation
  Protons

Miscellaneous
  Alcohol injection
  Hot saline injection
  Hyperthermia
  Cryosurgery
  Monoclonal antibodies

study[35] showing that 4 of 52 patients treated with more than 55 Gy had fatal hepatitis. These widely quoted early results have resulted in RT being placed on the "palliative" list of potential HCC therapies. More recent work has emphasized that although high doses of radiation cannot be administered to the whole liver, this does not necessarily imply that RT has no value, but rather that classic approaches to portals and fractionation must be abandoned and that innovative techniques should be evaluated. These fall into five categories: technical innovations designed to minimize normal hepatic irradiation, new fractionation protocols, new modalities, the use of radioisotopes, and the use of multimodality treatment.

A major innovation in portal approaches is CT-assisted three-dimensional conformal radiation therapy. Investigators at the University of Michigan have implemented a program consisting of high-dose, partial liver irradiation using conformal therapy in conjunction with intra-arterial chemotherapy. Their studies of 43 patients with unresectable hepatobiliary disease (27 with HCC) are instructive, although preliminary.[4,36,37] Doses ranged from 28.5 to 90 Gy and were based on the amount of normal liver tissue (evaluated by dose-volume histograms based on CT slices), which could be effectively excluded from the fields using three-dimensional treatment planning, multiple conformal portals, and immobilization. Initially patients received whole liver irradiation, a practice later abandoned because of toxicity and ineffectiveness. Of 25 assessable patients in whom partial liver was treated for local disease, there was a 68% overall response rate (one complete response). Nine patients failed in the treated site; the median potential follow-up is 26.5 months. In this series, there was one case of radiation hepatitis, and six cases of significant gastrointestinal toxicity when tumors and fields were near the stomach and duodenum. The median survival was 16 months overall, and 11 months for patients with local but unresectable HCC. For patients treated with 70 Gy or more, the median survival had not yet been reached at the time of publication of these results (16.4+ months compared with 11.6 months for those treated with lower doses, $P = 0.003$). These numbers exceed those quoted for radiation or regional chemotherapy alone and match most surgical series, and should serve as the basis for future studies using dose escalation and radiation sensitizers. A second major advance in treatment planning has been the development of gated treatments. Intra-abdominal organ motion has been shown to be a significant problem in the treatment of liver tumors; some series have found that the liver moves from 1 to 8 cm in the superior-inferior direction with respiration, and smaller shifts are noted in the anterior-posterior as well as left-right directions with breathing. Because of this significant displacement over time, standard (nongated) treatment techniques require large margins on the gross tumor volume to ensure full dose to the tumor throughout the respiratory cycle. However, with the advent of significantly improved conformal techniques, methods to account for internal organ motion are becoming increasingly important. Use of "gating" of respiration, whereby the delivery of dose is synchronized with patient respiration, has been proposed as one method to overcome the challenges posed by moving organs, and

has been shown to allow for sparing of normal tissues and for dose escalation.[38-40]

The primary alternative fractionation scheme used in this country has been hyperfractionation; twice-daily treatments were, in fact, used in the University of Michigan series.[4,36,37] The rationales for hyperfractionation are the rapid doubling time of HCC tumors (estimated at 41 days) and the shortened treatment times. In a nonrandomized study by the Radiation Therapy Oncology Group (RTOG),[41] 194 patients with advanced HCC (70% to 80% had metastases or had failed prior treatment) received treatment to the whole liver. Conventional fractionation (3 Gy four times per week to 21 Gy) was used in 135 patients, while 59 received 24 Gy in 1.2 Gy fractions twice a day. Concurrent doxorubicin and 5-FU were given intravenously every other day to both groups. The response rate for both was dismally low ($\approx$20%) and unaffected by fractionation scheme. Both acute esophagitis and thrombocytopenia occurred significantly more often in the group that received twice-daily radiation. It should also be noted that another RTOG study on patients with hepatic metastases found that 33 Gy given at 1.5 Gy twice a day resulted in an unacceptably high rate of liver injury; 27 and 30 Gy did not carry the same risk.[42] The role of twice-daily treatments in the work of Robertson and colleagues[4] cannot be elucidated at this time because of the preliminary nature of their results. Given the persuasive theoretical rationale for hyperfractionation and the need for decreased long-term morbidity, further studies seem worthwhile.

Charged particles have been shown, in reports of small, nonrandomized studies, to increase local control and survival rates in bile duct cancers.[43] A recent report[44] described a decreased tumor size in 92% of 15 HCC patients treated with 50 to 87 GyEq using protons in Japan; in 17 lesions treated with proton irradiation and "Lipiodol-targeted chemotherapy," 100% of patients had reduction in size of their tumor. These newer modalities may be able to minimize normal tissue effects via precise dose localization, and should be investigated further.

Much work has been done with various radioisotopes. Iodine-131-labeled (^{131}I) Lipiodol has considerable theoretical appeal given its avid uptake by HCC cells, and numerous small studies have shown it to be associated with a short-lived decrease in tumor size and AFP values.[22] A recent prospective randomized trial found significant improvement in local control, disease-free survival, and overall survival for patients who underwent curative resection followed by a single dose of intra-arterial ^{131}I-Lipiodol compared with postresection observation; with a median follow-up of 34.6 months, the recurrence rate for the adjuvant treatment group was 28.5% versus 59% for the control group ($P = 0.04$). Three-year overall survival in the treatment and control groups was 86.4% and 46.3%, respectively ($P = 0.039$).[45] Several institutions also plan to investigate Yttrium-90-labeled (^{90}Y) Lipiodol because of its advantages as a beta emitter. Another agent of interest has been ferritin, which is found in relatively high levels around HCC cells. ^{131}I-antiferritin and ^{125}I-antiferritin have been used alone or in combination with external beam radiation, chemotherapy, mixed bacterial vaccines, or hepatic artery ligation. A study from China of 41 patients

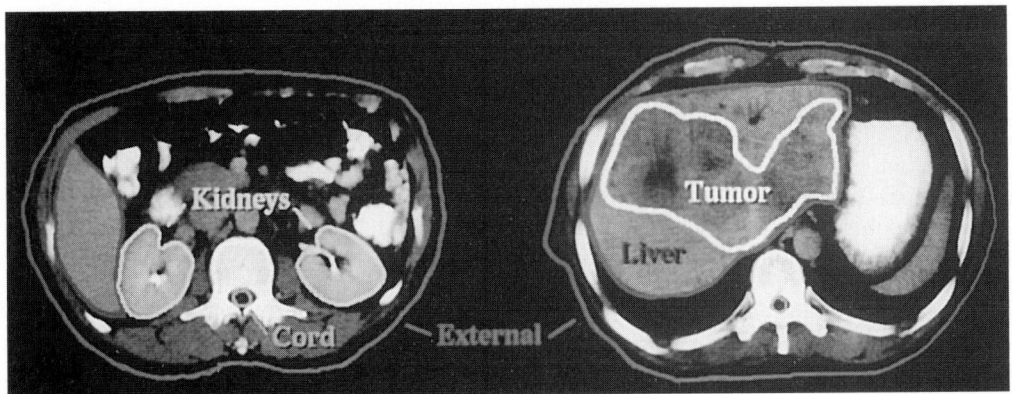

Figure 39–2. Contouring of critical structures for an external beam CT-guided radiotherapy plan (as used at the University of Michigan Medical Center). Contours are drawn on each computed tomography slice for tumor, liver, kidneys, spinal cord, skin, and, when appropriate, stomach and duodenum. See also Color Figure 39–2. (From Lawrence R, Kessler M, Robertson J: Conformal high-dose radiation plus intra-arterial floxuridine for hepatic cancer. *Oncology.* 1993;7:51.)

treated with hepatic artery ligation and intra-arterial antibody showed an increased resectability rate and higher 3-year overall survival rate compared with control subjects (25% vs. 7%).[46] A randomized RTOG trial[47] comparing IV chemotherapy with ^{131}I-antiferritin confirmed a comparable response rate (25%), a better response to antibody in patients whose AFP titers were low, and found a small but definable group of patients who became surgically resectable. Of note, in this series, all patients received "induction" whole liver irradiation (21 Gy in 7 fractions) and IV doxorubicin/5-FU chemotherapy 4 to 6 weeks before randomization. Also, radiolabeled monoclonal antibody work shows early promise. Zeng and coworkers[48] treated 23 unresectable patients with hepatic artery ligation and ^{131}I-Hepama-1, an anti-HCC monoclonal antibody. They found a 75% partial response rate as measured by tumor size and AFP level, and achieved a 48% resection rate.

Lastly, recent data suggests that the use of combined RT and embolization may give promising results. Seong et al. from South Korea evaluated 27 patients who had failed TACE (failure judged by incomplete tumor filling of Lipiodol Adriamycin on angiogram/CT), and went on to receive RT (51.8 Gy ± 7.9 Gy). They found objective responses in 67% of patients, and a median survival from RT start of 14 months, and 1-year overall survival of 85%.[49] In a separate review, Seong et al. evaluated 30 patients treated with TACE followed by *planned* RT, and noted a 63% objective response rate and a median survival of 17 months.[50] Cheng et al. reported similar results, with a median survival of 19.2 months in patients treated with combination radiation and TACE.[51]

Simulation

Immobilization can be made difficult by variations in patient size during a treatment course (e.g., resolution of ascites) and respiratory excursion. Commonly used immobilization methods include alpha cradles, Aquafoam casts, and low-density body cradles.

It is important to ascertain the location of *normal structures* during simulation, including the stomach,

duodenum, liver, kidneys, and spinal cord. These can be reconstructed by CT scans performed *in the treatment position,* and identification can be augmented through orally and intravenously administered contrast at the time of simulation.

CT treatment planning should be used, with IV and small bowel contrast to help define tumor and normal tissues. Landmarks are designated and entered into the computerized CT planning system. CT films are examined slice by slice, and tumor and critical structures are outlined. A formal, multiple-field treatment plan is devised, aiming for subtolerance irradiation (Fig. 39-2) of normal structures and a homogeneous dose distribution in the tumor volume (Fig. 39-3).

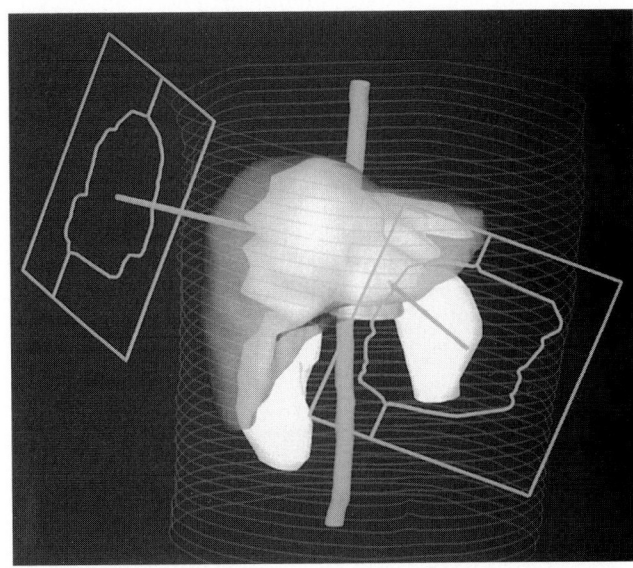

Figure 39–3. Multiple-beam conformal radiotherapy plan for hepatocellular carcinoma (as used at the University of Michigan Medical Center). A computer-generated plan showing varying angles and approaches to maximize tumor dose and minimize irradiation of the normal liver. See also Color Figure 39–3. (From Lawrence TS, Kessler M, Robertson J: Conformal high-dose radiation plus intra-arterial floxuridine for hepatic cancer. *Oncology.* 1993;7:51.)

Radiation Plans

Target volumes at the University of Michigan[36,37] included the CT-described tumor volume, a 1.5-cm margin in the AP and lateral directions to account for subclinical disease and patient position, and a 2.5- to 3.0-cm margin in the superior-inferior direction to account for respiratory excursion. Dose-volume histograms and normal tissue complication probability calculations were used in deciding upon the treatment dose.

Fractionation schemes have ranged from 21 Gy in 7 fractions[46] to varying hyperfractionation protocols. The University of Michigan[36,37] has used several dose schedules: 1.5 to 1.65 Gy twice a day to a total dose of 30 Gy, 1.5 Gy twice a day to 48 Gy (with a 16-day break after 18 Gy), and 1.5 to 1.65 Gy to 66 Gy (with a 16-day break after 36 Gy). Early on in their trials, the whole liver always received at least 30 Gy; but as noted earlier, this dose scheme is no longer in use. The RTOG, as reported by Stillwagon and associates,[41] used 1.2 Gy to 24 Gy to the whole liver in HCC and safely used 1.5 Gy twice a day to 27 to 30 Gy in the setting of liver metastases.[42] As noted earlier, investigators at the University of Michigan have described a dose-response pattern of patients with HCC treated with radiation, and have established that, with careful planning, high-dose irradiation can be delivered to parts of the liver safely; further studies are needed to confirm these findings.

Metastases

Radiation offers good palliation for HCC metastases. Anecdotal reports have revealed excellent relief of metastatic bone pain (80% to 100%), and Chen and colleagues[24] noted that good responses to radiation were seen in 33 patients with skin, nodal, pulmonary, and brain lesions, although recurrences were seen.

Follow-Up

After any treatment for HCC, patients should be closely followed with serial AFP titers, contrast-enhanced CT or MRI, and chest x-rays. Ikeda and coworkers[25] make a convincing case for aggressive treatment of recurrences with some of the best survival rates reported in the literature.

Summary

Hepatocellular carcinoma is a major health problem in much of the world. Patients often present with locally advanced disease in the setting of major hepatic compromise. Surgical resection seems to offer the only real hope for cure, but recurrences are often the rule, which has resulted in experimentation with a variety of systemic and local modalities. The role of radiation is unclear, although preliminary data suggests possible roles in both the ablative and adjunctive settings, with the use of varying fractionation schemes and sophisticated treatment planning systems to minimize damage to normal hepatic parenchyma. In the future, best results will probably be obtained with a multimodality program.

EXTRAHEPATIC BILE DUCT CARCINOMA

The term "extrahepatic bile duct carcinoma" (EHBDC) excludes tumors of the ampulla of Vater and gallbladder, intrahepatic adenocarcinomas, and hepatomas. EHBDCs are also known as cholangiocarcinomas. There are approximately 4500 new cases per year in the United States.[52,53] A host of predisposing factors have been proposed, as outlined in Table 39-6. The most widely accepted associations are with liver flukes, ulcerative colitis, and congenital biliary cysts. The tumor may be associated with several identified oncogenes. Voravud and coworkers[10] found that 63 cholangiocarcinomas stained positively for antibodies as follows: c-*myc*, 95% of tumors; c-*ras*, 75%; and *erbB*-2, 73%. There were no obvious differences in staining rates based on fluke infestation.

Anatomy

Bile duct anatomy follows fairly predictable general patterns, with variants that may be important to the surgeon and occasionally of interest to the radiation oncologist. The liver ductules gradually coalesce into right and left hepatic ducts, which then form the common hepatic duct (known as the "upper" or proximal third). Fused with the cystic duct from the gallbladder, they form the common bile duct (the middle third), which, as it draws nearer to the ampulla of Vater, becomes known as the distal common bile duct (the lower or distal third). This is a lymph-rich system: lymphatic channels course throughout the submucosa of bile ducts and eventually drain into the porta hepatis, the pancreaticoduodenal nodes, and the celiac axis.

Pathology

More than 90% of EHBDCs are adenocarcinomas of varying differentiations. Subclassifications include papillary, nodular, and sclerosing. The World Health Organization

Table 39–6 Carcinoma of the Bile Duct: Proposed Etiologic Factors and Associations

Flukes
  Clonorchis sinensis
  Opisthorchis viverrini
  Opisthorchis felineus
Ulcerative colitis
Crohn's disease
Congenital abnormalities
Choledochal cysts
Biliary atresia
Caroli's disease
Multiple biliary papillomatosis
Nitrosamines

Histological Classification[12] describes three grades and six variations of adenocarcinomas (papillary, intestinal type, mucinous, clear cell, signet ring, and adenosquamous). Special stains that help in the diagnosis include AFP, which is positive in 35% to 75% of hepatomas and almost never in EHBDC tumors; and CA 19-9 or CA-50, which is positive in 80% to 90% of cholangiocarcinomas and very rarely in hepatomas.[2] The remaining 10% of bile duct lesions include squamous cell, mucoepidermoid, granular cell, small cell, adenosquamous carcinoma, leiomyosarcoma, rhabdomyosarcoma, cystadenocarcinoma, carcinoid, Kaposi's sarcoma, angiosarcoma, melanoma, and lymphoma.

Clinical Presentation

On average, EHBDC tends to present in the seventh to eighth decades of life, although every report includes a few patients under 40. EHBDC is slightly more common in males, but the exact ratio varies from study to study. Initial signs and symptoms include jaundice, pruritus, right upper quadrant or epigastric pain, anorexia, weight loss, nausea, fever, hepatomegaly, and a right upper quadrant mass (Table 39-7). In end-stage disease, patients may have a periumbilical mass, massive ascites and limb edema, a rectal shelf, or supraclavicular lymphadenopathy.

Routes of Spread

When initially diagnosed, EHBDC tumors usually appear relatively small and circumscribed; patients rarely present with signs of overt metastatic disease. The bile duct tree is variably involved; 40% to 60% involve the hilus (upper third; Klatskin tumors), 10% to 15% involve the middle third, and 15% to 25% are in the distal third.[53,55] Less than 10% of patients present with multifocal/diffuse involvement of the biliary tree.[53-55] Although prognosis has historically been considered worse for hilar cholangiocarcinoma than for distal tumors, this is thought to represent the relatively later presentation and failure to institute effective therapy. Recent studies suggest that

Table 39–7   Carcinoma of the Bile Duct: Signs and Symptoms

Symptoms	Jaundice
	Pruritus
	Weight loss
	Anorexia
	Right upper quadrant pain
	Nausea
Signs	Icterus
	Right upper quadrant tenderness
	Fever
	Hepatomegaly
	Excoriations
Advanced disease	Right upper quadrant mass
	Periumbilical mass
	Rectal shelf
	Supraclavicular lymphadenopathy

location in the biliary tree has no impact on survival, provided that complete resection can be performed.[55]

Local-regional recurrences are exceedingly common, even in the fortunate few who are technically resectable, even with the use of aggressive adjuvant therapies. Prognostic factors for local failure include wall penetration and lymph node involvement; tumor location, grade, and perineural invasion may also have an influence on local relapse. Approximately 30% of patients have lymph node involvement at presentation[43,55]; the lymph nodes are a frequent site of recurrence owing to the extensive lymphatics in the bile duct submucosa. Intrahepatic involvement is extremely common at the time of failure, but is usually contiguous with the bile duct lesion itself. Metastases appear in the peritoneum, distant liver, bones, thoracic lymph nodes, and surgical or drain incisions[55,56]; but often, lethal local recurrence develops before systemic spread is clinically manifested.

Diagnostic Studies

Local imaging studies generally begin with ultrasonography to evaluate jaundice, and then proceed to CT scans, which often show dilated intrahepatic ducts and a normal-appearing extrahepatic biliary system. Historically, percutaneous transhepatic cholangiography (PTC), endoscopic retrograde cholangiopancreatography (ERCP), and angiography were considered standard investigations; currently, however, at Memorial Sloan-Kettering Cancer Center (MSKCC), magnetic resonance cholangiopancreatography (MRCP), CT, and duplex ultrasonography have replaced these invasive tests and can often provide the same information with less risk to the patient.[55] High-quality CT scans can provide indispensable information regarding vascular involvement, level of obstruction, and extent of liver atrophy. Similarly, in the hands of an experienced operator, duplex ultrasonography can provide information about not only vascular invasion, but also tumor extension within the bile duct and adjacent tissues. MRCP can provide information about the location of the tumor, level of biliary obstruction, presence of isolated ducts, patency of the hilar vascular structures, and the presence of nodal or distant metastases. Invasive cholangiography continues to have multiple uses, however, as it can serve to localize the tumor, act as a biopsy route, and allow for stent placement for biliary drainage or brachytherapy catheters; the need for an invasive procedure needs to be weighed with the risks of biliary intubation. Each modality can serve to pinpoint with considerable accuracy a site of stricture or obstruction, or intraductal disease extent. The primary metastatic study is a chest CT scan.

A tissue diagnosis is preferred, as several other conditions can mimic bile duct cancers, particularly sclerosing cholangitis. Cytology is accurate approximately 60% to 75% of the time.[2,52] The optimal method for obtaining tissue is controversial, however. Different institutions prefer brushings, CT-guided needle biopsies, or controlled open procedures. Buskirk and coworkers[6] have shown a 37% incidence of peritoneal seeding if there is violation of the lesion, and they recommend the use of transabdominal fine-needle biopsies following stent placement.

Laboratory studies include a full liver function panel including assessment of the transaminases, alkaline phosphatase, lactate dehydrogenase, total and direct bilirubin levels, complete blood count, and PT/PTT. Other potential laboratory tests depend on the certainty of diagnosis and the width of the differential (Table 39-8).

The differential diagnosis includes sclerosing cholangitis, carcinoma of the gallbladder, duodenum, or pancreas with local extension; hepatoma, and benign stricture.

Staging

The AJCC TNM staging classification for extrahepatic bile duct carcinoma is provided in Table 39-9. It has limited applicability in evaluating the older medical literature due to its modified and inconsistent use. In addition, pathologists apply and report these criteria inconsistently, biopsy-only specimens can include insufficient tissue for full T-staging, and lymph nodes are often not resected, even during curative procedures. Lastly, as this staging system is based upon pathologic criteria, it has little value in preoperative staging and prediction of resectability.

THERAPEUTIC MODALITIES

Surgery

The primary curative modality for EHBDC tumors is surgery. However, the "hostile anatomical arrangements ... make this ... challenging to the surgeon and dangerous to the patient."[52] Tumor location can be a critical factor in resectability, applicable surgical procedure, and survival. Resectability rates are low, ranging from 5% to 47%. The operability rates appear to be falling as preoperative diagnostic expertise increases, but the ensuing ability to safely perform complete resections grows as patient selection improves, particularly with Klatskin tumors.[53,57] Contraindications to "curative" surgical resection include hepatic duct involvement up to secondary biliary radicles bilaterally, encasement/occlusion of the main portal vein

Table 39–8   Carcinoma of the Bile Duct: Workup

Laboratory Tests
   Liver function tests, including
      transaminases
      alkaline phosphatase
      lactate dehydrogenase
      total and direct bilirubin
   Complete blood count
   PT/PTT
Imaging Studies
   Ultrasonography
   CT scan
   Percutaneous transhepatic cholangiography
   Endoscopic retrograde cholangiopancreatography
   Angiography
Histologic or Cytologic Material

Table 39–9   Classification of Carcinoma of the Bile Duct

Primary Tumor (T)

TX	Primary tumor cannot be assessed
T0	No evidence of primary tumor
Tis	Carcinoma in situ
T1	Tumor confined to the bile duct histologically
T2	Tumor invades beyond the wall of the bile duct
T3	Tumor invades the liver, gallbladder, pancreas, and/or unilateral branches of the portal vein (right or left) or hepatic artery (right or left)
T4	Tumor invades any of the following: main portal vein or its branches bilaterally, common hepatic artery, or other adjacent structures, such as the colon, stomach, duodenum, or abdominal wall

Regional Lymph Nodes (N)

NX	Regional lymph nodes cannot be assessed
N0	No regional lymph node metastasis
N1	Regional lymph node metastasis

Distant Metastasis (M)

MX	Distant metastasis cannot be assessed
M0	No distant metastasis
M1	Distant metastasis

From Greene FL, Page DL, Fleming JD, et al, eds. *AJCC Cancer Staging Manual*, 6th ed. New York: Springer; 2002.

proximal to its bifurcation, atrophy of one hepatic lobe with encasement of the contralateral portal venous branch or with contralateral involvement of secondary biliary radicles, distant metastases (peritoneum, liver, lung), and significant medical comorbidities.[55] EHBDC resections demand considerable skill and experience on the part of the surgeon. Klatskin tumors, that is, those at the bifurcation, can require lobectomy. Distal bile duct tumors are often treated with a Whipple procedure (pancreaticoduodenectomy). The primary goal of palliative procedures is to improve the quality of life through resolution of jaundice and pruritus, prevention of infection, and improvement in pain. Options include palliative debulking, external or internal stent placement, and bypass operations, including hepaticojejunostomies for proximal disease. Palliative procedures are accompanied by high 30-day mortality rates and short survivals with inconsistent improvements in quality of life.

Survival rates after any surgical resection, even curative ones, are low. Median survivals after gross total resection and palliative surgery have been remarkably consistent over the past decade with values of 17 versus 8.5 months,[58] 22 versus 7 months,[54] 32 versus 8 months,[57] and 23 months versus 8 months,[53] respectively. Likewise, Boerma,[59] in an analysis of more than 1000 patients treated worldwide, found a mean survival of 21 versus 11 months. Cameron and associates[60] showed a 32% 2-year survival after gross resection and 6% survivorship after stenting; University of California, San Francisco (UCSF) rates were 44% and 11%. Tompkins and associates[61] found a 27% 5-year survival rate after resection and 7% to 9% after bypass.

Local recurrence is the most common site of failure and cause of mortality: After potentially curative resections, the local failure rate was 59% in the study by Kopelson and associates[62] and 53% in the study by Cameron and associates.[60]

Complete resections were performed on 21% of patients treated at UCSF in the years 1977 to 1987.[41] This is similar to that of other major biliary centers where resectability rates range from 5% to 47%.[52,53,60,61,63] The finding of tumor at the margins of macroscopically resected specimens is the rule, however, rather than the exception.[56,63] Among UCSF patients, 5% of the total group had microscopically negative margins (22% of those with complete resections), with median survivals of 39 months. Patients with microscopically positive margins fared less well than those with negative margins but significantly better than those with gross tumor (median survivals of 11 vs. 5 months).[54] Over the past 20 years, an increase in the use of hepatic resection, especially for patients with hilar cholangiocarcinoma, has been noted; some believe that this is responsible for the increase in the percentage of negative margin resections, and an observed improvement in survival in some series.[55]

Wide variations in morbidity and mortality are seen because of variabilities in tumor site, disease extension, medical condition, referral patterns, and institutional expertise. An acceptable mortality rate for Whipple procedures is under 5%. A recent review[59] of the world's literature on hilar bile duct cancer management since 1980 described an overall mortality rate of 8% after local resection and 15% after hepatic resection. Regarding all bile duct sites, Reding and colleagues[53] reported a 26% hospital mortality rate in a summary of the experience at 55 centers over several decades. At UCSF, Princess Margaret Hospital, and Johns Hopkins Hospital, similar crude mortality rates of 4.8%, 3%, and 4%, respectively, were observed.[54,57,60] Other recent reports indicate that mortality rates are higher after palliative procedures, a finding that confirms intuition.[52,57] Postoperative complication rates are high (39% at Johns Hopkins,[60] 25% at UCLA[64]), and can include wound infection, liver or subphrenic abscess, cholangitis, pulmonary embolus, gastrointestinal hemorrhage, and small bowel obstruction.

Liver transplantation has been performed at several centers. Investigators at the University of Pittsburgh[65] reported a 22% 4-year survival rate in nine patients who underwent orthotopic liver transplantation followed by RT (two are alive with no evidence of disease after 50 months). They found that transplant with postoperative RT was "the only treatment factor studied that improved survival." Patients treated by Ringe and associates[66] had an overall median survival of 16 months, but a subgroup with uninvolved lymph nodes had a 2-year actuarial survival rate of 64%. However, the reported high incidence of recurrence both in the allograft and in distant organs after transplant for EHBDC suggests that this should not be considered a standard treatment option.[55,67]

Chemotherapy

The use of chemotherapy has been described in multiple, small, single-institution studies. Lotze and associates[2] reviewed the literature and found a 16% response rate

with single-agent therapy, an 18% rate with multiple agents, and a 45% rate with hepatic artery infusion. More recently, gemcitabine has been evaluated and, in one series, a 30% overall response rate was seen in patients with cholangiocarcinoma, with relief of tumor symptoms or weight gain seen in 7 of 11 patients.[68] However, no effect on survival has been seen with any agents. The only randomized study, an Eastern Cooperative Oncology Group (ECOG) report examining combinations of 5-FU, semustine (methyl-CCNU), and streptozocin, concluded that "none of the regimens studied seems to be of sufficient value to justify use in clinical practice."[69] Furthermore, no study has shown any survival improvement for EHBDCs when chemotherapeutic agents (including 5-FU) are combined with radiation.[54,65]

Radiation Therapy

Historically, the use of external beam RT was largely limited to unresectable, recurrent, or gross residual disease treated in the pre-CT era, and this led to the conclusion that EHBDCs were radioresistant. There is, however, no evidence that bile duct tumor cells have an inherent radioresistance, but rather that the doses of radiation generally administered have been limited by the surrounding structures. Indeed, some recent reports indicate that radiation limited to relatively small fields but reaching higher dose levels, combined with more modern surgical approaches and techniques, may have a positive effect on outcome.[43,56,60] Generally, this improvement has been found to be most marked in the setting of minimal residual disease,[43] although occasionally an advantage is seen in unresectable patients treated with stents and radiation.[60] It should be kept in mind that all of these reports are of relatively small, nonrandomized, single-institution, historical experiences. One institution has discussed the initiation of a prospective randomized study.[60]

The indications for postoperative RT are not yet clear. There are no available data on the role of RT following complete resection with negative margins; these patients are rarely referred for consideration of radiation therapy, although the available data suggests isolated local-regional recurrence rates of up to 60% after curative resection alone (personal communication, W. Jarnagin, 2003). Some recent studies seem to indicate a potential role for postoperative RT when a tumor is grossly resected but positive margins are present. Cameron and coworkers[60] reported a 41% 2-year actuarial survival rate if the tumor is completely resected (33/39 had positive margins) and a 31% rate if radiation was added, but he also noted that the only survivors (3/53) at 5 years had all undergone radiation therapy, and that radiation was given to a mixture of patients with completely and partially resected tumors. The patients who underwent resection in a study by Gonzalez and associates[56] had median survivals of 19 and 8 months and 2-year survival rates of 42% and 18% with and without radiation, respectively ($P = 0.0005$). Schoenthaler and coworkers[54] reported that the median survival for patients with microscopic residual disease was 21.5 months when treated with adjuvant photon irradiation, and 11 months when RT was not

Table 39–10   Carcinoma of the Bile Duct: Impact of Radiation and Extent of Residual on Survival

	Median Survival, mo				
	S	S + X	S + CP	*Overall*	P Value
No microscopic disease	39	—	—	39	N/A
Microscopic disease	11	21.5	61	19	S vs S + X: *P* = 0.01
					S vs S + CP: *P* = 0.0005
Gross disease	5	9	10	7	S vs S + X: *P* = 0.05
					S vs S + CP: *P* = 0.04

S, surgery alone; S + X, postoperative photons; S + CP, postoperative charged particles.
Modified from Schoenthaler R, Phillips T, Castro J, et al: Carcinoma of the extrahepatic bile ducts: The UCSF experience. *Ann Surg.* 1994;219:267.

used (*P* = 0.0109; 61 months with charged particles, *P* = 0.0005) (Table 39-10). A large French study of 552 patients at 55 centers has been cited as showing no radiation effect, but, in fact, only 5% of these patients received any form of radiation therapy.[53]

The influence of adjuvant postoperative radiation on patients with gross disease has also been explored. Schoenthaler and colleagues[54] showed that radiation had a reduced but still statistically significant impact (median survival of 9 vs. 5 months with and without radiation, *P* = 0.05). Grove, as described by Lotze and coworkers,[2] reported a median survival of 12.2 versus 2.2 months (*P* = 0.005), while Reding and colleagues[53] had corresponding values of 13 versus 8 months, both groups with small patient numbers. In the study by Cameron and coworkers,[60] 10% of patients treated with stents and radiation were alive at 2 years, while none of the patients treated with stenting alone survived.

The majority of patients with EHBDC tumors die of their disease. At times, the exact cause of death can be difficult to document; abnormal radiographic findings are frequently present after the definitive therapy, disease progression is often evaluated clinically, intervening infections and treatment-related side effects can confuse the picture, and autopsies are infrequently performed or reported. Overall, the literature is full of considerable "best guess" work as to the cause of death. As an example, death due to "hepatic failure" may be secondary to local recurrence, sepsis, radiation hepatitis, surgical misadventure, biliary obstruction, liver abscess, bile duct sclerosis, cholangitis, hepatic metastases, and so on. However, it is generally agreed that local failure plays a significant role in many EHBDC deaths, and that this is a persistent problem after surgery with or without irradiation, and after irradiation alone, with recurrent or persistent local disease rates ranging from 50% to 83%.[43,56]

Prognostic factors that may assist in determining which patients might benefit from adjuvant therapy include age younger than 65 and small tumor size (Table 39-11).[54] The degree of differentiation, lymph node involvement, local invasiveness, and papillary characteristics may also serve as prognosticators. All of these factors must be weighed with the demands of upper quadrant irradiation, the patient's overall medical status, and the significant quality-of-life issues raised by this disease. As always, by far the most important prognosticator for survival is the extent of resection.

There is scant evidence for a dose-response relationship in the treatment of cholangiocarcinomas. One of the obstacles to its determination is the enormous number of local failures with few successes left for analysis. Flickinger and coworkers[65] and Schoenthaler and coworkers[43] attempted to overcome this difficulty by performing a reanalysis of their patients, eliminating those who died shortly after the initiation of treatment (e.g., within 1 or 2 months). Even after eliminating "dose-selection bias," however, there is no clear-cut evidence for an optimal RT dose; while some studies suggest improved outcome with higher dose, others report increased morbidity with increasing dose.

Short-term morbidity associated with standard external beam RT includes nausea, vomiting, malaise, fatigue, or weight loss, and many patients with in-dwelling catheters have intermittent fevers. Long-term post-RT complications, particularly duodenal, have been reported in the literature at rates that seem to vary with survival times, and are discussed in greater detail in later sections. Efforts to minimize dose to nearby radiosensitive structures, and hence to minimize complications, may include brachytherapy in combination with external beam therapy (potentially using the new technology of high-dose-rate

Table 39–11   Carcinoma of the Bile Duct: Prognostic Factors

Factor	Survival, mo	P Values
Age		0.0085
<65	13	
>65	7	
Gender		0.7166
T Classification		0.0001
T2	19	
T4	5	
N Classification		0.0036
N0	16	
N+	7.5	
Differentiation		0.0159
Well differentiated	13	
Moderately	13	
Poorly	5	
Location		0.4432
Chemotherapy		0.2269
Previous malignancy		0.4338

Modified from Schoenthaler R, Phillips T, Castro J, et al: Carcinoma of the extrahepatic bile ducts: The UCSF experience. *Ann Surg.* 1994;219:267.

brachytherapy), intraoperative radiation therapy, higher linear energy transfer modalities, radioprotectors, and the increasing use of CT-based conformal planning systems.

Brachytherapy has been used at numerous institutions. Overall, there appears to be a small trend toward improved survival with its use as a boost.[55] The potential advantages are clear: the area is reasonably accessible via stents placed during surgery or by the interventional radiologist; a high dose can be limited to a few surrounding centimeters; the risk of serious short-term toxicity is low, although most series report rates of cholangitis of 30% to 50%. Dose distributions can be quite satisfactory with the use of ^{192}Ir catheters (Fig. 39-4). Long-term complications secondary to the high doses and use of stents are common, and include stricture, bowel obstruction, and bleeding. In addition, the rapid dose falloff means that some of the high-risk area may well lie outside the high-dose area, so brachytherapy should only be used in conjunction with external beam radiation therapy; no study has shown that brachytherapy alone has anything but the briefest of palliative effects. Reports of high-dose rate brachytherapy are just beginning to appear in the literature.[70]

The use of charged particles has been reported by Lawrence Berkeley Laboratory, where 18 patients were treated with curative intent from 1977 to 1987 with helium or neon or both.[43] Two-year actuarial survival was 50% for particle-treated patients (compared with 18% for patients treated with photons; $P = 0.048$). Local control was also improved, although less significantly, in patients treated with particles (median local control 20 months vs. 4.5 months; $P = 0.054$). Multivariate analysis showed that only the extent of residual disease predicted outcome; median survival was 23 months for the whole group but 32 months if only microscopic residual disease remained after surgery. There was also a trend toward improved survival with neon: Median actuarial survival in the neon-treated patients was 25 months, whereas the patients treated with helium had a survival of 12.5 months. This pattern did not reach statistical significance ($P = 0.23$) because of small patient numbers, but the use of heavy charged particles has a sound theoretical basis, as it combines improved dose localization with increased relative biologic effectiveness and linear energy transfer.

There are currently 4 long-term survivors (6 to 9 year follow-up) in the Lawrence Berkeley Laboratory series of 18, for a crude rate of 22% (personal communication, J. Castro, 1995). This is one of the highest survival rates seen in the literature, and may be due to the combination of sophisticated treatment planning, higher dose (median dose 60 GyEq with a range of 48 to 68), and, in the case of the neon-treated patients, higher relative biologic effectiveness. Transient serious adverse sequelae occurred in the majority of patients who survived more than a year. Interestingly, the one patient to survive with no evidence of disease and no serious radiation-associated complications was treated with a brachytherapy implant in

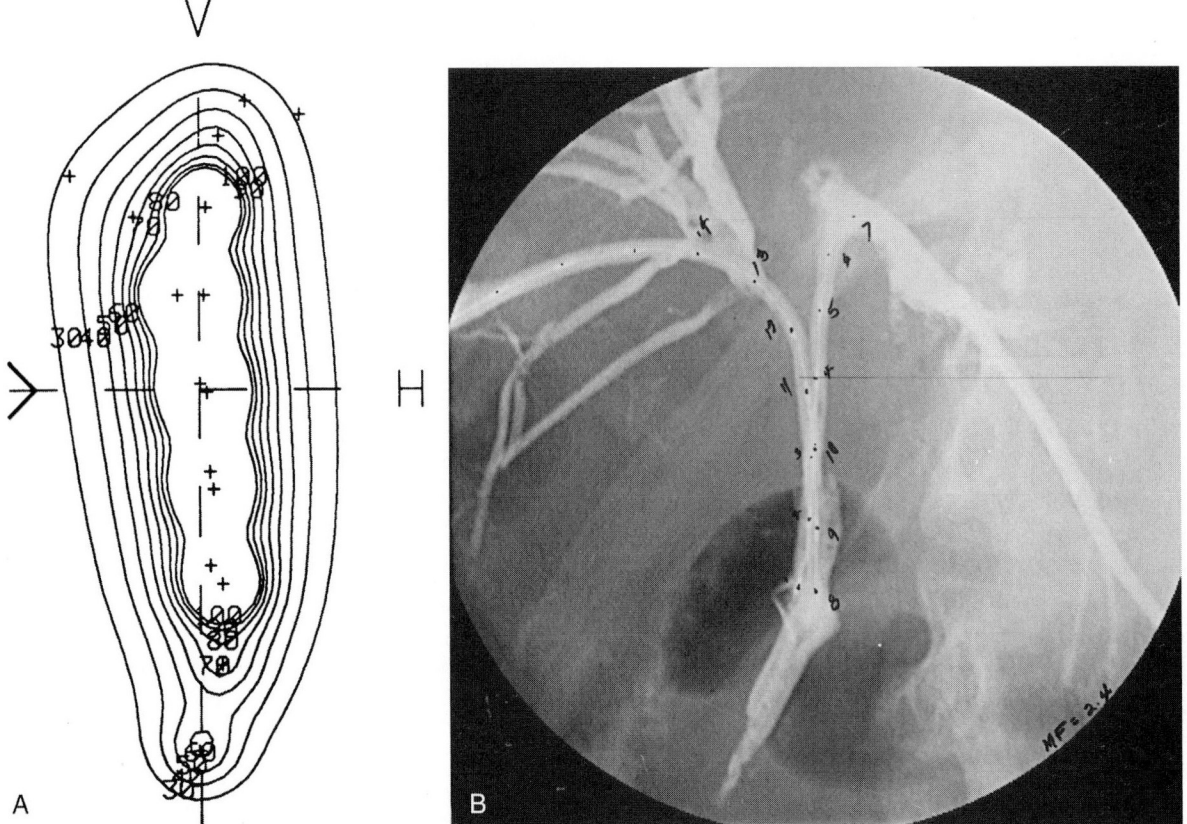

Figure 39–4. [192]Ir brachytherapy treatment for an extrahepatic bile duct carcinoma (as used at the University of California at San Francisco). **A,** Fourteen ^{192}Ir sources are used to create the dose distribution seen. **B,** Simulation film for brachytherapy treatment. (Courtesy of Mack Roach, MD, and Bob Roberts, RTT, Department of Radiation Oncology, University of California at San Francisco.)

addition to helium treatments, raising the possibility that combining radiation modalities may be a potentially useful tool.

Lawrence and colleagues[36] published the earliest reports on photon conformal therapy. There appears to be a trend for an improvement in disease-free survival, and two of the nine patients have lived for more than 2 years, but follow-up is too short for any definitive conclusions.

Intraoperative RT has been used on EHBDCs at several institutions. After promising preliminary work in Japan, an RTOG protocol (85-06) gave 14 to 22 Gy as intraoperative RT before 45 to 50 Gy external beam to eight evaluable patients with unresectable, unresected, or recurrent tumors. Two patients were alive (one with no evidence of disease) at the time of publication with a median follow-up of 10.5 months.[71] In their study of 15 patients, Busse and coworkers[72] had a median survival of 14 months with a 50% local control rate using 5 to 20 Gy. In the study by Buskirk and coworkers,[6] the only long-term survivors had either intraoperative RT or a brachytherapy boost. All of these reports involve the use of both intraoperative and external beam radiation therapy, as the use of the intraoperative RT alone (or brachytherapy alone) has not been shown to have a durable impact.

Simulation

Patients are generally placed supine; the treatment position should be reproducible, ideally through an immobilization device (Fig. 39-5). Critical structures to be identified include the tumor volume, kidneys, liver, stomach, duodenum, and spinal cord. IV contrast at the time of simulation (or an IV pyelogram done immediately before the simulation) identifies the kidneys on the simulation films; at MSKCC, we use a CT scan obtained in the treatment position to accurately identify tumor volume and adjacent normal tissues. Oral contrast material, ingested 10 to 30 minutes before simulation, allows for visualization of the stomach and proximal small intestine. Preoperative tumor volumes can be ascertained through diagnostic CT scans, ERCP, PTC, MRCP, ultrasound evaluations; physical examination findings should not be overlooked. Good documentation of the anterior-posterior and lateral-medial extent of disease requires review of the operative reports and consultation with the surgeon. Metallic clips placed intraoperatively in the tumor bed can also offer guidance, and the CT scan can sometimes be of further assistance in target localization. If stents are in place, contrast may be of help during the actual simulation process.

Kao and associates[73] did a helpful study of bony landmarks for the celiac axis. Based on their findings, the field should extend superiorly/inferiorly from at least the T11 to T12 interspace to L2 to L3 whenever radiologic data is uncertain.

Representative examples of typical treatment portals are shown in Figure 39-6. Table 39-12 gives a summary checklist for EHBDC simulations.

Radiation Plans

The standard fractionation protocol for typical three- or four-portal plans treating the tumor volume, draining lymph nodes (porta hepatis, pancreaticoduodenal, and celiac), and margin is 1.8 Gy per day, 5 days per week, to a total dose of 45 Gy. With very large tumors, a second smaller field may have to be designed to preserve normal liver. Thereafter, a cone-down treatment to a volume of tumor bed with a smaller margin is taken to 50 or 54 Gy depending on dose to the surrounding radiosensitive structures, particularly the stomach and duodenum. A few practitioners will use doses as high as 60 Gy if tumor location allows and the patient understands the additional risks. Margins for the original fields range from 3 to 5 cm, depending on the standards of the institution, and are usually reduced to 1.5 to 3 cm for the boost. An additional margin should be considered for the superior and inferior borders to account for diaphragmatic motion. Cone-down treatments can be given through reduced AP-PA–lateral portals, wedged pairs, arcs, or obliques. Three-dimensional CT conformal treatment planning can be invaluable in designing boost fields that minimize normal tissue dose deposition. In each of these fields, individually designed Cerrobend blocks or multileaf collimators are vital to preserve as much normal tissue as possible, and doses to liver, stomach, duodenum, both kidneys, and spinal cord should be monitored. Lateral fields and blocks help protect the spinal cord. Multiple fields help minimize doses to the liver and upper gastrointestinal tract (Figs. 39-7 and 39-8).

Another boost technique used at some institutions is brachytherapy. Ideally, an external beam dose designed to eradicate microscopic disease (i.e., 45 to 50 Gy) is given

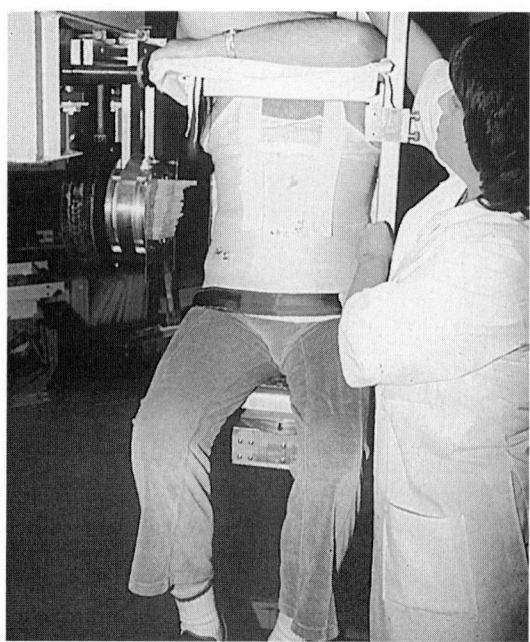

Figure 39–5. Immobilization device for external beam treatment for hepatobiliary carcinomas, with which increased accuracy of dose distribution can be obtained. (Courtesy of Joseph R. Castro, MD, Department of Radiation Oncology, University of California at San Francisco, and Lawrence Berkeley Laboratory, Berkeley, Calif.)

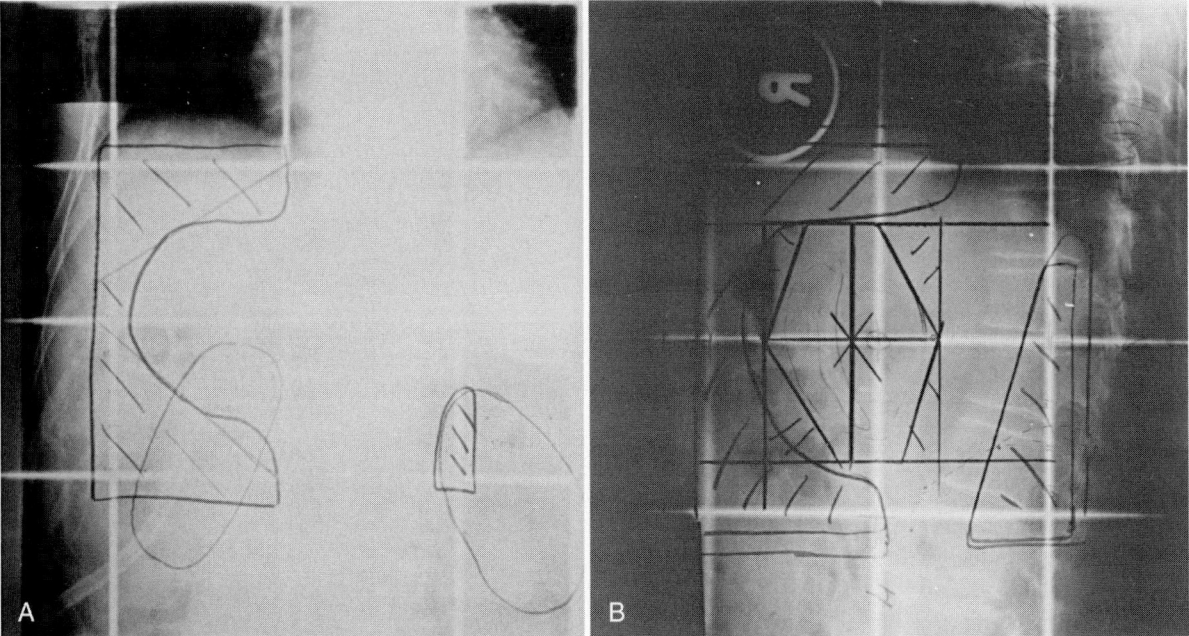

Figure 39–6. Anterior-posterior–posterior-anterior **(A)** and lateral **(B)** portals for extrahepatic bile duct carcinoma. Presimulation contrast aids in the localization of kidneys and stomach. Location of tumor and spinal cord can also be noted. (Courtesy of Christopher Willet, MD, Department of Radiation Oncology, Massachusetts General Hospital, Boston.)

first, followed by seed placement designed to give an additional high dose to the site of gross or highly suspect disease. Doses ranging from 15 to 100 Gy have been administered using [192]I, ^{131}I, and [198]Au. Dose is usually prescribed at 0.5 to 1.0 cm from the radiation sources (see Figs. 39-4A and 39-8A).

Intraoperative electron doses of 15 to 25 Gy have been given, again before external beam treatments of approximately 45 to 50 Gy. Buskirk and colleagues[6] leave transhepatic catheters in place after this procedure.

Treatment Complications

Significant gastrointestinal complications (hemorrhage and stenosis) are frequently seen following EHBDC treatment.[36,60] Gastrointestinal hemorrhage was observed in 21% of the patients studied by Buskirk's group,[6] and Flickinger and associates[65] found a 29% 2-year actuarial risk of symptomatic duodenal ulcer disease. These

Table 39–12   Carcinoma of the Bile Duct: Simulation Checklist

Patient supine
Immobilization device
Presimulation pyelogram *or* IV contrast at simulation
Oral contrast
Stent contrast
Physical exam for liver size, incisions, drain sites
CT scan for landmarks
Percutaneous transhepatic cholangiography or endoscopic retrograde
Cholangiopancreatography for tumor volume
Plain films for clips and stent location

complications are undoubtedly dose-related, but this is not absolutely clear from the literature, possibly because of survival selection bias or different treatment techniques. In the study from Buskirk and colleagues,[6] doses of greater than 55 Gy to the distal stomach and duodenum were associated with a higher rate of duodenal ulcers, but total tumor dose was not a risk factor in other reports.[54] Schoenthaler and colleagues[54] also found an increased complication rate in distal tumors compared with proximal, if resected rather than biopsied, if microscopically negative margins were obtained, and in patients with T2 compared with T4 disease, all of which are probably related to an increased survival time rather than an inherent tendency toward complications.

Quality of life should be a critical goal in the management of EHBDC, given the poor prognosis and treatment hazards associated with this disease, but the issue is unfortunately rarely discussed in the medical literature. Lai and coworkers[64] evaluated outcomes of surgical patients at the University of California, Los Angeles based on multiple factors including hospitalizations (frequency and percentage of days), catheter-related problems, duration of jaundice, and requirements for antibiotics and analgesics. As expected, outcome scores were better among patients who had undergone complete tumor resection. They also found a significantly improved outcome in patients in whom a stent was used as opposed to those who underwent surgical bypass: "good" or "fair" scores were seen in 76%, 68%, and 29% in the subpopulations who had resection, stent, and bypass, respectively. Likewise, Gonzalez and associates,[56] in their collective review of several surgical studies, showed improved quality of life or "comfort indexes" in patients after curative resections as opposed to palliative procedures. They also studied a subgroup (18 of 112) of their own patients who

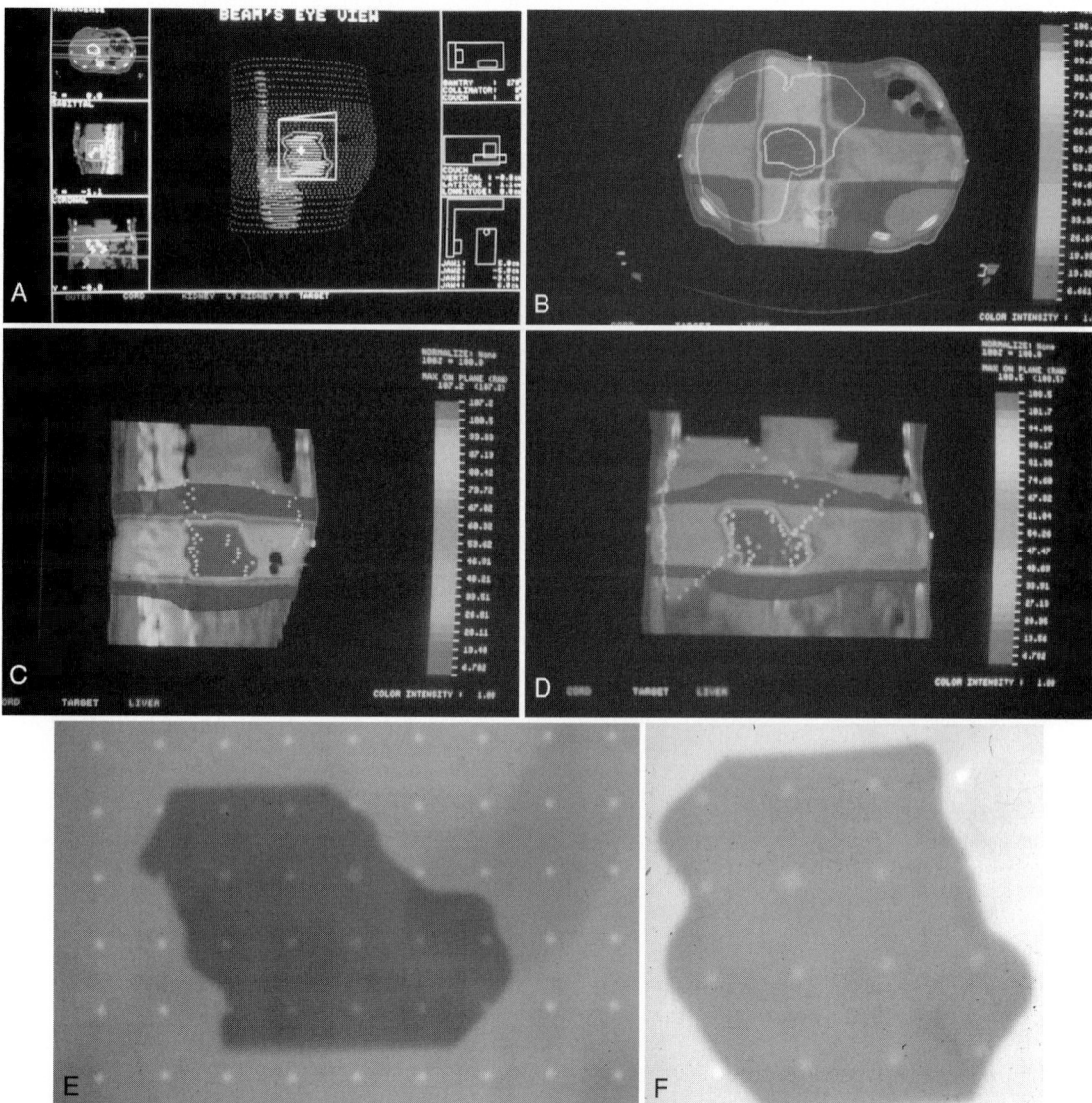

Figure 39–7. Boost portals for extrahepatic bile duct carcinoma (EHBDC) (external beam photons). The use of three-dimensional treatment planning allows for tight boosts and the potential for decreased morbidity. Shown are a beam's-eye view reconstruction **(A)**, and axial **(B)**, sagittal **(C)**, and coronal **(D)** color-wash displays of a four-field, three-dimensional boost plan for a patient with an unresectable EHBDC of the junction of the right and left hepatic ducts and common hepatic duct (Klatskin tumor). See also Color Figure 39–7A through D. Also shown are port films of the anterior **(E)** and right lateral **(F)** fields. (Courtesy of Steven A. Leibel, MD.)

underwent resection and radiation and found that, overall, Karnofsky performance status improved or was stable after irradiation in the 6 survivors compared with their immediate postoperative status. However, they also noted that 13 patients had cholangitis, 10 patients required hospitalization (4 more than once), and 5 patients required reoperation (reason not given). With the surgical literature as a basis for comparison, more work is needed to quantify the quality of life in irradiated patients (particularly compared to untreated patients) to provide an additional criterion on which to base therapeutic decisions.

Summary

Bile duct carcinomas are relatively rare but generally lethal solid tumors. Resections are infrequently achieved

and recurrences are common. RT may play a role in treatment, but higher doses than can be safely given with standard external beam radiation may be required. Specialized boost techniques should be used and studied whenever possible. The search for effective systemic therapies is ongoing. To improve long-term outcome, a highly skilled, specially trained multidisciplinary team (surgeon, radiation oncologist, interventional radiologist, medical oncologist) is required, and quality of life issues for the patient must be emphasized.

HEPATIC METASTASES

Liver metastases are exceedingly common, usually represent widespread systemic disease, adversely affect quality of life in many patients, and can contribute to

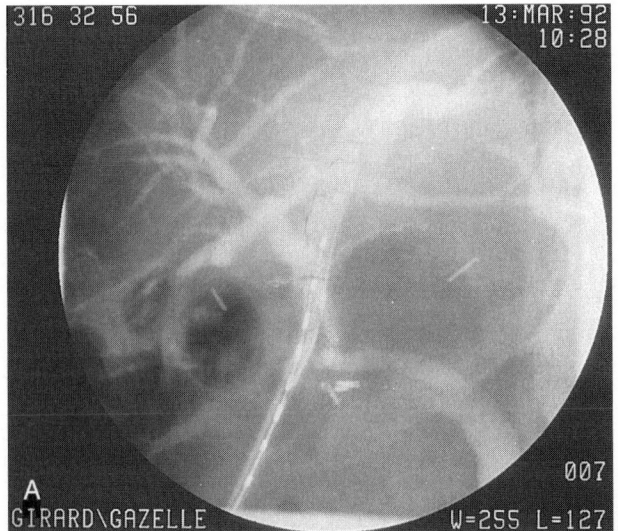

Figure 39–8. Specialized boost portals for extrahepatic bile duct carcinoma. **A,** High-dose-rate implants administered through percutaneous or endoscopically placed catheters can result in tightly circumscribed dose distributions with minimal patient discomfort. (Courtesy of Christopher Willett, MD, Department of Radiation Oncology, Massachusetts General Hospital, Boston.) **B,** Sophisticated treatment planning with charged particles (*left*, helium; *right*, neon) has resulted in some of the best results seen in the medical literature. See also Color Figure 39–8B. (Courtesy of Joseph R. Castro, MD, Department of Radiation Oncology, University of California at San Francisco, and Lawrence Berkeley Laboratory, Berkeley, Calif.)

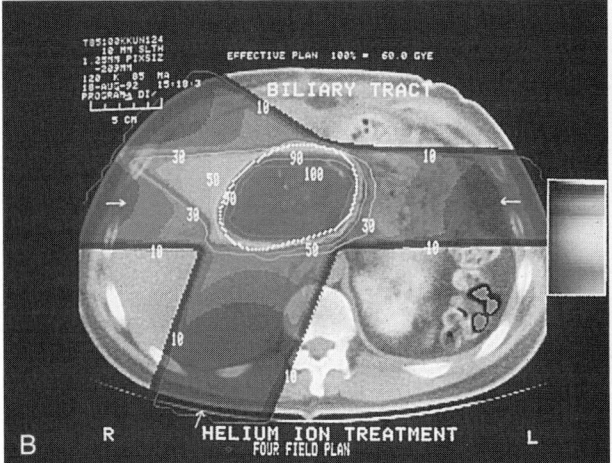

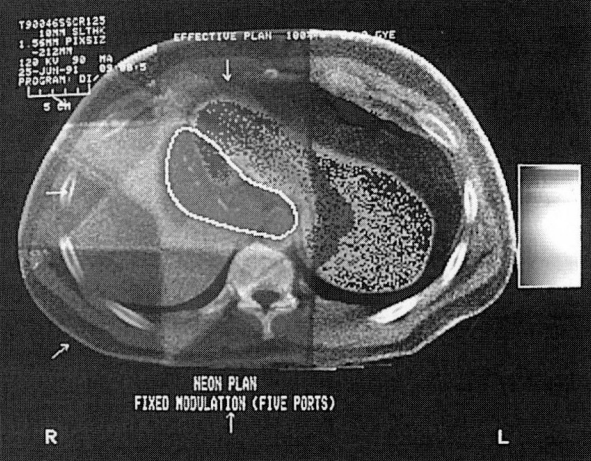

the cause of death. The average survival for patients with hepatic metastases from any source is approximately 5 months.[74] Treatment options have included surgical resection, devascularization, local or systemic chemotherapy, radiation therapy, and combinations of techniques.

Radiation efficacy is limited by liver tolerance and the gross, often multicentric nature of the disease. However, some studies, including RTOG reports,[75] have shown an improvement in quality of life (decreased pain, nausea, fever, and other symptoms) following the use of small whole liver radiation doses (21 to 30 Gy), although such treatment has no impact on survival. Many of the same local techniques (radioactive isotopes, particulates) used in the treatment of HCC have been used in the setting of metastases, with only minor responses seen.

An accelerated hyperfractionation dose-escalating protocol was studied by the RTOG.[42] Sequential groups of patients with hepatic metastases from various sites received 1.5 Gy fractions twice a day to total whole liver doses of 27, 30, and 33 Gy. No improvement was noted in median survival or the impact of the metastases on survival. However, a clear-cut increase in radiation hepatitis (clinical or biochemical) was noted in patients treated with 33 Gy compared with the lower doses, leading the authors to conclude that "33 Gy in fractions of 1.5 Gy (bid) is unsafe."

Regional infusion of various chemotherapeutic agents, particularly FUdR, has been demonstrated in several small randomized studies to result in higher local response rates than those associated with systemic therapy, at the cost of increased toxicity, greater expense, and no improvement in survival.[22,74]

Multiple nonrandomized studies of chemoradiation have been reported, but none has shown an improvement over single-modality trials. This was also borne out in a randomized trial.[76] The addition of a radiosensitizer has likewise not shown to be of greater efficacy than irradiation alone.[77]

In conclusion, in the fortunate few who qualify, surgical resection of hepatic metastases is the treatment of choice. In all other patients, treatment must be individualized depending on the burden of metastatic disease, status of the primary tumor, condition of the patient, and previous treatments. Combination therapies have not yet been demonstrated to be more efficacious than any single modality, and radiation is one of the demonstrated methods for providing palliation.

CARCINOMA OF THE GALLBLADDER

Epidemiology

Gallbladder cancer is the fifth most common cancer of the gastrointestinal tract. It is estimated that gallbladder cancer will be diagnosed in 6900 patients in the United States in 2001, of whom 3300 will die of their disease. There is significant regional variation in the incidence of gallbladder cancer: According to the American Cancer Society, the highest risk of developing gallbladder cancer in the United States is found in New Mexico, where it accounts for 9% of all cancers.[78] Gallbladder cancer is found almost three times more often in women than in men. Worldwide, the highest incidences of gallbladder cancer are reported in Chile, northeastern Europe, and Israel.[79] High incidences are also seen in American Indians and Americans of Mexican origin.[78] In the United States, the incidence of gallbladder cancer is higher in urban areas than in rural areas.[79] The incidence of gallbladder cancer increases steadily with age, and reaches its maximum in the seventh decade,[80] with a median age of occurrence of invasive carcinoma of 73 years, and of in situ carcinoma of 69 years. In fact, when stratified by age, of patients at New York Hospital undergoing biliary tract operations, gallbladder cancer was found in 0.3% of patients younger than 50 years of age, 3.8% of patients 50 to 65 years of age, and 8.8% in patients older than 65 years of age.[81] Over the past several decades, the incidence of gallbladder cancer in Canada, the United Kingdom, and the United States has stabilized or declined; this trend appears to be linked to the rising number of cholecystectomies. Of note, gallbladder cancer is found in about 1% of all routine cholecystectomy specimens, and it is estimated that 1 fewer death from gallbladder cancer occurs for about every 100 cholecystectomies done during the preceding year.[82]

Etiology

Although the cause of gallbladder cancer is unknown, a number of risk factors have been proposed, based on epidemiologic data. The most important risk factor for gallbladder cancer is a history of gallstone disease. Of patients with gallbladder cancer, more than 75% have cholelithiasis.[83] Overall, the risk of developing gallbladder cancer is approximately 4 to 5 times higher in patients with gallstones than in patients without gallstones.[84] In a large, collaborative, multicenter case-control study of cancer of the gallbladder, conducted in centers in Australia, Canada, the Netherlands, and Poland, from 1983 to 1988, a history of gallbladder symptoms requiring medical attention was the major risk factor associated with gallbladder cancer (odds ratio 4.4).[85] However, in autopsy series, gallbladder cancer is found in only 1% to 3% of patients with gallstones. Furthermore, in series following patients with silent gallstones over time, less than 1% developed gallbladder cancer.[86]

Other variables associated with elevated gallbladder cancer risk include an elevated body mass index, high total energy intake, high carbohydrate intake,[87] and anomalous junction of the pancreaticobiliary ducts (AJPBD).[88,89] Patients who suffer from Mirizzi syndrome (a rare complication of long-standing cholelithiasis, defined as obstructive jaundice caused by external compression of the common hepatic duct by an impacted stone in the gallbladder neck) may be at significant risk of developing a gallbladder cancer.[90] Gallstone size has also been implicated in increasing risk for gallbladder cancer; Diehl et al. found that patients with stone diameters of 2 to 2.9 cm as compared to less than 1 cm were at a 2.4-fold increased risk of developing gallbladder cancer; for stones 3 cm or larger, the relative risk was 10.1.[91] However, a recent case-control study evaluating 264 controls with cholelithiasis or choledocholithiasis in the absence of cancer, 126 controls with normal biliary tracts, and 84 cases of gallbladder cancer, found differing bile biochemistries in patients with gallbladder cancer, but no association with stone size.[92,93]

Carriers of typhoid suffer chronic inflammation of the gallbladder, and are at a six-times increased risk of developing gallbladder cancer.[94] Increased rates of gallbladder cancer are also found in patients with ulcerative colitis (relative risk [RR] 5 to 10),[95] history of porcelain gallbladder (RR 13.89),[96] and in those with a family history of gallbladder cancer (RR 3.0).[97] Other risk factors include tobacco exposure, use of certain medications and industrial chemicals (especially in the rubber and metal industries), and exposure to nitrosamines.[81,98]

Anatomy

The gallbladder is a conical or pear-shaped sac located in a fossa on the undersurface of the right lobe of the liver. It measures about 4 inches in length, and 1 inch in breadth at its widest part. It is divided into three parts— a fundus, body, and neck—and is attached to the liver by connective tissue and blood vessels. The under surface is covered by peritoneum. The body of the gallbladder sits adjacent to the origin of the transverse colon and to the duodenum. The fundus of the gallbladder is completely covered by peritoneum, and sits immediately below the ninth costal cartilage.[99]

The gallbladder is composed of three layers: 1) The external coat, or serosa, is derived from the peritoneum, and completely covers the fundus, as noted earlier, but covers the body and neck only on their undersurfaces; 2) The fibrous muscular coat consists of dense fibrous tissue, interlaced in all directions, mixed with muscular fibers oriented primarily in a longitudinal manner; 3) The internal layer, the mucosa, connects loosely with the fibrous layer, and forms small rugae. This layer has a lining of columnar epithelium and secretes thick mucus. At the neck of the gallbladder, this membrane projects inward and forms a screw-like valve. The wall of the gallbladder is much thinner than that of the intestine as it lacks a circular and transverse muscle layer.[99]

The cystic duct is comprised of a dense fibrous and a mucosal layer, and measures about 1½ inches in length; the cystic duct joins the hepatic duct to form the common bile duct. The common bile duct is approximately 3 inches in length; it descends behind the first part of the duodenum, in front of the portal vein, to its entry point into the small intestine, the ampulla of Vater.

The function of the gallbladder is to concentrate and store bile, a substance produced in the liver that helps to digest fat in the small intestine. When food enters the small intestine, the gallbladder contracts and releases bile into the small intestine via the common bile duct.[100]

Lymphatic drainage from the gallbladder is first to the cystic and pericholedochal lymph nodes, which are involved in more than 70% of cancers overall, and 20% of resectable cancers,[101] followed by drainage to the posterosuperior pancreaticoduodenal, superior mesenteric, celiac, and retroportal lymph nodes, then to the interaortocaval nodes. In some series, lymphatic drainage directly from the pericholedochal lymph nodes to the interaortocaval lymph nodes has been reported.[102,103]

Histology

Classification of primary cancers of the gallbladder is provided in Table 39-13. More than 95% of gallbladder cancers are carcinomas, of which adenocarcinomas comprise 89%. In some series, anaplastic carcinomas are the second most common type (4.6% of cases), while others have found papillary adenocarcinoma to be the second most common type. Mucinous carcinoma, squamous cell carcinoma, and adeno-acanthoma occur with descending frequency. Sarcomas and other unspecified histologies occur less than 2% of the time.[81,103-111]

Prognostic factors for gallbladder cancers include histologic type, histologic grade, and vascular invasion. Among carcinomas, unfavorable histologic types include small cell carcinomas and undifferentiated carcinomas. Papillary adenocarcinomas typically grow intraluminally, with less aggressive invasion of the gallbladder wall; this histology has been reported to have a better prognosis overall, possibly due to its tendency to present earlier while still localized to the gallbladder.[81] In terms of histologic grade, gallbladder cancers range from grade 1 (well-differentiated) to grade 4 (undifferentiated). While for unspecified adenocarcinomas in the Surveillance, epidemiology, and End Results data, there was a statistically significant association between grade and survival, with higher-grade tumors having a worse prognosis,[109] the majority of patients present with grade 3 disease. Overall, the stage of disease appears to be the most reliable predictor of outcome, regardless of histology or grade.[109-114]

Molecular Genetics

Multiple genetic changes are associated with development of gallbladder cancer. It is known that many gallbladder cancers are the endpoint of a sequence that starts with dysplasia, followed by progression to carcinoma in situ, followed lastly by development of frank invasive cancer.[115] In cases of gallbladder cancer, sectioning of the entire gallbladder shows severe dysplasia and carcinoma in situ in the majority of cases. It is thought that dysplasia progresses to carcinoma in situ over a period of 5 years, and to invasive cancer over a period of 10 to 15 years.[116]

In contrast to colonic lesions, adenomas are not thought to be the precursor lesions to gallbladder carcinomas in the majority of cases. Studies of molecular changes in gallbladder cancers have identified that, while mutations in *p53* are found commonly in dysplasia, carcinoma in situ, and gallbladder cancer, they are uncommonly found in adenomas.[117-119] Similarly, the occurrence of K-*ras* mutations in 25% of adenomas, with only rare occurrence in carcinoma or precursor lesions, supports the theory that adenomas are not precursors for invasive gallbladder cancer.[118,119] However, some papillary cancers are thought to represent malignant degeneration of papillary adenomas.

As noted earlier, recent studies have identified intracellular accumulation of *p53* in gallbladder cancers[117-119]; Wee et al. found this in 92% of the invasive carcinomas they studied, compared with 86% of carcinoma in situ, and 28% of dysplastic epithelium.[117]

Similarly, positive staining for carcinoembryonic antigen is found in 86% of invasive cancers studied, and in 89% of in situ cancers; tumors with an increased expression of carcinoembryonic antigen are associated with low median survivals.[120]

Lastly, cyclin D1 *over*-expression has been found to be a critical event in gallbladder carcinogenesis, and independently predicts for decreased survival for patients with gallbladder cancer.[121] In contrast, *decreased* p27(kip1) expression significantly correlates with tumor progression, and predicts poor prognosis.[122]

Presentation and Evaluation

Carcinoma of the gallbladder occurs rarely, and clinical symptoms often mimic benign gallbladder disease until invasion of surrounding structures causes increasingly severe symptoms. The most frequent presenting symptom, occurring in 80% of patients, is right upper quadrant abdominal pain.[123] Many patients report symptoms of biliary colic, which have become more continuous, localized, of progressive intensity, and are aggravated by meals.[124] In advanced disease, jaundice (present in 38% to 48% of patients at presentation), anorexia, weight loss (present in 40% to 68%), nausea and vomiting (30% to 60%), and a palpable right upper quadrant mass (Courvoisier's sign, found in 42% of patients at presentation) may be found.[81,124,125] Physical examination findings

Table 39–13   Gallbladder Cancer: Distribution by Histology*

Histologic Type	Subtypes, %	5-Yr OS, %
Carcinoma	99.0	12.1
Adenocarcinoma (all types)	89.4	13.0
Adenocarcinoma (NOS)	73.9	32.0
Papillary adenocarcinoma	5.5	40.0
Mucinous adenocarcinoma	5.3	7.8
Other adenocarcinomas	4.7	13.0
Other carcinomas	7.8	13.0
Squamous cell carcinoma	1.8	8.8
Sarcoma	0.2	NR
Carcinoid	<1.0	NR
Primary melanoma	<1.0	NR
Basal cell carcinoma	<1.0	NR

*Data from references 81, 104, 106-109.
NOS, Not Otherwise Specified; NR, Not Reported; OS, Overall Survival.

in advanced disease also can include a periumbilical mass (Sister Mary Joseph node), hepatomegaly, a rectal shelf (Blumer's shelf, due to peritoneal seeding), or supraclavicular lymphadenopathy.[125,126,127] Due to the vague symptoms with which it presents, carcinoma of the gallbladder is extremely difficult to diagnose early, and a high index of suspicion is recommended, especially for patients older than 70 years of age who present with recent weight loss and prolonged right upper quadrant pain. In the majority of patients at presentation, resection is made impossible by virtue of local invasion of the liver, biliary ducts, and adjacent structures.[124-127]

Laboratory evaluation should include a complete blood count, screening profile, and liver function tests. A high alkaline phosphatase with minimal rise in bilirubin can be found with limited obstruction of the intrahepatic bile ducts. Many patients with advanced disease have anemia, hypoalbuminemia, and abnormal liver function tests.[101,125] If the index of suspicion is high, serum carcinoembryonic antigen or CA19-9 can be considered. These studies have been evaluated with regard to potential use as screening agents for gallbladder cancer. According to Strom et al., a carcinoembryonic antigen of greater than 4 ng/mL is 93% specific and 50% sensitive for the diagnosis of gallbladder cancer, compared to controls undergoing cholecystectomy for benign conditions.[128] Similarly, Ritts et al. found that elevation of CA19-9 of greater than 20 units/mL in the setting of ambiguous imaging was 79% sensitive and specific for the diagnosis of gallbladder cancer.[129]

Ultrasound or CT scan are often the first studies obtained in evaluation of a patient with jaundice or right upper quadrant pain or both. These studies may reveal dilated intrahepatic bile ducts, a mass replacing the normal gallbladder, diffuse or focal thickening of the gallbladder wall, or a polypoid mass within the gallbladder lumen. Often, adjacent organ invasion (e.g., the liver) is seen. As most patients present with advanced disease, it is important to evaluate for periportal and peripancreatic lymphadenopathy, hematogenous metastases, and peritoneal carcinomatosis. The radiologic differential diagnosis includes inflammatory conditions of the gallbladder, xanthogranulomatous cholecystitis, adenomyomatosis, other hepatobiliary malignancies, and metastatic disease.[130] According to one series in which ultrasound was used preoperatively with findings compared to pathologic findings at surgery, ultrasound was able to correctly identify gallbladder masses in 85%, liver metastases in 67%, and portal venous involvement in 67% of cases. However, ultrasound was able to identify lymph node involvement in only 36%, and peritoneal seeding in 0% of cases identified at surgery to have peritoneal involvement. These authors conclude that ultrasound is a reliable test in the detection of a primary gallbladder mass or of local extension of tumor into the liver but is limited in the diagnosis of metastases to the peritoneum and lymph nodes.[131] Donohue et al. report a false-negative rate for ultrasound of 2% and a diagnostic accuracy for gallbladder cancer in 22%. In their series, 98% of patients with gallbladder cancer were noted to have abnormalities on ultrasound, including cholelithiasis, thickened gallbladder wall, a mass in the gallbladder, or a combination of these findings.[126]

CT identifies 60% to 80% of primary tumors.[132,133] Advances in magnetic resonance imaging may offer more detailed information than either CT scan or ultrasound,[134,135] and can be used to identify the level of obstruction and the site of underlying tumor in neoplastic pancreaticobiliary duct obstruction.[135] Endoscopic or percutaneous cholangiograms may be used for evaluation of obstructive jaundice, or in cases where vague symptoms and abnormal blood work prompt further workup and other imaging modalities are nondiagnostic. A correct preoperative diagnosis is made in less than 50% of cases, depending upon location and stage of tumor.[133] The most common preoperative diagnosis is benign biliary tract disease (76%); the second most common is cancer of the pancreas or bile ducts.[125]

The role of preoperative pathologic diagnosis in management of gallbladder cancer is unclear; many studies suggest that these tumors seed and grow along needle biopsy tracts and along drain tracts after cholecystectomy, and even in port sites after laparoscopy.[136,137] However, bile cytology can be obtained via ERCP without violating the tumor or risking peritoneal or incisional seeding. Although earlier studies suggested that the accuracy of combined ERCP and bile cytology was only 50%,[138] more recent data has found that the sensitivity of bile cytology alone in diagnosis of cancer of the gallbladder is up to 90%.[139,140] If lesions are not considered amenable to surgical resection, percutaneous fine-needle aspiration is recommended over core needle biopsy, due to decreased risk of needle-tract seeding. The accuracy of this approach is up to 90%, with a negligible false-negative rate.[137-141]

Staging

The AJCC/International Union Against Cancer (UICC) staging system for gallbladder cancer is provided in Table 39-14[142]; the TNM stage has been found to be a strong predictor of patient outcome in many series. The risk of lymph node metastases increases with increasing depth of tumor invasion. Tsukada et al. reviewed their experience with 106 patients with gallbladder cancer treated with radical surgery and found that lymph node metastases were present in 0% of T1 tumors, 48% of T2 tumors, 72% of T3 tumors, and 80% of T4 tumors.[143]

At diagnosis, involvement of the liver is found in 22% to 69% of cases,[81,125,126] peritoneal seeding is found in 10% to 24% of cases,[125,126] and distant metastases are found in under 10% (bone: 3%, central nervous system: 4%, lung: 1%).[125] Duodenal or hepatic flexure invasion is found in 10% to 15% at diagnosis.[101,125] In autopsy series, 91% of patients have metastases to the liver, 82% to intra-abdominal lymph nodes, and 60% to the upper gastrointestinal tract. Metastases to extra-abdominal organs are less common (lung 32%, central nervous system 5%).[124] Overall, according to Surveillance, Epidemiology, and End Results data, 25% of gallbladder cancers are "localized" at diagnosis, and 40% have distant metastases.[109] Many reports also use the Nevin staging, as modified by Donohue et al. (Table 39-15).[126,144]

Management of High-Risk Patients

As noted previously, there is a broad range of differential diagnoses of gallbladder lesions. Several series have

Table 39–14   Classification of Cancer of the Gallbladder

Primary Tumor(T)

TX	Primary tumor cannot be assessed
T0	No evidence of primary tumor
Tis	Carcinoma in situ
T1	Tumor invades lamina propria or muscle layer
T1a	Tumor invades lamina propria
T1b	Tumor invades muscle layer
T2	Tumor invades perimuscular connective tissue; no extension beyond serosa or into liver
T3	Tumor perforates the serosa (visceral peritoneum) and/or directly invades the liver and/or one other adjacent organ or structure, such as the stomach, duodenum, colon, or pancreas, omentum or extrahepatic bile ducts
T4	Tumor invades main portal vein or hepatic artery or invades multiple extrahepatic organs or structures

Regional Lymph Nodes (N)

NX	Regional lymph nodes cannot be assessed
N0	No regional lymph node metastasis
N1	Regional lymph node metastasis

Distant Metastases (M)

MX	Distant metastases cannot be assessed
M0	No distant metastases
M1	Distant metastases

Stage Grouping

Stage 0	Tis	N0	M0
Stage IA	T1	N0	M0
Stage IB	T2	N0	M0
Stage IIA	T3	N0	M0
Stage IIB	T1	N1	M0
	T2	N1	M0
	T3	N1	M0
Stage III	T4	Any N	M0
Stage IV	Any T	Any N	M1

From Greene FL, Page DL, Fleming ID, et al, eds: *AJCC Cancer Staging Manual*, 6th ed. New York: Springer; 2002:139.

Table 39–15   Modified Nevin Staging

Stage I	In situ carcinoma
Stage II	Involvement of the mucosa and muscularis
Stage III	Transmural invasion or direct liver invasion
Stage IV	Lymph node metastases
Stage V	Distant metastases

From Donohue JH, Nagorney DM, Grant CS: Carcinoma of the gallbladder: Does radical resection improve outcome? *Arch Surg.* 1990;125:237 and Nevin JE, Moran TJ, Kay S, et al: Carcinoma of the gallbladder: Staging, treatment, and prognosis. *Cancer.* 1976;37:141.

gallbladder cancer, in patients with a diagnosis of porcelain gallbladder or pancreaticobiliary maljunction, cholecystectomy should be done.[88,89,96,98]

Prophylactic cholecystectomy for asymptomatic gallstones cannot be justified for control of gallbladder cancer. However, careful ultrasound screening for abnormalities in the gallbladder wall, and CA19-9 determination before routine cholecystectomy of symptomatic patients, or in the high-risk asymptomatic population, may improve outcome in patients found to have gallbladder cancer.

MANAGEMENT OF GALLBLADDER CANCER

Overall, the curative resection rates for gallbladder cancer range from 10% to 30%.[148] Outcome in gallbladder cancer is closely related to tumor stage. According to a National Cancer Data Base report based on information collected from hospital registries across the United States from 1989 to 1995, the 5-year survivals for patients with stage 0, I, II, III, and IV tumors were 60%, 39%, 15%, 5%, and 1%, respectively. Overall, 5-year survival was less than 5%, with a median survival of 5 to 8 months. According to this report, many patients diagnosed with gallbladder carcinoma between 1989 and 1995 received no definitive therapeutic intervention because of the advanced stage of disease at presentation.[149] According to Piehler and Crichlow, after curative resection, 5-year overall survival is 16.5%, while after any kind of surgery, 5-year overall survival is 4.1%, and after no surgery, median survival is 2 to 6 months.[81] According to Beltz et al., mean survival for patients with "inapparent" disease after simple cholecystectomy is 16.7 months; with localized disease, mean survival is 24.7 months. After palliative surgical therapy, mean survival is 15.4 weeks, and after no operative therapy, mean survival is 8.5 weeks.[101]

AJCC STAGE IA AND IB. By virtue of its poor prognosis, late presentation, and rarity, there is a lack of consensus about surgical management of gallbladder cancer. In general, simple cholecystectomy is thought to be curative for lesions confined to the mucosal layer of the gallbladder,[150,151] but these represent less than 20% of all gallbladder cancers.[86] Results of the French Surgical Association Survey suggest that only in situ carcinoma can be treated adequately by simple cholecystectomy; in this series, 5-year survivals after simple cholecystectomy for Tis, T1, and T2 disease were 93%, 18%, and 10%, respectively.[152] Other authors suggest that, while pT1a disease can be managed safely with simple cholecystectomy as long as negative margins are obtained,[150,151,153] pT1b disease (invasion of the *muscularis propria*) necessitates

reported results on resections of polypoid lesions of the gallbladder, in an attempt to clarify indications for surgical management. Terzi et al. reviewed their experience with 100 patients who underwent cholecystectomy for polypoid lesions. In their series, 27% of patients with benign polyps and 73% of patients with malignant polyps were older than 60 years of age. The polypoid lesions were greater than 10 mm in 88% of malignant polyps, and in only 15% of benign polyps. The authors therefore concluded that the risk factors for malignancy include age older than 60 years, polypoid lesion size greater than 10 mm, and coexistence of gallstones and recommend cholecystectomy for patients with these risk factors.[145] Other authors recommend cholecystectomy for any patient with fewer than three polyps, regardless of size.[146] For lesions that do not fit these criteria, appropriate follow-up consists of follow-up imaging studies every 6 to 12 months, with further work-up indicated for any suspicious findings.[147] Alternately, in high-risk patients who do not meet the standard criteria, prophylactic cholecystectomy can be considered. Also, given the high incidence of associated extended cholecystectomy.[154,155] If suspicious nodes are seen at the time of surgery, removal for frozen section is recommended.[136] Piehler et al. recommend that all resected gallbladders be opened and inspected within the operating room, with an attempt made to visualize any gross suspicious lesion; also, frozen section analysis should be done to evaluate the extent of invasion. After simple cholecystectomy, if pathologic resection shows invasion beneath the mucosa, consideration of reoperation and hepatic wedge resection and regional lymphadenectomy is recommended.[81] As for T1b disease, for T2 disease, recent surgical series suggest that aggressive surgical resection can achieve 3-year survival rates of 90% to 100%.[143,156-159] Considering the frequent spread of disease to adjacent liver and regional lymph nodes, many have advocated en bloc resection of the gallbladder, liver resection (ranging from wedge resection of the liver to en bloc resection of segments IVb and V of the liver), and regional lymphadenectomy (including the porta hepatis, posterior pancreaticoduodenal and interaortocaval lymph nodes) in any case where there is uncertainty about the extent of invasion, or if the tumor is located adjacent to the liver for any stage II or III tumor and for select stage IVa tumors.[81,104,154] Shirai et al. have correlated the extent of microscopic angiolymphatic portal tract invasion with the gross depth of direct liver invasion and suggest that this should be used to estimate adequate hepatectomy margins.[160] Similarly, there is disagreement about the extent of lymph node dissection; however, most authors agree that there is little benefit to resection of disease beyond the regional lymph nodes, and significant added morbidity.[126,136,156-158,161]

AJCC STAGE IIA TO IV. Management of patients with stage II to IV disease is highly controversial; the benefit of radical surgery is unclear given the dismal long-term survival. Some recent data suggest that long-term survival can be achieved even in select patients with stage III and IV tumors, although the data is difficult to interpret in light of the recent changes in the staging system[143,152,161,162]; Bartlett et al. reported a 67% actuarial 5-year survival for patients with completely resected stage III disease and a 35% 5-year survival for patients with completely resected stage IV tumors.[158] Similarly, Tsukuda et al. have found a 40% 5-year survival rate in patients with stage III tumors, and a 19% survival in patients with stage IV tumors. For stage III and IV tumors in their series, the 5-year survival rate was significantly better after curative resection than after noncurative resection (52% vs. 5%, respectively).[143] Todoroki et al. also found that prognosis, even for stage IV disease, was significantly improved by gross total resection combined with radiotherapy.[163] Of note, these series use older versions of the AJCC staging; thus, many of the patients most likely had stage II to III disease, not stage IV disease.

THE ROLE OF ADJUVANT RADIATION THERAPY

A review of the literature by Kopelson and Gunderson found that up to 86% of patients with gallbladder cancer treated curatively failed with locoregional disease.[164] Piehler and Crichlow, in their exhaustive review of the literature, noted that the majority of deaths from gallbladder cancer are from obstructive failure from local recurrence.[81] Furthermore, even after aggressive resection, the majority of patients with stage IV disease have microscopic disease left behind. According to Todoroki et al., in only 15% of all patients with stage IV disease were negative margins obtained with aggressive resection, and 56% of patients had positive margins that subsequently became the apparent source of locoregional failure.[165] Similarly, a report from the Massachusetts General Hospital on their experience with gallbladder cancer patients treated with curative resection, without adjuvant chemotherapy or irradiation, found that locoregional failure occurred in 7 of 11 patients (64%).[166]

The use of adjuvant RT has been proposed as a method to decrease local-regional failure. Despite a number of largely retrospective series reporting a benefit to adjuvant radiotherapy (Table 39-16), the small number of patients with mixed diagnoses, stages, and treatments make it difficult to draw any significant conclusions.[104,167-176] The largest series, reported by Todoroki et al., evaluated 93 patients with stage III to IV gallbladder cancer, 50 of whom had been treated with RT after resection. Forty of these patients received intraoperative RT (range: 15 to 30 Gy, mean dose 20.9 Gy) just after resection, 21 received additional external beam RT (range: 12 to 54 Gy; mean dose 40.1 Gy), and 10 received external beam irradiation alone. On multivariate analysis, adjuvant RT significantly predicted for increased survival.[165] These authors reported that patients treated with adjuvant RT had a significantly higher 5-year survival rate (8.9% vs. 2.9%, respectively; $P = 0.0023$), and a higher local control rate (59.1% vs. 36.1%, $P = 0.0467$) than those managed with resection alone. On subset analysis, those patients who received adjuvant RT for microscopic residual disease had a 5-year survival rate of 17.2%, while for patients with macroscopic residual disease or without residual microscopic disease, there was no benefit to adjuvant radiation therapy.[167] Similarly, Hanna and Rider from the Princess Margaret Hospital evaluated outcomes in 51 patients treated with gallbladder cancer, 35 of whom also received RT (range: 34.88 to 60 Gy; mean dose 40 Gy), and found that RT increased the total survival of patients who received curative or palliative surgery: Median survivals in patients treated with radical radiation and surgery, palliative radiation and surgery, and surgery alone were 9.8, 10.6, and 5.3 months, respectively.[168]

Kresl et al. reported their prospective experience with 21 patients at the Mayo Clinic who were diagnosed with gallbladder cancer. Of the 21 patients, 20 had stage III to IV disease, and, after surgical resection, 57.1% had negative margins, 23.8% had microscopic residual disease, and 19% had gross residual disease. All patients received external beam RT (median total dose: 54 Gy), with concurrent 5-FU–based chemotherapy. In this series, the 5-year local control rate was 73% overall, 88% for those with no residual disease, and 80% after gross total resection with microscopic residual disease, a significant improvement in locoregional control over most surgery-alone series. Furthermore, median survivals of stage IV patients and patients less than stage IV were 16 months and 60 months, respectively. This is an improvement

Table 39–16 Adjuvant Radiation Therapy for Gallbladder Cancer

Study	Pts	Surgery	EBRT dose (No. of pts)	IORT dose	Chemo	LC	OS	Med Surv	Comments
Sasson[170]	10 GB	GTR	46.8 (median), (10)	1 pt	9-5 FU, 1-gem	NR	40% (4 yr)	53.6 mo	4 alive, NED (@8,33,49,73 mo)
Kresl[169]	21 GB	GTR	54 Gy (median), (21)	1 pt, 15 Gy	21 - 5-FU	NR	33% (5 yr)	2.6 yr	5 yr LC for EBRT> vs <54 Gy: 100% vs 65% (NSS)
Todoroki[167]	85 GB	50 - GTR	40 Gy (mean), (28)	21 Gy (mean), 37 pts	none	NR	6.3% (5 yr)	NR	All stage IV dz; 5y OS + RT 8.9% vs 2.9% –RT (p = 0.0023)
						59/36%, +RT/–RT			
Kraybill[171]	38 GB, 58 BD	49 (GTR-27)	48 Gy (mean), (80)	18 pts	31 pts	NR	10% vs 0% (+ vs –rsxn, 5 y)	11 mo	GTR + RT: Improved OS with >40 Gy vs <40 Gy (p = 0.003); on MVA only GTR & RT dose significant
Mahe[172]	19 GB	11 CR, 6 GTR, 2 pall surg	46 Gy (median), (19)	N/A	none	NR	CR: 36%, GTR/PS: 0% (5 y)	48 mo (CR), 6 mo (GTR/PS)	
Houry[173]	20 GB	20 (GTR-4)	42 Gy (mean), (20)	N/A	7 - 5 FU	NR	10% (2 yr)	8 mo	GTR - 1/4 NED (@84 mo), 3/4 DOD; mean surv 6.2 mo
Bosset[174]	7 GB	GTR	46 Gy + 9 Gy boost (7)	N/A	none	NR	NR	NR	5 NED (@5, 9, 11, 31, 58 mo), 2 abd/LR
Fields[175]	3 GB	GTR	45 Gy (3)	N/A	1 pt	NR	NR	NR	2 NED (22 mo, 27 mo), 1 LR, DOD 5.5 mo
Hanna[168]	51 GB, 17 BD	17- GTR	40 Gy (mean), (68)	N/A	none	NR	1 y OS = 50%	NR	MS significantly longer for curative RT vs no RT (p = 0.018)
Treadwell[176]	43 GB	43 (GTR-21)	10–45 Gy (9)	N/A	6 pts	NR	17% (5 yr)	NR	Longer surv in pts with adjuv tx (p < 0.05)
Vaittinen[104]	31 GB	GTR	NR (7 pts)	N/A	1 pt	NR	NR	63 mo	MS cur surg alone: 29 mo, +RT: 63 mo

GB, gallbladder; BD, bile duct; GTR, gross total resection; CR, complete resection; 5-FU, 5-fluorouracil; gem, gemcitabine; N/A, not applicable; NR, not reported.

over the results seen in reported pooled surgical series (3 and 6 months, respectively).[125,126,132,152,169]

Sasson et al. from Fox Chase Cancer Center recently reported a retrospective review of 10 patients with gallbladder cancer (9—stage III to IV, 1—locally recurrent), 9 of whom received definitive surgery, RT (range 37.8 to 60 Gy; median dose 48.6 Gy), and chemotherapy (5-FU in 8, gemcitabine in 1; given concurrently with radiation in 8 patients). Of these patients, the median survival was 53.6 months, and four continue to be without evidence of disease with follow-up ranging from 8 to 73 months.[170]

De Aretxabala et al. also recently reported encouraging data on the use of preoperative chemoradiation for gallbladder cancer. In their series, 18 patients who had undergone cholecystectomy for cholelithiasis/acute cholecystitis and were found to have a gallbladder cancer (AJCC 6th edition stage IB to III) were treated with continuous infusion of 5-FU with concomitant RT (45 Gy). Of these 18 patients, 15 underwent a reoperation, and resection was performed in 13. Residual tumor was found in the liver and lymph nodes in 3 patients. With a median follow-up of 24 months, 7 patients are alive, and all 7 are without evidence of disease. Of the 11 patients who have died after curative resection, isolated local recurrence was found in only one, with findings of peritoneal dissemination, liver metastasis, and brain metastasis in the remainder.[177]

Because of the relative rarity of gallbladder cancer, and the difficulty in diagnosis while still locally confined, there are no prospective, randomized studies examining the role of radiation and chemotherapy in this disease. However, given its propensity for local failure, some have suggested that a multimodality approach with effective chemotherapy and radiotherapy may provide the best chance for long-term survival. Certainly, the previously mentioned retrospective data, as well as recent data in gastric and gastroesophageal junction carcinomas[178] and pancreas cancers[179] suggest that there may be a benefit for chemoradiation in these tumors. Therefore, it may not be unreasonable to recommend adjuvant RT for resected, locally advanced gallbladder cancers (e.g., with invasion of the perimuscular connective tissue, hepatic invasion, or positive regional lymph nodes), or for unresectable disease. However, it is important to note that, in contrast to bile duct tumors, gallbladder cancers are much more likely to fail distantly in addition to locally, thus implying an even greater need for improvements in systemic therapy (*isolated* local/regional local failure was seen in only 15% of gallbladder patients after curative resection in one large series, compared with findings of distant failure ± local failure in 85%; personal communication, W. Jarnagin, 2003). Based on this limited data, a prospective multi-institutional phase III study would be of significant value; without this information, no standard treatment recommendations can be given, and treatment decisions must be made on a case-by-case basis.

RADIATION THERAPY FOR UNRESECTABLE DISEASE

RT has been used as primary treatment for unresectable gallbladder cancers for relief of jaundice (usually after percutaneous transhepatic biliary drainage has been established) and pain.[180-182] In a report by Pilepich and Lambert, 11 patients with carcinoma of the extrahepatic biliary system were treated (gallbladder: 5, cholangiocarcinoma: 6) with 25 to 60 Gy external beam irradiation; palliation was achieved in the 5 patients treated with palliative intent (relief of jaundice: 3, decreased T-tube drainage: 1, pain relief: 1). Survivals in this group of palliatively treated patients ranged from 1 to 8 months (median: 3 months).[181] Miura et al. reviewed the efficacy of adjuvant therapy on stent patency in malignant biliary obstruction. In their series of 29 patients (gallbladder cancer: 11, hilar ductal carcinoma: 8, pancreatic carcinoma: 10), 17 patients received radiotherapy, and 16 received chemotherapy. The median stent patency and median survival times were significantly greater (182 vs. 68 days, $P = 0.017$, and 261 vs. 109 days, $P = 0.0337$, respectively) in the chemoradiation group than in the no chemoradiation group.[183] Uno et al. found several long-term survivors among 17 patients treated with external beam RT alone (median dose: 50 Gy); in their series, median survival was 6 months (range: 1 to 99 months).[184] In comparison, as noted earlier, mean survival after palliative surgery alone or with no operative therapy after diagnosis is 15.4 weeks and 8.5 weeks, respectively.[101,185]

SIMULATION

If patients have adverse prognostic features after surgery, including invasion of the perimuscular connective tissue, liver, or involvement of the regional lymph nodes, adjuvant RT should be considered. Similarly, for unresectable disease, palliative radiation may be used. At simulation, the patient should be positioned supine, with his arms at the side of the head; an immobilization device should be used to ensure treatment position reproducibility. Oral contrast should be given approximately one half hour before simulation to allow for visualization of the small bowel and stomach. IV contrast can be used for better tumor and lymph node delineation, and CT images should be obtained from the dome of the diaphragm to the bottom of the kidneys. The tumor volume, liver, kidneys, and nodal regions of concern (porta hepatis, celiac axis) should be defined on the scan. If the gallbladder has been removed, preoperative studies are helpful to define the gallbladder fossa. Surgical clips can also help to define the tumor volume. Doses of 45 to 50 Gy (1.8 to 2.0 Gy fractions) are recommended for microscopic disease; areas of residual disease may be boosted to 54 to 60 Gy, if normal tissue tolerance can be respected.

ROLE OF CHEMOTHERAPY

The role of chemotherapy in management of gallbladder cancer has not been well defined. Multiple agents have been tried, including 5-FU, Adriamycin, methyl-CCNU, irinotecan, mitomycin C, and cisplatin, with few objective responses.[86,186-188] The Eastern Cooperative Oncology Group conducted a prospective three-arm randomized trial comparing oral 5-FU, oral 5-FU and streptozocin, and oral 5-FU and methyl-CCNU. There was no significant difference among treatments with respect to response or survival.[189] Hepatic arterial infusion with 5-FU–based chemotherapy has been used, with mixed results.[190,191] Early experience with gemcitabine suggests promising response rates.[192-194] Further prospective trials are needed to assess the role of chemotherapy in gallbladder carcinoma.

SUMMARY

Gallbladder cancers are relatively rare tumors with a dismal prognosis. Most gallbladder cancers are unresectable at diagnosis due to advanced local disease. Surgical resection is the preferred method of treatment, if technically feasible, although management of advanced disease (stage III and IV) with surgery is controversial. Data from single institution series suggests an improvement in local control and survival for resected, locally advanced gallbladder cancers with multi-modality treatment. Also, RT has been effectively used for palliation of jaundice and pain in unresectable patients. The search for effective systemic therapies is ongoing.

REFERENCES

1. Stevens K Jr: The liver and biliary system. In Cox JD, ed. *Moss' Radiation Oncology: Rationale, Technique, Results.* St. Louis: Mosby-Year Book; 1994:452.
2. Lotze M, Flickinger J, Carr B: Hepatobiliary neoplasms. In DeVita V Jr, Hellman S, Rosenberg S, eds. *Cancer: Principles and Practice of Oncology.* Philadelphia: JB Lippincott; 1993;883.
3. Austin-Seymour M, Chen G, Castro J, et al: Dose volume histogram analysis of liver radiation tolerance. *Int J Radiat Oncol Biol Phys.* 1986;12:31.
4. Robertson J, Lawrence T, Andrews J, et al: Long-term results of hepatic artery fluorodeoxyuridine and conformal radiation therapy for primary hepatobiliary cancers. *Int J Radiat Oncol Biol Phys.* 1997;37:325.
5. Iwasaki Y, Todoroki T, Fukao K, et al: The role of intraoperative radiation therapy in the treatment of bile duct cancer. *World J Surg.* 1988;12:91.
6. Buskirk J, Gunderson L, Schild S, et al: Analysis of failure after curative irradiation of extrahepatic bile duct carcinoma. *Ann Surg.* 1991;215:125.
7. Rubin P: The law and order of radiation sensitivity: Absolute vs relative. In Vaeth J, Meyer J, eds. *Radiation Tolerance of Normal Tissues.* Basel, Switzerland: Karger; 1989.
8. Oberfield R, Steele G Jr, Gollan J, et al: Liver cancer. *CA Cancer J Clin.* 1989;39:206.
9. Tsukuma H, Hiyama T, Tanaka S, et al: Risk factors for hepatocellular carcinoma among patients with chronic liver disease. *N Engl J Med.* 1993;328:1797.
10. Voravud N, Foster C, Gilbertson J, et al: Oncogene expression in cholangiocarcinoma and in normal hepatic development. *Hum Pathol.* 1989;20:1163.
11. Guo Y, Wu M, Chen H, et al: Effective tumor vaccine generated by fusion of hepatoma cells with activated B cells. *Science.* 1993;263:518.
12. Albores-Saavedra J, Henson D, Sobin L: The WHO histological classification of tumors of the gallbladder and extrahepatic bile ducts. *Cancer.* 1992;10:410.
13. Dusheiko G, Hobbs K, Dick R, et al: Treatment of small hepatocellular carcinomas. *Lancet.* 1992;340:285.
14. Wong LL, Limm WM, Severino R, et al: Improved survival with screening for hepatocellular carcinoma. *Liver Transpl.* 2000;6:320.
15. Heiken J, Weyman P, Lee J, et al: Detection of focal hepatic masses: Prospective evaluation with CT, delayed CT, CT during arterial portography, and MR imaging. *Radiology.* 1989;171:47.
16. Okuda K, Ohtuski T, Obata H, et al: Natural history of hepatocellular carcinoma and prognosis in relation to treatment. *Cancer.* 1985;56:918.
17. Baron R, Peterson M: Screening the cirrhotic liver for hepatocellular carcinoma with CT and MR imaging: Opportunities and pitfalls. *Radiographics.* 2001;21:S117.

18. Rode A, Bancel B, Douek P, et al: Small nodule detection in cirrhotic livers: Evaluation with US, spiral CT, and MRI and correlation with pathologic examination of explanted liver. *J Comput Assist Tomogr.* 2001:25:327.
19. Vogl TJ, Hammerstingl R, Schwarz W: Diagnostic imaging of hepatocellular carcinoma. *Radiologie.* 2001;41:895.
20. Johnson PJ: The role of serum alpha-fetoprotein estimation in the diagnosis and management of hepatocellular carcinoma. *Clin Liver Dis.* 2001;5:145.
21. Levy I, Greig P, Gallinger S, et al: Resection of hepatocellular carcinoma without preoperative tumor biopsy. *Ann Surg.* 2001;234:206.
22. Kemeny N, Schneider A: Regional treatment of hepatic metastases and hepatocellular carcinoma. *Curr Prob Cancer.* 1989;13:253.
23. Lawrence T, Ten Haken R, Kessler M, et al: The use of 3-D dose volume analysis to predict radiation hepatitis. *Int J Radiat Oncol Biol Phys.* 1992;23:781.
24. Chen M, Hwang T, Jeng L, et al: Hepatic resection in 120 patients with hepatocellular carcinoma. *Arch Surg.* 1989;124:1025.
25. Ikeda K, Saitoh S, Tsubota A, et al: Risk factors for tumor recurrence and prognosis after curative resection of hepatocellular carcinoma. *Cancer.* 1993;71:19.
26. El-Serag H, Mason A, Key C. Trends in survival of patients with hepatocellular carcinoma between 1977 and 1996 in the United States. *Hepatology.* 2001;33:62.
27. Iwatsuki S, Starzl T, Sheahan D, et al: Hepatic resections versus transplantation for hepatocellular carcinoma. *Ann Surg.* 1991;214:221.
28. Ringe B, Pichlmayr R, Wittekind C, et al: Surgical treatment of hepatocellular carcinoma: Experience with liver resection and transplantation in 198 patients. *World J Surg.* 1991;15:270.
29. Leung T, Patt Y, Lau W, et al: Complete pathological remission is possible with systemic combination chemotherapy for inoperable hepatocellular carcinoma. *Clin Cancer Res.* 1999;5:1676.
30. Venook A: Regional strategies for managing hepatocellular carcinoma. *Oncology.* 2000;14:347.
31. Pelleter G, Roche A, Ink O, et al: A randomized trial of hepatic arterial chemoembolization in patients with unresectable hepatocellular carcinoma. *J Hepatol.* 1990;11:181.
32. Groupe d'Etude de Traitement du Carcinome Hepatocellulaire. A comparison of Lipiodol chemoembolization and conservative treatment for unresectable hepatocellular carcinoma. *N Engl J Med.* 1995;332:1256.
33. Kim B, Chun, H, Seong J, et al: Phase II trial for combined external radiotherapy and hyperthermia for unresectable hepatoma. *Cancer Chemother Pharmacol.* 1992;31(suppl):1119.
34. Honda N, Guo Q, Uchida H, et al: Percutaneous hot saline injection therapy for hepatic tumors: An alternative to percutaneous ethanol injection therapy. *Radiology.* 1994;190:53.
35. Finney R: An evaluation of postoperative radiotherapy in hypernephroma treatment: A clinical trial. *Cancer.* 1973;32:1332.
36. Lawrence R, Kessler M, Robertson J: Conformal high-dose radiation plus intra-arterial floxuridine for hepatic cancer. *Oncology.* 1993;7:51.
37. Dawson L, McGinn C, Normolle D, et al: Escalated focal liver radiation and concurrent hepatic artery fluorodeoxyuridine for unresectable intrahepatic malignancies. *J Clin Oncol.* 2000;18:2210.
38. Ten Haken R, Balter J, Marsh L, et al: Potential benefits of eliminating planning target volume expansions for patient breathing in the treatment of liver tumors. *Int J Radiat Oncol Biol Phys.* 1996;36:167.
39. Wong J, Sharpe M, Jaffray D, et al: The use of active breathing control (ABC) to reduce margin for breathing motion. *Int J Radiat Oncol Biol Phys.* 1997;38:613.
40. Wagman R, Yorke E, Giraud P, et al: Reproducibility of organ position with respiratory gating for liver tumors: Use in dose escalation. *Int J Radiat Oncol Biol Phys.* 2001;51:28. Abstract.
41. Stillwagon G, Order S, Guse C, et al: 194 hepatocellular cancers treated by radiation and chemotherapy combinations: Toxicity and response: An RTOG study. *Int J Radiat Oncol Biol Phys.* 1989;17:1223.
42. Russell AH, Clyde C, Wasserman TH: Accelerated hyperfractionated hepatic irradiation in the management of patients with liver metastases: Results of the RTOG dose-escalating protocol. *Int J Radiat Oncol Biol Phys.* 1993;27:117.

43. Schoenthaler R, Castro J, Halberg F, et al: Definitive postoperative irradiation of bile duct carcinoma with charged particles and/or photons. *Int J Radiat Oncol Biol Phys.* 1992;27:75.

44. Matsuzaki Y, Osuga T, Saito Y, et al: A new, effective, and safe therapeutic option using proton irradiation for hepatocellular carcinoma. *Gastroenterology.* 1994;106:1032.

45. Lau W, Leung T, Ho S, et al: Adjuvant intra-arterial iodine-131 labeled Lipiodol for resectable hepatocellular carcinoma: A prospective randomized trial. *Lancet.* 1999;353:797.

46. Fan Z, Tang Z, Zhou D, et al: Radioiodinated anti-hepatocellular carcinoma (anti-HCC) ferritin. Targeting therapy, tumor imaging and anti-antibody response in HCC patients with hepatic arterial infusion. *J Cancer Res Clin Oncol.* 1992;118:371.

47. Order S, Pajak T, Leibel S, et al: A randomized prospective trial comparing full dose chemotherapy to [131]Iantiferritin: An RTOG study. *Int J Radiat Oncol Biol Phys.* 1991;20:953.

48. Zeng Z, Tang Z, Xie H, et al: Radioimmunotherapy for unresectable hepatocellular carcinoma using ^{131}I-Hepama-1 mAb: Preliminary results. *J Cancer Res Clin Oncol.* 1993;119:257.

49. Seong J, Park H, Han K, et al: Local radiotherapy for unresectable hepatocellular carcinoma patients who failed transcatheter arterial chemoembolization. *Int J Radiat Oncol Biol Phys.* 2000; 47:1331.

50. Seong J, Keum K, Han K, et al: Combined transcatheter arterial chemoembolization and local radiotherapy of unresectable hepatocellular carcinoma. *Int J Radiat Oncol Biol Phys.* 1999;43:393.

51. Cheng J, Chuang V, Cheng S, et al: Local radiotherapy with or without transcatheter arterial chemoembolization for patients with unresectable hepatocellular carcinoma. *Int J Radiat Oncol Biol Phys.* 2000;47:435.

52. Blumgart L, Thompson J: The management of malignant strictures of the bile duct. *Curr Probl Surg.* 1987;24:69.

53. Reding R, Buard J, Lebeau G, et al: Surgical management of 552 carcinomas of the extrahepatic bile ducts (gallbladder and peri-ampullary tumors excluded). *Ann Surg.* 1991;213:236.

54. Schoenthaler R, Phillips T, Castro J, et al: Carcinoma of the extrahepatic bile ducts: The University of California at San Francisco experience. *Ann Surg.* 1994;219:267.

55. Jarnagin WR. Cholangiocarcinoma of the extrahepatic bile ducts. *Semin Surg Oncol.* 2000;19:156.

56. Gonzalez D, Gerard J, Maners A, et al: Results of radiation therapy in carcinoma of the proximal bile duct (Klatskin tumor). *Semin Liver Dis.* 1990;10:131.

57. Langer J, Langer B, Taylor B, et al: Carcinoma of the extrahepatic bile ducts: Results of an aggressive surgical approach. *Surgery.* 1985;98:752.

58. Blumgart L, Hadjis N, Benjamin I, et al: Surgical approaches to cholangiocarcinoma at confluence of hepatic ducts. *Lancet.* 1984;1:66.

59. Boerma EJ: Research into the results of resection of hilar bile duct cancer. *Surgery.* 1990;103:572.

60. Cameron J, Pitt H, Zinner M, et al: Management of proximal cholangiocarcinomas by surgical resection and radiotherapy. *Am J Surg.* 1990;159:91.

61. Tompkins R, Thomas D, Wile A, et al: Prognostic factors in bile duct carcinoma. *Ann Surg.* 1981;194:447.

62. Kopelson G, Galdabini J, Warshaw A, et al: Patterns of failure after curative surgery for extra-hepatic biliary tract carcinoma: Implications for adjuvant therapy. *Int J Radiat Oncol Biol Phys.* 1981;7:413.

63. Ouchi K, Matsuno S, Sato T: Long-term survival in carcinoma of the biliary tract. *Arch Surg.* 1989;124:248.

64. Lai E, Tompkins R, Mann L, et al: Proximal bile duct cancer: Quality of survival. *Ann Surg.* 1987;205:111.

65. Flickinger J, Epstein A, Iwatsuki S, et al: Radiation therapy for primary carcinoma of the extrahepatic biliary system. *Cancer.* 1991;68:289.

66. Ringe B, Wittekind C, Bechstein W, et al: The role of liver transplantation in hepatobiliary malignancy: A retrospective analysis of 95 patients with particular regard to tumor stage and recurrence. *Ann Surg.* 1989;209:88.

67. Meyer CG, Penn I, James L: Liver transplantation for cholangiocarcinoma: Results in 207 patients. *Transplant.* 2000;69:1633.

68. Kubicka S, Rudolph KL, Tietze MK, et al: Phase II study of systemic gemcitabine chemotherapy for advanced unresectable hepatobiliary carcinomas. *Hepatogastroenterlogy.* 2001;48:783.

69. Falkson G, MacIntyre J, Moertel C: Eastern Cooperative Oncology Group experience with chemotherapy for inoperable gallbladder and bile duct cancer. *Cancer.* 1983;54:965.

70. Kurisu K, Hishikawa Y, Taniguchi M, et al: High-dose-rate intraluminal brachytherapy for bile duct carcinoma after surgery. *Radiother Oncol.* 1991;21:65.

71. Wolkov H, Graves G, Won M, et al: Intraoperative radiation therapy of extrahepatic biliary carcinoma: A report of RTOG-8605. *Am J Clin Oncol.* 1992;15:323.

72. Busse P, Stone M, Sheldon T, et al: Intraoperative radiation therapy for biliary tract carcinoma: Results of a 5-year experience. *Surgery.* 1989;105:724.

73. Kao G, Whittington R, Coia L: Anatomy of the celiac axis and superior mesenteric artery and its significance in radiation therapy. *Int J Radiat Oncol Biol Phys.* 1992;25:131.

74. Hamilton J, Nerenstone S, Friedman M: Liver. In John M, ed. *Chemoradiation: An Integrated Approach to Cancer Treatment.* Philadelphia: Lea & Febiger; 1993:315.

75. Leibel S, Pajak T, Massullo V: A comparison of misonidazole sensitized radiation therapy to radiation therapy alone for the palliation of hepatic metastases: Results of a RTOC randomized prospective protocol. *Int J Radiat Oncol Biol Phys.* 1987;13:1057.

76. Friedman M, Phillips T, Hannigan J: Phase III trial of irradiation plus chemotherapy for patients with hepatic metastases and hepatoma: Experience of the NCOG. *Natl Cancer Inst Monogr.* 1988;6:259.

77. Tsujii D, Okumura T, Marushashi A, et al: Potential efficacy of proton therapy in thoraco-abdominal tumors. In proceedings of the 18th Annual Particle Therapy Cooperative Oncology Group Meeting, 1993, Nice, France.

78. Greenlee RT, Murray T, Bolden W, et al: Cancer statistics, 2000. *CA Cancer J Clin.* 2000;50:7.

79. Diehl AK: Epidemiology of gallbladder cancer: A synthesis of recent data. *J Natl Cancer Inst.* 1980;65:1209.

80. Nakayama F: Recent progression of the diagnosis and treatment of carcinoma of the gallbladder -introduction. *World J Surg.* 1991; 15:313.

81. Piehler JM: Primary carcinoma of the gallbladder. *Surg Gynecol Obstet.* 1978;147:929.

82. Diehl AK, Beral V: Cholecystectomy and changing mortality from gallbladder cancer. *Lancet.* 1981;2:187.

83. Wanebo HJ, Vezeridis MP: Treatment of gallbladder cancer. *Cancer Treat Res.* 1994;69:97.

84. Lowenfels AB, Maisonneuve P, Boyle P, et al: Epidemiology of gallbladder cancer. *Hepatogastroentology.* 1999;46;1529.

85. Zatonski WA, Lowenfels AB, Boyle P, et al: Epidemiologic aspects of gallbladder cancer: A case-control study of the SEARCH program of the International Agency for Research on Cancer. *J Natl Cancer Inst.* 1997;89;1132.

86. Abi-Rached B, Neugut AI: Diagnostic and management issues in gallbladder carcinoma. *Oncology.* 1995;9:19.

87. Lazcano-Ponce EC, Miquel JF, Munoz N, et al: Epidemiology and molecular pathology of gallbladder cancer. *CA Cancer J Clin.* 2001;51:349.

88. Kobayashi S, Asano T, Yamasaki M, et al: Prophylactic excision of the gallbladder and bile duct for patients with pancreaticobiliary maljunction. *Arch Surg.* 2001;136:759.

89. Chijiiwa K, Kimura H, Tanaka M: Malignant potential of the gallbladder in patients with anomalous pancreaticobiliary ductal junction. The difference in risk between patients with and without choledochal cyst. *Int Surg.* 1995;80:61.

90. Redaelli CA, Buchler MW, Schilling MK, et al: High coincidence of Mirizzi syndrome and gallbladder carcinoma. *Surgery.* 1997; 121:58.

91. Diehl AK: Gallstone size and the risk of gallbladder cancer. *JAMA.* 1983;250:2323.

92. Strom BL, Soloway RD, Rios-Dalenz J, et al: Biochemical epidemiology of gallbladder cancer. *Hepatology.* 1996;23:1402.

93. Chow WH, Johansen C, Gridley G, et al: Gallstones, cholecystectomy and risk of cancers of the liver, biliary tract, and pancreas. *Br J Cancer.* 1999;79:640.

94. Welton JC, Marr JS, Friedman SM: Association between hepatobiliary cancer and typhoid carrier state. *Lancet.* 1979;1:791.

95. Joffe N, Antonioli DA: Primary carcinoma of the gallbladder associated with chronic inflammatory bowel disease. *Clin Radiol.* 1981;32:319.

96. Stephen AE, Berger DL: Carcinoma in the porcelain gallbladder; a relationship revisited. *Surgery*. 2001;129:699.

97. Fernandez E, la Vecchia C, D'Avanzo B, et al: Family history and the risk of liver, gallbladder, and pancreatic cancer. *Cancer Epidemiol Biomarkers Prev*. 1994;3:209.

98. Sheth S, Bedford A, Chopra S: Primary gallbladder cancer: Recognition of risk factors and the role of prophylactic cholecystectomy. *Am J Gastroenterol*. 2000;95:1402.

99. Gray H: In Pickering Pick T, Howden R, eds: *Gray's Anatomy*, 1901 ed: Philadelphia: Running Press; 1974:942.

100. Blumgart LH, Hann LE: Surgical and radiologic anatomy of the liver and bile duct. In Blumgart LH, Fong Y, eds. *Surgery of the Liver and Biliary Tract*, 3rd ed, vol 1; New York: WB Saunders; 2000:3.

101. Beltz WR: Primary carcinoma of the gallbladder. *Ann Surg*. 1973; 180:180.

102. Tsukada K, Kurosaki I, Uchida K, et al: Lymph node spread from carcinoma of the gallbladder. *Cancer*. 1997;80:661.

103. Bartlett DL, Fong Y: Tumors of the gallbladder. In Blumgart LH, Fong Y, eds. *Surgery of the Liver and Biliary Tract*, 3rd ed, vol. 1. New York: WB Saunders; 2000:995.

104. Vaittinen E: Carcinoma of the gallbladder: A study of 390 cases diagnosed in Finland 1953-1967. *Ann Chir Gynaecol*. 1970;59:1.

105. Henson DE, Albores-Saavedra J, Corle D: Carcinoma of the gallbladder: Histologic types, stage of disease, grade and survival rates. *Cancer*. 1992;70:1492.

106. Gruttadauria S, Doria C, Minervini MI, et al: Malignant fibrous histiocytoma of the gallbladder: Case report review of the literature. *Am Surg*. 2001;67:714.

107. Yokoyama Y, Fujioka S, Kato K, et al: Primary carcinoid tumor of the gallbladder: Resection of a case metastasizing to the liver and analysis of outcomes. *Hepatogastroenterology*. 2000; 47:135.

108. Dong XC, Dematos P, Prieto VG, et al: Melanoma of the gallbladder: A review of cases seen at Duke University Medical Center. *Cancer*. 1999;85:32.

109. Carriaga MT, Henson DE: Liver, gallbladder, extrahepatic bile ducts, and pancreas. *Cancer*. 1995;75(1 suppl):171.

110. Albores-Saavedra, Cruz-Ortiz H, Alcantara-Vazquez A, et al: Unusual malignant epithelial tumors of the gallbladder carcinoma. *Semin Diagn Pathol*. 1996;13:326.

111. Albores-Saavedra J, Henson DE: The WHO histological classification of tumors of the gallbladder and extrahepatic bile ducts. A commentary on the second edition. *Cancer*. 1992;70:410.

112. Friedman RB, Anderson RE, Gilchrest KW, et al: Prognostic factors in invasive gallbladder carcinoma. *J Surg Oncol*. 1983; 23:189.

113. Guo K-J, Yamaguchi K, Enjoji M: Undifferentiated carcinoma of the gallbladder. A clinicopathologic, histochemical, and immunohistochemical study of 21 patients with a poor prognosis. *Cancer*. 1988;61:1872.

114. Hisatomi K, Haratake J, Horie A, et al: Relation of histopathologic features to prognosis of gallbladder cancer. *Am J Gastroenterol*. 1990;85:567.

115. Albores-Saavedra J, Alcantra-Vasquez A, Cruz-Ortiz H, et al: The precursor lesions of invasive gallbladder carcinoma. Hyperplasia, atypical hyperplasia and carcinoma in situ. *Cancer*. 1980;45:919.

116. Roa I, Araya JC, Willaseca M, et al: Preneoplastic lesions and gallbladder cancer: An estimate of the period required for progression. *Gastroenterology*. 1996;111:232.

117. Wee A, The M, Raju GC: Clinical importance of p53 protein in gallbladder carcinoma and its precursor lesions. *J Clin Pathol*. 1994;47:453.

118. Wistuba II, Miquel JF, Gazdar AF, et al: Gallbladder adenomas have molecular abnormalities different from those present in gallbladder carcinomas. *Hum Pathol*. 1999;30:21.

119. Wistuba II, Albores-Saavedra J: Genetic abnormalities involved in the pathogenesis of gallbladder carcinoma. *J Hepatobiliary Pancreat Surg*. 1999;6:237.

120. Kanthan R, Radhi JM, Kanthan SC: Gallbladder carcinomas: An immunoprognostic evaluation of p53, Bcl-2, CEA, and alpha-fetoprotein. *Can J Gastroenterol*. 2000;14:181.

121. Hui AM, Li x, Shi YZ, et al: Cyclin D1 overexpression is a critical event in gallbladder carcinogenesis and independently predicts decreased survival for patients with gallbladder carcinoma. *Clin Cancer Res*. 2000;6;4272.

122. Hui AM, Li X, Shi YZ, et al: p27(Kip1) expression in normal epithelia, precancerous lesions, and carcinomas of the gallbladder: Association with cancer progression and prognosis. *Hepatology*. 2000;31:1068.

123. North JH, Pack MS, Hong C, et al: Prognostic factors for adenocarcinoma of the gallbladder: An analysis of 162 cases. *Am Surg*. 1998;64:437.

124. Perpetuo M, Valdivieso M, Heilbrun LK, et al: Study of gallbladder cancer. A review of 36 years experience at MD Anderson Hospital and Tumor Institute. *Cancer*. 1978;42:330.

125. Arnaud J, Graf P, et al: Primary carcinoma of the gallbladder—Review of 143 cases. *Hepatogastroenterology*. 1995;42:811.

126. Donohue JH, Nagorney DM, Grant CS: Carcinoma of the gallbladder: Does radical resection improve outcome? *Arch Surg*. 1990;125:237.

127. Shieh CJ, Dunn E, Standard JE: Primary carcinoma of the gallbladder: A review of a 16-year experience at the Waterbury Hospital Health Center. *Cancer*. 1981;47:996.

128. Strom BL, Soloway RD, Rios-Dalenz J, et al: Serum CEA and CA19-9: Potential future diagnostic or screening tests for gallbladder cancer? *Int J Cancer Prevention*. 1990;2:155.

129. Ritts RE, Nagorney DM, Jacobson DJ, et al: Comparison of preoperative CA19-9 levels with results of diagnostic imaging modalities in patients undergoing laparotomy for suspected pancreatic or gallbladder disease. *Pancreas*. 1999;9:707.

130. Levy AD, Murakata LA, Rohrmann CA Jr: Gallbladder carcinoma: Radiologic-pathologic correlation. *Radiographics*. 2001; 21:295.

131. Bach AM, Loring LA, Hann LE, et al: Gallbladder cancer: Can ultrasonography evaluate extent of disease? *J Ultrasound Med*. 1998;17:303.

132. Chijiwa K, Sumiyoshi K, Nakayama F: Impact of recent advances in hepatobiliary imaging techniques on the preoperative diagnosis of carcinoma of the gallbladder. *World J Surg*. 1991;15:322.

133. Campbell WL, Peterson MS, Federle MP, et al: Using CT and cholangiography to diagnose biliary tract carcinoma complicating primary sclerosing cholangitis. *Am J Roentgenol*. 2001;177:1095.

134. Yoshimitsu K, Honda H, Jimi M, et al: MR diagnosis of adenomyomatosis of the gallbladder and differentiation from gallbladder carcinoma: Importance of showing Rokitansky-Aschoff sinuses. *Am J Roentgenol*. 1999;172:1535.

135. Schwartz LH, Coakley FV, Sun Y, et al: Neoplastic pancreaticobiliary duct obstruction: Evaluation with breath-hold MR cholangiopancreatography. *Am J Roentgenol*. 1998;170:1491.

136. Fong Y, Brennan MR, Turnbull A, et al: Gallbladder cancer discovered during laparoscopic cholecystectomy: Aggressive reresection is beneficial. *Cancer*. 1998;83:423.

137. Winston CB, Chen JW, Fong Y, et al: Recurrent gallbladder carcinoma along laparoscopic cholecystectomy port tracks: CT demonstration. *Radiology*. 1999;212:439.

138. Harada H, Sasaki T, Yamamoto N, et al: Assessment of endoscopic aspiration cytology and endoscopic retrograde cholangiopancreatography in patients with cancer of the hepatobiliary tract. Part II. *Gastroenterologia Japonica*. 1977;12:59.

139. Akosa AB, Barker F, Desa L, et al: Cytologic diagnosis in the management of gallbladder carcinoma. *Acta Cytol*. 1995;39:494.

140. Krishnani N, Shukla S, Jain M, et al: Fine needle aspiration cytology in xanthogranulomatous cholecystitis, gallbladder adenocarcinoma and coexistent lesions. *Acta Cytol*. 2000;44:508.

141. Zargar SA, Khuroo MS, Mahajan R, et al: US-guided fine-needle aspiration biopsy of gallbladder masses. *Radiology*. 1991;179:275.

142. Greene FL, Page DL, Fleming JD, et al, (eds). Gallbladder. In *AJCC Cancer Staging Manual*, 6th ed. New York: Springer; 2002:139.

143. Tsukada K, Hatakeyama K, Kuroaki I, et al: Outcome of radical surgery for carcinoma of the gallbladder according to TNM stage. *Surgery*. 1996;120:816.

144. Nevin JE, Moran TJ, Kay S, et al: Carcinoma of the gallbladder: Staging, Treatment, and Prognosis. *Cancer*. 1976;37:141.

145. Terzi C, Sokmen S, Seckin S, et al: Polypoid lesions of the gallbladder: Report of 100 cases with special reference to operative indications. *Surgery*. 2000;127:622.

146. Shinkai H, Kimura W, Muto T: Surgical indications for small polypoid lesions of the gallbladder. *Am J Surg*. 1998;175:114.

147. Bartlett DL, Fong Y: Tumors of the gall bladder. In Blumgart LH, Fong Y (eds): *Surgery of the Liver and Biliary Tract*, 3rd ed., vol. 1. New York: WB Saunders; 2000:1002.

148. Levin B: Gallbladder carcinoma. *Ann Oncol.* 1999;10 (suppl 4):129.

149. Donohue JH, Steward AK, Menck HR: The National Cancer Data Base report on carcinoma of the gallbladder, 1989-1995. *Cancer.* 1998;83:2618.

150. Bartlett DL: Gallbladder cancer. *Semin Surg Oncol.* 2000;19:145.

151. Benoist S, Panis Y, Fagniez PL: Long-term results after curative resection for carcinoma of the gallbladder. French University Association for Surgical Research. *Am J Surg.* 1998;175:118.

152. Cubertafond P, Gainant A, Cucchiaro G: Surgical treatment of 724 carcinomas of the gallbladder. Results of the French Surgical Association Survey. *Ann Surg.* 1994;219:275.

153. Wakai T, Shirai Y, Yokoyama N, et al: Early gallbladder carcinoma does not warrant radical resection. *Br J Surg.* 2001;88:675.

154. Ouchi K, Sugawara T, Ono H, et al: Diagnostic capability and radical resectional surgery for early gallbladder carcinoma. *Hepatogastroenterology.* 1999;46:1557.

155. Bartlett DL, Fong Y: Tumors of the gall bladder. In Blumgart LH, Fong Y (eds): *Surgery of the Liver and Biliary Tract,* 3rd ed., vol. 1. New York: WB Saunders; 2000:1003.

156. Shirai Y, Yoshida K, Tsukada K, et al: Radical surgery for gallbladder cancer. Long-term results. *Ann Surg.* 1992;216:565.

157. Bartlett DL, Fong Y, Fortner JG, et al: Long-term results after resection for gallbladder cancer. *Ann Surg.* 1996;224:639.

158. Bartlett DL, Fong Y: Tumors of the gall bladder. In Blumgart LH, Fong Y (eds): *Surgery of the Liver and Biliary Tract,* 3rd ed., vol. 1. New York: WB Saunders; 2000:1003.

159. Oertli D, Herzog U, Tondelli P: Primary carcinoma of the gallbladder: Operative experience during a 16 year period. *Eur J Surg.* 1993;159:415.

160. Shirai Y, Tsukada K, Ohtani T, et al: Hepatic metastases from carcinoma of the gallbladder. *Cancer.* 1995;75:2063.

161. Kondo S, Nimura Y, Hayakawa N, et al: Regional and para-aortic lymphadenectomy in radical surgery for advanced gallbladder carcinoma. *Br J Surg.* 2000;87:418.

162. Schauer RJ, Meyer G, Baaretton G, et al: Prognostic factors and long-term results after surgery for gallbladder carcinoma: A retrospective study of 127 patients. *Langenbecks Arch Surg.* 2001; 386:110.

163. Todoroki T, Kawamoto T, Takahashi H, et al: Treatment of gallbladder cancer by radical resection. *Br J Surg.* 1999;86:622.

164. Kopelson G, Harisiadis L, Tretter P, et al: The role of radiation therapy in cancer of the extra-hepatic biliary system. *Int J Radiat Oncol Biol Phys.* 1977;2:883.

165. Todoroki T, Takahashi H, Koike N, et al: Outcomes of aggressive treatment of stage IV gallbladder cancer and predictors of survival. *Hepatogastroenterology.* 1999;46:2114.

166. Kopelson G, Galdabini J, Warshaw A, et al: Patterns of failure after curative surgery for extra-hepatic biliary tract carcinoma: Implications for adjuvant therapy. *Int J Radiat Oncol Biol Phys.* 1981;7:413.

167. Todoroki T, Kawamoto T, Otsuka M, et al: Benefits of combining radiotherapy with aggressive resection for stage IV gallbladder cancer. *Hepatogastroenterology.* 1999;46:1585.

168. Hanna SS, Rider WD: Carcinoma of the gallbladder or extrahepatic bile ducts: The role of radiotherapy. *Can Med Assoc J.* 1978; 118:59.

169. Kresl JJ, Schild SE, Henning GT, et al: Adjuvant external beam radiation therapy with concurrent chemotherapy in the management of gallbladder carcinoma. *Int J Radiat Oncol Biol Phys.* 2002;52:167.

170. Sasson AR, Hoffman JP, Ross E, et al: Trimodality therapy for advanced gallbladder cancer. *Am Surg.* 2001;67:277.

171. Kraybill WG, Lee H, Picus J, et al: Multidisciplinary treatment of biliary tract cancers. *J Surg Oncol.* 1994;55:239.

172. Mahe M, Stampfli C, Romestaing P, et al: Primary carcinoma of the gallbladder: Potential for external radiation therapy. *Radiother Oncol.* 1994;33:204.

173. Houry S, Schlienger M, Huguier M, et al: Gallbladder carcinoma: Role of radiation therapy. *Br J Surg.* 1989;76:1578.

174. Bosset J, Mantion G, Gillet M, et al: Primary carcinoma of the gallbladder: Adjuvant postoperative external irradiation. *Cancer.* 1989;64:1843.

175. Fields JN, Emama B: Carcinoma of the extrahepatic biliary system—Results of primary and adjuvant radiotherapy. *Int J Radiat Oncol Biol Phys.* 1986;13:331.

176. Treadwell TA, Hardin WJ: Primary carcinoma of the gallbladder. *Am J Surg.* 1976;132:703.

177. De Aretxabala X, Roa I, Burgos L, et al: Preoperative chemoradiotherapy in the treatment of gallbladder cancer. *Am Surg.* 1999; 65:241.

178. Macdonald JS, Smalley SR, Benedetti J, et al: Chemoradiotherapy after surgery compared with surgery alone for adenocarcinoma of the stomach or gastroesophageal junction. *N Engl J Med.* 2001; 345:725.

179. Foo M, Gunderson LL, Urrutia R, et al: Pancreas cancer. In Gunderson LL, Tepper J, eds. *Clinical Radiation Oncology.* New York: Churchill Livingstone; 2000:687.

180. Kopelson G, Gunderson LL, et al: Primary and adjuvant radiation therapy in gallbladder and extrahepatic biliary tract carcinoma. *J Clin Gastroenterol.* 1983;5:43.

181. Pilepich MV, Lambert PM: Radiotherapy of carcinomas of the extrahepatic biliary system. *Radiology.* 1978;127:767.

182. Smoron GL: Radiation therapy in carcinoma of the gallbladder and biliary tract. *Cancer.* 1977;40:1422.

183. Miura Y, Endo I, Togo S, et al: Adjuvant therapies using biliary stenting for malignant biliary obstruction. *J Hepatobiliary Pancreat Surg.* 2001;8:113.

184. Uno T, Itami J, Aruga M, et al: Primary carcinoma of the gallbladder: Role of external beam radiation therapy in patients with locally advanced tumor. *Strahlenther Onkol.* 1996;172:496.

185. Suzuki S, Kurachi K, Yokoi Y, et al: Intrahepatic cholangiojejunostomy for unresectable malignant biliary tumors with obstructive jaundice. *J Hepatobiliary Pancreat Surg.* 2001;8:124.

186. Sanz-Altamira PM, O'Reilly E, Stuart KE, et al: A phase II trial of irinotecan (CPT-11) for unresectable biliary tree carcinoma. *Ann Oncol.* 2001;12:501.

187. Gebbia V, Majello E, Testa A, et al: Treatment of advanced adenocarcinoma of the exocrine pancreas and gallbladder with 5-fluorouracil, high dose levofolinic acid and oral hydroxyurea on a weekly schedule. Reports of a multicenter study of the Southern Italy Oncology Group (GOIM). *Cancer.* 1996;78:1300.

188. Taal BG, Audisio RA, Bleiberg H, et al: Phase II trial of mitomycin C (MMC) in advanced gallbladder and biliary tree carcinoma. An EORTC Gastrointestinal Tract Cancer Cooperative Group Study. *Ann Oncol.* 1993;4:607.

189. Falkson G, MacIntyre JM, Moertel CG: Eastern Cooperative Oncology Group experience with chemotherapy for inoperable gallbladder and bile duct cancer. *Cancer.* 1984;54:965.

190. Ishizaki M, Akiyama N, Tanaka S, et al: Long-term survival of a patient with postoperative liver metastasis of stage IVa gallbladder cancer responding to hepatic arterial infusion chemotherapy. *Gan To Kagaku Ryoho.* 2001;28:395.

191. Ohta K, Sawamura A, Miyahara E, et al: A case of inoperable advanced gallbladder cancer responding to intra-arterial infusion of 5-fluorouracil (5-FU) and leucovorin (LV). *Gan To Kagaku Ryoho.* 2001;28:516.

192. Gallardo J, Rubio B, Ahumada M, et al: Efficacy of gemcitabine in gallbladder cancer. Initial experience in 4 cases. *Rev Med Chil.* 2000;128:1025.

193. Castro MP: Efficacy of gemcitabine in the treatment of patients with gallbladder cancer. A case report. *Cancer.* 1998;82:639.

194. Verderame F, Mandina P, Abruzzo F, et al: Biliary tract cancer: Our experience with gemcitabine treatment. *Anticancer Drugs.* 2000;11:707.

Cancer of the Colon

Bruce D. Minsky, MD

The sections in this chapter on Epidemiology and Genetics, Pathology, Routes of Spread, and Diagnostic and Staging Studies pertain to both colon and rectal cancer. The remainder of the chapter focuses exclusively on colon cancer.

EPIDEMIOLOGY, ETIOLOGY, GENETICS, AND CYTOGENETIC ABNORMALITIES

Epidemiology

In 2003 there will be an estimated 105,500 new cases of colon cancer in the United States with 49,000 occurring in men and 56,500 occurring in women. Approximately 48,100 deaths are expected.[1] The median age at diagnosis is 62 years. Patients younger than age 40 have a less favorable prognosis; however, it is unclear if this is independent of the stage of their cancer.

It has been postulated that colorectal cancer is caused or promoted by environmental factors and especially by dietary factors that affect the enteric milieu.[2] A number of studies reveal an association of human colorectal cancer with certain diets (such as those rich in animal fats and meat and poor in fiber) and certain high-risk populations.[3]

In general, the affluent Western diet (high fat, low fiber, high phosphate, and low calcium) is associated with an increased risk of colorectal cancer. However, there have not been any clear studies demonstrating whether dietary factors increase the risk in patients with an underlying genetic susceptibility. There are various risk factors for colorectal cancer, as shown in Table 40-1. Approximately 75% of colorectal cancers are sporadic.

Molecular Genetics

Only recently have the genetic basis of colorectal cancer and its precursors begun to be understood.[4,5] The current data suggest that the development of colorectal cancer is a multistep process that involves a successive activation or deletion of genes and their protein products.[6] This is mediated by regulatory genes. Advances in molecular biology techniques have allowed characterization of the genetic changes thought to be responsible for this multistep process.[4]

Of the numerous molecular markers examined to date, microsatellite instability (MSI),[7,8] 18q,[7] and thymidylate synthase[9] appear to have the most prognostic impact in colon cancer. Although they are not currently incorporated in the staging system, they should be noted.

ANATOMY

The large bowel is divided into the colon and rectum.[10,11] The cecum, transverse colon, and sigmoid loop are mobile structures that lie free in the peritoneal cavity and are completely covered with serosa (visceral peritoneum). The dorsal or posterior aspect of the ascending and descending colon and both flexures are frequently without serosa. Tumor spread from these segments may involve the retroperitoneal soft tissues, kidney, ureter, and pancreas. Although the rectum is frequently considered to be extraperitoneal, the anterior surface of the proximal third of the rectum is covered with serosa and is therefore intraperitoneal. Anatomically, the transition from sigmoid colon to rectum is marked by the fusion of the tenia of the sigmoid colon to the circumferential longitudinal muscle of the rectum. This occurs approximately 12 to 15 cm from the dentate line. Patterns of recurrence of proximal rectal cancer may depend on whether the location of the tumor is anterior or posterior.

The overall rationale for the use of adjuvant radiation therapy in colon cancer is based on the patterns of failure following potentially curative surgery. The primary

Table 40–1   Clinical Risk Factors for Colorectal Cancer

General
  Age older than 40
Genetic Syndromes
  Peutz-Jeghers
  Familial adenomatous polyposis
  Gardner's
  Turcot's
  Oldfield's
Familial
  Family history
  Lynch I: Familial colorectal cancer syndrome
  Lynch II: Hereditary adenocarcinomatosis syndrome
Other Diseases
  Prior colorectal cancer
  Malignant colorectal polyps
  Inflammatory bowel disease

determinant of failure patterns in colorectal cancer is the location of the tumor in reference to the peritoneal reflection. In contrast with tumors located at or below the peritoneal reflection (rectosigmoid and rectum), most tumors located above the peritoneal reflection (cecum-sigmoid) have a higher incidence of failure within the abdominal cavity.[12-15] This is because colon tumors have easier access to a free peritoneal surface.

Representative series examining the patterns of failure after potentially curative surgery are provided in Table 40-2. There is much variation as to what defines failure, the method by which failure is determined, the staging system used, and whether patients with metastatic disease are excluded from analysis. Failure patterns will be lowest in series that use clinical or radiographic evidence of first failure,[12] whereas they will be highest in series that use reoperation or autopsy evidence of cumulative failure.[15]

Treatment recommendations are based on the stage of the patient's cancer and tumor location in reference to the peritoneal reflection. If the tumor is completely above the reflection, it is treated as a colon cancer. If any portion is at or below the reflection, it is treated as a rectal cancer.

PATHOLOGY

Gross Appearance

Tumor configuration may be divided into fungating (exophytic), ulcerating, stenosing, or constricting (annular, circumferential). Although there are data to suggest that ulcerative tumors have a worse prognosis compared with exophytic tumors, it is unclear if this is independent of stage.

Histologic Subtypes

The most common histologic type of large bowel cancer is adenocarcinoma, which accounts for 90% to 95% of all large bowel tumors.[10] It is the only histologic type further classified by grade. A number of histologic types of large bowel cancer have been identified. The World Health Organization has developed a classification of both benign and malignant tumors. Colloid or "mucinous" adenocarcinomas represent approximately 17% of large bowel tumors.[16] These adenocarcinomas are defined by large amounts of extracellular mucin retained within the tumor. A separate classification is the rare signet-ring cell carcinoma (2% to 4% of mucinous carcinomas), which contains abundant intracellular mucin, pushing the nucleus to one side. Some signet-ring tumors form a linitis plastica appearance and have a poor prognosis.

Other rare variants of epithelial tumors include squamous cell carcinomas, adenosquamous carcinoma (adenoacanthoma), undifferentiated carcinomas, and carcinoids. Gastrointestinal stromal tumors should be treated as sarcomas.[17] Sarcomas account for 0.1% to 0.3% of all malignancies of the colorectum.[18] The most common type is leiomyosarcoma. It may arise from the smooth muscle of the muscularis propria, muscularis mucosa, or blood vessels.[19] Primary colorectal malignant lymphomas are usually diffuse histiocytic (large-cell) lymphomas.[20] Squamous cell cancers of the rectum should be treated as anal cancer with 5-FU/mitomycin-C and radiation, saving surgery for salvage.[21]

Grade

Broders classified adenocarcinomas by their degree of differentiation. He designated four grades, based on the percentage of differentiated tumor cells. "Well differentiated" in Broders' system meant well formed glands, resembling an adenoma. Broders included the mucinous carcinomas in his system. Dukes considered mucinous carcinomas separately.[22] There is no uniform agreement on the grading criteria, but most investigators agree on the use of a three-grade system, similar to that described in other adenocarcinomas.

Other Clinicopathologic Factors

The influence of clinical and pathologic factors on the patterns of failure and survival following surgery for

Table 40–2 Failure Patterns Following Potentially Curative Surgery for Colon Cancer (All Stages)

Series	Detection and Definition of Failure	Stage	Patients, n	Local Failure, %		Abdominal Failure, %*		Distant Failure, %	
				Only	Component	Only	Component	Only	Component
Gunderson et al[15]	Reoperation, cumulative failure	All T3-4 and/or N1-2	91 72	22 (0-30) 17	48 (0-64) 49	4 (0-9) 6	21 (0-36) 26	7 (0-16) 7	30 (0-38) 35
Willett et al[13,14,]	Clinical, cumulative failure	All T3-4 and/or N1-2	533 395	6 (0-12) 8	19 (0-49) 26	11 (2-24) 14	21 (3-43) 25 5	4 (0-10)	13 (0-25) 16
Minsky et al[12]	Clinical, first failure	All T3-4 and/or N1-2	284 229	6 (0-8) 4	9 (0-25) 10	8 (0-29) 10	13 (0-57) 15	3 (0-11) 5	6 (0-25) 9

*In the Gunderson series, liver metastasis is considered distant failure whereas in the series by the Willett and Minsky groups, liver metastasis is considered abdominal metastasis.

colorectal cancer has been the subject of numerous investigations. By univariate analysis, numerous factors have been reported to be of prognostic importance. Many of these factors are interrelated and merely reflections of the same overall characteristic of the cancer. Using a multivariate (proportional hazards) analysis, various independent factors for survival have been reported. However, the majority of investigators agree that the most important independent pathologic factor for survival or recurrence following surgery is stage (depth of penetration through the bowel wall and the presence and number of positive lymph nodes).[23,24] Prognosis is related to the number rather than the volume of tumor present in the nodes.[25] The presence of lymphatic vessel (L) or venous (V) invasion is now indicated as an additional descriptor in the TNM staging system.

Select adverse clinical factors include: age younger than 40, blood transfusions, long duration of symptoms, obstruction or perforation, ulcerative, and various primary tumor locations. Select adverse pathologic/molecular factors include: perineural invasion, high grade, colloid, signet ring cell, blood vessel invasion, lymphatic vessel invasion, aneuploidy, elevated carcinoembryonic antigen (CEA), collagen, local immune response, cell surface antigen 19-9, and various growth factors, receptors, oncogenes, and blood group antigens.[10] Except for CEA, none of these tumor markers have been helpful in prospective follow-up following treatment.[26]

In summary, it is difficult to draw firm conclusions from the data, and treatment recommendations based solely on the presence or absence of the pathologic features mentioned earlier should be made with caution. Prospective trials are needed in order to determine if these pathologic factors should be used to select patients for adjuvant therapy.

CLINICAL PRESENTATION

Symptoms of colon cancer include intermittent abdominal pain, nausea, or vomiting. These are secondary to bleeding, obstruction, or perforation. Bleeding may be acute and most commonly appears as red blood mixed with stool. Dark blood is most commonly secondary to diverticular bleeding.

ROUTES OF SPREAD

After the initial mucosal growth, there are several directions in which colorectal cancer may progress.

BOWEL WALL. The tumor penetrates through the bowel wall and extracolonic tissues and then directly invades adjacent organs or structures. An additional pattern of local spread is perineural invasion, which may extend as far as 10 cm from the primary tumor.

LYMPH NODES. The risk of lymph node metastases increases with increasing tumor grade. In addition, there is a clear relationship between lymphatic vessel invasion and the incidence and number of lymph node metastases

in colorectal cancer.[27,28] At least 12 to 14 lymph nodes must be examined for an accurate classification of nodal status.[29,30] Although they may be confused as lymph nodes, pericolonic tumor deposits are a harbinger of intra-abdominal metastasis in colon cancer.[31] In the sixth edition of the American Joint Committee on Cancer TNM Staging System, smooth metastatic nodules in the pericolic or perirectal fat are considered lymph node metastasis, whereas irregularly contoured metastatic nodules in the fat are considered vascular invasion.[32]

In *colon* cancer, the normal lymphatic flow is through the lymphatic channels along the major arteries, with three echelons of lymph nodes: pericolic, intermediate, and principal (Table 40-3).[10] If tumors lie between two major vascular pedicles, lymphatic flow may drain in either or both directions. If the central lymph nodes are blocked by tumor, lymphatic flow can become retrograde along the marginal arcades both proximally and distally.

In *rectal* cancer, the disease first metastasizes to the perirectal nodes at the level of the primary tumor or immediately above it.[33] Then the chain accompanying the superior hemorrhoidal vessels is involved. Discontinuous or skip metastases are rare. Usually, the pericolic lymph nodes along the mesenteric border of the pelvis are not involved by these rectal tumors unless there is extensive tumor with lymphatic blockage. In late stages of the disease, when the hemorrhoidal lymphatics are blocked, there is lateral or downward spread.

DISTANT METASTASIS. The liver is the primary site of hematogenous metastases, followed by the lung. In approximately 40% of autopsy studies, the liver is the only site involved.[34] Involvement of other distant sites in the absence of liver or lung involvement is rare.

DIAGNOSTIC AND STAGING STUDIES

The workup for colon carcinoma is presented in Table 40-4. Positron emission tomography (PET) scanning shows promise; however, it remains investigational.[35,36] The staging of colorectal carcinoma has been complicated by the fact that it has evolved over a century and various authors have developed systems that use the same terms to represent different stages. Because of these discrepancies in coding for the same stages, the comparison of clinical studies reported in the literature is often impossible.

Table 40–3   Regional Lymph Nodes in Colon Cancer

Site	Regional Nodes
Cecum	Anterior and posterior cecal, ileocolic, right colic
Ascending colon	Ileocolic, right and middle colic
Hepatic flexure	Middle and right colic
Transverse colon	Middle colic
Splenic flexure	Middle and left colic, inferior mesenteric
Descending colon	Left colic, inferior mesenteric, sigmoid
Sigmoid loop	Inferior mesenteric, superior rectal (hemorrhoidal), sigmoid, sigmoid mesenteric

Table 40-4   Workup for Colon Cancer

History—including family history of colorectal cancer or polyps
Physical examination
Colonoscopy (preferred) or barium enema
Biopsy of the primary tumor
Chest x-ray
Abdominal/pelvic CT scan or MRI
Screening profile
Carcinoembryonic antigen
Complete blood count
PET Scan (investigational)

The first practical staging system was Dukes' classification. This system classified colorectal tumors from A to C, with stage A indicating penetration into but not through the bowel wall; stage B representing penetration through the bowel wall; and stage C representing involvement of lymph nodes, regardless of the extent of bowel wall penetration. However, it has since been modified by many authors including Dukes to reflect finer levels of penetration and nodal metastases and has been extended to include the colon as well as the rectum.

The Astler-Coller staging system allowed separation of wall penetration and nodal status. The Gunderson-Sosin modification of the Astler-Coller staging system subdivided T3 tumors into those with microscopic (B_{2m} or C_{2m}) or gross (B_{2m+g} or C_{2m+g}) penetration of tumor through the bowel wall.[15,37] It also defined tumors adherent to or invading an adjacent organ or structure as B_3 if the nodes were negative and C_3 if the nodes were positive. Several studies have analyzed both local failure and survival using the modified Astler-Coller staging system.[12,13,15,37-39] Most have confirmed the predictive capability of this staging system.

In 1988 the AJCC[40] and the Union Internationale Contre le Cancer (UICC)[41] proposed a joint TNM staging system, based on the fifth edition of the AJCC TNM staging system. The sixth edition of the AJCC TNM staging system is presented in Table 40-5.[32] Major changes from the fifth edition are:

1. A revised description of the anatomy of the colon and rectum, which better delineates the data regarding the boundaries between the colon, rectum, and anus. Adenocarcinomas of the veriform appendix are classified with the TNM system, but should be recorded separately.
2. Smooth metastatic nodules in the pericolic or perirectal fat are considered nodal metastasis. In contrast, irregularly contoured metastatic nodules in the peritumoral fat are considered vascular invasion and are coded as a subcategory of the T stage as V1 (microscopic vascular invasion) if microscopically visible or V2 (macroscopic vascular invasion) if grossly visible.
3. Stage group II is subdivided into IIA (T3 disease) and IIB (T4 disease).
4. Stage group III is subdivided into IIIA (T1-2N1M0 disease), IIIB (T3-4N1M0 disease), and IIIB (TanyN2M0 disease). Additional descriptors do not affect the stage grouping, but do indicate cases needing separate analysis. The AJCC TNM staging system

Table 40-5   Classification of Colorectal Cancer

Primary Tumor (T)

Tx	Primary tumor cannot be assessed
T0	No evidence of primary tumor
Tis	Carcinoma in situ: intraepithelial or invasion of the lamina propria*
T1	Tumor invades submucosa
T2	Tumor invades muscularis propria
T3	Tumor invades through the muscularis propria into the subserosa, or into nonperitonealized pericolic or perirectal tissues
T4	Tumor directly invades other organs or structures or perforates the visceral peritoneum or both.†‡

Regional Lymph Nodes (N)

Nx	Regional nodes cannot be assessed
N0	No regional nodes
N1	Metastasis to 1-3 regional lymph nodes
N2	Metastasis to >4 regional lymph nodes

Distant Metastasis (M)

Mx	Distant metastasis cannot be assessed
M0	No distant metastasis
M1	Distant metastasis

*Tis includes cancer cells confined within the glandular basement membrane (intraepithelial) or lamina propria (intramucosal) with no extension through the muscularis mucosa into the submucosa.
†Direct invasion in T_4 includes invasion of other segments of the colorectum by way of the serosa; for example, invasion of the sigmoid colon by a carcinoma of the cecum.
‡Tumor that is adherent to other organs or structures, macroscopically, is classified as T_4. However, if no tumor is present in the adhesion, microscopically, the classification should be pT_3. The V and L substaging should be used to identify the presence or absence of vascular or lymphatic invasion.
NOTE: A tumor nodule in the pericolonic adipose tissue of a primary carcinoma without histologic evidence of residual lymph node in the nodule is classified in the pN category as a regional lymph node metastasis if the nodule has the form and smooth contour of a lymph node. If the nodule has an irregular contour, it should be classified in the T category and also coded as V1 (microscopic venous invasion) or as V2 (if it was grossly evident), because there is a strong likelihood that it represents venous invasion.

Stage Groupings

Stage	T	N	M
0	Tis	N0	M0
I	T1-2	N0	M0
IIA	T3	N0	M0
IIB	T4	N0	M0
IIIA	T1-2	N1	M0
IIIB	T3-4	N1	M0
IIIC	Tany	N2	M0
IV	Tany	Nany	M1

NOTE: Although additional descriptors do not affect the stage grouping, additional prefixes are used to indicate the need for additional analysis:

Suffix	Reason
m	The presence of multiple primary tumors in a single site, recorded in parentheses: pT(m)NM.
y	When classification is performed during or following initial radiation or chemotherapy or both and is based on the amount of tumor present at the time of the examination, and not an estimate of tumor before therapy: ycTNM or ypTNM.
r	Indicates recurrent tumor: rTNM.

Continued

Table 40–5   Classification of Colorectal Cancer—Cont'd

a   Indicates the stage at autopsy: aTNM.

Lymphatic Vessel Invasion (L)

Lx	Cannot be assessed
L0	No lymphatic vessel invasion
L1	Lymphatic vessel invasion present

Venous Invasion (V)

Vx	Cannot be assessed
V0	No venous invasion
V1	Microscopic venous invasion present
V2	Macroscopic venous invasion present

From Greene FL, Page DL, Fleming ID, et al, eds: *AJCC Cancer Staging Manual*, 6th ed, New York: Springer, 2002.

should be used routinely for staging and treatment purposes. Although CEA has prognostic importance, it is not a requirement of the staging system.[42]

If the pretreatment CEA is greater than 100 and the abdominal/pelvic CT does not reveal evidence of metastatic disease, a liver MRI should be performed to exclude liver metastasis.

Clinical staging is designated as yTNM and is based on physical examination, radiologic imaging, endoscopy, biopsy, and laboratory findings. Pathologic staging is designated as pTNM and depends on data acquired clinically in addition to surgical and pathologic findings. Tumors that have recurred are designated with the *r* prefix. If there is uncertainty regarding the appropriate T, N, or M staging, the lower (less advanced) category should be used.

STANDARD THERAPEUTIC APPROACHES

Surgery

Surgery is the standard treatment for both colon and rectal cancer. The successful management of this disease depends on careful surgical techniques[43] and the surgeon's experience.[44,45] Preliminary results of the Intergroup randomized comparison of open versus laparoscopic surgery in colon cancer do not reveal a clear benefit of laparoscopy.[46] The final results are pending.

Chemotherapy

The standard adjuvant therapy for node-positive (T1-4 N1-2 M0) resectable colon cancer is 6 cycles of postoperative 5-FU and leucovorin.[47,48] The role of adjuvant therapy in a patient with high-risk T3 N0 M0 disease remains controversial. For patients with advanced or metastatic disease, the standard is 5-FU, leucovorin, and irinotecan.[49,50] For patients who fail this regimen, oxaliplatin plus continuous infusion 5-FU is recommended.[51] Oral chemotherapeutic agents are being used more frequently,[52,53] and a number of targeted therapies are under development.[54]

The remainder of the discussion focuses on the rationale and results of adjuvant radiation therapy in colon cancer.

Radiation Therapy

LOCAL/REGIONAL RADIATION THERAPY

Radiation therapy is an effective but local modality. Its use in the adjuvant setting should be limited to (1) those clinical presentations where the risk of local failure is sufficiently high enough (10%) to justify its use, and (2) when an adequate dose can be delivered to the site at the highest risk for failure. In patients with stages T3-4 N0 M0 or T1-4 N1-2 M0 rectal cancer, radiation therapy is reasonable since the risk of local failure, depending on the stage, is 15% to 67% and an adequate dose to control microscopic disease (>45 Gy) can be delivered safely to the pelvis.

In contrast to rectal cancer, the role of adjuvant radiation therapy in colon cancer is less well defined. As discussed earlier, this is due to differences in the natural history of colon cancer compared with rectal cancer. All stages combined, the most common failure site in colon cancer is abdominal rather than local. Furthermore, when local failure occurs outside the pelvis, it usually does not produce the same degree of debilitating symptoms as those seen in rectal cancer.

Although the overall incidence of local failure is relatively low in colon cancer, some data suggest that, depending upon the anatomic location and selected pathologic features, there are subsets of patients in whom the incidence of local failure is increased. However, there is no uniform agreement on how to define these subsets. Gunderson et al.[15] divided the colon into two regions. Anatomically immobile (or mainly retroperitoneal) included the ascending colon, hepatic flexure, splenic flexure, and descending colon. Anatomically mobile (or mainly intraperitoneal) included the cecum and transverse colon. The highest incidence of local failure occurred in the cecum (30%); however, the other intraperitoneal site, the transverse colon, had one of the lowest rates of local failure (13%).

In contrast, Minsky et al.[12] reported a general trend of increased local failure with more distal colon sites. Patients with cecal cancer had a significantly lower incidence of local failure (3%) compared to those with cancer of the transverse (15%) or descending colon (25%). These data do not support the notion that bowel mobility is predictive of local failure.

Willett et al.[13,14] divided the colon into two groups. Group 1 included the cecum, ascending, midsigmoid, transverse, and descending colon. Group 2 included the high and low sigmoid colon, the splenic flexure, and the hepatic flexure. In stage T1-2 N0 M0 disease, there was a higher incidence of local failure in group 1 tumors (16% to 24%) compared with group 2 tumors (0 to 11%).

In summary, from series to series, there is no consistency as to which anatomic sites have the highest local failure rates. This inconsistency may reflect the differences in methods used to determine failure rather than the true natural history of the disease.

In addition to stage and site, pathologic features may be helpful in predicting those patients with a higher risk of local or distant failure. Although some pathologic features, by multivariate analysis, have a significant impact on local failure or survival or both, the primary decision for adjuvant therapy should be based primarily on stage. Molecular markers may be helpful and are under active investigation.

WHOLE ABDOMINAL RADIATION THERAPY

The rationale of whole abdominal radiation therapy is based on the high incidence of abdominal failure in colon cancer. With this technique, the whole abdomen receives 30 Gy, and in select series, is followed by a cone-down to the primary tumor bed. The results are discussed later in the Outcomes section.

TECHNIQUES OF RADIATION THERAPY

Introduction

The design and delivery of radiation therapy for colon cancer requires knowledge of the natural history of the disease, patterns of failure, anatomy, identification of surrounding structures, and radiobiologic principles. Furthermore, the use of proper equipment, implementation of methods to decrease treatment-related toxicity, and a close collaboration with the physics and technology staff are essential.

The biologic mechanisms of acute and delayed toxicity, as well as dietary interventions, have been previously published.[55,56] This review is limited to the technical aspects of the design of local/regional radiation therapy fields for colon cancer. It includes idealized treatment fields for various common clinical presentations. These techniques are modified from Gunderson, Martenson, and Willett.

General Treatment Techniques

For nonsigmoid primaries, patients should initially be placed in the lateral decubitus position. Immobilization devices are recommended to help stabilize the patient. The lateral decubitus position may help exclude small bowel from the treatment field. In the majority of cases, parallel opposed fields are recommended. Wedges or compensation devices should be used as needed.

In most cases where the majority of the pelvis is being treated (i.e., sigmoid primaries), treatment in the prone position and a three-field technique (if possible) should be used to help exclude the small bowel and maximize homogeneity within the treatment volume. These techniques are outlined in Chapter 41, Cancer of the Rectum.

Definition of the Treatment Field

The tumor bed is defined as the involved segment of large intestine and, when present, the adjacent organ or structure to which it was adherent or invading. If the tumor was adherent to an organ that was only partially resected (e.g., bladder, stomach), all or a majority of that organ should be treated to 45 Gy providing this does not exceed tolerance of critical structures. If the adherence was to a structure (e.g., pelvic sidewall, diaphragm, psoas muscle), a 3 to 5 cm margin beyond the area of adherence is recommended. When tumor adherence to an organ or structure places nodal groups at risk, the acceptable superior-inferior extent of node inclusion is the same as tumor bed plus margin. For example, adherence to the posterior abdominal wall would include the para-aortic nodes plus margin.

INITIAL FIELD

The tumor bed and the immediately adjacent para-aortic or pelvic nodes (depending on the site of the primary tumor) are treated to 45 Gy in 25 fractions. A margin of 3 cm of normal tissue should surround the tumor bed.

BOOST FIELD

If small bowel contrast studies demonstrate the exclusion of small bowel from the tumor bed such that no small bowel receives greater than 45 Gy, a boost of 5.4 Gy in 3 fractions should be delivered to the tumor bed plus a 2 cm margin.

IDEALIZED TREATMENT FIELDS

The diagrams in Figures 40-1 to 40-8 are general guidelines for designing radiation therapy fields for patients with primary lesions in various locations. In individual cases the actual design of the field will depend on a number of factors. These include assessment of tumor volume from preoperative studies (e.g., barium enema and abdominal CT scan), information from the operative and pathology reports, and the position of clips marking the tumor bed and sites of adherence to adjacent organs or structures.

In each diagram, the initial treatment area (tumor bed plus local/regional nodes) is indicated by the large field. The boost area, where applicable, is indicated by the small field.

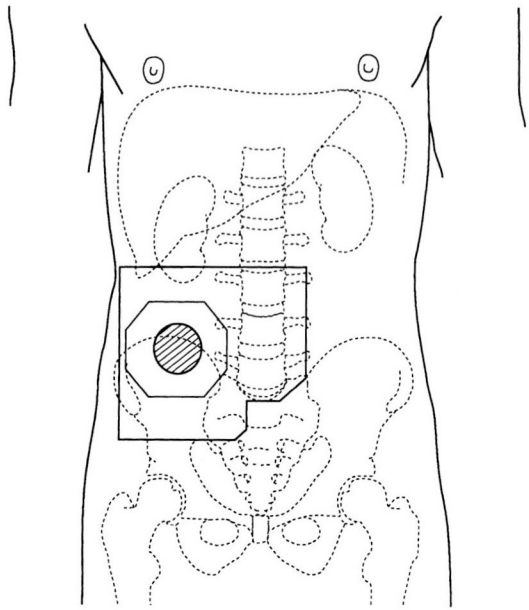

Figure 40–1. Idealized radiation treatment field for the cecum and proximal ascending colon.

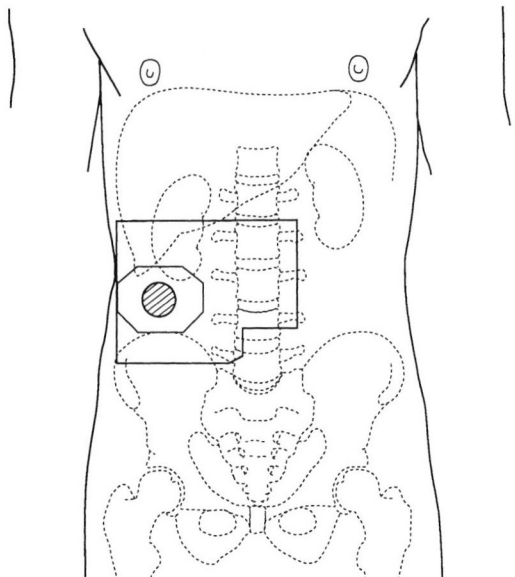

Figure 40–2. Idealized radiation treatment for the middle ascending colon.

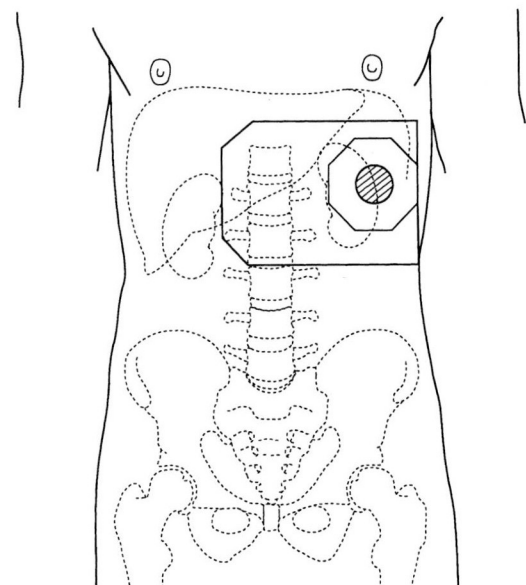

Figure 40–4. Idealized radiation treatment field for the splenic flexure and proximal descending colon.

CRITICAL NORMAL TISSUES

The primary dose-limiting structures in patients receiving local/regional radiation therapy for colon cancer commonly include the small bowel, liver, kidney, and spinal cord. The tolerance of these organs when conventional fractionation is used is as follows:

- Small bowel: maximum 45 Gy (30 Gy in patients receiving whole abdomen radiation).
- Liver: at least two thirds of the total liver volume must receive less than 30 Gy.
- Kidney: at least two thirds of one kidney must not receive a dose higher than 20 Gy. Depending on the field size and anatomic location, most or all of one

kidney may be in the radiation field. In such cases, a renal scan should be obtained to ensure that the contralateral kidney has adequate function.
- Spinal cord: the maximum dose to the spinal cord must be less than 50 Gy.

OUTCOMES

Local/Regional Radiation Therapy

Although all the series are retrospective and were performed in the era before effective chemotherapy,[49-51] the most comprehensive one examining the role of

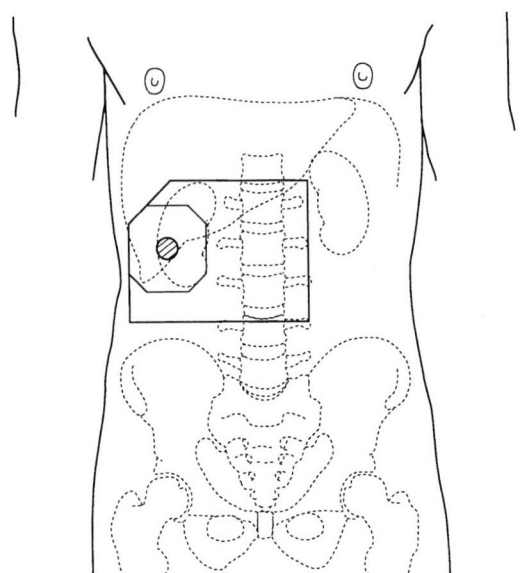

Figure 40–3. Idealized radiation treatment field for the distal ascending colon and hepatic flexure.

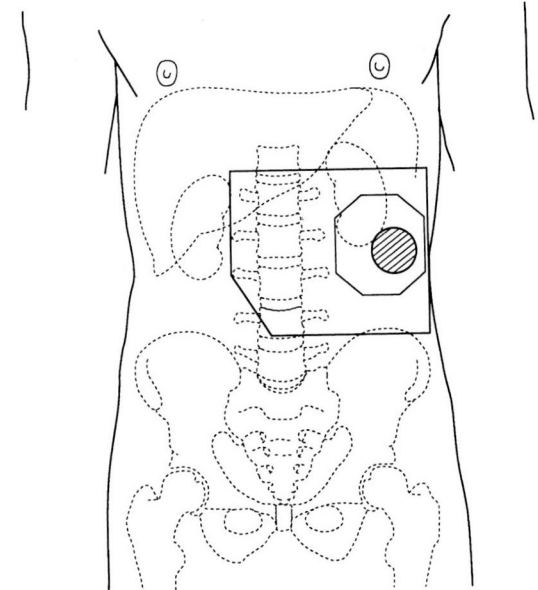

Figure 40–5. Idealized radiation treatment field for the middle descending colon.

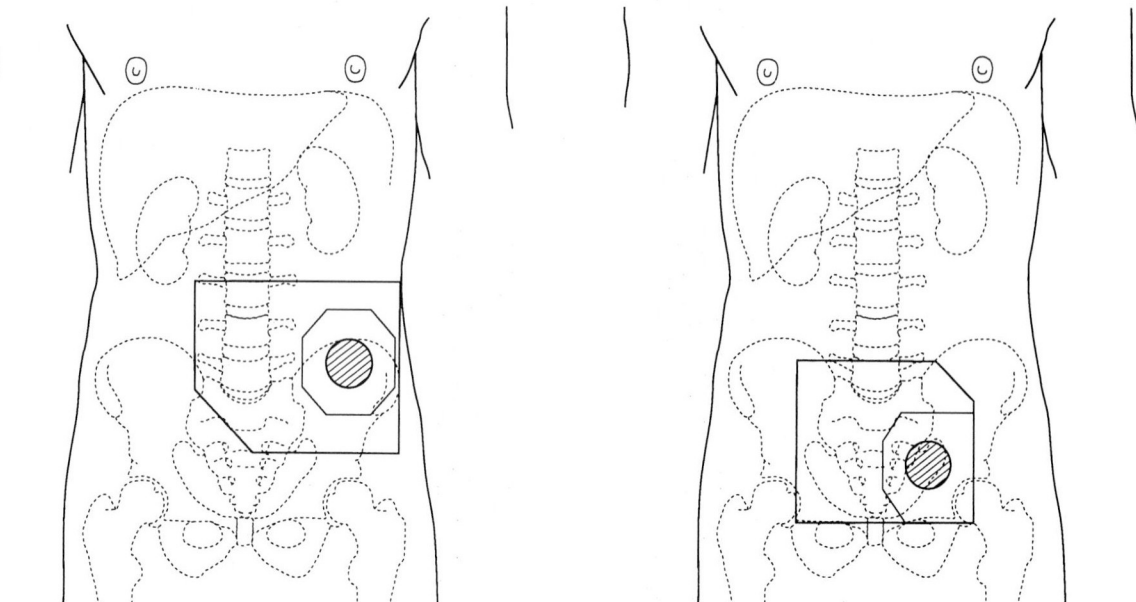

Figure 40–6. Idealized radiation treatment field for the distal descending colon. The ipsilateral common and external iliac nodes at the distal end of the tumor as well as the para-aortic nodes at the level of the proximal tumor bed should be included.

Figure 40–7. Idealized radiation treatment field for the middle sigmoid colon adherent to left pelvic sidewall or proximal sigmoid. As with other sites in the colon, placement of fields varies depending on the exact site of the tumor volume or the tumor bed.

local/regional radiation in colon cancer is from the Massachusetts General Hospital.[57,58] Following potentially curative surgery for stages T3-4 N0-2 M0 colon cancer, 203 patients received postoperative adjuvant radiation therapy. Eligibility included patients with the following stages: T4 N0-2 M0 regardless of anatomic site, T3 N1-2 M0 excluding mid-sigmoid and transverse colon, and select high-risk T3 N0 M0 tumors with close margins. Patients received 45 Gy to the primary tumor bed with a 5-cm margin as well as the primary draining lymph nodes. This was followed by a shrinking field technique to 50.4-55 Gy depending on the volume of small bowel, which could be excluded from the high-dose field. Of the

203, 173 were treated in the adjuvant setting and 30 after a subtotal resection. Sixty-three received bolus 5-FU with various doses and schedules.

The results at 5 years were compared with a historic control group of 395 patients who underwent surgery only.[57] As presented in Table 40-6, three groups of patients appeared to benefit from postoperative radiation therapy. First, there was a significant improvement in local control and disease-free survival for patients with stages T4 N0 M0 or T4 N1-2 M0 disease. Second, patients with stage T4 N0 M0 disease with a perforation or fistula had improved local control and disease-free survival. Third, radiation therapy salvaged some patients

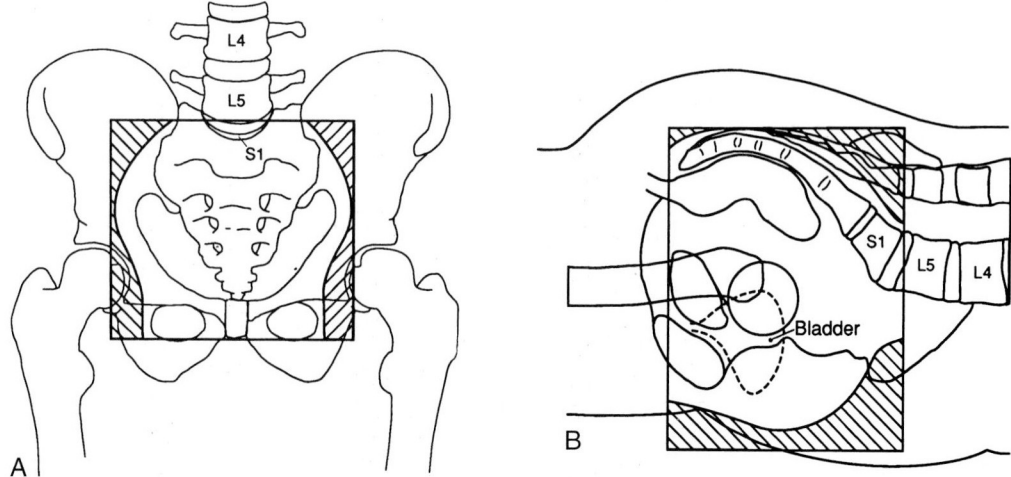

Figure 40–8. A and **B,** Idealized radiation treatment field for the sigmoid colon adherent to the bladder. A three- or four-field technique is recommended. At the time of simulation, 30 to 50 mL of contrast material should be introduced into the bladder via a Foley catheter as well as 10 to 15 mL of air to help define its anterior extent. The entire bladder and pelvis, including external and internal iliac nodes, should be included in the radiation field. For patients with distal sigmoid primary tumors, a three- or four-field technique similar to the one shown here is used except the bladder does not need to be included in the field. Techniques of pelvic radiation therapy are outlined in Chapter 41, Cancer of the Rectum.

Table 40–6 Local Adjuvant Radiation Therapy in Colon Cancer

Group	Stage	n	5-Yr Local/Regional Failure Surgery	n	Surgery + Radiation	5-Yr Disease-Free Survival Surgery	Surgery + Radiation
Adjuvant	T3N0	163	10%	23	9%*	70%	72%
	T4N0	83	31%	54	7%	63%	79%
	T3N1-2	100	35%	55	30%	44%	47%
	T4N1-2	49	53%	39	28%	37%	53%
Perforation/fistula	T4N0	21	48%	23	6%	43%	91%
Residual disease	All	—	—	30	47%	—	37%

*Actuarial component of total failure.
DFS, disease-free survival; —, data not available.
From Willett CG, Fung CY, Kaufman DS, et al: Postoperative radiation therapy for high-risk colon cancer. *J Clin Oncol.* 1993;11:1112.

with residual disease following subtotal resection (37% 5-year disease-free survival). There was no benefit in local control or disease-free survival in patients with stage T3 N0 M0 or T3 N1-2 M0 disease. It must be emphasized that the results may be biased against radiation therapy since many were high-risk patients referred because of concerns about margins.

With 10-year follow-up, local control in patients with T$_4$ disease was 78% with negative margins and 53% with positive margins.[58] For the 42 patients with positive margins, local control was 56% for the 30 with microscopically positive and 42% for the 12 with grossly positive margins.

Complications of treatment were acceptable. For the total patient group, the incidence of grade 3$^+$ acute bowel toxicity was 8%. Grade 3$^+$ long-term bowel toxicity was 4.5%. These toxicity results are similar to those reported from the Mayo Clinic/North Central Cancer Treatment Group postoperative adjuvant rectal trial 79-41-51.[24] Therefore, with careful treatment techniques, the acute and long-term bowel toxicity of postoperative local/regional radiation therapy (+ chemotherapy) for colon cancer are comparable to those reported for rectal cancer.

Based on the retrospective data from the Massachusetts General Hospital, a randomized phase III Intergroup trial coordinated by the Mayo/North Central Cancer Treatment Group (INT 0130) was developed. Patients with T4 or selected T3 N1-2 colon tumors were randomized to 12 cycles of bolus 5-FU + levamisole with or without local/regional radiation (45-50.4 Gy in 25-28 fractions) beginning with cycle 2 of chemotherapy. The trial was closed early due to poor accrual with only 222 of the anticipated 400 patients randomized, leaving 189 eligible patients.[59] Grade 3$^+$ toxicity was modestly higher in the combined modality therapy arm (43% vs. 35%, *P* = NS). With a median follow-up of 35 months, there was no significant difference in survival between the 2 arms. The patterns-of-failure data have not been reported.

In a phase I trial of 21 patients (4 with colon cancers) who received upper abdominal radiation plus continuous infusion 5-FU, Martenson and associates reported a 40% grade 3$^+$ toxicity rate.[60] Due to the large radiation field sizes, the dose of continuous infusion 5-FU must be attenuated in patients receiving combined modality therapy for upper abdominal malignancies.

Palermo and associates treated 45 patients with intraperitoneal 5-FU plus radiation to the tumor bed and para-aortic nodes.[61] Although local failure was only 11%, the 10-year survival was 53%, which is not superior to conventional approaches.

In summary, the retrospective data from the Massachusetts General Hospital suggest that there are subsets of colon cancer patients with high local failure rates in whom the addition of postoperative local/regional radiation therapy may improve local control and disease-free survival. The randomized INT 0130 trial did not show a survival advantage with combined modality therapy versus chemotherapy alone. It must be emphasized, however, that the INT 0130 trial was closed before meeting its accrual goals and has not yet reported local control results, although postoperative local/regional radiation in colon cancer remains investigational. Furthermore, more effective chemotherapeutic agents are now available.[49-51] However, there are two clinical situations where it is reasonable to use it. The first is in patients with close or positive resection margins. The second is in a patient who has undergone a resection of a T4 colon cancer adherent to pelvic structures. These cancers (most commonly sigmoid or cecal primaries) have local failure rates similar to rectal cancers, and it is reasonable to treat them as such with adjuvant combined modality therapy with 6 cycles of 5-FU based chemotherapy plus concurrent pelvic radiation.[62]

Whole Abdominal Radiation Therapy

The use of whole abdominal radiation therapy is limited by dose considerations. To treat the volume at risk with a potentially curative dose of radiation required for microscopic disease, the whole abdomen would need to receive 45 Gy. Although limited portions of the abdomen can tolerate this dose, the tolerance of the whole abdomen with conventional fractionation is 30 Gy. Based on the high incidence of abdominal failure in some colon cancers, a number of phase II adjuvant trials were designed to examine the efficacy of whole abdominal radiation therapy.[63-67]

In general, patients received 20 to 30 Gy to the whole abdomen with or without a boost to the primary tumor bed. In three of the series, 5-FU was delivered with various doses and schedules. The combined results revealed an in-field (abdominal) failure rate of 12% to 50%. Significant toxicity varied from 5% to 38%. Although the initial phase II results appeared promising, three of the series (Brenner,[64] Meek,[65] and Wong[63]) have never been updated.

The most encouraging data have been reported by Fabian et al. from the Southwest Oncology Group (SWOG 8572).[66] In this phase II adjuvant pilot trial, 41 patients with T3 N1-2 M0 disease received whole abdominal radiation therapy plus continuous infusion 5-FU followed by 9 monthly cycles of continuous infusion 5-FU. Due to unacceptable toxicity in the first 6 patients, the protocol was modified such that (1) the 5-FU was started day 1 and radiation began concurrently on day 8, and (2) a 1-week treatment break from both the 5-FU and radiation was required at day 42. The tumor bed boost (1.6 Gy × 10) was delivered first, followed by whole abdominal radiation therapy (1 Gy/day × 30) for a total dose of 30 Gy to the whole abdomen and 46 Gy to the tumor bed.

With a median follow-up of 5 years, the 5-year disease-free and overall survival rates were 58% and 67%, respectively. Limiting the analysis to the 20 patients with more than 4 positive nodes, the 5-year disease-free and overall survival rates were 55% and 74%, respectively. For the total patient group, patterns of failure included local, 12%; liver, 22%; and peritoneal and other abdominal, 15%. In contrast with other whole abdomen radiation therapy trials, toxicity during the combined modality segment was tolerable (17%: grade 3, 7%: grade 4). These results are encouraging but need further follow-up. At present, whole abdominal radiation remains investigational.

In summary, following resection for colon cancer, the primary failure pattern is abdominal. Although local failure does occur, it is less frequent, more difficult to detect, and usually does not result in the same degree of morbidity as a local failure in rectal cancer. Retrospective data from the Massachusetts General Hospital suggest some benefit of local/regional radiation therapy on local control and disease-free survival in select patients with T4 disease. The phase III Intergroup trial 0130 did not reveal a survival advantage for the addition of local/regional radiation therapy to 5-FU/levamasole. In contrast to rectal cancer, where radiation plus chemotherapy is standard treatment in the adjuvant setting, the use of radiation therapy (either local/regional or whole abdominal) in colon cancer remains investigational.

FOLLOW-UP FOR COLORECTAL CANCER

Significant controversy exists as to the recommended follow-up for patients after they are treated for colorectal cancer. Evidence-based clinical practice guidelines have been published by the American Society of Clinical Oncology.[68] However, these can be modified based on risk and individual patient and clinician requirements. Isolated liver, lung, and pelvic recurrences should be considered for aggressive treatment.[69]

REFERENCES

1. Jemal A, Murray T, Samuel A, et al: Cancer Statistics, 2003. *CA Cancer J Clin.* 2003;53:5.
2. Weisburger JH, Wynder EL: Etiology of colorectal cancer with emphasis on mechanism of action and prevention. In DeVita V, Hellman S, Rosenberg SA, eds. *Important Advances in Oncology.* Philadelphia: JB Lippincott; 1987:197.
3. Michels KB, Giovannucci E, Joshipura KJ, et al: Prospective study of fruit and vegetable consumption and incidence of colon and rectal cancers. *J Natl Cancer Inst.* 2000;92:1740.
4. Nicholl ID, Dunlop MG: Molecular markers of prognosis in colorectal cancer. *J Natl Cancer Inst.* 1999;91:1267.
5. Ogunbiyi OA, Goodfellow PJ, Herfarth K, et al: Confirmation that chromosome 18q allelic loss in colon cancer is a prognostic indicator. *J Clin Oncol.* 1998;16:427.
6. Leslie A, Carey FA, Pratt NR, et al: The colorectal adenoma-carcinoma sequence. *Br J Surg.* 2002;89:845.
7. Watanabe T, Wu TT, Catalano PJ, et al: Molecular predictors of survival after adjuvant chemotherapy for colon cancer. *N Engl J Med.* 2001;344:1196.
8. Gryfe R, Kim H, Hsieh ETK, et al: Tumor microsatellite instability and clinical outcome in young patients with colorectal cancer. *N Engl J Med.* 2000;342:69.
9. Lenz HJ, Danenberg KD, Leichman CG, et al: *p53* and thymidylate synthase expression in untreated stage II colon cancer: Associations with recurrence, survival, and site. *Clin Cancer Res.* 1998;4:1227.
10. Skibber JM, Minsky BD, Hoff PM: Cancer of the colon. In Devita VT, Hellman S, Rosenberg SA, eds. *Cancer: Principles and Practice of Oncology.* 6th ed. Philadelphia: Lippincott, Williams & Wilkins; 2001:1216.
11. Skibber JM, Hoff PM, Minsky BD: Cancer of the rectum. In Devita VT, Hellman S, Rosenberg SA, eds. *Cancer: Principles and Practice of Oncology.* 6th ed. Philadelphia: Lippincott, Williams & Wilkins; 2001:1271.
12. Minsky BD, Mies C, Rich TA, et al: Potentially curative surgery of colon cancer: 1. Patterns of failure and survival. *J Clin Oncol.* 1988;6:106.
13. Willett CG, Tepper JE, Cohen AM, et al: Failure patterns following curative resection of colonic carcinoma. *Ann Surg.* 1984;200:685.
14. Willett C, Tepper JE, Cohen AM, et al: Local failure following curative resection of colonic adenocarcinoma. *Int J Radiat Oncol Biol Phys.* 1984;10:645.
15. Gunderson LL, Sosin H, Levitt S: Extrapelvic colon—Areas of failure in a reoperation series: Implications for adjuvant therapy. *Int J Radiat Oncol Biol Phys.* 1985;11:731.
16. Minsky BD: Clinicopathologic impact of colloid in colorectal carcinoma. *Dis Colon Rectum.* 1990;33:714.
17. Pidhorecky I, Cheney RT, Kraybill WG, et al: Gastrointestinal stromal tumors: Current diagnosis, biologic behavior, and management. *Ann Surg Oncol.* 2000;7:705.
18. Hatch KF, Blanchard DK, Hatch GF, et al: Tumors of the rectum and anal canal. *World J Surg.* 2000;24:437.
19. Grann A, Paty PB, Cohen AM, et al: Sphincter preservation of leiomyosarcoma of the rectum and anus with local excision and brachytherapy. *Dis Colon Rectum.* 1999;42:1296.
20. Doolabh N, Anthony T, Simmang C, et al: Primary colonic lymphoma. *J Surg Oncol.* 2000;74:257.
21. Frizelle FA, Hobday KS, Batts KP, et al: Adenosquamous and squamous carcinoma of the colon and upper rectum. *Dis Colon Rectum.* 2001;44:341.
22. Dukes CE: The classification of cancer of the rectum. *J Pathol.* 1932;35:323.
23. Minsky BD, Mies C, Rich TA, et al: Potentially curative surgery of colon cancer. The influence of blood vessel invasion. *J Clin Oncol.* 1988;6:119.
24. Krook JE, Moertel CG, Gunderson LL, et al: Effective surgical adjuvant therapy for high-risk rectal carcinoma. *N Engl J Med.* 1991;324:709.
25. Wong JH, Steinemann S, Tom P, et al: Volume of lymphatic metastasis does not independently influence prognosis in colorectal cancer. *J Clin Oncol.* 2002;20:1506.
26. Bast RC, Ravdin P, Hayes DF, et al: 2000 update of recommendations for the use of tumor markers in breast and colorectal cancer: Clinical practice guidelines of the American Society of Clinical Oncology. *J Clin Oncol.* 2001;19:1865.

27. Davis NC, Evans EB, Cohen JR, et al: Staging of colorectal cancer: The Australian Clinico-Pathological Staging (ACPS) system compared with the Dukes' system. *Dis Colon Rectum.* 1984;27:707.

28. Minsky BD, Mies C, Rich TA, et al: Lymphatic vessel invasion is an independent prognostic factor for survival in colorectal cancer. *Int J Radiat Oncol Biol Phys.* 1989;17:311.

29. Tepper JE, O'Connell MJ, Niedzwiecki D, et al: Impact of number of nodes retrieved on outcome in patients with rectal cancer. *J Clin Oncol.* 2001;19:157.

30. Wong JH, Severino R, Honnebier MB, et al: Number of nodes examined and staging accuracy in colorectal cancer. *J Clin Oncol.* 1999;17:2896.

31. Goldstein NS, Turner JR: Pericolonic tumor deposits in patients with T3N+M0 colon adenocarcinomas. Markers of reduced disease free survival and intra-abdominal metastases and their implications for TNM classification. *Cancer.* 2000;88:2228.

32. Colon and Rectum. In Green FL, Page DL, Fleming ID, et al., eds. *AJCC Cancer Staging Manual.* 6th ed. New York: Springer; 2002:113.

33. Cohen AM, Minsky BD, Friedman MJ: Cancer of the rectum. In Devita VT, Hellman S, Rosenberg SA, eds. *Cancer: Principles and Practice of Oncology.* 4th ed. Philadelphia: JB Lippincott; 1993:978.

34. Weiss L, Grundmann E, Torhorst J, et al: Haematogenous metastatic patterns in colonic carcinoma: An analysis of 1541 necropsies. *J Pathol.* 1986;150:195.

35. Whiteford MH, Whiteford HM, Yee LF, et al: Usefulness of FDG-PET scan in the assessment of suspected metastatic or recurrent adenocarcinoma of the colon and rectum. *Dis Colon Rectum.* 2000;53:759.

36. Flamen P, Stroobants S, van Cutsem E, et al: Additional value of whole-body positron emission tomography with fluorine-18-2-fluoro-2-deoxy-D-glucose in recurrent colorectal cancer. *J Clin Oncol.* 1999;17:894.

37. Gunderson LL, Sosin H: Areas of failure found at reoperation (second or symptomatic look) following "curative surgery" for adenocarcinoma of the rectum: Clinicopathologic correlation and implications for adjuvant therapy. *Cancer.* 1974;34:1278.

38. Minsky BD, Mies C, Recht A, et al: Resectable adenocarcinoma of the rectosigmoid and rectum: 1. Patterns of failure and survival. *Cancer.* 1988;61:1408.

39. Rich T, Gunderson LL, Lew R, et al: Patterns of recurrence of rectal cancer after potentially curative surgery. *Cancer.* 1983;52:1317.

40. Weitz J, Kienle P, Lacroix J, et al: Dissemination of tumor cells in patients undergoing surgery for colorectal cancer. *Cancer Res.* 1998;4:343.

41. Obrand DI, Gordon PH: Continued change in the distribution of colorectal carcinoma. *Br J Surg.* 1998;85:246.

42. Compton C, Fenoglio-Preiser CM, Pettigrew N, et al: American Joint Committee on Cancer prognostic factors consensus conference. Colorectal Working Group. *Cancer.* 2000;88:1739.

43. Nelson H, Petrelli N, Carlin A, et al: Guidelines 2000 for colon and rectal surgery. *J Natl Cancer Inst.* 2001;93:583.

44. Schrag D, Cramer LD, Bach PB, et al: Influence of hospital procedure volume on outcomes following surgery for colon cancer. *J Amer Med Assoc.* 2000;284:3028.

45. Stocchi L, Nelson H, Sargent DJ, et al: Impact of surgical and pathologic variables in rectal cancer: A United States community and cooperative group report. *J Clin Oncol.* 2001;19:389.

46. Weeks JC, Nelson H, Gelber S, et al: Short-term quality-of-life outcomes following laparoscopic-assisted colectomy vs. open colectomy for colon cancer. *J Amer Med Assoc.* 2002;287:321.

47. O'Connell MJ, Laurie JA, Kahn M, et al: Prospectively randomized trial of postoperative adjuvant chemotherapy in patients with high-risk colon cancer. *J Clin Oncol.* 1998;16:295.

48. O'Connell MJ, Mailliard JA, Kahn MJ, et al: Controlled trial of fluorouracil and low-dose leucovorin given for 6 months as postoperative adjuvant therapy for colon cancer. *J Clin Oncol.* 1997;15:246.

49. Saltz LB, Cox JV, Blanke C, et al: Irinotecan plus fluorouracil and leucovorin for metastatic colorectal cancer. *N Engl J Med.* 2000;343:905.

50. Rothenberg MA, Meropol NJ, Poplin E, et al: Mortality associated with irinotecan plus bolus fluorouracil/leucovorin: summary findings of an independent panel. *J Clin Oncol.* 2001;19:3801.

51. Goldberg RM, Morton RF, Sargent DJ, et al: N9741: oxaliplatin (oxal) or CPT-11 + 5-fluorouracil (5FU)/leucovorin (LV) or oxal + CPT-11 in advanced colorectal cancer (CRC). Initial toxicity and response data from a GI Intergroup study. *Proc ASCO.* 2002;21:128a [abstract].

52. Eng C, Kindler HL, Schlisky RL: Oral fluoropyrimidine treatment of colorectal cancer. *Clin Colorec Cancer.* 2001;1:95.

53. van Cutsem E, Twelves C, Cassidy J, et al: Oral capecitabine compared with intravenous fluorouracil plus leucovorin in patients with metastatic colorectal cancer: Results of a large phase III study. *J Clin Oncol.* 2001;19:4097.

54. DeMario MD, Ratain MJ: Oral chemotherapy: Rationale and future directions. *J Clin Oncol.* 1998;16:2557.

55. Kinsella TJ, Bloomer WD: Tolerance of the intestine to radiation therapy. *Surg Gynecol Obstet.* 1980;151:273.

56. Klimberg VS, Souba WW, Dolson DJ, et al: Prophylactic glutamine protects the intestinal mucosa from radiation injury. *Cancer.* 1990;66:62.

57. Willett CG, Fung CY, Kaufman DS, et al: Postoperative radiation therapy for high-risk colon cancer. *J Clin Oncol.* 1993;11:1112.

58. Willett CG, Goldberg S, Shellito PC, et al: Does postoperative irradiation play a role in the adjuvant therapy of stage T4 colon cancer. *Cancer J Sci Am.* 1999;5:242.

59. Martenson J, Willett C, Sargent D, et al: A phase III study of adjuvant radiation therapy (RT), 5-fluorouracil (5-FU) and levamisole (LEV) vs. 5-FU and LEV in selected patients with resected high risk colon cancer: Initial results of INT 0130. *Proc ASCO.* 1999;18:235a [abstract].

60. Martenson JA, Swaminathan R, Burch PA, et al: Pilot study of continuous-infusion 5-fluorouracil, oral leucovorin, and upper-abdominal radiation therapy in patients with locally advanced residual or recurrent upper gastrointestinal or extrapelvic colon cancer. *Int J Radiat Oncol Biol Phys.* 1997;37:615.

61. Palermo JA, Richards F, Lohman KK, et al: Phase II trial of adjuvant radiation and intraperitoneal 5-fluorouracil for locally advanced colon cancer: results with 10 year follow-up. *Int J Radiat Oncol Biol Phys.* 2000;47:725.

62. Tepper JE, O'Connell MJ, Petroni GR, et al: Adjuvant postoperative fluorouracil-modulated chemotherapy combined with pelvic radiation therapy for rectal cancer: Initial results of Intergroup 0114. *J Clin Oncol.* 1997;15:2030.

63. Wong CS, Harwood AR, Cummings BJ, et al: Total abdominal irradiation for cancer of the colon. *Radiother Oncol.* 1984;2:209.

64. Brenner HJ, Bibi C, Chaitchik S: Adjuvant therapy for Dukes' C adenocarcinoma of the colon. *Int J Radiat Oncol Biol Phys.* 1983;8:1789.

65. Meek AG, Lam WC, Order SE: Carcinoma of the colon: Irradiation by delayed split whole-abdominal technique. *Radiology.* 1983;148:845.

66. Fabian C, Shankar S, Estes N, et al: Adjuvant continuous infusion 5-FU, whole-abdominal radiation, and tumor bed boost in high-risk stage III colon carcinoma; a Southwest Oncology Group pilot study. *Int J Radiat Oncol Biol Phys.* 1995;32:457.

67. Ben-Joseph E, Court WS: Whole abdominal radiotherapy and concomitant 5-fluorouracil as adjuvant therapy in advanced colon cancer. *Dis Colon Rectum.* 1995;38:1088.

68. Benson III AB, Desch CE, Flynn PJ, et al: 2000 update of American Society of Clinical Oncology colorectal cancer surveillance guidelines. *J Clin Oncol.* 2000;18:3586.

69. Hamy A, Baron O, Bennouna J, et al: Resection of hepatic and pulmonary metastases in patients with colorectal cancer. *Am J Clin Oncol.* 2001;24:607.

Cancer of the Rectum

41

Bruce D. Minsky, MD

The sections in this chapter on Epidemiology and Genetics, Pathology, Routes of Spread, and Diagnostic and Staging Studies apply to both colon cancer and rectal cancer and are discussed in Chapter 40, Cancer of the Colon. This chapter focuses exclusively on rectal cancer.

EPIDEMIOLOGY, ETIOLOGY, GENETICS, AND CYTOGENETIC ABNORMALITIES

Information on epidemiology and genetics is covered in Chapter 40, Cancer of the Colon. In 2003 there will be an estimated 42,000 new cases of rectal cancer in the United States with 23,800 occurring in men and 18,200 occurring in women. Approximately 8500 deaths are expected.[1]

ANATOMY

The rectum is approximately 15 cm in length. As shown in Figure 41-1, it is divided into three 5-cm segments in relation to the anal verge (upper third, middle third, and lower third). However, the actual rectal length and division into surgical segments reflect various features such as height, body habitus, pelvic width, and curve of the sacral hollow. For treatment purposes, large bowel cancers located at or below the peritoneal reflection (rectosigmoid plus rectum) are collectively defined as rectal cancer.

The major portion of the lymphatic drainage of the rectum passes along the superior hemorrhoidal arterial trunk toward the inferior mesenteric artery.[2] Only a few lymphatics follow the inferior mesenteric vein. The pararectal nodes above the level of the middle rectal valve drain exclusively along the superior hemorrhoidal lymphatic chain. Below this level (approximately 7 to 8 cm above the anal verge), some lymphatics pass to the lateral rectal pedicle. These lymphatics are associated with nodes along the middle hemorrhoidal artery, obturator fossa, and hypogastric and common iliac arteries. Extensive lymphatics are also present in women contiguous with the rectovaginal septum, and in men along Denonvilliers' fascia. The entire extraperitoneal soft tissue (mesorectum) is permeated with lymphatics.

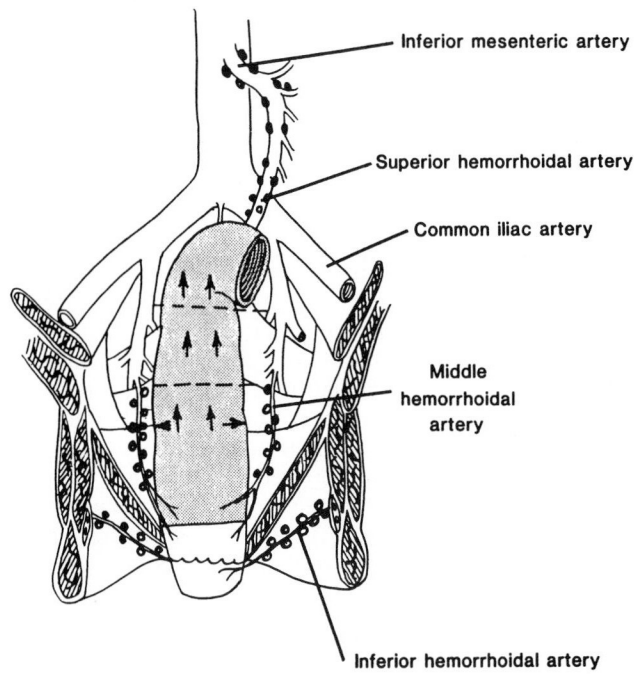

Figure 41–1. Anatomy and lymphatic drainage of the rectum. (From Pemberton JH: Anatomy and physiology of the anus and rectum. In Zuidema GD, ed. *Shackelford's Surgery of the Alimentary Tract.* 2nd ed. Philadelphia: WB Saunders; 1991:253.)

PATHOLOGY

The majority of this information is covered in Chapter 40, Cancer of the Colon. However, the issue of lateral margins, which is most relevant to rectal cancer, is discussed here.

In general, when pathologists describe negative margins of resection, they are referring to the proximal and distal margins. Since the staging of rectal cancer depends on the penetration of tumor through the bowel wall, it is rational to examine the lateral (or circumferential or radial) margin. Birbeck and associates reviewed surgical specimens of 586 patients and found that 28% had a positive circumferential margin.[3] There was a significant increase in local recurrence (38% vs. 10%) and decrease in 5-year survival (40% vs. 79%) in patients with positive versus negative circumferential margins. In contrast, Cawthorn et al. found no correlation between lateral margins and local failure.[4] Of 167 patients with rectal cancer, 13 developed local failure and 12 of the 13 had negative lateral margins. Likewise, 11 patients had positive lateral margins and only 1 (9%) developed local failure.

The conflicting results may be a function of how meticulous the pathologic examination is performed. For example, the incidence of positive lateral margins was 28% in the series by Quirke et al. as compared with 7% in the series by Cawthorn et al. In addition, some patients in Cawthorn's series received postoperative radiation therapy. In summary, although there is controversy regarding the impact of lateral margins, most clinicians accept their clinical importance.

CLINICAL PRESENTATION

Rectal cancer is usually symptomatic before diagnosis. Common symptoms include gross red blood (mixed or covering stool, or by itself), unexplained constipation, or reduction in stool caliber. Hemorrhoidal bleeding should always be a diagnosis of exclusion. Obstructing rectal cancers frequently present with diarrhea rather than constipation.

In cases of locally advanced rectal cancer with circumferential growth and extensive transmural penetration, urgency, inadequate emptying, and tenesmus are seen. This is usually a grave sign. Urinary symptoms or buttock/perineal pain from posterior extension are also grave signs.

ROUTES OF SPREAD

This information is covered in Chapter 40, Cancer of the Colon.

DIAGNOSTIC AND STAGING STUDIES

The standard workup for rectal cancer is presented in Table 41-1. The primary imaging modalities to assess the extent of the primary tumor are computed tomography (CT), magnetic resonance imaging (MRI), and transrectal ultrasound. The overall accuracy in predicting T stage is approximately 50% to 90% with transrectal ultrasound[5,6] and 50% to 70% with CT or MRI.[7-9] Preliminary data suggest that positron emission tomography (PET) may offer a higher sensitivity compared with CT.[10,11] PET is also helpful in predicting patients who will achieve negative margins at surgery.[12]

The identification of positive lymph nodes is more difficult. The overall accuracy in detecting positive lymph nodes with the techniques just mentioned is approximately 50%. The accuracy of MRI is similar to CT; however, it may be further enhanced with the use of Helmholtz or endorectal coils or both.[9] Both CT and MRI can identify lymph nodes that measure 1 cm or more, although enlarged lymph nodes are not pathognomonic of tumor involvement. Furthermore, using a nodal clearing technique, Herrera et al. found that 78% of positive lymph nodes in rectal cancer occur most frequently in lymph nodes measuring less than 5 mm.[13]

STAGING SYSTEMS

Pathologic

The sixth edition of the American Joint Commission on Cancer (AJCC) TNM staging system, as well as details regarding the evolution of pathologic staging of rectal cancer, are discussed in Chapter 40, Cancer of the Colon.

Clinical

A number of clinical staging systems for rectal cancer have been developed. Clinical stages I and II commonly include cases in which local curative excision may be possible. Nicholls et al. tested the accuracy of the digital examination by comparing it with the final pathologic stage. They reported that clinical determination of the local extent and penetration correlated positively with survival.[14]

None of these clinical staging systems have been widely accepted. Therefore, most investigators recommend the TNM staging system with the notation based on clinical or radiographic findings or both (i.e., uT3 or cT4). The sixth edition of the AJCC TNM staging system recommends the y prefix (ycTNM or ypTNM) when the tumor is staged during or after radiation or chemotherapy or both.[15]

STANDARD THERAPEUTIC APPROACHES

Two conventional treatments for clinically resectable rectal cancer are: (1) surgery and, if the tumor is T3 or N1-2 or both, postoperative combined modality therapy,[16] and (2) if the tumor is ultrasound T3 or clinical T4, preoperative combined modality therapy followed by surgery and postoperative chemotherapy.[17] In patients with recurrent or clinically unresectable disease, intraoperative radiation therapy is added at the time of surgery.[18,19] In select patients with T1-2 disease, a local excision with or without postoperative combined modality therapy has been used.[20] Radiation therapy alone has been used for patients who refuse surgery or are medically inoperable.[21] The selection and results of these approaches are discussed in the Outcomes section.

TECHNIQUES OF RADIATION THERAPY

The design and delivery of pelvic radiation therapy for rectal cancer requires knowledge of the patterns of failure, anatomy, identification of pelvic structures, and

---

Table 41–1   Workup for Rectal Cancer

History—including family history of colorectal cancer or polyps

Physical examination—including assessment of mobility, minimum diameter of the lumen, and distance from the anal verge

Proctoscopy—including assessment of mobility, minimum diameter of the lumen, and distance from the anal verge

Colonoscopy or barium enema

Biopsy of the primary tumor

Chest x-ray

Abdominal/pelvic computed tomography scan or magnetic resonance imaging

Screening profile

Carcinoembryonic antigen

Complete blood count

Transrectal ultrasound (if considering a local excision or preoperative therapy)

Pelvic magnetic resonance imaging (optional, preferably with an endorectal or Helmholtz coil or both)

Positron emission tomography (PET) (investigational)

radiobiologic principles. Furthermore, the use of proper equipment, implementation of methods to decrease treatment-related toxicity, and a close collaboration with the physics and technology staff are essential.

The biologic mechanisms of acute and delayed toxicity as well as dietary interventions have been well described.[22] Acute complications such as diarrhea and increased bowel frequency (small bowel), acute proctitis (large bowel), thrombocytopenia, leukopenia, and dysuria are common during treatment. These conditions are usually transient and resolve within a few weeks following completion of radiation. The symptoms appear to be a function of the dose rate and fraction size rather than the total dose. The mechanism is primarily the depletion of actively dividing cells in what is otherwise a stable cell renewal system. In the small bowel, loss of the mucosal cells results in malabsorption of various substances including fat, carbohydrate, protein, and bile salts. Sigmoidoscopy during treatment frequently reveals an inflamed, edematous, and friable rectal mucosa. The bowel mucosa usually recovers completely in 1 to 3 months following radiation. Management usually involves the use of antispasmodic or anticholinergic medications or both.

Delayed complications occur less frequently but are substantially more serious. The initial symptoms commonly occur 6 to 18 months following completion of radiation. Complications include: persistent diarrhea and increased bowel frequency, proctitis, small bowel obstruction not requiring surgery, perineal/scrotal tenderness, delayed perineal wound healing, urinary incontinence, and bladder atrophy/bleeding. Injury to the vascular and supporting stromal tissues is the presumed pathophysiology.

The most common, delayed, severe complications are due to small bowel damage and include small bowel enteritis, adhesions, and small bowel obstruction requiring surgical intervention. The incidence of small bowel obstruction requiring surgery following postoperative pelvic radiation for rectal cancer is 4% to 12% in modern series and as high as 17.5% in historical series. In the Massachusetts General Hospital (MGH) series the incidence of small bowel destruction with postoperative radiation therapy was 6% as compared with 5% with surgery alone.[23]

Toxicity of Pelvic Radiation Therapy

This section focuses on the technical aspects of the design of pelvic radiation therapy—first on general methods to decrease treatment-related toxicity in patients receiving radiation for various pelvic malignancies, then on the design of treatment fields for patients receiving pelvic radiation specifically for rectal cancer.

Complications of pelvic radiation therapy are a function of the volume of the radiation field, overall treatment time, fraction size, radiation energy, total dose, and technique. A number of simple radiotherapeutic techniques are available to decrease radiation-related small bowel toxicity (Table 41-2).[24,25] For example, the use of multiple-field techniques (preferably a three-field) allows a larger amount of small bowel to be blocked from the pelvis compared with an anterior-posterior–posterior-anterior (AP–PA) (two-field) technique. The treatment of all fields each day

Table 41–2   Techniques to Decrease Radiation Toxicity in Small Bowel

1. High-energy (15 MV) linear accelerators.
2. Treatment 5 days per week and all fields each day.
3. Port films once per week or more often if clinically indicated.
4. Pelvic field: multiple-field technique (posterior-anterior plus laterals or posterior-anterior–anterior-posterior plus laterals) is recommended. If the patient is male (the genitalia are commonly in the treatment field), there is a large volume of small bowel in the pelvis, or if a colostomy is present, a three-field technique (posterior-anterior plus laterals) is recommended.
5. Boost field: opposed laterals.
6. Computerized dosimetry optimizing between minimizing the lateral hot spots and small bowel dose and increasing the homogeneity within the target volume (see Fig. 41-8). In thin patients, a combination of 6 MV for the posterior fields and 10 to 15 MV for the lateral fields may result in more homogeneous dosimetry.
7. Shaped blocks and, if needed, wedges on the lateral fields.
8. Small bowel contrast. Shield as much small bowel as possible in the lateral parts.
9. Rectal contrast. Barium sulfate is injected with a 16-French Foley catheter. A wire is placed on the catheter to identify the anal verge.
10. Prone position.
11. Full bladder, only if it does not make the patient so uncomfortable as to cause movement.
12. The only portion of the perineum at risk for recurrence after an abdominoperineal resection is the scar. The remaining perineum can be blocked. The entire perineum can be blocked after a low anterior resection. Use wire to outline the portion of the perineum that is not at risk for recurrence and block it on the lateral fields (see Fig. 41-7).
13. Immobilization molds (belly boards) and abdominal wall compression may be helpful.
14. Dose considerations:
    A. Limit whole pelvis dose to 45 to 46.8 Gy.
    B. Limit boost to 50 to 50.4 Gy if the small bowel is in the boost field.
    C. Total dose: preoperative, 50.46 Gy; postoperative, 50.4 Gy, or if the small bowel is excluded from the high-dose field, the boost dose can be increased to 54 Gy. If there is microscopic or gross residual disease, then higher doses (55 Gy–60 Gy) are needed; however, this may be associated with increased toxicity.
    D. Standard fractionation in patients receiving combined-modality therapy is 1.8 Gy per day and in patients receiving radiation therapy alone is 1.8 Gy–2 Gy per day.

results in a lower integral dose and more homogeneous dose distribution. The use of lateral fields for the boost as well as positioning the patient in the prone position further decreases the volume of small bowel in the lateral radiation fields. The treatment should be designed with the use of computerized radiation dosimetry and be delivered by high-energy linear accelerators (15 MV), which, by nature of their depth dose characteristics, deliver a higher dose to the tumor volume while sparing the surrounding normal structures. When the perineal scar needs to be treated, it should be included in the pelvic radiation fields. The use of a separate perineal field is associated with an increased risk of overlap of the radiation fields and should be avoided. Split-course pelvic radiation is associated with increased chronic bowel complications.[26] Patients with active inflammatory bowel disease should not receive pelvic radiation.[27] Pelvic fractures following pelvic radiation are rare.[28] Even with appropriate doses and techniques of radiation, approximately 1% of patients will have significant long-term toxicity to pelvic organs.

SMALL BOWEL CONTRAST

Small bowel-related complications are directly proportional to the volume of small bowel in the radiation field. The incidence and clinical consequences of bowel injury have been reviewed by Miller and colleagues.[29] In patients receiving combined radiation and chemotherapy, the volume of small bowel in the radiation field limits the ability to escalate the dose of 5-FU.[30-32] Small bowel contrast is essential in order to determine the position of the small bowel during simulation. It should be used routinely during the simulation in patients receiving curative pelvic radiation therapy. Herbert et al. found that in patients with endometrial and rectal cancer who had small bowel contrast used at the time of radiation simulation, there was a change in the treatment field as well as a lower incidence of complications.[33] Nonfixed small bowel normally moves and CT scan may be more accurate than traditional small bowel series in detecting the position and volume of small bowel.[34]

PHYSICAL MANEUVERS

Various physical maneuvers to exclude the small bowel from the pelvis have been examined. Gallagher et al. reported a significant decrease in the average small bowel volume when the patients were treated in the prone position with the combination of abdominal wall compression and bladder distention compared with the supine position.[35] Use of a four-field technique further decreased the volume of small bowel. Treatment in the prone position without abdominal wall compression was not consistently effective in displacing small bowel and, in some patients, most commonly obese, the volume of small bowel increased.

Caspers and Hop performed a similar study in 50 patients who received pelvic radiation for bladder or prostate cancer.[36] Using the Trendelenburg or inclined procubitus positions was helpful in excluding small bowel from the pelvic radiation fields, especially for obese patients. While the prone position was less effective than these inclined positions, it was superior to the supine position.

Using a three-dimensional (3-D) planning system, Koelbl and associates found that in patients who received postoperative radiation, the use of the prone position plus a belly board versus the supine position decreased the small bowel volume treated.[32]

IMMOBILIZATION MOLDS

The effectiveness of custom bowel immobilization molds (belly boards) has been documented in a number of series.[32,37] Shanahan et al. reported that the combination of the prone position and immobilization mold decreased the mean small bowel volume in the radiation field by 66% compared with patients treated in the supine position without the immobilization mold.[37]

It must be emphasized that any physical maneuver beyond the use of the prone position may be associated with patient discomfort, thereby leading to increased

movement and daily setup errors. Brierley et al. analyzed the variation of small bowel volume in the pelvis before and during adjuvant pelvic radiation therapy for rectal cancer and reported that the displacement of small bowel from the posterior pelvis by bladder distention was not reliably maintained throughout the treatment course.[38] Therefore, physical maneuvers beyond the prone position may not be beneficial in all patients. The use of such techniques should be tailored to the individual patient.

RADIOPROTECTORS/RADIOSENSITIZERS

Patients with gynecologic malignancies who receive pelvic radiation therapy may have lower long-term severe toxicity with increased caffeine consumption.[39] Nonrandomized data from Rhomberg et al. suggest that razoxane may improve local control and median survival in patients who receive radiation for inoperable recurrent rectal cancer.[40]

Although nonrandomized trials suggest a benefit to select radioprotectors, randomized trials of radioprotectors do not confirm these findings.[41-45] For example, Liu et al. performed a randomized trial of pelvic radiation therapy (2.25 Gy/day to 45 Gy) + WR-2721 in patients with inoperable or unresectable rectal cancer.[44] There was no difference in acute radiation toxicity. The incidence of Radiation Therapy Oncology Group (RTOG) long-term grade 3+ GI, GU, and skin toxicity was 3% in the radiation-alone arm compared with 0% in the radiation + WR-2721 arm.

In a randomized trial from the North Central Cancer Treatment Group, sucralfate had no benefit in decreasing pelvic radiation-related toxicity.[46] In a separate trial, patients receiving 5-aminosalicylic acid were found to have an increased rather than decreased incidence of acute radiation enteritis.[45] Rectally administered amifostine is well tolerated; however, its efficacy remains to be determined.[47] In patients with prostate cancer, rectally administered sucralfate did not reduce late rectal toxicity.[48]

ALTERED RADIATION FRACTIONATION SCHEMES

Various fractionation strategies have evolved with the goal of enhancing tumor cell damage by radiation without augmenting normal tissue injury.[49] The repair of subcellular injury, regeneration, cell cycle redistribution, and reoxygenation are all factors at the cellular level contributing to differences in how various normal tissues and tumors respond to fractionated radiation therapy. The use of hyperfractionation and accelerated fractionation schemes takes advantage of some of these factors. The major limitation of accelerated hyperfractionation is acute normal tissue toxicity. However, late effects should be the same as or, more likely, less than in conventional fractionation schemes.

Data on the use of twice a day (BID) radiation therapy in the pelvis are limited. In a phase I/II trial from the RTOG, 54 patients with advanced bladder cancer received 1.2 Gy BID to a pelvic dose of 50.4 Gy followed by a boost to 60 to 69 Gy.[50] The actuarial incidence of grade 3 to 4 complications was 11% at 2 years, which was no different than the incidence with conventional fractionation in prior RTOG protocols. Investigators from Laussane reported a phase I trial of accelerated hyperfractionation (1.6 Gy BID to 48 Gy) and found this approach tolerable.[51] Investigators from Laussane advocate BID radiation delivered preoperatively as opposed to postoperatively.[52,53] In the series by Janjan and associates, the use of a concomitant boost BID during standard combined modality therapy increased the incidence of perioperative morbidity.[54] Movsas et al. recommend limiting the BID component to the boost,[55,56] whereas Myerson and colleagues deliver a concomitant 3-D boost once or twice a week.[57] The RTOG R-0012 phase II randomized trial compared BID radiation with conventional fractionation plus 5-FU/irinotecan. BID radiation, especially in combination with chemotherapy, remains investigational.

3-D TREATMENT PLANNING

Innovative techniques using 3-D treatment planning were investigated.[57,58] The most important contribution of 3-D treatment planning is the ability to plan and localize the target and normal tissues at all levels of the treatment volume, rather than using the traditional method of planning with only a single central transverse slice and simulation films.[59] An analysis of 3-D treatment planning techniques at the MGH suggested that the volume of small bowel in the radiation field is decreased with protons as compared with photons.[60] The results of a randomized trial of conformal versus conventional treatment planning techniques are pending.[58]

OTHER INVESTIGATIONAL APPROACHES

Investigational radiation therapy approaches such as neutrons[61] and hyperthermia[62-64] have been examined. None have shown a clear advantage compared with conventional pelvic radiation therapy.

SURGICAL TECHNIQUES

The two most useful surgical techniques to minimize small bowel injury in the postoperative setting are (1) placing clips in the high-risk areas in order to better define the tumor volume; and (2) the use of absorbable Dexon or Vicryl mesh, which temporarily removes the small bowel from the pelvis.[24] Rodier et al. reported that in 60 patients, Vicryl mesh excluded small bowel from the pelvis in 93% of cases and there was complete reabsorption by 3 to 5 months.[65] The incidence of mesh-related complications was 8%. It should be noted that since the radiation component of postoperative combined modality therapy does not begin until 4 months after surgery, the mesh may have already resorbed. Other techniques such as an inflatable pelvic/small bowel displacement prosthesis,[66] reconstruction of the pelvic floor, construction of an omental pedicle flap,[67] and retroversion of the uterus have had variable success.

Design of Radiation Therapy Fields for Rectal Cancer

The design of pelvic radiation therapy fields for rectal cancer is based on knowledge of the patterns of failure and the primary nodal drainage. The majority of local failures are in the posterior one half to two thirds of the true pelvis.[24] Furthermore, since the internal iliac and presacral nodes are posterior in reference to the external iliac nodes, much of the normal structures in the anterior pelvis can be spared with the use of lateral fields.

General guidelines for the design of pelvic radiation therapy fields are listed in Table 41-3. The whole pelvic radiation field should adequately cover the primary bed as well as the primary nodes at risk. The intent of the boost is to treat the primary tumor and not to include the nodes. Therefore, the exact size is determined by the size and location of the primary tumor. Specific examples of field arrangements for various clinical presentations are presented in Figures 41-2 to 41-7.

OUTCOMES

Patterns of Failure

Despite radical surgery, local-regional failure occurs frequently in patients with T3 and/or node-positive rectal cancers. The incidence of treatment failure in the pelvis is directly related to the extent of transmural penetration (microscopic vs. gross) and the additive risks of lymph node metastases. Local recurrence is the most common

Table 41–3   General Guidelines for Pelvic Radiation Therapy for Rectal Cancer

1. Whole pelvic field:
   A. Posterior-anterior
      Lateral borders: 1.5 cm lateral to the widest bony margin of the true pelvic side walls.
      Distal border: 3 cm below the primary tumor or at the inferior aspect of the obturator foramina, whichever is the most inferior.
      Superior border: L5-S1 junction.
   B. Laterals
      Posterior border: 1 to 1.5 cm behind the anterior bony sacral margin.
      Anterior border:
      T3 disease: Posterior margin of the symphysis pubis (to treat only the internal iliac nodes).
      T4 disease: Anterior margin of the symphysis pubis (to include the external iliac nodes).
2. Blocks are used to spare the posterior muscle and soft tissues behind the sacrum, to reduce the amount of dose inferior to the symphysis pubis, and to decrease the amount of small bowel treated both superiorly and anteriorly.
3. Boost field:
   A. Treat the primary tumor bed plus a 3-cm margin (not the nodes).
   B. In general, field sizes measure 10 × 10 or 12 × 12 cm.
   C. Corner blocks as needed.
4. After an abdominoperineal resection:
   A. Wire the perineal scar and create a 1.5-cm margin beyond the wire in all fields.
   B. Never use an electron or photon boost for the perineum—there will be overlap between the fields.
   C. Bolus the perineal scar every other day to bring the dose to 100%.

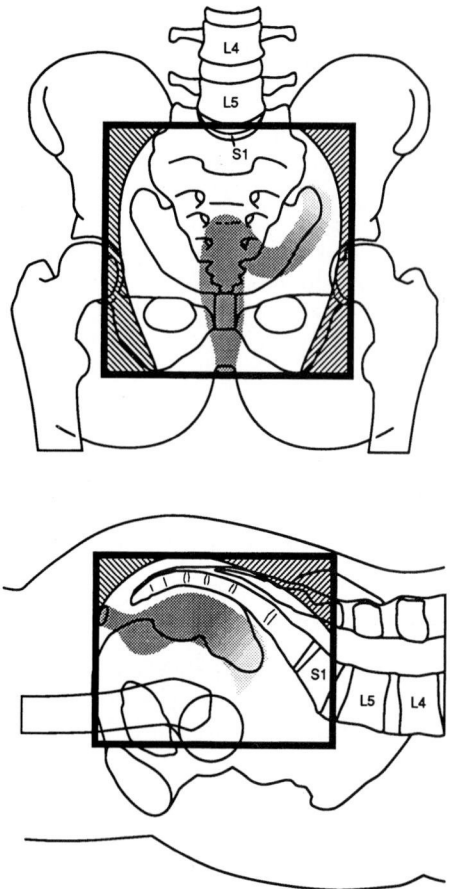

Figure 41–2. Treatment fields after a low anterior resection for a T3N1M0 rectal cancer 8 cm from the anal verge. In this example, the distal border is at the bottom of the obturator foramen and the perineum is blocked. Since the tumor was a T3, the anterior field is at the posterior margin of the symphysis pubis (to treat only the internal iliac nodes).

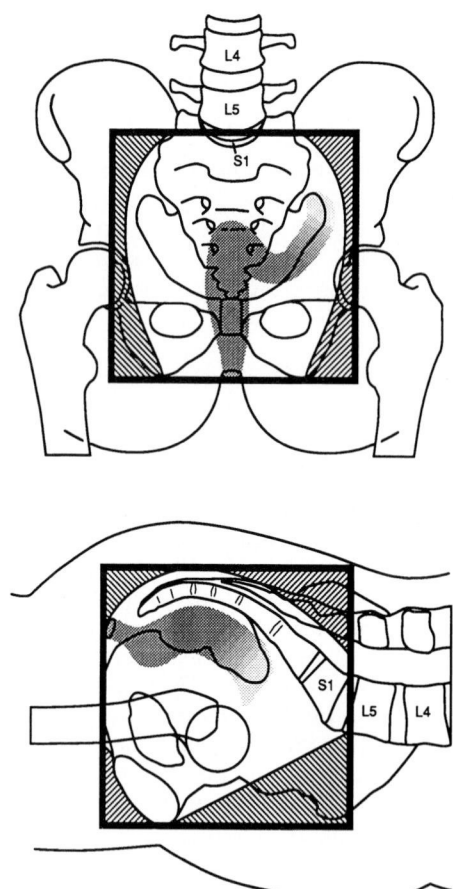

Figure 41–3. Treatment fields after a low anterior resection for a T4N1M0 rectal cancer 8 cm from the anal verge. In this example, the distal border is at the bottom of the obturator foramen and the perineum is blocked. Since the tumor was a T4, the anterior field is at the anterior margin of the symphysis pubis (to include the external iliac nodes).

site of failure in rectal cancer. The most common metastatic site is liver followed by lung. Brain[68] and inguinal node[69] metastasis are uncommon.

Resectable Rectal Cancer

POSTOPERATIVE THERAPY

The National Cancer Institute Consensus Conference concluded in 1990 that combined modality therapy was the standard postoperative adjuvant treatment for patients with T3 or N1-2 disease.[16] Pelvic radiation therapy decreases local recurrence, but does not improve survival. As would be predicted, randomized data do not reveal a survival advantage of pelvic radiation plus elective para-aortic and liver radiation versus pelvic radiation alone.[70]

For patients treated with postoperative combined modality therapy and who received 5-FU as a single agent, there was a 10% survival advantage with continuous infusion 5-FU versus bolus 5-FU.[71] Whether continuous infusion 5-FU for G cycles is superior to bolus 5-FU/leucovorin for cycles 1, 2, 5, and 6, and continuous infusion for cycles 3 and 4 (with radiation) is being tested in the INT 0144 postoperative adjuvant rectal trial. Until these

results are available, either of the above regimens are reasonable approaches.

It is the addition of 5-FU–based chemotherapy to pelvic radiation that further decreases local recurrence to approximately 10% and increases the overall 5-year survival of surgery by approximately 10% to 15%. The NSABP R-02 trial reported a local recurrence rate of only 13% with postoperative chemotherapy alone; however, it was further decreased to 8% with postoperative combined modality therapy ($P = 0.02$).[72]

Associated with this improvement in local control and survival with postoperative combined modality therapy is an increase in acute toxicity. For example, the incidence of grade 3+ toxicity in the combined modality arms of the Gastrointestinal Tumor Study Group (GITSG) and Mayo/North Central Cancer Treatment Group 79-47-51 trials was 25% to 50%. Furthermore, the percentages of patients finishing the prescribed 6 cycles of chemotherapy in those trials were only 65% and 50%, respectively. Retrospective data suggest that the acute toxicity with preoperative combined modality therapy may be less than in the postoperative setting.[73] Randomized trials in progress will provide a more definitive answer to this question.[74,75]

Numerous new chemotherapeutic agents have been developed for the treatment of patients with colorectal

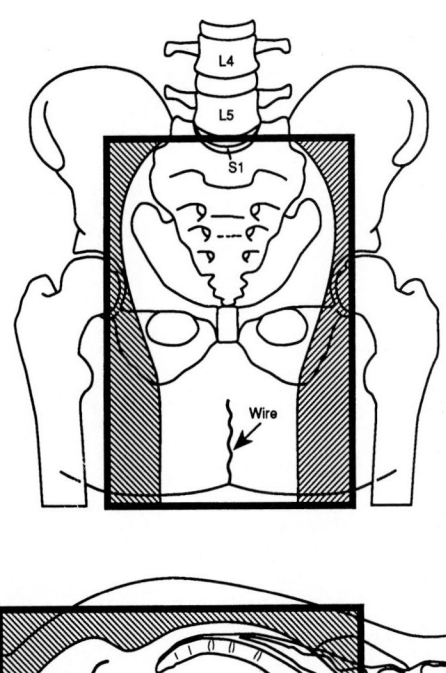

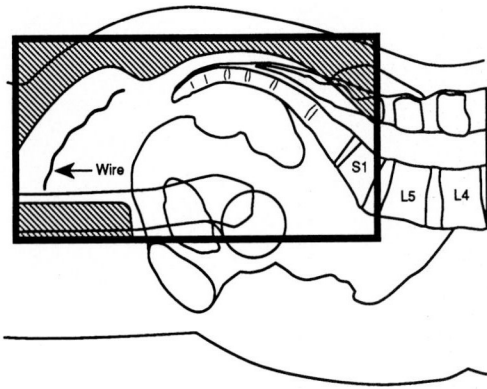

Figure 41–4. Treatment fields after an abdominoperineal resection for a T3N1M0 rectal cancer 2 cm from the anal verge. In this example the distal border is extended to include the perineal scar. Since the distal border is being extended only to include the scar, the remaining normal tissues can be blocked.

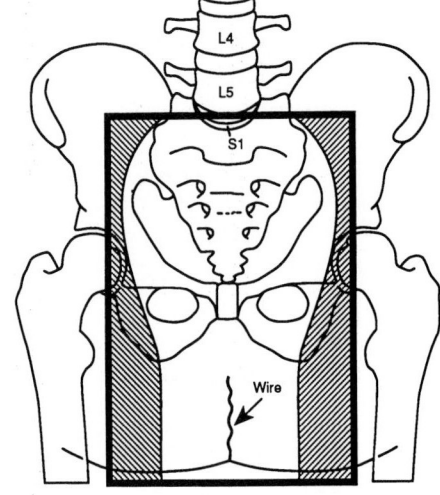

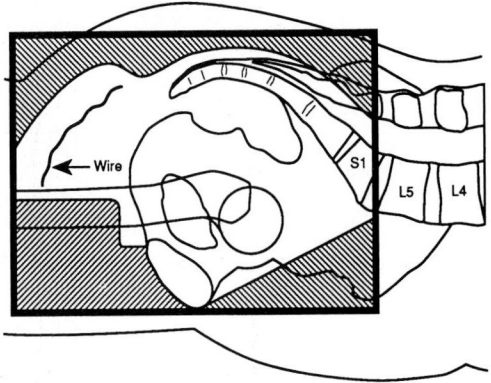

Figure 41–5. Treatment fields following an abdominoperineal resection for a T4N1M0 rectal cancer 2 cm from the anal verge. In this example, because the tumor was a T4, the anterior field is at the anterior margin of the symphysis pubis (to include the external iliac nodes). Since the distal border is being extended only to include the scar and external iliac nodes, the remaining normal tissues can be blocked.

cancer.[76] Phase I/II trials are examining the use of new chemotherapeutic agents in combination with pelvic radiation therapy. Selected agents include uracil and tegafur (UFT),[77,78] Tomudex,[79] oxaliplatin,[80,81] CPT-11,[82] Iressa,[83] and capecitabine[84] with pelvic radiation therapy. Phase III trials are needed to determine if these regimens offer an advantage compared with 5-FU–based combined modality therapy regimens.

Do Some Patients Not Require Postoperative Adjuvant Therapy?

Retrospective data suggest that there may be a subset of patients with T3 N0 disease who may *not* require adjuvant therapy, as well as patients with stage I disease who *should* be considered for adjuvant therapy. Retrospective trials examining patients at both the MGH[85] and Memorial Sloan-Kettering Cancer Center[86] have identified favorable subsets of patients with T3 N0 disease who, following surgery alone, had a 10-year actuarial local recurrence rate of less than 10%. A pooled analysis of 3 Intergroup postoperative adjuvant trials revealed that the subset of patients with stages T3 N0 or T1-2 N1 disease had a 5-year local

failure rate of 6% to 8% and a survival rate of 74% to 81%.[87] These results must be confirmed in a randomized trial before a change in the standard of care of combined modality therapy can be recommended.

PREOPERATIVE THERAPY

Rationale and Results

Preoperative therapy (most commonly combined modality therapy) has gained acceptance as a standard adjuvant therapy. The potential advantages of the preoperative approach include decreased tumor seeding, less acute toxicity, increased radiosensitivity due to more oxygenated cells, and enhanced sphincter preservation.[17] The primary disadvantage of preoperative radiation therapy is possibly overtreating patients with either early-stage (T1-2 N0) or undetected metastatic disease. However, the imaging techniques discussed earlier allow more accurate selection, thereby decreasing the number of patients who are overtreated.

Retrospective data suggest that preoperative combined modality therapy increases pathologic downstaging compared with preoperative radiation without chemotherapy[88]

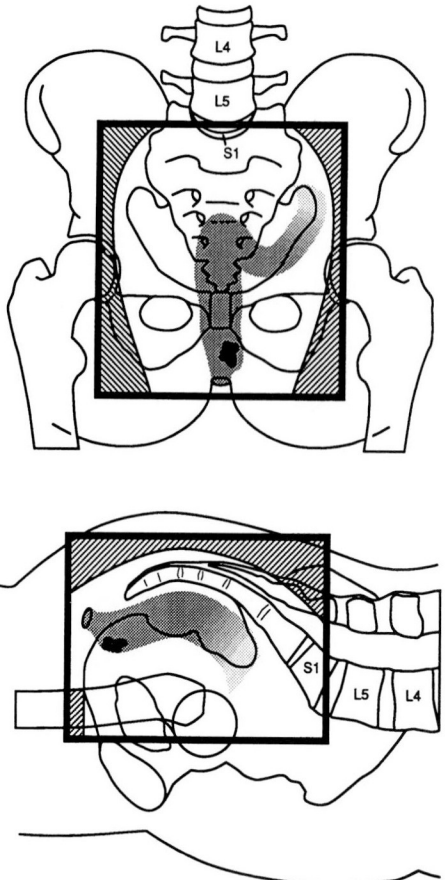

Figure 41–6. Treatment fields for preoperative radiation therapy for a low-lying T3NXM0 rectal cancer. In this example the distal border is extended 3 cm beyond the primary tumor and the perineum is blocked. Since the tumor was a T3, the anterior field is at the posterior margin of the symphysis pubis (to treat only the internal iliac nodes).

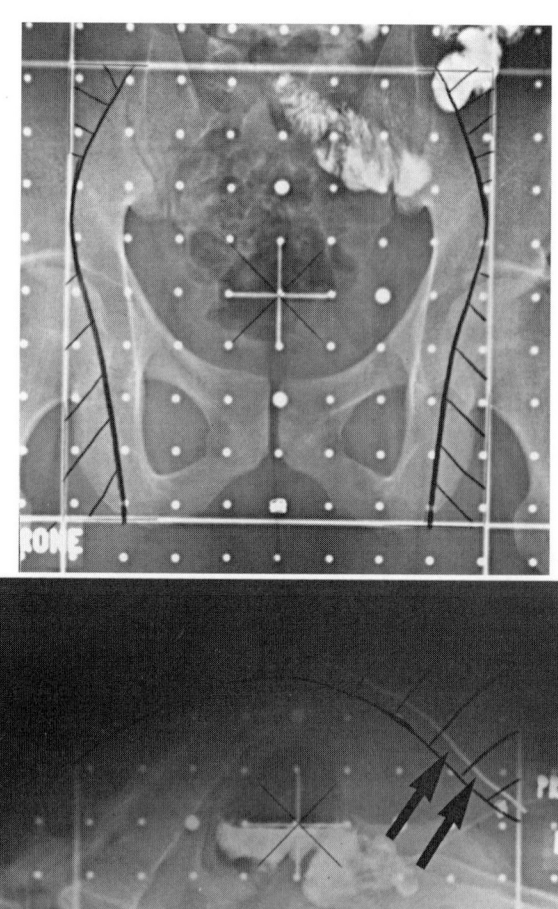

Figure 41–7. Lateral field for preoperative radiation therapy for a low-lying T3NXM0 rectal cancer. This example illustrates the position of the wire on the Foley catheter outlining the anal verge as well as a separate wire outlining the perineum, which is blocked (*arrows*).

and is associated with a lower incidence of acute toxicity compared with postoperative combined modality therapy.[73] In general, the incidence of grade 3+ acute toxicity during the combined modality segment is 15% to 25%, the complete response rates are 10% to 30% pathologic and 10% to 20% clinical, and the incidence of local recurrence is 0 to 10%. Whether preoperative combined modality therapy is more effective than preoperative radiation therapy and if the postoperative chemotherapy component is necessary is being addressed in the ongoing randomized European Organization for the Research and Treatment of Cancer (EORTC) trial 22921.

There have been 12 modern randomized trials of preoperative radiation therapy (without chemotherapy) for clinically resectable rectal cancer.[17] All have used low to moderate doses of radiation. Overall, most of the trials showed a decrease in local recurrence, and in five of the trials this difference reached statistical significance. Although in some trials a subset analysis has revealed a significant improvement in survival, the Swedish Rectal Cancer Trial is the only one that reported a survival advantage for the total treatment group. Two meta-analyses report conflicting results. While both reveal a decrease in local recurrence, the analysis by Camma et al.[89] reported a survival advantage, whereas the analysis by the Colorectal Cancer Collaborative Group[90] did not.

Intensive Short Course Preoperative Radiation

The Swedish Rectal Cancer Trial is the only randomized trial of preoperative radiation therapy to report a significant improvement in survival. Patients with clinically resectable (T1-3) rectal cancer were randomized to receive 25 Gy in 1 week followed by surgery 1 week later versus surgery alone.[91] Those who received preoperative radiation had a significant decrease in local recurrence (12% vs. 27%) and a corresponding significant improvement in 5-year survival (58% vs. 48%).

It is important to analyze these positive results in context with the remainder of the literature. First, given that the other 11 randomized trials of preoperative radiation therapy do not report a survival benefit, these data clearly must be confirmed by additional studies.

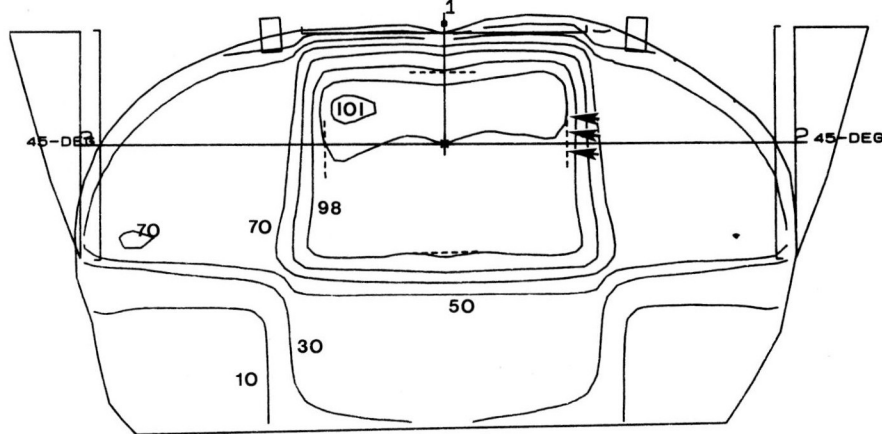

Figure 41–8. Dosimetry of a representative three-field pelvic treatment plan. The arrows indicate the prescription point located 1.5 cm inside the edge of the field. Since the volume inside this point should receive at least 100% of the dose, the dose is prescribed to 98%.

The most recent trial to report results was the Dutch CKVO 95-04 trial, which randomized 1805 patients with clinically resectable (T1–3) disease to surgery alone (with a total mesorectal excision [TME]) or intensive short course preoperative radiation followed by TME.[92] Although radiation significantly decreased local recurrence (8% vs. 2%) there was no difference in 2-year survival (82%). Second, even if future trials confirm a survival benefit, there are other equally important endpoints in rectal cancer that must be addressed. These include acute toxicity, sphincter preservation and function, and quality of life. For example, acute toxicity in the Dutch CKVO 95-04 trial included 10% neurotoxicity, 29% perineal wound complications, and 12% postoperative leaks.[93] In the patients who developed postoperative leaks, 80% required surgery resulting in 11% mortality.

It is not possible to accurately compare the local control and survival results of intensive short-course radiation with conventional preoperative combined modality therapy. This is due to selection bias in favor of the series using intensive short-course radiation. The conventional preoperative combined modality therapy regimens are limited to patients with clinical T3 disease, whereas most trials that use intensive short-course preoperative radiation include patients with clinical T1-3 disease.

SPHINCTER PRESERVATION WITH PREOPERATIVE RADIATION

A major goal of preoperative therapy is sphincter preservation. From the viewpoint of sphincter preservation, the advantage of preoperative therapy is to decrease the volume of the primary tumor. When the tumor is located in close proximity to the dentate line, this decrease in tumor volume may allow the surgeon to perform a sphincter-conserving procedure that would not otherwise be possible. However, if the tumor directly invades the anal sphincter, sphincter preservation is unlikely even when a complete response is achieved.

One of the most important controversies with preoperative therapy is whether the degree of downstaging is adequate to enhance sphincter preservation. Furthermore, if preoperative radiation therapy is effective, what regimen (intensive short-course vs. conventional course) is preferred?

An analysis of 1316 patients treated with intensive short-course radiation during 2 previously published Scandinavian trials revealed that downstaging was most pronounced when the interval between the completion of radiation and surgery was at least 10 days.[94] In the Dutch CKVO 95-04 trial, where the interval was 1 week, there was no downstaging.[95] None of the other randomized trials of intensive short-course preoperative radiation address the issue of sphincter preservation, and it is not an endpoint of the trials.

When the goal of preoperative therapy is sphincter preservation, conventional doses and techniques of radiation are recommended. These include multiple-field techniques to a total dose of 45 to 50.4 Gy at 1.8 Gy/ fraction. Surgery should be performed 4 to 7 weeks following the completion of radiation. Unlike the intensive short-course radiation regimen, this conventional design allows for two important events to occur. First is the recovery from the acute side effects of radiation, and second is adequate time for tumor downstaging. Data from the Lyon R90-01 trial of preoperative radiation suggest that an interval longer than 2 weeks following the completion of radiation increases the chance of downstaging.[96] Whether increasing the interval between the end of intensive short-course radiation and surgery to more than 4 weeks will increase downstaging is not known. This question is being addressed in an ongoing Stockholm III randomized trial from Sweden.

Preoperative, Prospective Clinical Assessment

The most accurate method by which to determine if preoperative therapy increases sphincter preservation is to perform a prospective clinical assessment. In this setting, the operating surgeon examines the patient before the start of preoperative therapy and declares the type of operation required. It should be noted that this assessment is based on an office examination and may not accurately reflect the assessment when the patient is relaxed under general anesthesia. The only method by which to account for this potential bias is to perform a randomized trial of preoperative versus postoperative therapy. A preliminary report from the German CAO/ARO/AIO 94 randomized trial of preoperative versus postoperative combined modality therapy suggests that this assessment is accurate approximately 80 percent of the time.[97]

Clinical Experience with Sphincter Preservation

Seven series have reported results in patients with clinically resectable rectal cancer whose surgeons conducted a prospective clinical assessment before preoperative therapy and recommended an abdominoperineal resection. All series use conventional doses and techniques of radiation therapy. Three use radiation therapy alone,[96,98,99] and four use combined modality therapy.[100-103] The incidence of sphincter preservation is only 23% in the National Surgical Adjuvant Breast and Bowel Project (NSABP) series[100] and 44% in the Lyon series.[96] In the remaining 5 series it is approximately 70%.

Sphincter Function

Sphincter preservation without good function is of questionable benefit. In a series of 73 patients who underwent surgery, Grumann and associates reported that the 23 patients who underwent an abdominoperineal resection had a more favorable quality of life compared with the 50 who underwent a low anterior resection.[104]

Although preoperative combined modality therapy may adversely affect sphincter function, the impact is most likely less than postoperative combined modality therapy.[105] Of the seven preoperative series discussed previously, four report functional outcome, indicating that the majority of patients (approximately 75%) have good to excellent sphincter outcome. Functional results continue to improve up to 1 year after surgery.

Randomized Trials

Three randomized trials of preoperative versus postoperative combined modality therapy for clinically resectable, T_3 rectal cancer have been developed. Two are from the United States (INT 0147, NSABP R0-3), one from Germany (CAO/ARO/AIO 94). All 3 use conventional doses and techniques of radiation therapy and concurrent 5-FU–based chemotherapy. They also require a preoperative clinical assessment declaring the type of operation required. Unfortunately, low accrual has resulted in early closure of both the NSABP R-03 and INT 0147 trials. A preliminary report of the NSABP R-03 trial (with a median follow-up of only 1 year) revealed that the percent of patients who underwent sphincter-sparing surgery and were without evidence of disease was higher in the preoperative versus the postoperative arm (44% vs. 34%).[75] Fortunately, the German CAO/ARO/AIO 94 trial has completed the planned accrual of more than 800 patients and will have adequate statistic power to address the issues of toxicity, efficacy, and sphincter preservation.[74,97]

Response of the Primary Tumor

Although some series show no correlation,[106] most suggest that there is improved outcome with increasing pathologic response to preoperative therapy.[107-112] Analyses of biopsies examining select molecular markers such as c-K-ras,[113] thymidylate synthase,[114] p27kip1,[115] p53,[116-118] apoptosis,[119,120] and Ki-67[121] have had varying success in helping to select patients who may best respond to preoperative therapy.

In one series the value of radical surgery in patients with T1-3 disease who had a biopsy-proved complete response was questioned.[122] However, in series limited to patients with T3 disease who received preoperative therapy, radical surgery is still necessary to fully evaluate whether a pathologic response has been achieved. Neither post-treatment ultrasound[123,124] nor physical examination (which is only 25% accurate)[110] is sufficiently adequate. The use of PET scan as a noninvasive measure of response is being investigated.[11]

The Impact of Total Mesorectal Excision on Adjuvant Therapy

Some clinicians contend that adjuvant therapy is not necessary if patients undergo resection with a TME. In one series, TME, which involves sharp dissection around the integral mesentery of the hindgut, decreased the local recurrence rate to 5%.[125] These data must be interpreted with caution for a number of reasons. First is selection bias. TME allows the identification and exclusion of patients with more advanced disease as compared with patients treated in the adjuvant trials, in which more conventional surgery is performed. Second, some patients received radiation therapy with or without chemotherapy (e.g., 15% in the series by Leong et al.,[126] 18% in the series by Haas-Kock et al.,[127] 28% in the series from Enker and associates,[128] and 58% in the series from Arenas et al.[129]). In a combined analysis of 1411 patients from 5 international centers, an undisclosed number received adjuvant radiation or combined modality therapy.[130] Third, some series (e.g., Aitken et al.) exclude operative deaths.[131] Fourth, TME is associated with high anastomotic leak rates (12% in the Dutch CKVO 95-04 TME trial[92] and 16% at the Basingstoke Hospital).[132] Poon and colleagues recommend the creation of a defunctioning stoma to decrease the high leak rate with TME.[133] Lastly, in the Dutch CKVO trial, the 324 patients with stage III disease who underwent a TME alone with negative margins had a local recurrence rate of 20%.[134]

Dahlberg and colleagues report a 3% local recurrence rate in patients with resectable rectal cancer with the combination of TME and intensive short-course preoperative irradiation.[135] As with most trials that use intensive short-course preoperative radiation, patients with clinical stages T1-3 disease were included. Therefore, it is difficult to compare these results with the preoperative combined modality therapy series that are limited to patients with T3 disease.

In summary, the use of TME has increased awareness of the importance of surgical technique. Careful surgical techniques such as sharp dissection are central to the successful management of rectal cancer. However, the results of the Dutch CKVO 95-04 trial confirm that despite TME surgery, radiation therapy is still a necessary component in the adjuvant management of rectal cancer.

Alternative Methods for Sphincter Preservation

ENDOCAVITARY RADIATION

Early localized tumors (3% to 5% of rectal cancers) include small, exophytic, mobile tumors without adverse pathologic factors (e.g., high grade, blood vessel invasion, lymphatic vessel invasion, colloid histology, or the penetration of tumor into or through the bowel wall) and are adequately treated with various local therapies such as local excision or endocavitary radiation. In 22 patients who were stage T1 N0 by rectal ultrasound, Gerard et al. reported no local failures with endocavitary radiation.[136] Aumock and associates advocated adding external beam radiation therapy (EBRT) for T2-T3 tumors and reported local control rates of T1:100%, mobile T2:85%, and T3 or tethered T2:56%.[137]

LOCAL EXCISION AND RADIATION THERAPY

Local excision has been performed before and after radiation therapy.[20] Some investigators have used preoperative therapy followed by local excision.[138,139] This approach remains investigational. The advantage of performing a local excision before irradiation is that pathologic details such as margins, depth of bowel wall penetration, and histologic features can be well characterized. Patients with T1 tumors without adverse pathologic factors have a low enough incidence of local failure (5% to 10%) and positive nodes (<10%) that they do not require adjuvant therapy. However, once adverse pathologic factors are present (high grade, lymphatic vessel invasion, or signet-ring cells) or the tumor invades into or through the muscularis propria, the local failure rate is at least 17% and the incidence of positive mesorectal or pelvic nodes or both is at least 10% to 15%.

Survival

Since the pelvic lymph nodes are not pathologically examined at the time of a local excision, it is not possible to accurately compare, stage for stage, the results of this approach with radical surgery. Data from phase I/II trials reveal that a 5-year actuarial survival in these select series is approximately 80% (range: 70% to 94%). In most series, patients had T1-3 tumors and underwent a local excision followed 4 to 6 weeks later by 45 to 50 Gy to the pelvis. Some patients received an EBRT or brachytherapy boost. In most series, a limited number of patients received 5-FU. Although not randomized, these survival data appear comparable with the results of radical surgery alone for stage T1-2 N0 disease.

Local Failure

When the series are combined, the average crude local failure rate increases with T classification—T1: 5%, T2: 14%, and T3: 22%. A full-thickness local excision is recommended since patients who undergo a piecemeal excision usually have higher local failure rates.[140] Most investigators would recommend that negative margins be obtained if technically feasible, and a re-excision performed if needed, providing that it does not compromise

sphincter function. If this is impossible, doses of greater than 50.4 Gy, if the small bowel is excluded from the high dose field, are probably necessary.

The mature or local excision and postoperative therapy are not as favorable as previously reported. In the local excision series with longer than 4-year follow-up (MGH,[141] Memorial Sloan-Kettering,[142] cancer and Leukemia Group B (CALGB) 8984,[143] Princess Margaret Hospital,[144] and RTOG 89-02[145]) the incidence of local failure for T2 disease was 14% to 24%. Therefore, patients who are treated with local excision and postoperative adjuvant therapy require close follow-up beyond 5 years. Salvage of local failures is possible with most series reporting that approximately half the patients who undergo a salvage abdominoperineal resection can be cured. The few series that measure sphincter function report favorable outcomes. All patients should receive 5-FU–based therapy concurrently with radiation. For patients with T2-T3 disease where the incidence of pelvic lymph nodes is at least 20%, an additional 4 cycles of adjuvant chemotherapy for a total of 6 cycles is recommended. Transmural (T3) tumors have a 25% local failure rate and are treated more effectively with radical surgery and pre- or postoperative combined modality therapy.

Unresectable or Recurrent Disease

INTRODUCTION

In patients with primary, resectable T3 rectal cancer, combined modality therapy significantly improves local control and survival. It is more difficult to obtain these same results for patients with more advanced (T4 or recurrent or both) disease. The heterogeneity of the disease and absence of a uniform definition of resectability may explain some of the variation in results seen among the series. With the exception of the uncommon suture line-only recurrence, all patients with primary or recurrent unresectable disease should receive preoperative combined modality therapy as described earlier (45 to 50.4 Gy plus 5-FU–based chemotherapy). Although 50% to 90% will be able to undergo a resection with negative margins, depending on the degree of tumor fixation, 24% to 55% still develop a local recurrence.[17]

INTRAOPERATIVE RADIATION THERAPY

The primary advantage of intraoperative radiation therapy (IORT) is that radiation can be delivered at the time of surgery to the site with the highest risk of local failure (the tumor bed) while decreasing the dose to the surrounding normal tissues. IORT can be delivered by two techniques: electron beam and brachytherapy. Brachytherapy is most commonly delivered by the high-dose rate (HDR) technique, and the dose rate is similar to that used for electron beam IORT.[19,146]

The results (and recommended dose) of IORT depend on whether the patient has primary unresectable or recurrent disease and on whether the margins of resection are negative or there is microscopic or gross residual disease. In general, series have used 10 to 20 Gy.

PRIMARY UNRESECTABLE DISEASE

The largest experience and longest median follow-up of patients receiving preoperative therapy followed by IORT has been reported by the MGH.[18] In that series, local failure in patients with negative margins decreased from 18% without IORT to 11% with IORT. In patients with positive margins, local failure decreased from 83% without IORT to 43% with IORT if there was gross residual disease, and to 32% with IORT if there was microscopic residual disease. For all patients in the series (with or without IORT), the 5-year disease-free survival was 63% for patients with negative margins and 32% for patients with positive margins. These results underscore the importance of delivering preoperative therapy in order to help achieve negative margins. If negative margins cannot be obtained, then microscopic residual disease is still preferable to gross residual disease. Reports from the Mayo Clinic[147] and Memorial Sloan-Kettering[148] revealed similar local failure rates in patients with negative margins (7% and 8%, respectively). Similar series from Munich,[149] Heidelberg,[150] and Eindhoven[151] have been reported.

RECURRENT DISEASE

In contrast with primary disease, some patients in these series had prior EBRT and received either a limited dose or no EBRT. In the MGH series of 40 patients, the overall 5-year local control was 35% and was higher with negative margins (56%) versus positive margins (13%).[152] The overall 5-year survival was 27% and was higher with negative margins (40%) versus positive margins (12%). Similar results were reported in 74 patients from Memorial Sloan-Kettering, where the overall 5-year local control was 39% and was higher in patients with negative margins (43%) versus positive margins (26%).[146] The overall 5-year survival was 23% and was higher with patients with negative margins (36%) versus positive margins (11%). In contrast, the Mayo Clinic reported no difference by margin status, but reported a higher 5-year local control (63% vs. 34%) and survival (20% vs. 12%) in patients who received EBRT versus those who did not receive additional EBRT. Investigators at the MD Anderson Center also report no benefit of IORT for patients with positive margins.[153] In summary, in contrast to patients who have negative or microscopically positive margins, it is unclear if those with positive margins benefit from aggressive therapy.

TOXICITY OF IORT

It is difficult to clearly separate treatment-related complications from disease-related complications in patients with unresectable primary or recurrent rectal cancers or both. The total incidence ranges from 15% to 50% in most series and is highest in patients with the most advanced disease (recurrent unresectable). Complications such as delayed healing, an increase in infection, fistula formation, and neuropathy may be the result of recurrent tumor, aggressive surgery, irradiation, or a combination of these. The incidence of IORT-related toxicity increases with IORT doses greater than 20 Gy.

In contrast with patients undergoing sphincter preservation for primary resectable disease, due to the extensive surgery and higher dose of radiation (IORT), patients considered for colo-anal anastomosis or a very low anterior resection may have a better functional outcome with a permanent colostomy.[154]

Radiation Therapy Alone

Some investigators have advocated the use of radiation therapy alone.[155-159] Various techniques have been used, including combinations of EBRT, brachytherapy, and intracavitary radiation.

Patients selected for radiation therapy alone are usually medically inoperable or have such advanced local disease that resection would compromise a vital structure. In most series, patients received pelvic radiation therapy followed by a boost with either EBRT or brachytherapy or both. Brierley et al. from the Princess Margaret Hospital reported the results of EBRT alone (40 to 60 Gy) in patients who refused surgery or had unresectable or medically inoperable disease.[21] The overall 5-year survival was 27%. The primary tumor was mobile in 47% of the patients, partially fixed in 27%, and fixed in 4%. These data suggest that patients with mobile or partially fixed rectal cancers who are medically inoperable should be treated aggressively with pelvic radiation therapy as a component of their therapy.

Gerard and associates reported the results of the combination of EBRT, intracavitary, and brachytherapy in 63 patients with uT2-3 tumors.[159] For patients with uT3 disease, the 5-year local failure and survival rates were 20% and 35%, respectively.

Pelvic radiation offers highly effective palliation. In a subset of 80 patients with metastatic disease who received pelvic radiation, 94% had complete resolution of pelvic symptoms and the 2-year pelvic symptom-free control was 82%.[160] The Princess Margaret Hospital series reported similar palliative benefits.[21] In the subset of 84 patients who received greater than 45 Gy, the following presenting symptoms were palliated by 6 to 8 weeks following the completion of radiation: pain, 89%; bleeding, 79%; neurologic, 52%; mass effect, 71%; discharge, 50%; urologic, 22%; and other, 42%.[161] In the Thomas Jefferson University series, complete plus partial symptomatic relief was achieved in the following categories: pain (65% + 28%), bleeding (100%), and mass effect (24% + 64%), respectively.[162] The duration of palliation was 8 to 10 months. In patients who are unable to receive radiation, laser or stents[163] offer some palliative benefit.

REFERENCES

1. Jemal A, Murray T, Samuel A et al: Cancer Statistics, 2003. *CA Cancer J Clin.* 2003;53:5.
2. Cohen AM, Minsky BD, Friedman MJ: Cancer of the Rectum. In Devita VT, Hellman S, Rosenberg SA, eds. *Cancer: Principles and Practice of Oncology.* 4th ed. Philadelphia: JB Lippincott; 1993:978.
3. Birbeck KF, Macklin CP, Tiffin NJ, et al: Rates of circumferential resection margin involvement vary between surgeons and predict outcomes in rectal cancer surgery. *Ann Surg.* 2002;235:449.

4. Cawthorne SJ, Parmus DV, Gibbs NM, et al: Extent of mesorectal spread and involvement of lateral resection margin as prognostic factors after surgery for rectal cancer. *Lancet.* 1990;335:1055.

5. Gualidi GF, Casciani E, Guadalaxara A, et al: Local staging of rectal cancer with transrectal ultrasound and endorectal magnetic resonance imaging. Comparison with histologic findings. *Dis Colon Rectum.* 2000;43:338.

6. Garcia-Aguilar J, Pollack J, Lee SH, et al: Accuracy of endorectal ultrasonography in preoperative staging of rectal tumors. *Dis Colon Rectum.* 2002;45:10.

7. Heriot AG, Grundy A, Kumar D: Preoperative staging of rectal carcinoma. *Br J Surg.* 1999;86:17.

8. Kim NK, Kim MJ, Park JK, et al: Preoperative staging of rectal cancer with MRI: Accuracy and clinical usefulness. *Ann Surg Oncol.* 2000;7:732.

9. Kim NK, Kim MJ, Yun SH, et al: Comparative study of transrectal ultrasonography, pelvic computerized tomography, and magnetic resonance imaging in preoperative staging of rectal cancer. *Dis Colon Rectum.* 1999;42:770.

10. Whiteford MH, Whiteford HM, Yee LF, et al: Usefulness of FDG-PET scan in the assessment of suspected metastatic or recurrent adenocarcinoma of the colon and rectum. *Dis Colon Rectum.* 2000;53:759.

11. Guillem JG, Puig-La Calle J, Akhurst T, et al: Prospective assessment of primary rectal cancer response to preoperative radiation and chemotherapy using 18-fluorodeoxyglucose positron emission tomography. *Dis Colon Rectum.* 2000;43:18.

12. Beets-Tan RGH, Beets GL, Vliegen RFA, et al: Accuracy of magnetic resonance imaging in prediction of tumor-free resection margin in rectal cancer surgery. *Lancet.* 2001;357:497.

13. Herrera L, Villarreal JR, Cert RT: Incidence of metastasis from rectal adenocarcinoma in small lymph nodes detected by a clearing technique. *Dis Colon Rectum.* 1992;35:783.

14. Nicholls RJ, York Mason A, Morson BC, et al: The clinical staging of rectal cancer. *Br J Surg.* 1982;69:404.

15. Colon and Rectum. In Green FL, Page DL, Fleming ID, et al., eds. *AJCC Cancer Staging Manual.* 6th ed. New York: Springer; 2002:113.

16. National Institutes of Health Consensus Conference: Adjuvant therapy for patients with colon and rectal cancer. *J Amer Med Assoc.* 1990;264:1444.

17. Skibber JM, Hoff PM, Minsky BD: Cancer of the rectum. In Devita VT, Hellman S, Rosenberg SA, eds. 6th ed. *Cancer: Principles and Practice of Oncology.* Philadelphia: Lippincott, Williams & Wilkins; 2001:1271.

18. Nakfoor BM, Willett CG, Shellito PC, et al: The impact of 5-fluorouracil and intraoperative electron beam radiation therapy on the outcome of patients with locally advanced primary rectal and rectosigmoid cancer. *Ann Surg.* 1998;228:194.

19. Strassmann G, Walter S, Kolotas C, et al: Reconstruction and navigation system for intraoperative brachytherapy using the flab technique for colorectal tumor bed irradiation. *Int J Radiat Oncol Biol Phys.* 2000;47:1323.

20. Wagman RT, Minsky BD: Conservative management of rectal cancer with local excision and adjuvant therapy. *Oncology.* 2001;15:513.

21. Brierley JD, Cummings BJ, Wong CS, et al: Adenocarcinoma of the rectum treated by radical external radiation therapy. *Int J Radiat Oncol Biol Phys.* 1995;31:255.

22. Klimberg VS, Souba WW, Dolson DJ, et al: Prophylactic glutamine protects the intestinal mucosa from radiation injury. *Cancer.* 1990;66:62.

23. Willett CG, Tepper JE, Kaufman DS, et al: Adjuvant postoperative radiation therapy for rectal adenocarcinoma. *Am J Clin Oncol.* 1992;15:371.

24. Gunderson LL, Russell AH, Llewellyn HJ, et al: Treatment planning for colorectal cancer: Radiation and surgical techniques and value of small-bowel films. *Int J Radiat Oncol Biol Phys.* 1985;11:1379.

25. Minsky BD, Cohen AM: Minimizing the toxicity of pelvic radiation therapy. *Oncology.* 1988;2:21.

26. Sigmon WR, Randall ME, Olds WE, et al: Increased chronic bowel complications with split-course pelvic irradiation. *Int J Radiat Oncol Biol Phys.* 1993;28:349.

27. Willett CG, Ooi CJ, Zeitman AL, et al: Acute and late toxicity of patients with inflammatory bowel disease undergoing irradiation for abdominal and pelvic neoplasms. *Int J Radiat Oncol Biol Phys.* 2000;46:995.

28. Tai P, Hammond A, Dyk JV, et al: Pelvic fractures following irradiation of endometrial and vaginal cancers—A case series and review of literature. *Radiother Oncol.* 2000;56:23.

29. Miller AR, Martenson Jr. JA, Nelson H, et al: The incidence and clinical consequences of treatment-related bowel injury. *Int J Radiat Oncol Biol Phys.* 1999;43:817.

30. Minsky BD, Conti JA, Huang Y, et al: The relationship of acute gastrointestinal toxicity and the volume of irradiated small bowel in patients receiving combined modality therapy for rectal cancer. *J Clin Oncol.* 1995;13:1409.

31. Baglan KL, Frazier RC, Yan D, et al: The dose-volume relationship of acute small bowel toxicity from concurrent 5-FU-based chemotherapy and radiation therapy for rectal cancer. *Int J Radiat Oncol Biol Phys.* 2002;52:176.

32. Koelbl O, Richter S, Flentje M: Influence of patient positioning on dose-volume histogram and normal tissue complication probability for small bowel and bladder in patients receiving pelvic irradiation: A prospective study using a 3D planning system and a radiobiological model. *Int J Radiat Oncol Biol Phys.* 1999;45:1193.

33. Herbert SH, Curran WJ, Solin LJ, et al: Decreasing gastrointestinal morbidity with the use of small bowel contrast during treatment planning for pelvic radiation. *Int J Radiat Oncol Biol Phys.* 1991;20:835.

34. Nuyttens JJ, Robertson JM, Yan D, et al: The position and volume of the small bowel during adjuvant radiation therapy for rectal cancer. *Int J Radiat Oncol Biol Phys.* 2001;51:1271.

35. Gallagher MJ, Brereton HD, Rostock RA, et al: A prospective study of treatment techniques to minimize the volume of pelvic small bowel with reduction of acute and late effects associated with pelvic irradiation. *Int J Radiat Oncol Biol Phys.* 1986;12:1565.

36. Caspers RJL, Hop WCJ: Irradiation of true pelvis for bladder and prostatic carcinoma in supine, prone, or Trendelenburg position. *Int J Radiat Oncol Biol Phys.* 1983;9:589.

37. Shanahan TG, Mehta MP, Bertelrud KL, et al: Minimization of small bowel volume within treatment fields utilizing customized "belly boards." *Int J Radiat Oncol Biol Phys.* 1990;19:469.

38. Brierley JD, Cummings BJ, Wong CS, et al: The variation of small bowel volume within the pelvis before and during adjuvant radiation for rectal cancer. *Radiother Oncol.* 1994;31:110.

39. Stelzer KJ, Koh WJ, Kurtz H, et al: Caffeine consumption is associated with decreased severe late toxicity after radiation to the pelvis. *Int J Radiat Oncol Biol Phys.* 1994;30:411.

40. Rhomberg W, Eiter H, Hergan K, et al: Inoperable recurrent rectal cancer: Results of a prospective trial with radiation therapy and razoxane. *Int J Radiat Oncol Biol Phys.* 1994;30:419.

41. Talley NA, Chen F, King D, et al: Short-chain fatty acid in the treatment of radiation proctitis. A randomized, double-blind, placebo-controlled, cross-over pilot trial. *Dis Colon Rectum.* 1997;40:1046.

42. Resbeut M, Marteau P, Cowen D, et al: A randomized double blind placebo controlled multicenter study of mesalazine for the prevention of acute radiation enteritis. *Radiother Oncol.* 1997;44:59 [abstract].

43. Martenson JA, Hyland G, Moertel CG, et al: Olsalazine is contraindicated during pelvic radiation therapy: Results of a double-blind randomized clinical trial. *Int J Radiat Oncol Biol Phys.* 1996;35:299.

44. Liu T, Liu Y, He S, et al: Use of radiation with or without WR-2721 in advanced rectal cancer. *Cancer.* 1992;69:2820.

45. Baughan CA, Canney PA, Buchanan RB, et al: A randomized trial to assess the efficacy of 5-aminosalicylic acid for the prevention of radiation enteritis. *Clin Oncol.* 1993;5:19.

46. Martenson Jr. JA, Bollinger JW, Sloan JA, et al: Sucralfate in the prevention of treatment-induced diarrhea in patients receiving pelvic radiation therapy: A North Central Cancer Treatment Group Phase III double-blind placebo-controlled trial. *J Clin Oncol.* 2000;18:1239.

47. Ben-Joseph E, Han S, Tobi M, et al: A pilot study of topical intrarectal application of amifostine for prevention of late radiation rectal injury. *Int J Radiat Oncol Biol Phys.* 2002;53:1160.

48. O'Brien PC, Franklin CI, Poulsen M, et al: Acute symptoms, not rectally administered sucralfate, predict for late radiation proctitis: Longer term follow-up of a phase III trial—Trans-Tasman Radiation Oncology Group. *Int J Radiat Oncol Biol Phys.* 2002;54:442.

49. Withers HR: Biological basis for altered fractionation schemes. *Cancer.* 1985;55:2086.

50. Cox JD, Guse C, Asbell S, et al: Tolerance of pelvic normal tissues to hyperfractionated radiation therapy: Results of protocol 83-08 of the Radiation Therapy Oncology Group. *Int J Radiat Oncol Biol Phys.* 1988;15:1331.

51. Coucke PA, Cuttat JF, Mirimanoff RO: Adjuvant postoperative accelerated hyperfractionated radiotherapy in rectal cancer: A feasibility study. *Int J Radiat Oncol Biol Phys.* 1993;27:885.

52. Coucke PA, Sartorelli B, Cuttat JF, et al: The rationale to switch from postoperative hyperfractionated accelerated radiotherapy to preoperative hyperfractionated accelerated radiotherapy in rectal cancer. *Int J Radiat Oncol Biol Phys.* 1995;32:181.

53. Stupp R, Matter M, Volter V, et al: Preoperative hyperfractionated accelerated radiotherapy (HART) and concomitant CPT-11 in locally advanced rectal cancer (LARC): A phase I study. *Int J Radiat Oncol Biol Phys.* 2001;51:11 [abstract].

54. Janjan NA, Crane C, Feig BW, et al: Prospective trial of preoperative concomitant boost radiotherapy with continuous infusion 5-fluorouracil for locally advanced rectal cancer. *Int J Radiat Oncol Biol Phys.* 2000;47:713.

55. Movsas B, Hanlon A, Lanciano R, et al: Phase I dose escalating trial of hyperfractionated pre-operative chemoradiation for locally advanced rectal cancer. *Int J Radiat Oncol Biol Phys.* 1998;42:43.

56. Diratzouian H, Movsas B, Hanlon AL, et al: Phase II trial of preoperative chemoradiation with a hyperfractionated RT boost in locally advanced rectal cancer. *Int J Radiat Oncol Biol Phys.* 2001;51:10 [abstract].

57. Myerson RJ, Valentini V, Birnbaum EH, et al: A phase I/II trial of three-dimensionally planned concurrent boost radiotherapy and protracted venous infusion of 5-FU chemotherapy for locally advanced rectal carcinoma. *Int J Radiat Oncol Biol Phys.* 2001;50:1299.

58. Tait DM, Nahum AE, Meyer LC, et al: Acute toxicity in pelvic radiotherapy; a randomised trial of conformal versus conventional treatment. *Radiother Oncol.* 1997;42:121.

59. Shank B, LoSasso T, Brewster L, et al: Three-dimensional treatment planning for post-operative treatment of rectal carcinoma. *Int J Radiat Oncol Biol Phys.* 1991;21:253.

60. Tatsuzaki H, Urie MM, Willett CG: 3-D comparative study of proton vs. x-ray radiation therapy for rectal cancer. *Int J Radiat Oncol Biol Phys.* 1991;22:369.

61. Duncan W, Arnott SJ, Jack WJL, et al: Results of two randomized trials of neutron therapy in rectal adenocarcinoma. *Radiother Oncol.* 1987;8:191.

62. Anscher MS, Lee C, Hurwitz HI, et al: A pilot study of preoperative continuous infusion 5-fluorouracil, external microwave hyperthermia, and external beam radiotherapy for treatment of locally advanced, unresectable, or recurrent rectal cancer. *Int J Radiat Oncol Biol Phys.* 2000;47:719.

63. Rau B, Wust P, Tilly W, et al: Preoperative radiochemotherapy in locally advanced or recurrent rectal cancer: Regional radiofrequency hyperthermia correlates with clinical parameters. *Int J Radiat Oncol Biol Phys.* 2000;48:381.

64. van der Zee J, Gonzalez DG, van Rhoon GC, et al: Comparison of radiotherapy alone with radiotherapy plus hyperthermia in locally advanced pelvic tumors: A prospective, randomised, multicenter trial. *Lancet.* 2000;355:1119.

65. Rodier JF, Janser JC, Rodier D, et al: Prevention of radiation enteritis by an absorbable polyglycolic acid mesh sling. A 60-case multicentric study. *Cancer.* 1991;68:2545.

66. Hoffman JP, Sigurdson ER, Eisenberg BL: Use of saline-filled expanders to protect the small bowel from radiation. *Oncology.* 1998;12:51.

67. Chen JS, Chang Chien CR, Wang JY, et al: Pelvic peritoneal reconstruction to prevent radiation enteritis in rectal carcinoma. *Dis Colon Rectum.* 1992;35:897.

68. Michels KB, Giovannucci E, Joshipura KJ, et al: Prospective study of fruit and vegetable consumption and incidence of colon and rectal cancers. *J Natl Cancer Inst.* 2000;92:1740.

69. Tocchi A, Lepre L, Costa G, et al: Rectal cancer and inguinal metastasis. Prognostic role and therapeutic indications. *Dis Colon Rectum.* 1999;42:1464.

70. Bosset JF, Horiot JC, Hamers HP, et al: Postoperative pelvic radiotherapy with or without elective irradiation of para-aortic nodes and liver in rectal cancer patients. A controlled clinical trial of the EORTC Radiotherapy Group. *Radiother Oncol.* 2001;61:7.

71. Krook JE, Moertel CG, Gunderson LL, et al: Effective surgical adjuvant therapy for high-risk rectal carcinoma. *N Engl J Med.* 1991;324:709.

72. Wolmark N, Weiand HS, Hyams DM, et al: Randomized trial of postoperative adjuvant chemotherapy with or without radiotherapy for carcinoma of the rectum: National Surgical Adjuvant Breast and Bowel Project protocol R-02. *J Natl Cancer Inst.* 2000;92:388.

73. Minsky BD, Cohen AM, Enker WE, et al: Combined modality therapy of rectal cancer: Decreased acute toxicity with the preoperative approach. *J Clin Oncol.* 1992;10:1218.

74. Sauer R, Fietkau R, Wittekind C, et al: Adjuvant versus neoadjuvant radiochemotherapy for locally advanced rectal cancer. *Strahlenther Onkol.* 2001;177:173.

75. Roh MS, Petrelli N, Weiand H, et al: Phase III randomized trial of preoperative versus postoperative multimodality therapy in patients with carcinoma of the rectum (NSABP R-03). *Proc ASCO.* 2001;20:123a [abstract].

76. Botwood N, James R, Vernon C, Price P: A phase I study of "Tomudex" (raltitrexed) with radiotherapy (RT) as adjuvant treatment in patients (pt) with operable rectal cancer. *Proc ASCO.* 1998;17:277a [abstract].

77. Fernandez-Martos C, Aparicio J, Bosch C, et al: Preoperative therapy (PT) with oral uracil and tegafur (UFT) and concomitant irradiation (RT) in operable rectal cancer (RC). Preliminary results of a multicenter phase II study. *Proc ASCO.* 2001;20:148a [abstract].

78. Uzcudun AE, Batlle JF, Velasco JC, et al: Efficacy of preoperative radiation therapy for resectable rectal adenocarcinoma when combined with oral tegafur-uracil modulated with leucovorin. *Dis Colon Rectum.* 2002;45:1349.

79. Valentini V, Morganti AG, Luzi S, et al: Chemoradiation with raltitrexed (Tomudex) and oxaliplatin in preoperative treatment of stage II/III resectable rectal cancer: A dose finding study. *Proc ASCO.* 2001;20:131a [abstract].

80. Freyer G, Bossard N, Romestaing P, et al: Addition of oxaliplatin to continuous infusion fluorouracil, l-folinic acid, and concomitant radiotherapy in rectal cancer: The Lyon R 97-03 phase I trial. *J Clin Oncol.* 2001;19:2433.

81. Carraro S, Roca EL, Cartelli C, et al: Radiochemotherapy with short daily infusion of low-dose oxaliplatin, leucovorin, and 5-FU in T3-T4 unresectable rectal cancer: A phase II IATTGI study. *Int J Radiat Oncol Biol Phys.* 2002;54:397.

82. Klautke G, Kirchner R, Hopt U, Fietkau R: Continuous infusion of 5-FU and weekly irinotecan with concurrent radiotherapy as neoadjuvant treatment for locally advanced or recurrent rectal cancer. *Proc ASCO.* 2001;20:140a [abstract].

83. Ranson M, Hammond LA, Ferry D, et al: ZD1839, a selective oral epidermal growth factor receptor-tyrosine kinase inhibitor, is well tolerated and active in patients with solid, malignant tumors: results of a phase I trial. *J Clin Oncol.* 2002;20:1512.

84. Dunst J, Reese T, Sutter T, et al: Phase I trial evaluating the concurrent combination of radiotherapy and capecitabine in rectal cancer. *J Clin Oncol.* 2002;20:3983.

85. Willett CG, Badizadegan K, Ancukiewicz M, et al: Prognostic factors in stage T3N0 rectal cancer. Do all patients require postoperative pelvic irradiation and chemotherapy? *Dis Colon Rectum.* 1999;42:167.

86. Merchant NB, Guillem JG, Paty PB, et al: T3N0 rectal cancer: Results following sharp mesorectal excision and no adjuvant therapy. *J Gastrointest Surg.* 1999;3:642.

87. Gunderson LL, Sargent DJ, Tepper JE, et al: Impact of T and N substage on survival and disease relapse in adjuvant rectal cancer: a pooled analysis. *Int J Radiat Oncol Biol Phys.* 2002;54:386.

88. Minsky BD: Multidisciplinary management of resectable rectal cancer. *Oncology.* 1996;10:1701.

89. Camma C, Giunta M, Fiorica F, et al: Preoperative radiotherapy for resectable rectal cancer. A meta-analysis. *J Amer Med Assoc.* 2000;284:1008.

90. Colorectal Cancer Collaborative Group: Adjuvant radiotherapy for rectal cancer: A systematic overview of 22 randomised trials involving 8507 patients. *Lancet.* 2001;358:1291.

91. Swedish Rectal Cancer Trial: Improved survival with preoperative radiotherapy in resectable rectal cancer. *N Engl J Med.* 1997;336:980.

92. Kapiteijn E, Marijnen CAM, Nagtegaal ID, et al: Preoperative radiotherapy combined with total mesorectal excision for resectable rectal cancer. *N Engl J Med.* 2001;345:638.

93. Marijnen CAM, Kapiteijn E, van de Velde CJH, et al: Acute side effects and complications after short-term preoperative radiotherapy combined with total mesorectal excision in primary rectal cancer: Report of a multicenter randomized trial. *J Clin Oncol.* 2002;20:817.

94. Graf W, Dahlberg M, Osman MM, et al: Short-term preoperative radiotherapy results in down-staging of rectal cancer: A study of 1316 patients. *Radiother Oncol.* 1997;43:133.

95. Marijnen CAM, Nagtegaal ID, Kranenbarg EK, et al: No downstaging after short-term preoperative radiotherapy in rectal cancer patients. *J Clin Oncol.* 2001;19:1976.

96. Francois Y, Nemoz CJ, Baulieux J, et al: Influence of the interval between preoperative radiation therapy and surgery on downstaging and on the rate of sphincter-sparing surgery for rectal cancer: The Lyon R90-01 randomized trial. *J Clin Oncol.* 1999;17:2396.

97. Sauer R, Fietkau R, Martus P, et al: Adjuvant and neoadjuvant radiochemotherapy for advanced rectal cancer—First results of the German multicenter phase-III-trial. *Int J Radiat Oncol Biol Phys.* 2000;48:119 [abstract].

98. Wagman R, Minsky BD, Cohen AM, et al: Sphincter preservation with preoperative radiation therapy and coloanal anastomosis: Long term follow-up. *Int J Radiat Oncol Biol Phys.* 1998;42:51.

99. Rouanet P, Saint Aubert B, Lemanski C, et al: Restorative and nonrestorative surgery for low rectal cancer after high dose radiation. Long term oncologic and functional results. *Dis Colon Rectum.* 2002;45:305.

100. Hyams DM, Mamounas EP, Petrelli N, et al: A clinical trial to evaluate the worth of preoperative multimodality therapy in patients with operable carcinoma of the rectum. A progress report of the National Surgical Adjuvant Breast and Bowel Project protocol R0-3. *Dis Colon Rectum.* 1997;40:131.

101. Valentini V, Coco C, Cellini N, et al: Preoperative chemoradiation for extraperitoneal T3 rectal cancer: acute toxicity, tumor response, and sphincter preservation. *Int J Radiat Oncol Biol Phys.* 1998;40:1067.

102. Grann A, Feng C, Wong D, et al: Pre-op combined modality therapy (CMT) for uT3 rectal cancer. *Proc ASCO.* 2000;19:249a [abstract].

103. Maghfoor I, Wilkes J, Kuvshinoff B, et al: Neoadjuvant chemodiotherapy with sphincter-sparing surgery for low lying rectal cancer. *Proc ASCO.* 1997;16:274 [abstract].

104. Grumann MM, Noack EM, Hoffman IA, et al: Comparison of quality of life in patients undergoing abdominoperineal extirpation or anterior resection for rectal cancer. *Ann Surg.* 2001;233:149.

105. Kollmorgen CF, Meagher AP, Pemberton JH, et al: The long term effect of adjuvant postoperative chemoradiotherapy for rectal cancer on bowel function. *Ann Surg.* 1994;220:676.

106. Onaitis MW, Noone RB, Fields R, et al: Complete response to neoadjuvant chemoradiation for rectal cancer does not influence survival. *Ann Surg Oncol.* 2001;8:801.

107. Janjan NA, Crane C, Feig BW, et al: Improved overall survival among responders to preoperative chemoradiation for locally advanced rectal cancer. *Am J Clin Oncol.* 2001;24:107.

108. Mohiuddin M, Hayne M, Regine WF, et al: Prognostic significance of postchemoradiation stage following preoperative chemotherapy and radiation for advanced/recurrent rectal cancers. *Int J Radiat Oncol Biol Phys.* 2000;48:1075.

109. Read TE, Ogunbiyi OA, Fleshman JW, et al: Neoadjuvant external beam radiation and proctectomy for adenocarcinoma of the rectum. *Dis Colon Rectum.* 2001;44:1778.

110. Hiotis SP, Weber SM, Cohen AM, et al: Assessing the predictive value of clinical complete response to neoadjuvant therapy for rectal cancer: An analysis of 488 patients. *J Am Coll Surg.* 2002;194:131.

111. Ruo L, Tickoo S, Klimstra DS, et al: Long-term prognostic significance of extent of rectal cancer response to preoperative radiation and chemotherapy. *Ann Surg.* 2002;236:75.

112. Valentini V, Coco C, Picciocchi A, et al: Does downstaging predict improved outcome after preoperative chemoradiation for extraperitoneal locally advanced rectal cancer? A long term analysis of 165 patients. *Int J Radiat Oncol Biol Phys.* 2002;53:664.

113. Luna-Perez P, Segura J, Alvarado I, et al: Specific *c-K-ras* gene mutations as a tumor-response marker in locally advanced rectal cancer treated with preoperative chemoradiotherapy. *Ann Surg Oncol.* 2000;7:727.

114. Villafranca E, Okruzhnov Y, Dominguez MA, et al: Polymorphisms of the repeated sequences in the enhancer region of the thymidylate synthase gene promoter may predict downstaging after preoperative chemoradiation in rectal cancer. *J Clin Oncol.* 2001;19:1779.

115. Esposito G, Pucciarelli S, Alaggio R, et al: p27kip1 Expression is associated with tumor response to preoperative chemoradiotherapy in rectal cancer. *Ann Surg Oncol.* 2001;8:311.

116. Elsaleh H, Robbins P, Joseph D, et al: Can p53 alterations be used to predict tumor response to pre-operative chemoradiotherapy in locally advanced rectal cancer? *Radiother Oncol* 2000;56:239.

117. Kandioler D, Zwrtek R, Ludwig C, et al: TP53 genotype but not p53 immunohistochemical result predicts response to preoperative short-term radiotherapy in rectal cancer. *Ann Surg.* 2002;235:493.

118. Schwander O, Bruce HP, Broll R: p21, p27, cyclin D1, and p53 in rectal cancer: immunohistology with prognostic significance? *Int J Colorec Dis.* 2002;17:11.

119. Adell GCE, Zhang H, Evertsson S, et al: Apoptosis in rectal cancer. Prognosis and recurrence after preoperative radiotherapy. *Cancer.* 2001;91:1870.

120. Rodel C, Grabenbauer GG, Papadopoulos T, et al: Apoptosis as a cellular predictor for histopathologic response to neoadjuvant radiochemotherapy in patients with rectal cancer. *Int J Radiat Oncol Biol Phys.* 2002;52:294.

121. Adell G, Zhang H, Jansson A, et al: Decreased tumor cell proliferation as an indicator of the effect of preoperative radiotherapy of rectal cancer. *Int J Radiat Oncol Biol Phys.* 2001;50:659.

122. Habr-Gama A, Santinho B, de Souza PM, Ribeiro U, et al: Low rectal cancer. Impact of radiation and chemotherapy on surgical treatment. *Dis Colon Rectum.* 1998;41:1087.

123. Barbaro B, Schulsinger A, Valentini V, et al: The accuracy of transrectal ultrasound in predicting the pathological stage of low-lying rectal cancer after preoperative chemoradiation therapy. *Int J Radiat Oncol Biol Phys.* 1999;43:1043.

124. Gavioli M, Bagni A, Piccagli I, et al: Usefulness of endorectal ultrasound after preoperative radiotherapy in rectal cancer. *Dis Colon Rectum.* 2000;43:1075.

125. MacFarlane JK, Ryall RD, Heald RJ: Mesorectal excision for rectal cancer. *Lancet.* 1993;341:457.

126. Leong APK: Selective total mesorectal excision for rectal cancer. *Dis Colon Rectum.* 2000;43:1237.

127. Haas-Kock DFM, Baeten CGMI, Jager JJ, et al: Prognostic significance of radial margins of clearance in rectal cancer. *Br J Surg.* 1996;83:781.

128. Enker WE, Thaler HT, Cranor ML, et al: Total mesorectal excision in the operative treatment of carcinoma of the rectum. *J Am Coll Surg.* 1995;181:335.

129. Arenas RB, Fichera A, Mhoon D, et al: Total mesenteric excision in the surgical treatment of rectal cancer. A prospective study. *Arch Surg.* 1998;133:608.

130. Havenga K, Enker WE, Norstein J, et al: Improved survival and local control after total mesorectal excision or D3 lymphadenectomy in the treatment of primary rectal cancer: An international analysis of 1411 patients. *Eur J Surg Oncol.* 1999;25:368.

131. Aitken RJ: Mesorectal excision for rectal cancer. *Br J Surg.* 1996;83:214.

132. Carlsen E, Schlichting E, Guldvog I, et al: Effect of the introduction of total mesorectal excision for the treatment of rectal cancer. *Br J Surg.* 1998;85:526.

133. Poon RTP, Chu KW, Ho JWC, et al: Prospective evaluation of selective defunctioning stoma for low anterior resection with total mesorectal excision. *World J Surg.* 1999;23:463.

134. van de Velde CJH: Preoperative radiotherapy and TME-surgery for rectal cancer: detailed analysis in relation to quality control in a randomized trial. *Proc ASCO.* 2002;21:127a [abstract].

135. Dahlberg M, Glimelius B, Pahlman L: Changing strategy for rectal cancer is associated with improved outcome. *Br J Surg.* 1999;86:379.

136. Gerard JP, Ayzac L, Coquard R, et al: Endocavitary irradiation for early rectal carcinomas T1 (T2). A series of 101 patients treated with the Papillon's technique. *Int J Radiat Oncol Biol Phys.* 1996;34:775.

137. Aumock A, Birnbaum EH, Fleshman JW, et al: Treatment of rectal adenocarcinoma with endocavitary and external beam radiotherapy: results for 199 patients with localized tumors. *Int J Radiat Oncol Biol Phys.* 2001;51:363.

138. Bonnen M, Crane C, Feig BW, et al: Long term results using local excision after preoperative chemoradiation among selected T3 rectal cancer patients. *Int J Radiat Oncol Biol Phys.* 2001;51:12 [abstract].

139. Ruo L, Guillem JG, Minsky BD, et al: Preoperative radiation with or without chemotherapy and full-thickness transanal excision for selected T2 and T3 distal rectal cancers. *Int J Colorec Dis.* 2002;17:54.

140. Willett CG: Local excision followed by postoperative radiation therapy. *Sem Radiat Oncol.* 1998;8:24.

141. Chakravarti A, Compton CC, Shellito PC, et al: Long-term follow-up of patients with rectal cancer managed by local excision with and without adjuvant irradiation. *Ann Surg.* 1999;230:49.

142. Wagman R, Minsky BD, Cohen AM, et al: Conservative management of rectal cancer with local excision and post-op radiation + chemotherapy. *Int J Radiat Oncol Biol Phys.* 1999;44:841.

143. Steele GD, Herndon JE, Bleday R, et al: Sphincter-sparing treatment for distal rectal adenocarcinoma. *Ann Surg Oncol.* 1999;6:433.

144. Benson R, Wong CS, Cummings BJ, et al: Local excision and postoperative radiotherapy for distal rectal cancer. *Int J Radiat Oncol Biol Phys.* 2001;50:1309.

145. Russell AH, Harris J, Rosenberg PJ, et al: Anal sphincter conservation for patients with adenocarcinoma of the distal rectum: Long-term results of Radiation Therapy Oncology Group protocol 89-02. *Int J Radiat Oncol Biol Phys.* 2000;46:313.

146. Alekitar KM, Zelefsky MJ, Paty PB, et al: High dose rate intraoperative brachytherapy for recurrent colorectal cancer. *Int J Radiat Oncol Biol Phys.* 2000;48:219.

147. Gunderson LL, Nelson H, Martenson JA, et al: Locally advanced primary colorectal cancer: intraoperative electron and external beam irradiation + 5-FU. *Int J Radiat Oncol Biol Phys.* 1997;37:601.

148. Harrison LB, Minsky BD, Enker WE, et al: High dose rate intraoperative radiation therapy (HDR-IORT) as part of the management strategy for locally advanced primary and recurrent rectal cancer. *Int J Radiat Oncol Biol Phys.* 1998;42:325.

149. Huber FT, Stepan R, Zimmermann F, et al: Locally advanced rectal cancer: Resection and intraoperative radiotherapy using the flab method combined with preoperative or postoperative radiochemotherapy. *Dis Colon Rectum.* 1996;39:774.

150. Kallinowski F, Eble MJ, Buhr HJ, et al: Intraoperative radiotherapy for primary and recurrent rectal cancers. *Eur J Surg Oncol.* 1995;21:191.

151. Mannaerts GHH, Martijn H, Crommelin MA, et al: Feasibility and first results of multimodality treatment combining EBRT, extensive surgery, and IORET in locally advanced primary rectal cancer. *Int J Radiat Oncol Biol Phys.* 2000;47:425.

152. Lindel K, Willett CG, Shellito PC, et al: Intraoperative radiation therapy for locally advanced recurrent rectal or rectosigmoid cancer. *Radiother Oncol.* 2001;58:83.

153. Sanfilippo NJ, Crane CH, Skibber J, et al: T4 rectal cancer treated with preoperative chemoradiation to the posterior pelvis followed by multivisceral resection: patterns of failure and limitations of treatment. *Int J Radiat Oncol Biol Phys.* 2001;51:176.

154. Shibata D, Guillem JG, Lanouette NM, et al: Functional and quality of life outcomes in patients with rectal cancer after combined modality therapy, intraoperative radiation therapy, and sphincter preservation. *Dis Colon Rectum.* 2000;43:752.

155. Papillon J: Present status of radiation therapy in the conservative management of rectal cancer. *Radiother Oncol.* 1990;17:275.

156. Myerson RJ, Walz BJ, Kodner IJ, et al: Endocavitary radiation therapy for rectal cancer: Results with and without external beam. *Endocurie Hypertherm Oncol.* 1989;5:195.

157. Horiot JC, Roth SL, Calais G, et al: The Dijon clinical staging system for early rectal carcinomas amenable to intracavitary treatment techniques. *Radiother Oncol.* 1990;18:329.

158. Roth SL, Horiot JC, Calais G, et al: Prognostic factors in limited rectal cancer treated with intracavitary irradiation. *Int J Radiat Oncol Biol Phys.* 1989;16:1445.

159. Gerard JP, Chapet O, Ramaioli A, et al: Long-term control of T2-T3 rectal adenocarcinoma with radiotherapy alone. *Int J Radiat Oncol Biol Phys.* 2002;54:142.

160. Crane CH, Janjan NA, Abbruzzese JL, et al: Effective pelvic symptom control using initial chemoradiation without colostomy in metastatic rectal cancer. *Int J Radiat Oncol Biol Phys.* 2001;49:107.

161. Wong CS, Cummings BJ, Brierley JD, et al: Treatment of locally recurrent rectal carcinoma—Results and prognostic factors. *Int J Radiat Oncol Biol Phys.* 1998;40:427.

162. Lingareddy V, Ahmad NR, Mohiuddin M: Palliative reirradiation for recurrent rectal cancer. *Int J Radiat Oncol Biol Phys.* 1997;38:785.

163. Liberman H, Adams DR, Blatchford GJ, et al: Clinical use of the self-expanding metallic stent in the management of colorectal cancer. *Am J Surg.* 2001;180:407.

Cancer of the Anal Canal

Bruce D. Minsky, MD

42

EPIDEMIOLOGY, ETIOLOGY, GENETICS, AND CYTOGENETIC ABNORMALITIES

Cancers of the anal region account for 1% to 2% of all large bowel cancers and 4% of all anorectal carcinomas. The majority of these patients (75% to 80%) have squamous cell carcinomas.[1] Approximately 15% have adenocarcinomas.

In 2002 there were an estimated 3900 new cases in the United States, 1700 occurring in men and 2200 in women. Approximately 500 deaths occurred.[2] Anal cancers, while still uncommon tumors, have increased substantially in incidence over the last several decades.[3] This increase may be due to sexual transmission of human papilloma virus (HPV), especially HPV-16.[4] It is postulated that, similar to cervical carcinoma, in which HPV is strongly associated and may be a necessary factor for development of the disease, high-grade atypical intraepithelial neoplastic lesions are the immediate precursors to anal cancer.[5] The association between AIDS and an increased risk for anal canal cancer is thought to be related to immunodeficiency, perhaps increasing susceptibility to HPV infection. A similar increase in risk has been noted in patients with severe immunodeficiency (e.g., CD4 counts, <200/µL) and for renal transplant patients undergoing immunosuppression.[6]

Various molecular and chromosomal abnormalities may be associated with anal cancer. In an analysis of Radiation Therapy Oncology Group (RTOG) protocol 87-04, there was a trend toward decreased local control and survival in patients overexpressing *p53*; however, this did not reach statistic significance.[7]

ANATOMY

Cancers of the anus can occur in three regions: the perianal skin, the anal canal, and the lower rectum (Fig. 42-1). The anal canal is 3 to 4 cm long and extends from the anal verge to the pelvic floor.[8] A clear anatomic distinction between the anal canal and the anal margin is needed because of the different natural histories of cancers that arise in these two distinct anatomic areas. There is considerable confusion when comparing series in the literature because of the use of different definitions of the anal canal and the anal margin.

To clarify this issue, the American Joint Committee on Cancer (AJCC) and the Union Internationale Contra le Cancer (UICC) formed a consensus that the anal canal extends from the anorectal ring (dentate line) to the anal verge.[9,10] This is an important distinction, since these two governing bodies agree that anal margin tumors behave in a similar fashion to skin cancers, and therefore should be classified as skin tumors and treated as such. However, if there is any involvement of the anal verge by tumor, then it should be treated as an anal canal cancer.

The anal region has an extensive lymphatic system, and there are many connections between the various levels (Fig. 42-2). The three main pathways are: (1) superiorly from the rectum along the superior hemorrhoidal vessels to the inferior mesenteric lymph nodes, (2) from the upper anal canal and superior to the dentate line along the inferior and middle hemorrhoid vessels to the hypogastric lymph nodes; and (3) inferior from the anal margin and anal canal to the superficial inguinal lymph nodes.

PATHOLOGY

Various histologic cell types are present in the anal area (Table 42-1).[11] The most common is squamous cell carcinoma. Since the mucosal epithelium over the rectal columns is cuboidal, transitional (cloacogenic) carcinomas can arise. Most investigators agree that prognosis is more dependent on stage than histologic subtype. Adenocarcinomas can arise from anal crypts and should

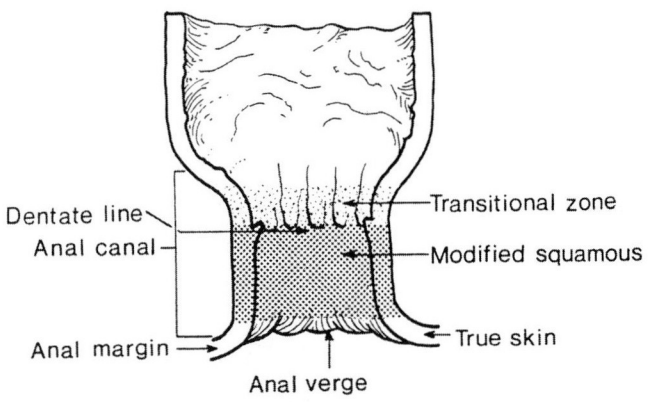

Figure 42–1. Anatomy of the anal region. (From Nigro ND: Neoplasms of the anus and anal canal. In Zuidema GD, ed. *Shackelford's Surgery of the Alimentary Tract.* 2nd ed. Philadelphia: WB Saunders; 1991:319.)

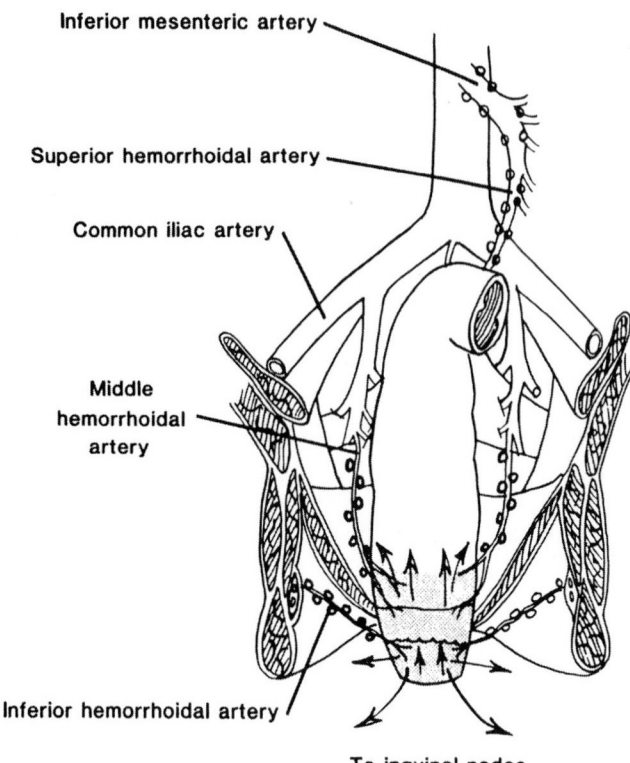

Figure 42–2. Lymphatic drainage of the anal region. (From Pemberton JH: Anatomy and physiology of the anus and rectum. In Zuidema GD, ed. *Shackelford's Surgery of the Alimentary Tract.* 2nd ed. Philadelphia: WB Saunders; 1991:253.

be treated as rectal cancer.[12] In this chapter squamous cell basaloid and cloacogenic histologies are collectively defined as *anal canal cancers.* Less common cancers, such as melanoma, lymphoma, and sarcoma are not discussed.[13]

CLINICAL PRESENTATION

The most common presenting symptoms are bleeding and anal pain. Other less common symptoms include pruritus and a palpable mass.

ROUTES OF SPREAD

The primary routes of spread of anal canal cancer are direct extension into soft tissues and lymphatic pathways (Fig. 42-2). Hematogenous spread is less common. At the

time of presentation, pelvic lymph node metastases occur in 30% of patients and inguinal lymph node metastases in 15% to 35%.[14] The incidence of synchronous and metachronous inguinal node metastasis in patients who initially present with clinically negative nodes and are not treated to the inguinal nodes is T1:10%, T2:8%, T3:16%, and T4:11%.[15] Most inguinal lymph node metastases are unilateral. Only 10% of patients present with extrapelvic visceral metastases at the time of presentation. These metastases occur most commonly in the liver and lungs.

DIAGNOSTIC AND STAGING STUDIES

Required as well as *optional* diagnostic and staging studies for anal cancer are presented in Table 42-2. Transanal ultrasound may help identify the depth of tumor penetration.[16] The preferred imaging study is abdominal/pelvic computed tomography (CT) scan or magnetic resonance imaging (MRI).

Surgery for the initial diagnosis and staging of anal canal tumors should be limited to a biopsy of the primary tumor and evaluation of the inguinal lymph nodes. Clinically enlarged lymph nodes should be aspirated. If the cytology is nondiagnostic or demonstrates only benign disease, an open excisional biopsy of one or two lymph nodes should be performed. *Under no circumstances should a formal lymph node dissection be performed for the initial evaluation of suspicious nodes.*

STAGING

In 1997 the AJCC and UICC developed a common staging system. This system takes into account the fact that anal canal carcinoma is primarily treated by combined modality therapy (or in select cases by radiation alone). Abdominoperineal resection (APR) is reserved for patients failing initial treatment. Thus, the TNM classification for anal canal cancers is clinical. The primary tumor is assessed for size and, for T4 tumors, invasion of local structures such as the vagina, urethra, or bladder. The sixth edition of the AJCC staging system is presented in Table 42-3.[17] There were no major changes from the fifth edition. Although additional descriptors do not affect the stage grouping, they *do* indicate cases needing separate analysis.

Table 42–1   Histologic Types of Anal Cancer

Type of Cancer	%
Squamous cell	63
Transitional (cloacogenic)	23
Adenocarcinoma	7
Paget's disease	2
Basal cell	2
Melanoma	2

Modified from Peters RK, Mack TM: Patterns of anal carcinoma by gender and marital status in Los Angeles County. *Br J Cancer.* 1983;48:629.

Table 42–2   Workup for Anal Canal Cancer

History
Physical examination
Proctoscopy
Biopsy of primary tumor
Biopsy of inguinal nodes if clinically suspicious
Chest x-ray film
Abdominal/pelvic computed tomography or magnetic resonance imaging
Screening profile
Complete blood count
Transanal ultrasonography (*optional*)

Table 42–3   Classification of Anal Canal Cancer

Primary Tumor (T)

TX	Primary tumor cannot be assessed
T0	No evidence of primary tumor
Tis	Carcinoma in situ
T1	Tumor ≤2 cm in maximum diameter
T2	Tumor >2 cm but ≤5 cm in maximum diameter
T3	Tumor >5 cm in maximum diameter
T4	Tumor of any size that invades an adjacent structure or structures; involvement of the sphincter muscles alone is not classified as T4

Regional Lymph Nodes (N)

NX	Regional lymph nodes cannot be assessed
N0	No regional lymph node metastasis
N1	Perirectal lymph node metastasis
N2	Unilateral internal iliac or inguinal node metastasis or both
N3	And/or perirectal and inguinal node, bilateral internal iliac, or inguinal node metastasis

Distant Metastasis (M)

MX	Distant metastasis cannot be assessed
M0	No distant metastasis
M1	Distant metastasis

Stage Groupings

Stage

0	Tis	N0	M0
I	T1	N0	M0
II	T2-3	N0	M0
IIIA	T4	N0	M0
	T1-3	N1	M0
IIIB	T4	N1	M0
	T1-4	N2-3	M0
IV	T1-4	N0-3	M1

Note: Anal margin cancers are classified as skin cancers.
Note: Although additional descriptors do not affect the stage grouping, additional prefixes are used to indicate the need for additional analysis:

Suffix	Reason
m	The presence of multiple primary tumors in a single site, recorded in parentheses: pT(m)NM.
y	When classification is performed during or following initial radiation or chemotherapy or both, based on the amount of tumor present at the time of the examination, and not an estimate of tumor before therapy: ycTNM or ypTNM.
r	Indicates recurrent tumor: rTNM.
a	Indicates the stage at autopsy: aTNM.

Lymphatic Vessel Invasion (L)

Lx	Cannot be assessed
L0	No lymphatic vessel invasion
L1	Lymphatic vessel invasion present

Venous Invasion (V)

Vx	Cannot be assessed
V0	No venous invasion
V1	Microscopic venous invasion present
V2	Macroscopic venous invasion present

From Greene FL, Page DL, Fleming ID, et al., eds. *AJCC Cancer Staging Manual.* 6th ed. New York: Springer; 2002.

STANDARD THERAPEUTIC APPROACHES

Surgery

LOCAL EXCISION

Local excision has been used in highly selected patients with tumors that are less than 2 cm in diameter, well differentiated, or found incidentally at the time of hemorrhoidectomy. Of 188 patients with anal canal carcinoma treated at the Mayo Clinic, a subset of 19 were treated with local excision.[18] For the 12 patients with tumors confined to the epithelium and subepithelial connective tissues, 11 had tumors less than 2 cm in size and 1 patient had 2 lesions. Overall survival for these patients was 100%. In one of 12 patients the tumor recurred, and this patient was without evidence of disease 5 years after an APR. Patients with tumors penetrating into muscle who refused a colostomy had a higher recurrence rate. Often, these patients can be salvaged with an APR or combined modality therapy.

Results of local treatment for tumors less than 2 cm were not as favorable at Memorial Sloan-Kettering Cancer Center (MSKCC), where only 3 of 8 patients with local excisions had prolonged survival.[19] In summary, local excision alone for anal canal cancer is considered an investigational approach.

ABDOMINOPERINEAL RESECTION

Radical surgery (APR) is reserved for salvage in patients who have failed radiation or in patients who have received prior pelvic radiation therapy.

Combined Modality Therapy

Until the late 1970s, the conventional treatment for anal canal cancer was an APR. Nigro et al. challenged this practice with a report of 3 patients with squamous cell carcinoma of the anal canal who, following preoperative treatment with 30 Gy plus concurrent 5-FU and mitomycin-C, were found to have a pathologically complete response at the time of surgery.[20]

Since that time, increasing evidence from single-arm phase II studies has indicated that initial combined modality therapy (chemotherapy plus concurrent external beam radiation therapy [EBRT]) yields a complete response rate of approximately 80% to 90% in most patients with squamous cell carcinomas of the anal canal. Surgery, most commonly an APR, is reserved for salvage. Even in patients with large (≥5-cm) primary cancers, although the complete response rates are lower (50% to 75%), the majority of patients may be spared a colostomy and have an excellent overall survival. The results of these trials will be discussed in the Outcomes section.

TECHNIQUES OF RADIATION THERAPY

Introduction

The design and delivery of pelvic radiation therapy for anal cancer requires a knowledge of the natural history of the disease, patterns of failure, anatomy, and radiobiologic principles. Furthermore, the use of proper equipment, implementation of methods to decrease treatment-related toxicity, and a close collaboration with the physics and technology staff are essential.

A comprehensive discussion of techniques to decrease the toxicity of pelvic irradiation, such as physical maneuvers, immobilization molds, dietary supplements and radioprotectors, three-dimensional treatment planning, and other investigational approaches, is presented in Chapter 41, Cancer of the Rectum. However, some general principles specific to the design and delivery of radiation for anal cancer are presented in this chapter.

Design of Radiation Therapy Fields for Anal Cancer

The design of pelvic radiation therapy fields for anal cancer is based on knowledge of the natural history of the disease and the primary nodal drainage. Since the internal iliac and presacral nodes are posterior in reference to the external iliac nodes, much of the normal structures in the anterior pelvis can be spared with the use of lateral fields. This approach will underdose the inguinal nodes; however, they can be supplemented with electrons. General guidelines for the design of pelvic radiation therapy fields for anal cancer are listed in Table 42-4.

PELVIC FIELD

A prone three-field technique (posterior-anterior + opposed laterals) is recommended. Figures 42-3 and 42-4 provide examples. This arrangement results in the lowest dose to the anterior structures, such as the genitalia and bladder. The underdosed inguinal nodes are then treated concurrently with electrons to bring the dose up to 100% of the prescription dose. An alternative method is to use an anterior-posterior–posterior-anterior (AP–PA) technique. Although this technique treats the pelvic and inguinal nodes in the same field, it results in the highest dose to the anterior pelvic structures and skin, thereby increasing toxicity. An electron boost for the perineum is not recommended since there will be overlap between the electron and photon fields. The portion of the perineum that needs to be treated should be included in the photon fields. The whole pelvis receives 30.6 Gy followed by a 14.4 Gy conedown to the true pelvis for a total dose of 45 Gy. Dosimetry from a representative three-field plan is seen in Figure 42-5.

PRIMARY TUMOR BOOST FIELD FOR COMBINED MODALITY THERAPY SALVAGE

If clinicians elect to follow the RTOG recommendations for combined modality therapy "salvage" of patients with biopsy residual disease 6 weeks after initial therapy, then an additional 9 Gy (concurrent with 5-FU/cisplatin) are delivered. Using opposed laterals, the field includes the primary tumor plus a 2 to 3 cm margin in all directions. As an alternative at MSKCC, patients with T3 tumors can receive an additional 5.4 Gy to the primary tumor plus a 2 to 3 cm margin for a total dose of

Table 42–4   General Guidelines for Radiation Therapy in Anal Cancer

1. Whole Pelvic Field
   A. *Posterior-anterior*
      Superior border: L5/S1 junction for the first 30.6 Gy. This is then decreased to the inlet of the true pelvis (bottom of the sacroiliac joints) for the remaining 14.4 Gy.
      Inferior border: 3 cm below the anal verge or the inferior extent of the primary tumor—whichever is most inferior.
      Lateral borders: 1.5 cm lateral to the widest bony margin of the true pelvic side walls. The lateral border is then extended to include the lateral inguinal nodes. These nodes should be outlined with wire in order to help identify them.

   B. *Laterals*
      Superior border: Same as posterior-anterior field.
      Inferior border: Same as posterior-anterior field.
      Posterior border: 1-1.5 cm behind the anterior body sacral margin.
      Anterior border: Posterior margin of the symphysis pubis (to treat only the internal iliac nodes).

   C. *Blocking*
      Blocks are used to spare the posterior muscle and soft tissues behind the sacrum, to reduce the amount of dose inferior to the symphysis pubis, and to decrease the amount of small bowel treated both superiorly and anteriorly.

   D. *Perineum*
      1. Never use an electron or photon boost for the perineum—there will be overlap between the electron and photon fields. The perineum should be treated in the photon fields.

2. Inguinal Nodes Boost Field
   While the patient is in the supine position, the medial and lateral inguinal nodes are outlined with a 2-cm margin in all directions.

3. Primary Tumor Boost for Combined-Modality Therapy Salvage
   If the Radiation Therapy Oncology Group recommendations for combined-modality therapy salvage are followed, then an additional 9 Gy (concurrent with 5-fluorouracil-cisplatin) are delivered. With a multiple-field technique, the field includes the primary tumor plus a 3-cm margin in all directions.

50.4 Gy, which is delivered immediately following the 45 Gy of pelvic radiation.

MEDIAL AND LATERAL INGUINAL LYMPH NODES

Following treatment of the pelvis in the prone position, the patient is placed in the supine position and the inguinal nodes are treated with electrons. The medial and lateral inguinal nodes are outlined with a 2-cm margin in all directions. The inguinal nodes are included in the PA pelvic photon field. They receive only exit dose from this field, usually approximately 30% to 40% of the pelvic field prescription. This is determined from the treatment plan. Since they need to receive a total of 1.8 Gy/day, the remaining dose should be given concurrently with electrons. The depth of the inguinal nodes can be determined from a CT scan.[21,22] If this is unavailable, then a clinical estimate may be used. If the inguinal lymph nodes are biopsy positive, a three-field technique is still recommended. However, a four-field technique (AP–PA plus opposed laterals) may be needed in order to adequately treat the external iliac nodes. In this setting, the inguinal node dose should be 50.4 Gy.

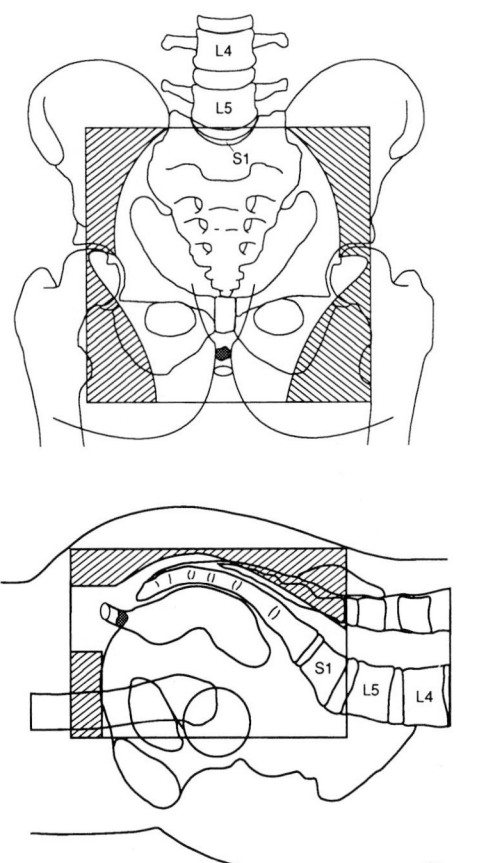

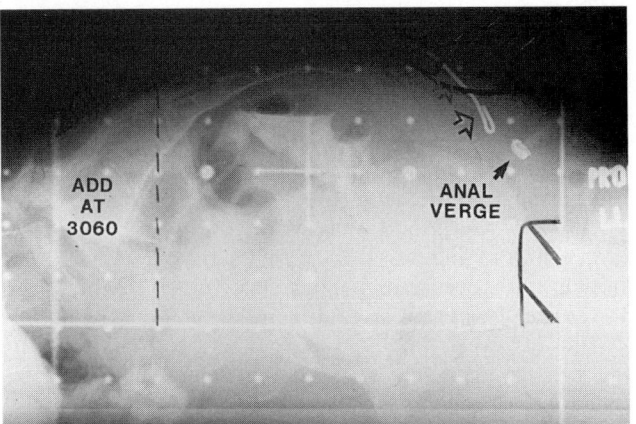

Figure 42–4. Example illustrating the position of the wire on the Foley catheter outlining the anal verge (*arrow*). The *open arrows* identify a separate wire outlining the perineum.

Figure 42–3. Idealized treatment fields for a clinical T2N0M0 squamous cell carcinoma of the anal canal. The inguinal nodes are included in the posterior-anterior field and are supplemented with electrons.

BRACHYTHERAPY

In contrast with treatment programs in the United States and Canada, in which patients receive combined EBRT plus chemotherapy, many patients treated in select European centers receive EBRT alone, with or without brachytherapy. The nonrandomized data suggest that the results of radiation therapy alone are comparable to combined radiation therapy plus chemotherapy.[23] Brachytherapy techniques commonly involve afterloading ^{192}Ir. A frequent treatment approach is EBRT for the first 45 Gy followed by an additional 15 to 20 Gy with a perineal boost or brachytherapy. These techniques are discussed in the Outcomes section.

CRITICAL NORMAL TISSUES

As with other cancer therapies, pelvic radiation is associated with acute and long-term toxicity. Complications of pelvic radiation therapy are a function of the volume of the radiation field, overall treatment time, fraction size, radiation energy, total dose, and technique. Large field sizes, a short overall treatment time, large fraction sizes (>2.0 Gy/day), orthovoltage or low energy megavoltage radiation (Cobalt-60), doses of >50.4 Gy when there is small bowel in the field, the use of an AP–PA technique, treatment of only one field/day, a direct perineal boost field, and the lack of computerized dosimetry all contribute to an increased incidence of radiation complications. Split-course pelvic radiation is associated with an increase in chronic bowel complications and, in one series, a

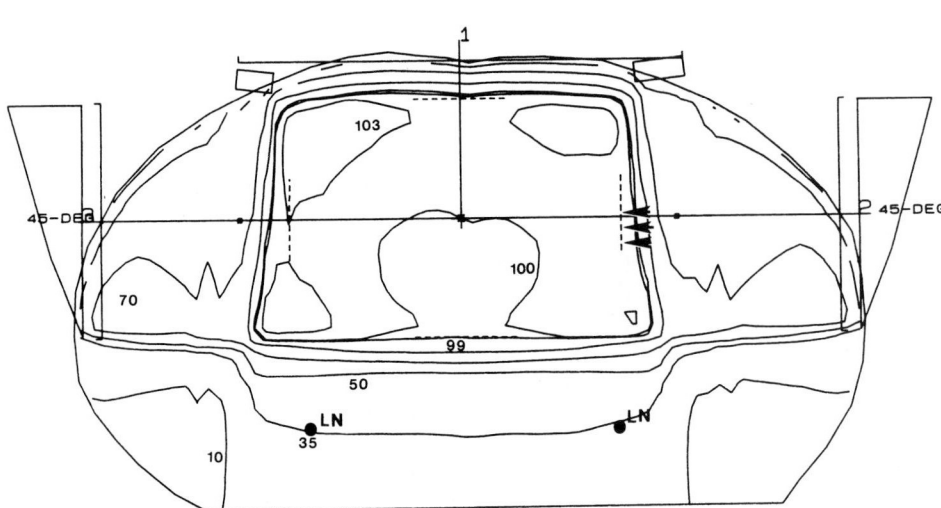

Figure 42–5. Dosimetry of a three-field plan for anal canal cancer. In this case, because of the patient's large body habitus, the inguinal nodes are 4 cm below the anterior skin surface. They receive 35% of 18 Gy from the posterior-anterior field. Therefore, an additional 65% (1.17 Gy) needs to be delivered with 12 MeV electrons prescribed to 90%. The *arrows* indicate the prescription point located 1.5 cm inside the edge of the field. Since the volume inside this point should receive at least 100% of the dose, the dose is prescribed to the 99% isodose line.

lower local control rate.[24] Critical normal tissues that must be considered in the treatment of anal canal cancer include bone marrow, rectum, small bowel, bladder, and skin. The acute toxicity is due to a combination of chemotherapy and radiation therapy. Toxicities include leukopenia, thrombocytopenia, proctitis, diarrhea, cystitis, and perineal erythema. It must be emphasized that even when pelvic radiation is delivered with appropriate doses and techniques, almost all patients receiving combined modality therapy for anal cancer will develop acute grade 3+ toxicity requiring a treatment break at some point (commonly week three) in their treatment course. Even when appropriate radiation techniques are used, approximately 1% of patients will develop severe long-term toxicity.

Unless there is a contraindication, the most simple techniques to decrease radiation toxicity, such as the use of small bowel contrast, multiple field techniques, high energy linear accelerators, custom blocks, avoiding a direct perineal boost, and treatment in the prone position should be part of the standard treatment of patients receiving curative pelvic radiation therapy. These are outlined in Table 42-5. Small bowel contrast is essential in order to determine the position of the small bowel during simulation. Any physical maneuver beyond the use of the prone position, such as a belly board, abdominal wall compression, or a full bladder, may be associated with patient discomfort, thereby leading to increased movement and daily setup errors.

Radiation therapy can affect sphincter function. There is an increasing body of literature reporting the impact of radiation therapy on functional results in rectal cancer.[25] However, it is not directly applicable to anal cancer since patients do not undergo pelvic surgery. Reports of functional outcome are limited in the anal cancer literature. One series reports that full function was maintained in 93% of patients,[26] and a second series that used anorectal manometry reported complete continence in 56%.[27] Another reported good to excellent function in 93% of patients with a minimum follow-up of 1 year.[28]

OUTCOMES

The Role of Chemotherapy

Results of two prospective randomized trials from Europe regarding combined modality therapy versus radiation alone (EORTC[29] and UKCCCR[30]) support the use of combined modality therapy. In the UKCCCR trial, although the improvement in 4-year survival with combined modality therapy did not reach statistic significance (65% vs. 58%), there was a significant improvement in 3-year actuarial local control (61% vs. 29%).[30] In the EORTC trial, combined modality therapy resulted in a higher complete response rate (80% vs. 54%), and a significantly higher 5-year actuarial local control rate (68% vs. 50%) and colostomy-free survival rate (72% vs. 40%), but no difference in survival (57% vs. 52%).[29] Although neither trial revealed a significant overall survival advantage, given the improvement in local control and colostomy-free survival, they helped to establish combined modality therapy as the standard of care.

Table 42–5 Techniques to Decrease Toxicity for Anal Cancer

1. High-energy (15 MV) linear accelerator.
2. Treatment 5 days per week and all fields each day.
3. Port films once per week or more often if clinically indicated.
4. Pelvic field: A three-field technique (posterior-anterior + two laterals) is recommended. This arrangement results in the lowest dose to the anterior structures. The underdosed inguinal nodes then need to be treated concurrently with electrons to bring the dose up to 100% of the prescription dose. An alternative method is to use an anterior-posterior–posterior-anterior technique. Although this treats the pelvic and inguinal nodes in the same field, it results in the highest dose to the anterior pelvic structures such as the genitalia.
5. Inguinal lymph nodes: As discussed in item 4, the technique that delivers the least amount of dose to the anterior pelvic structures is a three-field. The patient is treated in the prone position for pelvic radiation followed by treatment in the supine position for the inguinal electrons.
6. Computerized dosimetry optimizing between minimizing the lateral hot spots and small bowel dose and increasing the homogeneity within the target volume (see Fig. 42-5). In thin patients, a combination of 6 MV for the posterior fields and 10-15 MV for the lateral fields may result in more homogeneous dosimetry.
7. Shaped blocks and, if needed, wedges on the lateral fields.
8. Small bowel contrast.
9. Rectal contrast. Barium sulfate is injected with a 16-French Foley catheter (see Table 42-4). A wire is placed on the catheter to identify the anal verge (see Fig. 42-4).
10. Full bladder, only if it does not make the patient so uncomfortable as to cause movement.
11. Wire to outline the perineum. The perineum within a minimum 3-cm radius of the anal verge must be included in the pelvic radiation field. The remainder can be blocked (see Fig. 42-4).
12. Immobilization molds (belly boards) and abdominal wall compression may be helpful.
13. Dose considerations:
    A. Whole pelvis: 45 Gy.
    B. Medial and lateral inguinal nodes: 45 Gy. The inguinal nodes are in the posterior-anterior pelvic field. They receive only exit dose, usually approximately 30% to 40% of the pelvic field prescription. This is determined from the treatment plan (see Fig. 42-5). Since they need to receive a total of 1.8 Gy per day, the remaining dose should be given concurrently with electrons. The depth of the inguinal nodes is best determined from a computed tomography scan.[21] If this is unavailable, then a clinical estimate may be used.
    C. Standard fractionation is 1.8 Gy per day.

In North America, combined modality therapy has been well established and randomized trials focus on defining the ideal combined modality therapy regimen. The role of mitomycin-C as a necessary component of combined modality therapy was established by the Intergroup trial RTOG 87-04.[31] Patients were randomized to 45 Gy plus continuous infusion 5-FU with or without mitomycin-C. At 6 weeks after completion of treatment, patients with less than a complete response had an additional 9 Gy to the primary tumor plus concurrent 5-FU/cisplatin as salvage therapy. If there was still less than a complete response 6 weeks after the completion of this salvage therapy, an APR was performed. Patients who received mitomycin-C had a higher complete response rate (92% vs. 85%). They had a significantly lower colostomy rate (9% vs. 22%) and a corresponding significant increase in colostomy-free survival (71% vs. 59%). There was little difference in overall 4-year survival (75% vs. 70%). Early grade 4+ toxicity was significantly increased in the mitomycin-C arm (23% vs. 7%). Although overall survival was not significantly increased given the advantage in colostomy-free survival, mitomycin-C is considered a necessary component of combined modality therapy.

The combined modality therapy arm using radiation/5-FU/mitomycin-C arm from RTOG 87-04 is the most common treatment approach. Patients received continuous course pelvic radiation for a total dose of 45 Gy (30.6 Gy whole pelvis followed by 14.4 Gy true pelvis) and two cycles (weeks 1 and 5) of concurrent continuous infusion 5-FU (1000 mg/m² days 1 through 4) and bolus mitomycin-C (10 mg/m² bolus day 1). If 6 weeks following completion of the initial treatment there was persistent disease, patients received 1 week of salvage therapy. Salvage therapy involved 1 cycle of chemotherapy (continuous infusion 5-FU: 1000 mg/m² day × 4, bolus cisplatin 100 mg/m² day 2) and concurrent 9 Gy (limited to the primary tumor). If there was biopsy residual disease 6 weeks following the salvage therapy, then an APR was recommended.

Is Biopsy Necessary at 6 Weeks?

There is considerable controversy as to the need for the first biopsy at 6 weeks following initial treatment. Data from the Princess Margaret Hospital suggest that squamous cell carcinomas of the anus regress slowly and continue to decrease in size for 3 to 12 months after the completion of combined modality treatment.[32] Based on these data, an increasing number of investigators advocate a more conservative approach and do not recommend a post-treatment biopsy. In the Intergroup trial, of the 25 patients with biopsy residual disease after 45 Gy and 5-FU/mitomycin-C who then received salvage therapy with 9 Gy plus 5-FU/cisplatin, 55% achieved a complete response 6 weeks later (a total of 12 weeks following the completion of the initial 45 Gy).[31] It is unclear if the complete response was a result of the "salvage" therapy or was due to an additional 6 weeks of tumor regression following initial therapy.

At many institutions including MSKCC, if there is residual disease at the 6-week post-treatment evaluation, patients do not receive the 1 week of "salvage" therapy. The patients are examined every 6 weeks and, providing the tumor continues to decrease in size, no salvage therapy is performed. However, if there is progression of disease or no response at 6 weeks following initial therapy, APR is necessary. In addition to careful physical examination, anal ultrasound may be helpful in following the tumor. In the current Intergroup phase III anal canal cancer protocol RTOG 98-11, biopsy at 6 weeks following the initial 45 Gy is optional (Fig. 42-6).

For certain subgroups of high-risk patients (e.g., T3-4 tumors), induction chemotherapy followed by concurrent chemotherapy and radiation to higher doses may prove

RTOG 98-11

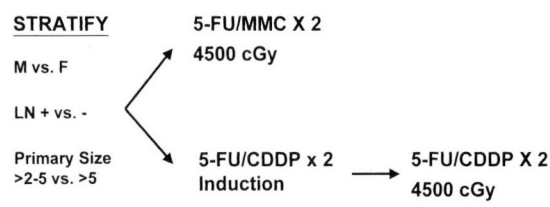

Figure 42–6. Radiation Therapy Oncology Group (RTOG) 98-11 phase III trial for anal cancer.

to be a useful option. This is currently being tested in a single-arm Cancer and Leukemia Group B (CALGB) trial for advanced anal canal tumors.[33] Combined modality therapy trials can be broadly divided into those that use either 5-FU/mitomycin-C chemotherapy or, more recently, 5-FU/cisplatin chemotherapy. At Memorial Sloan-Kettering, all patients with T3-4 disease receive 2 cycles of induction 5-FU/cisplatin.

Mitomycin-C versus Cisplatin

For patients who receive mitomycin-C–based regimens, the average results in the literature include a complete response rate of 84% (81% to 87%), a local control rate of 73% (64% to 86%), and a 5-year survival rate of 77% (66% to 92%). For patients with T1-2 disease the complete response rates are in excess of 90%, with ultimate local control rates following surgical salvage of 80% to 90%. In patients with T3-4 disease approximately 50% will require a salvage APR. If they achieve a complete response following the completion of combined modality therapy, then only 25% will require a salvage APR.

Although the results of 5-FU, mitomycin-C, and concurrent 45 Gy are impressive, there is room for improvement, especially in patients with T3-4 disease. Various treatment approaches have been tested. These include the use of 5-FU and cisplatin (as induction therapy or concurrently with radiation or both) and intensifying the radiation dose beyond 45 Gy using EBRT or brachytherapy. The combination of 5-FU plus cisplatin is an attractive regimen since: (1) patients who have failed 5-FU/mitomycin-C still respond to 5-FU cisplatin and (2) cisplatin is a radiation sensitizer.

Most cisplatin-based trials use higher radiation doses compared with the mitomycin-C–based trials. Although the numbers are small, the data suggest that the results may be better than the mitomycin-C–based regimens. However, these differences may be due to other factors such as patient selection bias and higher radiation doses.

Meropol et al. reported the results of the Cancer and Leukemia Group B (CALGB) pilot trial.[33] Patients with stages T3–4 disease received induction 5-FU/cisplatin and concurrent 5-FU/cisplatin plus radiation. The complete response rate was 80%, colostomy-free survival was 56%, and crude survival was 78%. The Intergroup has developed a randomized trial (RTOG 98-11) to compare this approach with conventional 5-FU, mitomycin-C, and 45 Gy (see Fig. 42-6).

Intensification of the Radiation Dose

EXTERNAL BEAM

In an attempt to improve local control and survival, two parallel pilot trials of radiation dose intensification were designed. In both trials patients received 36 Gy to the pelvis (30.6 whole pelvis plus 5.4 Gy to the true pelvis). Following a 2-week break, they received an additional 23.4 Gy to the primary tumor with a 2 to 3 cm margin for a total dose of 59.4 Gy. The main difference between the two trials was the type of chemotherapy. The RTOG 9208 trial[34] used concurrent 5-FU and mitomycin-C whereas the ECOG 4292 trial used 5-FU and cisplatin.

The RTOG 9208 trial reported similar results to the standard regimen of 45 Gy plus 5-FU/mitomycin-C used in RTOG 89-04 except for a higher 2-year colostomy rate (30% vs. 7%). Likewise, the ECOG 4292 trial did not reveal a benefit compared with conventional treatment.[35] Other series have reported higher complete response rates.[15]

BRACHYTHERAPY

Brachytherapy is an ideal method by which to deliver conformal radiation for anal cancer while sparing the surrounding normal structures such as small intestine and bladder. In most series, patients received 30 to 55 Gy of pelvic radiation with or without 5-FU/mitomycin-C or cisplatin followed by a 15-25 Gy boost with ^{192}Ir afterloading catheters. Most use low dose rate; however, some investigators have advocated high dose rate.[36,37]

Combining the series, the mean results include a complete response rate of 83% (73% to 91%), local control rates of 81% (73% to 89%), and a 5-year survival rate of 70% (60% to 84%). The primary concern is anal necrosis, with reports varying from 2% to as high as 76%.[37] The average is 5% to 15%.

In summary, it is unclear if increasing the radiation dose in patients receiving combined modality therapy improves the results compared with conventional doses of 45 to 50 Gy. Although there are no randomized data, the phase II trials suggest that even in experienced hands, brachytherapy is associated with higher complication rates than is EBRT.

The ideal combined modality therapy regimen and the most appropriate radiation dose to use for patients with anal canal tumors have not yet been defined. Currently in North America, the standard of care is the RTOG combined modality therapy regimen of continuous course radiation (45 Gy in 1.8 Gy fractions) plus 2 cycles of concurrent continuous infusion 5-FU weeks 1 and 5 plus mitomycin-C bolus days 1 and 29. This is the control arm of RTOG 98-11. For patients with T3-4 disease (primary tumors >5 cm) it is reasonable to boost with an additional 5.4-9.0 Gy. In the RTOG 98-11 trial, the experimental arm uses the same design except for 5-FU/cisplatin both as induction (2 cycles) and concurrently with radiation (2 cycles). The post-treatment biopsy at 8 weeks is optional.

Radiation Therapy Alone

EXTERNAL BEAM

Patients who receive radiation alone have an average local control rate of 74% (61% to 100%) and a 5-year survival rate of 63% (50% to 94%). Although the series of 18 patients from the Mayo Clinic had the highest survival and local control rate, they also had a high rate of complications requiring surgery (17%).[38] Overall, the results are comparable to patients who receive combined modality therapy with 45 Gy plus 5-FU and mitomycin-C. However, the average incidence of complications requiring surgery is 10% (range: 3% to 17%), which probably reflects the high radiation doses that must be delivered to the primary site to control this disease when radiation therapy is the sole treatment modality.

BRACHYTHERAPY—EXTERNAL BEAM

The largest experience is from the Centre Leon Berard in which 221 patients were treated over a 15-year period with external radiation therapy (Cobalt-60) to a dose of 35 Gy, followed 2 months later by an additional 15 to 20 Gy with a ^{192}Ir implant.[39] There was a 3% rate of serious complications, and patients achieved a 65% 5-year disease-free survival and a 79% local-regional control rate. Another study from France confirmed a high 5-year survival rate (61%) and good local control (75%), but a 6% rate of complications requiring surgery.[40]

In summary, radiation therapy alone with either EBRT or combined with brachytherapy may yield comparable local control and survival rates to combined modality therapy. However, since it is associated with an increase in anal necrosis even in experienced hands, it should be used with caution.

Prognostic Factors

As with most gastrointestinal cancers, the most important prognostic factors in anal cancer are T classification and lymph node status. In patients treated with radiation with or without chemotherapy, the most striking difference in results is seen when comparing T1-2 primary cancers (<5 cm) versus T3-4 primary cancers (>5 cm). The local failure rates with T3-4 primary cancers are approximately 50% following combined modality therapy. When a complete response is achieved, the local failure rate is 25%.

T-CLASSIFICATION

For example, Peiffert et al. reported an increase in local failure with T classification (T1: 11%, T2: 24%, T3: 45%, and T4: 43%) and a corresponding decrease in

5-year survival (T1: 94%, T2: 79%, T3: 53%, and T4: 19%).[41] A similar decrease in 5-year colostomy-free survival with T1-2 tumors versus T3-4 tumors was reported by Gerard and colleagues (T1: 83% and T2: 89% vs. T3: 50% and T4: 54%).[15]

N-CLASSIFICATION

In contrast to T classification, the impact of positive lymph nodes is less clear. Unlike rectal cancer, inguinal lymph nodes in anal cancer are considered nodal metastasis rather than distant metastasis, and patients should be treated in a curative fashion. Cummings et al. reported that patients with negative nodes who received combined modality therapy had a higher 5-year cause-specific survival compared with those with positive nodes (81% vs. 57%).[32] By univariate analysis, Allal and colleagues reported a significant increase in local failure in patients with positive versus negative nodes who received 5-FU, mitomycin-C, and radiation (36% vs. 19%, $P = 0.03$); however, this difference was not found to be significant by multivariate analysis.[42]

The RTOG 87-04 randomized trial reported a higher colostomy rate (which is an indirect measurement of local failure) in N1 versus N0 patients (28% vs. 13%).[31] In node-negative patients, and possibly node-positive patients, the addition of mitomycin-C decreased the overall colostomy rates. The EORTC randomized trial of 45 Gy + 5-FU/mitomycin-C also reported that patients with positive nodes experienced significantly higher local failure ($P = 0.035$) and lower survival ($P = 0.038$) rates compared to those with negative nodes. However, there was no difference in prognosis between N1 versus N2–3 disease.[29]

By multivariate analysis, Allal and associates found that the only variable for which there was a possible impact was overall treatment time ($P = 0.09$).[24] In the EORTC randomized trial, multivariate analysis identified that positive nodes, skin ulceration, and male gender were independent, negative prognostic factors for local control and survival.[29] Goldman and coworkers also found that women had a more favorable outcome compared with men.[43] Other authors have reported that T stage, radiation dose, and percent hemoglobin were significant.

Histologic cell type for squamous cancers of the anal canal (squamous vs. cloacogenic vs. basaloid) has not been found to be of major prognostic relevance. Studies examining DNA content (i.e., whether tumors were diploid or nondiploid)[44] and *p53* expression[45,46] have conflicting results.

Treatment of the Patient with Human Immunodeficiency Virus

In general, patients with human immunodeficiency virus (HIV+) have received lower doses of radiation and chemotherapy due to a concern that standard therapy may not be tolerated.[47] With a better understanding of the immunologic deficiencies seen in HIV+ patients, more recent reports have recommended therapy based on clinical and immunologic parameters such as a history of

prior opportunistic infections and CD4 counts.[48,49] The limited experience suggests that in patients with a CD4 count >200 μL who do not have signs or symptoms of other HIV-related diseases, standard combined modality therapy is appropriate. However, they must be followed carefully, and frequent modifications during therapy are likely necessary. For those patients with a CD4 count <200μL or who have signs or symptoms of other HIV-related diseases, attenuated doses of radiation or chemotherapy or both are recommended at the start of treatment.

Treatment of Anal Margin Cancer

A more comprehensive discussion of the treatment of anal margin cancers will be covered in Chapter 66, Cancer of the Skin. In brief, a reasonable approach is to recommend a local excision for smaller tumors (<4 cm) that are not in direct contact with the anal verge. If the patient requires an APR due to anatomic constraints or if a local excision would compromise sphincter function, or if the tumor is >4 cm and node positive or both, then nonoperative treatment is an appropriate alternative. Based on the randomized trial from the UKCCCR, which had 23% of patients with anal margin cancers, combined modality therapy rather than radiation therapy alone is recommended.

Follow-up After Treatment

Patients treated for anal cancer must be followed carefully since those with local failure are amenable to salvage APR and can achieve long-term survival. Most recurrences occur within the first 3 years. Patients should be examined by physical examination and anoscopy every 6 weeks until a complete response is achieved, then every 3 months for a total of 2 years. As previously discussed, biopsy is recommended only if the tumor stops responding, or there is evidence of a local recurrence. Follow-up examinations can then be decreased to every 6 months for the next 3 years and then yearly after 5 years. The usefulness of computed tomography of the abdomen and pelvis for follow-up is unclear. Transrectal ultrasound may be of value. Since the most common site of failure is at the primary tumor site, there is no substitute for physical examination.

REFERENCES

1. Myerson RJ, Karnell LH, Menck HR: The National Cancer Data Base report on carcinoma of the anus. *Cancer*. 1997;80:805.
2. Jemal A, Thomas A, Murray T, et al: Cancer Statistics, 2002. *CA Cancer J Clin*. 2002;52:23.
3. Landis SH, Murray T, Bolden S, et al: Cancer statistics, 1999. *CA Cancer J Clin*. 1999;49:8.
4. Frisch M, Fenger C, van den Brule AJ, et al: Variants of squamous cell carcinoma of the anal canal and perianal skin and their relation to human papillomaviruses. *Cancer Res*. 1999;59:753.
5. Freidman HB, Saah AJ, Sherman ME, et al: Human papillomavirus, anal squamous intraepithelial lesions, and human immunodeficiency virus in a cohort of gay men. *J Infect Dis*. 1998;178:45.

6. Penn I: Cancers of the anogenital region in renal transplant recipients. *Cancer.* 1986;58:611.

7. Bonin SR, Pajak TJ, Russell AH, et al: Overexpression of *p53* protein and outcome of patients with chemoradiation for carcinoma of the anal canal: A report of the randomized trial RTOG 87-04. Radiation Therapy Oncology Group. *Cancer.* 1999;85:1226.

8. Cummings BJ: Anal canal. In Perez C, Brady L, eds. *Principles and Practice of Radiation Oncology.* 2nd ed. Philadelphia: JB Lippincott; 1993:1015.

9. American Joint Committee on Cancer: Anal canal. In Fleming ID, Cooper JS, Henson DE, et al., eds. *AJCC Cancer Staging Manual.* 5th ed. Philadelphia: Lippincot-Raven; 1997:91.

10. Anal Canal. In Sobin LH, Wittekind CH, eds. *TNM Classification of Malignant Tumors.* 5th ed. New York: Wiley-Liss; 1997:70.

11. Peters RK, Mack TM: Patterns of anal carcinoma by gender and marital status in Los Angeles County. *Br J Cancer.* 1983;48:629.

12. Joon DL, Chao MWT, Ngan SYK, et al: Primary adenocarcinoma of the anus: A retrospective analysis. *Int J Radiat Oncol Biol Phys.* 1999;45:1199.

13. Minsky BD, Kelsen DP, Hoffman JP: Cancer of the anal region. In DeVita V, Hellman S, Rosenberg SA, eds. *Cancer: Principles and Practice of Oncology.* 6th ed. Philadelphia: Lippincott, Williams & Wilkins; 2001:1319.

14. Berard P, Papillon J: Role of pre-operative irradiation for anal preservation in cancer of the low rectum. *World J Surg.* 1992;16:502.

15. Gerard JP, Ayzac L, Hun D, et al: Treatment of anal canal carcinoma with high dose radiation therapy and concomitant fluorouracil-cisplatin. Long term results in 95 patients. *Radiother Oncol.* 1998;46:249.

16. Tarantino D, Bernstein MA: Endoanal ultrasound in the staging and management of squamous-cell carcinoma of the anal canal. Potential implications of a new ultrasound staging system. *Dis Colon Rectum.* 2002;45:16.

17. Anal Canal. In Greene FL, Page DL, Fleming ID, et al., eds. *AJCC Cancer Staging Manual.* 6th ed. New York: Springer; 2002:125.

18. Boman BM, Moertel C, O'Connell M, et al: Carcinoma of the anal canal, a clinical and pathologic study of 188 cases. *Cancer.* 1984;54:114.

19. Greenall M, Quan SHQ, Urmacher C, et al: Treatment of epidermoid carcinoma of the anal canal. *Surg Gynecol Obstet.* 1985;161:509.

20. Nigro ND, Vaitkevicius VK, Considine B: Combined therapy for cancer of the anal canal: A preliminary report. *Dis Colon Rectum.* 1974;17:354.

21. Koh WJ, Chiu M, Stelzer KJ, et al: Femoral vessel depth and the implications for groin node radiation. *Int J Radiat Oncol Biol Phys.* 1993;27:969.

22. Wang CJ, Chin YY, Leung SW, et al: Topographic distribution of inguinal lymph nodes metastasis: Significance in determination of treatment margin for elective inguinal lymph nodes irradiation of low pelvic tumors. *Int J Radiat Oncol Biol Phys.* 1996;35:133.

23. Touboul E, Schlienger M, Buffat L, et al: Epidermoid carcinoma of the anal canal. Results of curative-intent radiation therapy in a series of 270 patients. *Cancer.* 1994;73:1569.

24. Weber DC, Kurtz JM, Allal AS: The impact of gap duration on local control in anal canal carcinoma treated by split-course radiotherapy and concomitant chemotherapy. *Int J Radiat Oncol Biol Phys.* 2001;50:675.

25. Kollmorgen CF, Meagher AP, Pemberton JH, et al: The long term effect of adjuvant postoperative chemoradiotherapy for rectal cancer on bowel function. *Ann Surg.* 1994;220:676.

26. Kapp KS, Geyer E, Gebhart FH, et al: Evaluation of sphincter function after external beam irradiation and Ir-192 high-dose-rate (HDR) brachytherapy plus chemotherapy in patients with carcinoma of the anal canal. *Int J Radiat Oncol Biol Phys.* 1999;45s:339 [abstract].

27. Vordermark D, Sailer M, Flentje M, et al: Continence and anorectal manometry after curative-intent radiation therapy for anal carcinoma. *Int J Radiat Oncol Biol Phys.* 1999;45s:340 [abstract].

28. Weber DC, Nouet P, Kurtz JM, et al: Assessment of target dose delivery in anal cancer using in vivo thermoluminescent dosimetry. *Radiother Oncol.* 2001;59:43.

29. Bartelink H, Roelofsen F, Eschwege F, et al: Concomitant radiotherapy and chemotherapy is superior to radiotherapy alone in the treatment of locally advanced anal cancer: Results of a phase III randomized trial of the European Organization for Research and Treatment of Cancer radiotherapy and gastrointestinal cooperative groups. *J Clin Oncol.* 1997;15:2040.

30. UKCCCR Anal Cancer Trial Working Party: Epidermoid anal cancer: Results from the UKCCCR randomised trial of radiotherapy alone versus radiotherapy, 5-fluorouracil, and mitomycin. *Lancet.* 1997;348:1049.

31. Flam M, John M, Pajak T, et al: Role of mitomycin in combination with fluorouracil and radiotherapy, and salvage chemoradiation in the definitive nonsurgical treatment of epidermoid carcinoma of the anal canal: Results of a phase III randomized intergroup study. *J Clin Oncol.* 1996;14:2537.

32. Cummings BJ, Keane TJ, O'Sullivan B, et al: Epidermoid anal cancer: Treatment by radiation alone or by radiation and 5-fluorouracil with and without mitomycin-C. *Int J Radiat Oncol Biol Phys.* 1991;21:1115.

33. Meropol NJ, Niedzwiecki D, Shank B, et al: Combined-modality therapy of poor risk anal canal carcinoma; A phase II study of the Cancer and Leukemia Group B (CALGB). *Proc ASCO.* 1999;18 [abstract].

34. John M, Pajak T, Flam M, et al: Dose escalation in chemoradiation for anal cancer: Preliminary results of RTOG 92-08. *Cancer J Sci Am.* 1996;2:205.

35. Martenson JA, Lipsitz SR, Wagner H, et al: Initial results of a phase II trial of high dose radiation therapy, 5-fluorouracil, and cisplatin for patients with anal cancer (E4292): An Eastern Cooperative Oncology Group study. *Int J Radiat Oncol Biol Phys.* 1996;35:745.

36. Gerard JP, Mauro F, Thomas L, et al: Treatment of squamous cell anal canal carcinoma with pulsed dose rate brachytherapy. Feasibility study of a French cooperative group. *Radiother Oncol.* 1999;51:131.

37. Roed H, Engelholm SA, Svendsen LB, et al: Pulsed dose rate (PDR) brachytherapy of anal carcinoma. *Radiother Oncol.* 1996;41:131.

38. Martenson JA, Gunderson LL: External radiation therapy without chemotherapy in the management of anal cancer. *Cancer.* 1993;71:1736.

39. Papillon J, Montbarbon JF: Epidermoid carcinoma of the anal canal. *Dis Colon Rectum.* 1987;30:324.

40. Ng Ying, Kin KNY, Pigneux J, et al: Our experience of conservative treatment of anal canal carcinoma combining external irradiation and interstitial implants: 32 cases treated between 1973 and 1982. *Int J Radiat Oncol Biol Phys.* 1988;14:253.

41. Peiffert D, Bey P, Pernot M, et al: Conservative management by irradiation of epidermoid cancers of the anal canal: Prognostic factors of tumor control and complications. *Int J Radiat Oncol Biol Phys.* 1997;37:313.

42. Allal AS, Mermillod B, Roth AD, et al: The impact of treatment factors on local control in T2-T3 anal carcinomas treated by radiotherapy with or without chemotherapy. *Cancer.* 1997;79:2329.

43. Goldman S, Glimelius B, Glas U, et al: Management of anal epidermoid carcinoma: An evaluation of treatment results in two population-based series. *Int J Colorect Dis.* 1989;4:234.

44. Dalby JF, Pointon RS: The treatment of anal carcinoma by interstitial irradiation. *Am J Radiol.* 1961;85:515.

45. Bonin SR, Qian C, Russell AH, et al: Overexpression of p53 protein is associated with decreased local disease-free survival in patients treated with chemoradiation for anal canal cancer: A report of RTOG 87-04. *Int J Radiat Oncol Biol Phys.* 1996;36:210 [abstract].

46. Wong CS, Tsao MS, Sharma V, et al: Prognostic role of p53 protein expression in epidermoid carcinoma of the anal canal. *Int J Radiat Oncol Biol Phys.* 1999;45:309.

47. Melbye M, Cote T, Kessler L, et al: AIDS/Cancer Working Group. High incidence of anal cancer among AIDS patients. *Lancet.* 1994;343:636.

48. Hoffman R, Welton ML, Klencke B, et al: The significance of pretreatment CD4 count on the outcome and treatment tolerance of HIV-positive patients with anal cancer. *Int J Radiat Oncol Biol Phys.* 1999;44:131.

49. Place RJ, Gregorcyk SG, Huber PH, et al: Outcome analysis of HIV-positive patients with anal squamous cell carcinoma. *Dis Colon Rectum.* 2001;44:512.

Cancer of the Kidney

Tracey Schefter, MD and Rachel Abrams Rabinovitch, MD

43

EPIDEMIOLOGY AND RISK FACTORS

There were an estimated 31,900 new cases of kidney cancer diagnosed in 2003 in the United States, with an estimated 11,900 deaths from this disease.[1] More than 85% of these tumors were predicted to be renal cell carcinoma (RCC), with the remainder consisting of transitional cell carcinomas of the renal pelvis and Wilms' tumors. Approximately half of these cases have metastatic disease on presentation.[2] RCC accounts for 3% of all adult malignancies and demonstrates a slight male predominance, with 60% of the diagnoses and deaths occurring in men. With a peak incidence in the sixth to eighth decades, RCC is a tumor of older adults, although presentation at other ages is not uncommon.

Numerous risk factors have been associated with the development of RCC, many of which are listed in Table 43-1. Cigarette smoking has a well-established association, with the risk of RCC increasing proportionately with pack-years of use. Patients with end-stage renal failure on long-term hemodialysis are at risk for developing acquired cystic disease of the kidney. It is this latter condition, and not hemodialysis per se, that appears to be the etiologic factor for the development of RCC in this subpopulation. There is accumulating evidence that chronic diuretic therapy may be a risk factor for development of renal cell carcinoma.[3-5]

There is growing evidence for the presence of an allele on the short arm of chromosome 3 that acts as a suppressor gene against the development of RCC. Deletion of this sequence results in a loss of protection and the development of RCC. In 1979, Cohen and colleagues[6] reported a familial pattern of RCC that appeared to be transmitted via an autosomal dominant gene pattern. A 3;8 translocation was found in numerous family members, and all RCC cases occurred only in those members with the translocation. Pathak and colleagues[7] described a second family pedigree

with RCC in 1982; however, the translocation occurred between chromosomes 3 and 11 and was present only within tumor tissue. Patients with von Hippel–Lindau (VHL) disease develop retinal angiomas, hemangioblastomas of the central nervous system, and clear cell renal carcinoma. This disease is transmitted in an autosomal dominant pattern and is associated with the development of RCC in 25% to 45% of those afflicted.[8-10] Cohen has shown that the human VHL gene maps to chromosome 3p25.[11] Studies analyzing the polymorphism of restriction fragment lengths have revealed 3p deletions in nonfamilial cases of RCC. Overall, there appears to be a consistent relationship between a deletion on the 3p chromosome and the presence of RCC in several studies. Further clinical-genetic correlation will be necessary to determine what fraction of diagnosed RCC patients are affected with this genetic abnormality and whether karyotype analysis will select a high-risk population to target for screening.

ANATOMY

The kidneys are paired retroperitoneal organs, the medial edges of which lie parallel to the psoas muscles. Each kidney is typically 11 to 12 cm in length, corresponding radiographically to 3 to 3.5 vertebral bodies. Although there is some variation, the kidney is usually centered at L1 or L2 and extends from T12 to L3 (Fig. 43-1). Due to diaphragmatic contracture, the kidneys may move caudally by as much as 2.5 cm with inhalation. The right kidney is depressed by the liver 1 to 2 cm relative to the left and is in association with the second part of the duodenum, the right colic flexure, and the posterior portions of the right eleventh and twelfth ribs (Fig. 43-2). The left kidney is adjacent to the spleen, stomach, pancreas, left colic flexure, and left 11th and 12th ribs.

Each kidney is surrounded by a fibrous capsule, over which lies a covering of perinephric fat. The kidney, perinephric fat, and adrenal gland are all entirely encased by a fascial layer, known as Gerota's fascia. All these structures are removed en bloc in a radical nephrectomy.

Draining lymph nodes originate within the renal hilus and follow the renal artery to the para-aortic and paracaval chains (Fig. 43-3). Regional nodal drainage extends from the crus of the diaphragm to the bifurcation of the aorta, varying somewhat with tumor laterality. For a right-sided tumor, this specifically includes the paracaval, retrocaval, precaval, interaortocaval, and preaortic lymph nodes. The para-aortic, preaortic,

Table 43–1 Risk Factors for Cancer of the Kidney

Factor	Reference Number
Cigarette smoking	74-76
Obesity	74-76
Phenacetin abuse	74-76
Asbestos exposure	77, 78
Leather tanning	77, 78
Shoe repair	77, 78
Chronic hemodialysis	79-81
Von Hippel-Lindau disease	8, 9

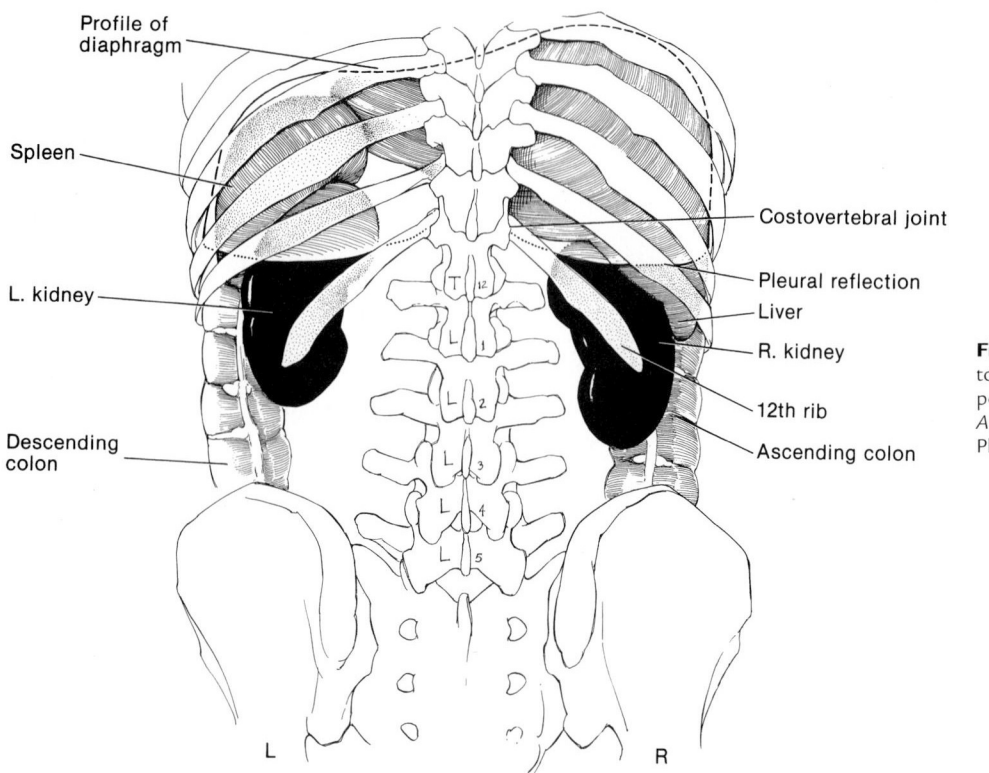

Figure 43–1. Relation of the kidneys to the thorax and vertebral bodies, posterior view. (From Hinman F Jr: *Atlas of Urosurgical Anatomy*. Philadelphia: WB Saunders; 1993:260.)

retroaortic, interaortocaval, and precaval lymph nodes are at risk for a left-sided tumor.

PATHOLOGY

Renal cell carcinoma is a neoplasm arising from proximal renal tubular epithelium. Historically, this tumor was erroneously considered to arise from adrenal rests within the kidney and thereby acquired the name "hypernephroma," titled by Grawitz in 1883.[12] Recent immunohistologic

and ultrastructural analysis confirms the true renal origin of RCC,[13,14] validating its more common and correct name.

Gross sectioning of RCC tumors often reveals the classic yellow-tan fatty appearance with occasional focal areas of hemorrhage and necrosis (Fig. 43-4). Calcifications, fluid-filled cysts, and areas of fibrosis may also be apparent. Although not truly encapsulated, these lesions are often surrounded by a pseudocapsule due to their expansile growth pattern, which results in compression of surrounding renal parenchyma.

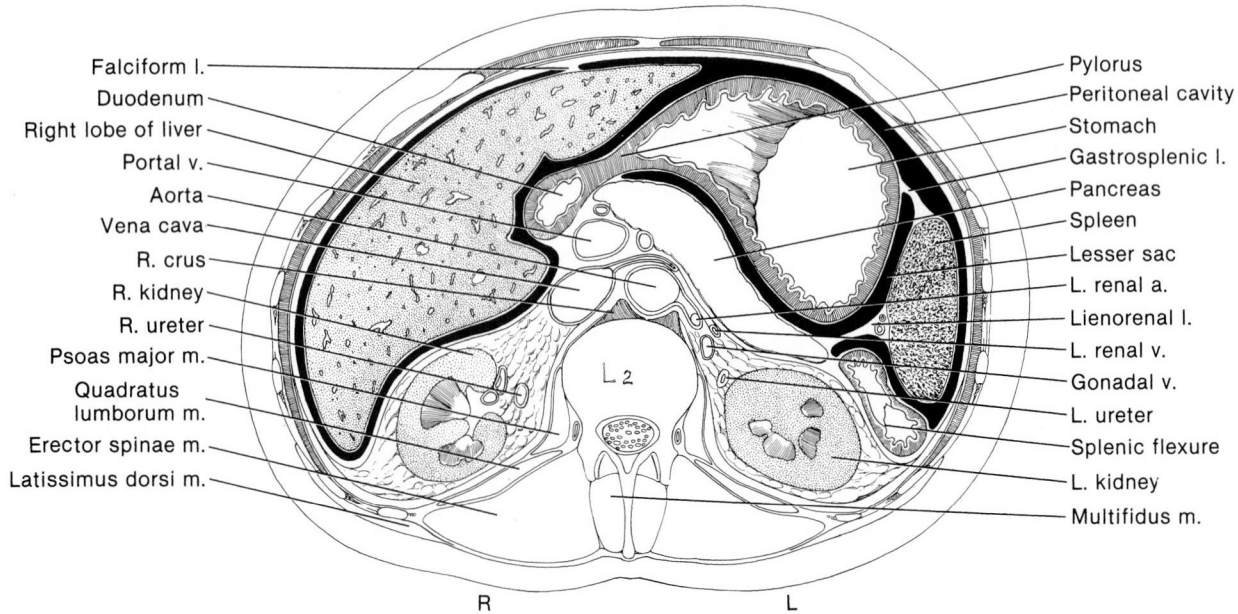

Figure 43–2. Transverse section of the kidney at the L2 level. (From Hinman F Jr: *Atlas of Urosurgical Anatomy*. Philadelphia: WB Saunders; 1993:262.)

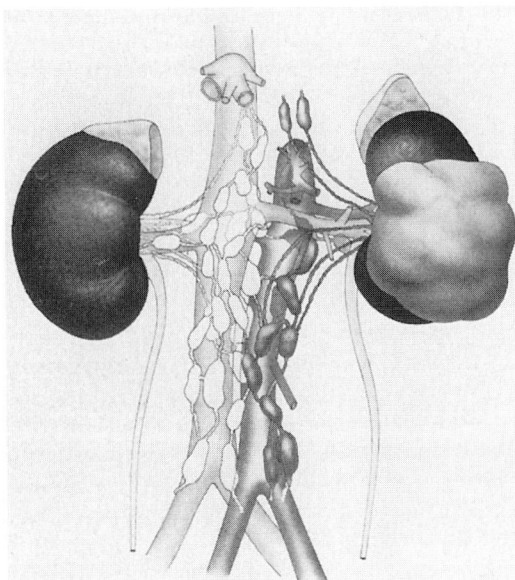

Figure 43–3. Lymphatic drainage of the kidneys. The dark lymph nodes represent drainage from the left kidney, and white lymph nodes represent drainage from the right. Note the hilar lymph nodes located along the renal arteries. (From Wood DP Jr: Role of lymphadenectomy in renal cell carcinoma. *Urol Clin North Am.* 1991;18:421.)

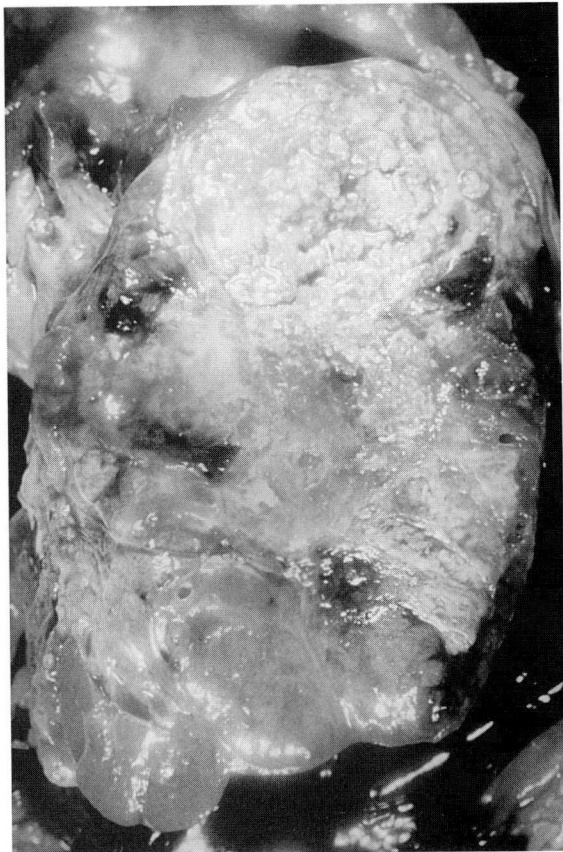

Figure 43–4. Section through an upper pole clear cell carcinoma. Note the characteristic dark areas of focal necrosis and hemorrhage, as well as the light, fatty appearance of this tumor.

There has been a long-standing controversy as to the existence of a benign entity called renal adenoma, defined as lesions less than 3 cm in diameter. Although histologically indistinguishable from RCC, these lesions were considered benign since the 1938 publication of Bell's classic paper,[15] in which he described the absence of metastatic spread in lesions smaller than 3 cm. Although it is not uncommon for such lesions to be detected incidentally or at autopsy without clinical evidence of spread, there is an increased number of reports of tumors fulfilling the size criterion of renal adenoma, but with nodal and distant metastases (DM) present.[16] Furthermore, when one contemplates the natural history of a large RCC lesion, it is illogical to conclude that it had never once measured less than 3 cm. It is generally now advocated that renal neoplasms be defined as malignant or benign based on their histologic appearance and not size.

The histologic appearance of RCC is variable, with three main cell types predominating: (1) clear cell, (2) granular cell, and (3) spindle cell or sarcomatoid variant (Figs. 43-5 to 43-7). Clear cell RCC is by far the most common, constituting approximately 75% of all tumors.[17] Histologically, these cells contain lightly staining cytoplasm, and are rich in glycogen and lipid material. The cell of origin for clear cell carcinomas is thought to be proximal tubular epithelium. Granular cells demonstrate more variation in cell and nuclear size. They have abundant and often abnormal mitochondria, and mitotic figures are not uncommon. Sarcomatoid or spindle cell tumors resemble mesenchymal cells. They are frequently high grade and demonstrate an aggressive clinical course with 70% to 80% presenting with metastases.[18] An individual tumor may demonstrate one or a combination of these cell types.

Aside from classification by histologic cell type, RCC may be further classified by the microscopic patterns formed by groups of cells: solid, papillary, and spindle.

CLINICAL PRESENTATION

Renal cell carcinoma has been described as "the internist's tumor" because of the myriad of signs and symptoms that may be noted at presentation (Table 43-2), some of which are due to the direct effects of an invasive renal mass, and others of which are considered paraneoplastic in origin. The most common symptoms are gross hematuria, flank pain, and a flank mass. Together, these symptoms are known as the *classic triad* and are noted in approximately

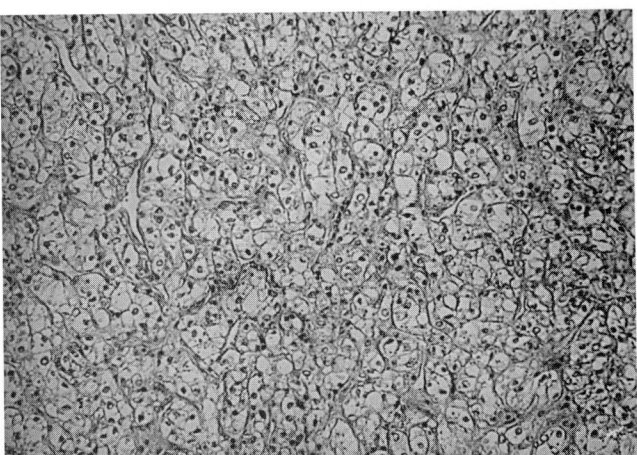

Figure 43–5. Clear cell subtype on light microscopy.

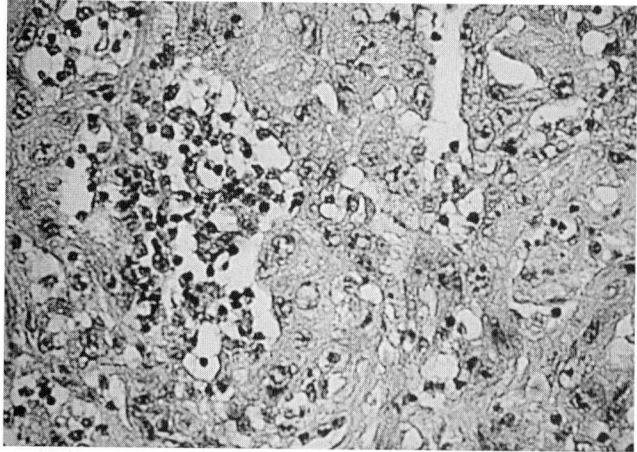

Figure 43–6. Granular cell subtype, light microscopy.

Table 43–2   Presenting Signs and Symptoms

	Skinner 1971[29]	Chisolm 1971[82]	Boxer 1979[35]	Ramon 1991[43]	Sene 1992[34]
Patients, n	309	119	96	112	155
Flank pain	41	—	32	28	46
Flank mass	45	—	35	12	47
Hematuria	59	—	35	34	68
Classic triad	9	—	6	—	12
Anemia	21	33	23	—	30
Erythrocytosis	3	4	—	—	—
Weight loss	28	—	30	24	—
Hypercalcemia	3	—	12	—	—
Hypertension	—	37	21	4	15
Fever	—	18	14	8	11
Varicocele	2	—	4	—	—

10% of presenting patients. Whether gross or microscopic, hematuria presents primarily when the collecting system has been invaded. Flank masses resulting from RCC are firm, nontender, and homogeneous. The sudden onset of a varicocele in a male, particularly on the left, should raise the possibility of a renal neoplasm obstructing the gonadal vein at its entry point into the left renal vein.

Anemia is generally considered a paraneoplastic process, as it is often out of proportion to the degree of hematuria. Conversely, erythrocytosis is a well-recognized phenomenon; however, it is much less common. Ectopic production of a parathyroid hormone-like material is responsible for the rare finding of hypercalcemia.

With increased use of diagnostic and staging abdominal computed tomography (CT) and ultrasound, there has been an increase in detection of incidental RCCs. There is some controversy about whether these incidentally detected asymptomatic renal carcinomas are of earlier stage and thus associated with better prognosis. This has relevance if one considers a screening program aimed at detecting more curable renal cancers. Tsui reported on the University of California at Los Angeles experience.[19] Retrospective analysis of 633 consecutive RCC cases treated by radical or partial nephrectomy showed that 54% of patients with symptomatic

disease had stage IV disease versus 27.4% in incidentally detected cases. These authors concluded that incidentally detected tumors are of lower grade and stage and result in better survival and decreased mortality; therefore, a screening program aimed at detecting early lesions should be developed. Five-year survival rates improved from 51% between 1980 and 1982 to 62% between 1989 and 1996,[20] but other authors point out that 5-year survival is not an accurate surrogate outcome measure due to lead-time bias and that disease-specific age-adjusted mortality should be used.[21,22] It is clear that the increased detection of incidental renal carcinomas has contributed to the rising incidence of renal carcinoma. However, a corresponding decrease in age-specific renal carcinoma mortality rates has not been observed in the United States.

ROUTES OF SPREAD

RCC spreads by direct extension, as well as by lymphatic and hematogenous routes. Peripheral lesions are more likely to extend through the renal capsule, while central lesions have more direct access to the renal vein. Renal vein involvement includes both tumor thrombi "floating" within the renal vein and actual invasion of the vessel wall. The nodal drainage for renal tumors was discussed previously in the section on anatomy.

One quarter to one third of all patients are found to have DM at presentation. Furthermore, among patients treated for localized disease, the primary cause of RCC death is metastatic tumor burden and not local failure.[23] Approximately 50% of initial metastatic sites are to the lung. The common involvement of the renal vein by this tumor gives direct evidence for the early hematogenous spread commonly seen in this disease.

STAGING WORKUP

Standard evaluation for patients suspected of having a renal mass includes a complete history and physical examination; routine blood work (a complete blood cell count, liver function tests, and measurements of levels of electrolytes, blood urea nitrogen, creatinine, alkaline phosphatase, and

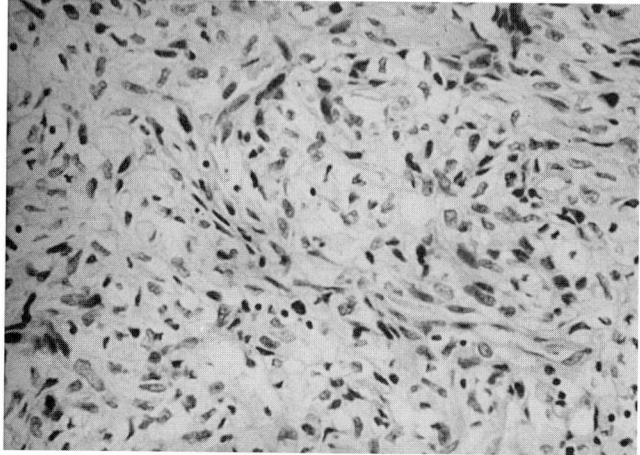

Figure 43–7. Sarcomatoid subtype, light microscopy.

calcium); and initial renal evaluation with urinalysis and intravenous pyelography (IVP), or preferably, a CT scan of the abdomen with intravenous contrast material. These latter two tests (IVP and CT) are important not only for verifying the presence of a renal mass, but also for determining the position of the contralateral kidney and making an assessment of overall renal function. CT examination is also useful for evaluation of regional lymph nodes.

Once the presence of a renal mass has been documented, a chest x-ray film and bone scan are required. If there is no evidence of DM or impaired renal function, no further tests are required, and patients are generally brought to the operating room for definitive resection. For patients in whom a partial nephrectomy is being considered (see later discussion of indications), or a locally advanced lesion is identified, a selective renal arteriogram may be obtained to better delineate tumor extent and vascular anatomy (Figs. 43-8 to 43-11).[24] Inferior venacavography is a useful tool for evaluating renal vein and inferior vena cava (IVC) extension. Preoperative needle biopsies of the renal mass for the purpose of obtaining a tissue diagnosis may be indicated in patients with evidence of metastatic disease, but they are not required in a patient who is a candidate for definitive resection. Other complementary radiologic tests include ultrasonography, magnetic resonance imaging (MRI), and percutaneous puncture of a renal cyst.

STAGING SYSTEMS

The oldest and most commonly used staging system is Robson's classification (Table 43-3), which was proposed by Charles Robson and colleagues[25] in 1969 as a modification of the system presented by Flocks and Kadesky[26] in 1958.

The American Joint Committee on Cancer's (AJCC) latest definition of TNM classification (Table 43-4) provides more detailed information by separating

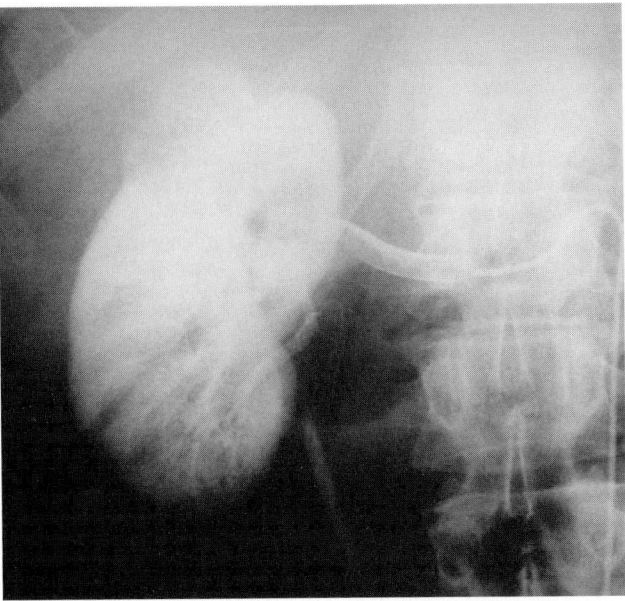

Figure 43–9. Selective renal arteriogram of the patient whose scan is shown in Figure 40-8. Note the highly vascular appearance of these tumors.

characteristics of the primary lesion from those of regional nodes.[27] These definitions can be used as either a clinical or a pathological staging system.

There is very poor correlation between the Robson and AJCC staging systems, as demonstrated in Table 43-5, making comparisons quite confusing.

Distribution of patients by Robson's stage at presentation is listed in Table 43-6. One must bear in mind that nearly all studies defining tumor stage at presentation are surgical series, resulting in a slight downward stage migration. It must be presumed that many patients with widespread disease at presentation (i.e., stage 4) would not be surgical candidates and would therefore be excluded from these reports. Overall, approximately 40% of patients have disease confined to the kidney, 12% have perinephric extension, 20% have renal vein extension, 5% have lymph node involvement, and 20% have extension to adjacent organs or distant disease.

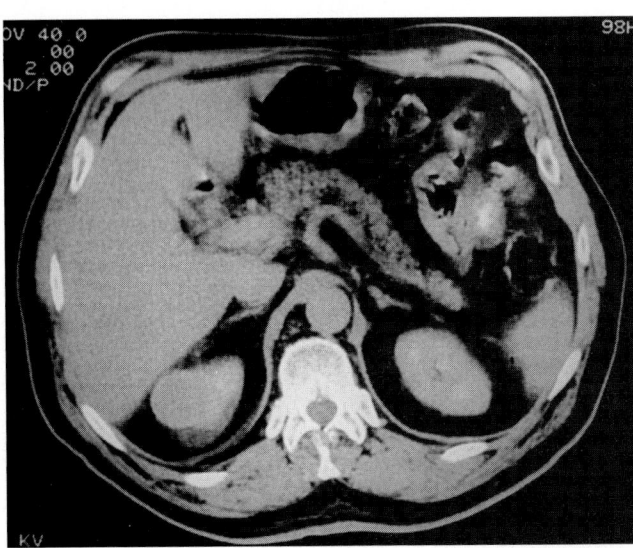

Figure 43–8. Computed tomographic examination of a 4-cm right upper pole renal mass with probable perinephric extension. There is no evidence of regional adenopathy.

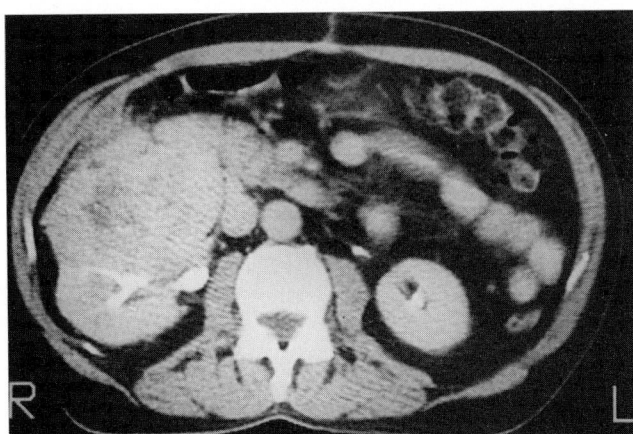

Figure 43–10. Computed tomographic (CT) examination of a massive right renal mass with perinephric extension. Other CT cuts were highly suggestive of renal vein extension. There is no evidence of regional adenopathy.

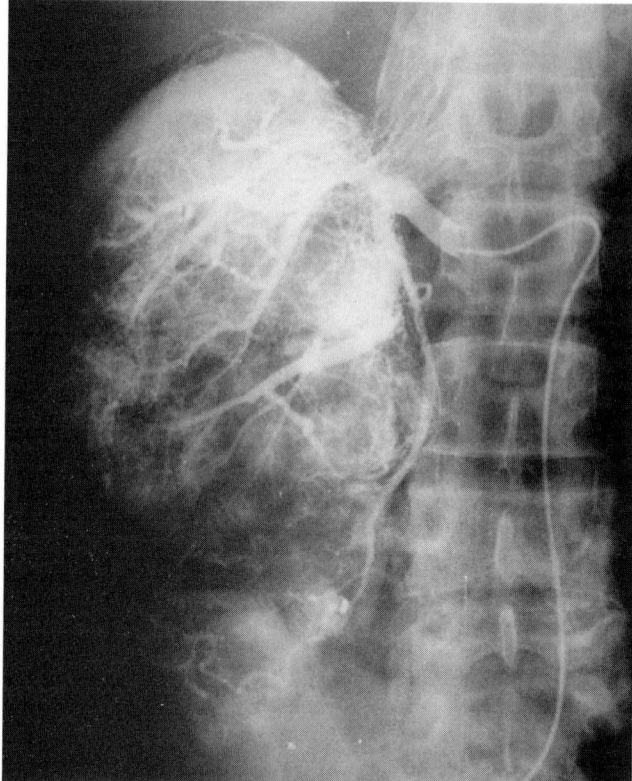

Figure 43–11. Selective renal arteriogram of the patient whose scan is shown in Figure 43–10, performed to confirm the suspicion of renal vein extension. During the outflow phase of the study, tumor vascularity rising into the inferior vena cava became readily apparent.

PROGNOSTIC FACTORS

A myriad of features, both clinical and pathological, have been analyzed for the determination of their prognostic significance. The great majority of studies analyze individual factors by univariate analysis, ignoring the potential interdependence of factors on patient outcome. A thorough discussion of the relative importance of all such features is beyond the scope of this chapter; however, the interested reader is referred to an exhaustive review by Thrasher and Paulson.[28]

The most commonly evaluated prognostic factors relate to the gross anatomic extent of the primary lesion at the time of diagnosis; perinephric extension, renal vein extension, lymph node involvement, and metastatic disease

Table 43–3   Robson's Staging Classification

Stage 1	Tumor confined to kidney, negative lymph nodes
Stage 2	Perirenal fat involvement (but confined to Gerota's fascia), negative lymph nodes
Stage 3	
3a	Gross renal vein or inferior vena cava involvement, negative lymph nodes
3b	Lymph node involvement (primary tumor as in 1–3A)
3c	Renal vein involvement *and* positive lymph nodes
Stage 4	
4a	Tumor involves adjacent organs other than adrenal
4b	Distant metastases

TABLE 43–4   Classification of Renal Cancer

Primary Tumor (T)

TX	Primary tumor cannot be assessed
T0	No evidence of primary tumor
T1	Tumor 7 cm or less in greatest dimension, limited to the kidney
T1a	Tumor 4 cm or less in greatest dimension, limited to the kidney
T1b	Tumor more than 4 cm but not more than 7 cm in greatest dimension, limited to the kidney
T2	Tumor more than 7 cm in greatest dimension, limited to the kidney
T3	Tumor extends into major veins or invades adrenal gland or perinephric tissues but not beyond Gerota's fascia
T3a	Tumor directly invades adrenal gland or perirenal and/or renal sinus fat but not beyond Gerota's fascia
T3b	Tumor grossly extends into the renal vein or its segmental (muscle-containing) branches, or vena cava below the diaphragm
T3c	Tumor grossly extends into vena cava above diaphragm or invades the wall of the vena cava
T4	Tumor invades beyond Gerota's fascia

Regional Lymph Nodes (N)*

NX	Regional lymph nodes cannot be assessed
N0	No regional lymph node metastases
N1	Metastasis in a single regional lymph node
N2	Metastasis in more than one regional lymph node

*Laterality does not affect the N classification.
Note: If a lymph node dissection is performed, then pathologic evaluation would ordinarily include at least eight nodes.

Distant Metastasis (M)

MX	Distant metastasis cannot be assessed
M0	No distant metastasis
M1	Distant metastasis

Stage Grouping

Stage I	T1	N0	M0
Stage II	T2	N0	M0
Stage III	T1	N1	M0
	T2	N1	M0
	T3	N0	M0
	T3	N1	M0
	T3a	N0	M0
	T3a	N1	M0
	T3b	N0	M0
	T3b	N1	M0
	T3c	N0	M0
	T3c	N1	M0
Stage IV	T4	N0	M0
	T4	N1	M0
	Any T	N2	M0
	Any T	Any N	M1

From Greene FL, Page DL, Fleming ID, et al (eds): *AJCC Cancer Staging Manual*, 6th ed. New York: Springer 2002.

have all been demonstrated by numerous authors[25,29-33] to negatively affect patient survival. Pathologic features detectable by light microscopy have been evaluated, and several—tumor histologic type, grade, and cellular pattern—have repeatedly been found to have prognostic import.[29,30,34] Patient features, such as age, sex, and race,

TABLE 43-5 Comparison of Staging Systems

| | AJCC Stage | | | |
	T	N	M	Robson's Stage
I	T1	N0	M0	1
II	T2	N0	M0	1
III	T1	N1	M0	3a
	T2	N1	M0	3b
	T3a	N0	M0	2
	T3a	N1	M0	3b
	T3b	N0	M0	3a
	T3b	N1	M0	3c
	T3c	N0	M0	3a
	T3c	N1	M0	3c
IV	T4	Any N	M0	3b–4a
	Any T	N2	M0	3b–4a
	Any T	Any N	M1	4b

From Greene FL, Page DL, Fleming ID, et al (eds): *AJCC Cancer Staging Manual*, 6th ed. New York: Springer 2002.

and performance status have been considered relevant clinical prognostic factors by other authors.[35-37]

Rabinovitch and colleagues[23] performed a multivariate analysis on a population of 172 surgically treated patients at Memorial Sloan-Kettering Cancer Center and demonstrated that only renal vein extension ($P = 0.001$) and lymph node involvement ($P = 0.026$) were independent prognosticators for the development of distant metastases.[23] Although positive margins and perinephric extension were considered significant on univariate analysis, these factors lost significance on multivariate analysis. Patient sex, radical versus partial nephrectomy, age, histologic type, and tumor size were not prognosticators on either univariate or multivariate analysis.

SURGICAL MANAGEMENT

Surgery is the only treatment modality with proved efficacy in curing patients of RCC. The earliest nephrectomies were performed in the late 1800s, and the procedure came into widespread use by 1900. Current surgical controversies revolve around both the appropriate management of the primary renal tumor (i.e., radical vs. partial nephrectomy) and its regional nodal stations.

Radical Nephrectomy

The radical nephrectomy (RN) defines the procedure in which the kidney, along with Gerota's fascia and its contents, are removed en bloc from the retroperitoneum. This procedure, first described by Mortensen[38] in 1948, became the standard surgical technique beginning in the following decade, and is the standard of care today. The RN allows a more reliable margin around the known tumor than does a simple nephrectomy. Although the RN has never been compared with the simple nephrectomy in a randomized fashion, Robson in 1963 was the first to propose that the RN confers the best survival results.[39]

The RN can be performed through various approaches, the selection of which is determined by the patient's body habitus, as well as the position and extent of the renal lesion. Common approaches include the anterior transperitoneal approach, the flank approach (which may include a portion of the 10th or 11th rib), and the thoracoabdominal approach.

The standard RN is modified in situations of locally advanced primary lesions. When a tumor thrombus exists within the renal vein, ligation of the vessel can be performed beyond the known tumor extent. Tumor within the vena cava does not preclude curative resection. A simple partial vena cava wall resection can be performed if the tumor thrombus minimally extends into the lumen of this vessel. However, if there is actual vena cava wall involvement or extensive tumor bulk, a portion of the vena cava itself may need to be excised with graft reconstruction. Lesions that directly extend to adjacent organs should be resected en bloc whenever possible, and this may involve splenectomy, partial colectomy, pancreatectomy, hepatectomy, or diaphragmatic resection. The guiding principle is to remove all gross disease whenever possible.

A summary of the results from surgical management of RCC is presented in Table 43-7. Despite the differences among published reports, the overall 5-year survival rates have changed little since Robson's report in 1963. The relative constancy in outcome reflects not so much any *factor* regarding surgical management, but rather the *lack of progress* in any adjuvant treatment modality.

Surgical outcomes from the past 2 decades defined as 5-year overall survival are approximately 80% to 100% for stage 1, 60% to 70% for stage 2, 35% to 50% for stage 3, and 10% for stage 4.

Table 43-6 Robson's Stage at Presentation Among Surgical Series (%)

Reference	n	Yr	Stage 1	Stage 2	Stage 3 (3a + 3b)	Stage 4
Rabinovitch et al[23]	172	1994	63	17	19 (13 + 6)	<1
Sene et al[34]	152	1992	45	10	24 (18 + 6)	20
Ramon et al[43]	112	1991	51	8	28	13
Medeiros et al[30]	121	1988	40	7	38	16
Siminovitch et al[31]	246	1983	32	16	23 (19 + 4)	29
Selli et al[83]	115	1983	63	7	13	17
Waters and Richie[44]	130	1979	28	20	28 (22 + 6)	25
Boxer et al[35]	96	1979	36	10	19	35
Skinner et al[29]	309	1971	33	7	35	25
Robson et al[25]	87	1969	38	17	31	14
Total	1540		Average 41	12	26	20

Table 43-7   Radical Nephrectomy, 5-Year Survival Rates by Robson's Stage, %

Reference	Yrs	n	Stage 1	Stage 2	Stage 3 (3a, 3b)	Stage 4	All	Notes
Robson et al[25]	1949-1964	88	66	64	42	11	52	Crude
Skinner et al[29]	1935-1965	203	68	50	49	—	57	Crude
Middleton & Presto[48]	1950-1967	61	59	48	—	—	59	Crude
Waters & Richie[44]	1957-1977	130	51	59	(53, 12)	0	—	Majority are RN
Boxer et al[35]	1956-1976	96	56	100	50	8	37	RN and PN
Siminovitch et al[31]	1968-1978	175	82	58	(31, 11)	—	—	NED rates
Medeiros et al[30]	1960-1978	121	82	50	46	0	—	90/121 are RN
Selli et al[83]	1970-1981	115	93	63	80	13	73	Includes 20 patients with DM
Giuliani et al[32]	1970-1987	200	80	70	(5, 52)	0-7	—	All RN
Sene et al[34]	1965-1985	155	81	65	39	6	—	
Rabinovitch et al[23]	1978-1988	172	—	—	—	—	87	

DM, distant metastases; NED, no evidence of disease; PN, partial nephrectomy; RN, radical nephrectomy.

Partial Nephrectomy

Partial nephrectomies (PNs) have been performed for the treatment of RCC since the beginning of the 20th century. When Robson reported his improved results with RN, however, this became the new surgical standard and nephron-sparing procedures fell out of favor. Although the RN remains the standard of care regarding surgical management, the PN plays an important role when preservation of functional renal parenchyma is important. There has been a recent revival of the PN due primarily to improved imaging with CT and MRI, presenting the potential for preoperative identification of small peripheral lesions. This is an important consideration in patients with bilateral RCC, von Hippel-Lindau disease, unilateral renal agenesis, prior nephrectomy, diabetic nephropathy, horseshoe kidney, renal artery stenosis, hydronephrosis, ureteral reflux, and nephrosclerosis.

Most published series on PN consist of patients with bilateral RCC or unilateral disease in the presence of impaired contralateral renal function. Despite this unfavorable baseline, the overall results are quite acceptable (Table 43-8). Local failure (LF) is a significant concern in this conservative procedure; however, in well-selected cases, recurrence within the residual renal parenchyma is less than 10%. The 5-year cause-specific survival is approximately 85%, although overall survival is poorer because of the concurrent diseases that necessitate the conservative procedures.

It is reasonable to assume that the PN performed on a healthy group of well-selected patients with peripheral stage I lesions, as determined by preoperative evaluation, without contralateral tumors or renal dysfunction, would result in improved overall survival rates compared with existing PN series. A prospective trial comparing RN to PN is required, although the benefit for renal-conserving surgery in the otherwise healthy patient is unclear. PN is a more complicated surgical procedure than RN with a greater risk of bleeding complications and longer operative times.[40]

Patients who develop LF after PN are still eligible for surgical salvage with an RN, assuming the absence of distant disease. Novick and Straffon[41] from the Cleveland Clinic have proposed salvage of such patients with a second partial nephrectomy, although longer follow-up in greater numbers of patients is needed.

LF after radical nephrectomy is uncommon, but in the absence of concomitant distant disease, patients should be considered for salvage surgery.[42]

Lymph Node Dissection

The role of regional lymph node dissection (LND) in RCC remains a controversial issue. A randomized trial to settle this ongoing question has never been performed. The theoretical advantage of a complete LND is the removal of gross or microscopic nodal disease in patients

Table 43-8   Renal-Conserving Surgery (Partial Nephrectomies and Enucleations)

Reference	Yrs	n	Stage 1, %	LF	5-Yr Survival, %	Follow-up, Mo	Notes
Novick & Straffon[41]	1956-1987	100	75	9/100	84	50	23% enuc.
Morgan & Zincke[84]	1965-1987	104	90	6/104	89-92*	59	60% enuc.
Provet et al[45]	1974-1988	44	90	3/44	80-100†	36	all PN
Herr[85]	1979-1981	41	90	1/41	95	36	all PN
Total		289		Average 7%			

*Cause-specific survival rates.
†Disease-free survival rates.
enuc., enucleations; LF, local failure; PN, partial nephrectomies.

without distant metastases, thus improving the overall cure rate. Unfortunately, this simple concept is difficult to demonstrate clinically.

A second potential value for an extended LND is to better define those patients at greatest risk for developing metastatic disease who would then benefit most from systemic therapy. This would be analogous to the axillary node dissections considered standard in the management of breast cancer in order to obtain prognostic information and identify those patients who would benefit from systemic therapy. Unfortunately, there is currently no effective chemotherapy or immunotherapy for RCC, and certainly none that is considered standard in the adjuvant setting. So at the present time, this argument is moot.

With regard to anatomic extent, a complete regional LND defines a procedure in which draining lymph nodes from the crus of the diaphragm to the bifurcation of the aorta are removed. Hilar dissections include only those lymph nodes surrounding the renal vessels. These latter lymph nodes are taken automatically as part of an RN specimen. Therefore, when PNs are performed, no lymph nodes are necessarily taken, and lymph node sampling depends completely on the operating surgeon.

The argument against performing a complete LND revolves around the lack of proven benefit in the face of prolonged anesthesia time, increased risk of bleeding from lumbar vessels, and lack of adjuvant treatment options in node-positive patients.

PATTERNS OF FAILURE AFTER SURGICAL RESECTION

An understanding of the patterns of failure after definitive surgical management is essential to determine the value of any potential adjuvant treatment. Surprisingly few of the surgical series report the incidences of both local and distant failure.

Review of the literature reveals LF rates of 2% to 14% after PN or RN in a widely heterogeneous population of patients.[32,41,43-47] Most of these data are derived from crude rather than actuarial numbers. Only the study from Memorial Sloan-Kettering presented actuarial LF (Fig. 43-12) and analyzed the pathologic features that predict LF.[23] The actuarial LF was only 5% at 7 years among the 172 surgically treated patients. Univariate analysis found LF significantly increased in the presence of either lymph node involvement (21% vs. 4%, $P = 0.0002$) or positive margins (21% vs. 4%, $P = 0.002$).

The development of DM varies from 9% to 36%,[23,43-45,48,49] depending primarily on the stage of disease at presentation, and whether CT technology was available during the study period. Rabinovitch and colleagues[23] reported an actuarial incidence of 26% at 7 years (Fig. 43-13). Most importantly, no clear causal relationship has ever been demonstrated between LF and DM. The Memorial Sloan-Kettering experience found 32 patient-failures among 172 surgically managed

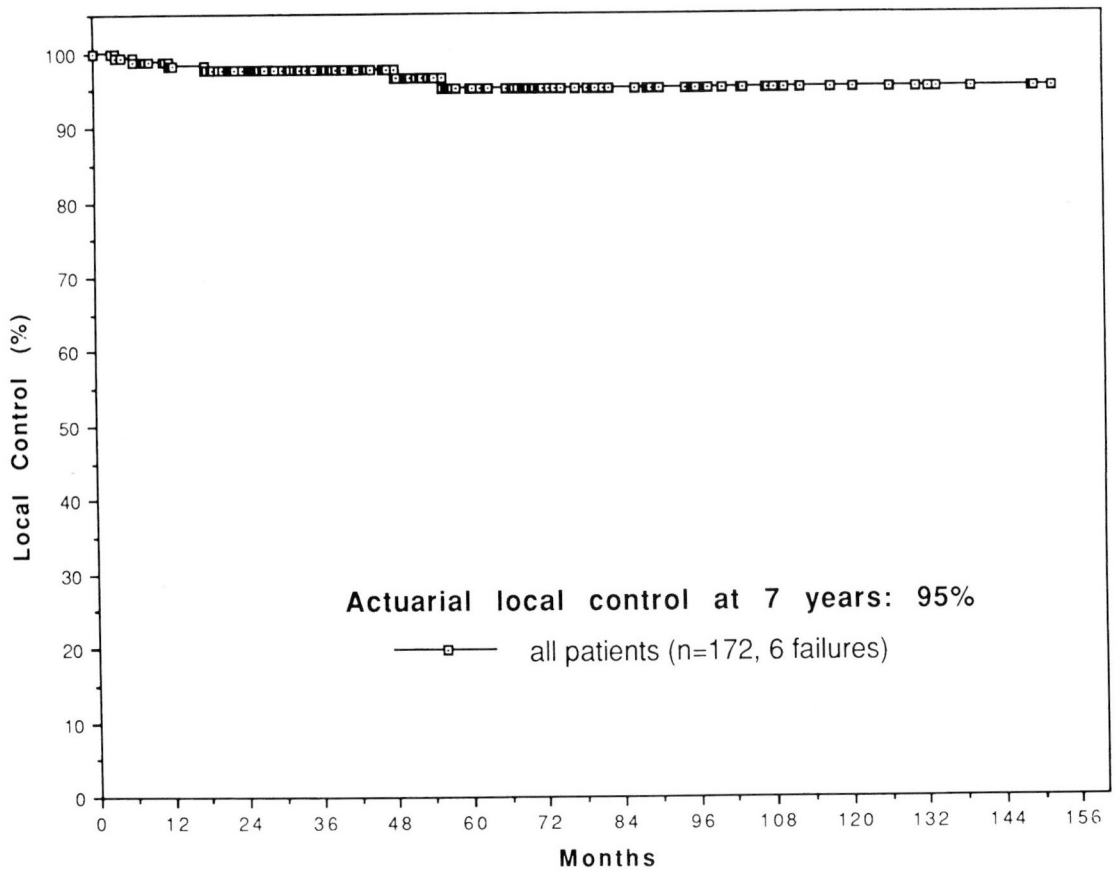

Figure 43–12. Actuarial local control for 172 surgically managed patients from Memorial Sloan-Kettering Cancer Center. (From Rabinovitch RA, Zelefsky MJ, Gaynor JJ, et al: Patterns of failure following surgical resection of renal cell carcinoma: Implications for adjuvant local and systemic therapy. *J Clin Oncol.* 1994;12:206.)

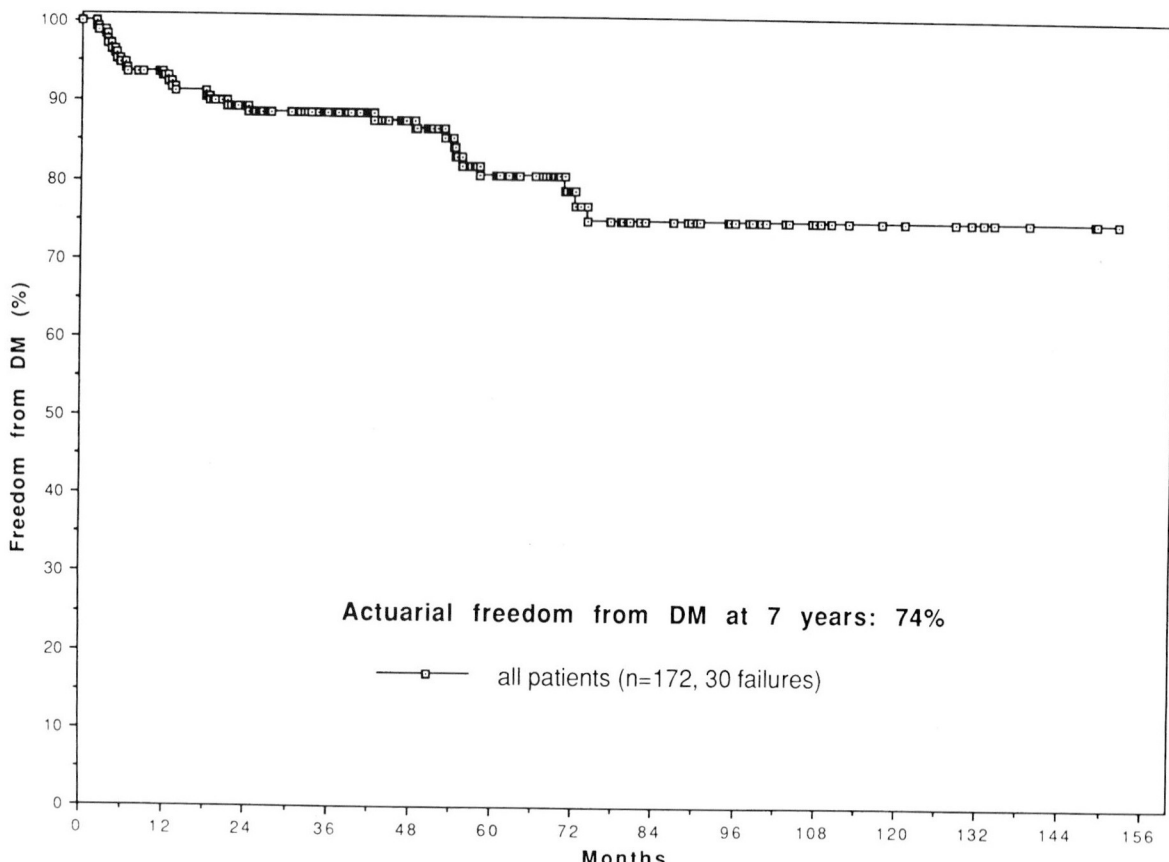

Figure 43–13. Actuarial freedom from distant metastases (DM) for 172 surgically managed patients from Memorial Sloan-Kettering Cancer Center. (From Rabinovitch RA, Zelefsky MJ, Gaynor JJ, et al: Patterns of failure following surgical resection of renal cell carcinoma: Implications for adjuvant local and systemic therapy. *J Clin Oncol.* 1994;12:206.)

patients.[23] Of these, only one patient first developed LF and later developed DM. Twenty-six patients were found to have DM without ever having failed locally. Occult DM at the time of presentation is the primary mode of treatment failure, and the lack of causality between local and distant failure argues against the use of local adjuvant treatment (i.e., radiotherapy).

ADJUVANT RADIATION THERAPY

Nonrandomized Data

Radiation therapy (RT) has been investigated as an adjuvant treatment for RCC since the 1930s. Several series were published in the 1950s and 1960s comparing nonrandomized groups of patients treated with surgery (Sx) and surgery with adjuvant RT (Sx/RT), most of which suggested a survival advantage to patients treated with adjuvant RT.[26,50-52] Several more recent series have suggested a local control advantage (Table 43-9). These studies served as the foundation upon which the randomized trials were based (see later). Rafla[53] published the experience of the Winnipeg General Hospital in 1970. He claimed that postoperative RT improved overall survival at 5 years. Subgroup analysis revealed this survival benefit to be limited only to those patients with "renal pelvis" or "capsular tissue" involvement. Unfortunately, the paper does not include any details of the radiation technique, target volume, total dose delivered, fractionation scheme, beam energy, or treatment toxicity. A significant reduction in the LF rate was obtained in the Sx/RT group: 25% versus 7%.

Table 43–9   Adjuvant Radiation Therapy—Retrospective Data

Reference	Yr	Timing	n	Dose, cGy	5-Yr Survival, %		LF, %	
					Sx	Sx/RT	Sx	Sx/RT
Cox et al[86]	1970	Post	120	—	38	20	—	—
Rafla[53]	1970	Post	190	?	37	56	25	7
Stein et al[47]	1992	Post	123	3600-5000	110	50	21	9

LF, local failure; Pre, preoperative; Post, postoperative; Sx, surgical therapy; Sx/RT, surgery with radiotherapy.

The most recent retrospective series were published in 1992 by Stein and colleagues[47] from the Rambam Medical Center in Israel and in 1997 by Aref and colleagues from Ottawa Regional Cancer Center in Canada.[54] In Stein's series, evaluation of 123 patients treated with and without adjuvant postoperative RT resulted in no significant difference in overall survival or LF, but there was a trend toward improved outcome in the combined modality patients. Of the 19 LFs among both groups, 3 were scar recurrence. There was, however, a significant decrease in LF for patients with T3 tumors. The authors therefore recommend inclusion of the scar within the treatment volume whenever such patients are treated. Aref evaluated the pattern of failure in patients with resected renal cell carcinoma and found that locoregional failure alone was rare following nephrectomy. DM was the predominant failure and therefore these authors concluded that postoperative radiotherapy is not indicated.

Randomized Trials

The role of adjuvant RT has been evaluated in four prospective randomized trials (Table 43-10), all conducted in Europe. Two examined preoperative RT, and two examined postoperative RT. The information gleaned from these studies is clouded by various issues. The first three trials were conducted in the 1960s and early 1970s, before the development of CT technology (which is today considered essential for accurate staging of the primary tumor and the regional lymph nodes, and evaluation of suspicious chest x-ray lesions that are suggestive of metastatic disease). These same three studies were also nondiscriminating with regard to which patients were appropriate candidates for study inclusion; that is, even patients with small T1N0 tumors were eligible for enrollment. With such trial design, it would be difficult to detect a benefit from adjuvant therapy if, for example, only patients with T3-T4 tumors demonstrated an advantage. Only the most recently published study, by Kjaer and colleagues,[55] was performed in the CT era, and it excluded patients with early-stage lesions.

PREOPERATIVE RADIOTHERAPY. Both preoperative trials reported no difference in 5-year overall survival between the two arms of the study.[49,56] Neither study, however, used doses considered adequate to sterilize even microscopic disease by current standards. Patients were eligible for participation, regardless of the stage of their lesions.

Surprisingly, neither study gives any information regarding LF, a logical endpoint for studies evaluating a local therapy.

POSTOPERATIVE RADIOTHERAPY. Finney's study[46,57] is difficult to evaluate because it was published in two journals in the same year and cited different results in each. The results given are crude, not actuarial, further making comparisons between studies difficult. In both postoperative studies, however, doses adequate for microscopic residual disease were delivered. These studies concur with the preoperative studies, demonstrating no survival advantage after adjuvant RT. LF was determined to be unusual regardless of treatment, with no apparent impact of the local treatment.

The postoperative trials both emphasize the toxicity encountered in patients receiving adjuvant RT. Interestingly, the severe complications observed in each study differed. Finney documented four deaths due to hepatic toxicity among the 51 patients treated on the experimental arm of the study.[46] All four patients were treated for right-sided renal tumors, and no such deaths were encountered in patients treated with surgery alone. Kjaer and colleagues[55] describe significant toxicity in 12 of 27 patients treated with postoperative RT. Of these, three were due to hepatic dysfunction; however, all improved with conservative management. The remaining nine patients developed stenosis or bleeding within the duodenum, and five of them died directly as a result of small bowel toxicity. This study has been criticized for delivering relatively large fraction sizes (250 cGy) to a total dose of 5000 cGy to volumes that include small bowel. Of the 32 patients randomly assigned to receive postoperative treatment, 4 were never irradiated and 1 had no follow-up.

Despite the many flaws of these trials and the difficulty of making comparisons, all found no survival advantage to administration of adjuvant RT. Local failure, as documented by the postoperative studies, is unusual and is not affected by local irradiation. Both reports make note of the significant incidence of DM in the absence of LF, indicating the presence of occult distant disease at the time of treatment, precluding a potential survival advantage from adjuvant RT.

Conclusions

It is unlikely that future trials evaluating adjuvant RT, even if well designed, will be performed. Although it has

Table 43–10 Adjuvant Radiation Therapy—Prospective Randomized Data

Reference	Yr	Timing	n	Dose, cGy	5-Yr Survival, %		LF, %	
					Sx	Sx/RT	Sx	Sx/RT
Van der Werf-Messing[49]	1973	Pre	126	3000 (200 ×15)	*		—	—
Juusela et al[56]	1977	Pre	88	3000 (220 × 15)	63	47	—	—
Finney[46]	1973	Post	100	5500 (204 × 27)	47	36	13	13
Kjaer[55]	1987	Post	65	5000 (250 × 20)	64	38	3	0

*No value given, but difference not statistically significant. LF, local failure; Pre, preoperative; Post, postoperative; Sx, surgical therapy; Sx/RT, surgical therapy with radiotherapy.

never proved beneficial in completed randomized trials, a definitive conclusion regarding the use of RT in the adjuvant setting would require a multi-institutional study with hundreds of patients with advanced lesions. These patients would have to be treated with meticulous treatment planning and a well-thought-out fractionation scheme. Clearly, modern three-dimensional conformal radiation therapy (3DCRT) and intensity modulated radiotherapy (IMRT) techniques would reduce complications and increase effective dose. As of 2002, standard treatment of RCC did not include adjuvant RT. Based on several retrospective series, an argument can nevertheless be made for treating positive margins, positive lymph nodes, or unresected disease in medically inoperable patients. As there are no ongoing randomized trials in which to enroll such patients, in these situations it is not unreasonable to treat with RT. A sample CT-based treatment plan for a patient with a T3aN0 tumor with positive margins is demonstrated in Figure 43-14.

PALLIATIVE RADIATION THERAPY

Brain Metastases

Brain metastases occur in approximately 10% of RCC patients and are associated with a poor prognosis. There have been a number of retrospective reports and most conclude that surgical resection is the most effective treatment associated with the best outcome. One such series was reported by Shibui and colleagues in 1990.[58] In this series median survival time from diagnosis of brain metastases was 17 months for patients who underwent resection compared to 4 months for patients who did not undergo surgery. The median survival for patients who received postoperative radiotherapy was 20 months, compared with 10.5 months for patients who received radiotherapy alone. It is noteworthy that patients who are candidates for craniotomy and whose lesions are resectable are likely to have better outcomes independent of therapeutic modality, and this series, like other retrospective series, has inherent biases associated with selection of patients for specific therapies. Wronski and colleagues reported the MD Anderson Cancer Center experience using whole brain radiotherapy for patients with RCC metastatic to brain.[59] One-hundred nineteen patients received whole brain radiotherapy only and form the cohort of study. Median survival for the entire cohort was only 4.4 months. Sixty percent of patients had multiple metastases and 40% had solitary metastases. The authors concluded that these poor results should be impetus to use more aggressive approaches such as surgery and stereotactic radiosurgery. The study period spans almost 2 decades, however, and it is not stated how these patients were selected for whole brain radiotherapy alone. During the study period 79 patients underwent resection and thus were not included in this report.

Yoshimasa reported their single institution results using stereotactic radiosurgery for brain metastases from RCC.[60] Thirty-five patients with 52 brain metastases were treated. The median survival was 14 months. The local control rate was 90% for 39 cases evaluated by imaging. These results are comparable to surgical series. There have been no randomized trials comparing surgical metastasectomy to stereotactic radiosurgery. Retrospective reports support comparable outcomes; therefore, selecting one modality over the other should depend on patient and disease-related factors.

Bone Metastases

To date there are no reports assessing radiation therapy specifically for bone metastases from RCC. The Radiation Therapy Oncology Group showed that higher doses of radiotherapy are required for palliation of symptoms related to bone metastases from RCC, but the number of patients with RCC was small.[61]

Total Body Irradiation

Nonmyeloablative bone marrow or stem cell transplant is showing promise in metastatic RCC and is further discussed in the systemic therapy section of this chapter. Low-dose total body irradiation (TBI) (200cGy) is being explored as a preparative regimen for mini-allogeneic transplant. It is well tolerated and can be given on an outpatient basis.

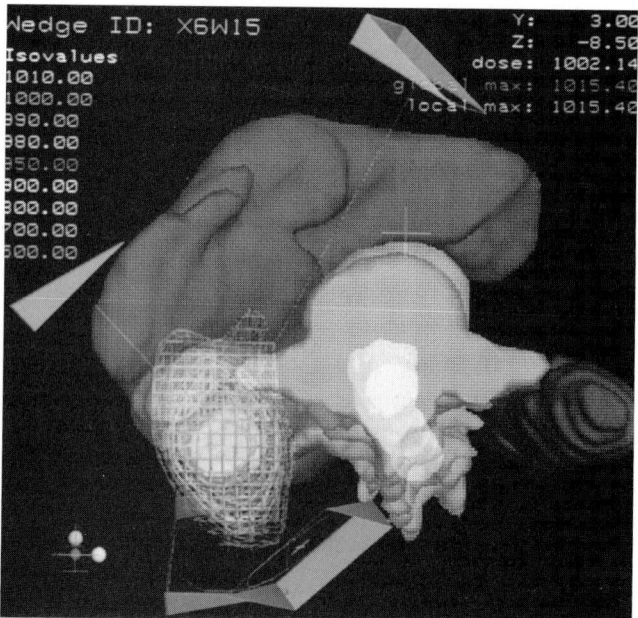

Figure 43–14. Isodose cloud displaying coverage of right lower pole carcinoma of the kidney in a 63-year-old woman who was medically ineligible for surgical therapy. Lesion is covered with a 1.5-cm margin and spares contralateral kidney, upper ipsilateral kidney, and spinal cord. Isovalues displayed represent percent × 10 (i.e., the 1000 isovalue = 100% isodose line). The plan uses a four-field noncoplanar mixed-beam technique combining both 6 and 18 MV photons. (Planned on the FOCUS 3D treatment planning system from Computerized Medical Systems.)

SYSTEMIC THERAPY

Like RT, systemic treatment (whether chemotherapy or immunotherapy) is not a standard part of the overall management of patients with localized and resectable disease.

Chemotherapy

In the past 30 years, no cytotoxic agent or combination of agents with activity against RCC has been identified. Nearly all the reported experience with chemotherapy results from the treatment of patients with measurable metastatic disease, in which activity is measured by complete responses (CRs), partial responses (PRs), and overall response rates (RR = CR + PR). More than 40 single agents have been evaluated, all with RRs of 0% to 16%.[62]

Yagoda and colleagues[62] pooled all patients treated since 1983 in trials with single-agent chemotherapy. Of the 3502 patients adequately treated, only 5.6% responded. The authors point out that because of the dismal rate of response with these agents, they have no role as a neoadjuvant or adjuvant treatment. For patients with advanced disease, chemotherapeutic choices are limited to (1) no treatment, (2) participation in an experimental trial, or (3) administration of vinblastine or a nitrosourea (both of which are approved by the Food and Drug Administration for use in patients with RCC). Combination chemotherapy should not be used, as toxicity is increased without any evidence of benefit.

Immunotherapy

Treatment of metastatic RCC with immunotherapy has a more recent history than cytotoxic chemotherapy. The two primary immunotherapeutic agents that have been extensively studied are interferon (IFN) and interleukin 2 (IL-2). IFN demonstrates antiproliferative, antiviral, and immunoregulatory activity and is subdivided into IFN-α, -β, and -γ. Response to any of the IFNs ranges from 0% to 38%, with an average response rate of 14%.[63] Response is usually demonstrated within 3 months, and lack of response to treatment within this interval is an indication for cessation of treatment. The duration of response is generally less than 2 years.

The T-cell growth factor IL-2, when given alone, demonstrates slightly lower RRs than IFN-α. In an effort to improve results, IL-2 has been combined with either lymphokine-activated killer (LAK) cells, tumor-infiltrating lymphocytes, or IFN-α with differing results. The administration of LAK cells is associated with significant side effects, whereas the administration of IL-2 with IFN-α subcutaneously has resulted in fewer side effects, with the advantage that it can be delivered as an outpatient treatment.[64]

Overall, treatment with any of the immunotherapeutic agents, whether alone or in combination, rarely yields RRs greater than 20% to 30%. Recent trials have focused on combining IL-2, IFN, and 5-fluorouracil, as well as the use of IL-2 in lower doses.[65] Administration is indicated only in the setting of clinical trials.

Nonmyeloablative Bone Marrow or Stem Cell Transplant

Metastatic RCC has a poor prognosis, and although responses of approximately 20% have been obtained with IL-2 and IFN-α, there is no associated improvement in survival, and treatment toxicity can be substantial. Allogeneic transplant for hematogenous malignancies can result in profound *graft versus tumor effect*. Based on the observation that RCC can spontaneously regress, the importance of the immune system was realized. Childs first explored the therapeutic approach of immunosuppressive but nonmyeloablative preparative regimens followed by peripheral-blood stem cell allogeneic transplantation in a patient with metastatic RCC. The goal was to exploit the donor T-cell graft versus tumor effect.[66] Childs further reported on 19 consecutive patients with refractory metastatic RCC who were treated with mini-allogeneic peripheral stem cell transplant.[67] The cumulative probability of response was 53%, and 3 of 19 patients had a complete response that lasted longer than 16 months. The median time to regression was 4 months after transplant. This delay in response is associated with limitations in patients with rapidly progressive metastatic disease who may not live long enough to develop graft versus tumor effect. This approach is still considered experimental, but these early results are promising.

RENAL RADIATION TOLERANCE

The effects of radiation on the kidney were first described in 1952 in a classic paper by Kunkler, Farr, and Luxton[68] analyzing patients treated for testicular seminoma with orchiectomy and abdominal irradiation. A clinical syndrome of radiation-induced nephritis developed in 20 patients, resulting in renal failure and death in 50% of those afflicted. Hypertension, anemia, elevated blood urea nitrogen levels, and albuminuria were the hallmarks of this syndrome and developed after an average latency period of 8 months. Severe cases included signs and symptoms of severe fluid overload, including peripheral edema, cardiomegaly, and pleural effusions. Death was due to malignant hypertension in six patients, and renal failure in the remaining four. Analysis of the various irradiation techniques in the 93 patients reviewed revealed the greatest risk to those receiving bilateral whole kidney irradiation to greater than 2300 cGy. They proposed, more than 4 decades ago, limiting the renal dose to below this level and excluding at least one third of the total kidney volume from the radiation fields whenever possible.

Whole abdominal radiotherapy has been used in the adjuvant treatment of intermediate risk ovarian cancer. The total dose that can be given is limited by the radiation tolerance of the kidney. Irwin and colleagues reviewed the Princess Margaret Hospital (PMH) experience over a 5-year period and identified 60 analyzable patients who had received whole abdominal radiotherapy, had *not* received chemotherapy, and had at least 5 years of follow-up since therapy.[69] The total dose to the kidneys was limited to less than 20 Gy over 4.5 weeks. The following analyses were done: complete blood count, urinalysis, urine microscopy, serum creatinine, urine osmolarity following an overnight fast and 24-hour urine collection for creatinine clearance, phosphorous and uric acid, and quantitative estimation of protein excretion. There was no evidence of renal dysfunction more than 5 years following

Table 43–11   Sequelae of Partial Renal Irradiation

Reference	n	Disease Treated	Renal Volume Irradiated & Dose, cGy	Abnormal Renal Scan	Creatinine Clearance, mL/min	Increased Blood Pressure	Malignant Hypertension
Birkhead et al[87]	23	Hodgkin's disease	Partial left kidney 4000	6/16	—	1/23	0/23
Kim et al[88]	18	Non-Hodgkin's	Both kidneys Right ≤1500 Left ≥2299	9/18	Decreased, av. 52	5/18	0/18
Willet et al[70]	86	Gastrointestinal tumors	≥1/2 of one kidney ≥2600	—	17% decrease, av. 62	6/6	1/86
Thompson et al[89]	67	Gastric hypersecretion	Entire left kidney 1500–2000	—	—	10/67	4/67
LeBourgeois et al[90]	74	Lymphoma	30–80% of left kidney 4000	—	Normal in all patients	0/74	0/74

bilateral kidney irradiation to doses in the 15 to 20 Gy range as a result of whole abdominal radiotherapy for ovarian cancer.

Fortunately, clinical manifestations of renal irradiation are now unusual because of our increased awareness of the marked sensitivity of this organ and subsequent care in treatment planning. Although the syndrome described by Kunkler and colleagues is rarely reported, evidence of renal damage can be documented even when the volume of one kidney or more is excluded from the treatment portals and clinical symptoms are not clinically evident (Table 43-11). Renal scan abnormalities corresponding to the region of irradiated kidney are seen in at least one third of patients when such tests are performed.

Decreases in average creatinine clearance have been documented; however, there have been no reports of such patients requiring dialysis or developing overt renal failure in the absence of malignant hypertension. Willet and colleagues[70] nicely demonstrated that the mean percentage decrease in creatinine clearance corresponds to the percentage of kidney irradiated: 10% decrease when 50% of the kidney is irradiated, 19% when 60% to 85% is irradiated, and 24% when 90% to 100% is treated.

The most common and clinically relevant sequela of renal irradiation is the development or worsening of pre-existent hypertension. It is reasonable to conclude that up to 10% of patients may require medication for control of newly diagnosed or worsening hypertension in the years after renal irradiation. The incidence of malignant hypertension or other serious sequelae of irradiation is 2% or less when all 268 patients from these series are pooled.

Histologically, radiation-induced renal damage is manifested by glomerular endothelial cell swelling, glomerular hyalization, interstitial edema or fibrosis or both, and basement membrane thickening and splitting. Electron microscopy reveals marked subendothelial accumulation of electron-lucent material with deposition of basement membrane material subjacent to the endothelial cells.[71-73]

In summary, doses to both kidneys that would result in permanent renal function impairment with a probability of 5% and 50% at 5 years are 2000 and 2500 cGy,

respectively (TD 5/5, TD 50/5).[71] Ideally, every attempt should be made to ensure that at least one third of the total renal mass is shielded from the treatment portals and receives less than 1500 cGy.

REFERENCES

1. Jemal A, Murray T, Samuels A et al: Cancer statistics. A cancer journal clinicians. 2003;53:5.
2. McLaughlin JK, Lipworth L: Epidemiologic aspects of renal cell carcinoma. *Semin Oncol.* 2000; 27:115.
3. Reddan DN, Raj GV, Polascik TJ: Management of small renal tumors: an overview. *Am J Med.* 2001;110:558.
4. Grossman E, Messerli FH, Goldbourt U: Does diuretic therapy increase the risk of renal cell carcinoma? *Am J Cardiol.* 1999;83:1090.
5. Grossman E, Messerli FH, Goldbourt U: Antihypertensive therapy and the risk of malignancies. *Eur Heart J.* 2001;22:1343.
6. Cohen AJ, Li FP, Berg S, et al: Hereditary renal-cell carcinoma associated with a chromosomal translocation. *N Engl J Med.* 1979;301:592.
7. Pathak S, Stron LC, Ferrell RE, et al: Familial renal cell carcinoma with a 3:11 chromosome translocation limited to tumor cells. *Science.* 1982;217:939.
8. Glenn GM, Choyke PL, Zbar B, et al: Von Hippel-Lindau disease: Clinical aspects and molecular genetics. In Anderson EE, ed. *Problems in Urologic Surgery: Benign and Malignant Tumors of the Kidney.* Philadelphia: JB Lippincott; 1990.
9. Solomon D, Schwartz A: Renal pathology in von Hippel-Lindau disease. *Hum Pathol.* 1988;19:1072.
10. Karumanchi SA, Merchan J, Sukhatme VP: Renal cancer: Molecular mechanisms and newer therapeutic options. *Curr Opin Nephrol Hypertens.* 2002;11:37.
11. Cohen HT: Advances in the molecular basis of renal neoplasia. *Curr Opin Nephrol Hypertens.* 1999;8:325.
12. Grawitz P: Die sogennanten Lipoma der Niere. *Virchows Arch Pathol Anat.* 1883;93:39.
13. Fisher DR, Horvat B: Comparative ultrastructural study of so-called renal adenoma and carcinoma. *J Urol.* 1972;108:382.
14. Holthofer H: Immunohistology of renal cell carcinoma. *Eur Urol.* 1990;18:15.
15. Bell ET: A classification of renal tumors with observations on the frequency of the various types. *J Urol.* 1938;39:238.
16. Curry NS, Schabel SI, Betsill WL Jr: Small renal neoplasms: Diagnostic imaging, pathologic features, and clinical course. *Radiology.* 1986;158:113.
17. O'Toole KM, Brown M, Hoffman P: Pathology of benign and malignant kidney tumors. *Urol Clin North Am.* 1993;20:193.
18. Mian BM, Bhadkamkar N, Slaton JW, et al: Prognostic factors and survival of patients with sarcomatoid renal cell carcinoma. *J Urol.* 2002;167:65.

19. Tsiu K, Shvarts O, Smith R, et al: Renal cell carcinoma: Prognostic significance of incidentally detected tumors. *J Urol.* 2000;163:426.

20. *Cancer Facts and Figures—2001.* Atlanta: American Cancer Society; 2001:18.

21. Parsons JK, Schoenberg MS, Carter HB: Incidental renal tumors: Casting doubt on the efficacy of early intervention. *Urology.* 2001;57:1013.

22. Luciani LG, Tsui KH, Shvarts O, et al: Renal cell carcinoma: Prognostic significance of incidentally detected tumors [letter]. *J Urol.* 2001;165:1223.

23. Rabinovitch RA, Zelefsky MJ, Gaynor JJ, et al: Patterns of failure following surgical resection of renal cell carcinoma: Implications for adjuvant local and systemic therapy. *J Clin Oncol.* 1994;12:206.

24. Mauro MA, Wadsworth DE, Stanley RJ, et al: Renal cell carcinoma: Angiography in the CT era. *AJR.* 1982;139:1135.

25. Robson CJ, Churchill BM, Anderson W: The results of radical nephrectomy for renal cell carcinoma. *J Urol.* 1969;101:297.

26. Flocks RH, Kadesky MC: Malignant neoplasms of the kidney: An analysis of 353 patients followed 5 years or more. *J Urol.* 1958;79:196.

27. American Joint Committee on Cancer: Kidney. In Fleming ID, Cooper JS, Henson DE, et al, eds: *AJCC Cancer Staging Manual.* 5th ed. Philadelphia: Lippincott-Raven; 1997:231.

28. Thrasher JB, Paulson DF: Prognostic factors in renal cancer. *Urol Clin North Am.* 1993;20:247.

29. Skinner DG, Colvin RB, Clinton DV, et al: Diagnosis and management of renal cell carcinoma: A clinical and pathologic study of 309 cases. *Cancer.* 1971;28:1165.

30. Medeiros LJ, Gelb AB, Weiss LM: Renal cell carcinoma: Prognostic significance of morphologic parameters in 121 cases. *Cancer.* 1988;61:1639.

31. Siminovitch JMP, Montie JE, Straffon RA: Prognostic indicators in renal adenocarcinoma. *J Urol.* 1983;130:20.

32. Giuliani L, Giberti C, Martorana G, et al: Radical extensive surgery for renal cell carcinoma: Long-term results and prognostic factors. *J Urol.* 1990;143:468.

33. Golimbu M, Al-Astari J, Tesler A, et al: Renal cell carcinoma: Survival and prognostic factors. *Urology.* 1986;27:291.

34. Sene AP, Hunt L, McMahon RFT, et al: Renal carcinoma in patients undergoing nephrectomy: Analysis of survival and prognostic factors. *Br J Urol.* 1992;70:125.

35. Boxer RJ, Waisman J, Lieber FM, et al: Renal carcinoma: Computer analysis of 96 patients treated by nephrectomy. *J Urol.* 1979;122:598.

36. Chasan SA, Pothel LR, Huben RP: Management and prognostic significance of hypercalcemia in renal cell carcinoma. *Urology.* 1989;33:167.

37. Lieber M, Tomera F, Taylor W, et al: Renal adenocarcinoma in young adults: Survival and variables affecting prognosis. *J Urol.* 1981;125:164.

38. Mortensen H: Thoracic nephrectomy. *J Urol.* 1948;60:855.

39. Robson C: Radical nephrectomy for renal cell carcinoma. *J Urol.* 1963;89:37.

40. Shekarriz B, Upadhyay J, Shekarriz H, et al: Comparison of costs and complications of radical and partial nephrectomy for treatment of localized renal cell carcinoma. *Urology.* 2002;59:211.

41. Novick AC, Straffon RA: Management of locally recurrent renal cell carcinoma after partial nephrectomy. *J Urol.* 1987;138:607.

42. Wiesner C, Jjakse G, Rohde D: Therapy of local recurrence of renal cell carcinoma. *Oncol Rep.* 2002;9:189.

43. Ramon J, Goldwasser B, Raviv G, et al: Long-term results of simple and radical nephrectomy for renal cell carcinoma. *Cancer.* 1991;67:2506.

44. Waters WB, Richie JP: Aggressive surgical approach to renal cell carcinoma: Review of 130 cases. *J Urol.* 1979;122:306.

45. Provet J, Tessler A, Brown J, et al: Partial nephrectomy for renal cell carcinoma: Indications, results and implications. *J Urol.* 1991;145:472.

46. Finney R: The value of radiotherapy in the treatment of hypernephroma. A clinical trial. *Br J Urol.* 1973;45:258.

47. Stein M, Kuten A, Halpern J, et al: The value of postoperative irradiation in renal cell cancer. *Radiother Oncol.* 1992;24:41.

48. Middleton RG, Presto AJ III: Radical thoracoabdominal nephrectomy for renal cell carcinoma. *J Urol.* 1973;110:36.

49. Van der Werf-Messing B: Carcinoma of the kidney. *Cancer.* 1973;32:1056.

50. Riches EW, Griffiths IH, Thackray AC: New growths of the kidney and ureter. *Br J Urol.* 1951;23:297.

51. Bratherton DG: The place of radiotherapy-The treatment of hypernephroma. *Br J Urol.* 1964;37:141.

52. Peeling WB, Mantell BS, Shepheard BGF: Postoperative irradiation in the treatment of renal cell carcinoma. *Br J Urol.* 1969;41:23.

53. Rafla S: Renal cell carcinoma: Natural history and results of treatment. *Cancer.* 1970;25:26.

54. Aref I, Bociek RG, Salhani D: Is post-operative radiation for renal cell carcinoma justified? *Radiother Oncol.* 1997;43:155.

55. Kjaer M, Frederiksen PL, Engelholm SA: Postoperative radiotherapy in stage II and III renal adenocarcinoma: A randomized trial by the Copenhagen renal cancer study group. *Int J Radiat Oncol Biol Phys.* 1987;13:665.

56. Juusela H, Malmio K, Alfthan O, et al: Preoperative irradiation in the treatment of renal adenocarcinoma. *Scand J Urol Nephrol.* 1977;11:277.

57. Finney R: An evaluation of postoperative radiotherapy in hypernephroma treatment: A clinical trial. *Cancer.* 1973;32:1332.

58. Shibui S, Nishikawa R, Nomura K: Treatment of metastatic brain tumor from renal cell carcinoma [Japanese]. *No Shinkei Geka.* 1990;18:935.

59. Wronski M, Maor MH, Davis BJ, et al: External radiation of brain metastases from renal cell carcinoma: A retrospective study of 119 patients from the M.D. Anderson Cancer Center. *Int J Radiat Oncol Biol Phys.* 1997; 37:753.

60. Yoshimasa M, Kondziolka D, Flickinger J, et al: Stereotactic radiosurgery for brain metastases from renal cell carcinoma. *Cancer.* 1998;83:344.

61. Tong D, Gillick L, Henrickson FR: The palliation of symptomatic osseous metastases: Final results of the study by the Radiation Therapy Oncology Group. *Cancer.* 1982;50:893.

62. Yagoda A, Petrylak D, Thompson S: Cytotoxic chemotherapy for advanced renal cell carcinoma. *Urol Clin North Am.* 1993; 20:303.

63. Wirth MP: Immunotherapy for metastatic renal cell carcinoma. *Urol Clin North Am.* 1993;20:283.

64. Pierce WC, Belldegron A, Figlin RA: Cellular therapy, scientific rationale and clinical results in the treatment of metastatic renal-cell carcinoma. *Semin Oncol.* 1995;22:74.

65. Vogelzang NJ, Lipton A, Figlin RA: Subcutaneous interleukin-2 plus interferon alfa-2a in metastatic renal cancer: An outpatient multicenter trial. *J Clin Oncol.* 1993;11:1809.

66. Childs RW, Clave E, Tisdale J, et al: Successful treatment of metastatic renal cell carcinoma with a nonmyeloablative allogeneic peripheral-blood progenitor-cell transplant: evidence for a graft-versus-tumor effect. *JCO.* 1999;17:2044.

67. Childs RW, Chernoff A, Contentin N, et al: Regression of metastatic renal-cell carcinoma after nonmyeloablative allogeneic peripheral-blood stem-cell transplantation. *NEJM.* 2000;343:750.

68. Kunkler PB, Farr RF, Luxton RW: The limit of renal tolerance tox-rays. *Br J Radiol.* 1952;25:190.

69. Irwin C, Fyles A, Wong CS, et al: Late renal function following whole abdominal irradiation. *Radiother Oncol.* 1996;38:257.

70. Willett CG, Tepper JE, Orlow BA, et al: Renal complications secondary to radiation treatment of upper abdominal malignancies. *Int J Radiat Oncol Biol Phys.* 1986;12:1601.

71. Rubin P, Cooper RA, Phillips TL, eds: *Radiation Biology and Radiation Pathology Syllabus.* (SET RT1: *Radiation Oncology.*) Chicago: American College of Radiology; 1975.

72. Keane WF, Crosson JT, Staley NA: Radiation-induced renal disease: A clinicopathologic study. *Am J Med.* 1976;60:127.

73. Pearse HD: The kidney. In Moss WT, Cox JD, eds. *Radiation Oncology.* 6th ed. St Louis: CV Mosby; 1989;416.

74. McLaughlin JK, Mandell JS, Blot WJ, et al: A population-based case control study of renal cell carcinoma. *J Natl Cancer Inst.* 1984;72:275.

75. Yu MC, Mack TM, Hanisch R, et al: Cigarette smoking, obesity, diuretic use, and coffee consumption as risk factors for renal cell carcinoma. *J Natl Cancer Inst.* 1986;77:351.

76. Whittemore AS, Paffenbarger RS, Anderson K, et al: Early precursors of urogenital cancers in former college men. *J Urol.* 1984;132:1256.

77. Malker HR, Malker BK, McLaughlin JK, et al: Kidney cancer among leather workers. *Lancet.* 1984;1:56.

78. Ross RK, Pagannini-Hill A, Landolph J, et al: Analgesics, cigarette smoking and other risk factors for cancer of the renal pelvis and ureter. *Cancer Res.* 1989;49:1045.

79. Chung-Park M, Parveen T, Lam M: Acquired cystic disease of the kidneys and renal cell carcinoma in chronic renal insufficiency without dialysis treatment. *Nephron.* 1989;53:157.

80. Matson MA, Cohen EP: Acquired cystic kidney disease: Occurrence, prevalence, and renal cancers. *Medicine.* 1990;69:217.

81. Bretan PN, Busch MP, Hricak H: Development of acquired renal cysts and renal cell carcinoma. *Cancer.* 1986;57:1871.

82. Chisolm GD, Roy RR: The systemic effects of malignant renal tumours. *Br J Urol.* 1971;43:687.

83. Selli C, Hinshaw WM, Woodard BH, et al: Stratification of risk factors in renal cell carcinoma. *Cancer.* 1983;52:899.

84. Morgan W, Zincke H: Progression and survival after renal-conserving surgery for renal cell carcinoma: Experience in 104 patients and extended follow-up. *J Urol.* 1990;144:852.

85. Herr H: Partial nephrectomy for renal cell carcinoma with a normal opposite kidney. *Cancer.* 1994;73:160.

86. Cox CE, Lacy SS, Montgomery WG, et al: Renal adenocarcinoma: 28-year review, with emphasis on rationale and feasibility of pre-operative radiotherapy. *J Urol.* 1970;104:53.

87. Birkhead BM, Dobbs CE, Beard MF, et al: Assessment of renal function following irradiation of the intact spleen for Hodgkin's disease. *Radiology.* 1979;130:473.

88. Kim TH, Somervilee PJ, Freeman CR: Unilateral radiation nephropathy—The long term significance. *Int J Radiat Oncol Biol Phys.* 1984;10:2053.

89. Thompson PL, Mackay IR, Robson GSM, et al: Late radiation nephritis after gastric x-irradiation for peptic ulcer. *Q J Med.* 1971;40:145.

90. LeBourgeois JP, Meignan M, Parmentier C, et al: Renal consequences of irradiation of the spleen in lymphoma patients. *Br J Radiol.* 1979;52:56.

Cancer of the Bladder

44

Michael J. Zelefsky, MD, Jonathan E. Rosenberg, MD, and Eric J. Small, MD

ETIOLOGY

Bladder cancer is estimated to have an annual incidence in the United States of 57,400 cases, accounting for 4% of all cancers and 19% of all genitourinary cancers. Approximately 12,500 people per year will die of this disease, accounting for 2% of all cancer-related mortality in the United States.[1] At diagnosis, 73% of patients have localized disease only, 19% have regional disease, and 8% present with distant metastases.[1] Two thirds of all diagnosed cases occur among persons 65 years of age or older. The male/female ratio is 3:1. From the early 1970s to the mid-1980s the incidence of this cancer has risen while mortality has fallen. This phenomenon is likely attributable to the increased detection of localized lesions.[2]

Cigarette smoking is the single most significant known cause of bladder cancer, as demonstrated by both cohort and case-control studies.[2-7] The risk of bladder cancer appears to be related to the number of pack-years, and such an individual's risk of bladder cancer declines if smoking is ceased.[8] It is estimated that 50% of bladder cancers diagnosed in the United States can be linked to a smoking history.[9] In a case-controlled study of more than 1500 patients with bladder cancer and a large control group matched for age, sex, and race, there was a statistically higher risk of bladder cancer observed in female smokers when compared to male smokers with similar smoking habits.[8b] It appears that the relationship of smoking to bladder cancer development stems from exposure to selected arylamines. Studies have demonstrated that smokers have higher levels of 3- and 4-aminobiphenyl hemoglobin adducts, which are increased 10-fold and 3-fold, respectively, compared to nonsmokers.[10] Cytogenetic analyses indicate a direct relationship between smoking and suppressor gene p53 nuclear overexpression.[11]

Exposure to industrial chemicals and the high rates of bladder cancer in specific occupations have been a major focus of epidemiologic investigation. Individuals in contact with chemicals necessary for the production of dyes, rubber, plastics, and synthetic materials are at increased risk for development of bladder cancer.[2,11-15] Dye workers may be particularly at risk owing to exposure to aromatic amines, specifically 2-naphthylamine and benzidine, which have been shown to be bladder carcinogens.[16] Rubber workers are also exposed to 2-naphthylamine, and benzidine is found in paints.[2] Dry cleaners may have an increased risk of bladder cancer from exposure to organic solvents, including perchloroethylene.[17] Hair dyes are known to contain arylamines, and a recent study demonstrated an increased risk of bladder cancer among users of hair dyes and an additive effect for bladder cancer development among smokers who use hair dyes.[18]

Schistosoma haematobium is presumed to be the primary cause of endemic squamous cell carcinoma common in Egypt.[19] This form of bladder cancer is recognized to occur in patients 10 to 20 years younger than patients with typical cases of transitional cell carcinoma diagnosed in the United States.[20] It has been hypothesized that the parasite may induce an inflammatory response with the release of reactive oxygen radicals that results in genetic damage, leading to carcinogenesis.[21] Patients with chronic urinary tract infections or with the need to frequently self-catheterize after spinal cord injury are also predisposed to squamous cell carcinomas.[22-24]

The role of diet in the predisposition or reduction of risk of developing bladder cancer remains unclear. There have been conflicting data about the role of coffee consumption and an association with bladder cancer development. A summary of 35 case-control studies of the etiologic role of coffee showed no evidence of a relationship between the beverage and the development of bladder cancer.[25,26] On the other hand, a recent meta-analysis for urinary tract cancers estimated a 20% increase of bladder cancers among coffee drinkers irrespective of dose or duration of consumption.[27] It is now believed that there is no relationship between artificial sweeteners and the development of bladder cancer.[28] Some studies have shown a minimal protective effect with vitamin A, fruits, and vegetables.[29,30] People who drink fresh well water were found to have lower rates of bladder cancer than those drinking chlorinated municipal water.[31] A higher incidence of bladder cancer has been noted in agricultural areas where fertilizers seep into water supplies, raising the level of nitrates in drinking water.[32]

Iatrogenic causes of bladder cancer include radiation exposure, chronic phenacetin usage, and administration of cyclophosphamide.[2,33] Patients with rheumatoid arthritis were shown to have an increased rate of bladder cancer for as long as 17 years after taking oral cyclophosphamide.[34]

A genetic predisposition to bladder cancer in certain families has been described. It is likely that there is an interaction between hereditary predisposition of oncogenes and tumor suppressor genes that are amplified or deleted due to environmental stimuli.[2] The interplay between environment and genetic predisposition is exemplified by the reduction of glutathione S-transferase activity with the loss of the *GSTM1* gene. The glutathione enzyme appears to play a role in modulating the carcinogenic effects of tobacco smoke.[35,36]

CYTOGENETICS

Scientific inquiry has concentrated on the molecular biology and cytogenetics of bladder cancer with the expectation that insight into the natural history of the disease will translate into clinical advances. An attempt is under way to define independent prognostic factors that predict which of two similar superficial lesions is destined to relapse as muscle invasive disease. Flow cytometry has shown that lesions with an increased chromosome number and aneuploidy were associated with higher-grade tumors destined to be invasive.[37-39] One study showed that the percentages of hyperdiploid cells for chromosomes 7, 11, and 17 were predictive of grade and stage.[40] A model of an orderly progression of alteration in genetic material involving oncogenes and tumor suppressor genes is being elucidated.[41]

An early occurrence that may be critical in distinguishing Tis and T1 from normal bladder epithelium and the less aggressive papillary tumors (Ta) appears to involve loss of a tumor suppressor gene on chromosome 9.[41-44] Progression to muscle invasive disease appears to require loss of the tumor suppressor gene *p53* on chromosome 17, shown to be present in 65% of Tis compared with 3% of Ta tumors.[45] Other intermediate events in the progression to invasive disease likely involve deletions in 5q, 3p, and 17p, which are not present in Ta lesions.[46,47] No single oncogene has been found in the majority of tumors, although c-*erb* B2, H-*ras*, c-*src*, and c-*jun* have been expressed and likely play a role in the intermediate progression to muscle invasive lesions.[48-50] Late events may involve loss of suppressor genes on 11p, 6q, 13q, and 18q.[37,41,51] In particular, the loss of the retinoblastoma gene on chromosome 13 likely has a role in bladder cancer similar to its role in other malignancies.[52,53] Investigators have also suggested additional loci of tumor suppressor genes, including 4p, 8p, 14q, and 12q.[54,55] Others have recently demonstrated a strong association with 6p+ and high tumor cell proliferation rate, which was noted to be an independent variable in addition to grade and tumor stage.[56]

A prognostic factor for transitional cell carcinoma confined to the bladder independent of grade, stage, and lymph node status is the accumulation of the p53 protein in the nucleus. With mutation of the wild-type p53, the protein product has a longer half-life and can be detected by immunohistochemistry.[57] After radical cystectomy, patients with stages pT1, pT2, and pT3a who had p53 detected by immunohistochemistry had a shorter relapse-free and overall survival.[58] Similarly, an analysis of p53 nuclear overexpression in 33 patients with carcinoma in situ showed disease progression in 13 of 15 p53-positive patients compared with 3 of 18 p53-negative patients.[59] The potential clinical implications of using the p53 status as a marker are far reaching and include in the future the selection of lower-risk patients for bladder conservation and patients with early-stage disease who may benefit from adjuvant radiotherapy or chemotherapy.[60-64]

ANATOMY

Both for the radiation oncologist and for the surgeon, the relationship between the bladder and neighboring structures is critical in treatment planning. The bladder functions as a muscular reservoir and is anatomically divided into a fundus, apex, body, trigone, and neck. Empty, the bladder is confined to the true pelvis. As the organ fills, it expands anterosuperiorly into the abdominal cavity. The fundus or base faces posteriorly and in males is separated from the rectum superiorly by the rectovesical pouch and inferiorly by the seminal vesicles (Figs. 44-1 and 44-2). In the female, the bladder faces the uterus and the anterior vaginal wall. The neck is located 3 to 4 cm behind the symphysis pubis. This lowest and most fixed part of the bladder is pierced by the urethra and in males approximates the prostate. A remnant of the median umbilical ligament called the urachus links the apex of the bladder (which lies posterior to the cranial section of the symphysis pubis) to the umbilicus. The superior surface of the bladder is covered by peritoneum and may approximate the sigmoid colon or ileum and the uterus in females. Fascia forms the pubovesical ligaments that suspend the bladder between the pubic bones, anterior abdominal wall, and pelvic side walls. An empty bladder is characterized by a mucosa with folds except for a smooth triangular region called the trigone. The superior border of the trigone is characterized by its appearance as a pale band on cystoscopy and is called the interureteral crest. This band separates the ureteral openings. At the trigonal apex is the internal urethral orifice completing the triangle.[65]

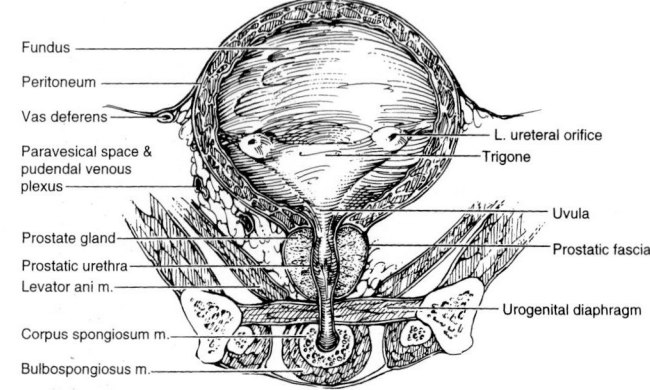

Fundus
Peritoneum
Vas deferens
Paravesical space & pudendal venous plexus
Prostate gland
Prostatic urethra
Levator ani m.
Corpus spongiosum m.
Bulbospongiosus m.

L. ureteral orifice
Trigone
Uvula
Prostatic fascia
Urogenital diaphragm

Figure 44–1. Sagittal view in the male demonstrates that the full bladder expands into the lower abdominal cavity. Tumors occur in all five regions of the bladder and are often multifocal.

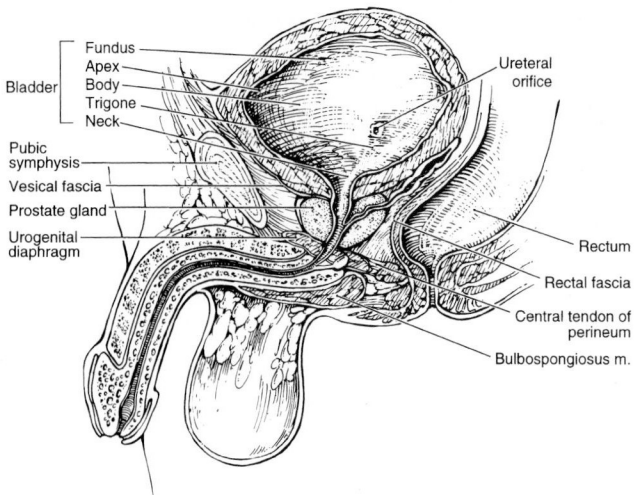

Figure 44–2. Cross sectional view in the male of the bladder and surrounding anatomy. The proximity of the bladder to the prostate and rectum explains the occurrence of locally advanced invasion into these structures.

The arterial supply to the bladder arises from the anterior division of the hypogastric artery. Branches from the obturator and inferior gluteal arteries contribute to the rich vascular supply. In the female, additional vessels include the uterine and vaginal arteries. An important venous plexus exists between the bladder wall and the adventitial layer that drains into the hypogastric veins.[65] Lymphatics from the mucosa and muscular layer drain to the surface of the bladder and form three collecting ducts at the trigone, anterior, and posterior walls. The trigone collecting duct drains into the external iliac nodes (Fig. 44-3). Hypogastric and common iliac lymph nodes are the destination of lymph collected in the anterior and posterior ducts. Some of the lymph also flows through the route of the anterior bladder wall collecting ducts to external iliac nodes.[66]

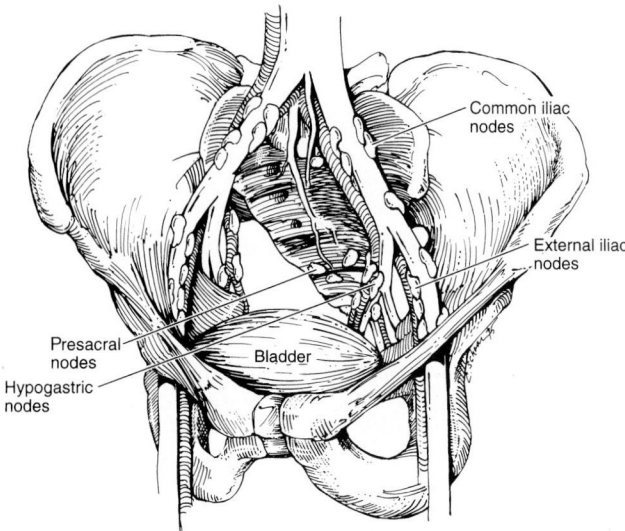

Figure 44–3. Lymphatic drainage of the bladder. Involvement of the common iliac nodes is considered a manifestation of distant metastatic and not regional disease.

The internal anatomy of the bladder can be viewed as consisting of three layers with a nerve supply. The mucosa consists of an epithelium of transitional cells supported by a lamina propria of loose connective tissue. The second layer consists of nonstriated muscle cells that form the detrusor muscle. This muscle is composed of two layers of longitudinally directed muscle bundles surrounding a layer of circular bundles. The third layer is adventitia, and for certain sections of the bladder a serosal covering of peritoneum is also present.

Innervation of the bladder can be divided into a parasympathetic nerve supply arising from S2-4 and a sympathetic supply that originates mainly in T11-12 and L1-2. Sympathetic nerves are found primarily in the trigone, and in the male these nerves stimulate closure of the bladder neck sphincter to prevent reflux ejaculation. Parasympathetic nerves play a large role in detrusor muscle constriction. A small group of autonomic nerves can be found scattered in the bladder wall. The adult male bladder has a normal capacity of 120 to 320 mL, with pain due to stretch sensations mediated by parasympathetic nerve fibers when distention beyond 500 mL occurs.[65,67]

Bladder tumors are often multifocal, reflecting a field cancerization defect. Of the tumors that have a subsite listed at diagnosis, the majority occur on the bladder walls. The lateral walls account for 40% of malignancies, with posterior involvement of 11% and anterior involvement of 3%. As much as 17% of tumors are known to arise adjacent to the ureteral orifice, whereas the trigone, dome, and neck account for 13%, 9%, and 7%, respectively, of sites from which the cancers arise.[2]

PATHOLOGY

Transitional cell carcinomas account for approximately 93% of all bladder cancer in the United States.[2] Pattern of tumor growth can take one of four forms: papillary, noninvasive carcinoma in situ, invasive, or invasive with scattered foci of carcinoma in situ. Tumors range from well-differentiated grade I lesions with cellular architecture resembling normal urothelium with mild cytologic atypia to anaplastic grade III. Immunohistochemical analysis of microvessel density has been shown to be an independent prognostic indicator demonstrating a relationship between tumor angiogenesis, nodal metastasis, and survival.[68,69]

Carcinoma in situ on cystoscopy often appears as multiple erythematous patches without a gross structural component. Histologic examination reveals an increase in the number of cell layers, lack of cohesion between cells resulting in shedding into the urine, disordered architecture, and increased number of mitotic figures. The basement membrane confines the tumor to the mucosa. Papillary carcinomas are exophytic stalks protruding into the lumen of the bladder. Invasive lesions show involvement of the muscular layer and are often palpable on examination.[70,71]

Transitional cell carcinomas with squamous or glandular components are classified as transitional tumors with a similar natural history to those of pure histology.

Squamous cell carcinomas comprise 5% to 8% of primary bladder malignancies in the United States. In Egypt and other areas endemic with *Schistosoma haematobium*, squamous cell tumors are the predominant histology. Appearance on cytoscopic evaluation is one of ulceration and invasion. Adenocarcinomas account for 1% to 2% of bladder tumors. They predominantly arise in the urachus or less frequently in the trigone.[71,72]

A variety of rare histologic findings account for less than 2% of all primary bladder cancers. Extrapulmonary small cell carcinoma can occasionally originate in the bladder, and because of its aggressive and high metastatic potential, it is often treated with chemotherapy generally used for small cell carcinomas of the lung.[73] Rhabdomyosarcoma of the bladder occurs in children but rarely present in adults.[74] Other rare histologies include lymphoma, leiomyosarcoma, melanoma, and primary bladder pheochromocytoma.[75-78] In addition, adenocarcinomas can metastasize to the bladder from the colon, rectum, endometrium, prostate, ovary, breast, and lung.[79]

CLINICAL PRESENTATION AND ROUTES OF SPREAD

Gross or microscopic hematuria is a presenting sign in 75% of patients with bladder cancer. Approximately 25% of patients present with symptoms of vesical irritation and 20% are asymptomatic. The majority of patients with carcinoma in situ have urinary frequency, urgency, dysuria, and microscopic hematuria. Advanced tumors may present as pelvic pain, ureteral obstruction, hydronephrosis, or rectal obstruction.[80,81]

The regional lymph nodes at risk are those in the true pelvis below the bifurcation of the common iliac arteries. These lymph nodes include the hypogastric, obturator, internal and external iliac, perivesical, pelvic, sacral, and presacral chains. Staging is dependent on the size and number of nodes and not on whether they are unilateral or ipsilateral (Table 44-1). Spread to the common iliac nodes is considered a manifestation of distant metastases and not regional disease.[82] Skinner and colleagues[83] correlated the depth of bladder wall invasion to involvement of lymph nodes. In their study, 5% of patients with pT1, 30% with pT2, 31% with pT3a, 64% with pT3b, and 50% with pT4 disease had nodal metastases. The most common sites of distant metastatic disease are the lung, bone, and liver.

DIAGNOSTIC AND STAGING STUDIES

The initial formulation of an organized staging system reproducible in predicting survival dates back to the work of Jewett and Strong in the 1940s. Primary bladder tumors were classified as *stage A* when involvement was limited to the submucosa, as *stage B* when tumor penetrated into the muscularis, and as *stage C* with evidence of perivesical fat involvement. Stage A tumors had no evidence of metastases compared with 13% of stage B tumors and 74% of stage C tumors. In 1951, Jewett

Table 44–1 Classification of Bladder Cancer

Primary Tumor (T)

TX	Primary tumor cannot be assessed
T0	No evidence of primary tumor
Ta	Non-invasive papillary carcinoma
Tis	Carcinoma in situ: "flat tumor"
T1	Tumor invades subepithelial connective tissue
T2	Tumor invades muscle
pT2a	Tumor invades superficial muscle (inner half)
pT2b	Tumor invades deep muscle (outer half)
T3	Tumor invades perivesical tissue
pT3a	Microscopically
pT3b	Macroscopically (extravesical mass)
T4	Tumor invades any of the following: prostate, uterus, vagina, pelvic wall, abdominal wall
T4a	Tumor invades prostate, uterus, vagina
T4b	Tumor invades pelvic wall, abdominal wall

Regional Lymph Nodes (N)

Regional lymph nodes are those within the true pelvis; all others are distant lymph nodes.

NX	Regional lymph nodes cannot be assessed
N0	No regional lymph node metastasis
N1	Metastasis in a single lymph node, 2 cm or less in greatest dimension
N2	Metastasis in a single lymph node, more than 2 cm but not more than 5 cm in greatest dimension; or multiple lymph nodes, none more than 5 cm in greatest dimension
N3	Metastasis in a lymph node, more than 5 cm in greatest dimension

Distant Metastasis (M)

MX	Distant metastasis cannot be assessed
M0	No distant metastasis
M1	Distant metastasis

Stage Grouping

Stage 0a	Ta	N0	M0
Stage 0is	Tis	N0	M0
Stage I	T1	N0	M0
Stage II	T2a	N0	M0
	T2b	N0	M0
Stage III	T3a	N0	M0
	T3b	N0	M0
Stage IV	T4a	N0	M0
	T4b	N0	M0
	Any T	N1	M0
	Any T	N2	M0
	Any T	N3	M0
	Any T	Any T	M1

From Greene FL, Page DL, Fleming ID, et al., eds: *AJCC Cancer Staging Manual*, 6th ed. New York: Springer; 2002.

proposed a division of stage B into *B1* and *B2* to correspond with superficial and deep muscle penetration. The following year, Marshall added a *stage 0* to include tumors not infiltrating the lamina propria and *stage D* for metastatic disease.[84]

The current Tumor Node Metastasis (TNM) staging system standardized by the American Joint Committee on Cancer (AJCC) and the TNM Committee of the International Union Against Cancer (UICC) continues to reflect the importance of depth of bladder wall invasion. The *T* stands for depth of tumor in relation to the mucosa, muscularis, and the perivesical fat. Regional nodes include those of the true pelvis, whereas *M* disease involves nodes above the bifurcation of the common iliac arteries or distant visceral metastasis.[82]

The current TNM staging system (see Table 44-1) recognizes that Ta papillary growths convey a significantly better prognosis than Tis (carcinoma in situ) or T1 lesions. Also recognized is that either microscopic or gross involvement of perivesical fat (T3b) is more important than the distinction between superficial (T2) or deep muscle invasion (T3a). Stage T4 includes locally advanced tumors that directly adhere to the pelvic or abdominal wall.[82]

Bladder cancer may be staged clinically (TNM) or pathologically (pTNM). Clinical staging is defined by the extent of tumor on physical examination, bimanual examination under general anesthesia before and after cystoscopic biopsy or transurethral resection, urine cytology, biochemical studies, and radiographic imaging. The upper urinary tract should be imaged with intravenous urography or contrast CT to rule out concurrent lesions. Muscle must be seen by the pathologist in a biopsy or transurethral resection for it to be an adequate indicator of prognosis. The cystoscopic examination includes documentation on a bladder diagram of tumor location, number of lesions, pattern of growth, and tumor size. A transurethral bladder resection (TURB) is diagnostic and often therapeutic in superficial lesions. Biopsy specimens of surrounding and apparently unaffected areas are taken because carcinoma in situ may be visibly indistinguishable from normal mucosa. Persistence of a palpable mass on examination under anesthesia after TURB identifies a poor prognostic group, usually with T3b disease.[85] Patients with muscle invasive disease require a screening workup for metastatic disease that includes chest radiography and computed tomography (CT) or magnetic resonance imaging (MRI) of the pelvis extending into the abdomen if there is pelvic nodal disease or abnormal results of liver biochemistry studies. Elevation of the serum alkaline phosphatase level or bone pain requires a bone scan to rule out metastases.[85,86]

Imaging with CT or MRI has an important role in defining the extent of disease for locally advanced bladder lesions. Mural and mucosal lesions are distinguishable from perivesical fat and urine, allowing visualization of papillary and extravesical lesions (Fig. 44-4). Important diagnostic information that can be demonstrated with CT is the presence of gross perivesical extension or lymphadenopathy.[87]

Although not always as available as CT, MRI has been suggested to be more accurate in staging bladder tumors.[88] Tachibana and coworkers[89] correlated imaging with histologic staging for 57 bladder tumors. The sensitivity and specificity for differentiating superficial and invasive tumor were 96% and 83% for gadolinium-enhanced MRI, 96% and 58% for CT, and 88% and 67% for transurethral ultrasonography. The contrast between tumor and fat is critical for evaluating locally advanced lesions and is best detected on T1-weighted images. It is important to recognize in the post-treatment

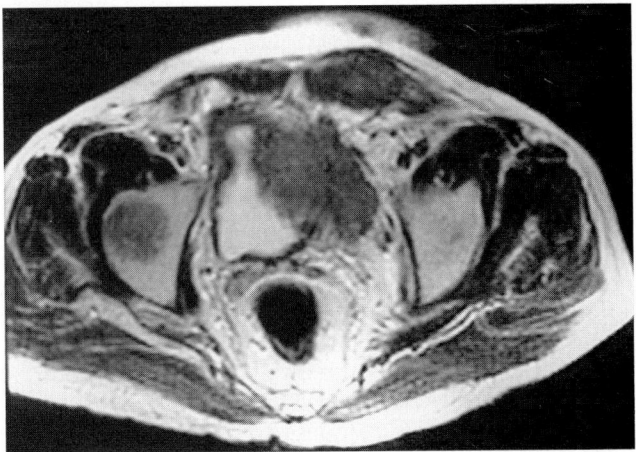

Figure 44–4. Axial *T1*-weighted images demonstrate a large left-sided bladder mass with extravesical extension into the perivesical fat. Axial *T2*-weighted images show the mass to be of intermediate signal intensity, but darker than the urine-filled bladder and displacing it to the right.

management of the patient that changes in signal intensity of normal bladder wall 3 to 4 months after irradiation limit the usefulness of MRI in detecting tumor recurrences.[90] Reports indicate improved accuracy in staging muscle invasive tumors when MRI is performed with gadolinium-enhanced images. Tanimoto and associates[91] showed that for 86 tumors, MRI with gadolinium enhancement had a staging accuracy of 85%, in comparison with 55% for CT scan and 58% for conventional MRI. Detection of superficial lesions was improved and there was a decrease in the overstaging of T1 tumors. Sensitivity and specificity of MRI for staging bladder tumors have been improved with the advent of imaging with oblique planes, smaller pixel size, and three-dimensional (3D) technology. Applying 3D technology to MRI was associated with improved accuracy of local staging from 78% to 93% and nodal staging from 86% to 93%.[90,92,93] The detection of nodal involvement with clinical staging has obvious treatment planning implications for the radiation oncologist. One report from the Christie Hospital in the United Kingdom demonstrated that preradiotherapy staging with MRI was helpful in providing more anatomic detail and clarifying the extent of disease. In that series, 39 of 71 patients with clinical T2a tumors were upstaged. Among the 27 patients in that series upstaged to T3b, this group experienced a significantly worse local control and overall survival outcomes. A multivariate analysis demonstrated that among other variables, the tumor stage based on the MRI was a significant factor predicting for treatment failure and overall survival.[94]

Pathologic staging requires either a partial or total cystectomy and lymph node dissection. Suspected metastatic disease on imaging studies can often be confirmed by CT-guided biopsies. Staging error between clinical and pathologic stages has been shown to be as high as 50%.[82] Survival is lower for each stage when grouped clinically as opposed to pathologically. It is for this reason that comparing outcome of radiotherapy series based on clinical staging with surgical series based on pathologic staging is fraught with difficulties. Nevertheless, with both modalities, survival decreases with increasing stage. This provides the clinician with the necessary prognostic information to formulate a treatment approach.[85]

Identification of prognostic factors allows the clinician to select those patients who would potentially benefit from bladder conservation approaches. Advanced-stage disease has been shown to be an accurate predictor for a high risk of developing early distant metastases.[86] In addition to the depth of invasion and the presence or absence of nodal involvement reflected in the stage, other prognostic variables have been defined. Low-grade and papillary growth have been shown to represent good prognostic indicators for survival.[95] Tumors characterized as larger than 5 cm, with associated carcinoma in situ, with evidence of vascular invasion, and with failure to obtain a complete response to chemoradiation have been shown to have a poor outcome.[96] Researchers have indicated that a tumor with a high degree of angiogenesis may have a poorer prognosis.[69] It is likely that in the future prognostic factors will be increasingly identified at the cytogenetic level.

TREATMENT OF SUPERFICIAL BLADDER CARCINOMA

Three fourths of bladder carcinomas present as Ta, T1, or Tis superficial lesions that do not extend farther than the lamina propria. Although the majority of such tumors are controlled by transurethral resection, more than 30% may recur. Prognostic factors for recurrence include grade, depth of penetration, multifocality, and presence of carcinoma in situ. The management of superficial bladder carcinoma involves TURB and, in many cases, adjuvant therapy to prevent recurrence and potential development of muscle invasive disease.[80,97,98]

Low-grade Ta papillary lesions without multifocality and without associated carcinoma in situ can be treated with a diagnostic and therapeutic resection using a resectoscope, followed by close monitoring including repeat cystoscopies. Muscle must be seen in this specimen before ruling out invasive disease. For patients with persistent tumor cells on urine cytology after TURB, multifocal lesions, grades II or III histology, or evidence of carcinoma in situ, adjuvant intravesical therapy is indicated. If all visualized superficial lesions are not excised, there is also a need for further therapy. Adjuvant therapy is given in the form of intravesical administration of immunotherapy or chemotherapy. Bacillus Calmette-Guérin (BCG) is administered adjuvantly weekly for 6 weeks. The chemotherapeutic agents of greatest known efficacy are mitomycin C, doxorubicin, and thiotepa. These three agents have all demonstrated efficacy in the reduction of disease recurrence.[98] Thiotepa causes the most systemic toxicity, including myelosuppression in 20% of patients owing to its low molecular weight, which allows absorption. Doxorubicin creates the greatest local reaction, which may predispose the patient to urinary urgency. The three drugs have nearly identical efficacy in prolonging the time to recurrence.[80]

A randomized trial of intravesical doxorubicin versus BCG in 262 patients with superficial transitional cell carcinoma showed an advantage in the complete response and 5-year disease-free survival rates for those treated with adjuvant BCG.[80] A classic series of 86 patients with recurrent superficial bladder cancer prospectively randomized to TURB plus BCG or TURB alone was reported by Herr and colleagues.[99] Patients treated with BCG had a prolonged median disease-free interval of 24 months compared with 8 months for those patients treated with TURB alone.[99] An update of the data has revealed a 10-year disease-specific survival rate of 75% in the group that received TURB plus BCG compared with 55% in those treated with TURB alone. The majority of recurrences were discovered within the first 5 years. Of the 61 patients who received BCG, 33 (54%) were disease free with their bladders preserved.[100,101]

In a recent of review of 11 clinical trials consisting of 2749 patients treated with BCG or mitomycin C, a greater incidence of tumor recurrence was observed for patients treated with mitomycin C compared to BCG (46% vs. 36%, respectively). This review also demonstrated improved results with BCG maintenance therapy for reducing the risk of tumor recurrence. The incidence of associated cystitis related to intravesical therapy was more prevalent, however, among BCG treated patients (54% vs. 39%, respectively).[102]

The standard of care for superficial bladder cancer with a high risk of recurrence has been established as intravesical BCG. Histologic persistence after 6 months indicates the need to change the intravesicular agent. Disease beyond 1 year indicates the need for a different treatment approach to prevent progression to muscle invasive cancer. Investigators are testing the application of interferon alpha.[98,103] The role of external-beam radiation in the treatment of carcinoma in situ is unclear. Especially among patients previously treated with multiple resections and intravesical therapy, the tolerance of external irradiation may be poor because of the preexisting chronic irritation within the bladder mucosa. Van der Werf-Messing and Hop[104] have reported excellent control rates (>90%) for limited T1 tumors using interstitial therapy through an open cystotomy approach. In that report, interstitial radium-226 was used with an intended dose of 60 Gy delivered to the visualized bladder tumor. This approach, however, is generally not used in the United States. Patients with persistent carcinoma in situ or refractory Ta/T1 disease ultimately require cystectomy.

SURGICAL TREATMENT OF MUSCLE INVASIVE BLADDER CANCER

The current standard of care for muscle invasive bladder cancer in the United States is radical cystectomy. The use of neoadjuvant or adjuvant chemotherapy is investigational. In the United Kingdom and Europe the prevailing primary treatment is definitive external-beam radiation therapy with the option of salvage cystectomy.

Radical cystectomy in the male implies the en bloc removal of the bladder (with its peritoneal covering), perivesical adipose tissue, lower ureters, prostate gland and seminal vesicles, pelvic vas deferens, proximal urethra, and pelvic lymph nodes (Fig. 44-5). A total urethrectomy is performed for patients with carcinoma in

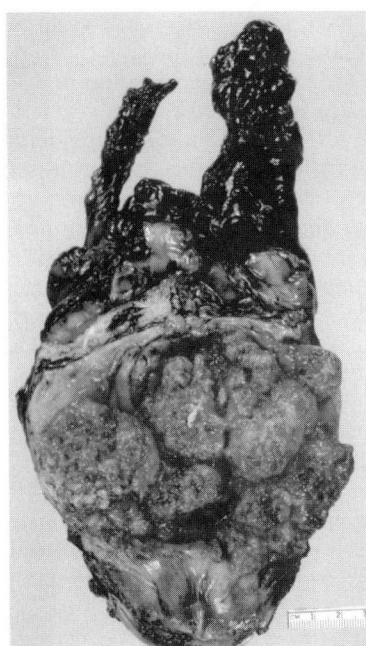

Figure 44–5. Multifocal bladder tumor with papillary growth patterns. The cystectomy specimen includes en bloc removal of the bladder, lower ureters, prostate, seminal vesicles, proximal urethra, and pelvic lymph nodes.

situ, multicentric tumors, and involvement of the bladder neck or prostatic urethra. A radical cystectomy in female patients is an anterior exenteration with sacrifice of the bladder (with its peritoneal covering), entire urethra, uterus, fallopian tubes, ovaries, anterior vaginal wall, and pelvic lymph nodes. A bilateral pelvic lymph node dissection encompasses the common iliac, external iliac, hypogastric, and obturator nodes. The dissection extends from the aortic bifurcation superiorly to the inguinal ligament and node of Cloquet inferiorly and the genitofemoral nerve laterally.[105,106]

Herr recently reported on the prognostic impact of nodal status in 637 patients who underwent radical cystectomy and pelvic lymph node dissection.[107] For both node-negative and node-positive patients, improved survival and reduced local recurrence related to negative surgical margins correlated with the number of lymph nodes removed at the time of the node dissection. The 5-year survival rates for patients who had 0 to 5, 6 to 10, 11 to 14, and more than 14 lymph nodes removed were 79%, 73%, 44%, and 33%, respectively. The corresponding local relapse rates in these aforementioned nodal groups were 4%, 7%, 8.5%, and 17%. A multivariate analysis demonstrated that the number of nodes removed was an independent predictor of survival outcome.

Attempts to reduce the morbidity of radical cystectomy have focused on preserving potency in the male and developing urinary diversion alternatives that maximize continence and cosmesis. A nerve-sparing radical cystectomy requires preservation of the neurovascular bundles and the dorsal-venous complex surrounded by the lateral prostatic fascia located posterolateral to the prostatic capsule and membranous urethra.[106,108]

There are two types of urinary diversions after cystectomy. The standard urinary diversion, an incontinent diversion, is accomplished with a conduit derived from 15 cm of distal ileum to which the ureters are anastomosed. An ostomy is created by attachment of the distal end of the ileum to the defect in the anterior abdominal wall.[106] More recently, a second type of urinary diversion, the creation of *neobladders*, has become available to allow the patient to retain continence. Two classes of alternative diversions of the urinary flow are stomal reservoirs that require intermittent catheterization and orthotopic reservoirs that connect neobladders to the remaining distal male urethra. Patients must be carefully chosen for the orthotopic reservoirs to avoid incontinence, particularly during sleep. The three techniques of creating a neobladder with a stoma that can be catheterized are the cecoappendicostomy, the cecoileostomy (Indiana pouch), and the ileostomy (Kock pouch). All involve constructing a detubularized pouch from intestine that becomes a spherical neobladder with a constructed sphincter to maintain continence. The most popular technique is the Kock pouch with improved continence by adaptations in the stoma suggested by Skinner. By 3 to 4 months the average catheterization interval is decreased to 6 to 8 hours. Nevertheless, the pouch is associated with a 2% mortality, a 5% incidence of serious complications, and a reoperative rate of 30%. For this reason the majority of patients who undergo cystectomy still require urinary diversion through an ileal conduit.[106]

Five-year survival rates for early-stage T2 tumors were often reported to be as low as 17% to 36% before 1980. Patients with stage T3a and T3b tumors had 5-year rates ranging from 18% to 31% and 20% to 25%, respectively. However, more recent studies of cystectomy using modern surgical techniques report survival rates as high as 50% to 88% for T2, 36% to 69% for T3a, and 11% to 47% for T3b tumors.[105,109] The overall local control rates with radical cystectomy alone have been reported to be as high as 95%[110,111]; however, in particular, patients with locally advanced-stage disease treated with radical cystectomy alone do not fare as well. In one study reported by Greven and associates,[112] 39% of patients with clinical stage T3 disease failed locally. Similarly, other investigators reported that the likelihood of local failure at 5 years for patients with T3b lesions was approximately 30%.[113]

In an effort to improve the outcome for patients with locally advanced bladder cancers treated with surgery, preoperative radiotherapy was commonly used from 1960 to 1980. The rationale for using this neoadjuvant irradiation was to reduce the incidence of tumor bed failures and potential seeding of malignant cells from the operation. Although some retrospective studies have suggested that the addition of preoperative radiotherapy improves the overall outcome,[114,115] other series have found no benefit when results are compared with modern surgical series.[116-118] Several randomized prospective trials that compared preoperative radiotherapy plus radical cystectomy to radical cystectomy alone have demonstrated no significant differences between the treatment arms.[119-121] Nevertheless, it must be pointed out that these trials were performed before the improvement in surgical techniques and suffered as well from limited accrual, compromising their power to detect significant differences between the study arms. A review from the M.D. Anderson Hospital supports the notion that preoperative irradiation improves the outcome in a select cohort of patients.[122] In this report, 338 patients treated with preoperative radiotherapy between 1960 and 1983 were retrospectively compared with 232 patients treated at the same institution between 1985 and 1990. The majority of the latter group were treated with neoadjuvant or adjuvant chemotherapy. Despite this apparent advantage, there was a significant improvement in local control among patients with T3b disease who received preoperative irradiation. Within this cohort of patients, there was a trend for improved disease-free survival and overall survival, although no significant differences were seen. The use of preoperative radiotherapy remains unclear, and at this time radical cystectomy alone remains the standard of care for patients who are surgical candidates.

DEFINITIVE RADIOTHERAPY FOR MUSCLE INVASIVE BLADDER CANCER

There are no modern prospective randomized studies comparing definitive irradiation with surgery. Patients offered definitive irradiation are usually nonsurgical candidates with poorer prognoses than those selected for surgery. Comparison of cystectomy to radiotherapy series must be interpreted with the understanding of inherent selection bias and stage migration differences between these groups of patients as well as the differences in overall performance status. External-beam radiotherapy is, however, often first-line therapy in Great Britain and Europe, with salvage cystectomy reserved for treatment failures.

The 5-year survival rate for muscle invasive bladder cancer treated with definitive external-beam radiotherapy is 20% to 40%. Most series report complete response rates of approximately 50%. Although often staged clinically, survival rates have been higher in patients with invasion limited to the bladder compared with those with extravesical (T3b or T4) disease.[110,123,124] Analysis of clinical characteristics has defined several prognostic factors that predict for local control, freedom from metastasis, and survival in patients treated with definitive irradiation. Most series show that depth of tumor invasion defined by stage is an important prognostic indicator.[113,124-126] Patients with stage T4 disease have been shown to have 5-year survival rates often lower than 10%, indicating irradiation alone is likely to benefit only a minority of those with advanced disease. In addition to advanced T stage, other poor prognostic signs include tumors greater than 5 cm, residual disease after TURB, and radiographic evidence of ureteral obstruction with hydronephrosis.[126] A multivariate analysis of 116 patients treated at Fox Chase Cancer Center showed that both local control and survival were dependent on the pretreatment clinical T stage and hemoglobin levels.[113] Grade was also shown to influence prognosis, with a 5-year survival of 43% in patients with grade I or II carcinoma versus 27% in those with grade III or IV histology.[113] Patients with a papillary or mixed tumor

morphology have been shown to have higher local control rates and survival than those with solid lesions.[127] A report from M.D. Anderson Hospital of 135 patients, of whom the majority underwent an attempt at complete transurethral resection of tumor before definitive irradiation, indicated the importance of a cystoscopically verified complete response 2 to 6 months after the completion of therapy.[128] Multivariate analysis showed that a clinically complete response was the most important independent prognostic factor for survival and local pelvic control.[128,129] A study from Scotland of 333 patients with stage T3 disease confirmed the correlation of a documented complete response to improved survival.[129] The presence or absence of histologic evidence of vascular invasion has not been shown to influence prognosis in the majority of series.[113,125,126]

In an effort to improve local control rates with external-beam radiotherapy for patients with invasive bladder cancers, hyperfractionated treatment schedules have been used.[114,123,130-132] Edsmyr and coworkers[131] reported a Swedish trial of 168 patients with T2 to T4 disease randomly assigned to receive either 1 Gy three times a day to a total of 84 Gy or 2 Gy once a day to a total of 64 Gy. Both regimens were given over 8 weeks, with an imposed mid-course 2-week treatment interruption. The 5-year survival for the group receiving 84 Gy was 37%, and for those receiving 64 Gy it was 16%.[123] Patients with T3 disease particularly appeared to benefit from the hyperfractionated schedule. An update with a follow-up period of at least 10 years shows the benefit in survival for the entire group, and specifically for those with T3 lesions, has persisted. A study in Great Britain has tested an accelerated hyperfractionated regimen in 24 patients with muscle invasive bladder cancer.[114] Over a 22-day period, patients received doses of 1.8 to 2.0 Gy per fraction to total doses of 54 to 64 Gy to the bladder and 39.6 to 44 Gy to the whole pelvis. Local control was 56%, and survival was 35% at 2 years. However, acute toxicity included a patient with an intestinal obstruction requiring a colostomy and a treatment-related death. Treatment with accelerated and hyperfractionated schedules remains investigational and should be conducted in a protocol setting.

Radiotherapy is generally well tolerated; most patients experience dysuria, urgency, urinary frequency, and diarrhea as acute self-limiting symptoms. The incidence of long-term complications is acceptable when proper treatment techniques are used. In general, such complications become clinically manifest within the first 3 years after radiotherapy. Shipley reported an 11% incidence of chronic grade III to IV genitourinary complications among 35 patients with locally advanced bladder cancer treated with conventional fractionated therapy. A range of toxicities was reported in a series of 135 patients treated at M.D. Anderson Hospital between 1960 and 1984 in which the majority were treated to a dose of 40 to 50 Gy with a cone-down technique for a median total dose of 66 Gy.[128,129] Late complications included hematuria, bladder contracture, bladder and rectal ulceration, rectal stricture, and small bowel obstruction. Severe complications requiring surgery occurred in 12%. Analysis indicated that patients treated with a four-field technique versus arc rotation, higher energy machines as opposed to cobalt, and less than 70 Gy had a significantly lower rate of severe complications. A measurement of quality of bladder function on a more modern series of patients was performed by Lynch and colleagues[133] at the Royal London Hospital. The 72 patients who showed an initial complete response to radiotherapy for muscle invasive bladder cancer were assessed for hematuria, frequency, incontinence, and rectal symptoms. The bowel and bladder symptomatology scores were found to be similar to a group of 55 inpatients in other surgical wards who did not have a history of urinary or bowel disease. Cox and coworkers[123] reported the results of a phase I study in which patients were treated with 1.2 Gy fractions twice daily to a cumulative dose of 60 to 69.6 Gy. Treatment was well tolerated, whereas the incidence of grade III or IV late toxicity was 11% for patients treated at the highest dose level. Most recently, investigators from the Massachusetts General Hospital reported the results of a retrospective quality of life evaluation performed on 21 women who underwent bladder preservation therapy for invasive bladder cancer.[134] Nineteen of 21 patients reported no change or improvement of their baseline bladder capacity and function. No patient reported any symptoms of bowel incontinence. With the advent of new imaging modalities and 3D conformal treatment planning technologies that allow for enhanced accuracy of radiation delivery and further limit the volume of normal organs exposed to the doses of therapy, improved results are likely with a further reduction in treatment-related toxicity.

BLADDER PRESERVATION THERAPY

Several reports now substantiate the efficacy of combined chemotherapy and radiotherapy as an organ preservation alternative for patients with localized transitional cell carcinoma of the bladder.[135-144] The preliminary results suggest that this chemoradiation approach provides comparable survivorship to that expected for similar patients treated with radical cystectomy with a high rate of bladder preservation. The success of this treatment approach is predicated on the meticulous selection of patients with known favorable prognostic factors that are associated with improved response rates. This section summarizes the experience with combined modality therapy and discusses current trials that attempt to further explore this approach.

One of the earliest reports using combined modality therapy as a means for bladder preservation was conducted by the National Bladder Cancer Cooperative Group.[143] Seventy patients with T2 to T4 bladder cancer were enrolled in a prospective study, all with medical contraindications for radical cystectomy. Cisplatin was given at a dose of 70 mg/m² every 3 weeks concurrent with external-beam radiotherapy to a total dose of 64.8 Gy. Initially, 45 Gy of radiation was directed to the entire bladder, perivesicular tissues, and adjacent lymph nodes using a four-field plan. This was followed by a boost to the tumor within the bladder for an additional 19.8 Gy in 11 fractions delivered in 2 weeks. The overall complete

response rate was 70%, and the 4-year survival among the complete responders to therapy was 57%, compared with 11% among patients who did not achieve a complete response.

These highly encouraging results were the impetus for a phase II chemoradiation bladder preservation study for patients with localized bladder cancer who were otherwise eligible for radical cystectomy.[144] In this study, transurethral resection was incorporated as a critical component in the treatment regimen based on several reports indicating higher complete response rates in irradiated patients who underwent this procedure as a debulking maneuver before therapy. Frequent cystoscopic evaluations were performed throughout the therapy to further assess the response as a means of selecting the most optimal patients for this treatment approach. Fifty-three patients were enrolled in this study, of whom 15 had clinical T2, 29 had T3, and 9 had T4 disease. Treatment consisted of a transurethral resection followed by two cycles of neoadjuvant methotrexate, cisplatin, and vinblastine and then 45 Gy to the pelvis with two concomitant doses of cisplatin. The 36 patients with a complete response at 40 Gy (as demonstrated by repeat urologic examination including cystoscopy, examination under anesthesia, and urine cytology) were allowed to complete the pelvic radiation and proceed to a 24.8 Gy tumor boost with a final dose of cisplatin. Radical cystectomy was performed for 15 patients who could not tolerate the combined chemoradiation, had an incomplete response at the repeat urologic evaluation, or required salvage after completion of the entire treatment plan. This study demonstrated that a multimodality approach resulted in a 5-year survival rate of 48%, comparable to the expected outcome after radical cystectomy based on historic controls. There were no major complications involving the bladder or rectum, with only two patients experiencing intermittent hematuria. Toxicity associated with chemotherapy included nausea and vomiting (73%), stomatitis (24%), and diarrhea (10%). A 58% rate of bladder conservation was achieved at median follow-up of 48 months without an apparent compromise in survival. Of 27 patients who were complete responders after neoadjuvant chemotherapy and 40 Gy of radiation, 81% maintained a normal, functioning bladder.[144] Similar findings have been reported for Radiation Therapy Oncology Group (RTOG) protocol 85-12, which used the same concurrent cisplatin-radiation regimen. Complete response to therapy was observed in 66% of patients. At 3 years the survival rate was 64%, with 40% of evaluable patients achieving bladder preservation.[135]

Shipley et al.[136] recently updated the results of 190 patients treated on various institutional protocols with a combined modality bladder preservation approach. With a median follow-up time of 6.7 years, the 5- and 10-year overall survival rates were 54% and 36%, respectively. For patients with clinically staged T2 disease, the 5- and 10-year survival rates were 62% and 41%, respectively. For patients with clinically staged T3 to T4 disease, the 5- and 10-year survival rates were 47% and 31%, respectively. Disease-free survival outcome with an intact bladder was also excellent in this group of selected patients. The 5- and 10-year disease-free survival rates with an

Table 44–2   Bladder Conservation Trials

Reference	Patients, n	Total/Dose, Gy	Chemotherapeutic Regimen	Patients in Clinical Remission, n (%)	Patients with Organ Intact, n (%)	Patients alive, % (y)
Shipley[136]	53	64.8	MCV	28 (53)	20 (38)	45 (5)
Dunst*†	245	56	Cisplatin or CARBO	—	98 (40)	47 (5)
Housset[139]*	54	44	5-FU + cisplatin	40 (74)	—	59 (3)
Tester[135]	48	64	Cisplatin	31 (66)	—	64 (3)
Cervek[137]*	47	66	MCV	28 (62)	24 (53) 2 y	73 (2)
Rotman[141]	20	65	5FT ± mitomycin C	14 (74)	—	39 (5)
Eapen*‡	25	60	Cisplatin IA	23 (96)	1.5 y	90 (2)
Vikram[142]	21	60	MVAC	16 (89)	15 (71)	60 (3)
Sumiyoshi[140]*	60	24	Adriamycin IA	36 (60)	—	49 (5)

*A transurethral resection was done before chemoradiation.
†From Dunst J, Saver R, Schrott KM, et al: Organ-sparing treatment of advanced bladder cancer: A 10-year experience. *Int J Radiat Oncol Biol Phys:* 1994;30:261.
‡From Eapen L, Stewart D, Danjoux C, et al: Intraarterial cisplatin and concurrent radiation for locally advanced bladder cancer. *J Clin Oncol:* 1989 Feb; 7(2):230-235.
CARBO, carboplatin; 5-FU, 5-fluorouracil; IA, intra-arterially; MCV, methotrexate, cisplatin, vinblastine; MVAC, methotrexate, vinblastine, doxorubicin (Adriamycin), cisplatin.

intact bladder were 57% and 50%, respectively. For patients with clinically staged T3 to T4 disease, the 5- and 10-year disease-free survival with an intact bladder rates were 35% and 34%, respectively. Bladder contractures requiring cystectomy were not observed in these patients.

Additional phase II studies and retrospective reports of patients with invasive bladder cancer treated conservatively with combined modality therapy have been reported (Table 44-2). Cervek and colleagues[137] reported a series from Ljubljana in which 47 patients were treated with three to four cycles of methotrexate, vinblastine, and cisplatin after a transurethral resection.[137] Patients with a complete response to chemotherapy were selected for bladder preservation with radiation. The responses were higher in those with T2/T3 compared with T4 tumors, and with a preliminary report at a median follow-up of 23 months, 68% had bladders preserved.

The largest series of patients treated with a combined modality approach has been recently reported by Rodel and colleagues at the University of Erlangen.[138] In that report, 289 patients were treated with locally advanced tumors with transurethral resection, simultaneous cisplatin, and pelvic radiotherapy plus a tumor boost for a cumulative dose of 54 Gy. Chemotherapy was administered during the first and fifth week of radiotherapy and consisted of cisplatin 25 mg/m^2 daily for 5 days. Carboplatin was used for those patients with creatinine clearance less than 60 mL per minute or congestive heart disease. In 68% the full dose chemotherapy was able to be administered, while in 32% the doses needed to be curtailed secondary to hematologic toxicity, gastrointestinal toxicity, or nephrotoxicity. For this treatment program, a re-staging TURB was performed 6 weeks after completion of radiotherapy. Patients who had a complete response were followed while those with residual disease were advised to undergo a salvage cystectomy. The median follow-up in the study was 60 months. The complete response (CR) rates at the 6 week re-staging

TURB for patients treated with RT in combination with cisplatin and 5-fluorouracil (5-FU), cisplatin alone, and carboplatin was 87%, 82%, and 66% respectively. The rates of response were significantly higher than the CR rate (61%) observed among 126 patients who were treated with radiotherapy alone (*P* = 0.001). Among all patients who achieved a CR, the 10-year local control rate was 64%. The overall likelihoods of distant metastases development and disease-specific survival were 35% and 42%, respectively, at 10 years. Eighty percent of long-term surviving patients maintained a functioning bladder, and cystectomy was only required in 2% of patients secondary to a contracted bladder after radiotherapy. In a multivariate analysis, early tumor stage and the performance of a complete TURB before radiochemotherapy were predictors of a higher complete response rate and improved overall survival. The 5-year survival rates among patients who had a complete TURB, microscopic residual disease, and gross residual disease after resection were 76%, 52%, and 34%, respectively (Fig. 44-6). The data also suggested that adjuvant radiotherapy is of benefit even among selected patients who

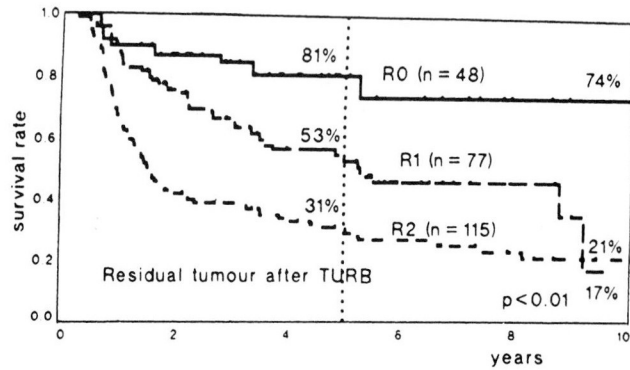

Figure 44–6. Data from the University of Erlangen demonstrating the impact of having a complete transurethral resection among patients treated with chemoradiation.

had complete TURB. In this latter group, the incidence of bladder preservation was 85%, compared with 75% reported by Herr[145] for highly selected patients with muscle invasive tumors treated with TURB alone.

The efficacy of the chemoradiation approach in eradicating disease has been corroborated by pathologic documentation of tumor clearance after therapy. Investigators from the University of Paris reported on 54 patients with stage T2 to T4 operable, invasive bladder cancer treated with TURB, neoadjuvant cisplatin and 5-FU, and hyperfractionated split-course pelvic irradiation.[139] Cystoscopy was performed 6 weeks after completion of treatment. Patients who had persistent disease underwent cystectomy, and those with complete responses were treated with additional chemoradiation or cystectomy. Forty of 54 (74%) were classified as complete responders after initial therapy. The 3-year overall disease-free survival rate was 77% for complete responders, compared with 21% for nonresponders. Most interestingly, among the 18 complete responders who underwent planned surgery after chemoradiation, no residual tumor was found in the cystectomy specimens in all cases. As in the Erlangen study, preserved bladders remained functional and no chronic treatment sequelae (i.e., contracted bladder, chronic cystitis, or small bowel obstruction) were observed.

Identification of prognostic factors is important for the selection of patients who are most likely to benefit from this multimodality approach. The Massachusetts General Hospital group analyzed clinicopathologic characteristics in 40 patients treated with their combined modality bladder preservation program.[97] Based on a multivariate analysis, tumor stage and absence of carcinoma in situ were significant predictors of complete response. Failure to obtain a complete response to therapy was strongly predictive of distant metastatic development and a short survival duration. For this reason, repeat cystoscopy to evaluate for complete response has been routinely incorporated into bladder preservation treatment programs to select out, before completion of chemoradiation, those patients likely to suffer recurrence. High-risk patients should proceed directly to cystectomy without the added toxicity that would result from completion of the chemoradiation therapy.

The optimal chemotherapy regimen and the sequencing of radiation to maximize bladder preservation rates while minimizing toxicity are not defined. One of the most potent single agents in bladder cancer is cisplatin, which is also an attractive drug to use for bladder preservation therapy because of its radiation-enhancing properties. In patients with advanced/metastatic bladder cancer, results of randomized trials have demonstrated superior response rates with combination regimens such as cisplatin, methotrexate, and vinblastine (CMV) or methotrexate, vinblastine, doxorubicin (Adriamycin), and cisplatin (MVAC) compared with cisplatin alone, although the survival rates were not significantly improved with more therapy.[146-148] As noted earlier, excellent responses have also been reported with cisplatin and 5-FU in combination with radiotherapy for patients with muscle invasive disease.[139] Limited data employing alternative drug regimens and route of delivery are described in the bladder conservation literature. Rotman and colleagues have used 5-FU infusion alone concurrent with irradiation and reported excellent long-term bladder preservation rates.[141] In a larger Japanese study with 60 patients, 60% achieved a complete response with TURB, intra-arterial doxorubicin, and irradiation.[140] A femoral artery catheter delivered three doses of doxorubicin within 48 hours in 3- to 4-week intervals for four cycles. Pelvic radiation was 6 Gy in three fractions per chemotherapy cycle. Tumor stage, size, and grade significantly predicted response.

The optimal sequence and integration of chemotherapy with radiotherapy is also not established. The RTOG has completed a phase III trial that randomly assigned patients to a neoadjuvant CMV regimen for two cycles followed by the bladder preservation regimen compared with concurrent cisplatin and radiotherapy without neoadjuvant chemotherapy. The results of this study are not yet available. Preliminary results of alternate fractionation schedules of radiotherapy have been reported by Vikram and colleagues.[142] In their report, 21 patients with T2 or T3 disease were treated with three cycles of MVAC, rapidly alternating with three cycles of accelerated irradiation. Three cycles of twice-a-day irradiation of 20 Gy in 10 fractions was administered with the first two cycles to the true pelvis and the last with a cone-down approach. At a median follow-up of 2 years, the observed survival rate is 72%, with normal bladder function in 84% of evaluable patients.

Bladder preservation accomplished with combined modality therapy is an acceptable treatment option for selected patients with muscle invasive bladder cancer. Critics of this approach have raised concerns about the possible risks of a greater number of deaths associated with this treatment program compared to patients treated with up-front cystectomy. However, there is no evidence that there is any diminution in survival rates from any of the published studies among patients who underwent radiotherapy and subsequently required a salvage cystectomy. Although concerns have also been raised regarding the extended treatment time and morbidity associated with combined modality chemotherapy, these are unfounded as the long-term toxicity outcomes have been minimal. Indeed, there appears to be great potential for integrating conformal-based treatment delivery approaches such as 3D conformal radiotherapy and intensity modulated radiotherapy for dose escalation trials in the future. While improved continent diversion techniques such as the use of neo-bladders are available for patients undergoing surgery, quality of life studies have demonstrated superior satisfaction when patients can maintain their own bladders. Nevertheless, combined modality radiotherapy-chemotherapy programs require very careful patient selection, and only those patients who demonstrate a complete response to initial therapy are the optimal candidates to complete the treatment program as they have a high likelihood of bladder preservation without compromise of their survival.

Best results are achieved when the tumor burden is completely reduced with aggressive TURB and when cisplatin-based chemotherapy is used. Because patients with initial complete responses are more likely to have durable local control rates, careful selection based on prognostic factors and frequent evaluations in conjunction with the urologist and medical oncologist are critical to increase the likelihood of preserving bladder function without compromising survival rates.

SIMULATION AND TREATMENT

During simulation and treatment, the patient is supine and the bladder is emptied to ensure reproducibility. At the time of simulation, a Foley catheter is inserted and 25 to 30 mL of radiopaque contrast material is instilled in addition to 10 to 15 mL of air for bladder visualization. A rectal tube with barium contrast medium is placed to visualize the rectum. In general, a four-field box approach is used (anterior, posterior, and lateral fields) delivered through 15- to 25-MV x-rays. The initial fields encompass the entire bladder and the first echelon draining lymph nodes. The superior border of the anterior-posterior–posterior-anterior fields is the L5 to S1 interspace; however, especially among patients treated with combined modality therapy, the true pelvic inlet can be used to minimize potential morbidity of therapy. The inferior border of these fields is at the level of the bottom of the obturator foramina, and the lateral fields generally extend 2 cm beyond the bony pelvic side walls. The anterior border of the lateral fields can be recognized as the air bubble and should be included with a 2 to 3 cm margin. Often, the anterior border may extend several centimeters beyond the symphysis pubis. The posterior border of the lateral fields can be placed with a 2 to 3 cm margin posterior to the bladder, which will incorporate the presacral lymph nodes.

To properly plan the boost portion of therapy, which is limited to the involved area within the bladder, the radiation oncologist will need to know the location of the tumor based on the pretreatment cystoscopy and findings from the examination under anesthesia. A treatment planning CT scan can be obtained and a multifield technique can be used that minimizes the volume of normal bladder exposed to the prescription radiation dose. In some cases based on the location of the bladder tumor (i.e., limited to the dome or anterior-posterior wall), lateral fields alone may be sufficient for this phase of the

therapy. More recently, the authors have incorporated 3D treatment planning for planning the cone-down phase of therapy (Fig. 44-7). A multifield plan can be used in an effort to minimize the dose to uninvolved regions of the bladder as well as other normal tissue structures such as the rectum, bowel, and femoral heads. Care must be taken to assure similar degrees of bladder filling during the planning process and during treatment. Ultrasound verification is advised.

Treatment is initiated with four fields delivering daily 1.8-Gy fractions five times a week for a total dose of 45 Gy. At this dose the 3D plan is initiated for the cone-down approach and is directed to the tumor-containing normal bladder. The total dose is brought to 64.8 Gy using daily 1.8-Gy fractions.

BRACHYTHERAPY

Although the experience with brachytherapy for localized bladder cancer has been a limited one in the United States, an extensive experience with radium needle implants has been reported by Van der Werf-Messing and colleagues from Rotterdam.[149] Three hundred and twenty-eight patients with T2 disease and 63 patients with T3 muscle invasive bladder cancer were treated with preoperative radiation of three fractions each at a dose of 3.5 Gy followed by radium implantation. Local recurrence at 5 years was 16% for T2 tumors and 28% for T3 tumors. Survival was similar to historic controls undergoing definitive external-beam radiotherapy or cystectomy, with 56% of patients with T2 disease and 37% of those with T3 disease alive at 5 years.

Other investigators have reported their experience with other isotopes, including cesium and iridium.[150-153] Mazeron[152] treated 30 patients with T2 disease and 5 with T3 disease using a single fraction of 8.5 Gy, followed by partial cystectomy and iridium implantation, and attained excellent local control. Rozan and colleagues[153] reported a multicenter French experience that included 98 pT1, 66 pT2, 26 pT3a, 9 pT3b, and 1 pT4 disease treated by preoperative external-beam irradiation, partial cystectomy with lymphadenectomy, and placement of an iridium implant into the tumor bed. Preoperative radiation was targeted to the bladder in 44 patients and to the

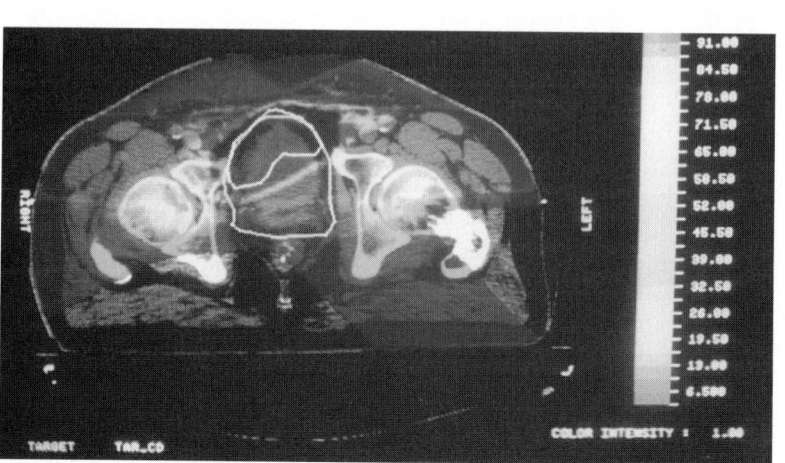

Figure 44–7. Three-dimensional conformal plan for the cone-down phase of therapy. Note the high-dose region confined to a small volume of bladder (site of known initial disease). See also Color Figure 44-7.

pelvis in 161 patients for a mean total dose of 11 Gy and a mean dose per fraction of 5.4 Gy. Of the 36 tumor recurrences, 9 were located at the original site and 19 occurred in a different site. They reported an overall 5-year survival of 67%. Survival was 77% for pT1, 63% for pT2, and 47% for pT3a disease. Serious complications included 8 patients with hematuria, 17 patients with chronic cystitis, and 11 with fistulas.

Neoadjuvant (Preoperative) and Adjuvant (Postoperative) Chemotherapy for Muscle Invasive Bladder Cancer

The majority (70%) of urothelial cancers are superficial, without invasion of the lamina propria or muscle.[154] Despite initially adequate treatment of superficial bladder cancers with transurethral endoscopic resection, up to 70% recur, with a third of these progressing to a higher grade or stage. Between 10% and 20% of superficial cancers will ultimately progress to muscle invasive bladder cancer despite aggressive resection.

Mortality rates with cystectomy alone for muscle invasive bladder cancer can be high. Survival in muscle invasive bladder cancer is a function of stage. The 5-year survival for patients with pathologically staged T2 (pT2) tumors is 60% to 75%. pT3 tumors are associated with a 36% to 58% five-year survival, and pT4 or node-positive tumors with a 4% to 30% five-year survival. This stage-dependent reduction in survival is believed to be due to the presence of micrometastases at the time of cystectomy. Thus, long-term survival depends on prevention of distant metastasis.

Bladder cancer is a chemotherapy-sensitive cancer. A wide variety of agents with varying mechanisms of action all have activity against bladder cancer. In metastatic disease, objective response proportions of 50% to 70%, and complete response rates of 20% to 30% have been reported (see later). This chemosensitivity provides the rationale for employing adjuvant and neoadjuvant chemotherapy in an effort to reduce the incidence of distant metastases to improve long-term survival. The success of adjuvant and neoadjuvant chemotherapy in other cancers to eradicate micrometastases has led to the application of these strategies in bladder cancer.

Neoadjuvant (preoperative) treatment offers the advantage of in vivo drug sensitivity testing, which may provide prognostic information. In addition, preoperative chemotherapy has the advantage of shrinking and downstaging tumors, potentially allowing for easier surgery and raising the potential of a bladder sparing approach. Furthermore, neoadjuvant chemotherapy delivers full dose systemic chemotherapy, with the intent of allowing early treatment of micrometastases and reducing the incidence of subsequent metastatic disease. Various preoperative (neoadjuvant) regimens have been evaluated in a number of prospective randomized trials. The Nordic Cystectomy I trial evaluated neoadjuvant chemotherapy in combination with low dose irradiation and cystectomy.[155] Patients with T1G3, T2-T4a NXM0 tumors were randomly assigned to either two cycles of chemotherapy with cisplatin and doxorubicin or no chemotherapy

before cystectomy. In addition, all patients in this study received radiotherapy (4 Gy/day × 5 days) following the second cycle of chemotherapy. Initial results appeared to show a benefit for neoadjuvant chemotherapy. However, longer follow-up failed to demonstrate a statistically significant difference in overall survival between the two groups (59% vs. 51%, $P = 0.1$).[156] Subgroup analysis also demonstrated no survival benefit for patients with T1 and T2 tumors, although patients with T3 and T4a tumors did show a 5-year survival benefit of 52% vs. 37% ($P = 0.03$).

The largest neoadjuvant trial to date was a European study involving more than 900 patients. Between 1989 and 1995, patients with T2 G3, T3, and T4a, N0 to NX, or M0 tumors were randomized to receive either three cycles of CMV (cisplatin, methotrexate, and vinblastine) neoadjuvant chemotherapy ($n = 491$) or no chemotherapy ($n = 485$) before planned cystectomy or definitive radiation therapy.[157] Chemotherapy mortality was 1% and cystectomy operative mortality was 3.7%. Although at 4 years no significant difference in overall survival was seen, after longer follow-up (median 7.4 years), a statistically significant 6% absolute survival benefit was found in favor of the chemotherapy-treated patients.[158] In addition, the rate of pathological CR was found to be dramatically higher in the primary tumors of chemotherapy-treated patients.

A similar, but smaller, randomized phase III trial of neoadjuvant MVAC plus cystectomy ($n = 153$) versus cystectomy alone ($n = 154$) was conducted by the U.S. Intergroup in patients with T2 to T4a N0M0 bladder cancer. After a median follow-up of 8.5 years, survival in the MVAC arm was marginally superior, with a hazard ratio of 0.74 (95% CI 0.55-0.99, $P = 0.06$). The estimated median survival of the MVAC arm was 77 months, while the no-MVAC arm was 46 months.[159] A recent meta-analysis of trials using cisplatin combination chemotherapy has shown that neoadjuvant therapy may provide a moderate benefit in patients with T2-T4a disease. Patients who received neoadjuvant combination chemotherapy experienced a 13% reduction in the risk of death (Hazard Ratio = .87 [CI = .78-.98]).[160]

Overall, data from phase II and III trials of neoadjuvant chemotherapy for bladder cancer suggest that the pT0 rate is about 30% to 40% in patients receiving neoadjuvant chemotherapy. Unfortunately, this pT0 rate has not translated into a dramatic survival advantage for neoadjuvant chemotherapy. Neoadjuvant chemotherapy is generally well tolerated, and does not appear to increase the rate of surgical complications. Regimens currently in use are tolerable and safe. Older regimens for neoadjuvant treatment (e.g., single-agent cisplatin, CISCA) have not been proven to reduce the risk of death. However, modern regimens (MVAC and CMV) have shown a potential modest improvement in survival (6%-15% at 5 years). More recently, in metastatic disease, the use of gemcitabine/cisplatin (GC) rather than MVAC has become common (see later), although GC has not yet been formally tested in the neoadjuvant or adjuvant setting. The preponderance of evidence demonstrates that neoadjuvant therapy is well tolerated, prolongs time to relapse, provides an overall modest survival benefit, and does not negatively impact on surgical complications. Neoadjuvant therapy achieves high rates of pathologic complete responses out of proportion to the clinical benefit, suggesting that distant metastasis is an early event in locally advanced bladder cancer which is only modestly impacted by chemotherapy. Use of less toxic regimens such as GC is gaining acceptance in the neoadjuvant setting as trials proceed.

In contrast to neoadjuvant chemotherapy, adjuvant (postoperative) chemotherapy allows for earlier cystectomy without the delay of preoperative chemotherapy, resulting in immediate local therapy and tumor debulking. In addition, risk stratification of patients based on pathological examination of cystectomy specimens can guide subsequent adjuvant treatment. Therefore, only higher-risk patients (T3-T4a or node positive) would be considered for chemotherapy.

Several prospective randomized trials have been undertaken to address whether adjuvant chemotherapy improves survival after cystectomy. An early trial using single-agent cisplatin was unable to detect any advantage for adjuvant therapy.[161] Subsequently, a prospective randomized trial using combination chemotherapy was undertaken in patients with pT3, pT4, or node-positive transitional cell carcinoma of the bladder. Between 1980 and 1988, 91 patients were randomly assigned to adjuvant chemotherapy or observation. CISCA (cisplatin, cyclophosphamide, and doxorubicin) was the predominant chemotherapy administered on this trial, although some patients received other chemotherapy agents and regimens. This trial showed a significant increase in time to progression (6.58 vs. 1.92 years, $P = 0.011$), although overall survival was not significantly different at 5 years. In retrospective subgroup analyses, patients with a single positive lymph node appeared to derive the most benefit from adjuvant chemotherapy. Interestingly, patients with two or more positive lymph nodes did not appear to benefit from adjuvant chemotherapy.[162] This study has been criticized for the lack of standard treatment, as well as failure to receive assigned therapy in a significant proportion of the patients.

In a study from Stanford University, 55 patients who underwent cystectomy and were found to have pT3 and T4 tumors with or without lymph node involvement were randomized to four cycles of CMV chemotherapy or observation. This study was halted early due to the observation of significant benefit in favor of patients receiving chemotherapy. With a median follow-up of 62 months, freedom from progression was superior in patients receiving adjuvant chemotherapy (37 vs. 12 months, $P = 0.01$). Patients who developed progressive disease and who had not received adjuvant therapy subsequently received systemic therapy, perhaps accounting for the fact that overall survival was not significantly improved by the use of adjuvant therapy.[163]

A third prospective randomized trial involved 49 patients with pT3b, pT4a, or pelvic lymph node involvement without any evidence of tumor remaining after cystectomy. These patients were randomized to three cycles of adjuvant MVAC or MVEC (methotrexate, vinblastine, epirubicin, cisplatin) (26 patients) or observation (23 patients). Only 18 of the 26 patients randomized to adjuvant

chemotherapy actually went on to receive adjuvant chemotherapy. The study was designed to show a 35% improvement in disease-free survival at 5 years. However, an interim analysis showed a significant increase in disease-free survival among patients in the chemotherapy arm, resulting in early stopping of the study. In intent-to-treat analysis, at 3.5 years, 63% of patients in the chemotherapy arm were disease-free, compared with 13% in the observation arm, in an intent-to-treat analysis. The benefit of adjuvant therapy appeared strongest for those patients whose lymph nodes were involved with cancer.[164]

Taken together, these studies demonstrate that in the appropriate patients (T3, T4, or node positive), adjuvant therapy appears to prolong time to progression and may potentially improve survival. The question of whether or not adjuvant chemotherapy confers an overall survival benefit remains unanswered. Chemotherapy administered at the time of relapse with metastatic disease is quite effective at salvaging patients. This may explain the apparent lack of efficacy of neoadjuvant and adjuvant strategies in improving overall survival. Studies are ongoing to evaluate early vs. delayed chemotherapy using MVAC, high dose MVAC, or GC.

CHEMOTHERAPY FOR METASTATIC DISEASE

Reported survival for patients with metastatic bladder cancer treated on chemotherapy trials varies widely. This wide variation can be explained by pretreatment disease and patient-related factors. In an effort to define the effect of pretreatment patient characteristics on clinical outcome, Bajorin and colleagues conducted a multivariate analysis evaluating 18 variables in 203 patients treated with MVAC. In this analysis, the only variables that were prognostic of survival were Karnofsky Performance Status (KPS) less than 80% and presence of visceral metastases. Patients with a KPS less than 80% and visceral metastases had a median survival of 9.3 months, compared with patients who had no adverse prognostic factors and whose median survival was 33 months.[165] An understanding of these prognostic features allows interpretation of outcomes reported in phase 2 clinical trials. Identification of additional pretreatment prognostic factors will allow more accurate identification of patients at high risk for death from their cancer.

Historically, MVAC had been considered the standard therapy for treating advanced bladder cancer patients. The efficacy of MVAC was first reported in 1989 when Sternberg and colleagues treated 121 patients with advanced urothelial tract cancers and demonstrated a 72% response rate.[166] MVAC was subsequently compared to single-agent cisplatin and shown to be superior in terms of response rate and overall survival in patients with advanced bladder cancer.[167] MVAC has also been compared to a previously used multi-agent regimen, CISCA (cisplatin, cyclophosphamide, doxorubicin). One hundred and ten patients were randomized to either MVAC or CISCA. MVAC was found to have both a higher objective response rate and a longer median survival.[168] Despite superior outcome with MVAC, significant limitations include its severe toxicity (mucositis, infectious complications, and a 3% toxic death rate are consistently seen in randomized trials). In addition, only a very small percentage of patients with metastatic bladder cancer have long-term disease-free survival (3.7% at 6 years).[167]

The GC regimen has largely replaced MVAC as the standard of care, based on a recently reported randomized trial comparing the two regimens.[169] Although the trial was not sufficiently powered to prove equivalence of GC to MVAC, this 405-patient trial showed similar antitumor efficacy (equal complete response rate and similar partial response rate) and a hazard ratio for survival approaching 1.0. An overall response proportion of around 50% was observed with either regimen. However, toxicity in GC-treated patients was substantially lower than observed in patients treated with MVAC, including a lower death rate, fewer infections, and less mucositis. This markedly superior therapeutic index has led to fairly wide acceptance of GC as the standard first-line therapy for metastatic bladder cancer.

Unfortunately, many patients with advanced transitional cell carcinoma have concurrent renal insufficiency and are unable to undergo therapy with cisplatin or other potentially nephrotoxic agents. Consequently, regimens with less nephrotoxic drugs have been developed. These have included single-agent treatments with non-nephrotoxic drugs such as the taxanes, gemcitabine, and carboplatin.[170-179] The median survival reported for patients with renal insufficiency (in predominantly single-institution studies) ranges from 8 to 10 months, and is generally inferior to the results of the large multicenter trial ($n = 405$) comparing GC to MVAC in patients with nonimpaired renal function, which found median survivals of 13.8 and 14.8 months, respectively.[169] Whether this is attributable to a fundamentally worse prognosis in patients with renal insufficiency or to the use of less effective regimens is not known. Frequently used combinations in metastatic transitional cell carcinoma patients with renal insufficiency include GC and carboplatin/paclitaxel.

New drug targets have been identified, and novel agents against these targets are currently being tested. These targets include EGFR, HER2, the proteasome, and vascular endothelial growth factor (VEGF) receptor, among others. Drugs that interfere with these targets have been designed, and clinical trials are ongoing. In addition, dose-dense regimens with different combinations of existing agents, such as AG-ITP (Adriamycin and gemcitabine alternating with ifosfamide, paclitaxel, and cisplatin) are being tested.[180] Although much progress has made in improving combination chemotherapy, there is still much room for progress.

PALLIATIVE RADIOTHERAPY

Bladder cancer can metastasize to various visceral organs, causing symptoms that require palliation. The treatment approach in advanced disease is dictated by a desire to deliver therapy for rapid relief of pain or hematuria with minimal inconvenience to the patient. This can be accomplished with a short course with a high dose per fraction. Srinivasan and associates[181] compared in 41 patients a conventional regimen of 45 Gy in 12 fractions over 26 days to a hypofractionated treatment of 17 Gy in 2 fractions over 3 days.[181] In patients receiving the hypofractionated regimen, 59% had a clearance of hematuria and 73% had an improvement in pain. This was superior to the conventional treatment that resulted in a 16% clearance of hematuria and a 37% improvement in pain. Median survival was higher at 14 months for those treated conventionally compared with 10 months for those receiving the hypofractionated treatment.

A palliative regimen of 30 Gy in six fractions of two fractions per week was reported by Salminen and colleagues[182] in 94 patients. Forty attained complete palliation and 27 had partial improvement, although many suffered acute side effects, including diarrhea in nearly 60% of patients. A regimen of 21 Gy in three fractions over 5 days resulted in palliation of 75 of 102 patients but at a cost of significant acute toxicity.[183] External-beam irradiation has had mixed results in relieving ureteral obstruction.[164] The obstruction was relieved for 20%, unchanged in 24%, and worse in 56% after a 60 Gy course in 2 Gy fractions for 55 patients with 68 obstructed kidneys. This limited success was at a cost of vesicovaginal fistulas in one patient, contracted bladders in 22 patients, and diarrhea in 25 patients. Median survival was 11 months, with a median of 9.5 months spent at home.

REFERENCES

1. Jemal A, Murray T, Samuel A, et al: Cancer statistics, 2003. *CA Cancer J Clin.* 2003;53:5.
2. Silverman D, Hartge P, Morrison A, et al: Epidemiology of bladder cancer. *Hematol Oncol Clin North Am.* 1992;6:1.
3. Sorahan T, Lancashire R, Sole G: Urothelial cancer and cigarette smoking: Findings from a regional case-controlled study. *Br J Urol.* 1994;74:753.
4. Momas I, Daures JP, Festy B, et al: Bladder cancer and black tobacco cigarette smoking: Some results from a French case-control study. *Eur J Epidemiol.* 1994;10:599.
5. Anton-Culver H, Lee-Feldstein A, Taylor TH: The association of bladder cancer risk with ethnicity, gender, and smoking. *Ann Epidemiol.* 1993;3:429.
6. Chyou PH, Nomura AM, Stemmermann GN: A prospective study of diet, smoking, and lower urinary tract cancer. *Ann Epidemiol.* 1993;3:211.
7. Siemiatycki J, Dewar R, Krewski D, et al: Are the apparent effects of cigarette smoking on lung and bladder cancers due to uncontrolled confounding by occupational exposures? *Epidemiology.* 1994;5:57.
8. Salminen E, Pukkala E, Teppo L: Bladder cancer and the risk of smoking-related cancers during followup. *J Urol.* 1994;152:1420.
9. Yu MC, Skipper PL, Tannenbaum SR, et al: Arylamine exposures and bladder cancer risk. *Mutation Res* 2002;506;21.
10. Esteban Castelao JE, Yuan JM, Skipper PL, et al: Gender- and smoking-related bladder cancer risk. *J Natl Cancer Inst.* 2001;93;538.
11. Kunze E, Chang-Claude J, Frentzel-Beyme R: Life style and occupational risk factors for bladder cancer in Germany: A case-control study. *Cancer.* 1992;69:1776.
12. Tremblay C, Armstrong B, Theriault G, et al: Estimation of risk of developing bladder cancer among workers exposed to coal tar pitch volatiles in the primary aluminum industry. *Am J Ind Med.* 1995;27:335.
13. Barbone F, Franceschi S, Talamini R, et al: Occupation and bladder cancer in Pordenone (north-east Italy): A case-control study. *Int J Epidemiol.* 1994;23:58.

14. Zheng W, McLaughlin J, Gao Y, et al: Bladder cancer and occupation in Shanghai. *Am J Indust Med.* 1992;21:877.

15. Bi W, Hayes R, Feng P, et al: Mortality and incidence of bladder cancer in benzidine-exposed workers in China. *Am J Indust Med.* 1992;21:481.

16. Vineis P: Epidemiology of cancer from exposure to arylamines. *Environ Health Perspect.* 1994;102:7.

17. Weiss NS: Cancer in relation to occupational exposure to perchloroethylene. *Cancer Causes Control.* 1995;6:257.

18. Gago-Dominguez M, Castelao JE, Yuan JM, et al: Use of permanent hair dyes and bladder cancer risk. *Int J Cancer.* 2001;94;903

19. Badawi AF, Mostafa MH, Probert A, et al: Role of schistosomiasis in human bladder cancer: Evidence of association, etiological factors, and basic mechanisms of carcinogenesis. *Eur J Cancer Prevent.* 1995;4:45.

20. Warren W, Biggs PJ, el-Baz M, et al: Mutations in the p53 gene in schistosomal bladder cancer: A study of 92 tumours from Egyptian patients and a comparison between mutational spectra from schistosomal and non-schistosomal urothelial tumours. *Carcinogenesis.* 1995;16:1181.

21. Rosin MP, Anwar WA, Ward AJ: Inflammation, chromosomal instability, and cancer: The schistosomiasis model. *Cancer Res.* 1994;54:1929.

22. Shirai T: Etiology of bladder cancer. *Semin Urol.* 1993;11:113.

23. Gonzalez C, Errezola M, Izarzugaza I, et al: Urinary infection, renal lithiasis and bladder cancer in Spain. *Eur J Cancer.* 1991;27:498.

24. Bickel A, Culkin DJ, Wheeler JS: Bladder cancer in spinal cord injury patients. *J Urol.* 1991;146:1240.

25. Viscoli C, Lachs M, Horwitz R: Bladder cancer and coffee drinking: A summary of case-control research. *Lancet.* 1993;341:1432.

26. Stensvold I, Jacobsen BK: Coffee and cancer: A prospective study of 43,000 Norwegian men and women. *Cancer Causes Control.* 1994;5:401.

27. Zeegers MP, Dorant E, Goldbohm RA, van den Brandt PA: Are coffee, tea and total fluid consumption associated with bladder cancer risk? Results from the Netherlands Cohort Study. *Cancer Causes Control.* 2001;12:231.

28. Elcock M, Morgan R: Update on artificial sweeteners and bladder cancer. *Regul Toxicol Pharmacol.* 1993;17:35.

29. Vena J, Graham S, Freudenheim J, et al: Diet in the epidemiology of bladder cancer in western New York. *Nutr Cancer.* 1992; 18:255.

30. Nomura A, Kolonel L, Hankin J, et al: Dietary factors in cancer of the lower urinary tract. *Int J Cancer.* 1991;48:199.

31. McGeehin MA, Reif JS, Becher JC, et al: Case-control study of bladder cancer and water disinfection methods in Colorado. *Am J Epidemiol.* 1993;138:492.

32. Morales S, Llopis G, Tejerizo P: Concentration of nitrates in drinking water and its relationship with bladder cancer. *J Environ Pathol Toxicol Oncol.* 1993;12:229.

33. Petersen I, Ohgaki H, Ludeke BI, et al: p53 mutations in phenacetin-associated human urothelial carcinomas. *Carcinogenesis.* 1993; 14:2119.

34. Radis CD, Kahl LE, Baker GL, et al: Effects of cyclophosphamide on the development of malignancy and on long-term survival of patients with rheumatoid arthritis: A 20-year followup study. *Source.* 1995;38:1120.

35. Bell D, Taylor J, Paulson D, et al: Genetic risk and carcinogen exposure: A common inherited defect of the carcinogen-metabolism gene glutathione S-transferase M1 (*GSTM1*) that increases susceptibility to bladder cancer. *J Natl Cancer Inst.* 1993;85:1159.

36. Wijkstrom H, Naslund I, Ekman P: Short-term radiotherapy as palliative treatment in patients with transitional cell bladder cancer. *Br J Urol.* 1991;67:74.

37. Sandberg AA, Berger CS: Review of chromosome studies in urological tumors. *J Urol.* 1994;151:545.

38. Schapers RF, Smeets AW, Pauwels RP: Cytogenetic analysis in transitional cell carcinoma of the bladder. *Br J Urol.* 1993; 72:887.

39. Lipponen PK, Eskelinen MJ, Nordling S: Progression and survival in transitional cell bladder cancer: A comparison of established prognostic factors, S-phase fraction and DNA ploidy. *Eur J Cancer.* 1991;27:877.

40. Nemoto R, Nakamura I, Uchida K, et al: Numerical chromosome aberrations in bladder cancer detected by in situ hybridization. *Br J Urol.* 1995;75:470.

41. Borland RN, Brendler CB, Isaacs WB: Molecular biology of bladder cancer. *Hematol Oncol Clin North Am.* 1992;6:31.

42. Sauter G, Moch H, Carroll P, et al: Chromosome-9 loss detected by fluorescence in situ hybridization in bladder cancer. *Int J Cancer.* 1995;64:99.

43. Matsuyama H, Bergerheim US, Nilsson I, et al: Nonrandom numerical aberrations of chromosomes 7, 9, and 10 in DNA-diploid bladder cancer. *Cancer Genet Cytogenet.* 1994;77:18.

44. Cairns P, Shaw ME, Knowles MA: Initiation of bladder cancer may involve deletion of a tumour-suppressor gene on chromosome 9. *Oncogene.* 1993;8:1083.

45. Spruck CH III, Ohneseit PF, Gonzalez-Zulueta M, et al: Two molecular pathways to transitional cell carcinoma of the bladder. *Cancer Res.* 1994;54:784.

46. Voorter C, Joos S, Bringuier PP, et al: Detection of chromosomal imbalances in transitional cell carcinoma of the bladder by comparative genomic hybridization. *Am J Pathol.* 1995;146:1341.

47. Dalbagni G, Presti J, Reuter V, et al: Genetic alterations in bladder cancer. *Lancet.* 1993;342:469.

48. Tiniakos DG, Mellon K, Anderson JJ, et al: C-*jun* oncogene expression in transitional cell carcinoma of the urinary bladder. *Br J Urol.* 1994;74:757.

49. Burchill SA, Neal DE, Lunec J: Frequency of H-*ras* mutations in human bladder cancer detected by direct sequencing. *Br J Urol.* 1994;73:516.

50. Lipponen P: Expression of c-*erb*B-2 oncoprotein in transitional cell bladder cancer. *Eur J Cancer.* 1993;29A:749.

51. Presti JC, Reuter VE, Galan T, et al: Molecular genetic alterations in superficial and locally advanced human bladder cancer. *Cancer Res.* 1991;51:5405.

52. Kubota Y, Miyamoto H, Noguchi S, et al: The loss of retinoblastoma gene in association with c-*myc* and transforming growth factor-beta 1 gene expression in human bladder cancer. *J Urol.* 1995;154:371.

53. Dalbagni G, Cordon-Cardo C, Reuter V, et al: Tumor suppressor gene alterations in bladder carcinoma. *Surg Oncol Clin North Am.* 1995;4:231.

54. Chang WY, Cairns P, Schoenberg MP, et al: Novel suppressor loci on chromosome 14q in primary bladder cancer. *Cancer Res.* 1995; 55:3246.

55. Kallioniemi A, Kallioniemi OP, Citro G, et al: Identification of gains and losses of DNA sequences in primary bladder cancer by comparative genomic hybridization. *Genes Chromosomes Cancer.* 1995;12:213.

56. Tomovska S, Richter J, Suess K et al: Molecular cytogenetic alterations associated with rapid tumor cell proliferation in advanced urinary bladder cancer. *Int J Oncol.* 2001;18:1239.

57. Esrig D, Sprick CH, Nichols PW, et al: p53 nuclear protein accumulation correlates with mutations in the p53 gene, tumor grade, and stage in bladder cancer. *Am J Pathol.* 1993;143:1389.

58. Esrig D, Elmajian D, Groshen S, et al: Accumulation of nuclear p53 and tumor progression in bladder cancer. *N Engl J Med.* 1994; 331:1259.

59. Sarkis AS, Dalbagni G, Cordon-Cardo C, et al: Association of p53 nuclear overexpression and tumor progression in carcinoma in situ of the bladder. *J Urol.* 1994;152:388.

60. Uchida T, Wada C, Ishida H, et al: p53 mutations and prognosis in bladder tumors. *J Urol.* 1995;153:1097.

61. Kusser WC, Miao X, Glickman BW, et al: p53 mutations in human bladder cancer. *Environ Mol Mutagen.* 1994;24:156.

62. Lianes P, Orlow I, Zhang ZF, et al: Altered patterns of *MDM2* and *TP53* expression in human bladder cancer. *J Natl Cancer Inst.* 1994;86:1325.

63. Dalbagni G, Presti JC, Reuter VE, et al: Molecular genetic alterations of chromosome 17 and p53 nuclear overexpression in human bladder cancer. *Diagn Mol Pathol.* 1993;2:4.

64. Fujimoto K, Yamada Y, Okajima E, et al: Frequent association of p53 gene mutation in invasive bladder cancer. *Cancer Res.* 1992;52:1393.

65. Williams PL, Warwick R, Dyson M, Bannister LH: *Gray's Anatomy*, 37th ed. New York: Churchill Livingstone; 1989:1416.

66. Lerner SP: Lymphadenectomy for bladder cancer. In *Atlas of the Urologic Clinics of North America: Lymphadenectomy for Urologic Cancers*. Philadelphia: WB Saunders; 1995:52.

67. Tanagho E: Anatomy of the lower urinary tract. In Walsh P, ed. *Campbell's Urology*, 6th ed. Philadelphia: WB Saunders; 1992:40.

68. Dickinson AJ, Fox SB, Persad RA, et al: Quantification of angiogenesis as an independent predictor of prognosis in invasive bladder carcinomas. *Br J Urol.* 1994;74:762.

69. Jaeger TM, Weidner N, Chew K, et al: Tumor angiogenesis correlates with lymph node metastases in invasive bladder cancer. *J Urol.* 1995;154:69.

70. Kissane JM: *Anderson's Pathology,* 9th ed. St. Louis: CV Mosby, 1990:857.

71. Someren A: *Urologic Pathology With Clinical and Radiologic Correlations.* New York: Macmillan; 1989:363.

72. Burnett AL, Epstein JI, Marshall FF: Adenocarcinoma of urinary bladder: Classification and management. *Urology.* 1991; 37:315.

73. Holmang S, Borghede G, Johansson SL: Primary small cell carcinoma of the bladder: A report of 25 cases. *J Urol.* 1995; 153:1820.

74. Aydoganli L, Tarhan F, Atan A, et al: Rhabdomyosarcoma of the urinary bladder in an adult. *Int Urol Nephrol.* 1993;25:159.

75. Suzuki Y, Nakada T, Suzuki H, et al: Primary bladder pheochromocytoma without hypertension. *Int Urol Nephrol.* 1993;25:153.

76. Bitker MO, Bagnis C, Mouquet C, et al: Primary bladder lymphoma in kidney transplant recipients: Report of a case. *Prog Urol.* 1992;2:908.

77. Kawamura J, Sakurai M, Tsukamoto K, et al: Leiomyosarcoma of the bladder eighteen years after cyclophosphamide therapy for retinoblastoma. *Urol Int.* 1993;51:49.

78. Lange-Welker U, Papadopoulos I, Wacker HH: Primary malignant melanoma of the bladder. *Urol Int.* 1993;50:226.

79. Williams JR, Stott MA, Moisey CU: Bilateral hydronephrosis secondary to breast carcinoma metastasising to the bladder. *Br J Urol.* 1992;69:97.

80. Fair W, Fuks Z, Scher H: Cancer of the bladder. In Devita V, Hellman S, Roenberg S, eds. *Cancer: Principles and Practice of Oncology,* 4th ed. Philadelphia: JB Lippincott; 1993:1052.

81. Parsons J, Million R: Bladder. In Perez C, Brady L, eds. *Principles and Practice of Radiation Oncology,* 2nd ed. Philadelphia: JB Lippincott; 1992:1036.

82. American Joint Committee on Cancer: Urinary bladder. In Fleming ID, Cooper JS, Henson DE, et al, eds: *AJCC Cancer Staging Manual,* 5th ed. Philadelphia: Lippincott-Raven; 1997:195.

83. Skinner DG, Tift JP, Kaufman JJ: High dose, short course preoperative radiation therapy and immediate single stage radical cystectomy with pelvic node dissection in the management of bladder cancer. *J Urol.* 1982;127:671.

84. Lieskovsky G, Ahlering T, Skinner D: Diagnosis and staging of bladder cancer. In Skinner D, Lieskovsky G, eds. *Diagnosis and Management of Genitourinary Cancer.* Philadelphia: WB Saunders; 1988.

85. Gospodarowicz MK: Staging of bladder cancer. *Semin Surg Oncol.* 1994;10:51.

86. Denis L: Clinical staging: Its importance in therapeutic decisions and clinical trials. *Hematol Oncol Clin North Am.* 1992;6:41.

87. Goldman S, Gatewood O: *CT and MRI of the Genitourinary Tract.* New York: Churchill Livingstone; 1990:209.

88. Kim B, Semelka RC, Ascher SM, et al: Bladder tumor staging: Comparison of contrast-enhanced CT, T1- and T2-weighted MR imaging, dynamic gadolinium-enhanced imaging, and late gadolinium-enhanced imaging. *Radiology.* 1994;193:239.

89. Tachibana M, Baba S, Deguchi N, et al: Efficacy of gadolinium-diethylenetriaminepentaacetic acid-enhanced magnetic resonance imaging for differentiation between superficial and muscle invasive tumor of the bladder: A comparative study with computerized tomography and transurethral ultrasonography. *J Urol.* 1991;145:1169.

90. Hawnaur JM, Johnson RJ, Read G: Magnetic resonance imaging with gadolinium-DTPA for assessment of bladder carcinoma and its response to treatment. *Clin Radiol.* 1993;47:302.

91. Tanimoto A, Yuasa Y, Imai Y, et al: Bladder tumor staging: Comparison of conventional and gadolinium-enhanced dynamic MR imaging and CT. *Radiology.* 1992;185:741.

92. Narumi Y, Kadota T, Inoue E, et al: Bladder tumors: Staging with gadolinium-enhanced oblique MR imaging. *Radiology.* 1993; 187:145.

93. Maeda H, Kinukawa T, Hattori R, et al: Detection of muscle layer invasion with submillimeter pixel MR images: Staging of bladder carcinoma. *Magn Reson Imaging.* 1995;13:9.

94. Robinson R, Collins CD, Ryder WDJ et al. Relationship of MRI and clinical staging to outcome in invasive bladder cancer treated by radiotherapy. *Clin Radiol.* 2000:55;301.

95. Angulo JC, Lopez JI, Flores N, et al: The value of tumour spread, grading and growth pattern as morphological predictive parameters in bladder carcinoma: A critical revision of the 1987 TNM classification. *J Cancer Res Clin Oncol.* 1993;119:578.

96. Fong C, Shipley W, Young R, et al: Prognostic factors in invasive bladder carcinoma in a prospective trial of preoperative adjuvant chemotherapy and radiotherapy. *J Clin Oncol.* 1991;9:1533.

97. Itoku KA, Stein BS: Superficial bladder cancer. *Hematol Oncol Clin North Am.* 1992;6:99.

98. Herr H: Intravesical therapy. *Hematol Oncol Clin North Am.* 1992;6:117.

99. Herr H, Laudone V, Badalament R, et al: Bacillus Calmette-Guérin therapy alters the progression of superficial bladder cancer. *J Clin Oncol.* 1988;6:1450.

100. Herr H, Schwalb D, Zhang Z, et al: Intravesical bacillus Calmette-Guérin therapy prevents tumor progression and death from superficial bladder cancer: Ten-year follow-up of a prospective randomized trial. *J Clin Oncol.* 1995;13:1404.

101. Herr H, Wartinger D, Fair W, et al: Bacillus Calmette-Guérin therapy for superficial bladder cancer: A 10-year followup. *J Urol.* 1992;147:1020.

102. Bohle A, Jocham D, Bock PR. Intravesical bacillus Calmette-guerin versus mitomycin C for superficial bladder cancer: A formal meta-analysis of comparative studies on recurrence and toxicity. *J Urol.* 2003;169:90.

103. Molto L, Alvarez-Mon M, Carballido J, et al: Use of intracavitary interferon-alpha-2b in the prophylactic treatment of patients with superficial bladder cancer. *Cancer.* 1995;75:2720.

104. van der Werf-Messing B, Hop WCJ: Carcinoma of the urinary bladder (category T1NXM0) treated either by radium or by transurethral resection only. *Int J Radiat Oncol Biol Phys.* 1982; 8:1849.

105. Freiha F: Open bladder surgery. In Walsh P, ed. *Campbell's Urology,* 6th ed. Philadelphia: WB Saunders; 1992:2750.

106. Richie J: Surgery for invasive bladder cancer. *Hematol Oncol Clin North Am.* 1992;6:129.

107. Herr H: Extent of surgery and pathology evaluation has an impact on bladder outcomes after radical cystectomy. *Urology.* 2003: 61;105.

108. Brendler C, Steinberg G, Marshall F, et al: Local recurrence and survival following nerve-sparing radical cystoprostatectomy. *J Urol.* 1990;144:1137.

109. Wang CC: *Clinical Radiation Oncology: Indications, Techniques, and Results.* Littleton, MA, Publishing Company; 1988:273.

110. Montie J, Straffon R, Stewart B: Radical cystectomy without radiation therapy for carcinoma of the bladder. *J Urol.* 1984;131:477.

111. Wishnow K, Dmochowski R: Pelvic recurrence after radical cystectomy without preoperative radiation. *J Urol.* 1988;140:42.

112. Greven K, Solin L, Hanks G: Prognostic factors in patients with bladder carcinoma treated with definitive irradiation. *Cancer.* 1990;65:908.

113. Cole D, Durrant R, Roberts J, et al: A pilot study of accelerated fractionation in the radiotherapy of invasive carcinoma of the bladder. *Br J Radiol.* 1992;65:792.

114. Boileau MA, Johnson DE, Chan RC, et al: Bladder carcinoma: Results with preoperative radiation therapy and radical cystectomy. *Urology.* 1980;16:569.

115. Herr HW: Preoperative irradiation with and without chemotherapy as adjunct to radical cystectomy. *Urology* 1985;25:127.

116. Skinner DG, Lieskovsky G: Contemporary cystectomy with pelvic node dissection compared to preoperative radiation therapy plus cystectomy in management of invasive bladder cancer. *J Urol.* 1984; 131:1069.

117. Montie JE, Straffon RA, Stewart BH: Radical cystectomy without radiation therapy for carcinoma of the bladder. *J Urol.* 1984;131:477.

118. Blackard CE, Byar DP, and The Veterans Administration Cooperative Urological Research Group: Results of a clinical trial of surgery and radiation in stages II and III carcinoma of the bladder. *J Urol.* 1972;198:875.

119. Anderström C, Johansson S, Nilsson S, et al: A prospective randomized study of preoperative irradiation with cystectomy or cystectomy alone for invasive bladder carcinoma. *Eur Urol.* 1983;9:142.

120. Crawford ED, Das S, Smith JA Jr: Preoperative radiation therapy in the treatment of bladder cancer. *Urol Clin North Am.* 1987; 14:781.

121. Slack NH, Bross IDJ, Prout GR Jr: Five-year follow-up results of a collaborative study of therapies for carcinoma of the bladder. *J Surg Oncol.* 1977;9:393.

122. Cole CJ, Pollack A, Zagars GK, et al: Local control of muscle invasive bladder cancer: Preoperative radiotherapy and cystectomy versus cystectomy alone. *Int J Radiat Oncol Biol Phys.* 1995;32:331.

123. Cox JD, Guse C, Asbell S: Tolerance of pelvic normal tissues to hyperfractionated radiation therapy: Results of protocol 83-08 of the Radiation Therapy Oncology Group. *Int J Radiat Oncol Biol Phys.* 1988;15:1331.

124. Gospodarowicz M, Warde P: The role of radiation therapy in the management of transitional cell carcinoma of the bladder. *Hematol Oncol Clin North Am.* 1992;6:147.

125. Bessell E, Taylor J, Moloney A: Regression of transitional cell carcinoma of the bladder with radiotherapy: Progression-free control in the bladder at 5 years. *Radiother Oncol.* 1993;29:344.

126. Shipley W, Prout G, Kaufman D, et al: Invasive bladder carcinoma: The importance of initial transurethral surgery and other significant prognostic factors for improved survival with full-dose irradiation. *Cancer.* 1987;60:514.

127. Gospodarowicz M, Hawkins N, Rawlings G: Radical radiotherapy for muscle invasive transitional cell carcinoma of the bladder: Failure analysis. *J Urol.* 1989;142:1448.

128. Pollack A, Zagars G, Swanson D: Muscle-invasive bladder cancer treated with external beam radiotherapy: Prognostic factors. *Int J Radiat Oncol Biol Phys.* 1994;30:267.

129. Pollack A, Zagars GK: Radiotherapy for stage T3b transitional cell carcinoma of the bladder. *Semin Urol Oncol.* 1996;14:86.

130. Quilty P, Duncan W: Primary radical radiotherapy for T3 transitional cell cancer of the bladder: An analysis of survival and control. *Int J Radiat Oncol Biol Phys.* 1986;12:853.

131. Edsmyr F, Andersson L, Esposti L, et al: Irradiation therapy with multiple small fractions per day in urinary bladder cancer. *Radiother Oncol.* 1985;4:197.

132. Naslund I, Nilsson B, Littbrand B: Hyperfractionated radiotherapy of bladder cancer. *Acta Oncol.* 1994;33:397.

133. Lynch W, Jenkins B, Fowler G, et al: The quality of life after radical radiotherapy for bladder cancer. *Br J Urol.* 1992;70:519.

134. Kachnic LA, Shipley WU, Griffin PP, et al: Combined modality treatment with selective bladder conservation for invasive bladder cancer: Long-term tolerance in the female patient. *Cancer J Sci Am.* 1996;2:79.

135. Tester W, Porter A, Asbell S, et al: Combined modality program with possible organ preservation for invasive bladder carcinoma: Results of RTOG protocol 85-12. *Int J Radiat Oncol Biol Phys.* 1992;25:783.

136. Shipley WU, Kaufman DS, Zehr E, et al. Selective bladder preservation by combined modality protocol treatment: Long-term outcomes of 190 patients with invasive bladder cancer. *Urology.* 2002;60;62.

137. Cervek J, Cufer T, Kragelj B, et al: Sequential transurethral surgery, multiple drug chemotherapy and radiation therapy for invasive bladder carcinoma: Initial report. *Int J Radiat Oncol Biol Phys.* 1993;25:777.

138. Rodel C, Grabenbauer GG, Kuhn RE, et al: Combined-modality treatment and selective organ preservation in invasive bladder cancer: Long-term results. *J Clin Oncol.* 2002;230:3061.

139. Housset M, Maulard C, Chretien Y, et al: Combined radiation and chemotherapy for invasive transitional-cell carcinoma of the bladder: A prospective study. *J Clin Oncol.* 1993;11:2150.

140. Sumiyoshi Y, Yokota K, Akiyama M, et al: Neoadjuvant intra-arterial doxorubicin chemotherapy in combination with low dose radiotherapy for the treatment of locally advanced transitional cell carcinoma of the bladder. *J Urol.* 1994;152:362.

141. Rotman M, Macchia R, Silverstein N, et al: Treatment of advanced bladder carcinoma with irradiation and concomitant 5-fluorouracil infusion. *Cancer.* 1987;59:710.

142. Vikram B, Malamud S, Silverman P, et al: A pilot study of chemotherapy alternating with twice-a-day accelerated radiation therapy as an alternative to cystectomy in muscle infiltrating (stages T2 and T3) cancer of the bladder: Preliminary results. *J Urol.* 1993;151:602.

143. Shipley WU, Prout GR, Einstein AB, et al: Treatment of invasive bladder cancer by cisplatin and radiation in patients unsuited for surgery. *JAMA.* 1987;258:931.

144. Kaufman DS, Shipley WU, Griffin PP, et al: Selective bladder preservation by combination treatment of an invasive bladder cancer. *N Engl J Med.* 1993;329:1377.

145. Herr HW: Conservative management of muscle-infiltrating bladder cancer: Prospective experience. *J Urol.* 1987;138:1162.

146. Khandekar JD, Elson PJ, DeWys WD, et al: Comparative activity and toxicity of *cis*-diamminedichloroplatinum (DDP) and a combination of doxorubicin, cyclophosphamide and DDP in disseminated transitional cell carcinomas of the urinary tract. *J Clin Oncol.* 1985;3:539.

147. Loehrer PJ, Einhorn LH, Elson PJ, et al: A randomized comparison of cisplatin alone or in combination with methotrexate, vinblastine, and doxorubicin in patients with metastatic urothelial carcinoma: A cooperative group study. *J Clin Oncol.* 1992; 10:1066.

148. Soloway MS, Einstein A, Corder MP, et al: A comparison of cisplatin and the combination of cisplatin and cyclophosphamide in advanced urothelial cancer. *Cancer.* 1983;52:767.

149. van der Werf-Messing B, van Putten W: Carcinoma of the urinary bladder category T2,3NxM0 treated by 40 Gy external irradiation followed by cesium implant at reduced dose (50%). *Int J Radiat Oncol Biol Phys.* 1989;16:369.

150. Grossman H, Sandler H, Perez-Tamayo C: Treatment of T3a bladder cancer with iridium implantation. *Urology.* 1993;41:217.

151. Straus KL: Treatment of bladder cancer with interstitial iridium-192 implantation and external beam irradiation. *Int J Radiat Oncol Biol Phys.* 1988;14:265.

152. Mazeron J: Conservative treatment of bladder carcinoma by partial cystectomy and interstitial iridium 192. *Int J Radiat Oncol Biol Phys.* 1988;15:1323.

153. Rozan R, Albuisson E, Donnarieix D: Interstitial iridium-192 for bladder cancer (a multicentric survey: 205 patients). *Int J Radiat Oncol Biol Phys.* 1992;24:469.

154. Cookson MS, Herr HW, Zhang ZF, et al: The treated natural history of high risk superficial bladder cancer: 15-year outcome. *J Urol.* 1997;158:62.

155. Rintala E, Hannisdahl E, Fossa SD, et al: Neoadjuvant chemotherapy in bladder cancer: A randomized study. Nordic Cystectomy Trial I. *Scand J Urol Nephrol.* 1993;27:355.

156. Malmstrom PU, Rintala E, Wahlqvist R, et al: Five-year followup of a prospective trial of radical cystectomy and neoadjuvant chemotherapy: Nordic Cystectomy Trial I. The Nordic Cooperative Bladder Cancer Study Group. *J Urol.* 1996;155:1903.

157. Neoadjuvant cisplatin, methotrexate, and vinblastine chemotherapy for muscle-invasive bladder cancer: A randomized controlled trial. International collaboration of trialists. *Lancet.* 1999; 354:533.

158. Hall RR: Updated results of a randomised controlled trial of neoadjuvant cisplatin (C), methotrexate (M) and vinblastine (V) chemotherapy for muscle-invasive bladder cancer. *Proc Am Soc Clin Oncol.* 2002;710.

159. Grossman HB, Natale, RB, Tanagen CT, et al: Neoadjuvant chemotherapy plus cystectomy compared with cystectomy alone for locally advanced bladder cancer. *New Eng J Med.* 2003; 349:859.

160. Advaned Bladder Cancer Meta-Analysis: Collaboration: Neoadjuvant chemotherapy in invasive bladder cancer: A systematic review and meta-analysis. *Lancet.* 2003;361:1972.

161. Studer UE, Bacchi M, Biedermann C, et al: Adjuvant cisplatin chemotherapy following cystectomy for bladder cancer: Results of a prospective randomized trial. *J Urol.* 1994;152:81.

162. Skinner DG, Daniels JR, Russell CA, et al: The role of adjuvant chemotherapy following cystectomy for invasive bladder cancer: A prospective comparative trial. *J Urol.* 1991;145:459.

163. Freiha F, Reese J, Torti FM: A randomized trial of radical cystectomy versus radical cystectomy plus cisplatin, vinblastine and methotrexate chemotherapy for muscle invasive bladder cancer. *J Urol.* 1996;155:495.

164. Stockle M, Meyenburg W, Wellek S, et al: Advanced bladder cancer (stages pT3b, pT4a, pN1 and pN2): Improved survival after radical cystectomy and 3 adjuvant cycles of chemotherapy. Results of a controlled prospective study. *J Urol.* 1992; 148:302.

165. Bajorin DF, Dodd PM, Mazumdar M, et al: Long-term survival in metastatic transitional-cell carcinoma and prognostic factors predicting outcome of therapy. *J Clin Oncol.* 1999;17:3173.

166. Sternberg CN, Yagoda A, Scher HI, et al: Methotrexate, vinblastine, doxorubicin, and cisplatin for advanced transitional cell carcinoma of the urothelium. Efficacy and patterns of response and relapse. *Cancer.* 1989;64:2448.

167. Saxman SB, Propert KJ, Einhorn LH, et al: Long-term follow-up of a phase III intergroup study of cisplatin alone or in combination with methotrexate, vinblastine, and doxorubicin in patients with metastatic urothelial carcinoma: a cooperative group study. *J Clin Oncol.* 1997;15:2564.

168. Logothetis CJ, Dexeus FH, Finn L, et al: A prospective randomized trial comparing MVAC and CISCA chemotherapy for patients with metastatic urothelial tumors. *J Clin Oncol.* 1990; 8:1050.

169. von der Maase H, Hansen SW, Roberts JT, et al: Gemcitabine and cisplatin versus methotrexate, vinblastine, doxorubicin, and cisplatin in advanced or metastatic bladder cancer: Results of a large, randomized, multinational, multicenter, phase III study. *J Clin Oncol.* 2000;18:3068.

170. Petrioli R, Frediani B, Manganelli A, et al: Comparison between a cisplatin-containing regimen and a carboplatin- containing regimen for recurrent or metastatic bladder cancer patients. A randomized phase II study. *Cancer.* 1996;77:344.

171. Waxman J, Barton C: Carboplatin-based chemotherapy for bladder cancer. *Cancer Treat Rev.* 1993;19:21.

172. Raabe NK, Fossa SD, Paro G: Phase II study of carboplatin in locally advanced and metastatic transitional cell carcinoma of the urinary bladder. *Br J Urol.* 1989;64:604.

173. Small EJ, Fippin LJ, Ernest ML, et al: A carboplatin-based regimen for the treatment of patients with advanced transitional cell carcinoma of the urothelium. *Cancer.* 1996;78:1775.

174. Dreicer R, Gustin DM, See WA, et al: Paclitaxel in advanced urothelial carcinoma: Its role in patients with renal insufficiency and as salvage therapy. *J Urol.* 1996;156:1606.

175. Dimopoulos MA, Deliveliotis C, Moulopoulos LA, et al. Treatment of patients with metastatic urothelial carcinoma and impaired renal function with single-agent docetaxel. *Urology.* 1998;52:56.

176. Yang MH, Yen CC, Chang YH, et al: Single agent paclitaxel as a first-line therapy in advanced urothelial carcinoma: Its efficacy and safety in patients even with pretreatment renal insufficiency. *Jpn J Clin Oncol.* 2000;30:547.

177. Bellmunt J, de Wit R, Albanell J, et al: A feasibility study of carboplatin with fixed dose of gemcitabine in "unfit" patients with advanced bladder cancer. *Eur J Cancer.* 2001;37:2212.

178. Carles J, Nogue M, Domenech M, et al: Carboplatin-gemcitabine treatment of patients with transitional cell carcinoma of the bladder and impaired renal function. *Oncology.* 2000;59:24.

179. Vaughn DJ: Paclitaxel and carboplatin in bladder cancer: Recent developments. *Eur J Cancer.* 2000;36(suppl 2):7.

180. Bajorin DF: Exploring sequenced chemotherapy regimens in the treatment of transitional cell carcinoma of the urothelial tract. *Eur J Cancer.* 2000;36(suppl 2):26.

181. Srinivasan V, Brown CH: A comparison of two radiotherapy regimens for the treatment of symptoms from advanced bladder cancer. *Clin Oncol.* 1994;6:11.

182. Salminen E: Unconventional fractionation for palliative radiotherapy of urinary bladder cancer: A retrospective review of 94 patients. *Acta Oncol.* 1992;31:449.

183. Aass N, Fossa S: Aims and results of palliative radiotherapy in urological cancer. *Curr Opin Oncol.* 1994;6:308.

184. Honnens de Lichtenberg M, Miskowiak J, Rolff H: Results of radiotherapy on ureteric obstruction in muscle-invasive bladder cancer. *Br J Urol.* 1995;75:197.

Cancer of the Prostate

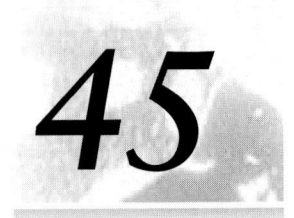

Mack Roach III, MD, and Kent Wallner, MD

For no other common, primary, solid neoplasm has more been learned in the past 10 years. This increase in knowledge has improved our ability to select the most appropriate therapies for subsets of patients and to better define the efficacy of treatment. This rapid expansion of information initially resulted from the availability of the serum marker *prostate-specific antigen* (PSA). More recently, prospective randomized trials and large post-treatment databases have allowed us to define prognostic risk groups, improving our ability to counsel patients, select therapy, and design clinical trials. From these trials and retrospective studies we have also learned much about the importance of PSA and its limitations as a prognostic marker.

This chapter focuses on the curative treatment of men with clinically localized prostate cancer. Although most data published to date emphasize the use of the serum marker PSA (a major determinant of the disease-free status), overall and disease-specific survival are also discussed. The outcomes of radiation are compared with surgery. No attempt is made to comprehensively address "watchful waiting" or deferred treatment or the impact of treatment decisions on health care costs. These topics lend themselves to philosophical discussion, such as "how much is it worth for a 70-year-old man to live longer?" Instead, this chapter focuses on the treatment of prostate cancer with various forms of radiation therapy, with and without hormonal therapy.

EPIDEMIOLOGY

Incidence, Etiology, and Genetics

An estimated 189,000 men were diagnosed as having prostate cancer in 2002.[1] This represents roughly 30% of all cancers diagnosed in men, with the next most common site (lung) being diagnosed less than half as often. It was also estimated that approximately 30,200 men would die of prostate cancer, making prostate cancer the second cause of cancer death in men.[1] The estimated lifetime risk was 1 in 6 based on men diagnosed from 1996 through 1998. The annual age-adjusted cancer incidence lifetime risk of a man developing prostate cancer appeared to peak in 1991, reflecting the initial "harvesting effect" from widespread screening in the early to mid-1990s (Fig. 45-1*A* and *B*).

Prostate cancer is generally considered a disease of "older men," with the average age historically being 72 years at diagnosis.[2] In 1990, less than 10% of men with prostate cancer were younger than 60 years of age, whereas more than one third were older than 75 years of age. With routine screening, the number of men diagnosed at younger than 60 years of age will increase.[2] There are wide variations in the incidence of prostate cancer internationally, with men from Scandinavian countries experiencing the highest rates and men from Asia the lowest (Fig. 45-2).[3] The highest incidence of prostate cancer in the United States is in African Americans (the ratio of blacks to whites is 1.5 to 2.0:1). Diet, obesity, or environmental exposures related to urban living may account for a portion of the predisposition noted among African American men. African Americans also tend to present with more advanced disease.[4] Biologic differences have been proposed by some investigators; however, socioeconomic and lifestyle factors are a more likely basis for this phenomenon. It appears to be reasonably well established that the incidence of short CAG repeats is higher in African Americans.[5] However, this does not necessarily correlate with other important clinical parameters. Variations in polymorphisms in different populations are expected and alone are not proof of a cause-and-effect relationship. Most studies based on data from prospective randomized trials fail to identify race as an independent prognostic factor, and therapy should not be modified based on race considerations alone.[4]

A genetic predisposition has a major impact on the risk of developing prostate cancer.[6] Screening first-degree relatives of prostate cancer patients may improve the cost-effectiveness of this practice.[7] It is clear from the long list of potential factors that the precise cause of prostate cancer is unknown, but it is likely to be multi-factorial. Prostate cancer does not appear to be related to benign prostatic hypertrophy (BPH).[8] However, having BPH increases the risk of having a high PSA, which may lead incidentally to a diagnosis of disease.[9] Vasectomy does not appear to be a risk factor.[10-13] The number of sexual partners, venereal disease, dietary fat, alcohol, cadmium, and exercise have inconsistently been supported by studies as risk factors.[14-19] Several epidemiologic and in vitro studies support the possible role of vitamin D and calcium, but other studies do not.[20-22] A high intake of vitamin E was associated with a lower incidence of prostate cancer in one prospective randomized trial, but other recent

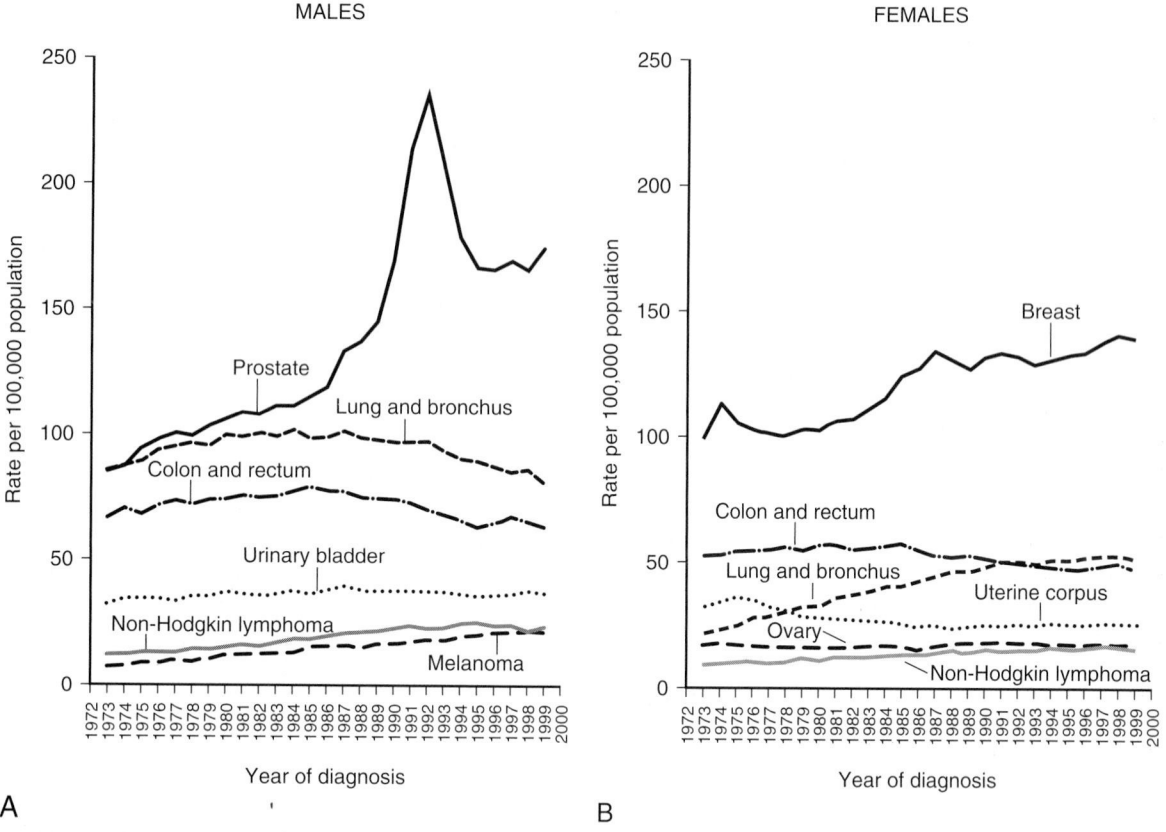

MALES

FEMALES

Figure 45–1. A and **B,** Annual age-adjusted cancer incidence and death rates among males for selected cancer types in the United States from 1973 to 1999 from prostate cancer by year. (From Jemal A, Murra T, Samuels A, et al: Cancer Statistics 2003. *CA Cancer J Clin.* 2003;53:5.)

studies suggest little or no relationship between diet and the risk of prostate cancer.[23-26] Several studies suggests that smoking may be associated with more extensive and aggressive disease cancer.[27-29] In general, smoking appears to be at most weakly related to the risk factor of developing prostate cancer.[30-34]

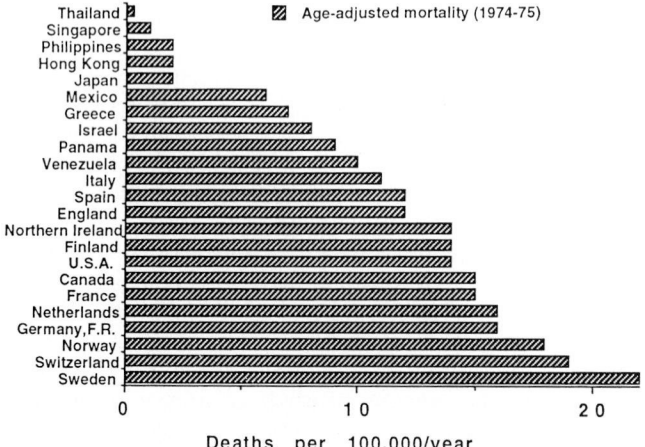

Figure 45–2. International prostate cancer mortality rates. Note the wide range, with the lowest rates in Asia and the highest rates in Scandinavian countries. (From Silverberg E: Cancer Statistics. *Cancer Statistics.* 1980;30:23.)

NATURAL HISTORY

The controversies surrounding the management of prostate cancer arise largely as a result of the long natural history of the disease in untreated patients, the competing causes of mortality in this population, and a lack of prospective randomized trials comparing modalities. Many men may not benefit from treatment because the risk of death from early-stage, low-stage, low-grade disease has been estimated to be approximately 10% at 10 years.[35] Conservative management and delayed hormone therapy are reasonable initial options for such men, if their life expectancy is less than 10 years.[36,37] However, local progression to clinical stage C (T3) disease approaches 50% at 10 years, and beyond 10 years the risk of death seems to climb substantially.[38] Among such patients, 50% are likely to die either directly or indirectly from prostate cancer. The cause-specific survival for these patients has been estimated to be 80%, 50%, 30%, and 10% at 5, 10, 15, and 20 years, respectively.

Patients at a reduced risk for death due to prostate cancer were those with T1a stage disease (10%), low grade (43%), and age of 75 or older. Historically, before routine PSA screening, patients with small palpable nodules experienced a mortality of 20% at 10 years; ultimately 52% of these patients died due to prostate cancer. The survival of such patients is likely to be improved significantly due to PSA screening and improvement in results associated with more contemporary series. For patients with higher stage and grade disease, the need for treatment would appear to be less controversial. Such patients have a higher risk of death and the benefits of therapy have now been well established.[39-45]

Trials conducted in Canada and Europe support the argument for PSA screening and early treatment.[46-48] Additional randomized trials are under way and should allow us to determine the impact of early versus delayed treatment on patients with low-risk disease. These trials will be difficult to complete because they need to be large, require that few patients "change their minds," and take a long time to complete (>10 years). In addition, some clinicians may see inclusion of patients who are likely to benefit from early therapy as unethical. Without better modeling of the expected cure rates and more accurate assessments of the true extent of disease, it may not be possible yet to design a "great study."

ANATOMY

External Anatomy

The normal prostate in a young man has been described as a walnut-sized gland with similar consistency to the tip of the nose. In a young man the prostate volume is approximately 20 mL. The average gland in a patient of 65 years with prostate cancer is approximately 40 mL. The prostate is penetrated by the urethra as the urethral canal proceeds or descends to the urogenital diaphragm and then to the bulb of the penis. The distal (apical) portion of the prostate rests against the urogenital diaphragm and the proximal (base) portion of the prostate rests against the bladder. The surface anatomy of the prostate is shown diagrammatically in Figure 45-3.[49] The prostate is surrounded by a complex array of fibro-connective tissue that is penetrated by bundles of nerves and vessels running superior-laterally and inferior-laterally. These bundles, called the *superior and inferior pedicles*, are attached to the pubic symphysis by puboprostatic ligaments.

As the prostate narrows distally, the inferior pedicles course medially. It becomes increasingly difficult to spare these nerves at the time of radical prostatectomy without increasing the risk of positive apical margins. Efforts to obtain wide margins in this region are likely to result in a shortened external sphincter and a higher risk of urinary incontinence. Since up to 80% of the time the apical portion of the prostate is involved by tumor, positive margins in this region following radical prostatectomy are not infrequent.[50] Suboptimal surgical technique is the cause of positive apical margins in 50% of patients, whereas the remaining cases are attributed to extracapsular extension in association with the neurovascular bundles.[51] Because of scant coverage of the apex by capsule, true extracapsular extension may be difficult to recognize with reliability in this region. True extracapsular extension is most common at the base of the prostate in the rectolateral region and in the region of the superior pedicle. Extracapsular extension tends to occur in association with regions of the capsule that are penetrated by nerves. These regions can be considered "routes of least resistance."

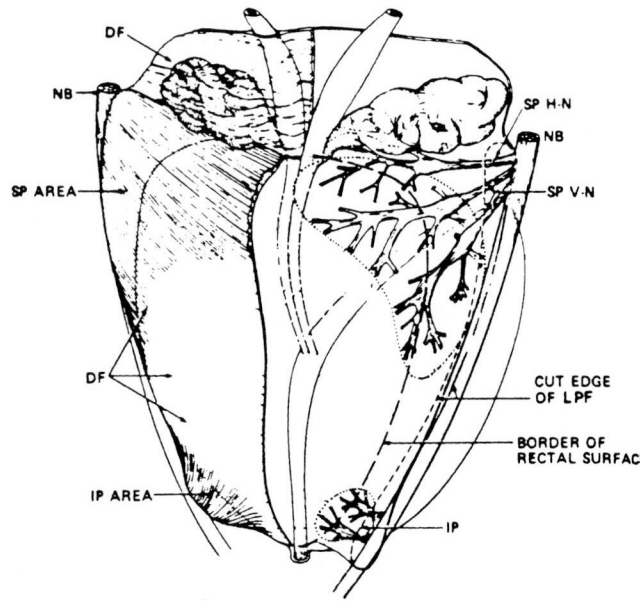

Figure 45–3. Distribution of nerve branches to prostate—right posterolateral view. Nerves within neurovascular bundle (*NB*) branch to supply prostate in large superior pedicle (*SP*) at prostate base and small inferior pedicle (*IP*) at prostate apex. Branches leave lateral pelvic fascia (*LPF*) to travel in Denonvilliers' fascia (*DF*), which has been cut away from right half of prostate. Nerve branches from superior pedicle fan out over large pedicle area (thickened area of *DF*). Small horizontal subdivision (*H-N*) crosses base to midline; large vertical subdivision (*V-N*) fans out extensively over prostate surface as far distally as midprostate. Branches continue their course within prostate after penetrating capsule within large nerve penetration area (*dotted line*). Small inferior pedicle has limited ramification and nerve penetration area (*dotted line*). (From Villers A, McNeal JE, Redwine EA, et al: The role of perineural space invasion in the local spread of prostate adenocarcinoma. *J Urol.* 1989;142:63.)

Although it would seem like a straightforward histopathologic diagnosis, the definition of extracapsular extension is not uniformly established in the literature. Investigators from Johns Hopkins University argue that focal penetration in association with low-grade disease is of little clinical significance.[52] These investigators have noted that "established extracapsular extension" (defined as a penetration of approximately 1 cm into surrounding fat) is a major unfavorable prognostic factor if the tumor Gleason score (GS) is grade 7 or higher. Because of the extremely favorable nature of the patients in the Johns Hopkins series, it is unclear whether their generalizations hold true for patients with favorable pretreatment characteristics, for whom less rigorous histopathologic evaluations are conducted.

Internal Anatomy

The prostate is frequently described as being made up of four distinct zones.[53] Anteriorly, fibromuscular stroma constitutes nearly one third of the prostate. The anterior zone is nonglandular and extends superiorly from the smooth muscle of the bladder neck and inferiorly to the urethra, apex, and external sphincter. This collection of fibromuscular tissue results in the characteristic *anterior prostatic convexity*. The central zone normally makes up 25% of the glandular prostate and is associated with a duct system that has orifices surrounding the ejaculatory duct on the convexity of the verumontanum. This portion of the prostate is both central and proximal to most of the remaining gland. The peripheral zone makes up nearly 70% of the glandular prostate, corresponding to the palpable portion of the gland and the source of most prostate cancers. The periurethrally located transitional zone makes up the remaining 5% of the glandular prostate. Histologically, the transitional zone resembles the peripheral zone but behaves differently and is the major site for the development of BPH.

The distribution of carcinoma within the prostate does not appear to be random, with adenocarcinoma involving the first 5 to 8 mm of the apical portion of the gland in up to 80% and being multifocal in up to 85% of patients. Even among the earliest cases, with mean volumes of only 0.11 mL, 40% are multifocal.[53] Historically, perineural invasion (PNI) has been a fairly common finding, with 84% of patients manifesting some degree of such involvement. Due to stage migration and a higher incidence of pathologically confined disease, this incidence of PNI may be decreasing as well.[54] In a study of stage B (T2) patients, Villers and associates reported extracapsular extension within perineural spaces in 50% and in the remaining cases it occurred in combination with PNI.[49] Figure 45-4 demonstrates the relationship between positive surgical margins and perineural space invasion. These authors concluded, "The penetration of carcinoma through the prostate capsule may depend almost entirely on the ability of the cancer to invade and travel along perineural spaces." This fact is partly responsible for the very cautious use of nerve sparing in patients with adverse pretreatment features.

PATHOLOGIC CONSIDERATIONS

Nearly 95% of all prostate cancers are adenocarcinomas. Small cell anaplastic carcinomas with neuroendocrine features and lymphomas are best managed with chemotherapy plus or minus radiation therapy, whereas sarcomas and various other types of carcinomas are frequently managed by surgery with or without radiation therapy. In general, patients with these unusual histologic types do poorly. Tumors displaying a signet ring pattern, for example, represent an uncommon subtype with a 3-year survival as low as 16.7%.[55] Several classification systems have been used to define the histologic grade for adenocarcinomas of the prostate. Tumors are frequently described as *well*, *moderately*, or *poorly differentiated* (grades I, II, and III, respectively).

The most widely accepted (and respected) grading system was described by Gleason.[56] The total *Gleason pattern score*, a sum of the two most common histologic patterns ("primary" and "secondary"), was shown to correlate with cancer-specific survival. Using this approach, the possible total GS may range from 2 to 10. Based on studies from the early 1990s, five major categories—2 to 4, 5, 6, 7, and 8 to 10—have been used classically for prognostic risk groups based on GS. Cruder grading systems using three groupings (e.g., well, moderate, and poor) suffer from the fact that moderately differentiated tumors usually include grades that are comparable

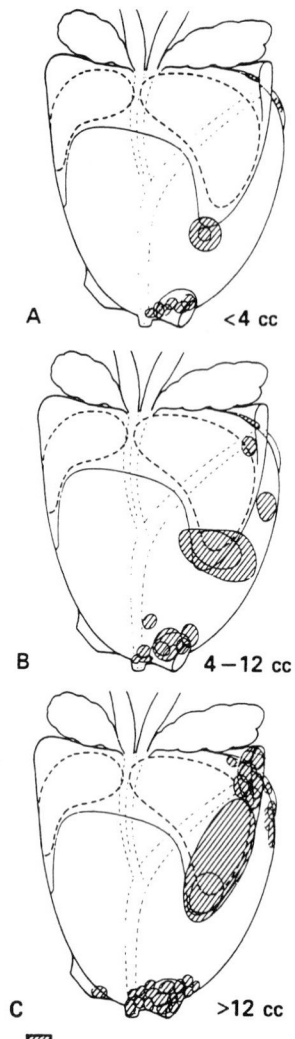

Figure 45–4. Distribution of areas of surgical margin positive for 156 stage B carcinomas in three consecutive volume ranges. Nerve penetration area is indicated by dotted lines. When bilateral, smallest area is represented on left side. **A,** ≤4 mL. **B,** 4 to 12 mL. **C,** >12 mL. (From Villers A, McNeal JE, Redwine EA, et al: The role of perineural space invasion in the local spread of prostate adenocarcinoma. *J Urol.* 1989;142:763-8.)

to GS's of 5, 6, or 7. Most contemporary series divide patients into GS less than or equal to 6, GS equal to 7, and GS 8 to 10.[45,54,57] If a patient presents with what is reported to be an unusually low GS (e.g., ≤4), his slides should be re-reviewed by an expert pathologist. When this is done, some will have no cancer, but most will have higher-grade cancers.[58]

Fine-needle aspiration of the prostate is very specific (false-positive rate, 0% to 2%) but not nearly as sensitive as once thought when six or fewer biopsies are taken.[59,60] There is a good correlation between cytologic grade and GS. Table 45-1 combines data reported by Benson with a series by Johnstone.[61,62] For low-grade tumors (GS 2 to 4) there is roughly a 50% chance of under-grading. For intermediate tumors there is a 15% chance of under-grading but a nearly equal chance of over-grading (10%). For high-grade tumors there is roughly a 25% chance of over-grading. The likelihood of under-grading decreases with the use of more biopsies and increases as the PSA

Table 45–1   Relationship Between Biopsy Stage and Final Pathologic Stage

Biopsy Grade	Pathologic Gleason Score			No. of Patients[†]
	2–4*	5–7*	8–10*	
Well (2–4)	50%	48%	2%	*n* = 122
Moderate (5–7)	10%	74%	15%	*n* = 258
Poor (8–10)	1%	25%	74%	*n* = 81

*Modified from the review by Johnstone et al (1995)[61] and from Benson (1988).[59]
†Number of patients in series by Benson and review of five series by Johnstone. Underlined numbers reflect understaging, and boldface numbers reflect overstaging.

level increases, with under-grading uncommon in patients with normal PSAs. As a result of these changes in biopsy practice patterns, Table 45-1 may not reflect the distribution in contemporary patients, but this table is still relevant to contemporary series reporting results out at 10 years.

There has been a gradual and rather dramatic increase in the number of biopsies taken over the past 10 years.[63] In the mid-1980s most patients had a single biopsy taken based on a palpable abnormality. By the early to mid-1990s, urologists began obtaining random or "blind" biopsies in response to an elevated PSA in addition to those areas resulting from a palpable abnormality. Sextant biopsy became standard in the 1990s. By the late 1990s it became clear that sextant biopsies are probably no longer adequate for diagnosing patients with an elevated PSA.[64,65] It now appears that obtaining two additional lateral cores substantially reduces that risk of missing foci of disease, while midline biopsies increase morbidity without significantly increasing the yield. In addition to reducing the number of false-negative biopsies, obtaining six or more cores may provide prognostic information (see later discussion).[66-68]

The clinical significance of PNI remains controversial. Some, but not all, studies attribute prognostic importance to this PNI.[69-78] Part of this controversy arises from the fact that pathologists do not uniformly comment on the presence or absence of PNI or distinguish between intraprostatic and extraprostatic PNI or the extent of nerve involvement. The significance may also be different for patients treated by surgery and radiotherapy and may be dependent on the dose of radiation delivered.[74,77,79,80] In a "borderline patient" (i.e., a patient with features straddling between low- and intermediate-risk disease) it may be prudent to consider it as a possible prognostic factor or "tie-breaker."

PROGNOSTIC FACTORS

Prostate-Specific Antigen, Gleason Score, Stage, and Risk Stratification Schemes

The most frequently used predictors for the extent of disease for clinically localized prostate cancer are pretreatment PSA, histologic grade (GS), and clinical stage. Additional pathologic features such as the percent or number of positive biopsies and the presence of perineural invasion have gained recognition as potentially

important prognostic factors.[66,67,81,82,69,72-74] Of these various factors, pretreatment PSA is the most important predictor of PSA failure, while GS followed by T stage appear to be the more important predictors of survival (see later discussion). Theoretically, the staging system used should divide patients into *low-*, *intermediate-*, and *high-risk* subsets of patients in such a way that prognosis is predicted and treatment guidelines can be evidence based. Table 45-2 summarizes the 2002 American Joint Committee on Cancer (AJCC) staging system.[83] The major revision compared with the earlier staging system is reinstatement of the category T2c category. A major shortcoming to the revised system includes the fact that it virtually ignores both PSA and GS. These factors have been shown to be important predictors of death from prostate cancer.[57,103] The 2002 AJCC staging system also fails to specify the imaging studies required before assigning clinical stage.

The biggest change in the management of prostate cancer over the past 5 years has been the development of a number of risk stratification schemes and predictive

Table 45–2   Classification of Cancer of The Prostate

Primary Tumor (T)

Clinical

TX	Primary tumor cannot be assessed
T0	No evidence of primary tumor
T1	Clinically inapparent tumor neither palpable nor visible by imaging
T1a	Tumor incidental histologic finding in ≤5% of tissue resected
T1b	Tumor incidental histologic finding in >5% of tissue resected
T1c	Tumor identified by needle biopsy (e.g., because of elevated PSA)
T2	Tumor confined within prostate*
T2a	Tumor involves one half of one lobe or less
T2b	Tumor involves more than one half of one lobe but not both lobes
T2c	Tumor involves both lobes
T3	Tumor extends through prostate capsule†
T3a	Extracapsular extension (unilateral or bilateral)
T3b	Tumor invades seminal vesicle(s)
T4	Tumor is fixed or invades adjacent structures other than seminal vesicles: bladder neck, external sphincter, rectum, levator muscles, or pelvic wall

*Tumor found in one or both lobes by needle biopsy but not palpable or reliably visible by imaging; classified as T1c.
†Invasion into the prostatic apex or into (but not beyond) the prostatic capsule is classified not as T3 but as T2.

Regional Lymph Nodes (N)

Clinical

NX	Regional lymph nodes were not assessed
N0	No regional lymph node metastasis
N1	Metastasis in regional lymph nodes

Pathologic

PNX	Regional nodes not sampled
PN0	No positive regional nodes
PN1	Metastases in regional nodes

From Greene FL, Page DL, Fleming ID, et al, eds. *AJCC Cancer Staging Manual*, 6th ed. New York: Springer; 2002.

algorithms based on combining the various prognostic factors. An increasing number of predictive algorithms are available to practicing clinicians. For example, Ross and investigators from Memorial Sloan-Kettering Cancer Center (MSKCC) cataloged 42 different predictive algorithms or nomograms described between 1966 and April 2000.[84] As summarized in Table 45-3, these predictive algorithms predict many different things ranging from the likelihood of a positive biopsy to pathologic stage, to the risk of PSA recurrence after "salvage" therapy delivered following failure of primary therapy. Just which is best and how to use them in clinical practice remains controversial, and a detailed discussion of these and newer algorithms is beyond the scope of this chapter. The next section focuses on the algorithms, nomograms, and risk group classification schemes that are currently most relevant to the use of radiotherapy in the treatment of localized prostate cancer.

SELECTED ALGORITHMS, NOMOGRAMS, AND RISK GROUP CLASSIFICATION SCHEMES

The available predictive algorithms appear to fall into four major categories: (1) simple additive models, predicting PSA failure; (2) models based on computational approaches, predicting PSA failure; (3) models based on computational approaches, predicting pathologic end points; and (4) models based on the computational approaches, predicting disease-specific and overall survival. There is overlap between these models because factors that predict PSA failure may predict survival with longer follow-up, pathologic stage correlates with PSA failure and survival, and models that predict overall and disease-specific survival also predict PSA failure.

The simple additive models are based on well-recognized prognostic factors that predict for PSA failure (± modifiers). The most commonly used risk stratification schemes were popularized by D'Amico and co-investigators from Harvard and Zelefsky and investigators from MSKCC.[85,86] These two risk systems are similar in that both define "low risk" as GS = 2 to 6, PSA less than 10 ng/mL, T1c-T2a; "intermediate risk" as including patients with any one of these: T2b, GS = 7 or PSA = 10 to 20; and "high

risk" as GS = 8 to 10, T2c or T3, or PSA greater than 20 ng/mL. Thus, both systems assume that the clinical significance of a GS of 7 is similar to having a PSA between 10 and 20 ng/mL and that a GS of 8 is similar in importance to having a PSA greater than 20 ng/mL. This assumption may or may not be a good one as discussed later. The major distinction between these two models is that Zelefsky et al. were among the first to report that patients with two intermediate factors behaved more like a high-risk patient (see Fig. 45-5). Le et al. carried this concept one step forward by demonstrating that patients with three adverse features did worse than those with two.[87] D'Amico et al. have championed the concept that the percentage of positive biopsies can be added to his risk classification system to improve its predictive ability for intermediate-risk patients (Fig. 45-6).[66] These *percent positive biopsies* may correlate with overall or disease-specific survival when additional modifications are made.[82] The importance of the percent positive biopsies may also depend on the type of therapy rendered. In at least one series, percent positive biopsies did not correlate with outcome when higher doses of radiotherapy are delivered.[81]

In an effort to address these issues, more complex models using multivariate statistical approaches that predict PSA failure have been developed by numerous investigators.[88-90] Several of the most widely recognized nomograms were developed by Kattan et al. from MSKCC. Inclusive in this list of nomograms are those that predict the risk of recurrences following three-dimensional conformal radiotherapy (3DCRT), radical prostatectomy, or brachytherapy (Fig. 45-7A and B). Several nomograms have been validated and some have been incorporated into the design of clinical trials.[91] The major strengths of these nomograms include: they were developed using well established statistical methods, they are based on the results of a relatively large number of patients, they have been validated by several other institutions, and they are available on the Internet. The Kattan nomograms (as they are frequently called) are also valuable because they incorporate additional factors such as the dose of radiation and the use of hormonal therapy. These nomograms are useful tools for providing estimates of

Table 45-3   Various Types of Nomograms for Prostate Cancer from 1966 to February 2000

Tables	End Point	Comments
1	Initial prostate evaluation predicting positive biopsies	Three studies: (ROC curve analysis, validated, and validated neural network)
2	Clinically localized predicting final pathologic stage	Four studies: (two of four validated) using pretreatment features
3	Clinically localized predicting specific path features	13 studies: insignificant disease (2); capsular penetration or extracapsular extension (2); organ confined (1); seminal vesicle involvement (2); lymph node (3); positive margins (2); and tumor volume (1)
4	Pretreatment variables to predict PSA recurrence after radical prostatectomy	Four studies: neural network (1); probability tables (1); risk groups (2); nomogram (1)
5	Pretreatment variables to predict PSA recurrence after EBRT	Six studies: probability tables (2); probability graph (2); risk groups (2)
6	Pretreatment variables to predict PSA recurrence after BT	Two studies: probability graph (2); risk groups (2)
7	Post-treatment variables to predict PSA recurrence after RP	Seven studies: probability formula (1); probability graph (1); risk groups (4); probability nomogram (1)
8	Increasing PSA to predict metastatic disease	Two studies: probability graph (1); probability table (1)

BT, brachytherapy; EBRT, external beam radiotherapy; PSA, prostate-specific antigen; ROC, receives operating curve; RP, radical prostatectomy.
Modified from Ross PL, Scardino PT, Kattan MW: A catalog of prostate cancer nomograms. *J Urol.* 2003;165:1562.

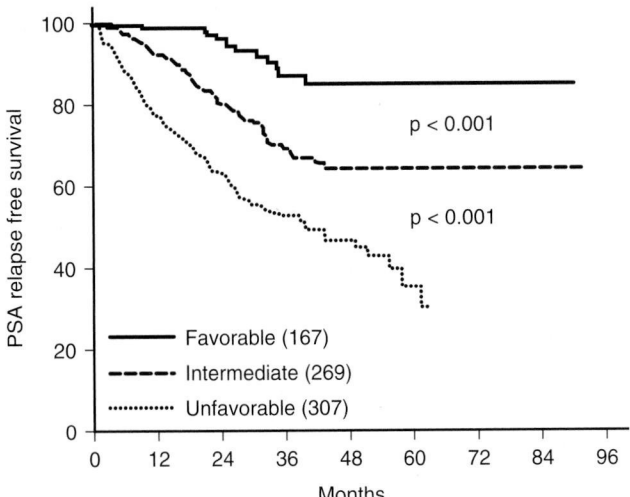

Figure 45–5. Actuarial (Kaplan-Meier) probability of achieving PSA relapse-free survival by prognostic subgroups. Patients with and without neoadjuvant androgen deprivation therapy were included in this analysis. PSA failure was defined as three consecutive elevations of serum PSA observed from post-treatment nadir, and the date of failure was recorded as the date of the first PSA rise. The numbers in parentheses indicate the number of patients included in each group. The number of patients at risk at 5 years for the favorable, intermediate, and unfavorable prognostic risk groups were 12, 17, and 6, respectively. (From Zelefsky MJ, Leibel SA, Gaudin PB, et al: Dose escalation with three-dimensional conformal radiation therapy affects the outcome in prostate cancer. *Int J Radiat Oncol Biol Phys.* 1998;41:491.)

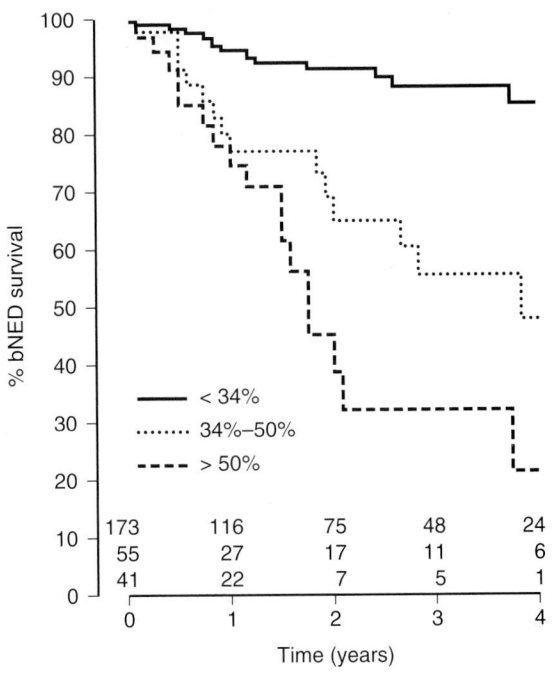

Figure 45–6. PSA failure-free survival stratified by the risk group defined using the PSA value, biopsy Gleason score, and 1992 American Joint Committee on Cancer clinical T stage for validation patients managed using a radical retropubic prostatectomy. Pair-wise *P* values: low versus intermediate risk, *P* < .0001; intermediate versus high risk, *P* < .0001; low versus high risk, *P* < .0001. (From D'Amico AV, Whittington R, Malkowicz SB, et al: Clinical utility of the percentage of positive prostate biopsies in defining biochemical outcome after radical prostatectomy for patients with clinically localized prostate cancer. *J Clin Oncol.* 2000;18:1164.)

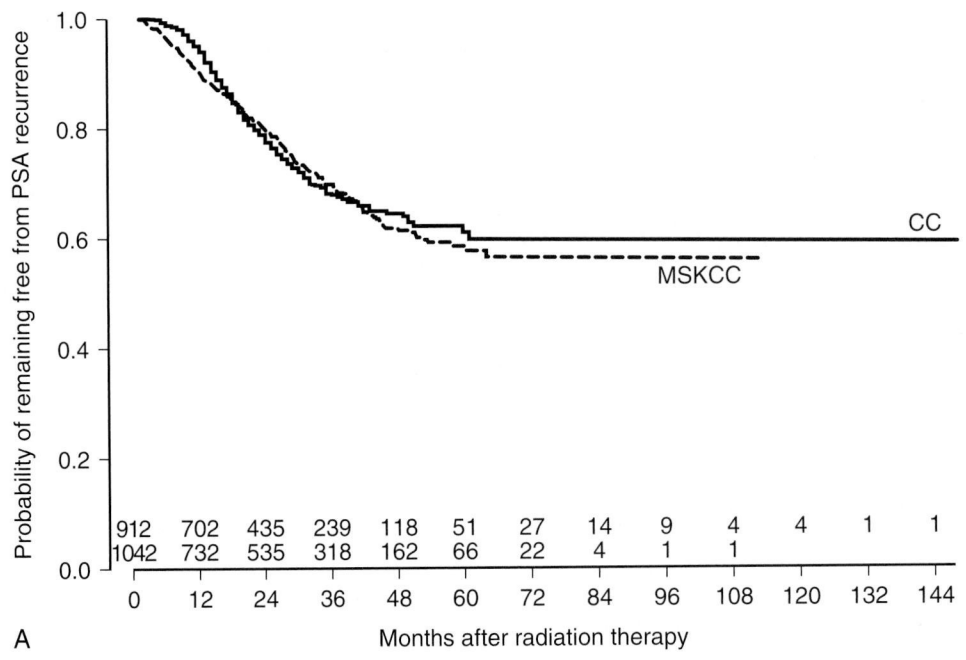

Figure 45–7. A, Kaplan-Meier estimates of disease-free probability for the Memorial Sloan-Kettering Cancer Center (MSKCC) and Cleveland Clinic series of 1042 and 912 patients, respectively. Numbers above the months indicate patients at risk for recurrence within each series. Abbreviation: CC, Cleveland Clinic.

Continued

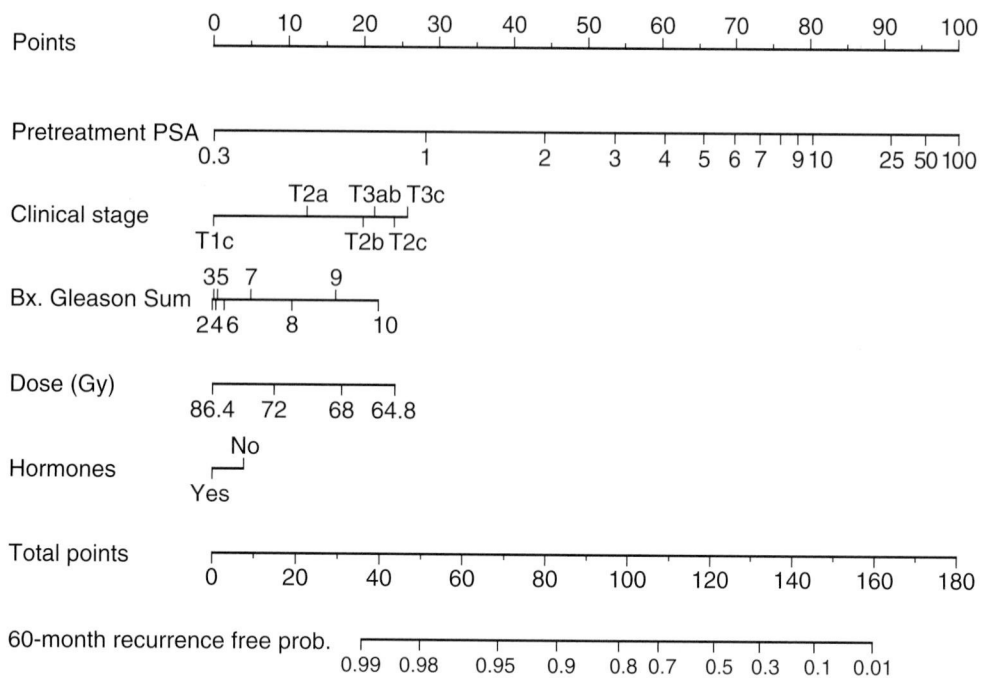

3D CONFORMAL RADIATION THERAPY NOMOGRAM FOR PSA RECURRENCE

Instructions for physician: Locate the patient's PSA on the **PSA** axis. Draw a line straight upwards to the **Points** axis to determine how many points towards recurrence the patient receives for his PSA. Repeat this process for the other axes, each time drawing straight upward to the **Points** axis. Sum the points achieved for each predictor and locate this sum on the **Total Points** axis. Draw a line straight down to find the patient's probability of remaining recurrence free for 60 months assuming he does not die of another cause first.

Note: This nomogram is not applicable to a man who is not otherwise a candidate for radiation therapy. You can use this only on a man who has already selected radiation therapy as treatment for his prostate cancer.

Instruction to patient: "Mr. X, if we had 100 men exactly like you, we would expect between <predicted percentage from nomogram – 10%> and <predicted percentage + 10%> to remain free of their disease at 5 years following conformal radiation therapy, and recurrence after 5 years is very rare."

B

Figure 45–7, cont'd. B, Radiotherapy nomogram based on 1042 patients treated at MSKCC for predicting PSA recurrence after radiation therapy. (From Kattan MW, Zelefsky MJ, Kupelian PA, et al: Pretreatment nomogram for predicting the outcome of three-dimensional conformal radiotherapy in prostate cancer. *J Clin Oncol.* 2000;18:3352.)

expected outcomes for the average patient. However, these nomograms should be used cautiously because the follow-up is limited; the data are not based on the results of prospective trials; and most importantly, these nomograms do not address survival. These nomograms are based on PSA failure, which has yet to be validated as a surrogate for important clinically meaningful end points.

Several investigators have described nomograms that predict the probability of pathologic end points.[92-94] Among these empirically derived models, the one proposed by Partin et al. from Johns Hopkins is the most widely recognized and used. Originally published in 1993, it allowed estimates of the risk of extra-capsular extension (ECE), seminal vesicle involvement (+SV), and lymph node involvement (+LN) based on pretreatment stage, PSA, and biopsy GS.[92] This nomogram was based on approximately 700 patients undergoing radical prostatectomy between 1982 and 1996 and was later validated by others. Partin et al. have updated their nomogram based on patients operated on from 1994 through 2000,

reflecting the changing patterns of presentation and clinical outcomes of more contemporary patients.[54]

Based on Partin's original report, Roach described three relatively simple equations that allowed estimates to be made of the risk of ECE, +SV, and +LN.[95] The simplicity of these equations in part comes from the fact that each uses a very similar format.

The equation used for estimating the risk of ECE is:

$$ECE = (3/2) \times PSA + [(GS - 3) \times 10]$$

The equation used for estimating the risk of +SV is:

$$+SV = (3/3) \times (PSA) + [(GS - 6) \times 10]$$

The equation used for estimating the risk of lymph node involvement is:

$$+LN = 2/3 \times (PSA) + [(GS - 6) \times 10]$$

Major advantages associated with using these equations include: they are simple enough to memorize, they have been validated, and they have been shown to predict

Table 45–4A   Overall Survival Rates (95% CI) by Risk and Age Groups

Risk Group	Age Group*	Death/n	5-yr (CI)	10-yr (CI)	15-yr (CI)	Median (yr)
1	≤ 65	60/136	86% (80–92)	66% (59–75)	52% (43–62)†	
T1–2 & GS = 6	65–75	96/185	85% (80–90)	58% (51–66)	35% (27–46)*	10.9
or T3 GS <6	>75	27/42	86% (76–97)	43% (30–62)	NS	9.0
	ALL	183/363	85% (82–89)	59% (54–65)	39% (32–47)*	11.2
2	≤65	65/144	87% (81–93)	62% (54–72)	31% (20–46)	12.7
T3 & GS = 6	65–75	137/239	80% (75–85)	44% (37–52)	21% (14–29)	9.2
or T1–2 & GS = 7	>75	30/60	81% (71–92)	40% (26–60)	18% (6–52)*	8.9
	ALL	232/443	82% (79–86)	50% (45–56)	24% (18–32)	10.0
3	≤65	53/90	67% (58–78)	36% (25–50)	18% (8–39)	8.5
T3 & GS = 7	65–75	104/187	67% (60–74)	36% (28–46)	19% (8–45)	7.8
or T1–2 & GS >7	>75	42/61	70% (59–83)	15% (7–34)	NS	7.1
	ALL	199/338	68% (63–73)	32% (26–39)	16% (9–27)	7.6
4	≤65	62/91	54% (45–66)	23% (14–36)	15% (8–29)†	6.3
T3 & GS = 8	65–75	135/184	48% (41–56)	17% (11–26)	11% (6–20)†	4.8
or N + GS = 8	>75	32/49	62% (49–77)	20% (10–42)	NS	5.8
	ALL	229/324	52% (47–58)	19% (14–25)	12% (8–19)*	5.3

*Extrapolated from 13-year results.
†Extrapolated from 12-year results. From Roach M, Lu J, V. Pilepich M, et al: Four prognostic groups predict long-term survival from prostate cancer following radiotherapy alone on Radiation Therapy Oncology Group clinical trials. *Int J Radiat Oncol Biol Phys.* 2000;47:609.
CI, Confidence interval; GS, Gleason score; NS, Not sufficient number of patients for accurate estimates.

biochemical failure in patients undergoing external beam radiotherapy.[96-99] These equations also formed the basis for stratification in a large phase I to II 3D dose escalation trial (9406) and defined eligibility for a large phase III Trial (9413) conducted by the Radiation Therapy Oncology Group (RTOG).[100,101] A potential disadvantage is the fact that patients with similar calculated risk for pathologic extent of disease may not have uniform outcomes. For example, a risk of 10% could result from having a GS of 7 or a PSA of 15 ng/mL. Of note, recent data from Stanford University suggest that the correlation coefficient between serum PSA and tumor volume is relatively poor for patients with PSAs less than 9 ng/mL.[9] Thus, at the lower PSA values this equation might underestimate the actual risk in patients with extensive high-grade disease (which tends to be associated with a lower PSA per gram of tissue). In addition, these equations don't include confidence intervals and don't take into account other factors such as the percent positive biopsies. These equations also tend to give higher calculated risk than the more recent updated Partin nomogram.[54] This may or may not be a problem, however, depending on how the information is used clinically (see results of RTOG 9413 later).

All of the models, algorithms, nomograms, and risk groups described earlier are used to predict either pathologic extent of disease or risk of PSA failure. Empirical

models that predict overall and disease-specific survival have been described by investigators from the RTOG.[57] These RTOG risk groups were derived based on a large collection of patients treated on phase III prospective randomized trials with long follow-up. These risk groups were developed using GS, T-stage, and lymph node status. The RTOG risk groups with overall survival by age are summarized in Table 45-4 and the disease-specific survival curves are shown in Figure 45-8. Pretreatment PSA was not included because most patients were treated before the availability of this marker. The beauty of this model is that it can be used to estimate survival as well as the benefits of hormonal therapy (see discussion on use of hormonal therapy).[45] Additional strengths are that it has been validated by investigators from the University of California at San Francisco (UCSF) and the University of Michigan using independent data based on contemporary patients, and it maintains its ability to predict overall and disease-specific survival (Fig. 45-9A–C).[102,103] Furthermore, using this risk scheme, these investigators have demonstrated the impact of pretreatment PSA on failure and overall survival (Fig. 45-10A, B). Based on these data, the investigators have modified the RTOG risk groups by adding in pretreatment PSA to develop a "new" staging system, and work is under way to validate its use in a larger data set.[104]

Table 45–4B   Disease-Specific Survival (95% CI) by Risk Groups

Risk Group	Death/n	5-yr (CI)	10-yr (CI)	15-yr (CI)
1	53/363	96% (94–98)	86% (82–90)	72% (62–83)
2	84/232	94% (92–97)	75% (70–81)	61% (51–72)
3	92/338	83% (79–87)	62% (55–70)	39% (26–60)
4	154/324	64% (58–70)	34% (27–42)	27% (20–37)*

*Extrapolated from 12-year results.
CI, Confidence interval.
From Roach M, Lu J, V. Pilepich M, et al: Four prognostic groups predict long-term survival from prostate cancer following radiotherapy alone on Radiation Therapy Oncology Group clinical trials. *Int J Radiat Oncol Biol Phys.* 2000;47:609.

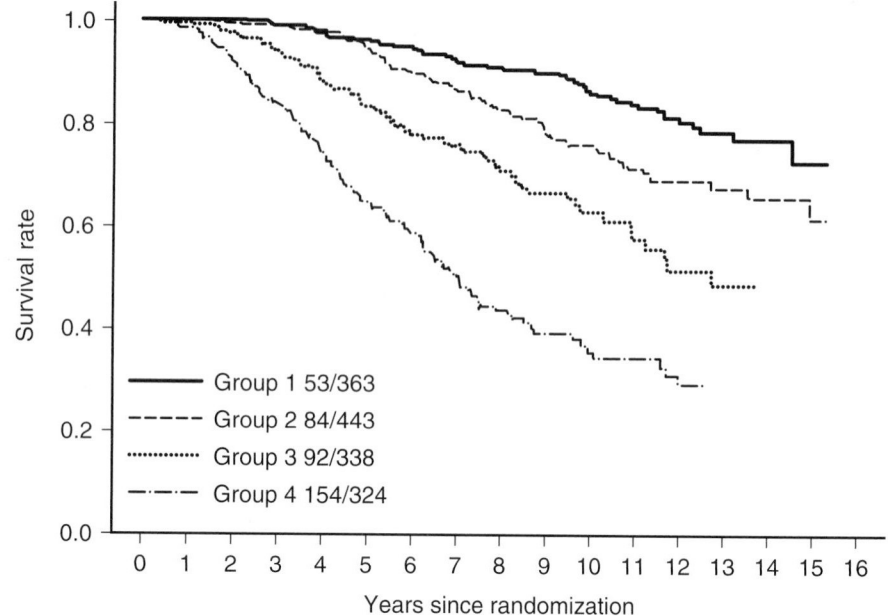

Figure 45–8. Disease-specific survival, respectively, by four risk groups. From top to bottom: (1) group 1 patients had a GS = 2–6, and clinical stage T1–2Nx; (2) group 2 patients had a GS = 2–6, and T3Nx or N+ or GS = 7, T1–2Nx; (3) group 3 patients were clinically staged as T3Nx, with a GS = 7, or T1–2Nx, GS = 8–10; and (4) group 4 patients were clinically staged as T3Nx, S = 8–10, or N+, GS = 8–10. (From Roach M, Lu J, V. Pilepich M, et al: Four prognostic groups predict long term survival from prostate cancer following radiotherapy alone on Radiation Therapy Oncology Group clinical trials. *Int J Radiat Oncol Biol Phys.* 2000;47:609.)

There are advantages and disadvantages to each of the available algorithms. Some are simpler than others, some are more logical reflections of the extent of disease. Each is like a different language, religion, or style of art. Clinicians must decide which nomogram, algorithm, or risk group classification scheme they find useful in their practice. The routine use of cytogenetic markers are not yet ready for "prime time" and readers are invited to review this extensive and growing body of literature on their own if they wish. By the next edition of this text, this area may well be the "new frontier" for truly understanding the risk of death from prostate cancer, perhaps making much of the section just covered obsolete.

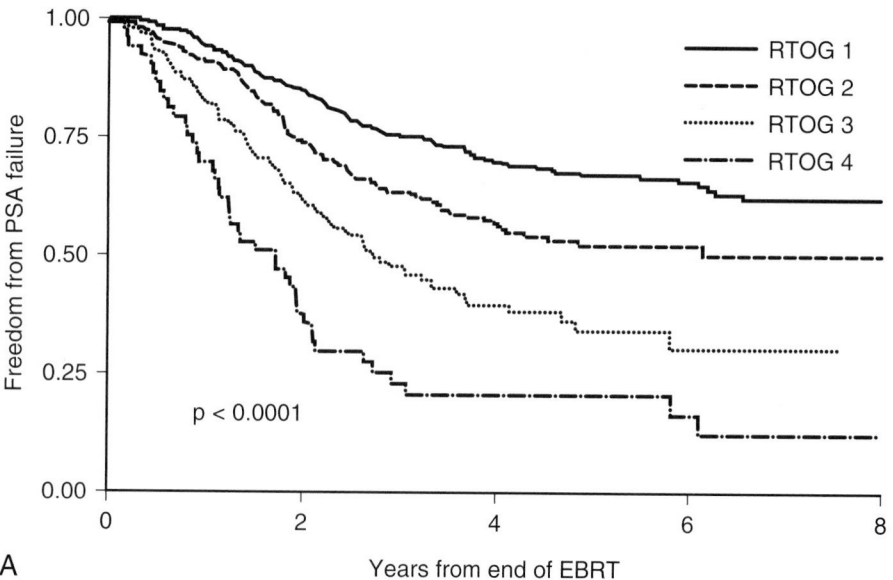

Figure 45–9. A, B, C. Relationship between Radiation Therapy Oncology Group risk groups and freedom from PSA failure. **A,** Freedom from PSA failure (FFPF); **B,** progression-free survival defined as death after PSA failure; and **C,** overall survival (OS) rates. Each sequential pairwise comparison of FFPF also differed significantly, indicating that the risk groups designed using the RTOG criteria are also relevant to contemporary patients (risk 1 vs. 2, P = 0.0002; risk 2 vs. 3, P = 0.0005; risk 3 vs. 4, P = 0.002). All pairwise comparisons of PFS were significantly different, with the one exception of the two intermediate risk groups 2 and 3 (risk 1 vs. 2, P = 0.008; risk 2 vs. 3, P = 0.11; risk 3 vs. 4, P = 0.007). The same effect of increasing risk on OS as observed with risk group 1 differing from groups 3 and 4 (P = 0.006 and <0.0001, respectively) and risk group 2 differing from group 4 (P = 0.001). (From Roach M, Weinberg V, McLaughlin P, et al: Serum prostate specific antigen (PSA) and survival following external beam radiotherapy for carcinoma of the prostate. *Urology.* 2003; Apr, 61(4):730-5).

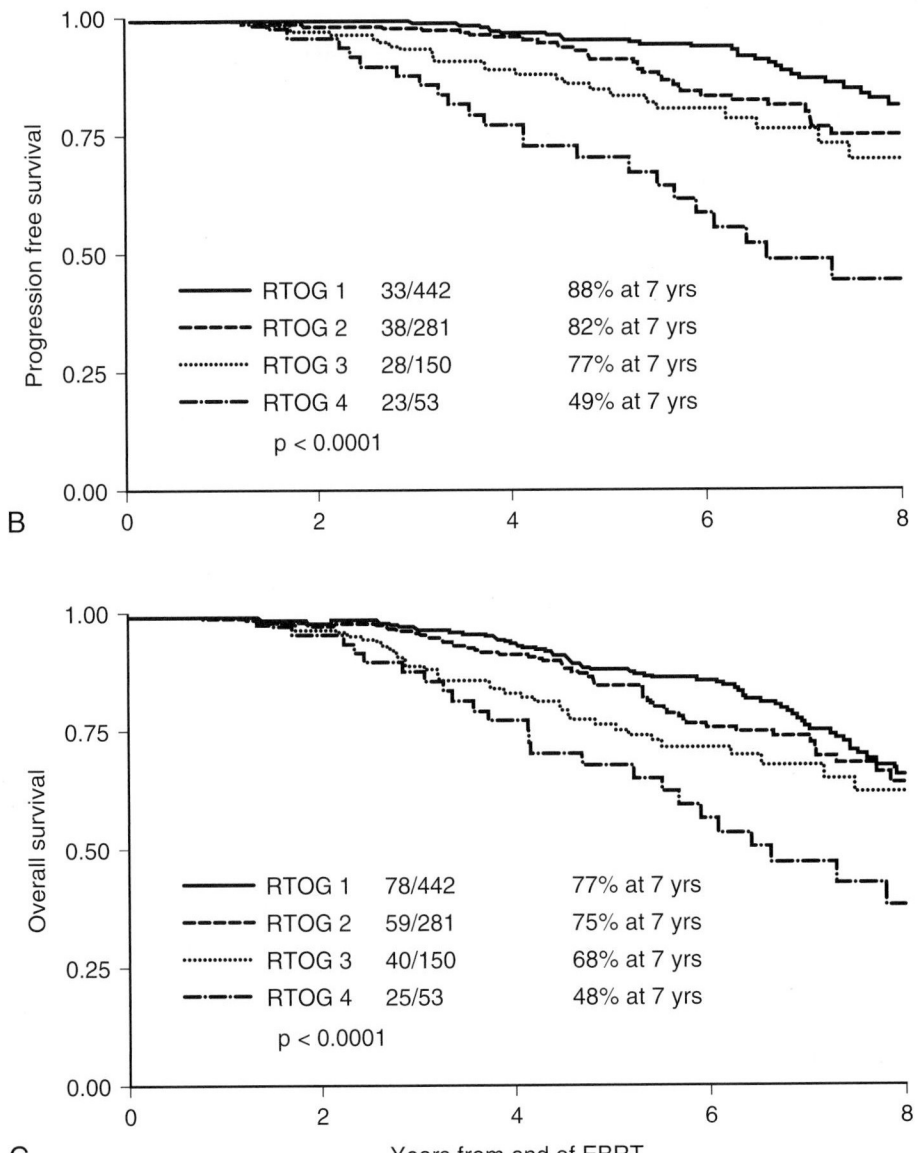

Figure 45–9, cont'd. For legend see opposite page.

CLINICAL PRESENTATION

Most men presenting with prostate cancer are asymptomatic and diagnosed only because of an elevated PSA or an incidentally noted abnormality on digital rectal examination. Occasionally a diagnosis is made following a transurethral resection of the prostate (TURP) for obstructive symptoms due to BPH. Rarely, patients with locally advanced disease present with obstructive symptoms due to bulky tumor. Some men develop locally advanced or metastatic disease without ever manifesting obstructive symptoms.[105]

A number of investigators have reported a poorer outcome among patients who receive a TURP before radiation therapy.[106,107] However, an equal number of reports have concluded that there is no difference in outcome following a TURP.[108,109] Reports suggesting the possible dissemination of cancer cells (detected by RT-PCR) at the time of radical prostatectomy, brachytherapy, or

biopsies have revived concern over the potential for systemic spread resulting from TURPs.[110-112] However, more recent studies suggest that RT-PCR–based detection methods are overly sensitive and should be ignored, thus alleviating some concerns about dissemination of disease secondary to these procedures.[113]

ROUTES OF SPREAD

Tumor volume, grade, location, and serum PSA are considered independent risk factors for ECE. The initial enthusiasm for PSA as a marker resulted from the belief that the serum PSA correlated roughly with the volume of tumor in the prostate.[114] More recent data suggest that the correlation between PSA and tumor volume is poor for patients with PSAs less than 9 ng/mL.[9] Stamey et al. noted that the correlation between cancer volume and preoperative serum PSA in 875 men was driven by large

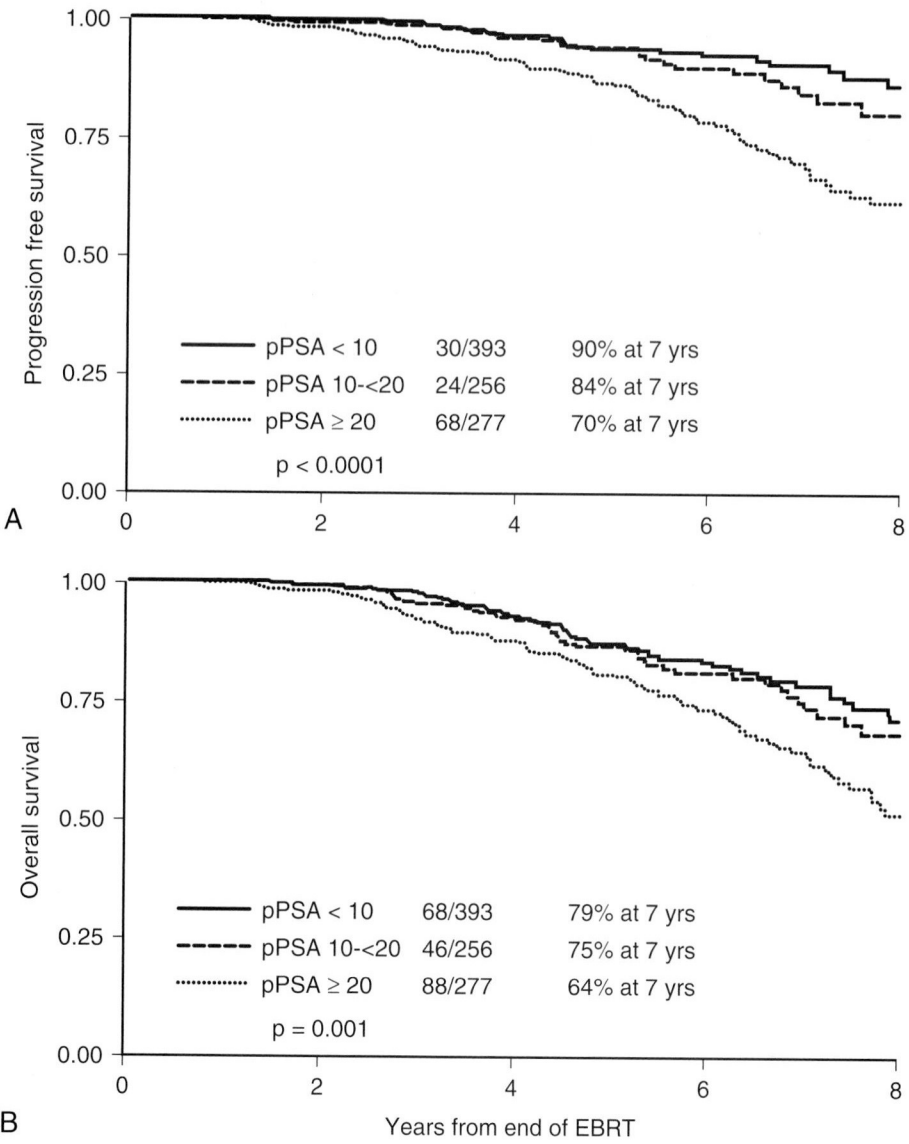

Figure 45–10. A, Progression-free survival (PFS) defined as death after PSA failure and **B,** overall survival (OS) for patients treated with radiotherapy alone by pretreatment PSA (pPSA), respectively. (From Roach M, Weinberg V, McLaughlin P, et al: Serum prostate specific antigen (PSA) and survival following external beam radiotherapy for carcinoma of the prostate. *Urology.* 2003; Apr, 61(4):730-5.)

cancers with serum PSAs greater than 22 ng/mL. They concluded that below 9 ng/mL, BPH was the major cause of PSA elevation and the primary reason for diagnosis of prostate cancer.[9]

After local extension beyond the capsule of the prostate and seminal vesicles, the next major sites recognized for tumor spread are the pelvic lymph nodes. Table 45-5 summarizes the distribution of lymph nodes reported in surgical series as reviewed by Golimbu and coworkers.[115] This review is unusual because it evaluates the incidence of involvement of presacral and presciatic nodes. In addition to the classic involvement of the obturator nodes, patients were found to have frequent metastasis to the external iliac, presacral, and presciatic nodes. These last two sites are noteworthy because patients occasionally manifest single lymph node metastasis to these two nodal drainage areas. Figure 45-11 demonstrates by lymphangiography the location of the major nodal drainage areas.

Prostate-Specific Antigen, Lymphadenectomy, and Laparoscopic Nodal Sampling

There is no universal agreement on the indications for a lymphadenectomy or laparoscopic nodal sampling. It is clear that certain subgroups of patients can be spared this procedure because they are at very low risk for lymph node involvement. If a patient plans to undergo a radical prostatectomy only if the nodes are negative, then the information could be perceived as useful. High-risk patients who are found to have positive lymph nodes may benefit because of the potential benefits associated with early androgen deprivation.[116] If a high-risk patient will undergo long-term androgen suppression and whole-pelvic irradiation, it may not be worth the cost and morbidity for him to undergo node sampling.

The standard lymph node dissection is generally described as extending from the bifurcation of the

Table 45–5   Distribution of Node Metastasis in Clinically Localized Prostate Cancer

Nodal Sites	Involved, %	Single, %
#1 External iliac	60	0
#2 Obturator	53	20
#3 Presacral	53	7
#4 Presciatic	47	7
#5 Common iliac	27	0
#6 Hypogastric	14	0
#1 + 2 External iliac/obturator	86	NA
#3 + 4 Presacral-presciatic	80	NA

NA, not available.

Modified from Golimbu M, Morales P, Al-Askari S, et al: Extended pelvic lymphadenectomy for prostate cancer. *J Urol.* 1979;121:617-620.

common iliac vessels medially to the pelvic floor and to the inferior border of the prostate, and then superiorly along the hypogastric vessels back to the bifurcation of the common iliac vessels. If pelvic lymph nodes are negative, periaortic nodes are generally assumed to be negative, although skip metastases have been reported.[117] There is a clear correlation between the side of palpable tumor and the side that metastatic nodes are likely to occur.[118] Frozen sections are highly specific (100%) but

the sensitivity is modest at 65% or less.[119] Although a standard lymph node dissection is usually considered the most sensitive method of establishing lymph node status, it is also not 100% sensitive. In the series reported by Freeman and colleagues, 16% of patients who by standard approaches were defined as being pathologic stage T3N0 were found by a monoclonal epithelial PSA assay to have occult metastases.[120] This estimate is also likely to be an underestimation of the true incidence because not all of the nodes were sampled and occult nodal involvement may be much more common than previously recognized.[121] One recent trial suggested that extended node dissections did not increase the yield compared to a more limited sampling, but it included patients with very early disease.[122] Studies including patients with more extensive disease tend to confirm the problem with sampling error and a significant incidence of false-negatives when only limited sampling is done.[123,124] These studies may underestimate the true incidence of metastatic disease, based on assays thought to be more sensitive than a histopathologic evaluation. However, most urologists seem to consider a node sampling adequate even for high-risk patients.[121,125]

One of the most compelling studies addressing the issue of occult nodal involvement is the recent report by Shariat et al. They compared the detection of human glandular kallikrein 2 (hK2) mRNA expression in archival

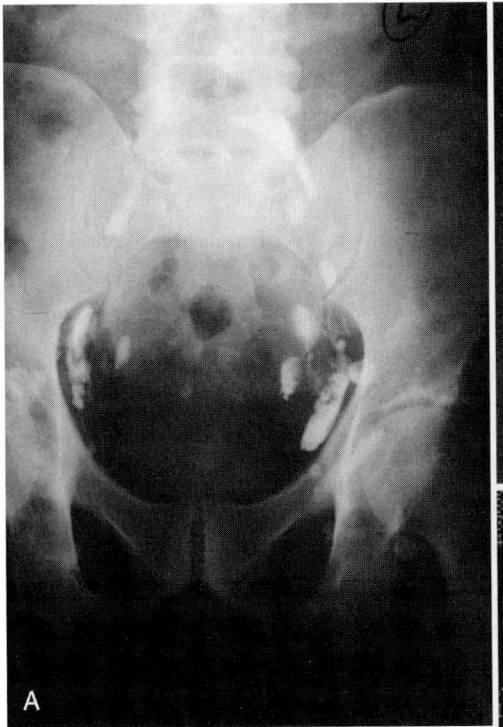

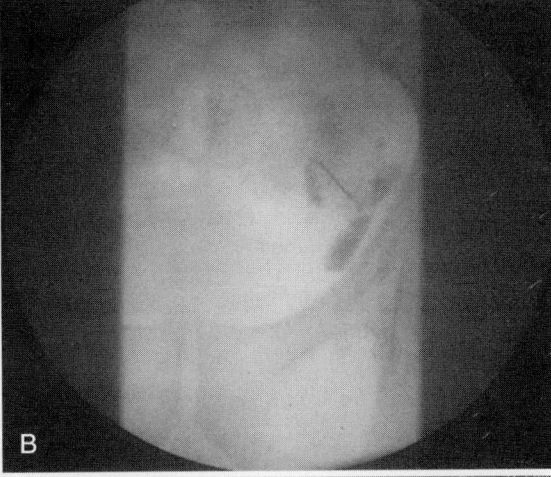

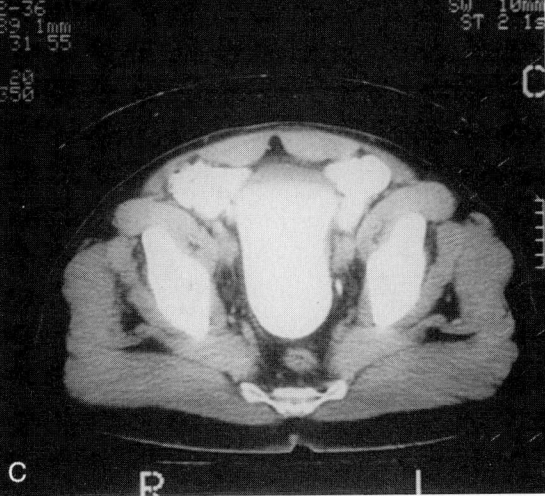

Figure 45–11. A, Anterior view of a lymphangiogram in a patient with prostate cancer. Note the enlarged external iliac node. **B,** Needle-directed biopsy of that node. Fluoroscopy demonstrates needle placement into external iliac node. **C,** Axial CT of nodes seen on lymphangiogram. (Courtesy of Sucha Asbell, MD, Albert Einstein Medical Center, Philadelphia, PA.)

lymph nodes and the risk of progression of disease and survival in patients who were found to have pathologically unfavorable but node-negative disease following radical prostatectomy.[126] They evaluated total RNA extracted from fixed, paraffin-embedded, histopathologically normal pelvic lymph nodes from 199 pT3N0 prostate cancer patients for hK2-expressing cells using a reverse transcriptase polymerase chain reaction (RT-PCR)/hK2 assay. In postoperative multivariable models, the RT-PCR/hK2 result was associated with disease progression ($P = 0.001$), development of distant metastases ($P = 0.001$), and prostate cancer–specific survival ($P = 0.005$). The authors concluded that RT-PCR/hK2 could be used to detect biologically and clinically significant occult prostate cancer metastases in histopathologically normal lymph nodes in patients with adverse pathology.[126] These data taken as a whole suggest that the reported incidences of lymph node involvement in multiple surgical series must be taken with "a grain of salt" and provide a rationale for prophylactic pelvic nodal radiotherapy.[54,127]

The Significance of Lymph Node Involvement

Nearly all patients with lymph node involvement eventually fail. Leibel and associates demonstrated that while local control tended to decrease the risk of distant failure for node-negative patients, obtaining local control did not appear to reduce the risk of distant metastasis in node-positive patients (Fig. 45-12).[128] As with other studies, they noted that the extent of lymph node involvement correlated with how soon failure is likely to occur. These patients did not receive early adjuvant hormonal therapy, however. Ten-year survivors have been noted among patients with pathologically proven positive lymph nodes despite initial treatment with radiotherapy with and without hormonal therapy, with the former generally doing substantially better than the latter group.[45,57,129-131] The recent results of RTOG 9413 (demonstrating the benefits of whole pelvic irradiation when combined with neoadjuvant hormonal therapy) suggest that there may be a sub-population of patients with nodal disease that is controllable.[127]

STAGING STUDIES

Standard staging studies for prostate cancer should include a pretreatment PSA, transrectal ultrasound-directed multiple core biopsies (generally eight or more cores), and a digital rectal examination. Routine chest x-ray studies or cystoscopic examinations are unwarranted unless accompanied by the presence of a smoking history or urinary symptoms. Bone scans are not justified if the PSA is less than or equal to 10 ng/mL with a relatively poor yield for this test until the PSA exceeds 50 ng/mL when the serum alkaline phosphatase is normal. The routine use of lymphangiograms has no role in the management of prostate cancer because of the failure to define the architecture for commonly involved lymph nodes. Neither abdominal-pelvic computed tomography (CT) nor conventional magnetic resonance imaging (MRI) are warranted if the

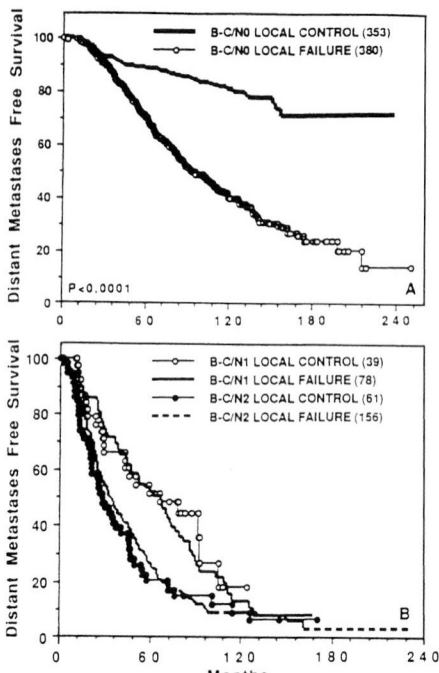

Figure 45–12. **Top,** Kaplan-Meier time-adjusted analysis of distant metastases–free survival by local tumor status in 679 patients with stage B-C/N0 carcinoma of the prostate treated with pelvic lymphadenectomy and retropubic ^{125}I implantation. The actuarial distant metastases–free survival for locally controlled patients was significantly improved compared to those who developed a local recurrence ($P < 0.00001$). **Bottom,** Kaplan-Meier time-adjusted analysis of distant metastases–free survival by local tumor status in 334 patients with stage B-C/N1-2 carcinoma of the prostate treated with pelvic lymphadenectomy and retropubic ^{125}I implantation. Control of the primary tumor had no impact on subsequent development of distant metastases in the N1 or N2 subgroup of patients. However, the distant metastases–free survival for locally controlled N1 patients was significantly improved, compared with locally controlled N2 patients ($P < 0.004$). (From Leibel SA, Fuks Z, Zelefsky MJ, et al: The effects of local and regional treatment on the metastatic outcome in prostatic carcinoma with pelvic lymph node involvement. *Int J Radiat Oncol Biol Phys.* 1994;28:7.)

PSA is less than 20 ng/mL.[132,133] These scans may be of limited value in this setting because there appears to be a poor correlation between the size of the lymph node and the presence of cancer. For example, Teguert et al. measured the axial and longitudinal dimensions of the nodes in 980 patients who underwent radical retropubic prostatectomy with bilateral pelvic lymph node dissection for clinically localized prostate cancer. Patients with and without metastases were analyzed to assess the significance of lymph node size in predicting the presence of metastases.[134] All patients had negative preoperative CT and bone scans. The mean longitudinal and axial nodal size was $1.65 \text{ cm} \times 0.8 \text{ cm}$ and $3.50 \text{ cm} \times 1.0 \text{ cm}$ for positive and negative nodes, respectively. They concluded that lymph node size should not be used as a surrogate for the presence of lymph node metastases.[134] Of course, there may have been some selection bias whereby patients with poor risk features and increased nodes on CT scan did not undergo surgery.

Recent work conducted at UCSF suggests that endorectal MRI combined with magnetic resonance spectroscopy imaging (MRSI) may prove to be useful in staging and treatment planning for selected patients.[135] The metabolic information provided by MRSI combined with the morphologic information provided by MRI can significantly improve the assessment of ECE.[136,137] In a study of 62 patients undergoing radical prostatectomy followed by an evaluation of histopathologic step-sections, UCSF researchers reported that the addition of MRSI (high specificity) to MRI (high sensitivity) resulted in improved localization of prostate cancer within the prostate. Combined MRI/MRSI allowed localization of cancer to a sextant of the prostate with a sensitivity of up to 95% ($P < 0.05$ to MRI alone) when either MRI or MRSI were positive. When both MRI and MRSI were positive, they reported a specificity of up to 91% ($P < 0.05$ vs. MRI alone). MRSI may also improve the accuracy of cancer detection by MRI in patients with postbiopsy hemorrhage.[138] Postbiopsy hemorrhage is present in a large percentage of newly diagnosed patients and causes the overestimation of intra-glandular cancer extent and the assessment of extracapsular spread.

An improvement in sensitivity and specificity of cancer localization can be attained when MRI/MRSI data are combined with biopsy data.[139] The addition of a positive sextant biopsy to concordant MRI/MRSI findings may increase the specificity (98%) and the sensitivity (94%) of cancer localization obtained compared to when any of the tests alone were positive for cancer. A small study also indicated that MRSI might provide new insights into tumor aggressiveness, leading to an improvement in risk assessment in patients with clinically localized prostate cancer.[140] Based on a preliminary analysis of 26 patients who underwent prostatectomy, there appeared to be a strong linear correlation between the decrease in citrate and the elevation of choline with cancer aggressiveness (GS).[141] While histologic scores will remain the standard, the potential of MRSI to provide additional information is exciting because of the potential for biopsy sampling errors. Patient management is critically dependent on the GS, so perhaps this technology could be used to identify patients who might benefit from repeat biopsies to selected regions of the gland (see Fig. 45-15 later).

DEFINITIONS OF FAILURE FOLLOWING DEFINITIVE LOCAL THERAPIES

Definitions of Failure Following Radiation Therapy

The long natural history of prostate cancer and imprecise methods of gauging local control have hampered an accurate assessment of the efficacy of treatment. It is generally assumed that effective local therapy can reduce mortality if the patient survives other comorbid conditions. Until the early 1990s, local control following irradiation was based on regression of palpable tumor. However, some tumors (stage T1a-T1c) are nonpalpable at diagnosis, and the true extent of involvement among patients with palpable disease is frequently underestimated. Significant interobserver differences and the possibility that palpable nodules may not be cancerous also compromise the validity of using this end point alone. To further confound the problems associated with specificity of digital rectal exams, benign prostate nodules associated with a slight rise in the PSA, despite several negative biopsies, have occasionally been observed (Roach personal communication, 2001).

Post-treatment biopsies have been used selectively in hopes of obtaining a more objective measure of local tumor eradication. Biopsies show a much higher incidence of residual tumor than palpation. The identification of histologically viable tumor is reflective of ineffective local treatment. A wide range of results in the incidence of positive biopsies following radiotherapy can be found in the literature, with the differences seen probably reflecting major selection bias. Table 45-6 summarizes data from a selected number of these series and the relationship of the PSA level to the likelihood of a positive biopsy. If patients with locally advanced disease or with palpable re-growth of disease are biopsied, the incidence of positive biopsies approaches 90%.[142] If patients with low pretreatment PSAs or patients with clinically controlled disease and nonrising PSAs are biopsied, the incidence of positive biopsies is much lower.[143-145] Routine post-treatment biopsies may be conceptually appealing, but the adoption of this policy is hampered by reluctance of patients to undergo this

Table 45–6   Selected Biopsy Results After Radiotherapy for Localized Prostate Cancer by Clinical Stage

First Author (yr)	T1/T2a/T2b-c/T3	Patients, *n*	+ Biopsy %	Comments
Crook (2000)*	96/115/170/108	489	≈15/28/34/42	Only PSA nadir and Bx status at 24–36 months were independent predictors of outcome
Martineli (1992)	16/30/32/14	81	22	Temporary implants
Kabalin (1989)	11/11/44/22	27	93	How were they selected?
Scardino (1988)	16/40/18/26	140	32	+ Bx predicts local recurrences
Schellhammer (1987)	10/6/51/34	126	33[†]	+ Bx predicts for distant recurrences
Freiha (1984)	2/3/47/48	64	61[†]	89% + if abnormal exam
Leach (1982)	11/7/14/68	107	≈65	—
Nactsheim (1978)	0/10/24/66	32	52[†]	How were they selected?

*Modified from Crook J, Malone S, Perry G, et al: Postradiotherapy prostate biopsies: What do they really mean? Results for 498 patients. *Int J Radiat Oncol Biol Phys.* 2000;48:355.
[†]Greater than or equal to 12 to 18 months.
Bx, biopsies; PSA, prostate-specific antigen.

invasive procedure for which a certain course of action is lacking. Cost considerations and ambiguity in interpretation of biopsy samples have also tended to discourage the routine use of post-treatment biopsies.

Crook et al. have extensively studied the issue of post-treatment biopsies following conventional EBRT.[144] A cohort of 498 men were followed prospectively with systematic transrectal ultrasound (TRUS)-guided post-RT prostate biopsies, starting 12 to 18 months after treatment with conventional RT. Patients with negative biopsies were re-biopsied at 36 months while those with a positive biopsy but a declining PSA underwent additional biopsies every 6 to 12 months. They reported an actuarial freedom from local failure at 5 years ranging from 85% for T1b/T1c; to 72% for T2a; to 60% for T2b/c/T3; to 0% for T4. After a multivariate analysis, only PSA nadir ($P = 0.0002$) and biopsy status at greater than 24 months ($P = 0.0005$) were independent predictors of outcome. The authors concluded that "Post-RT prostate biopsies were not a gold standard of treatment efficacy, but are an independent predictor of outcome." Kestin et al. demonstrated a relationship between the dose of radiation delivered and the risk of a positive biopsy, but Pollack et al. did not, leaving this issue unresolved.[145,146] These conflicting results may reflect problems with sample size, duration of follow-up, differences in patient selection, or the number of biopsies obtained.

The use of the serum PSA has improved our ability to identify treatment failure much earlier than before using the digital rectal exam. Eradication of local tumor results in a substantial decline (>90% reduction) in the serum PSA. An empirical "rule of thumb" is that the PSA half-life following external beam radiotherapy (EBRT) is approximately 3 months. The lowest PSA value achieved following EBRT is typically reached at 24 to 36 months, but continued declines may be seen at 4 to 5 years and beyond and may be indicative of cure.[168] The rate of decline following brachytherapy tends to be more variable, but the median nadir tends to be lower and occur later (beyond 40 months) compared to EBRT.

As with radical prostatectomy, the definition of biochemical (PSA) failure following radiotherapy has evolved over the past 10 years.[147] Most early definitions were based on the notion that a value exceeding a specific threshold could be used to determine when treatment had failed. For example, Geist recommended that the upper limits of PSA for biochemical control be less than 2.0 ng/mL.[148] Hanks et al. initially defined biochemical failure as a PSA of greater than 1.5 ng/mL.[149] Several other investigators suggested that a PSA of greater than 1 ng/mL be considered evidence of biochemical failure.[150,151] Obviously, the decision as to which PSA level is used for defining biochemical failure has a substantial impact on the percentage of patients defined as being free of disease at 5 years.[152]

Some investigators also observed that the PSA nadir value (the lowest level achieved or the lowest before rising) correlated with the risk of failure and thus suggested that a definition of biochemical failure should be based on the nadir. Most early reports tended to emphasize a nadir as less than 1.0 ng/mL as critical based on the observation that in patients treated with EBRT, the risk of relapse

rises progressively as nadir values increase to greater than 1.0 ng/mL.[153] Some investigators have argued that a PSA nadir less than or equal to 0.5 ng/mL provides a more accurate estimate of long-term outcome. For example, Zietman et al. performed a retrospective analysis on the biochemical outcome in men with T1 to T2 disease treated by conventional EBRT at the Massachusetts General Hospital.[154] Ninety percent of those who achieved a PSA nadir of less than or equal to 0.5 ng/mL were disease free at 5 years compared to 55% for those with a nadir of 0.6 to 1.0 ng/mL and 34% for nadirs greater than 1.0 ng/mL. They concluded that a PSA nadir of less than or equal to 0.5 ng/mL represented the earliest end point predictive of a favorable outcome following conventional EBRT. In contrast, Critz and colleagues, using a combination of brachytherapy and EBRT, initially reported that a nadir below 0.5 and later less than 0.2 ng/mL was required for cure.[155] He also concluded that all patients with a nadir exceeding 1.0 ng/mL failed within 5 years.

The requirement for relatively low values following EBRT is likely to result in a high incidence of false-positive failures.[156] The series reported by Doyle et al. from UCSF provides a useful insight into the relative importance of PSA nadir.[157] First, she selected only patients who were unlikely to fail early with distant disease, by eliminating patients whose nadirs were very likely to be influenced by PSA contributed from metastasis. Next, rather than choosing arbitrary cut points such as 0.2, 0.5, 1.0, or 1.5 ng/mL, she divided PSA nadirs into quartiles based on the distribution of nadirs in a large population of patients with long follow-up treated with radiotherapy alone. Finally, not only was PSA failure used as an end point, but death after PSA failure ("progression-free survival") and overall survival were determined as well. In contrast to the results reported by Critz et al., her analysis demonstrated that, although PSA nadir correlated with each of these end points, there was no absolute quartile that guaranteed a favorable or unfavorable outcome.[155] Comparing the results reported by the UCSF group with those reported by Critz suggests that the nadirs following brachytherapy-based treatments tend to be lower than those seen after EBRT. This observation is supported by a monograph comparing PSA responses.[158] This observation supports the notion that if a patient receives brachytherapy and EBRT and continues to have a PSA greater than 1.0 ng/mL at 5 years, he is likely to have had micro-metastatic disease, a "cold spot" in his implant, or both. This speculative conclusion is consistent with the recent observations made using serial MRI/MRSI to follow patients completing brachytherapy at UCSF.[159] The fraction of patients having greater than 95% of their voxels showing no metabolic signal increases from approximately 46% within the first 6 months following PPI to nearly 100% at 48 months. The point is that the dose with brachytherapy is so high that residual normal prostate tissue is less likely than seen after EBRT.[159]

Although controversies regarding the optimal definition for PSA continue, it is clear that a rising PSA is the most agreed-on characteristic of progression. Based on this point, a consensus conference held by the American Society for Therapeutic Radiology and Oncology (ASTRO) defined

PSA failure as three consecutive rises.[160] Although this is the most widely accepted definition of PSA failure, it is far from perfect. First, the ASTRO consensus definition does not specify how much of a rise is significant. Due to random variations, occasionally three consecutive rises may occur by chance alone. It is well known that the PSA tends to increase normally with age, so very small increases (e.g., 0.03 ng/mL) separated over a long time period might not represent progression. The ASTRO definition also fails to specify whether the lowest value ever achieved should be used to define the nadir or whether the lowest value before rising should be used to calculate the time to failure. The ASTRO definition also does not address tied values (e.g., 0.1, 0.2, 0.3, 0.3, 0.7, and 0.9 ng/mL) or the slope of the PSA. The rate at which the PSA rises may help distinguish between local and distant failures, with rapidly rising PSAs more likely to reflect distant metastases.[161-163] Despite its flaws, however, the ASTRO definition has been shown to correlate with progression-free, cause-specific, and overall survival.[103,164,165] Using the ASTRO definition after brachytherapy is particularly problematic because "PSA blips" or benign bounces are known to occur in 20% of patients. This problem is not addressed in the ASTRO definition. Thus, papers published on brachytherapy claiming to use the ASTRO definition but ignoring bounces may not actually be using this definition correctly unless multiple nadirs are used as longer follow-up is achieved. This could be a source of bias because bounces alone occur after EBRT as well, just less frequently.

One of the most critical considerations when using the ASTRO definition is the importance of the duration of follow-up. Several studies have shown that when using the ASTRO consensus definition, an accurate outcome requires 5 years or more median follow-up.[166,167] As shown in Figure 45-13, investigators from William Beaumont

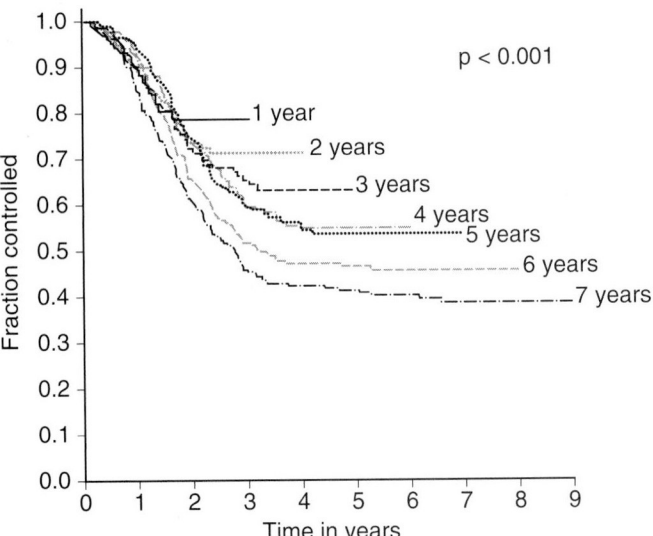

Figure 45–13. Actuarial biochemical control for patient cohorts with varying median follow-up intervals. Demonstrates how duration of follow-up impacts the interpretation of long-term control rate effects. (From Vicini FA, Kestin LL, Martinez AA: The importance of adequate follow-up in defining treatment success after external beam irradiation for prostate cancer. *Int J Radiat Oncol Biol Phys*. 1999;45:553.)

demonstrated that, using the ASTRO definition, the median follow-up should exceed the estimated date of biochemical control (BC) by at least 2 years before estimates of control stabilize.[166] For example, if the median follow-up is 5 years, only estimates out at 3 years or less are likely to be accurate!

Some have even argued that the rate of rise might be used as a surrogate end point in patients failing radiotherapy.[161,168,169] This would seem logical; however, additional confirmatory studies are needed before the long-term prognosis associated with specific PSA doubling times is precisely defined. Of note, although the PSA doubling time is slightly longer following radiotherapy than after prostatectomy, after year 2, there appear to be no significant differences between the two groups, suggesting that the rate of regrowth of cancers that recur after either therapy is similar.[170,171] This observation is an important one to bear in mind as we address definitions of failure following surgery.

Definitions of Disease-Free Survival Following Surgery

In the mid-1990s it became clear that the failure rates following radical prostatectomy were also much higher than previously believed. For example, Stein and colleagues were among the first to acknowledge that at least 60% of patients with clinically staged T1 or T2, N0 disease undergoing prostatectomy had detectable PSA within 10 years of surgery.[172] This was in marked contrast to a clinical failure rate of only 25%. Other prostatectomy series, even with less follow-up, also show surprisingly high chemical failure rates with only 2 to 4 years of follow-up.[173]

The most appropriate definition for biochemical (PSA) failure following a radical prostatectomy is just as controversial as it is after radiation therapy. Some investigators have defined a PSA failure as a PSA greater than 0.5 ng/mL, while others have used greater than 0.4 or greater than 0.3 ng/mL, although 0.2 ng/mL is perhaps the commonly used in the literature.[174-176] Amling et al. recently convinced many urologists that a PSA greater than 0.4 ng/mL should become the new standard (Fig. 45-14).[177] They analyzed the effect of using various PSA end point definitions for defining biochemical progression after radical prostatectomy and attempted to determine the best PSA cut point to use. Biochemical progression-free percent after radical prostatectomy was determined using several PSA cut points, including 0.2, 0.3, 0.4, and 0.5 ng/mL or greater, as well as 0.4 ng/mL or greater and increasing. To determine which PSA level was most appropriate to define progression after radical prostatectomy, they determined the percentage of patients with a continued PSA increase after reaching each cut point. The 5-year biochemical progression-free percentages ranged from 62% for cut points 0.2 to 78% for 0.5 ng/mL or greater. The 10-year biochemical progression-free percentages ranged from 43% for 0.2 ng/mL to 61% for 0.5 ng/mL or greater. A subsequent increase in PSA was noted in 49%, 62%, and 72% of patients who had PSA 0.2, 0.3, and 0.4 ng/mL, respectively. They concluded that a PSA 0.4 ng/mL or greater was the most appropriate cut point to use, since a

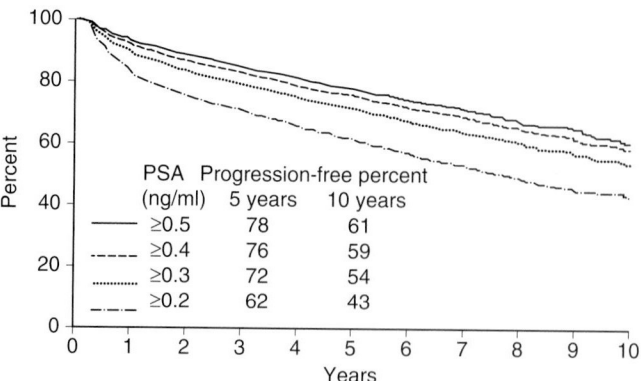

Figure 45–14. Biochemical progression-free percent using different PSA cut points to define progression after radical prostatectomy. Number of patients at risk for progression at 5, 7, and 10 years ranged 1354 to 1728, 497 to 703, and 53 to 83, respectively. (From Amling CI, Bergstralh EJ, Blute ML, et al: Defining prostate specific antigen progression after radical prostatectomy: What is the most appropriate cut point? *J Urol.* 2001;165:1146.)

significant number of patients with lower PSA do not have a continued increase in PSA. Earlier, however, Zincke et al. (same institution) had demonstrated that the relative risk of failure was 1.3 times higher at 5 years if failure was defined as greater than 0.2 ng/mL compared to greater than 0.4 ng/mL and recommended the PSA greater than 0.2 ng/mL for PSA failure.[178] The authors tend to agree with Zincke. Many normal men have PSAs of 0.4 ng/mL with an intact prostate. Such a high value is inconsistent with the notion of a "radical prostatectomy with curative intent" or complete removal of the gland.

Investigators from Stanford have shown that using an "ultra-sensitive" PSA assay can substantially shorten the time to identify biochemical failure.[179] They evaluated the clinical applicability of serum concentration techniques to enhance the detection of PSA in men with recurrent prostate cancer after radical prostatectomy. All serum samples of less than 0.07 ng/mL were concentrated by lyophilization or ultrafiltration. Serum concentrated by lyophilization and filtration detected PSA recurrence significantly earlier than did un-concentrated serum in up to 94% of patients. The mean advantage for detecting early recurrences exceeded 362 days for these patients. They concluded that concentrated serum provides a specific and sensitive technique that yields a significant lead-time of an additional 12 months in detecting cancer recurrence after radical prostatectomy when compared with nonconcentrated serum. They also concluded that when run in the ultra-sensitive mode and with modifications, they could detect recurrences about 2 years earlier than using the standard approach (residual cancer detection limit of 0.2 ng/mL).[179] These data suggest that the reports of surgical results using higher PSA failure definitions must be "taken with a grain of salt," because many of them use definitions of PSA failure that may result in a delay in the detection of failure by 1 to 2 years or more. However, investigators from Stanford recently characterized a subset of patients with biochemical failure after radical prostatectomy but with little or no subsequent rise in PSA and no clinical progression with long follow-up.[180] Serum PSA was measured using an ultrasensitive assay with failure

defined as a serum PSA of 0.07 ng/mL or greater. They identified 14 patients (8.8% of PSA failures) with a detectable serum PSA level and a mean PSA velocity after recurrence of 0.028 ng/mL per year after radical prostatectomy but without clinical or continued PSA progression at 10 years. They concluded that there is a subset of patients with PSA failure after prostatectomy who will not progress and cautioned against the use of early salvage therapy without first observing the kinetics of PSA progression.

Some investigators have even argued that it is appropriate to use the ASTRO consensus definition in surgically treated patients.[181] However, there are numerous methodological reasons why such an approach appears unjustified at this time.[182] If an "ASTRO-style" definition is adopted for PSA failure following prostatectomy, it would seem most reasonable to require the use of an ultrasensitive definition so that the date of first rise is not missed due to an insensitive assay.[179]

STANDARD THERAPEUTIC APPROACHES

Radical Prostatectomy

The radical perineal prostatectomy (RPP) was the first surgical approach used to completely remove the prostate. Unfortunately, the first two patients died within 14 months of surgery. It was not until 1949 that Memmelaar first reported the successful use of the retropubic approach for treatment of prostate cancer.[184] However, in the 1950s and 1960s it was believed that radiotherapy provided comparable results with less morbidity. In late 1970s and early 1980s, Walsh and others demonstrated the potential value of the radical retropubic prostatectomy to reduce blood loss, minimize the risk of incontinence, and preserve potency.[185,186] With this advancement, the radical retropubic prostatectomy became the surgical approach of choice in the eyes of most urologists. Thus, the modern anatomic retropubic prostatectomy is only a few years older than 3D conformal radiotherapy. Brachytherapy has been around longer than both!

Based on a comparison of treatment patterns from 1986 to 1987 and 1992, the percentage of patients receiving radical prostatectomy increased nearly 2.5 times (from 11.4% to 29.1%).[191] In contrast, during the same period the percentage of patients treated with radiotherapy went up approximately 20% (from 27.6% to 31%). Several years ago, less than half of patients undergoing surgery had organ-defined disease, but today the incidence of confined disease is much higher.[187,188] Among patients with organ-confined disease, as many as 25% will fail (with detectable PSA) within 5 to 10 years.[189] Most series report failures occurring well beyond 10 years consistent with late local recurrences, resulting in late PSA failures.[176,190] Alternatively, these "late failures" may be artifacts resulting from the definition chosen for PSA failure (see previous discussion of PSA failure after surgery).

Patients who are treated with surgery are usually younger, have lower initial PSAs, are more likely to have well-differentiated tumors, tend to have earlier-stage disease, and are generally healthier than patients treated with irradiation. These tendencies make outcome after surgery difficult to compare with outcome following radiation therapy. These differences in pretreatment characteristics may explain the fact that the results of many radical prostatectomy series appear to be more favorable than the typical radiation therapy series. Based on such data, many urologists believe that surgery is more likely to be curative than radiation therapy, perhaps explaining the surge in radical prostatectomies.[191]

SURGICAL TECHNIQUE AND COMPLICATIONS

Pelvic pain, impotence, transient incontinence, and slight shortening of the penile length are the most common immediate complications associated with radical prostatectomy.[192] The reported intraoperative blood loss is typically on the order of 500 mL to 1 L (range, 300 to 4320 mL). Techniques that minimize injury to the anterior periprostatic veins, the dorsal vein complex, and the numerous small branches from the neurovascular bundles, the seminal vesicles, and the base of the bladder reduce the risk of blood loss. Among most urologists, the retropubic radical prostatectomy appears to be favored because of the reduced risk of rectal injury and the ease of completing a pelvic lymphadenectomy.

A major criticism of the results of radical prostatectomy is that although it is a widely performed procedure, the results usually quoted by urologists are those of a relatively small handful of experts. Begg et al. demonstrated that the rates of postoperative and late urinary complications are significantly reduced if the procedure is performed in a high-volume hospital and by a surgeon who performs a large number of prostatectomies. They used the Surveillance, Epidemiology, and End Results (SEER) Medicare-linked database to evaluate health-related outcomes after radical prostatectomy in relation to hospital volume and surgeon volume. Unfortunately, less than 10% of urologists qualified as high-volume surgeons; thus, the results reported by a relatively small handful of surgeons are unlikely to be representative of the results of the other 90% of urologists![193] Given this limitation, it is clear that numbers quoted based on the published literature once again must be "taken with a grain of salt."

The randomized trial of watchful waiting versus prostatectomy provides an important assessment of the impact of surgery on the overall quality of life.[194] Urinary leakage occurred in 49% vs. 21% after radical prostatectomy compared to watchful waiting; however, bowel dysfunction, anxiety, depression, well-being, and the subjective quality of life were similar in the two groups.

Operative mortality nationally has been reported to be nearly 2%, but in the hands of an experienced surgeon, the risk is reported to be lower.[191] Similarly, rectal injury may occur as infrequently as less than 1% when reported by experienced surgeons but is substantially more common based on national statistics. Thromboembolic events have been reported to occur in approximately 1% to 3% of patients, whereas myocardial infarctions and wound infections are reported to occur in 1% or less in selected series. However, based on a national sample of 20% of Medicare beneficiaries aged 65 and older, nearly 8% suffered major myocardial infarctions within 30 days of surgery.[191] Urinary stress incontinence is reported by experienced surgeons to occur in 5% to 14% of patients but is much more common based on national statistics or surveyed patients. Impotence is the most common long-term complication associated with radical prostatectomy.

POTENCY AFTER RADICAL PROSTATECTOMY

Several caveats should be considered when comparing surgical and radiation series. First, the generalization of surgical series should be viewed cautiously, as there could be a substantial effect of patient self-selection, with men more concerned about potency seeking the highest profile surgical centers. The most widely quoted results of potency preservation after nerve-sparing radical prostatectomy have been reported in series from Johns Hopkins School of Medicine and Washington University. Potency was reportedly maintained in approximately 60% of patients, with markedly better results in younger patients. At Washington University, patients younger than 60 years of age were reported to have a 68% likelihood of maintaining potency, versus 55% in patients 60 years or older. This patient selection phenomenon is highlighted by the prostatectomy series from Johns Hopkins, in which 86% of treated patients were potent preoperatively compared to only 50% of patients in radiation series. It only follows that as with other types of surgically induced morbidity, it is likely that the maintenance of potency depends on the skill and experience of the surgeon.[193]

In contrast to these most optimistic reports, Robinson et al. recently updated a 1997 meta-analysis of rates of erectile function after treatment of localized prostate cancer.[195] They conducted a comprehensive literature review and meta-analysis of the rates of erectile dysfunction associated with the use of nerve-sparing and non–nerve-sparing prostatectomies, brachytherapy (permanent seed implants) with and without EBRT, and cryosurgery for localized prostate cancer. The predicted probability of maintaining erectile function after brachytherapy, brachytherapy plus EBRT, EBRT alone, nerve sparing and non–nerve sparing prostatectomy, and cryosurgery were 0.76, 0.60, 0.55, 0.34, 0.25, and 0.13, respectively. A similar pattern was seen when only studies reporting more than 2 years follow-up were considered, except that no brachytherapy studies had a follow-up this far out.

The randomized trial of watchful waiting versus prostatectomy provides an important multi-center assessment of the impact of surgery on potency.[194] These investigators surveyed 376 men treated on this trial, and 87% of the men responded to the survey. All patients included were younger than 75 years of age with the mean age approximately 64.5 and 68.5 years at time of surgery and surveyed, respectively. All were followed in excess of 1 year with the median follow-up approximately 49 months, ample time for full recovery of function. In this study erectile dysfunction occurred in 80% of men after radical prostatectomy compared to 45% on the watchful waiting arm.

To complicate matters further, potency is not an all-or-none phenomenon after prostatectomy. For example, in one report the authors noted that "no patient could get a 100% rigid penis any more ... " or "experience the exquisite sensation of inevitability, the so-called point 'of no return', which is caused by contractions of seminal vesicles and prostate capsule."[196] These authors noted that it was not uncommon for men to abandon sexual intercourse because of orgasm-induced acute urinary incontinence. Clearly more research is needed in this area, but potency rates generally appear to be lower with surgery than with radiotherapy-based approaches.

Cryosurgery

Cryosurgery is in a sense another form of "brachytherapy" in which freezing is used to ablate prostatic tissue. The efficacy of cryosurgery in ablating tissues is well established based on histopathologic studies. To avoid unacceptable toxicity, the urethra is spared from the full cryosurgical effect by using a warming device. However, the degree of warming may be variable, resulting in the undertreatment of periurethral tissues. Sparing the urethra from a full cryosurgical dose will as a matter of course spare portions of the apex, which is likely to result in persistent microscopic disease. Like other forms of brachytherapy, nonuniform dose (temperature) distributions are a potential shortcoming of cryosurgery. The failure to achieve a uniformly ablating dose is borne out by the fact that post-treatment biopsies showed a high incidence of persistent viable-appearing prostatic tissue, and few patients have undetectable PSAs following a single session of cryosurgery. The use of multiple cryosurgery sessions appears to provide more complete ablation of the gland complicated by a higher incidence of impotence than any other major treatment option for localized disease.[195] Recent series suggest that in the hands of some surgeons, cryosurgery may compete favorably with radiotherapy.[71,197-199]

With the recognition of the high failure rate associated with the style of cryosurgery used in the mid 1980s, adjuvant radiation therapy has been added with favorable results. Mobley and others reported their experience using a combination of cryosurgery and radiation therapy (C-RT) in 14 patients with prostate cancer.[200] In most cases radiation therapy was recommended due to evidence of local tumor recurrence following cryosurgery. Eleven patients (79%) were clinical stage C, two patients (14%) were stage B2, and a single patient was stage B1. Ten patients (71%) presented with obstructive symptoms. The average time from cryosurgery to radiation therapy was 21.8 months (three patients received irradiation in the immediate postoperative period before recurrence). Two patients (14%) subsequently developed radiation cystitis and one patient who had undergone a lymphadenectomy had persistence of penile edema. Only one patient was documented to have local tumor recurrence. They concluded that cryosurgery followed by RT was "safe and effective" and that the "complications of local growth of the primary tumor are reduced dramatically when this bimodal form of therapy is used."

Cryosurgical salvage of radiation therapy failures has been tried with mixed results. The high incidence of urinary incontinence and rectal injury has discouraged many investigators from routinely recommending cryosurgery for salvage of radiation therapy failures.

Recently several investigators have claimed more encouraging results.[197,199,201] The group from Columbia reported their series of 38 men treated between October 1997 and September 2000. All patients had negative bone scans, but positive biopsies and a biochemical disease recurrence, defined as an increase in PSA of greater than 0.3 ng/mL above the post-radiation PSA nadir. In their series patients received 3 months of neoadjuvant androgen deprivation therapy before cryotherapy. Biochemical recurrence-free survival was 74% at 2 years. Rectal pain occurred in 39.5%, scrotal edema in 10.5%, and incontinence in 7.9%, but none of their patients developed rectourethral fistula, urethral sloughing, or urinary retention. The authors concluded that using their equipment and technique, cryosurgery can be performed safely and effectively in men with locally recurrent prostate cancer that radiotherapy failed to cure.

Radiation Therapy

CONVENTIONAL EXTERNAL BEAM RADIATION THERAPY

A number of retrospective and prospective studies support the long-term efficacy of radiation therapy in the management of clinically localized prostate cancer.[57,202] These older studies are particularly valuable because they document the impact of treatment on long-term survival. Based on physical examination alone, these studies suggested that the local control rate following EBRT was between 70% and 90%. These end points are now known to underestimate the incidence of local failure.[144] The long natural history observed in patients who receive no initial treatment makes an accurate assessment of the impact of treatment on survival difficult. Patients with high-grade tumors may be most likely to benefit from treatment because of the high mortality associated with this histologic type.

Local failure rate following conventional radiation therapy is likely to be due in large part to tumor-related factors and in part to technical factors related to the delivery of the radiation. Recent studies have demonstrated that these older techniques were associated with inadequate coverage of the target volume in at least 20% to 41% of the patients treated.[203] These "old" techniques were characterized by the use of relatively small boost fields, routinely using bony landmarks to define treatment borders. Early conventional series used total doses in the range of 60 to 70 Gy because it was believed that this dose was sufficient and close to the maximum dose allowed by the surrounding normal tissues. These problems are currently being addressed by the use of 3D treatment planning technology (3DCRT) and, more recently, intensity-modulated radiotherapy (IMRT).[204-208]

"Conventional" versus Conformal Blocking Radiation Therapy

In the 1980s the most popular techniques included the use of a "four-field box" or bilateral 120-degree arcs. These "conventional," nonconformal techniques used open square or rectangular fields with minimal to no blocking and were based on bony landmarks or a single CT slice. Conformal blocking attempts to make the radiation dose distribution correspond to the shape of the target volume. Conformal blocking was usually designed using manually reconstructed, and, less frequently, computer-reconstructed CT images. When these images are displayed on the simulation film as viewed from the vantage point of the central axis of the radiation beam, they are usually referred to as a "beam's-eye view." A display that allows viewing of the treatment setup from the vantage point of an observer in the room who is *not* visually aligned with the beam's central axis is commonly referred to as a "room's-eye view" display.

Manually reconstructed images generally result in blocks that are limited to the axial plane usually using anteroposterior/posteroanterior (AP/PA) and lateral beam arrangements. When this approach is used to draw blocks conforming to the shape of the target volume, it is traditionally classified as "conformal radiation therapy." By manually stacking these two-dimensional (2D) images, volumes are created that approximate the three-dimensional (3D) volumes. The term *two and one-half dimensional conformal radiation therapy* (2.5DCRT) usually refers to the use of computerized stacking of 2D images. This approach allows beam's-eye views to be generated and used to design oblique beam arrangements, but these plans are still usually restricted to the axial plane. 3DCRT involves the use of computer-generated beam's-eye views that can be used to design beam arrangements that are noncoplanar (including beams outside the axial plane). 3DCRT allows greater flexibility in beam arrangements. Additional benefits of 3DCRT include the ability to make 3D dose calculations and generate 3D dose displays and dose-volume histograms that allow different techniques to be compared and ranked.

THREE-DIMENSIONAL CONFORMAL RADIATION THERAPY

3DCRT allows delivery of higher doses of radiation to the target volume of interest while sparing more of the surrounding normal tissues than is possible using conventional techniques. At the University of California, San Francisco (UCSF), six-field and seven-field techniques were adopted in the early 1990s.[209,210] These investigators noted that placing the oblique fields at 35 degrees (from the lateral field), and delivering 50% of the dose by laterals, 25% by anterior obliques, 15% to 20% from posterior obliques, and 5% to 10% from an anterior field created an excellent dose distribution.[211] Using conformally blocked arcs to deliver radiation therapy to the prostate only for patients at very low risk for seminal vesicle involvement may simplify and shorten treatment time.[212]

Compared with treating a patient by standard technique, 3DCRT is associated with a nearly 30% reduction in the dose received by 50% of the rectum. Based on this kind of analysis, an estimated increase in minimum tumor dose of greater than or equal to 10% is possible without an increase in acute or chronic toxicity.[213] An even greater increase is likely to be safely achieved if dose inhomogeneity constraints are relaxed, as is common with IMRT.

INTENSITY-MODULATED RADIATION THERAPY

Following the plethora of retrospective and prospective studies demonstrating that higher doses are better and complications can be reduced, 3DCRT became the standard of care in nearly every major academic center in the U.S. in the mid 1990s. To extend the principles learned from 3DCRT (more dose is better and sparing normal tissues is a good thing), various investigators began to apply IMRT to the treatment of prostate cancer. Simply put, IMRT is a more sophisticated type of 3DCRT. Exactly at what point in the spectrum of EBRT 3DCRT becomes IMRT remains somewhat controversial. To address this controversy, the National Cancer Institute formed an IMRT working group composed of radiation physicists and oncologists with experience using this technology.

The NCI-IMRT Working Group Consensus Paper: Complex Conclusions Simplified

The NCI-IMRT Collaborative Working Group (NCI-IMRT-CWG) set out to define an agreed-upon set of jargon, provide standards for quality assurance, and provide a clinical context through which this technology might be viewed.[205] When the NCI-IMRT-CWG consensus paper was written, there were three major types of IMRT in common use (Table 45-7). The authors acknowledge that

Table 45–7   Conformal Therapy Techniques

Type of Conformal Therapy	Minimum Dose Calculation Requirements	Minimum Imaging Requirements	Treatment Delivery Requirements	Degree of Conformality*
Conventional 3DCRT	3D with DVHs	Full set of CT or MRI images	Cerrobend blocks or MLC	2H
Forward planned SMLC IMRT	3D with DVHs	Full set of CT or MRI images	Computer-controlled MLC	3H
Inverse planned SMLC IMRT	3D with DVHs	Full set of CT or MRI images	Computer-controlled MLC	2H to 4H
DMLC IMRT	3D with DVHs	Full set of CT or MRI images	Dynamic MLC	2H to 4H
Tomotherapy IMRT	3D with DVHs	Full set of CT or MRI images	Tomotherapy device or a Linac with binary MLC	2H to 4H

*Conformality is subjectively rated on a scale of 1H to 5H, (higher number indicating a higher degree of conformality). This is to point out that inversed-planned IMRT can either be better or worse than forward-planned techniques, depending on the objective function or the input parameters used in the inverse planning process, or both, and on technical details related to various delivery techniques. Note that no attempt was made to distinguish how well the three inversed planned IMRT methods would compare among each other.
CT, computed tomography; 3DCRT, three-dimensional conformal radiotherapy; DVH, dose-volume histogram; IMRT, intensity-modulated radiation therapy; MLC, multi-leaf collimation; MRI, magnetic resonance imaging; SMLC, segmental multi-leaf collimation.
Modified from Boyer A, Butler EB, Dipetrillo TA, et al: Intensity-modulated radiotherapy: Current status and issues of interest. *Int J Radiat Oncol Biol Phys.* 2001;51:880.

there are several other exciting forms of IMRT currently being developed, but the following discussion is limited to the three most common types used today.

Dynamic multi-leaf collimation (DMLC) IMRT is used to describe a complex delivery approach in which the gantry and leaves move simultaneously and inverse planning is incorporated. This approach has been popularized at MSKCC, where investigators have demonstrated the feasibility of high-dose IMRT in a large number of patients.[206,214,215] Based on this pioneering work, this type of IMRT has been incorporated into routine practice at numerous U.S. centers. Only time will tell exactly how this technology should be used for treating prostate cancer.

The second type of inverse planning–based IMRT, tomotherapy, involves the use of a rotating multi-segmented delivery system. Tomotherapy delivers radiation via either sequential or continuous arcs much like a CT scanner. Sequential tomotherapy is most commonly delivered using the so-called *MiMic* device developed by the NOMOS corporation.[216] Using such a device to treat prostate cancer was first popularized by investigators from Baylor University in Texas.[217,218] They have treated more than 1000 patients for prostate cancer using this device. They routinely implemented IMRT incorporating a Vac-Lok bag-and-box system to immobilize the patient and a rectal balloon for immobilization of the prostate gland. They also concluded that the overall toxicity profile for these patients treated with IMRT was very favorable.

The most common misconception about IMRT is that it requires inverse treatment planning. At least five problems are associated with this assumption, however. First, the practical dose/volume constraints typically specified for inverse plans by the planner are not intuitive. Obviously we would all prefer to give a full dose to the tumor and no dose to surrounding normal tissues, but this is impossible. This problem is compounded by the fact that the mathematical parameters used in the inverse algorithm have not been validated to properly weight the risk of complications versus tumor control. Most importantly, inverse planning algorithms usually do not select the optimal number of beams or beam angles. If the selection of the beam angles is poor, the inverse plan may not be as good as one generated using forward planning. Furthermore, in contrast to some other sites (e.g., head and neck), most patients with prostate cancer have a similar anatomy (oval-shaped prostate in the midline, in front of the rectum and above the penis), and thus may be particularly amenable to the use of "a class solution." That is, once an optimized inverse plan with a set of beam weights, angles, and margins has been identified, there may be little additional value to running an inverse plan for each and every patient. Finally, rarely is a "pure" inverse plan used to design an IMRT treatment for any cancer site. In fact, most plans are generated using multiple iterations ("backward and forward planning"). Thus, to define IMRT as requiring inverse plan is not logical.

Figure 45-15 provides an example of a site of dominant intra-prostatic disease or a so-called "dominant intra-prostatic lesion" or "DIL" as defined by Roach and others. Figure 45-16A–C shows axial, sagittal, and coronal distributions associated with tomotherapy, forward-planned segmental MLC (SMLC), and inverse-planned SMLC, all targeting a DIL to 90 Gy while treating the entire prostate to 75.6 Gy.[207]

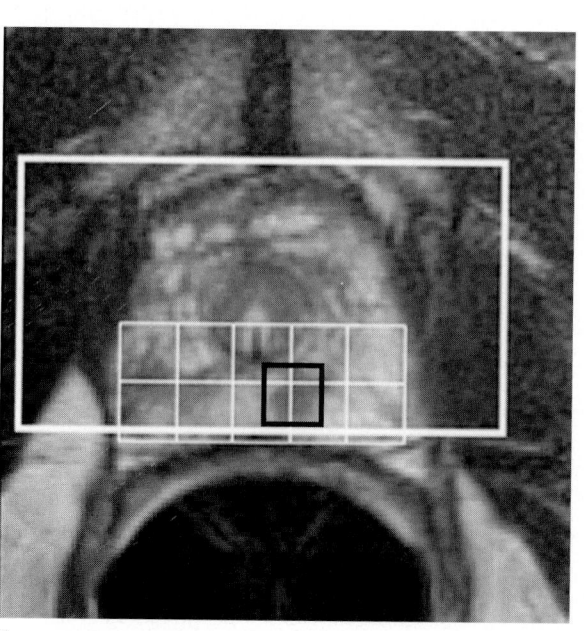

A

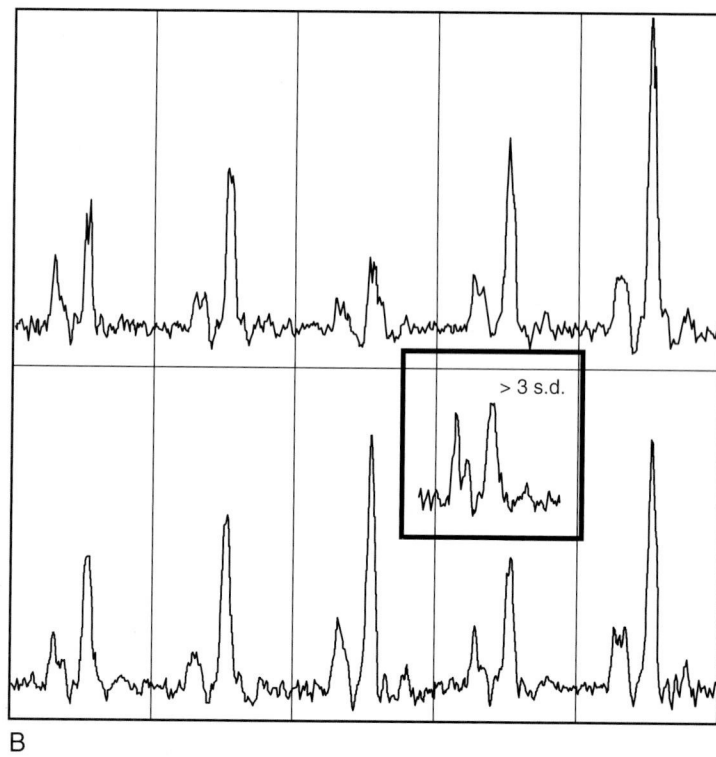

B

Figure 45–15. Example of a site of dominant intra-prostatic disease or a so-called *dominant intra-prostatic lesion or DIL* as defined by Roach and others. **A,** Image of voxels with spectroscopy at the apex of the prostate. **B,** Magnetic resonance spectra for voxels shown in A.

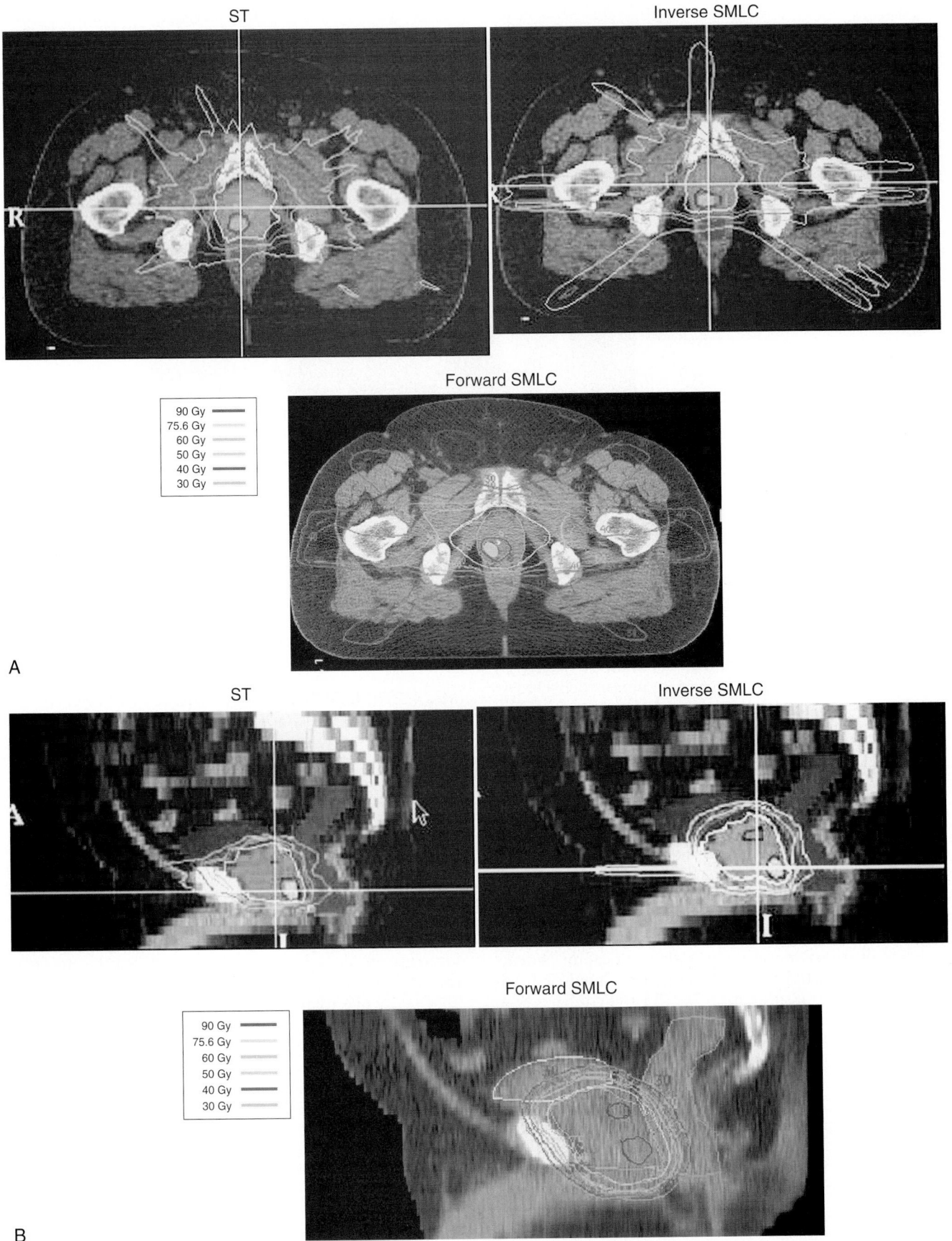

Figure 45–16. A, Axial, **B,** sagittal, and **C,** coronal distributions associated with tomotherapy, forward planned segmental multi-leaf collimator (SMLC) intensity-modulated radiotherapy (IMRT) and inverse planned SMLC IMRT, all targeting a dominant intra-prostatic lesion to 90 Gy while treating the entire prostate to 75.6 Gy. See also Color Figure 45–16. (From Xia P, Pickett B, Vigneault E, et al: Forward or inversely planned segmental multileaf collimator IMRT and sequential tomotherapy to treat multiple dominant intraprostatic lesions of prostate cancer to 90 Gy. *Int J Radiat Oncol Biol Phys.* 2001;51:244.)

ST

Inverse SMLC

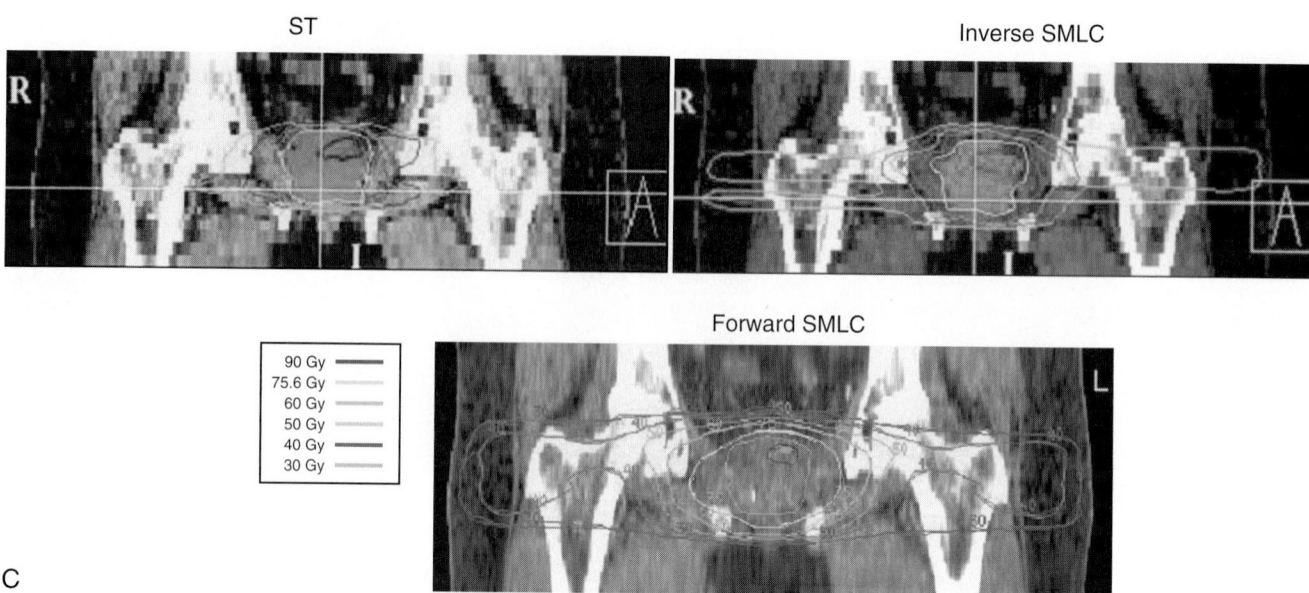

Forward SMLC

90 Gy
75.6 Gy
60 Gy
50 Gy
40 Gy
30 Gy

C

Figure 45–16, cont'd. For legend see previous page.

IMRT delivered using static fields is the simplest form used to treat prostate cancer. The vast majority of patients treated for prostate cancer with IMRT at UCSF in recent years have been treated using a technique originally called *static field IMRT* (SF-IMRT).[204] IMRT at UCSF evolved from a previously described six-field 3DCRT technique.[211,219] By incorporating partial transmission blocks generated using a beam's-eye-view (BEV), the intensity of the posterior oblique beams could be selectively attenuated to reduce the dose of radiation delivered to the anterior rectal wall. Partial transmission blocks were routinely incorporated into the SF-3DCRT technique at UCSF in January 1992.[220] This technique initially required the use of hand-cut partial transmission blocks to modulate the dose from the posterior obliques. Hand-cut blocks were replaced with MLC in 1994. As with hand-cut blocks, MLC allowed partial transmission of dose by selectively blocking a portion of the field after a fraction (e.g., ≈80%) of the dose had been delivered. A lightly weighted anterior field was added to complete the "standard" seven-field technique used at UCSF through the end of 1999. Although delivered differently, the plans, goals, and dose distribution were essentially identical for patients treated using partial blocks generated by hand or using MLC. Thus, the transition from 3DCRT to IMRT has been as a continuum rather than an abrupt "leap forward" in the application of technology.

Based on conventions proposed by the NCI IMRT working group, SF-IMRT is now considered a type of "SMLC IMRT" or "SMLC-IMRT." The term *SMLC*, without specifying whether it was accomplished by inverse or forward planning, generally refers to the inverse treatment planning method. SF-IMRT can also be called "forward planned SMLC IMRT (F-SMLC)" using the NCI IMRT working group convention, since it was developed empirically using forward planning. This approach involves the use of multiple static segments, which can be put together to generate complex dose distributions.[204,221] There are advantages and disadvantages to each form of

IMRT, but all can deliver very complex dose distributions.[205] The advantages associated with F-SMLC include: the ability to generate port films that resemble conventional films from a 3D plan, more intuitive planning, and manual editing of blocks can be carried out relatively easily. Using automated sequence software, SMLC IMRT treatment can be delivered within a similar time line as with DMLC or tomotherapy-based IMRT.

MAGNETIC RESONANCE SPECTROSCOPY IMAGING AND INTENSITY-MODULATED RADIOTHERAPY

The encouraging preliminary data from work demonstrating that endorectal MRI/MRSI could improve the accuracy of defining the intra-prostatic extent of disease brought additional possibilities for the use of IMRT for prostate cancer. Investigators at UCSF and MSKCC demonstrated that it was feasible to selectively intensify the dose to selected regions of the prostate.[204,222] Investigators at MSKCC popularized the concept of "dose painting." Investigators at UCSF popularized the concept of DILs. Using F-SMLC and online portal imaging, these investigators demonstrated that it was feasible to treat the entire prostate at 180 cGy daily, to a dose exceeding 73.8 Gy, while treating a single tumor-bearing region of the prostate simultaneously to 90 Gy.[204] Later they showed it was feasible to treat multiple DILs using F-SMLC, SMLC, or sequential tomotherapy (ST).[207] All three IMRT techniques were capable of ensuring that 90 Gy could be delivered to two DILs, while treating the entire prostate to 75.6 Gy without exceeding normal tissue tolerance. This approach begged the question: "If the disease is not uniformly distributed throughout the gland, why uniformly distribute the dose?" Uniformly delivering a high dose to the entire prostate uniformly increases the risk of complications to surrounding normal tissues.

Previous studies conducted at UCSF had shown that MRI/MRSI could be used to define regions within the prostate that are at high risk for involvement by tumor.[135,223] Selective targeting is best accomplished by combining endorectal MRI/MRSI with biopsy information. Traditional sextant biopsies may have relatively low sensitivity.[64,224,225] A number of studies suggest that MRI combined with MRSI can potentially enhance the sensitivity of biopsies.[137,139,226] Thus, by combining information from multiple (more than sextant) biopsies and MRI/MRSI, the sensitivity and specificity for defining DILs should improve.

The Challenges of Day-to-Day Setup Variation and Organ Movement and IMRT

The ability to take full advantage of IMRT depends on the accuracy of reproducing the desired dose distribution from a computerized plan in the patient. A beautiful dose distribution delivered even 5 mm posterior to the intended location can have a substantial impact on the dose delivered to surrounding normal tissues.[207,227] It is now abundantly clear that although the current standard of care involves the use of weekly port films, this is probably inadequate for the accurate delivery of highly conformal dose distributions.[203] Numerous studies have now demonstrated that organ movement and day-to-day setup variations can result in significant treatment errors.[228,229] The use of a rectal balloon, an ultrasound localization system, or an electronic portal imaging device (EPID) in conjunction with implanted markers are options in use at centers using IMRT.[217,230-232] Investigators at UCSF have compared these options and found the EPID-based process to be reproducible, fast, and accurate.[233,234] Neither intrafraction movement or seed migration appear to be limiting factors in the application of the EPID-based approach.[208,235] Figure 45-17A and B demonstrate examples of lateral EPID images for whole pelvic and prostate-only (PO)

radiotherapy, respectively. We expect that in the next few years, daily monitoring by one of these methods will replace weekly port films as the standard of care.[228] The major disadvantage of the EPID-based approach is the requirement for an invasive procedure to place the markers.

RATIONALE AND INDICATIONS FOR PELVIC IRRADIATION

Nonrandomized Studies

Despite the uncertainty about the cure rates of patients with lymph node involvement, survival may be prolonged by prophylactic lymph node irradiation. That whole-pelvic radiotheraphy (WPRT) might be associated with a prolongation would not be completely surprising. The survival of women treated to para-aortic lymph nodes for cervical cancer, and with groin and pelvic radiotherapy in cancer of the vulva, is associated with a prolongation in survival.[236,237] Furthermore, prophylactic nodal radiotherapy in women with breast cancer (a disease that biologically more closely resembles prostate cancer) has been shown to prolong survival.[238,239]

At least four groups have reported retrospective studies demonstrating an improvement in disease-free survival for a subset of patients treated with WPRT when compared to PO radiotherapy (PORT).[240-244] The two reports by Seaward et al. from UCSF and the report by Pan et al. from the University of Michigan were based on patients treated in the PSA era. The UCSF group concluded that patients with an estimated risk of lymph node involvement of 15% to 35% (based on the risk equation: $+LN = 2/3 (PSA) + \{(GS-6) \times 10\}$) benefited the most from

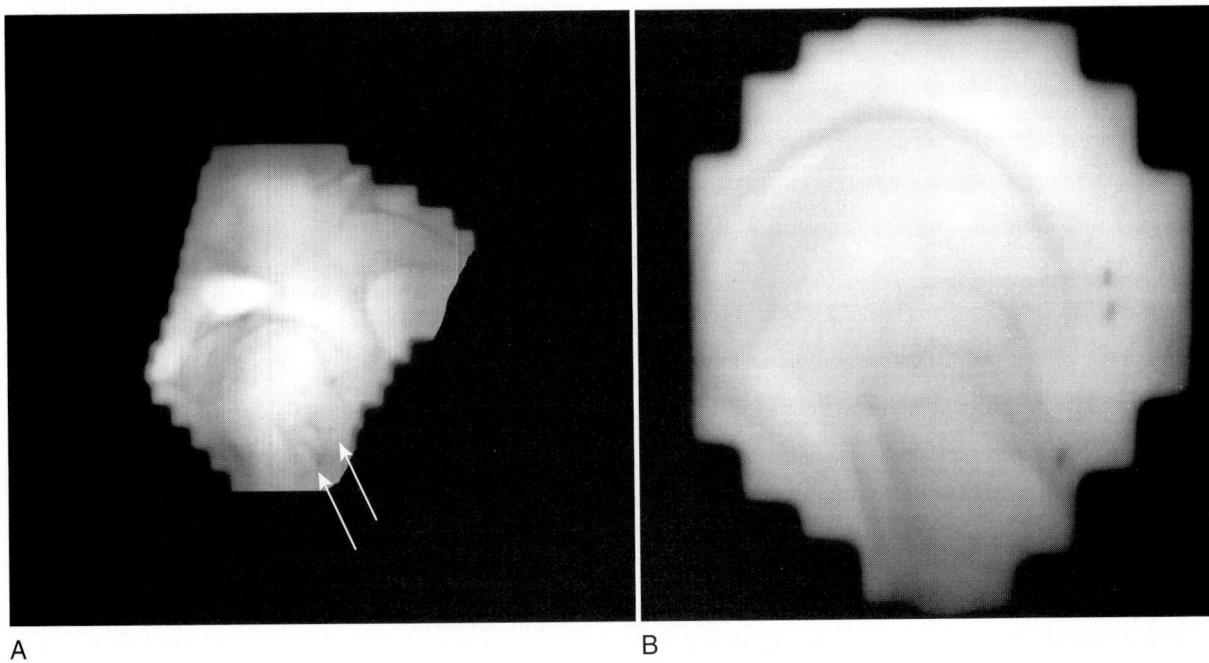

A   B

Figure 45–17. **A,** Example of a lateral EPID image for whole pelvic radiotherapy with gold mark *(arrows)* and **B,** example of image for prostate-only radiotherapy.

prophylactic pelvic radiotherapy. In contrast, the analysis by Pan estimated the risk of each patient's percentage of risk of lymph node (%rLN) involvement based on the updated Partin tables. They divide their patients into three different categories based on %LN involvement: low, 0% to 5%; intermediate, greater than 5% to 15%; and high, greater than 15%. Multivariate analysis demonstrated a statistically significant benefit for the entire population treated with WPRT, with a relative risk reduction of 0.72 (95% confidence interval 0.54 to 0.97). Again, the greatest benefit to WPRT was seen in the intermediate risk (5% to 15%) group. They concluded that WPRT appears to improve biologic no evidence of disease in prostate cancer patients and that additional studies are needed to define the optimal group for WPRT. The preliminary report (abstract) by Rasp et al. (Mayo Clinic) is the only analysis based on patients treated in the PSA era that we know of that fails to show a benefit for a subset of patients treated with WPRT.[245] Like the UCSF group, they evaluated patients with an estimated risk of lymph node involvement of greater than or equal to 15%. The negative findings from their report could have been due to the fact that patients treated with WPRT tended to have more advanced tumors with a poorer prognosis, or other factors (sample size, follow-up, method of estimating risk).

RANDOMIZED TRIALS

We are aware of three prospective randomized trials published to date that have compared WPRT to PORT. The oldest study conducted at Stanford was very small (*n* = 57), included only patients who were pathologically proven to be node negative, and was completed in the pre-PSA era. A small but statistically insignificant difference (perhaps due to sample size) in disease-free survival of 70% versus 53% favoring patients who received WPRT compared to PORT is noteworthy. RTOG 7706 also compared whole-pelvic irradiation with prostate irradiation alone in patients at low risk for lymph node involvement (stages A2, B1, and B2; node negative by imaging or pathologically).[246] No differences in outcome were noted between the two arms. The major problems with these studies are that even if pelvic irradiation were beneficial, the very low incidence of lymph node involvement in these patients and the small number of patients probably would not allow such a benefit to be recognized. It should not be surprising that WPRT is of little or no benefit in patients at low risk for lymph node involvement.

The most important phase III prospective randomized trial completed to date addressing the issue of prophylactic pelvic nodal irradiation is RTOG 9413.[127] This large, recently reported four-arm trial assessed the value of whole pelvic irradiation as well as the impact of the timing of combined androgen suppression therapy in patients with an estimated risk of lymph node involvement exceeding 15%. More than 1300 men were accrued to this study in just over 4 years. This was the first major trial to use PSA to define progression-free survival as the primary end point. At the time of the initial analysis the follow-up for this study was too short to expect a difference in the secondary end points such as overall and disease-specific survivals. However, since having earlier progression is never more desirable and all patients received the same total dose of radiation and duration of hormonal therapy, a primary end point of progression-free survival was considered an appropriate intermediate end point.

Eligibility for 9413 included localized adenocarcinoma of the prostate with an elevated PSA of less than 100 ng/mL. Patients were stratified by clinical T stage, PSA, and GS and required to have an estimated risk of lymph node (LN) involvement greater than 15%. Patients were randomized to one of four arms designed in a two by two fashion to receive neoadjuvant (before) and concurrent (N&CHT) combined androgen blockade (CAB) or the same regimen given as adjuvant hormonal therapy (AHT) after the completion of radiotherapy. CAB was either delivered in combination with whole pelvic (WP) radiotherapy followed by a boost to the prostate (including the seminal vesicles) or with PO (including the seminal vesicles) EBRT. In all cases CAB consisted of luteinizing hormone-releasing hormone (LHRH) and flutamide for 4 months. Thus, the four arms consisted of WP + N&CHT, PO + N&CHT, WP + AHT, and PO + AHT, and included more than 300 patients per arm. The median PSA was 22.6 ng/mL, 67% of patients had T2c to T4 disease, and 72% had a GS of 7 to 10. Failure for progression-free survival was defined as the first occurrence of local progression, regional nodal failure, distant failure, biochemical (PSA) failure, or death due to any cause.

With a median follow-up of nearly 5 years, patients treated with WPRT experienced a 4-year progression-free survival of 54% compared to 47% in patients treated with PORT (*P* = 0.022). When simultaneously comparing all four arms, there was a progression-free difference among WPRT + N&CHT, PORT + N&CHT, WPRT + AHT and PORT + AHT (60% vs. 44%, 49% and 50% respectively, *P* = 0.008). The results of 9413 are more impressive when viewed as pairs of curves as shown in Figure 45-18*A–D*. Thus, this phase III trial demonstrated that WPRT + N&CHT is associated with an improvement in freedom from progression compared to PORT and N&CHT or AHT, and WPRT + AHT in patients with a risk of lymph node involvement greater than 15%. Because of the long follow-up required to determine the impact of treatment on survival in prostate cancer patients, as expected, no survival difference has been seen.

RTOG 9413 also suggests that the greatest benefit to WPRT + N&CHT is in patients with intermediate- to high-risk disease (GS = 7 & PSA <20ng/mL or GS = 6 & PSA >30 ng/mL), compared to those with lower or higher risk of disease. This observation is consistent with retrospective data from the UCSF.[243] This finding has major implications for the large number of patients receiving radiotherapy and CAB for clinically localized prostate cancer. However, the failure to identify an apparent benefit of pelvic nodal treatment in the lower risk patients could have been due to sample size, since relatively few patients in this category were included in this study.

CLINICAL GUIDELINES FOR WHOLE PELVIC RADIOTHERAPY

At UCSF whole-pelvic irradiation is used only for patients perceived to be at significant risk for lymph node

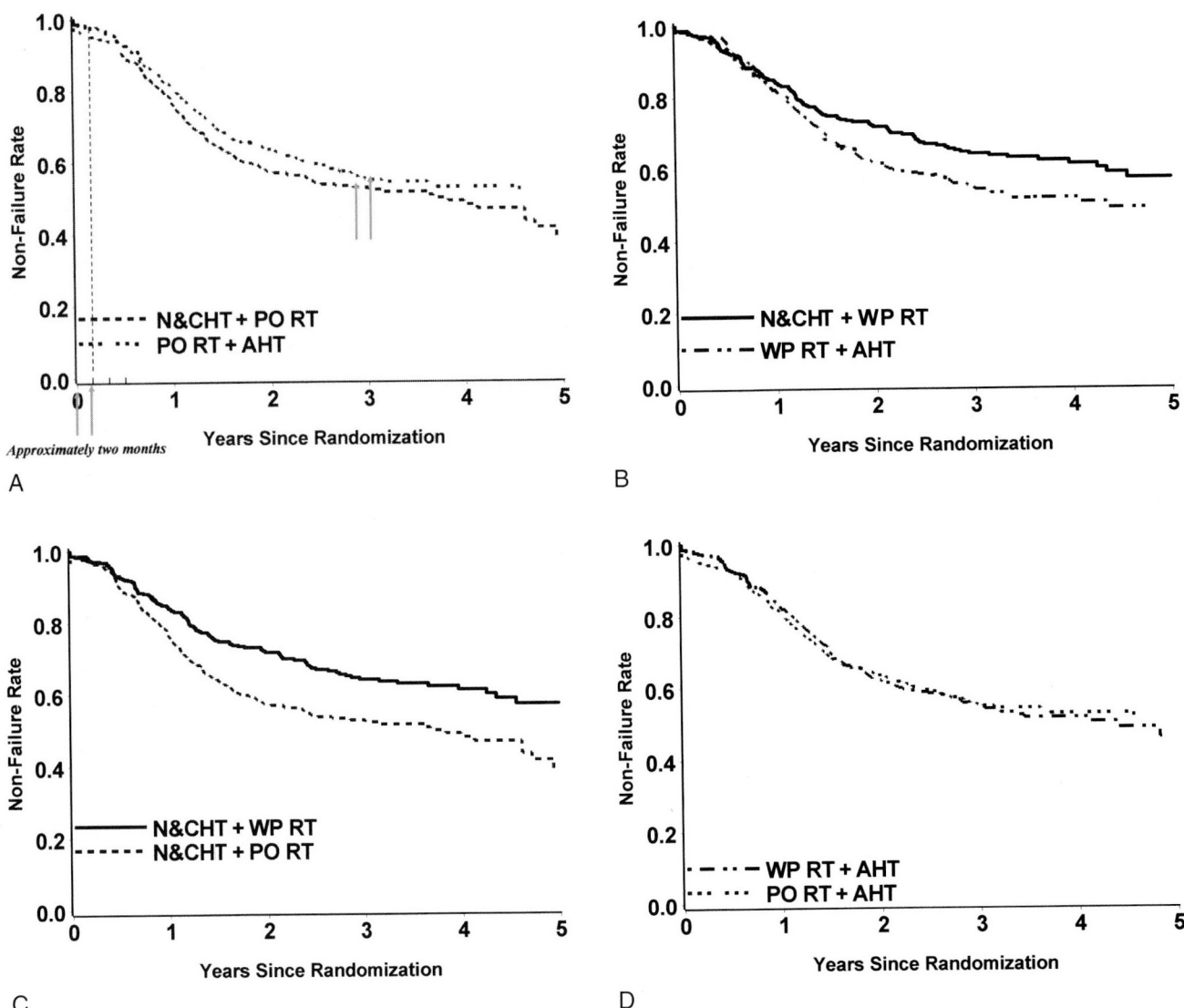

Figure 45–18. A, Compares patients treated on arm 2 and arm 4 (both prostate-only arms). These curves are consistent with a 2 month time-to-failure bias in favor of adjuvant hormonal therapy (AHT) compared to neoadjuvant (before) and concurrent hormone therapy (N&CHT) and suggest there is no difference in biologic interactions if only the prostate is irradiated. **B,** Compares the two whole-pelvic arms, the one receiving N&CHT (arm 1) and the other receiving AHT (arm 3). Despite the bias in timing in completion of hormonal therapy, the early part of the curves are superimposed but separate with longer follow-up, suggesting that there is a greater biologic interaction when hormonal therapy is given before and during rather than whole pelvic radiotherapy. **C,** Compares arms 1 and 2, both using N&CHT. Arm 1 included the whole pelvis while arm 2 includes only prostate. **D,** Compares arm 3 and arm 4, both of which used AHT, but arm 3 had whole-pelvis and arm 4, prostate-only radiotherapy. These curves suggest that there is no evidence of benefit to whole-pelvic radiotherapy if given with AHT. (Modified from Roach M, Di Silvo M, Lawton C, et al: A phase III trial comparing whole-pelvic versus prostate-only radiotherapy and neoadjuvant versus adjuvant combined androgen suppression. Radiation Therapy Oncology Group (RTOG) 9413. *J Clin Oncol.* 2003;21:1904-1911.)

involvement. The indications for whole-pelvic irradiation are:

1. Proof of lymph node involvement by node sampling.
2. Documented seminal vesicle involvement.
3. A risk of lymph node involvement greater than or equal to 15%.

   The equation used for estimating the risk of lymph node involvement is:

$$+LN = 2/3 \ (PSA) + \{(GS - 6) \times 10\}$$

4. GS = 7 and greater than 50% of biopsies positive (or predominantly Gleason grade 4 disease) or GS = 6 and clinical T3.

Based on the results of RTOG 9413 in general, WPRT is recommended in combination with neoadjuvant hormonal therapy and, conversely, neoadjuvant hormonal therapy is recommended when WPRT is planned. Although it is recognized that when using traditional treatment fields to deliver whole-pelvic irradiation, some lymph node groups may not be adequately encompassed, most experts believe that the first nodes are probably the most important to cover.[247]

SEMINAL VESICLE IRRADIATION

At UCSF, our philosophy toward seminal vesicle irradiation is similar to that for lymph node involvement.

We recommend treating them if positive by biopsy or as defined by transrectal ultrasound or endorectal MRI. In the absence of these findings, at UCSF patients are considered high risk if the calculated risk of seminal vesicle invasion (+SV) is greater than or equal to 15%. Other investigators seem to share a similar philosophy toward treatment of the seminal vesicles.[248] For example, Kestin et al. performed a complete pathology review of prostatectomy specimens to determine when the seminal vesicles should be irradiated and the appropriate length of seminal vesicles that should be included within the CTV. They concluded that only 1% of low-risk patients (PSA <10 ng/mL, Gleason ≤6, and clinical stage ≤T2a) were found to have seminal vesicle involvement compared to 27% of high-risk patients. Patients with only one high-risk feature reached the 15% risk threshold for seminal vesicle involvement, while 58% of patients with all three high-risk features had seminal vesicle involvement. They reported that the median length of SV involvement was 1.0 cm (90th percentile: 2.0 cm, range: 0.2 to 3.8 cm) while the risk of involvement beyond 2 cm was approximately 1%. They concluded that a portion of the seminal vesicles should be included in the CTV for higher-risk patients, but only the proximal 2.0 to 2.5 cm corresponding to approximately 60% of the seminal vesicle should be included within the CTV (high dose area).

Even if the calculated risk is low, if the primary tumor is located at the base of the prostate (immediately adjacent to the seminal vesicles), SV irradiation may be appropriate. At UCSF a prophylactic dose for patients at risk for SV involvement is 54 to 55.8 Gy. Patients with documented involvement received full dose to all or the proximal portion of the SV. A single seminal vesicle is treated if there is a well-lateralized, low-volume lesion. If the calculated risk exceeds the threshold for high risk for SV involvement but the tumor is apical in origin and imaging studies and SV biopsies are negative, omitting elective SV irradiation would also seem reasonable in some cases. Omitting SV radiation therapy, when possible, should theoretically allow us to treat the prostate to a higher dose because of the rectal sparing resulting from this policy.[249]

GUIDELINES FOR TREATMENT PLANNING AND SETUP

The standard terms recommended by The International Commission for Radiation Units (ICRU 50) for defining target volumes during treatment planning are summarized in Table 45-8. Correlative pathologic studies have demonstrated that MRI is slightly more accurate in assessing volume than transrectal ultrasonography (TRUS), and both are superior to CT.[250,251] When assessed by non–contrast CT, the prostate appears somewhat larger posteriorly and inferiorly than when assessed by MRI or TRUS. This region of discrepancy appears to correspond to the anterior wall of the rectum and the region of the levator ani muscles. Inclusion of peri-prostatic fat or blood vessels anteriorly, or both, may also contribute to over-estimates of the prostatic volume when defined by CT. Lack of image resolution and not understanding these

Table 45–8 Definitions for Treatment Planning

Volume	General Definitions and Comments
Gross tumor volume—GTV	Tumor only, no margin (the prostate gland in this example as determined by a computed tomography scan).
Clinical target volume—CTV	Includes margin around the GTV for regions of microscopic risk.
Planning target volume—PTV	Includes margin around the CTV accounting for beam penumbra, patient movement, setup error, and organ movement.

anatomic landmarks probably explain the tendencies for the discrepancies noted. Discrepancies in prostate volumes may also result in part from inaccurate assumptions about the length of the external sphincter when a retrograde urethrogram is used to assist in defining the apical portion of the prostate. Interobserver variability in defining the prostate size on CT probably also contributes to this problem.[252]

Bony Anatomy-Based and Retrograde Urethrography-Based Simulation

Bony anatomy-based x-ray simulation (BAXS) has long been the most widely used approach for defining the treatment volume for prostate cancer. Pilepich and collaborators correlated CT scans with bony anatomy in 100 consecutive patients and described guidelines for assuring adequate coverage of the prostate.[253] However, because of variations in prostatic volume, shape, and location, the volume of normal tissue irradiated may be excessive in patients with small glands and inadequate in patients with large or unusually located glands.

The value of retrograde urethrography during treatment planning is not universally agreed on in the radiation therapy literature. At UCSF, retrograde urethrography is used in conjunction with CT for identifying the inferior border of the prostate. Retrograde urethrography can provide independent confirmation, since the images are generated in a plane that is perpendicular (coronal and sagittal) to the axial CT slices. Because of the abruptly rounded shape of the apical portion of the prostate, the most inferior portion of the gland cannot always be easily defined by CT. Typically the location of the apex can be resolved to within one, two, or three CT slice intervals. Because of this difficulty, retrograde urethrography is often used as a sort of "tie breaker." In the past, the inferior border of the ischial tuberosities was used as the landmark for defining the inferior treatment field margin. Using the ischial tuberosities to define the lower border of the field results in an inferior margin that is excessive in some patients and inadequate in others. Retrograde urethrography more accurately defines the inferior border of the prostate than BAXS alone, because it takes into account large variations found in individuals who either have a high or low pelvic floor. At UCSF the location of the prostate is assumed to be 1 to 1.5 cm superior to the point at which the dye narrows on the retrograde urethrography (called the *apex of the urethra* by some).

For patients receiving radiation therapy in the postoperative setting, retrograde urethrography can be particularly useful because the sphincter tends to be lower and generally there is no identifiable prostatic tissue. Despite these apparent benefits, the routine use of urethrograms continues to be controversial.

Malone et al. recently reported that performing a urethrogram may introduce errors during treatment simulation by inducing displacement of the prostate.[254] These investigators reported that performing a urethrogram induced a mean superior shift of 6.1 mm and that this might result in inadequate coverage of the prostate. This conclusion has been challenged by investigators from Fox Chase Cancer Center.[255] These investigators used sagittal MRI scans acquired immediately before and after a localization urethrogram to assess the degree of displacement. They had the prostate contoured by 3 different observers and found no significant systematic motion of either the prostate or its apex in either the anterior-posterior or superior-inferior directions. They concluded that a 2 mm margin was sufficient to compensate for 95% of the motion that might result from using urethrograms. Investigators from UCSF have also demonstrated that the prostate does not exhibit significant displacement following urethrography.[256] Using fiducial markers placed before simulation and an electronic portal imaging device, they compared the position of the prostate before and after simulation, and daily during the course of treatment. Based on this analysis, they concluded that the magnitude of displacement induced by performing a urethrogram was clinically insignificant. Malone et al. did not take into account random or "natural" movement that might occur unrelated to the urethrogram. The type of penile clamp used, the volume of contrast, and other differences in patient preparation such as the routine use of an enema before simulation could also have contributed to the differences observed between the two studies. At UCSF urethrograms are still used and recommended, particularly in postoperative patients.

Patient Immobilization

Large day-to-day setup errors (>0.5 mm) can be significantly reduced with the use of patient immobilization devices. Reducing the frequency of setup errors reduces the likelihood of underdosing the tumor, allows the use of "tighter margins," and reduces the dose unintentionally received by surrounding normal tissues. Although the use of immobilization devices appears to reduce the risk of large errors, small errors (<2.5 mm) still occur. Regardless of the degree of patient immobilization, the potential for organ movement limits the advisability of using "very tight margins." (See Treatment Verification section later.)

Commonly used immobilization devices are constructed of a melted plastic mold material, a solidified Styrofoam mold, or reusable inflatable mold devices.[257,258] Patients may be simulated and treated supine or prone.[259] The prone position in combination with a thermoplastic shell tends to be associated with less setup error but may be more prone to organ movement error due to respirations.[257,259,260] Some patients (particularly obese ones) find the prone position less comfortable and it is more difficult to perform retrograde urethrograms in this position. Simulating and treating patients in a standardized set of conditions should reduce the variations in prostate position errors during the course of treatment. Regardless of the type of immobilization device used, or the treatment position chosen, there is no replacement for a careful three-point setup and clear instructions to patients on how to assume the same position every day.[258]

Setup and Simulation

Before simulation, an immobilization device is usually made. Implementation of daily monitoring via a transabdominal ultrasound-based system or intraprostatic markers combined with EPIDs may eliminate the need to use immobilization devices.[232] The following directions explain how UCSF treats patients beginning whole-pelvic irradiation before CT.

1. A week or more before simulation, two gold marker seeds are placed in the base and one in the apex. The patient is placed in the supine position with a full bladder and the rectum empty (following an enema).
2. To define the isocenter in the lateral projection (under fluoroscopy), the grid may be placed 3 cm posterior to the most anterior portion of the femoral heads. The gantry is then rotated 90 degrees, an AP film is taken, and superior and inferior borders are set, as defined further on the lateral view.
3. At UCSF, urethrograms are performed as follows: After a sterile preparation, contrast (≈10 mL) is injected into the penile urethra and a penile clamp immediately applied to minimize leakage of contrast from the urethra. The inferior border is placed 0.5 to 1 cm below the area where the dye narrows to a point on the urethrogram ("the apex of the urethra"). In the postoperative setting with positive apical margins or recurrent disease, the inferior border is generally placed 1.0 to 1.5 cm below the "apex of the urethra." The superior border is placed at the L5-S1 junction. The lateral margins of the AP/PA field are symmetrical and should extend 1.5 cm lateral to the bony margin of the pelvic inlet at the widest point. Corners are blocked to decrease the dose to the femoral heads, bowel, and bone marrow.
4. The gantry is rotated 90 degrees and a lateral film is taken with the superior and inferior border set, as defined earlier. The field is then opened symmetrically until the anterior portion of the pubic synthesis and middle of the sacrum are incorporated into the field. The shaped field spares the posterior wall of the rectum and splits the sacrum along its long axis, extending inferiorly (usually down to approximately the S2 to S3 interspace). Instillation of a large volume of contrast into the rectum is discouraged because of the risk of organ displacement.

When planning to use 3DCRT it is best to have the dosimetrist generate the BEV and draw the rectal block. This ensures that the resulting dose distribution provides adequate coverage yet does not result in excessive irradiation of normal tissues. At UCSF patients receiving whole-pelvic irradiation receive 180 cGy daily, prescribed to the 92% to 95% isodose line by a four-field box technique to 45 to 50 Gy using 3DCRT. Occasionally patients with lymph nodes that are obviously bulky on CT are treated using IMRT to ensure that a higher dose (50 to 65 Gy) can be safely delivered to such regions. All fields are treated daily with the bladder full. Whole-pelvic irradiation should be followed by a cone-down boost using 3DCRT, IMRT, or brachytherapy.

Treatment Planning and the Cone-Down Boost

Treatment planning CT scans should be obtained with the patient on a flat table with images obtained from the lower border of the sacroiliac joints, using 2 to 5 mm slices inferiorly to 1 cm below the ischial tuberosities. At UCSF we prefer to obtain the treatment planning CT with the rectum empty and the bladder full based on the assumption that this results in the prostate being in its most posterior inferior position. Nonuniform field-edge margins varying from 0.75 to 2.0 cm are used to take into account the dose distribution associated with the technique used, day-to-day setup variation, beam penumbra, and movement error. Nonuniform margins should allow the greatest opportunity for escalation of dose to the prostate, while maximizing tumor control probability and minimizing the normal tissue complication probability. Theoretically, when anterior movement occurs, the post margins become slightly larger, but in the absence of movement they are still adequate. When intraprostatic markers and an EPID-based system are used, all of these field edge margins may be decreased because errors due to day-to-day setup variation and organ movement will also be reduced.

Boosts are usually prescribed at 180 to 200 cGy daily to the 92% to 95% (range 90% to 100%) isodose line such that it encompasses the entire prostate with a small margin. At UCSF the minimum prostatic dose for low-risk patients being treated off study with an intact gland is 72 Gy with a central axis dose of 78 Gy. For patients receiving treatment to the seminal vesicles, partial transmission blocks or multi-leaf blocking are used to keep the dose under the blocks (including the seminal vesicles and anterior rectal wall) to 54 Gy at 180 cGy/day. When IMRT is used, greater dose inhomogeneity is frequently allowed such that the daily dose rate to portions of the prostate significantly exceeds 200 cGy. Some investigators believe that doses in excess of 81 Gy may be considered desirable. This question is the subject of RTOG 0126. Readers at all but selected research institutions are cautioned to avoid excess morbidity by *not* treating patients to doses greater than 78 Gy until phase III trials have been completed.

Treatment Verification

Monitoring treatment alignment by weekly port films is a customary practice. Significant gradual isocenter displacement may occur during the course of treatment in approximately 25% of patients.[261] The magnitude of setup error described is sufficient to reduce the tumor control probability and increase the normal tissue complication probability. Daily monitoring has been shown to reduce the magnitude of these errors and should allow the use of "tighter" margins. Endorectal balloons, ultrasound localization systems, or electronic portal imaging in conjunction with implanted markers are currently the major options for addressing the problem of organ movement (see The Challenges of Day- to-Day Setup Variation and Organ Movement earlier in this chapter).[217,230-232]

BRACHYTHERAPY

Introduction to Permanent and Temporary Implants

Prostate brachytherapy, in various forms, has fluctuated in popularity for more than 100 years. Interstitial prostate brachytherapy was first reported by Barringer in 1917, at what is now MSKCC.[262] Its first widespread adoption occurred in the 1970s, when the retropubic method was popularized.[263,264] In the 1970s, permanent implants were performed by the retropubic approach. A laparotomy was done for lymph node dissection and exposure of the prostate. ^{125}I sources were implanted under direct visualization. The procedure was technically difficult to perform, in part because of limited working space in the pelvis. ^{125}I implantation lost popularity in the 1980s because of the requirement for laparotomy, competition from emergence of modern prostatectomy and CT-based EBRT, and inferior local control rates reported in some series.[265,266]

The past 15 years witnessed a tremendous surge in prostate brachytherapy, due primarily to the introduction of TRUS technology in the early 1980s.[267,268] In 1983, Holm and coworkers reported the use of TRUS for transperineal implantation at the University of Copenhagen in Denmark. TRUS allowed visualization of the needle location within the prostate, allowing for readjustment of needle position as necessary. Implants could be computer preplanned using the transverse ultrasound images. Transperineal implants also could be done on an outpatient basis, without laparotomy. Combined with modern computer-based treatment planning, technological advances allowed for high-quality outpatient prostate brachytherapy.[268-270]

While enthusiasm remains high, there are still vexing discrepancies in reported cure rates and morbidities. It is becoming clearer that such discrepancies result partly from different technical and patient management policies.[271-273] There is little question that there is more to practicing optimal brachytherapy than is currently generally appreciated. Identifying ways to improve and standardize outcomes is a slow and complicated process, and to some, achieving optimal results is looking more and more like "rocket science."

Brachytherapy offers potential biologic advantages over external beam irradiation in terms of dose localization, higher total doses, and higher dose rates (depending on the time interval over which the rate is calculated).[274] All three factors may be significant advantages, but data regarding their clinical relevance are scarce. A modification of the TDF tables (time, dose, fractionation) has been made to allow interconvertability between beam radiation and low dose rate brachytherapy.[275] While it reflects current prescription doses, its clinical applicability is unclear. And long-standing controversies regarding the radiobiologic differences between beam radiation and brachytherapy are unlikely to be resolved soon.[276,277] While the radiobiologic and physical advantages of beam radiation versus brachytherapy are likely to be argued for many years to come, there are substantial practical advantages of brachytherapy, including vastly shorter treatment times, and when performed as monotherapy, lower costs—especially when done efficiently.[278] These practical advantages have helped maintain widespread interest in brachytherapy, despite continuous improvements in beam radiation.

Patient Selection

Cancer status and the risk of morbidity are the two principal criteria by which patients' suitability for brachytherapy is judged. All patients with clinical stage T1/T2 could be considered good candidates for brachytherapy, with or without supplemental beam radiation. Contraindications to brachytherapy include metastatic disease (including lymph node involvement), gross seminal vesicle involvement, or large T3 disease that cannot be adequately implanted due to geometrical impediments to adequate tumor mass implantation (a very unusual presentation). The rationale for excluding patients with seminal vesicle invasion is that radioactive seeds are unlikely to be capable of sterilizing more than the most proximal 1.0 cm of seminal vesicle tissue.[279]

There is general agreement that cancer control in patients with low pretreatment PSA and GS's is similar between modalities, and that brachytherapy without supplemental beam radiation is sufficient. In contrast, there is a common perception that patients with a higher PSA or GS should receive beam radiation or surgery based on their poorer outcomes in some brachytherapy series. In fact, patients with higher indices are at greater risk of cancer recurrence regardless of therapy, due primarily to their higher likelihood of subclinical metastatic disease at presentation. With good quality brachytherapy, implant-based therapy is an acceptable component of treatment for higher risk patients.[280,281] Isolated series with inferior results in higher risk patients have been widely promulgated,[282] but inferior results may very well be due to inadequate treatment planning, especially failure to use proper treatment margins.[273]

Morbidity profiles are the second basis by which to judge patients' suitability for brachytherapy versus other modalities. There is little question that brachytherapy patients experience more short-term urinary morbidity than do external beam radiation patients. Prospective patients should be warned that substantial, though temporary, urinary obstructive symptoms are likely. Patients unlikely to cope well with a temporary exacerbation of obstructive symptoms might be better served with beam radiation or prostatectomy.

While most brachytherapy-related morbidities are self-limited, there is a small likelihood of severe long-term complications, including rectal ulceration, refractory urinary retention, and urinary incontinence. Particular pretreatment conditions may predispose patients to implant-related problems. Unfortunately, we still lack a reliable set of criteria to identify patients who are at substantial risk of morbidity. In addition to general considerations regarding brachytherapy-related short-term morbidity, there are a number of specific conditions that have been widely considered to be relative contraindications to brachytherapy: large prostate size (50 mL), pretreatment urinary obstructive symptoms (American Urological Association [AUA] score >15), prostatitis, and median lobe hypertrophy.

BIG PROSTATES

Large prostate size is probably the most common and least understood alleged contraindication to brachytherapy, due to technical concerns and the perception that such patients are at a higher risk of morbidity. Patients with large prostates are at higher risk of acute postimplant retention, but such retention is typically short-lived, rapidly resolving after several days of an indwelling catheter or self-catheterization.[283] In the past, patients with prostate volumes greater than 50 to 60 mL were commonly advised against brachytherapy or were placed on androgen therapy to implant to shrink their gland before implantation. Some series suggest, however, that hormonal ablation does *not* decrease the risk of retention, and may increase the risk of rectal complications.[283-285]

The primary technical concern regarding implantation of large prostates is that the anterior/lateral portion of the gland may be inadequately covered due to pubic arch interference of needle placement. In fact, pubic arch interference is largely a function of arch anatomy, and less dependent on gland size.[286] Additionally, pubic arch interference is readily circumvented with technical maneuvers.[287,288] With good technique, adequate coverage of large prostate glands is readily achievable.[289,290] With increasing experience, prostate size is less likely to be perceived by brachytherapists as a technical contraindication. On the other extreme, small prostate volume should also not be considered a contraindication to brachytherapy.[291]

PREIMPLANT RETENTIVE SYMPTOMS

After prostate size, preimplant urinary retentive symptoms (high AUA score) is probably the most commonly cited contraindication to brachytherapy. Preimplant retentive symptoms may predispose to postimplant urinary retention or excessive obstructive symptoms, or both. In most cases, however, retention lasts only a few days and is of little or no long-term consequence (Fig. 45-19).[284,292,293] Although it is logical that patients with substantial pretreatment obstructive symptoms would be more prone to brachytherapy-related problems, Terk, Stock, and Stone showed that AUA scores are only a weak predictor of the risk of postimplant urinary retention (Fig. 45-20). Urodynamic studies, postvoid residual urine volume maximum flow rate, or cystoscopy are poor predictors for postimplant retention.[284,294,295] Oddly enough, patients with higher preimplant scores experience less change in their scores compared to those with low preimplant scores, one simplistic explanation being that patients

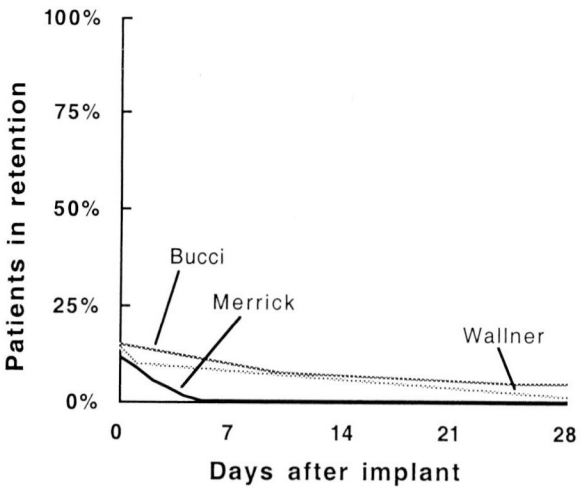

Figure 45–19. Percentage of patients still in urinary retention following brachytherapy. Of note is that postimplant retention is typically short-lived, and perhaps undeserving of the countless publications that it will likely generate. (Data from 273, 496, 497).

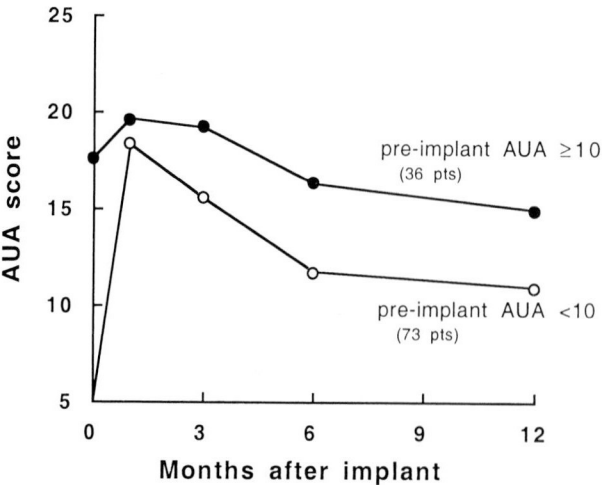

Figure 45–21. Mean American Urological Association (AUA) scores after implantation in patients with pretreatment AUA scores greater or less than 10. Note that patients with higher preimplant scores were already "maxed out," and typically did not get substantially worse, at least as portrayed in their AUA scores. (From Wallner K: Prostate brachytherapy under local anesthesia: Lessons from the first 600 patients. *Brachytherapy*. 2002;1:145.)

with urinary obstructive symptoms are already having trouble and won't get much worse (Fig. 45-21).[296] So while it is unpleasant to have substantial obstructive symptoms, such symptoms are not necessarily, in themselves, contraindications to brachytherapy. The relationship between pre- and postimplant obstructive symptoms is complex, and should be considered on an individual basis, taking into account how willing a patient is to accept a temporary exacerbation of urinary symptoms.

Prior TURP

In an early report from Blasko and colleagues, approximately 50% of TURP patients developed postimplant incontinence.[297] In contrast, the risk of incontinence in TURP patients has been low in more recent experience, probably due to the adoption of peripheral source loading patterns that avoid excessive urethral doses.[298,299]

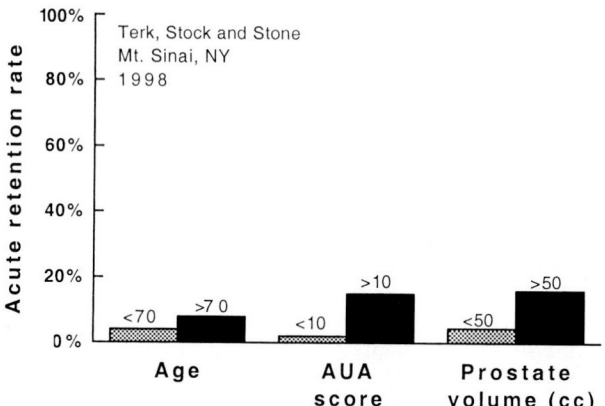

Figure 45–20. Likelihood of post-implant urinary retention versus age, American Urological Association (AUA) scores, and prostate volume. In multivariate analysis, only AUA score was predictive of retention. (From Terk MD, Stock RG, Stone NN: Identification of patients at increased risk for prolonged urinary retention following radioactive seed implantation of the prostate. *J Urol.* 1998;160:1379.)

If brachytherapy is performed for a patient with prior TURP, there should probably be at least a 1.0 cm rim of tissue left around the defect, to ensure sufficient tissue to hold the sources. CT, MRI, or TRUS are generally adequate to assess remaining tissue.

AGE

There has been a reluctance among oncologists to recommend brachytherapy for younger patients, primarily due to the lack of long-term tumor control data. However, with longer follow-up showing high tumor control rates in all ages, reluctance to implant young patients is waning.[300] Although postimplant morbidity is not clearly higher in older patients, it is possible that more elderly patients would have more trouble coping with radiation prostatitis. The possibility of a more difficult postimplant course should be considered when deciding between brachytherapy and external beam radiation for older patients.

Other Alleged Contraindications

Prostatitis is a poorly understood condition often treated empirically with antibiotics. Hughes and colleagues saw no relationship between preimplant clinical or pathologic findings of prostatitis and postimplant urinary morbidity.[301] The presence of a penile prosthesis is a potential contraindication to brachytherapy, due to the possibility of periprosthetic infection or physical damage to the prosthesis. However, concerns over prosthesis-related complications may be exaggerated. No unusual complications were seen in four patients with preexisting penile prosthesis.[302] Median lobe hyperplasia (MLH) refers to protrusion of transitional zone tissue into the bladder.[303-306] It has been considered by some to be a contraindication to brachytherapy, due to an increased risk of postimplant urinary morbidity or because of technical difficulties implanting intravesicular tissue. On the contrary, there appears to be little association between MLH and postimplant morbidity.[304] Intraoperatively, MLH is readily viewed by TRUS, and there is little difficulty placing sources in the MLH tissue. There is no documented justification for prophylactic resection of hypertrophic tissue.

Considering the high prevalence of obesity, surprisingly little has been reported regarding treatment of prostate cancer in such patients. Heavy patients pose a relatively minor problem for brachytherapy. Operative setup can take longer, and there is less room to maneuver between the patient's legs, but this has not presented a huge problem.[307] Standard 20 cm brachytherapy needles are almost always sufficient to reach the prostate. Clinical outcomes appear to be unaffected.[308]

Inflammatory bowel disease (IBD), including ulcerative colitis and regional enteritis (Crohn's disease), has long been believed to be a contraindication to radiation, despite scant documentation of IBD-related complications.[309,310] IBD patients treated with brachytherapy have not experienced unusual gastrointestinal morbidity.[311] The use of supplemental beam radiation in the setting of IBD has not specifically been addressed, but data from patients treated with beam radiation alone suggest that it is not strongly contraindicated.

Patients with prior therapeutic pelvic radiation are presumably at higher risk for radiation-related complications. Reirradiation in other sites has generally been better tolerated than predicted radiobiologically, and it is likely reasonably safe in the setting of prostate cancer.[312] Data regarding brachytherapy in previously irradiated prostatic regions are fragmentary, but suggestive that it is generally safe.[313-315]

TREATMENT PLANNING

Treatment planning refers to the determination of what type of seed and how many will be used, and where they will be placed. Growing evidence suggests that planning and implementation have a significant effect on the likelihoods of cure.[316-318] Implants are typically planned from TRUS images of the prostate, taken at 5 mm intervals from the base through the apex (Fig. 45-22). The patient should be in the lithotomy position, similar to that for the implant procedure itself (Fig. 45-23). It's important that the prostate is not deformed by excessive probe pressure.

The most proximal image is considered the *0.0 plane* or *zero plane*. It is located by visualizing the most proximal image or base, usually including a portion of the seminal vesicles (Figs. 45-24 to 45-29). Images and source positions are typically specified by their caudal distance from the 0.0 plane. The most caudal images, through the prostatic apex, are frequently indistinct on transverse imaging but can be verified on sagittal imaging.

TARGET DEFINITIONS

The gross target volume (GTV) is the prostate itself, as visualized on the TRUS images. The treatment margin (TM) is the perpendicular distance between the GTV and the prescription isodose (Fig. 45-30).[319,320] The treated volume (TV) is that enclosed by the prescription isodose. To start the treatment planning process, the prostatic margin (GTV) is identified on the TRUS images and transferred into a planning program. The margins appear fuzzy, especially at the apex, where the prostatic tissue blends into the nearly isodense pelvic floor musculature. When in doubt, it is probably best to err on the side of being too generous rather than too skimpy in identifying the prostatic borders. The goal of treatment planning is to deliver a cancerocidal dose to the prostate, with a sufficient margin to encompass the likely extent of extracapsular disease extension (ECE), keeping in mind the high incidence of early EPE even in patients with low PSA and GS's.[92] The goal of treatment planning should be to cover the prostate itself and periprostatic tissue, remembering that EPE is nearly always limited to within 3 mm of the prostatic edge, so a 3 to 5 mm postimplant TM should suffice.[321,322]

Unfortunately, achieving a sufficient postimplant TM is complicated by the substantial and unpredictable degree of implant-related prostate swelling. The prostate volume increases by approximately 20% by the completion of the implant procedure, but with a large degree of variability between patients.[323] Predicting swelling in the individual patient has proven impossible, being unrelated to the prostate size or number of sources. To achieve adequate postimplant TMs, some allowance must be made for source placement error and implant-related swelling that continues over much of the active life of the isotopes.[324,325] Adequate postimplant TMs are readily achievable using a heavily peripheral source placement, large planning treatment margins, and a central dose of 150% to 200% of the prescription dose.[273,326,327] Achieving sufficient postimplant TMs is facilitated by placement of extraprostatic sources (see Fig. 45-30).[328,329]

Cancers occur more frequently in the posterior-lateral regions, where EPE is also more common.[330] There is some rationale for lesser TMs anteriorly.[322,330] However, cancer regionalization is still not thoroughly understood. It is probably better to minimize margin variability, especially considering that apart from rectal doses and strictures, morbidity is probably little affected by TMs.

Early reports of correlations between central doses and urinary morbidity have not been corroborated in more recent series, probably due to adoption of peripheral loading patterns without the central dose extremes of early use of homogeneous placement patterns.[292,331] A simple rule of thumb is to keep the urethral dose between 150% and 250% of the prescription dose, a goal that is easily met using modified peripheral source placement patterns.[273]

Much has been said regarding the importance of dose homogeneity, and detailed recommendations have been made regarding allegedly optimal V150, V200, and so on.[332] In fact, the relationship between morbidity and dose homogeneity per se is unproven.[333] Homogeneity indices appear to be of little use, as long as guidelines for treatment margins and urethral and rectal doses are followed.

A wide variety of source strengths have been used for prostate brachytherapy, with no clinical evidence of any

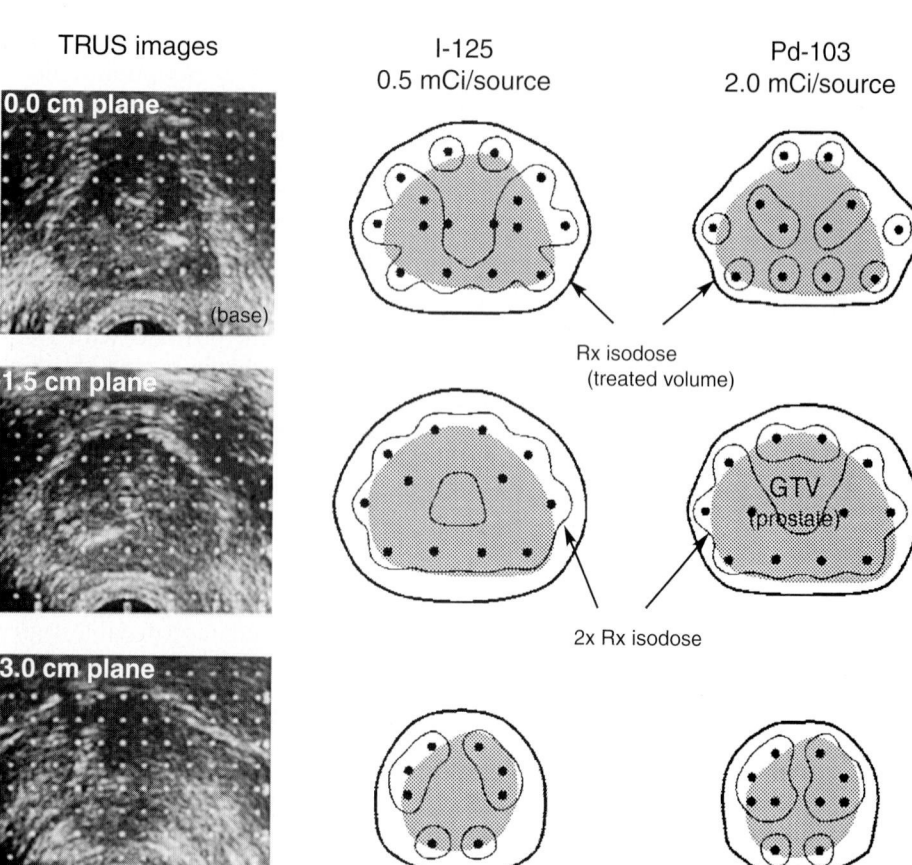

TRUS images

0.0 cm plane
(base)

1.5 cm plane

3.0 cm plane
(Apex)

I-125
0.5 mCi/source

Pd-103
2.0 mCi/source

Rx isodose
(treated volume)

GTV
(prostate)

2x Rx isodose

Figure 45–22. Pre-implant transrectal ultrasound images and plans for I-125 (144 Gy) or Pd-103 implant (124 Gy) by K. Wallner. Note the generous treatment margins and peri-prostatic sources, particularly at the prostatic base and apex. The V200s (twice prescription dose) cover 50% to 75% of the preplan prostate volume but are less on the postplan due to implant-related swelling. High V200s, in the absence of excessive urethral or rectal doses, are not related to urinary or rectal morbidity. (From Jones S, Wallner K, Merrick G, et al: Clinical correlates of high brachytherapy dose regions within the prostate. *Int J Radiat Oncol Biol Phys.* 2002; 53(2):328.) Plane numbers refer to distance (cm) from the prostatic base.

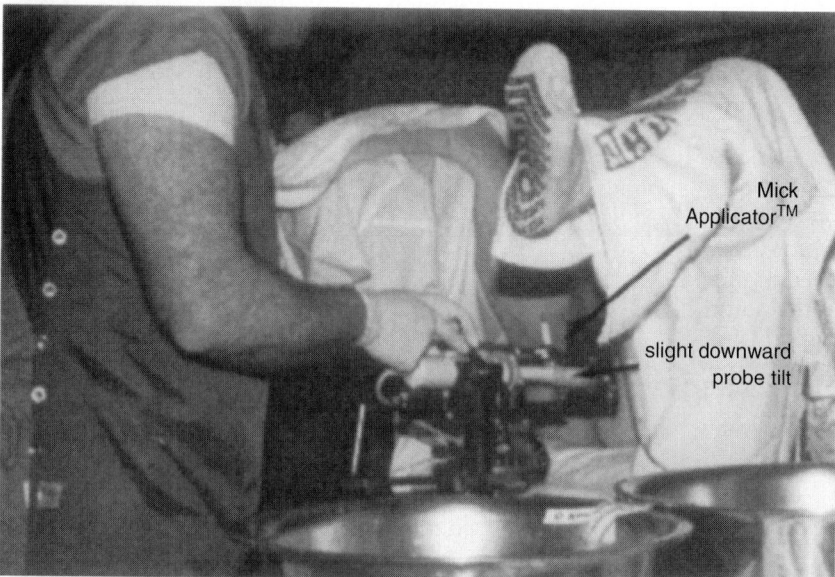

Mick Applicator™

slight downward probe tilt

Figure 45–23. Patient positioning—the legs can be moved to a more extended lithotomy position if pubic arch interference is a problem.

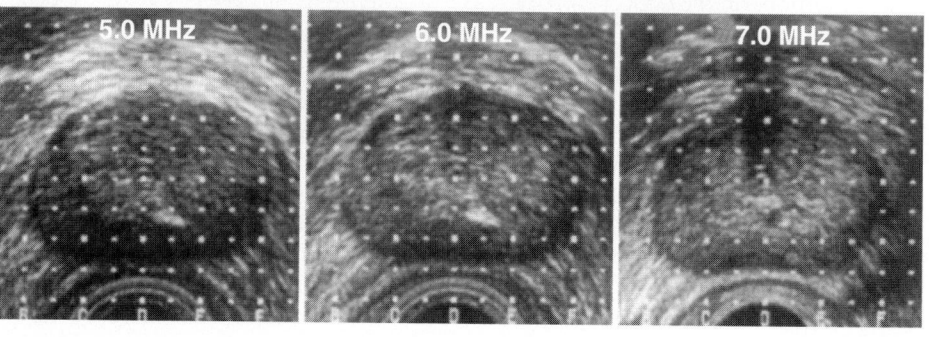

5.0 MHz   6.0 MHz   7.0 MHz

Figure 45–24. Increasing transrectal ultrasound frequencies typically improves near-probe imaging, so that the rectal wall is most sharply seen with higher frequency. However, the visualization difference varies from patient to patient.

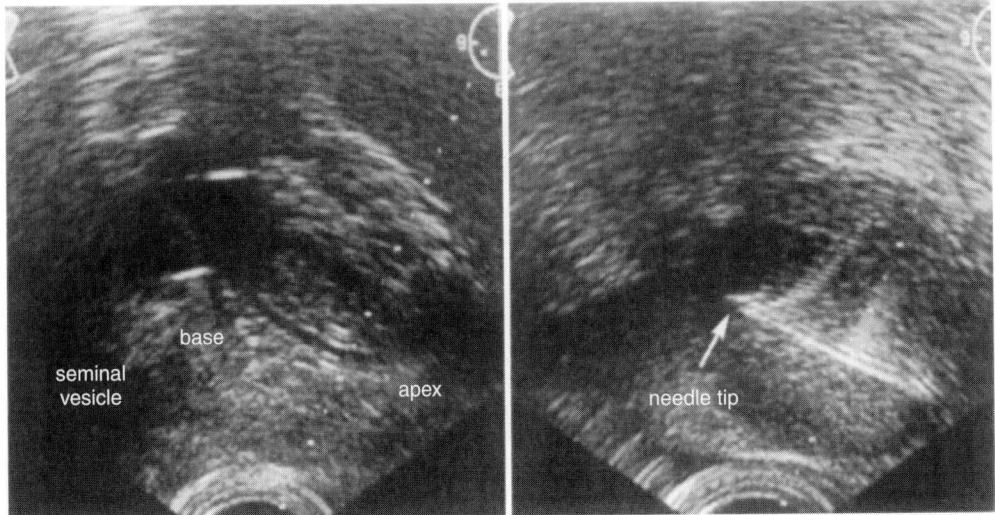

Figure 45–25. Sagittal imaging helps verify the base and apical planes. It can be helpful in verifying proper needle depth. Note that the sagittal image in the right panel is off midline, to show a laterally placed needle.

effect on outcomes.[331] [125]I sources typically vary in strength from 0.2 to 0.9 mCi and Pd-103 sources vary from 1.1 to 2.5 mCi (NIST-99). Using higher activity sources reduces the number required.[334] Arguments that high activity sources could lead to a higher complication rate or less adequate target coverage are based on a small number of patients implanted at Stanford with the retropubic method.[335] There is no evidence that end-to-end seed placement has any detrimental effect. However, when fewer seeds are used, each makes up a higher percentage of the total dose so that seed loss into the bladder or into the vasculature will have more impact on the dose.

HORMONAL DOWNSIZING

Androgen deprivation typically reduces the prostate volume by approximately 25% to 50%.[336] When pretreatment androgen deprivation is used, dosimetry should be based on the reduced prostate volume. Sufficient time should be given to allow near maximal shrinkage before obtaining the planning images. Most shrinkage occurs in

the first 2 months of androgen deprivation, although additional shrinkage beyond this point is also seen.[336]

PREPLANNING VERSUS INTRAOPERATIVE PREPLANNING

In early versions of intraoperative preimplant treatment planning, the prostate size was estimated from preimplant TRUS imaging and the approximate number of sources needed was determined from a nomogram.[337] At the time of the procedure, two thirds of the activity is placed at the prostatic periphery, and the remainder in the interior of the gland. More recently, faster treatment-planning systems allow intraoperative preplanning based on intraoperative image capture.[338-340]

The most touted advantage of intraoperative preplanning is better matching of the planning and implementation images, circumventing the potential problem of a

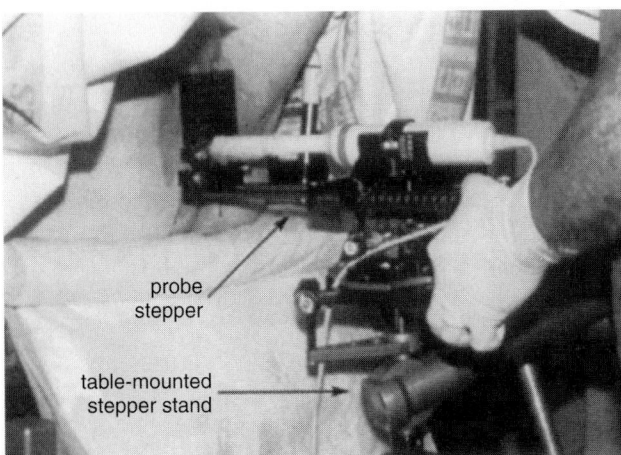

Figure 45–26. Stepping units facilitate precise movement of the transrectal ultrasound probe at 5 mm increments.

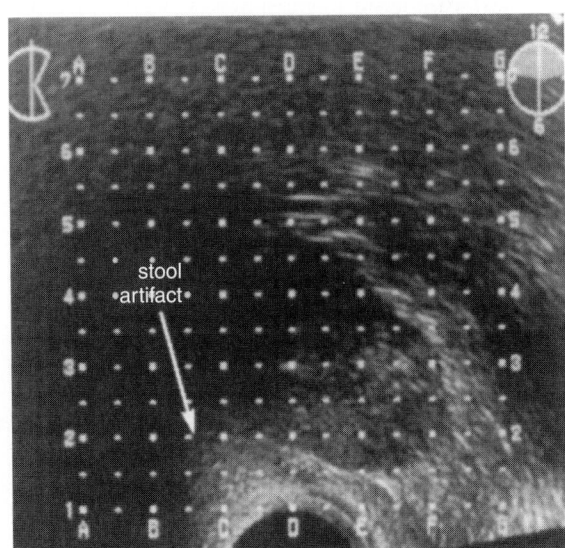

Figure 45–27. Stool artifact obscuring the prostatic image. If you do not get a good image of the entire prostate, stop and fix the situation.

pre-implant   post-implant

Figure 45–28. Pre- and postimplant transrectal ultrasound images at mid prostate. Source insertion leads to degeneration in prostatic edge visualization. The degree of image degradation varies from patient to patient and at different levels in the same patient, these examples being fairly typical. (From Smith S, Wallner K, Merrick G, et al: Interpretation of pre- versus post-implant TRUS images. *Med Phys.* 2003 May, 30(5):920.)

discrepancy between the planning versus the intraoperative images some weeks later. However, in experienced hands such discrepancies are minimal and likely inconsequential. Reports of improved results with one technique over the other likely reflect evolving brachytherapy skill levels rather than a true advantage of one over the other. From a purely practical standpoint, intraoperative preplanning has some substantial disadvantages. It can increase operating time by 20 to 30 minutes or more and requires a greater degree of physics support intraoperatively. Additionally, it requires extra sources on hand, in case the intraoperative plan calls for more seeds than were anticipated.

SUPPLEMENTAL EXTERNAL BEAM RADIATION

The use of supplemental beam radiation to cover the prostate with a 1 to 2 cm margin has been widely practiced since the use of low dose rate Ir-192.[341] In the TRUS era, the generally accepted policy has been to add external beam radiation for patients with a pretreatment PSA above 10 or a GS above 6. While favorable tumor control rates have resulted from this policy, results with implant alone, even in patients with higher PSA and GS's, have been remarkably good in most series.[281,342-344] Additionally, detailed pathology studies have revealed that the radial extent of extraprostatic cancer extension, even in patients with higher PSA and GS's, is surprisingly limited and within reach of treatment margins achievable with a peripherally loaded implant.[272,321,322,327] As such, the need for supplemental beam radiation is coming under increasing question. Wallner, Merrick, and colleagues are conducting a large, randomized study comparing moderate-dose (44 Gy) versus low-dose (20 Gy) supplemental beam radiation for intermediate-risk patients. The rationale behind the trial is that large brachytherapy treatment margins obviate the need for higher dose supplemental beam radiation.[345]

Beyond the basic question of whether or not to use supplemental beam radiation, there are a dizzying menu of ways to combine brachytherapy and supplemental radiation, with little data to support one policy over another. Basic issues including sequencing, time gaps, isotope choice, and beam field sizes have been arrived at empirically, with no basis in comparative trials. Optimal ways to combine radiation modalities should be a subject of intense future clinical investigation.[346,347]

Patient Preparation

Preoperative patient preparation should facilitate the implant procedure and decrease the risk of postoperative

Undesirable
(excessive peri-apical sources)

Desirable

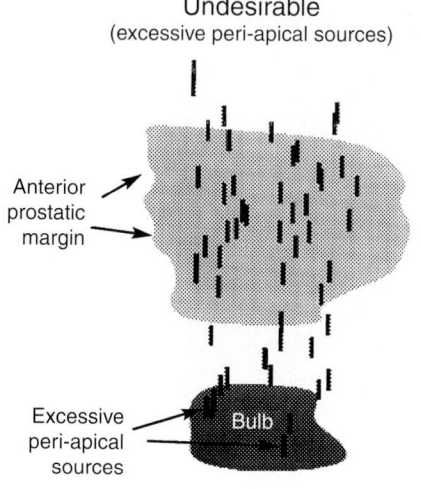

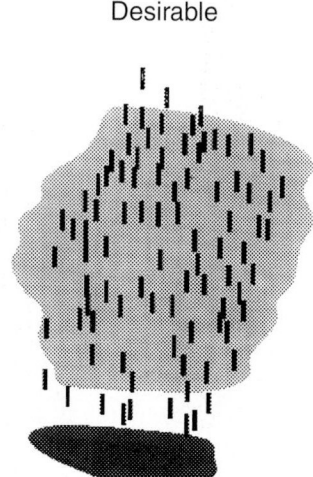

Anterior prostatic margin

Excessive peri-apical sources

Bulb

Figure 45–29. Sagittal view of two implants—the patient on the left has excessive peri-apical sources, due either to poor planning or poor implementation. (From Wallner K, Blasko J, Dattoli M: Technique. In Waller K, Blasko J, Dattoli M, eds. *Prostate Brachytherapy Made Complicated,* 2nd ed. Seattle: SmartMedicine; 2001;8:1.)

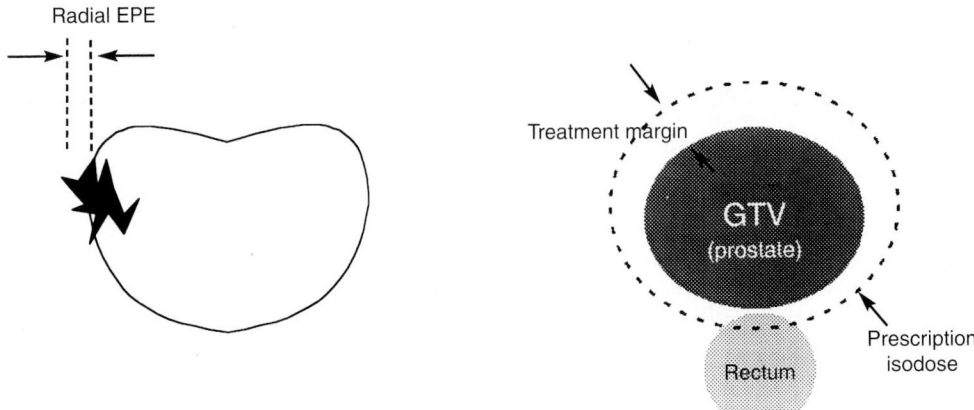

Figure 45–30. Schematic of extraprostatic cancer extension (EPE) and radiation treatment margin (TM).

morbidity. Preparatory practices vary widely, some being more onerous than others.

BOWEL PREPARATION

The rectum should be clear of feces to facilitate proper TRUS imaging. Various enemas, diets, and laxative cocktails can be used. Many brachytherapists have abandoned the use of laxatives—an early morning enema is usually sufficient. At the Puget Sound VA, patients are simply instructed to try to have unassisted bowel movement the morning of the implant: if unable, rectal feces are rarely a problem.

ANESTHESIA

Spinal (epidural) or general anesthesia are routinely used. However, local anesthesia is being increasingly adopted. Surprisingly well tolerated, local anesthesia is accomplished with parenteral lidocaine given in a 0.5% solution.[348] Immediately following injection into the subcutaneous tissues, the pelvic floor and prostate are anesthetized by injecting lidocaine solution with small-gauge needles. Patients tolerate brachytherapy under local anesthesia surprisingly well, and its use may increase, considering the patient convenience and cost savings.[278,349]

PERIOPERATIVE CORTICOSTEROIDS

Prophylactic corticosteroids have been proposed to decrease the likelihood of postoperative urinary retention. In a preliminary trial, corticosteroids did not appreciably alter the risk of retention or implant-related prostatic size changes.[323,350] Randomized, controlled trials are warranted.

Patient Positioning

After induction of anesthesia, place the patient in the lithotomy position (see Fig. 45-23). Try to reproduce the positioning of the planning scan, realizing that there will usually be minor differences. The legs should be symmetrically rotated and extended at the hips and at the knees to avoid rotating the pelvis on the head-to-toe axis. In patients with pubic arch interference, the extended lithotomy position moves the pubic bones away from the anterior portion of the prostate.[288]

Urethral Visualization

Most brachytherapists use a catheter or aerated gel to visualize the urethra during the procedure—a catheter is the simplest, most reliable method. Alternatively, aerated gel can be instilled through the urethra, using a penile clamp to prevent leaking.[351]

TRUS frequencies of 5.0, 6.0, and 7.0 MHz are standard. Higher frequencies give better tissue visualization closer to the probe. The optimal MHz varies from patient to patient (see Fig. 45-24). The probe should be covered generously with lubricant. A probe cover (condom) is used to facilitate postprocedure cleaning; water-filled covers are unnecessary.

Transverse imaging alone is sufficient in most cases, but sagittal imaging helps visualize the prostatic base and apex and verify proper needle location and depth (see Fig. 45-25). Biplane probes, capable of transverse and sagittal imaging, are standard in newer machines.

STEPPING UNIT AND STABILIZER

The TRUS probe is supported on a stepping unit, allowing it to be moved caudal or cephalad at 0.5 cm intervals. The unit should hold the probe steady, without obstructing access to the perineum (see Fig. 45-26). An easily adjustable stepping unit (and stabilizer) facilitates the procedure, and is well worth the initial investment. The stepping unit is supported by a stabilizing table-mounted or floor-mounted stand (see Fig. 45-26). Table-mounted stands are typically lighter and move with the procedure table if the table position is changed during the case. They also tend to allow more foot space in front of the table, which can be a major advantage at teaching institutions.

PROBE POSITIONING

To begin imaging the prostate, place the probe tip against the anus and press gently until the sphincter gives way. The probe should advance easily and the prostate will come into view. Make gross probe adjustments by moving the stand itself. Make small changes with the fine adjusters on the stepping unit/stand. If the image is not clear, move the probe in and out to clear gas from the interface between the probe and the anterior rectal wall. If unsuccessful, completely withdraw and reinsert the probe.

If gas or fecal artifact persists, an intraoperative enema or rectal tube may be needed (see Fig. 45-27).

DUPLICATE THE PREPLANNING IMAGES

If using a preplan, check that the intraoperative images match the preoperative ones; they may not match exactly, but should be very close. An example of an important landmark for matching is the space between the seminal vesicles and the base of the gland. The probe tip should be angled slightly toward the floor. Gentle probe pressure against the prostate allows good coupling with the tissue, but too much pressure distorts the image, leading to artifactual flattening of the prostate (see Figs. 45-25 and 45-27).

NEEDLE INSERTION

Once the probe is properly positioned, needles are inserted through the template holes and through the perineal skin until visible on the TRUS template grid. Needles can be deflected by material used to drape the patient, the skin, the tissue planes, or by the pubic bones, causing them to appear off their mark on the template coordinates. Excessively deflected needles should be withdrawn and reinserted. Image degradation typically occurs in the course of the implant, but images are still adequate to evaluate the prostatic edges (see Fig. 45-28).[352] A look at more proximal images will generally help clarify a needle's position on the template. Determining needle depth is as important to proper source placement as is correct positioning in the transverse images. Proper depth is typically determined by inserting the needle until it is viewed on the desired plane. When the tip of the needle is exactly at the same plane of the probe, rotating the needle generally allows two distinct lines to be seen, corresponding to the point at the bevel of the needle. If in doubt, sagittal imaging can be helpful (see Fig. 45-28).

Some patients' prostates are highly mobile.[353] Tissue-gripping needles hold the prostate and decrease motion along the needle tracks, but most brachytherapists prefer simply to monitor motion and adjust the probe accordingly.[354]

DEPOSITING SOURCES

A growing variety of tools and techniques for source placement is available. The two most common modes are preloaded needles and the Mick applicator. Radioactive seeds on a strand are also being used at a number of centers. Observing placement under fluoroscopy is a good way to guard against source misplacement because you can usually see when sources are not staying put after they should have left the needle tip.

PUBIC ARCH INTERFERENCE

A sometimes vexing technical problem, pubic arch interference, can usually be readily circumvented by changing the patient to a more extended lithotomy position, rotating the pubic arch superiorly (see Fig. 45-23).[288] In most cases, simply changing the probe angulation allows needles to be inserted just behind the arch. However, such maneuvers can alter the relationship of the probe to the prostate—be sure to recheck the prostate's positioning on the TRUS grid. Occasionally, if the seed loading pattern allows (e.g., most at base), pubic arch interference can be circumvented by using more medial holes in the template while diverging the needle laterally. With some experience, occasionally a needle can be curved so as to hook around and under the pubic bone.

Implant Quality

A critical assessment of postimplant dosimetry is the key to delivering good therapy—it is the cornerstone of quality assurance. Optimal dosimetric parameters are key for maximizing cure rates.[317,355] CT currently is the standard dosimetric imaging modality. Its principal advantages include wide availability and easy source identification. Admittedly, the prostatic margins are typically indistinct on CT, in part due to scatter artifact, especially near the prostatic apex. However, if anatomic landmarks are used, excluding the levator ani musculature from the prostate volume, CT is a more accurate modality than some investigators have claimed.[356] Nevertheless, it is possible that there will be a switch to MR- or TRUS-based dosimetry imaging in the future.[352,357,358]

ISODOSE OVERLAYS

The simplest way to evaluate an individual implant is visual inspection of the isodose overlays on the prostate (see Fig. 45-29). Despite the emphasis on dosimetric parameters, looking at the seed positions is also the best way to evaluate the clinical significance of underdosed regions. That's because dose parameters like D90 or V100 are geographically nonspecific—they don't tell the magnitude of a particular cold spot, and they don't take into account the relationship between underdosed regions and where cancers are more likely to be (posteriorly and laterally).

QUANTIFYING PROSTATE COVERAGE

The simplest index to quantify prostate coverage is the *V100*, or the percent of the postimplant prostate volume covered by the prescription dose. Roy and colleagues first used postimplant CTs to calculate *V100s*, reporting typical values of only about 80%.[359] It later became apparent that lesser values were due primarily to implant-related prostate swelling.[324,325,360] In fact, *V100s* of 80% to 95% are typical among even experienced implant teams.

The second most widely used dosimetric parameter is the D90—the dose that covers 90% of the postimplant prostate volume. D90s can be expressed either in Gy or as a percent of the prescription dose. Based on retrospective studies, tumor control appears better with a D90 greater than 90% of the prescription dose. D90 and V100 values are closely correlated, so that both are commonly used; the principal advantage of the V100 is that it's easier to conceptualize. The advantage of the D90 is that it is less sensitive to a wider dose range, and seems to give a better picture of the overall coverage, since it does not depend on the upper limit of 100% coverage that V100 does. The minimum prostatic dose (Dmin) is not useful because it is too sensitive to minor variations in source placement or target definitions.[359]

Another parameter of increasing interest is the treatment margin (TM), defined as the distance between the prostatic edge and the prescription isodose (see Fig. 45-30).[272,326,327] TMs can vary markedly between implant patients, even when their V100s and D90s are similar. Because the radial extent of extraprostatic cancer extension (EPE) is typically limited to 3 to 5 mm, it seems logical that achieving a minimum 3 mm TM would increase the likelihood of eradicating EPE and maximize the chance for cure.[321,322,345] Several authors have shown that 3 mm TMs are achievable with current implant techniques.[272,326,327] Because of their direct relation to EPE coverage, assessment of TMs is theoretically appealing. The limited data currently available correlating TMs with clinical outcomes suggest that TMs will be incorporated into clinical practice in the future.[318]

PROSTATE SWELLING

Postimplant dosimetry is complicated by the fact that the prostate volume increases by 20% or more during the implant procedure, with substantial variability among patients; also seeds in the prostate degrade the image (Fig. 45-30).[324,325,361] Implant-related swelling increases the prostate volume on which postimplant evaluation is based, making target coverage inferior to what would be determined if it were based on the smaller, preimplant prostate size. Target coverage decreases by 5% to 20%, depending on what indices are used.[362] One way to account for the degree of swelling is to base the postimplant dosimetry on the preimplant volume, somehow registered with the postimplant source locations. Doing so may be the most realistic way to assess how well the preplan was executed. But such a solution would likely be of little clinical use because much of the dose would be delivered while the prostate was still larger than the pretreatment volume.

Some have argued in favor of waiting 1 month to obtain postimplant dosimetry films, to allow implant-related swelling to resolve. The practical limitation of such a policy is that if target coverage is determined at that time to be inadequate, adding sources so long after the initial procedure would probably be radiobiologically suboptimal. Elegant formulas have been devised to account for the degree of swelling resolution over time.[363] However, correction factors are impractical in clinical practice because of inconsistent edema resolution rates among patients.[325]

INADEQUATE IMPLANTS

Regardless of one's technique, there will be cases in which the degree of prostate coverage appears insufficient. Probably the best way to supplement an inadequate implant is to return to the operating room to add more sources to the underdosed region. Use the postimplant CT to determine the dose to be delivered by the sources already implanted, and then prepare a plan to adequately supplement where needed, without excessive rectal or urethral doses. Alternatively, supplemental external beam radiation could be added. However, using beam radiation to bring the dose to therapeutic levels in the most under-dosed regions may mean overtreating other regions. Labeling an implant as inadequate is a murky endeavor, one for which there are currently no published data regarding how best to proceed.

Postoperative Care

Perioperative care is relatively simple—complications calling for readmissions are infrequent.[364] However, for several months, patients typically experience marked urinary and rectal symptoms that can usually be addressed effectively. Postoperative pain (apart from dysuria) is usually limited to minor perineal discomfort. More significant postoperative pain is unusual. Narcotic analgesics should not be routinely prescribed. Patients who experience pain requiring narcotics should be carefully assessed for an unusual circumstance. Urinary retention is the most common acute implant-related complication and almost impossible to predict for an individual patient.[283] Fortunately, it typically resolves rapidly, with or without institution of alpha-1 blockers.[292] In cases of protracted retention, surgical interventions or suprapubic tubes should be avoided in favor of long-term intermittent self-catheterization.[284,365] Most patients have a minor degree of postimplant gross hematuria, lasting for a few days. Occasional patients will report late, episodic hematuria, of little or no clinical significance.[366] Diagnostic procedures should be considered on an individual basis.

OBSTRUCTIVE SYMPTOMS

Nearly all patients develop symptoms of radiation prostatitis, including dysuria, daytime frequency, nocturia, and urgency. Symptoms generally peak at 2 to 4 weeks following implantation and are due to urethral inflammation, not to cystitis.[367] If no medications are routinely prescribed at the time of implantation, about half of patients will end up on them due to increasing symptoms.[368] Selective alpha-1 adrenergic blockers are by far the most effective treatment. Early, aggressive use of blockers is probably most effective in relieving symptoms and may hasten their resolution. Most patients stop their alpha-blockers within 6 to 24 months.

Monitoring Treatment Response

PSA has dramatically decreased the time to detect cancer persistence, rendering routine follow-up digital rectal examination nearly obsolete. In the absence of a rising PSA, repeat prostatic biopsies rarely show residual cancers, and palpable tumor recurrence in the absence of a rising PSA is virtually unseen.[369,370] Although still a subject of controversy, postimplant nadir PSA correlates with the likelihood of long-term biochemical control; while there is no single nadir PSA value that guarantees against late biochemical failure, the lower the better.[154,157] Because of the great variability in the rate and consistency of PSA declines after brachytherapy, the optimal time to allow for nadiring to occur is unknown—some patients nadir at 6 months, while others take 6 years. The rate of decline is

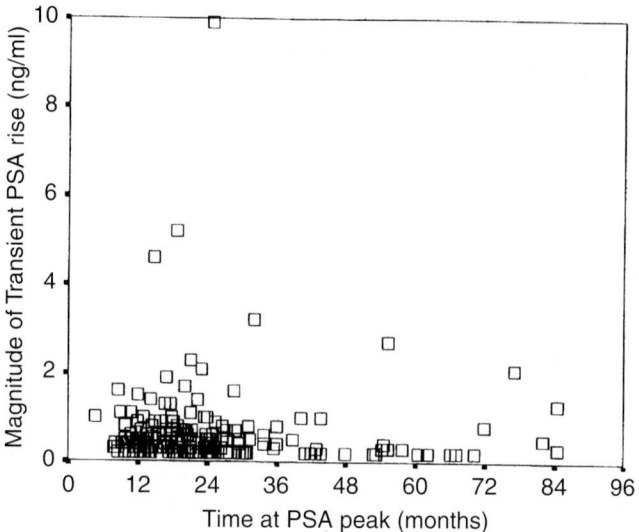

Figure 45–31. Magnitude of the temporary serum PSA increase plotted against maximum time noted for 191 patients who exhibited a serum PSA "spike." (From Cavanaugh W, Blasko JC, Grimm PD, et al: Transient elevation of serum prostate-specific antigen following I-125/Pd-103 brachytherapy for localized prostate cancer. *J Urol.* 2000;163:1085.)

prognosis for PSA spike patients appears similar to patients without a spike.[372,373]

POST-TREATMENT BIOPSIES

Postradiation biopsy has been used sporadically to assess intraprostatic tumor eradication. Patients with histologically viable tumor have a greater likelihood of developing local recurrence and distant metastases.[374,375] Postimplant biopsies are conceptually appealing, but their routine use is limited by ambiguous interpretation and the fact that biopsies are almost always negative in patients with a low postradiation PSA.[376,377] The clinical dilemma of a rising PSA in the first 3 postimplant years is made doubly confusing when a postimplant biopsy in the same period is positive, because biopsies may take 2 years or more to revert to negative.[376,378,379]

Isotopes

I-125 and Pd-103 are commonly used radioisotopes for prostate brachytherapy. The sources are the same size (4.5 × 0.8 mm) but appear differently on radiographs, depending on the manufacturer's radiographic marker inside the titanium capsule. The isotopes differ substantially in their half-life and photon energy, factors that may influence their biologic effects. I-125 has been the most widely used radionuclide. Its relatively long half-life of sixty days is a practical advantage, allowing it to be stored for several weeks if a case is postponed. The difference in average energy between I-125 and Pd-103 has only minor effects on most treatment planning parameters.[380] Pd-103's shorter half-life of 17 days may be a radiobiologic advantage, with a shorter duration of radiation-related urinary symptoms and a suggestion of lower postimplant PSA values (Fig. 45-32).[296]

SUTURE-MOUNTED SOURCES

Suture-mounted I-125 sources (RAPID Strand, Nycomed-Amersham) are mounted in #1 Vicryl (polyglactin 910), which dissolves in 1 to 3 months. Suture-mounted sources are more likely to maintain their position, and decreases

highly variable and has not, in itself, been correlated with prognosis after beam radiation. In the post-brachytherapy setting, any relation between the rate of decline and prognosis is made especially murky by the occurrence of temporary PSA rises.

Temporary PSA rises, also referred to as PSA *bumps*, *blips*, or *spikes*, occur typically between 6 and 36 months after implantation (Fig. 45-31). The magnitude of most temporary rises is less than 2.0 ng/mL, but rises as high as 10 ng/mL or more are seen.[371-373] If PSAs are taken at the typical 4 to 6 month intervals and any increase is considered, about a third of patients will experience a spike or bump. Their likelihood is independent of pretreatment PSA, GS, isotope, or use of supplemental external beam radiation. Some relationship to intraprostatic higher dose regions and age has been shown.[371] The long-term

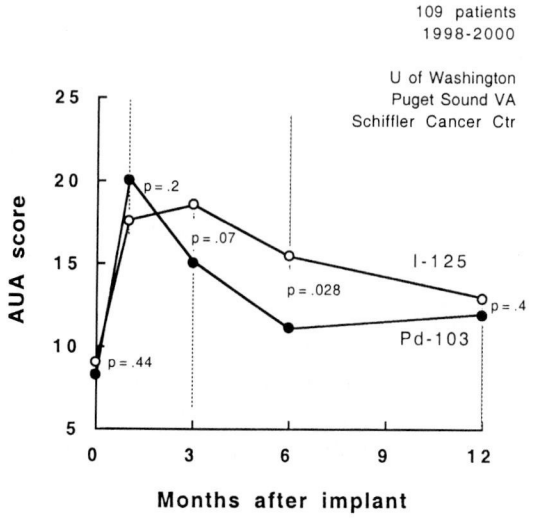

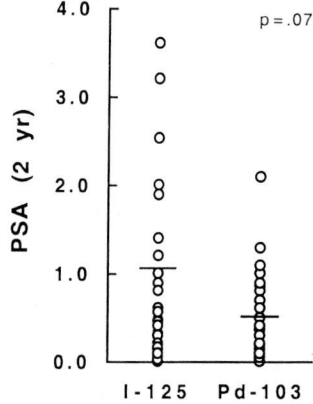

Figure 45–32. Mean American Urological Association scores (left panel) or 2-year PSAs (right panel) after I-125 versus Pd-103 implantation. (From Wallner K: Prostate brachytherapy under local anesthesia: Lessons from the first 600 patients. *Brachytherapy.* 2002;1:145.)

source migration. Theoretically, they could allow for wider periprostatic coverage, but their true clinical benefit is unclear. Their primary disadvantage has been their tendency to stick inside the needles, a technical problem that requires some attention.[381] Newer versions of stranded seeds are being introduced.

Temporary Implants

Although temporary implants are performed less frequently, a body of evidence suggests that this approach is also an effective treatment option for clinically localized prostate cancer. Temporary prostate implants are also a TRUS-based procedure. Afterloading catheters are inserted under TRUS guidance and typically secured into position using a perineal template. The position of the catheter is then usually captured by a CT scan and transferred into a treatment planning system. Each catheter is then sequentially loaded with a radioactive source (typically Iridium Ir-192). Treatment planning software is then used to determine the optimal loading or duration that the radioactive source is left in a given position. Computer-driven stepping motors control the placement of a high activity Ir-192 source located at the end of a cable coming from the afterloading machines. By controlling the amount of time the source spends at points along the catheter (dwell time), various dose distribution can be generated. Modern treatment planning software also allows the dwell time to be optimized using mathematical algorithms to produce better coverage of the implant volume while minimizing doses to critical normal structure.[382,383] The radioactive sources are removed after a predetermined dose is delivered. The time required to deliver a given dose can range from hours to days when low dose rate therapy is used, to minutes when high dose rate (HDR) therapy is used. After treatment is completed, the afterloading catheters are removed and the patient is discharged. Temporary prostate implants are usually administered using multiple fractionated treatments delivered over one to three outpatient or inpatient visits. The radiation exposure to personnel is minimized, since the radioactive sources are loaded outside the treatment room. The ability to load the sources after placement of the catheters and to use computer control to place the radioactive source make HDR brachytherapy extremely flexible.

Over the past several years there has been an increase in the enthusiasm for HDR brachytherapy supported by a flurry of recent publications touting the theoretical reasons for radiobiologic advantages associated with HDR. These recent reports have centered around the notion that the alpha-beta value for prostate cancer has been estimated to be as low as 1.5 Gy.[384-386] This low alpha-beta ratio has been interpreted as providing a rationale for treating prostate cancer using HDR radiotherapy.[387,388] Due to the logistic and financial advantages of using fewer numbers of fractions, some have argued this could well become the preferred approach. Fowler, Chappell, and Ritter and, more recently, King and Fowler reviewed a large collection of papers published from 1995 to 2000 and estimated PSA control rates following EBRT, I-125, or Pd-103 PPI. They concluded that a hypofractionated regimen might be most logical.[384-386]

Not all experts agree that this is a clinically relevant observation, however.[389] One argument against the use of hypofractionation is that it is likely the control rates used for the analysis conducted by Fowler and others significantly overestimated control rates due to the inadequacy of follow-up. For example, although the follow-up was considered "mature" in the paper by Brenner et al., in fact the data were not. The follow-up extended to 5 years, but the median follow-up for the study reported to was only 32 months for brachytherapy patients. In particular, the patients receiving the highest doses, 140 Gy, had substantially shorter follow-up than those who received lower doses. In the report by Fowler et al., the 2-year PSA control rates were used. Several studies have shown that using the ASTRO consensus definition to define an accurate outcome required follow-up at least 2 years beyond the median follow-up.[166,167] Furthermore, Fowler et al. analyzed "intermediate" risk patients. The definition used was based on eligibility PSA 10 to 20, or T2b disease or GS = 7. However, GS is the most important predictor of survival. Higher GS's are associated with shorter survivals and more rapidly dividing tumors. Thus, this "intermediate-risk group" is actually a heterogeneous population that may have different α/β ratios. Their assumptions are probably most accurate for patients with a GS less than 7.

One of the strongest arguments against hypofractionated regimens is the fact that intermediate-risk patients appear to benefit from pelvic radiotherapy (see discussion of RTOG 9413 later). It is unlikely that a hypofractionated regimen would be well tolerated by the gut. Since HDR has not proven to be more effective than EBRT, it is likely to be more expensive to add anesthesia and operating room time than 2 weeks of EBRT to prostate-only boost. Furthermore, to date, rates of stricture and incontinence appear to be higher in patients treated with HDR than seen in patients treated with EBRT (see complications later). Only time and more studies can sort these issues out.

NEUTRONS, PROTONS, AND HEAVY CHARGED PARTICLES

Heavy particles (e.g., neutrons), charged particles (e.g., protons) and heavy charged particles (e.g., neon, carbon) are alternative forms of external beam irradiation. The theoretical advantage of neutron irradiation relates to its relative lack of dependence on the presence of oxygen, and its relative resistance to the repair of sublethal radiation-induced damage. In a prospective randomized trial reported by Russell and coworkers, fast neutrons were associated with a lower clinical local failure rate and a lower incidence of PSA failures compared to x-ray therapy.[390] An earlier trial (RTOG 7704) suggested an improvement in survival. The results of this trial were questioned, however, because the patients on the photon-only arm had larger tumors, and a worse survival than expected based on other contemporary series of the time (e.g., Patterns of Care data and data from Stanford) for comparable-stage disease.

The major theoretical advantage to the use of protons and other charged particles is the dose distribution associated with this type of radiation. The only randomized trial completed to date demonstrated that there was an increase in local control only in the subset of patients with high-grade tumors.[391] Perhaps earlier-stage patients would have benefited from the use of this technology, but at present, there is no evidence that proton-based radiotherapy, even when delivered to higher doses, is superior to conventional radiotherapy. Heavy charged particles are thought to have the advantages of both neutrons and protons. Early studies using this technology have been very limited. Longer follow-up will be required to assess the impact of these alternative types of irradiation on survival.

COMPLICATIONS

Complications Associated with External Beam Radiation Therapy

TYPICAL CLINICAL COURSE DURING TREATMENT

During the delivery of radiation most patients note some dysuria, and many experience mild diarrhea. Dysuria is generally mild and often responds to nonsteroidal anti-inflammatory drugs. Patients who complain of moderate to severe discomfort, frequency, urgency with or without incontinence, or gross hematuria should be sent for a urine analysis as well as culture and sensitivity, in order to detect the occasional patient with a urinary tract infection. Patients who are documented to have a bacterial infection frequently are at risk for a recurrent infection during the course of treatment and need to be monitored more closely. Severe urinary symptoms may suggest a fungal urinary tract infection or an error in delivered dose.

Patients receiving whole-pelvic irradiation are more likely to require medication for diarrhea than patients being treated only to the prostate. Rectal bleeding ("just a few spots") occurs in up to 10% of patients during the course of treatment and may not correlate with a late risk of bleeding. When they have completed and recovered from their course of treatment, a workup for an occult gastrointestinal primary may be indicated. At least three patients in the past 4 years have been diagnosed with colon cancer at UCSF within a few years after completing a course of radiation. Patients who experience tenesmus during treatment should have all of their films, CT scans, and treatment plans carefully re-evaluated. For patients receiving irradiation to the prostate with or without the seminal vesicles, tenesmus during treatment may imply that the patient has an unusually mobile prostate such that the isocenter may now be in the anterior rectal wall, instead of being in the posterior portion of the gland.

CLINICIAN-REPORTED COMPLICATIONS

Most of the published literature on complications related to radiotherapy is based on clinician-reported toxicity. Unfortunately, such data are likely to underestimate the incidence and severity of complications experienced by patients. Despite these limitations, it is instructive to summarize the incidence of moderate to severe complications from patients treated on prospective randomized trials

and large multi-institutional databases. For example, Shipley et al. reviewed long-term treatment-related sequelae in 2611 men.[392] Based on such data, treatment-related mortality, severe complications, and incontinence rates are 0.2%, 1.9%, and 0.9%, respectively, while the incidence of genitourinary strictures, hematuria, and rectal bleeding is 5.4%, 5.1%, and 5.4%, respectively. With a minimum follow-up of 7 years, grade 3 or 4 (moderate to severe) urinary complications occurred in 7.7% of patients. The range of time to develop grade 4 complications was 3.4 to 18.3 months with a median of 14.1 months. Only 3.3% of patients experienced grade 3 to 5 intestinal toxicity. The median time to developing grade 4 or 5 toxicity was 17.9 months (range, 2 to 52 months). Although there was a higher risk of grade 3 urinary complications in patients who received greater than 70 Gy, this was not true of grade 4 or 5 urinary complications, nor was it true for grades 3, 4, or 5 gastrointestinal complications. Urinary or fecal incontinence, or both, are uncommon following radiotherapy and are usually related to prior TURPs. Rectal bleeding is not infrequent (occurring in ≈10% of patients) following external beam irradiation, but it is usually mild, self-limited, and dose and volume related. Reduction in the volume of the ejaculate is noted in most patients who receive definitive radiotherapy even if potency is preserved.

Complications Following Conformal and Intensity-Modulated Radiotherapy

Retrospective studies from a number of institutions suggest that acute toxicity is reduced with the use of conformal radiation therapy compared with conventional therapy. The earliest prospective trials used relatively crude techniques but provide useful insights into dose response and morbidity from radiotherapy.[393,394] Investigators from the United Kingdom treated patients to the same dose, 64.8 Gy, and observed that lower toxicity was seen in the patients treated with a 3D technique that would be considered crude by today's standards.[393] However, the side-effect profile of both groups appeared higher than usually reported in the United States, making it more difficult to interpret their results. In a trial conducted at MD Anderson Hospital, initially there also appeared to be a reduction in toxicity despite using higher doses, 78 versus 70 Gy.[394] Unfortunately, with longer follow-up it has become clear that when using relatively crude techniques only during the boost, the late effects were actually higher in the 78 Gy 3D arm.[395] The rectal side effects were significantly greater in the 78 Gy group with grade 2 or higher rectal toxicity rates at 6 years of 26% compared to 12% for the 70 Gy group ($P = 0.001$) (Fig. 45-33). Further study is warranted before the limits of normal tissues and the question of the optimal dose and technique are defined.

When 3DCRT is used to deliver higher doses of radiation than are typically used with "conventional" non–3D-based techniques, the risk of late complications may be increased if the 3D radiotherapy technique is not sophisticated enough to compensate for the additional dose.[213,395,396] Using more sophisticated techniques, late

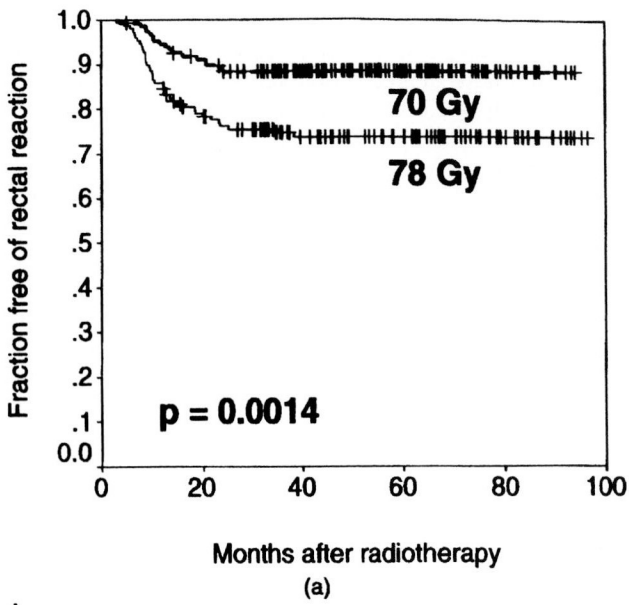

(a)

A

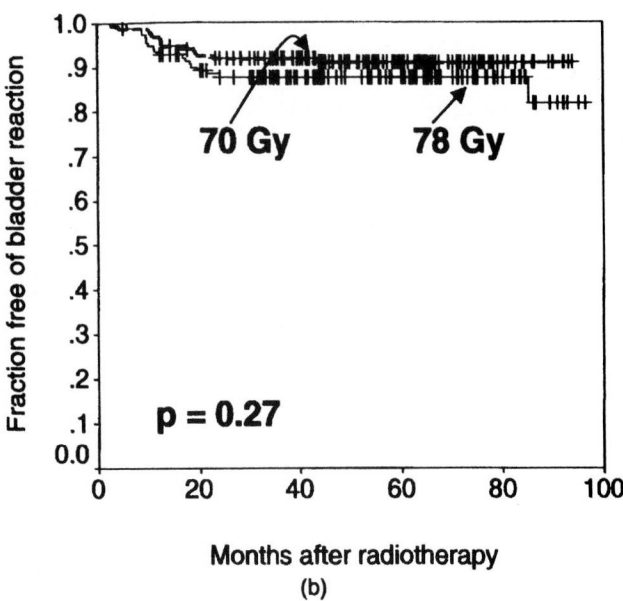

(b)

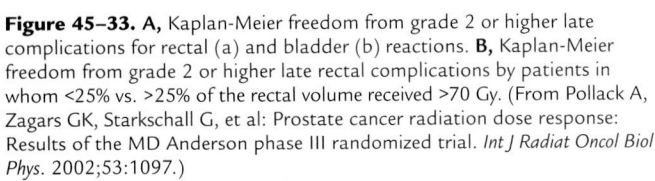

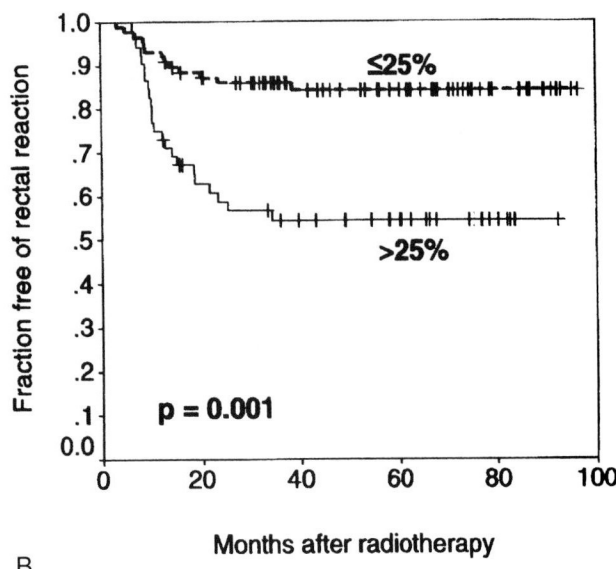

B

Figure 45–33. A, Kaplan-Meier freedom from grade 2 or higher late complications for rectal (a) and bladder (b) reactions. **B,** Kaplan-Meier freedom from grade 2 or higher late rectal complications by patients in whom <25% vs. >25% of the rectal volume received >70 Gy. (From Pollack A, Zagars GK, Starkschall G, et al: Prostate cancer radiation dose response: Results of the MD Anderson phase III randomized trial. *Int J Radiat Oncol Biol Phys.* 2002;53:1097.)

complications appear to be reduced despite the higher doses in patients managed in a multi-institutional setting.[100,101,213,397]

More than 1000 patients have been treated to doses exceeding 73.8 Gy using F-SMLC at UCSF and the complication rates have been low. An analysis of a subset of these patients who received doses in excess of 82 Gy to portions of the prostate has been reported.[398] With a median follow-up of 23 months and a median Dmax 84.5 Gy (range: 82.0 to 96.7 Gy), the 2-year actuarial rates for freedom from late grade 2 gastrointestinal and genitourinary morbidity are 76.5% (95% CI: 59.5% to 87.1%) and 81.3% (95% CI: 64.4% to 90.7%), respectively. At the time of analysis, no grade 3 or greater late genitourinary morbidity has been observed; however, three patients experienced grade 3 gastrointestinal late morbidity. The authors concluded that doses greater than or equal to 82 Gy can be delivered by external beam

radiotherapy to at least a portion of the prostate gland and are tolerated with acceptable morbidity. However, to lower morbidity further, great effort must be made to compensate for day-to-day setup variation and organ movement (see earlier discussion in Challenges of Day-to-Day Setup Variation and Organ Movement).

Investigators at MSKCC were among the first to demonstrate that moving from 3DCRT to IMRT resulted in a reduction in morbidity.[206,215] Zelefsky et al. reported the acute and late toxicity in 772 patients treated for clinically localized prostate cancer with high-dose IMRT between April 1996 and January 2001. Ninety percent of their patients were treated to 81.0 Gy, and 10% to 86.4 Gy. With a median follow-up time of 24 months, 4.5% developed acute grade 2 rectal toxicity, and 0% greater than acute grade 3 toxicity. Late grades 2, 3, and 4 rectal toxicity occurred in 1.5%, 0.1%, and 0%, respectively. While the 3-year actuarial likelihood of greater than or equal to late grade 2 rectal toxicity was 4%, late grade 2 urinary toxicity was 15%. These researchers concluded that it was feasible to use high-dose IMRT to treat a large number of patients and toxicities seem to be significantly reduced compared to standard 3DCRT techniques. Based on these preliminary data, IMRT has become the standard therapy for localized prostate cancer at a number of institutions. The critical questions that remain to be determined are what dose should be used for which patients and does this dose require IMRT or is 3DCRT sufficient?

MORBIDITY AFTER PERMANENT IMPLANTS

Despite the assumption by many clinicians and prospective patients that highly localized brachytherapy will result in lesser treatment-related morbidity, brachytherapy typically causes more marked urinary symptoms, at least in the first 6 to 12 postimplant months. Fortunately, nearly all implant-related symptoms resolve spontaneously. Most patients return to their baseline AUA scores within 1 year.[284,292,367] Prophylactic institution of alpha-blockers substantially decreases the intensity and time-to-resolution of radiation-related symptoms. Although spontaneous resolution of radiation prostatitis is the norm, there is some chance of more serious complications, including superficial urethral necrosis and incontinence. Superficial urethral necrosis (SUN), associated with severe dysuria and urinary incontinence, occurred in up to 4% of patients treated by Blasko and colleagues in the late 1980s.[297] It is currently an uncommon complication, likely due to adoption of peripheral seed loading patterns that avoid excessive urethral doses and the avoidance of TURPs.[299]

Reports regarding the incidence of postimplant urinary incontinence are mixed, with rates dependent on the measurement instrument, follow-up instrument, and implant technique. There is no obvious difference in incontinence risk for patients treated with implant alone versus those treated with implant and supplemental external beam radiation.[347] The homogeneous source loading pattern that led to an increased incidence of SUN in some early patients likewise resulted in an increased risk of long-term incontinence. With longer follow-up of the early NWTI patients, a relatively high rate of incontinence was seen even in patients without a prior TURP.[399] More recent experience, using modified peripheral loading (that has been standard since 1995) has been that urinary incontinence is unusual.[273] Urethral stricture is an uncommon complication of modern brachytherapy, probably related to excessive apical radiation doses.[271] When stricture does occur, it typically is successfully managed with one or more urethral dilations.

Proctitis

Some degree of postimplant radiation proctitis is almost inevitable, given the proximity of the prostate to the rectum. Symptoms usually resolve within a few months. Rectal function typically returns to the preimplant level by 1 to 2 years.[400] Rectal bleeding occurs in 2% to 10% of patients, and nearly always manifests between 6 and 18 months of implantation.[400-402] It is partly related to rectal wall doses, and is more common in patients with lesser amounts of peri-rectal fat.[402,403] Endoscopy typically reveals a circumscribed area of intense erythema, telangiectasia, and friability on the anterior rectal wall, overlying the prostate.[404] Rectal ulceration, occurring in less than 1% of patients, is a more ominous complication that may lead to temporary or permanent colostomy.[405-407] Surprisingly, fistulas appear not to be secondary to excessive rectal doses but might be explained by a predisposition of some patients to rectal complications, perhaps due to inherent radiation sensitivity or some other disease process.[406,408] Reports regarding the effects of supplemental external beam radiation on rectal morbidity are mixed.[347,409,410]

Most patients who develop bleeding after external beam radiation or brachytherapy do not progress to rectal ulceration or fistula. Given enough time, most will heal spontaneously.[405,411,412] However, healing is typically slow, sometimes requiring years. In contrast to medical therapies, more invasive therapies with electrocoagulation, laser, argon plasma coagulation (APC), or topical formalin have been highly effective therapy for bleeding from radiation proctitis.[404] Invasive therapies, however, might exacerbate radiation damage, so they should be undertaken with caution. Patients who undergo rectal wall biopsy in the course of evaluation for implant-related proctitis may be at higher risk of fistula formation.[407] It appears that spontaneous healing of fistulas is unlikely, even with a diverting colostomy. Data regarding their surgical repair are limited, and an optimal management policy has not been determined.[413]

Quality of Life Methodology

Partly in reaction to past inconsistencies in morbidity reports, there is a growing effort to quantify morbidities with far more detailed survey instruments, attempting to make lifestyle effects more uniformly reported. While admirable in their intent, such efforts have culminated in scores like *urinary bother, functional well-being,* or *EPIC scores,* indices so nebulous that they are almost meaningless to patients and clinicians.[414-417] While more standardized approaches to quality of life measures are warranted, some degree of common sense seems to be in order. Making matters worse, brachytherapy-related sexual symptoms, especially, are different in nature to those of prostatectomy or even beam radiation, and are not accurately portrayed in generic quality of life scales.[418,419]

COMPLICATIONS AFTER HDR

The incidence of grade 3 complications noted after HDR includes 1% urethral necrosis and urethral strictures in approximately 5% of patients. Incontinence, particularly in association with TURPs, has been reported in up to 5% of patients. Grade 3 proctitis has been reported to occur in approximately 2%. The incidence of posttreatment impotence has not been studied as extensively as other forms of radiotherapy but is generally thought to be slightly worse as a result of high-dose-per-fraction effects on nerves and blood supply. Overall, approximately 80% of the patients from these various series appear to be disease free at 5 years. Positive biopsy rates ranged from 4% to 18%. The RTOG is launching a phase I to II trial to determine whether the encouraging results reported by a relatively small number of institutions can be reproduced in a multi-institutional setting.

Complications with Protons and Neutrons

Benk and coworkers, using protons to boost the prostate to higher than usual doses, reported rectal bleeding in more than 70% of men at 4 years if 40% or more of the anterior rectal wall received greater than or equal to 75 Gy.[420] The median time to the onset of rectal bleeding in their series exceeded 2 years. Complications following neutron and heavy charged particle–based radiotherapy generally have been more severe than with protons.[226] These alternative forms of radiotherapy remain to be proven as superior to forms of external beam radiotherapy to justify the cost associated with each. Comparisons between conventional 3DCRT (and IMRT) and protons or neutrons have been made, but the inherent biases in the comparisons make it difficult to reach conclusions about which we can have great confidence.[421]

Impotence Following Radiotherapy

Loss of potency is the most common, permanent morbidity resulting from radiation therapy. Even when potency is maintained, the frequency and quality of intercourse and the volume of the ejaculate tends to be reduced. A definition used frequently to define the potent state is "the ability to maintain an erection, sufficient for intercourse." Unfortunately, this definition leaves considerable room for interpretation on the part of the patient and the investigator. Analysis of the effect of treatment on potency is also clouded by the fact that prostate cancer patients are frequently in an older age group, for whom there is an approximately 50% incidence of impotency before treatment, and for whom there is some natural loss of potency with time.

One common suggestion regarding the analysis of potency rates is that the spouses should be interviewed, the implication being that patients are not realistic or honest in reporting their erectile capacity. However, the limited data available suggest that patients and spouses report similar function. Physiologic monitoring before and after treatment would be ideal, but from a practical standpoint, it would be difficult to arrange and pay for physiologic testing for the large number of patients involved.

One of the earliest series reporting the effect of EBRT on potency is from Stanford.[422] Based on questionnaires mailed to patients, short-term potency appears to be preserved in approximately 85% of patients at 15 to 21 months after treatment.[423,424] While rarely mentioned in the literature, the increased loss of potency with time probably represents a combination of natural loss with aging and long-term, radiation-induced normal tissue changes. Banker reported on potency in 83 patients,

approximately 12 months following external beam radiation therapy.[425] Potency was maintained in 73% of patients who were potent and sexually active before treatment, but in only 40% of patients who were potent but not sexually active. Partial loss of potency in most patients might be expected; microvascular and neurologic compromise following external beam radiation therapy is probably a continuum rather than an all-or-nothing effect. The high likelihood of at least partial loss of erectile function should be expected and conveyed to patients before treatment.

Robinson et al. recently published a meta-analysis comparing the rates of erectile function after EBRT, radical prostatectomy (RP) (with or without nerve sparing), brachytherapy with or without EBRT, and cryotherapy.[195] Rates of potency were 76%, 60%, 55%, 34%, 25%, and 13% for brachytherapy alone, brachytherapy + EBRT, EBRT alone, nerve-sparing RP, non–nerve-sparing RP, and cryosurgery, respectively. Of note, contrary to the commonly held beliefs when analyzing only studies reporting greater than or equal to 2 years' follow-up, the only significant change was a decline in the probability of maintaining potency following nerve-sparing radical prostatectomy. Also of note when the probabilities were adjusted for age, potency advantage favoring EBRT over surgery was even greater.[195] In contrast to the findings of this meta-analysis, Litwin et al. reported that potency declined more with radiation over time than with surgery.[426] Whether the different inclusions between these studies reflect different patient populations, selection bias, or other unidentified factors, the fact is that most men have declining sexual function over time. The apparent lower impotence rate following ^{125}I implants must be viewed cautiously because patients treated with implants tend to have smaller tumors and, thus, smaller volumes may be treated.[195] More importantly, because it is commonly believed (although not proved) that ^{125}I implants result in less impotence, there may be self-selection for more potent and sexually active patients to pursue getting an implant.

Based initially on animal work, an evolving body of evidence suggests a relationship between the dose to the bulb of the penis and radiation-induced impotence.[427-431] It is unclear whether the bulb itself is the dose-limiting structure. It may well be that neurovascular structures immediately adjacent to the bulb are the true dose-limiting source of morbidity. However, because the bulb of the penis is a midline structure immediately below the prostate, the dose to the bulb is likely to be a good surrogate for doses to structures lateral to and below the prostate. The importance of this observation lies in the fact that the results historically associated with EBRT and brachytherapy could be significantly improved without compromising cure or cost! In addition, the response rate to sildenafil, already reported to be as high as 75%, might actually be higher if adjacent structures were spared.[432,433]

SEXUAL DYSFUNCTION AFTER BRACHYTHERAPY

Despite some early claims, brachytherapy, like surgery and beam radiation, carries a high risk of long-term sexual dysfunction. While most discussion of treatment-related sexual dysfunction has focused on impotence, various sexual dysfunctions follow brachytherapy that are not even mentioned in popular quality of life scales. Patients commonly experience burning with orgasm (orgalmasia) in their first 6 to 12 post-implant months.[418,434] Bloody ejaculate is very common in the first several weeks after implantation, and patients commonly report a diminished amount of ejaculate fluid. Intermittent hematospermia may occur for years after implantation.[418] Approximately 10% of patients develop impotence immediately after their implant procedure, presumably due to needle trauma to the neurovascular bundles or venous bodies.[418] Patients with acute postimplant impotence may spontaneously improve over time.

As with EBRT, there is increasing evidence that potency loss may be ameliorated with greater care to limit doses to the proximal penis. Merrick and colleagues found no relationship between neurovascular bundle doses and impotence among patients followed up to 4 years postimplant, consistent with growing evidence that neurovascular bundle doses are not as crucial to potency as alleged by investigators at Johns Hopkins University Hospitals.[435] In contrast, radiation-induced impotence may be related to venous insufficiency from damage to the proximal corpus spongiosum, or bulb, of the penis.[431,436] Separated from the prostate by the striated urethral sphincter, the bulb typically lies 1.5 cm below the prostatic apex and is fairly well visualized on CT, TRUS, or MRI (Fig. 45-34).[437] The bulb typically receives a maximal radiation dose of about 50% of the brachytherapy prescription dose. Because of the proximity of the bulb to the prostatic apex, excessive radiation dosage has been fairly common. Increased effort to limit proximal penile doses in the planning and implementation processes would likely result in a lower likelihood of implant-related impotence.

Response rates to sildenafil appear to be partially dependent on the prior use of hormonal therapy and the degree of potency.[432,438] For example, Weber et al. noted that only 15% of patients failed to respond without hormonal therapy compared to 50% receiving it. What is not commonly appreciated is that the time course of response was gradual, with responses increasing from 40% at week 1 to 74% by week 5. Patients with partial erections following radiotherapy may have responses as high as 90%.[433,439] Response rates to sildenafil following brachytherapy appear to be similar to slightly lower than those associated with EBRT. Potter et al. reported their experience with 482 men who were potent before undergoing brachytherapy for clinically localized prostate cancer.[438] With a median follow-up of 34 months and a median age of 68 years, the 5-year actuarial potency rate was 76%, 56%, and 52% for brachytherapy alone, in combination EBRT and brachytherapy, with neoadjuvant androgen deprivation, respectively. However, only 29% of patients treated with brachytherapy, EBRT, and neoadjuvant androgen deprivation maintained potency. They reported that 62% (52/84) of patients treated with sildenafil responded successfully, with a higher percentage responding if not treated with neoadjuvant androgen deprivation (P = 0.04). The slightly lower responses to sildenafil in brachytherapy patients could be due to patient selection bias. *If* brachytherapy is potentially more potency sparing, sexual dysfunction after brachytherapy could reflect poorer baseline function or a high bulb dose compromising the response potential to drug therapy.

Complications of Hormonal Therapy

Following the favorable results of several phase III prospective randomized trials demonstrating improved survival with the use of hormonal therapy and EBRT for subsets of patients with locally advanced prostate cancer, this practice became widespread in the mid-1990s. As increasing numbers of patients receive neoadjuvant

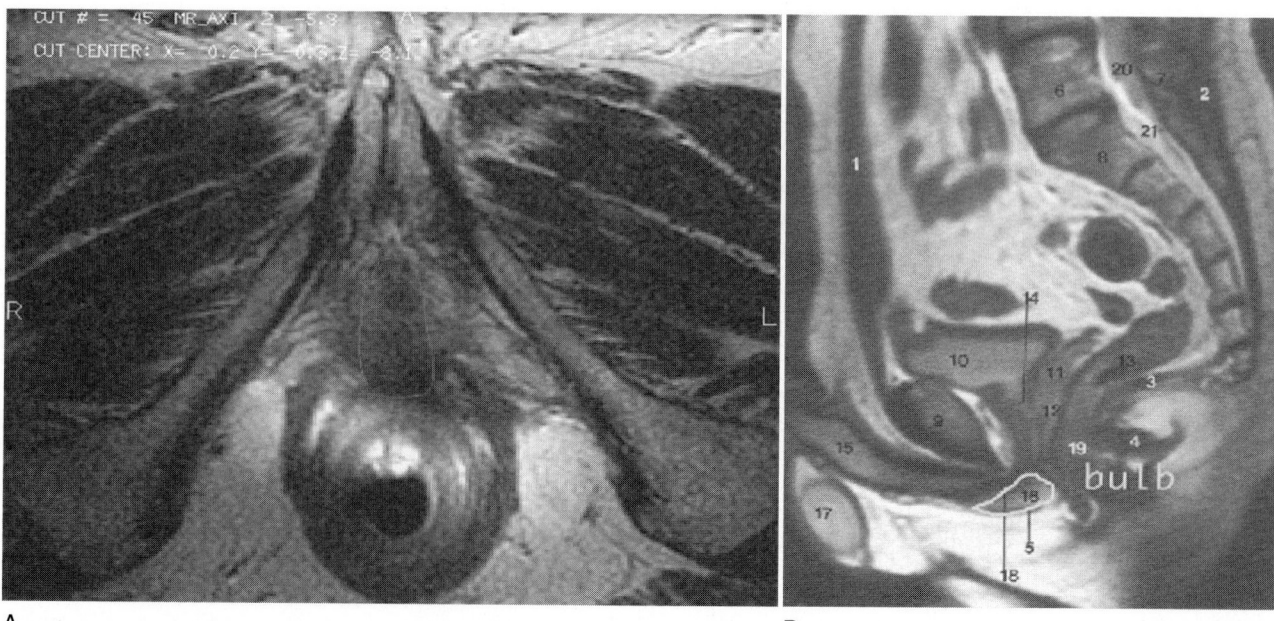

A   B

Figure 45–34. A, Axial view of bulb of penis circled in red and **B,** sagittal view. (*B* from Hricak H, Carrington BM: MRI of the Pelvis: A Text Atlas. Norwalk CT: Appleton & Lange, 1991.)

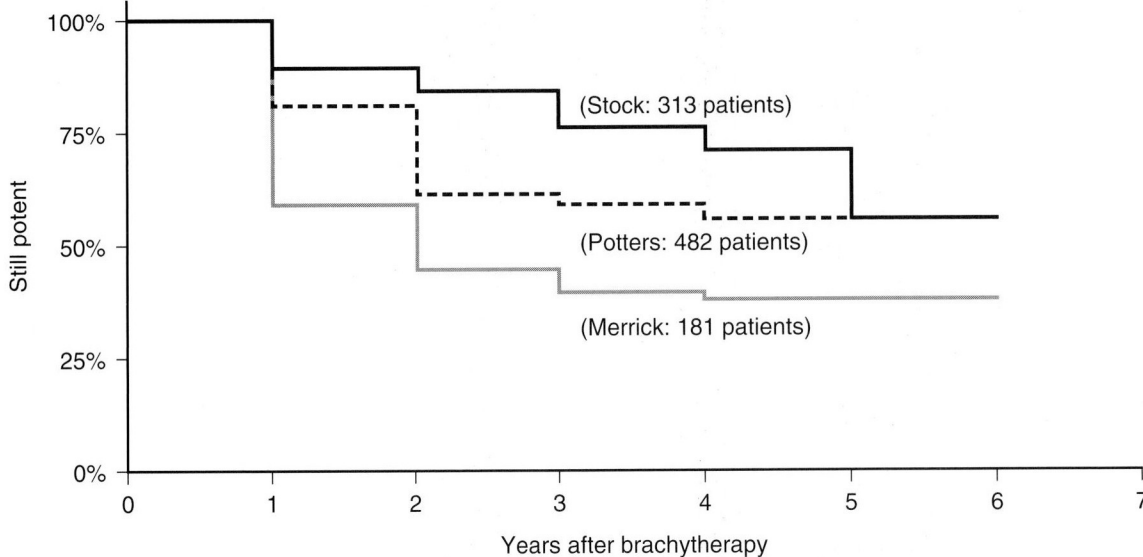

Figure 45–35. Potency following brachytherapy-based treatment. Differences between series may result from differing use of adjuvant hormone therapy, supplemental beam radiation, and data collection. The lowest potency rates, reported by Merrick, were in the only series to use a validated patient-reported questionnaire. (From Merrick GS, Wallner KE, Butler WM: Management of sexual dysfunction after prostate brachytherapy. Oncology (Huntingt.) 2003;1:52-62.)

hormonal therapy as a component of their treatment course, knowledge of management of drug-related toxicity has become important. Most commonly, leuprolide, 7.5 mg or goserelin acetate, 3.6 mg (both luteinizing hormone-releasing hormone [440] agonists) are administered monthly instead of surgical castration (orchiectomy) or diethylstilbestrol to block testicular production of testosterone. For CAB, anti-androgens such as flutamide or bicalutamide are frequently added to prevent the so-called *flare phenomena* and to block androgens arising from the adrenal glands. This "flare" is due to a surge in serum testosterone that is known to occur within a week or two after administration of an LHRH. The clinical manifestations of the "flare" are thought to be blocked by the use of anti-androgens. The most common complaint voiced by patients receiving CAB are "hot flashes." Although these are generally mild, occasionally patients find this side effect intolerable. For such patients, megestrol, 20 mg orally twice daily is effective.[441] Impotence is common following hormonal ablation. Because as many as half the patients undergoing radiation therapy are impotent before treatment, it is not as common a complaint during treatment (perhaps due to the reduced libido). Liver dysfunction due to the anti-androgen, although uncommon and reversible, can be life threatening. It is prudent to consider obtaining liver function tests (LFTs) at 2- to 4-week intervals during the first 6 weeks of CAB. It is common for the LFTs to rise slightly above the normal limits within a few weeks of initiating hormonal therapy. Usually, despite continued therapy, these chemical abnormalities plateau or decline without sequelae. However, if the LFTs rise to reach two to four times normal, the anti-androgen should be discontinued, but the LH-RH agonist can usually be continued.

The use of CAB is also associated with anemia, particularly when combined with irradiation. Although CAB-induced anemia is also a reversible phenomenon, it may take up to a year or more for the patient to return to his baseline hematocrit. Osteoporosis, which is its related sequelae, is a potential complication of surgical or medical castration.[442-446] Vitamin D with calcium at 800 international units each should generally be administered to patients on long-term therapy. Bisphosphates can prevent or reverse this problem and can reduce the risk of skeletal-related events.[444]

SELECTED OUTCOMES

Surgery: Selected Outcomes without and with Postoperative Radiation Therapy

Table 45-9 summarizes the characteristics of patients and outcomes from selected surgical series at several major institutions. Based on a review of the major surgical series completed and published as of 1994, approximately 75% (56% to 91%) and 50% (40% to 65%) of patients with stage T1 to T2 disease were free from failure at 5 and at 10 years, respectively.[447] Nearly 75% of the patients treated with surgery had GS's of less than or equal to 6, and roughly two thirds of patients (56% to 78%) making up these series had PSAs less than 10 ng/mL. Outcomes are significantly more unfavorable in patients with higher GS's. For example, 75% of patients undergoing prostatectomy with a GS of 8 to 10 had recurrence rates at 4 years in the major surgical series published in the mid-1990s.[448-450] Even when patients with pathologically confined disease were considered, patients with GS's of 7 had a recurrence rate of 40% and those with scores of 8 to 10 had failure rates exceeding 50% within 5 years.[451]

A more contemporary assessment of results associated with radical prostatectomy can be found in a number of recent reports. One large study based on a pooled analysis of 6754 patients validated the use of the Kattan

Table 45–9 Patient Characteristics from Selected Surgical and Radiation Therapy Series

Prognostic Factor	Surgical Average, % (range)*	Radiation Therapy Average, % (range)†	Major Differences	Comments
0–4	26 (15–43)	21 (11–33)	PSV <10 ng/mL	Patients treated by surgery tend to have lower grade
4.1–10.0	41 (35–52)	30 (27–32)	56–78%	(Gleason score ≥7 ≈27% vs 42%) and lower
10.1–20.0	26 (16–32)	21 (18–22)	vs.	T-stage tumors than patients included in radiation
10–30	—	29	27–64%	therapy series (≈1/3 T3) and node-positive
>20	13 (6–20)	35 (18–50)		patients are frequently excluded.
>30	—	7		
2–4	22 (10–16)	30 (23–42)‡	GS ≥7	Larger percentages of surgical patients have lower
5	25	NA	21–29%	PSAs (<10 ng/mL average 67% vs 51%) and
6	36 (28–44)	20 (15–25)	vs	lower T-stages than radiation therapy series (≈1/3
7	17 (14–20)	22 (15–32)	21–55%	T3) and node-positive patients are frequently
8–10	10 (7–13)	20 (6–37)		excluded.
T1a–T2a	53 (35–67)	36 (20–61)	T2c	Larger percentages of surgical patients have lower
T2b–T2c	47 (33–65)	39 (33–39)	0–6% vs 9% +	PSAs (<10 ng/mL, average 67% vs 51%) and
T3/4	≈0	25–48	and	lower tumor grades (Gleason score ≥7 ≈27% vs
N+	≈0	0–?	T3	42%) and node-positive patients are frequently
			≈0%vs to 52%	excluded.

*Most surgical series exclude node-positive patients and PSA failures >0.2–0.6 ng/mL.
†Clinical staging includes node-positive T3/4 patients and PSA failures >1.0–4.0 ng/mL or rising.
‡With the exception of MD Anderson, other institutions have very few patients with Gleason scores of 2 to 4.
NA, Not available; PSA, prostate-specific antigen.

nomogram for predicting the risk of recurrences after radical prostatectomy (Fig. 45-36A–B).[452] The results of the published surgical series have been somewhat of "a moving target" with the results of more contemporary series being somewhat more favorable with 85% and 75% disease free at 5 and 10 years, respectively.[176,452] The recent results of patients with high-grade disease also seem to be improving whether treated with surgery or radiotherapy, with the latter apparently dependent on the dose of radiation used.[39,453,454] The improvement in the surgical results is probably due to the improved patient selection and the addition of postoperative radiotherapy.[455] Given the apparent impact of treatment era on outcome, it is very important not to mix comparisons of results for patients treated with radiotherapy and surgery from different treatment periods.

Among patients with capsular penetration (up to 50% of all patients undergoing surgery), the local failure rate has been estimated to be from 25% to 68%.[456] The high incidence of positive surgical margins and frequency of occult residual disease (as evidenced by late local failures) suggest that postoperative radiation therapy may be underused in the treatment of prostate cancer. External beam irradiation appears to reduce the local recurrences after radical prostatectomy (Fig. 45-37).[457-460] Patients who are treated before demonstrating a local recurrence appear to have an improvement in disease-free survival as well as the time to distant metastasis. The vast majority of patients experience a marked reduction in their PSA levels when irradiated postoperatively. Patients who never obtain an undetectable PSA postoperatively or who develop a detectable PSA within the first 6 months are somewhat more likely to have occult metastases than those who demonstrate a rising PSA later.

Although the impact of postoperative irradiation on survival remains unproved, it seems reasonable to assume that patients whose only remaining disease consists of microscopic residual disease may benefit from treatment. A number of factors have been shown to predict the likelihood of salvage, with the most important being the preop PSA, preradiation PSA, and postrecurrence PSA doubling time.[460] The patients with a local recurrence who are most likely to benefit from radiation therapy are those with a PSA of less than 1 ng/mL.[461] Even if biopsies are negative, if pathologic features place a patient at a high risk for local recurrence or the pattern of PSA rise is consistent with a local recurrence, postoperative radiation therapy should be considered. This aggressive posture is based on the fact that it is not uncommon for multiple sets of biopsies to be negative before a positive biopsy is obtained, and the lower the PSA, the better the chances are for control. Patients with a documented local recurrence who have a PSA greater than 1 ng/mL should be considered for neoadjuvant total androgen ablation before high-dose irradiation because of their relatively unfavorable outcome with conventional radiation therapy alone.[461,462]

RADIATION THERAPY: SELECTED OUTCOMES

Conventional External Beam Irradiation: PSA Failure and Survival

Published results from selected series following conventional external beam irradiation and radical prostatectomy through 1994 are shown in Tables 45-9 and 45-10. The survival results at 10 to 15 years appear to be similar for patients treated with surgery or irradiation who are comparably staged despite the fact that men who undergo surgery are usually younger and healthier than age-matched

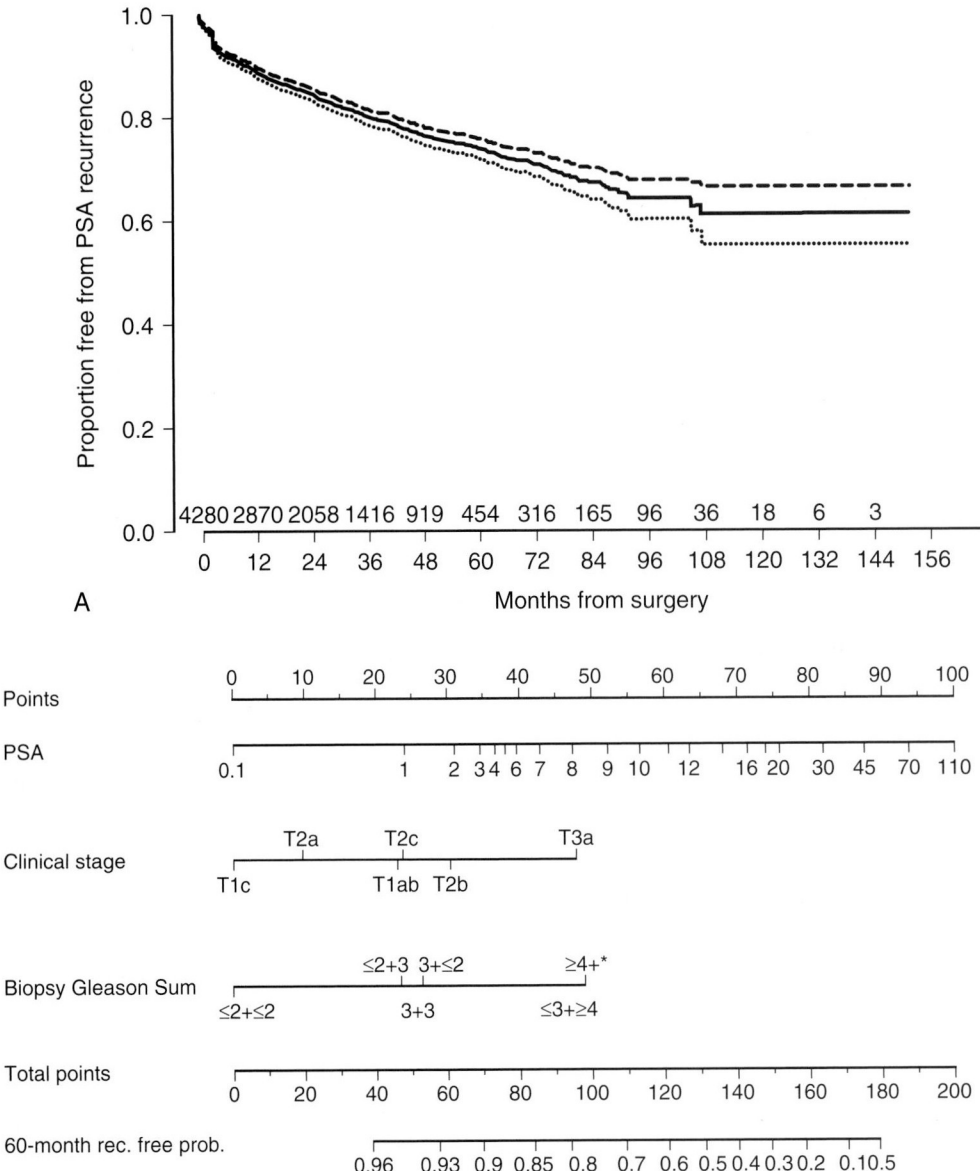

A

Points

PSA

Clinical stage

Biopsy Gleason Sum

Total points

60-month rec. free prob.

Instructions for physician: Locate the patient's PSA on the **PSA** axis. Draw a line straight upwards to the **Points** axis to determine how many points towards recurrence the patient receives for his PSA. Repeat this process for the **Clinical Stage** and **Biopsy Gleason Sum** axes, each time drawing straight upward to the **Points** axis. Sum the points achieved for each predictor and locate this sum on the **Total Points** axis. Draw a line straight down to find the patient's probability of remaining recurrence free for 60 months assuming he does not die of another cause first.

Note: This nomogram is not applicable to a man who is not otherwise a candidate for radical prostatectomy. You can use this only on a man who has already selected radical prostatectomy as treatment for his prostate cancer.

Instruction to patient: "Mr. X, if we had 100 men exactly like you, we would expect between <predicted percentage from nomogram – 10%> and <predicted percentage + 10%> to remain free of their disease at 5 years following radical prostatectomy, and recurrence after 5 years is very rare."

B

Figure 45–36. A, Freedom from recurrence in 4280 patients; patients had both primary and secondary Gleason grades assigned, did not receive neoadjuvant hormones, and did not have an aggressive adjuvant radiation therapy policy (*dotted lines,* 95% confidence bounds; *numbers above months,* patients at risk). (From Graefen M, Karakiewicz PI, Cagiannos I, et al: International validation of a preoperative nomogram for prostate cancer recurrence after radical prostatectomy. *J Clin Oncol.* 2002;20:3206.) **B,** Preoperative nomogram based on 983 patients treated at Baylor College of Medicine, Houston, Texas, for predicting freedom from recurrence after radical prostatectomy. (Adapted from Kattan, et al.)

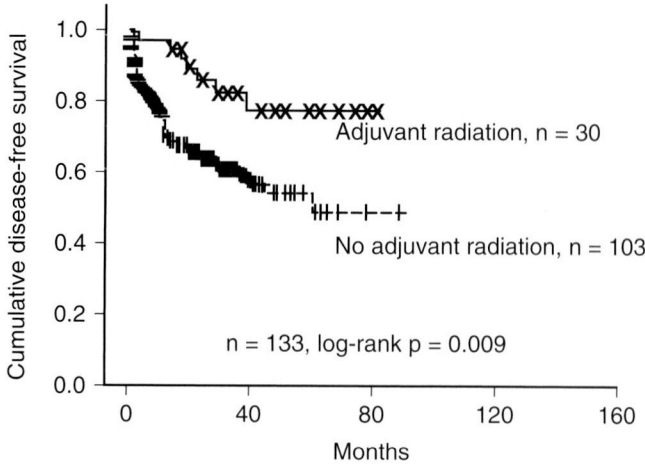

Figure 45–37. Demonstrates benefits of adjuvant radiotherapy on risk of recurrences in patients with multiple positive margins. (From Quinn DI, Henshall SM, Haynes AM, et al: Prognostic significance of pathologic features in localized prostate cancer treated with radical prostatectomy: Implications for staging systems and predictive models. *J Clin Oncol.* 2001;19:3692.)

controls.[174,202] A comparison of the pretreatment characteristics of patients from major series treated surgically with those treated with radiation therapy is summarized in Table 45-9. Note that patients included in surgical series tend to have lower PSAs, fewer patients have tumors with GS's greater than or equal to 7, and a larger percentage of patients have lower clinical stages (<T2c). Furthermore, many surgical series exclude node-positive patients, while few radiation therapy series do. Considering these obvious differences, there is still considerable overlap in freedom from PSA failure at 5 to 10 years, suggesting similar efficacy for surgery and radiation therapy (Table 45-10). The slightly better outcome

among some of the surgical subgroups shown in this table can be explained by the fact that all three factors (PSA, GS, and stage) favor surgical series. Thus, when matched for any one of the factors, the other two factors still favor surgical series over radiation therapy series. As discussed earlier, given the apparent impact of era of treatment on outcome, it is also very important not to mix comparisons of patients treated with radiotherapy and surgery from different eras.

Shipley conducted a large multi-institutional assessment of the results of EBRT alone for patients with T1 to T2 disease.[463] This retrospective, nonrandomized pooled analysis included a total of 1765 patients. A minimum of 2 years' subsequent follow-up was required for participation. The patients were treated between 1988 and 1995 at six U.S. medical centers. Of note, 24% had initial PSA values of 20 ng/mL or higher. The 5-year estimates of overall survival, disease-specific survival, and the freedom from biochemical failure are 85%, 95%, and 65.8%, respectively. The PSA failure-free rates 5 and 7 years after treatment for patients presenting with a PSA of less than 10 ng/mL were 78% and 73%, respectively.[463] Of the 302 patients followed up beyond 5 years who were free of biochemical disease, only 5% relapsed from the fifth to the eighth year, suggesting that the results with radiotherapy are durable. The notion that radiotherapy is associated with a relatively low risk of late failures is supported by the long-term results reported by other series as well.[58,149,464]

Estimated PSA control rates in this pooled analysis are similar to those of single institutions. These results based on patients treated at multiple different institutions are considered by many to represent a benchmark for evidence-based counseling of prostate cancer patients when they are treated with radiotherapy alone. Several large single institution comparisons have found that the

Table 45–10 Summary of PSA Results for Selected Surgical and Radiation Therapy Series

Prognostic Factor	Surgical Series PSA NED, %* (5/10 yr)	RT Series PSA NED, %† (5/10 yr)	Comments
0–4	85–95/	80–86/	Patients treated by surgery tend to have lower grade (Gleason score ≥7 ≈27% vs. 42%) and lower T-stage tumors than patients included in radiation therapy series (≈1/3 T3) and node-positive patients are frequently excluded.
4.1–10.0	55–93/	42–67/	
10.1–20.0	56–/	30–75/	
10–30	—	45/	
2–4	<75–98/82	68–75/	Surgical patients have lower PSAs (<10 ng/mL, average 67% vs. 51%) and lower T-stages than radiation therapy series (≈1/3 T3) and node-positive patients are frequently excluded.
5–6	85–92/53–88‡	60/	
7	62/50	63§/	
8–10	<20–46/15§	10¶–33/9	
T1a	74–100/100	—	In addition to differences in T-stage a larger percentage of surgical patients have lower PSAs (<10 ng/mL, average 67% vs. 51%) and lower tumor grades (Gleason score ≥7 ≈27% vs. 42%) and node-positive patients are frequently excluded.
T1b	74–91/70–91	66–72/32–47	
T1c	100/	—	
T2a	56–87/56–76	63/18–47	
T2b/T2c	56–70/47–60	60/21–29	
T3/4	—	30**–34/10–21	

Based on Tables 42–12 through 42–18.
*PSA failure defined as 0.2 to 0.6 ng/mL.
†PSA failure 1.0 to 4.0 ng/mL.
‡Zincke GS = 4–6.
§Excludes node-positive patients.
¶At 3 years.
**Greater than 1 ng/mL at 4 years.
NED, no evidence of disease; PSA, prostate-specific antigen; RT, radiation therapy.

results following treatment by surgery or radiation are very similar.[181,465]

3D CONFORMAL AND INTENSITY-MODULATED RADIATION THERAPY

A limited number of institutions are treating large numbers of patients with 3DCRT and IMRT. In the mid- to late-1980s, investigators at the University of Michigan pioneered the use of 3D conformal treatment planning technology. By the late 1980s to early 1990s, investigators from several other institutions including the University of Chicago, MSKCC, Fox Chase Cancer Center, and UCSF were reporting their experiences with this technology. By the mid-1990s the RTOG had mounted a phase I to II 3D dose escalation trial, initially including only nine institutions. Later, as the technology became more widely available, RTOG 9406 expanded to include more than 25 institutions and more than 900 patients.

Evidence for improved freedom from PSA failure results associated with the use of 3DCRT comes from both retrospective and prospective studies. These retrospective studies have demonstrated that doses in excess of 70 to 72 Gy are associated with a reduction in the risk of recurrence compared to lower doses.[39,143,454,466-469] These series must be viewed cautiously, however, because the duration of follow-up is shorter for the patients treated with 3D compared to conventional radiotherapy, and duration of follow-up can have a major impact on the estimated risk of biochemical failure.[166] The prospective randomized trial reported by Pollack et al. demonstrated that using 3DCRT to deliver a boost to 78 Gy (central axis dose) improved PSA control for patients with PSAs greater than 10 ng/mL compared to 70 Gy (central axis dose) using conventional planning (Fig. 45-38).[395]

Investigators from MSKCC have demonstrated the feasibility of high-dose IMRT in a large number of patients.[206,214,215] These investigators described their experience in 772 patients treated with high-dose IMRT between April 1996 and January 2001. Ninety percent of these men were treated to 81.0 Gy, and 10% were treated to 86.4 Gy. The authors concluded that the acute and late rectal toxicities appeared to be less than had

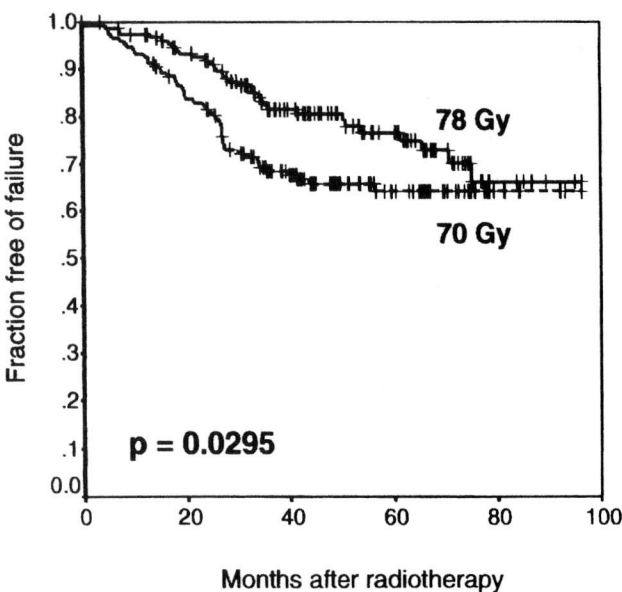

Figure 45–38. Kaplan-Meier freedom-from-failure curves for all patients by dose randomization (70 Gy vs. 78 Gy). Results of a randomized trial 70 vs. 78 Gy, the latter delivered with a boost using 3DCRT. (From Pollack A, Zagars GK, Starkschall G, et al: Prostate cancer radiation dose response: Results of the MD Anderson Phase III randomized trial. *Int J Radiat Oncol Biol Phys.* 2002;53:1097.)

been observed with conventional 3DCRT techniques. With respect to freedom from biochemical failure, the authors concluded that "Short-term PSA control rates seem to be at least comparable to those achieved with 3DCRT at similar dose levels." They reported 3-year actuarial PSA relapse-free survival rates for favorable, intermediate, and unfavorable risk group patients as 92%, 86%, and 81%, respectively (Fig. 45-39). They argued that "based on this favorable risk:benefit ratio, IMRT has become the standard mode of conformal treatment delivery for localized prostate cancer at our institution." What remains to be proven is whether the long-term outcomes will be better than those reported by series using 3DCRT to deliver doses in excess of 72 Gy (Fig. 45-40).[465]

Figure 45–39. Actuarial (Kaplan-Meier) probability of achieving PSA relapse-free survival for the favorable, intermediate, and unfavorable prognostic risk subgroups. Favorable risk, intermediate risk, and unfavorable risk patients treated with intensity-modulated radiotherapy doses of 81 to 86 Gy. (From Zelefsky MJ, Fuks Z, Hunt M, et al: High-dose intensity modulated radiation therapy for prostate cancer: Early toxicity and biochemical outcome in 772 patients. *Int J Radiat Oncol Biol Phys.* 2002;53:1111.)

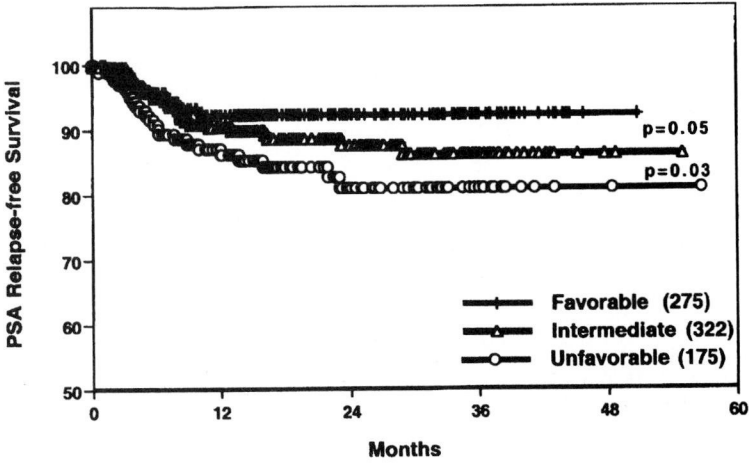

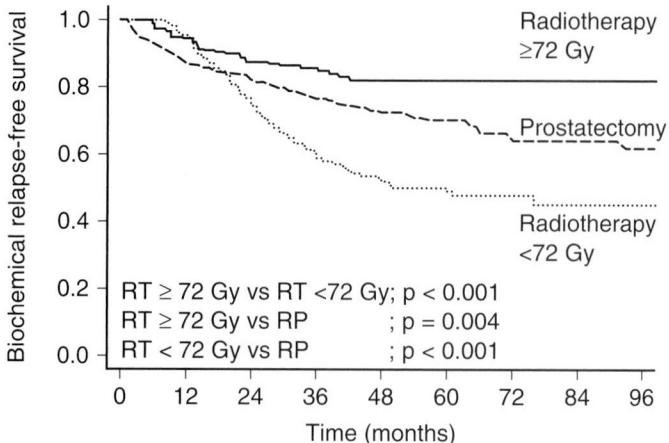

Figure 45–40. Biochemical relapse-free survival for patients with unfavorable tumors (stage T2B to T2C lesions, or biopsy Gleason scores >7, or pretreatment prostate-specific antigen levels >10 ng/mL) by treatment modality: radiotherapy (RT) to doses <72 Gy, RT to doses >72 Gy, and radical prostatectomy. (From Kupelian PA, Elshaikh M, Reddy CA, et al: Comparison of the efficacy of local therapies for localized prostate cancer in the prostate-specific antigen era: A large single-institution experience with radical prostatectomy and external-beam radiotherapy. *J Clin Oncol.* 2002;20:3376.)

Selected Results Associated with Brachytherapy

PERMANENT IMPLANTS

With the widespread adoption of prostate brachytherapy during the past 5 years, the body of literature regarding tumor control rates has grown rapidly.[280,470-473] Investigators from MSKCC have provided a nomogram that can be used to predict PSA failure after brachytherapy (Fig. 45-41A–B).[474] Perhaps the simplest way to evaluate

these brachytherapy results is to divide them into low-risk and "higher-risk" disease. High-risk patients like those treated on RTOG series (i.e., clinical T3 and GS >7 and median PSA >20 ng/mL) have not frequently been treated with permanent implants, and, with limited exceptions, are generally not considered ideal candidates for PPI alone.

Low-Risk Patients (PSA <10, Gleason Score = 6)

There are several reported series of patients treated with I-125 or Pd-103 alone, with median follow-up approaching 10 years. Ten-year actuarial biochemical control rates are in the 70% to 90% range, comparing favorably to those reported from premier surgical series (Fig. 45-42A).[342,475,476] To date, in most series, there is no evidence of excessive late failures (beyond 10 years).[58] However, caution is still in order when making claims about long-term efficacy. But caution is equally in order when considering long-term effectiveness of prostatectomy, for which some surprisingly poor long-term control rates have been reported.[172,282]

Higher-Risk Patients

As with low-risk patient groups, there are rapidly increasing reports showing high biochemical cure rates using brachytherapy-based treatment for patients with PSAs of 10 to 20 ng/mL or GS = 7, or both (Fig. 45-42B). The most remarkable aggregate finding is a relatively high percent of patients who appear to be cured, evidenced by flattening of the freedom-from-failure curves past the 2-year follow-up period.[280,342,473,476] Again, longer follow-up is required to confirm that these results will hold up.

One brachytherapy series of note, reported by Dattoli and colleagues, included patients with higher PSAs or GS's

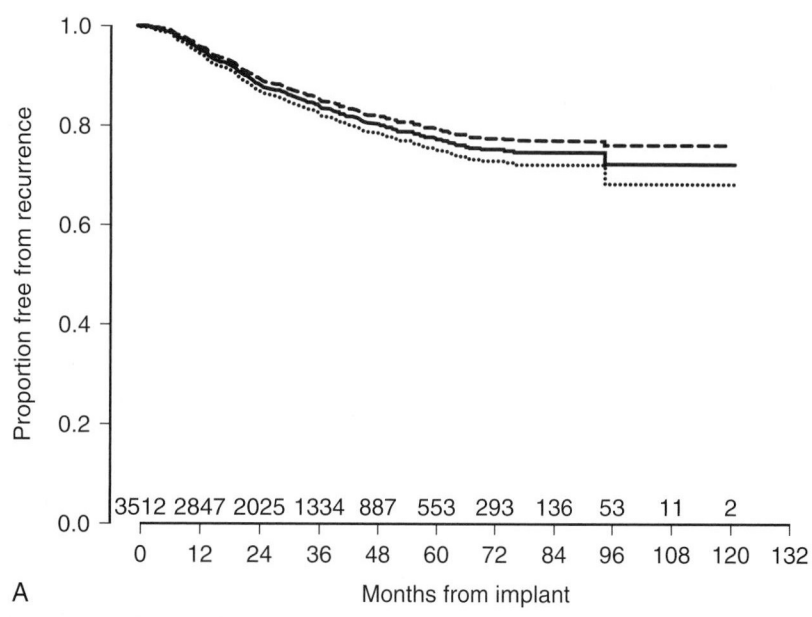

A

Figure 45–41. A, Kaplan-Meier estimates of disease-free probability with 95% confidence bounds for all cohorts combined (*n* = 3512). Numbers above the months indicate patients at risk of recurrence. Although many of the failures were observed before 60 months, recurrence beyond this point did occur.

Continued

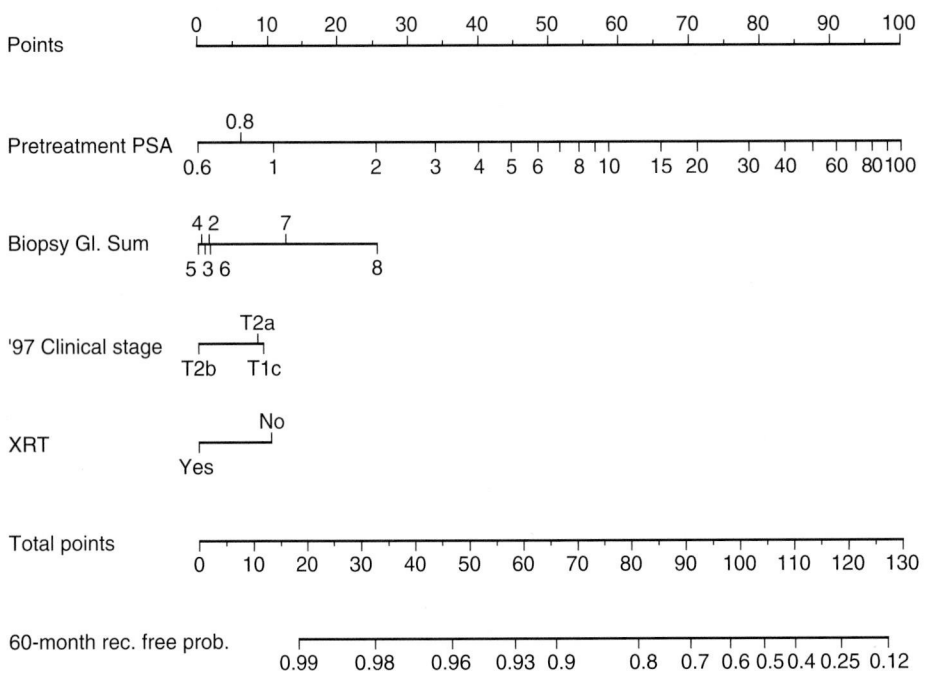

Instructions for physician: Locate the patient's PSA on the **Pretreatment PSA** axis. Draw a line straight upwards to the **Points** axis to determine how many points towards recurrence the patient receives for his PSA. Repeat this process for the other axes, each time drawing straight upward to the **Points** axis. Sum the points achieved for each predictor and locate this sum on the **Total Points** axis. Draw a line straight down to find the patient's probability of remaining recurrence free for 60 months assuming he does not die of another cause first.

Note: This nomogram is not applicable to a man who is not otherwise a candidate for permanent prostate brachytherapy. You can use this only on a man who has already selected permanent prostate brachytherapy as treatment for his prostate cancer. You must decide upon use of adjuvant XRT prior to consulting this nomogram.

Instruction to patient: "Mr. X, if we had 100 men exactly like you, we would expect between <predicted percentage from nomogram – 30%> and <predicted percentage + 5%> to remain free of their disease at 5 years following permanent prostate brachytherapy, and recurrence after 5 years is very rare."

B

Figure 45–41, cont'd. B, Nomogram for predicting 5-year freedom from PSA recurrence after permanent prostate brachytherapy without neoadjuvant androgen ablative therapy. (From Kattan MW, Potters L, Blasko JC, et al: Pretreatment nomogram for predicting freedom from recurrence after permanent prostate brachytherapy in prostate cancer. *J Urol.* 2001;166:876.)

treated with implant and supplemental beam radiation.[280] The unique aspect of their series is that all patients' biopsies were reviewed by a single, highly regarded uropathologist, making analysis of the role of GS's more reliable. All patients had at least one adverse risk factor: a pretreatment PSA = 10 or GS of 7 or higher. From 1992 through 1995, 142 consecutive patients were treated. Their ages ranged from 49 to 88 years (median: 71 years). Patients received 41 Gy external beam radiation to a limited pelvic field, followed 2 to 4 weeks later by a Pd-103 boost (80 Gy, pre-NIST-99).

Twenty-five patients developed biochemical failure, which was defined as a PSA greater than 0.5 ng/mL at last follow-up. The overall actuarial freedom from biochemical progression at 5 years is 82%, with 81 patients followed beyond that time, particularly encouraging for patients with higher pretreatment PSAs or GS's. No clinically evident local failures occurred. Progressively more elevated pretreatment PSA, GS, or prostatic acid phosphatase were each associated with a progressively higher

failure rate (Fig. 45-42C). In Cox proportional hazards model multivariate analysis, considering each factor as a continuous variable, the strongest predictor of failure was elevated acid phosphatase (*P* = 0.02), followed by GS (*P* = 0.1) and PSA (*P* = 0.14). There was little correlation among pretreatment PSA, GS, or PAP.

The Dattoli series shows the high rate of cancer control achievable in even more unfavorable cancers, along with the importance of serum PAP. The high rate of control at 5 to 10 years suggests that even patients with GS's above 7, or with PSAs above 20 ng/mL, still have a good chance of being nonmetastatic and are still curable. There is an increasing number of series corroborating high cancer eradication rates, even in patients with high preimplant PSA or Gleason scores.[342,473]

Outliers

The majority of brachytherapy reports have been surprisingly favorable. But like any modality, there are scattered

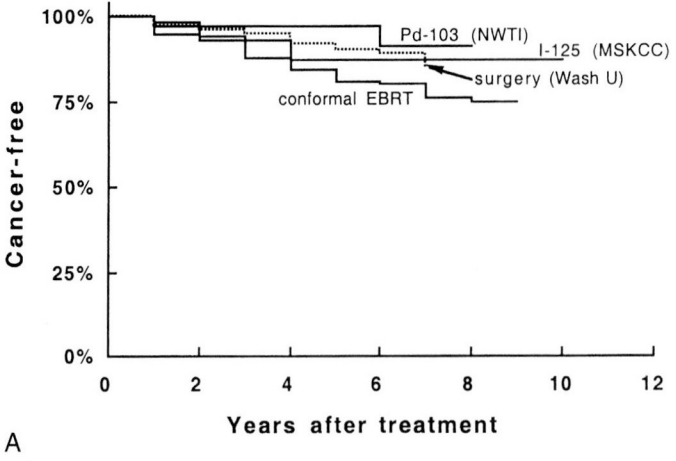

A

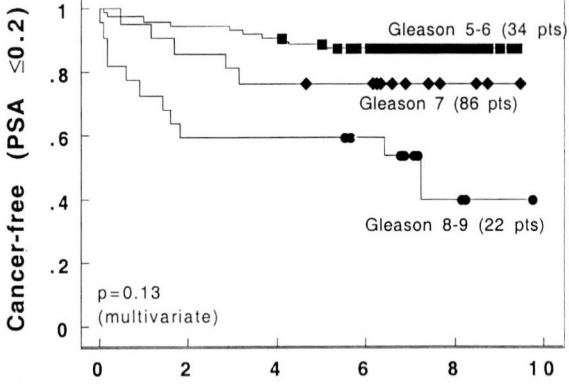

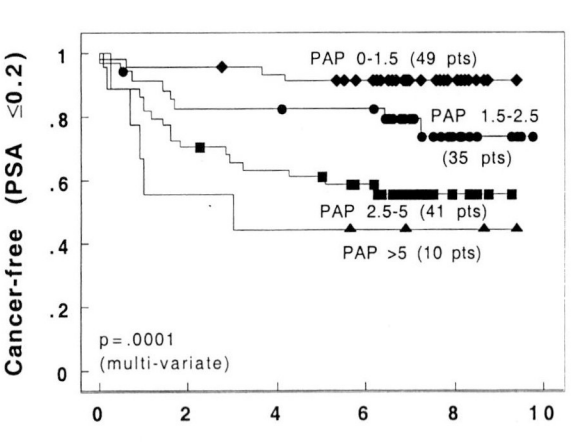

B

Figure 45–42. A, Biochemical freedom-from-failure rates for low-risk patients in selected series after beam radiation, surgery, or brachytherapy. Cancer control rates for low-risk patients appear very similar among series and are likely explained by minor differences in patient selection or PSA failure definitions. **B,** Freedom from biochemical failure for patients treated with Pd-103 + beam radiation, stratified by PSA, Gleason score, or prostatic acid phosphatase. (Total number of patients in each group shown in parentheses.) (From Dattoli M, Wallner K, True L, et al: Long-term outcomes following EBRT + Pd-103 for higher risk prostatic carcinoma: Influence of prostatic acid phosphatase. *Cancer*. 2003;97:979-93.)

reports to the contrary. The most publicized outliers for prostate brachytherapy are reported by D'Amico and colleagues (Fig. 45-43).[282] Poor results, far inferior to the norm, likely reflect poor technique or poor patient selection rather than inherent flaws in the modality. Unfortunately, aggressive publication of inferior outcomes may lead the casual observer to conclude that poor results are representative of other practitioners.

IMPLANTS AS SALVAGE THERAPY. There is substantial interest in the use of brachytherapy as salvage for patients with local tumor persistence after external beam irradiation. Two optimistic reports regarding salvage brachytherapy

for failed external beam patients have appeared. Grado reported on 49 patients salvaged with either I-125 or Pd-103 between 1990 and 1996.[315] Biochemical freedom from failure in salvaged patients was 33% at 5 years, similar to that reported in surgical salvage series. In a similarly optimistic publication, Beyer reported 17 patients treated with reduced dose I-125 or Pd-103 salvage implants with an overall freedom from second relapse of 53%.[313] In contrast to salvage prostatectomy, the reported risk of incontinence has been relatively low after salvage brachytherapy. Even more surprising, no severe rectal complications were reported. However, it is possible that the incidence could rise with longer follow-up.

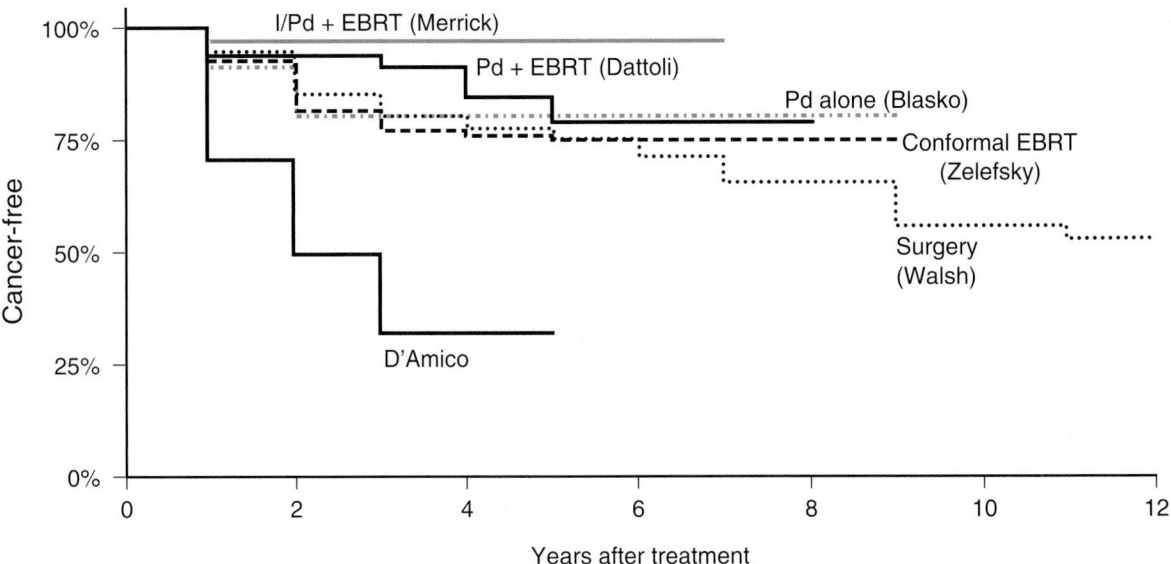

Figure 45–43. Intermediate-risk patients (PSA 10-20, Gleason score ≥7). Biochemical freedom-from-failure rates for intermediate risk patients in selected series after beam radiation, surgery, or brachytherapy. The D'Amico series results, probably the most widely quoted, are far worse than any other, and should not be used to make recommendations regarding optimal forms of therapy in the hands of experienced practitioners.

While published results with salvage brachytherapy are mildly encouraging, caution is in order, primarily because dosimetric details are missing from both reports. Simply stating the prescription dose of a salvage implant does not tell enough about the implant technique to safely duplicate it at other centers. The treatment margins used in the planning process, for instance, might have a substantial impact on the true dose to adjacent normal tissues. More meticulous information regarding salvage planning parameters is needed.[477] Use of brachytherapy in the post-prostatectomy setting has not been reported, and would be considered unconventional.

Results of High Dose Rate Brachytherapy

Most reported results of HDR brachytherapy cover boost in combination with EBRT. Major series that are highly quoted include the University of Kiel, the Swedish Medical Center in Seattle, the William Beaumont Group outside Detroit, as well as groups from Goteborg University in Sweden and the University of Berlin.[478-486] Patient selection has been variable as well, with some series including a relatively large number of patients with T3 disease while others selected almost exclusively patients with T1 to T2 patients. Follow-up has also been highly variable, ranging from 2 to 3 years to beyond 10 years. Different fractionation schemes and doses have been used by each of these groups. Fractionation schemes have been as aggressive as 9.5 Gy × 2 to 5.0 Gy × 3 combined with EBRT from 45 to 50 Gy. Treatment results and complications from HDR brachytherapy boost in combination with EBRT are summarized in Table 45-11.[487]

Cost of Therapies for Localized Disease

Cost considerations are not a major focus of this chapter, and different conclusions can be found in different studies.[334,488-493] Making an accurate estimate of the cost of treatment depends on the distribution of risk factors within a given population.[489] Two studies have shown the cost of brachytherapy and radical prostatectomy to be similar, while another found brachytherapy to be more expensive.[488,492,493] Based on 1996 Medicare reimbursement rates, the charge for an I-125 prostate implant totals approximately $12,000, 80% of which represents hospital charges and 20% clinician charges. The cost of the sources themselves is a substantial portion of the bill. The typical I-125 or Pd-103 cost to the provider is about $2500 to $5000. Several reports comparing the charges for brachytherapy versus radical prostatectomy have appeared, generally concluding that brachytherapy costs about 105 to 20% more than surgery.[492-494] When making such comparisons, however, it should be kept in mind that authors who calculated the comparisons were all practicing in a fee-for-service setting in which inefficiencies, if billable, are encouraged. In contrast, Seddon, Wallner, and Walker showed that in a managed care setting, the cost of brachytherapy is likely to be far lower than competing modalities (Fig. 45-44).[349] While implant alone is cost-competitive with prostatectomy or external radiation, the addition of supplemental external beam radiation increases the cost substantially. If supplemental beam radiation increases cure rates, combined modality could still be a bargain in the long run. Only randomized trials will answer this issue definitively.[347]

Other series find brachytherapy to be cheaper but discourage its use.[490] Based on SEER-Medicare data, one study found EBRT to be substantially (23%) cheaper than radical prostatectomy.[495] All that can be stated with confidence is that because differences in outcomes appear to be small between treatments, any treatment that is poorly performed (resulting in more complications and failure) is likely to be far more expensive than other therapies when well done (associated with fewer complications and fewer failures).

Table 45-11 Selected Series Using High-Dose-Rate Brachytherapy in Combination with External Beam Radiotherapy

Institution	Patients	Treatment	Follow-up, *n*	Results	Complications
University of Kiel	T1–T3 G1–G3	EB (30) 50 Gy IS 15 Gy × 2	171 55 mo	78% clinical disease free	5/1717 G3 proctitis 3/1717 G3 dysuria cystitis 9/171 incontinence
Swedish Tumor Institute	T1–T3 PSA 12.9 GS 3–9	EB 50.4 Gy IS 3–4 Gy × 4	104 46 mo	84% at 5 yr actuarial (3 increases)	6.7% stricture 1% necrosis
William Beaumont Hospital	T2b–T3 PSA GS ≥7	EB 46 IS 5.5–6.5 Gy × 3 8.25–9.5 Gy × 2	142 2.1 yr	89% DFS at 5yr 95% OS at 5 yr	5% G3 acute toxicity 9% 5 yrs actuarial G3 late toxicity
Goteborg University	T1– T3pN0 G1–3	EB 50 Gy IS 10–15 Gy × 2	50 45 mo	84% PSA ≤1.0 4% positive Bx at 18 mo	4% dysuria 6% frequency 8% diarrhea 2% proctitis 12% impotence
University of Berlin	T2–T3pN0 G1–3 PSA 14.0	EB 40–45 Gy IS 9–10 Gy × 2	82 24 mo	52.9% PSA <1.0 26.9% positive Bx at 24 mo	7/82 G3 stricture 6/82 G3 incontinence 3/82 G4 proctitis

NS, not stated.
Modified from Hsu I-C III MR: Brachytherapy. In Grossfield CA, ed. *Prostate Cancer.* Hamilton, Ontario, Canada: Decker; 2002.

MAJOR CLINICAL TRIALS USING RADIATION THERAPY AND HORMONAL THERAPY

The largest phase III prospective randomized trials evaluating the use of radiation therapy for the treatment of clinically localized prostate cancer have been conducted by the RTOG. A summary of these trials is shown in Table 45-12. These trials can be divided into three major periods, those conducted in the late 1970s to the mid-1980s (RTOG 7506, 7706, and 8307), or the "pre-PSA era" studies. The RTOG trials conducted from the mid- to late 1980s to the early 1990s (RTOG 8531, 8610,

and the intergroup study 9019) may be considered the "peri-PSA era" trials. The "PSA era" studies began in the early to mid-1990s and include RTOG 9202, 9406, 9408, 9412, 9413, 9601, and 9910, for which pretreatment PSA is available for all of these patients. At press time, the "final reports" of all pre- and peri-PSA RTOG trials and the initial reports of RTOG 9202 and 9413 were available.

The addition of hormonal manipulation to radiation therapy is now a standard approach for selected patients. In the first edition of this chapter, much was made of the

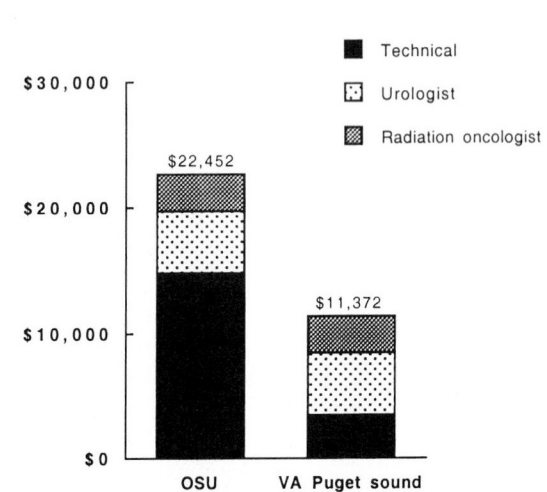

Figure 45–44. Technical charges at Ohio State University (OSU, 1999), compared to those calculated for the VA Puget Sound Health Care System. Clinician charges were assumed to be unchanged. (From Seddon R, Wallner K, Walker J: Revisiting the cost of prostate brachytherapy: VAPSHCS experience. *Oncol News Internat.* 2002;11:37 and Wagner TT, Young D, Bahnson RR: Charge and length of hospital stay analysis of radical retropubic prostatectomy and transperineal prostate brachytherapy. *J Urol.* 1999;161:1216.)

Table 45-12   Completed and Ongoing Major Phase III Radiation Therapy Oncology Group Prostate Cancer Trials

Trial	Study Question	Conclusions	Comments
RTOG 7506	± Para-aortic irradiation in addition to pelvic and prostate RT	No benefit to para-aortic RT	No hormonal therapy used and pre-PSA era
RTOG 7706	± Pelvic irradiation in addition to prostate RT	No benefit to pelvic RT	No hormonal therapy used and pre-PSA era
RTOG 8307	4 mo of diethylstilbestrol or Megestrol Acetate plus RT using either	Diethylstilbestrol and Megestrol Acetate have similar efficacy	No radiotherapy-alone control arm. When matched by Gleason and stage, results worse than CAB and RT alone?
RTOG 8531	± Adjuvant LH-RH following pelvic and prostate RT	Survival advantage for Gleason scores 8–10	Update demonstrates and overall survival advantage
RTOG 8610	± Neoadjuvant LH-RH and flutamide (CAB) 2 mo before and during RT	Survival advantage for Gleason scores <7	Very high risk patients require longer-term hormonal therapy
RTOG 9202	Randomized to neoadjuvant (NHT) (2 mo before and during RT) ± 2 years of adjuvant (AHT) LH-RH alone	Survival advantage for Gleason scores 8–10	Very high risk patients require longer-term hormonal therapy
RTOG 9408	± Neoadjuvant LH-RH and flutamide 2 mo before and during RT	Not yet available	Closed results pending
RTOG 9413	Four arms randomized to NHT (2 mo before and during RT) vs. AHT (4 mo immediately after RT) LH-RH & flutamide and to receive prostate & seminal vesicle ± whole pelvic RT	Whole pelvic RT beneficial if given with NHT HT	No evidence of a benefit to NHT if only the prostate is treated. No evidence that there is a benefit to pelvic RT without pelvic NHT
RTOG 9601	RT alone vs. RT plus bicalutamide 150 mg prostate only in patients with a rising PSA after prostatectomy	Not yet available	Closed results pending
RTOG 9902	Neoadjuvant CAB 2 mo before and during RT + adjuvant LH-RH × 2 yr ± chemotherapy with Taxol estramustin etoposide	Not yet available	Ongoing
RTOG 9910	8 vs 28 weeks of neoadjuvant CAB before and during RT	Not yet available	Closed results pending
RTOG 0011	RT vs. RT and LH-RH agonist: for 2 yr after 1 mo of anti-androgen for patients with pT2-3N0M0 at high risk for PSA relapse	Not yet available	Ongoing
RTOG 0014	After failure of surgery and/or radiation (a rising PSA of >2.0 and a doubling time of <8 mo): CAB plus concurrent chemo × 4 cycles vs. initial CAB, then chemo at clinical failure.	Not yet available	Ongoing
RTOG 0126	Three-dimensional conformal radiotherapy 72.9 in 39 fx vs. 82.28 in 44 fx	Not yet available	Ongoing

AHT, adjuvant hormonal therapy; CAB, combined androgen blockade; LH-RH, luteinizing hormone–releasing hormone; NHT, neoadjuvant hormonal therapy; RT, radiotherapy.

animal models, the concept of "debulking" as supported in the initial reports of neoadjuvant hormonal therapy before radical prostatectomy. We emphasized the preliminary findings of RTOG 8610, 8531, and the EORTC trial reported by Bolla et al. Things are much clearer now. The use of neoadjuvant hormonal therapy before radical prostatectomy has failed to translate into an improvement in freedom from biochemical failure. Similarly, the routine use of hormonal therapy before EBRT has begun to be questioned because of reports of increased radiotherapy-related morbidity, including GU and GI symptoms. Because hormonal therapy may increase the risk of impotence, is expensive, and fails to improve the outcomes of low-risk patients, we discourage the indiscriminant use of this modality in these patients. What seemed like a simple

story, "hormonal therapy won't hurt and might help," has changed to "do the right thing" for the right patient.

More retrospective studies with longer follow-up, a meta-analysis of RTOG trials, and two recently completed phase III trials (9202 and 9413) have brought new insights. The problem has been the interpretation of the major trials. Several phase III trials reached what appeared to be conflicting conclusions about the role of hormonal therapy and radiotherapy. RTOG 8531, a trial including approximately 900 patients with locally advanced prostate cancer treated with or without long-term adjuvant LH-RH–based hormonal therapy, concluded that the major benefit was seen in patients with GS's greater than 7. In contrast, RTOG 8610 (n = 471) patients with locally advanced prostate cancer randomized

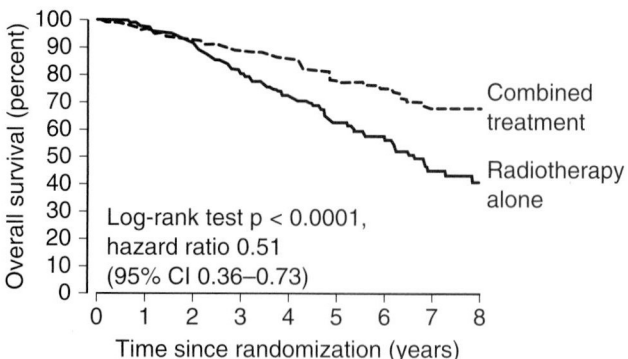

Figure 45–45. Kaplan-Meier estimates of overall survival by treatment group. (From Bolla M, Collette L, Blank L, et al: Long-term results with immediate androgen suppression and external irradiation in patients with locally advanced prostate cancer (an EORTC study): A phase III randomized trial. *Lancet.* 2002;360:103.)

to receive radiation therapy alone or with CAB 2 months before and during radiation therapy demonstrated a survival benefit only for patients with a GS of less than 7. The European Oncology Radiotherapy Therapy Committee (EORTC) Trial reported by Bolla et al. compared EBRT alone versus EBRT with 3 years of adjuvant hormonal therapy for patients with T3 (any GS) or GS's of 8 to 10 and concluded that all benefited (Fig. 45-45).

Unfortunately, when these three trials were designed, the relative importance of race, age, lymph node status, pretreatment PSA, GS, and T stage on overall survival were not well defined. In an attempt to model the relative importance of these factors, the RTOG defined four prognostic subgroups that allowed overall and disease-specific survival to be predicted at 5, 10, and 15 years.[57] These investigators based their model on data from 1500 patients treated with radiation alone on several prospective trials (RTOG 7506, 7706, 8531, and 860)

with long follow-up. Using this model, they next performed a meta-analysis including 900 additional patients treated with hormonal therapy in an attempt to assess the possible impact of short-term or long-term hormonal therapy survival. This meta-analysis demonstrated that apparently conflicting results could be explained by a unifying hypothesis, summarized as follows: low-risk, intermediate-, and high-risk patients were best served by the use of no hormonal therapy, short-term neoadjuvant plus concurrent hormonal therapy, and long-term adjuvant hormonal therapy, respectively (Table 45-13 and Fig. 45-46A–B).[45]

This hypothesis is explained by the fact that patients with low-risk disease appear to be at such a low risk for lymph node involvement and death due to prostate cancer, and the potential benefits of hormonal therapy are lost in the "noise of competing causes of death and time." Patients with intermediate-risk disease have a significant risk of occult lymph node involvement and thus benefit from neoadjuvant hormonal therapy combined with whole pelvic radiotherapy. But these patients are at a relatively low risk for micro-metastatic disease and thus do not benefit much from long-term hormonal therapy. High-risk patients are at a substantial risk for micro-metastatic disease and thus require neoadjuvant and long-term adjuvant hormonal therapy to increase survival. This hypothesis is consistent with recent findings of RTOG 9413 and 9202.

The Future of Radiotherapy for Prostate Cancer

In this chapter we have attempted to summarize "the state of the art" of managing prostate cancer with radiotherapy. We believe that chemotherapy will eventually play a greater role as it has for cancers of the cervix, breast, lung, head and neck, and bladder. Organ preservation will be enhanced by the availability of such agents. The routine use of technology that allows more accurate delivery combined with a higher degree of quality assurance and a better understanding of dose response relationship is likely to result in the increased use of radiotherapy for patients with clinically localized prostate cancer.

Table 45-13   Disease-Specific Survival Rates

Risk Group	Statistics	RT Alone	Short DES/Megestrol	Short Goserelin + Flutamide	Long Hormone	p Value*
2	Death/N	84/443	25/55	1/70	9/114	D/M vs RT
T3 & GS = 6	5-yr rate	94%	74%	100%	93%	0.0001
or T1–2 &	8-yr rate	83%	57%	98%	89%	G&F vs RT, 0.003
GS = 7						Long vs RT, 0.13
3	Death/N	96/338	15/45	25/88	16/132	D/M vs RT, 0.28
T3 & GS = 7	5-yr rate	83%	83%	80%	93%	G&F vs RT, 0.49
or T1–2 & GS >7	8-yr rate	70%	64%	67%	88%	Long vs RT, 0.004
4	Death/N	154/324	15/25	20/45	25/103	D/M vs RT, 0.36
T3 & GS = 8	5-yr rate	64%	50%	64%	81%	G&F vs RT, 0.63
or N + GS = 8	8-yr rate	42%	35%	49%	69%	Long vs RT, 0.001

*RT vs long HT in group 3 and 4 patients, $P < 0.0001$.
DES, diethylstilbestrol; G&F, goserelin and flutamide; HT, hormonal therapy; NA, not available; RT, radiotherapy alone.
From Roach M, Lu J, Pilepich MV, et al: Predicting long-term survival, and the need for hormonal therapy: A meta-analysis of RTOG prostate cancer trials. *Int J Radiat Oncol Biol Phys.* 2000;47:617.

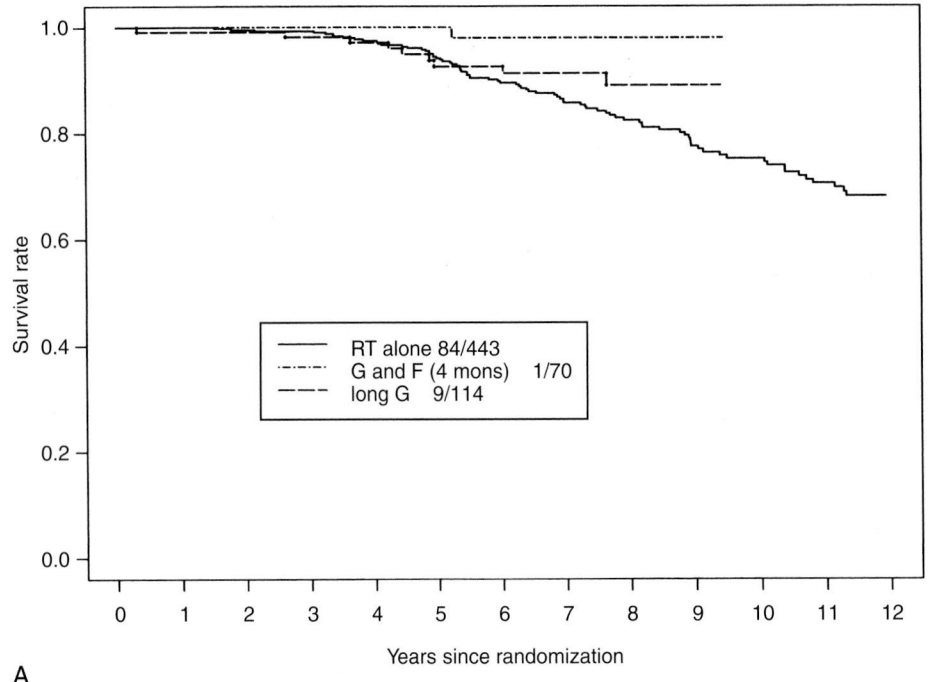

A

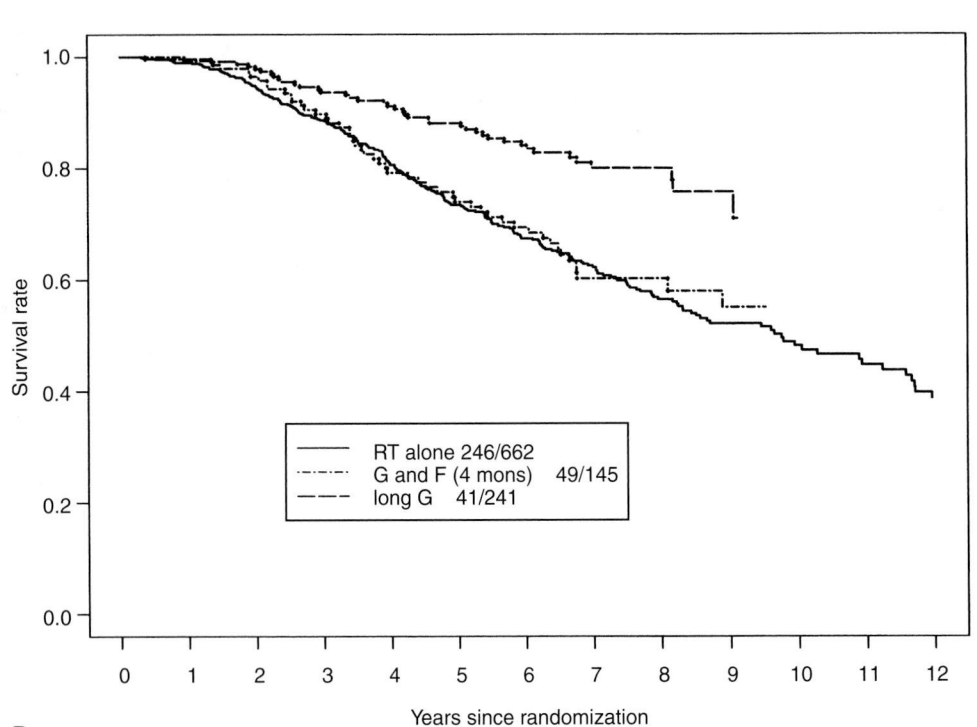

B

Figure 45–46. A, Overall and disease-specific survival for groups 1 and 2 by treatment type. **B,** Overall and disease-specific survival for groups 3 and 4 by treatment type. (From Roach M, Lu J, Pilepich MV, et al: Predicting long-term survival, and the need for hormonal therapy: A meta-analysis of RTOG prostate cancer trials. *Int J Radiat Oncol Biol Phys.* 2000;47:617-627.)

REFERENCES

1. Jemal A, Murra T, Samuels A, et al: Cancer Statistics 2003. *CA Cancer J Clin.* 2003;53:5.
2. Mettlin CJ, Murphy GP, Rosenthal DS, et al: The National Cancer Data Base report on prostate carcinoma after the peak in incidence rates in the U.S. The American College of Surgeons Commission on Cancer and the American Cancer Society. *Cancer.* 1998;83:1679.
3. Silverberg E: Cancer Statistics. *Cancer Stat.* 30:23, 1980.
4. Roach M III, Lu J, Pilepich MV, et al: Race and survival of men treated for prostate cancer on radiation therapy oncology group phase III randomized trials. *J Urol.* 2003;169:245.
5. Bennett CL, Price DK, Kim S, et al: Racial variation in CAG repeat lengths within the androgen receptor gene among prostate cancer patients of lower socioeconomic status. *J Clin Oncol.* 2002; 20:3599.
6. Lichtenstein P, Holm NV, Verkasalo PK, et al: Environmental and heritable factors in the causation of cancer—Analyses of cohorts of twins from Sweden, Denmark, and Finland. *N Engl J Med.* 2000;343:78.

7. McWhorter WP, Hernandez AD, Meikle AW, et al: A screening study of prostate cancer in high risk families. *J Urol*. 1992; 148:826.

8. Hutchison GB: Incidence and etiology of prostate cancer. *Urol*. 1981;XVII(suppl):4.

9. Stamey TA, Johnstone IM, McNeal JE, et al: Preoperative serum prostate specific antigen levels between 2 and 22 ng/mL correlate poorly with post-radical prostatectomy cancer morphology: Prostate specific antigen cure rates appear constant between 2 and 9 ng/mL *J Urol*. 2002;167:103.

10. Giovannucci E, Ascherio A, Rimm EB, et al: Vasectomy and prostate cancer: Chance, bias, or a causal relationship. *JAMA*. 1993;269:913.

11. Lynge E: Prostate cancer is not increased in men with vasectomy in Denmark. *J Urol*. 2002;168:488.

12. Dennis LK, Dawson DV, Resnick MI: Vasectomy and the risk of prostate cancer: A meta-analysis examining vasectomy status, age at vasectomy, and time since vasectomy. *Prostate Cancer Prostatic Dis*. 2002;5:193.

13. Cox B, Sneyd MJ, Paul C, et al: Vasectomy and risk of prostate cancer. *JAMA*. 2002;287:3110.

14. Steele R, Lees REM, Kraus AS, et al: Sexual factors in the epidemiology of cancer of the prostate. *J Chron Dis*. 1971;24:29.

15. Hiatt RA, Armstrong MA, Klatsky AL, et al: Alcohol consumption, smoking, and other risk factors and prostate cancer in a large health plan cohort in California (United States). *Cancer Causes Control*. 1994;5:66.

16. Schuurman AG, van den Brandt PA, Dorant E, et al: Association of energy and fat intake with prostate carcinoma risk: Results from The Netherlands Cohort Study. *Cancer*. 1999;86:1019.

17. Shike M, Latkany L, Riedel E, et al: Lack of effect of a low-fat, high-fruit, -vegetable, and -fiber diet on serum prostate-specific antigen of men without prostate cancer: Results from a randomized trial. *J Clin Oncol*. 2002;20:3592.

18. Moyad MA: Dietary fat reduction to reduce prostate cancer risk: Controlled enthusiasm, learning a lesson from breast or other cancers, and the big picture. *Urology*. 2002;59:51.

19. Giovannucci E, Leitzmann M, Spiegelman D, et al: A prospective study of physical activity and prostate cancer in male health professionals. *Cancer Res*. 1998;58:5117.

20. Chan JM, Stampfer MJ, Ma J, et al: Dairy products, calcium, and prostate cancer risk in the Physicians' Health Study. *Am J Clin Nutr*. 2001;74:549.

21. Konety BR, Getzenberg RH: Vitamin D and prostate cancer. *Urol Clin North Am*. 2002;29:95.

22. Berndt SI, Carter HB, Landis PK, et al: Calcium intake and prostate cancer risk in a long-term aging study: The Baltimore Longitudinal Study of Aging. *Urology*. 2002;60:1118.

23. Alpha-T, Beta, Carotene, Cancer, Prevention, Study Group: The effect of vitamin E and beta carotene on the incidence of lung cancer and other cancers in male smokers. *N Engl J Med*. 1994; 330:1029.

24. Giovannucci E, Rimm EB, Liu Y, et al: A prospective study of tomato products, lycopene, and prostate cancer risk. *J Natl Cancer Inst*. 2002;94:391.

25. Schuurman AG, Goldbohm RA, Brants HA, et al: A prospective cohort study on intake of retinol, vitamins C and E, and carotenoids and prostate cancer risk (Netherlands). *Cancer Causes Control*. 2002;13:573.

26. Moyad MA: Selenium and vitamin E supplements for prostate cancer: Evidence or embellishment? *Urology*. 2002;59:9.

27. Hussain F, Aziz H, Macchia R, et al: High grade adenocarcinoma of prostate in smokers of ethnic minority groups and Caribbean island immigrants. *Int J Radiat Biol Phys*. 1992;24:451.

28. Daniell HW: A worse prognosis for smoker with prostate cancer. *J Urol*. 1995;154:153.

29. Roberts WW, Platz EA, Walsh PC: Association of cigarette smoking with extraprostatic prostate cancer in young men. *J Urol*. 2003;169:512; discussion 516.

30. Hickey K, Do KA, Green A: Smoking and prostate cancer. *Epidemiol Rev*. 2001;23:115.

31. Goodman GE, Schaffer S, Bankson DD, et al: Predictors of serum selenium in cigarette smokers and the lack of association with lung and prostate cancer risk. *Cancer Epidemiol Biomarkers Prev*. 2001;10:1069.

32. Sharpe CR, Siemiatycki J: Joint effects of smoking and body mass index on prostate cancer risk. *Epidemiology*. 2001;12:546.

33. Giles GG, Severi G, McCredie MR, et al: Smoking and prostate cancer: Findings from an Australian case-control study. *Ann Oncol*. 2001;12:761.

34. Levi F, La Vecchia C: Tobacco smoking and prostate cancer: Time for an appraisal. *Ann Oncol*. 2001;12:733.

35. Johansson J-E, Adami H-O, Andersson S-O, et al: High 10-year survival rate in patients with early, untreated prostatic cancer. *JAMA*. 1992;267:2191.

36. Fleming C, Wasson JH, Albertsen PC, et al: A decision analysis of alternative treatment strategies for clinically localized prostate cancer. *JAMA*. 1993;269:2650.

37. Chodak GW, Thisted RA, Gerber GS, et al: Results of Conservation Management of Clinically Localized Prostate Cancer. *N Engl J Med*. 1994;330:242.

38. Aus G, Hugosson J, Norlen L: Long-term survival and mortality in prostate cancer treated with noncurative intent. *J Urol*. 1995; 154:460.

39. Roach M, Meehan S, Kroll S, et al: Radiotherapy (XRT) for high-grade (HG) clinically localized adenocarcinoma of the prostate (CAP). *J Urol*. 1996;156:1719.

40. (MRC) MRC: Immediate versus deferred treatment for advanced prostatic cancer: initial results of the Medical Research Council trial. *Br J Urol*. 1997;79:235.

41. Albertsen PC, Hanley JA, Gleason DF, et al: Competing risk analysis of men aged 55 to 74 years at diagnosis managed conservatively for clinically localized prostate cancer [see comments]. *JAMA*. 1998;280:975.

42. Bolla M, Collette L, Blank L, et al: Long-term results with immediate androgen suppression and external irradiation in patients with locally advanced prostate cancer (an EORTC study): A phase III randomized trial. *Lancet*. 2002;360:103.

43. Pilepich MV, Winter K, John MJ, et al: Phase III radiation therapy oncology group (RTOG) trial 86-10 of androgen deprivation adjuvant to definitive radiotherapy in locally advanced carcinoma of the prostate. *Int J Radiat Oncol Biol Phys*. 2001;50:1243.

44. Pilepich MV, Caplan R, Byhardt RW, et al: Phase III trial of androgen suppression using goserlin in unfavorable-prognosis carcinoma of the prostate treated with definitive radiotherapy: report of Radiation Oncology Group Protocol 85-31. *J Clin Oncol*. 1997; 15:1013.

45. Roach M, Lu J, Pilepich MV, et al: Predicting long term survival, and the need for hormonal therapy: a meta-analysis of RTOG prostate cancer trials. *Int J Radiat Oncol Biol Phys*. 2000; 47:617.

46. Labrie F, Dupont A, Candas B, et al: Decrease of prostate cancer death by screening: First data from the Quebec prospective and randomized trial. *Proc ASCO*. 1998;17:2a.

47. Bartsch G, Horninger W, Klocker H, et al: Prostate cancer mortality after introduction of prostate-specific antigen mass screening in the Federal State of Tyrol, Austria. *Urology*. 2001;58:417.

48. Holmberg L, Bill-Axelson A, Helgesen F, et al: A randomized trial comparing radical prostatectomy with watchful waiting in early prostate cancer. *N Engl J Med*. 2002;347:781.

49. Villers A, McNeal JE, Redwine EA, et al: The role of perineural space invasion in the local spread of prostate adenocarcinoma. *J Urol*. 1989;142:63.

50. Byar DP, Mostofi FK, Veterans Administration Cooperative Urological Research Group: Carcinoma of the prostate: Prognostic evaluation of certain pathologic features in 208 radical prostatectomies. *Pathol Prost Cancer*. 1972;29:5.

51. Voges GE, McNeal JE, Redwine EA, et al: Morphologic analysis of surgical margins with positive findings in prostatectomy for adenocarcinoma of the prostate. *Cancer*. 1992;69:520.

52. Epstein JI, Pizov G, Steinberg GD, et al: Correlation of prostate cancer nuclear deoxyribonucleic acid, size, shape and Gleason grade with pathological stage at radical prostatectomy. *J Urol*. 1992; 148:87.

53. McNeal JE, Price HM, Redwine EA, et al: Stage A versus stage B adenocarcinoma of the prostate: Morphological comparison and biological significance. *J Urol*. 1988;139:61.

54. Partin AW, Mangold LA, Lamm DM, et al: Contemporary update of prostate cancer staging nomograms (Partin Tables) for the new millennium. *Urology*. 2001;58:843.

55. Saito S, Iwaki H: Mucin-producing carcinoma of the prostate: Review of 88 cases. *Urology.* 1999;54:141.

56. Gleason DF, Mellinger GT, Group VCUR: Prediction of prognosis for prostatic adenocarcinoma by combined histological grading and clinical staging. *J Urol.* 1974;111:58.

57. Roach M, Lu J, V.Pilepich M, et al: Four prognostic groups predict long term survival from prostate cancer following radiotherapy alone on Radiation Therapy Oncology Group clinical trials. *Int J Radiat Oncol Biol Phys.* 2000;47:609.

58. Schellhammer PF, Moriarty R, Bostwick D, et al: Fifteen-year minimum follow-up of a prostate brachytherapy series: Comparing the past with the present. *Urology.* 2000;56:436.

59. Benson MC: Fine-needle aspiration of the prostate. *NCI Monogr:* 1988;7:19.

60. Crawford ED, Hirano D, Werahera PN, et al: Computer modeling of prostate biopsy: Tumor size and location—not clinical significance—determine cancer detection [see comments]. *J Urol.* 1998;159:1260.

61. Johnstone PAS, Riffenburgh R, Saunders EL, et al: Grading inaccuracies in diagnostic biopsies revealing prostatic adenocarcinoma: Implications for definitive radiation therapy. *Int J Radiat Oncol Biol Phys.* 1995;32:479.

62. Benson MC: Application of flow cytometry and automated image analysis to the study of prostate cancer. *NCI Monogr.* 1988;7:25.

63. Lewis P, Bloemers M, Weinberg V, Roach M: Prognostic value of biopsy extent and era on the outcome of patients with prostate cancer treated with radiotherapy. In Cox J, ed. *Proceedings of the American Society for Therapeutic Radiology and Oncology, 40th Annual Meeting. Int J Radiat Oncol Biol.* Phoenix: Elsevier; 1998:308.

64. Chang JJ, Shinohara K, Hovey RM, et al: Prospective evaluation of systematic sextant transition zone biopsies in large prostates for cancer detection. *Urology.* 1998;52:89.

65. Presti JC, Chang JJ, Bhargava V, et al: The optimal systematic prostate biopsy scheme should include 8 rather than 6 biopsies: Results of a prospective clinical trial. *J Urol.* 2000;163:163.

66. D'Amico AV, Whittington R, Malkowicz SB, et al: Clinical utility of the percentage of positive prostate biopsies in defining biochemical outcome after radical prostatectomy for patients with clinically localized prostate cancer. *J Clin Oncol.* 2000;18:1164.

67. Grossfeld GD, Latini DM, Lubeck DP, et al: Predicting disease recurrence in intermediate and high-risk patients undergoing radical prostatectomy using percent positive biopsies: Results from CaPSURE. *Urology.* 2002;59:560.

68. Moul JW, Connelly RR, Lubeck DP, et al: Predicting risk of prostate specific antigen recurrence after radical prostatectomy with the Center for Prostate Disease Research and Cancer of the Prostate Strategic Urologic Research Endeavor databases. *J Urol.* 2001;166:1322.

69. Anderson PR, Hanlon AL, Patchefsky A, et al: Perineural invasion and Gleason 7-10 tumors predict increased failure in prostate cancer patients with pretreatment PSA <10 ng/ml treated with conformal external beam radiation therapy. *Int J Radiat Oncol Biol Phys.* 1998;41:1087.

70. Narayan P, Tewari A: Systematic biopsy-based staging of prostate cancer: Scientific background, individual variables, combination of parameters, and current integrative models. *Semin Urol Oncol.* 1998;16:172.

71. Wurzer JC, Al-Saleem TI, Hanlon AL, et al: Histopathologic review of prostate biopsies from patients referred to a comprehensive cancer center: Correlation of pathologic findings, analysis of cost, and impact on treatment. *Cancer.* 1998; 83:753.

72. Algan O, Pinover WH, Hanlon AL, et al: Is there a subset of patients with PSA > or = 20 ng/ml who do well after conformal beam radiotherapy? *Radiat Oncol Investig.* 1999;7:106.

73. Vargas SO, Jiroutek M, Welch WR, et al: Perineural invasion in prostate needle biopsy specimens. Correlation with extraprostatic extension at resection. *Am J Clin Pathol.* 1999;111:223.

74. Merrick GS, Butler WM, Galbreath RW, et al: Perineural invasion is not predictive of biochemical outcome following prostate brachytherapy. *Cancer J.* 2001;7:404.

75. Sebo TJ, Cheville JC, Riehle DL, et al: Predicting prostate carcinoma volume and stage at radical prostatectomy by assessing needle biopsy specimens for percent surface area and cores positive

76. Kaminski JM, Hanlon AL, Horwitz EM, et al: Relationship between prostate volume, prostate-specific antigen nadir, and biochemical control. *Int J Radiat Oncol Biol Phys.* 2002;52:888.

77. Horwitz EM, Hanlon AL, Pinover WH, et al: Defining the optimal radiation dose with three-dimensional conformal radiation therapy for patients with nonmetastatic prostate carcinoma by using recursive partitioning techniques. *Cancer.* 2001;92:1281.

78. O'Malley KJ, Pound CR, Walsh PC, et al: Influence of biopsy perineural invasion on long-term biochemical disease-free survival after radical prostatectomy. *Urology.* 2002;59:85.

79. Rubin MA, Bassily N, Sanda M, et al: Relationship and significance of greatest percentage of tumor and perineural invasion on needle biopsy in prostatic adenocarcinoma. *Am J Surg Pathol.* 2000; 24:183.

80. Kestin LL, Goldstein NS, Vicini FA, et al: Percentage of positive biopsy cores as predictor of clinical outcome in prostate cancer treated with radiotherapy. *J Urol.* 2002;168:1994.

81. Merrick GS, Butler WM, Galbreath RW, et al: Relationship between percent positive biopsies and biochemical outcome after permanent interstitial brachytherapy for clinically organ-confined carcinoma of the prostate gland. *Int J Radiat Oncol Biol Phys.* 2002;52:664.

82. D'Amico AV, Keshaviah A, Manola J, et al: Clinical utility of the percentage of positive prostate biopsies in predicting prostate cancer-specific and overall survival after radiotherapy for patients with localized prostate cancer. *Int J Radiat Oncol Biol Phys.* 2002;53:581.

83. Greene FL, Page DL, Fleming ID, et al: *AJCC Cancer Staging Manual,* 6th ed. New York: Springer; 2002.

84. Ross PL, Scardino PT, Kattan MW: A catalog of prostate cancer nomograms. *J Urol.* 2001;165:1562.

85. D'Amico AV, Whittington R, Malkowicz SB, et al: Biochemical outcome after radical prostatectomy, external beam radiation therapy, or interstitial radiation therapy for clinically localized prostate cancer. *JAMA.* 1998;280:969.

86. Zelefsky MJ, Leibel SA, Gaudin PB, et al: Dose escalation with three-dimensional conformal radiation therapy affects the outcome in prostate cancer [see comments]. *Int J Radiat Oncol Biol Phys.* 1998;41:491.

87. Le Q-T, Weinberg V, Ryu J, et al: An analysis of patients with clinically localized high-risk prostate carcinoma. *Prostate J.* 2000; 2:146.

88. Pisansky TM, Kahn MJ, Rasp GM, et al: A multiple prognostic index predictive of disease outcome after irradiation for clinically localized prostate cancer. *Cancer.* 1997;79:337.

89. Kattan MW, Potters L, Blasko JC, et al: Pretreatment nomogram for predicting freedom from recurrence after permanent prostate brachytherapy in prostate cancer. *Urology.* 2001;58:393.

90. Kattan MW, Zelefsky MJ, Kupelian PA, et al: Pretreatment nomogram for predicting the outcome of three-dimensional conformal radiotherapy in prostate cancer. *J Clin Oncol.* 2000; 18:3352.

91. Garzotto M, Higano CS, Lowe BA, et al: Neoadjuvant weekly docetaxel and mitoxantrone in patients with high risk prostate cancer, Proc ASCO. Orlando, Fla: 2002;155b.

92. Partin AW, Yoo J, Carter HB, et al: The use of prostate specific antigen, clinical stage and Gleason score to predict pathologic stage in men with localized prostate cancer. *J Urol.* 1993;150:10.

93. Blute ML, Bergstralh EJ, Iocca A, et al: Use of Gleason score, prostate specific antigen, seminal vesicle and margin status to predict biochemical failure after radical prostatectomy. *J Urol.* 2001; 165:119.

94. Blute ML, Bergstralh EJ, Partin AW, et al: Validation of Partin tables for predicting pathological stage of clinically localized prostate cancer. *J Urol.* 2000;164:1591.

95. Roach M: Equations for predicting the pathologic stage of men with localized prostate cancer using the preoperative prostate specific antigen (PSA) *and* Gleason score. *J Urol.* 1993;150:1923.

96. Spevack L, Killion LT, West JC Jr, et al: Predicting the patient at low risk for lymph node metastasis with localized prostate cancer: An analysis of four statistical models. *Int J Radiat Oncol Biol Phys.* 1996;34:543.

97. Polascik TJ, Manyak MJ, Haseman MK, et al: Comparison of clinical staging algorithms and 111indium-capromab pendetide immunoscintigraphy in the prediction of lymph node involvement in high risk prostate carcinoma patients. *Cancer*. 1999;85:1586.

98. Medica M, Giglio M, Germinale F, et al: Roach's mathematical equations in predicting pathological stage in men with clinically localized prostate cancer. *Tumori*. 2001;87:130.

99. Roach M III, Chen A, Song J, et al: Pretreatment prostate-specific antigen and Gleason score predict the risk of extracapsular extension and the risk of failure following radiotherapy in patients with clinically localized prostate cancer. *Semin Urol Oncol*. 2000; 18:108.

100. Ryu JK, Winter K, Michalski JM, et al: Interim report of toxicity from 3D conformal radiation therapy (3D-CRT) for prostate cancer on 3DOG/RTOG 9406, level III (79.2 Gy). *Int J Radiat Oncol Biol Phys*. 2002;54:1036.

101. Michalski JM, Purdy JA, Winter K, et al: Preliminary report of toxicity following 3D radiation therapy for prostate cancer on 3DOG/RTOG 9406. *Int J Radiat Oncol Biol Phys*. 2000;46:391.

102. Roach M, Weinberg V, McLaughlin P, et al: *Death Due to Prostate Cancer Following Radiotherapy (XRT) Alone: Defining Candidates For Early "Salvage" Trials, Proceedings of American Society of Clinical Oncology*. San Francisco: 2001;176a.

103. Roach M, Weinberg V, McLaughlin P, et al: Serum prostate specific antigen (PSA) and survival following external beam radiotherapy for carcinoma of the prostate. *Urology*. (In Press), 2003.

104. Weinberg V, Roach M, McLaughlin P, Sandler H: A new staging system for prostate cancer based on T-Stage, Gleason score, and PSA improves the prediction of survival. In Cox J, ed. *Proceedings of ASTRO*. San Francisco: Elsevier: 2001.

105. Brawn PN, Johnson EH, Speights DO, et al: Incidence, racial differences, and prognostic significance of prostate carcinomas diagnosed with obstructive symptoms. *Cancer*. 1994;74:1607.

106. Pilepich MV, Krall JM, Hanks GE, et al: Correlation of pretreatment transurethral resection and prognosis in patients with stage C carcinoma of the prostate treated with definitive radiotherapy—RTOG experience. *Int J Radiat Oncol Biol Phys*. 1987;13:195.

107. Landmann C, Hunig R, Rutishauser G: Adverse effect of transurethral resection on disease-free survival in locally advanced prostatic cancer treated with irradiation. *Int J Radiat Oncol Biol Phys*. 1992;26:217.

108. Kuban D, El-Mahdi AM, Schellhammer PF: Effect of local tumor control on distant metastasis and survival in prostatic adenocarcinoma. *Urology*. 1987;30:420.

109. Zelefsky MJ, Whitmore WF Jr, Leibel SA, et al: Impact of transurethral resection on the long-term outcome of patients with prostatic carcinoma. *J Urol*. 1993;150:1860.

110. Goldman HB, Israeli RS, Lerner JL, et al: Effect of prostate biopsy on the results of the PSA RT-PCR test. *Urology*. 1998;52:1073.

111. Ghossein RA, Carusone L, Bhattacharya S: Review: Polymerase chain reaction detection of micrometastases and circulating tumor cells: application to melanoma, prostate, and thyroid carcinomas. *Diagn Mol Pathol*. 1999;8:165.

112. Eschwege P, Dumas F, Blanchet P, et al: Haematogenous dissemination of prostatic epithelial cells during radical prostatectomy. *Lancet*. 1995;346:1528.

113. Thomas J, Gupta M, Grasso Y, et al: Preoperative combined nested reverse transcriptase polymerase chain reaction for prostate-specific antigen and prostate-specific membrane antigen does not correlate with pathologic stage or biochemical failure in patients with localized prostate cancer undergoing radical prostatectomy. *J Clin Oncol*. 2002;20:3213.

114. Stamey TA, Kabalin JN, McNeal JE, et al: Prostate specific antigen in the diagnosis and treatment of adenocarcinoma of the prostate. II. Radical prostatectomy treated patients. *J Urol*. 1989; 141:1076.

115. Golimbu M, Morales P, Al-Askari S, et al: Extended pelvic lymphadenectomy for prostate cancer. *J Urol*. 1979;121:617.

116. Messing EM, Manola J, Sarosdy M, et al: Immediate hormonal therapy compared with observation after radical prostatectomy and pelvic lymphadenectomy in men with node-positive prostate cancer. *N Engl J Med*. 1999;341:1781.

117. Murphy GP, Elgamal AA, Troychak MJ, et al: Follow-up ProstaScint scans verify detection of occult soft-tissue recurrence

after failure of primary prostate cancer therapy. *Prostate*. 2000; 42:315.

118. Harrison SH, Seale-Hawkins C, Dunn JK, et al: Correlation between size of palpable tumor and size of pelvic lymph node metastasis in clinically localized prostate cancer. *Cancer*. 1992;69:750.

119. Davis GL: Sensitivity of frozen section examination of pelvic lymph nodes for metastatic prostate carcinoma. *Cancer*. 1995;76:661.

120. Freeman JA, Esrig D, Grossfeld GD, et al: Incidence of occult lymph node metastases in pathological stage C (pT3N0) prostate cancer. *J Urol*. 1995;154:474.

121. Ferrari AC, Stone NN, Eyler JN, et al: Prospective analysis of prostate-specific markers in pelvic lymph nodes of patients with high-risk prostate cancer. *J Natl Cancer Inst*. 1997;89:1498.

122. Clark T, Parekh DJ, Cookson MS, et al: Randomized prospective evaluation of extended versus limited lymph node dissection in patients with clinically localized prostate cancer. *J Urol*. 2003; 169:145; discussion 147.

123. Bader P, Burkhard FC, Markwalder R, et al: Is a limited lymph node dissection an adequate staging procedure for prostate cancer? *J Urol*. 2002;168:514; discussion 518.

124. Wawroschek F, Wagner T, Hamm M, et al: The influence of serial sections, immunohistochemistry, and extension of pelvic lymph node dissection on the lymph node status in clinically localized prostate cancer. *Eur Urol*. 2003;43:132.

125. Parkin J, Keeley FX Jr, Timoney AG: Laparoscopic lymph node sampling in locally advanced prostate cancer. *BJU Int*. 2002; 89:14; discussion 17.

126. Shariat SF, Kattan MW, Erdamar S, et al: Detection of clinically significant, occult prostate cancer metastases in lymph nodes using a splice variant-specific rt-PCR assay for human glandular kallikrein. *J Clin Oncol*. 2003;21:1223.

127. Roach M, Di Silvo M, Lawton C, et al: A phase III trial comparing whole pelvic versus prostate only radiotherapy and neoadjuvant concurrent versus adjuvant combined androgen suppression: Radiation Therapy Oncology Group (RTOG) 9413. *J Clin Oncol*. 2003;21.

128. Leibel SA, Fuks Z, Zelefsky MJ, et al: The effects of local and regional treatment on the metastatic outcome in prostatic carcinoma with pelvic lymph node involvement. *Int J Radiat Oncol Biol Phys*. 1994;28:7.

129. Lawton CA, Cox JD, Glisch C, et al: Is long-term survival possible with external beam irradiation for stage D1 adenocarcinoma of the prostate? *Cancer*. 1992;69.

130. Whittington R, Malkowicz B, Barnes MM, et al: Combined hormonal and radiation therapy for lymph node-positive prostate cancer. *Urology*. 1995;46:213.

131. Hanks GE, Buzydlowski JW, Perez CA, et al: The ten year outcome of pathologic and imaging node positive patients treated with irradiation in Radiation Therapy Oncology Group (RTOG)-7506. *J Urol*. 1996;155:611A.

132. Huncharek M, Muscat JK: Serum prostate-specific antigen as a predictor of radiographic staging studies in newly diagnosed prostate cancer. *Cancer Invest*. 1995;13:31.

133. Wolf JS Jr, Cher M, Dall'era M, et al: The use and accuracy of cross-sectional imaging and fine needle aspiration cytology for detection of pelvic lymph node metastases before radical prostatectomy. *J Urol*. 1995;153:993.

134. Tiguert R, Gheiler EL, Tefilli MV, et al: Lymph node size does not correlate with the presence of prostate cancer metastasis. *Urology*. 1999;53:367.

135. Roach M III, Kurhanewicz J, Carroll P: Spectroscopy in prostate cancer: Hope or hype? *Oncology (Huntingt)*. 2001;15:1399; discussion 1415, 1418.

136. Yu KK, Scheidler J, Hricak H, et al: Prostate cancer: Prediction of extracapsular extension with endorectal MR imaging and three-dimensional proton MR spectroscopic imaging. *Radiology*. 1999; 213:481.

137. Scheidler J, Hricak H, Vigneron DB, et al: Prostate cancer: Localization with three-dimensional proton MR spectroscopic imaging—Clinicopathologic study. *Radiology*. 1999;213:473.

138. Kaji Y, Kurhanewicz J, Hricak H, et al: Localizing prostate cancer in the presence of postbiopsy changes on MR images: Role of proton MR spectroscopic imaging. *Radiology*. 1998;206:785.

139. Wefer AE, Hricak H, Vigneron DB, et al: Sextant localization of prostate cancer: Comparison of sextant biopsy, magnetic resonance imaging and magnetic resonance spectroscopic imaging with step section histology. *J Urol.* 2000;164:400.

140. Kurhanewicz J, Vigneron DB, Males RG, et al: The prostate: MR imaging and spectroscopy—Present and future. *Radiol Clin North Am.* 2000;38:115,VIII, IX.

141. Kurhanewicz J, Vigneron DB, Nelson SJ: Three-dimensional magnetic resonance spectroscopic imaging of brain and prostate cancer. *Neoplasia.* 2000;2:166.

142. Kabalin JN, Hodge KK, McNeal JE, et al: Identification of residual cancer in the prostate following radiation therapy: Role of transrectal ultrasound guided biopsy and prostatic specific antigen. *J Urol.* 1989;142:326.

143. Zelefsky MJ, Leibel SA, Gaudin PB, et al: Dose escalation with three-dimensional conformal radiation therapy affects the outcome in prostate cancer. *Int J Radiat Oncol Biol Phys.* 1998;41:491.

144. Crook J, Malone S, Perry G, et al: Postradiotherapy prostate biopsies: What do they really mean? Results for 498 patients. *Int J Radiat Oncol Biol Phys.* 2000;48:355.

145. Pollack A, Zagars GK, Antolak JA, et al: Prostate biopsy status and PSA nadir level as early surrogates for treatment failure: Analysis of a prostate cancer randomized radiation dose escalation trial. *Int J Radiat Oncol Biol Phys.* 2002;54:677.

146. Kestin LL, Goldstein NS, Vicini FA, et al: Pathologic evidence of dose-response and dose-volume relationships for prostate cancer treated with combined external beam radiotherapy and high-dose-rate brachytherapy. *Int J Radiat Oncol Biol Phys.* 2002;54:107.

147. Small EJ, Roach M III: Prostate-specific antigen in prostate cancer: A case study in the development of a tumor marker to monitor recurrence and assess response. *Semin Oncol.* 2002;29:264.

148. Geist RW: Reference range for prostate-specific antigen levels after external beam radiation therapy for adenocarcinoma of the prostate. *Urology.* 1995;45:1016.

149. Hanks GE, Perez CA, Kozar M, et al: PSA confirmation of cure at 10 years of T1b, T2, N0, M0 prostate cancer patients treated in RTOG protocol 7706 with external beam irradiation. *Int J Radiat Oncol Biol Phys.* 1994;30:289.

150. Zietman AL, Coen JJ, Shipley WU, et al: Radical radiation therapy in the management of prostatic adenocarcinoma: The initial prostate specific antigen value as a predictor of treatment outcome. *J Urol.* 1994;151:640.

151. Zelefsky MJ, Leibel SA, Wallner KE, et al: Significance of normal serum prostate-specific antigen in the follow-up period after definitive radiation therapy for prostate cancer. *J Clin Oncol.* 1995;13:459.

152. Horwitz EM, Vicini FA, Ziaja EL, et al: Assessing the variability of outcome for patients treated with localized prostate irradiation using different definitions of biochemical control. *Int J Radiat Oncol Biol Phys.* 1996;36:565.

153. Lee WR, Hanlon AL, Hanks GE: Prostate specific antigen nadir following external beam radiation therapy for clinically localized prostate cancer: The relationship between nadir level and disease-free survival [see comments]. *J Urol.* 1996;156:450.

154. Zietman AL, Tibbs MK, Dallow KC, et al: Use of PSA nadir to predict subsequent biochemical outcome following external beam radiation therapy for T1-2 adenocarcinoma of the prostate. *Radiother Oncol.* 1996;40:159.

155. Critz FA, Williams WH, Holladay CT, et al: Post-treatment PSA < or = 0.2 ng/mL defines disease freedom after radiotherapy for prostate cancer using modern techniques. *Urology.* 1999;54:968.

156. Crook JM, Choan E, Perry GA, et al: Serum prostate-specific antigen profile following radiotherapy for prostate cancer: Implications for patterns of failure and definition of cure. *Urology.* 1998;51:566.

157. Doyle KL, Roach III M, Weinberg V, et al: What does the post radiotherapy prostate specific antigen (PSA) nadir tell us about progression free survival in patients with localized prostate cancer? In Cox JD, ed. *Proceedings of the 43rd Annual ASTRO Meeting.* San Francisco: Elsevier; 2001:279.

158. Stamey T: A comparison of different irradiation therapies for prostate cancer. In Stamey T, ed. *Monographs in Urology.* Montverde, Fla: Medical Directions; 1997:121.

159. Pickett B, Ten Haken RK, Kurhanewicz J: Time course to metabolic atrophy following permanent prostate seed implantation based on magnetic resonance spectroscopic imaging. In Cox JD, ed. *Proceeding of the 44th Annual ASTRO Meeting.* New Orleans: Elsevier; 2003:31.

160. ASTRO: Consensus Statement: Guidelines for PSA Following Radiation Therapy. *Int J Radiat Oncol Biol Phys.* 1997;37:1035.

161. Sartor CI, Strawderman MH, Lin XH, et al: Rate of PSA rise predicts metastatic versus local recurrence after definitive radiotherapy. *Int J Radiat Oncol Biol Phys.* 1997;38:941.

162. Taylor JMG, Griffith KA, Sandler HM: Definitions of biochemical failure in prostate cancer following radiation therapy. *Int J Radiat Oncol Biol Phys.* 2001;50:1212.

163. Hanlon AL, Diratzouian H, Hanks GE: Posttreatment prostate-specific antigen nadir highly predictive of distant failure and death from prostate cancer. *Int J Radiat Oncol Biol Phys.* 2002;53:297.

164. Horwitz EM, Vicini FA, Ziaja EL, et al: The correlation between the ASTRO Consensus Panel definition of biochemical failure and clinical outcome for patients with prostate cancer treated with external beam irradiation. American Society of Therapeutic Radiology and Oncology. *Int J Radiat Oncol Biol Phys.* 1998;41:267.

165. Hanlon AL, Hanks GE: Scrutiny of the ASTRO consensus definition of biochemical failure in irradiated prostate cancer patients demonstrates its usefulness and robustness. American Society for Therapeutic Radiology and Oncology. *Int J Radiat Oncol Biol Phys.* 2000;46:559.

166. Vicini FA, Kestin LL, Martinez AA: The importance of adequate follow-up in defining treatment success after external beam irradiation for prostate cancer. *Int J Radiat Oncol Biol Phys.* 1999;45:553.

167. Connell PP, Ignacio L, McBride RB, et al: Caution in interpreting biochemical control rates after treatment of prostate cancer: Length of follow-up influences results. *Urology.* 1999;54:875.

168. Takamiya R, Weinberg V, Roach M, et al: A "zero slope" in post-treatment prostate specific antigen (PSA) supports "cure" of patients with long term follow-up after external beam radiation therapy (EBRT) for localized prostate cancer. In Cox, ed. *Int J Radiat Oncol Biol Phys.* San Francisco: Elsevier; 2001:298.

169. D'Amico AV, Cote K, Loffredo M, et al: Determinants of prostate cancer-specific survival after radiation therapy for patients with clinically localized prostate cancer. *J Clin Oncol.* 2002;20:4567.

170. Leibman BD, Dillioglugil O, Scardino PT, et al: Prostate-specific antigen doubling times are similar in patients with recurrence after radical prostatectomy or radiotherapy: A novel analysis. *J Clin Oncol.* 1998;16:2267.

171. Fowler JE Jr, Pandey P, Braswell NT, et al: Prostate specific antigen progression rates after radical prostatectomy or radiation therapy for localized prostate cancer. *Surgery.* 1994;116:302; discussion 305.

172. Stein A, DeKernion JB, Smith RB, et al: Prostate specific antigen levels after radical prostatectomy in patients with organ confined and locally extensive prostate cancer. *J Urol.* 1992;147:942.

173. Smitt MC, Heltzel M: The results of radical prostatectomy at a community hospital during the prostate specific antigen era. *Cancer.* 1996;77:928.

174. Iselin CE, Robertson JE, Paulson DF: Radical prostatectomy: Oncological outcome during a 20-year period. *J Urol.* 1999;161:163.

175. Ramos CG, Carvalhal GF, Smith DS, et al: Retrospective comparison of radical retropubic prostatectomy and 125iodine brachytherapy for localized prostate cancer. *J Urol.* 1999;161:1212.

176. Han M, Partin AW, Pound CR, et al: Long-term biochemical disease-free and cancer-specific survival following anatomic radical retropubic prostatectomy. The 15-year Johns Hopkins experience. *Urol Clin North Am.* 2001;28:555.

177. Amling CL, Bergstralh EJ, Blute ML, et al: Defining prostate specific antigen progression after radical prostatectomy: What is the most appropriate cut point? *J Urol.* 2001;165:1146.

178. Zincke H, Oesterling JE, Blute ML, et al: Long-term (15 years) results after radical prostatecomy for clinically localized (staged T2c or lower) prostate cancer. *J Urol.* 1994;152:1850.

179. Pruthi RS, Haese A, Huland E, et al: Use of serum concentration techniques to enhance early detection of recurrent prostate cancer after radical prostatectomy. *Urology.* 1997;49:404.

180. Shinghal R, Yemoto C, McNeal JE, et al: Biochemical recurrence without PSA progression characterizes a subset of patients after radical prostatectomy. Prostate-specific antigen. *Urology.* 2003; 61:380.

181. D'Amico AV, Whittington R, Malkowicz SB, et al: Biochemical outcome after radical prostatectomy or external beam radiation therapy for patients with clinically localized prostate carcinoma in the prostate specific antigen era. *Cancer.* 2002;95:281.

182. Roach III M: Radical prostatectomy or external beam radiotherapy: One step forward or two steps back? *Cancer.* 2002;95.

184. Memmelaar J: Total prostatovesiculectomy-retropubic approach. *J Urol.* 1949;62:340.

185. Elder JS, Jewett HJ, Walsh PC: Radical perineal prostatectomy for clinical stage B2 carcinoma of the prostate. *J Urol.* 1982; 127:704.

186. Reiner WG, Scott WW, Eggleston JC, et al: Long-term survival after hormonal therapy for stage D prostatic cancer. *J Urol.* 1979; 122:183.

187. Bianco FJ Jr, Wood DP Jr, Grignon DJ, et al: Prostate cancer stage shift has eliminated the gap in disease-free survival in black and white American men after radical prostatectomy. *J Urol.* 2002; 168:479.

188. Penson DF, Grossfeld GD, Li YP, et al: How well does the Partin nomogram predict pathological stage after radical prostatectomy in a community based population? Results of the cancer of the prostate strategic urological research endeavor. *J Urol.* 2002; 167:1653; discussion 1657.

189. Lerner SE, Blute ML, Zincke H: Risk factors for progression in patients with prostate cancer treated with radical prostatectomy. *Semin Urol Oncol.* 1996;14:12.

190. Swanson GP, Riggs MW, Earle JD, et al: Long-term follow-up of radical retropubic prostatectomy for prostate cancer. *Eur Urol.* 2002;42:212.

191. Lu-Yao GL, McLerran D, Wasson J, et al: An assessment of radical prostatectomy: Time trends, geographic variation, and outcomes. *JAMA.* 1993;269:2633.

192. Savoie M, Kim SS, Soloway MS: A prospective study measuring penile length in men treated with radical prostatectomy for prostate cancer. *J Urol.* 2003;169:1462.

193. Begg CB, Riedel ER, Bach PB, et al: Variations in morbidity after radical prostatectomy. *N Engl J Med.* 2002;346:1138.

194. Steineck G, Helgesen F, Adolfsson J, et al: Quality of life after radical prostatectomy or watchful waiting. *N Engl J Med.* 2002; 347:790.

195. Robinson JW, Moritz S, Fung T: Meta-analysis of rates of erectile function after treatment of localized prostate carcinoma. *Int J Radiat Oncol Biol Phys.* 2002;54:1063.

196. Koeman M, van Driel MF, Schultz WC, et al: Orgasm after radical prostatectomy. *Br J Urol.* 1996;77:861.

197. Katz AE, Rukstalis DB: Introduction. Recent scientific and technological advances have challenged the traditional treatment options for patients with localized prostate cancer. *Urology.* 2002;60:1.

198. Seltzer MA, Barbaric Z, Belldegrun A, et al: Comparison of helical computerized tomography, positron emission tomography and monoclonal antibody scans for evaluation of lymph node metastases in patients with prostate specific antigen relapse after treatment for localized prostate cancer. *J Urol.* 1999; 162:1322.

199. Ghafar MA, Johnson CW, De La Taille A, et al: Salvage cryotherapy using an argon based system for locally recurrent prostate cancer after radiation therapy: The Columbia experience. *J Urol.* 2001;166:1333; discussion 1337.

200. Mobley WC, Loening SA, Narayana AS: Combination perineal cryosurgery and external radiation therapy for adenocarcinoma of prostate. *Urology.* 1984;24:11.

201. Burton S, Brown DM, Colonias A, et al: Salvage radiotherapy for prostate cancer recurrence after cryosurgical ablation. *Urology.* 2000;56:833.

202. Roach M III, Lu J, Pilepich MV, et al: Long-term survival after radiotherapy alone: radiation therapy oncology group prostate cancer trials. *J Urol.* 1999;161:864.

203. Roach M III, Blasko JC, Perez CA, et al: Treatment planning for clinically localized prostate cancer. American College of Radiology. ACR appropriateness criteria. *Radiology.* 2000; 215(suppl):1441.

204. Pickett B, Vigneault E, Kurhanewicz J, et al: Static field intensity modulation to treat a dominant intra-prostatic lesion to 90 Gy compared to seven field 3-dimensional radiotherapy. *Int J Radiat Oncol Biol Phys.* 1999;44:921.

205. Boyer A, Butler EB, Dipetrillo TA, et al: Intensity-modulated radiotherapy: Current status and issues of interest. *Int J Radiat Oncol Biol Phys.* 2001;51:880.

206. Zelefsky MJ, Fuks Z, Hunt M, et al: High-dose intensity modulated radiation therapy for prostate cancer: early toxicity and biochemical outcome in 772 patients. *Int J Radiat Oncol Biol Phys.* 2002;53:1111.

207. Xia P, Pickett B, Vigneault E, et al: Forward or inversely planned segmental multileaf collimator IMRT and sequential tomotherapy to treat multiple dominant intraprostatic lesions of prostate cancer to 90 Gy. *Int J Radiat Oncol Biol Phys.* 2001; 51:244.

208. Huang E, Dong L, Chandra A, et al: Intrafraction prostate motion during IMRT for prostate cancer. *Int J Radiat Oncol Biol Phys.* 2002;53:261.

209. Roach M, Pickett B, Phillips TL: The Advantages and Limitation of Three-Dimensionally (3-D) Based Coplanar Conformal External Beam Irradiation (XRT) in the Treatment of Localized Prostate Cancer. European Association of Radiology, 1993.

210. Roach M, Pickett B, Rosenthal S, et al: Defining treatment margins for 3-D based six field conformal (SFC) irradiation of localized prostate cancer. *Int J Radiat Oncol Biol Phys.* 1994; 28:267.

211. Pickett B, Roach M, Horine P, et al: Optimization of the oblique angles in the treatment of prostate cancer during six-field conformal radiotherapy. *Med Dosim.* 1994;19:237.

212. Weil M, Pickett B, S K, et al: A three field ARC technique (3-FAT) for treating prostate cancer. *Int J Radiat Oncol Biol Phys.* 1998; 40:733.

213. Roach M, Pickett B, Weil M, et al: The "Critical Volume Tolerance Method" for estimating the limits of dose escalation during three-dimensional conformal radiotherapy for prostate cancer. *Int J Radiat Oncol Biol Phys.* 1996;35:1019.

214. Ling CC, Burman C, Chui CS, et al: Conformal radiation treatment of prostate cancer using inversely-planned intensity-modulated photon beams produced with dynamic multileaf collimation [see comments]. *Int J Radiat Oncol Biol Phys.* 1996; 35:721.

215. Zelefsky MJ, Fuks Z, Happersett L, et al: Clinical experience with intensity modulated radiation therapy (IMRT) in prostate cancer. *Radiother Oncol.* 1999; (In Press).

216. Low DA, Gerber RL, Mutic S, et al: Phantoms for IMRT dose distribution measurement and treatment verification. *Int J Radiat Oncol Biol Phys.* 1998;40:1231.

217. Teh BS, Woo SY, Mai WY, et al: Clinical experience with intensity-modulated radiation therapy (IMRT) for prostate cancer with the use of rectal balloon for prostate immobilization. *Med Dosim.* 2002;27:105.

218. Teh B, Woo SY, Butler B: Intensity modulated radiation (IMRT): A new promising technology in radiation oncology. *The Oncologist 4:* 1999;4:433.

219. Pickett B, Roach M, Verhey L, et al: The value of non-uniform margins for six-field conformal irradiation of localized prostate cancer. *Int J Radiat Oncol Biol Phys.* 1995;32:211.

220. Roach M, Pickett B, Phillips TL: *The Advantages and Limitations of Three-Dimensionally (3-D) Based Coplanar Conformal External Beam Irradiation (XRT) in the Treatment of Localized Prostate Cancer.* Geneva: European Association of Radiology 5th Workshop on 3-D Treatment Planning; 1993.

221. Shu HK, Lee TT, Vigneauly E, et al: Toxicity following high-dose three-dimensional conformal and intensity-modulated radiation therapy for clinically localized prostate cancer. *Urology.* 2001; 57:102.

222. Ling CC, Humm J, Larson S, et al: Towards multidimensional radiotherapy (MD-CRT): biological imaging and biological conformality. *Int J Radiat Oncol Biol Phys.* 2000;47:551.

223. Kurhanewicz J, Vigneron DB, Hricak H, et al: Three-dimensional H-1 MR Spectroscopic Imaging of the in Situ Human Prostate with High (0.24-0.7 cm³) Spatial Resolution. *Radiology.* 1996; 198:795.

224. Terris MK: Sensitivity and specificity of sextant biopsies in the detection of prostate cancer: Preliminary report. *Urology.* 1999; 54:486.

225. Bauer JJ, Zeng J, Zhang W, et al: Lateral biopsies added to the traditional sextant prostate biopsy pattern increases the detection rate of prostate cancer. *Prostate Cancer Prostat Dis.* 2000;3:43.

226. Tsuda K, Yu KK, Coakley FV, et al: Detection of extracapsular extension of prostate cancer: Role of fat suppression endorectal MRI. *J Comput Assist Tomogr.* 1999;23:74.

227. Pickett B, Roach M: The impact of isocenter placement errors associated with dose distributions used in irradiating prostate cancer. *Med Dosim.* 1996;21:61.

228. Roach M, Faillace-Akazawa P, Malfatti C: Prostate volumes and organ movement defined by serial CT scans during 3D conformal radiotherapy. *Radiat Oncol Investig.* 1997;5:187.

229. Langen KM, Jones DT: Organ motion and its management. *Int J Radiat Oncol Biol Phys.* 2001;50:265.

230. Lattanzi J, McNeeley S, Pinover W, et al: A comparison of daily CT localization to a daily ultrasound-based system in prostate cancer [see comments]. *Int J Radiat Oncol Biol Phys.* 1999; 43:719.

231. Balter JM, Lam KL, Sandler HM, et al: Automated localization of the prostate at the time of treatment using implanted radiopaque markers: Technical feasibility. *Int J Radiat Oncol Biol Phys.* 1995;33:1281.

232. Litzenberg D, Dawson LA, Sandler H, et al: Daily prostate targeting using implanted radiopaque markers. *Int J Radiat Oncol Biol Phys.* 2002;52:699.

233. Michèle Aubin Y-ML, Katja Langen, Katsuto Shinohara, et al: Set-up verification using portal images of implanted markers: An inter-observer study. In Cox JD, ed. *44th Annual Meeting of ASTRO.* New Orleans: ASTRO; 2002:269.

234. Langen KM PJ, Angzinos C, Aubin M, et al: Investigation of the BAT system's efficacy for daily prostate localization and repositioning. In Cox JD, ed. *44th Annual ASTRO Meeting.* New Orleans: ASTRO; 2002:317.

235. Pouliot J AM, Langen K, Liu YM, et al: Non-migration of radiopaque markers used for on-line localization of the prostate with EPID. *Int J Radiat Oncol Biol Phys.* 2003;56(3):862.

236. Homesley HD, Bundy BN, Sedlis A, et al: Radiation therapy versus pelvic node resection for carcinoma of the vulva with positive groin nodes. *Obstet Gynecol.* 1986;68:733.

237. Rotman M, Pajak TF, Choi K, et al: Prophylactic extended-field irradiation of para-aortic lymph nodes in stages IIB and bulky IB and IIA cervical carcinomas: Ten-year treatment results of RTOG 79-20. *JAMA.* 1995;274:387.

238. Ragaz J, Jackson S, Le N, et al: Adjuvant radiotherapy and chemotherapy in node-positive premonopausal women with breast cancer. *N Engl J Med.* 1997;337:956.

239. Overgaard M, Hansen P, Overgaard J, et al: Postoperative radiotherapy in high-risk premenopausal women with breast cancer who receive adjuvant chemotherapy. *N Engl J Med.* 1997;337:949.

240. Ploysongsang S, Aron B, Seiiata W, et al: Comparison of whole pelvis versus small-field radiation therapy for carcinoma of prostate. *Urology.* 1986;17:10.

241. McGowan DG: The value of extended field radiation therapy in carcinoma of the prostate. *Int J Radiat Oncol Biol Phys.* 1981; 7:1333.

242. Seaward S, Weinberg V, Lewis P, et al: Improved freedom from PSA failure with whole pelvic irradiation for high risk prostate cancer. *Int J Radiat Oncol Biol Phys.* 1998;42:1055.

243. Seaward SA, Weinberg V, Lewis P, et al: Identification of a high-risk clinically localized prostate cancer subgroup receiving maximum benefit from whole-pelvic irradiation. *Cancer J of Sci Am.* 1998;4(6):370.

244. Pan CC, Kim KY, Taylor JM, et al: Influence of 3D-CRT pelvic irradiation on outcome in prostate cancer treated with external beam radiotherapy. *Int J Radiat Oncol Biol Phys.* 2002; 53:1139.

245. Rasp G, Pisansky T, Haddock M, et al: Elective pelvic nodal irradiation in patients with clinically localized prostate cancer at high risk for pelvic nodal involvement. *Int J Radiat Oncol Biol Phys.* 1996;36:245, #1003.

246. Asbell SO, Krall JM, Pilepich MV, et al: Elective pelvic irradiation in stage A2, B carcinoma of the prostate: Analysis of RTOG 77-06. *Int J Radiat Oncol Biol Phys.* 1988;15:1307.

247. Forman JD, Lee Y, Roberson P, et al: Advantages of CT and beam's eye view display to confirm the accuracy of pelvic lymph node irradiation in carcinoma of the prostate. *Radiology.* 1993; 186:889.

248. Kestin L, Goldstein N, Vicini F, et al: Treatment of prostate cancer with radiotherapy: should the entire seminal vesicles be included in the clinical target volume? *Int J Radiat Oncol Biol Phys.* 2002; 54:686.

249. Diaz AZ, Roach M, Marquez C, et al: Indications for and significance of including the seminal vesicles during 3-D conformal radiotherapy in men with clinically localized prostate cancer. *Int J Radiat Oncol Biol Phys.* 1994;30:323.

250. Hricak H, Jeffrey B, Dooms GC, et al: Evaluation of prostate size: A comparison of ultrasound and magnetic resonance imaging. *Urol Radiol.* 1987;9:1.

251. Roach M, Faillace-Akazawa P, Malfatti C, et al: Prostate volumes defined by magnetic resonance imaging and computerized tomographic scans for three-dimensional conformal radiotherapy. *Int J Radiat Oncol Biol Phys.* 1996;35:1011.

252. Lee WR, Roach M III, Michalski J, et al: Interobserver variability leads to significant differences in quantifiers of prostate implant adequacy. *Int J Radiat Oncol Biol Phys.* 2002;54:457.

253. Pilepich MV, Prasad SC, Perez CA: Computed tomography in definitive radiotherapy of prostatic carcinoma, Part 2: Definition of target volume. *Int J Radiat Oncol Biol Phys.* 1982;8:235.

254. Malone S, Donker R, Broader M, et al: Effects of urethrography on prostate position: Considerations for radiotherapy treatment planning of prostate carcinoma. *Int J Radiat Oncol Biol Phys.* 2000;46:89.

255. Mah D, Freedman G, Movsas B, et al: To move or not to move: Measurements of prostate motion by urethrography using MRI. *Int J Radiat Oncol Biol Phys.* 2001;50:947.

256. Liu Y-M, Ling SM, Shinohara K, et al: *Prostate Movement During Simulation Due to Retrograde Urethrography Compared with "Natural" Prostate Movement.* 88th Scientific Assembly and Annual Meeting Radiological Society of North America, 2002, Chicago.

257. Malone S, Szanto J, Perry G, et al: A prospective comparison of three systems of patient immobilization for prostate radiotherapy. Int J Radiat Oncol Biol Phys. 2000;48:657.

258. Song PY, Washington M, Vaida F, et al: A comparison of four patient immobilization devices in the treatment of prostate cancer patients with three dimensional conformal radiotherapy. *Int J Radiat Oncol Biol Phys.* 1996;34:213.

259. Malone S, Crook JM, Kendal WS, et al: Respiratory-induced prostate motion: Quantification and characterization. *Int J Radiat Oncol Biol Phys.* 2000;48:105.

260. Kitamura K, Shirato H, Seppenwoolde Y, et al: Three-dimensional intrafractional movement of prostate measured during real-time tumor-tracking radiotherapy in supine and prone treatment positions. *Int J Radiat Oncol Biol Phys.* 2002; 53:1117.

261. El-Gayed AAH, Bel A, Vijlbrief R, et al: Time trend of patient setup deviations during pelvic irradiation using electronic portal imaging. *Radiother Oncol.* 1993;26:162.

262. Barringer B: Radium in the treatment of carcinoma of bladder and prostate: Review of one year's work. *JAMA.* 1917; 68:1227.

263. Aronowitz JN: Dawn of prostate brachytherapy: 1915-1930. *Int J Radiat Oncol Biol Phys.* 2002;54:712.

264. Whitmore WF, Hilaris B, Grabstald H: Retropubic implantation of Iodine 125 in the treatment of prostatic cancer. *J Urol.* 1972; 108:918.

265. Kuban DA, El-Mahdi A, Schellhammer PF: I-125 interstitial implantation for prostate cancer. What have we learned 10 years later? *Cancer.* 1989;63:2415.

266. Fuks Z, Leibel SA, Wallner KE, et al: The effect of local control on metastatic dissemination in carcinoma of the prostate: Long term results in patients treated with 125-I implantation. *Int J Radiat Oncol Biol Phys.* 1991;21:337.

267. Holm HH, Juul N, Pederson JF, et al: Transperineal 125-Iodine seed implantation in prostatic cancer guided by transrectal ultrasonography. *J Urol.* 1983;130:282.

268. Blasko JC, Ragde H, Schumacher D: Transperineal percutaneous iodine-125 implantation for prostatic carcinoma using transrectal ultrasound and template guidance. *Endo Hypertherm Oncol.* 1987;3:131.

269. Charyulu KKN: Transperineal interstitial implantation of prostate cancer: A new method. *Int J Radiat Oncol Biol Phys.* 1980; 6:1261.

270. Osian AD, Anderson LL, Linares LA, et al: Treatment planning for permanent and temporary percutaneous implants with custom made templates. *Int J Radiat Oncol Biol Phys.* 1989; 16:219.

271. Merrick GS, Butler WM, Tollenaar BG, et al: The dosimetry of prostate brachytherapy-induced urethral strictures. *Int J Radiat Oncol Biol Phys.* 2002;52:461.

272. Merrick GS, Butler WM, Wallner KE, et al: Extracapsular radiation dose distribution after permanent prostate brachytherapy. *Am J Clin Oncol.* 2003;26:178.

273. Merrick GS, Butler WM: Modified uniform seed loading for prostate brachytherapy: rationale, design, and evaluation. *Tech Urol.* 2000;6:78.

274. Wallner K, Blasko J, Dattoli M: Radiobiology. In Wallner K, Blasko J, Dattoli M, eds. *Prostate Brachytherapy Made Complicated*, 2nd ed. Seattle: SmartMedicine Press; 2001:3.1.

275. Orton CG, Webber BM: Time-dose factor (TDF) analysis of dose rate effects in permanent implant dosimetry. *Int J Radiat Oncol Biol Phys.* 1977;2:55.

276. Ling CC: Permanent implants using Au-198, Pd-103 and I-125: Radiobiological considerations based on the linear quadratic model. *Int J Radiat Oncol Biol Phys.* 1992;23:81.

277. Wang JZ, Guerrero M, Li A: How low is the alpha/beta ratio for prostate cancer? *Int J Rad Oncol Biol Phys.* 2003;55:194.

278. Wallner K: Prostate brachytherapy under local anesthesia: Lessons from the first 600 patients. *Brachytherapy.* 2002;1:145.

279. Stock RG, Lo Y, Gaildon M, et al: Does prostate brachytherapy treat the seminal vesicles: A dose-volume histogram analysis of seminal vesicles in patients undergoing combined Pd-103 prostate implantation and external beam irradiation. *Int J Radiat Oncol Biol Phys.* 1999;45:385.

280. Dattoli M, Wallner K, True L, et al: Long-term outcomes following EBRT + Pd-103 for higher risk prostatic carcinoma: Influence of prostatic acid phosphatase. *Cancer.* 2003;97:979.

281. Blasko JC, Grimm PD, Sylvester JE, et al: The role of external beam radiotherapy with I-125/Pd-103 brachytherapy for prostate carcinoma. *Radiother Oncol.* 2000;57:273.

282. D'Amico AV, Whittington R, Malkowicz SB, et al: Biochemical outcome after radical prostatectomy, external beam radiation therapy, or interstitial radiation therapy for clinically localized prostate cancer. *JAMA.* 1998;280:969.

283. Terk MD, Stock RG, Stone NN: Identification of patients at increased risk for prolonged urinary retention following radioactive seed implantation of the prostate. *J Urol.* 1998;160:1379.

284. Landis D, Wallner K, Locke J, et al: Late urinary morbidity after prostate brachytherapy. 2002;1:21.

285. Sanguineti G, Agostinelli S, Foppiano F, et al: Adjuvant androgen deprivation impacts late rectal toxicity after conformal radiotherapy of prostate carcinoma. *Br J Cancer.* 2002;86:1843.

286. Bellon J, Wallner K, Ellis W, et al: Use of pelvic CT scanning to evaluate pubic arch interference of transperineal prostate brachytherapy. *Int J Radiat Oncol Biol Phys.* 1999;43:579.

287. Wallner K, Blasko J, Dattoli M: Technique. In Wallner K, Blasko J, Dattoli M, eds. *Prostate Brachytherapy Made Complicated*, 2nd ed. Seattle: SmartMedicine Press; 2001:8,1.

288. Tincher SA, Kim RY, Ezekiel MP, et al: Effects of pelvic rotation and needle angle on pubic arch interference during transperineal prostate implants. *Int J Radiat Oncol Biol Phys.* 2000;47:361.

289. Stone NN, Stock RG: Prostate brachytherapy in patients with prostate volumes >/= 50 cm(3): Dosimetic analysis of implant quality. *Int J Radiat Oncol Biol Phys.* 2000;46:1199.

290. Wang H, Wallner K, Sutlief S, et al: Transperineal brachytherapy in patients with large prostate glands. *Int J Cancer.* 2000; 90:199.

291. Loblaw DA, Wallner K, Dibiase S, et al: Brachytherapy in patients with small prostate glands. *Tech Urol.* 2000;6:64.

292. Merrick GS, Butler WM, Lief JH, et al: Temporal resolution of urinary morbidity following prostate brachytherapy. *Int J Radiat Oncol Biol Phys.* 2000;47:121.

293. Wallner K, Roy J, Harrison L: Tumor control and morbidity following transperineal Iodine 125 implantation for stage T1/T2 prostatic carcinoma. *J Clin Oncol.* 1996;14:449.

294. Yap J, Wallner K, Gray G: Cystourethroscopic findings and long-term urinary function after prostate brachytherapy. *J Brachytherapy Int.* 2000;16:257.

295. Gray G, Wallner K, Roof J, et al: Cystourethroscopic findings before and after prostate brachytherapy. *Tech Urol.* 2000; 6:109.

296. Wallner K, Merrick G, True L, et al: I-125 versus Pd-103 for low risk prostate cancer: Morbidity outcomes from a prospective randomized multicenter trial. *Ca J Sci American.* 2002;8:67.

297. Blasko JC, Ragde H, Grimm PD: Transperineal ultrasound-guided implantation of the prostate: Morbidity and complications. *Scand J Urol Nephrol Suppl.* 1991;137:113.

298. Wallner K, Lee H, Wasserman S, et al: Low risk of urinary incontinence following prostate brachytherapy in patients with a prior TURP. *Int J Radiat Oncol Biol Phys.* 1997;37:565.

299. Stone NN, Ratnow ER, Stock RG: Prior transurethral resection does not increase morbidity following real-time ultrasound-guided prostate seed implantation. *Tech Urol.* 2000;6:123.

300. Merrick GS, Butler WM, Galbreath RW, et al: Five year biochemical outcome after prostate brachytherapy for hormone-naive men ≤62 years of age. *Int J Radiat Oncol Biol Phys.* 2001;51:41.

301. Hughes S, Wallner K, Miller G, et al: Pre-existing histologic evidence of prostatitis is unrelated to post-implant urinary morbidity. *Radiat Oncol Invest.* 2001;96(suppl):79.

302. Li P, Wallner K, Ellis W, et al: Prostate brachytherapy in patients with a penile prosthesis. *Br J Urol.* 2001;7:712.

303. Watson LR: Ultrasound anatomy for prostate brachytherapy. *Semin Urol Oncol.* 1997;13:391.

304. Nguyen J, Wallner K, Han B, et al: Increased long-term urinary morbidity in brachytherapy patients with median lobe hyperplasia. *Brachytherapy.* 2002;1:42.

305. Din K, Wildt M, Wijkstra H, et al: The correlation between urodynamic and cystoscopic findings in elderly men with voiding complaints. *J Urol.* 1996;155:1018.

306. Wallner KE, Smathers S, Sutlief S, et al: Prostate brachytherapy in patients with median lobe hyperplasia. *Int J Cancer.* 2000;90:152.

307. Rockhill J, Wallner K, Hoffman C, et al: Prostate brachytherapy in massively obese patients. *Brachytherapy.* 2002;1:54.

308. Merrick G, Butler W, Wallner K, et al: Permanent prostate brachytherapy-induced morbidity in patients with grade II and III obesity. *Urology.* 2002;60:104.

309. Willett CG, Ooi C, Zietman AL, et al: Acute and late toxicity of patients with inflammatory bowel disease undergoing irradiation for abdominal and pelvic neoplasms. *Int J Radiat Oncol Biol Phys.* 2000;46:995.

310. Leibel SA, Heimann R, Kutcher GJ: Three-dimensional conformal radiation therapy in locally advanced carcinoma of the prostate: Preliminary results of a phase I dose-escalation study. *Int J Radiat Oncol Biol Phys.* 1993;26:55.

311. Grann A, Wallner K: Prostate brachytherapy in patients with inflammatory bowel disease. *Int J Radiat Oncol Biol Phys.* 1998; 40:135.

312. Wong WW, Schild SE, Sawyer TE, et al: Analysis of outcome in patients reirradiated for brain metastases. *Int J Radiat Oncol Biol Phys.* 1996;34:585.

313. Beyer DC: Permanent brachytherapy as salvage treatment for recurrent prostate cancer. *Urology.* 1999;54:880.

314. Battermann JJ: Feasibility of permanent implants for prostate cancer after previous radiotherapy in the true pelvis. *Radiother Oncol.* 2000;57:297.

315. Grado GL, Collins JM, Kriegshauser JS, et al: Salvage brachytherapy for localized prostate cancer after radiotherapy failure. *Urology.* 1999;53:2.

316. Potters L, Cao Y, Calugaru E, et al: A comprehensive review of CT-based dosimetry parameters and biochemical control in patients treated with permanent prostate brachytherapy. *Int J Radiat Oncol Biol Phys.* 2001;50:605.

317. Stock RG, Stone NN, Dahlal M, et al: What is the optimal dose for 125-I prostate implant? A dose-response analysis of biochemical control, posttreatment prostate biopsies, and long-term symptoms. *Brachytherapy.* 2002;1:83.

318. Choi S, Wallner KE, Merrick G, Butler W: Treatment margins predict PSA outcome after Pd-103 prostate brachytherapy. *Brachytherapy.* 2004: (In press).

319. ICRU: Prescribing, recording, and reporting photon beam therapy. ICRU Report 50:1-8, 1993.

320. Mueller A, Wallner K, Merrick G, et al: Modification of prostate implants based on post-implant treatment margin assessment. *Med Phys.* 2003;29:2782.

321. Davis BJ, Pisansky TM, Wilson TM, et al: The radial distance of extraprostatic extension of prostate carcinoma: implications for prostate brachytherapy. *Cancer.* 1999;85:2630.

322. Sohayda C, Kupelian PA, Levin JS, et al: Extent of extracapsular extension in localized prostate cancer. *Urology.* 2000; 55:382.

323. Speight JL, Shinohara K, Pickett B, et al: Prostate volume change after radioactive seed implantation: Possible benefit of improved dose volume histogram with perioperative steroid. *Int J Radiat Oncol Biol Phys.* 2000;48:1461.

324. Willins J, Wallner KE: Time-dependent changes in CT-based dosimetry of I-125 prostate brachytherapy. *Radiat Oncol Invest.* 1998;6:157.

325. Waterman FM, Yue N, Corn BW, et al: Edema associated with I-125 or Pd-103 prostate brachytherapy and its impact on postimplant dosimetry: an analysis based on serial CT acquistion. *Int J Radiat Oncol Biol Phys.* 1998;41:1069.

326. Han B, Wallner K, Aggarwal S, et al: Treatment margins for prostate brachytherapy. *Semin Urol Oncol.* 2000;18:137.

327. Butzbach D, Waterman FM, Dicker AP: Can extraprostatic extension be treated by prostate brachytherapy? An analysis based on postimplant dosimetry. *Int J Radiat Oncol Biol Phys.* 2001; 51:1196.

328. Dattoli MJ, Wallner KE, Sorace R, et al: Planned extracapsular seed placement using palladium-103 for prostate brachytherapy. *J Brachyther Int.* 2000;16:35.

329. Davis BJ, Haddock MG, Wilson TM, et al: Treatment of extraprostatic cancer in clinically organ-confined prostate cancer by permanent interstitial brachytherapy: Is extraprostatic seed placement necessary? *Tech Urol.* 2000;6:70.

330. D'Amico AV, Davis A, Vargas SO, et al: Defining the implant treatment volume for patients with low risk prostate cancer: Does the anterior base need to be treated? *Int J Radiat Oncol Biol Phys.* 1999;43:587.

331. Wallner KE, Roy J, Harrison L: Dosimetry guidelines to minimize urethral and rectal morbidity following transperineal I-125 prostate brachytherapy. *Int J Radiat Oncol Biol Phys.* 1995; 32:465.

332. Nag S, Beyer D, Friedland J, et al: American Brachytherapy Society (ABS) recommendations for transperineal permanent brachytherapy of prostate cancer. *Int J Radiat Oncol Biol Phys.* 1999;44:789.

333. Jones S, Wallner K, Merrick G, et al: Clinical correlates of high brachytherapy dose regions within the prostate. IJROBP 2002; 53:328-33.

334. Maguire PD, Waterman FM, Dicker AP: Can the cost of permanent prostate implants be reduced? An argument for peripheral loading with higher strength seeds. *Tech Urol.* 2000; 6:85.

335. Cumes DM, Goffinet DR, Martinez A, et al: Complications of 125-Iodine implantation and pelvic lymphadenectomy for prostatic cancer with special reference to patients who had failed external beam therapy as their initial mode of therapy. *J Urol.* 1981;126:620.

336. Shearer RJ, Davies JH, Gelister JSK, et al: Hormonal cytoreduction and radiotherapy for carcinoma of the prostate. *Br J Urol.* 1992;69:521.

337. Stock RG, Stone NN, Wesson MF, et al: A modified technique allowing interactive ultrasound-guided three-dimensional transperineal prostate implantation. *Int J Radiat Oncol Biol Phys.* 1995;32:219.

338. Gewanter RM, Wuu C, Laguna JL, et al: Intraoperative preplanning for transperineal ultrasound-guided permanent prostate brachytherapy. *Int J Radiat Oncol Biol Phys.* 2000;48:377.

339. Messing EM, Zhang JBY, Rubens DJ, et al: Intraoperative optimized inverse planning for prostate brachytherapy: early experience. *Int J Radiat Oncol Biol Phys.* 1999;44:801.

340. Beyer DC, Shapiro RH, Puente F: Real-time optimized intraoperative dosimetry for prostate brachytherapy: A pilot study. *Int J Radiat Oncol Biolo Phys.* 2000;48:1583.

341. Syed AM, Puthawala A, Austin P, et al: Temporary iridium-192 implant in the management of carcinoma of the prostate. *Cancer.* 1992;69:2515.

342. Grimm PD, Blasko JC, Sylvester JE, et al: 10-year biochemical (prostate specific antigen) control of prostate cancer with I-125 brachytherapy. *Int J Radiat Oncol Biol Phys.* 2001; 51:31.

343. Zelefsky MJ, Hollister T, Raben A, et al: Five-year biochemical outcome and toxicity with transperineal CT-planned permanent I-125 prostate implantation for patients with localized prostate cancer. *Int J Radiat Oncol Biol Phys.* 2000;47:1261.

344. Sharkey J, Chovnick SD, Behar RJ, et al: Minimally invasive treatment for localized adenocarcinoma of the prostate: Review of 1048 patients treated with ultrasound-guided palladium-103 brachytherapy. *J Endourol.* 2000;14:343.

345. Wallner K, Blasko J, Dattoli M: Supplemental beam radiation. In Wallner K, Blasko J, Dattoli M, eds. *Prostate Brachytherapy Made Complicated*, 2nd ed. Seattle: SmartMedicine Press; 2001:11.1.

346. Corriveau J, Wallner K, Merrick G, et al: Morbidity effect of the time gap between supplemental beam radiation and Pd-103 prostate brachytherapy. *Brachytherapy.* 2003;2:118.

347. Ghaly M, Wallner K, Merrick G, et al: The effect of supplemental beam radiation on prostate brachytherapy-related morbidity: Morbidity outcomes from two prospective randomized multicenter trials. *Int J Radiat Oncol Biol Phys.* in press, 2003.

348. Mueller A, Wallner K, Corriveau J, et al: A reappraisal of local anesthesia for prostate brachytherapy. *Radiother Oncol.* in press, 2003.

349. Seddon R, Wallner K, Walker J: Revisiting the cost of prostate brachytherapy: VAPSHCS experience. *Oncol News Internat.* 2002;11:37.

350. Merrick GS, Butler WM, Dorsey AT, et al: Influence of prophylactic dexamethasone on edema following prostate brachytherapy. *Tech Urol.* 2000;6:117.

351. Sylvester J, Grimm P, Blasko J, et al: Urethral visualization during transperineal interstitial brachytherapy for early stage prostate cancer. *J Brachytherapy Int.* 2000;16:145.

352. Smith S, Wallner K, Merrick G, et al: Interpretation of pre- versus post-implant TRUS images. *Med Phys.* in press, 2003.

353. Lattanzi J, McNeely S, Hanlon A, et al: Daily CT localization for correcting portal errors in the treatment of prostate cancer. *Int J Radiat Oncol Biol Phys.* 1998;41:1079.

354. Taschereau R, Pouliet J, Roy J, et al: Seed misplacement and stabilizing needles in transperineal permanent prostate implants. *Radiother Oncol.* 2000;55:59.

355. Potters L, Cao YJ, Calugaru E, et al: A comprehensive review of CT-based dosimetry parameters and biochemical control in patients treated with permanent prostate brachytherapy. *Int J Radiat Oncol Biol Phys.* 2001;50:605.

356. Badiozamani KR, Wallner KE, Cavanagh W, et al: Comparability of CT-based and TRUS-based prostate volumes. *Int J Radiat Oncol Biol Phys.* 1999;43:375.

357. Amdur RJ, Gladstone D, Leopold KA, et al: Prostate seed implant quality assessment using MR and CT image fusion. *Int J Radiat Oncol Biol Phys.* 1999;43:67.

358. Gong L, Cho P, Han B, et al: Registration of prostate brachytherapy seeds with prostate anatomy for postimplant dosimetry. *Int J Rad Oncol Biol Phys.* 2002;54:1322.

359. Roy JN, Wallner KE, Harrington PJ, et al: A CT-based evaluation method for permanent implants: Application to prostate. *Int J Radiat Oncol Biol Phys.* 1993;26:163.

360. Prestidge BR, Bice WS, Kiefer EJ, et al: Timing of computed tomography-based postimplant assessment following permanent

transperineal prostate brachytherapy. *Int J Radiat Oncol Biol Phys.* 1998;40:1111.

361. Merrick GS, Butler WM, Dorsey AT, et al: Influence of timing on the dosimetric analysis of transperineal ultrasound-guided, prostatic conformal brachytherapy. *Radiat Oncol Invest.* 1998; 6:182.

362. Waterman FM, Dicker AP: Impact of postimplant edema on V100 and D90 in prostate brachytherapy: Can implant quality be predicted on day 0? *Int J Radiat Oncol Biol Phys.* 2002; 53:610.

363. Chen Z, Yue N, Wang X, et al: Dosimetric effects of edema in permanent prostate seed implants: A rigorous solution. *Int J Radiat Oncol Biol Phys.* 2000;47:1405.

364. Han BH, Demel KC, Wallner KE, et al: Patient reported short-term complications after prostate brachytherapy. *J Urol.* (in press), 2001.

365. Hu K, Wallner KE: Urinary incontinence in patients who have a TURP/TUIP following prostate brachytherapy. *Int J Radiat Oncol Biol Phys.* 1998;40:783.

366. Barker J, Wallner K, Merrick G: Gross hematuria after prostate brachytherapy. *Urology.* in press, 2003.

367. Gelblum DY, Potters L, Ashley R, et al: Urinary morbidity following ultrasound-guided transperineal prostate seed implantation. *Int J Radiat Oncol Biol Phys.* 1999;45:59.

368. Merrick GS, Butler WM, Wallner KE, et al: Prophylactive versus therapeutic alpha blockers following permanent prostate brachytherapy. *Urology.* 2002;60:650.

369. Obek C, Neulander E, Sadek S, et al: Is there a role for digital rectal examination in the follow-up of patients after radical prostatectomy? *J Urol.* 1999;162:762.

370. Pound CR, Christens-Barry OW, Gurganus RT, et al: Digital rectal examination and imaging studies are unnecessary in men with undetectable prostate specific antigen following radical prostatectomy. *J Urol.* 1999;162:1337.

371. Merrick GS, Butler WM, Wallner KE, et al: Prostate specific antigen (PSA) spikes following permanent prostate brachytherapy. *Int J Radiat Oncol Biol Phys.* 2002;54:450.

372. Cavanagh W, Blasko JC, Grimm PD, et al: Transient elevation of serum prostate-specific antigen following I-125/Pd-103 brachytherapy for localized prostate cancer. *Semin Urol Oncol.* 2000;18:160.

373. Critz FA, Williams WH, Benton JB, et al: Prostate specific antigen bounce after radioactive seed implantation followed by external beam radiation for prostate cancer. *J Urol.* 2000;163:1085.

374. Kuban DA, El-Mahdi AM, Schellhammer P: The significance of post-irradiation prostate biopsy with long-term follow-up. *Int J Radiat Oncol Biol Phys.* 1992;24:409.

375. Scardino PT, Wheeler TM: Prostatic biopsy after irradiation therapy for prostatic cancer. *Urology.* 1985;25:39.

376. Prestidge BR, Hoak DC, Grimm PD, et al: Posttreatment biopsy results following interstitial brachytherapy in early-stage prostate cancer. *Int J Radiat Oncol Biol Phys.* 1997;37:31.

377. Zelefsky MJ, Leibel SA, Gaudin PB, et al: Dose escalation with three-dimensional conformal radiation therapy affects the outcome in prostate cancer. *Int J Radiat Oncol Biol Phys.* 1998; 41:491.

378. Smathers S, Wallner K, Sprouse J, et al: Temporary PSA rises and repeat prostate biopsies after brachytherapy. *Int J Radiat Oncol Biol Phys.* 2001.

379. Reed D, Wallner K, Merrick G, et al: Clinical correlates to PSA spikes and positive repeat biopsies after prostate brachytherapy. Submitted, 2003.

380. Dicker AP, Lin C-C, Leeper DB, et al: Isotope selection for permanent prostate implants? An evaluation of 103-Pd versus 125-I based on radiobiological effectiveness and dosimetry. *Semin Urol Oncol.* 2000;18:152.

381. Butler WM, Merrick GS: I-125 Rapid Strand* loading technique. *Radiat Oncol Invest.* 1996;4:48.

382. Lessard E, Pouliot J: Inverse planning anatomy-based dose optimization for HDR-brachytherapy of the prostate using fast simulated annealing algorithm and dedicated objective function. *Med Phys.* 2001;28:773.

383. Kolkman-Deurloo IKK, Visser AG, Niël CGJH, et al: Optimization of interstitial volume implants. *Radiother Oncol.* 1994;31:229.

384. Brenner DJ, Hall EJ: Fractionation and protraction for radiotherapy of prostate carcinoma. *Int J Radiat Oncol Biol Phys.* 1999;43:1095.

385. King CR, Fowler JF: A simple analytic derivation suggests that prostate cancer alpha/beta ratio is low. [Comment In: *Int J Radiat Oncol Biol Phys.* 2001;51:1 UI: 21407940]. *Int J Radiat Oncol Biol Phys.* 2001;51:213.

386. Fowler J, Chappell R, Ritter M: Is alpha/beta for prostate tumors really low? *Int J Radiat Oncol Biol Phys.* 2001;50:1021.

387. Duchesne GM, Peters LJ: What is the alpha/beta ratio for prostate cancer? Rationale for hypofractionated high-dose-rate brachytherapy [editorial]. *Int J Radiat Oncol Biol Phys.* 1999;44:747.

388. D'Souza WD, Thames HD: Is the alpha/beta ratio for prostate cancer low? [Comment On: *Int J Radiat Oncol Biol Phys.* 2001;51:213 UI: 21407968]. *Int J Radiat Oncol Biol Phys.* 2001;51:1.

389. Gottschalk A, Roach M: Radiobiology: Old, present, future, and practical considerations. In Grossfeld CA, ed. *Prostate Cancer.* Hamilton, Ontario: BC Decker; 2002.

390. Russell KJ, Caplan RJ, Laramore GE, et al: Photon versus fast neutron external beam radiotherapy in the treatment of locally advanced prostate cancer: Results of a randomized prospective trial. *Int J Radiat Oncol Biol Phys.* 1994;28:47.

391. Shipley WU, Verhey LJ, Munzenrider JE, et al: Advanced prostate cancer: The results of a randomized comparative trial of high dose irradiation boosting with conformal protons compared with conventional dose irradiation using photons alone. *Int J Radiat Oncol Biol Phys.* 1995;32:3.

392. Shipley WU, Zietman AL, Hanks GE, et al: Treatment related sequelae following external beam radiation for prostate cancer: A review with an update in patients with stages T1 and T2 tumor [see comments]. *J Urol.* 1994;152:1799.

393. Dearnaley DP, Khoo VS, Norman AR, et al: Comparison of radiation side-effects of conformal and conventional radiotherapy in prostate cancer: A randomised trial. *Lancet.* 1999;353:267.

394. Nguyen LN, Pollack A, Zagars GK: Late effects after radiotherapy for prostate cancer in a randomized dose-response study: results of a self-assessment questionnaire. *Urology.* 1998;51:991.

395. Pollack A, Zagars GK, Starkschall G, et al: Prostate cancer radiation dose response: Results of the M. D. Anderson phase III randomized trial. *Int J Radiat Oncol Biol Phys.* 2002;53:1097.

396. Lee WR, Hanks GE, Hanlon AL, et al: Lateral rectal shielding reduces late rectal morbidity following high dose three-dimensional conformal radiation therapy for clinically localized prostate cancer: Further evidence for a significant dose effect [see comments]. *Int J Radiat Oncol Biol Phys.* 1996;35:251.

397. Michalski JM, Winter K, Purdy JA, et al: Trade-off to low-grade toxicity with conformal radiation therapy for prostate cancer on Radiation Therapy Oncology Group 9406. *Semin Radiat Oncol.* 2002;12:75.

398. Shu H-KG, Lee TT, Vigneualt E, et al: Toxicity following high dose three-dimensional conformal and intensity modulated radiation therapy (IMRT) for clinically localized prostate cancer. *Urology.* 2001;57:102.

399. Talcott JA, Clark JC, Start P, et al: *Long-Term Treatment-Related Complications of Brachytherapy for Early Prostate Cancer: A Survey of Treated Patients.* Atlanta: Proceedings of ASCO; 1999:311a.

400. Merrick GS, Butler WM, Dorsey AT, et al: Rectal function following prostate brachytherapy. *Int J Radiat Oncol Biol Phys.* 2000;48:667.

401. Gelblum DY, Potters L: Rectal complications associated with transperineal interstitial brachytherapy for prostate cancer. *Int J Radiat Oncol Biol Phys.* 2000;48:119.

402. Han B, Wallner K: Dosimetric and radiographic correlates to prostate brachytherapy-related rectal complications. *Int J Cancer.* 2002;96:372.

403. Snyder KM, Stock RG, Hong SM, et al: Defining the risk of developing grade 2 proctitis following 125-I prostate brachytherapy using a rectal dose-volume histogram analysis. *Int J Rad Oncol Biol Phys.* 2001;50:335.

404. Smith S, Wallner K, Han B, et al: Argon plasma coagulation for rectal bleeding following prostate brachytherapy. *Int J Radiat Oncol Biol Phys.* 2001;51:636.

405. Hu K, Wallner K: Clinical course of rectal complications following I-125 prostate brachytherapy. *Int J Radiat Oncol Biol Phys.* 1998;41:263.

406. Howard A, Wallner K, Han B, et al: Clinical course and dosimetry of rectal fistulas after prostate brachytherapy. *J Brachytherapy Int.* 2001;17:37.

407. Theodorescu D, Gillenwater JY, Koutrouvelis PG: Prostatourethral-rectal fistula after prostate brachytherapy: Incidence and risk factors. *Cancer.* 2000;89:2085.

408. Wallner K, Blasko J, Dattoli M: Morbidity. In Wallner K, Blasko J, Dattoli M, eds. *Prostate Brachytherapy Made Complicated*, 2nd ed. Seattle: SmartMedicine Press; 2001:15.1.

409. Patel J, Worthen R, Abadir R, et al: Late results of combined Iodine-125 and external beam radiotherapy in carcinoma of prostate. *Urology.* 1990;36:27.

410. Zeitlin SI, Sherman J, Raboy A, et al: High dose combination radiotherapy for the treatment of localized prostate cancer. *J Urol.* 1998;160:91.

411. Teshima T, Hanks GE, Hanlon AL, et al: Rectal bleeding after conformal 3D treatment of prostate cancer: Time to occurrence, response to treatment and duration of morbidity. *Int J Radiat Oncol Biol Phys.* 1997;39:77.

412. Crook J, Esche B, Futter N: Effect of pelvic radiotherapy for prostate cancer on bowel, bladder, and sexual function: The patient's perspective. *Urology.* 1996;47:387.

413. Jordan GH, Lynch DF, Warden SS, et al: Major pelvic complications following interstitial implantation of Iodine-125 for carcinoma of the prostate. *J Urol.* 1985;134:1212.

414. Krupski T, Petroni GR, Bissonette EA, et al: Quality-of-life comparison of radical prostatectomy and interstitial brachytherapy in the treatment of clinically localized prostate cancer. *Urology.* 2000;55:736.

415. Brandeis JM, Litwin MS, Burnison CM, et al: Quality of life outcomes after brachytherapy for early stage prostate cancer. *J Urol.* 2000;163:851.

416. Lim AJ, Brandon AH, Fiedler J, et al: Quality of life: Radical prostatectomy versus radiation therapy for prostate cancer. *J Urol.* 1995;154:1420.

417. Wei JT, Dunn RL, Litwin MS, et al: Development and validation of the expanded prostate cancer index composite (EPIC) for comprehensive assessment of health-related quality of life in men with prostate cancer. *Urology.* 2000;56:899.

418. Merrick GS, Wallner K, Butler WM, et al: Short-term sexual function after prostate brachytherapy. *Int J Cancer.* 2001;96:313.

419. Merrick G, Bulter W, Wallner K, et al: Dysuria following permanent prostate brachytherapy. *Int J Radiat Oncol Biol Phys.* in press, 2003.

420. Benk VA, Adams JA, Shipley WU, et al: Late rectal bleeding following combined X-ray and proton high dose irradiation for patients with stages T3-T4 prostate cancer. *Int J Radiat Oncol Biol Phys.* 1993;26:551.

421. Rossi CJ Jr, Slater JD, Reyes-Molyneux N, et al: Particle beam radiation therapy in prostate cancer: Is there an advantage? *Semin Radiat Oncol.* 1998;8:115.

422. Bagshaw MA, Cox RS, Ray GR: Status of prostate cancer at Stanford University. *NCI Monogr.* 1988;7:47.

423. Roach M III, Chinn DM, Holland J, et al: A pilot survey of sexual function and quality of life following 3D conformal radiotherapy for clinically localized prostate cancer. *Int J Radiat Oncol Biol Phys.* 1996;35:869.

424. Chinn DM, Holland J, Crownover RL, et al: Potency following high-dose three-dimensional conformal radiotherapy and the impact of prior major urologic surgical procedures in patients treated for prostate cancer. *Int J Radiat Oncol Biol Phys.* 1995;33:15.

425. Banker RL: The preservation of potency after external beam irradiation for prostate cancer. *Int J Radiat Oncol Biol Phys.* 1988;15:219.

426. Litwin MS, Flanders SC, Pasta DJ, et al: Sexual function and bother after radical prostatectomy or radiation for prostate cancer: multivariate quality-of-life analysis from CaPSURE. Cancer of the Prostate Strategic Urologic Research Endeavor. *Urology.* 1999;54:503.

427. Carrier S, Hricak H, Lee SS, et al: Radiation-induced decrease in nitric oxide synthase-containing nerves in the rat penis. *Radiology.* 1995;195:95.

428. Pickett B, Fisch BM, Weinburg V, et al: Dose to the bulb of the penis is associated with the risk of impotence following radiotherapy for prostate cancer. In Cox, ed. *Proceedings of ASTRO*. San Antonio, Texas: Elsevier; 1999:263.

429. Fisch BM, Pickett B, Weinberg V, et al: Dose of radiation received by the bulb of the penis correlates with risk of impotence after three-dimensional conformal radiotherapy for prostate cancer. *Urology.* 2001;57:955.

430. Merrick GS, Butler WM, Wallner KE, et al: The importance of radiation doses to the penile bulb vs. crura in the development of postbrachytherapy erectile dysfunction. *Int J Radiat Oncol Biol Phys.* 2002;54:1055.

431. Merrick GS, Wallner K, Butler WM, et al: A comparison of radiation dose to the bulb of the penis in men with and without prostate brachytherapy-induced erectile dysfunction. *Int J Radiat Oncol Biol Phys.* 2001;50:597.

432. Weber DC, Bieri S, Kurtz JM, et al: Prospective pilot study of sildenafil for treatment of postradiotherapy erectile dysfunction in patients with prostate cancer. *J Clin Oncol.* 1999;17:3444.

433. Zelefsky MJ, McKee AB, Lee H, et al: Efficacy of oral sildenafil in patients with erectile dysfunction after radiotherapy for carcinoma of the prostate. *Urology.* 1999;53:775.

434. Kleinberg L, Wallner K, Roy J, et al: Treatment-related symptoms during the first year following transperineal I-125 prostate implantation. *Int J Radiat Oncol Biol Phys.* 1994;28:985.

435. Merrick GS, Butler WM, Dorsey AT, et al: A comparison of radiation dose to the neurovascular bundles in men with and without prostate brachytherapy induced erectile dysfunction. *Int J Radiat Oncol Biol Phys.* 2000;48:1065.

436. Kiteley RA, Lee WR, deGuzman AF, et al: Radiation dose to the neurovascular bundles or penile bulb does not predict erectile function after prostate brachytherapy. *Brachytherapy.* 2002;1:90.

437. Wallner K, Merrick G, Benson ML, et al: Penile bulb imaging. *Int J Radiat Oncol Biol Phys.* 2002;53:928.

438. Potters L, Torre T, Fearn PA, et al: Potency after permanent prostate brachytherapy for localized prostate cancer. *Int J Radiat Oncol Biol Phys.* 2001;50:1235.

439. Valicenti RK, Choi E, Chen C, et al: Sildenafil citrate effectively reverses sexual dysfunction induced by three-dimensional conformal radiation therapy. *Urology.* 2001;57:769.

440. Matzkin H, Rangel MC, Soloway MS: Relapse on endocrine treatment in patients with stage D2 prostate cancer. Does second-line hormonal therapy affect survival? *Urology.* 1993;41:144.

441. Loprinzi CL, Michalak JC, Quella SK, et al: Megestrol acetate for the prevention of hot flashes. *N Engl J Med.* 1994;331:347.

442. Orwoll E, Ettinger M, Weiss S, et al: Alendronate for the treatment of osteoporosis in men. *N Engl J Med.* 2000;343:604.

443. Smith MR, McGovern FJ, Zietman AL, et al: Pamidronate to prevent bone loss during androgen-deprivation therapy for prostate cancer. *N Engl J Med.* 2001;345:948.

444. Lipton A, Small E, Saad F, et al: The new bisphosphonate, Zometa (zoledronic acid), decreases skeletal complications in both osteolytic and osteoblastic lesions: A comparison to pamidronate. *Cancer Invest.* 2002;20(suppl 2):45.

445. Fournier P, Boissier S, Filleur S, et al: Bisphosphonates inhibit angiogenesis in vitro and testosterone-stimulated vascular regrowth in the ventral prostate in castrated rats. *Cancer Res.* 2002;62:6538.

446. Lee MV, Fong EM, Singer FR, et al: Bisphosphonate treatment inhibits the growth of prostate cancer cells. *Cancer Res.* 2001;61:2602.

447. Roach M, Wallner K: Prostate cancer. In Leibel S, Phillips T, eds. *Textbook of Radiation Oncology*, 1st ed. Philadelphia: WB Saunders; 1998:741.

448. Partin AW, Lee BR, Carmichael M, et al: Radical prostatectomy for high grade disease: A reevaluation 1994. *J Urol.* 1994;151:1583.

449. Oefelein MG, Grayhack JT, McVary K: Survival after radical prostatectomy of men with clinically localized high grade carcinoma of the prostate. *Cancer.* 1995;76:2535.

450. Ohori M, Goad JR, Wheeler TM, et al: Can radical prostatectomy alter the progression of poorly differentiated prostate cancer? *J Urol.* 1994;152:1843.

451. Lerner SE, Blute ML, Bergstralh EJ, et al: Analysis of risk factors for progression in patients with pathologically confined prostate cancers after radical retropubic prostatectomy. *J Urol.* 1996; 156:137.

452. Graefen M, Karakiewicz PI, Cagiannos I, et al: International validation of a preoperative nomogram for prostate cancer recurrence after radical prostatectomy. *J Clin Oncol.* 2002; 20:3206.

453. Kupelian PA, Buchsbaum JC, Elshaikh M, et al: Factors affecting recurrence rates after prostatectomy or radiotherapy in localized prostate carcinoma patients with biopsy Gleason score 8 or above. *Cancer.* 2002;95:2302.

454. Fiveash JB, Hanks G, Roach M, et al: 3D conformal radiation therapy (3DCRT) for high grade prostate cancer: A multi-institutional review. *Int J Radiat Oncol Biol Phys.* 2000; 47:335.

455. Do TM, Parker RG, Smith RB, et al: High-grade carcinoma of the prostate: A comparison of current local therapies. *Urology.* 2001; 57:1121.

456. Connolly JA, Shinohara K, Presti J, et al: Local recurrence after radical prostatectomy: Characteristics in size, location, and relationship to prostate-specific antigen and surgical margins. *Urology.* 1996;47:225.

457. Valicenti RK, Gomella LG, Ismail M, et al: The efficacy of early adjuvant radiation therapy for pT3N0 prostate cancer: A matched-pair analysis. *Int J Radiat Oncol Biol Phys.* 1999; 45:53.

458. Quinn DI, Henshall SM, Haynes AM, et al: Prognostic significance of pathologic features in localized prostate cancer treated with radical prostatectomy: implications for staging systems and predictive models. *J Clin Oncol.* 2001;19:3692.

459. Catalona WJ, Smith DS: Cancer recurrence and survival rates after anatomic radical retropubic prostatectomy for prostate cancer: Intermediate-term results. *J Urol.* 1998;160:2428.

460. Leventis AK, Shariat SF, Kattan MW, et al: Prediction of response to salvage radiation therapy in patients with prostate cancer recurrence after radical prostatectomy. *J Clin Oncol.* 2001; 19:1030.

461. Nudell DM, Grossfeld GD, Weinberg VK, et al: Radiotherapy after radical prostatectomy: Treatment outcomes and failure patterns. *Urology.* 1999;54:1049.

462. Eulau SM, Tate DJ, Stamey TA, et al: Effect of combined transient androgen deprivation and irradiation following radical prostatectomy for prostatic cancer. *Int J Radiat Oncol Biol Phys.* 1998; 41:735.

463. Shipley WU, Thames HD, Sandler HM, et al: Radiation therapy for clinically localized prostate cancer: A multi-institutional pooled analysis. *JAMA.* 1999;281:1598.

464. Yock TI, Zietman AL, Shipley WU, et al: Long-term durability of PSA failure-free survival after radiotherapy for localized prostate cancer. *Int J Radiat Oncol Biol Phys.* 2002;54:420.

465. Kupelian PA, Elshaikh M, Reddy CA, et al: Comparison of the efficacy of local therapies for localized prostate cancer in the prostate-specific antigen era: A large single-institution experience with radical prostatectomy and external-beam radiotherapy. *J Clin Oncol.* 2002;20:3376.

466. Hanks GE, Lee WR, Hanlon AL, et al: Conformal technique dose escalation for prostate cancer: Biochemical evidence of improved cancer control with higher doses in patients with pretreatment prostate-specific antigen > or = 10 NG/ML [see comments]. *Int J Radiat Oncol Biol Phys.* 1996;35:861.

467. Pollack A, Zagars G: External beam radiotherapy dose-response of prostate cancer. *Int J Radiat Oncol Biol Phys.* 1997; 39:1011.

468. Perez CA, Michalski JM, Purdy JA, et al: Three-dimensional conformal therapy or standard irradiation in localized carcinoma of prostate: Preliminary results of a nonrandomized comparison. *Int J Radiat Oncol Biol Phys.* 2000;47:629.

469. Kupelian PA, Buchsbaum JC, Reddy CA, et al: Radiation dose response in patients with favorable localized prostate cancer (Stage T1-T2, biopsy Gleason < or = 6, and pretreatment prostate-specific antigen < or = 10). *Int J Radiat Oncol Biol Phys.* 2001;50:621.

470. Brachman DG, Thomas T, Hilbe J, et al: Failure-free survival following brachytherapy alone or external beam irradiation alone for T1-2 prostate tumors in 2222 patients: Results from a single practice. *Int J Radiat Oncol Biol Phys.* 2000;48:111.

471. Blasko JC, Grimm PD, Sylvester JE, et al: Palladium-103 brachytherapy for prostate carcinoma. *Int J Radiat Oncol Biol Phys.* 2000;46:839.

472. Polascik TJ, Pound CR, DeWeese TL, et al: Comparison of radical prostatectomy and iodine 125 interstitial radiotherapy for the treatment of clinically localized prostate cancer: A 7-year biochemical (PSA) progression analysis. *Urology.* 1998;51:884.

473. Potters L: Permanent prostate brachytherapy: Lessons learned, lessons to learn. *Oncol-NY.* 2000:14:981.

474. Kattan MW, Potters L, Blasko JC, et al: Pretreatment nomogram for predicting freedom from recurrence after permanent prostate brachytherapy in prostate cancer. *Urology.* 2001;58:393.

475. Zelefsky MJ, Fuks Z, Hunt M, et al: High dose radiation delivered by intensity modulated conformal radiotherapy improves the outcome of localized prostate cancer. *J Urol.* 2001;166:876.

476. Merrick G, Butler W, Lief JH, et al: Biochemical outcome for hormone-naive intermediate-risk prostate cancer managed with permanent interstitial brachytherapy and supplemental external beam radiation. *Brachytherapy.* 2002;1:95.

477. Bice WS, Freeman JE, Russell LF, et al: Use of image coregistration in salvage prostate brachytherapy. *Tech Urol.* 2000; 6:151.

478. Kovacs G, Wirth B, Bertermann H, et al: Prostate preservation by combined external beam and HDR brachytherapy at nodal negative prostate cancer patients—An intermediate analysis after ten years experience. *Int J Radiat Oncol Biol Phys.* 1996; 36:198.

479. Kovács G, Galalae R, Loch T, et al: Prostate preservation by combined external beam and HDR brachytherapy in nodal negative prostate cancer. *Strahlentherapie und Onkologie.* 1999;175 (suppl 2):87.

480. Mate TP, Gottesman JE, Hatton J, et al: High dose-rate afterloading 192-Iridium prostate brachytherapy: Feasibility report. *Int J Radiat Oncol Biol Phys.* 1998;41:525.

481. Martinez A, Gonzalez J, Stromberg J, et al: Conformal prostate brachytherapy: Initial experience of a phase I/II dose-escalating trial. *Int J Radiat Oncol Biol Phys.* 1995;33:1019.

482. Martinez AA, Kestin LL, Stromberg JS, et al: Interim report of image-guided conformal high-dose-rate brachytherapy for patients with unfavorable prostate cancer: The William Beaumont phase II dose-escalating trial. *Int J Radiat Oncol Biol Phys.* 2000;47:343.

483. Martinez AA, Pataki I, Edmundson G, et al: Phase II prospective study of the use of conformal high-dose-rate brachytherapy as monotherapy for the treatment of favorable stage prostate cancer: A feasibility report. *Int J Radiat Oncol Biol Phys.* 2001;49:61.

484. Borghede G, Hedelin H, Holmäng S, et al: Combined treatment with temporary short-term high dose rate iridium-192 brachytherapy and external beam radiotherapy for irradiation of localized prostatic carcinoma. *Radiother Oncol.* 1997;44:237.

485. Borghede G, Hedelin H, Holmäng S, et al: Irradiation of localized prostatic carcinoma with a combination of high dose rate iridium-192 brachytherapy and external beam radiotherapy with three target definitions and dose levels inside the prostate gland. *Radiother Oncol.* 1997;44:245.

486. Dinges S, Deger S, Koswig S, et al: High-dose rate interstitial with external beam irradiation for localized prostate cancer—Results of a prospective trial. *Radiother Oncol.* 1998;48:197.

487. Hsu I-C, III MR: Brachytherapy. In Grossfeld CA, ed. *Prostate Cancer.* Hamilton, Ontario: BC Decker; 2002.

488. Makhlouf AA, Boyd JC, Chapman TN, et al: Perioperative costs and charges of prostate brachytherapy and prostatectomy. *Urology.* 2002;60:656.

489. Goharderakhshan RZ, Grossfeld GD, Kassis A, et al: Additional treatments and reimbursement rates associated with prostate cancer treatment for patients undergoing radical prostatectomy, interstitial brachytherapy, and external beam radiotherapy. *Urology.* 2000;56:622.

490. Alexianu M, Weiss GH: Radical prostatectomy versus brachytherapy for early-stage prostate cancer. *J Endourol.* 2000;14:325.

491. Hayman JA, Lash KA, Tao ML, et al: A comparison of two methods for estimating the technical costs of external beam radiation therapy. *Int J Radiat Oncol Biol Phys.* 2000;47:461.

492. Ciezki JP, Klein EA, Angermeier KW, et al: Cost comparison of radical prostatectomy and transperineal brachytherapy for localized prostate cancer. *Urology.* 2000;55:68.

493. Kohan AD, Armenakas NA, Fracchia JA: The perioperative charge equivalence of interstitial brachytherapy and radical prostatectomy with 1-year followup. *J Urol.* 2000;163:511.

494. Wagner TT, Young D, Bahnson RR: Charge and length of hospital stay analysis of radical retropubic prostatectomy and transperineal prostate brachytherapy. J Urol. 1999;161:1216.

495. Burkhardt JH, Litwin MS, Rose CM, et al: Comparing the costs of radiation therapy and radical prostatectomy for the initial treatment of early-stage prostate cancer. *J Clin Oncol.* 2002; 20:2869.

496. Bucci J, Morris WJ, Keyes M, et al: Predictive factors of urinary retention following prostate brachytherapy. *Int J Radiat Oncol Biol Phys.* 2002;53:91.

497. Wallner KE, Roy J, Harrison L: Tumor control and morbidity following transperineal I-125 implantation for stage T1/T2 prostatic carcinoma. *J Clin Oncol.* 1996;14:449.

Cancer of the Testis

46

Dan P. Garwood, MD

INCIDENCE AND EPIDEMIOLOGY

Testicular cancer accounted for an estimated 7600 new cancer cases in men in 2003, with 400 estimated deaths.[1] Although it accounts for only about 1% of all cancers in males, it is the most common cancer in men aged 20 to 34 years, with an age-adjusted incidence rate of about 4 per 100,000. Testicular cancers are also the most curable malignancies in men of this age group. Seminomas, the testicular neoplasm of greatest interest to radiation oncologists, may well be the most curable of all solid tumors. The peak incidence of nonseminoma germ cell tumors (NSGCTs) falls in the 20 to 29 age range, whereas the incidence of seminomas is greatest in the 30 to 39 age range and is more represented in the older age groups, with spermatocytic seminomas most common in those older than 60.[2] The incidence of testicular cancer appears to be increasing over time.[3] From 1% to 3% of testicular neoplasms are bilateral, with either synchronous or metachronous (usually within 2 years) presentations.[4]

The origin of testicular neoplasia is unclear, but it may be related to gonadal atrophy or dysgenesis. A review of the literature on patients with testicular tumors found that the cancer arose in atrophic testes in 1.5% of cases.[5] Cryptorchidism increases the risk of malignancy some 10 to 40 times and is the major identified risk factor, with roughly 12% of all germ cell tumors coming from undescended testes.[6] The risk of developing a testicular neoplasm was estimated at 1 out of 20 for a testis retained intra-abdominally and 1 out of 80 if it was within the inguinal canal. The risk is still elevated in a testicle after orchiopexy, although it is decreased if the operation is performed before age 10.[7] One in 10 of the germ cell tumors that develop in patients with a history of cryptorchidism arise in the contralateral, descended testis. Maternal hormone usage has been linked, although less clearly, to an increased risk of testicular cancer.[8] Patients with multiple atypical nevi, such as the dysplastic nevus syndrome, have been shown to be at increased risk of developing germ cell tumors.[9] Trauma to the testis has also been suggested as a risk factor but may instead be associated with increased rates of discovery. The incidence of testicular cancer in whites is more than five times that seen in blacks.[2] Men infected with the human immunodeficiency virus (HIV) may have a higher incidence of testis tumors; a review of 3015 men followed in an immunodeficiency clinic showed an incidence 57 times the United States average.[10]

Chromosomal abnormalities are being recognized in germ cell tumors with increasing frequency, most commonly involving chromosomes 1 and 12.[11,12] Changes in chromosome 1 involved both arms, with both deletions and rearrangements being noted. The most frequent alteration, however, seems to be an isochromosome of the short arm of chromosome 12, noted as i(12p), which has been reported to be present in up to 90% of germ cell tumors.[13,14] This particular abnormality has been reported in all subtypes of germ cell tumors and is believed to be nearly diagnostic for germ cell neoplasms, although it has also been rarely reported in gastric cancer. It has been reported in carcinoma in situ of the testis as well, suggesting an early role in the development of germ cell malignancies.[15] The i(12p) abnormality may be present multiple times in the tumor cell, with a poor prognosis demonstrated when three or more copies are seen.[16] Exactly which genes are involved in the neoplastic transformation has not yet been elucidated, although c-ki-ras_2, a recognized oncogene, is known to be located on the short arm of chromosome 12. Amplification or overexpression of this oncogene may contribute to tumorigenesis.[17] Up to 44% of germ cell tumors have also been found to have deletions of the terminal portion of chromosome 12.[18]

ANATOMY

The testis is a roughly oval-shaped organ that usually measures 4 to 5 cm in length and 2 to 3 cm in thickness (Fig. 46-1). It is composed of many convoluted seminiferous tubules, which develop spermatozoa from their inner epithelial lining. The seminiferous tubules are arranged in wedge-shaped compartments, which unite at the upper posterior portion of the testis, the mediastinum testis or hilum, to form the rete testis. The seminiferous tubule compartments are formed by connective tissue septa, which connect with the tunica albuginea, a fibrous capsule that encases the testis and is itself contained by the tunica vaginalis, forming a double-layered structure like the abdominal peritoneum. This is surrounded by the internal spermatic fascia, the cremasteric fascia, external spermatic fascia, dartos muscle, and finally the scrotal skin. Efferent ducts from the rete testis penetrate the tunica albuginea to join the epididymis, which bends upward at the caudal pole of the testis to form the vas deferens. The seminiferous tubules are lined with stem

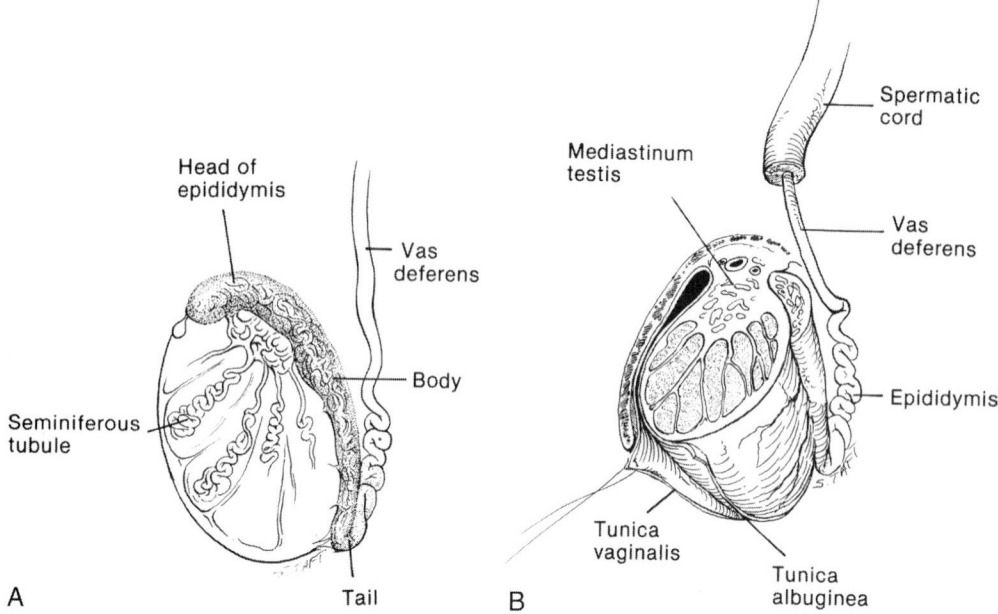

Figure 46–1. Diagram of testicular anatomy. **A,** Testis and epididymis. **B,** Cross section of testis. (From Tanagho EA: Anatomy of the lower urinary tract. In Walsh PC, Retik AB, Stamey TA, Vaughan, ED, eds. *Campbell's Urology*, 6th ed. Philadelphia: WB Saunders; 1992.)

cells, or spermatogonia, which produce spermatocytes, which become spermatids and finally spermatozoa. Admixed with the spermatogonia are Sertoli's cells, which provide support to the developing spermatozoa. The process from stem cell to mature spermatozoa takes around 67 days in humans.[19] Interspersed within the connective tissue surrounding the seminiferous tubules are Leydig's cells, which produce testosterone.

Lymphatic vessels collect from the hilum of the testis and pass through the internal inguinal ring along with the spermatic cord, following the testicular veins. These vessels drain to lymph nodes that lie in the retroperitoneum, generally from the level of the first through third lumbar vertebral bodies. Lymphatics from the testicle do not, as a rule, go to the inguinal or iliac nodes, but lymphatics from the skin and subcutaneous tissues of the scrotum do, and prior surgical disturbance of the scrotum or inguinal region can redirect drainage to these areas.

PATHOLOGY

Of all the organs in the body, the testis can fall prey to a wider variety of neoplasia than most (Table 46-1). The vast majority of primary tumors are of germ cell origin, accounting for about 95% of testicular cancers. Classification schemes abound, with substantial variability among them. In the United States, testicular germ cell tumors are usually classified along the lines of the system adopted by the Armed Forces Institute of Pathology, which is similar to that of the World Health Organization.[20] Tumors of germ cell origin can be predominantly of a single histologic type or can be mixtures of types, with more than one histologic pattern seen in about 40% of testicular tumors.[21] From the perspective of therapy, germ cell tumors are broadly divided into two groups,

seminomas and nonseminoma germ cell tumors (NSGCT), with pure seminomas constituting roughly 40%. This chapter concentrates on germ cell tumors, with emphasis on seminomas, as NSGCTs are comparatively much less sensitive to radiation.

Since the advent of effective chemotherapy for NSGCTs, the role of radiation in these neoplasms has been very limited. About 85% of pure seminomas are classic, or typical, seminomas. These tumors generally diffusely enlarge the testis (although they may be nodular), with

Table 46–1   Pathology of Testicular Neoplasms

Primary testicular neoplasms
  95% Germinal cells
    ~40% Pure seminoma
    85% Classic seminoma
    10% Anaplastic seminoma
    5% Spermatocytic seminoma
    ~60% Nonseminoma
    Embryonal carcinoma
    Teratoma
    Choriocarcinoma
    Mixed germ cell neoplasms
  5% Nongerminal neoplasms
    Stromal tumors
      Sertoli's cell tumors
      Leydig's cell tumors
      Gonadoblastomas
      Granulosa-theca tumors
    Lymphoma
    Sarcoma
    Melanoma
    Mesothelioma
Metastatic tumors
Involvement from systemic disease (lymphoma,
  leukemia, multiple myeloma)

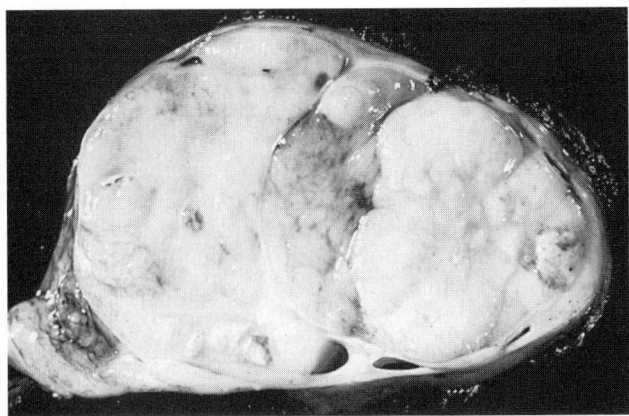

Figure 46–2. Cut section of seminoma replacing a testis. (Courtesy of Kyle Molberg, M.D., Department of Pathology, University of Texas, Southwestern Medical Center at Dallas.)

Table 46–2   Serum Markers in Testicular Neoplasms

Histology	AFP, %	β-HCG, %
Seminoma	0	9
Teratoma	38	25
Embryonal carcinoma	70	60
Choriocarcinoma	0	100
Yolk sac tumor	75	25

Data from Javadpour N: Current status of tumor markers in testicular cancer. *Eur Urol.* 1992;21(suppl 1):34.

the entire testis replaced by tumor in more than half the cases, showing a bulging, grayish, usually largely homogeneous tissue on cross section (Fig. 46-2). Microscopically, the cells are relatively uniform, large, and polygonal or round, with clear cytoplasm and hyperchromatic nuclei, supported by a delicate connective tissue stroma and admixed with varying amounts of lymphocytes (Fig. 46-3). Mitoses are uncommon. Anaplastic seminomas account for around 10% and show greater cellular and nuclear irregularity, with more frequent mitoses. The spermatocytic pattern, seen in about 5% of seminomas, is somewhat mucoid and grossly yellow and may show areas of cystic necrosis and occasionally focal hemorrhage. These neoplasms contain a mixture of small cells resembling spermatocytes, scattered giant cells, and a majority of medium-sized cells. In the majority of cases, seminomas do not penetrate the tunica albuginea, but extension to the epididymis or spermatic cord occurs in 10% to 15% of patients with early-stage disease.[22] Carcinoma in situ appears to precede invasive testicular germ cell tumors (except for spermatocytic seminoma), with a median time for progression to invasive cancer of 3 to 5 years.[23] Non–germ cell tumors include embryonal

cancer, which is the most common type; teratomas; yolk sac or endodermal sinus tumors (considered a subtype of embryonal tumors); and choriocarcinoma, which is rare and shows a high rate of dissemination. As noted earlier, a significant fraction of NSGCTs are mixtures of different elements and may contain seminomatous elements as well.

Germ cell tumors frequently produce proteins that can be detected in the blood at very low levels. These proteins serve as markers for disease burden beyond the ability of current imaging technology to detect; allow for the assessment of response to therapy and follow-up; and, on occasion, offer clues to the diagnosis and histologic makeup of the neoplasm. The most clinically applicable markers in testicular germ cell tumors are alpha-fetoprotein (AFP) and the beta subunit of human chorionic gonadotropin (β-HCG) (Table 46-2). Lactate dehydrogenase (LDH) can be increased. Placental alkaline phosphatase, gamma-glutamyl transpeptidase, pregnancy-specific beta$_1$-glycoprotein, and basic fetoprotein can also be elevated in germ cell tumors, but the usefulness and role of these markers have not been established.[24] It is important for the clinician to ascertain the consistency of the laboratory performing the analysis, as different assays may measure different things, such as the free beta-subunits versus the intact molecule, or have differing sensitivities. Clinical judgments should be made based on consistent laboratories using consistent assays. AFP is a protein made by the fetal yolk sac, liver, and gastrointestinal tract and is a large component of serum protein in the fetus, acting in the same role as albumin. The serum half-life of AFP is 4 to 6 days.[25] AFP is also elevated in hepatocellular carcinomas, often to extreme levels; to a lesser extent in benign hepatic disease; and occasionally in malignancies of the stomach, pancreas, biliary tree, and lung. HCG is a glycoprotein made by trophoblastic tissue and is elevated in conditions such as pregnancy, hydatidiform mole, and choriocarcinoma. It is composed of alpha and beta subunits, the alpha subunit being homologous with subunits of the following pituitary hormones: thyroid-stimulating hormone, luteinizing hormone, and follicle-stimulating hormone. The beta subunit is less closely related; hence, most radioimmunoassays for HCG are directed against the beta subunit portion of the molecule, to minimize cross-reactivity. The serum half-life for the free beta subunit is only about 45 minutes, but the half-life for the intact HCG molecule is 24 to 36 hours.[26-28]

Different clones within the tumor may secrete markers in differing proportions, and the primary tumor may have a different profile than the metastases. Seminomas may show a modestly elevated β-HCG in 10% to 30% of

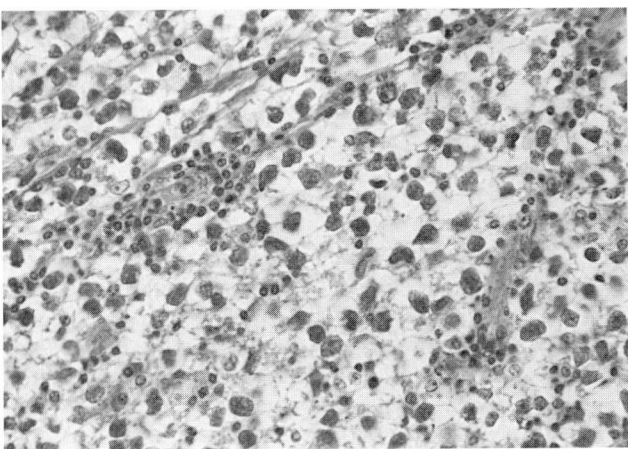

Figure 46–3. Photomicrograph of classic seminoma. (Courtesy of Kyle Molberg, M.D., Department of Pathology, University of Texas, Southwestern Medical Center at Dallas.)

cases, with a review of 20 publications finding an average of 21%, but seldom do levels exceed 100 ng/mL, unless there is bulky abdominal lymphadenopathy.[29,30] AFP, in contrast, should not be elevated in a pure seminoma, and the finding of this marker should lead one to question the pathologic diagnosis. Elevation of AFP or β-HCG or both is seen in 80% to 90% of patients with NSGCTs.[31] Tumor cells that produce HCG are thought to be considerably more sensitive to chemotherapy than those that produce AFP.[32] In NSGCTs, elevation of AFP is associated with 70% of embryonal carcinomas, 75% of yolk sac tumors, and 38% of teratomas and is absent in choriocarcinomas. β-HCG is elevated in 100% of choriocarcinomas, 60% of embryonal carcinomas, and 25% of teratomas and yolk sac tumors.[30] LDH is much less specific and less sensitive than AFP or β-HCG, but it has been shown to be an independent marker for prognosis.[33] Approximately 50% of germ cell tumors show elevation of LDH.[34]

An assortment of less common non–germ cell tumors make up the remaining 5% after germ cell neoplasms are considered.[35] Lymphomas of the testicle, although constituting only a small minority compared with germ cell neoplasms, are the most common testicular cancer in men older than age 60.[36] Leukemias can also involve the testis as a sanctuary site. Various primary intratesticular sarcomas, most commonly rhabdomyosarcoma, may also be seen.[37] Gonadal stromal tumors, known as Leydig's or interstitial cell tumors and Sertoli's cell tumors, are benign in about 90% of cases. Leydig's cell tumors, which tend to present in adult life, are capable of secreting testosterone, as well as lesser amounts of estrogens. Sertoli's cell tumors also present throughout the life span, although a considerable fraction develop in the first decade. Gonadoblastoma refers to a tumor combining gonadal stromal elements with germ cell elements. Granulosa-theca tumors are also stromal tumors. Adenocarcinomas, mesotheliomas of the tunica vaginalis, melanomas, angiomas, and neuromas may all rarely occur. Tumors from other sites can metastasize to the testis, most commonly from prostate, lung, kidney, and melanoma.[38] Rarely, tumors from the bowel may spread to the testis, homologous to Krukenberg's tumors of the ovary.[39] The management of non–germ cell tumors is beyond the scope of this chapter, but in general, the main approach is surgical.

Different histologies of neoplasms of the testis have prognostic significance. As far as seminomas are concerned, however, any difference among the subtypes is controversial and probably minimal. Anaplastic seminomas do not appear to be different from typical seminomas when compared stage for stage.[40,41] Spermatocytic seminomas are most common in men older than age 40, and some authors suggest that they have a lower metastatic potential and a favorable prognosis. Production of HCG does not appear to be an adverse prognostic feature for seminomas.[42] Seminomas are localized to the testis in around 70% of patients, with metastases to the lymph nodes in about 25% at presentation and visceral metastases in around 5%, often manifesting late in the course of the disease.[43] NSGCTs have a higher tendency toward dissemination, with 60% to 70% showing metastatic disease at presentation.[44] Pure teratomas are somewhat less

aggressive than other NSGCTs with a lower propensity for metastases.[45] The behavior of testicular tumors in patients infected with HIV is controversial but may not be intrinsically different from that in the uninfected, beyond general effects of immunocompromise. Some data have supported a comparable natural history to that in non-HIV infected men and comparable tolerance to therapies. Given that germ cell tumors can be controlled in a substantial fraction of these patients who would otherwise have their lives significantly shortened over and above the course of HIV infection, a number of authors have advocated that the standard therapeutic approaches be offered.[46,47]

CLINICAL PRESENTATION

The classic presentation of testicular neoplasia is said to be that of a painless testicular mass, which may be noted by either the patient or his sexual partner. This enlargement is generally gradual, although on occasion it may be quite abrupt. Trauma may also lead to the incidental discovery of a preexisting tumor. Pain, however, is not unknown and can be seen in up to 45% of patients.[48-50] A sensation of heaviness or fullness in the scrotum may also be reported. Delay in diagnosis is not uncommon and may be exacerbated by either patient fear or lack of concern owing to the absence of pain. Confusion with epididymitis, orchitis, or hydrocele is a factor that can also contribute to delay. Periods of 3 to 6 months from symptoms to diagnosis are not uncommon and have been shown to correlate with increased metastatic risk.[51] Signs and symptoms of metastatic disease are the presenting complaint in roughly 10% of cases. The patient may note a mass in the neck from lymphadenopathy, respiratory complaints from mediastinal nodes, or gastrointestinal symptoms or back pain stemming from retroperitoneal involvement. Even less commonly, evaluation of infertility may lead to the diagnosis. Gynecomastia or tenderness of the breasts, seen in around 5% of patients with testicular germ cell tumors owing to production of estradiol in response to elevated HCG, may also be the initial clue.[52]

ROUTES OF SPREAD

As noted previously, the predominant route of lymphatic drainage for testicular tumors is orderly spread to the retroperitoneal lymph nodes. Lymphatic drainage from the testicle is generally not to the inguinal or iliac regions, unless inguinal or scrotal surgery has disrupted the normal lymphatic drainage and collaterals have formed.[53] The lymphatics of the scrotum, however, do drain to the superficial inguinal nodes. Four to eight lymphatic vessels collect from the hilum of the testis and accompany the testicular veins up to their termination. The right testicular vein joins the inferior vena cava a few centimeters below where the right renal vein enters the inferior vena cava; the left testicular vein enters the left renal vein. The path of the lymphatics on the left side often swings out wider than on the right as they cross over the region of the sacroiliac joint.[53] The lymphatics drain into the retroperitoneum from the eleventh thoracic to the

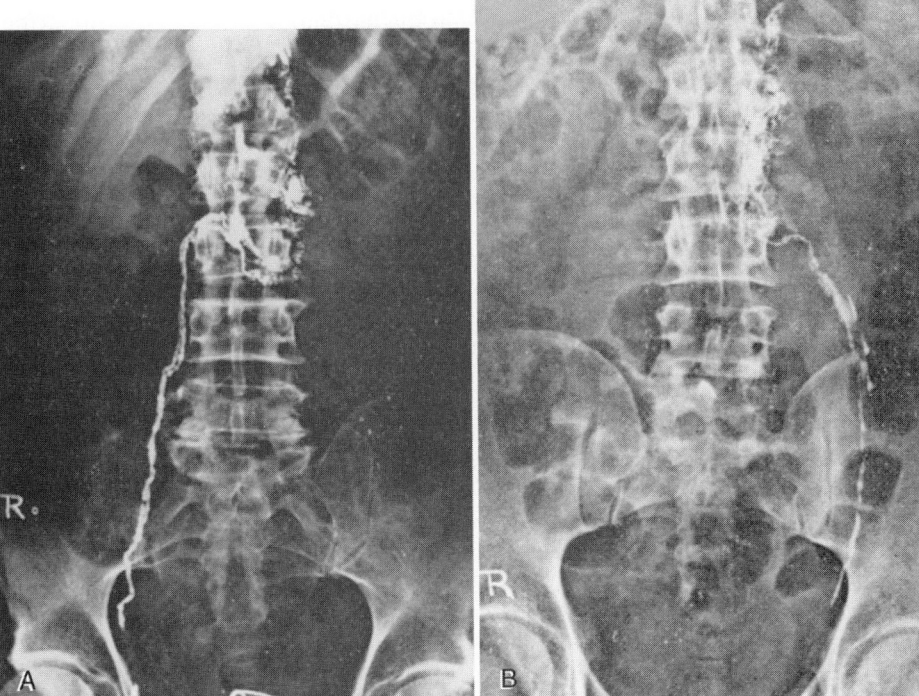

Figure 46–4. Testicular lymphangiograms. **A,** Right. **B,** Left. (From Busch FM, Sayegh ES: Roentgenographic visualization of human testicular lymphatics: A preliminary report. *J Urol.* 1963;89:106.)

fourth lumbar vertebral bodies; in the majority of cases, this occurs between L1 and L3. Testicular lymphangiography has shown that the primary draining node is generally located lateral to the vertebral bodies from L1 to L3 for left-sided tumors and at L2 for those on the right (Fig. 46-4).[54] Right-sided drainage is most commonly to the lymph nodes lateral, anterior, and medial to the vena cava (interaortocaval) and anterior, but not lateral, to the aorta. Left-sided nodes are generally lateral and anterior to the aorta but are usually not medial to the aorta.[55,56] Crossover from the right side to the left is consistently demonstrated by lymphangiography, but crossover from the left to the right is rare and occurs only when the primary nodes are filled. Awareness of the patterns of drainage can help detect smaller lymph nodes when reviewing computed tomography (CT) scans (Fig. 46-5). After involvement of the sentinel nodes, spread is to the lumbar retroperitoneal nodes, followed by metastases to supradiaphragmatic nodes in the mediastinal and supraclavicular regions and by hematogenous dissemination. An autopsy series has demonstrated the most common sites of spread to be the lung, liver, brain, viscera, and bone.[57]

DIAGNOSTIC AND STAGING STUDIES

When faced with a testicular mass, one should consider the possibility of tumor until it is proved otherwise. The most common differential diagnosis of a testicular mass is epididymitis or orchitis. With epididymitis, the swollen epididymis can usually be separated from the testis if the patient is seen early. If enough time has passed for inflammation to set in, the examination may not be sufficient to distinguish the different structures. In the

past, a trial of antibiotics was often used to clarify the picture if epididymitis was suspected; now ultrasonography is frequently helpful. Sonography has become a valuable diagnostic procedure in the workup of testicular masses and can generally distinguish intratesticular lesions from extratesticular problems. Hydroceles may also be confused with testicular neoplasms, but the failure to transmit light on scrotal transillumination indicates a solid mass and calls for exploration. Positive cytologic fluid has been reported from aspiration of hydroceles associated with testicular neoplasms; thus, aspiration of

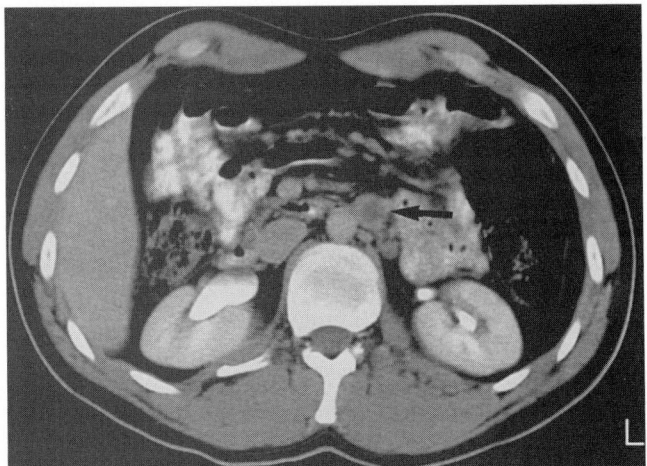

Figure 46–5. Computed tomography scan of nodal metastasis from left-sided testicular tumor, marked by *black arrow*, located immediately below the renal vessels, anterior and lateral to the aorta. Note that left-sided lymph nodes generally are anterior and lateral, but not medial, to the aorta and may extend farther out toward the renal hilum, whereas nodes from right-sided tumors are lateral or anterior to the vena cava, or between the vena cava and aorta, and anterior, but not lateral, to the aorta.

a questionable hydrocele is contraindicated.[58] Magnetic resonance imaging may play a larger role in the workup of testicular masses in the future, but at present, the use of this modality is not established. If physical examination, transillumination, and ultrasonography fail to satisfactorily identify the problem as benign and a high clinical suspicion for testicular tumor exists, an inguinal orchiectomy (or at least exploration) is indicated. Incisions through the scrotum are contraindicated, because of concern about altering the lymphatic drainage of the testicle. Serum markers should be obtained *before surgery* to establish baseline values.

Once the diagnosis of testicular germ cell tumor is established, the workup includes a history and physical examination, with attention to prior scrotal or inguinal surgery or history of cryptorchidism; attention to lymph nodes, particularly the left supraclavicular and inguinals; abdominal examination for abdominal masses or hepatomegaly; examination of the breasts for gynecomastia; and examination of the scrotum and contralateral testis. Serum chemistries and complete blood count; postoperative markers; chest radiography and possibly chest CT; and radiographic assessment of the retroperitoneal lymph nodes, now usually by CT, should also be performed. If the tumor markers were elevated preoperatively, their rate of fall postoperatively relative to their half-lives gives some indication as to the presence of metastatic disease. The classic way of detecting retroperitoneal lymphadenopathy, bipedal lymphangiography, has essentially been replaced in most centers by CT scanning, and it is increasingly difficult to find radiologists skilled at the performance and interpretation of the procedure. Lymphangiography has the advantage of being able to detect distortions of internal nodal architecture, which can allow the detection of metastatic involvement not causing nodal enlargement and thus not visible to CT. Foot lymphangiography, however, often does not opacify the lymph nodes that testicular neoplasms drain to first[54,59]; thus testicular lymphangiography is required for the greatest sensitivity, a procedure that is unappealing to both patients and most radiologists. A review of the literature found that the sensitivity, specificity, and accuracy of CT scanning were comparable to that of lymphangiography.[44] A report from the MD Anderson Cancer Center described a change in policy for evaluating retroperitoneal nodes in patients with testicular seminoma.[60] The use of CT rather than lymphangiogram led to no increase in relapse, with 1 of 74 patients (1.4%) evaluated with CT having distant relapse, as compared with 7 of 172 (4%) who were staged with lymphangiogram. None of the relapses were in-field or marginal. The possible increase in sensitivity to small-volume nodal involvement gained through lymphangiography appears not to translate into improved clinical outcome. If available, lymphangiography may be useful for patients with stage I NSGCTs who are considering observation without retroperitoneal lymph node dissection; the sensitivity to architecturally abnormal lymph nodes may increase the overall sensitivity for early metastases.

Newer imaging modalities have yet to have significant impact on the evaluation of testicular malignancy.

Magnetic resonance imaging (MRI), like CT, detects retroperitoneal lymphadenopathy as abnormal only when the nodes are enlarged. MRI has not consistently demonstrated superiority to CT; while it can be useful to distinguish vascular structures from lymph nodes, no oral contrast agent exists clinically to enable the separation of small bowel from nodal masses with MRI. Recent reports suggest that MRI of lymph nodes after injection of a paramagnetic contrast agent can be very accurate in diagnosing nodal involvement by prostate cancer. This method has not been reported yet for testis cancer. (ref needed here, NEJM 2003) Positron emission tomography (PET) scanning may prove useful as an imaging modality that can detect metabolic activity, as opposed to being limited to measuring geometry. PET may be found to have a role in staging, detection of relapse, and in distinguishing fibrosis from viable tumor,[61,62,63] although as yet availability is limited in most regions.

STAGING SYSTEMS

Staging of testicular cancers may be the only area in which the number of different classifications at different institutions approaches the variations in pathologic classification. Many systems have in common the division into three stages, as initially described by Boden and Gibb,[64] with stage I being tumor limited to the testicle, stage II metastases to subdiaphragmatic lymph nodes, and stage III involvement of supradiaphragmatic lymph nodes or distant or extranodal metastases. The Walter Reed Hospital staging system is a modification of this approach.[65] The Royal Marsden Hospital system subdivides stage II into IIA, with lymph nodes less than 2 cm; IIB, 2 to 5 cm; IIC, 5 to 10 cm; and IID, greater than 10 cm, as well as designating stage III for supradiaphragmatic node metastases and stage IV for extralymphatic spread (Table 46-3). This staging system was adopted at a consensus conference on testicular cancer held in England in 1989 and is the basis for the staging approach used in this chapter.[66] The American Joint Committee on Cancer (AJCC) has also adopted a staging system that incorporates serum markers (Table 46-4); it is published in the sixth edition of the *Manual for Staging of Cancer*.

Table 46–3 Modified Royal Marsden Hospital Staging System

Stage I	No clinical evidence of metastases beyond the testicle
Stage II	Infradiaphragmatic lymph node metastases
	IIA Maximum diameter <2 cm
	IIB Maximum diameter >2 but <5 cm
	IIC Maximum diameter >5 but <10 cm
	IID Maximum diameter >10 cm
Stage III	Supradiaphragmatic nodal involvement
Stage IV	Parenchymal metastatic disease

From Thomas G, Jones W, VanOosterom A, Kawai T: Consensus statement of the investigation and management of testicular seminoma 1989. In Newling DW, Jones WG, eds. *EORTC Genitourinary Group Monograph 7: Prostate Cancer and Testicular Cancer.* New York: Wiley-Liss; 1990:288.

Table 46–4 Classification of Cancers of the Testis

Primary Tumor (T)

The extent of primary tumor is usually classified after radical orchiectomy, and for this reason, a *pathologic* stage is assigned.

*pTX	Primary tumor cannot be assessed
pT0	No evidence of primary tumor (e.g., histologic scar in testis)
pTis	Intratubular germ cell neoplasia (carcinoma *in situ*)
pT1	Tumor limited to the testis and epididymis without vascular/lymphatic invasion; tumor may invade into the tunica albuginea but not the tunica vaginalis
pT2	Tumor limited to the testis and epididymis with vascular/lymphatic invasion, or tumor extending through the tunica albuginea with involvement of the tunica vaginalis
pT3	Tumor invades the spermatic cord with or without vascular/lymphatic invasion
pT4	Tumor invades the scrotum with or without vascular/lymphatic invasion

Note: Except for pTis and pT4, extent of primary tumor is classified by radical orchiectomy. TX may be used for other categories in the absence of radical orchiectomy.

Regional Lymph Nodes (N)

Clinical

NX	Regional lymph nodes cannot be assessed
N0	No regional lymph node metastasis
N1	Metastasis with a lymph node mass 2 cm or less in greatest dimension; or multiple lymph nodes, none more than 2 cm in greatest dimension
N2	Metastasis with a lymph node mass more than 2 cm but not more than 5 cm in greatest dimension; or multiple lymph nodes, any one mass greater than 2 cm but not more than 5 cm in greatest dimension
N3	Metastasis with a lymph node mass more than 5 cm in greatest dimension

Pathologic (pN)

pNX	Regional lymph nodes cannot be assessed
pN0	No regional lymph node metastasis
pN1	Metastasis with a lymph node mass 2 cm or less in greatest dimension and less than or equal to 5 nodes positive, none more than 2 cm in greatest dimension
pN2	Metastasis with a lymph node mass more than 2 cm but not more than 5 cm in greatest dimension; or more than 5 nodes positive, none more than 5 cm; or evidence of extranodal extension of tumor
pN3	Metastasis with a lymph node mass more than 5 cm in greatest dimension

Distant Metastasis (M)

MX	Distant metastasis cannot be assessed
M0	No distant metastasis
M1	Distant metastasis
M1a	Non-regional nodal or pulmonary metastasis
M1b	Distant metastasis other than to non-regional lymph nodes and lungs

Serum Tumor Markers (S)

SX	Marker studies not available or not performed
S0	Marker study levels within normal limits
S1	LDH $<1.5 \times$ N* AND hCG (mIu/ml) <5000 AND AFP (ng/ml) <1000
S2	LDH 1.5–$10 \times$ N OR hCG (mIu/ml) 5000–$50,000$ OR AFP (ng/ml) 1000–$10,000$
S3	LDH $>10 \times$ N OR hCG (mIu/ml) $>50,000$ OR AFP (ng/ml) $>10,000$

*N indicates the upper limit of normal for the LDH assay.

Stage Grouping

Stage 0	pTis	N0	M0	S0
Stage I	pT1–4	N0	M0	SX
Stage IA	pT1	N0	M0	S0
Stage IB	pT2	N0	M0	S0
	pT3	N0	M0	S0
	pT4	N0	M0	S0
Stage I	Any pT/Tx	N0	M0	S1–3
Stage II	Any pT/Tx	N1–3	M0	SX
Stage IIA	Any pT/Tx	N1	M0	S0
	Any pT/Tx	N1	M0	S1
Stage IIB	Any pT/Tx	N2	M0	S0
	Any pT/Tx	N2	M0	S1
Stage IIC	Any pT/Tx	N3	M0	S0
	Any pT/Tx	N3	M0	S1
Stage III	Any pT/Tx	Any N	M1	SX
Stage IIIA	Any pT/Tx	Any N	M1a	S0
	Any pT/Tx	Any N	M1a	S1
Stage IIIB	Any pT/Tx	N1–3	M0	S2
	Any pT/Tx	Any N	M1a	S2
Stage IIIC	Any pT/Tx	N1–3	M0	S3
	Any pT/Tx	Any N	M1a	S3
	Any pT/Tx	Any N	M1b	Any S

From Greene FL, Page DL, Fleming ID, et al, eds. *AJCC Cancer Staging Manual*, 6th ed. New York: Springer; 2002.

STANDARD THERAPEUTIC APPROACHES

This chapter discusses only the therapy of germ cell tumors of the testis, particularly seminoma. The standard initial therapy for a suspected testicular neoplasm, as noted earlier, is inguinal orchiectomy. The surgical approach to the testicle is through an inguinal incision, to avoid the risk of interruption of the testicular lymphatics. The incision is made in the skin at a spot overlying the internal inguinal ring, and the external oblique aponeurosis is incised. The testicular vessels and vas deferens are mobilized, and a noncrushing clamp is placed across the cord structures to help decrease the theoretical risk of spreading the tumor by manipulation. The testicle is delivered to the operative field and examined. If a mass can be clearly identified in the testicle itself, the orchiectomy is performed, with separation of the cord structures at the internal inguinal ring. If there is a question about the location of the mass, the tunica vaginalis can be opened to allow more direct inspection; rarely, a biopsy is performed. Any doubt as to the nature of the problem should lead to orchiectomy, as retention of a testis with a malignant neoplasm is worse than removal of a testis with a benign problem.

Once the testis has been removed and the diagnosis of malignancy confirmed, the therapeutic branch point comes with the determination of the pathology, specifically, whether the cancer is seminoma or NSGCT. In early-stage seminomas, the role of radiation therapy is well established and is discussed later. In more advanced stages (bulky abdominal lymphadenopathy) and with disseminated disease, the trend has been toward chemotherapy, with radiation reserved for persistent or recurrent disease in focal areas. The agents active in seminoma include cisplatin and analogues, etoposide, bleomycin, vinblastine, and ifosfamide. These agents are also active against NSGCT.

Standard therapy for stage I NSGCT, after inguinal orchiectomy has been performed, has been retroperitoneal lymph node dissection. This procedure has relatively low morbidity, but ejaculatory dysfunction is high, although newer surgical approaches seek to minimize this risk.[67] Chemotherapy is used if there is evidence of relapse. About 15% of patients with negative lymph nodes suffer recurrence, usually within 18 months, with the most common site being the lungs.[68] A current controversy involves observation after orchiectomy as opposed to lymph node dissection. As with seminomas (discussed later), surveillance is probably acceptable in selected patients—those with negative serum markers, negative radiologic imaging, and a willingness to comply with regular follow-up and imaging. Histologic evidence of lymphatic or venous invasion may also portend a higher risk of relapse and may mark a patient as unsuitable for surveillance.[50] Chemotherapy is also being considered as an option for stage I NSGCT after orchiectomy.[69] Radiation therapy can control microscopic nonseminomatous disease in the retroperitoneum, but the higher propensity for hematogenous spread has largely led to the abandonment of adjuvant irradiation for stage I NSGCT, favoring either surveillance in low-risk patients or chemotherapy.[70]

For pathologic stage II NSGCT, standard therapy is again retroperitoneal lymph node dissection, with chemotherapy at relapse. Patients whose markers do not return to normal after lymph node dissection usually are treated with chemotherapy. The issue of adjuvant chemotherapy versus chemotherapy at relapse is controversial.[71,72] Patients with radiographically bulky lymph nodes are often treated with chemotherapy instead of lymph node dissection. Unlike seminoma, where resection of residual masses is difficult, residual disease after chemotherapy for NSGCT is often resected, with a significant probability of finding teratomatous elements. Various factors can be used to predict the risk of residual disease.[73] Persistent elevations of AFP and HCG after chemotherapy are considered to be markers for viable, unresectable disease, and salvage chemotherapy is generally recommended.[74,75] More advanced NSGCTs are treated with chemotherapy as well. Radiation is used occasionally for patients with bulky disease that is not resectable, often after chemotherapy. Full discussion of the issues relating to the therapy of NSGCT is beyond the scope of this chapter.

ROLE OF RADIATION THERAPY

Postoperative irradiation of the para-aortic and ipsilateral pelvic lymph nodes, as detailed later, is standard therapy for stage I seminomas. Because only about 20% of the patients treated actually harbor disease, however, there has been great interest in whether a policy of observation rather than immediate adjuvant radiation could be followed to spare the majority of patients unnecessary radiation.[76] Patients relapsing in the retroperitoneum may be salvaged with radiation; those failing in the mediastinum or elsewhere would receive chemotherapy. A number of reports have shown that surveillance appears to be a safe management policy, with a review of data from three different institutions for a total of 583 patients showing a combined rate of relapse of 15% and an overall survival of 99.7%.[77] Relapses in seminoma often occur later than in NSGCT, making longer intensive follow-up necessary.[78] Frequent radiologic examinations are necessary if surveillance is selected. Continuing with this degree of follow-up may be difficult outside of a study setting.[79] The relatively slow growth rate of seminoma compared with other NSGCTs, the longer period of intensive surveillance, and the lack of a sensitive tumor marker to select those patients most at risk for relapse increase the difficulty as well. Finally, a study from the University of Wisconsin demonstrated 39% greater medical costs per patient with a policy of surveillance over a 5-year follow-up period than with the standard therapy of adjuvant irradiation to the pelvic and para-aortic regions, with no noted difference in outcome.[80] An alternative approach being explored involves the use of initial adjuvant chemotherapy in stage I seminoma.[81] Surveillance appears to be a safe approach, but whether the small reduction in potential toxicity justifies the increased vigilance and cost of observation remains to be seen.

Stage II seminomas may also be managed with radiotherapy after orchiectomy, provided the retroperitoneal disease is not excessively large. The risk of subsequent failure after abdominal irradiation is directly related to the initial bulk of disease.[82,83] Stage IIA disease (<2 cm) is managed in the same fashion as stage I; stage IIB (2-<5 cm) patients receive the same initial radiotherapy, with an additional boost to the site of gross disease. The optimal treatment for patients with stage IIC disease (5-10 cm) is controversial. Thomas[84] published a review of collected data showing a risk of recurrence of 8% for patients with abdominal masses between 5 and 10 cm, but rising to 35% for masses greater than 10 cm. The likelihood of control of stage IIC masses with platinum-containing chemotherapy is probably equivalent to control with radiotherapy, sometimes requiring additional chemotherapy or surgery.[85-87] An important consideration when selecting therapy is the location of the mass; bulky disease overlying the majority of a kidney or a significant fraction of the liver is much less attractive for radiation than is centrally located disease. Primary irradiation of patients with retroperitoneal masses greater than 10 cm has been abandoned in most institutions in favor of chemotherapy.[82,88-90]

In patients with bulky abdominal lymphadenopathy, careful radiographic investigation demonstrates a residual mass after chemotherapy in as many as 75% of patients.[87] Resection of these masses is technically difficult, with dense fibrosis and a severe scirrhous reaction to chemotherapy causing adherence to surrounding structures and attendant increased morbidity.[85,91,92] The size of the residual mass may have prognostic implications.[74] One study found that 6 of 14 patients (42%) with a residual mass greater than 3 cm had viable tumor on surgical resection, whereas none of the patients with residual masses less than 3 cm had viable tumor.[93] Others have not seen this relationship.[94,95] Routine irradiation for the residual mass after chemotherapy is thought to be unnecessary in the majority of patients, and at this time, careful observation appears to be a reasonable course.[96]

For stage III and IV seminomas, chemotherapy has supplanted radiation. The role of radiation in advanced seminomas is unclear, but it may be used for sites that have not demonstrated complete regression following chemotherapy, as discussed earlier. In the past, focal radiation was used as salvage after failure in a localized region, such as supraclavicular lymph nodes, but chemotherapy is now increasingly employed as salvage for patients with recurrent seminoma after radiotherapy. Patients who develop a second seminoma after orchiectomy and radiation for an initial seminoma can be considered for re-irradiation of the retroperitoneum, with a portion of the dose delivered through lateral fields and careful attention to the total renal dose. Surveillance is also an attractive option in this setting.

The role of radiation therapy in NSGCT is very limited. Some have advocated the use of radiation to the retroperitoneal lymph nodes after orchiectomy,[97,98] but the higher likelihood of relapse in distant sites with NSGCT makes this approach less attractive than in seminoma. Radiation therapy has no role in the management of patients with disseminated NSGCT, with the exception of palliative irradiation of local problems such as brain metastases.

SIMULATION

Before the initiation of therapy, inquiry should be made regarding the patient's desire to retain fertility. Given the young age of many patients with this disease, this question is often of great interest, either at the time of treatment or at some point in the future. Sperm banking and semen analysis may be offered as a precautionary measure. Because many patients with seminomas have diminished fertility before treatment—about 40% are azoospermic at presentation[77]—it can be useful to discover this before the radiation. Gonadal shielding of the contralateral testis (the evocatively named "clamshell") can be used, particularly if fertility is desired. This can reduce the dose to the remaining testicle to 1% to 2% of the prescribed dose, or 25 to 50 cGy over the course of therapy.[99] If a further dose reduction is desired, a dose on the order of one tenth of 1% can be achieved by extending the custom block used in the linear accelerator blocking tray 5 cm below the edge of the field; adding a 10 cm-thick lead scrotal block below the inferior field edge, supported over the patient on a stand; and using a gonadal shield designed to minimize internal scattered radiation.[100]

For simulation, the patient is placed in the supine position (Fig. 46-6). No special immobilization devices are generally necessary. An intravenous pyelogram was

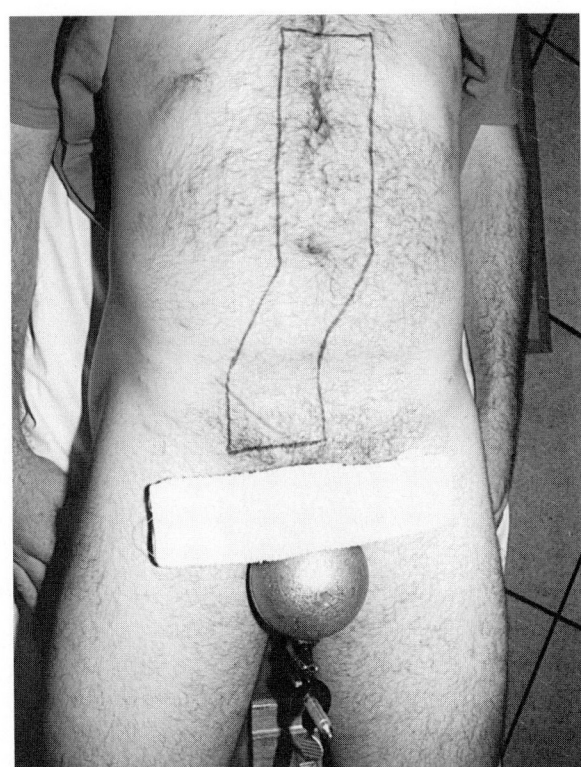

Figure 46–6. Patient at treatment for right-sided seminoma, with clamshell.

traditionally performed to delineate the renal tissue, but in the modern era of CT-based simulators, this is often not necessary. Whichever means is chosen, it is essential to verify exclusion of adequate kidney volume from the treated fields. When intravenous contrast is administered, adequate equipment and personnel to respond to severe contrast allergies must be on hand. The superior margin of the field is at minimum the T10 to T11 interspace,[101] as T11 is the highest level of lymphatic drainage as visualized on testicular lymphangiograms, and the level of the cisterna chyli.[102] Other authors advocate the superior border at the T9 to T10 interspace.[103] The inferior border is usually in the region of the top of the obturator foramen. Unless there is tumor invasion of the spermatic cord, inclusion of the entire orchiectomy scar does not appear to be necessary.[43,66] The field is usually 10 to 12 cm wide, although care must be taken to cover the left renal hilum, which may necessitate wider fields in this area. Nodes that are not pathologically enlarged generally do not extend laterally beyond the transverse process of the lumbar vertebral bodies. At least the lateral two thirds of both kidneys should be shielded whenever possible. Generally, no special effort is made to extend the fields wide enough in the pelvis to cover the farthest possible reach of the transit of the lymphatics from the testicle to their landing sites in the retroperitoneum as demonstrated on lymphangiogram, as failure in these sites is uncommon.[56] More space is usually allowed for left-sided tumors, however. The ipsilateral iliac and pelvic nodes are included. Custom field blocking should be used to exclude irradiation of unnecessary tissue (Figs. 46-7 and 46-8).

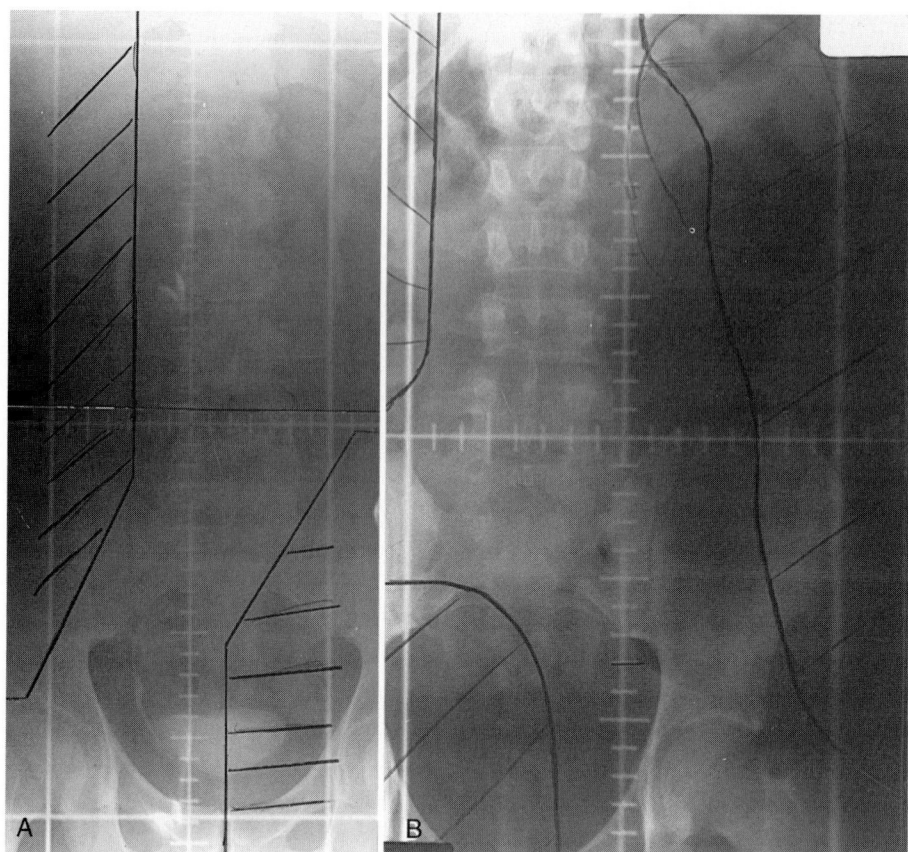

Figure 46–7. A, Example of simulation field for right-sided tumor. **B,** Example of simulation field for left-sided tumor. (Courtesy of L. Chinsoo Cho, M.D., Department of Radiation Oncology, University of Texas, Southwestern Medical Center at Dallas.)

RADIATION TREATMENT PLAN

Patients should be treated with megavoltage photons, using parallel opposed anterior and posterior custom-shaped fields as outlined earlier, taking into account CT or lymphangiogram data, or both. Both fields are treated

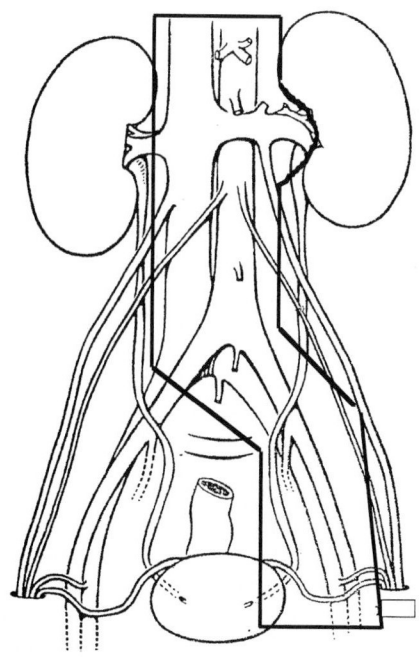

Figure 46–8. Diagram of field for left-sided tumor.

daily, 5 days per week. Seminomas are very radiosensitive, and doses of 25 to 30 Gy appear to be adequate. For a patient with stage I seminoma, it has been the author's practice to give 25.5 Gy in 15 fractions of 1.7 Gy each; if gastrointestinal tolerance is an issue, this can be decreased to 1.5 Gy or even 1.25 Gy. In the past, higher doses up to 40 Gy were often used, but there appear to be no data that higher doses are necessary for control in patients without macroscopic retroperitoneal disease. Thomas[104] reported a series of 150 patients treated at the Princess Margaret Hospital treated with 25 Gy in 20 fractions, with no in-field failures. Higher doses, however, appear to be associated with increased risk of side effects such as gastric ulceration.[105] Prophylactic mediastinal radiation for stage I seminoma patients is generally not recommended, as the risk of failure is very low.[83,106] Because less than 3% of patients with stage I seminomas have disease in the pelvis,[107] there is growing discussion of omitting the pelvic portion of the radiotherapy field and treating only the para-aortics (Fig. 46-9).[108] This field is currently used at the University of California–San Francisco for patients believed to be at low risk. The morbidity from including the ipsilateral hemipelvis is very low, however, providing little motivation to change what has been a highly successful therapeutic approach. The omission of the pelvic portion of the radiation field is currently a matter of some debate.[109] The Medical Research Council has published a multicenter randomized trial of 478 men with stage I seminoma comparing conventional "dog-leg" irradiation, including the ipsilateral hemipelvis and the para-aortic nodes, with para-aortic treatment only,

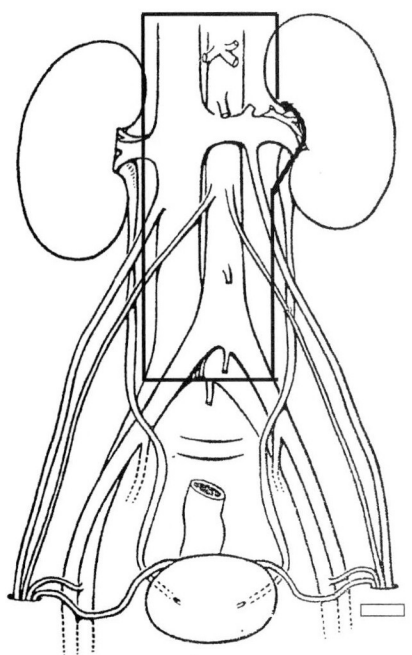

Figure 46–9. Diagram of para-aortic field for low-risk patients.

showing equivalent relapse-free survival in the two groups, and reduced toxicity with the more limited fields.[110]

Another area of controversy involves how to approach a patient with prior scrotal violation. Traditional teaching has been to avoid trans-scrotal biopsy or scrotal incisions, on the assumption that alteration of lymphatic drainage may lead to increased risk of local or inguinal failure. When the scrotum has been disturbed, the standard recommendation has been to treat the ipsilateral hemiscrotum with a local electron field, generally employing 12 to 15 MeV electrons, matched to the inferior edge of the photon field. The contralateral testis is retracted up toward the inguinal canal under lead shielding to attempt to minimize the dose to the remaining testicle. If the patient has had prior orchiopexy or inguinal herniorrhaphy, traditional treatment has included the contralateral inguinal and iliac regions. It has been reported, however, that scrotal surgery at the time of the primary treatment did not predispose to disease recurrence in the abdomen, pelvis, or scrotum, with the finding that the incidence of abdominopelvic or scrotal recurrence in patients with a history of previous scrotal surgery and without additional radiation to the inguinoscrotal region was not significantly different from the rate of recurrence in those patients without such surgery.[83] The number of patients given additional radiation was too small to tell whether there was any benefit. Other reviews have confirmed that spread to the inguinal nodes is unusual, even in a patient who has had prior inguinal or scrotal surgery or when tumor invades into structures involved with the testicle.[111-113] A report from the University of California–Los Angeles described 14 patients with violated scrotums, 5 of whom received prophylactic irradiation to the scrotum; 2 of these 5 relapsed in the abdomen.[115] Of the nine patients who did not receive prophylactic irradiation to the scrotum, three relapsed in the abdomen. None of the patients failed in the scrotum or inguinal nodes.

Twenty-one patients had previous pelvis surgery, and four had the whole pelvis treated. Two of these patients failed in the abdomen, and both had bulky lymphadenopathy (stage IIC). Of the 17 patients not receiving whole pelvis radiotherapy, none failed. Given the low risk of scrotal failure in patients with disturbance of the scrotum, it would be reasonable to omit radiation to the involved hemiscrotum, particularly if the patient is interested in retaining fertility. The 1989 consensus conference on seminoma management in England recommended that inguinal or scrotal irradiation be omitted even if interference with the scrotum has occurred.[67] A massive primary tumor invading into the scrotum but not requiring a hemiscrotectomy would be an indication to include the ipsilateral hemiscrotum. Whether radiation to the contralateral pelvis in a patient with a history of orchiopexy or herniorrhaphy is wise is also unclear, but there appears to be little firm evidence to support this as a universal approach.

For stage II patients (radiographic evidence of spread to retroperitoneal lymph nodes), treatment is based on the bulk of disease. For patients with minimal lymphadenopathy (stage IIA, nodes <2 cm), no modification to fields or doses is used. For patients with more significant nodes (stage IIB, nodes 2-<5 cm), radiation is employed using the same fields as in stage I, although a 2 to 3 cm margin around the enlarged nodes as visualized on CT should be provided. Because of concern about retrograde lymphatic drainage into the pelvis, bilateral pelvic nodal irradiation is sometimes recommended. If this is done, shielding over the midline of the pelvis may be used to reduce toxicity. The initial fields are treated as in stage I disease, to a dose on the order of 25 Gy, followed by field reduction to boost the enlarged nodes plus at least 2 cm margins, for an additional 5 to 10 Gy. Residual masses at the site of bulk disease after radiation are not uncommon; observation is recommended unless serial imaging studies show enlargement.

Whether to administer prophylactic mediastinal and supraclavicular radiation for stage II seminomas is controversial. Thomas and colleagues[83] published the results of a study of 86 patients with stage II seminoma treated at Princess Margaret Hospital and found that prophylactic mediastinal irradiation appeared to be unnecessary. Gregory and Peckham[82] found no benefit to supradiaphragmatic irradiation in a review of 53 patients with stage II seminoma treated at Royal Marsden Hospital; relapse was 14% for those patients receiving infradiaphragmatic irradiation only, compared with 19% for those who had radiation above the diaphragm as well. Other series have confirmed the lack of benefit from mediastinal and supraclavicular radiation.[88,115-119] Dosmann and Zagars[64] reported the results obtained after abandoning elective mediastinal irradiation in stage II patients at MD Anderson Cancer Center. They found that omission of mediastinal irradiation increased the 5-year actuarial risk of failure in the left supraclavicular fossa to 20% (3 of 16 patients), compared with a 0% 5-year actuarial risk for patients treated with prophylactic radiation to the mediastinum and supraclavicular region. However, all patients failing were salvaged, and the prophylactic irradiation of the mediastinum appeared to be associated with an increase in death from intercurrent illness, most marked in patients older than 40 years of age, possibly owing to cardiac toxicity. This increased mortality is supported by the Patterns of Care study, which showed an increase in cardiac and pulmonary deaths in patients older than 40 when prophylactic mediastinal irradiation was used.[120] A retrospective analysis from the Joint Center for Radiation Therapy also showed a higher incidence of cardiac complications in patients receiving supradiaphragmatic radiation.[121] The recommendation was for elective radiation to the left supraclavicular region only, sparing the mediastinum.[60] A report from the University of Florida recommended the omission of elective supradiaphragmatic irradiation in stage II patients, unless there were three or more lymph node metastases or metastases larger than 3 cm.[122] The arguments against prophylactic mediastinal irradiation in the current era can be summed up as follows: The risk of failure is low for most patients; if failure does occur, the likelihood of salvage with chemotherapy is good; side effects of the radiation may be increased by the expanded volume of tissue treated; and irradiation of these areas may decrease the patient's ability to tolerate subsequent chemotherapy if needed. If primary radiation therapy is used for patients with more bulky retroperitoneal disease in the 5 to 10 cm range, this subset of patients has a higher risk of failure, and the arguments for prophylactic supradiaphragmatic irradiation have greater weight. If elective radiation is given to the mediastinum and supraclavicular area, the dose is generally in the range of 25 Gy.

After the conclusion of treatment, the patient should be followed for the development of recurrent or metastatic disease. Patients who will have recurrences often do so within 2 years.[105,123] Because of the possibility of developing a second tumor, the risk of which can be as high as 3%,[124] self-examination of the remaining testicle may also be helpful.

CRITICAL NORMAL TISSUES

Acute side effects of radiation therapy for testicular cancer are usually modest, with the most common being gastrointestinal. Nausea, vomiting, and diarrhea during the course of therapy occur in at least 20% to 50% of patients.[123,125,126] One study from the Norwegian Radium Hospital found that all 39 patients required sick leave from work during treatment, with a median period of leave after radiotherapy of 5 weeks; the dose given for stage I patients was 36 Gy, and 40 Gy for stage II.[127] Because of the large volume of bone marrow irradiated, estimated at 35% to 40% for an adult,[128] transient declines in blood counts may be seen.

The typical radiation treatment approach, which gives 1% to 2% of the prescribed dose to the contralateral remaining testis, often leads to a significant temporary reduction in sperm production and fertility.[129] Over 2 to 3 years, however, fertility is generally restored in those patients who were fertile before the radiotherapy.[130,131] If fertility before this time interval is desired, sperm banking should be considered. Avoiding fatherhood for 6 to 12 months after therapy, to avoid possible insemination

by sperm that have been damaged by radiation, also seems prudent.

Chronic toxicity is difficult to assess; most of the longer-term information deals with patients treated with outdated techniques or equipment. The most frequent long-term complications are gastric. Radiation therapy for stage I seminoma has been reported to result in a 6% incidence of peptic ulceration, compared with none in patients managed by observation.[105] Another study showed that 6% of patients developed significant dyspepsia, with frank ulceration in 3%, after doses of 35 to 40 Gy in 2 Gy fractions.[111] This can be compared, however, with a retrospective review from Toronto, which found no late gastrointestinal toxicity using lower doses of 25 Gy over 20 fractions.[83] Late nephrotoxicity or myelitis should be minimal.[132,133] Psychosocial problems can result after therapy. Up to 40% of patients may note difficulties with sexual function,[134-136] but some patients report an improvement following therapy.[135,137] One study found that 14% of patients suffered symptoms of anxiety, and 8% had symptoms of depression, within 5 years of treatment.[136] The most worrisome risk is the development of second malignancies as a result of the radiation exposure. A number of studies have reported a small increased risk of second solid tumors, largely gastrointestinal malignancies and sarcomas,[138-140] but others have not shown an increased incidence.[141] The exact risk of secondary tumors is uncertain but is probably modestly increased.[142]

OUTCOME

Testicular tumors as a group represent one of the greatest triumphs of modern oncology, with the vast majority of patients able to enjoy long-term survival. The overall survival in patients with seminoma is excellent, probably because most patients present without disseminated disease, the spread of nodal metastases is predictable, and the tumor is radiosensitive. With modern treatment, the cure rate for stage I seminoma should approach 99%, with relapse-free survival rate exceeding 95%.[104,105,111] Patients with stage IIA disease should also have long-term survival in the range of 95%.[88,104] More bulky disease has a less optimistic prognosis and a higher risk for relapse, but with chemotherapy salvage, approximately 85% of patients with masses between 5 and 10 cm should be long-term survivors.[107] Treatment of stage I NSGCT should also yield survival rates near 100%.[69] For more advanced stages, overall about 70% to 80% survive.

REFERENCES

1. Jemal A, Murray T, Samuels A, et al: Cancer statistics, 2003. *CA Cancer J Clin.* 2003;53:5.
2. Gilliland FD, Key CR: Male genital cancers. *Cancer.* 1995;75:295.
3. Zheng T, Holford T, Ma Z: Continuing increase in incidence of germ cell testis cancer in young adults: Experience from Connecticut, USA, 1935-1992. *Int J Cancer.* 1996;65:723.
4. Sokol M, Peckham MI, Hendry WF: Bilateral germ cell tumors of the testis. *Br J Urol.* 1979;52:158.
5. Gilbert JB: Tumors of the testis following mumps orchitis: Case report and review of 24 cases. *J Urol.* 1944;51:296.

6. Gilbert JB, Hamilton JB: Incidence and nature of tumors in ectopic testes. *Surg Gynecol Obstet.* 1940;71:731.

7. Martin DC: Germinal cell tumors of the testis after orchiopexy. *J Urol.* 1979;121:422.

8. Henderson BE, Benton B, Jing J, et al: Risk factors for cancer of the testis in young men. *Int J Cancer.* 1979;23:598.

9. Raghavan D, Zalcberg JR, Grygiel JJ, et al: Multiple atypical nevi: A cutaneous marker of germ cell tumors. *J Clin Oncol.* 1994; 12:2284.

10. Wilson WT, Frenkel E, Vuitch F, et al: Testicular tumors in men with human immunodeficiency virus. *J Urol.* 1992;147:1038.

11. Rodriguez E, Mathew S, Reuter V, et al: Cytogenetic analysis of 124 prospectively ascertained male germ cell tumors. *Cancer Res.* 1992;52:2285.

12. Chaganti RSK, Rodriguez E, Bosl GJ: Cytogenetics of male germ cell tumors. *Urol Clin North Am.* 1993;20:55.

13. Kurie JM, Bosl GJ, Dmitrovsky E: Genetic and biologic aspects of treatment response and resistance in male germ cell cancer. *Semin Oncol.* 1992;19:197.

14. Atkin NB, Baker MC: i(12p): Specific chromosomal marker in seminoma and malignant teratoma of the testis. *Cancer Genet Cytogenet.* 1983;10:199.

15. Vos A, Oosterhuis JW, deJong B, et al: Cytogenetics of carcinoma in situ of the testis. *Cancer Genet Cytogenet.* 1990;46:75.

16. Bosl G, Dmitrovsky E, Reuter VE, et al: Isochrome of chromosome 12: Clinically useful marker for male germ cell tumors. *J Natl Cancer Inst.* 1989;81:1874.

17. Wang L-C, Vass W, Gao C, et al: Amplification and enhanced expression of the c-ki-*ras* 2 proto-oncogene in human embryonal carcinomas. *Cancer Res.* 1987;47:4192.

18. Saminiego F, Rodriguez E, Houldsworth J, et al: Cytogenetic and molecular analysis of human male germ cell tumors: Chromosome 12 abnormalities and gene amplification. *Genes Chromosomes Cancer.* 1990;1:289.

19. Rowley MJ, Leach DR, Warner GA, et al: Effect of graded doses of ionizing radiation on the human testis. *Radiat Res.* 1974;59:665.

20. Mostofi FK, Price EB: Tumors of the male genital system. In *Atlas of Tumor Pathology,* 2nd series, fascicle 8. Washington, DC: AFIP; 1973:16.

21. Mostofi FK, Price EB: Tumors of the male genital system. In *Atlas of Tumor Pathology,* 2nd series, fascicle 8. Washington, DC: AFIP; 1973:68.

22. Babaian RJ, Zagars GK: Testicular seminoma: The M. D. Anderson experience: An analysis of pathological and patient characteristics, and current recommendations. *J Urol.* 1988;139:311.

23. Skakkebaek NE: Carcinoma in situ of the testis: Frequency and relationship to invasive germ cell tumors in infertile men. *Histopathology.* 1978;2:157.

24. Bartlett NL, Freiha FS, Torti FM: Serum markers in germ cell neoplasm. *Hematol Oncol Clin North Am.* 1991;5:1245.

25. Gitlin D, Boesman M: Serum alpha-fetoprotein, albumin, and gamma G-globulin in the human conceptus. *J Clin Invest.* 1966;45:1826.

26. Lange PH, Raghavan D: Clinical applications of tumor markers in testicular cancer. In Donohue JD, eds. *Testis Tumors.* Baltimore: Williams & Wilkins; 1983:111.

27. Rizkallah T, Gurpide E, Vandeweile RL: Metabolism of HCG in man. *J Clin Endocrinol.* 1969;29:92.

28. Bower M, Rustin GJS: Serum tumor markers and their role in monitoring germ cell cancers of the testis. In Vogelzang NJ, Scardino PT, Shipley WU, Coffey DS, eds. *Comprehensive Textbook of Genitourinary Oncology.* Baltimore: Williams & Wilkins; 1996:970.

29. Weissback L, Bussar-Maatz R: HCG-positive seminoma. *Eur Urol.* 1993;23(suppl 2):29.

30. Javadpour N: Current status of tumor markers in testicular cancer. *Eur Urol.* 1992;21(suppl 1):34.

31. Javadpour N: Applications of biologic tumor markers to testicular cancer. *Cancer Treat Rep.* 1979;63:1643.

32. Carl J, Christensen TB, van der Maase H: Cisplatinum dose-dependent response in germ cell cancer evaluated by tumour marker modeling. *Acta Oncol.* 1992;31:749.

33. Stoter G, Bosl GJ, Droz JP, et al: Prognostic factors in metastatic germ cell tumours. In Newling DW, Jones WG, eds. *EORTC Genitourinary Group Monograph 7: Prostate Cancer and Testicular Cancer.* New York: Wiley-Liss; 1990:313.

34. Von Eyben FE: Lactate dehydrogenase and its isoenzymes in testicular germ cell tumors: An overview. *Oncodev Biol Med.* 1983;4:395.

35. Hamilton CR, Horwich A: Rare tumors of the testis and paratesticular tumors. In Williams CJ, Krikorian JG, Green MR, Raghavan D, eds. *Textbook of Uncommon Cancer.* Chichester: John Wiley & Sons; 1988:225.

36. Doll DC, Weiss RB: Malignant lymphoma of the testis. *Am J Med.* 1986;81:515.

37. Washecka RM, Mariani AJ, Zuna RE, et al: Primary intratesticular sarcoma. *Cancer.* 1966;77:1524.

38. Tiltman AJ: Metastatic tumors in the testis. *Histopathology.* 1979;3:31.

39. London MZ, Grossman SN: Secondary testicular tumor resembling Krukenberg tumor: A case report. *J Urol.* 1949;62:713.

40. Percapio B, Clements JC, McLeod DG, et al: Anaplastic seminoma: An analysis of 77 patients. *Cancer.* 1979;43:2510.

41. Cockburn A, Vugrin D, Batala M, et al: Poorly differentiated (anaplastic) seminoma of the testis. *Cancer.* 1984;53:1991.

42. Mirimanoff RO, Sinzia M, Kruger M, et al: Prognosis of human chorionic gonadotropin producing seminoma treated by postoperative radiotherapy. *Int J Radiat Oncol Biol Phys.* 1993;27:17.

43. Horwich A, Dearnaley DP: Treatment of seminoma. *Semin Oncol.* 1992;19:171.

44. Fung AW, Garnick MB: Clinical stage I carcinoma of the testis: A review. *J Clin Oncol.* 1988;6:734.

45. Leibovitch H, Foster RS, Ulbright TM, et al: Adult primary pure teratoma of the testis: The Indiana experience. *Cancer.* 1995;75:2244.

46. Timmerman JM, Northfelt DW, Small EJ: Malignant germ cell tumors in man infected with the human immunodeficiency virus: Natural history and results of therapy. *J Clin Oncol.* 1995;13:1391.

47. Bernardi D, Salvioni R, Vaccher E, et al: Testicular germ cell tumors and human immunodeficiency virus infection: A report of 26 cases. *J Clin Oncol.* 1995;13:2705.

48. Kennedy BJ, Schmidt JD, Winchester DP, et al: National survey of patterns of care for testis cancer. *Cancer.* 1987;60:1921.

49. Bosl GJ, Vogelzang NJ, Goldman A, et al: Impact of delay in diagnosis on clinical stage of testicular cancer. *Lancet.* 1981;2:970.

50. Sesterhenn IA, Weiss RB, Mostofi FK, et al: Prognosis and other clinical correlates of pathologic review in stages I and II testicular carcinoma: A report from the testicular cancer intergroup study. *J Clin Oncol.* 1992;10:69.

51. Oliver RTD: Factors contributing to delay in diagnosis of testicular tumors. *Br Med J.* 1985;290:356.

52. Stepanas AV, Samaan NA, Schultz PN, et al: Endocrine studies in testicular tumor patients with and without gynecomastia: A report of 45 cases. *Cancer.* 1978;41:369.

53. Busch FM, Sayegh ES, Chenault OW: Some uses of lymphangiography in the management of testicular tumors. *J Urol.* 1965;93:490.

54. Chiappa S, Uslenghi C, Bonadonna G, et al: Combined testicular and foot lymphangiography in testicular carcinomas. *Surg Gynecol Obstet.* 1966;123:10.

55. Ray B, Hajdu SI, Whitmore WF: Distribution of retroperitoneal lymph node metastases in testicular germinal tumors. *Cancer.* 1974; 33:340.

56. Donohue JP, Zachary JM, Maynard BR: Distribution of nodal metastases in nonseminomatous testis cancer. *J Urol.* 1982;128:315.

57. Johnson DE, Appelt G, Samuels ML, et al: Metastases from testicular carcinoma: Study of 78 autopsied cases. *Urology.* 1976; 8:234.

58. Orecklin JR: Testicular tumor occurring with hydrocele and positive cytologic fluid. *Urology.* 1974;3:232.

59. Lee JKT, McClennan BL, Stanley R, et al: Computed tomography in the staging of testicular neoplasms. *Radiology.* 1979;130:387.

60. Dosmann MA, Zagars MA: Postorchiectomy radiotherapy for stages I and II testicular seminoma. *Int J Radiat Oncol Biol Phys.* 1993;26:381.

61. Hain S, O'Doherty M, Timothy A, et al: Fluorodeoxyglucose PET in the initial staging of germ cell tumours. *Eur J Nucl Med.* 2000; 27:590.

62. Hain D, O'Doherty M, Timothy A, et al: Fluorodeoxyglucose positron emission tomography in the evaluation of germ cell tumours at relapse. *Brit J Cancer.* 2000;83:863.

63. De Santis M, Bokemeyer C, Becherer A, et al: Predictive impact of 2-18fluoro-2deoxy-D-glucose positron emission tomography for residual postchemotherapy masses in patients with bulky seminoma. *J Clin Oncol.* 2001;19:3740.

64. Boden G, Gibb R: Radiotherapy and testicular neoplasms. *Lancet.* 1951;2:1195.

65. Maier JG, Sulak MH: Proceedings: Radiation therapy in malignant testis tumors: Part II. Carcinoma. *Cancer.* 1973;32:1212.

66. Thomas GM, Jones W, VanOosterom A, et al: Consensus statement on the investigation and management of testicular seminoma 1989. In Newling DW, and Jones WG, eds. *EORTC Genitourinary Group Monograph 7: Prostate Cancer and Testicular Cancer.* New York: Wiley-Liss; 1990:285.

67. Donohue JP, Thornhill JA, Foster RS, et al: Retroperitoneal lymphadenectomy for clinical stage A testis cancer (1965 to 1989): Modifications of technique and impact on ejaculation. *J Urol.* 1993;149:237.

68. Klepp O, Olsson AM, Hendrikson H, et al: Prognostic factors in clinical stage I nonseminomatous germ cell tumors of the testis: Multivariate analysis of a prospective multicenter study. *J Clin Oncol.* 1990;8:503.

69. Rorth M: Therapeutic alternatives in clinical stage (nonseminomatous) disease. *Semin Oncol.* 1992;19:190.

70. Rorth M, Jacobsen GK, von der Maase H, et al: Surveillance alone versus radiotherapy after orchiectomy for clinical stage I nonseminomatous testicular cancer. *J Clin Oncol.* 1991;9:1543.

71. Bosl GJ, Gluckman R, Geller NL, et al: VAB-6: An effective chemotherapy regimen for patients with germ-cell tumors. *J Clin Oncol.* 1986;4:1493.

72. Williams SD, Stablein DM, Einhorn LH, et al: Immediate adjuvant chemotherapy versus observation with treatment at relapse in pathological stage II testicular cancer. *N Engl J Med.* 1987;317:1433.

73. Steyerberg EW, Keizer HJ, Fossa D, et al: Prediction of residual retroperitoneal mass histology after chemotherapy for metastatic nonseminomatous germ cell tumor: Multivariate analysis of individual patient data from six study groups. *J Clin Oncol.* 1995;13:1177.

74. Sheinfeld J, Bajorin D: Management of the postchemotherapy residual mass. *Urol Clin North Am.* 1993;20:133.

75. Bajorin D, Herr H, Motzer R, et al: Current perspectives on the role of adjunctive surgery in combined modality treatment of patients with germ cell tumors. *Semin Oncol.* 1992;19:148.

76. Warde P, Jewett M: Surveillance for stage I testicular seminoma. Is it a good option? *Urol Clin North Am.* 1998;25:425.

77. Thomas GM: Surveillance in stage I seminoma of the testis. *Urol Clin North Am.* 1993;20:85.

78. Peckham M: Testicular cancer. *Acta Oncol.* 1988;27:439.

79. Thomas GM, Sturgeon JF, Alison R, et al: A study of post orchiectomy surveillance in stage I testicular seminoma. *J Urol.* 1989;142:313.

80. Sharda NN, Kinsella TI, Ritter MA: Adjuvant radiation versus observation: Cost analysis of alternate management schemes in early-stage testicular seminoma. *J Clin Oncol.* 1996;14:2933.

81. Oliver RTD, Edmonds PM, Ong JYH, et al: Pilot studies of 2 and 1 course carboplatin as adjuvant for stage I seminoma: Should it be tested in a randomized trial against radiotherapy? *Int J Radiat Oncol Biol Phys.* 1994;29:3.

82. Gregory C, Peckham MJ: Results of radiotherapy for stage II testicular seminoma. *Radiother Oncol.* 1986;6:285.

83. Thomas GM, Rider WD, Dembo AJ, et al: Seminoma of the testis: Results of treatment and patterns of failure after radiation therapy. *Int J Radiat Oncol Biol Phys.* 1982;8:165.

84. Thomas GM: Management of metastatic seminoma: Role of radiotherapy. In Horwich A, ed. *Testicular Cancer: Clinical Investigation and Management.* New York: Chapman and Hall Medical; 1991:211.

85. Fossa SD, Borge L, Aass N, et al: The treatment of advanced metastatic seminoma: Experience in 55 cases. *J Clin Oncol.* 1987; 5:1071.

86. Loehrer PJ, Birch R, Williams SD, et al: Chemotherapy of metastatic seminoma: The southeastern cancer study group experience. *J Clin Oncol.* 1987;5:1212.

87. Peckham MJ, Horwich A, Hendry WF: Advanced seminoma: Treatment with cisplatinum-based chemotherapy or carboplatin (JM8). *Br J Cancer.* 1985;52:7.

88. Evensen JF, Fossa SD, Kjellevold K, et al: Testicular seminoma: Analysis of treatment and failure for stage II disease. *Radiother Oncol.* 1985;4:55.

89. Zagars GK, Babaian RJ: The role of radiation in stage II testicular seminoma. *Int J Radiat Oncol Biol Phys.* 1987;13:163.

90. Mason BR, Kearsley JH: Radiotherapy for stage 2 testicular seminoma: The prognostic influence of tumor bulk. *J Clin Oncol.* 1988;6:1856.

91. Herr HW, Bosl G: Residual mass after chemotherapy for seminoma: Changing concepts of management. *J Urol.* 1987;137:1234.

92. Friedman El, MB Garnick, Stomper PC, et al: Therapeutic guidelines and results in advanced seminoma. *J Clin Oncol.* 1985;3:1325.

93. Motzer R, Bosl G, Heelan R, et al: Residual mass: An indication for further therapy in patients with advanced seminoma following systemic chemotherapy. *J Clin Oncol.* 1987;5:1064.

94. Horwich A, Dearnaley DP, Duchesne GM, et al: Simple non-toxic treatment of advanced metastatic seminoma with carboplatin. *J Clin Oncol.* 1989;7:1150.

95. Schultz SM, Einhorn LH, Conces DJ, et al: Management of postchemotherapy residual mass in patients with advanced seminoma: Indiana University experience. *J Clin Oncol.* 1989; 7:1497.

96. Thomas GM: Refining the therapy of testicular seminoma. *Eur Urol.* 1993;23(suppl 2):24.

97. Tyrrell CJ, Peckham MJ: The response of lymph node metastases of testicular teratoma to radiation therapy. *Br J Urol.* 1976; 48:363.

98. Rorth M, von der Maase H, Neilsen ES, et al: Orchidectomy alone versus orchidectomy plus radiotherapy in stage I non-seminomatous testicular cancer: A randomized study by the Danish Testicular Carcinoma Study Group. *Int J Androl.* 1987;10:255.

99. Frass BA, Kinsella TJ, Harrington, et al: Peripheral dose to the testes: The design and clinical use of a practical and effective gonadal shield. *Int J Radiat Oncol Biol Phys.* 1985;11:609.

100. Kubo H, Shipley WU: Reduction of the scatter dose to the testicle outside the radiation treatment field. *Int J Radiat Oncol Biol Phys.* 1982;8:1741.

101. Einhorn LH, Richie JP, Shipley WU: Cancer of the testis. In DeVita VT, Hellman S, Rosenberg SA, eds. *Cancer: Principles and Practice of Oncology,* 4th ed. Philadelphia: JB Lippincott; 1993:1133.

102. Busch FM, Sayegh ES: Roentgenographic visualization of human testicular lymphatics: A preliminary report. *J Urol.* 1963;89:106.

103. Thomas GM, Williams SD: Testis. In Perez CA, Brady LW, eds. *Principles and Practice of Radiation Oncology.* Philadelphia: JB Lippincott; 1992:1125.

104. Thomas GM: Controversies in the management of testicular seminoma. *Cancer.* 1985;55:2296.

105. Hamilton C, Horwich A, Easton D, et al: Radiotherapy for stage I seminoma testis: Results of treatment and complications. *Radiother Oncol.* 1986;6:115.

106. Lester SG, Morphis J, Hornback NB: Testicular seminoma: Analysis of treatment results and failures. *Int J Radiat Oncol Biol Phys.* 1986;12:353.

107. Thomas GM: Progress and controversies in the management of seminoma. In Newling DW, Jones WG, eds. *EORTC Genitourinary Group Monograph 7: Prostate Cancer and Testicular Cancer.* New York: Wiley-Liss; 1990:217.

108. Kiricuta IC, Sauer J, Bohndorf W: Omission of the pelvic irradiation in stage I testicular seminoma: A study of postorchiectomy paraaortic radiotherapy. *Int J Radiat Oncol Biol Phys.* 1996; 35:293.

109. Thomas GM: Para-aortic radiotherapy for stage I seminoma: A new standard. *Int J Radiat Oncol Biol Phys.* 1996;35:413.

110 Fossa S, Horwich A, Russell J, et al: Optimal planning target volume for stage I testicular seminoma: A Medical Research Council randomized trial. *J Clin Oncol.* 1999;17:1146.

111. Fossa SD, Aass N, Kaaluhus O: Radiotherapy for testicular seminoma stage I: Treatment results and long term post-irradiation morbidity in 365 patients. *Int J Radiat Oncol Biol Phys.* 1989; 16:383.

112. Kennedy CL, Hendry F, Peckham MJ: The significance of scrotal interference in stage I testicular cancer managed by orchiectomy and surveillance. *Br J Urol.* 1986;58:705.

113. Lanteri VJ, Choudhury M, Pontes JE, et al: Treatment of testicular tumors arising in patients with previous inguinal and/or scrotal surgery. *J Urol.* 1982;127:58.

114. Ellerbroek NA, Tran LM, Selch MT, et al: Testicular seminoma: A study of 103 cases treated at UCLA. *J Clin Oncol.* 1988;11:93.

115. Abdeen N, Souhami L, Freeman C, et al: Radiation therapy of testicular seminoma: A 15 year survey. *Am J Clin Oncol.* 1992; 15:87.

116. Bayens YC, Helle PA, VanPutten WLJ, et al: Orchidectomy followed by radiotherapy in 176 stage I and II testicular seminoma patients: Benefits of a 10 year follow-up study. *Radiother Oncol.* 1992;25:97.

117. Willan BD, McGowan DG: Seminoma of the testis: A 22 year experience with radiation therapy. *Int J Radiat Oncol Biol Phys.* 1985;11:1769.

118. Sause WT: Testicular seminoma-analysis of radiation therapy for stage II disease. *J Urol.* 1983;130:702.

119. Skinner DG, Scardino PT, Daniels JR: Testicular cancer. *Ann Rev Med.* 1981;32:543.

120. Hanks G, Peters T, Owen J: Seminoma of the testis: Long term beneficial and deleterious results of radiation. *Int J Radiat Oncol Biol Phys.* 1992;24:913.

121. Lederman GS, Sheldon TA, Chaffey JT, et al: Cardiac disease after mediastinal irradiation for seminoma. *Cancer.* 1987;60:772.

122. Speer TW, Sombeck MD, Parsons JT, et al: Testicular seminoma: A failure analysis and literature review. *Int J Radiat Oncol Biol Phys.* 1995;33:89.

123. Dosoretz DE, Shipley WU, Blitzer PH, et al: Megavoltage irradiation for pure testicular seminoma: Results and patterns of failure. *Cancer.* 1981;48:2184.

124. Peckham MJ, McElwani TJ, Hendry FW: Testicle and epididymis. In Hallman KE, Boak JL, Crowther D, eds. *The Treatment of Cancer.* New York: Chapman & Hall; 1982:501.

125. Duncan W, Munro AJ: The management of testicular seminoma: Edinburgh 1970-1981. *Br J Cancer.* 1987;55:443.

126. Sommer K, Brockmann WP, Hubener KH: Treatment results and acute and late toxicity of radiation therapy for testicular seminoma. *Cancer.* 1990;66:259.

127. Aass N, Fossa SD, Host H: Acute and subacute side effects due to infradiaphragmatic radiotherapy for testicular cancer: A prospective study. *Int J Radiat Oncol Biol Phys.* 1992;22:1057.

128. Ellis RE: The distribution of active bone marrow in the adult. *Phys Med Biol.* 1960;5:255.

129. Smithers DW, Wallace DM, Austin DE: Fertility after unilateral orchiectomy and radiotherapy for patients with malignant tumors of the testis. *Br Med J.* 1973;4:77.

130. Amelar RD, Dubin L, Hotchkiss RS: Restoration of fertility following unilateral orchiectomy and radiation therapy for testicular tumors. *J Urol.* 1971;106:714.

131. Shapiro E, Kinsella TJ, Markuch RW, et al: Effects of fractionated irradiation on endocrine aspects of testicular function. *J Clin Oncol.* 1985;3:1232.

132. Coia LR, Hanks GE: Complications from large field intermediate dose infradiaphragmatic radiation: An analysis of the patterns of care outcome studies for Hodgkin's disease and seminoma. *Int J Radiat Oncol Biol Phys.* 1988;15:29.

133. Aass N, Fossa SD, Aas M, et al: Renal function related to different treatment modalities for malignant germ cell tumors. *Br J Cancer.* 1990;62:842.

134. Bissett D, Kunkeler L, Zwanenburg L, et al: Long term sequelae of treatment for testicular germ cell tumors. *Br J Cancer.* 1990; 62:655.

135. Stoter G, Koopman A, Verdrik CPJ, et al: Ten year survival and late sequelae in testicular cancer patients treated with cisplatin, vinblastine, and bleomycin. *J Clin Oncol.* 1989;7:1099.

136. Moynihan C: Testicular cancer: The psychological problems of patients and their relatives. *Cancer Surg.* 1987;6:477.

137. Fossa SD, Kreuser ED, Roth GJ, et al: Long-term side effects after treatment of testicular cancer. *Prog Clin Biol Res.* 1990; 357:321.

138. Bokemeyer C, Schmoll HJ: Treatment of testicular cancer and the development of secondary malignancies. *J Clin Oncol.* 1995; 13:283.

139. Hellbardt A, Mirimanoff RO, Obradovic M, et al: The risk of second cancer in patients treated for testicular seminoma. *Int J Radiat Oncol Biol Phys.* 1990;18:1327.

140. van Leeuwen FE, Stiggelbout AM, van den Belt-Dusebout AW, et al: Second cancer risk following testicular cancer: A follow-up study of 1909 patients. *J Clin Oncol.* 1993;11:415.

141. Chao CKS, Lai PP, Michalski JM, et al: Secondary malignancy among seminoma patients treated with adjuvant radiation therapy. *Int J Radiat Oncol Biol Phys.* 1995;33:831.

142. Kollmannsberger C, Kuzcyk M, Mayer F, et al: Late toxicity following curative treatment of testicular cancer. *Sem Surg Oncol.* 1999;17:275.

Cancer of the Male Urethra and Penis

47

Yoshiya Yamada, MD

In 2001 approximately 1.26 million people were diagnosed with cancer in the United States. Only 1200 cases were classified as cancers of the penis or male genitourinary malignancies (not bladder, ureter, prostate, or testis).[1] The overall incidence based upon the SEER (Surveillance, Epidemiology, and End Results) database is 0.6 per 100,000 for penile cancers and 0.3 per 100,000 for male urethral cancers. Analysis of the SEER database indicates that the incidence increases with age. Primary cancers of the penis and male urethra are extremely uncommon before the age of 55 (<1/100,000).[2] Overall, primary penile and male urethral malignancies are relatively uncommon.

PRIMARY CARCINOMA OF THE MALE URETHRA

Incidence by Age

Primary carcinoma of the male urethra is extremely rare. Although cases have been reported in the literature as young as age 13, the SEER database records no cases in patients younger than the age of 20. The incidence increases with advancing age from 0.1 per 100,000 in those ages 20 to 34, to a peak incidence of 2.6 per 100,000 in those older than age 85.[2]

Etiology

No specific etiologic factors have been identified. However, chronic inflammation likely plays a role in the development of urethral cancers. Patients diagnosed with urethral cancers often have a history of prior sexually transmitted disease, urethritis, or urethral stricture. The incidence of urethral stricture in men diagnosed with carcinoma of the urethra ranges from 24% to 76%.[3] The site of stricture is also the most likely site of malignancy.[4] Approximately 10% of patients who undergo cystectomy for invasive bladder cancer also develop a urethral cancer distal to the urogenital diaphragm.

Anatomy

The male urethra, composed of a mucosa and submucosa, is approximately 20 cm in length and extends from the neck of the bladder to the external meatus of the glans penis. The prostatic urethra begins at the bladder neck and lies within the prostate. It is usually 3 cm long. It is the widest and most readily dilated portion of the urethra. It typically emerges anterior to the prostatic apex and merges with the membranous urethra. The membranous urethra lies within the urogenital diaphragm surrounded by the sphincter urethrae muscle and is the least dilatable portion of the urethra. The prostatic and membranous urethra are lined with transitional epithelium. The spongy (cavernous) urethra is enclosed in the corpus spongiosum. It is further subdivided into urethra confined by the penile bulb (bulbous urethra) and urethra distal to the bulb (penile or pendulous urethra). The narrowest portion of the urethra is the external meatus. The bulbomembranous urethra is known as the posterior urethra, while the penile urethra is referred to as the anterior urethra. Pseudostratified columnar epithelium lines the bulbous and penile urethra. Stratified squamous epithelium lines the urethra defined by the glans penis (Fig. 47-1). Numerous glands can be found in the submucosa of the urethra.

The bulbomembranous urethra is the most common site of primary malignancies (60%). Thirty percent occur in the penile urethra, and 10% originate in the prostatic urethra.[5]

The anterior urethra drains into the superficial and deep inguinal lymph nodes. The bulbomembranous and prostatic urethra drain into the pelvic lymph nodes. Posterior lesions may drain to the external and internal iliac, obturator, and presacral lymph nodes.[6]

Pathology

Transitional cell carcinomas that arise in the prostatic urethra are clinically and histologically similar to those that arise in the bladder. Transitional cell carcinomas that originate in the bladder neck that extend into the

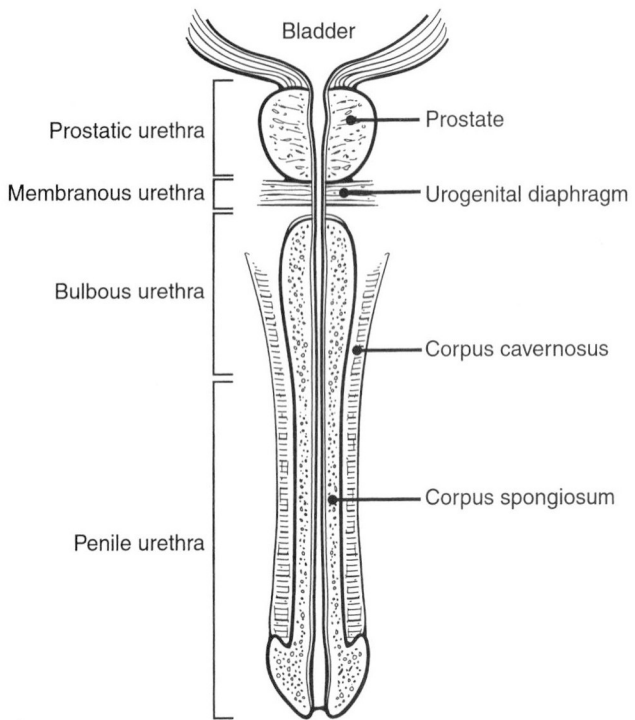

Figure 47–1. Anatomy of the penis and urethra.

urethra may be mistaken for a primary urethral cancer. Eighty percent of male urethral cancers are squamous cell carcinomas, and 15% of male urethral cancers are transitional cell carcinomas. Only 5% are either adenocarcinomas, which are thought to arise in the submucosal glandular tissue, or undifferentiated tumors.

Natural History

Primary urethral cancers are often insidious, and symptoms are often present only when the disease is locally advanced.[7] The most common presenting symptoms include a palpable urethral mass, obstructive urinary symptoms, pain, urethral fistula or abscess, hematuria, or a palpable inguinal mass.[8] Because many symptoms are not specific, symptoms have been reported to be present on average 5 months before diagnosis (range 1 day to 15 years).[9] Urethral carcinoma often directly invades adjacent structures such as the corpus spongiosum and periurethral tissues. Bulbomembranous lesions can extend into the urogenital diaphragm and prostate. Invasion into the corpora cavernosa is common at the time of diagnosis. Hematogenous spread (lung, brain, bone, lymph nodes) is relatively uncommon, except in locally advanced cases.[10]

Prognosis of male urethral carcinomas depends primarily on location and the degree of invasion. Anterior superficial lesions generally present earlier and carry the best prognosis, while deeply invasive lesions or those located posteriorly are rarely curable. Posterior lesions tend to be deeply invasive at the time of diagnosis. Histology is thought to be less significant as a prognostic factor.[11]

Staging

Diagnosis is established with a transurethral biopsy. Urine cytology may also be helpful. The extent of disease is determined by careful inspection and palpation of the external genitalia and perineum as well as cystourethroscopy. Bimanual examination under anesthesia may also be indicated for posteriorly located lesions. Computed tomography (CT) and magnetic resonance imaging (MRI) of the pelvis may help to evaluate the extent of disease and the status of lymph nodes. MRI should be performed whenever possible to document the extent of local soft tissue extension. Positron emission tomography (PET) and lymphangiograms may also help in evaluating the true extent of disease.

The Tumor Node Metastasis (TNM) staging system set forth by the American Joint Committee on Cancer (AJCC) allows data collected by both physical examination and imaging in the staging of urethral cancers. T staging is determined mainly by the depth of invasion. Regional lymph nodes are considered to be the pelvic and inguinal nodal beds. Laterality does not affect the N status (Table 47-1).[12]

Management

The primary modalities of therapy for male urethral carcinomas include surgery, radiation therapy, and chemotherapy.

In most cases, surgery is the primary therapy for urethral carcinomas. Surgical approaches include transurethral resection (TUR), local excision, partial amputation, or radical amputation of the penis. For superficial papillary or in situ disease, TUR and fulguration are deemed adequate therapy. For anterior lesions in the distal half of the penis, a partial resection with 2 cm margins should be attempted. Local recurrences after partial amputation are uncommon. Conservative surgical therapy is generally only considered for solitary, low-grade, low-stage lesions. For invasive lesions in the more proximal portion of the penis, a radical amputation is indicated. If the lesion is extensive and involves the scrotum, emasculation may be necessary. Ilioinguinal lymph node dissection is carried out if the nodes are palpable or appear to be involved on imaging studies (after confirmation in frozen sections). In cases of limited regional lymph node involvement, node dissection may still be curative. In cases where no lymph node involvement is evident, groin dissection is not indicated but should still be watched carefully in follow-up visits.

The role of radiation therapy alone for lesions in the distal urethra is not well defined but provides the option of organ preservation. Radiation therapy alone can be curative for distal lesions, with long-term cure rates similar to those reported for surgery. The most common approach uses external beam radiotherapy with doses between 50 and 75 Gy.[13]

Various techniques for treating male urethral cancers with radiotherapy have been described. The "crossfire" technique, commonly used for distal lesions, involves positioning the penis vertically by suspending it with a Foley

Table 47-1   Classification of Primary Urethral Carcinomas

Primary Tumor

Tx	Primary tumor cannot be assessed
T0	No evidence of primary tumor
Ta	Noninvasive papillary, polypoid, or verrucous carcinoma
Tis	Carcinoma in situ
T1	Tumor invades subepithelial connective tissue
T2	Tumor invades any of the following: corpus spongiosum, prostate, periurethral muscle
T3	Tumor invades any of the following: corpus cavernosum, beyond prostatic capsule, anterior vagina, bladder neck
T4	Tumor invades other adjacent organs

Transitional cell carcinoma of the prostate (prostatic urethra)

Tis pu	Carcinoma in situ, involvement of the prostatic urethra
Tis pd	Carcinoma in situ, involvement of the prostatic ducts
T1	Tumor invades subepithelial connective tissue
T2	Tumor invades any of the following: corpus spongiosum, prostate, periurethral muscle
T3	Tumor invades any of the following: corpus cavernosum, beyond prostatic capsule, anterior vagina, bladder neck (extraprostatic extension)
T4	Tumor invades other adjacent organs (invasion of the bladder)

Regional Lymph Nodes (N)

Nx	Regional lymph nodes cannot be assessed
N0	No regional lymph node metastasis
N1	Metastasis in a single lymph node ≤2 cm in greatest dimension
N2	Metastasis in a single lymph node >2 cm in greatest dimension, or multiple lymph nodes

Distant Metastasis (M)

Mx	Distant metastasis cannot be assessed
M0	No distant metastasis
M1	Distant metastasis

Stage Grouping

Stage 0a	Ta	N0	M0
0is	Tis	N0	M0
	Tis pu	N0	M0
	Tis pd	N0	M0
Stage 1	T1	N0	M0
Stage 2	T2	N0	M0
Stage 3	T1–2	N1	M0
	T3	N0–1	M0
Stage 4	T4	N0–1	M0
	Any T	N2	M0
	Any T	Any N	M1

From Greene FL, Page DL, Fleming ID, et al (eds): *AJCC Cancer Staging Manual*, 6th ed. New York: Springer, 2002.

catheter and using parallel opposed external beam fields without bolus. Prophylactic lymph node irradiation is generally not advocated. Prostatic urethra patients can be treated in similar fashion to prostatic adenocarcinomas.

Penile radiotherapy often produces a brisk acute skin reaction and edema. These effects generally subside over a 2 to 4 week period. Skin necrosis or ulceration is uncommon. Significant edema and strictures can develop as a result of radical radiotherapy.

Local control may be more difficult to achieve in the bulbomembranous urethra because these lesions tend to be more locally aggressive (Fig. 47-2). Because metastasis

tends to be a late event, aggressive combined approaches to local therapy should be considered.

Similar to the treatment of epidermoid lesions in other tumor sites, it is recommended to treat microscopical/subclinical disease to about 50 Gy. Gross tumor should be irradiated to doses up to 70 Gy in standard fractionation. The Memorial Sloan-Kettering Cancer Center (MSKCC) experience has found that those who received salvage surgery after radiotherapy fared worse than those who were treated with surgery upfront, although only six patients were reported in this category. None of these patients received chemoradiotherapy.[10]

Chemoradiation has been described for both female and male urethral cancers. Case series have reported the use of fluorouracil, mitomycin, and external beam radiation for squamous cell cancers of the male urethra.[14] When chemotherapy is used in conjunction with radiation, the radiation doses have been typically lower than those with radiation alone. More modest doses (45 Gy to 55 Gy) may be sufficient in the setting of combined modality therapy, with surgery reserved for salvage.[15] Encouraging results have been reported at MSKCC for transitional cell carcinomas in both men and women using combined modality therapy that includes chemotherapy, radiotherapy, and surgery.[16]

Chemotherapy, acting as a radio enhancer and a deterrent to distant metastasis, has been used successfully in conjunction with radiotherapy in other sites such as esophagus, head and neck malignancies, vulva, and anal canal. Failure after radiation therapy is often central, whereas surgical failures are due to inability to achieve sufficiently wide margins. Given the rarity of urethral cancers in men, there are no reports with patients in significant enough numbers to draw conclusions. Most of the literature consists of case reports. However, in advanced tumors, the use of combined modality therapy has yielded 60% to 100% disease-free survivals.[14,17-20] Not only is multimodality therapy (chemoradiation and surgery) conceptually appealing in the management of urethral cancers, but initial experiences have been encouraging, and should be explored further as an aggressive management option.

PRIMARY CARCINOMA OF THE PENIS

Incidence

Primary carcinoma of the penis is an uncommon diagnosis, accounting for less than 2% of urogenital malignancies. The SEER database has no cases of primary penile cancer in men younger than age 25. Incidence appears to be age related. The incidence of primary penile cancer between the ages of 25 and 30 is 0.1 per 100,000 and rises to an incidence of 5.8 per 100,000 for those between the ages of 80 and 84.[2]

Etiology

In areas of the world where circumcision is not a common practice, primary penile cancers make up 10%

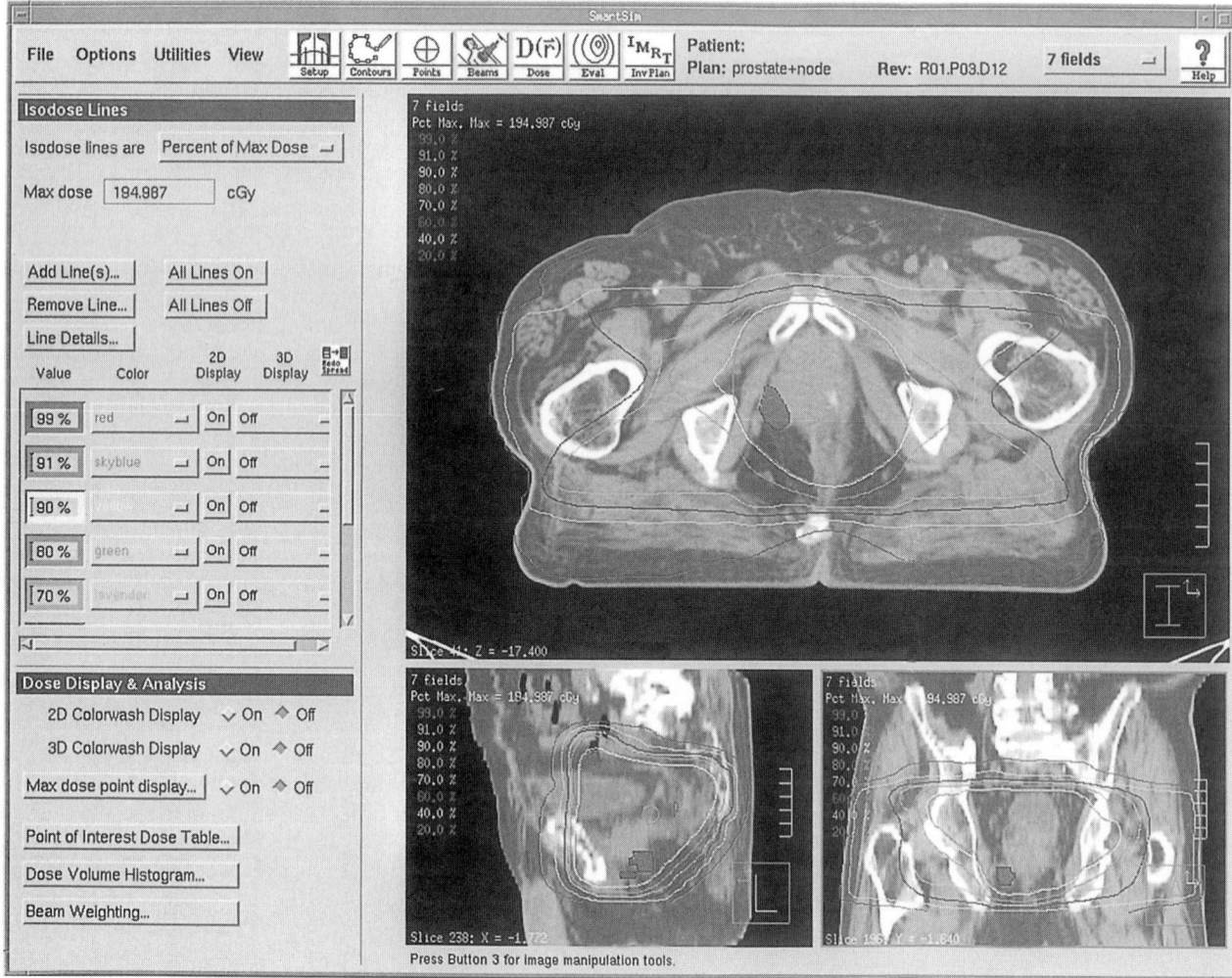

Figure 47–2. Conformal external beam radiotherapy for a lesion of the bulbo membrane urethra. See also Color Figure 47-2.

to 12% of cancers diagnosed in men.[21] Penile cancers are exceedingly rare in North America, but account for 45% to 76% of all genitourinary malignancies in Paraguay. In Uganda, it is the most commonly diagnosed malignancy in men.[22] Overall, the incidence of primary penile cancer in the SEER database is less than 1 per 100,000. However, the lifetime risk of developing penile cancer in an uncircumcised male is estimated to be as high as 1 per 600. Also, it appears that circumcision at an early age is more likely to be protective against cancer of the penis than circumcision at the time of puberty or later.[23] Penile cancer is extremely uncommon in Jewish populations that practice infant circumcision, and rarely seen in Moslems who delay circumcision to age 3 to 13.[24] Given this association with being uncircumcised, it has been postulated that smegma, which has been found to be carcinogenic in animals, may play a role in penile carcinogenesis. There is no conclusive evidence to suggest that a causative relationship exists with sexually transmitted diseases. It has also been observed to occur more commonly in the partners of women with cancer of the cervix, suggesting that human papilloma virus (HPV), which has been shown to possibly promote carcinogenesis in vitro, may be a possible etiology.

Anatomy

The penis (see Fig. 47-1) is composed of the corpus spongiosum and two corpora cavernosa bound together in Buck's fascia. The corpus spongiosum expands distally into the glans penis, which is covered by the prepuce (foreskin). The lymph from the skin of the penis, including foreskin, drains into the superficial inguinal nodes. Because of lymphatic cross drainage, penile cancers do not localize inguinal drainage to just one side. Lymphatics from the glans penis may drain to either superficial inguinal nodes or follow the lymphatics of the corpora to the iliac nodes in the pelvis. Corporal tissue drains to the deep inguinal and iliac lymph nodes.

Pathology

Although histologies including malignant melanoma, lymphoma, basal cell carcinoma, and connective tissue malignancies (Kaposi's sarcoma) have been noted, 95% of primary penile cancers are squamous cell carcinoma. Eighteen percent of patients with AIDS who have Kaposi's sarcoma have lesions on the penis or genitals.[25]

Natural History

The most common early symptoms include itching or burning under the foreskin with erythema, which may progress to areas of induration and ulceration of the glans or prepuce. Given time, these lesions progressively enlarge into palpable masses. If allowed to grow, they can progress into ulcerative masses with purulent discharge and a phimotic nonretractable, distorted prepuce. Pain may not be a dominant feature of the presentation. Occasionally, an ulcerative inguinal lymph node may be the presenting complaint. Half of patients with penile cancer present with a palpable lymph node. However, only approximately 50% of palpable lymph nodes will harbor metastatic disease, and 20% of clinically negative lymph nodes will contain disease. The most common sites of distant metastasis are the lungs, liver, and bone.[26]

Early-stage lesions are very curable. Nodal involvement reduces the likelihood of cure. The risk of lymph node involvement increases with the invasiveness of the primary lesion. The most common site of involvement is the glans penis.

Staging

The TNM staging system, shown in Table 47-2, allows the use of findings from endoscopy, imaging, and physical examination in determining the stage of disease. Regional lymph node drainage is considered to be the superficial and deep inguinal lymph nodes, as well as pelvic nodes.[12]

Physical examination of the penis and inguinal lymph nodes is crucial to correct staging. Ultrasound or MRI or both may be useful in determining the extent of disease. Computed tomographic (CT) scans of the pelvis and abdomen provide additional data regarding lymph node status. The usefulness of lymphangiograms is controversial.

Management

Surgical management of primary penile cancers yields excellent local control rates and should always be discussed with patients as a treatment option. However, the potential functional loss and impact upon psychosocial concerns has made organ-sparing therapy an attractive alternative to surgery.

Circumcision is recommended before initiating radiotherapy. This allows for a more complete evaluation of the extent of disease and will reduce the likelihood of significant treatment-related morbidity, including swelling, desquamation, secondary infections, and the risk of phimosis.

Various techniques using both brachytherapy and external beam radiotherapy have been described in the literature.[27]

For external beam techniques using megavoltage radiation beams, tissue equivalent bolus is required (usually wax, plastic, or a water bath is used) to provide sufficient dose buildup to the surface of the lesion. The penis is suspended and surrounded by bolus above the abdomen and radiation beams treat the whole length of the penis. When

Table 47-2 Classification of Penile Cancers

T Primary Tumor

Tx	Tumor cannot be assessed
T0	No evidence of tumor
Tis	Carcinoma in situ
Ta	Noninvasive verrucous carcinoma
T1	Tumor invades subepithelial connective tissue
T2	Tumor invades corpus spongiosum or cavernosa
T3	Tumor invades urethra or prostate
T4	Tumor invades other adjacent structures

Regional Lymph Nodes (N)

Nx	Regional lymph nodes cannot be assessed
N0	No regional lymph node metastasis
N1	Metastasis in a single superficial inguinal lymph node
N2	Metastasis in multiple or bilateral superficial inguinal lymph nodes
N3	Metastasis in deep inguinal or pelvic lymph nodes, unilateral or bilateral

Distant Metastasis (M)

Mx	Distant metastasis cannot be evaluated
M0	No distant metastasis
M1	Distant metastasis

Stage Grouping

Stage 0	Tis	N0	M0
	Ta	N0	M0
Stage 1	T1	N0	M0
Stage 2	T1	N1	M0
	T2	N0–1	M0
Stage 3	T1–2	N2	M0
	T3	N0–2	M0
Stage 4	T4	Any N	M0
	Any T	N3	M0
	Any T	Any N	M1

From Greene FL, Page DL, Fleming ID, et al (eds): *AJCC Cancer Staging Manual*, 6th ed. New York: Springer, 2002.

the pelvic lymph nodes are being treated, the penis can be secured cranially into the pelvic field and irradiated. Typical doses are 65 to 70 Gy to the gross tumor volume (GTV) in standard fractionation. This is usually accomplished by treating the entire length of the penis initially to a dose of 45 to 50 Gy, and performing a 10 to 20 Gy cone-down boost to the GTV. Acute reactions such as swelling, discomfort, and desquamation are usually self limiting. Care should be taken to avoid secondary infections that may result from skin breakdown. The use of large fraction sizes should be avoided to reduce the risk of late radiation effects such as fibrosis. The incidence of stricture or stenosis has been reported to be 16% to 49%. The majority of patients (up to 90%) will maintain sexual potency.[28,29] The published local control rates for stages I and II cancers of the penis range from 65% to 90%, with a mean of 75%.[24] Table 47-3 provides a summary of outcomes of external beam radiotherapy.

Brachytherapy is indicated in lesions less than 4 cm in diameter and less than 1 cm of invasion into the corpora cavernosa. There are generally two techniques employed: molds (plesiobrachytherapy) and interstitial implants. When using molds, radioactive sources (generally

Table 47–3   External Beam Radiotherapy and Brachytherapy Outcomes for Primary Penile Cancer

Author	TNM Stage	n	Median Follow-up (mo)	Local Control with Penile Preservation, %
External Beam Radiotherapy[29]				
Grabstald	I–II	10		90
Krieg	I–II–III	12		75
Fossa	I–II	12		73
Sageman	I–II	12		66
McLean	I–II	17		65
Brachytherapy[31]				
Crook	I–II–III	30	34	83
Kiltie	—	31	61.5	74.8
Chaudhary	I–II	23	24	70.5
Mazeron	I–II–III	50	>36	74*
Soria	—	111	72	82 (2 yr) 72 (8 yr)
Rozan	I–II–III	184	139	78*
Delannes	I–II–III	51	83.5	67*

*Some patients had external beam radiation or partial penectomy.
Adapted from Crook J, Grimard L, Tsihlias J, Morash C, Panzarella T: Interstitial brachytherapy for penile cancer: An alternative to amputation.
J Urol. 2002;167:506 and Krieg R, Luk K: Carcinoma of the penis: Review of cases treated by surgery and radiation therapy 1960-1970. *Urology.* 1981;18:149.

Ir-192) are placed into contact with the lesion and tissue to be irradiated. The mold holds the sources and the patient wears the mold for a calculated amount of time daily (usually 12 hours a day for 1 week). The penis is placed in a cylinder loaded with Ir-192 sources. The target dose to the target is 60 Gy, while the urethra should receive less than 50 Gy. Typically, this technique is reserved for superficial tumors only and requires a competent brachytherapist and a high degree of patient cooperation.[30]

Interstitial implants are generally performed under a spinal or general anesthetic. A Foley catheter is introduced and kept in place for the duration of the implant. Metal or plastic catheters are placed perpendicular to the long axis of the penis and spaced parallel to each other, 1 to 1.5 cm apart, held in place with acrylic templates located at the entry and exit points of the catheters. Radioactive sources, typically Ir-192, are afterloaded into each catheter to deliver the prescribed dose of radiation. Prescribed doses range from 55 to 60 Gy, with a mean dose of 60 Gy given at a dose rate of 68 cGy/hour.[31] It has been recommended that no more than 65 Gy be prescribed for T1 or T2 tumors because of the risk of significant necrosis.[30] Local control rates between 78% and 95% have been reported. Significant increases in urethral strictures have been noted when treating T3 tumors that invade the urethra. In such cases, surgery is advisable over brachytherapy. The rate of penile preservation ranges between 74% and 95% for T1 and T2 lesions. Approximately 10% to 40% of patients will experience urethral stenosis that requires dilation (usually at the meatus) after interstitial brachytherapy. Potency is preserved in 80% to 90% of patients.[24,30-32] It has been observed that diabetic patients are more likely to experience radiation therapy–related toxicity.[30]

Prophylactic groin node irradiation is generally not recommended. Lymph nodes may be enlarged secondarily to infection and may reduce in size with a course of antibiotics. Cooperative patients with well-differentiated tumors confined to the glans are well suited for observation. The management of clinically N0 groins in patients with poorly differentiated tumors or deeply invasive lesions is controversial.

Although no randomized trials regarding the efficacy of radiation therapy versus surgery for the management of primary penile carcinoma have been conducted, radiation therapy appears to be a reasonable consideration for T1 and T2 tumors less than 4 cm in size. Table 47-3 summarizes the reported results of radiotherapy as primary therapy for penile cancers.

There is significant experience with the use of brachytherapy in the management of penile carcinomas, particularly in Europe. In France, brachytherapy has been the treatment of choice for clinically localized squamous cell carcinomas of the penis for several decades.[31] Although late effects such as strictures or stenosis may occur in up to 40% of patients, these are usually easily remedied with simple dilation. Sexual function is also preserved in most men. Thus, the penis can remain functional and be spared amputation in greater than 80% of cases without sacrificing control rates, while surgery can be reserved for salvage of persistent or recurrent disease.

REFERENCES

1. American Cancer Society: *Cancer Facts and Figures.* Atlanta: American Cancer Society; 2001:5.
2. Surveillance, Epidemiology, and End Results (SEER) Program Public-Use Data (1973-1999), National Cancer Institute, DCCPS, Surveillance Research Program, Cancer Statistics Branch, released April 2002, based on the November 2001 submission.
3. Herr HW, Fuks Z, Scher HI: Cancer of the urethra and penis. In Devita V, Hellman S, Rosenberg SA, eds. *Cancer. Principles and Practices of Oncology.* Philadelphia: Lipincott, 1997:1386.

4. Konnack JR: Conservative management of low grade neoplasms of the male urethra: A preliminary report. *J Urol.* 1980;123:175.

5. Grabsalt H: Tumors of the urethra in men and women. *Cancer.* 1973;32:1236.

6. Hand JR: Surgery of the penis and urethra. In Campbell MF, Harrison JH, eds. *Urology.* Philadelphia: WB Sanders; 1970:2541.

7. Mandeler JT, Pool TL: Primary carcinoma of the male urethra. *J Urol.* 1966;96:67.

8. Fair WR, Yang CR: Urethral carcinoma in males. In Resnick M, Kursch E, eds. *Current Therapy in Surgery.* Toronto: BC Decker; 1987.

9. Kaplan GW, Bulkley GH, Grayhack JT: Carcinoma of the male urethra. *J Urol.* 1967;134:753.

10. Dalbagni G, Zhang ZF, Lacombe L: Male urethral carcinoma: Analysis of treatment outcome. *Urol.* 1999;53:1126.

11. Grigbsy PW, Corn BW: Localized urethral tumors in women: Indications for conservative versus exenterative therapies. *J Urol.* 1992;147:1516.

12. Greene FL, Page DL, Fleming ID, et al: *AJCC Cancer Staging Manual.* 6th ed. New York: Springer-Verlag; 2002.

13. Heysek RV, Parsons JR, Drylie DM: Carcinoma of the male urethra. *J Urol.* 1985;197:753.

14. Licht M, Klein E, Bukowski R: Combination radiation and chemotherapy for the treatment of squamous cell carcinoma of the male and female urethra. *J Urol.* 1995;153:1918.

15. Krieg R, Hoffman R: Current Management of Unusual Genitourinary Cancers. Part 2: Urethral Cancer. *Oncology.* 1999;13:1511.

16. Scher HI, Ygoda A, Herr HW: Neoadjuvant MVAC chemotherapy for extravesical urinary tract tumors. *J Urol.* 1998;139:475.

17. Baskin LS, Turzan C: Carcinoma of the male urethra: Management of locally advanced disease with combined chemotherapy, radiotherapy, and penile-preserving surgery. *Urology.* 1992;39:21.

18. Johnson DW, Kessler JF, Ferrigni RG: Low dose combined chemotherapy/radiotherapy in the management of locally advanced urethral squamous cell carcinoma. *J Urol.* 1989;142:615.

19. Tran LN, Krieg RM, Szabo RJ: Combination chemotherapy and radiotherapy for the treatment of squamous cell carcinoma of the urethra: a case report. *J Urol.* 1995;153:422.

20. Oberfield RA, Zinman LN, Leibenauth M, et al: Management of invasive squamous cell carcinoma of the bulbomembranous male urethra with coordinated chemoradiotherapy and genital preservation. *Br J Urol.* 1996;78:573.

21. Hanash K, Furlow W, Utz D: Carcinoma of the penis: A clinicopathologic study. *J Urol.* 1970;140:291.

22. Riveros M, Lebrone RF: Geographical pathology of cancer of the penis. *Cancer.* 1963;16:798.

23. Koenen M, McCurdy S: Circumcision and the risk of cancer of the penis: A lifetable analysis. *Am J Dis Child.* 1980;134:484.

24. Krieg R, Hoffman R: Current management of unusual genitourinary cancer: Part 1: Penile cancers. *Oncology.* 1999;13:1347.

25. Grossman H: Premalignant carcinomas of the penis and scrotum. *Urol Clin North Am.* 1992;19:221.

26. Burgers J, Badalament R, Drago J: Penile cancer: Clinical presentation, diagnosis and staging. *Urol Clin North Am.* 1992;19:247.

27. McClean M, Akl A, Ward P, et al: The results of primary radiation therapy in the management of squamous cell carcinoma of the penis. *Int J Radiat Oncol Biol Phys.* 1993;5;623.

28. Grabstald H, Kelley C: Radiation therapy of penile cancer six to ten year follow up. *Urology.* 1980;15:575.

29. Krieg R, Luk K: Carcinoma of the penis: Review of cases treated by surgery and radiation therapy 1960-1970. *Urology.* 1981;18:149.

30. Gerbaulet A, Lambin P: Radiation therapy of cancer of the penis. Indications, advantages and pitfall. *Urol Clin North Am.* 1992;19:325.

31. Crook J, Grimard L, Tsihlias J, et al: Interstitial brachytherapy for penile cancer: An alternative to amputation. *J Urol.* 2002;167:506.

32. Delannes M, Malavaud B, Douchez J, et al: Iridium-192 interstitial therapy for squamous cell carcinoma of the penis. *Int J Radiat Oncol Biol Phys.* 1992;24:479.

Cancer of the Uterine Cervix

48

Patrick S. Swift, MD, and I-Chow Joe Hsu, MD

EPIDEMIOLOGY

In 2003 an estimated 13,000 new cases of invasive carcinoma of the uterine cervix were diagnosed in the United States, representing 2% of all cancers in women.[1] An estimated 4100 deaths from cervical cancer were expected in 2003, accounting for 1.5% of all female cancer deaths. The average age for patients with invasive disease is in the mid- to late 40s, with approximately 25% of cases and 50% of deaths occurring in patients older than 65. At the time of presentation, 45% of women have localized disease, 34% have regional spread, and 10% have disseminated disease.

During the past five decades, the incidence of invasive cervical carcinoma has dropped dramatically, from 32.6 (late 1940s) to 8.3 (mid-1980s) per 100,000 women in the United States.[2] Much of this improvement is attributable to the development of effective screening techniques for the identification of preinvasive lesions. Incidence varies worldwide, with the highest rates found in Latin America and the lowest prevalence found among Jewish women in Israel. Over the past decade, there has been a noticeable increase in the incidence of preinvasive lesions reported in many nations, and an actual increase in mortality rates in young women in Canada, Great Britain, New Zealand, and Australia.[2] This increase in incidence is due in part to changes in the classification of these lesions, but it is likely that a true increase is attributable to the sexual transmission of human papillomavirus (HPV), a contributing factor in the development of cervical carcinoma.

Lower socioeconomic status is associated with an increased risk of frankly invasive disease, partially because of ineffective or absent screening programs in many parts of the world.[3] Although in developed nations there appears to be an increased incidence among black and Latino people as compared with white or Asian people, Surveillance Epidemiology End Results (SEER) data from 1987 showed that black people had twice the incidence of invasive cervical cancer as white people,[2] although socioeconomic factors cloud the issue. When evaluated in a multifactorial analysis, race drops significantly as a major factor.[3]

As of January 1, 1993, the Centers for Disease Control and Prevention modified their reporting guidelines to state that the presence of cervical carcinoma in the setting of infection with the human immunodeficiency virus (HIV) establishes the diagnosis of acquired immunodeficiency syndrome (AIDS), regardless of CD4 count or absence of prior opportunistic infections. The incidence of infection with HPV is higher in HIV-positive women than in their HIV-negative counterparts.[5] Likewise, since T-cell immunity is essential in maintaining control of HPV infection, an increase in the incidence of cervical intraepithelial neoplasia (CIN) and invasive cervical carcinoma is seen in this population.[6]

RISK FACTORS

Two strains of human papillomavirus (HPV 16 and 18) are considered to have a high malignant potential, while strains 31, 33, 35, 39, 40, 45, 51 to 56, and 58 have a moderate malignant potential.[7] HPV DNA sequences are identified in 80% to 100% of cervical carcinomas evaluated by polymerase chain reaction (PCR).[5,8-12] The epidemiologic characteristics of HPV closely resemble those of CIN and invasive cancer, lending weight to the theory that infection with certain strains of HPV can lead to the development of invasive disease. The development of vaccines against the various strains of HPV holds great promise that the numbers of patients worldwide with HPV-initiated malignancies could drop within the next decade.

Attention has returned to the role of herpes simplex virus type 2 (HSV2) as a potential cofactor with HPV in the initiation of malignant degeneration.[2] Women with HSV2 alone have a 1.2 relative risk (RR) compared with women negative for both HPV and HSV2. Those positive for HPV 16/18 DNA alone had an RR of 4.3, but those positive for HPV 16/18 and HSV2 had an RR of 8.8. Additional studies using PCR techniques are needed to confirm this finding.

Early age at initiation of sexual activity and multiple sexual partners are associated with increased risk.[2] Girls who begin engaging in intercourse before the age of 16 have a two-fold increase in risk over those who begin after age 20. Exceptionally low rates are found in Catholic nuns and Mormon and Amish women. A relative decrease in risk has been reported when a comparison is made of women with male partners afflicted with genital warts who routinely use condoms and those who do not use condoms. Long-term use of oral contraceptives may increase the risk of cervical cancer. Compared with never-users, patients who had used oral contraceptives for fewer than 5 years did not have increased risk of cervical cancer. However, the relative risk is 2.82 for 5 to 9 years and 4.03 for use for 10 years or longer.[13] Long-term use of oral contraceptives may be a cofactor in woman who are HPV positive.

Cigarette smoking has been implicated,[2] with most studies revealing a twofold increase in incidence in smokers compared with nonsmokers. Multiple dietary elements are currently being investigated for their potentially protective effects, including vitamins A, C, and E, as well as beta-carotene.

Diethylstilbestrol (DES), a nonsteroidal estrogen developed in the 1940s and used in the prevention of recurrent or threatened miscarriages, was administered to between 0.5 and 2 million women in the United States before it was banned for this purpose by the FDA in 1971. Intrauterine exposure to DES was found to be associated with the development of clear cell adenocarcinoma of the cervix and vagina.[14,15] In reports from the Registry for Research on Hormonal Transplacental Carcinogenesis, 60% of 519 cases of clear cell adenocarcinoma of the vagina or cervix were found to be related to DES exposure or related compounds, with an estimated risk after exposure of 1 in 1000 up to the age of 34.[16] Ninety-one percent of patients were diagnosed between the ages of 15 and 27, with more than 90% presenting with early (stage I or II) disease.

A number of suspected proto-oncogenes have been identified for various tumor sites, using the technique of restriction fragment length polymorphism (RFLP) analysis to identify regions of loss of heterozygosity (LOH) or allele loss.[11,17-19] For cervical carcinoma, however, the numbers of cases studied to date are small, and the findings are rather inconclusive.[10,18,20,21] Reports of loss of *p53* on chromosome 17p in HPV-negative patients show a limited frequency in invasive cervical tumors. Upon infection of human epithelial keratinocytes by HPV subtypes 16 and 18, the open reading frames (ORFs) of early proteins E6/E7 remain intact.[11,18] These proteins are required, but not sufficient, for the development of immortalization of the cells. Intracellular compartment localization studies support a mechanism in which the E6 protein forms a complex with the P53 (tumor suppressor gene) protein in the cytoplasm, thereby interfering with the entry of the P53 protein into the nucleus, where it would normally function as a negative growth controller. Such a model could explain the interaction of HPV 16 and 18, P53, and immortalization of keratinocytes. Other reviews reveal a wide variety of chromosomal aberrations without dominance of any specific karyotypic abnormalities to date.[19,22]

ANATOMY

A clear understanding of the anatomic relationships of the uterine cervix and surrounding structures is essential for maximizing the therapeutic ratio in the management of cervical carcinoma.[23] The cervix is sandwiched between the trigone of the bladder, the ureters, the anterior wall of the rectum, and the sigmoid colon, so that these critical organs are by necessity exposed to the interventions used to control neoplasms of the cervix (Figs. 48-1 and

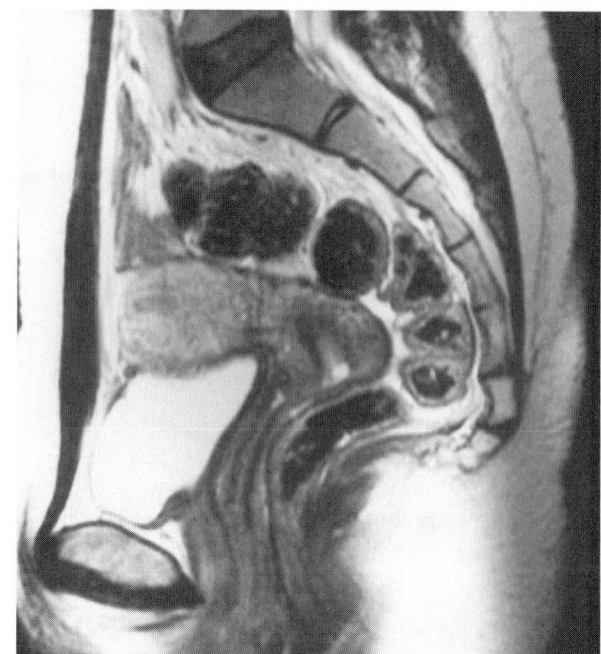

Figure 48–1. Normal anatomy of the uterus as visualized by magnetic resonance imaging: sagittal view.

48-2). The uterus itself is a hollow, muscular organ divided functionally into two parts, the fundus and cervix, separated by a constriction known as the isthmus. The upper portion, the body or corpus uteri, is covered by the reflection of the peritoneum, which anteriorly becomes the peritoneal reflection over the bladder and posteriorly extends down over the cervix and posterior fornix of the vagina before covering the anterior portion of the rectum and sigmoid colon. The broad ligament is a double layer of peritoneum through which the blood supply, lymphatics, and nerves of the uterus course. These ligaments connect the lateral aspects of the uterus with the pelvic sidewalls. They contain three

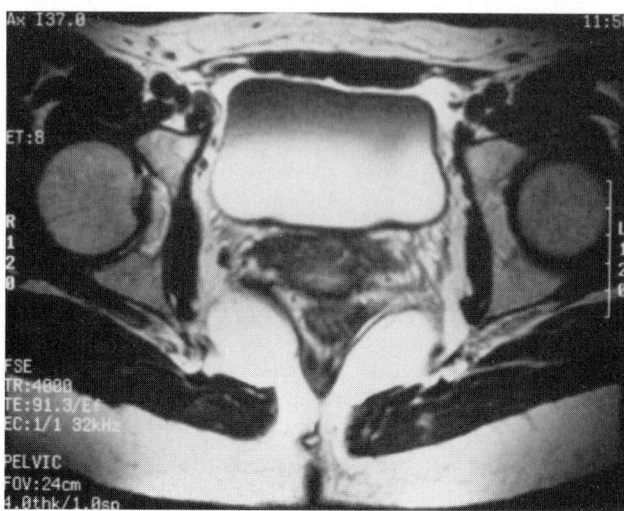

Figure 48–2. Normal anatomy of the uterus as visualized by magnetic resonance imaging: axial view.

ligaments: (1) the round ligament anteriorly, which courses out through the abdominal inguinal ring; (2) the ovarian ligament posteriorly connecting the uterine pole of the ovary and the lateral uterus; and (3) the suspensory ligament of the ovary between the two layers of the broad ligament connecting the lateral pole of the ovary and the pelvic side wall. Atop the broad ligament lie the fallopian tubes. Posteriorly located are the ovaries.

The uterus is supported in the pelvis above the pelvic diaphragm (mainly the levator ani muscle) by two ligaments. The cardinal ligament is composed of the fascias of the cervix and vagina at the lateral margins of these organs, combined with the paravesical fascias that surround the cervix, upper vagina, bladder base, and urethra before extending laterally to the pelvic side walls. The cardinal ligament forms the bottom of the broad ligament. Posteriorly, the same tissues that make up the cardinal ligament course backwards to form the uterosacral ligaments (the lateral boundaries of the cul-de-sac of Douglas) and insert into the periosteum of the fourth sacral vertebra. These ligaments serve to pull the cervix and lower uterine segment backward, maintaining an anteflexed position for the uterus.

Resting on the urogenital diaphragm anterior to the cervix, the trigone of the bladder is continuous with the upper third of the vagina and the anterior fornix. The remainder of the base presses against the anterior cervix and lower uterine segment. The ureters, leaving the renal pelvis, run caudally along the psoas muscle and along the anterior border of the greater sciatic notch. They enter the pelvis by crossing the iliac vessels at the bifurcation of the common iliacs into the external and internal branches, and pass along the posterolateral pelvic walls. They then enter the cardinal ligament (base of the broad ligament), pass beneath the uterine arteries, and travel immediately around the cervix and vaginal fornices, inserting into the trigone of the bladder. Their location on the lateral aspect of the cervix and cardinal ligaments and along the uterine artery make them prone to injury from expanding tumor in the cervix, as well as from both surgical and radio-therapeutic interventions.

Posterior to the uterus, the sigmoid colon dives below the peritoneal reflection to become the rectum and is closely related to the uterus and posterior fornix of the vagina. The rectum is separated from the posterior vagina by only a thin wall of loose areolar tissue. The thickness of the rectovaginal septum is approximately 5 mm.

The lymphatics of the cervix course in three separate routes. Laterally, they pass along the uterine artery to the external iliac lymph nodes. Posterolaterally, they pass behind the ureters to the internal iliac nodes. Posteriorly, they enter the common iliac and lateral sacral nodal groups. The fundus of the uterus drains mainly to the internal iliac nodes via lymphatics in the broad ligament, although some drainage occurs to the para-aortic chain via the ovarian vessels, to the external iliac chain, and to the inguinal nodes via the round ligament. The upper vagina drains laterally to both the internal and external iliac nodal groups, whereas the middle third tends to drain to the internal iliac group alone. The lower third of the vagina has lymphatic channels that merge with those of the vulva and lead to the superficial inguinal region. Depending on the local growth characteristics of cervical tumors, therefore, involvement of the internal and external iliac, para-aortic, sacral, and inguinal nodes is possible and must be taken into consideration when a treatment strategy is planned.

The sympathetic nervous supply of the bladder, rectum, and female genitalia (with the exception of the ovary) descends from the superior hypogastric plexus (the presacral nerve) with input from L1 to L4, spreads out in the retroperitoneum over the fourth and fifth lumbar vertebrae, and forms the bilateral hypogastric nerves. Additional sacral sympathetic fibers and parasympathetic fibers from S2 to S4 arising from the sacral plexus join the hypogastric nerves to become the inferior hypogastric plexus and eventually the pelvic plexus. From the pelvic plexus, the uterine vaginal and vesical plexuses arise to supply the uterus, vagina, and bladder. The uterine plexus enters the uterus via the base of the broad ligament along with the uterine artery. The major sensory nerves to the uterus traverse along with the autonomic sympathetic fibers, proceeding to the L1 to L4 level for the corpus and to the S2 to S4 level for the cervix. Therefore, cervical pain is often experienced as referred low back pain.

Of clinical relevance in patients with recurrent cervical cancer or enlarged pelvic lymph nodes are the lumbosacral nerve trunks, the sacral plexus, and the sciatic nerve, which may be damaged due to disease progression. The lumbosacral nerve trunk rests on the pyriform muscle in the posterolateral pelvis where it joins the sacral nerves to form the sacral plexus, which in turn gives rise to the sciatic nerve. The sciatic nerve passes through the greater sciatic foramen on its way to innervate the muscles of the lower extremity.

PATHOLOGY

In 2001 the National Cancer Institute (NCI) convened a workshop to update modern guidelines for cytopathologic reporting of cervical specimens to replace the outdated Papanicolaou (Pap) classification, resulting in the Bethesda classification system for cytopathology reports (Table 48-1).[24] For those lesions considered to be possible precursors of invasive carcinoma, the previously used CIN (levels I, II, III) and dysplasia (mild, moderate, severe, carcinoma in situ [CIS]) grading systems had been replaced in the 1988 system with a two-tier designation. Low-grade squamous intraepithelial lesions (LSILs) include those lesions previously referred to as cellular changes associated with HPV infection or mild dysplasia (CIN I). High-grade squamous intraepithelial lesions (HSILs) include moderate or severe dysplasia (CIN II or III) or CIS.

Invasive cervical cancers are composed of approximately 85% squamous cell varieties, 15% adenocarcinomas, and a rare collection of other entities.[25] Squamous cell carcinoma (SCC) has been classified according to a new system by the International Society of Gynecological Pathologists to include keratinizing, nonkeratinizing, verrucous, papillary transitional, and lymphoepithelial types

Table 48–1 Bethesda System for Reporting Cervical/Vaginal Cytological Diagnoses

I. Statement on specimen adequacy
II. General categorization (WNL or other)
III. Descriptive diagnosis
   A. Infection
   B. Reactive or reparative changes
   C. Epithelial cell abnormalities
      1. Squamous cell
         a. atypical
         b. squamous intra-epithelial lesions (SIL)
            i. low grade (LSIL)
               cellular changes assoc. with HPV
               mild dysplasia grade 1 (CIN 1)
            ii. high grade (HSIL)
               moderate dysplasia (CIN 2)
               severe dysplasia (CIN 3)
               carcinoma in situ
            iii. squamous cell carcinoma
      2. Glandular cell
         a. atypical
         b. adenocarcinoma
         c. other epithelial malignant neoplasms
      3. Other nonepithelial malignant neoplasms

WNL, within normal limit; SIL, squamous intra-epithelial lesions; HPV, human papilloma virus; CIN 1, cervical intraepithelial neoplasm grade 1; CIN 2, cervical intraepithelial neoplasm grade 2; CIN 3, cervical intraepithelial neoplasm grade 3. Data from National Cancer Institute Workshop: The 1988 Bethesda System for reporting cervical/vaginal cytologic diagnoses. *JAMA*. 1989;262:931.

Table 48–2 International Society of Gynecological Pathologists Classification of Uterine Cervix Epithelial Tumors

A. Squamous cell carcinoma varieties
   1. microinvasive
   2. invasive
   3. verrucous
   4. warty (condylomatous)
   5. papillary
   6. lymphoepithelial-type
B. Adenocarcinoma varieties
   1. mucinous types
      endocervical
      intestinal
      signet-ring
   2. endometrioid ± squamous metaplasia
   3. clear cell
   4. minimal deviation
      endocervical (adenoma malignum)
      endometrioid
   5. serous
   6. mesonephric
   7. well-differentiated villoglandular
C. Other carcinomas
   1. adenosquamous
   2. glassy cell
   3. mucoepidermoid
   4. adenoid cystic
   5. adenoid basal
   6. carcinoid
   7. small cell
   8. undifferentiated

Data from Wright TC, Ferenczy A, Kurman RJ: Carcinomas and other tumors of the cervix. In Kurman RJ, ed: *Blanstein's Pathology of the Female Genital Tract*. New York: Springer-Verlag; 1994:280.

(Table 48-2).[26] Adenocarcinomas include the following subtypes: mucinous (endocervical, intestinal, and signet ring types), endometrioid, clear cell, minimal deviation (adenoma malignum), papillary villoglandular, serous, and mesonephric. The remaining tumor types include adenosquamous, glassy cell, adenoid cystic, adenoid basal, carcinoid, small cell, and undifferentiated carcinomas (Fig. 48-3).

Squamous Cell Carcinoma

Several different classification systems have been suggested over the past 60 years, including the early Broders/Warren classification (based on differentiation, mitotic activity, keratinization, and pearl formation) and that of Reagan and Ng (based on size, keratinization, and nuclear pleomorphism).[27] In an analysis of patients entered into the Gynecologic Oncology Group (GOG) prospective treatment protocol for stage Ib cervix carcinoma, none of the histologic grading systems for SCCs were found to correlate with incidence of lymph node metastasis or progression-free interval.[28]

Variants of SCC of the cervix exist, although it is unclear whether any of these variations affect the response to therapy. Verrucous carcinoma is a very well differentiated carcinoma lacking cellular atypia and possessing orderly elements of maturation. It can achieve massive exophytic proportions and be extensively invasive, in contrast to the bland microscopic appearance. Verrucous carcinomas are differentiated from condylomata by the presence of invasion in addition to a lack of

fibrovascular cores in the papillae and by the exophytic expansion of surrounding normal tissue.[27,29,30] Spread to lymph nodes is quite rare. Concern is expressed by many authors that the use of radiation in these lesions may contribute to malignant degeneration, but this point is contestable.[31,32]

Papillary SCC differs from the verrucous form in that its cells show a high degree of nuclear atypia. Although grossly the tumor may have a warty, exophytic appearance, on microscopic examination papillae are found with atypical immature basaloid cells reminiscent of transitional cell carcinoma of the bladder. The determination of invasion requires full-thickness biopsy, since a large exophytic component may be associated with a minimal amount of invasion.[27]

Lymphoepithelioma-like carcinoma is characterized by solid cords of cells with minimal squamous differentiation resting like islands in a diffuse stromal chronic inflammatory reaction, with lymphocytes, plasma cells, and eosinophils. As in their counterparts in the nasopharynx, thymus, larynx, stomach, and salivary glands, well-circumscribed margins are found around nests of poorly differentiated cells with uniform vesiculated nuclei. Unlike the nasopharyngeal variety, Epstein-Barr virus–specific genomic DNA sequences have not been identified in the cervical form.[33]

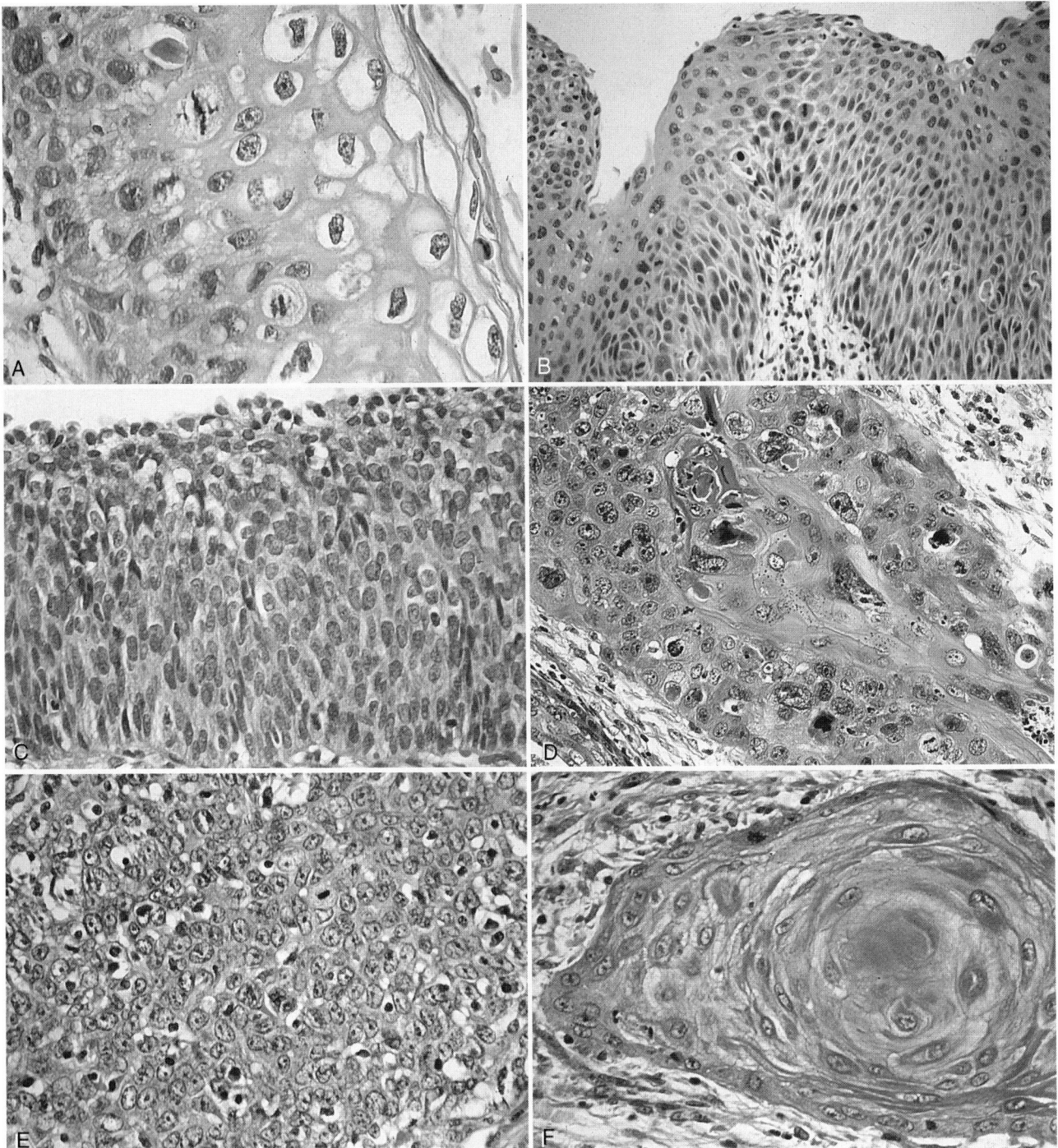

Figure 48–3. Pathologic types of carcinoma of the uterine cervix. **A,** Low-grade squamous intra-epithelial lesions; **B,** high-grade squamous intra-epithelial lesions (severe dysplasia); **C,** high-grade squamous intra-epithelial lesions (carcinoma in situ); **D,** squamous cell, keratinizing; **E,** squamous cell, poorly differentiated; **F,** verrucous.

Adenocarcinoma

Adenocarcinomas account for 10% to 20% of cervical neoplasms in the literature.[34] This would appear to represent an increase from older data that showed the incidence to be in the range of 5% to 10%, possibly because of a decline in the incidence in invasive SCC secondary to effective screening programs, although the possibility remains that the incidence of adenocarcinoma is actually on the rise.[34,35] The most common type, endocervical adenocarcinoma, is generally composed of mucin-producing glands of varying differentiation, within a fibrous stroma that sets it apart from normal endometrial stroma. It may be difficult to differentiate from adenocarcinoma of uterine corpus origin, increasing the necessity of a proper fractional dilatation and curettage (D&C) to establish the actual origin of the disease. It appears in an admixture with other variants in a large number of cases.

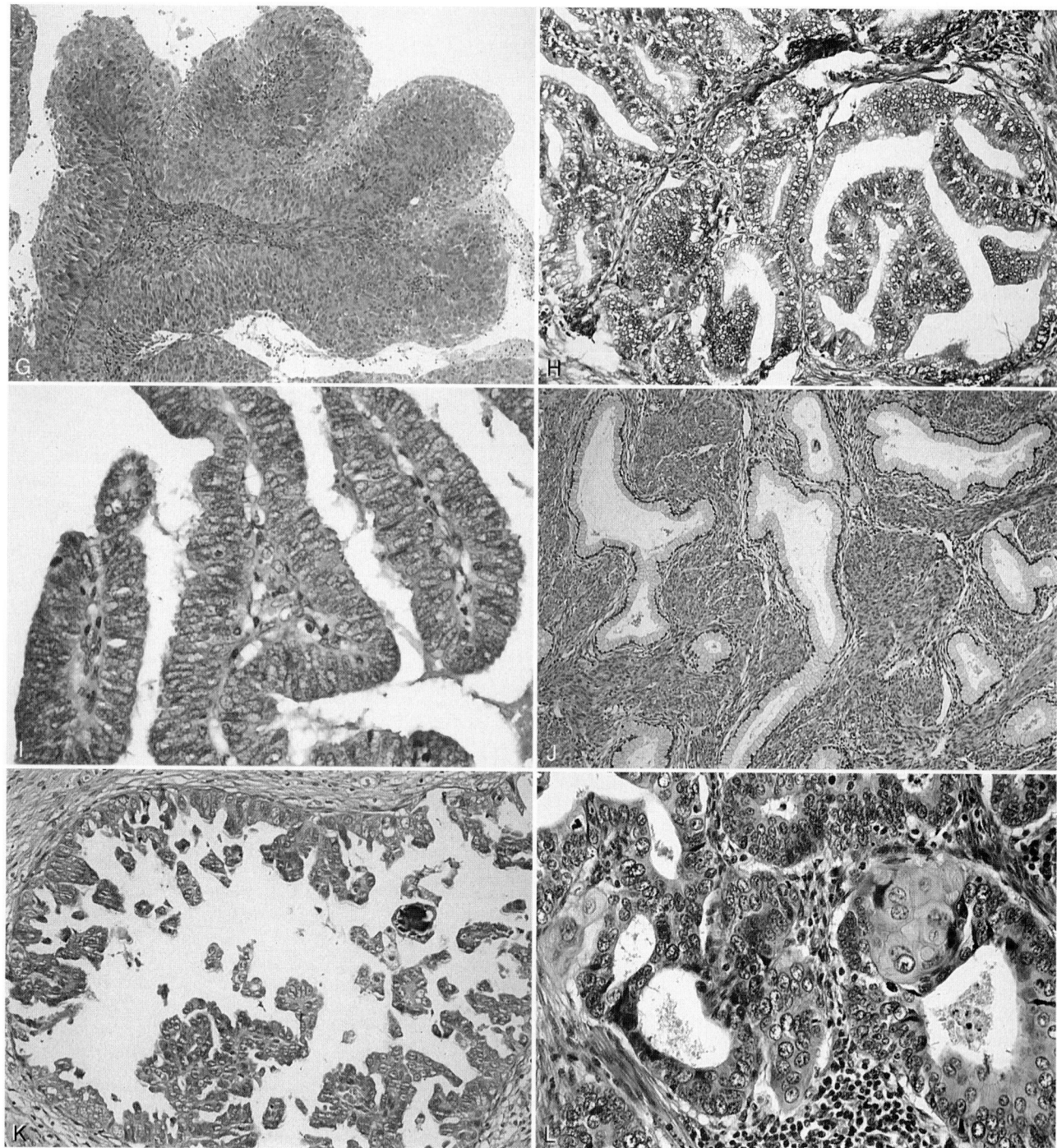

Figure 48–3. *Continued* **G,** papillary squamous; **H,** adenocarcinoma; **I,** villoglandular adenocarcinoma; **J,** minimum deviation adenocarcinoma; **K,** papillary serous adenocarcinoma; **L,** adenocarcinoma with squamous metaplasia.

Minimal deviation adenocarcinoma (MDA) is a variant that is an extremely well differentiated lesion composed of endocervical glands with basal nuclei and low nuclear/cytoplasmic ratios.[36-38] The nuclei appear minimally atypical, belying the aggressive clinical nature. On extensive sampling, markedly dysplastic cells can be identified. These malignant glands can be helpful in differentiating these lesions from other benign conditions such as adenomatous hyperplasia or deep nabothian cysts. They are almost uniformly deeply invasive and are associated with

a very poor prognosis. A high frequency of associated mucinous tumors of the ovary has also been reported.

Villoglandular papillary adenocarcinoma is generally found in younger women (average age 33) and consists of a surface papillary component with fibrous stroma.[37] Unless there is clear evidence of vascular involvement or deep invasion, conservative management may be warranted owing to the excellent prognosis.

Endometrioid adenocarcinoma of the cervix is difficult to distinguish histologically from uterine adenocarcinoma.

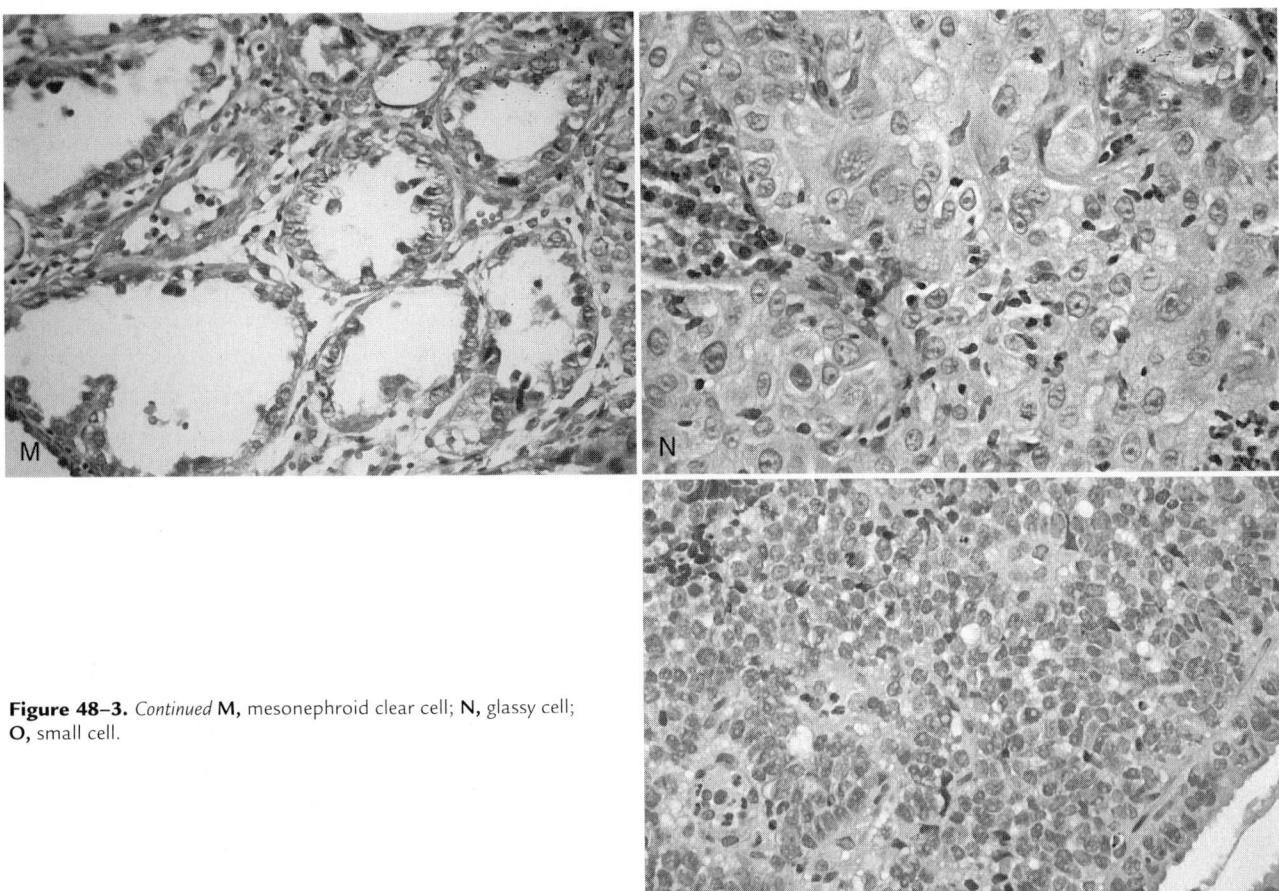

Figure 48–3. *Continued* **M**, mesonephroid clear cell; **N**, glassy cell; **O**, small cell.

The clinical activity is similar to the endocervical variety.[25,34,39-44]

Clear cell adenocarcinomas of the cervix, most commonly seen in young women exposed to DES in utero, are identical to the lesions that show up in the vagina, endometrium, and ovary. They can be seen in women of any age in the absence of DES exposure history. Three patterns have been described (tubulocystic, solid, and papillary), with the appearance of cells bearing a "hobnail" configuration that clearly sets them apart from other variants of adenocarcinoma.[15,16,45-49]

Serous papillary adenocarcinoma is a rare subtype, which histologically looks similar to its namesake in the uterus and ovary.[50,51] A search must be carried out to ensure that it is not a metastatic deposit from another site in the pelvis. Too few cases have been reported to state whether or not this entity in the cervix is prone to intraperitoneal dissemination like the uterine variety. Mesonephric, signet-ring cell, and intestinal-type adeno-carcinomas are additional extremely rare subtypes, for which care must be taken to rule out metastases from other locations.[34]

Adenosquamous and Glassy Cell Carcinoma

Adenosquamous carcinomas are tumors that contain mucin or glands in an admixture with clearly recognizable squamous elements.[34,39,52,53] Any pattern of squamous cell may appear in this setting, usually in conjunction with poorly differentiated adenocarcinoma. Once again, care should be taken to establish that this is truly adenosquamous carcinoma and not two separate primary tumors of the cervix and corpus ("collision" tumors). A particularly aggressive form of poorly differentiated adenosquamous carcinoma is the glassy cell carcinoma, so called because of a ground-glass appearance to the finely granulated cytoplasm in conjunction with clearly defined cell walls and large nuclei with prominent nucle-oli.[53-56] These tumors, representing about 1% to 2% of all cervical neoplasms, have a high mitotic rate and a particularly aggressive course.

Small Cell (Neuroendocrine) Carcinoma

Small cell carcinoma is a neuroendocrine tumor similar to small cell tumors of the lung, believed to arise from APUD cells (amine precursor uptake and decarboxylation).[55,57-59] It accounts for less than 2% of all cervical neoplasms. These lesions may have been lumped in with other small cell variants of squamous cell in the classification of Reagan mentioned earlier, giving rise to the differences seen in clinical outcome using that schema. Histologically, however, the picture seen is a sea of small monomorphous cells with a high nuclear/cytoplasmic ratio, with an occasional minimal element of glandular or squamous differentiation. Neuroendocrine granules may be identified on electron microscopy or immunohistochemical analysis. Up to one half may stain for markers such as serotonin, corticotropin (ACTH), somatostatin, or gastrin, although clinical syndromes associated with the production of these markers are very unusual. A hallmark of this disease is its systemic nature early on. Any meaningful intervention must take into account the high propensity for early dissemination and include chemotherapeutic approaches similar to those used for oat cell carcinoma of the lung.

Other rare cervical tumors include carcinoid, adenoid basal, adenoid cystic, sarcomas (mixed müllerian, endocervical stromal), embryonal rhabdomyosarcoma, and melanoma. The interested reader is referred to an excellent review article by Clement.[57] Uncommonly, the cervix may also be a site of metastatic disease.

CLINICAL PRESENTATION

Extensive data support the theory that malignant lesions arise from the precursor lesions described as HSIL.[25] On reviews of earlier biopsies of patients found to have invasive disease, severe dysplasia and CIS are often found.[60] Similarly, patients followed up with serial biopsies after discovery of HSIL show subsequent development of frank invasion. The two lesions are often found concurrently in specimens, and both arise most frequently from the squamocolumnar junction or the transformation zone.[61] Most significantly, however, incidence rates and death rates due to invasive cancer of the cervix have dropped dramatically over the past years in those regions where effective detection and treatment of HSIL occurred.[62-66]

Once the disease has broken through the basement membrane, the possibility of metastatic spread exists. Carcinoma of the cervix is divided into microinvasive (minimally invasive) or invasive. The former, making up approximately 10% of all carcinomas of the cervix, is defined as any tumor with no evidence of vascular or lymphatic invasion and less than or equal to 3 mm deepest invasion below the superficial stromal-epithelial interface.[67] The depth of invasion necessary to satisfy the criteria for this diagnosis has been the subject of considerable controversy, varying from 1 to 5 mm, with most authors preferring the 3 mm mark, since lesions with this degree of invasion have less than 1% risk of lymph node metastases. In cases with invasion from 3.1 to 5 mm, 12 of 146 patients (8%) had pelvic lymph node metastases at lymphadenectomy.[68] Although technically not a part of the definition of microinvasive carcinoma, the extent of lateral spread of the tumor has considerable prognostic significance, with lesions greater than 7 mm being associated with a greater lymph node metastatic rate.[69]

As disease progresses within the cervix, common symptoms of cervical pain, dyspareunia, vaginal discharge, or frank bleeding are reported. Pain referred to the low back or gluteal region may be present, either because of locally aggressive disease or involvement of pelvic adenopathy with pressure on the lumbosacral nerves or hypogastric plexus. Bleeding, from minor spotting to life-threatening hemorrhage, may occur. A prolonged history of intermittent bleeding may be associated with significant anemia and depletion of iron stores in the marrow. Bleeding may be emergent in some cases and can be associated with small as well as large lesions. Local progression of disease may result in invasion of surrounding organs. Hematuria and dysuria secondary to bladder invasion, rectal pain, bright red blood per rectum or change of stool caliber due to rectal involvement, or hydronephrosis and uremia secondary to ureteral obstruction by tumor may occur. In seriously neglected cases, fistula formation may already be present, with fecal or urinary diversion into the vagina. Fever secondary to local infection of the cervix, vagina, and vulva, or urinary tract infections with the possibility of pyelonephritis may be seen.

Dissemination of disease occurs either mainly through lymphatic channels or hematogenously, although intraperitoneal spread may occur in advanced disease. The lymphatic spread of disease tends to be orderly and predictable, with internal and external iliac nodes first involved, followed by common iliac and para-aortic spread. Involvement of the lower third of the vagina is associated with spread to the inguinofemoral lymph nodes. The incidence of nodal involvement is correlated significantly with the stage and volume of local disease, as well as depth of invasion.[70] Stage I disease has an 11% to 18% risk of pelvic nodal involvement, stage II, 32% to 45%, and stage III, 46% to 66%.[70-74] Para-aortic nodal involvement can also be associated with early-stage disease and has been found to be a powerful prognosticator. The incidence of para-aortic nodal involvement is 0% to 18% for stage IB/IIA disease, 13% to 33% for stage IIB, up to 46% for stage III disease, and as high as 57% for stage IVA disease.[75-82]

Hematogenous spread occurs late in the course of disease, with metastases most commonly found in the lungs, bone, and liver. Patients with metastatic disease may present with palpable supraclavicular adenopathy, painful bony metastases, nausea and anorexia due to liver involvement, or pulmonary insufficiency secondary to lung metastases. Rapid enlargement of para-aortic lymph nodes can lead to pain in the upper gastric region or pain radiating into the back.

STAGING AND WORKUP

Screening

The introduction of widespread Pap smear screening has led to a dramatic reduction in the incidence of invasive carcinoma on a worldwide level,[2,83] although a significant need remains to further extend this testing to patients of low socioeconomic status who are at high risk for dissemination of HPV, HIV, and HSV. False-negative rates of 25% to 50% have been reported with Pap smears.[84] Current recommendations for screening include annual Pap smears at the age of 18 or at initiation of sexual intercourse, whichever occurs earlier.[83]

After three consecutive yearly normal Pap smears, the frequency of Pap smears may be reduced at the discretion of the clinician, but intervals beyond 3 years are not recommended. If high-risk behavior continues, it is probably wiser to continue with yearly testing. Pap smears are currently reported using the revised Bethesda classification system. Since one quarter of cases of invasive cervical carcinoma occur in patients older than 60 and these same patients make up 40% of the mortalities, screening with routine pelvic examinations and Pap smears should continue into the later years of life. The routine use of HPV DNA testing is undergoing extensive scrutiny as a means of improving the sensitivity of screening over Pap tests alone.[85] PCR evaluation for HPV-DNA substantially increases the sensitivity of the screening procedure and helps to identify high-risk strains of HPV that require close follow-up.

Colposcopy and Biopsy

In the face of a Pap smear suspicious for malignancy (HSIL by the Bethesda classification),[24,86,87] or the presence of a high risk strain of HPV in patients classified as ASCUS, a search is performed to look for possible invasion. Colposcopy is performed to visibly evaluate the cervix to define the extent of any lesion and to allow directed biopsies of abnormal-appearing regions. In cases in which the initial biopsies show no invasion but the transformation zone was not well visualized, the entire lesion was not identified due to extension into the canal, or the endocervical curettage specimens are positive for dysplasia, the clinician cannot be sure that the biopsied portion is representative of the entire lesion, and a conization is required to rule out invasive disease. Cone specimens should include the entire transformation zone as well as a significant portion of the endocervical canal. Techniques that will allow accurate assessment of the margins of the specimen should be used. A cone specimen with no evidence of invasion but positive margins may indicate residual disease in the endocervical canal, which may harbor invasive foci and require more extensive treatment.

Large loop excision of the transformation zone, or LEEP,[88] involves the use of thin wire loop electrodes to remove the transformation zones in patients with LSIL. As opposed to ablative techniques such as cryotherapy, laser ablation, and electrocautery, LEEP produces a histologically evaluable specimen. When LEEP is correctly performed, some information will be available regarding proximity of lesions to the margins. Generally these procedures are not performed if there is suspicion of invasive disease, but they occasionally provide evidence of unsuspected invasion requiring additional intervention.

Diagnostic Workup and Staging

Once a biopsy has established the presence of invasive disease, the extent of the disease must be determined. The use of a fractional D&C is useful to rule out endometrial extension, particularly in cases of adenocarcinoma in which the origination of the disease may actually be the uterine corpus with extension into the cervix.

The current International Federation of Gynecology and Obstetrics (FIGO) staging system has evolved over the past 60 years from its initial form as the League of Nations Health Organization system in 1929.[89] Various changes have been made over that interval to incorporate applicable information, such as the removal of corpus extension from staging consideration (1950) and the creation of stage IA in 1962 and its later subdivision into IA1 and IA2 (1972), among other modifications.[90] The current system fails to incorporate some critically important information, most notably tumor volume and the presence of nodal disease. The 5-year survival rate for patients with stage Ib disease can vary from less than 20% for patients with bulky disease and both pelvic and para-aortic adenopathy to greater than 90% for those with lesions less than 2 cm in maximum diameter and no involved nodes (Fig. 48-4).[90] Survival rates for patients with higher staged disease also vary within each stage depending on primary tumor volume and nodal status.[91,92] In the Patterns of Care report on uterine cervix, the differentiation between Ia and Ib was not found to predict for either 5-year actuarial survival or pelvic control, whereas the presence of bulky disease did correlate with a higher pelvic failure rate in stage Ib disease.[92] In stage II disease, unilateral versus bilateral disease impacted significantly on both actuarial survival and pelvic control rates, a significance that persisted on multivariate analysis. In the analysis of stage III disease, the differentiation between unilateral or bilateral sidewall or lower third vaginal involvement was highly significant in both actuarial survival and pelvic control results. The GOG findings regarding the great prognostic significance of para-aortic adenopathy and tumor volume also point out the shortcomings of the current system.[93]

The American Joint Committee on Cancer (AJCC) has devised a TNM system closely modeled after the FIGO system, with the addition of nodal and metastatic categories, but fails to differentiate between pelvic and para-aortic adenopathy.[94] At present, the FIGO staging system is most widely used (Table 48-3) despite its shortcomings. For practical purposes of reporting, it is imperative that the clinical staging rules be adhered to in order to ensure accurate comparisons of therapeutic interventions. The rules for clinical staging according to FIGO state that

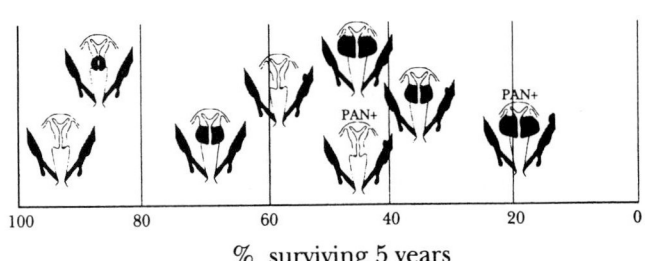

% surviving 5 years

Figure 48–4. Approximate survival rates of eight International Federation of Gynecology and Obstetrics (FIGO) stage IB cervical cancers of varying size and extent of regional spread. (From Eifel PJ: Problems with the clinical staging of carcinoma of the cervix. *Semin Radiat Oncol.* 1994;4:1.)

Table 48–3   Classification of Uterine Cervix Cancer

TNM Categories	FIGO Stages	
Primary Tumor (T)		
TX		Primary tumor cannot be assessed
T0		No evidence of primary tumor
Tis	0	Carcinoma *in situ*
T1	I	Cervical carcinoma confined to uterus (extension to corpus should be disregarded)
*T1a	IA	Invasive carcinoma diagnosed only by microscopy. Stromal invasion with a maximum depth of 5.0 mm measured from the base of the epithelium and a horizontal spread of 7.0 mm or less. Vascular space involvement, venous or lymphatic, does not affect classification
T1a1	IA1	Measured stromal invasion 3.0 mm or less in depth and 7.0 mm or less in horizontal spread
T1a2	IA2	Measured stromal invasion more than 3.0 mm and not more than 5.0 mm with a horizontal spread 7.0 mm or less
T1b	IB	Clinically visible lesion confined to the cervix or microscopic lesion greater than T1a/IA2
T1b1	IB1	Clinically visible lesion 4.0 cm or less in greatest dimension
T1b2	IB2	Clinically visible lesion more than 4.0 cm in greatest dimension
T2	II	Cervical carcinoma invades beyond uterus but not to pelvic wall or to lower third of vagina
T2a	IIA	Tumor without parametrial invasion
T2b	IIB	Tumor with parametrial invasion
T3	III	Tumor extends to pelvic wall and/or involves lower third of vagina, and/or causes hydronephrosis or non-functioning kidney
T3a	IIIA	Tumor involves lower third of vagina, no extension to pelvic wall
T3b	IIIB	Tumor extends to pelvic wall and/or causes hydro-nephrosis or non-functioning kidney

TNM Categories	FIGO Stages	
T4	IVA	Tumor invades mucosa of bladder or rectum, and/or extends beyond true pelvis (bullous edema is not sufficient to classify a tumor as T4)
Regional Lymph Nodes (N)		
NX		Regional lymph nodes cannot be assessed
N0		No regional lymph node metastasis
N1		Regional lymph node metastasis
Distant Metastasis (M)		
MX		Distant metastasis cannot be assessed
M0		No distant metastasis
M1	IVB	Distant metastasis

Stage Grouping

Stage 0	Tis	N0	M0
Stage I	T1	N0	M0
Stage IA	T1a	N0	M0
Stage IA1	T1a1	N0	M0
Stage IA2	T1a2	N0	M0
Stage IB	T1b	N0	M0
Stage IB1	T1b1	N0	M0
Stage IB2	T1b2	N0	M0
Stage II	T2	N0	M0
Stage IIA	T2a	N0	M0
Stage IIB	T2b	N0	M0
Stage III	T3	N0	M0
Stage IIIA	T3a	N0	M0
Stage IIIB	T1	N1	M0
	T2	N1	M0
	T3a	N1	M0
	T3b	Any N	M0
Stage IVA	T4	Any N	M0
Stage IVB	Any T	Any N	M1

*All macroscopically visible lesions—even with superficial invasion—are T1b/IB.
From Greene FL, Page DL, Fleming ID, et al, eds: *AJCC Cancer Staging Manual*, 6th ed. New York: Springer; 2002.

staging is to be based on careful clinical examination, before intervention, preferably an examination under anesthesia. Once established, the stage is not to be changed by later findings or therapeutic interventions. Palpation, inspection, colposcopy, endocervical curettage, hysteroscopy, cystoscopy, proctoscopy, intravenous pyelography, chest x-ray, and bone scan are allowed. Specifically excluded from the clinical staging system are the results of such tests as lymphangiography (LAG), magnetic resonance imaging (MRI), computed tomography (CT), arteriography, laparoscopy, and laparotomy.[90,95] These tests are not allowed to influence the clinical stage for reporting purposes but obviously may play a critical role in the treatment of the patient.

Locally, it is important to fully describe the extent of palpable disease through the use of extensive diagrams and descriptions of the three-dimensional characteristics of the lesion. The degree of parametrial (medial or lateral, unilateral or bilateral) or vaginal (upper two-thirds, lower one-third) extension should be clearly defined, as should the presence or absence of hydronephrosis, rectal invasion, bladder mucosal invasion, bullous edema, uterosacral ligament involvement, or extension to the pelvic sidewall

(bilateral or unilateral). The use of MRI evaluation of the pelvis is not allowed by the current staging system in determining the clinical stage but has proved to be of benefit in defining the extent of disease locally as well as regionally.[96-101] It also provides information that is useful in optimizing brachytherapy planning. Cystoscopy and proctosigmoidoscopy are routinely called for by the FIGO system, but in cases of early disease in which MRI shows no suspicion of local extension, these more invasive procedures may not be necessary. On the other hand, if an MRI scan raises the question of bladder or rectal involvement, endoscopic evaluation is essential to rule out pathologic involvement of these organs. An IVP or a CT scan with contrast can provide information as to the presence of hydroureterosis or hydronephrosis.

Pelvic evaluation with CT or MRI, or alternatively laparoscopic nodal dissection, may provide invaluable information for radiation treatment planning. The finding of abnormal lymph nodes in the pelvis or para-aortic region on an MRI or a CT scan should be followed with a CT-guided fine needle aspiration of the suspicious nodes.

LAG is less useful in evaluation of the pelvis because of its failure to highlight internal iliac nodes. On the other hand, evaluation of the para-aortic nodes by LAG is found to be more sensitive than either CT or ultrasonography.[93] Current randomized protocols of the GOG include evaluation of the para-aortic lymph nodes by either LAG or extraperitoneal lymph node dissection due to the import of extension to these nodes. Outside the trial setting, however, it is not clear that routine evaluation of these nodes by invasive means is justified.[92,102]

Positron emission tomography (PET) holds promise as a useful staging modality for locally advanced cervical cancer. It may be an accurate noninvasive method of evaluating nodal status, tumor volume, and prognosis.[103-105] These preliminary studies must be validated in prospective trials before routine application of PET can be recommended.

Further routine workup should include a complete blood count, liver function tests, renal function tests, and a chest x-ray. In patients believed to be at risk for exposure to HIV, testing for antibodies to HIV should be discussed with the patient before the initiation of therapy. If the patient is HIV-antibody positive, the CD4 count is currently recommended as a rough indicator of the immune status and of the patient's likelihood to be able to tolerate therapy.[6,106-108] The usefulness of a bone scan is limited to patients with advanced disease with symptoms suggestive of dissemination and is not routinely obtained. In cases in which there is evidence of spread to pelvic lymph nodes on pelvic CT or MRI scan, evaluation of the abdomen to rule out higher adenopathy or liver involvement is recommended.

Blind scalene node biopsy performed in the setting of positive para-aortic lymphadenopathy has a positive rate of 0% to 35%.[109,110] In a prospective evaluation of biopsies of nonpalpable scalene nodes in 55 patients with positive para-aortic (48) or high common iliac nodes (8), only 4 were confirmed positive (14%).[111] The routine use of such biopsies is not warranted. Prior to the initiation of para-aortic radiation for patients with known retroperitoneal disease, CT scan of the chest to rule out disease missed on plain chest x-rays may be a more useful test than biopsy of clinically negative nodes.

PROGNOSTIC FACTORS

Tumor volume is directly related to the incidence of spread to pelvic and para-aortic lymph nodes, as well as inversely related to local control and actuarial survival. In a retrospective review by Piver and Chung[78] of 289 patients who underwent a radical hysterectomy for stages IB/IIA or recurrent cervical carcinoma at Roswell Park, patients with tumors 3 cm or less had a 21% incidence of pathologically involved nodes, compared with 35% to 42% for those patients with tumors greater than 3 cm. In a prospective GOG surgical pathologic study of patients with stage I SCC of the cervix treated with a radical hysterectomy and pelvic lymph node dissection, tumors up to 1.0 cm in maximum diameter had a 12% incidence of involved pelvic lymph nodes, compared with 23% for those tumors greater than 3 cm.[112] A separate analysis of patients entered into three consecutive radiation trials for stages I to IVA cervical cancer by the GOG found tumor size to be a significant predictor for progression-free

interval.[113] In a retrospective review of 1526 patients with MD Anderson Cancer Center stage IB (confined to cervix, <1 quadrant involved), IC (>1 quadrant), and IIB barrel (>6 cm), all treated with radiation and adjuvant hysterectomy, maximum tumor diameter correlated significantly with central control of disease, pelvic control, and disease-specific survival, with the risk of pelvic recurrence increasing markedly with tumors greater than 5 cm.[114] A review of 1178 patients with stages IB to IVA cervical cancer at Mallinckrodt identified a strong relationship between tumor size and local control, distant metastases, disease-free survival, and actuarial survival in patients with early-stage disease.[115]

In a retrospective review of 625 patients with stages IB to IIB cervical cancer treated with a radical hysterectomy between 1965 and 1977, Inoue[70] found a significant correlation between the depth of invasion and the incidence of pelvic nodal involvement and parametrial involvement. Of 97 tumors less than 5 mm deep, there was only one with pathologic evidence of involvement of pelvic nodes. Other investigators have reported that tumors measuring less than 3 mm in maximum depth have a less than 1% risk of spread to pelvic lymph nodes,[68] while tumors in the range of 3 to 5 mm deep have up to an 8% incidence of nodal involvement.[95,116] Depth of invasion was a potent prognosticator for spread to pelvic lymph nodes in the GOG surgical pathologic study of patients with stage I cancer ($P < 0.0001$) (Table 48-4).[112]

Table 48-4   Incidence of Positive Pelvic Nodes

		Incidence, %	Reference
Stage	I	11–18	Guttman[71]
	II	32–45	Meigs[72]
	III	46–66	Brunschweig & Barber[73]
			Inoue & Morita[140]
			Inoue & Okumura[329]
Depth of invasion, mm	≤3	<1	Coppleson[68]
			Ueki et al[172]
			Sevin et al[173]
			Johnson et al[174]
			Schink & Lurain[175]
	3–5	1–8	Coppleson[68]
			FIGO[95]
			Ruch et al[116]
	≤5	<1–3.5	Inoue[70]
			Delgado et al[112]
	6–10	15.1	Delgado et al[112]
	11–15	22.2	Delgado et al[112]
	16–20	38.8	Delgado et al[112]
	>20	22.6	Delgado et al[112]
Maximum tumor dimension (IB/II), cm	0.1–1.0	12.7	Delgado et al[112]
	1.1–2.0	15.8	Delgado et al[112]
	2.1–3.0	16.3	Delgado et al[112]
	≤3 cm	21	Delgado et al[112]
	>3 cm	23–42	Piver & Chung[78]
			Delgado et al[112]
Grade	I	9.7	Delgado et al[112]
	II	13.9	Delgado et al[112]
	III	21.8	Delgado et al[112]
LVSI	Absent	8.2	Delgado et al[112]
	Present	25.4	Delgado et al[112]

LVSI, lymphatic vascular space invasion.

Histologic grade of squamous cell carcinoma does not appear to influence the response to primary surgery, as indicated by the GOG study of patients with stage I disease.[28] There is debate, however, as to what impact the squamous cell subtype may have on the responsiveness of the tumor to primary radiation treatment.[117,118] Most authors have failed to establish such a connection.[119,120] Adenocarcinomas appear to have a reduced actuarial survival compared with squamous cell cancers,[42,114,121,122] although this has been disputed.[123] The annual report of the FIGO results of 30,322 patients treated for cervix cancer between 1982 and 1986 showed superior 3- and 5-year survival rates for patients with squamous cell lesions versus those with adenocarcinoma, regardless of the modality used (surgery or radiation) and within each stage.[124] Among the subtypes of adenocarcinomas, however, certain types clearly do carry a worse prognosis, notably papillary serous and minimal deviation adenocarcinoma.

Despite its imperfections, the FIGO staging system has been effective in dividing patients into groups with different prognoses.[125-132] The FIGO report of 8538 patients treated with either radiation or surgery between 1982 and 1986 showed the following 5-year actuarial survival rates: stage I, 81.6%; stage II, 61.5%; stage III, 36.7%; stage IV, 12.1%.[124] According to the Patterns of Care Study, 5-year survival rates for stages I, II, and III cancers of the cervix treated with radiation were 74%, 56%, and 33%, respectively (Fig. 48–5).[133] The French Cooperative Group report in 1988 stated survival rates of 89% for patients with stage IB disease, 85% for IIA, 76% for IIB, 62% for IIIA, 50% for IIIB, and 20% for stage IV.[91]

Metastatic disease in the pelvic nodes is a powerful prognostic factor, as evidenced by multivariate analyses in both retrospective and prospective reports. The presence of disease in pelvic lymph nodes in stage I disease decreases the survival into the 50% to 60% range.[70,74,78,125,130,134-142] In FIGO's annual report regarding cervical cancer results, patients with stage IB disease with negative nodes had an 89.5% 5-year survival versus 59% for those with histologically positive nodal involvement.[124] Inoue,[140] in a retrospective review of 875 patients with stage IB to IIB resected cases found survival rates of 89%, 81%, 63%, and 41% for patients with no nodes, 1 node, 2 to 3 nodes, and 4 to 18 nodes positive, respectively. In a separate multi-institutional review, Alvarez and associates[125] found the number of nodes involved to have a significant impact on survival in a multivariate analysis. The presence of extracapsular extension further increased the risk of recurrence in the study by Tinga and associates.[143] Terada and associates[144] identified the level of the node (obturator, external iliac, common iliac, or para-aortic) as a separate prognostic indicator. In the GOG analysis of patients treated with definitive radiation, the presence of para-aortic adenopathy was found to be the most potent prognostic factor evaluated.[93]

Anemia has been associated with decreased local control in patients with locally advanced cervical carcinoma in many series.[131,145-148] In the excellent review of the topic by Dische, however, it is made clear that the issue is quite complex because of the varying levels of hemoglobin used to define anemia and the association of anemia with more advanced disease at presentation.[148,149] In a multivariate analysis of prognostic factors in a retrospective review of 2800 patients with cervical carcinoma of all stages treated for cure performed at Princess Margaret Hospital, Bush and associates[147,150] found that anemia achieved a high level of significance, particularly at levels below 12 g%. It is not clear, however, that performing transfusions on patients to bring them up to a hemoglobin level of 12 g% alters outcome. In the only prospective published study to date, from the Princess Margaret Hospital, 132 patients with stage IIB or III disease were initially randomly assigned either to receive transfusions to keep their hemoglobin above 12.5 or not receive transfusions until the hemoglobin fell below 10 g%.[150] Patients in either arm with hemoglobin greater than 12.5 did not receive transfusions. A subgroup analysis done retrospectively showed a significant decrease in local failure and disease-specific death rates for patients who received transfusions to keep their hemoglobin above 12 compared with anemic patients who did not receive transfusions. This information, although suggestive of a benefit for transfusion, is not conclusive.[149] Several authors have failed to find a correlation between anemia and response to radiation.[148,151] The suggested benefit of correction of the anemia must be weighed against the attendant risks of routine transfusions.[148] Before the initiation of radiation, it is reasonable to correct severe anemia (hemoglobin below 10 g%) or transfuse the patient with borderline anemia who continues to actively bleed while attempts are made to control the bleeding with packing, the use of Monsel's ferric subsulfate solution, and radiation intervention.

The questionable influence of endometrial extension on outcome is interrelated with the volume of tumor as well as the issue of parametrial extension (stage). Several retrospective reports identify endometrial stromal invasion as having a negative impact on survival,[152,153] possibly because of an increase in distant metastases rather than an increased incidence of local failure after definitive irradiation.

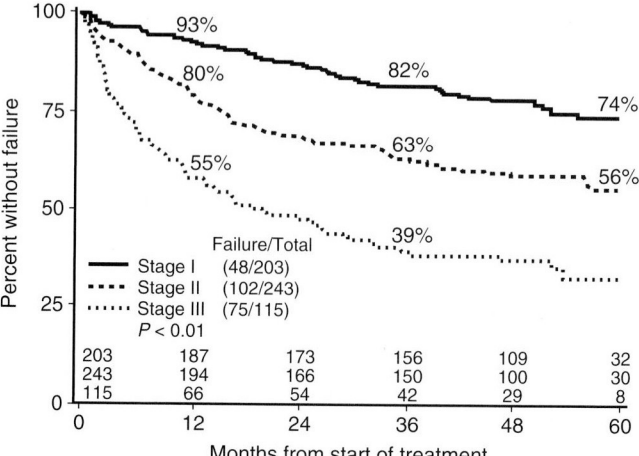

Figure 48–5. Actuarial no-evidence-of-disease survival by stage from the Patterns of Care Study. (From Coia L, Won M, Lanciano R, et al: The Patterns of Care Outcome Study for cancer of the uterine cervix: Results of the Second National Practice Survey. *Cancer.* 1990;66:2451.)

Young age at diagnosis appears to carry with it a worse prognosis.[93,131,151,154-159] Karnofsky performance status (KPS) has been identified as an independent prognostic factor of actuarial survival in the GOG analysis of 606 patients entered into three consecutive radiation therapy trials[160] as well as in the Patterns of Care studies.[161]

Women with cervical cancer and HIV disease tend to present with more advanced disease compared with seronegative patients.[106,107,142] In a report of 84 patients evaluated and treated for cervical cancer at the State University of New York (SUNY), 16 patients were known to be HIV positive.[106] Only one of these patients presented with early-stage disease, compared with 40% of the remaining 68 HIV-negative women. Ten of the 16 suffered recurrences after a brief interval, 4 were either lost to follow-up or died shortly after therapy, and only 2 experienced long-term control. The mean CD4 count, a crude indicator of the immune status of the patient, was 360 compared with 830 for the HIV-negative group. The only two long-term survivors were patients with initial CD4 counts greater than 600. HIV status, taken in conjunction with other measures of the immunocompetence of the patient (such as frequency of opportunistic infections, CD4 count) has a profound influence on tolerance to therapy and overall survival.

The DNA ploidy, DNA index, and S phase fraction (SPF) information has been shown to have prognostic importance in a number of malignancies.[162,163] Their significance is less well established in patients with early-stage carcinoma of the uterine cervix. For each article reporting a correlation between flow cytometric data and outcome endpoints,[162-165] there is an article with opposing results.[128,166-169] Part of the problem appears to arise from the variation in techniques used and the difficulty in identifying a cutoff point for the level of the DNA index that is truly significant.[163] DNA ploidy by itself appears to have little value in predicting outcome,[169] although taken in conjunction with SPF, a subgroup with a particularly bad outcome has been identified. Strang and coworkers,[162] in a prospective evaluation of SPF and ploidy status in 307 patients with early-stage cervical carcinoma, found that patients with an elevated SPF, particularly if it exceeded 20%, and a near diploid DNA content had a significantly decreased recurrence-free survival rate. This information was reaffirmed in a prospective series of 310 patients carried out by Willen and coworkers.[170] Overall, however, this subgroup represents less than 10% of all patients with early-stage disease. In general, flow cytometric data are less helpful than established prognosticators such as nodal involvement, parametrial extension, or tumor size.

MANAGEMENT AND RESULTS BY STAGE AND SIZE

Carcinoma In Situ and Stage IA Disease

Carcinoma in situ and disease with early stromal invasion isolated to buds of neoplastic cells that penetrate the basement membrane but remain immeasurable macroscopically (true IA1 disease)[171] have essentially a 0% incidence of involvement of the lymph nodes.[172-177] In the absence of disease at the cone biopsy margins, a recurrence rate of 0% would be expected after simple hysterectomy. Conization itself represents adequate therapy in these cases, as long as the margins are definitely clear. A lesion cannot be classified as stage IA disease unless all margins of the cone biopsy are free of disease, since the entirety of the lesion may not have been identified.[175] Alternative approaches such as laser vaporization and cryotherapy[172,178,179] have success rates in excess of 95%, although obliteration of the margins may make it difficult to identify those patients with residual disease.

Patients with stage IA2 disease with maximum depth of invasion of 3 mm or less and no evidence of lymphatic vascular space invasion also have a risk of lymph node involvement that is less than 1%.[172-175] A simple hysterectomy with no lymph node dissection and optional oophorectomy is standard therapy, although more conservative therapy such as conization may be considered in the patient who is interested in further childbearing.

The presence of lymphatic vascular space invasion (LVSI) or invasion to a depth greater than 3 mm is associated with a slight increase in the risk of spread to pelvic nodes or recurrence after hysterectomy. Up to 13% of patients with these findings may have lymphatic spread at the time of hysterectomy (range 2% to 13%),[173,175-177] arguing for more aggressive local therapy tailored to the histologic findings. Patients with LVSI but invasion to less than 3 mm and clear margins after cone resection might be suitable for a simple hysterectomy and pelvic node dissection to reduce morbidity. If, however, the depth of invasion is from 3.1 to 5 mm and LVSI is present, an extended or radical hysterectomy should be performed. Under these conditions, if the patient strongly desires to maintain her ability to bear children, a therapeutic conization may be considered, but close follow-up is essential as invasive recurrences are reported in up to 5% of cases.[173,175-177]

Surgical approaches are preferred for such minimal disease. In cases of medical inoperability, definitive radiation is an acceptable alternative with outstanding results.[177,180] One or two intracavitary insertions are employed to deliver a dose of 60 to 70 Gy to point A. External beam radiation is not routinely employed for stage IA disease, unless the risk of pelvic nodal spread is considered to be substantial, such as in a case with greater than 3 mm invasion, LVSI, and poorly differentiated histology.

Surgery alone for stage IA disease has resulted in local recurrence rates of 2% to 5%, with the majority of recurrences being noninvasive and amenable to effective salvage. Depriest[171] found no invasive recurrences in 145 patients treated with hysterectomy at the University of Kentucky. Kolstad,[177] reporting on 496 cases of microinvasive disease treated with surgery in Norway, had recurrences in only 15 patients, all of whom were cured with further surgery. In a review by Sevin and coworkers[173] of six major series in the literature, 0.2% of 513 cases with disease invasion less than 3 mm recurred, versus 5.4% of 166 cases with invasion of 3.1 to 5.0 mm.

The results with radiation alone are comparable to those found with surgery. In Kolstad's series, an additional

136 patients were treated with brachytherapy alone, and none had recurrences.[177] Of 32 patients with IA disease treated at Mallinckrodt with radiation alone (either with brachytherapy alone or in combination with external beam therapy), there was only one failure reported at 15 years.[180]

Stage IB/IIA

Stage IB cases include a wide variety of tumors, ranging from the smallest visible tumors with no pathologically involved lymph nodes to bulky endophytic endocervical tumors greater than 6 cm in diameter with positive pelvic and periaortic nodes. It is obvious that no one approach is suitable for all patients with stage IB disease. The treatment must be tailored to the physical characteristics of the lesion and the overall medical condition of the patient.

Stage IB/IIA lesions that measure 3 cm or less can be managed with either definitive surgery or radiation. The decision usually hinges on the side effects and complications associated with each procedure and the medical condition of the patient. The standard surgical approach is the radical hysterectomy with pelvic and para-aortic lymph node dissection. Five-year disease-free survival rates of 80% to 92%[73,181-183] are reported after radical hysterectomy, while for radiation, the actuarial 5-year survival rates vary from 78% to 90% (Table 48-5).[91,184-189]

For patients with centrally located tumors limited to 3 cm or less in maximum dimension; no evidence of spread to lymph nodes on scans, the geometry of which allows placement of colpostats into the fornices; and in whom hemorrhaging is not a critical issue, immediate

brachytherapy is desirable (Table 48-6). The entire tumoricidal dose may be administered using two insertions, thereby increasing the chance of local control and reducing the risk of morbidity. Paracervical doses—best conceived of as minimal tumor doses rather than a dose to a specific point, such as point A, as tumors get larger than 4 cm in size or are eccentrically located (see "Dose Specifications" later)—of 75 to 80 Gy may be delivered through brachytherapy alone, followed by 45 Gy external beam therapy to the pelvic lymph nodes using a midline shield to protect the bladder and rectum from further injury. In cases in which bleeding must first be controlled or arrangements made for operating room time, external beam may be started to the whole pelvis, with the insertion planned after 20 Gy has been delivered. (Bleeding may be adequately controlled through the judicious use of packing and Monsel's ferric subsulfate solution.) External beam therapy should be continued between the two insertions with a midline bar in place. Every effort must be made to minimize the total duration of the external beam therapy once it has been started. Lesions measuring greater than 3 cm that are significantly eccentric or endophytic in their entirety are best approached with external beam therapy initially to allow shrinkage before brachytherapy, since the isodose distribution may not adequately encompass the tumor at initial presentation.

Caution must be used when comparing results with surgery and radiation in the treatment of early-stage disease. Younger patients, in better medical condition and with a smaller burden of disease, tend to be referred for surgery, whereas older or medically challenged patients and those with a larger central burden of disease are referred for radiation. In addition, in a significant proportion of patients who have worrisome findings at

Table 48–5   Results of Treatment by Stage and Modality

Stage	Modality	Patients, n	5-Yr Survival, %	Parameter	Reference
IB–IIA	Surgery	213	92	Cumulative	Hopkins & Morley[196]
		978	90	Actuarial	Averette et al[197]
	Radiation	97	86	Cumulative	Hopkins & Morley[196]
		197	83	Cumulative	Montana et al[198]
		701 (<4 cm)	89.6	Disease-free	Eifel et al[201]
		1526	81	Disease-free	Eifel et al[201]
		130	81	Relapse-free	Lowrey et al[151]
IB bulky	Radiation	38 (>5 cm)	61	CSS	Perez et al[330]
		75 (≥6 cm)	60	CSS	Mendenhall et al[213]
		402 (>5 cm)	58–69	Disease-free	Eifel et al[201]
	Radiation + Surgery	35 (>5 cm)	66	CSS	Perez et al[330]
		75 (≥6 cm)	55	CSS	Mendenhall et al[213]
IIB	Radiation	629	76–85	Actuarial	Horiot et al[91]
		214	58	Actuarial	Kovalic et al[227]
		143	76	Actuarial	Kraiphibul et al[226]
III	Radiation	203	33	Cumulative	Montana et al[228]
		271	25–47	Actuarial	Komaki et al[331]
		482	50–62	Actuarial	Horiot et al[91]
		66	32	Actuarial	Kovalic et al[227]
		17 (IIIA)	58	Disease-free	Cardinale et al[231]
		42 (IIIA)	37	Actuarial	Kavadi & Eifel[332]
IVA	Radiation	32	20	Actuarial	Horiot et al[91]
		48	18	Actuarial	Kramer et al[236]

CSS, cause-specific survival.

Table 48–6   Dose Recommendations for Radiation Therapy

Stage	Nodal Status	Paracervical Dose, Gy	Minimum Tumor Dose	Parametrial Dose, Gy	Pelvic Lymph Node Dose, Gy	Para-aortic Lymph Node Dose, Gy
IA1		60–70[†]		(brachytherapy only)	0[†]	0[†]
IA2		60–70[†]		45–50	45[†]	0[†]
IB/IIA ≤2 cm		75–85[†]		50	45[†]	0[†]
IB/IIA 2–4 cm		80–90[†]		50–55	45[†]	0[†]
	+				50–60*	45[†]
IB/IIA ≥4 cm, no surgery	–	85–90[†]		55–60	45[†]	45[†]
	+			50–60*		
IB/IIA ≥4 cm, adjuvant hysterectomy	±	75[†]		55	45[†]	0[†]
IIB		85–90[†]	70–75[‡]	60	45[†]	45[†]
	+			50–60*		
IIIA	–/+	85–90[†]	70–75[‡]	60–65	50–60*	0–50[§]
IIIB	–/+	85–90[†]	70–75	60–65	50–60*	0–50[§]
IVA[¶]	–/+	85–90[†]	70–75[‡]	60	50–60*	0–50[§]

*Conformal approaches are used to eliminate small bowel from field beyond 50 Gy.
[†]Recommended doses if tandem and colpostats are used (intracavitary therapy).
[‡]Recommended minimum tumor doses if an interstitial implant is used (interstitial therapy).
[§]Prophylactic para-aortic radiation is not of proven benefit beyond stage IIB. Doses depend on level of clinical suspicion.
[¶]Alternatively, palliative doses, using 370 cGy bid approach described in text.

exploratory laparotomy, such as positive pelvic lymph nodes, parametrial extension, or surgical complications, the hysterectomy is not completed, and the patients are referred for definitive radiation. Because the clinical stage of these patients is unchanged by the surgical findings, they are lumped together in most reports of patients with early-stage disease treated with radiation.

With that prelude, the retrospective reports reveal a notable similarity in results for radiation and surgery. In a review of surgical series carried out in the post-1970 era,[182,190-196] Averette[197] found an average 5-year overall survival rate of 87.9% for patients with stage IB/IIA disease treated surgically (range, 80.7% to 92.5%). Operative mortality for a total of 26 series was 0.72%. Reporting on 978 consecutive patients with early-stage disease who underwent radical hysterectomy between 1965 and 1990 at the University of Miami, Averette[197] had a 90.1% 5-year actuarial survival overall, 90.5% for stage IB, and 65.7% for stage IIA. Breaking them down by histology, SCC had a 90.7% 5-year survival; adeno-carcinoma, 80.5%; and adenosquamous carcinoma, 63.5%. Of the 17.7% of patients who had positive pelvic lymph nodes, the 5-year survival was 63.5%, 40.8% for those with positive para-aortic lymph nodes. Overall complications in this series were as follows: 0.8% urinary fistulae, 8.5% wound-related problems, 20.5% bladder dysfunction, 6% ileus, and 2.6% chronic lymphedema. Hopkins and Morley[196] at the University of Michigan reported a 92% 5-year overall survival rate in 213 patients treated between 1970 and 1985 with surgery alone. Lee[183] reported a survival rate of 86.1% for 237 patients with stage IB disease and a 71.7% survival for 106 patients with stage IIA disease.

Radiation results in reports on 5-year survival rates of patients with clinical stage IB alone range from 67.2% to 91.5%[91,184,186-188,198-200] and are predominantly in the 80% to 85% range for most modern series.[91,186,187,194,201,202] The Patterns of Care reports revealed an 81% 4-year actuarial survival rate for all stage I patients treated with radiation alone.[161] Stage IIA results range from 70% to 76%.[91,184,187] Considering the previous statements about treatment selection bias, these results compare quite favorably with those seen with surgery.

Central disease control rates of 92% to 94% are reported for patients with stage IB cervical cancers treated with radiation alone.[91,201,203] Eifel analyzed the results of radiation treatment of 1526 stage IB squamous cell cancers of the cervix treated at MD Anderson Hospital between 1960 and 1989.[201] Central disease control was achieved in 95% of patients at 10 years, and 98.9% of those with tumors less than 4 cm in size. Pelvic tumor control was established in 92% of all cases at 10 years, and in 97% of tumors less than 4 cm in size (Fig. 48-6). The influence of brachytherapy technique on local control has been assessed. Jampolis[204] found only 11 central failures out of 494 patients with stage IB/IIA disease, 8 of which could be correlated with improper placement of the colpostats during brachytherapy. Perez found a correlation of poor insertion technique with increased risk of central failure.[205] It is difficult to define the relationship between central dose and central recurrence rates because of the retrospective nature of the reviews.[187,203,206,207] Differing doses often reflect larger initial tumor bulk, the nature of regression patterns, and the clinical concern of the clinician, and dose-searching studies have not been reported.

In a separate report on 88 patients from the University of Miami who had adenocarcinoma stage IB, radical hysterectomy resulted in an 81% overall survival.[208] Reviewing the reported results from 24 series, with a total of 1669 patients with stage IB adenocarcinoma, Steren and associates[208] found a 79% 5-year survival rate

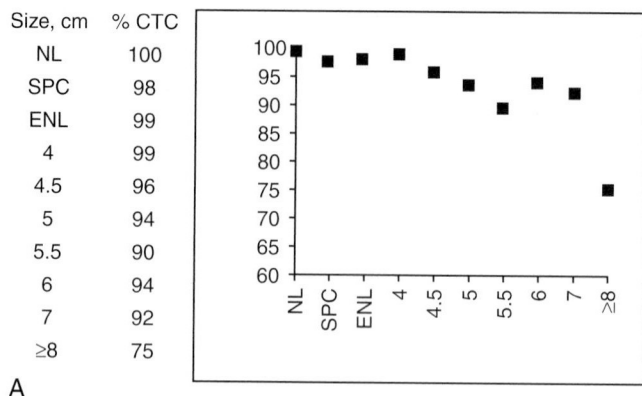

Size, cm	% CTC
NL	100
SPC	98
ENL	99
4	99
4.5	96
5	94
5.5	90
6	94
7	92
≥8	75

A

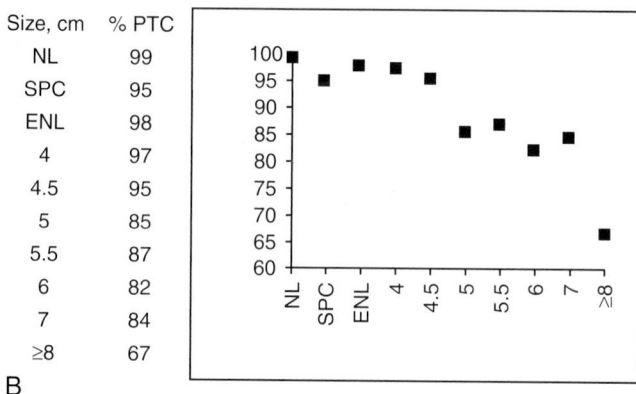

Size, cm	% PTC
NL	99
SPC	95
ENL	98
4	97
4.5	95
5	85
5.5	87
6	82
7	84
≥8	67

B

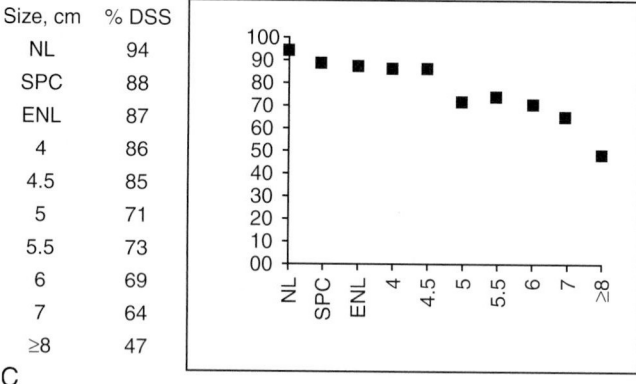

Size, cm	% DSS
NL	94
SPC	88
ENL	87
4	86
4.5	85
5	71
5.5	73
6	69
7	64
≥8	47

C

Figure 48–6. A, Central tumor control (CTC); **B,** pelvic tumor control (PTC); and **C,** disease-specific survival (DSS) for 1526 patients who received radiation for stage IB cervical carcinoma treated at MD Anderson Hospital from 1960 to 1989. ENL, enlarged cervix less than 4 cm; NL, normal-sized cervix; SPC, small cervix after cone biopsy. (Data from Eifel PJ, Morris M, Wharton JT, et al: The influence of tumor size and morphology on the outcome of patients with FIGO stage IB squamous cell carcinoma of the uterine cervix. *Int J Radiat Oncol Biol Phys.* 1994;29:9.)

among 487 patients treated with surgery alone. An additional 398 patients were approached with definitive radiation, with a 67% survival. Of 449 patients treated with a combined approach, a 74% 5-year survival rate was noted.

The only prospective randomized trial comparing surgery and radiotherapy was reported by Landoni et al. in 1997.[209] Over a period of 5 years, 343 patients with stage IB and IIA cervical carcinoma were randomized between surgery and radiotherapy. Adjuvant radiotherapy was given for patients found to have pathologic stage T2b or greater at surgery, less than 3 mm of margin, cut-through, or positive lymph nodes (64% of the surgical cases received adjuvant radiotherapy). The result was analyzed based on intention to treat. With a median follow-up of 87 months, the 5-year overall and disease-free survivals were identical between the two groups (83% and 74%, respectively). When analyzed in terms of tumor size greater than or less than 4 cm, there was also no difference in overall survival. Twenty-eight percent of the surgery group had severe morbidity compared with 12% in radiotherapy-alone group of patients ($P = 0.0004$). Given that patients receiving combined surgery and radiotherapy had the worst morbidity, this study suggests that only patients with limited disease that can be completely excised should be offered the option of surgery.

STAGE IB/IIA, BULKY LESIONS

Bulky lesions, those exceeding 4 cm in maximum dimension, and endophytic lesions with significant extension into the lower uterine segment can be approached in various ways. It is imperative, however, to first fully establish the shape and direction of growth of disease at the onset, especially in adenocarcinomas. A fractional D&C is needed to rule out uterine corpus involvement, and an MRI scan is helpful in determining the geometry of the lesion beyond what is palpable on examination.

If radiation is the treatment of choice, external beam therapy is necessary at the outset to allow tumor shrinkage for proper placement of tandem and colpostats. Weekly pelvic examinations are essential to determine the point in time when brachytherapy should be performed. It is advisable to proceed with brachytherapy when the tumor has shrunk to less than 4 cm in diameter unless the tumor is eccentrically located to one side. A balance is necessary between tumor shrinkage and the inevitable restriction of the vaginal fornices that occurs with increasing external beam dose. Doses as high as 40 Gy may be required to allow enough reduction in tumor size to proceed with an insertion, but doses in excess of 40 Gy before placement of a midline bar should be avoided because the risk of damage to the bladder and rectum is directly related to the external dose to these organs.[155,184,200,210] For larger lesions confined to the cervix, doses to point A in the 85 to 90 Gy region are recommended if no adjuvant surgery is planned. In cases in which an extrafascial hysterectomy is deemed necessary, the total dose to point A should be confined to 75 Gy and the pelvic nodal dose should be held at 45 Gy to lower the risk of complications.

The decision to proceed with definitive irradiation or to add an extrafascial hysterectomy for patients with bulky disease (disease >4 cm in maximum dimension in this discussion) is ideally made midway through the treatment program. A routine hysterectomy in all cases of bulky disease is not justifiable. Citing an increased risk of central failure after radiation therapy alone, Rutledge[211] in 1976 published recommendations for adjuvant extrafascial hysterectomy after radiation therapy for patients with bulky cervical cancers measuring 6 cm or greater in diameter with lower uterine segment involvement, presenting the results of 212 patients so treated at MD Anderson Hospital from 1954 to 1967. A vesicovaginal fistula rate of 4.1% was reported after the combined procedures in a later report (four times the rate seen with radiation therapy alone), and the approach was changed to eliminate routine surgery in patients with a history of pelvic inflammatory disease or parametrial involvement with a subsequent fall in complication rates.[212] Mendenhall[202,213] reported the results of 150 patients with cervix tumors 6 cm or greater in diameter treated at the University of Florida from 1964 to 1983. Seventy-five of the patients received radiation therapy alone, and 75 received radiation followed by an extrafascial hysterectomy. There was no significant difference seen in pelvic disease control (70% to 76% at 5 years), cause-specific survival (55% to 60%), or absolute survival (48% to 52%) between the two groups (Fig. 48-7). In a separate review, Mendenhall reported a pelvic tumor control rate of 84% for patients with stage IB tumors measuring 4 to 5 cm and 76% for those with tumors 6 cm or greater who were treated with radiation alone (Fig. 48-8).[202] Perez[214] reviewed 128 patients with tumors 5 cm or greater in diameter, stages IB/IIA/IIB, treated with either radiation alone or with extrafascial hysterectomy. The judicious use of higher doses of radiation therapy in patients treated with radiation therapy alone appeared to produce similar control rates compared with those who added adjuvant surgery. Among 44 patients with tumors larger than 5 cm treated with radiation alone, Perez[114] reported a 20% 5-year actuarial pelvic failure rate and a disease-free survival rate of only 60%. In a report on 361 patients with stage IB tumors 6 cm or greater in diameter treated at MD Anderson Hospital, Thoms[215] reported that 244 patients received radiation

therapy alone while 117 received radiation therapy plus surgery. With a median follow-up of 130 months, no difference was seen in actuarial survival or pelvic disease control rates for lesions less than 8 cm in size treated with either approach. In the overall group, however, a bias existed in older patients and in those with lesions greater than 8 cm, abnormal lymphangiograms and parametrial extension being more heavily represented in the radiation-alone group. This resulted in a slightly improved 10-year actuarial survival rate (59% vs. 42%) and pelvic control rate (85% vs. 72%) for the combined modality group. The pelvic control rate was 93% for patients with no residual disease in the surgical specimen, 91% for those with focal residual disease, and 59% for those with nonfocal residual disease. Although the overall complication rates did not differ between the two groups (22% at 10 years), the incidence of fistula formation was twice as great in the combined modality group (9% vs. 4%) as in the radiation-alone group. An analysis by Eifel and colleagues[201] of 280 patients with lesions of 6 cm or greater, all of whom were treated primarily by irradiation and some of whom underwent an extrafascial hysterectomy, found a 5-year central control rate of 89.2%, pelvic control rate of 79.1%, and disease-specific survival rate of 62.5% (Fig. 48-9).

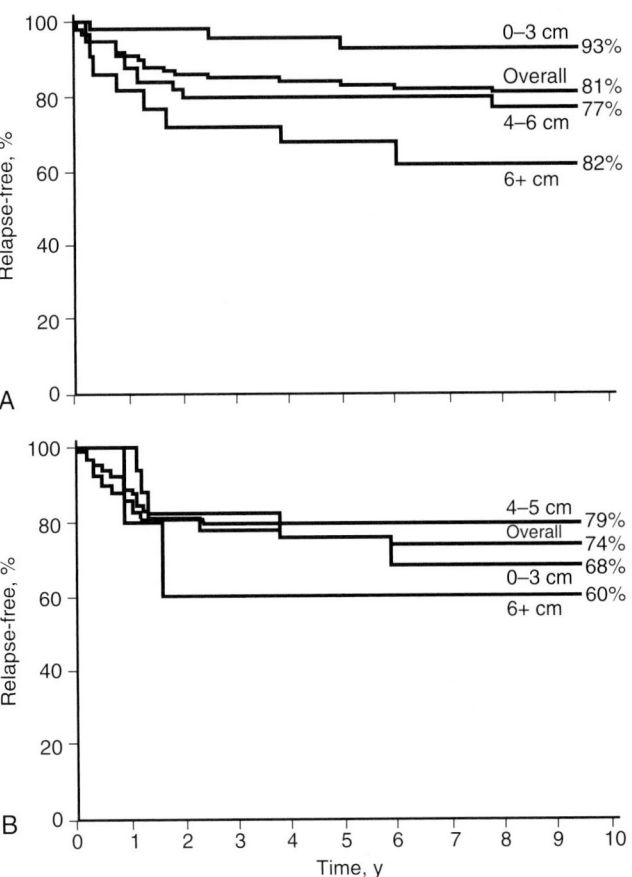

Figure 48–8. Actuarial relapse-free survival stratified by tumor size for stage IB (**A**) and stage IIA (**B**) carcinoma of the uterine cervix. (From Mendenhall WM, Sombeck MD, Freeman DE, et al: Stage IB and IIA-B carcinoma of the intact uterine cervix: Impact of tumor volume and the role of adjuvant hysterectomy. *Semin Radiat Oncol.* 1994;4:16.)

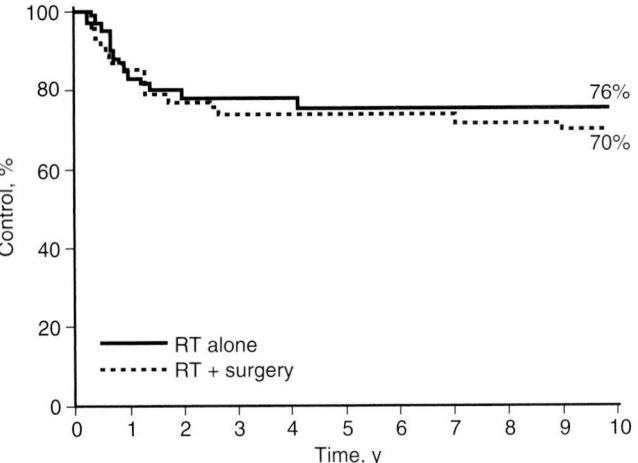

Figure 48–7. Control of disease in the pelvis (product limit method) for patients with stage IB-IIA uterine cervix carcinoma 6 cm or greater in maximum diameter, treated with radiation alone or with adjuvant hysterectomy. (From Mendenhall WM, McCarty PJ, Morgan LS, et al: Stage IB or IIA-B carcinoma of the intact uterine cervix greater than or equal to 6 cm in diameter: Is adjuvant extrafascial hysterectomy beneficial? *Int J Radiat Oncol Biol Phys.* 1991;21:899.)

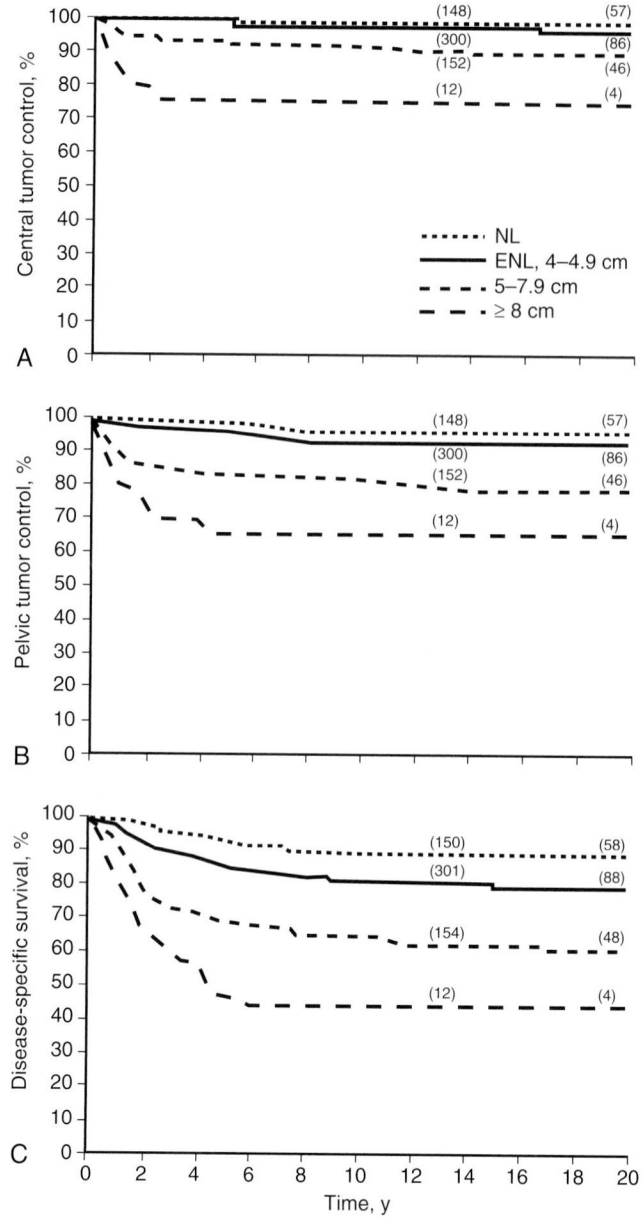

Figure 48–9. Central tumor control (**A**), pelvic tumor control (**B**), and disease-specific survival (**C**) for patients with stage IB cervical carcinoma grouped by size. (From Eifel PJ, Morris M, Wharton JT, et al: The influence of tumor size and morphology on the outcome of patients with FIGO stage IB squamous cell carcinoma of the uterine cervix. *Int J Radiat Oncol Biol Phys.* 1994;29:9.)

Bloss described 84 patients with lesions greater than 4 cm who were treated primarily with radical hysterectomy. Only 10 of these lesions were 6 cm or less in size.[216] Forty-two of these patients were treated with postoperative radiation due to high-risk features such as the presence of positive nodes, positive margins, or invasion of deep third of the cervix. The actuarial 5-year survival rate was 70.4% with a small bowel obstruction incidence of 8.5% in those who received combined modality treatment (a sixfold increase over the use of surgery alone). These results are comparable to those seen with radiation alone.[201]

A prospective randomized trial, initiated by the GOG and Radiation Therapy Oncology Group (RTOG) in 1984 and closed in 1991, randomly assigned patients with lesions 4 cm or greater in maximum diameter to receive radiation alone (80 Gy to point A, 55 Gy to point B) or reduced radiation (75 Gy to point A), followed in 6 weeks by an extrafascial hysterectomy.[202] No results have been released to date on the results of this trial.

The GOG trial preoperative radiation versus preoperative radiation plus cisplatinum (40 mg/m² weekly) for patients with bulky IB disease showed a statistically significant benefit to the addition of chemotherapy in terms of progression-free survival and overall survival (see Table 48-7).[217] It is not clear, however, that the addition of surgery was an essential component of this treatment.

Distant dissemination of disease remains a problem in larger tumors. Perez reported that IB/IIA patients with 3 to 5 cm lesions had pelvic failure rates of 15% to 28% and distant metastatic rates of 27% to 30%.[115] These numbers rose to 20% to 30% and 37% to 57% for patients with tumors 5 cm or greater in size. Eifel found that disease-free survival dropped to 71% for patients with tumors 5 cm or greater in diameter, although pelvic tumor control rates remained at 85%.[207]

A rational approach is to begin with external beam radiation therapy and closely evaluate the response of the tumor. If at the time of the first planned insertion, there has been considerable shrinkage of tumor (>50% reduction) and the geometry will allow an adequate intracavitary placement, it would be appropriate to proceed with definitive high-dose irradiation to point A with doses in excess of 85 Gy. The final dose chosen must also take into account the maximal bladder and rectal doses. The parametria should be boosted to a dose of 55 Gy with external beam and midline bar between insertions. If, however, there remains considerable bulk of disease at the time of the first insertion after 40 Gy external beam, and the vaginal geometry precludes an adequate isodose coverage of the tumor, it would be appropriate to proceed with reduced doses of radiation (75 Gy to point A) with a planned extrafascial hysterectomy 6 weeks later. Parametrial extension, presence of para-aortic nodal involvement, or history of pelvic inflammatory disease would tend to lead one toward definitive radiation therapy alone. On the other hand, the presence of grossly enlarged pelvic lymph nodes and the absence of para-aortic nodal enlargement might cause one to lean toward adjuvant surgery to remove both essential bulk of disease as well as the involved nodes.

The duration of the treatment time should be kept as short as possible, respecting the individual levels of adverse reactions experienced by the patient. Treatment times in excess of 8 weeks are associated with a decrease in local control rates as well as overall survival.[218]

PROPHYLACTIC PARA-AORTIC RADIATION

Two major prospective randomized studies have been carried out to determine the efficacy of treating the para-aortic nodes prophylactically in patients with cervical cancer. The European Organization for Research and

Treatment of Cancer (EORTC) randomly assigned 441 patients with stage IB through IVA disease, with no clinical or radiographic evidence of para-aortic spread, to receive pelvic radiation either alone or in conjunction with 45 Gy para-aortic radiation.[219] No improvement was seen in local control or survival with the addition of para-aortic radiation, although there was a decrease in para-aortic and distant recurrence rates seen in the extended field group. Small bowel injury was 0.9% for the pelvic-only group versus 2.3% in the extended field group. The severe complication rate in the para-aortic radiation arm was approximately twice that of the pelvis-only arm.

The RTOG study was limited to patients with bulky stage IB/IIA disease and those with any stage IIB disease, eliminating those patients with low-volume disease who might not be expected to benefit from the prophylactic extension of the field, as well as those with more advanced stage III disease in whom both local control and distant dissemination might mask any potential benefit of para-aortic radiation.[220] The 5-year survival rate was significantly better in those patients who received prophylactic para-aortic radiation, 66% versus 55% (P = 0.043). The incidence of severe and life-threatening complications was similar for both groups. The extended field arm became the control arm in the next RTOG trial comparing extended field radiation to pelvic radiation plus concomitant chemotherapy with fluorouracil (5-FU) and cisplatin.

The RTOG successfully completed a prospective randomized trial of 403 patients with stage IIB-IVA, or lesser stage with tumors greater than 5 cm in size, with no evidence of para-aortic nodal involvement.[221] The two arms were pelvic plus para-aortic radiation (including two intracavitary insertions) versus pelvic radiotherapy (external plus brachytherapy) with concurrent cisplatin and fluorouracil. Overall survival rates at 5 years (73% vs. 58%) and disease-free survival rates (67% vs. 40%) favored the combined modality arms. This approach of concurrent chemoradiotherapy is preferred over the use of para-aortic radiation alone in the prophylactic setting.

Stage IIB

Disease extension into the parametria is a contraindication to radical hysterectomy, since the chance of cutting through tumor is high. These patients are ideally managed by definitive radiation in conjunction with cisplatin-based chemotherapy, as discussed later in the section on concurrent chemoradiotherapy. As in cases of large IB tumors, external beam is first administered to allow tumor shrinkage. Generally, 40 Gy is administered via whole pelvis fields, followed by two insertions to bring the paracervical dose to 85 to 90 Gy total, with parametrial boosts to the involved sides of 60 Gy, 55 Gy to uninvolved sides. This final parametrial dose must take into account the dose administered externally as well as the dose from the brachytherapy. The whole pelvis dose can be reduced if there is considerable early reduction in tumor burden, once again pointing out the importance of routine evaluation of the tumor during therapy. In

patients whose disease is massive, bordering on IIIB, treatment with an interstitial template may be more appropriate. Central control rates of 78% to 86%[91,203] and pelvic control rates of 69% to 83%[91,203,222-224] have been reported with concurrent chemoradiotherapy. Overall survival rates of radiation alone are 60% to 68%.[91,200,203,222-227]

Stage III/IVA

Patients with stage III disease have a 17% to 67% chance of pelvic failure when treated with radiation alone.[204,205,228,229] These results differ according to the bulk of disease, the presence of unilateral versus bilateral pelvic sidewall involvement, the presence or absence of lower vaginal involvement, and the type of brachytherapy used.[161] Involvement of the lower portion of the vagina represents one of the most challenging situations encountered by the radiation oncologist; fortunately, it is a rare condition, comprising only 1% to 3% of all cases of stage III disease.[204,205,228,229] As with stage IIB disease, cisplatin-based chemotherapy in conjunction with radiation is essential. The radiation approach is dependent on the extent and location of vaginal involvement, as well as the initial response to external beam radiotherapy. Extension into the middle or lower third of the vagina is not adequately encompassed by standard loadings of the tandem and colpostats. After initial external beam therapy, the response is assessed and the residual disease clearly defined in terms of its thickness and location. Brachytherapy plays an essential role in managing this portion of the disease, but care must be taken to respect the normal tissue tolerances of surrounding structures, most notably the urethra and rectum. Minimal tumor doses, in addition to the doses to the vaginal surface and normal tissues, must be followed closely.

After 40 Gy external beam, if the residual disease thickness is circumferential and 5 mm or less (the average thickness of the rectovaginal septum), sources may be placed in the tandem below the level of the colpostats. The tandem is not loaded at the level of the colpostats, since this would unacceptably increase the dose rate to the bladder and rectum at this level. A special applicator with cylindrical sleeves in addition to vaginal apex caps and tandem was designed by Perez at Mallinckrodt for this situation.[230] For thicker residua, or disease that is either anterior or posterior only, however, this approach is not optimal, since it would require excessive rectal or urethral irradiation to ensure sufficient dose to the tumor.

Disease that is confined to one or two walls of the vagina is best approached with interstitial implantation, allowing maximal coverage of the tumor itself with careful tailoring of the treatment to involved regions. One approach is to perform a volume implant using a perineal template, with coverage of the parametria and vagina via afterloading catheters. If the use of a tandem is possible, the first ring of needle locations is left vacant to improve dose homogeneity in the manually afterloaded situation. Additional needles are inserted based on an MRI scan obtained for treatment planning, adequately covering the areas of residual vaginal involvement. An attempt is made to deliver a vaginal surface dose of 60 Gy total to all areas of clinically uninvolved vagina and a minimum tumor dose of 75 Gy to involved areas. This latter dose is not the surface dose, but rather the true minimum tumor dose. Since these target volumes may include portions of the rectum or urethra, a decision must be made as to the acceptable risk to these organs associated with the increasing doses necessary to achieve local control. With the template, every attempt must be made to keep uninvolved areas of the vagina, as well as rectum, urethra, and bladder, from exceeding tolerance doses.

Pelvic control rates of 71% to 72% were reported for two small series of patients with IIIA disease from MD Anderson Hospital and Yale, in which most patients received a combination of external beam and intracavitary or interstitial brachytherapy.[229,231] Five-year actuarial survival rates ranged from 37% to 58%.[91,229,231]

Disease with extension to the sidewalls (stage IIIB) has a 45% to 50% chance of locoregional failure when treated with standard tandem and colpostats in addition to external beam therapy.[133,228] One or two volume implants using a perineal template with angled holes to permit placement of catheters or needles into the lateral parametria allows delivery of a more homogeneous dose throughout the tumor bed without exposing the rectum and bladder to unreasonably high doses. Once again, a minimum tumor dose of 75 Gy is the goal. Alternatively, two insertions may be attempted to deliver a paracervical dose of 90 Gy, followed with parametrial boosts to 60 to 65 Gy on the involved sides. In patients not amenable to implant or insertion, external beam therapy to a dose of 65 Gy, coming off all small bowel after 50 Gy, may have to suffice. Pelvic control rates for all stage III disease presentations are in the range of 50% to 60%, with overall survival rates of 30% to 55%.[91,133,187,222,228,232-235] Prempree[156] reported an improved local control rate of 97% in 23 patients with stage IIIB disease who underwent perineal interstitial implantation as part of their therapy, but the 5-year disease-free survival rate was a disappointing 61% in this highly selected group.

For patients with bladder invasion but minimal or no parametrial invasion (stage IVA), an aggressive approach, including an anterior exenteration, is warranted. Likewise, those with extension into the rectum are candidates for posterior exenteration. Alternatively, definitive irradiation has been successful. Reports from Yale[236] and MD Anderson Hospital[237] revealed a low but significant cure rate of 18% to 46% depending on the aggressiveness of the treatment and the lateral extent of tumor. The dose to the bladder is higher than would be acceptable in cases without bladder involvement, since the risk of fistula formation is weighed against the prospects of an anterior exenteration. Those patients in whom a fistula has already occurred or who have bilateral hydronephrosis due to obstruction may be best served with an exenteration, although extension into the lateral parametria precludes such an approach. In cases of rectal invasion, a posterior exenteration is the preferred approach, since the rectovaginal fistula rate is quite high at doses necessary to control disease. If more extensive parametrial extension is noted, definitive irradiation

would be the preferred treatment. The decision to proceed with palliative or curative radiation must be based upon an awareness of the full extent of disease (nodal spread, distant metastases), local aggressiveness (existence of fistulae or ureteral obstruction), the patient's overall medical status, and the patient's desires.

The management of patients with locally far-advanced cervical cancer ("frozen pelvis," massive stage IIIB or IVA disease) or those with metastatic disease at presentation must be tempered by an understanding of the likelihood of local control, the effect of local progression on quality of life, and the morbidity of aggressive intervention. Although it may be reasonable not to place ureteral stents in the patient with bilateral ureteral obstruction and hydronephrosis who also has distant disease and consequently no meaningful hope for long-term survival, it may be quite justifiable to intervene in a similarly obstructed patient who has no distant disease. In the former case, the chance of cure is negligible and a death due to renal failure may be preferred by the patient to one due to continued spread of the disease both locally and distantly. In the latter case, however, locally aggressive management may result in an extended period of life with disease control. The issues of quality of life and morbidity of treatment must be addressed with the patient.

Palliative radiotherapy in the setting of advanced carcinoma of the cervix should be tailored to the patient's overall condition. The rapid fractionation approach tested by the RTOG in protocol 85-02 involved the delivery of 3.7 Gy twice daily for two days for a total dose of 14.8 Gy.[238] This is repeated after a 2- to 4-week break. After a final 2- to 4-week break, the field is reduced to exclude all small bowel and a third session of four treatments is administered for a total dose of 44.4 Gy. A tumor response rate of 42% was seen after completion of all three courses with response rates (complete and partial) of 75% for pain, 98% for bleeding, and 83% for tenesmus. The treatment course was well tolerated with a severe complication rate of only 5/132 (4%).

Disease in a patient with a frozen pelvis but no signs of spread elsewhere may be approached more aggressively, since the patient may live long enough to develop local progression after the rapid course just described. The impact of locally uncontrolled disease on quality of life is tremendous. Fistula formation, severe pain, and bleeding severely compromise a patient's dignity and ability to interact with family and friends during her final months. It is not unusual to have a patient linger for many months with local progression before death occurs from systemic involvement, uremia, sepsis, or bleeding. Therefore, consideration should be given to aggressive radiotherapeutic palliation in patients who are likely to survive longer than 6 months. External beam alone to doses of 60 to 65 Gy may be considered, as long as the small bowel is removed from the field after 50 Gy is administered. Alternatively, the judicious use of interstitial implantation may play a role in select cases. Entry into protocols evaluating combined modality therapy or radiation with hyperthermia may also be warranted. In any such circumstance, however, the patient must be allowed to make the decision for herself after she has received sufficient information regarding her long-term prognosis, the possibilities for quality of life, and the expected morbidity of any proposed intervention.

Positive Para-Aortic Node Disease

Patients found to have positive para-aortic nodes at the time of sampling have a poor prognosis, with survival rates as low as 9% to 29% at 3 years.[81,93,239] In a review of 98 patients with pathologically positive para-aortic lymph nodes in GOG surgical studies who had clinically undetectable para-aortic node metastases, median survival was 15.2 months with a 3-year actuarial survival rate of only 25%.[240] A majority of these patients were treated with postoperative para-aortic radiation to doses of 40 to 60 Gy. A trial of the use of hyperfractionated radiation therapy to the nodal areas resulted in a rate of 27% late complications at 5 years without a significant improvement in survival over earlier reports.[241] RTOG protocol 92-10 attempted to improve on these results. Patients with positive para-aortic lymph nodes were treated with concomitant 5-FU and cisplatin with twice-daily fractionation of 1.2 Gy delivered to the pelvis (60 Gy) and para-aortic (48 Gy) regions, followed by brachytherapy. Unfortunately, this combination resulted in an unacceptably high rate of grade 4 late toxicity (50%) and did not show superior survival results.[103,242,243] Varia et al. reported on a GOG trial of standard fractionation radiation plus 5-FU and cisplatin in 95 patients with documented para-aortic involvement that resulted in a 3-year progression-free survival rate of 33%, with a 14% rate of severe late complications at 4 years.[244] Given the results of the prospective randomized trials showing improvement in outcome with the use of concurrent chemoradiotherapy in pelvic disease, the use of concurrent chemoradiotherapy in these patients with para-aortic nodal involvement is a reasonable approach. Consideration is being given to try lowering the small bowel toxicity of radiation through the use of three-dimensional conformal or intensity-modulated radiation therapy (IMRT) techniques.

ADJUVANT CHEMOTHERAPY

In 1999 a series of positive prospective randomized trials documented the advantage of adjuvant cisplatin-based chemotherapy in conjunction with radiation for patients with high-risk cervical cancer. Concurrent chemoradiotherapy has become the standard treatment of locally advanced cervical cancer.

Based on prior small randomized studies of patients with stages IIB to IIIB cervical carcinoma treated at Roswell Park looking at the addition of hydroxyurea,[245] the GOG initiated a group-wide phase III study of patients with stages IIIB to IVA disease (surgically staged and negative para-aortic nodes), randomly assigning patients to receive radiation therapy alone or radiation plus hydroxyurea.[246] The analysis pertained to only 97 of the original 190 patients entered; approximately half of the patients were considered inevaluable. Results of this study showed a marginal improvement in complete clinical response and superiority in disease-free survival and

overall survival rates in those receiving hydroxyurea. Significant toxicity was seen in the hydroxyurea arm (47%). These results have been criticized because of inadequate radiation portals and doses administered as well as the large percentage of inevaluable patients.[247]

The RTOG randomly assigned patients with stages IIIB to IVA disease to receive radiation therapy with or without misonidazole, a radiation sensitizer, and found that misonidazole may have had a deleterious effect on overall survival compared with radiation therapy alone.[248] The median survival in the control arm was 1.9 years, compared with 1.6 years for the misonidazole arm, and the study was terminated early. A GOG study randomly assigned patients with stages IIB to IVA disease to receive radiation therapy plus hydroxyurea or misonidazole from 1981 to 1985.[160] No difference was observed between the two arms in terms of progression-free survival or overall survival rates, although there was a trend favoring the hydroxyurea arm. Their conclusion was that "misonidazole was not superior to hydroxyurea as an adjunct to radiation."[249] The failure of hydroxyurea to show a clear superiority over misonidazole calls into question the inherent benefit of hydroxyurea, although this arm remained the control arm for other GOG studies to date.[249]

As a single agent, cisplatin acts as a potent radiation enhancer.[250,251] Two small prospective randomized studies looking at the addition of cisplatin to radiation therapy indicated improvement in local control of disease but failed to show a survival benefit.[252,253] A subsequent prospective nonrandomized study carried out by Souhami with radiation therapy plus cisplatin (30 mg/m² given weekly during the radiation treatment) had an impressive 88% complete response rate in patients with bulky stages IIB to IVA disease and an actuarial survival rate of 65% at 4 years.[254] Mickiewicz[255] randomly assigned patients with stages IIB to IVA disease to receive radiation therapy alone or with 5-FU, mitomycin-C, and cisplatin, but failed to show an overall survival benefit in the combined modality group. An additional four randomized trials of neoadjuvant chemotherapy and radiation therapy versus radiation therapy alone with various regimens failed to show either a local control benefit or an overall survival benefit.[256-258] In fact, survival was significantly worse with the neoadjuvant therapy in at least one of these trials.[258]

A series of landmark randomized trials comparing radiotherapy alone with concurrent chemoradiotherapy were published in 1999 (Table 48-7). RTOG 90-01 randomized 403 patients with locally advanced cervical cancer stage to radiotherapy to pelvis and para-aortic lymph nodes or pelvis radiotherapy with three cycles of fluorouracil (4 mg/m² in a continuous infusion over 96 hours) and cisplatin (75 mg/m²). Patients randomized included stages IIB to IVA, and stages IB to IA with tumor diameter at least 5 cm or involvement of pelvic lymph nodes. With a median follow-up of 43 months, there were statistically significant improvements in survival and disease-free survival at 5 years favoring the chemoradiotherapy group. Local-regional recurrences and distant metastases were significantly less in the chemoradiotherapy group.[221]

Table 48–7   Results of Trials Comparing Radiotherapy Alone with Concurrent Chemoradiotherapy

Group/Reference	Study Group	Arms	Eligible	Med. F/U	Survival	DFS/PFS
RTOG[221]	IIB-IVA, IB >5 cm	XRT alone vs. XRT + CDDP 75 mg/m² + 5-FU	388	43 mo	5 yr OS 63% vs. 76% (P = 0.004)	5 yr. DFS 58% vs. 73% (P < 0.001)
GOG[259]	IIB-IVA	XRT + 1. CDDP 40 mg/m² weekly 2. CDDP 50 mg/m² + 5-FU + HU 3. HU	526	35 mo	RR of death 1. 0.61 2. 0.58 3. 1.00 (P = 0.002–0.004)	2 yr. PFS 1. 67% 2. 64% 3. 47% (P < 0.001)
GOG/SWOG[333]	IIB-IVA	XRT + HU vs. XRT + CDDP 50 mg/m² + 5-FU	368	8.7 yr	8 yr. OS 43% vs. 55% (P = 0.018)	8 yr. PFS 47% vs. 57% (P = 0.033)
GOG preop[217]	Bulky IB	Preop XRT vs. Preop XRT + CDDP 40 mg/m² weekly	373	36 mo	3 yr OS 74% vs. 83% (P < 0.001)	3 yr PFS 74% vs. 83% (P = 0.008)
GOG/SWOG/RTOG postop[267]	IA2, IB, IIA + pelvic LN or + parametrium or + margins	Postop XRT alone vs. Postop XRT + CDDP 50 mg/m² + 5-FU	243	42 mo	4 yr OS 71% vs. 81% (P = 0.007)	4 yr. PFS 63% vs. 80% (P = 0.003)

CDDP, cisplatin; DFS, disease-free survival; F/U, follow-up; HU, LN, lymph nodes; OS, PFS, progression free survival; RR, relative risk; XRT, radiotherapy.

A GOG protocol randomized patients with locally advanced cervical cancer (stages IIB to IVA, with no para-aortic nodal involvement) to radiotherapy plus one of three chemotherapy regimens (cisplatin 40 mg/m² weekly for six cycles; cisplatin 50 mg/m² twice during radiation along with 5-FU 4 gm as a 96-hour infusion and hydroxyurea; or oral hydroxyurea alone). Patients who received either of the two platinum-containing regimens had significantly higher overall survival rates and progression-free survival rates.[259]

Another GOG protocol evaluated the role of adjuvant chemotherapy in patients with bulky stage IB cervical cancers (tumor diameter ≥4 cm). All patients were treated with radiotherapy followed by adjuvant hysterectomy. Patients were randomized to weekly cisplatin (40 mg/m²) versus radiotherapy alone. The 3-year overall survival and progression-free survival were significantly better in the group that received chemotherapy (83% vs. 74% overall survival).[217] Results of these trials have established the role of concurrent chemoradiotherapy in the treatment of locally advanced cervical cancer. The optimal chemotherapy regimen has yet to be clarified, although it would seem that a platinum-based approach is preferred.

Hyperthermia

The role of combined hyperthermia with radiotherapy has not been clearly established. An early prospective trial did not show any benefit of adding hyperthermia with radiotherapy.[260] Failure to demonstrate the benefit of hyperthermia was proposed to be the result of inadequate delivery of hyperthermia to deep-seated tumor. Using a different hyperthermia delivery system, the Dutch Deep Hyperthermia Group conducted a prospective randomized trial. One hundred fourteen patients with stages IIB to IV cervical cancer were randomized to radiotherapy alone or radiotherapy with hyperthermia. There was a significant difference in 3-year overall survival and local control favoring the hyperthermia group.[261] The result of this trial has revived interest in hyperthermia with radiotherapy for treatment of cervical cancer, although the concurrent use of chemotherapy with radiation has received greater attention.

ADJUVANT RADIATION AFTER HYSTERECTOMY

Patients who have undergone radical hysterectomy for early-stage disease are at variable risk for recurrent disease, depending on factors that include tumor size, nodal status, parametrial extension, adequacy of margins, histology, lymphatic space invasion, and depth of penetration of the cervical stroma. A rational approach depends on the definition of those subgroups at greatest risk for recurrence and therefore most likely to show a regional control benefit and potentially a survival benefit.

Patients at low risk for pelvic recurrence after radical hysterectomy who would not be expected to benefit from postoperative radiotherapy are those whose pelvic lymph nodes are negative and those with tumors less than 4 cm in maximum dimension, no evidence of lymphatic vascular invasion, and less than one third of the thickness of the surgical stroma involved. The risk of microscopically involved nodes in these patients is less than 15%.[125,181-183,195,262-265] The group of patients who might be expected to have improved local control (although it has been difficult to show a survival benefit) are those found to have involved pelvic lymph nodes or positive parametrial or vaginal margins.

An intermediate risk group may be more likely to show a benefit of adjuvant radiation, since their disease is in an earlier stage than those with positive nodal spread.[112] Patients in this group include those who have positive lymphatic vascular space involvement and at least one of the following characteristics: deep third penetration of the cervix, middle third penetration with a tumor 2 cm or greater in diameter, or superficial third penetration with clinical tumor size 5 cm or greater. Alternatively, those with no lymphatic vascular space invasion with tumors 4 cm or greater in size with deep or middle third invasion of the cervix are considered intermediate risk.

The Gynecologic Oncology Group performed a randomized study to address the role of postoperative radiotherapy in such patients (see Table 48-7). The study enrolled 277 patients who had at least two of the following risk factors: greater than one third stromal invasion, capil-lary lymphatic space involvement, and large clinical tumor diameter. Patients were randomized to postoperative radiotherapy or no further treatment. Adjuvant pelvic radiotherapy significantly reduced the risk of recurrence in these patients from 27.9% in the observation arm to 15.3% in the radiated arm.[266] For patients who are found to have high-risk features, postoperative chemoradiotherapy has also been shown to improve survival.

The role of adjuvant therapy in high-risk patients was validated in a Southwest Oncology Group trial. High-risk features were defined as one or more of the following: positive pelvic lymph nodes, positive margins, or microscopic involvement of the parametrium. Two hundred sixty-eight patients were randomized to concurrent chemoradiotherapy with cisplatin and 5-FU or radiotherapy alone. The chemoradiotherapy arm had a significantly improved overall survival and progression-free survival.[267] The American Brachytherapy Society panel on the use of radiation for cervix cancer recommends the use of postoperative radiation in intermediate-risk patients with at least two of the three factors identified by the GOG study, namely invasion of greater than one third of the cervical stroma, lymphovascular space invasion, and tumor size greater than 4 cm.[218] Those patients with pelvic nodal involvement, positive margins, or microscopic parametrial involvement should be treated with chemoradiation.

CERVICAL STUMP

The performance of a supracervical hysterectomy is controversial in the management of benign diseases. Although it may be a less extensive surgery than a simple hysterectomy with less risk of urinary complications and fewer changes in the patient's sexual activity,[268] it is associated with the development of cervical malignancies (either SCC or adenocarcinoma).[268-271] Although surgery may be feasible if the disease occurs as stage I, the risk of metastatic disease remains. The ability to deliver curative radiation with brachytherapy is obviously hampered by the lack of a normal uterine canal for tandem placement. In a multi-institutional study of 213 cases of cancer of the cervical stump in France from 1970 to 1987, 50% were found to be CIS/stage I/stage IIA.[271] The majority of patients were treated with external beam radiation and brachytherapy consisting of a short tandem (when possible) with vaginal colpostats, or vaginal cylinders for more extensive disease in the vagina. Early stages (I to IIA) had an 80% local regional control rate at 5 years. Stages IIB to IIIA had a 70% local regional control rate and stage IIIB, only 55%. Overall, distant metastases developed in 19% of patients. Stage II patients who received external beam radiation alone had only a 38.5% local regional control as opposed to 81.5% for those who received external beam radiation and brachytherapy. Grade 3 to 4 complications were seen in 13% to 23% of cases depending on the stage, with three fatal complications reported, indicating the increased risk associated with aggressive intervention when compared with similar treatment in patients with an intact uterine corpus. Kovalic[270] reported on 70 patients treated at Mallinckrodt from 1956 to 1986, 67 of whom received brachytherapy as part of their treatment, 16 of whom also underwent surgery. The 10-year actuarial survival rate was lower in patients with stage IB disease of the stump compared with similar patients with stage IB disease of the intact uterus (50% vs. 76%), but for all stages, the actuarial survival rates were comparable. Through the use of appropriate rectal and bladder shielding, the complication rate was lower in those patients treated only with radiation and no surgery, compared with other studies.

CERVICAL CANCER AND PREGNANCY

The incidence of cervical cancer during pregnancy varies from 1.6 to 10.6 cases per 10,000 pregnancies.[272-276] The treatment approach differs depending on the gestational age of the fetus and the stage of disease at diagnosis as well as the informed consent of the patient. In the first two trimesters, the standard recommendation is termination of the pregnancy and immediate hysterectomy or radiation for all but the most limited cases of invasive disease (microinvasive), which has been approached with cautious conization, very rigorous follow-up, and hysterectomy after a full-course delivery in isolated cases. For patients in the late third trimester, early delivery via cesarean section at the time of fetal maturity may cause only minimal delay in dealing with the cancer. The difficulty arises in patients in the early part of the third trimester who are desirous of maintaining the fetus, but in whom a delay in intervention may decrease the expected survival rate. The survival for stage I patients using immediate intervention is excellent.[274] In a small series of patients with early-stage disease who elected to continue their pregnancies, delaying their therapeutic intervention, delay did not have a negative impact. In a series of eight patients with stage IA/B disease who had delays from 53 to 212 days, no progression of disease was documented. In a historical review of 51 patients in the literature who delayed therapy, 77% of stage IA cases had attained no-evidence-of-disease (NED) status and 80% of stage IB cases were NED, although the follow-up was short in some cases.[274] In patients whose pregnancies are in early stages and who desire intervention to terminate the pregnancy, surgery or radiation may be selected based on the stage of disease, with cure rates similar to those expected in the nonpregnant patient.

RADIOTHERAPY AFTER SIMPLE HYSTERECTOMY

A simple hysterectomy is inadequate treatment for cervical cancer that invades deeper than 5 mm (stage IA2) or that invades deeper than 3 mm in the presence of lymphatic vascular space invasion. Unfortunately, some patients who undergo simple hysterectomies for benign conditions may be found to have invasive cancer at the time of pathologic examination.[277] Two treatment options are available, immediate reoperation with radical parametrectomy and pelvic lymph node dissection[278] or postoperative radiation. Surgery will result in a 5-year disease-free survival rate of 82% to 96% in patients with no gross residual disease.[277,279,280] The radiation approach is dependent upon the volume and location of residual disease. Patients with no disease or microscopic disease only at the margins are approached with whole pelvis radiation to a total dose of 45 to 50 Gy, followed by intracavitary treatment with colpostats or a vaginal cylinder to boost the dose at the vaginal apex to 60 to 65 Gy (total dose). Five-year disease-free survival rates of 71% to 90% are reported using this approach.[279] For patients with gross residual disease, exenteration has produced approximately a 39% disease control,[281] versus 23% to 43% for aggressive radiation intervention.[279] Gross residual disease, which responds well to external beam radiation therapy, may be treated with intracavitary brachytherapy, whereas greater residual volumes of disease should be considered for perineal interstitial templates to boost the residual disease sites to 65 to 70 Gy minimum tumor dose.

SURGICAL TECHNIQUE

An excellent review of the classes of hysterectomy was published by Piver and colleagues in 1974.[282] These procedures differ in the handling of the uterine arteries, the ureters, the cardinal and utero sacral ligaments, and the vaginal cuff, as well as adjacent organs. The morbidity and mortality rates increase gradually with the more extensive resections. The gynecologic oncologist adopts the procedure that is appropriate for the size and extent of the cervical neoplasm.

The class I or extrafascial hysterectomy is considered adequate for patients with microinvasive disease or CIS or as adjunctive therapy after radiation for patients with bulky primary tumors. Minimal manipulation of the ureter and bladder thereby reduces the risk of ureteral damage or fistula formation. The class II modified hysterectomy is appropriate for patients with early invasive disease and is often accompanied by a pelvic lymph node dissection. In this procedure, the ureters are dissected in the paracervical region to the entry into the bladder.

The traditional Meigs' or Wertheim's radical hysterectomy plus pelvic lymph node dissection is the standard approach for patients with stage IB disease. The ureters are mobilized completely from their bed to allow for total removal of the parametria to the pelvic sidewalls. The more extensive resections listed in class IV or V procedures, with additional portions of vagina and bladder removed, are reserved for patients with anteriorly extending disease in whom bladder preservation is considered possible, to prevent the need for an anterior exenteration.

RADIATION TECHNIQUE

Cure cannot be accomplished without local control of disease. In the treatment of carcinoma of the cervix, the ability to achieve local control is dependent on the appropriate use of external beam irradiation and brachytherapy. No set schedule for the interweaving of external beam therapy and brachytherapy is useful for all cases. Each patient's disease requires individualization of the schedule based on the local characteristics of the tumor, the suspected risk of nodal involvement, repeated evaluation of response to therapy, and the patient's overall medical condition.

External Beam Therapy: Simulation

PELVIC FIELD

For patients in whom the *pelvis only* is to be treated, the patient is given 135 mL of barium to drink approximately 1 hour before simulation for best visualization of the small intestine. The patient is placed in the prone position, a vaginal marker firmly mounted on an external stand is placed in the vagina, and an anal marker is placed externally. Ideally, a gold seed is placed in the lowest vaginal extent of tumor at the time of initial examination. The upper border should be at the L4 to L5 interspace to completely cover the common iliac nodes (Figs. 48-10 and 48-11). The lower border of the field is set approximately 5 cm beneath the lowest extent of vaginal involvement, as marked by the gold seed. Caution must be used if a vaginal marker alone is used, since it may extend into the posterior vaginal fornix and be above the most distal extent of disease. The lateral borders are set 1.5 to 2 cm beyond the edge of the pelvic brim.

The decision to use either two or four fields must be individualized, taking into account the size of the patient, the shape of the pelvis, and the extent of disease. MRI or CT data are very helpful in determining the safety of proceeding with a four-field arrangement,[283] as is obvious in the MRI slices shown in Figure 48-12 and the CT reconstructions shown in Figure 48-13. A patient with significant uterosacral ligament involvement, a significantly anteflexed or retroflexed uterus, lower uterine segment involvement, or extension into the endometrial cavity, or an extremely thin patient with a small pelvis may be better approached with a two-field technique, since the use of blocking on lateral fields may shield tumor. The majority of patients, however, are best treated with a four-field plan, since small bowel and a portion of the low rectum can be shielded on the lateral fields. Borders for the lateral fields are 1 cm in front of the anterior edge of the symphysis pubis to ensure coverage of the external iliac nodes and S2 to S3 posteriorly (except in cases of

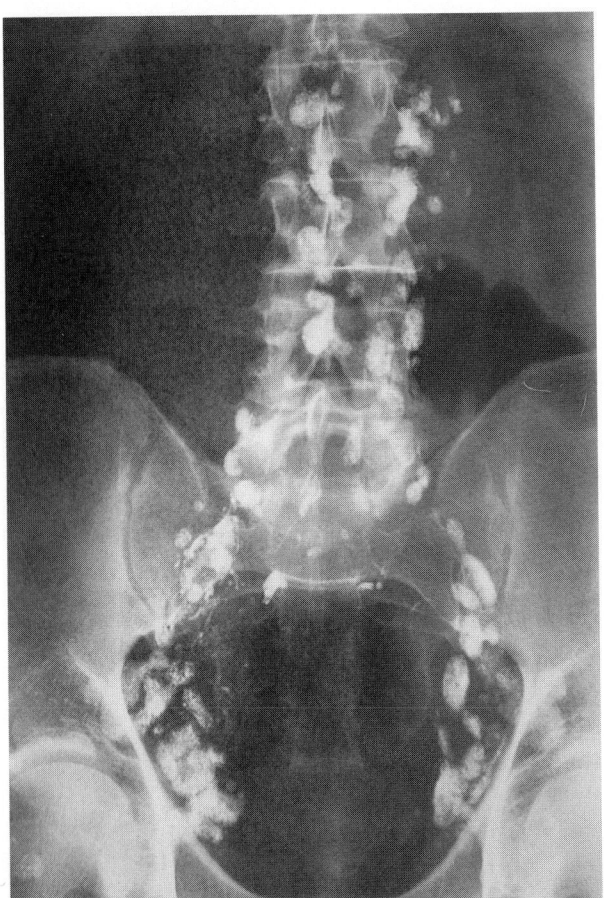

Figure 48–10. Anterior view of a lymphangiogram showing location of primary pelvic lymph nodes.

uterosacral ligament involvement, where the entire sacrum may need to be covered).

In cases with extension into the lower portion of the vagina, where the inguinal nodes are considered to be at risk, the inguinal nodes should be covered as well. Acceptable approaches for their coverage include an anterior-posterior–posterior-anterior (AP–PA) plan with partial transmission block over the pelvic portion anteriorly, allowing treatment of the inguinal nodes with the AP photon field only, or electron fields matched to the AP photon field.

A novel approach that appears promising is the use of intensity-modulation as a means of reducing the amount of normal small bowel exposed to the full doses of radiation in pelvic nodal irradiation. Researchers at the University of Chicago have reported on a decrease in the intensity and incidence of small bowel toxicity during pelvic radiation using IMRT compared to whole-pelvic irradiation, and an increased ability to tolerate chemotherapy concurrent with radiation due to reduced dose to the iliac crests.[284,285] Early work at Mallinckrodt, comparing the isodose distributions attainable with IMRT in conjunction with IMRT-compatible vaginal applicators, suggests a possibility for improvement of isodose distributions over those attainable with brachytherapy for locally advanced cervical cases and a major improvement in

terms of reducing small bowel dose for patients requiring para-aortic irradiation.[286,287] Issues regarding internal organ motion within the female pelvis and proper target delineation must be resolved before this can be considered for routine use.

PARA-AORTIC FIELD

If the para-aortic lymph nodes are to be treated simultaneously, the field is generally raised to the T11 to T12 interspace, although the upper border may be individualized, depending on the patient's known extent of disease (Fig. 48-14). The use of barium should be avoided so that the kidneys can be better visualized. The availability of a lymphangiogram will allow for the creation of adequate blocks to ensure inclusion of the para-aortic nodes. In the absence of an LAG, the field should encompass the tips of the transverse processes. If there is adequate renal function (normal blood urea nitrogen and creatinine levels, no history of serious dye allergy with hypoallergenic dye), 50 mL of Omnipaque hypoallergenic intravenous dye is administered, after setting the borders on a test film or under fluoroscopy, to determine the exact position of the kidneys for precise blocking. A CT scan with the patient in the treatment position is preferable for kidney localization. The pelvic and para-aortic fields may also be treated using a four-field approach. On the lateral fields, the anterior blocks are placed approximately 3.5 cm in front of the vertebral bodies (or anterior to the nodes as seen on LAG) for coverage of the para-aortic nodes, and the posterior blocks split the vertebral bodies. Care must be taken, however, to ensure that this approach does not irradiate a significant portion of the kidneys. A CT scan in the treatment position is extremely useful in planning the isodose distributions to assess the dose to renal tissue.

If the use of multi-leaf collimators with independent jaws is possible, another approach is to simulate the entire field from obturator foramina to T11 to T12. The pelvic field may then be treated with a four-field approach, using the independent jaws to beam-split the pelvis from the para-aortic field. The para-aortics may then be treated with AP–PA fields, similarly using the independent jaws to beam-split the pelvis from the field, a six-field approach with a single patient set-up, and no problems of field matching.

At the time of daily treatment, the patient should be instructed to keep her bladder full, preferably by drinking several glasses of fluid before treatment (if her fluid and renal status permit), thereby removing more bowel from the treatment field. A daily dose of 1.8 to 2 Gy, using 6 to 25 MeV photons, is delivered.

In circumstances of excessive bleeding at presentation, adequate control of bleeding can usually be attained with the judicious use of vaginal packing and application of Monsel's ferric subsulfate solution. For patients with exophytic bleeding lesions that can be completely encompassed within a transvaginal orthovoltage cone, one or two large fractions of 5 Gy surface dose with a 100 kVp (0.4 mm Cu half-value layer) beam can be used, with the dose disregarded in the final tally due to the near total absorption of dose within the tumor itself. Similarly,

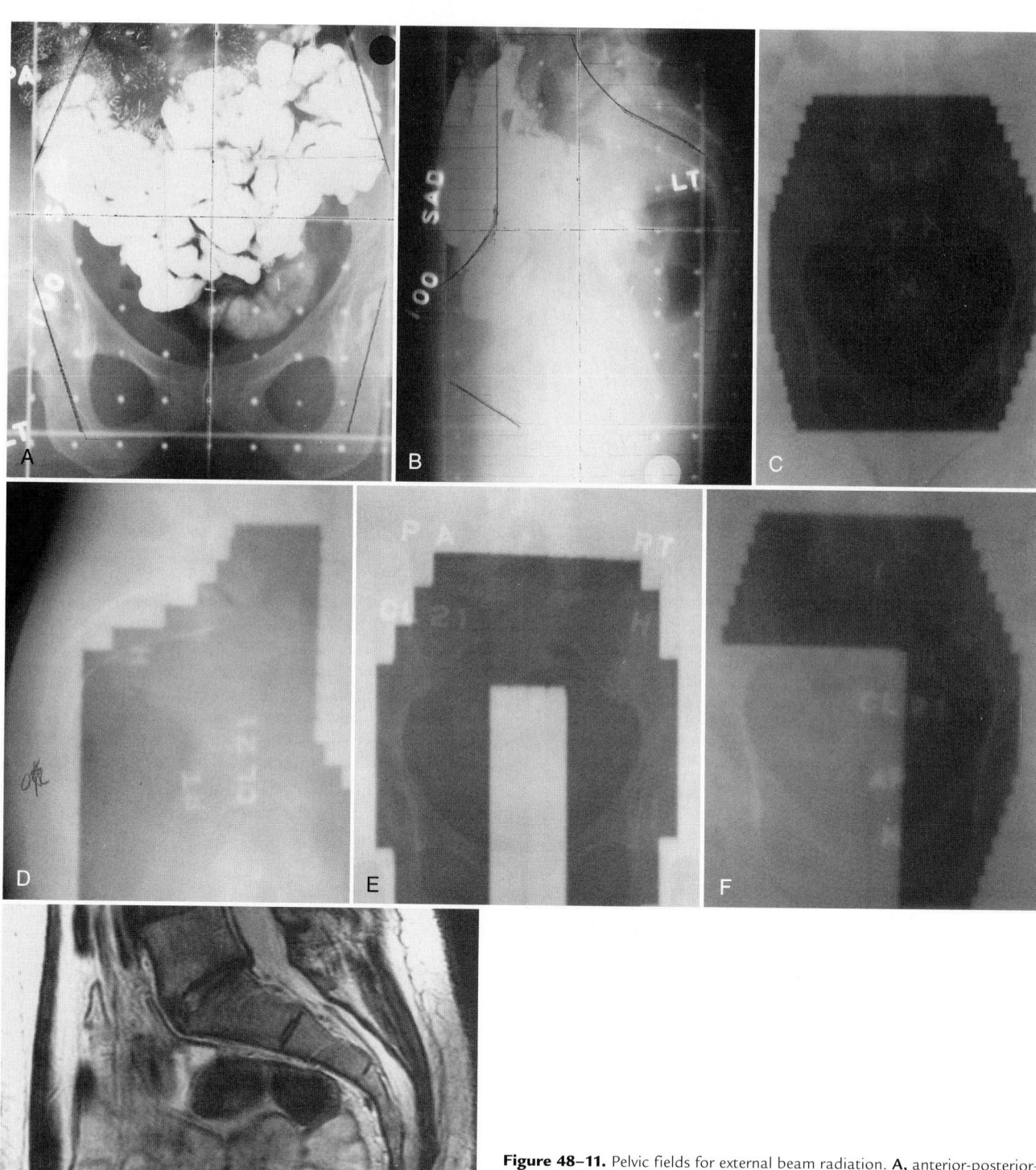

Figure 48–11. Pelvic fields for external beam radiation. **A,** anterior-posterior-posterior-anterior (AP–PA) simulation film; **B,** lateral simulation film; **C,** AP port film; **D,** lateral port film; **E,** AP port film with midline block; **F,** AP port film with unilateral parametrial block; **G,** sagittal magnetic resonance image of tumor.

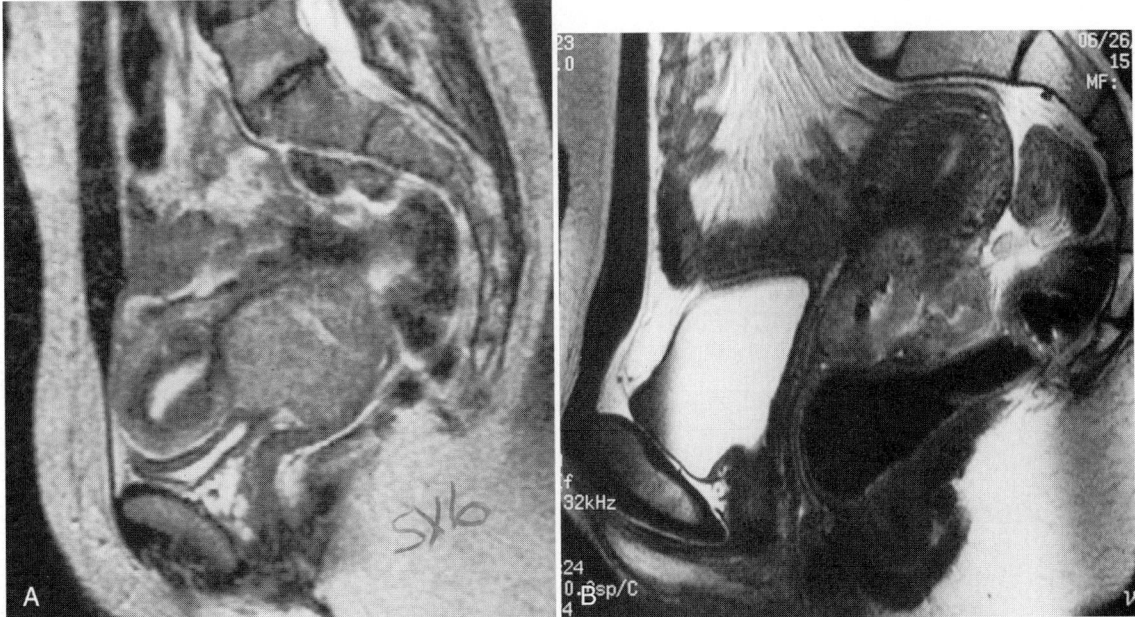

Figure 48–12. Sagittal magnetic resonance slices of two different patients with cervical carcinoma demonstrating variability in location of the uterus and its influence in designing lateral ports. **A,** Anteflexed uterus with bulky cervical tumor. **B,** Upright to slightly retroflexed uterus with cervical tumor.

delivery of these doses with appropriately selected electron energies may be used. The use of large individual fractions of external photon therapy should be avoided unless absolutely necessary. An external beam daily dose of 3 Gy for 3 days is generally adequate to stop the bleeding. The daily dose should be reduced as soon as possible, to save as much bladder and rectal tolerance as possible.

Weekly pelvic examinations should be performed to assess the response to therapy and to determine the timing of the first brachytherapy insertion. The earlier the first insertion is performed in the course of treatment, the less radiation-induced vaginal geometry distortion is expected. In cases of early disease, generally less than 2 to 3 cm, the insertions may be carried out initially, with the external beam initiated between the two insertions.

MIDLINE BLOCKING

A decision must often be made as to what level of risk to bladder and rectum is acceptable to achieve local control. When bladder and rectal tolerance have been reached in the opinion of the clinician, the plan reverts to a two-field approach, and the placement of a midline block is necessary to protect these organs from further radiation (Fig. 48-14). The block is designed with the tandem and colpostat placement positions from the insertions taken into consideration, as well as the isodose distributions selected for each insertion. The upper edge of the block should approximate the upper extent of the tandem, not higher. A central block that traverses the entire field is unacceptable because this blocks a portion of the iliac nodes from further treatment. The block, although most commonly centrally located, may extend to one side or the other depending on how eccentrically located the insertions were. Typically, a 4 cm block is used, but the width may be greater if the isodose line chosen for

the insertion was wider than 4 cm at the bladder base level. Some authors advocate the use of a step-wedge.[224] Additionally, one of the parametria may reach the desired dose earlier than the opposite side because of asymmetry of tumor or eccentric insertions, requiring unilateral parametrial blockage (see Fig. 48-14).

Brachytherapy

TANDEM AND COLPOSTAT PROCEDURES

A preoperative bowel regimen is generally started 3 days before the procedure. A half bottle (150 mL) of magnesium citrate is taken on the afternoons of the Friday and Saturday preceding a Monday morning procedure. A Fleet enema is used on Saturday and Sunday evenings. Starting on Saturday, the patient is instructed to begin a clear liquid diet, and the patient receives nothing by mouth after midnight on Sunday.

Once the patient is under anesthesia (general or spinal) and placed in the lithotomy position, a careful examination is carried out with attention to the extent of disease (parametrial, sidewall, vaginal, uterosacral ligamentous involvement), position of the uterus (anteflexed or retroflexed), dimensions of the tumor, status of the normal vaginal anatomy (forniceal effacement), and response to initial therapy. A decision must be made at this time as to whether the insertion can proceed or must be delayed until further shrinkage has occurred. Generally, tumors measuring greater than 4 cm in maximum diameter may be too bulky for early insertion, especially if eccentric in location, since the standard pear-shaped isodose distribution of the tandem and colpostats may not adequately encompass the tumor. These tumors may be best approached with additional external beam

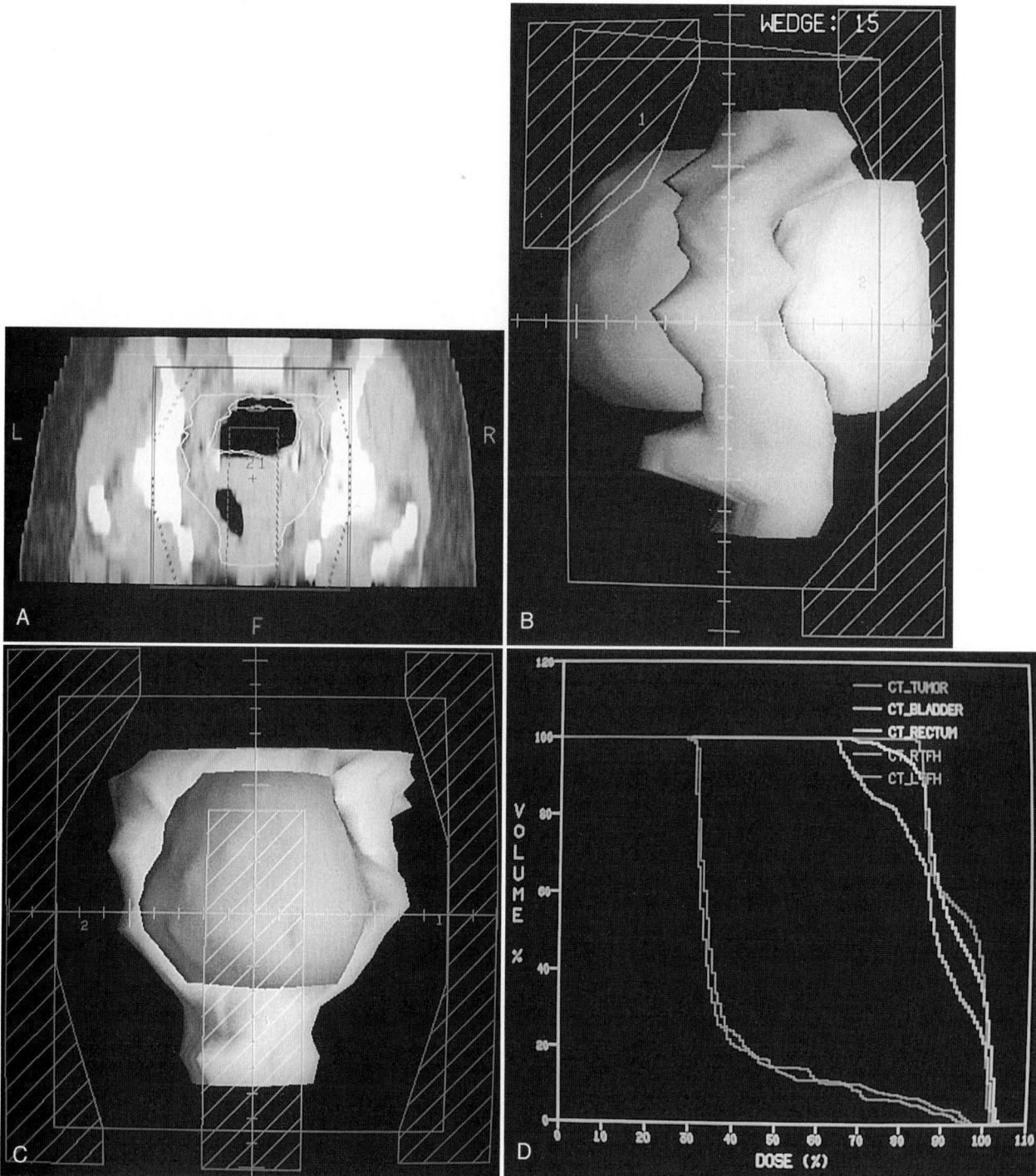

Figure 48–13. A, Field outline with blocks superimposed on coronal computed tomographic reconstruction; **B,** lateral three-dimensional (3D) reconstruction of bladder, rectum, and target volume of primary tumor plus regional nodes, with field and block outlines superimposed; **C,** Anterior-posterior 3D reconstruction of bladder and target volume (rectum concealed behind target) with superimposed field and block outlines; **D,** dose-volume histogram for initial 45 Gy (including addition of midline bar). RTFH and LTFH indicate doses to femoral heads.

radiation in an attempt to further reduce the tumor burden before brachytherapy. The tradeoff, however, is that the vaginal geometry may be further altered with the additional external beam radiation, making an insertion more difficult to carry out.

Before the procedure, the patient should have pneumatic compression stockings applied, and consideration should be given to administering low-dose heparin (5000 units subcutaneously, twice daily)[218] in order to lower the risk of thrombophlebitis. The patient is prepped with an external Betadine wash and vaginal Betadine douche and draped. Suction is desirable to assure good visualization before packing. Establishment of optimal lighting is essential from the outset, using either multiple ceiling-mounted

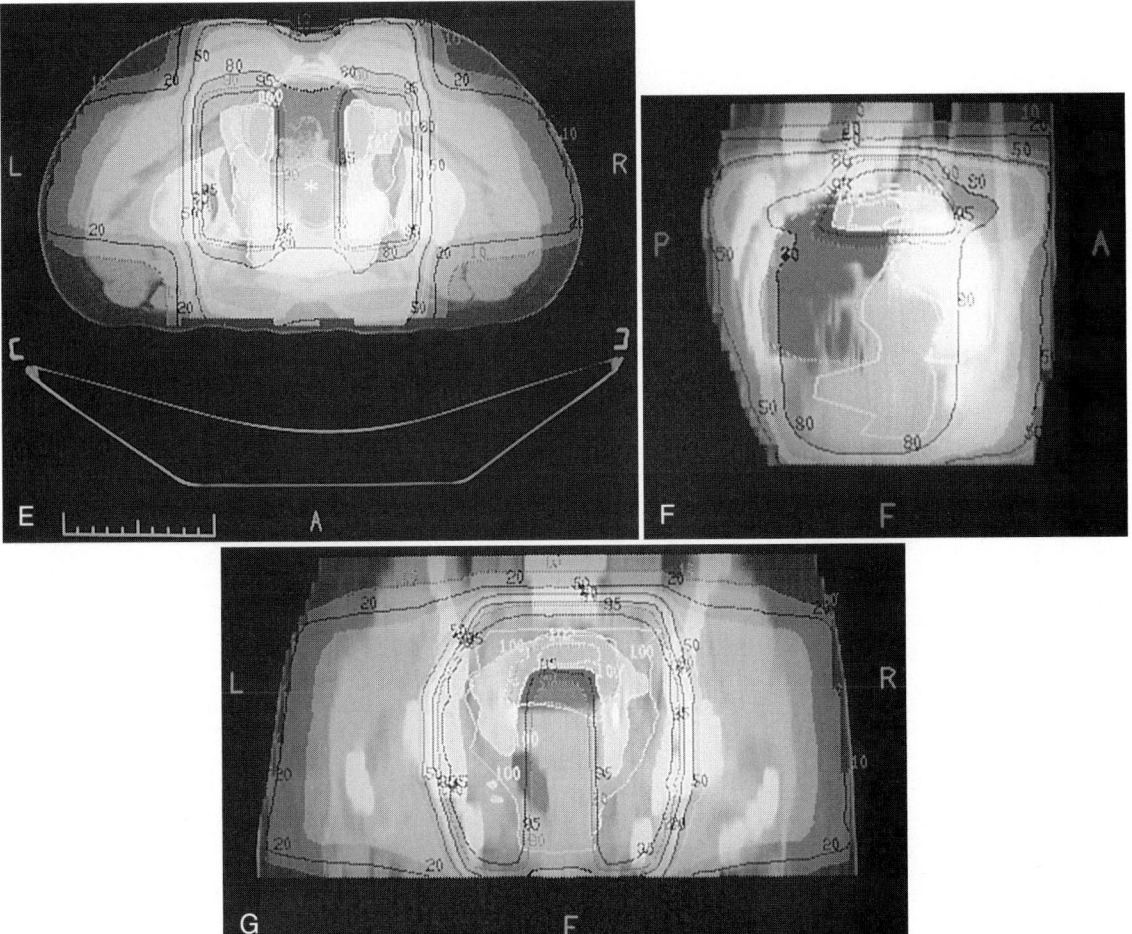

Figure 48–13. *Continued* **E,** Composite axial isodose distributions of initial 45 Gy; **F,** sagittal isodose distributions; **G,** coronal isodose distributions. See also Color Figure 48-13.

lights alone or in combination with headlamps, with the table raised to the level at which visualization is best. A weighted speculum with a blade deep enough for the vault is placed. Some clinicians prefer to avoid the use of the weighted speculum due to the risk of vaginal tears, but this has not been a problem in our experience. An additional right-angle Deaver retractor is used to raise the anterior portion of the vagina for maximal cervical visualization. The anterior lip of the cervix is firmly grasped using a single-toothed tenaculum. In cases in which the anterior lip is extremely friable due to tumor involvement or is effaced, an alternative approach is the placement of a heavy suture through the superior aspect of the cervix for the needed traction. Pulling forward and upward on the tenaculum, the cervical os is located and carefully sounded. *At this point, the risk of perforation of the uterus or lower uterine segment is significant, so care must be taken not to create a false canal through necrotic tissue, especially in the case of a retroflexed uterus.* A blunt probe is preferred to lower this risk. If, after careful probing, a canal cannot be identified, ultrasonography can be used to identify the appropriate orifice. Once identified, the uterine canal is sounded, the depth of the uterus is recorded by grasping the exposed portion of the sound immediately adjacent to the cervical

os with a clamp, and the sound is withdrawn. The sound is measured from the clamp to the tip with a ruler.

A keel, any of several radiopaque devices affixed to the tandem at the position along the tandem that correlates with the sounded depth of the uterus, has a metal ring on one side that faces the cervix (Fig. 48-15). The keel is generally fixed at a distance approximately 0.5 cm less than the length of the uterus to reduce the risk of inadvertent perforation during placement. The keel is positioned with the radiopaque marker facing the cervix, and the orientation of the keel is aligned with the curvature of the tandem. Observation of the keel during the procedure is important to ensure that the tandem has not rotated to one side or the other. In the case of a large os or necrotic tumor, *care must be taken that the tandem is not pushed too far into the uterus.*

Selection of the appropriate curvature of tandem is based on the position of the uterus on initial examination and the desired location for the brachytherapy treatment. A tandem is selected to attempt to straighten the uterus, allowing reduction of dose to the bladder during treatment by drawing the uterus into more of a midline position. Care must be taken, however, since a straight tandem may perforate an anteflexed uterus. Likewise, a too-straight uterus may cause the rectal dose to be

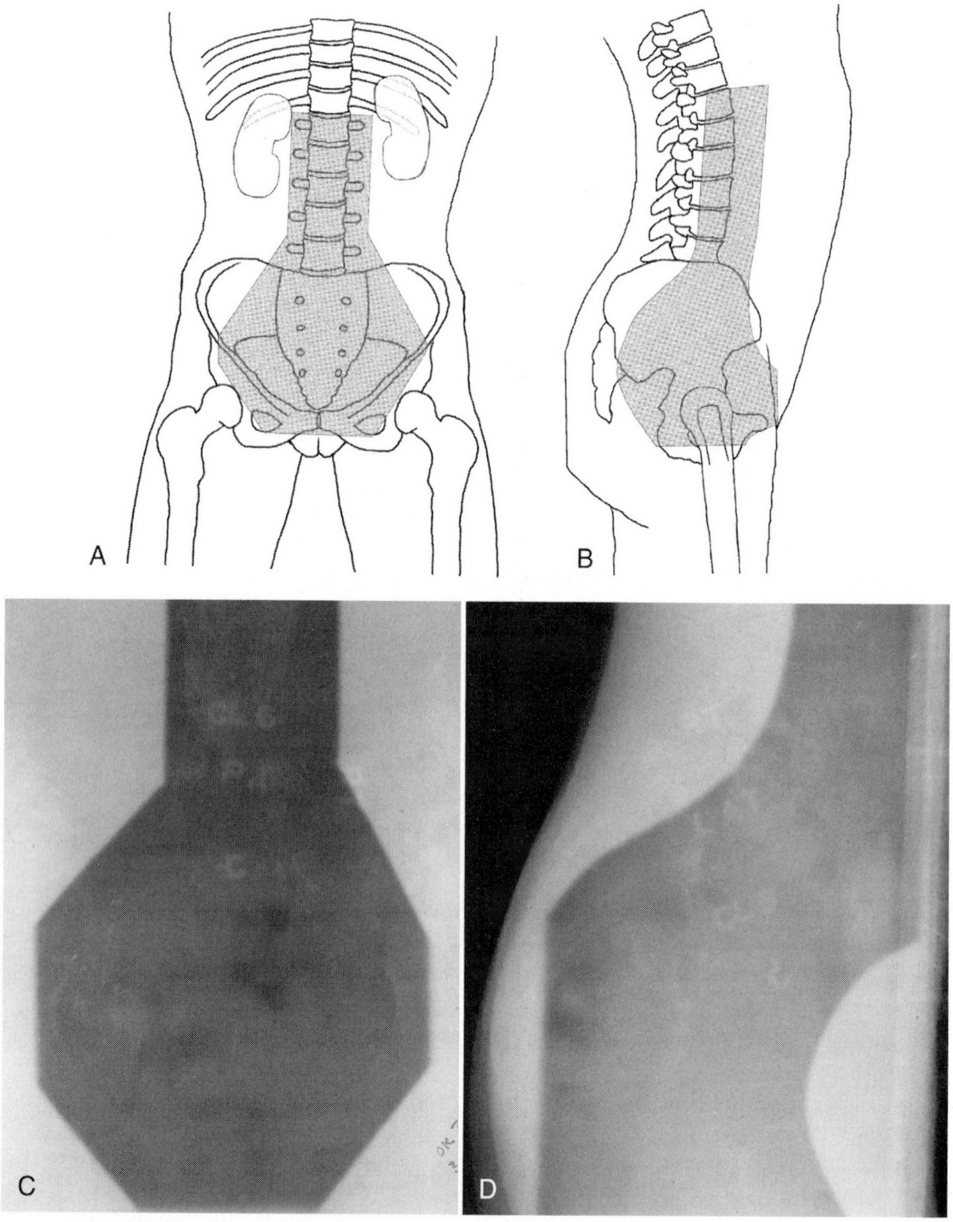

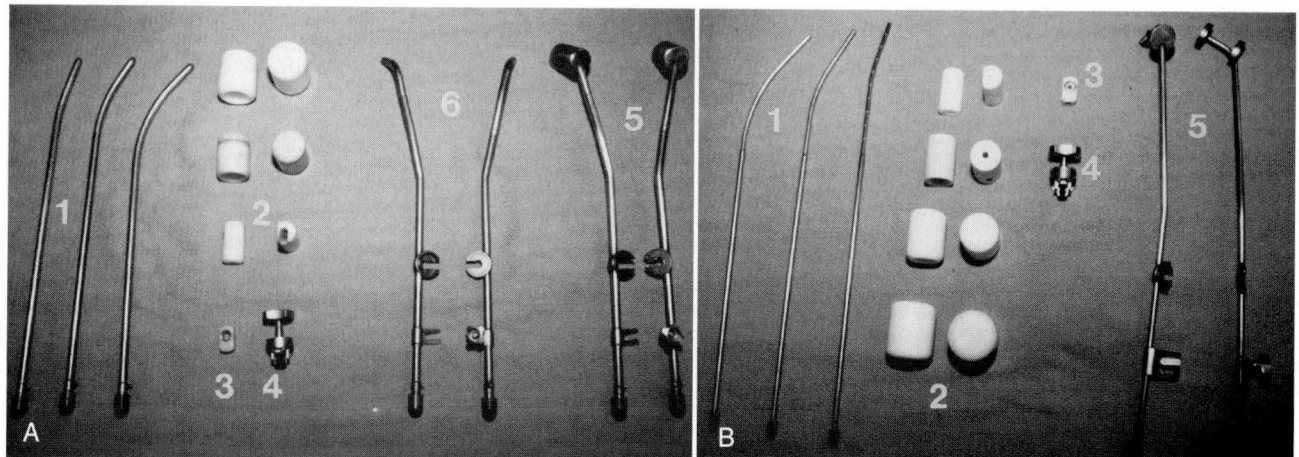

Figure 48–14. Extended-field irradiation to top of L2 vertebral body in patient s/p radical hysterectomy for IB cervix carcinoma with positive common iliac nodes. **A,** Diagram of extended para-aortic anterior-posterior (AP) simulation field to cover up to bottom of T12; **B,** lateral field; **C,** AP port film; **D,** lateral port film.

Figure 48–15. Tandem and colpostat sets for regular Selectron (**A**) and pulsed microselectron (**B**). 1 = tandems of differing curvatures; 2 = plastic caps for colpostats; 3 = keel with radio-opaque ring; 4 = locking mechanism for fixing colpostats to tandem; 5 = colpostats with inherent shielding; 6 = mini-colpostats without additional shielding for use with smallest caps.

increased beyond acceptable limits. Most often, a tandem with a minor amount of curvature is the ideal selection.

Radiopaque markers, such as gold seeds, are then placed into the cervix at two or three positions for identification of location on radiographs. These seeds should be embedded in the cervix at locations off midline to prevent their being obscured behind the tandem (e.g., at the 2 and 8 o'clock positions). The cervical canal is dilated using Hegar's dilators up to a size slightly greater than the diameter of the tandem, which varies significantly depending on the instruments used (see Fig. 48-15).

Once the cervical canal is dilated, the tandem is placed in the canal so that the keel is flush with the cervical surface. From this point on, it is important to maintain firm traction on the tenaculum or suture to assure that the keel remains in contact with the cervix. The success of the brachytherapy depends on the appropriate juxtaposition of the keel, colpostats, and cervical tumor. This point cannot be overstated.

Ideally, the largest colpostat caps that will fit into the fornices are used to optimize the dose to the vaginal surface relative to the lateral margins of tumor. Colpostats (or ovoids) fall into two general categories. Standard colpostats have built-in tungsten shielding in the top and bottom portions that provides partial dose reduction to the adjacent bladder and rectum. Smaller colpostats (so-called mini-colpostats) have no inherent shielding and were designed to accommodate narrow vaginal vaults with minimal forniceal space. Caps of various diameters (2.5 cm medium and 3.0 cm large caps) are available to fit over the standard 2.0 cm diameter colpostats to increase the distance between the sources and the vaginal mucosa in patients with roomier fornices. The shielding arrangements within standard colpostats can vary significantly between applicators from different manufacturers.[288] It is incumbent on the clinician to become familiar with the shielding characteristics and alteration of the isodose distributions of the applicators in use, since these shields may provide a 10% to 25% dose reduction to nearby rectal and bladder tissues.[288]

The colpostats are placed into the fornices one at a time, with care to avoid vaginal lacerations. If caps that are too large are used, the colpostats may be forced down and away from the cervix and tumor. Smaller caps may be required to assure that the colpostats remain astride the tumor. In situations in which one fornix has been effaced, caps of two different sizes may be needed. Depending on the instrumentation, the colpostats may be either locked together or left unattached. In either situation, it is important to maintain the positioning of the colpostats and tandem keel so that the keel bisects the colpostats, the keel remains unrotated, and the colpostats rest on either side of the cervical tumor within the residual fornices.

Packing is carried out using 1-inch wide vaginal packs and a packing forceps. It is our preference to use an agent such as triple sulfa cream to saturate the packing (if the patient is not allergic to sulfa drugs) to decrease the discomfort of packing removal later. Other lubricating agents, such as K-Y jelly, are too slick and make handling the apparatus very difficult. Packing is essential to maintain the ideal geometry of the tandem and colpostats as described. Slow, firm packing behind and above the

colpostats distends the posterior vaginal wall/anterior rectal wall as far posterior as possible and the bladder anteriorly, thereby reducing the relative exposure dose rates to these structures. During packing, traction must be maintained on the tenaculum at all times to prevent the tandem from slipping down into the vagina and the colpostats from being moved away from the fornices. It is very important to assure that packing does not extend between the colpostat and the tumor or cervix.

After packing is done halfway down the vagina, the tenaculum or suture is gently removed from the cervix, with care that the packing does not slip. A Foley catheter is placed after the urethral meatus is cleaned with Betadine. Seven milliliters of a radiopaque dye are used to inflate the balloon. Packing is then completed, and the speculum is removed carefully. A rectal tube is inserted, and the patient is removed from the lithotomy position. It is our practice to obtain orthogonal radiographs in the operating suite while the patient is still under anesthesia, to check the instrument positioning and for use for dosimetric calculations. The films must be exactly orthogonal and extend from the bottom of the tandem to the level of the L4 vertebral body. Dummy markers compatible with the remote afterloading system are placed in the tandem and colpostats, and the Foley balloon is tugged securely down into the bladder base before filming.

In the classic analysis of central treatment failures after brachytherapy by Fletcher,[197] a majority of the failures could be attributed to improper placement of the tandem or colpostats in relation to the cervix and tumor. A placement must have several characteristics to be considered acceptable (Fig. 48-16, Table 48-8). If it is unacceptable, the packing is removed and the procedure is repeated to improve the situation. On the anterior film, the clinician checks to assure that the keel is up against the cervical surface as evidenced by the proximity of the keel to the gold seeds. The tandem should bisect the angle between the colpostats. The colpostats also should be up at the level of the cervix. On the lateral film, the tandem should pass through the center of the colpostats, neither too far anterior nor too far posterior. Under certain circumstances, eccentric location may, however, be acceptable if it conforms to the geometry of the tumor. The adequacy of the packing is also assessed. Inadequate packing increases the dose to the rectum and bladder and lowers the therapeutic ratio and is a common reason for repacking the vagina. Once the placement is judged acceptable, the patient is taken out of anesthesia and returned to the postoperative unit.

Postoperative orders must give attention to diet (clear liquids, advance to low residue as tolerated), fluid management, bed positioning (head of bed at or below 30 degrees during insertion), incentive spirometry, pain and symptom management, maintenance of the patient's routine medications, and antithromboembolic precautions. The development of deep venous thrombosis is a serious concern in patients undergoing surgical procedures for gynecologic malignancies. Pulmonary embolism is a leading cause of death in such patients.[289,290] Although embolism is infrequently reported in brachytherapy procedures,[291] the result may be devastating. Prospective randomized studies looking at several preventive measures,

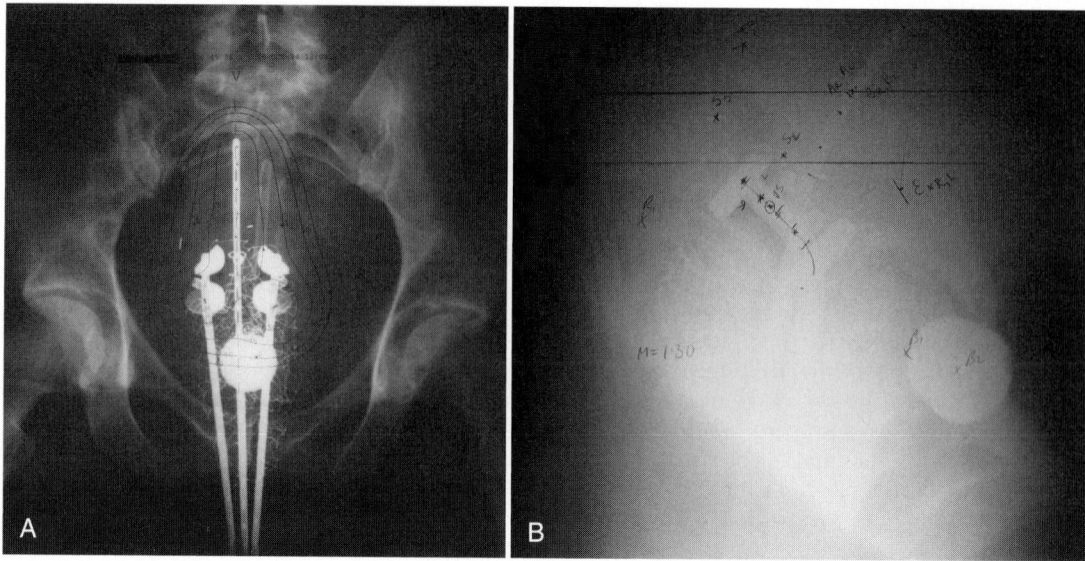

Figure 48–16. Anterior-posterior (**A**) and lateral (**B**) radiographs of tandem and colpostat insertion.

such as mini-dose heparin administration and external pneumatic calf compression of short and long duration, have been carried out.[292,293] Extended use of the compression devices (perioperatively plus 5 days postoperatively) was superior to perioperative use only in decreasing thromboembolic events after gynecologic surgical procedures.[293] The preoperative and postoperative use of low-dose heparin (5000 U subcutaneously) every 8 hours was superior to 12-hour dosing regimens and to no heparin regimens (in control subjects),[292] with no concomitant increase seen in bleeding complications. We standardly administer an initial dose of 5000 U of heparin subcutaneously 2 hours before the procedure, then every 8 hours thereafter until removal of the instruments. In addition, we use external pneumatic calf compression devices for the hospital stay.

DOSE SPECIFICATIONS

Dose reporting in the brachytherapy management of gynecologic malignancies has a complex history, with several major approaches that have their own vehement advocates. Whether an institution uses the mg-hrs system originally used in the Paris and Stockholm systems, the Manchester system with its classic reference points, or the reference volume system recommended by the

International Commission on Radiation Units and Measurements (ICRU) report 38,[294] it is critical that the selected system be used consistently by the practitioner (clinician and physicist alike), with careful attention paid to the rules established for that system. It is confusing to compare delivered doses between systems, and switching between systems may inadvertently result in significant under- or over-dosing in individual cases. For a detailed discussion of the different systems available, the interested reader is referred to the discussion in the chapter by Khan.[295]

The classic definition of point A from 1938 was a point 2 cm superior to the top of the lateral vaginal fornix and 2 cm lateral to the middle of the cervical canal.[296] This was revised in 1953[297] by moving the vertical origin from the vaginal mucosa to the external cervical os. Although originally used in the Manchester method to define levels of tolerance,[296] point A has gradually been converted to a reference for target doses, a rather unwise development.[298] This single point cannot be expected to represent a true minimum tumor dose since it can vary considerably in its true location due to multiple factors, including applicator types, tumor bulk (intracervical, parametrial extent, exophytic vaginal component), or forniceal effacement secondary to radiation effect. Given the fact that this point falls in the high-dose-gradient region of the isotopes, lateral or vertical displacement of the point by only a few millimeters will lead to significant differences in dose rate and total dose applied.[298] To prescribe doses to point A alone, therefore, without consideration of these factors, is to ignore the impact of tumor and anatomical geometry on the brachytherapy application.

The particular system advocated by the author is a combination of the ICRU 38 recommendations,[294] the ABS recommendations,[218] and a computer optimization program designed for use with remote afterloading systems but that is adaptable for use with standard manual afterloading systems as well. At the time of completion of the insertion of tandem and colpostats, orthogonal

Table 48–8   Characteristics of Good Insertion in Brachytherapy

Anterior-Posterior View
1. Tandem midline, unrotated
2. Tandem midway between colpostats
3. Keel in close proximity to gold seed markers
4. Colpostats high in the fornices along cervix

Lateral View
1. Tandem bisects the colpostats
2. Sufficient anterior and posterior packing
3. Foley balloon firmly tugged down

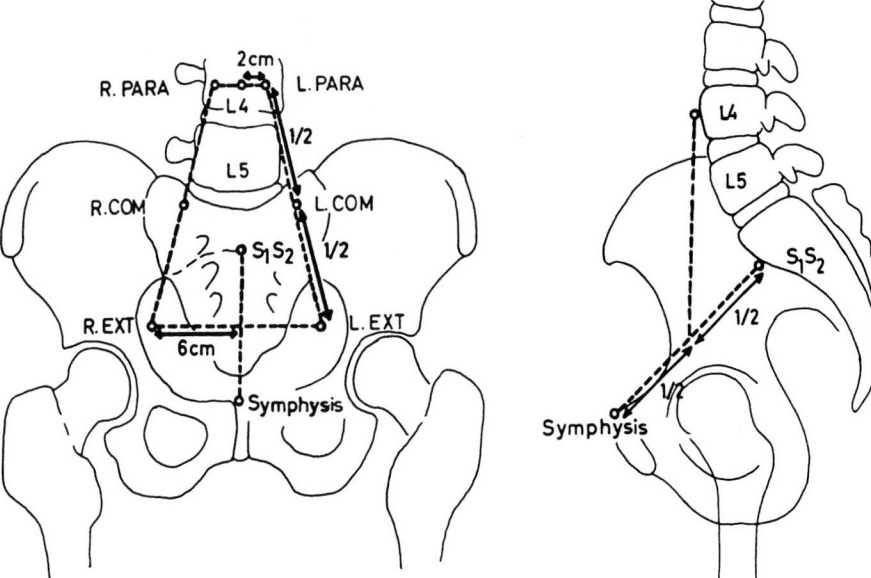

Figure 48–17. Lymphatic trapezoid for calculation of brachytherapy doses to pelvic lymph nodes. (From Dose and volume specifications for reporting intracavitary therapy in gynecology. ICRU Report #38; 1985.)

radiographs are obtained, and the rectal and bladder points are selected using the ICRU recommendations (Figs. 48-16 and 48-17). The bladder point is located on the lateral radiograph on an AP line drawn through the center of the balloon, at the posterior-most location on the balloon. The balloon must be snugly pulled down before filming. On the AP film, the point is located in the center of the balloon. In addition, a separate bladder point is recorded at the center of the balloon on the lateral film. The rectal point is found on the AP film at the midpoint of the colpostats (or at the lower end of the lowest uterine source), and on the lateral film is located 5 mm behind the posterior vaginal wall, on an AP line drawn from the middle of the colpostats. Using the recommendations of Pourquier and coworkers[299] and Crook and colleagues,[300] additional rectal points may be recorded along the anterior rectal wall parallel to the tandem, with attention paid to the highest dose rate recorded. Awareness of the dose rates along the entire length of the rectosigmoid is more helpful than awareness of a single-point dose rate, especially when optimization programs are used to adapt the isodose distributions to tumor geometry with remote afterloading systems that do not necessarily use standard loading arrangements. A vaginal surface dose rate is taken at the surface of the colpostats. Other points may be recorded on a case-by-case basis depending on the peculiarities of the tumor.

Dose rates are calculated at a number of points in the pelvis. Point A is herein defined as the point located 2 cm cephalad from the exocervix (as visualized by the radiopaque ring in the keel affixed to the tandem, if it has not slipped away from the cervix during packing) and 2 cm lateral to the tandem, taking into consideration the angle of the tandem. Whether or not this point represents the dose delivered to the tumor depends on the lateral and cephalocaudad dimensions of the tumor within the cervix, as well as the positioning of the instruments. It should not, therefore, be routinely considered to represent

the minimum tumor dose. Point B is defined as a point 2 cm up from the exocervix and 5 cm lateral to midline (*not* the tandem) and represents the lateral parametrial tissue. An additional point E is 1 cm lateral to point B and approximates the location of the sidewall. The lymphatic trapezoid of Fletcher is used to calculate doses to the external iliac, common iliac, and para-aortic nodes (see Figs. 48-17 and 48-18).[295] Additionally, the ICRU calls for information regarding the technique used (radionuclide characteristics, applicator type, source arrangement), total source strength in terms of total reference air kerma, and the three-dimensional description of the reference volume encompassed by the reference isodose surface (height/width × thickness).

The significance of all these points is that they define a true three-dimensional volume that can be related to

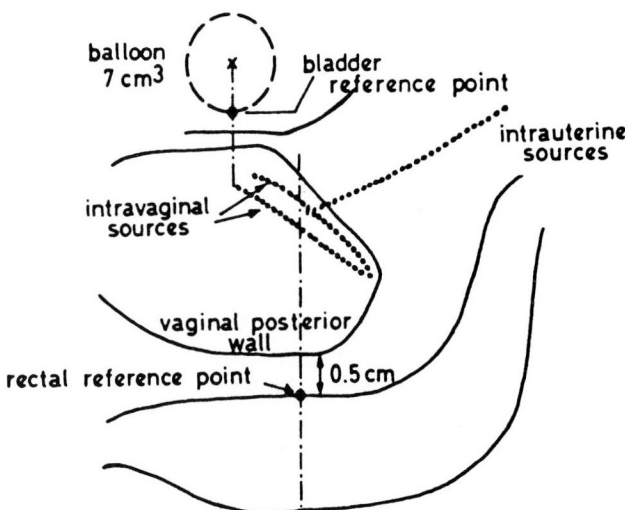

Figure 48–18. Point definitions for bladder and rectum reference points from ICRU #38. (From Dose and volume specifications for reporting intracavitary therapy in gynecology. ICRU Report #38; 1985.)[294]

the known tumor geometry (as seen with MRI and palpated by the clinician) and acknowledge the degree to which normal tissue is being irradiated by the insertion. The computer-generated three-dimensional isodose distributions are evaluated before selection of final loading of sources to maximize the therapeutic ratio. For reporting purposes, the ABS recommends documentation of the following parameters: prescribed dose to point A; rectal/bladder, vaginal, and pelvic wall points; dose rate; duration of implant; radionuclide used; source strength and loading pattern; and type of applicator selected.[218]

REMOTE AFTERLOADING SYSTEMS

Two different remote afterloading systems are in use at the University of California at San Francisco, in addition to the HDR unit described separately. The first is the low-dose-rate Selectron (made by Nucletron), which uses cesium-137 pellets and spacers that can be assigned to locations at 0.25 cm intervals along the length of the tandem, from a distance of 0.8 cm from the tip, as well as at 0.25 cm intervals from the tip of each of the colpostats. The sources are spherical and have a nominal source strength of 6 to 10 mgRaEq. The sources are most commonly spaced at 1 cm intervals along the length of the tandem from the tip down to the external os (without protruding) but may be spaced differently in cases of endocervical bulky disease to match the isodose distribution more closely to the geometry of the tumor. The number of pellets loaded into colpostats is based on the size of the caps and colpostats used. For mini-colpostats (1.5 cm diameter and no inherent shielding), the sources are limited to two or less than 15 mgRaEq maximum to keep the vaginal surface dose rates within acceptable limits (ideally below 1 Gy/hour); for regular 2.0 cm colpostats, up to three sources or a maximum of 20 mgRaEq; for 2.5 cm medium caps, three sources or maximum 25 mgRaEq; for large 3.0 cm caps, four sources or maximum 30 mgRaEq. The use of different source locations within the colpostats can provide a small amount of dose redistribution to more closely follow the tumor geometry or to alter the dose to bladder and rectum reference points. For instance, there are 5 positions available within the colpostats. Selection of the most anterior or posterior positions will result in modifications of the relative bladder and rectal doses. An attempt is made to achieve close to a 1:1 ratio between numbers of sources in the two colpostats and in the tandem, but the assessment of the isodose distribution and dose to normal tissue points is critical in choosing the final loading of the source positions and dwell times.

Alternatively, patients are treated using the Nucletron pulsed-dose rate MicroSelectron. The pulsed low-dose-rate unit has several advantages including the ability to deliver the dose in a pulsed fashion for a fraction of each hour (generally between 10 and 15 minutes), with the remainder of the hour available for the safe entry of medical support staff into the patient's room. The dose optimization program allows improved tailoring of the isodose distributions to the geometric proportions of the tumor to a degree not possible with manual afterloading systems or even the regular multiple source Selectron.

The pulsed unit has a single ^{192}Ir source (0.3 to 1.0 Ci), which is replaced every 3 months to make up for decay. Positions are located at 2.5 mm intervals along the length of the tandem and colpostats, starting at 8 mm from the tip of the tubes. The clinician and physicist/dosimetrist select not only the positions to be filled but also the actual time the source spends at each position (the dwell time). The combination of these two factors allows optimization of dose to target and normal tissues. In the process of optimization, source positions and dwell times at each position are manipulated to arrive at an isodose volume that gives the best conformation to the perceived target volume (using information from the examination under anesthesia as well as any CT and MRI data available) and the least possible dose rate to normal tissues. The dwell time in various positions can be altered to allow isodose lines to approximate the dimensions of the tumor as seen on coronal and sagittal magnetic resonance slices. This is especially useful in cases with significant endocervical extension. In the colpostats, there are multiple source positions. The choice of which positions to use depends on the size of the caps used, the relation of the final colpostat position to the tumor, and the need for reduction of dose to bladder or rectum. The smaller the cap, the fewer the positions chosen or the shorter the duration of the dwell time accepted to reduce the vaginal surface dose rate. The aim is to arrive at an isodose distribution, assessed in all three planes, classically pear-shaped but ideally matched to the tumor geometry, that incorporates the entire target volume without significant cold spots or hot spots, with the greatest reduction of rectal and bladder dose rates possible. Although the packing and placement of the instruments are the major determinants of the therapeutic ratio, careful manipulation of source positions and relative dwell times may improve this ratio. It is critical to point out, however, that dose optimization cannot make a bad insertion good. Efforts to further reduce the bladder and rectal dose rates may significantly reduce the tumor dose rate as well. Great caution must be used in working with the dose optimization program.

In the pulsed system, once an acceptable relative isodose distribution geometry has been attained (as assessed in each of the three major planes), a decision is made as to the desired dose rate to the isodose volume. Traditionally, a dose rate of 45 to 60 cGy/hr has been selected, based on the considerable amount of data available from these dose rates with manual afterloading systems. Under certain circumstances, such as advanced age or severe obesity, higher dose rates of 70 to 85 cGy/hr have been used without noticeable increase in morbidity. Dose rates above this level are discouraged, however, due to lack of information on the late effects of the pulsed approach. The dwell times at each position are then manipulated to arrive at the desired dose rate to the target isodose. This information is programmed into the computer at the patient's bedside, and treatment is initiated.

From May 11, 1992, to February 6, 1995, 62 patients underwent 73 pulsed brachytherapy procedures as part of their treatment regimen for pelvic malignancies.[301] Forty-two intracavitary and 30 interstitial procedures were performed. With a median follow-up of 10.4 months, grade 2 or 3 acute toxicities (requiring medical or surgical intervention) occurred in 6 of 73 procedures (8.2%) and delayed complications in 8 of 62 patients (12.9%). Of 30 intracavitary insertions for cervical cancer in 24 patients, there was one case of acute toxicity requiring medical intervention and two cases of delayed toxicity. Of 31 interstitial templates performed on 30 patients for pelvic malignancies, there were three incidences of significant acute toxicity and three of delayed toxicities. There appears to be no significant increase in acute toxicity above that seen with the standard continuous low-dose-rate approach. Longer follow-up is required for full assessment of local control and late toxicity with the pulsed approach.

Rogers et al. reported on 52 cervical cancer patients treated with pulsed low-dose-rate radiotherapy, with tumor control outcomes comparable to those reported using low-dose-rate insertions and complication rates that were quite acceptable.[302]

The isodose distributions of the regular Selectron, the pulsed Selectron, and standard cesium tubes show a great deal of similarity in the case of a patient with stage IIB cervical carcinoma (see Fig. 48-12*B*). In a patient with centrally bulky disease, each of the afterloading approaches can be adjusted to increase the central dose rate. In the case of cesium tubes, a loading of the tandem with 10-10-15 mgRaEq tubes causes a central bulging of the distribution (Fig. 48-19*A*). With the regular Selectron, the closer spacing of sources in the lower portion of the intrauterine tandem has the same effect (Fig. 48-19*B*), as does the increase of dwell time of the source location 2 cm above the keel in the pulsed system (see Fig. 48-19*C*).

PERINEAL INTERSTITIAL IMPLANTATION

Under certain circumstances, standard tandem and colpostat placement is not feasible or is not sufficient for adequate delivery of dose to tumor, and consideration is given to interstitial implantation. These conditions include disease extending to the sidewall or into the lower half of the vagina or complete eradication of the fornices with a constricted vaginal space, which prevents placement of colpostats. An interstitial implant is carried out to allow a more homogeneous distribution of radiation to the entire tumor volume, taking into consideration the normal tissues adjacent to the tumor (Fig. 48-20). After approximately 40 Gy has been delivered with external beam therapy, the patient is reassessed to determine if there is adequate space for the placement of tandem and colpostats and that the disease has regressed enough to allow appropriate coverage by the pear-shaped isodose distribution attainable with an insertion. If an implant is deemed necessary, one approach is to obtain an MRI scan with gadolinium enhancement, with a MUPIT (Martinez universal perineal interstitial template) and vaginal obturator in place. The vaginal obturator is placed as deeply as possible into the vagina, and the template is secured to the perineum with tape for the procedure. MRI scans (T_1-weighted and T_2-weighted with and without gadolinium) are obtained in coronal, axial, and sagittal planes, with the template visible on each of the cuts. The residual tumor is defined and its relationship to the

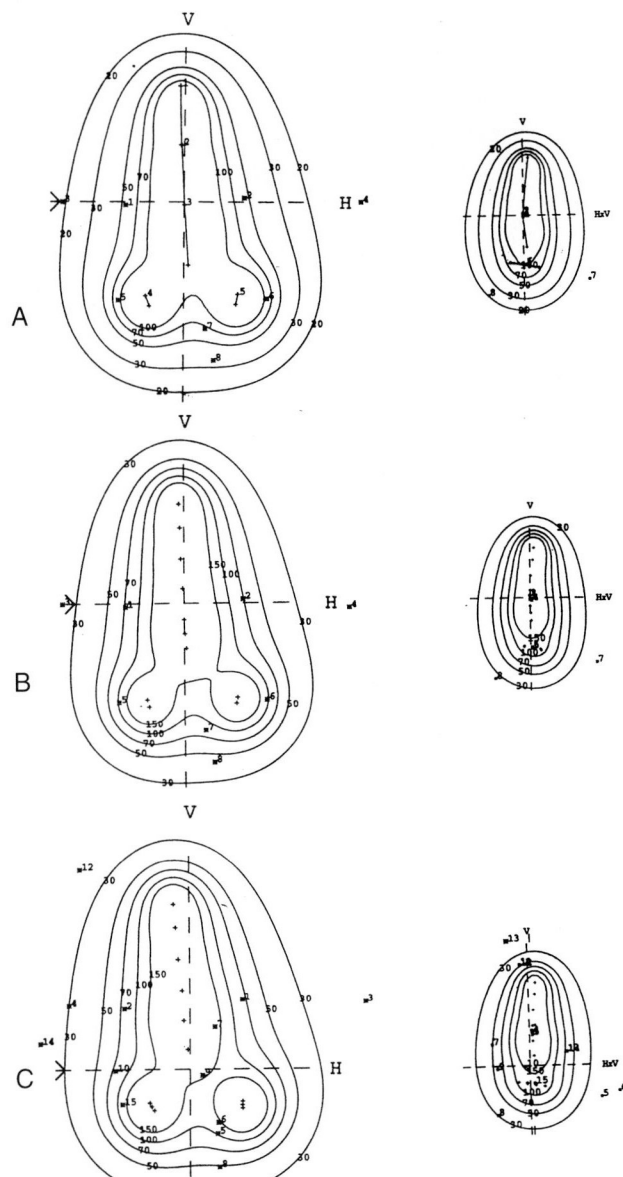

Figure 48–19. Coronal and sagittal isodose distributions for patient with magnetic resonance slices in Fig. 48-12*B* using three different systems. **A,** Manual afterloaded cesium tubes, with 10-10-15 mgRaEq in tandem and 15 mgRaEq in each colpostat with 2.5 cm. caps; **B,** Regular Selectron with seven 6 mgRaEq sources in the tandem and two each in the colpostats; **C,** pulsed microSelectron with six source dwell positions in the tandem and three in each colpostat. In examples *A* and *B*, points have the following identification: 1 = point A right, 2 = point A left, 3 = point B right, 4 = point B left, 5 & 6 = vaginal surface points, 7 = bladder, 8 = rectum. In example *C*, 1 = A left, 2 = A right, 3 = B left, 4 = B right, 5 = bladder, 7 = rectum, and 15 = vaginal surface.

obturator and template is assessed. Measurements are taken to assess the depth to which needles need to be inserted through the template to adequately encompass the tumor. The number of needles necessary to cover the entire target volume is determined, as is the need for straight or angled needles to allow optimal coverage of the lateral-most extent of tumor. Needle locations are selected at 1.0 cm intervals throughout the tumor volume for a multiplane implant. A decision is made regarding

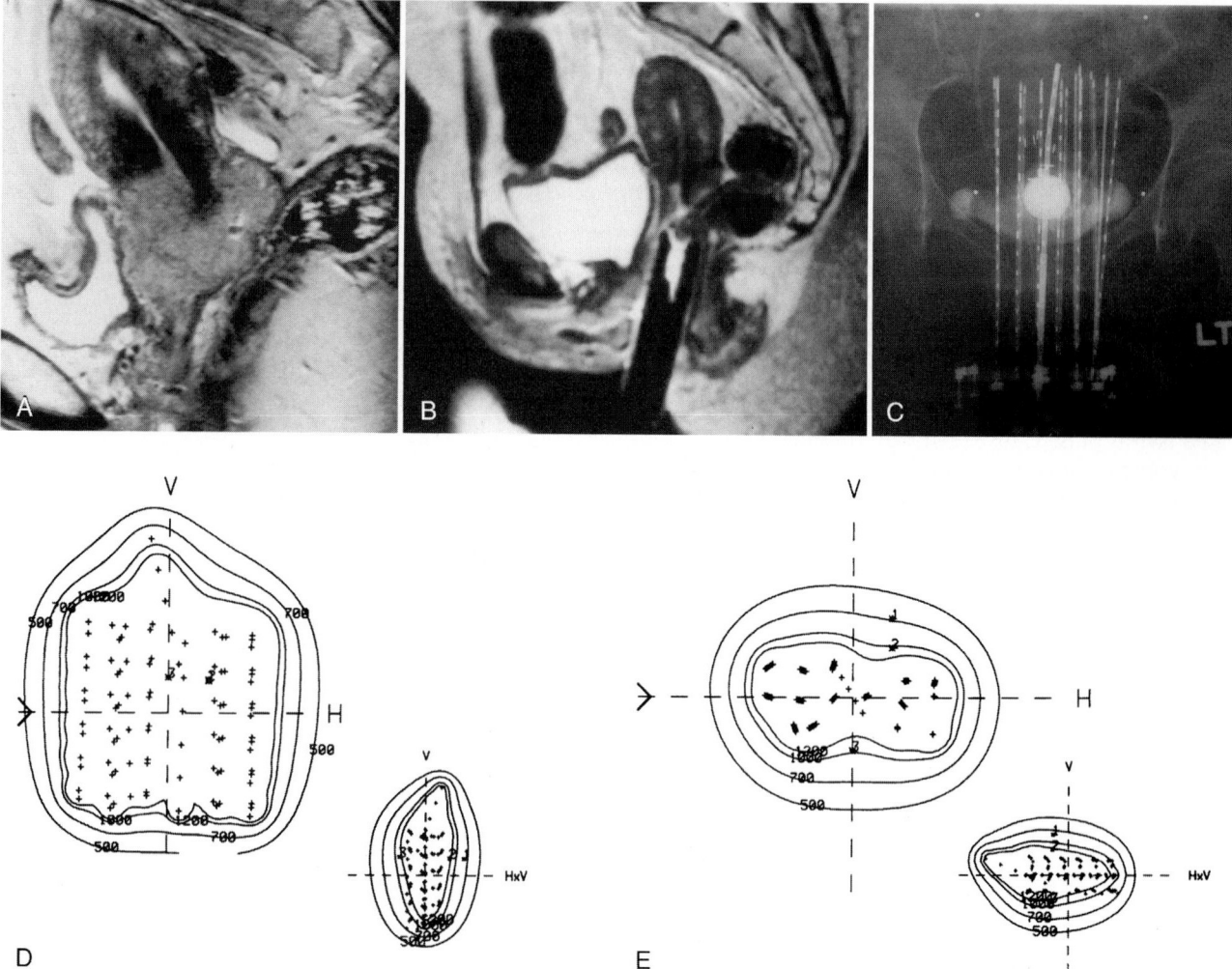

Figure 48–20. A, Pretreatment sagittal magnetic resonance image of a patient with stage IIIA cervical carcinoma. **B,** Same patient after 30 Gy external beam therapy and one course of cisplatin plus 5-FU. **C,** Anterior-posterior film of implant. **D,** Coronal isodose distributions of implant. **E,** Axial isodose distribution of implant.

the use of the tandem for loading with sources or the need for the central circle of needles around the obturator. The central ring of needles should not be loaded simultaneously with the tandem unless a remote afterloading system with optimization capability is available, since this would unnecessarily increase the dose to the bladder and rectum. Careful attention must be given to the location of the bladder, urethra, and rectum, as well as any small bowel adjacent to the tumor, when planning for needle placement and eventual loading in an effort to minimize the risk to these organs. MRI is superior to CT for delineating normal from malignant tissue.

Once the number and position of needles has been preplanned, the patient is taken to the operating room, where the template placement is performed under general or spinal anesthesia. We prefer the use of spinal anesthesia, since pain management via epidural catheter has markedly improved our patients' ability to tolerate the procedure. Intraoperatively, the patient is given a loading dose of a third-generation cephalosporin, and antithrombus precautions are taken as discussed earlier. A Foley catheter is placed. If possible, a tandem is placed in the cervical os for stabilization. If not possible, a suture is

placed through the anterior lip of the cervix and used for traction during the procedure to maintain the position of the cervix relative to the obturator. The template and obturator are placed against the perineum (with the tandem through the central hole of the obturator if a tandem is present) as in the preplan. The needles are then carefully inserted to the predetermined depth, starting with those adjacent to the rectum. The clinician is double-gloved, with the index finger of one hand inserted in the rectum and feeling along the anterior rectal wall as the first needles are inserted to ensure that no needle penetrates the rectum. Once the needles along the rectum are in place, the outer pair of gloves is carefully removed to prevent contamination of the remainder of the procedure. Working from the inner core outwards, the planned needles are inserted to the predetermined depth. Care must be taken during the insertion of needles that the template does not change position, to ensure that the needles are adequately spaced in the planned fashion. The template is then secured to the skin with several sutures to reduce the risk of slippage. Orthogonal radiographs are obtained in the operating room to look for any severely angled needles, needles penetrating the bladder, or needles that have entered too deeply and may be adjacent to small bowel. These needles are readjusted before the patient comes out of anesthesia.

Dosimetry is carried out after either stereo-shift or orthogonal radiographs are obtained, and digital entry of the locations of dummy strings placed in the needles to identify positions available for source placement (in static afterloading systems using iridium ribbons) or dwell positions (in pulsed remote afterloading systems) has been accomplished. Isodose distributions are obtained, and the line chosen is generally the first unbroken line that surrounds the tumor volume as defined by clinical and radiographic criteria, with close attention paid to doses to normal adjacent structures. The duration of the implant is dependent on the desired doses to tumor and normal tissues in the clinical setting. Ideally, a dose rate of 0.5 to 0.7 Gy/hour is selected if using a low-dose-rate system. ICRU #58 lays out the dose and volume specifications for use with interstitial implants.[303] Information on the use of high-dose-rate systems for interstitial implants is limited but shows intriguing results.[304]

Integration of Brachytherapy, External Beam Therapy, and Chemotherapy

Locoregional control is inversely related to the total duration of radiation treatment (Fig. 48-21).[305,306] Therefore, every effort should be made to minimize the period from initiation of therapy to completion. Waiting 2 weeks after completion of external beam therapy before starting brachytherapy, ostensibly to allow tumor shrinkage, in fact allows time for tumor repopulation. Such breaks in therapy compromise control rates. Therefore, a treatment schedule needs to be flexible enough to adapt to the response of tumor, normal tissue reactions, and hematologic parameters while at the same time minimizing treatment interruptions. For instance, in the period between two insertions, it is preferable to proceed with

external beam radiation, either whole pelvis or with a midline block depending on the doses to normal structures. Likewise, an insertion should proceed immediately after external beam therapy with no break planned. A typical scenario for a small (<3 cm) stage IB cervical tumor might be 20 Gy external beam therapy to the whole pelvis, succeeded immediately by an initial 60-hour insertion, resumption of external beam therapy in the 10 days between insertions, second insertion, followed by external beam with a midline block (total duration, 6.5 weeks). In addition to using chemotherapy during the external beam component of therapy, the prospective randomized trials of chemotherapy and radiation integrated a course of chemotherapy with one of the planned insertions with reasonable tolerance.[221]

Complications

Rectal irritation due to radiation may range from episodic diarrhea, rectal spasm, and occasional bleeding to localized ulceration and partial stenosis, recurrent and abundant hemorrhage with necrosis and obstruction, and finally rectovaginal fistula formation. Similarly, bladder irritation varies from mild dysuria with infrequent hematuria to protracted bladder spasm with continuous hematuria to necrosis and eventual vesicovaginal or urethrovaginal fistula formation. Diarrhea and pelvic cramping secondary to small bowel irritation may progress to intermittent small bowel obstruction and eventual complete obstruction or fistula formation with peritonitis.

Reports of incidence of severe complications requiring medical intervention, hospitalization, or surgical intervention or resulting in death provide conflicting evidence as to what factors are the most important in predicting adverse sequelae.[185,206,210,223,291,307] Most commonly discussed are brachytherapy doses, doses to various rectal/bladder/paracervical points, and history of prior procedures or illness. The comparison of brachytherapy doses between separate institutions is made difficult by the various manners in which the normal tissue dose points are defined.

Using the reference points defined in the ICRU 38 report,[294] Perez[308] described the incidence of major sequelae in 1456 patients treated at Mallinckrodt between 1959 and 1993. Those patients who received a dose of less than or equal to 8000 Gy to the rectal point had a 1% to 4% incidence of major rectal complications, compared with a rate of 9% at doses greater than 8000 Gy. Urinary sequelae did not correlate well with dose to the bladder point, with a range of 3% to 5% at all doses analyzed. Small bowel injury increased as total dose to the lateral pelvic wall rose above 6000 Gy (2% to 4%). Looking at the ratio of the rectal dose to the point A dose revealed a significant difference in the severe rectal complication rate for those cases where the ratio was 0.8 or less (0.3%) compared to those with a ratio greater than 0.8 (5%). In an earlier report, Perez[291] had pointed out that age, prior surgery, history of pelvic inflammatory disease, external beam dose, and type of midline block used all failed to correlate with the major sequelae rate.

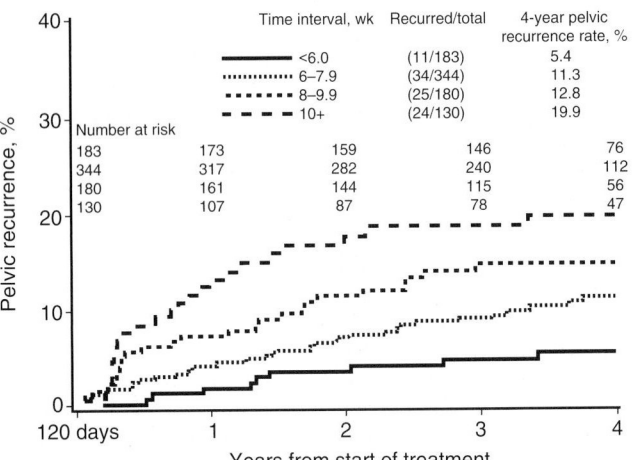

Figure 48–21. Actuarial pelvic recurrence after radiation therapy for cervical carcinoma by treatment duration, from the Patterns of Care Study. (From Lanciano RM, Pajak TF, Martz K, et al: The influence of treatment time on outcome for squamous cell cancer of the uterine cervix treated with radiation: A Patterns-of-Care Study. *Int J Radiat Oncol Biol Phys.* 1993;25:391.)

Montana reported on 527 cervical cancer patients treated at Duke from 1969 to 1980.[185] A total incidence of 6% (4% severe) for cystitis and 11% (8% severe) for proctitis was reported. The incidence correlated significantly with a total dose to each organ and, unlike with the Perez data, the whole pelvis radiation dose. As whole pelvic dose increased from 2000 to 4000 Gy or greater, the frequency of rectal complications rose from 3% to 14%. Bladder complications did not correlate with external beam dose or total dose to the bladder.

Lanciano[155] in the Patterns of Care Study reported a crude complication rate of 9.8% with 3- and 5-year actuarial rates of 10% and 14%, respectively, in 1558 patients treated only with radiation for all stages of disease at a large number of institutions in the United States. Sixty-one percent of complications occurred in the large and small bowel, 21% in the bladder, and 10% in the vagina. Sixty-four percent of these complications required surgical correction, and 9% of these were fatal (total of 0.8% fatal complication rate). The median time to development of complications in the bowel was 13.5 months, bladder 23.2 months, and vagina 17.4 months. In this multivariate analysis, five factors were associated with an increased risk of major complications: the use of external beam therapy, dose per fraction in excess of 2 Gy, the use of radium rather than cesium, paracentral dose, and dose to the lateral parametrium.

Target organ threshold doses are not by themselves reliable predictors of the risk of serious radiation sequelae because they fail to take into account the volume of the organ incorporated in the high dose region. This volume will vary significantly based on the total external beam contribution to the organ and on the manipulation of source locations and dwell times possible with currently remote afterloading optimization systems. Pourquier and colleagues[299] and Crook and colleagues[300] have each recommended the use of a mean rectal dose (the average of the doses received at four different rectal points along the axis of the anterior rectal wall, in addition to the maximum rectal dose) to identify groups at low, intermediate, and high risk for major rectal sequelae. The critical dose is not a simple value at a point; rather, it is an estimate of the volume of tissue exposed to a high radiation dose from both the external and intracavitary components of treatment. Ideally, CT-based three-dimensional dosimetry and inverse optimized planning with dose volume histograms for tumor and normal tissues will allow more accurate prediction of and avoidance of major complications.

The risk of damage to the small bowel is related to the total dose delivered to the pelvis, the fraction size per dose, and the presence of physical factors such as multiple abdominal surgical procedures or pelvic inflammatory disease.[80,155,210,291,309-312] Technical factors such as the treatment of one field per day, lower energy machines, or extended field coverage of the para-aortic nodes have also been implicated.[210,313] Doses above 45 Gy to the entire pelvis are associated with a rising incidence of the development of intermittent or surgical small bowel obstruction.[210,309] Methods proposed for the reduction in risk of small bowel morbidity include the treatment of all fields each day,[210] the use of megavoltage equipment,[210] treatment with the bladder full, and the placement of an omental or mesh sling to remove bowel from the field of radiation at the time of preradiation surgical exploration or lymphadenectomy.[314-316] The use of an extraperitoneal rather than a transperitoneal approach for para-aortic lymph node sampling is associated with a reduction in radiation risk to small bowel[220,317,318] and is the recommended approach in patients entered into GOG studies requiring para-aortic lymph node sampling. Overall, for patients treated with radiation for carcinoma of the uterine cervix, the crude incidence of small bowel obstruction was 2% to 3% in the Perez report,[206] 4% in the Patterns of Care Study,[155] and 4% in the pelvic radiation therapy–alone arm of the RTOG para-aortic study.[313] This incidence increases, however, with extended field radiation to cover the para-aortics in 9%, and to 17% in patients so treated who had a prior history of abdominal surgery.[313] Studies that have pushed the dose to 60 Gy have resulted in severe gastrointestinal complication rates of as high as 57%.[240,319]

Other risks associated with the treatment of cervical cancer include the development of thromboembolic phenomena or major cardiac complications during or immediately after brachytherapy procedures for cervical carcinoma, although the reported incidence is quite low at 0% to 4%.[289,290,292,320,321] One particularly bothersome side effect of radiation for cervical cancer is the development of vaginal adhesions, vaginal shortening, and, potentially, total agglutination of the vagina. Small adhesions form quickly in the irradiated patient, which can make sexual intercourse and future pelvic examinations quite painful. Therefore, at the completion of therapy, the patient is instructed in the use of a vaginal dilator, to be used on a daily or every other day basis for 5 to 10 minutes. The patient is started with a small dilator, instructed in its use with lubricating jelly, and encouraged to begin using it on a very regular basis. Dryness of the irradiated vagina is a common side-effect, due to a combination of direct radiation effect and the onset of menopause. Vaginal lubricants and topical estrogen creams are beneficial in partially relieving these symptoms.

The risk of second malignancies rises over time after radiation for carcinoma of the cervix, although the exact increase over the rate expected in the general population is difficult to assess. Several reports suggest that the increase is not significant overall,[322-324] although some specific subtypes of cancer are seen with an increased rate over expected incidence rates.[325] Analyzing data from a combination of the Connecticut Tumor Registry and SEER data bases, Rabkin[325] reported on close to 25,000 women treated for cervical carcinoma with either surgery or radiation who were long-term survivors. The relative risk of developing a second tumor after radiation was greater than 2.5 for the development of carcinoma of the anus, (RR 4.6), larynx (RR 3.3), lung (RR 3.0), vulva/vagina (RR 5.6), bladder (RR 2.7), and bone (RR 2.7). However, the presence of shared etiologic factors, such as HPV in anal, vulvar, and cervical malignancies, or excess smoking in the population of cervix and lung cancer patients,[322,323] makes it unclear that the treatment contributed to this excess risk.[322,325] Information from the Danish Cancer Registry in approximately 45,000 patients treated between 1943 and 1982 revealed an excess of only 64 cases per 10,000 women per year of tumors in the pelvises of irradiated patients,[326] reaching a maximum at 30 years, indicating the need for prolonged follow-up in assessing the true increased incidence of second malignancies.

The RTOG and EORTC collaborated to develop a uniform staging system for late effects to normal tissues using a subjective/objective/management/analytic scale system (LENT/SOMA) for all organ sites.[327,328] This system uses SOMA scales derived in a site-specific fashion. These scales (grades 1 to 4) include the patient's assessment of the condition (subjective), the specific physically assessable deficits associated with the condition (objective), the intervention required to ameliorate the condition (management), and the radiologic or laboratory evaluation of the problem (analytic). These grades are combined to give a total LENT score. Scales have been established for all sites, including vulvovaginal, uterine, ovarian, bladder, rectal, and urethral for sexual dysfunction relevant to patients with cervical carcinoma. These scales may prove important over time in the comparisons of effects of various treatment regimens in the gynecologic arena.

FUTURE DIRECTIONS

Systemic failure of cervical carcinoma remains a considerable challenge to the gynecologic oncologist. Local and regional control, however, is being aided by technologic developments that will result in an improvement in the therapeutic ratio. MRI provides superior differentiation of normal from macroscopically abnormal tissue, information that is crucial for the optimization of brachytherapy and external beam therapy approaches. The development of treatment planning software that can merge information from multiple scans (MRI, CT) with the production of isodose distributions for brachytherapeutic interventions will allow improved dose-volume analysis of tumor and normal tissues. Integration and fusion of scans such as PET in the treatment planning process will further allow the ideal delineation of true target volumes for both external irradiation and brachytherapy. The use of intensity-modulated radiation treatment planning of external beam therapy may allow delivery of higher doses of radiation to involved or clinically relevant pelvic nodes in an attempt to improve regional control. Identifying the previously subclinical areas of spread with PET, and modulating the radiation beam with IMRT will potentially reduce the risk of recurrence and lower the morbidity rates in cervical carcinoma. The integration of newer agents such as irinotecan and the taxanes as concurrent sensitizers is under way in hopes of improving both local control and overall survival.

REFERENCES

1. Jemal A, Thomas A, Murray T, Thun M: Cancer statistics, 2002. *CA Cancer J Clin.* 2002;52:23.
2. Brinton LA: Epidemiology of cervical cancer: Overview. *IARC Sci Publ.* 1992;1992:3.
3. Cancer Statistics, 1995. *CA Cancer J Clin.* 1995;45:8.
4. Devesa S, Diamond E: Association of breast cancer and cervical cancer incidences with income and education among whites and blacks. *J Natl Cancer Inst.* 1980;65:515.
5. Feingold A, Vermund S, Burk R: Cervical cytologic abnormalities and human papillomavirus in women infected with HIV. *J Acquir Immune Defic Syndr.* 1990;3:896.
6. Levine AM: AIDS-related malignancies: The emerging epidemic. *J Natl Cancer Inst.* 1993;85:1382.
7. Judson FN: Interactions between human papillomavirus and human immunodeficiency virus infections. *IARC Sci Publ.* 1992;1992:199.
8. Arends MJ, Donaldson YK, Duvall E, et al: Human papillomavirus type 18 associates with more advanced cervical neoplasia than human papillomavirus type 16. *Hum Pathol.* 1993;24:432.
9. Beral V, Day NE: Screening for cervical cancer: Is there a place for incorporating tests for the human papillomavirus? *IARC Sci Publ.* 1992;1992:263.
10. Crook T, Wrede D, Tidy JA, et al: Clonal *p53* mutation in primary cervical cancer: Association with human-papillomavirus-negative tumors. *Lancet.* 1992;339:1070. See comments.
11. Gissmann L: Papillomaviruses and human oncogenesis. *Curr Opin Genet Dev.* 1992;2:97.
12. Inman GJ, Cook ID, Lau RK: Human papillomaviruses, tumor suppressor genes and cervical cancer. *Int J STD AIDS.* 1993;4:128. Editorial.
13. Moreno V, Bosch FX, Munoz N, et al: Effect of oral contraceptives on risk of cervical cancer in women with HPV infection: The IARC multi-centric case-control study. *Lancet.* 2002;359:1085.
14. Herbst A, Ulfelder H, Poskranzer D: Adenocarcinoma of the vagina. *N Engl J Med.* 1971;284:878.
15. Hill E: Clear cell carcinoma of the cervix and vagina in young women. *Am J Obstet Gynecol.* 1971;116:470.
16. Melnick S, Cole P, Anderson D, et al: Rates and risks of diethylstilbestrol-related clear-cell adenocarcinoma of the vagina and cervix: An update. *N Engl J Med.* 1987;316:514.
17. Couturier J, Sastre GX, Schneider MS, et al: Integration of papillomavirus DNA near *myc* genes in genital carcinomas and its consequences for proto-oncogene expression. *J Virol.* 1991;65:4534.
18. Liang XH, Volkmann M, Klein R, et al: Co-localization of the tumor-suppressor protein p53 and human papillomavirus E6 protein in human cervical carcinoma cell lines. *Oncogene.* 1993; 8:2645.
19. Nair BS, Pillai R: Oncogenesis of squamous carcinoma of the uterine cervix. *Int J Gynecol Pathol.* 1992;11:47.
20. Lo KW, Mok CH, Chung G, et al: Presence of *p53* mutation in human cervical carcinomas associated with HPV-33 infection. *Anticancer Res.* 1992.
21. Kaelbling M, Burk RD, Atkin NB, et al: Loss of heterozygosity on chromosome 17p and mutant *p53* in HPV-negative cervical carcinomas. *Lancet.* 1992;340:140.
22. Atkin NB, Baker MC, Fox MF: Chromosome changes in 43 carcinomas of the cervix uteri. *Cancer Genet Cytogenet.* 1990;44:229.
23. Mattingly R: Anatomy. In Mattingly R, ed. *TeLinde's Operative Gynecology.* Philadelphia: JB Lippincott; 1977:25.
24. Solomon D, Davey D, Kurman R, et al: The 2001 Bethesda System: Terminology for reporting results of cervical cytology. *JAMA.* 2002;287:2114.
25. Gompel C, Silverberg S: *Pathology in Gynecology and Obstetrics.* Philadelphia: JB Lippincott; 1994:36.
26. Kurman R, Norris H, Wilkinson E: Tumors of the cervix, vagina and vulva. *Atlas of Tumor Pathology,* 3rd series, 1992. Fascicle 4.
27. Robert ME, Fu YS: Squamous cell carcinoma of the uterine cervix: A review with emphasis on prognostic factors and unusual variants. *Semin Diagn Pathol.* 1990;7:173.
28. Zaino RJ, Ward S, Delgado G, et al: Histopathologic predictors of the behavior of surgically treated stage IB squamous cell carcinoma of the cervix. A Gynecologic Oncology Group study. *Cancer.* 1992; 69:1750.
29. Buckley CH, Beards CS, Fox H: Pathological prognostic indicators in cervical cancer with particular reference to patients under the age of 40 years. *Br J Obstet Gynaecol.* 1988;95:47.
30. Kraus F, Perez-Mesa C: Verrucous carcinoma: Clinical and pathologic study of 105 cases involving oral cavity, larynx and genitalia. *Cancer.* 1966;19:26.
31. Dische S, Saunders M, Bennett M, et al: Cell proliferation and differentiation in squamous cancer. *Radiother Oncol.* 1984; 15:19.

32. Wong W, Ng C, Lee C: Verrucous carcinoma of the cervix. *Arch Gyn Obstet*. 1990;241:47.

33. Weinberg E, Hoisington S, Eastman AY, et al: Uterine cervical lymphoepithelial-like carcinoma. Absence of Epstein-Barr virus genomes. *Am J Clin Pathol*. 1993;99:195.

34. Young R, Scully R: Invasive adenocarcinoma and related tumors of the uterine cervix. *Semin Diag Pathol*. 1990;7:205.

35. Anderson M: Premalignant and malignant disease of the cervix. In Fox H, ed. *Haines and Taylor Obstetrical and Gynecological Pathology*. London: Churchill Livingstone; 1987:255.

36. Gilks C, Young R, Aguirre P, et al: Adenoma malignum (MDA) of the uterine cervix. *Am J Surg Path*. 1989;13:717.

37. Young RH, Scully RE: Villoglandular papillary adenocarcinoma of the uterine cervix. A clinicopathologic analysis of 13 cases. *Cancer*. 1989;63:1773.

38. Michael H, Grawe L, Kraus FT: Minimal deviation endocervical adenocarcinoma: Clinical and histologic features, immunohistochemical staining for carcinoembryonic antigen, and differentiation from confusing benign lesions. *Int J Gynecol Pathol*. 1984;3:261.

39. Buckley C, Fox H: Pathology of clinical invasive carcinoma of cervix. In Coppleson M, ed. *Gynecologic Oncology*. London: Churchill Livingstone; 1992:649.

40. Berek JS, Hacker NF, Fu YS, et al: Adenocarcinoma of the uterine cervix: Histologic variables associated with lymph node metastasis and survival. *Obstet Gynecol*. 1985;65:46.

41. Donadello N, Balestreri D, Fasola M, et al: Adenocarcinoma of the uterine cervix. *Eur J Gynaecol Oncol*. 1991;12:133.

42. Eifel PJ, Morris M, Oswald MJ, et al: Adenocarcinoma of the uterine cervix. Prognosis and patterns of failure in 367 cases. *Cancer*. 1990;65:2507.

43. Kleine W, Rau K, Schwoeorer D, et al: Prognosis of the adenocarcinoma of the cervix uteri: A comparative study. *Gynecol Oncol*. 1989;35:145.

44. Resta L, Scordari MD, Mastrogiulio RS, et al: Endocervical adenocarcinoma. Clinico-pathologic and histochemical study of 29 cases. *Eur J Gynecol Oncol*. 1989;10:49.

45. Herbst AL, Anderson D: Clear cell adenocarcinoma of the vagina and cervix secondary to intrauterine exposure to diethylstilbestrol. *Semin Surg Oncol*. 1990;6:343.

46. Horwitz RI, Viscoli CM, Merino M, et al: Clear cell adenocarcinoma of the vagina and cervix: Incidence, undetected disease, and diethylstilbestrol. *J Clin Epidemiol*. 1988;41:593.

47. Jones WB, Koulos JP, Saigo PE, et al: Clear-cell adenocarcinoma of the lower genital tract: Memorial Hospital 1974-1984. *Obstet Gynecol*. 1987;70:573.

48. Sharp GB, Cole P, Anderson D, et al: Clear cell adenocarcinoma of the lower genital tract. Correlation of mother's recall of diethylstilbestrol history with obstetrical records. *Cancer*. 1990;66:2215.

49. Herbst AL, Anderson S, Hubby MM, et al: Risk factors for the development of diethylstilbestrol-associated clear cell adenocarcinoma: A case-control study. *Am J Obstet Gynecol*. 1986;154:814.

50. Gilks CB, Clement PB: Papillary serous adenocarcinoma of the uterine cervix: A report of three cases. *Mod Pathol*. 1992;5:426.

51. Shintaku M, Ueda H: Serous papillary adenocarcinoma of the uterine cervix. *Histopathology*. 1993;22:506.

52. Tsukahara Y, Kato J, Sakai Y, et al: Clinicopathologic study of adenosquamous carcinoma of the uterine cervix. *Nippon Sanka Fujinka Gakkai Zasshi*. 1983;35:2387.

53. Littman P, Clement PB, Henriksen B, et al: Glassy cell carcinoma of the cervix. *Cancer*. 1976;37:2238.

54. Lotocki RJ, Krepart GV, Paraskevas M, et al: Glassy cell carcinoma of the cervix: A bimodal treatment strategy. *Gynecol Oncol*. 1992;44:254.

55. van Nagell JR Jr, Powell DE, Gallion HH, et al: Small cell carcinoma of the uterine cervix. *Cancer*. 1988;62:1586.

56. Talerman A, Alenghat E, Okagaki T: Glassy cell carcinoma of the uterine cervix. *APMIS Suppl*. 1991;23:119.

57. Clement P: Miscellaneous primary and metastatic tumors of the uterine cervix. *Sem Diag Pathol*. 1990;7:228.

58. Groben P, Reddick R, Askin F: The pathologic spectrum of small cell carcinoma of the cervix. *Int J Gynecol Pathol*. 1985;4:42.

59. van Nagell JR Jr, Donaldson ES, Wood EG, et al: Small cell cancer of the uterine cervix. *Cancer*. 1977;40:2243.

60. Jones H, Ga G, TeLinde R: Reexamination of biopsies taken prior to the development of invasive carcinoma of the cervix. In Proceedings of the Third National Cancer Conference; 1957; Philadelphia. p 678.

61. Carson R, Gall E: Preinvasive carcinoma and precancerous metaplasia of cervix: Serial block survey. *Am J Pathol*. 1954;30:15.

62. Christopherson W, Parker J, Mendez W, et al: Cervix cancer death rates and mass cytologic screening. *Cancer*. 1970;21:808.

63. Boon M, DeGraaf-Gouillard J: Cost effectiveness of population screening and rescreening for cervical cancer in the Netherlands. *Acta Cytol*. 1981;25:539.

64. Eddy D: Appropriateness of cervical cancer screening. *Gynecol Oncol*. 1981;12:s168.

65. Beilby J, Guillebaud J, Steele S: Paired cervical smears: A method of reducing the false-negative rate in population screening. *Obstet Gynecol*. 1982;60:46.

66. Parkin D, Collins W, Clayden A: Cervical cytology screening in two Yorkshire areas: Pattern of service. *Public Health*. 1981;95:311.

67. Nuovo G: *Cytopathology of the Lower Female Genital Tract*. Baltimore: Williams & Wilkins; 1994:294.

68. Coppleson M: Early invasive squamous and adenocarcinoma of cervix: (FIGO stage Ia) clinical features and management. In Coppleson M, ed. *Gynecologic Oncology*. Edinburgh: Churchill Livingstone; 1992:639.

69. Larsson G, Alm P, Gullberg B, et al: Prognostic factors in early invasive carcinoma of the uterine cervix. A clinical, histopathologic, and statistical analysis of 343 cases. *Am J Obstet Gynecol*. 1983;146:145.

70. Inoue T: Prognostic significance of the depth of invasion relating to nodal metastases, parametrial extension, and cell types. A study of 628 cases with stage IB, IIA, and IIB cervical carcinoma. *Cancer*. 1984;54:3035.

71. Guttmann R: Significance of postoperative radiation in carcinoma of the cervix: A 10 year study. *Am J Roentgen Radium Ther Nucl Med*. 1970;108:102.

72. Meigs J: *Radical Hysterectomy with Bilateral Dissection of Pelvic Lymph Nodes: Surgical Treatment of Cancer of the Cervix*. New York: Grune and Stratton; 1954:50.

73. Brunschweig A, Barber H: Surgical treatment of carcinoma of the cervix. *Obstet Gynecol*. 1966;27:21.

74. Tanaka Y, Sawada S, Murata T: Relationship between lymph node metastases and prognosis in patients irradiated postoperatively for carcinoma of the uterine cervix. *Acta Radiol (Oncol)*. 1984;23:455.

75. Wharton JT, Jones HW III, Day TG Jr, et al: Preirradiation celiotomy and extended field irradiation for invasive carcinoma of the cervix. *Obstet Gynecol*. 1977;49:333.

76. Sudarsanam A, Charyulu K, Jea Belinson: Influence of exploratory celiotomy on the management of carcinoma of the cervix: A preliminary report. *Cancer*. 1978;41:1049.

77. Nelson J, Macaset M, Tea LU: The incidence and significance of para-aortic lymph node metastases in late invasive carcinoma of the cervix. *Am J Obstet Gynecol*. 1974;118:749.

78. Piver MS, Chung WS: Prognostic significance of cervical lesion size and pelvic node metastases in cervical carcinoma. *Obstet Gynecol*. 1975;46:507.

79. Piver M, Barlow J: Para-aortic lymphadenectomy in staging patients with advanced local cervical cancer. *Obstet Gynecol*. 1974;43:544.

80. Lagasse L, Creasman W, Shingleton H: Results and complications of operative staging in cervical cancer: Experience of the GOG. *Gynecol Oncol*. 1980;9:90.

81. Berman ML, Keys H, Creasman W, et al: Survival and patterns of recurrence in cervical cancer metastatic to periaortic lymph nodes (a Gynecologic Oncology Group study). *Gynecol Oncol*. 1984;19:8.

82. Welander C, Pierce V, Nori D: Pretreatment laparotomy in carcinoma of the cervix. *Gynecol Oncol*. 1981;12:336.

83. Dewar MA, Hall K, Perchalski J: Cervical cancer screening. Past success and future challenge. *Prim Care*. 1992;19:589.

84. Mandelblatt J, Lawrence WF, Womack SM, et al: Benefits and cost of using HPV testing to screen for cervical cancer. *JAMA*. 2002;287:2372.

85. Kulasingam S, Hughes JP, Kiviat NB, et al: Evaluation of HPV testing in primary screening for cervical abnormalities. *JAMA*. 2002;288:1749.

86. Ferenczy A: Management of the patient with an abnormal Papanicolaou test. Recent developments. *Obstet Gynecol Clin North Am*. 1993;20:189.

87. Fowler J: Screening for cervical cancer: Current terminology, classification, and technique. *Postgrad Med.* 1993;93:57.

88. Luesley DM, Cullimore J, Redman CW, et al: Loop diathermy excision of the cervical transformation zone in patients with abnormal cervical smears. *Br Med J.* 1990;301:343.

89. LoNH Organization: *Inquiry into the Results of Radiotherapy in Cancer of the Uterus.* Stockholm, Sweden: Kungl. Botryckeriet P. A. Norstedt & Soner; 1938.

90. Eifel PJ: Problems with the clinical staging of carcinoma of the cervix. *Semin Radiat Oncol.* 1994;4:1.

91. Horiot J-C, Pigneux J, Pourquier H, et al: Radiotherapy alone in carcinoma of the intact uterine cervix according to G H Fletcher guidelines: A French Cooperative study of 1383 cases. *Int J Radiat Oncol Biol Phys.* 1988;14:605.

92. Lanciano RM, Won M, Hanks GE: A reappraisal of the International Federation of Gynecology and Obstetrics staging system for cervical cancer. A study of patterns of care. *Cancer.* 1992;69:482.

93. Stehman FB, Bundy BN, DiSaia PJ, et al: Carcinoma of the cervix treated with radiation therapy: I. A multi-variate analysis of prognostic variables in the Gynecologic Oncology Group. *Cancer.* 1991;67:2776.

94. American Joint Committee on Cancer: Cervix uteri. In Fleming ID, Cooper JS, Henson DE, et al, eds: *AJCC Cancer Staging Manual,* 5th ed. Philadelphia: Lippincott-Raven; 1997:189.

95. International Federation of Gynecologists and Obstetricians (FIGO): Changes in the definitions of clinical staging for the cervix and ovary. *Am J Obstet Gynecol.* 1987;56:263.

96. Kim SH, Choi BI, Han JK, et al: Preoperative staging of uterine cervical carcinoma: Comparison of CT and MRI in 99 patients. *J Comput Assist Tomogr.* 1993;17:633.

97. Hawnaur JM, Johnson RJ, Hunter RD, et al: The value of magnetic resonance imaging in assessment of carcinoma of the cervix and its response to radiotherapy. *Clin Oncol (R Coll Radiol).* 1992;4:11.

98. Soeters RP, Beningfield SJ, Dehaeck K, et al: The value of magnetic resonance imaging in patients with carcinoma of the cervix (a pilot study). *Eur J Surg Oncol.* 1991;17:119.

99. Brodman M, Friedman FJ, Dottino P, et al: A comparative study of computerized tomography, magnetic resonance imaging, and clinical staging for the detection of early cervix cancer. *Gynecol Oncol.* 1990;36:409.

100. Schoeppel SL, Ellis JH, LaVigne ML, et al: Magnetic resonance imaging during intracavitary gynecologic brachytherapy. *Int J Radiat Oncol Biol Phys.* 1992;23:169.

101. Hricak H, Lacey CG, Sandles LG, et al: Invasive cervical carcinoma: Comparison of MR imaging and surgical findings. *Radiology.* 1988;166:623.

102. Lanciano RM, Corn BW: The role of surgical staging for cervical cancer. *Semin Radiat Oncol.* 1994;4:46.

103. Grigsby PW, Siegel BA, et al: Lymph node staging by positron emission tomography in patients with carcinoma of the cervix. *J Clin Oncol.* 2001;19:3745.

104. Narayan K, Hicks RJ, et al: A comparison of MRI and PET scanning in surgically staged loco-regionally advanced cervical cancer: Potential impact on treatment. *Int J Gynecol Cancer.* 2001; 11:263.

105. Miller TR, Grigsby PW: Measurement of tumor volume by PET to evaluate prognosis in patients with advanced cervical cancer treated by radiation therapy. *Int J Radiat Oncol Biol Phys.* 2002; 53:353.

106. Maiman M, Fruchter RG, Guy L, et al: Human immunodeficiency virus infection and invasive cervical carcinoma. *Cancer.* 1993;71:402.

107. Schwartz LB, Carcangiu ML, Bradham L, et al: Rapidly progressive squamous cell carcinoma of the cervix coexisting with human immunodeficiency virus infection: Clinical opinion. *Gynecol Oncol.* 1991;41:255.

108. Mandelblatt JS, Fahs M, Garibaldi K, et al: Association between HIV infection and cervical neoplasia: Implications for clinical care of women at risk for both conditions. *AIDS.* 1992;6:173.

109. Perez-Mesa C, Spratt J: Scalene node biopsy in the pretreatment staging of carcinoma of the cervix uteri. *Am J Obstet Gynecol.* 1976;125:93.

110. Ketcham A, Chretien P, Rea Hoye: Occult metastases to the scalene lymph nodes in patients with clinically operable carcinoma of the cervix. *Cancer.* 1973;31:180.

111. Stehman FB, Bundy BN, Hanjani P, et al: Biopsy of the scalene fat pad in carcinoma of the cervix uteri metastatic to the periaortic lymph nodes. *Surg Gyn Obstet.* 1987;165:503.

112. Delgado G, Bundy BN, Fowler WCJ, et al: A prospective surgical pathological study of stage I squamous carcinoma of the cervix: A Gynecologic Oncology Group Study. *Gynecol Oncol.* 1989; 35:314.

113. Stehman FB, Bundy BN: Carcinoma of the cervix treated with chemotherapy and radiation therapy. Cooperative studies in the Gynecologic Oncology Group. *Cancer.* 1993;71:1697.

114. Eifel P: Carcinoma of the Cervix (ASTRO Refresher Course). ASTRO; New Orleans: 1993.

115. Perez CA, Grigsby PW, Nene SM, et al: Effect of tumor size on the prognosis of carcinoma of the uterine cervix treated with irradiation alone. *Cancer.* 1992;69:2796.

116. Ruch R, Pitcock J, Ruch W: Microinvasive carcinoma of the cervix. *Am J Obstet Gynecol.* 1976;125:87.

117. Randall ME, Constable WC, Hahn SS, et al: Results of the radiotherapeutic management of carcinoma of the cervix with emphasis on the influence of histologic classification. *Cancer.* 1988;62:48.

118. Reagan J, Fu Y: Histologic types and prognosis of cancers of the uterine cervix. *Int J Radiat Oncol Biol Phys.* 1979;5:1015.

119. Crissman JD, Budhraja M, Aron BS, et al: Histopathologic prognostic factors in stage II and III squamous cell carcinoma of the uterine cervix. An evaluation of 91 patients treated primarily with radiation therapy. *Int J Gynecol Pathol.* 1987;6:97.

120. Gunderson L, Weems W, Hebertson R, et al: Correlation of histopathology with clinical results following radiation therapy for carcinoma of the cervix. *Am J Roentgen Radium Ther Nucl Med.* 1974;120:74.

121. Kjorstad KE, Bond B: Stage IB adenocarcinoma of the cervix: Metastatic potential and patterns of dissemination. *Am J Obstet Gynecol.* 1984;150:297.

122. Matthews CM, Burke TW, Tornos C, et al: Stage I cervical adenocarcinoma: Prognostic evaluation of surgically treated patients. *Gynecol Oncol.* 1993;49:19.

123. Grigsby PW, Perez CA, Kuske RR, et al: Adenocarcinoma of the uterine cervix: Lack of evidence for a poor prognosis. *Radiother Oncol.* 1988;12:289.

124. Pettersson F: Annual report on the results of treatment in gynecological cancer. *Int J Gynecol Obstet.* 1992;21:27.

125. Alvarez RD, Soong SJ, Kinney WK, et al: Identification of prognostic factors and risk groups in patients found to have nodal metastasis at the time of radical hysterectomy for early-stage squamous carcinoma of the cervix. *Gynecol Oncol.* 1989;35:130.

126. Benedetti Panici P, Di Roberto PF, Greggi S, et al: Squamous cervical cancer at stage IB and II: A ten year experience, analysis of 231 cases. *Eur J Gynecol Oncol.* 1987;8:76.

127. Calais G, Le FO, Chauvet B, et al: Carcinoma of the uterine cervix stage IB and early stage II. Prognostic value of the histological tumor regression after initial brachytherapy. *Int J Radiat Oncol Biol Phys.* 1989;17:1231.

128. Davis JR, Aristizabal S, Way DL, et al: DNA ploidy, grade and stage in prognosis of uterine cervical cancer. *Gynecol Oncol.* 1989;32:4.

129. Delgado G, Bundy B, Zaino R, et al: Prospective surgical-pathological study of disease-free interval in patients with stage IB squamous cell carcinoma of the cervix: A Gynecologic Oncology Group study. *Gynecol Oncol.* 1990;38:352.

130. Heller PB, Malfetano JH, Bundy BN, et al: Clinical-pathologic study of stage IIb, III and IVa carcinoma of the cervix: Extended diagnostic evaluation for para-aortic node metastasis—A GOG study. *Gynecol Oncol.* 1990;38:425.

131. Kapp DS, Fischer D, Gutierrez E, et al: Pretreatment prognostic factors in carcinoma of the uterine cervix: A multivariable analysis of the effect of age, stage, histology and blood counts on survival. *Int J Radiat Oncol Biol Phys.* 1983;9:445.

132. Shelton D, Paturzo D, Flannery J, et al: Race, stage disease of, and survival with cervical cancer. *Ethn Dis.* 1992;2:47.

133. Coia L, Won M, Lanciano R, et al: The Patterns of Care Outcome Study for cancer of the uterine cervix. Results of the Second National Practice Survey. *Cancer.* 1990;66:2451.

134. Baltzer J, Koepcke W: Tumor size and lymph node metastases in squamous cell carcinoma of the uterine cervix. *Arch Gynecol.* 1979;227:271.

135. Berman ML, Bergen S, Salazar H: Influence of histological features and treatment on the prognosis of patients with cervical cancer metastatic to pelvic lymph nodes. *Gynecol Oncol.* 1990; 39:127.

136. Bonanno JP, Boyce J, Fruchter R, et al: Involvement of para-aortic lymph nodes in carcinoma of the cervix. *J Am Osteopath Assoc.* 1980;79:567.

137. Burnett AF, Barnes WA, Johnson JC, et al: Prognostic significance of polymerase chain reaction detected human papillomavirus of tumors and lymph nodes in surgically treated stage IB cervical cancer. *Gynecol Oncol.* 1992;47:343.

138. Chung CK, Nahhas WA, Zaino R, et al: Histologic grade and lymph node metastasis in squamous cell carcinoma of the cervix. *Gynecol Oncol.* 1981;12:348.

139. Giaroli A, Sananes C, Sardi JE, et al: Lymph node metastases in carcinoma of the cervix uteri: Response to neoadjuvant chemotherapy and its impact on survival. *Gynecol Oncol.* 1990; 39:34.

140. Inoue T, Morita K: The prognostic significance of number of positive nodes in cervical carcinoma stages IB, IIA, and IIB. *Cancer.* 1990;65:1923.

141. Lanza A, Re A, D'Addato F, et al: Lymph nodal metastases and pathological patterns in cervical cancer: A critical review. *Eur J Gynecol Oncol.* 1989;10:3.

142. Schafer A, Friedmann W, Mielke M, et al: The increased frequency of cervical dysplasia-neoplasia in women infected with the human immunodeficiency virus is related to the degree of immunosuppression. *Am J Obstet Gynecol.* 1991;164:593.

143. Tinga DJ, Timmer PR, Bouma J, et al: Prognostic significance of single versus multiple lymph node metastases in cervical carcinoma stage IB. *Gynecol Oncol.* 1990;39:175.

144. Terada KY, Morley GW, Roberts JA: Stage IB carcinoma of the cervix with lymph node metastases. *Gynecol Oncol.* 1988;31:389.

145. Vigario G, Kurohara SS, George FW: Association of hemoglobin levels before and during radiotherapy with prognosis in uterine cervix cancer. *Radiology.* 1973;106:649.

146. Overgaard J, Bentzen SM, Kolstad P, et al: Misonidazole combined with radiotherapy in the treatment of carcinoma of the uterine cervix. *Int J Radiat Oncol Biol Phys.* 1989;16:1069.

147. Bush RS, Jenkin RD, Allt WE, et al: Definitive evidence for hypoxic cells influencing cure in cancer therapy. *Br J Cancer Suppl.* 1978;37:302.

148. Dische S: Radiotherapy and anaemia: The clinical experience. *Radiother Oncol.* 1991;1:35.

149. Thomas GM: Hypoxia and carcinoma of the cervix. *Semin Radiat Oncol.* 1994;4:9.

150. Bush RS: The significance of anemia in clinical radiation therapy. *Int J Radiat Oncol Biol Phys.* 1986;12:2047.

151. Lowrey GC, Mendenhall WM, Million RR: Stage IB or IIA-B carcinoma of the intact uterine cervix treated with irradiation: A multivariate analysis. *Int J Radiat Oncol Biol Phys.* 1992;24:205.

152. Grimard L, Genest P, Girard A, et al: Prognostic significance of endometrial extension in carcinoma of the cervix. *Gynecol Oncol.* 1988;31:301.

153. Perez CA, Camel HM, Kao MS, et al: Randomized study of preoperative radiation and surgery or irradiation alone in the treatment of stage IB and IIA carcinoma of the uterine cervix: Final report. *Gynecol Oncol.* 1987;27:129.

154. Dattoli MJ, Gretz HF, Beller U, et al: Analysis of multiple prognostic factors in patients with stage IB cervical cancer: Age as a major determinant. *Int J Radiat Oncol Biol Phys.* 1989;17:41.

155. Lanciano RM, Martz K, Montana GS, et al: Influence of age, prior abdominal surgery, fraction size, and dose on complications after radiation therapy for squamous cell cancer of the uterine cervix. A Patterns of Care study. *Cancer.* 1992;69:2124.

156. Prempree T, Patanaphan V, Sewchand W, et al: The influence of patients' age and tumor grade on the prognosis of carcinoma of the cervix. *Cancer.* 1983;51:1764.

157. Kaplan M: Investigation of age as a prognostic factor in early stage invasive cancer of the cervix: Implications for nursing. *Cancer Nurs.* 1989;12:177.

158. Robertson D, Fedorkow DM, Stuart GC, et al: Age is prognostic variable in cervical squamous cell carcinoma. *Eur J Gynecol Oncol.* 1993;14:283.

159. Spanos WJJ, King A, Keeney E, et al: Age as a prognostic factor in carcinoma of the cervix. *Gynecol Oncol.* 1989;35:66.

160. Stehman FB, Bundy BN, Keys H, et al: A randomized trial of hydroxyurea versus misonidazole adjunct to radiation therapy in carcinoma of the cervix. A preliminary report of a Gynecologic Oncology Group study. *Am J Obstet Gynecol.* 1988;159:87. See comments.

161. Lanciano RM, Won M, Coia LR, et al: Pretreatment and treatment factors associated with improved outcome in squamous cell carcinoma of the uterine cervix: A final report of the 1973 and 1978 Patterns of Care studies. *Int J Radiat Oncol Biol Phys.* 1991;20:667.

162. Strang P, Stendahl U, Bergstrom R, et al: Prognostic flow cytometric information in cervical squamous cell carcinoma: A multivariate analysis of 307 patients. *Gynecol Oncol.* 1991;43:3.

163. Nguyen HN, Sevin BU, Averette HE, et al: The role of DNA index as a prognostic factor in early cervical carcinoma. *Gynecol Oncol.* 1993;50:54.

164. Leminen A, Paavonen J, Forss M, et al: Adenocarcinoma of the uterine cervix. *Cancer.* 1990;65:53.

165. Sorensen FB, Bichel P, Jakobsen A: DNA level and stereologic estimates of nuclear volume in squamous cell carcinomas of the uterine cervix. A comparative study with analysis of prognostic impact. *Cancer.* 1992;69:187.

166. Braly SP: The current status of flow cytometry in gynecologic oncology. *Oncology.* 1992;6:23.

167. Connor JP, Miller DS, Bauer KD, et al: Flow cytometric evaluation of early invasive cervical cancer. *Obstet Gynecol.* 1993;81:367.

168. Kenter GG, Cornelisse CJ, Aartsen EJ, et al: DNA ploidy level as prognostic factor in low stage carcinoma of the uterine cervix. *Gynecol Oncol.* 1990;39:181.

169. Strang P: Cytogenetic and cytometric analyses in squamous cell carcinoma of the uterine cervix. *Int J Gynecol Pathol.* 1989;8:54.

170. Willen R, Himmelmann A, Langstrom EE, et al: Prospective malignancy grading, flow cytometry DNA-measurements and adjuvant chemotherapy for invasive squamous cell carcinoma of the uterine cervix. *Anticancer Res.* 1993;13:1187.

171. DePriest PD, Nagel JR Jr, Powell DE: Microinvasive cervical cancer. *Clin Obstet Gynecol.* 1990;33:846.

172. Ueki M, Okamoto Y, Misaki O, et al: Conservative therapy for microinvasive carcinoma of the uterine cervix. *Gynecol Oncol.* 1994;53:109.

173. Sevin BU, Nadji M, Averette HE, et al: Microinvasive carcinoma of the cervix. *Cancer.* 1992;70:2121.

174. Johnson N, Lilford RJ, Jones SE, et al: Using decision analysis to calculate the optimum treatment for microinvasive cervical cancer. *Br J Cancer.* 1992;65:717.

175. Schink JC, Lurain JR: Microinvasive cervix cancer. *Int J Gynecol Obstet.* 1991;36:5.

176. Burghardt E, Girardi F, Lahousen M, et al: Microinvasive carcinoma of the uterine cervix (International Federation of Gynecology and Obstetrics Stage IA). *Cancer.* 1991;67:1037.

177. Kolstad P: Follow-up study of 232 patients with stage Ia1 and 411 patients with stage Ia2 squamous cell carcinoma of the cervix (microinvasive carcinoma). *Gynecol Oncol.* 1989;33:265.

178. Popkin DR, Scali V, Ahmed MN: Cryosurgery for the treatment of cervical intraepithelial neoplasia. *Am J Obstet Gynecol.* 1978;130:551.

179. Bryson SCP, Lenehan P, Lickrish GM: The treatment of grade 3 intraepithelial neoplasia with cryotherapy: An 11 year experience. *Am J Obstet Gynecol.* 1985;151:201.

180. Grigsby PW, Perez CA: Radiotherapy alone for medically inoperable carcinoma of the cervix: Stage IA and carcinoma in situ. *Int J Radiat Oncol Biol Phys.* 1991;21:375.

181. Artman LE, Hoskins WJ, Bibro MC, et al: Radical hysterectomy and pelvic lymphadenectomy for stage IB carcinoma of the cervix: 21 years experience. *Gynecol Oncol.* 1987;28:8.

182. Lee Y-N, Wang KL, Lin M-H, et al: Radical hysterectomy with lymph node dissection for treatment of cervical carcinoma: A clinical review of 954 cases. *Gynecol Oncol.* 1989;32:135.

183. Fuller AFJ, Elliott N, Kosloff C, et al: Determinants of increased risk for recurrence in patients undergoing radical hysterectomy for stage IB and IIA carcinoma of the cervix. *Gynecol Oncol.* 1989;33:34.

184. Perez CA, Camel HM, Walz BJ, et al: Radiation therapy alone in the treatment of carcinoma of the cervix: A 20 year experience. *Gynecol Oncol.* 1986;23:127.

185. Montana GS, Fowler WC: Carcinoma of the cervix: Analysis of bladder and rectal radiation dose and complications. *Int J Radiat Oncol Biol Phys*. 1989;16:95.

186. Lanciano RM, Won M, Coja LR, et al: Pretreatment and treatment factors associated with improved outcome in squamous cell carcinoma of the uterine cervix: A final report of the 1973 and 1978 Patterns of Care studies. *Int J Radiat Oncol Biol Phys*. 1990;19(suppl 1):126.

187. Kim RY, Tiort A, Wu CJ, et al: Radiation alone in the treatment of carcinoma of the uterine cervix: Analysis of pelvic failure and dose response relationship. *Int J Radiat Oncol Biol Phys*. 1989;17:973.

188. Kottmeier HL: Annual report on the results of treatment in carcinoma of the uterus, vagina, and ovary. *Gynecol Oncol*. 1976;4:13.

189. Fletcher G: Cancer of the uterine cervix: Janeway lecture. *J Roentgen Radium Ther Nucl Med*. 1971;111:225.

190. Park RC, Patow WE, Rogers RE, Zimmerman EA: Treatment stage I carcinoma of the cervix. *Obstet Gynecol*. 1973;41:117.

191. Morley GW, Seski JC: Radical pelvic surgery vs radiation therapy for stage I carcinoma of the cervix. *Am J Obstet Gynecol*. 1976;125:785.

192. Hoskins WJ, Ford JH, Lutz MH, et al: Radical hysterectomy and pelvic lymphadenectomy for the management of early invasive carcinoma of the cervix. *Gynecol Oncol*. 1976;4:278.

193. Lerner HM, Jones HW, EC Hill: Radical surgical treatment for early invasive cervical carcinoma (stage Ib): Review of 15 years' experience. *Obstet Gynecol*. 1980;56:413.

194. Powell JL, Burrell MO, Franklin EW: Radical hysterectomy and pelvic lymphadenectomy. *South Med J*. 1984;77:596.

195. Kenter GG, Ansink AC, Heintz AP, et al: Carcinoma of the uterine cervix stage I and IIA: Results of surgical treatment: Complications, recurrence and survival. *Eur J Surg Oncol*. 1989;15:55.

196. Hopkins MP, Morley GW: Radical hysterectomy versus radiation therapy for stage IB squamous cell cancer of the cervix. *Cancer*. 1991;68:272.

197. Averette HE, Nguyen HN, Donato DM, et al: Radical hysterectomy for invasive cervical cancer. A 25-year prospective experience with the Miami technique. *Cancer*. 1993;71:1422.

198. Montana GS, Fowler WC, Varai MA, et al: Analysis of results of radiation therapy for stage Ib cervix carcinoma. *Cancer*. 1987;60:2195.

199. Fletcher GH: Squamous cell cancer of the uterine cervix. In Fletcher GH, ed. *Textbook of Radiotherapy*. Philadelphia: Lea & Febiger; 1980:726.

200. Hanks G, Kerring D, Kramer S: Patterns of Care outcome studies: Results of the national practice in cancer of the cervix. *Cancer*. 1983;51:959.

201. Eifel PJ, Morris M, Wharton JT, et al: The influence of tumor size and morphology on the outcome of patients with FIGO stage IB squamous cell carcinoma of the uterine cervix. *Int J Radiat Oncol Biol Phys*. 1994;29:9.

202. Mendenhall WM, Sombeck MD, Freeman DE, et al: Stage IB and IIA-B carcinoma of the intact uterine cervix: Impact of tumor volume and the role of adjuvant hysterectomy. *Semin Radiat Oncol*. 1994;4:16.

203. Montana GS, Martz KL, Hanks GE: Patterns and sites of failure in cervix cancer treated in the U.S.A. in 1978. *Int J Radiat Oncol Biol Phys*. 1991;20:87.

204. Jampolis S, Andras J, Fletcher G: Analysis of sites and causes of failures of irradiation in invasive SCC of the intact uterine cervix. *Radiology*. 1975;15:681.

205. Perez C, Breaux S, Madoc-Jones H: Radiation therapy alone in the treatment of carcinoma of the uterine cervix: Analysis of tumor recurrence. *Cancer*. 1983;51:1393.

206. Perez CA, Fox S, Lockett MA, et al: Impact of dose in outcome of irradiation alone in carcinoma of the uterine cervix: Analysis of two different methods. *Int J Radiat Oncol Biol Phys*. 1991;21:885.

207. Eifel PJ, Thoms WWJ, Smith TL, et al: The relationship between brachytherapy dose and outcome in patients with bulky endocervical tumors treated with radiation alone. *Int J Radiat Oncol Biol Phys*. 1994;28:113.

208. Steren A, Nguyen HN, Averette HE, et al: Radical hysterectomy for stage IB adenocarcinoma of the cervix: The University of Miami experience. *Gynecologic Oncology*. 1993;48:355. Review.

209. Landoni F, Maneo A, Colombo A et al: Randomized study of radical surgery versus radiotherapy for stage IB-IIA cervical cancer. *Lancet*. 1997;350:535.

210. Hamberger A, Unal A, Gershenson D, et al: Analysis of the severe complications of irradiation of carcinoma of the cervix: Whole pelvis irradiation and intracavitary radium. *Int J Radiat Oncol Biol Phys*. 1983;9:367.

211. Rutledge F, Wharton J, Fletcher G: Clinical studies with adjunctive surgery and irradiation in the treatment of carcinoma of the cervix. *Cancer*. 1976;38:596.

212. O'Quinn A, Fletcher G, Whartton J: Guidelines for conservative hysterectomy after irradiation. *Gynecol Oncol*. 1980;9:68.

213. Mendenhall WM, McCarty PJ, Morgan LS, et al: Stage IB or IIA-B carcinoma of the intact uterine cervix greater than or equal to 6 cm in diameter: Is adjuvant extrafascial hysterectomy beneficial? *Int J Radiat Oncol Biol Phys*. 1991;21:899.

214. Perez CA, Kao MS: Radiation therapy alone or combined with surgery in the treatment of barrel-shaped carcinoma of the uterine cervix (stages IB, IIA, IIB). *Int J Radiat Oncol Biol Phys*. 1985;11:1903.

215. Thoms WWJ, Eifel PJ, Smith TL, et al: Bulky endocervical carcinoma: A 23-year experience. *Int J Radiat Oncol Biol Phys*. 1992;23:491. See comments.

216. Bloss JD, Berman ML, Mukhererjee J, et al: Bulky stage IB cervical carcinoma managed by primary radical hysterectomy followed by tailored radiotherapy. *Gynecol Oncol*. 1992;47:21.

217. Keys HM, Bundy BN, et al: Cisplatin, radiation, and adjuvant hysterectomy compared with radiation and adjuvant hysterectomy for bulky stage IB cervical carcinoma. *N Engl J Med*. 1999;340:1154.

218. Nag S, Chao C, Enickson B, et al: The American Brachytherapy Society recommendations for low-dose-rate brachytherapy for carcinoma of the cervix. *Int J Radiat Oncol Biol Phys*. 2002;52:33.

219. Haie C, Pejovic MH, Gerbaulet A, et al: Is prophylactic para-aortic irradiation worthwhile in the treatment of advanced cervical carcinoma? Results of a controlled clinical trial of the EORTC radiotherapy group. *Radiother Oncol*. 1988;11:101.

220. Rotman M, Choi K, Guse C, et al: Prophylactic irradiation of the para-aortic lymph node chain in stage IIB and bulky stage IB carcinoma of the cervix, initial treatment results of RTOG 7920. *Int J Radiat Oncol Biol Phys*. 1990;19:513. See comments. Published erratum appears in *Int J Radiat Oncol Biol Phys*. 1991;20:193.

221. Morris M, Eifel PJ, et al: Pelvic radiation with concurrent chemotherapy compared with pelvic and para-aortic radiation for high-risk cervical cancer. *N Engl J Med*. 1999;340:1137.

222. Lanciano RM, Martz K, Coia LR, et al: Tumor and treatment factors improving outcome in stage III-B cervix cancer. *Int J Radiat Oncol Biol Phys*. 1991;20:95.

223. Perez CA: Radiation therapy in the management of cancer of the cervix. *Oncology (Huntingt)*. 1993;7:89.

224. Kim RY, Trotti A, Wu CJ, et al: Radiation alone in the treatment of cancer of the uterine cervix: Analysis of pelvic failure and dose response relationship. *Int J Radiat Oncol Biol Phys*. 1989;17:973.

225. Heller PB, Maletano JH, Bundy BN, et al: Clinical-pathologic study of stage IIB, III, and IVA carcinoma of the cervix: Extended diagnostic evaluation for paraaortic node metastasis—a Gynecologic Oncology Group study. *Gynecol Oncol*. 1990;38:425.

226. Kraiphibul P, Srisupundit S, Pairachvet V, et al: Results of treatment in stage IIB squamous cell carcinoma of the uterine cervix: Comparison between two and one intracavitary insertion. *Gynecol Oncol*. 1992;45:160.

227. Kovalic JJ, Perez CA, Grigsby PW, et al: The effect of volume of disease in patients with carcinoma of the uterine cervix. *Int J Radiat Oncol Biol Phys*. 1991;21:905.

228. Montana G, Fowler W, Varia M, et al: Carcinoma of the cervix, stage III: Results of radiation therapy. *Cancer*. 1986;57:148.

229. Kavadi VS, Eifel PJ: FIGO stage IIIA carcinoma of the uterine cervix. *Int J Radiat Oncol Biol Phys*. 1992;24:211.

230. Perez C, Slessinger E, Grigsby P: Design of an afterloading vaginal applicator (MIRALVA). *Int J Radiat Oncol Biol Phys*. 1990;18:1503.

231. Cardinale JG, Peschel RE, Gutierrez E, et al: Stage IIIA carcinoma of the uterine cervix. *Gynecol Oncol*. 1986;23:199.

232. Aramburo P, Otero J, Paredes MC: Stage III carcinoma of the cervix treated with whole pelvis irradiation and four brachytherapy applications. *Int J Radiat Oncol Biol Phys*. 1981;7:403.

233. Averette HE, Jobson VW: Current concepts in cancer: Updated cervix cancer. Stages III and IV. The role of exploratory laparotomy in the staging and treatment of invasive cervical carcinoma. *Int J Radiat Oncol Biol Phys.* 1979;5:2137.

234. Hiilesmaa VK, Vesterinen E, Nieminen U, et al: Carcinoma of the uterine cervix stage III: A report of 311 cases. *Gynecol Oncol.* 1981;12:99.

235. Souhami L, Melo JA, Pareja G: The treatment of stage III carcinoma of the uterine cervix with telecobalt irradiation. *Gynecol Oncol.* 1987;28:262.

236. Kramer C, Peschel RE, Goldberg N, et al: Radiation treatment of FIGO stage IVA carcinoma of the cervix. *Gynecol Oncol.* 1989; 32:323.

237. Million R, Rutledge F, Fletcher G: Stage IV carcinoma of the cervix with bladder invasion. *Am J Obstet Gynecol.* 1972; 113:239.

238. Spanos W, Perez C, Marcus S, et al: Effect of rest interval on tumor and normal tissue response: A report of phase III study of accelerated split course palliative radiation for advanced pelvic malignancies (RTOG-8502). *Int J Radiat Oncol Biol Phys.* 1993;25:399.

239. Manetta A, Delgado G, Petrilli E, et al: The significance of paraaortic node status in carcinoma of the cervix and endometrium. *Gynecol Oncol.* 1986;23:284.

240. Malfetano JH, Keys H: Aggressive multimodality treatment for cervical cancer with paraaortic lymph node metastases. *Gynecol Oncol.* 1991;42:44.

241. MacLeod C, Bernshaw D, Leung S, et al: Accelerated hyperfractionated radiotherapy for locally advanced cervix cancer. *Int J Radiat Oncol Biol Phys.* 1999;44:519.

242. Grigsby PW, Lu JD, Mutch DG, et al: Twice-daily fractionation of external irradiation with brachytherapy and chemotherapy in carcinoma of the cervix with positive para-aortic lymph nodes: Phase II study of the Radiation Therapy Oncology Group 92-10. *Int J Radiat Oncol Biol Phys.* 1998;41:817.

243. Grigsby PW, Heydon K, Mutch DG, et al: Long-term follow-up of RTOG 92-10: Cervical cancer with positive para-aortic lymph nodes. *Int J Radiat Oncol Biol Phys.* 2001;51:982.

244. Varia MA, Bundy BN, Deppe G, et al: Cervical carcinoma metastatic to para-aortic nodes: Extended field radiation therapy with concomitant 5-fluorouracil and cisplatin chemotherapy: A Gynecologic Oncology Group study. *Int J Radiat Oncol Biol Phys.* 1998;42:1015.

245. Piver MS: Is there a role for adjuvant chemotherapy in cervical cancer? *J Clin Oncol.* 1985;3:899.

246. Hreschyshyn M, Aron B, Boronow R: Hydroxyurea or placebo combined with radiation to treat stages IIIB/IVA cervical cancer confined to the pelvis. *Int J Radiat Oncol Biol Phys.* 1979;5:317.

247. Grigsby PW: Lack of proven efficacy of chemotherapy for patients with carcinoma of the uterine cervix. *Semin Radiat Oncol.* 1994;4:30.

248. Leibel S, Bauer M, Wasserman T, et al: Radiotherapy with or without misonidazole for patients with stage IIIB or stage IVA squamous cell carcinoma of the uterine cervix: Preliminary report of a Radiation Therapy Oncology Group randomized trial. *Int J Radiat Oncol Biol Phys.* 1987;13:541.

249. Stehman F, Bundy B: Carcinoma of the cervix treated with chemotherapy and radiation therapy: Cooperative studies in the GOG. *Cancer.* 1993;71:1697.

250. Bonomi P, Blessing J, Stehman F: A randomized trial of three cisplatinum dose schedules in SCC of the uterine cervix. *J Clin Oncol.* 1985;3:1079.

251. Alberts DS, Kronmal R, Baker LH, et al: Phase II randomized trial of cisplatin chemotherapy regimens in the treatment of recurrent or metastatic squamous cell cancer of the cervix. *J Clin Oncol.* 1987;5:1791.

252. Wong L, Choo Y, Choy DT: Long term follow-up of potentiation of radiotherapy by cis-platinum in advanced cervical cancer. *Gynecol Oncol.* 1989;35:159.

253. Choo Y, Choy DT, Wong L: Potentiation of radiotherapy by cis-DDP (II) in advanced cervical carcinoma. *Gynecol Oncol.* 1986;23:94.

254. Souhami L, Seymour R, Roman TN, et al: Weekly cisplatin plus external beam radiotherapy and high dose rate brachytherapy in patients with locally advanced carcinoma of the cervix. *Int J Radiat Oncol Biol Phys.* 1993;27:871.

255. Mickiewicz E, Roth B, Alvarez A: Chemotherapy and radiotherapy vs. radiotherapy alone in cervical cancer stage IIA-IVA, a randomized study. *Proc ASCO.* 1991;10:192. Abstract.

256. Cardenas J, Olguin A, Figueroa F, et al: Randomized neoadjuvant chemotherapy in cervical carcinoma stage IIb: PEC + RT versus RT (abstract). *Proc Am Soc Clin Oncol.* 1991;10:620.

257. Souhami L, Gil RA, Allan SE, et al: A randomized trial of chemotherapy followed by pelvic radiation therapy in stage IIIB carcinoma of the cervix. *J Clin Oncol.* 1991;9:970.

258. Tattersall MH, Ramirez C, Coppleson M: A randomized trial of adjuvant chemotherapy after radical hysterectomy in stage Ib-IIa cervical cancer patients with pelvic lymph node metastases. *Gynecol Oncol.* 1992;46:176.

259. Whitney CW, Sause W, Bundy BN, et al: Randomized comparison of fluorouracil plus cisplatin versus hydroxyurea as an adjunct to radiation therapy in stage IIB-IVA carcinoma of the cervix with negative para-aortic lymph nodes: A Gynecologic Oncology Group and Southwest Oncology Group study. *J Clin Oncol.* 1999;17:1339.

260. Emami B, Scott C, Perez CA, et al: Phase III study of interstitial thermoradiotherapy compared with interstitial radiotherapy alone in the treatment of recurrent or persistent human tumors. A prospectively controlled randomized study by the Radiation Therapy Group. *Int J Radiat Oncol Biol Phys.* 1996;34:1097.

261. van der Zee J, Gonzalez D, van Rhoon GC, et al. Comparison of radiotherapy alone with radiotherapy plus hyperthermia in locally advanced pelvic tumors: A prospective, randomized, multicentre trial. Dutch Deep Hyperthermia Group. *Lancet.* 2000;355:1119.

262. Hoskins WJ: Prognostic factors for risk of recurrence in stages Ib and IIa cervical cancer. *Baillieres Clin Obstet Gynecol.* 1988; 2:817.

263. Shingleton HM, Soong SJ, Gelder MS, et al: Clinical and histopathologic factors predicting recurrence and survival after pelvic exenteration for cancer of the cervix. *Obstet Gynecol.* 1989;73:1027.

264. Smiley LM, Burke TW, Silva EG, et al: Prognostic factors in stage IB squamous cervical cancer patients with low risk for recurrence. *Obstet Gynecol.* 1991;77:271.

265. Soisson AP, Soper JT, Clarke A, et al: Adjuvant radiotherapy following radical hysterectomy for patients with stage IB and IIA cervical cancer. *Gynecol Oncol.* 1990;37:390.

266. Sedlis A, Bundy BN, Rotman MZ, et al: A randomized trial of pelvic radiation therapy versus no further therapy in selected patients with stage IB carcinoma of the cervix after radical hysterectomy and pelvic lymphadenectomy: A Gynecologic Oncology Group Study. *Gynecol Oncol.* 1999;73:177.

267. Peters WA III, Liu PY, Barrett RJ, et al: Concurrent chemotherapy and pelvic radiation therapy compared with pelvic radiation therapy alone as adjuvant therapy after radical surgery in high-risk early-stage cancer of the cervix." *J Clin Oncol.* 2000;18:1606.

268. Petersen LK, Mamsen A, Jakobsen A: Carcinoma of the cervical stump. *Gynecol Oncol.* 1992;46:199.

269. Goodman HM, Niloff JM, Buttlar CA, et al: Adenocarcinoma of the cervical stump. *Gynecol Oncol.* 1989;35:188.

270. Kovalic JJ, Grigsby PW, Perez CA, et al: Cervical stump carcinoma. *Int J Radiat Oncol Biol Phys.* 1991;20:933.

271. Barillot I, Horiot JC, Cuisenier J, et al: Carcinoma of the cervical stump: A review of 213 cases. *Eur J Cancer.* 1993;29A:1231.

272. Burger MP, Wilterdink JB: Age at first pregnancy and the viral etiology of cervical neoplasia. *Acta Obstet Gynecol Scand.* 1988;67:689.

273. Duggan B, Muderspach LI, Roman LD, et al: Cervical cancer in pregnancy: Reporting on planned delay in therapy. *Obstet Gynecol.* 1993;82:598.

274. Hopkins MP, Morley GW: The prognosis and management of cervical cancer associated with pregnancy. *Obstet Gynecol.* 1992;80:9.

275. Monk BJ, Montz FJ: Invasive cervical cancer complicating intrauterine pregnancy: Treatment with radical hysterectomy. *Obstet Gynecol.* 1992;80:199.

276. Sivanesaratnam V, Jayalakshmi P, Loo C: Surgical management of early invasive cancer of the cervix associated with pregnancy. *Gynecol Oncol.* 1993;48:68.

277. Roman LD, Morris M, Eifel PJ, et al: Reasons for inappropriate simple hysterectomy in the presence of invasive cancer of the cervix. *Obstet Gynecol.* 1992;79:485.

278. Orr J, Ball G, Soong S, et al: Surgical treatment of women found to have invasive cervix cancer at the time of total hysterectomy. *Obstet Gynecol.* 1986;68:353.

279. Roman LD, Morris M, Mitchell MF, et al: Prognostic factors for patients undergoing simple hysterectomy in the presence of invasive cancer of the cervix. *Gynecol Oncol.* 1993;50:179.

280. Davy M, Bentzen H, Jahren R: Simple hysterectomy in the presence of invasive cervical cancer. *Acta Obstet Gynecol Scand.* 1977;56:105.

281. Barber H, Pece G, Brunschwig A: Operative management of patients previously operated on for benign lesion with a cervical cancer as a surprise finding. *Am J Obstet Gynecol.* 1968;101:960.

282. Piver M, Rutledge F, Smith J: Five classes of extended radical hysterectomy for women with cervical cancer. *Obstet Gynecol.* 1974;44:265.

283. Russell AH: Contemporary radiation treatment planning for patients with cancer of the uterine cervix. *Semin Oncol.* 1994;21:30.

284. Roeske JC, Lujan A, Rotmensch J, et al: Intensity-modulated whole pelvic radiation therapy in patients with gynecologic malignancies. *Int J Radiat Oncol Biol Phys.* 2000;48:1613.

285. Mundt AJ, Lujan AE, Rotmensch J, et al: Intensity-modulated whole pelvic radiotherapy in women with gynecologic malignancies. *Int J Radiat Oncol Biol Phys.* 2002;52:1330.

286. Portelance L, Chao KS, Grigsby PW, et al: Intensity-modulated radiation therapy (IMRT) reduces small bowel, rectum, and bladder doses in patients with cervical cancer receiving pelvic and para-aortic irradiation. *Int J Radiat Oncol Biol Phys.* 2001;51:261.

287. Low DA, Grigsby PW, Dempsey JF, et al: Applicator-guided intensity-modulated radiation therapy. *Int J Radiat Oncol Biol Phys.* 2002;52:1400.

288. Haas JS, Dean RD, Mansfield CM: Dosimetric comparison of the Fletcher family of gynecologic colpostats, 1950-1980. *Int J Radiat Oncol Biol Phys.* 1985;11:1317.

289. Clarke PDL, Olt G: Thromboembolism in patients with GYN tumors: Risk factors, natural history, and prophylaxis. *Oncology (Williston Park).* 1989;3:39.

290. Clarke PDL, DeLong ER, Synan IS, et al: Variables associated with postoperative deep venous thrombosis: A prospective study of 411 gynecology patients and creation of a prognostic model. *Obstet Gynecol.* 1987;69:146.

291. Perez CA, Breaux S, Bedwinek JM, et al: Radiation therapy alone in the treatment of carcinoma of the uterine cervix: II. Analysis of complications. *Cancer.* 1984;54:235.

292. Clark-Pearson DL, DeLong E, Synan IS, et al: A controlled trial of two low-dose heparin regimens for the prevention of postoperative deep vein thrombosis. *Obstet Gynecol.* 1990;75:684.

293. Clark-Pearson DL, DeLong ER, Synan IS, et al: Complications of low-dose heparin prophylaxis in gynecologic oncology surgery. *Obstet Gynecol.* 1984;64:689.

294. Dose and volume specifications for reporting intracavitary therapy in gynecology. ICRU Report #38; 1985.

295. Khan F: Brachytherapy: Rules of implantation and dose specification. In Levitt SH, Khan FM, Potish RA, eds. *Levitt and Tapley's Technological Basis of Radiation Therapy: Practical Clinical Applications.* Philadelphia: Lea & Febiger; 1992:113.

296. Tod MC, Meredith WJ: A dosage system for use in the treatment of cancer of the uterine cervix. *Br J Radiol.* 1938;11:809.

297. Tod MC, Meredith WJ: Treatment of cancer of the cervix uteri: A revised "Manchester" method. *Br J Radiol.* 1953;26:252.

298. Potish RA: Cervix cancer. In Levitt SH, Khan FM, Potish RA, eds. *Levitt and Tapley's Technological Basis of Radiation Therapy: Practical Clinical Applications.* Philadelphia: Lea & Febiger; 1992:289.

299. Pourquier H, Dubois JB, Delard R: Cancer of the uterine cervix: Dosimetric guidelines for prevention of late rectal and rectosigmoid complications as a result of radiotherapeutic treatment. *Int J Rad Oncol Biol Phys.* 1982;8:1887.

300. Crook JM, Esche BA, Chaplain G, et al: Dose-volume analysis and the prevention of radiation sequelae in cervical cancer. *Radiother Oncol.* 1987;8:321.

301. Swift PS, Purser P, Roberts LW, et al: Pulsed low dose rate brachytherapy for pelvic malignancies. *Int J Radiat Oncol Biol Phys.* 1997;37:811.

302. Rogers CL, Freel JH, Speiser BL, et al: Pulsed low dose rate brachytherapy for uterine cervix carcinoma. *Int J Radiat Oncol Biol Phys.* 1999;43:95.

303. Measurements, International Commission on Radiation Units and Measurements. *Report #58: Dose and Volume Specifications for Reporting Interstitial Therapy.* Bethesda, Md: International Commission on Radiation Units and Measurements; 1997.

304. Demanes DJ, Rodriguez RR, Bendre DD, et al. High dose rate transperineal interstitial brachytherapy for cervical cancer: High pelvic control and low complication rates. *Int J Radiat Oncol Biol Phys.* 1999;45:105.

305. Perez CA, Grigsby PW, Castro-Vita H, et al: Impact of prolongation of irradiation and tumor size in carcinoma of the uterine cervix. *Int J Radiat Oncol Biol Phys.* 1994;30:191.

306. Lanciano RM, Pajak TF, Martz K, et al: The influence of treatment time on outcome for squamous cell cancer of the uterine cervix treated with radiation: A Patterns-of-Care study. *Int J Radiat Oncol Biol Phys.* 1993;25:391.

307. Magrina JF: Complications of irradiation and radical surgery for gynecologic malignancies. *Obstet Gynecol Surv.* 1993;48:571.

308. Perez CA, Grigsby PW, et al: Radiation therapy morbidity in carcinoma of the uterine cervix: Dosimetric and clinical correlation. *Int J Radiat Oncol Biol Phys.* 1999;44:855.

309. Strockbine MF, Hancock JE, Fletcher GH: Complications in 831 patients with SCC of the intact uterine cervix treated with 3000 rads or more whole pelvis irradiation. *Am J Roentgen Radium Ther Nucl Med.* 1970;108:293.

310. Cunningham MJ, Dunton CJ, Corn B, et al: Extended-field radiation therapy in early-stage cervical carcinoma: Survival and complications. *Gynecol Oncol.* 1991;43:51.

311. Gaspar LE, Cheung AY, Allen HH: Cervical carcinoma: Treatment results and complications of extended-field irradiation. *Radiology.* 1989;172:271.

312. Sinistrero G, Sismondi P, Rumore A, et al: Analysis of complications of cervix carcinoma treated by radiotherapy using the Franco-Italian glossary. *Radiother Oncol.* 1993;26:203.

313. Komaki R, Pajak TF, Marcial VA, et al: Twice-daily fractionation of external irradiation with brachytherapy in bulky carcinoma of the cervix. Phase I/II study of the Radiation Therapy Oncology Group 88-05. *Cancer.* 1994;73:2619.

314. van Kasteren YM, Burger CW, Meijer OW, et al: Efficacy of a synthetic mesh sling in keeping the small bowel in the upper abdomen to prevent radiation enteropathy in gynecologic malignancies. *Eur J Obst Gynecol Reprod Biol.* 1993;50:211.

315. Devereux DF, Kavanah MT, Feldman MI, et al: Small bowel exclusion from the pelvis by a polyglycolic acid mesh sling. *J Surg Oncol.* 1984;26:107.

316. Rodier JF, Janser JC, Rodier D, et al: Prevention of radiation enteritis by an absorbable polyglycolic acid mesh sling. A 60-case multicentric study. *Cancer.* 1991;68:2545.

317. Potish RA, Twiggs LB, Prem KA, et al: The impact of extraperitoneal surgical staging on morbidity and tumor recurrence following radiotherapy for cervical carcinoma. *Am J Clin Oncol.* 1984;7:245.

318. Weiser EB, Bundy BN, Hoskins WJ, et al: Extraperitoneal versus transperitoneal selective paraaortic lymphadenectomy in the pretreatment surgical staging of advanced cervical carcinoma (a Gynecologic Oncology Group study). *Gynecol Oncol.* 1989;33:283.

319. Nori D, Valentine E, Hilaris BS: The role of paraaortic node irradiation in the treatment of cancer of the cervix. *Int J Radiat Oncol Biol Phys.* 1985;11:1469.

320. Clarke PDL, Synan IS, Creasman WT: Anticoagulation therapy for venous thromboembolism in patients with gynecologic malignancy. *Am J Obstet Gynecol.* 1983;147:369.

321. Clarke PDL, Synan IS, Hinshaw WM, et al: Prevention of postoperative venous thromboembolism by external pneumatic calf compression in patients with gynecologic malignancy. *Obstet Gynecol.* 1984;63:92.

322. Pettersson F, Fotiou S, Einhorn N, et al: Cohort study of the long-term effect of radiation for carcinoma of the uterine cervix. Second primary malignancies in the pelvic organs in women irradiated for cervical carcinoma at Radiumhemmet 1914-1965. *Acta Radiol Oncol.* 1985;24:145.

323. Lee JY, Perez CA, Ettinger N, et al: The risk of second primaries subsequent to irradiation for cervix cancer. *Int J Radiat Oncol Biol Phys.* 1982;8:207.

324. Kapp DS, Fischer D, Grady KJ, et al: Subsequent malignancies associated with carcinoma of the uterine cervix: Including an analysis of the effect of patient and treatment parameters on incidence and sites of metachronous malignancies. *Int J Radiat Oncol Biol Phys.* 1982;8:197.
325. Rabkin CS, Biggar RJ, Melbye M, et al: Second primary cancers following anal and cervical carcinoma: Evidence for shared etiologic factors. *Am J Epidem.* 1992;136:54.
326. Storm HH: Second primary cancer after treatment for cervical cancer: Late effects after radiotherapy. *Cancer.* 1988;61:679.
327. Rubin P, Constine LS, Fajardo LF, et al: Overview of late effects normal tissues (LENT) scoring system. *Radiother Oncol.* 1995;35:9.
328. Pavy J-J, Denekemp J, Letscher J: Late effects toxicity scoring: The SOMA scale. *Radiother Oncol.* 1995;35:11.
329. Inoue T, Okumura M: Prognostic significance of parametrial extension in patients with cervical carcinoma stages IB, IIA, and IIB. A study of 628 cases treated by radical hysterectomy and lymphadenectomy with or without postoperative irradiation. *Cancer.* 1984;54:1714.
330. Perez CA, Grigsby PW, Camel HM, et al: Irradiation alone or combined with surgery in stage IB, IIA, and IIB carcinoma of uterine cervix: Update of a nonrandomized comparison. *Int J Radiat Oncol Biol Phys.* 1995;31:703.
331. Komaki R, Brickner TJ, Hanlon AL, et al: Long-term results of treatment of cervical carcinoma in the US in 1973, 1978, and 1983: Patterns of Care Study (PCS). *Int J Radiat Oncol Biol Phys.* 1995;31:973.
332. Kavadi VS, Eifel PJ: FIGO stage IIIA carcinoma of the uterine cervix. *Int J Radiat Oncol Biol Phys.* 1992;24:211.

Cancer of the Endometrium

49

Kaled M. Alektiar, MD, and Dattatreyudu Nori, MD

EPIDEMIOLOGY

Endometrial cancer is the most common gynecologic cancer and the fourth most frequently diagnosed cancer in women in the United States. According to the 2003 cancer statistics, the estimated number of newly diagnosed cases is 40,100, with a probability of 1 of every 37 women (2.7%) developing it during their lifetime.[1] Endometrial cancer occurs most commonly in postmenopausal women, although 25% of cases occur in women before menopause and 5% in patients younger than 40 years of age.[2] Worldwide, the incidence of endometrial cancer is higher in North America and Western Europe than in developing countries and Japan. Immigrant populations generally assume the risk of native ones, reflecting the importance of environmental factors in this disease. In the United States, Caucasian women have a twofold higher risk of developing this disease than African-American women, and it is more common among urban than rural residents. The expected number of deaths from endometrial cancer in 2003 is 6,800, making it the seventh leading cause of death from cancer in women. According to the Surveillance, Epidemiology, and End Results (SEER) program, there has been a statistically significant decrease in the 5-year relative cancer survival rate from 88% during the 1974-1976 time period to 84% during the 1992-1997 period.[1]

ANATOMY

The uterus is a hollow muscular organ situated in the pelvis between the urinary bladder anteriorly and the rectum posteriorly. Structurally and functionally, it is divided into two parts—the body and the cervix. At the transition between these two, there is a slight narrowing called the isthmus, which is the location of the internal os of the cervix. It is this region that differentiates into the lower uterine segment during parturition. The body of the uterus is made up of three layers—the *endometrium*, consisting of a complex glandular lamina functionalis and a basal layer, which is closely applied to the underlying *myometrium*, consisting of smooth muscle fibers, and the outer *serosa*, which is essentially the visceral peritoneum. The nulliparous uterus is about 7.5 cm long, the upper two thirds (5.0 cm) being the corpus and the lower one third (2.5 cm), the cervix. The uterine cavity is about 6.0 cm in length and the wall is approximately 1.2 cm in thickness. After menopause, the uterus gradually atrophies, the myometrium thins out, and the cavity may be less than 5.0 cm in length, with a markedly attenuated cervix.

The main supports of the uterus are fibromuscular condensations of tissue in the pelvic fascia, namely the broad ligaments, the round ligaments, the uterosacral ligaments, and the transverse or Mackenrodt's cardinal ligaments. The arterial supply is from the paired uterine arteries, which usually arise from the anterior division of the internal iliac arteries. The uterine artery enters the uterine wall at the isthmus, after crossing the ureter, and has free anastomoses with the ovarian and vaginal arteries. The venous drainage follows the arterial supply. There are relatively few lymphatics in the endometrium, but the myometrium and the subserosa have a rich lymphatic network. The uterine body drains primarily to the external and internal iliac lymph nodes, which then drain to the lateral aortic nodes. When the cervix is involved by disease, the pattern of spread of cancer parallels that of cervical cancer. Anastomoses between lymphatics from the body of the uterus and those in the round ligament provide a pathway for the rare metastasis to the inguinal lymph nodes. Similarly, there is a direct pathway for the lymphatics from the fundus of the uterus to the lateral aortic nodes, bypassing the iliac nodes (Fig. 49–1).

RISK FACTORS

The true cause of endometrial cancer remains unknown. However, it is safe to say that in a large proportion of patients, the cancer seems to be related to estrogen stimulation.

Hormones

Alterations in the hormonal milieu are closely associated with an increased risk of developing endometrial cancer. The interaction between estrogens and endometrial cancer has been discussed for several decades.[3] The coexistence of hyperplasia and adenocarcinoma and the apparent evolution of adenomatous hyperplasia into florid adenocarcinoma have been recognized by pathologists for more than 3 decades,[4] and cytopathologists have long reported on the increased prevalence of well-cornified vaginal epithelium, indicating high levels of estrogens, in women with endometrial cancer.[5] The clinical counterpart

1101

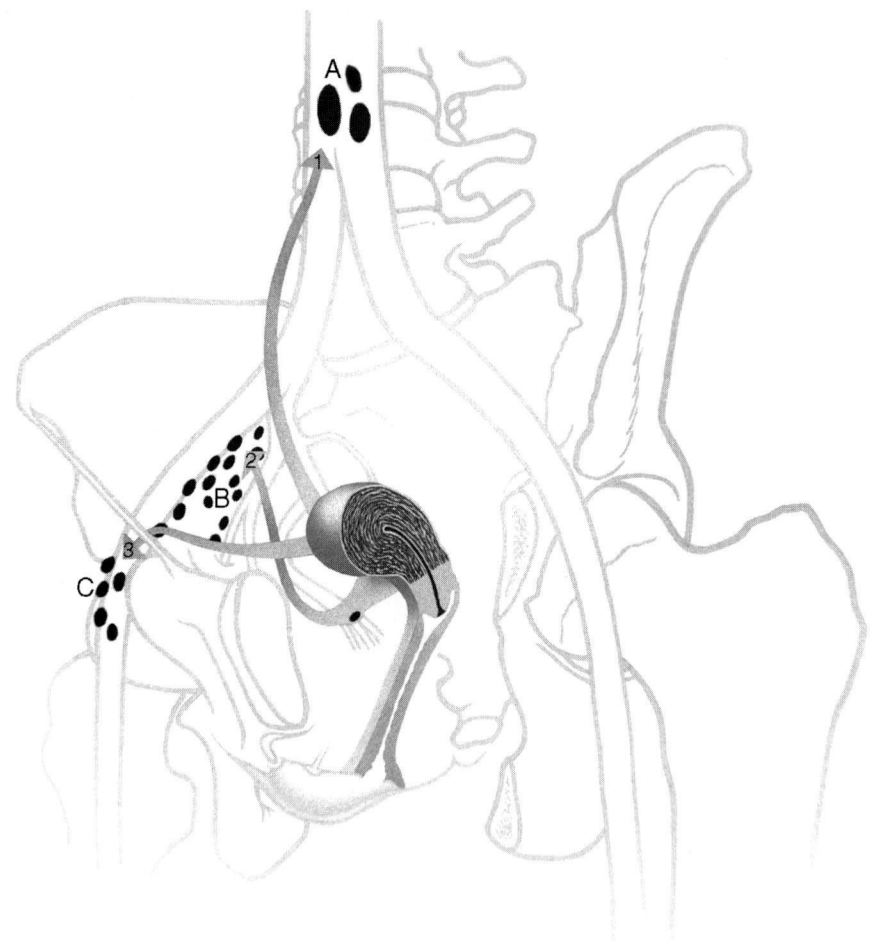

Figure 49–1. Lymphatic drainage pathways from the uterine body. **A,** Aortic nodes: all nodes anterior to the lumbar spine, which lie anteriorly, posteriorly, and laterally to the abdominal aorta, superior to its bifurcation. These drain the cornual and fundal region of the uterus via the lymphatics of the ovarian pedicle.[1] **B,** Interiliac nodes: nodes lying within the pyramidal space bounded by the medial surface of the external iliac artery, the internal iliac (hypogastric) artery and its anterolateral branches, and the lateral pelvic wall. The middle and lower portions of the body of the uterus drain here via the broad ligament lymphatics.[2] **C,** Deep femoral nodes: all nodes within the fatty tissue of the femoral triangle, which lie beneath the fascia lata. The most medial of these is the Cloquet's (Rosenmüller's) node. This constitutes an alternative pathway for drainage of the cornual region, via the lymphatics of the round (teres) ligament.[3]

of these pathologic findings is the increased risk for endometrial cancer in several conditions associated with abnormally high levels of estrogens. Thus, Stein-Leventhal syndrome, or polycystic ovarian syndrome, has traditionally been associated with a very high risk (up to 25%) of endometrial cancer. Although this number may be somewhat of an overestimate, these cancers account for a large proportion of cases in young women.[6] Similarly, a fairly large number of patients with granulosa or theca cell tumors of the ovary, or both, also develop a concomitant endometrial carcinoma. This association was first described by Novak and Yui[7] in 1936 and it is now recognized that the probability of developing endometrial carcinoma is related to the predominance of theca cells in the ovarian tumor, since these are the important source of feminizing estrogens.[3] It is also interesting to note that the prognosis of endometrial cancer in either of these settings is more favorable than for endometrial cancer in general.[8]

Late menopause, nulliparity, and obesity are classically associated with the development of endometrial cancer. Thus, delayed menarche is associated with a lower risk of endometrial cancer, whereas menopause after 52 years of age results in a 2.5-fold increase in the risk. The effect of delayed menopause (and to a lesser extent, early age at menarche) may reflect prolonged exposure of the endometrium to unopposed estrogen

stimulation in the presence of anovulatory cycles.[9] Similarly, nulliparous women have the highest risk, with 25% to 30% of all endometrial cancers occurring in nulliparous women. Having one child reduces this risk by half, and quintipara have less than 20% the risk faced by nulliparous women.[10] This adverse effect of nulliparity may also be a manifestation of prolonged periods of infertility.[11] In one study, nulliparous women who sought advice for infertility were at an almost eightfold excess risk compared with nulliparous women without an infertility problem.[12] A number of biologic mechanisms have been proposed for this increased risk with infertility: anovulatory menstrual cycles resulting in prolonged exposure to estrogens without sufficient progesterone, high serum levels of androstenedione, lower levels of serum sex-hormone binding globulin (with resultant high levels of free estrogen), and the absence of the monthly sloughing of the endometrial lining (allowing the residual tissue to become hyperplastic).[13] Finally, obesity is a well-recognized risk factor for endometrial cancer, possibly accounting for up to 25% of the disease.[14,15] Obesity affects the incidence of both premenopausal and postmenopausal endometrial cancer.[14-16] Being 21 to 50 pounds overweight increases the risk by almost threefold, and women who are more than 50 pounds overweight may have as high as a 10-fold increase in risk of developing endometrial cancer.[17] The increased peripheral conversion of androstenedione to estrone may be the underlying pathophysiologic mechanism for this risk. Apart from the absolute increase in weight, the duration of obesity[15] and the distribution of body fat may also play an important role.[15,18,19] Conversely, physical activity may exert a protective effect on the risk of endometrial carcinoma.[20,21] This association is biologically quite feasible, since physical activity is well known to effect changes in hormone levels and menstrual cycles.

Exogenous estrogens, in the form of estrogen replacement therapy, are also implicated in endometrial carcinoma. Several studies have looked at this correlation, and case reports have existed in the literature for 40 years.[22] These studies have been performed in at least eight countries, under a wide spectrum of medical care systems and conventions, in urban and rural settings, in high-usage and low-usage populations, using cohort and case-control designs, and with population-based and hospital-based comparison groups. Most of the studies have shown a strong association between past estrogen use and the development of endometrial cancer. The biologic plausibility of this association is further enhanced by the positive correlations between the dose of estrogen used, the duration of use, and the risk of subsequent endometrial cancer. At least 2 to 3 years' use was required to develop an increased risk, and the highest relative risks of 10 to 20 are observed after at least 10 years of estrogen use.[23-25] The relative risk is highest among thin, nondiabetic, normotensive women.[23,25,26] This may hint at a difference in estrogen metabolism in this group of patients, or that the risk in the typical obese, diabetic, hypertensive patient is already high enough as to not be affected by additional exogenous estrogens. Like the tumors arising in the setting of high levels of endogenous estrogen, most of these tumors are also relatively nonaggressive: They are generally diagnosed at an early stage, are well differentiated, and have little myometrial penetration[26,27] and a relatively small impact on mortality.[28,29]

Further evidence for the role of estrogens comes from the studies evaluating the effects of oral contraceptives. These studies have demonstrated significantly higher risks in users of the sequential oral contraceptives—which have a relatively high dose of estrogen with a weak progestin—and substantially lower risks of endometrial cancer in the women using estrogen-progestin combination pills, which have a higher dose of progestins.[11,16,30,31] The protective effect of the combination "pill" may be most marked in nulliparous women and in nonobese patients who have not been exposed to noncontraceptive estrogens.[32]

Progesterone is known to produce regressive changes in endometrial hyperplasia, and recently there has been an upsurge in enthusiasm for combining estrogen therapy with progestin to counteract the carcinogenic effects.[23,33,34] The recently published Women's Health Initiative randomized trial of healthy postmenopausal women showed that estrogen and progestin did not increase the risk of endometrial or colorectal cancers, but it did significantly increase the risk of invasive breast cancer.[35]

The risk of endometrial cancer from tamoxifen use has been the subject of many studies in light of its widespread use for breast cancer treatment and prevention.

The mechanism of action is competition with endogenous estrogen for estrogen receptors. In premenopausal women, tamoxifen has an antiestrogenic effect, but in postmenopausal women it has a weak estrogenic effect because of the up-regulation of estrogen receptors. In an overview of the breast cancer prevention trials, Cuzich et al. reported that the rates of endometrial cancer were increased with tamoxifen in all prevention trials (relative risk 2.4, 95% confidence interval [CI]: 1.5-4; $P = 0.0002$). Most of the excess risk was seen in women 50 years old or older.[36] Most authors[37-39] believe that there is no real difference in the stage, grade, or prognosis of endometrial cancers associated with tamoxifen, although there are emerging data to the contrary.[40]

Diet

In contrast to cervical cancer, uterine cancer is a disease of the Western countries; even there, it is more common in the urban population belonging to the higher socioeconomic strata of society. The rates are highest in North America and Northern Europe; intermediate in Israel, Southern Europe, and Latin America; and lowest in Africa and Asia.[41] This geographic difference may be a reflection of the high content of animal fat in the Western diets,[42] since both observational and interventional studies have shown a higher level of plasma estrone, estradiol, and prolactin among women consuming a high-fat diet.[43,44] Diet probably plays a multifaceted role in the risk of developing endometrial cancer, as other studies have shown a protective effect of high levels of micronutrients[45] and diets high in fruits and vegetables.[46]

Other Comorbidity

Endometrial carcinoma is also known to be associated with several other medical conditions. Diabetes and hypertension have long been related to a significant increase in the endometrial cancer risk, and recent reports confirmed that this risk persisted over time and was independent of the patient's weight.[47,48] Other interesting correlations include the interrelationship with smoking. The bulk of evidence from epidemiological studies suggests that smoking reduces the risk of developing endometrial cancer. The exact cause is not clear, but mechanisms such as the antiestrogenic effect of smoking on circulating estrogen concentrations, a reduction in relative body weight, and earlier age at menopause have been suggested.[49] Alcohol also has been associated with a reduction in the risk of endometrial cancer, perhaps by attenuating the endogenous estrogens.[50]

Genetics

Genetic predisposition to endometrial carcinoma occurs primarily within the context of HNPCC (hereditary nonpolyposis colorectal cancer), which probably accounts for less than 5% of all endometrial cancer cases. In patients with HNPCC there is increased risk of developing not only colon cancer but other cancers as well. The latter (Lynch syndrome II) includes endometrial cancers; ovarian cancers; gastric adenocarcinomas; carcinomas of the small bowel, pancreas, and biliary tree; transitional cell carcinomas of the ureters and renal pelvis; and tumors of the skin (Muir-Torre syndrome).[51] The lifetime risk estimates for endometrial carcinoma range from 40% to 60%, corresponding to a relative risk of 13 to 20. These estimates are not population based but derived from analyses of HNPCC families and thus may be higher than expected in the population generally. The genes involved in HNPCC include *MSH2*, *MLH1*, and *MSH6*. Tumors from patients with HNPCC syndrome are characterized by genetic instability that leads to error-prone DNA replication-RER⁺ phenotype, also referred to as *microsatellite instability*.[52] Apart from the special considerations of colorectal cancer, screening for endometrial and ovarian cancers should also be carried out. Currently for endometrial cancer, this consists of assessment of the endometrial stripe at the time of transvaginal ultrasonography as well as endometrial aspiration for cytology and histology. With respect to risk-reducing surgery, there are no data on the efficacy of hysterectomy and bilateral salpingo-oophorectomy (BSO) for cancer prevention in women at risk for HNPCC, and no recommendation was made for or against risk-reducing surgery by the Cancer Genetics Studies Consortium that addressed this issue.[53] Nevertheless, it is reasonable to assume that hysterectomy would be completely preventive for endometrial carcinoma, and there are no published case reports to the contrary.

PATHOLOGY

Hyperplasia

On gross inspection, hyperplastic endometrium has no distinctive features. There is a diffuse thickening resulting in an increase in the amount of endometrial tissue. The endometrium appears pale and knobby, and has a spongy, velvety feel. Microscopically, the diagnostic criterion for hyperplasia is an increase in the number and size of proliferating glands. The International Society of Gynecologic Pathologists has standardized the subclassification of endometrial hyperplasia.[54] In *simple hyperplasia*, there is only glandular proliferation and enlargement with increased stromal cellularity. This rarely progresses to carcinoma (<1%). *Complex hyperplasia* is characterized by back-to-back proliferation of glands with intraluminal papillae, epithelial pseudostratification, and few mitotic figures. If there is no cytologic atypia, the risk of malignant degeneration is again quite low, on the order of 3%. Any proliferation demonstrating cytologic abnormalities (in cellular or nuclear morphology) is classified as *atypical hyperplasia*. Atypical hyperplasia has a much higher risk of progression to an invasive carcinoma—8% for simple atypical hyperplasia, increasing to almost 30% for complex hyperplasia associated with atypia. Based on the histologic type and the patient's age and general medical condition, treatment options for endometrial hyperplasia include periodic endometrial curettage, high-dose progestin, ovulation induction, total abdominal hysterectomy

with bilateral salpingo-oophorectomy, and even intracavitary radiotherapy.

Carcinomas

On gross inspection most endometrial cancer involves the endometrial surface diffusely and is found frequently in the upper part of the uterine body, especially on the posterior wall. Only 40% of endometrial cancers are localized, which may take the form of a polyp or a localized, flattened, pyramidal thickening involving a part of the endometrial surface. The tumor obtained from endometrial curettage has a typical firm feel with a dry, granular, and often friable appearance. Necrotic areas may be yellow, white, or red. The International Society of Gynecologic Pathologists has proposed a classification for endometrial carcinomas (Table 49-1). Although the typical carcinoma is easy to diagnose, it may not always be easy to distinguish between a well-differentiated adenocarcinoma and an advanced atypical hyperplasia.[55,56] The chief feature that helps in this distinction is the *extent* of the proliferative changes: To diagnose a specimen as well-differentiated adenocarcinoma, the proliferative changes must be widespread and involve at least one half of a low-power microscopic field, 4.2 mm in diameter. Nuclear atypia is not required for this distinction.

ENDOMETRIOID ADENOCARCINOMA. Endometrioid adenocarcinoma is the most common endometrial carcinoma, constituting 75% to 80% of all cases. The classic histologic appearance is that of marked glandular proliferation with *back-to-back* proliferation of glands and little intervening stroma. The name *endometrioid* is derived from resemblance to proliferative phase endometrium. These tumors are graded according to the architectural pattern of the glands and nuclear features. Architectural grading is determined by the amount of solid masses of tumor cells compared to well-defined glands. Grade 1 is an endometrioid cancer in which less than 5% of the tumor growth is in solid sheets. Grade 2 is an adenocarcinoma in which 6% to 50% of the tumor is composed of solid sheets of cells. Grade 3 occurs when greater than 50% of the tumor is made up of solid sheets. The differentiation of the carcinoma is expressed as its *grade*. Nuclear grading is determined by the nuclear shape, size, chromatin

Table 49–1 Classification of Endometrial Carcinoma

Endometrial adenocarcinoma
    Papillary villoglandular
    Secretory
    Ciliated cell
    Adenocarcinoma with squamous differentiation
Mucinous carcinoma
Serous carcinoma
Clear-cell carcinoma
Squamous carcinoma
Undifferentiated carcinoma
Mixed types
Miscellaneous carcinoma
Metastatic carcinoma

distribution, and size of the nucleoli. The grading is primarily driven by the architectural grading but if there is marked nuclear atypia in an otherwise grade 2 architectural grading, it should be increased to grade 3.

Most of the endometrioid adenocarcinomas are designated *NOS* (not otherwise specified). Foci of squamous differentiation are often found with endometrioid adenocarcinoma. The squamous component could be benign with the designation of adenoacanthoma or malignant where it is called adenosquamous carcinoma. But such designations have not been very useful because the degree of differentiation of the squamous component parallels that of the glandular architectural grading. Therefore, most gynecologic pathologists use the term *adenocarcinoma with squamous differentiation*. Other subtypes of endometrioid adenocarcinoma include the relatively common *villoglandular carcinoma*, which grows in papillary fashion. The prognosis of this subtype is similar to that of low-grade endometrioid cancer and must not be confused with serous carcinoma because of its papillary features. *Secretory carcinoma*, which represents less than 2% of all endometrial carcinomas, is characterized by a very well differentiated glandular pattern with a lot of intracellular glycogen, thus resembling early secretory endometrium. Although the cells have clear cytoplasm, their histological and cytological features are different from clear cell carcinoma. Included is also *ciliated carcinoma*, which is a very rare subtype, characterized by the presence of ciliated cells composing more than 75% of the tumor specimen.[57] It is usually associated with a history of prior estrogen usage, and the prognosis is quite good, since most are well differentiated.

MUCINOUS CARCINOMA. Composing about 9% of all endometrial cancers, this designation requires more than 50% of the tumor cells to be mucinous. These cells are carcinoembryonic antigen (CEA) positive and are laden with mucin that stains positively with mucicarmine and periodic acid–Schiff (PAS) stains but is diastase resistant. Because this subtype is more commonly seen as an endocervical primary tumor, it is essential to establish the endometrial origin of the tumor. This is done by excluding an endocervical tumor on endocervical curettage. Mucinous carcinomas are usually well differentiated and have the same prognosis as ordinary endometrioid carcinomas.[58]

SEROUS CARCINOMAS. Serous carcinomas, also known as *papillary serous cancer*, resemble that of ovary cancer in terms of histology and to some extent in terms of behavior. The mere presence of papillary structure is not diagnostic because other histologic types may have papilla as well. But the presence of marked cellular atypia in addition to papilla is what distinguishes serous carcinoma from others. Psammoma bodies are found in up to 33% of cases. In most single large institution series, the prevalence is about 10%, but in a population-based study from Norway it was only 1%, reflecting perhaps the patterns of referrals.[59] This is a very aggressive subtype with a high propensity for early lymphatic and intraperitoneal dissemination, often despite little myometrial penetration.[60] The overall relapse rates are very high—up to 50%, even in stage I to II tumors.[61]

CLEAR CELL CARCINOMA. Clear cell carcinoma of the endometrium resembles renal carcinoma. Previously believed to arise from the mesonephric duct remnants (hence the synonyms *mesonephroma* or *adenocarcinoma of mesonephric origin*), its origin from müllerian structures is now well established.[62] Unlike vaginal and cervical clear cell carcinoma, it is not related to intrauterine DES (diethylstilbestrol) exposure. The microscopic structure may vary from solid patterns to glandular differentiation. In the latter pattern, the small cells resembling "hobnail" cells line spaces and glands. These are cells that have extruded their cytoplasm, leaving bare nuclei that protrude into the glandular lumens. The prognosis of this cancer is somewhat similar to that of serous cancer.[63]

MIXED HISTOLOGY. Mixed cell type endometrial cancer composed of two or more pure types is not uncommon. By convention in order to be designated *mixed*, the other cell type component has to compose at least 10% of the tumor. Except for mixed endometrioid and serous or clear cell carcinoma, the clinical significance of mixed cell type is questionable.

SIMULTANEOUS TUMORS. Cancers of an identical type may be discovered in the ovary and endometrium simultaneously.[64] Usually, the site of the largest tumor is assigned the primary origin, but occasionally true primary endometrial and ovarian malignancies may coexist. This *field effect* of the müllerian system may occur in as much as 15% to 20% of the ovarian endometrioid tumors.[65] If the endometrial tumor is less than 5 cm in diameter, well differentiated, with no vascular invasion and limited to less than the middle third of the myometrium, and the ovarian lesions are bilateral, it is more likely that there are two concomitant primary tumors.[66]

MOLECULAR BIOLOGY

Several investigators in the past pointed out that there are two distinct types of endometrial cancer.[67,68] In type I endometrial cancer there is strong correlation with prior estrogen stimulation. The cancers in this category are often indolent in nature, with minimal myometrial invasion and low-grade histology. They affect premenopausal and perimenopausal women. Type II endometrial cancer often affects postmenopausal women with no prior history of estrogen stimulation. The histology of the tumors is often high grade, such as serous or clear cell cancers with deep invasion, and at a more advanced stage at the time of presentation. What is intriguing is the fact that at the molecular level, the existence of two distinct types of endometrial cancer seems to be validated.[69]

Inactivation of the *p53 tumor suppressor gene* is seen in almost 90% of cases of serous carcinoma.[70,71] Mutation in the *p53* gene, however, is encountered in only 10% of endometrioid adenocarcinoma, with most occurring in International Federation of Gynecology and Obstetrics (FIGO) grade 3 tumors. Several studies have also demonstrated that *p53* mutation is an independent predictor of poor outcome.[72,73] In contrast, mutation in the *PTEN tumor suppressor gene* is found in 30% to

50% of endometrioid adenocarcinoma.[74,75] *PTEN* mutation is also associated with early-stage, nonmetastatic disease and more favorable survival.[76] *Microsatellite instability*, which is found in patients with HNPCC, is also seen in approximately 20% of "sporadic" endometrial cancers.[77] Data in the literature suggest a favorable survival associated with microsatellite instability in endometrioid endometrial cancers.[78] Mutation in k-*ras proto-oncogene* is seen in 10% to 30% of endometrial cancer patients,[79] but it seems that there is no correlation between k-*ras* mutation and clinical outcome. Overexpression of *HER-2/NEU* is also seen in 10% to 15% of endometrial cancers and is associated with more advanced disease and poor outcome.[80,81] Other oncogenes[82-85] that have been found to be overexpressed or amplified include c-*myc*, *bcl-2*, *c-fms*, and *B-catenin*. Microarray analysis has further revealed distinct gene expression profiles among different histologic types of endometrial cancer.[86]

MODE OF SPREAD

Endometrial cancer tends to remain confined to the body of the uterus for a long time. In most cases, the initial spread is by local extension, along the endometrial surface with or without enlargement of the uterus. Subsequent growth continues in radial and longitudinal directions. Longitudinal growth results in cervical involvement, initially through the openings of the endocervical glands, and later with frank cervical stromal infiltration. The tumor can also extend along the cornua to involve the fallopian tubes (although ovarian involvement is more often embolic in nature). As the tumor grows radially, it penetrates the myometrium and makes its way toward the subserosa and serosa. In a small number of cases, following extensive penetration through the myometrium or the cervix, the tumor involves the pelvic soft tissues and continues to reach the pelvic sidewall; the tumor may also directly invade the bladder or the rectum. Once the tumor breaches the serosa, transperitoneal dissemination can occur, resulting in a pattern of dissemination much like that of ovarian cancer. Overall, of the clinical stage I tumors, 15% are limited to the endometrium, 45% penetrate the inner third of the myometrium, 20% reach the middle third of the myometrium, and only about 20% reach the subserosa. The extent of myometrial penetration correlates very well with the histologic grade of the tumor (Table 49-2). Peritoneal seeding can result from transmural spread of the tumor once the serosa is breached, or because of transtubal spillage of tumor cells into the general peritoneal cavity.

The endometrium proper has few lymphatics. However, once the tumor penetrates the myometrium, and especially when it reaches the lymphatic-rich subserosa, spread via lymphatic embolization is common. Overall, only about 11% of patients with clinical stage I and occult stage II endometrial carcinoma have pelvic or para-aortic lymph node involvement.[87] However, a number of adverse pathologic factors can affect this number, as shown in Table 49-3. There is a close correlation between the tumor grade and the depth of myometrial invasion, as discussed earlier. This risk of pelvic and para-aortic lymph node involvement as related to grade and depth of myometrial invasion is given in Tables 49-4 and 49-5. Lymph node involvement also increases with increasing surgical stages. Thus, about 10% to 15% of all patients with stage I disease have pelvic lymph node involvement; this rises to 30% to 40% in stage II.

Lymph node involvement in endometrial cancer is of immense prognostic importance. Whereas stage I endometrial carcinoma is generally associated with a 5-year disease-free survival (DFS) rate in excess of 90%, patients with pelvic lymph node involvement have a 5-year DFS rate of only 65% to 70%, and the minority with para-aortic

Table 49–2 Correlation of Tumor Grade with Extent of Myometrial Invasion

Depth of Penetration	Grade, %		
	G1	G2	G3
Endometrium	24	11	7
Inner third	53	45	35
Middle third	12	24	16
Outer third	10	20	42

From Creasman WT, Marrow CP, Bundy BN, et al: Surgical pathologic spread patterns of endometrial cancer (a Gynecologic Oncology Group Study). *Cancer.* 1987;60:2035. Copyright © 1987 American Cancer Society. Reprinted by permission of Wiley-Liss Inc, a subsidiary of John Wiley & Sons.

Table 49–3 Frequency of Nodal Metastases as a Function of Various Risk Factors

Risk Factor	Patients, n	Pelvic, n (%)	Para-aortic, n (%)
Histology			
Endometrioid	599	56 (9)	30 (5)
Others	22	2 (9)	4 (18)
Grade			
1 Well	180	5 (3)	3 (2)
2 Moderate	288	25 (9)	14 (5)
3 Poor	153	28 (18)	17 (11)
Myometrial invasion			
Endometrial	87	1 (1)	1 (1)
Superficial	279	15 (5)	8 (3)
Middle	116	7 (6)	1 (1)
Deep	139	35 (25)	24 (17)
Tumor location			
Fundus	524	42 (8)	20 (4)
Isthmus/Cervix	97	16 (16)	14 (14)
Capillary-like space involvement			
Negative	528	37 (7)	19 (4)
Positive	93	21 (23)	15 (16)
Other extrauterine metastasis			
Negative	586	40 (7)	19 (4)
Positive	35	18 (51)	15 (16)
Peritoneal cytology			
Negative	537	38 (7)	20 (4)
Positive	75	19 (25)	14 (19)

From Creasman WT, Marrow CP, Bundy BN, et al: Surgical pathologic spread patterns of endometrial cancer (a Gynecologic Oncology Group Study). *Cancer.* 1987;60:2035. Copyright © 1987 American Cancer Society. Reprinted by permission of Wiley-Liss Inc, a subsidiary of John Wiley & Sons.

Table 49–4   Grade, Depth of Invasion, and Pelvic Node Involvement

	Grade, n (%)		
Depth of Invasion	G1 (n = 180)	G2 (n = 288)	G3 (n = 153)
Endometrium (n = 86)	0 (0)	1 (3)	0 (0)
Inner (n = 281)	3 (3)	7 (5)	5 (9)
Middle (n = 115)	0 (0)	6 (9)	1 (4)
Outer (n = 139)	2 (11)	11 (19)	22 (34)

From Creasman WT, Marrow CP, Bundy BN, et al: Surgical pathologic spread patterns of endometrial cancer (a Gynecologic Oncology Group Study). *Cancer.* 1987;60:2035. Copyright © (1987) American Cancer Society. Reprinted by permission of Wiley-Liss Inc, a subsidiary of John Wiley & Sons.

lymph node involvement have only a 30% to 35% 5-year DFS rate. Lymphatic spread is also believed to be responsible for involvement of the vagina, without contiguous cervical involvement (relapse in the distal vagina following a prior hysterectomy, without a vault recurrence) and for the isolated adnexal involvement often seen in stage IIIA disease.

Hematogenous spread is infrequent in endometrial cancer, occurring mainly in high-grade tumors or tumors with an unfavorable histology (e.g., serous adenocarcinoma). The common sites of metastases include the lungs, liver, and bones.

CLINICAL PRESENTATION

Early endometrial cancer has few symptoms, and a high index of suspicion is necessary to avoid any delay in diagnosis. The perimenopausal phase has only one normal pattern: menstrual periods that get progressively lighter and further apart. Any variant of this should always sound a warning note in the treating clinician. Although postmenopausal bleeding can have several nonmalignant causes,[88] abnormal bleeding is the presenting symptom in more than 80% of cases of endometrial cancer. Another fairly frequent (≈10%), but rather nonspecific, symptom is that of leukorrhea. Pain or other symptoms of pelvic pressure are rarely present in early-stage disease.

Table 49–5   Grade, Depth of Invasion, and Aortic Node Involvement

	Grade, n (%)		
Depth of Invasion	G1 (n = 180)	G2 (n = 288)	G3 (n = 153)
Endometrium (n = 86)	0 (0)	1 (3)	0 (0)
Inner (n = 281)	1 (1)	5 (4)	2 (4)
Middle (n = 115)	1 (5)	0 (0)	0 (0)
Outer (n = 139)	1 (6)	8 (14)	15 (23)

From Creasman WT, Marrow CP, Bundy BN, et al: Surgical pathologic spread patterns of endometrial cancer (a Gynecologic Oncology Group Study). *Cancer.* 1987;60:2035. Copyright © (1987) American Cancer Society. Reprinted by permission of Wiley-Liss Inc, a subsidiary of John Wiley & Sons.

Physical examination is also not helpful in the early stages, as uterine enlargement or extrauterine spread usually implies advanced disease. Any pyometra in a postmenopausal woman warrants an exclusion of an underlying endometrial cancer.

The diagnosis is usually established by endometrial sampling, usually via a fractional dilation and curettage (D&C) or an office biopsy. The first step in the D&C procedure is curettage of the endocervix. This is followed by sounding of the uterus, cervical dilation, and a systematic curettage of the entire endometrium. Cervical and endometrial specimens should be labeled and processed separately. The fractional D&C also provides an opportunity to examine the relaxed patient under anesthesia and allows for a cystoscopy or proctoscopy in the rare cases in which bladder or rectal involvement is suspected. Outpatient procedures, such as an endometrial biopsy or aspiration curettage with endocervical sampling, are diagnostic only if positive for cancer (≈10% false negative). If these are negative, a formal fractional D&C must be carried out.

Following histologic confirmation of the diagnosis, patients must undergo a thorough evaluation and staging workup. It is important to realize that these are often frail, elderly patients. They may have a number of concurrent medical problems that can affect the potential treatment-related morbidity and thus influence selection of the appropriate treatment modality. Routine blood and urine studies are obtained, as is a chest x-ray (to rule out metastases and evaluate the cardiopulmonary status of the patient). Other studies, including a cystoscopy, proctosigmoidoscopy, and barium enema may be required in selected patients in whom more extensive disease is suspected.

Several imaging studies are being evaluated for their ability to accurately define the disease extent preoperatively. The typical finding on ultrasonogram is a thickened endometrium. It is suggested that less differentiated tumors may be hypoechoic[89] or that distinct sonographic patterns allow one to distinguish among hyperplasia, polyps, and carcinoma.[90] In this respect, transvaginal ultrasonography (TVS) is believed to be superior to conventional transabdominal sonography.[91] TVS is also useful in determining the depth of myometrial invasion.[92] Its overall accuracy in determining invasion is 79% and its accuracy is in determining the degree of myometrial invasion is 60% to 76%. Good-quality pelvic computed tomography (CT) scans obtained with oral and intravenous contrast can demonstrate the extent of the endometrial tumor. The endometrial carcinoma is a hypodense mass relative to the normal myometrium[93] and may be seen as a diffuse, circumscribed vegetative or polypoidal mass within the uterine cavity. If myometrial invasion is seen, it usually implies involvement of greater than one third to one half of the myometrial thickness.[94] Endometrial involvement of the cervix is seen on CT as cervical enlargement greater than 3.5 cm in diameter with heterogeneous low-attenuation areas within the fibromuscular stroma.[95] Parametrial or sidewall extension is seen by the loss of periureteral fat in the former and less than 3 mm of intervening fat between the soft tissue mass and the pelvic sidewall in the latter.[96]

Involvement of the fallopian tubes, ovaries, and lymph nodes is detected in the usual fashion.

Although the largest study looking at the ability of CT to detect myometrial invasion by dynamic and delayed images reported an overall accuracy of about 76%, the authors noted that CT did provide clinically useful information in almost 90% of cases.[94] The major limitation of CT is the failure to detect microscopic parametrial, lymph nodal, bladder, or rectal invasion.[95,97] Other problems include an unreliability in assessing myometrial invasion in the atrophic uteri of postmenopausal women and an occasional difficulty in differentiating a uterine from an adnexal mass.[93,94,97] Because of these problems, and since surgical staging is the standard approach in most patients, CT is not routinely recommended in clinical stage I or II disease. Its greatest impact may lie in clinical stage III patients, in whom it may confirm extrauterine spread, detect pelvic lymphadenopathy, or reclassify the disease as stage IV by detecting extrapelvic involvement.[95,97] It may also help in staging a patient with an equivocal pelvic examination or a contraindication to surgery and in confirming advanced stage III or IV disease.[93-95,97] CT scanning is also useful in the evaluation of recurrent disease by helping to define the extent of disease at relapse and in facilitating a directed biopsy for histologic confirmation of relapse.[95,97,98]

Magnetic resonance imaging (MRI) is increasingly being recommended as part of the preoperative evaluation of endometrial carcinoma.[99-102] Since unenhanced T1- and T2-weighted images lack specificity in diagnosing endometrial cancer, use of intravenous contrast is necessary.[91,103] Following contrast injection, even small tumors contained within the endometrium can be diagnosed by their enhancement relative to the normal endometrium, and dynamic MRI with rapid administration of Gd-DTPA (gadolinium diethylenetriaminepentaacetic acid) using the turbo-FLASH technique can delineate the inner myometrium from the outer layers even in postmenopausal women.

Magnetic resonance images have been correlated to the FIGO subdivisions of stage I endometrial cancer.[104] Stage IA tumors typically show a clear junctional zone or preservation of a sharp delineation between the tumor and the myometrium; IB disease is characterized by disruption of the junctional zone or increased signal-intensity tumor in the inner half of the myometrium with preservation of the outer myometrium, or both. Finally, in stage IC patients, there is extension of the high-signal-intensity tumor into the outer myometrium with preservation of a peripheral rim of normal, intact myometrium.[105] MRI also helps delineate stage II disease by showing an expansion of the cervical canal with stromal heterogeneity. Similarly, imaging of extrauterine spread is facilitated, although lymph node involvement is limited to the criterion of increased size. State-of-the-art MRI using gadolinium chelates is probably accurate in more than 90% of cases.[106,107] It definitely outperforms CT in determining myometrial invasion[103,107,108] and is possibly better than TVS.[109,110]

Tumor markers such as CA-125 have been shown to be elevated in 63% to 67% of patients with advanced or metastatic disease compared to 10% to 19% in those with early-stage disease. Whether CA-125 is a useful tool in screening for endometrial cancer is not determined, but most authors agree about its potential in patients with aggressive histologies, advanced disease, or pretreatment elevated levels.[111,112]

STAGING AND PROGNOSTIC FACTORS

The Gynecologic Oncology Group (GOG) conducted two large prospective trials[87,113] in 1984 and 1987. The major prognostic factors in endometrial cancer were defined from these studies, and surgical staging has gradually become the standard in this disease. This surgical approach led FIGO, in 1988, to design a surgical staging scheme for endometrial cancer, incorporating most of the known prognostic factors (Table 49-6).[114] For the small minority of patients who are not surgical candidates and are treated with primary radiotherapy, the earlier clinical staging system is still applied (Table 49-7).[115]

Several clinicopathologic factors have been identified in patients with endometrial carcinoma to help predict the prognosis and individualize the treatment plan. Based on clinical experiences, Nolan and Huen[116] developed a mathematical model for prognostication, wherein patient

Table 49–6 Corpus Cancer Surgical Staging (FIGO 1988)

Stage		Definition
IA	G123	Tumor limited to the endometrium
IB	G123	Invasion to <50% of the myometrium
IC	G123	Invasion to >50% of the myometrium
IIA	G123	Cervical involvement restricted to the endocervical glands
IIB	G123	Cervical stromal invasion
IIIA	G123	Tumor invades uterine serosa, or adnexae, or positive peritoneal cytology
IIIB	G123	Tumor involving the vagina
IIIC	G123	Pelvic or para-aortic lymph nodal involvement
IVA	G123	Invasion of bladder, bowel mucosa, or both
IVB		Distant metastases, including intra-abdominal spread or inguinal lymph nodes

Table 49–7 Clinical Staging of Endometrial Cancer (FIGO 1971)

Stage	Definition
I	Carcinoma confined to the uterus
IA	Length of uterine canal is ≤8 cm
IB	Length of uterine canal is >8 cm
Histologic Subtypes of Adenocarcinoma	
G1	Highly differentiated adenomatous carcinoma
G2	Differentiated adenomatous carcinoma with partly solid areas
G3	Predominantly solid or entirely undifferentiated carcinoma
II	Carcinoma involves the corpus and the cervix
III	Carcinoma extends outside the uterus but is confined to the true pelvis
IV	Carcinoma extends outside the true pelvis or involves the bladder, rectum, or both

prognosis is directly proportional to host resistance, inversely related to tumor virulence, and positively affected by appropriate treatment factors.

Prognosis = k {(Resistance/Virulence) × Treatment}

Host Resistance Factors

AGE. The importance of age has been well documented in endometrial cancer. Frick and associates,[117] in 1973, reported a better outcome for patients under the age of 59 with stage I endometrial cancer, even after correcting for comorbid medical conditions. This was subsequently confirmed by other investigators.[118-120] The adverse impact of advanced age on outcome persists even when elderly patients are treated as aggressively as their younger counterparts.[121] The improved survival in younger patients may reflect the tendency toward earlier, better differentiated tumors with less myometrial invasion in these patients; in older postmenopausal women with atrophic uteri, relatively little myometrial penetration brings the tumor close to the lymphatic-rich subserosa, with a correspondingly high risk of lymph node metastases.[122] Better host immunocompetence may be an additional factor in the younger patients.

RACE. Caucasian women tend to fare better than African-Americans independent of other prognostic factors.[123] It is important to note that while the prevalence of endometrial cancer is lower in African-American women, the incidence of high-risk tumors in this group is higher.[124] The influence of histologic type and differentiation on outcome is discussed earlier.

PERFORMANCE STATUS AND ANEMIA. A poor performance status and anemia, which may predict a poorer response to radiotherapy, are other adverse host-related "resistance" factors.

Tumor Virulence Factors

STAGE AT DIAGNOSIS. Since the very concept of stage grouping is based on creating groups with similar prognoses, it is not surprising that the outcome gets less favorable with advancing stage. Reported results of stage-based survival are remarkably consistent, with stages I, II, III, and IV disease having 5-year survival rates of 92%, 80%, 40%, and 5% respectively.[125]

SIZE OF THE UTERUS. This has long been recognized as a predictor of survival and was incorporated in the earlier clinical staging for endometrial cancer. Creasman and associates[85] showed a direct correlation between uterine size and the incidence of para-aortic and pelvic nodal metastases.[87] It has been pointed out, however, that uterine size may not always reflect tumor volume, since a number of benign conditions can cause enlargement of the uterus.[126] Furthermore, since the size of the uterus correlates with tumor grade and myometrial penetration, it is very possible that size merely acts as a surrogate for these far more significant prognostic factors.

LOWER UTERINE SEGMENT INVOLVEMENT. Although 92% of stage I endometrial carcinomas lie in the fundus, it has been proposed that cancers involving the isthmus or lower uterine segment may have a worse prognosis.[127] The GOG study of surgical-pathologic spread patterns found a doubling of the incidence of pelvic nodal involvement from 8% to 16% and an increase in para-aortic nodal involvement from 4% to 14% when the tumor arose from or involved the isthmus.[87] Mayr and associates[128] found that lower uterine segment involvement, in the absence of any other adverse prognostic factors, resulted in an almost 50% local failure rate when postoperative radiotherapy was omitted; in patients receiving postoperative radiotherapy, the relapse rates dropped to 3%.

CERVICAL INVOLVEMENT. It is important to separate pathologic (occult) from clinical involvement of the cervix in endometrial cancer since only occult cervical involvement is recognized in the 1988 FIGO staging system. Prognosis for patients with cervical involvement (stage II) is much poorer than for those with earlier-stage lesions. Surwit and associates[122] reported that cervical stromal involvement dropped the survival rate to less than 50%, as compared with almost 75% with tumor involvement limited to the endocervical glands; access to the cervical stroma probably increases the propensity for lymphatic dissemination, as positive pelvic lymph nodes are seen in about 35% of the patients.[129] Similarly, Rubin and associates reported on the Memorial Sloan-Kettering Cancer Center experience with stage II endometrial cancer.[130] At 60 months, the actuarial disease-free survival rate was 39% in patients with gross cervical involvement, 62% in those with clinically occult stromal involvement (detected only on a fractional D&C), and 88% in the subset having only detached tumor fragments on fractional D&C.

HISTOLOGIC SUBTYPES. While the most common subtype—endometrioid adenocarcinoma—has a worse prognosis with increasing grade,[87,131] there are cell types that have a high propensity to early systemic dissemination with a uniformly bad prognosis, regardless of the pathologic grade. These include the serous, clear-cell, squamous, and undifferentiated subtypes. The overall survival rate in this group is less than 35%.[132,133]

TUMOR GRADE. Tumor grade is one of the most sensitive indicators of prognosis. Grade directly affects the depth of myometrial penetration and the frequency of lymph node involvement (see Table 49-3).[87,131,134,135] Thus, most grade 1 tumors are limited to the endometrium or have superficial myometrial penetration, and the overall risk of pelvic and para-aortic lymph nodal metastases is 3% and 1.5%, respectively; however, 10% of grade 1 tumors have deep myometrial penetration, and the pelvic and para-aortic lymph nodal involvement in these are 12% and 6%, respectively. Similarly, more than 50% of grade 3 tumors have a greater than 50% myometrial penetration, and these have pelvic and para-aortic nodal involvement on the order of 30% and 20%, respectively.[87]

MYOMETRIAL INVASION. Myometrial invasion is probably the factor most consistently identified with treatment failures. Conventionally, the depth of invasion has been reported as *inner, middle,* or *outer* thirds of the myometrium. The FIGO staging system, however, refers only to inner and outer halves, and the pathologic reporting should change to incorporate this recommendation. In patients with stage IB disease (<50% invasion), it seems that invasion to less than versus greater than one third is not a significant predictor of outcome.[136] Lutz and associates also noted that proximity to the serosa may be more important than absolute depth of penetration.[126] They found a 65% survival rate for patients whose tumors had invaded to within 5 mm of the serosa, compared with a 97% survival rate for patients with tumors more than 10 mm from the serosa. Both grade and depth of penetration are predictive for lymph nodal involvement; however, depth is more influential in determining lymphatic and extrauterine spread, treatment failure, and relapse. Thus, regardless of grade, only 1% of tumors limited to the endometrium had lymph nodal involvement, as compared with 25% pelvic and 17% para-aortic involvement with deep penetration.[87]

VASCULAR OR CAPILLARY-LIKE SPACE INVASION. This is seen in about 15% of the cases of endometrial cancer.[87,137,138] The GOG study found that capillary-like space (CLS)–positive tumors were associated with a 27%, or fourfold, increase in the pelvic lymph nodal metastases, and a 19%, or sixfold, increase in para-aortic nodal metastases.[87] This translates into more frequent relapses and a poorer survival for the CLS-positive patients.[137]

ADNEXAL INVOLVEMENT. About 5% of patients with stage I and occult stage II disease have adnexal involvement.[87] This is associated with a fourfold increase in lymph node metastases; thus, pelvic lymph nodal positivity rises to 32% (as compared with 8% without adnexal spread) and para-aortic nodal involvement is seen in 20% (as opposed to only 5% in patients with no adnexal spread). The depth of myometrial invasion is still an important factor: Patients with adnexal spread but less than 50% myometrial involvement have a 5-year survival rate of about 80%, as compared with a 45% 5-year survival rate when adnexal involvement is associated with deep myometrial invasion. The extent of adnexal involvement is also of prognostic significance. Patients with occult, microscopic invasion do far better (5-year survival rate >80%) than those with gross adnexal involvement (5-year survival rate <40%).[139]

PERITONEAL CYTOLOGY. Peritoneal fluid positive for malignant cells is found in 12% to 15% of all patients undergoing surgical staging. This is associated with 25% pelvic lymph nodal involvement and 19% para-aortic nodal involvement. However, only about 5% of patients with positive peritoneal cytologic finding have no extrauterine disease,[87] and the literature regarding the true impact of positive peritoneal cytology is mixed. Several small series indicate that a positive peritoneal cytologic finding has no independent prognostic value.[140-142] On the other hand, two relatively large series show a distinct adverse effect from positive peritoneal cytology.[143,144] One confounding factor, mainly in patients with no other risk factors, is whether all endometrial cancer cells that gained access to the peritoneal cavity are capable of independent growth. The meta-analysis by Milosevic and associates concluded that, while malignant cytology was strongly associated with disease recurrence (odds ratio of 4.7 with 95% CI of 3.5-6.3), this was largely due to the association of malignant cytology with other adverse prognostic factors, which dominate the clinical presentation.[145] In the absence of any other adverse features, the true incidence of malignant cytology is quite low and is unlikely to act as an independent predictor for relapse. Recent data suggest a higher rate of positive cytology for patients undergoing laparoscopic-vaginal hysterectomy, in which there is manipulation of the uterine cavity, compared to total abdominal hysterectomy, in which there is no such manipulation.[146]

SEROSAL INVOLVEMENT. This is the least studied feature of all stage III-A subsets. Its incidence ranges from 7% to 16% and it is often associated with other poor prognostic factors.[147] But even when it is isolated, the 5-year disease-free survival is only 41.5%.

GROSS INTRAPERITONEAL SPREAD. This again correlates very highly with lymph nodal metastases. Pelvic lymph nodal positivity increased to 51% in the presence of gross intraperitoneal spread as compared with only 7% without such dissemination; similarly, para-aortic nodal involvement rises to 23% with intraperitoneal spread, as compared with only 4% without this spread.

PELVIC AND PARA-AORTIC LYMPH NODES. Overall, about 11% of patients with stage I and occult stage II endometrial cancer have pelvic nodal involvement.[87] This increases to 25%, 30%, and 50% with deep myometrial penetration, adnexal involvement, and extrauterine spread, respectively. Lymph nodal involvement is a major predictor for distant disease: the 5-year disease-free survival rates drop to 65% to 70% in patients with pelvic lymph nodal involvement as their only risk factor.[148] Similarly, while para-aortic nodal metastases are seen in about 5% of all patients with stage I and occult stage II disease, the biggest risk factor for para-aortic node involvement is the presence of pelvic nodal metastases; more than 30% of patients with pelvic nodal involvement have para-aortic disease. The pattern of lymphatic spread in endometrial cancer is different than in cervical cancer. In endometrial cancer, a simultaneous spread to both pelvic and para-aortic nodes could occur, while in cervical cancer the spread to para-aortic nodes is almost always secondary to pelvic lymph nodal involvement. Despite optimal debulking and radiation, 5-year disease-free survival rates drop to about 30% in this subpopulation.

Other Significant Prognostic Factors

PLOIDY. There are several studies now to indicate that aneuploid tumors correlate with advanced surgical stage, higher grade, and a poorer clinical outcome. Multivariate analysis has identified ploidy as an independent risk factor. In fact, a recent review on this subject notes that "DNA ploidy is an independent, broadly applicable, quantifiable predictor of progression-free survival in patients with endometrial cancer and, therefore, warrants designation as a major prognostic factor or therapeutic determinant."[149] There appears to be an association between DNA ploidy and the overexpression of several regulatory genes, such as c-*fms*, k-*ras*, HER-2/*neu*, and *p53*. Although overexpression of these oncogenes and tumor suppressor genes harbors prognostic significance in endometrial cancer, the ploidy status of the tumor appears to represent the most objective prognostic variable.[149-158] In fact, there are data to suggest that ploidy may be an independent prognosticator with greater predictive power than tumor grade.[159,160] As a variant of ploidy, the DNA index (DI) has also been evaluated for prognostic importance in endometrial cancer. A DI greater than 1.2 was found to be strongly predictive of recurrent disease, independent of other conventional risk factors, including histologic subtype, depth of myometrial penetration, and lymphovascular invasion.[161]

S-PHASE. As a marker of tumor proliferation, the fraction of tumor cells in S-phase has been extensively studied. The results so far are mixed; at one extreme, S-phase is believed to have a very high prognostic value, while other investigators claim that S-phase is not shown to add to the risk-modeling based on conventional surgicopathologic factors.[151,156,159,162,163]

HORMONE RECEPTORS. The physiology of the normal endometrium is closely regulated by estrogens and progesterone, and it is not surprising that expression of hormone receptors by endometrial carcinoma is of prognostic value. In general, patients with receptor-positive tumors have a significantly better disease-free survival, with receptor status acting as an independent risk factor.[150,164-167] The receptor status is also important in predicting the likelihood of response to hormonal therapy in patients who have relapsed.

PROGNOSTIC INFORMATION FROM MOLECULAR BIOLOGY. The application of molecular biology tools to endometrial cancer has provided insights into the pathophysiology of the disease and may reveal new avenues for early diagnoses as well as development of therapeutic strategies based on newer models of risk stratification. Mutations and overexpression of the tumor suppressor gene *p53* have been most extensively studied. There is a consistent observation linking the overexpression of *p53* with advanced stage and a poorer outcome. In most studies, *p53* maintained an independent prognostic value separate from the conventional clinicopathologic risk factors.[149,151,152,168-176] A study from Duke University also reported an increased frequency of *p53* overexpression in black women, which may account for the racial disparity in survival.[168] Hamel and associates,[155] from the Mayo Clinic, reported on a retrospective analysis of 221 patients managed surgically for endometrial carcinoma.

Their multivariate analysis identified four independent prognostic factors for progression-free survival: intense *p53* expression (defined as staining of 66% or more of the nuclear area), histologic subtype, DNA ploidy status, and HER-2/*neu* expression. When none of these were present, the 4-year progression-free survival rate was 96%; in contrast, it dropped to 63% in the presence of one of these factors and was only 40% when two or more factors were present.

Several other prognostic factors have been identified, including c-*fms*,[84] HER-2/*neu*,[151,152,158,160,171,172,177,178] epidermal growth factor receptor,[152,171,172,179,180] k-*ras* activation,[181] Nm23,[182,183] and macrophage colony-stimulating factor 1.[184] Although a lot of the information regarding these newer prognostic factors is preliminary, it is likely that molecular abnormalities are the fundamental mechanisms underlying malignant transformation and further progression of the established neoplasm-tumor grade. Myometrial penetration and the other gross prognostic factors may be mere epiphenomena, that is, the secondary results of the molecular changes. As the knowledge regarding the molecular biology of endometrial cancer matures, the risk stratification may soon be based on cytogenetic and molecular abnormalities rather than on pathologic variables. This may be particularly useful in devising treatment strategies for patients who would currently be classified as belonging to the intermediate-risk group.

Treatment-Related Prognostic Factors

RESIDUAL TUMOR AFTER PREOPERATIVE RADIOTHERAPY. In their study of 91 patients with early endometrial cancer treated with two intracavitary insertions, Macasaet and associates found residual tumor in almost 50% of cases.[185] These patients had a 19% relapse rate and a 23% probability of dying from their tumor, compared with only 6% in patients without residual cancer.

DELAY IN INITIATING POSTOPERATIVE ADJUVANT THERAPY. A recent report from the Fox Chase Cancer Center concluded that prolonging the surgery-to-radiation interval beyond 6 weeks has an adverse effect on disease-specific survival and may also influence local control.[186] In light of this, it was surprising that overall treatment time and external beam treatment time did not emerge as significant prognostic factors.

TREATMENT

Endometrial cancer is perhaps unique in having more treatment options advocated by different clinicians than any other malignancy of the female pelvis. This is especially the case for stage I/II tumors, which constitute more than 75% of all endometrial cancers. A summary of the current approach to managing the various stage presentations of endometrial carcinoma is outlined in the critical pathway flow diagrams (Fig. 49-2).

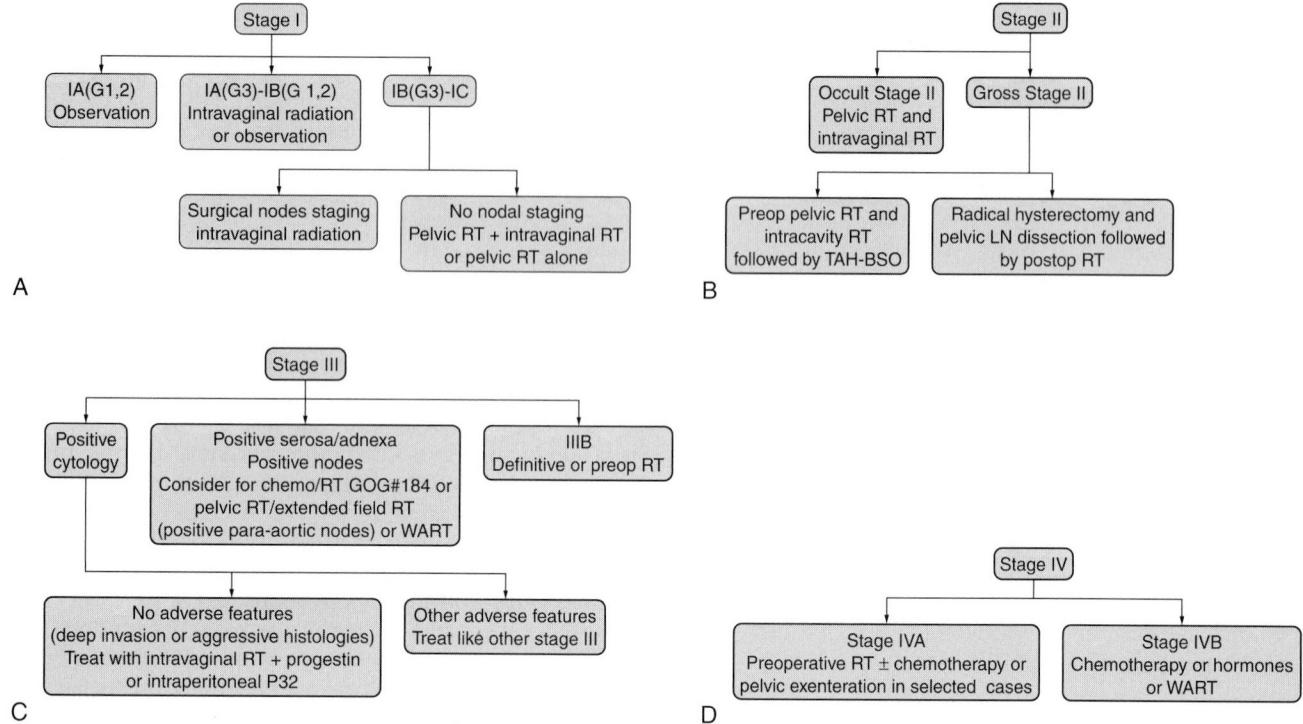

Figure 49–2. (A–D). Critical pathways for workup and stage-based management of endometrial carcinoma. GOG, Gynecologic Oncology Group; LN, lymph node; P32, RT, radiation therapy; TAH/BSO, total abdominal hysterectomy and bilateral salpingo-oophorectomy.

Surgery

Surgery is the mainstay treatment for most patients with endometrial cancer. In a small subset of patients who present with unresectable disease or those whose disease is resectable but medically inoperable, definitive radiation is used instead as the primary treatment. The surgical management of endometrial cancer often involves simple hysterectomy and bilateral salpingo-oophorectomy with or without lymph node staging. Although pelvic and para-aortic lymph nodal sampling/ dissection (as part of a surgical staging) is fast becoming routine, especially for patients operated on by gyneco-logic oncologists, there are no objective data from randomized trials to support the contention that lymph node dissection is of any benefit in terms of survival to the patient. On the other hand, emerging data suggest that pelvic radiation following lymph nodal sampling may be associated with a higher than expected (7% vs. 1%) risk of severe complications.[187] Unfortunately, despite lack of objective benefit from surgical staging, it has already sig-nificantly influenced the likelihood of patients being referred for postoperative radiotherapy. Thus, the knowledge of pathologically negative lymph nodes has reduced the likelihood of patients being referred for post-operative radiotherapy, especially in the subgroup with 50% to 66% myometrial invasion.[188,189] This is unfortu-nate, since the adequacy of a lymph node dissection varies greatly among different surgeons. Whether the procedure is being performed by a gynecologist or a gynecologic oncologist, the patient's general condition, the habitus of the patient, and several other factors affect the thoroughness of the lymphadenectomy. The minimum number of lymph nodes that need to be retrieved for the dissection to be representative has yet to be determined,

and the final evaluation of a lymphadenectomy specimen will also depend on how meticulously the specimens are examined by the pathologist. Also, pelvic lymph nodal involvement is likely a marker for a biologically aggres-sive disease with a propensity for distant failures; any pelvic radiation offered in that setting is aimed at essen-tially optimizing local control.[148] On the other hand, patients with high-risk uterine factors without lymph nodal involvement may be the very subpopulation at greatest risk for an isolated local relapse, and radiation could have the maximum curative potential in this sub-group. Finally, patients with endometrial cancer often have a multitude of comorbid conditions that put them at a higher than normal risk for complications related to major or prolonged surgery, such as an extended lym-phadenectomy. Thus, it is imperative that the role of extensive surgical staging procedures be critically evalu-ated in well-conducted trials before we institute major changes in the management of these patients.

SURGICAL TECHNIQUE

After an appropriate preoperative workup—aimed at establishing the disease extent and evaluating any concur-rent medical problems that these patients often have—a plan is made for the patient to undergo a hysterectomy with bilateral salpingo-oophorectomy and surgical staging.

HYSTERECTOMY. Total abdominal hysterectomy and bilateral salpingo-oophorectomy (TAH-BSO) is still considered the standard operative procedure for patients with endometrial cancer. The first successful total abdominal hysterectomy for this disease was performed by W. A. Freund[190] in 1878. Usually, an adequate midline incision is employed to allow thorough intra-abdominal exploration and lymph nodal sampling. Upon entry into the peritoneal cavity, fluid samples are obtained for cytology. This is followed by a thorough intra-abdominal exploration with a biopsy or excision of any suspicious areas. The uterus is then evaluated for any breach in the serosa, the distal ends of the fallopian tubes are ligated, and an extrafascial hysterectomy with bilateral salpingo-oophorectomy is performed. The operative plane of dissection lies outside the pubocervical fascia and does not require any unroofing of the ureters. The excised uterus is then opened away from the surgical field and an assessment is made regarding the depth of myometrial penetration.[191] Frozen sections may be employed in doubtful cases.[192] A new approach that is gaining popularity is the laparoscopically assisted vaginal hysterectomy and bilateral salpingo-oophorectomy (LAVH-BSO). The use of laparoscopy enables the surgeon to have a thorough intra-abdominal exploration and to be able to perform bilateral salpingo-oophorectomy, which is difficult to perform with just a vaginal hysterectomy. The potential advantages of this approach include significantly shorter hospitalization stays and fewer complications, resulting in fewer overall hospital charges when compared to patients treated by TAH.[193] Currently, the GOG is conducting a prospective randomized trial comparing TAH/BSO to LAVH/BSO in early-stage endometrial cancer. Radical hysterectomy (RH) is not routinely performed in endometrial cancer due to low incidence of parametrial involvement. There is no evidence to show that the cure rates are any better with such radical operations.[194] The possible exception to this might be in patients with gross cervical involvement.[195]

LYMPH NODAL STAGING. Who needs routine lymph nodal staging is still a matter of great debate. Some advocate full nodal staging for all patients regardless of stage or grade while others don't employ it even for high-risk patients since they will be getting radiation anyhow. The middle of the road approach includes lymph nodal sampling for patients with aggressive histologies or more than 50% myometrial invasion (Table 49-8). The degree of lymph nodal staging also varies, but at a minimum it should include inspection and removal of any enlarged

Table 49–8   Indications for Lymph Node Sampling in Endometrial Cancer

Clinically enlarged pelvic/para-aortic lymph nodes
>50% Myometrial invasion
Extrauterine spread
Involvement of the isthmus/cervix
Serous, clear, squamous, or undifferentiated cell types

pelvic or para-aortic nodes. Pelvic and para-aortic sampling includes removal of the fat pads surrounding the major vessels in the abdomen and pelvis without skeletonizing them. According to the GOG surgical guidelines, in order for the sampling to be adequate, five lymphatic stations need to be removed. These include para-aortic nodes, common iliac, internal iliac, external iliac, and obturator. Lymph nodal dissection involves not only removal of the fat but also skeletonization of the vessels in similar fashion to pelvic lymph nodal dissection in cervical cancer. The surgical approach for pelvic/para-aortic lymph nodal sampling or dissection is still an intra-abdominal approach, but there is growing interest in evaluation laparoscopic retroperitoneal approach in an attempt to reduce the morbidity.

Adjuvant Radiation Therapy

Radiation therapy plays a significant role in the management of endometrial cancer either in the adjuvant setting or as a definitive treatment for those patients with unresectable disease or who are medically inoperable. The bulk of this section focuses on the role adjuvant radiation plays for patients with stage I to III endometrioid adenocarcinoma. The three main issues with regard to adjuvant radiation relate to its sequencing with surgery (i.e., preoperative vs. postoperative); indication; and, if indicated, the type of radiation that should be used.

Historically, radiation therapy was given preoperatively using various techniques (Fig. 49-3) followed by an extrafascial hysterectomy. Supplemental postoperative

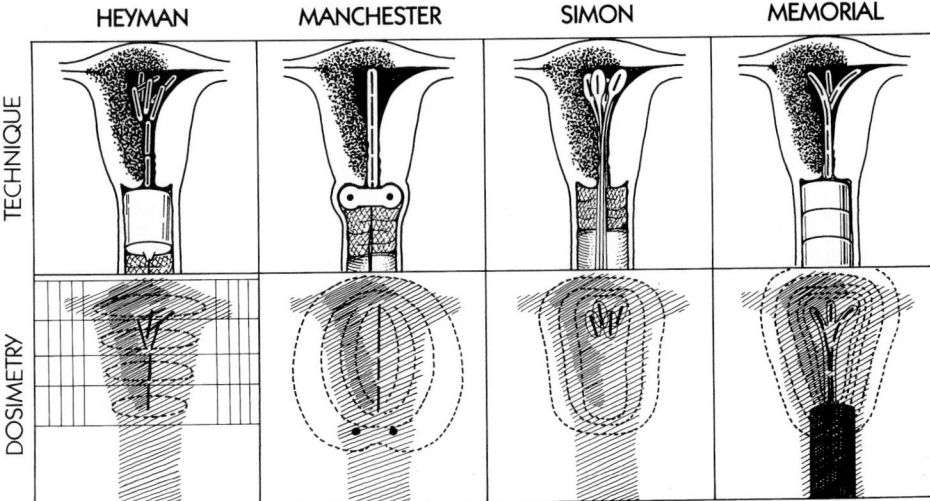

Figure 49–3. Selected intracavitary techniques used for preoperative radiation for endometrial cancer.

radiotherapy was added in select cases based on the pathologic risk factors. Proposed advantages to the use of preoperative radiotherapy include: (1) delivery of radiation to a well-oxygenated tumor, (2) cytoreduction (especially of the superficial tumor mass) to facilitate surgical resection and reduce the likelihood of intraoperative implantation, (3) minimizing the risk of tumor embolization, (4) eradication of microscopic tumor extensions to ensure a pathologically clear resection margin, and (5) potentially lowering the overall complication rate, resulting in better patient outcome. This approach[196] has yielded excellent long-term results, with 5-year survival rates of 85% to 90%. The major disadvantages of this approach include the unnecessary treatment of patients who are at a low risk for recurrence and would have been cured by surgery alone. There is also the concern about downstaging the tumor and thus losing valuable pathologic prognostic information on which further adjuvant treatment would be based. Current treatment policies for endometrial carcinoma aim to minimize the use of preoperative radiation. All patients' disease is preferably surgically staged and postoperative treatment is employed selectively for those patients deemed to be at a significant risk for relapse based on clinicopathologic prognostic factors (Table 49-9).

The *low-risk* group includes patients with stage IA G1, G2 tumors. The risk of pelvic lymph nodal positivity[87] is less than or equal to 3%, and the 5-year progression-free survival rate in this group is on the order of 90% to 96%. It is unlikely that postoperative pelvic external beam radiation would add anything to the final outcome, and therefore radiation is not routinely recommended to this group of patients.[197-200] The role of intravaginal radiation in these patients is also of questionable benefit due to a very low rate of vaginal recurrence with surgery alone.

The *intermediate-risk* group has been defined by the GOG as those with pathologic stage IB to IIB (occult cervical involvement). It is in this risk category where most of the controversy resides about the indication and type of radiation needed. With regard to the *indication* of adjuvant radiation in intermediate risk patients, the controversy relates to the lack of improvement in overall survival with the use of adjuvant radiation compared to surgery alone. The two recently completed randomized trials demonstrating lack of survival advantage leads to the conclusion on the part of many gynecologic oncologists that adjuvant radiation is not needed. The first trial was conducted by the GOG No. 99 and presented only in abstract form; 390 patients with stage IB to IIB endometrial cancer who underwent TAH/BSO and pelvic and para-aortic lymph nodal sampling were randomized to

observation ($n = 200$) or postoperative pelvic radiation ($n = 190$) to a total dose of 50.4 Gy in 28 fractions.[201] With a median follow-up of 56 months, the 3-year survival rate was 96% in the irradiation arm, compared with 89% in the observation arm ($P = 0.09$). The 2-year estimated progression-free survival rate was 96% versus 88% in favor of the irradiation arm ($P = 0.004$). The second trial was the Postoperative Radiation in Endometrial Cancer (PORTEC) trial in which 714 patients with stage IB G2,3 and IC G1,2 were randomized after TAH/BSO and without lymph nodal sampling to observation ($n = 360$) or pelvic radiation ($n = 354$) to a total dose of 46 Gy in 23 fractions.[120] With a median follow-up of 52 months, the 5-year locoregional control was 96% in the radiation arm compared to 86% in the observation arm ($P < 0.001$). The corresponding 5-year survival rates were 81% and 85% respectively ($P = 0.37$). While overall survival is the ultimate endpoint of any randomized trial in cancer treatment in general, it is important to point out that in patients with endometrial cancer there are other competing causes of death such as diabetes, hypertension, and obesity, to name a few. Furthermore, the cause of death from endometrial cancer is often distant relapse, which adjuvant radiation obviously can't control. It is essential to take those facts into an account when deciding on the benefit of adjuvant radiation in endometrial cancer, which is of the same magnitude of adjuvant chemotherapy for node-negative breast cancer patients.

With regard to *the type of radiation* to be used, there are three options: intravaginal brachytherapy, pelvic external beam radiation, or a combination of both. Only one prospective randomized trial has tried to determine the optimal type of postoperative radiation in this group of patients.[202] Aalders et al. reported on 540 patients with stage IB to IC endometrial cancer who underwent TAH/BSO without lymph nodal sampling, and postoperative intravaginal brachytherapy to 60 Gy to vaginal mucosa. Then the patients were randomized to observation ($n = 277$) or to supplemental pelvic radiation to 40 Gy ($n = 263$). A significant reduction in local recurrence rates was seen with the addition of pelvic radiation (1.9% vs. 6.9%, $P < 0.01$). With regard to overall survival, there was no significant difference between the two arms of the study, but in the subset of patients with grade 3 disease and deep myometrial penetration, there was a survival advantage (cause-specific survival) of 18% versus 7% in favor of the pelvic radiation arm.

The data from this trial contributed somewhat to the shift in treatment policies from intravaginal brachytherapy alone to external beam pelvic radiation alone. But whether pelvic radiation alone is equivalent to a combination of pelvic and intravaginal radiation has never been compared in a randomized fashion. Greven et al. reviewed the experience of two institutions in order to compare the outcome of the two approaches. In that study, there were 270 patients with stage I to II endometrial cancer—173 were treated with postoperative pelvic radiation alone and 97 with a combination of intravaginal and pelvic radiation.[203] The corresponding 5-year pelvic control and disease-free survival rates were 96% vs. 93% ($P = 0.32$) and 88% vs. 83% ($P = 0.41$). This study as well as others called into question whether the addition of vaginal

Table 49–9   Risk Grouping Following Surgical Staging

Low Risk	Intermediate Risk	High Risk
IA (Grades 1 & 2)	IA, G3	IIIA, IIIB, IIIC (All grades)
	IB, IC (All grades)	IVA, IVB (All grades)
	IIA, IIB (All grades)	
	IIIA (Positive cytology)	

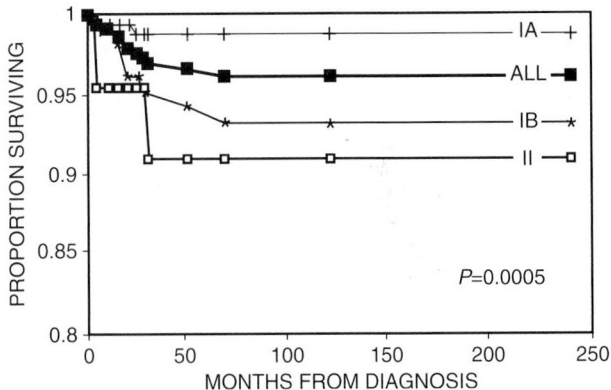

Figure 49–4. Long-term disease-free survival of low-risk and intermediate-risk patients with endometrial carcinoma treated with a combination of surgery and postoperative radiotherapy.

radiation is needed.[204,205] A number of other reports,[199,206] however, suggest that vaginal vault radiation can be added to pelvic radiation with minimal morbidity and a very low rate of recurrence (Fig. 49-4).

While such debate is intriguing to radiation oncologists, the changes in the management of these patients made this debate less pressing. The two randomized trials[120,201] comparing surgery to adjuvant radiation both employed pelvic radiation alone with a local recurrence of only 2% to 4%. On the other hand, with the increase of surgical lymph nodal staging, the use of postoperative intravaginal brachytherapy alone regained its appeal, the rationale being that full surgical lymph nodal staging could potentially eliminate the need for pelvic radiation while vaginal brachytherapy could still address the risk of vaginal cuff recurrence. Several reports in the past 5 years have indeed shown a very low rate of recurrence either in the vagina or the pelvis with such an approach.[207-209]

From this discussion, it is clear that different treatment options exist for patients with intermediate-risk disease. This makes the treatment decision for clinicians as well as patients difficult and at times confusing. But it is important to note that there are subgroups within the intermediate-risk category that need to be considered and are discussed here.

STAGE IA G3. Even though this group of patients was not included in the GOG definition of intermediate risk, from a treatment point of view this group should be treated in a similar fashion. These patients constituted less than 10% of all grade 3 patients in the GOG study,[87] and while they have a very low risk of lymph nodal metastasis (see Table 49-5), there were no relapses in the three patients receiving postoperative radiation as compared with one failure out of the five patients who received no postoperative therapy. These patients could be offered either intravaginal brachytherapy alone or observation.

STAGE IB G1,2. This group of patients constitutes the most common stage subgroup of all endometrial cancers. The outcome of patients who had lymph nodal dissection and no adjuvant radiation seems to be very good. Straughn et al. reported on 296 patients with IB G1,2 and found

only 9 (3%) vaginal recurrences and 1 (0.3%) pelvic recurrence.[210] In comparison, data from Memorial Sloan-Kettering Cancer Center on 233 patients with IB G1,2 showed a vaginal recurrence rate of only 1% and pelvic recurrence of 2% using postoperative intravaginal brachytherapy alone without routine surgical lymph nodal staging.[211] Other investigators reported a vaginal recurrence rate of 0% to 1% and pelvic recurrence rate of 1% to 2%, also using intravaginal brachytherapy.[212-214] Horowitz et al. reported on 62 patients who had surgical lymph nodal staging and received adjuvant intravaginal brachytherapy. There was one (1.6%) vaginal recurrence and zero pelvic recurrence.[209] Based on data from the Aalders randomized trial, it seems that pelvic radiation is not needed in this group of patients, even without surgical lymph nodal staging. When the subset of patients with stage IB G1,2 was evaluated (*n* = 257), the rate of local recurrence either in the vagina or pelvis was 4% (5/126) in those treated with intravaginal brachytherapy compared to 2.3% (3/131) for those treated with brachytherapy and external radiation.[202]

Thus it seems reasonable to suggest that either observation or intravaginal brachytherapy are reasonable options. But when deciding whether adjuvant radiation is needed, it is important to address two issues. First, older patients tend to have higher rates of relapse. In the study by Straughn et al., 8 of the 10 vaginal/pelvic recurrences were in patients 60 years old or older.[210] Second, often the indications for adjuvant radiation are rather arbitrarily based on the depth of myometrial invasion defined in thirds and on grade 1 versus 2. Yet the amount of myometrial invasion in this group of patients and whether an endometrial cancer is assigned to grade 1 as opposed to 2 in general doesn't appear to be a significant predictor of outcome.[136,215]

STAGE IB G3-IC G1,2,3. Until the past 5 years, most data in the literature on this group of patients are based on pelvic radiation either alone or in combination with intravaginal brachytherapy.[199,204,206,216,217] Weiss et al. reported on 61 patients with stage IC endometrial cancer who were treated with postoperative pelvic radiation alone. With a median follow-up of 69.5 months, there was only one recurrence in the pelvis (1.6%). Their review of the published data from the literature on patients with IC showed a pelvic recurrence of 1.04% in 240 patients treated with pelvic radiation alone compared to 0.97% in 301 patients treated with pelvic and intravaginal vaginal radiation. Their conclusion was that pelvic radiation alone is sufficient and effort should focus instead on trying to reduce the risk of distant relapse in this group of patients.[218]

With the increase in surgical lymph nodal staging, a shift is occurring with regard to the role of radiation even in stage IC disease. A recent multi-institutional review of 220 patients with stage IC endometrial cancer by Straughn et al. compared adjuvant radiation to no radiation in patients with negative nodes on surgical staging.[219] The authors concluded that adjuvant radiation is not needed even though the 5-year disease-free survival was 74.5% for those treated with surgery alone compared to 92.5% for those treated with adjuvant radiation

(P = 0.0134). It is unlikely that observation alone, even in those patients with full surgical staging, will be accepted by the radiation oncology community or even the patients when they see an 18% statistically significant difference in disease-free survival from a retrospective study in which, most likely, those patients with the worst prognostic features were the ones who received radiation.

Perhaps a reasonable alternative to observation or even pelvic radiation is intravaginal brachytherapy. In the Aalders randomized trial, the rate of local recurrence in the subset of patients with IB G3 to IC G 1,2,3 was 9.3% (13/137) for those treated with brachytherapy alone compared to 1.3% (2/146) for those treated with brachytherapy and external radiation.[202] While subset analysis should be interpreted with caution, it seems that the addition of external beam did have an impact, in terms of local recurrence, on patients with stage IB G3 to stage IC. This is not surprising since no lymph nodal sampling was done in that trial. But if one evaluates the data on patients with surgical lymph nodal staging and who received intravaginal brachytherapy alone, it becomes evident that the rate of local recurrence is lower. Horowitz et al. reported on 81 patients who were IB G3-IC. Only 2 patients (2.4%) had vaginal recurrences and 1 (1%) had a pelvic recurrence.[209] Similarly, Chada et al. and Fanning reported no vaginal or pelvic recurrence in 38 and 39 patients, respectively.[220,221]

Thus, in this group of patients the most accepted treatment recommendation is pelvic radiation alone. The addition of intravaginal radiation to pelvic radiation doesn't seem to increase the rate of local control, albeit there is no randomized trial comparing the two approaches to guide us in our decision making. The second emerging alternative to pelvic radiation is intravaginal brachytherapy *if* the patient had surgical lymph nodal staging of all five lymphatic stations as described by the GOG. What impact lymphovascular invasion may have on the outcome needs to be determined if the omission of pelvic radiation is to be become the standard of practice in this group of patients.

STAGE II. There are very little data regarding the optimal treatment of stage II patients. It is important to recognize the distinction between gross and occult cervical involvement and that these patients have a risk of parametrial involvement as well as a pelvic lymph nodal positivity of 25% to 50%. Preoperative radiation is generally preferred in patients with gross cervical involvement. This is usually given as a combination of external beam pelvic radiotherapy and intracavitary radiotherapy, followed by an extrafascial total abdominal hysterectomy and bilateral salpingo-oophorectomy. An alternative approach involves surgery upfront: A modified or radical hysterectomy with bilateral salpingo-oophorectomy and pelvic lymph nodal dissection is first employed and is followed by postoperative pelvic and intravaginal radiation based on pathologic findings. For occult cervical involvement, the combination of preoperative radiation and surgery may still be employed, although most centers would prefer a formal surgical staging followed by postoperative pelvic and intravaginal brachytherapy.[206,222] A review of the literature fails to support any one approach over the other (Table 49-10). Five-year survival rates in the

Table 49–10   Stage I Endometrial Carcinoma: Survival Rates

Reference	Patient, *n*	5-Year Survival, %
Wharam et al*	269	81 (NED)
Graham et al*	123	74 (Crude)
Malkasian et al*	409	82 (Actuarial)
Underwood et al*	220	91 (Actuarial)
Frick et al*	239	78 (Crude)
Salazar et al*	307	84 (Actuarial)
Brady et al*	99	88 (Crude)
Stokes et al*	304	87 (Actuarial)
Ritcher et al*	161	95 (Actuarial)
Nori et al*	278	85 (Actuarial—10 y)
Grigsby et al*	858	89 (NED)

NED, no evidence of disease.
*From Glassburn JR, Brady LW, Grigsby PW: Endometrium. In Perez CA and Brady LW, eds. *Principles and Practice of Radiation Oncology*, 2nd ed. p 1214, 1992. Reproduced with permission from J. B. Lippincott Company, Philadelphia.

range of 70% to 80% can be obtained if these principles are adhered to. Data are emerging on the role of intravaginal brachytherapy alone in patients with occult cervical involvement who also had surgical lymph nodal staging. The rate of pelvic recurrence in four such series ranged from 0% to 6%, but the data need confirmation on a larger number of patients and longer follow-up.[209,214,221,233]

HIGH RISK. The high-risk group consists of all patients with stage III and IV disease, regardless of grade, with the possible exception of patients who are stage III (positive peritoneal cytology) but without deep invasion or aggressive histology. Though the overall outcome is far from satisfactory, this is a very heterogeneous group and the therapy has to be individualized according to the patient's presentation. In general, for stage III patients, the outcome is much better for patients presenting with pathologic stage III disease than for those who present with clinical stage III disease.[234] While vascular space involvement, tumor grade, and myometrial invasion are still important prognostic factors, the number and site of extrauterine involvement, the ability to maximally debulk, and the presence or absence of nodal metastases have far greater prognostic importance.[197,234-236]

STAGE III. In patients with stage IIIA disease (positive cytology), the presence of other adverse features should be determined. If they are *present*, then the patients should be considered true high risk and be treated as such. On the other hand, if they are *absent*, then the true prognostic value of positive peritoneal cytology is still unclear.[145] The literature regarding the benefits of treatment in this setting is mixed; even if treatment is beneficial, the appropriate modality still must be defined. Based on the concept that the entire peritoneal cavity is at risk, intraperitoneal radioactive colloidal P32 has been used by some with results that were better than in historic controls.[144] One of the important lessons learned early in the experience with P32 was that its use should not be combined with that of external beam radiation because of a high complication rate. Soper and associates[237] reported 29% bowel complications requiring surgical intervention in such patients, with two patients dying of operative complications. In a similar setting of positive peritoneal cytology, Piver and associates[238] have employed systemic therapy with megestrol acetate (Megace) in 45 patients. The treatment was given for 1 year, and only 2 of the 36 patients who underwent a second-look laparotomy had persistence of positive peritoneal cytology. These two patients underwent continued therapy for another year and both were negative at a third-look laparotomy. However, even when no therapy was given, disease recurred in only 10% of similar patients with a minimum follow-up of 10 years; thus, the true status of adjuvant treatment in this subgroup is still a subject of considerable debate.

Patients with stage IIIA disease (positive adnexa or serosa) usually undergo surgical staging as the initial part of their therapy. Postoperative pelvic with or without intravaginal radiation is offered to patients with disease limited to the adnexa; these form the most favorable subset, with a 5-year survival rate of about 80% (Table 49-11). Stage IIIB is a very uncommon presentation; these patients are not surgical candidates and are generally treated with a combination of external beam and intracavitary/interstitial radiotherapy tailored to the extent of their disease. Following a good response to radiation, the treatment may be consolidated with an extrafascial hysterectomy. Patients with *stage IIIC disease* usually have the staging established at surgery when they are discovered to have positive pelvic or para-aortic nodes. If pelvic nodal involvement is the only major risk factor, treatment with postoperative pelvic radiotherapy can yield a 60% to 72% long-term survival rate in these patients.[197,236]

Patients with stage IIIC disease, by virtue of para-aortic nodal involvement, represent a particularly high-risk group. Following optimal debulking, these patients are generally treated with extended field radiation to encompass the pelvis and the para-aortic regions (with a carefully designed boost to any gross residual disease). With this aggressive approach, several authors have reported 30% to 40% survival rates in small patient populations.[197,248-254]

The recognition that a significant number of patients with stage III disease fail in the abdomen[234,255] has prompted numerous investigators to evaluate whole abdominal radiotherapy in these patients.[256,257] The GOG also did a pilot study, No. 94, on patients with maximally debulked stages III and IV disease using whole abdominal radiotherapy to a total dose of 30 Gy at 1.5 Gy per fraction followed by a pelvic boost for additional 19.8 Gy at 1.8 Gy per fraction. The 3-year disease-free and overall survival rates for the 58 patients with stage III endometrioid histology were 42.2% and 34.5%, respectively. The incidence of late gastrointestinal morbidity was 6%.[258] Using a different technique capable of delivering higher doses of radiation to the areas at risk for relapse in the abdomen, Stewart et al. reported 5-year disease-free and overall survival rates of 62% and 67%, respectively, in 62 patients with stage III endometrioid adenocarcinoma.[259]

STAGE IV. Stage IV disease usually has a dismal outcome, with survival rates in the range of 5% to 15%. Even in patients with tumors that can be thoroughly and optimally debulked, the results of whole abdominal radiation are still much inferior to those with stage III disease.[256] In the earlier mentioned GOG trial, 19 patients with stage IV endometrioid adenocarcinoma were treated with whole abdomen radiation after maximal debulking. The 3-year disease-free and overall survival rates were 12.5% and 21.1%, respectively.[258]

Table 49–11   Survival of Patients with Clinical/Pathologic Stage II Endometrial Cancer

	Preoperative RT		Postoperative RT	
Reference	Patients, n	5-Year Actuarial, %	Patients, n	5-Year Actuarial, %
Lanciano et al[223]	100	77*	68	87*
Podczaski et al[224]	36	58	—	—
Ahmad et al[225]	35	71	10	78
Larson et al[226]	64	68	5	60
Greven et al[227]	—	—	26†	86
Calkins et al[228]	28	57	39	52
Grigsby et al[229]	90‡	78*	—	—
Onsrud et al[230]	85§	85	—	—
Kinsella et al[231]	55¶	75	—	—
Surwit et al[129]	73**	70*	—	—
Bruckman et al[232]	40	80	—	—
Rubin et al[130]	77††	72	—	—

RT, radiotherapy.
*Disease-free survival.
†Three patients received preoperative radiotherapy.
‡Twenty-three patients may have had a component of postoperative radiotherapy.
§All patients had Heyman packing preoperatively with postoperative vaginal radiotherapy; 50% had external beam radiation.
¶Eight patients received postoperative radiotherapy.
**Fourteen patients received postoperative radiotherapy.
††Preoperative whole pelvic radiation + postoperative intravaginal radiation; 97 months, mean follow-up.
From Lanciano RM, Curan WJ, Greven KM, et al: Influence of grade, histologic subtype and timing of radiotherapy on the outcome among patients with stage II carcinoma of the endometrium. *Gynecol Oncol.* 1990;39:368. Reprinted with permission from Academic Press, Inc.

RADIATION THERAPY TECHNIQUES

External Beam Radiation

PELVIC RADIATION. Most patients are treated in the postoperative setting. The clinical target volume consists of the areas at risk, including the pelvic lymph nodes (external, internal, and lower common iliac groups) and the proximal two thirds of the vagina (since the treatment is generally delivered in the adjuvant setting without any residual tumor, there is no real gross tumor volume). The planning target volume is derived by ensuring an appropriate margin beyond the anatomic location of these structures to allow for variability in daily setup and beam penumbra. High-energy linear accelerators are preferred, and the four-field pelvic-box technique is employed (Figs. 49-5 and 49-6). The conventional field borders are as follows:

Superior: Interspace between L5 and S1 vertebrae
Inferior: Usually at the bottom of the obturator foramina
Lateral: 2 cm beyond the widest point of the inlet of the
  true bony pelvis
Anterior: In front of the pubic symphysis
Posterior: At a minimum through the S2 to S3 interspace.

During the simulation or CT-simulation, the small bowel is opacified using oral contrast, a vaginal marker is used to define the vault and outline the vagina, and the rectum is opacified with barium or other CT-compatible contrasts. Customized blocks or multi-leaf collimators are used to shield as much of the small bowel, rectum, and other soft tissues as possible without compromising on the target tumor volume. For example; there should be a 3 cm margin around the upper two thirds of the vagina, and in some patients the posterior border needs to be extended toward the sacral hollow in order to provide adequate coverage of internal iliac lymph nodes.

All fields are treated daily to a minimum target dose of 1.8 Gy. A total dose of 50.4 Gy is generally used when pelvic radiation is used alone or 45 Gy when combined with intravaginal brachytherapy.

EXTENDED FIELD. This technique is mainly used for patients with documented positive para-aortic nodes. The preferred approach is the four-field box technique in order to lower the dose to the small intestines. However, attention should be paid to the dose that the kidneys might receive with the four-field arrangement. The lower border is the same as in pelvic radiation, but the upper border is extended usually to the T11 to T12 interspace. The typical dose is 45 Gy at 1.8 Gy or 1.5 Gy if patients have developed gastrointestinal acute toxicity.

WHOLE ABDOMEN RADIATION. The standard approach is anterior-posterior–posterior-anterior (AP–PA) open fields with five half-value layer kidney blocks placed over the PA field only (if the patient is lying supine) from the start of the treatment. The dose is usually 30 Gy at 1.5 Gy per fraction followed by 19.8 Gy boost to the pelvis at 1.8 Gy per fraction. The upper border is usually placed 1 cm above the diaphragm, and the lateral borders should extend beyond the peritoneal reflections. The lower border is usually at the bottom of the obturator foramen. The alternative approach advocated

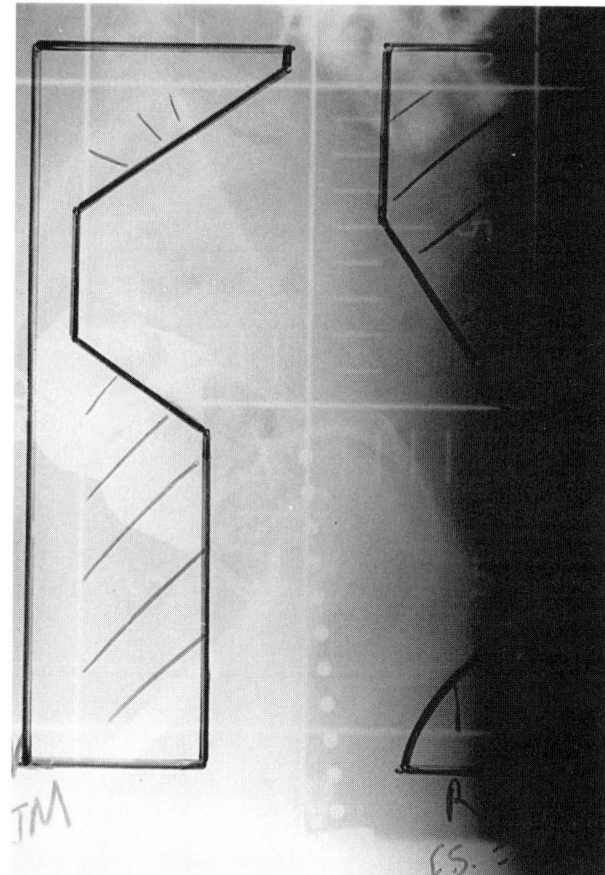

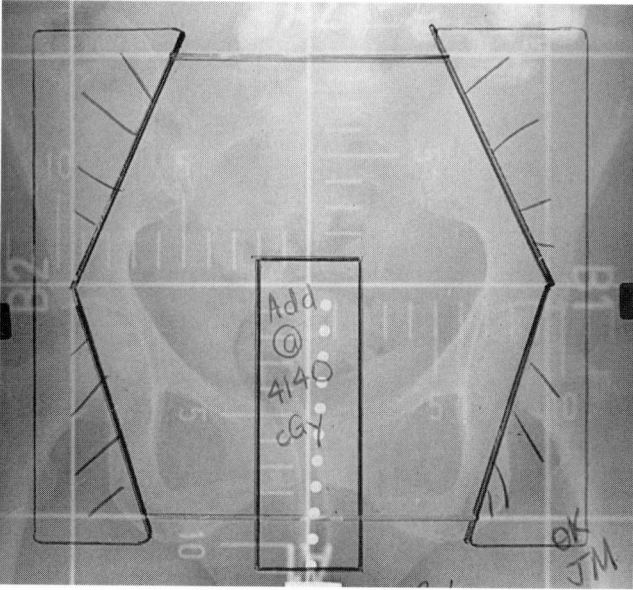

Figure 49–5. Simulation film for the AP–PA fields with the vaginal marker and the midline block.

Figure 49–6. Simulation film of the lateral fields, showing the fields shaped to protect the small bowel and the rectum.

by Martinez is shown in Chapter 50, Cancer of the Ovary, Figure 50-6, where after 30 Gy to the whole abdomen, an additional 12 Gy are given to the pelvic/para-aortic nodes and diaphragm.

Intravaginal Brachytherapy

Intravaginal brachytherapy has conventionally been delivered using *low-dose-rate* manual or remote afterloaders, employing either vaginal cylinders or colpostats. Based on the relapse patterns, the proximal two thirds of the vagina is considered the target volume for early-grade disease; in patients with high-grade disease, the entire length of the vagina is at risk and is accordingly treated. The conventional dose is 30 to 35 Gy prescribed at a depth of 0.5 cm from the vaginal mucosa if the planning is also done for external pelvic radiation, or 40 to 45 Gy at a similar depth if the patient is not to receive any external radiation.

There is now a considerable body of experience with the use of *high-dose-rate* remote afterloaders for vaginal vault irradiation (Fig. 49-7). This offers several advantages over the conventional low-dose-rate treatments in that the entire course of therapy can be delivered on an outpatient basis, the patients are far more comfortable during the short treatment time at each session, and there is a much better optimized dose distribution. The dose distribution with the low-dose-rate applicators often shows a relatively cold spot at the apex and at the distal end of the treatment volume due to anisotropy.[260] The intravaginal brachytherapy is usually delivered about 4 to 6 weeks postoperatively or a week after completion of the external beam radiotherapy and is given in three fractions every 1 to 2 weeks. This is best delivered with a vaginal cylinder rather than the conventional colpostats—

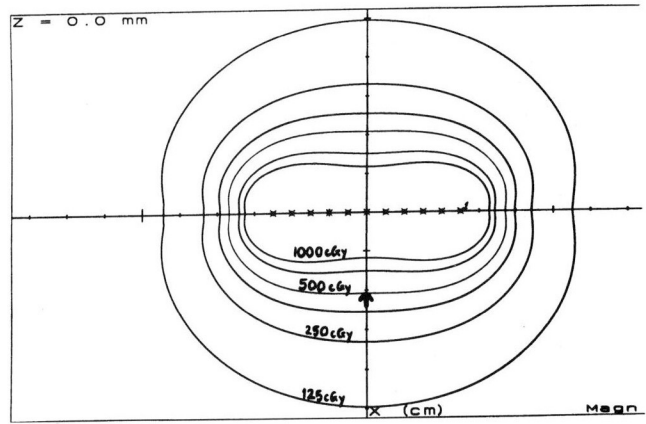

Figure 49–8. Isodose distribution using a 3.0 cm vaginal cylinder for high-dose-rate vaginal vault irradiation.

the geometry of the cylinder conforms much better to the posthysterectomy vagina than the colpostat; the cylinder also gives a better dose distribution in this setting (Fig. 49-8). The largest possible cylinder that fits the vagina snugly is selected. This allows for uniform mucosal apposition and ensures an optimal depth-dose distribution without overdosing the vaginal mucosa. An empirical study of different fraction sizes showed that a dose per fraction of greater than 7.5 Gy was associated with an unacceptable level of both early and late bladder and bowel toxicity.[261] Based on the long-term results of different fractionation schemes[262] and radiobiologic modeling using the linear-quadratic equation, we prescribe three fractions of 7 Gy each if the intravaginal radiation is used alone or 5 Gy if supplemented with external beam radiation. This dose is prescribed at a depth of 0.5 cm from the vaginal mucosa. Dose prescriptions at greater depths (with the same, or even smaller, fraction sizes) result in much higher vaginal mucosal doses, with a much higher incidence of late vaginal stenosis and other side-effects.[261] If the diameter of the cylinder is less than 3 cm, then the dose per fraction is reduced from 7 Gy to 6 Gy when intravaginal radiation is used alone or from 5 Gy to 4 Gy when combined with pelvic radiation. Such reduction is necessary to avoid an excessive dose to the vaginal mucosa. Our current approach to intravaginal radiation is given in Table 49-12.

ADJUVANT SYSTEMIC THERAPY

Endocrine Therapy

Several hormonal agents have been studied in patients with endometrial carcinoma. Initial studies showing tumor response to alpha-hydroxy-progesterone stimulated the development of a number of clinical trials. Although early, uncontrolled trials using progestational agents in an adjuvant setting suggested a reduction in the relapse rates in patients with stages I and II disease, these results have not been borne out in the three randomized trials that studied progesterone in the adjuvant

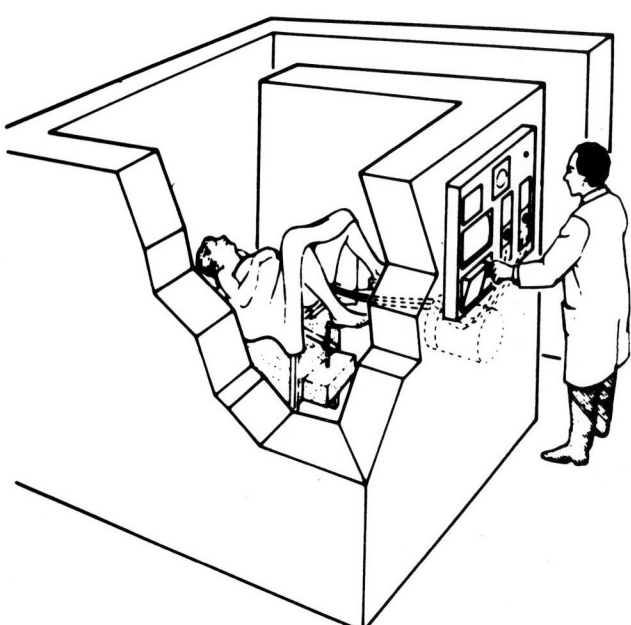

Figure 49–7. Schematic diagram of a high-dose-rate remote afterloader set up for vaginal vault irradiation.

Table 49–12   Outcome of Patients with Isolated Adnexal Involvement

Reference	Patients, n	Adjuvant Therapy	Results
Antoniades et al[239]	7	Pelvic RT	71% RFS
Bruckman et al[240]	15	Pelvic RT	80% actuarial 5-year RFS
Danoff et al[241]	5	Pelvic RT	60% 5-year survival
Greven et al[242]	42	Pelvic RT	60% actuarial 5-year RFS
Mackillop et al[243]	18	Pelvic RT (n = 12)	82% 5-year survival
		No RT (n = 6)	
Milton et al[244]	17	RT (not WAI)	80% 5-year RFS
Greer et al[245]	9	WAI	88% 5-year survival
Potish et al[246]	9	WAI	100% RFS (median FU 3 yrs)
Nori et al[247]	21 (microscopic)	Pelvic + Intravaginal RT	80% 5-year survival
	12 (gross)	Pelvic + Intravaginal RT	40% 5-year survival

FU, follow up; RFS, relapse-free survival; RT, radiotherapy; WAI, whole abdominal irradiation.
From Randall ME, Reisinger S: Radiation therapy and combined chemo-irradiation in advanced and recurrent endometrial carcinoma. *Semin Oncol.* 1994;21:91. Reproduced with permission from WB Saunders.

setting.[263-265] Two of these failed to show any advantage for progesterone,[263,264] while one showed a reduction in cancer-related deaths at the expense of an increase in non–cancer-related deaths, resulting in no net benefit from the treatment.[265] The problems of obtaining statistically meaningful data from randomized trials in the adjuvant setting are highlighted by the fact that these patients have an approximately 75% cure rate, and more than 40% of the deaths are from nonmalignant causes. Thus, detection of a treatment-related benefit of even 5% would require more than 2000 patients, a goal that has not been met in any of the studies.[266] Thus, adjuvant progestin therapy cannot be recommended as a standard treatment. The situation can only be clarified by further trials focusing on high-risk patients, and stratifying for receptor status so that we can define a subpopulation that *may* benefit from this therapy.

Chemotherapy

The only large randomized trial using adjuvant chemotherapy in pathologic stage I to III disease that has been completed to date is the GOG trial that treated patients who had poor prognostic factors with postoperative radiation and then randomized them to no further therapy or intravenous doxorubicin. At 5 years' follow-up, there were no differences between the two groups.[267] Based on the positive outcome of a pilot study from MD Anderson Hospital,[268] the GOG launched study No. 156 looking at patients with stages IB, IC, IIA, and IIB with high-risk features. Patients must have two or more of the following characteristics: grade 3, clear cell, or papillary serous histology, greater than one-third myometrial penetration, and vascular space invasion. Following postoperative pelvic irradiation, patients are randomized to doxorubicin, cisplatin, and cyclophosphamide or observation. Unfortunately, the study was closed due to lack of accrual.

Although radiotherapy can help patients with stage III disease, and even cure select subgroups (such as those with only adnexal involvement, or with microscopic disease limited to a few extrauterine sites that are all optimally debulked), advances in systemic therapy may hold the key to improving cures in these patients. The GOG launched study No. 122 in 1992, randomizing patients with advanced stages III/IV disease to whole abdominal irradiation versus systemic therapy with doxorubicin and cisplatin. The preliminary data presented in abstract form showed statistically significant improvement in disease-free and overall survival in favor of chemotherapy, yet cancer in 55% of patients in the trial recurred.[269] Thus, the current direction is to combine chemotherapy and radiation. Hoskins et al. reported on 21 patients with primary advanced endometrioid adenocarcinoma treated with adjuvant radiation and six cycles of carboplatin and taxol given sequentially.[270] The 3-year overall survival was 62%.

RECURRENT ENDOMETRIAL CANCER

Despite the fact that most patients with endometrial cancer are cured with standard therapy, disease does recur both locally and systemically. Of the patients with stage I disease treated with a combination of surgery and postoperative radiotherapy, about 3% have an isolated pelvic relapse, 7% have only distant disease, and another 2% have both. For stage II patients who are optimally treated, pelvic (including cuff) failures occur in about 3%, isolated distant failures occur in 10.5%, and another 8% have a component of both. Overall, recurrent endometrial carcinoma is confined to the pelvis in about half of the patients, with half of these having disease limited to the vagina. Factors predictive of salvage include vaginal vault versus pelvic relapse, lack of prior radiation, tumor size greater than 2 cm, and longer disease-free intervals.[271,272] There is also a suggestion that apical vaginal relapses fare better than distal relapses, although there are reports to the contrary.[273] Depending on the location of the recurrence, the extent of disease, and prior therapy, patients may be treated for palliation or with a curative intent. The treatment plan may include irradiation, surgery, endocrine therapy, or cytotoxic chemotherapy.

Radiation Therapy

Radiation therapy can be curative in a select group of patients with small vaginal recurrences who have not received prior radiation. The 5-year local control rate ranges from 42% to 65% and the 5-year overall survival rate from 31% to 53%.[271,274,275] The etiology of vault recurrences is still uncertain. Upper vaginal recurrences have been variously attributed to spill or implantation at the time of surgery or positive surgical margins, whereas lower vaginal relapses are often believed to represent retrograde lymphatic or vascular embolization and are especially associated with high-grade tumors. Almost 90% of the relapses occur within the first 3 years after hysterectomy. The vault and the upper third of the vagina are twice as often involved as the distal vagina, and vaginal relapses account for 20% to 25% of all failures in patients treated with surgery alone.[193]

With the impetus to try to eliminate any adjuvant radiation for early-stage endometrial cancer, the issue of radiation for salvage has become a very intriguing topic. Creutzberg et al. reported on survival after relapse in the PORTEC randomized trial.[276] In patients who were initially randomized to surgery alone, the 5-year survival after vaginal relapse was 65%. Thus, the conclusion that some are drawing is that we should accept the higher rate of relapse with surgery alone because the majority of patients could be salvaged with radiation.

But before adopting such an approach it is important to address certain pertinent issues. First, this high rate of salvage pertains only to isolated vaginal recurrence and not pelvic recurrence. In fact, the rate of survival for pelvic recurrence in the PORTEC trial was 0% at 3 years. On the one hand we are being asked to omit adjuvant radiation despite its significant improvement in local control because overall survival was not improved (i.e., we need to look at the big picture), yet on the other hand we are being asked to focus only on the high rate of salvage in those with isolated vaginal recurrence and not pelvic recurrences. Second, there is no mention in the trial of how salvage radiation was given and what the potential complications were. In addition to the lack of survival advantage, the high rate of complications from adjuvant radiation in the PORTEC trial was the second impetus to recommend omitting adjuvant radiation. It is not unreasonable to expect that the rate of complications from the definitive radiation used for salvage is much higher than just adjuvant radiation. Third, the extent of vaginal recurrence is a significant predictor of outcome.[274] The question then becomes how comparable is this salvage rate in the setting of a randomized trial where patients are vigorously followed and recurrences are detected early to that in a routine clinical setting where patients are seen by their general gynecologists perhaps once or twice a year? Fourth, as alluded to by Drs. Cardenes and Randall in their editorial, many advocates of omitting any type of adjuvant radiation in patients who are surgically staged use the data from the PORTEC trial to justify their conclusion. But if we were to accept the findings of this trial, then why recommend surgical lymph nodal staging? None of the patients in the PORTEC trial had it.[277]

Surgery

The rare patient who has an isolated central recurrence after prior irradiation may benefit from pelvic exenteration. One of the largest series of pelvic exenterations for endometrial carcinoma comes from Barakat and associates,[278] who reviewed the Memorial Sloan-Kettering Cancer Center experience from 1947 to 1994. Of the 44 patients so treated, 20% were long-term survivors, with a median survival of only 10.2 months. Almost half the patients needed a total exenteration, and the complication rate was very high (>80% major complications). However, the procedure remains the only potentially curative option for patients with a central pelvic recurrence following prior surgery and radiotherapy.

Hormonal Therapy

Progestational agents have been extensively used in recurrent disease. If objective and rigorous criteria are used to evaluate the response, response rates range from 15% to 20%.[279,280] The average time to progression following an initial response is about 4 months; patients achieving a partial or complete response may remain stable for 6 months to several years. The overall survival is about 1 year, although there are reports of up to 15% 5-year survival rates.[279-281] Patients with well-differentiated tumors that are receptor positive and who have a long disease-free interval (2 to 3 years) appear to have a higher response rate and a better overall outcome.[281-283]

Cytotoxic Chemotherapy

A number of single agents and combination regimens show objective responses in endometrial carcinoma; however, most responses are partial and last only an average of 3 to 6 months, with a median survival of only 7 to 10 months. The rare patient who attains a complete remission may have a progression-free interval of 1 to 2 years, but that is more a reflection of the biology of the disease process than an attribute of the therapy. Doxorubicin, cisplatin, carboplatin, and taxol are the main single agents with activity in endometrial carcinoma.[284-287] The response rates range from 20% to 36%. Among the combinations used, regimens of doxorubicin-cisplatin and doxorubicin-cisplatin-cyclophosphamide have response rates varying from 30% to 80%. This variation in response rates is probably affected by the patient's performance status, prior therapy, extent of disease, and the criteria used to evaluate response. Most of the responses are partial, with durations ranging from 4 to 8 months, and a median survival of less than 12 months. While several agents are being evaluated by the GOG, EORTC, and others, the doxorubicin-cisplatin-taxol carboplatin and taxol combinations are probably the most active regimens available today. The addition of hormones to chemotherapy does not seem to improve the outcome. Also, prior hormonal therapy does not influence the response rates to subsequent chemotherapy; this means that all patients should have a trial of hormonal therapy first, reserving the more toxic chemotherapy for endocrine treatment failures.

In summary, systemic therapy with progestogens remains the mainstay of patients with recurrent endometrial cancer. In patients with an isolated local relapse, carefully tailored radiotherapy can achieve local control in a fair proportion, if they have not received radiation in the postoperative period. In patients who have been previously irradiated, the rare isolated, central relapse may be evaluated for an exenteration, but the potential for cure must be tempered by the considerable morbidity associated with the operation. Cytotoxic chemotherapy is usually reserved for patients who do not respond to, or progress despite, hormonal therapy.

TREATMENT OF MEDICALLY INOPERABLE PATIENTS

Almost 10% of patients with endometrial cancer are not surgical candidates because of major comorbid medical conditions. These patients can be successfully treated with radiotherapy alone.[288,289] Patients with clinical stage I disease are treated with a curative intent using a combination of external beam therapy and intracavitary brachytherapy. The outcome of curative radiotherapy in these patients depends on the tumor-related prognostic factors as well as the severity of the underlying medical conditions. While it is generally believed that radiation alone may yield slightly lower local control rates, a significant proportion of the mortality in this population is due to the patients' intercurrent medical problems.[290,291] Grigsby et al.[290] reported that the 5-year progression-free survival rate of patients with clinical stage I disease treated with a combination of external and intracavitary radiotherapy was 94% for grade 1 disease, 92% for grade 2 disease, and 78% for grade 3 disease. At the New York Hospital, the external beam component is delivered as in the adjuvant setting, and we prefer high-dose-rate intracavitary brachytherapy, delivered using a tandem and vaginal cylinders for the "boost" to the site of initial disease. A pretreatment ultrasonogram or preferably magnetic resonance image is used to determine the myometrial thickness. Because these patients usually have intercurrent medical problems that make them a poor anesthetic risk, the intracavitary portion of the therapy may be delivered in two fractions of 10 Gy each, prescribed at an appropriate depth from the source center to encompass the entire myometrial thickness (generally 2.0 cm). For clinical stage II presentations, the parametria also need to be adequately treated. We deliver the intracavitary portion using a tandem and ovoids, prescribing the dose to Point A. The results in stage II disease are less encouraging: almost 25% of patients have a component of pelvic failure, whereas distant metastases are seen in about 35% of cases.

POOR-PROGNOSIS HISTOLOGIC SUBTYPES

Given the aggressive nature and the relapse patterns of papillary serous (PS) and clear cell cancers, both systemic chemotherapy and whole abdominal radiation have been tried, following maximal surgical debulking.[259,292-294] Lim et al.[294] reported on 78 patients with stage I to IIIA PS carcinoma, 58 of whom were treated with whole abdomen radiation and 20 of whom were not. The corresponding 5-year disease-specific survival rates were 74.9% and 41.3%, respectively (P = 0.04). In GOG No. 94, the 3-year disease-free and overall survival rates for the 60 patients with stage III PS or clear cell carcinomas were 40.9% and 45%, respectively.[258] The data on whole abdomen are somewhat encouraging, but the rate of relapse is still substantial, indicating the need for effective systemic therapy.

SEQUELAE OF TREATMENT

A TAH/BSO has an operative mortality, in general, of less than 1%. However, a significant number of patients with endometrial carcinoma are elderly and have various comorbid medical conditions (diabetes, hypertension, heart disease, obesity), which places them at a higher than usual risk of perioperative morbidity and mortality. It is especially important to remember this while contemplating extended surgical staging procedures in these patients.

Pelvic external beam radiotherapy may cause transient, self-limiting diarrhea or cystitis, but these are rarely a problem if megavoltage units and judicious field-shaping are employed. Late (chronic) small bowel toxicity, proctitis, or cystitis are also uncommon (less than 5%) with modern techniques and standard dose/fractionation regimens. In the PORTEC randomized trial,[295] the overall (grades 1 to 4) rate of late complications was 26% in the RT group compared to 4% in the observation group (P < 0.0001). Most of the late complications in the RT group were grades 1 to 2 (22%) and only 3% were grades 3 to 4. It is important to note that many patients in this trial were treated with AP–PA fields, where the overall rate of complications was 30% compared to 21% for those treated with a four-field box (P = 0.06). *Whole abdomen radiation* toxicity is more pronounced than pelvic radiation but not as high as expected. In GOG study No. 94, the rate of grade 4 gastrointestinal toxicity was seen in six patients (3.8%). Severe liver toxicity was seen in 3 of 158 evaluable patients (2%), with two thirds recovering without sequelae. And there was no grade 3 to 4 genitourinary toxicity.[258]

Intravaginal brachytherapy's main advantage is its ability to deliver a relatively high dose of radiation to the vagina while limiting the dose to the surrounding normal structures such as bowels and bladder. This advantage is manifested with the low rate of severe late toxicity seen with this treatment technique, ranging from 0% to 1%.[209,211,212] But such very low rates of severe complications can't be taken for granted because special attention must be paid to the depth of prescription, dose per fraction, the length of vagina treated, and the diameter of the cylinder used. Sorbe and Smeds[296] reported a 15% late complication rate and a very high incidence of vaginal stenosis following postoperative high-dose-rate intravaginal irradiation. This was attributed to the high dose per

Table 49–13 Treatment Policy for Vault Irradiation

Category	Surgery	External Radiation	High-Dose-Rate Intravaginal Radiation
Operable Cases			
Intermediate/High Risk	TAH/BSO	45 Gy	5 Gy × 3, at 0.5 cm from the vaginal mucosa
Low Risk (PS 1, Gr 2)	TAH/BSO	None	7 Gy × 3, at 0.5 cm from the vaginal mucosa
Low Risk (PS 1, Gr 1)	TAH/BSO	None	Most centers would elect to observe; may be offered vault radiation (7 Gy × 3 at 0.5 cm)
Inoperable Cases	None	45 Gy	10 Gy × 2, at 2 cm from the central axis of the uterus, using a tandem & cylinders
Recurrent Cases	None	Depends on prior RT	Individualize use of shielded applicators based on extent of disease

BSO, bilateral salpingo-oophorectomy; RT, radiotherapy; TAH, total abdominal hysterectomy.

fraction of 6 to 9 Gy; moreover, this dose was prescribed at a depth of 10 mm from the surface of the cylinder, resulting in very high vaginal mucosal, bladder, and rectal doses.

FUTURE DIRECTIONS

The role of radiation in endometrial cancer is at a critical crossroad. The significant increase in the use of surgical lymph nodal staging seems to be heavily encroaching on the role of adjuvant radiation in early-stage endometrial cancer. But some advances in surgical techniques such as laparoscopy may prove advantageous for radiation in the long run. With a potential decrease in surgical complications with laparoscopic-assisted vaginal hysterectomy, the complications from radiation will potentially decrease as well. Similarly, with laparoscopic lymph nodal dissection, the potential complications from postoperative external beam radiation will also be more acceptable. The emphasis on the role of adjuvant radiation should be on how to improve the therapeutic ratio. The judicious use of intravaginal brachytherapy in patients with adequate surgical lymph nodal staging should be an area of intense investigation. Surgical lymph nodal staging has decreased the rate of pelvic recurrence to an extremely low rate, but obviously it has no impact on vaginal recurrence. Thus, intravaginal radiation with its low morbidity is the best approach with the best therapeutic ratio that is currently being studied in the PORTEC II trial.

The high rate of relapse in high-risk endometrial cancer or those with poor histologies indicate the need for systemic therapy. The data from GOG No. 122 showed promising results for combination chemotherapy in the adjuvant setting. But it is unlikely that chemotherapy alone is going to be sufficient, especially with more than 55% of patients still relapsing. Therefore, the most logical conclusion is to try to integrate radiation and chemotherapy better. Currently, the GOG study No. 184 is evaluating pelvic ± para-aortic radiation followed by either Adriamycin/cisplatin or Adriamycin/cisplatin/taxol in patients with stage III disease. Future studies will focus on trying to use concurrent radiation and chemotherapy rather than sequential treatment. Advances in intensity-modulated radiation therapy will further facilitate the integration of concurrent chemotherapy and radiation.

Ultimately, we need to incorporate the data from molecular studies to help us better stratify the patients into appropriate risk categories and develop treatment schedules based on these "primary" prognostic factors.

ACKNOWLEDGMENT

To the late Dr. Suhrid K. Parikh, for his immense contributions to this chapter in the first edition of this book.

REFERENCES

1. Jemal A, Murray T, Samuels A, et al: Cancer statistics. *CA Cancer J Clin.* 2003;53:5.
2. Gallup DG, Stock RJ: Adenocarcinoma of the endometrium in women 40 years of age or younger. *Obstet Gynecol.* 1984;64:417.
3. Lucas WE: Causal relationships between endocrine-metabolic variables in patients with endometrial carcinoma. *Obstet Gynecol Survey.* 1974;29:507.
4. Sommers SC, Meissner WA: Endocrine abnormalities accompanying human endometrial cancer. *Cancer.* 1957;10:516.
5. Rosenblum JM, Hendricks CH: Estrogenated vaginal epithelium. *Obstet Gynecol.* 1954;3:535.
6. Farhi DC, Nosanchuk J, Silverberg SG: Endometrial adenocarcinoma in women under 25 years of age. *Obstet Gynecol.* 1986; 68:741.
7. Novak E, Yui E: Relation of endometrial hyperplasia to adenocarcinoma of the uterus. *Am J Obstet Gynecol.* 1936;32:674.
8. McDonald TW, Malkasian GE, Gaffey TA: Endometrial cancer associated with feminizing ovarian tumor and polycystic ovarian disease. *Obstet Gynecol.* 1977;49:654.
9. Elwood JM, Cole P, Rothman KJ, et al: Epidemiology of endometrial cancer. *J Natl Cancer Inst.* 1977;59:1055.
10. MacMahon B: Risk factors for endometrial cancer. *Gynecol Oncol.* 1974;2:122.
11. Henderson BE, Casagrande JT, Pike MC, et al: The epidemiology of endometrial cancer in young women. *Br J Cancer.* 1983;47:749.
12. Brinton LA, Berman RJ, Mortel R, et al: Reproductive, menstrual and medical risk factors for endometrial cancer: Results from a case-control study. *Am J Obstet Gynecol.* 1992;167:1317.
13. Brinton LA, Hoover RN: Epidemiology of gynecologic cancers. In Hoskins WJ, Perez CA, Young RC, eds. *Principles and Practice of Gynecologic Oncology,* 2nd ed. Philadelphia: Lippincott-Raven; 1997:3.
14. Swanson CA, Potischman N, Wilbanks GD, et al: Relation of endometrial cancer risk to past and contemporary body size and body fat distribution. *Cancer Epidemiol Biomark Prev.* 1993; 2:231.
15. La Vecchia C, Parazzini F, Negri E: Anthropometric indicators of endometrial cancer risk. *Eur J Cancer.* 1991;27:487.

16. Kelsey JL, LiVolsi VA, Holford TR, et al: A case-control study of cancer of the endometrium. *Am J Epidemiol.* 1982;116:333.
17. Wynder EL, Escher GC, Mantel N: An epidemiological investigation of cancer of the endometrium. *Cancer.* 1966;19:489.
18. Shu XO, Brinton LA, Zheng W, et al: Relation of obesity and body fat distribution to endometrial cancer in Shanghai, China. *Cancer Res.* 1992;52:3865.
19. Schapira DV, Kumar NB, Lyman GH, et al: Upper body fat distribution and endometrial cancer risk. *JAMA.* 1991;266:1808.
20. Sturgeon SR, Brinton LA, Berman ML, et al: Past and present physical activity and endometrial cancer risk. *Br J Cancer.* 1993; 68:585.
21. Shu XO, Hatch MC, Zheng W, et al: Physical activity and risk of endometrial cancer. *Epidemiology.* 1993;4:342.
22. Gusberg SB, Hall RE: Precursors of corpus cancer: III. The appearance of cancer of the endometrium in estrogenically conditioned patients. *Obstet Gynecol.* 1961;17:397.
23. Brinton LA, Hoover RN, The Endometrial Cancer Collaborative Group: Estrogen replacement therapy and endometrial cancer risk: Unresolved issues. *Obstet Gynecol.* 1993;81:265.
24. Hulka BS, Fowler WC, Kaufman DG, et al: Estrogen and endometrial cancer: Cases and two control groups from North Carolina. *Am J Obstet Gynecol.* 1980;137:92.
25. Weiss NS, Szeleky DR, English DR, et al: Endometrial cancer in relation to patterns of menopausal estrogen use. *JAMA.* 1979; 242:261.
26. Mack TM, Pike MC, Henderson BE, et al: Estrogens and endometrial cancer in a retirement community. *N Engl J Med.* 1976; 294:1262.
27. Underwood PB, Miller MC, Kreutner A, et al: Endometrial carcinoma: The effect of estrogens. *Gynecol Oncol.* 1979;8:60.
28. La Vecchia C, Franceschi S, Gallus G, et al: Prognostic features of endometrial carcinoma in estrogen users and obese women. *Am J Obstet Gynecol.* 1982;144:387.
29. Chu J, Schweid AI, Weiss NS: Survival among women with endometrial cancer: A comparison of estrogen users and non-users. *Am J Obstet Gynecol.* 1982;143:569.
30. Weiss NS, Sayvetz TA: Incidence of endometrial cancer in relation to use of oral contraceptives. *N Engl J Med.* 1980;302:551.
31. Voigt LF, Deng Q, Weiss NS: Recency, duration and progestin content of oral contraceptives in relation to the incidence of endometrial cancer (Washington, USA). *Cancer Causes Control.* 1994;5:227.
32. Cancer and Steroid Hormone Study of the Centers for Disease Control and The National Institute of Child Health and Human Development: Combination oral contraceptive use and the risk of endometrial cancer. *JAMA.* 1987;257:796.
33. Gambrell RD Jr, Bagnell CA, Greenblatt RB: Role of estrogens and progesterone in the etiology and prevention of endometrial cancer: Review. *Am J Obstet Gynecol.* 1983;146:696.
34. Voigt LF, Weiss NS, Chu J, et al: Progestagen supplementation of exogenous estrogens and the risk of endometrial cancer. *Lancet.* 1991;338:274.
35. Writing Group for the Women's Health Initiative Investigators. Risks and benefits of estrogen plus progestin in healthy postmenopausal women: Principal results From the Women's Health Initiative randomized controlled trial. *JAMA.* 2002;288:321.
36. Cuzick J, Powles T, Veronesi U, et al: Overview of the main outcomes in breast-cancer prevention trials. *Lancet.* 2003;361:296.
37. Fisher B, Constantino JP, Redmond CK, et al: Endometrial cancer in tamoxifen-treated breast cancer patients: Findings from the National Surgical Adjuvant Breast and Bowel Project (NSABP)-B14. *J Natl Cancer Inst.* 1994;86:527.
38. Barakat RR, Wong G, Curtin JP, et al: Tamoxifen use in breast cancer patients who subsequently develop corpus cancer is not associated with a higher incidence of adverse histological features. *Gynecol Oncol.* 1994;55:164.
39. Fornander T, Hellstrom A-C, Moberger B: Descriptive clinicopathologic study of 17 patients with endometrial cancer during or after adjuvant tamoxifen in early breast cancer. *J Natl Cancer Inst.* 1993;85:1850.
40. Bergman L, Beelen ML, Gallee MP, et al: Risk and prognosis of endometrial cancer after tamoxifen for breast cancer. Comprehensive Cancer Centres' ALERT Group. Assessment of liver and endometrial cancer risk following tamoxifen. *Lancet.* 2000;356:881.

41. Parker SL, Tong T, Bolden S, et al: Cancer statistics, 1997. *CA Cancer J Clin.* 1997;47:5.
42. Potischman N, Swanson CA, Brinton LA, et al: Dietary associations in a case-control study of endometrial cancer. *Cancer Causes Control.* 1993;4:239.
43. Barbosa JC, Shultz TD, Fillery SJ, et al: The relationship among adiposity, diet and hormone concentrations in vegetarian and nonvegetarian postmenopausal women. *Am J Clin Nutr.* 1990; 51:798.
44. Prentice R, Thompson D, Clifford C, et al: Dietary fat reduction and plasma estradiol concentration in healthy postmenopausal women. *J Natl Cancer Inst.* 1990;82:129.
45. Barbone F, Austin H, Partridge EE: Diet and endometrial cancer: A case-control study. *Am J Epidemiol.* 1993;137:393.
46. Levi F, Franceschi S, Negri E, et al: Dietary factors and the risk of endometrial cancer. *Cancer.* 1993;71:3575.
47. Parazzini F, La Vecchia C, Negri E, et al: Diabetes and endometrial cancer: An Italian case-control study. *Int J Cancer.* 1999;81:539.
48. Soler M, Chatenoud L, Negri E, et al: Hypertension and hormone-related neoplasms in women. *Hypertension.* 1999;34:320.
49. Terry PD, Rohan TE, Franceschi S, Weiderpass E: Cigarette smoking and the risk of endometrial cancer. *Lancet Oncol.* 2002; 3:470.
50. Webster LA, Weiss NS: The Cancer and Steroid Hormone Study Group: Alcoholic beverage consumption and the risk of endometrial cancer. *Int J Epidemiol.* 1989;18:786.
51. Lynch HT, Smyrk TC, Watson P, et al: Genetics, natural history, tumor spectrum and pathology of hereditary nonpolyposis colorectal cancer: An updated review. *Gastroenterology.* 1993;104:1535.
52. Parsons R, Li G-M, Longley MJ, et al: Hypermutability and mismatch repair deficiency in RER+ tumor cells. *Cell.* 1994;75:1227.
53. Burke W, Petersen G, Lynch P, et al: Recommendations for follow-up care of individuals with an inherited predisposition to cancer. I. Hereditary nonpolyposis colon cancer. Cancer Genetics Studies Consortium. *JAMA.* 1997;277:915.
54. Kurman RJ, Kaminski PF, Norris HJ. The behavior of endometrial hyperplasia. A long-term study of "untreated" hyperplasia in 170 patients. *Cancer.* 1985;56:403.
55. Norris HJ, Tavassoli FA, Kurman RJ: Endometrial hyperplasia and carcinomas, diagnostic considerations. *Am J Surg Pathol.* 1988;7:839.
56. Silverberg SG: Hyperplasia and carcinoma of the endometrium. *Semin Diagn Pathol.* 1988;5:135.
57. Ng AB, Reagan JW, Hawliczek S, et al: Significance of endometrial cells in the detection of endometrial carcinoma and its precursors. *Acta Cytol.* 1974;18:356.
58. Ross JC, Eifel PJ, Cox RS, et al: Primary mucinous adenocarcinoma of the endometrium: A clinicopathologic and histochemical study. *Am J Surg Pathol.* 1983;7:715.
59. Abeler VM, Kjorstad KE. Endometrial adenocarcinoma in Norway: A study of a total population. *Cancer.* 1991;67:3093.
60. Cirisano FD Jr, Robboy SJ, Dodge RK, et al: Epidemiologic and surgicopathologic findings of papillary serous and clear cell endometrial cancers when compared to endometrioid carcinoma. *Gynecol Oncol.* 1999;74:385.
61. Hendrickson M, Ross J, Eifel P, et al: Uterine papillary serous carcinoma: A highly malignant form of endometrial adenocarcinoma. *Am J Surg Pathol.* 1982;6:93.
62. Kurman RJ, Scully RE: Clear-cell carcinoma of the endometrium: An analysis of 21 cases. *Cancer.* 1976;37:872.
63. Cirisano FD Jr, Robboy SJ, Dodge RK, et al: The outcome of stage I-II clinically and surgically staged papillary serous and clear cell endometrial cancers when compared with endometrioid carcinoma. *Gynecol Oncol.* 2000;77:55.
64. Piura B, Glezerman M: Synchronous carcinomas of the endometrium and ovary. *Gynecol Oncol.* 1989;33:261.
65. Scully RE: Tumors of the ovary and maldeveloped gonad. AFIP pamphlet No. 16. Washington, DC: Armed Forces Institute of Pathology; 1982:92.
66. Ulbright T, Roth L: Metastatic and independent cancers of the endometrium and ovary: A clinicopathologic study of 34 cases. *Human Pathol.* 1985;16:28.
67. Bokhman JV. Two pathogenetic types of endometrial carcinoma. *Gynecol Oncol.* 1983;15:10.
68. Deligdisch L, Holinka CF. Endometrial carcinoma: Two diseases? *Cancer Detect Prev.* 1987;10:237.

69. Lax SF, Kendall B, Tashiro H, et al: The frequency of *p53*, K-*ras* mutations, and microsatellite instability differs in uterine endometrioid and serous carcinoma: Evidence of distinct molecular genetic pathways. *Cancer.* 2000;88:814.

70. Tashiro H, Isacson C, Levine R, et al: *p53* gene mutations are common in uterine serous carcinoma and occur early in their pathogenesis. *Am J Pathol.* 1997;150:177.

71. Moll UM, Chalas E, Auguste M, et al: Uterine papillary serous carcinoma evolves via a *p53*-driven pathway. *Hum Pathol.* 1996;27:1295.

72. Sung CJ, Zheng Y, Quddus MR, et al: *p53* as a significant prognostic marker in endometrial carcinoma. *Int J Gynecol Cancer.* 2000;10:119.

73. Geisler JP, Geisler HE, Wiemann MC, et al: *p53* expression as a prognostic indicator of 5-year survival in endometrial cancer. *Gynecol Oncol.* 1999;74:468.

74. Tashiro H, Blazes MS, Wu R, et al: Mutations in *PTEN* are frequent in endometrial carcinoma but rare in other common gynecological malignancies. *Cancer Res.* 1997;57:3935.

75. Risinger JI, Hayes AK, Berchuck A, Barrett JC. *PTEN/MMAC1* mutations in endometrial cancers. *Cancer Res.* 1997;57:4736.

76. Risinger JI, Hayes K, Maxwell GL, et al: *PTEN* mutation in endometrial cancers is associated with favorable clinical and pathologic characteristics. *Clin Cancer Res.* 1998;4:3005.

77. Duggan BD, Felix JC, Muderspach LI, et al: Microsatellite instability in sporadic endometrial carcinoma. *J Natl Cancer Inst.* 1994;86:1216.

78. Maxwell GL, Risinger JI, Alvarez AA, et al: Favorable survival associated with microsatellite instability in endometrioid endometrial cancers. *Obstet Gynecol.* 2001;97:417.

79. Boyd J, Risinger JI. Analysis of oncogene alterations in human endometrial carcinoma: Prevalence of *ras* mutations. *Mol Carcinog.* 1991;4:189.

80. Berchuck A, Rodriguez G, Kinney RB, et al: Overexpression of *HER-2/neu* in endometrial cancer is associated with advanced stage disease. *Am J Obstet Gynecol.* 1991;164:15.

81. Hetzel DJ, Wilson TO, Keeny GL, et al: *HER-2/neu* expression: A major prognostic factor in endometrial cancer. *Gynecol Oncol.* 1992;47:179.

82. Berchuck A, Boyd J. Molecular basis of endometrial cancer. *Cancer.* 1995;76(suppl 10):2034.

83. Taskin M, Lallas TA, Barber HR, Shevchuk MM. *bcl-2* and *p53* in endometrial adenocarcinoma. *Mod Pathol.* 1997;10:728.

84. Leiserowitz GS, Harris SA, Subramaniam M, et al: The proto-oncogene *c-fms* is overexpressed in endometrial cancer. *Gynecol Oncol.* 1993;49:190.

85. Kobayashi K, Sagae S, Nishioka Y, et al: Mutations of the beta-catenin gene in endometrial carcinomas. *Jpn J Cancer Res.* 1999;90:55.

86. Risinger JI, Maxwell GL, Chandramouli GV, et al: Microarray analysis reveals distinct gene expression profiles among different histologic types of endometrial cancer. *Cancer Res.* 2003;63:6.

87. Creasman WT, Morrow CP, Bundy BN, et al: Surgical pathologic spread patterns of endometrial cancer (a Gynecologic Oncology Group Study). *Cancer.* 1987;60:2035.

88. Caspi E, Perpinial S, Reif A: Incidence of malignancy in Jewish women with post-menopausal bleeding. *Israel J Med Sci.* 1977;13:299.

89. Fleisher AC, Dudley BS, Entman SS, et al: Myometrial invasion by endometrial carcinoma: Sonographic assessment. *Radiology.* 1987;162:307.

90. Hulka CA, Hall DA, McCarthy K, et al: Endometrial polyps, hyperplasia, and carcinoma in post-menopausal women: Differentiation with endovaginal sonography. *Radiology.* 1994;191:755.

91. Mendelson EB, Bohm-Velez M, Joseph N, et al: Endometrial abnormalities: Evaluation with transvaginal sonography. *Am J Roentgenol.* 1989;150:139.

92. DelMaschio A, Vanzulli A, Sironi S, et al: Estimating the depth of myometrial involvement of endometrial carcinoma: Efficacy of transvaginal sonography vs. MR imaging. *Am J Roentgenol.* 1993;160:533.

93. Hamlin DJ, Burgener FA, Belcham JB: CT of intramural carcinoma: Contrast enhancement is essential. *Am J Roentgenol.* 1981;137:551.

94. Dore R, Moro B, D'Andrea F, et al: CT evaluation of myometrial invasion in endometrial carcinoma. *J Comput Assist Tomogr.* 1987;11:282.

95. Balfe DM, Van Dyke J, Lee JKT, et al: Computerized tomography in endometrial neoplasms. *J Comput Assist Tomogr.* 1982;7:677.

96. Walsh JW, Vick CW: Staging of female genital tract cancer. In Walsh JW, ed. *Computerized Tomography of the Pelvis.* New York: Churchill Livingstone; 1985:163.

97. Walsh JW, Goplerud DR: Computerized tomography of primary, persistent and recurrent endometrial malignancy. *Am J Roentgenol.* 1982;139:1149.

98. Franchi M, LaFianza A, Babilonti L, et al: Clinical value of computerized tomography (CT) in assessment of recurrent uterine cancers. *Gynecol Oncol.* 1989;35:31.

99. Chen SS, Rumanik WM, Spiegel G: Magnetic resonance imaging in stage I endometrial carcinoma. *Obstet Gynecol.* 1990;75:274.

100. Hricak H, Rubinstein LV, Gherman GM, et al: MR imaging evaluation of endometrial carcinoma: Results of an NCI cooperative study. *Radiology.* 1991;179:829.

101. Pellorito JS, Taylor KJ, Quedenas-Case C, Hammers LW: Endovaginal color flow scoring system: A sensitive indicator of pelvic malignancy [abstract]. *Radiology.* 1994;193(P):276.

102. Weber TM, Sostman DH, Spritzer CE, et al: Cervical carcinoma: Determination of recurrent tumor versus radiation changes with MR imaging. *Radiology.* 1995;194:135.

103. Hricak H, Stern JL, Fisher MR, et al: Endometrial carcinoma staging by MR imaging. *Radiology.* 1987;162:297.

104. Joja I, Asakawa M, Nakagawa T, et al: Endometrial carcinoma: Dynamic MRI with turbo-FLASH technique. *J Computer Assist Tomogr.* 1996;20:878.

105. Carrington B, Hricak H: The uterus and vagina. In Hricak H, Carrington BM, eds: *MRI of the Pelvis: A Text Atlas.* London: Martin Dunitz; 1991:93.

106. Hirano Y, Kubo K, Hirai Y, et al: Preliminary experience with gadolinium-enhanced dynamic MR imaging for uterine neoplasms. *Radiology.* 1992;12:243.

107. Sironi S, Mellone R, Venzulli A, et al: Assessment of the myometrial infiltration of endometrial carcinoma (FIGO stage I-II): The accuracy of magnetic resonance. *Radiol Med (Torino).* 1989;77:386.

108. Fishman-Javitt MC, Stein HL, Lovecchio JL: MRI in staging endometrial and cervical carcinoma. *Magn Reson Imaging.* 1987;5:83.

109. DelMaschio A, Vanzulli A, Sironi S, et al: Estimating the depth of myometrial involvement of endometrial carcinoma: Efficacy of transvaginal sonography vs. MR imaging. *Am J Roentgenol.* 1993;160:533.

110. Gordon AN, Fleisher AC, Dudley BS: Preoperative assessment of myometrial invasion of endometrial adenocarcinoma by sonography (US) and magnetic resonance imaging. *Gynecol Oncol.* 1989;34:175.

111. Berchuck A, Soisson AP, Clarke-Pearson DL, et al: Immunohistochemical expression of CA 125 in endometrial adenocarcinoma: Correlation of antigen expression with metastatic potential. *Cancer Res.* 1989;49:2091.

112. Rose PG, Sommers RM, Reale FR, et al: Serial serum CA 125 measurements for evaluation of recurrence in patients with endometrial carcinoma. *Obstet Gynecol.* 1994;84:12.

113. Boronow RC, Morrow CP, Creasman WT, et al: Surgical staging in endometrial cancer: Clinicopathological findings of a prospective study. *Obstet Gynecol.* 1984;63:825.

114. International Federation of Gynecology and Obstetrics: Corpus cancer staging. *Int J Gynecol Obstet.* 1989;28:190.

115. International Federation of Gynecology and Obstetrics: Classification and staging of malignant tumors in the female pelvis. *Int J Gynecol Obstet.* 1971;9:172.

116. Nolan JF, Huen A: Prognosis in endometrial cancer. *Gynecol Oncol.* 1976;4:384.

117. Frick HC, Munnell EW, Richart RM, et al: Carcinoma of the endometrium. *Am J Obstet Gynecol.* 1973;115:663.

118. Creasman WT, Odicino F, Maisonneuve P, et al: Carcinoma of the corpus uteri. *J Epidem Biostat.* 2001;6:45.

119. Kosary CL: FIGO stage, histology, histologic grade, age and race as prognostic factors in determining survival for cancers of the female gynecological system: An analysis of 1973-87 SEER cases of cancers of the endometrium, cervix, ovary, vulva, and vagina. *Semin Surg Oncol.* 1994;10:31.

120. Creutzberg CL, van Putten WL, Koper PC, et al: Surgery and postoperative radiotherapy versus surgery alone for patients with stage-1 endometrial carcinoma: Multicentre randomized trial. PORTEC Study Group. Post Operative Radiation Therapy in Endometrial Carcinoma. *Lancet.* 2000;355:1404.

121. Alektiar KM, Abu-Rustum N, Venkatraman E, et al: Is endometrial cancer intrinsically more aggressive in elderly patients. Cancer, in press.

122. Nori D, Hilaris B: Principles of radiation therapy in the treatment of carcinoma of the endometrium. In Nori D, Hilaris B, eds. *Radiation Therapy of Gynecologic Cancer.* Alan R. Liss, New York; 1987:121.

123. Connell PP, Rotmensch J, Waggoner SE, Mundt AJ: Race and clinical outcome in endometrial carcinoma. *Obstet Gynecol.* 1999;94:713.

124. Hicks ML, Phillips JL, Parham G, et al: The National Cancer Data Base report on endometrial carcinoma in African-American women. *Cancer.* 1998;83:2629.

125. Nori D, Hilaris BS, Batata MA, et al: Clinical application of remote afterloaders with special reference to endometrial cancer. In Brachytherapy Oncology, Memorial Hospital Annual Brachytherapy Proceedings, pp. 101-118. New York: MSKCC Publishers; 1983.

126. Lutz MH, Underwood PB Jr, Kreutner A Jr, et al: Endometrial carcinoma: A new method of classification of therapeutic and prognostic significance. *Gynecol Oncol.* 1978;6:83.

127. Boente MP, Yordan EL Jr, McIntosh DG, et al: Prognostic factors and long-term survival in endometrial adenocarcinoma with cervical involvement. *Gynecol Oncol.* 1993;51:316.

128. Mayr NA, Wen BC, Benda JA, et al: Postoperative radiotherapy in clinical stage I endometrial cancer—corpus, cervical and lower uterine segment involvement: Patterns of failure. *Radiology.* 1995; 196:323.

129. Surwit EA, Fowler WC Jr, Rogoff EE, et al: Stage II adenocarcinoma of the endometrium. *Int J Radiation Oncol Biol Phys.* 1979; 5:323.

130. Rubin SC, Hoskins WJ, Saigo PE, et al: Management of endometrial adenocarcinoma with cervical involvement. *Gynecol Oncol.* 1992;45:294.

131. Chambers SK, Kapp DS, Peschel RE, et al: Prognostic factors and sites of failure in FIGO stage I, grade 3 endometrial cancer. *Gynecol Oncol.* 1987;27:180.

132. Wilson TO, Podratz KC, Gaffey TA, et al: Evaluation of unfavorable histologic subtypes in endometrial adenocarcinoma. *Am J Obstet Gynecol.* 1990;162:418.

133. Nicklin JL, Copeland LJ: Endometrial papillary serous carcinoma: Patterns of spread and treatment. *Clin Obstet Gynecol.* 1996; 39:686.

134. Sutton GP, Geiser HE, Stehman FB, et al: Features associated with survival and disease-free survival in early endometrial cancer. *Am J Obstet Gynecol.* 1989;160:1385.

135. Wharton JT, Kikuta JJ, Mettlin C, et al: Risk factors and current management in carcinoma of the endometrium. *Surg Gynecol Obstet.* 1986;162:515.

136. Alektiar KM, McKee A, Lin O, et al: The significance of the amount of myometrial invasion in patients with Stage IB endometrial carcinoma. *Cancer.* 2002;95:316.

137. Hanson MB, van Nagell JR Jr, Powell DE, et al: The prognostic significance of lymph-vascular space invasion in stage I endometrial cancer. *Cancer.* 1985;55:1753.

138. Sivridis E, Buckley CH, Fox H: The prognostic significance of lymphatic vascular space invasion in endometrial adenocarcinoma. *Br J Obstet Gynecol.* 1987;94:991.

139. Nori D, Hilaris B: Principles of radiation therapy in the treatment of carcinoma of the endometrium. In *Radiation Therapy of Gynecologic Cancer.* New York: Alan R. Liss; 1987:122.

140. Konski A, Poulter C, Keys H, et al: Absence of prognostic significance, peritoneal dissemination and treatment advantage in endometrial cancer patients with positive peritoneal cytology. *Int J Radiation Oncol Biol Phys.* 1988;14:49.

141. Lurain JR, Ramsey NK, Schink JC, et al: Prognostic significance of positive peritoneal cytology in clinical stage I adenocarcinoma of the endometrium. *Obstet Gynecol.* 1989;74:175.

142. Yazigi R, Piver MS, Blumenson L: Malignant peritoneal cytology as prognostic indicators in stage I endometrial cancer. *Obstet Gynecol.* 1983;62:359.

143. Turner DA, Gershenson DM, Atkinson N, et al: The prognostic significance of peritoneal cytology for stage I endometrial cancer. *Obstet Gynecol.* 1989;74:775.

144. Creasman WT, DiSaia PJ, Blessing J, et al: Prognostic significance of peritoneal cytology in patients with endometrial cancer and

preliminary data concerning therapy with intraperitoneal radiopharmaceuticals. *Am J Obstet Gynecol.* 1981;141:921.

145. Milosevic MF, Dembo AJ, Thomas GM: The clinical significance of malignant peritoneal cytology in stage I endometrial carcinoma. *Int J Gynecol Cancer.* 1992;2:225.

146. Sonoda Y, Zerbe M, Smith A, et al: High incidence of positive peritoneal cytology in low-risk endometrial cancer treated by laparoscopically assisted vaginal hysterectomy. *Gynecol Oncol.* 2001;80:378.

147. Ashman JB, Connell PP, Yamada D, et al: Outcome of endometrial carcinoma patients with involvement of the uterine serosa. *Gynecol Oncol.* 2001;82:338.

148. Descamps P, Calais G, Moire C, et al: Predictors of distant recurrence in clinical stage I or II endometrial carcinoma treated by combination surgical and radiation therapy. *Gynecol Oncol.* 1997;64:54.

149. Evans MP, Podratz KC: Endometrial neoplasia: Prognostic significance of ploidy status. *Clin Obstet Gynecol.* 1996;39:696.

150. Lindahl B, Ranstam J, Norgren A, Willen R: Identification of high-risk groups in endometrial carcinoma stage I-II: A combination of DNA- and steroid-receptor measurements identifies early deaths from the disease. *Anticancer Res.* 1995;15:1095.

151. Pisani AL, Barbuto DA, Chen D, Ramos L, et al: *HER-2/neu, p53* and DNA analyses as prognosticators for survival in endometrial carcinoma. *Obstet Gynecol.* 1995;85:729.

152. Lukes AS, Kohler MF, Pieper CF, et al: Multivariate analysis of DNA ploidy, *p53* and *HER-2/neu* as prognostic factors in endometrial cancer. *Cancer.* 1994;73:2380.

153. Coleman RL, Schink JC, Miller DS, et al: DNA flow cytometric analysis of clinical stage I endometrial carcinoma with lymph node metastasis. *Gynecol Oncol.* 1993;50:20.

154. Melchiorri C, Chieco P, Lisignoli G, et al: Ploidy disturbances as an early indicator of intrinsic malignancy in endometrial carcinoma. *Cancer.* 1993;72:165.

155. Hamel NW, Sebo TJ, Wilson TO, et al: Prognostic value of *p53* and proliferating cell nuclear antigen expression in endometrial carcinoma. *Gynecol Oncol.* 1996;62:192.

156. Kaleli S, Kosebay D, Bese T, et al: A strong prognostic variable in endometrial carcinoma: Flow cytometric S-phase fraction. *Cancer.* 1997;79:944.

157. Nordstrom B, Strang P, Lindgren A, et al: Endometrial carcinoma: The prognostic impact of papillary serous carcinoma (UPSC) in relation to nuclear grade, DNA ploidy and *p53* expression. *Anticancer Res.* 1996;16:899.

158. Ferrara F, De Santis L, Mangili F, et al: Role of DNA ploidy and *ERB-B2* oncogene expression in the prognosis of endometrial carcinoma. *Pathol Res Pract.* 1994;190:1039.

159. Friberg LG, Noren H, Delle U: Prognostic value of DNA ploidy and S-phase fraction in endometrial cancer stage I and II: A prospective 5-year survival study. *Gynecol Oncol.* 1994;53:64.

160. Nazeer T, Ballouk F, Malfetano JH, et al: Multivariate survival analysis of clinicopathologic features in surgical stage I endometrial carcinoma including analysis of *HER-2/neu* expression. *Am J Obstet Gynecol.* 1995;173:1829.

161. Geisler JP, Weimann MC, Zhou Z, et al: DNA index by image analysis in advanced endometrial carcinoma. *J Surg Oncol.* 1996; 63:91.

162. Nordstrom B, Strang P, Bergstrom R, et al: A comparison of proliferation markers and their prognostic value for women with endometrial carcinoma: Ki-67, proliferating nuclear antigen and flow cytometric S-phase fraction. *Cancer.* 1996;78:1942.

163. Pfisterer J, Kommoss F, Sauerbrei W, et al: The prognostic value of DNA ploidy and S-phase fraction in stage I endometrial carcinoma. *Gynecol Oncol.* 1995;58:149.

164. Creasman WT: Prognostic significance of hormone receptors in endometrial cancer. *Cancer.* 1995;71(4 suppl):1467.

165. Nyholm HC, Christensen IJ, Nielsen AL: Progesterone receptor levels independently predict survival in endometrial adenocarcinoma. *Gynecol Oncol.* 1995;59:347.

166. Vecek N, Nola M, Marusic M, et al: Prognostic value of steroid hormone receptors concentration in patients with endometrial carcinoma. *Acta Obstet Gynecol Scand.* 1994;73:730.

167. Wang D, Konishi I, Koshiyama M, et al: Expression of c-erb-2 protein and epidermal growth receptor in endometrial carcinomas: Correlation with clinicopathologic and sex steroid receptor status. *Cancer.* 1993;72:2628.

168. Kohler MF, Carney P, Dodge R, et al: *p53* Overexpression in advanced stage endometrial adenocarcinoma. *Am J Obstet Gynecol.* 1996;175:1246.

169. Kohlberger P, Gitsch G, Loesch A, et al: *p53* Protein overexpression in early stage endometrial cancer. *Gynecol Oncol.* 1996; 62:213.

170. Sherman ME, Bur ME, Kurman RJ: *p53* in endometrial cancer and its putative precursors: Evidence for diverse pathways of tumorigenesis. *Hum Pathol.* 1995;26:1268.

171. Reinartz JJ, George E, Lindgren BR, et al: Expression of *p53*, transforming growth factor alpha, epidermal growth factor receptor, and *c-erb-2* in endometrial carcinoma and correlation with survival and known predictors of survival. *Hum Pathol.* 1994;25:1075.

172. Khalifa MA, Mannel RS, Haraway SD, et al: Expression of *EGFR*, *HER-2/neu*, *p53* and *PCNA* in endometrioid, serous papillary, and clear-cell endometrial adenocarcinomas. *Gynecol Oncol.* 1994;53:84.

173. Ito K, Watanabe K, Nasim S, et al: Prognostic significance of *p53* overexpression in endometrial cancer. *Cancer Res.* 1994;54:4667.

174. Berchuck A, Boyd J: Molecular basis of endometrial cancer. *Cancer.* 1995;76:2034. Review.

175. Kihana T, Hamada K, Inoue Y, et al: Mutation and allelic loss of the *p53* gene in endometrial carcinoma: Incidence and outcome in 92 surgical patients. *Cancer.* 1995;76:72.

176. Honda T, Kato H, Imamura T, et al: Involvement of *p53* gene mutations in human endometrial carcinomas. *Int J Cancer.* 1993; 53:963.

177. Saffari B, Jones LA, el-Naggar A, et al: Amplification and overexpression of *HER-2/neu* in endometrial cancers: Correlation with overall survival. *Cancer Res.* 1995;55:5693.

178. Kohlberger P, Loesch A, Koelbl H, et al: Prognostic value of immunohistochemically detected HER-2/neu oncoprotein in endometrial cancer. *Cancer Lett.* 1996;98:151.

179. Jassoni VM, Amadori A, Santini D, et al: Epidermal growth factor receptor (EGF-R) and transforming growth factor alpha (TGFA) expression in different endometrial cancers. *Anticancer Res.* 1995; 15:1327.

180. Watanabe J, Sato Y, Kuramoto H, et al: Expression of nm23-H1 and nm23-H2 protein in endometrial carcinoma. *Br J Cancer.* 1995;72:1469.

181. Ito K, Watanabe K, Nasim S, et al: K-*ras* point mutations in endometrial carcinoma: Effect on outcome is dependent on the age of the patient. *Gynecol Oncol.* 1996;63:238.

182. Marone M, Scambia G, Ferrandina G, et al: Nm23 expression in endometrial and cervical cancer: Inverse correlation with lymph node involvement and myometrial invasion. *Br J Cancer.* 1996; 74:1063.

183. Niikura H, Sasano H, Matsunaga G, et al: Prognostic value of epidermal growth factor receptor expression in endometrioid endometrial carcinoma. *Hum Pathol.* 1995;26:892.

184. Hakala A, Kacinski BM, Stanley ER, et al: Macrophage colony-stimulating factor 1, a clinically useful tumor marker in endometrial adenocarcinoma: Comparison with CA 125 and the aminoterminal propeptide of type III procollagen. *Am J Obstet Gynecol.* 1995;173:112.

185. Macasaet M, Brigati D, Boyce J, et al: The significance of residual disease after radiotherapy in endometrial carcinoma: Clinicopathologic correlation. *Am J Obstet Gynecol.* 1980;138:557.

186. Ahmad NR, Lanciano RM, Corn BR, Schultheiss T: Postoperative radiation therapy for surgically staged endometrial cancer: Impact of time factors (overall treatment time, and surgery-to-radiation interval) on outcome. *Int J Radiat Oncol Biol Phys.* 1995;33:837.

187. Corn BW, Lanciano RM, Greven, KM, et al: Impact of improved irradiation technique, age and lymph node sampling on the severe complication rate of surgically staged endometrial cancer patients: A multivariate analysis. *J Clin Oncol.* 1994;12:510.

188. Gretz HF 3rd, Economos K, Husain A, et al: The practice of surgical staging and its impact on adjuvant treatment recommendations in patients with stage I endometrial carcinoma. *Gynecol Oncol.* 1996;61:409.

189. Fanning J, Nanavati PJ, Hilgers RD: Surgical staging and high dose-rate brachytherapy for endometrial cancer: Limiting external radiotherapy to node-positive patients. *Obstet Gynecol.* 1996; 87:1041.

190. Freund WA: A new method for extirpation of the whole uterus. *Berl Klin Wochenschr.* 1878;18:275.

191. Doering DL, Barnhill DR, Weiser EB, et al: Intraoperative evaluation of depth of myometrial invasion in stage I endometrial adenocarcinoma. *Obstet Gynecol.* 1989;74:930.

192. Malviya VK, Deppe G, Malone JM Jr, et al: Reliability of frozen section examination in identifying poor prognostic indicators in Stage I endometrial adenocarcinoma. *Gynecol Oncol.* 1989; 34:299.

193. Gemignani ML, Curtin JP, Zelmanovich J, et al: Laparoscopic-assisted vaginal hysterectomy for endometrial cancer: Clinical outcomes and hospital charges. *Gynecol Oncol.* 1999;73:5.

194. Homesley HF, Boronow RC, Lewis JL: Treatment of adenocarcinoma of the endometrium at Memorial-James Ewing Hospitals: 1946-1965. *Obstet Gynecol.* 1976;47:100.

195. Mariani A, Webb MJ, Keeney GL, et al: Role of wide/radical hysterectomy and pelvic lymph node dissection in endometrial cancer with cervical involvement. *Gynecol Oncol.* 2001;83:72.

196. Grigsby PW, Perez CA: Clinical stage I endometrial cancer: Results of adjuvant irradiation and patterns of failure. *Int J Radiat Oncol Biol Phys.* 1991;21:379.

197. Morrow CP, Bundy BN, Kumar RJ, et al: Relationship between surgical-pathologic risk factors and outcome in clinical stages I and II carcinoma of the endometrium: A Gynecologic Oncology Group study. *Gynecol Oncol.* 1991;40:55.

198. Carey M, O'Connell G: Good outcome associated with a standardized treatment protocol using selective post-operative radiation with clinical stage I adenocarcinoma of the endometrium. *Gynecol Oncol.* 1995;57:138.

199. Kucera H, Vaura N, Weghoupt K: Benefit of external irradiation in pathologic Stage I endometrial carcinoma: A prospective clinical trial of 605 patients who received postoperative vaginal irradiation and additional pelvic irradiation in the presence of unfavorable prognostic factors. *Gynecol Oncol.* 1990;38:99.

200. Elliot P, Green D: The efficacy of postoperative vaginal irradiation in preventing vaginal recurrence in endometrial cancer. *Int J Gynecol Cancer.* 1994;4:84.

201. Roberts JA, Brunetto, Keyes HM, et al: A phase III randomized study of surgery vs. surgery plus adjunctive radiation therapy in intermediate-risk endometrial carcinoma (GOG 99) abstract 35. *Proc Soc Gynecol Oncol.* 70, 1998.

202. Aalders J, Abeler V, Kolstad P, et al: Postoperative external irradiation and prognostic parameters in stage I endometrial carcinoma: Clinical and histopathologic study of 540 patients. *Obstet Gynecol.* 1980;56:419.

203. Greven KM, D'Agostino RB Jr, Lanciano RM, Corn BW: Is there a role for a brachytherapy vaginal cuff boost in the adjuvant management of patients with uterine-confined endometrial cancer? *Int J Radiat Oncol Biol Phys.* 1998;42:101.

204. Rush S, Gal D, Potters L, et al: Pelvic control following external beam radiation for surgical stage I endometrial adenocarcinoma. *Int J Radiat Oncol Biol Phys.* 1995;33:851.

205. Randall ME, Wilder J, Greven K, et al: Role of intracavitary cuff boost after adjuvant external irradiation in early endometrial carcinoma. *Int J Radiat Oncol Biol Phys.* 1990;19:49.

206. Nori D, Merimsky O, Batata M, et al: Postoperative high dose-rate intravaginal brachytherapy combined with external irradiation for early stage endometrial cancer: A long-term followup. *Int J Radiat Oncol Biol Phys.* 1994;30:831.

207. Mohan DS, Samuels MA, Selim MA, et al: Long-term outcomes of therapeutic pelvic lymphadenectomy for stage I endometrial adenocarcinoma. *Gynecol Oncol.* 1998;70:165.

208. Orr JW Jr, Holimon JL, Orr PF. Stage I corpus cancer: Is teletherapy necessary? *Am J Obstet Gynecol.* 1997;176:777.

209. Horowitz NS, Peters WA III, Smith MR, et al: Adjuvant high dose rate vaginal brachytherapy as treatment of stage I and II endometrial carcinoma. *Obstet Gynecol.* 2002;99:235.

210. Straughn JM Jr, Huh WK, Kelly FJ, et al: Conservative management of stage I endometrial carcinoma after surgical staging. *Gynecol Oncol.* 2002;84:194.

211. Alektiar KM, McKee A, Venkatraman E, et al: Intravaginal high-dose-rate brachytherapy for stage IB (FIGO grade 1, 2) endometrial cancer. *Int J Radiat Oncol Biol Phys.* 2002;53:707.

212. Petereit DG, Tannehill SP, Grosen EA, et al: Outpatient vaginal cuff brachytherapy for endometrial cancer. *Int J Gynecol Cancer.* 1999;9:456.

213. Anderson JM, Stea B, Hallum AV, et al: High-dose-rate postoperative vaginal cuff irradiation alone for stage IB and IC endometrial cancer. *Int J Radiat Oncol Biol Phys.* 2000;46:417.

214. MacLeod C, Fowler A, Duval P, et al: High-dose-rate brachytherapy alone post-hysterectomy for endometrial cancer. *Int J Radiat Oncol Biol Phys.* 1998;42:1033.

215. Scholten AN, Creutzberg CL, Noordijk EM, Smit VT: Long-term outcome in endometrial carcinoma favors a two- instead of a three-tiered grading system. *Int J Radiat Oncol Biol Phys.* 2002; 52:1067.

216. Irwin C, Levin W, Fyles A, et al: The role of adjuvant radiotherapy in carcinoma of the endometrium—results in 550 patients with pathologic stage I disease. *Gynecol Oncol.* 1998;70:247.

217. Piver M, Hempling R: A prospective trial of post-operative vaginal radium/cesium for grade 1-2 less than 50% myometrial invasion and pelvic radiation therapy for grade 3 or deep myometrial invasion in surgical stage I endometrial adenocarcinoma. *Cancer.* 1990;66:133.

218. Weiss MF, Connell PP, Waggoner S, et al: External pelvic radiation therapy in stage IC endometrial carcinoma. *Obstet Gynecol.* 1999;93:599.

219. Straughn JM, Huh WK, Orr JW Jr, et al: Stage IC adenocarcinoma of the endometrium: Survival comparisons of surgically staged patients with and without adjuvant radiation therapy. *Gynecol Oncol.* 2003;89:295.

220. Chadha M, Nanavati PJ, Liu P, et al: Patterns of failure in endometrial carcinoma stage IB grade 3 and IC patients treated with postoperative vaginal vault brachytherapy. *Gynecol Oncol.* 1999;75:103.

221. Fanning J. Long-term survival of intermediate risk endometrial cancer (stage IG3, IC, II) treated with full lymphadenectomy and brachytherapy without teletherapy. *Gynecol Oncol.* 2001;82:371.

222. Pitson G, Colgan T, Levin W, et al: Stage II endometrial carcinoma: Prognostic factors and risk classification in 170 patients. *Int J Radiat Oncol Biol Phys.* 2002;53:862.

223. Lanciano RM, Curran WJ, Greven KM, et al: Influence of grade, histologic subtype and timing of radiotherapy on the outcome among patients with stage II carcinoma of the endometrium. *Gynecol Oncol.* 1990;39:368.

224. Podczaski ES, Kaminski P, Manetta A, et al: Stage II endometrial carcinoma treated with external beam radiotherapy, intracavitary application of cesium, and surgery. *Gynecol Oncol.* 1989;35:251.

225. Ahmad K, Kim YH, Deppe G, et al: Radiation therapy in stage II carcinoma of the endometrium. *Cancer.* 1989;63:854.

226. Larson DM, Copeland LJ, Gallagher HS, et al: Stage II endometrial carcinoma: Results and complications of a combined radiotherapeutic-surgical approach. *Cancer.* 1988;61:1528.

227. Greven K, Olds W: Radiotherapy in the management of endometrial carcinoma with cervical involvement. *Cancer.* 1987;60:1737.

228. Calkins AR, Stehman FB, Sutton GP, et al: Adenocarcinoma corpus et colli: Analysis of diagnostic variables. *Int J Radiat Oncol Biol Phys.* 1986;12:911.

229. Grigsby PW, Perez CA, Camel HM, et al: Stage II carcinoma of the endometrium: Results of therapy and prognostic factors. *Int J Radiat Oncol Biol Phys.* 1985;11:1915.

230. Onsrud M, Aalders J, Abeler V, et al: Endometrial carcinoma with cervical involvement (stage II): Prognostic factors and value of combined radiological-surgical treatment. *Gynecol Oncol.* 1982; 13:76.

231. Kinsella TJ, Bloomer WD, Lavin PT, et al: Stage II endometrial carcinoma: 10 year followup of combined radiation and surgical treatment. *Gynecol Oncol.* 1980;10:290.

232. Bruckman JE, Goodman RL, Murthy A, et al: Combined irradiation and surgery in the treatment of stage II carcinoma of the endometrium. *Cancer.* 1978;42:1146.

233. Ng TY, Nicklin JL, Perrin LC, et al: Postoperative vaginal vault brachytherapy for node-negative stage II (occult) endometrial carcinoma. *Gynecol Oncol.* 2001;81:193.

234. Greven K, Corn B, Lanciano RM: Pathologic stage III endometrial carcinoma. *Cancer.* 1993;71:3697.

235. Mariani A, Webb MJ, Keeney GL, et al: Stage IIIC endometrioid corpus cancer includes distinct subgroups. *Gynecol Oncol.* 2002; 87:112.

236. Nelson G, Randall M, Sutton G, et al: FIGO stage IIIC endometrial carcinoma with metastases confined to pelvic lymph nodes: Analysis of treatment outcomes, prognostic variables, and failure patterns following adjuvant radiation therapy. *Gynecol Oncol.* 1999;75:211.

237. Soper JT, Creasman WT, Clarke-Pearson DL, et al: Intraperitoneal chromic phosphate P-32 suspension therapy of malignant peritoneal cytology in endometrial carcinoma. *Am J Obstet Gynecol.* 1985;153:191.

238. Piver MS, Recio FO, Baker TL, et al: A prospective trial of progesterone therapy for malignant peritoneal cytology in patients with endometrial cancer. *Gynecol Oncol.* 1993;47:373.

239. Antoniades J, Brady LW, Lewis GC: The management of stage III carcinoma of the endometrium. *Cancer.* 1976;38:1838.

240. Bruckman JE, Bloomer WD, Marck A, et al: Stage III adenocarcinoma of the endometrium: Two prognostic groups. *Gynecol Oncol.* 1980;9:12.

241. Danoff BF, McDay J, Louka M, et al: Stage III endometrial carcinoma: Analysis of patterns of failure and therapeutic implications. *Int J Radiat Oncol Biol Phys.* 1980;6:1491.

242. Greven KM, Curran WJ, Whittington R, et al: Analysis of failure patterns in stage III endometrial carcinoma and therapeutic implications. *Int J Radiat Oncol Biol Phys.* 1989;17:35.

243. Mackillop WJ, Pringle JF: Stage III endometrial carcinoma: A review of 90 cases. *Cancer.* 1985;56:2519.

244. Milton PJ, Metters J: Endometrial carcinoma: An analysis of 355 cases treated at St. Thomas' Hospital, 1945-1969. *J Obstet Gynecol Br Commonwealth.* 1972;79:455.

245. Greer BE, Hamberger AD: Treatment of intraperitoneal metastatic adenocarcinoma of the endometrium by the whole abdomen moving-strip technique and pelvic boost irradiation. *Gynecol Oncol.* 1983;16:365.

246. Potish RA, Twiggs LB, Adcock LL, et al: Role of whole abdominal radiation therapy in the management of endometrial cancer: Prognostic importance of factors indicating peritoneal metastases. *Gynecol Oncol.* 1985;21:80.

247. Nori D, Hilaris BS, Tome M, et al: Combined surgery and radiation in endometrial carcinoma: An analysis of prognostic factors. *Int J Radiat Oncol Biol Phys.* 1987;13:489.

248. Potish RA, Twiggs LB, Adcock LL, et al: Para-aortic lymph node radiotherapy in cancer of the uterine corpus. *Obstet Gynecol.* 1985;654:251.

249. Komaki R, Mattingly RF, Hoffman RG: Irradiation of para-aortic lymph node metastases from carcinoma of the cervix or endometrium: Preliminary results. *Radiology.* 1983;147:245.

250. Blythe JG, Hodel KA, Wahl TB, et al: Para-aortic lymph node biopsy in cervical and endometrial cancer: Does it affect survival? *Am J Obstet Gynecol.* 1986;155:306.

251. Feuer GA, Calnog A: Endometrial carcinomas: Treatment of positive para-aortic nodes. *Gynecol Oncol.* 1987;27:106.

252. Corn BW, Lanciano RM, Greven KM, et al: Endometrial carcinoma with para-aortic lymphadenopathy: Patterns of failure and opportunity for cure. *Int J Radiat Oncol Biol Phys.* 1992;24:223.

253. Hicks ML, Piver S, Jeffrey LP, et al: Survival in patients with paraaortic lymph node metastases from endometrial adenocarcinoma clinically limited to the uterus. *Int J Radiat Oncol Biol Phys.* 1993;26:607.

254. Rose PG, Cha SD, Tak WK, et al: Radiation therapy for surgically proven para-aortic node metastasis in endometrial carcinoma. *Int J Radiat Oncol Biol Phys.* 1992;24:229.

255. Mariani A, Webb MJ, Keeney GL, Aletti G, Podratz KC. Endometrial cancer: Predictors of peritoneal failure. *Gynecol Oncol.* 2003;89:236.

256. Martinez A, Podratz K: Results of whole abdomino-pelvic radiation with nodal boost for patients with endometrial cancer at high risk of failure in the peritoneal cavity. *Hematol Oncol Clin North Am.* 1988;2:431.

257. Gibbons S, Martinez A, Schary M, et al: Adjuvant whole abdominopelvic irradiation for high-risk endometrial carcinoma. *Int J Radiat Oncol Biol Phys.* 1991;21:1019.

258. Sutton G, Axelrod JH, Bundy BN, et al: Whole abdominal radiotherapy in the adjuvant treatment of patients with stage III and IV endometrial cancer: A Gynecologic Oncology Group Study. In press.

259. Stewart KD, Martinez AA, Weiner S, et al: Ten-year outcome including patterns of failure and toxicity for adjuvant whole abdominopelvic irradiation in high-risk and poor histologic feature patients with endometrial carcinoma. *Int J Radiat Oncol Biol Phys.* 2002;54;527.

260. Gore G, Gillin MT, Albano K: Comparison of high dose-rate and low dose-rate dose distributions for vaginal cylinders. *Int J Radiat Oncol Biol Phys.* 1995;31:165.

261. Nori D: High dose rate brachytherapy in endometrial cancer. *Selectron Brachyther J.* 1991;2:5.

262. Reisinger S, Nori D, Lewis JL: Postoperative intravaginal radiation therapy as an adjunct to external irradiation in high-risk endometrial adenocarcinoma: An evaluation of two different dose schedules. *Endocuriether Hyperther Oncol.* 1991;7:35.

263. Lewis GC Jr, Slack NH, Mortel R, et al: Adjuvant progestogen therapy in the primary definitive treatment of endometrial cancer. *Gynecol Oncol.* 1974;2:368.

264. MacDonald RR, Thorogood J, Mason MK: A randomized trial of progestogens in the primary treatment of endometrial carcinoma. *Br J Obstet Gynecol.* 1988;95:166.

265. Vergote I, Kjorstad K, Abeler V, et al: A randomized trial of adjuvant progestogen in early endometrial cancer. *Cancer.* 1989; 64:1011.

266. Kneale BL, Quinn MA, Rennie GC, et al: A randomized trial of progestogens in the primary treatment of endometrial cancer. *Br J Obstet Gynecol.* 1988;95:828. Letter.

267. Morrow C, Bundy B, Holmesley H, et al: Doxorubicin as an adjuvant following surgery and radiation therapy in patients with high-risk endometrial carcinoma, stage I and occult stage II: A Gynecologic Oncology Group study. *Gynecol Oncol.* 1990; 36:166.

268. Burke TW, Gershenson DM, Morris M, et al: Postoperative adjuvant cisplatin, doxorubicin and cyclophosphamide (PAC) chemotherapy in women with high-risk endometrial carcinoma. *Gynecol Oncol.* 1994;55:47.

269. Randall ME, Brunetto G, Muss H, et al. Whole abdominal versus combination doxorubicin-cisplatin chemotherapy in advanced endometrial carcinoma: A randomized phase III trial of the Gynecologic Oncology Group Study. ASCO 39th annual meeting; 2003, 22: page 2.

270. Hoskins PJ, Swenerton KD, Pike JA, et al: Paclitaxel and carboplatin, alone or with irradiation, in advanced or recurrent endometrial cancer: A phase II study. *J Clin Oncol.* 2001; 19:4048.

271. Sears J, Greven K: Prognostic factors and treatment outcome for patients with locally recurrent endometrial cancer. *Cancer.* 1994;74:1303.

272. Aalders J, Abeler V: Recurrent adenocarcinoma of the endometrium: A clinical and histopathological study of 379 patients. *Gynecol Oncol.* 1984;17:85.

273. Ackerman I, Malone S, Thomas G, et al: Endometrial carcinoma: Relative effectiveness of adjuvant irradiation vs therapy reserved for relapse. *Gynecol Oncol.* 1996;60:177.

274. Curran WJ, Whittington R, Peters AJ, et al: Vaginal recurrences of endometrial carcinoma: The prognostic value of staging by a primary vaginal carcinoma system. *Int J Radiat Oncol Biol Phys.* 1988;15:803.

275. Wylie J, Irwin C, Pintilie M, et al: Results of radical radiotherapy for recurrent endometrial cancer. *Gynecol Oncol.* 2000; 77:66.

276. Creutzberg CL, van Putten WL, Koper PC, et al: Survival after relapse in patients with endometrial cancer: Results from a randomized trial. *Gynecol Oncol.* 2003;89:201.

277. Cardenes H, Randall ME: Is observation and salvage (when necessary) an appropriate approach to intermediate risk endometrial cancer? *Gynecol Oncol.* 2003;89:199.

278. Barakat RR, Goldman NA, Patel DA, et al: Pelvic exenteration for recurrent endometrial cancer. *Gynecol Oncol.* 1999;75:99.

279. Thigpen JT, Blessing J, DiSaia P: Oral medroxyprogesterone acetate in advanced or recurrent endometrial carcinoma: Results of therapy and correlation with estrogen and progesterone levels. The Gynecologic Oncology Group experience. In Baulieu EE, Slacobelli S, McGuire WL, eds. *Endocrinology of Malignancy.* Park Ridge, NJ: Parthenon; 1986:446.

280. Thigpen JT, Homesley HD: A randomized study of medroxyprogesterone acetate (MPA) 200 mg vs 1000 mg in the treatment of advanced, persistent or recurrent carcinoma of the endometrium. In: *Gynecologic Oncology Group Statistical Report.* Buffalo, NY: Gynecologic Oncology Group; 1990:177.

281. Reifenstein EC Jr: The treatment of advanced endometrial cancer with hydroxyprogesterone caproate. *Gynecol Oncol.* 1974;2:377. Review.

282. Piver MS, Barlow JJ, Lurain JR, et al: Medroxyprogesterone acetate (depo-Provera) vs hydroxyprogesterone caproate (Delalutin) in women with metastatic endometrial adenocarcinoma. *Cancer.* 1980;45:268.

283. Podratz KC, O'Brien PC, Malkasian GD Jr, et al: Effects of progestational agents in the treatment of endometrial carcinoma. *Obstet Gynecol.* 1985;66:106.

284. Thigpen JT, Buchsbaum HJ, Mangan C, Blessing JA: Phase II trial of Adriamycin in the treatment of advanced or recurrent endometrial carcinoma: A Gynecologic Oncology Group study. *Cancer Treat Rep.* 1979;63:21.

285. Thigpen JT, Blessing JA, Homesley H, et al: Phase II trial of cisplatin as first-line chemotherapy in patients with advanced or recurrent endometrial carcinoma: A Gynecologic Oncology Group study. *Gynecol Oncol.* 1989;33:68.

286. Long HJ, Pfeifle DM, Wieand HS, et al: Phase II evaluation of carboplatin in advanced endometrial carcinoma. *JNCI.* 1988; 80:276.

287. Ball HG, Blessing JA, Lentz SS, Mutch DG: A phase II trial of paclitaxel in patients with advanced and recurrent adenocarcinoma of the endometrium: A Gynecologic Oncology Group study. *Gynecol Oncol.* 1996;62:278.

288. Knocke TH, Kucera H, Weidinger B, et al: Primary treatment of endometrial carcinoma with high-dose-rate brachytherapy: Results of 12 years of experience with 280 patients. *Int J Radiat Oncol Biol Phys.* 1997;37:359.

289. Nguyen TV, Petereit DG. High-dose-rate brachytherapy for medically inoperable stage I endometrial cancer. *Gynecol Oncol.* 1998;71:196.

290. Grigsby P, Kuske R, Perez CA, et al: Medically inoperable stage I adenocarcinoma of the endometrium treated with radiotherapy alone. *Int J Radiat Oncol Biol Phys.* 1986;13:483.

291. Rose P, Baker S: Primary radiation therapy for endometrial carcinoma: A case-controlled study. *Int J Radiat Oncol Biol Phys.* 1993;27:585.

292. Smith RS, Kapp DS, Chen Q, Teng NN: Treatment of high-risk uterine cancer with whole abdominopelvic radiation therapy. *Int J Radiat Oncol Biol Phys.* 2000;48:767.

293. Levenback C, Burke T: Uterine papillary serous carcinoma: Treatment with cisplatin, doxorubicin and cyclophosphamide. *Gynecol Oncol.* 1992;46:317.

294. Lim P, Al Kushi A, Gilks B, et al: Early stage uterine papillary serous carcinoma of the endometrium: Effect of adjuvant whole abdominal radiotherapy and pathologic parameters on outcome. *Cancer.* 2001;91:752.

295. Creutzberg CL, van Putten WL, Koper PC, et al: The postoperative radiation therapy in endometrial carcinoma. The morbidity of treatment for patients with stage I endometrial cancer: Results from a randomized trial. *Int J Radiat Oncol Biol Phys.* 2001; 51:1246.

296. Sorbe BG, Smeds AC: Postoperative vaginal irradiation with high dose-rate afterloading technique in endometrial carcinoma Stage I. *Int J Radiat Oncol Biol Phys.* 1990;18:305.

Cancer of the Ovary

Kaled M. Alektiar, MD and *Zvi Fuks, MD*

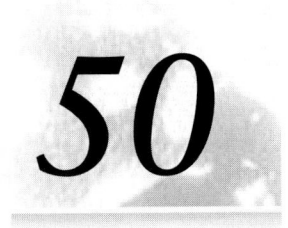

The role of radiation in the management of ovarian carcinoma continues to represent a topic of considerable controversy, and the indications for its use are not fully established. Ovarian tumor cells are sensitive to the lethal effects of radiation. High-dose radiation to the pelvis is effective in permanently eradicating ovarian tumors, providing an approach to cure early-stage disease.[1-3] However, the curative potential of whole abdominal irradiation for advanced-stage disease is limited due to high sensitivity of the normal organs of the abdomen to the radiation doses required to cure peritoneal metastases.[1-3] Because of these limitations, combination chemotherapy has been increasingly used as alternative curative therapy for ovarian cancer. Paclitaxel and platinum-based combinations, albeit highly toxic, induce clinical remissions in the excess of 90% of advanced-stage patients.[4-7] However, responses are frequently not durable, even when an apparently complete pathologic remission is initially achieved.[4,5] Reports on long-term survival after chemotherapy for advanced-stage disease[8,9] have indicated that the long-term outcome is similar to that observed with whole abdominal irradiation.[10] This chapter reviews the basic policies and therapeutic strategies that dominate the current management of ovarian cancer, with an emphasis on the role of radiotherapy.

EPIDEMIOLOGY AND RISK FACTORS

In the United States, ovarian cancer is the fourth most common type of female cancer and the fifth leading cause of cancer death in women.[11] In 2003, an estimated 25,400 U.S. women were diagnosed with ovarian cancer and 14,300 succumbed to the disease, representing more than half of all deaths from gynecologic cancers. When initially diagnosed with ovarian cancer, more than half of the patients have advanced-stage disease and nearly 20% have intermediate stage (regional) disease. The age-adjusted lifetime risk is about 1.9%, although for women with a family history of ovarian cancer, the lifetime risk may be as high as 9.4%.[12]

Epithelial ovarian cancer is infrequent below the age of 40 and increases in incidence from 15.7 per 100,00 in the 40 to 44 age group to 54 per 100,00 at 75 to 79 years of age.[13] The incidence is about 50% greater for white than black women, although 20% of the difference can

be attributed to differences of risk factors.[14] The etiology of ovarian cancer remains unknown. But several environmental, physiologic, and genetic factors have been identified as risk factors (Table 50-1). These include residence in North America and northern Europe, nulliparity,[16] infertility,[17] use of fertility drugs,[16] fat consumption,[18] milk products,[19] consumption of coffee,[17] and the use of perineal talc.[20] Multiple pregnancies (regardless of gestational length or outcome), long-term use of oral contraceptives, extended duration of breast-feeding, and tubal ligation or hysterectomy have been shown to have a protective effect.[16]

Genetic factors are also associated with increased risk for developing ovarian cancer. Increases of 2- to 20-fold in risk for ovarian cancer have been reported for familial clusters.[21,22] Pedigree analysis has led to recognition of several familial ovarian cancer syndromes associated with autosomal dominant patterns of inheritance.[21,23] Approximately 5% to 10% of all ovarian cancers are thought to be associated with these genetic syndromes.

Table 50–1 Factors Influencing the Risk for Ovarian Cancer

	Estimated Risk, %	Estimated Relative Risk
Baseline Lifetime Risk	1.4 to 1.8	1
Risk Factors		
BRCA1 mutation	30-40	18-29
BRCA2 mutation	27	16-19
HNPCC	10	6-7
Family history	9.4	5-7
Infertility		2-5
Nulliparity		2-3
Late menopause		1.5-2
Early menarche		1-1.5
Protective Factors		
Oral contraceptive use		
× 4 years		0.6
× 8 years		0.5
× 12 years		0.4
Multiparity		0.4-0.6
Hysterectomy or tubal ligation		0.4-0.6

HNPCC, hereditary nonpolyposis colorectal cancer.
Modified from Holschneider CH, Berek JS: Ovarian cancer: Epidemiology, biology, and prognostic factors. *Semin Surg Oncol.* 2000;19:4.

Three familial ovarian cancer syndromes have been identified. The most common syndrome is the hereditary breast/ovarian cancer (HBOC) syndrome, which accounts for 65% to 75% of hereditary ovarian cancers. The hereditary nonpolyposis colorectal/ovarian cancer (HNPCC, also known as Lynch II syndrome), accounts for 10% to 15% of hereditary ovarian cancers, and the hereditary site-specific ovarian carcinoma accounts for the remaining 10% to 15% of cases.[21]

The use of polymorphic DNA markers has facilitated linkage analysis of specific syndromes with specific genes. Linkage of HBOC has been identified with the long arm of chromosome 17,[21,24-26] localized between the polymorphic marker loci D17S702 and D17S78, and involving a tumor suppressor gene known as the *BRCA1* gene. Tumors from affected patients carry an inherited *BRCA1* mutation in at least one copy of the gene, but for tumors to develop the second wild type, allele must be lost.[27] *BRCA1* mutations have been linked to 80% to 90% of HBOC families.[28] Women carrying a germline mutation of *BRCA1* have a significantly higher risk of developing both ovarian and breast cancer than the general population. The average risk in the public for breast cancer is 12.5% and for ovarian cancer 1.5%. But with *BRCA1* mutation and a strong family history of cancer, these risks increase to 90% and 65%, respectively. The risk is much lower, however, in women with less impressive family history. The *BRCA2* tumor suppressor gene on chromosome 13q is also associated with high rates of breast and ovarian cancer. It is estimated that this gene is linked to 15% of breast-ovarian cancer families.[28] Linkage studies have identified loci on chromosomes 2 and 3 as associated with colon and ovarian tumors in HNPCC families.[29-31] The genes involved belong to the family of DNA mismatch repair genes. Germline mutations of these genes cosegregate with the disease phenotype in affected families, displaying dominant inheritance with high penetration. The identification of the *BRCA1/2* and *HNPCC* genes should make it possible to accurately predict ovarian cancer susceptibility in women from high-risk families.

ANATOMY AND TUMOR PATHOLOGY

Normal Anatomy

The normal adult ovary measures approximately 4 cm in length, 3 cm in width, and 1.5 to 3 cm in thickness. The size of the ovary changes during a normal menstrual cycle and may enlarge to 5 cm or more. With advancing age, the size and weight of the ovary slowly decreases. The average postmenopausal ovary is $1.5 \times 1 \times 0.5$ cm and is not palpable through a vaginal examination. A postmenopausal ovary that can be palpated is a significant clinical finding and the possibility of malignancy must be considered.

The ovaries develop during embryonic life as a stratification of the coelomic epithelium of the medial aspect of the urogenital ridge. The surface epithelium of the ovary originates from this mesothelial lining and in adult life represents a single layer of cuboidal or low columnar epithelium that is continuous with the peritoneum at the mesovarium. The mesothelial lining of the urogenital ridge also gives rise to the müllerian ducts, from which the fallopian tubes, uterus, and vagina subsequently develop. When the epithelium of the ovary becomes malignant, it exhibits a variety of müllerian-type differentiation, such as serous (resembling the fallopian tube), mucinous (resembling the endocervix), endometrioid (resembling endometrium), and clear cell (glycogen-rich cells resembling endometrial glands in pregnancy). The ovarian surface epithelium may also exhibit urothelial differentiation in the form of transitional cells. At adult life the ovaries consist of an outer cortex and an inner medulla. The outer cortex consists of a condensed connective tissue stroma named the tunica albuginea, and of follicles in various stages of development surrounded by tightly packed stromal (theca) cells. The medulla is highly vascular and consists of specialized polyhedral cells that are similar to testicular interstitial cells.

The ovaries are attached to the posterior lateral walls of the pelvis by the infundibulopelvic ligament, to the lateral pelvic wall by the mesovarian (broad) ligament, and to the uterus by the utero-ovarian ligament. In the nulliparous patient, the ovary is located in the ovarian fossa, an indentation in the posterior peritoneum. The main blood supply is via the ovarian artery, which originates from the aorta below the renal artery and courses in the retroperitoneum to enter the ovary at the hilum. A second major source of blood supply is through the ovarian branch of the uterine artery, which courses through the utero-ovarian ligament into the hilum and anastomoses with the ovarian artery supply. The veins course alongside the arteries and drain into the inferior vena cava on the right and into the renal vein on the left.

The lymphatic drainage follows the vascular supply. Lymphatic capillaries and vessels of the ovary collect the lymph into a subovarian lymphatic plexus in the hilum, which gives rise to three lymphatic systems (Fig. 50-1). The main drainage system consists of six to eight large collecting trunks, which ascend bilaterally along the ovarian blood vessels and terminate in para-aortic lymph nodes between the bifurcation of the aorta and the renal pedicles. A second system is the accessory efferent system, which courses within the broad ligament toward the lateral and posterior pelvic wall and terminates in the uppermost external iliac and hypogastric nodes. From there the lymph drains along the external, internal, and common iliac nodes into the para-aortic region. A third collecting system runs along the round ligament and drains into the external iliac and inguinal nodes. Drainage via the latter route is rare and accounts for the appearance of metastases in inguinal nodes.

Histopathologic Classification of Ovarian Tumors

Most ovarian neoplasms are of coelomic epithelial origin, but other ovarian cell types also give rise to malignant neoplasm. Table 50-2 shows the classification of ovarian tumors as recommended by the World Health Organization.[32] The surface epithelial tumors account for

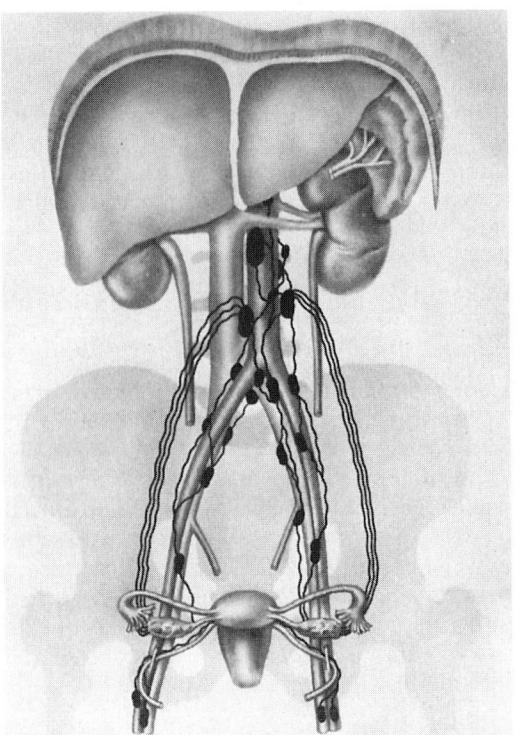

Figure 50–1. Schematic presentation of the routes of lymphatic drainage of the ovaries. (Reproduced with permission from Fuks Z, Bagshaw MA: The rationale for curative radiotherapy for ovarian carcinoma. *Int J Radiat Oncol Biol Phys.* 1975;1:21.)

Table 50–2   World Health Organization (WHO) Classification of Malignant Ovarian Tumors

A. Common (Surface) Epithelial Tumors
    Malignant serous tumors
    Malignant mucinous tumors
    Malignant endometrioid tumors
    Clear cell (mesonephroid) tumors
    Brenner tumors, malignant
    Mixed epithelial tumors, malignant
    Undifferentiated carcinoma
    Unclassified
B. Sex Cord–Stromal Tumors
    Granulosa-stromal cell tumors
    Androblastomas: Sertoli-Leydig cell tumors
    Gynandroblastoma
    Unclassified
C. Lipid (Lipoid) Cell Tumors
    Germ cell tumors
        Dysgerminoma
        Endodermal sinus tumor
        Embryonal carcinoma
        Polyembryoma
        Choriocarcinoma
        Teratomas
        Mixed forms
    Gonadoblastoma

Modified from Serov SF, Scully RE, Solvin LH: *Histological Typing of Ovarian Tumors*, vol. 9. Geneva: World Health Organization; 1973.

approximately two thirds of all ovarian neoplasms (Table 50-3), and their malignant forms for about 85% of ovarian cancers. Surface tumors are predominantly epithelial, with only a minor portion derived from the ovarian stroma. When a tumor has a predominant stromal component, the term "fibroma" is added (e.g., cystadenofibroma, serous adenofibroma).

The malignant surface epithelial tumors consist of tumors of borderline malignancy and of invasive tumors. The borderline tumors are characterized by an indolent clinical course and excellent prognosis.[34-36] Histologically, these tumors exhibit cellular proliferation to a higher degree than in the benign tumors, but without destructive invasion of the stroma. The distinction between borderline and the invasive variants is frequently unclear, particularly in nonserous tumors.[35] Distinction from invasive variants is, nonetheless, important because patients with borderline tumors require minimal treatment, significantly less aggressive than would be required for the corresponding invasive tumors. Some studies have suggested that flow cytometry and morphometric analysis may be useful in this regard.[36,37]

Serous carcinoma is the most common subtype of invasive ovarian tumors (see Table 50-3). These tumors are frequently bilateral and widely disseminated at diagnosis.

Table 50–3   Frequency Distribution of Benign and Malignant Tumors of the Ovary

Type	All Tumors, %	Benign Tumors, %	Malignant Borderline, %	Malignant Invasive, %	Malignant Tumors Only, %
Surface epithelial	59	33	8	18	
Serous	27	13	4	10	46
Mucinous	21	17	3	1	13
Endometrioid	5	<1	1	1	16
Clear cell	2	<1		<1	6
Brenner	1			1	<1
Mixed	2			2	2
Undifferentiated	1			1	3
Germ cell	27				6
Sex cord–stromal	10				4
Steroid cell	1				<1
Metastatic	1				3
Other	2				<1

Modified from Ozols RF, Rubin SC, Dembo AJ, Roboy S: *Epithelial Ovarian Cancer.* Philadelphia: JB Lippincott; 1993.

The tumors are usually solid, but sometimes they do contain cystic components and often exhibit areas of hemorrhage and necrosis. Typical findings on microscopic examination are slit-like glandular spaces, small deposits of tumor cells within dense fibrous or hyalinized stroma, frequent psammoma bodies, and irregular small cellular papillae (Fig. 50-2). Serous tumors are regarded as aggressive and overall 5-year survival rates have been reported to range from 20% to 35%.[38,39]

Mucinous invasive tumors are significantly less common (see Table 50-3) and are frequently confined to one ovary at the time of initial diagnosis.[40] On microscopic examination these tumors are characterized by a prominent cribriform mucinous pattern lined with epithelial cells with prominent mitotic activity (see Fig. 50-2). Differential diagnosis from mucinous adenocarcinomas arising in other organs and metastasizing to the ovaries occasionally represents a diagnostic challenge. A high proportion of mucinous tumors are detected at an early stage of disease, contributing to a relatively favorable prognosis.[38,41,42]

Endometrioid tumors histologically resemble tumors of the endometrium. Tubular glands are frequently lined by pseudostratified epithelium with occasional basal vacuolization (see Fig. 50-2). Some tumors contain abundant mucin in the lumen of glands, but the lack of intracytoplasmic mucin differentiates this tumor from gastrointestinal tumors. In about one third of the cases, foci of squamous differentiation are also found. Endometrioid carcinoma appears to have a better prognosis than serous carcinomas, with 40% to 60% of patients surviving more than 5 years.[42-44]

Clear cell carcinomas (also known as mesonephroid tumors) are characterized histologically by abundant clear and glycogen-rich cytoplasm and eccentric nuclei (see Fig. 50-2). The cytoplasmic glycogen may be scanty in poorly differentiated areas. The overall prognosis approximates that of endometrioid and mucinous carcinomas, with 50% to 70% of the patients surviving 5 or more years.[44,45]

Molecular Pathology and Tumor Markers

Although the histological type and tumor grade are the most common guidelines for the selection of treatment, these parameters are inconsistent predictors of the outcome. Tumor grade is a powerful independent predictor of relapse in early-stage disease,[44,46,47] but not in advanced-stage disease.[48,49] Further, in advanced-stage disease, even the histologic subtype does not represent a consistent independent variable in predicting response to treatment.[48-52] Therefore, there has been a great deal of interest in molecular and cellular markers as predictors of the outcome and as guides in the selection of the most appropriate treatment for a given patient.

DNA PLOIDY

Of several emerging cellular markers, DNA ploidy is the most useful marker, particularly in early-stage disease. DNA ploidy is derived from measurements of the DNA content by flow cytometry. The term *DNA euploidy* refers to diploid content, as exists in G0/G1 cells, or tetraploid, as exists in S/G2/M cells. Aneuploidy is defined

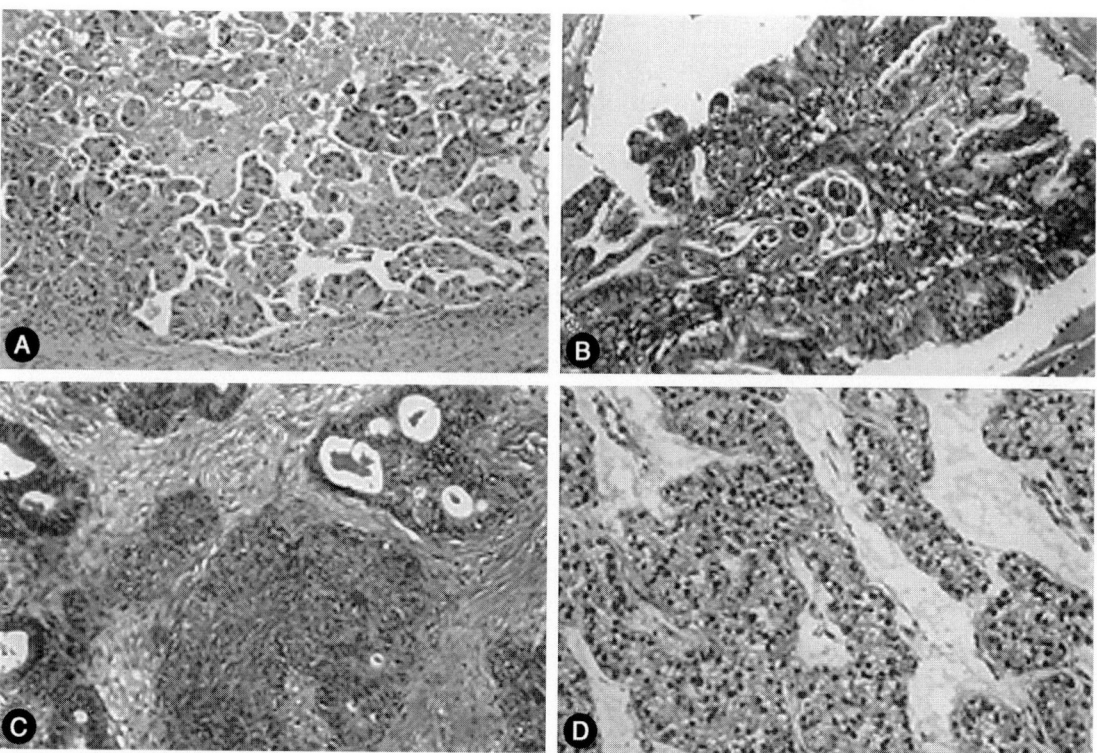

Figure 50–2. Serous papillary (**A**), mucinous (**B**), endometrioid (**C**) and clear cell (**D**) tumors of the ovary (H&E stain, magnified ×400).

as DNA content that deviates from euploidy. Kaern et al.[53] reported that in 315 patients rendered tumor-free by surgery, the risk of succumbing to ovarian carcinoma was 19 times higher for patients with aneuploid than diploid tumors. Several investigators have suggested that conservative surgery with a potential for fertility preservation may be sufficient for stage I patients with euploid tumors, but that more aggressive surgery and postoperative treatment is required for patients with aneuploid tumors.[53-55] In early-stage disease, DNA ploidy indeed seems to have an important predictive role. In advanced-stage III to IV patients, however, univariate analysis suggested that DNA ploidy was a significant predictor of outcome,[40,56-58] but multivariate studies mostly reported that DNA ploidy was not an independent prognostic variable.[54,58,59]

HER2-neu GENE AMPLIFICATION

HER2-neu belongs to the epidermal growth factor (EGF) receptor gene family and is a potent oncogene when overexpressed in various cells.[60,61] *HER2-neu* is overexpressed in approximately 42% of ovarian cancers and is associated with an unfavorable outcome, especially in patients with more than five copies of the *HER2-neu* gene.[62-66] Berchuck et al.[62] reported that patients with increased *HER2-neu* expression had a survival median of 15.7 months, compared with 32.8 months in patients with normal *neu* expression. Further, patients whose cancers had normal *HER2-neu* were fivefold more likely to achieve a negative second-look laparotomy. Some studies, however, failed to demonstrate an adverse effect of *HER2-neu* expression on survival.[66,67] The frequency with which *HER2-neu* amplification and overexpression are observed in a single ovarian tumor is variable. The variability and the lack of consistency in predicting the outcome raise questions regarding the potential as of *HER2-neu* as a prognostic indicator.

MUTATIONS OF THE p53 GENE

The *p53* gene belongs to the family of tumor-suppressor genes, and mutations in these genes have been implicated in malignant transformation and tumor progression.[68] The *p53* gene is located on chromosome 17p. Loss of heterozygosity of chromosome 17 was described in 78% of ovarian tumor specimens.[69] Polymerase chain reactions have disclosed diverse types of *p53* mutations, occurring frequently in exons 5 to 8.[70] Allelic deletion of one of the *p53* genes was found in 67% of ovarian cancers in which a *p53* mutation was present.[70] Overexpression of mutated p53 protein has been detected by immunohistochemistry in 43% to 62% of ovarian cancer tumors.[71-74] Univariate analysis showed that a mutation of *p53* was associated with a significant adverse effect on survival, but this association was no longer observed on multivariate analysis.[73-75] Furthermore, a study reported that *p53* mutation correlated with reduced response of ovarian tumor cells to drugs.[76]

SERUM TUMOR MARKER

Circulating proteins shed from ovarian tumor cells can be detected in the serum by radioimmunoassays. Detection of human chorionic gonadotrophin, or its beta subunit, serves as a serum marker for germ cell tumors with choriocarcinomatous elements,[77] while alpha-fetoprotein is a marker for patients with endodermal sinus tumors.[78] Serum carcinoembryonic antigen (CEA) is elevated in approximately two thirds of patients with advanced-stage ovarian cancer,[79] most frequently associated with the mucinous subtype. For patients with ovarian cancer who have elevated CEA levels before therapy, serial CEA measurements may be valuable in monitoring subclinical relapse.

The most useful serum marker for epithelial ovarian carcinoma is CA-125. Quantitative radioimmunoassay measurement of this marker uses antibodies raised against cell surface antigens of ovarian cell lines.[80] The normal serum level of CA-125 is ≤30 U/ml. Several malignant and nonmalignant conditions may produce nonspecific serum CA-125 elevation (Table 50-4). Approximately 20% of patients with benign ovarian diseases will have CA-125 values above 35 U/mL,[81] while in patients with invasive tumors CA-125 is elevated in approximately 85%. The incidence of elevation by stage is 50% in stage I, 90% in stage II, 92% in stage III, and 94% in stage IV.[82]

CA-125 measured in stored samples was found to be elevated in half of women who eventually developed ovarian cancers.[83] Even 5 years before diagnosis, 24% of individuals who eventually develop epithelial ovarian cancer had increased CA-125, compared with 7% of age-matched controls. These studies suggested that CA-125 can serve as a marker for the early detection of ovarian carcinoma. In a pilot study from the United Kingdom, Jacobs et al. reported on 22,000 women who were randomized to a control group or to screening that entailed CA-125 measurement and transvaginal ultrasound and referral for gynecologic examination, if needed. The results showed an improvement in survival in the screened group (72.9 months vs. 41.8 months) and a positive predictive value of 21%. The number of deaths from cancer of the ovary or fallopian tube did not vary significantly between the control and screened groups.[84] Several investigators have suggested improving the sensitivity by concomitant use of other markers. In a study of 192 patients with ovarian cancer and 273 patients with benign ovarian diseases, Woolas et al.[85] found that evaluating CA-125 in conjunction with any two of a panel of the

Table 50–4   Causes of Elevated Serum CA-125

Benign Conditions	Malignant Conditions
Benign ovarian cystic and solid tumors	Ovarian cancer
Leiomyomata uteri	Metastatic cancer to the ovary
Endometriosis	Metastatic endometrial cancer
Adenomyosis	Metastatic cervical cancer
Peritoneal, pleural, or pericardial inflammation	Breast cancer
Intraperitoneal adhesions	Pancreatic cancer
Tuberculous peritonitis	Gastrointestinal cancers
Pregnancy	Lung cancer
Liver disease	Plasma cell dyscrasias

markers OVX1, LASA, CA-15-3, and CA-72.4 increased the sensitivity of early detection to 83% and the specificity to 84%.

CA-125 is also useful for monitoring ovarian cancer relapse after completion of treatment. Persistent abnormal or increasing levels of CA-125 after surgery are almost invariably associated with residual disease at second-look laparotomy,[86,87] although more than half of advanced stage patients with normal CA-125 after surgery may have residual disease at second-look surgery. Several studies have also reported that CA-125 predicts the response to chemotherapy.[80,86,88] Patients whose CA-125 values decrease to normal during therapy often exhibit CA-125 elevation as the earliest sign of relapse.[89] It is generally accepted that a CA-125 rise to levels exceeding 70 to 100 U/mL after treatment indicates a high probability of relapse.

Routes of Metastatic Spread

Hematogenic spread is extremely rare in ovarian cancer, although metastases to the brain, lung, and liver have been occasionally reported.[90,91] The main routes of metastatic spread are via the lymphatic system and by transcoelomic dissemination.

SPREAD TO ADJACENT PELVIC ORGANS

The earliest and most common sites of ovarian tumor spread are the pelvic reproductive organs. Approximately 10% of ovarian cancer patients present with tumors in both ovaries (stage IB or IC). Bilaterality of involvement is regarded as a state of metastatic spread from the primary tumor into the contralateral ovary. In fact, old series reported metachronous spread to the contralateral ovary in 12% to 17.5% of stage Ia patients undergoing unilateral oophorectomy.[92,93] In advanced-stage disease, the incidence of bilateral ovarian involvement is 50% to 70%.[94,95] Gross involvement of the uterus and the fallopian tubes without evidence of other extraovarian spread occurs in 5% of the patients (stage IIa), while in advanced-stage disease, the uterus is involved in about one fourth of the cases.[96] Metastatic spread to the pelvic reproductive organs may occur by transperitoneal dissemination, but spread via lymphatic channels connecting the subovarian lymphatic plexuses with the uterus is an alternative mechanism. Because of the high frequency of synchronous and metachronous involvement of both ovaries, the uterus, and fallopian tubes, total abdominal hysterectomy and bilateral salpingo-oophorectomy has been accepted as the routine surgical procedure in ovarian cancer.[92,97,98]

SPREAD TO RETROPERITONEAL LYMPH NODES

Metastatic spread into the retroperitoneal lymph nodes follows the routes of lymphatic drainage of the ovaries (see Fig. 50-1). In surgical series of patients undergoing pelvic and para-aortic lymphadenectomy, 25% of stage I patients, 50% of stage II patients, and 64% to 74% of stage III to IV patients were found to have metastatic lymph node involvement.[99-101] Similar results were reported in lymphangiography series.[102-106] Positive lymphographic findings were confined to para-aortic nodes in approximately 20% of the patients, but in the majority of cases, positive nodes were identified in the pelvis, with or without concomitant involvement of para-aortic nodes.[102,104]

TRANSCOELOMIC SPREAD

Transcoelomic (transperitoneal) dissemination is the most common mode of metastatic spread. Ovarian tumors shed cells into the peritoneal cavity, and are frequently identified in peritoneal washings even in early clinical stages.[104] It is generally assumed that free-floating tumor cells are capable of random implantation on the omentum or other regions of the peritoneum to produce metastatic deposits. However, cell migration within the peritoneal cavity is not random. It occurs via specific routes, directed by shifts of the intraperitoneal pressure. Cells and fluids accumulate by gravity in the pelvis, which even in the supine position is the lowest compartment of the peritoneal cavity.[107] The movement of the diaphragm during respiration produces a typical pattern of hydrostatic pressure in the subphrenic compartment of the peritoneal cavity. During inspiration the pressure falls precipitously, creating a momentary negative pressure, which serves as a pump and directs the movement of intraperitoneal fluid through the lateral paracolic gutters toward the diaphragm.[107-110] Having reached the diaphragm, fluid and cells are trapped in lymphatic lacunae located beneath the mesothelial cell lining,[111] and are drained via a network of lymphatic capillaries (Fig. 50-3) that penetrate through the muscle into diaphragmatic lymph nodes.[112] The subsequent drainage is via the internal mammary chain and the thoracic duct into the venous blood system.

Data on anatomic distribution of peritoneal metastases correspond to the routes of drainage of intraperitoneal fluids and cells. Laparoscopic studies demonstrated that approximately 25% of otherwise stage I and II patients will have involvement of the undersurface of the diaphragm.[113,114] Dissemination to other parts of the peritoneal surface lags significantly behind the spread to the undersurface of the diaphragm, because the uptake of cells by the diaphragmatic lymphatic system is highly efficient. When a partial or complete obstruction of the diaphragmatic drainage occurs, conditions are created for implantation of tumor cells on the omentum and other peritoneal sites and for the accumulation of malignant ascites.[110] Lymph node involvement in the cardiophrenic angle has also been described in advanced ovarian cancer[115] and in autopsy series.[116]

CLINICAL PRESENTATION AND DIAGNOSTIC STUDIES

Ovarian cancer has no specific signs or symptoms, particularly in early-stage disease, and is frequently missed until relatively advanced stages of the disease. As the ovary is loosely attached to its pelvic ligaments, ovarian masses can grow to relatively large sizes without producing

Figure 50–3. Schematic presentation of the lymphatic drainage of the diaphragms. Posterior view of a transverse section of the chest is shown at the level of the diaphragm. The subpleural diaphragmatic lymph trunks converge on the diaphragmatic lymph nodes located adjacent to the pericardium. Retrosternal efferent trunks connect these nodes with the internal mammary group of lymph nodes. (Reproduced with permission from Fuks Z, Bagshaw MA: The rationale for curative radiotherapy for ovarian carcinoma. *Int J Radiat Oncol Biol Phys.* 1975;1:21.)

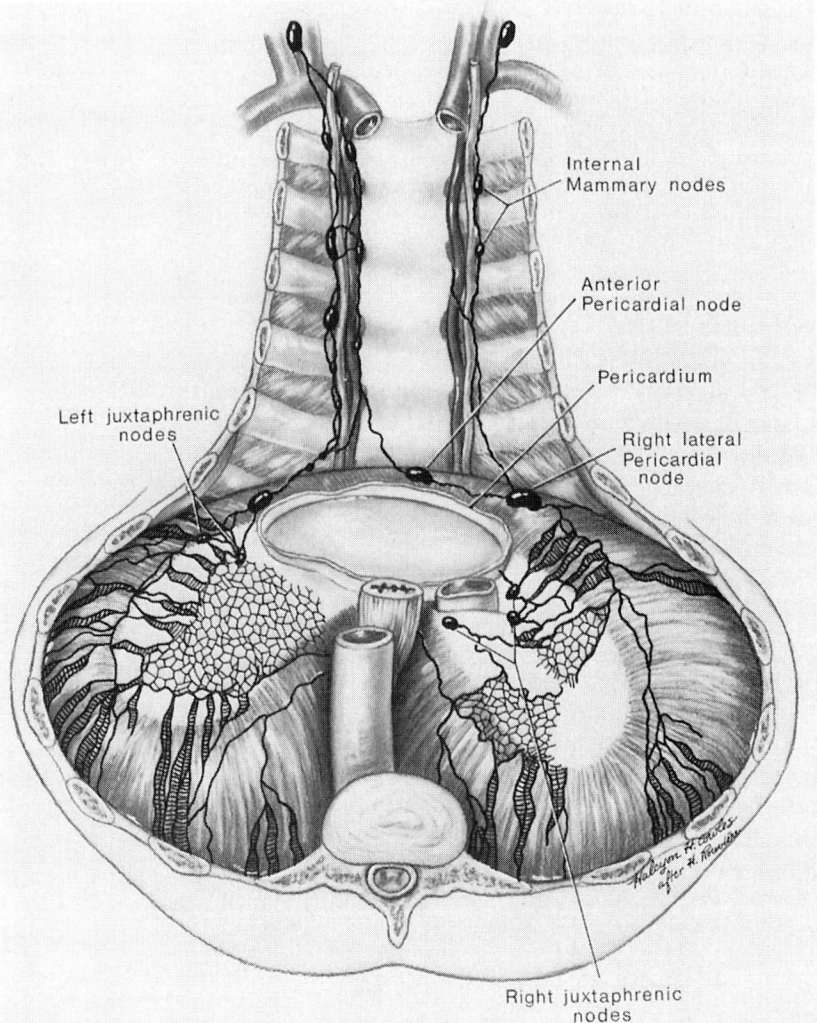

symptoms. Presenting symptoms are usually vague and nonspecific, including abdominal discomfort, nausea, dyspepsia, constipation, urinary frequency, or dysuria.[117] When more obvious symptoms arise, they are usually associated with advanced disease. Pain and abdominal distention are the presenting symptoms in approximately one half of the patients and are frequently associated with malignant ascites or large intra-abdominal masses. Vaginal bleeding occurs in 25% of the patients and is associated with locally invasive tumors. Since symptoms are nonspecific, a recto-vaginal examination with careful assessment of the adnexal region should be part of the clinical evaluation of every woman presenting with pelvic or abdominal symptoms. However, only 13% to 21% of adnexal masses turn out to be malignant.[118,119] Functional ovarian cysts constitute the majority of adnexal masses in reproductive-age women, and 70% regress spontaneously.[120] Benign functional cysts are rare in postmenopausal females, and an adnexal mass in these age groups should be regarded as malignant until proven otherwise.

Table 50-5 shows the most commonly used procedures for evaluation of the extent of involvement with ovarian cancer. Ultrasonography frequently detects irregular borders of tumors, solid elements, papillary projections, or bilateral involvement.[121] Masses that are greater than 10 cm are best evaluated with transabdominal sonography, but a transvaginal approach is more useful for smaller tumors and is increasingly used in the workup of adnexal masses. Computed tomography (CT) and magnetic resonance imaging (MRI) provide useful diagnostic and staging information, especially in delineating abdominal and pelvic masses and in the diagnosis of retroperitoneal nodal involvement. However, none of the

Table 50–5   Diagnostic Procedures in the Diagnosis and Staging of Patients with Ovarian Carcinoma

Patient medical history and physical examination
Complete blood count and biochemical profile
Serum CA-125 and other serum markers
Papanicolaou smear and cytology of ascitic fluids
Transabdominal and transvaginal ultrasonography
Cystoscopy and proctoscopy
Radiographic studies (chest, intravenous pyelogram, upper GI, and barium enema)
Abdominal computed tomography and magnetic resonance imaging
Laparotomy/laparoscopy

procedures listed in Table 50-5 are sufficient for accurate staging, and laparotomy remains the single most important method for assessing the stage of disease and the design of treatment. The role of positron emission tomography (PET) is under investigation[122] and the introduction of combined CT and PET imaging will markedly expand the role of PET in the diagnosis and post-treatment evaluation of ovarian cancer.

STAGING CLASSIFICATION

The purpose of classification by stage is to assign patients to clinical and prognostically homogeneous subgroups, ideally characterized by specific patterns of response to treatment and survival. Because ovarian cancer has no specific signs or symptoms, clinical staging has a low specificity, and the initial laparotomy serves as the most effective staging procedure. Table 50-6 shows the staging classification system introduced by the International Federation of Gynecology and Obstetrics (FIGO).[123] The "c" category in stages I and II identifies malignant cytology or tumor rupture. In stage III, categories a, b, or c address the location and size of abdominal metastatic disease, as determined before surgical debulking. Lymph node metastases, regardless of location, define the patient as in stage IIIc. In the past, routine staging procedures have frequently missed occult tumors on the undersurface of the diaphragm.[113,114] Therefore, routine staging includes multiple biopsies of retroperitoneal nodes, the diaphragm, and the peritoneum. Table 50-7 shows the distribution and survival of patients by the FIGO staging. Approximately 25% of the patients present with stage I disease, 10% with stage II, 50% with stage III, and 15% with stage IV disease.

Although the FIGO staging classification roughly correlates with prognosis (Table 50-8), there have been concerns over whether it adequately addresses *all* relevant tumor-related parameters that affect the outcome. Univariate statistical studies confirm the validity of the FIGO system,[125] but multivariate studies showed that other variables, in particular the size of residual tumor after initial surgery, are more powerful independent covariates than the FIGO stage in predicting the therapeutic outcome.[42,44,48,126-131] Because FIGO stage does not adequately address the issue of tumor residuum, there has been an increasing tendency to use the absence or presence of residual disease after initial surgery and its size as guidelines for selection of treatment. Markers such as nuclear ploidy, *HER2-neu*, *p53*, and serum CA-125, are additional parameters used. Hence, there is an apparent need for revision of the staging classification system in ovarian carcinoma to provide a more adequate basis for therapeutic decisions and for comparison of treatment results.

TECHNIQUES OF TREATMENT

Surgery

Surgery is the mainstay of the initial treatment of epithelial ovarian cancer. The goals of surgery are to establish the diagnosis, provide staging data, and carry out a maximal

Table 50–6 The International Federation of Gynecology and Obstetrics Staging Classification of Malignant Ovarian Tumors

Stage I	Growth limited to the ovaries
Ia	Growth limited to one ovary; no ascites; no tumor on the external surface; capsule intact
Ib	Growth limited to both ovaries; no ascites; no tumor on the external surfaces; capsules intact
Ic	Tumor either stage Ia or Ib but with tumor on the surface of one or both ovaries, or with capsule ruptured, or with ascites present containing malignant cells, or with positive peritoneal washings
Stage II	Growth involving one or both ovaries with pelvic extension
IIa	Growth involving one or both ovaries with pelvic extension
IIb	Extension and/or metastases to the uterus and/or tubes
IIc	Tumor either stage IIa or IIb but with tumor on the surface of one or both ovaries, or with capsules ruptured, or with ascites present containing malignant cells, or with positive peritoneal washings
Stage III	Tumor involving one or both ovaries with peritoneal implants outside the pelvis and positive retroperitoneal or inguinal nodes, or both. Superficial liver metastases equal stage III. Tumor is limited to the true pelvis but with histologically verified malignant extension to small bowel or omentum.
IIIa	Tumor grossly limited to the true pelvis with negative nodes but with histologically confirmed microscopic seeding of abdominal peritoneal surfaces
IIIb	Tumor of one or both ovaries with histologically confirmed implants of abdominal peritoneal surfaces, none >2 cm in diameter; nodes negative
IIIc	Abdominal implants >2 cm in diameter and/or positive retroperitoneal or inguinal nodes
Stage IV	Growth involving one or both ovaries with distant metastasis. If pleural effusion is present, there must be positive cytologic test results to allot a case to stage IV. Parenchymal liver metastasis equals stage IV.

Modified from International Federation of Gynecology and Obstetrics. Changes in definitions of clinical staging for carcinoma of the cervix and ovary. *Am J Obstet Gynecol.* 1986;156:263.

tumor cytoreduction in preparation for postoperative therapy. The Gynecologic Oncology Group (GOG) has published guidelines for the initial surgical approach.[132] A sufficiently extended vertical incision of the abdominal wall is recommended to permit visual exploration of the entire abdomen and facilitate maximal tumor resection. Free peritoneal fluid and peritoneal washings are obtained for cytology. Careful inspection of the entire abdominal content and the undersurfaces of the diaphragm is performed to identify all tumor deposits. Extrafascial total abdominal hysterectomy, bilateral salpingo-oophorectomy and resection of the infracolic omentum are routinely carried out. If gross disease still exists, a maximal cytoreductive effort is made to remove

Table 50–7 Stage Distribution and Survival

Stage	Patients, n	Distribution, %	5-Yr Survival, %
IA	421	13	90
IB	46	1	85
IC	436	13	80
IIA	55	2	70
IIB	108	3	64
IIC	154	5	67
IIIA	118	4	59
IIIB	264	8	40
IIIC	1330	40	29
IV	396	12	17

From Heintz APM, Odicino F, Maisnneuve P, et al: Carcinoma of the Ovary. In Pecorelli S, Beller U, Heintz APM, et al, eds: *FIGO Annual Report on the Results of Treatment in Gynecologic Cancer*, vol 24. Oxford: Isis Medical Media Limited; 2000.

as much of the remaining tumor as feasible. In addition, blind peritoneal biopsies are obtained from the cul-de-sac, right and left pelvic sidewalls, right and left paracolic gutters, and the diaphragm, tracing the known routes of transperitoneal spread of ovarian cancer to detect microscopic dissemination. Sampling of pelvic and para-aortic lymph nodes is also performed (Table 50-9).

When these surgical procedures are implemented, a successful complete removal of visible tumor is achieved in the great majority of stage I to II patients. However, in stage III to IV disease, optimal cytoreduction to tumor masses less than 2 cm in diameter is accomplished in only 20% to 40% of the patients.[10] More aggressive surgery that leads to higher rates of optimal debulking is technically feasible, albeit for the price of excessive peritoneal stripping, resection of a portion of the bowel and bladder, and increased postoperative morbidity.[133] Multiple studies have demonstrated that *cytoreduction* is a critical component of any approach to cure ovarian cancer.[48,97,132,134-138] Table 50-10 summarizes some of the data that demonstrate the impact of cytoreduction on survival in stage III patients. When all visible tumor is removed, 38% to 91% (mean 64%) of the patients survive

Table 50–8 Survival of 4809 Ovarian Cancer Patients by the FIGO Staging Classification

Substage	Cases, n	5-Yr Survival	P value*
IA	926	92 ± 0.9	
IB	131	85 ± 3.4	0.02
IC	391	82 ± 2.0	NS†
IIA	130	67 ± 4.3	0.0002
IIB	205	56 ± 3.6	0.03
IIC	146	51 ± 4.5	NS†
IIIA	333	41 ± 2.8	0.006
IIIB	317	26 ± 2.6	0.0004
IIIC	868	21 ± 1.4	0.005
IV	1362	12 ± 0.9	0.00001

*Survival comparisons were made between the listed substage and its immediate less advanced substage.
†NS, nonsignificant.
Modified from Nguyen HN, Averette HE, Hoskins W, et al: National survey of ovarian carcinoma. VI. Critical assessment of current International Federation of Gynecology and Obstetrics staging system. *Cancer.* 1993;72:3007.

Table 50–9 Recommended Comprehensive Surgical Staging for Ovarian Cancer

- Vertical midline abdominal incision to allow adequate visualization and palpation of structures in the upper abdomen, peritoneum, and retroperitoneum
- Total abdominal hysterectomy with bilateral salpingo-oophorectomy (unilateral salpingo-oophorectomy may be considered for fertility sparing in select patients with apparent stage Ia disease)
- Bilateral pelvic and para-aortic lymph node sampling
- Peritoneal washings (pelvis, paracolic gutters, hemidiaphragms)
- Infracolic (partial) omentectomy
- Biopsy of any lesions or adhesions
- Multiple biopsies from:
  Cul-de-sac
  Rectal and bladder serosa
  Right and left pelvic sidewalls
  Right and left paracolic gutters
  Right and left hemidiaphragms
  Any adhesions

5 to 10 years after treatment, compared to 16% to 57% (mean 36%) in patients with minimal (<2 cm) residua and 7% to 30% (mean 18%) in patients with larger residua. This overall trend was confirmed by a meta-analysis of 58 publications covering 6962 patients.[147] However, a multiple linear regression analysis revealed that the use of platinum-based chemotherapy and dose intensity were also independent variables impacting on survival. When corrected for these variables, maximum cytoreduction was associated with only a small improvement in median survival. Therefore, the benefit of a highly aggressive approach to maximal cytoreduction should be carefully weighed against the risk of sacrificing normal bowel and urinary function.

Second-look laparotomy is more controversial. The procedure was originally introduced to assess the results of chemotherapy and to determine whether treatment can be discontinued.[52] Noninvasive techniques such as sonography, CT, and MRI generally fail to detect small intraperitoneal masses (<2cm) that are found during laparotomy. However, when second-look laparotomy is performed in patients with complete clinical response after chemotherapy, only 45% are found to be without histopathologic evidence of residual tumors.[142,148] Further, several studies have shown that only 50% of patients with pathologically complete remission as assessed during second-look surgery remain free of relapse.[130,140-142,148,149] Therefore, the benefits of second-look laparotomy as a diagnostic technique have recently been questioned. It had, nonetheless, been suggested that secondary debulking should be attempted during the second-look procedure with the hope that it may improve survival if debulking is successful.

The validity of the second debulking approach was addressed by Creasman.[148] In a retrospective review of the literature, he reported that it was possible to completely debulk residual disease at second-look surgery in 188 of 600 patients, although only 31% survived at long-term. Investigators from the European Organization for Research on Treatment of Cancer (EORTC)[150] treated patients with initial suboptimally reduced tumors with

Table 50–10   Long-term (5-10 Yr) Survival in Stage III Ovarian Carcinoma: Correlation of Survival with the Size of the Residual Tumor Remaining After Initial Surgery

Author	Year	Treatment	No Residual Tumor		Minimal Residual Tumor (<2 cm)		Large Residual Tumor (>2 cm)	
			n	*Surviving, %*	*n*	*Surviving, %*	*n*	*Surviving, %*
Dembo[139]	1985	Radiation	46	48	55	43	71	18
Martinez[129]	1985	Radiation	30	68	42	54	54	20
Louie[140]	1986	Chemotherapy	3	66	10	16	28	7
Neijt[141]	1987	Chemotherapy	21	71	41	57	12	30
Weiser*	1988	Radiation	37	59	24	42	23	10
Fuks[142]	1988	Chemo + rad	6	38	10	20	22	20
Belinson[143]	1990	Chemotherapy	13	91	27	24	63	8
Hoskins[144]	1994	Chemotherapy	70	60	140	35	138	20
Del Campo[145]	1994	Chemotherapy	7	75	18	49	66	5
Baker[146]	1994	Chemotherapy	55	50	58	19	23	13

*From Weiser EB, Burke TW, Heller PB, et al: Determinants of survival of patients with epithelial ovarian carcinoma following whole abdomen irradiation (WAR). *Gynecol Oncol.* 1988;30;201.

three courses of cyclophosphamide-cisplatin chemotherapy and subsequently randomized the patients to have, or not to have, a planned interval (second) debulking operation. Both groups subsequently received an additional three courses of the same chemotherapy. Progression-free survival and overall survival rates were statistically improved in the patients who had an interval cytoreduction, with a 33% improvement in survival. Vaccarello[151] reported results of debulking during a third operation in patients who developed recurrent tumor after a negative second-look laparotomic examination. Although the procedure was associated with significant morbidity, 47% of the patients were alive at 20 months, compared with a median survival of 9 months in patients who were not explored. Altogether, these data provide a basis for the current generally accepted practice of aggressive cytoreduction to maximize the probability of survival with postoperative therapy, but the issue of increased toxicity with each consecutive operation remains a disadvantage that limits the general use of this approach. Second-look laparoscopy may represent an attractive alternative to laparotomy in patients who already have had prior laparotomy and chemotherapy.[152]

Radiation Therapy

TUMORICIDAL DOSE LEVELS

There is conclusive evidence that radiation can permanently eradicate ovarian epithelial tumors, although the tumoricidal dose levels may be tumor-size dependent. Schray et al.[153] reported that pelvic irradiation at doses of 50 to 60 Gy was associated with a 16% local relapse when given to patients with minimal residual tumors (<2 cm), compared with 45% in patients with larger pelvic tumors. When lower doses (45 Gy to the pelvis and 22.5 Gy to the upper abdomen) were given by Dembo[139,154] to patients with stages I, II, and IIIa disease, the 5-year survival in 50 patients with small or no residual tumors was 78%, compared with 19% in 26 patients with larger residua. These data suggest that for large

tumors the tumoricidal doses probably exceed 50 to 60 Gy, whereas for small tumors (<2 cm diameter) it is probably 45 to 50 Gy. The tumoricidal dose for microscopic tumors is probably lower. The Princess Margaret Group[139] reported that a dose of 22.5 Gy, given by the hypofractionated moving strip technique, can control occult disease in the upper abdomen. Stages I to III patients without detectable tumors after initial surgery treated with 45 Gy to the pelvis and 22.5 Gy to the upper abdomen had an approximately 30% higher control of the upper abdomen, as compared with patients who received 45 Gy to the pelvis only. Similarly, Delclos and Smith[155,156] reported that only 17% of stage II patients treated with 50 to 55 Gy to the pelvis were disease free at 5 years, compared with 49% of those treated to the pelvis plus 26 to 28 Gy to the upper abdomen by the moving strip technique. These data indicate that 22.5 to 30 Gy given by the fractionation scheme of the moving strip technique (daily fractions of 2.25 to 3 Gy), or their biologically equivalent doses when given at standard daily fractions of 1.8 to 2 Gy, are effective and sufficient for permanent eradication of microscopic ovarian tumor deposits.

NORMAL TISSUE TOLERANCE

The probability of tumor control with radiation is dependent not only on the delivery of tumoricidal doses, but also on the feasibility of encompassing all sites of disease with sufficient radiation doses, without significantly injuring normal tissues. Table 50-11 shows the tolerance of the critical normal organs encompassed by whole abdominal irradiation, expressed in terms of the TD 5/5 and TD 5/50 according to Rubin et al.[157] The data indicate that when whole abdominal fields are used, the limited tolerance of the liver, kidneys, and spinal cord would practically rule out eradication of visible tumor masses in the upper abdomen, regardless of tumor size. For pelvic fields, the tolerance of the intestines, rectum, and bladder would restrict the delivery of tumoricidal doses to tumors of less than 2 cm in size. This analysis suggests that only patients with minimal or microscopic residua would be candidates for cure by radiotherapy.

Table 50–11   Radiation Tolerance of Normal Organs Included in Whole Abdominal Radiation Fields*

Organ	Injury	TD 5/5	TD 50/5
Kidney	Nephrosclerosis	20	25
Liver	Veno-occlusive disease	25	40
Bone marrow	Aplasia	30	40
Spinal cord	Radiation myelitis	45	50
Stomach	Bleeding, ulcer, perforation	45	50
Intestines	Bleeding, ulcer, stricture	50	65
Rectum	Bleeding, ulcer, stricture	55	80
Urinary bladder	Bleeding, contracture	60	80

*Data are expressed as TD 5/5 and TD 50/5 doses in Gy according to Rubin et al.[157]

TREATMENT FIELDS

Because the entire peritoneal cavity is at risk for metastatic dissemination, treatment fields encompass either the whole or major portions of the abdominal cavity. Whole abdominal irradiation is given either by the open field technique (Fig. 50-4)[104] or by the moving strip technique (Fig. 50-5).[56,156] The open field technique is employed via anterior and posterior ports shaped to encompass the entire peritoneal cavity.[104,157] The treatment fields extend from above the domes of the diaphragm to below the obturator foraminae and laterally beyond the peritoneal reflection. The use of CT-based planning to accurately visualize the peritoneal reflections is very helpful.[159] Radiation is delivered at a rate of 1.2 to 1.5 Gy/day. The total dose to this field is 30 Gy in 20 fractions over 33 days, although the kidneys are shielded at 20 Gy and the

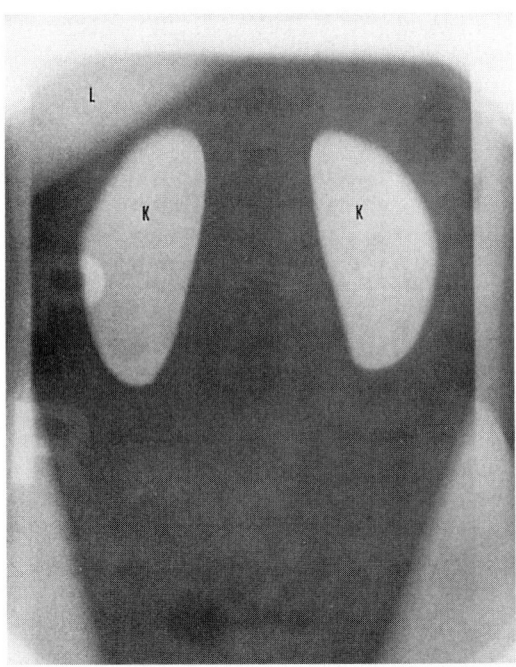

Figure 50–4. Treatment portal film demonstrating the open-field technique for whole abdominal irradiation. The field encompasses the entire peritoneal cavity and extends from the lower border of the obturator foramina up to 1 cm above the domes of the diaphragms. Lead blocks shield the liver (*L*) and the kidneys (*K*). (Reproduced with permission from Fuks Z, Bagshaw MA: The rationale for curative radiotherapy for ovarian carcinoma. *Int J Radiat Oncol Biol Phys.* 1975;1:21.)

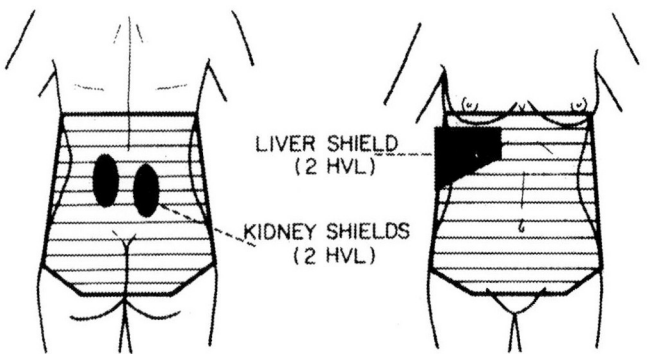

Figure 50–5. Schematic presentation of the moving strip technique for whole abdominal irradiation. The kidneys are shielded from the posterior and the liver from the anterior with two half-value layer lead blocks. To compensate for the lower dose at both ends of the irradiated volume, treatment is started one strip below the lower margin of the pelvic field and one strip above the diaphragm. (Reproduced with permission from Delclos L, Smith J: *Tumors of the Ovary.* Philadelphia: Lea & Febiger; 1973:670.)

liver at 25 Gy to protect these organs from radiation damage. The para-aortic region is usually carried to an additional 15 Gy and the lower abdomen to an additional 20 to 25 Gy. Several studies have described the use of hyperfractionated dose schedules to improve the tolerance of whole abdominal irradiation.[160,161] This technique uses differences in cell kinetics and radiation damage repair between normal and tumor cells. The delivery of low dose per fraction (8 to 1.25 Gy) twice or three times daily, 6 hours apart, is associated with decreased damage to late-responding normal tissues without compromising the lethal effects on the rapidly growing tumor cells.[162]

The moving strip technique (see Fig. 50-5) divides the peritoneal cavity into horizontal 2.5 cm segments.[155,156] Treatment starts by irradiation of the four lowest pelvic segments, and is moved upward by one strip at a time until the whole abdominal cavity is covered. Each strip receives 10 fractions of 2.5 Gy, to a total dose of 25 to 30 Gy in 10 to 12 fractions. The kidneys and liver are usually shielded by partial-thickness lead blocks to restrict the dose to 15 Gy. An additional dose of 20 Gy in 10 fractions over 12 days is usually delivered to the pelvis by an open field. When calculated by the nominal standard dose (NSD) method of Ellis,[163] the dose delivered by this technique is roughly equivalent to the dose delivered by the open field technique. Dembo et al.[154] compared the moving strip and the open field technique and found that the relapse-free and overall survival rates and the acute toxicities were similar, but severe late complications requiring bowel surgery were observed approximately five times more frequently with the moving strip technique. On the basis of these data, the open field technique currently serves as the standard technique of whole abdominal irradiation.

There have been several modifications to the open field technique, mostly designed to increase the dose to areas of high risk, such as the para-aortic region and the diaphragms. The technique described by Martinez[129] responds to these criteria and also implements a fractionation scheme that improves the tolerance of treatment.

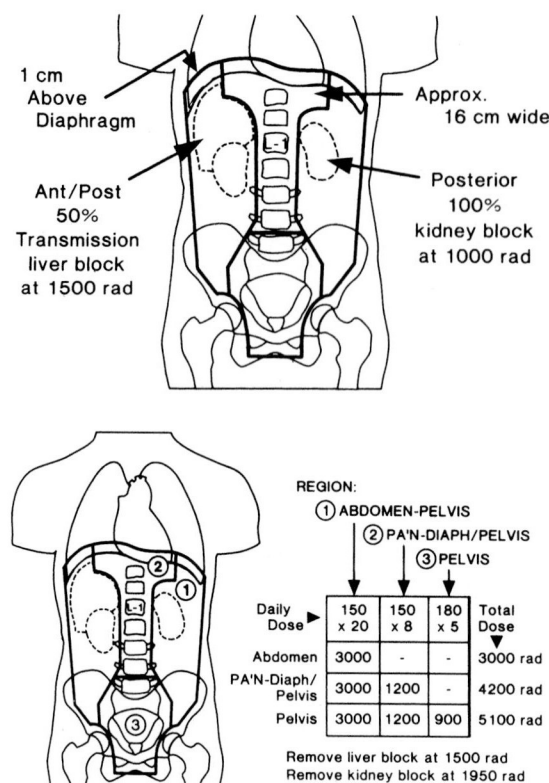

Figure 50–6. Schematic presentation of treatment fields and dose schedules for the Martinez technique of radiation therapy for ovarian cancer. (Reproduced with permission from Martinez A, Schray MF, Howes AE, Bagshaw MA: Postoperative radiation therapy for epithelial ovarian cancer: The curative role based on a 24-year experience. *J Clin Oncol.* 1985;3:901.)

Treatment according to the Martinez technique (Fig. 50-6) is initiated with 9 Gy to the true pelvis via anterior and posterior open fields at daily fractions of 1.5 to 1.8 Gy. Subsequently, 30 Gy are given at this fractionation scheme to a classic whole abdominal field, and then 12 Gy through a "T-shaped" field, which includes the para-aortic and the medial diaphragmatic regions.[1] Reports on the use of this technique have demonstrated it to be well tolerated.[129]

TOLERANCE OF TREATMENT

The acute toxicity is dose-dependent and consists mainly of gastrointestinal symptoms and marrow suppression. Diarrhea, vomiting, and weight loss during the course of treatment have been reported in 62% to 90% of patients receiving 45 to 60 Gy to the pelvis.[104,164,165] These symptoms mostly subside within a few weeks after the completion of treatment. Subacute enteritis with or without bleeding persists, however, in 14% to 29% over a period of a few months after treatment.[104,165] Bowel stenosis and bleeding, which require surgical intervention, were reported in 4% to 14% of treated patients.[104,165-168]

Leukopenia or thrombocytopenia or both are nearly always observed during the course of radiation,[104] although treatment needs to be interrupted in only 23% to 27% because of marrow toxicity.[165] The counts usually return to normal after completion of treatment, but

the activity of the irradiated marrow was shown to remain impaired for extended periods of time.[169] Radiation hepatitis and nephritis may occur with doses exceeding 25 Gy.[156,170-173] More recently, however, these complications have not been observed because of the careful application of appropriate shielding of the liver and kidneys.

INTRAPERITONEAL RADIOISOTOPES

The radioisotope most commonly used for the treatment of ovarian cancer is ^{32}P in the form of chromic phosphate colloid. The ^{32}P isotope is a pure beta emitter and has a half-life time of 14.3 days. Its beta particles have a mean energy of 0.69 MeV and tissue penetration of 3 to 5 mm. The fact that there is no gamma emission provides significant safety to the treating staff. The standard dose of ^{32}P is 15 mCi given in a single intraperitoneal application. The colloidal phase increases the isotope uptake by macrophages and by the mesothelial peritoneal cells, and decreases systemic elution. Boye et al.[174] reported dose calculations assuming a uniform distribution of ^{32}P in the mesothelial layer of the peritoneum. The estimated surface dose to the peritoneum from 10 mCi of ^{32}P is approximately 30 Gy. The uptake and distribution of ^{32}P in the peritoneal cavity is, however, inhomogeneous,[175,176] as it follows the patterns of peritoneal drainage. The distribution is optimized by instillation of the isotope in a large volume of fluid and by frequent changes of patient positioning during the first several hours after treatment. Eventually, the highest concentrations of the colloid particles are found on the peritoneum of the diaphragm, liver, and omentum. The range of the beta particles of ^{32}P in tissue suggests that it would effectively sterilize microscopic peritoneal implants, but may be inadequate for larger tumors. The pattern of isotope distribution, which parallels the pattern of transcoelomic spread of ovarian cancer, would suggest that the best therapeutic effect would be on micrometastases that are frequently present at the sites of maximal isotope accumulation.

The use of intraperitoneal ^{32}P appears to be safe and well tolerated. Acute toxicity is minimal and uncommon if the administration is done properly. The most common long-term complication is small-bowel obstruction and stenosis. It occurs in 10% to 20% of treated patients,[161,177,178] depending on the tumor stage, the number of surgical procedures performed, and whether external beam therapy is also given. A study of 69 patients with early-stage disease[179] reported that 6 had severe acute gastrointestinal symptoms, 1 had a small bowel perforation 20 months after ^{32}P treatment, and 3 required surgery for small bowel obstruction. No patients had suppression of marrow and there were no deaths attributed to treatment with ^{32}P.

Chemotherapy

SYSTEMIC CHEMOTHERAPY

Ovarian tumor cells are highly sensitive to drugs, responding to various chemotherapeutic agents with prompt shrinkage and partial to complete clinical

Table 50–12   Initial Response Rates (Complete and Partial Remissions) in Stage III-IV Ovarian Carcinoma Patients Treated with Single-Agent Chemotherapy

Drug	Patients, n (Response, %)
Cisplatin	190 (32)
Carboplatin	82 (24)
Taxol	189 (29)
Doxorubicin	102 (33)
Alkylating agents	1371 (33)
Isophosphamide	37 (22)
Hexamethylmelamine	215 (24)
5-fluorouracil	26 (29)
Methotrexate	34 (18)
Mitomycin-C	49 (16)

*Modified from Thigpen JT, Blessing JA, Vance RB, et al: Chemotherapy in ovarian carcinoma: Present role and future prospects. *Semin Oncol.* 1989;16(suppl 6):58.

responses. Table 50-12 lists the most active drugs and the rates of response when given as single agents. The response to any agent differs depending on the volume of residual disease, the dose intensity of treatment, and whether there has been prior chemotherapy, which may have induced a cross-resistance to a given drug.

The platinum analogs are considered the most active agents in ovarian carcinoma. Cisplatin, delivered at a dose of 50 to 75 mg/m^2 every 4 weeks, has been reported to induce a 20% surgical complete response in chemotherapy-naive stage III and IV patients and a 19.4-month median survival.[149,181,182] The dose-limiting side effects are nephrotoxicity and neurotoxicity, but vomiting is also a serious side effect that requires special attention. Carboplatin is another active platinum analog that has a similar anti-tumor activity, but is associated with minimal or no nephrotoxicity and neurotoxicity, and with decreased vomiting. The tradeoff, however, is greater myelosuppression than is seen with cisplatin.

One of the main adverse effects of cisplatin is the relative frequent and fast induction of multidrug resistance, which is associated with cross-resistance to radiation and a number of drugs active against ovarian cancer. Paclitaxel (Taxol) is among the few that do not exhibit cross-resistance with platinum. Paclitaxel is a diterpenoid, originally extracted from the bark of the western yew tree *Taxus brevifolia*. It acts by stabilizing cellular microtubules, thereby interfering with cell replication.[183] Responses to paclitaxel were reported in both platinum-sensitive and platinum-resistant patients. Phase II studies showed 24% to 30% response rates in women with platinum-resistant advanced-stage disease and 37% in less heavily pretreated women who received higher starting paclitaxel doses.[183-186] The drug is usually given by 24-hour infusion at a dose of 135 mg/m^2 or over 3 hours at 175 mg/m.^{2} Adverse effects include myelosuppression, hypersensitivity reactions, and arrhythmias. The dose-limiting toxicity is myelosuppression, which is severe, albeit short in duration.

Alkylating agents are among the first used in the treatment of ovarian carcinoma. The most active alkylating agents are melphalan (L-PAM), cyclophosphamide, chlorambucil, and thiotepa. A GOG study reported an overall response rate of 37.5%, with a 20% clinical complete response for oral melphalan in bulky stage III and stage IV disease.[187] Alkylating agents, in particular cyclophosphamide, are most commonly used in combination with cisplatin. The major toxicities are myelosuppression and bladder toxicity, especially with high-dose cyclophosphamide.

Doxorubicin is also active in ovarian carcinoma, but has mostly been used in drug combinations. Its use has decreased because it appears to be cross-resistant with platinum. However, a meta-analysis of four randomized studies involving 1194 patients[8] reported a small, albeit significant, survival benefit for the combination of cyclophosphamide, doxorubicin, and cisplatin (CAP) as compared to cyclophosphamide and cisplatin (C-P) alone. In addition, there was a significant advantage for CAP in the frequency of negative second-look laparotomies. More recently, liposomal doxorubicin has been used, especially in patients who failed platinum-based chemotherapy.[188-190]

COMBINATION CHEMOTHERAPY

The basic guidelines for the design of a protocol of multi-agent chemotherapy include the selection of drugs that do not have overlapping toxicities and cross-resistance, and an attempt to achieve maximal dose intensification. Because of the availability of numerous drugs that differ in the mechanism of action and toxicity, multiagent schemes have gradually become the standard of care in ovarian cancer. Despite the fact that most patients with advanced ovarian cancer in the United States receive combination therapy of paclitaxel and carboplatinum,[191] the debate on whether single agent therapy is better than combination therapy is far from over. In the GOG-132 trial, 614 patients with suboptimally debulked stage III to IV disease were randomized to cisplatin alone (100 mg/m^2), paclitaxel alone (200 mg/m^2), or a combination (75 mg/m^2 and 135 mg/m,^{2} respectively). Cisplatin alone or in combination yielded superior response rates and disease-free survival relative to paclitaxel. However, overall survival was similar in all three arms, and the combination therapy had a better toxicity profile due to difference in the prescribed dose.[192] The International Collaborative Ovarian Neoplasm (ICON) group reported on two randomized trials comparing single-agent carboplatin to combination chemotherapy. ICON2 was a randomized trial of 1526 patients comparing carboplatin to CAP (cyclophosphamide, doxorubicin, and cisplatin). There was no significant difference in disease-free or overall survival between the two arms of the trial.[193] ICON3 was a randomized trial of 2074 patients who were randomly assigned to paclitaxel plus carboplatin or control, the control (carboplatin alone or CAP) being chosen by the patient and clinician before randomization. Single-agent carboplatin and CAP were as effective as paclitaxel and carboplatin in terms of disease-free and overall survival.[194] While the data from individual randomized trials may seem contradictory, several meta-analyses have shown the following. Aabo et al., in a review of 37 randomized trials, demonstrated a trend in favor of platinum combinations over single-agent platinum.[195]

Covens et al., in a similar review, demonstrated the superiority of combination platinum/paclitaxel over single-agent platinum.[196] Perhaps some of the inconsistency of the data relate to the nature of the control arm of each individual trial as demonstrated by Sandercock et al.[197]

INTRAPERITONEAL CHEMOTHERAPY

One approach to achieve dose intensification is the instillation of chemotherapeutic drugs intraperitoneally.[198] The intraperitoneal concentration of drugs feasible with this method has been shown to exceed the plasma levels when maximally tolerable drug concentrations are given intravenously. Some studies have demonstrated that paclitaxel can be delivered safely intraperitoneally, with a 3 log or higher pharmacokinetic advantage for peritoneal cavity exposure over that achieved by systemic administration.[199]

TREATMENT OF EARLY-STAGE DISEASE

Observation

Not all early-stage patients require postoperative therapy.[200] Tumor variables that predict a high risk of relapse after complete resection include low differentiation, the presence of dense tumor adhesions, and the presence of extensive ascites.[47] In a GOG randomized trial, 81 patients with well or moderately differentiated cancers confined to the ovaries (*surgical* stage IA and IB) were assigned to receive 12 cycles of melphalan or no further therapy.[201] With a median follow-up of more than 6 years, there were no significant differences between the patients given no chemotherapy and those treated with melphalan with respect to either 5-year disease-free survival (91% vs. 98%; $P = 0.41$) or overall survival (94% vs. 98%; $P = 0.43$).[199] Dembo et al.[154] randomized 54 stage IA patients between no postoperative treatment and pelvic irradiation and observed that all the relapses occurred among the patients with poor prognosis variables. Based on these observations, it is generally accepted that stage IA and IB patients with well- or moderately differentiated tumors and without positive peritoneal cytology or densely adherent tumors do not require postoperative therapy.

Chemotherapy

The success of combination chemotherapy in advanced-stage ovarian cancers prompted the adoption of these combinations for further study in early-stage, unfavorable-prognosis ovarian cancer. Bolis et al. reported on 85 patients with stage Ia and Ib FIGO grade II or III who were randomized to observation or 6 cycles of cisplatin.[202] The 5-year disease-free survival was 65% in the observation arm compared to 83% in the chemotherapy arm ($P = 0.028$). The 5-year overall survival, however, was not significantly different, 82% in the control arm vs. 88% in the chemotherapy arm ($P = 0.773$). The EORTC recently reported the results of a randomized trial[203] in 448 patients with stages Ia to Ib, grades II to III, and all stages Ic to IIa. Patients were assigned to either observation or

platinum-based chemotherapy. With a median follow-up of 5.5 years, the 5-year disease-free survival rate was 68% in the observation arm compared to 76% in the chemotherapy arm ($P = 0.02$). This difference, however, did not translate into overall survival advantage (78% for observation vs. 85% for chemotherapy; $P = 0.1$). Not all patients in this trial were optimally debulked; therefore, when the subset of patients who were optimally debulked was analyzed, adjuvant chemotherapy lost its impact on disease-free or overall survival ($P = 0.73$ and 0.65, respectively). The only trial that showed improvement in overall survival[204] was that reported by the International Collaborative Ovarian Neoplasm (ICON) 1. There were 477 patients with early-stage disease including grade 1 who were randomized to no further therapy or 6 cycles of chemotherapy. The 5-year overall survival rate was 70% in the observation arm compared to 79% in the chemotherapy arm ($P = 0.03$). Some of the shortcomings of this trial involve the inclusion of patients with low-risk disease (Ia to Ib, FIGO grade I or II) where adjuvant chemotherapy is not needed. It used an unusual entry criterion that allowed entry into the trial "if, in the opinion of the responsible clinician, it was uncertain whether the patients would benefit from immediate adjuvant chemotherapy." In addition, the type of chemotherapy was to some extent left to the discretion of the treating clinician. This assumes that the various chemotherapy regimens used in this trial are interchangeable and equally effective.[205] In the United States, most experts recommend adjuvant chemotherapy for patients with high-risk, early-stage disease. The emphasis, therefore, has been on how much chemotherapy is needed in this group of patients. In the GOG-157 trial, patients with stages Ia to Ib, FIGO grade 3, and all stages IC to II, were randomized to three versus 6 cycles of carboplatin/paclitaxel. Preliminary data indicated that the probability of recurrence at 5 years was 27% in the 3-cycles arm compared to 19% in the 6-cycles arm, which was not significantly different. The toxicity, however, was higher with 6 cycles.[206]

Radiation Therapy

Stage I patients with adverse prognostic features, as well as stage II and III patients without residual tumor after initial surgery, are generally classified as intermediate-risk patients.[207] These patients benefit from radiation therapy. Patterns of failure in this class of patients (Table 50-13) have indicated that the application of radiation decreases the rates of local relapse.[153,154,208,209]

INTRAPERITONEAL^{32}P

Several prospective randomized trials have looked at ^{32}P versus chemotherapy and all have shown equivalent survival rates. The GOG randomized 141 patients with poorly differentiated stage I and stage II tumors to melphalan or 15 mCi of intraperitoneal ^{32}P. With a median follow-up of more than 6 years, the outcome for the two treatment groups was similar with respect to 5-year disease-free survival (80% in both groups) and overall survival (81% with melphalan vs. 78% with ^{32}P,

Table 50–13 Correlation of Sites of Relapse with Radiation Treatment Fields in Patients with Early-Stage Ovarian Carcinoma

Author	Yr Published	Stage	Treatment	Total Relapses, n (%)	Pelvic ± Upper Abdomen	Upper Abdomen ± Distant
Dembo[154]	1984	IA	None	4/27 (15)	3/4	1/4
			Pel-xRT	5/27 (18)	1/5	4/5
		IB+II+III0	Pel-xRT ± CHB	39/82 (47)	19/39	21/39
			WAR	11/50 (22)	11/11	0/11
Hershchyshyn[208]	1980	IA+IB	None	5/29 (175)	4/5	1/5
			Pelvic xRT	7/23 (30)	3/7	4/7
			Melphalan	2/34 (6)	1/2	1/2
Schray[153]	1983	I+II	Pel xRT	19/61 (31)	5/19	14/19
		IIIA	Pel xRT	14/21 (66)	6/14	8/14
Macbeth[209]	1988	I+II+IIIA	WAR	25/57 (44)	14/25	11/25

Pel-xRT, pelvic field radiotherapy; WAR, whole abdominal radiotherapy; CHB, chlorambucil.

$P = 0.4$). In the ^{32}P arm, 6% of patients required laparotomy for bowel obstruction compared to a 3% leukemia rate in the melphalan arm.[201] The critics of this study point that ^{32}P was not compared to cisplatin-based chemotherapy, which represents the standard chemotherapy approach. The GOG recently reported on a second trial that randomized 205 patients with stages I to IIA (high risk) to 15 mCi intraperitoneal ^{32}P versus 3 cycles of cyclophosphamide and cisplatin. With a median follow-up of 6 years, there was no statistically significant difference in overall 5-year survival rates (84% chemotherapy arm vs. 76% ^{32}P arm). The authors concluded that chemotherapy is better because of the better progression-free interval.[210] Several studies have confirmed this rate of relapse after intraperitoneal ^{32}P of treatment for intermediate-risk ovarian cancer.[178,211] Soper[212] reported that the overall 5-year survival rates among 49 stage I and II patients were 84% and 86%, respectively, with disease-free survival rates of 79% and 57%, respectively. Forty-two percent of the recurrences had a component of failure in the lymph nodes, indicating the inability of ^{32}P to sterilize microscopic disease at retroperitoneal nodal sites.

WHOLE ABDOMEN RADIATION

Unlike ^{32}P, with whole abdomen radiation (WAR), not only the peritoneal surface is treated but the pelvic and para-aortic lymph nodes, as well. Several randomized trials have compared WAR to chemotherapy, including two trials with cisplatin-based chemotherapy. Most of these trials showed no statistically significant difference in survival but a trend toward improvement in disease-free survival in some. The Princess Margaret Hospital (PMH) group in Toronto reported on a group of 190 patients with stages Ib and II and asymptomatic stage III disease who were randomized to receive adjuvant pelvic irradiation, pelvic irradiation plus oral chlorambucil for 2 years, or WAR.[139,170] Survival differences were observed only in those patients who had a complete resection of disease. In this group, whole abdominal irradiation achieved a 78% 5-year and 64% 10-year survival

rate, compared with 51% and 40%, respectively, in patients receiving pelvic irradiation with or without chlorambucil. The improved survival of patients treated with whole abdominal irradiation appeared to be due to a 30% decrease of relapses in the upper abdomen. Two other randomized trials compared WAR (moving-strip technique) to melphalan. One, from M.D. Anderson Cancer center,[213] compared WAR to 12 cycles of melphalan with no difference in 5-year survival (71% vs. 72%). The other was from the National Cancer Institute of Canada,[214] which compared three arms: WAR, pelvic radiation and melphalan, or pelvic radiation and intraperitoneal ^{32}P. The corresponding 5-year overall survival rates were 62%, 61%, and 66%, respectively ($P = 0.34$). Sell et al. compared WAR (open field) to pelvic radiation and cyclophosphamide.[215] There was no significant difference in disease-free survival or overall survival between the two arms. Two other randomized trials compared cisplatin to WAR. Redman et al.[216] reported on 40 patients randomized to 5 cycles of cisplatin or WAR (moving strip) with 5-year survival rates of 62% and 58%, respectively ($P = 0.66$). Chiara et al. reported on 70 patients randomized to WAR or 6 cycles of cisplatin + cyclophosphamide.[217] The 5-year survival rate was 71% and 53% ($P = 0.16$), while disease-free survival was 74% and 50% ($P = 0.07$). Interestingly, both trials were closed prematurely due to lack of accrual, perhaps reflecting bias on the part of the treating clinicians. The opponents of WAR point out that some of these trials showed a superior therapeutic ratio since the complication rate with chemotherapy was lower. It is important to note, however, that the overlap of abutting fields with the moving strip technique may have contributed significantly to the high incidence of gastrointestinal damage. When meticulous attention is paid to treatment techniques, the rate of serious toxicity should be low. In a recent randomized trial from Canada, 125 patients with optimally debulked stage I, II, and III disease were randomized to two different doses of WAR.[218] The rate of any grade 3 complication in that trial was 4%. Most authors today use the open field technique with appropriate shielding of the kidneys.

The total dose is usually 25 to 30 Gy given at 1 to 1.5 Gy per fraction.

In summary, intraperitoneal ^{32}P or WAR as an adjuvant therapy for high-risk, early-stage patients seems to offer similar survival rates to chemotherapy. Therefore, it should be considered at least as an alternative to chemotherapy in patients who refuse or are not good candidates for chemotherapy. Special attention, however, needs to be paid to assure adequate distribution of ^{32}P throughout the peritoneal cavity and to the treatment techniques with WAR.

TREATMENT OF ADVANCED-STAGE DISEASE

Upfront Therapy

Treatment results in advanced-stage disease have been significantly less favorable. In the past, these patients were treated with whole abdominal irradiation, and old series reported 10% to 20% survival rates at 5 to 10 years.[104] In the past 3 decades there has been a shift to the use of chemotherapy in this group of patients, in search of a combination that might enhance the cure of advanced-stage disease (Table 50-14). Currently in the United States, the standard treatment approach for advanced-stage ovarian cancer consists of Total Abdominal Hysterectomy and Bilateral Salpingo-oophorectomy (TAH/BSO), staging, and an attempt at maximal surgical debulking followed by 6 cycles of carboplatin/paclitaxel. Two landmark trials (GOG 111 and Intergroup/EORTC) demonstrated that paclitaxel plus cisplatin improved response rates, progression-free survival, and overall survival compared to treatment with cyclophosphamide and cisplatin.[191,219] But as mentioned earlier in the chapter, the cisplatin analog carboplatin is associated with less toxicity than cisplatin. GOG 158 compared cisplatin/paclitaxel to carboplatin/paclitaxel and found no difference in outcome but less toxicity with carboplatin/paclitaxel.[220] Two other randomized trials comparing the same regimens demonstrated identical results.[221,222] These results make paclitaxel (175 mg/m^2 over 3 hours plus carboplatin 5 to 7.5 AUC (area under the curve) with both drugs delivered intravenously every 3 weeks for a total of 6 cycles) a reasonable standard approach for most patients with advanced ovarian cancer following cytoreductive surgery. Before the availability of paclitaxel, a randomized trial by the GOG compared intravenous cisplatin and cyclophosphamide to intraperitoneal cisplatin plus intravenous cyclophosphamide in patients with optimal debulked stage III ovarian cancer. The risk of death was lower in the intraperitoneal group (hazard ratio, 0.76; 95% CI: 0.61 to 0.96; P = 0.02) and the toxicity was less compared to the intravenous arm.[223] An intergroup trial compared intravenous cisplatin plus paclitaxel to intravenous carboplatin followed by intravenous paclitaxel plus intraperitoneal cisplatin. This study also demonstrated a trend toward improvement in survival.[224] Preliminary results from the most recent GOG-172 trial comparing intravenous paclitaxel and cisplatin to intravenous paclitaxel plus intraperitoneal cisplatin and

Table 50–14 Median Survival Of Chemotherapy Randomized Trials for Advanced Ovarian Cancer

A. Paclitaxel vs. Cisplatin Trials

Trial	Chemo	Progression-Free Survival	Overall Survival
GOG[191]	Paclitaxel/cisplatin	18 mo	38 mo
	Cyclophosphamide/cisplatin	13 mo	24 mo
OV[219]	Paclitaxel/cisplatin	15.5 mo	35.6 mo
	Cyclophosphamide/cisplatin	11.5 mo	25.8 mo

B. Carboplatin vs. Cisplatin Trials

Trial	Chemo	Progression-Free Survival	Overall Survival
GOG[220]	Carboplatin-AUC 7.5 Paclitaxel-175 mg/m^2	20.7 mo	57.4 mo
	Cisplatin-75 mg/m^2 Paclitaxel-135 mg/m^2	21.7 mo	48.7 mo
Dutch/Danish[221]	Carboplatin-AUC 5 Paclitaxel-175 mg/m^2	—	32 mo
	Cisplatin-75 mg/m^2 Paclitaxel-175 mg/m^2	—	30 mo

C. Intraperitoneal vs. Intravenous Cisplatin Trials

Trial	Chemo	Progression-Free Survival	Overall Survival
INT[224]	I.V. Carboplatin-9 AUC I.V. Paclitaxel-135 mg/m^2 I.P. Cisplatin-100 mg/m^2	28 mo	63 mo
	I.V. Cisplatin-75 mg/m^2 I.V. Paclitaxel-135 mg/m^2	22 mo	52 mo
GOG[223]	I.V. Cyclophosphamide-600 mg/m^2 I.P. Cisplatin-100 mg/m^2	—	49 mo
	I.V. Cyclophosphamide-600 mg/m^2 I.V. Cisplatin-100 mg/m^2	—	41 mo

intraperitoneal paclitaxel are showing similar trends.[225] Based on these trials, it seems that intraperitoneal chemotherapy is a reasonable alternative to intravenous chemotherapy in patients with optimally debulked stage III ovarian cancer. But the familiarity and ease of administration of intravenous paclitaxel and carboplatin, both given on an outpatient basis, makes it more appealing to many medical oncologists.

Although some patients respond favorably to chemotherapy, a close examination of the data indicates that the rates of cure have not changed substantially. Several meta-analysis studies conducted, involving more than 50 randomized chemotherapy trials,[8,49,147,182,226,227] have provided an insight into this issue. Cisplatin was identified as the most effective single agent, associated with a 2-year survival rate of 64%, but survival rates at 6 and 8 years were only 17% and 14%, respectively.[182] Platinum combinations improved survival rates over those observed with combinations that did not include cisplatin and produced an absolute survival advantage over single-agent platinum of 7% to 10% at 4 to 8 years.[182] It should be noted that long-term results of two large series of whole abdominal irradiation have been similar to those reported so far with cisplatin combinations

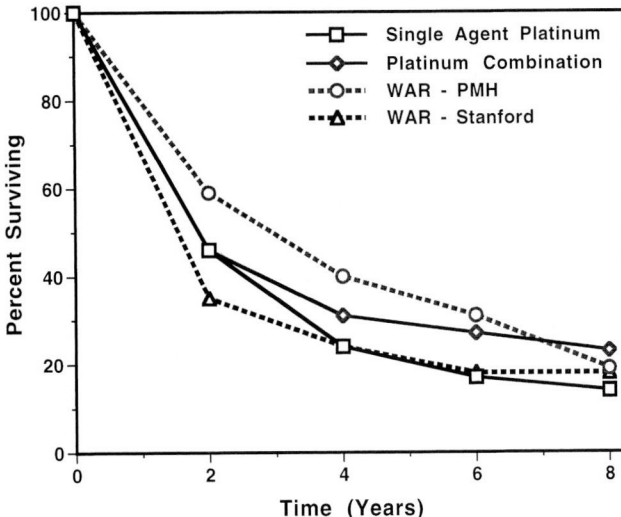

Figure 50–7. Comparison of long-term survival of advanced-stage ovarian cancer treated with single-agent cisplatin, cisplatin-based combination chemotherapy, or whole abdominal irradiation. Data for the survival curves of cisplatin and cisplatin combination chemotherapy were derived from a meta-analysis reported by Williams et al.,[228] for the Princess Margaret Hospital series from Dembo et al.,[139] and for the Stanford series from Martinez et al.[129]

(Fig. 50-7).[129,139,228] This observation is of particular interest in view of the fact that the PMH and Stanford radiotherapy series involved mostly patients treated and followed before the era of cisplatinum. Hence, an effect on survival from treatment of radiation-failing patients with cisplatin-based combinations is ruled out in these series.

CONSOLIDATION THERAPY

While the overall results of treatment with chemotherapy or radiation in advanced-stage disease are poor, survival of patients optimally cytoreduced during initial surgery is significantly improved compared to patients with suboptimally reduced tumors (see Table 50-10). Bristow et al. reported on 6885 patients with stages III and IV ovarian cancer treated in the platinum era. The study demonstrated a statistically significant positive correlation between percent maximal cytoreduction and log median survival time, and this correlation remained significant after controlling for other variables ($P < 0.001$). Each 10% increase in maximal cytoreduction was associated with a 5.5% increase in median survival time.[229] However, approximately one half of optimally cytoreduced patients who exhibit a complete pathologic response to chemotherapy eventually fail and succumb to ovarian cancer.[130,140-142,148,149]

Several approaches to treatment intensification have been tested in an attempt to improve the outcome.

SYSTEMIC CHEMOTHERAPY

The GOG tested the effect of doubling the dose of cyclophosphamide-cisplatin but failed to demonstrate a therapeutic advantage, although toxicity was significantly increased.[230] A study from Scotland,[231] which kept the dose of cyclophosphamide constant but tested the doubling of the cisplatin dose, initially demonstrated a significant increase in the median survival (114 weeks for the high dose vs. 69 weeks for the low dose; $P = 0.0008$), but this significant difference diminished on a longer follow-up.[232] The issue of dose intensity thus remains open, although it is clear that tolerance may limit its use. Increasing the duration of chemotherapy from five to six courses of the CAP combination to 10 to 12 courses failed to confer any survival advantage.[233,234] The recent GOG/SWOG trial comparing 3 vs. 12 months of paclitaxel in patients with advanced ovarian cancer who attain a clinically defined complete response following platinum/paclitaxel-based chemotherapy had to be closed prematurely due to significant improvement in disease-free survival (28 months for 12 monthly cycles compared to 21 months for 3 monthly cycles, $P = 0.023$). The data on overall survival in this trial await longer follow-up.[235]

Another approach to dose intensification is *intraperitoneal chemotherapy*. Barakat et al. reported on a phase II trial of intraperitoneal cisplatin and etoposide as consolidation therapy in patients with stage II to IV ovarian cancer following negative surgical assessment.[236] With a median follow-up of 36 months, 61% (22/36) of the treated patients were without evidence of recurrent disease. This group of patients was compared to a cohort of 46 contemporaneous patients who underwent observation only. The recurrence rate in this group was 54% (25/46), and when the protocol patients and the cohort were combined, the only predictor of improved disease-free survival was protocol treatment ($P < 0.01$). One important aspect of intraperitoneal chemotherapy as consolidation is the size of disease at the time of initiation of intraperitoneal chemotherapy. In a review of 433 patients who received intraperitoneal chemotherapy at the Memorial Sloan-Kettering Cancer Center, the median survival was 8.7 years for patients with negative second-look laparotomy, 4.8 years microscopic, 3.3 years for less than 1 cm, and 1.2 years for greater than 1 cm.[237] Currently no phase III data exist on intraperitoneal chemotherapy for consolidation and since many of the patients who get this type of consolidation tend to have a more favorable prognosis to begin with, it becomes difficult to determine its proper role.

Radiation Therapy

Several studies have attempted to consolidate complete responses to chemotherapy with radiation therapy.

INTRAPERITONEAL ^{32}P

The GOG recently completed a prospective randomized trial in 202 patients with negative second-look laparotomy.[238] All patients were treated with postoperative platinum-based chemotherapy and then were randomized to observation or 15 mCi of ^{32}P. There was no significant difference in disease-free survival (42% in ^{32}P arm vs. 36% in observation; $P = 0.27$) or in overall survival (67% vs. 63%, respectively; $P = 0.19$).

WHOLE ABDOMEN RADIATION

Most protocols have used WAR, delivered after several courses of combination chemotherapy and a second-look cytoreductive effort. Fuks et al.[142] reported the results in 38 stage III patients induced with 3 to 14 courses of the Cyclophosphamide Hexamethylmelamine Adriamycin Cisplatin (CHAD) combination chemotherapy. After the second cytoreductive operation, 76% of the patients were without gross residual tumors. WAR was relatively well tolerated. However, the actuarial 5-year survival and disease-free survival rates for the whole group were 27% and 17%, respectively. These survival data were similar to those observed in patients receiving the same chemotherapy without WAR. One randomized trial compared WAR to no further therapy in 64 patients with no residual disease following carboplatin-based chemotherapy.[239] There was a significant difference in 5-year disease-free survival (49% in WAR arm vs. 26% no WAR arm; $P = 0.013$) and overall survival (59% vs. 26%, respectively; 0.012). At least five prospective, randomized trials have investigated the value of consolidation following chemotherapy with WAR or further chemotherapy. Two of these trials had such small sample sizes that no meaningful conclusions could be drawn from them,[240,241] and the third trial used chlorambucil chemotherapy.[242] Lambert et al. reported on a randomized trial of 254 patients with advanced ovarian cancer who were treated with 5 cycles of carboplatin. Of the 254 patients, 117 patients with residual disease less than or equal to 2 cm were then randomized to WAR or another 5 cycles of carboplatin. There was no significant difference in disease-free or overall survival between the two arms.[243] Sorbe et al. reported on 742 patients with stage III ovarian cancer who received 4 cycles of cisplatin-based chemotherapy.[244] Patients with complete pathologic response ($n = 172$) were randomized to no further therapy, 6 cycles of cisplatin-based chemotherapy, or WAR. In patients with microscopic residual disease ($n = 74$), the randomization was between WAR and chemotherapy. The disease-free survival rate in the group of patients with complete pathologic response was better in the WAR than the chemotherapy on observation arms ($P = 0.032$). The overall survival for WAR was also better ($P = 0.084$). This difference in disease-free survival did not translate into survival improvement; the 3-year overall survival rate was 83% after WAR, 76% after chemotherapy, and 73% after observation ($P = 0.11$). In the group of patients with residual microscopic disease, there was no difference in overall survival; the 3-year survival rate was 46% after WAR and 56% after chemotherapy ($P = 0.57$).

In summary, consolidation with WAR seems to be at least equivalent to further chemotherapy. But if such investigations continue, two aspects of WAR need to be addressed. First, attention to dose and techniques in this subset of patients is very important since most of them have had multiple laparotomies and several cycles of chemotherapy. Whelan et al. reported on 105 patients treated with WAR following chemotherapy for advanced ovarian cancer.[245] The 5-year actuarial rate of severe bowel complication (requiring surgery or obstruction or both) was 13% ± 3.5%. The presence of both a dose of WAR greater than 22.5 Gy, as well as a second-look laparotomy before radiation, was associated with an increased risk of serious bowel complications ($P = 0.006$). Second, the reasons why consolidation WAR seems to be less effective than upfront WAR need to be investigated. In fact, the radiation doses employed in many studies were considered tumoricidal, at least for microscopic disease. One possible explanation relates to the emergence of acquired resistance to radiation, induced by the preceding chemotherapy. In vitro studies have demonstrated that several drugs, such as cisplatin and alkylating agents, lead to development of pleiotropic drug resistance and cross-resistance to radiation.[246,247] The mean values of radiation dose survival curves for cell lines derived from ovarian cancer patients after cisplatin therapy were significantly higher than in cell lines obtained from untreated patients. Further, when pleiotropic drug resistance was induced experimentally in ovarian tumor cell lines developed from untreated patients, it was accompanied by acquired cross-resistance to radiation.[246]

TREATMENT OF RELAPSE

Salvage therapy after chemotherapy failure has also been unsuccessful in most patients. *Palliative surgery* might benefit patients with bowel obstruction due to progression of disease. Most patients, however, receive further chemotherapy for their recurrent disease. It is important to keep in mind that, while cure is unlikely, the goal of continuing chemotherapy is to control tumor-related symptoms, limit disease progression if possible, and try to improve the quality of life in this patient population. Patients who initially responded to platinum-based therapy can be retreated with platinum agents. Response rates of 20% to 60% may be expected, especially if the interval between initial platinum therapy and relapse was more than 6 months.[248] For patients who have failed prior platinum therapy, several chemotherapy agents can be used with objective response rates of 20% to 30%. These agents include oral etoposide, Topotecan, liposomal doxorubicin, and Gemcitabine (Table 50-15).

The role of radiation as a *salvage* treatment after chemotherapy relapse is of limited value. In addition to failure to control relapsing disease, radiation was poorly tolerated in these heavily pretreated patients. Early

Table 50–15 Salvage Chemotherapy

Agent	Platinum Sensitive(S)/ Resistant(R)	Response Rate, %	Survival Duration
Topotecan[249-252]	S	19.2-28.8	
	R	5.9-13.3	10 mo
Oral etoposide[253]	S	34.1	16.5+ mo
	R	26.8	10.8 mo
Liposomal doxorubicin[188-190]	R	9-25	11.0 mo
Docetaxel[254,255]	R	35-40	10 mo
Vinorelbine[256,257]	R	21-30	11.2 mo
Gemcitabine[258,259]	R	13-19	6.2-9 mo
Ifosfamide[260]	R	12	9.0 mo
Tamoxifen[261]	S	15	—
	R	13	

discontinuation of radiotherapy because of marrow toxicity was reported in 30% to 53%, and chronic radiation enteritis requiring surgery in 27% to 63% of those who survived long enough to develop this complication.[262-264] Several studies have attempted to improve tolerance of WAR in patients previously treated with chemotherapy by using hyperfractionated radiation schemes.[159,160] These studies used low radiation doses per fraction (0.8 to 1.25 Gy), given at intervals of 6 hours twice or three times daily. These treatments were well tolerated, but tumor control was not improved.[265] While the role of radiation as a salvage treatment may not be promising, its use as a *palliative* treatment is of value. Several investigators have reported a 50% to 70% complete resolution of symptoms after palliative radiation. The duration of palliation could be up to 1 year in about one third of patients.[266,267] The recommended dose range is usually from 35 to 45 Gy, depending on the patient's performance status and the types of treatments received in the past.

GERM CELL AND STROMAL TUMORS

Germ cell tumors comprise less than 5% of ovarian malignancies but draw a great deal of attention because they occur in young patients. The most common germ cell tumor is dysgerminoma, which accounts for 50% of all germ cell tumors in women. Cytologically, dysgerminoma is similar to seminoma of the testis. These tumors are often localized, but bilateral ovarian involvement is seen in up to 20% of cases. Endodermal sinus tumors, also known as yolk sac tumors, account for 20% of all germ cell tumors in women. They are derived from extraembryonic tissues and are characterized by papillary formations known as Schiller-Duval bodies and intracellular and extracellular hyaline droplets. Immature teratoma accounts for another 20% of germ cell tumors in women. These tumors are graded as low or high based on the amount of immature neural tissue seen. Other less common types of germ cell tumors in women include embryonal carcinoma, nongestational choriocarcinoma, and polyembryoma.

The most common presentations are vague abdominal pain and a palpable pelvic mass. Elevated serum human chorionic gonadotropin (hCG) is seen in some dysgerminomas and most nongestational choriocarcinoma. High levels of α-fetoprotein (AFP) indicate the presence of yolk sac elements and are mostly elevated in endodermal sinus tumors. At the time of diagnosis, most women with germ cell tumors present with stage I disease (70%) and 25% to 30% with stage III. The main treatment is surgery, which includes unilateral salpingo-oophorectomy, to preserve fertility,[268,269] and full surgical staging. For patients with surgical stage I disease, the decision on whether adjuvant chemotherapy is needed depends on the histology and grade of the tumors. Observation is a valid option for stage I dysgerminoma or low-grade immature teratoma. But for those with high-grade teratoma, endodermal sinus tumors, nongestational choriocarcinoma, or embryonal carcinoma, chemotherapy is recommended. Typically 3 to 4 cycles of bleomycin, etoposide, and cisplatin (BEP) are given every 21 days. For several

decades, radiation therapy has been the traditional postoperative treatment for patients with dysgerminoma.[270,271] Although dysgerminoma is exquisitely radiosensitive and survival rates are excellent, fertility is almost always destroyed. To achieve equal efficacy with acceptable toxicity and also preserve fertility, chemotherapy has become the standard of care in these patients. For advanced-stage disease, the surgery should include maximal cytoreduction followed by 4 to 6 cycles of BEP. With the use of combination chemotherapy, cure rates of 90% and 60% to 80% are achievable in early-stage and advanced-stage, respectively.[272-274]

Sex cord–stromal tumors consist of granulosa-stromal-cell tumors (juvenile and adult types), thecoma, fibroma, Sertoli-Leydig cell tumors, sex cord tumors with annular tubules (SCTAT), gynandroblastoma, and steroid-cell tumors. These tumors account for only 7% of all ovarian tumors. But of the functioning ovarian tumors, 90% are sex cord–stromal tumors. There is also some association between certain rare syndromes with reduced penetrance and sex cord–stromal tumors. Peutz-Jeghers syndrome and SCTAT, multiple nevoid basal cell carcinoma (Gorlin's) syndrome and fibromas, and Olier's and Maffucci's syndromes are associated with juvenile granulosa cell tumor of the ovary.[21] In the juvenile type of granulosa-stromal-cell tumors, the diagnosis is often made before the age of 10 and is frequently associated with precocious puberty resulting from estrogen secretion by the tumor cells. The average age of the adult type is 54 years and 22% of cases might be associated with endometrial cancer due to endogenous estrogen secretion. Sertoli-Leydig cell tumors are rare and usually present in the second or third decade of life. Excess androgen production is seen in 50% of cases. These tumors are characterized by differentiation toward testicular structures and contain Sertoli and Leydig cells that resemble the fetal testis. The gynandroblastomas contain granulosa cell elements combined with tubules and Leydig cells characteristic of the arrhenoblastoma and represent a rare form of mixed stromal tumors.

The surgical approach in patients with sex cord–stromal tumors is similar to that of epithelial tumors except in young patients where fertility-sparing procedures should be considered. There is no role for adjuvant therapy in completely resected stage I disease. The role of chemotherapy in more advanced stages is not well defined. The GOG studied the influence of BEP on outcome in 57 patients with incompletely resected sex cord–stromal tumors, but the results were not as encouraging as those with germ cell tumors using the same regimen.[275] The data suggest that radiation therapy can induce a clinical response with occasional long-term remission in patients with persistent or recurrent granulosa cell tumors.[276]

FUTURE DIRECTIONS

With the large body of data on chemotherapy in ovarian cancer, it seems that the role of radiation has been completely abandoned. This is an unfortunate development, especially since radiation has been shown to be very effective. While it is unlikely for radiation to regain the upper hand, the focus should be on how best to integrate radiation and chemotherapy. As we have shown in this chapter, it is clear that about 50% of patients with locally advanced disease will still relapse even after achieving a complete response to paclitaxel/platinum-based chemotherapy. Recent data from the Gray Laboratory suggest that the initial shoulder of the cell survival curve is made of a hypersensitive initial slope to 0.6 to 0.8 Gy followed by a plateau to 1 to 1.2 Gy followed by a straight-line portion.[277] This potential hyper-killing of tumor cells at low doses of radiation could be used in addition to standard chemotherapy without potentially increasing the risk of complications from radiation. Currently, the GOG is considering a phase I/II trial using WAR (0.8 Gy twice daily) as a chemosensitizer for stage III ovarian cancer. With intensity-modulated radiation therapy, WAR could be delivered more accurately since no kidney blocks are required.[278] But more importantly, the dose to the bone marrow, a dose-limiting structure for chemotherapy, is much lower with intensity-modulated radiation therapy than conventional radiation. Such innovative approaches may allow radiation to gain back some of its preeminence in the multimodality management of this disease.

REFERENCES

1. Fuks Z, Bagshaw MA: The rationale for curative radiotherapy for ovarian carcinoma. *Int J Radiat Oncol Biol Phys.* 1975;1:21.
2. Mychalczak BR, Fuks Z: The current role of radiotherapy in the management of ovarian cancer. [Review]. *Hematol—Oncol Clin North Am.* 1992;6:895.
3. Thomas GM, Dembo AJ: Integrating radiation therapy into the management of ovarian cancer. [Review]. *Cancer.* 1993;71:1710.
4. Ozols RF, Young RC: Ovarian cancer. [Review]. *Current Problems in Cancer.* 1987;11:57.
5. Ozols RF, Young RC: Chemotherapy of ovarian cancer. [Review]. *Semin Oncol.* 1991;18:222.
6. Ozols RF: Carboplatin and paclitaxel in ovarian cancer. *Semin Oncol.* 1995;22:78.
7. Reed E, Kohn EC, Sarosy G, et al: Paclitaxel, cisplatin, and cyclophosphamide in human ovarian cancer: Molecular rationale and early clinical results. [Review]. *Semin Oncol.* 1995;22:90.
8. Cyclophosphamide plus cisplatin versus cyclophosphamide, doxorubicin, and cisplatin chemotherapy of ovarian carcinoma: A meta-analysis. The Ovarian Cancer Meta-Analysis Project. *J Clin Oncol.* 1991;9:1668.
9. Long-term results of a randomized trial comparing cisplatin with cisplatin and cyclophosphamide with cisplatin, cyclophosphamide, and Adriamycin in advanced ovarian cancer. GICOG (Gruppo Interregionale Cooperativo Oncologico Ginecologia), Italy. *Gynecol Oncol.* 1992;45:115.
10. Fuks Z: Ovarian carcinoma. In Horwich A, ed: *Combined Radiotherapy and Chemotherapy in Clinical Oncology.* London: Edward Arnold; 1992:165.
11. Jemal A, Murray T, Samuels A, et al: Cancer statistics, 2003. *CA Cancer J Clin.* 2003;53:5.
12. Hartge P, Whittemore AS, Itnyre J, et al: Rates and risks of ovarian cancer in subgroups of white women in the United States. The Collaborative Ovarian Cancer Group [see comments]. *Obstet Gynecol.* 1994;84:760.
13. Yancik R, Ries LG, Yates JW: Ovarian cancer in the elderly: An analysis of Surveillance, Epidemiology, and End Results Program data. *Am J Obstet Gynecol.* 1986;154:639.
14. John EM, Whittemore AS, Harris R, Itnyre J: Characteristics relating to ovarian cancer risk: Collaborative analysis of seven U.S. case-control studies. Epithelial ovarian cancer in black women.
Collaborative Ovarian Cancer Group. *J Natl Cancer Instit.* 1993;85:142.
15. Holschneider CH, Berek JS: Ovarian cancer: Epidemiology, biology, and prognostic factors. *Semin Surg Oncol.* 2000;19:3.
16. Whittemore AS, Harris R, Itnyre J: Characteristics relating to ovarian cancer risk: Collaborative analysis of 12 US case-control studies. II. Invasive epithelial ovarian cancers in white women. Collaborative Ovarian Cancer Group [see comments]. *Am J Epidemiol.* 1992;136:1184.
17. McGowan L, Parent L, Lednar W, Norris HJ: The woman at risk for developing ovarian cancer. *Gynecol Oncol.* 1979;7:325.
18. La Vecchia C, Decarli A, Negri E, et al: Dietary factors and the risk of epithelial ovarian cancer. *J Natl Cancer Instit.* 1987;79:663.
19. Mettlin CJ, Piver MS: A case-control study of milk-drinking and ovarian cancer risk [see comments]. *Am J Epidemiol.* 1990;132:871.
20. Whittemore AS, Wu ML, Paffenbarger RS Jr, et al: Personal and environmental characteristics related to epithelial ovarian cancer. II. Exposures to talcum powder, tobacco, alcohol, and coffee. *Am J Epidemiol.* 1988;128:1228.
21. Lynch HT, Lynch JF: Hereditary ovarian carcinoma. [Review]. *Hematol—Oncol Clin North Am.* 1992;6:783.
22. Schildkraut JM, Thompson WD: Familial ovarian cancer: A population-based case-control study [see comments]. *Am J Epidemiol.* 1988;128:456.
23. Bewtra C, Watson P, Conway T, et al: Hereditary ovarian cancer: A clinicopathological study. *Int J Gynecol Pathol.* 1992;11:180.
24. Easton DF, Bishop DT, Ford D, Crockford GP: Genetic linkage analysis in familial breast and ovarian cancer: Results from 214 families. The Breast Cancer Linkage Consortium. *Am J Hum Genet.* 1993;52:678.
25. Hall JM, Lee MK, Newman B, et al: Linkage of early-onset familial breast cancer to chromosome 17q21. *Science.* 1990; 250:1684.
26. Narod SA, Feunteun J, Lynch HT, et al: Familial breast-ovarian cancer locus on chromosome 17q12-q23 [see comments]. *Lancet.* 1991;338:82.
27. Smith SA, Easton DF, Evans DG, Ponder BA: Allele losses in the region 17q12-21 in familial breast and ovarian cancer involve the wild-type chromosome. *Nat Genet.* 1992;2:128.
28. Ford D, Easton DF, Stratton M, et al: Genetic heterogeneity and penetrance analysis of the BRCA1 and BRCA2 genes in breast cancer families. The Breast Cancer Linkage Consortium. *Am J Hum Genet.* 1998;62:676.
29. Aaltonen LA, Peltomaki P, Leach FS, et al: Clues to the pathogenesis of familial colorectal cancer [see comments]. *Science.* 1993; 260:812.
30. Peltomaki P, Aaltonen LA, Sistonen P, et al: Genetic mapping of a locus predisposing to human colorectal cancer [see comments]. *Science.* 1993;260:810.
31. Hemminki A, Peltomaki P, Mecklin JP, et al: Loss of the wild type MLH1 gene is a feature of hereditary nonpolyposis colorectal cancer. *Nat Genet.* 1994;8:405.
32. Serov SF, Scully RE, Solvin LH: *Histological Typing of Ovarian Tumors,* vol 9. Geneva: World Health Organization; 1973.
33. Ozols RF, Rubin SC, Dembo AJ, Roboy S: *Epithelial Ovarian Cancer.* Philadelphia: JB Lippincott; 1993:731.
34. Seidman JD, Kurman RJ: Ovarian serous borderline tumors: A critical review of the literature with emphasis on prognostic indicators. *Hum Pathol.* 2000;31:539.
35. Zanetta G, Rota S, Chiari S, et al: Behavior of borderline tumors with particular interest to persistence, recurrence, and progression to invasive carcinoma: A prospective study. *J Clin Oncol.* 2001;19:2658.
36. Baak JP, Chan KK, Stolk JG, Kenemans P: Prognostic factors in borderline and invasive ovarian tumors of the common epithelial type. [Review]. *Pathol Res Pract.* 1987;182:755.
37. Friedlander ML, Russell P, Taylor IW, et al: Flow cytometric analysis of cellular DNA content as an adjunct to the diagnosis of ovarian tumours of borderline malignancy. *Pathology.* 1984;16:301.
38. Aure JC, Hoeg K, Kolstad P: Clinical and histologic studies of ovarian carcinoma. Long-term follow-up of 990 cases. *Obstet Gynecol.* 1971;37:1.
39. Sorbe B, Frankendal B, Veress B: Importance of histologic grading in the prognosis of epithelial ovarian carcinoma. Obstet Gynecol. 1982;59:576.

40. Marsoni S, Torri V, Valsecchi MG, et al: Prognostic factors in advanced epithelial ovarian cancer. (Gruppo Interregionale Cooperativo di Oncologia Ginecologica (GICOG)). *Br J Cancer.* 1990;62:444.

41. Hart WR, Norris HJ: Borderline and malignant mucinous tumors of the ovary. Histologic criteria and clinical behavior. *Cancer.* 1973;31:1031.

42. Bjorkholm E, Pettersson F, Einhorn N, et al: Long-term follow-up and prognostic factors in ovarian carcinoma. The radiumhemmet series 1958 to 1973. *Acta Radiol—Oncol.* 1982;21:413.

43. Czernobilsky B, Silverman BB, Mikuta JJ: Endometrioid carcinoma of the ovary. A clinicopathologic study of 75 cases. *Cancer.* 1970;26:1141.

44. Swenerton KD, Hislop TG, Spinelli J, et al: Ovarian carcinoma: A multivariate analysis of prognostic factors. *Obstet Gynecol.* 1985;65:264.

45. Norris HJ, Robinowitz M: Ovarian adenocarcinoma of mesonephric type. *Cancer.* 1971;28:1074.

44. Williams SD: Germ cell tumors. [Review]. *Hematol Oncol Clin North Am.* 1992;6:967.

46. Sevelda P, Vavra N, Schemper M, Salzer H: Prognostic factors for survival in stage I epithelial ovarian carcinoma. *Cancer.* 1990;65:2349.

47. Dembo AJ, Davy M, Stenwig AE, et al: Prognostic factors in patients with stage I epithelial ovarian cancer. *Obstet Gynecol.* 1990;75:263.

48. Redman JR, Petroni GR, Saigo PE, et al: Prognostic factors in advanced ovarian carcinoma. *J Clin Oncol.* 1986;4:515.

49. Voest EE, van Houwelingen JC, Neijt JP: A meta-analysis of prognostic factors in advanced ovarian cancer with median survival and overall survival (measured with the log [relative risk] as main objectives [see comments]). *Eur J Cancer Clin Oncol.* 1989;25:711.

50. Klein B, Falkson G, Smit CF, et al: Advanced ovarian carcinoma. Factors influencing survival. Prognostic factors in advanced ovarian carcinoma. *Cancer.* 1985;55:1829.

51. Krag KJ, Canellos GP, Griffiths CT, et al: Predictive factors for long-term survival in patients with advanced ovarian cancer. *Gynecol Oncol.* 1989;34:88.

52. Lund B, Williamson P: Prognostic factors for outcome of and survival after second-look laparotomy in patients with advanced ovarian carcinoma. *Obstet Gynecol.* 1990;76:617.

53. Kaern J, Trope CG, Abeler V, Pettersen EO: Cellular DNA content: The most important prognostic factor in patients with borderline tumors of the ovary. Can it prevent overtreatment? In Sharp F, Mason P, Blackett T, Berek J, eds. *Ovarian Cancer*, vol. 3. New York: Chapman and Hall Medical; 1995:181.

54. Gajewski WH, Fuller AF Jr, Pastel-Ley C, et al: Prognostic significance of DNA content in epithelial ovarian cancer [see comments]. *Gynecol Oncol.* 1994;53:5.

55. Wagner TM, Adler A, Sevelda P, et al: Prognostic significance of cell DNA content in early-stage ovarian cancer (FIGO stages I and II/A) by means of automatic image cytometry. *Int J Cancer.* 1994;56:167.

56. Friedlander ML, Hedley DW, Swanson C, Russell P: Prediction of long-term survival by flow cytometric analysis of cellular DNA content in patients with advanced ovarian cancer. *J Clin Oncol.* 1988;6:282.

57. Kaern J, Trope CG, Kristensen GB, Pettersen EO: Flow cytometric DNA ploidy and S-phase heterogeneity in advanced ovarian carcinoma. *Cancer.* 1994;73:1870.

58. Pfisterer J, Kommoss F, Sauerbrei W, et al: Cellular DNA content and survival in advanced ovarian carcinoma. *Cancer.* 1994;74:2509.

59. Bertelsen K, Hansen MK, Pedersen PH, et al: The prognostic and therapeutic value of second-look laparotomy in advanced ovarian cancer. *Br J Obstet Gynaecol.* 1988;95:1231.

60. Di Fiore PP, Pierce JH, Kraus MH, et al: *erbB-2* is a potent oncogene when overexpressed in NIH/3T3 cells. *Science.* 1987;237:178.

61. Schechter AL, Hung MC, Vaidyanathan L, et al: The *neu* gene: An *erbB*-homologous gene distinct from and unlinked to the gene encoding the EGF receptor. *Science.* 1985;229:976.

62. Berchuck A, Rodriguez GC, Kamel A, et al: Epidermal growth factor receptor expression in normal ovarian epithelium and ovarian cancer. I. Correlation of receptor expression with prognostic factors in patients with ovarian cancer. *Am J Obstet Gynecol.* 1991;164:669.

63. Slamon DJ, Godolphin W, Jones LA, et al: Studies of the HER-2/neu proto-oncogene in human breast and ovarian cancer. *Science.* 1989;244:707.

64. Bast RC Jr, Boyer CM, Jacobs I, et al: Cell growth regulation in epithelial ovarian cancer. [Review]. *Cancer.* 1993;71:1597.

65. Fan QB, Bian ML, Huang SZ, et al: Amplification of the C-erbB-2(HER-2/neu) proto-oncogene in ovarian carcinomas. *Chin Med J.* 1994;107:589.

66. Rubin SC, Finstad CL, Wong GY, et al: Prognostic significance of HER-2/neu expression in advanced epithelial ovarian cancer: A multivariate analysis. *Am J Obstet Gynecol.* 1993;168:162.

67. Rubin SC, Finstad CL, Federici MG, et al: Prevalence and significance of HER-2/neu expression in early epithelial ovarian cancer. *Cancer.* 1994;73:1456.

68. Finlay CA, Hinds PW, Levine AJ: The p53 proto-oncogene can act as a suppressor of transformation. *Cell.* 1989;57:1083.

69. Foulkes WD, Black DM, Stamp GW, et al: Very frequent loss of heterozygosity throughout chromosome 17 in sporadic ovarian carcinoma. *Int J Cancer.* 1993;54:220.

70. Kohler MF, Marks JR, Wiseman RW, et al: Spectrum of mutation and frequency of allelic deletion of the p53 gene in ovarian cancer. *J Natl Cancer Inst.* 1993;85:1513.

71. Marks JR, Davidoff AM, Kerns BJ, et al: Overexpression and mutation of p53 in epithelial ovarian cancer. *Cancer Res.* 1991;51:2979.

72. Green JA, Robertson LJ, Campbell IR, Jenkins J: Expression of the p53 gene and presence of serum autoantibodies in ovarian cancer: Correlation with differentiation. *Cancer Detect Prev.* 1995;19:151.

73. Hartmann LC, Podratz KC, Keeney GL, et al: Prognostic significance of p53 immunostaining in epithelial ovarian cancer. *J Clin Oncol.* 1994;12:64.

74. Levesque MA, Katsaros D, Yu H, et al: Mutant p53 protein overexpression is associated with poor outcome in patients with well or moderately differentiated ovarian carcinoma. *Cancer.* 1995; 75:1327.

75. Kohler MF, Kerns BJ, Humphrey PA, et al: Mutation and overexpression of p53 in early-stage epithelial ovarian cancer. *Obstet Gynecol.* 1993;81:643.

76. Vikhanskaya F, D'Incalci M, Broggini, M: Decreased cytotoxic effects of doxorubicin in a human ovarian cancer-cell line expressing wild-type p53 and WAF1/CIP1 genes. *Int J Cancer.* 1995;61:397.

77. Goldstein DP: Chorionic gonadotropin. *Cancer.* 1976;38:453.

78. Kurman RJ, Norris HJ: Endodermal sinus tumor of the ovary: A clinical and pathologic analysis of 71 cases. *Cancer.* 1976;38:2404.

79. DiSaia PJ, Morrow CP, Haverback BJ, Dyce BJ: Carcinoembryonic antigen in cancer of the female reproductive system. Serial plasma values correlated with disease state. *Cancer.* 1977;39:2365.

80. Bast RC Jr, Klug TL, St JE, et al: A radioimmunoassay using a monoclonal antibody to monitor the course of epithelial ovarian cancer. *N Engl J Med.* 1983;309:883.

81. Einhorn N: Ovarian cancer. Early diagnosis and screening. [Review]. *Hematol Oncol Clin North Am.* 1992;6:843.

82. Jacobs I, Bast RC Jr: The CA 125 tumour-associated antigen: A review of the literature. [Review]. *Hum Reprod.* 1989;4:1.

83. Zurawski VR Jr, Orjaseter H, Andersen A, Jellum E: Elevated serum CA 125 levels prior to diagnosis of ovarian neoplasia: relevance for early detection of ovarian cancer. *Int J Cancer.* 1988;42:677.

84. Jacobs IJ, Skates SJ, MacDonald N, et al: Screening for ovarian cancer: A pilot randomised controlled trial. *Lancet.* 1999;353:1207.

85. Woolas RP, Xu FJ, Jacobs IJ, et al: Elevation of multiple serum markers in patients with stage I ovarian cancer. *J Natl Cancer Inst.* 1993;85:1748.

86. Rubin SC, Hoskins WJ, Hakes TB, et al: Serum CA 125 levels and surgical findings in patients undergoing secondary operations for epithelial ovarian cancer. *Am J Obstet Gynecol.* 1989;160:667.

87. Berek JS, Knapp RC, Malkasian GD, et al: CA 125 serum levels correlated with second-look operations among ovarian cancer patients. *Obstet Gynecol.* 1986;67:685.

88. Vergote IB, Kaern J, Abeler VM, et al: Analysis of prognostic factors in stage I epithelial ovarian carcinoma: Importance of degree of differentiation and deoxyribonucleic acid ploidy in predicting relapse. *Am J Obstet Gynecol.* 1993;169:40.

89. Podczaski E, Whitney C, Manetta A, et al: Use of CA 125 to monitor patients with ovarian epithelial carcinomas. *Gynecol Oncol.* 1989;33:193.

90. Dvoretsky PM, Richards KA, Bonfiglio TA: The pathology and biologic behavior of ovarian cancer. An autopsy review. [Review]. *Pathol Ann.* 1989;24:1.

91. Dauplat J, Hacker NF, Nieberg RK, et al: Distant metastases in epithelial ovarian carcinoma. *Cancer.* 1987;60:1561.

92. Norris C, Vogt M: Malignant ovarian neoplasms. *Am J Obstet Gynecol.* 1925;10:684.

93. Munnell EW: Is conservative therapy ever justified in stage I (IA) cancer of the ovary? *Am J Obstet Gynecol.* 1969;103:641.

94. Bergman F: Carcinoma of the ovary. A clinicopathological study of 86 autopsied cases with special reference to mode of spread. *Acta Obstetricia et Gynecologica Scandinavica.* 1966;45:211.

95. Tweeddale LP, Pederson BL: Serous neoplasma of the ovary. *Am J Med Sciences.* 1965;249:701.

96. Plentl AA, Friedman EA: Clinical Significance of Ovarian Lymphatics. Lymphatic System of the Female Genitalia. Philadelphia: WB Saunders; 1971;B173.

97. Munnell EW: The changing prognosis and treatment in cancer of the ovary. A report of 235 patients with primary ovarian carcinoma 1952-1961. *Am J Obstet Gynecol.* 1968;100:790.

98. Tobias JS, Griffiths CT: Management of ovarian carcinoma. Current concepts and future prospects (first of two parts). [Review]. *N Engl J Med.* 1976;294:818.

99. Spirtos NM, Gross GM, Freddo JL, Ballon SC: Cytoreductive surgery in advanced epithelial cancer of the ovary: The impact of aortic and pelvic lymphadenectomy. *Gynecol Oncol.* 1995;56:345.

100. Petru E, Lahousen M, Tamussino K, et al: Lymphadenectomy in stage I ovarian cancer. *Am J Obstet Gynecol.* 1994;170:656.

101. Burghardt E, Girardi F, Lahousen M, et al: Patterns of pelvic and paraaortic lymph node involvement in ovarian cancer. *Gynecol Oncol.* 1991;40:103.

102. Musumeci R, Banfi A, Bolis G, et al: Lymphangiography in patients with ovarian epithelial cancer: An evaluation of 289 consecutive cases. *Cancer.* 1977;40:1444.

103. Athey PA, Wallace S, Jing BS, et al: Lymphangiography in ovarian cancer. *Am J Roentgenol Rad Ther Nucl Med.* 1975;123:106.

104. Fuks Z: External radiotherapy of ovarian cancer: Standard approaches and new frontiers. *Semin Oncol.* 1975;2:253.

105. Musumeci R, De PG, Kenda R, et al: Retroperitoneal metastases from ovarian carcinoma: Reassessment of 365 patients studied with lymphography. *Am J Roentgenol.* 1980;134:449.

106. Parker BR, Castellino RA, Fuks ZY, Bagshaw MA: The role of lymphography in patients with ovarian cancer. *Cancer.* 1974;34:100.

107. Meyers MA: The spread and localization of acute intraperitoneal effusion. *Radiology.* 1970;95:547.

108. Overholt PH: Intraperitoneal pressure. *Arch Surg.* 1931;22:691.

109. Drye JC: Intraperitoneal pressure in the human. *Surg Gynecol Obstet.* 1948;87:472.

110. Feldman GB, Knapp RC: Lymphatic drainage of the peritoneal cavity and its significance in ovarian cancer. *Am J Obstet Gynecol.* 1974;119:991.

111. French JE, Florey HW, Morris BL: The absorption of particles by the lymphatics of the diaphragm. *Q J Exp Biol.* 1960;45:88.

112. Courtice PH, Steinbeck AW: The lymphatic drainage of plasma from the peritoneal cavity of the cat. *Aust J Exp Biol.* 1950;28:161.

113. Monga M, Carmichael JA, Shelley WE, et al: Surgery without adjuvant chemotherapy for early epithelial ovarian carcinoma after comprehensive surgical staging [see comments]. *Gynecol Oncol.* 1991;43:195.

114. Young RC, Decker DG, Wharton JT, et al: Staging laparotomy in early ovarian cancer. *JAMA.* 1983;250:3072.

115. Vock P, Hodler J: Cardiophrenic angle adenopathy: Update of causes and significance. *Radiology.* 1986;159:395.

116. Holm-Nielsen P: Absorption of exudate from the peritoneal cavity in man. Elucidated by the distribution of implantation metastases on the peritoneum. *Acta Pathologica.* 1947;24:575.

117. Brooks SE: Preoperative evaluation of patients with suspected ovarian cancer. [Review]. *Gynecol Oncol.* 1994;55:S80.

118. Killackey MA, Neuwirth RS: Evaluation and management of the pelvic mass: A review of 540 cases. *Obstet Gynecol.* 1988;71:319.

119. Koonings PP, Campbell K, Mishell DR Jr, Grimes DA: Relative frequency of primary ovarian neoplasms: A 10-year review. [Review]. *Obstet Gynecol.* 1989;74:921.

120. Spanos WJ: Preoperative hormonal therapy of cystic adnexal masses. *Am J Obstet Gynecol.* 1973;116:551.

121. Buy JN, Ghossain MA, Sciot C, et al: Epithelial tumors of the ovary: CT findings and correlation with US. *Radiology.* 1991;178:811.

122. Kubik-Huch RA, Dorffler W, von Schulthess GK, et al: Value of (18F)-FDG positron emission tomography, computed tomography, and magnetic resonance imaging in diagnosing primary and recurrent ovarian carcinoma. *Eur Radiol.* 2000;10:761.

123. International Federation of Gynecology and Obstetrics. Changes in definitions of clinical staging for carcinoma of the cervix and ovary. *Am J Obstet Gynecol.* 1986;156:263.

124. Heintz APM, Odicino F, Maisnneuve P, et al: Carcinoma of the ovary. In Pecorelli S, Beller U, Heintz APM, et al, ed: *FIGO Annual Report on the Results of Treatment in Gynecologic Cancer,* vol 24. Oxford: Isis Medical Media Limited; 2000:107.

125. Nguyen HN, Averette HE, Hoskins W, et al: National survey of ovarian carcinoma. VI. Critical assessment of current International Federation of Gynecology and Obstetrics staging system. *Cancer.* 1993;72:3007.

126. Levin L, Lund B, Heintz APM: An overview of multi-variate analyses of prognostic variables with special reference to the role of cytoreductive surgery. *Ann Oncol.* 1993;4:23.

127. Einhorn N, Nilsson B, Sjovall K: Factors influencing survival in carcinoma of the ovary. Study from a well-defined Swedish population. *Cancer.* 1985;55:2019.

128. Dembo AJ, Bush RS: Current concepts in cancer: Ovary— Treatment of stages III and IV. Choice of postoperative therapy based on prognostic factors. *Int J Radiat Oncol Biology, Physics.* 1982;8:893.

129. Martinez A, Schray MF, Howes AE, Bagshaw MA: Postoperative radiation therapy for epithelial ovarian cancer: The curative role based on a 24-year experience. *J Clin Oncol.* 1985;3:901.

130. Rubin SC, Hoskins WJ, Saigo PE, et al: Prognostic factors for recurrence following negative second-look laparotomy in ovarian cancer patients treated with platinum-based chemotherapy. *Gynecol Oncol.* 1991;42:137.

131. Unzelman RF: Advanced epithelial ovarian carcinoma: Long-term survival experience at the community hospital. *Am J Obstet Gynecol.* 1992;166:1663; discussion 1671.

132. Hoskins WJ: Epithelial ovarian carcinoma: Principles of primary surgery. [Review]. *Gynecol Oncol.* 1994;55:S91.

133. Rubin SC: Surgery for ovarian cancer. [Review]. *Hematol Oncol Clin North Am.* 1992;6:851.

134. Heintz AP, Hacker NF, Berek JS, et al: Cytoreductive surgery in ovarian carcinoma: Feasibility and morbidity of surgical resection of tumor bulk in the primary treatment of ovarian carcinoma. *Obstet Gynecol.* 1986;67:783.

135. Griffiths CT: Surgical resection of tumor bulk in the primary treatment of ovarian carcinoma. *NCI Monographs.* 1975;42:101.

136. Hacker NF, Berek JS, Lagasse LD, et al: Primary cytoreductive surgery for epithelial ovarian cancer. *Obstet Gynecol.* 1983;61:413.

137. Delgado G, Oram DH, Petrilli ES: Stage III epithelial ovarian cancer: The role of maximal surgical reduction. *Gynecol Oncol.* 1984;18:293.

138. Rubin P, Griese J, Terry R: Has postoperative irradiation proved itself? *Am J Roentgenol Radium Ther Nucl Med.* 1962;89:849.

139. Dembo AJ: Abdominopelvic radiotherapy in ovarian cancer. A 10-year experience. *Cancer.* 1985;55:2285.

140. Louie KG, Ozols RF, Myers CE, et al: Long-term results of a cis-platin-containing combination chemotherapy regimen for the treatment of advanced ovarian carcinoma. *J Clin Oncol.* 1986;4:1579.

141. Neijt JP, Ten Bokkel Huinink WW, van der Burg ME, et al: Randomized trial comparing two combination chemotherapy regimens (CHAP-5 v CP) in advanced ovarian carcinoma. *J Clin Oncol.* 1987;5:1157.

142. Fuks Z, Rizel S, Biran S: Chemotherapeutic and surgical induction of pathological complete remission and whole abdominal irradiation for consolidation does not enhance the cure of stage III ovarian carcinoma. *J Clin Oncol.* 1988;6:509.

143. Belinson JL, Lee KR, Jarrell MA, McClure M: Management of epithelial ovarian neoplasms using a platinum-based regimen: A 10-year experience. *Gynecol Oncol.* 1990;37:66.

144. Hoskins WJ, McGuire WP, Brady MF, et al: The effect of diameter of largest residual disease on survival after primary cytoreductive surgery in patients with suboptimal residual epithelial ovarian carcinoma. *Am J Obstet Gynecol.* 1994;170:974; discussion 979.

145. Del Campo JM, Felip E, Rubio D, et al: Long-term survival in advanced ovarian cancer after cytoreduction and chemotherapy treatment. *Gynecol Oncol.* 1994;53:27.

146. Baker TR, Piver MS, Hempling RE: Long term survival by cytoreductive surgery to less than 1 cm, induction weekly cisplatin and monthly cisplatin, doxorubicin, and cyclophosphamide therapy in advanced ovarian adenocarcinoma. *Cancer.* 1994;74:656.

147. Hunter RW, Alexander ND, Soutter WP: Meta-analysis of surgery in advanced ovarian carcinoma: Is maximum cytoreductive surgery an independent determinant of prognosis? [see comments]. *Am J Obstet Gynecol.* 1992;166:504.

148. Creasman WT: Second-look laparotomy in ovarian cancer. [Review]. *Gynecol Oncol.* 1994;55:S122.

149. Omura G, Blessing JA, Ehrlich CE, et al: A randomized trial of cyclophosphamide and doxorubicin with or without cisplatin in advanced ovarian carcinoma. A Gynecologic Oncology Group Study. *Cancer.* 1986;57:1725.

150. van der Burg ME, van Lent M, Buyse M, et al: The effect of debulking surgery after induction chemotherapy on the prognosis in advanced epithelial ovarian cancer. Gynecological Cancer Cooperative Group of the European Organization for Research and Treatment of Cancer [see comments]. *N Engl J Med.* 1995;332:629.

151. Vaccarello L, Rubin SC, Vlamis V, et al: Cytoreductive surgery in ovarian carcinoma patients with a documented previously complete surgical response. *Gynecol Oncol.* 1995;57:61.

152. Husain A, Chi DS, Prasad M, et al: The role of laparoscopy in second-look evaluations for ovarian cancer. *Gynecol Oncol.* 2001;80:44.

153. Schray MF, Cox RS, Martinez A: Lower abdominal radiotherapy for stages I, II, and selected III epithelial ovarian cancer: 20 years experience. *Gynecol Oncol.* 1983;15:78.

154. Dembo AJ: Radiotherapeutic management of ovarian cancer. [Review]. *Semin Oncol.* 1984;11:238.

155. Delclos L, Barun EJ, Herrera JER, et al: Whole abdominal irradiation by cobalt-60 moving strip technique. *Radiology.* 1963;81:632.

156. Delclos L, Smith J: *Tumors of the Ovary.* Philadelphia: Lea & Febiger; 1973:670.

157. Rubin P, Cooper R, Phillips T: *Radiation Biology and Radiation Pathology Syllabus.* Chicago: American College of Radiology, 1974.

158. Hanks G, Bagshaw M: Megavoltage radiation therapy and lymphangiography in ovarian cancer. *Radiology.* 1969;93:649.

159. LaRouere J, Perez-Tamayo C, Fraass B, et al: Optimal coverage of peritoneal surface in whole abdominal radiation for ovarian neoplasms. *Int J Radiat Oncol Biol Phys.* 1989;17:607.

160. Kong JS, Peters LJ, Wharton JT, et al: Hyperfractionated split-course whole abdominal radiotherapy for ovarian carcinoma: Tolerance and toxicity. *Int J Radiat Oncol Biol Phys.* 1988;14:737.

161. Morgan L, Chafe W, Mendenhall W, Marcus R: Hyperfractionation of whole-abdomen radiation therapy: Salvage treatment of persistent ovarian carcinoma following chemotherapy. *Gynecol Oncol.* 1988;31:122.

162. Peters LJ, Ang KK: Unconventional fractionation schemes in radiotherapy. [Review]. *Import Advances Oncol.* 1986;269.

163. Ellis F: Dose-time fractionation. A clinical hypothesis. *Clin Radiol.* 1969;20:1.

164. Schray MF, Martinez A, Howes AE: Toxicity of open-field whole abdominal irradiation as primary postoperative treatment in gynecologic malignancy. *Int J Radiat Oncol Biol Phys.* 1989;16:397.

165. Fyles AW, Dembo AJ, Bush RS, et al: Analysis of complications in patients treated with abdomino-pelvic radiation therapy for ovarian carcinoma. *Int J Radiat Oncol Biol Phys.* 1992;22:847.

166. Goldberg N, Peschel RE: Postoperative abdominopelvic radiation therapy for ovarian cancer. *Int J Radiat Oncol Biol Phys.* 1988;14:425.

167. van Bunningen B, Bouma J, Kooijman C, et al: Total abdominal irradiation in stage I and II carcinoma of the ovary. *Radiother Oncol.* 1988;11:305.

168. Fuller DB, Sause WT, Plenk HP, Menlove RL: Analysis of postoperative radiation therapy in stage I through III epithelial ovarian carcinoma. *J Clin Oncol.* 1987;5:897.

169. Kjellgren O, Jonsson L: Bone marrow depression in the pelvis after megavoltage irradiation. A study with radioisotope scanning. *Am J Obstet Gynecol.* 1969;105:849.

170. Dembo AJ, Bush RS, Beale FA, et al: The Princess Margaret Hospital study of ovarian cancer: Stages I, II, and asymptomatic III presentations. *Cancer Treat Rept.* 1979;63:249.

171. Ingold J, JB R, HS K: Radiation hepatitis. *J Roentgenol.* 1965;93:200.

172. Luxton R: Radiation nephritis. *Q J Med.* 1953;22:215.

173. Perez CA, Korba A, Zivnuska F, et al: 60Co moving strip technique in the management of carcinoma of the ovary: Analysis of tumor control and morbidity. *Int J Radiat Oncol Biol Phys.* 1978;4:379.

174. Boye E, Lindegaard MW, Paus E, et al: Whole-body distribution of radioactivity after intraperitoneal administration of 32P colloids. *Br J Radiol.* 1984;57:395.

175. Coats G, Bush RS, Aspin NA: Study of ascites using lymphoscintigraphy with 99Tc-sulfur colloid. *Radiology.* 1973;107:577.

176. Leichner PK, Rosenshein NB, Leibel SA, Order SE: Distribution and tissue dose of intraperitoneally administered radioactive chromic phosphate (32P) in New Zealand white rabbits. *Radiology.* 1980;134:729.

177. Spanos WJ Jr, Day T, Abner A, et al: Complications in the use of intra-abdominal 32P for ovarian carcinoma. *Gynecol Oncol.* 1992;45:243.

178. Vergote IB, Winderen M, De Vos LN, Trope CG: Intraperitoneal radioactive phosphorus therapy in ovarian carcinoma. Analysis of 313 patients treated primarily or at second-look laparotomy. *Cancer.* 1993;71:2250.

179. Walton LA, Yadusky A, Rubinstein L: Intraperitoneal radioactive phosphate in early ovarian carcinoma: An analysis of complications. [Review]. *Int J Radiat Oncol Biol Phys.* 1991;20:939.

180. Thigpen JT, Blessing JA, Vance RB, Lambuth BW: Chemotherapy in ovarian carcinoma: Present role and future prospects. *Semin Oncol.* 1989;16(suppl 6):58.

181. Wiltshaw E, Kroner T: Phase II study of cis-dichlorodiammine-platinum (II) (NSC-119875) in advanced adenocarcinoma of the ovary. *Cancer Treat Repts.* 1976;60:55.

182. Williams CJ, Stewart L, Parmar M, Guthrie D: Meta-analysis of the role of platinum compounds in advanced ovarian carcinoma. The Advanced Ovarian Cancer Trialists Group. *Semin Oncol.* 1992;19:120.

183. Rowinsky EK, Donehower RC: Paclitaxel (Paclitaxel) [published erratum appears in *N Engl J Med* 1995;July 6;333:75]. [Review]. *N Engl J Med.* 1995;332:1004.

184. Thigpen JT, Blessing JA, Ball H, et al: Phase II trial of paclitaxel in patients with progressive ovarian carcinoma after platinum-based chemotherapy: A Gynecologic Oncology Group study. *J Clin Oncol.* 1994;12:1748.

185. McGuire WP, Rowinsky EK, Rosenshein NB, et al: Paclitaxel: A unique antineoplastic agent with significant activity in advanced ovarian epithelial neoplasms. *Ann Intern Med.* 1989;111:273.

186. McGuire WP: Paclitaxel: A new drug with significant activity as a salvage therapy in advanced epithelial ovarian carcinoma. *Gynecol Oncol.* 1993;51:78.

187. Omura GA, Morrow CP, Blessing JA, et al: A randomized comparison of melphalan versus melphalan plus hexamethylmelamine versus adriamycin plus cyclophosphamide in ovarian carcinoma. *Cancer.* 1983;51:783.

188. Muggia FM, Hainsworth JD, Jeffers S, et al: Phase II study of liposomal doxorubicin in refractory ovarian cancer: Antitumor activity and toxicity modification by liposomal encapsulation. *J Clin Oncol.* 1997;15:987.

189. Markman M, Kennedy A, Webster K, et al: Phase 2 trial of liposomal doxorubicin (40 mg/m^2) in platinum/paclitaxel-refractory ovarian and fallopian tube cancers and primary carcinoma of the peritoneum. *Gynecol Oncol.* 2000;78:369.

190. Gordon AN, Granai CO, Rose PG, et al: Phase II study of liposomal doxorubicin in platinum- and paclitaxel-refractory epithelial ovarian cancer. *J Clin Oncol.* 2000;18:3093.

191. McGuire WP, Hoskins WJ, Brady MF, et al: Cyclophosphamide and cisplatin compared with paclitaxel and cisplatin in patients with stage III and Stage IV ovarian cancer. *N Engl J Med.* 1996;334:1.

192. Muggia FM, Braly PS, Brady MF, et al: Phase III randomized study of cisplatin versus paclitaxel versus cisplatin and paclitaxel in patients with suboptimal stage III or IV ovarian cancer: A gynecologic oncology group study. *J Clin Oncol.* 2000;18:106.

193. The ICON Collaborators. ICON2: Randomised trial of single-agent carboplatin against three-drug combination of CAP (cyclophosphamide, doxorubicin, and cisplatin) in women with ovarian cancer. ICON Collaborators. International Collaborative Ovarian Neoplasm Study. *Lancet.* 1998;352:1571.

194. International Collaborative Ovarian Neoplasm Group. Paclitaxel plus carboplatin versus standard chemotherapy with either single-agent carboplatin or cyclophosphamide, doxorubicin, and cisplatin in women with ovarian cancer: The ICON3 randomised trial. *Lancet.* 2002;360:505.

195. Aabo K, Adams M, Adnitt P, et al: Chemotherapy in advanced ovarian cancer: Four systematic meta-analyses of individual patient data from 37 randomised trials. Advanced Ovarian Cancer Trialists' Group. *Br J Cancer.* 1998;78:1479.

196. Covens A, Carey M, Bryson P, et al: Systematic review of first-line chemotherapy for newly diagnosed postoperative patients with stage II, III, or IV epithelial ovarian cancer. *Gynecol Oncol.* 2002;85:71.

197. Sandercock J, Parmar MK, Torri V, Qian W: First-line treatment for advanced ovarian cancer: Paclitaxel, platinum and the evidence. *Br J Cancer.* 2002;87:815.

198. Markman M, Reichman B, Hakes T, et al: Intraperitoneal chemotherapy in the management of ovarian cancer. [Review]. *Cancer.* 1993;71:1565.

199. Markman M, Francis P, Rowinsky E, Hoskins W: Intraperitoneal paclitaxel: A possible role in the management of ovarian cancer? [Review]. *Semin Oncol.* 1995;22:84.

200. Ahmed FY, Wiltshaw E, A'Hern RP, et al: Natural history and prognosis of untreated stage I epithelial ovarian carcinoma. *J Clin Oncol.* 1996;14:2968.

201. Young RC, Walton LA, Ellenberg SS, et al: Adjuvant therapy in stage I and stage II epithelial ovarian cancer. Results of two prospective randomized trials [see comments]. *N Engl J Med.* 1990;322:1021.

202. Bolis G, Colombo N, Pecorelli S, et al: Adjuvant treatment for early epithelial ovarian cancer: Results of two randomised clinical trials comparing cisplatin to no further treatment or chromic phosphate (32P). G.I.C.O.G.: Gruppo Interregionale Collaborativo Oncologica Ginecologia. *Ann Oncol.* 1995;6:887.

203. Trimbos JB, Vergote I, Bolis G, et al; EORTC-ACTION collaborators. European Organization for Research and Treatment of Cancer-Adjuvant ChemoTherapy in Ovarian Neoplasm. Impact of adjuvant chemotherapy and surgical staging in early-stage ovarian carcinoma: European Organization for Research and Treatment of Cancer—Adjuvant ChemoTherapy in Ovarian Neoplasm trial. *J Natl Cancer Inst.* 2003;95:113.

204. International Collaborative Ovarian Neoplasm (ICON 1) Collaborators. International Collaborative Ovarian Neoplasm Trial 1: A randomized trial of adjuvant chemotherapy in women with early-stage ovarian cancer. *J Natl Cancer Inst.* 2003;95:125.

205. Young RC: Early-stage ovarian cancer: To treat or not to treat. *J Natl Cancer Inst.* 2003;95:94.

206. Bell J, Brady M, Lage J, et al: A randomized phase III trial of three versus six cycles of carboplatin and paclitaxel as adjuvant treatment in early stage ovarian epithelial carcinoma: A gynecologic Oncology Group Study. *Gynecol Oncol.* 2003;88:156.

207. Dembo AJ: Epithelial ovarian cancer: The role of radiotherapy. [Review]. *Int J Radiat Oncol Biol Phys.* 1992;22:835.

208. Hreshchyshyn MM, Park RC, Blessing JA, et al: The role of adjuvant therapy in Stage I ovarian cancer. *Am J Obstet Gynecol.* 1980;138:139.

209. Macbeth FR, Macdonald H, Williams CJ: Total abdominal and pelvic radiotherapy in the management of early stage ovarian carcinoma. *Int J Radiat Oncol Biol Phys.* 1988;15:353.

210. Young RC, Brady MF, Nieberg RK, et al: Adjuvant treatment for early ovarian cancer: A randomized phase III trial of intraperitoneal P32 or intravenous cyclophosphamide and cisplatin—A Gynecologic Oncology Group Study. *I Clin Oncol* 2003;21:4350–4355.

211. Rosenshein NB: Radioisotopes in the treatment of ovarian cancer. *Clin Obstet Gynaecol.* 1983;10:279.

212. Soper JT, Berchuck A, Clarke-Pearson DL: Adjuvant intraperitoneal chromic phosphate therapy for women with apparent early ovarian carcinoma who have not undergone comprehensive surgical staging. *Cancer.* 1991;68:725.

213. Smith JP, Rutledge FN, Delclos L: Postoperative treatment of early cancer of the ovary: A random trial between postoperative irradiation and chemotherapy. *Natl Cancer Inst Monogr.* 1975;42:149.

214. Dent SF, Klaassen D, Pater JL, et al: Second primary malignancies following the treatment of early stage ovarian cancer: Update of a study by the National Cancer Institute of Canada—Clinical Trials Group (NCIC-CTG). *Ann Oncol.* 2000;11:65.

215. Sell A, Bertelsen K, Andersen JE, et al: Randomized study of whole-abdomen irradiation versus pelvic irradiation plus cyclophosphamide in treatment of early ovarian cancer. *Gynecol Oncol.* 1990;37:367.

216. Redman CW, Mould J, Warwick J, et al: The West Midlands epithelial ovarian cancer adjuvant therapy trial. *Clin Oncol (R Coll Radiol).* 1993;5:1.

217. Chiara S, Bruzzone M, Merlini L, et al: Randomized study comparing chemotherapy plus radiotherapy versus radiotherapy alone in FIGO stage IIB-III cervical carcinoma. GONO (North-West Oncologic Cooperative Group). *Am J Clin Oncol.* 1994;17:294.

218. Fyles AW, Thomas GM, Pintilie M, et al: A randomized study of two doses of abdominopelvic radiation therapy for patients with optimally debulked Stage I, II, and III ovarian cancer. *Int J Radiat Oncol Biol Phys.* 1998;41:543.

219. Piccart MJ, Bertelsen K, James K, et al: Randomized intergroup trial of cisplatin-paclitaxel versus cisplatin-cyclophosphamide in women with advanced epithelial ovarian cancer: Three-year results. *J Natl Cancer Inst.* 2000;92:699.

220. Ozlos RF, Bundy BN, Greer BE, et al: Phase III trial of carboplatin and paclitaxel compared with cisplatin and paclitaxel in patients with optimally resected stage III ovarian cancer: A Gynecologic Oncology group study. *J Clin Oncol.* 2003; early release.

221. Neijt JP, Engelholm SA, Tuxen MK, et al: Exploratory phase III study of paclitaxel and cisplatin versus paclitaxel and carboplatin in advanced ovarian cancer. *J Clin Oncol.* 2000;18:3084.

222. Du Bois A, Lueck HJ, Meier W, et al: AGO ovarian cancer study group. Cisplatin/paclitaxel vs carboplatin/paclitaxel in ovarian cancer: Update of an Arbeitsgemeinschaft Gynaekologie (AGO) study group trial. *Proceed ASTRO.* 1999;18:356a.

223. Alberts DS, Liu PY, Hannigan EV, et al: Intraperitoneal cisplatin plus intravenous cyclophosphamide versus intravenous cisplatin plus intraperitoneal cyclophosphamide for stage III ovarian cancer. *N Engl J Med.* 1996;335:1950.

224. Markman M, Bundy BN, Alberts DS, et al: Phase III trial of standard-dose intravenous cisplatin plus paclitaxel versus moderately high-dose carboplatin followed by intravenous paclitaxel and intraperitoneal cisplatin in small-volume stage III ovarian carcinoma: an intergroup study of the Gynecologic Oncology Group, Southwestern Oncology Group, and Eastern Cooperative Oncology Group. *J Clin Oncol.* 2001;19:1001.

225. Armstrong DK, Bundy BN, Baergen R, et al: Randomized phase III study of intravenous (IV) paclitaxel and cisplatin versus IV paclitaxel, intraperitoneal (IP) cisplatin and IP paclitaxel in optimal stage III epithelial ovarian cancer (OC): A Gynecologic Oncology Group trial (GOG 172). *Proceed ASCO.* 2002; 21:201a.

226. Chemotherapy in advanced ovarian cancer: an overview of randomised clinical trials. Advanced Ovarian Cancer Trialists Group [see comments]. *BMJ.* 1991;303:884.

227. Fanning J, Bennett TZ, Hilgers RD: Meta-analysis of cisplatin, doxorubicin, and cyclophosphamide versus cisplatin and cyclophosphamide chemotherapy of ovarian carcinoma [see comments]. *Obstet Gynecol.* 1992;80:954.

228. Williams CJ, Stewart L, Parmar M, Guthrie D: Meta-analysis of the role of platinum compounds in advanced ovarian carcinoma. The Advanced Ovarian Cancer Trialists Group. *Semin Oncol.* 1992;19(suppl 2):120.

229. Bristow RE, Tomacruz RS, Armstrong DK, et al: Survival effect of maximal cytoreductive surgery for advanced ovarian carcinoma during the platinum era: A meta-analysis. *J Clin Oncol.* 2002;20:1248.

230. McGuire WP, Hoskins WJ, Brady MF, et al: Assessment of dose-intensive therapy in suboptimally debulked ovarian cancer: A Gynecologic Oncology Group study. *J Clin Oncol.* 1995;13:1589.

231. Kaye SB, Lewis CR, Paul J, et al: Randomised study of two doses of cisplatin with cyclophosphamide in epithelial ovarian cancer [see comments]. *Lancet.* 1992;340:329.

232. Kaye SB, Paul J, Cassidy J, et al: Mature results of a randomized trial of two doses of cisplatin for the treatment of ovarian cancer. Scottish Gynecology Cancer Trials Group. *J Clin Oncol.* 1996; 14:2113.

233. Hakes TB, Chalas E, Hoskins WJ, et al: Randomized prospective trial of 5 versus 10 cycles of cyclophosphamide, doxorubicin, and cisplatin in advanced ovarian carcinoma. *Gynecol Oncol.* 1992;45:284.

234. Bertelsen K, Jakobsen A, Stroyer J, et al: A prospective randomized comparison of 6 and 12 cycles of cyclophosphamide, adriamycin, and cisplatin in advanced epithelial ovarian cancer: A Danish Ovarian Study Group trial (DACOVA). *Gynecol Oncol.* 1993;49:30.

235. Markman M, Liu PY, Wilczynski S, et al: Phase III randomized trial of 12 versus 3 months of maintenance paclitaxel in patients with advanced ovarian cancer after complete response to platinum/paclitaxel-based chemotherapy. A Southwest Oncology Group and Gynecologic Oncology Group Trial. *J Clin Oncol.* 2003;(13): 2460.

236. Barakat RR, Almadrones L, Venkatraman ES, et al: A phase II trial of intraperitoneal cisplatin and etoposide as consolidation therapy in patients with Stage II–IV epithelial ovarian cancer following negative surgical assessment. *Gynecol Oncol.* 1998;69:17.

237. Barakat RR, Sabbatini P, Bhaskaran D, et al: Intraperitoneal chemotherapy for ovarian carcinoma: Results of long-term follow-up. *J Clin Oncol.* 2002;20:694.

238. Varia MA, Stehman FB, Bundy BN, et al: Intraperitoneal radioactive phosphate (^{32}P) versus observation after negative second-look laparotomy for stage III ovarian carcinoma: A Gynecologic Oncology Group Study. *J Clin Oncol.* 2003;(21):2849.

239. Pickel H, Lahousen M, Petru E, et al: Consolidation radiotherapy after carboplatin-based chemotherapy in radically operated advanced ovarian cancer. *Gynecol Oncol.* 1999;72:215.

240. Bruzzone M, Repetto L, Chiara S, et al: Chemotherapy versus radiotherapy in the management of ovarian cancer patients with pathological complete response or minimal residual disease at second look. *Gynecol Oncol.* 1990;38:392.

241. Mangioni C, Epis A, Vassena L, et al: Radiotherapy (RT) versus chemotherapy (CH) as second line treatment of minimal residual disease (MRD) in advanced ovarian cancer (AOC). *Proc Int Gynecol Cancer Soc.* 1987;49.

242. Lawton F, Luesley D, Blackledge G, et al: A randomized trial comparing whole abdominal radiotherapy with chemotherapy following cisplatinum cytoreduction in epithelial ovarian cancer. West Midlands Ovarian Cancer Group Trial II. *Clin Oncol (R Coll Radiol).* 1990;2:4.

243. Lambert HE, Rustin GJ, Gregory WM, Nelstrop AE: A randomized trial comparing single-agent carboplatin with carboplatin followed by radiotherapy for advanced ovarian cancer: A North Thames Ovary Group study. *J Clin Oncol.* 1993;11:440.

244. Sorbe B: On behalf of the Swedish-Norwegian cancer study group. Consolidation treatment of advanced (FIGO stage III) ovarian cancer in complete surgical remission, after induction chemotherapy: A randomized, controlled trial comparing whole abdominal radiotherapy, chemotherapy, and no further therapy. *Int J Gynecol Cancer.* 2003;(13), 278.

245. Whelan TJ, Dembo AJ, Bush RS, et al: Complications of whole abdominal and pelvic radiotherapy following chemotherapy for advanced ovarian cancer. *Int J Radiat Oncol Biol Phys.* 1992;22:853.

246. Louie KG, Behrens BC, Kinsella TJ, et al: Radiation survival parameters of antineoplastic drug-sensitive and -resistant human ovarian cancer cell lines and their modification by buthionine sulfoximine. *Cancer Res.* 1985;45:2110.

247. Wolf CR, Hayward IP, Lawrie SS, et al: Cellular heterogeneity and drug resistance in two ovarian adenocarcinoma cell lines derived from a single patient. *Int J Cancer.* 1987;39:695.

248. Dizon DS, Hensley ML, Poynor EA, et al: Retrospective analysis of carboplatin and paclitaxel as initial second-line therapy for recurrent epithelial ovarian carcinoma: Application toward a dynamic disease state model of ovarian cancer. *J Clin Oncol.* 2002;20:1238.

249. Kudelka AP, Tresukosol D, Edwards CL, et al: Phase II study of intravenous topotecan as a 5-day infusion for refractory epithelial ovarian carcinoma. *J Clin Oncol.* 1996;14:1552.

250. Ten Bokkel, Huinink W, Gore M, et al: Topotecan versus paclitaxel for the treatment of recurrent epithelial ovarian cancer [see comments]. *J Clin Oncol.* 1997;15:2183.

251. Creemers GJ, Bolis G, Gore M, et al: Topotecan, an active drug in the second-line treatment of epithelial ovarian cancer: Results of a large European phase II study. *J Clin Oncol.* 1996; 14:3056.

252. Bookman MA, Malmstrom H, Bolis G, et al: Topotecan for the treatment of advanced epithelial ovarian cancer: An open-label phase II study in patients treated after prior chemotherapy that contained cisplatin or carboplatin and paclitaxel. *J Clin Oncol.* 1998;16:3345.

253. Rose PG, Blessing JA, Mayer AR, Homesley HD: Prolonged oral etoposide as second-line therapy for platinum-resistant and platinum-sensitive ovarian carcinoma: A Gynecologic Oncology Group study. *J Clin Oncol.* 1998;16:405.

254. Kavanagh JJ, Kudelka AP, de Leon CG, et al: Phase II study of docetaxel in patients with epithelial ovarian carcinoma refractory to platinum. *Clin Cancer Res.* 1996;2:837.

255. Francis P, Schneider J, Hann L, et al: Phase II trial of docetaxel in patients with platinum-refractory advanced ovarian cancer. *J Clin Oncol.* 1994;12:2301.

256. Bajetta E, Di Leo A, Biganzoli L, et al: Phase II study of vinorelbine in patients with pretreated advanced ovarian cancer: Activity in platinum-resistant disease. *J Clin Oncol.* 1996;14:2546.

257. Gershenson DM, Burke TW, Morris M, et al: A phase I study of a daily x3 schedule of intravenous vinorelbine for refractory epithelial ovarian cancer. *Gynecol Oncol.* 1998;70:404.

258. Shapiro JD, Millward MJ, Rischin D, et al: Activity of gemcitabine in patients with advanced ovarian cancer: Responses seen following platinum and paclitaxel. *Gynecol Oncol.* 1996; 63:89.

259. Lund B, Neijt JP: Gemcitabine in cisplatin-resistant ovarian cancer. *Semin Oncol.* 1996;23(suppl 10):72.

260. Markman M, Kennedy A, Sutton G, et al: Phase 2 trial of single agent ifosfamide/mesna in patients with platinum/paclitaxel refractory ovarian cancer who have not previously been treated with an alkylating agent. *Gynecol Oncol.* 1998;70:272.

261. Markman M, Iseminger KA, Hatch KD, et al: Tamoxifen in platinum-refractory ovarian cancer: A Gynecologic Oncology Group Ancillary Report. *Gynecol Oncol.* 1996;62:4.

262. Hoskins WJ, Lichter AS, Whittington R, et al: Whole abdominal and pelvic irradiation in patients with minimal disease at second-look surgical reassessment for ovarian carcinoma. *Gynecol Oncol.* 1985;20:271.

263. Hainsworth JD, Malcolm A, Johnson DH, et al: Advanced minimal residual ovarian carcinoma: Abdominopelvic irradiation following combination chemotherapy. *Obstet Gynecol.* 1983; 61:619.

264. Hacker NF, Berek JS, Burnison CM, et al: Whole abdominal radiation as salvage therapy for epithelial ovarian cancer. *Obstet Gynecol.* 1985;65:60.

265. Fein DA, Morgan LS, Marcus RB Jr, et al: Stage III ovarian carcinoma: An analysis of treatment results and complications following hyperfractionated abdominopelvic irradiation for salvage. *Int J Radiat Oncol Biol Phys.* 1994;29:169.

266. Gelblum D, Mychalczak B, Almadrones L, et al: Palliative benefit of external-beam radiation in the management of platinum refractory epithelial ovarian carcinoma. *Gynecol Oncol.* 1998; 69:36.

267. Cmelak AJ, Kapp DS: Long-term survival with whole abdominopelvic irradiation in platinum-refractory persistent or recurrent ovarian cancer. *Gynecol Oncol.* 1997;65:453.

268. Low JJ, Perrin LC, Crandon AJ, Hacker NF: Conservative surgery to preserve ovarian function in patients with malignant ovarian germ cell tumors. A review of 74 cases. *Cancer.* 2000; 89:391.

269. Zanetta G, Bonazzi C, Cantu M, et al: Survival and reproductive function after treatment of malignant germ cell ovarian tumors. *J Clin Oncol.* 2001;19:1015.

270. Bjorkholm E, Lundell M, Gyftodimos A, Silfversward C: Dysgerminoma: The Radiumhemmet series 1927–1984. *Cancer.* 1990;65:38.

271. Zaghloul MS, Khattab TY: Dysgerminoma of the ovary: Good prognosis even in advanced stages. *Int J Radiat Oncol Biol Phys.* 1992;24:161.

272. Williams S, Blessing JA, Liao SY, et al: Adjuvant therapy of ovarian germ cell tumors with cisplatin, etoposide, and bleomycin: A trial of the Gynecologic Oncology Group. Adjuvant therapy of ovarian germ cell tumors with cisplatin, etoposide, and bleomycin: A trial of the Gynecologic Oncology Group. *J Clin Oncol.* 1994;12:701.

273. Williams SD, Blessing JA, Hatch KD, Homesley HD: Chemotherapy of advanced dysgerminoma: Trials of the Gynecologic Oncology Group. *J Clin Oncol.* 1991;9:1950.

274. Gershenson DM, Morris M, Cangir A, et al: Treatment of malignant germ cell tumors of the ovary with bleomycin, etoposide, and cisplatin. *J Clin Oncol.* 1990;8:715.

275. Homesley HD, Bundy BN, Hurteau JA, Roth LM: Bleomycin, etoposide, and cisplatin combination therapy of ovarian granulosa cell tumors and other stromal malignancies: A Gynecologic Oncology Group study. *Gynecol Oncol.* 1999;72:131.

276. Wolf JK, Mullen J, Eifel PJ, et al: Radiation treatment of advanced or recurrent granulosa cell tumor of the ovary. *Gynecol Oncol.* 1999;73:35.

277. Short SC, Joiner MC: Cellular response to low-dose irradiation (Review). *Clin Oncol (R Coll Radiol).* 1998;10:73.

278. Hong L, Alektiar K, Chui C, et al: IMRT of large fields: Whole-abdomen irradiation. *Int J Radiat Oncol Biol Phys.* 2002;54:278.

Cancer of the Vagina

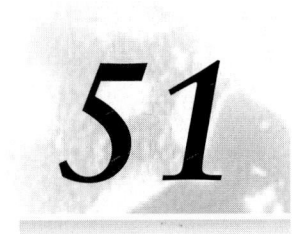

Richard G. Stock, MD, and Sheryl Green, MBBch

EPIDEMIOLOGY

Primary carcinoma of the vagina, a rare malignancy found primarily in older women, constitutes 1% to 2% of all gynecologic malignancies. The majority of women with diagnosed vaginal cancer range in age from 50 to 70 years.[1,2] Most malignant lesions detected in the vagina are metastases from other primary gynecologic malignancies. In one study of 141 cases of vaginal carcinoma, 37 were primary lesions and 104 were classified as secondary.[3] For this reason, strict criteria are necessary to classify a vaginal neoplasm as primary. Tumors that involve both the vagina and cervix or the vagina and vulva are classified as cervical and vulvar lesions, respectively. In addition, vaginal tumors detected less than 5 years after the diagnosis of a previous gynecologic malignancy are considered metastatic. Although various intervals of time have been used to separate primary from secondary carcinomas, Murad and colleagues[3] found that subsequent vaginal lesions detected after treatment for cervical cancer occurred either within the first year or after 5 years. Vaginal lesions detected 5 years or more after treatment for cervical cancer more closely resembled, histologically, primary carcinomas than did vaginal lesions detected within 1 year after treatment for cervical cancer. They concluded that lesions detected more than 5 years after treatment for cervical cancer were primary vaginal carcinomas.

Because of its rare occurrence, risk factors relating to primary vaginal carcinoma have been elusive. As with other squamous cell cancers of the gynecologic tract, human papillomavirus (HPV) has been implicated in the development of both in situ and invasive squamous cell carcinomas of the vagina. Ostrow and colleagues[4] examined 14 biopsies of invasive squamous cell carcinoma of the vagina using in situ hybridization and found that 21% of the samples contained the HPV DNA.[4] Using Southern blot hybridization with P32 labeled HPV DNA, Ikenberg and colleagues identified HPV DNA in 55% of patients with vaginal cancer. HPV-positive patients were noted to have improved survival rates as compared with HPV-negative patients.[5] An HPV association of the same order of magnitude has been found in cervical cancer.[6,7] HIV-infected women also appear to be at increased risk for development of vaginal carcinoma, which may demonstrate more aggressive behavior and less response to therapy as compared with HIV-negative patients.[8]

Chronic irritation of the vaginal mucosa can lead to hyperkeratosis, thickening, acanthosis, and inflammation.[9] These changes may progress to metaplastic and dysplastic changes. Earlier studies noting a predominance of posterior wall lesions gave rise to the theory that pooling of irritating substances in the posterior fornix led to chronic irritation and the development of vaginal cancers on the posterior wall. Recent series weaken this theory by finding approximately equal distribution of lesions on the anterior and posterior vaginal walls.[10-14] The use of a vaginal pessary for uterine prolapse can cause chronic vaginitis, which has also been implicated in the development of vaginal cancer.[9]

Hysterectomy has also been linked to the development of vaginal cancer. Patients with vaginal cancer have a history of prior hysterectomy, for both benign and malignant disease, that ranges from 47% to 60%.[10,11,13,15,16] The interval of time from hysterectomy to the diagnosis of vaginal cancer can be many years, with a median time of 10 years.[11] The case-control study of Brinton and colleagues found that hysterectomy was associated with a 6.7-fold excess risk for the subsequent development of vaginal cancer.[17] Herman and associates[18] challenged this association. They compared 49 patients with vaginal cancer with 49 matched control subjects and found that the incidence of prior hysterectomy was 49% in both groups.[18]

In utero exposure to the synthetic estrogen diethylstilbestrol (DES) has been linked to the development of clear cell adenocarcinoma of the vagina and cervix. DES was prescribed in the mid-1940s to 1950s to manage high-risk pregnancies. Clear cell adenocarcinoma of the vagina was virtually unknown until 1970, when Herbst and Scully[19] reported six cases of primary vaginal clear cell adenocarcinoma. These patients were 15 to 22 years of age; five of the six had been exposed to DES in utero in the first trimester. In 1986, Melnick and colleagues[20] reported on 519 cases of clear cell adenocarcinoma of the vagina and cervix. In 60% of all cases, the patient's mother received DES during pregnancy. In an additional 12% of patients, the mothers were treated with another hormone or an unidentified medication. These patients ranged in age from 15 to 27, with a median age of 19 years in 91% of patients exposed to DES. The risk of developing clear cell adenocarcinoma in exposed females from birth to age 34 was estimated to be 1 case per 1000. This low risk suggested that DES is not a complete carcinogen and that other factors probably contribute to the pathogenesis of these cancers. Other factors thought to increase risk were DES exposure before the 12th week of pregnancy, a maternal history of prior miscarriage, birth in autumn, and prematurity.[21]

ANATOMY

The vagina is a fibromuscular tube lined with a mucous membrane, extending from the uterus superiorly down to the vestibule, or the cleft between the labia minora (Fig. 51-1). It lies between the rectum posteriorly and the urethra and bladder anteriorly. Superiorly, the vagina joins the uterus at an angle of more than 90 degrees. Because of the angle of the junction, the posterior wall, which measures about 9 cm, is longer than the anterior wall, which measures approximately 7 cm. The cervix projects into the lumen of the vagina, resulting in a

circular invagination between the walls of the vagina and the cervix. These invaginations are called the anterior, posterior, and lateral fornices. The walls of the vagina are usually in contact and form a lumen with the shape of the letter *H* on transverse section. Running in a longitudinal direction along the midline of the anterior and posterior walls are ridges called the vaginal columns. From these columns originate transverse rugae, which extend laterally on each side.

As the vagina extends caudally, it passes through the urogenital diaphragm. At its opening it is partially covered by a fold of connective tissue covered by a mucous membrane known as the hymen. Posteriorly the vagina is covered by peritoneum in its upper fourth and is separated from the rectum in this area by the rectouterine pouch (pouch of Douglas). As the vagina extends caudally, it is directly adjacent to the rectum until its most caudal aspect, where it is separated from the anal canal by fibrous and muscular tissue known as the perineal body.

Anteriorly the vaginal wall is directly adjacent to the urethra and bladder. The lateral walls are adjacent to

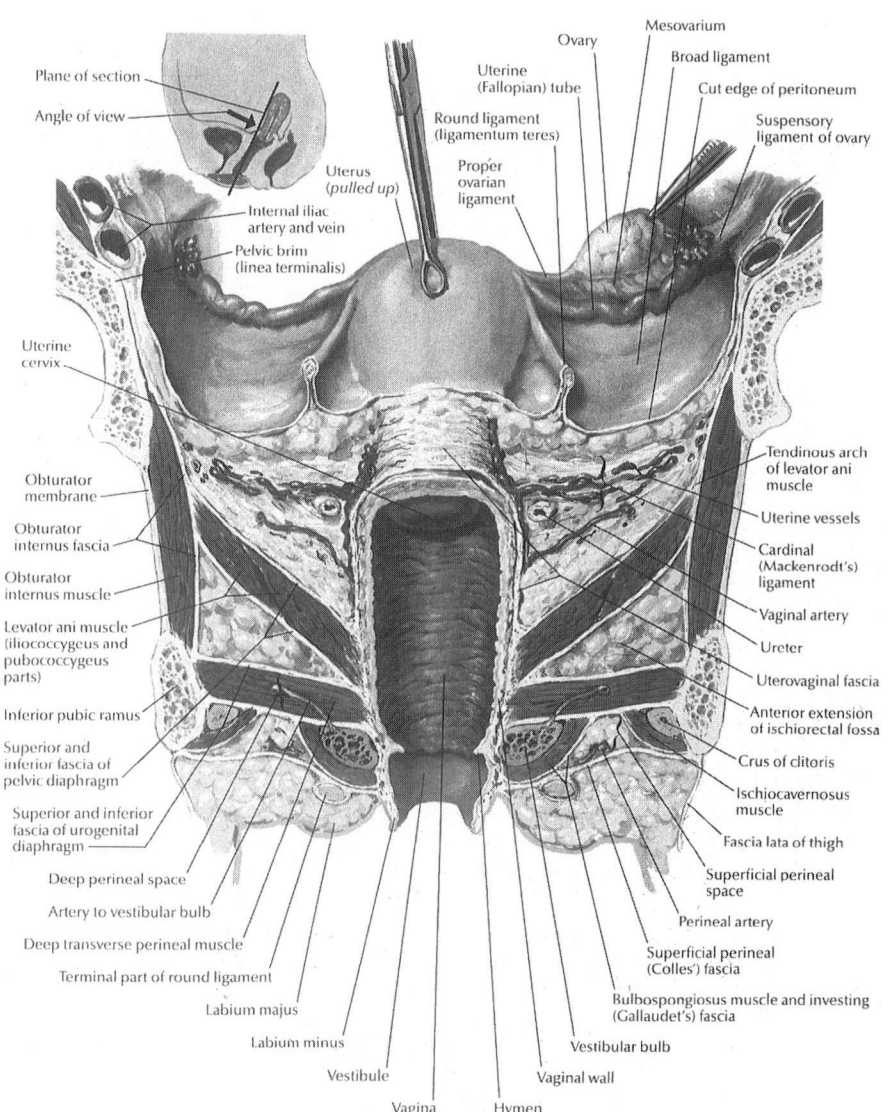

Figure 51–1. Standard diagram of the vaginal anatomy. (© Copyright 1989. CIBA-GEIGY Corporation. Reprinted with permission from the *Atlas of Human Anatomy* illustrated by Frank Netter, MD. All rights reserved.)

the pelvic fascia and levator ani muscles. The ureters cross the lateral walls as they travel forward and medially to join the bladder.

The lining of the vagina is formed by an inner layer of a nonkeratanizing, stratified squamous epithelium covering a basement membrane. The epithelium contains no glands but receives its lubrication from glands in the cervix and uterus. Beneath the mucosa is the lamina propria, which consists of connective tissue. Underlying this is a muscular layer consisting of two layers of nonstriated smooth muscle. The smooth muscle fibers of the inner layer are arranged circularly, whereas the outer layer consists of smooth muscle fibers arranged longitudinally. The muscular layer is covered by a thin adventitia.

PATHOLOGY

Carcinoma In Situ

Carcinoma in situ (CIS), or vaginal intraepithelial neoplasia (VAIN), is a preinvasive lesion seen with much less frequency than invasive vaginal cancer. The relationship between VAIN and invasive vaginal cancer is similar to the relationship of cervical CIS and invasive cervical cancer, although VAIN is a less frequent finding than CIS of the cervix. Histopathologically, most of the lesions are epidermoid and demonstrate full-thickness alterations in maturation with atypical mitoses, individual cell maturation, and hyperchromatism.[22] The majority of lesions are multifocal and can involve all the vaginal surfaces, although the most common site of involvement is in the superior one third of the vaginal canal.[23,24]

Squamous Cell Carcinoma

Invasive squamous cell carcinoma is found in 75% to 95% of primary vaginal carcinomas (Fig. 51-2). The majority of these lesions tend to be nonkeratinizing and moderately differentiated.[25] The well-differentiated

lesions may demonstrate keratinization, manifested by squamous pearls and intracellular bridges.[26]

Vaginal Adenosis and Adenocarcinoma

Adenocarcinoma is found in 5% to 10% of all vaginal cancers.[2,11,13,27-29] The non–clear cell adenocarcinoma frequently arises in the submucosa. When a biopsy of a vaginal lesion reveals adenocarcinoma, it is important to look for a primary lesion, such as endometrial cancer, elsewhere.

Vaginal adenosis defines the abnormal presence of glandular epithelium in the vagina, which is normally devoid of glandular elements (Fig. 51-3). The glandular epithelial cells may line glands in the submucosa or cover or replace surface squamous cells and are usually located near the surface epithelium.[30] Three types of epithelial cells have been observed: mucinous, which resemble endocervical glandular elements; tubo-endometrial; and embryonic. Histologic changes in the female genital tract in women exposed to DES in utero include vaginal adenosis, vaginal and cervical ridges, and cervical erosion.[31]

Vaginal adenosis has been found in one third of patients exposed to DES.[31] The microscopic appearance of the adenosis in this subset of patients is identical to the adenosis seen in patients born before the DES era.[32] Vaginal adenosis is intimately associated with the presence of clear cell adenocarcinoma of the vagina (Fig. 51-4). Robboy and colleagues[33] found that 95% of cases of vaginal clear cell adenocarcinoma were associated with vaginal adenosis. Of the three types of epithelium seen in vaginal adenosis, the tubo-endometrial type was most commonly associated with clear cell adenocarcinoma, suggesting that this type of epithelium provides the bed from which clear cell adenocarcinoma develops.[34] Clear cell adenocarcinoma is found in zero to 12% of all vaginal cancers, depending on the study, but has been recognized less often during the past 15 years.[2,10,35,36] These lesions tend to arise in the upper one third of the vaginal canal and involve the anterior wall.[33,35,37] The most common histologic pattern is tubulocystic,[37,38] followed by a solid pattern. The most common cells noted are the clear cell, hobnail cell, and endometrioid cell.[38]

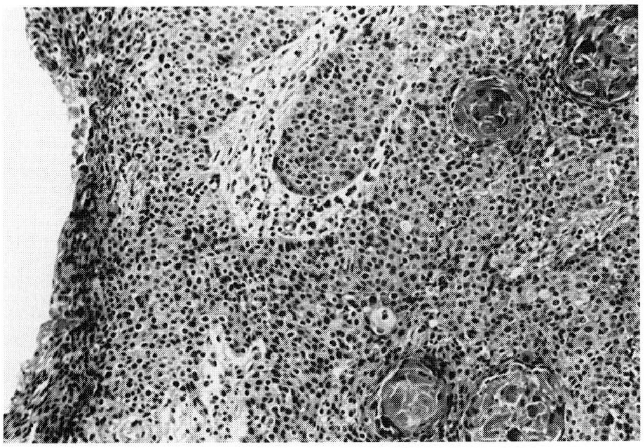

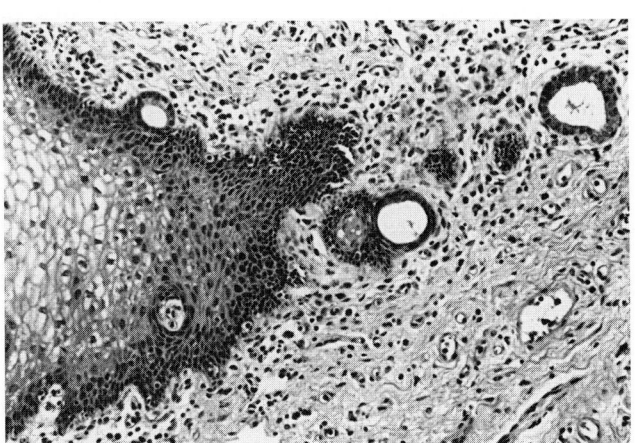

Figure 51–2. Photomicrograph of an invasive squamous cell carcinoma of the vagina. (Courtesy of Tamara Kalir, MD, PhD.)

Figure 51–3. Photomicrograph of vaginal adenosis. (Courtesy of Tamara Kalir, MD, PhD.)

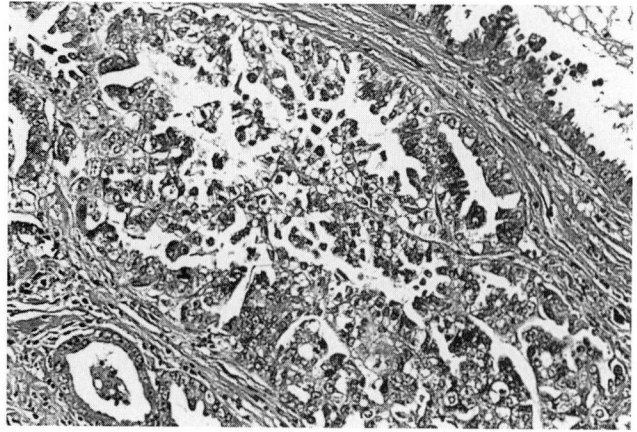

Figure 51–4. Photomicrograph demonstrating clear cell adenocarcinoma. (Courtesy of Tamara Kalir, MD, PhD.)

Melanoma

Malignant melanoma of the vagina represents approximately 5% of all vaginal neoplasms and approximately 0.7% of all melanomas.[36,39,40] Most of these mucosal lesions project into the vaginal lumen, and there is greater involvement along the mucosal surface rather than penetration into the vaginal wall. These tumors are characterized by the presence of melanin and marked cellular pleomorphism. Since spindle cell transformation can occur, the presence of melanin and junctional changes in these lesions is important in differentiating them from sarcomas.[41]

Lymphomas and small cell carcinomas may also arise in the vagina. Small cell carcinomas behave in an aggressive manner, similar to small cell carcinomas arising in other parts of the body.

Nonepithelial Tumors

Nonepithelial tumors of the vagina are extremely rare. Spindle cell epithelioma has been described by Branton and Tavassoli[42] as a vaginal mixed tumor composed predominantly of spindle cells but often containing elements of glandular and squamous differentiation. Smooth muscle tumors of the vagina manifest as submucosal bulges. They are identified microscopically by interlacing bundles of spindle cells with elongated round-ended nuclei. The majority of these lesions are benign or only locally aggressive. Tavassoli and Norris[43] described 60 cases of vaginal smooth muscle tumors and found that only 5 recurred locally after a wide local excision, and only 1 metastasized.

Rhabdomyosarcoma

Rhabdomyosarcoma primarily affects children younger than 5 years of age. Sarcoma botryoides, a variant of embryonal rhabdomyosarcoma, is the most common malignant neoplasm of the vagina in infants and children. It has the characteristic gross appearance of grape-like masses that are exophytic and can protrude from the vagina. These tumors are composed of ovoid and spindle-shaped undifferentiated cells.

LOCATION

Vaginal carcinomas involve the anterior and posterior walls with equal frequencies.[10-14] The lateral walls are less frequently involved. Vaginal carcinoma more frequently involves the superior one third of the vaginal canal compared with the middle or inferior thirds.[2,10,12,13,16,28,44,45] The middle and inferior thirds are involved with approximately equal frequencies.[2,10,12,46] A factor contributing to this distribution may be the high percentage of patients with a history of prior hysterectomy and the increased incidence of upper one-third lesions in this subset of patients.[11]

CLINICAL PRESENTATION

The majority of patients with vaginal cancer are symptomatic, and vaginal bleeding is the most common presenting symptom, occurring in 50% to 65% of patients.[13,27,44,47] The next most common presenting symptom is vaginal discharge, which occurs in 10% to 15% of patients.[13,16,19,27,47] Other signs and symptoms that occur less frequently are postcoital bleeding, pain, urinary symptoms, and the presence of a mass. Urinary symptoms are more common in vaginal cancer than in cervical cancer because of the proximity of anterior vaginal wall lesions to the urethra and bladder. Vaginal lesions in asymptomatic patients are often discovered by abnormal cytological findings on a Papanicolaou (Pap) smear or by the presence of a mass on speculum examination.

ROUTES OF SPREAD

Local Invasion

Lesions arising in the vaginal mucosa can extend into the lumen and form exophytic masses or can penetrate the vaginal wall and invade the surrounding musculature. Lesions of the inferior two thirds of the vaginal canal can penetrate the vaginal wall and involve the urogenital diaphragm, levator ani muscles, or pelvic fascia. As these lesions continue growing, they can fix to the pelvic sidewall. Lesions of the superior one third of the vagina often behave like cervical cancer and grow beyond the vaginal wall into the parametria and eventually to the pelvic sidewall. Lesions of the anterior and posterior vaginal wall can extend beyond the confines of the vaginal walls and invade the bladder and rectum, respectively.

Lymphatics

Lymphatic channels in the mucosa run parallel to a network of lymphatic channels in the submucosa and muscular layer, converging to form trunks at the periphery of the vaginal wall. These trunks drain to the major pelvic nodal groups. The upper vagina's lymphatic drainage pattern is similar to that of the cervix, draining to the obturator, hypogastric, external iliac, and common iliac nodal groups. The lower vagina has trunks that drain to the inguinal, femoral, and external iliac nodes.[48] Since there is considerable crossover drainage as well as atypical drainage patterns, any pelvic lymph node group can serve as a drainage site (Fig. 51-5).

The true incidence of positive lymph nodes is difficult to determine, since the majority of patients are treated with radiation therapy and do not undergo surgical exploration. Most of the information concerning nodal metastases derives from series in which exploratory laparotomies and lymph node dissections were performed. Table 51-1 lists the occurrence of positive nodes in series that recorded this finding. Lymph node involvement in patients with stage I and II disease has been reported in zero to 6%, and 21% to 26% of cases, respectively.[14,37] The incidence of nodal involvement increases with stage and has been reported at 78% and 83% for stages III and IV, respectively.[14]

PROGNOSTIC FACTORS

The most important factor influencing survival is, the stage of disease at the time of intervention.[2,11,35.44,45] Increasing stage is associated with a decrease in complete response rates to radiation therapy and an increase in local, pelvic, and distant failure. In addition to the International Federation of Gynecology and Obstetrics (FIGO) stage, several authors have shown that the FIGO modification by Perez,[49] which divides stage II disease into stage IIa (paravaginal extension) and IIb (parametrial extension), is also of prognostic significance. Patients with stage IIb disease have a poorer outcome than patients with stage IIa disease.[47,50] The presence of symptoms carries an unfavorable prognosis, since larger tumors are more likely to cause symptoms than smaller lesions. Tumor histology has also been identified as an important prognostic factor, with (non–clear cell) adenocarcinoma having more than twice the rates of local and metastatic relapse of squamous cell carcinoma.[51]

The extent of vaginal canal involvement also affects prognosis. Lesions limited to one third of the vaginal length carry a better prognosis than lesions extending farther.[11,52] In the series of Stock and colleagues,[11] of 100 cases, 64 patients with involvement of only one third of the vaginal canal had a significantly improved 5-year disease-free survival (DFS) rate of 61% compared with 36 patients with a more extensive involvement (25% 5-year DFS). In addition, patients with lesions of the upper one third of the vaginal canal have a better

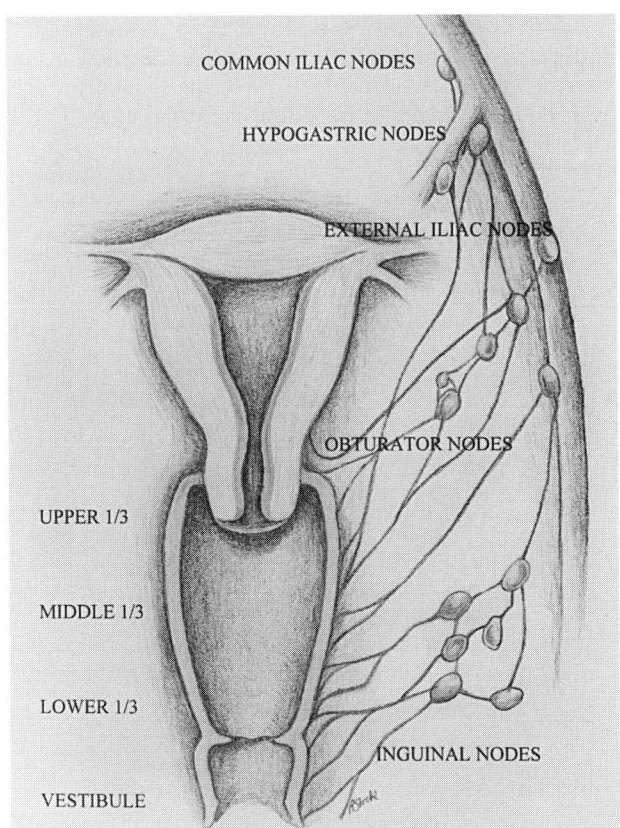

Figure 51–5. Lymphatic drainage of the vagina.

prognosis than patients with involvement of other areas of the vaginal canal. In an analysis of 110 patients, Kucera and Vavra[2] found 5-year survival rates of 60%, 37.5%, and 37% for patients with lesions involving the upper, middle, and lower one third, respectively. Chyle et al. also found the tumor circumferential location to be of independent prognostic significance, with lesions involving the posterior wall faring worse than lesions located elsewhere in the vagina.[51] Lymph node involvement carries an unfavorable prognosis.[2,53]

DIAGNOSIS AND STAGING

DIAGNOSIS. A complete history and physical examination should initiate the diagnostic workup. Careful attention should be given to the pelvic examination. When a

Table 51–1   Lymph Node Metastasis

Reference	Institution	Patients, n	Loc	Nodes, n	Positive Nodes, %	Method of Detection
Herbst et al[53]	Mass. General	23	P, I	10	43	LND
Rubin et al[14]	U. Pennsylvania	38	N	16	42	Lymphangiogram
Stock et al[11]	U. Pittsburgh	32	P, I	13	41	LND
Stock et al[10]	Memorial	22	P, I, A	7	32	LND
Kucera & Vavra[2]	U. of Vienna	110	I	21	19	Physical examination
Davis et al[35]	Mayo Clinic	48	P, A	9	19	LND

A, para-aortic nodes; I, inguinal nodes; Loc, location of positive nodes; LND, lymph node dissection; N, not specified; P, pelvic nodes.

speculum examination is performed, it is essential to rotate the speculum carefully to visualize the anterior and posterior vaginal walls, which are usually obscured by the speculum blades. A thorough bimanual examination should be performed.

Ultimately, an examination under anesthesia is required to delineate the extent of the tumor. Adequate biopsies of the tumor should include biopsies of the cervix as well, to rule out a cervical primary. A Schiller test using Lugol's solution, which stains normal mucosal cells but not malignant cells, and colposcopy can be useful in identifying lesions, which are difficult to visualize on speculum examination. The workup should include a chest x-ray film, intravenous pyelography (IVP), barium enema, cystoscopy, and proctosigmoidoscopy. Although not officially sanctioned by FIGO as a staging tool, computed tomographic (CT) imaging is commonly used instead of IVP to evaluate kidney function. Pelvic CT and magnetic resonance imaging (MRI) studies are not part of the FIGO clinical staging system but can be very important in defining the extent of disease. MRI technology produces excellent images of the pelvis and, unlike CT scans, often can differentiate malignant tissue from normal structures or fibrosis (Fig. 51-6).[54,55]

Positron emission tomography (PET) with the glucose analogue [18F]-fluoro-2-deoxy-D-glucose (FDG) has recently been demonstrated to be the most sensitive and specific imaging test for detecting lymph node tumor involvement in patients with stage I to IV carcinoma of the cervix.[56] Because of the many similarities of carcinomas of the cervix and vagina, particularly regarding patterns of spread, whole body FDG-PET should strongly be considered as a standard imaging evaluation for patients with carcinoma of the vagina.[57]

STAGING. Vaginal carcinomas are staged by either the American Joint Committee on Cancer (AJCC) system or the FIGO system (Tables 51-2 and 51-3).[58,59]

TREATMENT

When a treatment strategy is constructed, it is important to consider anatomic location and routes of local spread. Vaginal tumors in various anatomic sites present different clinical problems. Lesions on the anterior wall are often in close proximity to the bladder or urethra. Relatively small lesions on the anterior wall can thus invade the urethra early before they grow large. Lesions on the posterior wall can likewise invade the rectovaginal septum and the rectum. Similarly, relatively small lesions can invade the rectum early in their disease course. Tumors located in the vaginal fornices of patients with an intact uterus and cervix frequently behave like cervical cancers and can often be treated in a similar manner. Patients who have had a hysterectomy can have altered anatomic structures. Loops of small bowel can adhere to the apex of the vagina. Beyond anatomic considerations, the overall medical condition and age of the patient must be taken into account when a treatment plan is chosen.

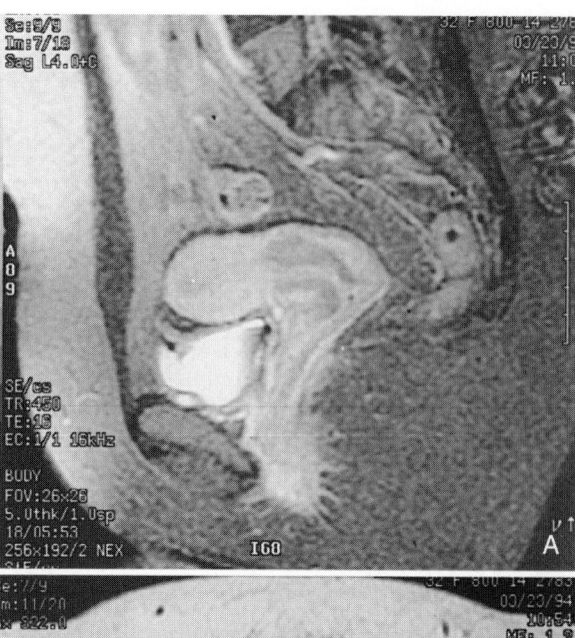

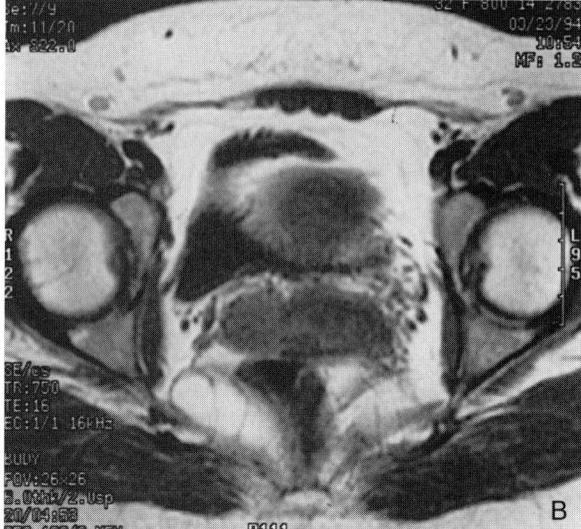

Figure 51–6. Sagittal **(A)** and transverse **(B)** T1-weighted magnetic resonance images of a patient with stage II squamous cell cancer of the vagina located in the left vaginal fornix with involvement of the left parametria. Multiple biopsies of the cervix and endocervical canal were negative for tumor.

These many factors preclude defining strict treatment guidelines. Each case requires an individualized optimal therapeutical evaluation. The limitations as well as benefits of surgery and radiation therapy must be considered.

Surgery

Surgical treatment for this disease varies from local excision to total exenteration. Wide local excision is usually reserved for localized CIS or well-demarcated, superficially invasive lesions. This technique can be used when adequate margins are possible without compromising the anatomical structure of the vagina. In patients with an intact uterus and lesions located in the superior one third of the vaginal canal, particularly on the posterior or lateral walls, radical hysterectomy extending inferiorly to include a partial

Table 51–2   Classification of Cancer of the Vagina

Primary Tumor (T)

TX	Primary tumor cannot be assessed
T0	No evidence of primary tumor
Tis	Carcinoma in situ
T1	Tumor confined to the vagina
T2	Tumor invades paravaginal tissues but not to the pelvic wall
T3	Tumor extends to the pelvic wall
T4*	Tumor invades the mucosa of the bladder or rectum and/or extends beyond the true pelvis

Regional Lymph Nodes (N)

NX	Regional lymph nodes cannot be assessed
N0	No regional lymph node metastasis
N1	Pelvic or inguinal lymph node metastasis

Distant Metastasis (M)

MX	Presence of distant metastasis cannot be assessed
M0	No distant metastasis
M1	Distant metastasis

*The presence of bullous edema is not sufficient evidence to classify a tumor as T4. If the mucosa is not involved, the tumor is stage III.
From Greene FL, Page DL, Fleming ID, et al, eds. *AJCC Cancer Staging Manual*, 6th ed. New York: Springer, 2002.

Table 51–3   International Federation of Gynecology and Obstetrics Staging System

0	Carcinoma in situ (intraepithelial)
I	Tumor confined to vaginal mucosa
II	Tumor infiltration into subvaginal or parametrial tissue not extending to pelvic wall
III	Tumor extending to pelvic wall
IVa	Tumor extension to bladder or rectum or outside true pelvis
IVb	Distant metastasis

From Kottmeier HL: The classification and clinical staging of carcinoma of the uterus and vagina. *J Int Fed Gynecol Obstet.* 1963;83:1.

vaginectomy can be performed. Radical hysterectomy and total vaginectomy are usually required to excise lesions that extend down to the inferior one third of the vagina. In patients with a prior hysterectomy and lesions limited to the superior one third of the vaginal canal, an upper partial vaginectomy may be performed unless the tumor is adherent to the bladder. An anterior exenteration that removes the vagina, urethra, and bladder is often required to achieve negative margins for invasive anterior wall lesions in proximity to the urethra and bladder. A posterior exenteration that removes the vagina and rectum is often required to resect invasive lesions on the posterior wall, because of the proximity of these lesions to the rectum. Tumors that are deeply invasive and circumferential may require a total exenteration to obtain negative margins.

Radiation Therapy

Radiation therapy is the most common treatment for this disease. Both external beam radiation therapy and brachytherapy are used as part of the treatment plan.

External beam therapy is usually delivered by a whole pelvic field, to treat the vaginal tumor and for prophylaxis of the entire vaginal mucosa. In addition, the pelvic lymph nodes are treated in most cases, because of the relatively high incidence of positive pelvic nodes found on pelvic lymph node dissections.[10,11,35,53] Inguinal lymph nodes are usually included in a modified whole pelvic field for lesions involving the distal vaginal canal. External beam therapy alone is inferior to combined external beam therapy and brachytherapy or brachytherapy alone.[10,12,60,61]

Many forms of brachytherapy have been used in the treatment of vaginal cancer and include a tandem and colpostat system (as employed to treat cervical cancer), vaginal cylinders, vaginal plaques, and interstitial needle implants. There are no accepted guidelines for the treatment of vaginal cancer with those various techniques. Treatment with brachytherapy is individualized based on the clinical stage, tumor location, and extent. A summary of external beam therapy and brachytherapy by stages, showing the total doses used in the radiotherapeutic management of vaginal cancer, is provided in Table 51-4.

Chemotherapy

Chemotherapy has been ineffective in the treatment of vaginal cancer. Small phase II trials using only chemotherapy for advanced, metastatic, persistent, or recurrent vaginal cancer have shown uniformly poor results. Thigpen and colleagues[62] employed cisplatin in 16 patients with recurrent or advanced squamous cell vaginal cancers; only 1 patient had an objective response, which lasted just 3 months. Muss and colleagues[63] treated eight patients with advanced or metastatic lesions with mitoxantrone and found that no patient had even a partial response to treatment. The experience of

Table 51–4   External Beam, Brachytherapy, and Total Doses (cGy) in the Treatment of Vaginal Carcinoma by Stage

Stage	External Beam	Low-Dose-Rate Brachytherapy		Total
		Intracavitary	*Interstitial*	
I				
<0.5 cm depth	—	7000	—	7000
>0.5 cm depth	—	4500	2500-3500	7000-8000
>2/3 involvement of length	4500	—	3000-4000	7500-8000
II	4500-5040	—	3500-4500	8000-9500
III + IV	4500-5400	—	3500-4500	8000-9500

Slayton and colleagues[64] in 19 patients given etoposide for recurrent or advanced lesions was equally dismal. Neither chloroethyl-cyclohexyl-nitrosourea (CCNU) nor methyl CCNU favorably influenced the course of the disease in nine patients with persistent vaginal cancers after initial treatment.[65]

Chemotherapy administered concurrently with radiation therapy has produced no clear added benefit in reported trials. Evans and colleagues[61] gave 5-fluorouracil (5-FU) and mitomycin concurrently with radiation in seven patients with vaginal cancer (two stage II, four stage III, and one stage IV). Four out of the seven achieved a complete response (CR) and were free of disease recurrence (NED) from 19 to 39 months. Two of these four responders had stage II disease. Roberts and colleagues[67] used cisplatin and 5-FU with radiation therapy in five stage III patients and two patients with recurrent lesions. Local recurrence developed in three patients, and one developed distant metastases.

Concurrent cisplatin-based chemotherapy with irradiation is now considered standard therapy for patients with advanced carcinoma of the cervix. Since the incidence of vaginal carcinoma is low, it is highly unlikely that prospective randomized trials evaluating the role of chemotherapy in these patients could be completed. Considering that the etiology, histological features, and natural history of vaginal carcinoma are essentially identical to that of invasive carcinoma of the uterine cervix, some authors are advocating the use of concurrent cisplatin-based chemotherapy and irradiation as standard therapy for patients with advanced (i.e., stages II, III and IVa) carcinoma of the vagina.[57]

Carcinoma In Situ

Many forms of therapy have been tried in the treatment of CIS, including surgical excision, carbon dioxide laser therapy, radiation therapy, and topical 5-FU. None has proved superior to the others. Surgical excision is usually accomplished with a wide local excision or partial vaginectomy, which provides a pathological specimen to rule out invasive disease.[26] Limited surgical procedures fail to treat the entire vaginal surface. Since this disease is frequently multifocal, areas of CIS may be overlooked. A Schiller's mucosa test is mandatory to define abnormal mucosa. If there are multiple areas of abnormal mucosa, other treatment options must be considered, since a total vaginectomy is often necessary.

Carbon dioxide laser ablation has been used to treat multifocal disease. It has the advantage of precise microscopic control of tissue destruction with minimal destruction of normal tissue.[68] The procedure may also be repeated for persistent or recurrent disease and carries a failure rate ranging from 10% to 50%.[68-70]

Radiation therapy is effective but less often employed. Treatment involves the use of an intravaginal cylinder to deliver radiation to the entire vaginal mucosa. Doses of 6000 to 8000 cGy can be delivered to the mucosal surface using a low-dose-rate brachytherapy system. In addition, in cases with discrete lesions, small portions of the mucosa can be boosted with a shielded cylinder to deliver

an additional 1000 to 2000 cGy. Perez and colleagues[60,71] reported that disease recurred in only 1 of 20 patients after intravaginal therapy, and Prempree and Amornmarn[72] reported that disease was controlled in all their eight patients with CIS using intravaginal brachytherapy.

Stage I

Both radiation therapy and surgical excision are treatment options for stage I disease. Surgical excision can yield results equivalent to those obtained with radiation therapy.[11,14,35] Limited surgical procedures can often provide adequate margins.[11] Although these lesions are limited to the vaginal wall, involvement of the entire length of the vagina or extensive involvement of the anterior wall often requires a more radical surgical approach such as a total vaginectomy or anterior exenteration, respectively. Treatment must be individualized and surgical treatment selected only if the expected morbidity is limited. Younger patients with clear cell adenocarcinoma and smaller lesions are often candidates for limited surgical resection, which has the added advantage of preserving ovarian function in these patients.

An alternative and often preferred treatment for stage I disease is radiation therapy, directed toward controlling the local disease. Treatment of the pelvic lymph nodes is not indicated in most cases. For this reason, stage I disease is treated with brachytherapy alone. Stage I patients can be divided into two groups, based on the depth of tumor invasion. Lesions that are less than 0.5 cm in depth can be treated with an intracavitary vaginal cylinder. Intravaginal brachytherapy can be delivered by either a traditional low-dose-rate system or a high-dose-rate system.

With a low-dose-rate system, treatment is given in two separate applications. The first application is designed to treat the entire vaginal wall to a dose of 4500 cGy at a depth of 0.5 cm into the vaginal mucosa. This delivers a vaginal mucosal surface dose of 6000 to 6500 cGy, adequate to provide prophylactic treatment to control microscopic mucosal disease to the entire mucosa. The second application delivers an additional 2500 cGy to a depth of 0.5 cm to cover the tumor volume. This can be given with a shielded vaginal cylinder to treat the tumor with a 2 cm margin and block the uninvolved mucosal surfaces.

Superficial lesions can also be treated with high-dose-rate brachytherapy, avoiding a 2- to 4-day hospital stay and confinement to bed rest. High-dose-rate brachytherapy can be particularly useful in obese patients or individuals with other medical problems at risk for the development of a pulmonary embolism. Unfortunately, there are few published data describing this form of treatment for vaginal cancer. Stock and colleagues[10] reported 15 patients treated with a fractionated high-dose-rate system. Fourteen of the 15 were treated with high-dose-rate vaginal brachytherapy combined with whole pelvic external beam irradiation. The median whole pelvic dose was 4000 cGy, and the median brachytherapy dose was 2100 cGy. This was delivered using a median dose per fraction of 700 cGy given 1 to 2 weeks apart. Nanavati and colleagues[73] also reported on the combined use of whole pelvic irradiation and high-dose-rate vaginal cylinder therapy. External doses of 4500 cGy were used in combination with high-dose-rate doses of 2000 to 2800 cGy given in three to four weekly doses.

When treatment consists of high-dose-rate brachytherapy alone, doses of 2100 to 2500 cGy prescribed to a depth of 0.5 cm are given to the entire vaginal mucosa by means of weekly fractions of 500 to 700 cGy. This prophylactic dose is designed to control microscopic disease. This fractionation regimen has been successfully and safely used to prophylactically treat the vaginal cuff after hysterectomy for endometrial cancer.[74] An additional 2100 to 2500 cGy prescribed to a depth of 0.5 cm is delivered to the tumor via a shielded vaginal cylinder; weekly fractions of 500 to 700 cGy are used. This boost brings the total dose to 4200 to 5000 cGy.

Kucera et al. reported on 80 patients with invasive carcinoma of the vagina who were treated with high-dose-rate brachytherapy (HDRB) with or without external beam therapy.[90a] These patients were compared with a historical group of 110 patients treated with intracavitary low-dose-rate (LDRB) radium-226 or cesium-137 brachytherapy with or without external beam irradiation. There were no significant differences in local and distant recurrences between the treatment modalities. The comparison of treatment with or without external beam radiation and of complications showed no significant differences between the HDRB and LDRB series. HDRB would appear to be the preferred treatment modality due to the decreased radiation exposure, less variability in patient positioning, and better dose distribution, as compared to LDRB.[91a]

In the second group of stage I patients, with lesions whose depth of invasion is greater than 0.5 cm, brachytherapy should be delivered using both an intracavitary and an interstitial system. Using a vaginal cylinder, the first application should deliver 4500 cGy (low dose rate) or 2100 to 2500 cGy (high dose rate) to a depth of 0.5 cm into the vaginal mucosal surfaces. Because of the increased depth, the second application should be delivered with an interstitial implant. The tumor depth should be estimated, and the dose given to the tumor volume by the vaginal cylinder treatment should be calculated. The second implant with an interstitial system (low dose rate) should deliver an additional dose of 2500 to 3500 cGy to the tumor volume.

Combined external beam irradiation and brachytherapy is indicated in stage I lesions that are large and more invasive, occupy extended areas of vaginal mucosa (greater than two-thirds involvement of vaginal length), or are indeterminate between stages I and II. Whole-pelvis irradiation or a modified field including the inguinal regions can be used to deliver a dose of 4500 cGy with a 180 cGy fraction size. This should be followed by one or two interstitial implants to deliver an additional 3000 to 4000 cGy to the tumor volume.

Stage II

Radiation therapy is the primary treatment for stage II disease. Surgery is infrequently indicated since radical

procedures are usually required to excise these lesions adequately. Stock and colleagues[11] noted that 23 of 33 (70%) stage II patients treated with surgery required either a total vaginectomy or an exenterative procedure. Radical surgical procedures such as these are often associated with significant morbidity and functional impairment. Herbst and colleagues[53] reported that 27% of patients undergoing this type of radical surgery developed serious complications that were often fatal. For this reason surgical treatment is usually reserved for radiation therapy failures.

Treatment with radiation therapy involves a combination of external beam therapy and brachytherapy. External beam therapy covers a whole or a modified pelvic field that includes the inguinal region. Doses of 4500 to 5040 cGy are given to the pelvic field by means of 180 cGy fractions. If there is metastatic disease to the pelvic or groin lymph nodes, these regions should receive an external beam boost to 60 to 66 Gy.

The next stage of treatment should be delivered with brachytherapy. Unlike stage I lesions, stage II lesions should be treated with an interstitial implant. Because these are deeper lesions, an intracavitary system is inadequate as it fails to provide the needed dose to the deepest part of the tumor volume without exceeding the tolerance of the mucosal surface. Interstitial brachytherapy has been shown to improve local control when compared with intracavitary therapy.[10,29] Perez[26] recommends total tumor doses of 7500 to 8000 cGy given to the tumor volume by combined external beam irradiation and interstitial implant, but Perez and colleagues[60] acknowledge relatively high failure rates with these doses, with local and parametrial failure rates of 39% for stage IIa and 46.1% for stage IIb. Fleming and colleagues[75] and Puthawala and colleagues[76] recommend higher total doses of 8000 to 10,000 cGy of combined external beam irradiation and brachytherapy with 4500 to 5000 cGy of the dose delivered with two interstitial implants. Puthawala and associates[76] report improved local control with seven of seven stage IIa and seven of nine stage IIb patients locally controlled with total doses of 8000 to 10,000 cGy. These data suggest improved local control with higher doses of interstitial therapy. Based on these data, a recommended dose to be delivered to the tumor volume with interstitial therapy is 3500 to 4500 cGy, given in one or two applications. Two applications are usually scheduled, with a 1- to 2-week break between applications when higher interstitial doses are delivered.

Stage III

Stage III disease is treated like stage II. If the goal is cure, one should try not to exceed doses of 5040 to 5400 cGy of external beam therapy to the central vaginal area, since an integral part of the treatment will be the subsequent brachytherapy. The tolerance of the bladder and rectum should be respected and not jeopardized by the external beam portion of the therapy. If the dose given with external beam radiation is excessive, then the dose given by brachytherapy will be limited. The interstitial implant should deliver a dose of 3500 to 4500 cGy given in one or two applications.

Stage IVa

A similar radiotherapeutic approach can be taken with stage IV disease. One must keep in mind that the use of high-dose brachytherapy in combination with external beam therapy to areas of tumor volume that invade bladder or rectum will be associated with a high incidence of fistula formation if local control is achieved. If a curative approach is taken, then treatment may involve an exenterative surgical procedure either for persistent disease or for complications.

Vaginal Melanoma

There are relatively few reports on the management of vaginal melanoma, which is a rare lesion. Treatment has varied and has included wide local excision, radical surgery, radiation therapy, or combinations of these treatments. The limited data available preclude definitive treatment recommendations. The overall prognosis for patients with vaginal melanoma is extremely poor, with reported 5-year survival rates of 5% to 29%.[77-79] Distant metastases, with rates ranging from 66% to 100%, contribute to the poor outcome.[39,41,77,78,80] Patients with primary tumor size of less than 3 cm appeared to have improved survival rates.[77a,78a]

Morrow and Disaia,[79] in a review of the literature, recommend radical surgery for these patients. Chung and colleagues[78] reported local vaginal control in six of eight patients treated with radical surgery. Radical surgical procedures can still be associated with a high local failure rate, especially when pelvic failure including inguinal and pelvic nodal failure is considered. Bonner and colleagues[77] treated five patients with radical surgery; four developed pelvic lesions as their first site of recurrence.

Radiation therapy has also been employed, particularly when more advanced lesions or lesions to be treated only for palliative intent are selected for radiotherapeutic management.[36] This may explain the poor results reported with radiation therapy.[78] In earlier-stage disease, radiation therapy may provide adequate local control. Harrison and colleagues[39] reported on three cases of vaginal melanoma, two stage I cases and one isolated vaginal recurrence after local excision. Disease in all three patients was locally controlled with radiation therapy.

Given the high rate of distant metastases and the limited overall survival rate, radical surgical procedures are difficult to justify when there is no clear evidence that this approach provides increased local control or increased survival. Bonner and associates[77] suggest adding pelvic radiation therapy to radical surgical procedures to increase local control. A less morbid treatment schema combines a wide local excision followed by postoperative whole pelvic irradiation and intravaginal brachytherapy.

Radiation therapy alone can also be used. Some evidence suggests that high doses per fraction may be more beneficial in treating melanomas because of the large shoulder demonstrated in dose-response curves of cells in vitro. These data suggest a greater ability of these cells to undergo sublethal damage repair.[81] The clinical relevance of these findings is unclear. Radiation Therapy Oncology Group (RTOG) 83-05, a prospective randomized trial, compared a standard fractionation scheme for the treatment of melanomas (5000 cGy in 20 daily fractions) to 3200 cGy by means of 800 cGy fractions given once a week and found no difference in response rates between the two arms of the study.[82] Because of these data, it is reasonable to treat vaginal melanomas using a dose and fractionation scheme similar to that employed in the treatment of squamous cell vaginal carcinomas of comparable stages.

EXTERNAL BEAM RADIATION THERAPY

If external beam therapy is employed in the treatment plan, a whole pelvic field or pelvic field modified to include the inguinal nodes is used. Techniques include a four-field plan with an anterior, a posterior, and two lateral fields. Alternatively, a parallel opposed, anterior and posterior field plan can also be applied. In general these techniques are best done with high energy x-rays of 15 to 18 MeV. At the time of simulation, the patient should be given radiographic oral contrast material, allowing an estimation of the amount of small bowel in the pelvis. This information is needed to determine the position of simulation (prone vs. supine), the technique (four-field vs. anterior-posterior–posterior-anterior), and the energy. Additionally, a marker should be placed in the vagina to identify the canal and its apex. A frequently used marker is a thin acrylic (Lucite) cylinder with inner metallic markings at 1 cm intervals, and an adjustable metallic ring to mark the introitus. A small Foley catheter placed in the rectum permits filling with contrast material to identify the rectum on a lateral film.

The treatment technique and the selection of the appropriate energy level must be individualized. In the presence of significant loops of small bowel in the field, a four-field plan may be preferable, since the small bowel can be blocked on the lateral fields. Energies from 6 to 18 MV photons can be selected, based on the patient's size and isodose treatment plan. If the inguinal nodes are to be included in an anterior-posterior plan or a four-field technique, then the dose to the inguinal nodes (which usually lie 3 to 5 cm below the skin surface) should be calculated by means of a treatment plan. An inadequate dose to the inguinal nodes can be compensated by concurrent electron boosts to the inguinal regions. If there is no small bowel in the pelvic field, then an anterior-posterior plan (using 15 to 18 MV photons) may be preferable, especially if the inguinal nodes are to be treated. A standard whole pelvic field should extend superiorly to the L5-S1 interspace and inferiorly to cover the inferior extent of the vagina. The lateral borders should be 1.5 to 2.0 cm lateral to the pelvic brim. If lateral fields are used, the posterior border should lie at the S2-S3 interspace and the anterior border 1 cm anterior to the symphysis pubis (Fig. 51-7). These fields are designed to treat the vagina and the common iliac, external iliac, hypogastric, and obturator lymph nodes. If positive pelvic lymph nodes have been identified, the superior border is raised to the L4-L5 interspace to include the proximal common iliac nodes. If the inguinal nodes are to be treated, the lateral border should be extended to

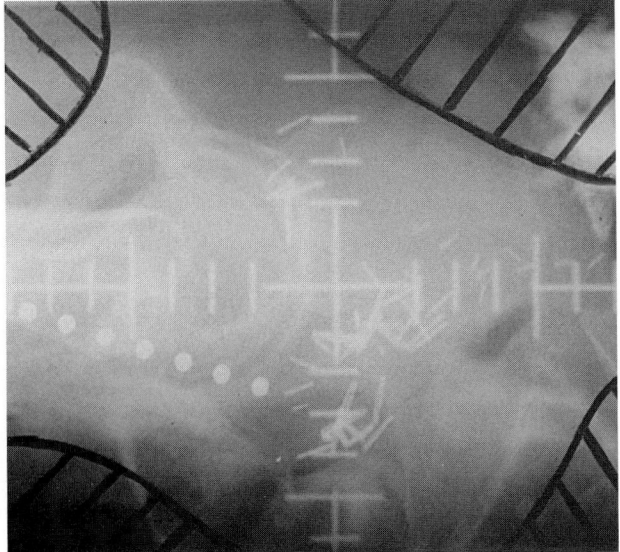

Figure 51–7. Simulation film of a lateral port used in a four-field plan.

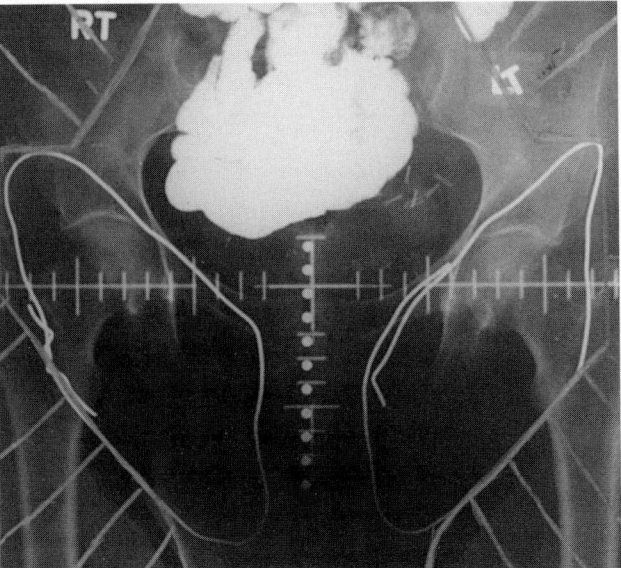

Figure 51–9. Corresponding simulation film for the field shown in Figure 51-8. A wire has been placed around the inguinal-femoral region with a margin.

include these nodes. The inguinal nodes lie beneath and inferior to the inguinal ligament, which runs from the pubic tubercle to the anterior superior iliac spine. Figures 51-8 and 51-9 show a patient setup and simulation for an anterior pelvic-inguinal field.

BRACHYTHERAPY

Intracavitary

Intracavitary therapy is indicated primarily for superficial lesions. The most commonly employed intracavitary system used is the vaginal cylinder. Many vaginal applicators are available, including the Bloedorn, Burnett, and Delclos cylinders. In addition, vaginal cylinders are available for use with high-dose-rate units (Figs. 51-10

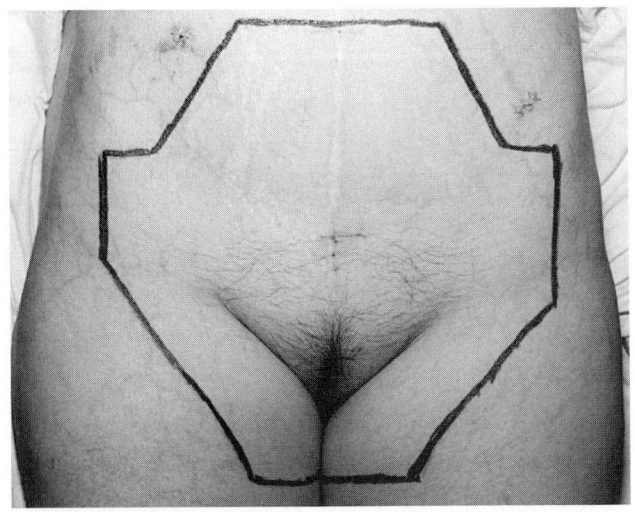

Figure 51–8. Photograph of a patient in the supine setup position. The anterior treatment field to include the inguinal nodes has been outlined on the patient in black.

and 51-11). Most of these applicators are available in different diameters. The largest-diameter cylinder that fits comfortably into the vaginal canal should be used. A 3 cm-diameter cylinder is the size most commonly used. The center of these cylinders contains a hollow tandem, through which the radioactive sources are inserted. The most common isotope employed for a low-dose-rate system is cesium-137 and for a high-dose-rate system, iridium-192. Usually two to three cesium sources are placed in the central tandem of the cylinder, determined by the extent of the vaginal canal to be treated. In a high-dose-rate system, one iridium source is used. It travels along the length of the central tandem, occupying specific dwell locations for prescribed times, determined by the extent of vaginal canal to be treated and the dose to be delivered. The dose delivered declines rapidly as the distance from the source increases. The differential between the dose delivered to the vaginal mucosa that lies adjacent to the vaginal cylinder and the prescription depth varies with the length of vaginal canal treated and the diameter of the cylinder. The larger the length of the canal treated and the diameter of the cylinder, the smaller the differential between mucosal and prescription dose. The prescription depth should be based on the estimated depth of tumor involvement. Doses are usually prescribed up to a depth of 1 cm into the mucosa. A depth of 0.5 cm is the most commonly prescribed depth. In patients with an intact cervix and superficial lesions in the fornices, vaginal ovoids can be employed.

Interstitial

The two most commonly used applicators for transperineal interstitial brachytherapy are the Syed-Neblett template and the multiple-site perineal applicator (MUPIT) (Figs. 51-12 and 51-13).[83,84] These applicators contain a template that is placed adjacent to the perineum

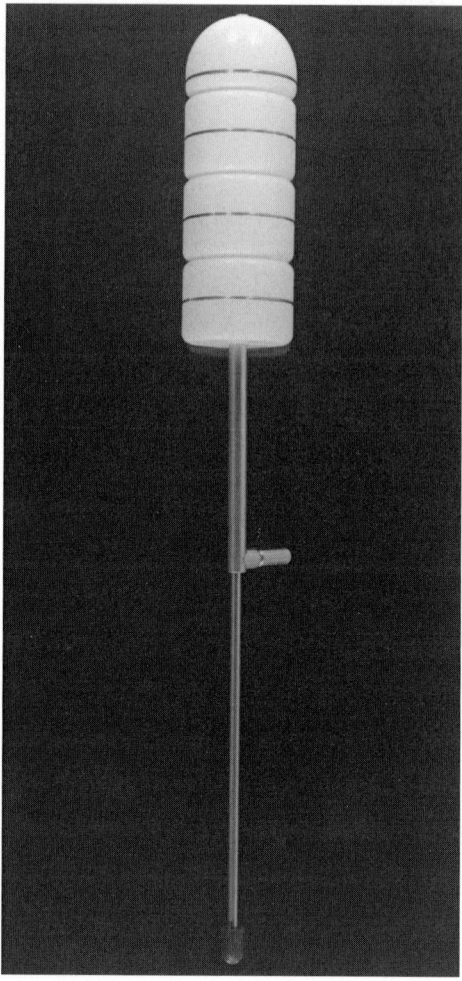

Figure 51–10. Vaginal cylinder used for high-dose-rate applications.

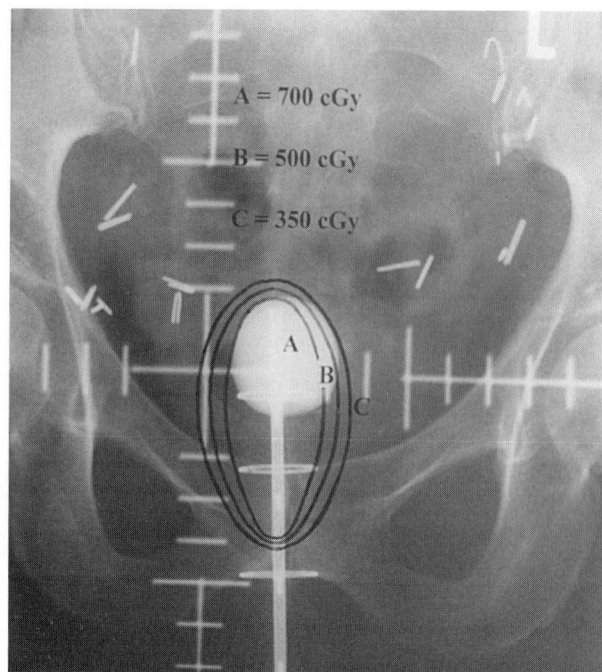

Figure 51–11. Simulation film of a pelvis with an intravaginal cylinder used with a high-dose-rate system in place. Isodose curves have been superimposed for a plan that delivers a dose of 700 cGy to the vaginal mucosal surface and a dose of 500 cGy to a depth of 0.5 cm.

circles 1 cm apart. Planning an interstitial implant requires a three-dimensional concept. The goal of the implant is to cover the tumor volume with a 1 to 2 cm margin by placing needles into a three-dimensional volume. The needles are placed 1 to 2 cm apart, superior

and vulva. Through the center of this template runs an opening through which a cylinder inserts into the vaginal canal. The template contains holes through which needles can be inserted and guided along the vaginal mucosa and into the paravaginal space, parametria, cervix, and uterus. In the operating room the patient is placed in the dorsal-lithotomy position, anesthetized with either general or spinal anesthesia, and then prepared and draped. A careful speculum and bimanual examination is performed to assess the tumor's dimensions and location. Small hemostat clips or titanium seeds are used to mark the vaginal mucosal component of the tumor. A diagram of the area to be implanted should be drawn. In patients with an intact uterus, the cervical os should be identified and dilated. By means of the Syed-Neblett applicator, the central tandem is inserted into the uterus through the dilated cervix. The vaginal cylinder is placed over the tandem by guiding the tandem through the central hole in the cylinder. A needle is then placed into one of the grooves on the cylinder and inserted into the cervix. This secures the central cylinder. If the patient has had a hysterectomy, the central tandem is not used. Rather, the template is inserted over the cylinder and secured in place by tightening the screws around the cylinder. The tumor volume is implanted by inserting needles through the holes in the template, which are arranged in concentric

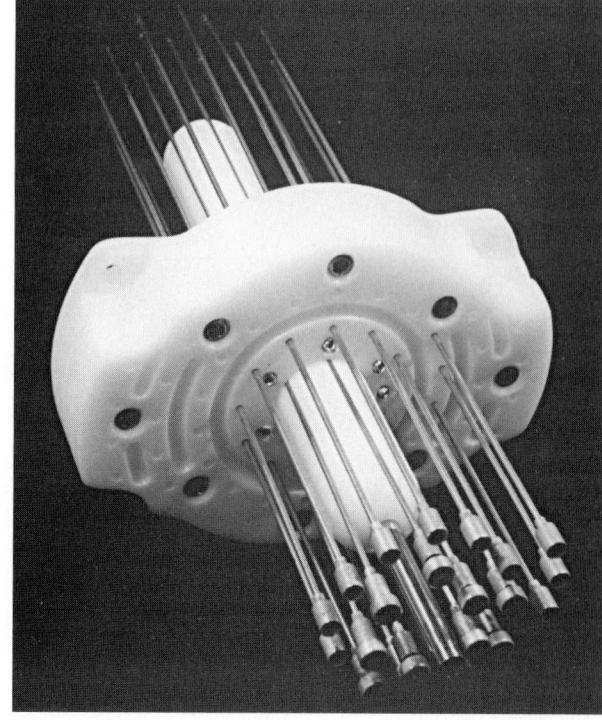

Figure 51–12. Syed-Neblett template with obturator and needles in place.

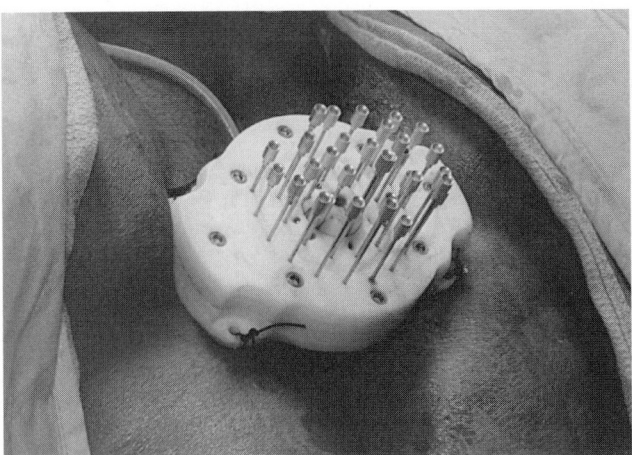

Figure 51–13. Syed-Neblett template used to perform an interstitial implant in a patient with prior hysterectomy who presented with a large stage II vaginal cancer located at the vaginal apex.

to the original tumor volume. The needles in the grooves of the cylinder will lie just outside the mucosal component of the tumor. Needles placed in the outer rows should implant an area at least 1 cm deep to the original volume. Once the needles are in place, they are secured by tightening the screws in the periphery of the template (Fig. 51-14). These implants can be optimally preplanned using CT scans and a template and cylinder placed in the vagina for the scan.

After the implant is complete, localization films are taken of the implanted area (Figs. 51-15 and 51-16). The information from the original simulation film, pelvic examination, and pretreatment CT scans is used to map out the original tumor volume. By providing a 1 to 2 cm margin to this volume, one can determine the number of needles to be implanted as well as the active length of each needle. Iridium-192 is the most common isotope used with this type of implant. Iridium-192 ribbons can be ordered with radioactive seeds placed 1 cm apart.

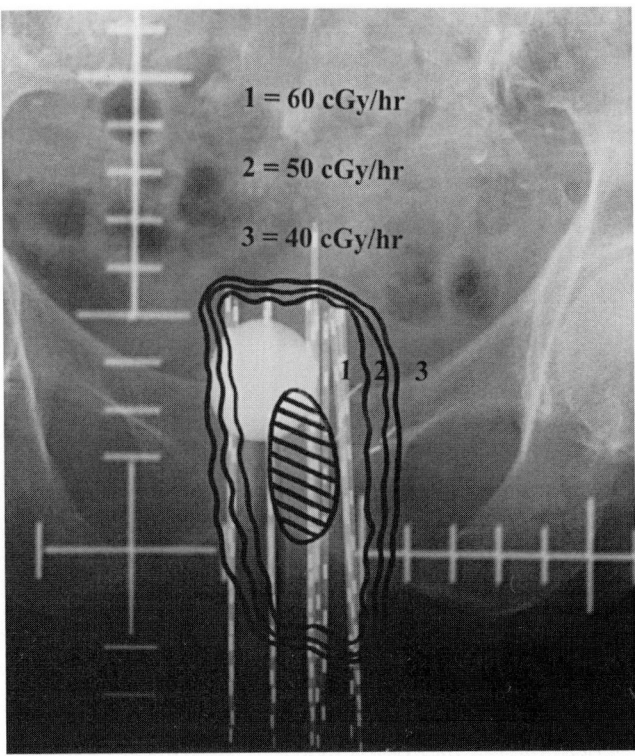

Figure 51–15. Anterior localization film of an interstitial implant used to treat a deeply invasive stage I lesion. Isodose curves representing dose rates and the tumor volume have been superimposed.

Activities of 0.25 to 0.35 mgRaEq per seed are used. The lower-activity ribbons are usually placed in the center of the implant to decrease central hot spots and create a uniform dose distribution. These lower-strength ribbons can also be placed in needles close to the urethra or rectum to decrease the dose delivered to these adjacent structures. The central tandem can be loaded with cesium-137 if needed. If the central tandem is loaded with cesium-137, the six central needles that lie in the obturator grooves should not be loaded in order to avoid hot spots in the bladder and rectum.[83] The goal is a uniform dose distribution that covers the treatment volume with a dose rate of 50 to 70 cGy/hour.

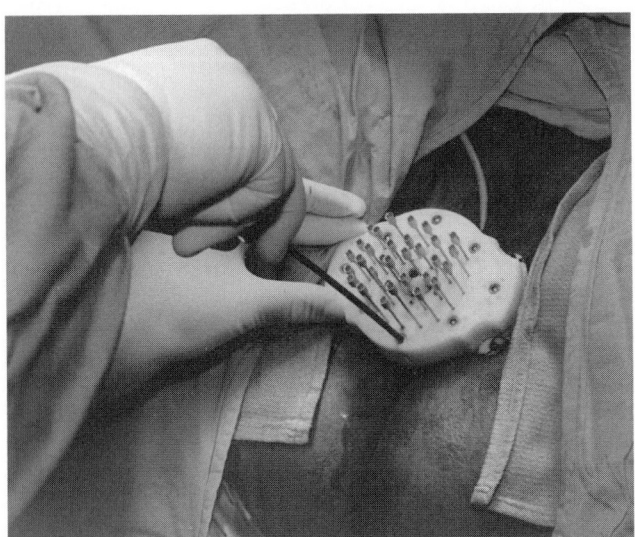

Figure 51–14. Securing the needle template system by tightening the screws in the periphery of the template.

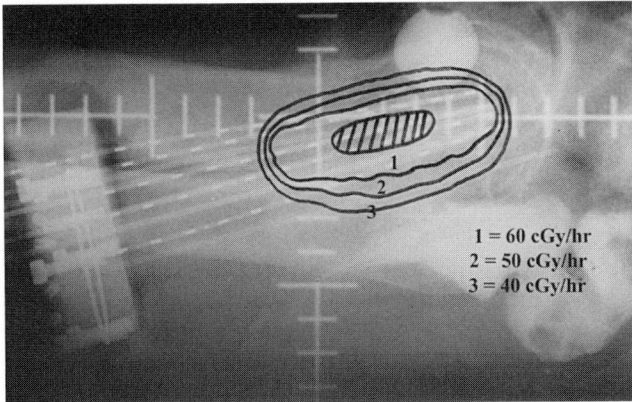

Figure 51–16. Lateral localization film of an interstitial implant showing its position relative to the bladder and rectum. Isodose curves representing dose rates and the tumor volume have been superimposed.

The inability to visualize the tumor and surrounding normal structures during interstitial implantation has hampered the accuracy and safety of such implants.[85] Consideration should be made to performing these implants with imaging guidance or under direct visualization, particularly in patients with a prior hysterectomy. When the implant is performed in conjunction with an open laparotomy, the needles can be visualized entering the tumor volume as well as the adjacent normal structures. This procedure can help avoid small bowel or bladder perforation. The surgeon can assist in guiding the needles into the tumor volume and determining the depth of needle placement. The major problem with laparotomy-guided implants is that structures can only be visualized from an intraperitoneal view. Extraperitoneal structures, such as parts of the bladder, uterus, and cervix, as well as the vagina and paravaginal tissues, cannot be visualized. At the time of laparotomy, placement of an intraperitoneal sling can prevent small bowel loops from contacting the top of the implant. Disaia and Creasman[86] describe creating an "omental carpet" at the time of laparotomy. A section of omentum is placed along the descending colon into the pelvis; it separates the bladder and rectum from the implant and prevents small bowel from adhering to the implant. Laparotomy is usually not performed for the second implant in a two-application treatment.[87]

Laparoscopic visualization of needle placement is an alternative to open laparotomy. Although laparoscopy is less invasive, it suffers the same limitations as the open laparotomy in its inability to visualize extraperitoneal structures.

Other methods have been attempted to improve the accuracy of needle placement. Both CT and MRI preplanning have been used.[88] These systems rely on accurate imaging of the target volume with the template and obturator in place. The limited accuracy of CT in visualizing pelvic structures has rendered this method to be of marginal value. MRI has been shown to be more accurate than CT in assessing tumor size and locoregional disease extent in cervical carcinoma.[89] However, there are significant limitations in using MRI for preplanning, primarily since patients cannot be scanned through the MRI in the dorsal lithotomy position, which is the position of template insertion. For this reason, exact duplication of the plan is difficult. In addition, the position of the pelvic structures changes continually with filling and emptying of the bladder as well as changes in rectal fullness. Changes in body position can also alter the position of these organs.

To overcome the inaccuracies and limitations mentioned earlier, Stock et al. developed a system that relies on real-time transrectal ultrasound for guidance.[85] Transrectal ultrasound, as opposed to transabdominal imaging, was used because it brings the ultrasound probe in closer proximity to the structures of interest (cervix, parametria, vagina) than abdominal ultrasound. The ultrasound probe can visualize all of the pelvic structures during the implant and allows for placement of needles into the target volume under direct visualization. Transverse ultrasound imaging is used to assure that needles cover the target area and do not enter the bladder, rectum, or small bowel. The longitudinal mode of the ultrasound probe is extremely useful and accurate in determining the optimum depth of needle insertion. Needles can be inserted under direct guidance and placed at the appropriate depth. In addition, these images can be used to assess the overall length of the target volume, which will help to determine the active length of the implant. Using this technique, complicated preplanning or invasive laparotomy or laparoscopy can be avoided. CT scans with the needles in place can be used to optimize the dwell times and the plan when HDRB is used.

CRITICAL NORMAL TISSUES—RADIATION INJURY

Complications can range from the acute side effects of external beam radiation therapy, which resolve shortly after treatment, to those that develop 6 months to 2 years after completion of therapy. Most late complications develop within the first 2 years after treatment, with a median time of 1 year.[11,52] Evaluating complication rates from the literature is problematic; most studies report crude complication rates. Such figures fail to provide a true account of the risk of developing complications, since a large percentage of patients develop recurrences and die of their disease and thus would no longer be at risk for developing treatment complications. Thus, most reports tend to underestimate the actual risk, which is more accurately calculated by using an actuarial complication rate. Chyle et al. reported an actuarial incidence of serious complications of 19% at 20 years.[51] This illustrates the importance of prolonged follow-up in determining the true incidence of late complications. Although most complications were evident by 5 years, a significant fraction appeared beyond this time, even up to nearly 16 years after treatment.

One of the most common treatment sequelae is vaginal stenosis. The incidence of vaginal stenosis ranges from 10% to 50%.[1,12,13,47,90] Among 16 disease-free patients, Hintz and colleagues[90] found 50% with some degree of vaginal stenosis. To avoid or minimize this problem, patients are encouraged to use vaginal dilators post-treatment since many women in this age group are sexually inactive. Vaginal stenosis interferes with follow-up examinations and may hinder discovery of local recurrences. Injury to the vulva and introitus can occur if the vaginal cylinder is loaded below the introitus. Care should be taken not to deliver high doses to this area unless it is involved with tumor.

Major complications requiring hospitalization or surgical intervention occur in 5% to 19% of patients.[1,39,47,51,60,61,72,76,91] The most common serious complications from radiation therapy are cystitis, proctitis, rectovaginal and vesicovaginal fistula formation, and vaginal necrosis. Kucera and Vavra[2] reported a 40% incidence of proctitis and cystitis, although they did not comment on the extent of these complications. The incidence of fistula formation ranges from 1% to 7%.[1,2,52,60] This serious complication may not resolve with conservative management. Exenterative surgical procedures are often necessary to prevent septicemia. Vaginal necrosis has been reported in 4% to 15% of cases.[12,76,92]

The distal vagina has a lower radiation tolerance than the upper vagina with both HDR and LDR brachytherapy.[93] Hintz and colleagues[87] found that none of their 16 patients developed vaginal necrosis in the upper vagina with summated doses up to 14,000 cGy. The lower vagina was more susceptible to vaginal necrosis when summated doses exceeded 9800 cGy. Cases of vaginal necrosis refractory to conservative management have been managed with hyperbaric oxygen treatments.[94] In a series from the MD Anderson Cancer Center, the only significant determinants of complications in multivariate analysis were pelvic lymphadenectomy and FIGO stage.[51]

PATTERNS OF RECURRENCE

Local recurrence is the most common pattern of treatment failure. In addition, persistent disease after radiation therapy is often a problem in more advanced lesions. In the series of Dixit and colleagues,[52] 68% of local failures in stage III patients were due to persistent disease. Although complete response rates are higher in earlier-stage disease, vaginal failure continues to be the main pattern of failure. Overall crude local failure rates range from 15% to 45%.[1,11,28,29,52,76] Extravaginal, intrapelvic failure, including nodal failure, is less common, seen in 7% to 18% of cases.[1,11,35] A list of pelvic and local control rates by stage can be found in Table 51-5. Most locoregional recurrences and distant failures are noted in the first 2 years following treatment.[95] Distant failures can also represent a significant problem, particularly in advanced disease.

Distant failure tends to occur later in the course of the disease than does local or pelvic recurrence. Reported incidences of distant failures vary widely. This is due to the difficulty, in retrospective reviews, of assessing the true incidence of distant failure, since thorough metastatic workups are seldom done in the setting of an incurable local failure. Distant failure rates range from 7% to 33%.[1,11,28,29,35,52] At least half of all distant failures demonstrate concurrent local failure.[29,53,60] The ability to accurately assess the various failure rates is also hampered by the use of crude recurrence rate figures. Ten-year actuarial recurrence rates for local, pelvic, and distant failures of 26%, 30%, and 18%, respectively, have been reported.[51]

QUALITY OF LIFE ISSUES

Minimal data have been reported regarding quality of life issues for women with carcinoma of the vagina.[57] Preservation of the anatomy and function of the vagina have been the reported advantage of radiation therapy versus surgical management of vaginal carcinomas. In addition, it has been presumed that preservation of the vagina confers a psychological benefit. However, it is unclear as to the percentage of women who actually maintain a functional vagina following definitive therapy for an invasive vaginal cancer.

Quality of life assessments in women with cervical carcinoma have demonstrated equivalent outcomes whether they are treated with primary irradiation or surgery. These treatments, however, are primarily directed to the cervix and upper vagina. Patients with vaginal cancer may present with tumor involvement of the upper, middle, and distal vagina, and tumor may spread to involve the urinary bladder and urethra. Therefore, depending on the tumor location and extent, vaginal function may be differentially affected.[57]

Both surgery and irradiation may lead to significant anatomical changes in the vagina and adjacent structures. The majority of patients with vaginal cancers are elderly with an atrophic vagina and are likely to experience poor anatomical and functional outcomes following treatment. Younger patients, with small invasive cancers, are likely to attain anatomical and functional preservation. Tumor involvement of adjacent structures (bladder, urethra, and rectum) may require surgical resection of these structures or may yield dysfunction of these organs following definitive irradiation.

In an attempt to maintain vaginal functioning following definitive irradiation, the use of a vaginal dilator (two to three times per week) is strongly recommended. Topical intravaginal estrogen therapy and lubrication during intercourse is also advised. Some authors advocate the use of a vaginal douche during radiation therapy. A mixture of hydrogen peroxide and water (1:10 mixture) on a twice-daily basis is prescribed.[57] After completion of irradiation, patients are instructed to continue to douche with this mixture.

Ultimately, functional outcome is dependent upon the initial tumor size and extent, type of therapy, personal hygiene, the addition of hormone replacement therapy,

Table 51-5   Local and Pelvic Control Rates After Radiation Therapy

| Reference | Control | Control Rate, % (Patients, *n*) | | | |
		Stage I	*Stage II*	*Stage III*	*Stage IV*
Chu[50]	L	87 (8)	68 (19)	57 (7)	0 (3)
Dancuart[1]	P	79 (71)	83 (42)	74 (38)	73 (11)
Leung[29]	L	77 (44)	67 (9)	57 (21)	50 (10)
Perez[60]	P	86 (50)	IIa61 (49)	62 (16)	25 (8)
			IIb52 (26)		
Prempree[72]	P	89 (9)	IIa87 (13)	65 (26)	12 (8)
			IIb64 (14)		
Stock[10]	L	50 (6)	47 (27)	40 (10)	0 (6)

L, local; P, pelvic.

and compliance with the prescribed post-treatment regimen.[57]

RESULTS

Overall survival rates by stage are listed in Table 51-6. Figure 51-17 shows the actuarial survival of patients by stage from an analysis by Stock and colleagues[11] from the University of Pittsburgh.

Stage I

Actuarial survival rates for stage I disease range from 60% to 82%.[11,29,35,44,60,71] The results of treatment for stage I patients support the use of local therapy directed to the vagina and tumor volume and reveal local failure to be the primary site of recurrence. Among the 71 stage I patients of Dancourt and colleagues,[1] of whom 36 were treated with local therapy alone (brachytherapy [intracavitary or interstitial] or transvaginal cone irradiation), the local failure rate was 18%. In only 2 of their 71 patients did the recurrence occur outside the central vaginal area. Perez and associates[60] reported a pelvic failure rate of 14% for 50 stage I patients. The addition of external beam therapy to local brachytherapy did not improve pelvic control. Distant metastases in this stage of disease are uncommon, occurring in about 5% of patients.[1,35]

Stage II

The actuarial survival rates for stage II disease range from 48% to 55%.[10,11,35,60,71] Among stage II patients, disease can vary in extent. There can be minimal extension beyond the wall of the vagina or there can be extensive spread with involvement of the rectovaginal septum, parametria, bladder wall, or rectal wall (excluding mucosal involvement). These varied presentations are all considered stage II disease. Perez and colleagues[49] suggested a modification of the FIGO staging system, dividing stage II into IIa (subvaginal involvement) and stage IIb (parametrial involvement). They found an improved 10-year disease-free survival of 55% in 49 stage IIa patients compared with 43% in 26 stage IIb patients.[60] Other data to support this modification reveal survival rates of 51% to 66% for stage IIa patients

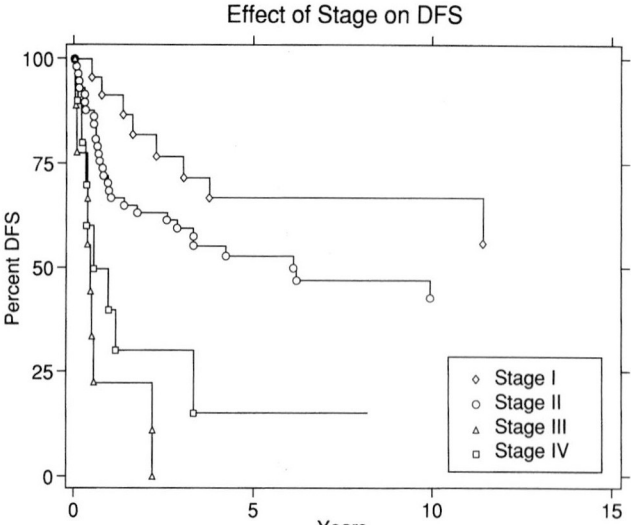

Figure 51–17. Overall disease-free survival by stage. (Data from Magee-Women's Hospital, University of Pittsburgh School of Medicine.[11])

compared with rates of 24% to 31% for stage IIb.[47,52] Local recurrence continues to be the main site of failure. Stock and associates,[10] in a series from Memorial Sloan-Kettering Cancer Center, recorded an actuarial local failure rate of 53% for 27 patients with stage II disease. In a series from Magee-Women's Hospital, the actuarial local failure rate in 58 stage II patients was 38%.[11] Compared with stage I, patients with stage II disease, in addition to demonstrating increased local failure, have a higher likelihood of developing distant metastases, with reported rates ranging from 22% to 46.1%.[35,60] The distant metastasis rate has been shown to be higher in stage IIb lesions when compared with stage IIa.[60,72]

Stages III and IV

The actuarial survival rates for stage III disease range from 29% to 40%.[10,29,36,44,52,60,71] The local failure rates for stage III lesions range from 35% to 75%, reflecting the extent of disease as well as the treatment intent.[10,47,60,72] Treatment with external beam therapy alone has been associated with a poorer outcome than treatment with external beam therapy combined with brachytherapy, or brachytherapy alone.[10,47,53] Many stage III lesions are often managed with palliative intent and treated with

Table 51–6 Actuarial 5-Year Survival by Stage

Reference	Survival, % (Patients, *n*)			
	Stage I	*Stage II*	*Stage III*	*Stage IV*
Davis[35]	82 (44)	53 (45)	—	—
Eddy[44]	75 (25)	IIa47 (17)	40 (15)	25 (12)
		IIb35 (22)		
Macnaught[36]	68 (14)	34 (22)	29 (18)	14 (7)
Perez[60]	75 (50)	IIa55 (49)	45 (16)	IVa38 (8)
		IIb35 (26)		
Stock[11]	67 (23)*	53 (58)*	0 (9)*	15 (10)*

*Disease-free survival.

external beam irradiation alone. This partially accounts for the high reported local failure rates. In addition to an increasing local failure rate, distant failure is also increased. Reported distant failure rates have ranged from 23% to 50%.[29,60,71,72]

The actuarial survival rates for stage IV disease range from zero to 25%.[10,11,36,44,52,60,61,71] This high incidence of distant metastases and decreased survival rates emphasizes the need for earlier diagnosis and effective systemic cytotoxic agents. These uniformly poor results reflect the inability of radiation therapy to control these lesions, with doses limited by the tolerance of the adjacent pelvic organs. Occasionally, lesions that have spread to the bowel or bladder but are not yet fixed to the pelvic sidewall can be treated or salvaged with a partial or total exenteration.[11,44]

Salvage Treatment

Theoretically, stage I and stage II lesions that fail radiation therapy might be salvaged with radical surgical procedures such as total vaginectomy, anterior or posterior exenteration, or total pelvic exenteration. Likewise, early lesions that recur after limited surgical procedures could theoretically be salvaged with more radical surgical procedures or radiation therapy. Unfortunately, salvage results have been uniformly poor. Stock and colleagues[11] found that in only 5 of 50 patients with local failures (10%) was salvage possible. These five patients had stage I or stage II disease at presentation. Chu and Beechinor[50] reported a 15% salvage rate. These poor results reflect the fact that local recurrences are often more advanced and aggressive than the disease at initial presentation.

FUTURE DIRECTIONS IN TREATMENT

Due to the low incidence of vaginal carcinoma, it is unlikely that significant prospective clinical trials will be conducted. Based on the similarities with the etiological factors and treatment approaches for patients with carcinoma of the uterine cervix, it is likely that new treatment approaches for patients with vaginal cancer will parallel those designed for patients with cervical cancer. Current clinical trials in patients with advanced cervical cancer are evaluating the status of hemoglobin levels during therapy, the role of chemical radioprotectors such as Amifostine) and new chemotherapeutic agents. The role of external beam irradiation with intensity-modulated radiotherapy in patients with vaginal cancer has yet to be defined.

REFERENCES

1. Dancuart F, Delclos L, Wharton JT, Silva EG: Primary squamous cell carcinoma of the vagina treated by radiotherapy: A failures analysis—the M D Anderson Hospital experience 1955-1982. *Int J Radiat Oncol Biol Phys.* 1988;14:745.
2. Kucera H, Vavra N: Radiation management of primary carcinoma of the vagina: Clinical and histopathological variables associated with survival. *Gynecol Oncol.* 1991;40:12.
3. Murad TM, Durant JR, Maddox WA, Dowling EA: The pathologic behavior of primary vaginal carcinoma and its relationship to cervical cancer. *Cancer.* 1975;35:787.
4. Ostrow RS, Manias DA, Clark BA, et al: The analysis of carcinoma of the vagina for human papillomavirus DNA. *Int J Gynecol Pathol.* 1988;7:308.
5. Ikenberg H, Runge M, Goppinger A, et al: Human papillomavirus DNA in invasive carcinoma of the vagina. *Obstet Gynecol.* 1990;76:432.
6. Ostrow RS, Manias DA, Clark BA, et al: Detection of human papillomavirus DNA in invasive carcinomas of the cervix by in situ hybridization. *Cancer Res.* 1987;47:47.
7. Fukushima M, Okagaki T, Twiggs LB, et al: Histologic types of carcinoma of the uterine cervix and the detectability of human papillomavirus DNA. *Cancer Res.* 1985;45:45.
8. Lee YC, Holcomb K, Buhl A, et al: Rapid progression of primary vaginal squamous cell carcinoma in a young HIV-infected woman. *Gynecol Oncol.* 2000;78:380.
9. Merino MJ: Vaginal cancer: The role of infectious and environmental factors. *Am J Obstet Gynecol.* 1991;165:1255.
10. Stock RG, Mychalczak B, Armstrong JG, et al: The importance of brachytherapy technique in the management of primary carcinoma of the vagina. *Int J Radiat Oncol Biol Phys.* 1992;24:747.
11. Stock RG, Chen ASJ, Seski J: A thirty-year experience in the management of primary carcinoma of the vagina: Analysis of prognostic factors and treatment modalities. *Gynecol Oncol.* 1995;56:45.
12. Benedet JL, Murphy KJ, Fairey RN, Boyes DA: Primary invasive carcinoma of the vagina. *Obstet Gynecol.* 1983;62:715.
13. Gallup DG, Talledo OE, Shah KJ, Hayes C: Invasive squamous carcinoma of the vagina: A 14-year study. *Obstet Gynecol.* 1987;69:782.
14. Rubin SC, Young J, Mikuta JJ: Squamous cell carcinoma of the vagina: Treatment, complications, and long-term follow-up. *Gynecol Oncol.* 1985;20:346.
15. Bell J, Sevin BU, Averette H, Nadjl M: Vaginal cancer after hysterectomy for benign disease: Value of cytologic screening. *Obstet Gynecol.* 1984;64:699.
16. Manetta A, Gutrecht EL, Berman ML, Disaia PJ: Primary invasive carcinoma of the vagina. *Obstet Gynecol.* 1990;76:639.
17. Brinton LA, Nasca PC, Malein K, et al: Case-control study of in situ and invasive carcinoma of the vagina. *Gynecol Oncol.* 1990;38:49.
18. Herman JM, Homesly HD, Dignan MB: Is hysterectomy a risk factor for vaginal cancer? *JAMA.* 1986;256:601.
19. Herbst AL, Scully RE: Adenocarcinoma of the vagina and cervix. A report of 7 cases including 6 clear cell carcinomas. *Cancer.* 1970;25:745.
20. Melnick S, Cole P, Anderson D, Herbst A: Rates and risks of diethylstilbestrol-related clear-cell adenocarcinoma of the vagina and cervix. An update. *N Engl J Med.* 1987;316:514.
21. Herbst AL, Anderson S, Hubby MM, et al: Risk factors for the development of diethylstilbestrol-associated clear cell adenocarcinoma: A case-controlled study. *Am J Obstet Gynecol.* 1986;154:814.
22. Woodruff JD: Carcinoma in situ of the vagina. *Clin Obstet Gynecol.* 1981;24:485.
23. Aho M, Vesterinen E, Meyer B, et al: Natural history of vaginal intraepithelial neoplasia. *Cancer.* 1991;68:195.
24. Lenehan PM, Meffe F, Lickrish GM: Vaginal intraepithelial neoplasia: Biologic aspects and management. *Obstet Gynecol.* 1986;68:33.
25. Perez CA, Arneson AN, Dehner LP, Galakatos A: Radiation therapy in carcinoma of the vagina. *Obstet Gynecol.* 1974;44:862.
26. Perez CA: Vagina. In Hoskins WJ, Perez CA, Young RC, eds: *Principles and Practice of Gynecologic Oncology.* Philadelphia: JB Lippincott; 1992:567.
27. Frick HC, Jacox HW, Taylor HC: Primary carcinoma of the vagina. *Am J Obstet Gynecol.* 1968;101:695.
28. Houghton CRS, Iversen T: Squamous cell carcinoma of the vagina: A clinical study of the location of the tumor. *Gynecol Oncol.* 1982;13:365.
29. Leung S, Sexton M: Radical radiation therapy for carcinoma of the vagina—impact of treatment modalities on outcome: Peter MacCallum Cancer Institute experience 1970-1990. *Int J Radiat Oncol Biol Phys.* 1993;25:413.

30. Kurman RJ, Scully RE: The incidence and histogenesis of vaginal adenosis. *Hum Pathol.* 1974;5:265.

31. Robboy SJ, Scully RE, Herbst AL: Pathology of vaginal and cervical abnormalities associated with prenatal exposure to diethylstilbestrol (DES). *J Reprod Med.* 1975;15:13.

32. Robboy SJ, Hill EC, Sandberg EC: Vaginal adenosis in women born prior to the diethylstilbestrol era. *Hum Pathol.* 1986;17:488.

33. Robboy SJ, Young RH, Welch WR, et al: Atypical vaginal adenosis and cervical ectropion. *Cancer.* 1984;54:869.

34. Robboy SJ, Welch WR, Young RH, et al: Topographic relation of cervical ectropion and vaginal adenosis to clear cell adenocarcinoma. *Obstet Gynecol.* 1982;60:546.

35. Davis KP, Stanhope R, Garton GR, et al: Invasive vaginal carcinoma: Analysis of early-stage disease. *Gynecol Oncol.* 1991;42:131.

36. Macnaught R, Symonds RP, Hole D, Watson ER: Improved control of primary vaginal tumors by combined external-beam and interstitial radiotherapy. *Clin Radiol.* 1986;37:29.

37. Senekjian EK, Frey BA, Stone C, Herbst AL: An evaluation of stage II vaginal clear cell adenocarcinoma according to substages. *Gynecol Oncol.* 1988;31:56.

38. Jones WB, Koulos JP, Saigo PE, Lewis JL: Clear-cell adenocarcinoma of the lower genital tract: Memorial Hospital 1974-1984. *Obstet Gynecol.* 1987;70:573.

39. Harrison LB, Fogel TD, Peschel RE: Primary vaginal cancer and vaginal melanoma: A review of therapy with external beam radiation and a simple intracavitary brachytherapy system. *Endocurie Hypertherm.* 1987;3:67.

40. Iversen K, Robins RE: Mucosal malignant melanomas. *Am J Surg.* 1980;139:660.

41. Norris HJ, Taylor HB: Melanomas of the vagina. *Am J Clin Pathol.* 1966;46:420.

42. Branton PA, Tavassoli FA: Spindle cell epithelioma, the so-called mixed tumor of the vagina. A clinicopathologic, immunohistochemical, and ultrastructural analysis of 28 cases. *Am J Surg Pathol.* 1993;17:509.

43. Tavassoli FA, Norris HJ: Smooth muscle tumors of the vagina. *Obstet Gynecol.* 1979;53:689.

44. Eddy GL, Marks RD, Miller C, Underwood PB: Primary invasive vaginal carcinoma. *Am J Obstet Gynecol.* 1991;165:292.

45. Peters WA, Kumar NB, Morley GW: Carcinoma of the vagina: Factors influencing treatment outcome. *Cancer.* 1985;55:892.

46. Rutledge F: Cancer of the vagina. *Am J Obstet Gynecol.* 1967;97:635.

47. Pride GL, Schultz AE, Chuprevich TW, Buchler DA: Primary invasive squamous carcinoma of the vagina. *Obstet Gynecol.* 1979;53:218.

48. Plentl AA, Friedman EA: *Lymphatic System of the Female Genitalia: The Morphologic Basis of Oncologic Diagnosis and Therapy.* Philadelphia: WB Saunders; 1971:51.

49. Perez CA, Arneson AN, Galakatos A, Samanth HK: Malignant tumors of the vagina. *Cancer.* 1973;31:36.

50. Chu AM, Beechinor R: Survival and recurrence patterns in the radiation treatment of carcinoma of the vagina. *Gynecol Oncol.* 1984;19:298.

51. Chyle V, Zagars GK, Wheeler JA, et al: Definitive radiotherapy for carcinoma of the vagina: Outcome and prognostic factors. *Int J Radiat Oncol Biol Phys.* 1996;35:891.

52. Dixit S, Singhal S, Baboo HA: Squamous cell carcinoma of the vagina: A review of 70 cases. *Gynecol Oncol.* 1993;48:80.

53. Herbst AL, Thomas GH, Ulfelder H: Primary carcinoma of the vagina. *Am J Obstet Gynecol.* 1970;106:210.

54. Chang YCF, Hricak H, Thurnher S, Lacey CG: Vagina: Evaluation with MR imaging. *Radiology.* 1988;169:175.

55. Ebner F, Kressel HY, Mintz MC, et al: Tumor recurrence versus fibrosis in the female pelvis: Differentiation with MR imaging at 1.5 T1. *Radiology.* 1988;166:333.

56. Grigsby PW, Siegal BA, Dehdashti F: Lymph-node staging by positron emission tomography in patients with carcinoma of the cervix. *J Clin Oncol.* 2001;19:3745.

57. Grigsby PW: Vaginal cancer. Current treatment options in oncology. *Curr Treat Options Oncol.* 2002;3:125.

58. Greene FL, Page DL, Fleming ID, et al, eds: *AJCC Cancer Staging Manual.* 6th ed. New York: Springer-Verlag; 2002.

59. Kottmeier HL: The classification and clinical staging of carcinoma of the uterus and vagina. *J Int Fed Gynecol Obstet.* 1963;1:83.

60. Perez CA, Camel M, Galakatos AE, et al: Definitive irradiation in carcinoma of the vagina: Long-term evaluation of results. *Int J Radiat Oncol Biol Phys.* 1988;15:1283.

61. Spiritos NM, Doshi BP, Kapp DS, Teng N: Radiation therapy for primary squamous cell carcinoma of the vagina: Stanford University experience. *Gynecol Oncol.* 1989;35:20.

62. Thigpen JT, Blessing JA, Homesley HD, et al: Phase II trial of cisplatin in advanced or recurrent cancer of the vagina: A Gynecologic Oncology Group study. *Gynecol Oncol.* 1986;23:101.

63. Muss HB, Bundy BN, Christoferson WA: Mitoxantrone in the treatment of advanced vulvar and vaginal carcinoma: A Gynecologic Oncology Group study. *Am J Clin Oncol.* 1989;12:142.

64. Slayton RE, Blessing JA, Beecham J, Disaia P: Phase II trial of etoposide in the management of advanced or recurrent squamous cell carcinoma of the vulva and carcinoma of the vagina: A Gynecologic Oncology Group Study. *Cancer Treat Rep.* 1987;71:869.

65. Omura GA, Shingleton HM, Creasman WT, et al: Chemotherapy of gynecologic cancer with nitrosoureas: A randomized trial of CCNU and methyl-CCNU in cancers of the cervix, corpus, vagina and vulva. *Cancer Treat Rep.* 1978;62:833.

66. Evans LS, Kersh CR, Constable WC, Taylor PT: Concomitant 5-fluorouracil, mitomycin-C, and radiotherapy for advanced gynecologic malignancies. *Int J Radiat Oncol Biol Phys.* 1988;15:901.

67. Roberts WS, Hoffman MS, Kavanagh JJ, et al: Further experience with radiation therapy and concomitant intravenous chemotherapy in advanced carcinoma of the lower female genital tract. *Gynecol Oncol.* 1991;43:233.

68. Jobson VW, Homesley HD: Treatment of vaginal intraepithelial neoplasia with the carbon dioxide laser. *Obstet Gynecol.* 1983;62:90.

69. Lenehan PM, Meffe F, Lickrish GM: Vaginal intraepithelial neoplasia: Biologic aspects and management. *Obstet Gynecol.* 1986;68:33.

70. Petrilli ES, Townsend DE, Morrow CP, Nakao CY: Vaginal intraepithelial neoplasia: Biologic aspects and treatment with topical 5-fluorouracil and the carbon dioxide laser. *Am J Obstet Gynecol.* 1980;138:321.

71. Perez CA, Grigsby PW, Garipagaoglu M, et al: Factors affecting long-term outcome of irradiation in carcinoma of the vagina. *Int J Radiat Oncol Biol Phys.* 1999; 44:37.

72. Prempree T, Amornmarn: Radiation treatment of primary carcinoma of the vagina. *Acta Radiol Oncol.* 1985;24:51.

73. Nanavati PJ, Fanning J, Hilgers RD, et al: High-dose rate brachytherapy in primary stage I and II vaginal cancer. *Gynecol Oncol.* 1993;51:67.

74. Mandell L, Nori D, Anderson L, Hilaris B: Postoperative vaginal radiation in endometrial cancer using a remote afterloading technique. *Int J Radiat Oncol Biol Phys.* 1985;11:473.

75. Fleming P, Syed N, Neblett D, et al: Description of an afterloading Ir-192 interstitial-intracavitary technique in the treatment of carcinoma of the vagina. *Obstet Gynecol.* 1980;55:525.

76. Puthawala A, Syed N, Nalick R, et al: Integrated external and interstitial radiation therapy for primary carcinoma of the vagina. *Obstet Gynecol.* 1983;62:367.

77. Bonner JA, Perez-Tamayo C, Reid GC, et al: The management of vaginal melanoma. *Cancer.* 1988;62:2066.

77a. Petru E, Nagele F, Czerwerka K, et al: Primary malignant melanoma of the vagina: Long-term remission following radiation therapy. *Gynecol Oncol.* 1998;70:23.

78. Chung AF, Casey MJ, Flannery JT, et al: Malignant melanoma of the vagina—report of 19 cases. *Obstet Gynecol.* 1980;55:720.

78a. Buchanan DJ, Schlaerth J, Kurasaki T: Primary vaginal melanoma: Thirteen-year disease-free survival after wide local excision and review of recent literature. *Am J Obstet Gynecol.* 1998;178:1177.

79. Morrow CP, Disaia PJ: Malignant melanoma of the female genitalia: A clinical analysis. *Obstet Gynecol Surv.* 1976;31:233.

80. Jentys W, Sikorowa L, Morkrzanowsk A: Primary melanoma of the vagina. *Oncology.* 1975;31:83.

81. Barranco SC, Romsdahl MM, Humphrey RM: The radiation response of human malignant melanoma cells grown in vitro. *Cancer Res.* 1971;31:830.

82. Sause WT, Cooper JS, Rush S, et al: Fraction size in external beam radiation therapy in the treatment of melanoma. *Int J Radiat Oncol Biol Phys.* 1991;20:429.

83. Syed AMS, Puthawala AA, Neblett D, et al: Transperineal interstitial-intracavitary "Syed-Neblett" applicator in the treatment of carcinoma of the uterine cervix. *Endocurie Hypertherm Oncol.* 1986;2:1.

84. Martinez A, Cox RS, Edmunson GK: A multiple-site perineal applicator (MUPIT) for treatment of prostatic, anorectal, and gynecologic malignancies. *Int J Radiat Oncol Biol Phys.* 1984;10:297.

85. Stock RG, Chan K, Terk M, et al: A new technique for performing Syed-Neblett template interstitial implants for gynecologic malignancies using transrectal-ultrasound guidance. *Int J Radiat Oncol Biol Phys.* 1997;37:819.

86. Disaia PJ, Creasman WT: *Clinical Gynecologic Oncology.* 4th ed. St. Louis: Mosby-Year Book; 1993:273.

87. Monk BJ, Walker JL, Tewari K, et al: Open interstitial brachytherapy for the treatment of local-regional recurrences of the uterine corpus and cervix cancer after primary surgery. *Gynecol Oncol.* 1994;52:222.

88. Corn BW, Lanciano RM, Rosenblum N, et al: Improved treatment planning for the Syed-Neblett template using endorectal-coil magnetic resonance and intraoperative (laparotomy/laparoscopy) guidance: A new integrated technique for hysterectomized women with vaginal tumors. *Gynecol Oncol.* 1995;56:255.

89. Subak LL, Hricak H, Powell CB, et al: Cervical carcinoma: Computed tomography and magnetic resonance imaging for preoperative staging. *Obstet Gynecol.* 1995;86:43.

90. Hintz BL, Kagan AR, Chan P, et al: Radiation tolerance of the vaginal mucosa. *Int J Radiat Oncol Biol Phys.* 1980;6:711.

90a. Kucera H, Mock U, Knocke TH, et al: Radiotherapy for invasive vaginal cancer: Outcome with intracavitary high dose rate brachytherapy versus conventional low dose rate brachytherapy. *Acta Obstet Gynecol Scand.* 2001;80:355.

91. Marcus RB, Million RR, Daly JW: Carcinoma of the vagina. *Cancer.* 1978;42:2507.

91a. Gore E, Gillin MT, Albano , et al: Comparison of high dose rate and low dose rate dose distribution for vaginal cylinders. *Int J Radiat Oncol Biol Phys.* 1995;31:165.

92. Reddy S, Lee MS, Graham JE, et al: Radiation therapy in primary carcinoma of the vagina. *Gynecol Oncol.* 1987;26:19.

93. Tyree WE, Cardenes H, Randall M, et al: High dose rate brachytherapy for vaginal cancer: Learning from treatment complications. *Int J Gynecol Cancer.* 2002;12:27.

94. Williams JA, Clarke D, Dennis WA, et al: The treatment of pelvic soft tissue radiation necrosis with hyperbaric oxygen. *Am J Obstet Gynecol.* 1992;167:412.

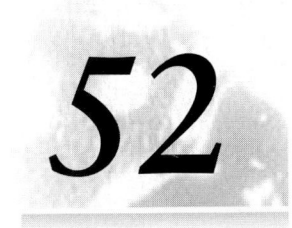

Cancer of the Vulva

Anthony H. Russell, MD

The middle third of the 20th century witnessed remarkable progress in the surgical treatment of vulvar cancer. During the 1940s and 1950s, radical vulvectomy in continuity with bilateral inguinal, femoral, and selective pelvic lymphadenectomy emerged as the standard of operative therapy and succeeded in more than doubling the cure rates previously obtained by less comprehensive surgical strategies.[1-4] Initially, this operation was accompanied by substantial risk of perioperative mortality, as well as long, difficult periods of recuperation. Refinements in surgical technique, including primary closure of the perineal wound, shortened the duration of hospitalization and recovery. Reported at rates of 6% to 19% by the pioneers of radical vulvar surgery,[3,5] total operative and postoperative deaths had declined to a rate less than 4% by the 1970s,[6,7] and select patients with locally extensive disease were being treated by anterior, posterior, or total pelvic exenteration with salvage rates exceeding 50% when regional nodes were found to be free of metastatic involvement.[8] Radiation was infrequently used and largely restricted to palliative treatment. In retrospect, radiotherapy was administered using naive dose and fractionation schedules as well as techniques of limited sophistication.[9-11]

The past 30 years have witnessed a series of remarkable transformations in the treatment of this disease. Due to the success of radical vulvar surgery, substantial numbers of patients treated and followed in large regional referral centers became available for the assessment of treatment outcomes, including chronic morbidities of surgical therapy. Leg lymphedema following radical groin and pelvic node dissection may be temporary, lasting a year or longer, or may be permanent, massive, and disabling.[6,12] Pelvic relaxation, organ prolapse, and urinary incontinence can develop in some patients, particularly when removal of the distal urethra or a portion of the lower vagina is required. Significant vaginal introital stenosis can occur. Absence of the vulva and venereal fat can have the functional consequence of shortening the effective vaginal depth and removing a protective cushion from the pubic arch, contributing to dyspareunia in many patients. Clitorectomy will profoundly diminish capacity for arousal and climax. The psychosexual consequences of vulvectomy are frequently devastating.[13-15]

The clinical extent of vulvar cancer at the time of diagnosis may be decreasing, possibly consequent to enlightened attitudes toward the pathogenesis of the disease and improved use of health care resources.

Among operable patients undergoing radical groin dissection, the frequency of lymph node metastasis has fallen from 50% to 60% at mid-20th century[2,4] to 30% in surgical literature from the 1980s.[16-20] Younger, sexually active patients are being diagnosed with preinvasive disease or unifocal disease of minimal volume and depth of invasion, often with regional nodes free of metastatic contamination.[21] Modifications in the surgical approach to vulvar cancer have been provoked by concerns about the chronic morbidities of ablative surgery in patients with disease of limited extent. In select individuals, limited vulvar and groin surgery can accomplish equivalent cancer control as more extensive surgery, with less functional loss and mutilation.[22-24] Judicious use of adjuvant postoperative radiation has reduced regional relapse, improved survival, and decreased the indications for pelvic lymphadenectomy.[25] Planned in coordination with surgery of reduced extent, preoperative or postoperative radiation (alone or with concurrent chemotherapy) has permitted salvage of patients who would otherwise have required exenterative surgery for cure, thus preserving sexual, urinary, and anorectal function often sacrificed in the era of radical surgical monotherapy.[25-40] Extrapolating from the success achieved in fashioning effective conservative therapy for patients with carcinoma of the anal canal, synchronous chemotherapy and radiation in reduced dose have accomplished curative nonsurgical management of some patients with massive, unresectable vulvar disease and of other patients judged too frail for extensive surgical intervention.[40-45] A proliferation of management options now permits treatment responsibly tailored to the initial volume and extent of disease; the presence or absence of defined clinical and histopathological prognostic factors; and the age, anatomy, personality, and priorities of the individual patient. This chapter reviews the essential elements of these contemporary therapeutic strategies.

EPIDEMIOLOGY

Vulvar malignancies constitute less than 5% of female genital tract cancer, and only 1% to 2% of cancer in women. Cancer of the vulva is most commonly observed in the seventh and eighth decades of life, but the age-specific incidence rates in the United States rise steeply at age 70 and continue to rise beyond age 80.[46] The coincidence of vulvar intraepithelial neoplasia (VIN) or invasive squamous carcinoma of the vulva with in situ or invasive epidermoid carcinoma of the cervix has long been noted, and synchronous or sequential (usually antecedent) cervical lesions may be present in as many as 20% of women with primary vulvar lesions, suggesting a common etiology in at least some patients.[47-53] Following conservative local excision, local-regional cancer re-growth, sometimes at anatomically distinct structures within conserved vulvar tissues and therefore plausibly representing metachronous appearance of independent primaries, lends credence to the so-called "field change" model of oncogenesis.[54] Additional risk factors for the development of invasive vulvar cancer include a history of condyloma acuminatum, VIN, smoking, and chronic vulvar dystrophies, particularly lichen sclerosus.[55-58]

A rising incidence of VIN and reports of invasive vulvar cancer in young patients may reflect changing sexual mores and transmission of the human papilloma virus (HPV). Detection of HPV in VIN or invasive disease is most common in young patients and less frequent as a function of advancing age.[59,60] Invasive vulvar cancer has been reported in young patients with both naturally occurring and iatrogenic immune compromise.[61-65] Patients infected with the human immunodeficiency virus (HIV) are much more likely to have HPV infection than HIV-uninfected women and may be more vulnerable to development of VIN than HIV negative controls. VIN may be more difficult to clear in HIV-infected women and may progress to invasive disease with greater rapidity.[66,67] Recent detection of HIV in 4 of 18 young (age younger than 50) vulvar cancer patients from an inner city population raises the spectre of rising rates of vulvar as well as cervical cancer as the AIDS epidemic unfolds.[68]

Vulvar carcinoma frequently coexists with vulvar dystrophy, particularly in older women.[70,71] However, it is unknown whether lesions such as lichen sclerosus and typical or atypical hyperplastic dystrophy are true precursor lesions. Cancers in these older patients are much less commonly associated with HPV infection, leading to the hypothesis that patients with vulvar cancer may be segregated into two broad groups: an older population with cancer arising in association with vulvar dystrophy and unassociated with HPV, and a younger population with HPV-associated tumors frequently adjacent to areas of VIN.[58,72]

ANATOMY

The vulva is composed of the mons veneris; labia majora; labia minora; clitoris, and vulvar vestibule, which harbors the urethral meatus and is bounded by the vaginal introitus (Fig. 52-1). The labia, limited laterally by the labiocrural folds, are the female analogue of the male scrotum and are pigmented and covered by hair lateral to the crests of the labia majora. Medially, the skin of the labia majora is smooth and hairless, with underlying sebaceous glands. Between the labia majora lie the hairless labia minora, whose medial skin also contains multiple sebaceous glands. Coursing posteromedially, the labia minora taper and join in a fold called the posterior fourchette. Anteriorly, the labia minora taper, then split

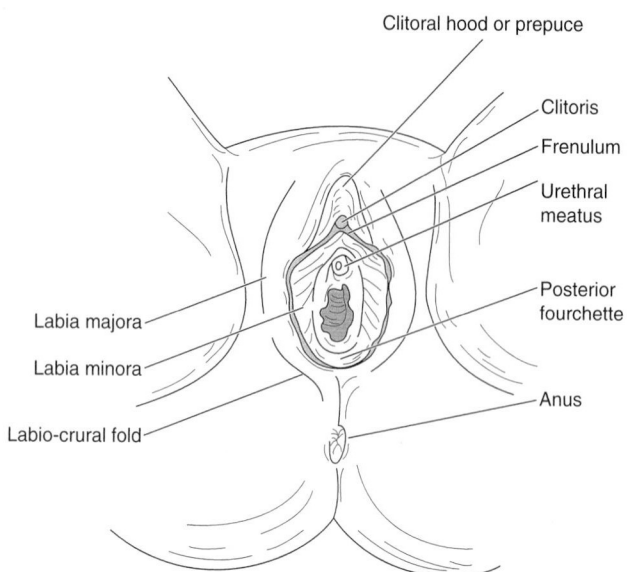

Figure 52–1. External anatomy of the vulva and perineum.

to envelop the clitoris, fusing in front of the clitoris to form the prepuce, and behind the clitoris to form the frenulum. The clitoris, an erectile organ analogous to the penis in the male, is composed of the glans and a body consisting of two corpora cavernosa that diverge into the two crura which lie attached to the undersurface of the pubic rami. The paired, mucus-secreting Bartholin glands lie deep to the posterior labia majora and drain by a simple duct to the vulvar vestibule between the hymenal membrane and the medial borders of the labia minora. The arterial supply of the vulva is formed by branches of the pudendal artery, and the innervation of the vulva and adjacent perineum is by the second through fourth sacral nerves via the pudendal nerves and the first and second lumbar nerves via genitofemoral and ileoinguinal nerves.

The lymphatics of the vulva are constituted by a network that covers the entire labia minora, fourchette, prepuce, and distal vagina below the hymenal membrane. These coalesce anteriorly, forming larger trunks, which run lateral to the clitoris to the mons veneris, acquiring tributaries from the lymphatics of the labia majora, which run in a parallel fashion anteriorly from the perineal body (Fig. 52-2). The vulvar lymphatics run through the vulva and do not cross the labiocrural fold. The lymphatics of the perineum, however, course lateral to the labiocrural fold through the superficial tissues of the upper medial thigh. In the treatment of patients with advanced vulvar cancer that extends beyond the vulva to the perineal skin or anus, these more lateral channels must be addressed. Similarly, extension of an advanced vulvovaginal cancer along the vaginal cylinder proximal to the hymenal ring implies attention to the direct pelvic lymphatic flow of the middle and upper vagina. At the mons veneris, the vulvar lymphatic trunks deviate laterally to the primary regional nodes, the ipsilateral or contralateral inguinal nodes. Study of the localization of radiolabeled tracer in regional lymph nodes after focal injection of discrete sites in the vulva and on the perineum reveals that the lymphatic drainage of the perineum, clitoris, and anterior labia minora is bilateral,

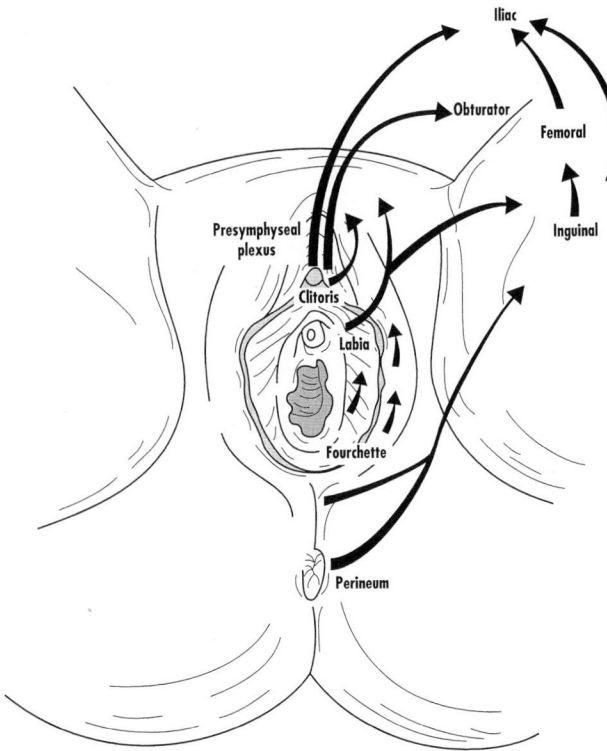

Figure 52-2. Lymphatic channels of the vulva and perineum.

direct lymphatic channels from the clitoris and anterior vulva to the femoral nodes exist, and although occasional patients with metastatic spread to the femoral nodes without inguinal nodal metastasis have been reported,[75,80-82] this is rare. Metastatic spread to pelvic nodes will be found in approximately 15% to 25% of patients with groin node metastasis, but only very rarely without involvement of the inguinal or femoral nodes.[6,7,17,24,73-88] The node of Cloquet, also called Rosenmüller's node, is the most cephalad of the femoral nodes, often lying in the femoral canal below Poupart's (inguinal) ligament. Metastasis to Cloquet's node is considered a herald of pelvic node contamination and a harbinger of distant dissemination.

PATHOLOGY

Malignant melanoma, adult and embryonal sarcomas of varied histologies, Merkel cell tumors, histiocytosis X, Kaposi's sarcoma, hemangiopericytoma, lymphoma, eccrine carcinoma, primary breast cancers, basal cell carcinomas, adenocarcinomas, and adenoid cystic carcinomas (usually arising within Bartholin's glands), as well as other histological tumor types have all been reported as primary malignancies arising from the vulva.[89] However, more than 85% of invasive vulvar malignancies are epidermoid carcinomas,[90] leading to the common practice of using the terms *squamous carcinoma of the vulva* (Fig. 52-4) and *vulvar carcinoma* synonymously. Because of distinctive histopathology and characteristic clinical behaviors, it is important to recognize verrucous carcinoma (Fig. 52-5)[91-94] and so-called "spray" pattern carcinomas (Fig. 52-6)[95,96] as variants of squamous carcinoma representing polar extremes in biological behavior. Verrucous cancer may resemble cauliflower in gross appearance, with a predominantly exophytic pattern of growth. Histologically characterized by well differentiated cells with a broad, pushing interface between cancer and surrounding stroma, verrucous cancer uncommonly metastasizes to regional lymph nodes, even when quite

whereas the lymph flow from well-lateralized sites in the vulva is, predominantly, to the ipsilateral groin.[73] Discrete (≤2 cm-diameter), well-lateralized primary cancers limited to the vulva and not approaching midline structures rarely manifest spread to contralateral groin nodes in the absence of spread to ipsilateral nodes.[23,24,74-77] From the superficial inguinal nodes, secondary lymphatic drainage is through the cribriform fascia to the deep inguinal or femoral nodes, with subsequent tertiary flow under the inguinal ligaments to the deep pelvic (external iliac) nodes (Fig. 52-3). Although direct lymphatic channels from the clitoris to the deep pelvic nodes have been described, these pathways are of limited clinical significance.[16,78,79] Similarly,

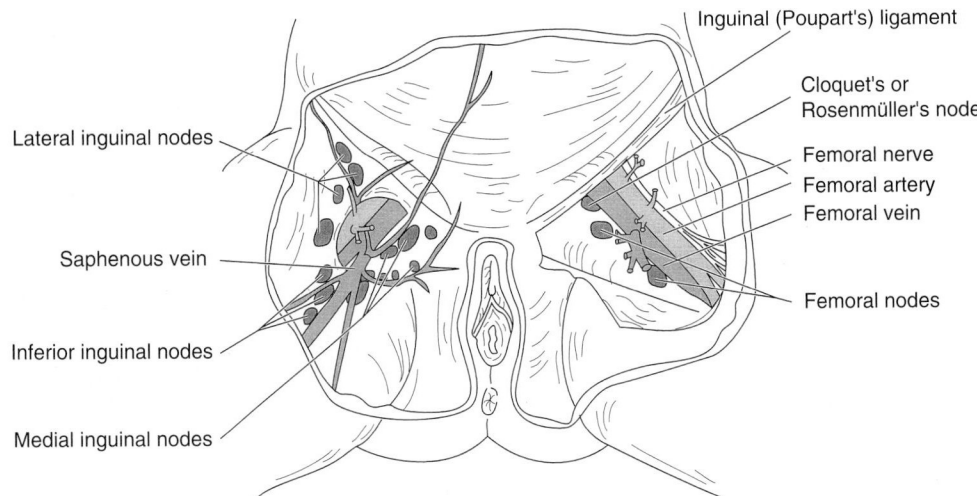

Figure 52-3. Superficial and deep groin dissections illustrating the relationship between nodal groups and major vessels, femoral nerves, and inguinal ligaments.

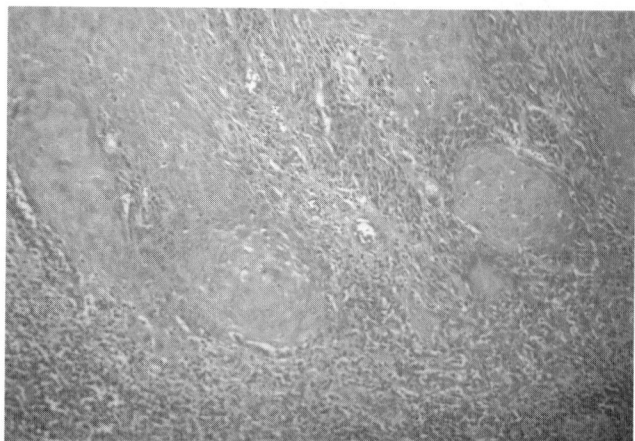

Figure 52–4. Photomicrograph of well-differentiated squamous cancer of the vulva. (Courtesy of Dr. Richard Oi.)

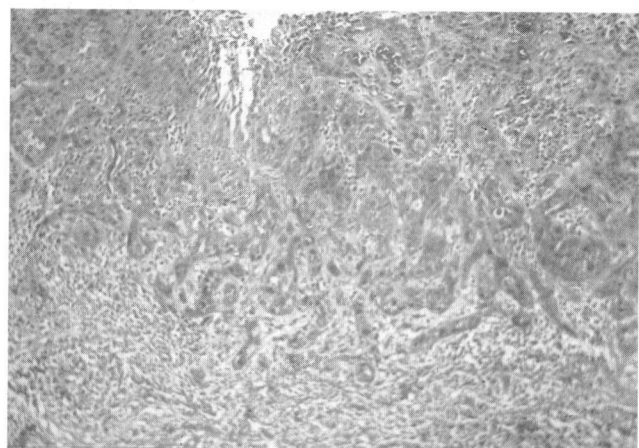

Figure 52–6. Photomicrograph of squamous cancer of the vulva with an infiltrative pattern of invasion. A trabecular growth architecture often associated with finger-like projections of tumor into surrounding stroma and discontiguous islands or satellites of malignant cells, this type of invasion is sometimes called a "spray" pattern, and is associated with a high risk of dissemination to lymph nodes and satellite metastases within dermal lymphatic channels. (Courtesy of Dr. Richard Oi.)

large, but often recurs locally after surgical therapy. Squamous cancers with finger-like microscopic projections, or a "spray" histological appearance, often have a trabecular architecture of poorly differentiated cells with separate islands or discontiguous satellites of tumor cells in proximity to the infiltrative interface between the main tumor mass and surrounding stroma. These cancers may metastasize to regional nodes even when quite small and may recur at the skin margins of surgical resection as well as relapsing distantly.

CLINICAL PRESENTATION

Pruritis or a localized sore are common presenting symptoms. Burning after urination may occur when urine comes in contact with areas of epithelial destruction and inflammation. Spotting and serous oozing may be noticed by the patient, but major hemorrhage is unusual. Most vulvar cancers arise in the labia, with only 15% involving the clitoris. The tumor is often exophytic, with a raised velvety red appearance, although centrally ulcerated lesions undermining surrounding skin may also be seen. Vulvar cancer may coexist with and mimic the gross appearance of

venereal warts (condyloma acuminatum), which may result in neglect by the patient or delay in diagnosis (Fig. 52-7).

ROUTES OF SPREAD

Vulvar cancer involves adjacent structures by direct extension. Invasion of the vagina is common (stage T3), often in conjunction with involvement of the distal urethra. When vaginal involvement is extensive, invasion of the bladder may be observed, or destruction of the

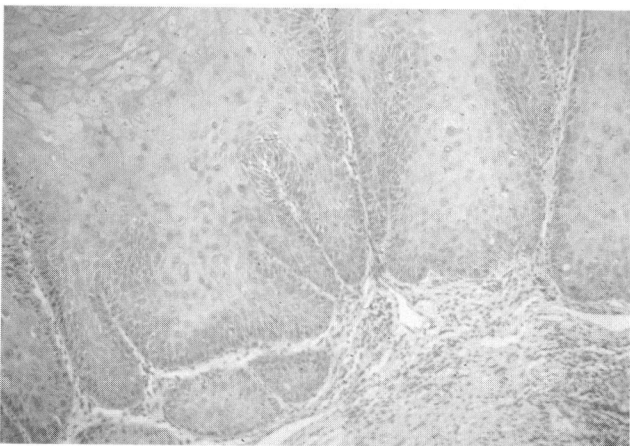

Figure 52–5. Photomicrograph of verrucous cancer of the vulva. The interface of the tumor and surrounding stroma is characterized by a broad, bulbous, pushing front. (Courtesy of Dr. Richard Oi.)

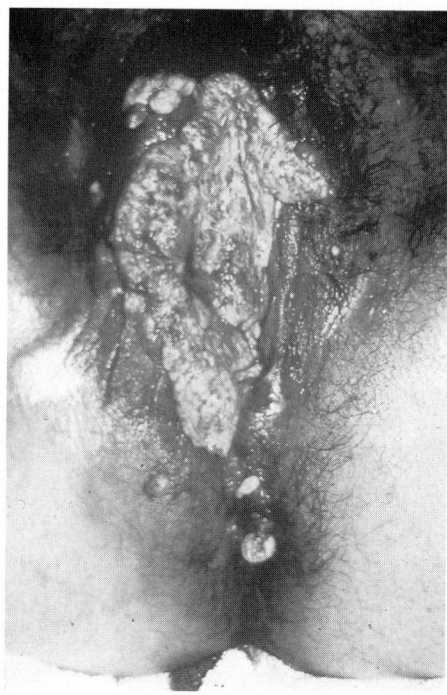

Figure 52–7. Clinical appearance of locally advanced vulvar cancer in association with condyloma acuminatum. Prior diagnosis of venereal warts resulted in delay in the diagnosis of subsequent malignancy.

rectovaginal septum with involvement of the rectal mucosa (stage T4). Extension to the perineum is frequent, often with involvement of anal or perianal skin. Extensive lesions may invade the anal sphincter. Satellite lesions in adjacent skin may occur, presumably by transit through dermal lymphatics. Rarely, extensive permeation of regional dermal lymphatics presents a picture analogous to peau d'orange of the skin of the breast (Fig. 52-8). The earliest non-contiguous spread is to regional lymph nodes in the groin, which will be contaminated in approximately 30% of patients with operable vulvar cancer. Pelvic lymph nodes represent the second echelon of lymphatic spread and are involved in 15% to 25% of patients with groin node metastasis but rarely in the absence of metastasis to inguinofemoral nodes. Remote, hematogenous dissemination is infrequent at the time of diagnosis. The lung is the most frequent site of distant metastatic spread; however, pulmonary metastases are rare in the absence of extensive primary or regional nodal disease. Following initial therapy, most treatment failures are local-regional. Distant metastasis without prior local-regional recurrence is uncommon.

DIAGNOSTIC ASSESSMENTS

The joint 2002 staging system (Table 52-1) of the Fédération Internationale de Gynécologie et d'Obstétrique (FIGO), the American Joint Committee on Cancer (AJCC), and the Union Internationale Contre le Cancer (UICC) is a mixed clinical, surgical, and histopathological staging system that relies on clinical examination and selected biopsies for the assignment of T stage and the results of biopsies or therapeutic node dissection for the assignment of N stage. In patients with potentially operable squamous vulvar cancer, preoperative assessment is limited to routine blood work and chest radiography. For patients with clinically apparent groin node metastases, an abdominopelvic computed tomography (CT) scan is used to assess possible spread to pelvic or upper retroperitoneal lymph nodes. A patient who will be treated with all or partial initial radiation must undergo a pelvic

Table 52–1 Classification of Cancer of the Vulva

T: Primary Tumor

TX	Primary tumor cannot be assessed
T0	No evidence of primary tumor
Tis	Carcinoma in situ (preinvasive carcinoma)
T1	Tumor confined to the vulva and perineum* ≤2 cm in greatest dimension
T1a	Tumor confined to the vulva or vulva and perineum, ≤2 cm in greatest dimension, and with stromal invasion ≤1 mm†
T1b	Tumor confined to the vulva or vulva and perineum, ≤2 cm in greatest dimension, with stromal invasion >1 mm†
T2	Tumor confined to the vulva and perineum* >2 cm in greatest dimension
T3	Tumor of any size with adjacent spread to one or more of the following: lower urethra, vagina, or anus
T4	Tumor of any size invading any of the following: the upper urethral mucosa, the bladder mucosa, the rectal mucosa, or tumor fixed to the bone

N: Regional Lymph Nodes‡

N0	No nodal metastases
N1	Unilateral regional lymph node metastasis
N2	Bilateral regional lymph node metastasis

M: Distant Metastasis

M0	No evidence of distant metastasis
M1	Any distant metastasis including pelvic lymph nodes

FIGO/AJCC/UICC	Stage Grouping
0	TisN0M0
I	T1N0M0
II	T2N0M0
III	T3N0M0
	T1,2,3N1M0
IVA	T1,2,3N2M0
	T4NxM0
IVB	TxNxM1

*Note that lesions extending onto the perineum were previously classified as T3.
†The depth of invasion is defined as the measurement of the tumor from the epithelial-stromal junction of the adjacent most superficial dermal papilla to the deepest point of invasion.
‡Note that assessment of inguinofemoral nodes is now histological.
From Greene FL, Page DL, Fleming ID, et al (eds): *AJCC Cancer Strains Manual*, 6/E. New York, Springer-Verlag, 2002; FIGO, Fédération Intérnationale de Gynécologie et d'Obstétrique; UICC, Union Internationale Contre le Cancer; x, any T or N category.

CT scan both to screen for gross pelvic adenopathy and to conduct dosimetric planning of radiotherapy directed to the inguinofemoral nodes. Magnetic resonance imaging (MRI) may be helpful in establishing extent of invasion of the primary tumor. No other radiographic imaging studies have an established role in the routine management of squamous vulvar cancer.

Identification of sentinel lymph nodes by lymphoscintigraphy or isosulfan blue intradermal injection or both is an area of active clinical investigation.[97-100] Lymphatic mapping may be helpful for selection of patients with lateralized primary cancers in whom treatment of the ipsilateral groin may suffice. Depending on surgical philosophy and the threshold for use of adjunctive therapies, confirmation of sentinel lymph node metastasis may alter the extent of surgical therapy both for patients with squamous cancers

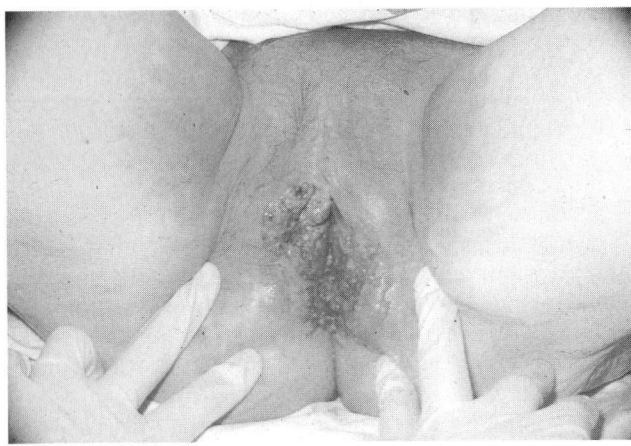

Figure 52–8. Pretreatment photograph of a patient with locally advanced squamous cancer of the vulva and extensive, biopsy-confirmed infiltration of the dermal lymphatics of the perineum, upper medial thighs, and mons (peau d'orange).

of the vulva and those with melanoma. However, credible consensus treatment algorithms, based on sentinel node identification and biopsy, are not yet developed.

Positron emission tomography (PET) may be useful in evaluating patients with vulvar melanoma for distant metastases. A role for PET in squamous cancer has not been established. Preliminary evidence suggests relative insensitivity in detection of nodal metastases in the groins (67%), but a high specificity (95%).[101] A negative groin PET alone should thus not exempt a patient from some form of therapy directed to the regional nodes. A positive study, particularly in a patient to be treated with definitive or preoperative radiation-based therapy, may assist in the selection of target volume and radiotherapy dose.

STANDARD THERAPEUTIC APPROACHES

Surgery

For approximately 40 years, en bloc radical vulvectomy and bilateral regional lymphadenectomy (inguinofemoral ± pelvic), using a single "butterfly" or trapezoidal incision, was the standard of care for patients with operable carcinoma of the vulva. The most common postoperative complication, frequently responsible for prolonged hospitalization and delayed recovery, is breakdown of the surgical wound in the groin. This complication is markedly reduced in frequency and severity by performance of the vulvectomy and the groin dissections through separate incisions, which serves to reduce tension on the skin flaps, preserve vascular supply, and improve the probability of primary healing.[102,103] This refinement in technique, customarily reserved for patients with clinically uninvolved groins, comes at the price of the rare recurrence in the preserved bridge of tissue between the separate incisions. These failures may represent in-transit or retrograde lymphatic metastasis, unlikely events unless groin nodes are contaminated.[102] It is essential to appreciate that much of the classic surgical literature analyzes results using the 1969 staging system of FIGO, which employed clinical evaluation of both the primary tumor and the groin nodes (Table 52-2). In 1989, FIGO adopted modifications to this staging system, resulting in a hybrid, clinicopathologic staging system that incorporated the results of histological assessment of regional nodes, thus acknowledging the importance of nodal status in determining prognosis and therapy and recognizing the inaccuracies of clinical assessment of the regional lymph nodes by palpation. Approximately 20% of patients with clinically uninvolved groin nodes (1969 FIGO N0,1) have histological evidence of groin metastasis if subjected to radical groin dissection.[3,7,17,83,85,104] Approximately 22% of patients with clinically suspicious groin nodes (1969 FIGO N2,3) show no histological evidence of nodal spread if the groin nodes are dissected (Table 52-3).[3,7,83,85,104] The risk of clinically occult involvement of inguinofemoral nodes in patients with palpably normal groins is tabulated by primary tumor size and T category in Table 52-4.

The prognosis of surgically treated vulvar cancer is directly related to the presence or absence of regional

Table 52–2 FIGO 1969 TNM Classification and Stage Grouping

T:	Primary Tumor
Tis	Preinvasive carcinoma (carcinoma-in-situ)
T1	Tumor confined to the vulva, ≤2 cm in greatest dimension
T2	Tumor confined to the vulva, >2 cm in greatest dimension
T3	Tumor of any size with adjacent spread to one or more of the following: the urethra, vagina, perineum, or anus
T4	Tumor of any size invading any of the following: the upper urethral mucosa, the bladder mucosa, the rectal mucosa; or tumor fixed to the bone
N:	**Regional Lymph Nodes**
N0	No nodes palpable
N1	Nodes palpable in either groin, not enlarged, mobile (not clinically suspicious of neoplasm)
N2	Nodes palpable in one or both groins, enlarged, firm, and mobile (clinically suspicious of neoplasm)
N3	Fixed or ulcerated nodes
M:	**Distant Metastases**
M0	No clinical metastases
M1a	Palpable pelvic lymph nodes
M1b	Other distant metastases
FIGO	**Stage:**
0:	Tis
I:	T1N0,1M0
	T2N0,1M0
III:	T1,2N2M0
	T3N0,1,2M0
IV:	TxN3M0
	T4N0,1,2M0
	TxNxM1a
	TxNxM1b

x, denotes any T or N category.

node metastasis, the extent of lymph node infestation, and the anatomic level of nodal involvement. Five-year disease-free survival probability is approximately 95% for patients with T1,2N0 tumors,[7,105] decreasing to approximately 70% for stage T3N0.[7] Metastasis to a single node is prognostically less ominous than involvement of multiple nodes.[16,18] Patients with unilateral node metastasis fare better than those with bilateral spread,[104] and 5-year disease-free survival drops to approximately 40% when multiple nodes are involved. Approximately 20% of patients with pelvic (iliac) node metastasis can be cured by locoregional therapies (surgery, radiation, or combined modality therapy).[6,7,16,83,84,87,106]

Tumor size, depth of invasion, presence of vascular or lymphatic space invasion, pattern of tumor growth and invasion, and histologic grade seem to be important predictors of lymph node spread as well as prognosis, although there is no consensus concerning the relative importance of each parameter in multivariant analysis.[81,88,100,105,107] Surgical specimens from patients with primary tumors 2 cm or less in diameter (T1) clearly show escalating risk of node metastasis with progressive depth of invasion (Table 52-5).[24,75,76,82,101,108] Probability of finding groin node metastasis is related to the size of the primary tumor, as shown in Table 52-6.[109,110]

Table 52–3   Assessment of Inguinofemoral Nodes by Palpation*

	Histologically (−), n (%)	Histologically (+), n (%)
Clinically (−)		
1969 FIGO N0,1 n = 451 patients	363 (80.5)	88 (19.5)
Clinically (+)		
1969 FIGO N2,3 n = 243 patients	53 (21.8)	190 (78.2)

*Pooled data, six institutions.[3,7,17,83,85,104]

Table 52–5   Incidence of Groin Node Metastasis Correlated with Depth of Invasion for Primary Tumors ≤2 cm*

Depth of Invasion, mm	Patients, n	Positive Nodes, n	%
≤1	120	0	0
1.1-2	121	8	6.6
2.1-3	97	8	8.2
3.1-4	50	11	22
4.1-5	40	10	25
>5	32	12	37.5

*Pooled data, six series.[24,75,76,82,96,108]
Modified from Hacker NF: Current treatment of small vulvar cancers. *Oncology.* 1990;4:21.

An infiltrative pattern of growth correlates with nodal spread,[81,100] and the presence of vascular or lymphatic space invasion substantially escalates the probability of finding metastases in dissected nodes.[109] The presence of metastatic spread to contralateral groin nodes in the absence of disease in ipsilateral nodes occurs in 15% or less of all patients with metastases to groin nodes,[86] generally in patients with larger lesions. Although described in two patients with lateralized T1 lesions,[51] the risk of contralateral nodal spread in the absence of ipsilateral metastasis is less than 1%.[22,24,74,75,77,82] When metastatic disease is present in multiple groin nodes, pelvic lymphadenectomy will detect disease in 15% to 25% of patients,[6,7,17,25,83-88] but rarely when only one groin node is microscopically contaminated.[16,18] A thoughtful appraisal of the risk of nodal spread and the anatomical level of potential contamination is an essential part of determining target volume, dose, and technique for a course of radiation therapy, whether the radiation is given preoperatively, postoperatively, or as primary treatment.

Integration of radiation and surgery for optimal outcomes requires an understanding of the strengths and limitations of primary surgical treatment and the extent of operative therapy to be performed. Surgical strategy is predicated on primary tumor parameters, clinical assessment of the groin nodes, the status of adjacent tissues, patient age and vigor, and patient preference. Based on an appreciation of clinicopathologic risk factors and an ability to identify patients who have minimal risk of nodal spread, wide local excision (employing a clinical margin of at least 1.0 cm in all dimensions) without node dissection has been reported to be a sensible surgical option for select patients with discrete tumors, 2 cm or less in diameter, with 1 mm or less of invasion and without an infiltrating or "spray" pattern of growth. Provided the surgical margins are adequate, local recurrence will be observed in only 5% of such patients.[22,24,75,77] Wide local excision may be appropriate for patients with larger or more deeply invasive primary tumors, but it should be accompanied by at least ipsilateral groin dissection. For patients with well-lateralized T1 primary tumors, contralateral groin dissection may be omitted unless there is spread to more than one node in the ipsilateral groin.[23-25,74-77,111] Unless conservation of the clitoris and sexual function are of major importance to the patient, radical vulvectomy will generally be the most appropriate surgical management of the primary tumor for patients with multifocal invasive vulvar cancer, extensive VIN, or vulvar dystrophy that has been unresponsive to topical steroids.

The best clinical predictor of local recurrence is the adequacy of the surgical margin.[112] An 8-mm margin in fixed tissue, corresponding to a clinical margin of 1 cm, is a useful guide in planning conservative surgery for

Table 52–4   Probability of Clinically Occult Metastasis to Inguinofemoral Lymph Nodes Correlated with Primary Tumor Category and Size

T Stage (1992 FIGO)	N0* (1969 FIGO) n (%)	N1* (1969 FIGO) n (%)	Total n (%)
T1	13/84 (15.5)	3/21 (14.3)	16/105 (15.2)
T2	17/56 (30.4)	4/14 (28.5)	21/70 (30)
T3	11/38 (28.9)	1/11 (9.1)	12/49 (24.4)
T4	0/1	0/0	0/1
Total	41/179 (22.9)	8/46 (17.4)	49/225 (21.7)
Clinical Tumor Size cm			
0-1.0	3/39 (7.7)	0/4	3/43 (7)
1.1-2.0	11/46 (23.9)	3/17 (17.6)	14/63 (22.2)
2.1-3.0	13/42 (31)	1/10 (10)	14/52 (26.9)
3.1-5.0	12/33 (36.4)	2/8 (25)	14/41 (34.1)
>5.0	1/10 (10)	2/5 (40)	3/15 (20)
Total†	40/170 (23.5)	8/44 (18.2)	48/214 (22.4)

*N0 denotes no palpable inguinal nodes; N1 denotes nodes palpable, nonsuspicious.
†Clinical tumor measurements not available for all patients.
Data from Gonzalez-Bosquet J, Kinney WK, Russell AH, et al: Risk of occult inguinofemoral lymph node metastasis from squamous carcinoma of the vulva. *Int J Radiat Oncol Biol Phys.* (submitted for publication 2002)

Table 52–6   Primary Tumor Size and Risk of Groin Node Metastasis*

Primary Size, cm	Patients, n	Positive Nodes, n	%
≤2	75	5	6.7
2-4	78	19	24.4
>4	79	26	32.9

*Pooled data, two series.[109,110]

patients with primary tumors that approach or extend to critical normal structures such as the anus, urethra, distal vagina, and clitoris. The distal urethra can be removed with preservation of urinary continence in most patients, although removal of only a portion of the anal sphincter may compromise fecal continence.[113] The risks of both local recurrence and loss of normal tissue function must be judiciously assessed and compared with risks associated with alternative strategies, such as those employing preoperative radiation or chemoradiation with less extensive surgery or chemoradiation alone. Exenterative surgery, even for massive primary disease, should seldom be chosen as initial therapy unless the cancer has already destroyed the functions of the critical normal tissues that might otherwise be preserved. It is rarely appropriate when regional node metastases are present.[8]

Approximately 80% of patients in whom surgical therapy fails suffer recurrences in the residual vulva, on the perineum, at the vaginal introital margin, in the groins or upper thighs, or in the pelvis, and less than 20% have recurrences distantly (Table 52-7).[24,114-119] Parameters that are predictive of locoregional recurrence include the width of the surgical margin, the presence of groin node metastasis, vascular or lymphatic space invasion, and an infiltrative pattern of growth. The presence of one or more of these factors should prompt consideration of adjuvant radiation.

Radiation Therapy

Radiotherapy is increasingly employed in the curative management of vulvar cancer,[26-32] often in conjunction with synchronous administration of radiation potentiating chemotherapy (chemoradiation).[33-44] Radiation salvages some patients with locoregional recurrence after radical vulvectomy and regional node dissection.[120] Postoperative radiation directed to the groins and pelvic nodes improves disease-free survival in patients with metastatic spread to two or more inguinofemoral nodes[25] and may further improve results if residual vulva and perineum are included within the irradiated volume.[121] Preoperative radiation or chemoradiation have reduced the indications for exenterative surgery and may permit a substantial decrease in the volume of normal tissue that must be removed in patients with tumors invading or intimately approximating the anus, clitoris, urethra, and distal vagina.[26-29,31,39,40] Radical chemoradiation provides sensible alternative therapy for patients who are technically unresectable or medically inoperable.[41-44]

Table 52–7 Pattern of Recurrence* in 267 Patients Failing Regional Therapy† for Carcinoma of the Vulva‡

Vulva/Perineum n (%)	Groin n (%)	Pelvis n (%)	Distant n (%)
162 (60.7)	62 (23.2)	42 (15.7)	51 (19.1)

*Due to some patients manifesting recurrence at more than 1 site, the total recurrences exceed 267 and the total of the percentages exceeds 100%.
†The majority of patients underwent radical surgery. Adjunctive radiation was administered in some, and a small number were treated with radiation alone.
‡Pooled data, seven series.[24, 114-119]

SALVAGE RADIATION THERAPY

Postsurgical, central, limited-volume, local recurrence in the residual vulva—at the introital margin or on the perineum—will often be salvaged with secondary surgery, radiation, or combined-modality therapy.[110,114,118-120,122] A disease-free interval of 2 or more years and lack of involvement of regional nodes portend a favorable outcome with salvage therapy.[118] Under circumstances in which the anticipated surgical margin is less than that of the original surgery, when recurrence approaches or involves critical structures, or when the pattern of recurrence is multifocal, it is prudent to plan for delivery of radiation as *at least* a component of the salvage strategy. Regional relapse in the groin or in pelvic nodes is much less likely to be salvaged, regardless of the combination of modalities used.[110,114,118-120] Radiation alone, in doses ranging from 63 Gy to 72 Gy employing progressive volume reductions or partial treatment with brachytherapy, often controls small-volume recurrence. Preoperative radiation ranging in dose from 45 Gy to 54 Gy followed by local excision may be less injurious in terms of delayed normal tissue effects than a high radiation dose to a large perineal volume in the absence of surgery. The majority of patients with vulvar cancer who develop clinical recurrence do so within 2 years of initial therapy,[118] and recurrent disease may grow rapidly. Thus, when a combined approach employing surgery and radiation is planned, it is best to commence with radiation, as residual occult cancer may proliferate more rapidly than the wound heals.

ADJUVANT POSTOPERATIVE RADIOTHERAPY

The Gynecologic Oncology Group conducted a randomized trial comparing pelvic lymphadenectomy with radiotherapy directed to the bilateral groins and pelvic nodes (but not the tumor bed or perineum) in patients who were found to have groin node metastasis. A total of 114 eligible patients were randomized, 40 of whom had only 1 positive groin node. In 15 patients of 53 undergoing pelvic lymphadenectomy, disease had spread to pelvic nodes (28.3%); 9 of these patients (60%) died of cancer within 1 year of study entry. The overall survival advantage for radiation at 2 years (68% for radiation, 54% for pelvic node dissection) was limited to patients with 2 or more involved groin nodes (63% for radiation, 37% for pelvic node dissection) and was attributable to a decrease in recurrence in the groin among the irradiated patients (5.1%) compared with those patients treated by surgery alone (23.6%). Lymphedema was reported in 19% of irradiated patients compared to 11% of patients treated with surgery alone. Of the 44 patients who had recurrence, only 11 patients failed with a component of "distant" disease (including 3 patients with relapse in the thigh, periaortic nodes, and abdominal skin), whereas 75% of relapsing patients failed with locoregional disease alone (vulvar area, groins, or pelvis). Eleven patients experienced recurrence in the unirradiated vulvar area (25%); 10 of these had no other apparent sites of failure. As a consequence of this study, pelvic lymphadenectomy is less likely to be performed and regional adjuvant radiation has become the standard of additional care for patients with metastasis to two or more regional nodes.[25] Because many patients in whom disease spread to regional nodes also have adverse prognostic factors predictive of local relapse, it is sensible to consider inclusion of the primary tumor bed and perineum in the treatment volume when postoperative radiation is administered.[121]

PREOPERATIVE RADIATION THERAPY

Under circumstances in which the extent of the primary disease indicates postoperative radiation, it is reasonable to consider preoperative radiation, particularly if it has the potential to reduce the scope of surgery and to conserve normal tissue structure and function or to convert the status of the patient from unresectable to operable.[26-31,39,40] An anticipated clinical margin of 1 cm or less from structures that will not be removed surgically is a useful guide for selecting patients for preoperative radiation. Tumors that encroach on the anal sphincter, abut the pubic arch, or involve more than the distal urethra should be considered for preoperative therapy. Patients with tumors that approach the clitoris or extend more than minimally past the vaginal introitus should also be considered for preoperative irradiation if conservation of sexual function is desired. Moderate-dose radiation (36 Gy to 54 Gy) has been given, followed by excision of residual palpable abnormalities that revealed no evidence of persistent cancer in 50% of cases (Table 52-8).[28-30] External beam radiation is most commonly employed, but interstitial or intracavitary brachytherapy may apply a higher dose to a discrete tissue volume where a surgical margin is anticipated to be inadequate.[27]

The Gynecologic Oncology Group studied 73 patients with stage III to IV squamous cancers of the vulva who were judged not amenable to resection due to local disease extent beyond the conventional boundaries of radical vulvectomy. Preoperative chemoradiation, consisting of 47.6 Gy delivered in fractions of 1.7 Gy, coordinated with 2 cycles of synchronous cisplatin and 5-fluorouracil, converted 69 of 71 patients medically fit for surgery to having lesions considered amenable to resection. Ultimately, urinary and fecal continence was conserved in all but 3 patients. With the use of this approach, local tumor control has been excellent, with conservation of normal tissue integrity in many patients who would otherwise have required exenterative surgery for tumor clearance.[40] Employing the identical regimen in 46 patients with extensive (matted, fixed, or ulcerated) and unresectable groin metastases, clinicians of the Gynecologic Oncology Group were ultimately able to resect groin nodes in 37 patients, 15 of whom had histologically negative groin specimens.[123] The observation of complete histological clearance of malignancy following moderate-dose preoperative radiation (alone or coordinated with synchronous chemotherapy) serves to encourage efforts to control vulvar cancer with radiation-based therapy under circumstances in which surgery is either technically unfeasible or medically contraindicated.

Radical Radiotherapy and Chemoradiation

Definitive radiation has been used to treat medically inoperable or technically unresectable patients. Historically, results have been poor, in terms of both tumor control and normal tissue sequelae, although the tumor control probability for patients with disease of limited volume has approached that of surgery.[11,31,124] The favorable experience with chemotherapy and reduced-dose radiation in the treatment of cancers of the anal canal has prompted increasing use of this approach in the treatment of advanced vulvar cancer. Most published experiences employed fluorouracil (5-FU), with or without cisplatin or mitomycin.[32-41,125-128] Small numbers of reported patients with heterogeneous disease undergoing individualized and quite variable management with chemoradiation, coupled with the small number of such patients available for long-term surveillance, necessarily render any conclusions preliminary. Retrospective study of treatment outcomes comparing chemoradiation with radiation alone suggests improved cancer control with chemoradiation,[128] but prospective randomized data do not exist to validate the clinical impression of better results. Unquestionably, the administration of concurrent chemotherapy augments the acute reaction in normal tissues. Moist desquamation of the vulva necessitates treatment interruption in most patients. Hybrid dose/fractionation regimens have been developed to preserve dose intensity and to maximize potential synergistic effects. Twice-daily fractionation has become a popular strategy to exploit the radiation-drug interaction while minimizing the theoretic disadvantages of split-course radiation that is made mandatory by the enhanced effects in normal tissue.[41,43,44] Frequently, the additional patient and clinician effort necessitated by combined-modality therapy is rewarded by dramatic, rapid tumor regression (Figs. 52-9 and 52-10). Fraction size should not exceed 1.8 Gy, and a fraction size aslow as 1.6 Gy has been recommended to reduce late sequelae.[129] Because of potential enhancement of late normal tissue effects, and because full radiation dose must be administered to some skin when treating what is fundamentally a skin cancer, it is advisable that total dose not exceed approximately 54 Gy in 30 fractions, 59.5 Gy in 35 fractions, or 64 Gy in 40 fractions to gross disease when chemoradiation is used, and that the volume receiving the full dose be as small as possible, while including all areas of initial measurable clinical involvement. Results of 5-FU–based chemoradiation for locally advanced or recurrent vulvar cancer are presented in Table 52-9.

Table 52–8   Histological Tumor Clearance by Preoperative Radiation

Authors	Patients, n	Dose (Gy)	Negative Specimen, n	%
Hacker et al[28]	8*	44-54	4	50
Acosta et al[29]	14	36-55	5	36
Jafari et al[30]	4	30-42	4	100
Total	26	30-55	13	50

*Includes 1 patient who received additional 24 Gy by intravaginal mold.

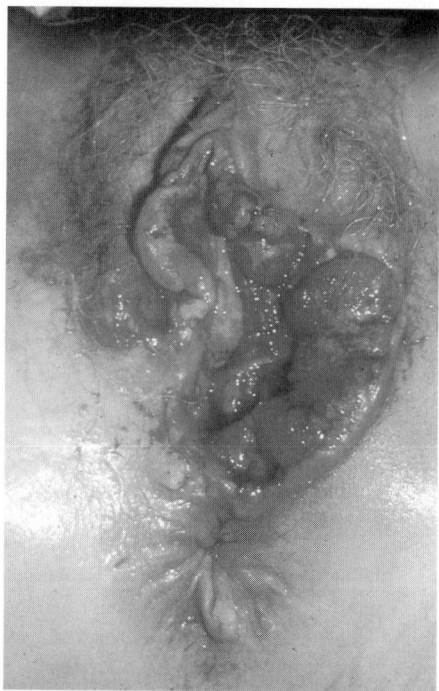

Figure 52–9. Pretreatment photograph of a 57-year-old woman with locoregionally advanced squamous cancer of the vulva. Tumor circumferentially involved the vulva and extended both anteriorly and posteriorly up the vaginal canal almost to the vault. Cancer was adherent to the anal sphincter, but fecal continence was not impaired. Anoscopy revealed tumor extension through the rectovaginal septum to involve a small area of anterior rectal mucosa proximal to the sphincter. Inguinal nodes were considered suspicious for metastasis, and the patient's disease was staged T4N2M0 (1969 FIGO). Total pelvic exenteration and bilateral inguinofemoral lymphadenectomy would have been indicated to attempt surgical clearance. Treatment with chemoradiation was initiated as alternative management.

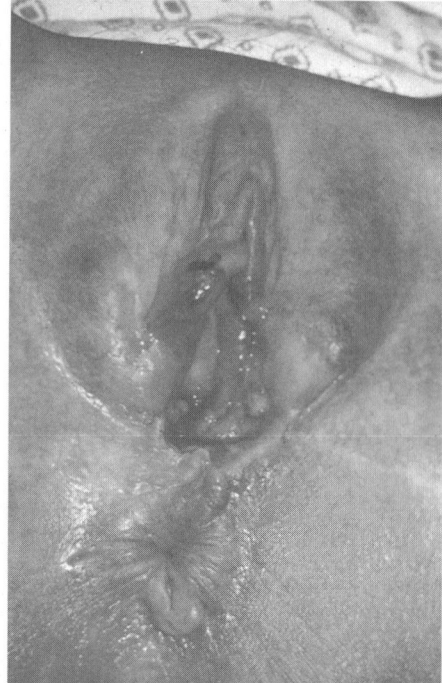

Figure 52–10. Post-treatment photograph of the same patient shown in Figure 52-9 5 weeks following chemoradiation. A dose of 36 Gy was administered to a volume at risk for occult, microscopic disease. With reduced volumes, 50 Gy was administered to the initial volume of gross disease. Three cycles of fluorouracil and cisplatin were administered concurrent with radiation. Suspected residual disease involving the posterior fourchette was removed by limited local excision sparing the anal sphincter. Scattered foci of neoplastic cells of questionable viability were found surrounded by a primarily fibrous stroma. The patient remained continent and continuously cancer-free more than 10 years following completion of treatment.

Elective Groin Radiation

A contributing factor to perioperative complications and chronic morbidity is the dissection of the inguinofemoral nodes. Postoperative wound breakdown is frequent, and chronic lymphedema is a common consequence of radical surgical treatment of the groins.[130] In select patients with limited primary tumors, omission of the node dissection is prudent. In others, limiting the groin dissection to nodes superficial to the cribriform fascia (if clinically and histopathologically negative) has been an effective strategy for reducing acute and chronic surgical morbidity. Dissection of the groin nodes through a separate incision from that used to remove the vulvar primary tumor substantially reduces the probability of wound dehiscence. Elective irradiation of clinically negative groins is an alternative strategy that has the theoretical advantage of treating *all* of the regional nodes rather than leaving all, or some portion, untreated. This approach may also be applicable to patients with locally advanced primary tumors, in whom less than radical bilateral groin dissection would be inadequate surgical therapy. Several series[27,32,131-134] have reported favorable results with elective or prophylactic groin irradiation (Table 52-10) but frequently in the setting in which groin nodes would be expected to be histologically uninvolved if treated surgically (e.g., T1,2 primary tumors of limited extent) (see Table 52-4).[134,135]

The Gynecologic Oncology Group, in a randomized trial, compared groin irradiation with groin surgery in select patients with vulvar cancer.[136] The study was terminated early because of an unacceptable rate of groin node failures (5/27 patients, 18.5%) observed in the group assigned to radiation. Technical inadequacies in radiation administration may have inadvertently caused substantial underdosage of inguinofemoral nodes, resulting in the observed failures.[137] Chemoradiation[138,139] may be a mechanism to improve the results of elective groin irradiation (see Table 52-10), but the simplest expedient is to deliver treatment with adequate dose distribution to the tissues at risk. At the Radiation Oncology Center in Sacramento, 23 previously untreated patients with locally advanced primary squamous cancers of the vulva (stages T2 [n = 2], T3 [n = 20], T4 [n = 1]) and clinically negative groin nodes have electively undergone chemoradiation to a volume that included the inguinofemoral nodes, without subsequent surgical therapy to the groins. No patient has suffered relapse in an irradiated groin.[138] Among 17 similar patients (stages T2 [n = 4], T3 [n = 13]) undergoing elective groin chemoradiation at Loma Linda University Medical Center, no patient has experienced groin relapse.[139] Elective groin irradiation is likely

Table 52–9 Results of Radical Chemoradiation for Locoregionally Advanced or Recurrent Cancers of the Vulva

Authors	Patients, Stages (n)	Drugs	Radiation Dose, Gy	Complete Response, n (%)	Subsequent Failure, n (%)*	NED F/U, mo†
Previously Untreated Patients						
Thomas et al[41]	9 Advanced	F,M	40-64	6 (67)	3 (50)	N/A
Berek et al[42]	12 III (8) IV (4)	F,P	44-54	8 (67)	0	7-60
Russell et al[43]	18‡ II (1) III (10) IV (6)	F,P M	46.8-56	16 (89)	2 (13)	2-52
Koh et al[44]	14‡ III (4) IV (10)	F,P M	34-63.1	8§ (57)	1 (17)	5-75
Eifel et al[125]	12 II (1) III, IV (11)	F,P	40-50	6§ (50)	1 (16)	17-37
Cunningham et al[126]	14 III (9) IV (5)	F,P	50-65	9 (64)	1 (11)	7-81
Akl et al[127]	12 I (3) II (5) III (4)	F,M	30-36	12 (100)	1 (8)	8-125
Total	91			65 (71)	9 (14)	
Patients with Recurrent Disease						
Thomas et al[41]	15	F,M	40-64	8 (53)	0	N/A
Russell et al[43]	7	F,P	54-72	4 (57)	1 (25)	2-35
Total	22			12 (55)	1 (13)	

*Recurrence within the irradiated volume.
†Length of follow-up in patients continuously cancer free.
‡Includes one patient in each series dying of treatment-related complications (neutropenia and sepsis).
§Includes patients who underwent surgery following completion of chemoradiation because of clinically suspected residual disease. Surgical specimens were without residual cancer.
F, 5-Flourouracil; F/U, follow-up; M, mitomycin; N/A, not available; NED, no evidence of disease; P, cis-platinum.

Table 52–10 Results of Elective Groin Radiation or Chemoradiation in Patients with Vulvar Cancer and Clinically Negative Inguinofemoral Lymph Nodes*

Authors	Patients	Groin Failure	%
Radiation Alone			
Frankendal et al[131]	12	0	0
Simonsen et al[132]	65	11	16.9
Boronow et al[27]	13	0	0
Perez et al[32]	39	2	5.1
Lee et al[133]	16	3	18.8
Petereit et al[134]	23	2	8.7
Stehman et al[136]	27	5	18.5
Total	195	23	11.8
Chemoradiation			
Leiserowitz et al[138]	19	0	0
Wahlen et al[139]	17	0	0
Total	36	0	0

*Patients with FIGO 1969 N0,1 clinically evaluated groin nodes.

to remain a controversial issue in the therapy of patients with limited-volume operable primary tumors and clinically negative nodes in whom radiation may be avoided if histopathological results of radical surgery are favorable. For patients who are already undergoing preoperative or definitive radiation or chemoradiation, either because of the extent of the primary tumor or because of medical inoperability, extension of the treatment volume to encompass the regional nodes may be a sensible alternative to groin dissection. Elective nodal irradiation to a volume encompassing the groins and the low pelvic nodes may be associated with less acute and chronic morbidity than bilateral groin dissection, particularly if postoperative groin and pelvic node irradiation becomes necessary because the groin nodes are found to be microscopically involved.

Techniques of Radiotherapy

There is no standard approach to the treatment of vulvar cancer with radiation. The circumstance of radiation (postoperative, preoperative, or as definitive treatment) will influence the designation of target volume, fractionation, and dose. Clinical and histopathologic characteristics of the primary and regional nodes may independently affect the selection of treatment parameters, which depends further on the scope of any coordinated surgery and whether chemotherapy is to be administered with radiation. Comorbidities in elderly patients may constrain the volume and intensity of treatment. Conservation of ovarian function and possible reproductive integrity in younger patients may also influence the technique of treatment.[140]

TARGET VOLUME

Selection of an appropriate target volume necessitates appraisal of the patient's general condition and the presence or absence of comorbidities that may compromise the optimal use of radiation. The health of all of the normal tissues (small and large bowel, blood vessels, nerves, bones, bladder, vulvar and perineal skin) that might be included in the treatment volume should be assessed; such an assessment may indicate alterations in treatment volume and technique. Figure 52-11 depicts treatment volumes that may be selectively modified as clinical circumstances dictate.

Volume for Postoperative Radiation

The target volume in patients undergoing treatment for groin node involvement detected at the time of radical vulvectomy should, in general, include both groin areas and the caudal pelvic nodes. If there has been no surgical assessment of the pelvic nodes, a CT scan or equivalent imaging modality should be used to define whether pelvic nodes are grossly enlarged, and a fine-needle aspiration (FNA) biopsy should be performed if suspicious nodes are detected. In the absence of clinical pelvic node involvement, the superior border of the treatment volume should encompass the caudal external iliac nodes and will not usually extend higher than the middle of the sacroiliac joints. When node involvement cephalad to the inguinal ligament has been documented at surgery or by

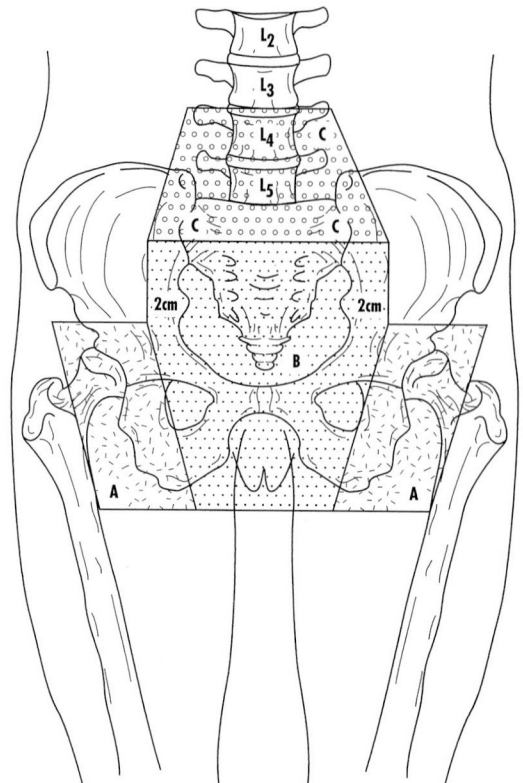

Figure 52–11. Target volumes for treatment of vulvar cancer with teletherapy. Volumes labeled *A* encompass lateral inguinofemoral nodes, which may lie superficial to the femoral necks. Treatment of these volumes may be accomplished with anterior photons or electrons in a manner that will limit dose deep to the femoral arteries (see Figs. 52-12 and 52-13). The volume labeled *B* is intended to encompass the vulva (or operative bed), the medial groin nodes, and the caudal pelvic nodes in patients in whom there is no clinical evidence of node involvement superior to the inguinal ligament. The superior border of this volume may be placed at the middle of the sacroiliac joints. The volume labeled *C* is an extended volume employed in the treatment of patients with pelvic lymph node involvement and is intended to include common iliac nodes.

postoperative imaging, the superior border of the treatment volume may be extended to the level of the L3-L4 interspace to encompass the common iliac nodes. The extent of the nodal treatment volume need not be symmetric in patients with only unilateral groin or pelvic node metastasis.

A 2-cm margin lateral to the medial bony margin of the pelvis assures adequate coverage of the lymphatics lateral to the external iliac vessels. If there has been invasion of overlying skin, inclusion of an additional 5 cm of the skin flaps is prudent to encompass potential contamination of dermal lymphatics. In the groins, the lateral border of the treatment volume should extend close to the anterior iliac crest and encompass the full extent of the operative dissection. If there has been extensive nodal involvement (more than microscopic, subcapsular embolization of the medial inguinal nodes), the caudal border of the treatment volume should encompass the inferior inguinal node chain lying along the saphenous vein in the upper medial thigh. Accumulating evidence suggests that under circumstances dictating irradiation of the groin and pelvic nodes, it is usually wise to include the vulvar tumor bed and adjacent perineal skin, because of the substantial risk of recurrence in this volume when midline shielding has been employed.[25,121] When an infiltrating, or "spray," pattern of tumor growth is detected in the primary site, wider margins of clinically normal tissue should be included around the tumor bed and perineum. If the primary tumor has grown across the labiocrural fold, treatment volume should include the lymphatics that run through the upper medial thighs. Occasional patients with negative, fully dissected groin nodes have indications for local tumor bed irradiation only. Gratuitous extension of the treatment volume to encompass the groins or pelvic nodes only increases the risk of subsequent lymphedema or other late sequelae and should be avoided.

Volume for Preoperative Radiation

Use of radiation before surgery should be considered either when surgical margins are anticipated to be inadequate (1 cm or less of clinically normal tissue) or when the scope of initial surgery would compromise the functional integrity of important normal tissues (anus, urethra, clitoris, bladder). Usually patients with these conditions have T3,4 primary tumors, but occasionally patients, particularly thin ones, have predictably inadequate margins with T2 primary tumors. Fixed or matted groin nodes or nodes invading or ulcerating through overlying skin are additional indications for preoperative radiation. If preoperative radiation is to be used, the histopathological status of groin and pelvic nodes should be assessed before treatment by fine needle aspiration (FNA) of palpable groin nodes exceeding 1 cm in size, or by excisional biopsy if they are superficial and accessible. CT through the pelvis and inguinal areas should be used both diagnostically and for treatment planning, with FNA assessment of abnormal findings. At the Radiation Oncology Center in Sacramento, it has become standard practice to include groin and caudal external iliac nodes in the initial target volume for most patients undergoing preoperative chemoradiation, even if these structures are clinically uninvolved. Generally, the extent of the primary lesion suggests a substantial possibility of occult nodal contamination.[134] Moderate dose radiation (36 Gy to 48 Gy) is applied synchronously with chemotherapy, with the intention of sterilizing occult micrometastases. The groins are not dissected when the primary tumor is removed. If groin nodes are histologically confirmed to be involved, preoperative chemoradiation is administered and limited dissection of residual palpable nodes is carried out at the same time as removal of the primary tumor. The anatomic extent of the target volume is determined in a fashion similar to that used to define the target volume for postoperative radiation, with the exception that a larger pelvic node volume may be treated if the primary tumor extends to involve the middle or upper vagina, proximal urethra, bladder, or rectum, or if groin nodes are extensively involved.

Volume for Radical Radiation

Nonsurgical treatment with radiation alone, or with concurrent chemotherapy, should generally be reserved for patients who have advanced locoregional disease that cannot be converted to resectable status with preoperative

therapy. Patients for whom resection by exenterative procedures is possible may choose radiation-based therapy as an alternative, as may the sexually active patients among the approximately 15% of vulvar cancer patients whose primary tumor involves the clitoris. Treatment volume considerations are similar to those for patients undergoing preoperative radiation, with the exception that in patients in whom resection is not possible because of extensive skin involvement with dermal lymphatic invasion (peau d'orange) or satellite skin nodules, inclusion of larger areas of clinically uninvolved skin is required to achieve secure lateral margins.

TECHNIQUE

Selection of technique depends on the availability of equipment and the sophistication of medical dosimetry support. Attention must be directed not only to defining rational target volumes for potential occult microscopic disease as well as clinically apparent gross disease, but also to the composition and volume of normal tissue that is unavoidably included. Critical normal tissues include the femoral necks (which are posterior to groin nodes that lie lateral to the femoral vessels), femoral and external iliac arteries, small bowel, bladder, urethra, clitoris, and anus. For patients who may be undergoing radiation therapy without surgery, an essential step will be a meticulous written record of the anatomical extent of initial disease involvement, which may be supplemented by clinical photographs and, in select circumstances, placement of small tattoos. This permits accurate volume reductions and sensible selection of limited, high-dose volumes even when there has been rapid tumor shrinkage.

Reasonable techniques include the use of a large anterior photon field designed to encompass the entire target volume, a smaller posterior photon field designed to encompass the perineum, pelvic nodes, and medial inguinofemoral nodes while excluding the femurs, and use of supplemental anterior electron fields to bring up the dose to the lateral inguinofemoral node areas that overlie the femoral heads and necks (Fig. 52-12).[43]

Alternatively, a large anterior photon field can be used to encompass the entire target volume and to deliver the full dose to the groin areas, employing a partial transmission block centrally to attenuate dose to the midplane of the low pelvis (central axis) to 50% of the daily dose, the remaining 50% being administered through a smaller posterior pelvic photon port, which excludes the femoral necks.[141] When available, use of different photon energies further reduces dose to the femurs (Fig. 52-13).

Because of the contour of the perineum in the sagittal plane, patients treated with parallel opposed anterior and posterior ports that encompass the pelvis as well as the perineum should have a treatment plan that reflects the fact that the dose to the vulva may be as much as 20% higher with each fraction than the midplane (central axis) pelvic dose, depending on the patient's size and the beam energy employed. The use of tissue-equivalent bolus or compensators may be advisable to minimize this effect, and thermoluminescent dosimetry (TLD) may be helpful to clarify dose ambiguities. Successful use of these

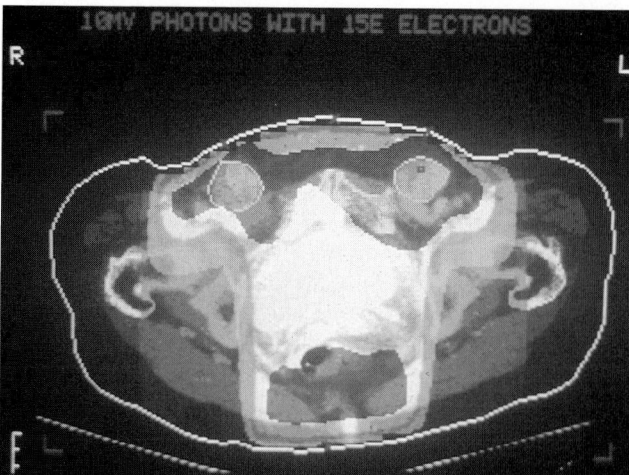

Figure 52–12. Computed tomography-based treatment plan illustrating a transverse dose distribution at the level of the femoral necks and pelvic floor in a patient with biopsy-confirmed bilateral inguinal node metastases (*white circles*) from a squamous cancer of the vulva staged T3N2M0 (1988 FIGO). The treatment plan makes use of a wide anterior 10 MV photon field and a narrower, opposed posterior 10 MV photon field excluding the femoral necks but including the low pelvic nodes. Dose to the involved inguinal nodes is supplemented by bilateral anterior 15 MeV electron fields, which overlie the femoral necks and abut the exit beam from the posterior photon field. Gradations in shade represent 10% increments in dose.

techniques requires that the dose to the groin area be applied at an appropriate depth in tissue,[137] which is defined by the depth of the femoral arteries, as determined by CT or ultrasonography, and depends markedly on patient size and body fat, whether nodes are grossly enlarged, and whether groin dissection has been previously accomplished. Depending on treatment technique,

the potential for "cold" or "hot" areas exists at the abutment of the inguinofemoral node treatment volumes and the primary tumor treatment volume. The potential hazard of these focal areas of dose inhomogeneity may be mitigated through the use of moving junctions or "feathering" the field abutments. Treatment to a reduced volume limited to gross primary disease can be accomplished by small opposed anterior and posterior photon fields, but usually excludes more normal tissue if accomplished with an en face perineal electron or orthovoltage port (Figs. 52-14 and 52-15). Under some circumstances, such as significant vaginal mucosal extension, interstitial or intracavitary brachytherapy may be useful to carry a discrete tumor volume to high dose. Intensity modulated radiation therapy may ultimately lead to more refined dose distributions with greater sparing of vulnerable normal tissues including bone, bladder, urethra, and bowel (Figs. 52-16 through 52-19). This technology may also reduce potential focal "cold" or "hot" areas at the abutment of portals targeting the groin nodes and the primary tumor. The heterogeneity of patients with vulvar cancer precludes a facile class solution for treatment with intensity modulated radiation therapy technique. The requirement to deliver therapeutic dose to the skin implies additional complexity in treatment planning with software algorithms that are imprecise for calculation of dose in the buildup region. Designation of the at-risk skin as a clinical target volume or gross tumor volume target can be very helpful. In addition to the ordinary intensity modulated radiation therapy requirements for meticulous patient positioning and immobilization, reproducible application of custom-designed bolus material may be required for accurate dose delivery.

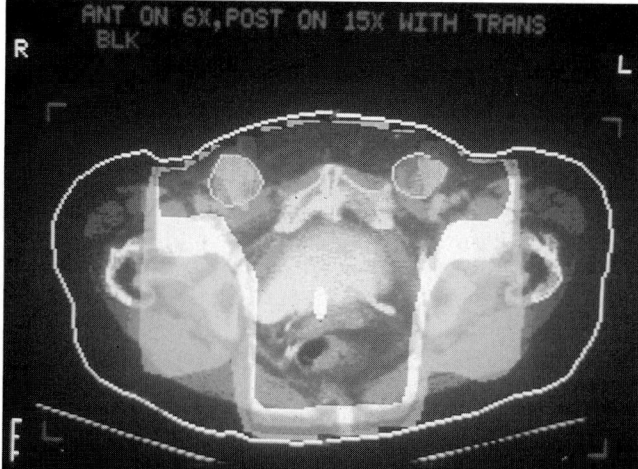

Figure 52–13. Computed tomography-based treatment plan of an alternative transverse dose distribution for the same patient as shown in Figure 52-3. This plan makes use of opposed anterior 6 MV and posterior 15 MV photon beams. Dose is prescribed at depth to the inguinal nodes from the anterior using the wider 6 MV photon field. Dose contribution to the midplane central axis is calculated and a partial transmission block is introduced in the beam over the central pelvis of sufficient thickness to reduce the central axis dose to 50% of the prescribed inguinal dose. A narrow, posterior 15 MV photon field, shaped to match the central partial transmission block and to exclude the femoral necks, is used to supplement the dose to the midplane central axis to a full therapeutic level. Gradations in shade represent 10% increments in dose. See also Color Figure 52-13.

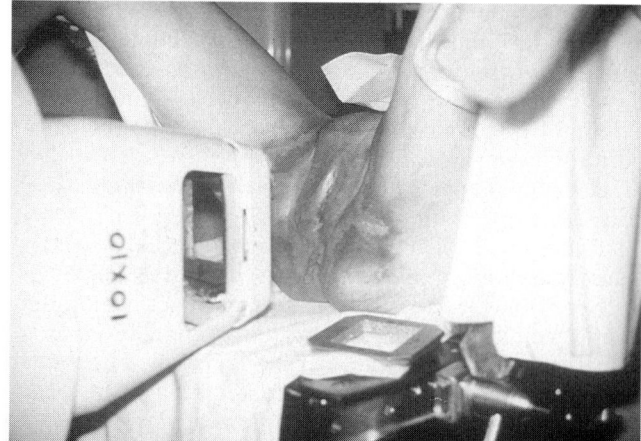

Figure 52–14. En face perineal electron beam therapy employed to carry a limited vulvar volume to a radical dose employing a 10 cm × 10 cm electron cone with a custom low melting point alloy block contoured to encompass the residual volume of gross disease. This 90-year-old patient, treated for T3N0M0 squamous cancer of the vulva, had previously received 36 Gy in 20 fractions of 1.8 Gy each over 4 weeks delivered with two 96-hour cycles of continuous-infusion 5-FU. Acute radiation dermatitis can be seen over the vulva and perineum as the patient's legs are abducted and suspended by operating room stirrups under the knees. Orthovoltage x-rays may be applied in a similar fashion. Biopsy confirmed that complete response was achieved after an additional 18 Gy was administered with this technique in concert with a third cycle of chemotherapy. The patient died of intercurrent illness 4 years after finishing cancer therapy.

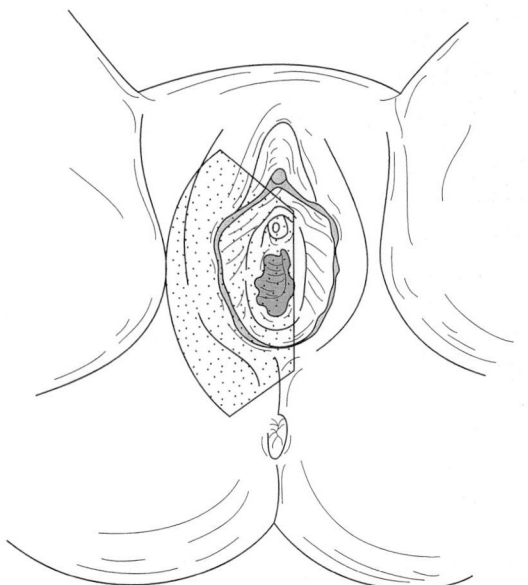

Figure 52–15. Perineal electron port for treatment of a reduced volume in a patient with locally extensive vulvar cancer involving the right labia and encroaching on the distal urethra. The port is shaped to encompass residual tumor while sparing the anus and clitoris.

FRACTIONATION AND DOSE

Definitive radiation-based therapy for vulvar cancer is difficult to do because of the requirement to administer a high dose to what is fundamentally a skin tumor, involving tissue that is frequently moist from perspiration and lack of ventilation and that is subject to continual friction through walking and other normal activities. Acute radiation dermatitis is worse in the vulva, perineum, and groins, with moist desquamation and pain the inevitable consequence of a continuous course of conventionally fractionated radiation. Interruption of therapy, either mandated by skin reaction or planned to avoid severe acute effects, is the rule and may prolong the elapsed time required to complete a course of radiation by 2 or more weeks, prompting consideration of compensatory increase in the total dose. Topical application of granulocyte-macrophage colony-stimulating factor impregnated gauze has been reported to decrease the severity and duration of acute radiation dermatitis and may reduce the duration of treatment interruption.[142]

Although radiation doses of 63 Gy to 72 Gy can often control gross vulvar cancer, the late sequelae induced by non–skin-sparing treatment, even when administered in fractions of 1.8 Gy, render such an approach problematic. Thin, atrophic skin with prominent telangiectasis, vulnerable to interruption of the epithelial integrity and formation of so-called "greasy ulcers," with chronic weeping of serum and infection as well as dense subcutaneous fibrosis and contracture are the late effects of high-dose radiation in this area and may be quite limiting if a large volume has been necessarily treated to the total dose. Topical application of testosterone (2% testosterone in a water-soluble base such as Eucerin) to the vulva may thicken and toughen vulvar skin rendered atrophic by radiation in a fashion analogous to the use of topical estrogen for radiation vaginitis.

Chemoradiation complicates the treatment program and substantially increases the potential for acute effects on all cycling cell systems (cancer and normal epithelia), as well as subjecting the patient to the hazards of systemic treatment. However, the total radiation dose employed is 15% to 20% less than might otherwise be employed with radiation alone, and effects on the infrequently cycling cell populations responsible for late radiation injury do not appear to be as pronounced as effects in the frequently cycling cell populations responsible for acute effects. Acute skin reactions and the need for treatment interruption have led to the use of hybrid fractionation regimens employing twice-daily fractionation for all or a portion of the treatment, as well as planned treatment interruptions both for skin and hematological recovery.[40,41,43,44] Multiple daily fractions during chemotherapy infusion will, theoretically, maximize radiation-drug synergism.

The chemotherapy agent most commonly used has been 5-FU, in doses from 750 mg/m² per 24 hours to 1000 mg/m² per 24 hours for 72 to 120 continuous hours. Cisplatin at 50 mg/m² to 100 mg/m² has been used as a second agent (renal function permitting), as well as mitomycin C at 6 mg/m² to 12.5 mg/m² (see Table 52-9). The preoperative fractionation scheme recently employed by the Gynecologic Oncology Group (Table 52-11) is a rational approach to preserving dose intensity, maximizing radiation-drug synergy, minimizing treatment interruption, and minimizing late effects in normal tissue through the use of reduced dose-per-fraction, twice-daily radiation.[40] However, the author recommends limiting cumulative dose for patients who remain unresectable to 59.5 Gy in fractions of 1.7 Gy when concurrent chemotherapy is used. Guidelines for radiation dose, alone or in combination with concurrent chemotherapy, are summarized in Table 52-12 and are compartmentalized for volume of disease (microscopic vs. gross) and treatment intent (preoperative, adjuvant postoperative, or radical).

CRITICAL NORMAL TISSUES

Radiation Injury

Skin sequelae are minimal and usually asymptomatic in patients receiving moderate-dose adjuvant preoperative or postoperative radiation coordinated with surgery. Some degree of chronic skin injury is inevitable in patients undergoing radical radiotherapy to high dose, and skin changes are progressive for 5 or more years after completion of therapy (Fig. 52-20). Skin and subcutaneous sequelae can be minimized by the use of lower doses per treatment fraction and judicious restriction of the volume to be carried to high dose for gross disease (see Fig. 52-15). Dose to clinically uninvolved skin rarely needs to exceed 45 Gy in 25 fractions, with or without concurrent chemotherapy.

Special care should be taken to exclude perianal, anal, and clitoral skin from high-dose volumes to minimize the hazard of late functional sequelae. Dose to the small intestine should not exceed 50.4 Gy in 28 fractions, even if only small volumes are to be treated. At the Radiation Oncology Center in Sacramento, small bowel dose is

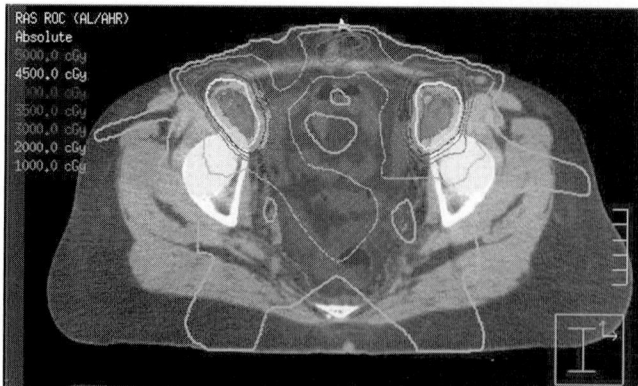

Figure 52–16. Transverse isodose distribution at the level of the mid-pelvis. Deep blue coloration corresponds to large and small bowel. High-dose volume is confined to caudal external iliac nodes. See also Color Figure 52–16.

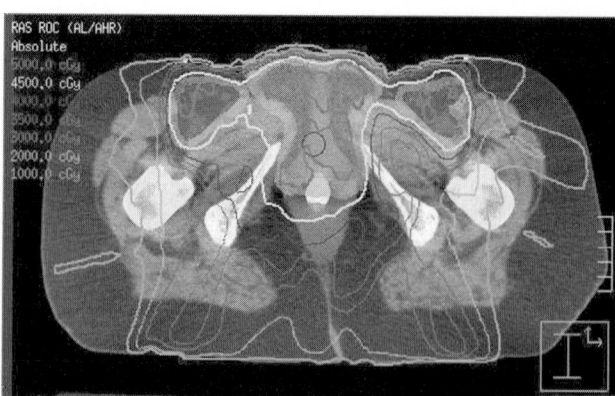

Figure 52–18. Transverse isodose distribution at the level of the anterior (superior) vulva at the level of the inferior ischial rami. High-dose volume is confined to the vulva and groin nodes and interconnecting skin. See also Color Figure 52–18.

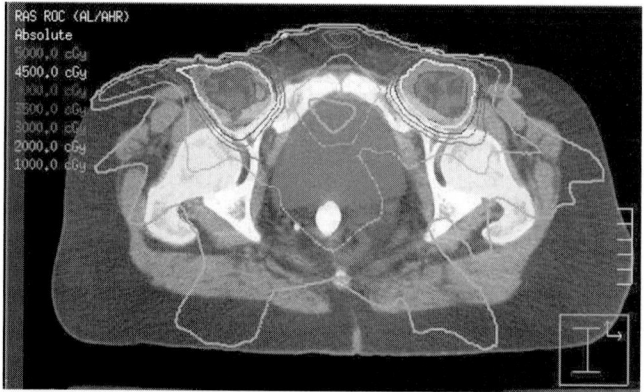

Figure 52–17. Transverse isodose distribution at the level of the urinary bladder (purple) and acetabulae. High dose volume is confined to the femoral vessels and associated lymph node tissue underlying the inguinal ligament. See also Color Figure 52–17.

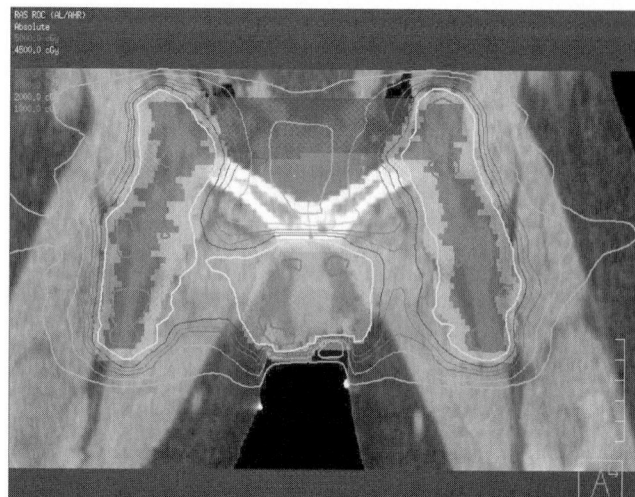

Figure 52–19. Coronal isodose distribution at the depth of the pubic symphysis illustrating selective dose deposition in the vulva, inguinofemoral, and caudal pelvic (external iliac) lymph nodes. See also Color Figure 52–19.

Figures 52–16 through 52–19. Intensity-modulated radiation therapy (IMRT) treatment plan for a patient with clinical stage T0N0M0 squamous carcinoma of the vulva undergoing radical chemoradiation with elective inclusion of the inguinofemoral lymph nodes and caudal pelvic nodes. Philips/ADAC *Pinnacle3 version 6.2b with IMRT version 1.2b* was used to plan a 7-field, 6 MV x-ray "step and shoot" plan for the patient in supine position using the following field arrangement: anterior 180°, right anterior oblique 225°, left anterior oblique 135°, right posterior oblique 285°, right posterior oblique 330°, left posterior oblique 75°, and left posterior oblique 30°. A 1-cm bolus was applied uniformly over the skin anteriorly, assuring adequate dose delivery to the approximate skin area customarily excised with an en-bloc radical vulvectomy and bilateral inguinofemoral lymphadenectomy. Application of bolus additionally assures accuracy of the dose calculation algorithm in the skin and immediately adjacent subcutaneous tissues. Treatment plan courtesy of Mr. Ali Layeghi.

limited to 36 Gy in 20 fractions when concurrent chemotherapy is administered.

Femoral neck fracture (avascular necrosis) can be a consequence of irradiation of inguinofemoral nodes lateral to the femoral vessels. At the Radiation Oncology Center in Sacramento, dose to the anterior cortical bone of the femoral neck has been limited to 45 Gy. Spontaneous microfractures of other bones may be seen when these bones have been included within high-dose volumes, particularly the pubic and ischial rami. Focal injury to femoral arteries may occur, particularly if there are "hot" areas of dose inhomogeneity at the abutment of portals targeted to the groin nodes and the primary vulvar tumor. Late sequelae in bladder, rectum, and pelvic nerves can be expected to be rare when the dose

guidelines shown in Table 52-12 are observed. Radiation vaginitis with atrophy, itching, and discharge is usually mild and can be ameliorated with topical estrogen unless a substantial length of vagina has been included within a high-dose volume. Regular use of a vaginal dilator should be strongly encouraged in all patients who wish to retain the capacity for vaginal intercourse.

Bartholin's Gland Carcinoma

Malignancy arising from the Bartholin's gland constitutes approximately 4% to 7% of vulvar malignancy. The criteria established by the Armed Forces Institute of Pathology for the diagnosis of Bartholin's gland carcinoma

Table 52–11   Time/Dose/Fractionation Schedule: Phase II Evaluation of Preoperative* Chemoradiation for Advanced Vulvar Cancer

Cycle #1

	MON				FRI			MON				FRI
Day	1	2	3	4	5	6	7	8	9	10	11	12
Radiation	R	R	R	R	R	0[†]	0[†]	R	R	R	R	R
1.7 Gy/Fx	R	R	R	R								
5-FU	F	F	F	F								
1000 mg/m^2 per24 hr												
Cisplatin		P										
50 mg/m^2												

1½-2½ Week Planned Rest

Cycle #2

	MON				FRI			MON				FRI
Day	1	2	3	4	5	6	7	8	9	10	11	12
Radiation	R	R	R	R	R	0[†]	0[†]	R	R	R	R	R
1.7 Gy/Fx	R	R	R	R								
5-FU	F	F	F	F								
1000 mg/m^2 per 24 hr												
Cisplatin		P										
50 mg/m^2												

*Patients who are judged to be unresectable following completion of 47.6 Gy preoperative chemoradiation receive additional 20 Gy in fractions of 1.7 Gy-2.0 Gy with reduced treatment volume encompassing gross residual disease, or may receive additional radiation dose via brachytherapy. A third cycle of chemotherapy is recommended if teletherapy is employed. The author suggests restricting the cumulative dose to 59.5 Gy/35 fractions in the interest of avoiding severe late skin effects.
[†]A day without radiation treatment.
F, 5-fluorouracil by continuous intravenous infusion; Fx, fraction; P, bolus cisplatin administration; R, a fraction of external radiation. A 4-hour minimum inter-treatment interval is mandatory, but 6 or more hours are suggested when practically feasible.
From Moore DH, Thomas GM, Montana GS, et al: Preoperative chemoradiation for advanced vulvar cancer: A phase II study of the Gynecologic Oncology Group. *Int J Radiat Oncol Biol Phys.* 1998;42:79.

enjoy the broadest contemporary acceptance.[143] A primary Bartholin's cancer should show areas of apparent transition from normal elements to neoplastic ones on histologic study, should be histologically compatible with origin from Bartholin's gland, and should exist without evidence of primary cancer elsewhere. The Bartholin's complex comprises a duct that is lined by squamous epithelium as it enters the distal vagina. The more proximal portions of the ductal system are lined by transitional epithelium and may be lined by columnar epithelium before arborization into secretory glandular elements. Various histological tumor types may arise. Squamous carcinoma constitutes approximately 35% to 50% of cases, with adenocarcinoma only slightly less common.[143-147] Adenosquamous carcinomas and transitional cell carcinomas make up a small minority of cases. Adenoid cystic carcinoma (cylindroma) represents

a distinct subset thought to be less likely to spread to regional nodes and associated with a long natural history and late recurrences, which may be either local or hematogenous.[148]

Bartholin's gland carcinomas have been reported in younger women and in association with pregnancy,[143,144] although an etiologic relationship is not apparent. Often presenting with a mass deep in the labia with intact overlying skin, Bartholin's gland carcinomas may be confused with a Bartholin's cyst or abcess, particularly if the patient is young. There is no persuasive evidence that squamous carcinomas of Bartholin's gland behave differently or should be managed differently than squamous cancers arising from other vulvar structures. However, it may be more difficult to accomplish conservative excision with adequate surgical margins in patients with Bartholin's

Table 52–12   Dose Guidelines*

Cancer Volume Treatment Intent	Radiation Alone		Chemoradiation	
	Microscopic	*Gross*	*Microscopic*	*Gross*
Preoperative	45-56	45-56	36-48	36-48
Postoperative	45-56	54-64 (+ margin)	36-48	45-56 (+ margin)
Radical	45-56	63-72	36-48	45-64

*All doses expressed in Gray. Dose guidelines assume that treatment will be administered in fractions of 1.6 Gy to 1.8 Gy and that multiple daily fractions may be employed for all or part of the treatment. Higher total doses imply fraction size of 1.6 Gy, and lower total doses imply fraction size of 1.8 Gy. Dose guidelines should be interpreted in the contexts of tumor bulk, health of normal tissues unavoidably included within the treatment volume, tolerance, and response to treatment. Use of doses in the lower end of the range for gross disease is predicated on a biopsy at the completion of treatment confirming histological clearance. Doses for gross disease should be applied with progressively shrinking volumes that confine high dose to not more, and possibly less, than the original volume of measurable disease.

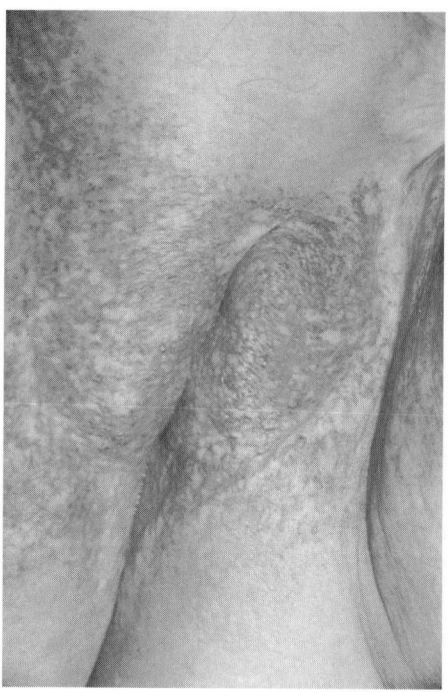

Figure 52–20. Severe late skin sequelae in a patient treated for T3N2M0 cancer of the vulva with external radiation and 3 courses of synchronous chemotherapy (5-FU and cisplatin). A dose of 54.0 Gy was prescribed in 30 fractions of 1.8 Gy each, administered twice daily in a planned split-course fashion concurrently with administration of drugs. Dose was prescribed to the midplane separation ($D_{1/2}$) of the low pelvis with the use of opposed 10 MV photon fields with volume reduction after 36.0 Gy, but without adequate compensation for diminished patient thickness and beam attenuation at the level of the vulva and perineum. The photograph was obtained 32 months after completion of chemoradiation.

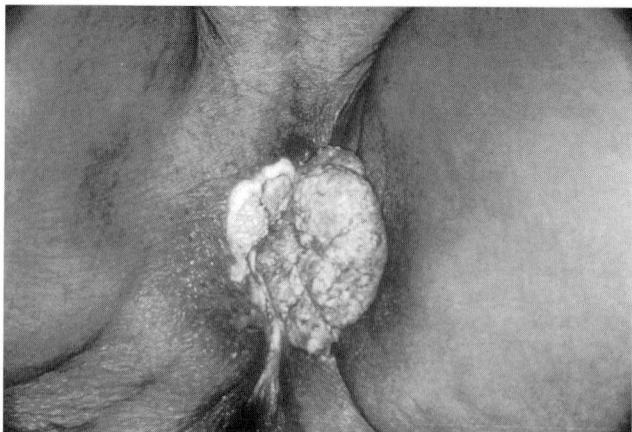

Figure 52–21. Locally recurrent verrucous cancer of the vulva following radical vulvectomy and bilateral inguinofemoral lymphadenectomy. Lymph nodes were uninvolved. Recurrence was confined to the primary operative bed. Gross morphology resembles a cauliflower.

gland cancers, and the majority of patients who fail surgical therapy have a component of locoregional recurrence.[146,147] The use of adjuvant postoperative radiation is common.[149,150] A retrospective review of 36 nonrandomized patients at MD Anderson Hospital and Tumor Institute revealed that 6 of 22 patients (27%) treated with surgery alone developed local recurrence, whereas only 1 of 14 higher risk patients (7%) selected to receive adjuvant radiation manifested local failure.[147]

VERRUCOUS CARCINOMA

Verrucous carcinoma is a variant of squamous cancer that frequently occurs after, or concurrent with, condylomata acuminatum.[94] Generally large, pearly gray to white in color, and with gross morphology similar to a cauliflower (Fig. 52-21), this cancer characteristically invades with a sharply circumscribed pushing margin. While locally destructive, this cancer rarely metastasizes to regional lymph nodes or distantly[92-94] but often recurs locally.

Radiation therapy of verrucous carcinoma has generally been considered ineffective and possibly dangerous. Transformation of verrucous lesions to more anaplastic histology following unsuccessful radiation has been attributed to radiation mutagenesis or accelerated repopulation, although the evidence for this is anecdotal. However, as reports of any favorable outcomes after radiotherapy are infrequently encountered,[91] it seems

prudent to limit the use of radiation to circumstances in which potentially curative surgery cannot be performed.

Melanoma

Vulvar melanoma occurs in a small minority of patients with mucocutaneous melanoma (approximately 2%) as well as a minority of patients with primary malignancies of the vulva (10% or less). The Mayo Clinic reported only 48 patients seen between 1950 and 1980.[151] Memorial Sloan-Kettering Cancer Center recorded 44 patients between 1934 and 1973.[152] MD Anderson saw 51 patients between 1970 and 1997.[153] Retrospective reviews have revealed several clear clinical parameters that distinguish this disease from squamous cancer. Patients are more likely to have nodal and hematogenous metastases at the time of diagnosis. Although an overall 5-year survival rate as high as 50% has been reported,[154] most series record 5-year survival rates between 15% and 30% except for patients with stage I disease.[153] Patients with nodal spread are uncommonly cured.[152] As with melanoma arising at other sites, the spectrum of biological virulence is broad.

Recurrences and metastases 10 years or longer after initial treatment are not uncommon.[151,152,155,156] The reported patterns of recurrence reveal a high frequency of relapse locally, in the groins, and in pelvic soft tissues, which often predates the clinical appearance of hematogenous metastases.[151,152,154-156] Prognosis can be correlated with the level of invasion using Clark's methodology[158] or the depth of invasion using Breslow's classification[159] which may be useful tools in selecting prognostically unfavorable node-negative patients for adjuvant therapies.

A role for radiation therapy has not been established, although anecdotal information suggests that melanoma arising in this location may be more radiosensitive than melanoma from other cutaneous sites.[157] Given the high locoregional recurrence rate following what is often extensive and sometimes mutilating surgery, prospective investigation of adjuvant regional radiotherapy or chemoradiation, either preoperatively or postoperatively, appears warranted.

CONCLUSION

The management of carcinoma of the vulva is in transition. The past 30 years have seen major modifications in treatment techniques, reflecting alterations in the goals of therapy. No longer is cancer eradication the sole objective. Preservation of normal tissue integrity and associated function has become equally important as results of therapy have improved. As clinical experience with newer combinations of treatment modalities accumulates and matures, guidelines for patient selection, treatment volume, technique, dose, fractionation, and use of adjunctive therapies are anticipated to become increasingly refined. In an era of evolutionary change, rigid adherence to the treatment algorithms of the past is a formula for inevitable obsolescence. Given the heterogeneity of patients afflicted with vulvar cancer, individualized treatment plans constitute the essence of excellence in clinical management.

REFERENCES

1. Taussig FJ: Cancer of the vulva: An analysis of 155 cases. *Am J Obstet Gynecol.* 1940;40:764.
2. Way S: The anatomy of the lymphatic drainage of the vulva and its furtherance on the radical operation for carcinoma. *Ann R Coll Surg Engl.* 1948;3:187.
3. Way S: Carcinoma of the vulva. *Am J Obstet Gynecol.* 1960;79:692.
4. Green TH Jr, Ulfelder H, Meigs JV: Epidermoid carcinoma of the vulva: An analysis of 238 cases. Parts I and II. *Am J Obstet Gynecol.* 1958;73:834.
5. Collins CG, Collins JH, Barclay DL, et al: Cancer involving the vulva: A report on 109 consecutive cases. *Am J Obstet Gynecol.* 1963;87:62.
6. Green TH Jr: Carcinoma of the vulva: A reassessment. *Obstet Gynecol.* 1978;52:462.
7. Morley GW: Infiltrative carcinoma of the vulva: Results of surgical treatment. *Am J Obstet Gynecol.* 1976;124:874.
8. Cavanagh D, Shepherd JH: The place of pelvic exenteration in the primary management of advanced carcinoma of the vulva. *Gynecol Oncol.* 1982;13:318.
9. Helgason NM, Hass AC: Radiation therapy in carcinoma of the vulva: A review of 53 patients. *Cancer.* 1972;30:997.
10. Kuipers T: Carcinoma of the vulva. *Radiol Clin.* 1975;44:475.
11. Frischbier HJ, Thomsen K: Treatment of cancer of the vulva with high energy electrons. *Am J Obstet Gynecol.* 1971;111:431.
12. McKelvey JL, Adcock LL: Cancer of the vulva. *Obstet Gynecol.* 1965;26:455.
13. Andersen BL, Hacker NF: Psychosexual adjustment after vulvar surgery. *Obstet Gynecol.* 1983;62:457.
14. Stellman RE, Goodwin JM, Robinson J, et al: Psychological effects of vulvectomy. *Psychosomatics.* 1984;25:779.
15. Green MS, Naumann RW, Elliot M, et al: Sexual dysfunction after vulvectomy. *Gynecol Oncol.* 2000;77:73.
16. Curry SL, Wharton JT, Rutledge F: Positive lymph nodes in vulvar squamous carcinoma. *Gynecol Oncol.* 1980;9:63.
17. Iversen T, Aalders JG, Christensen A, et al: Squamous cell carcinoma of the vulva: A review of 424 patients, 1956-1974. *Gynecol Oncol.* 1980;9:271.
18. Hacker NF, Berek JS, Lagasse LD, et al: Management of regional lymph nodes and their prognostic influence in vulvar cancer. *Obstet Gynecol.* 1983;61:408.
19. Podratz KC, Symmonds RE, Taylor WF, et al: Carcinoma of the vulva: Analysis of treatment and survival. *Obstet Gynecol.* 1983;61:63.
20. Monaghan JM, Hammond IG: Pelvic node dissection in the treatment of vulval carcinoma: Is it necessary? *Br J Obstet Gynaecol.* 1984;91:270.
21. Woodruff JD, Julian C, Puray T, et al: The contemporary challenge of carcinoma in situ of the vulva. *Am J Obstet Gynecol.* 1973;115:677.
22. DiSaia PJ, Creasman WT, Rich WM: An alternative approach to early cancer of the vulva. *Am J Obstet Gynecol.* 1979;133:825.
23. Iversen T, Abeler V, Aalders J: Individualized treatment of stage I carcinoma of the vulva. *Obstet Gynecol.* 1981;57:85.
24. Hacker NF, Berek JS, Lagasse LD, et al: Individualization of treatment for stage I squamous cell vulvar carcinoma. *Obstet Gynecol.* 1984;63:155.
25. Homesley HD, Bundy BN, Sedlis A, et al: Radiation therapy versus pelvic node resection for carcinoma of the vulva with positive groin nodes. *Obstet Gynecol.* 1986;68:733.
26. Boronow RC: Therapeutic alternative to primary exenteration for advanced vulvo-vaginal cancer. *Gynecol Oncol.* 1973;1:223.
27. Boronow RC, Hickman BT, Reagan MT, et al: Combined therapy as an alternative to exenteration for locally advanced vulvovaginal cancer. *Am J Clin Oncol.* 1987;10:171.
28. Hacker NF, Berek JS, Juillard GJF, et al: Preoperative radiation therapy for locally advanced vulvar cancer. *Cancer.* 1984;54:2056.
29. Acosta AA, Given FT, Frazier AB, et al: Preoperative radiation therapy in the management of squamous cell carcinoma of the vulva: Preliminary report. *Am J Obstet Gynecol.* 1978;132:198.
23. Jafari K, Magalotti M: Radiation therapy in carcinoma of the vulva. *Cancer.* 1981;47:686.
31. Fairey RN, MacKay PA, Benedet JL, et al: Radiation treatment of carcinoma of the vulva, 1950-1980. *Am J Obstet Gynecol.* 1985;151:591.
32. Perez CA, Grigsby PW, Galakatos A, et al: Radiation therapy in management of carcinoma of the vulva with emphasis on conservation therapy. *Cancer.* 1993;71:3707.
33. Kalra JK, Grossman AM, Krumholz BA, et al: Preoperative chemoradiotherapy for carcinoma of the vulva. *Gynecol Oncol.* 1981;12:256.
34. Levin W, Goldberg G, Altaras M, et al: The use of concomitant chemotherapy and radiotherapy prior to surgery in advanced stage carcinoma of the vulva. *Gynecol Oncol.* 1986;25:20.
35. Whitaker SJ, Kirkbride P, Arnott SJ, et al: A pilot study of chemoradiotherapy in advanced carcinoma of the vulva. *Br J Obstet Gynaecol.* 1990;97:436.
36. Evans LS, Kersh CR, Constable WC, et al: Concomitant 5-fluorouracil, mitomycin-C, and radiotherapy for advanced gynecologic malignancies. *Int J Radiat Oncol Biol Phys.* 1988;15:901.
37. Carson LF, Twiggs LB, Adcock LL, et al: Multimodality therapy for advanced and recurrent vulvar squamous cell carcinoma. *J Reprod Med.* 1990;35:1029.
38. Roberts WS, Hoffman MS, Kavanagh JJ, et al: Further experience with radiation therapy and concomitant intravenous chemotherapy in advanced carcinoma of the lower female genital tract. *Gynecol Oncol.* 1991;43:233.
39. Landoni F, Maneo A, Zanetta G, et al: Concurrent preoperative chemotherapy with 5-fluorouracil and mitomycin C and radiotherapy (FUMIR) followed by limited surgery in locally advanced and recurrent vulvar carcinoma. *Gynecol Oncol.* 1996;61:321.
40. Moore DH, Thomas GM, Montana GS, et al: Preoperative chemoradiation for advanced vulvar cancer: A phase II study of the Gynecologic Oncology Goup. *Int J Radiat Oncol Biol Phys.* 1998;42:79.
41. Thomas G, Dembo A, DePetrillo A, et al: Concurrent radiation and chemotherapy in vulvar carcinoma. *Gynecol Oncol.* 1989;34:263.
42. Berek JS, Heaps JM, Fu YS, et al: Concurrent cisplatin and 5-flourouracil chemotherapy and radiation therapy for advanced-stage squamous carcinoma of the vulva. *Gynecol Oncol.* 1991;42:197.
43. Russell AH, Mesic JB, Scudder SA, et al: Synchronous radiation and cytotoxic chemotherapy for locally advanced or recurrent squamous cancer of the vulva. *Gynecol Oncol.* 1992;47:14.
44. Koh WJ, Wallace JH III, Greer BE: Combined radiotherapy and chemotherapy in the management of local-regionally advanced vulvar cancer. *Int J Radiat Oncol Biol Phys.* 1993;26:809.
45. Plentl AA, Friedman EA: *Lymphatic System of the Female Genitalia.* Philadelphia: WB Saunders; 1971.
46. Henson D, Tarone R: An epidemiologic study of cancer of the cervix, vagina, and vulva based on the Third National Cancer Survey in the United States. *Am J Obstet Gynecol.* 1977;129:525.
47. Marcus SL: Multiple squamous cell carcinomas involving the cervix, vagina, and vulva: The theory of multicentric origin. *Am J Obstet Gynecol.* 1960;80:802.

48. Stern BD, Kaplan L: Multicentric foci of carcinomas arising in structures of cloacal origin. *Am J Obstet Gynecol.* 1969;104:255.

49. Jimerson GK, Merrill JA: Multicentric squamous malignancy involving both the cervix and vulva. *Cancer.* 1970;26:150.

50. Franklin EW, Rutledge FD: Epidemiology of epidermoid carcinoma of the vulva. *Obstet Gynecol.* 1972;39:165.

51. Figge DC, Gaudenz R: Invasive carcinoma of the vulva. *Am J Obstet Gynecol.* 1974;119:382.

52. Choo YC, Morley GW: Double primary epidermoid carcinoma of the vulva and cervix. *Gynecol Oncol.* 1980;9:324.

53. Sherman KJ, Daling JR, Chu J, et al: Multiple primary tumours in women with vulvar neoplasms: A case-control study. *Br J Cancer.* 1988;57:423.

54. Microinvasive cancer of the vulva: Report of the ISSVD Task Force. *J Reprod Med.* 1984;29:454.

55. Daling JR, Chu J, Weiss NS, et al: The association of condylomata acuminata and squamous carcinoma of the vulva. *Br J Cancer.* 1984;50:533.

56. Newcomb PA, Weiss NS, Daling JR: Incidence of vulvar carcinoma in relation to menstrual, reproductive, and medical factors. *J Natl Cancer Inst.* 1984;73:391.

57. Mabuchi K, Bross DS, Kessler II: Epidemiology of cancer of the vulva: A case-control study. *Cancer.* 1985;55:1843.

58. Brinton LA, Nasca PC, Mallin K, et al: Case-control study of cancer of the vulva. *Obstet Gynecol.* 1990;75:859.

59. Crum CP: Carcinoma of the vulva: Epidemiology and pathogenesis. *Obstet Gynecol.* 1992;79:448.

60. Ansink AC, Heintz APM: Epidemiology and etiology of squamous cell carcinoma of the vulva. *Eur J Obstet Gynecol Reprod Biol.* 1993;48:111.

61. Porreco R, Penn I, Droegmuller W, et al: Gynecologic malignancies in immunosuppressed organ homograft recipients. *Obstet Gynecol.* 1975;45:359.

62. Caterson RJ, Furber J, Murray J, et al: Carcinoma of the vulva in two young renal allograft patients. *Transplant Proc.* 1984;16:559.

63. Halpert R, Fruchter RG, Sedlis A, et al: Human papillomavirus and lower genital neoplasia in renal transplant patients. *Obstet Gynecol.* 1986;68:251.

64. Giaquinto C, Del Mistro A, De Rossi A, et al: Vulvar carcinoma in a 12-year old girl with vertically acquired human immunodeficiency virus infection. *Pediatrics.* 2000;106:E57.

65. Wright TC, Koulos JP, Liu P, et al: Invasive vulvar carcinoma in two women infected with the human immunodeficiency virus. *Gynecol Oncol.* 1996;60:500.

66. Korn AP, Abercrombie PD, Foster A: Vulvar intraepithelial neoplasia in women infected with human immunodeficiency virus-1. *Gynecol Oncol.* 1996;61:384.

67. Kuhn L, Sun XW, Wright TC Jr: Human Immunodeficiency virus infection and female lower genital tract malignancy. *Curr Opin Obstet Gynecol.* 1999;11:35.

68. Abercrombie PD, Korn AP: Vulvar intraepithelial neoplasia in women with HIV. *AIDS Patient Care STDS.* 1998;12:251.

69. Levine P, Maiman M, Zavalas E, et al: Invasive vulvar cancer and HIV infection. In *Proceedings of the 25th Annual Meeting of the Society of Gynecologic Oncologists,* Orlando, Fla.; Feb. 6-9, 1994. Abstract 1.

70. Buscema J, Stern J, Woodruff JD: The significance of the histologic alterations adjacent to invasive vulvar carcinoma. *Am J Obstet Gynecol.* 1980;137:902.

71. Zaino RJ, Husseinzadeh N, Nahhas W, et al: Epithelial alterations in proximity to invasive squamous carcinoma of the vulva. *Int J Gynecol Pathol.* 1982;1:73.

72. Neill SM, Lessana-Leibowitch M, Pelisse M, et al: Lichen sclerosus, invasive squamous cell carcinoma and human papillomavirus. *Am J Obstet Gynecol.* 1990;162:1633.

73. Iversen T, Aas M: Lymph drainage from the vulva. *Gynecol Oncol.* 1983;16:179.

74. Wharton JT, Gallagher S, Rutledge FN: Microinvasive carcinoma of the vulva. *Obstet Gynecol.* 1974;118:159.

75. Parker RT, Duncan I, Rampone J, et al: Operative management of early invasive epidermoid carcinoma of the vulva. *Am J Obstet Gynecol.* 1975;123:349.

76. Magrina JF, Webb MJ, Gaffey TA, et al: Stage I squamous cell cancer of the vulva. *Am J Obstet Gynecol.* 1979;134:453.

77. Buscema J, Stern JL, Woodruff JD: Early invasive carcinoma of the vulva. *Am J Obstet Gynecol.* 1981;140:563.

78. Way S: *Aspects and Treatment of Vulvar Cancer.* Basel, Switzerland: Karger; 1972;18.

79. Piver MS, Xynos FP: Pelvic lymphadenectomy in women with carcinoma of the clitoris. *Obstet Gynecol.* 1977;49:592.

80. Chu J, Tamimi HK, Figge DC: Femoral node metastases with negative superficial inguinal nodes in early vulvar cancer. *Am J Obstet Gynecol.* 1981;140:337.

81. Hacker NF, Nieberg RK, Berek JS, et al: Superficially invasive vulvar cancer with nodal metastases. *Gynecol Oncol.* 1983;15:65.

82. Hoffman JS, Kumar NB, Morley GW: Microinvasive squamous carcinoma of the vulva: Search for a definition. *Obstet Gynecol.* 1983;61:615.

83. Rutledge F, Smith JP, Franklin EW: Carcinoma of the vulva. *Am J Obstet Gynecol.* 1970;106:1117.

84. Dean RE, Taylor ES, Weisbrod DM, et al: The treatment of premalignant and malignant lesions of the vulva. *Am J Obstet Gynecol.* 1974;119:59.

85. Morris JM: A formula for selective lymphadenectomy: Its application to cancer of the vulva. *Obstet Gynecol.* 1977;50:152.

86. Krupp PJ, Bohm JW: Lymph gland metastases in invasive squamous cell carcinoma of the vulva. *Am J Obstet Gynecol.* 1978;130:943.

87. Benedet JL, Turko M, Fairey RN, et al: Squamous carcinoma of the vulva: Results of treatment, 1938-1976. *Am J Obstet Gynecol.* 1979;134:201.

88. Boyce J, Fruchter RG, Kasambilides E, et al: Prognostic factors in carcinoma of the vulva. *Gynecol Oncol.* 1985;20:364.

89. Figge DC: Rare vulvar malignancies. In Greer BE, Berek JS, eds. *Gynecologic Oncology: Treatment Rationale and Techniques.* New York: Elsevier; 1991:239.

90. Hunter DJS: Carcinoma of the vulva: A review of 361 patients. *Gynecol Oncol.* 1975;3:117.

91. Foye G, Marsh MR, Minkowitz S: Verrucous carcinoma of the vulva. *Obstet Gynecol.* 1969;34:484.

92. Gallousis S: Verrucous carcinoma: Report of three vulvar cases and review of the literature. *Obstet Gynecol.* 1972;40:502.

93. Lucas WE, Benirschke K, Lebherz TB: Verrucous carcinoma of the female genital tract. *Am J Obstet Gynecol.* 1974;119:435.

94. Japaze H, Van Dinh T, Woodruff JD: Verrucous carcinoma of the vulva: A study of 24 cases. *Obstet Gynecol.* 1982;60:462.

95. Crissman JD, Azoury RS: Microinvasive carcinoma of the vulva. A report of two cases with regional lymph node metastasis. *Diag Gynecol Obstet.* 1981;3:75.

96. Wilkinson EJ, Rico MJ, Pierson KK: Microinvasive carcinoma of the vulva. *Int J Gynecol Pathol.* 1982;1:29.

97. Sideri M, De Cicco C, Maggioni A, et al: Detection of sentinel nodes by lymphoscintography and gamma probe guided surgery in vulvar neoplasia. *Tumori* 2000;86:359.

98. Levenback C, Coleman RL, Burke TW, et al: Intraoperative lymphatic mapping and sentinel node identification with blue dye in patients with vulvar cancer. *Gynecol Oncol.* 2001;83:276.

99. Sliutz G, Reinthaller A, Lantzsch T, et al: Lymphatic mapping of sentinel nodes in early vulvar cancer. *Gynecol Oncol.* 2002;84:449.

100. de Hullu JA, Hollema H, Hoekstra HJ, et al: Vulvar melanoma: Is there a role for sentinel lymph node biopsy? *Cancer.* 2002;94:486.

101. Cohn DE, Dehdashti F, Gibb RK, et al: Prospective evaluation of positron emission tomography for the detection of groin node metastases from vulvar cancer. *Gynecol Oncol.* 2002;85:179.

102. Byron RL, Mishell DR, Yonemoto RH: The surgical treatment of invasive carcinoma of the vulva. *Surg Gynecol Obstet.* 1965; 121:1243.

103. Hacker NF, Leuchter RS, Berek JS, et al: Radical vulvectomy and bilateral inguinal lymphadenectomy through separate groin incisions. *Obstet Gynecol.* 1981;58:574.

104. Goplerud DR, Keetel WC: Carcinoma of the vulva: A review of 156 cases from the University of Iowa Hospitals. *Am J Obstet Gynecol.* 1968;100:550.

105. Rutledge FN, Follen Mitchell M, Munsell MF: Prognostic indicators for invasive carcinoma of the vulva. *Gynecol Oncol.* 1991;42:239.

106. Boutselis JG: Radical vulvectomy for squamous cell carcinoma of the vulva. *Obstet Gynecol.* 1972;39:827.

107. Binder SW, Huang I, Fu YS, et al: Risk factors for the development of lymph node metastasis in vulvar squamous cell carcinoma. *Gynecol Oncol.* 1990;37:9.

108. Kneale BLG, Elliott PM, McDonald IA: Microinvasive carcinoma of the vulva: Clinical features and management. In Coppleson M, ed. *Gynecologic Oncology.* Edinburgh: Churchill Livingstone; 1981:320.

109. Franklin EW, Rutledge FN: Prognostic factors in epidermoid carcinoma of the vulva. *Obstet Gynecol.* 1971;37:892.

110. Krupp PJ, Lee FYL, Bohm JW: Prognostic parameters and clinical staging criteria in epidermoid carcinoma of the vulva. *Obstet Gynecol.* 1975;46:84.

111. Dvoretsky PM, Bonfiglio TA, Helmkamp F, et al: The pathology of superficially invasive thin vulvar squamous cell carcinoma. *Int J Gynecol Pathol.* 1984;3:331.

112. Heaps JM, Fu YS, Montz FJ, et al: Surgical-pathologic variables predictive of local recurrence in squamous cell carcinoma of the vulva. *Gynecol Oncol.* 1990;38:309.

113. Hoffman MS, Roberts WS, LaPolla JP, et al: Carcinoma of the vulva involving the perianal or anal skin. *Gynecol Oncol.* 1989;35:215.

114. Podratz KC, Symmonds RE, Taylor WF: Carcinoma of the vulva: Analysis of treatment failures. *Am J Obstet Gynecol.* 1982;143:340.

115. Malfetano J, Piver MS, Tsukada Y: Stage III and IV squamous cell carcinoma of the vulva. *Gynecol Oncol.* 1986;23:192.

116. Cavanagh D, Fiorica JV, Hoffman MS, et al: Invasive carcinoma of the vulva: Changing trends in surgical management. *Am J Obstet Gynecol.* 1990;163:1007.

117. Bryson SCP, Dembo AJ, Colgan TJ, et al: Invasive squamous cell carcinoma of the vulva: Defining low and high risk groups for recurrence. *Int J Gynecol Cancer.* 1991;1:25.

118. Tilmans AS, Sutton GP, Look KY, et al: Recurrent squamous carcinoma of the vulva. *Am J Obstet Gynecol.* 1992;167:1383.

119. Piura B, Masotina A, Murdoch J, et al: Recurrent squamous cell carcinoma of the vulva: A study of 73 cases. *Gynecol Oncol.* 1993;48:189.

120. Prempree T, Amornmarn R: Radiation treatment of recurrent carcinoma of the vulva. *Cancer.* 1984;54:1943.

121. Dusenbery KE, Carlson JW, LaPorte JJ, et al: Radical vulvectomy with postoperative nodal radiotherapy: A reappraisal of the vulvar central block. *Int J Radiat Oncol Biol Phys.* 1993;27:199.

122. Buchler DA, Kline JC, Tunca JC, et al: Treatment of recurrent carcinoma of the vulva. *Gynecol Oncol.* 1979;8:180.

123. Montana GS, Thomas GM, Moore DH, et al: Preoperative chemo-radiation for carcinoma of the vulva with N2/N3 nodes: a Gynecologic Oncology Group study. *Int J Radiat Oncol Biol Phys.* 2000;48:1007.

124. Pirtoli L, Rottoli ML: Results of radiation therapy for vulvar carcinoma. *Acta Radiol Oncol.* 1982;21:45.

125. Eifel PJ, Morris M, Burke TW, et al: Prolonged continuous infusion cisplatin and 5-fluorouracil with radiation for locally advanced cancer of the vulva. *Gynecol Oncol.* 1995;59:51.

126. Cunningham MJ, Goyer RP, Gibbons SK, et al: Primary radiation, cisplatin, and 5-fluorouracil for advanced squamous carcinoma of the vulva. *Gynecol Oncol.* 1997;66:258.

127. Akl A, Akl M, Boike G, et al: Preliminary results of chemoradiation as a primary treatment for vulvar carcinoma. *Int J Radiat Oncol Biol Phys.* 2000;48:415.

128. Han SC, Kim DH, Higgins SA, et al: Chemoradiation as primary or adjuvant treatment for locally advanced carcinoma of the vulva. *Int J Radiat Oncol Biol Phys.* 2000;47:1235.

129. Thomas GM, Dembo AJ, Bryson SCP, et al: Review: Changing concepts in the management of vulvar cancer. *Gynecol Oncol.* 1991;42:9.

130. Gould N, Kamelle S, Tillmanns T, et al: Predictors of complications after inguinal lymphadenectomy. *Gynecol Oncol.* 2001;82:329.

131. Frankendal B, Larsson L-G, Westling P: Carcinoma of the vulva: Results of an individualized treatment schedule. *Acta Radiol Ther Phys Biol.* 1973;12:165.

132. Simonsen E, Nordberg U-B, Johnsson J-E, et al: Radiation therapy and surgery in the treatment of regional lymph nodes in squamous cell carcinoma of the vulva. *Acta Radiol Oncol.* 1984;23:433.

133. Lee WR, McCollough WM, Mendenhall WM, et al: Elective inguinal lymph node irradiation for pelvic carcinomas. *Cancer.* 1993;72:2058.

134. Petereit DG, Mehta MP, Buchler DA, et al: Inguinofemoral radiation of N0,N1 vulvar cancer may be equivalent to lymphadenectomy if proper radiation technique is used. *Int J Radiat Oncol Biol Phys.* 1993;27:963.

135. Gonzalez Bosquet J, Kinney WK, Russell AH, et al: Risk of occult inguinofemoral node metastasis from squamous carcinoma of the vulva. *Int J Radiat Oncol Biol Phys.* (submitted for publication 2002)

136. Stehman FB, Bundy BN, Thomas G, et al: Groin dissection versus groin radiation in carcinoma of the vulva: A Gynecologic Oncology Group study. *Int J Radiat Oncol Biol Phys.* 1992;24:389.

137. Koh WJ, Chiu M, Stelzer KJ, et al: Femoral vessel depth and the implications for groin node radiation. *Int J Radiat Oncol Biol Phys.* 1993;27:969.

138. Leiserowitz GS, Russell AH, Kinney WK, et al: Prophylactic chemoradiation of inguino-femoral lymph nodes in patients with locally advanced vulvar cancer. *Gynecol Oncol.* 1994;54:112.

139. Wahlen SA, Slater JD, Wagner RJ, et al: Concurrent radiation therapy and chemotherapy in the treatment of primary squamous cell carcinoma of the vulva. *Cancer.* 1995;75:2289.

140. Serkjes K, Wysocka B, Emerich J, et al: Salvage hemipelvis radiotherapy with fertility preservation in an adolescent with recurrent vulvar carcinoma. *Gynecol Oncol.* 2002;85:381.

141. King GC, Sonnik DA, Kalend AM, et al: Transmission block technique for the treatment of the pelvis and perineum including the inguinal lymph nodes: Dosimetric considerations. *Int J Radiat Oncol Biol Phys.* 1993;18:7.

142. Kouvaris JR, Kouloulias VE, Plataniotis GA, et al: Dermatitis during radiation for vulvar carcinoma: Prevention and treatment with granulocyte-macrophage colony-stimulating factor impregnated gauze. *Wound Repair Regen.* 2001;9:187.

143. Chamlian DK, Taylor HB: Primary carcinoma of Bartholin's gland: A report of 24 patients. *Obstet Gynecol.* 1972;39:489.

144. Barclay DL, Collins CG, Macey HB: Cancer of the Bartholin gland: A review and report of 8 cases. *Obstet Gynecol.* 1964;24:329.

145. Leuchter RS, Hacker NF, Voet RL, et al: Primary carcinoma of the Bartholin gland: A report of 14 cases and review of the literature. *Obstet Gynecol.* 1982;60:361.

146. Wheelock JB, Goplerud DR, Dunn LJ, et al: Primary carcinoma of the Bartholin gland: A report of ten cases. *Obstet Gynecol.* 1984;63:820.

147. Copeland LJ, Sneige N, Gershenson DM, et al: Bartholin's gland carcinoma. *Obstet Gynecol.* 1986;67:794.

148. Copeland LJ, Sneige N, Gershenson DM, et al: Adenoid cystic carcinoma of Bartholin's gland. *Obstet Gynecol.* 1986;67:115.

149. Cardosi RJ, Speights A, Fiorica JV, et al: Bartholin's gland carcinoma: A 15-year experience. *Gynecol Oncol.* 2001;82:247.

150. Balat O, Edwards CL, Delclos L, et al: Advanced primary carcinoma of the Bartholin gland: Report of 18 patients. *Eur J Gynaecol Oncol.* 2001;22:46.

151. Podratz KC, Gaffey TA, Symmonds RE, et al: Melanoma of the vulva: An update. *Gynecol Oncol.* 1983;16:153.

152. Chung AF, Woodruff JM, Lewis JL Jr: Malignant melanoma of the vulva: A report of 44 cases. *Obstet Gynecol.* 1975;45:638.

153. Verschraegen CF, Benjabipal M, Supakarapongkul W, et al: Vulvar melanoma at the M.D. Anderson Cancer Center: 25 years later. *Int J Gynecol Cancer.* 2001;11:359.

154. Morrow CP, Rutledge FN: Melanoma of the vulva. *Obstet Gynecol.* 1972;39:745.

155. Fenn ME, Abell MR: Melanomas of vulva and vagina. *Obstet Gynecol.* 1973;41:902.

156. Brand E, Fu YS, Lagasse LD, et al: Vulvovaginal melanoma: Report of seven cases and literature review. *Gynecol Oncol.* 1989;33:54.

157. Cascinelli N, Di Re F, Lupi G, et al: Malignant melanoma of the vulva. *Tumori.* 1970;56:345.

158. Clark WH Jr., From L, Bernardino EA, et al: The histogenesis and biologic behavior of primary human malignant melanomas of the skin. *Cancer Res.* 1969;29:705.

159. Breslow A: Thickness, cross-sectional areas, and depth of invasion in the prognosis of cutaneous melanoma. *Ann Surg.* 1970;172:902.

53

Pediatric Central Nervous System Tumors

Michael D. Weil, MD,   Daphne A. Haas-Kogan, MD,
and   William M. Wara, MD

EPIDEMIOLOGY

The ordeal of a child with a brain tumor most frequently begins without antecedent. At present there is no known cause of these tumors. Tumors can appear in association with genetic syndromes (Table 53-1) but most frequently arise spontaneously. SV40, a simian virus and frequent contaminant of early polio vaccines, has been found in association with ependymomas as well as choroid plexus tumors.[1] Exposure to x-rays during development seems to increase the incidence of gliomas and meningiomas.[2,3] Table 53-2 is a chart of statistics for pediatric central nervous system (CNS) tumors.

ANATOMY

The surface anatomy of the brain is of minimal import, as pediatric brain tumors are best evaluated and treated by correlation of a magnetic resonance image or planning computed tomographic scan with a plain radiograph.[4] The normal internal anatomy of the brain is schematically outlined and the sites of tumor origin are correlated in Figure 53-1. The circulation of the cerebrospinal fluid from its origins in the choroid plexus through the ventricular system and then on to the arachnoid granules via the subdural space is an important route for tumor dissemination. Disease that often involves the ventricles, such as medulloblastoma and germ cell tumors, readily spreads beyond the primary site.

Table 53–1   Syndromes Associated with Pediatric Central Nervous System Tumors

Syndrome	Associated Tumors
Basal cell nevus	Medulloblastomas
Li-Fraumeni	Astrocytomas
Neurofibromatosis	Visual pathway gliomas, meningiomas
Tuberous sclerosis	Periventricular giant cell astrocytomas
Turcot's	Medulloblastomas
von Hippel-Lindau	Cerebellar hemangioblastomas

Table 53–2   Epidemiology of Pediatric Central Nervous System Tumors

Number of Cases	
United States	1500
Worldwide	40,000
Gender Ratio	
Male:female	1.2:1
Location	
Supratentorial:infratentorial	1:1

PATHOLOGY

The division of primary pediatric brain tumors is listed in Table 53-3, and photomicrographs of these lesions are shown in Figures 53-2 through 53-5. The ontogeny of the brain appears to result in a greater number of astrocytes than other cell types. However, there is only minimal correlation between the incidence of particular histologic types of cancer in the brain and the absolute number of potential precursor cells in that region.[5]

Nearly half of the malignancies found in the pediatric age group are derived from the supporting glial cells. The grading of these tumors probably represents a spectrum of the same disease. Discrepancies between the pathologic grading and clinical outcome can result from sampling errors associated with biopsy of a heterogeneous tumor mass.

The second major pathologic division of pediatric brain tumors is the small, round blue cell tumor. The most common representative of this group is medulloblastoma. There is some controversy in the classification of these tumors and similar tumors found in the pineal region and cortex; therefore, the term *primitive neuroectodermal tumor* has been used to distinguish them from other tumor types.

Germ cell tumors are likely to develop in the midline paraventricular region after abnormal migration of primitive germ cells. Primary pituitary lesions and

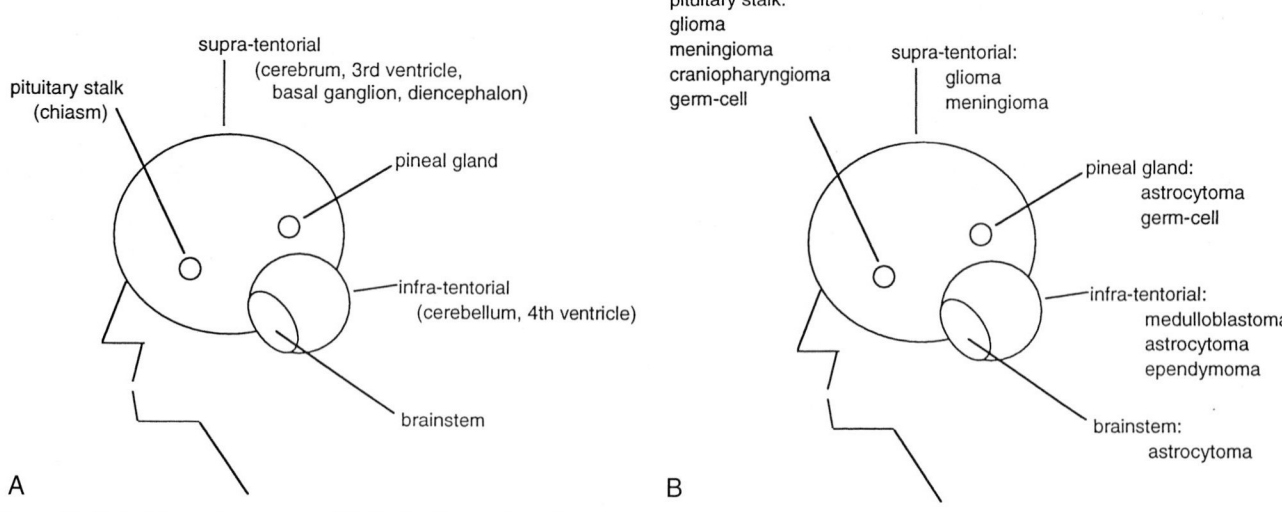

Figure 53–1. A, Schematic anatomy of the brain. **B,** Location of tumors and histologies by site.

craniopharyngiomas are benign lesions that can produce hormonal and visual aberrations.

The influence of histologic type on outcome is important in several sites.[6] The low-grade astrocytomas, such as the pilocytic astrocytomas, rarely evolve into high-grade lesions and can be successfully treated with surgery alone. Ependymoblastomas have a tendency to metastasize early and are treated with craniospinal irradiation, whereas low-grade lesions are treated with involved field therapy only. Germ cell tumors are divided into germinomas and nongerminomatous germ cell tumors. The former are highly radiosensitive and are treated with whole ventricular irradiation followed by a boost to the primary lesion. Nongerminomatous germ cell tumors require platinum-based chemotherapy in addition to radiotherapy.

Table 53–3   Nomenclature of Brain Tumors

Glioma

Astrocytoma (e.g., juvenile pilocytic, glioblastoma multiforme)
Oligodendroglioma
Ependymoma (and ependymoblastoma)
Choroid plexus tumor

Primitive Neuroendocrine Tumor

Medulloblastoma
Pineoblastoma?

Germ Cell Tumor

Germinoma
Nongerminomatous (e.g., teratoma, embryonal,
  endodermal sinus)

Miscellaneous

Craniopharyngioma
Meningioma
Hemangiopericytoma
Hemangioblastoma

CLINICAL PRESENTATIONS

The presenting signs and symptoms of intracranial lesions in the developing child vary depending on the location of the tumor (which is often related to histology) and age at presentation (Table 53-4). These factors also influence the time to diagnosis. Supratentorial lesions manifest with seizures, headaches, and disturbances related to the area of anatomic involvement. Involvement of the optic tracts, nerves, or chiasm produces visual field cuts.[10,11] In a child younger than 2 years of age, developmental delays and euphemistically described "failure to thrive" are seen with diencephalic lesions, and involvement of the hypothalamus or pituitary can produce endocrinologic aberrations (diabetes insipidus, precocious puberty, loss of menses, acromegaly, and galactorrhea). Lesions of the posterior fossa most often produce symptoms related to obstructions of the flow of cerebrospinal fluid through the ventricles. Increased intracranial pressure can result in headaches, nausea, and vomiting. Papilledema may be present. Involvement of the cerebellum can result in truncal ataxia and dysmetria. Lesions in the pineal area can cause pressure on the tectal plate, resulting in gaze abnormalities known as Parinaud's syndrome (paralysis of conjugate upward gaze).[7,8] Brainstem lesions typically produce cranial nerve palsies and motor and sensory deficits. In several series, the rapidity of the onset of symptoms was shown to be related to survival.[9] More slowly growing tumors, those that produce symptoms of more than 2 months' duration before diagnosis, are associated with longer median survivals.

ROUTES OF SPREAD

Primary malignancies of the CNS generally do not relapse or recur far from the primary lesion.[8] Unfortunately, as vital structures are compressed within the confines of the skull, it is destruction of the primary organ, rather than metastasis, that results in great

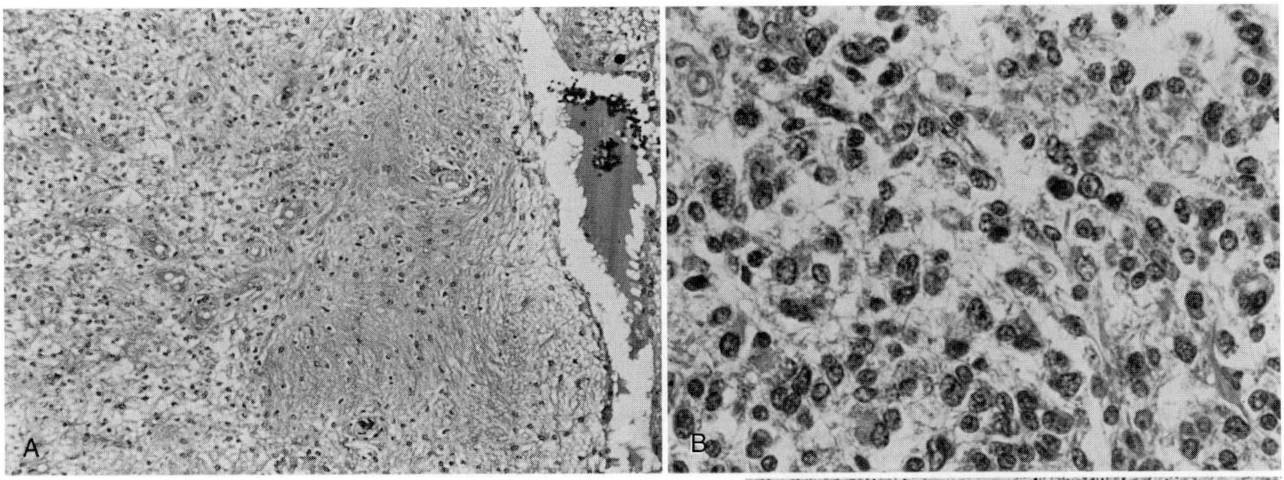

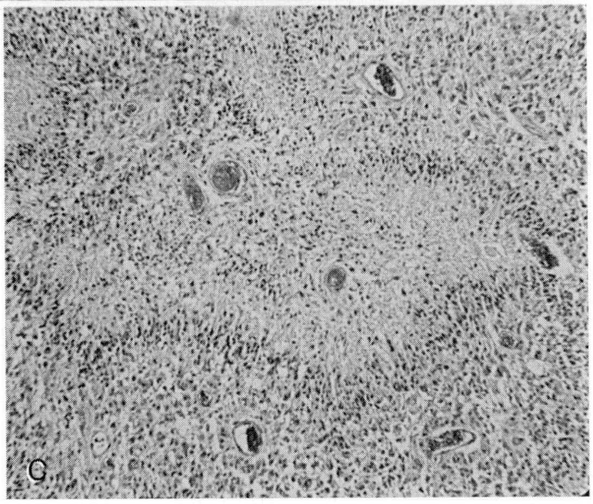

Figure 53–2. Astrocytoma. **A,** Grade I; **B,** grade II; **C,** grade III. (Courtesy of Dr. Richard Davis, University of California–San Francisco.)

morbidity and mortality. Lesions such as medulloblastomas[10] and germ cell tumors[11] can spread through the ventricular system and metastasize beyond the primary brain tissue of origin. It is common for medulloblastoma to metastasize beyond the posterior fossa to involve the entire contents of the spinal compartment or the brain or both. Although CNS tumors metastasize outside the CNS, this is currently thought to be a rare occurrence, and the documentation of such events in earlier reports may have been the result of tumor cells that spread through unfiltered shunts.[12]

DIAGNOSTIC AND STAGING STUDIES

With the exception of germ cell tumors, there are no biochemical markers for brain tumors that can be evaluated from the blood. Germinomas may produce beta-chorionic

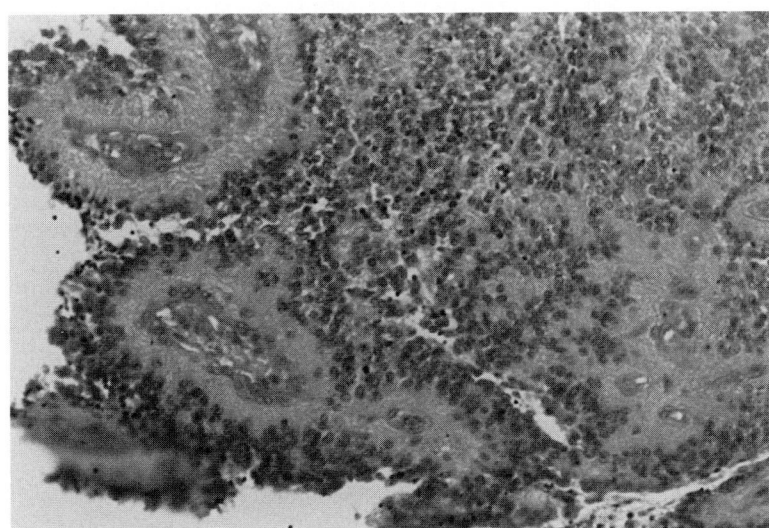

Figure 53–3. Ependymoma. (Courtesy of Dr. Richard Davis, University of California–San Francisco.)

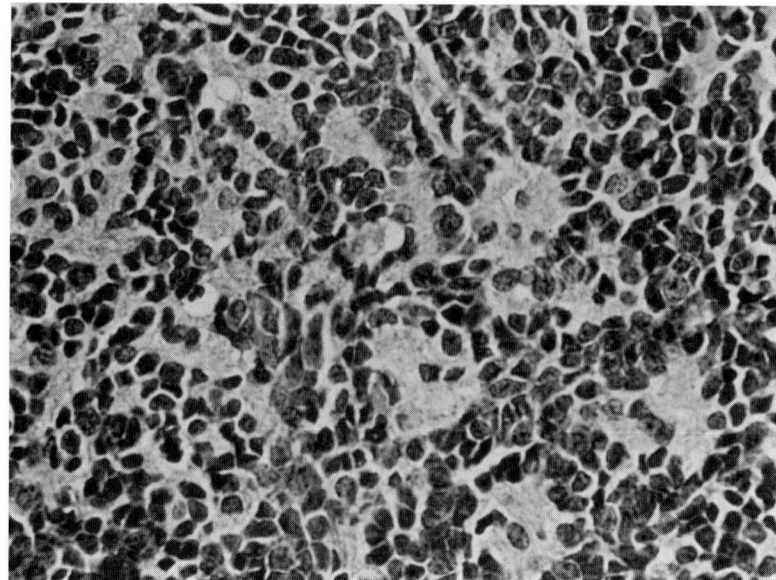

Figure 53–4. Medulloblastoma: Homer-Wright rosettes. (Courtesy of Dr. Richard Davis, University of California–San Francisco.)

gonadotropin in 15% of the cases, but the presence of alpha fetoprotein is always indicative of nongerminomatous germ cell tumors. The cerebrospinal fluid should be evaluated in all patients with medulloblastoma, ependymoma, and germ cell tumors. Cytology and biochemical studies of the cerebrospinal fluid should be performed 2 to 3 weeks after surgical extirpation to avoid misinterpretation. Patients with lesions involving the optic nerve, chiasm, or pituitary gland should undergo formal neuro-ophthalmologic examination and visual field testing after surgery and before radiation therapy.[13] Furthermore, all lesions in the region of the hypothalamus or pituitary require careful pretreatment as well as post-treatment evaluation of hormonal function.[14] Pediatric patients who undergo cranial irradiation should be evaluated for cognitive function before and after treatment. Documentation of growth and hearing should be performed as well. In addition to these studies, the emotional needs of the family, parents, and siblings,

as well as the patient, should not be overlooked. There is a high incidence of divorce following the treatment of pediatric malignancy.[15]

The dramatic advances in imaging over the past 2 decades have resulted in a major improvement in diagnosis and targeting of therapy for lesions of the CNS.[10] Young children often require sedation for any study, but magnetic resonance imaging (MRI) yields the best definition of parenchymal lesions, as well as clear views of the posterior and middle cranial fossa. It is superior to myelography for evaluation of the spine and therefore the modality of choice for evaluation of the craniospinal axis. MRI scans are routinely ordered within 48 hours of surgery to evaluate the extent of resection prior to the formation of a hematoma. The results of therapy are followed by routine MRI scans, and in cases of ambiguous findings, positron emission tomography is used to distinguish between necrosis and recurrent tumor. Figure 53-6 demonstrates the common lesions on magnetic resonance

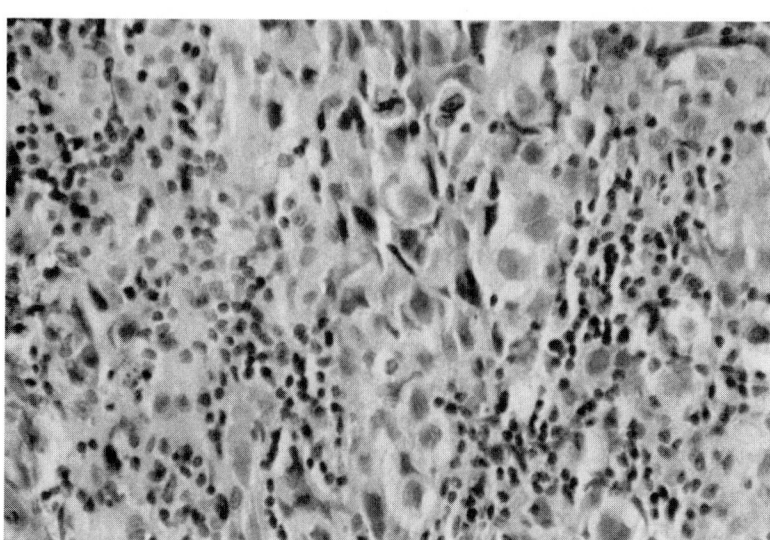

Figure 53–5. Germinoma. (Courtesy of Dr. Richard Davis, University of California–San Francisco.)

Table 53–4 Signs and Symptoms of Pediatric Central Nervous System Tumors

Infants	Children
Failure to thrive	Headaches
Bulging fontanels	Nausea and vomiting
Arrested development	Lethargy
Head nodding	Ataxia
Nystagmus	Cranial nerve palsies
	Seizures
	Visual field abnormalities

images. The information is of critical importance for planning further treatment and for defining the gross tumor volume and the clinical treatment volume.

STAGING SYSTEM

Several staging systems are used to guide the management of primary pediatric brain tumors.[3] In contrast to staging systems for other types of cancer, these are often based on the postoperative imaging of the surgical site and the presence of lesions outside the primary area. Table 53-5 lists the most commonly used systems for medulloblastoma. In medulloblastoma, the *Chang* staging system has been widely referred to in the literature[16] but has not been used recently for clinical studies. Rather, the extent of surgical resection, the patient's age, and the presence of disease outside the primary region are considered to be important.[10] For most CNS tumors in the pediatric age group, the histologic type and the location of the tumor are critical to the outcome.

STANDARD THERAPEUTIC APPROACHES

Pediatric brain tumors require initial surgical evaluation in almost all cases.[6,17] Over the past 2 decades, the availability of computed tomography (CT) and MRI scans has improved the ability to diagnose and localize an intracranial tumor mass, and thereby improve the operative approach.[18] Surgical intervention provides a histologic diagnosis and the opportunity to place a shunt and allows the excision of as much tumor mass as is safely possible.[5] It is now possible to decompress hydrocephalus

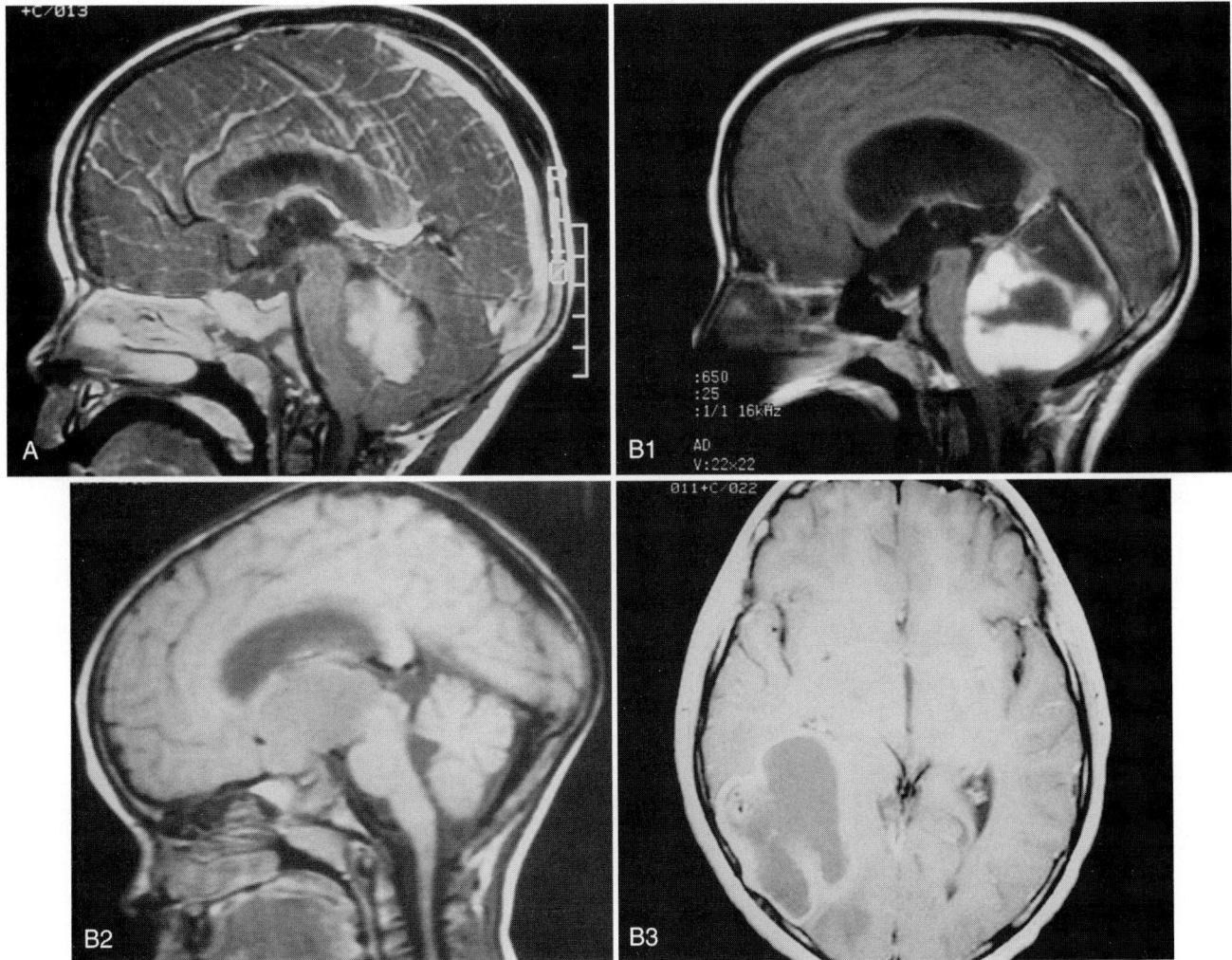

Figure 53–6. Magnetic resonance images of common lesions. **A,** Medulloblastoma; **B,** astrocytoma: 1, juvenile pilocytic astrocytoma; 2, anaplastic astrocytoma; and 3, glioblastoma multiforme.

Continued

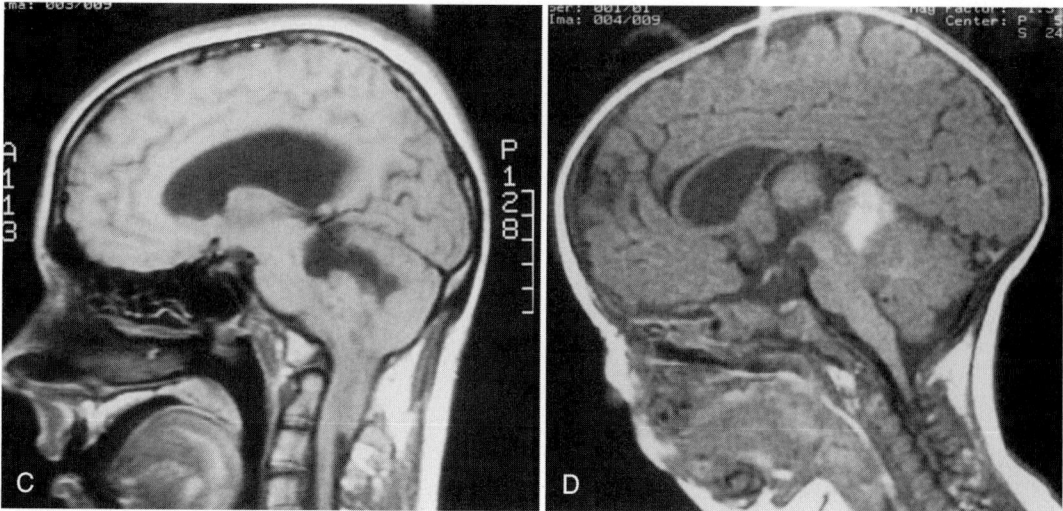

Figure 53–6. cont'd C, ependymoma; and **D,** germinoma. (Courtesy of Dr. A. James Barkovitch, University of California–San Francisco.)

by an external ventricular drain or by percutaneous endoscopic ventriculostomy. These procedures minimize the requirement for a permanent shunt following surgical extirpation. Endoscopy can also be used to take biopsy samples of paraventricular tumors, although inaccessible tumors are best biopsied stereotactically.

Functional mapping to distinguish the motor and sensory cortex permits the identification of critical brain structures to be avoided. In addition, stereotactic radiosurgery and techniques using hand-held, computer-guided instruments offer the opportunity to localize the surgical procedure with much greater accuracy than previously possible. Surgical resection using ultrasonic aspirators improves the probability of achieving a gross total resection and decreases the risk of damage to normal tissue.

The benefit of performing maximal debulking of the tumor mass in all cases remains controversial.[8,20,22,23] Except in very young children, incomplete surgical resection requires postoperative radiotherapy. Table 53-6 lists the scheduling of combined modalities for various malignant pediatric CNS tumors.

Chemotherapy offers the opportunity to delay radiation therapy and to potentiate the effects of radiation. Except for germ cell tumors, chemotherapy has not been proved beneficial in prospective, randomized trials. However, chemotherapy is commonly used to treat astrocytomas in young children and to treat medulloblastoma. In theory, treatment can be equally effective with lower total doses of each modality.

Radiotherapy continues to be the second line of treatment for pediatric CNS tumors. Although planning

Table 53–6   Scheduled Postoperative Therapy by Histologic Type

Medulloblastoma

Low-risk: craniospinal axis to 36 Gy and posterior fossa boost to 54 Gy. On protocol, lower craniospinal axis dose (23.4 Gy) with chemotherapy (cisplatin, vincristine, and CCNU or cytoxan).

High-risk: craniospinal axis to 36 Gy and posterior fossa boost to 54 Gy, with chemotherapy (cisplatin, vincristine, and CCNU or cytoxan). Gross disease is boosted to higher doses.

Astrocytoma

Juvenile pilocytic: observation

Anaplastic: 54 Gy; protocols are studying observation as well as higher doses.

Glioblastoma multiforme/brainstem: 59.4 Gy with standard fractions, up to 70.4 Gy with 1.6 Gy bid. Chemotherapy per protocol.

Germ Cell Tumor

Germinoma: whole ventricle to 19.8 Gy; boost primary to 50.4 Gy.

Nongerminomatous: Chemotherapy (cisplatin, etoposide, and bleomycin), then whole ventricle to 19.8 Gy; boost primary to 54 Gy.

Ependymoma

Tumor plus margin to 54 Gy; ependymoblastoma is treated with craniospinal axis irradiation similar to medulloblastoma.

Craniopharyngioma

Tumor plus tight margin to 54 Gy.

CCNU, chloroethyl-cyclohexyl-nitrosourea (Lomustine).

Table 53–5   Staging of Medulloblastoma

Chang Staging		UCSF System
T1	Tumor <3 cm	**Low-risk:**
T2	Tumor >3 cm	no spread beyond primary
T3a	Extension into the aqueduct of foramen	*and*
		gross total resection
T3b	Invasion of brain stem	*and*
T4	Midbrain, third ventricle, or upper cord involved	age greater than 3 y
M0	No metastasis	
M1	Microscopic cerebrospinal fluid involvement	**High-risk:**
M2	Gross seeding of third ventricle	spread outside of primary area
		or
M3	Gross seeding of cord	less than gross total resection
		or
M4	Extra–central nervous system metastasis	age less than 3 y

techniques and the ability to localize the tumor volume have significantly improved over the past 2 decades, it is difficult to correlate this progress with improvements in survival. Despite the more sophisticated treatment planning and the apparent sparing of normal tissues, the long-term sequelae of radiotherapy to the brain of a developing child have not yet been shown to decrease. Likewise, it is difficult to prove any benefit from altered fractionation schemes that have come from radiobiologic studies.

TECHNIQUES OF RADIOTHERAPY

Radiotherapy of pediatric brain tumors should be performed at centers with dedicated pediatric oncology departments. While radiation therapy plays a key role in the treatment of pediatric brain tumors, delivery of adequate therapy must always be balanced against potential treatment-related toxicity. Both biologic and physical techniques can maximize the therapeutic ratio of radiation, thus enhancing tumor kill while protecting normal tissues. Precise planning and delivery of radiation have evolved rapidly in the past decade.

Improved imaging technology, specifically MRI and CT, and biological, metabolic imaging such as positron emission tomography (PET), have improved delineation of tumor and surrounding critical structures. Novel techniques capitalize on an improved definition of tumor volumes, allowing clinicians to decrease the doses delivered to critical structures while maintaining or increasing the dose to tumor. The advent of other technical advances such as multi-leaf collimation (MLC), digitally reconstructed radiographs (DRRs), and electronic portal imaging have contributed to the integration of conformal radiation delivery. Intensity-modulated radiotherapy (IMRT) has the potential to reduce morbidity (e.g., sparing the inner ear in posterior fossa treatment).

CT images are analyzed jointly by radiation oncologists, diagnostic radiologists, and occasionally by other treating clinicians such as pediatric oncologists and pediatric neurosurgeons. The treatment volume is dictated by the natural history of the tumor. Gross tumor volume (GTV) is defined by physical examination and imaging studies and encompasses the macroscopic extent of the tumor. Clinical target volume (CTV) contains both the GTV and areas at risk for microscopic spread of disease. The planning target volume (PTV) is defined as the CTV surrounded by adequate margin to account for variation in patient position, organ motion, and other movement.

Once target volumes and critical structures are defined, beam geometry and weighting are defined and dose distribution is calculated. Selection of beam angles can be done by referencing axial images or by use of beam's-eye view (BEV) (Fig. 53-7). BEV allows visualization of the relationship of tumor volumes to the volumes of critical normal tissues as if looking from the origin of the beam. This allows beam angles and beam shaping to be selected more intelligently. Once an initial plan has been developed, the resulting dose distributions are calculated and evaluated by the clinician. The plan can then be altered to improve on initial results, if necessary.

The beam directions as well as their relative weights and shapes are modified to finally optimize the three-dimensional (3D) plan (see Fig. 53-7).

The last decade has seen rapid development of novel technical approaches to radiotherapy and its application to pediatric CNS malignancies. These include 3D conformal radiotherapy (3D-CRT), IMRT, proton beam radiotherapy, intraoperative radiotherapy, radiosurgery, and temporary or permanent interstitial brachytherapy.

Interstitial brachytherapy allows for the delivery of high doses of radiation to a tumor region. A recent retrospective study reports the largest series of pediatric brain tumors treated with ^{125}I brachytherapy. Twenty-eight children were treated with temporary, high-activity ^{125}I brachytherapy for recurrent or persistent supratentorial tumors. The study is most useful in its documentation of acute and late toxicities. No grade 3 or grade 4 acute or late toxicities occurred. However, 22 patients (79% of 28 total patients) required at least one reoperation following brachytherapy, and 17 of these 22 patients had evidence of necrosis in the resected specimen.

SPECIFIC RADIOTHERAPY TECHNIQUES

Posterior Fossa and Brainstem

The patient is simulated in the prone position. The head is secured in a "doggie dish" with tape across the back of the head and is maintained with slight extension. The posterior clinoid is the most forward insertion of the tentorium. The apex of the tentorium is at a point approximately halfway between the foramen magnum and a vertical line drawn to the top of the skull. The tentorium inserts posteriorly at the inion. Lesions of the posterior fossa should be treated to the contents of the posterior fossa, with at least a 1 cm margin and the inferior border at C2.[9,21] For boost fields, the inferior border is brought up to the C1-2 interspace. The accuracy of the simulation is verified during the simulation by projection of a sagittal, contrast-enhanced magnetic resonance image onto the port film. This is performed by first outlining features on the port film with a wax pencil for orientation. The entire scalp is outlined along with the pituitary fossa and the vertebral bodies. An overhead projector is used to superimpose the magnetic resonance image at equal magnification onto the port film by matching the outlined anatomy between the two films. The proper magnification is assured by matching the ruler on the MR image to the grid on the port film. The anatomy of the normal structures and the tumor is then outlined on the port film, and blocking is performed by providing at least a 2 cm margin around the tumor. This technique is to be employed if neither 3DCRT nor IMRT is available.

Sellar and Suprasellar Region

Lesions in the region of the sella turcica, such as germinomas and craniopharyngiomas, are treated with arcs or multi-field plans based on CT treatment planning.[11] If the patient is not scheduled to undergo treatment

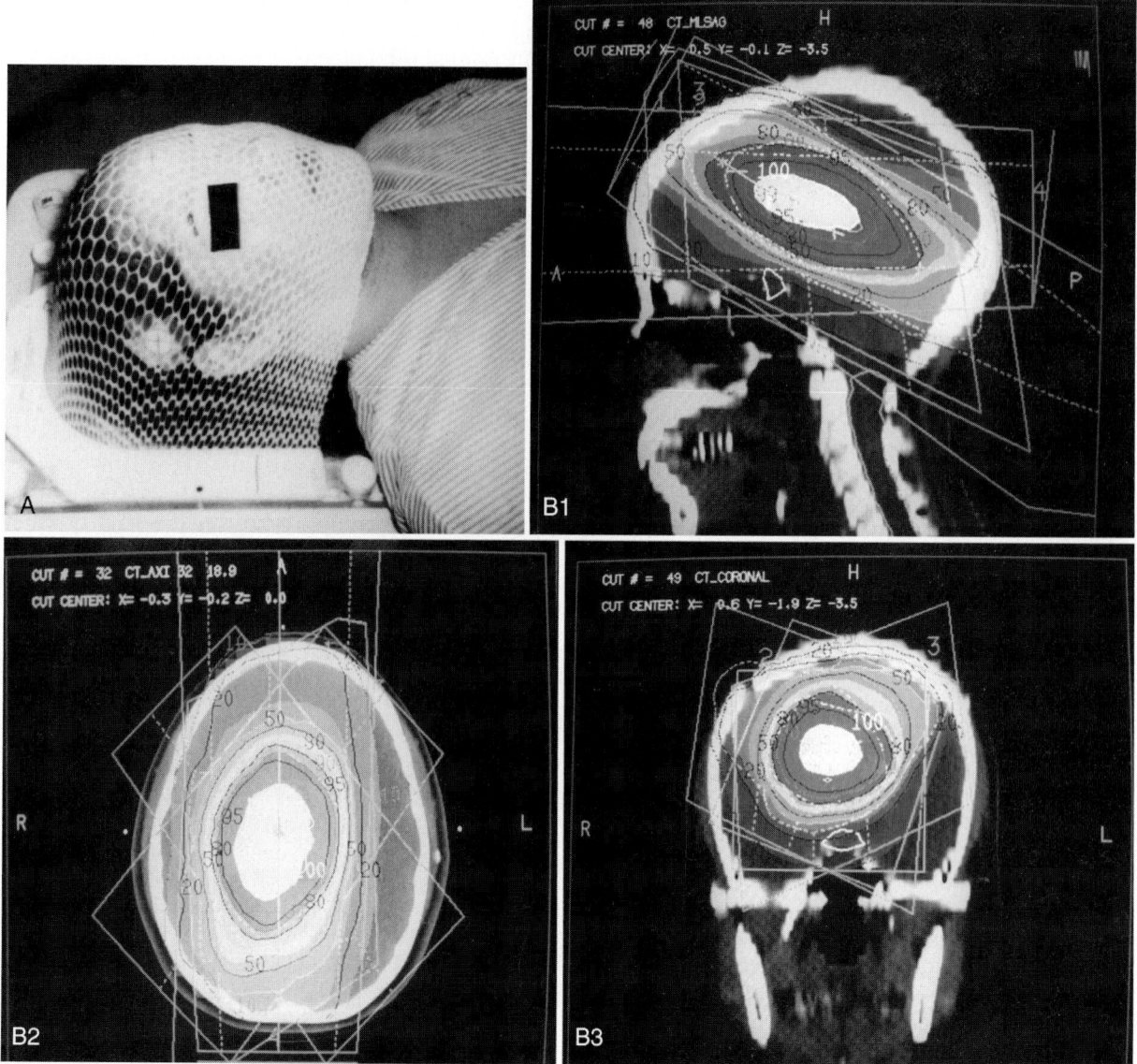

Figure 53–7. Three-dimensional conformal, noncoplanar treatment plan. The patient, a 21-year-old student, became increasingly disoriented over several days. Magnetic resonance imaging revealed a 5 cm intraventricular mass, which was subtotally resected because of involvement of the thalamus. Pathologic examination revealed an intraventricular neurocytoma. **A,** Simulation and planning computed tomography were performed with the head immobilized by a plastic mask. **B,** CT and MR images were merged to define the tumor volume, and a three-field, noncoplanar plan was devised, employing one posterior and two anterior, superior oblique beams. The plan's isodose curves are shown superimposed on the sagittal (*B1*), axial (*B2*), and coronal (*B3*) views.

with arcs, simulation is performed with the patient supine with the head in the neutral position to try to duplicate the position of the patient's head during the MRI scan. For treatment with arcs, the patient is placed on a slant board with the head in maximum flexion. In both cases, a plastic mask is then contoured to maintain the head in the same position and to avoid having to place marks on the patient's face. The isocenter is evaluated during the simulation by projection of the contrast-enhanced, sagittal magnetic resonance image onto the port film during simulation. In the case of arcs, a plaster of Paris contour is then taken through the isocenter in the coronal plane, perpendicular to the tabletop. The field size is usually 5 × 5 cm. It is preferable to use CT-based 3DCRT. In this case the patient is positioned and immobilized in a face mask, and a CT

scan is taken in that position after simulation. The CT scan can then be merged with an MRI scan using the planning computer.

Lesions of the Cerebrum

Tumors of the cerebral parenchyma[22] are simulated with the patient in the supine position with the head neutral, as in the MRI scan. Contrast enhancing and preoperative and postoperative images are then used to generate CT-based plans. Although many midline lesions can be adequately treated with opposed lateral beams, every attempt is made to reduce the dose to normal intervening structures by optimizing the volume of the dose distribution, often with the use of multiple beams.

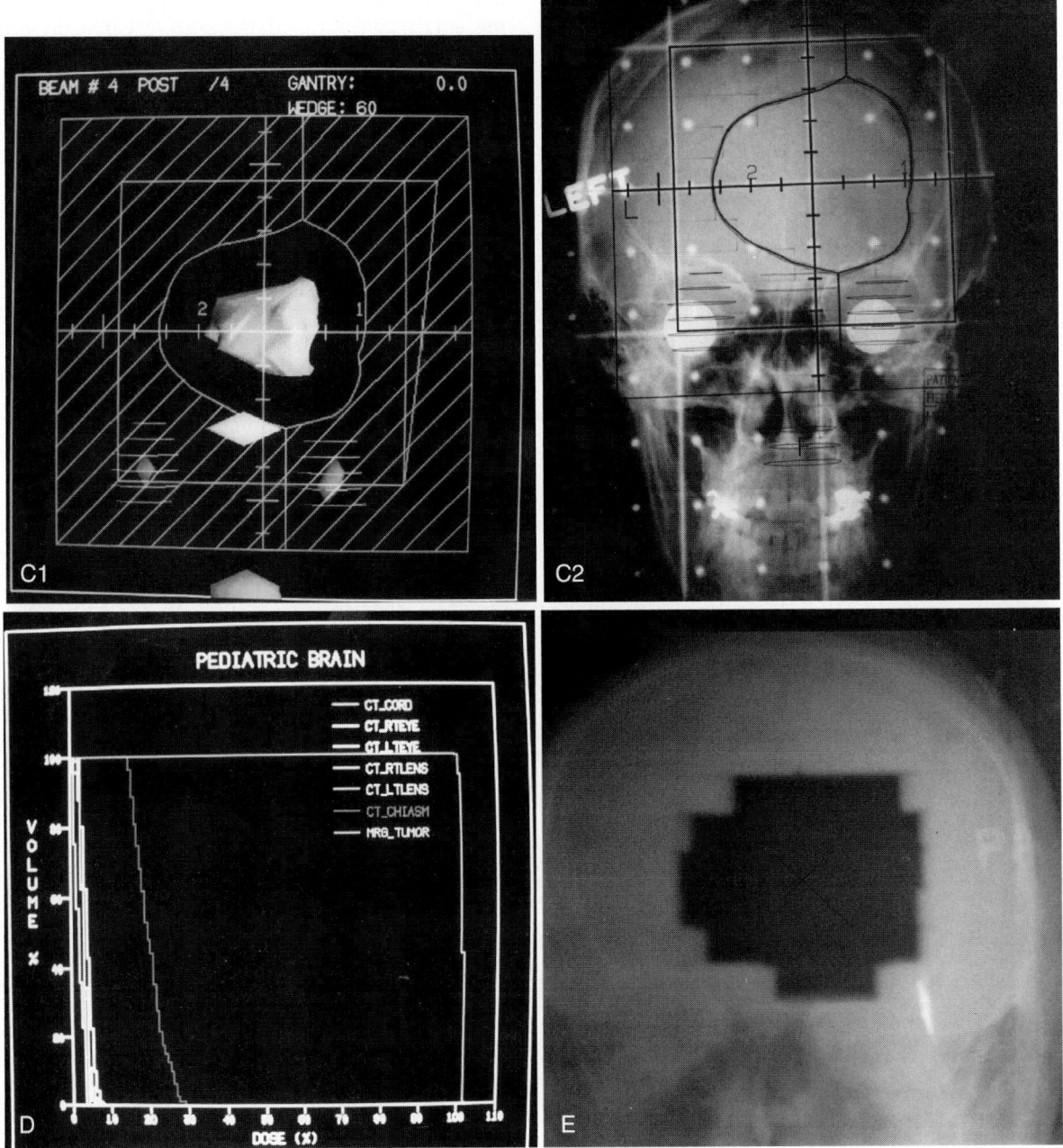

Figure 53–7. cont'd C, Beam's eye views were employed to design the blocking and to verify the plan. **D,** Dose-volume histograms were calculated and revealed satisfactory coverage of the planning treatment volume, and the dose to the chiasm was less than 30%. **E,** The treatment was performed with multi-leaf collimation and the setup was checked with weekly port films. Total dose was 54 Gy. See also Color Figure 53-7B, C, D.

Craniospinal Axis Irradiation

In all cases of medulloblastoma and ependymoblastoma, treatment is given to the craniospinal axis.[5,23,24] The patient is simulated in the prone position with the face in a concave holder ("doggie dish"). The spinal field is simulated with a posterior field from C2 down to S3 and covering the transverse spinal processes. It is unnecessary to widen the lower portion of the field to cover the cauda equina, although many clinicians routinely treat with a flared, inferior spinal portal. The whole brain field is treated with opposed laterals.[25] Diversion between the brain and spinal field is accounted for by appropriate rotation of the collimator and angling of the foot of the treatment table toward the lateral fields. This is calculated

in a similar fashion to a gap between adjacent fields. The collimator is rotated by an angle subtended by the arc tangent of half the length of the spinal field divided by the source-skin distance (SSD). Similarly, the table is moved toward the gantry by the angle subtended by the arc tangent of half the length of the cranial field divided by its SSD. The resultant match line should be moved 1 cm after each 10 Gy of dose.

TOXICITY OF RADIATION THERAPY

A wide range of potential toxicities complicates the implementation of radiation therapy in the treatment of tumors of the craniospinal axis. These toxicities can be

Table 53-7 Late Toxicities of Central Nervous System Irradiation

Structure	Late Effect	Threshold Dose
Spinal cord	Chronic progressive myelitis	45 Gy
Brain	Radiation necrosis	54 Gy
	Intellectual deficits	12–18 Gy
Lens of eye	Cataract formation	8 Gy
Retina	Radiation retinopathy	45 Gy
Optic nerve	Optic neuritis	50 Gy
Inner ear	Sensorineural hearing loss	40–50 Gy

severe and debilitating, particularly in pediatric patients. Care should be taken to minimize these effects. Treatment of intracranial tumors can result in damage to the eye, ear structures, brain, and hypothalamic-pituitary axis, as well as growth abnormalities. Treatment of the spine can result in growth deficits and damage to the spinal cord. Specific potential acute side effects of radiation to the CNS include epilation, skin reactions, otitis, hematopoietic depression, and somnolence. Specific late toxicities of such radiation include radionecrosis, myelopathy, leukoencephalopathy, vascular injury, neuropsychologic sequelae, endocrine dysfunction, bone and tooth abnormalities, ocular complications, ototoxicity, and induction of second primary tumors. Table 53-7 delineates the radiation doses associated with late toxicities that may result from radiation therapy to the CNS.

Spinal Cord

Severe damage to the spinal cord can result following radiation therapy, with transection of the cord at the affected level being the direct result. Radiation damage takes the form of chronic progressive myelitis. The 5% incidence of radiation myelopathy probably lies between 57 Gy and 61 Gy in the absence of chemotherapy, using standard fractionation. At <45 Gy the risk of myelitis is less than 0.2%. At 73 Gy the risk of myelitis approaches 50%.[26,27] A number of reports have indicated that tolerance of the cervical spinal cord to radiation toxicity is somewhat higher than 45 Gy in adults. However, it is unclear what the cervical spinal cord tolerance is in pediatric patients.

Radiation to the spinal cord can also result in Lhermitte's syndrome, which is characterized by tingling, numbness, and a sensation of electric shock. Symptoms are often present only with neck flexion. Lhermitte's syndrome is typically self-limiting, presenting within the first 1 to 3 months following radiation and having an average duration of 3 to 4 months. Craniospinal radiation can result in decreased truncal, or sitting, height. This is due to decreased growth of the vertebral bodies following radiation therapy, and becomes clinically evident at doses greater than 20 Gy.

Brain

Acute reactions during radiation therapy, thought to result from disruption of the blood-brain barrier, are uncommon. However, there are reports of edema following single conventional fractions.[28] Clinically apparent acute changes are more common with hypofractionated doses, such as used in radiosurgery.[29] Subacute reactions are more common and are thought to be due to transient demyelination.[30] These effects typically occur within the first few months following radiation and usually resolve within 6 to 9 months. Cranial nerve palsies have also been reported.[31] Severe subacute effects such as rapidly progressive ataxia are rarer and are generally associated with fractions larger than 2.0 Gy and total doses larger than 50 Gy.[32]

The late effects of radiation are primarily due to radiation necrosis. Symptoms are related to the neuroanatomic location of necrosis (sensory, motor, speech/receptive deficits, seizures) and may, in addition, be due to increased intracranial pressure. Focal necrosis is uncommon with doses below 60 Gy given with conventional fractionation.[33]

With large volume radiation therapy, diffuse white matter changes can be seen. Clinically, these can result in lassitude, personality change, or neurocognitive deficits. Multiple studies have examined the effect of whole brain radiation therapy on intellect in patients treated for leukemia. Radiation-associated depression in intelligence quotient (IQ) has been noted by a number of authors.[34,35] Halberg et al. compared three groups of patients. The first group received 18 Gy (1.8 Gy per fraction) cranial irradiation, while the second received 24 Gy cranial irradiation. The third group consisted of other oncology patients who did not receive cranial irradiation. Lower IQ scores were noted in the group receiving 24 Gy.[36] High-dose methotrexate and female sex appear to increase risk of intellectual deficits.[37,38] The effects of cranial irradiation are also more severe the younger the child. Intellectual deficits resulting from radiation most commonly result in difficulty acquiring new knowledge, decreased processing speed, and memory deficits (most frequently short-term).[39]

Studies of children irradiated for primary brain tumors have also shown intellectual deficits. Effects of radiation are more difficult to evaluate in this setting, as most of these patients also have had surgical resection. However, as with acute lymphoblastic leukemia (ALL) patients, younger age appears to result in a higher rate of neurocognitive deficits. Larger fields and higher doses also appear to cause a higher rate of toxicity.

Eye

The lens of the eye is exquisitely sensitive to radiation. Radiation-induced cataracts are caused by damage to the germinal zone at the equator of the lens. Initially, this results in a central opacity, which progresses to an opaque cortex. The threshold for radiation damage is 8 Gy in a single fraction, or 10 Gy to 15 Gy in fractionated doses. More rapid cataract formation is associated with higher doses of radiation.

Radiation-induced retinopathy appears to have a threshold of 46 Gy at conventional fractionation (1.8 to 2.0 Gy per fraction). Retinopathy is typically seen beginning from 6 months to 3 years following radiation. It is characterized by macular edema, nonperfusion, and neovascularization.

The optic nerves and chiasm are also at risk for damage from radiation. Damage to the optic nerve is characterized by a pale optic disc, abnormal papillary response, and visual deficits. Damage to the optic nerve or chiasm is potentially blinding. The threshold for damage is 50 Gy with fractions of 1.8 Gy. Every effort should be made to keep these structures below their tolerated doses.

Ear

Radiation-induced sensorineural hearing loss is dose dependent and is more severe in younger patients. Hearing loss can result from doses greater than 40 to 50 Gy, usually developing within 6 to 12 months of treatment.[40] High frequency hearing loss is seen in 25% to 50% of patients who received greater than 50 to 60 Gy to inner ear structures.[41-43] Hearing loss is typically attributed to radiation changes induced in the cochlea and vasculature. Ototoxicity related to cisplatinum chemotherapy is well documented.[44,45] Cranial irradiation before or concurrent with cisplatinum chemotherapy enhances ototoxicity.[44,46] Chronic otitis can also develop following radiation therapy, due to obstruction of the eustachian canal.

Endocrine

Whole cranial irradiation or more focal radiation that includes the hypothalamic-pituitary axis can result in neuroendocrine abnormalities. The neuroendocrine complications that can result from radiation therapy are summarized in Table 53-8. Growth hormone (GH) production appears to be the most prone to disruption by radiation therapy. GH deficiency worsens over time and may follow radiation doses as low as 12 Gy.[47] This appears to be a result of decreased growth hormone–releasing hormone (GH-RH) in the hypothalamus, as GH deficiency is seen in patients undergoing hypothalamic radiation with pituitary sparing. Clinically, GH deficiency can result in short stature, bone loss, and metabolic abnormalities. Treatment with synthetic GH can allow children to maintain their expected growth percentile despite irradiation.

Other endocrine deficiencies, including decreased thyroid stimulating hormone, corticotropin, follicle-stimulating hormone, and luteinizing hormone appear to have a higher threshold. These effects are typically seen following doses greater than 40 Gy. It is important that children treated for tumors in the region of the hypothalamic-pituitary axis be followed closely for endocrine abnormalities, so that replacement therapy can be initiated in a timely fashion.

RESULTS IN SELECTED SPECIFIC CENTRAL NERVOUS SYSTEM TUMORS

It can be assumed that the reported outcomes of treatment for pediatric tumors of the CNS are somewhat better than the actual outcome.[48] This is because the most aggressive presentations of the various histologic types disable or kill the patient before therapy is completed, and therefore the very worst cases are excluded from most studies. Summaries of survival are listed according to treatment and histology in Table 53-9.

Medulloblastoma

Medulloblastoma is the most common pediatric brain tumor and the tumor for which staging seems to be most useful for determining subsequent outcome. Up to one third of medulloblastomas in children are associated with dissemination beyond the primary site at the time of diagnosis.[49] Age younger than 3 years and inability to perform a gross total surgical removal of tumor are associated with poor survival. Historically, standard treatment delivered 36 Gy to the brain and spine and a total dose to the posterior fossa of 54 Gy. Significant abnormalities in intellectual development, growth, and hormonal function commonly occurred after craniospinal irradiation.[50-53]

Table 53–8 Endocrine Abnormalities Resulting from Radiation

Hormone Abnormality	Threshold Dose to Hypothalamic Axis
Growth hormone deficit	18–25 Gy
ACTH deficit	40 Gy
TRH/TSH deficit	40 Gy
Precocious puberty	20 Gy
LH/FSH deficit	40 Gy
Hyperprolactinemia	40 Gy

ACTH, corticotropin; TRH/TSH, thyrotropin-releasing hormone/thyrotropin; LH/FSH, luteinizing hormone/follicle-stimulating hormone.

Table 53–9 Selected Outcome from University of California–San Francisco

Histology	5-Yr Survival, %
Gliomas	
Diffuse, brainstem	0
Medulloblastoma	
Low risk	59
High risk	22
Ependymoma	67
Germ cell	
Germinoma	100
Nongerminomatous	80

Data from Shrieve DC, Wara WM, Edwards MS, et al: Hyperfractionated radiation therapy for gliomas of the brain stem in children and adults. *Int J Radiat Oncol Biol Phys*. 1992;24:599; Wolden SL, Wara WM, Larson DA, et al: Radiation therapy for primary intracranial germ-cell tumors. *Int J Radiat Oncol Biol Phys*. 1995;32:943; and Wara WM, Le QT, Sneed PK, et al: Pattern of recurrence of medulloblastoma after low-dose craniospinal radiotherapy. *Int J Radiat Oncol Biol Phys*. 1994;30:551.

The Pediatric Oncology Group and Children's Cancer Group jointly examined the role of reduced-dose neuroaxis irradiation in low-stage medulloblastoma. A planned interim analysis resulted in early closure of this trial when it documented that reduced-dose neuroaxis irradiation resulted in increased rates of isolated neuroaxis failure. Although an update of this study revealed that the differences between standard-dose and reduced-dose craniospinal irradiation became less pronounced with time, the update did confirm the inferiority of 23.4 Gy to the craniospinal axis. Reduced-dose craniospinal irradiation resulted in increased risk of early relapse, early isolated neuroaxis failure, and lower event-free and overall survival rates compared with 36 Gy.[54]

Although reduced-dose craniospinal irradiation proved inadequate in the treatment of low-stage medulloblastoma, the addition of chemotherapy to reduced-dose irradiation has shifted the standard-of-care paradigm. Treatment of children 3 to 10 years of age with non-disseminated medulloblastoma using chemotherapy, reduced-dose craniospinal irradiation, and 55.8 Gy of local radiation resulted in excellent clinical outcome. At 3 years, the progression-free survival rate was 86%.[55]

Over the past 25 years, children with high-stage medulloblastoma have achieved 5-year survival rates of 50% to 80%. The standard of care includes combined-modality chemotherapy and radiation therapy. For children older than 3 years, the craniospinal dose is 36 Gy and the posterior fossa dose is 54 to 55.8 Gy. For younger children, consideration should be given to lowering the craniospinal and local radiation doses. In one trial the Children's Cancer Group evaluated two different chemotherapeutic regimens for the treatment of high-stage medulloblastoma. The superior arm of this prospective, randomized trial consisted of weekly vincristine during radiotherapy, followed by eight 6-week cycles of vincristine, lomustine, and prednisone. This regimen resulted in 5-year progression-free survival of 63%.[56] The major benefit of combined modality therapy with reduced radiation dose is the decrease in subsequent sequelae.

Cerebellar Astrocytomas

The majority of cerebellar astrocytomas carry a good prognosis when treated with surgery alone and are often of the pilocytic type.[18,57] Even with subtotally resected tumors, irradiation is withheld until evidence of progression is seen on an MRI or CT scan.

Brainstem Gliomas

In contrast to the juvenile pilocytic astrocytomas, diffuse brainstem gliomas are nearly universally fatal within 3 years of diagnosis.[33,58-60] Except for dorsally exophytic lesions, which can be cured by surgery alone, these lesions are usually treated with radiation only. Lesions that are more focal, of a lower grade, involve the thalamus or midbrain, and have a slower onset of symptoms progress more slowly than the diffuse variety. Although radiotherapy is often performed without biopsy, the influence of surgical intervention on this disease (excluding dorsally exophytic lesions) is uncertain. Hyperfractionated radiotherapy of 1 Gy twice a day to a total dose of 72 Gy has been shown to produce similar survival to that of other treatment schemes, with an acceptable rate of morbidity.[9,61]

Cerebral Astrocytomas

The prognosis for astrocytomas is much better for children than for adults.[22] However, the role of radiotherapy following surgery is controversial and is currently the object of several protocols.

Ependymomas

Ependymomas occur most frequently in the posterior fossa and are treated with 54 Gy with a local field, achieving relatively good 5-year survival rates.[62] There is some controversy as to the need for craniospinal radiotherapy in addition to local field treatment. Most centers treat with local therapy only. There is no proven benefit from chemotherapy in children with ependymoma.

Germ Cell Tumors

Intracranial germ cell tumors (GCT) represent 3% to 11% of pediatric and 1% of adult brain tumors.[63] Intracranial GCTs compose two distinct histologic groupings: Germinomas are the most common histologic subtype, while nongerminomatous germ cell tumors (NGGCT) represent one third of intracranial GCTs and consist of embryonal carcinoma, endodermal sinus (yolk sac) tumor, choriocarcinoma, teratoma, and GCT of mixed cellular origin.[63,64] Historically, radiation alone, frequently encompassing a large treatment volume, has constituted the gold standard of treatment for intracranial GCTs.[11,63,65,66] However, the morbidity of radiation therapy in children,[67-72] particularly craniospinal irradiation (CSI), has prompted many investigators to explore approaches that reduce the volume and dose of radiotherapy while preserving high cure rates.

The development of strategies to reduce the morbidity of radiotherapy has been hampered by an absence of randomized trials comparing treatment approaches. Several large retrospective studies have shed light on persistent controversies in the management of intracranial GCTs. Current literature supports distinct therapeutic approaches for germinomas versus NGGCT. Although many published studies group germinomas with NGGCT, their distinct prognosis points to the need to approach these clinical entities individually.

Published reports corroborate poorer prognosis for patients with NGGCT compared with those with germinomas.[64,73] Radiation alone produces 5-year survival rates of only 30% to 40%.[74] More recent studies that demonstrate excellent response rates to chemotherapy have shifted the standard treatment of NGGCT to combined modality therapy consisting of chemotherapy and radiation.

Of the various histologic subtypes of intracranial GCTs, germinomas represent the most common and prognostically favorable subgroup. Historically, intracranial germinoma has been treated with radiation alone, producing excellent cure rates.[11,63,66] The significant long-term toxicity of radiation, particularly in children,[67-72] has prompted investigation to explore alternative treatment that minimizes the dose and volume of irradiation. However, these alternative approaches must preserve the high cure rates established with radiation alone.

Several series have reported excellent clinical outcome with preirradiation chemotherapy followed by focal irradiation.[4,75-80] The appeal of this approach lies in lower radiation dose and smaller radiation fields that presumably translate into reduced long-term toxicity. Radiation alone continues to be the gold standard for the treatment of intracranial germinoma. Promising approaches such as combined chemotherapy and focal, reduced-dose irradiation must be compared to radiation alone in a prospective, randomized trial.

In addition to the role of chemotherapy, a point of controversy in the treatment of localized germinoma has been the appropriate field of radiation.[81] Current evidence substantiates omitting CSI from the treatment of localized germinoma. Spinal failure rates of less than 10% in the absence of CSI, reported in most contemporary series, do not justify routine incorporation of CSI into the treatment strategy for localized germinoma.[65,73,82-85] Nevertheless, the precise irradiation field appropriate for localized germinoma remains unclear. Several studies report higher recurrence rates associated with radiation targeting the tumor volume only.[65,73,86,87] We recommend whole ventricular irradiation, followed by a boost to the primary tumor for localized germinoma when using radiation alone. The literature supports a dose of greater than or equal to 45 Gy to the primary tumor for germinomas treated with radiation alone. In the context of combined chemotherapy and radiation, many investigators have tailored the dose of radiation to the tumor response observed following chemotherapy. Doses of radiation following chemotherapy range from 24 to 40 Gy.

Craniopharyngiomas

These lesions are not malignant but, because of their location in the suprasellar region, are often associated with high morbidity. The judgment and skill of the operating surgeon is therefore critical if significant endocrine and visual problems are to be avoided. It appears that subtotal resection followed by local irradiation to 54 Gy offers progression-free survival similar to that of gross total resection with a much lower rate of morbidity.

Miscellaneous: Meningiomas and Hemangiopericytomas

Meningiomas are rare in children but are treated in similar fashion to meningiomas in adults, with maximal surgical resection followed by radiotherapy for subtotal resections. Hemangiopericytomas are like meningiomas but appear to be more aggressive and are treated to a total dose of 60 Gy.

REFERENCES

1. Bergsagel DJ, et al: DNA sequences similar to those of simian virus 40 in ependymomas and choroid plexus tumors of childhood. *N Engl J Med.* 1992;326:988.
2. Ghim TT, Finegold MJ, Butel JS, et al: Childhood intracranial meningiomas after high-dose irradiation. *Cancer.* 1993;71:4091.
3. Kuijten RR, Bunin GR: Risk factors for childhood brain tumors. *Cancer Epidemiol Biomarkers Prev.* 1993;2:277.
4. Kollias SS, Barkovich AJ, Edwards MS: Magnetic resonance analysis of suprasellar tumors of childhood. *Pediatr Neurosurg.* 1991;17:284.
5. Packer RJ: Brain tumors in children. *Curr Opin Pediatr.* 1995;7:64.
6. Conway PD, et al: Importance of histologic condition and treatment of pediatric cerebellar astrocytoma. *Cancer.* 1991;67:2772.
7. Bernstein M, Laperriere NJ: A critical appraisal of the role of brachytherapy for pediatric brain tumors. *Pediatr Neurosurg.* 1990;16:213.
8. Ceddia A, Di Rocco C, Iannelli A: Epilepsy and low grade gliomas in pediatric neurosurgery. *J Neurosurg Sci.* 1993;37:91.
9. Shrieve DC, et al: Hyperfractionated radiation therapy for gliomas of the brainstem in children and in adults. *Int J Radiat Oncol Biol Phys.* 1992;24:599.
10. Neumann E, Kalousek DK, Norman MG, et al: Cytogenetic analysis of 109 pediatric central nervous system tumors. *Cancer Genet Cytogenet.* 1993;71:40.
11. Wolden SL, et al: Radiation therapy for primary intracranial germ-cell tumors. *Int J Radiat Oncol Biol Phys.* 1995;32:943.
12. Tamura M, Kohga H, Ono N, et al: Calcified astrocytoma of the amygdalo-hippocampal region in children. *Childs Nerv Syst.* 1995;11:141.
13. Kivela T, Tarkkanen A: Orbital germ cell tumors revisited: A clinicopathological approach to classification. *Surv Ophthalmol.* 1994;38:541.
14. Butler D, Jose B, Summe R, et al: Pediatric astrocytomas. The Louisville experience: 1978-1988. *Am J Clin Oncol.* 1994;17:475.
15. Freeman CR, Souhami L, Caron JL, et al: Stereotactic external beam irradiation in previously untreated brain tumors in children and adolescents. *Med Pediatr Oncol.* 1994;22:510.
16. Chang CH, Housepian EM, Herbert C Jr: An operative staging system and a megavoltage radiotherapeutic technic for cerebellar medulloblastomas. *Radiology.* 1969;93:1351.
17. Cochrane DD, Gustavsson B, Poskitt KP, et al: The surgical and natural morbidity of aggressive resection for posterior fossa tumors in childhood. *Pediatr Neurosurg.* 1994;20:19.
18. Rekate HL, Rakfal SM: Low-grade astrocytomas of childhood. *Neurol Clin.* 1991;9:423.
19. Bourne JP, Geyer R, Berger M, et al: The prognostic significance of postoperative residual contrast enhancement on CT scan in pediatric patients with medulloblastoma. *J Neurooncol.* 1992;14:263.
20. Friedman HS, Oakes WJ: New therapeutic options in the management of childhood brain tumors. *Oncology (Huntingt).* 1992;6:27; discussion 36, 39.
21. Halperin EC, Wehn SM, Scott JW, et al: Selection of a management strategy for pediatric brainstem tumors. *Med Pediatr Oncol.* 1989;17:117.
22. Pollack IF, Claassen D, al-Shboul Q, et al: Low-grade gliomas of the cerebral hemispheres in children: An analysis of 71 cases. *J Neurosurg.* 1995;82:536.
23. Hart RM, Kimmler BF, Evans RG, Park CH: Radiotherapeutic management of medulloblastoma in a pediatric patient with ataxia telangiectasia. *Int J Radiat Oncol Biol Phys.* 1987;13:1237.
24. Wara WM, Le QT, Sneed PK, et al: Pattern of recurrence of medulloblastoma after low-dose craniospinal radiotherapy. *Int J Radiat Oncol Biol Phys.* 1994;30:551.
25. Duffner PK, Burger PC, Cohen ME, et al: Desmoplastic infantile gangliogliomas: An approach to therapy. *Neurosurgery.* 1994;34:583; discussion 589.
26. Schultheiss TE, Kun LE, Ang KK, et al: Radiation response of the central nervous system. *Int J Radiat Oncol Biol Phys.* 1995;31:1093.

27. Wong CS, Van Dyke J, Milosevic M, et al: Radiation myelopathy following single courses of radiotherapy and retreatment. *Int J Radiat Oncol Biol Phys*. 1994;30:575.

28. Kramer S, Lee KF: Complications of radiation therapy: The central nervous system. *Semin Roentgenol*. 1974;9:75.

29. Loeffler JS, Siddon RL, Wen PY, et al: Stereotactic radiosurgery of the brain using a standard linear accelerator: A study of early and late effects. *Radiother Oncol*. 1990;17:311.

30. Boldrey E, Sheline G: Delayed transitory clinical manifestations after radiation treatment of intracranial tumors. *Acta Radiol Ther Phys Biol*. 1966;5:5.

31. Littman P, Rosenstock J, Gale G, et al: The somnolence syndrome in leukemic children following reduced daily dose fractions of cranial radiation. *Int J Radiat Oncol Biol Phys*. 1984;10:1851.

32. Lampert H, Alegria A: Treatment of post-poliomyelitis paralysis of long duration. *Acta Neurol Latinoam*. 1964;10:160.

33. Halperin EC: Pediatric brain stem tumors: Patterns of treatment failure and their implications for radiotherapy. *Int J Radiat Oncol Biol Phys*. 1985;11:1293.

34. Rowland JH, Glidewell OJ, Sibley RF, et al: Effects of different forms of central nervous system prophylaxis on neuropsychologic function in childhood leukemia. *J Clin Oncol*. 1984;2:1327.

35. Copeland DR, Fletcher JM, Pfefferbaum-Levine B, et al: Neuropsychological sequelae of childhood cancer in long-term survivors. *Pediatrics*. 1985;75:745.

36. Halberg FE, Kramer JH, Moore IM, et al: Prophylactic cranial irradiation dose effects on late cognitive function in children treated for acute lymphoblastic leukemia. *Int J Radiat Oncol Biol Phys*. 1992;22:13.

37. Waber DP, Tarbell NJ, Kahn LM, et al: The relationship of sex and treatment modality to neuropsychologic outcome in childhood acute lymphoblastic leukemia. *J Clin Oncol*. 1992;10:810.

38. Hardenbergh PH, et al: Intracranial germinoma: The case for lower dose radiation therapy. *Int J Radiat Oncol Biol Phys*. 1997;39:419.

39. Mulhern RK, Ochs J, Fairclough D: Deterioration of intellect among children surviving leukemia: IQ test changes modify estimates of treatment toxicity. *J Consult Clin Psychol*. 1992;60:477.

40. Grau C, Overgaard J: Postirradiation sensorineural hearing loss: A common but ignored late radiation complication. *Int J Radiat Oncol Biol Phys*. 1996;36:515.

41. Anteunis LJ, Engel JA, Hendriks JJ, Manni JJ: A prospective longitudinal study on radiation-induced hearing loss. *Am J Surg*. 1994;168:408.

42. Kwong DL, Wei WI, Sham JS, et al: Sensorineural hearing loss in patients treated for nasopharyngeal carcinoma: A prospective study of the effect of radiation and cisplatin treatment. *Int J Radiat Oncol Biol Phys*. 1996;36:281.

43. Low WK, Fong KW: Long-term hearing status after radiotherapy for nasopharyngeal carcinoma. *Auris Nasus Larynx*. 1998;25:21.

44. Schell MJ, McHaney VA, Green AA, et al: Hearing loss in children and young adults receiving cisplatin with or without prior cranial irradiation. *J Clin Oncol*. 1989;7:754.

45. McHaney VA, Thibadoux G, Hayes FA, Green AA: Hearing loss in children receiving cisplatin chemotherapy. *J Pediatr*. 1983;102:314.

46. Walker DA, Pillow J, Waters KD, Keir E: Enhanced cis-platinum ototoxicity in children with brain tumors who have received simultaneous or prior cranial irradiation. *Med Pediatr Oncol*. 1989;17:48.

47. Merchant TE, Goloubeva O, Pritchard DL, et al: Radiation dose-volume effects on growth hormone secretion. *Int J Radiat Oncol Biol Phys*. 2002;52:1264.

48. Novakovic B: U.S. childhood cancer survival, 1973-1987. *Med Pediatr Oncol*. 1994;23:480.

49. Nebeling LC, Miraldi F, Shurin SB, Lerner E: Effects of a ketogenic diet on tumor metabolism and nutritional status in pediatric oncology patients: Two case reports. *J Am Coll Nutr*. 1995;14:202.

50. Agard ET, Ehlers G, Kirchberg S: Scattered radiation doses to some critical organs during pediatric radiotherapy. *Health Phys*. 1985;48:447.

51. Moss SD, Rockswold GL, Chou SN, et al: Radiation-induced meningiomas in pediatric patients. *Neurosurgery*. 1988;22:758.

52. Silber JH, Radcliffe J, Peckham V, et al: Whole-brain irradiation and decline in intelligence: The influence of dose and age on IQ score. *J Clin Oncol*. 1992;10:1390.

53. Duffner PK, Cohen ME, Thomas PR, Lansky SB: The long-term effects of cranial irradiation on the central nervous system. *Cancer*. 1985;56(7 suppl):1841.

54. Thomas PR, Deutsch M, Kepner JL, et al: Low-stage medulloblastoma: Final analysis of trial comparing standard-dose with reduced-dose neuraxis irradiation. *J Clin Oncol*. 2000;18:3004.

55. Packer RJ, Goldwein J, Nicholson HS, et al: Treatment of children with medulloblastomas with reduced-dose craniospinal radiation therapy and adjuvant chemo-therapy: A Children's Cancer Group Study. *J Clin Oncol*. 1999;17:2127.

56. Zeltzer PM, Boyett JM, Finlay JL, et al: Metastasis stage, adjuvant treatment, and residual tumor are prognostic factors for medulloblastoma in children: Conclusions from the Children's Cancer Group 921 randomized phase III study. *J Clin Oncol*. 1999;17:832.

57. Lee YY, Van Tassel P, Bruner JM, et al: Juvenile pilocytic astrocytomas: CT and MR characteristics. *AJR Am J Roentgenol*. 1989;152:1263.

58. Epstein F, McCleary EL: Intrinsic brain-stem tumors of childhood: Surgical indications. *J Neurosurg*. 1986;64:11.

59. Raffel C, McComb JG, Bodner S, Giles FE: Benign brain stem lesions in pediatric patients with neurofibromatosis: Case reports. *Neurosurgery*. 1989;25:959.

60. Robertson PL, Muraszko KM, Brunberg JA, et al: Pediatric midbrain tumors: A benign subgroup of brainstem gliomas. *Pediatr Neurosurg*. 1995;22:65.

61. Freeman CR, Muraszko KM, Brunberg JA, et al: Hyperfractionated radiotherapy in brain stem tumors: Results of a Pediatric Oncology Group study. *Int J Radiat Oncol Biol Phys*. 1988;15:311.

62. Mastrangelo R, Marmiroli L, Tomesello A, Ausili-Celaro G: Radiation and chemotherapy in pediatric infratentorial tumors. *Rays*. 1993;18:471.

63. Hoffman HJ, Otsubo H, Hendrick EB, et al: Intracranial germ-cell tumors in children. *J Neurosurg*. 1991;74:545.

64. Kretschmar CS: Germ cell tumors of the brain in children: A review of current literature and new advances in therapy. *Cancer Invest*. 1997;15:187.

65. Aoyama H, Shirato H, Yoshida H, et al: Retrospective multi-institutional study of radiotherapy for intracranial non-germinomatous germ cell tumors. *Radiother Oncol*. 1998;49:55.

66. Bamberg M, Kortmann RD, Caliminus G, et al: Radiation therapy for intracranial germinoma: Results of the German cooperative prospective trials MAKEI 83/86/89. *J Clin Oncol*. 1999;17:2585.

67. Chapman CA, Waber DP, Bernstein JH, et al: Neurobehavioral and neurologic outcome in long-term survivors of posterior fossa brain tumors: Role of age and perioperative factors. *J Child Neurol*. 1995;10:209.

68. Ellenberg L, McComb JG, Siegel SE, Stowe S: Factors affecting intellectual outcome in pediatric brain tumor patients. *Neurosurgery*. 1987;21:638.

69. Moore BD, Ater JL, Copeland DR: Improved neuropsychological outcome in children with brain tumors diagnosed during infancy and treated without cranial irradiation. *J Child Neurol*. 1992;7:281.

70. Packer RJ, Sutton LN, Atkins TE, et al: A prospective study of cognitive function in children receiving whole-brain radiotherapy and chemotherapy: 2-year results. *J Neurosurg*. 1989;70:707.

71. Radcliffe J, Packer RJ, Atkins TE, et al: Three- and four-year cognitive outcome in children with noncortical brain tumors treated with whole-brain radiotherapy. *Ann Neurol*. 1992;32:551.

72. Waber DP, Tarbell NJ, Fairclough D, et al: Cognitive sequelae of treatment in childhood acute lymphoblastic leukemia: cranial radiation requires an accomplice. *J Clin Oncol*. 1995;13:2490.

73. Matsutani M, Sano K, Takakura K, et al: Primary intracranial germ cell tumors: A clinical analysis of 153 histologically verified cases. *J Neurosurg*. 1997;86:446.

74. Fuller BG, Kapp DS, Cox R: Radiation therapy of pineal region tumors: 25 new cases and a review of 208 previously reported cases. *Int J Radiat Oncol Biol Phys*. 1994;28:229.

75. Baranzelli MC, Patte C, Bouffet E, et al: Nonmetastatic intracranial germinoma: The experience of the French Society of Pediatric Oncology. *Cancer*. 1997;80:1792.

76. Bouffet E, Baranzelli MC, Patte C, et al: Combined treatment modality for intracranial germinomas: Results of a multicentre SFOP experience. Société Française d'Oncologie Pédiatrique. *Br J Cancer*. 1999;79:1199.

77. Buckner JC, et al: Phase II trial of primary chemotherapy followed by reduced-dose radiation for CNS germ cell tumors. *J Clin Oncol.* 1999;17:933.

78. Fouladi M, Grant R, Baruchel S, et al: Comparison of survival outcomes in patients with intracranial germinomas treated with radiation alone versus reduced-dose radiation and chemotherapy. *Childs Nerv Syst.* 1998;14:596.

79. Kitamura K, Shirato H, Sawamura Y, et al: Preirradiation evaluation and technical assessment of involved-field radiotherapy using computed tomographic (CT) simulation and neoadjuvant chemotherapy for intracranial germinoma. *Int J Radiat Oncol Biol Phys.* 1999;43:783.

80. Sawamura Y, Shirato H, Ikeda J, et al: Induction chemotherapy followed by reduced-volume radiation therapy for newly diagnosed central nervous system germinoma. *J Neurosurg.* 1998; 88:66.

81. Paulino AC, Wen BC, Mohideen MN: Controversies in the management of intracranial germinomas. *Oncology.* 1999;13:513; discussion 521.

82. Dattoli MJ, Newall J: Radiation therapy for intracranial germinoma: The case for limited volume treatment. *Int J Radiat Oncol Biol Phys.* 1990;19:429.

83. Haddock MG, Schild SE, Scheithaver BW, Schomburg PJ: Radiation therapy for histologically confirmed primary central nervous system germinoma. *Int J Radiat Oncol Biol Phys.* 1997;38:915.

84. Linstadt D, Wara WM, Edwards MS, et al: Radiotherapy of primary intracranial germinomas: The case against routine craniospinal irradiation. *Int J Radiat Oncol Biol Phys.* 1988;15:291.

85. Sugiyama K, Uozumi T, Arita K, et al: Clinical evaluation of 33 patients with histologically verified germinoma. *Surg Neurol.* 1994;42:200.

86. Shibamoto Y, Abe M, Yamashita J, et al: Treatment results of intracranial germinoma as a function of the irradiated volume. *Int J Radiat Oncol Biol Phys.* 1988;15:285.

87. Shirato H, Nishio M, Sawamura Y, et al: Analysis of long-term treatment of intracranial germinoma. *Int J Radiat Oncol Biol Phys.* 1997;37:511.

54

Pediatric Leukemias and Lymphomas

Barbara Asselin, MD, Melissa Hudson, MD,
Lynda Mandell, MD, PhD, and Louis S. Constine, MD

The evolution of curative treatment of pediatric leukemias and lymphomas reflects the success and, consequently, the changing focus in the management of childhood cancers in general. With the advent of effective multiagent chemotherapy, combined modality regimens were devised that dramatically improved the dismal survival rates associated with the use of local therapy alone. Scientific progress in immunophenotyping, cytogenetics, and cytochemistry generated the tools necessary to determine prognostic factors and risk-adapted therapeutic approaches. The major efforts of investigative trials over the past 20 years have focused on: (1) deintensifying therapy in low-risk patients, with the aim of improving quality of life in the increasing number of surviving patients; and (2) exploring alternative and innovative ways to improve the cure rate in those patients considered to be at high risk for relapse with standard therapeutic regimens. As a corollary, in depth investigations into the acute and chronic normal tissue effects have become a priority.

This chapter is a guide to the management of childhood leukemias and lymphomas, with a special emphasis on the current use of radiotherapy. Historically used treatment approaches are presented to create a framework for understanding the rationale of the current treatment protocols and also for future trials, as the evolution of treatment continues. As with most pediatric malignancies during the past 3 decades, the role of radiotherapy in the treatment of leukemias and lymphomas has become increasingly restricted in light of the continued success of chemotherapy and the growing concern about long-term treatment-related morbidity in children surviving cancer. Therefore, the changes in therapeutic approaches that have been prompted by our recognition of associated adverse effects will be emphasized.

CHILDHOOD LEUKEMIAS

Leukemia is the most common form of malignancy seen in the pediatric age group, comprising 30% of cancer cases in children.[1] The vast majority of childhood leukemia cases are acute, unlike those in adults.

Acute lymphoblastic leukemia (ALL) is most common, accounting for 80% of all cases of childhood leukemia.

Acute nonlymphoblastic leukemia, most often acute myelogenous leukemia (AML), constitutes almost 20% of cases, and chronic myelogenous leukemia (CML) approximately 3% of all leukemia cases. Over the past 2 decades in the United States, an unexplained increase in leukemia rates among children younger than 15 years of age has been observed. This trend results primarily from an increase in ALL incidence since the rates of leukemias other than ALL did not appear to increase from 1977 to 1995.[2]

ACUTE LYMPHOBLASTIC LEUKEMIA

Epidemiology and Etiology

ALL accounts for more than 2400 of the 3250 new cases of childhood leukemia diagnosed each year in the United States.[1] In the United States, childhood ALL has a peak incidence between 3 and 5 years of age, and is more common in boys than in girls and in whites more than in blacks.[1] The frequency of ALL is increased in certain genetic disorders including Down's syndrome (DS), congenital immunodeficiency diseases (e.g., Wiskott-Aldrich syndrome, congenital hypogammaglobulinemia), and chromosomal fragility syndromes (e.g., Fanconi's anemia, ataxia telangiectasia).[3] Molecular studies of identical twins suggest a prenatal origin for acute leukemia, both lymphoid and myeloid subtypes.[4,5]

These epidemiologic observations suggest an important role for genetic factors, host immunocompetence, as well as prenatal and postnatal events in the development of leukemia. However, most cases of ALL remain unexplained.

Clinical Presentation

The common presenting signs and symptoms reflect the degree of bone marrow compromise, the extent and location of leukemic cell infiltration, and the general systemic effects of these processes. Fever, the most common feature, is caused most often by the leukemia itself rather than by infection.[6,7] Bleeding symptoms with bruising or petechiae and pallor with fatigue are among the common complaints resulting from the thrombocytopenia and anemia, respectively. Bone pain is common due to leukemic periosteal infiltration and marrow expansion. Lymphadenopathy and hepatosplenomegaly result from extramedullary infiltration of leukemic cells, occurring in 60% of children with ALL.[6,7] An anterior mediastinal mass is present in up to 10% of newly diagnosed patients, making a chest roentgenogram crucial in the initial evaluations. Central nervous system (CNS) involvement occurs in about 5% of patients at diagnosis. Children younger than age 2 and those with T-cell ALL have a higher incidence of CNS leukemia. Testicular leukemia manifest as painless enlargement of one or both testes is rare, occurring in less than 5% of patients. A mild to moderate degree of anemia and thrombocytopenia are common hematologic abnormalities. The white blood cell count (WBC) may be normal, decreased, or increased. A relatively small proportion of patients (14%) have hyperleukocytosis with a WBC greater than 100,000/mm³.[7] Blasts frequently, but not always, are found in the peripheral blood smear.

Diagnosis and Extent of Disease Evaluation

Examination of the bone marrow is essential to confirm the diagnosis of leukemia. Bone marrow aspirate usually provides sufficient material for successful diagnosis including flow cytometry and cytogenetic studies for complete classification (see later). Hematologic and chemical laboratory studies are performed routinely to assess a patient's status for the dual purpose of obtaining prognostic information (e.g., WBC for risk assignment) and elucidating hemodynamic and metabolic abnormalities in order to correct them before cytotoxic therapy.

A thorough physical examination is required to determine the extent of the disease and detect lymphadenopathy, abdominal organomegaly, and testicular involvement. CNS involvement is suspected in the presence of cranial nerve palsies, papilledema, a history of headaches, or vomiting, although asymptomatic pleocytosis is the most common presentation of CNS ALL. The traditional definition of CNS disease requires the presence of lymphoblasts in a cytocentrifuged sample of cerebrospinal fluid (CSF) along with at least 5 WBC per microliter of CSF or the presence of a cranial nerve palsy.[8] Studies to evaluate the clinical significance of lymphoblasts in diagnostic CSF samples with less than 5 WBC/µl have been inconclusive and therefore remain under scrutiny.[9,10] In addition, the finding of blast cells in CSF with fewer than 5 WBC/µl obtained during treatment is not conclusive of CNS relapse.[11] Chest roentgenograms are essential to document mediastinal mass and potential risk of airway or vascular compromise before invasive procedures, sedation, or definitive therapy.

Classification

It is now well recognized that pediatric ALL is a heterogeneous disease. Originally, lymphoblasts were classified solely by morphologic criteria and cytochemical staining characteristics. These methods were sufficient to distinguish ALL from AML. More recently, classification of ALL has expanded to include immunologic and cytogenetic criteria. These criteria are useful in defining lineage and maturational stage of the leukemic clone for prognostic and therapeutic purposes as well as contributing to our understanding of important mechanisms of leukemogenesis. Classification of the different types of ALL with the characteristic phenotypes and associated immunologic and cytogenetic features is presented in Table 54-1.

MORPHOLOGY

In 1976, the French-American-British Cooperative Group (FAB) devised a classification system for ALL

Table 54–1 Classification of Acute Lymphoblastic Leukemia

Common Name	Frequency, %	Morphology	Cytochemistry		Immunophenotype	Frequent Cytogenetic Abnormalities	Clinical Features
			MP	TdT	ALL HLA-DR+		
Early pre-B cell	70	L1 or L2	(−)	+	+CD 10, 19, 20, 22	Hyperdiploid, t(12;21), t(11;19)	Peak incidence age 2–5 yr
							Infants <1 yr usually CD 10−, t(4;11), poor prognosis
Pre-B cell	15	L1 or L2	(−)	+	±CD 10, 19, 20, 22 +cIg	t(1;19)	Clinically indistinguishable from early pre-B cell
							May carry worse prognosis
T cell	12	L1 or L2	(−)	+	+CD 2, 5, 7 ±CD 3, CD 1	TCR gene rearrangement t(11;14), t(7;9)	More common in boys, teens, with mediastinal mass, bulky adenopathy, organomegaly, and high WBC
Mature B cell	2	L3	(−)	(−)	+sIg	Pathognomonic t(8;14), t(2;8) or t(8;22)	Clinically indistinguishable from Burkitt's lymphoma with marrow involvement Treated very differently than ALL

cIg, cytoplasmic immunoglobulin; MP, myeloperoxidase; sIg, surface immunoglobulin; TdT, terminal deoxynucleotidyl transferase; HLA-DR+, HLA-DR positive.
Modified from Asselin, BL: Leukemias. In Hoekelman RA, Adam HM, Nelson NM, et al, eds: *Primary Pediatric Care*, 4th ed. St Louis: Mosby; 2001:1609.

based on the morphologic features of bone marrow lymphoblasts.[12] This system divided ALL into three subtypes (L1, L2, and L3). Application of this system has been limited because the distinction between the most common subtypes, L1 and L2, (98% of cases) is somewhat arbitrary, results are difficult to reproduce between different observers, and neither L1 or L2 subtypes correlate with immunologic, genetic, or clinical features.[13,14] This is in contrast to the L3 subtype, which predicts the mature B-cell ALL phenotype and translocations involving the MYC oncogene on chromosome 8. Thus, excluding the L3 subtype, the FAB classification system for ALL has been replaced by immunophenotype and cytogenetic-based systems.[15]

CYTOCHEMISTRY

Cytochemical staining properties of blast cells can be used to distinguish ALL from AML.[16] Myeloperoxidase staining detects myeloperoxidase in the granules of neutrophilic, eosinophilic, and monocytic precursors. Lymphoblasts are uniformly negative, making this an important distinguishing feature of ALL versus AML. Terminal deoxynucleotidyl transferase (TdT), a DNA polymerizing enzyme, is specific to lymphoblasts of precursor B-cell or T-cell origin; mature B-cell lymphoblasts are negative, as are myeloid precursors. The lack of B- or T-cell lineage-specific cytochemical staining characteristics has limited the usefulness of these techniques. In clinical practice they have been largely replaced by immunologic methods.

IMMUNOPHENOTYPE

Normal hematopoietic cells undergo changes in expression of cell differentiation genes recognized as cell surface antigens as they mature from stem cells into cells of a distinct lineage. The pattern of expression of these antigens detected by flow cytometry with a panel of lineage-associated antibodies is called immunophenotype. The immunophenotype of ALL confirms the lymphoid origin and indicates lineage (B- or T-cell), as well as stage of lymphoid maturation at which the malignant transformation occurred. Current therapeutic strategies for ALL require the immunophenotype as part of the diagnostic evaluation.[17]

Immunophenotype studies of cell surface antigens have defined four subsets of ALL: early pre-B, pre-B, mature B-cell, and T-cell. As detailed in Table 54-1, each immunologic subtype is associated with specific clinical and cytogenetic features. The majority of ALL cases are of immature B-lineage expressing the common ALL antigen, CALLA or CD10. T-cell ALL can also be subclassified according to the stage of thymocyte maturation; however, for therapeutic purposes, only the differentiation between T-cell, mature B-cell, and B-precursor ALL is important for risk stratification and treatment assignment. More recently, measurements of these panels of immunologic markers have been adapted to allow very sensitive monitoring of minimal residual disease.[18]

CYTOGENETICS

Improvements in cytogenetic and molecular technologies now make it possible to identify abnormalities in chromosome number or structure in more than 90% of ALL cases.[19] The most common abnormality, hyperdiploidy, is associated with B precursor ALL and correlates with a good prognosis. A number of these abnormalities are detectable only at the molecular level; the TEL/AML1 fusion t(12;21) is an example of such an abnormality.[20] Cytogenetics and molecular genetics play an important role in the classification of leukemias and correlate significantly with the outcome of the treatment.[21] It is now well recognized that the morphology, immunophenotype, and drug responsiveness of the leukemic blast cell are a direct reflection of its genetic characteristics.[22,23]

Prognostic Factors

Interest in prognostic factors arose in the late 1970s as therapy became successful in many patients who had ALL. Pediatric oncologists began looking for common features among groups of patients who did well compared with patients whose disease relapsed. Through retrospective analysis of disease-free survival, certain features present at the time of diagnosis of ALL were identified that were useful in predicting which patients had a good, fair, or poor prognosis[8,24,25] (Table 54-2). The initial WBC and the age of the child at diagnosis have been the two

Table 54–2 Most Commonly Reported Poor Prognostic Features in Pediatric Lymphoblastic Leukemia

Morphology	FAB L_2
	FAB L_3
	Hand mirror cell
Immunophenotype	Surface immunoglobulin [+] (B-cell)
	Cytoplasmic immunoglobulin [+] (pre–B-cell)
	Common ALL antigen [−] = CD10 [−]
	T-cell
Cytogenetics	Translocations
	t(9;22): Philadelphia chromosome
	t(4;11)
	t(8;22)
	t(8;14)
	t(1;19)
	Hypoploidy and pseudoploidy (DNA index <1.16 × normal)
Clinical (at diagnosis)	Age <2 yr; >10 yr
	Black race
	Male sex
	Bulky mediastinal mass
	Massive adenopathy
	Massive organomegaly
	Central nervous system leukemia at diagnosis
Laboratory (at diagnosis)	Elevated leukocyte count
	Elevated hemoglobin
	Low platelet count
	Elevated lactic dehydrogenase
	Presence of human leukocyte antigen types B12, B18, A11/B35
Response to therapy	Low glucocorticoid receptor content
	Slow response to therapy; day 7, 14, or 28

FAB, French-American-British.
Modified from Bleyer WA: Acute lymphoblastic leukemia in children: Advances and prospectus. *Cancer.* 1990;65:689.

most reliable indicators of prognosis, both for duration of remission and survival.[24,26]

Higher leukocyte counts, more frequent in T-cell disease and infants, are strongly correlated with a worse prognosis although the biologic rationale for this is not clear. Children who are younger than 1 year of age or older than 10 years of age have a relatively poor prognosis compared to those in the intermediate age group. The majority of infants have 11q23 rearrangements, primarily the t(4;11) translocation, which creates an MLL-AF4 fusion gene and is associated with hyperleukocytosis and a poor prognosis.[27]

The prognostic importance of other clinical features such as gender, race, degree of organomegaly, presence of a mediastinal mass, initial platelet count, and DNA index is not reproducible among different study groups. As a result, the National Cancer Institute (NCI) sponsored a workshop in September 1993 to define uniform criteria to be used for risk-based treatment assignment for children with ALL. Workshop participants agreed on uniform age and WBC count criteria (Table 54-3) and a common set of prognostic factors to be evaluated prospectively as the prognostic factors of the future including cytogenetics, early response to treatment, and minimal residual disease status.[26]

Risk-Targeted Therapy

With the advent of improved outcomes for an increasing number of children with leukemia and lymphoma came the realization that successful therapy was associated with significant costs in terms of late sequelae. These observations are the basis for current treatment strategies with risk-directed therapy; that is, the intensity of required treatment is adjusted for a patient or group of patients according to the clinical features of the disease and whether it is associated with a higher or lower risk of relapse. Such a tailored approach means that patients who have a good outcome with modest therapy can be spared more intensive and thus more toxic therapy. Furthermore, in an attempt to improve chances for cure, patients with more aggressive disease and higher risk of relapse may require more intensive therapy with a higher risk of side effects. This is justified if the disease-free survival and overall outcome can be improved. In the cohort of patients considered to be at low risk for relapse with standard therapy, clinical trials have focused on quality-of-life issues. Designing treatment regimens that decrease the potential for long-term toxicities

without compromising cure rates in these patients became the goal.

Chemotherapy has been implicated in the development of significant long-term morbidities associated with ALL treatment, including leukoencephalopathy associated with high dose methotrexate, secondary leukemias related to epipodophyllotoxins or alkylating agents, cardiomyopathy following anthracycline use, and avascular necrosis of the bone or osteoporosis related to corticosteroids.

Common Elements of Therapy

Most ALL treatment regimens divide therapy into four phases: initial remission induction, intensification (consolidation), CNS prophylaxis, and continuation (maintenance) therapy. Induction treatment typically includes prednisone, vincristine, and asparaginase and intrathecal therapy. With this three drug regimens, complete remission is achieved in 97% of children.[28] Treatment for prevention of overt CNS disease is initiated early and continues at intervals throughout the other phases of therapy. Most centers continue treatment for 2.5 to 3 years.

Mature B-Cell ALL

Similar to Burkitt's lymphoma, mature B-cell ALL is more common in boys, with a median age of 8 years. It frequently is associated with bulky abdominal tumor and a very high rate of cell proliferation, factors that can result in the metabolic complications associated with tumor lysis syndrome. When treated with traditional ALL therapy, patients with B-cell ALL had a grim prognosis. This has changed dramatically with the development of short-term (6 to 8 month) regimens of extremely intensive therapy that incorporate fractionated high-dose cyclophosphamide, high-dose methotrexate, and cytarabine.[29,30] These regimens have been adopted by virtually all centers with event-free survival of up to 80%. Some groups are looking at the benefits of addition of ifosfamide, etoposide, or both in these regimens.[31,32]

T-Cell ALL

Historically, T-cell ALL in children has been associated with a worse prognosis than other subtypes of childhood ALL. Patients with T-ALL are more likely to present with high-risk features of older age, high leukocyte count,

Table 54-3   Uniform Age and WBC Count Criteria for B-Precursor All Standard- and High-Risk Cohorts Adopted at the CTEP/NCI Workshop

Risk	Definition	4-Yr EFS, %	B-Precursor Patients, %
Standard	WBC count <50,000/µl and age 1–<10 yr	80.3	68
High	WBC count ≥50,000/µl or age ≥10 yr	63.9	32

CTEP/NCI, Cancer Therapy Evaluation Program/National Cancer Institute; EFS, event-free survival; WBC, white blood cell.
Data derived from children treated by the Pediatric Oncology Group (AlinC-14) and CCG (–100 and –1800 series) protocols.
From Smith M, Arthur D, Camitto B, et al: Uniform approach to risk classification and treatment assignment for children with acute lymphoblastic leukemia. *J Clin Oncol.* 1996;14:20.

mediastinal mass, bulky organomegaly, and lymph-adenopathy often termed "lymphomatous presentation" as well as testicular involvement. T-cell ALL can be successfully treated according to the same regimens as B-lineage ALL although the majority of patients will have one or more high risk features, thus requiring treatment on a high-risk arm.[29,33,34] High doses of methotrexate (5 grams/m[2]) appear to improve the outcome in patients with T-cell ALL.[29,35]

ALL in Infants

Among children younger than 1 year of age, in whom the prognosis is poor, 80% have rearrangements of the MLL gene.[25,36] Most cooperative groups have designed treatment regimens specifically for infants, which include high-dose cytarabine, high-dose methotrexate, etoposide, and cyclophosphamide combined with elements of high-risk ALL therapy such as vincristine, corticosteroid, asparaginase, and anthracyclines. Allogeneic bone marrow transplantation (BMT) is considered in first remission when a matched-related donor is available.

THE EVOLVING ROLE OF RADIOTHERAPY

Historically, the role of radiotherapy in ALL has been in the management of extramedullary disease. Trials that compared its efficacy to that of alternative therapy for both prophylaxis and treatment of extramedullary leukemia addressed the growing concern about the potential long-term toxic effects of radiation in young children.[37-40] The findings of these trials have resulted in a reduction in the use of radiotherapy in the treatment of extramedullary pediatric ALL. More recently, radiation has played a significant role in BMT cytoreductive therapy designed for patients with a poor prognosis or relapse. The various total body irradiation regimens and techniques employed are presented in detail in Chapter 14, Total Body Irradiation, along with the rationale for and results of BMT in pediatric ALL.

Central Nervous System Prophylaxis

With the advent of effective CNS prophylaxis, the survival rates associated with ALL improved dramatically. Improving the quality of life in the increasing number of survivors became a main focus of CNS prophylaxis trials of the 1970s and 1980s. Ways to modify the delivery of CNS radiotherapy to potentially decrease the incidence and severity of treatment-related late toxicity were explored. Reduction of the cranial irradiation dose from 24 Gy to 18 Gy was tested successfully in the Children's Cancer Group (CCG) 143 trial (1974-1975),[41] and by the mid 1970s the lower dose was preferred by most investigators for cranial prophylaxis in pediatric ALL.[42,43] Although subsequent attempts have been made to further reduce the potential for late morbidity associated with cranial irradiation,[44,45] current investigative efforts have centered principally on finding effective strategies for CNS prophylaxis that do not require the use of radiotherapy.[46-53]

In current practice, cranial irradiation has been eliminated from CNS prophylactic therapy regimens in patients with B-precursor ALL who are between the ages of 1 and 9, with an initial leukocyte count of less than 50,000/μL and no evidence of lymphomatous or CNS involvement. The elimination of cranial irradiation in the treatment of so-called "high-risk" patients remains a controversial issue. In this setting, the need for cranial radiation as part of prophylaxis is highly dependent on the intensity of intrathecal medications and systemic medications that have CNS activity[54-57] and which are administered as part of the chemotherapy regimen.

Of note is a recent collaborative meta-analysis of pre-1993 trials performed to clarify the relative effects on relapse and survival of different types of therapies directed at the CNS in childhood acute lymphoblastic leukemia.[58] Radiotherapy and long-term intrathecal therapy gave similar outcomes, with no significant difference in event-free survival despite random assignment of treatment to 2848 patients, 1001 of whom suffered relapse or death. Intravenous methotrexate reduced nonCNS rather than CNS relapses, and hence, the addition of intravenous methotrexate to a treatment regimen including radiotherapy or long-term intrathecal therapy improved event-free survival, with a 17% reduction in the event rate. The event-free survival at 10 years in these trials was 61.9% without intravenous methotrexate and 68.1% with intravenous methotrexate. There was no significant difference in survival. No evidence was found regarding differences, between trials or between subgroups of different types of patients, in the relative effects of treatment. The conclusion was that radiotherapy could be replaced by long-term intrathecal therapy, and intravenous methotrexate gives some additional benefit by reducing nonCNS relapses.

Meningeal Leukemia

Various therapies have been employed for the management of overt meningeal leukemia; however, given the small number of patients with CNS leukemia, definitive, statistically valid conclusions as to the superiority of one approach over another are precluded. Nevertheless, there appears to be enough evidence in the literature to make some generalizations and to support some recommendations with regard to therapy of meningeal leukemia.

Craniospinal axis radiotherapy has been shown to be successful in controlling meningeal leukemia, producing long-term CNS control rates as high as 90%.[59-63] Its associated toxicities, however, both to the CNS and to the hematopoietic tissue (producing immunosuppression and thus a compromise in systemic chemotherapy delivery), have prompted investigators to develop other treatment strategies aimed at decreasing the role of radiotherapy, either by eliminating it entirely or by modifying the dosing regimen or volume, or both. Attempts at curing meningeal leukemia with chemotherapy alone, initiated in the 1970s, have been unsuccessful to date.[64] Regardless of the drug combination or route of administration employed, there is no convincing evidence to support the use of chemotherapy alone in the eradication of overt CNS leukemia. Although excellent remission rates are achieved with chemotherapy, both intrathecal and systemic, they are usually of short duration.[64-66] Currently, new intrathecal agents are being studied, the long-term results of which are forthcoming.[67,68]

Based on the results obtained to date for chemotherapy alone, CNS radiotherapy should be part of any regimen designed for the treatment of overt meningeal leukemia, regardless of prior CNS radiation exposure.[69] Since the number of leukemic patients who exhibit meningeal disease is small, and since the systemic and intrathecal chemotherapy employed in the trials designed to deliver CNS radiotherapy is variable, definitive conclusions cannot yet be made with regard to the optimal dosing regimen (hyperfractionated[70] vs. conventional radiotherapy), field extent (craniospinal vs. cranial irradiation), and timing (early vs. delayed) of the radiotherapy for all scenarios of CNS disease presentation. Recent reports of success in patients who present with CNS disease and are treated with low-dose cranial irradiation (6 Gy)[71] or no spinal radiation at all,[72] however, do clearly challenge the necessity of spinal irradiation in meningeal leukemia, especially for chemotherapy-naive patients in whom drug-resistant clones have not yet developed. For this group of patients, cranial irradiation of 18 to 24 Gy has become a widely accepted form of CNS radiotherapy, although controversy still exists about the appropriate timing of the delivery of cranial irradiation.[9] For those patients who develop a relapse either during or off therapy, cranial irradiation (craniospinal axis radiation) remains the most widely used form of CNS radiotherapy.[63,73] The commonly employed total dose for the cranial irradiation is 18 to 24 Gy. Although some investigators suggest that a spinal dose of 18 Gy may be necessary for optimal CNS control, there is sufficient evidence to support the use of a lower dose of 12 Gy.[61,74] Currently, there is no ongoing CCG CNS relapse trial. The Pediatric Oncology Group (POG) continues to study the effects of delayed craniospinal irradiation in patients with CNS relapse.[75] Of interest are the results of the CCG 105 study, which question the need to alter or intensify therapy in those patients considered to be in remission during therapy but who are found to have blast cells, albeit with normal cell count on routine cytocentrifuge examination.[11]

For the small group of patients who present with symptomatic cranial nerve deficits, an immediate course of CNS radiation is a consideration. Since the goal of such therapy is to salvage nerve function, the use of as low a dose as possible to produce the desired effect is advocated. Although irradiation of the entire cranial contents is often used for this purpose, treatment to a more limited field to include only the base of the skull, to total doses of 10 to 15 Gy, is recommended. If cranial irradiation is used, it is important that the patient be treated in a prone position, so that the subsequent craniospinal irradiation treatment may be planned appropriately. Completion of the curative CNS radiotherapy, that is, craniospinal irradiation, may be initiated once hematologic remission has been achieved and the chance of reseeding of the CNS from medullary leukemia has been reduced. After low-dose emergent radiotherapy, an additional course of 12 to 18 Gy to the cranial contents is administered.

TECHNIQUES OF CENTRAL NERVOUS SYSTEM RADIOTHERAPY

Cranial Irradiation

When cranial irradiation is indicated, the intent is to deliver a full dose to the subarachnoid spaces, including the superficial meninges and the majority of the retina and orbital apex. By providing a 1 to 2 cm field margin around the skull and restricting the beam energy to 6 MeV or less (necessary for treatment of the lateral meninges, which are close to the skull surface), one can deliver a full dose as planned with opposed lateral photon beams.[76] To assure adequate margin inferiorly on the base of the skull, the bottom edge of the second cervical vertebra is used. Special attention is needed when designing the blocking to ensure an adequate margin on the cribriform plate and temporal fossa.

Craniospinal Axis Irradiation

When craniospinal irradiation is indicated, the treatment volume extends to include the entire CNS subarachnoid space. This volume is most often treated with lateral cranial fields and one or more posterior spine fields. The inferior border for the spinal field extends below S2 to include the thecal sac. The fiducial field markers used for designing the lens block may be set up as previously described for cranial irradiation. However, matching the cranial and spinal fields requires careful technical planning and is dependent on several physical factors, including the modality chosen for the spinal field treatment. Photon therapy is most widely used for the spine fields; however, electrons may be used when the depth of the anterior surface of the spinal cord is situated within the maximum range of available electrons, after the bone attenuation is accounted for. Although the dosimetry of electrons in regions of inhomogeneities is quite complex, the sparing of anterior structures can be substantial, as shown in a comparison of the dose distributions generated with photon and with electron spinal fields (Fig. 54-1). The spine, indicated on the illustration by a dashed line, is adequately covered using either modality. The electrons, however, deliver less than 10% of the dose anteriorly, while the photon beam delivers 70% to 90% of the prescription dose. Depending on the location of the cranium-spine field match planes, the reduction in dose to the thyroid may be substantial.

Simulation Setup

The clinician begins the simulation by preparing the appropriate immobilization devices with the patient lying in a prone position, taking care to keep the patient's chin down to avoid folds in the neck and to align the body in such a way as to minimize changes in source-skin distance along the length of the spine. It is essential to determine the length and depth of the spinal fields from C2 to S2 early in the simulation process. This information is used to determine prescription depths and the need for a

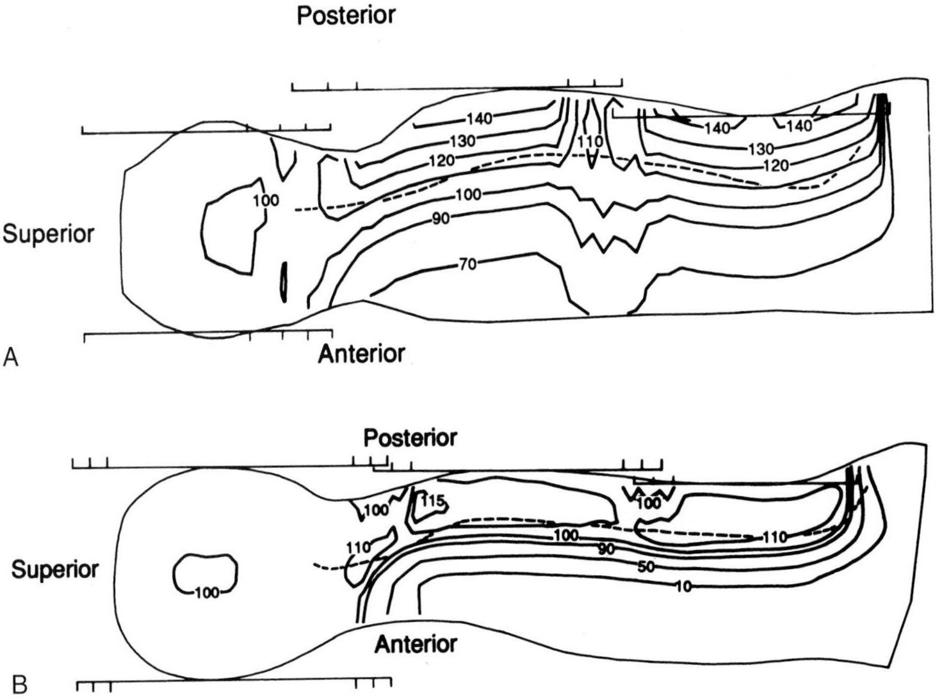

Posterior

Figure 54–1. Mid-sagittal contour plane of a patient in prone position, with spine indicated by the *dashed line*. Cranial contour is a coronal contour rotated about the body axis to align with sagittal body contour. **A**, Cobalt-60 photon beams for spinal fields and cranial fields. **B**, Electron beams for spinal fields and cranial fields.

second spine field. The simulation proceeds in a caudal to cephalad direction; the parameters of the spinal fields are established first, followed by the cranial fields.

Spinal Fields

If two spinal fields are indicated, a scheme must be worked out for matching the two fields and reducing the dose inhomogeneities that occur in the match region. The fields must be separated on the skin by a gap calculated such that the borders of the two spine fields intersect at a point deep within the patient along the anterior surface of the spinal cord. Posterior to the intersection is a region that is not included in either field and is therefore underdosed, while below (more anterior to) this intersection is a region of high dose where the two fields overlap and both beams contribute to the dose. To reduce the dose inhomogeneity in both regions, the point along the spine where the two fields intersect is moved on different treatment days.

Craniospinal Field Matching

The matching of the posterior spine field with the cranial fields adds technical complexities to the alignment of the cranial fields as discussed for cranial irradiation. One approach to handling this junctioning problem is to accept a slight overlap due to beam divergence (Fig. 54-2*A*); another is to attempt to create a match plane, accomplished by pedestal rotation, which abuts to both fields (Fig. 54-2*B*); yet another approach is to create a gap between the cranial and spinal fields (Fig. 54-2*C*). In all approaches, however, the collimator is rotated for the cranial fields to create a field edge, which follows the

divergence of the upper spine field (Fig. 54-2*D*), and the juncture where all three fields come together is shifted or moved daily to allow for an averaging out of the high-dose and low-dose regions in the junction (feathering). For any cranial field, the inferior border should never be higher than the bottom of C2 to assure complete coverage of the base of the skull; however, caudally it is limited by the presence of the shoulders. In general, the cranial field length should change by 2 to 4 cm each day of a 4-day cycle, which is equivalent to shifting the field edge by 1 to 2 cm daily.

Although gapping is a common practice, it has been shown that improved dose distributions over the junction region are achieved when fields are matched on the skin such that all three fields intersect along the mid-sagittal plane.[77] Regardless of whether gapping is used, however, significant problems with dose inhomogeneity arise from variability in the daily treatment setup.[78] When gapping is used, feathering the fields reduces the extent of inhomogeneity resultant not only from errors in the daily setup but also from the inherent underdosage in the gapped region.

Recommended Technique For Photon Craniospinal Irradiation

The problem of determining a collimator, gantry, and pedestal angle when planning photon craniospinal irradiation is quite complex.[79] A recommended approach is to situate the central axes of the lateral cranial fields along the line bisecting the globes; to rotate the collimator of the cranial fields to follow the divergence of the upper spine field (abutting the upper spine field with the cranial fields on the posterior surface of the neck using the light field); and to feather the junction daily.

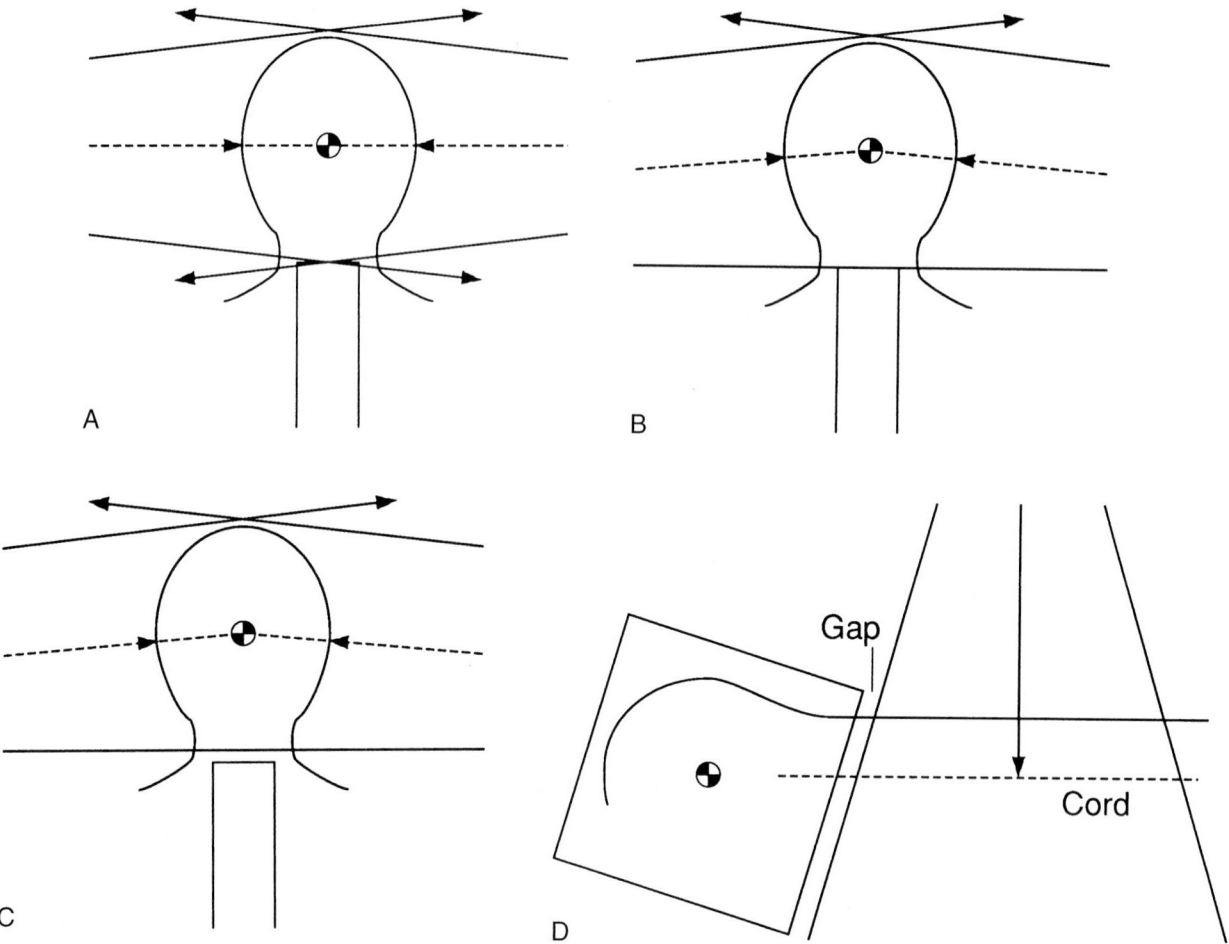

Figure 54–2. Field arrangements for craniospinal irradiation. **A,** Coronal plane with overlap between cranial and spinal fields indicated by *darkened triangles*. **B,** Coronal plane with pedestal rotation for cranial fields. **C,** Coronal plane with pedestal rotations and a gap between the cranial and spinal fields. **D,** Mid-sagittal plane indicating the collimator rotation on the cranial fields that follows the divergence of the spinal field and the gap between the cranial fields and the spinal field.

Electron Spinal Fields

As previously discussed, electrons may be used to treat the spine where the maximum depth of the spine is within the range of the 80% to 90% depth dose of the most energetic electron beam available, including corrections for the bone heterogeneity. The dosimetry of the electron beams must be carefully examined, as algorithms for handling the presence of the bone heterogeneity within the field may use one-, two-, or three-dimensional corrections. With the use of computed tomography (CT) scanning to generate isodose curves, it has been reported that the 90% isodose curves shift toward the patient's posterior surface on the order of 4 mm due to bone absorption and scatter.[80] An additional 3 mm geometric margin is added to give a total shift of the 90% isodose line of 7 mm posteriorly.

Testicular Leukemia

Clinically evident testicular disease at diagnosis is a rare event.[81,82] Before the advent of modern-day chemotherapy regimens, testicular relapse was a significant obstacle to cure.[82,83] Because of the high rate of relapse and because of the high frequency of leukemic infiltration of testes (64% to 92%) demonstrated in autopsy series,[84-86] testicular biopsies at completion of therapy became a routine practice for many investigators, as did the delivery of testicular irradiation to those boys with positive findings. Although the approach of administering presymptomatic testicular irradiation to high-risk males reduced the incidence of testicular relapse, the ultimate survival was not significantly improved.[40,87-90] Since the introduction of aggressive regimens, not only have disease-free survival rates improved, but isolated testicular relapse has become a rare event.[90] As a result, testicular biopsies at completion of therapy in high-risk patients are no longer performed, and prophylactic testicular radiation is no longer necessary.

Confirmation of clinically suspected testicular leukemia is done by wedge biopsy. Bilateral biopsies should be performed, since studies have shown that involvement is bilateral.[87,89] At diagnosis, testicular involvement is most often treated with systemic chemotherapy and rarely requires testicular radiation. Testicular relapse requires a course of testicular irradiation in combination with intensive salvage systemic chemotherapy. Because of the bilateral nature of testicular leukemia, the target volume should include the entire scrotum to encompass both the testes and epididymis. Although the exact total dose required for local control has not been established, it is clear that doses of less than 12 Gy are suboptimal,[83,91] and those of 18 to 24 Gy (at 1.8 to 2 Gy/fraction) are effective.[91-94] Reports of prolonged disease-free survival after testicular relapse with aggressive salvage therapy have been encouraging, especially for those patients with an isolated testicular relapse occurring 6 months or longer after completion of therapy.[95,96]

Testicular radiation, at doses used for ALL, independent of any contribution of chemotherapy effect, is associated with sterility and altered Leydig cell function; the latter could result in delayed sexual maturation and the need for appropriate androgen replacement.[97,98]

Technique of Testicular Radiotherapy

Testicular irradiation is administered via a single anterior portal with the use of an electron beam of appropriate energy or low-energy photons, with the patient in a supine position and the penile shaft taped up and over the symphysis pubis. The treatment field is rectangular and should include a minimum 5 mm margin around the scrotum. Usually a 10×10 cm cone provides adequate coverage.

The electron beam, as administered in the energy range most often appropriate for testicular irradiation (9 to 12 MeV), offers the distinct advantage over photon modalities of a region of high-dose uniformity followed by a rapid dose falloff. There should not be more than a $\pm 10\%$ variance in dose homogeneity within the treated volume, and the underlying perineal tissues should be spared. A polystyrene/lead combination block is used to

support the testicles posteriorly and shield the perineum (Fig. 54-3A). For electron energies of 9 to 12 MeV, 5 mm lead is adequate for shielding and the overlying 5 mm polystyrene dissipates the effect of electron backscatter. Skin apposition of the beam is achieved by angling the gantry so that the end of the cone is parallel to the treatment surface (Fig. 54-3B).

In the absence of an electron beam of appropriate energy, low-energy photons (4 to 6 MV) may be used. The criteria for treatment volume—that is, bilateral testes and epididymis—dose homogeneity, and treatment position are the same as for treatment with electrons. To achieve dose homogeneity, 0.5 to 1.0 cm of bolus over the entire scrotal area may be necessary. Shielding the underlying soft tissue is more problematic, however, with photon beam treatment, since the required full thickness block of about 7.5 cm cannot be placed underneath the testes. The exit dose to the perineal area with such treatment is therefore approximately equal to the prescription dose.

THE CURRENT ERA

Recently reported results of major cooperative group studies demonstrate that childhood ALL is currently curable in approximately 80% of cases (Table 54-4). This level of success has resulted from the collaborative efforts of clinical oncologists and laboratory researchers over several decades. Each group has made significant contributions to the design of the sequential clinical trials that have identified increasingly effective treatments and deepened our understanding of the heterogenous nature of leukemia. The treatment strategies responsible for these high cure rates for ALL are listed in Table 54-4.

Vincristine, prednisone, methotrexate, and mercaptopurine have been the backbone to virtually all successful

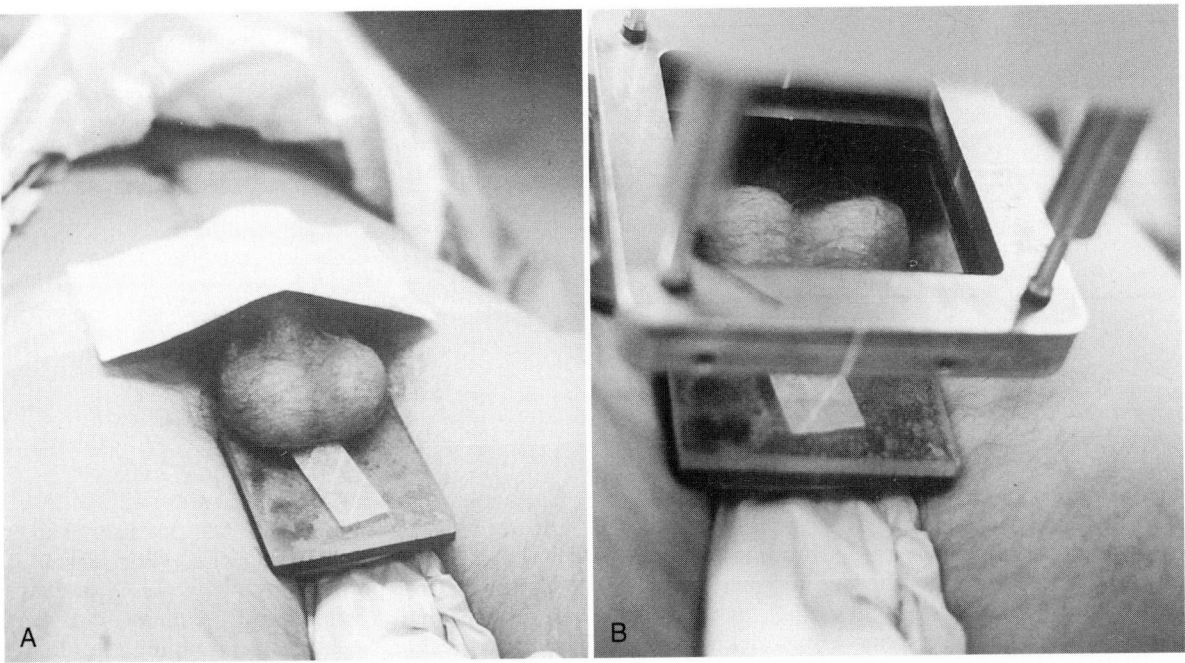

Figure 54–3. A, The patient in position for testicular radiation with the scrotum supported on a polystyrene/lead block and the penis taped up and out of the field of treatment. **B,** Positioning of the gantry angle so that the end of the cone is parallel to the treatment field.

Table 54–4   Results of Recently Completed ALL Clinical Trials

Study	Patient Accrual, Yr	Evaluable Patients, n	Eligibility Criteria	Event-Free Survival Rate (±SE), %	Effective Treatment Component Identified	Reference
AIEOP-ALL88	1988–92	396	All risk groups, <15 yr	66.4 ± 2.4 at 5 yr	Extended intrathecal treatment and intensive systemic chemotherapy may replace cranial irradiation for subclinical CNS therapy in intermediate-risk ALL	Conter et al[99]
BFM-86	1986–90	998	All risk groups, <18 yr	72 ± 2 at 6 yr	Intensive reinduction therapy benefits even low-risk patients; high-dose methotrexate (5 g/m²) improves outcome of T-cell ALL	Reiter et al[29]
BFM-90	1990–95	1950	All risk groups, <19 yr	76 ± 1 at 5 yr	A cranial radiation dose of 12 Gy appears to provide adequate treatment for subclinical CNS leukemia, even in high-risk cases	Conter et al[34]
CCG-105	1983–89	1388	Intermediate risk, <21 yr	64 to 68 at 7 yr	Intrathecal methotrexate and intensive chemotherapy can replace cranial irradiation in children <10 yr old; delayed intensification (weeks 16–24) improves clinical outcome	Tubergen et al[100,101]
CCG-1882	1991–95	311	High risk, <21 yr	75.0 ± 3.8 at 5 yr	Prolonged second reinduction/intensification phase ("augmented post induction therapy") can abolish the adverse prognostic impact of a poor early response	Nachman et al[102]
Dana Farber 85-01	1985–87	220	All risk groups, <18 yr	73 ± 3 at 7 yr	Early intensive treatment including l-asparaginase, doxorubicin, and cranial irradiation is effective treatment for childhood ALL, including T-cell cases	Schorin et al[33]
Dutch VI	1984–88	291	All risk groups, <15 yr	72 ± 3 at 6 yr	Combination of dexamethasone, intermediate-dose methotrexate (2 g/m²), and triple intrathecal therapy is effective treatment, especially in preventing CNS relapse in "non-high-risk" ALL	Veerman et al[52]
FRALLE-8	1983–87	559	All risk groups	57 ± 2 at 7 yr	Intermediate-dose methotrexate (500 mg/m²) is insufficient to prevent CNS relapse	Schaison et al[103]
MRC UKALLX	1985–90	1612	All risk groups, <15 yr	62 ± 2 at 5 yr	Early (week 5) and delayed (week 20) intensification therapy improves treatment outcome for all patients, even those with lower-risk ALL	Chessells et al[104]
POG AlinC-14	1986–90	2404	All risk groups, <21 yr	66.4 ± 2.4 at 4 yr	Moderate-dose methotrexate (1 gm/m²) benefits lower-risk B-lineage ALL cases, especially those with hyperdiploidy >50 chromosomes	Trueworthy et al[105]
POG 9005	1991–93	609	Lower risk, <21 yr	79.6 ± 2.9 at 4 yr	Moderate-dose methotrexate (1 gm/m²) benefits lower-risk B-lineage ALL cases	Chessells et al[104]
SJCRH-XI	1984–88	358	All risk groups, <18 yr	71 ± 4 at 8 yr	Early intensive chemotherapy improves outcome for all patients	Rivera et al[107]
SJCRH-XII	1988–91	188	All risk groups, <18 yr	67 ± 4 at 5 yr	Individualized therapy based on pharmacokinetic characteristics improves outcome	Evans et al[108]
SJCRH-XIIIA	1991–94	165	All risk groups, <18 yr	80.2 ± 9.2 at 5 yr	Early intensification of intrathecal chemotherapy reduces risk of CNS relapse	Pui et al[56]

AIEOP, Italian Association of Pediatric Hematology Oncology; BFM, Berlin-Frankfurt-Münster; CCG, Children's Cancer Group (Arcadia, Calif.); CNS, central nervous system; Dana Farber, Dana Farber Cancer Institute/Children's Hospital Acute Lymphoblastic Leukemia Consortium (Boston); Dutch, Cutch Childhood Leukemia Study Group; FRALLE, French Acute Lymphoblastic Leukemia Cooperative Group; MRC, Medical Research Council (UK); UKALLX, United Kingdom Acute Lymphoblastic Leukemia X; POG, Pediatric Oncology Group (Chicago); AlinC, Acute Leukemia in Childhood; SJCRH, St. Jude Children's Research Hospital (Memphis, Tenn.).
From Pui CH, Crist WM: Acute lymphoblastic leukemia. In Pui CH, ed. *Childhood Leukemias.* Cambridge, Mass: Cambridge University Press; 1999:298.

ALL treatments for 30 years. The dosage and schedule varies among specific protocols. Additional effective antileukemic drugs have been discovered and incorporated into the current regimens. The role and common complications of the common agents used in ALL therapy are listed in Table 54-5. The development of these intensive systemic combination chemotherapy regimens has resulted in marked improvement in outcomes especially in patients presenting with unfavorable immunophenotypic and biologic features (see Table 54-2).

THE NEW ERA: FUTURE DIRECTIONS

The evolution of curative therapy in ALL continues, with the ultimate goal of increasing the cure rate of all children with ALL, regardless of risk group, while at the same time decreasing the potential for adverse treatment-related sequelae. One direction being taken is to develop more sensitive techniques to detect minimal residual disease in patients who are apparently in complete remission, according to current criteria, and thus may benefit from

Table 54–5   Use and Complications of Chemotherapeutic Agents in Acute Leukemia

Drug	Route	Common Use	Acute Toxicity	Delayed Toxic Effects
Methotrexate, cytosine arabinoside, or both	Intrathecal	CNS prophylaxis of ALL and ANLL	Nausea, vomiting, headache, stiff neck, arachnoiditis, seizures	Cortical atrophy, leukoencephalopathy
L-Asparaginase	IM	Induction and consolidation of ALL	Anaphylaxis, nausea, vomiting, fever, chills, hyperglycemia, diabetes, abdominal pain, pancreatitis (increased amylase), CNS depression, coagulation defects with thrombosis or hemorrhage (i.e., stroke), hypoproteinemia, hepatic damage	Pancreatic or hepatic damage, diabetes mellitus
Methotrexate	PO, IM, IV	Maintenance of ALL	Nausea, vomiting, mucositis, rash, myelosuppression, hepatic damage, renal toxicity	Hepatic damage, neurotoxicity
Prednisone	PO	Induction and maintenance of ALL	Hyperglycemia, hypertension, emotional lability, increased appetite, fluid retention, weight gain, striae, cushingoid facies, peptic ulcer, diabetes mellitus	Osteoporosis, growth retardation, aseptic necrosis, cataracts, glaucoma, diabetes mellitus
6-Thioguanine	PO	Induction and maintenance of ANLL	Same as for mercaptopurine but less hepatic toxicity	
Trans-retinoic acid (ATRA)	PO	Induction and maintenance of APML	Myelosuppression, fever, hyperleukocytosis, fluid retention, pulmonary edema, respiratory distress, pseudo-tumor cerebri	None known
6-Mercaptopurine	PO, IV	Maintenance of ALL	Alopecia, nausea, vomiting, diarrhea, myelosuppression, hepatic damage, cholestasis	Hepatic disease, cholestasis
Vincristine	IV	Induction and maintenance of ALL	Alopecia, constipation, paralytic ileus, peripheral neuropathy, jaw pain, SIADH, danger with extravasation, myelosuppression in rare cases	Peripheral neuropathy
Doxorubicin	IV	Induction and consolidation of ALL	Myelosuppression, alopecia, nausea, vomiting, mucositis, anorexia, hepatic damage, cardiac arrhythmias, red urine, danger with extravasation	Cardiomyopathy, hepatic damage
Daunorubicin	IV	Induction and maintenance of ALL and ANLL	Myelosuppression, alopecia, nausea, vomiting, cardiac arrhythmias, hepatic damage, red urine, danger with extravasation	Cardiomyopathy
Cytosine arabinoside	IV	Induction and maintenance of ANLL; Consolidation of high-risk ALL	Myelosuppression, alopecia, nausea, vomiting, diarrhea, mucositis, conjunctivitis, fever, neurotoxicity	Hepatic damage, neurotoxicity
Etoposide/teniposide	IV	Induction and maintenance of ANLL; Consolidation of high-risk ALL	Hypotension, anaphylaxis, myelosuppression, nausea, vomiting, alopecia, mucositis, danger with extravasation	Second malignancy, most commonly ANLL
Radiation		ALL; CNS prophylaxis	Alopecia, nausea, vomiting, skin hypersensitivity, mild myelosuppression	Sleeping syndrome, seizures, leukoencephalopathy, growth retardation

ALL, acute lymphoblastic leukemia; ANLL, acute nonlymphoblastic leukemia; APML, acute promyelocytic leukemia; CNS, central nervous system; SIADH, syndrome of inappropriate secretion of antidiuretic hormone.
Data compiled from Perry MC, ed. *The Chemotherapy Source Book*. Baltimore: Williams & Wilkins; 1997.
Modified from Asselin, BL: Leukemias. In Hoekelman RA, Adam HM, Nelson NM, et al, eds. *Primary Pediatric Care*, 4th ed. St Louis: Mosby; 2001:1615.

additional therapy to prevent relapse. Another direction is to discover new, effective antileukemic drugs and treatment approaches. Several new anticancer agents are currently being studied for ALL. They include such families as the cytokines (interferon-α, interleukin-4, and tumor necrosis factor) and the antibody-toxin conjugates.[109,110] Innovative treatment regimens are being designed to better address the needs of the continuously evolving biologic subtypes and risk groups of ALL, including the use of hematopoietic growth factors to permit further intensification of therapy. Still another direction is to devise effective salvage therapy for those children who do not achieve remission or who relapse on current protocols.

With the fields of cytogenetics and immunology growing exponentially, coupled with the inexhaustible energy and enthusiasm invested in finding a cure for children with ALL on the parts of both basic scientists and clinicians, the next decade should be an exciting and productive era for pediatric ALL.

ACUTE NONLYMPHOCYTIC LEUKEMIA

Epidemiology and Etiology

Acute nonlymphocytic leukemia (ANLL) represents 20% of acute leukemias in children, accounting for approximately 650 of the 3250 new cases of childhood leukemia diagnosed each year in the United States.[1] This is a striking contrast to the prevalence of ANLL or AML in adults, where it accounts for 80% of acute leukemias or approximately 10,000 new cases a year. The incidence of ANLL remains steady from birth to adulthood with only a slight peak in late adolescence. The median age of onset of ANLL is generally older than that of ALL, approximately 8 to 10 years.

Like in ALL, the frequency of ANLL is increased in patients with DS, Fanconi's anemia, Bloom's syndrome, neurofibromatosis, and other genetic disorders. Several causative factors have been implicated in the development of ANLL, including genetic predisposition, chronic exposure to benzene and prior treatment with chemotherapy, or radiotherapy. In the majority of cases, however, the cause is unknown.

Clinical Presentation and Diagnosis

The clinical presentation of ANLL is very similar to that of ALL. Pallor, fatigue, skin or mucosal bleeding, and fever are present in the majority of children at initial presentation.[111] Infection at diagnosis is also common. Bone pain, lymphadenopathy, and marked hepatosplenomegaly are less common in ANLL than in ALL. Chloromas are solid tumor collections of immature myeloid cells that can occur in patients with ANLL. Leukemia cutis is more common in infants than older children. Almost all patients have some degree of anemia and thrombocytopenia. Twenty percent of patients present with hyperleukocytosis with a WBC greater than 100,000/mm^3. Bleeding secondary to a coagulopathy is more common in ANLL and results in an increased risk of early death from hemorrhage, especially intracranial bleeding. This is particularly true of patients with acute promyelocytic leukemia, the majority of whom have a coagulopathy at diagnosis.

The diagnosis of ANLL is confirmed by bone marrow aspirate showing greater than 25% blasts. Cytochemical staining and immunophenotyping of the leukemic blast cells are important to distinguish between the two forms of acute leukemia and help to distinguish among the different subtypes of ANLL (see Table 54-1). In young infants with DS, true ANLL must be differentiated from transient myeloproliferative syndrome.[112] No single test is available to distinguish infants who have this transient myeloproliferative disorder from those who have true

congenital leukemia, so conservative therapy with close monitoring for 6 to 8 weeks is the recommended approach in this situation.

Classification

The blast cell population in patients with ANLL can be characterized by morphology, cytochemistry, immunophenotype, and cytogenetics as detailed in Table 54-6. The current system of classification, defined by the FAB working group in 1976, recognizes eight subtypes of ANLL based on degree of cellular expression of granulocytic, monocytic, erythroid, or megakaryocytic features.[113]

Acute myeloid leukemia (M1 and M2) is the most common form of ANLL, representing almost 50% of all cases of pediatric ANLL.[114] Among patients younger than 2 years of age, the majority have either myelomonocytic or monocytic leukemia (M$_4$ or M$_5$ subtype) and frequently present with high WBC, leukemia cutis, and CNS disease.[115] Acute megakaryocytic leukemia (M$_7$) is seen most frequently in infants, especially those with DS.[116]

A definitive immunologic classification of ANLL is not yet available; megakaryocytic leukemia is the only subtype with type-specific immunophenotype (CD41 positive). Development of monoclonal antibodies to these myeloid and monocytic markers has been used to develop targeted therapies such as gemtuzamab and agents for purging of marrow in preparation for autologous BMT.

Cytogenetic abnormalities have been observed in the majority of patients with ANLL.[117] Of these, the t(15;17) pattern is the only one associated with a particular FAB subtype, namely acute promyelocytic leukemia (M$_3$). The presence of the PML-RARα fusion gene is pathognomic for M$_3$ subtype and is thought to be crucial to pathogenesis as well.[118] A unique translocation, t(1;22), has been described in infants with M$_7$ megakaryocytic leukemia.[119] The t(8;21), which produces a fusion gene of the AML1 and ETO genes from chromosomes 21 and 8, respectively, is the most common gene abnormality in AML, usually the M$_2$ subtype, and is associated with better remission rates and prognosis.[120] Translocations involving the 11q23 band with a breakpoint involving the MLL gene are common in M$_4$ and M$_5$ subtypes, as well as infant leukemias and secondary leukemias following epipodophyllotoxin therapy.[121] Deletions of single chromosomes, either 5 or 7, are not specific to an FAB subtype but predict a poor prognosis.[117,120]

Prognostic Factors

The evolution of curative therapy for ANLL has not progressed as rapidly as that for ALL. Because of the relative scarcity of effective treatment options for patients with ANLL, there has been limited clinical application of the information obtained from immunophenotype or cytogenetics studies in terms of identifying prognostic indicators. Initial leukocyte count, age at diagnosis, and FAB classification appear to be the most significant factors related to treatment outcome. High WBC, age older than 14 years, infancy (age younger than 1 year),

Table 54–6   Classification of Acute Nonlymphoid Leukemia

Common Name (Subtype)	Frequency, %	Morphology	Cytochemistry			Immunophenotype	Frequent Cytogenetic Abnormalities	Clinical Features
			MP	NSE	Other			
FAB (M$_0$)	2	>90% blasts often without diff. features				+CD 34 +TdT (sometimes)	del (5) del (7) common	Rare in children
AML without maturation (M$_1$)	24	>90% myeloblasts Auer rods	+	(−)		+CD 15, 33, 34 +HLA-DR		
AML with maturation (M$_2$)	23	30%–90% blasts Auer rods	+	(−)		+CD 15, 33, 34 +HLA-DR	t(8;21)	
Promyelocytic (M$_3$)	5	Hypergranular promyelocyte Many Auer rods	+	(−)		+CD 11, 13, 34 (−) HLA-DR	Pathognomonic t(15;17)	Often DIC at diagnosis Trans-retinoic acid part of Rx
Myelomonocytic (M$_4$)	27	>30% myeloblasts >30% monoblasts >80% monoblasts	+	+		+CD 11, 13, 14, 15, 33, 34	Common t(9;11) t(11;19) t(10;11)	Common in children <2 yr, M$_4$EO ~inv 16 has better px
Monocytic (M$_5$)	10		(−)	+		+CD 11, 13, 14, 15, 33, 34	Common t(9;11) t(11;19) t(10;11)	Common in children <2 yr Worse prognosis, extramedullary leukemia, secondary leukemia after epipodophyllotoxins
Erythroleukemia (M$_6$)	2		(−)	(−)	Pas+	+CD 13, 22, 34 + glycophorin		Very rare in children
Megakaryocytic (M$_7$)	7	>30% megakaryoblasts, cytoplasmic blebs, myelofibrosis	(−)	(−)	Plat PO+	+CD 13, 33, 34 +CD 41, 42, 61	t(1;22)	Most common in children with Down's syndrome Rare in teens, adults

MP, myeloperoxidase stain; NSE, nonspecific esterase stain; Pas, periodic acid-Schiff stain; Plat PO, platelet peroxidase stain.
Modified from Asselin, BL: Leukemias. In Hoekelman RA, Adam HM, Nelson NM, et al, eds. *Primary Pediatric Care*, 4th ed. St Louis: Mosby; 2001:1609.

and FAB M$_5$ subtype have been associated with worse prognosis in most studies.[114,122] The era of tailoring therapy to meet the specific needs of different risk groups has not been reached in AML.

TREATMENT

Chemotherapy

The majority of patients with ANLL are treated according to one standard therapeutic regimen. In contrast to the marked improvements in survival outcome in pediatric ALL, long-term event-free survival rates in ANLL have not increased dramatically over the past few decades. Although response rates may reach levels of 75% to 85%, the median duration of remission rarely exceeds 2 years.[123] Relapse occurs frequently during the first 6 to 12 months on therapy, and early deaths due to treatment-related complications such as sepsis and bleeding reach levels as high as 5% to 15%. The 2-year event-free survival rate with current therapy remains modest, with reported values of 35% to 45%.[124,125] With growing recognition of the importance of morphology, cytogenetics, and immunology in distinguishing subtypes of ANLL with respect to the selection of chemotherapeutic agents, investigators have initiated subtype-specific therapeutic

trials. The results of such trials are promising.[126-136] At present, allogeneic transplantation is the recommended choice for postremission induction therapy in newly diagnosed patients with ANLL who have an available matched, related donor, unfortunately the minority of patients. The role of allogeneic transplantation using unrelated donor sources is controversial for patients in first remission.

Acute Promyelocytic Leukemia

Acute promyelocytic leukemia (APML) is the only subtype of ANLL for which there is type-specific therapy. The t(15;17) translocation, which characterizes APML blasts, produces a PML/RARα fusion gene resulting in disruption of the retinoic acid receptor and blockade of normal cellular differentiation pathways. All-*trans*-retinoic acid (ATRA) binds to the chimeric RARα and overcomes the differentiation blockade, resulting in cell maturation, then apoptosis.[137,138] The best results have been obtained with the combination of ATRA and chemotherapy with induction rates of 90% and disease-free survival of greater than 70%.[138,139] Arsenic trioxide, also a differentiating agent, has been effective in treatment of APML, especially when resistance to ATRA develops.[140] Ongoing clinical trials are designed to determine how the differentiating agents, ATRA and arsenic, can best be combined with cytotoxic drugs for the safe and effective treatment of APML.

Down's Syndrome and Acute Nonlymphocytic Leukemia

Although rare in children without DS, megakaryocytic (M7) leukemia is the most common form of AML in young children with DS.[141] Interestingly, children with DS and AML have been observed to have better responses and superior outcomes (event-free survival rate ≈80%) with standard AML therapy than other children with AML, even the M_7 subtype. This has been shown to be a characteristic of the patient, not of the leukemia. Most treatment failures in patients with DS are a result of treatment-related mortality.[142,143] Thus, increased intensity regimens and allogeneic BMT are not recommended for these patients.

Secondary Leukemia

The association between treatment with the epipodophyllotoxins, etoposide or teniposide, and development of secondary ANLL is now well established.[144] The epipodophyllotoxin-induced leukemias are characterized by a short latency period (2 to 4 years) and a myelomonocytic or monocytic phenotype with a translocation involving band 11q23 with MLL gene rearrangement.[145] In contrast, secondary leukemia that develops after therapy with alkylating agents is characterized by a longer latency period (≈10 years), a prodrome of myelodysplasia and monosomy 5 or 7 genotype.[146] Secondary leukemias are not responsive to traditional chemotherapy and BMT holds the only hope for cure.

THE ROLE OF RADIOTHERAPY

Radiotherapy has always played a minor role in the overall management of pediatric ANLL. It has classically been used in the treatment of chloromas, management of acute leukocytosis, and in the cytoreductive regimen of BMT (in the form of total body irradiation, discussed in Chapter 14, Total Body Irradiation).

Chloromas, also known as myeloblastomas and granulocytic sarcomas, are extramedullary masses of malignant myeloid cells associated most commonly with ANLL (especially FAB M_2), but also observed in patients with chronic myelogenous leukemia.[147] Doses of 24 Gy, at 2 Gy per fraction, are highly effective in eradicating the local masses of malignant infiltrates refractory to chemotherapy.

Excessive leukocytosis, defined as a white cell count above 150,000 to 200,000/μL, may produce cerebral vaso-occlusion, which, if untreated, may lead to infarction. Although excessive leukocytosis is most commonly managed with chemotherapy, leukapheresis, and hydration, radiotherapy is recommended by some investigators. Low-dose cranial irradiation of 1.5 to 2 Gy in two to four fractions is usually successful in reversing the process.

FUTURE THERAPIES

One of the exciting new areas of research is in the use of targeted immunotherapies.[110] Gemtuzamab ozogamicin (myeloTang), a humanized antiCD33 conjugated to calicheamicin, is an example of such an agent. Clinical trials with this immunoconjugate have shown an approximate 37% remission rate in adults with relapsed AML.[148,149] In addition, a CD-45 monoclonal antibody has been radiolabeled with I^{131} for use during BMT as a means of delivering focused bone marrow irradiation.[150] Mutation of the *ras* oncogene is common in AML. The *ras* product must be farnesylated for it to function properly as a growth signal transduction protein. A new class of compounds called *farnesyl transferase inhibitors* has been developed and clinical trials are under way.[151]

CHRONIC MYELOGENOUS LEUKEMIA

Chronic myelogenous leukemia (CML) is rare in childhood, representing 3% to 5% of all pediatric leukemias.[1] In childhood the disorder may appear as two distinct clinical syndromes: adult-type CML, which is virtually indistinguishable from that seen in older patients, and juvenile myelomonocytic leukemia (JMML; formerly known as juvenile CML), a disease relatively restricted to very young children that has distinct clinical, laboratory, and cytogenetic features.[152]

The classic adult-type is characterized by the presence of the Philadelphia chromosome, a reciprocal translocation t(9;22) (q34;q11). The resultant fusion gene formed, *bcr/abl*, appears to have a major role in the pathogenesis of CML. It is typically seen in adolescents with a peak incidence between 10 and 14 years of age. Treatment and outcomes of CML in childhood parallels that of the adult patient.[153] Allogeneic BMT is the only curative approach now available for patients who have CML. The disease status at the time of transplantation is the most powerful predictor of disease-free survival. Thus, most centers recommend allo-BMT for any child who has adult-type CML in the chronic phase, preferably within 1 year from diagnosis.

The introduction of STI-571 (Gleevec) as an *abl*-specific tyrosine kinase inhibitor will have a significant impact on the natural history, treatment, and survival rates of CML in the near future. As a single agent, it has shown significant activity in patients in the chronic phase who are refractory to interferon[154] as well as patients in blast crisis.[155]

JMML is a clonal disorder that begins at the pluripotent stem cell level. Although the predominant abnormality is observed in the monocyte, JMML is also associated with disordered erythrocyte, platelet, and lymphocyte function.[156] Common clinical features at diagnosis include age under 2 years, persistent respiratory infection (with tachypnea, cough, wheezing), prominent lymphadenopathy, splenomegaly, skin rash (eczema, xanthomata, and café-au-lait spots), bleeding, and failure to thrive. In addition, anemia, leukocytosis, thrombocytopenia, monocytosis, and nucleated RBCs in the peripheral blood are common laboratory findings.[157,158] Cytogenetic analysis may be abnormal (e.g., monosomy 7), but the Philadelphia chromosome is never found. The disease is generally more aggressive than CML with a median survival of 9 months; most patients die of infection.[159] Traditional chemotherapy with single agents (e.g., busulfan, hydroxyurea) or intensive multiagent regimens have been unsuccessful. BMT is currently the standard choice of treatment of JMML. There is currently a clinical trial sponsored by the International JMML Registry that is testing the efficacy and safety of farnesyl transferase inhibitors for this patient population.

NON-HODGKIN'S LYMPHOMA

Epidemiology and Etiology

Non-Hodgkin's lymphoma (NHL) is the third most common cancer seen in children, comprising 8% of malignancies seen in the pediatric age group.[160] In the United States, approximately 800 children and adolescents younger than 20 years of age are diagnosed with NHL each year. The incidence peaks between 5 and 15 years of age and is higher in males than in females and in Caucasians than in African-Americans. In younger children NHL is more frequent than Hodgkin's disease (HD), while in adolescents HD is the more common type of lymphoma. Congenital immunodeficiency syndromes and acquired immunodeficiency syndrome (AIDS) are associated with an increased risk of NHL.[161-163] The association of immunosuppressive drug therapy including corticosteroids and androgens with development of malignant lymphomas is well described.[163] With the increasing rate of successful organ or marrow transplantation, the number of children with post-transplant lymphoproliferative disease (PTLD) represents an increasingly significant proportion of patients with NHL.[164,165] Cases that are seen associated with diseases known to carry an increased risk still represent the minority of NHL diagnoses; overall, the cause is unknown in most cases.

Classification

These lymphomas are a heterogeneous group of malignancies arising from transformation of cells of lymphocytic origin, but are quite variable in terms of clinical manifestations, site of origin, histopathology, immunophenotype, and cytogenetic abnormalities. Pediatric NHL is an aggressive disease with diffuse, high grade, histologic features in which the malignant cells appear undifferentiated or poorly differentiated.[166,167] NHL in children is characterized by disseminated disease at diagnosis, frequent extranodal involvement (tonsils, thymus, or Peyer's patches), and commonly, involvement of the bone marrow and the CNS. This is in notable contrast to the NHL seen in adults, where localized, low or intermediate grade, intranodal tumors predominate.

Pediatric NHL can be classified into three major categories based on predominant cell type and architectural pattern: small, noncleaved cell, large cell, and lymphoblastic lymphoma. All three histologic subtypes are classified as high grade according to the NCI Working Formulation for Clinical Usage.[166] These three major subtypes also can be categorized further according to immunophenotype, cytogenetic abnormalities, and molecular features as shown in Table 54-7.[168] Several chromosomal abnormalities have been shown to be pathognomic for certain subtypes of NHL. For example, the translocation t(8;14) correlates with Burkitt's cells[169] and the nonrandom chromosomal translocation t(2;5) is expressed by the Ki-1 (CD30) positive anaplastic large cell lymphoma.[170] These genetic abnormalities are useful primarily in classification but not predicting outcome or modifying therapy.[171] Along with stage of disease, the classification according to histology and immunophenotype is the most important factor in determining appropriate therapy and predicting outcome.[172-175]

Table 54–7   Clinical and Biologic Characteristics of Childhood non-Hodgkin's Lymphoma

Histology Subtype*	Cases†, %	Common Sites	Immunophenotype	Cytogenetics‡	Molecular Genetics‡
Small non–cleaved cell (SNCC) (Burkitt's and Burkitt-like)	39	Abdomen Head and neck	B-cell	t(8;14), t(8;22) t(2;8)	c-myc with Ig H, Ig κ, or Ig λ
Lymphoblastic Lymphoma	28	Mediastinum Head and neck	Immature T-cell Rarely pre-B-cell	t(10;14), t(11;14) t(1;14), t(1;19) and others	TCR with Tal-1, Rhomb-2, or LCK
Large cell (LCL) Anaplastic ALCL (Ki-1+, CD 30+) B-LCL	26	Mediastinum, abdomen, head and neck, skin, bone, soft tissue, or lymph nodes	T-cell or null B-cell	t(2;5), t(1;5)	NPM/ALK

*The subtypes are classified according to the National Cancer Institute's Working Formulation.[166]
†Proportion at St. Jude Children's Research Hospital; other histiotypes account for approximately 7%.[177]
‡Not all tumors will have a cytogenetic or molecular genetic abnormality.
ALCL, anaplastic large cell lymphoma; NPM/ALK.
Data compiled from references 168,176–178.

Clinical Presentation

All childhood lymphomas are rapidly growing and thus the interval between onset of symptoms and diagnosis is short, averaging 2 to 6 weeks. The majority of children have widespread disease at the time of diagnosis with involvement of the bone marrow, CNS, or both. Signs of bone marrow involvement are similar to leukemia with bone pain, neutropenia, anemia and pallor, thrombocytopenia, and associated bruising or petechiae. CNS involvement may present with cranial nerve palsies or signs of increased intracranial pressure including headache, vomiting, and visual changes. Systemic symptoms such as fever, night sweats, malaise, anorexia, and weight loss are generally mild, except in anaplastic large cell lymphoma, where 50% of patients will present with one or more of these symptoms.

The signs and symptoms at diagnosis of NHL in pediatric patients are dependent on the anatomic site and the extent of disease.[176-178] The abdomen is the most common site of disease seen in 35% of cases and frequently presents with nausea and vomiting; abdominal pain, swelling, or both; change in bowel habits; and ascites. The symptoms may mimic intussusception with bloody diarrhea or appendicitis since a common site of tumor infiltration is the distal ileum, appendix, or large bowel, resulting in bowel obstruction by extrinsic compression or intussusception. Primary involvement with a mediastinal mass occurs in about 25% of cases and may be accompanied by pleural effusions. Symptoms may include chest pain, dyspnea and cough, dysphagia, and swelling of the neck and face. The head and neck region, including Waldeyer's ring and cervical lymph nodes, is involved in up to 30% of cases. Presenting features include unilateral tonsillar enlargement and orbital or jaw masses.

The presenting site of disease and thus clinical features also correlate with the histopathologic subtype as shown in Table 54-7.[177] The majority of the abdominal lymphomas are small non–cleaved cell type or Burkitt's lymphoma. In the lymphoblastic lymphomas the typical primary site is the mediastinum. Large cell lymphomas can present with an anterior mediastinal mass, abdominal primary tumor, or head and neck involvement. Anaplastic large cell lymphoma frequently involves the lymph nodes and can involve other atypical sites such as the skin, lung, thyroid, soft tissues, and bone. Relative to the other subtypes of pediatric NHL, marrow and CNS involvement are uncommon. Tumors presenting in the head and neck are seen with any of the three major histologic types.

Diagnosis

The differential diagnosis of NHL includes both benign and malignant conditions. Initial laboratory evaluation should include a complete blood count with differential, a chemistry profile including creatinine, uric acid, calcium, phosphorus, and lactic dehydrogenase to rule out metabolic abnormalities of tumor lysis syndrome (TLS) and immediate chest x-ray or abdominal series if there is supraclavicular adenopathy, respiratory symptoms, facial swelling, or abdominal mass. If the diagnosis of NHL is suspected, consultation with a pediatric oncologist is imperative before biopsy or corticosteroid therapy.

The diagnosis of NHL requires examination of tissue obtained by either open or needle biopsy of an involved site. Sufficient tissue should be obtained by either biopsy method to allow for not only histology but also for immunophenotype, cytogenetics analysis, and molecular studies. In cases with pleural effusions or ascites, examination of the fluid obtained by thoracentesis or paracentesis may be diagnostic, avoiding the need for more invasive procedures such as mediastinal or abdominal mass sampling. In the same way in children with clinical evidence of marrow or CNS involvement, a bone marrow and CSF fluid examination may be diagnostic. Initial evaluation must distinguish NHL from the other small, blue, round cell tumors, including rhabdomyosarcoma, Ewing sarcoma, and neuroblastoma, as well as other conditions such as HD or histiocytosis.

Staging

In a newly diagnosed patient, essential laboratory investigations for staging purposes include the complete blood cell count (CBC), chemistry profile (electrolytes, calcium, phosphorus, creatinine, urate, liver panel), chest x-ray, CT imaging or magnetic resonance imaging of the primary site, bone scan, CT of chest/abdomen/pelvis, bone marrow examination, and CSF cytology. Gallium scanning has also been shown to be helpful, particularly in follow-up evaluation of residual masses that were gallium avid at diagnosis. Positron emission tomography (PET) scans, which are increasing in availability, may replace gallium scans in diagnostic and restaging evaluations of lymphomas in children and adults.[179,180] Staging laparotomy is not advocated in children with NHL since chemotherapy is the primary therapeutic modality for both low-stage and advanced-stage disease.

The most widely used staging system in childhood NHL is St. Jude Children's Research Hospital's Staging System, described by Murphy (Table 54-8).[181] It is applicable to all histologic types of childhood lymphoma. For treatment purposes, patients often are stratified into treatment groups based on whether they have limited-stage or advanced-stage disease that corresponds to stages I/II and III/IV, respectively, of the St. Jude system.

Treatment and Results

Recognition of the propensity for early widespread dissemination of pediatric NHL, regardless of stage or histology, formed the basis for development of systemic therapy regimens with combination chemotherapy and cranial nervous system prophylaxis that has dramatically improved the outcomes of children with NHL.[174,176,182-186] The significant increase in event-free survival over 2 decades is demonstrated by the results of successive trials at St. Jude Children's Research Hospital (Fig. 54-4).[177] Currently, cure rates of 85% to 90% in patients with

Table 54–8   The St. Jude Staging System for Childhood Non-Hodgkin's Lymphoma

Stage	Description
I	A single tumor (extranodal) or single anatomic area (nodal), excluding the mediastinum or abdomen
II	A single tumor (extranodal) with regional lymph node involvement on same side of the diaphragm:
	Two or more nodal areas
	Two single (extranodal) tumors with or without regional node involvement
	A primary gastrointestinal tract tumor (usually ileocecal) with or without associated mesenteric node involvement, grossly completely resected
III	On both sides of the diaphragm:
	Two single tumors (extranodal)
	Two or more nodal areas
	All primary intrathoracic tumors (mediastinal, pleural, thymic)
	All extensive primary intra-abdominal disease; unresectable
	All primary paraspinal or epidural tumors regardless of other sites
IV	Any of the above with initial central nervous system or bone marrow involvement (<25% blasts)

With permission from Murphy SB: Classification, staging and end results of treatment of childhood non-Hodgkin's lymphomas; Dissimilarities from lymphomas in adults. *Semin Oncol.* 1980;7:332.

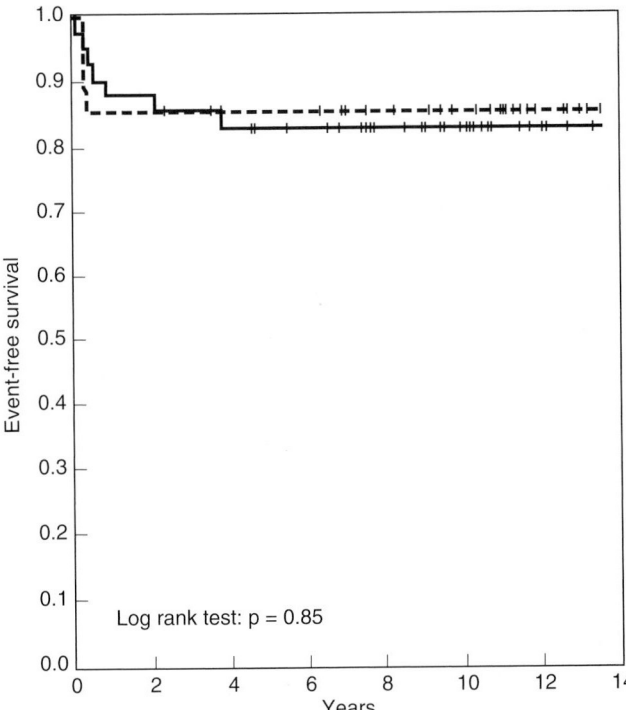

Figure 54–4. EPS for 68 localized disease patients by treatment group. (—), COMP (41 patients); (---), LSA₂L₂ (27 patients). (From Anderson JR, Jenkins RDT, Wilson JF, et al: Long-term follow-up of patients treated with COMP or LSA₂-L₂ therapy for childhood non-Hodgkin's lymphoma: A report of CCG-551 from the Children's Cancer Group. *J Clin Oncol.* 1993;11:1024.)

limited disease and 60% to 80% in those with extensive involvement are reported.[178] Two-year event-free survival rates are equaled with cure in pediatric NHL, since relapse beyond 2 years from diagnosis is uncommon.

Chemotherapy

In modern day regimens, chemotherapy is the primary therapeutic modality for all histologies and stages of childhood NHL. Surgery is indicated only for diagnostic purposes or in the case of an abdominal emergency such as intussusception, acute appendicitis, or intestinal obstruction.[176,187] In patients who present with life-threatening situations such as airway obstruction, superior vena cava syndrome, or spinal cord compression, low-dose focal radiation therapy (RT) may be helpful in alleviating critical symptoms while maximal supportive care measures and specific chemotherapy are instituted.[178]

Early in the evolution of NHL therapy it became evident that not only stage but also histologic subtype must be taken into consideration in selecting the most appropriate treatment regimen. This was most dramatically demonstrated in a randomized trial of the 4-drug COMP (cyclophosphamide, vincristine [Oncovin], methotrexate, prednisone) regimen[188] versus the 10-drug LSA₂L₂ regimen (cyclophosphamide, vincristine, prednisone, daunomycin, methotrexate, cytarabine, thioguanine, asparaginase, BCNU, hydroxyurea), a regimen designed for treatment of ALL.[172,175] The results of this CCG study confirmed the efficacy of the COMP regimen for patients with advanced-stage disease of small non–cleaved cell type, whereas patients with advanced stage lymphoblastic NHL fared significantly better with the more aggressive LSA₂L₂ regimen. Neither therapy was statistically superior in

treatment of advanced-stage large cell lymphoma. In this trial, children with localized NHL had excellent outcomes, regardless of histology or treatment group. These findings have been confirmed with long-term follow-up as shown in Figure 54-5.[189] Today, the choice of specific

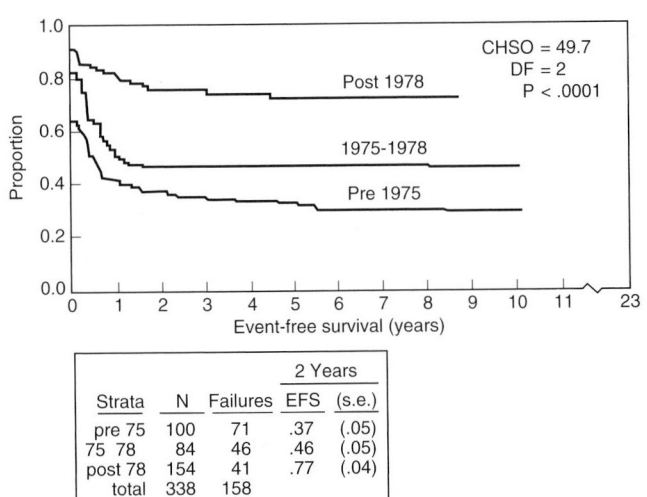

Strata	N	Failures	2 Years EFS	(s.e.)
pre 75	100	71	.37	(.05)
75 78	84	46	.46	(.05)
post 78	154	41	.77	(.04)
total	338	158		

Figure 54–5. The overall event-free survival as a function of the treatment eras for all cases are indicated. There is a successive and significant increase in the proportion of patients who are event free (*P* < .0001). (From Murphy SB, Fairclough DL, Hutchinson RE, Berard CW: Non-Hodgkin's lymphomas of childhood: An analysis of the histology, staging, and response to treatment of 338 cases at a single institution. *J Clin Oncol.* 1989;7:186.)

chemotherapy regimens and duration of treatment are determined based on stage and histology of the disease.

Successful treatment of advanced stage small non–cleaved cell (Burkitt's or nonBurkitt's) consists of repetitive dose intensive cycles including cyclophosphamide, high-dose methotrexate, and cytarabine given over 3 to 6 months (Table 54-9). This therapy is in sharp contrast to regimens used for lymphoblastic lymphomas, which, similar to high risk ALL therapy, use multiple chemotherapy agents and last anywhere from 24 to 36 months (Table 54-9). The optimal therapy for advanced-stage large cell lymphoma has been difficult to define because of the biologic heterogeneity of this histologic subtype of tumors.[201,203] Generally speaking, regimens that include cyclophosphamide, vincristine, prednisone, and doxorubicin have been successful (Table 54-9). In addition to intensive systemic chemotherapy, intrathecal therapy is with some exceptions an integral part of all treatment protocols for prevention of CNS disease regardless of histology.

More recent data suggests that therapy based on immunophenotype may result in improved survival. The POG recently reported that among children with large cell lymphoma (LCL) treated with the same regimen, those with B-cell LCL had better outcomes than patients with non–B-cell LCL.[183] European investigators have had excellent results in children with LCL when the treatment regimen is determined by immunophenotype (B vs. T cell). Children with B-cell LCL have excellent outcomes when treated according to small non–cleaved cell regimens and those with T-cell LCL treated according to T-ALL protocols. The best therapy for the treatment of anaplastic

Table 54–9 Treatment Outcomes for Advanced Stage Non-Hodgkin's Lymphoma Based on Histologic Subtype

Protocol	Stage	Patients, n	Event-Free Survival	Reference
Small Non–Cleaved Cell (Burkitt's and Burkitt-like) Lymphoma				
SJCRH-Total B	III	17	2 yr = 81%	Murphy et al[190]
	IV/B-ALL	4/8	2 yr = 17%	
POG-8617	IV	34	4 yr = 79%	Bowman et al[191]
	B-ALL	47	4 yr = 65%	{Fontanesi, Bowman, et al. 1992 #286}
LMB 89*	III	279	3 yr = 93%	Patte et al[192]
	IV/ALL	165	3 yr = 88%	
BFM 90	III	171	6 yr = 86%	Reiter et al[28]
	IV	23	6 yr = 83%	
	B-ALL	56	6 yr = 76%	
CCG LSA$_2$L$_2$	III/IV/B-ALL	44	5 yr = 29%	Anderson et al[189]
vs. COMP	III/IV/B-ALL	93	5 yr = 50%	
CCG				Chilcote et al[193]
COMP vs. D-COMP	III/IV/B-ALL	175	2 yr = 65%	
NCI*	III	30	3 yr = 57%	Magrath et al[194]
77-04	IV	9	3 yr = 13%	
DFCI	III	12	2 yr = 95%	Schwenn et al[195]
HIC-COM	IV/B-ALL	8	2 yr = 50%	
Lymphoblastic Lymphoma				
CCG 551	III/IV	124	5 yr = 64%	Anderson et al[189]
LSA$_2$L$_2$ (modified)				
BFM 86/90	III	119	EFS† = 87%	Schrappe et al[196]
	IV	30	EFS† = 90%	
SJCRH – Total X	III/IV	22	4 yr DFS = 73%	Dahl et al[197]
DFCI – APO	III/IV	21	3 yr DFS = 58%	Weinstein et al[198]
NCI – 77-04	III	10	4 yr EFS = 70%	Magrath et al[194]
POG – ACOP+	III	33	3 yr DFS = 54%	Hvizdala et al[173]
Large Cell Lymphoma				
CCG LSA$_2$L$_2$	III/IV	18	5 yr = 43%	Anderson et al[189]
vs. COMP		42	5 yr = 52%	
DFCI-APO	III/IV	—	3 yr = 65%	Weinstein et al[200]
POG-ACOP+	III/IV	22	4 yr = 67%	Hvizdala et al[173]
CCG	III	86	2 yr = 66%	Chilcote et al[193]
COMP vs. D-COMP				
SJCRH-CHOP	III/IV	21	3 yr = 62%	Sandlund et al[201]
SJCRH-MACOP-B	III/IV	11	3 yr = 55%	Santana et al[202]

*Includes patients with B-cell, large cell, non-Hodgkin's lymphoma.
†Median observation time 4.3 years.

CD30+ LCL is now known; a variety of approaches such as specific anaplastic large cell lymphoma (ALCL) and B-cell specific therapy have been tried with good results.[204-206] Trials to evaluate the efficacy of immuno-phenotype-directed therapy for pediatric large cell lymphoma are under way in Europe and the United States.

Outcomes in children diagnosed with early-stage 1 or 2 NHL are excellent with cure rates of 85% to 95%. The POG conducted two consecutive studies to determine if the intensity and duration of therapy could be safely reduced without decreasing the excellent prognosis. The first trial demonstrated that an 8-month chemotherapy regimen without involved field radiation of the primary sites was as effective as chemotherapy plus radiotherapy.[207] In the second trial they concluded that 9 weeks of chemotherapy was adequate therapy for early-stage, nonlymphoblastic lymphoma; continuation therapy for 8 months was beneficial only in patients with lymphoblastic lymphoma.[182] Although this group still had a higher relapse than patients with other histologic subtypes, salvage therapies were quite successful and overall survival remained good. Other groups have also observed higher relapse rates in children with early-stage lymphoblastic lymphoma compared to patients with nonlymphoblastic histology; thus, many investigators choose to treat these children with localized lymphoblastic lymphoma according to the same protocols used for ALL or advanced-stage lymphoblastic lymphoma with prolonged maintenance therapy for up to 2 years.[208]

THE ROLE OF RADIOTHERAPY

The role of radiotherapy has been continuously redefined over the past 2 decades. With the development of effective multiagent chemotherapy regimens, local field irradiation for primary disease control is not indicated. Cranial irradiation for CNS prophylaxis has also been eliminated from essentially all modern-day protocols, although it is still considered for some patients with lymphoblastic histology, or with overt CNS disease, as discussed later. Thus, radiotherapy currently is reserved primarily for the ancillary treatment of life-threatening mass effect. At very low total doses of 6 to 10 Gy, radiotherapy is often quite successful in producing rapid relief from the symptoms associated with the superior vena cava syndrome, acute respiratory distress, spinal cord compression, and orbital proptosis. Palliation of cranial nerve deficits may require higher doses of local field radiation in the range of 20 to 30 Gy.[209]

Primary-Site/Involved-Field Irradiation (Exclusive of Bone Primary Tumors)

Because of the excellent local control rates achieved with radiotherapy in pediatric NHL before the era of chemotherapy,[186,210,211] radiotherapy to the primary site was incorporated into the design of early chemotherapy trials.[172,175,199,200,212] Typically, doses ranging from 30 to 40 Gy were used. Because of concern for the significant acute as well as long-term toxicities observed with

combined modality therapy, a re-evaluation of the role of radiotherapy in pediatric NHL was undertaken. Original attempts at minimizing the potential adverse effects of RT were directed at reducing the local field dose to 20 Gy and the volume of tissue irradiated from a 5 cm to a 2 to 3 cm margin around the tumor site.[213-216] Since results of the reduced therapy trials in patients with early-stage disease were similar to those achieved with more aggressive therapy, investigators proceeded to question the need for radiotherapy at all in the context of effective multiagent chemotherapy. The POG addressed this question of the independent contribution of radiotherapy to an effective multiagent chemotherapy regimen in children with localized NHL of all histologies exclusive of primary tumor of the bone. In a randomized trial comparing induction therapy of CHOP (cyclophosphamide, hydroxydaunomycin, vincristine [Oncovin], prednisone) alone with CHOP plus 27 Gy involved-field-radiotherapy, no difference in results was observed, and a 4-year event-free survival rate of approximately 87% was projected for both arms.[207] Although some investigators still advocate involved-field radiotherapy (IFRT) for patients with localized NHL, the vast majority have abandoned its use based on the results of this well-designed study.

To date, the use of local-field radiotherapy in advanced-stage disease has not been shown to be of benefit. In a randomized trial that studied the use of chemotherapy with or without involvement radiotherapy,[184] the 2-year event-free survival rate in both treatment arms was only 38%, a value so low that the potential contribution of radiotherapy may have been masked by the ineffective systemic control. Nonetheless, with no concrete evidence to justify its use, because of concern for the potential of radiotherapy to compromise the effective delivery of chemotherapy in a disease that is inherently systemic, IFRT has been eliminated from the design of advanced-stage pediatric NHL trials. Recent results of the chemotherapy-alone trials tend to support this practice.[190,195,197,217]

Primary Non-Hodgkin's Lymphoma of Bone

The high rate of systemic spread in patients with clinically apparent early-stage primary NHL of bone (PBL) has confirmed that this extranodal presentation, as all other presentations of NHL, is a disseminated disease at diagnosis and as such requires systemic therapy.[218,219] Local-field radiotherapy to the involved bone was included in the early pediatric NHL chemotherapy trials. However, because of the increased incidence of second primary bone tumors observed with the combined modality therapy,[220] as well as the potential for increased morbidity in growing children, radiation is no longer a component of therapy in the setting of primary bone disease in children. This is supported by recent POG and Children's Cancer Group trials, which reported the experience with treatment of PBL in children for the past 15 to 20 years.[221,222] Both groups observed excellent outcomes with chemotherapy regimens and therefore conclude that radiotherapy is unnecessary.

Central Nervous System Preclinical and Overt Disease

Early in the evolution of pediatric NHL therapy, CNS relapse was recognized to be an obstacle to cure in about 30% to 35% of children.[174] As in leukemia, CNS prophylactic therapy was incorporated into the treatment of NHL of childhood and achieved excellent results; also, as in leukemia, CNS radiotherapy played an integral role in the early trials. The combination of cranial irradiation and intrathecal methotrexate resulted in a less than 10% incidence of CNS relapse.[174] In the only randomized trial of CNS presymptomatic therapy in pediatric NHL, conducted at the SJCRH in patients with stage II to IV NHL, 6% (1/18) of children randomly assigned to receive cranial irradiation and intrathecal methotrexate developed an isolated CNS relapse, as compared with 25% (4/16) who did not receive any specific form of CNS prophylactic therapy.[184]

Concern for the increased risk of neurotoxicity associated with the use of cranial irradiation in children prompted investigators to test the efficacy of using intrathecal chemotherapy alone for CNS prophylaxis. Results of modern chemotherapeutic regimen trials with intrathecal chemoprophylaxis have been successful in preventing isolated CNS relapse in approximately 95% of children with NHL.[189,223] Radiotherapy is thus no longer indicated for CNS prophylaxis with the possible exception of lymphoblastic (T-cell) disease, where it retains a role in some centers, and where it may also be appropriate in patients who have undergone leukemic transformation.[224-226] Although high-dose systemic and intrathecal chemotherapy (Ara-C and methotrexate) are effectively used to treat overt CNS NHL, RT remains a consideration and is a component of treatment in some centers.[227]

Testicular Lymphoma

Testicular involvement at diagnosis is uncommon (5% to 10% of children with disseminated small non–cleaved cell NHL). Most of these patients undergo orchiectomy, and the efficacy of scrotal irradiation is unclear. Although the prolonged remissions seen in children with chemosensitive disease suggest that scrotal irradiation may not be necessary, the poor prognosis of patients with testicular involvement and the occurrence of relapses in the testes argue in favor of local therapy with orchiectomy or irradiation as a component of therapy.[228-230] Thus, some protocols continue to employ scrotal irradiation for testicular involvement despite recent data that question its value.[231] Testicular relapse on therapy appears to indicate drug-resistant disease and a poor prognosis, despite testicular irradiation and chemotherapy.

FUTURE DIRECTIONS

The successful treatment of pediatric NHL has been achieved by the refinement of multiagent chemotherapy protocols. Future trials will be aimed at further refinement of therapy regimens with identification of better prognostic factors[232] and active agents, with the goal that patients will not be over- or undertreated. In patients with localized disease, the excellent survival rates (>90%) support the strategy of reducing therapy in our effort to minimize adverse effects without compromising efficacy.[182] In patients with advanced-stage NHL, future trials must aim at better identification of patients destined to do poorly and more effective therapy regimens. The increasing understanding of molecular genetic pathogenesis of lymphomas has made it possible to develop sensitive techniques of measurement of minimal residual disease during clinical remission as a way of identifying patients at high risk of relapse as well as highly specific therapy targeted to the tumor cells.[233] Recent successful trials with the use of Rituxan, a monoclonal antibody directed against CD20, a B-cell antigen,[234,235] demonstrate the importance of continued study of novel approaches. Future clinical trials will likely include the use of (1) immunotherapy with monoclonal antibodies[236-238]; (2) stem cell transplantation[239]; (3) antisense oligonucleotides[240]; and (4) cytotoxic T-lymphocytes[241] or tumor vaccines.[242,243]

HODGKIN'S DISEASE

Epidemiology and Biology

Lymphomas, which constitute about 15% of cancer diagnoses in patients younger than 20 years of age, are the third most common form of childhood cancer. In the United States, approximately 1700 children and adolescents under age 20 years are diagnosed with lymphoma each year.[244] Overall, children with HD are slightly more common than NHL, with an annual incidence rate of 12.8/1 million children newborn to 19 years of age. For unapparent reasons, the incidence rates of HD have declined slightly between 1975 and 1995.[244] However, during this same period, the 5-year survival rate for Hodgkin's has increased to 91%.

At least two different presentations of HD in the early age groups are apparent: a childhood form developing in patients 14 years of age or younger, and a young adult form affecting patients 15 to 34 years of age.[245,246] HD is rarely diagnosed in children younger than 5 years of age. In a recently conducted clinical trial for children and adolescents with HD, 3% of patients were between newborn and 4 years of age; 12% of patients were between 5 and 9 years of age; 44% of patients were between 10 and 14 years of age, and 41% were older than 15 years of age.[247] In children and younger adolescents, the disease occurs more frequently in males; in older adolescents the incidence among males and females is roughly equal. Also, most adolescent patients diagnosed with HD are white. The biology and natural history of HD in children is similar to that in adults, and thus will not be discussed here at length. However, it is of interest that in the United States, Epstein-Barr virus (EBV) tumor cell positivity is common in children younger than 10 years of age, with only a 15% to 20% rate in adolescents and young adults.[248] Thus, the presence of EBV genome in Hodgkin's and Reed-Sternberg cells is not a prognostic factor in children.[249]

Detection and Diagnosis

Clinical presentations fall in rather predictable patterns. Most children are diagnosed on the basis of supradiaphragmatic lymph nodes, with painless cervical adenopathy in 80%. Mediastinal involvement occurs in 76% of adolescents, but in only 33% of 1- to 10-year-olds. Mediastinal disease may produce symptoms such as dyspnea, cough, or superior vena cava (SVC) syndrome. Axillary adenopathy is less common.[250]

Clinical Staging

After pathologic confirmation, the patient undergoes an extensive "clinical" staging, as is true for adults. This includes a thorough history and physical examination, laboratory testing, and imaging studies as follows.

Imaging of the Thorax

This should include a chest radiograph and CT scan. Distinguishing normal (or hyperplastic) thymus from nodes in children can be problematic. The usefulness of PET scanning in childhood in evaluating supradiaphragmatic nodes is under evaluation. The procedure is useful in adults, particularly in assessing the response of mediastinal adenopathy to treatment.[251-253]

Imaging of the Abdomen and Pelvis

This should include an abdominal/pelvic CT scan. Distinction of reactive lymph node hyperplasia from HD is problematic, and is more common in younger children than in adolescents.[254] Since essentially all patients are treated with chemotherapy, staging laparotomies are rarely used. In situations where equivocal imaging abnormalities exist and require resolution for therapy, isolated nodal sampling is generally performed. Complications following staging laparotomy include immediate postoperative morbidity (rare infection, bowel or ureteral obstruction), and a less than 4% risk of small bowel obstruction due to adhesion. Postoperative mortality is essentially unreported in the past 15 years,[255-257] although historically, a high rate of post-splenectomy sepsis in children (especially younger than 5 years old) was reported.[256] Administration of pneumococcal vaccination before surgery and daily prophylactic antibiotics appears to have decreased this risk.[258] Regardless, laparotomies rarely have a role in the current staging of children with HD.

Classification and Staging

Histopathology and staging is described in the section on adults. Of interest in pediatric HD is that the relative distribution of the subtypes in younger children differs from that in adolescents and adults, as shown in Table 54-10, which combines a recent Children's Cancer Study Group and the European GPOH-95 data. The distribution of stages observed in children is also somewhat different than that observed in adults, again described in Table 54-10.

Evolution of Therapy

When irradiation techniques and doses suitable for controlling disease in adults were used in the pediatric setting, substantial morbidities were produced.[256,261] It is within this context that treatment strategies specific to HD in the pediatric age group are discussed.[262] Overall survival rates for children with HD approach 85% to 95% (Tables 54-11 and 54-12). The desire to cure children with minimal treatment-related toxicity provided the stimulus to limit staging procedures and reduce the intensity and types of chemotherapeutic regimens as well as the dose and volume of radiotherapy used. Historically, treatment of adults with early-stage HD often was with radiotherapy alone, reserving chemotherapy for salvage of recurrent disease.[280-282] This approach was initially extended to the pediatric population.[263,264,283,284] Radiation treatment regimens used primarily prescribed standard doses of 35 to 44 Gy to extended fields, regardless of the patient's age. Impairment of soft tissue and skeletal growth including intraclavicular narrowing, shortened sitting height, decreased mandibular growth, and decreased muscle development became readily apparent as young patients matured after curative therapy.[256,283] Concerns about growth impairment led to the development of clinical trials designed to specifically address the

Table 54–10   Patient Characteristics

	Children, %*	Adults, %†
Number of patients	1659	1912
<10 yrs	269 (16.2)	
≥10 yrs	1385 (83.5)	
>17 yrs		1912 (100)
Gender		
Male	909 (54.8)	1147 (60.0)
Female	750 (45.2)	765 (40.0)
Histology		
Lymphocyte predominate	161 (9.7)	96 (5.0)
Mixed cellularity	251 (15.1)	325 (17.0)
Nodular sclerosing	1210 (72.9)	1377 (72.0)
Not classified and lymphocyte depleted	37 (2.2)	115 (6.0)
Stage		
I	194 (11.7)	210 (11.0)
II	922 (55.6)	899 (47.0)
III	294 (17.7)	593 (31.0)
IV	249 (15.0)	210 (11.0)
B Symptoms		
present	884 (53.3)	612 (32.0)
absent	775 (46.7)	1300 (68.0)

*Data taken from Rühl et al[260] and Nachman et al.[247]
†Data taken from Cleary et al.[259]

Table 54-11 Treatment Results in Children with Early-Stage Hodgkin's Disease

Group/Institution	Patients, n	Stage	Chemotherapy Regimen	Radiation Dose, Gy, and field	Survival, % Overall	Survival, % Relapse-free	Follow-up Interval, yr	Reference
Joint Center/Harvard	50	PS I, IIA	None	36–44, IF	97	82	11	Mauch et al[261]
Stanford University	48	PS* I, II	None	40–44, IF	86	82	10	Donaldson et al[263]
Stanford University	27	PS* I, II	6 MOPP	15–25, IF	100	96	10	Donaldson et al[262]
Germany-Austria HD-82	100	IA/IB–IIA	2 OPPA	35, IF	100	98	9	Schellong et al[270]
	53	IIB–IIIA	2 OPPA/2 COPP	30, IF	96	94	9	
Germany-Austria HD-85	275	IA/IB–IIA	2 OPA	35, IF	98	85	6	Schellong et al[270]
	124	IIB–IIIA	2 OPA/2 COMP	30, IF	95	55	6	
Germany-Austria HD-90	85	IA/IB–IIA	2 OEPA/OPPA	25, IF	99	94/95	5	Schellong et al[271]
	21	IIB–IIIA	2 OEPA/OPPA + 2 COPP	25, IF	97	90/96	5	
GPOH-HD95	326	I, IIA	2 OEPA/OPPA	None for CR, 20–35, IF for PR	97	94	3	Ruhl et al[260]
	224	IIB, IIIA	2 OEPA/OPPA + 2 COPP		97	91	3	
UKCCSG	125	II	6–10 ChlVPP	35, IF	92	85	10	Shankar et al[265]
SFOP MDH-82	79	CS I–IIA	4 ABVD	20–40, IF	90	89	6	Oberlin et al[262]
	67	CS I–IIA	2 MOPP/2 ABVD	20–40, IF	87	89	6	
	31	CSIB–IIB	3 MOPP/3 ABVD	20–40, EF		89	6	
SFOP MDH-90	171	I–II	4 VBVP	20, IF	97.5	91	5	Landman-Parker et al[268]
	27	I–II	4 VBVP + 1–2 OPPA	20, IF		78	5	
AEIOP-MH-83	83	IA	3 ABVD	20–40, IF	95	86	7	Vecchi et al[269]
	83	IIA (M/T <0.33)	3 ABVD	20–40, R	81		7	
		IIA (M/T ≥0.33)	3 MOPP/3 ABVD	20–40, R				
		IIIA	3 MOPP/3 ABVD	20–40, EF				
Stanford/St. Jude/ Dana Farber CI	110	CSI/II†	4 VAMP	15–25.5	99	93	5	Donaldson et al[267]
CCG Group 1	294	CS IA, B, IIA‡	4 COPP/ABVD	none vs. 21 Gy if CR, 21 Gy if PR	100	95	3	Nachman et al[247]
Uganda	18	CS I–IIIA	6 MOPP	None	75	74	5	Olweny et al[272]

*Some patients clinically staged.
†No bulk.
‡Without adverse features, (= +hila, >4 sites, bulk).
AEIOP, Italian Association of Hematology and Pediatric Oncology; CCG, Children's Cancer Group; CS, clinical stage; EF, extended field; GPOH, The Society for Pediatric Oncology and Haematology; IF, involved field; PS, pathologic stage; SFOP, French Society of Pediatric Oncology; UKCCSG, United Kingdom Children Cancer Study Group.
ABVD, doxorubicin, bleomycin, vinblastine and dacarbazine; ChlVPP, chlorambucil, vinblastine, procarbazine, and prednisolone; COMP, cyclophosphamide, vincristine, methotrexate, and prednisolone; COP(P), cyclophosphamide, vincristine, prednisone, and procarbazine; MOPP, nitrogen mustard, vincristine, procarbazine, and prednisone; OEPA, vincristine, etoposide, prednisone, doxorubicin; OPPA, oncovin, procarbazine, prednisolone, and Adriamycin; VAMP, vinblastine, doxorubicin, methotrexate, and prednisone; VBVP, vinblastine, bleomycin, etoposide, and prednisone. Modified from Constine LS, Qazi R, Rubin P: Malignant lymphomas. In Rubin P, McDonald S, Qazi R, eds. *Clinical Oncology: A Multidisciplinary Approach for Physicians and Students.* Philadelphia: WB Saunders; 1993:217.

needs of children with HD. These protocols evaluated lower radiation doses (15 to 25.5 Gy) to reduced (involved) treatment fields combined with multiagent chemotherapy.[247,258,260,266-269,271,273,275,277,284-293] Numerous studies subsequently established the efficacy of this treatment approach, after which the primary use of standard-dose radiation was reserved for skeletally mature patients with localized disease.

With more prolonged follow-up, reports implicating radiation as a causative factor for excess cardiovascular disease and subsequent malignancy risk in long-term pediatric Hodgkin's survivors motivated further therapeutic refinements.[146,276,294-310] The use of standard-dose, extended-field radiation in mature adolescents with localized HD has been abandoned at most centers because this treatment approach predisposes to a greater risk of cardiovascular disease and secondary solid tumor carcinogenesis. Contemporary risk-adapted treatment protocols have focused on further limiting radiation exposure of uninvolved tissues, especially the breast, and identifying

Table 54–12 Treatment in Children with Advanced-Stage Hodgkin's Disease

Group/Institution	Patients, n	Stage*	Chemotherapy Regimen	Radiotherapy Dose, Gy, and Field	Survival, % Overall	Survival, % Relapse-free	Follow-up Interval, yr	Follow-up Reference
Germany-Austria HD-82	50	IIIB–IV	2 OPPA/4 COPP	25, IF	85	86	9 / 9	Schellong et al[270]
Germany-Austria HD-85	24	IIIB–IV	2 OPA/4 COMP	25, IF	100	49	6 / 6	Schellong et al[270]
German (DAL)	179	IIIB/IV	2 OEPA/OPPA + 4 COPP	20, IF	94	84/89	5	Schellong et al[271]
GPOH-HD95	280	IIIB, IV	2 OEPA/OPPA + 4 COPP	None for CR, 20–35, IF for PR	97	84	3	Rühl et al[260]
SFOP MDH-82	40	CS III	3 MOPP/3 ABVD	20–40 EF		85	6	Oberlin et al[262]
	21	CS IV	3 MOPP/3 ABVD	20–40, EF		62		
St. Jude	85	CS II–IV	4–5 COP(P)/3–4 ABVD	20 Gy, IF	93	93	5	Hudson et al[300]
AEIOP-MH-83	49	IIIB–IV	5 MOPP/5 ABVD	20–40, EF	60		7	Vecchi et al[269]
CCG	54	PS–III/IV	6 ABVD	21, EF	90	87	4	Hutchinson et al[293]
UKCCSG	80	III	6–10 ChlVPP	35, IF	84	73	10	Shankar et al[265]
	27	IV	6–10 ChlVPP	35, IF	71	38	10	
Pediatric Oncology Group	80	IIB–IV	4 MOPP/4 ABVD	21, EF	87	80	3	Weiner et al[292]
Joint Center/Harvard	96	III–IV	6 MOPP	25–40	8	—	11	Mauch et al[267] Tarbell et al[276]
Stanford/St. Jude/ Dana Farber	56	CSI/II bulky (n = 26), CSIII/IV (n = 30)	6 VEPA	15–25.5	81.9	67.8	5	Friedmann et al[277]
CCG Group 2	394	CS I/II[†],	6 COPP/ABV	if CR none vs.	93	82	3	Nachman et al[247]
	141	CS IIB, CS III		21, IF if PR 21, IF	93	83	3	
Group 3		CS IV	COPP/ABV + CHOP + Ara-C/VP-16					
UKCCSG	67	IV	6–8 ChlVPP	none[‡]	80.8	55.2	5	Atra et al[279]
Australia/New Zealand	8	III/IV	6–12 MOPP	none	92	80	5	Ekert et al[278]

*Unless specified, surgically staged; P = 0.53.

[†]Adverse features = +hila, >4 sites, bulk.

[‡]12 patients received 20-35 Gy IF; 2 received whole lung irradiation.

AEIOP, Italian Association of Hematology and Pediatric Oncology; CCG, Children's Cancer Group; CS, clinical stage; EF, extended field; GPOH, The Society for Pediatric Oncology and Haematology; IF, involved field; PS, pathologic stage; SFOP, French Society of Pediatric Oncology; UKCCSG, United Kingdom Children Cancer Study Group.

Modified from Constine LS, Qazi R, Rubin P: Malignant lymphomas. In Rubin P, McDonald S, Qazi R, eds. *Clin Oncol: A Multidisciplinary Approach for Physicians and Students.* Philadelphia: WB Saunders; 1993:217.

patients for whom the addition of radiation optimizes disease-free survival.

In summary, devising the optimal therapeutic approach for children with HD is complicated by the increased risk for adverse treatment-related side effects. Radiotherapy doses and fields safely used in adults, when used in children, can often lead to significant musculoskeletal growth retardation and excess risk for the development of life-threatening cardiovascular dysfunction and subsequent malignancies.[146,256,276,283,294-298, 300,302-308,310-314] Because of differences in the developmental status of children of varying ages, there is, unfortunately, no single method of ideal treatment for all children.

Therapy in pediatric HD continues to vary widely among investigators with regard to the modality or modalities used, as well as to the specifics of chemotherapeutic regimens and radiotherapeutic doses and techniques. Currently, most prepubertal children with HD are managed with combined multiagent chemotherapy alone or combined with low-dose, IFRT radiotherapy.

Combination Chemotherapy

The prototypic chemotherapy regimen for HD is MOPP (mechlorethamine, vincristine [Oncovin], procarbazine, and prednisone). The well-recognized major toxicities observed with its use include an increased risk of acute leukemia,[146,300,312] azoospermia in up to 90% of males treated at any age,[315-318] and a risk of sterility in females that increases with age.[258,319-321] The development of the ABVD (doxorubicin [adriamycin], bleomycin, vinblastine, and dacarbazine) regimen in the 1970s provided an effective alternative to MOPP chemotherapy that was not associated with an increased risk of secondary AML or infertility.[322,323] Compared to MOPP, ABVD produced superior treatment outcomes and lacked leukemogenic and permanent gonadal toxicity.[324] For these reasons, ABVD is a standard front-line therapy for adults with newly diagnosed HD. However, reservations about potential cardiopulmonary toxicity, sequelae related to the doxorubicin and bleomycin in the combination, have influenced its use in children with HD. The severity of these complications may be exacerbated by the addition of mediastinal or mantle irradiation, in which a portion of the lungs and heart is included in the treatment field.[294,297,298,311]

Contemporary pediatric trials typically use ABVD or similar hybrid combinations, in risk-adapted treatment regimens prescribing fewer chemotherapy cycles for patients with favorable localized disease presentations.[247,260,267,268,271,277,325] For children with advanced or unfavorable disease, ABVD is often alternated or combined with alkylating agent regimens such as COPP (cyclophosphamide, vincristine [Oncovin], procarbazine, and prednisone), in an effort to reduce exposure of agents with dose-related toxicity and improve disease control.

Combined Modality Versus Chemotherapy Alone

Children and adolescents with HD may be cured using combination chemotherapy alone or a combined modality approach using chemotherapy and RT. Contemporary therapy produces long-term remission in 70% to 90% of patients with advanced, unfavorable HD and 85% to 100% of patients with localized favorable disease. The chemotherapy regimens employed largely include MOPP, ABVD, or therapies derived from one of the combinations. Chemotherapy-alone trials typically prescribe more cycles of chemotherapy, while combined modality protocols administer low-dose, IFRT in lieu of several chemotherapy cycles.[247,272,278,279,292,326-334] The limited number of randomized pediatric trials prospectively evaluating combined modality therapy versus chemotherapy alone has not definitely established the superiority of one treatment approach over the other, although the results of some trials suggest that the addition of RT may improve outcome in unfavorable and advanced-stage patients.[247, 292]

Consequently, debate continues among pediatric investigators regarding optimal therapy for newly diagnosed children. Treatment with chemotherapy alone eliminates the risk of radiation-associated adverse sequelae including musculoskeletal growth impairment, cardiovascular dysfunction, and solid tumor carcinogenesis. However, these sequelae are less substantial than in earlier

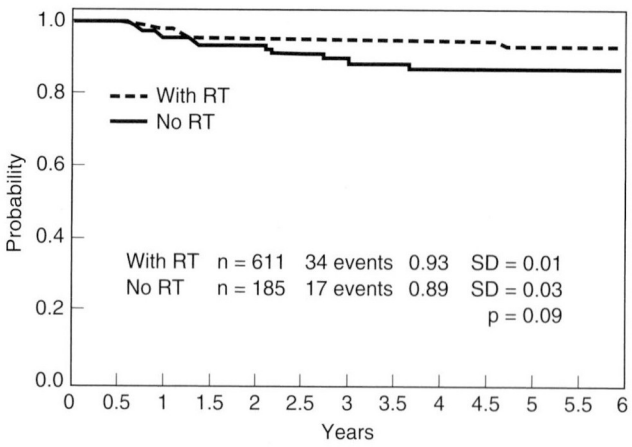

Figure 54–6. Relapse-free survival for 185 patients without radiation therapy (RT) after chemotherapy-induced complete remission in comparison to 611 patients with RT after partial remission postchemotherapy (median follow-up time 38 months). (From Rühl U, Albrecht M, Dieckmann K, et al: Response-adapted radiotherapy in the treatment of pediatric Hodgkin's disease: An interim report at 5 years of the German GPOH-HD 95 trial. *Int J Radiat Oncol Biol Phys.* 2001;51:1209.)

eras due to the use of low-dose IFRT. Moreover, chemotherapy-alone protocols rely on higher cumulative doses of agents with established dose-related toxicity, especially alkylators, which may also predispose to acute and late treatment effects. The identification of prognostic features of patients who may benefit from omission or addition of RT continues to be a primary objective of contemporary pediatric Hodgkin's trials.

For example, in the recent German GPOG-HD 95 trial, relapse-free survival was superior for patients treated with RT after partial response (93%) than for those without RT after CR (89%). The difference was significant for patients treated for advanced-stage but not early-stage disease (Fig. 54-6).[260] Similarly, in a recent CCG trial, low-dose IFRT after an initial complete response to risk-adapted chemotherapy improved event-free survival but not survival.[247]

RISK-ADAPTED THERAPY

Favorable Localized Disease

More recent pediatric trials have evaluated the efficacy of risk-adapted therapy using fewer cycles of multiagent chemotherapy and lower radiation doses and treatment volumes in clinically staged patients with favorable disease presentations. A favorable presentation is defined as a limited number of sites (usually less than four) of localized "nonbulky" nodal involvement in an asymptomatic patient (without constitutional systems like fever, sweats, or weight loss). Mediastinal masses are considered "bulky" if they measure greater than 33% of the maximum intrathoracic cavity; the definition of peripheral lymph node bulk varies from 4 to 6 cm, depending on the study center. Most protocols prescribe two to four cycles of novel chemotherapy combinations, which omit or reduce the amount of the more toxic agents in the original

MOPP and ABVD regimens.[260,267,268,271,335] The excellent treatment results of these trials affirm the concept that patients with localized disease could be cured with minimal therapy.

Advanced and Unfavorable Disease

Clinical presentations associated with symptomatic disease, bulky lymphadenopathy, extranodal extension, and advanced stage (IIIB-IV) are designated unfavorable. Two treatment approaches have been used in patients with unfavorable presentations of HD. The chemotherapy prescribed in both approaches is derived from the MOPP and ABVD combinations. Conventional treatment approaches use combination chemotherapy administered on a twice-monthly schedule for 6 to 8 months.[260,271,277,289,292,336] The second strategy uses abbreviated, dose-intensive, multi-agent chemotherapy delivered in a compacted schedule over 3 to 5 months.[247,325,336] Myelosuppressive and non-myelosuppressive chemotherapy is alternated in a weekly schedule with the intent to reduce the development of resistant disease. Low-dose, IFRT may be used to consolidate remission after completion of chemotherapy. Both treatment approaches produce comparable early treatment outcomes. Long-term follow-up of the abbreviated dose-intensive approach is required to establish its superiority over conventional treatment approaches in maintaining long-term disease control.

Results of Therapy

In assessing the literature pertaining to pediatric HD, several factors must be considered: (1) the endpoints used to evaluate treatment efficacy; (2) the definitions of survival (e.g., event-free, relapse-free, freedom from progression, overall); (3) the treatment regimens and techniques used; and (4) the therapy-related morbidity rate.

The actuarial 10-year survival rate for children with early-stage disease is reported to range from 85% to 97%, and for those with advanced-stage disease, from 70% to 90% (see Tables 54-11 and 54-12). Regardless of stage, the size of the mediastinal disease continues to influence the choice of therapy in most clinical trials. In studies in which patients are not stratified according to the mediastinal bulk, patients with residual mediastinal disease following the preselected number of chemotherapy cycles may receive higher radiation doses, obviating the ability to conclude that the bulk of disease did not influence treatment.[260] The relapse-free and overall survival rates for children with stage III disease are excellent; however, the outcome for stage IV patients remains poor.[279,337]

Refractory or Relapsed Disease

Historically, most treatment failures in patients with HD occur within the first 3 years. The prognosis following relapse depends on the primary therapy and timing of relapse. Salvage rates are very good if relapse develops after primary therapy with RT alone. As many as 50% to 80% of these patients can be salvaged with chemotherapy or combined modality therapy.[338-343] Conversely, patients with early-stage disease who recur in areas of initial disease after chemotherapy alone may also have an excellent salvage rate without myeloablative approaches.[247] Second remissions may also be achieved in up to 50% of patients who relapse after maintaining their first remission for 1 year or longer. Patients who develop refractory disease during or within 1 year of primary therapy have a very poor prognosis, particularly if they recur in irradiated sites following combined modality therapy. Intensive cytoreductive chemotherapy followed by consolidation with myeloablative therapy and hematopoietic stem cell transplantation produces the most durable remissions in these very high-risk patients. Overall, this approach may salvage 30% to 50% of patients with refractory disease, but acute and late treatment toxicity predisposes these patients to early mortality. IFRT to sites of recurrent disease is generally appropriate if these sites have not been previously irradiated. IFRT can be administered before the high-dose chemotherapy program in order to place patients in a minimal disease state. More often, RT is administered after the high-dose chemotherapy program in order to decrease the potential for disease progression elsewhere during the time RT is being administered, and RT-related peritransplant morbidity such as esophagitis, pneumonitis, cardiomyopathy, and veno-occlusive disease.[344,345] It is noteworthy that patients treated with hematopoietic stem cell transplant may experience relapse as late as 5 years after the procedure and should be monitored for relapse as well as late treatment sequelae.

TECHNIQUES OF RADIOTHERAPY

Most children with HD will be treated with combined chemotherapy and low-dose IFRT. Meticulous and judiciously designed fields are necessary for maximum success in terms of both disease control and normal tissue damage. Data from the Patterns of Care studies document the relationship between technique and outcome.[346] Because technique is discussed elsewhere, only select points applicable to children are discussed here.

A linear accelerator with a beam energy of 6 MV is desirable due to its penetration, well-defined edge, and homogeneity throughout an irregular treatment field. Excellent immobilization techniques are necessary for children in order to ensure accuracy and reproducibility. The appropriate treatment volume is often protocol specific but generally includes the initially involved lymph node regions. Additional considerations relate to the location of disease (e.g., pericardium, chest wall). Low-dose radiation is also variously defined and often protocol specific. In general, doses of 15 Gy to 25 Gy are used, with modifications based on patient age, the presence of bulk or residual (post-chemotherapy) disease, and normal tissue concerns. In some situations, a boost of 5 Gy is appropriate.

The definitions of such fields depend on the anatomy of the region in terms of lymph node distribution, patterns of disease extension into regional areas, and consideration for match line problems should disease recur. Field definitions are often protocol specific, but excessively small fields are usually inappropriate. In a child younger than age 5, consideration may be given to treating bilateral areas (e.g., both sides of the neck) to avoid growth asymmetry. However, this is less of a concern with low radiation doses and thus unilateral fields are usually appropriate if the disease is unilateral. Efforts to avoid unnecessary irradiation of contiguous normal tissues are important (e.g., breast tissue in a child with isolated mediastinal disease and no axillary involvement). Treatment of *involved supradiaphragmatic fields* or a *mantle field* requires precision because of the distribution of lymph nodes and the critical adjacent normal tissues. These fields can be simulated with the arms up over the head, or down with hands on the hips. The former pulls the axillary lymph nodes away from the lungs, allowing greater lung shielding. However, the axillary lymph nodes then move into the vicinity of the humeral heads, which should be blocked in growing children. Thus the position chosen involves weighing concerns regarding lymph nodes, lung, and humeral heads. Attempts should be made to exclude or position breast tissue under the lung/axillary blocking. When the decision is made to include some or all of a critical organ in the radiation field, such as liver, kidney, or heart, then normal tissue constraints, depending on the chemotherapy used and patient age, are critical.

COMPLICATIONS OF RADIOTHERAPY

ACUTE EFFECTS. Acute side effects most often associated with mantle irradiation are the same as those experienced in the adult population and include temporary loss or change in taste, xerostomia, sore throat, esophagitis, low posterior scalp epilation, skin erythema, and occasionally dyspepsia and nausea and vomiting. Acute effects of para-aortic irradiation include early-onset nausea and vomiting, which usually abates after the second or third treatment without antiemetic therapy.

LONG-TERM EFFECTS. Long-term adverse sequelae specific to irradiation to the pediatric age group include impairment of muscle, bone, and dental development[256,283,347-350] and injury to the lungs,[256,287,351,352] heart,[294,296-298,353] thyroid gland,[354,355] and reproductive organs.[315,316,318-321,356-358] Survivors who underwent surgical staging with splenectomy also have a life-long risk of overwhelming sepsis from encapsulated bacterial organisms.[359] Cardiovascular dysfunction and secondary carcinogenesis may result in early mortality in long-term survivors.[294,313,353]

Acute and chronic pneumonitis, pulmonary fibrosis, and spontaneous pneumothorax are pulmonary sequelae observed in survivors of HD. Predisposing therapies include thoracic radiation and ABVD chemotherapy.[256,287,288,351,352] The bleomycin in ABVD produces pulmonary fibrosis and may be responsible for veno-occlusive disease in rare cases. ABVD may also predispose to pneumonitis by inducing a "radiation recall" phenomena related to the doxorubicin. Most reports describe pulmonary dysfunction in survivors treated before the

era of risk-adapted therapy. Asymptomatic pulmonary dysfunction that improves over time has been commonly observed after more contemporary combined modality treatment approaches.[288,352] Symptomatic pulmonary toxicity is uncommon and more often develops in patients treated with pulmonary irradiation and bleomycin.[256,287,351]

Chemotherapeutic agents and RT used in the treatment of pediatric HD predispose to cardiovascular disease. Cardiac dysfunction is most commonly observed after anthracycline therapy, particularly doxorubicin.[294,296,298] In adults, the risk of congestive heart failure related to anthracycline-induced cardiomyopathy increases when cumulative doses exceed 550 mg/m². Young children may be at risk for anthracycline injury at lower cumulative doses because of the drug's adverse effect on cardiac myocyte growth. This is suggested by studies of childhood leukemia survivors who demonstrate a high frequency of abnormalities of afterload and contractility.[360] Mediastinal irradiation and other chemotherapeutic agents (e.g., cyclophosphamide) may predispose pediatric Hodgkin's survivors who received lower cumulative anthracycline doses in the range of 350 to 400 mg/m².[294,296,298] Acute anthracycline cardiotoxicity is rare with contemporary therapy that limits doses to 300 mg/m² or lower. However, the risk of delayed subclinical cardiac dysfunction, which may become clinically significant with cardiac senescence, is not yet established.

Radiation also injures the pericardium and myocardium in a dose-related fashion.[297,298,353] High-dose (35 to 44 Gy) mantle irradiation produces cardiac injury in 13% of children and adults, most commonly manifest as constrictive pericarditis or accelerated coronary atherogenesis. Stanford investigators reported that the actuarial risk of developing cardiac disease requiring pericardectomy was 4% at 17 years in a series of long-term survivors of childhood HD.[298] Most patients with severe pericardial complications were irradiated before the introduction of subcarinal shielding and received little or no cardiac blocking. Premature coronary artery disease and acute myocardial infarction may also contribute to excess mortality risk in patients treated with mediastinal radiation in doses more than 30 Gy before 20 years of age.[294] With the introduction of radiation techniques that reduce the radiation dose to the heart, the rates of radiation-associated cardiac injury have declined dramatically. Likewise, myocardial infarctions have not been reported in children treated with combined modality regimens using lower radiation doses and volumes and protective cardiac shielding. Again, the impact of subclinical cardiac injury after low-dose radiation may not become apparent until larger cohorts of survivors treated with these regimens begin to age. Thyroid sequelae are common after RT for pediatric HD. Hypothyroidism, hyperthyroidism, thyroid nodules, and thyroid cancer have been observed in long-term survivors.[354,361] Of these, hypothyroidism, particularly compensated hypothyroidism, defined as thyroid stimulating hormone (TSH) elevation in the presence of a normal thyroxine (T4) level, is the most frequently described thyroid abnormality. Risk factors for hypothyroidism include younger age at treatment and higher cumulative radiation dose. As many as 78% of patients treated with radiation doses exceeding 26 Gy demonstrate thyroid dysfunction, as indicated by elevated TSH levels.[351,354] Because persistent TSH elevation most often signals impending gland failure and may be a carcinogenic stimulus to the gland, thyroid hormone replacement therapy should be instituted. Gland suppression with thyroid hormone replacement is also recommended for patients who develop thyroid nodules after radiation. Replacement therapy should suppress gland function, as indicated by a TSH of 0.5 to 1.5 uIU/mL. Periodic withdrawal of hormonal therapy in asymptomatic patients will permit assessment of gland recovery, which has been observed in some patients serially monitored after RT. Persistent and enlarging nodules should be monitored with ultrasound and periodic biopsies for malignant degeneration, as thyroid carcinoma is a common second malignancy following HD.[355]

The risk of gonadal injury following HD is related to the type and intensity of treatment. In males, high-dose pelvic radiation may produce a transient oligospermia or azoospermia, but spermatogenesis typically recovers.[357,362] Six to eight cycles of MOPP (or similar hybrid chemotherapy containing alkylators) produces irreversible sterility in 80% to 90% of males; fertility may be preserved if treatment is limited to three or fewer cycles.[363] Recovery of gonadal function 10 to 15 years following MOPP chemotherapy has been rarely reported. Anthracycline-based regimens like ABVD (or similar hybrid) are usually associated with full recovery of spermatogenesis following a temporary period of azoospermia.[316,317] In contrast, testicular Leydig cell function is more resistant to the effects of antineoplastic treatment, so growth and puberty are adversely affected only in boys treated with very high cumulative doses of alkylating agent chemotherapy. Risk-adapted therapies reducing or eliminating gonadotoxic alkylating agent chemotherapy offer young men with newly diagnosed HD excellent prospects to maintain fertility.[358]

Young women have a higher chance of maintaining regular menses after treatment for HD compared to older women. The risk of ovarian failure after pelvic radiation is high, but can be reduced by midline ovarian transposition (oophoropexy).[356] Although most young women maintain or resume menses after MOPP (or similar hybrid) chemotherapy, they are predisposed to early menopause, particularly if they also received abdominal-pelvic radiation.[319-321] In a report of female Hodgkin's survivors by the Late Effects Study Group, 42% of women treated with alkylating agent chemotherapy and subdiaphragmatic radiation had experienced menopause by age 31 years compared to 5% of controls.[321] Reports by other groups have not indicated an excessive risk of premature menopause in young women treated with supradiaphragmatic RT alone.[320]

The overall cumulative risk of developing a subsequent malignancy following treatment for pediatric HD ranges from 7% to 8% at 15 years from diagnosis and rises to 16% to 28% by 20 years.[146,295,302-310,364]

Tumor histologies comprise two main types: acute myeloid leukemia (including a pancytopenic myelodysplastic syndrome) and solid tumors. Secondary leukemias exhibit a relatively brief latency with a peak frequency in the first 5 to 10 years after treatment. The risk plateaus to less than 2% after 10 years from diagnosis. Clinical and treatment factors correlated with secondary leukemogenesis include older age at treatment, history of splenectomy, presentation with advanced disease, treatment with high cumulative doses of alkylating agents, and history of relapse.[300] In contrast to secondary hematopoietic malignancies, the risk of developing a second solid tumor increases with the passage of time from diagnosis, with a latency usually exceeding 10 years from diagnosis. Various solid tumors have been observed, most commonly involving the breast, thyroid, bone, and soft tissues.[146,295,301-310,364]

FUTURE INVESTIGATIONS

The ability to conduct clinical trials in HD, where differences in survival among treatment arms are projected to be small, is compromised by the large patient numbers necessary to detect such differences. Furthermore, if a reduction in treatment toxicity is the intended goal of a new regimen, many years of follow-up are often necessary to prove effectiveness. Devising new strategies for the treatment of children with HD is problematic, owing to the overall success of current treatment regimens. However, grouping patients into different risk categories should allow investigators to develop protocols aimed at reducing therapy-induced toxicity for low-risk patients and improving the treatment effectiveness for the high-risk cohort.

REFERENCES

1. Smith MA, Ries LA, Gurney JG, et al: Leukemia. In Ries LA, Smith MA, Gurney JG, et al, eds. *Cancer Incidence and Survival Among Children and Adolescents: United States SEER Program 1975-1995, SEER Program.* Bethesda, Md: National Cancer Institute, 1999.
2. Gurney JG, Davis S, Severson RK, et al: Trends in cancer incidence among children in the U.S. *Cancer.* 1996;78:532.
3. Miller RW: Persons with exceptionally high risk of leukemia. *Cancer Res.* 1967;27:2420.
4. Greaves MF: Aetiology of acute leukemia. *Lancet.* 1997;349:344.
5. Wiemels JL, Ford AM, Van Wering ER, et al: Protracted and variable latency of acute lymphoblastic leukemia after TEL-AML1 gene fusion in utero. *Blood.* 1999;94:1057.
6. Miller DR: Acute lymphoblastic leukemia. *Pediatr Clin North Am.* 1980;27:269.
7. Pui CH, Crist WM: Acute lymphoblastic leukemia. In Pui CH, ed. *Childhood Leukemia.* New York: Cambridge University Press, 1999.
8. Mastrangelo R, Poplack D, Bleyer WA, et al: Report and recommendations of the Rome workshop concerning poor prognosis acute lymphoblastic leukemia in children: Biologic bases for staging stratification and treatment. *Med Pediatr Oncol.* 1986;14.
9. Mahmoud HH, Rivera GK, Hancock ML, et al: Low leukocyte counts with blast cells in cerebrospinal fluid of children with newly diagnosed acute lymphoblastic leukemia. *N Engl J Med.* 1993;329:314.
10. Odom LF, Wilson H, Cullen J: Significance of blasts of low-cell-count cerebrospinal fluid specimens from children with acute lymphoblastic leukemia. *Cancer.* 1990;66:1748.
11. Tubergen DG, Cullen JW, Boyett JM, et al: Blasts in CSF with a normal cell count do not justify alteration of therapy for acute lymphoblastic leukemia in remission: A Children's Cancer Group study. *J Clin Oncol.* 1994;12:273.
12. Bennett JM, Catovsky D, Daniel MT, et al: Proposals for the classification of the acute leukemias. French-American-British Cooperative Group. *Br J Haematol.* 1976;33:451.

13. Bennett JM, Catovsky D, Daniel MT, et al: The morphological classification of acute lymphoblastic leukemia: Concordance among observers and clinical correlations. *Br J Haematol.* 1981;47:553.

14. Miller DR, Leikin S, Albo V, et al: Prognostic importance of morphology (FAB classification) in childhood acute lymphoblastic leukemia (ALL). *Br J Haematol.* 1981;48:199.

15. Pui C: Childhood leukemias. *N Engl J Med.* 1995;332:1618.

16. Shaw MT: The cytochemistry of acute leukemia: A diagnostic and prognostic evaluation. *Semin Oncol.* 1976;3.

17. Pui CH, Behm FG, Crist WM: Clinical and biologic relevance of immunologic marker studies in childhood acute lymphoblastic leukemia. *Blood.* 1993;82:343.

18. Campana D, Pui CH: Detection of minimal residual disease in acute leukemia: Methodologic advances and clinical significance. *Blood.* 1995;85:1416.

19. Pui CH, Crist WM, Look AT: Biology and clinical significance of cytogenetic abnormalities in childhood acute lymphoblastic leukemia. *Blood.* 1990;76:1449.

20. Shurtleff SA, Buijs A, Behm FG, et al: TEL/AML1 fusion resulting from a cryptic t(12;21) is the most common genetic lesion in pediatric ALL and defines a subgroup of patients with an excellent prognosis. *Leukemia.* 1995;9:1985.

21. Pui CH: Acute lymphoblastic leukemia. *Pediatr Clin North Am.* 1997;44:831.

22. Pinkel D: Curing children of leukemia. *Cancer.* 1987;59:1683.

23. Pui CH, Williams DL, Roberson PK, et al: Correlation of karyotype and immunophenotype in childhood acute lymphoblastic leukemia. *J Clin Oncol.* 1988;6:56.

24. Hammond D, Sather H, Nesbit M, et al: Analysis of prognostic factors in acute lymphoblastic leukemia. *Med Pediatr Oncol.* 1986;14:124.

25. Pui CH, Kane JR, Crist WM: Biology and treatment of infant leukemias. *Leukemia.* 1995;9:762.

26. Smith M, Arthur D, Camitta B, et al: Uniform approach to risk classification and treatment assignment for children with acute lymphoblastic leukemia. *J Clin Oncol.* 1996;14:18.

27. Chen CS, Sorenson PHB, Domer PH: Molecular rearrangements on chromosome 11q23 predominate in infant acute lymphoblastic leukemia and are associated with specific biologic variables and poor outcome. *Blood.* 1993;81:2386.

28. Reiter A, Schrappe M, Ludwig WD, et al: Favorable outcome of B-cell acute lymphoblastic leukemia in childhood: A report of three consecutive studies of the BFM group. *Blood.* 1992;80:2471.

29. Reiter A, Schrappe M, Ludwig WD, et al: Chemotherapy in 998 unselected childhood acute lymphoblastic leukemia patients. Results and conclusions of the multicenter trial ALL-BFM 86. *Blood.* 1994;84:3122.

30. Patte C: Non-Hodgkin's lymphoma. *Eur J Cancer.* 1998;34:359.

31. Hoelzer D, Ludwig WD, Thiel E, et al: Improved outcome in adult B-cell acute lymphoblastic leukemia. *Blood.* 1996;87:495.

32. Schwenn MR, Mahmoud H, Bowman WP, et al: Addition of VP-Ifosfamide; intensification did no improve event-free survival for CNS-negative patients with advanced stage small noncleaved cell lymphoma or B-cell ALL: A Pediatric Oncology Group Study. *Proc ASCD.* 2001;20:366. Abstract.

33. Schorin MA, Blattner S, Gelber RD, et al: Treatment of childhood acute lymphoblastic leukemia: Results of Dana-Farber Cancer Institute/Children's Hospital Acute Lymphoblastic Leukemia Consortium Protocol 85-01. *J Clin Oncol.* 1994;12:740.

34. Conter V, Schrappe M, Arico M, et al: Role of cranial radiotherapy for childhood T-cell acute lymphoblastic leukemia with high WBC count and good response to prednisone. Associazione Italiana Ematologia Oncologia Pediatrica and the Berlin-Frankfurt-Munster groups. *J Clin Oncol.* 1997;15:2786.

35. Asselin B, Shuster J, Amylon M: Improved event-free survival with high dose methotrexate in T-cell lymphoblastic leukemia and advanced lymphoblastic lymphoma: A Pediatric Oncology Group study. *Proc ASCO.* 2001;20:367. Abstract.

36. Rubnitz JE, Link MP, Shuster JJ: Frequency and prognostic significance of HRx rearrangements in infant acute lymphoblastic leukemia: A Pediatric Oncology Group study. *Blood.* 1994;84:570.

37. Meadows AT, Gordon J, Massari DJ: Declines in IQ scores and cognitive dysfunctions in children with acute lymphocytic leukemia treated with cranial irradiation. *Lancet.* 1981;2:1015.

38. Bleyer WA: Neurologic sequelae of methotrexate and ionizing radiation: A new classification. *Cancer Treat Rep.* 1981;65(suppl 1):89.

39. Moss HA, Nannis ED, Poplack DG: The effects of prophylactic treatments of the central nervous system on the intellectual functioning of children with acute lymphoblastic leukemia. *Am J Med.* 1981;71:47.

40. Nesbit ME, Sather HN, Robison LL, et al: Sanctuary therapy: A randomized trial of 724 children with previously untreated acute lymphoblastic leukemia. *Cancer Res.* 1982;42:674.

41. Nesbit ME, Sather HN, Robison LL: Presymptomatic central nervous system therapy in previously untreated childhood acute lymphoblastic leukemia: Comparison of 1800 rad and 2400 rad. *Lancet.* 1981;1:461.

42. Bleyer WA, Poplack DG: Prophylaxis and treatment of leukemia in the central nervous system and other sanctuaries. *Semin Oncol.* 1985;12:131.

43. Chessels JM, Bailey CC, Richards S: MRC UKALLX The UK protocol for childhood ALL: 1985-1990. *Leukemia.* 1992;6(suppl 2):157.

44. Tarbell N, Waber D, Cohen H: Hyperfractionated cranial irradiation in childhood acute lymphoblastic leukemia: rationale and preliminary results. *Proc ASCO.* 1991;10:239. Abstract.

45. Schrappe M, Reiter A, Henze G: Prevention of CNS recurrence in childhood ALL: Results with reduced radiotherapy combined with CNS-directed chemotherapy in four consecutive ALL-BFM trials. *Klin Padiatr.* 1998;210:192.

46. Littman P, Coccia P, Bleyer WA, et al: Central nervous system prophylaxis in children with low-risk acute lymphoblastic leukemia. *Int J Rad Oncol Biol Phys.* 1987;13:1443.

47. Sullivan MP, Chen T, Dyment PG: Equivalence of intrathecal chemotherapy and radiotherapy as central nervous system prophylaxis in children with acute lymphatic leukemia: A Pediatric Oncology Group study. *Blood.* 1982;60:948.

48. van Eys J, Berry D, Crist W: A comparison of two regimens for high risk acute lymphoblastic leukemia in childhood: A Pediatric Oncology Group study. *Cancer.* 1989;63:23.

49. Pullen J, Boyett J, Shuster J, et al: Extended triple intrathecal chemotherapy trial for prevention of CNS relapse in good-risk and poor-risk patients with B-progenitor acute lymphoblastic leukemia: A Pediatric Oncology Group study. *J Clin Oncol.* 1993;11:839.

50. Freeman AI, Weinberg V, Brecher ML: Comparison of intermediate-dose methotrexate with cranial irradiation for the post-induction treatment of acute lymphoblastic leukemia in children. *N Engl J Med.* 1983;308:477.

51. Freeman AI, Boyett JM, Glicksman AS, et al: Intermediate-dose methotrexate versus cranial irradiation in childhood acute lymphoblastic leukemia: A ten-year follow-up. *Med Pediatr Oncol.* 1997;28:98.

52. Veerman AJ, Hahlen K, Kamps WA, et al: High cure rate with a moderately intensive treatment regimen in non-high-risk childhood acute lymphoblastic leukemia. Results of protocol ALL VI from the Dutch Childhood Leukemia Study Group. *J Clin Oncol.* 1996;14:911.

53. Pinkel D, Woo S: Prevention and treatment of meningeal leukemia in children. *Blood.* 1994;84:355.

54. Steinherz PG: Radiotherapy versus intrathecal chemotherapy for CNS prophylaxis in childhood ALL. *Oncology (Huntingt).* 1989;3:47.

55. Nachman J, Sather HN, Cherlow JM, et al: Response of children with high-risk acute lymphoblastic leukemia treated with and without cranial irradiation: a report from the Children's Cancer Group. *J Clin Oncol.* 1998;16:920.

56. Pui CH, Mahmoud HH, Rivera GK, et al: Early intensification of intrathecal chemotherapy virtually eliminates central nervous system relapse in children with acute lymphoblastic leukemia. *Blood.* 1998;92:411.

57. Silverman LB, Dederck L, Gelber RD, et al: Results of Dana-Farber Cancer Institute Consortium Protocols for children with newly diagnosed acute lymphoblastic leukemia (1981-1995). *Leukemia.* 2000;14:2247.

58. Clarke M, Gaynon P, Hann I, et al: CNS-Directed Therapy for Childhood Acute Lymphoblastic Leukemia: Childhood ALL Collaborative Group Overview of 43 Randomized Trials. *J Clin Oncol.* 2003;21.

59. Castro JR, Sullivan MP: Cerebrospinal axis radiation therapy for meningeal leukemia with tumor dose levels in the range of 2,000 rads. *Radiology.* 1972;104:643.

60. Gribbin MA, Hardisty RM, Chessells JM: Long-term control of central nervous system leukemia. *Arch Dis Child.* 1977;52:673.

61. Wells RJ, Weetman RM, Baehner RL: The impact of isolated central nervous system relapse following initial complete remission in childhood acute lymphocytic leukemia. *J Pediatr.* 1980;97:429.

62. Kun LE, Camitta BM, Mulhern RK, et al: Treatment of meningeal relapse in childhood acute lymphoblastic leukemia. I. Results of craniospinal irradiation. *J Clin Oncol.* 1984;2:359.

63. Land VJ, Thomas PR, Boyett JM, et al: Comparison of maintenance treatment regimens for first central nervous system relapse in children with acute lymphocytic leukemia. A Pediatric Oncology Group study. *Cancer.* 1985;56:81.

64. Poplack DG, Kun LE, Magrath IT, et al: Leukemias and lymphomas of childhood. In Devita VT Jr, Hellman S, Rosenberg SA, eds. *Cancer: Principles and Practice of Oncology.* Philadelphia: JB Lippincott; 1993.

65. Bleyer WA, Poplack DG: Intraventricular versus intralumbar methotrexate for central-nervous-system leukemia: Prolonged remission with the Ommaya reservoir. *Med Pediatr Oncol.* 1979; 6:207.

66. Balis FM, Savitch JL, Bleyer WA, et al: Remission induction of meningeal leukemia with high-dose intravenous methotrexate. *J Clin Oncol.* 1985;3:485.

67. Berg SL, Balis FM, Zimm S, et al: Phase I/II trial and pharmacokinetics of intrathecal diaziquone in refractory meningeal malignancies. *J Clin Oncol.* 1992;10:143.

68. Adamson PC, Balis FM, Arndt CA, et al: Intrathecal 6-mercaptopurine: Preclinical pharmacology, phase I/II trial, and pharmacokinetic study. *Cancer Res.* 1991;51:6079.

69. Gelber RD, Sallan SE, Cohen HJ, et al: Central nervous system treatment in childhood acute lymphoblastic leukemia. Long-term follow-up of patients diagnosed between 1973 and 1985. *Cancer.* 1993;72:261.

70. Kim TH, Ramsay NK, Steeves RA, Nesbit ME: Intermittent central nervous system irradiation and intrathecal chemotherapy for central nervous system leukemia in children. *Int J Radiat Biol Oncol Phys.* 1987;13:1451.

71. Cherlow JM, Steinherz P, Gaynon P, et al: Cranio-spinal radiation for CNS leukemia at presentation: How high does the spinal dose need to be? *Proc ASCO.* 1991;10:239. Abstract.

72. Patte C, Leverger G, Perel Y, et al: Results of LMB 86 and 89 protocols of the French Pediatric Oncology Society (S.F.O.P.) for children with B-cell lymphoma and leukemia with CNS involvement. *Med Pediatr Oncol* 1993;21:535. Abstract.

73. Willoughby ML: Treatment of overt meningeal leukemia in children: Results of second MRC meningeal leukemia trial. *Br Med J.* 1976;1:864.

74. Mandell LR, Steinherz P, Fuks Z: Delayed central nervous system (CNS) radiation in childhood CNS acute lymphoblastic leukemia. *Cancer.* 1990;66:447.

75. Winick NJ, Smith SD, Shuster J, et al: Treatment of CNS relapse in children with acute lymphoblastic leukemia: A Pediatric Oncology Group study. *J Clin Oncol.* 1993;11:271.

76. Gillin MT, Kline RW, Kun LE: Cranial dose distribution. *Int J Radiat Oncol Biol Phys.* 1979;5:1903.

77. Tatcher M, Glicksman AS: Field matching considerations in craniospinal irradiation. *Int J Radiat Oncol Biol Phys.* 1989;17:865.

78. Holupka EJ, Humm JL, Tarbell NJ, Svensson GK: Effect of set-up error on the dose across the junction of matching cranial-spinal fields in the treatment of medulloblastoma. *Int J Radiat Biol Oncol Phys.* 1993;27:345.

79. Siddon RL: Solution to treatment planning problems using coordinate transformations. *Med Phys.* 1982;8:766.

80. Maor MH, Fields RS, Hogstrom KR, et al: Improving the therapeutic ratio of craniospinal irradiation in medulloblastoma. *Int J Radiat Oncol Biol Phys.* 1985;11:687.

81. Miller LP, Miller DR: Acute lymphoblastic leukemia in children: Current status, controversies, and future perspective. *Crit Rev Oncol Hematol.* 1986;1:129.

82. Nesbit ME, Robinson LL, Ortega JA, et al: Testicular relapse in childhood acute lymphoblastic leukemia: Association with pre-treatment patient characteristics and treatment. A report for Children's Cancer Study Group. *Cancer.* 1980;45:2009.

83. Wong KY, Ballard ET, Strayer FH, et al: Clinical and occult testicular leukemia in long-term survivors of acute lymphoblastic leukemia. *J Pediatr.* 1980;96:569.

84. Finkelstein JZ, Dyment PG, Hammond GD: Leukemic infiltration of the testes during bone marrow remission. *Pediatrics.* 1969; 43:1042.

85. Nies BA, Bodey GP, Thomas LB, et al: The persistence of extramedullary leukemia infiltrates during bone marrow remission of acute leukemia. *Blood.* 1965;26:133.

86. Givlier RL: Testicular involvement in leukemia and lymphoma. *Cancer.* 1969;23:1290.

87. Medical Research Council: Testicular disease in acute lymphoblastic leukemia in childhood. *Br Med J.* 1978;1:334.

88. Ortega JJ, Javier G, Toran N: Testicular infiltrates in children with acute lymphoblastic leukaemia: A prospective study. *Med Pediatr Oncol.* 1984;12:396.

89. Bowman WP, Aur RJA, Hustu HO, et al: Isolated testicular relapse in acute lymphocytic leukemia of childhood: Categories and influence on survival. *J Clin Oncol.* 1984;2.

90. Pui CH, Dahl GV, Bowman WP, et al: Elective testicular biopsy during chemotherapy for childhood leukemia is of no clinical value. *Lancet.* 1985;2:410.

91. Byrd R: Testicular leukemia: Incidence and management results. *Med Pediatr Oncol.* 1981;9:493.

92. Hustu HO, Aur RJ: Extramedullary leukemia. *Clin Haematol.* 1978;7:313.

93. Atkinson K, Thomas PRM, Peckham MJ: Radiosensitivity of the acute leukaemic infiltrate. *Eur J Cancer.* 1976;12:535.

94. Sullivan MP, Perez CA, Herson J: Radiotherapy (2500 rad) for testicular leukemia: Local control and subsequent clinical events: A Southwest Oncology Group Study. *Cancer.* 1980; 46:508.

95. Frankel LS, Provisor A, Kletzel M, et al: Successful therapy for overt testicular relapse in childhood acute lymphocytic leukemia. *Proc ASCO.* 1984;3. Abstract.

96. Culbert S, Doering E, Jelden G, et al: Testicular leukemia relapse: A treatable entity *Proc ASCO.* 1983;2:79. Abstract.

97. Brauner R, Czernichow P, Cramer P: Leydig-cell function in children after direct testicular irradiation for acute lymphoblastic leukemia. *N Engl J Med.* 1983;309:25.

98. Leiper AD, Grant DB, Chessels JM: The effect of testicular irradiation on Leydig cell function in prepubertal boys with acute lymphoblastic leukemia. *Arch Dis Child.* 1983;58:906.

99. Conter V, Arico M, Valsecchi MG, et al: Extended intrathecal methotrexate may replace cranial irradiation for prevention of CNS relapse in children with intermediate-risk acute lymphoblastic leukemia treated with Berlin-Frankfurt-Munster-based intensive chemotherapy. The Associazione Italiana ed Ematologia ed Oncologia Pediatrica. *J Clin Oncol.* 1995;13:2497.

100. Tubergen DG, Gilchrist GS, O'Brien RT, et al: Improved outcome with delayed intensification for children with acute lymphoblastic leukemia and intermediate presenting features: A Children's Cancer Group phase III trial. *J Clin Oncol.* 1993;11:527.

101. Tubergen DG, Gilchrist GS, O'Brien RT, et al: Prevention of CNS disease in intermediate-risk acute lymphoblastic leukemia: Comparison of cranial radiation and intrathecal methotrexate and the importance of systemic therapy: A Children's Cancer Group report. *J Clin Oncol.* 1993;11:520.

102. Nachman JB, Sather HN, Sensel MG, et al: Augmented postinduction therapy for children with high-risk acute lymphoblastic leukemia and a slow response to initial therapy. *N Engl J Med.* 1998;338:1663.

103. Schaison G, Sommelet D, Bancillon A, et al: Treatment of acute lymphoblastic leukemia French protocol Fralle 83-87. *Leukemia.* 1992;6(suppl 2):148.

104. Chessells JM, Bailey C, Richards SM: Intensification of treatment and survival in all children with lymphoblastic leukemia: Results of UK Medical Research Council trial UKALL X. Medical Research Council Working Party on Childhood Leukemia. *Lancet.* 1995;345:143.

105. Trueworthy R, Shuster J, Look T, et al: Ploidy of lymphoblasts is the strongest predictor of treatment outcome in B-progenitor cell acute lymphoblastic leukemia of childhood: A Pediatric Oncology Group study. *J Clin Oncol.* 1992;10:606.

106. Land VJ, Shuster JJ, Crist WM, et al: Comparison of two schedules of intermediate-dose methotrexate and cytarabine consolidation therapy for childhood B-precursor cell acute lymphoblastic leukemia: A Pediatric Oncology Group study. *J Clin Oncol.* 1994;12:1939.

107. Rivera GK, Raimondi SC, Hancock ML, et al: Improved outcome in childhood acute lymphoblastic leukemia with reinforced early treatment and rotational combination chemotherapy. *Lancet.* 1991;337:61.

108. Evans WE, Relling MV, Rodman JH, et al: Conventional compared with individualized chemotherapy for childhood acute lymphoblastic leukemia. *N Engl J Med.* 1998;338:499.

109. Pui CH, Crist W: Biology and treatment of acute lymphoblastic leukemia. *J Pediatr.* 1994;124:491.

110. Ruffner KI, Matthews DC: Current uses of monoclonal antibodies in the treatment of acute leukemia. *Semin Oncol.* 2000;27:531.

111. Choi S, Simone JV: Acute nonlymphocytic leukemia in 171 children. *Med Pediatr Oncol.* 1976;2:119.

112. Homans AC, Verissimo AM, Vlacha V: Transient abnormal myelopoiesis of infancy associated with trisomy 21. *Am J Pediatr Hematol Oncol.* 1993;15:392.

113. Bennet JM, Catovsky D, Daniel MT, et al: Proposed revised criteria for the classification of acute myeloid leukemia. A report of the French-American-British Cooperative Group. *Ann Intern Med.* 1985;103:620.

114. Lampkin BC, Woods W, Strauss R: Current status of the biology and treatment of acute non-lymphocytic leukemia in children (Report from the ANLL strategy group of Children's Cancer Study Group). *Blood.* 1983;61:215.

115. Pui CH, Kalwinsky D, Schell M, et al: Acute nonlymphoblastic leukemia in infants: Clinical presentation and outcome. *J Clin Oncol.* 1988;6:1008.

116. Windebank KP, Tefferi A, Smithson W, et al: Acute megakaryocytic leukemia (M7) in children. *Mayo Clin Proc.* 1989;64:1339.

117. Bloomfield CTD, de la Chapelle A: Chromosome abnormalities in acute nonlymphocytic leukemia: Clinical and biologic significance. *Semin Oncol.* 1987;14:372.

118. Kakizuka A, Miller W, Umesuno K: Chromosome translocation t(15;17) in human acute promyelocytic leukemia fuses RAR alpha gene with a novel putative transcription factor PML. *Cell.* 1991; 66:663.

119. Carroll A, Civin C, Schneider N: The t(1;22) is nonrandom and restricted to infants with acute megakaryoblastic leukemia: A Pediatric Oncology Group study. *Blood.* 1991;78:748.

120. Woods WG, Nesbit ME, Buckley J, et al: Correlation of chromosome abnormalities with patient characteristics, histologic subtype and induction success in children with acute NLL. *J Clin Oncol.* 1985;3:3.

121. Sorenson P, Chen CS, Smith FO, et al: Molecular rearrangements of the MLL gene are present in most cases of infant acute myeloid leukemia and are strongly correlated with monocytic or myelomonocytic phenotypes. *J Clin Invest.* 1994;93:429.

122. Grier HE, Gelber RD, Camitta BM, et al: Prognostic factors in childhood acute myelogenous leukemia. *J Clin Oncol.* 1987;5:1026.

123. Champlin R, Gale RP: Acute myelogenous leukemia: Recent advances in therapy. Prolonged survival in acute myelogenous leukemia without maintenance chemotherapy. *Blood.* 1987; 69:1551.

124. Abromowitch M, Ochs J, Pui CH, et al: Efficacy of high-dose methotrexate in childhood acute lymphocytic leukemia: analysis by contemporary risk classifications. *Blood.* 1988;71:866.

125. Weinstein HJ, Mayer RJ, Rosenthal DS: Chemotherapy for acute myelogenous leukemia in children and adults. VAPA update. *Blood.* 1983;62:315.

126. Hurwitz CA, Schell MJ, Pui CH, et al: Adverse prognostic features in 251 children treated for acute myeloid leukemia. *Med Pediatr Oncol.* 1993;21:1.

127. Odom LF, Lampkin BC, Tannous R, et al: Acute monoblastic leukemia: A unique subtype—A review from the Children's Cancer Study Group. *Leuk Res.* 1990;14:1.

128. Kantarjian HM, Keating MJ, Walters RS, et al: Role of maintenance chemotherapy in acute promyelocytic leukemia. *Cancer.* 1987;59:1258.

129. Santana VM, Hurwitz CA, Blakley RL, et al: Complete hematologic remissions induced by 2-chlorodeoxyadenosine in children with newly diagnosed acute myeloid leukemia. *Blood.* 1994; 84:1237.

130. Santana VM, Mirro J Jr, Kearns C, et al: 2-Chlorodeoxyadenosine produces a high rate of complete hematologic remission in relapsed acute myeloid leukemia. *J Clin Oncol.* 1992;10:364.

131. Huang ME, Ye YC, Chen SR, et al: Use of all-trans retinoic acid in the treatment of acute promyelocytic leukemia. *Hamatologie und Bluttransfusion.* 1989;32:88.

132. Castaigne S, Chomienne C, Daniel MT, et al: All-trans retinoic acid as a differentiation therapy for acute promyelocytic leukemia. I. Clinical results. *Blood.* 1990;76:1704.

133. Amadori S, Testi AM, Arico M, et al: Prospective comparative study of bone marrow transplantation and postremission chemotherapy for childhood acute myelogenous leukemia. The Associazione Italiana Ematologia ed Oncologia Pediatrica Cooperative Group. *J Clin Oncol.* 1993;11:1046.

134. Reiffers J, Gaspard MH, Maraninchi D, et al: Comparison of allogeneic or autologous bone marrow transplantation and chemotherapy in patients with acute myeloid leukemia in first remission: a prospective controlled trial. *Br J Haematol.* 1989; 72:57.

135. Malik S, DeLaat C, Harris R: Allogeneic bone marrow transplantation versus autologous BMT vs chemotherapy in childhood acute myeloid leukemia. *Proc ASCO.* 1993;12:323. Abstract.

136. Nesbit M, Burkley L, Lampkin B, et al: Comparison of allogeneic bone marrow transplantation with maintenance chemotherapy in previously untreated childhood acute non-lymphocytic leukemia. *Proc ASCO.* 1987;6:163. Abstract.

137. Fenaux P, Chomienne C, Degos L: Acute pro-leukemia: Biology and treatment. *Semin Oncol.* 1997;24:92.

138. Tallman MS, Andersen JW, Schiffer CA: All-trans-retinoic acid in acute promyelocytic leukemia. *N Engl J Med.* 1997;337:1021.

139. Fenaux P, Chastang G, Chevret S: A randomized comparison of all-trans-retinoic acid (ATRA) followed by chemotherapy and ATRA plus chemotherapy and the role of maintenance therapy in newly diagnosed acute promyelocytic leukemia. The European APL Group. *Blood.* 1999;94:1192.

140. Calleja EM, Wamell RP: Differentiating agents in pediatric malignancies: All-trans-retinoic acid and arsenic in APML. *Curr Oncol Rep.* 2000;2:519.

141. Zipursky A, Thorner P, DeHarven E, et al: Myelodysplasia and acute megakaryocytic leukemia in Down's syndrome. *Leuk Res.* 1994;18:163.

142. Ravindranath Y, Abella E, Krischer JP, et al: Acute myeloid leukemia (AML) in Down's syndrome is highly responsive to chemotherapy: Experience on POG AML Study 8498. *Blood.* 1992;80:2210.

143. Lange BJ, Kobrinsky N, Barnard DR, et al: Distinctive demography, biology and outcome of acute myeloid leukemia and myelodysplastic syndrome in children with Down syndrome: CCSG studies 2861 and 2891. *Blood.* 1998;91:608.

144. Smith MA, Rubinstein L, Andersen JR: Secondary leukemia or myelodysplastic syndrome after treatment with epipodophyllotoxins. *J Clin Oncol.* 1999;17:569.

145. Felix CA: Secondary leukemias induced by topoisomerase-targeted drugs. *Biochim Biophys Acta.* 1998;1400:233.

146. Tucker MA, Meadows AT, Boice JD: Leukemia after therapy with alkylating agents for childhood cancer. *J Natl Cancer Inst.* 1987; 78:459.

147. Neiman RS, Barcos M, Berard C: Granulocytic sarcoma: A clinicopathologic study of 61 biopsied cases. *Cancer.* 1981; 48:1426.

148. Appelbaum FR: Antibody-targeted therapy for myeloid leukemia. *Semin Hematol.* 1999;36:2.

149. Sievers EL, Appelbaum FR, Spieberger RT, et al: Selective ablation of acute myeloid leukemia using antibody-targeted chemotherapy: A phase I study of an anti-CD33 calicheamicin immunoconjugate. *Blood.* 1999;93:3678.

150. Matthews DC, Appelbaum FR, Eary JF, et al: Phase I study of (131) I-anti-CD45-antibody plus cyclophosphamide and total body irradiation for advanced acute leukemia and myelodysplastic syndrome. *Blood.* 1999;94:1237.

151. Zujewski J, Horak ID, Bol CJ, et al: Phase I and pk study of farnesyl protein transferase inhibitor R115777 in advanced cancer. *J Clin Oncol.* 2000;18:927.

152. Smith KL, Johnson W: Classification of chronic myelocytic leukemia in children. *Cancer.* 1974;34:670.

153. Altman AJ: Chronic leukemias of childhood. *Pediatr Clin North Am.* 1988;35:765.

154. Druker BJ, Talpaz M, Resta D: Clinical efficacy and safety of an Abl specific tyrosine kinase inhibitor as targeted therapy for CML. *Blood*. 1999;94:368A.

155. Druker BJ, Kantarjian H, Sawyers CL: Activity of an Abl-specific tyrosine kinase inhibitor in patients with Bcr-Abl positive acute leukemias, including CML in blast crisis. *Blood*. 1999; 94:697A.

156. Altman AJ, Palmer G, Baehner RL: Juvenile "chronic granulocytic" leukemia: A panmyelopathy with prominent monocytic involvement and circulating monocyte colony-forming cells. *Blood*. 1974;43:341.

157. Arico M, Biondi A, Pui CH: Juvenile myelomonocytic leukemia. *Blood*. 1997;90:479.

158. Niemeyer CM, Arico M, Basso G, et al: Chronic myelomonocytic leukemia in childhood: A retrospective analysis of 110 cases. European Working Group on Myelodysplastic Syndromes in Childhood (EWOG-MDS). *Blood*. 1997;89:3534.

159. Mays JA, Neerhout RC, Bagby GC, et al: Juvenile chronic granulocytic leukemia: emphasis on cutaneous manifestations and underlying neurofibromatosis. *Am J Dis Child*. 1980;134:654.

160. Percy CL, Smith MA, Linet M, et al: Lymphomas and reticuloendothelial neoplasms. In Ries LAG, Smith MA, Gurney JG, et al, eds. *Cancer Incidence and Survival Among Children and Adolescents: United States SEER Program 1975-1995, National Cancer Institute, SEER Program*. Bethesda, Md: 1999.

161. Filipovich AH, Mathor A, Kamat D, et al: Lymphoproliferative disorders and other tumors complicating immunodeficiencies. *Immunodeficiency*. 1994;5:91.

162. Murphy SB, Jenson HB, McClain KL, et al: AIDS related tumors. *Med Pediatr Oncol*. 1997;29:381. Abstract.

163. Mueller BU: Lymphoproliferative disorders and malignancies related to immunodeficiencies. In Pizzo PA, Poplack DG, eds. *Principles and Practice of Pediatric Oncology*. Philadelphia: Lippincott Williams & Wilkins; 2002.

164. Swinnen LJ: Overview of post-transplant B-cell lymphoproliferative disorders. *Semin Oncol*. 1999;26:21.

165. Gross TG: Low-dose chemotherapy for children with posttransplant lymphoproliferative disease. *Recent Results Cancer Res*. 2002;159:96.

166. National Cancer Institute sponsored study of classifications of non-Hodgkin's lymphoma. Summary and description of a working formulation for clinical usage. The Non-Hodgkin's Lymphoma Pathologic Classification Project. *Cancer*. 1982; 49:2112.

167. Murphy SB, Frizzera G, Evans AF: A study of childhood non-Hodgkin's lymphoma. *Cancer*. 1975;36:3232.

168. Shad A, Magrath IT: Non-Hodgkin's lymphoma. *Pediatr Clin North Am*. 1997;44:863.

169. Dalla-Favera R, Bnegni M, Erikson J, et al: Human c-myc gene is located on the region of chromosome 8 that is translocated in Burkitt lymphoma cells. *Proc Natl Acad Sci*. 1982;79:7824.

170. Kadin ME: Ki-1-positive anaplastic large-cell lymphoma: A clinicopathologic entity? *J Clin Oncol*. 1991;9:533.

171. Kurtzberg J, Graham M: Non-Hodgkin's lymphoma: Biologic classification and implications of therapy. *Pediatr Clin North Am*. 1991;38:443.

172. Wollner N, Burchenal HJ, Leiberman P, et al: Non-Hodgkin's lymphoma in children: A comparative study of two modalities of therapy. *Cancer*. 1976;37:123.

173. Hvizdala EV, Berard C, Callihan T, et al: Non-lymphoblastic lymphoma in children: Histology and stage-related response to therapy. A Pediatric Oncology Group study. *J Clin Oncol*. 1991;9:1889.

174. Murphy SB: Prognostic features and obstacles to cure of childhood non-Hodgkin's lymphoma. *Semin Oncol*. 1977;4:265.

175. Anderson JR, Wilson JF, Jenkin RDT, et al: Childhood non-Hodgkin's lymphoma: The results of a randomized trial comparing a 4-drug regimen (COMP) with a 10-drug regimen (LSA2-L2). *N Engl J Med*. 1983;308:559.

176. Sandlund JT, Downing JR, Crist WM: Non-Hodgkin's lymphoma in childhood. *N Engl J Med*. 1996;331:1238.

177. Murphy SB, Fairclough DL, Hutchison RE, et al: Non-Hodgkin's lymphomas of childhood: An analysis of the histology, staging, and response to treatment of 338 cases at a single institution. *J Clin Oncol*. 1989;7:186.

178. Magrath IT: Malignant non-Hodgkin's lymphomas in children. In Pizzo PA, Poplack DG, eds. *Principles and Practice of Pediatric Oncology*. Philadelphia: Lippincott Williams & Wilkins; 2002.

179. Kostakoglu L, Leonard JP, Kuji I, et al: Comparison of fluorine-18 fluorodeoxyglucose positron emission tomography and Ga-67 scintigraphy in evaluation of lymphoma. *Cancer*. 2002;94:879.

180. Naumann R, Vaic A, Beuthien-Baumann B, et al: Prognostic value of positron emission tomography in the evaluation of post-treatment residual mass in patients with Hodgkin's disease and non-Hodgkin's lymphoma. *Br J Haematology*. 2001;115:793.

181. Murphy SB: Classification, staging and end results of treatment of childhood non-Hodgkin's lymphomas: Dissimilarities from lymphoma in adults. *Semin Oncol*. 1980;7:332.

182. Link MP, Shuster JJ, Donaldson SS, et al: Treatment of children and young adults with early-stage non-Hodgkin's lymphoma. *N Engl J Med*. 1997;337:1259.

183. Hutchison RE, Berard CW, Shuster JJ, et al: B-cell lineage confers a favorable outcome among children and adolescents with large-cell lymphoma: A Pediatric Oncology Group study. *J Clin Oncol*. 1995;13:2023.

184. Murphy SB, Hustu HO: A randomized trial of combined modality therapy of childhood non-Hodgkin's lymphoma. *Cancer*. 1980; 45:630.

185. Pinkel D, Johnson W, Aur RJ: Non-Hodgkin's lymphoma in children. *Br J Cancer*. 1975;31(suppl 2):298.

186. Sagerman RH, Wolff JA, Sitarz A, et al: Radiation therapy for lymphoma in children. *Radiology*. 1966;86:1096.

187. Whalen TV, La Quaglia MP: The lymphomas: An update for surgeons. *Semin Pediatr Surg*. 1997;6:50.

188. Ziegler JL: Treatment results of 54 American patients with Burkitt's lymphoma are similar to the African experience. *N Engl J Med*. 1977;297:75.

189. Anderson JR, Jenkin RDT, Wilson JF, et al: Long-term follow-up of patients treated with COMP or LSA2-L2 therapy for childhood non-Hodgkin's lymphoma: A report of CCG-551 from the Children's Cancer Group. *J Clin Oncol*. 1993;11:1024.

190. Murphy SB, Bowman WP, Abromowitch M, et al: Results of treatment of advanced-stage Burkitt's lymphoma and B cell (SIg+) acute lymphoblastic leukemia with high-dose fractionated cyclophosphamide and coordinated high-dose methotrexate and cytarabine. *J Clin Oncol*. 1986;4:1732.

191. Bowman WP, Shuster JJ, Cook B, et al: Improved survival for children with B-cell acute lymphoblastic leukemia and stage IV small noncleaved-cell lymphoma: a pediatric oncology group study. *J Clin Oncol*. 1996;14:1252.

192. Patte C, Michon J, Behrendt H, et al: Results of the LMB 89 protocol for childhood B-cell lymphoma and leukemia (ALL). SIOP XXIX. *Med Pediatr Oncol*. 1997;29:358.

193. Chilcote RR, Krailo M, Kjeldsberg C, et al: Daunomycin plus COMP vs COMP therapy in childhood non-lymphoblastic lymphoma. *Proc Am Soc Clin Oncol*. 1991;10:289. Abstract.

194. Magrath IT, Janus C, Edwards BK, et al: An effective therapy for both undifferentiated (including Burkitt's) lymphomas and lymphoblastic lymphomas in children and young adults. *Blood*. 1984;63:1102.

195. Schwenn MR, Blattner SR, Lynch E, et al: HiC-COM: A 2-month intensive chemotherapy regimen for children with stage III and IV Burkitt's lymphoma and B-cell acute lymphoblastic leukemia. *J Clin Oncol*. 1991;9:133.

196. Schrappe M, Tiemann M, Ludwig WD, et al: Risk-adapted therapy for lymphoblastic T-cell lymphomas: Results from trials NHL-BFM 86 and 90. SIOP XXIX. *Med Pediatr Oncol*. 1997; 29:356.

197. Dahl GV, Rivera G, Pui CH, et al: A novel treatment of childhood lymphoblastic non-Hodgkin's lymphoma: Early and intermittent use of teniposide plus cytarabine. *Blood*. 1985;66.

198. Weinstein HJ, Cassady JR, Levey R: Long-term results of the APO protocol (vincristine, doxorubicin [Adriamycin], and prednisone) for the treatment of mediastinal lymphoblastic lymphoma. *J Clin Oncol*. 1983;1:537.

199. Hvizdala EV, Berard C, Callihan T, et al: Lymphoblastic lymphoma in children: A randomized trial comparing LSA2-L2 with the ACOP+ therapeutic regimen: A Pediatric Oncology Group study. *J Clin Oncol*. 1988;6:26.

200. Weinstein HJ, Lack EE, Cassady JR: APO therapy for malignant lymphoma of large cell "histiocytic" type of childhood: Analysis of treatment results for 29 patients. *Blood.* 1984;64:422.

201. Sandlund JT, Santana V, Abromowitch M, et al: Large cell non-Hodgkin lymphoma of childhood: Clinical characteristics and outcome. *Leukemia.* 1994;8:30.

202. Santana VH, Abromowitch M, Sandlund JT, et al: MACOP-B treatment in children and adolescents with advanced diffuse large-cell non-Hodgkin's lymphoma. *Leukemia.* 1993;7:187.

203. Sandlund JT, Pui CH, Santana VM, et al: Clinical features and treatment outcome for children with CD30+ large-cell non-Hodgkin's lymphoma. *J Clin Oncol.* 1994;12:895.

204. Reiter A, Schrappe M, Tiemann M, et al: Successful treatment strategy for Ki-1 anaplastic large cell lymphomas of childhood: A prospective analysis of 62 patients enrolled in three consecutive Berlin-Frankfurt-Münster group studies. *J Clin Oncol.* 1994;12:899.

205. Murphy SB: Pediatric lymphomas: Recent advances and commentary on Ki-1 positive anaplastic large cell lymphomas of childhood. *Ann Oncol.* 1994;5(suppl 1):531.

206. Brugieres L, LeDeley MC, Pacquement H, et al: Anaplastic large cell lymphoma in children: analysis of 63 patients enrolled in two consecutive studies of the SFOP. *Med Pediatr Oncol.* 1997;29:237.

207. Link MP, Donaldson SS, Berard CW, et al: Results of treatment of childhood localized non-Hodgkin's lymphoma with combination chemotherapy with or without radiotherapy. *N Engl J Med.* 1990;322:1169.

208. Patte C, Kalifa C, Flamant F, et al: Results of the LMB81 protocol a modified LSA2L2 protocol with high dose methotrexate in 84 children with non–B-cell (lymphoblastic) lymphoma. *Med Pediatr Oncol.* 1992;20:105.

209. Ingram LC, Fairclough DL, Furman WL, et al: Cranial nerve palsy in childhood acute lymphoblastic leukemia and non-Hodgkin's lymphoma. *Cancer.* 1991;67:2262.

210. Glatstein E, Kim H, Donaldson S: Non-Hodgkin's lymphomas: VI. Results of treatment in childhood. *Cancer.* 1974;34:204.

211. Jenkin RDT, Sonley MJ, Stephens CA, et al: Primary gastrointestinal tract lymphoma in childhood. *Radiology.* 1969;92:763.

212. Jenkin RD, Anderson JR, Chilcote RR, et al: The treatment of localized non-Hodgkin's lymphoma in children: A report from the Children's Cancer Study Group. *J Clin Oncol.* 1984;2:88.

213. Wollner N, Mandell L, Filippa D, et al: Primary nasal-paranasal oropharyngeal lymphoma in the pediatric age group. *Cancer.* 1990;65:1438.

214. Meadows AT, Sposto R, Jenkin RDT, et al: Similar efficacy of 6 and 18 months of therapy with four drugs (COMP) for localized non-Hodgkin's lymphoma of children: A report from the Children's Cancer Study Group. *J Clin Oncol.* 1989;7:92.

215. Murphy SB, Hustu HO, Rivera G, et al: End results of treating children with localized non-Hodgkin's lymphomas with a combined modality approach of lessened intensity. *J Clin Oncol.* 1983;1:326.

216. Jereb B, Wollner N, Kosloff C, et al: The role of local radiation in the treatment of non-Hodgkin's lymphoma in children. *Med Pediatr Oncol* 1981;9:157.

217. Patte C, Philip T, Rodary C, et al: Improved survival rate in children with stage III and IV B cell non-Hodgkin's lymphoma and leukemia using multi-agent chemotherapy: Results of a study of 114 children from the French Pediatric Oncology Society. *J Clin Oncol.* 1986;4:1219.

218. Dosoretz DE, Murphy GF, Raymond AK, et al: Radiation therapy for primary lymphoma of bone. *Cancer.* 1983;51:44.

219. Boston MC, Dahlin DC, Ivins JC, et al: Malignant lymphoma (so-called reticulum cell sarcoma) of bone. *Cancer.* 1974;34:1131.

220. Loeffler JS, Tarbell NJ, Kozakewich H, et al: Primary lymphoma of bone in children: Analysis of treatment results with Adriamycin, prednisone, Oncovin (APO) and local radiation therapy. *J Clin Oncol.* 1986;4:496.

221. Suryanarayan K, Shuster JJ, Donaldson SS, et al: Treatment of localized primary non-Hodgkin's lymphoma of bone in children: A Pediatric Oncology Group study. *J Clin Oncol.* 1999;17:456.

222. Lones MA, Perkins SL, Sposto R, et al: Non-Hodgkin's lymphoma arising in bone in children and adolescents is associated with an excellent outcome: A Children's Cancer Group report. *J Clin Oncol.* 2002;20:2293.

223. Mandell LR, Wollner N, Fuks Z: Is cranial radiation necessary for CNS prophylaxis in pediatric NHL? *Int J Radiat Oncol Biol Phys.* 1987;13:359.

224. Murphy SB, Bleyer WA: Cranial irradiation is not necessary for central nervous system prophylaxis in pediatric non-Hodgkin's lymphoma. *Int J Radiat Oncol Biol.* 1987;13:467.

225. Reiter A, Schrappe M, Ludwig WD, et al: Intensive ALL-type therapy without local radiotherapy provides a 90% event-free survival for children with T-cell lymphoblastic lymphoma: A BFM group report. *Blood.* 2000;95:416.

226. Eden OB, Hann I, Imeson J, et al: Treatment of advanced stage T cell lymphoblastic lymphoma: Results of the United Kingdom Children's Cancer Study Group (UKCCSG) protocol 8503. *Br J Haematol.* 1992;310.

227. Patte C, Auperin A, Michon J, et al: The Societe Francais d'Oncologie Pediatrique LMB89 protocol: Highly effective multi-agent chemotherapy tailored to the tumor burden and initial reponse in 561 unselected children with B cell lymphomas and L3 leukemia. *Blood.* 2001;97:3370.

228. Reaman G, Zeltzer P, Bleyer WA, et al: Acute lymphoblastic leukemia in infants less than one year of age: A cumulative experience of the Children's Cancer Study Group. *J Clin Oncol.* 1985;3:1513.

229. Henze G, Fengler R, Hartman R, et al: Six-year experience with a comprehensive approach to the treatment of recurrent childhood acute lymphoblastic leukemia (ALL-REZ BFM 85). A relapse study of the BFM Group. *Blood.* 1991;78:1166.

230. Ch'ien LT, Aur RJA, Verzosa MS, et al: Progression of methotrexate-induced leukoencephalopathy in children with leukemia. *Med Pediatr Oncol.* 1981;9:133.

231. Dalle JH, Mechinaud F, Michon J, et al: Testicular disease in childhood B-cell non-Hodgkin's lymphoma: The French Society of Pediatric Oncology experience. *J Clin Oncol.* 2001;19:2397.

232. Weitzman S, Suryanarayan K, Weinstein HJ: Pediatric non-Hodgkin's lymphoma: Clinical and biologic prognostic factors and risk allocation. *Curr Oncol Rpts.* 2002;4:107.

233. Trainer KJ, Brisco MJ, Wan JH: Gene rearrangements in B- and T-lymphoproliferative disease detected by the polymerase chain reaction. *Blood.* 1991;78.

234. Czuczman MS, Grillo-Lopez AJ, White CA, et al: Treatment of patients with low-grade B-cell lymphoma with the combination of chimeric anti-CD20 monoclonal antibody and CHOP chemotherapy. *J Clin Oncol.* 1999;17:268.

235. Milpied N, Vasseur B, Parquet N, et al: Humanized anti-CD20 monoclonal antibody (Rituximab) in post transplant B-lymphoproliferative disorder: a retrospective analysis on 32 patients. *Ann Oncol.* 2000;11(suppl 1):113.

236. Maloney DG, Press OW: Newer treatments for non-Hodgkin's lymphoma: Monoclonal antibodies. *Oncology.* 1998;12:63.

237. Uckun FM, Reaman GH: Immunotoxins for treatment of leukemia and lymphoma. *Leuk Lymphoma.* 1995;18.

238. Ansell SM, Witzig TE, Kurtin PJ, et al: Phase 1 study of interleukin-12 in combination with rituximab in patients with B-cell non-Hodgkin lymphoma. *Blood.* 2002;99:67.

239. Kobrinsky NL, Sposto R, Narayan RS, et al: Outcomes of treatment of children and adolescents with recurrent non-Hodgkin's lymphoma and Hodgkin's disease with dexamethasone, etoposide, cisplatin, cytarabine, and L-Asparaginase, maintenance chemotherapy, and transplantation: Children's Cancer Group Study CCG-5912. *J Clin Oncol.* 2001;19:2390.

240. McManaway ME, Neckers LM, Loke SL, et al: Tumour-specific inhibition of lymphoma growth by an antisense oligodeoxynucleotide. *Lancet.* 1990;335:808.

241. Rooney C, Smith C, Ng C, et al: Use of viral-specific cytotoxic lymphocytes to control Epstein-Barr virus-related lymphoproliferation. *Lancet.* 1995;345:9.

242. Roberts WK, Livingston PO, Agus DB, et al: Vaccination with CD20 peptides induces a biologically active, specific immune response in mice. *Blood.* 2002;99:3748.

243. Davis TA, Hsu FJ, Caspar CB, et al: Idiotype vaccination following ABMT can stimulate specific anti-idiotype immune responses in patients with B-cell lymphoma. *Biol Blood Marrow Transplant.* 2001;7:517.

244. Ries LAG, Smith MA, Gurney JG, et al: Cancer Incidence and Survival among Children and Adolescents: United States SEER

Program 1975-1995, National Cancer Institute, SEER Program. NIH Pub. No. 99-4649, Bethesda, Md. 1999;1.

245. Grufferman S, Delzell E: Epidemiology of Hodgkin's disease. *Epidemiol Rev.* 1984;6:76.

246. Glaser SL, Jarrett RF: The epidemiology of Hodgkin's disease. *Baillieres Clin Hematol.* 1996;9:401.

247. Nachman JB, Sposto R, Herzog P, et al: Randomized comparison of low-dose involved-field radiotherapy and no radiotherapy for children with Hodgkin's disease who achieve a complete response to chemotherapy. *J Clin Oncol.* 2002;20:3765.

248. Armstrong AA, Alexander FE, Cartwright R: Epstein-Barr virus and Hodgkin's disease: Further evidence for the three disease hypothesis. *Leukemia.* 1998;12:1272.

249. Clavieza A, Tiemann M, Krams M, et al: Lack of prognostic significance of Epstein-Barr virus infection in children and adolescents with Hodgkin's disease. *Leuk Lymphoma.* 2001;42:41.

250. Kaplan HS: *Hodgkin's Disease.* Cambridge, Mass: Harvard University Press; 1980:689.

251. Hueltenschmidt B, Sauter-Bihl ML, Lang O, et al: Whole body positron emission tomography in the treatment of Hodgkin's disease. *Cancer.* 2001;91:302.

252. Lally KP, Arnstein M, Siegel S, et al: A comparison of staging methods for Hodgkin's disease in children. *Arch Surg.* 1986; 121:1125.

253. Salloum E, Brandt D, Caride V: Gallium scans in the management of patients with Hodgkin's disease: A study of 101 patients. *J Clin Oncol.* 1997;15:518.

254. Donaldson SS: Making choices in the staging of children with Hodgkin's disease. *Med Pediatr Oncol.* 1991;19:211.

255. Chilcote RR, Baehner RL, Hammond D: Septicemia and meningitis in children splenectomized for Hodgkin's disease. *N Engl J Med.* 1976;295:798.

256. Donaldson SS, Kaplan HS: Complications of treatment of Hodgkin's disease in children. *Cancer Treat Rep.* 1982;66:977.

257. Green DM, Ghoorah J, Douglass HO Jr, et al: Staging laparotomy with splenectomy in children and adolescents with Hodgkin's disease. *Cancer Treat Rev.* 1983;10:23.

258. Donaldson SS, Link MP: Combined modality treatment with low-dose radiation and MOPP chemotherapy for children with Hodgkin's disease. *J Clin Oncol.* 1987;5:742.

259. Cleary S, Link M, Donaldson S: Hodgkin's disease in the very young. *Int J Radiat Oncol Biol Phys.* 1994;28:77.

260. Rühl U, Albrecht M, Dieckmann K, et al: Response-adapted radiotherapy in the treatment of pediatric Hodgkin's disease: An interim report at 5 years of the German GPOH-HD 95 trial. *Int J Radiat Oncol Biol Phys.* 2001;51:1209.

261. Mauch PM, Weinstein H, Botnick L, et al: An evaluation of long-term survival and treatment morbidity in early-stage Hodgkin's disease. *Int J Radiat Oncol Biol Phys.* 1988;21:1157.

262. Donaldson SS, Link MP: Hodgkin's disease: treatment of the young child. *Pediatr Clin North Clin.* 1991;38:457.

263. Donaldson S, Whitaker S, Plowman N, et al: Stage I-II pediatric Hodgkin's disease: Long-term follow-up demonstrates equivalent survival rates following different management schemes. *J Clin Oncol.* 1990;8:1128.

264. Gehan EA, Sullivan MP, Fuller LM, et al: The intergroup Hodgkin's disease in children. A study of stage I and II. *Cancer.* 1990;65:1429.

265. Shankar A, Ashley S, Radford M, et al: Does histology influence outcome in childhood Hodgkin's disease? Results from the United Kingdom Children's Cancer Study Group. *J Clin Oncol.* 1997; 15:2622.

266. Oberlin O, Leverger G, Pacquement M, et al: Low-dose radiation therapy and reduced chemotherapy in childhood Hodgkin's disease: The experience of the French Society of Pediatric Oncology. *J Clin Oncol.* 1992;10:1602.

267. Donaldson SS, Hudson MM, Lamborn KR, et al: VAMP and low-dose, involved-field radiation for children and adolescents with favorable, early-stage Hodgkin's disease: Results of a prospective clinical trial. *J Clin Oncol.* 2002;20:3081.

268. Landman-Parker J, Pacquement M, Leblanc T, et al: Localized childhood Hodgkin's disease: Response-adapted chemotherapy with etoposide, bleomycin, vinblastine, and prednisone before low-dose radiation therapy—results of the French Society of Pediatric Oncology Study MDH90. *J Clin Oncol.* 2000; 18:1500.

269. Vecchi V, Burnelli R, DiFabio F, et al: Childhood Hodgkin's disease: Results of the Italian multicentric study AIEOP-MH'89-CNR. *Med Pediatr Oncol.* 1997;29:434.

270. Schellong G, Bramswig J, Hornig-Franz I: Treatment of children with Hodgkin's disease: Results of the German Pediatric Oncology Group. *Ann Oncol.* 1992;3:73.

271. Schellong G, Potter R, Bramswig J, et al: High cure rates and reduced long-term toxicity in pediatric Hodgkin's disease: The German-Austrian multicenter trial DAL-HD-90. The German-Austrian Pediatric Hodgkin's Disease Study Group. *J Clin Oncol.* 1999;17:3736.

272. Olweny CLM, Katongole-Mbidde E, Kiire C, et al: Childhood Hodgkin's disease in Uganda: A ten-year experience. *Cancer.* 1978; 42:787.

273. Dionet C, Oberlin O, Habriand JL, et al: Initial chemotherapy and low dose radiation in limited fields in childhood Hodgkin's disease: results of a joint cooperative study by the French Society of Radiation Oncology (SFOP) and Hospital Saint-Louis. Paris. *Int J Radiat Oncol Biol Phys.* 1988;15:341.

274. Hutchinson R, Krailo M, Fryer C: Prognostic factor analysis in advanced Hodgkin's disease (stages III and IV). Results of the CCG 521 trial. *Med Pediatr Oncol.* 1993;21:61. Abstract.

275. Weiner MA, Leventhal BG, Marcus R, et al: Intensive chemotherapy and low-dose radiotherapy for the treatment of advanced-stage Hodgkin's disease in pediatric patients: A Pediatric Oncology Group study. *J Clin Oncol.* 1991;9:1591.

276. Tarbell NJ, Gelber RD, Weinstein HJ, et al: Sex differences in risk of second malignant tumors after Hodgkin's disease in childhood. *Lancet.* 1993;341:1428.

277. Friedmann AM, Hudson MM, Weinstein HJ, et al: Treatment of unfavorable childhood Hodgkin's disease with VEPA and low-dose, involved-field radiation. *J Clin Oncol.* 2002;20:3088.

278. Ekert H, Waters KD, Smith PJ, et al: Treatment with MOPP or CHIVPP chemotherapy only for all stages of childhood Hodgkin's disease. *J Clin Oncol.* 1988;6:1845.

279. Atra A, Higgs E, Capra M, et al: ChlVPP chemotherapy in children with stage IV Hodgkin's disease: Results of the UKCCSG HD 8201 and HD 9201 studies. *Br J Hematol.* 2002; 119:647.

280. Mauch P, Tarbell N, Weinstein H, et al: Stage IA and IIA supra-diaphragmatic Hodgkin's disease: Prognostic factors in surgically staged patients treated with mantle and para-aortic irradiation. *J Clin Oncol.* 1988;6:1576.

281. Hoppe RT: Stage I-II Hodgkin's disease: Current therapeutic options and recommendations. *Blood.* 1983;62:32.

282. Barrett A, Crennan E, Barnes J, et al: Treatment of clinical stage I Hodgkin's disease by local radiation therapy alone. A United Kingdom Children's Cancer Study Group study. *Cancer.* 1990; 66:670.

283. Mauch PM, Weinstein H, Botnick L, et al: An evaluation of long-term survival and treatment complications in children with Hodgkin's disease. *Cancer.* 1983;51:925.

284. Maity A, Goldwein JW, Lange B, et al: Comparison of high-dose and low-dose radiation with and without chemotherapy for children with Hodgkin's disease: An analysis of the experience at the Children's Hospital of Philadelphia and the Hospital of the University of Pennsylvania. *J Clin Oncol.* 1992;10:929.

285. Oberlin O, Boilletot A, Leverger G, et al: Clinical staging, primary chemotherapy and involved-field radiotherapy in childhood Hodgkin's disease. *Eur Paediatr Oncol.* 1985;2:65.

286. Jenkin D, Doyle J, Berry M, et al: Hodgkin's disease in children: Treatment with MOPP and low-dose extended field irradiation without laparotomy late results and toxicity. *Med Pediatr Oncol.* 1990;18:265.

287. Fryer C, Hutchinson RJ, Krailo M, et al: Efficacy and toxicity of 12 courses of ABVD chemotherapy followed by low-dose regional radiation in advanced Hodgkin's disease in children: a report from the Children's Cancer Study Group. *J Clin Oncol.* 1990;8:1971.

288. Hudson M, Greenwald C, Thompson E: Efficacy and toxicity of multiagent chemotherapy and low-dose involved-field radiotherapy in children and adolescents with Hodgkin's disease. *J Clin Oncol.* 1993;11:100.

289. Hunger S, Link M, Donaldson S: ABVD/MOPP and low-dose involved-field radiotherapy in pediatric Hodgkin's disease: The Stanford experience. *J Clin Oncol.* 1994;12:2160.

290. Schellong G: The balance between cure and late effects in childhood Hodgkin's lymphoma: The experience of the German-Austrian Study-Group since 1978. *Ann Oncol.* 1996;7(suppl 4):67.

291. Schellong G, Bramswig J, Hornig-Franz I, et al: Hodgkin's disease in children: Combined modality treatment for stages IA, IB and IIA. Results of 356 patients of the German/Austrian Pediatric Study Group. *Ann Oncol.* 1994;5(suppl):113.

292. Weiner MA, Leventhal B, Brecher ML, et al: Randomized study of intensive MOPP-ABVD with or without low-dose total-nodal radiation therapy in the treatment of stages IIB, IIIA2, IIIB, and IV Hodgkin's disease in pediatric patients: A Pediatric Oncology Group study. *J Clin Oncol.* 1997;15:2769.

293. Hutchinson RJ, Fryer CJ, Davis PC, et al: MOPP or radiation in addition to ABVD in the treatment of pathologically staged advanced Hodgkin's disease in children: Results of the Children's Cancer Group Phase III Trial. *J Clin Oncol.* 1998;16:897.

294. Green DM, Hyland A, Chung CS, et al: Cancer and cardiac mortality among 15-year survivors of cancer diagnosed during childhood or adolescence. *J Clin Oncol.* 1999;17:3207.

295. Green DM, Hyland A, Barcos MP, et al: Second malignant neoplasms after treatment for Hodgkin's disease in childhood or adolescence. *J Clin Oncol.* 2000;18:1492.

296. Green D, Gingell R, Pearce J, et al: The effect of mediastinal irradiation on cardiac function of patients treated during childhood and adolescence for Hodgkin's disease. *J Clin Oncol.* 1987;5:239.

297. Scholz KH, Herrmann C, Tebbe U, et al: Myocardial infarction in young patients with Hodgkin's disease—Potential pathogenic role of radiotherapy, chemotherapy, and splenectomy. *Clin Investig.* 1993;71:57.

298. Hancock S, Donaldson S, Hoppe R: Cardiac disease following treatment of Hodgkin's disease in children and adolescents. *J Clin Oncol.* 1993;11:1208.

299. Tucker MA, Coleman CN, Cox RS, et al: Risk of second cancers after treatment for Hodgkin's disease. *N Engl J Med.* 1988; 318:76.

300. Hudson MM, Pratt CB: Risk of delayed second primary neoplasms after treatment of malignant lymphoma. *Surg Oncol Clin N Am.* 1993;2:319.

301. Clark D, Rubin P, Hutson A, et al: Increased incidence of second malignant neoplasms in Hodgkin's disease. *Int J Radiat Oncol Biol Phys.* 1993;27:233. Abstract.

302. Beaty O, Hudson M, Greenwald C, et al: Subsequent malignancies in children and adolescents after treatment for Hodgkin's disease. *J Clin Oncol.* 1995;13:603.

303. Bhatia S, Robison L, Oberlin O, et al: Breast cancer and other second neoplasms after childhood Hodgkin's disease. *N Engl J Med.* 1996;334:745.

304. Sankila R, Garwicz J, Olsen H, et al: Risk of subsequent malignant neoplasms among 1,641 Hodgkin's disease patients diagnosed in childhood and adolescence: A population-based cohort study in five Nordic countries. *J Clin Oncol.* 1996;14:1442.

305. Schellong G, Riepenhausen M, Creutzig U, et al: Low risk of secondary leukemias after chemotherapy without mechlorethamine in childhood Hodgkin's disease. German-Austrian Pediatric Hodgkin's Disease Group. *J Clin Oncol.* 1997;15:2247.

306. Swerdlow AJ, Barber JA, Hudson GV, Cunningham D, et al: Risk of second malignancy after Hodgkin's disease in a collaborative British cohort: The relation to age at treatment. *J Clin Oncol.* 2000;18:498.

307. Metayer C, Lynch CF, Clarke EA, et al: Second cancers among long-term survivors of Hodgkin's disease diagnosed in childhood and adolescence. *J Clin Oncol.* 2000;18:2435.

308. van Leeuwen FE, Klokman WJ, van't Veer MB, et al: Long-term risk of second malignancy in survivors of Hodgkin's disease treated during adolescence or young adulthood. *J Clin Oncol.* 2000;18:487.

309. Wolden SL, Hancock SL, Carlson RW, et al: Management of breast cancer after Hodgkin's disease. *J Clin Oncol.* 2000;18:765.

310. Wolden S, Lamborn K, Cleary S, et al: Second cancers following pediatric Hodgkin's disease. *J Clin Oncol.* 1998;16:536.

311. LaMonte CS, Yeh S, Straus D: Long-term follow-up of cardiac function in patients with Hodgkin's disease treated with mediastinal irradiation and combination chemotherapy including doxorubicin. *Cancer Treat Rep.* 1986;70:439.

312. Coleman CN, Williams CJ, Flint A, et al: Hematologic neoplasia in patients treated for Hodgkin's disease. *N Engl J Med.* 1977; 297:1249.

313. Hudson MM, Poquette CA, Lee J, et al: Increased mortality after successful treatment for Hodgkin's disease. *J Clin Oncol.* 1998; 16:3592.

314. Swerdlow AJ, Schoemaker MJ, Allerton R, et al: Lung cancer after Hodgkin's disease: A vested case-control study of the relation to treatment. *J Clin Oncol.* 2001;1610.

315. Chapman RM, Sutcliffe SB, Malpas JS: Male gonadal dysfunction in Hodgkin's disease. *JAMA.* 1981;245:1323.

316. Viviani S, Santoro A, Ragni G, et al: Gonadal toxicity after combination chemotherapy for Hodgkin's disease: Comparative results of MOPP vs ABVD. *Eur J Cancer Clin Oncol.* 1985;21:601.

317. Anselmo AP, Cartoni C, Bellantuono P, et al: Risk of infertility in patients with Hodgkin's disease treated with ABVD vs. MOPP vs. ABVD/MOPP. *Haematologica.* 1990;75.

318. Mackie E, Radford M, Shalet S: Gonadal function following chemotherapy for childhood Hodgkin's disease. *Med Pediatr Oncol.* 1996;27:74.

319. Horning SJ, Hoppe RT, Kaplan HS, et al: Female reproductive potential after treatment for Hodgkin's disease. *N Engl J Med.* 1981;304:1377.

320. Ortin TT, Shostak CA, Donaldson SS: Gonadal status and reproductive function following treatment for Hodgkin's disease in childhood: The Stanford experience. *Int J Radiat Oncol Biol Phys.* 1990;19:873.

321. Byrne J, Fears TR, Gail MH, et al: Early menopause in long-term survivors of cancer during adolescence. *Am J Obstet Gynecol.* 1992;166:788.

322. Bonadonna G: Chemotherapy strategies to improve the control of Hodgkin's disease. *Cancer Res.* 1982;42:4309.

323. Valagussa P, Santoro A, Fossati-Bellani F, et al: Second acute leukemia and other malignancies following treatment for Hodgkin's disease. *J Clin Oncol.* 1986;4:830.

324. Santoro A, Bonadonna G, Valagussa P, et al. Long-term results of combined chemotherapy-radiotherapy approach in Hodgkin's disease: Superiority of ABVD plus radiotherapy versus MOPP plus radiotherapy. *J Clin Oncol.* 1987;5:27.

325. Hamilton VM, Norris C, Bunin N, et al: Cyclophosphamide-based, seven-drug hybrid and low-dose involved field radiation for the treatment of childhood and adolescent Hodgkin's disease. *J Pediatr Hematol Oncol.* 2001;23:84.

326. Sackmann-Muriel F, Cebrian-Bonesana AC, Pavlovsky S, et al: Hodgkin's disease in childhood: Therapy results in Argentina. *Am J Pediatr Hematol Oncol.* 1981;3.

327. Bayle-Weisgerber C, Lemercier N, Teillet F, et al: Hodgkin's disease in children: Results of therapy in a mixed group of 178 clinically and pathologically staged patients over 13 years. *Cancer.* 1984;54:215.

328. Jacobs P, King HS, Karabus C, et al: Hodgkin's disease in children. A ten-year experience in South Africa. *Cancer.* 1984;53:210.

329. Behrendt H, van Bunningen BN, van Leeuwen EF: Treatment of Hodgkin's disease in children with or without radiotherapy. *Cancer.* 1987;59:1870.

330. Lobo-Sanahuja F, Garcia I, Barrantes J, et al: Pediatric Hodgkin's disease in Costa Rica: Twelve years' experience of primary treatment by chemotherapy alone without staging laparotomy. *Med Pediatr Oncol.* 1994;22:398.

331. Sripada PVSS, Tenali SG, Vasudevan M, et al: Hybrid (COPP/ABV) therapy in childhood Hodgkin's disease: A study of 53 cases during 1989-1993 at the Cancer Institute, Madras. *Pediatr Hematol Oncol.* 1995;12:333.

332. Behrendt H, Brinkhuis M, Van Leeuwen E: Treatment of childhood Hodgkin's disease with ABVD without radiotherapy. *Med Pediatr Oncol.* 1996;26:244.

333. Baez F, Ocampo E, Conter V, et al: Treatment of childhood Hodgkin's disease with COPP or COPP-ABV (hybrid) without radiotherapy in Nicaragua. *Ann Oncol.* 1997;8:247.

334. van den Berg H, Stuve W, Behrendt H: Treatment of Hodgkin's disease in children with alternating mechlorethamine, vincristine, procarbazine, and prednisone (MOPP) and Adriamycin, bleomycin, vinblastine, and dacarbazine (ABVD) courses without radiotherapy. *Med Pediatr Oncol.* 1997;29:23.

335. Tebbi C, Mendenhall N, Schwartz C: Response dependent treatment of stages IA, IIA and IIIA1 micro Hodgkin's disease with DBVE and low dose involved field irradiation with or without dexrazoxane. Fifth International Symposium on Hodgkin's Lymphoma. Harwood Academic, 2001.

336. Schwartz C, Constine L, et al: Intensive response-based therapy with or without dexrazoxane for intermediate/high-stage (I/HS) pediatric Hodgkin's disease (HD): A Pediatric Oncology Group (POG) study. Fifth International Symposium on Hodgkin's Lymphoma. Harwood Academic, 2001.

337. Bader S, Weinstein H, Mauch P, et al: Pediatric stage IV Hodgkin's disease: Long-term survival. *Cancer.* 1993;72:249.

338. Desch E, Lasala MR, Smith TJ, et al: The optimal timing of autologous bone marrow transplantation in Hodgkin's disease patients after a chemotherapy relapse. *J Clin Oncol.* 1992;10:200.

339. Williams C, Goldstone A, Pearce R, et al: Autologous bone marrow transplantation for pediatric Hodgkin's disease: A case-matched comparison with adult patients by the European Bone Marrow Transplant Group Lymphoma Registry. *J Clin Oncol.* 1993;11:2243.

340. Anderson JR, Litzow MR, Applebaum FR, et al: Allogeneic, syngeneic, and autologous marrow transplantation for Hodgkin's disease: The 21-year experience. *J Clin Oncol.* 1993;11:2342.

341. Baker S, Gordon B, Grass T, et al: Autologous hematopoietic stem-cell transplantation for relapsed or refractory Hodgkin's disease in children and adolescents. *J Clin Oncol.* 1999;17:825.

342. Alpek G, Ambinder RF, Piantadosi S, et al: Long-term results of blood and marrow transplantation for Hodgkin's lymphoma. *J Clin Oncol.* 2001;19:4314.

343. Sureda A, Arranz R, Iriondo A, et al: Autologous stem-cell transplantation for Hodgkin's disease: Results and prognostic factors in 494 patients from the Grupo Espanol de Linfomas/Transplante Autolog de Medula Osea Spanish Cooperative Group. *J Clin Oncol.* 2001;19:1395.

344. Constine L, Rapoport A: Hodgkin's disease, bone marrow transplantation, and involved field radiation therapy: Coming full circle from 1902 to 1996. *Int J Radiat Oncol Biol Phys.* 1996; 36:253.

345. Wadhwa P, Shina D, Shenkein D, et al: Should involved-field radiation therapy be used as an adjunct to lymphoma autotransplantation? *BMT.* 2002;29:183.

346. Hoppe RT, Hanlon AL, Hanks GE, et al: Progress in the treatment of Hodgkin's disease in the United States, 1973 versus 1983: The Patterns of Care study. *Cancer.* 1994;74:3198.

347. Willman K, Cox R, Donaldson S: Radiation induced height impairment in pediatric Hodgkin's disease. *Int J Radiat Oncol Biol Phys.* 1994;28:85.

348. Silverman CL, Thomas PR, McAlister WH, et al: Slipped femoral capital epiphysis in irradiated children: Dose, volume, and age relationships. *Int J Radiat Oncol Biol Phys.* 1981;7:1357.

349. Libshitz A, Edeikin BS: Radiotherapy changes of the pediatric hip. *AJR.* 1981;137:585.

350. Maguire A, Craft A, Evans R, et al: The long-term effects of treatment on the dental condition of children surviving malignant disease. *Cancer.* 1987;60:2570.

351. Mefferd JM, Donaldson SS, Link MP: Pediatric Hodgkin's disease: Pulmonary, cardiac, and thyroid function following combined modality therapy. *Int J Radiat Oncol Biol Phys.* 1989;16:679.

352. Marina NM, Greenwald CA, Fairclough DL, et al: Serial pulmonary function studies in children treated for newly diagnosed Hodgkin's disease with mantle radiotherapy plus cycles of cyclophosphamide, vincristine, and procarbazine alternating with cycles of doxorubicin, bleomycin, vinblastine, and dacarbazine. *Cancer.* 1995;75:1706.

353. Adams MJ, Hardenbergh PH, Constine LS, et al: Radiation-associated cardiovascular disease. *Crit Rev Oncol Hematol.* 2003; 45:55.

354. Constine LS, Donaldson SS, McDougall IR, et al: Thyroid dysfunction after radiotherapy in children with Hodgkin's disease. *Cancer.* 1984;53:878.

355. Sklar C, Whitton J, Mertens A, et al: Abnormalities of the thyroid in survivors of Hodgkin's disease: Data from the Childhood Cancer Survivor Study. *J Clin Endocrinol Metab.* 2000;85:3227.

356. LeFloch O, Donaldson SS, Kaplan HS: Pregnancy following oophoropexy and total nodal irradiation in women with Hodgkin's disease. *Cancer.* 1976;38:2263.

357. Pedrick TJ, Hoppe RT: Recovery of spermatogenesis following pelvic irradiation for Hodgkin's disease. *Int J Radiat Oncol Biol Phys.* 1986;12:117.

358. Bramswig J, Heimes U, Heiermann E, et al: The effects of different cumulative doses of chemotherapy on testicular function. Results in 75 patients treated for Hodgkin's disease during childhood or adolescence. *Cancer.* 1990;65:1298.

359. Jockovich M, Mendenhall NP, Sombeck MD, et al: Long-term complications of laparotomy in Hodgkin's disease. *Ann Surg.* 1994;219:615.

360. Lipshultz SE, Colan SD, Gelber RD, et al: Late cardiac effects of doxorubicin therapy for acute lymphoblastic leukemia in childhood. *N Engl J Med.* 1991;324:808.

361. Acharya S, Sarafoglou K, LaQuaglia M, et al: Thyroid neoplasms after therapeutic radiation for malignancies during childhood or adolescence. *Cancer.* 2003;97:2397.

362. Kinsella T, Trivette G, Rowland J, et al: Long-term follow-up of testicular function following radiation therapy for early-stage Hodgkin's disease. *J Clin Oncol.* 1989;7:718.

363. da Cunha M, Meistrich M, Fuller L, et al: Recovery of spermatogenesis after treatment for Hodgkin's disease: Limiting dose of MOPP chemotherapy. *J Clin Oncol.* 1984;2:571.

364. Tucker MA, Coleman CN, Cox RS, et al: Risk of second cancers after treatment for Hodgkin's disease. *N Engl J Med.* 1988;318:76.

Pediatric Bone and Soft Tissue Tumors

55

Moody D. Wharam, Jr., MD

Osteosarcoma and Ewing's sarcoma are first and second in incidence of childhood bone tumors and comprise 2.6% and 2.1% of pediatric solid tumors (approximately 260 and 200 cases annually), respectively.[1] Most primary osteosarcoma lesions are managed by amputation or limb-sparing procedures and intensive chemotherapy. Pulmonary metastases are managed by surgical excision. For primary lesions in an unresectable site, control with conventional photon radiotherapy is limited. With proton beam therapy, 60% local control was achieved for patients with axial skeletal tumors.[2] Hypofractionated, accelerated radiotherapy afforded durable response in 14 patients requiring palliation of primary or metastatic lesions.[3] For 17 patients with spine osteosarcoma, radiotherapy after intralesional surgery improved survival.[4] A dose escalation trial of Samarium ([153]Sm-EDTMP) followed by peripheral stem cell rescue demonstrated minimal toxicity and prolonged response in patients with recurrent or metastatic osteosarcoma.[5]

Other rare bone tumors may present in childhood. Non-Hodgkin's lymphoma of bone responds well to multiagent chemotherapy, and radiotherapy is required only for nonresponders.[6] Malignant fibrous histiocytoma of bone can be controlled with radiotherapy.[7] Hemangioendothelial sarcoma of bone has a variable presentation and natural history and may be multifocal in one limb or bone.[8] Radiotherapy to 40 to 60 Gy affords good local control.[8-11] Benign giant cell tumor of bone presents in the pediatric age group in locations not amenable to surgery.[12] Radiation to greater than 40 Gy resulted in a local control rate of 75% to 85% in two series.[13-14] Proton beam therapy has also been used with similar control rates.[2] Local control of aneurysmal bone cyst in three adolescents was achieved with 40 Gy.[15]

EWING'S SARCOMA OF BONE

Epidemiology and Cytogenetics

A case-control study of environmental and familial factors did not identify risk factors for Ewing's sarcoma.[16] A reciprocal translocation t(11;22)(q24;q12) characterizes Ewing's sarcoma of bone and is shared with extraosseous Ewing's sarcoma and peripheral primitive neuroectodermal tumor (of bone or soft tissue), and thus the concept of the Ewing's sarcoma family of tumors.[17,18] Mapping of the translocation break point indicates fusion of the *FLI-1* gene on 11q24 with the *EWS* gene of 22q12.[19] One function of the resulting fusion protein is repression of a tumor suppressor gene that encodes for the type II receptor of transforming growth factor beta.[20] Patients harboring the less frequent EWS-ERG fusion protein resulting from a t(21;22)(q22; q12) translocation were compared to patients with the EWS-FLI1 transcript. Differences in clinical phenotype and outcome were not observed.[21]

Clinical Presentation and Routes of Spread

Ewing's sarcoma of bone may present as late as the fourth and fifth decades of life, but the mean and median age (15 to 16 years) reflects the predominance of presentation between ages 10 and 20 years (about 65%).[22-24] Age at diagnosis of younger than 5 years is rare, as is diagnosis in blacks. The male/female ratio is 1.5:1. Pain is the most common presenting symptom (>90%), and two thirds of patients complain of a mass lesion. When a long bone is the primary site, the tumor is typically in the metaphysis or diaphysis. Three fourths of primary sites are extremities or pelvic bones, with the femur as the single bone most frequently involved (Fig. 55-1).[25] Other features at presentation include pathologic fracture (16%), systemic symptoms including fever (10% to 30%), and metastases (10% to 25%).[22] Of 122 patients in the Intergroup Ewing's Sarcoma Studies (IESS-I and IESS-II) with metastases at diagnosis, 53% had lung metastases with or without other metastases and 43% had bone metastases with or without other metastases.[26]

Pathology

The histogenesis of Ewing's sarcoma is uncertain. The classic or "typical" variant is shown in Figure 55-2A. A variant featuring greater range of cell size and more frequent mitoses has been termed *atypical* and may also have a lobular, alveolar, or organoid organizational pattern. The primitive round cell sarcoma of bone is less common and on light microscopy may have cells of greater size and shape, more pink cytoplasm, and a more

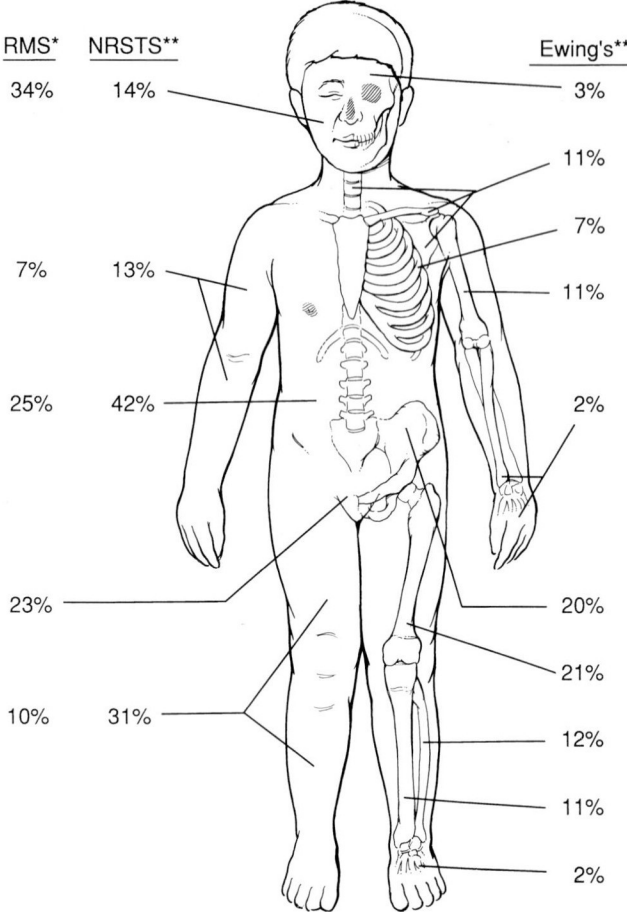

RMS*	NRSTS**	Ewing's***
34%	14%	3%
		11%
		7%
7%	13%	11%
25%	42%	2%
23%		20%
		21%
10%	31%	12%
		11%
		2%

Figure 55–1. Distribution of primary sites for rhabdomyosarcoma (RMS),[77] nonrhabdomyosarcoma soft tissue sarcoma (NRSTS),[159-161] and Ewing's sarcoma.[25] *For RMS, the head and neck site may be subdivided as: orbit, 8%; other head, 8%; parameningeal, 18%; and the pelvic sites as: bladder/prostate, 11%; and female genital/paratestis, 12%. **For NRSTS, the trunk data include pelvic sites. ***For Ewing's sarcoma, certain sites by subdivision are vertebral column, 5%; scapula, 4%; ilium, 12%; and sacrum/coccyx/pubis, 8%.

prominent matrix. Ultrastructural features are distinct from Ewing's sarcoma of bone and include the presence of cytoplasmic organelles, intracytoplasmic attachments, and developed intercellular attachments. Neurosecretory granules are not apparent in contrast to the peripheral primitive neuroectodermal tumor.[27] There is, at present, insufficient clinical experience to determine if the subtypes differ by age at diagnosis, site of presentation, probability of metastases, and response to therapy.

Diagnostic and Staging Studies

Laboratory studies at presentation, in addition to routine hematology and chemistry, should include serum lactase dehydrogenase level and histologic assessment of bone marrow. Chest computed tomography (CT) and bone scan are required. Imaging studies of the primary lesion include plain radiographs, which typically show a central destructive lesion with variable sclerosis and osteolysis. Periosteal elevation by the tumor mass stimulates calcium

deposition, which may form layers with an "onionskin" appearance and which may, at the periphery of the elevation, demonstrate the Codman triangle sign (Fig. 55-3). A soft-tissue component may show radiating calcium spicules. The bone scan will also show the extent of the primary lesion.[28] Although CT assessment of the primary site is superior to magnetic resonance imaging (MRI) for identification of tumor matrix calcification and periosteal reaction, MRI has several advantages. The assessment of bone cortex is best seen in the axial plane. Sagittal and coronal images show (on T1 sequences) the extent of marrow infiltration. Major blood vessels are well seen. Soft-tissue tumor mass and adjacent normal muscle are distinguished on T2-weighted images.[29] The coronal and sagittal images are best suited for determining the gross tumor volume (GTV), but correlation with the bone scan is mandatory.

After treatment, an elevated serum lactase dehydrogenase level may herald relapse.[30] Plain radiographs, CT, and MRI of the primary lesion will show primary site recurrence.[29,31] The bone scan should return to normal in 12 months median (range 6 to 18 months) after radiotherapy. Recurrence of uptake at 10 months median (range 6 to 12 months) or persistent uptake signals primary site tumor regrowth or, occasionally, pathologic fracture or ectopic bone formation.[28]

Staging System

No staging system is in common use for Ewing's sarcoma of bone. (see Chapter 59, Sarcomas of Bone.) Pretreatment tumor characteristics that portend a poor prognosis include presence of metastases,[22] proximal or central sites,[32] volume greater than either 100 or 500 mL,[32,33] and gross soft-tissue extension.[34]

Standard Treatment

Treatment of Ewing's sarcoma requires prompt initiation of chemotherapy at completion of diagnostic evaluation. Treatment of the primary site with radiotherapy, surgery, or both follows induction chemotherapy. Intergroup Study 0091 demonstrated the superiority of a six-drug regimen.[35] A modified regimen for patients receiving definitive radiotherapy on the subsequent Children's Oncology Group Study AEWS 0031 is shown in Table 55-1 and represents a contemporary standard.

The propensity for Ewing's sarcoma to extend within the medullary cavity or into adjacent soft tissue has limited the application of limb-sparing procedures successfully used for osteosarcoma patients. Historically, surgical resection was restricted to "expendable" bones (e.g., rib, clavicle, proximal fibula, scapula). The apparent benefit for the surgical approach in retrospective studies (in comparison to radiotherapy) resulted, in part, from selection bias, for which there was no reliable control.[36] The proportion of non-metastatic patients having surgery alone in Intergroup Study 0091 was 38%, with 23% having surgery and radiotherapy and 39%

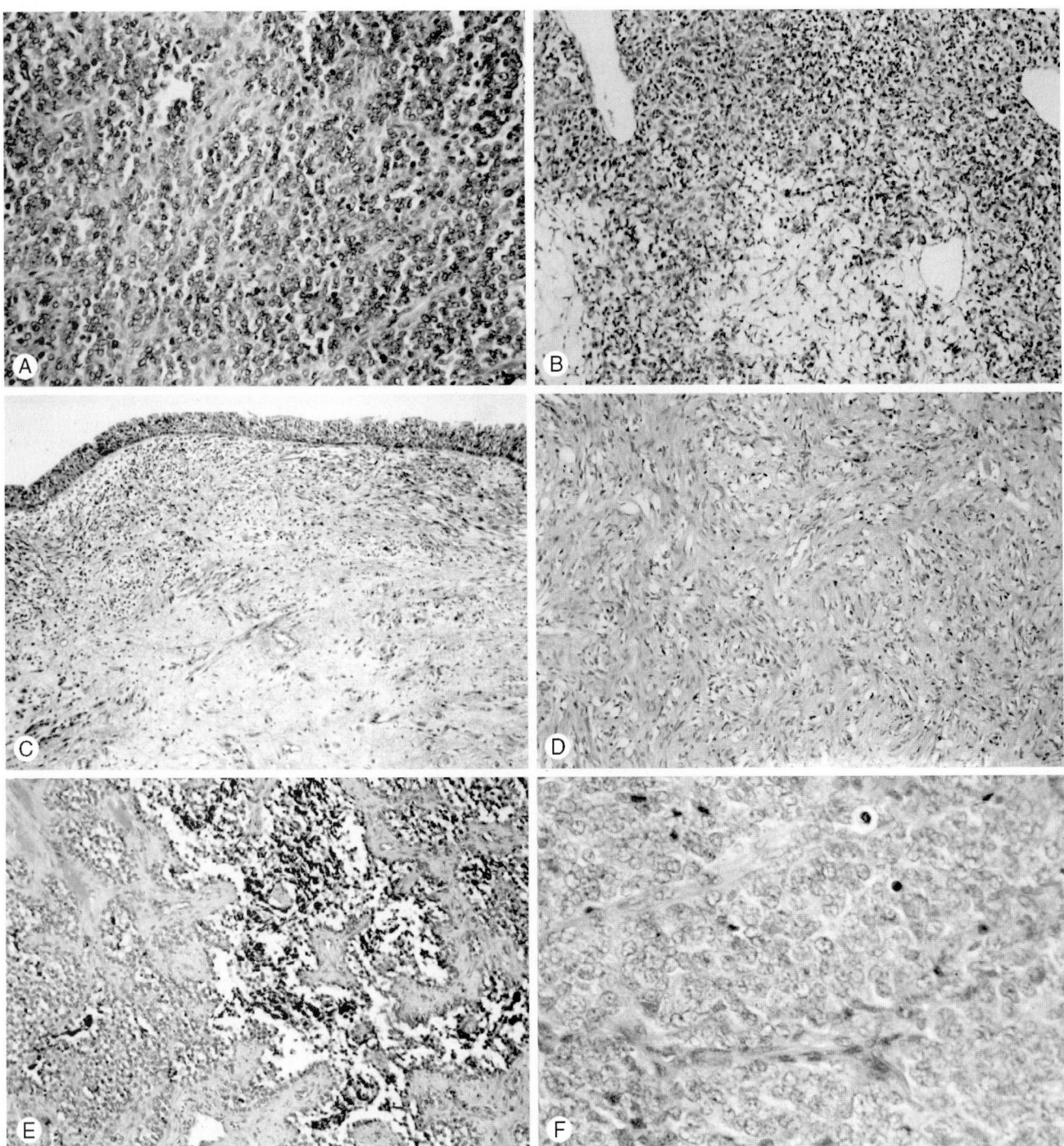

Figure 55–2. A, Ewing's sarcoma showing monotonous sheets of small, round, blue cells without evidence of differentiation. Mitotic figures are infrequent, and the periodic acid-Schiff stain will be positive. (Courtesy of Elizabeth J. Perlman, MD.) **B,** Embryonal rhabdomyosarcoma demonstrating classic features of small, primitive round cells that are elongated with eccentric pink cytoplasm and loose, edematous stroma. **C,** Botryoid rhabdomyosarcoma, a variant of embryonal rhabdomyosarcoma, which demonstrates a submucosal location (cambium layer) beneath a normal mucous membrane. **D,** Spindle cell variant of embryonal rhabdomyosarcoma showing whorls of medium-sized spindle cells admixed with abundant collagen. **E,** Alveolar rhabdomyosarcoma, composed of small undifferentiated cells with scant cytoplasm that line fibrovascular septa. **F,** Undifferentiated sarcoma, showing primitive cells that have varying degrees of cytoplasm and large, somewhat irregular nuclei. Cells suggestive of muscle differentiation are not seen. (**A** through **F,** hematoxylin and eosin stain.) (**B** through **F,** courtesy of William A. Newton, Jr., MD.)

having radiotherapy alone. In the first two European Cooperative Ewing's Sarcoma Studies (CESS 81 and 86), the proportion of patients having surgery with/without postoperative radiotherapy was 66%, and the number having preoperative radiotherapy was 5%. In the subsequent European Intergroup Cooperative Ewing's Sarcoma Study (EICESS 92), the proportions were 37% and 42%, respectively.[37]

Surgical technique varies with primary site. Resection without reconstruction can be done in small bones such as

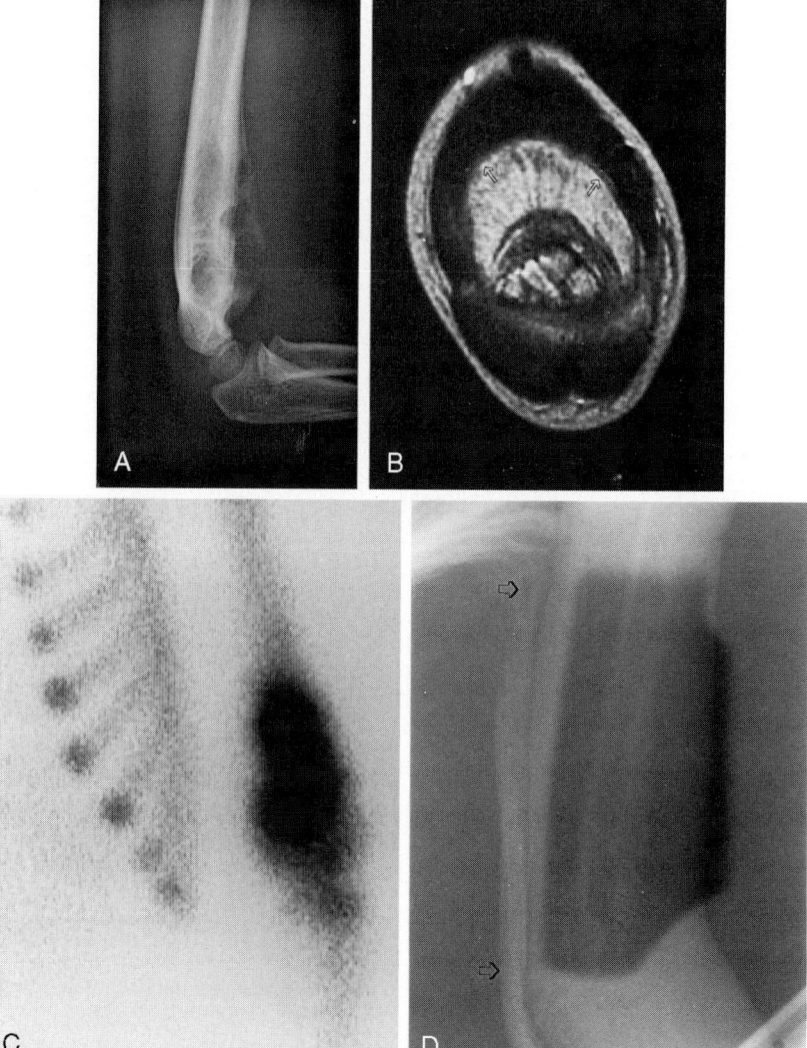

Figure 55–3. Imaging studies of a 6-year-old boy with Ewing's sarcoma of the distal left humerus. **A**, Lateral plain radiograph of the primary site demonstrating circumferential periosteal elevation with cortical destruction. **B**, Magnetic resonance imaging demonstrates significant soft tissue extension anteriorly (*arrow*). **C**, The bone scan is confirmatory. **D**, The patient is supine with left arm extended away from the thorax and immobilized with a cast. The portal verification film demonstrates the preservation of a posterior-lateral strip of skin and subcutaneous tissue and also shows the plaster of Paris cast (*arrows*).

rib, clavicle, proximal fibula, distal scapula, metatarsals, and metacarpals, and for the occasional, small lesion of the peripheral iliac wing or pubic bone. Large lesions or extremity primary lesions may require reconstruction using allograft or endoprosthetic methods.

Role of Radiotherapy

Radiotherapy is used pre- or postoperatively or definitively for the primary tumor and for treatment of pulmonary and skeletal metastases. Management of the primary tumor follows induction chemotherapy. The indications for surgery versus radiotherapy as initial local therapy are still evolving. For the very young child who would have significant leg-length discrepancy after definitive radiotherapy, amputation and prosthetic replacement may be preferred. Smaller lesions in expendable bones should also be considered for primary surgery, as should very large lesions (e.g., in the iliac wing). Sites with pathologic fracture can have definitive radiotherapy if healing occurs during induction

chemotherapy; otherwise, surgery is required. After primary surgery, adjuvant radiotherapy is indicated for intralesional resection or positive margins. In the three CESS/EICESS trials, local failure occurred in 20% of patients with intralesional resection who had postoperative radiotherapy. The same study showed a less than 5% local failure risk for patients who had good histologic response to initial chemotherapy followed by wide resection (with/without postoperative radiotherapy). The patients given preoperative radiotherapy had a local failure risk of 5%.[37]

Simulation

Ewing's sarcoma can occur in virtually any bone, and therefore the principles of simulation and treatment planning are site dependent. The initial decision for treatment planning is determination of optimal patient position. For an extremity lesion, a typical plan employs parallel opposed portals and the limb must be positioned so that the lesion, its adjacent soft-tissue extension, and the biopsy

Table 55–1   Chemotherapy Regimen for Ewing's Sarcoma Patients Receiving Definitive Radiotherapy

	Induction			Continuation			
	VDC	IE		VDC	RT	IE	VC
Week	1	4	Week	13	13-19	16,22	19
	7	10		25		28	
				31		34,40	37

C, cyclophosphamide 1200 mg/m² IV with MESNA; D, doxorubicin 75 mg/m² IV over 48 hours; E, etoposide 100 mg/m² per day IV, day 1-5; I, ifosfamide 1800 mg/m² per day IV, day 1-5 with MESNA; RT, radiotherapy; V, vincristine 2 mg/m² IV.
From Grier H, Krailo M, Tarbell N, et al: Addition of ifosfamide and etoposide to standard chemotherapy for Ewing's sarcoma and primitive neuroectodermal tumor of bone. *N Engl J Med.* 2003;348:694.

or surgical scar are encompassed while leaving a strip of soft tissue outside the port. The avoidance of circumferential irradiation facilitates lymphatic drainage and prevents the late appearance of distal edema. A combination of limb rotation and beam angulation (gantry rotation) will usually permit the necessary soft-tissue sparing for lesions that have mostly anterior or posterior extension. For the patient with an iliac or sacral primary lesion, the prone position, with or without the use of the "belly board" (which allows the gut to fall forward) will allow exclusion of small bowel from opposed oblique portals that parallel the plane of the iliac wing. Bladder distention will help keep the intestine away from the treated volume in patients with a pubic or ischial primary tumor. The patient with a scapular primary tumor may be positioned prone with the involved limb extending off the treatment couch and moved cephalad to place the scapula in a plane that accommodates opposed tangential ports and that maximally spares underlying lung. Immobilization of the treated limb should be done using plaster of Paris or commercially available thermal-reaction polymers. Figure 55-3 illustrates the imaging studies of a child with a primary tumor of the distal left humerus that had anterior soft tissue extension.

Portal margins are based on prechemotherapy imaging studies. Particular attention must be paid to soft-tissue extension in axial planes and intramedullary extension of long bones. The contribution of both MRI and bone scan imaging is essential. The typical presentation of the primary lesion in a long bone usually requires inclusion of the adjacent epiphysis in the port. Historically, the volume extended to include the opposite epiphysis, but this is no longer required.[38] For the Children's Oncology Group (COG) study AEWS 0031, the margin requirements were: clinical target volume (CTV) = GTV plus 1.5 cm; and planning target volume (PTV) = CTV plus 0.5 to 1 cm. A reduced portal (CTV = 1 cm) is based on the postinduction chemotherapy, preradiotherapy imaging if there has been regression of soft-tissue extension. The reduced portal maintains the same margin around the tumor extent in bone, but is planned to reflect the regression of the soft-tissue extension. This is done after a tumor dose of 45 Gy. Exceptions may be made to the rule that the CTV includes soft-tissue extension as it existed at the time of diagnosis. Examples include margins where the medial surface of primary lesions in the ileum or rib

have displaced bowel or lung (respectively), which then returned to a more anatomic location with regression. The same concept applies for low pelvic lesions that displace the bladder at the time of diagnosis, but do so to a lesser extent after induction chemotherapy. After resection of a primary lesion with microscopic residual, the margins are the original GTV plus 2 to 2.5 cm to 45 Gy; thereafter, a reduced port covers the area of residual tumor (CTV plus PTV = 1.5 to 2 cm) to 5.4 Gy (three fractions).

Radiation Treatment Plan

Plain radiographs, CT, MRI, and bone scan are used to determine GTV. Planar (two-dimensional) simulation is sufficient for primary tumors arising in long bones. A CT-based simulator facilitates planning of facial, vertebral, rib, scapular, and pelvic primary sites. The standard dose plan is 1.8 Gy per fraction, once a day, 5 days a week to 55.8 Gy. All fields are treated at each session. The energy selected should be 6 MV with higher energies reserved for central lesions in larger patients. After an initial 45 Gy to the original GTV, a reduced portal in the region of soft-tissue extension that has regressed after chemotherapy may be accomplished, based on postchemotherapy imaging with margins of 3 cm. The dose to the reduced portal is 10.8 Gy. The proximal and distal margin in bone is not changed.

If radiotherapy is given after resection of the primary lesion, the total dose may be limited to 50.4 Gy for the patient with positive margins. Gross residual tumor requires full dose (55.8 Gy). Single institution reports, however, suggest that the postoperative total dose may be reduced to 30 Gy.[39] For the patient with a rib primary tumor who has risk factors for pleural involvement, treatment should encompass the entire, ipsilateral hemithorax (1.5 Gy/day to 15 to 18 Gy) before reducing the port to a CTV appropriate to the rib primary tumor (Fig. 55-4).[40]

Critical Normal Tissues

Ewing's sarcoma can occur adjacent to virtually every important normal tissue. Figure 55-5 illustrates the treatment plan for a primary lesion in the third cervical vertebra using proton beam therapy to minimize dose to the spinal cord. When treating an extremity, the plan should spare a strip of normal tissue. The epiphyseal growth plate opposite the primary tumor can usually be excluded from treatment. Inclusion of only half the growth plate may lead to an exaggerated angle of the affected limb to its adjacent bone. Radiation-induced limb shortening is a function of age at diagnosis and radiotherapy dose. In a study from the orthovoltage era, growth loss for children receiving approximately 50 Gy was about 25% of the remaining (incremental) growth in the unaffected limb.[41] Leg dysfunction in patients treated at the National Cancer Institute was scored as minor or moderate in 18 of 22 patients. One patient required amputation.[42] Late functional results from a study of patients with primary

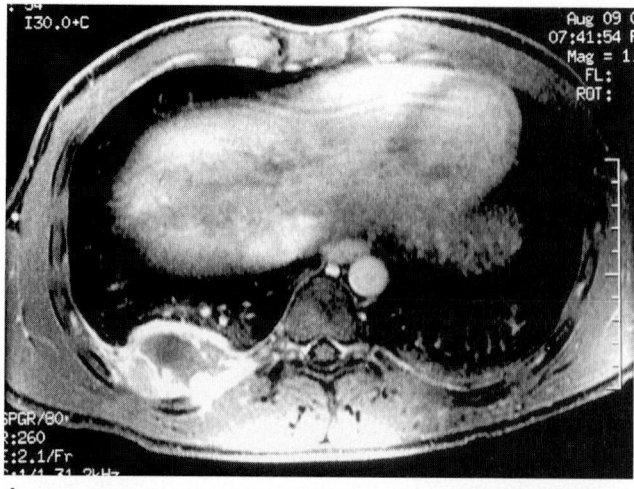

Figure 55–4. Imaging studies of a 19-year-old male with a primitive neuroectodermal tumor of the right thoracic wall. Following induction chemotherapy, chest wall resection (three ribs) was done and there was a positive margin. **A,** Magnetic resonance imaging scan (inverted) at time of diagnosis. **B,** After receiving 18 Gy (1.5 Gy/fraction) to the right hemithorax postoperatively, a reduced volume for the tumor bed (prone position) was planned using 10 off-axis beams, which follow the curvature of the chest wall. The plan reduces dose to lung, liver, and spinal cord compared with an opposed oblique plan. Total dose to tumor bed: 49.5 Gy. (Courtesy of Diane Latronico, MD.). See also Color Figure 55-4B.

tumors of an extremity who received hyperfractionated radiotherapy (1.2 Gy twice daily; total, 50.4 to 60 Gy) were very good and were subjectively improved over standard fractionation. No pathologic fractures occurred.[43] Five-year survivors of lower extremity osteosarcoma and Ewing's sarcoma were assessed for limb function and quality of life. Children treated after age 12 and females fared less well. No difference was observed between those having amputation or a limb-sparing procedure.[44]

The bladder should be avoided, if possible, when treating pelvic Ewing's sarcoma. Both cyclophosphamide and ifosfamide are bladder mucosal irritants that can cause hemorrhagic cystitis that is exacerbated by radiotherapy.

Reports of radiation-induced osteosarcomas usually describe patients whose tumor dose was 60 Gy or more. A multi-institutional report demonstrated no secondary sarcomas in patients receiving 48 Gy or less.[45] The National Cancer Institute (NCI) Surveillance, Epidemiology, and End Results Program included 595 patients with Ewing's sarcoma. One osteosarcoma and three soft tissue sarcomas developed in radiotherapy ports.[46] Secondary sarcomas developed in 3 of 674 patients enrolled in the CESS trials.[47]

After radiotherapy, widely distributed lytic changes of radiation osteitis will be seen on the plain radiograph in the initial 2 to 3 years. A localized area of lysis may herald recurrence of Ewing's sarcoma or, if at least 5 years have elapsed, a treatment-related bone sarcoma.[48]

Outcome

Several American institutions have reported treatment results for large patient numbers with 5- and 10-year follow-up. The Mayo Clinic report includes 105 patients with nonmetastatic disease treated from 1969 to 1982. Five-year survival was 42%, and local control was maintained in 73% of patients.[22] The NCI report included 80 patients with nonmetastatic disease treated between 1968 and 1980. The 5- and 10-year survival rates were 51% and 39%, respectively. Local control was 80%.[24] The IESS-I trial enrolled 342 patients with non-metastatic disease from 1973 to 1978 in a randomized trial of three treatment regimens. The 5- and 10-year survival rates for the best arm of the study were 65% and 60%, respectively. Local control was 85% and did not differ significantly by treatment assignment.[49] The failure pattern for non-metastatic patients on Intergroup Ewing's Sarcoma Study 0091 was local only, 5% (experimental arm); systemic, 20% (standard or experimental arm); and 2-5% (both arms).[35] The EICESS 92 trial enrolled 479 nonmetastatic patients. The 5-year relapse-free survival rate was 59%.[50]

Several patient and tumor characteristics affect outcome. Three that are interrelated are site, size, and extraosseous extension. Many studies indicate that pelvic, sacral, and other central sites have a worse prognosis. These lesions are typically larger than those at other sites and are more likely to have extraosseous extension. In IESS-I, patients with nonpelvic primary tumors had an overall 5-year survival rate of 57% and, on the superior treatment regimen, 72%. The 5-year survival for patients with a pelvic primary lesion was 34% (no difference by treatment arm), and relapses continued after 5 years. The survival rate was statistically significantly higher in IESS-II for patients with pelvic primary tumors, 63% at 5 years, and the local failure declined from 28% to 12%. The improvement was attributed to more intensive chemotherapy, more aggressive surgery, and the impact of CT on radiation treatment planning.[51] For patients with nonpelvic primary lesions, the IESS-II study (1978-1982) compared a regimen similar to the best arm of IESS-I (control arm) to a more intensive schedule of

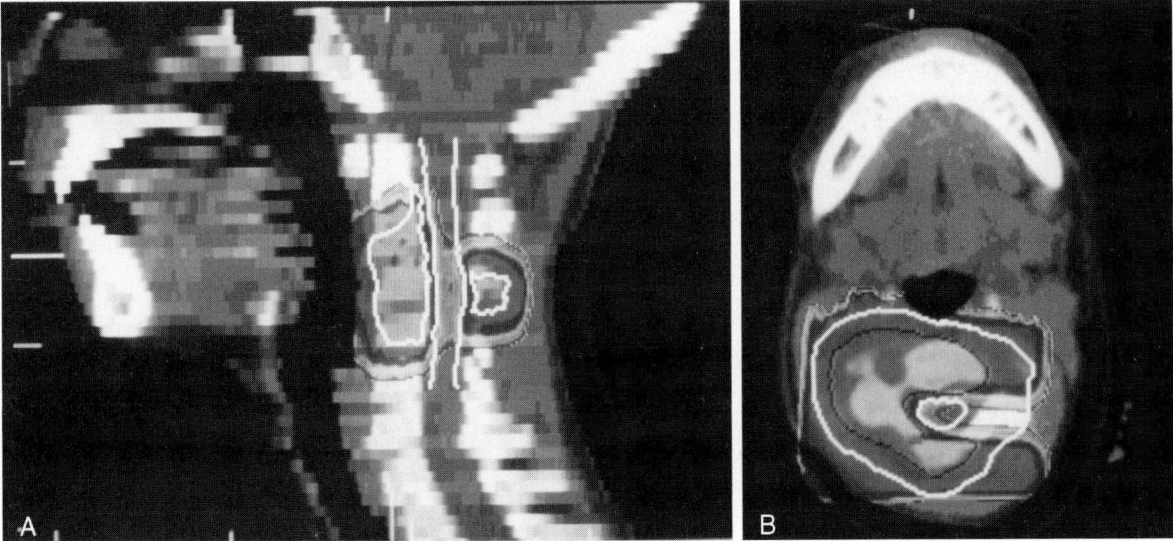

Figure 55–5. Isodose plan using proton beam therapy for Ewing's sarcoma of the third cervical vertebra in an 8-year-old boy. Sagittal (**A**) and axial (**B**) planes depict the volume receiving 55 cobalt GyEq. The majority of the cervical spinal cord received 50 cobalt GyEq or less. See also Color Figure 55-5. (Courtesy of Eugene B. Hug, MD, Department of Radiation Oncology, Massachusetts General Hospital, Boston.)

the same drugs. Five-year survival in the intensive arm was 77% and in the control arm was 63% ($P = 0.05$).[52] (The comparable figure for the best arm of IESS-I was 72%, as noted earlier.)[49] The local failure for IESS-II patients with nonpelvic disease was 9%. No site group (proximal, distal, rib, or other) was prognostic for an effect on survival.[52]

In another report, the presence of soft-tissue extension in patients with localized disease was more predictive of failure than large tumor size.[34] Significant prognostic factors (endpoint: 10-year event-free survival [EFS]) in CESS 86 included tumor size: greater than 200 mL (EFS 36%) and less than 200 mL (EFS 63%); also, poor histologic response (EFS 38%) and good response (EFS 64%).[53] To assess the relationship of these two variables, patients from the CESS and French EW88 trials were combined and the analysis restricted to 385 nonmetastatic patients who had initial chemotherapy followed by surgery (with/without postoperative radiotherapy). Histologic response (which was independent of tumor size) became the only significant prognostic factor. Based upon the percentage of viable cells in the surgical specimen, three prognostic groups were determined (endpoint: 5-year EFS): low risk (<10% cells), 73% EFS; intermediate risk (10% to 49% cells), 56% EFS; high risk (>50% cells), 37% EFS.[54]

Patients younger than age 3 constituted only 2.6% of the patients enrolled on five IESS protocols. Their 5-year survival rate was identical to that of older patients.[55]

Outcome of therapy at various uncommon sites has been published: rib, survival rate 50% to 60%[40,56]; vertebral column, 5-year EFS 36% to 44%[57,58]; small bones of the hands and feet, 6 of 7 alive and calcaneus, 1 of 5 alive[59];and bones of the head and neck, survival rate 80% (see Fig. 55-5).[60]

Patients with metastases at diagnosis do not have a uniformly fatal outcome. The CESS trials enrolled 114 patients with metastases confined to the lung and pleura.

The 10-year EFS for bilateral metastases was 24%; unilateral, 53%. Survival was better for patients who received whole lung irradiation.[61] When patients with skeletal metastases were included, the 4-year EFS was 27%.[62] Bone marrow ablative therapy (including total body irradiation) for patients with bone and marrow metastases did not improve outcome compared with conventional therapy in a report from the Memorial Sloan-Kettering Cancer Center.[63]

SOFT-TISSUE SARCOMA

Epidemiology

Soft-tissue sarcomas in children have an annual incidence of about 650 cases, or 6% of the approximate total of 10,500 new cancer cases per year in U.S. children younger than age 15.[1] They therefore rank among pediatric solid tumors after central nervous system and neuroblastoma, before bone tumors and retinoblastoma, and at about the same incidence as Wilms' tumor. Slightly more than half of patients have rhabdomyosarcoma (RMS). The remainder, nonrhabdomyosarcoma soft-tissue sarcomas (NRSTS), are many types of heterogeneous origin that are individually rare. For both types, the male/female ratio is about 1.2:1 and the incidence in both blacks and whites is 8 to 9 per million.[64]

The emphasis of the remainder of this chapter is on RMS. The role of radiotherapy in the management of NRSTS is briefly discussed at the end of the chapter.

Etiology and Genetics of Rhabdomyosarcoma

An environmental factors study of 322 children enrolled in Intergroup Rhabdomyosarcoma Study (IRS)-III found that parental use of marijuana and cocaine in the year before a child's birth was highly correlated with the subsequent diagnosis of RMS. The risk was greater (fivefold) for maternal use of cocaine.[65]

The normal development from uncommitted mesenchymal cell to myoblast (myogenesis) and its aberration to malignancy is being elucidated. Myogenic transcription factors are a group of DNA-binding proteins that bind to promoter regions for muscle-specific genes and promote their expression. Several of these factors (MyoD, Myf5, myogenin) are variably expressed in RMS and therefore help to identify a small, blue, round cell tumor without characteristic phenotypic features as RMS and not as another sarcoma such as extraosseous Ewing's sarcoma. Defects in the normal pathway are associated with the two major histologic subtypes of RMS: embryonal and alveolar. The embryonal type correlates with loss of heterozygosity at chromosome 11p15.5, with presumed loss of a tumor suppressor locus.[66,67] The alveolar subtype features a translocation t(2;13) (q35;q14) that results in the fusion of normally unassociated transcription factors (PAX 3) and the activation domain of FKHR. A variant translocation that produces the PAX 7-FKHR fusion transcript is associated with a better outcome.[68] A study of 45 tissue samples of RMS using comparative genomic hybridization and fluorescence in-situ hybridization methods demonstrated that genomic gains and losses were similar in alveolar and embryonal histologies, and that they did not differ between the two alveolar fusion transcript subtypes. Both histologies had a one-in-four rate of genomic amplification, which, for the embryonal subtype, was most common in those with anaplastic features. One locus of amplification included the gene for insulin-like growth factor type 1 receptor, which has been implicated in the induction of RMS.[69]

The cancer family syndrome of Li-Fraumeni includes childhood RMS and NRSTS and is characterized by the p53 suppressor gene germ line mutation.[70]

Pathology

An international committee of pathologists expert in RMS reviewed the histology of 800 randomly chosen cases from IRS-II.[71] The resulting classification retains the basic division between the embryonal and alveolar subtypes, omits the formerly used pleomorphic subtype, and further refines the embryonal category as follows: favorable prognosis, botryoid embryonal and spindle cell (SC) embryonal; intermediate prognosis, all other embryonal; and unfavorable prognosis, all alveolar subtypes (includes cases with any alveolar component) and undifferentiated sarcoma. Examples are shown in Figures 55-2B through F.

There are several anatomic site associations for the histologic types of RMS. The botryoid tumor occurs in the bladder and vagina, usually in infants and younger children, and 31% of SC variant cases occur in the paratesticular site. Other sites are head and neck, orbit, and extremity.[72] About half of patients have an embryonal type that is seen at every site. Alveolar RMS predominates in extremity and truncal sites. A rare, unfavorable variant containing anaplastic cells is found

most often in lower extremity, retroperitoneum/pelvis, and paratesticular sites.[73] Whether histology is an independent prognostic factor is uncertain. The IRS staging system uses primary site in preference to histology; however, all nonmetastatic patients with alveolar histology are assigned to the intermediate risk trial of IRS-V. The distribution of histologic types on IRS-IV for nonmetastatic patients was: embryonal, 70%; alveolar, 20%; undifferentiated sarcoma, 4%; and other, 6%.[74]

Clinical Presentation

Males with RMS predominate in the ratio of 3:2; and in IRS-I the race distribution was white, 80%; black, 12%; and other, 8%.[75] Median age at presentation is 5 years, and the distribution on IRS-III was less than 1 year, 6%; and less than 10 years, 66%.[76] The proportion of all patients presenting with dissemination is 17%.[77]

Symptoms at presentation relate to anatomic site of the primary tumor. Primary site distribution is shown in Figure 55-1. The parameningeal site is composed of four sites: nasopharynx/nasal cavity, paranasal sinuses, middle ear/mastoid, and infratemporal space/pterygopalatine fossa. Symptoms from a parameningeal primary tumor are protean and include cranial nerve palsy, facial pain and swelling, meningeal irritation, nasal voice, mouth breathing, trismus, and painless adenopathy.[78] Parameningeal primary tumors may erode skull base bone, transgress the dura, and invade brain; however, subarachnoid space dissemination is an uncommon event at diagnosis. Orbital tumors present with unilateral proptosis, chemosis, impaired mobility, ptosis, and lid or conjunctival mass.[79] The other head and neck lesions present as a superficial mass that may cause seventh nerve palsy if arising in the parotid region or a mass lesion that interferes with speech or swallowing.

The second most frequent primary site is genitourinary (23%) divided between bladder/prostate (11%) and other genitourinary sites (female genital tract and paratesticular) (12%).[75] The typical presentation is of bladder distention or outlet obstruction. The sarcoma botryoides may protrude from the vagina. The paratesticular presentation is as a painless mass. Next in frequency are extremity lesions (17%), which present with an enlarging, usually painless mass.

The remaining 25% of tumors are distributed among several sites including thorax, trunk, and intra-abdominal (including retroperitoneum). The history is usually of silent growth and presentation of a large mass associated with obstructive symptoms.

Routes of Spread

RMS is usually locally invasive and therefore frequently unresectable. In IRS-II patients with nonmetastatic tumor at presentation, 64% had only a biopsy or subtotal resection, approximately 20% had microscopic residual disease, and 16% had complete resection.[77] Lymphatic spread occurs. A retrospective review of IRS-I and IRS-II patients in clinical groups I and II provided data on lymphatic metastasis in 592 cases. Nodal spread was not influenced by gender, age, or histology. It was influenced by site as follows: prostate, 41%; paratesticular, 26%; extremity, 12%; trunk, 3%; head and neck, 7%; orbit, none; and all sites, 14%.[80] The inclusion of group I patients in the denominator minimizes the estimate of nodal involvement.

At presentation, 17% of IRS-II patients had hematogenous metastases (most common) or, less frequently, involvement of distant lymph node groups or malignant pleural or peritoneal effusion. Hematogenous metastases occur most frequently in lung. Both bone and bone marrow metastases are common.[81] Unusual sites (e.g., heart, breast, and subcutaneous tissues) can occur.[82,83] Brain metastases at diagnosis are rare.[84] The pattern and frequency of metastatic sites for IRS-IV patients are shown in Table 55-2.

Diagnostic and Staging Studies

Patients with RMS require diagnostic studies that consist of both standard and site-specific assessments. In addition to the routine history, detailed family history of cancer should be obtained. In addition to the routine physical examination, an examination under anesthesia may be required for genitourinary presentations, and direct nasopharyngoscopy and laryngoscopy may be needed for upper airway primary tumors. Routine blood cell count and a standard chemistry assay are done. Renal function is assessed. Detailed assessment of the primary tumor with MRI or CT is required to determine location, invasiveness, and size. For orbit and parameningeal primary sites, the MRI should include the brain to characterize intracranial extension. Sagittal and coronal views are useful for radiotherapy planning.[85] For genitourinary primary tumors, the entire urinary tract should be imaged with MRI or CT. Studies to assess dissemination include abdominal and chest CT and bone scan.[86] Bone marrow aspirate and biopsy are required, as is lumbar puncture for cerebrospinal fluid examination (chemistry and cytology) for parameningeal sites.

Before starting radiotherapy, children with head and neck sites should have evaluation by a dentist familiar with the effects of radiotherapy and who can supervise a program of dental prophylaxis. For patients with extremity lesions, a physical therapist should be consulted early in the course of treatment to determine the need for and to supervise a rehabilitation program.

Table 55–2   Pattern of Metastases, IRS-IV, Group IV

Metastatic Sites	%	Number of Sites	%
Lung	39	1	59
Bone Marrow	32	2	20
Lymph Nodes	30	3	16
Bone	27	4 or more	5
Omentum/Ascites	16		
Soft Tissue	16		

From Breneman JC, Lyden E, Pappo AS, et al: Prognostic factors and clinical outcome in children and adolescents with metastatic rhabdomyosarcoma—A report from the Intergroup Rhabdomyosarcoma Study IV. *J Clin Oncol.* 2003;21:78.

Table 55–3   Intergroup Rhabdomyosarcoma Study Clinical Group Classification

Group I	Localized disease, completely resected
a	Confined to muscle or organ of origin
b	Contiguous involvement—infiltration outside the muscle or organ of origin; as through fascial planes
Group II	Total gross resection with evidence of regional spread
a	Grossly resected tumor with microscopic residual disease; no evidence of regional nodal involvement
b	Regional disease with involved nodes, completely resected with no microscopic residual disease
c	Regional disease with involved nodes, grossly resected, but with evidence of microscopic residual disease and/or histologic involvement of the most distal regional node (from the primary site) in the dissection
Group III	Incomplete resection or biopsy with gross residual disease
Group IV	Distant metastases at diagnosis

Staging System

In the United States, 80% to 85% of patients with RMS are entered on the IRS trials, which have been ongoing since 1972. The IRS grouping system for classifying patients in prognostic categories and for determining therapy is thus a *de facto* national standard. The IRS groups are described in Table 55-3. The system, which is surgical/pathologic, assesses extent of resection for patients with localized disease. It is clearly prognostic for treatment outcome but does not account for the variation in surgical aggressiveness as a first therapeutic event. Accordingly, the IRS committee designed a pretreatment staging system that separately categorizes the primary tumor (T), the regional nodal status (N), the presence of metastases (M), and the primary anatomic site. The system (Table 55-4) was retrospectively assessed and found to be of prognostic significance and to be reproducible.[87,88] The TNM system was evaluated prospectively in IRS-III and was used to assign treatment in IRS-IV. The pretreatment staging system uses five features to determine stage: (1) primary site, (2) primary tumor invasiveness, (3) size, (4) nodal status, and (5) metastases. Primary sites are divided into favorable—orbit, nonparameningeal head and neck, biliary, and

Table 55–4   IRS Pretreatment Staging System

Stage	Site*	Invasiveness	Size	Nodal Status	Metastases
1	Favorable	T1 or T2	a or b	N0 or N1	M0
2	Unfavorable	T1 or T2	a	N0	M0
3	Unfavorable	T1 or T2	b	N0	M0
			a or b	N1	M0
4	Any site	T1 or T2	a or b	N0 or N1	M1

*Favorable sites: orbit, head and neck (nonparameningeal), genitourinary (non–bladder-prostate), biliary tract; unfavorable sites: genitourinary (bladder-prostate), extremity, parameningeal, other.

a, 5 cm or less; b, more than 5 cm; M0, no distant metastasis; M1, evidence of distant metastasis; N0, no evidence of regional node involvement; N1, evidence of regional node involvement; T1, tumor confined to site or organ of origin; T2, regional extension beyond the site or organ of origin.

Table 55–5   Standard VAC for Intermediate Risk* Patients Over Age 3 on IRS-V

		Induction					Continuation	
		VAC	V	RT	VC		VAC	V
Week	0		1, 2			Week	24, 27	
	3		4, 5				30	31, 32
	6		7, 8				33	34, 35
	9		10, 11				36, 39	
	12			12-18	15, 18			
			19, 20					
	21		22, 23					

*Intermediate risk: alveolar, stage 1, 2, and 3; groups I, II, and III. Embryonal, stage 2 and 3; group III. Embryonal, stage 4; group IV, age younger than 10. A, actinomycin D 0.045 mg/kg IV; C, cyclophosphamide 2.2 g/m^2 IV; RT, radiation therapy; V, vincristine 1.5 mg/m^2 IV.

genitourinary (but not bladder or prostate); and unfavorable—all others including bladder/prostate, extremity, and parameningeal. Invasiveness categories are T1, confined to anatomic site of origin, and T2, extension or fixation to surrounding tissues. T stage data are obtained, but they do not alter stage assignment. Size, rather than T stage, was believed to be a more reliable parameter and therefore affects stage assignment. Size (maximum tumor diameter) is divided into two categories: a, less than or equal to 5 cm; and b, greater than 5 cm. Nodal status is determined clinically: N0 indicates regional nodes clinically *uninvolved*, and N1 indicates regional nodes clinically *involved*. M staging assignment is M0, no distant metastases; and M1, indicating that metastases are present, often hematogenous, and including distant lymph nodes, pleural or peritoneal dissemination (or malignant effusion), and cytologically positive cerebrospinal fluid.

Standard Therapy

SURGERY

Treatment of RMS is multidisciplinary. The role of surgery in the therapeutic strategy is, in part, driven by primary site location. Many primary tumors are technically unresectable by virtue of site, size, and invasiveness. Resection of others would entail organ sacrifice, limb amputation, or cosmetic disfigurement. Among localized patients on IRS-IV, 62% of patients were in this category (group III). The use of surgery as a first therapeutic maneuver yielded margins as follows: group I (clear margins), 23%; and group II (microscopically positive margins), 15%.[74] Control of the primary site requires adjuvant radiotherapy for group II patients and definitive radiotherapy for the largest subset, group III. A subset of patients with incomplete resection (node-negative, group II) may be amenable to elective re-excision of the primary site before starting other treatment to achieve negative margins and thus restrict management to a group I approach. When this strategy was followed for patients with trunk and extremity primary tumors in IRS-I and IRS-II, there was an apparent survival benefit.[89] In addition to the initial diagnostic and therapeutic role for

surgery, the regression that occurs with induction chemotherapy (± radiotherapy) may render some group III primary tumors resectable. This opportunity was studied in IRS-III. A group of 83 patients (primary sites: extremity, trunk, retroperitoneum) had a second-look surgical procedure after induction chemotherapy and radiotherapy; 20% had complete resection of their initially unresected primary tumor. In addition, approximately 60% of partial responders and nonresponders had specimens from their second-look procedure consistent with pathologic complete response (E. Wiener, MD, personal communication).

CHEMOTHERAPY

Chemotherapy is essential since all patients with M0 stage disease are assumed to have occult metastatic spread. For all patients, multiagent chemotherapy is started postoperatively and when staging is complete and precedes radiotherapy. Virtually all patients will achieve at least a good partial response, which may facilitate radiotherapy planning.

The most effective chemotherapeutic agents for RMS are vincristine, actinomycin D, and cyclophosphamide (VAC). The schema and drug doses for VAC as used in the intermediate-risk IRS-V trial are shown in Table 55-5. That study compares VAC to a regimen wherein topotecan (a topoisomerase I inhibitor) replaces actinomycin. Irinotecan (CPT-11), also a topoisomerase I inhibitor, is being evaluated in a phase II, "upfront window" study of stage IV patients enrolled in IRS-V.

ROLE OF RADIOTHERAPY

Radiotherapy is not required for the patient with embryonal RMS who has surgery at diagnosis that yields negative margins and is node negative (group I).[75] Postoperative adjuvant radiotherapy is given to group I patients with alveolar histology and all group II patients.[90] Definitive radiotherapy is required for group III patients. It is also given with curative intent to the primary site in group IV patients along with treatment, when feasible, to metastatic sites (except bone marrow). An exception to the use of radiotherapy is for patients with vulvar or vaginal primary tumors (node negative, embryonal, group III) who have a second-look operation after induction chemotherapy, resulting in negative margins. The IRS-V protocol recommends withholding radiotherapy. There are no data to invalidate that recommendation.

Simulation

RMS occurs in every anatomic site, and the details of simulation and planning are site dependent. For all patients, whether or not sedation is required, immobilization in a reproducible, comfortable position is essential. Plaster of Paris, thermoplastic polymer, or vacuum-evacuated styrofoam bead bags are useful. Patient laser-beam setup points should be translated in the appropriate plane to the immobilization device to ensure reproducible positioning. Most patients can be positioned supine. For treatment of head and neck sites, a younger child should be elevated (below the neck) over the simulator table 2 to 3 inches to allow the neck to be extended. This will move structures of the oral cavity farther away from the thyroid gland and the pharynx. Principles for positioning and immobilizing a patient with a primary tumor of an extremity are the same as for Ewing's sarcoma. CT-based simulation is essential for three-dimensional treatment planning.[91] Sedation or anesthesia is required for many children younger than age 3.[92] A reward-based training and desensitization program by an experienced nurse will enable children in the 3- to 9-year age group to cooperate.[93]

Radiotherapy Plan

Many children with localized RMS will have had resection, exploratory surgery, or endoscopic evaluation. Data in the operation note, in addition to placement of radiopaque clips intraoperatively, should supplement the reconstruction of the GTV (time of diagnosis) from plain films, CT, and MRI scans. The CTV has a margin of 1.5 cm around the GTV. Adjacent lymphatic channels are not treated prophylactically. When involved, anatomic lymphatic pathways and regions are treated in contiguity with the primary tumor. This may not be feasible for primary tumors of an extremity. Patients with bladder/prostate tumors may present with gross bladder distention. The entire bladder is included in the CTV; however, the resolution that follows chemotherapy will allow the CTV to be reduced to the bladder's postinduction volume. Preradiotherapy CT or MRI is necessary for planning. Similarly, other lesions that displace bladder, lung, or intestine with a pushing, rather than an invasive, margin may also allow reduction of GTV based on chemotherapy-induced tumor response. Planned field reductions (cone-downs) are not used except to avoid exceeding the tolerances described later in the section on critical normal tissues. These reductions should reflect prior tumor response and may permit the usage of beam paths not employed initially as a method of minimizing normal tissue dose.

Patients with parameningeal primary tumors may have intracranial extension. This usually represents displacement of dura rather than brain parenchymal invasion. A 1.5-cm margin (CTV) above this extension is appropriate. Whole cranial radiotherapy is not needed unless there is evidence of hematogenous metastases, diffusely involved meninges, or cytologically positive cerebrospinal fluid (in which case, spinal subarachnoid space radiotherapy is required). Figure 55-6 shows the MRI and IMRT isodose plan for a child with parameningeal RMS arising in the pterygoid space.

Planning should always attempt to exclude cornea, lenses, and pituitary for orbit lesions. It may be possible to exclude only the pituitary from one beam of a wedged pair, but this may be sufficient to avoid hypothalamic/pituitary insufficiency. A proton beam plan elegantly excludes extra-orbital normal structures.[94] For a primary tumor of an extremity, inclusion of muscle from origin to insertion is not necessary. Figure 55-7 illustrates the combination of postoperative brachytherapy and external-beam radiotherapy for a 2-year-old boy with embryonal RMS of the right soleus muscle. Pleural or peritoneal involvement or malignant effusion requires that the initial port cover the hemithorax or entire peritoneal surface, respectively. For primary pelvic tumors, careful attention must be paid to the caudal (perineal) margin because it may not always be clearly seen on axial imaging studies.

Radiotherapy for group III patients on IRS-IV was a randomized comparison between an experimental arm (hyperfractionated RT) and a standard fractionation control arm.[95] No survival or local control advantage accrued to the twice-a-day radiotherapy patients and it was concluded that once-a-day fractionation remains the standard of care: Group III patients are treated once per day, all fields each session, 5 days per week, 1.8 Gy/fraction, total 50.4 Gy. Large volumes may be treated with a reduced daily dose of 1.5 Gy. The IRS-V protocol addresses the role of "second-look" surgery after 12 weeks of chemotherapy for most group III patients. Those patients with sufficient response to induction chemotherapy may have surgery if it is anticipated that form and function will be maintained and that surgical margins will be clear. The postoperative radiotherapy dose is reduced as determined by the margin status: negative margins, 36 Gy; microscopically involved margins, 41.4 Gy. For gross residual tumor, the total dose is maintained at 50.4 Gy. Patients not qualifying for second-look surgery can also have dose reduction to 41.4 Gy if they have clinical and biopsy evidence of complete response; otherwise, they receive 50.4 Gy.

In IRS-V, radiotherapy for group I patients (embryonal histology) is not given whereas it is for alveolar histology patients (41.4 Gy). Group II patients also receive 41.4 Gy if node positive and 36 Gy if node negative. Patients in group IV receive a daily and total dose to the primary tumor that would be used in the absence of dissemination (if a "local" group I, II, or III). Total dose to metastatic sites is 50.4 Gy, but should also account for the constraints of normal tissue tolerance (see Table 55-6).

Brachytherapy

Use of brachytherapy is restricted by the invasive character of localized RMS and the issues of confinement and nursing care for a radioactive child. The foremost proponent of brachytherapy has been the group at Institut Gustave-Roussy in Villejuif, France. Their early experience with small, subcutaneous sites (e.g., lip, nasolabial fold, perineum) led them to treat vagina and other gynecologic sites and head and neck sites. The technique was usually after loading ^{192}Ir at about 0.50 Gy/h to an average total of 60.8 Gy (pelvic sites) and 64 Gy (head and neck, perineum, extremities). Three fourths of patients had RMS. The survival rate of the entire group was 78%.[96] In an update that excluded pelvic primary sites, the 5-year local failure-free survival (FFS) rate was 66% in 72 children. There was a need for cosmetic rehabilitation in 24%, mainly for head and neck sites.[97] The same group achieved bladder preservation (mean dose 52 Gy) in 8 of 12 patients with bladder/prostate

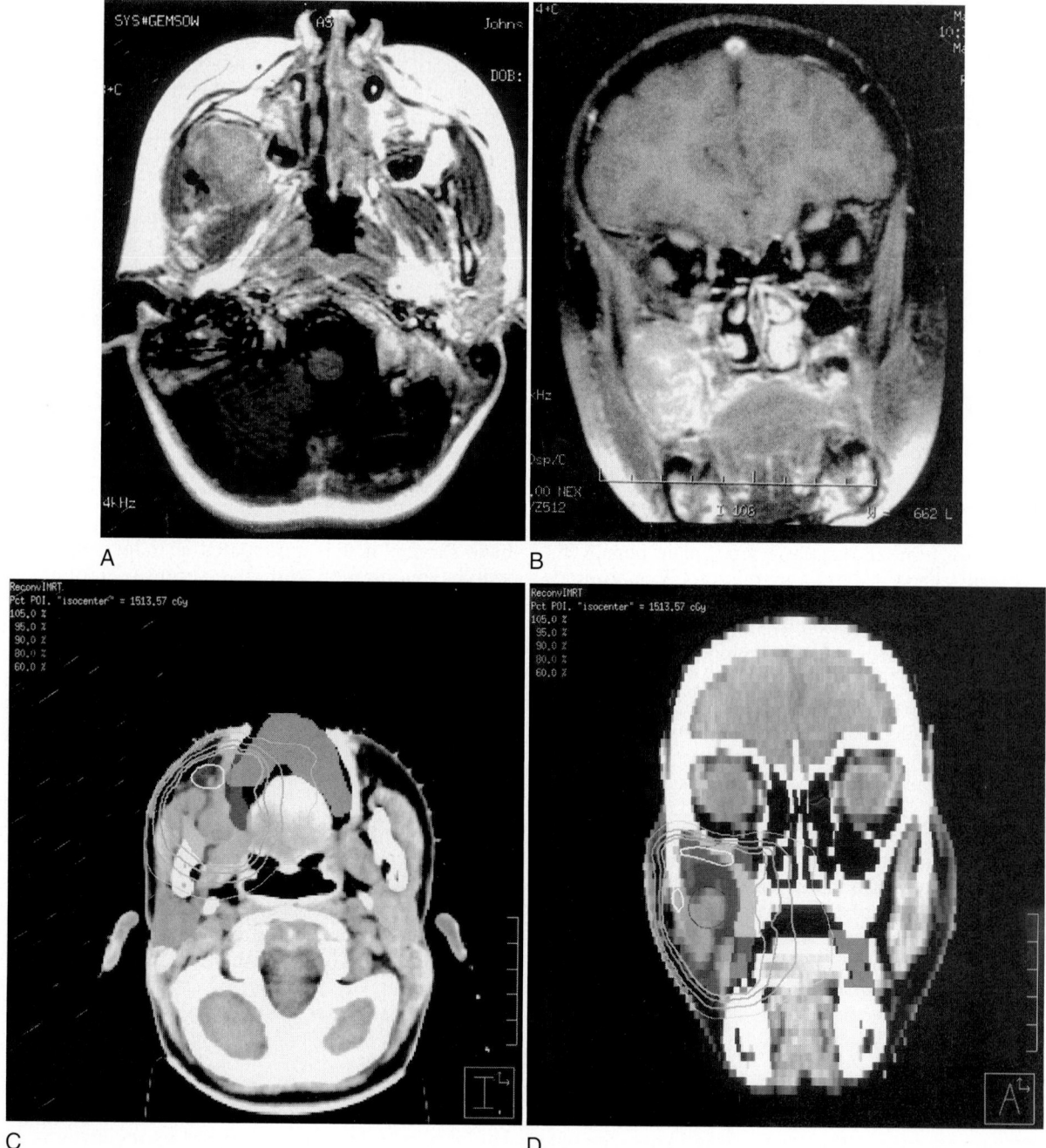

Figure 55–6. Eight-year-old male with a parameningeal rhabdomyosarcoma arising in the right pterygoid space. **A,** Axial and **B,** coronal magnetic resonance imaging scans at diagnosis. After 12 weeks of induction chemotherapy, his initial plan delivered 36 Gy to the gross target volume (GTV) plus 2 cm using a conformal, noncoplanar plan. **C,** Reduced field plan (axial view) to the initial GTV plus 1 to 1.5 cm using intensity-modulated radiation therapy. A dental prosthesis pushes the tongue posteriorly. The child is immobilized in a plastic facial cast. **D,** Coronal dose distribution. The depicted isodose curves (central to peripheral) are: 95%, 90%, 80%, and 60%. Total dose, 50.4 Gy at 1.8 Gy/fraction. (**C** and **D,** courtesy Terrance Teslow, PhD.). See also Color Figure 55-6C and D.

RMS. They recommend their approach in patients with tumor size of 4 cm or less.[98] Although late sequelae requiring surgical correction in vulvar and vaginal RMS occur, the French group reports successful childbearing in 2 of 17 patients.[99]

The University of Amsterdam group reports an intraoperative mold technique for head and neck sites. The mold is placed operatively in the surgical defect, and thereafter brachytherapy is accomplished using ^{192}Ir over 50 to 70 hours (dose, 40 to 50 Gy). Surgical removal

and plastic closure follows. Good healing and encouraging early cosmetic outcome were reported; however, 5 of 15 patients failed locally.[100]

The development of the remote afterloading high-dose-rate brachytherapy device preserves for pediatric patients the normal tissue-sparing advantage and eliminates the problem of nursing care for the radioactive child. It also permits the use of fractionated brachytherapy. Investigators at Ohio State University have used a regimen of 3 Gy twice a day (total dose, 36 Gy) to the postinduction

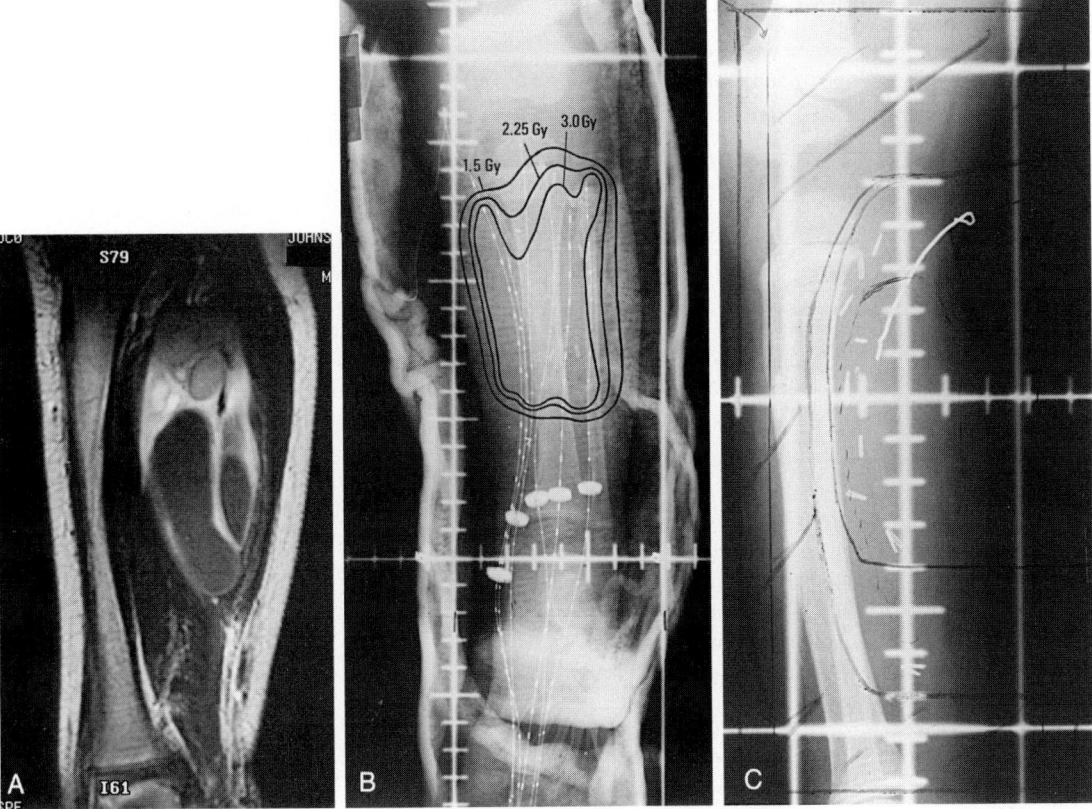

Figure 55–7. Twenty-two-month-old male with embryonal rhabdomyosarcoma of the right soleus muscle. **A,** Sagittal magnetic resonance imaging at diagnosis. **B,** After a partial response to induction chemotherapy, the tumor was conservatively resected. Surgical clips demarcate the gross tumor volume in the posterior-anterior simulator film. Also shown are blind-ended brachytherapy catheters that were used on postoperative day 5 for high-dose-rate brachytherapy. The isodose curves are superimposed. The child received treatments twice daily (3 Gy each at a 6-hour interval) on 3 consecutive days. **C,** Twelve days after the brachytherapy boost was completed, external-beam irradiation was initiated to the original GTV with a 1-cm margin. The patient's simulation film demonstrates that gantry rotation was done to align the tibia and fibula. This permitted inclusion of the posterior compartment using parallel-opposed beams. The external beam dose was 30 Gy.

chemotherapy volume. Patients were treated for primary tumors of the tongue, buccal mucosa, chest wall, clitoris, and vagina.[101] The indications for brachytherapy are evolving.[102] Conservative indications include group III patients with good response to induction chemotherapy and small residual tumor volume (see Fig. 55-7), and group II patients with an initial GTV less than 5 cm, with primary tumors in sites such as extremity, superficial trunk, scalp and face, oral cavity and oropharynx, uterus/vagina/vulva, and bladder/prostate. It may also be used after less than full-dose external-beam radiotherapy as a volume-restricted tumor bed boost.

Critical Normal Tissues

The growing normal tissues of a pediatric RMS patient should be shielded whenever possible, consistent with sufficient margin about the GTV. Examples of common problems include protection of contralateral lens (*always*), ipsilateral lens (*if possible*), and pituitary in patients with orbital and other head and neck tumors; unerupted molars in patients with head and neck tumors; larynx and thyroid gland when treating neck adenopathy; female breast buds when thorax lesions are present; epiphyseal growth plates and joints in extremity primary

tumor sites; kidneys in lower paravertebral sites; capital femoral epiphyses and rectum in pelvic sites; and the small intestine in abdominal sites. When a high dose of radiation to the abdomen is required, temporary surgically implanted tissue expanders to displace bowel should be considered. Controlled iatrogenic pneumothorax to avoid radiation pneumonitis has been successfully used for primary chest wall tumors.[103]

Tolerance doses as recommended in IRS-V using daily fractions of 1.8 Gy are listed in Table 55-6. These general guidelines may require modification for very young patients or those with a large CTV. For example, 45 Gy to a large volume of small intestine, particularly in a postlaparotomy patient, may lead to radiation enteritis or small bowel obstruction.

Outcome

Five-year survival of all patients in the IRS studies has shown improvement: IRS-I, 56%; IRS-II, 63%; and IRS-III, 72%. The 3-year FFS rate for nonmetastatic patients on IRS-IV was 77% (IRS-III, 76%). The pattern of failure (3-year cumulative incidence) was: local, 10%; regional, 4%; and distant, 7%. Prognostic factors for 3-year FFS included clinical group: I, 83%; II, 86%; and

Table 55–6 Normal Tissue Tolerance with Conventional Fractionation

Organ	Total Dose, Gy
Kidney	14.4
Whole liver	23.4
Bilateral lungs	14.4
Whole brain	
>3 yr	30.6
<3 yr	23.4
Optic nerve and chiasm	46.8
Spinal cord	45
Gastrointestinal tract	45
Whole abdomen and pelvis	30 at 1.50/day
Heart	30.6
Lens	14.4
Lacrimal gland/cornea	41.4

III, 73%. Also, age: younger than 1 year, 55%; 1 to 9, 83%; and 10 and older, 68%. Outcome by histology and risk group is shown in Table 55-7.[74] IRS-IV patients with metastatic disease (group IV) had 3-year FFS of 25%; however, a favorable subset with embryonal histology, age younger than 10 years, and one or two metastatic sites had 3-year FFS of 45%.[104]

The failure pattern for group II patients enrolled on IRS-I to IV was assessed: local failure, 8%; regional, 4%; and distant, 14%.[105] Local control in group III patients varies with site. The 5-year estimate of cumulative local failure risk on IRS-IV was: orbit, 5%; head and neck, 12%; parameningeal, 16%; bladder/prostate, 19%; extremity, 7%; and other sites, 14%.[95]

The special problems in management of infants younger than age 1 have been reviewed and the impact of age on outcome has been variable. Data to support omission of RT are lacking.[106-109] In general, there is a greater reliance on second-look surgery, and brachytherapy is encouraged.

The late sequelae of radiotherapy are site related and have been reviewed by Heyn.[110] Specific, site-related reports are noted in the following section. The risk for second malignant neoplasms in 1026 survivors enrolled on IRS-I and IRS-II was 1.7% at 10 years. Treatment with both an alkylating agent plus radiotherapy, compared with only one, carried increased risk, and a contributing factor was a family history of neurofibromatosis or Li-Fraumeni syndrome.[111] The 20-year cumulative risk of second malignant neoplasms in 4367 patients on IRS-I-IV

Table 55–7 Three-year Failure-Free Survival Rate for IRS-IV Patients (Without Metastases) by Risk Group and Histology

Histology	Risk Group*	
	Low	Intermediate
Embryonal	93%	76%
Alveolar/Undifferentiated	72%	55%

*Low risk: stage 1, clinical groups I, II, III; and stage 2 and 3, clinical groups I and II. Intermediate risk: stage 2 and 3, clinical group III.
From Crist WM, Anderson JR, Meza JL, et al: Intergroup Rhabdomyosarcoma Study-IV: Results for patients with nonmetastatic disease. *J Clin Oncol.* 2001;19:3091.

was 3.5%. Secondary leukemia/lymphoma and sarcoma were equally likely.[112]

Outcome by Site

HEAD AND NECK

The orbit is the most common single head and neck site for RMS. The history of improved outcome of these patients has been reviewed by Sagerman.[113] Patients with orbital tumors enrolled in IRS-I and II had 3-year local control of 94%.[114] For 186 patients enrolled on IRS studies through 1992, the 10-year EFS was 86%.[115] An early review of IRS-IV suggested improved 3-year EFS compared to IRS-III.[116] Five-year survival for patients with alveolar histology was 74%.[117] The recommended total dose is 45 Gy. A European cooperative group trial omitted radiotherapy for patients achieving complete remission with chemotherapy and 38% avoided radiotherapy; however, one third of patients failed locally with a 4-year EFS of 62%.[118] Late effects have been tabulated for patients on IRS-I: 90% had decreased vision, usually secondary to cataract formation; half of patients had facial asymmetry; and 61% had decreased stature due to radiotherapy.[119] Growth impairment was 24% for IRS-III patients, possibly reflecting improved treatment planning.[120]

Tumors of the four parameningeal sites are half of all head and neck primaries. An early IRS report noted that the pattern of failure in these patients included meningeal extension in 35% and that outcome thereafter was fatal in 90%.[121] Subsequent single-institution reports found a lesser risk.[122-123] The IRS strategy was altered in 1977 to include whole cranial prophylactic radiotherapy and intrathecal chemotherapy for patients who had cranial nerve palsy, skull base erosion, or intracranial extension. In addition, radiotherapy began concurrently with chemotherapy. Three-year survival improved from 41% to 68% and by site was: middle ear/mastoid, 73%; nasopharynx/nasal cavity, 69%; infratemporal fossa, 68%; and paranasal sinuses, 60%.[124] The subsequent IRS trials omitted prophylactic intrathecal methotrexate and cranial and spinal radiotherapy without a decline in outcome. Five-year EFS was influenced by histology and impingement of the primary tumor on adjacent meninges: alveolar and impingement present, 48%; embryonal and not present, 81%.[125] A trial was conducted to eliminate radiotherapy in patients under age 3. With intensified chemotherapy, only 11% avoided radiotherapy or radical surgery.[126] The remaining 25% of patients with head and neck RMS have involvement of the scalp, pinnae, face, parotid region, masseter muscle, cheek, buccal mucosa, oral cavity, oropharynx, hypopharynx, and larynx. Eighty-nine patients without metastases in IRS-I and IRS-II had a 3-year survival rate of 83%. Local control for the patients who received at least 40 Gy was 93%.[127]

An analysis of late effects of therapy in 213 patients with parameningeal and other nonorbital head and neck sites revealed growth retardation in 48%, with 19% receiving growth hormone. Facial and mandibular bone hypoplasia developed in 35%, of whom a fifth had reconstructive surgery. Other sequelae included poor dentition, decreased vision and hearing, and poor school performance.[128]

GENITOURINARY SITES

The treatment approach for patients with bladder/prostate tumors on IRS-I relied on radical surgery. In IRS-II, induction chemotherapy was used to delay radiotherapy or reduce radiotherapy dose. In each study, the proportion of patients alive and with a functional bladder at 3 years was about 23%.[129] For IRS-III, standard dose radiotherapy (45 Gy) was given at week 6. The proportion of patients alive with a functional bladder at 3 years was 60%.[130] The presence of postradiation maturing rhabdomyoblasts led to possibly unnecessary cystectomy in some IRS-III patients.[131] About 20% of bladder primary patients may have tumor confined to the bladder dome.[132] Forty such patients in IRS-I and IRS-II had partial cystectomy and 31 survived (24 bladder symptom-free). The benefit of radiotherapy was uncertain.[133]

Late sequelae in patients with bladder/prostate RMS were assessed in 54 patients with bladder preservation of 109 survivors enrolled on IRS-I and IRS-II. Bladder function was satisfactory in 73% of patients. Renal dysfunction and hypertension were uncommon. There was statural growth retardation in 10%.[134]

Paratesticular RMS is characterized by relatively early diagnosis, a predominance of embryonal histology (93%), and a 27% proportion of the more favorable SC variant histology. The patients with SC variant were more likely to be group I or II compared with the non-SC types (98% vs. 80%) and less likely to involve lymph nodes (16% vs. 36%). The overall rate of nodal involvement (determined pathologically) was 31%.[72] Retroperitoneal lymph node dissection was required for IRS-III, but not IRS-IV, which resulted in an increase in the proportion of IRS-IV patients in clinical group I. These patients therefore did not receive nodal radiotherapy and experienced a decrease in 3-year failure-free survival which was worse in boys age 10 and older: IRS-III, 78%; IRS-IV, 68%. The recommendation for retroperitoneal lymph node dissection was re-instituted for boys age 10 and older for IRS-V.[135] Group IV patients can have a protracted natural history, and cure is possible. The 3-year survival rate is 64%.[136,137] Radiotherapy should therefore be given to nodal and other metastatic sites as recommended for group IV patients.

Late sequelae attributable to radiotherapy in 86 IRS-I and IRS-II survivors included testicular dysfunction when testis shielding was not used, bone and soft tissue hypoplasia, and four instances of chronic diarrhea in 37 patients. Bladder function was unaffected by radiotherapy.[138] Another report confirmed the risk of gastrointestinal sequelae and impaired statural growth.[139]

The IRS protocols I-IV included 151 girls with genital tract primary tumors. Fifty-four percent occurred in the vagina, 64% were group III, and 87% were embryonal/ botryoid histology. Five-year survival was 87% for nonmetastatic patients, but was better (98%) for girls 1 to 9 years old. Radiation therapy was used in less than one third of patients.[140] Surgical resection for vaginal primaries has declined from IRS-I (100%) to IRS-IV (13%).[141] One third of girls enrolled in trials conducted by SIOP were cured with chemotherapy alone. The authors noted the efficacy of brachytherapy when local therapy was required.[142] Late effects were assessed in 12 girls who had attained pubertal age. Normal puberty occurred in 11, and 2 had three children. There were vaginal or other sequelae as follows: none in five; minimal in three who required surgery to allow intercourse; and serious in four (colorectal, vaginal, urethral, and ureteral stenosis).[99]

EXTREMITY SITES

Among 102 patients with an extremity primary tumor in IRS-I, 44% were of alveolar histology (25 of 48 in groups III and IV).[143] The 5-year survival in IRS-III was 74%.[76] In IRS-IV, 76 of 139 patients had surgical evaluation of regional lymph nodes and 38 (50%) were positive. The 5-year FFS for node-positive patients was 35% compared to 70% for node-negative patients.[144] The efficacy of radiation therapy in the control of node metastases from extremity primaries was demonstrated in IRS-II.[145] The local failure rate in Group III patients on IRS-IV was 7%.[95]

OTHER SITES

Thirty-six patients with primary tumors in the perineum were treated in IRS-I and IRS-II. For groups II and III, the number failing locally and 3-year survival rates were 2 of 11 and 46% in group II and 5 of 15 and 37% in group III.[146] RMS of the chest and abdominal wall was reported in 20 patients on IRS-I. Disease-free survival was attained in 6 of 11 (chest wall) and 2 of 9 (abdominal wall) patients.[147] Four teenage females have been enrolled on IRS protocols to 1992 with primary, locoregional breast RMS. All survive.[148] RMS in the paraspinal soft tissue was greater than 5 cm in diameter in half of patients and, in 55% of cases in IRS-I and IRS-II, was either undifferentiated histology or extraosseous Ewing's sarcoma. Fifty-six percent of patients required laminectomy for spinal cord compression at the time of diagnosis. Local or regional failure was a component of failure in 12 of 27 relapse patients.[149] Intrathoracic primary tumors (mediastinum, lung, pleura) occurred in 17 IRS-I and IRS-II patients. The benefit of radiotherapy was inconclusive.[150] Intra-abdominal RMS occurs in various sites. Embryonal or botryoid histology was present in 24 of 25 patients with a biliary tract RMS, and 17 were disease free. Aggressive surgery was not necessary and these patients are considered a "favorable" site in the IRS staging system.[151] Gastric RMS may present as an unknown primary lesion.[152] Radiotherapy contributed to survival in a report of hepatic RMS.[153] There were 101 patients enrolled on IRS-I and IRS-II with a retroperitoneal primary tumor. The median tumor size was 10 cm, and there was local or regional failure in 60% of evaluable patients. Five-year survival was 30%.[154]

NONRHABDOMYOSARCOMA SOFT TISSUE SARCOMA

Single-institution retrospective reviews of NRSTS report 5-year survival rates from 50% to 89%. Most confirm the substantial survival rate discrepancy between group I (IRS) patients (approximately 80%) and group III patients (12% to 30%).[155-162] In one report, 5-year relapse-free survival increased from 21% to 70% with postoperative radiotherapy (dose >45 Gy).[155] Another report showed the 5-year survival rate to vary by grade: low, 92%; high, 59%.[156] One series (*n* = 154) had the following site distribution: extremity, 45%; trunk, 35%; and head and neck, 15%. The primary site distribution compiled from five large series is depicted in Figure 55-1. The most common histology was synovial sarcoma (23%), followed by malignant fibrous histiocytoma and neurogenic sarcoma (16% each). Metastases were typically of trunk and lower extremity sites, whereas upper extremity tumors were usually in groups I or II (IRS). There was a strong correlation between invasiveness, histologic grade, and size greater than 5 cm, with, for example, a 12% disease-free survival rate in the 42% of patients with T2 lesions greater than 5 cm (all grades).[162] All of these studies confirm the lack of prognostic significance of primary site in contrast to RMS. A prospective trial conducted by the Pediatric Oncology Group concluded in 1994. There was no benefit of adjuvant chemotherapy for patients with NRSTS, group I or II (IRS), grade 1 or 2. Also, postoperative radiotherapy was not needed in group I patients, grade 1 or 2.[163,164]

The general principle for the use of postoperative radiotherapy in pediatric NRSTS is that it is indicated for the patient equivalent to IRS group II or III. For group I patients with clear but close margins, or uncertain margins, the adverse prognostic factors of higher T stage, larger size, and higher grade should influence the decision to treat. A report of 88 group I patients assessed outcome based on margin and grade. With margins less than 1 cm, high grade, and postoperative radiotherapy, none of seven recurred. Without radiotherapy, three of seven recurred. For 20 high-grade patients with margins of 1 cm or more, none received radiotherapy and four recurred.[165]

In a series of 121 group I and II children, factors predicting local failure were: positive surgical margins, intra-abdominal site, and omission of radiation therapy.[166] A report of local failure for group III patients showed improvement from 9 of 12 to 3 of 15 children when radiotherapy dose (median) was increased from 39.6 Gy to 59.4 Gy.[167]

For synovial sarcoma, histologic subtype (monophasic or biphasic) does not affect prognosis, but higher grade and size greater than 5 cm does. A multivariate analysis of 39 patients with localized synovial sarcoma demonstrated the significance of fusion transcript type on 5-year survival: *SYT-SSX2* (48%) *versus SYT-SSX1* (24%).[168] The 5-year survival for IRS group III and IV patients was 17% in one series that spanned 30 years but was 58% in a contemporary German cooperative group trial. In that trial, the median radiotherapy dose was 50 Gy and four of five patients not getting radiotherapy experienced local relapse.[169-171] Another report showed a reduced local failure rate with postoperative radiotherapy, but an unstated proportion were IRS group I.[172] The largest retrospective study of pediatric patients noted improved

overall survival in radiotherapy patients.[173] A high risk of local recurrence is associated with synovial sarcoma of pleuropulmonary primary site.[174]

Fibrosarcoma is usually low grade. In a series of 66 children, local recurrence was noted in one third, most of which were seen in the first 2 years (range, 1 month to 6 years). All patients with local recurrence had a positive margin, as did 46% of those with no recurrence.[175] A review of 110 children noted a metastasis rate of 7% in patients younger than age 5 despite a local recurrence rate of 43%. The metastatic rate in patients older than age 10 was 50%.[176] A related lesion of young adults, the desmoid tumor (aggressive fibromatosis), is occasionally seen in children. Definitive radiotherapy may be required for lesions of the shoulder girdle or head.[177-180] A dose of 50 to 55 Gy in standard fractions with generous margins is appropriate; however, alternative treatments including chemotherapy, hormonal therapy, and nonsteroidal anti-inflammatory drugs should be considered.[181-183]

Malignant fibrous histiocytoma occurred in the head and neck area in 6 of 16 children in two series. Postoperative radiotherapy (30 to 55 Gy) and chemotherapy were effective in three of five children.[184,185] A higher dose in a mainly adult series (60 Gy) resulted in a 68% (actuarial) rate of local control at 5 years.[186] The angiomatoid malignant fibrous histiocytoma is a variant seen in the age range of 5 to 25 years (median, 13 years). Its clinical presentation is usually as a painless, nodular, subcutaneous lesion thought to be a hematoma or hemangioma. Local recurrence was common and usually appeared within 1 year of diagnosis. Metastasis was uncommon.[187] In a series of 28 pediatric patients with malignant peripheral nerve sheath tumor, 39% had neurofibromatosis syndrome, type 1, which had no impact on outcome. Resectability was the prognostic factor most influencing 5-year survival: IRS group I and II, 65%; III and IV, zero. Radiotherapy was recommended for group II patients.[188] Liposarcoma is usually low grade and the benefit of chemotherapy is not apparent. Cure is accomplished by complete resection. Radiotherapy is effective against microscopic residual disease (42 to 60 Gy; median dose 57 Gy), but its role in pediatric patients with gross residual disease has not been adequately tested.[189,190]

The Askin tumor (malignant small cell tumor of the thoracopulmonary region of childhood) is recognized (along with extraosseous Ewing's sarcoma and peripheral primitive neuroectodermal tumor) to share the characteristic t(11:22) chromosomal translocation.[191-193] For patients with known or suspected pleural involvement, intrapleural colloidal ^{32}P should be considered in addition to external-beam radiotherapy.[194] In the IRS studies to 1991, 130 patients with extraosseous Ewing's sarcoma were registered. Primary site distribution was trunk, 32%; extremity, 26%; head and neck, 18%; retroperitoneal/GU, 20%; and other, 5%. Forty-six percent were in group III and their 10-year FFS rate was 55%.[195]

The alveolar soft part sarcoma occurs in the age range of 10 to 30. It arises primarily in the extremities (mainly the thigh) and has a predilection for the right side. The natural history is for the gradual evolution to distant metastases (lung, bone, brain) over a protracted time, ranging to 15 years.[196,197] In a pediatric series, 1 patient of 11 died of disease (6 of 11 received radiotherapy).[198] A review of epithelioid sarcoma noted a median age of 23 years with the lower age range of 4 years. The lesions usually arise in the hand, forearm, or pretibial region.[199] Lymph node involvement occurs. Four of five patients treated postoperatively to a median dose of 68 Gy were locally controlled and disease free.[200] Postoperative therapy may be useful for the intra-abdominal desmoplastic small round cell tumor that occurs mainly in adolescents. In one report, 2 of 17 patients survived.[201] The malignant melanoma of soft parts (clear cell sarcoma) may occur in older children. It usually involves tendons in the foot, knee, and other limb sites, and nodal metastases may occur. Radiotherapy may prevent local recurrence, but distant metastasis is common.[202] Other rare extremity sarcomas of childhood include the extraskeletal myxoid chondrosarcoma,[203] the malignant rhabdoid tumor,[204] and hemangiopericytoma.[205] Mesothelioma may occur in children.[206]

Children may develop various primary organ sarcomas for which radiotherapy may be required; however, the experience with radiotherapy is limited or anecdotal. Examples include the pleuropulmonary blastoma,[207] malignant rhabdoid tumor of the kidney,[208] clear cell sarcoma of the kidney,[209] and undifferentiated (embryonal) sarcoma of the liver.[210,211] Leiomyosarcoma of bowel has been reported in two girls with acquired immunodeficiency syndrome.[212]

REFERENCES

1. Gurney JG, Severson RK, Davis S, et al: Incidence of cancer in children in the United States. *Cancer.* 1995;75:2186.
2. Hug EB, Fitzek MM, Munzenrider JE, et al: Locally challenging osteo- and chondrogenic tumors of the axial skeleton: Results of combined proton and photon radiation therapy using three-dimensional treatment planning. *Int J Radiat Oncol Biol Phys.* 1995;31:467.
3. Lombardi F, Gandola L, Fossati-Bellani F, et al: Hypofractionated accelerated radiotherapy in osteogenic sarcoma. *Int J Radiat Oncol Biol Phys.* 1992;24:761.
4. Ozaki T, Flege S, Liljenqvist U, et al: Osteosarcoma of the Spine. *Cancer.* 2002;94:1069.
5. Anderson PM, Arndt CAS, Rodriquez V, et al: High-Dose[153] SM-EDTMP (Samarium Ethylenediaminetetramethylphosphonate) therapy in locally recurrent or metastatic osteosarcoma. *Med Pediatr Oncol.* 2001;37:183 [abstract O81].
6. Wollner N, Lane JM, Marcove RC, et al: Primary skeletal non-Hodgkin's lymphoma in the pediatric age group. *Med Pediatr Oncol.* 1992;20:506.
7. Nishida J, Sim FH, Wenger DE, et al: Malignant fibrous histiocytoma of bone. A clinicopathologic study of 81 patients. *Cancer.* 1997;79:482.
8. Campanacci M, Boriani S, Giunti A: Hemangioendothelioma of bone: A study of 29 cases. *Cancer.* 1980;46:804.
9. Wold LE, Unni KK, Beabout JW, et al: Hemangioendothelial sarcoma of bone. *Am J Surg Pathol.* 1982;6:59.
10. Finsterbush A, Husseini N, Rousso M: Multifocal hemangioendothelioma of bones in the hand: A case report. *J Hand Surg.* 1981;6:353.
11. Welles L, Dorfman H, Valentine ES, et al: Low grade malignant hemangioendothelioma of bone: A disease potentially curable with radiotherapy. *Med Pediatr Oncol.* 1994;23:144.
12. Dahlin DC: Giant-cell tumor of vertebrae above the sacrum: A review of 31 cases. *Cancer.* 1977;39:1350.
13. Schwartz LH, Okunieff PG, Rosenberg A, et al: Radiation therapy in the treatment of difficult giant cell tumors. *Int J Radiat Oncol Biol Phys.* 1989;17:1085.
14. Bennett CJ, Marcus RB, Million RR, et al: Radiation therapy for giant cell tumor of bone. *Int J Radiat Oncol Biol Phys.* 1993;26:299.
15. Marks RD, Scruggs HJ, Wallace KM, et al: Megavoltage therapy in patients with aneurysmal bone cysts. *Radiology.* 1976;118:421.
16. Buckley JD, Pendergrass TW, Buckley CM, et al: Epidemiology of osteosarcoma and Ewing's sarcoma in childhood. A study of 305 cases by the children's cancer group. *Cancer.* 1998;83:1440.
17. Turc-Carel C, Philip I, Berger MP, et al: Chromosomal translocations in Ewing's sarcoma. *N Engl J Med.* 1983;309:497.
18. Whang-Peng J, Triche TJ, Knutsen T, et al: Chromosome translocation in peripheral neuroepithelioma. *N Engl J Med.* 1984;311:584.
19. Delattre O, Zucman J, Melot T, et al: The Ewing family of tumors-a subgroup of small-round-cell tumors defined by specific chimeric transcripts. *N Engl J Med.* 1994;331:294.
20. Hahm K, Cho K, Lee C, et al: Repression of the gene encoding the TGF-β type II receptor is a major target of the EWS-FLI1 oncoprotein. *Nature Genetics.* 1999;23:222.
21. Ginsberg JP, de Alava E, Ladanyi M: EWS-FLI1 and EWS-ERG gene fusions are associated with similar clinical phenotypes in Ewing's sarcoma. *J Clin Oncol.* 1999;17:1809.
22. Wilkins RM, Pritchard DJ, Burgert EO, et al: Ewing's sarcoma of bone: Experience with 140 patients. *Cancer.* 1986;58:2551.
23. Mameghan H, Fisher RJ, O'Gorman-Hughes D, et al: Ewing's sarcoma: Long-term follow-up in 49 patients treated from 1967 to 1989. *Int J Radiat Oncol Biol Phys.* 1993;25:431.
24. Kinsella TJ, Miser JS, Waller B, et al: Long-term follow-up of Ewing's sarcoma of bone treated with combined modality therapy. *Int J Radiat Oncol Biol Phys.* 1991;20:389.
25. Kissane JM, Askin FB, Foulkes M, et al: Ewing's sarcoma of bone: Clinicopathologic aspects of 303 cases from the Intergroup Ewing's Sarcoma Study. *Hum Pathol.* 1983;14:773.
26. Cangir A, Vietti TJ, Gehan EA, et al: Ewing's sarcoma metastatic at diagnosis: Results and comparison of two Intergroup Ewing's Sarcoma studies. *Cancer.* 1990;66:887.
27. Horowitz ME, Malawer MM: Ewing's sarcoma family of tumors: Ewing's sarcoma of bone and soft tissue and the peripheral primitive neuroectodermal tumors. In Pizzo PA, Poplack DG, eds. *Principles and Practice of Pediatric Oncology.* 2nd ed. Philadelphia: JB Lippincott; 1993:795.
28. Hugenholtz EAL, Piers DA, Kamps WA, et al: Bone scintigraphy in nonsurgically treated Ewing's sarcoma at diagnosis and follow-up: Prognostic information of the primary tumor site. *Med Pediatr Oncol.* 1994;22:236.
29. Boyko OB, Cory DA, Cohen MD, et al: MR imaging of osteogenic and Ewing's sarcoma. *AJR.* 1987;148:317.
30. Farley FA, Healey JH, Caparros-Sison B, et al: Lactase dehydrogenase as a tumor marker for recurrent disease in Ewing's sarcoma. *Cancer.* 1987;59:1245.
31. Reinus WR, Gilula LA, Donaldson S, et al: Prognostic features of Ewing sarcoma on plain radiograph and computed tomography scan after initial treatment: A Pediatric Oncology Group Study (8346). *Cancer.* 1993;72:2503.
32. Jürgens H, Exner U, Gadner H, et al: Multidisciplinary treatment of primary Ewing's sarcoma of bone. A 6-year experience of a European Cooperative Trial. *Cancer.* 1988;61:23.
33. Sailer SL, Harmon DC, Mankin HJ, et al: Ewing's sarcoma: Surgical resection as a prognostic factor. *Int J Radiat Oncol Biol Phys.* 1988;15:43.
34. Mendenhall CM, Marcus RB, Enneking WF, et al: The prognostic significance of soft tissue extension in Ewing's sarcoma. *Cancer.* 1983;51:913.
35. Grier H, Krailo M, Tarbell N, et al: Addition of ifosfamide and etoposide to standard chemotherapy for Ewing's sarcoma and primitive neuroectodermal tumor of bone: *N Eng J Med.* 2003;348:694.
36. Barbieri E, Emiliani E, Zini G, et al: Combined therapy of localized Ewing's sarcoma of bone: Analysis of results in 100 patients. *Int J Radiat Oncol Biol Phys.* 1990;19:1165.
37. Shuck A, Ahrens S, Paulussen M, et al: Local therapy in localized Ewing tumors: Results of 1058 patients treated in the CESS 81, CESS 86 and EICESS 92 trials. *Int J Radiat Oncol Biol Phys.* 2003;55:168.
38. Donaldson SS, Torrey M, Link MP, et al: A multidisciplinary study investigating radiotherapy in Ewing's sarcoma: End results of POG #8346. *Int J Radiat Oncol Biol Phys.* 1998;42:125.

39. Merchant TE, Kushner BH, Sheldon JM, et al: Effect of low-dose radiation therapy when combined with surgical resection for Ewing sarcoma. *Med Pediatr Oncol.* 1999;33:65.

40. Schuck A, Dunst J, Ahrens S, et al: Hemithorax irradiation in Ewing tumors of the chest wall. *Med Pediatr Oncol.* 2001;37:177 [abstract O58].

41. Gonzalez D, Breur K: Clinical data from irradiated growing long bones in children. *Int J Radiat Oncol Biol Phys.* 1983;9:841.

42. Jentzsch K, Binder H, Cramer H, et al: Leg function after radiotherapy for Ewing's sarcoma. *Cancer.* 1981; 47:1267.

43. Marcus R, Cantor A, Heare TC, et al: Local control and function after twice a day radiotherapy for Ewing's sarcoma of bone. *Int J Radiat Oncol Biol Phys.* 1991;21:1509.

44. Nagarajan R, Clohisy DR, Greenberg M, et al: Function and quality of life (QOL) of survivors of pediatric lower extremity bone tumors: A report from the Childhood Cancer Survivor Study (CCSS). *Proc Am Soc Clin Oncol.* 2002;21:395a [abstract 1577].

45. Kuttesch JF, Wexler LH, Marcus RB. et al: Second malignancies after Ewing's sarcoma: Radiation dose-dependency of secondary sarcomas. *J Clin Oncol.* 1996;14:2818.

46. Travis LB, Curtis RE, Hankey BF, et al: [Letter to the editor]: Second cancers in patients with Ewing's sarcoma. *Med Pediatr Oncol.* 1994;22:296.

47. Dunst J, Ahrens S, Paulussen MP, et al: Second malignancies after treatment for Ewing's sarcoma: A report of the CESS-studies. *Int J Radiat Oncol Biol Phys.* 1998;42:379.

48. Ehara S, Kattapuram SV, Egglin TK: Ewing's sarcoma: Radiographic pattern of healing and bony complications in patients with long-term survival. *Cancer.* 1991;68:1531.

49. Nesbit ME, Gehan EA, Burgert EO, et al: Multimodal therapy for the management of primary, nonmetastatic Ewing's sarcoma of bone: A long-term follow-up of the First Intergroup Study. *J Clin Oncol.* 1990;8:1664.

50. Ahrens S, Paulussen M, Craft AW, et al: Ewing tumor of bone—Updated report of the European Intergroup Cooperative Ewing's Sarcoma Study EICESS 92. *Proc Am Soc Clin Oncol.* 2002;21:393a [abstract 1568].

51. Evans RG, Nesbit ME, Gehan EA, et al: Multimodal therapy for the management of localized Ewing's sarcoma of pelvic and sacral bones: A report from the Second Intergroup Study. *J Clin Oncol.* 1991;9:1173.

52. Burgert EO, Nesbit ME, Garnsey LA, et al: Multimodal therapy for the management of nonpelvic, localized Ewing's sarcoma of bone: Intergroup Study IESS-II. *J Clin Oncol.* 1990;8:1514.

53. Paulussen M, Ahrens S, Dunst J, et al: Localized Ewing tumor of bone: Final results of the Cooperative Ewing's Sarcoma Study CESS 86. *J Clin Oncol.* 2001;19:1818.

54. Le Deley MC, Ahrens S, Paulussen M, et al: Histological response is the main prognostic factor of survival in localized Ewing tumour (ET) treated with chemotherapy alone before surgery. *Med Pediatr Oncol.* 2001;37:178 [abstract O60].

55. Maygarden SJ, Askin FB, Siegal GP, et al: Ewing sarcoma of bone in infants and toddlers: A clinicopathologic report from the Intergroup Ewing's Study. *Cancer.* 1993;71:2109.

56. Thomas PRM, Foulkes MA, Gilula LA, et al: Primary Ewing's sarcoma of the ribs: A report from the Intergroup Ewing's Sarcoma Study. *Cancer.* 1983;51:1021.

57. Venkateswaran L, Rodriquez-Galindo C, Merchant TE, et al: Primary Ewing tumor of the vertebrae: Clinical characteristics, prognostic factors, and outcome. *Med Pediatr Oncol.* 2001;37:30.

58. Helfre S, Habrand JJ, Zucker JM, et al: Primary Ewing's sarcoma of the spine: Report of the French Society of Pediatric Oncology. *Med Pediatr Oncol.* 2001;37:178 [abstract O59].

59. Shirley SK, Askin FB, Gilula LA, et al: Ewing's sarcoma in bones of the hands and feet: A clinicopathologic study and review of the literature. *J Clin Oncol.* 1985;3:686.

60. Siegal GP, Oliver WR, Reinus WR, et al: Primary Ewing's sarcoma involving the bones of the head and neck. *Cancer.* 1987;60:2829.

61. Paulussen M, Ahrens S, Craft AW, et al: Ewing's tumors with primary lung metastases: Survival analysis of 114 (European Intergroup) cooperative Ewing's sarcoma studies patients. *J Clin Oncol.* 1998;16:3044.

62. Paulussen M, Ahrens S, Burdach S, et al: Primary metastatic (stage IV) Ewing tumor: Survival analysis of 171 patients from the EICESS studies. *Ann Oncol.* 1998;9:275.

63. Meyers PA, Krailo MD, Ladanyi M, et al: High-dose melphalan, etoposide, total-body irradiation, and autologous stem-cell reconstitution as consolidation therapy for high-risk Ewing's sarcoma does not improve prognosis. *J Clin Oncol.* 2001;19:2812.

64. Robison L: General principles of the epidemiology of childhood cancer. In Pizzo PA, Poplack DG (eds): *Principles and Practice of Pediatric Oncology.* 3rd ed. Philadelphia: JB Lippincott; 1997:1.

65. Grufferman S, Schwartz AG, Ruymann FB, et al: Parents' use of cocaine and marijuana and increased risk of rhabdomyosarcoma in their children. *Cancer Causes Control.* 1993;4:217.

66. Scrable HJ, Witte DP, Lampkin BC, et al: Chromosomal localization of the human rhabdomyosarcoma locus by mitotic recombination mapping. *Nature.* 1987;329:645.

67. Scrable HJ, Cavenee W, Ghavimi F, et al: A model for embryonal rhabdomyosarcoma tumorigenesis that involves genome imprinting. *Proc Natl Acad Sci USA.* 1989;86:7480.

68. Sorenson PH, Lynch JC, Qualman SJ, et al: PAX3-FKHR and PAX7-FKHR gene fusions are prognostic indicators in alveolar rhabdomyosarcoma: A report from the Children's Oncology Group. *J Clin Oncol.* 2002;20:2672.

69. Bridge JA, Liu J, Qualman SJ, et al: Genomic gains and losses are similar in genetic and histologic subsets of rhabdomyosarcoma, whereas amplification predominates in embryonal with anaplasia and alveolar subtypes. *Genes Chromosomes Cancer.* 2002;33:310.

70. Malkin D, Li FP, Strong LC, et al: Germ line p53 mutations in a familial syndrome of breast cancer, sarcomas, and other neoplasms. *Science.* 1990;250:1233.

71. Asmar L, Gehan EA, Newton WA, et al: Agreement among and within groups of pathologists in the classification of rhabdomyosarcoma and related childhood sarcomas: Report of an international study of four pathology classifications. *Cancer.* 1994:74:2579.

72. Leuschner I, Newton WA, Schmidt D, et al: Spindle cell variants of embryonal rhabdomyosarcoma in the paratesticular region: A report of the Intergroup Rhabdomyosarcoma Study. *Am J Surg Pathol.* 1993;17:221.

73. Kodet R, Newton WA, Hamoudi AB, et al: Childhood rhabdomyosarcoma with anaplastic (pleomorphic) features: A report of the Intergroup Rhabdomyosarcoma Study. *Am J Surg Pathol.* 1993;17:443.

74. Crist WM, Anderson JR, Meza JL, et al: Intergroup Rhabdomyosarcoma Study-IV: Results for patients with non-metastatic disease. *J Clin Oncol.* 2001;19:3091.

75. Maurer HM, Beltangady M, Gehan EA, et al: The Intergroup Rhabdomyosarcoma Study-I: A final report. *Cancer.* 1988;61:209.

76. Crist W, Gehan EA, Ragab AH, et al: The Third Intergroup Rhabdomyosarcoma Study. *J Clin Oncol.* 1995;13:610.

77. Maurer HM, Gehan EA, Beltangady M, et al: The Intergroup Rhabdomyosarcoma Study-II. *Cancer.* 1993;71:1904.

78. Wharam MD: Rhabdomyosarcoma of parameningeal sites. *Semin Radiat Oncol.* 1997;7:212.

79. Wharam MD, Maurer HM: Management of orbital rhabdomyosarcoma. In Jacobs C, ed. *Cancers of the Head and Neck.* Boston: Martinus Nijhoff; 1987:223.

80. Lawrence W, Hays DM, Heyn R, et al: Lymphatic metastases with childhood rhabdomyosarcoma: A report from the Intergroup Rhabdomyosarcoma Study. *Cancer.* 1987;60:910.

81. Raney RB, Tefft M, Maurer HM, et al: Disease patterns and survival rate in children with metastatic soft-tissue sarcoma: A report from the Intergroup Rhabdomyosarcoma Study (IRS)-I. *Cancer.* 1988;62:1257.

82. Pratt CB, Dugger DL, Johnson WW, et al: Metastatic involvement of the heart in childhood rhabdomyosarcoma. *Cancer.* 1973;31:1492.

83. Howarth CB, Caces JN, Pratt CB: Breast metastases in children with rhabdomyosarcoma. *Cancer.* 1980;46:2520.

84. Spunt SL, Anderson JR, Teot LA, et al: Routine brain imaging is unwarranted in asymptomatic patients with rhabdomyosarcoma arising outside the head and neck region that is metastatic at diagnosis. A report from the Intergroup Rhabdomyosarcoma Study Group. *Cancer.* 2001;92:121.

85. Yousem DM, Lexa FJ, Bilaniuk LT, et al: Rhabdomyosarcoma in the head and neck: MR imaging evaluation. *Radiology.* 1990;177:683.

86. Quddus FF, Espinola D, Kramer SS, et al: Comparison between x-ray and bone scan detection of bone metastases in patients with rhabdomyosarcoma. *Med Pediatr Oncol.* 1983;11:125.

87. Lawrence W, Gehan EA, Hays DM, et al: Prognostic significance of staging factors of the UICC staging system in childhood rhabdomyosarcoma: A report from the Intergroup Rhabdomyosarcoma Study (IRS-II). *J Clin Oncol.* 1987;5:46.

88. Rodary C, Flamant F, Donaldson SS: An attempt to use a common staging system in rhabdomyosarcoma: A report of an international workshop initiated by the International Society of Pediatric Oncology (ISPO). *Med Pediatr Oncol.* 1989;17:210.

89. Hays DM, Lawrence W, Wharam MD, et al: Primary reexcision for patients with "microscopic residual" tumor following initial excision of sarcomas of trunk and extremity sites. *J Pediatr Surg.* 1989;24:5.

90. Wolden SL, Anderson JR, Crist WM, et al: Indications for radiotherapy and chemotherapy after complete resection in rhabdomyosarcoma: A report from the Intergroup Rhabdomyosarcoma Studies I to III. *J Clin Oncol.* 1999;17:3468.

91. Michalski JM, Sur RK, Harms WB, et al: Three dimensional conformal radiation therapy in pediatric parameningeal rhabdomyosarcomas. *Int J Radiat Oncol Biol Phys.* 1995;33:985.

92. Bucholtz JD: Issues concerning the sedation of children for radiation therapy. *Oncol Nurs Forum.* 1992;19:649.

93. Slifer KJ, Bucholtz JD, et al: Behavioral training of motion control in young children undergoing radiation treatment without sedation. *J Pediatr Oncol Nursing.* 1994;11:55.

94. Hug EB, Adams J, Fitzek M: Fractionated, three-dimensional, planning-assisted proton-radiation therapy for orbital rhabdomyosarcoma: A novel technique. *Int J Radiat Oncol Biol Phys.* 2000;47:979.

95. Donaldson SS, Meza J, Breneman JC, et al: Results from the IRS-IV randomized trial of hyperfractionated radiotherapy in children with rhabdomyosarcoma—A report from the IRSG. *Int J Radiat Oncol Biol Phys.* 2001;51:718.

96. Flamant F, Chassagne D, Cosset JM, et al: Embryonal rhabdomyosarcoma of the vagina in children: Conservative treatment with curietherapy and chemotherapy. *Eur J Cancer.* 1979;15:527.

97. Habrand JL, Ganry O, Gerbaulet A, et al: Interstitial brachytherapy (IB) in the management of soft tissue sarcomas (STS) in children. *Med Pediatr Oncol.* 1994;23:188 [abstract 0-75].

98. Haie-Meder C, Flamant F, Revillon Y, et al: Brachytherapy in the multidisciplinary therapy of prostate and/or bladder rhabdomyosarcoma in children. *Med Pediatr Oncol.* 1994;23:188 [abstract 0-74].

99. Flamant F, Gerbaulet A, Nihoul-Fekete C, et al: Long-term sequelae of conservative treatment by surgery, brachytherapy, and chemotherapy for vulval and vaginal rhabdomyosarcoma in children. *J Clin Oncol.* 1990;8:1847.

100. Schouwenburg PF, Kupperman D, Bakker FP, et al: New combined treatment of surgery, radiotherapy, and reconstruction in head and neck rhabdomyosarcoma in children: The AMORE protocol. *Head and Neck.* 1998;20:283.

101. Nag S, Grecula J, Ruymann FB: Aggressive chemotherapy, organ-preserving surgery, and high-dose-rate remote brachytherapy in the treatment of rhabdomyosarcoma in infants and young children. *Cancer.* 1993;72:2769.

102. Nag S, Olson T, Ruymann R, et al: High-dose-rate brachytherapy in childhood sarcomas: A local control strategy preserving bone growth and function. *Med Pediatr Oncol.* 1995;25:463.

103. Ortega JA, Stowe SM, Shore NA, et al: Prevention of radiation pneumonitis by controlled pneumothorax in childhood rhabdomyosarcoma of the chest wall. *Int J Radiat Oncol Biol Phys.* 1985;11:2033 [letter].

104. Breneman JC, Lyden E, Pappo AS, et al: Prognostic factors and clinical outcome in children and adolescents with metastatic rhabdomyosarcoma—A report from the Intergroup Rhabdomyosarcoma Study IV. *J Clin Oncol.* 2003;21:78.

105. Smith LM, Anderson JR, Qualman SJ, et al: Which patients with microscopic disease and rhabdomyosarcoma experience relapse after therapy? A report of the Soft Tissue Sarcoma Committee of the Children's Oncology Group. *J Clin Oncol.* 2001;19:4058.

106. Ragab AH, Heyn R, Tefft M, et al: Infants younger than 1 year of age with rhabdomyosarcoma. *Cancer.* 1986;58:2606.

107. Koscielniak E, Harms D, Schmidt D, et al: Soft tissue sarcomas in infants younger than 1 year of age: A report of the German Soft Tissue Sarcoma Study Group (CWS-81). *Med Pediatr Oncol.* 1989;17:105.

108. Salloum E, Flamant F, Rey A, et al: Rhabdomyosarcoma in infants under 1 year of age: Experience of the Institut Gustave-Roussy. *Med Pediatr Oncol.* 1989;17:424.

109. Lobe TE, Wiener ES, Hays DM, et al: Neonatal rhabdomyosarcoma: The IRS experience. *J Pediatr Surg.* 1994;29:1167.

110. Heyn R: Late effects of therapy in rhabdomyosarcoma. *Clin Oncol.* 1985;4:287.

111. Heyn R, Haeberlen V, Newton WA, et al: Second malignant neoplasms in children treated for rhabdomyosarcoma. *J Clin Oncol.* 1993;11:262.

112. Spunt SL, Meza JL, Anderson JR, et al: Second malignant neoplasms (SMN) in children treated for rhabdomyosarcoma: A report from the Intergroup Rhabdomyosarcoma Studies (IRS) I-IV. *Proceedings Am Society of Clin Oncol.* 2001;20:369a [abstract 1473a].

113. Sagerman RH: Orbital rhabdomyosarcoma: A paradigm for irradiation. *Radiology.* 1993;187:605.

114. Wharam M, Beltangady M, Hays D, et al: Localized orbital rhabdomyosarcoma: An interim report of the Intergroup Rhabdomyosarcoma Study Committee. *Ophthalmology.* 1987; 94:251.

115. Oberlin O, Rey A, Anderson J, et al: Treatment of orbital rhabdomyosarcoma: Survival and late effects of treatment—Results of an international workshop. *J Clin Oncol.* 2001;19:197.

116. Wharam MD, Anderson JR, Laurie F, et al: Failure-free survival for orbit rhabdomyosarcoma patients on Intergroup Rhabdomyosarcoma Study IV (IRS-IV) is improved compared to IRS-III. *Proc Am Soc Clin Oncol.* 1997;16:578a [abstract 1864].

117. Kodet RI, Newton WA, Hamoudi AB, et al: Orbital rhabdomyosarcoma and related tumors in childhood: Relationship of morphology to prognosis—An Intergroup Rhabdomyosarcoma Study. *Med Pediatr Oncol.* 1997;29:51.

118. Rosseau P, Flamant F, Quintana E, et al: Primary chemotherapy in rhabdomyosarcoma and other malignant mesenchymal tumors of the orbit: Results of the International Society of Pediatric Oncology MMT 84 Study. *J Clin Oncol.* 1994;12:516.

119. Heyn R, Ragab A, Raney B, et al: Late effects of therapy in orbital rhabdomyosarcoma in children: A report from the Intergroup Rhabdomyosarcoma Study. *Cancer.* 1986;57:1738.

120. Raney RB, Anderson JR, Kollath J, et al: Late effects of therapy in 94 patients with localized rhabdomyosarcoma of the orbit: Report from the Intergroup Rhabdomyosarcoma Study (IRS)-III, 1984-1991. *Med Pediatr Oncol.* 2000;34:413.

121. Tefft M, Fernandez C, Donaldson M, et al: Incidence of Meningeal Involvement by Rhabdomyosarcoma of the Head and Neck in Children: A report of the Intergroup Rhabdomyosarcoma Study (IRS). *Cancer.* 1978;42:253.

122. Chan RC, Sutow WW, Lindberg RD: Parameningeal rhabdomyosarcoma. *Radiology.* 1979;13:211.

123. Berry MP, Jenkins RDT: Parameningeal rhabdomyosarcoma in the young. *Cancer.* 1981;48:281.

124. Raney RB, Tefft M, Newton WA, et al: Improved prognosis with intensive treatment of children with cranial soft tissue sarcomas arising in nonorbital parameningeal sites: A report from the Intergroup Rhabdomyosarcoma Study. *Cancer.* 1987;59:147.

125. Raney RB, Meza J, Anderson JR, et al: Treatment of children and adolescents with localized parameningeal sarcoma: Experience of the Intergroup Rhabdomyosarcoma Study Group protocols IRS-II through-IV, 1978-1997. *Med Pediatr Oncol.* 2002:38:22.

126. Spooner D, Gaze M, Habrand JL, et al: Treatment of young children (age <3 years) with parameningeal (PM) rhabdomyosarcoma (RMS): Experience of the SIOP MMT 89 study. *Med Pediatr Oncol.* 2001;37:182.

127. Wharam MD, Beltangady MS, Heyn RM, et al: Pediatric orofacial and laryngopharyngeal rhabdomyosarcoma: An Intergroup Rhabdomyosarcoma Study report. *Arch Otolaryngol Head Neck Surg.* 1987;113:1225.

128. Raney RB, Asmar L, Vassilopoulou-Sellin R, et al: Late complications of therapy in 213 children with localized, nonorbital soft-tissue sarcoma of the head and neck: A descriptive report from the Intergroup Rhabdomyosarcoma Studies (IRS) -II and -III. *Med Pediatr Oncol.* 1999;33:362.

129. Raney RB, Gehan EA, Hays DM, et al: Primary chemotherapy with or without radiation therapy and/or surgery for children with localized sarcoma of the bladder, prostate, vagina, uterus, and cervix. *Cancer.* 1990;66:2072.

130. Hays D, Raney RB, Crist W, et al: Improved survival and bladder preservation among patients with bladder/prostate primary tumors in Intergroup Rhabdomyosarcoma Study (IRS) III. *Proc Am Soc Clin Oncol.* 1991;10:318 [abstract 1119].

131. Heyn R, Newton WA, Raney RB, et al: Preservation of the bladder in patients with rhabdomyosarcoma. *J Clin Oncol.* 1997;15:69.

132. Hays DM, Lawrence W, Crist WM, et al: Partial cystectomy in the management of rhabdomyosarcoma of the bladder: A report from the Intergroup Rhabdomyosarcoma Study. *J Pediatr Surg.* 1990;25:719.

133. Hays DM, Raney RB, Wharam MD, et al: Children with vesical rhabdomyosarcoma (RMS) treated by partial cystectomy with neoadjuvant or adjuvant chemotherapy, with or without radiotherapy: A report of the Intergroup Rhabdomyosarcoma Study (IRS) Committee. *Am J Pediatr Hematol Oncol.* 1995;17:46.

134. Raney B, Heyn R, Hays DM, et al: Sequelae of treatment in 109 patients followed for 5 to 15 years after diagnosis of sarcoma of the bladder and prostate: A report from the Intergroup Rhabdomyosarcoma Study Committee. *Cancer.* 1993;71:2387.

135. Wiener ES, Anderson JR, Ojimba JI, et al: Controversies in the management of paratesticular rhabdomyosarcoma: Is staging retroperitoneal lymph node dissection necessary for adolescents with resected paratesticular rhabdomyosarcoma? *Semin Pediatr Surg.* 2001;10:146.

136. Curnes JT, Pratt CB, Hustu HO: Five-year survival after disseminated paratesticular rhabdomyosarcoma. *J Urol.* 1977;118:662.

137. Raney RB, Tefft M, Lawrence W, et al: Paratesticular sarcoma in childhood and adolescence: A report from the Intergroup Rhabdomyosarcoma Studies I and II, 1973-1983. *Cancer.* 1987;60:2337.

138. Heyn R, Raney RB, Hays DM, et al: Late effects of therapy in patients with paratesticular rhabdomyosarcoma. *J Clin Oncol.* 1992;10:614.

139. Hughes LL, Baruzzi MJ, Ribeiro RC, et al: Paratesticular rhabdomyosarcoma: Delayed effects of multimodality therapy and implications for current management. *Cancer.* 1994;73:476.

140. Arndt C, Donaldson S, Andrassy R, et al: What constitutes optimal therapy for rhabdomyosarcoma (RMS) of the female genitourinary tract? *Med Pediatr Oncol.* 2000;35:278 [abstract O-37].

141. Andrassy RJ, Wiener ES, Raney RB, et al: Progress in the surgical management of vaginal rhabdomyosarcoma: A 25-year review from the Intergroup Rhabdomyosarcoma Study Group. *J Pediatr Surg.* 1999; 34:731.

142. Martelli H, Oberlin O, Rey A, et al: Conservative treatment for girls with nonmetastatic rhabdomyosarcoma of the genital tract: A report from the Study Committee of the International Society of Pediatric Oncology. *J Clin Oncol.* 1999;17:2117.

143. Hays DM, Soule EH, Lawrence W, et al: Extremity lesions in the Intergroup Rhabdomyosarcoma Study (IRS-I): A preliminary report. *Cancer.* 1982;48:1.

144. Neville HL, Andrassy RJ, Lobe TE, et al: Preoperative staging, prognostic factors, and outcome for extremity rhabdomyosarcoma: A preliminary report from the Intergroup Rhabdomyosarcoma Study IV (1991-1997). *J Pediatr Surg.* 2000;35:317.

145. Heyn R, Beltangady M, Hays D, et al: Results of intensive therapy in children with localized alveolar extremity rhabdomyosarcoma: A report from the Intergroup Rhabdomyosarcoma Study. *J Clin Oncol.* 1989;7:200.

146. Raney RB, Crist W, Hays D, et al: Soft tissue sarcoma of the perineal region in childhood. *Cancer.* 1990;65:2787.

147. Raney RB, Ragab AH, Ruymann FB, et al: Soft-tissue sarcoma of the trunk in childhood: Results of the Intergroup Rhabdomyosarcoma Study. *Cancer.* 1982;49:2612.

148. Hays DM, Donaldson SS, Shimada H, et al: Primary and metastatic rhabdomyosarcoma in the breast: Neoplasms of adolescent females, a report from the Intergroup Rhabdomyosarcoma Study. *Med Pediatr Oncol.* 1997;29:181.

149. Ortega JA, Wharam M, Gehan EA, et al: Clinical features and results of therapy for children with paraspinal soft tissue sarcoma: A report of the Intergroup Rhabdomyosarcoma Study. *J Clin Oncol.* 1991;9:796.

150. Crist WM, Raney RB, Newton W, et al: Intrathoracic soft tissue sarcomas in children. *Cancer.* 1982;50:598.

151. Spunt SL, Lobe TE, Pappo AS, et al: Aggressive surgery is unwarranted for biliary tract rhabdomyosarcoma. *J Pediatr Surg.* 2000;35:309.

152. Fox KR, Moussa SM, Mitre RJ, et al: Clinical and pathologic features of primary gastric rhabdomyosarcoma. *Cancer.* 1990;66:772.

153. Horowitz ME, Etcubanas E, Webber BL, et al: Hepatic undifferentiated (embryonal) sarcoma and rhabdomyosarcoma in children: Results of therapy. *Cancer.* 1987;59:396.

154. Crist WM, Raney RB, Tefft M, et al: Soft tissue sarcomas arising in the retroperitoneal space in children: A report from the Intergroup Rhabdomyosarcoma Study (IRS) Committee. *Cancer.* 1985;56:2125.

155. Jenkin D, Sonley M: Soft-tissue sarcomas in the young: Medical treatment advances in perspective. *Cancer.* 1980;46:621.

156. Sollaccio RJ, Conrad C, Mendenhall NP, et al: Soft tissue sarcoma in children; analysis of prognostic factors. *Int J Radiat Oncol Biol Phys.* 1986;12:133 [abstract 82].

157. Horowitz ME, Pratt CB, Webber BL, et al: Therapy for childhood soft-tissue sarcomas other than rhabdomyosarcoma: A review of 62 cases treated at a single institution. *J Clin Oncol.* 1986;4:559.

158. Salloum E, Flamant F, Caillaud JM, et al: Diagnostic and therapeutic problems of soft tissue tumors other than rhabdomyosarcoma in infants under 1 year of age: A clinicopathological study of 34 cases treated at the Institut Gustave-Roussy. *Med Pediatr Oncol.* 1990;18:37.

159. Hayani A, Mahoney DH, Hawkins HK, et al: Soft-tissue sarcomas other than rhabdomyosarcoma in children. *Med Pediatr Oncol.* 1992;20:114.

160. Skene AI, Barr L, Robinson M, et al: Adult type (nonembryonal) soft tissue sarcomas in childhood. *Med Pediatr Oncol.* 1993;21:645.

161. Marcus KC, Grier HE, Shamberger RC, et al: Childhood soft tissue sarcoma: A 20-year experience. *J Pediatr.* 1997;131:603.

162. Rao BN: Nonrhabdomyosarcoma in children: Prognostic factors influencing survival. *Semin Surg Oncol.* 1993;9:524.

163. Dillon P, Maurer H, Jenkins J, et al: A prospective study of nonrhabdomyosarcoma soft tissue sarcomas in the pediatric age group. *J Pediatr Surg.* 1992;27:241.

164. Maurer HM, Cantor A, Salzberg A, et al: Adjuvant chemotherapy vs observation for localized nonrhabdomyosarcoma soft tissue sarcoma (NRSTS) in children. *Proc Am Soc Clin Oncol.* 1992;11:363 [abstract 1248].

165. Blakely ML, Spurbeck WW, Pappo AS, et al: The impact of margin of resection on outcome in pediatric nonrhabdomyosarcoma soft tissue sarcoma. *J Pediatr Surg.* 1999;34:672.

166. Spunt SL, Poquette CA, Hurt YS, et al: Prognostic factors for children and adolescents with surgically resected nonrhabdomyosarcoma soft tissue sarcoma: An analysis of 121 patients treated at St. Jude Children's Research Hospital. *J Clin Oncol.* 1999;17:3697.

167. Spunt SL, Hill DA, Motosue AM, et al: Clinical features and outcome of initially unresected nonmetastatic pediatric nonrhabdomyosarcoma soft tissue sarcoma. *J Clin Oncol.* 2002;20:3225.

168. Kawai A, Woodruff J, Healey JH, et al: *SYT-SSX* gene fusion as a determinant of morphology and prognosis in synovial sarcoma. *N Engl J Med.* 1998;338:153.

169. Schmidt D, Thum P, Harms D, et al: Synovial sarcoma in children and adolescents: A report from the Kiel Pediatric Tumor Registry. *Cancer.* 1991;67:1667.

170. Ladenstein R, Treuner J, Koscielniak E, et al: Synovial sarcoma of childhood and adolescence: Report of the German CWS-81 Study. *Cancer.* 1993;71:3647.

171. Pappo AS, Fontanesi J, Luo X, et al: Synovial sarcoma in children and adolescents: The St. Jude Children's Research Hospital Experience. *J Clin Oncol.* 1994;12:2360.

172. Okcu MF, Despa S, Choroszy M, et al: Synovial sarcoma in children and adolescents: Thirty-three years of experience with multimodal therapy. *Med Pediatr Oncol.* 2001;37:90.

173. Okcu MF, Treuner A, Mattke A, et al: Synovial sarcoma of childhood and adolescence: multicenter multivariate analysis of outcome of 220 patients. *Proc American Soc Clin Oncol.* 2002:21;391a [abstract 1560].

174. Essary LR, Vargas SO, Fletcher CD: Primary pleuropulmonary synovial sarcoma. Reappraisal of a recently described anatomic subset. *Cancer.* 2002;94:459.

175. Dehner LP, Askin FB: Tumors of fibrous tissue origin in childhood: A clinicopathologic study of cutaneous and soft tissue neoplasms in 66 children. *Cancer.* 1976;38:888.

176. Soule EH, Pritchard DJ: Fibrosarcoma in infants and children: A review of 110 cases. *Cancer.* 1977;40:1711.

177. Leibel SA, Wara WM, Hill DR, et al: Desmoid tumors: Local control and patterns of relapse following radiation therapy. *Int J Radiat Oncol Biol Phys.* 1983;9:1167.

178. Sherman NE, Romsdahl M, Evans H, et al: Desmoid tumors: A 20-year radiotherapy experience. *Int J Radiat Oncol Biol Phys.* 1990;19:37.

179. McCollough WM, Parson JT, Van Der Griend R, et al: Radiation therapy for aggressive fibromatosis: The experience at the University of Florida. *J Bone Joint Surg Am.* 1991;73:717.

180. Acker JC, Bossen EH, Halperin EC: The management of desmoid tumors. *Int J Radiat Oncol Biol Phys.* 1993;26:851.

181. Goepfert H, Cangir A, Ayala AG, et al: Chemotherapy of locally aggressive head and neck tumors in the Pediatric Age Group. *Am J Surg.* 1982;144:437.

182. Sportiello DJ, Hoogerland DL: A recurrent pelvic desmoid tumor successfully treated with tamoxifen. *Cancer.* 1991;67:1443.

183. Waddell WR: Treatment of intra-abdominal and abdominal wall desmoid tumors with drugs that affect the metabolism of cyclic 3′, 5′-adenosine monophosphate. *Ann Surg.* 1975;181:299.

184. Raney RB, Allen A, O'Neill J, et al: Malignant fibrous histiocytoma of soft tissue in childhood. *Cancer.* 1986;57:2198.

185. Cole CH, Magee JF, Gianoulis M, et al: Malignant fibrous histiocytoma in childhood. *Cancer.* 1993;71:4077.

186. Fagundes HM, Lai PP, Dehner LP, et al: Postoperative radiotherapy for malignant fibrous histiocytoma. *Int J Radiat Oncol Biol Phys.* 1992;23:615.

187. Enzinger FM: Angiomatoid malignant fibrous histiocytoma: A distinct fibrohistiocytic tumor of children and young adults simulating a vascular neoplasm. *Cancer.* 1979;44:2147.

188. DeCou JM, Rao BN, Parham DM, et al: Malignant peripheral nerve sheath tumors: The St. Jude Children's Research Hospital experience. *Ann Surg Oncol.* 1995;2:524.

189. Shmookler BM, Enzinger FM: Liposarcoma occurring in children: An analysis of 17 cases and review of the literature. *Cancer.* 1983;52:567.

190. La Quaglia MP, Spiro SA, Ghavimi F, et al: Liposarcoma in patients younger than or equal to 22 years of age. *Cancer.* 1993;72:3114.

191. Askin FB, Rosai J, Sibley RK, et al: Malignant small cell tumor of the thoracopulmonary region in childhood: A distinctive clinicopathologic entity of uncertain histogenesis. *Cancer.* 1979;43:2438.

192. Kinsella TJ, Triche TJ, Dickman PS, et al: Extraskeletal Ewing's sarcoma: Results of combined modality treatment. *J Clin Oncol.* 1993;1:489.

193. Jurgens H, Bier V, Harms D, et al: Malignant peripheral neuroectodermal tumors: A retrospective analysis of 42 patients. *Cancer.* 1988;61:349.

194. Shamberger RC, Grier HE, Weinstein HJ, et al: Chest wall tumors in infancy and childhoods. *Cancer.* 1989;63:774.

195. Raney RB, Asmar L, Newton WA, et al: Ewing's sarcoma of soft tissues in childhood: A report from the Intergroup Rhabdomyosarcoma Study, 1972 to 1991. *J Clin Oncol.* 1997; 15:574.

196. Lieberman PH, Foote FW, Stewart FW, et al: Alveolar soft-part sarcoma. *JAMA.* 1966;198:121.

197. Heller DS, Frydman CP, Gordon RE, et al: An unusual organoid tumor: Alveolar soft part sarcoma or paraganglioma? *Cancer.* 1991;67:1894.

198. Pappo AS, Parham DM, Cain A, et al: Alveolar soft part sarcoma in children and adolescents: Clinical features and outcome of 11 patients. *Med Pediatr Oncol.* 1996;26:81.

199. Enzinger FM: Epithelioid sarcoma: A sarcoma simulating a granuloma or a carcinoma. *Cancer.* 1970;26:1029.

200. Shimm DS, Suit HD: Radiation therapy of epithelioid sarcoma. *Cancer.* 1983;52:1022.

201. Gerald WL, Miller HK, Battifora H, et al: Intra-abdominal desmoplastic small round-cell tumor: Report of 19 cases of a distinctive type of high-grade polyphenotypic malignancy affecting young individuals. *Am J Surg Pathol.* 1991;15:499.

202. Sara AS, Evans HL, Benjamin RS: Malignant melanoma of soft parts (clear cell sarcoma): A study of 117 cases, with emphasis on prognostic factors. *Cancer.* 1990;65:367.

203. Hachitanda Y, Tsuneyoshi M, Daimaru Y, et al: Extraskeletal myxoid chondrosarcoma in young children. *Cancer.* 1988; 61:2521.

204. Kent AL, Mahoney DH, Gresik MV, et al: Malignant rhabdoid tumor of the extremity. *Cancer.* 1987;60:1056.

205. Ferrari A, Casanova M, Bisogno G, et al: Hemangiopericytoma in pediatric ages. *Cancer.* 2001;92:2692.

206. Kauffman SL, Stout AP: Mesothelioma in children. *Cancer.* 1964;17:539.

207. Manivel JC, Priest JR, Watterson J, et al: Pleuropulmonary blastoma. The so-called pulmonary blastoma of childhood. *Cancer.* 1988;62:1516.

208. Weeks DA, Beckwith JB, Mierau GW, et al: Rhabdoid tumor of kidney: A report of 111 cases from the National Wilms' Tumor Study Pathology Center. *Am J Surg Pathol.* 1989;13:439.

209. Sotelo-Avila C, Gonzalez-Crussi F, Sadowinski S, et al: Clear cell sarcoma of the kidney: A clinicopathologic study of 21 patients with long-term follow-up evaluation. *Hum Pathol.* 1986;16:1219.

210. Miettinen M, Kahlos T: Undifferentiated (embryonal) sarcoma of the liver: Epithelial features as shown by immunohistochemical analysis and electron microscopic examination. *Cancer.* 1989;64:2096.

211. Leuschner I, Schmidt D, Harms D: Undifferentiated sarcoma of the liver in childhood: Morphology, flow cytometry, and literature review. *Hum Pathol.* 1990;21:68.

212. Chadwick EG, Connor EJ, Hanson CG, et al: Tumors of smooth-muscle origin in HIV-infected children. *JAMA.* 1990;263:3182.

Neuroblastoma and Wilms' Tumor

Marnee Spierer, MD, Welela Tereffe, MD, and Suzanne Wolden, MD

NEUROBLASTOMA

Epidemiology, Etiology, Genetics, and Cytogenetic Abnormalities

Neuroblastoma is the most common extracranial solid tumor in children and the most common malignancy of infants with approximately 650 cases diagnosed annually in the United States.[1] The tumor accounts for 8% to 10% of all childhood cancers and is slightly more common in boys than in girls, with a male-to-female ratio of 1.1:1. Review of more than 3000 patients registered on studies at Pediatric Oncology Group (POG) institutions from 1990 to 2000 and at Children's Cancer Group (CCG) institutions from 1991 to 1995 show the median age at diagnosis is 17.3 months; 40.1% are younger than 1 year of age, 89.4% are younger than 5 years of age, and 97.8% are younger than 10 years of age.[2]

Neuroblastoma arises from primitive adrenergic neuroblasts of neural crest tissue. This tissue forms columns that are the precursors of spinal ganglia, dorsal spinal nerve roots, and chromaffin cells of the adrenal medulla. Thus, the majority of neuroblastoma cases occur in an anatomic distribution consistent with the location of neural crest tissue. The location of tumors at the time of

diagnosis varies with age (Table 56-1). The adrenal gland is the most common location for the development of neuroblastoma, accounting for 35% of cases (Figure 56-1). Paraspinal ganglia in the low thoracic and abdominal chains constitute 30% of all cases, the posterior mediastinum accounts for 19%, and pelvic and cervical ganglia account for 2% or fewer.[3] It has been reported that microscopic neuroblastic nodules, resembling neuroblastoma in situ, were found frequently at autopsy in infants younger than 3 months of age who died of unrelated causes.[4] Initially, this was believed to mean the incidence of neuroblastoma was much higher during early infancy, but these tumors regressed spontaneously and were never clinically detected. However, studies have demonstrated that these nodules occur uniformly in all fetuses, peaking between 17 and 20 weeks of gestation, and gradually regress by the time of birth or shortly thereafter.[5] Thus, the development and subsequent regression of neuroblastoma nodules most likely represents a normal embryologic event, and the development of clinically detectable neuroblastoma is a consequence of a disruption of this process.

The cause of neuroblastoma is unknown in most cases. No prenatal or postnatal exposure to drugs, chemicals,

Table 56–1 Primary Sites of Neuroblastoma According to Age

Site	Age at Diagnosis		
	≤1 year (%)	>1 year (%)	Total (%)
Cervical	4	0.5	1
Thoracic	29	14	19
Abdominal			
Adrenal	25	40	35
Nonadrenal	26	32	30
Pelvic	3	2.5	2
Other	13	9	12
Unknown	0	2	1

Data from Brodeur GM, Castleberry RP: Neuroblastoma. In Pizzo PA, Poplack DG, eds. *Principles and Practice of Pediatric Oncology*, 3rd ed. Philadelphia: Lippincott-Raven Publishers; 1997:761.

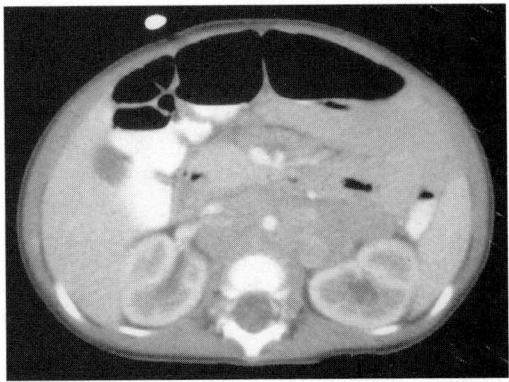

Figure 56–1. Axial computed tomography scan with contrast showing a typical adrenal primary tumor in a patient with high-risk neuroblastoma. The extensive tumor encases the major blood vessels and is inseparable from para-aortic lymph nodes. Adjacent organs are displaced but not invaded.

or radiation has unequivocally demonstrated an increased incidence of neuroblastoma.[2] Genetics, however, play an extremely important role. Knudson and Strong[6] estimated that as many as 22% of all neuroblastomas result from a germ line mutation, thus demonstrating an autosomal dominant pattern of inheritance. Because these patients inherit their first mutation, they only require one additional mutation to induce malignant transformation. Thus, their peak incidence is at an earlier age. Familial neuroblastoma is also well described and presents at an earlier median age (9 months vs. 22 months for sporadic cases). At least 20% of patients with familial neuroblastoma have bilateral or multifocal disease.[7]

Understanding neuroblastoma on the cellular and molecular level has helped to risk-stratify patients in terms of treatment options and predictability of response. For example, MYCN amplification and chromosomal ploidy (see later discussion) have been shown to correlate with outcome and are therefore included in the risk stratification that dictates treatment.

Deletion of the distal short arm of chromosome 1 (1p) was the first described genetic mutation in neuroblastoma tumors and is the most consistently reported abnormality, occurring in 70% to 80% of the karyotyped near-diploid tumors.[8] This most likely represents a deletion (and loss of heterozygosity, LOH) of a tumor suppressor gene and is found more commonly in advanced disease. Homogeneous staining regions (HSRs) and double-minute chromatin bodies (dmins) are a manifestation of gene amplification. Both of these are derived from the distal short arm of chromosome 2 (2p), which contains the proto-oncogene MYCN.[3]

MYCN amplification occurs in roughly 25% of primary neuroblastoma cases—5% to 10% in patients with low stages of disease and stage IV-S and 30% to 40% in patients with advanced disease.[9] The MYCN proto-oncogene is derived from the c-myc viral oncogene and, as mentioned previously, is located on 2p, thus correlating with the cytogenetic abnormalities of HSRs and dmins. If it is going to occur, MYCN amplification is almost always present by the time of diagnosis. This suggests that it is an intrinsic property of a subset of aggressive tumors with a poor prognosis.[2] Incidentally, molecular studies have shown a strong correlation between 1p LOH and MYCN, suggesting these two genetic events may be related.[8]

Chromosomal ploidy is another marker of prognosis that is particularly useful in infants younger than 18 months of age. Near-diploid or pseudodiploid tumors have near-normal nuclear DNA content but often have structural chromosomal abnormalities, including MYCN amplification. Hyperdiploid or near-triploid tumors typically lack MYCN amplification and 1p deletion and therefore have an excellent prognosis.[10]

Telomerase activity has been correlated with MYCN amplification and poor outcomes while increased expression of high-affinity nerve growth factor receptor (gp140TRK-A) has been associated with favorable outcomes. Conversely, the lack of expression of gp140TRK-A has been associated with MYCN amplification and poor survival.[10]

Pathology

Neuroblastoma is a classic "small round blue cell" tumor. Others include Ewing's sarcoma, non-Hodgkin's lymphoma, primitive neuroectodermal tumors (PNET), and rhabdomyosarcoma. Histologic subtypes, including neuroblastoma, ganglioneuroblastoma, and ganglioneuroma, represent different points along the maturation pathway in order of increasing differentiation. The typical neuroblastoma is composed of small, uniform cells containing dense, hyperchromatic nuclei and scant cytoplasm. The presence of neuritic processes (neuropil) is pathognomonic. Homer-Wright pseudorosettes, neuroblasts surrounding areas of eosinophilic neuropil, are seen in 15% to 50% of cases. Ganglioneuromas are composed primarily of mature ganglion cells, neuropil, and Schwann cells, and behave in a benign fashion. Ganglioneuroblastomas have histopathologic characteristics of both neuroblastomas and ganglioneuromas. Because histopathologic features may vary within any single tumor, multiple sections must be examined.[2] Distinguishing neuroblastomas from other small round blue cell tumors requires special techniques including immunohistochemistry and electron microscopy. Neuroblastoma stains with monoclonal antibodies that recognize neuron-specific enolase, synaptophysin, and neurofilament. Electron microscopy reveals neurosecretory granules that contain catecholamines, microfilaments, and parallel arrays of microtubules within the neuropil.[11]

Three major histopathologic classification systems exist for neuroblastomas, and they all assess pathology as a prognostic factor. The Shimada Classification is most widely used. It is divided into favorable and unfavorable prognostic groups based on age, amount of Schwann cell stroma, nodular versus diffuse histologic pattern, degree of differentiation, and mitotic-karyorrhectic index. Characteristics of the Shimada system are listed in Table 56-2. The Joshi System also uses characteristics to separate patients into favorable and unfavorable groups. Favorable prognosis is associated with grade 1, all ages or grade 2, younger than 1 year of age. Unfavorable prognosis is associated with grade 2, older than 1 year of age or grade 3, all ages. Grade 1 is defined as having a low mitotic rate (fewer than 10 mitotic figures per 10 high-power field) and calcification present; grade 2 is defined as having either a low mitotic rate or calcification present, and grade 3 is defined as having neither a low mitotic rate nor calcification present.[12] The International Neuroblastoma Pathology Committee classifies neuroblastoma based on: degree of differentiation toward ganglion cells; amount of Schwann cell stroma present; whether the tumor is nodular, noting particular macronodules (which tend to be associated with a poor prognosis compared with intermixed nodules); degree of calcification; and the mitosis-karyorrhexis Index (MKI).[3]

Clinical Presentation

As mentioned previously, primary tumor location varies with age (see Table 56-1). Extent of disease is also age-dependent; the majority of children younger than

Table 56–2   The Shimada System

Prognosis	Schwann Cell Stroma	Age (Yr)	Pattern	MKI
Favorable	Rich	All	No nodular	—
	Poor	1.5–5	Differentiated	<100
	Poor	<1.5	—	<200
Unfavorable	Rich	All	Nodular	—
	Poor	>5	—	—
	Poor	1.5–5	Undifferentiated	—
	Poor	1.5–5	Differentiated	>100
	Poor	<1.5	—	>200

MKI, mitosis-karyorrhexis index.
Data from Shimada H, Chatten J, Newton WA Jr, et al: Histopathologic prognostic factors in neuroblastic tumors: Definition of subtypes of ganglioneuroblastoma and an age-linked classification of neuroblastomas. *J Natl Cancer Inst.* 1984;73:405.

1 year of age have localized disease at the time of diagnosis, whereas the majority of children older than 1 year of age have disseminated disease (Table 56-3). Signs and symptoms of neuroblastoma depend on location of the primary tumor but can also reflect lymph node status and metastatic spread. Bone marrow, bone, liver, and skin are the most common sites for hematogenous spread. Rarely, disease spreads to the lungs and brain. Table 56-4 lists the associated signs and symptoms for each anatomic area of disease.[3] Because of the type of catecholamines secreted from most neuroblastomas, hypertension, flushing, and tachycardia are uncommon symptoms.

Diagnostic and Staging Studies

Diagnosing and staging neuroblastomas requires several imaging modalities. The primary tumor is typically imaged with plain films of the abdomen and thorax and computed tomography (CT) or magnetic resonance imaging (MRI).[13-16] The classic sign seen on an abdominal plain film is calcification within a suprarenal soft tissue mass. Calcifications are seen in roughly 85% of patients. A mediastinal mass will be evident on the thoracic plain film. An intravenous pyelogram (IVP) will show renal displacement without pelvicalyceal disruption. Both CT and MRI provide accurate three-dimensional measurements of tumor volume and can assess resectability.

In terms of regional and distant disease, CT and MRI can assess nodal disease, hepatic metastases, and intraspinal

Table 56–3   Extent of Disease at Diagnosis According to Age

Extent of Disease	≤1 year (%)	>1 year (%)	Total (%)
Localized	39	19	26
Regional	18	13	15
Disseminated	25	68	52
IV-S	18	0	7

The columns ≤1 year (%) and >1 year (%) fall under the spanning header **Age at Diagnosis**.

Data from Brodeur GM, Castleberry RP: Neuroblastoma. In Pizzo PA, Poplack DG, eds. *Principles and Practice of Pediatric Oncology*, 3rd ed. Philadelphia: Lippincott-Raven Publishers; 1997:761.

Table 56–4   Signs and Symptoms Based on Anatomic Location of Primary Tumor and Metastases

Primary Site	Signs and Symptoms
Abdomen	• abdominal distention and discomfort • large, irregular, firm palpable mass, often crossing midline
Cervical	• unilateral neck mass causing Horner's syndrome • often misdiagnosed as infection and diagnosed after incision and drainage
Thoracic	• often diagnosed incidentally on CXR that is done to evaluate infection or trauma • respiratory compromise • superior vena cava syndrome if tumor is large
Pelvis	• bowel and bladder disturbances
Paraspinal location in cervical, abdominal, thoracic or pelvic areas	• tumor may have a "dumbbell" configuration; tumor extends through the neural foramina and presents with a mass lesion in the spinal canal that may cause spinal cord compression
Metastatic Disease	
General	• fever, weight loss, weakness, failure to thrive
Liver	• respiratory compromise due to upward pressure on diaphragm (Pepper Syndrome); frequently in infants
Bone	• pain • refusal to walk • skull masses • proptosis with orbital ecchymosis (raccoon eyes) due to retrobulbar and orbital infiltration
Skin	• nontender, blue-tinged nodules (blueberry muffin sign); seen in infants with stage IV-S tumors
Bone marrow	• pancytopenia resulting in infection, pallor, lethargy, bleeding • bone pain
Brain	• typically meningeal, may have suture separation
Paraneoplastic Syndromes	
	• opsoclonus-myoclonus-truncal ataxia syndrome (myoclonic jerking and random eye movements); associated with early-stage neuroblastoma and may persist after cure • diarrhea associated with hypokalemia and dehydration due to tumor secretion of VIP, most common in ganglioneuroblastomas and ganglioneuromas

CXR, chest x-ray; VIP, vasoactive intestinal polypeptide.

extension. CT and MRI are also useful in determining whether metastases to the skull, orbit, mandible, or brain are present. Conventional radiographs are used to assess bone metastases in conjunction with either a 99mTc scan or a meta-iodobenzylguanidine (MIBG) scan. Metastatic lesions are most often located in the periorbital region, in the metaphases of long bones, and in the axial skeleton. MIBG is a sensitive and specific method (close to 90%) to assess the primary tumor and metastatic disease. A 99mTc bone scan is typically used for detection of bone metastases even if MIBG studies are used.[17-19] Complete staging includes two bilateral posterior iliac crest bone marrow aspirates and biopsies. A single positive result is sufficient for the documentation of bone marrow involvement.[20,21]

Excess catecholamines are produced in nearly 90% of cases. Therefore, part of the neuroblastoma workup includes measuring urine catecholamines and their metabolites, specifically norepinephrine, vanillylmandelic acid (VMA), 3-methoxy-4-hydroxylphenylglycol (MHPG), or homovanillic acid (HVA). Urine or serum dopamine may be measured. Urinary catecholamines are often given as ratios to urinary creatinine.[22]

According to the international criteria for diagnosing, staging, and assessing response to treatment, the diagnosis of neuroblastoma is established under one of the following circumstances: (1) An unequivocal pathologic diagnosis is made from tumor tissue by light microscopy (with or without immunohistology, electron microscopy, increased urine or serum catecholamines or metabolites), or (2) Bone marrow aspirate or trephine biopsy contains unequivocal tumor cells and urine or serum catecholamines or metabolites are increased.[20,21]

Staging and Prognostic Factors

Several different staging systems have been used in neuroblastoma. The Evans and D'Angio classification, historically used by the CCG classification, is the original system. It is based on the extent of the primary tumor and the presence or absence of distant disease. It includes stages I, II, III, IV, and IV-S.[23] The POG used an alternative staging system that included initial resectability of the primary and lymph node status, although the importance of lymph node involvement in neuroblastoma is unclear. It includes stages A, B, C, D, and D-S.[24,25] The differences between these two systems can be substantial, depending on the stage. Therefore, a group of investigators met at two international conferences in order to arrive at a consensus regarding neuroblastoma staging. Criteria for diagnosing, staging, and assessing response to treatment was set forth, and the International Neuroblastoma Staging System (INSS) is now generally accepted as the standard staging system (Table 56-5). In order to interpret the literature, it is important to recognize the similarities between the INSS and the other two major staging systems. Stage 1 is similar to stages I and A. Stage 4 is essentially the same as stages IV and D, and stage 4S is the same as IV-S and D-S. The greatest disagreement concerns the middle stages (II and III; B and C). Therefore, the INSS divided stage 2 into 2A

Table 56–5 International Neuroblastoma Staging System

STAGE 1:	Localized tumor with complete gross excision, with or without microscopic residual disease; representative ipsilateral lymph nodes negative for tumor (nodes adherent to and removed with the primary tumor may be positive).
STAGE 2A:	Localized tumor with incomplete gross excision; representative nonadherent lymph nodes negative for tumor microscopically.
STAGE 2B:	Localized tumor with or without complete gross excision, with ipsilateral nonadherent lymph nodes positive for tumor. Enlarged contralateral lymph nodes must be negative microscopically.
STAGE 3:	Unresectable unilateral tumor infiltrating across the midline,* with or without regional lymph node involvement; or localized unilateral tumor with contralateral regional lymph node involvement; or midline tumor with bilateral extension by infiltration (unresectable) or by lymph node involvement.
STAGE 4:	Any primary tumor with dissemination to distant lymph nodes, bone, bone marrow, liver, skin, or other organs (except as defined in stage 4S).
STAGE 4S:	Localized primary tumor (as defined for stage 1, 2A, or 2B), with dissemination limited to skin, liver, or bone marrow† (limited to infants younger than 1 year of age).

*The midline is defined as the vertebral column. Tumors originating on one side and crossing the midline must infiltrate to or beyond the opposite side of the vertebral column.
†Marrow involvement in stage 4S should be minimal (i.e., <10% of total nucleated cells identified as malignant on bone marrow biopsy or on marrow aspirate). More extensive marrow involvement would be considered to be stage 4. The MIGB scan (if performed) should be negative in the marrow.
Data from Brodeur GM, Seeger RC, Barrett A, et al: International criteria for diagnosis, staging and response to treatment in patients with neuroblastoma. *J Clin Oncol.* 1988;6:1874; and Brodeur GM, Pritchard J, Berthold F, et al: Revisions in the international criteria for neuroblastoma diagnosis, staging and response to treatment. *J Clin Oncol.* 1993;11:1466.

(incompletely excised tumor) and 2B (ipsilateral lymph node involvement) in order to evaluate whether patients with 2B disease behave more like stage 2A patients or stage 3 patients. In addition to revising staging, INSS delineated standard definitions of response to treatment (Table 56-6). These revisions and standard definitions were designed to make interpreting the literature and making management decisions uniform.[20,21]

Treatment for neuroblastoma is based on risk stratification. Therefore, it is essential to understand the clinical and biologic variables predictive of disease outcome. The most important clinical risk factors are disease stage and age at diagnosis. Infants younger than 12 to 18 months have a more favorable outcome compared with older children with the same disease stage. Greater than 85% of all children with POG stage A or B disease, as well as infants younger than 1 year of age with POG stage C disease, survive. Conversely, 60% to 80% of children older than 1 year with stage C disease and 10% to 30% of older children with POG stage D disease survive.[3] Similarly, several biologic variables have prognostic significance. A new histopathologic classification, the International Neuroblastoma Pathology Classification, based on the original Shimada system, is likely to become the new

Table 56-6 International Neuroblastoma Staging System Classification of Responses to Therapy

Response	Primary Tumor	Metastatic Sites/Markers
Complete response (CR)	No tumor	No tumor; catecholamines normal
Very good partial response (VGPR)	Decreased by 90%-99%	No tumor; catecholamines normal; ^{99}Tc bone changes allowed.
Partial response (PR)	Decreased by >50%	All sites decreased by >50%. Bones and bone marrow: number of positive bone sites decreased by >50%; no more than 1 positive bone marrow site allowed.*
Mixed response (MR)	No new lesions; >50% reduction of any measurable lesion (primary or metastases) with <50% reduction in any other; <25% increase in any existing lesion.	
No response (NR)	No new lesions; <50% reduction but <25% increase in any existing lesion.	
Progressive disease (PD)	Any new lesion; increase of any measurable lesion by >25%; previous negative marrow biopsy positive for tumor.	

*One positive marrow aspirate or biopsy allowed for PR if this response represents a decrease from the number of positive sites at diagnosis.
Data from Brodeur GM, Pritchard J, Berthold F, et al: Revisions in the international criteria for neuroblastoma diagnosis, staging and response to treatment. *J Clin Oncol.* 1993;11:1466.

international standard. Like the Shimada system, this classifies patients into favorable and unfavorable groups based on age, amount of Schwann cell stroma, degree of differentiation, and mitotic-karyorrhectic index. Serum markers including ferritin, neuron-specific enolase, lactate dehydrogenase, and GD2 each have prognostic value (increased levels associated with worse prognosis); however, they are not currently used in risk stratification. Genetic markers including MYCN amplification and hyperdiploid karyotype, are more prognostic than serum markers and are therefore used in risk stratification. MYCN amplification is associated with a poor prognosis whereas hyperdiploid karyotype is associated with a favorable outcome. 1p LOH, 11q LOH, and TRKA expression have been proposed to provide additional prognostic information but are not currently used in risk stratification.[2]

Standard Therapeutic Approaches

Treatment for neuroblastoma may include surgery, radiation therapy, and chemotherapy. The degree to which each is used is based on the risk-stratified group to which the patient belongs. General descriptions of the roles of all three modalities are presented, followed by detailed discussion on the subject of risk-stratified treatment.

SURGERY

Surgery is used to establish the diagnosis, provide tissue for biologic studies, stage, and resect the tumor. Second-look surgery is used to determine response to therapy and resect residual disease. INSS recommends an operative protocol for surgical-pathologic staging: (1) The resectability of the primary or metastatic tumor should be determined by tumor location, mobility, relationship to major vessels and nerves, ability to control blood supply, presence of distant metastases, and overall prognosis. Sacrifice of vital structures to achieve resection at diagnosis should be avoided. (2) Nonadherent, intracavitary lymph nodes should be sampled, including lymph nodes superior and inferior to the primary tumor. Lymph nodes adherent to the primary tumor have little relevance in predicting outcome. (3) Biopsy of the liver at the time of initial surgery is proposed for patients with abdominal tumors without clinical evidence of metastatic disease.[2]

RADIATION THERAPY

Neuroblastoma is a radiosensitive tumor. Historically, radiation therapy has been used in the management of bulky, unresectable, residual, and metastatic disease. Doses have ranged from 15 to 30 Gy in 1.5 to 4 Gy per fraction. The role of radiation therapy for patients with locoregional disease is not clearly defined. A study by Paulino and colleagues evaluated locoregional control in infants with neuroblastoma who received radiation therapy.[26] They reported 53 children younger than 1 year old who were retrospectively staged according to the INSS guidelines; 8 had stage 1, 7 stage 2A, 6 stage 2B, 15 stage 3, 6 stage 4, and 11 stage 4S. The primary tumor was located in the adrenal gland in 26 (49%), abdomen/nonadrenal in 14 (26%), thorax in 9 (17%), neck in 2 (4%), and pelvis in 2 (4%). All patients, except 11 with stage 4S and 4 with stage 4, had resection of the primary tumor. Postoperative doses ranged from 15 to 25 Gy whereas preoperative doses ranged from 12 to 31 Gy using a median fraction size of 1.5 Gy. Chemotherapy was employed in 22 of 53 patients (42%). The 5-year overall survival (OS), freedom from progression (FFP), and local control (LC) rates were 79%, 81%, and 88%, respectively. INSS stage was a prognostic factor for OS and FFP. There were no isolated locoregional relapses. The 15-year musculoskeletal toxicity rate was 47.3% for those receiving radiation and 3.3% for the group who did not receive radiation. The authors concluded that most LN+ infants achieve locoregional control without radiation and infants younger than 6 months of age who received radiation were the most susceptible to musculoskeletal abnormalities.[26]

For infants with stage 4S disease with respiratory distress secondary to hepatomegaly, radiation therapy is often indicated.[27] Effective doses are 3 to 6 Gy in single or multiple fractions. Radiation (alone or with surgery) may also be used for spinal cord compression secondary to dumbbell extension of the primary tumor; however, studies have shown that chemotherapy alone is equally efficacious with fewer long-term side effects. Doses range from 7.5 Gy to 30 Gy.[28-31] Total body irradiation (TBI) is often used for patients undergoing transplant. Doses are 7.5 to 12 Gy in 3 to 6 fractions.[32] Lastly, radiation is often used for symptomatic metastases including pain palliation. Doses of 4 to 32 Gy are typically used and may provide long-term pain control.[2] For rare patients who develop parenchymal brain metastases, unpublished experience at Memorial Sloan-Kettering Cancer Center has shown a significant risk for the development of leptomeningeal disease. It is therefore reasonable to consider prophylactic low-dose craniospinal radiation for these patients.

Radiation volume for localized neuroblastoma is determined by the surgeon's operative findings and presurgical imaging studies. Vertebral bodies should be covered in their entirety to minimize the risk of scoliosis and to ensure proper lymph node coverage.[3,33] Next-echelon lymph node stations are typically not included in the field. Special attention is paid to shielding the kidneys and, in girls, the ovaries when possible. For patients with metastatic disease who require radiation for palliation, portals include the problematic site with adequate margin.

With regard to technique, some sites are amenable to simple treatment with parallel-opposed anterior and posterior portals, whereas others require some form of three-dimensional planning. The goal is to minimize dose to normal tissues. Again, the surgeon's operative findings and presurgical imaging studies are integral for determining the best technique.

CHEMOTHERAPY

Chemotherapy is the principal modality used in intermediate and high-risk patients. Cyclophosphamide, cisplatin, doxorubicin, and the epipodophyllotoxins have proven efficacious in several phase II studies and have thus become the backbone of induction therapy.[34-37]

RISK-STRATIFIED THERAPY

The COG Risk Stratification System (Table 56-7) uses patient age, INSS stage, DI, and MYCN amplification to assign patients to low-, intermediate-, and high-risk groups. The assignments determine treatment.

Low Risk

Children with localized neuroblastoma and favorable tumor biology may be cured with surgery alone, and, unlike other tumors, complete resection is unnecessary in these patients. Chemotherapy and radiation are reserved for progressive or recurrent disease or local disease-related symptoms such as spinal cord compression or respiratory distress. The CCG recently reported on the outcome of Evans stages I to II neuroblastoma treated with surgery as primary therapy. Patients were also assigned an INSS stage—All Evans stage I patients were INSS stage 1; nearly half of Evans stage II patients were also INSS stage 1, with the other half being INSS stage 2b; few were INSS stage 2a. Event-free survival (EFS) and OS for all stage I patients were 93% and 99% and for stage II patients were 81% and 98%. Additional therapy (radiation, surgery, or chemotherapy) was needed in only 10% of stage I patients and 20% of stage II patients.[38]

MYCN amplification is rare in localized neuroblastoma. It remains controversial how to best manage low-risk patients who are MYCN amplified. In the aforementioned CCG study, seven patients had MYCN amplification. Four were INSS stage 1 and 3 were INSS stage 2b. Four of these patients relapsed 2 to 22 months from diagnosis and three died from progression of disease 8 to 25 months after relapse. Despite this, the conclusion was that stages I and II are a biologically favorable group

Table 56–7   Proposed Neuroblastoma Risk Groups Based on Clinical and Biologic Tumor Features

INSS Stage	Low Risk	Intermediate Risk	High Risk
1	All	None	None
2A, 2B	Age younger than 1 yr Age 1-21 yr; MYCN nonAMP* Age 1-21 yr; MYCN AMP; FH†	None	Age 1-21 yr; MYCN AMP; UH
3	None	Age younger than 1 yr; MYCN nonAMP Age 1-21 yr; MYCN nonAMP; FH	Age 0-21 yr; MYCN AMP Age 1-21 yr; MYCN nonAMP; UH
4	None	Age younger than 1 yr; MYCN nonAMP	Age younger than 1 yr; MYCN AMP Age 1-21 yr
4S	MYCN nonAMP; FH; DI >1‡	MYCN nonAMP; UH MYCN nonAMP; DI = 1	MYCN AMP

*MYCN amplification status: AMP = amplified, nonAMP = nonamplified.
†Histopathologic classification: FH = favorable, UH = unfavorable.
‡Ploidy status: DI >1 = hyperdiploid; DI = 1 = diploid.
DI = Diploid Index; INSS, International Neuroblastoma Staging System.
Data from Brodeur G, Maris J: Neuroblastoma. In Pizzo P, Poplack D, eds. *Principles and Practice of Pediatric Oncology*, 4th ed. Philadelphia: Lippincott Williams & Wilkins Publishers; 2002:895.

with an excellent prognosis. For stage II patients, MYCN amplification, Shimada unfavorable, age older than 2 years, or positive lymph nodes predicted for a lower OS. However, because most patients were salvaged, multimodality therapy was recommended only for those with progressive disease.[38] POG reported that the presence of MYCN amplification in localized neuroblastoma did not necessarily portend an adverse outcome. Only 2% of stage A (three patients) and 7% of stage B (three patients) were MYCN amplified. Four of the six were without evidence of disease for 16 to 38+ months. Two patients died of their disease; both had unfavorable histology (UH) and 1 had diploid DNA. The authors' concluded that the prognostic significance of MYCN amplification may vary according to histologic features.[39]

Patients who have localized neuroblastoma but UH are considered high risk. The French neuroblastoma study group reported that in multivariate analysis, MYCN amplification was the most powerful unfavorable predictive indicator in localized neuroblastoma. OS and EFS rates for these children were 36% and 32%, compared with 98% and 90% in nonamplified tumors ($P < .001$). Ten percent of all patients in this study had MYCN-amplified tumors and as in the POG study, very few of these patients had stage I or II disease (4/22 patients). Three of these patients died of disease progression.[40] Of the patients with MYCN amplification, most would not be considered low risk in the current INSS risk stratification.

Patients with INSS stage 4S usually fall into the low-risk category, with the exception of those patients with MYCN-amplified tumors, who are high risk, or with either UH or DI = 1, who are intermediate risk. Although these patients have metastatic disease on presentation, spontaneous regression occurs frequently and OS is very good. In a retrospective review, POG reported on the prognostic significance of age, MYCN amplification, ploidy, and histology in infants with stage D(S) disease. The estimated 3-year survival rate was 85% overall. When broken down with respect to prognostic indicators, estimated survival was 71% in infants 2 months or younger, 68% if diploid, 44% if MYCN amplified, and 33% if UH existed.[41]

Patients who have unfavorable biologic factors have a poorer prognosis and are now considered intermediate or high risk. The CCG recently reported on outcome and prognostic factors in infants treated prospectively with supportive care only or, in symptomatic patients, with low-dose cytotoxic therapy (radiation, chemotherapy, or a combination of the two). The 5-year EFS and OS were 86% and 92%, respectively. Fifty-five percent of the patients received supportive care only, and their 5-year OS was 100%, compared to 81% survival in those patients who required symptomatic treatment. Infants younger than 2 months old at diagnosis with rapidly progressive abdominal disease accounted for five of the six deaths. Such infants may benefit from more intensive treatment.[42]

Although not yet standardized, recommended management for 4S disease begins with a diagnostic biopsy only, as resection of the primary tumor does not influence outcome.[41-43] Patients with favorable biology are then observed for symptoms. Special attention is paid to infants younger than 2 months old. If respiratory compromise occurs, moderately intensive chemotherapy is used, with radiation therapy reserved for those who do not respond to chemotherapy. If radiation is needed, doses of 4.5 to 6 Gy in 3 to 4 fractions are usually sufficient.[2] Lastly, patients with 4S disease with intraspinal involvement are managed with chemotherapy. Several retrospective studies and a French prospective study have shown that chemotherapy alone is a safe and effective therapy for intraspinal disease.[28-31]

In a current phase III study (protocol P9641), the POG and CCG are evaluating primary surgical therapy in children with low-risk neuroblastoma. Their objectives are to determine whether low-risk stage 1, 2A/2B, and asymptomatic 4S neuroblastoma patients treated with surgery alone will have a 3-year survival of 95%. In addition, 3-year EFS of symptomatic patients treated with chemotherapy and EFS and OS of patients who relapse or progress after initial treatment with surgery alone will be estimated. All patients undergo maximal surgical resection and lymphadenectomy. Patients with at least 50% of their tumor resected are observed. Patients who have symptomatic 4S disease or whose disease is less than 50% resected receive four courses of chemotherapy including carboplatin, etoposide, cyclophosphamide, and doxorubicin. Patients with spinal cord compression may also receive chemotherapy, and those experiencing progressive or recurrent disease undergo repeat surgery or chemotherapy, or both, as described. Patients may also undergo radiation therapy if they do not respond to chemotherapy. The dose is 21 Gy in 1.5 Gy fractions (If 4S, 3 fractions of 1.5 Gy).[44]

Intermediate Risk

Patients in this risk group have regionally advanced disease (stage 3 or higher) and are MYCN nonamplified. CCG-3881 reported on the outcome of patients with Evans stage III disease; 92% of these patients fit the criteria for INSS stage 3, and 143 met the criteria for intermediate-risk disease. The patients were treated with chemotherapy including cyclophosphamide, doxorubicin, cisplatin, and etoposide followed by radiation for any gross residual disease following delayed surgery. The EFS rate at 4 years was 100% for patients with favorable biology regardless of age and 90% for those younger than 1 year of age with one unfavorable characteristic such as UH or MYCN amplification. The EFS for Evans stage III patients who were 1 year of age or greater with unfavorable biology was 54%. In multivariate analysis, only age and MYCN status were independent prognosticators.[45] These patients with the EFS of 54% and a portion of the patients with the EFS of 90% are thus appropriately considered high risk. Stage 4 patients were also analyzed in CCG-3881; before 1991, intermediate- and high-risk infants were treated in a similar fashion; after 1991, all high-risk infants were transferred to the high-risk protocol. The 3-year EFS and OS for all 134 infants were 63% and 71% respectively. The MYCN-nonamplified infants (true intermediate risk) had 93% EFS, whereas the MYCN-amplified infants (high risk) had 10% EFS.[46] These findings dramatically illustrate the prognostic significance of MYCN amplification status and support the need to stratify these infants into different risk groups.

The role of radiation therapy for intermediate-risk disease remains controversial; studies have provided conflicting results. POG found the percent of patients achieving a complete response (CR), EFS, and OS were significantly higher in the group that received chemotherapy and radiation as compared to chemotherapy alone in patients with POG stage C neuroblastoma.[47] Conversely, a randomized control trial conducted by de Bernardi and colleagues demonstrated no difference in relapse rates among those patients who received radiation therapy and those who did not.[48]

The COG is currently conducting a phase III study of combination chemotherapy in patients with intermediate-risk neuroblastoma. The objectives are to determine whether the use of select prognostic variables to assign treatment increases EFS and OS and to assess the relationship between extent of tumor resection and EFS and OS. All patients receive carboplatin, cyclophosphamide, doxorubicin, and etoposide. Patients who do not achieve a CR after four cycles with favorable biology undergo surgery to remove or debulk residual disease. Patients with unfavorable biology receive four additional cycles of chemotherapy and then undergo debulking surgery if they do not achieve a CR. The indications for radiation are: (1) progressive clinical deterioration despite chemotherapy or surgery, or both; (2) stage 4 infants with respiratory failure; (3) stage 3 or 4 patients with progressive neurologic decline; (4) partial response (PR) after eight cycles of chemotherapy and surgery in patients with unfavorable biology; and (5) PR after surgery for local recurrence greater than 3 months after completing protocol therapy. The radiation dose is 24 Gy in 1.5 Gy fractions; 4S patients with respiratory distress may receive 4.5 Gy to the liver in 3 fractions. The radiation volume includes viable gross or microscopic residual disease determined by CT/MR/MIBG imaging with 2 cm margins.[49]

The current practice is to reserve radiation for patients with disease progression despite surgery and chemotherapy or for persistent viable disease in patients with unfavorable biology after chemotherapy and second-look surgery or for PR after surgery for local recurrence greater than 3 months following completion of initial therapy.

High Risk

Survival rates for patients in this risk group have improved but remain unacceptably low despite aggressive treatment. The 4-year survival rate among the 507 stage 4 patients older than 1 year of age who were treated in the CCG studies from 1978 to 1985 was 9% compared to 30% among the 675 patients treated from 1991 to 1995.[50] The improvement may be attributable to chemotherapy dose intensification or to the increasing use of high-dose myeloablative therapy with autologous or allogenic bone marrow transplantation. The CCG completed a randomized control trial that demonstrated high-dose chemotherapy and radiation therapy followed by transplantation of autologous bone marrow is superior to conventional chemotherapy as consolidation therapy in children with high-risk neuroblastoma. The 3-year EFS rates were 34% and 22%, respectively. Furthermore, all patients who completed cytotoxic therapy without disease progression were then randomized to receive treatment with 13-cis-retinoic acid for 6 months or no further therapy. The 3-year EFS for those patients who received 13-cis retinoic acid was 46% as compared to 29% who received no further therapy.[51]

Current treatment approaches include intensive induction chemotherapy, myeloablative consolidation therapy with stem cell rescue, and targeted therapy for residual disease. The goal of induction therapy is to induce maximum reduction in tumor bulk. Studies have shown that response rates are the greatest with high-dose intensities, specifically high doses of platinum compounds.[52,53] The efficacy of induction therapy is typically assessed at the time of second-look surgery and is measured as a CR or a PR. Those who have a CR or very good partial response have a better chance of cure, although some patients with a PR can be converted to a CR with high-dose myeloablative therapy.[54] Other studies from Japan, the United States, and Europe suggest that alternative induction strategies may improve response rates.[55-58] The European Neuroblastoma Study Group (ENSG) recently performed a randomized control trial comparing two identical induction regimens that differ only in the rapidity of delivery. This directly tests the hypothesis that an increased dose intensity of induction chemotherapy improves response rate and overall survival. Results from this trial are pending.

The goal of subsequent therapy is to consolidate the response by eliminating any remaining tumor. This is usually accomplished with myeloablative chemotherapy with or without TBI and stem cell rescue.[2] Historically, autologous bone marrow was used as myeloablative rescue; however, using autologous peripheral blood stem cells is now a more common practice. Three-year EFS ranges from 38% to 62% in the most recent POG and CCG trials.[51,59-61] Investigations are under way to evaluate the efficacy of two myeloablative consolidations, known as "tandem transplants," rather than one.

External beam radiation therapy is generally used as consolidative treatment to initial sites of bulk disease including the primary site and large or persistent metastatic deposits. Specific indications for radiation therapy vary on different protocols. Excellent local control rates have been achieved when delivering 21 Gy to the primary site and regional lymph nodes after resection.[62,63] Bone metastases should be irradiated when they are persistent after chemotherapy or even after a CR if they were initially high volume (i.e., >3 cm).

The goal for using targeted therapy for residual disease is to eliminate any residual tumor cells that are chemoresistant. Although many patients are in a clinical and radiographic CR after consolidation, microscopic residual disease often remains, and thus many patients relapse. One agent that has proven effective is 13-cis-retinoic acid.[51] Immunotherapy is being investigated as a means of targeting residual disease after induction and consolidation therapy. Anti-GD2 antibodies, the murine monoclonal antibodies 3F8 and GD2a, and the human-mouse chimeric monoclonal antibody ch14.18 have shown the most promise.[64,65]

Lastly, the efficacy of intraoperative radiation therapy (IORT) was evaluated in a recent study by Haas-Kogan and colleagues. Twenty-three (21 of whom were considered high-risk) patients received IORT for neuroblastoma. Electron beam energies ranged from 4 MeV to 16 MeV and the median dose was 10 Gy (range 7 to 16 Gy). A gross total resection (GTR) was achieved in 18 patients. Of these patients, six experienced disease recurrence (two were locoregional recurrences). IORT was given to the 18 patients who had a GTR, and 14 were disease free at the time of publication. Five patients had subtotal resections (STRs), and all had recurrence locally and died of their disease. IORT was extremely well tolerated; surgical resection with IORT resulted in narrowing of the abdominal aorta and an atrophic kidney in one patient. The authors concluded that IORT for the primary tumor produced excellent local control after a GTR but was inadequate after an STR.[66]

Recurrent Disease

Current approaches for treating recurrent or refractory neuroblastoma include novel cytotoxic agents, targeted delivery of radionuclides, retinoids, and immunotherapy. Topotecan, paclitaxel, irinotecan, rebeccamycin, and oral etoposide are the most frequently investigated cytotoxic agents.[67-75] I[131] MIBG therapy is one example of targeted radiation. I[131] metaiodobenzylguanidine is bound at the cell membrane and is actively transported into cells by the majority of neuroblastoma tumors. Therapeutic use of I[131] IBG has been used in the upfront setting in patients with unresectable disease resulting in CR or in primary tumors becoming 95% resected. Trials combining I[131] with chemotherapy, surgery, and radiation therapy are currently in progress.[76,77] In addition to 13-cis-retinoic acid, new retinoids are being developed to treat recurrent or refractory disease. Fenretinide is one such compound that induces apoptosis even in cells resistant to 13-cis-retinoic acid.[78,79] Lastly, as mentioned in the section on high-risk disease, immune-mediated therapy, including anti-GD2 antibodies, the murine monoclonal antibodies 3F8 and GD2a, and the human-mouse chimeric monoclonal antibody ch14.18, are currently under investigation for their role in recurrent or refractory disease.[64,65]

Screening Studies

Neuroblastoma can be identified in the preclinical stage by detecting increased urine catecholamines. It is unclear whether screening in this fashion reduces mortality. Screening programs have been in place in Japan for nearly 25 years. Woods and colleagues recently conducted a trial in which screening for neuroblastoma was offered at 3 weeks and 6 months of age to all 476,654 children born in Quebec, Canada during a 5-year period (May 1989 to April 1994). Ninety-two percent of the children participated in the screening program. The rate of death due to neuroblastoma was determined and compared with rates in several unscreened populations during the same time period. No difference was found in mortality rates among those patients who were screened and those who were not.[80] Similar results were found in a recent German study. Routine urine screening was offered to 2.5 million children at 1 year of age from 1995 to 2000. A total of 1.4 million children actually underwent screening. A total of 2.1 million children served as controls. The screened group and the children in the control group had a similar incidence of stage 4 disease and a similar rate of death.[81]

Sequelae of Radiation Therapy

As holds true for radiation in all pediatric malignancies, consideration for long-term complications is of vital importance. Long-term survivors of neuroblastoma often suffer from spinal deformities secondary to surgery and radiation. Among the most common are kyphosis and scoliosis.[33] Factors that put the child at risk are: (1) very young age, (2) orthovoltage irradiation, (3) asymmetric irradiation of the spine, (4) epidural spread of tumor, and (5) laminectomy (see earlier discussion). However, spinal deformities are also seen in patients who received megavoltage symmetric radiation. It is essential that these children are followed closely; early and proper bracing may help considerably.

The infant kidney is more sensitive to radiation than the adult or older child's kidney. Abnormal creatine clearance has been reported in infants with stage IV-S disease who received 12.25 and 14 Gy. It has not been determined whether this is clinically significant.[82]

Other effects of treatment include infertility, neuropsychiatric sequelae, endocrinopathies, cardiac and pulmonary effects, fibrosis, bladder dysfunction, cataracts or decreased vision following orbital radiation, and second malignancies. These are due to one or all of the modalities used to treat the disease. Precautions should be made by the surgical, medical, and radiation oncologists to ensure the best outcome for long-term survivors.

WILMS' TUMOR

Wilms' tumor is the most common intra-abdominal tumor of childhood and the second most common extracranial solid tumor among children. It is a malignant neoplasm of the kidney believed to arise from persistent embryonal remnants known as nephrogenic rests.[83,84] Management of Wilms' tumor in the United States is based upon the National Wilms' Tumor Study (NWTS) group trials; similarly, in Europe the International Society of Pediatric Oncology trials have formed the basis of care for children with the disease. Wilms' represents a paradigm of multimodality treatment and multi-institutional study. The joint efforts of pediatric oncologists, radiation oncologists, surgeons, and pathologists have resulted in a dramatic improvement in survival of children with Wilms' tumor. Whereas the disease was once uniformly fatal, high cure rates have been achieved across all stages for patients

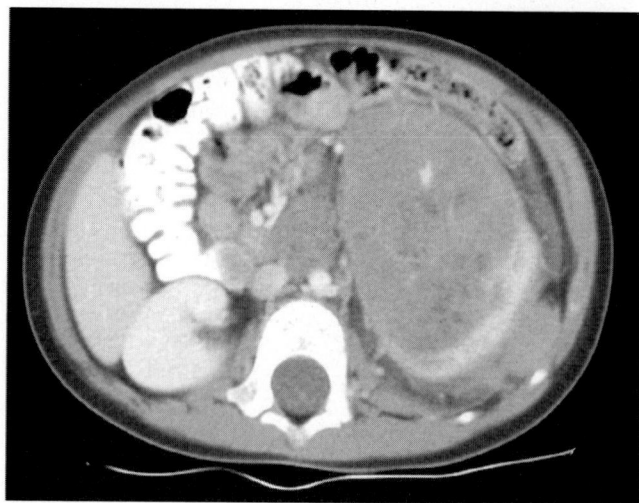

Figure 56–2. Axial computed tomography scan with contrast showing a typical Wilms' tumor. The large tumor arises from the parenchyma of the left kidney with destruction of the kidney. There is associated para-aortic lymphadenopathy.

with favorable histology disease, the most prevalent subtype. Advanced stages of Wilms' tumor with UH continue to pose major therapeutic challenges, however.

Epidemiology

Wilms' tumor accounts for 6% of all childhood cancers in the United States (Figure 56-2), where the estimated incidence is 470 cases per year,[85] or 8 per million children under the age of 16 years.[84,86] In the United States, the disease is slightly more prevalent among girls than boys (1:.92 for unilateral tumors, 1:.6 for bilateral tumors). This disparity is not maintained worldwide, however; the global incidence is 1 in 10,000 children with no sex predilection noted.[86] Racial and ethnic variations in incidence are noted throughout the world: The incidence of Wilms' is three times higher among Africans and African Americans than among East Asians, with the incidence among the European and American white population falling between these two extremes.[87]

Age at presentation is dependent upon gender and laterality. Males tend to present earlier than females, and bilateral tumors earlier than unilateral tumors. The median age at diagnosis of bilateral disease is 30 months (29.5 months for males and 32.6 months for females); in contrast, children with unilateral disease present at a median age of 40 months (41.5 months for males and 46.9 months for females).[88] Seventy-five percent of all patients present before 5 years of age.[89] Bilateral disease is noted in 4% to 8% of patients at presentation[90-92]; 7% to 12% of patients with unilateral Wilms' demonstrate multifocal disease in the affected kidney.[93]

The majority of cases are sporadic in origin. Wilms' tumor is thought to have a hereditary basis in 15% to 20% of affected patients.[94] Approximately 1.5% of patients have familial Wilms', wherein one or more family members has the disease (usually siblings or cousins, rarely parents); in these cases, the mode of inheritance is generally thought to be autosomal dominant with variable penetrance.[95]

Etiology, Genetics, and Cytogenetic Abnormalities

Investigation of the role of parental environmental exposures in the etiology of Wilms' tumor has yielded inconsistent findings. Case-control studies have suggested that paternal exposure to lead and hydrocarbons increases the incidence of Wilms' tumor in offspring, and that fathers employed as auto mechanics, welders, and machinists demonstrate an increased odds ratio for Wilms' tumor among their offspring.[96-99] However, other studies have failed to find any such correlation with paternal exposure or occupation.[100-102] Previously reported maternal associations (smoking during pregnancy, hypertension of pregnancy, tea consumption) were not confirmed in a large case-control study.[98,103]

Genetic explanations of the etiology of Wilms' tumor originated with Knudson's two-hit hypothesis, originally developed for retinoblastoma.[104,105] Briefly, the two-hit hypothesis proposes that tumors develop as a consequence of two mutational events in a single cell. If the first mutational event is prezygotic (or germ line), the tumor is potentially hereditary and affected individuals are at risk of developing multiple tumors. Conversely, sporadic cases occur as a result of two postzygotic (or somatic) mutations in a single cell; because two postzygotic events are unlikely to occur in more than one cell, these patients are unlikely to present with multiple tumors.[103] This hypothesis explains the earlier age of onset and bilateral presentation of familial Wilms' compared to sporadic cases.[95,106]

Whereas the two-hit hypothesis has been confirmed in retinoblastoma to occur via inactivation of both alleles of a tumor-suppressor gene on 13q, the genetic events that lead to the development of Wilms' tumor are less well-defined and appear to be more complex. Multiple genetic loci appear to play a role in the development of Wilms'. The best known of these are located on the short arm of chromosome 11.[107] Designated Wilms' Tumor-1 (WT-1, at 11p13) and WT-2 (at 11p15), mutations in these putative tumor suppressor genes are found in 30% to 40% of Wilms' tumors[103] and are associated with three well-described congenital anomaly syndromes:

1. Denys-Drash syndrome, linked to a point mutation at the WT-1 gene. This syndrome includes intersexual disorders (ambiguous genitalia, pseudohermaphrodism, and streak gonads), nephropathy, and a greater than 90% incidence of Wilms' tumor.[108]

2. WAGR syndrome, linked to a deletion at the WT-1 gene. The term is an acronym for **W**ilms' tumor susceptibility, **A**niridia, **G**enitourinary malformations, and mental **R**etardation. One third of children with this syndrome will develop Wilms' tumor.[108]

3. Beckwith-Wiedemann syndrome (BWS), linked to WT-2. These children demonstrate an overgrowth

complex including hemihypertrophy, organomegaly, macroglossia, and omphalocele and a predilection for the development of embryonal tumors including Wilms'.[84] The incidence of Wilms' tumor is less than 5% among these children,[108] but the risk of synchronous bilateral disease or metachronous contralateral recurrence is increased in comparison to non-BWS Wilms' cases.[109]

While evidence for the role of these genetic loci in the development of Wilms' is compelling, studies of affected pedigrees have failed to confirm either 11p13 or 11p15 as the location of the familial Wilms' tumor gene.[110] Based on epidemiologic and clinicopathologic analyses, NWTS group investigators have suggested that mechanisms other than germ line mutations (e.g., somatic mosaicism) are responsible for some bilateral and multicentric tumors.[88,111]

Other genetic mutations appear to contribute to adverse outcomes in children with Wilms' tumor, although they are not clearly causative of the disease. Alterations in chromosomes 1p and 16q are associated with poor prognosis in children with Wilms' tumor, implying that these genes are involved with tumor progression rather than tumor initiation[103]; hence they are referred to as Wilms' tumor *progressor genes*, to distinguish them from WT-1 and WT-2. In a study of 232 children registered on NWTS-3 and NWTS-4, loss of heterozygosity at either locus was associated with a poorer 2-year relapse-free and overall survival, even with adjustment for stage and histologic subgroup.[112]

Heterozygous mutations in *p53* are strongly associated with the anaplastic phenotype as compared with favorable histology,[113] suggesting that *p53* abnormalities result in more aggressive histologies. Overall, however, the incidence of *p53* mutations in Wilms' tumor is relatively low.[114,115]

Anatomy

Wilms' tumors can arise in any area of the renal parenchyma. There is no predilection for either side. Extrarenal Wilms' tumors are rare but can occur in the retroperitoneum, usually in the vicinity of the kidney. The tumor has occasionally been known to occur in the pelvis, inguinal region, or thorax, arising from displaced metanephric elements or teratomas.[116]

Pathology

Childhood kidney tumors are organized according to the NWTS pathologic classification system (Table 56-8), which includes favorable, as well as focal and diffuse anaplastic Wilms' tumors, as well as clear cell sarcoma of the kidney (CCSK) and rhabdoid tumor of the kidney. Although these are histologically distinct from Wilms' tumor, children with these diseases are included in NWTS trials due to the rarity of their occurrence, and treatment recommendations are based on NWTS findings.

Table 56-8 National Wilms' Tumor Study Pathologic Classification System of Pediatric Renal Tumors

Congenital mesoblastic nephroma
  Classical
  Cellular or atypical
Wilms' tumor
  Favorable histology
  Anaplastic
    Focal anaplasia
    Diffuse anaplasia
Clear cell sarcoma
Rhabdoid tumor

Congenital mesoblastic nephroma, which is included in the NWTS classification system, rests at the benign end of the spectrum of pediatric renal tumors. It is the most common renal tumor of infancy,[106] presenting at a median age of 2 to 3 months and occurring predominantly in males.[117] It is characterized by bundles of spindle cells resembling fibroblasts or smooth muscle; cells at the periphery frequently extend deeply into the parenchyma or perirenal tissues. Despite its tendency for local extension, local recurrence or distant metastasis is highly uncommon, and the tumor is curable by surgery alone (radical nephrectomy with wide margins). The cellular (or atypical) subclass of mesoblastic nephroma demonstrates increased cellularity and high mitotic rates. In older infants, this has been occasionally associated with local recurrence or the development of distant metastases.[118] However, in infants younger than 3 months, cellular congenital mesoblastic nephroma is not associated with a poorer prognosis.[119] Because there is no established role for radiation therapy in the management of mesoblastic nephroma, the subject is not discussed further in this chapter.

Wilms' tumor is derived from primitive metanephric blastema and is classically triphasic in composition, consisting of varying proportions of blastemic, stromal, and epithelial elements.[84] These elements appear to recapitulate normal renal embryogenesis. At the same time, Wilms' tumors often contain tissues not found in the kidney, such as skeletal muscle, cartilage, and squamous epithelium, reflecting the pluripotent nature of primitive metanephric cells.[103] Although triphasic composition is the classic norm, Wilms' tumor is characterized by tremendous structural and histologic diversity. Biphasic patterns are common, and tumors expressing predominantly or exclusively one element can still be categorized as Wilms' tumor.[120] Mixed composition is most common (41% of tumors), followed by blastemal predominant (39%) and epithelial predominant (18%); stromal predominant tumors are rare (1%). Although blastemal predominant tumors appear to be clinically more aggressive, these tumors are still classified as favorable histology unless diffuse anaplasia is noted.[121]

Wilms' tumors are classified as favorable histology unless they meet clearly defined criteria for anaplasia. These criteria were established by Beckwith and Palmer[122] following analysis of NWTS-1, and were refined by

Table 56–9 Anaplastic Wilms' Tumor: Definitions and Criteria

Definition of anaplasia	1. Nuclei with major diameters at least 3 times those of adjacent cells AND
	2. Hyperchromatism of the enlarged nuclei AND
	3. Multipolar or otherwise recognizably polypoid mitotic figures
Focal anaplasia: criteria	Anaplasia confined to a single region of the kidney
Diffuse anaplasia: criteria	Anaplasia present in more than one region of the kidney OR anaplasia in any extrarenal site (including vessels of the renal sinus, extracapsular infiltrates, or nodal or distant metastases) OR anaplasia in a random biopsy specimen

Modified from the National Wilms' Tumor Study-5: Therapeutic Trial and Biology Study. Unpublished. Activated June 16, 1995; last revised June 1998.

Faria and coworkers after analysis of NWTS-3 and 4 (Table 56-9). The original criteria did not account for location or multicentricity of anaplastic nests, and the distinction between focal and diffuse anaplasia lacked prognostic significance. In contrast, when Faria et al.'s strict criteria were applied in a review of NWTS-3 and 4 cases, patients with focal anaplasia were found to have a significantly superior 4-year survival as compared to patients with diffuse anaplasia; this difference was maintained stage for stage except for stage I tumors, in which survival was 100% for both focal and diffuse anaplasia.[123] This prognostic significance highlights the importance of thorough sampling of the gross specimen during pathologic evaluation, as well as meticulous documentation of the exact specimen site from which each slide is obtained.

Eighty-nine percent of Wilms' tumor cases in NWTS-3 were categorized as favorable histology; 5% were anaplastic. The likelihood of anaplasia increased with age in NWTS-3; it was noted in only 2% of children younger than age 2 but increased to 13% in children ages 5 and older. Anaplastic tumors are significantly more frequent in black children than white children.[124]

Clear cell sarcomas and rhabdoid tumors of the kidney were originally believed to be monophasic variants of Wilms' tumor; however, NWTS pathologists established both as unique tumors in 1978.[122,125] They have since been analyzed separately but remain within the NWTS trials. Both entities are associated with strikingly poorer outcomes than Wilms' tumor. CCSK is a primitive mesenchymal neoplasm distinguished by cells with poorly stained cytoplasm, prominent cytoplasmic vacuolation, and indistinct cell borders; groups of cells are often separated from one another by an arborizing network of thin-walled capillary vessels.[106,121] CCSK accounts for 4% of all childhood renal tumors. Like Wilms', its most common site of distant spread is to the lungs; however, CCSK is distinguished by its propensity for bone and brain metastases as well. Twenty-three percent of children with CCSK in NWTS-3 developed bone metastases, as compared with 0.3% of all other children entered in the study.[126,127]

Rhabdoid tumor of the kidney, in contrast to CCSK, is marked by strongly acidophilic cytoplasmic staining. The tumor cells thus resemble myoblasts, but skeletal muscle markers are negative and the cell of origin is unknown.[128,129] Like CCSK, rhabdoid tumors have a propensity for brain metastases; additionally, they are associated with separate primary CNS neoplasms,[130] particularly primitive neuroectodermal tumors; this finding suggests a possible neural crest origin for rhabdoid tumors, a hypothesis that has been supported by histochemical analysis.[129,131,132] Rhabdoid tumor occurs most commonly in male infants; median age at diagnosis is 13 months, and most cases are diagnosed in the first 2 years of life. In children older than 5 years diagnosed with rhabdoid tumor, pseudorhabdoid lesions (carcinomas, melanomas, histiocytic tumors, or myosarcomas) should be suspected.[133] Rhabdoid tumors carry the poorest prognosis of all childhood renal tumors due to propensity for both local relapse and distant metastases.

Clinical Presentation

Eighty-three percent of children with Wilms' present with a painless abdominal mass.[134] Other common presenting signs and symptoms include abdominal pain (37%), hypertension secondary to increased renin activity (25%), fever (23%), and hematuria (21%).[135] Abdominal pain due to any cause (local distention, intralesional hemorrhage, peritoneal rupture) has been correlated with poorer 5-year survival.[136] Acute subcapsular hemorrhage into the tumor results in a distinctive constellation of symptoms including rapid abdominal enlargement, anemia, hypertension, and sometimes fever; plain radiographs of the abdomen may demonstrate a thin rim of eggshell-like calcification.[137]

Less commonly, children may present with varicocele, enlarged testicle, hernia, pleural effusion, congestive heart failure, or hydrocephalus.[138] Several paraneoplastic syndromes have been reported in association with Wilms' tumor, including Cushing's syndrome, erythrocytosis, hypercalcemia, and acquired von Willebrand's disease.[139]

Screening for children with known phenotypic or genotypic risk factors for the development of Wilms' tumor is controversial. No randomized trials have been performed to address this question. Retrospective analyses of the NWTS registry and the National Childhood Cancer Registry of the United Kingdom failed to demonstrate a benefit to screening in children with aniridia, hemihypertrophy, or BWS.[140,141] However, these studies were limited by the variation in incidence and time intervals of screening, as well as the methods used. In contrast, a case series analysis of children with BWS or hemihypertrophy, in which the case group had undergone systematic ultrasound screening at intervals of 4 months or less, suggested that screening sonograms every 4 months decreased the incidence of late-stage disease in these children (42% stage III to IV disease in unscreened children vs. 0% in screened children, $P < 0.003$).[142] A simulation model of sonogram screening three times yearly for children with BWS suggested that such a program would be comparably cost-effective to mammographic screening if applied from birth to age 4, largely because detection of earlier-stage disease would obviate the expense associated with radiation therapy.[143] This hypothesis is supported by the finding that children with BWS in NWTS-3 and 4 were more likely to present with lower-stage tumors, although this may be a reflection of low biologic potential of Wilms' tumor in these children in addition to the effect of increased surveillance screening.[109]

Routes of Spread

The most common location of local spread in Wilms' is to the vessels of the renal sinus, which may be distended by tumor or demonstrate tumor thrombus. Penetration through the renal capsule is the second most common site of extrarenal spread. Not uncommonly, inflammation of the perirenal tissues can result in the formation of an inflammatory pseudocapsule, which may cause adhesions to adjacent organs such as the liver; yet on pathologic analysis, penetration of the true capsule by tumor is not demonstrated. Such cases are classified as stage I (limited to kidney, and completely resected, with negative margins).[103] Even when tumor is adherent to or directly invades the liver, analysis of favorable histology NWTS-3 cases demonstrated no detrimental effect on prognosis stage for stage.[144] Conversely, patients with renal vein involvement were much more likely to have metastatic disease at diagnosis.[145]

Metastatic spread occurs most commonly in the regional (renal hilar and para-aortic) lymph nodes, lung, and liver. Other metastatic sites are uncommon in Wilms' tumor. Bone metastases are a hallmark of CCSK, and both CCSK and rhabdoid tumor are associated with brain metastases.

Diagnostic and Staging Studies

The primary differential diagnosis of a pediatric abdominal mass is Wilms' tumor versus neuroblastoma; these can generally be distinguished on CT or MRI. Neuroblastoma arises from the adrenal gland or paravertebral sympathetic ganglia; as such, it compresses but does not distort the renal parenchyma. Conversely, Wilms' is an intrarenal tumor, and therefore is marked by distortion of kidney architecture. Furthermore, tumor calcification is more common in neuroblastoma (>50%) than in Wilms' (<10% to 15%). Ultimately, the determination of neuroblastoma versus Wilms' is pathologic.

The purpose of radiographic imaging in the workup of Wilms' tumor is to establish the presence of a functioning, normal contralateral kidney; identify tumor thrombus in the renal vein and inferior vena cava; and establish the presence or absence of pulmonary metastases. To this end, the NWTS-5 requires the following studies: abdominal ultrasound, CT of the abdomen, chest radiograph, and CT of the chest.

Abdominal ultrasound can fulfill several functions. It can establish the renal origin of the mass; demonstrate

whether the mass is solid or cystic; and identify the presence and extent of tumor thrombus in the renal vein and inferior vena cava.[116] Evaluation of the contralateral kidney is also possible, although this function is largely supplanted by CT. Contrast-enhanced CT imaging of the abdomen is recommended for further evaluation of the mass and adjacent viscera. CT can provide additional information on renal function, retroperitoneal lymphadenopathy, and extension to or invasion of adjacent organs, particularly hepatic metastases. Of note, however, in most cases where CT identifies hepatic invasion, subsequent surgical exploration reveals only compression by tumor.[147]

The use of preoperative CT or MRI to evaluate for tumor in the contralateral kidney has been advocated in some surgical literature. However, others believe that imaging cannot replace intraoperative exploration.[106] The NWTS-5 protocol requires surgical exploration to rule out contralateral disease. Debate also exists concerning the use of abdominal CT versus abdominal MRI in diagnosis of children with suspected Wilms' tumor—of primary concern is radiation exposure.[146]

Thoracic imaging is required to detect pulmonary metastases, the most likely site of extra-abdominal spread in Wilms' tumor. At a minimum, chest radiographs in posteroanterior and lateral views are required per NWTS-5, although two oblique views should probably also be obtained. The use of chest CT is controversial. In a small number of children with negative chest x-rays, abnormal chest CTs have been noted, leading to a treatment dilemma. The question of optimal therapy in these children was most recently addressed by Meisel et al. in an analysis of NWTS-3 and 4 data. The authors found no significant differences in EFS or OS among chest x-ray–positive/CT-negative children who received intensive doxorubicin-containing chemotherapy and whole lung irradiation (WLI) versus multidrug chemotherapy (with or without doxorubicin) and no WLI. Although WLI resulted in fewer pulmonary relapses, a greater number of deaths were attributed to pulmonary toxicity. The authors concluded that WLI was not clearly necessary in treatment of children with discordant chest x-ray/CT findings,[148] noting, however, that the small study numbers prevented a definitive recommendation. The current NWTS guidelines leave the decision to administer WLI in children with CT-only pulmonary metastases (and no other distant metastases) at the discretion of the overseeing clinician, but excisional biopsy to confirm metastatic disease is strongly recommended.[149]

Additional radiographic studies are required for children with CCSK or rhabdoid tumor of the kidney. CT or (preferably) MRI of the brain is required in both cases to rule out brain metastases and, in children with rhabdoid tumor, associated primary neuroectodermal tumors. Children with CCSK should also undergo skeletal survey and radionuclide bone scan to rule out bone metastases.

Laboratory studies should be obtained in all children with suspected Wilms' tumor, including urinalysis, complete blood count, blood chemistries, liver function tests, and alkaline phosphatase. Children with CCSK should also undergo bone marrow aspiration and biopsy.

Table 56–10 Wilms' Tumor Staging: NWTS-3 and 4, and Modifications per NWTS-5

Stage	NWTS-3 & 4	NWTS-5 Modifications
I	Tumor limited to kidney, complete resection; capsule intact. Tumor not biopsied before resection.	Protrusion of encapsulated tumor into or beyond sinus; <2 mm infiltration of tumor into the renal sinus without tumor thrombus in lymph or blood vessels; preoperative biopsy performed by FNA.
II	Tumor extends beyond kidney (through capsule, or infiltrating extrarenal vessels) but is completely resected with negative margins OR local flank spillage before or during surgery, not involving the peritoneal surface OR biopsy before resection.	Tumor infiltrates ≥2 mm into the renal sinus, or vessels outside kidney contain tumor thrombus. Preoperative biopsy performed by means other than FNA.
III	Residual nonhematogenous tumor confined to abdomen: A: Lymph nodes positive in renal hilum, para-aortics or beyond B: Diffuse peritoneal contamination from tumor spillage before or during surgery, or from penetration of tumor through the peritoneal surface C: Peritoneal implants D: Microscopic or gross extension beyond surgical margins E: Unresectable due to local infiltration of vital structures	A: Lymph nodes positive in renal hilar, para-aortic, or other abdominopelvic regions
IV	Hematogenous metastases in lung, liver, bone, or other distant sites	Lymph nodes positive outside the abdominopelvic region
V	Bilateral renal involvement at diagnosis (an attempt should be made to stage each side according to previous criteria)	

FNA, fine-needle aspiration; NWTS, National Wilms' Tumor Study.
Data from Lindsley KL, Smith SC, Douglas JG: Wilms' tumor and neuroblastoma. In Leibel SA, Phillips TL, eds. *Textbook of Radiation Oncology*, 1st ed. Philadelphia: WB Saunders; 1998:994; Halperin E, Constine LS, Tarbell NJ, Kun LE: *Pediatric Radiation Oncology*, 3rd ed. Philadelphia: Lippincott Williams & Wilkins; 1999:343; (Multiple authors). National Wilms' Tumor Study-5: Therapeutic Trial and Biology Study. Unpublished. Activated June 16, 1995; last revised June 1998.

Staging

Under the NWTS system, staging of Wilms' tumor is surgical (Table 56-10). The NWTS-3 and 4 staging system was significantly modified from NWTS-1 and 2, in which the categories were referred to as groups rather than stages. Specifically, para-aortic lymph nodes were classified as stage III rather than II; biopsy before resection automatically resulted in upstaging to stage II; and stage V disease was designated only when bilateral disease was noted at presentation, versus the NWTS-1 and 2 system in which eventual bilateral renal involvement resulted in upstaging to stage V. NWTS-3 and 4 staging also encouraged separate staging of each side in patients with bilateral disease. The current (NWTS-5) staging system is only slightly modified from that used in NWTS-3 and 4.

Standard Therapeutic Approaches

The treatment approach advocated by the NWTS involves upfront surgery consisting of a modified radical nephrectomy and selective lymph node sampling. Exceptions to this rule include cases with intravascular tumor thrombus above the level of the hepatic vein, tumor contiguous with other abdominal structures, or bilateral renal involvement. In these situations, initial surgical exploration is still recommended for accurate staging and to obtain biopsies (in these situations biopsy will not result in further upstaging), but definitive surgical resection is postponed until after the administration of preoperative chemotherapy.[149] Preoperative biopsy is not encouraged and results in automatic upstaging unless performed via fine-needle aspiration.

Preoperative sonography is strongly recommended to identify extensive intravascular thrombus, which can extend into the inferior vena cava to the right atrium, or in the case of left-sided tumors, down the gonadal vein. IVC extension occurs in only 6% of cases, and is usually asymptomatic. Attempts at primary excision of tumor and thrombus were associated with excessive surgical morbidity in NWTS-4[150]; however, if appropriate presurgical chemotherapy is given, even extensive intravascular thrombus does not adversely affect prognosis.[103,151,152]

Diagnostic imaging studies may reveal contiguity of tumor to adjacent structures such as the liver, spleen, or pancreas. If the surgeon is sure that all disease can be completely removed, radical en bloc resection of the affected kidney and adjacent nonessential structures is acceptable. However, if complete en bloc resection cannot be performed, the tumor will be considered *spilled*.[103,149,153]

Patients with bilateral Wilms' tumor have a good survival prognosis but increased risk of renal failure. This risk can be decreased through the use of preoperative chemotherapy and renal parenchymal-sparing surgical procedures. Upfront surgery is still recommended, at which time bilateral renal biopsies should be obtained, suspicious lymph nodes sampled, and a surgical stage assigned to each side. Radical excision should not be performed at the initial operation. Partial nephrectomy or wedge resection can be used only if all tumor can be removed with preservation of the majority of the renal parenchyma on both sides.

Preoperative chemotherapy is recommended by the NWTS in three distinct circumstances: tumors deemed unresectable at initial surgical exploration[154]; bilateral tumors at presentation[149]; and tumor extension into the inferior vena cava above the level of the hepatic veins.[152]

Table 56-11   Current Management of Wilms' Tumor by Stage and Histology

Stage	Favorable Histology	Focal Anaplasia	Diffuse Anaplasia	CCSK	Rhabdoid
I	Surgery + VA	Surgery + VA	Surgery + VA	Surgery + RT + CAVE	Surgery + RT + CEC
II	Surgery + VA	Surgery + RT + VAA	Surgery + RT + CAVE	↓	↓
III	Surgery + RT + VAA	↓	↓	↓	↓
IV	↓	↓	↓	↓	↓
	↓	↓	↓	↓	↓
	↓	↓	↓	↓	↓
	↓	↓	↓	↓	↓

CAVE, cyclophosphamide + Adriamycin + vincristine + etoposide; CCSK, clear cell sarcoma of the kidney; CEC, cyclophosphamide + etoposide + carboplatinum; RT, abdominal irradiation; VA, vincristine + actinomycin-D; VAA, vincristine + actinomycin-D + Adriamycin.
Notes:
1. Patients with bilateral tumors at presentation should receive preoperative chemotherapy with VAA, followed by resection of tumor but NOT nephrectomy. Postoperative radiation therapy should be guided by the stage of disease of each kidney.
2. Patients with stage IV FH disease whose primary lesions qualify as stage I receive no operative bed irradiation.
Data from the National Wilms' Tumor Study-5: Therapeutic Trial and Biology Study. Unpublished. Activated June 16, 1995; last revised June 1998.

Preoperative chemotherapy almost always reduces tumor bulk, which can facilitate complete removal of the tumor and decrease surgical complications. However, it has not been shown to improve OS and is not generally advocated by the NWTS because it results in loss of important staging information. Even in the circumstances outlined earlier where upfront chemotherapy is recommended, the NWTS strongly encourages surgical exploration for diagnosis and staging before chemotherapy.

The current NWTS-5 protocol requires postoperative chemotherapy for all children with Wilms' tumor, CCSK, or rhabdoid tumor of the kidney. A surgery-only arm of NWTS-5 for children younger than 24 months with stage I favorable histology (FH) disease and tumors weighing less than 550 grams was closed early when an interim analysis demonstrated an unacceptably poor 2-year relapse-free survival (RFS).[149]

Chemotherapy guidelines by stage and histology are briefly outlined in Table 56-11. Radiotherapy guidelines provided in the table are described in detail in the section Radiotherapy Techniques.

The evolution of Wilms' tumor management in North America is outlined in the following discussion of the NWTS. The International Society of Pediatric Oncology has conducted six clinical trials of Wilms' tumor management in Europe. This approach differs from that of NWTS primarily in its use of routine preoperative chemotherapy and radiation therapy. These trials are not discussed in this chapter.

National Wilms' Tumor Study-1

NWTS-1 (1969 to 1974) asked three major treatment questions: whether postoperative radiation therapy could be eliminated in children with stage I disease; whether actinomycin D or vincristine or the combination of both was superior in treatment of children with stage II and III disease; and whether preoperative vincristine was beneficial in the management of children with stage IV disease.[155] The study registered 606 patients and randomized 358 to the treatment schema outlined in Table 56-12.

The recommended surgical procedure involved a transabdominal approach. Chemotherapy was initiated within 48 hours of surgical diagnosis, and was given for a period of 15 months. The radiation dose was determined on an age-dependent scale, ranging from 18 Gy for children under 18 months to 40 Gy for children older than

Table 56-12   National Wilms' Tumor Study-1: Treatment Schema and Outcomes

Stage	Randomized Regimens	Treatment Outcomes at 2 Yr
I	A: SUR + RT + AMD B: SUR + AMD, NO RT	Children younger than 2 years: no benefit to RT (DFS 90% vs. 88%) Age 2 or older: DFS 77% vs. 58% without RT ($P = 0.04$)
II, III	A: SUR + RT + AMD B: SUR + RT + VCR C: SUR + RT + AMD + VCR	Combination chemotherapy (81% DFS) superior to AMD alone (57%) or VCR alone (55%) ($P = 0.002$)
IV	A: SUR + RT + AMD + VCR B: Pre-op VCR + SUR + RT + AMD + VCR	OS 83% without pre-op VCR, 29% with pre-op VCR ($P = 0.02$) (DFS not analyzed due to persistent disease after surgery in most patients)

AMD, actinomycin-D; RT, abdominal irradiation; SUR, surgery; VCR, vincristine.
Adapted from D'Angio GJ, Evans AE, Breslow N, et al: The treatment of Wilms' tumor: Results of the National Wilms' Tumor Study. *Cancer.* 1976;38:633.

40 months. Stage I and II patients received radiation to the site of the kidney and associated tumor as visualized on preoperative imaging. The field extended across the midline to encompass the vertebral bodies and minimize asymmetric growth deformities. Group III patients received either flank or whole abdomen radiation based on the extent of residual disease or tumor spillage at surgery. Patients with pulmonary metastases received whole lung irradiation to 14 Gy. Other sites of metastatic disease received higher doses, to a minimum of 30 Gy.

The results of NWTS-1 led to the following treatment recommendations. First, postoperative radiation could be eliminated in children under age 2 with stage I disease; among older children, radiation appeared to decrease the rate of abdominal recurrences. Second, combination chemotherapy with actinomycin-D and vincristine was preferred for children with stage II or III disease, rather than monotherapy with either agent alone. Lastly, preoperative vincristine was of no benefit to children with metastatic disease; indeed, children receiving preoperative therapy had an inferior OS. The latter conclusion must be tempered by the low statistical power of the analysis in stage IV patients. The majority of these patients had undergone surgery before registration on NWTS-1, and consequently could not be randomized. Therefore, the results cited represented a highly selected subsample. Nonetheless, there was no evidence that preoperative vincristine improved survival.[155]

Retrospective analyses of the NWTS-1 data demonstrated that initiation of radiation later than postoperative day 10 was associated with adverse outcomes,[156] a finding that was confirmed in NWTS-2 and 3.[153] Retrospective review also suggested that local spillage at surgery required flank irradiation only, rather than whole abdomen irradiation.[157]

Retrospective histologic analysis revealed significantly decreased survival for patients with anaplastic tumors or sarcomatous histology, including clear cell sarcoma and rhabdoid tumor, resulting in the designation of these three entities as *UH*.[84] Large tumor size, lymph node involvement, and age older than 2 years were also confirmed as poor prognostic factors.

NWTS-1 investigators also recorded the incidence of incorrect preoperative diagnoses in patients thought to have Wilms' tumor before pathologic confirmation. Thirty of the 606 patients registered (5%) were subsequently diagnosed with benign cysts or tumors (14 cases), neuroblastoma (9 cases), or other diseases (7 cases), providing support for the NWTS' advocacy of upfront surgery rather than preoperative chemotherapy.

It should be noted that 3% of the 358 children randomized (10 patients) died of complications of treatment; 5 of these children were disease free at the time of death. This highlights the importance of refining and minimizing therapeutic interventions, a major goal of the NWTS.

National Wilms' Tumor Study-2

NWTS-2 asked three major chemotherapeutic questions. First, could multi-agent chemotherapy replace radiation in older children with stage I disease? Second, did stage I

children require the protracted postoperative chemotherapy specified in NWTS-1? Third, did the addition of Adriamycin to actinomycin D and vincristine benefit children with stages II to IV disease?

In accordance with these questions, radiation therapy was eliminated for all stage I children. Flank irradiation was given to all stage II to IV children according to the same age-dependent scale used in NWTS-1; whole abdomen irradiation was reserved for children with diffuse peritoneal seeding. Children with lung metastases were initially treated with whole lung irradiation to 14 Gy, but the dose was scaled back to 12 Gy after a 10% incidence of pneumonitis was noted. No randomization was performed with regard to radiation. All patients were treated with actinomycin D and vincristine. Patients with stage I disease were randomized to receive either 6 or 15 months of chemotherapy. Patients with stage II to IV disease received 15 months of actinomycin D and vincristine with or without the addition of Adriamycin.

A total of 755 children were registered on NWTS-2; of these, 513 were eligible for randomization. Comparison of stage I outcomes with those recorded in NWTS-1 suggested that elimination of radiation in children age 2 and older did not adversely affect outcomes; the 2-year RFS in NWTS-2 children older than age 2 with stage I disease was 89%[158] as compared with 77% (irradiated) and 58% (unirradiated) 2-year RFS for the same children in NWTS-1. Data analysis showed no statistically significant difference in 3-year survival between children receiving 6 months of chemotherapy (97%) and children receiving 15 months of chemotherapy (92%). Addition of Adriamycin was shown to benefit children with stages II to IV disease. When analyzed by histology, this benefit was significant for FH patients. Patients with UH showed a trend toward improved survival with the addition of Adriamycin, but this did not reach statistical significance.[158]

National Wilms' Tumor Study-3

NWTS-3 (1979 to 1985) was the first of the cooperative group trials to use the modified staging system outlined in Table 56-10. It was also the first of the trials in which histology was used to stratify patients into treatment arms. The design of the study is outlined in Figure 56-3. The study enrolled 1489 patients and analyzed 1439; 50 patients were excluded from analysis either for lack of follow-up data or because they were retrospectively determined not to have been eligible for randomization.[91]

Results of randomization of stage I FH patients confirmed that these children could be successfully treated with surgery followed by an abbreviated course of chemotherapy (10 weeks vs. 6 months). The 4-year RFS and OS for children treated with short-course chemotherapy was 89% and 96%, respectively; this did not differ significantly from the outcomes of children treated with long-course chemotherapy.[91]

Regarding stage II FH patients, NWTS-3 asked two questions: (1) whether flank irradiation could be safely eliminated; and (2) whether addition of Adriamycin to

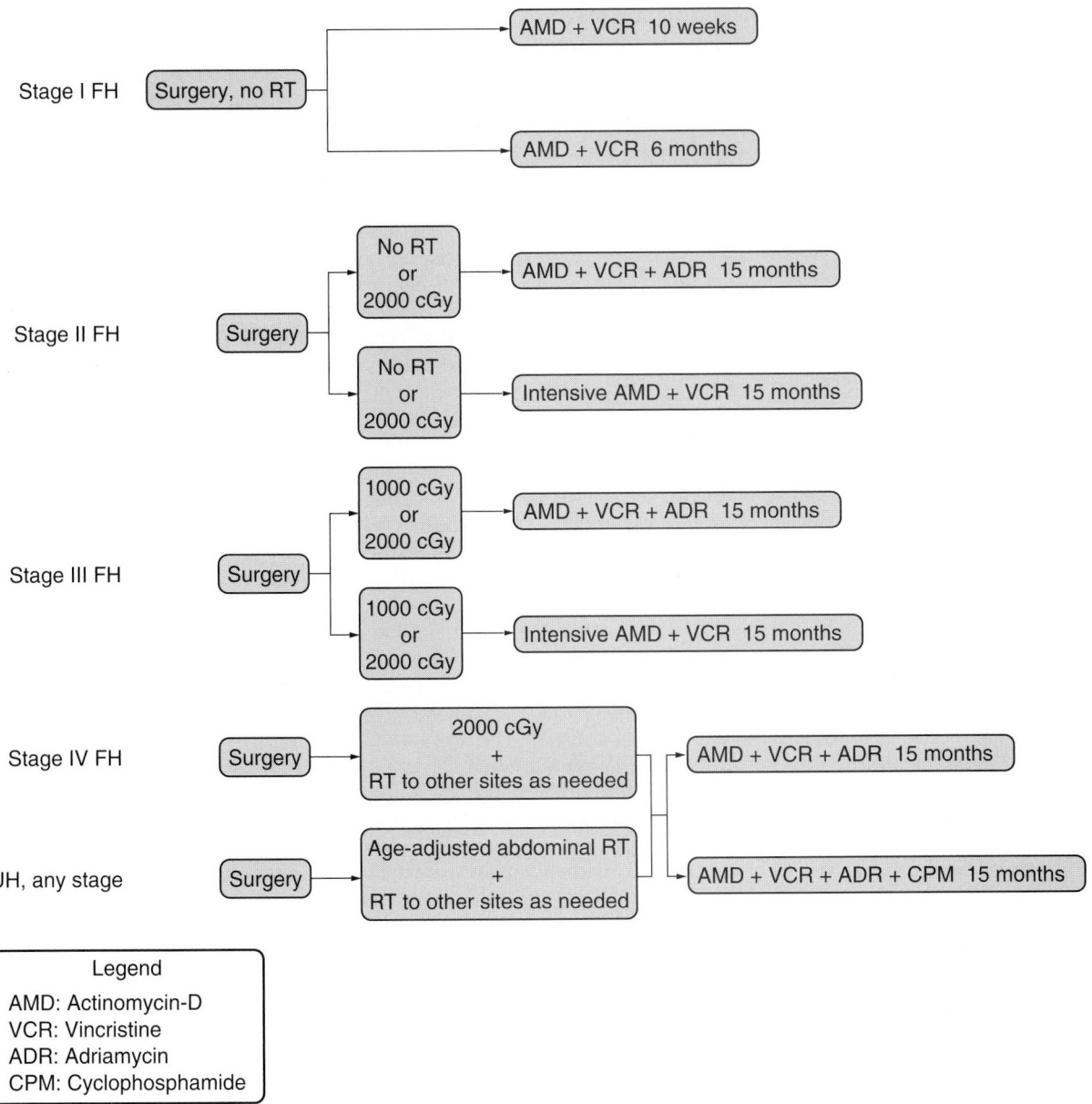

Figure 56–3. The design of the third National Wilms' Tumor Study. (From D'Angio GJ, Breslow N, Beckwith JB, et al: Treatment of Wilms' tumor: Results of the Third National Wilms' Tumor Study. *Cancer.* 1989;64:349.)

the standard regimen (actinomycin and vincristine) was beneficial. Children treated on the least intensive arm (actinomycin plus vincristine, without radiotherapy) demonstrated outcomes (87% 4-year RFS and 91% 4-year OS) that were statistically equivalent to those seen in the other three arms. Both Adriamycin and flank irradiation were thus shown to be unnecessary for children with stage II FH disease.[91]

Children with stage III FH disease were similarly randomized in a two-step fashion, to irradiation to 10 or 20 Gy and to chemotherapy with or without Adriamycin. In these children, addition of Adriamycin resulted in superior outcomes. There was no significant difference in rates of abdominal relapse between patients receiving 10 versus 20 Gy. However, a trend toward inferior

outcomes was noted among patients receiving 10 Gy in the absence of Adriamycin. This suggested the necessity of including either Adriamycin or full dose (20 Gy) irradiation in the treatment of stage III FH patients[91]; NWTS-4 subsequently prescribed Adriamycin plus 10 Gy for all stage III FH patients.

Patients with UH (any stage) or stage IV FH all underwent nephrectomy followed by tumor bed irradiation and radiotherapy to sites of metastatic disease. They were then randomized to receive actinomycin, vincristine, and Adriamycin with or without cyclophosphamide. Addition of cyclophosphamide did not result in a statistically significant improvement in RFS or OS.[91] However, subset analysis later suggested that when UH patients were further categorized as having either focal or diffuse anaplasia, those with stages II to IV diffuse anaplasia or CCSK (but not rhabdoid tumor) did benefit from the addition of cyclophosphamide.[159] For NWTS-4, the term "favorable histology" was thus amended to include focal anaplasia, and "unfavorable histology" was more strictly defined as diffuse anaplasia. Furthermore, stage I patients were grouped together in NWTS-4 regardless of histology, as neither focal nor diffuse anaplasia had a negative prognostic effect in the earliest stage of the disease.

National Wilms' Tumor Study-4

The primary intent of NWTS-4 (1986 to 1994) was to ascertain whether cost- and time-saving measures could be safely incorporated into the treatment regimens established in NWTS-3. To this end, 1687 patients across all stages were randomized to pulse-intensive (PI) versus standard-dose chemotherapy; for children with stages II to IV FH disease, a second randomization to 6 versus 15 months of chemotherapy was performed. As predicted, pulse-intensive chemotherapy was both cost- and time-effective, resulting in fewer clinic visits and lower treatment costs. The two-year RFS was equivalent between the PI and standard-dose arms (91.3% and 91.4%, respectively). Interestingly, the pulse-intensive regimen also resulted in less hematologic toxicity.[160] Analysis of short versus long course chemotherapy in stages II to IV FH patients similarly demonstrated no significant difference in 4-year RFS. The cost of treatment for patients treated with pulse-intensive short course chemotherapy was approximately one half that for patients treated on the standard-dose long course regimen.[161]

The focus on socioeconomic effects in NWTS-4 was made possible by the excellent treatment outcomes achieved in previous trials for children with favorable histology disease. However, outcomes for patients with stages II to IV diffuse anaplasia and children with CCSK remained relatively poor. Therefore, these children were also randomized to receive cyclophosphamide (in addition to actinomycin D, vincristine, and Adriamycin), in an attempt to improve outcomes and clarify the suggestion of benefit to cyclophosphamide, which was retrospectively noted in NWTS-3. Cyclophosphamide was shown to improve both RFS and OS for patients with stages II to IV diffuse anaplastic disease. The combined NWTS-3 and 4 results for this group of children revealed a 55% 4-year RFS and 52% 4-year OS for patients who received cyclophosphamide, approximately twice that of patients who did not receive the drug (27% 4-year RFS and OS) (P = 0.02).[84] However, even the improved outcomes noted in the cyclophosphamide group compared poorly with those of patients with FH disease.

Patients with CCSK (all stages) were randomized to PI versus standard-dose chemotherapy, followed by a second randomization to short (24 to 26 weeks) versus long (54 to 65 weeks) courses of chemotherapy. There was no statistically significant difference in outcomes between randomization arms, leading to the conclusion that pulse-intensive short course chemotherapy was also acceptable for children with CCSK.[160]

National Wilms' Tumor Study-5

The primary intent of NWTS-5 is to identify genetic prognostic factors (specifically, DNA ploidy and loss of heterozygosity at 16q or 1p) that predict for adverse outcomes, with the goal of targeting intensified therapies to patients at risk for relapse and minimizing treatment for the remainder of patients. To this end, urine, blood, and tumor tissue samples of enrolled patients are obtained for analysis, and blood samples are also obtained from both natural parents of each child.[149]

The NWTS-5 management guidelines by stage and histology represent the current standard of care in the United States and are outlined in Table 56-11. There are no treatment randomizations on NWTS-5. However, treatment recommendations have been modified from NWTS-4 for children with UH in an attempt to improve their historically poor outcomes. For children with stages II to IV diffuse anaplasia or CCSK, actinomycin has been replaced by etoposide, and cyclophosphamide has been dose-intensified. Children with rhabdoid tumors are now treated with a combination of cyclophosphamide, etoposide, and carboplatin, given that a neural crest origin has been postulated for rhabdoid tumor and that these agents have been previously employed for treatment of primitive neurogenic tumors.[60-62,149]

Another goal of NWTS-5 has been to minimize therapy (and thus decrease toxicity) for infants younger than 24 months with stage I FH disease. To this end, such patients were initially treated with surgery alone, provided that their tumors were less than 550 grams in weight. However, the protocol was revised to include postoperative chemotherapy in 1998, after increased pulmonary relapses were noted. NWTS-5 continues to advise that infants younger than 18 months with pulmonary metastases at presentation receive a trial of chemotherapy alone, with reservation of whole lung irradiation for persistent disease 4 weeks after initiation of chemotherapy.

Techniques of Radiotherapy

Indications and doses for flank versus whole abdomen irradiation are outlined in Table 56-13. Both regimens are delivered in an anteroposterior-posteroanterior fashion and are prescribed to midplane. For flank irradiation, the medial field border is extended across the midline to completely include the vertebral bodies at the levels concerned, but not far enough to overlap any portion of the contralateral kidney.[149] The lateral border extends to the abdominal wall, with a custom shield extending laterally from the external margin of the wall to prevent skin flashing. The superior and inferior borders are defined as the preoperative outline of the kidney and tumor, plus a 1 cm margin. Using this technique, the superior border should rarely approach the diaphragmatic dome.

In the case of whole abdomen irradiation, the portal extends from the diaphragmatic domes superiorly and to the bottom of the obturator foramina inferiorly, with shielding of the femoral heads. Bilateral abdominal wall shields are also employed, to prevent skin flashing.

Table 56–13   Abdominal Radiation: Fields and Doses

Extent of Disease	Radiotherapy Field	Dose
• Renal hilar nodes • Microscopic residuum confined to flank	Flank, crossing midline to include entire vertebral bodies	1.8 Gy × 6 = 10.8 Gy
• Positive para-aortic nodes	Include entire length of bilateral para-aortic chains	1.8 Gy × 6 = 10.8 Gy
• Peritoneal seeding	Whole abdomen	1.8 Gy × 6 = 10.8 Gy or 1.5 Gy × 7 = 10.5 Gy
• Preoperative intraperitoneal rupture • Diffuse operative spill • Gross residual disease >3 cm	Disease + 1 cm margin	10.8 Gy boost

Adapted from Grundy PE, Green DM, Coppes MJ, et al: In Pizzo PA, Poplack DG, eds. *Principles and Practice of Pediatric Oncology*, 4th ed. Philadelphia: Lippincott Williams & Wilkins. 2002;865; and (Multiple authors): National Wilms' Tumor Study-5: Therapeutic Trial and Biology Study. Unpublished. Activated June 16, 1995; last revised June 1998.

Abdominal irradiation should be initiated no later than 9 days postoperatively, provided the patient is stable, free of ileus or diarrhea, and has an absolute neutrophil count of at least 1000 and hemoglobin of at least 10.5. Rhabdoid tumor is the exception to this rule with abdominal irradiation delayed until week 6 of chemotherapy. The recommended schedule for both flank and whole abdomen irradiation is 1.8 Gy daily to 10.8 Gy; higher doses may be employed for CCSK and rhabdoid tumor. (Note that this represents a significant modification from all prior NWTS protocols, in which patients with UH received higher-dose radiotherapy (up to 40 Gy) on an age-dependent scale. This recommendation is based in part on retrospective analysis of prior NWTS studies, which failed to show a dose-response relationship for anaplastic Wilms'.[159] However, doses as low as 10.8 Gy have never been studied in this subgroup; the prior minimum dose was 18 Gy, for children 18 months or younger. An additional 10.8 Gy should be delivered to regions of gross (>3 cm) residual disease, with at least a 1 cm margin.

The treatment schedule may be modified to 1.5 Gy daily to 10.5 Gy in whole abdomen irradiation if the treating clinician is concerned about large-volume fields. This modification can also be used in either flank or whole abdomen therapy when simultaneous whole lung irradiation is required, to avoid disparate fractionation schedules to the two regions. Figure 56-4 displays an example of such a modification.

In patients older than 18 months with pulmonary metastases at diagnosis, both lungs are treated regardless of the number or location of visible metastases. (If metastases are seen on CT but not on chest x-ray, administration of whole lung irradiation is at the discretion of the treating clinician.) Treatment is delivered via anteroposterior-posteroanterior portals and is prescribed to midplane. The superior border extends above the clavicles to encompass the apices; the inferior border includes the posterior inferior portions of the lung. The humeral heads and extrathoracic scapulae and clavicles are shielded. No other shielding is employed. The recommended schedule is 1.5 Gy daily to 12 Gy, to commence simultaneously with abdominal irradiation. Localized foci of lung disease persisting 2 weeks after radiation may be either excised or treated with an additional 7.5 Gy (1.5 Gy/day × 5),[149] although caution is advised given the

potentially fatal risk of pulmonary toxicity in patients receiving combined modality therapy.

Patients younger than 18 months with pulmonary metastases at presentation should receive thoracic irradiation only if they have persistent metastases after 4 weeks of chemotherapy. In these children, whole lung irradiation should be delivered in 1.5 Gy daily fractions to 9 Gy, with a single 1.5 Gy boost to nodules that do not disappear after 9 Gy.[149]

If liver metastases are completely resected, hepatic irradiation is unnecessary. Treatment of residual or unresectable disease varies based on histology. For patients with favorable histology or focal anaplasia, focal unresectable liver metastases are treated with a 2 cm margin in 1.8 Gy daily fractions to 19.8 Gy. If diffuse liver involvement is known or suspected, the entire organ should receive 19.8 Gy. Additional boosting to focal

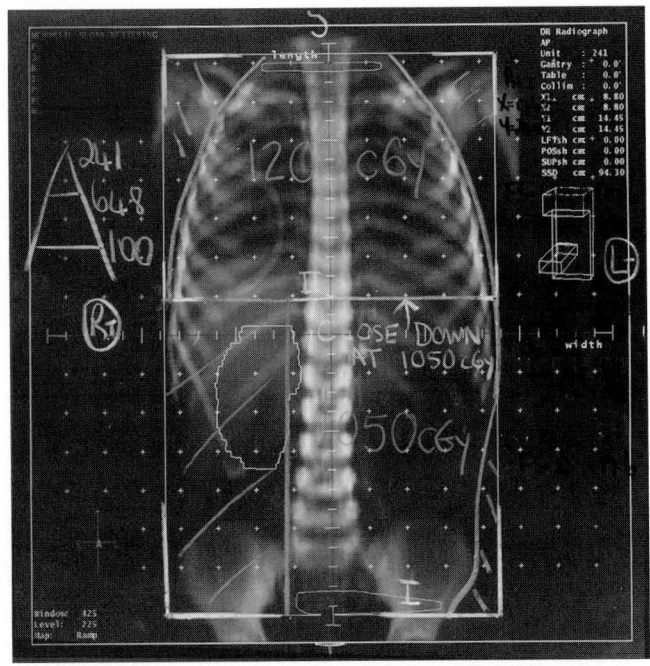

Figure 56–4. Simulation film showing typical combined whole lung and flank field. In this case, a single isocenter technique is used and an asymmetric jaw may be closed for the final fraction so that the lungs receive a total dose of 12 Gy and the flank receives 10.5 Gy in 1.5 Gy fractions.

regions (5.4 to 10.8 Gy) is at the discretion of the treating clinician, with the caveat that 75% of the whole liver should not receive more than 30.6 Gy as a result of all radiotherapy, including whole organ irradiation and overlap from abdominal or lung fields, or both. For patients with diffuse anaplasia, CCSK, or rhabdoid tumor, focal liver metastases are treated to 30.6 Gy. Whole liver irradiation for diffuse disease also requires a dose of 30.6 Gy, and supplemental boosting (5.4 to 10.8 Gy) to focal areas is permissible. In these children, the dose to the whole liver should not exceed 30.6 Gy.[149]

Other metastatic sites requiring radiation include lymph nodes outside of the abdomen or pelvis, bone, and brain. Metastatic nodes receive 19.8 Gy; bone metastases are treated with at least a 3 cm margin to a dose of 30.6 Gy. Cerebral metastases are treated with whole brain irradiation to 30.6 Gy.[149]

Radiotherapeutic management of metastatic Wilms' is outlined in Table 56-14. In all cases, care must be taken to limit the dose received by the normal kidney. NWTS-5 specifies that the dose to more than one third of the contralateral kidney (or to the residual normal kidney in children with bilateral Wilms') should not exceed 14.4 Gy. Use of brachytherapy in the management of Wilms' tumor has been anecdotally reported in fewer than 20 patients,[162-166] all of whom had either recurrent disease or residual tumor after standard therapy.

Management of Inoperable Disease

As previously described, patients with unresectable disease should undergo surgical exploration and biopsies for diagnosis and staging, followed by chemotherapy with vincristine, actinomycin, and Adriamycin. Radiographic re-evaluation should be performed at week 5, with surgery performed shortly thereafter. If a persistent inadequate response is noted, preoperative irradiation with concurrent vincristine may be considered. The suggested dose is 12 to 12.6 Gy in 1.5 to 1.8 Gy daily fractions. Postoperative radiotherapy should be administered to all children who did not receive it preoperatively. After completion of radiotherapy, the chemotherapy regimen for stage III disease should be completed.[116]

Management of Synchronous Bilateral Disease

After surgical exploration, bilateral biopsies, and staging of each kidney, children with bilateral Wilms' tumor should receive preoperative chemotherapy according to the highest stage of disease identified. Radiographic evaluation of response to therapy should begin at week 5, followed by a second-look procedure when the disease appears resectable; if serial imaging studies fail to show reduction in tumor, second-look surgery should still be performed, to distinguish between persistent viable tumor and residual benign tissue. At that time, bilateral partial nephrectomies or wedge excisions should be performed only if negative margins can be obtained. If one kidney has extensive tumor precluding partial resection, complete excision of tumor from the least involved kidney is performed; if this procedure leaves the partially resected kidney viable and functioning, the extensively involved kidney can be removed by radical nephrectomy.[149]

Table 56–14   Radiotherapy for Metastatic Disease

Disease Site	Radiotherapy Field	Dose
Lung		
Age 18 mo or older	WLI ± boost to residual foci post-RT	WLI: 1.5 Gy × 8 = 12 Gy
		Boost: 1.5 Gy × 5 = 7.5 Gy
Age younger than 18 mos	WLI if disease persists after week 4 of chemotherapy ± boost to residual foci post-RT	WLI: 1.5 Gy × 6 = 9 Gy
		Boost: 1.5 Gy × 1
Liver		
FH or focal anaplasia		
Focal metastases	Disease + 2 cm margin	1.8 Gy × 11 = 19.8 Gy
Diffuse involvement	Whole liver	1.8 Gy × 11 = 19.8 Gy
		± 5.4-10.8 Gy boost to focal areas
Diffuse anaplasia, CCSK, or rhabdoid tumor		
Focal metastases	Disease + 2 cm margin	1.8 Gy × 18 = 30.6 Gy
Diffuse involvement	Whole liver	1.8 Gy × 18 = 30.6 Gy
		± 5.4-10.8 Gy boost to focal areas
Lymph nodes outside the abdomen or pelvis		
	Involved nodes	1.8 Gy × 11 = 19.8 Gy
Bone	Lesion + 3 cm margin	1.8 Gy × 18 = 30.6 Gy
Brain	Whole brain	1.8 Gy × 18 = 30.6 Gy

CCSK, clear cell sarcoma of the kidney; FH, favorable histology; WLI, whole lung irradiation.
From Grundy PE, Green DM, Coppes MJ, et al: In Pizzo PA, Poplack DG, eds. *Principles and Practice of Pediatric Oncology*, 4th ed. Philadelphia: Lippincott Williams & Wilkins. 2002;865; and (Multiple authors): National Wilms' Tumor Study-5: Therapeutic Trial and Biology Study. Unpublished. Activated June 16, 1995; last revised June 1998.

Postoperatively, patients in whom complete resection was achieved should complete the chemotherapy regimen that corresponds to the highest stage of disease identified either initially or at second-look surgery. Radiotherapy is not indicated in the management of these patients.[149]

Patients with persistent gross disease after a second-look procedure should be considered for re-operation after further chemotherapy. If repeat abdominal explorations (the number and extent of which are at the discretion of the treating surgeon) fail to eradicate gross disease, patients should receive radiation to the involved kidney and tumor bed in the manner described earlier.[149]

Critical Normal Tissues—Radiation Injury

Musculoskeletal late effects in patients receiving combined modality treatment for Wilms' tumor can be directly attributed to radiation therapy.[167] These include scoliosis, kyphosis, muscular hypoplasia, and iliac wing hypoplasia in patients receiving flank or whole abdomen irradiation; and limb length inequalities in patients receiving radiotherapy to bone metastases in the extremities. Severe musculoskeletal complications are unlikely when doses under 24 Gy are used. Even in the setting of lower doses, however, radiation fields should be designed to minimize asymmetric development (e.g., treating the entire vertebral bodies in flank irradiation to avoid scoliosis).

Females who receive abdominal irradiation are at increased risk of late reproductive sequelae including ovarian failure[168] and adverse pregnancy outcomes such as fetal loss, premature delivery, and possibly birth defects.[169-171] In the largest series to date, Li and coworkers reported an excess risk of low birth weight (relative risk 4.0) and perinatal mortality (relative risk 7.9) in females who had received abdominal irradiation, as compared with white women in the United States.[171]

Radiation pneumonitis is a life-threatening consequence of whole lung irradiation, and is potentiated by concurrent chemotherapies. Twelve percent of patients on NWTS-3 who received pulmonary irradiation developed pneumonitis not due to *Pneumocystis carinii*, with an associated 75% mortality.[172] Reduction of the dose of concurrently administered Adriamycin and actinomycin-D has reduced the current incidence of radiation pneumonitis, although the risk of fatal pulmonary complications remains a major concern for children who receive supplemental radiation for residual lung disease after the standard 12 Gy.[149]

Chronic renal failure can occur as a consequence of radiation nephritis, but the reported incidence is less than 0.25% among children with unilateral disease and an apparently normal contralateral kidney at the time of diagnosis.[173] The risk of renal failure is higher in patients with bilateral disease, although the incidence has decreased over the span of the NWTS trials from 9.9% in NWTS-1 to 3.8% in NWTS-4. Most cases of renal failure in children with bilateral Wilms' are caused by either surgery or the sequelae of the Denys-Drash syndrome.[173]

Second malignancies are a potential complication of both chemotherapy and radiation therapy. The cumulative incidence of second malignancies among children followed by the NWTS is 1.6% at 15 years, and the risk appears to continuously increase.[174] Reviewers of the International Society of Pediatric Oncology experience reported a 0.65% cumulative incidence of second cancer at 15 years, with all second cancers occurring in the first 10 years after treatment. No excess risk was observed after 10 years, but this may have been a function of the length of follow-up.[175] The single most important risk factor appears to be radiation, and administration of Adriamycin potentiates the radiation-associated risk.[174] Notably, however, even patients who received only vincristine and actinomycin-D, without Adriamycin or radiation therapy, have an increased risk of second cancers as compared to the U.S. population when adjusted for age, sex, and race.[174] Furthermore, inherited predisposition to multiple cancers may contribute to the excess risk of second malignancies among children treated for Wilms' tumor.

Although late congestive heart failure is primarily due to Adriamycin toxicity, the risk of congestive heart failure is increased from 1% to 5.4% in patients receiving whole lung irradiation[176] and has been anecdotally reported in patients whose left ventricles received radiation during the course of left-sided abdominal therapy.[177]

Small bowel obstruction occurred in 6.9% of children enrolled in NWTS-3, primarily as a result of bowel adhesions after surgery. This incidence is comparable to that of other children undergoing major abdominal operations. A review of the NWTS-3 experience found that the incidence of small bowel obstruction was not increased by postoperative abdominal radiation therapy.[178]

REFERENCES

1. Smith M, Ries L, Gurney J: Cancer incidence and survival among children and adolescents: United States SEER program 1975-1995. Bethesda, MD, National Cancer Institute, SEER program, 1999.
2. Brodeur G, Maris J: Neuroblastoma. In Pizzo P, Poplack D, eds. *Principles and Practice of Pediatric Oncology*, 4th ed. Philadelphia: Lippincott Williams & Wilkins Publishers; 2002:895.
3. Halperin E, Constine L, Tarbell N, Kun L: Neuroblastoma. In *Pediatric Radiation Oncology*, 3rd ed. Philadelphia: Lippincott Williams & Wilkins; 1999:163.
4. Beckwith J, Perrin E: In situ neuroblastomas: A contribution to the natural history of neural crest tumors. *Am J Pathol.* 1963;43:1089.
5. Ikeda Y, Lister J, Bouton JM, Buyukpamukcu M: Congenital neuroblastoma, neuroblastoma in situ, and the normal fetal development of the adrenal. *J Pediatr Surg.* 1981;16:636.
6. Knudson AGJ, Strong LC: Mutation and cancer: Neuroblastoma and pheochromocytoma. *Am J Hum Genet.* 1972;24:514.
7. Kushner BH, Gilbert F, Helson L: Familial neuroblastoma: Case reports, literature review, and etiologic considerations. *Cancer.* 1986;57:1887.
8. Fong CT, Dracopoli NC, White PS, et al: Loss of heterozygosity for the short arm of chromosome 1 in human neuroblastomas: Correlation with N-myc amplification. *Proc Natl Acad Sci USA.* 1989;86:3753.
9. Brodeur GM, Seeger RC, Schwab M, et al: Amplification of N-myc in untreated neuroblastomas correlates with advanced disease stage. *Science.* 1984;224:1121.
10. Matthay KK: Neuroblastoma: Biology and therapy. *Oncology.* 1997;11:1857.
11. Delellis RA: The adrenal glands. In Sternbert SS, eds. *Diagnostic Surgical Pathology*, vol 1. New York: Raven Press; 1989:445.

12. Joshi V, Cantor A, Altshuler G, et al: Prognostic significance of histopathologic features of neuroblastoma: A grading system based on the review of 211 cases from the Pediatric Oncology Group. *Proc Am Soc Clin Oncol.* 1991;10:311. Abstract.

13. Couanet D, Hartmann O, Piekarski JD, et al: The use of computed tomography in the staging of neuroblastomas in childhood. *Arch Fr Pediatr.* 1981;38:315.

14. Golding SJ, McElwain TJ, Husband JE: The role of computed tomography in the management of children with advanced neuroblastoma. *Br J Radiol.* 1984;57:661.

15. Fletcher BD, Kopiwoda SY, Strandjord SE, et al: Abdominal neuroblastoma: Magnetic resonance imaging and tissue characterization. *Radiology.* 1985;155:699.

16. Smith FW, Cherryman GR, Redpath TW, et al: The nuclear magnetic resonance appearances of neuroblastoma. *Pediatr Radiol.* 1985;15:329.

17. Heisel MA, Miller JH, Reid BS, et al: Radionuclide bone scan in neuroblastoma. *Pediatrics.* 1983;71:206.

18. Podrasky AE, Stark DD, Hattner RS, et al: Radionuclide bone scanning in neuroblastoma: Skeletal metastases and primary tumor localization of 99mTc-MDP. *AJR Am J Roentgenol.* 1983;141:469.

19. Voute PA, Hoefnagel C, Marcuse HR, et al: Detection of neuroblastoma with [I-131]meta-iodobenzylguanidine. *Prog Clin Biol Res.* 1985;175:389.

20. Brodeur GM, Seeger RC, Barrett A, et al: International criteria for diagnosis, staging and response to treatment in patients with neuroblastoma. *J Clin Oncol.* 1988;6:1874.

21. Brodeur GM, Pritchard J, Berthold F, et al: Revisions in the international criteria neuroblastoma diagnosis, staging and response to treatment. *J Clin Oncol.* 1993;11:1466.

22. LaBrosse EH, Comay E, Bohuan C, et al: Catecholamine metabolism in neuroblastoma. *J Natl Cancer Inst.* 1976;57:633.

23. Evans AE, D'Angio G, Randolph J: A proposed staging for children with neuroblastoma. Children's Cancer Study Group A. *Cancer.* 1971;27:374.

24. Nitschke R, Smith EI, Shochat S, et al: Localized neuroblastoma treated by surgery. A Pediatric Oncology Group Study. *J Clin Oncol.* 1988;6:1271.

25. Hayes FA, Green A, Hustu HO, et al: Surgicopathologic staging of neuroblastoma: Prognostic significance of regional lymph node metastases. *J Pediatr.* 1983;102:59.

26. Paulino AC, Mayr NA, Simon JH, et al: Locoregional control in infants with neuroblastoma: Role of radiation therapy and late toxicity. *Int J Radiat Oncol Biol Phys.* 2002;52:1025.

27. McWilliams NB: Neuroblastoma in infancy. In Pochedly C, ed. *Neuroblastoma: Tumor Biology and Therapy.* Boca Raton, Fla: CRC Press; 1990:229.

28. Hayes FA, Green AA, O'Connor DM: Chemotherapeutic management of epidural neuroblastoma. *Med Pediatr Oncol.* 1989;17:6.

29. Hoover M, Bowman LC, Crawford SE, et al: Long-term outcome of patients with intraspinal neuroblastoma. *Med Pediatr Oncol.* 1999;32:353.

30. Plantaz D, Rubie H, Michon J, et al: The treatment of neuroblastoma with intraspinal extension with chemotherapy followed by surgical removal of residual disease. A prospective study of 42 patients—Results of the NBL 90 Study of the French Society of Pediatric Oncology. *Cancer.* 1996;78:311.

31. de Barnardi B, Pianca C, Pistamiglio P, et al: Neuroblastoma with symptomatic spinal cord compression at diagnosis: Treatment and results with 76 cases. *J Clin Oncol.* 2001;19:183.

32. August CS, Serota FT, Koch PA, et al: Treatment of advanced neuroblastoma with supralethal chemotherapy, radiation, and allogeneic autologous marrow reconstitution. *J Clin Oncol.* 1984; 2:609.

33. Mayfield JK, Riseborough EJ, Jaffe N, et al: Spinal deformity in children treated for neuroblastoma. *J Bone Joint Surg [Am].* 1981; 63a:183.

34. Thurman WG, Fernbach DJ, Sullivan MP, et al: Cyclophosphamide therapy in childhood neuroblastoma. *N Engl J Med.* 1964; 270:1336.

35. Green AA, Hayes FA, Pratt CB, et al: Phase II evaluation of cisplatin in children with neuroblastoma and other malignant solid tumors. In Prestyko AW, Crooke ST, Carter SK, eds. *Cisplatin: Current Status and New Developments.* New York: Academic Press; 1980:477.

36. Wang JJ, Cortes E, Sinks LF, et al: Therapeutic effect and toxicity of Adriamycin in patients with neoplastic disease. *Cancer.* 1971;28:837.

37. Rivera G, Green AA, Hayes F, et al: Epipodophyllotoxin VM-26 in the treatment of childhood neuroblastoma: *Cancer Treat Rep.* 1977;61:1243.

38. Perez CA, Matthay KK, Atkinson JB, et al: Biologic variables in the outcome of stages I and II neuroblastoma treated with surgery as primary therapy: A children's cancer study group study. *J Clin Oncol.* 2000;18:18.

39. Cohn SL, Look AT, Joshi VV, et al: Lack of correlation of N-myc gene amplification with prognosis in localized neuroblastoma: A Pediatric Oncology Group study. *Cancer Res.* 1995;55:721.

40. Rubie H, Hartmann O, Michon J, et al: N-Myc gene amplification is a major prognostic factor in localized neuroblastoma: Results of the French NBL 90 study. Neuroblastoma Study Group of the Societe Francaise d'Oncologie Pediatrique. *J Clin Oncol.* 1997; 15:1171.

41. Katzenstein HM, Bowman LC, Brodeur GM, et al: Prognostic significance of age, MYCN oncogene amplification, tumor cell ploidy, and histology in 110 infants with stage D(S) neuroblastoma: The pediatric oncology group experience—A pediatric oncology group study. *J Clin Oncol.* 1998;16:2007.

42. Nickerson HJ, Matthay KK, Seeger RC, et al: Favorable biology and outcome of stage IV-S neuroblastoma with supportive care or minimal therapy: A Children's Cancer Group Study. *J Clin Oncol.* 2000;18:477.

43. Guglielmi M, de Bernardi B, Rizzo A: Resection of primary tumor at diagnosis in stage IV-S neuroblastoma: Does it affect the clinical course? *J Clin Oncol.* 1996;14:1537.

44. Children's Oncology Group (COG) current study #P9641.

45. Matthay KK, Perez C, Seeger RC, et al: Successful treatment of stage III neuroblastoma based on prospective biologic staging: A Children's Cancer Group study. *J Clin Oncol.* 1998;16:1256.

46. Schmidt ML, Lukens JN, Seeger RC, et al: Biologic factors determine prognosis in infants with stage IV neuroblastoma: A prospective children's cancer group study. *J Clin Oncol.* 2000; 18:1260.

47. Castleberry RP, Kun LE, Shuster JJ, et al: Radiotherapy improves the outlook for patients older than 1 year with Pediatric Oncology Group stage C neuroblastoma. *J Clin Oncol.* 1991;9:789.

48. de Bernardi B, Rogers D, Carli M, et al: Localized neuroblastoma. Surgical and pathologic staging. *Cancer.* 1987;60:1066.

49. Children's Oncology Group (COG) current study #A3961.

50. Matthay KK, Lukens J, Stram D, et al: Improving survival from 1978-1995 using risk based treatment for neuroblastoma: Children's Cancer Group (CCG). *Med Pediatr Oncol.* 1996; 27:220.

51. Matthay KK, Villablanca JG, Seeger RC, et al: Treatment of high-risk neuroblastoma with intensive chemotherapy, radiotherapy, autologous bone marrow transplantation, and 13-cis-retinoic acid. Children's Cancer Group. *N Engl J Med.* 1999;341:1165.

52. Cheung NV, Heller G: Chemotherapy dose intensity correlates strongly with response, median survival, and median progression-free survival in metastatic neuroblastoma. *J Clin Oncol.* 1991; 9:1050.

53. Castleberry RP, Cantor AB, Green AA, et al: Phase II investigational window using carboplatin, iproplatin, ifosfamide, and epirubicin in children with untreated disseminated neuroblastoma: A Pediatric Oncology Group study. *J Clin Oncol.* 1994;12:1616.

54. Matthay KK, Castleberry RP: Treatment of advanced neuroblastoma: The U.S. experience. In Brodeur GM, Sawada T, Tsuchida Y, Voute PA, eds. Neuroblastoma. Amsterdam: Elsevier Science; 2000:437.

55. Kushner BH, LaQuaglia MP, Bonilla MA, et al: Highly effective induction therapy for stage 4 neuroblastoma in children over 1 year of age. *J Clin Oncol.* 1994;12:2607.

56. Kushner BH, Cheung NK, Kramer K, et al: Neuroblastoma and treatment-related myelodysplasia/leukemia: The Memorial Sloan-Kettering experience and a literature review. *J Clin Oncol.* 1998;16:3880.

57. Kaneko M, Tsuchida Y, Uchino J, et al: Treatment results of advanced neuroblastoma with the first Japanese study group protocol. Study group of Japan for treatment of advanced neuroblastoma. *J Pediatr Hematol Oncol.* 1999;21:190.

58. Hartmann O, Berthold F: Treatment of advanced neuroblastoma: The European experience. In Brodeur GM, Sawada T, Tsuchida Y, Voute PA, eds. Neuroblastoma. Amsterdam: Elsevier Science; 2000:437.

59. Graham-Pole J, Casper J, Elfenbein G, et al: High-dose chemotherapy supported by marrow infusions for advanced neuroblastoma: A Pediatric Oncology Group study. *J Clin Oncol.* 1991;152.

60. Stram DO, Matthay KK, O'Leary, et al: Consolidation chemoradiotherapy and autologous bone marrow transplantation versus continued chemotherapy for metastatic neuroblastoma: A report of two concurrent Children's Cancer Group studies. *J Clin Oncol.* 1996;14:2417.

61. Villablanca JG, Matthay KK, Swift PS, et al: Phase I trial of carboplatin, etoposide, melphalan and local irradiation (CEM-LI) with purged autologous bone marrow transplantation for children with high-risk neuroblastoma. *Med Pediatr Oncol.* 1999;33:170.

62. Wolden SL, Gollamudi SV, Kushner BH, et al: Local control with multi-modality therapy for stage 4 neuroblastoma. *Int J Radiat Oncol Biol Phys.* 2000;46:969.

63. Kushner BH, Wolden S, La Quaglia MP, et al: Hyperfractionated low-dose radiotherapy for high-risk neuroblastoma after intensive chemotherapy and surgery. *J Clin Oncol.* 2001;19:2821.

64. Yu AL, Batova A, Alvarada C, et al: Usefulness of a chimeric anti-GD2 (ch14.18) and GM-CSF for refractory neuroblastoma: A POG phase II study. *Proc Am Soc Clin Oncol.* 1997;16:513a.

65. Cheung NK, Kushner BH, Yeh SDJ, et al: 3F8 monoclonal antibody treatment of patients with stage 4 neuroblastoma: A phase II study. *Int J Oncol.* 1998;12:1299.

66. Haas-Kogan DA, Fisch BM, Wara WM, et al: Intraoperative radiation therapy for high-risk pediatric neuroblastoma. *Int J Radiat Oncol Biol Phys.* 2000;47:985.

67. Blaney SM, Balis FM, Cole DE, et al: Pediatric phase I trial and pharmacokinetic study of topotecan administered as a 24-hour continuous infusion. *Cancer Res.* 1993;53:1032.

68. Pratt CB, Stuart C, Santana VM, et al: Phase I study of topotecan for pediatric patients with malignant solid tumors. *J Clin Oncol.* 1994;12:539.

69. Kretschmar CS, Kletzel M, Murray K, et al: Phase II therapy with Taxol and topotecan in untreated children > 365 days with disseminated neuroblastoma. A POG study. *Med Pediatr Oncol.* 1995;24:243.

70. Blaney SM, Needle MN, Gillespie A, et al: Phase II trial of topotecan administered as a 72-hour continuous infusion in children with refractory solid tumors: A collaborative Pediatric Branch, National Cancer Institute, and Children's Cancer Group Study. *Clin Cancer Res.* 1998;4:357.

71. Nitschke R, Parkhurst J, Sullivan J, et al: Topotecan in pediatric patients with recurrent and progressive solid tumors: A Pediatric Oncology Group phase II study. *J Pediatr Hematol Oncol.* 1998;20:315.

72. Saylors RL III, Stewart CF, Zamboni WC, et al: Phase I study of topotecan in combination with cyclophosphamide in pediatric patients with malignant solid tumors: A Pediatric Oncology Group Study. *J Clin Oncol.* 1998;16:945.

73. Furman WL, Stewart CF, Poquette CA, et al: Direct translation of a protracted irinotecan schedule from a xenograft model to a phase I trial in children. *J Clin Oncol.* 1999;17:1815.

74. Weitman S, Moore R, Barrera H, et al: In vitro antitumor activity of rebeccamycin analog (NSC #655649) against pediatric solid tumors. *J Pediatr Hematol Oncol.* 1998;20:136.

75. Davidson A, Gowing R, Lowis S, et al: Phase II study of 21 day schedule oral etoposide in children. New Agents Group of the United Kingdom Children's Cancer Study Group (UKCCSG). *Eur J Cancer.* 1997;33:1816.

76. Matthay KK, DeSantes K, Hasegawa B, et al: Phase I dose escalation of I^{131} metaiodobenzylguanidine with autologous bone marrow support in refractory neuroblastoma. *J Clin Oncol.* 1998;16:229.

77. Tepmongkol S, Heyman S: I^{131} MIBG therapy in neuroblastoma: Mechanisms, rationale, and current status. *Med Pediatr Oncol.* 1999;32:427; discussion 432.

78. Mariotti A, Marcora E, Bunone G, et al: N-(4-hydroxyphenyl)-retinamide: A potent inducer of apoptosis in human neuroblastoma cells. *J Natl Cancer Inst.* 1994;86:1245.

79. Maurer BJ, Metelitsa LS, Seeger RC, et al: Increase of ceramide and induction of mixed apoptosis/necrosis by N-(4-hydroxyphenyl)-retinamide in neuroblastoma cell lines. *J Natl Cancer Inst.* 1999;91:1138.

80. Woods WG, Gao RN, Shuster JJ, et al: Screening infants and mortality due to neuroblastoma. *N Engl J Med.* 2002;346:1041.

81. Schilling FH, Spix C, Berthold F, et al: Neuroblastoma screening at one year of age. *N Engl J Med.* 2002;346:1047.

82. Peschel RE, Chen M, Seashore J: The treatment of massive hepatomegaly in stage IV-S neuroblastoma. *Int J Radiat Oncol Biol Phys.* 1981;7:549.

83. Paulino AC: Current issues in the diagnosis and management of Wilms' tumor. *Oncology (Huntington).* 1996;10:1553.

84. Lindsley KL, Smith SC, Douglas JG: Wilms' tumor and neuroblastoma. In Leibel SA, Phillips TL, eds. *Textbook of Radiation Oncology,* 1st ed. Philadelphia: WB Saunders; 1998:994.

85. Green, DM: Wilms' tumor. *Eur J Cancer.* 1997;33:409.

86. Breslow N, Olshan A, Beckwith JB, et al: Epidemiology of Wilms' tumor. *Med Pediatr Oncol.* 1993;21:172.

87. Stiller C, Parker DM: International variations in the incidence of childhood renal tumors. *Br J Cancer.* 1990;62:1026.

88. Breslow N, Beckwith JB, Ciol M, Sharples K: Age distribution of Wilms tumor: A report from the National Wilms Tumor Study. *Cancer Res.* 1988;48:1653.

89. D'Angio GJ: Informational bulletin #19. National Wilms' Tumor Study, 1991. Seattle: NWTS Data and Statistical Center.

90. Blute ML, Kelalis PP, Offord KP, et al: Bilateral Wilms' tumor. *J Urol.* 1991;146:514.

91. D'Angio GJ, Breslow N, Beckwith JB, et al: Treatment of Wilms' tumor: Results of the Third National Wilms' Tumor Study. *Cancer.* 1989;64:349.

92. Montgomery BT, Kelalis PP, Blute MD, et al: Extended follow-up of bilateral Wilms' tumor: Results of the National Wilms' Tumor Study. *J Urol.* 1991;146:514.

93. Bond JV: Bilateral Wilms' tumour: Age at diagnosis, associated congenital abnormalities, and possible pattern of inheritance. *Lancet.* 1975;2:482.

94. Knudson AG: Genetics and the child cured of cancer. In van Eys J, Sullivan MD, eds. *Status of the Curability of Childhood Cancers.* New York: Raven Press; 1980:295.

95. Matsunaga E: Genetics of Wilms' tumor. *Hum Genet.* 1981;57:231.

96. Kantor AF, Curnen MG, Meigs JW, Flannery JT: Occupations of fathers of patients with Wilms' tumour. *J Epidemiol Community Health.* 1979;33:253.

97. Sanders BM, White GC, Draper GJ: Occupations of fathers of children dying from neoplasms. *J Epidemiol Community Health.* 1981;35:245.

98. Olshan AF, Breslow NE, Daling JR, et al: Wilms' tumor and paternal occupation. *Cancer Res.* 1990;50:3212.

99. Bunin GR, Nass C, Kramer S, Meadows AT: Parental occupation and Wilms' tumor: Results of a case-control study. *Cancer Res.* 1989;49:725.

100. Fabia J, Thuy TD: Occupation of father at time of birth of children dying of malignant disease. *Br J Prev Soc Med.* 1974;28:98.

101. Hicks N, Zack M, Caldwell GG, et al: Childhood cancer and occupational radiation exposure in parents. *Cancer.* 1984;53:1637.

102. Zack M, Cannon S, Lloyd D, et al: Cancer in children of parents exposed to hydrocarbon-related industries and occupations. *Am J Epidemiol.* 1980;111:329.

103. Green DM, Coppes MJ, Breslow NE, et al: Wilms tumor. In Pizzo PA, Poplack DG, eds. *Principles and Practice of Pediatric Oncology,* 3rd ed. Philadelphia: Lippincott-Raven Publishers; 1997:733.

104. Knudson AG: Mutation and cancer: Statistical study of retinoblastoma. *Proc Nat Acad Sci USA.* 1971;68:820.

105. Knudson AG, Strong LC: Mutation and cancer: A model for Wilms' tumor of the kidney. *J Natl Cancer Inst.* 1972;48:313.

106. Halperin E, Constine LS, Tarbell NJ, Kun LE: *Pediatric Radiation Oncology,* 3rd ed. Philadelphia: Lippincott Williams & Wilkins; 1999:343.

107. Coppes MJ, Williams BR: The molecular genetics of Wilms' tumor. *Cancer Invest.* 1994;12:57.

108. Coppes MJ, Haber DA, Grundy PE: Genetic events in the development of Wilms' tumor. *N Eng J Med*. 1994;331:586.
109. Porteus MH, Narkool P, Neuberg D, et al: Characteristics and outcome of children with Beckwith-Wiedemann syndrome and Wilms' tumor: A report from the National Wilms' Tumor Study Group. *J Clin Oncol*. 2000;18:2026.
110. Grundy P, Koufos A, Morgan K, et al: Familial predisposition to Wilms' tumour does not map to the short arm of chromosome 11. *Nature*. 1988;336:374.
111. Breslow NE, Beckwith JB: Epidemiological features of Wilms' tumor: Results of the National Wilms' Tumor Study. *J Natl Cancer Inst*. 1982;68:429.
112. Coppes MJ, Ritchey ML, D'Angio GJ: Preface. *Hematol Oncol Clin North Am*. 1995;9:xiii.
113. Bardeesy N, Falkoff D, Petruzzi MJ, et al: Anaplastic Wilms' tumour, a subtype displaying poor prognosis, harbours p53 mutations. *Nature Genet*. 1994;7:91.
114. Malkin D, Sexsmith E, Yeger H, et al: Mutations of the p53 tumor suppressor gene occur infrequently in Wilms' tumor. *Cancer Res*. 1994;54:2077.
115. Waber PG, Chen J, Nisen PD: Infrequency of ras, p53, WT1, or RB gene alterations in Wilms tumors. *Cancer*. 1993;72:3732.
116. Grundy PE, Green DM, Coppes MJ, et al: In Pizzo PA, Poplack DG, eds. *Principles and Practice of Pediatric Oncology*, 4th ed. Philadelphia: Lippincott Williams & Wilkins; 2002:865.
117. Pettinato G, Manivel JC, Wick MR, Dehner LP: Classical and cellular (atypical) congenital mesoblastic nephroma: A clinico-pathologic, ultrastructural, immunohistochemical, and flow cyto-metric study. *Hum Pathol*. 1989;20:682.
118. Joshi VV, Kasnicka J, Walter TR: Atypical congenital mesoblastic nephroma: Pathologic characterization of a potentially aggressive variant of conventional congenital mesoblastic nephroma. *Arch Pathol Lab Med*. 1986;110:100.
119. Beckwith JB, Weeks DA: Congenital mesoblastic nephroma: When should we worry? *Arch Pathol Lab Med*. 1986;110:98.
120. Murphy WM, Beckwith JB, Farrow GM: Tumours of the kidney, bladder, and related urinary structures. In *Atlas of Tumor Pathology*, 3rd series, fascicle 11. Washington DC: Armed Forces Institute of Pathology; 1994.
121. Schmidt D, Beckwith JB: Histopathology of childhood renal tumors. *Hematol Oncol Clin North Am*. 1995;9:1179.
122. Beckwith JB, Palmer NF: Histopathology and prognosis of Wilms tumors: Results from the First National Wilms' Tumor Study. *Cancer*. 1978;41:1937.
123. Faria P, Beckwith JB, Mishra K, et al: Focal versus diffuse anaplasia in Wilms tumor—New definitions with prognostic significance: A report from the National Wilms' Tumor Study Group. *Am J Surg Pathol*. 1996;20:909.
124. Bonadio JF, Storer B, Norkool P, et al: Anaplastic Wilms' tumor: Clinical and pathologic studies. *J Clin Oncol*. 1985;3:513.
125. Marsden HB, Lawler W, Kumar PM: Bone metastasizing renal tumor of childhood: Morphological and clinical features and differences from Wilms' tumor. *Cancer*. 1978;42:1922.
126. Beckwith JB, Larson E: Clear cell sarcoma of the kidney. *Pediatr Pathol*. 1989;9:211.
127. Green DM, Breslow NE, Beckwith JB, et al: The treatment of children with clear cell sarcoma of the kidney: A report from the National Wilms' Tumor Study Group. *J Clin Oncol*. 1994; 12:2132.
128. Haas JE, Palmer NF, Weinberg AG, Beckwith JB: Ultrastructure of malignant rhabdoid tumor of the kidney: A distinctive renal tumor of children. *Hum Pathol*. 1981;12:646.
129. Weeks DA, Beckwith JB, Mierau GW, Luckey DW: Rhabdoid tumor of the kidney: A report of 111 cases from the National Wilms' Tumor Study pathology center. *Am J Surg Pathol*. 1989; 13:439.
130. Bonnin JM, Rubinstein LJ, Palmer NF, Beckwith JB: The associa-tion of embryonal tumors originating in the kidney and in the brain: A report of seven cases. *Cancer*. 1984;54:2137.
131. Fischer HP, Thomsen H, Altmannsberger M, Bertram U: Malignant rhabdoid tumor of the kidney expressing neurofila-ment proteins: Immunohistochemical findings and histogenic aspects. *Pathol Res Pract*. 1989;184:541.
132. Gururangan S, Bowman LC, Parham DM, et al: Primary extracra-nial rhabdoid tumors: Clinicopathologic features and response to ifosfamide. *Cancer*. 1993;71:2653.
133. Vogel AM, Gown AM, Caughlan J, et al: Rhabdoid tumors of the kidney contain mesenchymal specific and epithelial specific inter-mediate filament proteins. *Lab Invest*. 1984;50:232.
134. Green DM: *Diagnosis and Management of Malignant Solid Tumors in Infants and Children*. Boston: Martinus Nijhoff; 1985.
135. Ganguly A, Gribble J, Tune B, et al: Renin-secreting Wilms' tumor with severe hypertension: Report of a case and brief review of renin-secreting tumors. *Ann Intern Med*. 1973;79:835.
136. Leape L, Breslow N, Bishop H: Surgical resection of Wilms' tumor: Results of the National Wilms' Tumor Study. *Ann Surg*. 1978;181:351.
137. Ramsay NKC, Dehner LP, Coccia PF, et al: Acute hemorrhage into Wilms' tumor. *J Pediatr*. 1977;91:763.
138. Green DM, Jaffe N: Wilms' tumor—Model of a curable pediatric malignant solid tumor. *Cancer Treat Rev*. 1978;5:143.
139. Coppes MJ: Serum biological markers and paraneoplastic syndromes in Wilms' tumor. *Med Pediatr Oncol*. 1993;21:213.
140. Green DM, Breslow NE, Beckwith JB, Norkool P: Screening of children with hemihypertrophy, aniridia, and Beckwith-Weidemann syndrome in patients with Wilms tumor: A report from the National Wilms Tumor Study. *Med Pediatr Oncol*. 1993;21:188.
141. Craft AW, Parker L, Stiller C, Cole M: Screening for Wilms' tumour in patients with aniridia, Beckwith syndrome, or hemi-hypertrophy. *Med Pediatr Oncol*. 1995;24:231.
142. Choyke PL, Siegel MJ, Craft AW, et al: Screening for Wilms tumor in children with Beckwith-Wiedemann syndrome or idiopathic hemihypertrophy. *Med Pediatr Oncol*. 1999;32:196.
143. McNeil DE, Brown M, Ching A, DeBaun MR: Screening for Wilms tumor and hepatoblastoma in children with Beckwith-Wiedemann syndromes: A cost effective model. *Med Pediatr Oncol*. 2001;37:349.
144. Thomas PR, Shochat SJ, Norkool P, et al: Prognostic implications of hepatic adhesions, invasion, and metastases at diagnosis of Wilms' tumor. The National Wilms' Tumor Study Group. *Cancer*. 1991;68:2486.
145. Breslow NE, Churchill G, Nesmith B, et al: Clinicopathologic features and prognosis for Wilms' tumor patients with metastases at diagnosis. *Cancer*. 1986;58:2501.
146. (No author). Radiation and pediatric computed tomography: A guide for health care providers. Published by the National Cancer Institute in concert with the Society for Pediatric Radiology. Summer 2002.
147. Ng YY, Hall-Graggs MA, Dicks-Mireaux C, Pritchard J: Pre- and post-chemotherapy CT appearances. *Clin Radiol*. 1991;43:255.
148. Meisel JA, Guthrie KA, Breslow NE, et al: Significance and management of computed tomography detected pulmonary nodules: A report from the National Wilms Tumor Study Group. *Int J Radiat Oncol Biol Phys*. 1999;44:579.
149. (Multiple authors). National Wilms' Tumor Study-5: Therapeutic Trial and Biology Study. Unpublished. Activated June 16, 1995; last revised June 1998.
150. Ritchey ML, Kelalis PP, Breslow N, et al: Surgical complications after nephrectomy for Wilms' tumor. *Surg Gynecol Obstet*. 1992; 175:507.
151. Ritchey ML, Kelalis PP, Breslow N, et al: Intracaval and atrial involvement with nephroblastoma: Review of National Wilms' Tumor Study-3. *J Urol*. 1988;140:1113.
152. Ritchey ML, Kelalis PP, Haase GM, et al: Preoperative therapy for intracaval and atrial extension of Wilms' tumor. *Cancer*. 1993; 71:4104.
153. Thomas PR, Tefft M, Compaan PJ, et al: Results of two radiotherapy randomizations in the Third National Wilms' Study (NWTS-3). *Cancer*. 1991;68:1703.
154. Ritchey ML, Pringle KC, Breslow NE, et al: Management and outcome of inoperable Wilms' tumor. A report of National Wilms' Tumor Study-3. *Ann Surg*. 1994;220:683.
155. D'Angio GJ, Evans AE, Breslow N, et al: The treatment of Wilms' tumor: Results of the National Wilms' Tumor Study. *Cancer*. 1976;38:633.
156. D'Angio GJ, Tefft M, Breslow N, Meyer JA: Radiation therapy of Wilms' tumor: Results according to dose, field, post-operative timing and histology. *Int J Radiat Oncol Biol Phys*. 1978;4:769.
157. Tefft M, D'Angio GJ, Grant W III: Postoperative radiation therapy for residual Wilms' tumor: Review of Group III patients in the National Wilms' Tumor Study. *Cancer*. 1976;37:2768.

158. D'Angio GJ, Evans A, Breslow N, et al: The treatment of Wilms' tumor: Results of the second National Wilms' Tumor Study. *Cancer.* 1981;47:2302.

159. Green DM, Beckwith JB, Breslow NE, et al: Treatment of children with stages II to IV anaplastic Wilms' tumor: A report from the National Wilms' Tumor Study Group. *J Clin Oncol.* 1994; 12:2126.

160. Green DM, Breslow NE, Beckwith JB, et al: Comparison between single-dose and divided-dose administration of dactinomycin and doxorubicin for patients with Wilms' tumor: A report from the National Wilms' Tumor Study Group. *J Clin Oncol.* 1998; 16:237.

161. Green DM, Breslow NE, Beckwith JB, et al: Effect of duration of treatment on treatment outcome and cost of treatment for Wilms' tumor: A report from the National Wilms' Tumor Study Group. *J Clin Oncol.* 1998;16:3744.

162. Cooper CS, Jaffe WI, Huff D, et al: The role of renal salvage procedures for bilateral Wilms' tumor: A 15-year review. *J Urol.* 2000;163:265.

163. Duckett CP, Zderic S, Goldwein J, Duckett JW: Brachytherapy for residual intra-renal Wilms' tumor. *Med Pediatr Oncol.* 1997; 28:316.

164. Goodman KA, Wolden SL, LaQuaglia MP, et al: Intraoperative high-dose rate brachytherapy for pediatric solid tumors: A 10-year experience. *Brachytherapy* 2003;2(3):139.

165. McManus MC, Silliman C, Koyle MA: Combined endoscopic resection and brachytherapy for recurrent intrapelvic Wilms tumor. *J Urol.* 2002;167:2540.

166. Thoms WW, Goldwein JW, D'Angio G: A technique for the use of afterloading ^{137}Cs brachytherapy in renal-sparing irradiation of bilateral Wilms tumor. *Int J Radiat Oncol Biol Phys.* 1997; 39:1121.

167. Evans AE, Norkool P, Evans I, et al: Late effects of treatment for Wilms' tumor: A report from the National Wilms' Tumor Study Group. *Cancer.* 1991;67:331.

168. Shalet SM, Beardwell CG, Jones PH, et al: Ovarian failure following abdominal irradiation in childhood. *Br J Cancer.* 1976; 33:655.

169. Byrne J, Mulvihill JJ, Conelly RR, et al: Reproductive problems and birth defects in survivors of Wilms' tumor and their relatives. *Med Pediatr Oncol.* 1988;16:233.

170. Green DM, Fine WE, Li FP: Offspring of patients treated for unilateral Wilms' tumor in childhood. *Cancer.* 1982;49:2285.

171. Li FP, Gimbrere K, Gelber RD, et al: Outcome of pregnancy in survivors of Wilms' tumor. *JAMA.* 1987:257:216.

172. Green DM, Finklestein JZ, Tefft ME, Norkool P: Diffuse interstitial pneumonitis after pulmonary irradiation for metastatic Wilms' tumor. *Cancer.* 1989;63:450.

173. Ritchey ML, Green DM, Thomas PR, et al: Renal failure in Wilms' tumor patients: A report from the National Wilms' Tumor Study Group [comment]. *Med Pediatr Oncol.* 1997;26:75.

174. Breslow NE, Takashima JR, Whitton JA, et al: Second malignant neoplasms following treatment for Wilms' tumor: A report from the National Wilms' Tumor Study Group. *J Clin Oncol.* 1995;13:1851.

175. Carli M, Frascella E, Tournade MF, et al: Second malignant neoplasms in patients treated on SIOP Wilms tumour studies and trials 1, 2, 5, and 6. *Med Pediatr Oncol.* 1997;29:329.

176. Green DM, Donckerwolcke R, Evans AE, D'Angio GJ: Late effects of treatment for Wilms' tumor. *Hematol Oncol Clin North Am.* 1995;9:1317.

177. Pinkel D, Camitta B, Kun L, et al: Doxorubicin cardiomyopathy in children with left-sided Wilms' tumor. *Med Pediatr Oncol.* 1982;10:483.

178. Ritchey ML, Kelalis PP, Etzioni R, et al: Small bowel obstruction after nephrectomy for Wilms' tumor: A report of the National Wilms' Tumor Study-3. *Ann Surg.* 1993;218:654.

Cancer of the Breast

Allen S. Lichter, MD

57

EPIDEMIOLOGY AND GENETICS OF BREAST CANCER

Breast cancer is the most common cancer in women, accounting for a total of 211,300 cases and 39,800 deaths per year in the United States. This represents one third of all female cancer diagnoses and 15% of cancer deaths.[1] Worldwide, nearly 1 million cases are seen annually.[2]

Epidemiologists and statisticians have calculated that a woman born today in the United States has a 1 in 8 chance of developing breast cancer during her lifetime.[3] Breast cancer is a disease associated with increasing age, and a substantial portion of the risk occurs later in life, with nearly 70% of cases diagnosed in women aged 55 and older.[4] The chance of a woman being diagnosed with breast cancer before age 50 is 1 in 50. Other risk factors may be incorporated into prediction models to produce even more precise risk estimates.[5] A summary of the chances of being diagnosed with breast cancer as a function of age is presented in Table 57-1.

The epidemiology of breast cancer presents us with extraordinary opportunities to gain insight into who might be at increased risk of being diagnosed with the disease, and insight into the etiology of the disease itself. One cannot help but be struck by the pronounced variability in breast cancer incidence rates in different countries around the world. Such rates vary over 10-fold, with Western countries having breast cancer incidence rates of more than 100 cases per 100,000 women compared with 10 to 15 per 100,000 women in many Asian countries.[6] Even more intriguing is the fact that when women from low-risk areas migrate to high-risk areas, these populations gradually assume breast cancer incidence rates nearly identical with those of high-risk populations over one to two generations.[7,8] Women in rural areas have lower breast cancer rates than do women in urban areas.[9] These epidemiologic differences have focused our attention on the importance of environmental factors in the etiology of breast cancer, including alcohol consumption[10] and especially diet and the influence of diet on body habitus.[11] Endocrine factors are also critically important in the etiology of breast cancer.[12] For example, a woman who undergoes oophorectomy before age 40 reduces her breast cancer risk by approximately 50%.[9] Menstrual and reproductive history also play a role in influencing breast cancer incidence, with early menarche and late menopause being weak risk

factors.[9,13,14] Finally, we know that breast cancer is more common in women whose families have a history of breast cancer,[15-18] and that nearly 5% to 10% of breast cancers cluster tightly in families in what appears to be a hereditary pattern,[19] often associated with the appearance of ovarian carcinoma.[20] A summary of the major risk factors associated with the development of breast cancer is presented in Table 57-2.

There are several reasons why a radiation oncologist should be familiar with breast cancer risk factors and the overall epidemiology of the disease. Radiation oncologists commonly follow many patients who have been treated for breast cancer by radiation. These women frequently ask about breast cancer risks on behalf of other family members, such as sisters or daughters. In addition, radiation oncologists follow many women who have been successfully treated for nonbreast malignancies for whom breast cancer surveillance should become a routine part of their post-treatment follow-up, and radiation oncologists should have an understanding of the breast cancer risk that these women carry. Finally, exposure to radiation is, in itself, a risk factor for breast cancer. Many retrospective series involving a variety of populations, such as tuberculosis patients subjected to repeated chest fluoroscopy,[21] patients treated with radiation for post-partum mastitis,[22] survivors of atomic bomb explosions,[23] and patients irradiated for Hodgkin's disease,[24-29] have confirmed the association between radiation and breast cancer. It appears that the risk of a radiation-induced breast cancer is highly age-dependent, with women exposed at a young age having the greatest risk,[30] whereas women exposed beyond the age of 50 years have little or no risk increase.[31,32] The latent period for the induction of breast cancer is relatively long, 10 to 15 years or more in most studies.[24-26] All patients irradiated for Hodgkin's disease, but especially younger patients, require vigilant surveillance for the development of breast cancer.

The genetics of breast cancer has long been of interest to epidemiologists and clinicians involved in this disease. It is well established that a family history of breast cancer, especially in a first-degree relative (mother or sister), increases the risk of being diagnosed with breast cancer. However, a family history of the disease does not automatically imply genetic transmission of the disease. It is probable that mothers, daughters, and sisters share environmental risk patterns and dietary patterns, usually having lived together for many years. Thus, the appearance

Table 57-1 Chance of Being Diagnosed with Breast Cancer

Before Age	Risk
30	1:2525
40	1:217
50	1:50
60	1:24
70	1:14
80	1:10
Ever	1:8

From Feuer EJ, Wun LM, Boring CC, et al: The lifetime risk of developing breast cancer. *J Natl Cancer Inst.* 1993;85:892.

of breast cancer in certain families may reflect, in part, common environmental risk factors rather than genetic inheritance. But there are families in which a heritable form of breast cancer cannot be denied. These pedigrees show multiple cases of breast cancer (and frequently ovarian cancer as well) spread through many generations. Breast cancer not only occurs frequently in these heritable breast cancer families, but usually occurs at an early age. Genetic analysis of numerous families with this heritable breast cancer syndrome have traced the abnormality to the long arm of chromosome 17 (17q21).[33] The identity of the gene (called *BRCA1*) responsible for this inherited premenopausal form of breast cancer and ovarian cancer has been identified and confirmed.[34] Carriers of a *BRCA1* mutation appear to have a 36% to 56% risk of developing breast cancer during their lifetime,[35] and are also at high risk for the development of ovarian cancer.[36] But *BRCA1* accounts for only 40% to 50% of heredity breast cancer[37] and a second gene, *BRCA2*, has been

Table 57-2 Major Risk Factors for Breast Cancer

Category	Risk Factor	Relative Risk
Age at first birth	20 yr or younger	0.8
	Nulliparous	1.0
	35 yr or older	1.8
Age at menarche	Earlier	Risk increase ~ 5%/yr
Age at menopause	Later	Risk increase ~ 5%/yr
Alcohol consumption	Yes	1.3
Biopsied breast disease	Hyperplasia	1.5-2.0
	Atypia	3-5
Breast-feeding	Yes	0.8
Diet	High-fat	1.2 (?)
Family history	One first-degree relative with disease	1.5-2.0
	Two first-degree relatives with disease	5.0
Irradiation of breast	Age 10-20 yr	Over 20.0
	Age 20-30 yr	15.0
	Age older than 50 yr	1.0
Oral contraceptives	Use	1.0
	Use before first birth	1.5
Oophorectomy	Before age 40 yr	0.5
Estrogen replacement	Yes	1.1-1.4
Prior breast cancer	Yes	0.5-1.0%/yr

cloned and accounts for some, but not all, the additional heredity cases.[38] While numerous functions of *BRCA1* have been identified, exactly why loss of this gene leads to cancer and why this gene's increased cancer risk is overwhelmingly expressed in breast and ovarian epithelial cells is still a mystery.[39] Tamoxifen and prophylactic mastectomy reduce the subsequent appearance of breast cancer in women who carry breast cancer gene mutations and should be discussed with these women when they are detected by genetic testing.[40,41]

ANATOMY OF THE BREAST

The breast rests on the anterior chest wall, beginning below the level of the clavicular head and extending inferiorly to terminate at the inframammary fold. Superficially the breast extends to the dermis, and its deep extent lies on top of the pectoralis fascia. An extension of breast tissue known as the tail of the breast is located in the low axilla. The breast itself is composed largely of fat, in which are embedded lobules containing the milk-producing glandular tissue. These lobules are connected by an arborizing network of ducts that finally terminate at the nipple.

Lymphatic drainage of the breast moves primarily superiorly and laterally toward the axillary lymph nodes. For purposes of classification, the axilla is divided into three portions by the pectoralis minor muscle. This muscle has its origin in the third, fourth, and fifth ribs and inserts on the coracoid process. Portions of the axilla inferior to the muscle are referred to as level I, whereas the superior lymph nodes are referred to as level III. Lymph nodes that lie directly beneath the pectoralis minor muscles are designated as level II (Fig. 57-1). In general, lymphatic metastases to the axilla occur in an orderly fashion, with level I preceding level II, followed by level III, and it is relatively uncommon to see a patient with level III lymph node involvement with the absence of lymph node involvement at lower levels.[42-45] However, there are well-described routes of lymphatic spread that drain directly into the apical axillary lymph nodes. These lymphatic channels primarily drain the superior aspects of the breast and can account for the 2% to 5% of patients who have metastasis at level III without having disease detected in lower-level lymph nodes. A complete axillary dissection yields between 20 and 25 lymph nodes,[42] whereas a level I and II dissection yields a median of 15 lymph nodes.[46]

The other major route of lymphatic spread is to the internal mammary (IM) chain. These nodes are situated along the IM artery and vein, which runs parallel to the sternum and superficial to the pleura. They are primarily located in the first three intercostal spaces with far fewer nodes present as one moves inferiorly.[47,48] When pathologically enlarged, IM lymph nodes as well as axillary lymph nodes can be seen on computed tomography (CT) scans (Fig. 57-2).[49] Newer techniques, such as positron emission tomography (PET), can also illustrate pathologically involved lymph nodes in the axilla and in the IM chain (Fig. 57-3).[50-52] Understanding the anatomy of the breast and its routes of lymphatic spread is important to

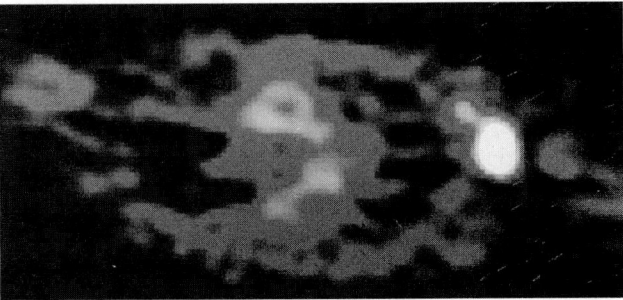

Figure 57–3. Cross-sectional slice from a positron emission tomogram (PET scan). The orientation of this slice is similar to that of a computed tomography (CT) scan. The activity in the center of the scan represents mediastinal uptake. The *dark areas* surrounding the mediastinum represent the lung shadows. In the left axilla is an exceedingly active area reflecting a substantial accumulation of the fluorodeoxyglucose tracer. Biopsy of this lymph node confirmed the presence of adenocarcinoma from a breast primary tumor.

Noninvasive Carcinomas

There are critically important differences between the two types of noninvasive cancer, ductal carcinoma in situ (DCIS) and lobular carcinoma in situ (LCIS). In the premammography era, DCIS was a relatively rare disease, often presenting as a palpable mass. Studies on the biological behavior of untreated DCIS were performed by reviewing thousands of benign breast biopsies, finding patients with previously undiagnosed DCIS, and reviewing their long-term outcome. Overall, approximately 25% to 30% of these inadvertently "untreated" DCIS patients developed subsequent invasive breast cancer. The median interval between biopsy and the subsequent development of invasive cancer was 7 to 10 years, and virtually all the cancers were in the same quadrant as the original lesion.[53-56] This suggests that DCIS is truly a preinvasive cancer that will, when left untreated, progress to invasive disease in a substantial number of patients. Molecular studies confirm this fact.

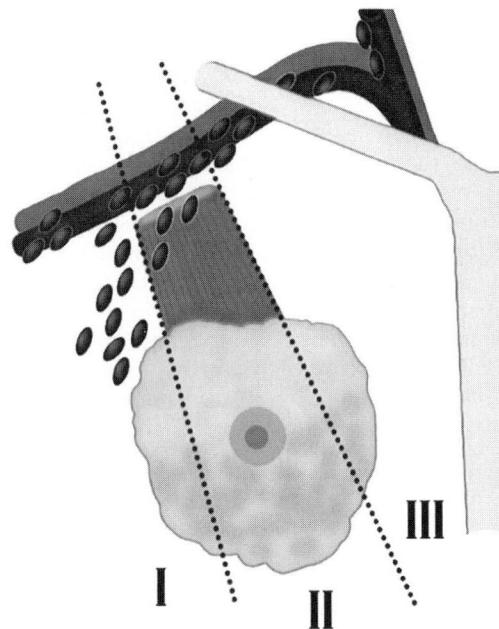

Figure 57–1. The three anatomic levels of the axillae are defined in relation to the pectoralis minor muscle. Nodes distal to the edge of the pectoralis minor are designated as level I, under the muscle as level II, and above the muscle as level III. The lymph node chain continues beneath the clavicle into the supraclavicular fossa.

the design of proper treatment strategies for breast carcinoma.

PATHOLOGY OF BREAST CANCER

Considering that it is composed of a limited number of cell types, the breast produces a wide variety of histopathologic cancers. Malignancies of the breast can be broadly divided into two categories: noninvasive and invasive. The major types of breast cancer are listed in Table 57-3.

Table 57–3   Histologic Types of Breast Cancer

In situ
    Lobular carcinoma in situ
    Ductal carcinoma in situ
        Cribriform
        Micropapillary
        Comedo
        Papillary
        Solid
Invasive
    Ductal carcinoma
    Lobular carcinoma
    Tubular carcinoma
    Medullary carcinoma
    Mucinous carcinoma
    Carcinoma with metaplasia
    Squamous cell carcinoma
    Papillary carcinoma
    Adenoid cystic carcinoma
    Secretory carcinoma
    Apocrine carcinoma
    Clear cell carcinoma

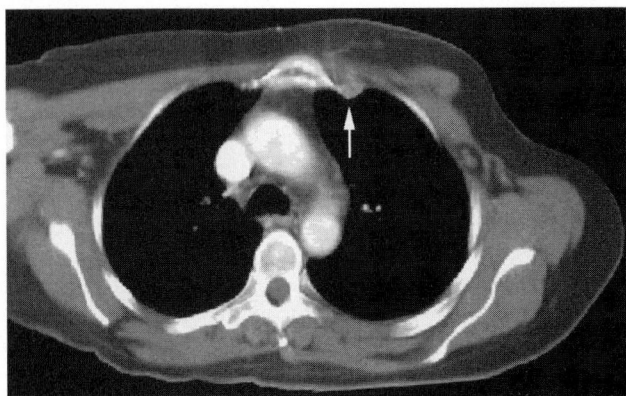

Figure 57–2. Enlarged internal mammary chain lymph nodes can, at times, be seen on computed tomographic scans (*arrow*). The nodes are typically located near the edge of the sternum and can enlarge by growing inward, displacing the pleura or growing more superficially and presenting as a visible and palpable mass in one of the upper intercostal spaces.

Genetic abnormalities can be detected in DCIS and these identical genetic changes can be found in nearby invasive carcinoma cells, confirming that the invasive component arose from DCIS.[57,58] There are five major histologically recognized architectural patterns of DCIS: (1) cribriform, (2) comedo, (3) micropapillary, (4) solid, and (5) papillary. Of these histopathologic subtypes, only comedo necrosis appears to behave differently from the other architectural patterns, displaying a somewhat more aggressive growth pattern with a slightly higher chance of lymph node involvement and a greater chance of local recurrence when lesions are treated with breast conservation.[59] It is worth pointing out that no cases of comedo DCIS were represented in the untreated series just mentioned, which likely causes the risk estimates for progression from DCIS to invasive cancer to be understated. DCIS has become a much more frequently diagnosed disease today with the advent of screening mammography. DCIS often presents with clustered microcalcifications on a mammogram, allowing early detection of this lesion (Fig. 57-4), and incidence rates of this disease have increased more than 10-fold in the last decade.[3,60] There is still a substantial amount of intraobserver variability in making the histologic diagnosis of noninvasive breast cancer, and close collaboration with one's pathologist is required before undertaking the management of these patients.[61] Pathologists should report not only the architectural type of DCIS, but its nuclear grade, degree of necrosis, and cell polarization as well in an effort to best estimate the biologic aggressiveness of the lesion.[62]

LCIS has an entirely different natural history. It is almost always an incidental diagnosis made on tissue that was obtained for another purpose.[63] The disease is, by definition, multifocal and is frequently found in both breasts.[64] Thus, obtaining negative surgical margins in LCIS is actually a misconception; the disease is so widely scattered bilaterally that the fact that LCIS is not present at an inked surgical margin does not mean that the lesion has been cleared from the breast. When patients with LCIS are followed conservatively without specific therapy, 20% to 30% of such patients eventually develop invasive breast cancer.[65,66] However, the subsequent cancers are equally divided between both breasts, and more than half of the lesions are invasive *ductal* carcinoma, not invasive *lobular* carcinoma.[66] The median interval to the development of invasive cancer is more than 15 years.[66,67] Most of these characteristics stand in sharp contradistinction to the biology of DCIS, and the two lesions must be regarded as completely separate entities.

A special type of noninvasive breast cancer that predominantly involves the nipple and underlying large ducts is Paget's disease of the breast. When the disease involves the nipple without an underlying palpable tumor, the disease is almost invariably intraductal on histopathologic examination.

Invasive Carcinomas

The most common form of invasive breast cancer is invasive ductal cancer. Accounting for approximately 80% of all invasive breast carcinomas, the malignant mass usually is seen as firm and gritty on gross examination. The cancer is frequently associated with a desmoplastic reaction accounting for the firm consistency of the mass and its irregular borders.[68] Infiltrating lobular carcinoma accounts for 5% to 10% of breast carcinomas.[64] These tumors arise from the lobules themselves and classically are seen to infiltrate the stroma of the breast with cords of cells lined up in a single-file pattern. Although such tumors may be associated with a higher frequency of multicentricity and bilaterality than invasive ductal carcinoma,[69,70] in general invasive lobular carcinoma is managed in exactly the same fashion as invasive ductal carcinoma.[71]

Some of the more uncommon histologic subtypes of breast cancer carry unusually favorable prognoses. These include tubular carcinoma, medullary carcinoma, and mucinous carcinoma. Each of these subtypes accounts for 1% to 2% of all invasive breast cancers, but appears to have outcomes that are substantially better than those of the typical infiltrating ductal carcinoma.[71-73]

CLINICAL PRESENTATION

In general, clinically detectable breast cancer presents as a painless mass, discovered by either the patient or the clinician on routine examination. At physical examination, the size of the mass, its texture, and any fixation to skin or underlying chest wall structures should be noted. On occasion, a painful breast mass turns out to be malignant, although painful masses are typically associated with cysts. A bloody nipple discharge sometimes heralds the onset of breast cancer, although most commonly this symptom is associated with a benign intraductal papilloma. Overall, any palpable breast mass should be evaluated until a diagnostic conclusion is reached and should not be passed off as benign or "nothing to worry about."

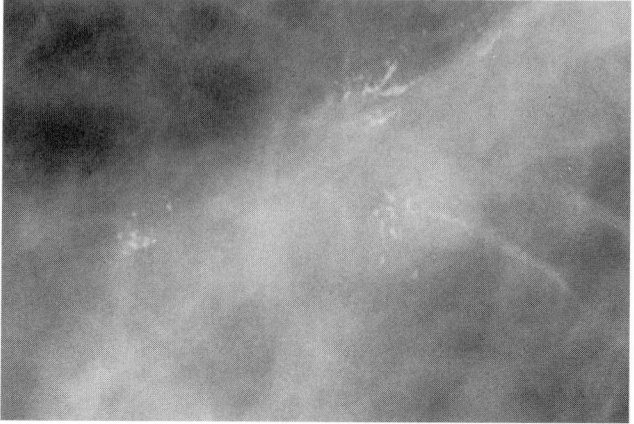

Figure 57–4. Magnification view of a mammogram showing microcalcifications. These calcifications vary in size and shape and are clustered together. These are typical of microcalcifications associated with malignancy.

In recent times, breast cancer has been diagnosed more frequently by mammography. In fact, virtually all the increase in breast cancer cases seen in recent years was in the categories *in situ* disease and small tumors less than 2 cm.[3] The majority of these small cancers are detected solely by mammography and emphasize the important role that mammography plays in the early detection of breast cancer.

Three other clinical presentations of breast cancer deserve special mention. Somewhat less than 1% of breast cancers present as axillary adenopathy.[74-76] Typically, these patients are managed for a short time with antibiotics to treat possible infectious causes of lymphadenopathy, but a biopsy subsequently reveals adenocarcinoma. These women should, of course, have routine mammography as part of their workup, and some of them will be found to have an occult breast cancer. Virtually all these women can be treated as though they had breast cancer, either with mastectomy or breast conservation,[76,77] once routine diagnostic studies, along with a history and physical examination, have ruled out any other obvious primary tumor. A second unusual presentation of breast cancer is that of Paget's disease of the breast.[78] Patients report pain, bleeding, or itching of the nipple and often have a red or eroded nipple lesion. These patients often are managed with topical creams for many months and have gone through several cycles of healing and further breakdown of the skin of the nipple. The diagnosis of Paget's disease is easily made by punch biopsy. These women are often managed by breast conservation.[79] Finally, some women present with an enlarged, swollen, warm, red breast that appears to have all the characteristics of a rapidly progressive infection. Often a discrete mass within the breast is not palpable, but along with erythema of the breast, the skin of the breast is edematous, showing an appearance much like that of the skin of an orange *(peau d'orange)*. These patients should immediately arouse the suspicion that they have inflammatory breast cancer, a particularly virulent form of the disease.[80] Biopsy of the breast itself along with overlying skin showing cancer cells in intradermal lymphatics confirms the diagnosis.

ROUTES OF SPREAD

Breast cancer can spread locally, regionally, and systemically. Locally the cancer can enlarge to involve the overlying skin or the underlying pectoralis musculature, even invading into the chest wall itself. The physical examination of the patient should always be designed to determine the local extent of disease. The tumor should be carefully measured, both on physical examination and on mammogram. The mobility of the tumor in relation to the overlying skin and the underlying chest wall musculature should be noted. Regional spread involves the axillary and IM lymph nodes. In general, the IM lymph nodes are less commonly involved in axillary node-negative breast cancer (involvement seen 5% to 15% of the time) than they are in axillary node-positive disease (involvement seen 25% to 35% of the time).[81-83] It has been relatively difficult to diagnose IM lymph node involvement, and it is not clear that treatment of these nodes improves patient outcome. Series of patients staged with IM lymph node dissections helped us learn the frequency with which these nodes are infiltrated, but also showed that their surgical removal did not change survival.[84,85] IM nodes are at times the drainage site of lymphatic flow as determined by sentinel lymph node mapping.[86] When the IM chain contains proven breast cancer cells, these nodes must be irradicated as part of the patient's initial management.

Far more common is spread to the axilla, which occurs in about 40% of breast cancer cases. Involvement of axillary lymph nodes is the most important prognostic factor in breast cancer, with survival decreasing in a fairly stepwise fashion as the number of involved lymph nodes increases, up to approximately 10 nodes, at which time the ultimate survival declines to the point that a further increase in lymph node number appears to have little influence on the outcome.[87] There are two ways to ascertain whether axillary lymph nodes are pathologically involved with tumor. Classically, one would perform an axillary lymph node dissection and examine 10 to 20 lymph nodes histopathologically. This operation was justified by the known inaccuracy of using clinical examination alone. Overall, approximately one third of patients who have clinically negative axillae have positive axillary lymph nodes found on axillary dissection, and approximately one fourth with clinically palpable lymph nodes prove to be lymph node-negative at the time of dissection.[88] Lymph node status is highly dependent on the size of the cancer and whether it is clinically palpable.[89]

Today, the newer technique of sentinel lymph node mapping is rapidly replacing formal axillary dissection as the method of choice to evaluate and initially stage the axilla. Based on work first done in cutaneous melanoma, the breast cancer tumor bed is injected with blue dye, radiocolloid, or both.[90] A small incision in the axilla is made and the dissection is advanced until the blue stained (or radioactive) nodes are encountered. These nodes (typically there is more than one)[91] are removed and sent for histopathologic examination and the procedure is terminated. If the sentinal nodes are negative, no further axillary surgery or treatment is performed. In experienced hands the overall accuracy of the procedure is 97% to 98% while the false-negative rates are in the 5% to 10% range.[92] If a sentinel node is positive for cancer, it is not clear what the optimal next step should be. The standard practice has been to take the patient through a formal axillary dissection. But since the majority of these subsequent dissections are negative,[93] clinical trials are now under way to determine whether full axillary dissection is warranted even in the face of a positive sentinel node.

Breast cancer recurrences can involve any area of the body. In general, approximately one third of all first recurrences after a mastectomy are locoregional,[94] and the remaining two thirds are systemic. Of the systemic metastases, approximately 60% are in bone, 10% in lung, 5% in liver, 5% in the central nervous system, and 15% to 20% in multiple sites.[95] This distribution differs from the sites of eventual metastatic spread found in autopsy series, which tend to show high values for all organs.[96] Knowledge of the distribution of first recurrences helps focus attention on specific areas in the follow-up of treated breast cancer patients. Locoregional sites should be carefully evaluated using physical examination and a bilateral mammogram in patients with an intact breast, and careful examination of the chest wall and regional lymph nodes along with contralateral mammography in patients who have had a mastectomy. The patient should be specifically interrogated about bone pain, especially in the spine, pelvis or hips, and ribs. Other symptoms such as unusual cough, shortness of breath, headache, dizziness, or a change in mental status should be noted. Routine mammography, however, is the only test that is justified in the follow-up of the asymptomatic patient. While other routine screening tests (chest x-ray, bone scan, blood work) can detect asymptomatic recurrences earlier, there are no data to indicate that early detection of metastatic disease improves outcome.[97]

One of the unique features of breast cancer that must be borne in mind when caring for patients with this disease is the time course of breast cancer recurrences. The median time to breast cancer recurrence is between 2 and 5 years, shortest for large, node-positive cases and longest for small, node-negative cases.[98] Overall, 75% to 80% of all patients in whom the disease will recur have had their recurrences by 5 years, but this leaves a substantial number of patients in whom the disease will recur beyond 5 years. More than 95% of recurrences have occurred by 10 years, but there is still a recurrence rate of breast cancer that goes out to 15 years and beyond. In fact, there is a debate on whether there is ever a point in time when a women can be told she is entirely risk-free in terms of a breast cancer recurrence,[99] and the

new appearance of metastatic disease has been observed 25 or more years beyond the original breast cancer treatment.

DIAGNOSTIC STUDIES

Mammography

All women with a suspicious breast mass should have bilateral mammography. This examination will, of course, help evaluate the index lesion itself. Is it smoothly marginated, suggestive of a benign lesion? Is it associated with suspicious-looking microcalcifications (Fig. 57-4)? Does it have an irregular speculated border, suggestive of a malignancy (Fig. 57-5)? The size of the lesion can often be measured on a mammogram. This aids in the clinical staging of disease. At times, axillary lymphadenopathy can be seen mammographically, and this can also aid in the clinical staging process (Fig. 57-6).

The mammographic appearance of the index lesion can also help determine whether the patient has an extensive intraductal component (EIC) associated with the primary invasive cancer, a factor useful for predicting a patient's risk of local failure after breast-conserving therapy (see later discussion). In retrospective and prospective studies, patients who have mammographic microcalcifications have EIC-positive disease about two thirds of the time, whereas those patients who present with a mass or architectural distortion without microcalcifications have an EIC-positive lesion only about one fifth of the time.[100] Lesions with microcalcifications larger than 3 cm are virtually always associated with an EIC, which can alert the surgeon to the possible need for

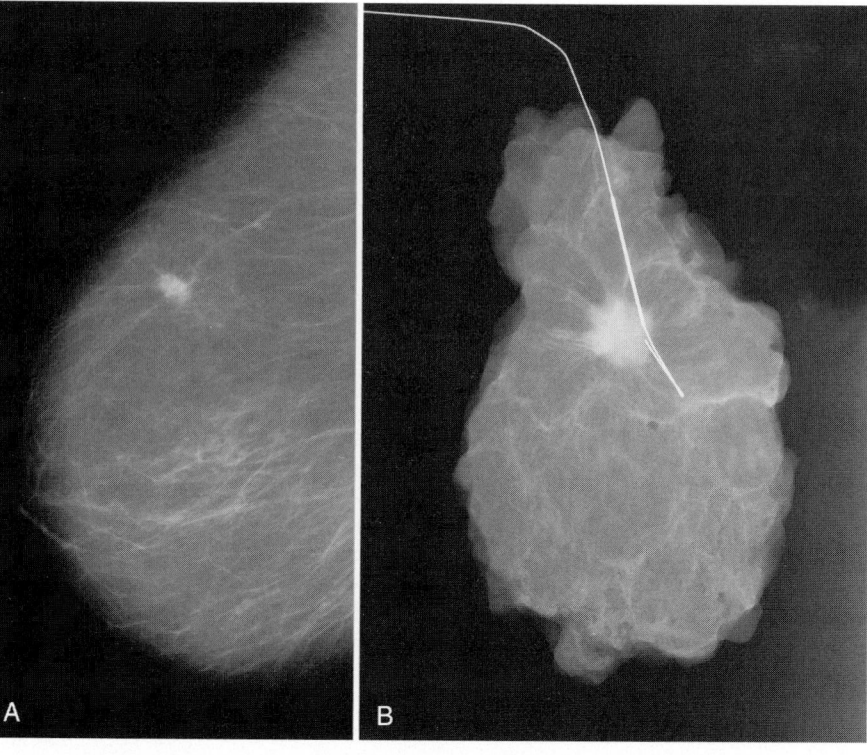

Figure 57–5. A, A dense mass, as seen in the upper aspect of this mammogram, is a sign of possible malignancy. **B,** A wire implanted in the breast under mammographic guidance was used to direct the surgeon in removal of this nonpalpable abnormality. A specimen radiograph, as seen here, shows that the abnormality has been completely removed. The speculated nature of this tumor can now be readily appreciated.

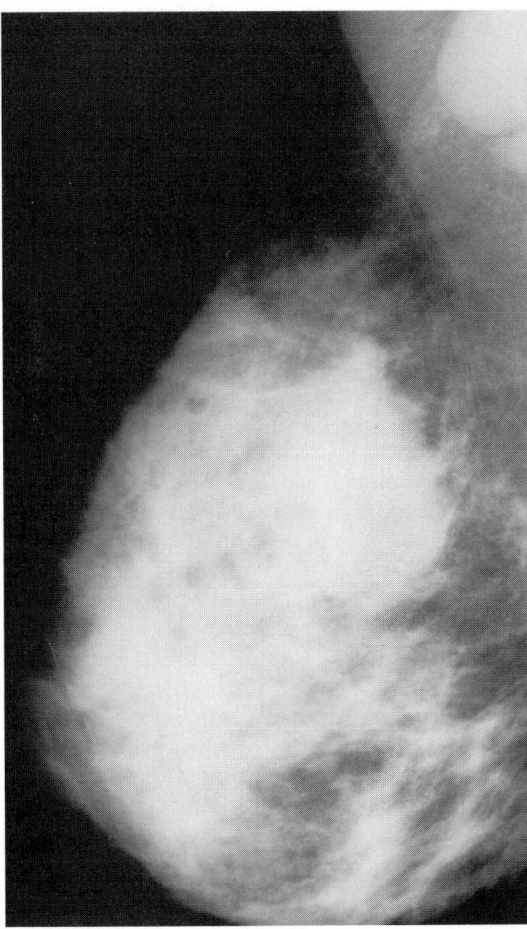

Figure 57–6. Occasionally, malignant lymph nodes can be appreciated on the mammogram. This breast is especially dense, making mammographic interpretation difficult. In the superior portion of the figure, behind the fold in the pectoralis major muscle, are two enlarged lymph nodes. In this patient with a known malignancy, these lymph nodes are suspicious for harboring metastatic disease.

wide lumpectomy margins and can alert the pathologist to carefully examine the specimen for the presence of widespread intraductal carcinoma.

The mammogram is useful to evaluate the remainder of the ipsilateral breast. If the primary treatment is to be mastectomy, such evaluation is relatively academic since the breast will be removed. But many women today are managed with conservative excision followed by radiation of the intact breast. In that case, evaluation of the remainder of the breast is critical in order to detect other suspicious lesions or microcalcifications in the remainder of the breast. If these are identified, they must be excised and proved benign before breast conservation therapy is instituted. The following rationale applies in these cases: (1) If there are other lesions in the breast that are malignant, then the patient is at higher risk for local recurrence after breast conservation therapy, and such therapy is often not pursued in favor of a mastectomy,[101,102] although some institutions do offer breast-conserving treatment to select patients with multiple lesions.[103,104] (2) Mammographic follow-up of the radiated breast is one of the most sensitive indicators of early recurrence.[105,106] If suspicious areas are left behind, the

ability for follow-up mammography to tell whether these lesions are progressing may be difficult, and thus an early recurrence may be missed.

The mammogram is also used to evaluate the contralateral breast. Although synchronous bilateral-lateral breast cancer occurs only in approximately 1% to 3% of cases,[107] it should not be forgotten that such cases do occur, and hence the contralateral breast must be examined carefully before primary treatment is undertaken. By the same token, the contralateral breast should be evaluated at least yearly for the appearance of a new contralateral breast cancer. Many studies have sought to ascertain the incidence of contralateral breast cancer, and it appears that the risk is approximately 0.75% per year (7.5% over 10 years).[108-111] The risk appears constant, and thus the cumulative risk increases with increasing years of follow-up.

Finally, mammography should be used after conservative excision of a lesion that contained microcalcification in order to determine that all suspicious-looking microcalcifications have been excised from the biopsy region. There are few things more disconcerting to the radiation oncologist than to obtain the first follow-up mammogram at approximately 6 months post-treatment and find that there are several malignant-looking microcalcifications present in the tumor bed. If a mammogram was not obtained after the initial excision, one has no way of knowing whether these are residual stable calcifications that can be managed with close follow-up or whether they are new calcifications associated with a rapid early recurrence. Thus, the author's institution obtains mammography postexcision in virtually all patients whose index lesion contained microcalcifications, and if residual microcalcifications are found, the mammogram is used to guide the re-excision that will clear them from the breast. The use of mammography in the management of breast cancer is summarized in Table 57-4.

Other Studies

Other staging tests that every breast cancer patient should undergo include a chest x-ray, blood cell count, and biochemical profile. Beyond that, additional staging studies are dictated by the patient's symptoms and stage of disease. Bone scanning in the asymptomatic patient with a node-negative breast cancer is of such low yield that its use should be strongly discouraged.[112,113] The

Table 57–4   Uses of Mammography in the Diagnosis and Management of Breast Cancer

Screening Asymptomatic Women
Age 40-50: every 1-2 yr.
Age 50 onward: yrly.

Symptomatic Women with New Mass
Mammogram should precede a diagnostic procedure.

Patient with Proven Cancer
Evaluate opposite breast.
Evaluate ipsilateral breast for presence of other suspicious areas.
Evaluate tumor bed for clearance of all suspicious microcalcifications.

highest yields of positive bone scans in asymptomatic breast cancer patients are in those with locally advanced breast cancer (T3 or T4 primary tumors). Since these patients usually receive systemic chemotherapy and since the treatment for metastatic breast cancer is systemic chemotherapy, it could be argued that treatment decisions are often not altered even if an occult metastatic bone deposit is missed. One should remember that the bone scan is a very *nonspecific* test, with 10% to 20% of patients having abnormalities noted. These bone scan abnormalities then call for additional staging workup including plain x-ray films, CT scans, magnetic resonance imaging (MRI), and possibly bone biopsy. For patients with stage I and stage II breast cancer, the chances of finding occult bone metastases pale in comparison to the chances of putting a patient through an unnecessary aggressive workup for what turns out to be a benign bone lesion. The yield from abdominal CT to screen for occult liver metastases is even lower than that of bone scanning, and such scans should not be routinely performed. On the other hand, any patient who has bone pain, especially if it is new or changing, or findings on physical examination or liver function studies suggestive of liver abnormalities should have these findings aggressively investigated. Recently, positron emission tomography (PET) scanning has been shown capable in solving specific diagnostic dilemmas in breast cancer staging and will, no doubt, have a role to play in the future.[114]

STAGING SYSTEM

The accurate staging of breast cancer is important if worthwhile data on results of treatment are to be recorded and compared among institutions and if uniform groups of patients are to be assembled for clinical trials. The current staging system in widespread use is a joint system from the American Joint Committee on Cancer (AJCC) and the Union Internationale Centre Cancer (UICC). It uses a classic TNM system, and patients may be staged by clinical criteria preoperatively or pathologic criteria postoperatively. Presented here is the new 6th edition of the staging system, effective as of January 2003.[115,116] The major changes to the staging system are as follows:

- Micrometastases are distinguished from isolated tumor cells on the basis of size and histologic evidence of malignant activity.
- Identifiers have been added to indicate the use of sentinel lymph node dissection and immunohistochemical or molecular techniques.
- Major classifications of lymph node status are designated according to the number of involved axillary lymph nodes as determined by routine hematoxylin and eosin staining (preferred method) or by immunohistochemical staining.
- The classification of metastasis to the infraclavicular lymph nodes has been added as N3.
- Metastasis to the IM nodes, based on the method of detection and the presence or absence of axillary nodal involvement, has been reclassified. Microscopic involvement of the IM nodes detected by sentinel

lymph node dissection using lymphoscintigraphy, but not by imaging studies or clinical examination, is classified as N1. Macroscopic involvement of the IM nodes as detected by imaging studies (excluding lymphoscintigraphy) or by clinical examinations is classified as N2 if it occurs in the absence of metastases to the axillary lymph nodes, or as N3 if it occurs in the presence of metastases to the axillary lymph nodes.

- Metastasis to the supraclavicular lymph nodes has been reclassified as N3 rather than M1.

The staging systems are presented in Tables 57-5 and 57-6. The TNM classification is further condensed into a stage grouping presented in Table 57-7.

Several points should be made about the staging system. At times, it is difficult to precisely gauge the size (T stage) of a tumor. For example, a lesion may measure 1.9 cm in the pathology laboratory, 2 cm on clinical examination, and 2.1 cm on mammography. Should such a patient be classified as having a T1 or a T2 primary tumor? In general, most clinicians believe that an accurate measurement of a fresh surgical specimen is the most reliable means of staging a breast cancer, and, as such, the patient would be classified as having a T1 primary tumor in the above example. However, what if a lesion measures 1.8 cm on physical examination and 2.2 cm on mammographic examination and the pathologist failed to perform a measurement? In this case, the decision would be an arbitrary one, but at the author's institution, the clinical size of the tumor would prevail. What about a tumor whose invasive component is 1.5 cm in diameter but in whom there is an adjacent area of intraductal carcinoma that would make the composite lesion greater than 2 cm? In this case, the author's institution stages patients by the size of the *invasive* component, and if this is clearly noted to be only a fraction of the entire lesion, the primary tumor size is adjusted accordingly.[117] When cancers are multifocal, the likelihood of lymph node metastases may correlate better with the combined diameters of the lesions rather than the size of the largest single lesion.[118]

In the absence of sentinel node biopsy, accurate lymph node staging requires that at least six lymph nodes be removed from the axilla. Beyond six lymph nodes, the percentage of patients with positive nodes changes little whether 10, 15, or 20 nodes have been removed.[88] In the National Surgical Adjuvant Breast and Bowel Project (NSABP) trial B-04, no patient with more than six nodes removed experienced a subsequent failure in the axilla.[119] However, the more lymph nodes removed, the more accurate the count of the absolute number of positive nodes becomes. If one wishes to ask whether the patient has one to three positive nodes, between 10 and 20 nodes should be examined, depending on the size of the primary and the number of positive nodes reported.[120]

STANDARD THERAPY

Carcinoma in Situ

Lobular carcinoma in situ is usually managed today by close observation.[121-123] There is no known role for breast

Table 57–5   **Classification of Breast Cancer**

T (Tumor)

TX	Primary tumor cannot be assessed
T0	No evidence of primary tumor
Tis	Carcinoma in situ
Tis (DCIS)	Ductal carcinoma in situ
Tis (LCIS)	Lobular carcinoma in situ
Tis (Paget's)	Paget's disease of the nipple with no tumor
	Note: Paget's disease associated with a tumor is classified according to the size of the tumor
T1	Tumor ≤2 cm in greatest dimension
T1mic	Microinvasion ≤0.1 cm in greatest dimension
T1a	Tumor >0.1 cm but not >0.5 cm in greatest dimension
T1b	Tumor >0.5 cm but not >1 cm in greatest dimension
T1c	Tumor >1 cm but not >2 cm in greatest dimension
T2	Tumor >2 cm but not >5 cm in greatest dimension
T3	Tumor >5 cm in greatest dimension
T4	Tumor of any size with direct extension to (a) chest wall or (b) skin, only as described below
T4a	Extension to chest wall, not including pectoralis muscle
T4b	Edema (including peau d'orange) or ulceration of the skin of the breast, or satellite skin nodules confined to the same breast
T4c	Both T$_{4a}$ and T$_{4b}$
T4d	Inflammatory carcinoma

N (Nodes)

NX	Regional lymph nodes cannot be assessed (e.g., previously removed)
N0	No regional lymph node metastasis
N1	Metastasis to movable ipsilateral axillary lymph nodes
N2	Metastasis in ipsilateral axillary lymph nodes fixed or matted, or in clinically apparent* ipsilateral internal mammary nodes in the *absence* of clinically evident axillary lymph node metastasis
N2a	Metastasis in ipsilateral axillary lymph nodes fixed to one another (matted) or to other structures
N2b	Metastasis only in clinically apparent* ipsilateral internal mammary nodes in the *absence* of clinically evident axillary lymph node metastasis
N3	Metastasis in ipsilateral infraclavicular lymph nodes, with or without axillary lymph node involvement, or in clinically apparent* ipsilateral internal mammary lymph nodes in the *presence* of clinically evident axillary lymph node metastasis; or metastasis in ipsilateral supraclavicular lymph nodes, with or without axillary or internal mammary lymph node involvement
N3a	Metastasis in ipsilateral infraclavicular lymph nodes
N3b	Metastasis in ipsilateral internal mammary lymph nodes and axillary lymph nodes
N3c	Metastasis in ipsilateral supraclavicular lymph nodes

M (Distant Metastasis)

MX	Distant metastases cannot be assessed
M0	No distant metastases
M1	Distant metastases present

Clinically apparent is defined as detected by imaging studies (excluding lymphoscintigraphy) or by clinical examination or grossly visible pathologically.

From Greene FL, Page DL, Fleming ID, et al, eds: *AJCC Cancer Staging Manual*, 6th ed. New York: Springer, 2002.

Table 57–6   **Pathologic Classification of Breast Cancer**

PNX	Regional lymph noses cannot be assessed (e.g., previously removed, or not removed for pathologic study).
PN0	No regional lymph node metatsasis histologically, no additional examination for isolated tumor cells (ITC).
pN0(i-)	No regional lymph node metastasis histologically, negative immunohistochemistry (IHC).
pN0(i+)	No regional lymph node metastasis histologically, positive IHC, no IHC cluster >0.2 mm.
pN0(mol-)	No regional lymph node metastasis histologically, negative molecular findings (RTPCR).
pN0(mol+)	No regional lymph node metastasis histologically, positive molecular findings (RTPCR).

^{a}RT-PCR: reverse transcriptase/polymerase chain reaction.

pN1	Metastasis in 1 to 3 axillary lymph nodes, or in internal mammary nodes with microscopic disease detected by sentinel lymph node dissection, or both, but not clinically apparent.*
pN1mi	Micrometastasis (>0.2 mm, none >2.0 mm).
pN1a	Metastasis in 1 to 3 axillary lymph nodes.
pN1b	Metastasis in internal mammary nodes with microscopic disease detected by sentinel lymph node dissection, but not clinically apparent.*
pN1c	Metastasis in 1 to 3 axillary lymph nodes and in internal mammary nodes, with microscopic disease detected by sentinel lymph node dissection, but not clinically apparent.* (If associated with more than 3 positive axillary lymph nodes, the internal mammary nodes are classified as pN$_{3b}$ to reflect increased tumor burden.)
pN2	Metastasis in 4 to 9 axillary lymph nodes, or in clinically apparent† internal mammary lymph nodes in the *absence* of axillary lymph nodes metastasis.
pN2a	Metastasis in 4 to 9 axillary lymph nodes (at least 1 tumor deposit >2.0 mm).
pN2b	Metastasis in clinically apparent† internal mammary lymph nodes in the *absence* of axillary lymph nodes metastasis.
pN3	Metastasis in 10 or more axillary lymph nodes, or in infraclavicular lymph nodes, or in clinically apparent† ipsilateral internal mammary lymph nodes in the *presence of* 1 or more positive axillary lymph nodes; or in more than 3 axillary lymph nodes with clinically negative microscopic metastasis in internal mammary lymph nodes; or in ipsilateral supraclavicular lymph nodes.
pN3a	Metastasis in 10 or more axillary lymph nodes (at least 1 tumor deposit >2.0 mm), or metastasis to the infraclavicular lymph nodes.
pN3b	Metastasis in clinically apparent† ipsilateral internal mammary lymph nodes in the *presence of* 1 or more positive axillary lymph nodes; or in more than 3 axillary lymph nodes and in internal mammary lymph nodes with microscopic disease detected by sentinel lymph node dissection, but not clinically apparent.*
pN3c	Metastasis in ipsilateral supraclavicular lymph nodes.

*Not *clinically apparent* is defined as not detected by imaging studies (excluding lymphoscintigraphy) or by clinical examination.
†*Clinically apparent* is defined as detected by imaging studies (excluding lymphoscintigraphy) or by clinical examination.

Table 57–7 Stage Grouping for Breast Cancer

Stage	Tumor	Nodes	Metastasis
0	Tis	N0	M0
I	T1	N0	M0
IIA	T0	N1	M0
	T1	N1	M0
	T2	N0	M0
IIB	T2	N1	M0
	T3	N0	M0
IIIA	T0	N2	M0
	T1	N2	M0
	T2	N2	M0
	T3	N1	M0
	T3	N2	M0
IIIB	T4	Any N	M0
	Any T	N3	M0
IV	Any T	Any N	M1

From Greene FL, Page DL, Fleming ID, et al, eds: *AJCC Cancer Staging Manual*, 6th ed. New York: Springer, 2002.

Table 57–8 Nonmastectomy Treatment of Ductal Carcinoma in Situ

Treatment	Patients n	Local Recurrence %	Local Recurrence Invasive, %
Excision	1148	22.5	43
Excision + radiation	1452	8.9	50

From Boyages J, Delaney G, Taylor R: Predictors of local recurrence after treatment of ductal carcinoma in situ: A meta-analysis. *Cancer.* 1999;85:616.

radiation in such patients. Since the disease is multifocal in both breasts at presentation in the majority of patients and subsequent cancers affect both breasts equally, surgical management requires bilateral mastectomies. Although some patients elect to undergo surgical treatment, the author's experience indicates that this group is a small minority of the patients seen today.

Ductal carcinoma in situ can be managed by mastectomy or with breast conservation. Mastectomy is extraordinarily effective in the treatment of DCIS. Reviews of aggregate surgical series with more than 1000 cases document a local recurrence rate of around 1% after mastectomy.[124,125] But over the last 2 decades, DCIS has dramatically changed its clinical presentation. In the past, the majority of DCIS patients presented with a palpable mass at a time when mastectomy was the preferred treatment for any form of breast cancer. Furthermore, DCIS was a relatively rare disease, accounting for 1% to 2% of all breast cancers, and thus research into the treatment of this disease was sparse. In recent years, in response to widespread mammographic screening, the diagnosis of DCIS has increased to the point at which 15% or more of all newly diagnosed breast cancer represents DCIS.[3] Furthermore, most of these mammographically detected lesions are nonpalpable. Many clinicians began to question whether mastectomy represented overtreatment of these small lesions. Today, the goal of treatment for DCIS is breast conservation when possible.[126]

Breast conservation for DCIS can be practiced with and without the use of postexcision irradiation. The results of excision alone for the treatment of DCIS are summarized in Table 57-8. Overall, approximately 20% of patients treated with excision alone have a recurrence and about half of these recurrences are invasive carcinoma. Furthermore, these studies show that the greatest risk of recurrence lies with larger, palpable lesions. The recurrence rate from excision alone appears to be relatively low for small lesions less than a few millimeters in size when excised with wide margins.[127]

The use of irradiation following excision of DCIS further reduces recurrence rates as shown in Table 57-8. While

some of these data were short term, today we have long-term data (10 years median follow-up) on larger series of patients demonstrating sustained effectiveness of excision plus radiation in the treatment of DCIS.[128]

Several randomized trials of breast conservation in DCIS have been performed. Three of these trials compared excision alone with excision plus radiation (Table 57-9). In all these trials, radiation when added to excision reduced the rate of subsequent ipsilateral breast cancers, both noninvasive and invasive events by 40% to 60%.[129-131] While subset analyses show that younger women, positive margins, and high-grade histology increase the recurrence risk, and one can define lower risk groups (older, low-grade histology, clear margins), all groups benefit from the addition of radiation following excision.[132,133]

However, it must be acknowledged that there are subgroups whose risk of recurrence following excision alone may be so small that the addition of radiation is not warranted. Silverstein and colleagues[127] analyzed a retrospective cohort of patients treated with breast conservation and showed that if the margin width was wide, greater than 10 mm, the addition of radiation did not decrease the already low rate of local recurrence. While the concept is provocative, it is based on the outcome of 40 women without radiation and a greater than 10 mm margin. The hypothesis that radiation can safely be avoided in select cases is the subject of further ongoing randomized trials.

Adding to the complexity of management decisions in DCIS are the results of NSABP B-24.[134] In this study, women with DCIS were treated with excision plus radiation with or without the addition of tamoxifen. Tamoxifen further reduced the number of subsequent ipsilateral breast cancer events (Table 57-10). In addition, tamoxifen reduced contralateral breast cancer

Table 57–9 Three Trials of Excision ± Radiation in Ductal Carcinoma in Situ

Trial	Hazard Ratio for Local Recurrence*
NSABP B-17[129]	0.43
EORTC[130]	0.62
UK[131]	0.41

*Ratios less than 1.0 mean a *reduction* in local recurrence with the addition of radiation.
EORTC, European Organization for Research and Treatment of Cancer; NSABP, National Surgical Adjuvant Breast and Bowel Project; UK, United Kingdom.

Table 57–10 Ipsilateral Breast Cancer Events in NSABP B-17 and B-24 (Crude Rates)

	Excision	E + XRT	E + XRT + Tamoxifen
B-17	31%	15%	
		52%↓	
B-24		11%	8%
		28%↓	
		74%↓	

From Fisher B, Land S, Mamounas E, et al: Prevention of invasive breast cancer in women with ductal carcinoma in situ: An update of the National Surgical Adjuvant Breast and Bowel Project experience. *Semin Oncol.* 2001;28:400.

by nearly 50%. If the goal of DCIS management is to preserve the breast and reduce the subsequent appearance of *any* further breast cancer, excision followed by radiation followed by 5 years of tamoxifen appears to be the best therapy. Whether subgroups will be defined whose outcome is excellent with less therapy or different therapy will be the subject of further clinical research.

T1 and T2 Breast Cancer

Localized breast cancer in stage I or stage II is managed today either by mastectomy with axillary sampling or dissection or by lumpectomy, axillary sampling, or dissection, and breast irradiation. Various factors enter into the decision to treat with mastectomy versus breast conservation:

Histopathology: presence of EIC
Age
Breast size
Nodal status
Tumor size
Margins of excision

HISTOPATHOLOGY

There is no particular histologic subtype of breast cancer that is more or less suitable for breast conservation treatment. Although infiltrating ductal carcinoma represents the vast majority of invasive breast cancers, studies of patients with less common forms of breast cancer such as lobular, tubular, and colloid fail to show any noteworthy excess risk of recurrence.[135,136] However, there is one histopathologic feature that does correlate with a higher risk of local recurrence after breast conservation therapy, the so-called *EIC*. Schnitt and colleagues[137] first drew attention to the fact that an invasive breast cancer could contain areas of intraductal carcinoma in the following four patterns: (1) no intraductal carcinoma at all (pure invasive carcinoma), (2) DCIS present in the primary tumor but not adjacent to the primary tumor, (3) intraductal carcinoma adjacent to the primary tumor but not present within the primary tumor and, (4) intraductal carcinoma present *both* within and adjacent to the

primary invasive tumor. They defined this latter category as representing an EIC. More definitively, they specified that the DCIS had to be more than minimally present in the invasive tumor, representing at least 25% of the main tumor mass. Similar quantitative restrictions were not placed on the DCIS component adjacent to the primary tumor, only the presence of DCIS. A special class of breast cancers that were predominantly DCIS with small areas of microinvasion were also classified as EIC-positive tumors.

When the risk of local breast failure after breast conservation therapy was studied as a function of each of the four subtypes of invasive cancer and DCIS, there were marked differences in the recurrence patterns for patients with EIC-positive tumors.[138] Specifically, 26% of EIC-positive patients had a local breast failure versus 7% for those women who were EIC-negative. These investigators went on to point out that the recurrence pattern was considerably different between the EIC-positive and EIC-negative patients.[138] Overall, 88% of the EIC-positive patients developed a "true recurrence" (recurrence in the quadrant involved with the original cancer) compared with 55% of the EIC-negative patients. This difference in the recurrence pattern suggested that the local tumor burden in EIC-positive patients might be greater than in EIC-negative patients. Additional evidence suggests that this hypothesis is true. Holland and colleagues[139] analyzed whole-organ sections of mastectomy specimens and plotted the location of malignant deposits using an elegant whole-organ mapping technique. A total of 217 mastectomy specimens were examined, and 30% met the Schnitt criteria for an EIC. Holland and colleagues were then able to show that the EIC-positive patients had significantly more tumor within their breast specimens than did EIC-negative patients. Specifically, if one looked 2 cm or more beyond the edge of the index lesion, residual histologic cancer could be identified in 59% of EIC-positive patients compared with 29% of EIC-negative patients. Of the EIC-positive patients, 20% had malignant cells present 6 cm or more beyond the edge of the invasive cancer.

It should be remembered, however, that the original work that identified EIC as a risk factor for local recurrence was based on patients treated in an era when careful histopathologic examination of lumpectomy surgical margins was not routinely performed. Most patients had only a gross excision of the primary tumor, and re-excisions were rarely done. Thus, although it is safe to conclude that EIC is a risk factor for local recurrence when surgical margins are not examined and re-excisions are not done, the issue today is whether EIC remains a risk factor when histologically negative margins are obtained either at the initial excision or at a subsequent re-excision. The Joint Center for Radiation Therapy in Boston examined this question in two ways. First, they correlated local breast failure with the volume of breast resected in 507 patients treated during the 1970s.[140] There was a strong relationship between the size of the excision, EIC status, and subsequent recurrence. For EIC-negative tumors, the size of the resection appeared to have little correlation with subsequent breast failure for either T1 or T2 tumors. On the other hand, there was a three- to fourfold higher rate of recurrence in EIC-positive patients who had "small" resections versus those who had "large" resections. This ties in with the data of Holland and colleagues, since patients with "large" resections probably had a greater portion of the occult residual DCIS excised than did patients with "small" excisions. In another study, the influence of margin negativity as a function of EIC was studied in 181 patients.[141] EIC-negative patients had little difference in the recurrence rate whether they were margin-negative, margin-close, or margin-positive. On the other hand, there was a substantial increase in the recurrence rate for EIC-positive patients who had margin positivity versus margin negativity. These data taken together allow one to formulate a treatment policy for the 25% to 30% of patients who have EIC-positive tumors. In such patients, re-excision of the tumor bed is almost always done. If no residual cancer is seen or only a limited amount of tumor is seen with negative margins on the re-excision, breast conservation is carried out. On the other hand, patients whose re-excision shows numerous areas of residual cancer, especially if those new areas involve the re-excision margin, are counseled that their local recurrence risk is higher and they are carefully considered for a mastectomy.

It is worth noting that not all institutions that have studied the influence of an EIC on local failure rates have seen a positive correlation.[142-145] Some of this apparent contradiction is due to differing definitions of EIC and to the amount of tissue removed during lumpectomy, since institutions routinely performing large excisions would tend to minimize the influence of an EIC. Overall, EIC should be considered a risk factor for local breast failure, and careful attention to excising this histopathologic entity with negative surgical margins should be employed.

PATIENT AGE

Local in-breast failures occur more often in patients under 35 years of age than in older patients, a situation observed in numerous retrospective analyses (Table 57-11).[146] The reasons for this high recurrence rate likely relate to the more aggressive nature of breast cancer in younger women such as a higher incidence of lymphatic space invasion, high nuclear grade, tumor necrosis,[147] and the frequent presence of an EIC.[148,149] It should be kept in mind that younger women have a higher rate of chest wall failure after mastectomy than do older patients.[150,151] Thus, in counseling young women concerning their options for primary breast cancer therapy, it should not be assumed that a mastectomy can allow a young woman to avoid the hazards of a local failure.

A factor that may reduce the risk of in-breast failure for younger women (and older women as well) is the use of adjuvant systemic chemotherapy. Without question, systemic therapy has the effect of reducing local breast failures after radiation.[152] Since most young women today receive adjuvant systemic chemotherapy or hormonal therapy or both, some of the risk associated with younger age in terms of local breast recurrence will be circumvented. In one study of young women with breast cancer, the local in-breast failure was reduced from 15% to 4% in patients who received chemotherapy/tamoxifen compared with those who did not.[153] Thus, with appropriate counseling it is still acceptable to offer breast-sparing therapy to young patients with primary breast cancer.

BREAST SIZE

The treatment of breast cancer with lumpectomy and radiation is far more challenging in women with large breasts than in other patients. A large, pendulous breast may be difficult to reposition each day for treatment. In some patients, the breast will partially rest on the upper abdominal wall, causing a bolus effect in the inframammary fold, thus producing a marked skin reaction. Substantial dose inhomogeneity can be observed when low-energy photons of 4 to 6 MV are used in the treatment of a breast with a large separation (distance from the edge of the medial tangent to the edge of the lateral tangent). The cosmetic effect achieved in women with large breasts may be inferior to that achieved in other patients.[154]

On the other hand, mastectomy represents a major problem for patients with large breasts. A substantial asymmetry on the chest wall is created by removing one breast in these patients. Furthermore, reconstruction is virtually impossible without undertaking a breast reduction on the opposite side. Overall, large-breasted patients do better with breast-conserving therapy than with mastectomy, and lumpectomy with radiation represents the treatment of choice for these women at the author's institution. At times, a higher-energy photon beam is used, or a mixture of low and high energy every other day in order to reduce "hot spots" in the treatment plan. Some special techniques for treating these patients have been described in the literature, such as treating with the patient in a lateral[155] or prone position.[156-159] Such techniques can be quite useful if the standard breast setup technique is problematic for a particular patient.

NODAL STATUS

Decisions about the use of mastectomy versus breast conservation should be made independent of the patient's nodal status. There is no reason to believe that lymph node-positive patients should more often be treated with

Table 57–11 Effect of Age on Local in-Breast Failure

Reference	Age Criterion	Recurrence, *n*/Treated, *n* (%)	
		Younger	*Older*
Boyages et al[138]	≤34	15/61 (25)	76/722 (11)
Clarke et al[339]	≤35	3/32 (9)	21/424 (5)
Delouche et al[143]	≤40	14/71 (20)	26/339 (8)
Forquet et al[340]	≤32	12/35 (34)	44/483 (9)
Fowble et al[124]	≤35	12/64 (19)	69/941 (7)
Haffty et al[341]	≤36	6/40 (15)	44/393 (11)
Kurtz et al 289[342]	≤39	52/243 (21)	133/1440 (9)
Matthews et al[150]	≤35	9/72 (13)	23/306 (8)
Ryoo et al[343]	≤40	8/51 (16)	18/342 (5)
Veronesi et al[344]	≤35	9/95 (9)	45/1137 (4)
TOTAL		140/764 (18.3)	499/6527 (7.6)

mastectomy than with lumpectomy and radiation. Furthermore, there is no reason to suspect that the status of the axillary lymph nodes would have an influence on local breast cancer failure and, since most node-positive patients receive adjuvant systemic therapy, node-positive patients actually have a somewhat reduced rate of local breast failure compared with their node-negative counterparts who do not receive systemic therapy. Data from various trials performed by the NSABP underscore this point, as summarized in Table 57–12.

Despite these data, analysis of clinical practice patterns reveals a substantial decrease in lumpectomy use in patients with positive nodes compared with patients with negative nodes.[160] At first glance, it might be assumed that nodal status is a surrogate for tumor size, since larger tumors are more likely to be node-positive than smaller tumors. Since larger tumors may be more difficult to excise with a cosmetically acceptable lumpectomy, a possible explanation for the declining use of breast conservation in lymph node-positive patients may thus be theorized. However, an analysis from the Breast Cancer Intergroup (a coalition of many national clinical trial organizations) reveals that this explanation is probably incorrect.[161] Even controlling for tumor size, patients with positive lymph nodes had a lower lumpectomy use than those with negative lymph nodes, and the more positive lymph nodes that were found, the lower the incidence of breast-sparing therapy. Thus, an interesting paradox is created since clinicians seem to believe that the greater the risk of *systemic* recurrence is, the greater the intensity of *local* therapy should be. This is clearly erroneous, and the misconception that node-positive patients are less suitable for breast conservation therapy should be dismissed.

If node-positive patients (or node-negative patients for that matter) are to receive adjuvant systemic chemotherapy, how should it be sequenced with the radiotherapy? As with most combined-modality therapy, there are three major sequencing methods: (1) deliver all the radiation followed by the chemotherapy, (2) deliver all the chemotherapy followed by the radiation, and (3) deliver the two concurrently. There are conflicting reports as to whether one or another of these sequences is preferable. Hartsell[162] suggested that delaying radiation for more

than four months or more increased the risk of local recurrence, while other studies did not see a similar effect.[163-165] In an effort to resolve this question, Recht[166] and colleagues performed a randomized trial of initial versus delayed chemotherapy. There were fewer distant metastases in the group of patients who received their chemotherapy up front, but there were fewer breast failures in the group who received the radiation first. Since the ultimate goal of breast cancer therapy is systemic cure, with breast conservation being an important secondary goal, most treatment today consists of delivery of all systemic treatment first, followed by radiation. The same is true when the primary treatment is mastectomy; chemotherapy precedes chest wall irradiation.[167]

Sequencing of chemotherapy *before* lumpectomy has been studied in single institutions[168,169] and in several randomized trials (Table 57–13).[170,171] Preoperative chemotherapy is as effective as postoperative treatment from an overall survival standpoint, so it can be administered with confidence in its safety. It has the distinct advantage of being able to produce objective shrinkage of tumor in about 80% of cases. Rates of lumpectomy increase in series of patients where chemotherapy is administered prior to surgical excision. This therapy should be employed in any woman who desires breast conservation, but whose primary tumor size precludes a cosmetically acceptable excision.

TUMOR SIZE

There is no evidence to suggest that the success of lumpectomy and radiation (in terms of local failure) is influenced by tumor size as long as a complete excision of the tumor has been performed. Obviously, as tumors become larger, the ratio of tumor size to breast size may mitigate against the performance of a lumpectomy. But assuming that a lumpectomy can be performed, the ultimate success of treatment is the same for small T1 tumors as it is for larger T2 tumors.[172] Interestingly, when patients are treated with lumpectomy alone *(without radiation)*, there is a profound influence of tumor size on the risk of subsequent breast cancer failure. When one analyzes the results from NSABP B-06, approximately 20% of patients with tumors of 1 cm or less had a local

Table 57–12   Local in-Breast Recurrence in NSABP Trials*

	Nodal Status	
	Negative	Positive
Patients, *n*	1309	836
Average time on study, mo	54	44
In-breast recurrences, *n*	45	32
In-breast recurrences, %	3.4	3.8

*B-13 N–, ER–; MF vs observation
B-14 N–, ER+; Tam vs placebo
B-15 N+, ER–; AC vs CMMF vs both
B-16 N+, ER+; Tam vs AC + Tam
A, doxorubicin (Adriamycin); C, cyclophosphamide (Cytoxan); ER, estrogen receptor; F, 5-fluorouracil; M, methotrexate; N, node; Tam, tamoxifen.
From Fisher B, Wickerham DL, Deutsch M, et al: Breast tumor recurrence following lumpectomy with and without breast irradiation: An overview of recent NSABP findings. *Semin Surg Oncol.* 1992;8:153.

Table 57–13   Randomized Trials of Neoadjuvant Chemotherapy

	Makris et al[345]	Broet et al[346]	Mauriac et al[347]	Wolmark et al[348]
Number of patients	309	390	272	1493
Med FU (mo)	48	105	124	114
Response rate	83%	65%	62%	79%
BCT				
Neoadjuvant	89%	82%	63%	68%
Adjuvant	78%	77%	0%	59%
Survival				
Neoadjuvant	78%	65%	"identical"	69%
	@ 5 yr	@ 10 yr		@ 9 yr
Adjuvant	78%	60%		70%

BCT, breast-conserving therapy; FU, follow-up.

breast failure within 5 years. For tumors between 1 and 2 cm, the rate increased to 30%, and for tumors greater than 2 cm, nearly 40% of patients had failures by 5 years.[152] On the other hand, in the same trial there was no influence of tumor size on the breast failure rate for those women treated with lumpectomy plus radiation (Table 57-14). As stated in the previous section on sequencing of chemotherapy, initial (neo-adjuvant) chemotherapy is so successful in reducing the size of the primary tumor that initial tumor size is beginning to have far less influence on the overall eligibility for breast conservation.

MARGINS

A great deal of attention has been paid to the influence of surgical margins on the outcome of breast-sparing therapy. While earlier studies were mixed in these conclusions, more recent studies indicate that margin status is one of the most important factors influencing the treatment outcome,[173-177] especially in mature series with longer median follow-up time. In patients whose surgical margins are positive or unknown, a re-excision is recommended to assure clear margins. Data suggest that a clear margin after re-excision confirms the same good prognosis as an initial clear excision.[174]

Divergent data exist concerning the influence of "close" surgical margins—often defined as less than 2 mm—on subsequent local failure, with some studies showing that close margins are similar to negative and others suggesting that close margins are intermediate between negative and positive margins in their influence on local failure. This issue may never be fully resolved since there are so many variables that can influence this result (e.g., follow-up time, number of distant failures, technique of margin examination, age of patients). The author believes that patients with close but negative margins can avoid re-excision if they are older, have pure invasive cancer, and have a mammogram that does not have widespread microcalcifications. It is probably safest to re-excise close surgical margins in younger women, women with an extensive intraductal component, and those whose mammograms suggest more diffuse disease. It is possible that higher doses of radiation[178,179] or the use of systemic therapy can overcome some or all of the adverse impact of a close or focally positive surgical margin. But the safest course of action is to clear the margins of excision widely. In women who cannot have this done, it does not automatically mean that mastectomy must be performed. Afterall, a close or focally positive margin may be associated with a recurrence risk in the 10% to 20% range, which may be acceptable to some patients and may be even less if systemic treatment is employed.

T3 and T4 Breast Cancer

A heterogeneous grouping of patients has been placed under the category of locally advanced breast cancer (LABC), or stage III disease. These include patients with noninflammatory, operable disease (T3N1), noninflammatory, inoperable disease (T4a, b, c; T3N2; or N3), or inflammatory carcinoma (T4d). If the wide spectrum of disease grouped under the heading *LABC* were not enough to render a study of this problem confusing, the AJCC changed the staging classification for this disease between the 1983[180] and 1987[181] staging manuals. As can be noted in Table 57-15, patients with T3N0 disease were classified as stage III disease in 1983, but reclassified to stage II disease in 1987. Furthermore, supraclavicular nodes were included in stage IIIB disease in 1983, but were considered a metastatic site after the 1987 staging classification. This issue will become ever more confusing as the new 2002 classification will move patients with supraclavicular nodes from the metastatic category into the locally advanced group. With this background, it is little wonder that the literature surrounding the treatment of LABC can be quite confusing. Some authors have grouped all their patients together, whereas others have separated stage IIIA from stage IIIB. Still others separate inflammatory stage IIIB from noninflammatory stage IIIB. Some papers have used the 1987 staging criteria, whereas others have used the earlier staging criteria and thus include patients with supraclavicular adenopathy. Many authors continue to report T3N0 cases in their LABC results, even though these patients are now recognized to have a relatively favorable outcome.

It is important to separate the treatment of noninflammatory from inflammatory breast carcinoma. The AJCC staging manual defines inflammatory carcinoma as

Table 57–14   In-Breast Failure as a Function of Tumor Size and Use of Radiation Therapy (XRT) in NSABP B-06

| Tumor Size, cm | Failed, *n*/Treated, *n* (%) | | |
	Lumpectomy	Lumpectomy + XRT	*P* Value
≤1.0	15/72 (21)	10/87 (11)	0.06
1.1-2.0	73/226 (32)	12/129 (5)	<0.000005
2.1-3.0	68/186 (37)	15/168 (9)	<0.000005
≥3.1	37/84 (44)	9/89 (10)	<0.000005

From Fisher B, Wickerham DL, Deutsch M, et al: Breast tumor recurrence following lumpectomy with and without breast irradiation: An overview of recent NSABP findings. *Semin Surg Oncol.* 1992;8:153.

Table 57–15   Changes in American Joint Committee on Cancer Staging of Locally Advanced Cancer of the Breast

Stage	1983[180]	1988,[181] 92, 97	2002[115]
IIIA	Any T, N2 T3, N0,1,2	Any T, N2 T3, N1,2	Any T, N2* T3, N1,2*
IIIB	Any T, N3† T4	Any T, N3† T4	T4, N0,1,2
IIIC	—	—	Any T, N3†
IV	Any M‡	Any M‡	Any M‡

*In 2002, N2 includes internal mammary nodes in the absence of clinical axillary involvement.
†In 1983 N3 = supraclavicular nodes; 1988 = internal mammary nodes; 2002 = see Table 57-5.
‡Supraclavicular nodes were M1 in 1988,92,97, but N3 in 1983 and 2002.

"a clinical pathologic entity characterized by diffuse brawny induration of the skin of the breast with an erysipeloid edge, usually without an underlying palpable mass. Radiologically, there may be a detectable mass and characteristic thickening of the skin over the breast. This clinical presentation is due to tumor embolization in dermal lymphatics." In general, inflammatory carcinoma of the breast is a clinical diagnosis supported by skin biopsy showing dermal lymphatic invasion by the breast cancer (Fig. 57-7). Several authors have reported that patients with dermal lymphatic carcinoma without the classic clinical signs of inflammatory breast cancer follow a clinical course that is similar to that of inflammatory carcinoma,[182-184] and most investigators would classify those patients along with their clinical inflammatory counterparts. Inflammatory breast cancer is universally metastatic when treated with local therapy alone,[80] whereas noninflammatory LABC can be cured in some patients with aggressive local treatment. Thus the two entities are discussed separately.

Noninflammatory Locally Advanced Breast Cancer

Historically, many patients with noninflammatory LABC, especially patients with stage IIIA disease, were treated with surgery. Results in the literature show 5-year survival rates ranging from 35% to 50%.[185-188] Some of the outcome differences relate to the proportion of T3N0 cases contained in the series. For example, Schottenfeld and colleagues[189] have shown that the 5-year survival for T3N0 is approximately 65% and is identical to the outcome in patients with T2N1 (stage IIB) disease. This fact led to the reclassification of patients with T3N0 breast cancer into stage IIB disease, as mentioned previously. When a patient with a T3 breast primary tumor is otherwise a candidate for mastectomy, surgical treatment up front (followed by adjuvant systemic therapy) is a perfectly reasonable treatment option. Local recurrence is seen in 20% to 30% of patients, and

these patients should receive postmastectomy chest wall irradiation.[190,191]

Radiotherapy alone has been used in the treatment of noninflammatory LABC, especially in patients with T4 primary tumors. Davila and Toonkel[192] reviewed 15 radiation series encompassing more than 2100 patients. Five-year survivals clustered in the 20% to 25% range, with local control achievable about 50% of the time. Many of these patients were treated with orthovoltage equipment. Some had gross tumor excisions, whereas others had endocrine or systemic chemotherapy manipulations. In general, very high doses of radiation, exceeding 70 Gy, and even 80 Gy in some instances, were needed to control these large breast masses. As the adverse long-term sequellae of high-dose radiation to the breast became clear,[193] the use of radiotherapy alone in the treatment of LABC was largely abandoned. In its place, combined treatment with surgery and radiation with or without chemotherapy took its place.[194]

Combinations of surgery and radiotherapy to treat LABC have a strong rationale. The doses needed to control large tumors with radiotherapy were prohibitive, and thus it made more sense to treat potential microscopic disease in the chest wall after the large breast mass and lymph nodes were removed. On the other hand, surgery alone had at least a 25% to 30% risk of local failure, and this could be reduced by the addition of radiation. Experience in the literature suggests that when radiation was added postmastectomy, locoregional recurrences were reduced in half to a level of approximately 15%, but that the 5-year survival was unaffected.[195-198] This focused attention on the need for chemotherapy to treat patients with LABC. There are several reasons for the use of chemotherapy, the most compelling of which is the effect it has in reducing the risk of dying from disseminated breast cancer. Since women with LABC have a high risk of occult disseminated disease, the need for systemic chemotherapy follows the same rationale as it does for node-positive stage II patients. One can now cite a number of retrospective, single-institution studies that show the benefit of chemotherapy added to the

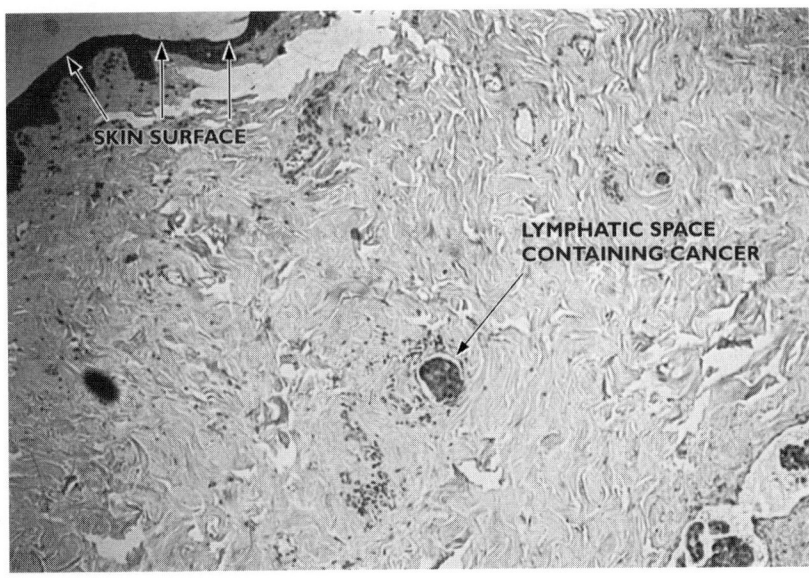

Figure 57-7. Involvement of the lymphatics directly under the skin, as seen in this specimen, is the pathologic correlate of inflammatory breast cancer. Although the diagnosis of inflammatory disease can be based solely on classic clinical features, seeing dermal lymphatic involvement further helps solidify the diagnosis.

therapy of patients with LABC compared with historic controls.[199-201] Several randomized trials testing the value of chemotherapy in noninflammatory LABC have been performed. Most of these randomized trials have failed to show a statistically significant survival advantage for the chemotherapy-treated group (Table 57-16). However, it must be acknowledged that most of these trials were rather small and thus had limited power to detect a survival difference. In addition, most of the studies showed a strong trend toward improved outcome when chemotherapy was added to local treatment. Despite the shortcomings in clinical research in the treatment of LABC, the use of systemic chemotherapy is virtually universally accepted today as an important component of the therapy of this condition. With a consensus established that the combined use of local and systemic treatment is required, treatment controversies revolve around the sequencing of the treatment and whether both local treatment modalities (radiotherapy and mastectomy) should be used along with chemotherapy in the treatment of these patients.

To address the sequencing question, many investigators have used chemotherapy as the initial treatment approach in the management of LABC.[202-205] Response rates to initial chemotherapy are high—70% to 80%—with 15% to 30% of patients having a complete clinical response to treatment. Although patients with T3N1 disease (and T3N0 disease) are technically operable and can be treated with standard mastectomy followed by adjuvant chemotherapy, most investigators treat LABC with at least three to four cycles of neoadjuvant chemotherapy before proceeding to local treatment. The local breast lesion becomes a good indicator of chemotherapy sensitivity, and patients with the most sensitive tumors, that is, those who have a complete response after chemotherapy, have the best overall survival outlook. Furthermore, a complete clearance of the tumor or reduction of the tumor size by a substantial amount, has allowed some investigators to practice breast-conserving therapy as part of the treatment of LABC.

The optimal local treatment for LABC has not been defined. Patients who have a complete response, especially if this response is confirmed by repeat biopsy, can be managed with local radiotherapy alone.[206-208] If the primary tumor does not exhibit a complete response, then most institutions would employ mastectomy followed by postoperative chest-wall irradiation. Retrospective reviews from the Mallinckrodt Institute have shown increased survival when mastectomy has been added to radiotherapy as part of the treatment program for LABC.[201] Investigators at the National Cancer Institute (NCI) have shown improved local control for patients treated with mastectomy plus radiation versus radiation alone, even though the latter group had a pathologically confirmed complete response, whereas the former group had pathologically confirmed residual disease.[209] But mastectomy in the NCI series did not improve survival, and the local failure rate of 15% to 20% is only marginally higher than that seen treating lower-stage disease, and in patients who have an in-breast failure, local control can often be restored with a salvage mastectomy. In general, although breast preservation is not the ultimate goal in the treatment of LABC, it can be practiced safely in patients who have had a complete or near-complete response to neoadjuvant chemotherapy. For those patients who have had a partial response, it is recommended that mastectomy be added to the treatment regimen.

Inflammatory Breast Cancer

Inflammatory breast cancer is almost always a systemic disease. In contrast to stage IIIA disease and some select cases of stage IIIB disease, inflammatory breast cancer has a dreadful outcome when treated with local therapy only. High rates of local recurrence are seen with mastectomy, with or without radiotherapy, or with radiotherapy alone.[80] Metastatic dissemination is virtually universal. Thus, the need for chemotherapy in the

Table 57–16   Randomized Trials Using Chemotherapy in Locally Advanced Breast Cancer

Reference	Patients, *n*	Treatment	Survival Disease-Free	Overall
Schaake-Konig et al[349]	118	RT	14 mo (med)	37% (5 yr)
		RT→→→→→CMF	26 mo (med)	37% (5 yr)
		AV–CMF →RT → AV–CMF–Tamoxifen	20 mo (med)	37% (5 yr)
Derman et al[350]	231	RT ± M →Observation	27 mo (med)	
		→CMF (dose level I)	53 mo (med)	
		→CMF (dose level II)	56 mo (med)	
Rubens et al[351]	368	RT	15% (5 yr)	35% (5 yr)
		RT + endocrine Rx	18% (5 yr)	33% (5 yr)
		RT + CMF	19% (5 yr)	33% (5 yr)
		RT + endocrine Rx + CMF	32% (5 yr)	54% (5 yr)
Klefstrom et al[352]	120	M →RT	32% (3 yr)	57% (3 yr)
		→VAC ± levamisole	47% (3 yr)	72% (3 yr)
		→RT + VAC	87% (3 yr)	90% (3 yr)

AV, doxorubicin, vincristine; BCG, bacillus Calmette-Guérin; CFV, cyclophosphamide; →, followed by.

treatment of inflammatory breast cancer is unquestioned, and chemotherapy as the first therapeutic maneuver in these patients is now widely accepted to be the treatment of choice. As with operable disease, inflammatory breast cancer has an 80% to 90% chance of responding to chemotherapy, and the chemotherapeutic response is an important predictor of ultimate outcome.[210,211] After chemotherapy is administered, local therapy is applied. Although some investigators have employed radiation alone in patients who had pathologically proven clinical responses, this therapy is difficult to employ. Inflammatory breast cancer often presents without a definable mass, making it difficult to boost the radiation dose to areas of high risk to 60 Gy or more, the dose often associated with curative treatment of the intact breast. Thus, one is faced with the dilemma of trying to treat the entire breast with a high dose, which can produce deleterious cosmetic effects in the long term, or trying to give a boost to a substantial portion of the breast with electrons or photons, which may have the same deleterious cosmetic consequences. Most investigators would advocate an aggressive local approach to inflammatory breast cancer that has been treated with chemotherapy, employing mastectomy followed by chest-wall, supraclavicular, and apex-of-axilla irradiation.[212] There is a suggestion that higher doses of radiation produce better results.[213] In inflammatory breast cancer, the advantage of combined-modality therapy compared with local therapy alone is unequivocal. From a disease with a historic 5-year survival rate in the range of zero to 10%, 5-year survival rates in the range of 30% to 50% can now be seen.[199,213-215] However, disease-free survival is 10% to 20% lower than overall survival, and survival curves in this disease continue a trend downward without an obvious plateau. Clearly, more effective systemic therapy will be necessary to increase the long-term cure rate in this disease.

Adjuvant Chemotherapy

Since the first experimental use of single-agent chemotherapy began in the 1960s, literally hundreds of clinical trials have been done testing the effects of cytotoxic chemotherapy, hormonal therapy, or both in the treatment of breast cancer. Virtually every therapeutic claim and counterclaim can be supported by one trial or another from the world's literature. In order to add as much order as possible to this chaos, all major breast cancer studies have been combined into a meta-analysis involving thousands of women allocated at random to different types of systemic therapy or observation.[216,217] These data support two major conclusions:

1. Adjuvant cytotoxic chemotherapy lowers the risk of recurrence in pre- and postmenopausal node-positive women and substantially lowers the risk of death in premenopausal women with positive nodes, with smaller effects seen in postmenopausal women as well.
2. Adjuvant tamoxifen reduces the risk of recurrence and the risk of death in estrogen receptor-positive breast cancer with either positive or negative nodes in both pre- and postmenopausal women.

Table 57–17 Changes in Survival Resulting from the Systemic Treatment of Breast Cancer

Age, Yr	Treatment	Nodal Status	10-Yr Survival, % No Chemotherapy	Chemotherapy
<50	Chemotherapy	neg	71	78
		pos	42	53
>50	Chemotherapy	neg	65	71
		pos	46	49
			No Tamoxifen	Tamoxifen
All	Tamoxifen	neg	73	79
ER+		pos	50	61

neg, negative; pos, positive.
Data from Early Breast Cancer Trialists' Collaborative Groups: Tamoxifen for early breast cancer: An overview of the randomized trials. *Lancet.* 1998;351:1451 and 352:930.

The magnitude of benefit from adjuvant therapy in pre- and postmenopausal node-positive patients is summarized in Table 57-17. It is unequivocal that node-positive patients should be treated with cytotoxic chemotherapy. Four to 6 months of therapy appears adequate, and standard regimens used today are summarized in Table 57-18. Women who are estrogen receptor-positive (the majority of women with postmenopausal breast cancer) should be treated with tamoxifen, 20 mg per day, for 5 years. Most node-negative women with cancer greater than 1 cm should receive chemotherapy as well.[218] Women with small node-negative cancers with tubular or mucinous histology can avoid chemotherapy. An overall framework for the use of systemic therapy is given in Table 57-19.

ROLE OF RADIATION THERAPY IN THE TREATMENT OF BREAST CANCER

Definitive Treatment of the Intact Breast

Radiation clearly plays an important role in the nonmastectomy therapy of breast cancer, both intraductal and invasive subtypes. The reduction of local breast cancer failures for patients with DCIS treated with radiation after excision versus those treated with excision alone has been detailed. The need for radiotherapy after local excision for patients with invasive breast cancer has been the subject of four major randomized prospective studies beyond NSAPB B-06 as summarized in Table 57-20. A statistically significant reduction in local breast failure was seen in each of the four studies. To date, only a single retrospective study reports that local control rates with lumpectomy alone are equivalent to the use of postlumpectomy radiation.[219] There is no suggestion to date that preventing in-breast failure improves overall survival,[220,221] and one might argue that local failure rates of 20% to 40% (or less than 10% with a quadrantectomy) after excision alone are acceptable in order to avoid treating all women with radiation. However, many local recurrences require a patient to undergo a mastectomy at the time of recurrence. Furthermore, as detailed

Table 57–18　Combination Chemotherapy Regimens Used in the Adjuvant Treatment of Breast Cancer

Regimen	Drugs	Dose, mg/m² (route)	Delivered on Day(s)	Repeat Cycle on Day
CMF – Classic[353]	Cyclophosphamide	100 (PO)	1 to 14	
	Methotrexate	40 (IV)	1 and 8	29
	5-Fluorouracil	600 (IV)	1 and 8	
CMF – IV[354]	Cyclophosphamide	600 (IV)	1	
	Methotrexate	40 (IV)	1	22
	5-Fluorouracil	600 (IV)	1	
CAF (ECOG)[355]	Cyclophosphamide	100 (PO)	1 to 14	
	Doxorubicin	30 (IV)	1 and 8	29
	5-Fluorouracil	500 (IV)	1 and 8	
AC[356]	Cyclophosphamide	600 (IV)	1	
	Doxorubicin	60 (IV)	1	22
FAC[357]	Cyclophosphamide	500 (IV)	1	
	Methotrexate	50 (IV)	1	22
	5-Fluorouracil	500 (IV)	1	
AC – Taxol[358]	Doxorubicin	60 (IV)	1	29
	Cyclophosphamide then	600 (IV)	1	(4 cycles)
	Paclitaxel	175 (IV)	1	22 (4 cycles)
CAF (CALGB)[359]	Cyclophosphamide	600 (IV)	1	
	Doxorubicin	60 (IV)	1	29
	5-Fluorouracil	600 (IV)	1 and 8	
CEF[360]	Cyclophosphamide	75 (PO)	1 to 14	
	Epirubicin	60 (IV)	1 and 8	
	5-Fluorouracil	500 (IV)	1 and 8	

CALGB, Cancer and Acute Leukemia Group B; ECOG, Eastern Cooperative Oncology Group.

later, breast radiotherapy is extremely well tolerated with very few complications. Thus, if the goal of nonmastectomy therapy is to provide a woman with the greatest chance of having an intact, cosmetically acceptable breast after the conclusion therapy, then the need for radiation is indisputable.[222] Tamoxifen does not appear to substitute for radiation, although the addition of tamoxifen to radiation further reduces local failure rates.[223]

Postmastectomy Chest Wall Irradiation

One of the most actively studied and controversial areas in the treatment of primary breast cancer is the use of postmastectomy chest-wall irradiation. In the first half of the 20th century, chest wall irradiation was applied to the majority of women undergoing mastectomies. This related to the fact that there were no good screening tests for breast cancer and women frequently presented with large node-positive tumors. Their risk for chest-wall failure was therefore high, and postmastectomy chest-wall irradiation became a routine part of breast cancer management. But as the years passed, surgical techniques improved, detection techniques improved, and investigators began to take a much closer look at the value of chest-wall irradiation. The technique has been tested in more than 20 randomized prospective trials, and it is noteworthy that possibly the original randomized prospective trial of any oncologic treatment was the first Manchester postmastectomy chest-wall trial begun in 1949.[224] A number of excellent reviews have both summarized and interpreted these studies, and

Table 57–19　Recommendations for Systemic Therapy of Breast Cancer

	Node-Negative			Node-Positive
	Low-Risk*	Intermediate-Risk†	High-Risk‡	
Premenopausal	Observation or tamoxifen	Tamoxifen ± CT	ER+ : CT (± T) ER− : CT	ER+ : CT (± T) ER− : CT
Postmenopausal	Observation or tamoxifen	Tamoxifen ± CT	ER+ : T (± CT) ER− : T (± CT)	ER+ : T (± CT) ER− : CT (± T)

*Low-risk = ductal cancer ≤1 cm; colloid, papillary, tubular ≤2 cm.
†Intermediate-risk = tumors 1-2 cm that are ER+ with low histologic grade.
‡High-risk = ER+ and ≥2 cm or ≥1 cm with high histologic grade; ER− ≥1 cm.
CT, chemotherapy; ER, estrogen receptor; T, tamoxifen.
Data from Goldhirsch A, Glick JH, Gelber RD, et al: Meeting highlights: International consensus panel on the treatment of primary breast cancer. *J Natl Cancer Inst.* 1998;90:1601.

Table 57-20 Randomized Trials of Excision Alone versus Excision Plus Radiation Therapy (XRT)

Reference	Patients, n	Largest Tumor size cm	In-Breast Failure Excision %	In-Breast Failure Excision + XRT %
Liljegren et al[362]	381	≤2	24.0	8.5
Veronesi et al[363]	579	<2.5	23.5	5.8
Clark et al[364]	837	<4	35.2	11.3
	93	≤1	28.5	
Forrest et al[365]	585	≤4	24.5	5.8

the interested reader is referred to them for more detail.[225-230]

While many early studies confirmed that the risk of a local failure on the chest was reduced by 60% to 70% with the addition of chest-wall irradiation,[231] survival was unaffected. This was due, in part, to toxicity balancing out benefit. Studies showed that breast cancer survival was improved, but that deaths from cardiac events were increased. This was possibly technique related as early trials used larger fraction size, older cobalt machines, and often treated the parasternal nodes with an enface photon field, treating the heart extensively.[229] Trials done by the Danish Breast Cancer Cooperative Group[232,233] and in British Columbia[234] strongly suggest a survival increase resulting from chest-wall radiation.

The issue of the use of postmastectomy chest-wall irradiation is still controversial and will likely be the subject of additional clinical trials in coming years. In the meantime, postmastectomy irradiation appears indicated in the following cases[235]:

1. Positive margins or gross residual disease
2. Any T3 or T4 tumor
3. Four or more positive axillary lymph nodes
4. Gross extracapsular disease in the axilla

The advantage of treating women postmastectomy who have one to three positive axillary nodes is not proved and is the subject of clinical research.

Palliative Care

One of the most important roles for radiotherapy relates to symptom palliation. Breast cancer can metastasize widely, especially to bone, frequently requiring palliative radiotherapy. Standard regimens of 20 Gy in 5 fractions or 30 Gy in 10 fractions are usually successful in relieving bone pain.[236] Similarly, brain metastases are often treated with 30 Gy in 10 fractions with a possible cone-down boost to a solitary metastasis. Breast cancer is one of the diseases that can metastasize to the choroid of the eye, with resulting visual compromise. This condition is often relieved with 30 Gy in 10 fractions to a small lateral field designed to treat the globe of the eye. Breast cancer also frequently recurs on the chest wall after mastectomy. In this setting, the favored treatment is excision of the recurrence (if possible) followed by chest-wall irradiation. It is the author's preference to treat the entire chest wall and supraclavicular nodes in response to any chest-wall failure. Data indicate that placing a small field around the lesion itself leaves the patient at high risk for re-recurrence on the chest wall.[237,238] Doses of 50 Gy are delivered with either tangential photon fields or en face electron fields. If the disease has been locally excised, a boost to 60 Gy is given to the bed of resection. If gross disease is left on the chest wall, 65 to 70 Gy of radiation are required to give the maximal chance for local disease control.

TECHNIQUES OF TREATMENT

Surgical Technique

Mastectomy is a treatment alternative for any woman with resectable breast cancer, either invasive or noninvasive. Frequently, the mastectomy is accompanied by an axillary lymph node dissection that typically removes lymph nodes at level I (inferior to the pectoralis minor muscle) and level II (beneath the pectoralis minor muscle). Lymph node dissection is often omitted today if the sentinel lymph nodes are negative. Several types of mastectomies have been described. The classic radical mastectomy, as described by Halstead,[239] involved the *en bloc* removal of the breast, the overlying skin, both the pectoralis major and minor muscles, and levels I, II, and III axillary lymph nodes. The modified radical mastectomy preserves the pectoralis minor muscle and a great deal of the skin of the chest wall.[240] Modified radical mastectomies are most often closed primarily, whereas radical mastectomies typically required a skin graft. In the modified radical mastectomy, the long thoracic and the thoracodorsal nerves are usually spared. This prevents the atrophy of the serratus anterior and latissimus dorsi muscles often seen after a radical mastectomy in which these nerves are sacrificed.[241] Even with the modified radical mastectomy, however, the intercostal brachial nerve, which provides sensory intervention to the medial aspect of the upper arm, is often transected, producing a characteristic numbness after the operation.

Today many patients are treated without mastectomy; instead, a surgical cancer removal that has been variously referred to as *lumpectomy, tylectomy,* or *segmental* or *partial mastectomy* is used. The incision for a lumpectomy should be directly over the tumor mass so that the surgeon has the most direct access to the tumor, can control margins with precision, and is not tunneling through many centimeters of normal breast tissue, as is often necessary for a circumareolar incision. Skin incisions in the inferior part of the breast should be radial, but all other incisions should be curvilinear to avoid breast deformity.[46] The cavity left by the lumpectomy should be closed without deep sutures or drains so that the cavity may fill in with fibrous and granulation tissue, restoring the contour of the breast. Several surgical clips should be left in the periphery of the excision bed to guide later boost treatment.[242-246] If an axillary dissection is performed, it is done through a separate incision and not by extending the lumpectomy incision into the axilla, which creates a great deal of breast deformity. The exceptions to this are in tumors located in the very tail of the breast, where two incisions would be impractical.

Radiation Technique

The intact breast is treated with a pair of photon fields directed tangentially to encompass the entire breast while missing as much lung and heart as possible.[247] A typical tangent field is illustrated in Figure 57-8. These fields can be set by palpation or more commonly today by outlining the breast target volume seen on a CT planning scan, a technique that can add accuracy to the process.[248] If one wishes to add the IM or axillary nodes into the volume, the radiation fields must be altered somewhat. Typically, a CT scan is required to define these nodal volumes, and additional static fields or intensity-modulated fields using a multileaf collimator are used.[249-251] Long-term sequellae of breast radiation can involve increased cardiac toxicity, and short-term complications can manifest as radiation pneumonitis. The volume of lung being seen on the tangent film correlates to the volume of lung treated, while the heart volume best correlates with gantry angles (the more vertical the field angle, the greater the heart volume).[252] Every effort

should be made to include the entire breast and nodal volume while minimizing lung and heart dose. Newer intensity-modulated radiation therapy techniques appear to offer a small but measurable improvement over standard fixed fields[253,254] and will likely dominate the technical treatment of breast cancer in the years ahead. Photon energies of 4 to 8 MV appear to provide equivalent results,[255] with 6 MV being a common prescription energy. Patients with full breasts can present a particularly troublesome problem of breast-conserving treatment. The breast has a large separation, which challenges dose homogeneity, and the breast often rests on the anterior abdominal wall creating a situation where skin toxicity due to lack of skin sparing can cause substantial acute and late skin changes. For these patients, one can consider treating the patient in the prone position.[159,256]

What follows is a discussion of how to set up standard fixed tangential fields, either shaped with fixed or multileaf collimators, and a summary of newer CT-based setup techniques.

Simulating Tangential Breast Fields

More than a dozen publications have described various techniques concerning the setup of the breast tangential fields.[257-270] Although each of these techniques presents

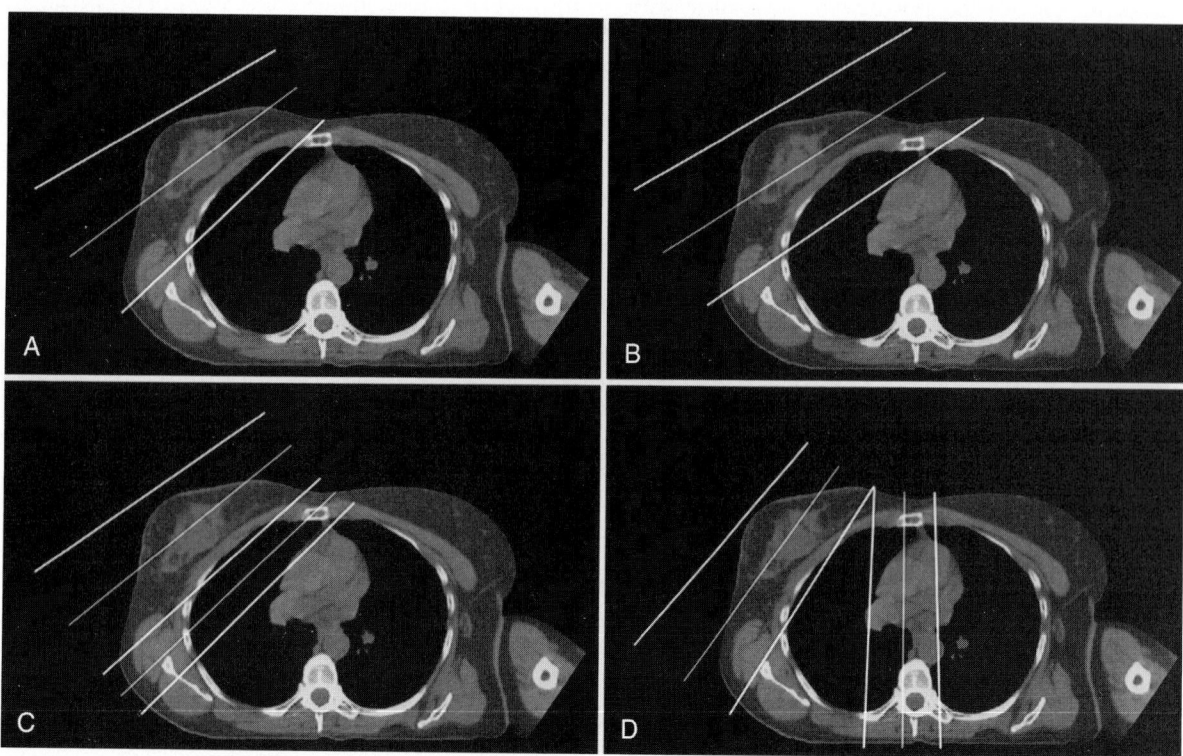

Figure 57–8. Four treatment techniques for irradiating the intact breast. **A,** "Standard" tangent fields. The medial field is illustrated here, entering at the midline and exiting in the posterior axillary fold. A small amount of lung is subtended by this field. An opposing lateral tangent field completes the field arrangement. The internal mammary lymph node chain next to the sternum is poorly covered with this technique. **B,** "Deep" tangential fields. The entrance point is moved several centimeters past the midline in order to treat the internal mammary lymph node region. As a consequence, extra lung is included in this field and, for left-sided lesions, additional heart volume. **C,** Shallow tangents matched to an angled electron field. This represents a good solution for treating the intact breast along with the internal mammary lymph nodes. Often a small amount of photon treatment is given to the internal mammary field so that the skin reaction is not too severe. **D,** The problem with a direct en face internal mammary field is illustrated in this picture. If the fields are matched on the skin, a "cold triangle" of tissue in between the internal mammary and tangential fields is left substantially underdosed.

a variation of how to perform the setup, there are a number of themes that run through all these techniques, such as:

1. The techniques are generally isocentric.
2. They generally do not use a half-beam block but rather use the primary collimator to define the deep (lung) portion of the field.
3. They keep the deep edges of the field coplanar, directing divergence into air rather than farther into the lung.
4. They attempt in some fashion to achieve a smooth match line between the tangential breast fields and the supraclavicular-axillary field if this field is used.

All good breast setups begin with careful immobilization of the patient. Some techniques use custom-made foam cradles for each patient, whereas other institutions use homemade or commercially available arm boards. Whatever device is chosen, it should be comfortable for the patient and should allow her to assume the same relative position of her body and her arm each day. The author prefers to treat breast cancer patients in the supine position rather than building them up on a tilt board. The advantage to a tilt board is that the sternum can be rendered level to the treatment couch, eliminating the need for a twist of the collimator on the tangential fields. This somewhat simplifies the match line between the breast tangential fields and the supraclavicular fields. However, positioning the patient on a tilt board each day may not be as reproducible as positioning the patient in the supine position, which is why our group has chosen to use a tilt board only when necessary. Furthermore, with today's asymmetric collimators, most patients who need a supraclavicular field can have a single isocenter placed at the match line, eliminating the complexity of the match. A tilt board is very helpful in treating a patient with a large breast that can tend to ride up high on the chest wall while the patient is lying supine. Also, our experience has shown that patients who have extremely steep chest wall angles (greater than 25 degrees from the horizontal) have a better setup on a tilt board than by rotating the collimator this large amount.

Once the patient is carefully and comfortably immobilized, various techniques can be used to set up the tangential fields. The interested reader is referred directly to a number of articles describing these techniques.[257-269] In our non–CT-based system, the superior and inferior extent of the field is marked on the patient's skin, and the appropriate length field is set on the simulator. We then mark where we would like the beam to enter medially over the sternum and where we would like the lateral field to enter near the midaxillary line. We then use a device called a *breast bridge* (Fig. 57-9) to determine:

1. The distance on a straight line that separates the medial and lateral entrance points
2. The angle from the horizontal that defines this connecting line
3. The width of the field necessary to flash over the surface of the breast

A fourth measurement, the angle that the sternum makes relative to the treatment table top, is taken by placing an inclinometer on the patient's sternum. With

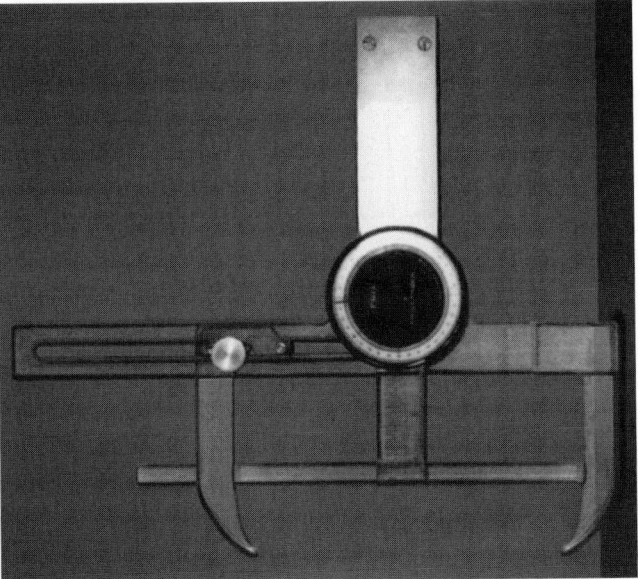

Figure 57–9. Version of a breast bridge used for setting up tangential treatments. The tips of the curved rods are placed at the entrance and exit points for the tangential fields, and their separation is read off a scale. The width of the field is measured by sliding the T-shaped bar higher or lower until the appropriate clearance beyond the breast is achieved. The inclinometer in the center of the device reads the angle of the line connecting the entrance and exit points. These numbers are fed into a simple computer program that determines the parameters of the treatment setup.

these four measurements, it is very simple to enter the data into a computer program that calculates the setup parameters relative to the medial entrance point.[271] The program calculates how deep below the medial entrance point the isocenter should lie and how far laterally the patient should be shifted on the table so that the isocenter lies in the appropriate position within the breast. Finally, the program computes the medial and lateral gantry angles that cause the fields to enter and exit through the medial and lateral entrance point (deep edges coplanar) (Fig. 57-10). A simulator film is then taken to confirm the accuracy of the setup (Fig. 57-11). If the fields do not line up correctly, it is relatively straightforward to note what type of correction should be applied, change the parameters entered into the computer program, and recalculate a new set of treatment angles and isocenter location quite quickly.

Many centers, including the author's, now use a CT simulator instead of a conventional simulator for breast cases. Once the patient is immobilized in the CT simulator, the clinical borders of the field are marked and a CT dataset is acquired. The patient can then leave and planning is accomplished on stored images. The external surface of the body is displayed and the field borders are easily seen (Fig. 57-12). Through an iterative process, the fields can be set and viewed from various angles, including the creation of a digitally reconstructed radiograph (DRR), which will serve as the reference film to guide the accuracy of the setup (Fig. 57-13).

A supraclavicular field is often treated when there are positive axillary lymph nodes. Some institutions treat the supraclavicular fossa when there are one or more positive

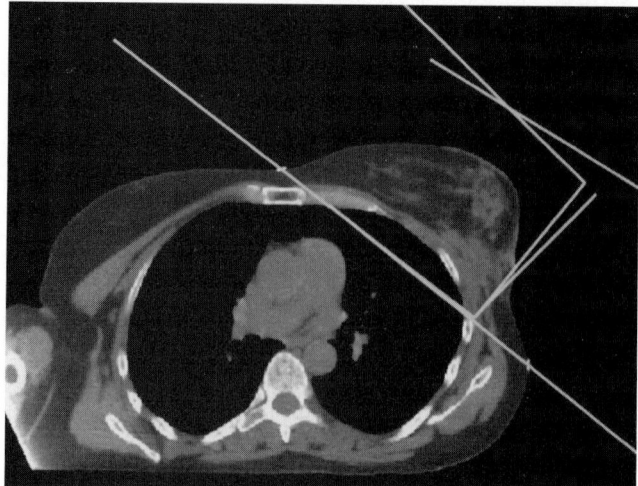

Figure 57–10. Standard set of tangential fields to cover a left-sided breast lesion. Catheters are placed on the entrance and exit points of the field, and the edges of the treatment beams are seen to pass through these points precisely. Note that the deep edges of the fields are made coplanar so that all divergence is directed into space, not into the underlying lung. A wedge filter, when used, is preferentially placed in the lateral tangential field where it has less effect on scattered dose to the opposite normal breast.

axillary nodes, whereas other institutions treat only when four or more lymph nodes are found to be positive.[272-274] In the setting of positive axillary lymph nodes, the supra-clavicular fossa is the site of first failure in between 5% and 10% of patients[94] and is an ultimate site of failure in 15% to 20% of patients.[275] These numbers are dramatically reduced with supraclavicular treatment. The field is also designed to treat the apex of the axilla (Fig. 57-14A). The apex of the axilla contains level III axillary lymph nodes, which usually are not dissected. Typically, the field measures approximately 8 cm in width, matches inferiorly to the tangential breast fields, and superiorly comes to just flashing the skin of the supraclavicular fossa. Medially, the field is placed along the lateral aspect of the cervical vertebral bodies. The field is often angled 10 degrees laterally so that there is no divergence into the

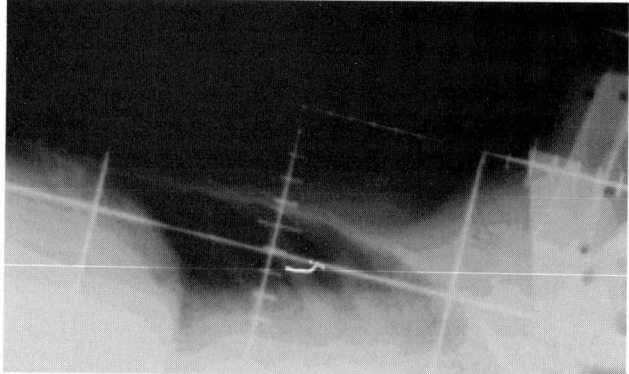

Figure 57–11. Typical simulator film for a tangential breast field. The medial field is shown here, and a BB dot is placed on the medial entrance point. A wire is placed on the lateral entrance point to confirm that the deep edge of the field has been angled properly and that no extra divergence reaches the lung. The collimator is angled to roughly parallel the chest wall.

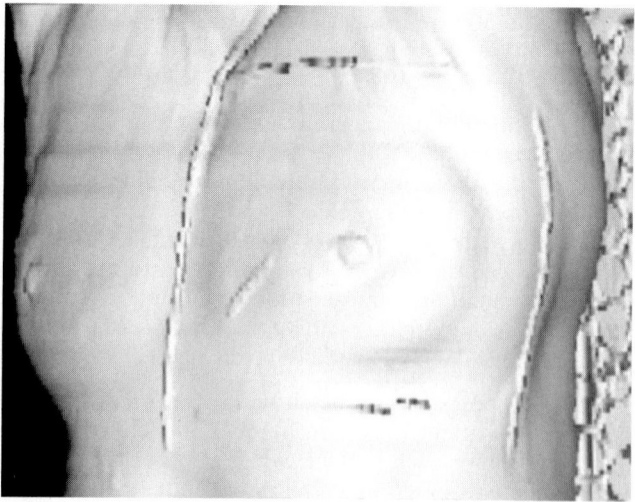

Figure 57–12. External contour generated from stored computed tomographic images with clinical field borders (medial, lateral, superior, inferior) defined using radiopaque catheters.

spinal cord, thus allowing a full radiation dose to be delivered later in the patient's illness should metastases occur in the cervical spine. It should be emphasized that it is rarely necessary to treat the dissected axilla. The axilla is the first site of failure after axillary lymph node dissection in approximately 1% of patients,[276] attesting to the fact that axillary irradiation itself is probably not warranted. Even if there is extension beyond the lymph node capsule in a microscopic fashion into the axillary fat, the incidence of axillary failure hardly changes, again allowing one to spare treatment of this region.[277,278] It is appropriate to irradiate the full axilla if no axillary lymph node dissection has been performed or if *gross* extracapsular lymph node disease has been encountered. In all the remaining patients, the bulk of the axilla itself is left largely unirradiated. The difference between a small supraclavicular field and the full supraclavicular-axillary field is illustrated in Figure 57-14B. Since the anterior field is usually dosed to a depth of 3 cm, the axillary lymph nodes in the full axillary field are under-dosed by 15% to 20% since they can lie at depths of 7 cm or so (near the midplane). To compensate for this underdosage, a small posterior axillary field is often used to supplement the midplane dose. In our hands, the posterior axillary field is set up by rotating the gantry 180 degrees from the anterior field and taking an x-ray film. A block is drawn to shape the field, and this isocentric field is treated daily, usually with doses in the 40 to 60 Gy range (Fig. 57-14C). An isocentric setup greatly facilitates the treatment of this field. These fields can be easily set using the CT data set.

RADIATION TREATMENT PLAN

Every primary breast cancer patient requires a customized treatment plan. A contour is taken manually or preferentially with a CT planning scan. It is obvious from looking at any port film that lung tissue is contained in the irradiated volume when the intact breast is treated.

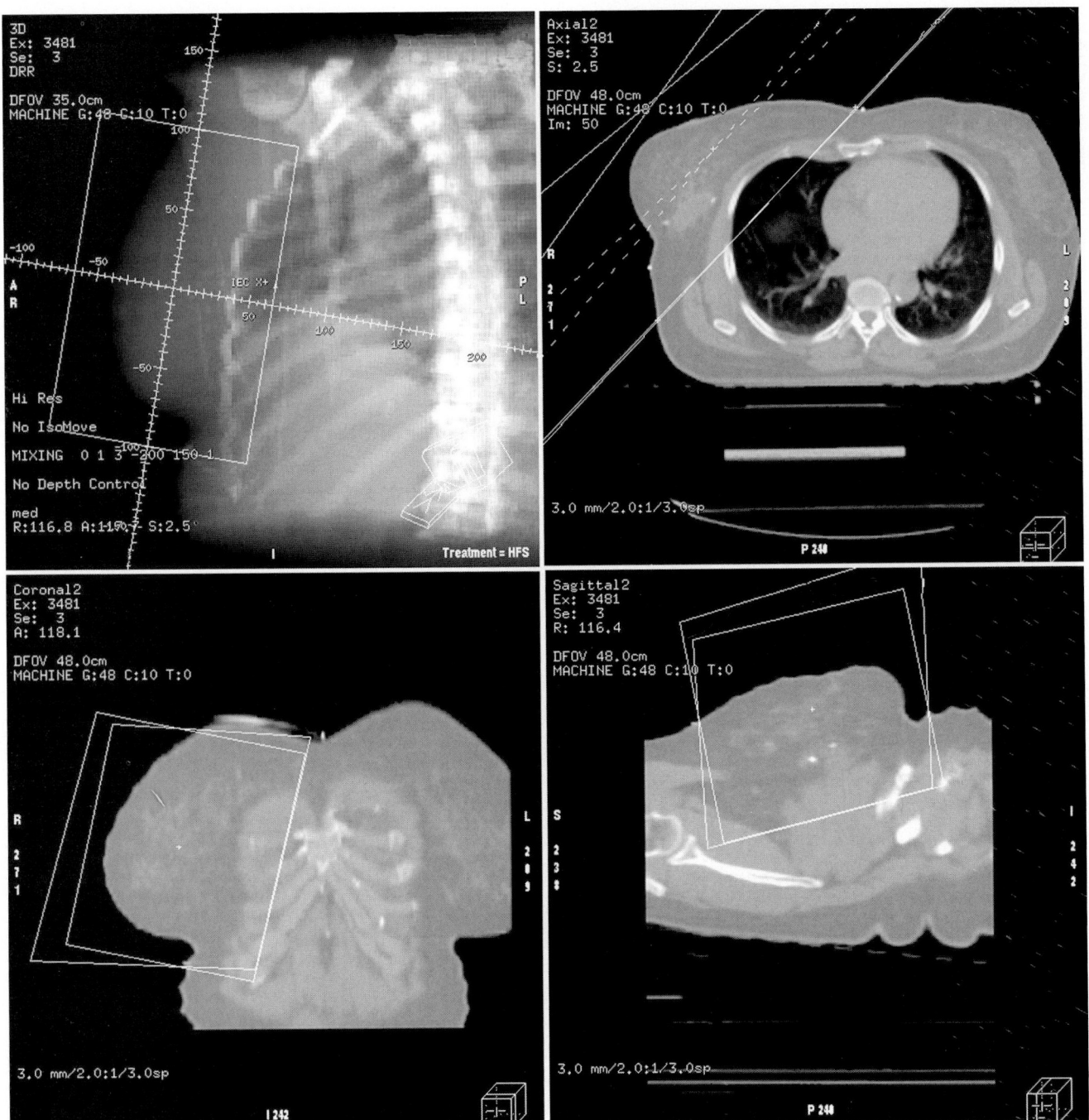

Figure 57–13. Field setting using computed tomographic data. Upper left: a digitally reconstructed radiograph of a tangent field. The other three panels show the field projected in the axial, coronal, and sagittal plane. The fields are adjusted until the optimal arrangement is produced.

Since lung tissue has a density of about 0.2 compared with soft tissues,[279] this lung tissue can create major dosimetric inhomogeneities unless its influence is taken into account.[280-282] Clinical results using treatment plans that are corrected for the density of lung are very satisfactory, indicating the safety of treating in this fashion.[283]

The contour or the CT scan is transferred to the treatment-planning computer, and the two tangential photon fields that have been simulated are placed. Most treatment-planning systems can correct isodose plans for lung tissue inhomogeneity, and we use a blanket value of 0.2 for lung tissue to make this correction. In doing this,

we find that the size of the wedge filters required to create a homogeneous dose within the conical-shaped breast volume diminishes and in some cases disappears.[280-282] We have also abandoned putting wedges in the medial tangential field and do all our wedge corrections in the lateral field. This is because the dose to the contralateral normal breast is increased severalfold by the presence of a wedge in the medial tangential field.[284-286] Not only is there more low-dose radiation scattered off this wedge, but the simple presence of the wedge requires the beam to be on for much longer periods of time, allowing more radiation leakage from the head of the machine to reach

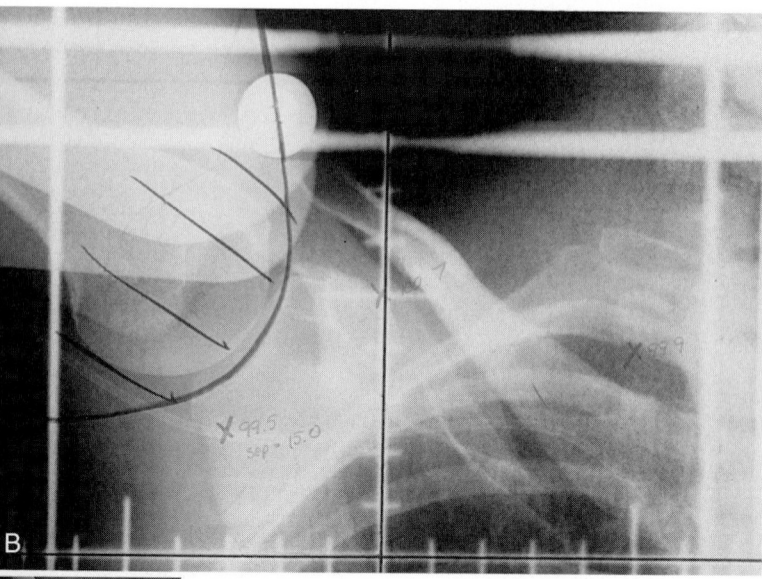

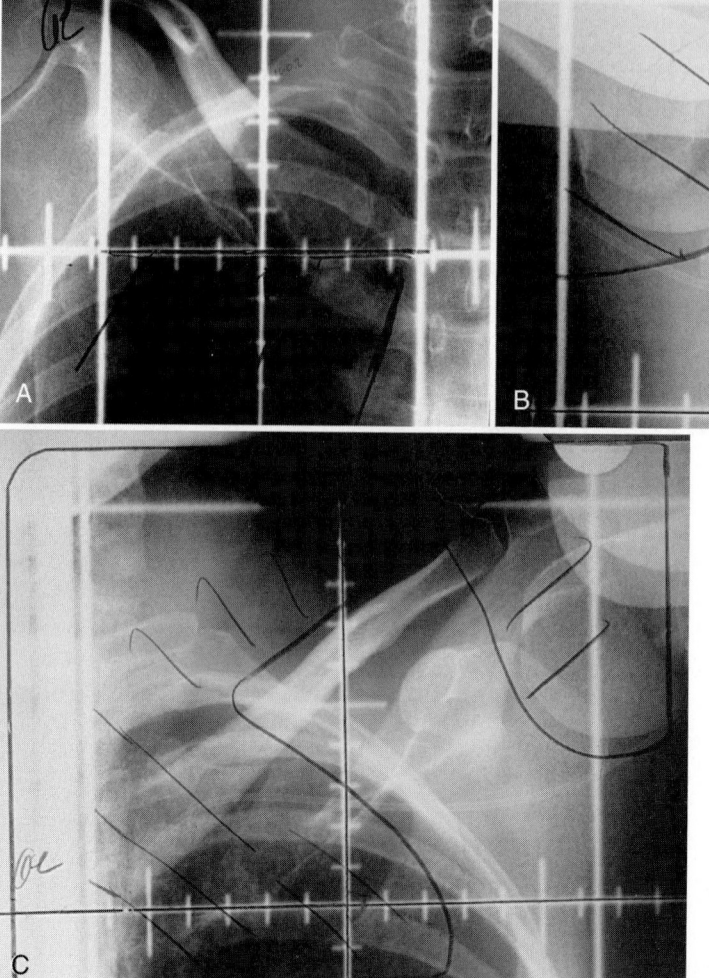

Figure 57–14. A, Typical supraclavicular field designed to treat the supraclavicular fossa and the superior portion of the axilla. The medial border is placed just outside the pedicles of the spine, and the field is angled 10 degrees away from the spine so that no divergence reaches the spinal cord. The field is typically 8 cm wide and extends inferiorly to the base of the clavicle and superiorly to just flashing the supraclavicular skin. The field is well medial to the humeral head. **B,** Full supraclavicular-axillary field. Here the field is extended well beyond the humeral head to include the entire axillary contents. The humeral head is shielded. As in *A,* the field is half-beam blocked so that its inferior edge is nondivergent. **C,** Posterior axillary boost field. This field is filmed and treated isocentrically. The block shields the humeral head, the supraclavicular fossa, and lung tissue. It is treated daily with typical doses ranging between 30 and 50 cGy at midplane of the axilla.

the contralateral breast. There is little question that breast cancer can be caused by relatively low doses of radiation.[21-23,31,32,287] Since many of our breast cancer patients will be living a long time and since the latent interval between radiation exposure and the appearance of breast cancer can be 15 to 20 years or more, we believe that it is important to try to minimize the dose to the contralateral breast as much as possible. A typical treatment plan for a breast cancer patient is presented in Figure 57-15.

It is well recognized that the breast is a complex three-dimensional conical structure. As one leaves the central axis and moves superiorly or inferiorly, the size of the breast diminishes and its shape changes. The dose distribution on off-axis slices has been calculated by a number of investigators, and one sees that there is substantial dose inhomogeneity as one moves from the carefully treatment-planned central axis.[288] It is not clear what one should do about this inhomogeneity. Certainly,

custom-built compensators could be created to eliminate many of the hot and cold spots.[289-291] However, it is not clear that a meaningful clinical problem is caused by this inhomogeneous dose distribution, especially when one considers that the total dose to the breast is only in the range of 46 to 50 Gy. Therefore, although the University of Michigan has a sophisticated three-dimensional treatment-planning system and can perform highly complex three-dimensional conformal radiotherapy, the author has not chosen to pursue this style of treatment routinely in breast cancer patients. The author plans carefully on the central axis slice, recognizing that there are inhomogeneities throughout the remainder of the breast, but also recognizing that few if any problems are created by this nonuniform dose distribution. However, the author continues to explore ways to improve upon breast radiation dosimetry, especially for treatment plans directed at the chest wall and IM nodes.[292] Using

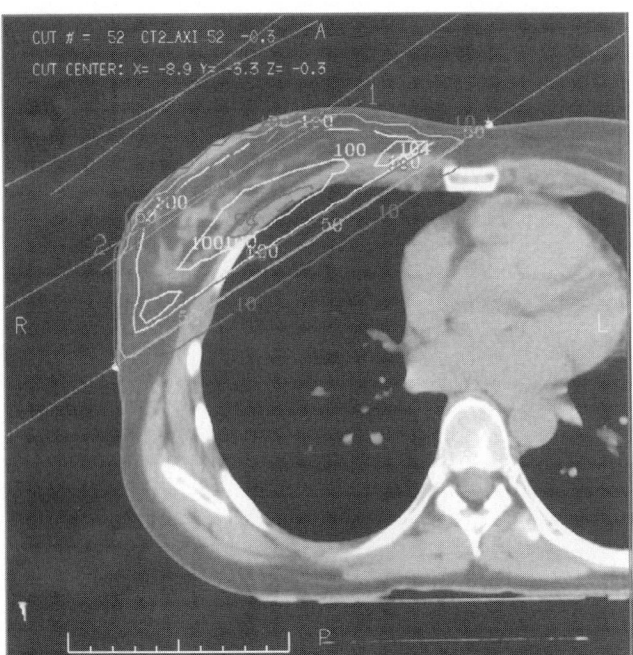

Figure 57–15. A typical treatment plan. The 100% line smoothly surrounds the breast except for a small cold area just above the lung. When lung density correction is used in breast treatment plans, this area just above the lung presents the greatest amount of tissue attenuation in the plan and thus often runs a few percentage points below the isocenter dose. The beams are weighted until the hot spots, in this case 104%, are equally balanced into the corners of the breast. See also Color Figure 57-15.

intensity-modulated radiation therapy some spectacular dose distributions can treat the left breast or chest wall and the IM nodes, and spare heart and lung (Fig. 57-16). Further research into treatment planning and treatment delivery of intensity-modulated radiation therapy for breast cancer is ongoing.

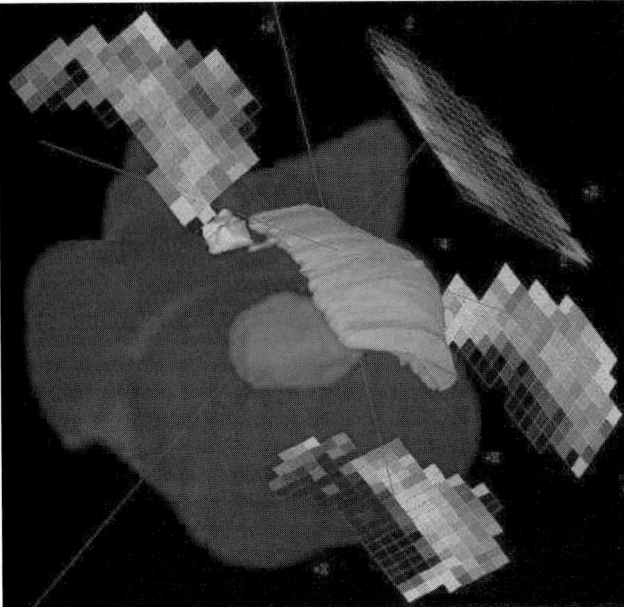

Figure 57–16. Example of intensity-modulated radiation therapy field arrangement. Each beam is divided into 1 × 1 cm beamlets of varying intensities. The breast (*violet*), supraclavicular region (*yellow*), internal mammary nodes (*green*), and heart (*red*) are shown. See also Color Figure 57-16.

Boost Field

Most institutions employ a boost dose to the tumor bed after whole-breast irradiation. The need for this boost is certainly debatable, especially in this era of pathologically controlled, margin-negative breast excisions. Today this debate is informed by the results of two randomized trials. In Lyon, France patients with a clear excision were given 50 Gy of whole breast radiation and then randomized to receive a 10 Gy boost or not. At 5 years follow-up, the boost treatment significantly reduced the in-breast failure rate (P = 0.04), but the absolute failure difference was 1% (3.6% vs. 4.5%).[293] In the second trial, from the European Organization for Research and Treatment of Cancer, patients were given 50 Gy to the whole breast and randomized to a 16 Gy boost. After 5 years median follow-up, the local failure rate was 7.3% in the observation group and 4.3% in the boost treatment group (P = 0.001).[294] Younger patients experienced the most benefit as their local recurrent rate without boost was the highest to begin with. Thus, it is clear that a radiation boost has a small but measurable effect on reducing local recurrence. Balanced against this goal is the knowledge that a breast boost can degrade the quality of the cosmetic outcome[295] and add costs that are not inconsequential.[296] Thus, even with two large trials, the decision to give a boost or not is less than clear. Certainly, women younger than 50 years old warrant a boost treatment. Whether older women, especially if they will receive systemic therapy, warrant a boost dose is a matter of individual opinion.

The boost can be done with brachytherapy implantation[297] or with electron beam.[247] The early experience with lumpectomy and radiation in the United States almost exclusively involved the use of interstitial boost treatment using iridium-192. In general, two-plane implants were used in an effort to give a boost of 15 to 20 Gy over 1 to 2 days. In some cases, the implantation was done before external beam radiation therapy, and the afterloading catheters were actually placed at the time of lumpectomy, thus ensuring very accurate coverage of the tumor bed.[298,299] More recently, most breast boosts have been performed with electron beam treatment. This therapy is certainly more convenient for the patient in that there is no need to be admitted for a hospital stay and no need for anesthesia and a potentially uncomfortable insertion of 10 to 20 needles in the breast. Some investigators actually believe that electron beam treatment is cosmetically superior to interstitial treatment, although this point is controversial.[300] With any boost technique, it is helpful to have clips left behind in the tumor bed to help guide the placement of the boost dose (Fig. 57-17). With electron beam treatment, the pedestal and gantry are angled until the electron field enters perpendicular to the breast tissue. An appropriate electron energy is selected to allow the 85% to 90% isodose line to encompass the target volume (Fig. 57-18). Some institutions set their electron beams clinically, whereas others use a more sophisticated CT or ultrasonography-based technique.[245,301,302] Finally, some investigators have begun to explore using a boost field, typically with a brachytherapy implant, as the sole treatment in breast

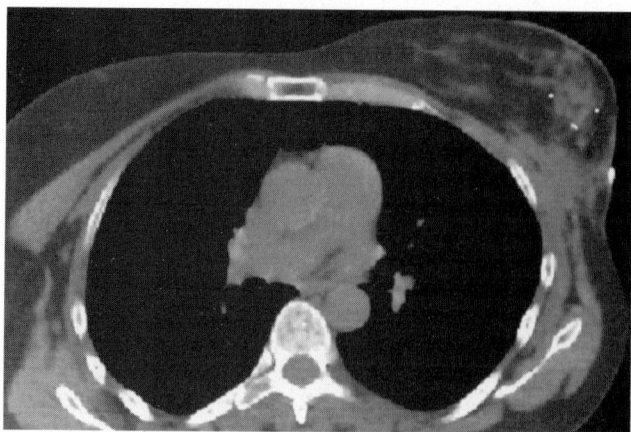

Figure 57–17. Clips left by the surgeon at the time of lumpectomy are invaluable in demarcating the tumor bed for subsequent electron beam or interstitial boost.

cancer. Recognizing that the majority of failures during the first 5 years of follow-up are in the vicinity of the tumor bed, this strategy makes sense. Early results look promising.[303,304] The possibility of reducing a 5 to 6 week course of treatment into a few days makes this an intriguing concept.

Time-Dose Fractionation

The breast is treated with 2 Gy fractions to a total dose of 46 to 50 Gy. The boost dose is then used to bring the total dose to the tumor bed to a minimum of 60 Gy. Some investigators have advocated giving higher doses if margins are close or positive.[305] It remains to be seen

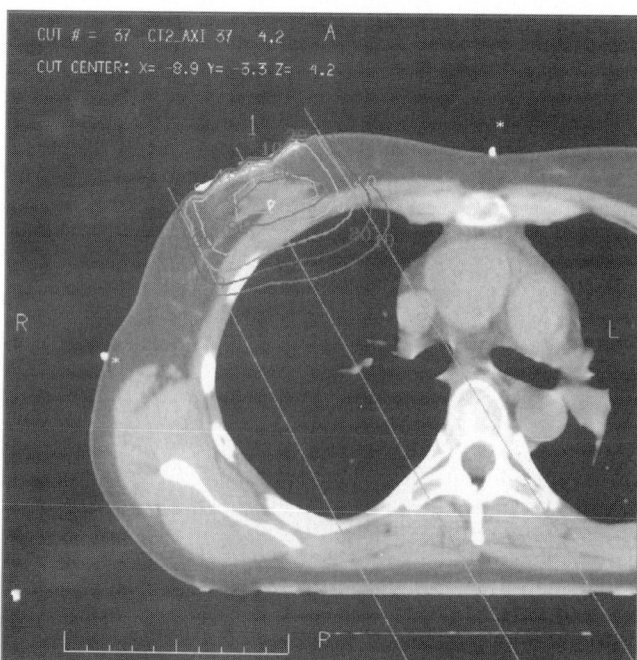

Figure 57–18. A suitable electron energy is used to cover the tumor bed with the 90% isodose line. Using electron energies of 16 MeV or greater can produce undesirable skin changes and such cases are often boosted with photons. See also Color Figure 57–18.

whether these nuances of technique improve results, but this tailoring of the ultimate dose based on the potential volume of residual disease appears appropriate.

Shorter fractionation schemes have been reported.[230,306-308] Whelan and colleagues[309] randomized more than 1200 patients to receive 50 Gy in 25 fractions or 42.5Gy in 16 fractions of 2.66 Gy. With a median follow-up of 5 years, no differences were seen in recurrence rate or cosmesis between the two groups. Longer follow-up will determine if late fibrosis will be seen in these cases. If not, shorter courses of treatment save time and cost less and should be kept in mind as an alternative to standard fractionation.

CRITICAL NORMAL TISSUES AND COMPLICATIONS

Complications of breast-sparing therapy are listed in Table 57-21. The most frequent complication associated with this treatment is arm edema, with between 5% and 20% of patients having this complication, depending on how stringent a definition of arm edema has been used in the study.[310,311] The incidence of arm edema is clearly related to the extent of axillary dissection[312] and to the use of direct axillary irradiation. In the randomized trial from the NCI, in which arm measurements were recorded at each follow-up visit, the incidence of arm edema in the lumpectomy and radiation group was identical to that in the mastectomy group (in which no radiation was given), strongly suggesting that the axillary surgery is the major determinant of risk of arm edema.[313] It is especially problematic to deliver full-course radiotherapy to an axilla that has been fully dissected. In this setting, the risk of arm edema can approach 40%.[311]

Radiation pneumonitis is now a rare complication of intact breast treatment, occurring in 1% to 2% of patients treated.[314,315] There is a slightly higher chance of a patient's developing symptomatic radiation pneumonitis if she is treated with chemotherapy or if the supraclavicular lymph nodes, with the underlying apex of the lung, are treated.[314,315] If the amount of lung tissue in the tangential breast fields is kept to less than 2 cm or less, the chance of producing symptomatic radiation pneumonitis is extremely small in the author's experience. Those patients who develop symptomatic pneumonitis in this setting usually have a relatively mild case that resolves either spontaneously or after a short course of steroids.

Radiation therapy can cause cardiac damage, and this has especially been noted in the postmastectomy chest-wall radiation literature.[316,317] An excess of cardiac

Table 57–21   Complications of Therapy

Complication	Frequency, %
Arm edema	5-20
Rib fractures	5
Radiation pneumonitis	1
Brachial plexus damage	<1
Second nonbreast malignancy	<0.1
Poor cosmetic outcome	5

deaths is seen in long-term survivors who received mastectomy plus chest-wall irradiation versus those treated with mastectomy alone. However, much of this excess cardiac mortality comes from earlier radiation series in which direct IM lymph node photon fields were frequently used. As mentioned previously, most IM lymph node treatment is now done with electrons and three-dimensional planning to spare as much cardiac radiation as possible. The morbidity of cardiac irradiation is seen long term, after 10, 15, or even 20 years of follow-up. Care should be taken to make sure that the amount of heart tissue in the radiation volume is as small as possible.[318] Recent series using modern techniques do not show an increase in cardiac events for women treated with lumpectomy and radiation.[319-321]

Rib fractures are also frequently seen after breast or chest-wall irradiation, with an incidence of approximately 2% to 5% after conventionally fractionated treatment.[322,323] In the author's experience, most of these fractures are asymptomatic and are found on bone scans or chest x-ray films taken for other purposes. There is no specific therapy indicated for these fractures, and they almost invariably heal spontaneously. A rare complication of treatment is brachial plexus injury, especially if large daily fractions of radiation have been used.[324-326] Troublesome cellulitis of the breast is also seen on occasion.[327-329] A very serious complication, and one that bears careful scrutiny in the upcoming years, is the appearance of a sarcoma in the radiated breast, especially angiosarcoma.[330-335] Although the absolute incidence among the large numbers of women being treated with breast-conserving therapy is relatively small, it is possible that more of these second malignancies will be seen in upcoming years.

OUTCOME OF THERAPY

Noninvasive Breast Cancer

The outcome of treatment for noninvasive breast cancer was discussed earlier in this chapter. Patients with LCIS are most frequently managed with observation. Their risk of developing invasive breast cancer later on in life approaches 30% over a 15-year time period. Their prognosis is clearly related to whether they develop a subsequent breast cancer and the stage of disease in which the cancer is detected. However, the risk of dying of breast cancer from an initial presentation of LCIS is extremely low. Patients with LCIS can be offered tamoxifen as a risk-reduction strategy.[336] Similarly, patients with DCIS have a relatively low chance of dying of breast cancer, although the rate is not zero. Mastectomy is, by definition, virtually 100% curative of DCIS, although patients still remain at risk for developing and dying of breast cancer because of the risk of developing cancer in the contralateral breast. The results of nonmastectomy treatment of DCIS were presented in Tables 57-8 and 57-9 earlier in this chapter.

Invasive Disease

The nonmastectomy treatment of breast cancer has been studied in multiple institutions. In general, the rate of local failure averages between 5% and 10% over the first 5 to 10 years of follow-up, and increases to approximately 15% by 10 to 15 years. Within the first 5 years, local recurrences tend to appear in the quadrant that was affected by the original tumor, suggesting that these are actual recurrences of the patient's original tumor. After 5 years, recurrences appear more often in other quadrants of the breast, suggesting that these may be new tumors that arose after the patient's treatment. Patients will clearly be at risk for the development of new tumors throughout the remainder of their lives, just as they are at risk for the development of contralateral breast cancer. This underscores the importance of regular follow-up examination and mammograms, since patients who do develop a reappearance of breast cancer in the treated breast can be effectively treated with mastectomy.

The survival of patients with invasive breast cancer is independent of whether they have had their primary disease managed with lumpectomy or mastectomy. Six randomized prospective studies have been performed testing this concept, and all of them have found identical survival rates when these two treatment strategies are compared (Table 57-22). The number of patients studied

Table 57-22   Randomized Trials of Mastectomy versus Breast-Sparing Therapy

Reference	Trial	Patients, n	Tumor Size (Max), cm	Median Follow-Up Yr	10-Yr Overall Survival, %	
					Lumpectomy + XRT	Mastectomy
Fisher et al[366]	NSABP	1217	4	>20	46*	47*
Jacobson et al[367]	NCI	237	5	10	77	75
van Dongen et al[368]	EORTC	8768	5	13	65	66
Blichert-Toft et al[369]	Danish	905	5	6	79†	82†
Arriagada et al[370]	French (Paris)	179	2	14	75	75
Veronesi et al[371]	Italian (Milan)	701	2	20	58*	59*

*20-year data
†6-year data
NSABP, National Surgical Adjuvant Breast and Bowel Project; NCI, National Cancer Institute; EORTC, European Organization for Research and Treatment of Cancer; XRT, radiation therapy.

and the long duration of follow-up have established the equivalence of these two treatments beyond a shadow of a doubt, and no further trials comparing lumpectomy to mastectomy are needed or planned.

Overall survival in breast cancer is highly dependent on the patient's nodal status, the size of the primary tumor, and whether or not systemic therapy has been employed. There is no question that the outcome for patients treated for breast cancer is improving. For example, between 1992 and 1999, there was a yearly decrease of 2.4% in breast cancer death rates.[3] With increasing use of mammography, earlier breast cancer detection, and the use of adjuvant systemic therapy, further reductions in deaths from breast cancer can be anticipated. To illustrate the progress, in 1985 the age-adjusted death rate from breast cancer was 33.0 per 100,000 women and in 1999 the rate was 27.0, a decline of nearly 20%. The 5-year survival rate has increased from 74% in 1975 to 87.1% in 1992-98. A woman diagnosed in 1975 had a 10-year survival rate of 63.8% compared with the same woman diagnosed in 1989 with a 10-year survival rate of 76.3%. The lifetime risk of being diagnosed with breast cancer today is 13.3% and the lifetime risk of dying of the disease is 3.1%. Thus, less than 25% of women diagnosed will die of their disease, which is a far cry from the early 1970s when 50% of women diagnosed would succumb to breast cancer. Although we are making slow but steady progress in improving the outlook for patients with breast cancer, node-positive patients, especially those with multiple lymph nodes, and patients with larger node-negative primary tumors still need further improvement in their recurrence-free and overall survival rates. This underscores the importance of clinical trials in adjuvant local and systemic therapy of breast cancer, and all patients who qualify should be encouraged to enter clinical trials in the treatment of this disease.

REFERENCES

1. Ahmedin J, Murray T, Samuels A, et al: Cancer statistics, 2003. *CA Cancer J Clin.* 2003;53:5.
2. Miller A, Bulbrook R: UICC multidisciplinary project on breast cancer: The epidemiology, actiology and prevention of breast cancer. *Int J Cancer.* 1986;37:173.
3. Ries L, Eisner M, Kosary C, et al., eds. *SEER Cancer Statistic Review, 1973-1999.* Bethesda, Md.: National Cancer Institute; 2002.
4. Hankey BF: Stat bite: Age distribution of breast cancer cases. *J Natl Cancer Inst.* 1994;86:1441.
5. Benichou J, Gail M, Mulvihill J: Graphs to estimate an individualized risk of breast cancer. *J Clin Oncol.* 1996;14:103.
6. Parkin DM, Muir CS, Whelan SL: Cancer incidence in five continents. Comparability and quality of data. *IARC Sci Publ.* 1992;120:45.
7. Deapen D, Liu L, Perkins C, et al: Rapidly rising breast cancer incidence rates among Asian-American women. *Int J Cancer.* 2002;99:747.
8. Ziegler RG, Hooever RN, Pike MC, et al: Migration patterns and breast cancer risk in Asian-American Women. *J Natl Cancer Inst.* 1993;85:1819.
9. Adami HO, Adams G, Boyle P: Breast cancer etiology. Report of a working party for the Nordic Cancer Union. *Int J Cancer.* 1990;5:22.
10. Smith-Warner S, Spiegelman D, Hunter D: Alcohol and breast cancer in women. *JAMA.* 1998;279:523.
11. Hankinson S, Willett W, Speizer F: Alcohol, height, and adiposity in relation to estrogen and prolactin levels in postmenopausal women. *J Natl Cancer Inst.* 1995;87:1297.
12. Clemons M, Goss P: Estrogen and the risk of breast cancer. *N Engl J Med.* 2001;344:276.
13. Kvale G, Heuch I, Eide GE: A prospective study of reproductive factors and breast cancer: I. Parity. *Am J Epidemiol.* 1987;126:831.
14. Kvale G, Heuch I: Menstrual factors and breast cancer risk. *Cancer.* 1988;62:1625.
15. Anderson DE, Badzioch MD: Risk of familial breast cancer. *Cancer.* 1985;56:383.
16. Bain C, Speizer FE, Rosner B, et al: Family history of breast cancer as a risk indicator for the disease. *Am J Epidemiol.* 1980;111:301.
17. Schneider NR, Williams WR, Chaganti RS: Genetic epidemiology of familial aggregation of cancer. *Cancer Res.* 1986;47:1.
18. Ottman R, Pike MC, King MC: Practical guide for estimating risk for familial breast cancer. Lancet;1983;2:556.
19. Martin A-M, Weber B: Genetic and hormonal risk factors in breast cancer. *J Natl Cancer Inst.* 2000;92:1126.
20. Claus E, Risch N, Thompson WD: The calculation of breast cancer risk for women with a first degree family history of ovarian cancer. *Breast Cancer Res Treat.* 1993;28:115.
21. Hrubec Z, Boice JJ, Monson RR, et al: Breast cancer after multiple chest fluoroscopies: Second follow-up of Massachusetts women with tuberculosis. *Cancer Res.* 1989;49:229.
22. Shore RE, Hildreth N, Woodard E, et al: Breast cancer among women given x-ray therapy for acute postpartum mastitis. *J Natl Cancer Inst.* 1989;77:689.
23. Tokunaga M, Land CE, Yamamote T, et al: Incidence of female breast cancer among atomic bomb survivors. *Radiat Res.* 1987;112:243.
24. Wolden S, Hancock S, Hoppe R: Management of breast cancer after Hodgkin's disease. *J Clin Oncol.* 2000;18:765.
25. van Leeuwen F, Klokman W, Aleman B: Long-term risk of second malignancy in survivors of Hodgkin's disease treated during adolescence or young adulthood. *J Clin Oncol.* 2000;18:487.
26. Aisenberg A, Finkelstein D, Willett C: High risk of breast carcinoma after irradiation of young women with Hodgkin's disease. *Cancer.* 1996;79:1203.
27. Tinger A, Wasserman T, Kucik N: The incidence of breast cancer following mantle field radiation therapy as a function of dose and technique. *Int J Radiat Oncol Biol Phys.* 1997;37: 865.
28. Cutuli B, Borel C, Velten M: Breast cancer occurred after treatment for Hodgkin's disease: Analysis of 133 cases. *Radiother Oncol.* 2001;59:247.
29. Bhatia S, Robison L, Meadows A: Breast cancer and other second neoplasms after childhood Hodgkin's disease. *N Engl J Med.* 1996;334:745.
30. Mattson A, Ruden BI, Hall P, et al: Radiation-induced breast cancer: Long-term follow-up of radiation therapy for benign breast disease. *J Natl Cancer Inst.* 1993;85:1679.
31. Boice J, Harvey E, Blettner M, et al: Cancer in the contralateral breast after radiotherapy for breast cancer. *N Engl J Med.* 1992; 326:781.
32. Boice J, Preston D, David F, et al: Frequent chest x-ray fluoroscopy and breast cancer incidence among tuberculosis patients in Massachusetts. *Radiat Res.* 1991;125:214.
33. Hall JM, Lee MK, Newman B, et al: Linkage of early-onset familial breast cancer to chromosome 17q21. *Science.* 1990;250:1684.
34. Miki Y, Swensen J, Shattuck-Eidens D: Isolation of BRCA1, the 17q-linked breast and ovarian cancer susceptibility gene. *Science.* 1993;266:66.
35. Burke W, Press N, Pinsky L: BRCA1 and BRCA2: A small part of the puzzle. *J Natl Cancer Inst.* 1999;91:904.
36. Nicoletto MO, Donach M, De Nicolo A: BRCA-1 and BRCA-2 mutations as prognostic factors in clinical practice and genetic counselling. *Cancer Treat Rev.* 2001;27:295.
37. Reynolds T: BRCA1: Lessons learned from the breast cancer gene. *J Natl Cancer Inst.* 2001;93:1200.
38. Carter RF: BRCA1, BRCA2 and breast cancer: A concise clinical review. *Clin Invest Med.* 2001;24:147.
39. Haber D: Roads leading to breast cancer. *N Engl J Med.* 2000; 343:1566.
40. King M-C, Wieand S, Fisher B: Tamoxifen and breast cancer incidence among women with inherited mutations in BRCA1 and BRCA2. *JAMA.* 2001;286:2251.

41. Meijers-Heijboer H, van Geel B, Klijn J: Breast cancer after prophylactic bilateral mastectomy in women with a BRCA1 or BRCA2 mutation. *N Engl J Med.* 2001;3:159.

42. Danforth D, Findlay P, McDonald H, et al: Complete axillary lymph node dissection for stage II-III carcinoma of the breast. *J Clin Oncol.* 1986;4:655.

43. Boova R, Bonnani R, Rosato F: Patterns of axillary nodal involvement in breast cancer: Predictability of level one dissection. *Ann Surg.* 1982;96:642.

44. Rosen P, Lesser M, Kinne D, et al: Discontinuous "skip" metastases in breast carcinoma: Analysis of 1228 axillary dissection. *Ann Surg.* 1983;97:276.

45. Veronesi U, Rilke F, Luini A, et al: Distribution of axillary node metastases by level of invasion: An analysis of 539 cases. *Cancer.* 1987;59:682.

46. Margolese R, Poisson R, Shibata H, et al: The technique of segmental mastectomy (lumpectomy) and axillary dissection: A syllabus from the National Surgical Adjuvant Breast Project workshops. *Surgery.* 1987;102:828.

47. Stibbe E: The internal mammary lymphatic glands. *J Anat.* 1981;52:258.

48. Turner-Warwick R: The lymphatics of the breast. *Br J Surg.* 1957;46:574.

49. Meyer J, Munzenrider J: Computed tomographic demonstration of internal mammary lymph node metastasis in patients with locally recurrent breast carcinoma. *Radiology.* 1981;139:661.

50. Wahl RL, Cody RL, Hutchins GD, et al: Primary and metastatic breast carcinoma: Initial clinical evaluation with PET with the radiolabeled glucose analogue 2-[f-18]-fluoro-2-deoxy-D-glucose 1. *Radiology.* 1991;179:765.

51. Wahl RL, Zasadny K, Helvie M, et al: Metabolic monitoring of breast cancer chemohormone therapy using positron emission tomography: Initial evaluation. *J Clin Oncol.* 1993;11:2101.

52. Bombardieri E, Crippa F: PET imaging in breast cancer. *Q J Nucl Med.* 2001;45:245.

53. Betsill WLJ, Rosen PP, Lieberman PH, et al: Intraductal carcinoma. Long-term follow-up after treatment by biopsy alone. *JAMA.* 1978;239:1863.

54. Eusebi V, Feudale E, Fosehini MP, et al: Long-term follow-up of in situ carcinoma of the breast. *Semin Diagn Pathol.* 1994;11:223.

55. Page D, Dupont W, Rogers l, et al: Intraductal carcinoma of the breast: Follow-up after biopsy only. *Cancer.* 1982;49:751.

56. Page DL, Dupont WD, Rogers LW, et al: Continued local recurrence of carcinoma 15-25 years after a diagnosis of low grade ductal carcinoma in situ of the breast treated only by biopsy. *Cancer.* 1995;76:1197.

57. O'Connell P, Pekkel V, Fuqua SA: Analysis of loss of heterozygosity in 399 premalignant breast lesions at 15 genetic loci. *J Natl Cancer Inst.* 1998;90:697.

58. Zhuang Z, Merino MJ, Chuaqui R: Identical allelic loss on chromosome 11q13 in microdissected in situ and invasive human breast cancer. *Cancer Res.* 1995;55:467.

59. Frykberg ER, Bland KI: Overview of the biology and management of ductal carcinoma in situ of the breast. *Cancer.* 1994;74:350.

60. Schnitt S, Silen W, Sadowsky N, et al: Ductal carcinoma in situ (intraductal carcinoma) of the breast. *N Engl J Med.* 1988;318:898.

61. Rosai J: Borderline epithelial lesions of the breast. *Am J Surg Pathol.* 1991;15:209.

62. The Consensus Conference Committee: Consensus Conference on the classification of ductal carcinoma in situ. *Cancer.* 1997;80:1798.

63. Rosen PP: Lobular carcinoma in situ and atypical lobular hyperplasia. In Rosen PP, ed. *Breast Pathology.* Philadelphia: Lippincott Williams & Wilkins; 2001:581.

64. Rosen P, Oberman H: *Tumors of the Mammary Gland.* Washington D.C.: Armed Forces Institute of Pathology; 1993:120.

65. Rosen P: Lobular carcinoma in situ: Recent clinicopathologic studies at Memorial Hospital. *Pathol Res Pract.* 1980;166:430.

66. Hutter R: The management of patients with lobular carcinoma in situ of the breast. *Cancer.* 1984;53:798.

67. Frykberg E, Santiago F, Betsill W, et al: Lobular carcinoma in situ of the breast. *Surg Gynecol Obstet.* 1987;164:285.

68. Schnitt SJ, Guidi AJ: The pathology of invasive breast carcinoma. In JR Harris, et al, eds. *Diseases of the Breast.* Philadelphia: Lippincott Williams & Wilkins; 2000:426.

69. Simkovich AH, Selafani LM, Masri M, et al: Role of contralateral breast biopsy in infiltrating lobular cancer. *Surgery.* 1993;114:555.

70. Broet P, de la Rochefordiere A, Scholl SM, et al: Contralateral breast cancer: Annual incidence and risk parameters. *J Clin Oncol.* 1995;13:1578.

71. Gallager H: Pathologic types of breast cancer: Their prognoses. *Cancer.* 1984;53:623.

72. Diab SG, Clark GM, Osborne CK, et al: Tumor characteristics and clinical outcome of tubular and mucinous breast carcinomas. *J Clin Oncol.* 1999;17:1442.

73. Page DL, Simpson JF: Pathology of preinvasive and excellent-prognosis breast cancer. *Curr Opin Oncol.* 2000;12:526.

74. Campana F, Fourquet A, Ashby MA, et al: Presentation of axillary lymphadenopathy without detectable breast primary (TO N1b breast cancer): Experience at Institut Curie. *Radiother Oncol.* 1989;15:321.

75. Baron PL, Moore MP, Kinne DW, et al: Occult breast cancer presenting with axillary metastases. Updated management. *Arch Surg.* 1990;125:210.

76. Forudi F, Tiver K: Occult breast carcinoma presenting as axillary metastases. *Int J Radiat Oncol Biol Phys.* 2000;47:143.

77. Merson M, Andreola S, Galimberti V, et al: Breast carcinoma presenting as axillary metastases without evidence of a primary tumor. *Cancer.* 1992;70:504.

78. Lichter AS, Lippman ME: Special situations in the treatment of breast cancer. In Lippman M, Lichter A, Danforth D, eds. *Diagnosis and Management of Breast Cancer.* Philadelphia: WB Saunders; 1988:407.

79. Pierce LJ, Haffty BG, Solin LJ, et al: The conservative management of Paget's disease of the breast with radiotherapy. *Cancer.* 1997;80:1065.

80. Waldman S, Toonkel LM, Davila E: Inflammatory Breast Cancer. In Ariel IM, ed. *High-Risk Breast Cancer.* Berlin: Springer-Verlag; 1991:319.

81. Cody HS, Urban JA: Internal mammary node status: A major prognosticator in axillary node-negative breast cancer. *Ann Surg Oncol.* 1995;2:32.

82. Veronesi U, Cascinelli N, Bufalino R: Risk of internal mammary lymph node metastases and its relevance on prognosis of breast cancer patients. *Ann Surg.* 1983;198:681.

83. Veronesi U, Cascinelli N, Greco M: Prognosis of breast cancer patients after mastectomy and dissection of internal mammary nodes. *Ann Surg.* 1985;202:702.

84. Lacour J, Le M, Caceres E, et al: Radical mastectomy versus radical mastectomy plus internal mammary dissection: Ten year results of an international cooperative trial in breast cancer. *Cancer.* 1983; 51:1941.

85. Veronesi U, Marubini E, Mariani L: The dissection of internal mammary nodes does not improve the survival of breast cancer patients. 30-year results of a randomised trial. *Eur J Cancer.* 1999; 35:1320.

86. Byrd DR, Dunnwald LK, Mankoff DA, et al: Internal mammary lymph node drainage patterns in patients with breast cancer documented by breast lymphoscintigraphy. *Ann Surg Oncol.* 2001;8:234.

87. Fisher B, Bauer M, Wickerham L, et al: Relation of number of positive axillary nodes to the prognosis of patients with primary breast cancer: An NSABP update. *Cancer.* 1983;52:1551.

88. Fisher B, Wolmark N, Bauer M, et al: The accuracy of clinical nodal staging and of limited axillary dissection as a determinant of histologic nodal status in carcinoma of the breast. *Surg Gynecol Obstet.* 1981;152:765.

89. Silverstein MJ, Gierson ED, Waisman JR, et al: Predicting axillary node positivity in patients with invasive carcinoma of the breast by using a combination of T category and palpability. *J Am Coll Surg.* 1995;180:700.

90. Reynolds C, Mick R, Donohue J: Sentinel lymph node biopsy with metastasis: can axillary dissection be avoided in some patients with breast cancer? *J Clin Oncol.* 1999;17:1720.

91. Guiliano A, Jones R, Brennan M, et al: Sentinel lymphadenectomy in breast cancer. *J Clin Oncol.* 1997;15:2345.

92. McMasters K, Guiliano A, Ross M, et al: Sentinel-lymph-node biopsy for breast cancer—Not yet the standard care. *N Engl J Med.* 1998;339:990.

93. Krag D, Weaver D, Asikaga T, et al: The sentinel node in breast cancer: A multicenter validation study. *N Engl J Med.* 1998; 339:941.

94. Crowe J, Gordon N, Antunez A, et al: Local-regional breast cancer recurrence following mastectomy. *Arch Surg.* 1991;126:429.

95. Hayes D: Evaluation after primary therapy. In J Harris, et al, eds. *Diseases of the Breast.* Philadelphia: Lippincott Williams & Wilkins; 2000:709.

96. Hagemeister J, Buzdar A, Luna M, et al: Causes of death in breast cancer: A clinicopathologic study. *Cancer.* 1980;46:162.

97. Smith TJ, Davidson NE, Schapira DV, et al: American Society of Clinical Oncology 1998 update of recommended breast cancer surveillance guidelines. *J Clin Oncol.* 1999;17:1080.

98. Hellman S, Harris JR: Natural history of breast cancer. In J Harris, et al, eds. *Diseases of the Breast.* Philadelphia: Lippincott Williams & Wilkins; 2000:407.

99. Joensuu H, Toikkanen S: Cured of breast cancer? *J Clin Oncol.* 1995;13:62.

100. Healey EA, Osteen RT, Schnitt SJ, et al: Can the clinical and mammographic findings at presentation predict the presence of an extensive intraductal component in early stage breast cancer? *Int J Radiat Oncol Biol Phys.* 1989;17:1217.

101. Kurtz JM, Jacquemier J, Amalric R, et al: Breast conserving therapy for macroscopically multiple cancers. *Ann Surg.* 1991;212:38.

102. Leopold K, Recht A, Schnitt S, et al: Results of conservative surgery and radiation therapy for multiple synchronous cancers of one breast. *Int J Radiat Oncol Biol Phys.* 1989;16:11.

103. Hartsell WF, Recine DC, Griem KL, et al: Should multicentric disease be an absolute contraindication to the use of breast-conserving therapy? *Int J Radiat Oncol Biol Phys.* 1994;30:49.

104. Cho LC, Senzer N, Peters GN: Conservative surgery and radiation therapy for macroscopically multiple ipsilateral invasive breast cancers. *Am J Surg.* 2002;183:650.

105. Solin LJ, Fowble BL, Troupin RH, et al: Biopsy results of new calcifications in the postirradiated breast. *Cancer.* 1989;63:1956.

106. Dershaw D, McCormick B, Osborne M: Detection of local recurrence after conservative therapy for breast carcinoma. *Cancer.* 1992;70:493.

107. Pressman PI: Treatment of bilateral breast cancer. In Roses DF, ed. *Breast Cancer.* Philadelphia: Churchill Livingstone; 1999.

108. Rosen PP, Groshen S, Kinne DW, et al: Contralateral breast carcinoma: An assessment of risk and prognosis in stage I (T1N0M0) and stage II (T1N1M0) patients with 20-year follow-up. *Surgery.* 1989;106:904.

109. Rutqvist LE, Cedermark B, Glas U, et al: Contralateral primary tumors in breast cancer patients in a randomized trial of adjuvant tamoxifen therapy. *J Natl Cancer Inst.* 1991;83:1299.

110. Horn PL, Thompson WD: Risk of contralateral breast cancer. Associations with histologic, clinical and therapeutic factors. *Cancer.* 1988;62:412.

111. Storm HH, Jensen OM: Risk of contralateral breast cancer in Denmark 1943-80. *Br J Cancer.* 1986;54:483.

112. Yeh KA, Fortunato L, Ridge JA, et al: Routine bone scanning in patients with T1 and T2 breast cancer: A waste of money. *Ann Surg Oncol.* 1995;2:319.

113. Coleman R, Rubens R, Fogelman I: Reappraisal of the baseline bone scan in breast cancer. *J Nucl Med.* 1988;29:1045.

114. Wahl RL: Current status of PET in breast cancer imaging, staging and therapy. *Semin Roentgenol.* 2001;36:250.

115. American Joint Committee on Cancer: *AJCC Cancer Staging Handbook.* 6th ed. New York: Springer-Verlag; 2002:255.

116. Singletary SE AC, Ashley P, et al: Revision of the American Joint Committee on Cancer staging system for breast cancer. *J Clin Oncol.* 2002;20:3628.

117. Seidman JD, Schnaper LA, Aisner SC: Relationship of the size of the invasive component of the primary breast carcinoma to axillary lymph node metastasis. *Cancer.* 1995;75:65.

118. Andea AA, Wallis T, Newman LA, et al: Pathologic analysis of tumor size and lymph node status in multifocal/multicentric breast carcinoma. *Cancer.* 2002;94:1383.

119. Wolmark N, Fisher B: Surgery in the primary treatment of breast cancer. *Breast Cancer Res Treat.* 1982;1:339.

120. Iyer R, Hanlon A, Fowble B, et al: Accuracy of the extent of axillary nodal positivity related to primary tumor size, number of involved nodes, and number of nodes examined. *Int J Radiat Oncol Biol Phys.* 2000;47:1177.

121. Osborne MP, Hoda SA: Current management of lobular carcinoma in situ of the breast. *Oncology (Huntingt).* 1994;8:45.

122. Fisher ER, Costantino J, Fisher B, et al: Pathologic findings from the National Surgical Adjuvant Breast Project (NSABP) Protocol B-17. Five-year observations concerning lobular carcinoma in situ. *Cancer.* 1996;78:1403.

123. Carson W, Sanchez-Forgach E, Stomper P, et al: Lobular carcinoma in situ: Observation without surgery as an appropriate therapy. *Ann Surg Oncol.* 1994;1:142.

124. Fowble B: Intraductal noninvasive breast cancer: A comparison of three local treatments. *Oncology.* 1989;3:51.

125. Boyages J, Delaney G, Taylor R: Predictors of local recurrence after treatment of ductal carcinoma in situ: a meta-analysis. *Cancer.* 1999;85:616.

126. Schwartz GF: The current treatment of ductal carcinoma in situ. *Breast J.* 2001;7:308.

127. Silverstein M, Lagios M, Groshen S, et al: The influence of margin width on local control of ductal carcinoma in situ of the breast. *N Engl J Med.* 1999;340:1455.

128. Solin LJ, Fourquet A, Vicini FA, et al: Mammographically detected ductal carcinoma in situ of the breast treated with breast-conserving surgery and definitive breast radiation: long term outcomes and prognostic significance of patient age and margin status. *Int J Radiat Oncol Biol Phys.* 2001;50:991.

129. Fisher B, Dignam J, Wolmark N, et al: Lumpectomy and radiation therapy for the treatment of intraductal breast cancer findings from National Surgical Adjuvant Breast and Bowel Project B-17. *J Clin Oncol.* 1998;16:441.

130. Julien JP, Bijker N, Fentiman IS, et al: Radiotherapy in breast-conserving treatment for ductal carcinoma in situ: First results of the EORTC randomised phase III trial 10853. EORTC Breast Cancer Cooperative Group and EORTC Radiotherapy Group. *Lancet.* 2000;355:528.

131. George W, Houghton J, Cuzick J, et al: Radiotherapy and tamoxifen following complete local excision (CLE) in the management of ductal carcinoma in situ (DCIS): Preliminary results from the UK DCIS Trial. *Proc ASCO.* 2000;19:70a [abstract].

132. Bijker N, Peterse JL, Duchateau L, et al: Risk factors for recurrence and metastasis after breast-conserving therapy for ductal carcinoma-in-situ: Analysis of European Organization for Research and Treatment of Cancer Trial 10853. *J Clin Oncol.* 2001;19:2263.

133. Fisher ER, Dignam J, Tan-Chiu E, et al: Pathologic findings from the National Surgical Adjuvant Breast Project (NSAB) eight-year update of Protocol B-17: Intraductal carcinoma. *Cancer.* 1999;86:429.

134. Fisher B, Dignam J, Wolmark N, et al: Tamoxifen in treatment of intraductal breast cancer: National Surgical Adjuvant Breast and Bowel Project B-24 randomised controlled trial. *Lancet.* 1999;353:1993.

135. Kurtz J, Jacquemier J, Torhurst J, et al: Conservation therapy for breast cancers other than infiltrating ductal carcinoma. *Cancer.* 1989;63:1630.

136. Weiss M, Fowble B, Solin L, et al: Outcome of conservative therapy for invasive breast cancer by histologic subtype. *Int J Radiat Oncol Biol Phys.* 1992;23:941.

137. Schnitt SJ, Connolly JL, Harris JR, et al: Pathologic predictors of early local recurrence in state I and II breast cancer treated by primary radiation therapy. *Cancer.* 1984;53:1049.

138. Boyages J, Recht A, Connolly J, et al: Early breast cancer: Predictors of breast recurrence for patients treated with conservative surgery and radiation therapy. *Radiother Oncol.* 1990;19:29.

139. Holland R, Connolly JL, Gelman R, et al: The presence of an extensive intraductal component following a limited excision correlates with prominent residual disease in the remainder of the breast. *J Clin Oncol.* 1990;8:113.

140. Vicini FA, Eberlein TJ, Connolly JL, et al: The optimal extent of resection for patients with stages I or II breast cancer treated with conservative surgery and radiotherapy. *Ann Surg.* 1991;214:200.

141. Schnitt SJ, Abner A, Gelman R, et al: The relationship between microscopic margins of resection and the risk of local recurrence in patients with breast cancer treated with breast-conserving surgery and radiation therapy. *Cancer.* 1994;74:1746.

142. Borger J, Kemperman H, Hart A, et al: Risk factors in breast-conservation therapy. *J Clin Oncol.* 1994;12:653.

143. Delouche G, Bachelot F, Premont M, et al: Conservation treatment of early breast cancer: Long-term results and complications. *Int J Radiat Oncol Biol Phys.* 1987;13:29.

144. van Limbergen E, van den Bogaert W, van der Schueren E, et al: Tumor excision and radiotherapy as primary treatment of breast cancer. Analysis of patient and treatment parameters and local control. *Radiother Oncol.* 1987;8:1.

145. Calle R, Vilcoq JR, Zafrani B, et al: Local control and survival of breast cancer treated by limited surgery followed by irradiation. *Int J Radiat Oncol Biol Phys.* 1986;12:873.

146. McCormick B: Selection criteria for breast conservation. *Cancer.* 1994;74:430.

147. Nixon AJ, Neuberg D, Hayes DF, et al: Relationship of patient age to pathologic features of the tumor and prognosis for patients with stage I or II breast cancer. *J Clin Oncol.* 1994;12:888.

148. Jacquemier J, Kurtz JM, Amalric R, et al: An assessment of extensive intraductal component as a risk factor for local recurrence after breast-conserving therapy. *Br J Cancer.* 1990;61:873.

149. Wazer DE, Schmidt-Ullrich RK, Ruthazer R: The influence of age and extensive intraductal component histology upon breast lumpectomy margin assessment as a predictor of residual tumor. *Int J Radiat Oncol Biol Phys.* 1999;45:885.

150. Matthews RH, McNeese MD, Montague ED, et al: Prognostic implication of age in breast cancer patients treated with tumorectomy and irradiation or with mastectomy. *Int J Radiat Oncol Biol Phys.* 1988;14:659.

151. de la Rochefordiere A, Asselain B, Campana F, et al: Age as a prognostic factor in premenopausal breast carcinoma. *Lancet.* 1993;341:1039.

152. Fisher B, Wickerham DL, Deutsch M, et al: Breast tumor recurrence following lumpectomy with and without breast irradiation: An overview of recent NSABP findings. *Semin Surg Oncol.* 1992;8:153.

153. Buchholz T, Tucker S, Erwin J, et al: Impact of systemic treatment on local control for patients with lymph node-negative breast cancer treated with breast-conservation therapy. *J Clin Oncol.* 2001;19:2240.

154. Gray JR, McCormick B, Cox L, et al: Primary breast irradiation in large-breasted or heavy women: Analysis of cosmetic outcome. *Int J Radiat Oncol Biol Phys.* 1991;21:347.

155. Cross M, Elson H, Aron B: Breast conservation radiation therapy technique for women with large breasts. *Int J Radiat Oncol Biol Phys.* 1989;17:199.

156. Bentel GC, Marks LB, Whiddon CS: Acute and late morbidity of using a breast positioning ring in women with large/pendulous breasts. *Radiother Oncol.* 1999;50:277.

157. Merchant TE, McCormick B: Prone position breast irradiation. *Int J Radiat Oncol Biol Phys.* 1994;30:197.

158. Zierhut D, Flentje M, Frank C, et al: Conservative treatment of breast cancer: Modified irradiation technique for women with large breasts. *Radiother Oncol.* 1994;31:256.

159. Grann A, McCormick B, Chabner ES, et al: Prone breast radiotherapy in early-stage breast cancer: A preliminary analysis. *Int J Radiat Oncol Biol Phys.* 2000;47:319.

160. Lazovich DA, White E, Thomas DB, et al: Underutilization of breast-conserving surgery and radiation therapy among women with stage I or II breast cancer. *JAMA.* 1991;266:3433.

161. Albain KS, Green SR, Lichter AS, et al: Influence of patient characteristics, socioeconomic factors, geography, and systemic risk on the use of breast-sparing treatment in women enrolled in adjuvant breast cancer studies: an analysis of two intergroup trials. *J Clin Oncol.* 1996;14:3009.

162. Hartsell WF, Recine DC, Griem KL, et al: Delaying the initiation of intact breast irradiation for patients with lymph node positive breast cancer increases the risk of local recurrence. *Cancer.* 1995;76:2497.

163. McCormick B, Norton L, Yao T, et al: The impact of the sequence of radiation and chemotherapy on local control after breast-conserving surgery. *Cancer J.* 1996;2:39.

164. Leonard C, Wood M, Zhen B, et al: Does administration of chemotherapy before radiotherapy in breast cancer patients treated with conservative surgery negatively impact local control? *J Clin Oncol.* 1995;13:2906.

165. Froud P, Mates D, Jackson J, et al: Effect of time interval between breast-conserving surgery and radiation therapy on ipsilateral breast recurrence. *Int J Radiat Oncol Biol Phys.* 2000;46:363.

166. Recht A, Come S, Henderson C, et al: The sequencing of chemotherapy and radiation therapy after conservative surgery for early-stage breast cancer. *N Engl J Med.* 1996;334:1356.

167. Metz J, Schultz D, Fox K, et al: Analysis of outcomes for high-risk breast cancer based on interval from surgery to postmastectomy radiation therapy. *Cancer.* 2000;6:324.

168. Touboul E, Lefranc JP, Blondon J, et al: Primary chemotherapy and preoperative irradiation for patients with stage II larger than 3 cm or locally advanced non-inflammatory breast cancer. *Radiother Oncol.* 1997;42:219.

169. von Minckwitz G, Costa S, Eirmann W, et al: Maximized reduction of primary breast tumor size using preoperative chemotherapy with doxorubicin and docetaxel. *J Clin Oncol.* 1999;17:1999.

170. Fisher B, Brown A, Mamounas E, et al: Effect of preoperative chemotherapy on local-regional disease in women with operable breast cancer: Findings from national surgical adjuvant breast and bowel project B-18. *J Clin Oncol.* 1997;15:2483.

171. Fisher B, Bryant J, Wolmark N, et al: Effect of preoperative chemotherapy on the outcome of women with operable breast cancer. *J Clin Oncol.* 1998;16:2672.

172. Eberlein T, Connolly J, Schnitt S, et al: Predictors of local recurrence following conservative breast surgery and radiation therapy: The influence of tumor size. *Arch Surg.* 1990;125:771.

173. Cowen D, Houvenaeghel G, Baqrdou V, et al: Local and distant failures after limited surgery with positive margins and radiotherapy for node-negative breast cancer. *Int J Radiat Oncol Biol Phys.* 2000;47:305.

174. Freedman G, Fowble B, Hanlon A, et al: Patients with early stage invasive cancer with close or positive margins treated with conservative surgery and radiation have an increased risk of breast recurrence that is delayed by adjuvant systemic therapy. *Int J Radiat Oncol Biol Phys.* 1999;44:1005.

175. Park CC, Mitsumori M, Nixon A, et al: Outcome at 8 years after breast-conserving surgery and radiation therapy for invasive breast cancer: Influence of margin status and systemic therapy on local recurrence. *J Clin Oncol.* 2000;18:1668.

176. Smitt MC, Nowels KW, Zdeblick MJ: The importance of the lumpectomy surgical margin status in long-term results of breast conservation. *Cancer.* 1995;76:259.

177. Wazer DE, Jabro G, Ruthazer R, et al: Extent of margin positivity as a predictor for local recurrence after breast conserving irradiation. *Radiat Oncol Investig.* 1999;7:111.

178. Assersohn L, Powles TJ, Ashley S, et al: Local relapse in primary breast cancer patients with unexcised positive surgical margins after lumpectomy, radiotherapy and chemoendocrine therapy. *Ann Oncol.* 1999;10:1451.

179. Wazer DE, Schmidt-Ullrich RK, Ruthazer R: Factors determining outcome for breast-conserving irradiation with margin-directed dose escalation to the tumor bed. *Int J Radiat Oncol Biol Phys.* 1998;40:851.

180. Beahrs OH, Myers MH: Breast cancer. In *Manual for Staging of Cancer.* Philadelphia: JB Lippincott; 1983:127.

181. Beahrs OH, Henson DE, Hutter RVP, et al: Breast cancer. In *Manual for Staging of Cancer.* Philadelphia: JB Lippincott; 1988:145.

182. Ellis D, Teitelbaum S: Inflammatory carcinoma of the breast: A pathologic definition. *Cancer.* 1974;33:1045.

183. Lucas F, Perez-Mesa C: Inflammatory carcinoma of the breast. *Cancer.* 1978;41:1595.

184. Saltzstein S: Clinically occult inflammatory carcinoma of the breast. *Cancer.* 1974;34:382.

185. Nemoto T, Vana J, Bedwani R, et al: Management and survival of female breast cancer: Results of a national survey by the American College of Surgeons. *Cancer.* 1980;45:2917.

186. Haybittle J: Results of treatment of female breast cancer in the Cambridge area 1960-71. *Br J Cancer.* 1979;40:56.

187. Fracchia A, Evans J, Eisenberg B: Stage III carcinoma of the breast: A detailed analysis. *Ann Surg.* 1980;192:705.

188. Arnold DJ, Lesnick GJ: Survival following mastectomy for stage III breast cancer. *Am J Surg.* 1979;137:362.

189. Schottenfeld D, Nash A, Robbins G, et al: Ten-year results of the treatment of primary operable breast carcinoma: A summary of 304 patients evaluated by the TNM System. *Cancer.* 1976; 38:1001.

190. Helinto M, Blomqvist C, Heikkila P, et al: Post-mastectomy radiotherapy in pT3N0M0 breast cancer: is it needed? *Radiother Oncol.* 1999;52:213.

191. Ragaz J, Spinelli J: Large breast cancer tumors and radiotherapy: Biology vs. chronology. *Radiother Oncol.* 1999;52:203.

192. Davila E, Toonkel LM: Locally advanced breast cancer. In Ariel IM, ed. *High-Risk Breast Cancer: Therapy*. Berlin: Springer-Verlag; 1991:357.

193. Spanos WJJ, Montague ED, Fletcher GH: Late complications of radiation only for advanced breast cancer. *Int J Radiat Oncol Biol Phys*. 1980;6:1473.

194. Recht A, Come S, Henderson C, et al: Locally advanced breast cancer and postmastectomy radiotherapy. *Surg Oncol Clin N Am*. 2000;9:603.

195. Strom EA, McNeese MD, Fletcher GH, et al: Results of mastectomy and postoperative irradiation in the management of locoregionally advanced carcinoma of the breast. *Int J Radiat Oncol Biol Phys*. 1991;21:319.

196. Graham MV, Perez CA, Kuske RR, et al: Locally advanced (noninflammatory) carcinoma of the breast: Results and comparison of various treatment modalities. *Int J Radiat Oncol Biol Phys*. 1991;21:311.

197. Zucali R, Uslenghi C, Kenda R, et al: Natural history and survival of inoperable breast cancer treated with radiotherapy and radiotherapy followed by radical mastectomy. *Cancer*. 1976;37:1422.

198. Pierce LJ, Lichter AS, Archer P: Indications, integration, and technical aspects of local-regional irradiation in the management of advanced breast cancer. *Semin Radiat Oncol*. 1994;4:242.

199. Ueno NT, Buzdar AU, Singletary SE, et al: Combined-modality treatment of inflammatory breast carcinoma: Twenty years of experience at M.D. Anderson Cancer Center. *Cancer Chemother Pharmacol*. 1997;40:321.

200. Armstrong DK, Fetting JH, Davidson NE: Sixteen week dose intense chemotherapy for inoperable, locally advanced breast cancer. *Breast Cancer Res Treat*. 1993;28:277.

201. Perez CA, Graham ML, Taylor ME, et al: Management of locally advanced carcinoma of the breast: Part I. Non-inflammatory. *Cancer*. 1994;74:453.

202. Duggan D: Local therapy of locally advanced breast cancer. *Oncology*. 1991;5:67.

203. Perloff M, Lesnick GJ, Korzun A, et al: Combination chemotherapy with mastectomy or radiotherapy for stage III breast carcinoma: A cancer and leukemia group B study. *J Clin Oncol*. 1988;6:261.

204. Merajver SD, Weber BL, Cody R, et al: Breast conservation and prolonged chemotherapy for locally advanced breast cancer: the University of Michigan experience. *J Clin Oncol*. 1997;15:2873.

205. Eltahir A, Heys SD, Hutcheon AW: Treatment of large and locally advanced breast cancers using neoadjuvant chemotherapy. *Am J Surg*. 1998;175:127.

206. Swain S, Lippman M: Locally advanced breast cancer: The National Cancer Institute experience. In Ariel IM, ed. *High-Risk Breast Cancer: Therapy*. Berlin: Springer-Verlag; 1991:416.

207. Touboul E, Buffat L, Lefranc JP, et al: Possibility of conservative local treatment after combined chemotherapy and preoperative irradiation for locally advanced noninflammatory breast cancer. *Int J Radiat Oncol Biol Phys*. 1996;34:1175.

208. Schwartz GF, Birchansky CA, Komarnicky LT, et al: Induction chemotherapy followed by breast conservation for locally advanced carcinoma of the breast. *Cancer*. 1994;73:362.

209. Pierce L, Lippman M, Ben-Baruch N, et al: The effect of systemic therapy on local-regional control in locally advanced breast cancer. *Int J Radiat Oncol Biol Phys*. 1992;23:949.

210. Strom EA, Dhingra K: Sequential therapy in the treatment of locally advanced noninflammatory breast cancer. *Semin Radiat Oncol*. 1994;4:217.

211. Kuske RR: Diagnosis and management of inflammatory breast cancer. *Semin Radiat Oncol*. 1994;4:270.

212. Fleming RY, Asmar L, Buzdar AU, et al: Effectiveness of mastectomy by response to induction chemotherapy for control in inflammatory breast carcinoma. *Ann Surg Oncol*. 1997;4:452.

213. Liao Z, Strom EA, Buzdar AU: Locoregional irradiation for inflammatory breast cancer: Effectiveness of dose escalation in decreasing recurrence. *Int J Radiat Oncol Biol Phys*. 2000;47:1191.

214. Perez CA, Fields JN, Fracasso PM, et al: Management of locally advanced carcinoma of the breast. Part II. Inflammatory carcinoma. *Cancer*. 1994;74:466.

215. Singletary SE, Ames FC, Buzdar AU: Management of inflammatory breast cancer. *World J Surg*. 1994;18:87.

216. Early Breast Cancer Trialists' Collaborative Group: Tamoxifen for early breast cancer: An overview of the randomised trials. *Lancet*. 1998;351:1451.

217. Early Breast Cancer Trialists' Collaborative Group: Polychemotherapy for early breast cancer: An overview of the randomised trials. *Lancet*. 1998;352:930.

218. National Institutes of Health: *Adjuvant Therapy for Breast Cancer. NIH Consensus Statement*. Bethesda, Md.: NIH; 2000:17:1.

219. Hermann RE, Esselstyn CBJ, Grundfest-Broniatowski S, et al: Partial mastectomy without radiation is adequate treatment for patients with stages 0 and I carcinoma of the breast. *Surg Gynecol Obstet*. 1993;177:247.

220. Fisher B, Anderson S, Fisher E, et al: Significance of ipsilateral breast tumor recurrence after lumpectomy. *Lancet*. 1991; 338:327.

221. Veronesi U, Marubini E, De Vecchio M, et al: Local recurrences and distant metastases after conservative breast cancer treatments: Partly independent events. *J Natl Cancer Inst*. 1995;87:19.

222. Lippman ME: How should we manage breast cancer in the breast, or Buddy, can you paradigm? *J Natl Cancer Inst*. 1995;87:3.

223. Fisher B, Bryant J, Dignam D, et al: Tamoxifen, radiation therapy, or both for prevention of ipsilateral breast tumor recurrence after lumpectomy in women with invasive breast cancers of one centimeter or less. *J Clin Oncol*. 2002;20:4141.

224. Cole M: The place of radiotherapy in the management of early breast cancer. *Br J Cancer*. 1964;51:216.

225. Overgaard M: Overview of randomized trials in high risk breast cancer patients treated with adjuvant systemic therapy with or without postmastectomy irradiation. *Semin Radiat Oncol*. 1999;9:292.

226. Arriagada R, Rutqvist LE, Le MG: Postmastectomy radiotherapy: Randomized trials. *Semin Radiat Oncol*. 1999;9:275.

227. Pierce LJ, Lichter AS: Defining the role of post-mastectomy radiotherapy: The new evidence. *Oncology*. 1996;10:991.

228. Marks LB, Hardenbergh P, Prosnitz LR: Mounting evidence for postmastectomy locoregional radiation therapy. *Oncology*. 1999;13:1123.

229. van de Steene J, Soete G, Storme G: Adjuvant radiotherapy for breast cancer significantly improves overall survival: The missing link. *Radiother Oncol*. 2000;55:263.

230. Whelan TJ, Julian J, Wright J, et al: Does locoregional radiation therapy improve survival in breast cancer? A meta-analysis. *J Clin Oncol*. 2000;18:1220.

231. Early Breast Cancer Trialists' Collaborative Group: Favourable and unfavourable effects on long-term survival of radiotherapy for early breast cancer: An overview of the randomised trials. *Lancet*. 2000;355:1757.

232. Overgaard M, Jensen MB, Overgaard J, et al: Postoperative radiotherapy in high-risk postmenopausal breast-cancer patients given adjuvant tamoxifen: Danish Breast Cancer Cooperative Group DBCG 82c randomised trial. *Lancet*. 1999;353:1641.

233. Overgaard M, Hansen PS, Overgaard J, et al: Postoperative radiotherapy in high-risk premenopausal women with breast cancer who receive adjuvant chemotherapy. Danish Breast Cancer Cooperative Group 82b Trial. *N Engl J Med*. 1997;337:949.

234. Ragaz J, Jackson SM, Le N, et al: Adjuvant radiotherapy and chemotherapy in node-positive premenopausal women with breast cancer. *N Engl J Med*. 1997;337:956.

235. Recht A, Edge SB, Solin LJ, et al: Postmastectomy radiotherapy: Clinical practice guidelines of the American Society of Clinical Oncology. *J Clin Oncol*. 2001;19:1539.

236. Kagan AR: Radiation therapy in the management of distant breast cancer metastases. *Semin Radiat Oncol*. 1994;4:283.

237. Halverson K, Perez C, Kuske RR, et al: Isolated local-regional recurrence of breast cancer following mastectomy: Radiotherapeutic management. *Int J Radiat Oncol Biol Phys*. 1990;19:851.

238. Bedwinek J: Natural history and management of isolated local-regional recurrence following mastectomy. *Semin Radiat Oncol*. 1994;4:260.

239. Halsted WS: The results of radical operations for the cure of cancer of the breast. *Ann Surg*. 1907;46:1.

240. Patey DH, Dyson WH: The prognosis of carcinoma of the breast in relation to the type of operation performed. *Br J Cancer*. 1948;2:7.

241. Lichter AS, Adler D, August D, et al: Breast cancer. In Hoskins W, Perez C, Young R, eds. *Principles and Practice of Gynecologic Oncology*. Philadelphia: JB Lippincott; 1992:847.

242. Bedwinek J: Breast conserving surgery and irradiation: The importance of demarcating the excision cavity with surgical clips. *Int J Radiat Oncol Biol Phys*. 1993;26:675.

243. Machtay M, Lanciano R, Hoffman J, et al: Inaccuracies in using the lumpectomy scar for planning electron boosts in primary breast tissue. *Int J Radiat Oncol Biol Phys*. 1994;30:43.

244. Rabinovitch R, Finlayson C, Pan Z, et al: Radiographic evaluation of surgical clips is better than ultrasound for defining the lumpectomy cavity in breast boost treatment planning: A prospective clinical study. *Int J Radiat Oncol Biol Phys*. 2000;47:313.

245. Harrington K, Harrison M, Bayle P, et al: Surgical clips in planning the electron boost in breast cancer: A qualitative and quantitative evaluation. *Int J Radiat Oncol Biol Phys*. 1996;34:579.

246. Hunter M, McFall T, Hehr K: Breast-conserving surgery for primary breast cancer: Necessity for surgical clips to define the tumor bed for radiation planning. *Radiology*. 1996;200:281.

247. Lichter AS, Fraass BA, Yanke B: Treatment techniques in the conservative management of breast cancer. *Semin Radiat Oncol*. 1992;2:94.

248. Bentel G, Marks L, Hardenbergh P, et al: Variability of the location of internal mammary vessels and glandular breast tissue in breast cancer patients undergoing routine CT-based treatment planning. *Int J Radiat Oncol Biol Phys*. 1999;44:1017.

249. Sprimger R, Connors S, Halls S, et al: CT-targeted irradiation of the breast and internal mammary lymph nodes using a 5-field technique. *Int J Radiat Oncol Biol Phys*. 2000;48:983.

250. Goodman R, Grann A, Saracco P, et al: The relationship between radiation fields and regional lymph nodes in carcinoma of the breast. *Int J Radiat Oncol Biol Phys*. 2001;50:99.

251. Cho J, Hurkmans C, Damen E, et al: Intensity modulated versus non-intensity modulated radiotherapy in the treatment of the left breast and upper internal mammary lymph node chain: A comparative planning study. *Radiother Oncol*. 2002;62:127.

252. Das I, Cheng E, Freedman G, et al: Lung and heart dose volume analyses with CT simulator in radiation treatment of breast cancer. *Int J Radiat Oncol Biol Phys*. 1998;42:11.

253. Li J, Williams S, Goffinet D, et al: Breast-conserving radiation therapy using combined electron and intensity-modulated radiotherapy technique. *Radiother Oncol*. 2000;56:65.

254. Zackrisson B, Arevarn M, Karlsson M: Optimized MLC-beam arrangements for tangential breast irradiation. *Radiother Oncol*. 2000;54:209.

255. Monson J, Chin L, Nixon A, et al: Is machine energy (4-8 MV) associated with outcome for stage I-II breast cancer patients? *Int J Radiat Oncol Biol Phys*. 1997;37:1095.

256. Algan O, Fowble B, McNeeley S, et al: Use of the prone position in radiation treatment for women with early stage breast cancer. *Int J Radiat Oncol Biol Phys*. 1998;40:1137.

257. Lichter AS, Fraass BA, van de Geijn J, et al: A technique for field matching in primary breast irradiation. *Int J Radiat Oncol Biol Phys*. 1983;9:263.

258. Siddon R, Tonnesen G, Svensson G: Three-field technique for breast treatment using a rotatable half-beam block. *Int J Radiat Oncol Biol Phys*. 1981;7:1473.

259. Siddon R, Buck B, Harris J, et al: Three-field technique for breast irradiation using tangential field corner blocks. *Int J Radiat Oncol Biol Phys*. 1983;9:583.

260. Podgorsak E, Gosselin M, Pla M, et al: A simple isocentric technique for irradiation of the breast, chest wall and peripheral lymphatics. *Br J Radiol*. 1984;57:57.

261. Buck B: Technical consideration of intact breast irradiation. *Radiol Technol*. 1980;51:743.

262. Buck B, Siddon R, Svensson G: A beam alignment device for matching fields. *Int J Radiat Oncol Biol Phys*. 1985;11:1039.

263. Hartsell W, Murthy A, Kiel K, et al: Technique for breast irradiation using custom blocks conforming to the chest wall contour. *Int J Radiat Oncol Biol Phys*. 1990;19:189.

264. Lebesque J: Field matching in breast irradiation: An exact solution to a geometrical problem. *Radiother Oncol*. 1986;5:47.

265. Rosenow U, Valentine E, Davis L: A technique for treating local breast cancer using a single set-up point and asymmetric collimation. *Int J Radiat Oncol Biol Phys*. 1990;19:183.

266. Chu J, Solin L, Hwang C, et al: A nondivergent three field matching technique for breast irradiation. *Int J Radiat Oncol Biol Phys*. 1990;19:1037.

267. Lagendijk J, Hofman P: A standardized multifield irradiation technique for breast tumors using asymmetrical collimators and beam angulation. *Br J Radiol*. 1992;65:56.

268. Marshall M: Three-field isocentric breast irradiation using asymmetric jaws and a tilt board. *Radiother Oncol*. 1993;28:228.

269. Brezovich K, Meredith R, Weppelmann B, et al: Expedient set-up of tangential breast fields with a simple gantry attachment. *Int J Radiat Oncol Biol Phys*. 1991;21:1073.

270. Galvin J, Powlis WP, Fowble BF, et al: A new technique for positioning tangential fields. *Int J Radiat Oncol Biol Phys*. 1993;26:877.

271. Lichter AS: Technical aspects of the treatment of breast cancer with radiation therapy. In Dabforth D, Lichter AS, Lippman ME, eds: *Diagnosis and Management of Breast Cancer*. Philadelphia: WB Saunders; 1988:208.

272. Halverson K, Taylor M, Perez C, et al: Regional nodal management and patterns of failure following conservative surgery and radiation therapy for stage I and II breast cancer. *Int J Radiat Oncol Biol Phys*. 1993;26:593.

273. Recht A, Pierce S, Abner A, et al: Regional nodal failure after conservative surgery and radiotherapy for early-stage breast carcinoma. *J Clin Oncol*. 1991;9:988.

274. Solin L: Regional lymph node management in conservation treatment of early stage invasive breast carcinoma. *Int J Radiat Oncol Biol Phys*. 1993;26:709.

275. Jackson S: Carcinoma of the breast—The significance of supraclavicular lymph node metastases. *Clin Radiol*. 1966;17:107.

276. Fisher B, Redmond C, Fisher E, et al: Ten-year results of a randomized clinical trial comparing radical mastectomy and total mastectomy with or without radiation. *N Engl J Med*. 1985;312:674.

277. Leonard C, Corkill M, Tompkin J, et al: Are axillary recurrence and overall survival affected by axillary extranodal tumor extension in breast cancer? Implications for radiation therapy. *J Clin Oncol*. 1995;13:47.

278. Pierce LJ, Oberman HA, Strawderman MH, et al: Microscopic extracapsular extension in the axilla: Is this an indication for axillary radiotherapy? *Int J Radiat Oncol Biol Phys*. 1995; 33:253.

279. Van Dyk J: Lung dose calculation using computerized tomography: Is there a need for pixel based procedures? *Int J Radiat Oncol Biol Phys*. 1983;9:1035.

280. Cross P, Joseph D, Cant Ja: Tangential breast irradiation: Simple improvements. *Int J Radiat Oncol Biol Phys*. 1992;23:433.

281. Fraass BA, Lichter AL, McShan DL, et al: The influence of lung density corrections on treatment planning for primary breast cancer. *Int J Radiat Oncol Biol Phys*. 1988;14:179.

282. Mijnheer B, Heukelom S, Lanson J, et al: Should inhomogeneity corrections be applied during treatment planning of tangential breast irradiation? *Radiother Oncol*. 1991;22:239.

283. Pierce L, Strawderman MS, Douglas K, et al: Conservative surgery and radiotherapy for early-stage breast cancer using a lung density correction: The University of Michigan Experience. *Int J Radiat Oncol Biol Phys*. 1997;39:921.

284. Muller-Runkel R, Kalokhe UP: Method for reducing scatter radiation dose to the contralateral breast during tangential breast irradiation therapy. *Radiology*. 1994;191:853.

285. Muller-Runkel R, Kalokhe UP: Scatter dose from tangential breast irradiation to the uninvolved breast. *Radiology*. 1990;175:873.

286. Fraass B, Roberson P, Lichter A: Dose to the contralateral breast due to primary breast irradiation. *Int J Radiat Oncol Biol Phys*. 1985;11:485.

287. Goss PE, Sierra S: Current perspectives on radiation-induced breast cancer. *J Clin Oncol*. 1998;16:338.

288. Chin L, Cheng C, Siddon R, et al: Three-dimensional photon dose distributions with and without lung corrections for tangential breast intact treatments. *Int J Radiat Oncol Biol Phys*. 1989; 17:1327.

289. Mayles W, Yarnold J, Webb S: Improved dose homogeneity in the breast using tissue compensators. *Radiother Oncol*. 1991;22:248.

290. Valdagni R, Ciocca M, Busana L, et al: Beam modifying devices in the treatment of early breast cancer: 3-D stepped compensating technique. *Radiother Oncol*. 1992;23:192.

291. Carruthers LJ, Redpath AT, Kunkler IH: The use of compensators to optimise the three dimensional dose distribution in radiotherapy of the intact breast. *Radiother Oncol.* 1999;50:291.

292. Pierce LJ, Butler JB, Martel MK, et al: Postmastectomy radiotherapy of the chest wall: Dosimetric comparison of common techniques. *Int J Radiat Oncol Biol Phys.* 2002;52:1220.

293. Romestaing P, Lehingue Y, Carrie C, et al: Role of a 10-Gy boost in the conservative treatment of early breast cancer: Results of a randomized clinical trial in Lyon, France. *J Clin Oncol.* 1997;15:963.

294. Bartelink H, Horiot JC, Poortmans P: Recurrence rates after treatment of breast cancer with standard radiotherapy with or without additional radiation. *N Engl J Med.* 2001;345:1378.

295. Vrieling C, Collette L, Fourquet A, et al: The influence of the boost in breast-conserving therapy on cosmetic outcome in the EORTC "boost versus no boost" trial. *Int J Radiat Oncol Biol Phys.* 1999;45:677.

296. Hayman J, Hillner B, Harris J, et al: Cost-effectiveness of adding an electron-beam boost to tangential radiation therapy in patients with negative margins after conservative surgery for early-stage breast cancer. *J Clin Oncol.* 2000;18:287.

297. Pierquin B, Huart J, Raynal M, et al: Conservative treatment for breast cancer: Long-term results (15 years). *Radiother Oncol.* 1990;20:16.

298. Mansfield CM, Komarnicky LT, Schwartz GF, et al: Perioperative implantation of iridium-192 as the boost technique for stage I and II breast cancer: Results of a 10-year study of 655 patients. *Radiology.* 1994;192:33.

299. Krishnan L, Jewell W, Mansfield C, et al: Early-stage breast cancer: Local control after conservative surgery and radiation therapy with immediate interstitial boost. *Radiology.* 1993;187:95.

300. Olivotto I, Rose M, Oteen R, et al: Late cosmetic outcome after conservative surgery and radiotherapy: Analysis of causes of cosmetic failure. *Int J Radiat Oncol Biol Phys.* 1989;17:747.

301. Gilligan D, Hendry JA, Yarnold JR: The use of ultrasound to measure breast thickness to select electron energies for breast boost therapy. *Radiother Oncol.* 1994;32:265.

302. Messer PM, Kirikuta IC, Bratengeier K, et al: CT planning of boost irradiation in radiotherapy of breast cancer after conservative surgery. *Radiother Oncol.* 1997;42:239.

303. Vicini FA, Baglan KL, Kestin LL, et al: Accelerated treatment of breast cancer. *J Clin Oncol.* 2001;19:1993.

304. King TA, Bolton JS, Kuske RR, et al: Long-term results of wide-field brachytherapy as the sole method of radiation therapy after segmental mastectomy for T (is, 1, 2) breast cancer. *Am J Surg.* 2000;180:299.

305. Solin L, Fowble B, Schultzx D, et al: The significance of the pathology margins of the tumor excision on the outcome of patients treated with definitive irradiation for early stage breast cancer. *Int J Radiat Oncol Biol Phys.* 1991;21:279.

306. Olivotto I, Weir L, Kim-Sing C, et al: Late cosmetic results of short fractionation for breast conservation. *Radiother Oncol.* 1996;41:7.

307. Schomberg P, Shanahan T, Ingle J, et al: Accelerated hyperfractionation radiation therapy after lumpectomy and axillary lymph node dissection in patients with stage I or II breast cancer: Pilot study. *Radiology.* 1997;202:565.

308. Shelley W, Brundage M, Hayter C, et al: A shorter fractionation schedule for postlumpectomy breast cancer patients. *Int J Radiat Oncol Biol Phys.* 2000;47:1219.

309. Whelan T, MacKenzie R, Julian J, et al: Randomized trial of breast irradiation schedules after lumpectomy for women with lymph node-negative breast cancer. *J Natl Cancer Inst.* 2002;94:1143.

310. Pezner RD, Patterson MP, Hill LR, et al: Arm lymphedema in patients treated conservatively for breast cancer: Relationship to patient age and axillary node dissection technique. *Int J Radiat Oncol Biol Phys.* 1986;12:2079.

311. Larson D, Weinstein M, Goldberg I, et al: Edema of the arm as a function of the extent of axillary surgery in patients with stage I-II carcinoma of the breast treated with primary radiotherapy. *Int J Radiat Oncol Biol Phys.* 1986;12:1575.

312. Liljegren G, Holmberg L, Group TU-OBCS: Arm morbidity after sector resection and axillary dissection with or without postoperative radiotherapy in breast cancer stage I. Results from a randomized trial. *Eur J Cancer.* 1997;33:193.

313. Lichter A, Lippman M, Danforth D, et al: Mastectomy versus breast-conserving therapy in the treatment of stage I and II carcinoma of the breast: A randomized trial at the National Cancer Institute. *J Clin Oncol.* 1992;10:976.

314. Lingos T, Recht A, Vicini F, et al: Radiation pneumonitis in breast cancer patients treated with conservative surgery and radiation therapy. *Int J Radiat Oncol Biol Phys.* 1991;21:355.

315. Lind P, Marks L, Hardenbergh P, et al: Technical factors associated with radiation pneumonitis after local + regional radiation therapy for breast cancer. *Int J Radiat Oncol Biol Phys.* 2002;52:137.

316. Rutqvist LE, Lax I, Fornander T, et al: Cardiovascular mortality in a randomized trial of adjuvant radiation therapy versus surgery alone in primary breast cancer. *Int J Radiat Oncol Biol Phys.* 1992;22:887.

317. Gyenes G, Fornander T, Carlens P, et al: Morbidity of ischemic heart disease in early breast cancer 15-20 years after adjuvant radiotherapy. *Int J Radiat Oncol Biol Phys.* 1994;28:1235.

318. Gyenes G, Gagliardi G, Lax I, et al: Evaluation of irradiated heart volumes in stage I breast cancer patients treated with postoperative adjuvant radiotherapy. *J Clin Oncol.* 1997;15:1348.

319. Vallis KA, Pintilie M, Chong N, et al: Assessment of coronary heart disease morbidity and mortality after radiation therapy for early breast cancer. *J Clin Oncol.* 2002;20:1036.

320. Rutqvist LE, Liedberg A, Hammar N, et al: Myocardial infarction among women with early-stage breast cancer treated with conservative surgery and breast irradiation. *Int J Radiat Oncol Biol Phys.* 1998;40:359.

321. Nixon AJ, Manola J, Gelman R, et al: No long-term increase in cardiac-related mortality after breast-conserving surgery and radiation therapy using modern techniques. *J Clin Oncol.* 1998;16:1374.

322. Overgaard M: Spontaneous radiation-induced rib fractures in breast cancer patients with postmastectomy irradiation. A clinical radiobiological analysis of the influence of fraction size and dose-response relationships on late bone damage. *Acta Oncol.* 1988;27:117.

323. Pierce S, Recht A, Lingos T, et al: Long-term radiation complications following conservative surgery (CS) and radiation therapy (RT) in patients with early stage breast cancer. *Int J Radiat Oncol Biol Phys.* 1992;23:915.

324. Olsen N, Pfeiffer P, Johanssen L, et al: Radiation-induced brachial plexopathy: Neurological follow-up in 161 recurrence-free breast cancer patients. *Int J Radiat Oncol Biol Phys.* 1993;26:43.

325. Olsen N, Mondrup K, Rose C: Radiation-induced brachial plexus neuropathy in breast cancer patients. *Acta Oncol.* 1990;29:885.

326. Salner AL, Botnick LE, Herzog AG, et al: Reversible brachial plexopathy following primary radiation therapy for breast cancer. *Cancer Treat Rev.* 1981;65:797.

327. Rescigno J, McCormick B, Brown AE, et al: Breast cellulitis after conservative surgery and radiotherapy. *Int J Radiat Oncol Biol Phys.* 1994;29:163.

328. Staren ED, Klepac S, Smith AP, et al: The dilemma of delayed cellulitis after breast conservation therapy. *Arch Surg.* 1996;131:651.

329. Bowers GJ, Prestidge B, Getz J, et al: Infectious complications in irradiated breasts following conservative breast therapy. *Br J.* 1995;1:295.

330. Otis C, Peschel R, McKhann C, et al: The rapid onset of cutaneous angiosarcoma after radiotherapy for breast carcinoma. *Cancer.* 1986;57:2130.

331. Wijnmaalen A, van Ooigen B, van Geel B, et al: Angiosarcoma of the breast following lumpectomy, axillary lymph node dissection, and radiotherapy for primary breast cancer: Three case reports and a review of the literature. *J Radiat Oncol Biol Phys.* 1993;26:135.

332. Edeiken S, Russo D, Knech J, et al: Angiosarcoma after tylectomy and radiation therapy for carcinoma of the breast. *Cancer.* 1992;70:644.

333. Bobin JY, Rivoire M, Delay E, et al: Radiation induced sarcomas following treatment for breast cancer: Presentation of a series of 14 cases treated with an aggressive surgical approach. *J Surg Oncol.* 1994;57:171.

334. Marchal C, Weber B, de Lafontan B, et al: Nine breast angiosarcomas after conservative treatment for breast carcinoma: A survey from French comprehensive cancer centers. *Int J Radiat Oncol Biol Phys.* 1999;44:113.

335. Strobbe L, Peterse H, van Tinteren H, et al: Angiosarcoma of the breast after conservation therapy for invasive cancer, the incidence and outcome. An unforeseen sequela. *Breast Cancer Res Treat.* 1998;47:101.

336. Chlebowski RT, Collyar DE, Somerfield MR, et al: American Society of Clinical Oncology technology assessment on breast cancer risk reduction strategies: Tamoxifen and raloxifene. *J Clin Oncol.* 1999;17:1939.

337. Feuer EJ, Wun LM, Boring CC, et al: The lifetime risk of developing breast cancer. *J Natl Cancer Inst.* 1993;85:892.

338. Fisher B, Land S, Mamounas E, et al: Prevention of invasive breast cancer in women with ductal carcinoma in situ: An update of the National Surgical Adjuvant Breast and Bowel Project experience. *Semin Oncol.* 2001;28:400.

339. Clarke D, Le M, Sarrazin D, et al: Analysis of local-regional relapses in patients with early breast cancers treated by excision and radiotherapy: experience of the Institut Gustave-Roussy. *Int J Radiat Oncol Biol Phys.* 1985;11:137.

340. Fourquet A, Campana F, Zafrani B, et al: Prognostic factors of breast recurrence in the conservative management of early breast cancer: A 25-year follow-up. *Int J Radiat Oncol Biol Phys.* 1989;17:719.

341. Haffty BG, Fischer D, Rose M, et al: Prognostic factors for local recurrence in the conservatively treated breast cancer patient: A cautious interpretation of the data. *J Clin Oncol.* 1991;9:997.

342. Kurtz J, Jacquemier J, Amalric R, et al: Risk factors for breast recurrence in premenopausal and postmonopausal patients with ductal cancers treated by conservation therapy. *Cancer.* 1990;65:1867.

343. Ryoo MC, Kagan AR, Wollin M, et al: Prognostic factors for recurrence and cosmesis in 393 patients after radiation therapy for early mammary carcinoma. *Radiology.* 1989;172:555.

344. Veronesi U, Salvadori B, Luini A, et al: Conservative treatment of early breast cancer. Long-term results of 1232 cases treated with quadrantectomy, axillary dissection, and radiotherapy. *Ann Surg.* 1990;211:250.

345. Makris A, Powles TJ, Ashley SE, et al: A reduction in the requirements for mastectomy in a randomized trial of neoadjuvant chemoendocrine therapy in primary breast cancer. *Ann Oncol.* 1998;9:1179.

346. Broet P, Scholl SM, de la Rochefordiere A, et al: Short and long-term effects on survival in breast cancer patients treated by primary chemotherapy: an updated analysis of a randomized trial. *Breast Cancer Res Treat.* 1999;58:151.

347. Mauriac L, MacGrogan G, Avril A, et al: Neoadjuvant chemotherapy for operable breast carcinoma larger than 3 cm: A unicentre randomized trial with a 124-month median follow-up. Institut Bergonie Bordeaux Groupe Sein (IBBGS). *Ann Oncol.* 1999;10:47.

348. Wolmark N, Wang J, Mamounas E, et al: Preoperative chemotherapy in patients with operable breast cancer: Nine-year results from National Surgical Adjuvant Breast and Bowel Project B-18. *J Natl Cancer Inst Monogr.* 2001;30:96.

349. Schaake-Koning C, van der Linden EH, Hart G, et al: Adjuvant chemo- and hormonal therapy in locally advanced breast cancer: A randomized clinical study. *Int J Radiat Oncol Biol Phys.* 1985;11:1759.

350. Derman DP, Browde S, Kessel IL, et al: Adjuvant chemotherapy (CMF) for stage III breast cancer: A randomized trial. *Int J Radiat Oncol Biol Phys.* 1989;17:257.

351. Rubens RD, Bartelink H, Engelsman E, et al: Locally advanced breast cancer: The contribution of cytotoxic and endocrine treatment to radiotherapy. An EORTC Breast Cancer Co-operative Group Trial (10792). *Eur J Cancer Clin Oncol.* 1989;25:667.

352. Klefstrom P, Grohn P, Heinonen E, et al: Adjuvant postoperative radiotherapy, chemotherapy, and immunotherapy in stage III breast cancer. II. 5-year results and influence of levamisole. *Cancer.* 1987;60:936.

353. Bonadonna G, Valagussa P: Dose-response effect of adjuvant chemotherapy in breast cancer. *N Engl J Med.* 1981;304:10.

354. Moliterni A, Bonadonna G, Valagussa P, et al: Cyclophosphamide, methotrexate, and fluorouracil with and without doxorubicin in the adjuvant treatment of resectable breast cancer with one to three positive axillary nodes. *J Clin Oncol.* 1991;9:1124.

355. Falkson G, Gelman RS, Tormey DC, et al: The Eastern Cooperative Oncology Group experience with cyclophosphamide, adriamycin, and 5-fluorouracil (CAF) in patients with metastatic breast cancer. *Cancer.* 1985;56:219.

356. Fisher B, Brown AM, Dimitrov NV, et al: Two months of doxorubicin-cyclophosphamide with and without interval reinduction therapy compared with 6 months of cyclophosphamide, methotrexate, and fluorouracil in positive-node breast cancer patients with tamoxifen-nonresponsive tumors: Results from the National Surgical Adjuvant Breast and Bowel Project B-15. *J Clin Oncol.* 1990;8:1483.

357. Hortobagyi GN, Bodey GP, Buzdar AU, et al: Evaluation of high-dose versus standard FAC chemotherapy for advanced breast cancer in protected environment units: A prospective randomized study. *J Clin Oncol.* 1987;5:354.

358. Henderson IC, Berry D, Demetri GD, et al: Improved disease-free and overall survival from the addition of sequential paclitaxel but not from the escalation of doxorubicin dose in an adjuvant chemotherapy regimen for patients with node positive primary breast cancer. *J Clin Oncol.* 2003;21:976.

359. Wood WC, Budman DR, Korzun AH, et al: Dose and dose intensity of adjuvant chemotherapy for stage II, node-positive breast carcinoma. *N Engl J Med.* 1994;330:1253.

360. Budman DR, Berry DA, Cirrincione CT, et al: Dose and dose intensity as determinants of outcome in the adjuvant treatment of breast cancer. The Cancer and Leukemia Group B. *J Natl Cancer Inst.* 1998;90:1205.

361. Goldhirsch A, Glick JH, Gelber RD, et al: Meeting highlights: International Consensus Panel on the Treatment of Primary Breast Cancer. *J Natl Cancer Inst.* 1998;90:1601.

362. Liljegren G, Holmberg L, Bergh J, et al: 10-Year results after sector resection with or without postoperative radiotherapy for stage I breast cancer: A randomized trial. *J Clin Oncol.* 1999;17:2326.

363. Veronesi U, Marubini E, Mariani L, et al: Radiotherapy after breast-conserving surgery in small breast carcinoma: Long-term results of a randomized trial. *Ann Oncol.* 2001;12:997.

364. Clark RM, Whelan T, Levine M, et al: Randomized clinical trial of breast irradiation following lumpectomy and axillary dissection for node-negative breast cancer: An update. Ontario Clinical Oncology Group. *J Natl Cancer Inst.* 1996;88:1659.

365. Forrest AP, Stewart HJ, Everington D, et al: Randomised controlled trial of conservation therapy for breast cancer: 6-Year analysis of the Scottish trial. Scottish Cancer Trials Breast Group. *Lancet.* 1996;348:708.

366. Fisher B, Anderson S, Bryant J, et al: Twenty-year follow-up of a randomized trial comparing total mastectomy, lumpectomy, and lumpectomy plus irradiation for the treatment of invasive breast cancer. *N Engl J Med.* 2002;347:1233.

367. Jacobson JA, Danforth DN, Cowan KH, et al: Ten-year results of a comparison of conservation with mastectomy in the treatment of stage I and II breast cancer. *N Engl J Med.* 1995;332:907.

368. van Dongen JA, Voogd AC, Fentiman IS, et al: Long-term results of a randomized trial comparing breast-conserving therapy with mastectomy: European Organization for Research and Treatment of Cancer 10801 trial. *J Natl Cancer Inst.* 2000;92:1143.

369. Blichert-Toft M, Rose C, Andersen JA, et al: Danish randomized trial comparing breast conservation therapy with mastectomy: Six years of life-table analysis. Danish Breast Cancer Cooperative Group. *J Natl Cancer Inst Monogr.* 1992;11:19.

370. Arriagada R, Le MG, Rochard F, et al: Conservative treatment versus mastectomy in early breast cancer: Patterns of failure with 15 years of follow-up data. Institut Gustave-Roussy Breast Cancer Group. *J Clin Oncol.* 1996;14:1558.

371. Veronesi U, Cascinelli N, Mariani L, et al: Twenty-year follow-up of a randomized study comparing breast-conserving surgery with radical mastectomy for early breast cancer. *N Engl J Med.* 2002;347:1227.

Sarcomas of Soft Tissue

Quynh-Thu Le, MD, Theodore L. Phillips, MD, and Steven A. Leibel, MD

58

Soft-tissue sarcomas are a group of rare tumors derived from mesenchymal cells. While these tumors were first described in ancient Egyptian papyrus, the word sarcoma (meaning "fish flesh") came from early Greek clinicians. Morgagni was the first to provide an accurate description of a soft-tissue sarcoma—a retroperitoneal liposarcoma—in 1761. Since then, knowledge of these tumors has exploded as evidenced by a large body of medical literature devoted to this field.

EPIDEMIOLOGY

An estimated 8300 new cases of soft-tisssue sarcoma will be diagnosed in the United States in 2003 and 3900 will die of the disease.[1] Soft-tissue sarcomas constitute approximately 0.6% of all malignancies diagnosed yearly in this country (excluding skin cancers and carcinomas in situ). They can occur at any age, and, like carcinomas, are more common in older patients. About 15% of affected persons are younger than age 16, and 40% are older than age 55. The male-to-female ratio is 1.12:1.

The pathogenesis of most soft-tissue tumors is still unknown. Trauma or past injuries, frequently implicated in the development of sarcomas, appear to be events that call attention to the underlying neoplasm. Rare cases of these tumors arising from scar tissue following surgery, a burn, or the site of a foreign body implantation have been reported.[2,3] Sarcomas (usually lymphangiosarcomas) have also been observed in the chronically edematous arm following breast cancer treatment as described in the Stewart-Treves syndrome. Chemical carcinogens, such as dioxin from herbicides and Agent Orange, have been linked to the development of soft-tissue tumors. Yet none of the case control studies carried out since 1980 has been able to substantiate the claim.[4-6] Olsson et al. showed a reduced risk of soft-tissue sarcoma development with an odd ratio of 0.57 with the chronic use (>2 years) of oral contraceptives in a population-based study.[7]

Past radiation exposure has been related to the development of soft-tissue and bone sarcomas. The interval between radiation and tumor development ranges from 2 to 25 years. The frequency of neoplasm increases with higher radiation dose and longer follow-up.[8] Taghian et al.[9] reported a 0.2% rate of radiation-induced sarcoma in 7620 women treated for breast cancer. The estimated actuarial frequency of sarcoma development at 15 to 20 years is approximately 0.5%. This number may be slightly higher with the addition of chemotherapy. A U.S. population-based study of 274,245 breast cancer patients showed that those who received breast irradiation had a higher risk of developing soft-tissue sarcoma than those not treated with radiation, although the excess risk with radiation was relatively small (incidence of 0.24 with radiation vs. 0.14 without radiation at 15 years).[10] The most common postradiation soft-tissue sarcoma is malignant fibrous histiocytoma (MFH), followed by fibrosarcoma and malignant nerve sheath tumor.

GENETICS, CYTOGENETICS, AND MOLECULAR BIOLOGY

Both osseous and soft-tissue sarcomas are included in the Li-Fraumeni cancer syndrome, which is characterized by a familial cluster of sarcomas, early breast cancers, brain tumors, leukemia, and adrenal carcinomas.[11] Germ line abnormalities of the *p53* tumor suppressor gene have been identified in the members of these families.[12] Neurofibromatosis type 1 (NF1), characterized by café-au-lait spots and numerous neurofibromas, is another genetic disorder classically linked to the development of soft-tissue tumors. Malignant peripheral nerve sheath tumors arise from malignant degeneration of neurofibromas in 1% to 5% of cases.[13] The gene for neurofibromatosis type 1 (NF1) has been cloned from the pericentromeric region of chromosome 17. The gene product (neurofibromin) appears to have tumor suppressor activities.[14] A slight increase in frequency of soft-tissue sarcomas has also been found in basal cell nevus syndrome, tuberous sclerosis, Werner's syndrome, intestinal polyposis, and Gardner's syndrome.

Cytogenetic studies have been carried out for many soft-tissue tumors. Table 58-1 lists characteristic chromosomal aberrations and their frequency for certain sarcomas. On the molecular level, alterations in the *Rb* and *p53* tumor suppressor genes have been found in soft-tissue sarcomas. Wunder et al. reported *Rb* changes in 5 of 12 high-grade and 1 of 11 low-grade soft-tissue tumors.[15] Toguchida discovered 42 somatic *p53* alterations in 127 cases of osseous and soft-tissue sarcomas.[16] Twenty-one were gross gene arrangements, and 21 had subtle changes (missense or nonsense mutations). Others have reported abnormal *p53* immunostaining in one third of the cases.[17,18] Of note, mutations of both *Rb* and

Table 58–1   Characteristic Cytogenetic Alterations in Soft-Tissue Sarcomas

Histology	Cytogenetic Events	Involved Genes	Frequency, %
Clear cell sarcoma	t(12;22)(q13;q12)	ATF1, EWS	>75
Dermatofibrosarcoma protuberans	Ring chromosome 17	Unknown	>75
Ewing's sarcoma of soft tissues	t(11;22)(q24;q12)	FLI, EWS	95
	t(22;22)(q22;q12)	ERG, EWS	
	t(7;22)(q22;q12)	ETV1, EWS	
	t(2;22)(q33;q12)	FEV, EWS	
	t(17;22)(q12;q12)	E1AF, EWS	
Leiomyosarcoma	Deletion of 1p	Not applicable	75
Liposarcoma			
Myxoid	t(12;16)(q13;p11)	CHOP, TLS	75
Well differentiated	ring chromosome 12	MDM2	80
Rhabdomyosarcoma			
Alveolar	t(2;13)(q35;q14)	PAX3, FKHR	80
	t(1;13)(p36;q14)	PAX7, FKHR	
Embryonal	+2q, +8, +12, +13	Unknown	80
Synovial sarcoma	t(X;18)(p11;q11)	SSX1 or 2, SYT	95

Adapted and modified from Enzinger FM, Weiss SW: *Soft Tissue Tumors*. 3rd ed. St. Louis: CV Mosby; 1994.

p53 genes were frequently seen in the same tumors. *MDM2* (located on chromosome 12q13-q14), an inhibitor of *p53* transcriptional activities, was found to be amplified in 8 of 24 soft-tissue tumors evaluated.[19] This suggests that *MDM2* amplification is an alternative mechanism for inactivating the cell cycle regulatory pathways. *SAS*, located in chromosome 12q13-q14 near a cyclin-dependent protein kinase gene, is thought to be involved in signal transduction and cell growth regulation. It was found to be amplified in 7 of 22 malignant fibrous histiocytomas (MFHs) and in three of three liposarcomas.[20] Its role as an oncogene has not been clearly established. More details of the cytogenetic changes and molecular biology of soft-tissue tumors can be found in an excellent review by Cyril Fisher.[21]

Transcriptional profiling using either oligonucleotide or complementary deoxyribonucleic acid (cDNA) microarrays has been employed to characterize soft-tissue tumors.[22] The authors analyzed 41 soft-tissue tumors, which provided more than 1.5 million data points for 5520 well-measured genes. Based on the level of gene expression, they found that these 41 specimens can be separated into five distinct groups: synovial sarcomas; gastrointestinal stromal tumors (GIST); benign peripheral nerve sheath tumors; half of the leiomyosarcomas; and a broad group containing all the MFHs, the liposarcomas, and the other leiomyosarcomas. In addition, they found that c-Kit and protein kinase C are highly expressed

in GIST, and cellular retinoic binding protein-1, retinoic acid receptor-γ, and the epidermal growth factor receptor are highly expressed in synovial sarcoma, suggesting that these can be exploited for molecular targeting of these tumors in the future.

ANATOMY

Embryologically, the soft-tissue structures arise from the primitive mesenchyme of the mesoderm with some contribution from the neuroectoderm. Soft-tissue structures consist of muscles, fat, fibrous tissues, blood vessels, and supporting cells of the peripheral nervous system. The frequency of involvement of different anatomic sites is shown in Table 58-2 and summarized in Figure 58-1. Soft-tissue sarcomas can arise in soft tissues in any part of the body.

PATHOLOGY

Each of the soft tissues can give rise to a group of malignant sarcomas. Tumor histology and their putative cells of origin (as suggested by Enzinger and Weiss[13]) are listed in Table 58-3. MFH and liposarcoma (Figs. 58-2 and 58-3) are the most common soft-tissue neoplasms in adults, accounting for 35% to 45% of all sarcomas.

Table 58–2   Anatomic Distribution of Soft-Tissue Sarcomas

Author	Yr	Tumors, *n*	Head and Neck	Trunk	Retroperitoneum	Upper Extremity	Lower Extremity	Other
Russell et al[172]	1977	1215	177	227	157	166	484	4
Potter et al[31]	1985	307	12	42	36	59	152	6
Lawrence et al[23]	1987	4550	406	814	568	594	2110	58
Suit and Spiro[88]	1993	788	94	79	47	166	347	55
Total (%)		6860	689 (10)	1162 (17)	808 (12)	985 (14)	3093 (45)	123 (2)

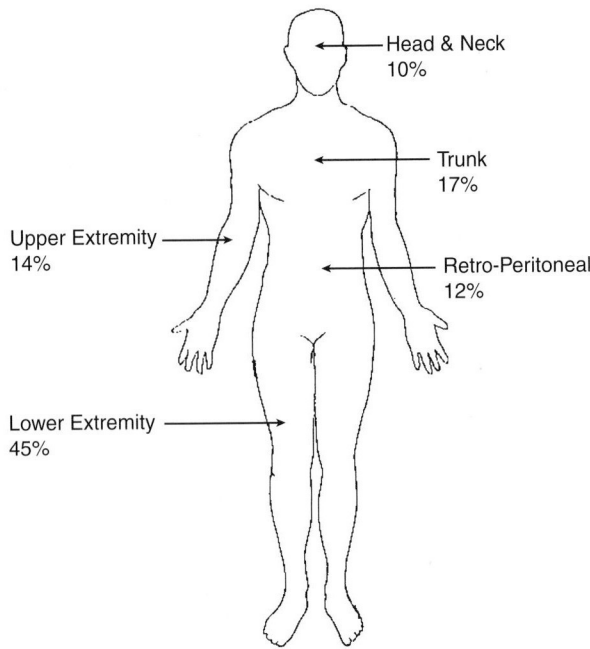

Head & Neck
10%

Trunk
17%

Upper Extremity
14%

Retro-Peritoneal
12%

Lower Extremity
45%

Figure 58–1. Anatomic distribution of soft-tissue sarcomas.

The three most common sarcomas found in U.S. hospital registries in the 1980s were MFH (26%), liposarcoma (18%), and leiomyosarcoma (15%).[23] Hashimoto and colleagues reported an incidence of 25% for MFH, 12% for liposarcoma, and 10% for rhabdomyosarcoma among 1116 cases evaluated.[24]

MFH was until recently considered the most common soft-tissue sarcoma among adults. Histologically, karyotypically, and clinically, this is by far the most heterogeneous group of sarcomas, and the concept of MFH as a histogenetically separate entity was called into question. An alternative hypothesis is that MFH is a poorly differentiated sarcoma and might represent a common endpoint for various other sarcomas. Fletcher et al. performed histologic, immunohistochemical, and, where available, ultrastructural reanalysis of 100 MHF cases of the extremity and trunk. In 84 cases, a specific line of differentiation was strongly suggested. The most common diagnosis was myxofibrosarcoma (22 cases) and leiomyosarcoma (20 cases). They also showed that myogenic sarcomas had a worse prognosis than nonmyogenic sarcomas.[25] Gene array analysis did not separate MFH from the liposarcomas, which strengthened the

Table 58–3 Histologic Classification of Soft-Tissue Sarcoma

Tissue	Sarcoma	Tissue	Sarcoma
I. Fibrous	Fibrosarcoma a. Adult b. Congenital or infantile c. Inflammatory	IX. Mesothelial	1. Malignant solitary fibrous tumor of pleura and peritoneum 2. Diffuse mesothelioma a. Epithelial b. Fibrous c. Biphasic
II. Fibrohistiocytic	Malignant fibrous histiocytoma a. Storiform-pleomorphic b. Myxoid c. Giant cell d. Xanthomatous	X. Neural	1. Malignant peripheral nerve sheath tumor (MPNST) (malignant schwannoma, neurofibrosarcoma) a. Malignant triton tumor (MPNST with rhabdomyosarcoma) b. Glandular c. Epithelioid
III. Lipomatous	Liposarcoma a. Well-differentiated b. Myxoid c. Pleomorphic d. Dedifferentiated		2. Malignant granular cell tumor 3. Clear cell sarcoma 4. Malignant melanocytic schwannoma 5. Gastrointestinal autonomous nerve tumor
IV. Smooth muscle	1. Leiomyosarcoma 2. Epithelioid leiomyosarcoma		6. Primitive neuroectodermal tumor a. Neuroblastoma
V. Skeletal muscle	1. Rhabdomyosarcoma a. Embryonal b. Botryoid c. Spindle cell d. Alveolar e. Pleomorphic 2. Rhabdomyosarcoma with ganglionic differentiation		b. Ganglioneuroblastoma c. Neuroepithelioma d. Extraskeletal Ewing's sarcoma
		XI. Paraganglionic	Malignant paraganglioma
		XII. Extraskeletal cartilaginous and osseous	1. Extraskeletal chondrosarcoma a. Well-differentiated b. Myxoid c. Mesenchymal 2. Extraskeletal osteosarcoma
VI. Vascular and lymphatic	1. Angiosarcoma 2. Lymphangiosarcoma 3. Kaposi's sarcoma	XIII. Pluripotential mesenchymal	Malignant mesenchymoma
VII. Perivascular	1. Malignant glomus tumor 2. Malignant hemangiopericytoma	XIV. Miscellaneous	1. Alveolar soft part sarcoma 2. Epithelioid sarcoma
VIII. Synovial	1. Synovial sarcoma a. Biphasic (fibrous and epithelial) b. Monophasic 2. Malignant giant cell tumor of tendon sheath		3. Malignant extrarenal rhabdoid tumor 4. Desmoplastic small cell tumor

Adapted and modified from Enzinger FM, Weiss SW: Soft tissue tumors. In Greene LG, Page DL, Fleming ID, et al., eds. *AJCC Cancer Staging Manual.* 6th ed. New York: Springer; 2002:193.

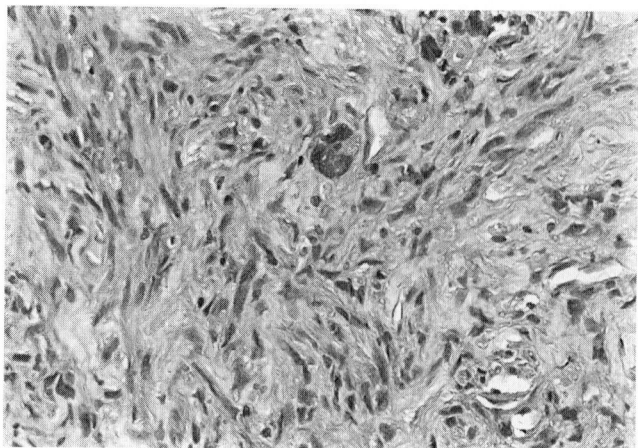

Figure 58–2. Malignant fibrous histiocytoma, storiform-pleomorphic variant. This variant is characterized by storiform cellular pattern and pleomorphic nuclei. (Hematoxylin and eosin. Original magnification ×40. Courtesy of Dr. Werner Roseneau, Dept. of Pathology, University of California at San Francisco.)

alternative view of MFH.[22] Further work is needed to clarify this controversy. The term MFH, however, continues to be well accepted and remains useful in diagnostic and clinical practice.

Sarcoma histology alone does not provide sufficient evidence for predicting the clinical course. Grading and staging are essential for accurate prognosis and treatment of these neoplasms. Unlike past classifications, each histology can be assigned a specific grade in the current system. When histologic grades are accounted for, with a few exceptions, most soft-tissue sarcomas have common biologic behaviors irrespective of histologic type. In a series of 211 high-grade sarcomas, Potter and coworkers showed that histology was not a significant determinant for either overall survival or disease-free survival.[26]

Traditionally, the designation of histopathologic grades depends on a combined assessment of several histologic features: degree of cellularity and pleomorphism, abundance of stroma, expansile or invasive growth, extent of differentiation, mitotic activity, and amount of necrosis. Mitotic count and necrosis appear to be the most significant prognostic factors in predicting the duration of survival and the time to developing distant metastasis.[27] There are at least four different grading systems in the literature, as summarized in Table 58-4. Despite their differences, all showed a strong correlation between grade and survival. The two systems most favored by pathologists are those designated as the National Cancer Institute (NCI) and the French Federation of Cancer Centers Sarcoma Group (FNCLCC). A direct comparison between these two systems in 410 patients with nonmetastatic soft-tissue sarcoma revealed that both systems were of prognostic value in predicting the risk of distant metastasis and tumor-related death, with the FNCLCC system providing a slightly better prediction.[28] Unfortunately, there is poor reproducibility of histologic diagnosis and tumor grading among trained pathologists. Coindre et al. found a crude agreement rate of only 61% for histology and 75% for tumor grade among 15 well-known sarcoma experts.[29]

CLINICAL PRESENTATION AND ROUTES OF SPREAD

The most common clinical presentation of soft-tissue sarcoma is a slow-growing, painless mass. The median period between detection of the lesion and presentation to the clinician is approximately 4 months, and the clinician's delay in establishing the diagnosis is about 1 month.[23] Pain, numbness, and swelling may result from tumor invasion of bone or neurovascular bundles.

Soft-tissue sarcomas are often surrounded by a pseudocapsule, composed of an inner rim of normal tissue, an outer rim of edema, and a reactive zone of small, newly formed vessels. They can invade muscles, nerves, vessels, and fascia and frequently envelop major neurovascular structures. Pseudopods of tumor can extend through the pseudocapsules and give rise to

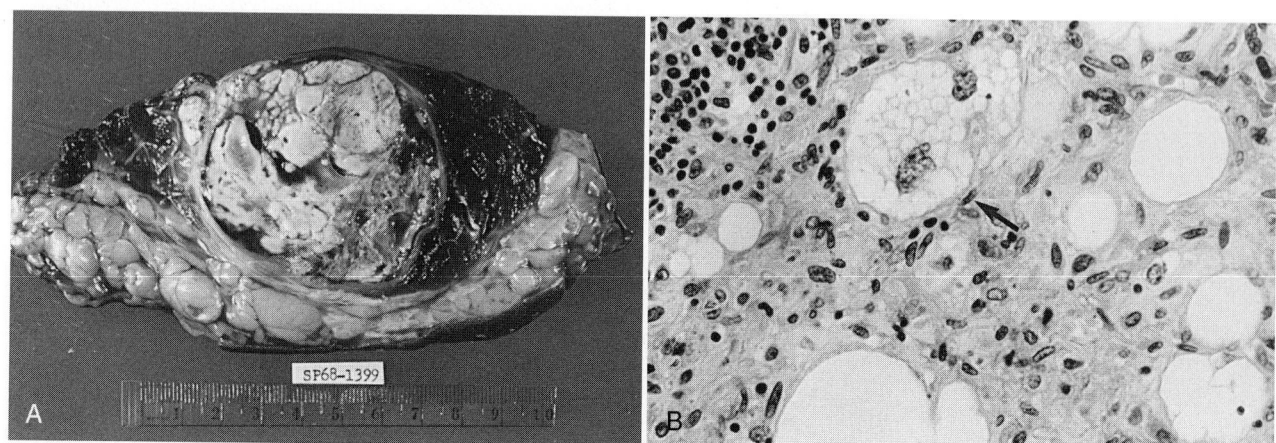

Figure 58–3. A, Liposarcoma: a cross section of a specimen. Note the appearance of the pseudocapsule around the tumor. **B,** Liposarcoma with a large lipoblast (*arrow*). (Hematoxylin and eosin. Original magnification ×40. Courtesy of Dr. Werner Roseneau, Dept. of Pathology, University of California at San Francisco.)

Table 58–4   Grading Systems of Sarcomas of Soft Tissue

Author	Yr	Dominant histologic variable	Grade	5-Yr Survival (%)
Markhede et al[66]	1982	Cellularity, mitosis, pleomorphism	1	100
			2	100
			3	68
			4	47
Myhre Jensen et al[173]	1983	Mitosis	1	97
			2	67
			3	38
Costa et al[174]	1984	Necrosis	1	100
			2	73
			3	46
Trojani (French Fed. System) et al[175]	1984	Differentiation, mitosis, necrosis	1	70
			2	43
			3	20

satellite lesions. Though locally aggressive, they rarely extend into adjacent tissue compartments until late in the course of disease. Local spread can, however, be facilitated by surgical violation of tissue planes.

Approximately 6% to 10% of patients have metastatic disease at diagnosis. Rydholm et al. reviewed the records of 278 patients with soft-tissue sarcomas of the extremities registered in the Southern District of the Swedish National Registry.[30] They found 19 cases (6.8%) with metastatic disease at diagnosis. In our review of 65 head and neck soft-tissue sarcomas treated primarily at the University of California, San Francisco (UCSF), four (6.1%) had distant metastases at presentation.

Hematogenous dissemination after diagnosis is common in high-grade lesions. Isolated pulmonary metastases are the most frequent, accounting for nearly 50% of all initial recurrence.[31] Bone, liver, and skin involvement occurred in less than 5% of patients.[32] Liposarcoma and retroperitoneal sarcomas display a different metastatic pattern. Although the lungs still predominate as a metastatic destination, liver involvement and peritoneal carcinomatosis do account for a small but significant number of deaths in these patients.[31,33] Approximately, 75% to 80% of distant metastases appear within 2 years of initial treatment.

Regional lymphatic dissemination is uncommon. In a comprehensive literature review, Weingrad observed a 5.8% incidence of nodal spread during the course of the disease.[34] Mazeron found that 5.9% of 323 patients without distant metastatic disease at presentation had nodal involvement.[35] There was a correlation between tumor grade and the frequency of nodal metastasis: 0% for grade 1, 2% for grade 2, and 12% for grade 3. Pooled data from published reports on 5257 patients treated for soft-tissue tumors showed a higher incidence of nodal spread in certain histologic subtypes: clear cell sarcoma (28%), epithelioid sarcoma (20%), angiosarcoma (23%), rhabdomyosarcoma (15%), and synovial sarcoma (14%).[35]

DIAGNOSTIC AND STAGING STUDIES

The history of patients suspected of having soft-tissue tumors should focus on the onset of symptoms, the rate of tumor progression, any evidence of neurovascular

bundle involvement, possible genetic predisposition (e.g., Li-Fraumeni syndrome, Gardner's syndrome, von Recklinghausen's disease) and history of past radiation exposure. The physical examination should detail the size and extent of the mass. Evidence of bony or neurovascular bundle invasion that may compromise the chance of performing an organ-sparing procedure should be assessed. Finally, a careful nodal evaluation should be carried out.

In addition to a thorough history and physical examination, a complete blood count and chemistry panels should be obtained to rule out occult metastases and to evaluate baseline organ functions for tolerance of future therapeutic treatments. An echocardiogram should be performed if the patient is being considered for Adriamycin-based chemotherapy.

Radiographic Imaging

Radiologic studies should preferentially be obtained before any surgical manipulation to avoid confusing postsurgical changes. Magnetic resonance imaging (MRI) is the preferred imaging modality for soft-tissue sarcomas because of its multiplanar imaging capability and superior soft-tissue contrast. Most musculoskeletal tumors have intermediate to low signal intensity in T1-weighted images and appear bright on T2-weighted images. Exceptions to these rules are tumors with high fat or blood product content such as liposarcomas and angiosarcomas, which appear as masses of high signal intensities on T1-weighted images (Fig. 58-4).[36] The use of contrast agents such as gadolinium has not been shown to improve the accuracy of tumor staging or lesion delineation.

Computed tomography (CT) remains the diagnostic modality of choice for detecting pulmonary metastases in high-grade tumors.[34] Yet the cost-effectiveness of routine chest CT for metastasis screening in patients with T1–2 soft-tissue sarcoma has been questioned. Fleming et al. showed that the routine use of chest CT in addition to a chest x-ray to screen for pulmonary metastasis in patients with T1 tumors of the extremity results in a substantial incremental cost of $2.9 million per case of pulmonary metastasis detected since less than 1% of the patients in

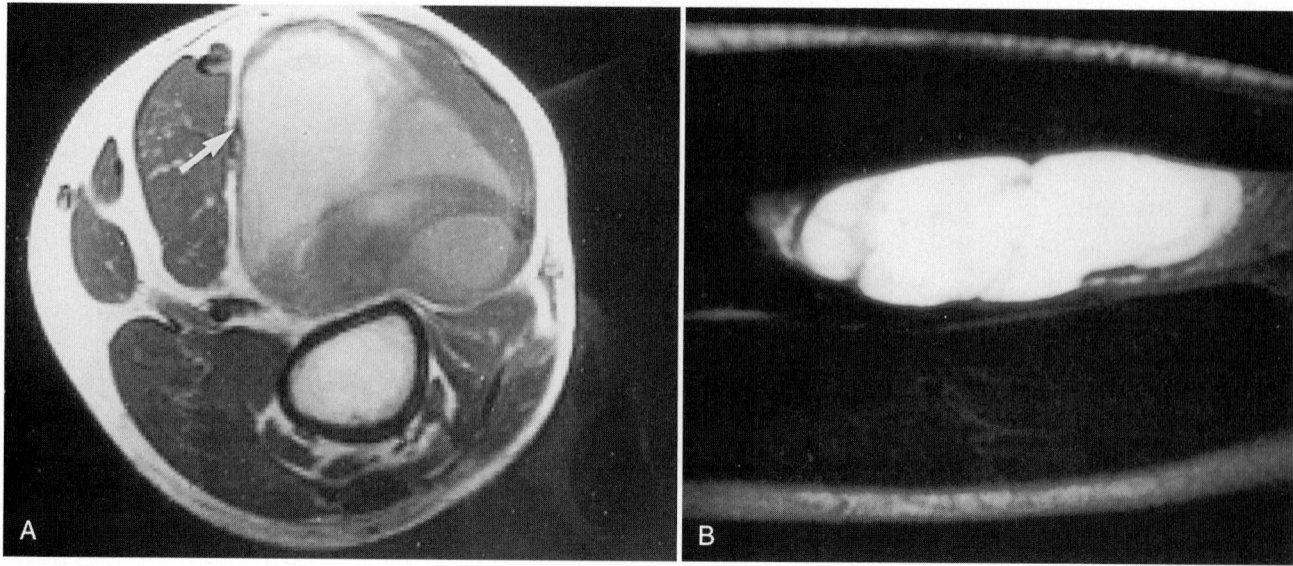

Figure 58–4. A, T1-weighted magnetic resonance image of a thigh liposarcoma: axial view. Note the high signal intensity of the tumor in relation to surrounding muscles. **B,** T2-weighted magnetic resonance image of the same thigh liposarcoma: coronal view. (Courtesy of Dr. Charles Peterfly, Dept. of Radiology, University of California at San Francisco.)

this group presented with lung metastasis at diagnosis.[37] Similarly Porter et al. found that the use of routine chest CT, when compared with selective CT, for evaluation of metastatic disease for T2 tumors is most cost-effective in patients with extremity and high-grade lesions.[38] For primary tumor evaluation, CT is a useful supplement to plain radiographs to evaluate for suspected bony invasion. Finally, CT is also widely used to image the tumor for three-dimensional treatment planning in radiation therapy.

Bone scans are not useful in the diagnostic workup of soft-tissue sarcomas. Bony metastases in the absence of visceral spread are rare. Bony invasion is best demonstrated by CT. Positron emission tomography (PET) scanning and magnetic resonance spectroscopy may help provide information on tumor metabolism and grade,[39] although the role of these studies is still undefined. Dimitrakopoulou-Strauss et al. studied the use of ^{18}F-FDG PET for the diagnosis of primary or recurrent soft-tissue sarcoma and found a sensitivity of 76%, specificity of 43%, and an accuracy of 68%.[40] It appeared to be most accurate in patients with high-grade tumors. Conrad et al. reported that the average standardized uptake values (SUV) obtained from PET scans were useful in differentiating high-grade and large tumors with high metabolism from low-grade and small tumors in 108 patients with bone sarcoma and soft-tissue sarcoma.[41] Finally, PET may serve as a useful predictor for response from neoadjuvant therapy. Schuetze et al. performed serial PET scans on 56 patients treated with two to three cycles of neoadjuvant Adriamycin-based chemotherapy. Patients with a greater than 50% reduction in maximal SUV had a longer time to recurrence (38 vs. 18 months, $P = 0.03$) and overall survival (not yet reached vs. 41 months, $P = 0.02$).[42]

Biopsy Considerations

Biopsy is a critical step in the evaluation of these neoplasms. Incisional biopsy is the preferred technique for diagnosis of most soft-tissue sarcomas. This technique involves a wedge removal of tissue with minimal surgical manipulation. The incision should be short, oriented in the same direction as the surrounding musculature, and situated so that it could easily be removed in future surgery without compromising limb-salvage or reconstructive options. Meticulous attention should be paid to hemostasis to prevent tumor dissemination by hematoma, and drains should not be used routinely. Occasionally, an excisional biopsy will suffice for lesions less than 3 cm in size, for which at least a 2-cm cuff of normal tissue around the tumor is resected. *True-cut core needle biopsy* is becoming an increasingly popular method for diagnosing soft-tissue tumors, particularly in situations where preoperative chemotherapy or radiotherapy or both are being considered for large accessible lesions.[43,44] Core needle biopsy and immunohistochemistry often confirm the diagnosis of sarcoma and shed light on the tumor grade even if exact classification of the tumor is not possible.[45] Many times this information is sufficient for clinicians to initiate preoperative therapy for high-grade tumors and resect the low-grade ones. Fine-needle aspiration is not routinely used to diagnose soft-tissue sarcomas due to the paucity of available tissues for examination and the loss of tissue architecture.

Histopathologic Studies

The pathologic evaluation of soft-tissue tumors should be carried out by an experienced pathologist due

Table 58–5   Commonly Used Immunohistochemical Antigens and Their Distribution in Normal Tissues and Soft-Tissue Tumors

Antigen	Cell Structure	Normal Tissue	Tumors
Vimentin	Intermediate filament	Most mesenchymal tissue	Almost all sarcomas, some carcinomas
Cytokeratin	Intermediate filament	Epithelium, mesothelium	Almost all carcinomas, some sarcomas (biphasic synovial sarcoma)
Desmin	Intermediate filament	Skeletal, cardiac, smooth muscles	Rhabdomyosarcoma, leiomyosarcoma, rare liposarcoma and malignant fibrous histiocytoma
Actin	Contractile protein	Skeletal, cardiac, smooth muscles, myofibroblasts, myoepithelium	Leiomyosarcoma, rhabdomyosarcoma, rare malignant fibrous histiocytoma
Myoglobin	Oxygen-binding protein	Skeletal muscles	Rhabdomyosarcoma
Factor VIII associated antigen	Antihemophilic factor	Vascular endothelium	Angiosarcoma, Kaposi's sarcoma
CD34	Cell surface protein	Hematopoietic stem cells, endothelium, dermal and periadnexal dendritic cells	Dermatofibroma protuberans, solitary fibrous tumors, spindle cell lipomas, gastrointestinal stromal tumors, epithelioid sarcoma, angiosarcomas
CD31	Membrane glycoprotein	Endothelium, hematopoietic cells	Angiosarcomas
S100	Cytoplasmic protein	Central nervous system, schwann cells, glial cells, chondrocytes, lipocytes	Malignant nerve sheath tumors, some chondrosarcomas, melanoma
Epithelial membrane antigen	Surface membrane glycoprotein	Epithelium, perineurium, meningothelial cells	Most carcinomas, biphasic synovial sarcomas and 50% monophasic ones, epithelioid sarcomas, mesotheliomas

to the vast diversity of sarcomas and their notoriety in mimicking other neoplasms. In addition to light microscopy, tools including electron microscopy, immunohistochemistry, cytogenetics, and molecular genetics are widely used to establish the diagnosis. Table 58-5 lists some commonly employed immunohistochemical antigens, their cellular origins, and distributions among certain types of soft-tissue sarcomas.

STAGING

The most frequently used staging system is that proposed by the American Joint Committee on Cancer (AJCC)[46] (Table 58-6). Table 58-7 summarizes the 5-year freedom from local recurrence, disease-free survival, and overall survival rates in more than 1000 patients treated at the Memorial Sloan-Kettering Cancer Center (MSKCC) by the new AJCC staging system. Histologic grade and tumor size are the primary determinants of clinical stage in the AJCC system. The T1 and T2 tumor sizes are further substaged based on tumor depth. Superficial tumors are defined as those located exclusively above the superficial fascia without fascial invasion and deep lesions are those that are deep to or invade or cross the investing fascia. For practical purposes, all retroperitoneal, visceral, mediastinal, intrathoracic, pelvic, and the majority of head and neck tumors are classified as deep lesions. The new staging system also accommodates a preferred "two-tiered" grading system (low vs. high grade). In the three-tiered system, grade 1 is considered "low grade" and grades 2 to 3,

"high grade." In the four-tiered system, grades 1 to 2 are considered "low grade" and grades 3 to 4, "high grade." The system is designed to stage extremity tumors optimally, but is also applicable to torso, head and neck, and retroperitoneal sarcomas. It should not be used to stage sarcomas arising within the confines of the dura mater, brain, parenchymatous organs and hollow viscera. All soft-tissue sarcoma histologies, including gastrointestinal stromal tumors and Ewing's sarcomas/primitive neuroectodermal tumors, are included except Kaposi's sarcomas, dermatofibrosarcoma protuberans, fibromatosis (desmoids), angiosarcomas, and malignant mesenchymomas.

A major pitfall of the current AJCC staging system is its failure to recognize the anatomic site of the tumor, which is an important determinant of prognosis. Although tumor site is not officially incorporated as a specific component of any present staging system, prospective data collection should include tumor site, and outcome data should be reported on a site-specific basis. The recommended groupings for tumor sites are: head and neck, extremity and superficial trunk, gastrointestinal, genitourinary, visceral, retroperitoneal, gynecological, breast, lung/pleural/mediastinal, and others.[46]

PROGNOSTIC FACTORS

Different prognostic factors exist for local recurrence, distant recurrence, and survival in patients with soft-tissue sarcoma. In a large analysis of prognostic factors in 1041 patients with extremity soft-tissue sarcoma,

Table 58–6 Classification of Soft-Tissue Sarcomas

Primary Tumor (T)

TX	Primary tumor cannot be assessed
T0	No evidence of primary tumor
T1	Tumor ≤5 cm in greatest dimension
T1a	Superficial
T1b	Deep
T2	Tumor >5 cm in greatest dimension
T2a	Superficial
T2b	Deep

Lymph Node (N)

NX	Regional lymph nodes cannot be assessed
N0	No regional lymph node metastasis
N1	Regional lymph node metastasis (presence of N1 is considered stage IV)

Distant Metastasis (M)

MX	Distant metastasis cannot be assessed
M0	No distant metastasis
M1	Distant metastasis

Histopathologic Grade (G)

GX	Grade cannot be assessed
G1	Well-differentiated
G2	Moderately differentiated
G3	Poorly differentiated
G4	Poorly differentiated or undifferentiated (4-tiered system only)

	Stage Grouping			4-tiered system	3-tiered system	2-tiered system
I	Any T (All tumors, low grade)	N0	M0	G1–2	G1	Low
II	T1a, 1b, 2a (All small tumors or large superficial tumors, high grade)	N0	M0	G3–4	G2–3	High
III	T2b (Large, deep tumors, high grade)	N0	M0	G3–4	G2–3	High
IV	Any T	N1	M0	Any G	Any G	High or low
	Any T (Nodal or distant metastasis)	Any N	M1	Any G	Any G	High or low

From Greene LG, Page DL, Fleming ID, et al., eds. *AJCC Cancer Staging Manual*. 6th ed. New York: Springer; 2002.

tumor grade, tumor size, and deep location were the strongest prognostic factors for disease-specific survival (Table 58-8).[47] These three factors were also confirmed independently by the FNCLCC study of 546 patients with soft-tissue sarcoma of the extremities, head and neck, trunk, pelvis, and retroperitoneum.[48] Other reported, unconfirmed prognostic factors for survival are gender, leiomyosarcoma or malignant peripheral nerve

Table 58–7 Five-Year Survival Rates in Extremity Soft-Tissue Sarcomas*

Stage	Patients, n	% FFLR	% DFS	% OS
I	137	88	86	90
II	491	82	72	81
III	469	83	52	56

*Source: Memorial Sloan-Kettering Cancer Center, July 1982 through June 2000. DFS, disease-free survival; FFLR, freedom from local recurrence; OS, overall survival.
From Greene LG, Page DL, Fleming ID, et al, eds. *AJCC Cancer Staging Manual*. 6th ed. New York: Springer; 2002.

sheath tumor, microscopically involved margins, no adjuvant chemotherapy, local recurrence at presentation, and lower extremity site.

For distant recurrence, tumor grade, tumor size, and deep location were significant prognostic factors in both large studies mentioned earlier (see Table 58-8). In addition, leiomyosarcoma or nonliposarcoma histology, local recurrence, and no adjuvant chemotherapy also appeared to impact the risk of distant metastasis to a lesser degree.

Unlike other solid tumors, local control appears to be influenced by a separate set of prognostic factors, different from those that predict survival and distant metastasis. Pisters et al. found that age older than 50 or local recurrence at diagnosis, microscopically involved surgical margins, fibrosarcoma, or peripheral nerve sheath tumor histology adversely influenced local control in 1041 patients treated for extremity soft-tissue sarcoma.[47] Approximately 40% of these patients received adjuvant radiotherapy and 23% had microscopic residual disease. In a different group of patients, including those with tumors outside the extremities, of whom 58% had adjuvant radiotherapy and only 69% had complete surgery,

Table 58–8 Prognostic Factors for Mortality, Distant Metastasis, and Local Recurrence in Soft-Tissue Sarcomas

Endpoint	Prognostic Factor	MSKCC[47]		FNCLCC[48]	
		Relative Risk	*P Value*	*Relative Risk*	*P Value*
Mortality (disease specific or overall)	Grade	4.0	0.0001	2.8	3×10^{-10}
	Size	2.1 (>10 cm)	0.0001	2.0 (≥5 cm)	0.004
	Depth	2.8	0.0002	2.1	0.005
	Recurrent*	1.5	0.0033		
	Lower extremity site	1.6	0.02		
	Leiomyosarcoma	1.9	0.01		
	MPNST	1.9	0.008		
	Male sex			1.9	0.00002
	Adjuvant chemotherapy			0.48	0.00005
Distant metastasis	Grade	4.3	0.0001	2.8	4×10^{-12}
	Size	1.9 (>5 cm)	0.0001	1.6 (>10 cm)	0.001
	Depth	2.5	0.0007	2.3	0.001
	Recurrent*	1.5	0.02		
	Liposarcoma	0.64	0.003		
	MPNST	1.7	0.02		
	Adjuvant chemotherapy			0.55	0.0006
	Surgical margin	1.8 (microscopic)	0.0001	2.0 (any residual)	0.0002
Local recurrence	Age older than 50	1.6	0.001		
	Recurrent*	2.0	0.0001		
	Fibrosarcoma	2.5	0.006		
	MPNST	1.8	0.001		
	Adjuvant radiotherapy			0.42	0.000004
	Grade			1.8	0.0002
	Depth			1.8	0.01

*Recurrent disease at presentation.

FNCLCC, French Federation of Cancer Centers Sarcoma Group; MPNST, malignant peripheral nerve sheath tumor; MSKCC, Memorial Sloan-Kettering Cancer Center.

Coindre et al. found that poor surgery (defined as local excision only), no adjuvant radiotherapy, grade 3, and deep location were adverse predictors for local control.[48]

Although rare, the presence of nodal metastasis is associated with poorer survival. Mazeron and Suit found that only 32% of patients with nodal involvement at presentation were alive more than 58 months after treatment.[35]

The location of primary tumors often influences the resectability of the lesion and the ability to deliver high dose radiation. Sarcomas of the head and neck, mediastinum, and retroperitoneum are more difficult to control locally due to their proximity to critical organs. Retroperitoneal sarcomas are often very large at the time of diagnosis. These adverse factors are reflected in the lower survival rates for patients with these tumors as compared to those found in the extremities.[23,49]

There is evidence that the status of surgical margins influences local control. Tanabe et al. reported a 5-year local disease-free survival of 91% for margin-negative patients, and 62% for margin-positive patients (P = 0.005).[50] Similarly, Suit et al. found that the 5-year local control rate for patients with negative margins was 97% compared to 81% for those with positive margins.[51] Interestingly, local control appears to be independent of the degree of margin negativity (negative at ≤1 mm or >1 mm). It is controversial whether tumor involvement at the surgical margins affects survival. Tanabe et al. reported similar 5-year survival rates for margin-negative

(65%) and margin-positive patients (70%), despite a higher local failure rate in the latter group.[50] However, Heslin et al. reported that a positive microscopic margin in patients with high risk soft-tissue sarcoma (high grade, deep, or ≥5 cm) is a predictor for biologically aggressive tumors and is associated with poorer survival.[52]

It is controversial whether achievement of local control after the first treatment affects long-term survival. Tanabe et al. found that local failure did not adversely affect overall survival.[50] They did emphasize that their number of local recurrences was too small to make a definite conclusion. In an NCI prospective randomized trial comparing amputation to limb-sparing surgery with radiotherapy, Rosenberg found no difference in survivals between the two groups, despite a higher local recurrence rate in the combined modality therapy arm.[53] In a prospective randomized study to evaluate the effectiveness of adjuvant brachytherapy (BRT) at MSKCC, Harrison et al. demonstrated an improvement in local control for patients with high-grade tumors receiving additional radiation. Unfortunately, this advantage in local control was not associated with an improvement in survival.[54] However, many other authors have concluded that local recurrences have a negative impact on survival.[31,55-57] Despite the difficulty in defining a relationship between local control and survival, every effort should be made to prevent local recurrences since salvage therapy often requires more mutilating surgery than would have been needed initially.

Attention is now focusing on molecular pathological prognostic factors. Ki-67, an antigenic measurement for cell proliferation, was shown to be an independent prognostic factor for soft-tissue sarcoma in at lease three separate studies.[58-60] Data on the underlying prognostic significance of *P53* and *MDM2* status are conflicting. Some investigators reported no independent adverse prognostic significance by regression analysis,[58] while others found a highly significant correlation with outcomes.[61] Plasma metalloprotease-9 (MMP) activity was shown to be elevated in patients with soft-tissue sarcoma when compared to healthy volunteers or patients with benign tumors in a small study.[62] In addition, MMP-9 circulating activity was decreased in nine patients after successful surgery and increased in three patients with relapsed tumor, suggesting that it may be a potential marker for tumor surveillance.

In synovial sarcomas, the t(X;18)(p11;q11) translocation fuses the *SYT* gene from chromosome 18 to either of two homologous genes at *Xp11*, *SSX1*, or *SSX2*. The fusion transcripts (*SYT-SSX1* or *SYT-SSX2*) are believed to function as aberrant transcriptional regulators. In a study of 45 patients, there was a significant correlation between histologic subtype and fusion transcript; all 12 biphasic tumors had *SYT-SSX1* fusion whereas only 17 (52%) of 33 monophasic tumors had the same transcript. Moreover, the presence of *STY-SSX1* transcript was associated with worse survival in this patient group.[63] This is an exciting observation suggesting that these fusion transcripts can be used as a prognostic marker for synovial sarcoma; however, these findings need to be confirmed in larger studies.

GENERAL MANAGEMENT

Surgery

Enneking and colleagues have defined four categories of surgical procedures used in the treatment of soft-tissue sarcomas based on surgical margins[64]:

1. *Intralesional biopsy*: As described earlier, this involves the removal of a portion of tumor through the pseudocapsule for diagnostic purposes. Gross residual tumor remains, and there is potential for contamination of surrounding tissues at the time of the procedure.
2. *Excisional biopsy*: The tumor and its pseudocapsule are removed. It is synonymous with marginal excision or "shelling out." There is potential for leaving microaggregates of tumor behind as well as contaminating the surrounding areas.
3. *Wide excision*: This involves resection of the tumor with a 2- to 3-cm rim of surrounding normal tissue. If an incisional biopsy was performed previously, the biopsy scar and crater should be excised. Microscopic disease may be left behind, but near normal functions are maintained by preserving muscles, neurovascular bundles, and bones.
4. *Radical local resection*: The tumor and all structures within the same anatomic compartment are extirpated en bloc. When the lesion is within an intrafascial compartment, surgery involves the removal of all musculoaponeurotic structures from the origin to the insertion as well as the neurovascular bundles, bones, or joint contained within the compartment. Amputation is included in this category for large extracompartmental lesions.

Traditionally, surgical resection has been the main treatment modality for soft-tissue sarcoma of all sites. Until the early 1950s, the surgical approach was a local excision or amputation. The local failure rate for local excision ranged from 60% to 90%.[65-67] Attempts to reduce local failures led to the introduction of radical soft-tissue compartmental resection (including amputation) in the 1960s. The local control rate increased to the 80% to 90% range at the expense of limb function.[68,69] Table 58-9 shows the local recurrence rates reported in the literature for different types of surgical procedures.

Radiation Therapy

RADIATION ALONE

Historically, the use of radiation treatment was limited to patients with locally advanced, inoperable, recurrent, or metastatic disease. The dose of radiation was usually low, and was reserved mainly for palliation. In 1951, Cade reported long-term disease-free survival (5 to 26 years) for 6 of 22 patients with unresectable tumors treated by radiation alone.[70] Between 1935 and 1959, McNeer et al. treated 25 patients with radiation alone at MSKCC.[71] Fourteen survived without disease for more than 5 years. Tepper and Suit reported on 51 patients treated with primary radiation at the Massachusetts General Hospital (MGH).[72] The overall 5-year survival and local control rates were 25% and 33%, respectively. For those who

Table 58–9 Local Recurrence for Different Types of Surgical Procedure

Author	Yr	Local Excision		Wide Excision		Radical Excision or Amputation	
		n	% LR	*n*	% LR	*n*	% LR
Shieber and Graham[67]	1962	46	87	23	39	ND	ND
Gerner et al[176]	1975	58	93	47	66	38	8
Markhede et al[66]	1982	19	74	ND	ND	78	9
Leibel et al[91]	1982	20	70	ND	ND	27	18

LR, local recurrence; ND, no data.

received a dose ≥64 Gy, the 5-year survival and local control rates were 28% and 44%, respectively. A 67% local control rate has also been observed in patients treated palliatively with fast neutron therapy.[73] These results indicate that patients may be cured by radiation alone if high doses are employed. The results also imply that sarcomas are not as radioresistant as previously thought. Primary radiation should be reserved for patients with unresectable lesions due to anatomic location, medical inoperability, or refusal to undergo surgery.

COMBINED CONSERVATIVE SURGERY AND RADIATION THERAPY

In 1951, Cade obtained a 61% survival rate in patients with wide excision and radiation therapy, compared to 27% with amputation with or without radiation.[70] He advocated combining radiation with surgery. In the 1960s, Suit investigated the role of radiation as an adjunct to limb-sparing surgery in an effort to preserve function and to reduce recurrence.[74] For the first 57 patients treated, a local control rate of 87% was achieved, comparable to that with radical resections. Between 1975 and 1981, the NCI conducted a prospective randomized study in which 43 patients with high-grade lesions of the extremities were randomized to either amputation or limb-sparing surgery with adjuvant radiation therapy. The radiation dose was 50 Gy to the anatomic area at risk, and 60 to 70 Gy to the tumor bed, delivered via a shrinking field technique. All patients had postoperative chemotherapy consisting of Adriamycin, Cytoxan, and high-dose methotrexate. With the median follow-up of 4 years and 10 months, none of the 16 tumors of patients undergoing amputation recurred locally. Four of 27 patients randomized to the limb-sparing arm relapsed locally. However, there was no difference in disease-free survival and overall survival

between the two arms. It was concluded that limb-sparing procedures in combination with radiation are effective for most patients with soft-tissue sarcomas, a practice widely in use at present.[53] The results of this small randomized trial, coupled with large reports from numerous institutions,[75-78] provided the impetus for the National Institutes of Health to publish a consensus statement recommending limb-sparing procedures.[79]

Many different strategies have been used to combine radiation and surgery. These included preoperative radiation, postoperative radiation, or intraoperative radiation with either BRT or electron beam techniques (IORT). The theoretic advantages and disadvantages of these treatment strategies are outlined in Table 58-10. Table 58-11 shows the results of the published randomized studies evaluating surgery alone versus surgery plus radiotherapy for local control in soft-tissue sarcoma. Although there was no direct comparison between postoperative external beam radiotherapy and BRT, the results suggest that both are equally effective for high-grade tumors, while external beam irradiation appeared to be more useful for local control in low-grade tumors. Controversies exist regarding the timing of delivering external beam irradiation in relation to surgery (i.e., whether it should be in the preoperative or postoperative settings). Recently, the National Cancer Institute of Canada (NCIC) conducted a randomized trial comparing these two approaches in patients with extremity soft-tissue sarcoma who would need combined surgery and radiotherapy. The trial was closed when an interim analysis showed a higher rate of acute wound complication with preoperative radiotherapy (35% vs. 17%).[80] However, there was no difference in function at 1 year of follow-up and an unexplained survival advantage with preoperative radiotherapy, presumably from less distant metastasis (Fig. 58-5). To date, there has been no difference in local control between the two strategies. At

Table 58–10 Advantages and Disadvantages of Different Combined Treatment Approaches

Treatment	Advantages	Disadvantages
1. Preoperative radiation	a. Smaller treatment volume b. Decreases risk of surgical implant or dissemination c. Smaller surgery d. Increases tumor resectability	a. Delay of surgery b. Delay of wound healing c. Diagnosis based on a small tissue specimen d. Need to rely on good radiographic images and physical examination to assess tumor extent
2. Postoperative radiation	a. Immediate surgery b. Tumor extent assessed directly with open surgery c. Larger specimen for pathologic diagnosis d. No radiation-induced wound healing delay	a. Larger treatment volume b. Delay of radiation
3. Brachytherapy/Intraoperative radiation	a. Radiation applied directly to tumor bed b. Minimizes radiation damage to surrounding tissue c. No delay in radiation to allow for tumor repopulation and hypoxia d. Shortens treatment time with possible cost reduction	a. Needs local expertise in IORT or brachytherapy b. Requires close cooperation between surgeon and oncologist c. Treatment volume is limited to direct tumor bed d. Radiation exposure to hospital staff.

IORT, intraoperative radiotherapy with electron beam techniques.

Table 58–11   Phase III Randomized, Controlled Trials in the Local Management of Soft-Tissue Sarcomas

Center	Period	Site	Schema	Grade	Patients, n	% Local Recurrence
NCI[53]	1975-1982	Extremity	Amputation vs. surg + EBRT	All	16	0
					27	15
NCI[81]	1983-1991	Extremity	Surg vs. surg + EBRT	High	44	20
					47	0
				Low	24	33
					26	4
MSKCC[114]	1982-1992	Extremity, trunk	Surg vs. surg + BRT	High	63	30
					56	9
				Low	23	26
					22	36
CSG/NCIC CTG[99]	1994-1997	Extremity	Pre- vs. post-operative EBRT		84	
					92	

BRT, brachytherapy; CSG/NCIC CTG, Canadian Sarcoma Group and NCI Canada Clinical Trials Group Study; EBRT, external beam radiotherapy; MSKCC, Memorial Sloan-Kettering Cancer Center; Surg, surgery; NCI, National Cancer Institute.

UCSF and Stanford, our policy is to employ preoperative external beam radiation for large (usually >5 cm) or unresectable lesions followed by IORT or BRT boost for microscopically positive margins. If gross residual disease remains and normal tissue tolerance has not been reached, external beam radiation delivered via three-dimensional treatment planning techniques can also be used to boost the tumor bed. For most small, resectable tumors, wide local excisions are performed followed by postoperative external beam radiotherapy. Again, IORT or BRT may be employed as a boost. We also use BRT, usually low dose rate, for recurrent disease in patients who had received radiation in the past. Chemotherapy is reserved for those with high-grade neoplasms.

The role of radiotherapy for small low-grade tumors is controversial. A small randomized study[81] and at least one retrospective study[82] suggested a local control benefit with the addition of postoperative radiotherapy, at least in larger tumors (>5 cm) with close surgical margins. Other studies indicated that in a subset of well-selected patients, radiotherapy may be omitted without compromising local control.[83-85] We do not typically recommend postoperative irradiation for small lesions that have been widely removed with negative margins since many are cured with surgery alone. Radiation therapy is used in patients with positive or close margins or in those with large tumors where local recurrence would require amputation.

RADIATION THERAPY TECHNIQUES

Close cooperation among the surgeon, radiation oncologist, medical oncologist, radiologist, pathologist, and physiotherapist is required for the management of

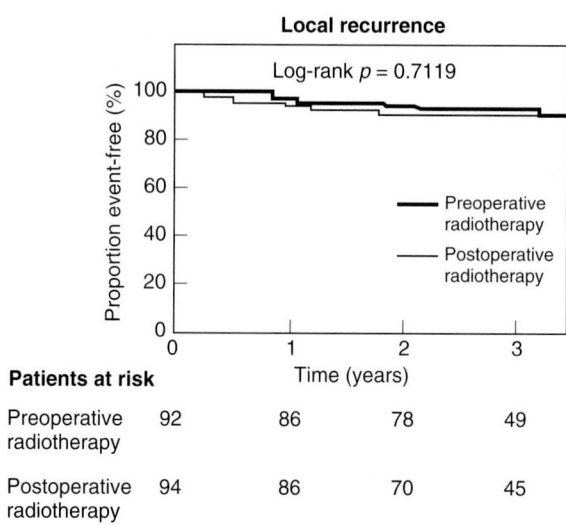
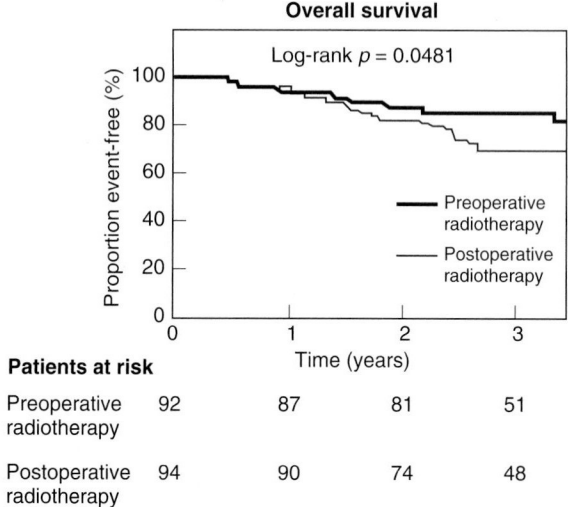

Figure 58–5. Local relapse-free survival and overall survival in patients treated with either preoperative or postoperative radiotherapy for soft-tissue sarcomas greater than 5 cm—Results from a phase III randomized study. (Adapted from O'Sullivan B, Davis AM, Turcotte R, et al: Preoperative versus postoperative radiotherapy in soft tissue sarcoma of the limbs: A randomized trial. *Lancet.* 2002;359:2235.)

soft-tissue sarcomas. Treatment planning mandates a thorough knowledge of the anatomy involved. The radiation oncologist should attempt to define a target volume before surgery from imaging studies and physical examination. Surgeons should be reminded to place metallic clips at the outer margins of the surgical field and the tumor bed to facilitate adequate coverage of the volume by radiation. The radiation oncologist should review the pathologic material and operative findings, including the tumor's location in relationship to the neurovascular bundles and bone, the presence of satellite nodules, the status of surgical margins, and the location of residual disease, if present. Radiation therapy, if given postoperatively, should start 10 to 20 days following surgery to allow time for sufficient healing. If radiation is delivered preoperatively, surgery should follow after an interval of 2½ to 3 weeks.

Simulation and Field Size

During simulation, the optimal position for the patient is determined. This involves rotating the extremity in order to treat the affected compartment while minimizing dose to surrounding tissues. Part of the thigh can be treated in the frog leg position. Elevation of one leg above the other allows for treatment of the posterior compartment. The "throwing" position,[86] which consists of abduction of the shoulder joint and flexion of the elbow joint, is an ideal position for treating part of the upper arms. Occasionally, patients may be treated in a sitting position while resting their extremities on the treatment couch. The lithotomy position is useful for treating perineal sarcomas, while prone positions are occasionally used for retroperitoneal lesions to minimize radiation exposure to the small bowel. Positioning of the patient can sometimes be difficult due to postsurgical fibrosis.

To ensure treatment reproducibility, the area treated should be immobilized. We employ devices such as a foam cradle (Fig. 58-6) or thermoplastic cast to provide special immobilization for individual patients.

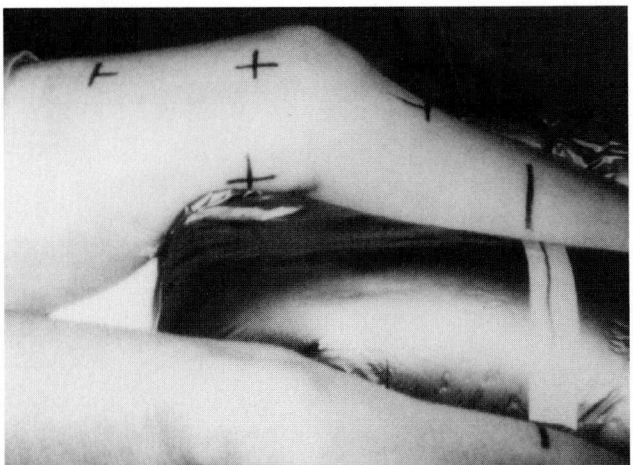

Figure 58–6. Foam cradle used to immobilize the lower extremity of a patient with a liposarcoma involving the distal posterior thigh compartment with surgical violation of the knee joint space.

CT treatment planning should be used in treating soft-tissue sarcoma. One must make sure that the CT is performed in the treatment position. In the preoperative setting, the gross tumor volume (GTV) typically represents the radiographically defined tumor. Peritumoral edema should be included when preoperative irradiation is given. Strictly speaking, there should not be a GTV for the postoperative setting. However, it is useful to designate a putative GTV for cone-down purposes. This GTV should encompass all the tissues handled during the surgery, including all tumor-related scars and draining sites. The optimal longitudinal margins that should be included around the GTV (i.e., the CTV or clinical target volume) is an area of controversy. At the MD Anderson Hospital (MDAH), a 5-cm longitudinal margin is used for grade 1 sarcomas, and a 7-cm margin is employed for grade 2 to 3 lesions (Matt Ballo, MD, personal communication).[87] No attempt is made to encompass the entire anatomic compartment. The large field is treated to a total dose of 50 Gy, followed by a boost field encompassing the primary lesion with 3- to 4-cm margins. The practice at MGH is to use ≤5 cm margins for small grade 1 tumors, 5- to 10-cm margins for large grade 1 and small grade 2 to 3 tumors, and 10- to 15-cm margins for larger high-grade lesions.[88] Again, a shrinking field technique is used with the large field size treated for the first 5 weeks, followed by field reductions at the sixth and the seventh week. At the NCI, initial radiation portals are designed to treat the muscle group from origin to insertion followed by shrinking volume as described.[89] The treatment policy at the Princess Margaret Hospital has been to place a field margin of 5 cm around the GTV, including any peritumoral edema, regardless of grade or size of the tumor.[90] At UCSF and Stanford, we generally follow the recommendation from MDAH and MGH. A 7- to 10-cm margin is used for large, high-grade tumors, and a margin of 5 cm is given for small low-grade lesions without attempting to cover the entire muscle compartment. In most cases, we use three-dimensional treatment planning to guide our field arrangement (Figs. 58-7 and 58-8). Since the incidence of nodal involvement is low, we do not recommend routine nodal prophylaxis. However, in the case of epithelioid sarcoma, clear cell sarcoma, high grade rhabdomyosarcoma, and synovial sarcoma, regional nodal treatment should be considered.

Circumferential irradiation of the extremity can result in severe fibrosis with pain, edema, and loss of function, which may necessitate amputation.[74] This should be avoided by sparing as many of the soft-tissue compartments as possible without missing the tumor bed. A portion of the circumference of the uninvolved bone should be spared to reduce the risk of a radiation-induced fracture. If the scar crosses the joint, part of the joint should be blocked out unless the joint space was violated surgically. A bolus should be placed over the surgical scar when it is not located in the tangential part of the beams to ensure adequate skin dose for the first part of treatment. Gonadal shielding should be considered in the treatment of thigh, groin, or pelvic lesions. If long fields are required, they must be gapped, and the match line needs to be moved weekly to avoid excessive hot or cold spots. Wedge filters and compensators should be

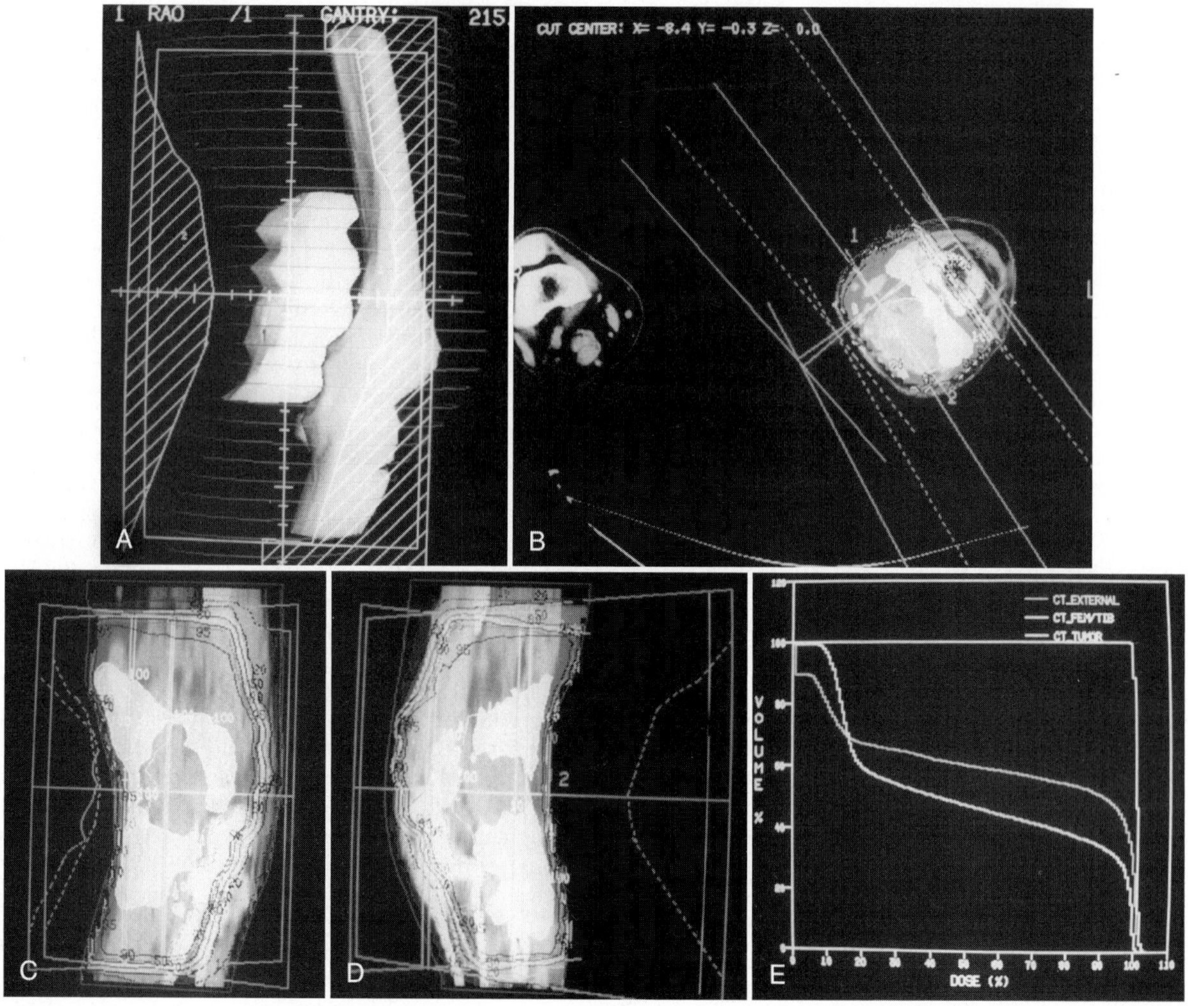

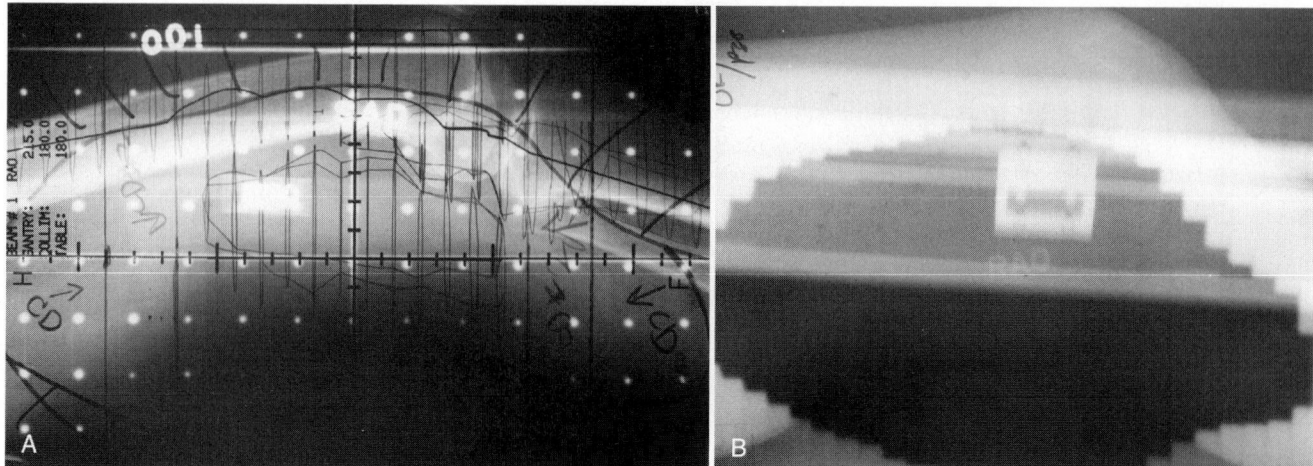

Figure 58–7. Computed tomography-based three-dimensional treatment plan using a right anterior oblique (RAO) and a left posterior oblique (LPO) field for the patient in Figure 58-6. **A,** Beam's eye view of the RAO field showing the tumor volume (*in pink*), the femur, the knee joint, the tibia (*in yellow*), and the computer-generated blocks (*in green*). **B,** Isodose distribution in relation to the tumor volume (*white line*) and surrounding structure—axial view, coronal view, and sagittal view. Note that the 95% isodose line (*in red*) encompasses all tumor volume. **C,** Dose volume histogram for the tumor volume (*white*), the surrounding skin (*green*), and adjacent bones (*yellow*) generated by three-dimensional computed tomography treatment planning. By using the plan, 40% to 60% of adjacent normal tissues will receive a full dose and the rest will receive 0% to 20% of the treatment dose from scatter radiation. See also Color Figure 58-7.

Figure 58–8. Simulation and port films of the right anterior oblique field for the patient in Figures 58-6 and 58-7. Note the sparing of the anterior half of the skin, knee joint, and bones.

employed regularly in treatment planning to enhance dose homogeneity.

RADIATION DOSE

In the past, sarcomas were thought to be radioresistant. Clinical and laboratory data have indicated otherwise. The radiation sensitivity of cell lines derived from human sarcomas appears to be the same as that for epithelial tumors.[51] In a retrospective study of 65 primary head and neck soft-tissue sarcomas at our institution, a dose-response relationship according to surgical margin status could not be demonstrated. Similarly, our review of extremity sarcomas failed to show a dose-response relationship.[91] In the 1970s, the MDAH reduced its total postoperative dose from 70 Gy to 60 Gy for low-grade lesions, and 65 Gy for high-grade lesions without an increased incidence of local recurrence.[77] At the NCI, a postoperative tumor dose of 63 Gy at 1.8 Gy per day is recommended. A dose of 70 to 75 Gy is used for gross residual disease.[89] At the MGH, preoperative radiation is advocated for large tumors. A dose of 50 Gy in 5 weeks is administered, followed by a 2 $\frac{1}{2}$ - to 3-week rest period before surgical resection. A boost of 15 Gy is given for microscopically positive margins, and 25 Gy is used for gross residual disease, delivered by external beam radiation, intraoperative electron beam radiation, or BRT. If administered postoperatively, 50 Gy is given to the large volume, followed by two field reductions to deliver a total dose of 60 Gy for negative margins, 66 Gy for microscopic residual disease, and 75 Gy for gross residual disease. The total dose is reduced by 10% in patients who also receive Adriamycin-based chemotherapy.[88] Our treatment policy at UCSF and Stanford is similar to that of the MGH. If radiation is to be given with Adriamycin, the starting time is delayed for 3 to 4 days after drug administration. The doses used in the treatment of sites other than the extremities, such as the head and neck, and the retroperitoneum, will depend on the volume of treatment and radiation tolerance of surrounding critical tissues.

BRACHYTHERAPY

At many institutions, BRT is generally used as a boost or for treatment of recurrent tumors following surgical re-resection for patients who have failed prior external beam irradiation. At MSKCC, BRT administered through afterloading catheters can be used either alone as definitive postoperative treatment for high-grade lesions or in combination with external beam radiotherapy in patients with multiple close or involved surgical margins, suboptimal dosimetry, or gross residual disease. The American Brachytherapy Society has published a comprehensive guideline and recommendations on the use of BRT for soft-tissue sarcoma.[92] Figure 58-9 shows catheter placements as recommended by the society. The target area, which includes the tumor bed plus a 2- to 3-cm margin, is defined intraoperatively by the radiation oncologist and the surgeon and should be delineated with radiopaque markers such as surgical clips. Afterloading catheters are placed percutaneously at 1- to 1.5-cm intervals, sutured in the target region to either underlying

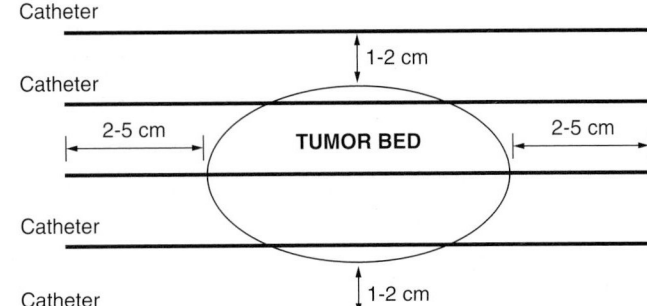

Figure 58–9. Recommended catheter placement and clinical target volume (CTV) for brachytherapy for soft-tissue sarcoma. Catheters are placed 1 to 2 cm beyond the lateral edge of the CTV and 2 to 5 cm beyond the CTV in the longitudinal direction. (Adapted with permission from Nag S, Shasha D, Janjan N, et al: The American Brachytherapy Society Recommendations for Brachytherapy of Soft Tissue Sarcomas. *Int J Radiat Oncol Biol Phys.* 2001;49:1033.)

fascia or muscles, and fixed to skin with buttons and silk sutures (Fig. 58-10). The skin entry point should be at least 1 cm away from the incision with consideration given to the ease of catheter loading. Whenever possible, normal structures at risk such as nerve bundles should be identified and marked with radiopaque markers different from those used to identify the target volume. Efforts should also be made to minimize doses to the nearby critical structures not directly involved with tumor by placing biodegradable spacers such as gelfoam layers between the catheters and these structures. The surgeon then places a drain in the implanted area and closes the skin. Care should be taken to ensure that the incision can be closed without tension to the wound. Plastic or metal wire inserts should be maintained within the catheter lumens until the treatment time to minimize the risk of catheter bending. Intraoperative radiographic localization is necessary if catheter movement after placement is suspected.

Generally, single plane implants are preferred because of less morbidity. If the implant crosses a joint, care must be taken to consider the postoperative position that

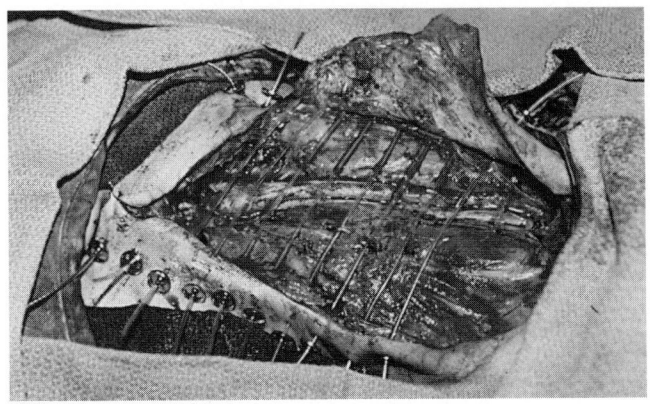

Figure 58–10. Brachytherapy using ^{192}Ir afterloading catheters for treatment of a recurrent malignant fibrous histiocytoma after the resection. A series of parallel catheters are inserted 1 cm apart percutaneously and secured onto the tumor bed with sutures and skin buttons.

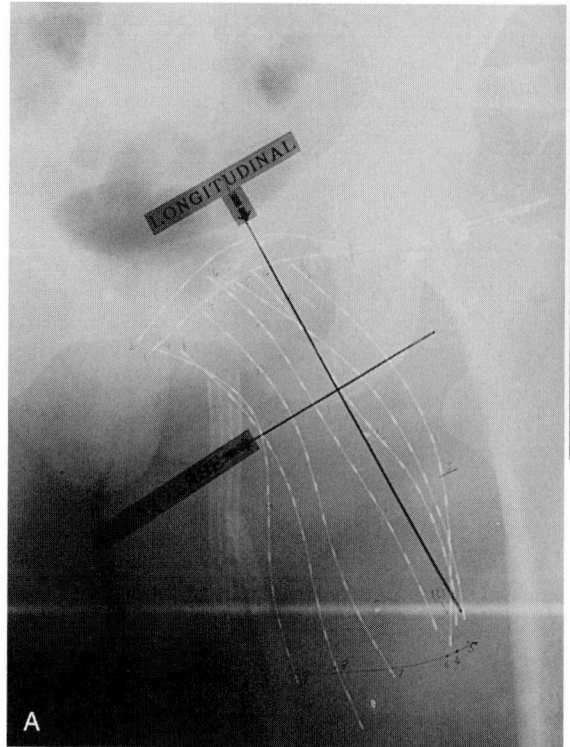

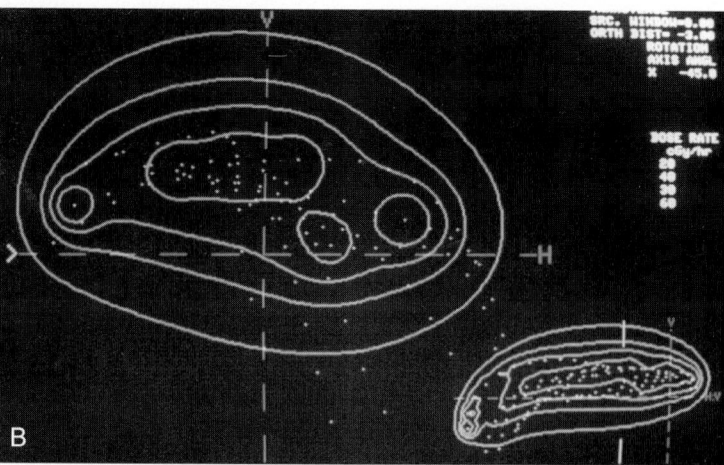

Figure 58-11. A, Anterior-posterior localization film for a different patient treated for a recurrent malignant fibrous histiocytoma of the proximal thigh and groin. **B,** Isodose distribution in a transverse central plane (large inset), and a longitudinal plane (small inset) of the implant. The outermost line represents 20cGy/hr isodose line, the next line: 30cGy/hr, the third line: 40cGy/hr, and the innermost line: 60cGy/hr. See also Color Figure 58-11B.

would minimize catheter movement if the limb is casted or braced into a position different from that of the time of implantation. In the retroperitoneal location, tissue expanders or peritoneal slings should be used by the surgeon to keep small bowels away from the implanted tumor bed.

On the first postoperative day, localization films are taken with dummy seeds within the catheters and computerized dosimetry performed (Fig. 58-11). If the orthogonal radiographic technique is used, a third film at a different angle should be taken to verify and improve delineation of source localization. Placement of a skin grid or radiopaque skin mark helps to define the skin dose. Catheters are loaded with ^{192}Ir between day 5 and day 14

to permit adequate wound healing if BRT is used as adjuvant monotherapy. However, the radioactive source can be loaded sooner (2 to 3 days after surgery) if BRT is used as a boost and the total BRT dose is ≤20 Gy. Times longer than 7 days can be associated with a higher risk of infection. Approximately 15 to 25 Gy at 40 to 50 cGy/hour can be safely given as a boost treatment. Alternatively, a dose of 45 Gy over 4 to 6 days, which is equivalent to 60 Gy of external beam radiation, is used for definitive postoperative radiation therapy or for the treatment of recurrent sarcomas. Loading of the catheters can be accomplished using standard iridium seeds, or afterloading iridium with the pulsed Selectron or fractionated high dose rate (HDR) BRT approach. Table 58-12 shows the

Table 58-12   Treatment Modalities Applicable for Brachytherapy of Soft-Tissue Sarcomas in Various Clinical Situations

Clinical Situation	LDR ^{192}Ir only	LDR ^{92}Ir + EBRT	Fx. HDR Only	Fx. HDR + EBRT	IOHDR +EBRT	IORT + EBRT
High grade, neg. or close margins	++	++	+	+	+	+
Low grade; neg. or close margins	-	+	-	+	+	+
Positive margin, all grade	-	++	-	+	-	-
Gross residual disease	+	++	-	+	-	-
Small volume recurrence	++	++	0	+	+	+
Large volume recurrence	-	++	-	+	+	+
Pediatric, small volume disease	++	+	++	0	+	+
Pediatric, extensive disease	-	++	-	++	++	++

++, recommended; +, used; 0, insufficient data; -, not recommended; EBRT, external beam radiotherapy; Fx, fractionated; HDR, high dose rate; IOHDR, intraoperative high dose rate; IORT, intraoperative radiotherapy (electron beam or orthovoltage); LDR, low dose rate; neg., negative.
Adapted and modified from Nag S, Shasha D, Janjan N, et al: The American Brachytherapy Society recommendations for brachytherapy of soft tissue sarcomas. *Int J Radiat Oncol Biol Phys.* 2001;49:1033.

BRT modalities considered applicable by the American Brachytherapy Society in various clinical situations.

Intraoperative high dose rate (IOHDR) BRT has been used as an alternative to low dose rate (LDR) BRT, fractionated HDR, or IORT. The IOHDR applicator, composed of Silastic, silicone, foam, or delcrin material, should be appropriate for the tumor bed. Delcrin is the most rigid material and more suitable for flat surfaces, whereas foam has the most flexibility, and the Silastic or silicone applicators (an example of which is the Harrison-Anderson-Mick or HAM applicator) have intermediate flexibility. The implant device is secured to the tumor bed with sutures without intervening air gap or fluid. Whenever possible, radiographs with dummy sources should be taken before treatment to document the site of treatment.

HDR BRT offers a number of theoretic advantages over LDR treatments. In addition to improved radiation protection for involved medical personnel, HDR can also facilitate the optimization of dose distribution. At present, the convenience of short treatment time for HDR is offset by the need for increased fractionation. In order to achieve clinical results comparable to LDR, most HDR treatments require multiple fractions, each in the range of 4 to 9 Gy.[93] At present, there is no consensus on an optimal number of HDR fractions or the total dose.

WOUND COMPLICATIONS AND FUNCTIONAL OUTCOME

Wound Complications

Quantitation of the individual impact of surgery, radiation, and chemotherapy on wound healing and limb function is quite difficult. Additionally, there is a large variability among sarcoma patients with respect to anatomic site, tumor size, tumor grade, treatment age, premorbid conditions (e.g., diabetes, vascular diseases), and type of treatment. Surgery alone renders a total complication rate of 30% to 35%, of which 3% to 10% are considered severe.[94,95] With the addition of external beam radiation, the overall complication rate ranges between 17% and 37%, and the severe complication rate

between 7% and 16.5%.[91,96] Significant factors that have been reported to increase wound healing problems include: lower extremity lesions, older age group, postoperative boost with interstitial implant, accelerated fractionation,[96] large specimen size, the use of preoperative radiation, and history of smoking or vascular disease.[97]

In the past, the use of BRT was connected to increased wound complication: 44% with interstitial implant versus 14% with surgery alone.[95] Further analysis of this problem showed a correlation between early loading time and the high incidence of wound breakdown. Delaying loading of radioactive seeds until after the fifth postoperative day resulted in a significant decrease in the complication rate in the BRT arm: 14% versus 10% for the surgery-alone group.[98]

Higher major acute wound complication rates have been observed with preoperative radiotherapy as compared to postoperative treatment in a phase III randomized study.[80] A similar high wound complication rate was seen in a single institution study, which reported a 31% incidence of major wound complications in 78 patients with extremity soft-tissue sarcoma treated with preoperative radiotherapy to 50 Gy.[100] Table 58-13 summarizes the incidence of wound morbidity for different treatment modalities.

Preoperative chemotherapy does not appear to influence morbidity in patients undergoing radical surgery for soft-tissue sarcoma. In a large series of 309 patients, of which 105 received neoadjuvant chemotherapy, there was no increase in the postoperative wound complication rates with neoadjuvant chemotherapy in either extremity (34% vs. 41%, $P = 0.37$) or retroperitoneal/visceral sites (29% vs. 34%, $P = 0.66$), even though patients treated with neoadjuvant chemotherapy had larger and more high-grade tumors.[101] Prospective randomized studies are needed to confirm these observations.

Functional Outcome in Extremity Tumors

Commonly reported functional impairments after treatment for extremity soft-tissue sarcoma are pain, loss of range of motion, muscle weakness, edema, and tissue fibrosis.[102] Pain was noted in 10% to 50% of the cases

Table 58–13   Wound Complication After Treatment of Soft-Tissue Sarcomas

Treatment	Authors	Patients, n	Complication (%) Overall	Severe
Surgery alone	Skibber et al[94]	93	34	10
	Arbeit et al[95]	64	33	3
Preoperative radiotherapy	Suit et al[177]	60	28	13
			NR	14
	Wayne et al[100]	78	NR	31
	NCIC[80]	88	NR	35
Postoperative radiotherapy	Leibel et al[91]	29	17	7
	Lindberg et al[77]	300	NR	6.5
	NCIC[80]	94	NR	17
Brachytherapy	Schray et al[115]	40	5	2
	Ormsby et al[98]	21	NR	14

NR, not reported.

with less than 10% of patients requiring pain medication on a regular basis. Joint motion restriction was noted in 33% to 50% of the patients, muscle weakness in 33%, moderate to severe edema in 25% and soft-tissue fibrosis in 50% to 60%.[102] Radiation parameters that can increase post-treatment impairment include: inclusion of the joint in radiation field (predictive of joint contracture), dose greater than 63 Gy at 1.8 Gy/fraction (predictive for pain, edema, muscle weakness), field greater than 35 cm and lower extremity location (predictive for edema, muscle weakness).[103] Other factors that have been shown to influence functional outcomes are tumor size, motor nerve sacrifice,[104] the use of adjuvant radiotherapy, and an older age group.[105] Finally, the IORT volume in patients treated with IORT and postoperative irradiation for extremity soft-tissue sarcoma is associated with the risk of soft-tissue fibrosis. The risk is ≤5% for IORT volumes ≤210 cm³, whereas it approaches 50% for volume ≥420 cm³.[106] Further details on the functional outcome after treatment of extremity soft-tissue sarcoma can be found in an excellent review written by Davis in the *Seminars in Radiation Oncology*.[102]

TREATMENT RESULTS

Surgery Alone

Several studies have suggested that surgery alone can result in excellent local control and survival in highly selected patients. Fabrizio et al. reported no local failure or distant relapse and a 96% survival rate in 18 patients with low-grade tumors treated with surgery alone after a median follow-up of 55 months.[83] Geer et al. reviewed 117 cases with T1 tumors treated with surgery alone and reported a local control rate of 92%.[85] Investigators from the University of Chicago used a wide-margin excision approach in 62 patients with subcutaneous sarcomas of the extremity.[107] The surgeons employed wide radial margins and resection of unviolated fascia. There were no local recurrences in the group of patients treated with surgery only. Alektiar et al. reviewed the records of 204 patients treated at MSKCC for stage IIB (high-grade histology and tumor size ≤5 cm) soft-tissue sarcoma of the extremity.[107] All had negative surgical margins and

43% received adjuvant radiotherapy (BRT in 26% and external beam irradiation in 17%); 17% also had adjuvant chemotherapy. The patients who did or did not receive radiation were well balanced with regard to age, tumor size, and location, with the exception of tumor depth with more deep tumors in the radiotherapy group. There was no difference in 5-year local control rates (84% vs. 80%) with the addition of radiotherapy. These data suggest that it is appropriate to consider withholding radiation in a select group of patients with low-grade tumors, widely negative surgical margins, and in whom a function preserving surgical salvage is possible in the event of a local relapse. The role of radiotherapy in small high-grade tumor is controversial; the findings from MSKCC are provocative and need confirmation in prospective randomized trials.

Preoperative Radiation

Many institutions advocate preoperative radiation treatment. Theoretic advantages of this approach are listed in Table 58-9. Nielsen et al. provided the first quantitative evidence that treatment field sizes can be smaller when radiation is given preoperatively.[108] They resimulated 26 patients who had received preoperative radiation treatments in the postoperative settings. Preoperatively, margins of 5 cm around the tumor were used for grade 1 to 2 disease and 7 cm for grade 3 sarcomas. The same margins were employed postoperatively, but around the surgical bed. The average preoperative field size was significantly smaller than that of the postoperative setting: 241 cm² versus 391 cm² ($P < 0.001$). Furthermore, more joints were included in the postoperative treatment volumes.

The outcome of preoperative radiation has been impressive. Barkley et al. reported on 110 patients treated with preoperative radiation followed by wide-local excision at the MDAH between 1970 and 1984.[109] Eighty-nine percent of the lesions were greater than 5 cm. With the minimal follow-up of 17 months, the local control and disease-free survival rates were 90% and 61%, respectively. Suit found a local control advantage for preoperative over postoperative radiation treatment, especially for larger lesions (Table 58-14).[51] The local control rates for

Table 58–14   Five-Year Actuarial Local Control for Primary Soft-Tissue Sarcoma According to Size and Radiotherapy Sequencing: the MGH Experience

Size (mm)	Postoperative Radiation		Preoperative Radiation	
	Patients, n	% Local Control	Patients, n	% Local Control
25	20	100	11	80
26-49	45	95	16	100
50-100	64	83	63	93
101-150	12	91	34	100
151-200	6	50	25	79
200	3	67	11	100
Total	150	87	160	92

MGH, Massachusetts General Hospital.
Adapted from Suit HD, Spiro IJ: The role of radiation in patients with soft tissue sarcomas. *Cancer Control.* 1994;592.

lesions greater than 15 cm were 56% for postoperative radiation and 86% for preoperative radiation. The conclusions from these studies can be subjected to biases due to the retrospective nature of the studies. The NCIC conducted a randomized study comparing preoperative and postoperative radiotherapy for soft-tissue sarcoma, with wound complication, local control, and overall survival rates as major endpoints. In addition, quality of physical function, economic cost, radiation planning parameters and treatment-related toxicity were evaluated. The study was closed when an interim analysis showed a higher acute wound complication rate with preoperative radiotherapy. With a median follow-up of more than 3.3 years, there was no difference in either the local control rates and in functional scores between the two treatment arms, but an unexplained survival advantage with preoperative radiotherapy.[80]

A number of investigators have studied preoperative chemotherapy either sequentially or in combination with preoperative radiotherapy. Based on promising results from single institution reports, the Radiation Therapy Oncology Group conducted an intergroup phase II trial of multi-agent chemotherapy (a modified MAID regimen with mesna, Adriamycin, ifosfamide, and dacarbazine) delivered concurrently with preoperative radiotherapy (44 Gy given in split courses of 22 Gy) followed by resection in patients with high-risk soft-tissue sarcoma (grade ≥II and ≥8 cm in maximal diameter).[110] This is followed by three cycles of postoperative chemotherapy with G-CSF. Eighty-eight percent of the patients completed preoperative chemotherapy and 93% completed radiation therapy. Delayed wound healing was observed in 26% of the patients. Of 45 patients with at least one year of follow-up, the estimated 2-year survival was 95%, which was encouraging. Edmonson et al. treated 49 patients with two cycles of ifosfamide, mesna, mitomycin, doxorubicin, and cisplatin (IMAP) followed by reduced dose ifosfamide, adriamycin, and cisplatin (MAP) chemotherapy concurrently with radiotherapy to 45 Gy, followed by limb-sparing surgery.[111] An additional 10 to 20 Gy boost was delivered to the tumor bed via IORT, BRT, or external beam radiotherapy at the completion of surgery. All but five patients had tumors greater than 5 cm. The estimated 5-year survival was 80%.

Eilber and colleagues have employed combined preoperative Adriamycin-based chemotherapy and radiation since 1974 at UCLA for the treatment of soft-tissue and bone sarcomas.[112] A list of the trials, the time frame, and the results for grade 3 lesions are shown in Table 58-15. In the initial trial, patients were treated with intra-arterial Adriamycin (30 mg/day × 3 days), followed by 35 Gy given in 10 fractions and conservative surgical resection. To reduce the 25% complication rate, a second trial, in which patients were given identical chemotherapy and surgery, but with a reduced radiation dose (17.5 Gy in 5 fractions), was opened. In the third trial, the radiation dose was raised to 28 Gy in 8 fractions because of poor local control in the second study. At the same time, this protocol compared the efficacy of intravenous (IV) versus intra-arterial Adriamycin. Since there was no difference in the complication or local control rates with the route of administration, a fourth trial evaluating the efficacy of IV Adriamycin, IV cisplatin, and 28 Gy radiation was started. The results were comparable to that of IV Adriamycin alone. The final protocol involved two courses of high-dose ifosfamide followed by 28 Gy radiation, Adriamycin, cisplatin, and conservative surgery. The last regimen improved local control rate to 95%. Treatment-induced pathologic necrosis, as determined from the tumor specimen after preoperative therapy, appeared to be an independent predictor for both local recurrence and overall survival in this group of 496 patients.[113] Patients with less than 95% pathologic necrosis were 2.5 times more likely to develop local recurrence and 1.9 times more likely to die of their disease as compared to those with ≥95% pathologic necrosis or a complete response.

Postoperative Radiation

The largest reported series on postoperative radiation treatment came from the MDAH.[77] Three hundred patients with soft-tissue tumors of the extremities, head and neck, and the retroperitoneum were treated with conservative excision, followed by radiation to a total dose of 60 to 75 Gy in 6 to 7½ weeks. No attempts were made to cover the entire muscle or anatomic compartment. The local recurrence rate was 20% for extremity, 38% for abdominal, and 23% for head and neck sarcomas. One third of the extremity failures occurred beyond margins of the irradiated field, and local control did not change with 10 Gy dose reduction in the later period. The 5-year disease-free survival was 61% for all sites.

Table 58–15 Preoperative Radiation and Chemotherapy for Soft-Tissue Sarcomas—the UCLA Experience

Period	Patients, *n*	Chemotherapy	Radiation (Gy)	LR (%)	Amputation	OS (G3) (%)	Complication
1974-1981	77	IA Adria	35	7 (9)	4	52	27
1981-1984	137	IA Adria	17.5	20 (15)	9	63	35
1984-1987	112	IA or IV Adria	28	10 (9)	6	64	26
1987-1990	46	IV Adria and CDDP	28	5 (11)	4	64	18
1990-1992	44	IV Ifos, Adria, CDDP	28	1 (2)	2	88	8
Total (%)	416			43 (10)	25 (6)		114 (27)

Adria, Adriamycin; CDDP, cisplatinum; Ifos, ifosfamide; IA, intraarterial; IV, intravenous; LR, local recurrence; OS, overall survival; G3, grade 3; UCLA, University of California at Los Angeles.
Adapted and modified from Eilber FR, Eckarett J, Rosen G, et al: Preoperative therapy for soft tissue sarcoma. *Hematol Clin North Am.* 1995;9:817-823.

At UCSF, 29 patients with extremity sarcomas were treated with conservative surgery and postoperative radiotherapy.[91] The majority of cases had grade 3 or larger than 5-cm tumors. The radiation dose ranged from 50 to 75 Gy. Eighty-two percent of the patients received more than 55 Gy. The local control rate with surgery and postoperative radiation was 90%, with a 5-year relapse-free survival of 68%. These results were superior to excisional surgery alone and comparable to radical surgery on a stage-by-stage basis. This study also demonstrated the ability of postoperative radiotherapy to sterilize microscopic disease. In the simple excision with positive margin group, the local recurrence rates were 14% (3 of 22) for patients receiving postoperative radiation versus 79% (11 of 14) for those with surgery alone. At the MGH, Suit et al. treated 150 patients with postoperative irradiation.[88] They achieved a local control rate of 87%. The results of these three series are summarized in Table 58-16.

Brachytherapy

Theoretic benefits for BRT include shorter treatment duration, relative sparing of normal tissues, and earlier delivery of radiation before fibrosis and hypoxia set in. Harrison and colleagues conducted a prospective randomized trial to evaluate the benefit of adjuvant BRT.[54] One hundred and twenty-six patients with soft-tissue sarcomas of the extremity and the superficial trunk underwent gross complete resection, with limb-sparing procedures. During the resection, they were randomized to either observation or adjuvant BRT to a total dose of 42 to 45 Gy over 4 to 6 days via ^{192}Ir afterloading implants. The target area was defined by adding a 2-cm margin in the cephalocaudal direction, and a 1.5- to 2-cm margin in the mediolateral direction around the tumor bed. No attempt was made to treat the surgical scar or drain site. With a median follow-up of 76 months, there was a significant improvement in local control in the high-grade tumor group with brachytherapy; the 5-year local control rates were 82% and 69% in the brachytherapy and no brachytherapy group, respectively (P = 0.04).[114] However, there was no difference in disease-specific survival or the rate of distant metastasis between the two groups. There was also no distinction in local control between the two arms for low-grade lesions.

Shray et al. evaluated the role of brachytherapy as a boost to the tumor bed in addition to external beam radiotherapy for nonretroperitoneal lesions treated at the Mayo Clinic.[115] A dose of 15 to 20 Gy via ^{192}Ir

afterloading catheters was combined with 45 to 50 Gy of external beam radiotherapy. With a median follow-up of 20 months, there were five local failures: one in the implant volume, two in the external beam volume, and two outside the radiation field. Delannes et al. reported a 5-year local control rate of 89% in 58 patients treated with external beam irradiation to 45 Gy with a 20 Gy LDR brachytherapy boost for predominantly large tumors.[116] Zelefsky employed BRT and conservative resection at MSKCC for the treatment of 45 locally advanced tumors involving the neurovascular bundles.[117] This was a group of poor-risk patients; more than 60% had high-grade lesions, positive margins, or tumor larger than 10 cm. ^{192}Ir afterloading catheters were placed directly over the neurovascular bundles in many cases. An average dose of 44 Gy/5 days was administered, and a number of patients (21 of 45) also received additional external beam irradiation. The 5-year actuarial local control and disease-free survival rates were 70% and 66%, respectively. After salvage treatments, 84% maintained functional extremities. Interestingly, they reported only a 9% incidence of neuritis, occurring in those who received a cumulative dose exceeding 90 Gy to the neurovascular bundles.

BRT has been advocated for retreatment of recurrent tumors after previous external beam radiation. Nori et al. reported their experience with 40 patients treated with 45 Gy via ^{192}Ir afterloading catheters for recurrent extremity sarcomas.[118] Half had evidence of bone, joint, or neurovascular bundle involvement. The 5-year actuarial local control rate with BRT and conservative resection was 68%. All local failures occurred in patients with more than two prior recurrences.

The use of fractionated HDR as a boost has also been popularized by a number of institutions.[119-121] Preliminary results suggested that local control and acute complications appear to be comparable to LDR brachytherapy. Unfortunately, most series are small and the dose-fractionation regimen are not uniform. In addition, the follow-up period is too short to make any definitive statement on treatment results or complication rates with fractionated HDR.

CHEMOTHERAPY

Approximately 50% of patients with high-grade sarcomas will die of distant disease despite adequate local control. To improve this rate, there have been intensive efforts in the last 3 decades to identify adjuvant systemic agents effective in preventing tumor dissemination. The most active single chemotherapeutic agents include ifosfamide and Adriamycin with single agent response rates of 15% to 30%.[122-124] Cyclophosphamide, dactinomycin, dacarbazine (DTIC), methotrexate, and cisplatin are also effective against soft-tissue sarcoma. These drugs have been used in combination with Adriamycin for metastatic disease as well as in the adjuvant setting for localized sarcomas. Temozolomide,[125] gemcitabine,[126] navelbine,[127] and Ecteinascidin (ET-743)—a cytotoxic alkaloid derived from a marine organism[128]—have also shown promising activity against soft-tissue sarcoma.

Table 58–16 Local Control with Conservative Surgery and Postoperative Radiation

Author	Yr	Patients, n	Dose (Gy)	Local Control (%)
Lindberg et al[77]	1981	300	60–75	78
Leibel et al[91]	1982	29	55–70	90
Suit and Spiro[51]	1994	150	60–68	87

Table 58–17   Adjuvant Chemotherapy: Summary of Randomized Trials of Adriamycin versus Control

Trial	Stage	Treatment	Patients, n	Med F/U (mo)	RFS (%)	OS (%)
Boston/ECOG[129] (1978-1985)	IIB-IVA	Adria Control	37 38	49	74 ⎤ NS 62 ⎦	68 ⎤ NS 68 ⎦
Scandinavian[131] (1981-1986)	High grade	Adria Control	93 88	40	62 ⎤ NS 57 ⎦	74 ⎤ NS 70 ⎦
UCLA[132] (1981-1984)	High-grade extremity only	Adria Control	56 63	28	58 ⎤ NS 54 ⎦	85 ⎤ NS 80 ⎦
Rizzoli Institute[134] (1981-1986)	High-grade extremity only	Adria Control	32 44	106	56 ⎤ $P = 0.015$ 32 ⎦	ND ⎤ $P = 0.006$ ND ⎦
ISSG[130] (1983-1987)	Intermediate and high grade	Adria Control	32 32	20	67 ⎤ NS 67 ⎦	82 ⎤ NS 77 ⎦

Adria, Adriamycin; ISSG, Intergroup Sarcoma Study Group; Med. F/U, median follow-up; ND, no data; NS, not statistically significant; OS, overall survival; RFS, relapse-free survival.

Adapted and modified from Mertens WC, Bramwell VHC: Adjuvant chemotherapy for soft tissue sarcomas. *Hematol Oncol Clin North Am* 1995;9:801.

Twelve prospective, randomized studies have reported on the role of adjuvant chemotherapy for M0 soft-tissue sarcomas. Five compared high-dose Adriamycin to untreated surgical controls (Table 58-17).[129-133] Most of these studies did not have enough power to detect small differences in results, and many are open to criticism on methodologic grounds. Antman et al. reported on 92 patients with localized large (>5 cm) intermediate and high-grade sarcomas of all sites treated in an intergroup trial.[130] After optimal local therapy, patients were randomized to either adjuvant Adriamycin (70 mg/m^2 × 6) or observation. With the median follow-up of 44 months, no difference in survival was observed between the two arms (see Table 58-17). One of the few trials that showed an advantage to adjuvant systemic treatment was the Bologna study, in which 77 patients with high-grade extremity sarcomas were evaluated.[133] Patients were treated with one of three local control procedures: amputation, preoperative radiation (45 Gy), and Adriamycin chemotherapy followed by conservative surgery, or re-excision of the scar and the surgical bed with radiation reserved for positive margins. They were then randomized to adjuvant Adriamycin or observation. With a median follow-up of 68 months, there was a disease-free survival advantage to the chemotherapy group, confined predominantly in the amputation and scar re-excision categories.[134] The group treated with conservative surgery and radiation had a poor survival rate due to a higher local recurrent rate. Criticisms of this study included: a high incidence of pelvic and thigh tumors in the control group compared to the experimental arm (54% vs. 38%), and a poorer disease-free survival for the control arm when compared to similar studies with the same follow-up.

Table 58-18 summarizes the results of six randomized studies using combination chemotherapy.[135-140] The MDAH trial opened 20 years ago. When results were reviewed with a median follow-up of 18 months, unacceptable toxicity and a lower disease-free survival rate for the experimental arm led to its early termination. However, after 10 years of follow-up, a significantly larger number of patients in the chemotherapy group were still alive and disease free compared to the controls.[135] The initial poor results could be accounted for by an imbalance in the treatment arms, particularly for tumor grades. At the NCI, 67 patients were randomized to either adjuvant chemotherapy or no further therapy after local treatments.[137] Chemotherapy consisted of high-dose Adriamycin, Cytoxan, and methotrexate. There was a superior disease-free survival (75% vs. 54%, $P = 0.04$) and local control (one local failure vs. four local failures, $P < 0.05$) in the chemotherapy arm. Toxicity was significant, however; 15% of the patients developed drug-induced congestive heart failure. In a subsequent study, 88 patients were randomized to receive either the same chemotherapy regimen (total Adriamycin dose: 500 to 550 mg/m^2) or a lower dose regimen of Adriamycin (350 mg/m^2). There was no difference in relapse-free survival and overall survival between the two arms. The largest published trial of adjuvant chemotherapy came from the European Organization for Tumor Control (EORTC).[136] Three hundred and seventeen patients were randomized to adjuvant CYVADIC chemotherapy (Cytophosphamicle, vincristine, Adriamycin, and DTIC) or no chemotherapy. With a median follow-up of 80 months, the 7-year relapse-free survival was higher (56% vs. 43%, $P = 0.007$)) and the local failure was lower (17% vs. 31%, $P = 0.004$) in the chemotherapy arm. The reduction in local recurrence was limited to tumors of the head, neck, and trunk. Criticisms of this study included a high ineligibility rate (33%) and a poor compliance rate (only 52% completed the planned eight courses of chemotherapy). Accrual spanned 11.5 years, during which new diagnostic and therapeutic techniques were developed.

Table 58–18   Adjuvant Chemotherapy: Summary of Randomized Trials of Combination Chemotherapy versus Control

Trial	Stage	Treatment	Patients, n	Med F/U (mo)	RFS (%)		OS (%)	
MDA[135]	IIB-IIIB	VACAd	20		54		65	
(1973-1976)	extremity	Control	23	120		$P = 0.04$		NS
					35		35	
Mayo Clinic[138]	I-IVA	VACACD	30				90	
(1975-1981)		Control	31	64	ND			NS
							77	
NCI[137]	IIA-IIIB	ACM	39		75		82	
(1977-1981)	extremity	Control	28	85		$P = 0.04$		NS
					54		60	
EORTC[136]	I-IVA	CAVD	145		56		63	
(1977-1988)		Control	172	80		$P = 0.007$		NS
					43		56	
Fondation	IIB-IVA	CAVD	31				87	
Bergonie[140]		Control	28	52	ND			$P = 0.002$
(1980-1988)							53	
INCR[139]	T2a, b, GIII-IV	IA Control	53	59	50		69	
(1992-1996)			51			$P = 0.04$		$P = 0.03$
					37		50	

A, Adriamycin; Ad, dactinomycin; C, Cytoxan; D, dacarbazine; EORTC, European Organization for Research and Treatment of Cancer; I, ifosfamide; INCR, Italian National Council for Research; M, methotrexate; Med F/U, median follow-up; MDA, MD Anderson Cancer Center; NCI, National Cancer Institute; ND, no data; NS, not statistically significant; OS, overall survival; Pt, patient; RFS, relapse-free survival; V, vincristine.
Adapted and modified from Mertens WC, Bramwell VHC: Adjuvant chemotherapy for soft tissue sarcomas. *Hematol Oncol Clin North Am.* 1995;9:801.

A study that showed an advantage in survival came from Fondation Bergonie in France.[140] The chemotherapy used was identical to, but in a more intense regimen than, that of the EORTC. With a median follow-up of 4.4 years, there was a significant improvement in the chemotherapy arm with respect to local control (97% vs. 85%, $P = 0.03$), freedom from metastases (84% vs. 43%, $P = 0.0003$), and overall survival (87% vs. 54%, $P = 0.002$). The study, however, failed to stratify patients according to known prognostic factors, resulting in a high proportion of patients with extremity sarcomas (a better prognostic group) in the treatment arm. Frustaci et al. conducted a phase III randomized study of 104 patients with T2 and grade 3 to 4 soft-tissue sarcoma treated with either 5 cycles of high-dose epirubicin (60 mg/m^2 on days 1 and 2) and ifosfamide (1.8 mg/m^2 on day 1 through 5) or no adjuvant chemotherapy.[139] There were three different primary treatment strategies (radical surgery vs. surgery + postoperative EBRT vs. preoperative EBRT + surgery) performed in at least six different treatment centers. Although the patients appear to be well balanced between the two groups, there were larger tumors in the control arm and more patients in the control arm required amputation, suggesting worse tumor biology. The trial was terminated early when an interim analysis revealed a significant disease-free and overall survival advantage with the addition of chemotherapy. With a median follow-up of 59 months, the median disease-free and overall survivals were 16 months and 46 months, respectively, for the control group and they were 48 months ($P = 0.04$) and 75 months for the treatment group ($P = 0.03$). The absolute survival benefit was 19% at 4 years with the addition of chemotherapy.

In an attempt to overcome the sample size limitations observed in the randomized studies, the Sarcoma Meta-Analysis Collaboration (SMAC) performed an individual data meta-analysis of the outcome for 1568 patients included in 14 randomized trials. The group compared adjuvant doxorubicin-based chemotherapy to no chemotherapy.[141] Significant improvements in local relapse-free interval (HR 0.73, $P = 0.016$), distant relapse-free interval (HR 0.70, $P = 0.0003$) and overall relapse-free interval (HR 0.75, $P = 0.0001$) were observed with adjuvant chemotherapy. In addition, there was a trend toward improved overall survival with an absolute survival benefit of 4% at 10 years (HR 0.89, $P = 0.12$). However, there was a significant 7% absolute survival benefit at 10 years (HR 0.80, $P = 0.029$) for soft-tissue sarcoma of the extremity with the addition of chemotherapy. Despite these encouraging results, additional well conducted, carefully planned multi-institutional prospective randomized trials will be needed before adjuvant chemotherapy can be considered the standard of care. It is reasonable to discuss the option of adjuvant systemic chemotherapy with patients younger than 65 who have high-grade large soft-tissue sarcoma. The treatment could delay distant recurrence and possibly prolong survival.

SURGICAL MANAGEMENT OF ISOLATED PULMONARY METASTASES

The most frequent site of distant metastasis in soft-tissue sarcomas is the lung. Despite a lack of randomized data on the use of neoadjuvant or adjuvant chemotherapy in the treatment of isolated pulmonary metastases, the most common approach today is systemic chemotherapy followed by surgical resection when the disease has stabilized for large lesions, or surgery followed by chemotherapy for smaller nodules. Candidates for pulmonary metastasectomy are patients who have: (1) control of the primary and no evidence of extrapulmonary metastases, (2) resectable lesions, (3) four or fewer nodules on imaging, (5) tumor doubling time of more than 40 days, and (6) a disease-free interval of more than 12 months. Numerous studies have shown that these patients have benefitted from surgical resection.[142,143] The 5-year survival for patients with complete resection is approximately 25% (range: 15% to 35%).[144]

SOME SPECIAL SARCOMA SUBGROUPS

Retroperitoneal Sarcomas

These rare tumors account for less than 15% of all adult soft-tissue sarcoma. Most retroperitoneal sarcomas are large (>10 cm) and locally infiltrative at diagnosis, making resection quite difficult. In a large series from MSKCC, only 49% of 158 lesions were amenable to complete resection.[145] The 5-year overall survival was 40% for patients with gross-total resection, and only 3% for those with incomplete tumor removal. Inability to obtain wide resection, high-grade lesions, and local recurrence negatively affected survival. There was a suggestion that adjuvant radiation improved 5-year survival (53% with radiation vs. 30% without); however, the gain was not statistically significant. The NCI prospectively evaluated the role of adjuvant radiation and chemotherapy to improve outcome.[146] They found no survival advantage with adjuvant chemotherapy. There was only one (3%) in-field failure with external beam radiation; however, the complication rate with this approach was high, with 22% of patients developing signs and symptoms of late radiation enteritis. To reduce bowel injury, a prospective randomized trial was conducted comparing IORT plus low-dose external beam irradiation versus high-dose external beam irradiation alone for resectable cases.[147] Fifteen patients received 20 Gy IORT with a single misonidazole infusion followed by external beam irradiation to 35 to 40 Gy postoperatively. Twenty had external beam irradiation alone to 50 to 55 Gy. In an updated analysis, the IORT arm had fewer local regional failures (40% vs. 75%, $P = 0.08$) and gastrointestinal complications (13% vs. 45%, $P < 0.05$) when compared to the control arm.[148] Four patients with IORT developed peripheral neuropathy with gradual recovery following conservative medical management. Gieschen et al. retrospectively compared 17 patients treated with preoperative external beam irradiation followed by surgery and IORT to the same number treated with external beam irradiation and surgery alone.[149] In patients who had gross total resections, the local control (83% vs. 61%) and overall survival rates (74% vs. 30%) were superior with the addition of IORT. Petersen et al. reported on 43 primary and 44 recurrent retroperitoneal sarcomas treated with 8.75 to 30 Gy IORT in addition to external beam irradiation (median dose 48.6 Gy) after partial or complete tumor resection.[150] There were 20 local failures: 4 within the IORT fields, 3 within IORT and external beam fields, and 13 within external beam

fields alone. Ten patients had gastrointestinal complications (seven fistulae and three severe proctitis) related to surgery, external beam irradiation, or both. Nine patients (10%) developed grade 3 peripheral neuropathy, but none had pain as a component of their neuropathy. In view of current results, IORT in conjunction with external beam radiotherapy is recommended for the treatment of retroperitoneal sarcomas.

IOHD is a new modality that has been applied to 32 patients (12 with primary and 20 with recurrent tumors) at MSKCC for the treatment of retroperitoneal soft-tissue sarcoma in conjunction with surgery and postoperative external beam irradiation.[151] The 5-year local control rate was 62% for the entire group, 74% for patients with primary tumors and 54% for patients with recurrent tumors. Treatment complications included gastrointestinal obstruction (18%), fistula formation (9%), peripheral neuropathy (6%), hydronephrosis (3%) and wound complication (3%). Further investigation of this novel modality is warranted.

Head and Neck Soft-Tissue Sarcomas

Soft-tissue sarcomas of the head and neck areas rarely occur in adults. They account for less than 1% of all malignant neoplasms and approximately 10% of all soft-tissue tumors.[152] Historically, they have been associated with poorer outcome when compared to sarcomas from other anatomic sites.[23,49] Reported 5-year disease-specific survival and local control rates ranged from 45% to 70%.[153-155] Tumor size, tumor grade, and the extent of surgical resection are important prognostic factors for survival and local control.[154,156-158] Age, tumor site, histology, and bony involvement have also been suggested to affect tumor control; however, their significance independent of other prognostic variables has not been firmly established. In reviewing 65 patients treated at UCSF for head and neck sarcomas, we found age, tumor grade, surgical margin status, and the extent of surgical resection to significantly influence disease-specific survival.[158] High tumor grade and large size also had an adverse impact on local control. The use of adjuvant radiation appeared to decrease local failure; however, it did not reach statistical significance due to the small sample size.

Technically, this is a challenging group of tumors to manage due to the difficulty in achieving a complete resection in this region without causing significant cosmetic impairment or functional morbidity. High local recurrence rates (up to 50%) have been reported with surgery alone.[159,160] Adjuvant radiotherapy, therefore, plays an essential part in the management of these sarcomas, particularly in cases of marginal surgical excision. Tran et al. reported a notable improvement in local control with radiation for 94 patients treated at UCLA.[154] Local failure was observed in 48% of patients treated with surgery alone compared to 10% of those treated with surgery and radiotherapy. Eeles and colleagues also found the use of adjuvant radiation to be superior to surgery alone.[161] The role of chemotherapy in the treatment of head and neck soft-tissue sarcoma remains undefined. The EORTC reported an improvement in local control with the addition of CYVADIC chemotherapy.[136] McKenna et al. treated 16 patients with aggressive surgery, high-dose postoperative radiation (60 to 63 Gy) and Adriamycin-based drugs.[162] With the median follow-up of 43 months, 64% were disease free, and 75% maintained local control. These encouraging results, however, have not been duplicated in other series.[156,160]

Fibromatosis (Desmoid Tumors)

Desmoid tumors—also known as aggressive fibromatoses—are rare, slowing growing benign fibrous neoplasms that arise from fascial or musculoaponeurotic structures. They are commonly associated with Gardner's syndrome. Although first described as tumors of the anterior abdominal wall in post-partum women, they may arise from any anatomic location, most commonly the shoulder girdle and thigh areas.[163] Histologically, they appear as well-differentiated fibrous neoplasms without associated cellular pleomorphism or mitotic activity (Fig. 58-12). These tumors rarely metastasize. Their natural history consists of slow, progressive invasion and destruction of contiguous structures by finger-like projections. This infiltrative behavior results in a high incidence of local recurrence (occasionally fatal) after conservative surgery.[163-165] Posner described 11 deaths from locally uncontrolled tumors of 138 patients treated at MSKCC.[166] Factors predictive of local failure were age between 18 and 30, recurrent disease, incomplete resection, close or microscopically positive margins, and no adjuvant radiation for gross residual disease.

The traditional treatment of desmoid tumors is aggressive surgical resection in effort to obtain a wide margin. However, radiation alone has been shown effective for the control of unresectable or recurrent lesions. Leibel et al. reviewed 19 cases of recurrent or residual tumors treated with radiation at UCSF.[167] At the time of treatment, eight patients had tumors larger than 10 cm, five with residuals between 4 and 6 cm. The majority received a tumor dose of 50 to 55 Gy at 1.6 to 1.8 Gy/fraction. With a median follow-up of 8 years, 13 patients remained free of disease. The 5-year relapse-free survival and overall survival rates were 73% and 88%, respectively. Complete tumor regression after radiation required 8 months to 2 years. There was only one true infield recurrence. Other centers have reported comparable results.[168,169] Adjuvant radiotherapy has been shown to improve local control, especially in patients with recurrent or involved surgical margins. Jelinek et al. showed that adjuvant radiotherapy was the only significant factor affecting local control in 54 patients treated for desmoid tumors at the University of Washington Medical Center.[170] The 5-year local control rate was 81% for patients receiving adjuvant radiotherapy compared to 53% for those treated with surgery alone. Nuyttens et al. reviewed the literature and concluded that the best local control rates were observed in patients treated with surgery and radiotherapy compared to surgery alone even after stratifying patients by surgical margin status and by primary versus recurrent tumors.[171]

We currently recommend a total dose of 54 to 60 Gy to a generous field for desmoid tumors. Indications for radiation treatment include: unresectable lesions, gross residual disease after resection, recurrent tumors or cases with involved surgical margins where future resection may not be feasible. In the special situation of an anterior abdominal wall desmoid with microscopic positive margin after the initial resection, we do not routinely use postoperative radiotherapy if the patient is reliable and agrees to close follow-up. For tumors involving other sites of the body, we recommend a dose of 50 to 54 Gy delivered in a generous field for microscopic residual disease.

Standard chemotherapeutic agents have been sporadically used, but reports are anecdotal and results inconclusive. Some complete responses have been observed with multi-agent chemotherapy. The roles of hormonal therapy (tamoxifen) and nonsteroidal anti-inflammatory drugs are similarly controversial.

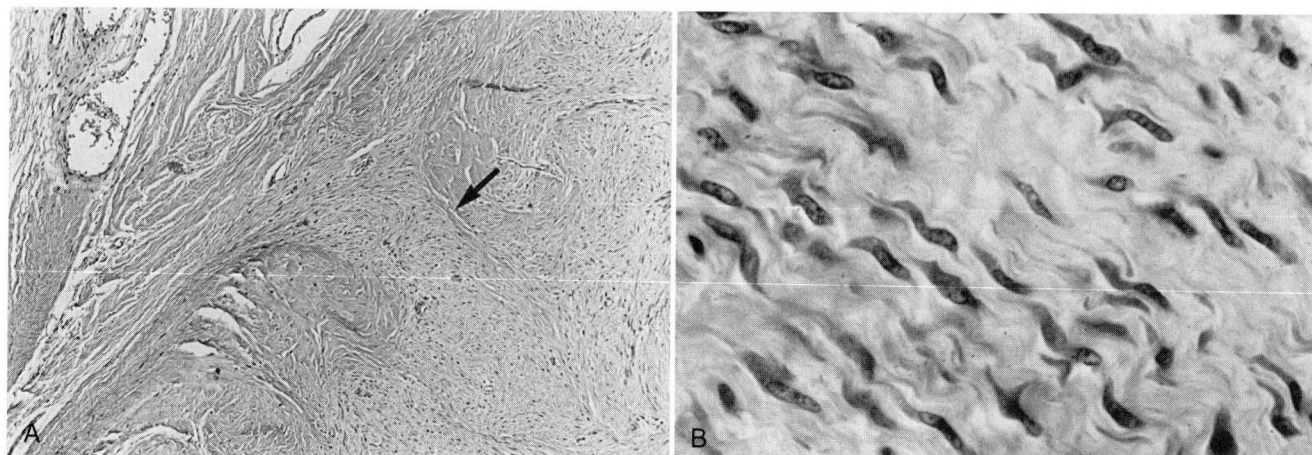

Figure 58-12. A, Desmoid tumor. Note the lack of encapsulation and extension into surrounding tissues (*arrow*) (Hematoxylin and eosin. Original magnification ×10.) **B,** Desmoid tumor at higher magnification (×40). Note the lack of cellular pleomorphism and mitotic activity. (Courtesy of Dr. Werner Roseneau, Dept. of Pathology, University of California at San Francisco.)

REFERENCES

1. Jemal A, Murray T, Samuels A, et al: Cancer statistics, 2002. *CA Cancer J Clin.* 2003;53:5.
2. Brand KG: Foreign body induced sarcomas. In Becker FF, ed. *Cancer.* New York: Plenum Press; 1975:485.
3. Dijkstra MD, Balm AJ, Gregor RT, et al: Soft tissue sarcomas of the head and neck associated with surgical trauma. *J Laryngol Otol.* 1995;109:126.
4. Bailar JC: How dangerous is dioxin? [editorial; comment] [see comments]. *N Engl J Med.* 1991;324:260.
5. Kang H, Enzinger FM, Breslin P, et al: Soft tissue sarcoma and military service in Vietnam: A case control study. *J Natl Cancer Inst.* 1987;79:693.
6. Suruda AJ, Ward EM, Fingerhut MA: Identification of soft tissue sarcoma deaths in cohorts exposed to dioxin and to chlorinated naphthalenes. *Epidemiology.* 1993;4:14.
7. Olsson HL, Perfekt R, Alvergard T, et al: Reduced risk for soft tissue sarcoma after oral contraceptive use—Results from population based studies. *Proceedings of ASCO.* 2001;20:363a.
8. Kim JH: Radiation induced soft tissue sarcoma and bone sarcoma. *Radiology.* 1978;129:501.
9. Taghian A, DeVathaire F, Terrier M, et al: Long-term risk of sarcoma following radiation treatment for breast cancer. *Int J Radiat Oncol Biol Phys.* 1991;21:361.
10. Yap J, Chuba PJ, Williams J, et al: Breast cancer and the incidence rates of sarcomas as subsequent malignant neoplasms: A US population-based analysis. *Proc ASCO.* 1999;18:549a.
11. Li FP, Fraumeni JFJ: Soft-tissue sarcomas, breast cancer, and other neoplasms. *Ann Intern Med.* 1969;71:747.
12. Malkin D, Li FP, Strong LC, et al: Germ line p53 mutations in a familial syndrome of breast cancer, sarcomas, and other neoplasms. *Science.* 1990;250:1233.
13. Enzinger EM, Weiss SW: General considerations. In Enzinger EM, Weiss SW, eds. *Soft Tissue Tumors.* St. Louis: CV Mosby; 1995:4.
14. Basu TN, Gutmann DH, Fletcher JA, et al: Aberrant regulation of ras proteins in malignant tumour cells from type 1 neurofibromatosis patients [see comments]. *Nature.* 1992;356:713.
15. Wunder JS, Czitron AA, Kandel R, et al: Analysis of alterations in the retinoblastoma gene and tumor grade in bone and soft tissue sarcomas. *J Natl Cancer Inst.* 1991;83:194.
16. Toguchida J, Yamaguchi T, Ritchie B, et al: Mutation spectrum of the p53 gene in bone and soft tissue sarcomas. *Cancer Res.* 1992;52:6194.
17. Porter PL, Gown AM, Kramp SG, et al: Widespread p53 overexpression in human malignant tumors. *Am J Pathol.* 1992;140:145.
18. Soini Y, Vahakangas K, Nuorva K, et al: p53 Immunohistochemistry in malignant fibrous histiocytomas and other mesenchymal tumors. *J Pathol.* 1992;168:29.
19. Leach FS, Tokino T, Meltzer P, et al: p53 Mutation and MDM2 amplification in human soft tissue sarcomas. *Cancer Res.* 1993;53:2231.
20. Smith SA, Weiss SW, Jankowski SA, et al: SAS amplification in soft tissue sarcomas. *Cancer Res.* 1992;52:3746.
21. Fisher C: Current aspects of the pathology of soft tissue sarcomas. *Semin Radiat Oncol.* 1999;9:315.
22. Nielsen TO, West RB, Linn SC, et al: Molecular characterisation of soft tissue tumours: A gene expression study. *Lancet.* 2002;359:1301.
23. Lawrence W, Donegan WL, Natarajan N, et al: Adult soft tissue sarcomas: Pattern of care survey of the American College of Surgeons. *Ann Surg.* 1987;205:349.
24. Hashimoto H, Daimaru Y, Takeshita S, et al: Prognostic significance of histologic parameters of soft tissue sarcomas. *Cancer.* 1992;70:2816.
25. Fletcher CD, Gustafson P, Rydholm A, et al: Clinicopathologic re-evaluation of 100 malignant fibrous histiocytomas: Prognostic relevance of subclassification. *J Clin Oncol.* 2001;19:3045.
26. Potter DA, Kinsella T, Glatstein E, et al: High grade soft tissue sarcomas of the extremities. *Cancer.* 1986;58:190.
27. van Unnik JAM, Coindre JM, Contesso C, et al: Grading of soft tissue sarcomas: Experience of the EORTC soft tissue and bone sarcoma group. *Eur J Cancer.* 1993;29A:2089.
28. Guillou L, Coindre JM, Bonichon F, et al: Comparative study of the National Cancer Institute and French Federation of Cancer Centers Sarcoma Group grading systems in a population of 410 adult patients with soft tissue sarcoma. *J Clin Oncol.* 1997;15:350.
29. Coindre JM, Trojani M, Contesso G, et al: Reproducibility of a histopathologic grading system for adult soft tissue sarcoma. *Cancer.* 1986;58:306.
30. Rydholm A, Berg NO, Gullberg B, et al: Epidemiology of soft-tissue sarcoma in the locomotor system. *Acta Path Microbiol Immunol Scand.* 1984;92:363.
31. Potter DA, Glenn J, Kinsella T, et al: Patterns of recurrence in patients with high-grade soft-tissue sarcomas. *J Clin Oncol.* 1985;3:353.
32. Vezeridis MP, Moore R, Karakousis CP: Metastatic patterns in soft-tissue sarcomas. *Arch Surg.* 1983;118:915.
33. Cheng EY, Springfield DS, Mankin HJ: Frequent incidence of extrapulmonary sites of initial metastasis in patients with liposarcoma. *Cancer.* 1995;75:1120.
34. Weingrad DN, Rosenberg SA: Early lymphatic spread of osteogenic and soft-tissue sarcomas. *Surgery.* 1978;84:231.
35. Mazeron JJ, Suit HD: Lymph nodes as sites of metastases from sarcomas of soft tissue. *Cancer.* 1987;60:1800.
36. Massengill AD, Seeger LL, Eckardt JJ: The role of plain radiography, computed tomography, and magnetic resonance imaging in sarcoma evaluation. *Hematol Oncol Clin North Am.* 1995;9:571.
37. Fleming JB, Holtz D, Cantor SB, et al: The utility and cost-effectiveness of computerized tomography (CT) to screen for pulmonary metastases in patients presenting with T1 extremity soft tissue sarcoma (STS). *Proc ASCO.* 1998;17:516a.
38. Porter GA, Ahmad SA, Cantor SB, et al: Cost-effectiveness of routine chest computed tomography (CT) in patients with T2 soft tissue sarcoma. *Proc ASCO.* 2000;19:553a.
39. Kern KA, Brunetti A, Norton JA, et al: Metabolic imaging of human extremity musculoskeletal tumors by PET. *J Nucl Med.* 1988;29:181.
40. Dimitrakopoulou-Strauss A, Strauss LG, Heichel T, et al: The role of quantitative (18)F-FDG PET studies for the differentiation of malignant and benign bone lesions. *J Nucl Med.* 2002;43:510.
41. Conrad EU, Eary JF, Van Linge J: FDG PET and "clinical grade" for treatment planning in sarcoma. *Proc ASCO.* 1999;18:548a.
42. Schueze S, Conrad E, Bruckner J, et al: FDG PET response to neoadjuvant chemotherapy predicts survival in patients with soft tissue sarcoma. *Proc ASCO.* 2001;20:348a.
43. Ayala AG, Ro JY, Fanning CV, et al: Core needle biopsy and fine-needle aspiration in the diagnosis of bone and soft-tissue lesions. *Hematol Oncol Clin North Am.* 1995;9:633.
44. Serpell JW, Fish SH, Fisher C, et al: The diagnosis of soft tissue tumors. *Ann R Coll Surg Engl.* 1992;74:277.
45. Kempson RL, Fletcher CD, Evans HL, et al: Tumor of the soft tissues. In Rosai J, Sobin LH, eds. *Atlas of Tumor Pathology.* Vol. 30. Washington D.C.: Armed Forces Institute of Pathology; 2001:17.
46. Soft tissue sarcoma. In Greene FI, Page DL, Fleming ID, et al., eds. *AJCC Cancer Staging Manual.* Chicago: Springer; 2002.
47. Pisters PW, Leung DH, Woodruff J, et al: Analysis of prognostic factors in 1,041 patients with localized soft tissue sarcomas of the extremities. *J Clin Oncol.* 1996;14:1679.
48. Coindre JM, Terrier P, Bui NB, et al: Prognostic factors in adult patients with locally controlled soft tissue sarcoma. A study of 546 patients from the French Federation of Cancer Centers Sarcoma Group. *J Clin Oncol.* 1996;14:869.
49. Ruka W, Emrich LJ, Driscoll DL, et al: Clinical factors and treatment parameters affecting prognosis in adult high-grade soft tissue sarcomas: A retrospective review of 267 cases. *Eur J Surg Oncol.* 1989;15:411.
50. Tanabe KK, Pollock RE, Ellis LM, et al: Influence of surgical margins on outcome in patients with preoperatively irradiated extremity soft tissue sarcomas. *Cancer.* 1994;73:1652.
51. Suit HD, Spiro IJ: The role of radiation in patients with soft tissue sarcomas. *Cancer Control.* 1994:592.
52. Heslin MJ, Woodruff J, Brennan MF: Prognostic significance of a positive microscopic margin in high-risk extremity soft tissue sarcoma: Implications for management. *J Clin Oncol.* 1996;14:473.
53. Rosenberg SA, Tepper J, Glatstein E, et al: The treatment of soft-tissue sarcomas of the extremities: Prospective randomized evaluations of (1) limb-sparing surgery plus radiation therapy

compared with amputation and (2) the role of adjuvant chemotherapy. *Ann Surg.* 1982;196.

54. Harrison LB, Franzese F, Gaynor JJ, et al: Long-term results of a prospective randomized trial of adjuvant brachytherapy in the management of completely resected soft tissue sarcomas of the extremity and superficial trunk. *Int J Radiat Oncol Biol Phys.* 1993;27:259.

55. Huth JF, Eilber FR: Patterns of metastatic spread following resection of extremity soft-tissue sarcomas and strategies for treatment. *Semin Surg Oncol.* 1988;4:20.

56. Williard WC, Hajdu SI, Casper ES, et al: Comparison of amputation with limb-sparing operations for adult soft tissue sarcomas of the extremity. *Ann Surg.* 1992;215:269.

57. Bramwell VHC, Rouesse J, Santoro A: Combined modality management of local and disseminated adult soft tissue sarcomas: A review of 257 cases seen over 10 years at the Christie Hospital and Holt Radium Institute, Manchester. *Br J Surg.* 1985;51:301.

58. Heslin MJ, Cordon-Cardo C, Lewis JJ, et al: Ki-67 detected by MIB-1 predicts distant metastasis and tumor mortality in primary, high grade extremity soft tissue sarcoma. *Cancer.* 1998;83:490.

59. Levine EA, Holzmayer T, Bacus S, et al: Evaluation of newer prognostic markers for adult soft tissue sarcomas. *J Clin Oncol.* 1997;15:3249.

60. Rudolph P, Kellner U, Chassevent A, et al: Prognostic relevance of a novel proliferation marker, Ki-S11, for soft-tissue sarcoma. A multivariate study. *Am J Pathol.* 1997;150:1997.

61. Wurl P, Meye A, Schmidt H, et al: High prognostic significance of Mdm2/p53 co-overexpression in soft tissue sarcomas of the extremities. *Oncogene.* 1998;16:1183.

62. Pallotta MG, Lastiri JM, Varela MS, et al: Plasma MMP-9 activity in soft tissue sarcomas. *Proc ASCO.* 2000;19:559a.

63. Kawai A, Woodruff J, Healey JH, et al: SYT-SSX gene fusion as a determinant of morphology and prognosis in synovial sarcoma. *N Engl J Med.* 1998;338:153.

64. Enneking WF, Spanier SS, Malawer MM: The effect of the anatomic setting on the results of surgical procedures for soft parts sarcoma of the thigh. *Cancer.* 1981;47:1005.

65. Brennhovd IO: The treatment of soft tissue sarcomas—A plea for a more urgent and aggressive approach. *Acta Chir Scand.* 1966;131:483.

66. Markhede G, Angervall L, Stener B: A multivariate analysis of the prognosis after surgical treatment of malignant soft tissue tumors. *Cancer.* 1982;49:1721.

67. Shieber W, Graham P: An experience with sarcomas of the soft tissues in adults. *Surgery.* 1962;52:295.

68. Simon MA, Enneking WF: The management of soft-tissue sarcomas of the extremities. *J Bone Joint Surg.* 1976;58:317.

69. Shiu MH, Hajdu SI: Management of soft tissue sarcoma of the extremity. *Semin Oncol.* 1981;8:172.

70. Cade SS: Soft tissue tumours: Their natural history and treatment. *Proc R Soc Med.* 1951;19.

71. McNeer GP, Cantin J, Chu F, et al: Effectiveness of radiation therapy in the management of sarcoma of the soft somatic tissues. *Cancer.* 1968;22:391.

72. Tepper JE, Suit HD: Radiation therapy alone for sarcoma of soft tissue. *Cancer.* 1985;56:475.

73. Schwartz DL, Einck J, Bellon J, et al: Fast neutron radiotherapy for soft tissue and cartilaginous sarcomas at high risk for local recurrence. *Int J Radiat Oncol Biol Phys.* 2001;50:449.

74. Suit HD, Russell WO, Martin RG: Management of patients with sarcoma of soft tissue in an extremity. *Cancer.* 1973;31:1247.

75. Hintz BL, Charyulu KK, Miller WE, et al: Adjuvant role of radiation in soft tissue sarcoma in adults. *J Surg Oncol.* 1977;9:329.

76. Eilber FR, Mirra JJ, Grant TT, et al: Is amputation necessary for sarcomas? A seven-year experience with limb salvage. *Ann Surg.* 1980;192:431.

77. Lindberg RD, Martin RG, Romsdahl MM, et al: Conservative surgery and postoperative radiotherapy in 300 adults with soft-tissue sarcomas. *Cancer.* 1981;47:2391.

78. Suit HD, Proppe KH, Mankin HJ, et al: Preoperative radiation therapy for sarcoma of soft tissue. *Cancer.* 1981;47:2269.

79. National Institutes of Health: Limb-sparing treatment of adult soft-tissue sarcomas and osteosarcomas. *Natl Inst Health Consens Dev Conf Consens Statement.* 1985;5:18.

80. O'Sullivan B, Davis AM, Turcotte R, et al: Preoperative versus postoperative radiotherapy in soft-tissue sarcoma of the limbs: a randomised trial. *Lancet.* 2002;359:2235.

81. Yang JC, Chang AE, Baker AR, et al: Randomized prospective study of the benefit of adjuvant radiation therapy in the treatment of soft tissue sarcomas of the extremity. *J Clin Oncol.* 1998;16:197.

82. Choong PF, Petersen IA, Nascimento AG, et al: Is radiotherapy important for low-grade soft tissue sarcoma of the extremity? *Clin Orthop.* 2001:191.

83. Fabrizio PL, Stafford SL, Pritchard DJ: Extremity soft-tissue sarcomas selectively treated with surgery alone. *Int J Radiat Oncol Biol Phys.* 2000;48:227.

84. Karakousis CP, Emrich LJ, Rao U, et al: Limb salvage in soft tissue sarcomas with selective combination of modalities. *Eur J Surg Oncol.* 1991;17:71.

85. Geer RJ, Woodruff J, Casper ES, et al: Management of small soft-tissue sarcoma of the extremity in adults. *Arch Surg.* 1992;127:1285.

86. Lawrence TS, Lichter AS: Soft tissue sarcomas (excluding retroperitoneum). In Perez CA, Brady LW, eds. *Principles and Practice of Radiation Oncology.* Philadelphia: JB Lippincott; 1992:1399.

87. Lindberg RD: Soft tissue sarcoma. In Fletcher GF, ed. *Textbook of Radiotherapy.* Philadelphia: Lea & Febiger; 1980:922.

88. Suit HD, Spiro I: Role of radiation in the management of adult patients with sarcoma of soft tissue. *Semin Surg Oncol.* 1994;10:347.

89. Yang JC, Rosenberg SA, Glatstein EJ, et al: Sarcomas of soft tissues. In DeVita VTJ, Hellman S, Rosenberg SA, eds. *Cancer: Principles and Practice of Oncology.* Philadelphia: JB Lippincott; 1993:1436.

90. O'Sullivan B, Wylie J, Catton C, et al: The local management of soft tissue sarcoma. *Semin Radiat Oncol.* 1999;9:328.

91. Leibel SA, Tranbaugh RF, Wara WM, et al: Soft tissue sarcomas of the extremities: Survival and patterns of failure with conservative surgery and postoperative irradiation compared to surgery alone. *Cancer.* 1982;50:1076.

92. Nag S, Shasha D, Janjan N, et al: The American Brachytherapy Society recommendations for brachytherapy of soft tissue sarcomas. *Int J Radiat Oncol Biol Phys.* 2001;49:1033.

93. Hilaris BS, Bodner WR, Mastoras CA: Role of brachytherapy in adult soft tissue sarcomas. *Semin Surg Oncol.* 1997;13:196.

94. Skibber JM, Lotze MT, Seipp CA, et al: Limb-sparing surgery for soft tissue sarcomas: Wound related morbidity in patients undergoing wide local excision. *Surgery.* 1987;102:447.

95. Arbeit JM, Hilaris BS, Brennan MF: Wound complications in the multimodality treatment of extremity and superficial truncal sarcomas. *J Clin Oncol.* 1987;5:480.

96. Bujko K, Suit HD, Springfield DS, et al: Wound healing after surgery and preoperative radiation for sarcoma of soft tissues. *Surg Gynecol Obstet.* 1992;176:124.

97. Peat BG, Bell RS, Davis A, et al: *Wound Healing Complications After Soft Tissue Sarcoma Surgery.* Washington, D.C.: American Academy of Orthopedic Surgeons; 1992.

98. Ormsby MV, Hilaris BS, Nori D, et al: Wound complications of adjuvant radiation therapy in patients with soft-tissue sarcomas. *Ann Surg.* 1989;210:93.

99. O'Sullivan B, Davis A, Bell R, et al: Phase III randomized trial of pre-operative versus post-operative radiothepy in the curative management of extremity sarcoma. A Canadian sarcoma group and NCI Canada clinical trials group study. *Proc ASCO.* 1999;18:535a.

100. Wayne JD, Langstein HN, Pollack A, et al: Preoperative radiotherapy for extremity soft tissue sarcoma (STS): Site specific wound complication rates and the impact of reconstructive surgery. *Proc ASCO.* 2000;19:558a.

101. Meric F, Milas M, Hunt KK, et al: Impact of neoadjuvant chemotherapy on postoperative morbidity in soft tissue sarcomas. *J Clin Oncol.* 2000;18:3378.

102. Davis AM: Functional outcome in extremity soft tissue sarcoma. *Semin Radiat Oncol.* 1999;9:360.

103. Stinson SF, DeLaney TF, Greenberg J, et al: Acute and long-term effects on limb function of combined modality limb sparing therapy for extremity soft tissue sarcoma. *Int J Radiat Oncol Biol Phys.* 1991;21:1493.

104. Bell RS, O'Sullivan B, Davis A, et al: Functional outcome in patients treated with surgery and irradiation for soft tissue tumours. *J Surg Oncol.* 1991;48:224.

105. Robinson MH, Spruce L, Eeles R, et al: Limb function following conservation treatment of adult soft tissue sarcoma. *Eur J Cancer.* 1991;27:1567.

106. van Kampen M, Eble MJ, Lehnert T, et al: Correlation of intraoperatively irradiated volume and fibrosis in patients with soft-tissue sarcoma of the extremities. *Int J Radiat Oncol Biol Phys.* 2001;51:94.

107. Gibbs CP, Peabody TD, Mundt AJ, et al: Oncological outcomes of operative treatment of subcutaneous soft-tissue sarcomas of the extremities. *J Bone Joint Surg Am.* 1997;79:888.

108. Nielsen OS, Cummings B, O'Sullivan B, et al: Preoperative and postoperative irradiation of soft tissue sarcomas: Effect on radiation field size. *Int J Radiat Oncol Biol Phys.* 1991;21:1595.

109. Barkley HT, Martin RG, Romsdahl MM, et al: Treatment of soft tissue sarcomas by preoperative radiation and conservative surgical resection. *Int J Radiat Oncol Biol Phys.* 1988;14:693.

110. Kraybill WG, Spiro I, Harris J, et al: Radiation Therapy Oncology Group (RTOG) 95-14: A phase II study of neoadjuvant chemotherapy (CT) and radiation therapy (RT) in high risk (HR), high grade, soft tissue sarcomas (STS) of the extremities and body wall: A preliminary report. *Proc ASCO.* 2001;20:348a.

111. Edmonson JH, Petersen IA, Shives TC, et al: Chemotherapy, irradiation, and surgery for function-preserving therapy of primary extremity soft tissue sarcomas: Initial treatment with ifosfamide, mitomycin, doxorubicin, and cisplatin plus granulocyte macrophage-colony-stimulating factor. *Cancer.* 2002;94:786.

112. Eilber F, Eckardt J, Rosen G, et al: Preoperative therapy for soft tissue sarcoma. *Hematol Oncol Clin North Am.* 1995;9:817.

113. Eilber FC, Rosen G, Eckardt J, et al: Treatment-induced pathologic necrosis: A predictor of local recurrence and survival in patients receiving neoadjuvant therapy for high-grade extremity soft tissue sarcomas. *J Clin Oncol.* 2001;19:3203.

114. Pisters PW, Harrison LB, Leung DH, et al: Long-term results of a prospective randomized trial of adjuvant brachytherapy in soft tissue sarcoma. *J Clin Oncol.* 1996;14:859.

115. Schray MF, Gunderson LL, Sim FH, et al: Soft tissue sarcoma: Integration of brachytherapy, resection, and external irradiation. *Cancer.* 1990;66:451.

116. Delannes M, Thomas L, Martel P, et al: Low-dose-rate intraoperative brachytherapy combined with external beam irradiation in the conservative treatment of soft tissue sarcoma. *Int J Radiat Oncol Biol Phys.* 2000;47:165.

117. Zelefsky MJ, Nori D, Shiu MH, et al: Limb salvage in soft tissue sarcomas involving neurovascular structures using combined surgical resection and brachytherapy. *Int J Radiat Oncol Biol Phys.* 1990;19:913.

118. Nori D, Shupak K, Shiu MH, et al: Role of brachytherapy in recurrent extremity sarcoma in patients treated with prior surgery and irradiation. *Int J Radiat Oncol Biol Phys.* 1991; 20:1229.

119. Koizumi M, Inoue T, Yamazaki H, et al: Perioperative fractionated high-dose rate brachytherapy for malignant bone and soft tissue tumors. *Int J Radiat Oncol Biol Phys.* 1999;43:989.

120. Crownover RL, Marks KE: Adjuvant brachytherapy in the treatment of soft-tissue sarcomas. *Hematol Oncol Clin North Am.* 1999;13:595.

121. Chun M, Kang S, Kim BS, et al: High dose rate interstitial brachytherapy in soft tissue sarcoma: technical aspects and results. *Jpn J Clin Oncol.* 2001;31:279.

122. Blum RH: An overview of studies of Adriamycin (NSC-123127) in the United States. *Cancer Chemother Rep.* 1975;6:247.

123. O'Bryan RM, Luce JK, Talley RW, et al: Phase II evaluation of adriamycin in human neoplasia. *Cancer.* 1973;32:1.

124. Borden EC, Amato D, Enterline HT, et al: Randomized comparison of adriamycin regimens for treatment of metastatic soft tissue sarcomas. *J Clin Oncol.* 1987;5:840.

125. Taub RN, Keohan M, Plitsas M, et al: Phase II study of temozolomide in advanced sarcomas. *Proc ASCO.* 2000;19:555a.

126. Spath-Schwalbe E, Koschuth A, Grunewald R, et al: Gemcitabine (GEM) in pretreated patients with advanced soft tissue sarcomas—Preliminary results from a phase II trial. *Proc ASCO.* 1998; 17:513a.

127. Fidias P, Demetri G, Harmon DC: Navelbine shows activity in previously treated sarcoma patients: Phase II results from MGH/Dana Farber/Partner's Cancercare study. *Proc ASCO.* 1998; 17:513a.

128. Demetri GD, Seiden M, Garcia-Carbonero R, et al: Exteinascidin (ET-743) shows promising activity in distinct populations of sarcoma patients: Summary of 3 U.S.-based phase II trials. *Proc ASCO.* 2000;19:553a.

129. Wilson RE, Wood WC, Lerner HL, et al: Doxorubicin chemotherapy in the treatment of soft-tissue sarcoma. *Arch Surg.* 1986; 121:1354.

130. Antman K, Suit H, Amato D, et al: Preliminary results of a randomized trial of adjuvant doxorubicin for sarcomas: Lack of apparent difference between treatment groups. *J Clin Oncol.* 1984;2:601.

131. Alvegard TA, Sigurdsson H, Mouridsen H, et al: Adjuvant chemotherapy with doxorubicin in high-grade soft tissue sarcoma: A randomized trial of the Scandinavian Sarcoma Group. *J Clin Oncol.* 1989;7:1504.

132. Eilber FR, Giuliano AE, Huth JF, et al: A randomized prospective trial using postoperative adjuvant chemotherapy (adriamycin) in high-grade extremity soft-tissue sarcoma. *Am J Clin Oncol.* 1988;11:39.

133. Picci P, Bacci G, Gherlinzoni F, et al: Results of a randomized trial for the treatment of localized soft tissue tumors (STS) of the extremities in adult patients. In Ryan HR, Baker LO, eds. *Recent Concepts in Sarcoma Treatment.* Dordrecht, The Netherlands: Kluwer Academic; 1988:144.

134. Gherlinzoni F, Picci P, Bacci G, et al: Late results of a randomized trial for the treatment of soft tissue sarcomas (STS) of the extremities in adult patients [abstract]. *Proc Am Soc Clin Oncol.* 1993;12:468.

135. Benjamin RS, Terjanian TO, Genoglio CJ, et al: The importance of combination chemotherapy for adjuvant treatment of high risk patients with soft tissue sarcomas of the extremities. In Salmon SE, ed. *Adjuvant Therapy of Cancer.* New York: Grune & Stratton; 1987:735.

136. Bramwell V, Rouesse J, Steward W, et al: Adjuvant CYVADIC chemotherapy for adult soft tissue sarcoma—Reduced local recurrence but no improvement in survival: A study of the European Organization for Research and Treatment of Cancer Soft Tissue and Bone Sarcoma Group. *J Clin Oncol.* 1994;12:1137.

137. Chang AE, Kinsella T, Glatstein E, et al: Adjuvant chemotherapy for patients with high-grade soft-tissue sarcomas of the extremity. *J Clin Oncol.* 1988;6:1491.

138. Edmonson JH, Fleming TR, Ivins JC, et al: Randomized study of systemic chemotherapy following complete excision of nonosseous sarcomas. *J Clin Oncol.* 1984;2:1390.

139. Frustaci S, Gherlinzoni F, De Paoli A, et al: Adjuvant chemotherapy for adult soft tissue sarcomas of the extremities and girdles: results of the Italian randomized cooperative trial. *J Clin Oncol.* 2001;19:1238.

140. Ravaud A, Bui NB, Coindre JM, et al: Adjuvant chemotherapy with CYVADIC in high risk soft tissue sarcoma: A randomized prospective trial. In Salmon SE, ed. *Adjuvant Therapy of Cancer VI.* Philadelphia: WB Saunders, 1990:556.

141. Adjuvant chemotherapy for localised resectable soft-tissue sarcoma of adults: Meta-analysis of individual data. Sarcoma Meta-analysis Collaboration. *Lancet.* 1997;350:1647.

142. Casson AG, Putnam JB, Natarajan G, et al: Five-year survival after pulmonary metastasectomy for adult soft tissue sarcoma. *Cancer.* 1992;69:662.

143. Jablons D, Steinberg SM, Roth J, et al: Metastasectomy for soft tissue sarcoma. *J Thorac Cardiovasc Surg.* 1989;97:695.

144. Frost DB: Pulmonary metastasectomy of soft tissue sarcomas: Is it justified? *J Surg Oncol.* 1995;59:110.

145. Cody HSI, Turnbull AD, Fortner JG, et al: The continuing challenge of retroperitoneal sarcomas. *Cancer.* 1981;47:2147.

146. Glenn J, Sindelar WF, Kinsella T, et al: Results of multimodality therapy of resectable soft-tissue sarcomas of the retroperitoneum. *Surgery.* 1985;97:316.

147. Kinsella TJ, Sindelar WF, Lack E, et al: Preliminary results of a randomized study of adjuvant radiation therapy in resectable adult retroperitoneal soft tissue sarcomas. *J Clin Oncol.* 1988;6:18.

148. Sindelar WF, Kinsella TJ, Chen PW, et al: Intraoperative radiotherapy in retroperitoneal sarcomas. Final results of a prospective, randomized, clinical trial. *Arch Surg.* 1993;128:402.

149. Gieschen HL, Spiro IJ, Suit HD, et al: Long-term results of intraoperative electron beam radiotherapy for primary and recurrent retroperitoneal soft tissue sarcoma. *Int J Radiat Oncol Biol Phys.* 2001;50:127.

150. Petersen IA, Haddock MG, Donohue JH, et al: Use of intraoperative electron beam radiotherapy in the management of retroperitoneal soft tissue sarcomas. *Int J Radiat Oncol Biol Phys.* 2002;52:469.

151. Alektiar KM, Hu K, Anderson L, et al: High-dose-rate intraoperative radiation therapy (HDR-IORT) for retroperitoneal sarcomas. *Int J Radiat Oncol Biol Phys.* 2000;47:157.

152. Hajdu SI: *Pathology of Soft Tissue Tumors.* Philadelphia: Lea & Febiger; 1979:14.

153. Kraus DH, Dubner S, Harrison LB, et al: Prognostic factors for recurrence and survival in head and neck soft tissue sarcomas. *Cancer.* 1994;74:697.

154. Tran LM, Mark R, Meier R, et al: Sarcomas of the head and neck. *Cancer.* 1992;70:169.

155. Willers H, Hug EB, Spiro IJ, et al: Adult soft tissue sarcomas of the head and neck treated by radiation and surgery or radiation alone: Patterns of failure and prognostic factors. *Int J Radiat Oncol Biol Phys.* 1995;33:585.

156. Farhood AI, Hajdu SI, Shiu MH, et al: Soft tissue sarcomas of the head and neck in adults. *Am J Surg.* 1990;160:365.

157. Le Vay J, O'Sullivan B, Catton C, et al: An assessment of prognostic factors in soft-tissue sarcoma of the head and neck. *Arch Otolaryngol Head Neck Surg.* 1994;120:981.

158. Le QT, Fu KK, Kroll S, et al: Prognostic factors in adult soft-tissue sarcomas of the head and neck. *Int J Radiat Oncol Biol Phys.* 1997;37:975.

159. Kowalski LP, San CI: Prognostic factors in head and neck soft tissue sarcomas: Analysis of 128 cases. *J Surg Oncol.* 1994;56:83.

160. Weber RS, Benjamin RS, Peters LJ, et al: Soft tissue sarcomas of the head and neck in adolescents and adults. *Am J Surg.* 1986;152:386.

161. Eeles RA, Fisher C, A'Hern RP, et al: Head and neck sarcomas: Prognostic factors and implications for treatment. *Br J Cancer.* 1993;68:201.

162. McKenna WG, Barnes MM, Kinsella TJ, et al: Combined modality treatment of adult soft tissue sarcomas of the head and neck. *Int J Radiat Oncol Biol Phys.* 1987;13:1127.

163. Enzinger FM, Shiraki M: Musculo-aponeurotic fibromatosis of the shoulder girdle (extra-abdominal desmoid). Analysis of thirty cases followed up for ten or more years. *Cancer.* 1967;20:1131.

164. Conley J, Healy WV, Stout AP: Fibromatosis of the head and neck. *Am J Surg.* 1966;112.

165. Das Gupta TK, Brasfield RD, O'Hara J: Extraabdominal desmoids: A clinicopathological study. *Ann Surg.* 1969;170:109.

166. Posner MC, Shiu MH, Newsome JL, et al: The desmoid tumor—Not a benign disease. *Arch Surg.* 1989;124:191.

167. Leibel SA, Wara WM, Hill DR, et al: Desmoid tumors: Local control and patterns of relapse following radiation therapy. *Int J Radiat Oncol Biol Phys.* 1983;9:1167.

168. Bataini JP, Belloir C: Desmoid tumors in adults: The role of radiotherapy in their management. *Am J Surg.* 1988;155:754.

169. Karakousis CP, Mayordomo J, Zografos GC, et al: Desmoid tumors of the trunk and extremity. *Cancer.* 1993;72:1637.

170. Jelinek JA, Stelzer KJ, Conrad E, et al: The efficacy of radiotherapy as postoperative treatment for desmoid tumors. *Int J Radiat Oncol Biol Phys.* 2001;50:121.

171. Nuyttens JJ, Rust PF, Thomas CR Jr, et al: Surgery versus radiation therapy for patients with aggressive fibromatosis or desmoid tumors: A comparative review of 22 articles. *Cancer.* 2000;88:1517.

172. Russel WO, Cohen J, Enzinger F, et al: A clinical and pathological staging system for soft tissue sarcomas. *Cancer.* 1977;40:1562.

173. Myhre Jensen O, Høgh J, Østgaard SE, et al: Histopathological grading of soft tissue tumors. Prognostic significance in a prospective study of 278 consecutive cases. *J Pathol.* 1991;163:19.

174. Costa J, Wesley RA, Glatstein E, et al: The grading of soft tissue sarcomas. Results of a clinicohistopathologic correlation in a series of 163 cases. *Cancer.* 1984;53:530.

175. Trojani M, Contesso G, Coindre JM, et al: Soft-tissue sarcomas of adults: Study of pathological prognostic variables and definition of a histopathological grading system. *Int J Cancer.* 1984;33:37.

176. Gerner RE, Moore GE, Pickren JW: Soft tissue sarcomas. *Ann Surg.* 1975;6.

177. Suit HD, Mankin HJ, Wood WC, et al: Treatment of the patient with stage M0 soft tissue sarcoma. *J Clin Oncol.* 1988;6:854.

Sarcomas of Bone

Karen Schupak, MD

Primary malignancies of the structural elements of bone include a diverse group of tumors with respect to patient age, incidence rates, skeletal sites of involvement, and biologic behavior. There are similarities, however, in the challenge that their multimodality management poses. Surgical resection remains the mainstay, with techniques of cryosurgery, autologous soft tissue and bone transfer, cadaveric allograph placement, and sophisticated customized biomechanical bone and joint prostheses extending the possibility of functional limb preservation to the majority of patients, even those who have not yet reached skeletal maturity.

Occasionally, amputative surgery is unavoidable or, in fact, may permit better function with advanced custom orthotics. Chemotherapy has resulted in a dramatically improved prognosis for patients with osteosarcoma, although its efficacy for other primary bone malignancies is yet to be demonstrated. Radiation therapy for primary, nonmetastatic bone malignancies has an established role in the case of chordoma, for example. Radiation therapy remains controversial in the modern management of the more common osteogenic or chondrosarcomas, but there is ample historic and growing modern evidence that these tumors are responsive to radiation, as well.

Above all, the care of the patient with a primary skeletal malignancy requires fastidious attention to early and complete bone and soft tissue imaging, biopsy location and technique, and complete extent of disease evaluation. Only then can collaboration between the surgical, medical, radiation oncology, and rehabilitation experts result in a treatment strategy that has the highest likelihood of cure with the least functional handicap.

This chapter reviews the techniques of treatment and the outcome for osteosarcoma, chondrosarcoma, malignant fibrous histiocytoma of bone, giant cell tumor, aneurysmal bone cyst, and chordoma.

NORMAL STRUCTURE AND FUNCTION OF BONE

The axial and appendicular skeleton is made up of dynamic, actively metabolic tissues. From early childhood, skeletal growth and maturation serve many functions besides the obvious means of locomotion. The dense temporal and calvarial bones protect the brain, while the delicate bones of facial structures have evolved to permit vocal resonance, air humidification, and maximal mobility of the skull on the vertebral column in an upright posture. Similarly, the spinal vertebral bodies articulate to permit maximum flexibility while securing the safety of the spinal cord within. Along with the brain, the evolution of the appendicular skeleton has permitted the eventual dominance of humans over their environment.

This complex living tissue is physically a composite of protein matrix, hydroxyapatite crystals, and the osteoclasts and osteoblasts that continually remodel the structure of bone. In addition, calcium and phosphorus metabolism are maintained through interactions among the parathyroid glands, calcitonin, vitamin D, and the skeletal system. Lastly, the progenitor cells of the hematopoietic system reside within the skeletal medullary cavity; their relative distribution changes during skeletal maturation and in response to radiation.[1]

In long bones, three anatomic zones are identified. The epiphysis is the broadened end of a bone that supports the articular surface. The metaphysis is the transition zone between the epiphysis and the shaft, or diaphysis. The metaphysis is the zone in which the majority of bone growth occurs. The diaphysis is the more slender shaft of long bones, and the cavity in this zone contains marrow. The calcified structure in each zone is different and gradually remodeled over time to match the interplay of muscle action, weight bearing, and stress with the necessary matrix arrangement to guarantee structural integrity.

Bones grow in two ways. Endochondral bone formation accounts for the lengthening of bones that have epiphyses. Continuous growth by the epiphyseal chondroblasts produces expansion of the cartilaginous plate, both toward the metaphysis and toward the epiphysis. The older cartilaginous growth on the metaphyseal side undergoes resorption and replacement as bone matrix, capillaries, and osteoblasts grow between the spicules left by the degenerating cartilage. The new bone at the distal metaphysis is actively remodeled in response to changes in weight bearing and stress.

In membranous bone formation, the mineralization of the osteoid matrix occurs directly by osteoblast activity. A cartilaginous template is not required. Membranous bone formation accounts for the growth of the calvaria, mandible, and other flat bones. In addition, long bones increase in diameter in this way. Specifically, the transverse growth of long bones occurs by bone formation at the subperiosteum with concomitant osteoclastic reabsorption at the endosteal surface, thereby enlarging the marrow space.[2]

The cellular activity that directs the growth and remodeling of the normal skeleton also explains the relative incidence of neoplastic transformation of these tissues with respect to skeletal site and age.

EPIDEMIOLOGY OF BONE TUMORS

Although multiple myeloma accounts for 50% of all primary bone tumors, it arises from the plasma cell, a hematopoietic cell within the marrow space, and not a true structural element of bone. Multiple myeloma is, therefore, not considered further in this chapter. True malignant bone tumors represent less than 1% of all malignant neoplasms.[3] Osteosarcoma is the most prevalent primary malignancy of bone; it is twice as common as chondrosarcoma, three times as common as Ewing's sarcoma, and 10 times more common than malignant fibrous histiocytoma of bone.[4]

Although osteosarcoma can occur at any age, nearly 60% of patients are between 10 and 20 years of age. Not surprisingly, the age peak is younger in females (17 years) than in males (18 years), mirroring the period of most active skeletal growth for each sex. An additional 10% of cases occur in patients older than 60 years of age. There is a slightly greater incidence in males, 1.3:1 at Memorial Sloan-Kettering Cancer Center (MSKCC) and 1.6:1 at the Mayo Clinic, perhaps reflecting the longer duration of skeletal growth in males and the greater skeletal bulk. Similarly, the distal femur and proximal tibia account for more than 50% of cases in adolescents, as this is the site of most rapid skeletal growth. Until epiphyseal closure, the long bones are involved in nearly 80% of cases, whereas after skeletal maturity, the incidence is about equal between the long and flat bones, with the skull and axial skeleton representing 40% of cases.[4]

Osteosarcoma has been noted to be more prevalent in taller children.[5,6] It is also more common in the giant breeds of dogs, with Great Danes, Saint Bernards, Great Pyrenees, and wolfhounds having up to 185 times the risk of small dogs.[7]

In patients older than 60, 56% of osteosarcomas are believed to arise as a consequence of other bone conditions, such as Paget's disease and fibrous dysplasia, or following irradiation. In this setting, response to chemotherapy is less likely,[8] with a 5-year survival rate of 15% in a review from MSKCC[9] and 10% at the Mayo Clinic.[9]

In a cohort of 900 patients followed at the National Cancer Institute (NCI) Epidemiology Branch who had received repeated injections of ^{224}Ra for the treatment of bone tuberculosis or ankylosing spondylitis, a 200-fold increased risk for developing bone sarcomas was noted.[10] The estimated cumulative skeletal dose was 4.2 Gy.

Glicksman and Fabrikant reviewed the current literature regarding postirradiation second neoplasms.[11] Bone sarcomas were the most common second malignancy reported. The authors noted that although doses ranged between less than 10 Gy and 80 Gy, only 21% of the secondary sarcomas were along the central axis of the radiation field and nearly 50% were on the field periphery. An additional 30% were located in the superficial tissues, superficial to d_{max}, causing the authors to speculate that the most likely regions of sarcoma induction received between 20% and 70% of the mid-plane dose.

In children with the germinal mutation resulting in retinoblastoma—a deletion in the 1-4 band on the long arm of chromosome 13 (13q14)—osteosarcoma of the extremity is 200 to 500 times more common than in the general population, and it is an additional 10-fold more prevalent in the skull in children who were irradiated.[12-14] Investigators at Stanford found a 38% actuarial incidence of secondary malignancies at 30 years among survivors of childhood retinoblastoma with a median latency of 16 years.[15] A review of more than 9000 survivors of childhood cancer[16] found that, in general, radiation caused a 2.7-fold increased risk of bone cancer. However, a sharp dose-response gradient was noted with doses in excess of 60 Gy resulting in a 40-fold risk. The cumulative risk for survivors of childhood retinoblastoma was higher. No difference in risk could be discerned based on the use of orthovoltage or megavoltage machinery. Treatment with alkylating agents was also associated with a 4.7 relative risk of bone cancer, with the risk increasing as cumulative drug exposure rose. It has been observed that mortality rates from secondary malignancies in this setting are significantly higher than in primary cases.[17]

The Cooperative German-Austrian-Swiss Osteosarcoma Study Group reviewed 1700 consecutive patients treated between 1980 and 1998 on neoadjuvant chemotherapy protocols for various prognostic factors. They found that axial tumor site (vs. appendicular), tumor size, presence of metastases at diagnosis, response to chemotherapy, and completeness of surgical resection were independent prognostic factors for survival. Interestingly, among the 32 patients identified in this cohort for whom osteosarcoma arose as a secondary malignancy, no significant negative impact upon survival could be identified.[18]

RADIOGRAPHIC FEATURES

When a malignant condition of bone is suspected, plain film radiographic evaluation will provide, in most instances, a highly reliable presumptive diagnosis and should not be overlooked in the current era of cross-sectional imaging. The age of the patient, location of the tumor within the bone (epiphysis, metaphysis, or diaphysis), and skeletal site (axial or appendicular) set the foundation for radiographic diagnosis.

Osteosarcomas commonly arise in the metaphyseal region and may extend into the diaphyseal or epiphyseal region, or both, of the affected bone.[19] Cortical bone is destroyed in a disorganized fashion, and the periosteal reaction, which is the effort of the native bone to restore cortical integrity, results in the radiographic appearance of the classic Codman's triangle and periosteal bone spicules (Fig. 59-1). The tumor itself images as a cloud-like density representing tumor osteoid. A soft tissue mass is usually present. Magnetic resonance imaging (MRI) is most useful for imaging soft tissue extension as well as identifying intramedullary skip metastases. The latter, which occur rarely, are also well detected on bone scintigraphy.

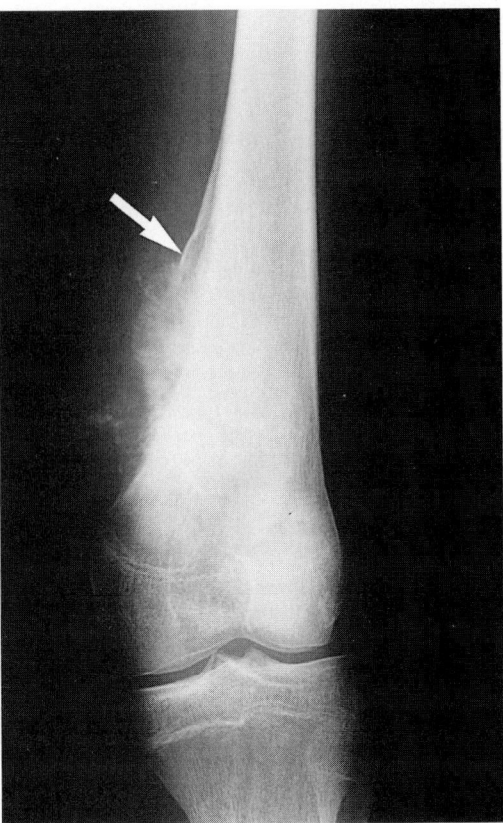

Figure 59–1. Osteosarcoma. This anterior-posterior view of the distal femur shows the typical bone-producing tumor in the distal diaphysis and metaphysis. There is ossification of the extraosseous soft tissue component and Codman's triangle (*arrow*) formation of the proximal aspect.

up to 2 years after therapy.[25-26] The short-term radiographic appearance may actually be confused with tumor progression as the original sclerotic rim involutes. Therefore, patience is required in the interpretation of radiographic studies in the short term after irradiation for giant cell tumors of bone.

PATHOLOGIC FEATURES

Histologic features that characterize malignant tissue, nuclear pleomorphism, cellular atypia, pathologic mitoses, and an infiltrative growth pattern may be variably expressed in bone malignancies. Frequently the age of the patient, skeletal location, and radiographic appearance of the tumor may be pivotal in rendering an accurate diagnosis. Therefore, the necessity of multimodality management, with collaboration among the clinician, pathologist, and skeletal radiologist is critical to the correct interpretation of the diagnostic material from the patient's initial presentation.

For example, in low-grade chondrosarcomas, mitoses are rare and the appearance of chondrocytes with a plump nucleus or moderate numbers of multinucleated cells may be diagnostic (Fig. 59-4). These histologic findings in association with an axial location in an adult would be more worrisome, whereas they would be of no particular importance in a child or in a distal location. As 10% of chondrosarcomas arise in preexisting, benign cartilaginous growths, extensive specimen sampling is necessary to avoid overlooking areas of malignant

As most cartilaginous lesions are typically slow growing and commonly arise from preexisting, benign cartilaginous lesions such as an enchondroma or an osteochondroma, the radiographic appearance of a chondrosarcoma may be only subtly different from that of a purely benign condition.[20] Although the cartilaginous matrix typically mineralizes in a benign growth, development of lucent areas within the matrix are worrisome for malignant degeneration (Fig. 59-2). Similarly, an enchondroma typically induces endosteal scalloping and gradual cortical remodeling, but when this picture evolves to include cortical destruction and penetration, malignancy is likely. Serial radiographs are recommended in monitoring apparently benign lesions, especially those in an axial location.

The most important radiographic features of giant cell tumors are their metaphyseal location and rather bland lytic appearance with little or no host response in the narrow transition zone between tumor and native bone.[21] Extension to the subarticular cortex in the epiphysis is common (Fig. 59-3). This has given rise to some dispute as to the site of origin, with some investigators citing the epiphysis.[22-24] These tumors usually cause cortical thinning, with frank breakthrough being a less common event.

Reports from institutions where the effects of radiation on giant cell tumors have been studied note that bone reparation may not be radiographically evident for

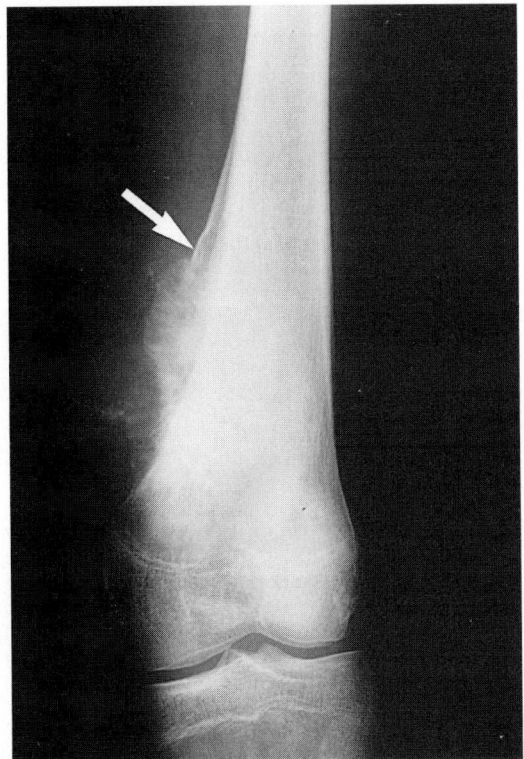

Figure 59–2. Chondrosarcoma. This lateral view of the femur demonstrates irregularly calcified cartilaginous matrix in the mid-diaphysis without gross cortical involvement.

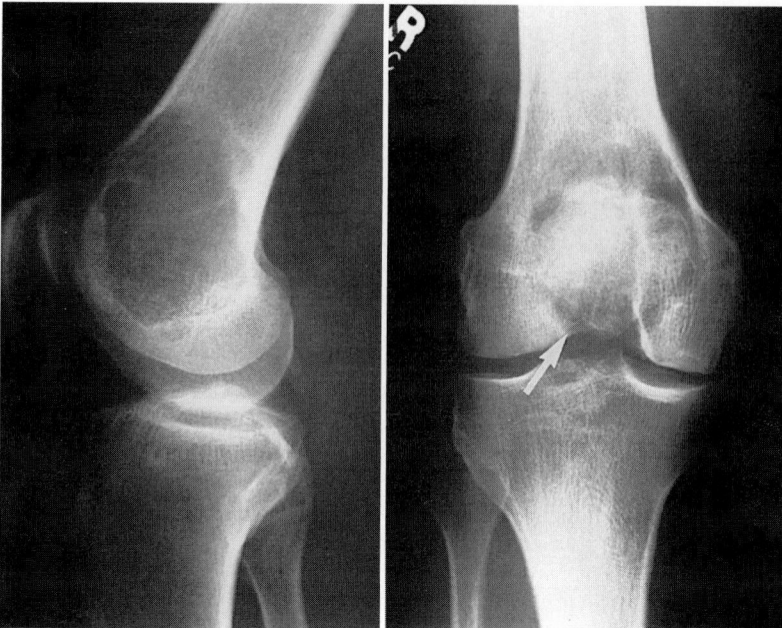

Figure 59–3. Giant cell tumor. These anterior-posterior (*right*) and lateral (*left*) views of the knee show a large, well-defined lytic lesion in the distal metaphysis and epiphysis with extension into the subarticular cortex (*arrow*).

degeneration. The periphery of the lesion is usually most revealing. Although the cartilaginous matrix may contain calcifications and ossifications, malignant osteoid is not seen.

Conversely, malignant osteoid is the hallmark of osteosarcoma. While it is logical to assume that the tumor arises from osteoblasts, the presence of other malignant mesenchymal tissues within osteosarcomas suggests that the precursor cell is actually of a more primitive mesenchymal, pluripotential origin. Therefore, the microscopic appearance is that of a sarcomatous stroma directly forming tumor osteoid or bone (Fig. 59-5). A large amount of atypical cartilage or fibrosarcomatous matrix may also be evident.

The physaliferous cell is the histologic hallmark of the chordoma. These so-called "bubbly cells" have abundant intracytoplasmic droplets of mucoid material and are usually seen in clusters surrounded by a sea of mucoid material (Fig. 59-6). They arise from the remnants of the notochord in the axial skeleton.[28] During embryonic development, the notochord undergoes gradual obliteration within the vertebral bodies during the second month of gestation. However, the central portion of the intervertebral disk, which contains notochordal tissue in the form of nucleus pulposus, may persist for an indefinite period of time. Experimentally, chordoma-like lesions have been produced in rabbits by piercing the anterior intervertebral ligaments with a needle and allowing the escape of nucleus pulposus.[29] In fact, 50% of patients with sacrococcygeal chordomas have a history of previous lower back trauma.[30]

Giant cell tumors are purely osteolytic and are said to arise from osteoclasts. The giant multinucleated osteoclast-like cell is the histologic hallmark of this growth.

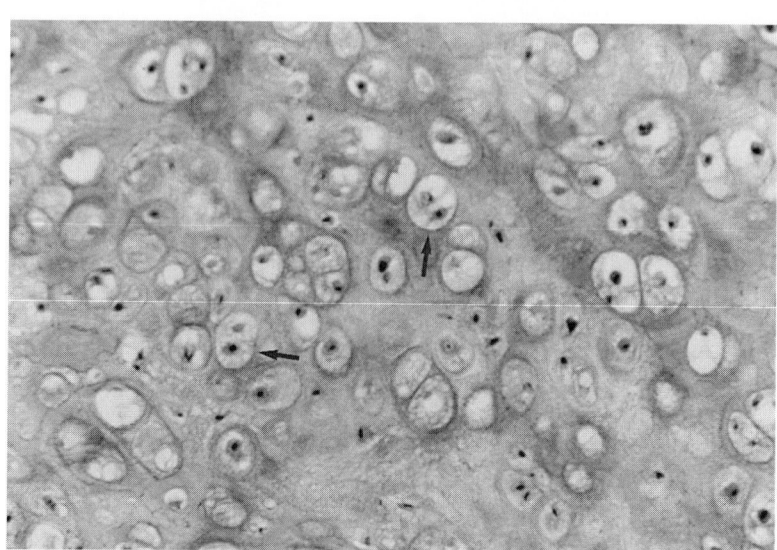

Figure 59–4. Low-grade chondrosarcoma. These mildly atypical chondrocytes display greater cellularity than is seen in benign cartilage. Some of the chondrocytes are binucleate (*arrows*).

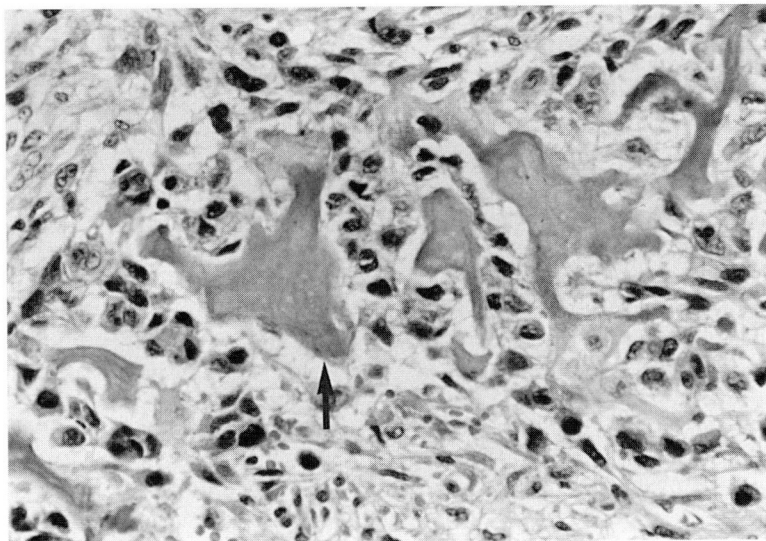

Figure 59–5. Osteosarcoma. These highly atypical cells make up the sarcomatous stroma adjacent to malignant osteoid (*arrow*).

OSTEOSARCOMA

Management

At least 50 years ago, it was evident that amputation alone was inadequate treatment for the majority of patients with osteosarcoma.[31-34] The fact that 80% of patients developed lung metastases within 2 years of diagnosis led to efforts to approach this disease in consideration of its likely systemic nature.

In the classic report by Cade in 1955,[35] doses of 70 to 90 Gy in 8 to 12 weeks were delivered to the primary tumor at diagnosis and those patients who were free of systemic metastases at 6 to 9 months underwent amputation. Cade's goal was to spare the children who were destined to develop pulmonary metastases from having an amputation. Among those patients who eventually underwent amputation after the course of radiation, many were found to have complete clearance of histologically viable tumor. Similarly, in 1973, Allen and Stevens[36]

reported on 10 patients with nonmetastatic osteosarcoma treated with 79 to 100 Gy with either ^{60}Co or 2 MV photons preoperatively. No histologic evidence of tumor was found in six of seven surgical specimens, and 6 of 10 patients were free of disease at a minimum follow-up of 30 months. The observation of improved survival compared with historic control subjects prompted the authors to speculate that tumors irradiated preoperatively were less likely to cause systemic metastases.

At the Princess Margaret Hospital, 29 patients with extremity osteosarcomas were treated between 1958 and 1970 with radical radiation. Only 3 patients obtained a complete response, with 17 achieving a partial response (defined as any decrease in tumor size). The primary tumor recurred in all patients at a mean time of 3.6 months; however, only three patients received more than 60 Gy.[37] The authors concluded that radiation achieved no more than transient control and neither meaningful local palliation nor a useful limb was obtained for any patient. Other investigators have noted that although massive

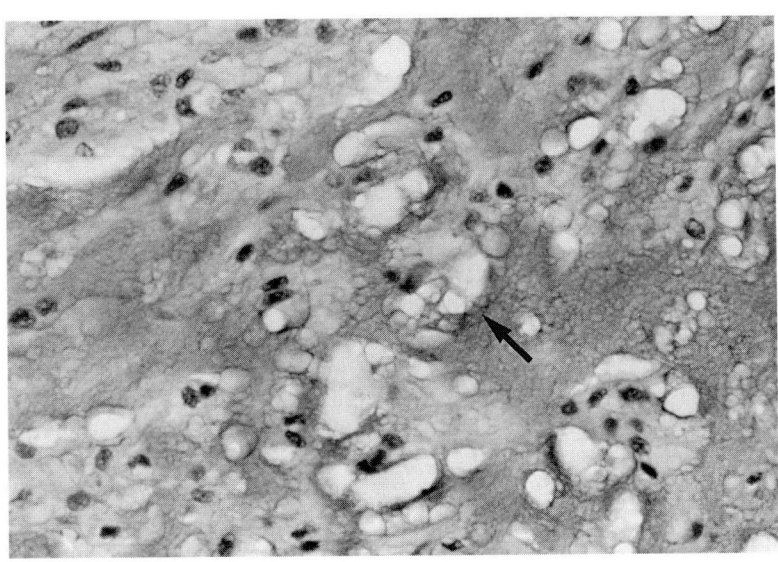

Figure 59–6. Chordoma. The physaliferous cells (*arrow*) display a bubbly cytoplasm due to copious intracytoplasmic mucoid droplets.

doses of preoperative radiation did regularly achieve significant tumor response and improved local control in some cases, overall survival was not improved.[38]

The Mayo Clinic,[39] among others,[40] investigated the efficacy of adjuvant pulmonary irradiation as part of the initial management of patients with osteosarcoma. Unfortunately, in no study was this modality found to be effective in preventing or even delaying the development of pulmonary metastases. An interesting study from the University of Florida[41] showed, through comprehensive pulmonary function testing, that adjuvant pulmonary irradiation caused a transient restrictive ventilatory defect between 6 and 12 months after treatment, which resolved by 2 years.

In 1975, Rosen and colleagues at MSKCC[42] proposed using high-dose methotrexate with vincristine, doxorubicin (Adriamycin), and cyclophosphamide on the "T-4 protocol" as adjuvant therapy following surgical ablation of primary osteosarcoma. This study was based on their promising results in children with metastatic disease, in which they found a median survival of 3 months without therapy and 15 months with the chemotherapy regimen and an overall response rate of 77%. They argued that local radiation followed by amputation for those patients who had not developed pulmonary metastases was no longer a tenable approach; rather, immediate amputation followed by adjuvant systemic chemotherapy held more hope for the majority, who were assumed to have microscopic dissemination at diagnosis.[43]

A review from the Mayo Clinic, however, found a striking improvement in survival for patients diagnosed after 1969 and treated only with surgery, with 35% to 40% surviving without recurrence.[44,45] Thus, the possibility that the natural history of osteosarcoma was changing prompted the evaluation of adjuvant chemotherapy within randomized trials with untreated control subjects. Indeed, a trial conducted at the Mayo Clinic[46] between 1976 and 1980 testing the efficacy of high-dose methotrexate could demonstrate no benefit from the adjuvant therapy, with a 44% relapse-free survival rate in both the treatment and control groups.

The Multi-Institutional Osteosarcoma Study[40] was initiated in 1982 and randomized 36 patients between intensive multiagent chemotherapy (high-dose methotrexate plus cyclophosphamide, Adriamycin, actinomycin-D, bleomycin, and cisplatin) and observation after definitive surgery had been completed. Chemotherapy started 2 weeks after surgery and continued for 1 year. An additional 77 patients who refused randomization elected therapy or observation. The results were similar for randomized and nonrandomized patients; at 2 years, the actuarial relapse-free survival rate was 17% in the control group and 66% in the adjuvant chemotherapy group ($P < 0.001$). The investigators further concluded that the natural history of osteosarcoma had not changed, with the observation arm experiencing the same dismal prognosis that had been seen in historic series.

The clear benefit of chemotherapy in an adjuvant setting led Rosen and colleagues at MSKCC to advocate using chemotherapy in a neoadjuvant fashion, thus permitting an "in vivo sensitivity test."[47,48] A good response, it was reasoned, would improve the opportunity to achieve better limb preservation with complete extirpation of the tumor and, moreover, could guide the selection of chemotherapy in the postoperative period.[49,50]

A system of pathologic grading of tumor response to preoperative, neoadjuvant chemotherapy has been developed by Huvos.[4] A grade I response denotes little or no discernible effect; grade II indicates an intermediate effect; grade III shows only scattered foci of viable tumor; and grade IV indicates no histologic evidence of viable tumor within the specimen. Forty percent of patients in the MSKCC series achieved a grade III or IV response. Those who do not have this level of response proceed to more intense postoperative chemotherapy.

Current Role of Radiation Therapy In Primary Management

Neoadjuvant chemotherapy remains the standard of care in the management of osteosarcoma with surgical resection, typically employed after 2 to 3 months of therapy. Adjuvant chemotherapy is then continued for an additional 4 to 6 months. Irradiation has not been considered part of the primary management of osteosarcoma for nearly 20 years.

Recent publications have identified a small group of patients for whom local adjuvant radiation therapy may, in fact, be useful. Ozaki and colleagues,[51] reporting for the Cooperative German/Austrian Osteosarcoma Study Group reviewed 1982 consecutive patients entered prospectively onto neoadjuvant chemotherapy studies between 1979 and 1998. Sixty-seven patients were identified with nonmetastatic, high-grade primary tumors of the pelvis (ilium, acetabulum, pubis, and ischium); sacral primaries were excluded. Eleven patients received radiation in some form to achieve local control: four postoperatively, and seven as definitive local management with doses between 56 and 68 Gy employed. The overall survival was statistically superior for this group of 11 patients when compared to 19 patients undergoing similar surgical management (intralesional surgery or no surgery) without radiation. The group of patients irradiated had a 29% 5-year overall survival compared to zero for the unirradiated group ($P = 0.0033$). The authors conclude that unresectable osteosarcomas or those operated on with inadequate margins should be treated with a regimen including radiotherapy.

Other investigators have noted that primary tumors of the pelvic bones pose a particular technical challenge in achieving a wide local resection while respecting the anatomic requirements to preserve structural and functional integrity.[52] Tumors in the sacral and para-acetabular regions especially may benefit from preoperative, intraoperative, or postoperative radiation, either alone or in combination.[53,54] Estrada-Aguilar and colleagues[55,56] reported achieving effective local control in five patients with unresectable pelvic osteosarcomas using intra-arterial chemotherapy (cisplatin and Adriamycin) concurrently with local irradiation (60 to 70 Gy). Local toxicity was reportedly minimal.

Stea and colleagues[57] at the NCI contend that the small cell variant of osteosarcoma may be as radiosensitive as

Ewing's sarcoma. They present both in vitro and clinical evidence for the radiation responsiveness of this tumor subtype and report 100% local control for five patients with gross disease treated with radiation alone.

Osteosarcoma of the axial skeleton presents considerable challenges in efforts toward local control. At the Mayo Clinic, 21 patients with osteosarcoma of the spine were treated with radiation after biopsy or decompression and all but 1 were dead of disease at a median of 10 months.[58] Only 5 patients received chemotherapy in this series. In a review from MSKCC of osteosarcoma of the spine, 13 patients underwent limited resection followed by radiation, whereas 11 patients, treated after 1978, underwent aggressive surgical resection, chemotherapy, and local radiation.[59] In the latter group there were five long-term survivors, and aggressive multimodality therapy was recommended.

Investigators from Russia reported that fractionated external beam radiation to a median dose of 60 Gy (range 40 to 68 Gy) was used after neoadjuvant chemotherapy in 31 patients who refused amputation for extremity osteosarcomas.[60] Eleven of these patients had a good response to therapy and none experienced local recurrence at the median follow-up of 67 months. Of 22 patients surviving without local disease progression, 86% had excellent limb function.

Osteosarcomas of the facial bones appear to have a different biology and natural history than those located elsewhere in the body. Numerous reports on small numbers of patients seem to consistently point to a lower tendency for distant metastases. Investigators from the Institut Gustave Roussy[61] obtained a clinically complete response after treating a young patient with osteosarcoma involving the nasal cavity, ethmoid, and maxilla with 45 Gy local radiotherapy followed by three cycles of high-dose ifosfamide. Radical ethmoid-maxillectomy revealed 100% tumor necrosis. Suit reported that high-dose radiation followed by resection was used to treat mandibular osteosarcomas with a resultant 5-year disease-free survival of 73%.[62] DeFries and colleagues[63] reported on two patients with osteosarcoma of the mandible treated with preoperative external radiation to 60 Gy, preoperative chemotherapy, resection, and postoperative chemotherapy. Both patients were disease free at 18 months.

Chambers and Mahoney,[64] reporting the results of 33 patients treated at Walter Reed over 23 years, used a technique of "intensive necrotizing irradiation" with radium needle interstitial implants to deliver 100 to 160 Gy, followed within days by surgical excision. They achieved a 5-year survival rate of 82% in the 27 patients treated with curative intent and with at least 5 years' follow-up. For the entire series of 33 patients, the overall 5-year survival rate was 76%.

Other investigators have also noted a lower rate of metastases and a superior 5-year disease-free survival rate compared with extra craniofacial osteosarcomas.[65-67] Conversely, in a review from UCLA,[68] only 6 of 18 patients with osteosarcomas in the head and neck region were free of disease at 5 years, but 4 of the 6 survivors had been treated with radical surgery, radiation, and chemotherapy initially, leading the authors to advocate multimodality therapy for all patients.

It is possible that the natural history of osteosarcoma of the facial bones is significantly different than that of the long bones. With current techniques of craniofacial reconstruction, adequate surgical margins for these tumors may be accomplished more frequently than in previous studies. However, the potential contribution of well-planned high-dose external or interstitial radiation should be brought to bear on the current multimodality management of such tumors.

Extracorporeal bone irradiation has been used with reported success where custom prostheses or allografts could not be used.[69] Hong and colleagues from Australia reported on extracorporeal radiation as the definitive local therapy for 16 patients with primary bone tumors between 1996 and 2000.[70] Eleven cases of Ewing's sarcoma, 4 osteosarcoma, and one chondrosarcoma constituted the study population. All patients received appropriate chemotherapy followed by en bloc resection of the affected bone. A single dose of 50 Gy was delivered to the resected specimen, which was then reimplanted using appropriate internal fixation. One patient received postoperative external beam radiation, as well. No cases of local recurrence or graft failure were noted at a median follow-up of 19 months. One patient required amputation for chronic osteomyelitis. Among the 10 patients with at least 18 months of follow-up, the functional outcome was graded as good to excellent.

In Milan, a technique of hypofractionated accelerated radiation was used as a single modality in 14 patients with osteosarcoma for palliative purposes.[71] Three weekly fractions of 6 Gy over 2 weeks to a total dose of 36 Gy were delivered. A durable response was obtained in 81% of irradiated sites, and when chemotherapy was added, a 92% response rate was observed. In seven patients who later underwent ablative surgery, six had 100% pathologic tumor necrosis. The investigators note that severe normal tissue damage was produced in a high proportion of patients treated in this manner.

Heavy ions (neon, helium, and carbon), neutrons, and protons have been used to improve locoregional control in patients with residual and unresectable bone sarcomas.[72-79] Promising data on the utility of high-dose Samarium-153 (^{153}Sm-EDTMP) for patients with osteosarcoma is emerging.[80] This isotope is currently approved for the palliation of bone metastases at modest doses (1 mCi/kg). Higher doses (30 mCi/kg) cause severe pancytopenias, and thus stem cell support was found to be necessary in the early trials of this agent. Nonhematologic toxicity was low and pain palliation was excellent. A single patient with a primary pelvic osteosarcoma and pulmonary metastases treated with aggressive chemotherapy, ^{153}Sm-EDTMP (4.5 mCi/kg), stem cell support, and external beam radiation to the pelvic tumor to 60 Gy was rendered disease free at 3 years, 4 months follow-up, the time of the report.[81]

Follow-Up and Rehabilitation

Since advances in the management of patients, especially pediatric patients, with bone tumors has resulted in improved survival and local control, the rehabilitation specialist must address the immediate rehabilitative needs incurred during the treatment period and anticipate future musculoskeletal sequelae.[82] Because dysfunction may evolve during a child's developmental period,[83] it is imperative that ongoing physical therapy assessment and intervention be provided until developmental maturity is achieved.

CHONDROSARCOMA

The MD Anderson experience with the use of radiotherapy in 20 patients with primary chondrosarcoma of bone for curative intent was reviewed.[84] Nine of 11 patients treated with radiation alone were controlled for 26 to 156 months. Doses ranged from 40 to 70 Gy in standard fractionation. The investigators believe that radiation is indicated in two settings: (1) as primary treatment when surgery is not possible, and (2) postoperatively when the surgical margins are either grossly or microscopically inadequate.

These concepts are in agreement with conclusions drawn from a 23-year experience in the irradiation of chondrosarcoma at the Princess Margaret Hospital.[85,86] No patient had complete surgery, and the majority presented with pain and tumors in an axial site—all poor prognostic features. Despite these facts, 50% of those whose tumors were irradiated with curative intent were controlled locally following treatment, and 25% were free of disease at 15 years. The majority received 50 to 55 Gy in 2.5 Gy fractions. The investigators point out that tumors in the head and neck and truncal regions have an 85% local recurrence rate with surgery alone, supporting the value of radiation in an adjuvant setting where surgical resection is judged to be inadequate.

Huvos and colleagues[87] reported a clinicopathologic analysis of 35 patients treated at Memorial Hospital for the mesenchymal variant of chondrosarcoma. They separated this group into patients with a predominant hemangiopericytomatoid component and those with a small cell undifferentiated pattern. These groups demonstrated responsiveness to both chemotherapy and radiation, in contrast to results with conventional chondrosarcoma.

Low-grade chondrosarcomas of the base of the skull have been treated with fractionated proton radiation therapy with a 5-year local control rate of 82%.[88] Investigators from the Proton Therapy facility in Orsay, France reported the results of combined proton/photon irradiation for 45 patients with base of the skull chordomas or chondrosarcomas.[89] The median dose to gross tumor was 67 CGE (cobalt gray equivalent) with one third of the dose being delivered with protons. Three-year local control and survival rates of approximately 90% were reported. Two patients experienced serious late symptoms from treatment—one had memory decline and the other had bilateral vision loss.

The series from Massachusetts General Hospital has published the results on treatment of 519 patients with chordomas and low-grade chondrosarcomas treated with proton therapy.[90] Five-year local control rates of 73% for chordomas and 98% for chondrosarcomas were achieved with tumor doses from 66 to 83 CGE. Results from Loma Linda show similar success, with five-year local control rates of 76% for chordomas and 92% for chondrosarcomas.[91]

CHORDOMA

According to Huvos,[28] 50% of chordomas arise in the sacrum, 35% in the clivus, and 15% in the true vertebrae. Between 5% and 43% eventually metastasize,[28,92,93] with the lungs being the most common metastatic site. Prolonged survival, even with metastatic disease, is not uncommon. Keisch and associates,[94] in their report on 21 patients treated at the Mallinckrodt Institute of Radiology, noted that no patient was controlled, regardless of initial therapy. The group treated with conventional radiation alone did most poorly, with no survivors. Patients with lumbosacral tumors treated with surgery plus radiation had a longer mean disease-free survival (6.6 years) than those treated with surgery alone (4.1 years). They recommend doses of 55 to 60 Gy in standard fractionation to respect normal tissue tolerance.

Fagundes and associates[93] reported a series of 204 patients with chordomas of the base of the skull and cervical spine treated with combined proton and photon radiation to a median dose of 70.1 CGE. Overall, 29% (60 patients) experienced local relapse. Although 10 of 60 who failed locally also recurred distantly, only 2 of 144 patients who were locally controlled developed distant metastases. Local control, therefore, proved to be a highly significant predictor of distant disease-free survival. Overall survival following local relapse was poor, with a 5% actuarial 5-year survival rate and no survivors at 7 years.

Complete surgical excision as the primary procedure with negative margins can be curative, but it is rarely possible. The poor long-term survival after local recurrence highlights the importance of a concerted approach by the surgical and radiation oncologists to achieve local control with combined modality therapy at the outset when negative margins cannot be attained. Local recurrence is the rule when the tumor is violated during resection, and a second radical resection will rarely achieve long-term local control. Heroic surgical procedures, such as hemicorporectomy,[95,96] have been advocated for locally extensive growths. However, if positive margins or gross residual disease are known to exist after the primary surgery, postoperative radiation therapy is indicated.

Adequate delivery of high-dose conventional photon irradiation is virtually impossible owing to the proximity to normal neural tissues and, in the sacrococcygeal region, to the bowel. Therefore, results with conventional photon irradiation have been unimpressive.[97] In contrast, proton beam therapy, using precise positioning and immobilization, is able to deliver doses as high as 74 CGE to chordomas and chondrosarcomas of the base of the skull and the cervical spine while respecting the normal tissue tolerance of the brainstem, spinal cord, optic structures, and temporal lobes. Investigators from Massachusetts General Hospital (MGH)[98,99] stress the importance of extreme positioning accuracy to extract the greatest advantage from the physical dosimetry characteristics of protons.

In addition, promising results with charged particle irradiation (helium and neon) in the treatment of sacral chordomas have been reported by the University of California Lawrence Berkeley Laboratory.[100] It is not clear whether charged particle therapy is superior to proton therapy, but there is no doubt that the physical characteristics and radiation biology of these modalities are superior to conventional photon irradiation. An approach using three-dimensional conformal radiation therapy may produce nearly equivalent dosimetric advantages (Fig. 59-7A–D). Such a technique requires fastidious attention to all phases of patient immobilization, fine cut–based computed tomography planning, and treatment delivery. For patients with these rare neoplasms,

efforts to optimize local control when planning primary management might be best served by early collaboration at a center with such specialized equipment.

MALIGNANT FIBROUS HISTIOCYTOMA OF BONE

This rare primary sarcoma of bone seems to behave similarly to its soft tissue counterpart. A review of 38 cases over a 15-year period in New South Wales[101] found that 26% of cases arose in a preexisting lesion. The 32 patients who underwent amputation or wide excision experienced a 5-year survival rate of 86%, whereas those who had a marginal or intralesional excision had a 30% 5-year survival rate. Adjuvant chemotherapy had no discernible effect on survival.

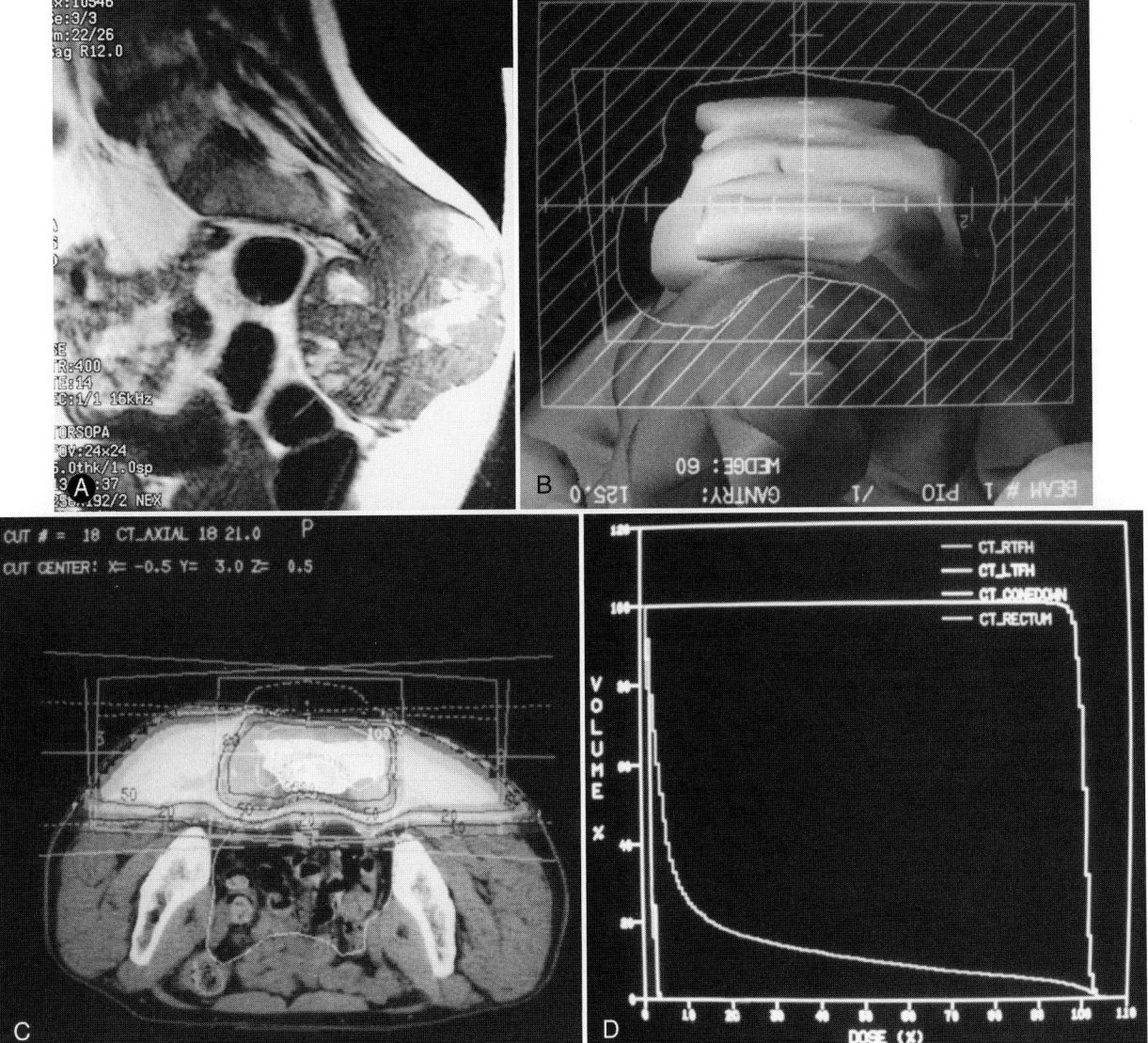

Figure 59–7. A, This T1-weighted sagittal image shows a heterogeneous mass arising from the distal sacrum. Note the clear separation between the anterior soft tissue component and the bowel. **B**, A three-dimensional (3D) reconstruction displays the sacral target volume and the bowel in close proximity. **C**, The dose distribution is projected on an axial computed tomographic slice for evaluation of beam arrangement and target coverage. **D**, Lastly, a dose-volume histogram is generated, indicating that the 3D plan achieves excellent sparing of the nearby bowel. See also Color Figure 59-7B–D.

GIANT CELL TUMOR OF BONE

Giant cell tumors are more prevalent in females and rarely occur before skeletal maturity is reached, the majority occurring between 20 and 40 years of age. Approximately three quarters of these tumors occur at the epiphysis of a long bone[24,102] of the extremities, almost always extending to the articular cartilage. Only 3% are in vertebral bodies. Consequently, the majority are managed surgically, with local control rates in the range of 85% to 90%.[24]

Dahlin and colleagues[24] reported the treatment results of 195 cases of giant cell tumor of bone treated at the Mayo Clinic between 1910 and 1969. They found the local failure rate to be nearly identical (43%) in primary tumors treated with surgical techniques alone and those treated by surgical removal followed by radiation therapy. The series, collected before the advent of custom allographs and joint prostheses, reveals the necessity of a wide en bloc resection leaving no residual tumor. In the surgery-alone group, 2 of 40 patients developed malignant degeneration at failure, and in the irradiated group, 5 of 61 had this event. Although the authors conclude that radiation is an important factor in the malignant transformation of giant cell tumors, they clearly report the occurrence of (1) malignant giant cell tumors at diagnosis, (2) malignant transformation at recurrence in unirradiated patients, and (3) metastases from "benign" giant cell tumors. Therefore, owing to the inherent selection bias in the aggressive treatment group, the contention that radiation causes malignant transformation is probably untenable. Unfortunately, such reports, when considered along with the young age of most affected patients, contribute to a reluctance to use radiation in many cases.

Series reporting the efficacy of radiation in the management of giant cell tumors always reflect the sites and nature of involvement that are unusual. For example, in the series reported by Chen and associates,[26] 30 of the 35 cases reported occurred in the skull or spinal axis. In only two cases was radiation delivered after complete surgical excision; 33 patients had gross tumor at the time of irradiation. Patients who received less than 30 Gy experienced local failure in the majority of cases (5/8), whereas at doses above 35 Gy, the majority (14/17) were controlled. Although they present no further dose-response data, the authors do recommend 50 to 60 Gy when radiation will be the sole treatment modality and 30 to 40 Gy in the postoperative setting. In addition, they suggest that a 1 to 2 cm margin be used when designing radiation fields.

Similarly, investigators at the Princess Margaret Hospital[103] report 21 patients treated over 42 years; 8 were treated at recurrence, but of the 13 primary cases, 11 were treated postoperatively for microscopic or grossly positive margins. Ten of these 11 patients were controlled with radiation doses between 10.8 and 50 Gy. For the eight patients treated at recurrence, seven were controlled with radiation doses between 35 and 55 Gy. The investigators concluded that even gross disease was readily controlled with moderate doses of radiation. They recommend 35 Gy in 15 fractions in situations in which

the probability of recurrence is high and the potential morbidity of further relapse is high. They do not go so far as to recommend that radiation be routinely employed after surgery with resultant positive margins, and, in fact, the results in the recurrent setting were as good as those in the primary setting.

The MD Anderson group[104] reported on 15 patients irradiated for giant cell tumors between 1948 and 1984, of whom 10 were evaluable. Three patients died of uncontrolled local and distant disease and 5 of the 10 had received chemotherapy as a component of their treatment course, attesting to the unrepresentative nature of the study population. Radiation doses ranged from 36 to 66 Gy, and the authors recommend 45 to 50 Gy when surgical excision cannot be performed.

In the University of Florida series spanning 15 years,[25] all 14 patients were treated for gross unresectable disease; 10 were in the axial skeleton and 6 were recurrent lesions. Nevertheless, 75% were controlled with radiation doses between 35 and 55 Gy, and the remainder were controlled with surgical salvage. The authors recommend doses in excess of 40 Gy.

In summary, giant cell tumors of bone are generally quite radioresponsive, with prolonged control of even gross disease likely with doses in the range of 40 to 50 Gy. Radiation would be indicated for unresectable lesions in the axial skeleton and after subtotal resection in any site. The role of radiation after surgical resection with microscopically positive margins is not established but may be appropriate in sites in which recurrent tumor would require major and potentially disabling surgical management for control.

REFERENCES

1. Robbins SL, Cotran RS: The musculoskeletal system. In Robbins SL, Cotran RS, eds. *Pathologic Basis of Disease*, 2nd ed. Philadelphia: WB Saunders; 1979:1477.
2. Vitale JJ: Nutritional disease. In Robbins SL, Cotran RS, eds. *Pathologic Basis of Disease*, 2nd ed. Philadelphia: WB Saunders; 1979:492.
3. Stanfill P, Pratt C: Bone tumors. In Hockenberry MJ, Coody DK, eds. *Pediatric Oncology and Hematology: Perspectives on Care*. St. Louis: CV Mosby; 1987:104.
4. Huvos AG: Osteogenic sarcoma. In *Bone Tumors: Diagnosis, Treatment and Prognosis*, 2nd ed. Philadelphia: WB Saunders; 1991:85.
5. Fraumeni JF: Stature and malignant tumors of bone in childhood and adolescence. *Cancer*. 1967;20:967.
6. Scranton PE, DeCicco FA, Totten RS, et al: Prognostic factors in osteosarcoma: A review of 20 years' experience at the University of Pittsburgh Health Center Hospitals. *Cancer*. 1975;36:2179.
7. Tjalma RA: Canine bone sarcoma: Estimation of relative risk as a function of body size. *J Natl Cancer Inst*. 1966;36:1137.
8. Healey JH, Buss D: Radiation and pagetic osteogenic sarcomas. *Clin Orthop*. 1991;270:128.
9. Frassica FJ, Sim FH, Frassica DA, et al: Survival and management considerations in postirradiation osteosarcoma and Paget's osteosarcoma. *Clin Orthop*. 1991;270:120.
10. Mays CW, Spiess H, Chmelevsky D: Cancers in patients injected with 224 Ra (meeting abstract). *Health Phys*. 1989;56 (suppl 1):S44.
11. Glicksman AS, Fabrikant J: Analysis of post-radiation sarcomas: Correlation of clinical data with experimental results (meeting abstract). *Proc Ann Meet Am Assoc Cancer Res*. 1987; 28:88.

12. Abramson DH: Retinoblastoma. In Skog DR, Buckley RH, DeVivo DC, et al, eds. *Pediatric Emergency Casebook*, vol 3. New York: World Health Communications; 1985.

13. Schwarz MB, Burgess LP, Fee WE Jr, et al: Postirradiation sarcoma in retinoblastoma: Induction or predisposition? *Arch Otolaryngol Head Neck Surg.* 1988;114:640.

14. Hawkins MM, Draper GJ, Kingston JE: Incidence of second primary tumors among childhood cancer survivors. *Br J Cancer.* 1987;56:339.

15. Smith LM, Donaldson SS, Egbert PR, et al: Aggressive management of second primary tumors in survivors of hereditary retinoblastoma. *Int J Radiat Oncol Biol Phys.* 1989;17:499.

16. Tucker MA, D'Angio GJ, Boice JD Jr, et al: Bone sarcomas linked to radiotherapy and chemotherapy in children. *N Engl J Med.* 1987;317:558.

17. Smith MB, Xue H, Strong L, et al: Forty-year experience with second malignancies after treatment of childhood cancer: Analysis of outcome following the development of the second malignancy. *J Pediatr Surg.* 1993;28:1342.

18. Bielack SS, Kempf-Bielack B, Delling G, et al: Prognostic factors in high-grade osteosarcoma of the extremities or trunk: An analysis of 1702 patients treated on neoadjuvant cooperative osteosarcoma study group protocols. *J Clin Oncol.* 2002;20:776.

19. Bloem JL, Kroon HM: Imaging of bone and soft tissue tumors: Osseous lesions. *Radiol Clin North Am.* 1993;31:261.

20. Giudici MA, Moser RP, Kransdorf MJ: Imaging of bone and soft tissue tumors: Cartilaginous bone tumors. *Radiol Clin North Am.* 1993;31:237.

21. Manaster BJ, Doyle AJ: Imaging of bone and soft tissue tumors: Giant cell tumors of bone. *Radiol Clin North Am.* 1993;31:299.

22. Hutter RVP, Worchester JN Jr, Francis KC, et al: Benign and malignant giant cell tumors of bone: A clinicopathological analysis of the natural history of the disease. *Cancer.* 1962;15:653.

23. Catto ME: Diseases of bone. In Anderson JR, ed. *Muir's Textbook of Pathology*, 12th ed. Baltimore: Edward Arnold; 1985:1.

24. Dahlin DC, Cupps RE, Johnson EW Jr: Giant cell tumor: A study of 195 cases. *Radiology.* 1986;161:537.

25. Bennett CJ Jr, Marcus RB Jr, Million RR, Enneing WF: Radiation therapy for giant cell tumor of bone. *Int J Radiat Oncol Biol Phys.* 1993;26:299.

26. Chen ZX, Gu DZ, Yu ZH, et al: Radiation therapy of giant cell tumor of bone: Analysis of 35 patients. *Int J Radiat Oncol Biol Phys.* 1986;12:329.

27. Bell RS, Harwood AR, Goodman SB, Fornasier VL: Supervoltage radiotherapy in the treatment of difficult giant cell tumors of bone. *Clin Orthop Rel Res.* 1983;174:208.

28. Huvos AG: Chordoma. In *Bone Tumors: Diagnosis, Treatment and Prognosis*, 2nd ed. Philadelphia: WB Saunders; 1991:599.

29. Congdon CC: Proliferative lesions resembling chordoma following puncture of nucleus pulposus in rabbits. *J Natl Cancer Inst.* 1952; 12:892.

30. Krayenbuhl H, Yasargil MG: Cranial chordomas. *Prog Neurol Surg.* 1975;6:380.

31. Dahlin DC, Coventry MB: Osteogenic sarcoma: A study of six hundred cases. *J Bone Joint Surg (Am).* 1967;49:101.

32. Lindbom A, Soderberg G, Spjut HJ: Osteosarcoma: A review of 96 cases. *Acta Radiol.* 1961;56:1.

33. Marcove RC, Mike V, Hajek JV, et al: Osteogenic sarcoma under the age of twenty-one: A review of 145 operative cases. *J Bone Joint Surg (Am).* 1970;52:411.

34. Weinfeld MS, Dudley HR: Osteogenic sarcoma: A follow-up study of the 94 cases observed at the Massachusetts General Hospital from 1920 to 1960. *J Bone Joint Surg (Am).* 1962;44:269.

35. Cade S: Osteogenic sarcoma: A study based on 133 patients. *J R Coll Surg Edinb.* 1955;1:79.

36. Allen CV, Stevens KR: Preoperative irradiation for osteogenic sarcoma. *Cancer.* 1973;31:1364.

37. Jenkin RDT, Allt WEC, Fitzpatrick PJ: Osteosarcoma: An assessment of management with particular reference to primary irradiation and selective delayed amputation. *Cancer.* 1972;30:393.

38. Caceres E, Zaharia M: Massive preoperative radiation therapy in the treatment of osteogenic sarcoma. *Cancer.* 1972;30:634.

39. Rab GT, Ivins JC, Childs DS, et al: Elective whole lung irradiation in the treatment of osteogenic sarcoma. *Cancer.* 1976;38:939.

40. Burgers JMV, VanGlabbeke M, Busson A, et al: Osteosarcoma of the limbs: Report of the EORTC-SIOP 03 Trial 20781 investigating the value of adjuvant treatment with chemotherapy and/or prophylactic lung irradiation. *Cancer.* 1988;61:1924.

41. Ellis ER, Marcus RB Jr, Cicale MJ, et al: Pulmonary function tests after whole-lung irradiation and doxorubicin in patients with osteogenic sarcoma. *J Clin Oncol.* 1992;10:459.

42. Rosen G, Tan C, Sanmaneechai A, et al: The rationale for multiple drug chemotherapy in the treatment of osteogenic sarcoma. *Cancer.* 1975;35:936.

43. Rosen G, Tefft M, Martinez A, et al: Combination chemotherapy and radiation therapy in the treatment of metastatic osteogenic sarcoma. *Cancer.* 1975;35:622.

44. Taylor WF, Ivins JC, Dahlin DC, et al: Trends and variability in survival from osteosarcoma. *Mayo Clin Proc.* 1978;53:695.

45. Taylor WF, Ivins JC, Pritchard DJ, et al: Trends and variability in survival among patients with osteosarcoma: A 7-year update. *Mayo Clin Proc.* 1985;60:91.

46. Edmonson JH, Green SJ, Ivins JC, et al: A controlled pilot study of high-dose methotrexate as post-surgical adjuvant treatment for primary osteosarcoma. *J Clin Oncol.* 1984;2:152.

47. Rosen G, Caparros B, Huvos AG, et al: Preoperative chemotherapy for osteogenic sarcoma: Selection of postoperative adjuvant chemotherapy based on the response of the primary tumor to preoperative chemotherapy. *Cancer.* 1982;49:1221.

48. Rosen G, Marcove RC, Caparros B, et al: Primary osteogenic sarcoma: The rationale for preoperative chemotherapy and delayed surgery. *Cancer.* 1979;43:2163.

49. Craft AW: Management of osteogenic sarcoma (abstract). *Br J Radiol.* 1988;61:730.

50. Meskens M, Burssens A, Hoogmartens M, et al: Osteogenic sarcoma in children: A retrospective study of 58 cases. *Acta Orthop Belg.* 1993;59:64.

51. Ozaki T, Flege S, Kevric M, et al: Osteosarcoma of the pelvis: Experience of the cooperative osteosarcoma study group. *J Clin Oncol.* 2003;21:334.

52. Fahey M, Spanier SS, Vander Griend RA: Osteosarcoma of the pelvis: A clinical and histopathological study of twenty-five patients. *J Bone Joint Surg (Am).* 1992;74:321.

53. Monticelli G, Santori FS, Ghera S, et al: Surgical problems in the treatment of pelvic tumors. *Monogr Ser Eur Org Res Treat Cancer.* 1986;16:101.

54. Calvo FA, Ortiz de Urbina D, Sierrasesumaga L, et al: Intraoperative radiotherapy in the multidisciplinary treatment of bone sarcomas in children and adolescents. *Med Pediatr Oncol.* 1991;19:478.

55. Estrada J, Greenberg H, Walling AK, et al: Control of pelvic osteosarcoma (OS) with intraarterial (IA) chemotherapy and radiation therapy (XRT) (meeting abstract). *Proc Annu Meet Am Soc Clin Oncol.* 1988;7:A1075.

56. Estrada-Aguilar J, Greenberg H, Walling AK, et al: Primary treatment of pelvic osteosarcoma: Report of five cases. *Cancer.* 1992;69:1137.

57. Stea B, Cavazzana A, Kinsella TJ: Small-cell osteosarcoma: Correlation of in vitro and clinical radiation response. *Int J Radiat Oncol Biol Phys.* 1988;15:1233.

58. Shives TC, Dahlin DC, Sim FH, et al: Osteosarcoma of the spine. *J Bone Joint Surg (Am).* 1986;68:660.

59. Sundaresan N, Rosen G, Huvos AG, et al: Combined treatment of osteosarcoma of the spine. *Neurosurgery.* 1988;23:714.

60. Machak GN, Tkachev SI, Solovyev YN, et al: Neoadjuvant chemotherapy and local radiotherapy for high grade osteosarcoma of the extremities. *Mayo Clin Proc.* 2003;78:147.

61. Gandia D, Domenge C, Schwaab G, et al: Radiotherapy followed by high-dose ifosfamide (HDI) in osteosarcoma of the facial bones (meeting abstract). *Ann Oncol.* 1992;3(suppl 5):169.

62. Suit HD: Role of therapeutic radiology in cancer of bone. *Cancer.* 1975;35:930.

63. DeFries HO, Perlin E, Leibel SA: Treatment of osteogenic sarcoma of the mandible. *Arch Otolaryngol.* 1979;105:358.

64. Chambers RG, Mahoney WD: Osteogenic sarcoma of the mandible: Current management. *Am Surgeon.* 1970;36:463.

65. Slootweg PJ, Muller H: Osteosarcoma of the jaw bones: Analysis of 18 cases. *J Maxillofac Surg.* 1985;13:158.

66. Bras J: Osteosarcoma of the jaws: Prognostic factors (meeting abstract). In: Proceedings of the Second International Conference on Head and Neck Cancer, American Society for Head and Neck Surgery. July 31-August 5, 1988; Boston. p 101.

67. Panizzoni GA, Gasparini G, Clauser L, et al: Osteosarcoma of the facial bones. *Ann Oncol.* 1992;3(suppl 2):s47.
68. Mark RJ, Sercarz JA, Tran L, et al: Osteogenic sarcoma of the head and neck: The UCLA experience. *Arch Otolaryngol Head Neck Surg.* 1991;117:761.
69. Myttendaele D, DeSchryver A, Claessens H, et al: Limb conservation in primary bone tumors by resection, extracorporeal irradiation and re-implantation. *J Bone Joint Surg.* 1988;70-B:348.
70. Hong A, Stevens G, Stalley P, Pendlebury S, et al: Extracorporeal Irradiation for Malignant Bone Tumors. *Int J Radiat Oncol Biol Phys.* 2001;50:441.
71. Lombardi F, Gandola L, Fossati-Bellani F, et al: Hypofractionated accelerated radiotherapy in osteogenic sarcoma. *Int J Radiat Oncol Biol Phys.* 1992;24:761.
72. Castro JR, Phillips TL, Collier JM, et al: A phase I–II trial of charged particle radiotherapy with neon ions: A northern California Oncology Group study (meeting abstract). *Proc Ann Meet Am Soc Clin Oncol.* 1989;8:A1237.
73. Linstadt DE, Castro JR, Phillips TL: Neon ion radiotherapy: Results of the phase I/II clinical trial. *Int J Radiat Oncol Biol Phys.* 1991;20:761.
74. Nowakowski VA, Castro JR, Petti PL, et al: Charged particle radiotherapy of paraspinal tumors. *Int J Radiat Oncol Biol Phys.* 1992;22:295.
75. Uhl V, Castro JR, Knopf K, et al: Preliminary results in heavy charged particle irradiation of bone sarcomas. *Int J Radiat Oncol Biol Phys.* 1992;24:755.
76. Schmitt G, Wambersie A: Review of the clinical results of fast neutron therapy. *Radiother Oncol.* 1990;17:47.
77. Chauvel P: Osteosarcomas and adult soft tissue sarcomas: Is there a place for high LET radiation therapy? *Ann Oncol.* 1992;3(suppl 2):s107.
78. Hug EB, Fitzek MM, Liebsch NJ, Munzenrider JE: Locally challenging osteo- and chrondrogenic tumors of the axial skeleton: Results of combined proton and photon radiation therapy using three-dimensional treatment planning. *Int J Radiat Oncol Biol Phys.* 1995;31:467.
79. Kamada T, Tsujii H, Yanagi T, et al: Efficacy and safety of carbon ion radiotherapy in bone and soft tissue sarcomas. *J Clin Oncol.* 2002;20:4466.
80. Anderson PM, Wiseman GA, Dispenzieri A, et al: High-dose samarium-153 ethylene diamine tetramethylene phosphonate: Low toxicity of skeletal irradiation in patients with osteosarcoma and bone metastases. *J Clin Oncol.* 2002;20:189.
81. Franzius C, Schuck A, Bielack SS: Correspondence: High dose samarium-153 ethylene diamine tetramethylene phosphonate: Low toxicity of skeletal irradiation in patients with osteosarcoma and bone metastases. *J Clin Oncol.* 2002;20:1953.
82. Lampert MH, Gahagen C: Rehabilitation of the sarcoma patient. In McGarvey CL, ed: *Clinics in Physical Therapy.* New York: Churchill Livingstone; 1988:111.
83. Butler MS, Robertson WW Jr, Rate W, et al: Skeletal sequelae of radiation for malignant childhood tumors. *Clin Orthop.* 1990;251:235.
84. McNaney D, Lindberg RD, Ayala AG, et al: Fifteen-year radiotherapy experience with chondrosarcoma of bone. *Int J Radiat Oncol Biol Phys.* 1982;8:187.
85. Harwood AR, Krajbich JI, Fornasier VL: Radiotherapy of chondrosarcoma of bone. *Cancer.* 1980;45:2769.
86. Krochak R, Harwood AR, Cummings BJ, Quirt IC: Results of radical radiation for chondrosarcoma of bone. *Radiother Oncol.* 1983;1:109.
87. Huvos AG, Rosen G, Dabska M, Marcove RC: Mesenchymal chondrosarcoma: A clinicopathologic analysis of 35 patients with emphasis on treatment. *Cancer.* 1983;51:1230.
88. Austin-Seymour M, Munzenrider J, Linggood R, et al: Fractionated proton radiation therapy of cranial and extracranial tumors. *Am J Clin Oncol.* 1990;13:327.
89. Noel G, Habrand JL, Mammar H, et al: Combination of photon and proton radiation therapy for chordomas and chondrosarcomas of the skull base: The Centre de Protontherapie D'Orsay Experience. *Int J Radiat Oncol Biol Phys.* 2001;51:392.
90. Munzingrider JE, Liebsch NJ: Proton therapy for tumors of the skull base. *Strahlenther Onkol.* 1999;175(suppl II):57.
91. Hug EB, Loredo LN, Slater JD, et al: Proton radiation therapy for chordomas and chondrosarcomas of the skull base. *J Neurosurg* 1999;91:432.
92. Wang CC, James AE Jr: Chordoma: Brief review of the literature and report of a case with widespread metastases. *Cancer.* 1968;22:162.
93. Fagundes MA, Hug EB, Liebsch NJ, et al: Radiation therapy for chordomas of the base of skull and cervical spine: Patterns of failure and outcome after relapse. *Int J Radiat Oncol Biol Phys.* 1995;33:579.
94. Keisch ME, Garcia DM, Shibuya RB: Retrospective long-term follow-up analysis in 21 patients with chordomas of various sites treated at a single institution. *J Neurosurg.* 1991;75:374.
95. Maroske D, Hupe K: Sacrococcygeal chordoma: Radical operation, a problem. *Chirurg.* 1977;48:118.
96. Miller TR, Mackenzie AR, Randal HT, et al: Hemicorporectomy. *Surgery.* 1966;59:988.
97. Watkins L, Khudados ES, Kaleoglu M, et al: Skull base chordomas: A review of 38 patients, 1958–88. *Br J Neurosurg.* 1993;7:241.
98. Tatsuzaki H, Urie MM: Importance of precise positioning for proton beam therapy in the base of skull and cervical spine. *Int J Radiat Oncol Biol Phys.* 1991;21:757.
99. Niemierko A, Urie M, Gotein M: Optimization of 3D radiation therapy with both physical and biological end points and constraints. *Int J Radiat Oncol Biol Phys.* 1992;23:99.
100. Schoenthaler R, Castro JR, Petti PL, et al: Charged particle irradiation of sacral chordomas. *Int J Radiat Oncol Biol Phys.* 1993;26:291.
101. Little DG, McCarthy SW: Malignant fibrous histiocytoma of bone: The experience of the New South Wales Bone Tumor Registry. *Aust N Z J Surg.* 1993;63:346.
102. Marcove RC, Weis LD, Vaghaiwalla MR, Pearson R: Giant cell tumors of bone: A report of 52 consecutive cases. *Clin Orthop Rel Res.* 1978;134:275.
103. Malone S, O'Sullivan B, Catton C, et al: Long-term follow-up of efficacy and safety of megavoltage radiotherapy in high-risk giant cell tumors of bone. *Int J Radiat Oncol Biol Phys.* 1995;33:689.
104. Seider MJ, Rich TA, Ayala AG, Murray JA: Giant cell tumors of bone: Treatment with radiation therapy. *Radiology.* 1986; 161:537.

Hodgkin's Disease

60

Richard T. Hoppe, MD

The management of Hodgkin's disease has evolved dramatically in the past 4 decades. Refined classification systems, advances in imaging technology, the identification of important prognostic factors, the development of improved radiation therapy techniques, and the discovery of effective combination chemotherapy have led to a marked improvement in patient survival. With improved outcome, the potential long-term complications of staging and treatment have become more apparent, and this has led to further refinement of management programs in order to maximize the likelihood of complication-free survival.

EPIDEMIOLOGY AND RISK FACTORS[1]

Hodgkin's disease accounts for less than 1% of cancers diagnosed in the United States each year.[2,3] There is a slight male predominance. The median age at the time of diagnosis is 26 to 30 years. The disease is uncommon in children younger than 10 years and the age-adjusted incidence is bimodal.[4] Both peaks, at ages 20 to 24 and 75 to 84, show an annual incidence of about 5.5 cases per 100,000. A decline in the height of the incidence peak for older adults may be attributed to improved diagnostic accuracy and the ability to differentiate mixed cellularity or lymphocyte depletion Hodgkin's disease from diffuse large cell or anaplastic large cell lymphomas.

There are no well-defined risk factors associated with the development of Hodgkin's disease.[5] Older reports associating an increased risk with tonsillectomy have been refuted. There are no definite associations between Hodgkin's disease and Human Leukocyte Antigen (HLA) loci. The slight increased risk associated with small sibship size and higher degree of education has not been explained, but contributes to the hypothesis of an infectious etiology. A relationship between Hodgkin's disease and prior infection with Epstein-Barr virus (EBV) has been proposed. Components of the EBV genome have been detected in the cellular DNA of Reed-Sternberg cells,[6] and elevated levels of immunoglobulin G (IgG) and IgA against the EBV capsid antigen and elevated levels of antibody against the EBV nuclear antigen and early antigen D have been detected in the serum of patients who later develop Hodgkin's disease.[7] The risk for developing Hodgkin's disease appears to be higher in the presence of a prior history of infectious mononucleosis.[8] Evidence of prior EBV infection is most common in mixed cellularity

Hodgkin's disease and in pediatric Hodgkin's disease in underdeveloped countries.[9]

ANATOMY

Hodgkin's disease arises primarily in lymph nodes. Solitary extralymphatic involvement in the absence of nodal disease is exceedingly rare. There is a general axial distribution of lymph node involvement. More than 80% of patients have cervical lymph node involvement at presentation, and more than half have mediastinal disease. The most common site of extranodal disease is the spleen. The lymphoid tissues of Waldeyer's ring or Peyer's patches are involved infrequently.

PATHOLOGY[10,11]

The diagnostic cell of Hodgkin's disease is the Reed-Sternberg cell; however, these cells account for less than 1% of the cells in a lymph node infiltrated by Hodgkin's disease. The majority of the cells are lymphocytes, eosinophils, and plasma cells. The Reed-Sternberg cell has a classic appearance that is binucleate, with two prominent nucleoli. There is a well-demarcated nuclear membrane, and eosinophilic cytoplasm with a perinuclear halo.

The cell of origin of the Reed-Sternberg cell is likely a precursor B-cell. In most instances, the Reed-Sternberg cells stain positively for CD30 and CD15. They also express the interleukin 2 (IL-2) receptor (TAC) and HLA-DR antigens. They stain negatively with the leukocyte common antigen; occasionally, they are positive for pan-B cell markers such as CD20.[12,13] However, the L and H (lymphocytic and histiocytic) cells (Reed-Sternberg equivalents) in lymphocyte predominance Hodgkin's disease are strongly positive for CD20 and CD45, but negative for CD15.[14] There are five histological subtypes of Hodgkin's disease, according to the World Health Organization modification of the Lukes and Butler system. These include nodular lymphocyte predominant Hodgkin's disease and four subtypes of classical Hodgkin's disease: nodular sclerosis, lymphocyte-rich, mixed cellularity, and lymphocyte depletion.[15]

Nodular lymphocyte predominance (Fig. 60-1) is characterized by an abundance of normal-appearing lymphocytes and a paucity of abnormal cells. Patients frequently present with limited disease (stage I-II), and

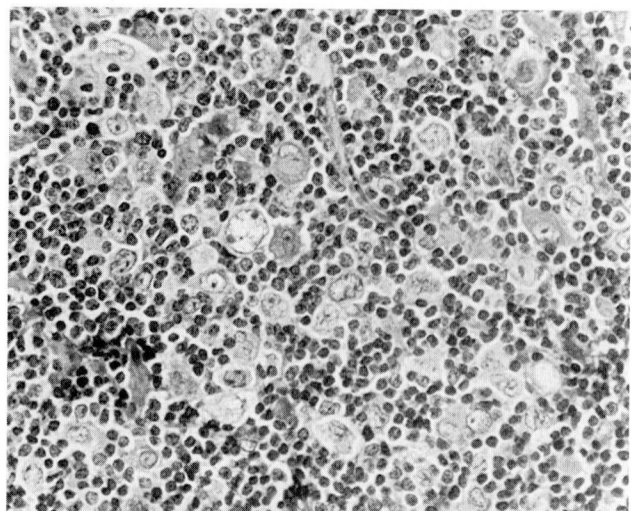

Figure 60–1. Nodular lymphocyte predominance. The abnormal large cells have pale-staining nuclei with lobulations that resemble popcorn (lymphocytic and histiocytic cells). The background is dominated by normal small lymphocytes admixed with occasional epithelioid histiocytes. (Courtesy of Roger A. Warnke, MD.)

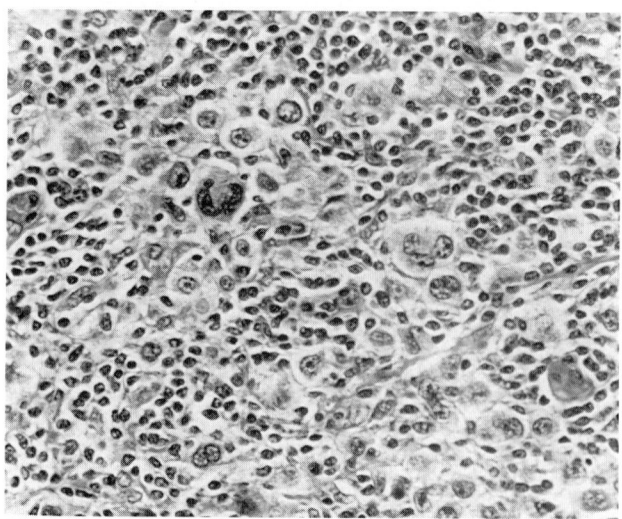

Figure 60–3. Nodular sclerosis. At high magnification, scattered neoplastic cells, some of which have multiple nuclei, are seen to be surrounded by a clear retraction space (lacunar cells). The non-neoplastic background is largely composed of normal lymphocytes and histiocytes. (Courtesy of Roger A. Warnke, MD.)

systemic symptoms are uncommon (<10%). The natural history of lymphocyte predominance is the most favorable among the histological subtypes. In some reports, the nodular form demonstrates a pattern of late relapse similar to that of the low-grade lymphomas.[16] However, the degree to which management programs should be influenced by this observation is not clear. In addition, these patients are at increased risk to develop transformation to other B-cell lymphomas, such as diffuse large cell lymphoma. These observations, coupled with the different staining characteristics of the L and H cells of nodular lymphocyte predominance Hodgkin's disease, suggest that this entity may actually be a form of B-cell non-Hodgkin's lymphoma.[14,16]

Patients affected by lymphocyte predominance Hodgkin's disease may have a history of a peculiar form

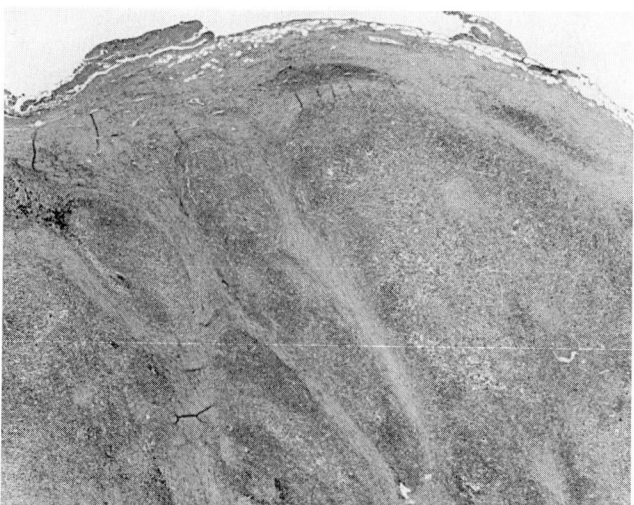

Figure 60–2. Nodular sclerosis. This low magnification of a lymph node replaced by nodular sclerosis shows sclerosis of the capsule at the top and well-demarcated nodules at the center surrounded by pale-staining collagen bands. (Courtesy of Roger A. Warnke, MD.)

of reactive hyperplasia termed *progressive transformation of germinal centers*. Progressive transformation of germinal centers may also occur concurrently or subsequently to a diagnosis of nodular lymphocyte predominance Hodgkin's disease.

Lymphocyte rich, classical Hodgkin's disease was previously considered a diffuse variant of lymphocyte predominance. However, unlike true lymphocyte predominance, lymphocyte rich, classical Hodgkin's disease includes Reed-Sternberg cells with the usual staining characteristics. The histology of this variant is marked by a diffuse effacement of the node by normal-appearing lymphocytes and occasional Reed-Sternberg cells.

Nodular sclerosis Hodgkin's disease (Figs. 60-2 and 60-3) is the most common histological subtype in the United States (>70%). Involved nodes are traversed by broad bands of birefringent collagen surrounding nodules of cells that include lymphocytes, eosinophils, plasma cells, tissue histiocytes, and a variable proportion of atypical mononuclear cells and Reed-Sternberg cells. Women are more commonly affected than men, and the median age is younger than for other histological subtypes. Clinically, the mediastinum and neck are often involved. One third of patients have B symptoms. The natural history is somewhat less favorable than that of lymphocyte predominance Hodgkin's disease.

Mixed cellularity Hodgkin's disease (Fig. 60-4) is characterized by a diffuse effacement of lymph nodes by lymphocytes, eosinophils, and plasma cells, and there are relatively abundant atypical mononuclear and Reed-Sternberg cells. Patients with mixed cellularity Hodgkin's disease tend to present with more advanced disease and tend to be slightly older than those with nodular sclerosing or lymphocyte predominance disease. The natural history of mixed cellularity Hodgkin's disease is less favorable than that of nodular sclerosing Hodgkin's disease.

Lymphocyte depletion Hodgkin's disease is characterized by a paucity of normal-appearing cells and an

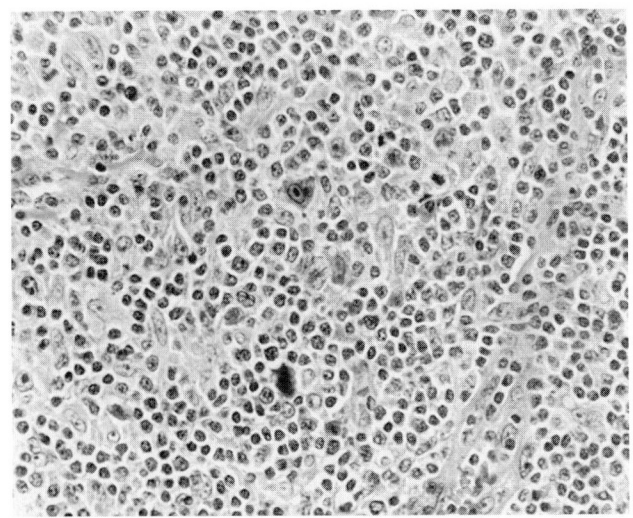

Figure 60–4. Mixed cellularity. This example shows a mixed inflammatory background of lymphocytes and histiocytes together with small numbers of eosinophils and plasma cells. A Reed-Sternberg cell is seen at the center of the field. (Courtesy of Roger A. Warnke, MD.)

abundance of abnormal mononuclear cells, Reed-Sternberg cells, and Reed-Sternberg variants. It may occasionally be difficult to distinguish lymphocyte depletion Hodgkin's disease from anaplastic large cell lymphoma. It is the least common histological subtype, tends to occur in older individuals, and is more likely to be associated with advanced disease and B symptoms. It has the worst prognosis of all histological subtypes.

Interfollicular Hodgkin's disease refers to a pattern of focal involvement of a lymph node in which there is a small focus of Hodgkin's disease in the interfollicular zone. It is easy to confuse these cases with reactive lymphoid hyperplasia.[17]

Table 60-1 summarizes the characteristics of 2590 patients treated at Stanford University from 1968 to 2001, according to histological subtype. Other large centers in the United States and Western Europe report a similar distribution of cases. However, the distribution of histological subtypes from South America, Asia, Africa, Eastern Europe, and even some parts of the United States includes a greater proportion of unfavorable histological types with a more aggressive clinical behavior.[18]

CLINICAL PRESENTATION/ROUTES OF SPREAD

Patients with Hodgkin's disease usually present with painless lymphadenopathy. Some report systemic symptoms including unexplained fevers, drenching night sweats, weight loss, generalized pruritus, or alcohol-induced pain (in tissues infiltrated by Hodgkin's disease). Occasionally, the diagnosis arises from an incidental finding noted on a routine chest x-ray.

Assuming contiguity between the supraclavicular lymph nodes and upper paraortic nodes–celiac axis–spleen (via the thoracic duct), 90% of patients with Hodgkin's disease present with contiguous sites of involvement.[19] The pattern of relapse among patients treated with irradiation alone also supports the concept of contiguity.[20] Visceral involvement may be secondary to direct extension (especially lung, bone, or soft tissue) or hematogenous spread (such as to liver or multifocal bone).

The mechanism of spread of disease to the spleen is unclear. However, there is a correlation between the burden of disease identified in the spleen and the likelihood of hematogenous dissemination. Nearly all patients with hepatic or bone marrow involvement by Hodgkin's disease have (or had) extensive involvement of the

Table 60–1   Clinical Characteristics and Outcome of 2590 Patients Treated for Hodgkin's Disease at Stanford (1968-2001)

	Lymphocyte Predominance	Nodular Sclerosis	Mixed Cellularity	Lymphocyte Depletion
Patients, *n* (% of total)	148 (6)	1980 (76)	433 (17)	29 (1)
Age, yr				
Range	4-77	1-82	2-81	11-65
Median	29	26	31	42
Male/female ratio	125:23	1018:962	338:95	20:9
Stage, %				
I	57 (39)	157 (8)	80 (18)	2 (7)
II	68 (46)	1160 (59)	167 (39)	8 (28)
III	22 (15)	489 (25)	148 (34)	9 (31)
IV	1 (1)	174 (9)	38 (9)	10 (34)
B symptoms, %	7 (5)	600 (30)	139 (32)	19 (66)
Actuarial survival, %				
5-year	96	89	79	38
10-year	87	81	67	27
15-year	81	75	55	23
20-year	71	67	49	17
Actuarial freedom from relapse, %				
5-year	91	75	70	26
10-year	84	72	66	22
15-year	80	71	65	17
20-year	79	71	65	17

spleen.[21] This observation supports the use of management programs with a systemic component when the spleen is involved extensively.

Hodgkin's disease only rarely involves the lymphoid tissues of Waldeyer's ring and Peyer's patches. In addition, although visceral involvement by Hodgkin's disease may be identified in the lungs, liver, bone marrow, and skeletal system, it uncommonly involves other organ systems such as the upper aerodigestive tract, central nervous system, skin, and gastrointestinal tract.[22]

The rapidity of growth and spread of Hodgkin's disease is variable. On occasion, a slow evolution of disease can be demonstrated on serial radiographs or suspected by clinical evolution over a period of several years. It is unusual for disease to progress during the evaluation and staging process.

One third of patients present with fever, night sweats, or weight loss (B symptoms). Fevers may have a classic intermittent Pel-Ebstein pattern. The night sweats may be drenching. The presence of B symptoms often signals more extensive disease; however, even patients with only one or two involved lymph node regions may have significant B symptoms. Patients who have both weight loss and fevers may have a particularly poor prognosis.[23]

Patient age may have an effect on the natural history of disease. In the elderly, the presence of intercurrent illness often affects the selection of staging and treatment procedures.[24]

Hodgkin's disease may be diagnosed during pregnancy, and it is common for pregnancy to follow successful treatment. However, there is no evidence that pregnancy has any effect on the natural history of Hodgkin's disease in these women.[25,26]

Although patients infected with human immunodeficiency virus (HIV-1) do not appear to be at increased risk for the development of Hodgkin's disease, patients infected with HIV-1 who develop Hodgkin's disease display an unusual natural history. The disease tends to present in a more advanced stage, is more likely to be associated with systemic symptoms, and often has unusual patterns of involvement.[27] Treatment is challenging because these patients have a poor tolerance for chemotherapy and opportunistic infections are common.

DIAGNOSTIC AND STAGING STUDIES[28,29]

Staging procedures commonly employed for Hodgkin's disease are listed in Table 60-2. Routine hematologic evaluation may reveal a mild anemia, leukopenia, or thrombocytosis. This is often a paraneoplastic effect, but in some cases may be indicative of bone marrow involvement. The erythrocyte sedimentation rate and alkaline phosphatase and lactate dehydrogenase (LDH) levels may be elevated and serve as useful markers to assess response to treatment and subsequent disease activity.[30] Serum albumin levels, white blood cell counts, and lymphocyte counts are all important prognostic factors, especially in advanced disease.[31]

Radiographic evaluation should include posterior-anterior and lateral chest radiographs. The extent of mediastinal adenopathy is measured as the maximum

Table 60–2 Staging Procedures in Hodgkin's Disease

Minimal Staging

Physical examination—careful attention to lymph node regions, chest, and abdominal examination
Blood work—CBC, differential platelet count, ESR, albumin, chemistry screen including liver function studies and LDH
Imaging—chest x-ray, chest/abdomen/pelvis CT scan
Biopsies—bone marrow (if B symptoms or clinical stage III disease)

Supplementary Staging

Blood work—serum copper, β2-microglobulin levels
Imaging—[18]FDG-PET scan, gallium scan (with SPECT imaging), lymphogram, MRI scan, bone scan

CBC, complete blood cell count; CT, computed tomography; ESR, erythrocyte sedimentation rate; [18]FDG-PET, 2-fluoro-2-deoxy-D-glucose positron emission tomography; LDH, lactate dehydrogenase; MRI, magnetic resonance imaging; SPECT, single photon emission CT.

single width of the mediastinal mass divided by the maximum intrathoracic diameter (near the level of the diaphragm), as shown in Figure 60-5. When this ratio exceeds 1:3, the disease is defined as bulky.[32] Other measurements have also been used to define bulky mediastinal disease, but this method is reproducible and reliable. A computed tomography (CT) scan of the chest should also be obtained if there is mediastinal disease, since it provides ancillary information regarding the extent of intrathoracic disease and assists in treatment planning.[33] Information derived from the chest CT scan

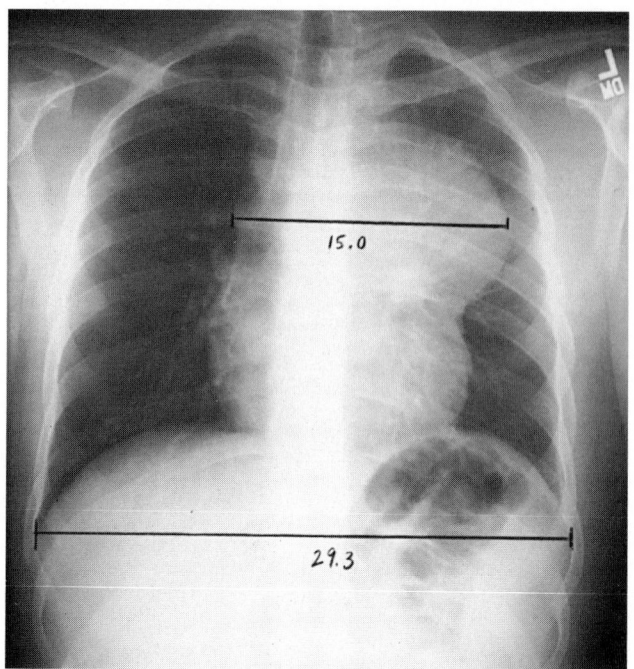

Figure 60–5. Mediastinal mass size. The most useful definition of mediastinal mass size is the ratio of the maximal width of the mediastinal mass divided by the maximal intrathoracic diameter (usually near the level of the diaphragm) on a standing posterior-anterior chest radiograph. In this case, the ratio is 0.51 (15.0:29.3). Masses with a ratio greater than 1:3 have a worse prognosis when treated with single-modality therapy than masses with a ratio less than 1:3.

may alter details of the radiation therapy plan in about 15% of patients, primarily due to identification of involvement of the pulmonary hilar or cardiophrenic lymph nodes or extension to the chest wall.

An abdominal and pelvic CT scan should be obtained with special attention paid to the retroperitoneal area, spleen, and liver. Lymph nodes are generally considered to be enlarged on a CT scan if their short axis measurement exceeds 1 cm.[34] Splenomegaly or hepatomegaly alone does not equate with involvement by Hodgkin's disease, since enlarged spleens are often uninvolved at the time of splenectomy; however, the presence of nodules visible on CT scan is considered indicative of involvement. The overall accuracy rate for detection of Hodgkin's disease in the spleen by CT was reported to be only 58% in a laparotomy series.[35] However, these data, obtained at a time when staging laparotomy was routine, may underestimate the detection rate with current CT scanning technology.

The retroperitoneal lymph nodes are evaluated best by bipedal lymphography, if the study can be obtained. The lymphogram reveals abnormalities not only in size but also in the internal architecture of lymph nodes. The lymphogram is especially helpful for subdiaphragmatic presentations. Unfortunately, skill in the performance and interpretation of this examination is diminishing, and access to the study generally is not available outside a few major academic centers. The sensitivity, specificity, and overall accuracy of the lymphogram for evaluation of retroperitoneal nodes are 85%, 98%, and 95%, respectively, versus 65%, 92%, and 87%, for CT scans.[35] Again, these data were based on confirmation by laparotomy.

Gallium imaging has proved useful in staging patients with Hodgkin's disease. High-dose gallium with single photon emission computed tomography (SPECT) provides the most valuable images. This technique is useful in evaluation of the mediastinum, especially the detection of residual disease after treatment.[36] Approximately two thirds of patients who have positive restaging gallium scans after completion of chemotherapy and who receive no further therapy experience a subsequent relapse, compared with less than 20% of those with negative studies.

Positron emission tomography (PET) using 2-fluoro-2-deoxy-D-glucose (18FDG) is replacing gallium imaging in many centers. FDG-PET is more sensitive than CT[37] scanning or gallium imaging[38] and is more convenient than gallium as a staging procedure due to the shorter interval between injection and scanning (1 hour vs. 48 to 72 hours). Like gallium, it may be particularly useful as a follow-up study to evaluate residual masses detected by CT scanning.[39]

Magnetic resonance imaging (MRI) may be an alternative to chest or abdominopelvic CT scanning for initial staging, but has not been employed widely. Its main value may be in the staging evaluation of pregnant women with Hodgkin's disease.[40]

A posterior iliac crest needle bone marrow biopsy should be performed in select patients. Since the yield is exceedingly low in asymptomatic patients with stage I-II disease, it should be restricted to patients who have B symptoms or stage III-IV disease. The overall frequency of bone marrow involvement in Hodgkin's disease is only 5%.

The use of laparotomy in the staging of Hodgkin's disease has been abandoned.[41] The procedure included a splenectomy, select lymph node biopsies, liver biopsies, and an open bone marrow biopsy.[22] Premenopausal women also underwent a bilateral midline oophoropexy. Laparotomy was routine in the early 1970s; however, the European Organization for Research and Treatment of Cancer (EORTC) H6F randomized trial, which tested the value of laparotomy in stage I-II disease, showed no difference in outcome with or without the procedure.[42] There were also potential long-term toxicities of splenectomy, including overwhelming sepsis.[43] Although the procedure has been abandoned, its enduring value is the knowledge it provided regarding the patterns of initial involvement and spread of disease and the risk for occult subdiaphragmatic disease.

The results of laparotomy in 915 patients with CS I-II Hodgkin's disease treated at Stanford have been analyzed in detail.[44] The overall yield of the procedure was 25% to 30%, with disease identified most commonly in the spleen. The likelihood of identifying subdiaphragmatic disease was related to age, gender, histologic type, and the number of supradiaphragmatic sites of involvement. Favorable groups of patients included those with clinical disease limited to intrathoracic sites (yield = 0%); women with CS I disease (yield = 6%); men with CS I lymphocyte predominance Hodgkin's disease (yield = 4%); and women with CS II disease who had three or fewer sites of supradiaphragmatic disease *and* were younger than 27 years (yield = 9%). These favorable subgroups accounted for about 25% of patients with supradiaphragmatic presentations of stage I-II disease.

STAGING SYSTEM

The Ann Arbor staging system for Hodgkin's disease is outlined in Table 60-3.[45] The lymphoid regions used in this system are displayed in Figure 60-6. The designation of clinical stage (CS) is based on results of the initial biopsy and clinical staging studies, while the pathologic stage (PS) is based on the results of any subsequent biopsies, including bone marrow biopsy and laparotomy and splenectomy. In the postlaparotomy era, the distinction between clinical and pathologic stage is rarely noted. Significant systemic (B) symptoms include fevers, night sweats, and weight loss. Other systemic symptoms of Hodgkin's disease, including pruritus, alcohol-induced pain, and fatigue, should be noted, but are not considered B symptoms. The E designation indicates extralymphatic disease, although the concept is very poorly defined. In practical clinical terms, an E lesion is often considered to be direct extension from involved lymph nodes and encompassable by a curative radiation field; however, the original description includes as an example "multiple nodules in the lung limited to one lobe." In addition, the Ann Arbor system fails to deal with the possibility of multiple E lesions, which can be identified quite clearly in the chest with the careful use of contemporary imaging studies such as CT and MRI. Some authors' inclusion of these patients in stage IV has led to a great deal of confusion in the literature. Another deficiency of the Ann

Table 60–3   Ann Arbor Staging Classification System

Stage I   Involvement of a single lymph node region

Stage II   Involvement of two or more lymph node regions on the same side of the diaphragm (II) or localized involvement of an extralymphatic organ or site and of one or more lymph node regions on the same side of the diaphragm (IIE)

Stage III   Involvement of lymph node regions on both sides of the diaphragm (III), which may also be accompanied by involvement of the spleen (IIIS) or by localized involvement of an extralymphatic organ or site (IIIE) or both (IIISE)

Stage IV   Diffuse or disseminated involvement of one or more extralymphatic organs or tissues, with or without associated lymph node involvement

The absence or presence of fever, night sweats, or unexplained loss of 10% or more of body weight in the 6 months before diagnosis is denoted by the suffix letter *A* or *B*, respectively.

Patients are assigned a clinical stage (CS) based on the initial biopsy and all subsequent nonsurgical staging studies. A pathologic stage (PS) is assigned based on all clinical studies as well as subsequent surgical staging procedures such as bone marrow biopsy, staging laparotomy, and splenectomy.

From Carbone PP, Kaplan HS, Mushoff K, et al: Report of the committee on Hodgkin's disease staging classification. *Cancer Res.* 1971;31:1860.

Arbor system is its failure to consider bulk of disease. This has been shown to be important, especially in the mediastinum. The presence of bulky disease in the mediastinum should be noted, together with the stage.

In addition to Ann Arbor stage, other indicators may be helpful in predicting prognosis or selecting therapy. An international study evaluated prognosis in advanced Hodgkin's disease by analyzing prognostic features among 5141 patients.[31] Seven factors were identified, each of which had a similar prognostic impact. These are summarized in Table 60-4.

STANDARD THERAPEUTIC APPROACHES

Radiation Therapy[46]

Radiation therapy is the most effective single agent for the treatment of Hodgkin's disease. As a single modality, it has provided the "gold standard" of curative therapy for patients with early-stage, favorable (nonbulky, asymptomatic) disease. Its efficacy has led to its incorporation into combined-modality therapy programs for all stages of disease.

Chemotherapy

Combination chemotherapy has excellent curative potential for patients with advanced-stage disease.[47] The initial drug combination that achieved substantial success in treating Hodgkin's disease was nitrogen mustard (mechlorethamine), vincristine (Oncovin), procarbazine, and prednisone (MOPP), reported by DeVita and associates[48] from the National Cancer Institute. The schedule of drug administration is shown in Table 60-5. The acute toxicities of MOPP include nausea, vomiting, peripheral neuropathy, constipation, leukopenia, and thrombocytopenia.

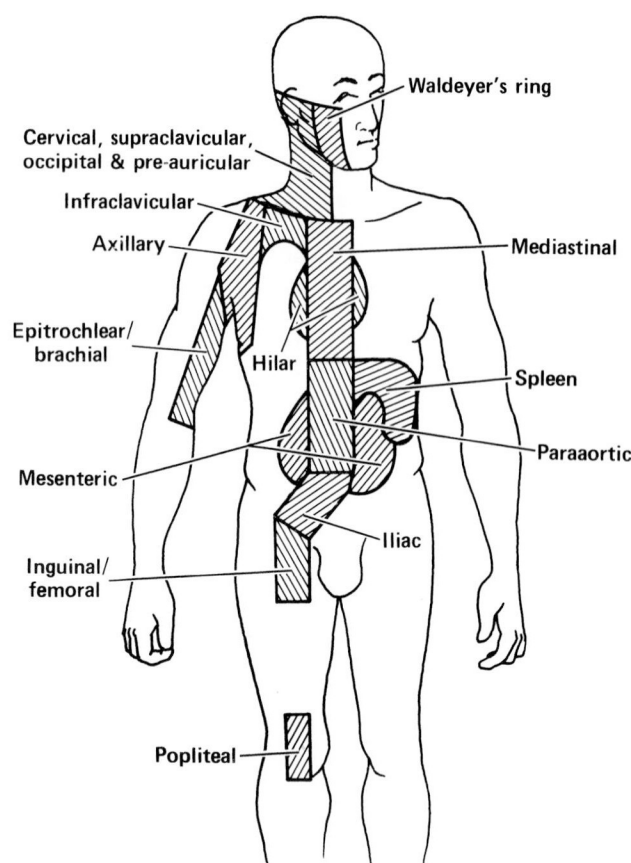

Figure 60–6. Ann Arbor lymphoid regions. Note that the cervical, supraclavicular, occipital, and preauricular areas compose a single region and that the mediastinum and bilateral hilar areas constitute three regions.

The major potential long-term toxicities are sterility (80% of men; in women it is directly linked to age) and secondary acute nonlymphocytic leukemia (usual latent period, 3 to 7 years; actuarial risk approximately 3% to 5% at 7 to 10 years). A number of MOPP-like programs achieve comparable results with less toxicity, including ChlVPP (chlorambucil, vinblastine, procarbazine, and prednisone), C-MOPP (cyclophosphamide, vincristine, procarbazine, and prednisone), and PAVe (procarbazine, L-phenylalanine mustard [Alkeran], and vinblastine); however, the largest experience is with traditional MOPP.

With the introduction of doxorubicin (Adriamycin), completely novel drug combinations were developed. The most successful of these is ABVD, which includes

Table 60–4   A Prognostic Score for Advanced Hodgkin's Disease

Factor	Unfavorable Covariate
Serum albumin	<4 g/dl
Hemoglobin	<10.5 g/dl
Gender	Male
Age	45 years and older
Stage	IV (Ann Arbor)
Leukocyte count	≥15,000/mm³
Lymphocyte count	<600/mm³ or <8% of white count

Table 60–5   Common Drug Combinations Used in the Treatment of Hodgkin's Disease

Drug Combination	Agents	Dose, mg/m²	Route	Treatment, days	Cycle Duration, days
MOPP	Nitrogen mustard	6	IV	1, 8	28
	Vincristine	1.4*	IV	1, 8	
	Procarbazine	100	PO	1-14	
	Prednisone	40	PO	1-14	
ABVD	Doxorubicin†	25	IV	1, 15	28
	Bleomycin	10	IV	1, 15	
	Vinblastine	6	IV	1, 15	
	Dacarbazine	375	IV	1, 15	
MOPP/ABVD	MOPP			1-14	56
	ABVD			29, 43	
MOPP-ABV	MOPP			1-7	28
	Doxorubicin†	35	IV	8	
	Bleomycin	10	IV	8	
	Vinblastine	6	IV	8	
	Prednisone	40	PO	8-14	
Stanford V	Nitrogen mustard	6	IV	1	28
	Doxorubicin	25	IV	1, 15	
	Vinblastine	6	IV	1, 15	
	Vincristine	1.4	IV	8, 22	
	Bleomycin	5	IV	8, 22	
	Etoposide	60	IV	15, 16	
	Prednisone	40	PO	qod	
BEACOPP	Bleomycin	10	IV	8	21
	Etoposide	100 (200)‡	IV	1-3	
	Doxorubicin	25 (35)‡	IV	1	
	Cyclophosphamide	650 (1250)‡	IV	1	
	Vincristine*	1.4*	IV	8	
	Procarbazine	100	PO	1-7	
	Prednisone	40	PO	1-14	

*Maximum = 2.0 mg.
†Adriamycin.
‡Higher doses for "BEACOPP-escalated"
IV, intravenous; PO, oral.

doxorubicin, bleomycin, vinblastine, and dacarbazine (see Table 60-5).[49] Acute toxicities include nausea and vomiting, hair loss, and blood count depression. The hematologic effects are less severe than with MOPP. Sterility is not usually a complication, and secondary leukemias have been reported only rarely. Important potential long-term risks include possible cardiac and pulmonary toxicity from the doxorubicin and bleomycin, respectively.

Different combinations of drugs have been combined in an alternating fashion, to address the problem of drug resistance. Most notable among "alternating non–cross-resistant" regimens is MOPP/ABVD, in which monthly cycles of MOPP are alternated with monthly cycles of ABVD.[50] A subsequent innovation was the MOPP-ABV hybrid program.[51] Table 60-5 summarizes the dosages and scheduling of these drug combinations.

An important clinical trial of the Cancer and Leukemia Group B (CALGB) compared the efficacy of MOPP, ABVD, and MOPP-ABVD in a prospective randomized study of patients with advanced-stage Hodgkin's disease.[52] The complete response rates and actuarial failure-free survivals were statistically superior for the two doxorubicin-containing arms of the trial (ABVD or MOPP-ABVD). Among the 115 patients

treated with ABVD chemotherapy, the complete response rate was 82%, the 5-year failure-free survival was 61%, and the 5-year survival was 73%.

In an effort to reduce toxicity or improve efficacy, new drug programs have been developed. These include Stanford V[53] and BEACOPP.[54]

Combined-Modality Therapy

Combined-modality therapy plays an essential role in the management of many patients with Hodgkin's disease.[55] In the past 10 years, there has been a rapid move to the adoption of combined-modality therapy programs for early-stage Hodgkin's disease. This has largely been due to the identification of significant late effects among patients who are long-term (>15 years) survivors after treatment with radiation therapy alone. These newer programs generally include modified chemotherapy regimens (different combinations of drugs or fewer cycles of established regimens) followed by limited radiation treatment. Clinical trials indicate that in this setting, involved field (IF) irradiation is sufficient. For example, in Milan, a randomized trial evaluated outcome for patients treated with four cycles of ABVD plus STLI versus four cycles of

ABVD plus IF. With a median follow-up in excess of 7 years, there was no significant difference in outcome for the two treatment approaches and patients treated with ABVD plus IF (36 Gy) had a survival and freedom-from-relapse of 94%.[56] At Stanford, 65 patients were treated with 8 weeks of Stanford V chemotherapy followed by IF (30 Gy). The 3-year freedom-from-progression was 96%.[57] Other similar programs are summarized in Table 60-6. Current clinical trials are studying variations in radiation dose and number of cycles of chemotherapy.

The treatment of choice for patients with bulky mediastinal Hodgkin's disease (mediastinal mass greater than one third of maximum intrathoracic diameter) is combined-modality therapy. Several reports show that patients with bulky mediastinal disease are at greater risk for relapse after treatment with irradiation alone than after treatment with combined-modality therapy.[58] Likewise, the risk of relapse is substantial in patients with large mediastinal masses treated with chemotherapy alone.[59] Although there is no difference in survival of patients treated initially with either approach, it is inappropriate to accept a relapse risk as high as 50%, and the general recommendation is that these patients be treated with combination chemotherapy and irradiation.

With respect to the choice of chemotherapy, the potential overlapping toxicities of doxorubicin and bleomycin with irradiation (cardiac and pulmonary effects) should be considered. The recommended radiation dose in this situation varies from 25 to 40 Gy, but most data cite doses of at least 30 to 36 Gy.[53,56] Doses in the higher part of the range should be used when the response to chemotherapy is incomplete, gallium or PET imaging remains positive after chemotherapy, or the chemotherapy course is abbreviated. The use of lower doses (as low as 20 Gy) should be restricted to clinical trials.[60]

Treatment may include all initially involved sites (sites <5 cm may be restricted to 20 Gy) or simply to the area of initial bulk (mediastinum). When treatment is limited to the mediastinum, it is preferable to include the bilateral supraclavicular areas. The irradiation fields should conform to the area of residual mediastinal disease with adequate margins laterally, not to the initial width of disease before chemotherapy. However, the fields generally extend at least 2 cm beyond the original extent of disease (Fig. 60-7).

Table 60–6 Chemotherapy Plus Involved Field Radiation Therapy for Stage I–II Favorable Prognosis Hodgkin's Disease

| | Chemotherapy | | Involved Field |
	Type	Duration	Radiation Dose
BNLI	VAPEC-B	1 mo	36 Gy
EORTC	EBVP II	4 mo	*20 Gy/36 Gy
GHSG	ABVD	*2 mo/4 mo	*20 Gy/30 Gy
Milan	ABVD	4 mo	36 Gy
Stanford	Stanford V	2 mo	20 Gy

BNLI, British National Lymphoma Investigation; EBVP II, epirubicin, bleomycin, vinblastine, and prednisone; EORTC, European Organization for Research and Treatment of Cancer; GHSG, German Hodgkin's Study Group; VAPEC-B, vincristine, doxorubicin, prednisone, etoposide, cyclophosphamide, bleomycin.
*Randomized trial.

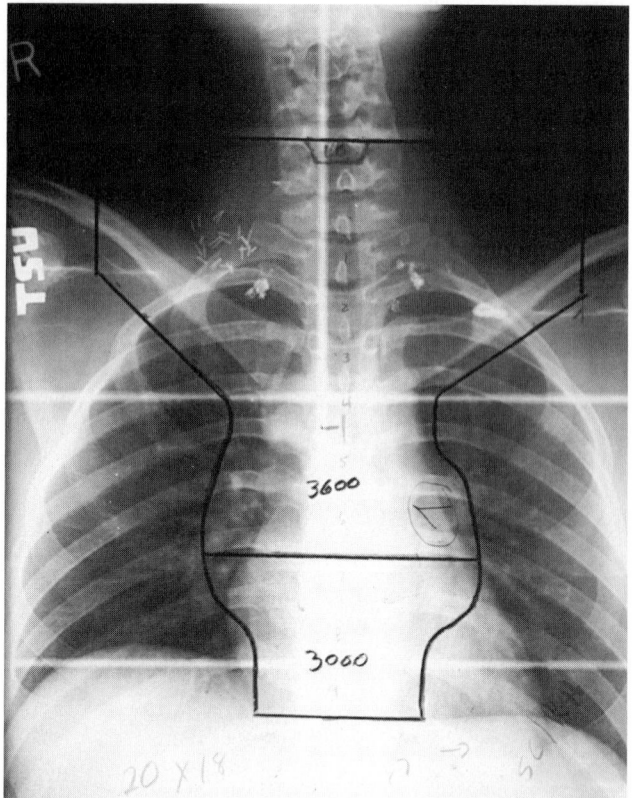

Figure 60–7. Simulator film of a mediastinal-supraclavicular field for planning consolidative radiation in a patient who has completed a course of chemotherapy. This patient initially had a large mediastinal mass (mediastinal mass ratio 0.39), and she had an excellent response to chemotherapy. Consolidative fields incorporate only the essential mediastinal, hilar, and supraclavicular regions, including areas of residual adenopathy. The entire initial tumor volume is not treated.

The use of combined-modality therapy for patients with stage III-IV Hodgkin's disease is rational, because most patients who relapse after treatment with chemotherapy alone do so in sites of initial disease.[61] However, many early randomized trials designed to resolve this issue were poorly designed or used chemotherapy programs that are no longer considered to be optimal.

Three trials that have addressed this question are important. The Southwest Oncology Group (SWOG) 7808 trial included patients with clinical stage III-IV disease.[62] All patients received induction chemotherapy with MOP-BAP (nitrogen mustard, vincristine, procarbazine, bleomycin, Adriamycin, prednisone) chemotherapy for 6 months. Complete responders were randomly assigned to receive either no further therapy or 20 Gy to the IF (except marrow). Of 530 patients included in the trial, 61% achieved a complete response. Of 285 patients randomly assigned, only 234 (73%) received the treatment to which they were assigned. The 5-year remission rate was 68% for patients who were assigned to no further therapy, compared with 79% for those assigned to involved-field irradiation (P = 0.09). The difference in outcome for patients with nodular sclerosing histology was more marked (60% vs. 82%, P = 0.02). When analysis was limited to patients who actually completed the assigned treatment, the 5-year remission rate was 67%

for those with no further therapy and 85% for those who received consolidative irradiation ($P = 0.002$). However, the difference did not translate into a survival benefit for any subset of patients.

Another trial, the German HD3 study, included patients with clinical stage IIIB-IV.[63] All patients were treated with 6 months of COPP/ABVD (cyclophosphamide, vincristine, procarbazine, and prednisone plus ABVD) induction chemotherapy followed by a randomization of patients who achieved a complete response to receive either 20 Gy involved-field irradiation (exclusive of bone marrow) or 2 months of additional COPP/ABVD chemotherapy. Of 288 patients included in the trial, 59% achieved a complete response. Among the 160 patients with a complete response, only 100 (58%) went on to receive consolidative treatment with *either* irradiation or additional chemotherapy. Five-year data showed no significant difference in relapse-free survival (79% with COPP/ABVD, 76% with combined modality, $P = 0.95$) or overall survival (95% with COPP/ABVD, 86% combined modality, $P = 0.22$).

A third trial with similar design is the EORTC-GPMC (Groupe Pierre-et-Marie Curie) H34 (#20884) trial. All patients were treated with MOPP-ABV chemotherapy and then randomly assigned to receive either no further therapy or treatment with IF irradiation (25 Gy). The preliminary results of this study, which included 736 patients, revealed no difference in survival, event-free survival, or relapse-free survival between the two groups.[64]

The general conclusion based upon these studies is that adjuvant radiation therapy in doses up to 25 Gy to involved sites is not warranted if patients have achieved a complete response to conventional chemotherapy. However, some question remains regarding patients with bulky disease, since the SWOG study showed an improvement in remission duration that was especially notable for patients with nodular sclerosing histology, patients who received the actual planned treatment, and patients with bulky disease. This question is being addressed in the GHSG HD12 trial. Patients with stage III-IV disease are treated with BEACOPP chemotherapy and then randomized after achieving a complete response. One group of patients receives no further therapy, while the other receives 30 Gy to initial sites of disease greater than 5 cm. Ultimately, improved imaging or marker studies for restaging of patients after completion of chemotherapy may prove helpful in identifying those who would truly benefit from consolidative irradiation.

In contrast to the previously mentioned studies, in which high cumulative doses of chemotherapy are administered and all initial sites of disease were irradiated to 20 to 25 Gy, the approach taken at Stanford has been to employ intense but low total dosage chemotherapy followed by radiation only to initially bulky sites (>5 cm), and at a higher dose (36 Gy). Irradiation is initiated 1 to 3 weeks after the completion of 12 weeks of Stanford V chemotherapy. With this approach, since the chemotherapy is abbreviated, the radiation is considered to be an integral part of the treatment, not simply an adjuvant therapy.[53] This approach is now being tested in a phase 3 intergroup trial.

Many salvage treatment programs also incorporate radiation therapy in a combined-modality approach. It may be used as an adjuvant to chemotherapy in patients who have localized relapse after primary treatment with irradiation,[65] with some data to support a superiority over treatment with chemotherapy alone in that setting. There is also a growing experience with total body irradiation or IF irradiation as a component of high-dose chemotherapy programs accompanied by autologous bone marrow or peripheral stem cell transplantation.[66]

Fractionated total body irradiation (TBI) is incorporated into a number of transplantation programs. Its value is unclear, and some series that have used regimens with or without fractionated TBI report similar outcomes for each.[67] TBI is probably not the most efficacious way to use irradiation in these patients. Recurrent Hodgkin's disease is often a locoregional problem, rather than a systemic one. In addition, data suggest that irradiation doses in the range used in TBI programs (12 to 15 Gy) are likely to eradicate disease in only about 20% of treated sites.[68] It is more logical to limit irradiation to sites of failure or those at high risk for disease. At the Memorial Hospital, investigators have reported the use of accelerated hyperfractionated total lymphoid irradiation in patients scheduled for high-dose therapy and bone marrow transplantation.[69] After standard induction chemotherapy and before transplantation, patients receive IF irradiation to 15 Gy (1.5 Gy twice a day) followed by total lymphoid irradiation to 20.04 Gy (1.67 Gy three times a day). They report a 6.5-year disease-free survival rate of 50%.

Irradiation may also be restricted to actual sites of relapse in high-dose therapy programs. This approach is supported by the observation that subsequent relapse among patients treated with high-dose therapy is often within sites of prior involvement.[70] Retrospective data from a number of institutions now point to better long-term disease control when these patients receive local irradiation.[71-73] For example, at Stanford, 24 of 100 patients received IF irradiation (median, 30 Gy) in addition to high-dose chemotherapy preparatory regimens.[73] For patients with relapsed stage I-III disease, the 3-year event-free survival rate was 84% when IF irradiation was included, compared with 55% for high dose therapy and transplant alone ($P = 0.13$). In patients who had received no previous irradiation, the 3-year event-free survival rate after high-dose therapy that incorporated consolidative irradiation was 79%, compared with 52% without irradiation ($P = 0.10$). For a subgroup of patients with stage I-III relapse and no history of irradiation, the event-free survival rate was 82% with consolidative irradiation and 43% without it ($P = 0.07$). This observation has led us to adopt programs that include consolidative irradiation in high-dose therapy programs.

ROLE OF RADIATION THERAPY

Radiation therapy has been used extensively in the management of patients with Hodgkin's disease. Until recently, it was the treatment of choice for the majority of patients with stage I-II disease. The gold standard of treatment until the mid-1980s was staging laparotomy followed by subtotal lymphoid irradiation. Based on studies of the EORTC H6F trial,[42] staging laparotomy was eliminated, and patients who had stage I-II disease were generally treated with subtotal lymphoid irradiation, including the spleen.

The issue of whether prophylactic treatment below the diaphragm is essential in clinically staged patients treated with radiation therapy alone has also been addressed by the EORTC. The EORTC H7VF trial was designed to include only the most favorable clinical presentations: women with stage IA nonbulky disease who had favorable histology (lymphocyte predominance or nodular sclerosis), erythrocyte sedimentation rate less than 50, and age younger than 40 years. These patients were treated with mantle irradiation alone. This group accounted for only 5% of patients with stage I-II Hodgkin's disease. At 3 years, the survival rate of 35 patients was 100%, but the relapse-free survival rate was only 82%.[74] Most patients failed in unirradiated subdiaphragmatic sites. This result in such a favorable subset of patients was deemed unacceptable by the EORTC group and this management approach was abandoned.

Palliative irradiation is not often employed for Hodgkin's disease, since primary and salvage treatment programs are usually effective. Nevertheless, it should not be overlooked as a potential important therapeutic intervention for patients with end-stage disease.

TECHNIQUES OF RADIOTHERAPY

SIMULATION

The mantle field includes all the major lymph node regions above the diaphragm (Fig. 60-8). These regions are involved or are at high risk for involvement in most patients with Hodgkin's disease. Although an entire classical mantle is not often treated, the supradiaphragmatic lymphoid regions that are included in IF protocols are all components of the mantle. Patients are simulated in the supine position, with the neck extended and arms akimbo or above the head. An "arms up" position pulls the axillary nodes farther from the chest wall and thereby permits more generous lung shielding. An "arms down" or "akimbo" position permits shielding of the humeral heads and minimizes the effect of tissue folds in the supraclavicular/low neck regions. Three-point setup technique or immobilization with foam body molds minimizes setup error due to "rotation." Palpable lymph node masses may be wired for visualization purposes. The superior border includes the inferior portion of the mandible and the mastoid. The inferior border should be near the insertion of the diaphragm. Laterally, the field should provide generous coverage of the axillae, extending just beyond the humeral heads. Lung blocks are designed to conform to the mediastinal contour, including no more than 0.5 cm margins around involved nodes. If there is extension of disease onto the anterior chest wall or other extranodal sites, CT-simulation is especially helpful in identifying the extent of disease. The pulmonary hilar lymph node regions are included routinely whenever the mediastinum is treated. The superior extent of the lung blocks is drawn to expose the infraclavicular region, through which lymphatic channels course between the axillary and supraclavicular regions.

Laterally, the lung blocks follow the inner rib margins. The apex of the heart may be shielded throughout or exposed for a portion of the treatment if the pericardium is considered to be "at risk," for example, in the setting of significant inferior extension of the mediastinal mass. Depending on the dose prescribed to the clinical target volume (CTV), it may be appropriate to shield the larynx anteriorly, the occiput and cervical spinal cord posteriorly, and the humeral heads both anteriorly and posteriorly.

If the treatment machine and couch permit, anterior and posterior treatments should be executed with the patient in the supine position. This minimizes anatomic variation between anterior and posterior fields and facilitates later matching of the subdiaphragmatic field.

The classic subdiaphragmatic irradiation field for Hodgkin's disease is the inverted Y, which includes the retroperitoneal and pelvic lymph nodes. With current treatment programs, a full inverted Y is rarely treated. More commonly, the inferior border of the subdiaphragmatic field is drawn at the L4-5 interspace or below the bifurcation of the aorta to include the common iliac nodes as well (spade field). Generally, the spleen is intact, and the entire spleen is included in the field (Fig. 60-9). When patients require sequential treatment to mantle and subdiaphragmatic fields, the calculation of field separation is exceedingly important in order to avoid field overlap and excessive dose to the spinal cord.[75]

The superior border of the subdiaphragmatic field is matched to the mantle with an appropriate skin gap. The paraortic portion of the field is defined best by CT-simulation and outlining of the retroperitoneal nodes, including 0.5- to 1.0-cm margins beyond visualized nodes. In the absence of CT simulation, the field may be drawn to the width of the transverse processes of the lumbar vertebral bodies, provided that the diagnostic CT scan does not show nodes in a more lateral position.

The inferior border of the paraaortic field may be drawn at the L4-5 interspace, at the level of the bifurcation of the large vessels. Alternatively, the field may be flared at that level and extended inferiorly to include the common iliac nodes (the *spade* field). In men, this field may extend to the widest portion of the pelvis without significant additional morbidity. In women, the inferior extent of the field should not be any lower than the superior level of the sacroiliac joints, unless an oophoropexy has been performed, in order to limit the scattered dose of irradiation to the ovaries.

The spleen is often treated in contiguity with the paraortic nodes. Treatment planning is best accomplished with CT-simulation (see Fig. 60-9). In order to accommodate respiratory movement, a 2-cm margin should be included superiorly and inferiorly.

The pelvic field, which includes the bilateral common and external iliac and inguinal-femoral nodes, requires careful blocking considerations (Fig. 60-10). If the pelvic field is treated concurrently with the para-aortic field, the term *inverted-Y* is used. If the fields are treated sequentially, the superior border of the pelvic field is matched to the inferior border of the para-aortic field. The inferior border is set by palpation to include the inguinal-femoral nodes, which may project radiographically at the inferior

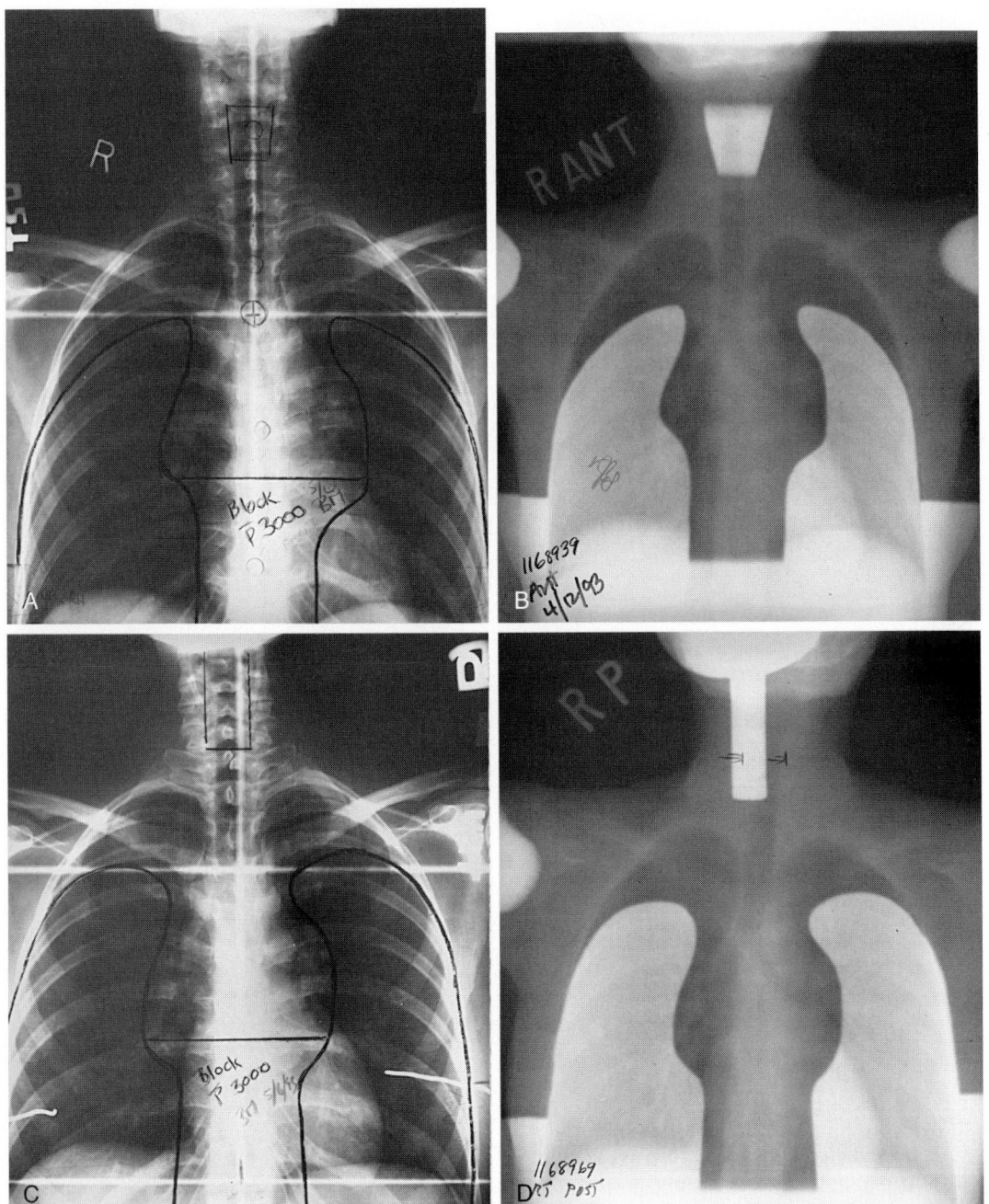

Figure 60–8. A, Anterior mantle simulator. **B,** Anterior port films. **C,** Posterior simulator. **D,** Posterior port films. The major difference between anterior and posterior films relates to larynx and cervical spinal cord blocking. The configuration of the lung blocks in the infraclavicular region may also differ and be individualized according to the presence of axillary, infraclavicular, or supraclavicular lymphadenopathy.

level of the lesser trochanter. Laterally, the field should include the iliac nodes as defined by lymphography or CT, with a 0.5-cm margin around these nodes. If radiographic studies are not available, the lateral extent of the field should be about 2 cm beyond the widest portion of the pelvis. Since the volume of pelvic marrow is substantial, the field must be shaped carefully, and this can best be achieved if a lymphogram has been performed.

In order to avoid irradiation-induced amenorrhea in women, an oophoropexy must be performed. This procedure is done by medial transposition of the ovaries. The surgeon marks the ovaries with radiopaque sutures or clips and locates them medially and as low as possible

behind the body of the uterus. A double-thickness (10 half-value layers [HVLs]) midline block is then used to shield the transposed ovaries. If the ovaries are at least 2 cm from the edge of this block, the dose is reduced to 8% of that delivered to the iliac nodes.[26] In males, the testicular dose may be as high as 10% of the dose delivered to the inguinal-femoral nodes. The use of a specially constructed testicular shield can reduce this dose to 0.75% to 3.0%, which is primarily due to internal scatter. The precise dose depends on the position of the testes relative to the inferior margin of the inguinal-femoral field.

In some patients, it is appropriate to treat a preauricular field (Fig. 60-11). Treatment is usually with 6 to

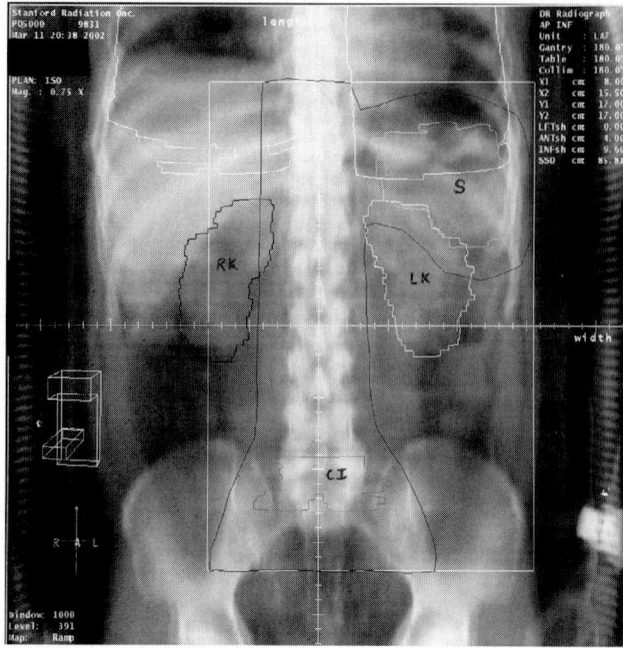

Figure 60–9. A digitally reconstructed radiograph for a three-dimensional planned spade-spleen field that includes the entire spleen (*S*), paraortic nodes, and proximal common iliac nodes (*CI*) A paraortic-spleen field would be truncated inferiorly at the L4-L5 interspace. Computed tomographic planning is performed to identify the location of the spleen and kidneys. A dose-volume histogram, not shown, demonstrates that 30% of the left kidney will receive a dose ≥ 50% of the dose delivered to the clinical target volume.

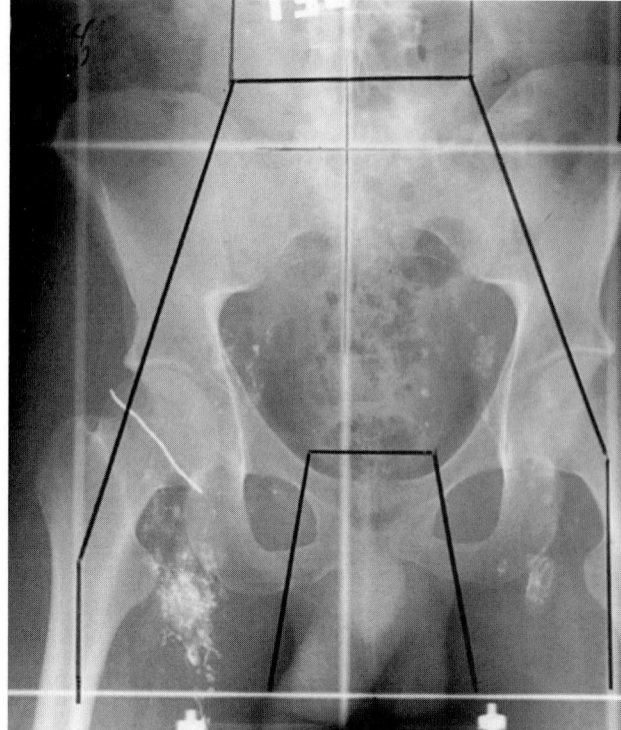

Figure 60–10. Typical design of a pelvic field in a male. Note how the opacified nodes from the lymphogram assist in design of the field. The position of the midline block is adjusted according to the extent of pelvic adenopathy.

9 MeV electrons. The inferior border is matched to the superior border of the mantle. Its posterior border is defined by the external auditory canal. The superior border is along the zygoma, and the anterior border is along the anterior masseter muscle.

RADIATION TREATMENT PLAN

Optimal irradiation technique requires the use of megavoltage photon beams, large fields contoured to the patient's anatomy and tumor configuration, a tumoricidal dose, opposed field fractionated treatment, pretreatment simulation, and port film verification. The presence of slanting body contours and variations in body thickness results in an inhomogeneous dose distribution. Treatment-planning computers facilitate these dose calculations and should include the effects of both primary and scattered radiation to each point of calculation.[76] The minimal dosimetry should include an irregular field point calculation for each important nodal region within the field. The dose variation determined by these calculations must be compensated for by individually designed compensators or selective area blocking.

Imaging studies are essential to the optimal design of the treatment fields for Hodgkin's disease. For patients with significant mediastinal adenopathy, a diagnostic chest CT scan or CT-simulation can provide important information regarding the extension of disease to the lung, pericardium, or chest wall, or involvement of

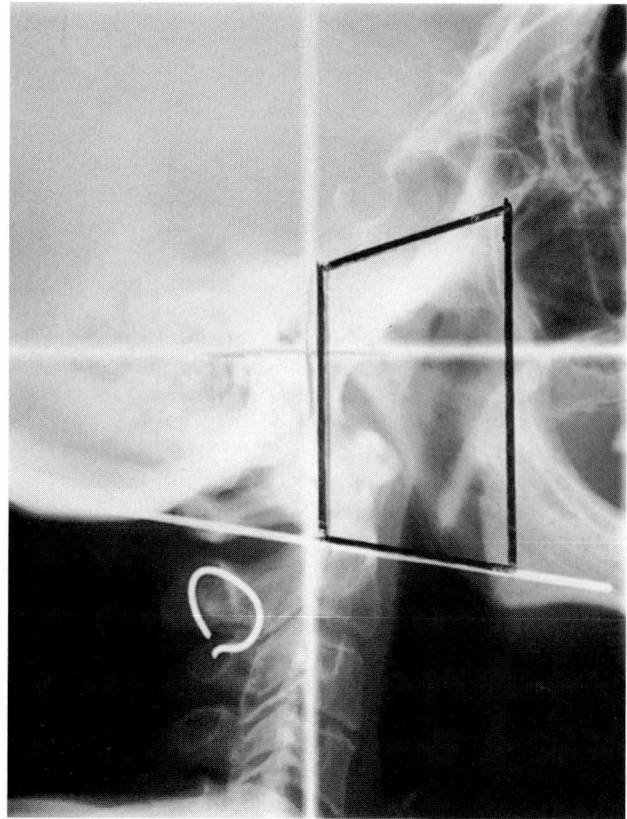

Figure 60–11. Simulator film for a preauricular field, usually treated with electrons.

internal mammary or pericardial lymph nodes that may have an impact on field design. For patients treated with radiation therapy alone, the incorporation of the CT scan into treatment-planning decisions results in changes in the treatment fields in about 15% of patients.[33] MRI scans of the chest may provide incremental information relevant to chest wall extension.[77]

A typical example of mantle field is shown in Figure 60-7. In addition to the lung blocks, blocks can be placed over the occipital region and spinal cord posteriorly, the larynx anteriorly, and the humeral heads both anteriorly and posteriorly. Special spinal cord shielding is not needed if the prescribed dose is 36 Gy but is indicated for doses greater than 40 Gy. The Patterns of Care Study guidelines recommend treatment to a dose of 36 to 44 Gy to involved portions of the field and 30 to 36 Gy to prophylactic fields.[78] At Stanford, the mantle is treated by evenly weighted anterior-posterior opposed technique, both fields treated daily, 1.5 to 1.8 Gy per fraction, 5 days a week. When a dose of 40 Gy or greater is prescribed, a posterior cord block (five HVLs) is inserted over the cervical cord from the outset of treatment (unless contraindicated) and is extended over the thoracic cord at a dose that limits the cord dose to 40 Gy or less. In the presence of inferior mediastinal disease or pericardial extension, the entire cardiac silhouette is irradiated to 15 Gy, with a block over the apex of the heart thereafter to shield that portion of the pericardium, if the planned management is with radiation therapy alone. After a dose of 30 to 35 Gy has been delivered, a block is placed in the subcarinal region (about 5 cm below the carina) in order to provide more cardiac and pericardial protection.[79] However, in no instance would areas of clinical involvement by Hodgkin's disease be treated with doses less than 36 Gy if radiation alone is planned for patient management.

Partial-transmission blocks can be used to deliver low-dose lung irradiation. If the pulmonary hilar lymph nodes are involved and irradiation is being used as a single modality, partial-transmission lung blocks can be used to deliver a dose of 15 to 16.5 Gy for the treatment of occult pulmonary disease, reducing the risk of failure in that site.[80,81] Areas of direct extension into lung should be treated to at least 36 Gy.

The mantle field may be modified during therapy. As mediastinal masses regress, wider blocks may be cut to protect more of the lungs (shrinking field technique).[79] Occasionally, an interruption in therapy after 10 or so fractions of treatment permits further shrinkage of disease.

When there is extranodal extension of disease, individualization of the mantle field is indicated. For example, disease may extend anteriorly into the chest wall. If this area is otherwise within the normal boundaries of the mantle, bolus may be used on the anterior field to build up the dose in that region. However, in some instances disease may extend more laterally in the chest wall, underneath the lung blocks. In this situation normal lung blocks can be used; however, the disease that extends under the lung blocks must be boosted with electrons or tangential photon fields if irradiation alone is to be used. CT simulation is extremely helpful in these circumstances.

In the setting of combined-modality therapy, substantial variation in treatment fields and dose delivered is appropriate. If a definitive course of chemotherapy is planned or completed, radiation treatment fields may be limited to clinically involved regions, and the dose may be reduced. The National Comprehensive Cancer Network (NCCN) guideline recommendations for radiation dose in combined-modality programs include a range of 30 to 36 Gy to involved regions for stage I-II disease or bulky sites and 20 to 36 Gy to involved regions in stage III-IV disease or nonbulky sites (NCCN Practice Guidelines in Oncology—Hodgkin's Disease—v.1.2002). In clinical practice, there may be minimal extension of the fields beyond the involved sites. For example, the pulmonary hilar regions and bilateral supraclavicular regions are generally included when the mediastinum is irradiated (Fig. 60-12).

In the abdomen and pelvis, a lymphogram is especially helpful in defining the location of the retroperitoneal nodes. When the intact spleen is to be treated, this is best achieved with CT planning. A limited number of CT cuts from the top of the diaphragm to the midabdomen is usually sufficient for defining the splenic and renal volumes. Dose and fractionation principles are the same for the subdiaphragmatic fields as they are for the mantle.

When treatment is indicated for the preauricular nodes, we generally use unilateral 6 to 9 MeV electrons (see Fig. 60-11). This region is treated if there is clinical involvement of the preauricular nodes. In addition, when the superior cervical lymph nodes are involved, the preauricular nodes are at risk for contiguous spread and the field is treated prophylactically to a dose of 30 to 36 Gy if radiation alone is planned as total management.

Occasionally, the primary site of enlarged nodes is in the high cervical area, extending near the upper border of the typical mantle field. In this setting, large opposed lateral *Waldeyer* fields can be employed to encompass the upper cervical and adjacent nodes and matched to a mantle with a lower superior border (Fig. 60-13).[82]

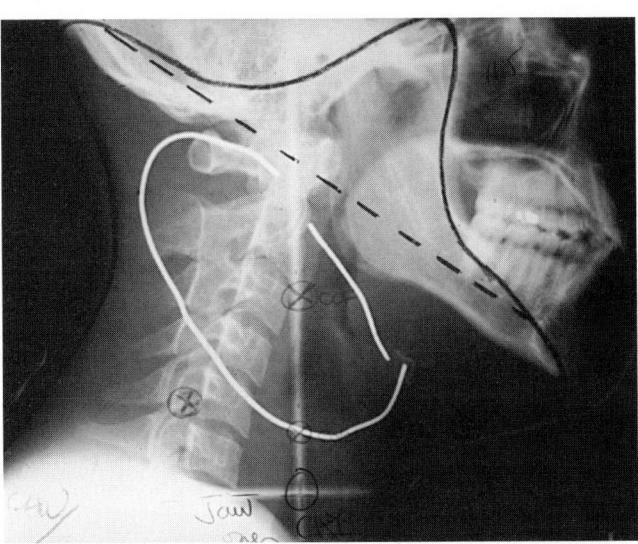

Figure 60–12. Large Waldeyer field designed to give adequate margin around bulky high cervical lymphadenopathy (*outlined by wire*). This is treated with opposed field photons. The inferior border of the field is matched to a mantle. The usual superior border of a standard mantle field is shown by the *broken line*.

① Stage I–II (295)
② Stage I–II, large mediastinal mass (84)
③ Stage III–IV (186)

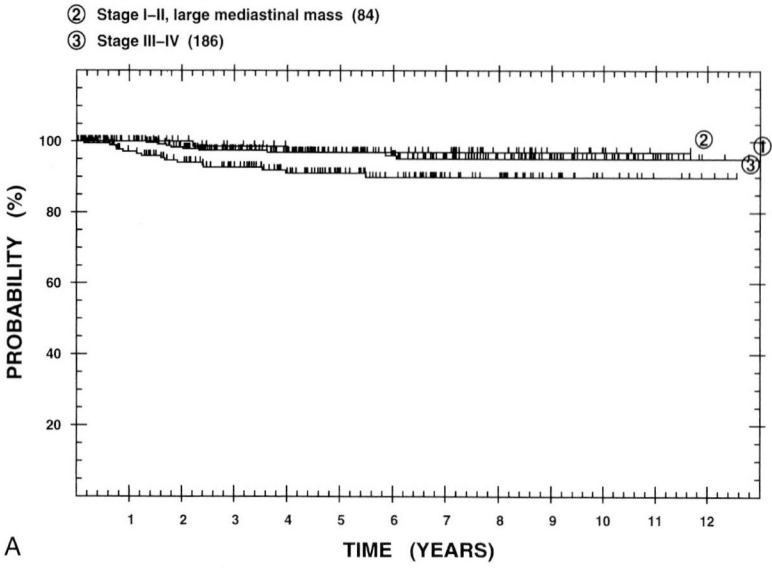

A

① Stage I–II (295)
② Stage I–II, large mediastinal mass (84)
③ Stage III–IV (186)

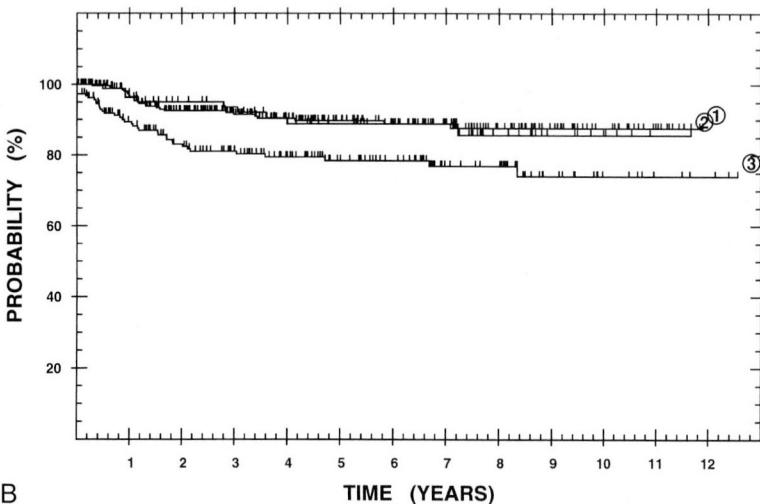

B

Figure 60–13. Survival (**A**) and freedom from relapse (**B**) of 565 patients treated for classical Hodgkin's disease (lymphocyte predominance is excluded) at Stanford University from 1989 through 2001. 1, favorable, stage I-IIA, or B (295); 2, stage I-II with a large mediastinal mass (n = 84); 3, stage III-IV (n = 186).

This field is treated with evenly weighted opposed lateral photons, generally to a dose of 30 Gy. Thereafter, a more traditional field arrangement may be employed to carry the dose to the involved area to 36 to 44 Gy.

CRITICAL NORMAL TISSUES

The number of organs and the volume of normal tissue within the treatment fields for Hodgkin's disease is substantial, and careful consideration of both short-term toxicity and long-term morbidity is essential in treatment planning. In the mantle field region, there is potential toxicity involving the salivary glands, thyroid, soft tissues of the neck and shoulder girdle (especially in younger people), brachial plexus, spinal cord, heart, and lungs. For subdiaphragmatic fields, dose-limiting organs include the kidneys, spinal cord, liver, bone marrow, gastrointestinal tract, and gonads. Specific discussion of radiation tolerance of many of these organs is included in the individual organ site chapters. Even modest doses of irradiation may be associated with potential long-term complications in some of these sites, especially considering the long duration of follow-up expected for the majority of patients.

In adults, the most sensitive of these organs are the lungs, where radiographic evidence of acute pulmonary reactions may be observed with doses as low as 15 Gy. Areas of lung treated to 40 to 44 Gy often demonstrate fibrosis during long-term follow-up; however, the severity varies remarkably among patients treated with similar technique. Both lungs may be treated safely to a dose of 16.5 Gy, especially if partial-transmission lung blocks (protracted fractionation) are employed. Function *may* be ablated in areas of lung treated to doses in excess of 25 Gy.

Subclinical injury to the pericardium may be present at lower doses, but symptomatic pericarditis is rare with doses of 30 Gy or less, even if the entire cardiac silhouette is treated. The use of partial-field blocking (apical portion of heart at 15 Gy, subcarinal portion of heart at 30 Gy) is associated with only a small risk of pericarditis. The myocardium is slightly more resistant than the pericardium, but doses of 35 Gy or more may be associated with minimal long-term risk of myocardial dysfunction. The coronary arteries are moderately radiation-resistant; however, doses in excess of 30 Gy are associated with an increased risk of coronary artery disease and myocardial infarction.[83]

Doses of 40 Gy or more may be associated with later soft tissue and muscle atrophy, even in adults. This is quite variable in expression. Children experience effects on growth or soft tissue development with doses as low as 15 Gy.

There are generally few long-term effects on salivary gland function after standard treatment for Hodgkin's disease. However, xerostomia may develop in patients treated to the Waldeyer region. Thyroid gland function may be diminished, despite partial thyroid shielding with a larynx block.[84] This is often manifest initially as an elevation of the sensitive thyroid-stimulating hormone (S-TSH), and exogenous replacement therapy is appropriate at that time.

Although spinal cord tolerance should not be an issue with standard Hodgkin's disease therapy, the length of spinal cord included in the field, expected success of treatment, long duration of follow-up, and use of contiguous fields that overlap the spinal cord demand conservative dose guidelines and extreme attention to treatment details. At Stanford, we use lateral simulator radiographs or CT simulation to calculate the cord dose and insert posterior spinal cord shielding to limit the cord dose to 40 Gy or less. Field separation for the mantle and paraortic fields is calculated carefully, and skin gap calculations are performed. In addition, a small block (1 to 2 cm in length) is inserted at the superior portion of the posterior paraortic field in order to further limit the dose to the cord in that area of field abutment.

With contemporary mantle therapy, injury to the brachial plexus should not be expected. However, with older techniques of treatment that employed larger daily doses or failed to take into account variations in body thickness, doses of 44 Gy have been associated with long-term brachial plexus injury.

In the abdomen, dose-limiting organ toxicity is not usually an issue in standard Hodgkin's disease therapy. Only a small portion of the total renal volume is within a standard paraortic-splenic pedicle field. If the spleen itself must be treated, the proportion of renal volume is much greater, but with CT planning, it is generally 30% of the left kidney or less. Although 30 to 36 Gy is sufficient to ablate renal function in that portion of kidney, this should not have any impact on normal renal function. However, the radiation oncologist must be alert to the presence of underlying renal disease, which may already compromise renal function.

A portion of the left lobe of liver is included in the paraortic field. This may cause transient hepatic dysfunction in that region of liver (accompanied by an elevation of the serum alkaline phosphatase level), but is not associated with long-term sequelae. The entire liver may be treated safely to a dose of 25 Gy using protracted fractionation, if necessary. Higher doses should be avoided.

The gastrointestinal tract generally tolerates doses up to 44 Gy. However, patients who have undergone abdominal surgical procedures such as staging laparotomy and have formed intra-abdominal adhesions may develop evidence of bowel injury with doses of 36 Gy or more.

In the pelvis, the gonads are the most sensitive organ of concern. The ovaries are exquisitely sensitive, especially in women 30 years and older. Fractionated doses of 4 Gy or more should be avoided. In women who require pelvic irradiation, this necessitates ovarian transposition and double-thickness blocking.

In addition to organ-specific complications, a significant risk for patients is the development of treatment-related malignancies. Long-term follow-up is essential to define this risk. Leukemia may develop in about 5% of patients with a latent period of 3 to 7 years after treatment with chemotherapy that includes an alkylating agent (e.g., MOPP). The occurrence of leukemia after treatment with irradiation alone is exceedingly rare, and it remains controversial whether the risk is greater after combined-modality therapy. Secondary solid tumors may be related to either chemotherapy or radiation and generally have a longer latent period (at least 7 to 10 years). Patients who smoke should be counseled to stop because of a high risk of lung cancer when smoking is combined with irradiation. Women should undergo mammography according to the usual American Cancer Society guidelines to detect early breast cancer, which may or may not be treatment-related. In addition, even younger women should begin mammogram screening 10 years after they have completed mantle irradiation. The relative risk that women will develop breast cancer after treatment for Hodgkin's disease is 4.1. This is manifest primarily in women who are younger than 30 years when they are treated.[85]

OUTCOME

An evaluation of outcome includes an assessment of survival, freedom from relapse, freedom from second relapse, and the risk of various complications. Survival and freedom from relapse for patients with classical Hodgkin's disease (lymphocyte predominance has been excluded) treated at Stanford using contemporary treatment techniques (between 1989 and 2000) are displayed in Table 60-7.

Stage I-IIA

Series that used subtotal lymphoid irradiation after staging laparotomy reported 10-year survival rates of almost 90% and 10-year relapse-free rates of 75% to 80%.

At Stanford, 73 patients with stage I-IIA favorable prognosis Hodgkin's disease (bulky mediastinal adenopathy was the only exclusion) were treated with STLI (including the spleen) following clinical staging only

Table 60–7 Ten-Year Outcome for 565 Patients with Classical Hodgkin's Disease Treated at Stanford, 1989-2001

Stage Grouping	Patients, n	Survival, %	Freedom from Relapse, %
Stage I-II	295	95	88
Stage I-II			
large mediastinal mass	84	97	86
Stage III-IV	186	90	74

during the 10-year period beginning in 1988. The 12-year survival is 99% and freedom from relapse is 91%, comparable to our previous data for laparotomy-staged patients.

Since 1995, we have treated these patients with the Stanford V program. After 8 weeks of chemotherapy, patients receive irradiation to the involved regions to a dose of 30 Gy. The 3-year freedom from progression is 95% and 3-year survival is 97%.[86]

Stage I-II, Subdiaphragmatic

Approximately 10% of patients with stage I-II Hodgkin's disease present with subdiaphragmatic disease. Lymphography is very helpful in staging these patients. The same general principles of management apply as for supradiaphragmatic disease. Combined-modality therapy is the treatment of choice. Alternatively, patients who have disease limited to the inguinal-femoral region may be effectively treated with radiation therapy alone, using an inverted-Y and spleen field. If involvement of iliac or paraortic nodes is detected by abdominal imaging, the spleen will be involved in about 40% of cases, and combined-modality therapy is appropriate. In general, the outcome of treatment for patients with subdiaphragmatic disease is equivalent to that for patients with supradiaphragmatic disease.[87,88]

Stage I-II with Bulky Mediastinal Involvement

Approximately 20% of patients with stage I-II Hodgkin's disease will present with a large mediastinal mass. As noted previously, single-modality therapy for these patients is generally considered to be inadequate and combined-modality treatment is the standard. During the 1980s, the conventional treatment at Stanford for these patients was a combination of 6 cycles of chemotherapy (MOPP, ABVD, or PAVe) followed by mantle irradiation to 44 Gy. The 9-year survival and freedom from relapse for these patients was 84% and 88%, respectively.[89] In the 1990s the Stanford V program was adopted, in which 12 weeks of chemotherapy were followed by radiation to the mantle to 44 Gy, later modified to 36 Gy to the mediastinum and bilateral supraclavicular areas. Not only is the Stanford V program of briefer duration, but the initial results appear to be better. The 5-year freedom from progression is 97% and the 5-year survival is 100%.[53]

Stage I-IIB

Approximately 15% to 20% of patients with stage I or II disease have B symptoms. In general, these patients should be managed in a fashion analogous to those with stage III-IV disease. However, given the limited anatomical extent of disease in stage I-II, one can make a strong argument to include consolidative IF irradiation for these patients. We currently include these patients in our protocols for stage III-IV disease.

Stage III-IV[90]

Systemic chemotherapy is the mainstay of treatment for patients with advanced-stage Hodgkin's disease. Although early clinical trials of systemic therapy for Hodgkin's disease often excluded patients with stage IIIA, these patients are now included as patients with "advanced Hodgkin's disease" in most clinical trials.

Since 1990, we have used the Stanford V program of combined-modality therapy for these patients. After 12 weeks of chemotherapy, they receive 36 Gy to initial sites of disease greater than 5 cm. With a median follow-up of more than 5 years, the 5-year freedom from progression is 85%, and survival is 96% for patients with stage III-IV disease.[53]

REFERENCES

1. Mueller NE, Grufferman S: The epidemiology of Hodgkin's disease. In Mauch P, Armitage JO, Diehl V, Hoppe R, Weiss LM, eds. *Hodgkin's Disease.* Philadelphia: Lippincott Williams & Wilkins; 1999:61.
2. Stat Bite. *J Natl Cancer Inst.* 1998:352.
3. Greenlee RT, Hill-Harmon, Murray T, Thun M: Cancer Statistics 2001. *CA Cancer J Clin 2001.* 2001;51.
4. Medeiros LJ, Greiner TC: Hodgkin's disease. *Cancer.* 1995;75:357.
5. Grufferman S, Delzell E: Epidemiology of Hodgkin's disease. *Epidemiol Rev.* 1984;6:76.
6. Weiss LM, Movahed LA, Warnke RA, Sklar J: Detection of Epstein-Barr viral genomes in Reed-Sternberg cells of Hodgkin's disease. *N Engl J Med.* 1989;320:502.
7. Mueller N, Evans A, Harris NL, et al: Hodgkin's disease and Epstein-Barr virus. Altered antibody pattern before diagnosis. *N Engl J Med.* 1989;320:689.
8. Hjalgrim H, Askling J, Sorensen P, et al: Risk of Hodgkin's disease and other cancers after infectious mononucleosis. *J Natl Cancer Inst.* 2000;92:1522.
9. Ambinder RF, Browning PJ, Lorenzana I, et al: Epstein-Barr virus and childhood Hodgkin's disease in Honduras and the United States. *Blood.* 1993;81:462.
10. Weiss LM, Chan JK, MacLennan KA, Warnke R: Pathology of classical Hodgkin's disease. In Mauch P, Armitage JO, Diehl V, et al, eds. *Hodgkin's Disease.* Philadelphia: Lippincott Williams & Wilkins; 1999:101.
11. Hansmann ML, Weiss LM, Stein H, et al: Pathology of lymphocyte predominance Hodgkin's disease. In Mauch P, Armitage JO, Diehl V, et al, eds. *Hodgkin's Disease.* Philadelphia: Lippincott Williams & Wilkins; 1999:169.
12. Chittal SM, Caveriviere P, Schwarting R, et al: Monoclonal antibodies in the diagnosis of Hodgkin's disease. The search for a rational panel. *Am J Surg Pathol.* 1988;12:9.
13. Rassidakis GZ, Medeiros LJ, Viviani S, et al: CD20 expression in Hodgkin and Reed-Sternberg cells of classical Hodgkin's disease: Associations with presenting features and clinical outcome. *J Clin Oncol.* 2002;20:1278.

14. Pinkus GS, Said JW: Hodgkin's disease, lymphocyte predominance type, nodular—A distinct entity? Unique staining profile for L&H variants of Reed-Sternberg cells defined by monoclonal antibodies to leukocyte common antigen, granulocyte-specific antigen, and B-cell-specific antigen. *Am J Pathol.* 1985;118:1.

15. Harris NL, Jaffe ES, Diebold J, et al: World Health Organization classification of neoplastic diseases of the hematopoietic and lymphoid tissues: Report of the Clinical Advisory Committee meeting—Airlie House, Virginia, November 1997. *J Clin Oncol.* 1999;17:3835.

16. Regula DP Jr, Hoppe RT, Weiss LM: Nodular and diffuse types of lymphocyte predominance Hodgkin's disease. *N Engl J Med.* 1988;318:214.

17. Doggett RS, Colby TV, Dorfman RF: Interfollicular Hodgkin's disease. *Am J Surg Pathol.* 1983;7:145.

18. Hu E, Hufford S, Lukes R, et al: Third-World Hodgkin's disease at Los Angeles County—University of Southern California Medical Center. *J Clin Oncol.* 1988;6:1285.

19. Rosenberg S, Kaplan HS: Evidence for an orderly progression in the spread of Hodgkin's disease. *Cancer Res.* 1966;26:1225.

20. Kaplan HS: The radical radiotherapy of regionally localized Hodgkin's disease. *Radiology.* 1962;78:553.

21. Hoppe RT, Cox RS, Rosenberg SA, Kaplan HS: Prognostic factors in pathologic stage III Hodgkin's disease. *Cancer Treat Rep.* 1982;66:743.

22. Kaplan HS: Patterns of anatomic distribution. In *Hodgkin's Disease.* Vol. 2. Cambridge, Mass.: Harvard University Press; 1980.

23. Crnkovich MJ, Hoppe RT, Rosenberg SA: Stage IIB Hodgkin's disease: The Stanford experience. *J Clin Oncol.* 1986;4:472.

24. Austin-Seymour MM, Hoppe RT, Cox RS, et al: Hodgkin's disease in patients over sixty years old. *Ann Intern Med.* 1984;100:13.

25. Jacobs C, Donaldson SS, Rosenberg SA, Kaplan HS: Management of the pregnant patient with Hodgkin's disease. *Ann Intern Med.* 1981;95:669.

26. Le Floch O, Donaldson SS, Kaplan HS: Pregnancy following oophoropexy and total nodal irradiation in women with Hodgkin's disease. *Cancer.* 1976;38:2263.

27. Schoeppel SL, Hoppe RT, Dorfman RF, et al: Hodgkin's disease in homosexual men with generalized lymphadenopathy. *Ann Intern Med.* 1985;102:68.

28. Gupta RK, Gospodarowicz MK, Lister TA: Clinical evaluation and staging of Hodgkin's disease. In Mauch PM, Armitage JO, Diehl V, et al, eds. *Hodgkin's Disease.* Philadelphia: Lippincott Williams & Wilkins; 1999:223.

29. Castellino RA, Podoloff DA: Diagnostic radiology and nuclear medicine imaging in Hodgkin's disease. In Mauch PM, Armitage JO, Diehl V, et al, eds. *Hodgkin's Disease.* Philadelphia: Lippincott Williams & Wilkins; 1999:241.

30. Friedman S, Henry-Amar M, Cosset JM: Evolution of erythrocyte sedimentation rate as predictor of early relapse in post-therapy early-stage Hodgkin's disease. *J Clin Oncol.* 1988;596.

31. Hasenclever D, Diehl V: A prognostic score for advanced Hodgkin's disease. International Prognostic Factors Project on Advanced Hodgkin's Disease. *N Engl J Med.* 1998;339:1506.

32. Piro AJ, Weiss DR, Hellman S: Mediastinal Hodgkin's disease: A possible danger for intubation anesthesia. Intubation danger in Hodgkin's disease. *Int J Radiat Oncol Biol Phys.* 1976;1:415.

33. Castellino RA, Blank N, Hoppe RT, Cho C: Hodgkin disease: Contributions of chest CT in the initial staging evaluation. *Radiology.* 1986;160:603.

34. Cheson BD, Horning S, Coiffier B, et al: Report of an International Workshop to Standardize Response Criteria for Non-Hodgkin's Lymphoma. *Clin Oncol (R Coll Radiol).* 1999;17:1244.

35. Castellino RA, Hoppe RT, Blank N, et al: Computed tomography, lymphography, and staging laparotomy: Correlations in initial staging of Hodgkin disease. *Am J Roentgenol.* 1984;143:37.

36. Front D, Israel O: The role of Ga-67 scintigraphy in evaluating the results of therapy of lymphoma patients. *Semin Nucl Med.* 1995;25:60.

37. Partridge S, Timothy A, O'Doherty MJ, et al: 2-Fluorine-18-fluoro-2-deoxy-D glucose positron emission tomography in the pretreatment staging of Hodgkin's disease: Influence on patient management in a single institution. *Ann Oncol.* 2000;11:1273.

38. Wirth A, Seymour JF, Hicks RJ, et al: F-18 fluorodioxyglucose positron emission tomography, gallium-67 scintigraphy, and conventional staging for Hodgkin's disease and non-Hodgkin's lymphoma. *Am J Med.* 2002;112:262.

39. de Wit M, Bohuslavizki KH, Buchert R, et al: 18FDG-PET following treatment as valid predictor for disease-free survival in Hodgkin's lymphoma. *Ann Oncol.* 2001;12:29.

40. Portlock CS, Yahalom J: The management of Hodgkin's disease during pregnancy. In Mauch P, Armitage JO, Diehl V, et al, eds. *Hodgkin's Disease.* Philadelphia: Lippincott Williams & Wilkins; 1999:693.

41. Carde P, Glatstein E: Role of staging laparotomy in Hodgkin's disease. In Mauch P, Armitage JO, Diehl V, et al, eds. *Hodgkin's Disease.* Philadelphia: Lippincott Williams & Wilkins; 1999:273.

42. Carde P, Hagenbeek A, Hayat M, et al: Clinical staging versus laparotomy and combined modality with MOPP versus ABVD in early-stage Hodgkin's disease: The H6 twin randomized trials from the European Organization for Research and Treatment of Cancer Lymphoma Cooperative Group. *J Clin Oncol.* 1993;11:2258.

43. Donaldson SS, Moore MR, Rosenberg SA, Vosti KL: Characterization of postsplenectomy bacteremia among patients with and without lymphoma. *N Engl J Med.* 1972;287:69.

44. Leibenhaut MH, Hoppe RT, Efron B, et al: Prognostic indicators of laparotomy findings in clinical stage I-II supradiaphragmatic Hodgkin's disease. *J Clin Oncol.* 1989;7:81.

45. Carbone PP, Kaplan HS, Musshoff K, et al: Report of the Committee on Hodgkin's Disease Staging Classification. *Cancer Res.* 1971;31:1860.

46. Mendenhall NP, Hoppe R, Prosnitz LR, Mauch P: Principles of radiation therapy in Hodgkin's disease. In Mauch P, Armitage JO, Diehl V, Hoppe R, et al, eds. *Hodgkin's Disease.* Philadelphia: Lippincott Williams & Wilkins; 1999:337.

47. Hough RE, Hancock BW: Principles of chemotherapy in Hodgkin's disease. In Mauch P, Armitage JO, Diehl V, Hoppe R, et al, eds. *Hodgkin's Disease.* Philadelphia: Lippincott Williams & Wilkins; 1999:377.

48. De Vita VT, Hubbard SM, Longo DL: The chemotherapy of lymphomas: Looking back, moving forward. The Richard and Hinda Rosenthal Foundation Award Lecture. *Cancer Res.* 1987;47:4810.

49. Bonadonna G: Chemotherapy strategies to improve the control of Hodgkin's disease: The Richard and Hinda Rosenthal Foundation Award Lecture. *Cancer Res.* 1982;42:4309.

50. Bonadonna G, Valagussa P, Santoro A: Alternating non-cross-resistant combination chemotherapy or MOPP in stage IV Hodgkin's disease. A report of 8-year results. *Ann Intern Med.* 1986;104:739.

51. Klimo P, Connors JM: MOPP/ABV hybrid program: Combination chemotherapy based on early introduction of seven effective drugs for advanced Hodgkin's disease. *J Clin Oncol.* 1985;3:1174.

52. Canellos GP, Anderson JR, Propert KJ, et al: Chemotherapy of advanced Hodgkin's disease with MOPP, ABVD, or MOPP alternating with ABVD. *N Engl J Med.* 1992;327:1478.

53. Horning SJ, Hoppe RT, Bueslin S, et al: Stanford V and radiotherapy for locally extensive and advanced HD: Mature results of a prospective clinical trial. *J Clin Oncol.* 2001;630.

54. Engel C, Loeffler M, Schmitz S, et al: Acute hematologic toxicity and practicability of dose-intensified BEACOPP chemotherapy for advanced stage Hodgkin's disease. German Hodgkin's Lymphoma Study Group (GHSG). *Ann Oncol.* 2000;11:1105.

55. Connors JM, Yahalom J, Noordijk E: Principles of combined-modality therapy in Hodgkin's disease. In Mauch P, Armitage JO, Diehl V, et al, eds. *Hodgkin's Disease.* Philadelphia: Lippincott Williams & Wilkins; 1999:395.

56. Bonfante V, Viviani S, Devizzi L, et al: Ten-years experience with ABVD plus radiotherapy: Subtotal nodal (STNI) vs involved field (IFRT) in early-stage Hodgkin's disease (Hd). *Proc ASCO.* 2001;20.

57. Horning SJ, Hoppe RT, Breslin S, et al: Very brief (8 weeks) chemotherapy and low dose (30 Gy) radiotherapy for limited stage Hodgkin's disease: Preliminary results of the Stanford-Kaiser G4 Study of Stanford V and Radiotherapy [Abstract]. *Blood.* 1999; 94:1;1;387a.

58. Hoppe RT, Coleman CN, Cox RS, et al: The management of stage I-II Hodgkin's disease with irradiation alone or combined modality therapy: The Stanford experience. *Blood.* 1982;59:455.

59. Longo DL, Russo A, Duffey PL, et al: Treatment of advanced-stage massive mediastinal Hodgkin's disease: The case for combined modality treatment. *J Clin Oncol.* 1991;9:227.

60. Hoppe RT, Cosset JM, Santoro A, Wolf J: Treatment of unfavorable prognosis stage I-II Hodgkin's disease. In Mauch P, Armitage JO, Diehl V, et al, eds. *Hodgkin's Disease*. Philadelphia: Lippincott Williams & Wilkins; 1999:459.

61. Young RC, Canellos GP, Chabner BA, et al: Patterns of relapse in advanced Hodgkin's disease treated with combination chemotherapy. *Cancer*. 1978;42:1001.

62. Fabian CJ, Mansfield CM, Dahlberg S, et al: Low-dose involved field radiation after chemotherapy in advanced Hodgkin disease. A Southwest Oncology Group randomized study. *Ann Intern Med*. 1994;120:903.

63. Diehl V, Loeffler M, Pfreundschuh M, et al: Further chemotherapy versus low-dose involved-field radiotherapy as consolidation of complete remission after six cycles of alternating chemotherapy in patients with advanced Hodgkin's disease. German Hodgkins' Study Group (GHSG). *Ann Oncol*. 1995;6:901.

64. Aleman BM, Raemaekers J, Henry-Amar M, et al: Involved-field radiotherapy in patients with stage III/IV Hodgkin's lymphoma: First results of the randomised EORTC trial # 20884. *Int J Radiat Oncol Biol Phys*. 2001;51.

65. Hoppe RT: The management of Hodgkin's disease in relapse after primary radiation therapy. *Eur J Cancer*. 1992;28A:1920.

66. Armitage JO, Goldstone AH, Carella AM, et al: Role of bone marrow transplantation in Hodgkin's disease. In Mauch P, Armitage JO, Diehl V, et al, eds. *Hodgkin's Disease*. Philadelphia: Lippincott Williams & Wilkins; 1999:521.

67. Nademanee A, O'Donnell MR, Snyder DS, et al: High-dose chemotherapy with or without total body irradiation followed by autologous bone marrow and/or peripheral blood stem cell transplantation for patients with relapsed and refractory Hodgkin's disease: Results in 85 patients with analysis of prognostic factors. *Blood*. 1995;85:1381.

68. Kaplan HS: Evidence for a tumoricidal dose level in the radiotherapy of Hodgkin's disease. *Cancer Res*. 1966;26:1221.

69. Yahalom J, Gulati SC, Toia M, et al: Accelerated hyperfractionated total-lymphoid irradiation, high-dose chemotherapy, and autologous bone marrow transplantation for refractory and relapsing patients with Hodgkin's disease. *J Clin Oncol*. 1993;11:1062.

70. Shamash J, Lee SM, Radford JA, et al: Patterns of relapse and subsequent management following high-dose chemotherapy with autologous haematopoietic support in relapsed or refractory Hodgkin's lymphoma: A two centre study. *Ann Oncol*. 2000;11:715.

71. Mundt AJ, Sibley G, Williams S, et al: Patterns of failure following high-dose chemotherapy and autologous bone marrow transplantation with involved field radiotherapy for relapsed/refractory Hodgkin's disease. *Int J Radiat Oncol Biol Phys*. 1995;33:261.

72. Pezner RD, Nademanee A, Niland JC, et al: Involved field radiation therapy for Hodgkin's disease autologous bone marrow transplantation regimens. *Radiother Oncol*. 1995;34:23.

73. Poen JC, Hoppe RT, Horning SJ: High-dose therapy and autologous bone marrow transplantation for relapsed/refractory Hodgkin's disease: The impact of involved field radiotherapy on patterns of failure and survival [see comments]. *Int J Radiat Oncol Biol Phys*. 1996;36:3.

74. Noordijk EM, Carde P, Mandard AM, et al: Preliminary results of the EORTC-GPMC controlled clinical trial H7 in early-stage Hodgkin's disease. EORTC Lymphoma Cooperative Group. Groupe Pierre-et-Marie-Curie. *Ann Oncol*. 1994;5:107.

75. Lutz WR, Larsen RD: Technique to match mantle and para-aortic fields. *Int J Radiat Oncol Biol Phys*. 1983;9:1753.

76. Smith AR: Treatment planning. In *Patterns of Care Newsletter*. Philadelphia: American College of Radiology; 1993.

77. Carlsen SE, Bergin CJ, Hoppe RT: MR imaging to detect chest wall and pleural involvement in patients with lymphoma: Effect on radiation therapy planning. *AJR Am J Roentgenol*. 1993;160:1191.

78. Hoppe R: Hodgkin's disease. In *Patterns of Care Study Newsletter 3*. American College of Radiology;1990-91;8:3.

79. Hoppe RT: Radiation therapy in the management of Hodgkin's disease. *Semin Oncol*. 1990;17:704.

80. Carmel RJ, Kaplan HS: Mantle irradiation in Hodgkin's disease. An analysis of technique, tumor eradication, and complications. *Cancer*. 1976;37:2813.

81. Palos B, Kaplan HS, Karzmark CJ: The use of thin lung shields to deliver limited whole-lung irradiation during mantle-field treatment of Hodgkin's disease. *Radiology*. 1971;101:441.

82. Hoppe RT, Burke JS, Glatstein E, Kaplan HS: Non-Hodgkin's Lymphoma. Involvement of Waldeyer's Ring. *Cancer* 1978;42:1096.

83. Hancock SL, Tucker MA, Hoppe RT: Factors affecting late mortality from heart disease after treatment of Hodgkin's disease. *JAMA*. 1993;270:1949.

84. Hancock SL, Cox RS, McDougall IR: Thyroid diseases after treatment of Hodgkin's disease. *N Engl J Med*. 1991;325:599.

85. Hancock SL, Tucker MA, Hoppe RT: Breast cancer after treatment of Hodgkin's disease. *J Natl Cancer Inst*. 1993;85:25.

86. Horning S, Hoppe R, Breslin S, et al: Very brief (8 week) chemotherapy (CT) and low dose (30 Gy) radiotherapy (RT) for limited stage Hodgkin's Disease (HD): *Preliminary Results of the Stanford-Kaiser G4 Study of Stanford V + RT*. 2000.

87. Leibenhaut MH, Hoppe RT, Varghese A, Rosenberg SA: Subdiaphragmatic Hodgkin's disease: Laparotomy and treatment results in 49 patients. *J Clin Oncol*. 1987;5:1050.

88. Liao Z, Ha CS, Fuller LM, et al: Subdiaphragmatic stage I & II Hodgkin's disease: Long-term follow-up and prognostic factors. *Int J Radiat Oncol Biol Phys*. 1998;41:1047.

89. Behar RA, Horning SJ, Hoppe RT: Hodgkin's disease with bulky mediastinal involvement: Effective management with combined modality therapy [see comments]. *Int J Radiat Oncol Biol Phys*. 1993;25:771.

90. Horning S, Yahalom J, Tesch H, et al: Treatment of stage III-IV Hodgkin's disease. In Mauch P, Armitage JO, Diehl V, et al, eds. *Hodgkin's Disease*. Philadelphia: Lippincott Williams & Wilkins; 1999:483.

Non-Hodgkin's Lymphoma

61

Joachim Yahalom, MD

he term *non-Hodgkin's lymphoma* (NHL) denotes a group of more than 30 lymphoproliferative malignancies that lack the pathologic characteristics of Hodgkin's disease (HD).[1,2] The common link for this diverse group of neoplasms is the monoclonal expansion of malignant B- or T-cells. Chronic lymphocytic leukemia, acute lymphoblastic leukemia, plasma cell disorders, mycosis fungoides, and HD are also malignancies of the immune system that occasionally display clinical and pathologic features that overlap with the "classic" nodal or extranodal NHLs.[1] This chapter focuses on the more common NHLs, particularly those that are commonly considered for radiation therapy. The leukemias, plasma cell disorders, mycosis fungoides, and HD are discussed elsewhere in this book.

Non-Hodgkin's lymphomas can appear at any age, although they are rare during the first year of life. Like HD, NHLs usually originate in lymphoid tissues and can spread to other organs. However, unlike HD, multiple sites are more frequently involved in NHL, and extranodal lesions are common, sometimes being the only site of disease. Progression of disease is less orderly than that of HD, and unlike HD, the prognosis of NHL strongly depends on histologic type. While the different lymphomas vary widely in natural history and response to therapy, they can still be categorized into two groups: indolent (low-grade) lymphomas and aggressive (intermediate- and high-grade) lymphomas. This categorization is useful and relevant to choice of therapy, including radiation therapy.

INCIDENCE

Approximately 53,000 new cases of NHL were diagnosed in the United States in 2003 and nearly 23,400 patients died of it, making NHL the fifth most common cancer in both incidence and mortality and the fourth most prevalent cancer.[3] Lymphomas are slightly more common in males (1.1:1) and the incidence is higher in white people than in black (1.6:1).[3,4]

The incidence of NHL has increased by 150% since 1950. An increase of 50% was documented between 1973 and 1988 (3% to 4% increase each year). This is one of the largest increases reported for any cancer over the past 2 decades.[5] Despite wide variations in data from different countries, ranging from approximately 2 per 100,000 per year in the Far East to 10 per 100,000 per

year in the United Kingdom and more than 15 per 100,000 per year in the United States, NHL incidence appears to be increasing in all parts of the world.[4] The increase in incidence has been most marked in elderly white males, in extranodal presentations, and in aggressive lymphomas.[6] Lymphomas associated with acquired immunodeficiency syndrome (AIDS) are responsible for some new lymphomas seen in young and middle-aged males since 1982; however, they represent only a small percentage of the total past increase.[4,6] The reasons for the increase are not clear; possible increase in occupational and environmental exposure to herbicides, solvents, and other suspected etiologic factors can account for only a small fraction of the observed increase.[4]

ETIOLOGY

Environmental exposures, viruses, congenital or acquired immunosuppression, collagen vascular diseases, and chromosomal aberrations have been associated with the development of NHL. These are summarized in Table 61-1.

Many of the conditions associated with NHL involve changes in the immune status: immunosuppression or immunostimulation. The Epstein-Barr virus (EBV) is commonly associated with lymphomas that develop in immunosuppressed patients.[7] In immunocompetent patients, EBV was implicated in the pathogenesis of endemic (African) Burkitt's lymphoma, in which 98% of patients contain the EBV genome.[8] The most convincing evidence for a viral cause of lymphoma is in a relatively rare type of lymphoma that is endemic to Japan and the Caribbean: adult T-cell leukemia-lymphoma. It is caused by a unique RNA retrovirus termed human T-cell leukemia virus-1 (HTLV-1) that is transmitted by the same routes as human immunodeficiency virus (HIV).[9]

Carriers of HIV have a higher risk of developing aggressive types of NHL, particularly primary central nervous system lymphoma. The cumulative incidence of NHL among the HIV-infected population is now 5% to 10% over a decade.[10] Molecular genetics studies indicate that more than one pathogenic mechanism is operative in HIV-associated NHL.[11,12]

Several epidemiologic studies have shown that agricultural workers have a high incidence of the disease.[13] Some researchers have attributed this to pesticide exposure.[14] There is also suggestive evidence that hair dyes may play a role in the etiology of lymphoma.[15] Ionizing

Table 61–1   Diseases and Chemical and Physical Agents Associated with Non-Hodgkin's Lymphoma

Inherited Immunodeficiency Diseases

Ataxia-telangiectasia
Chédiak-Higashi syndrome
Common variable immunodeficiency
Wiskott-Aldrich syndrome
Severe combined immunodeficiency
X-linked lymphoproliferative syndrome

Acquired Immunodeficiency States

Acquired immunodeficiency syndrome
Organ transplantation
Immunosuppression with cyclosporine, azathioprine, alkylating agents

Other Disorders

Sicca syndrome (Sjögren disease)
Rheumatoid arthritis and systemic lupus erythematosus
Hashimoto's thyroiditis
Nontropical sprue
Lymphomatoid papulosis

Chemical, Physical, and Biologic Agents

Agricultural chemicals
Hair darkening dyes
Radiation and chemotherapy treatment for Hodgkin's disease
Radiation exposure
Hydantoin anticonvulsants
Herbicides
Helicobacter pylori
Epstein-Barr virus
Human T-cell leukemia/lymphoma virus 1 (HTLV-1)

radiation alone has little or no effect on the risk of NHL,[16] but patients with HD treated with radiation therapy and chemotherapy have an increased risk of developing secondary large-cell lymphoma.

The presence of the bacteria *Helicobacter pylori* has been closely associated with the development of mucosa-associated lymphoid tissue (MALT) lymphoma of the stomach, and in some cases, eradication of *H. pylori* by antibiotic treatment resulted in lymphoma regression.[17]

CYTOGENETICS AND MOLECULAR BIOLOGY

Many lymphomas are associated with nonrandom chromosomal abnormalities that reflect molecular rearrangements involving specific oncogenes and one of the immunoglobulin genes. These abnormalities often correlate with the histologic type, immunophenotype, and clinical behavior. A typical example is the translocation t(14:18) (q32;q21) that occurs in approximately 90% of cases of follicular lymphoma. It results in the transposition of the *bcl-2* oncogene of chromosome 18 to become adjacent to the heavy chain immunoglobulin gene on chromosome 14. The *bcl-2* oncogene is essential for apoptosis or programmed cell death. The t(14:18) translocation interferes with the normal senescence and death of the follicular center cell and is possibly engaged in its malignant transformation.[18] Similarly, it was demonstrated that 90% of patients with Burkitt's lymphoma

have translocation t(8:14) or one of its variants and that *c-myc* was the relevant translocated oncogene. The *c-myc* product is an important transcription factor, and its dysregulation is probably involved in the proliferative process.[19] More recently, specific translocations have been characterized in other types of NHL. Translocation t(11:14) involving *bcl-1* has contributed to the recognition of mantle-cell lymphoma.[20] The gene product of *bcl-1*, cyclin D, is directly involved in the regulation of cell division. Trisomy 12 and *bcl-3* translocation t(14:19) were identified in small lymphocytic lymphoma/chronic lymphocytic leukemia.[21] Rearrangement of *bcl-6* has been reported recently in a third of patients with diffuse large-cell lymphoma.[22] The product of *bcl-6* resembles a class of zinc-finger transcription factors that regulates cell proliferation and differentiation. A translocation involving chromosomes 2 and 5 is characteristic of anaplastic large-cell lymphoma.[23] Trisomy 3 has been reported in 60% of MALT lymphomas and T(11:18) has also been detected in 25% to 40% of patients with MALT lymphoma.

IMMUNOPHENOTYPING

The detection of cell surface antigens using specific antibodies followed by immunoperoxidase staining or flow cytometry is termed immunophenotyping. In addition to allowing for a better understanding of the lymphoma cell origin, immunophenotyping is an invaluable diagnostic tool to distinguish lymphomas from myeloid and epithelial neoplasms and to define the specific type of lymphoma. It has become an important component of the new NHL classification.[1,2] Various surface antigens could be detected by several antibodies and are termed clusters of differentiation (CD). The lineage of the B-cell lymphomas, the most common type in adults, is confirmed by pan-B-cell markers (CD19, CD20, CD22). T-cell lineage is determined by the presence of pan-T-cell markers (CD2, CD3, CD7), and the T-cell subsets CD4 (inducer-helper) and CD8 (cytotoxic-suppressor) analysis. Further classification of indolent lymphomas is assisted by determination of CD5 and CD10. Among B-cell lymphomas, the CD5+, CD10– phenotype is characteristic of small lymphocytic lymphoma and mantle cell lymphoma. The CD5–, CD10+ phenotype is typical of the most common indolent lymphoma-follicular follicle center (small cleaved) lymphoma. The absence of CD5 and CD10 is important for the diagnosis of marginal zone lymphomas: MALT and its nodal variant. Anaplastic large-cell lymphoma typically displays CD30 (Ki-1) antigen and is also called Ki-1 lymphoma.

HISTOLOGIC CLASSIFICATION

Considering the clinical and histologic diversity of the lymphoid malignancies that are grouped under the generic title non-Hodgkin's lymphoma, it is crucial to obtain clear and detailed pathologic information about the biopsied specimen. This information should be interpreted carefully, recognizing the complexity and limitations of

Table 61–2 Histologic Classification of Non-Hodgkin's Lymphoma

WHO	Working Formulation	Rappaport
Indolent	**Low-grade**	
Follicular lymphoma (grade I)	Follicular small cleaved	Nodular poorly differentiated lymphocytic
Follicular lymphoma (grade II)	Follicular mixed, small cleaved, and large cell	Nodular mixed lymphocytic histiocytic
Small lymphocytic	Small lymphocytic	Diffuse well differentiated lymphocytic
Marginal zone: Extranodal (MALT)		
Nodal (monocytoid)		
Splenic		
Mycosis fungoides (T-cell)		
Aggressive	**Intermediate-grade**	
Diffuse large cell (including immunoblastic, mixed, and mediastinal B cell)	Diffuse large cell	Diffuse histiocytic
	Diffuse mixed small and large cell	Diffuse mixed lymphocytic and histiocytic
Follicular lymphoma (grade III)	Follicular large cell	Nodular histiocytic
Mantle cell lymphoma	Diffuse small cleaved cell differentiated lymphocytic	Diffuse poorly differentiated
T-cell lymphomas: Peripheral		
Angiocentric		
Angioimmunoblastic		
Anaplastic large cell		
Highly Aggressive	**High-grade**	
Lymphoblastic lymphoma	Lymphoblastic	Diffuse lymphoblastic
Burkitt's lymphoma	Small noncleaved: Burkitt's, nonBurkitt's Large cell immunoblastic	Diffuse undifferentiated

WHO, World Health Organization.

the present classification systems. An adequately processed pathologic specimen should be analyzed by a hematopathologist who is well versed in interpreting modern immunohistopathologic and molecular genetics techniques required for modern diagnosis and classification of NHL. Several pathologic classifications are currently in use, yet the most recent effort to develop a universally accepted classification was organized by the World Health Organization (WHO) and is presented in Table 61-2.[1,2] Table 61-3 may be helpful in translating between the different classifications and terminologies.

Over the past 40 years, the histologic classification of NHL has changed significantly. In the United States, the Rappaport classification was widely used during the 1960s and 1970s (see Table 61-3). Rappaport divided

Table 61–3 The Ann Arbor Staging Classification for Hodgkin's Disease and Non-Hodgkin's Lymphoma*

Stage I: Involvement of a single lymph node region (I) or single extra lymphatic organ or site (IE).

Stage II: Involvement of two or more lymph node regions on the same side of the diaphragm (II) or localized involvement of an extra lymphatic organ or site (IIE).

Stage III: Involvement of lymph node regions on both sides of the diaphragm (III) or localized involvement of an extra lymphatic organ or site (IIIE) or spleen (IIIS) or both (IIISE).

Stage IV: Diffuse or disseminated involvement of one or more extra lymphatic organs with or without associated lymph node involvement.

*The organs involved should be identified by a symbol: A, asymptomatic; B, fever, night sweats, weight loss of more than 10% of body weight.

lymphomas by pattern, whether nodular or diffuse, and then by cytologic shape using only basic staining morphology. Although the Rappaport classification gave no consideration to the emerging understanding of the immune system (i.e., B-cell or T-cell) and its malignant lymphoma counterparts, its simplicity and relative prognostic power made it popular among most clinicians. Nonetheless, during that period, five other classification systems (e.g., Kiel, Lukes-Collins) were also widely used in Europe and the United States. Communication between pathologists and clinicians as well as comparisons of clinical trials was extremely difficult.

In 1982, international collaborative efforts led to the Working Formulation for Clinical Usage that established terminology for "translation" among the different classifications and grouped the different subtypes into clinically relevant grades (see Table 61-3).[24] In spite of several deficiencies, the Working Formulation has become the most widely used method for lymphoma diagnosis in the United States and the basis for most American lymphoma clinical trials.

Over the past 15 years, new information has become available about lymphomas, leading to recognition of new entities and modifications of previously recognized lymphoma categories. An international group of hematopathologists (International Lymphoma Study Group) published a proposal for a Revised European-American Classification of Lymphoid Neoplasms (REAL). It has since been adapted with slight modification and is now termed the *WHO classification* (see Table 62-2).[2] The WHO classification described the morphologic, immunophenotypic, genetic, and clinical features of the different entities and divided all lymphoid malignancies into B-cell neoplasms, T-cell neoplasms, and Hodgkin's disease categories. In Table 61-3, the WHO entities for NHL are presented alongside the Working Formulation and the Rappaport classification.

In this table we maintained the basic categorization of three prognostic groups for both classifications. This grouping correlates relatively well with prognosis under current therapies and also properly corresponds with the general concepts of applying radiotherapy in these diseases. However, we changed the pathologic expression *(grade)* used by the Working Formulation to a clinical pattern term *(indolent or aggressive)* for WHO. The relatively new histologies, marginal zone (MALT) and mantle cell, are included in the indolent and aggressive groups, respectively. As recommended by other investigators,[1,2] we included the immunoblastic large-cell lymphoma in the intermediate group of the Working Formulation and not in the high-grade category as originally stated. The relatively uncommon T-cell lymphomas are categorized in the aggressive histology group.

Indolent Lymphomas

WHO: *Follicular Lymphoma—Grade I*
Follicular Lymphoma—Grade II

Working Formulation: Follicular small cleaved lymphoma
>Follicular mixed, small cleaved, and large cell lymphoma

Rappaport: Nodular lymphocytic, poorly differentiated
>Nodular mixed lymphocytic and histiocytic

Follicular lymphomas are the most common types of lymphoma in the United States. These closely related entities together constitute as much as 35% of the adult NHLs; the incidence is apparently lower in other parts of the world.[25] This is a disease of adults with a median age of 59 years and male-to-female ratio of 1:1.7. Follicular lymphomas, particularly of grade I, constitute a very

favorable prognostic subtype of lymphoma with a median survival of 8 to 10 years reported in selected populations.[26] Reproducible distinction between grades I and II is difficult and of questionable significance.

The disease involves predominantly lymph nodes; bone marrow is involved in approximately 40% of the patients. Of particular interest to the radiation oncologist is the fact that a third of the patients present with localized (stages I and II) disease. This group of localized disease patients is largely curable with radiation therapy.[27,28] Although patients with advanced-stage disease may have an indolent course, there is no curative treatment and there is an inexorable relapse rate of 15% to 20% per year.[29] In most patients, follicular lymphomas eventually evolve into aggressive and unresponsive disorders manifested by histologic transformation to diffuse pattern and large-cell morphology, clinical progression, and abnormal cytogenetic findings in addition to t(14;18). Diffuse large-cell lymphomas that evolve from follicular lymphomas lack the curability of diffuse large-cell neoplasms.

The follicular lymphomas exhibit follicular or nodular structures that reveal the origin of the cells: the follicle center (Fig. 61-1). There is usually a mixture of centrocytes (irregular or cleaved nuclei and weakly staining cytoplasm) and centroblasts (large noncleaved nuclei with multiple nucleoli and scant basophilic cytoplasm). The pattern is at least partially follicular, but diffuse areas may be present. This lymphoma shows B-cell–associated antigens (CD22, CS19, and CD20) and usually exhibits surface immunoglobulins that are IgM, IgD, or IgG.

In contrast to small lymphocytic lymphoma, the follicular lymphomas lack CD5 and often express CD10. Approximately 85% of the follicular follicle center lymphomas (grades I and II) genetically feature the transformation t(14;18), involving the rearrangement of the *bcl-2* gene. This results in expression of this "anti-apoptosis" gene, which is normally switched off at the translational level in normal germinal center cells.[30]

Rappaport first divided follicular lymphomas into three subgroups: small-cell, mixed small- and large-cell,

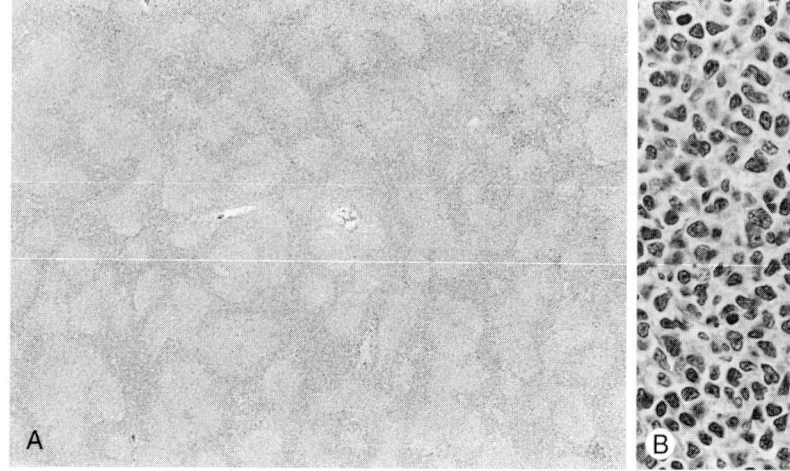
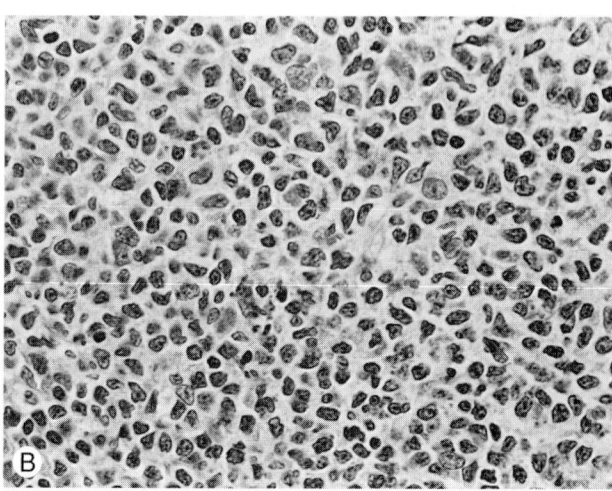

Figure 61–1. A, Follicular small cleaved cell lymphoma (low power). The lymph node architecture is effaced by back-to-back neoplastic follicles. **B,** Follicular small cleaved cell lymphoma (high power). Most of the cells in the neoplastic follicles are small cells with irregular (cleaved) nuclear contours.

and large-cell.[31] The proportion of centroblasts and the size of the centrocytes varies. It is hard to sharply divide those lymphomas into distinct subtypes and achieve reproducibility of these subdivisions among pathologists. Still, many individual pathologists can predict outcome by grading these lymphomas, and controversy exists over whether cases classified as follicular mixed-cell type are curable with aggressive therapy.[32-34] The REAL classification suggested the terms *grade I* for follicular lymphomas that are predominantly small, *grade II* for those that show a mixture of small and large cells, and *grade III* for those that are predominantly composed of large cells. At Memorial Sloan-Kettering Cancer Center (MSKCC) we regard grades I and II as indolent in our treatment approach and consider grade III as an aggressive lymphoma, similar to the diffuse large-cell type.

WHO: Small Lymphocytic Lymphoma/Chronic Lymphocytic Leukemia (SLL/CLL)

Working Formulation: Small lymphocytic lymphoma
Rappaport: Diffuse lymphocytic, well differentiated

In most cases, the disease predominantly involves the bone marrow and the peripheral blood in addition to involvement of multiple nodes, spleen, and liver and is called chronic lymphocytic leukemia (CLL). This is the most common form of leukemia in the Western world. The median age of onset is 61 years and the clinical course is indolent, with a median survival of 6 years. The term small lymphocytic lymphoma (SLL), consistent with CLL, is restricted to cases with tissue morphology and immunophenotype of CLL, but which are nonleukemic.

The lymph node exhibits a diffuse effaced pattern, although the presence of proliferation centers may give a vaguely nodular appearance. The predominant cell is a small lymphocyte with a round nucleus and clumped chromatin. The immunophenotype is characterized by the presence of CD5, an antigen usually associated with T-cells, but B-cell–associated antigens (CD19, CD20, CD22, CD23) are also present.[2] Whether adenopathy is a prominent part of the picture is apparently related to the expression of adhesion molecules (LFA-1).[35] Most patients who present with lymphadenopathy will prove to have bone marrow and peripheral blood involvement at the time of diagnosis or shortly thereafter. Some, however, may not develop leukemia, and a few (<10%) may even remain with a localized disease that will respond to radiation. In approximately 5% of cases, the tumor evolves into aggressive and highly lethal, clonally related, diffuse large-cell lymphoma. This transformation is called Richter's syndrome.[36]

WHO: Marginal Zone B-Cell Lymphomas:

>Extranodal:
>Mucosa-associated lymphoid tissue (MALT)
>Nodal:
>Monocytoid B-cell lymphomas

Marginal zone lymphomas were identified in 1983 and are not listed in the Rappaport classification or in the Working Formulation. They constitute 7% to 8% of all B-cell lymphomas. Most cases were probably described in the past as small lymphocytic lymphomas. The cells are thought to originate from the marginal zone of the follicle near the interface with the follicular mantle. When marginal zone lymphomas involve the nodes, they are called monocytoid B-cell lymphomas[37]; when they involve extranodal sites, they are called MALT lymphomas.[38] These are tumors of adults, most in the sixth to eighth decade of life with a 1.5:1 male predominance.

Marginal zone lymphomas are characterized by cellular heterogeneity, including marginal zone (centrocyte-like) cells, monocytoid B-cells, small lymphocytes, and plasma cells. In epithelial tissue, the marginal zone cells typically infiltrate the epithelium, forming *lymphoepithelial lesions* (Fig. 61-2). The immunophenotype of marginal zone lymphomas helps to distinguish them from other neoplastic proliferations of small lymphoid cells. Although

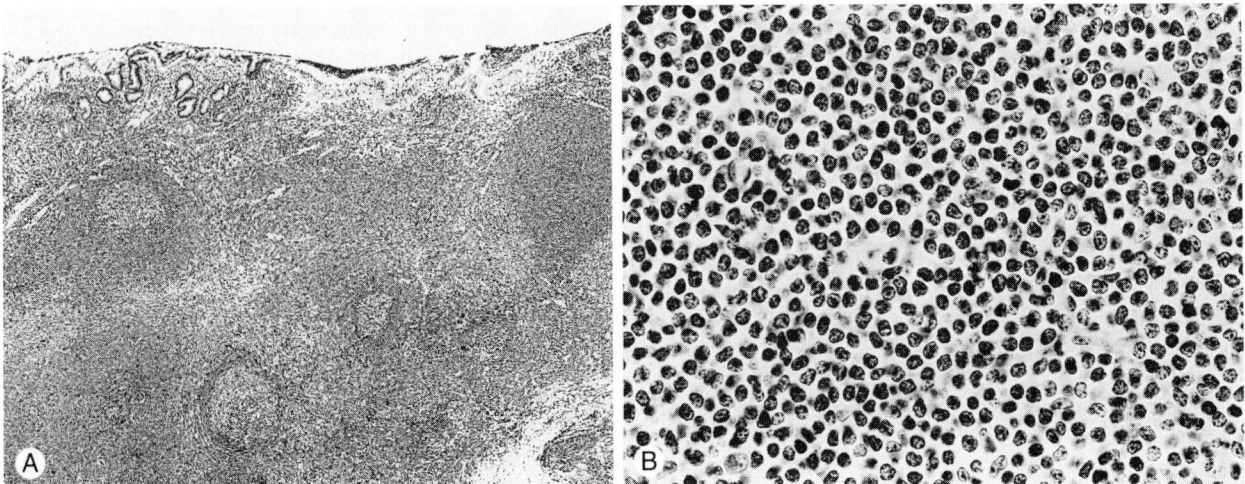

Figure 61–2. A, Mucosa-associated lymphoid tissue (MALT) lymphoma (low power). The gastric mucosa is involved by a dense, diffuse infiltrate of neoplastic lymphoid cells surrounding reactive germinal centers. **B,** MALT lymphoma (high power). The neoplastic cells are small and mature-appearing, with coarse chromatin and slightly irregular nuclear contours.

positive for pan-B-cell antigens and express surface immunoglobulin, they are negative for both CD5 (unlike small lymphocytic and mantle cell) and CD10 (unlike follicle center cells). No rearrangement of *bcl-2* or *bcl-1* is seen. Trisomy 3 has been detected in 60% of cases and T(11,18) has been observed in 25% to 50% of cases.[39]

The MALT lymphomas have been identified in many extranodal sites; most commonly in the stomach, but also in the salivary glands, Waldeyer's ring, large and small intestine, thyroid, eye (orbit and conjunctiva), lung, breast, and skin. Some of these sites do not have mucous membranes but contain columnar epithelium, which may be the common feature. Most of these lymphomas are limited to the involved site at diagnosis with occasional involvement of adjacent lymph nodes.[40,41] The clinical course is indolent in even advanced-stage patients.[42]

There is considerable evidence to suggest that MALT lymphoma develops as a result of prolonged antigenic stimulation and in some situations may depend on continuous stimulation. MALT lymphoma may develop in the thyroid gland of patients with Hashimoto's thyroiditis and in salivary glands of patients with Sjögren's syndrome. *Helicobacter pylori* infection of the stomach has been shown to be the etiologic factor in many patients with MALT lymphoma of the stomach and lymphoma regression has been documented following eradication of *H. pylori* with antibiotics.[17]

Aggressive Lymphomas

WHO: *Diffuse Large-B Cell Lymphoma (including immunoblastic, mixed, and mediastinal B-cell lymphomas)*

Working Formulation: Diffuse large-cell lymphoma
  >Diffuse large-cell immunoblastic
  >Diffuse mixed small- and large-cell
Rappaport: Diffuse histiocytic lymphoma
  >Diffuse mixed lymphocytic and histiocytic

Diffuse large-B cell lymphoma (DLBCL) is the most common aggressive lymphoma and constitutes approximately 30% of all NHLs. Its incidence has been increasing over the past few decades. The median age of patients is in the seventh decade, but the range is broad and includes children. Male/female ratio is equal. Most investigators recognize that subdividing this category into immunoblastic and nonimmunoblastic in the Working Formulation is neither reproducible nor clinically meaningful. The relatively rare Working Formulation category of diffuse mixed small and large cells is also similar clinically and pathologically to DLBCL and was not considered as a separate entity in the WHO classification. DLBCL is heterogeneous by morphologic, immunophenotypic, and molecular cytogenetic criteria. The characteristic cell of diffuse large cell lymphoma (DLCL) is large (nuclei at least twice the size of a small lymphocyte), with vesicular nuclei, prominent nucleoli, and basophilic cytoplasm (Fig. 61-3). Other cell types include large cleaved

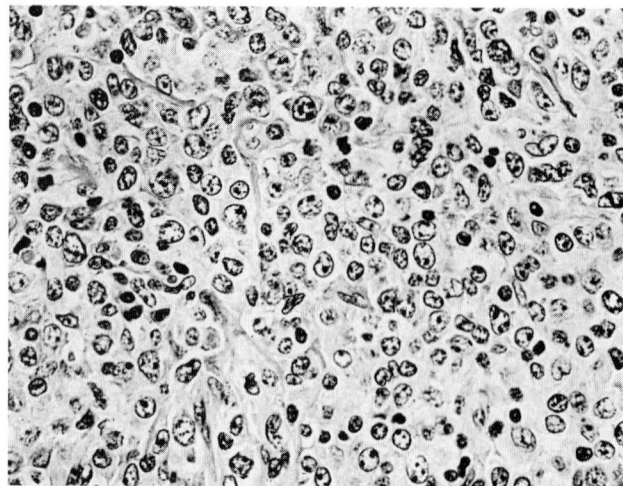

Figure 61–3. Diffuse large cell lymphoma (high power). The tumor comprises large neoplastic lymphoid cells with ovoid nuclei and peripheral nucleoli.

or anaplastic cells identical to those of T-cell or null-cell anaplastic large-cell lymphoma. Some cases are rich in small T-lymphocytes and may pathologically resemble lymphocyte-predominant HD or T-cell lymphoma but clinically are similar to the more typical DLBCL.

The immunophenotype is characterized by pan–B-cell markers (CD19, CD20, CD22) and clonal surface immunoglobulin (usually IgM) in about 75% of patients and CD10 in about 25% of patients. The *bcl-2* rearrangement and t(14;18) are found in about 30% of patients and probably represent transformation of CD10+ follicular lymphomas.[22] Recently, *bcl-6* rearrangements were identified in a significant subset of patients characterized by primary involvement of extranodal tissues, lack of bone marrow involvement, and favorable prognosis.[22,44]

Patients with DLBCL typically present with a rapidly enlarging, often symptomatic mass at a single nodal or extranodal site. Forty percent are, at least initially, confined to extranodal sites. Although DLBCL is an aggressive disease that, without treatment, has a rapidly lethal course with a median survival of 8 months, it is potentially curable in all stages. About 40% of patients in advanced-stage disease and approximately 80% to 90% of patients with stages I to II disease are curable with chemotherapy or with combined modality therapy, respectively. Almost half of the patients present with a localized disease. Radiation therapy, as part of a combined modality approach, has an important role in their treatment.

An important subset of patients with DLBCL present with predominant mediastinal disease. Patients with mediastinal B-cell lymphoma are usually young (fourth decade), and female sex predominates. The tumor usually involves the thymus at presentation and probably originates from rare B-cells in the thymus.[45] The tumor is associated with significant fibrosis, requiring differential diagnosis from nodular sclerosing HD. This lymphoma is locally invasive and may cause airway compromise and superior vena cava syndrome. The treatment approach is similar to that of other localized aggressive lymphomas: combination chemotherapy followed by involved-field radiotherapy.[46]

WHO: Mantle-Cell Lymphoma

Mantle-cell lymphoma is one of the "new" NHL entities that were not listed in the Working Formulation or Rappaport classification. It has been classified by different investigators as lymphocytic lymphoma of intermediate differentiation, intermediate lymphocytic lymphoma, centrocytic lymphoma, or mantle zone lymphoma. Many of the cases were termed *diffuse small cleaved cell lymphoma* in the Working Formulation. In a review of the Southwest Oncology Group (SWOG) advanced-stage NHL material, approximately 10% of cases were mantle-cell lymphoma.[42] Mantle-cell lymphoma is histologically, cytogenetically, and clinically distinct. This is a tumor of adults with a median age of 60 years and a high male/female ratio of at least 2:1.[42]

In most cases, the tumor is composed exclusively of small to medium-sized lymphoid cells, slightly larger than normal lymphocytes, with more dispersed chromatin, pale cytoplasm, and inconspicuous nucleoli (Fig. 61-4). Their immunophenotype shows positive B-cell–associated antigens, CD5+ (useful to distinguish from marginal zone lymphomas), CD23- (to distinguish from small lymphocytic), surface IgM+ and IgD+. Mantle-cell lymphomas often contain t(11;14), which involves the *bcl-1* gene and results in overexpression of cyclin D1, which may be related to the disease pathogenesis.[47] Overexpression of *p53* in mantle-cell biopsies was found to be associated with poor prognosis.[48]

The disease is usually widespread at diagnosis and is significantly more aggressive than other small lymphocytic lymphomas and other indolent lymphomas.[49-53] In the SWOG series of patients treated with doxorubicin-containing chemotherapy, the 10-year failure-free survival of patients with mantle cell lymphoma was only 6%, the lowest of all histologies analyzed in that study.[42]

WHO: Peripheral T-Cell Lymphoma, Unspecified

Lymphomas of mature (post-thymic) T-cells are termed *peripheral T-cell lymphomas*, since they express only CD4 or CD8, unlike thymocytes, which generally express both CD4 and CD8. Peripheral T-cell lymphomas were grouped in different categories (commonly included in diffuse, mixed small- and large-cell and in the immunoblastic categories) in the Working Formulation that did not identify T-cell lymphomas as separate entities. These lymphomas constitute less than 15% of adult lymphomas in the United States and Europe but are more common in other parts of the world. They have an aggressive natural history and are considered by some to have poorer prognosis than B-cell aggressive lymphomas.[54,55]

Diagnosis by morphologic criteria alone is difficult. The proliferation pattern is diffuse or interfollicular and the cells are often a mix of small and large atypical cells. The cells express a complete or imperfect mature T-cell phenotype: CD2, CD3, CD5, and more commonly CD4 rather than CD8. The WHO investigators commented that this category includes heterogeneous diseases that require further definition.[56]

WHO: Angioimmunoblastic T-Cell Lymphoma

This rare condition was originally called *angioimmunoblastic lymphadenopathy with dysproteinemia*. Although the median survival was approximately 16 months, the disease was thought to be an abnormal immune response. This entity is now generally accepted

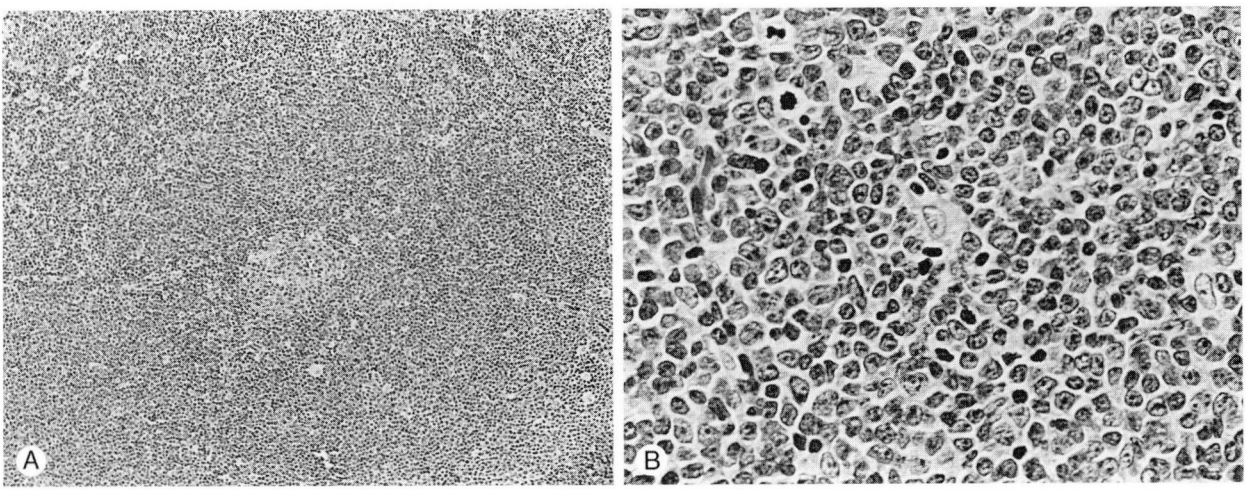

Figure 61–4. A, Mantle cell lymphoma (low power). There is a marked expansion of cells in the mantle zone surrounding a reactive germinal center. **B,** Mantle cell lymphoma (high power). The neoplastic cells are small and monomorphic, with ovoid to slightly irregular nuclear contours. Mitotic figures and scattered histiocytes are present.

as a T-cell lymphoma, since the cells show clonal T-cell gene rearrangements.[57] It is a rare but clinically distinctive disorder. Patients often have generalized lymphadenopathy, hepatosplenomegaly, B symptoms, skin rash, and a polyclonal increase in immunoglobulins. In about half of the cases, death is from infection rather than tumor progression. About one third of patients eventually develop a frank monoclonal T-cell lymphoma. The course is moderately aggressive, and treatment with doxorubicin-containing chemotherapy is recommended.[58]

WHO: Extranodal NK/T-Cell Lymphoma Nasal Type

This is a very rare disorder. Nasal NK/T-cell lymphoma is a tumor that commonly involves the nose, paranasal sinuses, nasopharynx, and other upper airway structures and was formerly included in the spectrum of diseases called lethal midline granuloma and midline malignant reticulosis.[59] This is a localized aggressive and destructive disease that rarely involves the lymph nodes. It is treated with combined modality therapy in which radiation therapy has a very important role.

WHO: Anaplastic Large-Cell Lymphoma (ALCL)

Anaplastic large-cell lymphoma is a T-cell lymphoma that was originally defined by its expression of the CD30 antigen.[62] ALCL accounts for approximately 3% of adult NHL and 10% to 30% of childhood lymphomas. It was not identified as a separate entity in the working formulation or in the Rappaport classification, but there is sufficient evidence that anaplastic large cell lymphoma is a distinct clinical and pathologic entity to warrant its inclusion in the WHO classification. Cases have been reported in all age groups; however, 15% to 30% of the cases are in patients younger than 20.[63]

Clinically, there appear to be two forms of disease: one limited to the skin and the other with systemic spread of disease including skin and lymph nodes.[64,65] Tumors that present with systemic disease (with or without skin involvement) have a bimodal age distribution in children and adults and are clinically aggressive. Primary cutaneous tumors occur predominantly in adults, may spontaneously regress, and generally have an excellent prognosis. Systemic disease may affect either children or adults, has a natural history similar to other aggressive lymphomas, and is usually responsive to combination chemotherapy.[65]

The tumor is composed of large blastic cells with pleomorphic, often horseshoe-shaped or multiple nucleoli with multiple or single prominent nucleoli. Immunophenotypically, the tumor cells are CD30+, EMA+ in most cases. Primary cutaneous cases are reported to lack EMA and express the cutaneous lymphocyte antigen. Cytogenetic studies on a small number of cases with the skin form show t(2;5) transformation.[66] Cytogenetic studies on primary cutaneous cases have not been reported. This translocation juxtaposes the anaplastic lymphoma kinase on chromosome 2 with nuclear nucleophosmin, and nucleoli phosphoprotein on chromosome 5.[67] These patients are positive for the anaplastic large cell

lymphoma kinase (ALK) protein. ALK positive patients have a better prognosis.

Highly Aggressive Lymphomas

WHO: Burkitt's Lymphoma

Working Formulation: Burkitt's lymphoma

Burkitt's lymphoma is a diffuse lymphoma composed of uniform, rapidly dividing, undifferentiated B-cells of uncertain derivation. It is most common in children (approximately one third of nonAfrican pediatric lymphomas). Adult cases are often associated with immunodeficiency. The male/female ratio is 2:1. In African (endemic) cases, the jaws and other facial bones are often involved. In nonAfrican (nonendemic) cases, jaw tumors are less common. The majority of patients present with disease in the abdomen, most often involving the distal ilium, sacrum or mesentery, ovaries, kidney, and breasts.[68] Rare cases present as acute leukemia with Burkitt's tumor cells. The tumor is highly aggressive but potentially curable. Prognosis in children correlates with the bulk of diseases at the time of diagnosis.[69]

Burkitt's tumor cells are monomorphic, medium-sized cells with round nuclei and multiple nucleoli and relatively abundant basophilic cytoplasm, which may give the cells a cohesive appearance. The tumor has an extremely high rate of proliferation as well as a high rate of spontaneous death. A "starry sky" pattern is usually present, in part due to numerous benign macrophages that have ingested apoptotic tumor cells. The immunophenotype is characterized by the presence of CD10, abundant clonal surface immunoglobulin, usually IgM, and the pan-B lineage markers (CD19, CD20, CD22). CD5 is negative.

Most cases have translocation of *c-myc* from chromosome 8 to the immunoglobulin heavy chain region on chromosome 14t(8;14) or less commonly t(2;8). EBV genes can be demonstrated in the tumor cells in most African cases and in 25% to 40% of cases associated with AIDS, but less frequently in nonAfrican nonimmune deficient cases.

WHO: Precursor B- or T-Lymphoblastic Leukemia/ Lymphoma/Lymphoblastic Lymphoma

Working Formulation: Lymphoblastic lymphoma

This disease was categorized as lymphoblastic lymphoma in the Working Formulation. The clinical distinction between lymphoblastic lymphoma and lymphoblastic leukemia can be made arbitrarily (usually on the basis of the percentage of bone marrow involvement). Both diseases, however, require a similar treatment approach, with high-dose induction chemotherapy usually with consolidation, maintenance therapy, and central nervous system prophylaxis.[71] Anatomic staging is not relevant to determining prognosis or selecting therapy. Children with lymphoblastic leukemia/lymphoma generally have a better treatment outcome than adults. This may be related in part to the more frequent derivation of childhood tumors from B-cells as well as to the metabolic differences in the tumor cells that make childhood tumors more responsive to therapy. The tumors are histologically indistinguishable from precursor T-lymphoblastic lymphoma. Of the B-cell lymphoblastic leukemia/lymphoma, a small proportion of patients present with solid tumors, most often in the skin, bone, and lymph nodes, with or without bone marrow or peripheral blood involvement. These solid tumors are histologically indistinguishable from precursor T-lymphoblastic lymphomas.[72] The disease is highly aggressive but frequently curable with chemotherapy. Cases with t(1;19) have the worst prognosis, as do cases with t(9;22).

Of the T-cell lymphoblastic lymphoma/leukemia, the patients are predominantly adolescent and young adult males, but older adults are occasionally affected.[73] Forty percent of childhood lymphomas and 15% of acute lymphoblastic lymphoma/leukemias are of precursor T-type. Patients present with rapidly enlarging symptomatic mediastinal (thymic) masses or peripheral lymphadenopathy. Untreated, it is a rapidly fatal disease, usually terminating in acute leukemia. Central nervous system involvement is common. The tumor is highly aggressive but potentially curable. Clinically important subtypes can be defined by immunophenotype profiles: leukemic cases tend to have a more immature phenotype than lymphoma cases.[72,74] Immunophenotyping studies are necessary to distinguish the T-cell tumor from precursor B lymphoblastic neuroplasms and occasionally from peripheral T-cell neuroplasms or granulocytic sarcoma. Immunophenotypically, most cases are CD7+ and CD3+. Expression of either T-cell–associated antigen, CD2 or CD5, is variable.

STAGING AND PROGNOSTIC FACTORS

Although histology is the predominant determinant of prognosis in this diverse group of lymphoid malignancies, stage remains important for selection of treatment strategy and predicting the prognosis in each histologic category. The Ann Arbor Staging Classification system, developed originally for HD, has been used also for NHL.[75] The staging system is described in Table 61-3.

This system reflects the number of sites of involvement and their relation to the diaphragm, the existence of B symptoms, and the presence of extranodal disease. Patients can be assigned a clinical stage or a pathologic stage. In NHL, most patients are staged clinically based on physical examination, imaging studies, and bone marrow biopsy. If additional biopsies are performed based on laparoscopy or during laparotomy, the patient is considered pathologically staged. Staging laparotomy and splenectomy are rarely performed in the evaluation of patients with NHL, and a distinction between clinical stage and pathologic stage is not commonly used in NHL. The Ann Arbor staging system is considered by many to be inadequate for NHL. Furthermore, the recent modification of the Ann Arbor staging system (Cotswolds modification)[76] addressed issues mostly relevant for HD, but not for NHL.

In addition to stage, other prognostic factors have been identified in patients with NHL. These prognostic factors frequently include patient parameters such as age (younger or older than 60 years) and performance status as well as tumor burden indicators such as bulk (< or > than 10 cm), number of involved sites (mostly extranodal), and lactate dehydrogenase (LDH) level. Mauch and coworkers[77] identified adverse prognostic factors in patients with aggressive lymphoma, stages I to II, that are of particular relevance to radiotherapy. They include bulky abdominal or thoracic disease and involvement of three or more sites.

An international team developed a prognostic model to predict outcome of patients with aggressive NHL (Table 61-4).[78,79] The international index (also known as the Shipp criteria) identified five significant risk factors prognostic of overall survival: age (younger than 60 vs. older than 60), serum LDH (normal vs. elevated), performance status (0 or 1 vs. 2 to 4), stage (I or II vs. III or IV) and extranodal site involvement (0 or 1 vs. 2 to 4). These features were incorporated into a model that identified four groups of patients with significantly different outcome following treatment. These were determined by adding the number of adverse risk factors, thus creating low-risk (0 to 1 factor), low-intermediate (2 factors), high-intermediate (3 factors), and high-risk (4 to 5 factors)

Table 61–4 International Prognostic Index for Aggressive Non-Hodgkin's Lymphoma

All Patients

- Age 60+
- Serum LDH above normal
- ECOG performance status = 2
- Ann Arbor clinical stage III or IV
- Number of involved extranodal sites >1

	IPI Score	5-Yr Survival, %
Low-risk	0-1	73
Low-intermediate	2	51
High-intermediate	3	43
High-risk	4-5	26

Patients = 60 Yr

Serum LDH above normal
ECOG performance = 2
Ann Arbor stage II or IV

	Age-Adjusted IPI Score	5-Yr Survival, %
Low-risk	0	83
Low-intermediate	1	69
High-intermediate	2	46
High-risk	3	32

Patients with Early-Stage (I-II) Disease

Age 60+
Serum LDH above normal
Stage II disease
ECOG performance status = 2

Modified IPI Score	10-Yr Survival, %
0	90
1-2	56
3	48

ECOG, Eastern Cooperative Oncology Group; IPI, International Prognostic Index; LDH, lactate dehydrogenase.

groups. The predicted 5-year survival rates for these groups were 73%, 51%, 43%, and 26%, respectively. When only patients younger than 60 years old were evaluated, stage, performance status, and LDH levels remained significant for poor prognosis (age-adjusted International Prognostic Index).[79] After validation by several centers, the major cooperative groups have accepted this index for the design of new protocols. The model is simple to apply, is reproducible, and predicts outcome even after patients have achieved complete response. Although originally designed for aggressive lymphomas, it has been shown to be of predictive value in low-grade lymphomas and in relapsing patients undergoing salvage therapy with or without high-dose therapy and stem-cell support.

Table 61-5 details the evaluation of patients with NHL. In the history, B symptoms should be reported and the rate of tumor growth should be assessed. In the physical examination, particular attention should be given to recording the size and site of all abnormal lymph nodes including the epitrochlear, femoral, and popliteal sites that are not usually involved in HD. Waldeyer's ring structures are often involved in NHL, and their evaluation should include direct or indirect laryngoscopy. Waldeyer's ring involvement is often associated with involvement of the intestine, and gastrointestinal studies are indicated if the patient appears to have localized disease. The basic initial evaluation includes a complete blood count, a chemistry screening profile including liver and renal function studies, serum LDH, computed tomography (CT) scan of the abdomen and pelvis, and bilateral bone marrow biopsy. The superior mediastinal (prevascular and paratracheal) lymph nodes are the most prevalent of thoracic disease sites.[80] The next most commonly involved lymph node sites were subcarinal, hilar, posterior mediastinal, and cardiophrenic angle. Whereas CT scan is positive when a chest x-ray is negative in only approximately 10% of the cases, it will demonstrate involvement of the thorax with one or more additional sites in approximately 75% of patients with a positive abnormal chest x-ray.[81] Parenchymal lesions and pleural effusions in patients with NHL do not necessarily indicate malignant involvement and may require pathologic verification. Chylous or transudative effusion that lacks malignant cells should not change the pathologic stage of the patient. As in HD, pulmonary lesions are usually associated with concurrent hilar or bulky mediastinal lymph node involvement.

The most informative noninvasive test for diagnosing lymphoma involvement of the abdomen and pelvis is the abdominal-pelvic CT scan. This test is particularly useful for patients with indolent lymphomas, in whom mesenteric nodal involvement is common. The abdominal-pelvic CT scan can also identify retrocrural disease and is more accurate than the lymphangiogram in determining the size of nodal disease. Although CT scan lacks the detailed architectural information obtained by a lymphangiogram, it offers imaging of mesenteric, portahepatic, and splenic hilar lymph nodes that are commonly involved in patients with indolent lymphoma. It also allows evaluation of involvement of the kidneys, bone, and bulky splenic or liver disease that may be present in patients with aggressive lymphomas.

Gallium-67 scanning is important for identifying sites of initial disease, for measuring response to treatment, and for detecting early recurrences. It is also a prognostic indicator of the response to treatment and of long-term prognosis. Of patients with positive gallium scans at mid-course of chemotherapy, only 25% had a durable response, compared with 70% of patients whose gallium scans were normal at the same time.[82]

Recently, positron emission tomography (PET) scanning using 18F-fluorodeoxyglucose was shown to be a sensitive tool for detecting both aggressive and indolent lymphomas. It is useful for initial staging, confirmation of response, and detection of relapse. It is quickly becoming an essential tool for making treatment decisions.[83]

Approximately 50% of patients with NHL have bone marrow or hepatic involvement at presentation. Incidence of bone marrow involvement is highest in patients with small lymphocytic lymphoma (70%), follicular lymphoma (50%), and lymphoblastic lymphoma (50%).

Table 61–5 Evaluation of New Patients with Non-Hodgkin's Lymphoma

Object of Evaluation	Mandatory Studies	Studies in Selected Situations
Confirm diagnosis	Adequate biopsy reviewed by experienced hematopathologist	Immunophenotyping, cytogenetics, molecular studies
General overview	History and physical examination	Blood coagulation tests
	Complete blood count	Immunoglobulins
	Chemistry screen	
Prognostic categorization	Serum lactate dehydrogenase	Erythrocyte sedimentation rate
		Serum β_2-microglobulin
Evaluation of chest, abdomen and pelvis	CT scan of chest, abdomen, pelvis	Lymphangiography
	PET scan	MRI
		Ultrasonography
Search of occult sites of involvement	Bone marrow biopsy	CT scan of the neck/MRI
	PET scan	Lumbar puncture
		Bone scan
		Gallium scan (if PET unavailable)
		Biopsy of suspicious sites

CT, computed tomography; MRI, magnetic resonance imaging; PET, positron emission tomography.

Approximately 10% of patients with diffuse large-cell lymphoma or marginal zone lymphoma show bone marrow involvement. The detection of bone marrow involvement is important, particularly in patients with follicular lymphoma who are potentially curable with radiation alone, if in early stage. It is also important in large B cell lymphoma because of the strong correlation with subsequent spread of disease to the central nervous system. Approximately 35% of patients with large-cell lymphoma and bone marrow involvement develop central nervous system disease. Cytologic examination of spinal fluid should be performed in all patients with the diffuse type of lymphoma and bone marrow involvement, because chemotherapy for the central nervous system is indicated if positive.

Since a second bone marrow biopsy is likely to increase the number of positive findings by up to 15%, bilateral bone marrow biopsy is recommended. Lymphomatous involvement of the bone marrow can be detected by morphologic assessment alone if there is 5% or greater infiltration by malignant cells. Newer techniques such as flow cytometry analysis may improve the detection level to 1%. The significance of the sensitive detection of marrow involvement by polymerase chain reaction (one in 10^5 to 10^6 cells) is still undetermined, and it is controversial whether this information should preclude patients with otherwise early-stage indolent disease from receiving localized treatment. Information regarding the prognostic significance of positive molecular studies is still evolving and may be important in determining the source, or purging, of stem-cell support for high-dose therapy.

Hepatic involvement has been found in 10% to 40% of patients with NHL. Frequency of identification of liver involvement increases as the size and number of biopsy specimens increase. Patients with diffuse large-cell lymphoma have a lower incidence of liver involvement than patients with other types of NHL. The need for liver biopsy should be determined by the likelihood that the finding will affect treatment.

TREATMENT

Indolent Lymphomas

Three types of lymphoma are considered to have an indolent clinical course: follicular follicle center cell lymphoma grades I and II, marginal zone (MALT lymphoma), and small lymphocytic lymphoma. While these lymphomas differ widely in their biologic characteristics, clinical presentation, and ultimate course, they all share a high sensitivity to ionizing radiation. Thus, radiation therapy has a potentially curative role in early-stage indolent lymphomas and plays an important palliative role in advanced and relapsed disease. It is important, however, to recognize that almost all small lymphocytic lymphomas involve the bone marrow and are rarely considered for primary radiotherapy, other than for palliation of symptoms. In contrast, the extranodal MALT lymphomas commonly remain localized to the involved organ and are highly responsive and potentially curable with RT.

Although in most series, all indolent (or low-grade) lymphomas were reported together,[84] most of the information is particularly relevant to the follicular histology. The follicular follicle center cell lymphoma is by far the most common indolent lymphoma, and a significant fraction (20%) of patients with a follicular histology present with stage I or II disease. In the absence of curative systemic therapies for these lymphomas, radiotherapy is the only treatment that offers a 20-year relapse-free survival to approximately half of all patients with early-stage disease (Table 61-6).

Results from large series of patients with stage I and II indolent lymphomas who were treated with radiotherapy alone are summarized in Table 61-6. The recent long-term follow-up study of patients with stage I and II low-grade follicular lymphoma from Stanford University indicated that a substantial number of patients in this category have, indeed, been "cured" by radiotherapy.[28] The median follow-up was 7.7 years and was maintained for up to 31 years in this series. The median survival after radiotherapy was 14 years. The actuarial survival rates at 5, 10, 15, and 20 years were 82%, 64%, 44%, and 35%, respectively. Freedom from relapse (FFR) at 5, 10, 15, and 20 years was 55%, 44%, 40% and 37%, respectively. Only 5 of 47 patients who reached 10 years without relapse suffered recurrence. There was no significant FFR difference between stage I and stage II or between nodal or extranodal disease. The survival of patients irradiated after the age of 60 years was significantly shorter than the survival of younger patients, but the decrease of survival in this age group was strongly affected by intercurrent deaths.

Most relapses in early-stage patients occur in unirradiated sites during the first 5 to 6 years following therapy.[85] In the Stanford series, administration of radiotherapy to nodal sites on both sides of the diaphragm was associated with a significantly better FFR compared with more localized treatment but did not translate into a clear survival benefit.[28] In the absence of a clear survival benefit for total lymphoid irradiation in this setting, the common involvement of mesenteric nodes that may require whole abdominal irradiation, and in consideration of the fact that almost half of the patients will eventually require chemotherapy for relapse, we currently employ involved or regional field irradiation for these patients. We normally design a minimantle field for supradiaphragmatic

Table 61–6   Radiotherapy Alone for Stage I and II Indolent Lymphomas

Reference	Patients, n	Stage	Relapse-free Survival, % (yr)	Overall Survival, % (yr)
Vaughn et al[84]	208	I	47 (10)	64 (10)
Suttcliffe et al[85]	190	I-II	53 (12)	58 (12)
MacManus[29]	177	I-II	44 (15)	40 (15)

disease that does not involve the mediastinum (an uncommon site for follicular lymphomas), a whole abdominal field for retroperitoneal and mesenteric involvement, and a pelvic-inguinal field for inguinal-femoral presentations. This approach allows treatment of adjacent uninvolved nodal sites, and in the dose range that we employ (30 to 40 Gy) is well tolerated by patients. Unfortunately, no study is available to determine whether extended-field irradiation has an advantage over a "pure" involved-site irradiation in this setting.

The optimal radiation dose for indolent lymphoma has not been determined in a prospective study. However, most current radiotherapy series for stage I and II indolent lymphomas usually employ 30 to 40 Gy, and in-field recurrences have been uncommon. Data from the Princess Margaret Hospital showed in-field disease control in 78% of patients treated with doses of less than 25 Gy and 91% control with doses greater than 25 Gy.[86] Fuks correlated relapse rate in regional areas of follicular lymphoma with the radiation dose delivered to these sites and showed 63% relapse in areas receiving less than 27.5 Gy, 27% relapse with a dose range of 30 to 35 Gy, 12% and 6% relapse rate for 40 Gy and 44 Gy, respectively.[87] We currently recommend 36 Gy (in 1.8 Gy daily fractions) to involved sites (40 Gy, if bulky) and 24 to 36 Gy to uninvolved adjacent sites.

Several prospective randomized trials failed to demonstrate that the use of radiation followed by chemotherapy was superior to radiation alone in early-stage indolent lymphoma.[88-92] Most studies used combinations of cyclophosphamide, vincristine, and prednisone (CVP),[88-90] while the British National Lymphoma Investigation (BNLI) studied chlorambucil[92] and MSKCC evaluated the cyclophosphamide, hydroxydaunomycin, vincristine (Oncovin), prednisone combination (CHOP).[91] Based on these studies, adjuvant chemotherapy has no role in the treatment of early-stage indolent lymphomas.

The role of radiotherapy in the treatment of stage III indolent lymphoma remains controversial. Several investigators treated patients with extensive irradiation fields that included mantle field, Waldeyer's ring, and the whole abdomen and pelvis, and were termed *comprehensive lymphatic irradiation*.[82,93,94] Radiation doses ranged from 20 to 40 Gy. The long-term results are summarized in Table 61-7.

The limited reported experience is favorable, with a 10-year relapse-free survival of 39% to 45%. Most relapses after 5 years have been transformations to a more aggressive histology, and salvage chemotherapy was well tolerated.[82] Favorable prognostic factors in

stage III disease treated with comprehensive lymphatic irradiation include fewer than five sites of involvement, absence of bulky disease, and B symptoms.[93,94] Other studies explored combined modality therapy in stage III indolent lymphomas. A small randomized study from Stanford found no advantage in survival or FFR to adding CVP chemotherapy to total lymphoid irradiation.[93] A study from Mexico City suggested that CVP combined with involved-field radiotherapy or with total lymphoid irradiation was better than CVP alone.[95] The 7-year relapse-free survival rate was 66%, 71% and 33%, respectively, and this advantage has also translated into a survival benefit. A study from the MD Anderson Cancer Center of combined modality therapy in stage III disease yielded results that were similar to those obtained with comprehensive lymphatic irradiation.[96] Although comprehensive lymphatic irradiation is a long, complex, and potentially toxic therapy for patients with an indolent disease, it should be considered for physiologically fit patients, particularly since no alternative strategy has been shown to be curative for disease in this stage.

Since there is no treatment that significantly affects the natural history of advanced-stage indolent lymphomas (mostly stage IV with bone marrow involvement), the optimal treatment strategy remains controversial.[26,34,97-100] Treatment recommendations usually follow one of two divergent courses: an aggressive approach that may include combination chemotherapy with or without extensive radiotherapy, including high-dose therapy with stem-cell support or a conservative approach that consists of no initial therapy followed by a palliative single-agent chemotherapy or palliative limited radiotherapy. The conservative approach was based on a Stanford study[101] that showed that selected asymptomatic patients with advanced-stage disease, who were assigned to a watch-and-wait approach in which treatment was deferred until disease progressed, had no inferior survival compared with patients who started therapy immediately following diagnosis. The National Cancer Institute (NCI) team directly tested the policy of deferred treatment in a randomized trial involving selected, asymptomatic patients.[102] Thus far no survival advantage to immediate intensive chemotherapy and extensive radiotherapy over deferred treatment has been found, although the complete response was higher among patients treated immediately.

For patients with advanced-stage disease who require treatment, alkylating agents are the gold standard of systemic therapy. As primary treatment, chlorambucil, cyclophosphamide alone or in combination with vincristine, and prednisone yield a response rate of 30%

Table 61–7 Results of Comprehensive Lymphatic Irradiation in Stage III Indolent Lymphomas

Institution	Patients, n	Median Follow-up, (yr)	Relapse-free Survival, % (yr)	Overall Survival, % (yr)
Paryani et al[94]	61	9.6	39 (10)	48 (10)
Jacobs et al[95]	34	9.6	40 (15)	28 (15)
Mendenhall & Lynch	11	25	45 (10)	49 (10)

Modified from Mendenhall NP, Lynch JW: The low-grade lymphomas. *Semin Radiat Oncol.* 1995;5:267.

to 80%. Unfortunately, the responses are not durable and last only a median of 2 years. Less than 10% of patients remain in remission for 5 years or more. The addition of doxorubicin has no significant impact on disease-free survival of patients with indolent lymphomas.[103]

The other class of agents that are effective in indolent lymphomas are the purine analogues such as fludarabine and 2-chlorodeoxyadenosine; however, these drugs have a significant myelosuppressive and immunosuppressive effect. They are usually reserved as a second-line therapy.[104,105,106] Of the biologic response modifiers, interferon alpha when used in combination with a chemotherapy program has shown a therapeutic benefit in recent trials.[107]

Monoclonal antibody therapy has received much attention for the treatment of NHL, particularly in the treatment of indolent lymphomas.[108] Most of the experience is with the use of "humanized" anti-CD20 monoclonal antibody rituximab (Rituxan).[108] In patients with previously treated follicular lymphoma, an overall response rate of 45% to 60%, with 3% to 6% complete response, and a median response duration of 9 to 11 months has been reported.[109,110] Retreatment with rituximab has also been successful in follicular lymphomas with an overall response rate of 40% and an estimated median time to progression of 18 months. Rituxan is currently approved for use in the treatment of relapsed or refractory, low-grade or follicular, CD20-positive B-cell non-Hodgkin's lymphomas, as well as for retreatment of such patients after an objective clinical response to an initial course of Rituxan. Two phase II trials have recently demonstrated the efficacy of rituximab as initial therapy in patients with indolent lymphoma. Most patients were in stages III and IV. The maximum response was 73% with 37% complete remissions. At the median follow-up of 30 months, the median progression-free survival was 34 months. Toxicity was mostly infusion-related and of brief duration. In another study of patients with follicular lymphoma stage II to IV and low tumor burden, the overall response was 73%, 31% of the patients obtaining polymerase chain reaction (PCR)-negativity for bcl2 in the bone marrow. At this point, it is not known if rituximab prolonged survival in this setting, and the use of rituximab as initial therapy is not considered standard.[111,112]

Recently, several anti-CD20 radioimmunoconjugates were investigated as treatment for indolent lymphomas. These agents delivered targeted radiation to tumor-bearing areas.[108,113] Zevalin (ibritumomab tiuxetan), a murine anti-CD20 monoclonal antibody with Yttrium-90 conjugated to the antibody, showed responses in patients with relapsed or refractory low-grade follicular, or transformed CD20 + NHL. Patients were randomly assigned to receive either rituximab or rituximab + Zevalin and the overall response rate to rituximab/Zevalin was significantly higher (56% vs. 80%, $P = 0.002$). The complete response rates were also significantly higher compared with rituximab alone. Zevalin is now FDA approved for treatment of patients with relapse or refractory low-grade, follicular or transformed B-cell NHL including patients with rituximab-refractory follicular

lymphoma.[114] The approved treatment program consists of a low dose of rituximab on day 1, followed by a dose of Indium-111–labeled Zevalin with two or three whole body scans to assist biodistribution. If biodistribution is normal, a second low dose of rituximab is given between days 7 and 9, followed by a therapeutic dose of itrium-90 labeled Zevalin. Prolonged and severe cytopenias have occurred after a therapeutic dose of Zevalin. This treatment is not recommended in patients with low platelet counts and should only be used by those qualified in the safe administration of therapeutic doses of radionuclides.

Another radionuclide antibody that has recently been approved by the FDA is Bexxar (tositumomab), a murine anti-CD20 monoclonal antibody conjugated with radioactive iodine-131. In various trials, treatment with Bexxar appeared to yield a high response rate in patients with relapsed, refractory, or transformed disease.[115]

Aggressive Lymphomas

This category includes mostly patients with diffuse large B-cell lymphoma. Additionally, patients with follicular lymphoma grade III (follicular large-cell lymphoma) and patients formerly classified as having immunoblastic large-cell lymphoma and anaplastic large-cell lymphomas as well as those with peripheral T-cell lymphoma are all managed with the same guidelines. Patients classified with the new entity, mantle-cell lymphoma, represent a relatively small group of patients that commonly present with an advanced-stage disease. Although their long-term response to chemotherapy may be inferior compared with patients with large-cell lymphoma, they are still managed with a similar treatment approach and will not be considered separately.[116-118] While most patients with advanced-stage (stages III to IV) aggressive lymphoma are treated with combination chemotherapy alone, and radiation therapy is rarely considered as primary or consolidation treatment for these patients, radiotherapy has an important role in the primary treatment of patients with early-stage (stages I to II) aggressive lymphoma.

Until the 1980s, the majority of patients with early-stage aggressive lymphoma were treated with radiotherapy alone. In clinically staged patients, the use of regional or extended field irradiation for stage I disease resulted in a cure rate of approximately 50%.[119] The survival of similarly treated stage II patients was only 20%. Most of the relapses in patients treated with radiotherapy alone were extranodal or occurred outside the irradiated field. More restrictive selection of patients (stage I only), using staging laparotomy, and treatment with extensive fields of radiation yielded a 10-year relapse-free survival rate of 90% to 100%. Still, even staging laparotomy and total lymphoid irradiation yielded unsatisfactory survival rates of 35% to 55% in patients with pathologic stage II disease.[120]

The advent of effective chemotherapy for aggressive NHL and the impracticality of staging laparotomy in relatively old patients with potentially progressive disease made radiotherapy alone obsolete for most patients with early-stage aggressive lymphoma. Several randomized studies indicated that adjuvant chemotherapy following involved or extended field radiotherapy results in significantly better relapse-free survival rates than treatment with radiation alone in early-stage aggressive lymphoma. In some studies, the improved relapse-free survival has translated into a survival advantage.[91] Most studies showed an advantage to combined modality using CVP chemotherapy (without doxorubicin).[88-90] In a more recent randomized study from MSKCC, patients with stage I were randomly assigned to receive either regional radiation therapy alone or radiation therapy followed by the commonly used CHOP regimen. The MSKCC study showed that in patients with aggressive NHL, the 7-year actuarial relapse-free survival rate for combined modality therapy was 86% compared with 20% for radiotherapy alone (P = 0.004). The corresponding actuarial survival rates were 92% and 47%, respectively (P = 0.08).[91]

The optimal sequence of modalities has not been studied in a randomized manner. Prestidge and associates[121] retrospectively analyzed the results of chemotherapy (CHT) combined with radiotherapy (RT) for stage I and II large-cell lymphoma patients treated at Stanford. Using both univariate and multivariate analyses, a favorable outcome was associated with a CHT-RT-CHT sequence of therapy (P = 0.001) compared with CHT-RT or RT-CHT. Initiating a combined modality program with systemic chemotherapy has the advantages of providing local control of both detected and undetected disease and preventing spread early in the course of therapy. Additionally, by shrinking the bulk of a sizable mass, the need for irradiating a large area at a critical site is spared. The value of adding more chemotherapy after CHT-RT ("sandwich" sequence) is not clear and may be difficult or associated with toxicity.[121] Using a short but effective course of chemotherapy is unlikely to affect the feasibility of administering involved-field radiation therapy.

Most current combined modality programs induce a complete response with a doxorubicin-containing chemotherapy (e.g., CHOP) followed by involved-field irradiation. Results of several nonrandomized combined modality programs are summarized in Table 61-8.

Some studies suggested that when chemotherapy is combined with involved-field radiotherapy, fewer than the standard six cycles of chemotherapy may be required for patients with good prognosis early-stage NHL (see Table 61-8). At the NCI, 49 patients with stage I or IE large-cell lymphoma were treated with four cycles of cyclophosphamide, etoposide, doxorubicin, nitrogen mustard, vincristine, procarbazine, high-dose methotrexate, and prednisone (ProMACE-MOPP) in reduced doses followed by involved-field radiotherapy to a dose of 40 Gy.[125] Forty-seven of 49 patients achieved a complete response, and all 47 patients remained free of disease with a median follow-up of 4 years. A similar prospective study in Vancouver, Canada treated 308 patients with aggressive lymphoma with three cycles of doxorubicin-containing chemotherapy followed by involved-field radiation therapy to a dose of 30 (10 fractions) to 35 (20 fractions) Gy. These patients achieved an 81% progression-free survival and 80% survival with a median at 5 years and 74% and 63% at 10 years.[126]

The question of whether the addition of radiotherapy improves the relapse-free survival rate and overall survival rate in patients with early-stage aggressive lymphoma who attained a complete response with chemotherapy was controversial until 15 years ago.[127] Two small, nonrandomized studies suggested that treatment with chemotherapy alone may yield results comparable to those obtained with combined modality therapy. At the MD Anderson Cancer Center, patients with stage I and II achieved a 10-year relapse-free survival rate of 83% and 65%, respectively.[128] At the University of Arizona, selected patients with stage I and II disease treated with CHOP alone attained a relapse-free survival rate of 75%.[129]

Adjuvant radiation therapy has become the standard of care in early-stage aggressive NHL. This is based on the analysis of two large randomized studies by the Eastern Cooperative Oncology Group (ECOG) and the Southwest Oncology Group (SWOG). These studies are summarized in Table 61-9. The ECOG study involved patients with bulky or extranodal stage I and stage II intermediate grade NHL (according to the Working Formulation). All patients received eight cycles of CHOP chemotherapy. Patients who attained only a partial response following chemotherapy received involved-field radiotherapy to 40 Gy, and 28% converted to complete-response status. Patients in complete response (61%) following chemotherapy alone were randomly assigned either to receive radiotherapy of 30 Gy to site pretreatment involvement or to observation alone. The recent 15-year update showed a statistically significant advantage to the adjuvant radiotherapy arm. The patients who received adjuvant radiotherapy attained a better

Table 61–8　Combined Modality Programs for Early-Stage Aggressive Lymphomas

Reference	Regimen	Patients, n	Stage	Relapse-Free Survival, %	Overall Survival, %
Kaminsky et al[123]	CHOP-EFRT	48	I	90	80
			II	70	68
Jones et al[124]	CHOP-IFRT	17	I-II	87	93
Stewart et al[53]	CHOP × 3–IFRT	78	I-II	84	85
Longo et al[125]	ProMACE–MOPP × 4–IFRT	49	I	100	100
Shenkier et al[126]	CHOP or CHOP-like × 3-4 + IFRT	308	I-II	81	80

CHOP, cyclophosphamide, hydroxydaunomycin, vincristine (Oncovin), and prednisone; EFRT, extended-field radiation therapy; IFRT, involved-field radiation therapy; ProMACE-MOPP, cyclophosphamide, etoposide, doxorubicin, nitrogen mustard, vincristine, procarbazine, high-dose methotrexate, and prednisone.

Table 61–9 Role of Radiotherapy in Stage I-II Aggressive Lymphomas: Randomized Studies

Reference	Patients, n	Progression-Free Survival, %		P value
		CHOP	CHOP + RT	
Horning et al[130]	345	39	54	0.06
Miller[131]	401	66	77	0.01

failure-free survival rate than those receiving CHOP alone (54% vs. 39%; P = 0.06).[130] Overall survival that included all causes of death in this aging population was better in the irradiated group (60% vs. 44%), but the difference was not statistically significant. Cause-specific survival was not reported.[130]

The SWOG study enrolled patients with stage I and nonbulky stage II aggressive NHL. The patients were randomly assigned to receive either eight cycles of CHOP chemotherapy alone or three cycles of CHOP followed by an involved field of 40 Gy (with an optional boost of up to 55 Gy). At a median follow-up of 4 years, the progression-free survival rate was significantly greater for the short-course CHOP plus radiotherapy group: 77% compared with 66% in the group receiving eight cycles of CHOP with no radiotherapy. The combined modality treatment also resulted in a superior overall survival rate (87% vs. 75%; P = 0.01). Additionally, reversible toxicity occurring during therapy also favored the combined-modality arm.[131] Recent analysis of the SWOG data suggested that patients with early-stage modified high International Prognostic Index had inferior survival and may require more than three cycles of chemotherapy.[132]

The results of both randomized studies confirm the importance of adjuvant radiation therapy to the involved field in patients who attained a complete response following short (three cycles) or long (eight cycles) chemotherapy. A relatively low dose of 30 Gy was adequate for patients who attained a complete response in the ECOG study (using eight cycles of CHOP), while a higher dose (40–55 Gy) was used in the short chemotherapy arm of the SWOG study. We currently advocate consolidation with a dose of 30 to 36 Gy for patients who attained an unquestionable complete response following three to six cycles of chemotherapy. This is based on our and others' excellent local control data at this dose range.[126,133,134] Yet other groups advocated dose in the range of 39 to 51 Gy for disease larger than 3.5 cm.[135] We advise a higher dose (40 to 50 Gy) for uncertain complete responses. For evaluating response, we recommend obtaining a PET scan before and after chemotherapy in addition to standard imaging tests, since a positive PET scan following chemotherapy may indicate an incomplete response that mandates a more aggressive approach.

The standard treatment for patients with advanced-stage (III or IV) aggressive lymphoma is combination chemotherapy. The most commonly used first-generation drug combination, CHOP, produced complete remission in the range of 45% to 55% and cured approximately one third of patients with advanced-stage disease. While some investigators considered more intensive regimens (second- and third-generation) to be more effective than CHOP, these claims could not be substantiated. A prospective randomized phase III study conducted by SWOG compared CHOP with third-generation regimens such as those consisting of low-dose methotrexate with leucovorin rescue, bleomycin, doxorubicin, cyclophosphamide, vincristine, and dexamethasone (m-BACOD); prednisone, doxorubicin, cyclophosphamide, and etoposide followed by cytarabine, bleomycin, vincristine, and methotrexate with leucovorin rescue (ProMACE/cytaBOM); and methotrexate with leucovorin rescue, doxorubicin, cyclophosphamide, vincristine, prednisone, and bleomycin (MACOP-B). No combination was better than CHOP. At 3 years, 44% of all patients were alive and free of disease, and the overall survival rate was 52%. CHOP remains the gold standard combination for patients with advanced, aggressive NHL.[136]

The role of radiation therapy in advanced-stage NHL is highly controversial. Most U.S. centers rarely recommend radiotherapy as an adjuvant following chemotherapy in stage III to IV intermediate-grade lymphoma, even for bulky disease or an incomplete response.[137] Unfortunately, while the superiority of combined modality over chemotherapy alone has been established for early stages, the concept and the feasibility have not been tested in trials for advanced-stage NHL in the United States. Yet recent data from other countries suggest that radiotherapy, particularly if administered to areas of originally bulky disease, may significantly improve the relapse-free survival and overall survival of patients who attained a complete response with chemotherapy.[138]

Investigators from Mexico City studied 218 patients with stage IV diffuse large cell lymphoma. Following chemotherapy, 155 patients (71%) achieved a complete response. Of the complete responders, 88 patients (56%) originally presented with bulky disease (>10 cm) and therefore were prospectively randomized to observation or to receive involved-field radiotherapy to a dose of 40 to 50 Gy. At 5 years, 72% of 43 patients randomized to receive radiotherapy were alive and disease free as compared with only 35% of the 45 patients who were not irradiated (P < 0.01). Most of the relapses occurred in the original site. Overall survival was also improved for the irradiated patients (81% vs. 55%; P < 0.01).[139]

In Milan, 97 patients with stages III and IV diffuse, large-cell lymphoma who were in complete response after chemotherapy were either observed or received consolidation radiotherapy. At 5 years, patients with bulky disease (= 10 cm) who received radiotherapy had a significantly longer time to relapse and a better overall survival (P = 0.05) compared with patients who were not irradiated. A multivariate analysis showed that the use of radiotherapy was an independent favorable prognostic factor before relapse (P = 0.001) and survival (P = 0.05).[140]

In Paris, patients with NHL who underwent high-dose chemotherapy with stem-cell transplantation as up-front treatment or treatment for relapse and received post-transplantation radiotherapy had a better event-free survival compared with patients who had not received radiotherapy (P = 0.02 in multivariate analysis). Other studies have also supported the use of consolidation radiotherapy after high-dose chemotherapy and bone-marrow transplantation.[141]

These data support the notion that although intermediate-grade NHL is a systemic disease, and all stages should primarily be treated with chemotherapy radiotherapy to bulky or residual disease may improve the outcome of the treatment program. More studies should address the potential benefit of radiation therapy in advanced-stage disease.

Mantle Cell Lymphoma

Although mantle cell lymphoma (MCL) was categorized in the past as an indolent lymphoma, it is now recognized to have a more aggressive behavior with an overall median survival of only 3 to 5 years. MCL almost always presents in an advanced stage (stage III or IV) and many times involves the gastrointestinal system in multiple places and the bone marrow. Mantle cell lymphoma remains an incurable disease. The treatment of MCL generally involves use of an alkylating agent, with or without other agents, to which 30% to 50% of the patients will have a complete response, but with a median duration of remission of only 1 to 3 years.[142] In general, single alkylating agents offer results similar to that of combination chemotherapy.[143] For example, a randomized trial comparing CVP (cyclophosphamide, vincristine, prednisone) to CHOP demonstrated no benefit for the addition of doxorubicin in terms of overall survival.[144] Recent studies indicated that even the attainment of molecular complete remission following chemotherapy is not sufficient to prevent relapse. In a phase II study employing CHOP + rituximab, progression-free survival was similar in those patients in complete remission who did or did not attain molecular complete response (16.5 vs. 18.5 months).[145] A more aggressive induction therapy followed by autologous or allogeneic stem cell transplantation has been attempted.[146] It is not clear as yet if this approach will result in extended survival.

It is of interest to note that mantle cell lymphoma is exquisitely sensitive to radiation therapy and often low doses in the range of 20 to 25 Gy will result in dramatic regression of the disease. When bulky disease is limited to a reasonable port, radiation therapy is an excellent palliative modality that may allow disease control for relatively long periods of time.

Highly Aggressive Lymphomas

The highly aggressive NHLs comprise the lymphoblastic lymphoma that is categorized as precursor B- or T-lymphoblastic leukemia/lymphoma by REAL, Burkitt's, and Burkitt's-like histologies. These diseases have a rapid growth rate and require prompt, vigorous intervention. Bulky localized presentations are common, particularly in the abdomen in children with Burkitt's lymphoma and in the mediastinum in adolescents with lymphoblastic lymphoma. But these diseases are almost always disseminated at presentation with common involvement of the

bone marrow, meninges, testes, and kidneys. Thus, radiation therapy is rarely indicated in the primary management of the highly aggressive lymphomas.[147,148] The treatment of choice, regardless of stage, is intensive chemotherapy patterned after the treatment of acute lymphoblastic lymphoma, including intrathecal methotrexate and often maintenance chemotherapy.[149,150] The cure rate with this approach is approximately 50% and is dependent on the presence of bone marrow or central nervous system involvement, bulky disease, and high LDH. The presence of these adverse prognostic factors can reduce the cure rate to 20% or less.

Treatment of Extranodal Lymphomas

Depending on the histologic subtype, 25% to 50% of NHLs arise in extranodal sites.[151,152] Since many patients with extranodal lymphomas present with localized disease, radiation therapy plays an important role in their management.[152] In general, most extranodal sites should be treated based on histologic subtype and stage as discussed earlier. In principle, the management of extranodal lymphomas is similar to the treatment of nodal presentations; namely, early-stage extranodal indolent lymphomas should be treated with radiation alone, and aggressive histologic subtypes involving an extranodal site should be managed with doxorubicin-containing chemotherapy followed by involved-field irradiation. Still, several extranodal sites require modified approaches: primary central nervous system lymphoma is addressed in Chapter 20, Primary and Metastatic Brain Tumors in Adults and the cutaneous lymphomas, including mycosis fungoides, are detailed in Chapter 62, Mycosis Fungoides. The management of gastrointestinal tract lymphoma, and particularly the treatment of gastric lymphoma, remains controversial.

Gastric Lymphoma

The gastrointestinal tract is the most common site for extranodal lymphomas, and gastric lymphomas account for approximately 65% of all primary gastrointestinal lymphomas.[154] Data from the Surveillance, Epidemiology, and End Results (SEER) study indicate an increase in the incidence of gastric lymphoma in the United States, particularly in people older than 60 years of age.[5] There is a significant variability in the incidence of gastric lymphoma between different geographical regions, which may be related to differences in the prevalence of *Helicobacter pylori* in gastric biopsies.[154,155]

The staging system commonly used for gastric lymphoma is based on the Ann Arbor system (see Table 61-3) with a modification introduced by Musshoff.[156] In brief, stage IE is defined as lymphoma involving the stomach, in the absence of any nodal involvement. Stage IIE1 includes patients with lymph node involvement in the perigastric area or at the level of L1 to L2, and stage IIE2 includes patients with lymph node involvement from L3 downward or in the mesentery. Stages IE and IIE1 are considered to represent truly localized disease and are associated with a significantly better prognosis than is stage IIE2.[154] Constitutional symptoms (particularly fever), abnormal LDH, and old age were found to be independent adverse prognostic factors in addition to advanced stage.[154]

In patients with localized disease, noninvasive staging (endoscopy supplemented with CT scan or lymphangiogram or both) was an adequate alternative to surgical staging and yielded equivalent staging accuracy and final outcome.[154] Endoscopic ultrasonography may improve the diagnostic yield and accuracy of staging in gastric lymphoma.[156]

In previous years, most researchers disregarded histology as an important determinant for treatment selection and advocated partial or total gastrectomy with or without adjuvant chemotherapy as the standard treatment. More recently, however, with the emergence of alternative nonsurgical approaches to diagnosis and treatment, and the recognition of the unique characteristics of MALT lymphoma, detailed histologic diagnosis has become critical for appropriate therapeutic decision making.

Approximately 60% of gastric lymphomas have an aggressive (intermediate-grade) histology; most commonly diffuse large-cell lymphoma with B-cell markers. Surgery alone, employing subtotal or total gastrectomy, has been reported to cure only a small proportion of patients with gastric lymphoma.[157] Most surgeons recommend subtotal gastrectomy as the procedure of choice, even if not all of the disease can be excised. This is because of the morbidity associated with total gastrectomy, including the dumping syndrome, malnutrition, pernicious anemia, and hypokalemia. A review of series in which curative gastrectomy was a component of treatment disclosed a 5-year survival rate between 38% and 75%.[158] Most series did not separate patients treated with surgery alone from those treated with surgery combined with adjuvant radiotherapy or chemotherapy and did not detail selection criteria for the different treatment modalities. The most benefit from adjuvant radiotherapy is expected in patients with incomplete resection or more extensive disease. An analysis of treatment outcome of 175 gastric lymphoma patients from Denmark indicated that patients who received radiotherapy as part of their therapy had a reduced relative risk of relapse.[152]

The experience of treating gastric lymphoma patients with radiotherapy alone is relatively limited, but a literature review of 170 patients with stage I and II gastric lymphoma showed that radiotherapy alone resulted in 54% to 58% freedom from relapse.[159] Taal and Burgers[160] reported a 64% disease-free survival rate in patients treated with radiotherapy alone. These data are similar to the outcome obtained in treatment of other extranodal or nodal sites with radiation alone and are also not significantly different from the outcome of surgery alone for stage I or II gastric lymphoma.

Analysis limited to patients with localized aggressive lymphoma who were treated primarily with surgery showed a 5-year survival of approximately 70% with no difference from a similar group of patients treated without gastric resection.[159] Although in the past, the nonsurgical approach was mostly reserved for patients who had unresectable disease or were poor surgical candidates, several recent reports have indicated that equivalent outcome can be attained without gastric resection using a combination of chemotherapy and radiotherapy. At the MD Anderson Cancer Center, a nonsurgical treatment program for localized gastric lymphoma yielded a 5-year disease-free survival rate of 62%.[161] In Amsterdam, treating gastric lymphoma with chemotherapy followed by radiation or with radiotherapy alone without surgical resection resulted in a relapse-free survival rate of 85% in stage I and 58% in stage II patients.[162] In Israel, Haim and associates[163] prospectively evaluated 26 patients with aggressive-histology gastric lymphoma treated with a stomach-conserving strategy. A complete response was endoscopically confirmed in 75% of patients and none of them relapsed; 17% had a partial response. Three patients had gastrointestinal bleeding during chemotherapy and one required surgical intervention, but no perforation or treatment-related mortality was observed.

The main argument against stomach-conserving therapies has been the risk of massive bleeding or perforation during chemotherapy or radiotherapy. A literature review of the reported experience of complications following nonsurgical therapies could not substantiate this concern.[158] Gastric hemorrhage or bleeding was reported in 3.5% of patients in stage I and II disease and in 10% of patients with advanced or unresectable disease.[158] Furthermore, an analysis of 106 patients with localized gastric lymphoma from Denmark showed that those treated with surgery had the highest risk of lethal (4.5%), early (21%), and major late complications (46%), including malabsorption, compared with patients treated primarily with radiotherapy or chemotherapy.[159]

Although many surgeons may still advocate stomach resection as the treatment of choice for patients with aggressive-histology, localized lymphoma, we consider the stomach-conserving approach using doxorubicin-containing chemotherapy followed by involved-field radiotherapy (30 to 36 Gy) to be safe and provide at least equivalent curative results and lower long-term morbidity compared with gastrectomy in this group of patients.

MALT LYMPHOMA OF THE STOMACH

The role of *H. pylori* infection in the pathogenesis of gastric MALT lymphoma has been well established. Antibiotic eradication of *H. pylori* is the standard primary treatment for patients with gastric MALT lymphoma and concomitant evidence for the presence of the bacteria in the stomach. Multiple series documented histologic regression of the gastric MALT lymphoma following successful eradication of *H. pylori* with a response ranging from 35% to 100%. Four relatively large series from Europe and North America documented responses of 50% to 80%. A treatment algorithm for patients presenting with or without *H. pylori* is outlined in Fig. 61-5.

Several effective anti-*H. pylori* programs are available.[164] It is expected that following 10 to 14 days of antibiotic treatment, *H. pylori* will be eradicated in 85% to 90% of the patients. Several factors predict the

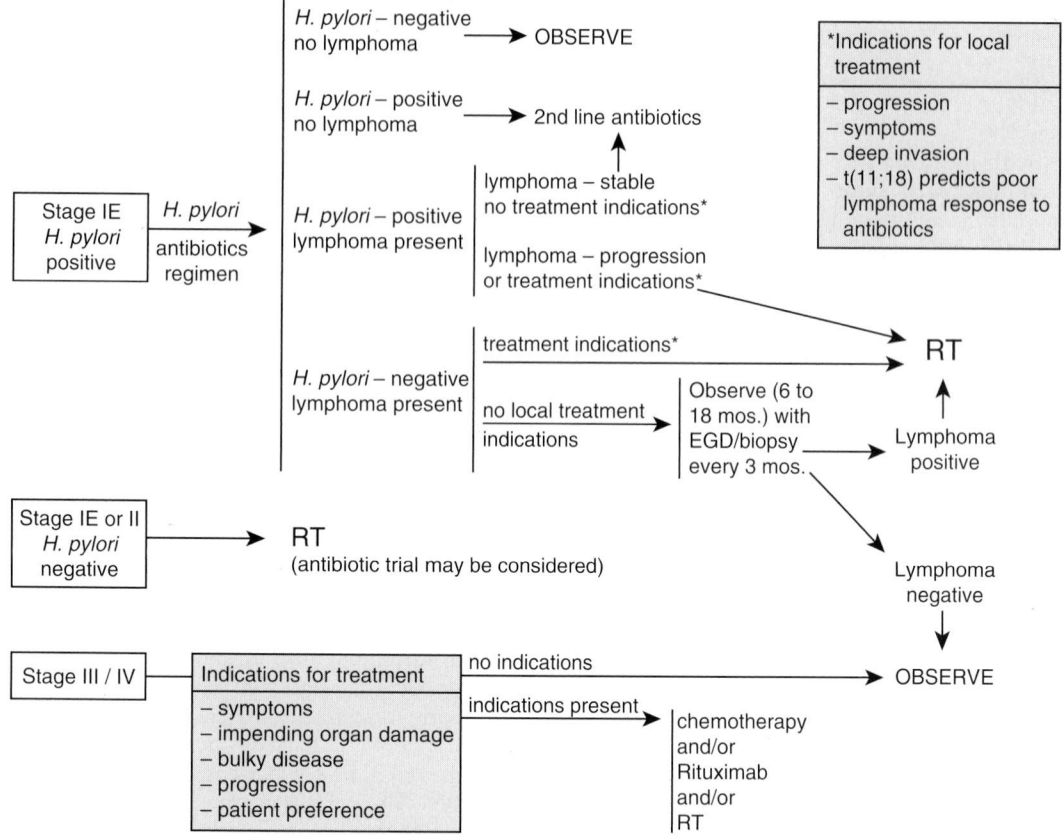

Figure 61–5. Treatment recommendations for MALT lymphoma of the stomach.

likelihood of gastric MALT lymphoma regression following antibiotic therapy. An obvious prerequisite for expecting a response to antibiotics is evidence of concomitant *H. pylori* infection. Indeed, in two series that included *H. pylori*-positive and negative patients, none of the *H. pylori*-negative lymphomas (16 patients) responded to antibiotic therapy.[165,166] Thus, it is highly questionable whether patients with no evidence of active *H. pylori* infection will benefit from a therapeutic trial with antibiotics.

Other factors have been associated with a low response of gastric MALT lymphoma to antibiotics treatment alone. A study from the French Groupe d'Etude Lymphome Digestif (GELD)[166] and MD Anderson Center[165] showed that in patients with *H. pylori*-positive gastric MALT lymphoma, the detection of nodal involvement by endoscopy with ultrasound or CT was associated with a significantly lower rate of lymphoma remission.[167] Likewise, penetration of lymphoma beyond the mucosa was also associated with a markedly decreased response.[167] These two features are related, as deep involvement is linked to increased risk of nodal involvement.[168] Furthermore, the likelihood of *H. pylori* presence is smaller when lymphoma involvement is found beyond the submucosa.[169] An additional (and not well explained) finding of the MD Anderson group is that the regression rate of tumors located in the distal part of the stomach was better than that of proximally located disease.[165] In a report from a German group, in four of

six patients whose lymphoma had not regressed following eradication of *H. pylori*, surgical resection showed the presence of high-grade lymphoma in deeper sections that were not appreciated during endoscopy.[170] This experience underlines the importance of multiple deep biopsies, particularly if endoscopy with ultrasound indicates deep penetration or lymph node enlargement or both. It also suggests that gastric MALT lymphoma with a high-grade component should be treated as intermediate-grade lymphoma with chemotherapy and involved-field radiotherapy.

While endoscopy with ultrasound could identify locally advanced disease that is unlikely to respond to antibiotics treatment, there are still a significant number of patients ($\approx$25%) with superficial lymphoma whose lymphoma will remain refractory even after *H. pylori* eradication. These antibiotic-resistant lymphomas are likely to demonstrate the chromosomal abnormality t(11;18)(q21;q21), a translocation involving approximately 40% of MALT lymphomas.[171-174] In analysis of biopsy material from 111 patients with *H. pylori*-positive gastric MALT lymphoma, only 2 of 48 (4%) of patients whose lymphoma completely regressed after *H. pylori* eradication showed that they had t(11;18), whereas 42 of 63 (67%) of the nonresponding patients demonstrated the translocation.[175] Thus, t(11;18) is a powerful indicator of response to *H. pylori* eradication and its presence at diagnosis should suggest that an alternative treatment (e.g., radiotherapy) be administered early, rather than waiting for regression with repeated endoscopies.[176] It has been suggested, however, that t(11;18) negative tumors have a higher risk of transformation into diffuse large B-cell lymphoma. Therefore, t(11;18)-negative tumors that have not completely regressed after antibiotics should be closely monitored for early alternative therapeutic intervention.

Approximately 30% to 50% of patients with H. pylori-positive gastric MALT lymphoma will show persistent or progressing lymphoma even after eradication of H. pylori with antibiotic therapy. Of the complete responders, almost 15% will relapse within 3 years, suggesting that about half of all patients with gastric MALT lymphoma will eventually be considered for additional therapies. Most of those will still have disease limited to the stomach. Patients who present with no evidence of H. pylori infection are unlikely to respond to antibiotics and should be considered for alternative treatments.

As a local therapy, surgery has been widely used in the past. Cogliatti et al.[177] reviewed 69 cases of low-grade gastric MALT lymphoma treated with surgery alone (45) or with surgery followed by either chemotherapy, radiotherapy, or both (24). The 5-year overall survival was 91% and no significant difference in survival was observed in patients selected for adjuvant therapy following surgery.

In recent years, the role of surgery in gastric MALT lymphoma has been questioned.[178-181] Gastric MALT lymphoma is a multifocal disease[182] and adequate gastrectomy needs to be quite extensive, severely impairing quality of life, and yet residual disease at the margins may still require additional radiation or chemotherapy or both.

Several institutions reported excellent results using involved-field radiotherapy of the stomach in H. pylori-independent gastric MALT lymphoma patients who either failed antibiotic therapy or had no evidence of H. pylori infection.[183,184-187] The recent update of the MSKCC experience included 51 patients with gastric MALT lymphoma (stage I—39; stage II—10; stage IV—2) who were either H. pylori-negative (30) or remained with persistent lymphoma after antibiotic therapies and adequate observation (21).[188] All patients were treated with radiation to the stomach and perigastric nodes; the median total dose was 30 Gy in 4 weeks. All patients had regular follow-up endoscopic evaluations and biopsies. 49 of 51 patients (96%) obtained a biopsy-proven complete response. Of three patients who relapsed, two were salvaged. Three patients died of other malignancies, all second tumors developed outside the radiation field. At a median follow-up of 4 years, freedom from treatment failure, overall survival, and cause-specific survival were 89%, 83% and 100%, respectively. Treatment was well tolerated, with no significant acute or chronic side effects. The experience from Toronto and Boston using the same radiation approach was equally successful,[183,185,186] supporting the approach that modest dose involved-field radiotherapy is the treatment of choice for patients with persistent gastric MALT lymphoma who have exhausted the antibiotic therapy approach or are unlikely to respond to it (H. pylori-negative patients).[189,190]

Patients with systemic disease should be considered for chemotherapy and immunotherapy (anti CD-20) or both.

Unfortunately, chemotherapy has never been adequately evaluated in gastric MALT lymphomas because it was usually not administered, or given after surgery or radiotherapy. Few compounds have been tested specifically in MALT lymphomas.[191] A nonrandomized study of 24 patients (17 in stage I and 7 in stage IV, most of them with primary gastric localization) reported that oral alkylating agents (either cyclophosphamide 100 mg/day or chlorambucil 6 mg/day, with a median treatment duration of 1 year) can result in a high rate of disease control with projected 5-year event-free and overall survival of 50% and 75%, respectively.[191] A more recent phase II study of 19 patients with gastric and 7 patients with nongastric MALT lymphoma demonstrated some anti-tumor activity of the purine analog cladribine (2-CDA, given as a 2-hour intravenous infusion at a dose of 0.12 mg/kg body weight on 5 consecutive days every 4 weeks) with a complete response rate of 84%. However, in this study, additional anti-*helicobacter* treatment might have contributed to the very high remission rate in patients with gastric lymphoma, since only 43% of patients with extragastric presentation achieved a complete response.[192]

In the presence of disseminated or advanced disease, chemotherapy may be an obvious choice. The activity of the anti-CD20 monoclonal antibody rituximab has also been shown in a phase II study (with a response rate of about 70%), and may represent an additional option for the treatment of systemic disease, but the efficacy of its combination with chemotherapy still needs to be explored in this histological type.[193] Depending on the response to systemic therapy, presence of bulky disease, and symptoms, selected patients with systemic disease may also benefit from irradiation of the stomach.

Nongastric MALT Lymphomas

MALT lymphomas have also been described in various nongastric sites, such as salivary glands, skin, orbit, conjunctiva, lung, thyroid, larynx, breast, kidney, liver, bladder, prostate, urethra, small intestine, rectum, pancreas, and even in the intracranial dura.[183,194-199] Nongastric MALT lymphomas have been difficult to characterize because these tumors, numerous when considered together, are distributed so widely throughout the body that it is difficult to assemble adequate series of any given site. Yet few series have recently addressed the characteristics of nongastric MALT lymphomas.[183,195,197] The International Extranodal Lymphoma Study Group (IELSG) published a retrospective survey of a large series of patients who were diagnosed with nongastric MALT lymphoma with the aim of better characterizing this disease entity.[194] The IELSG study confirmed the indolent course of nongastric MALT lymphomas despite the fact that one quarter of cases presented with stage IV disease, and regardless of treatment type, the 5-year survival was approximately 90%.[196] The finding that dissemination to multiple mucosal sites does not change the outcome has also been demonstrated in other series.[195,197] Nongastrointestinal MALT lymphoma patients seem to progress more often than those with gastric MALT lymphoma,[183,195] but whether different sites have a different natural history remains an open question. Location can be an important factor because of organ-specific problems, which result in particular management strategies. In the IELSG series, the patients with the disease initially presenting in the upper airways appeared to have a slightly poorer outcome, but their small number prevented any definitive conclusion.[194]

The optimal management of nongastric MALT lymphomas has not yet been clearly established. Retrospective series included patients treated with surgery, radiotherapy, and chemotherapy, alone or in combination.[183,185,190,194,196,197] In most patients, good disease control and excellent cause-specific and overall survival has been demonstrated, independent of the treatment modality selected. In a multivariate analysis of the IELSG data, the minority of patients (17%) with International Prognostic Index intermediate-high or high-risk groups had an inferior progression-free survival. Patients with stage IV due to disease at MALT sites plus bone marrow or lymph node involvement—but not those with multiple mucosal localizations only—had a lower overall survival rate, and presence of nodal involvement adversely affected cause-specific survival.[194] Thus, the treatment choice should be "patient-tailored," taking into account the site, the stage, and the clinical characteristics of the individual patient. In patients with localized disease, extensive surgery is unnecessary in most sites since marginal-zone lymphomas are exquisitely sensitive to relatively low doses of radiation. Specifically, MALT lymphoma in sites such as salivary glands, ocular, conjunctiva, thyroid, breast or bladder have been successfully eradicated with involved-field RT encompassing the involved organ alone with a dose of 24 Gy to 36 Gy.[183,185,190,200-207] Even unusual sites (such as larynx, base of the skull, urethra, prostate) not easily amenable to surgery have been well controlled by involved-field RT.[198,199,208,209] Patients with extensive lung disease or involvement of multiple sites or the bone marrow are likely to respond to various systemic chemotherapy regimens, although no specific chemotherapy regimen has been advocated.[194,196,197] Since responses to rituximab have also been reported,[193] the IELSG is planning a randomized trial to evaluate the benefit of the addition of rituximab to chlorambucil in either nongastric or gastric antibiotic-resistant MALT lymphoma.

REFERENCES

1. Longo DL: The REAL classification of lymphoid neoplasms: One clinician's view. *PPO Updates.* 1995;9:1.
2. Tumours of haematopoietic and lymphoid tissues: In Jaffe ES, Harris NL, Stein H, Vardiman JW, eds: *World Health Organization Classification of Tumours.* Lyon, France: IARC Press; 2001.
3. Jemal A, Murray T, Samuels A, et al: Cancer statistics, 2003. *CA Cancer J Clin.* 2003;53:5.
4. Hartge P, Devesa S, Fraumeni JF Jr: Hodgkin's and non-Hodgkin's lymphomas. *Cancer Surv.* 1994;19:423.
5. Miller B, Ries L, Hawkey B, et al: *SEER Cancer Statistics Review,* NIH Publication no. 93-2789, 1993.
6. Devesa S, Fears T: Non-Hodgkin's lymphoma time trends. *Cancer Res.* 1992;52:5432s.
7. Aisenberg AC: Coherent view of non-Hodgkin's lymphoma. *J Clin Oncol.* 1995;13:2656.
8. Young L, Rowe M: Epstein-Barr virus, lymphomas and Hodgkin's disease. *Semin Cancer Biol.* 1992;3:273.
9. Lenoir G: Role of the virus, chromosomal translocations and cellular oncogenes in the etiology of Burkitt's lymphoma. In Epstein MA, Achong BG, eds. *The Epstein-Barr Virus: Recent Advances.* London: Heinemann Medical Books; 1986:184.
10. Mueller N, Mohar A, Evans A: Viruses other than HIV and Non-Hodgkin's lymphoma. *Cancer Res.* 1992;52:5479s.
11. Obrams G, Grufferman S: Epidemiology of HIV-associated non-Hodgkin's lymphoma. *Cancer Surv.* 1991;10:91.
12. Ballerini P, Gaidano G, Gong J, et al: Multiple genetic lesions in acquired immunodeficiency syndrome-related non-Hodgkin's lymphoma. *Blood.* 1993;81:166.
13. Bashir R, Harris N, Hochberg F, et al: Detection of Epstein-Barr virus in primary CNS lymphomas in immunocompromised patients. *Neurology.* 1989;39:813.
14. Blair A, Zahm SH: Cancer among farmers. *Occupat Med.* 1991; 6:335.
15. Cantor KP, Blair A, Everett G, et al: Pesticides and other agricultural risk factors for non-Hodgkin's lymphoma among men in Iowa and Minnesota. *Cancer Res.* 1992;52:2447.
16. Cantor KP, Blair A, Everett G, et al: Hair dye use and risk of leukemia and lymphoma. *Am J Public Health.* 1988;78:570.
17. Boice JDJ: Radiation and non-Hodgkin's lymphoma. *Cancer Res.* 1992;52:5489s.
18. Wotherspoon AC, Doglinoni C, Diss TC, et al: Regression of primary low grade B cell lymphoma of mucosa-associated lymphoid tissue type after eradication of *Helicobacter pylori. Lancet.* 1993;342:575.
19. Rowley JD: Chromosomal studies in the non-Hodgkin's lymphomas: The role of the 14;18 translocation. *Clin Oncol.* 1988;6:919.
20. Dalla-Favera R: Chromosomal translocations involving the *c-myc* oncogene and their role in the pathogenesis of B-cell neoplasia. In Brugge J, Curran T, Harlow E, et al, eds. *Origins of Human Cancer: A Comprehensive Review.* Plainview, N.Y.: Coldspring Harbor Laboratory Press; 1991.
21. Rimokh R, Berger F, Delsol G, et al: Rearrangement and overexpression of the *bcl-1/PRAD-1* gene in intermediate lymphocytic lymphoma and in t(11q13)-bearing leukemias. *Blood.* 1993; 81:3063.
22. Escudier SM, Pereira-Leahy J, Drach JW, et al: Fluorescent in situ hybridization and cytogenetic studies of trisomy 12 in chronic lymphocytic leukemia. *Blood.* 1993;81:2702.
23. Remstein ED, Kurtin PJ, James CD, et al: Mucosa-associated lymphoid tissue lymphomas with t(11;18)(q21;q21) and mucosa-associated lymphoid tissue lymphomas with aneuploidy develop along different pathogenetic pathways. *Am J Pathol* 2002;161:63.
24. Rabbitts T: Chromosomal translocations in human cancer. *Nature.* 1994;372:143.
25. The Non-Hodgkin's Lymphoma Pathologic Classification Project: National Cancer Institute sponsored study of classifications of non-Hodgkin's lymphomas: Summary of a working formulation for clinical use. *Cancer.* 1982;49:2112.
26. Lennert K, Feller A: *Histopathology of Non-Hodgkin's Lymphomas.* New York: Springer-Verlag; 1992.
27. Rosenberg SA: The low grade non-Hodgkin's lymphomas: Challenges and opportunities. *J Clin Oncol.* 1985;3:299.
28. Paryani SB, Hoppe RT, Cox RS, et al: Analysis of non-Hodgkin's lymphomas with nodular and favorable histologies: Stage I and II. *Cancer.* 1983;52:2300.
29. MacManus MP, Hoppe RT: Is radiotherapy curative for stage I and II low-grade follicular lymphoma? Results of a long-term follow-up study of patients treated at Stanford University. *J Clin Oncol.* 1996;14:1282.
30. Ersboll J, Schultz HB, Pedersen-Bjergaard J, et al: Follicular low-grade non-Hodgkin's lymphoma: Long-term outcome with or without tumor progression. *Eur J Hematol.* 1989;42:155.
31. Tsujimoto T, Cossman J, Jaffe E, et al: Involvement of the *bcl-2* gene in human follicular lymphoma. *Science.* 1985;288:1440.
32. Rappaport H, Winter WJ, Hicks E: Follicular lymphoma: A reevaluation of its position in the scheme of malignant lymphomas based on a survey of 253 cases. *Cancer.* 1956;7:792.
33. Glick JH, Ezdinli EZ, Berard CW, et al: Nodular mixed lymphoma: Results of a randomized study failing to confirm prolonged disease-free survival with COPP chemotherapy. *Blood.* 1981;58:920.

34. Longo DL, Young RC, Hubbard SM, et al: Prolonged initial remission in patients with nodular mixed lymphoma. *Ann Intern Med.* 1984;100:651.

35. Longo DL: What's the deal with follicular lymphomas? *J Clin Oncol.* 1993;11:202.

36. Inghirami G, Wieczorek R, Zhu B, et al: Differential expression of LFA-1 molecules in non-Hodgkin's lymphoma and lymphoid leukemias. *Blood.* 1988;72:1431.

37. Robertson LE, Pugh W, O'Brien S, et al: Richter's syndrome: A report on 39 cases. *J Clin Oncol.* 1993;11:1985.

38. Nizze H, Cogliatti S, von Schilling C: Monocytoid B-cell lymphomas: Morphological variants and relationship to low-grade B-cell lymphoma of the mucosa-associated lymphoid tissue. *Histopathology.* 1991;18:409.

39. Isaacson PG, Spencer J: Malignant lymphoma of mucosa-associated lymphoid tissue: A distinctive B-cell lymphoma. *Cancer.* 1983; 52:1410.

40. Wotherspoon AC, Finn TM, Isaacson PG: Trisomy 3 in low-grade B-cell lymphoma of mucosa-associated lymphoid tissue. *Blood.* 1995;85:2000.

41. Montalban C, Castrillo JM, Serano M, et al: Gastric B-cell mucosa-associated lymphoid tissue lymphoma: Clinicopathological study and evaluation of the prognostic factors in 143 patients. *Ann Oncol.* 1995;6:355.

42. Isaacson PG, Spencer J: Gastric lymphoma and *Helicobacter pylori.* In DeVita VT, Hellman S, Rosenberg SA, eds. *Important Advances in Oncology 1996.* Philadelphia: Lippincott-Raven; 1996:111.

43. Fisher RI, Dahlberg S, Nathwani BN, et al: A clinical analysis of two indolent lymphoma entities: Mantle cell lymphoma and marginal zone lymphoma including mucosa-associated lymphoid tissue and monocytoid B-cell subcategories: A Southwest Oncology Group study. *Blood.* 1995;85:1075.

44. Wotherspoon AC, Ortiz-Hidalgo C, Falzon MR, et al: *Helicobacter pylori*-associated gastritis and primary B-cell gastric lymphoma. *Lancet.* 1991;338:1175.

45. Dalla-Favera R, Ye BH, Cattoretti G, et al: *BCL-6* in diffuse large-cell lymphomas. In DeVita VT, Hellman S, Rosenberg SA, eds. *Important Advances in Oncology 1996.* Philadelphia: Lippincott-Raven; 1996:139.

46. Addis B, Isaacson PG: Large cell lymphoma of the mediastinum: A B-cell tumor of probable thymic origin. *Histopathology.* 1986; 10:379.

47. Jacobson J, Aisenberg A, Lamarre L, et al: Mediastinal large cell lymphoma: An uncommon subset of adult lymphoma curable with combined modality therapy. *Cancer.* 1988;62:1893.

48. Williams M, Swerdlow S, Rosenberg C, Arnold A: Characterization of chromosome 11 translocation breakpoints at the bcl-1 and *PRAD1* loci in centrocytic lymphoma. *Cancer Res.* 1992; 52:5541.

49. Louie DC, Offit K, Jaslow R, et al: p53 overexpression as a marker of poor prognosis in mantle cell lymphomas with t(11;14) (q13;q32). *Blood.* 1995;86:2892.

50. Vandenberghe E: Mantle cell lymphoma. *Blood Rev.* 1994;8:79. (Review.)

51. Norton AJ, Matthews J, Pappa V, et al: Mantle cell lymphoma: Natural history defined in a serially biopsied population over a 20-year period. *Ann of Oncol.* 1995;6:249.

52. Zucca E, Roggero E, Pinotti G, et al: Patterns of survival in mantle cell lymphoma. *Ann Oncol.* 1995;6:257.

53. Stewart DA, Vose JM, Weisenburger DD, et al: The role of high-dose therapy and autologous hematopoietic stem cell transplantation for mantle cell lymphoma. *Ann Oncol.* 1995; 6:263.

54. Coiffier B, Hiddemann W, Stein H: Mantle cell lymphoma: A therapeutic dilemma. *Ann Oncol.* 1995;6:208. (Editorial.)

55. Armitage JO, Greer JP, Levine AM, et al: Peripheral T-cell lymphoma. *Cancer.* 1989;63:158.

56. Coiffier B, Brousse N, Peuchmaur M, et al: Peripheral T-cell lymphomas have a worse prognosis than B-cell lymphomas: A prospective study of 361 immunophenotyped patients treated with the LNH-84 regimen. *Ann Oncol.* 1990;1:45.

57. Harris NL: A practical approach to the pathology of lymphoid neoplasms: A revised European-American classification from the international lymphoma study group. In DeVita VT, Hellman S, Rosenberg SA, eds. *Important Advances in Oncology 1995.* Philadelphia: JB Lippincott; 1995:111.

58. Feller AC, Griesser H, Schilling CV, et al: Clonal gene rearrangement patterns correlate with immunophenotype and clinical parameters in patients with angioimmunoblastic lymphadenopathy. *Am J Pathol.* 1988;133:549.

59. Siegert W, Agathe A, Griesser H, et al: Treatment of angioimmunoblastic lymphadenopathy (AILD)-type T-cell lymphoma using prednisone with or without the COP-BLAM/IMVP-16 regimen. *Ann Intern Med.* 1992;117:364.

60. Lipford EH, Margolick JB, Longo DL, et al: Angiocentric immunoproliferative lesions: A clinicopathologic spectrum of post-thymic T-cell proliferations. *Blood.* 1988;72:1674.

61. Chott A, Dragosic B, Radazskievicz T: Peripheral T-cell lymphoma of the intestine. *Am J Pathol.* 1992;141:1361.

62. Murray A, Cuevas EC, Jones DB, Wright DH: Study of the immunohistochemistry and T-cell clonality of enteropathy-associated T-cell lymphoma. *Am J Pathol.* 1995;146:509.

63. Pileri S, Falini B, Delsol G, et al: Lymphohistiocytic T-cell lymphoma (anaplastic large cell lymphoma CD30+/Ki-1+ with a high content of reactive histiocytes). *Histopathology.* 1990;16:383.

64. Agnarsson B, Kadin M: Ki-1 positive large cell lymphoma: A morphologic and immunologic study of 19 cases. *Am J Surg Pathol.* 1988;12:264.

65. de Bruin P, Beljaards R, van Heerde P, et al: Differences in clinical behavior and immunophenotype between primary cutaneous and primary nodal anaplastic large cell lymphoma of T-cell or null cell phenotype. *Histopathology.* 1993;23:127.

66. Greer JR, Kinney MC, Collin RD, et al: Clinical features of 31 patients with Ki-1 anaplastic large-cell lymphoma. *Clin Oncol.* 1991;9:539.

67. Mason D, Bastard C, Rimokh R, et al: CD30-positive large cell lymphomas ("Ki-1 lymphoma") are associated with a chromosomal translocation involving 5q35. *Haematol.* 1990;74:161.

68. Kaneko Y, Frizzera G, Edamura S, et al: A novel translocation, t(2;5)(p23;q35), in childhood phagocytic large T-cell lymphoma mimicking malignant histiocytosis. *Blood.* 1989;73:806.

69. Magrath I, Shiramizu B: Biology and treatment of small non-cleaved cell lymphoma. *Oncology.* 1989;3:41.

70. Hutchison R, Murphy S, Fairclough D, et al: Diffused noncleaved cell lymphoma in children, Burkitt's versus non-Burkitt's types. *Cancer.* 1989;64:23.

71. Yano T, Van Krieken J, Magrath I, et al: Histogenetic correlations between subcategories of small noncleaved cell lymphomas. *Blood.* 1992;79:1282.

72. Hoelzer, DP: Therapy of the newly diagnosed adult with acute lymphoblastic leukemia. *Hematol Oncol Clin North Am.* 1993; 7:139.

73. Weiss L, Bindl J, Picozzi V, et al: Lymphoblastic lymphoma: An immunophenotype study of 26 cases with comparison to T cell acute lymphoblastic leukemia. *Blood.* 1986;67:474.

74. Nathwani B, Diamond L, Winberg C, et al: Lymphoblastic lymphoma: A clinicopathologic study of 95 patients. *Cancer.* 1981; 48:2347.

75. Bernard A, Boumsell L, Reinhertz L, et al: Cell surface characterization of malignant T cells from lymphoblastic lymphoma using monoclonal antibodies: Evidence of phenotypic differences between malignant T cells from patients with acute lymphoblastic leukemia and lymphoblastic lymphoma. *Blood.* 1981;57:1105.

76. Carbone P, Kaplan H, Musshoff K, et al: Report of the Committee on Hodgkin's Disease Staging Classification. *Cancer Res.* 1971; 31:1860.

77. Lister T, Crowther D, Sutcliffe S, et al: Report of a committee convened to discuss the evaluation and staging of patients with Hodgkin's disease: Cotswolds meeting. *J Clin Oncol.* 1989; 7:1630.

78. Mauch P, Leonard R, Skarin A, et al: Improved survival following combined radiation therapy and chemotherapy for unfavorable prognosis stage I-II non-Hodgkin's lymphomas. *J Clin Oncol.* 1985;3:1301.

79. Shipp MA, Harrington DP, Anderson JR, et al: A predictive model for aggressive NHL: The international NHL prognostic factors project. *N Engl J Med.* 1993;329:987.

80. Shipp MA: Prognostic factors in aggressive NHL, who has "high risk" disease? *Blood.* 1994;83:1165.

81. Castellino RA, Hilton S, O'Brien JP, Portlock CS: Non-Hodgkin's lymphoma: Contribution of chest CT in the initial evaluation. *Radiology.* 1996;199:129.

82. Kaplan W, Jochelson M, Herman T, et al: Gallium-67 imaging: A predictor of residual tumor viability and clinical outcome in patients with diffuse large-cell lymphoma. *J Clin Oncol.* 1990;8:1966.

83. Wirth A, Seymour J, Hicks R, et al. Fluorine-18 fluorodeoxy-glucose positron emission tomography, gallium-67 scintigraphy, and conventional staging for Hogkin's disease and non-Hodgkin's lymphoma. *Am J Med.* 2002;112:262.

84. Vaughan HB, Vaughan HG, MacLennan KA, et al: Clinical stage I non-Hodgkin's lymphoma: Long-term follow-up of patients treated by the British National Lymphoma Investigation with radiotherapy alone as initial therapy. *Br J Cancer.* 1994;69:1088.

85. Suttcliffe SB, Gospadarowicz MK, Bush RS, et al: Role of radiation therapy in localized non-Hodgkin's lymphoma. *Radiother Oncol.* 1985;4:211.

86. Lawrence TS, Urba WJ, Steinberg SM, et al: Retrospective analysis of stage I and II indolent lymphomas at the National Cancer Institute. *Int J Radiat Oncol Biol Phys.* 1988;14:417.

87. Bush RS, Gospadarowicz M, Sturgeon J, et al: Radiation therapy of localized non-Hodgkin's lymphoma. *Cancer Treat Rep.* 1977; 61:1129.

88. Fuks Z, Kaplan HS: Recurrence rates following radiation therapy of nodular and diffuse malignant lymphomas. *Radiology.* 1973; 108:675.

89. Nissen NI, Ersboll J, Hansen HS, et al: A randomized study of radiotherapy versus radiotherapy plus chemotherapy in stage I-II non-Hodgkin's lymphomas. *Cancer.* 1983;52:1.

90. Monfardini S, Banfi A, Bonadonna G, et al: Improved five year survival after combined radiotherapy-chemotherapy for stage I-II non-Hodgkin's lymphoma. *Int J Radiat Oncol Biol Phys.* 1980; 6:125.

91. Carde P, Burgers JMW, Glabbeke M, et al: Combined radiotherapy-chemotherapy for early stage non-Hodgkin's lymphoma: The 1975-1980 EORTC controlled lymphoma trial. *Radiother Oncol.* 1984;2:301.

92. Yahalom J, Varsos G, Fuks Z, et al: Adjuvant cyclophosphamide, doxorubicin, vincristine, and prednisone chemotherapy after radiation therapy in stage I low-grade and intermediate-grade non-Hodgkin lymphoma. Results of a prospective randomized study. *Cancer.* 1993;71:2342.

93. Kelsey SM, Newland AC, Vaughn HG, et al: A BNLI randomized trial of chlorambucil plus radiotherapy versus radiotherapy alone in low-grade, localized non-Hodgkin's lymphoma. *Radiat Oncol.* 1994;11:19.

94. Paryani SB, Hoppe RT, Cox RS, et al: The role of radiation therapy in the management of stage III follicular lymphomas. *J Clin Oncol.* 1984;2:841.

95. Jacobs JP, Murray KJ, Schultz CJ, et al: Central lymphatic irradiation for stage III nodular malignant lymphoma: Long-term results. *J Clin Oncol.* 1993;11:233.

96. Aviles A, Diaz-Maqueo JC, Sanchez E, et al: Long-term results in patients with low-grade nodular non-Hodgkin's lymphoma: A randomized trial comparing chemotherapy plus radiotherapy to chemotherapy alone. *Acta Oncol (Madrid).* 1991;30:329.

97. McLaughlin P, Fuller LM, Velasquez WS, et al: Stage III follicular lymphoma: Durable remissions with a combined chemotherapy-radiotherapy regimen. *J Clin Oncol.* 1987;5:867.

98. Horning SJ: Natural history of and therapy for the indolent non-Hodgkin's lymphomas. *Semin Oncol.* 1993;20(suppl 5):75.

99. Horning SJ: Low-grade lymphoma 1993: State of the art. *Ann Oncol.* 1994;5:23. (Review.)

100. Horning SJ: Treatment approaches to the low-grade lymphomas. *Blood.* 1994;83:881. (Review.)

101. Portlock CK: Management of the low-grade non-Hodgkin's lymphomas. *Semin Oncol.* 1990;17:51. (Review.)

102. Horning SJ, Rosenberg SA: The natural history of initially untreated low-grade non-Hodgkin's lymphomas. *N Engl J Med.* 1984;311:1471.

103. Young RC, Longo DL, Glatstein E, et al: The treatment of indolent lymphomas: Watchful waiting versus aggressive combined modality treatment. *Semin Hematol.* 1988;25:11.

104. Dana BW, Dahlberg S, Nathwani BN, et al: Long-term follow-up of patients with low-grade malignant lymphomas treated with doxorubicin-based chemotherapy or chemoimmunotherapy. *J Clin Oncol.* 1993;11:644.

105. Keating MJ, O'Brien S, Plunkett W, et al: Fludarabine phosphate: A new active agent in hematological malignancies. *Semin Hematol.* 1994;31:28.

106. Saven A, Piro LD: 2-chlorodeoxyadenosine: A newer purine analog active in the treatment of indolent lymphoid malignancies. *Ann Intern Med.* 1994;120:784.

107. Solal-Celigny P, Lepage E, Brousse N, et al: Recombinant interferon alpha-2b combined with a regimen containing doxorubicin in patients with advanced follicular lymphoma. *N Engl J Med.* 1993;329:1608.

108. Multani P, Grossbard M: Monoclonal antibody-based therapies for hematologic malignancies. *J Clin Oncol.* 1998;16:3691.

109. McLaughlin P, Grillo-Lopez AJ, Link BK, et al: Rituximab chimeric anti-CD20 monoclonal antibody therapy for relapsed indolent lymphoma: Half of patients respond to a four-dose treatment program. *J Clin Oncol.* 1998;16:2825.

110. Foran JM, Gupta RK, Cunningham D, et al: A UK multicentre phase II study of rituximab (chimaeric anti-CD20 monoclonal antibody) in patients with follicular lymphoma, with PCR monitoring of molecular response. *Br J Haematol.* 2000:109:81.

111. Hainsworth JD, Litchy S, Burris HAS III, et al: Rituximab as first-line and maintenance therapy for patients with indolent non-Hodgkin's lymphoma. *J Clin Oncol.* 2002;20:4261.

112. Colombat P, Salles G, Brousse N, et al: Rituximab (anti-CD20 monoclonal antibody) as single first-line therapy for patients with follicular lymphoma with a low tumor burden: Clinical and molecular evaluation. *Blood.* 2001;97:101.

113. Dillman RO: Radiolabeled anti-CD20 monoclonal antibodies for the treatment of B-cell lymphoma. *J Clin Oncol.* 2002;20:3545.

114. Witzig TE, White CA, Gordon L, et al: Response to zevalin is superior to response to rituximab regardless of age and extent of disease. *Proc Am Soc Clin Oncol.* 2001;20:2279a. Abstract.

115. Vose JM, Wahl RL, Saleh M, et al: Multicenter phase II study of iodine-131 tositumomab for chemotheapy-refractory low-grade or transformed low-grade B-cell non-Hodgkin's lymphomas. *J Clin Oncol.* 2000;18:1316.

116. Montserrat E, Bosch F, Lopez-Guillermo A, et al: CNS involvement in mantle-cell lymphoma. *J Clin Oncol.* 1996;14:941.

117. Teodorovic I, Pittaluga S, Kluin-Nelemans JC, et al: Efficacy of four different regimen in 64 mantle-cell lymphoma cases: Clinicopathologic comparison with 498 other non-Hodgkin's lymphoma subtypes. European Organization for the Research and Treatment of Cancer Lymphoma Cooperative Group. *J Clin Oncol.* 1995;13:2819.

118. Garcia-Conde J, Cabanillas P: Mantle cell lymphoma: A new lymphoproliferative entity with definite histopathological patterns, clinical characteristics and prognostic factors, and an investigational therapeutic approach. *Ann Oncol.* 1995;6:305.

119. Jones S, Fuks Z, Bull M, et al: Non-Hodgkin's lymphomas: IV. Clinicopathologic correlation in 405 cases. *Cancer.* 1973;31:806.

120. Chen MG, Prosnitz LR, Gonzalez-Serva A, Fisher DB: Results of radiotherapy in control of stage I and II non-Hodgkin's lymphoma. *Cancer.* 1979;43:1245.

121. Prestidge BR, Horning SJ, Hoppe RT: Combined modality therapy for stage I-II large-cell lymphoma. *Int J Radiat Oncol Biol Phys.* 1988;15:633.

122. Cosset JM, Henry-Amar M, Vuong T, et al: Alternating chemotherapy and radiology combination for bulky stage I and II intermediate and high grade non-Hodgkin's lymphoma: An update. *Radiother Oncol.* 1991;20:30.

123. Kaminski MS, Coleman CN, Colby TV, et al: Factors predicting survival in adults with stage I and II large-cell lymphoma treated with primary radiation therapy. *Ann Intern Med.* 1986; 104:747.

124. Jones S, Miller T, Connors J: Long-term follow-up and analysis for prognostic factors for patients with limited-stage diffuse large-cell lymphoma treated with initial chemotherapy with or without adjuvant radiotherapy. *J Clin Oncol.* 1989;7:1186.

125. Longo D, Glatstein E, Duffey P, et al: Treatment of localized aggressive lymphomas with combination chemotherapy followed by involved-field radiation therapy. *J Clin Oncol.* 1989;7:1295.

126. Shenkier TN, Voss N, Fairey R, et al: Brief chemotherapy and involved-region irradiation for limited-stage diffuse large-cell lymphoma: An 18-year experience from the British Columbia Cancer Agency. *J Clin Oncol.* 2002;20:197.

127. Longo DL: Combined modality therapy for localized aggressive lymphoma: Enough or too much? *J Clin Oncol.* 1989;7:1189.

128. Cabanillas S, Dody G, Freireich E: Management of chemotherapy only stage I and II malignant lymphoma of aggressive histologic types. *Cancer.* 1980;46:2356.

129. Miller T, Jones S: Initial chemotherapy for clinically localized lymphomas of unfavorable histology. *Blood.* 1983;62:413.

130. Horning SJ, Glick JH, Kim K, et al: Final report of E1484: CHOP v CHOP + radiotherapy (RT) for limited stage diffuse aggressive lymphoma. *Blood.* 2001;98:724a. Abstract.

131. Miller T, Dahlberg S, Cassady J, et al: Chemotherapy alone compared with chemotherapy plus radiotherapy for localized intermediate- and high-grade non-Hodgkin's lymphoma. *N Engl J Med.* 1998;339:21.

132. Miller TP, Leblanc M, Spier C, et al: CHOP alone compared to CHOP plus radiotherapy for early stage aggressive non-Hodgkin's lymphomas: Update of the Southwest Oncology Group (SWOG) randomized trial. *Blood.* 2001;98:724a. Abstract.

133. Roy I, Yahalom J: Excellent local control with involved-field radiotherapy following CHOP chemotherapy: Analysis of 145 patients with early-stage intermediate-grade non-Hodgkin's lymphoma. *Int J Radiat Oncol Biol Phys.* 2001;51:362a.

134. Kamath S, Marcus RJ, Lynch J, et al: The impact of radiotherapy dose and other treatment-related and clinical factors on in-field control in stage I and II non-Hodgkin's lymphoma. *Int J Radiat Oncol Biol Phys.* 1999;44:563.

135. Wilder RB, Tucker SL, Ha CS, et al: Dose-response analysis for radiotherapy delivered to patients with intermediate-grade and large-cell immunoblastic lymphomas that have completely responded to CHOP-based induction chemotherapy. *Int J Radiat Oncol Biol Phys.* 2001;49:17.

136. Fisher RI, Gaynor ER, Dahlberg S, et al: Comparison of a standard regimen (CHOP) with three intensive chemotherapy regimens for advanced non-Hodgkin's lymphoma. *New Engl J Med.* 1993;328:1002.

137. Shipp MA, Klatt MM, Yeap B, et al: Patterns of relapse in large-cell lymphoma patients with bulk disease: Implications for the use of adjuvant radiation therapy. *J Clin Oncol.* 1989;7:613.

138. Yahalom J: Radiation therapy in the treatment of lymphoma. *Curr Opin Oncol.* 1999;11:370.

139. Aviles A, Delgado S, Nambo MJ, et al: Adjuvant radiotherapy to sites of previous bulky disease in patients stage IV diffuse large cell lymphoma. *Int J Radiat Oncol Biol Phys.* 1994;30:799.

140. Ferreri AJM, Dell'Oro S, Reni G, et al: The role of consolidation radiotherapy in the management of stage III-IV diffuse large-cell lymphoma. *Oncology.* 2000;58:219.

141. Fouillard L, Laporte JP, Labopin M, et al: Autologous stem-cell transplantation for non-Hodgkin's lymphomas: The role of graft purging and radiotherapy posttransplantation-results of a retrospective analysis on 120 patients autografted in a single institution. *J Clin Oncol.* 1998;16:2803.

142. Campo E, Raffeld M, Jaffe E: Mantle-cell lymphoma. *Semin Hematol.* 1999;36:115.

143. Vandenberghe E, De Wolf-Peeters C, Vaughan Hudson G, et al: The clinical outcome of 65 cases of mantle cell lymphoma initially treated with non-intensive therapy by the British National Lymphoma Investigation Group. *Br J Haematol.* 1997; 99:842.

144. Meusers P, Engelhard M, Bartels H, et al: Multicentre randomized therapeutic trial for advanced centrocytic lymphoma: Anthracycline does not improve the prognosis. *Hematol Oncol.* 1989;7:365.

145. Howard OM, Gribben JG, Neuberg DS, et al: Rituximab and CHOP induction therapy for newly diagnosed mantle-cell lymphoma: Molecular complete responses are not predictive of progression-free survival. *J Clin Oncol.* 2002;20:1288.

146. Khouri I, Romaguera J, Kantarjian H, et al: Hyper-CVAD and high-dose methotrexate/cytarabine followed by stem-cell transplantation: An active regimen for aggressive mantle-cell lymphoma. *J Clin Oncol.* 1998;16:3803.

147. Slater DE, Mertelsmann R, Koziner B, et al: Lymphoblastic lymphoma in adults. *J Clin Oncol.* 1986;4:57.

148. Morel P, Lepage E, Brice P, et al: Prognosis and treatment of lymphoblastic lymphoma in adults: A report on 80 patients. *Clin Oncol.* 1992;10:1078.

149. Straus DJ, Wong GY, Liu J, et al: Small non-cleaved cell lymphoma (undifferentiated lymphoma, Burkitt's type) in American adults: Results with treatment designed for acute lymphoblastic leukemia. *Am J Med.* 1991;90:328.

150. Wollner N, Wachtel AE, Exelby PR, et al: Improved prognosis in children with intra-abdominal non-Hodgkin's lymphoma following LSA2-L2 protocol chemotherapy. *Cancer.* 1980; 45:3034.

151. d'Amore F, Christensen BE, Brinker H, et al: Clinicopathological features and prognostic factors in extranodal non-Hodgkin's lymphomas. *Eur J Cancer.* 1991;27:1201.

152. Otter R, Gerrits WB, Sandt MM, et al: Primary extranodal and nodal non-Hodgkin's lymphoma: A survey of population-based registry. *Eur J Cancer.* 1989;25:1203.

153. Gospadarowicz MK, Sutcliffe SB: The extranodal lymphomas. *Semin Radiat Oncol.* 1995;5:281.

154. d'Amore F, Brincker M, Gronbaek K, et al: Non-Hodgkin's lymphoma of the gastrointestinal tract: A population-based analysis of incidence, geographic distribution, clinicopathologic presentation features, and prognosis. *J Clin Oncol.* 1994;12:1673.

155. Doglioni C, Wotherspoon AC, Moschini A, et al: High incidence of primary gastric lymphoma in northeastern Italy. *Lancet.* 1992; 339:834.

156. Caletti G, Ferrari A, Brocchi E, Barbara L: Accuracy of endoscopic ultrasonography in the diagnosis and staging of gastric cancer and lymphoma. *Surgery.* 1991;113:14.

157. Thirlby RC: Gastrointestinal lymphoma: A surgical perspective. *Oncology.* 1993;7:29.

158. Varsos G, Yahalom J: Alternatives in the management of gastric lymphoma. *Leuk Lymph.* 1991;4:1.

159. Brincker H, D'Amore F: A retrospective analysis of treatment outcome in 106 cases of localized gastric non-Hodgkin lymphomas. *Leuk Lymph.* 1994;18:281.

160. Taal BG, Burgers JM: Primary non-Hodgkin's lymphoma of the stomach: Endoscopic diagnosis and the role of surgery. *Scand J Gastroenterol.* 1991;188:33.

161. Maor MH, Velasquez WS, Fuller LM, Silvermintz KB: Stomach conservation in stages IE and IIE gastric non-Hodgkin's lymphoma. *J Clin Oncol.* 1990;8:266.

162. Taal BG, Burgers JM, van Heerde P, et al: The clinical spectrum and treatment of primary non-Hodgkin's lymphoma of the stomach. *Ann Oncol.* 1993;4:839.

163. Haim N, Leviov M, Ben-Arieh Y, et al: Intermediate and high-grade gastric non-Hodgkin's lymphoma: A prospective study of non-surgical treatment with primary chemotherapy, with or without radiotherapy. *Leuk Lymph.* 1995;17:321.

164. Walsh JH, Peterson WL: The treatment of *Helicobacter pylori* infection in the management of peptic ulcer disease. *N Engl J Med.* 1995;333:984.

165. Steinbach G, Ford R, Glober G, et al: Antibiotic treatment of gastric lymphoma of mucosa-associated lymphoid tissue. An uncontrolled trial. *Ann Intern Med.* 1999;131:88.

166. Ruskone-Fourmestraux A, Lavergne A, Aegerter PH, et al: Predictive factors for regression of gastric MALT lymphoma after anti-*Helicobacter pylori* treatment. *Gut.* 2001;48:297.

167. Sackmann M, Morgner A, Rudolph B, et al: Regression of gastric MALT lymphoma after eradication of *Helicobacter pylori* is predicted by endosonographic staging. MALT Lymphoma Study Group. *Gastroenterology.* 1997;113:1087.

168. Eidt S, Stolte M, Fischer R: Factors influencing lymph node infiltration in primary gastric malignant lymphoma of the mucosa-associated lymphoid tissue. *Pathol Res Pract.* 1994; 190:1077.

169. Nakamura S, Yao T, Aoyagi K, et al: *Helicobacter pylori* and primary gastric lymphoma. A histopathologic and immunohistochemical analysis of 237 patients. *Cancer.* 1997;79:3.

170. Neubauer A, Thiede C, Morgner A, et al: Cure of *Helicobacter pylori* infection and duration of remission of low-grade gastric mucosa-associated lymphoid tissue lymphoma. *J Natl Cancer Inst.* 1997;89:1350.

171. Ott G, Katzenberger T, Greiner A, et al: The t(11;18)(q21;q21) chromosome translocation is a frequent and specific aberration in low-grade but not high-grade malignant non-Hodgkin's lymphomas of the mucosa-associated lymphoid tissue (MALT) type. *Cancer Res.* 1997;57:3944.

172. Dierlamm J, Baens M, Wlodarska I, et al: The apoptosis inhibitor gene API2 and a novel 18q gene, MALT, are recurrently rearranged in the t(11;18)(q21;q21)p6 associated with mucosa-associated lymphoid tissue lymphomas. *Blood.* 1999;93:3601.

173. Auer IA, Gascoyne RD, Connors JM, et al: t(11;18)(q21;q21) is the most common translocation in MALT lymphomas. *Ann Oncol.* 1997;8:979.

174. Akagi T, Motegi M, Tamura A, et al: A novel gene, MALT1 at 18q21, is involved in t(11;18) (q21;q21) found in low-grade B-cell lymphoma of mucosa-associated lymphoid tissue. *Oncogene.* 1999;18:5785.

175. Liu H, Ye H, Ruskone-Fourmestraux A, et al: T(11;18) is a marker for all stage gastric MALT lymphomas that will not respond to *H. pylori* eradication. *Gastroenterology.* 2002;122:1286.

176. Starostik P, Patzner J, Greiner A, et al: Gastric marginal zone B-cell lymphomas of MALT type develop along 2 distinct pathogenetic pathways. *Blood.* 2002;99:3.

177. Cogliatti SB, Schmid U, Schumacher U, et al: Primary B-cell gastric lymphoma: A clinicopathological study of 145 patients. *Gastroenterology.* 1991;101:1159.

178. Zucca E, Bertoni F, Roggero E, et al: The gastric marginal zone B-cell lymphoma of MALT type. *Blood.* 2000;96:410.

179. Zucca E, Cavalli F: Gut lymphomas. *Baillieres Clin Haematol.* 1996;9:727.

180. Schechter NR, Yahalom J: Low-grade MALT lymphoma of the stomach: A review of treatment options. *Int J Radiat Oncol Biol Phys.* 2000;46:1093.

181. Coiffier B, Salles G: Does surgery belong to medical history for gastric lymphomas? *Ann Oncol.* 1997;8:419.

182. Wotherspoon AC, Doglioni C, Isaacson PG: Low-grade gastric B-cell lymphoma of mucosa-associated lymphoid tissue (MALT): A multifocal disease. *Histopathology.* 1992;20:29.

183. Tsang RW, Gospodarowicz MK, Pintilie M, et al: Stage I and II MALT lymphoma: Results of treatment with radiotherapy. *Int J Radiat Oncol Biol Phys.* 2001;50:1258.

184. Schechter NR, Portlock CS, Yahalom J: Treatment of mucosa-associated lymphoid tissue lymphoma of the stomach with radiation alone. *J Clin Oncol.* 1998;16:1916.

185. Hitchcock S, Ng AK, Fisher DC, et al: Treatment outcome of mucosa-associated lymphoid tissue/marginal zone non-Hodgkin's lymphoma. *Int J Radiat Oncol Biol Phys.* 2002;52:1058.

186. Fung CY, Grossbard ML, Linggood RM, et al: Mucosa-associated lymphoid tissue lymphoma of the stomach: Long term outcome after local treatment. *Cancer.* 1999;85:9.

187. Park HC, Park W, Hahn JS, et al: Low grade MALT lymphoma of the stomach: Treatment outcome with radiotherapy alone. *Yonsei Med J.* 2002;43:601.

188. Yahalom J, Gulati P, Gonzales M, et al: *H. Pylori*-independent MALT lymphoma of the stomach: Excellent outcome with radiation alone. *Blood.* 2002;100:160a.

189. Gospodarowicz MK, Pintilie M, Tsang R, et al: Primary gastric lymphoma: Brief overview of the recent Princess Margaret Hospital experience. *Recent Results Cancer Res.* 2000;156:108.

190. Yahalom J: MALT lymphomas: A radiation oncology viewpoint. *Ann Hematol.* 2001;80:B100.

191. Hammel P, Haioun C, Chaumette MT, et al: Efficacy of single-agent chemotherapy in low-grade B-cell mucosa-associated lymphoid tissue lymphoma with prominent gastric expression. *J Clin Oncol.* 1995;13:2524.

192. Jager G, Neumeister P, Brezinschek R, et al: Treatment of extranodal marginal zone B-cell lymphoma of mucosa-associated lymphoid tissue type with cladribine: A phase II study. *J Clin Oncol.* 2002;20:3872.

193. Conconi A, Thieblemont C, Martinelli AJ, et al: IESLG Phase II Study of Rituximab in MALT Lymphomas. *Ann Oncol.* 2002;13 (Suppl 2):81.

194. Zucca E, Conconi A, Pedrinis E, et al: Non-gastric marginal zone B-cell lymphoma of mucosa-associated lymphoid tissue. *Blood.* 2003;7:2489. Prepublished online as Blood First Edition Paper, November 27, 2002; DOI 10.1182/blood-2002-04-1279.

195. Thieblemont C, Bastion Y, Berger F, et al: Mucosa-associated lymphoid tissue gastrointestinal and nongastrointestinal lymphoma behavior: Analysis of 108 patients. *J Clin Oncol.* 1997;15:1624.

196. Cavalli F, Isaacson PG, Gascoyne RD, et al: MALT lymphomas. *Hematology (Am Soc Hematol Educ Program).* 2001:241.

197. Zinzani PL, Magagnoli M, Galieni P, et al: Nongastrointestinal low-grade mucosa-associated lymphoid tissue lymphoma: Analysis of 75 patients. *J Clin Oncol.* 1999;17:1254.

198. Estevez M, Chu C, Pless M: Small B-cell lymphoma presenting as diffuse dural thickening with cranial neuropathies. *J Neurooncol.* 2002;59:243.

199. Masuda A, Tsujii T, Kojima M, et al: Primary mucosa-associated lymphoid tissue (MALT) lymphoma arising from the male urethra. A case report and review of the literature. *Pathol Res Pract.* 2002;198:571.

200. Suchy BH, Wolf SR: Bilateral mucosa-associated lymphoid tissue lymphoma of the parotid gland. *Arch Otolaryngol Head Neck Surg.* 2000;126:224.

201. Jhavar S, Agarwal JP, Naresh KN, et al: Primary extranodal mucosa associated lymphoid tissue (MALT) lymphoma of the prostate. *Leuk Lymphoma.* 2002;41:445.

202. Agulnik M, Tsang R, Baker MA, et al: Malignant lymphoma of mucosa-associated lymphoid tissue of the lacrimal gland: Case report and review of literature. *Am J Clin Oncol.* 2001;24:67.

203. Brogi E, Harris NL: Lymphomas of the breast: Pathology and clinical behavior. *Semin Oncol.* 1999;26:357.

204. Ansell SM, Grant CS, Habermann TM: Primary thyroid lymphoma. *Semin Oncol.* 1999;26:316.

205. Galieni P, Polito E, Leccisotti A, et al: Localized orbital lymphoma. *Haematologica.* 1997;82:436.

206. Balm AJ, Delaere P, Hilgers FJ, et al: Primary lymphoma of mucosa associated lymphoid tissue (MALT) in the parotid gland. *Clin Otolaryngol.* 1993;18:528.

207. Le QT, Eulau SM, George TI, et al: Primary radiotherapy for localized orbital MALT lymphoma. *Int J Radiat Oncol Biol Phys.* 2002;52:657.

208. Sanjeevi A, Krishnan J, Bailey PR, et al: Extranodal marginal zone B-cell lymphoma of malt type involving the cavernous sinus. *Leuk Lymphoma.* 2001;42:1133.

209. de Bree R, Mahieu HF, Ossenkoppele GJ, et al: Malignant lymphoma of mucosa-associated lymphoid tissue in the larynx. *Eur Arch Otorhinolaryngol.* 1998;255:368.

Mycosis Fungoides

Richard T. Hoppe, MD and Youn Kim, MD

62

EPIDEMIOLOGY, ETIOLOGY, GENETICS, AND CYTOGENETIC ABNORMALITIES

Mycosis fungoides is a rare lymphoma. The estimated annual incidence rate in the United States is 0.29 per 100,000, or fewer than 1000 new cases diagnosed each year.[1] It accounts for only 2% of new cases of non-Hodgkin's lymphoma. Although it is uncommon, it is the most common of the primary cutaneous T-cell lymphomas (CTCLs) and is distinguished from other CTCLs by its unique clinical and histologic features. It commonly affects older adults (median age 55 to 60 years); however, it may present in younger individuals with similar clinical findings and course.[2] There is a 2:1 male predominance, without an established racial predilection.

The etiologies of mycosis fungoides and Sézary syndrome are unknown. Some retrospective studies have suggested an etiologic role for environmental chemical exposure, as a source of either chronic antigenic stimulation or toxic exposure. However, recent case-controlled studies failed to reveal any relation between occupational or recreational exposures to chemicals and the development of mycosis fungoides, refuting this hypothesis.[3,4]

A viral etiology for mycosis fungoides was once proposed, based on the isolation of human T-cell leukemia/lymphoma virus 1 (HTLV-1) from the peripheral blood lymphocytes of a patient with a cutaneous lymphoma that resembled mycosis fungoides.[5] However, it was later demonstrated that this patient actually had a non–mycosis fungoides peripheral T-cell lymphoma with skin involvement. The clinical characteristics of this distinct entity, HTLV-1–associated T-cell lymphoma, have now been described more precisely and are quite different from those of typical mycosis fungoides.

A few studies have demonstrated histocompatibility antigen associations linked to mycosis fungoides and Sézary syndrome, in particular Aw31, Aw32, B8, Bw38, and DR5.[6,7] The significance of these immunogenetic findings is unclear but may suggest a genetic predisposition. Specific chromosomal abnormalities also have been demonstrated in some cases, mostly deletions and translocations in chromosome 1 or 6. In one series, the presence of clonal abnormalities in 11 of 19 patients correlated with advanced-stage disease and a significantly reduced survival.[8] In a second study, the detection of a chromosomal clone preceded relapse or progression of the disease.[9]

Cytokines have been implicated in the pathophysiology of mycosis fungoides and Sézary syndrome.[10-12] However, whether cytokine abnormalities are primarily involved or are secondary processes in the pathogenesis is unclear. Studies have reported that soluble interleukin-2 (IL-2) receptor (sIL-2R) values in Sézary syndrome were significantly higher than for other malignant or inflammatory T-cell diseases and that the serum levels correlated with clinical course and Sézary cell count. The highest sIL-2R levels were found in patients with advanced disease.[12] Other investigators have shown that peripheral blood mononuclear cells from patients with the Sézary syndrome expressed higher levels of IL-4 and lower levels of IL-2 and interferon gamma after phytohemagglutinin (PHA) stimulation, compared to normal controls.[10]

A number of studies have suggested that the malignant T-cells in Sézary syndrome account for aberrant cytokine production, with increased production of T helper type 2 cytokines (e.g., IL-4, IL-5, IL-10) and decreased production of T helper type 1 cytokines (e.g., IL-2 and interferon gamma).[13,14] Moreover, this aberrant cytokine production may cause the immune abnormalities seen occasionally in Sézary syndrome. These immune abnormalities may include decreased T-cell responses to antigens and mitogens, impaired cell-mediated cytotoxicity, including natural killer cell and lymphokine-activated killer cell activities, increased levels of serum IgE and IgA, and peripheral eosinophilia.

PATHOLOGY

A diagnosis of mycosis fungoides or Sézary syndrome may be suspected in patients who present with chronic, nonspecific dermatitis or generalized erythroderma. However, similar skin lesions can be seen in patients who have benign skin conditions, such as psoriasis, parapsoriasis, eczematous dermatitis, photodermatitis, or drug reactions. Rarely, patients can present initially with cutaneous tumors, referred to as *d'emblée* presentation. However, such a presentation is more suggestive of a non–mycosis fungoides CTCL.

Skin biopsy with routine histology is still considered the most important study to assist the clinician in establishing the diagnosis. The characteristic histopathology of mycosis fungoides demonstrates abnormal cells infiltrating the epidermis (epidermotropism) as single cells or in

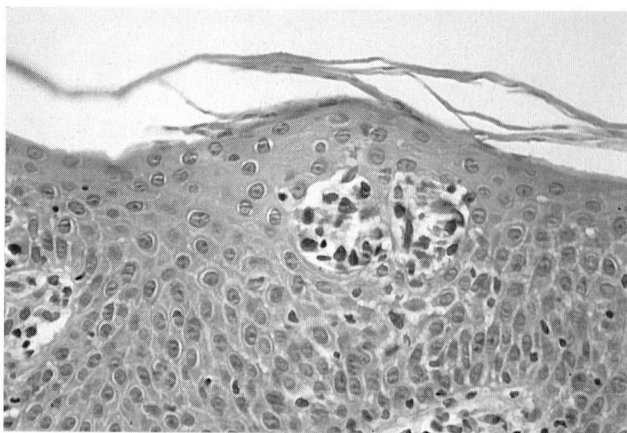

Figure 62–1. The classical biopsy findings in mycosis fungoides include atypical cells in the epidermis, sometimes forming clusters (Pautrier's microabscesses), and an infiltrate of similar cells in the upper dermis.

clusters (Pautrier's microabscesses) (Fig. 62-1). Typically, there is also an upper dermal infiltrate that includes cells similar to those seen in the epidermis, as well as variable proportions of histiocytes, eosinophils, and plasma cells. The criteria for a diagnosis of mycosis fungoides vary among pathologists. Based on the severity of the epidermal and dermal involvement, the categories "diagnostic of," "consistent with," and "suggestive of" mycosis fungoides have been recommended.[15] Treatment programs specific for mycosis fungoides should be considered only in patients who have a biopsy that is diagnostic of or consistent with, not merely suggestive of, mycosis fungoides.

The neoplastic cells of mycosis fungoides are mononuclear cells. Under oil immersion light microscopy, the nuclei of these cells have a hyperconvoluted surface. Electron microscopic studies demonstrate marked infolding of the nuclear membrane, and on three-dimensional reconstruction, there is a cerebriform appearance.

Immunoperoxidase staining indicates that the majority of cases of mycosis fungoides are associated with the helper T-cell phenotype (CD4+) and are also positive for CD2, CD3, CD45, and CD5. These cells may also be positive for CD25 and the p55 (alpha chain) subunit of the interleukin (IL)-2 receptor.[16] Usually, although the neoplastic cells of mycosis fungoides retain the CD4 antigen on their cell surface, they lose other mature T-cell antigens, such as Leu-8 or Leu-9 (CD7). The loss of these mature T-cell antigens may help in the differential diagnosis of mycosis fungoides from benign dermatoses. Rare cases of mycosis fungoides have been demonstrated to be CD8+ (cytotoxic/suppressor T-cell phenotype).

Evaluation of skin biopsies to detect T-cell receptor (TCR) gene rearrangements (genotyping) can be helpful in the differential diagnosis of early mycosis fungoides. TCR gene rearrangements can be detected by Southern blot analysis[17] or by methods using polymerase chain reaction (PCR) amplification.[18] PCR amplification methods for frozen or paraffin tissue analysis are widely available and affordable. Genotyping is becoming an important diagnostic procedure whenever the routine histology or immunophenotyping is equivocal in patients whose clinical presentation is strongly suggestive of mycosis fungoides or Sézary syndrome.

The pathology of extracutaneous disease poses special problems. In the most common situation, enlarged lymph nodes may be biopsied and demonstrate changes of dermatopathic lymphadenitis, including the presence of sinus histiocytosis and an abundance of pigment-laden macrophages. In addition, there may be a variable number of atypical lymphocytes with cerebriform nuclei. The prognostic relevance of different degrees of infiltration by these abnormal cells led to the development of a lymph node classification system. In this system, lymph nodes are classified as LN-0 to LN-4 to correspond with lymph node involvement ranging from "no atypical lymphocytes" (LN-0) to "complete replacement of nodal architecture by atypical lymphocytes or frankly neoplastic cells" (LN-4). This descriptive system for grading lymph node involvement has been shown to have prognostic relevance.[19] Detection of abnormal cells in the lymph node is facilitated by the use of Southern blot or PCR analysis. Potential neoplastic involvement with clonal TCR rearrangement may be demonstrated even in lymph nodes that show only dermatopathic changes in routine evaluation.[20] However, the clinical implication of lymph node involvement that is detectable only at the molecular level is unclear, and usually is not associated with as severe an impact on prognosis as when involvement is detected by routine light microscopy.

Flow cytometry studies of the peripheral blood may show expansion of the CD4+CD7-population reflective of circulating atypical lymphocytes of Sézary type.[21] Patients may have atypical lymphocytes with cerebriform nuclei, the Sézary cells, in their peripheral blood. It is controversial as to how many or what percentage of Sézary cells constitutes a significant level to define the Sézary syndrome, and low levels of Sézary-like cells can be detected in the peripheral blood of patients with benign skin conditions.[22] Although the original National Cancer Institute (NCI) classification used the criterion of greater than 5 percent of lymphocytes for significant blood involvement,[23] the current practice by many mycosis fungoides referral centers is to use an absolute Sézary cell count of >1000/μL or a CD4+:CD8+ T-cell ratio >10 for defining peripheral blood involvement.

CLINICAL PRESENTATION

Mycosis fungoides often has a long natural history, and the median duration from the onset of skin symptoms to a diagnosis of mycosis fungoides may be 5 years or longer.[24] In many patients, the disease presents initially in a premycotic phase with nonspecific, slightly scaling skin lesions that wax and wane over a period of years. Biopsies are generally nondiagnostic during this phase of disease, and patients may respond to treatment with topical corticosteroids. Some of these patients will experience an evolution of their disease and develop more typical patches or infiltrated plaques, from which a definitive diagnostic biopsy may be obtained. Repeated biopsies must be obtained from patients suspected of having mycosis fungoides, even when an initial biopsy is negative.

The most common initial cutaneous presentation is patch and plaque disease; however, some patients may present with tumors or generalized erythroderma.

There may be prominent poikiloderma (skin atrophy with telangiectasia) or associated alopecia or follicular mucinosis. Approximately 25% to 30% of patients will present with limited patch/plaque disease (<10% of the skin surface involved, T1), 35% to 40% with generalized patch/plaque (>10% of the skin surface involved, T2), 15% to 20% with tumorous (T3), and 15% to 20% with erythroderma (T4).

The typical patches of mycosis fungoides are slightly scaling and mildly erythematous. More infiltrated lesions evolve into palpable plaques. These plaques are erythematous and slightly scaling, with well-defined borders. The shape and distribution of lesions are variable. Many patients present with involvement in the "bathing trunk" distribution, although lesions may be present on any part of the body. Pruritus is the most common symptom, even in the early phases of the disease, and is often the problem that prompts a visit to the dermatologist.

Infiltrated plaques may evolve into ulcerating or fungating tumors. However, the majority of patients with initial patch or plaque disease treated at Stanford University never progressed to have more advanced cutaneous disease.[25,26] Tumors often become infected, and sepsis secondary to infection is often the cause of death in individuals so affected. Occasional patients present de novo with tumors, so-called *tumor d'emblee*. Generalized dermal thickening from infiltrative disease may cause the classic but very unusual leonine facies of mycosis fungoides.

Another manifestation of skin involvement in mycosis fungoides is generalized erythroderma. The erythema may be accompanied by either atrophic or lichenified skin, and plaques or tumors may also be present. These patients are almost always intensely symptomatic from pruritus and scaling, and often have lymphadenopathy due to diffuse and severe skin involvement. Many of these patients also have circulating abnormal cells in the peripheral blood that have the same microscopic appearance, immunophenotyping, and genotyping characteristics as the cells that infiltrate the epidermis. Patients with this complex of findings, generalized erythroderma, lymphadenopathy, and atypical T-cells (Sézary cells) in the peripheral blood have Sézary syndrome.[27] Patients with Sézary syndrome have a worse prognosis than erythrodermic patients with mycosis fungoides who do not have the other findings of the Sézary syndrome.

Although many patients demonstrate only the patch or plaque phase of skin involvement throughout the duration of their disease, some progress from patch/plaque to tumor phase. The rapidity of this progression is unpredictable. Patients with erythroderma usually present in that phase of skin involvement, but some may develop erythroderma superimposed over plaque or tumorous disease later during the course of their illness.

ROUTES OF SPREAD

Many patients with mycosis fungoides will have evidence of cutaneous disease only throughout the course of their disease. Although molecular studies may reveal extracutaneous disease to be present in a significant proportion of patients, only 15% to 20% of patients with mycosis fungoides will develop clinical problems related to extracutaneous disease during their lifetime. The likelihood of developing extracutaneous disease is related to the extent of skin involvement. In a series of patients at Stanford with extracutaneous disease, none had limited plaque disease, 11 had generalized plaque disease, 39 had cutaneous tumors, and 27 patients had erythroderma.[28] The most commonly identified route of extracutaneous spread of mycosis fungoides is to the regional lymphatics, usually in areas that drain significant sites of skin involvement. Visceral disease may be identified subsequently. The most common visceral sites of involvement identified are the lungs, oral cavity/pharynx, and the central nervous system, but virtually any organ may be involved at autopsy in patients who have died of the disease.[29]

The risk of disease progression in 525 patients with mycosis fungoides treated at Stanford has been analyzed. Patients were considered to have had disease progression when one of the following events occurred: progression of their mycosis fungoides to a more advanced tumor node metastases blood (TNMB) classification, a more advanced clinical stage, or death due to mycosis fungoides. The actuarial risk of disease progression at 10 years was 13% in limited plaque; 32% in generalized plaque; 72% in tumorous; and 57% for patients with erythroderma.[30]

The actuarial risk for developing extracutaneous disease in our 491 patients who presented with stage I to III disease was analyzed according to their initial T classification. The risk at 10 years was 2% in limited plaque, 9% in generalized plaque, 40% in tumorous, and 10% in patients with erythroderma. However, at the time these patients developed extracutaneous disease, none had limited plaque disease.[30]

DIAGNOSTIC AND STAGING STUDIES

The standard staging evaluation for patients with mycosis fungoides includes a comprehensive physical examination with careful examination of the skin (including the scalp, palms, soles, and perineum) and lymph nodes, a complete blood count with Sézary cell studies, screening chemistries (including lactate dehydrogenase [LDH]), and chest x-ray. Based on observations that it is unlikely for patients with T1 or T2 skin involvement to present with extracutaneous disease at diagnosis, additional imaging studies (computed tomography [CT] or magnetic resonance imaging [MRI]) or nuclear medicine scans (positron emission tomography [PET] or gallium) are not recommended unless the patient has lymphadenopathy. Since patients with T3 or T4 disease are at greater risk for extracutaneous involvement, further imaging studies should be considered. At Stanford we obtain a chest/abdomen/pelvis CT scan in these patients. The use of nuclear medicine scans such as PET have not been established but are being studied. Lymph node biopsies should be obtained if lymphadenopathy is present, since the presence of lymph node involvement affects the stage, prognosis, and management. Suspected sites of visceral involvement must be confirmed by appropriate imaging studies and biopsy when possible. Bone marrow involvement may often be detected in patients who meet the clinical criteria for Sézary syndrome[31] but is extremely uncommon in classical mycosis fungoides. Therefore, a bone marrow biopsy is not routinely used as part of the initial staging procedure for patients with mycosis fungoides.

STAGING SYSTEM

A tumor-node-metastasis-blood (TNMB) staging system that has proved useful for mycosis fungoides was proposed at the Workshop on Mycosis Fungoides held at the National Cancer Institute in 1978.[23] Tables 62-1 and 62-2 summarize the TNMB categories and staging classification.

The *T* classification reflects the extent and type of skin involvement. The *N* category indicates the presence or absence of lymph node involvement. Enlarged lymph nodes should always be biopsied, since palpable enlargement is often associated only with changes of dermatopathic lymphadenitis and not frank involvement by mycosis fungoides. In the *M* category, suspected disease should always be documented by biopsy. Treatment programs for visceral disease should be considered only if definite proof of such disease exists. In the *B* (blood) category, the absence or presence of a significant proportion of abnormal, cerebriform (Sézary) cells should be noted. Low levels of Sézary-like cells can be detected in the peripheral blood of patients with benign skin conditions. The current practice by many mycosis fungoides referral centers is to use a criterion of at least 20% lymphocytes an absolute Sézary count of at least 1000/mm^3, or a CD4+:CD8+ T-cell ratio >10 to define peripheral blood involvement.

STANDARD THERAPEUTIC APPROACHES

The nonspecific, symptomatic treatment of mycosis fungoides and Sézary syndrome is an integral component of the overall therapeutic regimen. Pruritus and xerosis,

Table 62–1 TNMB Classification for Mycosis Fungoides

T (Skin)

T1	Limited patch/plaque (<10% of total skin surface)
T2	Generalized patch/plaque (≥10% of total skin surface)
T3	Tumors
T4	Generalized erythroderma

N (Nodes)

N0	Lymph nodes clinically uninvolved
N1	Lymph nodes enlarged, histologically uninvolved (includes "reactive" and "dermatopathic" nodes)
N2	Lymph nodes clinically uninvolved, histologically involved
N3	Lymph nodes enlarged and histologically involved

M (Viscera)

M0	No visceral involvement
M1	Visceral involvement

B (Blood)

B0	No circulating atypical (Sézary) cells (<5% of total lymphocytes)
B1	Circulating atypical (Sézary) cells (≥5% of total lymphocytes)

Table 62–2 Clinical Staging System for Mycosis Fungoides

Clinical Stages	TNM Classification*		
IA	T1	N0	M0
IB	T2	N0	M0
IIA	T1–2	N1	M0
IIB	T3	N0–1	M0
IIIA	T4	N0	M0
IIIB	T4	N1	M0
IVA	T1–4	N2–3	M0
IVB	T1–4	N0–3	M1

*The B classification does not alter clinical stage.

either as a result of the disease or therapy, may be severe. Thus, supportive measures such as aggressive emolliation, topical steroids, and oral antipruritics should be used as necessary.

Multiple therapeutic options exist for mycosis fungoides and the Sézary syndrome. Selection of treatment is based primarily on the clinical stage of the disease (Fig. 62-2). However, factors such as access to special treatment approaches, the patient's age, other social and medical problems, and the cost-benefit ratio should also be taken into consideration. For patients with patch or plaque skin involvement (T1 and T2) without extracutaneous disease, the treatment plan may be limited to topical therapeutic measures, whereas patients with any extracutaneous disease should receive systemic (cytotoxic or biologic) therapy as part of their management. There is no evidence that early aggressive combined modality therapy is more effective than conservative sequential therapies in the management of limited or advanced disease.[32] Despite decades of experience in the treatment of mycosis fungoides and Sézary syndrome, well-designed, prospective, controlled clinical studies comparing the efficacy of various therapies are lacking.

TOPICAL CHEMOTHERAPY. Topical nitrogen mustard (mechlorethamine, nitrogen mustard) is a very effective form of topical management for patients with mycosis fungoides.[30,33,34] The activity of intravenous nitrogen mustard as an alkylating agent for the management of systemic malignancy is well documented. The mechanism of action when nitrogen mustard is applied topically for the management of mycosis fungoides is less certain and may not be related simply to its alkylating agent properties. Its activity may be mediated by immune mechanisms or by interaction with the epidermal cell–Langerhans cell–T-cell axis. It may be mixed in water or in an ointment base.

For the aqueous preparation, patients prepare the solution at a concentration of 10 to 20 mg per 100 mL of water and apply it to their skin with a cloth or brush. Nitrogen mustard ointment is prepared by the pharmacist at an initial concentration of 10 to 20 mg of nitrogen mustard per 100 grams of Aquaphor. The aqueous and ointment preparations appear to have similar clinical efficacy, although a prospective comparison has not been performed. The choice often depends on convenience, patient preference, or cost issues. The ointment preparation uses

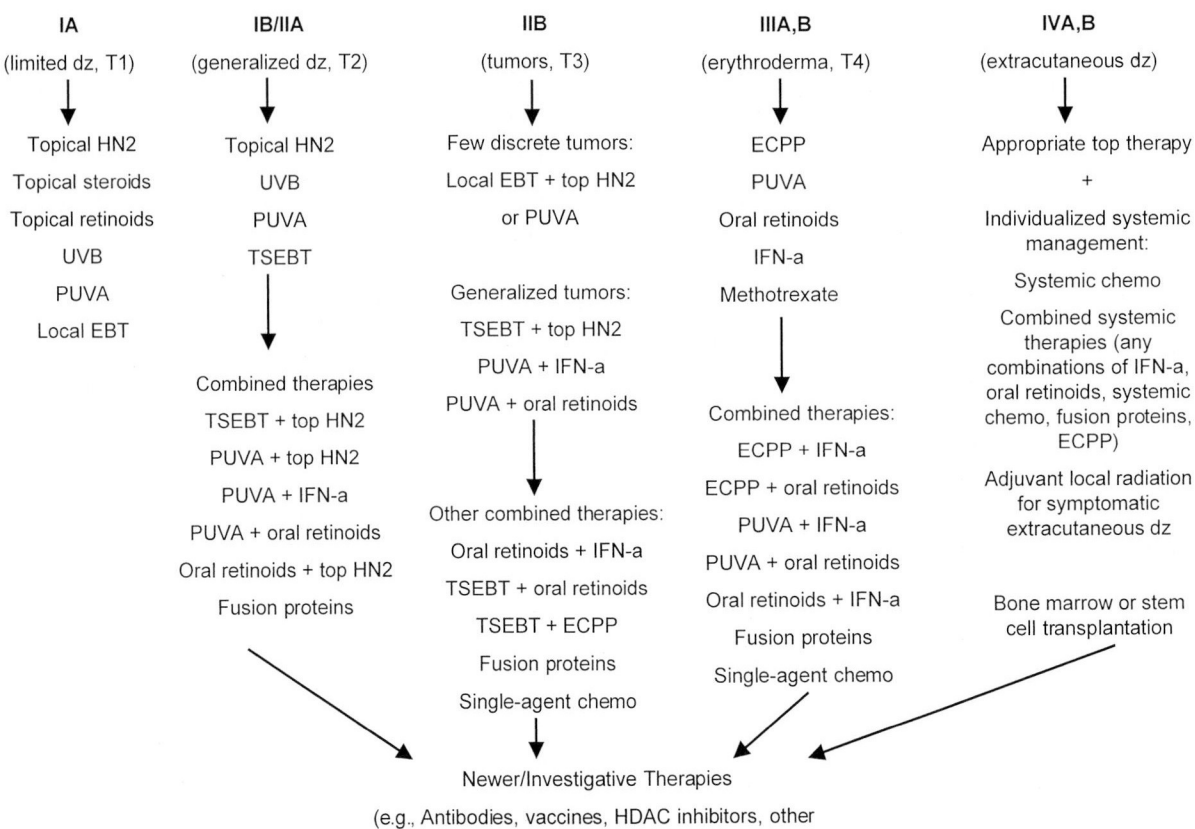

Figure 62–2. An algorithm summarizing management approaches for patients with all stages of mycosis fungoides. Chemo, chemotherapy; dz, disease; EBT, electron beam therapy; ECPP, extracorporeal photopheresis; HN2, nitrogen mustard; IFN-a, alpha interferon; PUVA, psoralens + ultraviolet wavelength A; top, topical; TSEBT, total skin electron beam therapy; UVB, ultraviolet wavelength B.

less nitrogen mustard for a similar response. In addition, the aqueous preparation is associated with much higher incidence (>30%) of hypersensitivity reaction compared with the low-rate (<5%) reported with the ointment preparation.

Nitrogen mustard may be applied locally or to the entire skin. It is applied at least once daily during the clearing phase. Other areas of disease activity may become evident secondary to the inflammatory reaction provoked by the nitrogen mustard. After several weeks, treatment may then be limited to the affected region. Alternatively, if the disease is very limited in distribution, the topical nitrogen mustard may be applied only to the affected anatomic region from the outset, with careful follow-up to detect any new areas of involvement. Treatment is continued on a daily basis until skin clearance is complete. This may require 6 months or longer and is then followed by a variable duration of maintenance therapy (3 to 6 months). There is no evidence that more prolonged maintenance therapy is beneficial. If response is particularly slow, the concentration of the topical nitrogen mustard may be increased to 30% to 40%, especially to small areas, or the frequency of application may be increased to twice a day. The complete response (CR) rate for topical nitrogen mustard for limited patch/plaque (T1) disease is 70% to 80%. The median time to skin clearance is 6 to 8 months. When treatment is discontinued, more than half of patients will relapse in the skin,

but most will respond to a resumption of therapy. The proportion of patients treated with topical nitrogen mustard who have a durable complete response (>10 years) is 20% to 25%.

The primary acute complication of topical nitrogen mustard is a cutaneous hypersensitivity reaction. As noted earlier, this is more common with the aqueous preparation. Desensitization may be achieved by various topical or systemic desensitization programs. There is no systemic absorption of topical nitrogen mustard, thus systemic complications such as bone marrow suppression or sterility are not observed toxicities. Occasional patients treated with topical nitrogen mustard develop secondary squamoproliferative lesions of the skin. This risk is the greatest among patients who have had long-term sequential therapy with multiple topical modalities.

Because of its efficacy and ease of application, topical nitrogen mustard is employed widely as primary or secondary therapy in the management of patients with mycosis fungoides, especially those who have a limited or generalized patch or plaque phase of skin involvement (Fig. 62-2). In patients with a discrete number of refractory lesions, treatment may be supplemented with local irradiation.

Another topical chemotherapeutic agent that has been used for patients with limited disease is carmustine (BCNU).[35] The efficacy of topical BCNU is similar to topical nitrogen mustard; however, because of the systemic absorption of BCNU, the potential hematologic complications are greater, and the maximum duration of treatment is limited. In addition, patients treated with BCNU tend to develop telangiectasia where the drug is applied.

PHOTOTHERAPY. Phototherapy involves using ultraviolet (UV) radiation in the form of UVA or UVB wavelengths, which can be used alone, together, or with psoralen, a photosensitizing agent, as psoralen plus UVA or PUVA. The long-wave UVA has the advantage over UVB in its greater depth of penetration into the dermal infiltrates of mycosis fungoides. For early limited diseases, UVB alone[36] or home UV phototherapy (UVA + UVB)[37] has been shown to be effective.

PUVA is the most commonly used form of phototherapy for mycosis fungoides and Sézary syndrome patients. It was first used in the treatment of psoriasis but has proved effective for patients with mycosis fungoides as well.[38-40] In the presence of UVA, the psoralen drug intercalates with DNA, forming both monofunctional and bifunctional adducts, which inhibit DNA synthesis.

The technique of treatment is for the patient to ingest the psoralen drug (usually 8-methoxypsoralen) followed by controlled exposure to UVA in a specially designed light box (PUVA box). Only the eyes are shielded routinely. All other body surfaces may be treated; however, selected areas can be shielded to minimize undesired photodamage. Certain "shadowed" areas such as the scalp, perineum, axillae, and other skin fold areas will not receive adequate exposure. During the clearing phase, which may require up to 6 months, patients are treated two to three times weekly. After the clearing phase has been completed, patients continue on a maintenance program with decreased frequency of treatment. If the disease begins to recur during the maintenance phase, then the frequency of treatment is increased in an effort to achieve better control.

With PUVA treatment, the complete clearance rate is 50% to 90% in patients with patch or plaque disease, with the likelihood of clearance dependent on the initial extent of skin involvement. The response is less impressive in patients with erythrodermic or tumor disease.

Indications for PUVA treatment include its use as the primary therapy for patients with limited or generalized patch or plaque disease or as a secondary therapy following the failure of other topical modalities. PUVA may also be effective for patients with erythroderma, provided that very low daily exposures are used to avoid phototoxic reactions. For patients with Sézary syndrome, PUVA may be supplemented by systemic biologic therapies, such as interferon alpha (IFN-alpha) or systemic retinoids.[41,42] The treatment of patients with more advanced cutaneous disease may be facilitated by the addition of localized irradiation to particular refractory plaques or tumors.

The primary acute complications of PUVA therapy include nausea and phototoxic reactions such as erythroderma and blistering as well as skin dryness. Patients should shield their skin and eyes from the sun for at least 24 hours following psoralen ingestion. The potential long-term complications of PUVA therapy include cataract formation (requiring the use of UVA-opaque goggles during therapy) and secondary cutaneous malignancies. Among patients treated for mycosis fungoides, this risk is greatest for patients who have undergone long-term treatment with multiple topical therapies.[43]

PUVA may often be used in combination with other therapies, such as interferon or retinoids. For the combined regimen with PUVA, IFN-alpha and PUVA therapy are initiated concurrently, each usually given thrice weekly. When skin clearance is complete, the frequency of PUVA treatment is reduced. Complete and partial response (PR) rates of 79% to 80% and 14% to 20% in patients with generalized patch/plaque (stages IB and IIA) disease treated with the combination of IFN-alpha and PUVA have been reported.[41] The clinical response and response duration results may be better with the combined regimen of PUVA and IFN-alpha compared to either treatment alone; however, prospective randomized clinical trials are needed to confirm this impression.[44,45]

When retinoids are used in combination with PUVA (RePUVA), the response rate is similar to that of PUVA alone; however, the responses may be achieved with fewer PUVA treatments and with lower cumulative UVA dose.[42] The duration of remission may be more prolonged if retinoids are given as maintenance therapy.

TOPICAL RETINOIDS. Bexarotene (Targretin) 1% gel is the most commonly used topical retinoid for treating mycosis fungoides. The reported overall response (OR) rate is 63% with a CR rate of 21%.[46] Due to the irritant effect of the retinoids, it is only feasible to use this agent when there are discrete patches or plaques. It is not intended for generalized application. Bexarotene gel is applied with a thin application to the patches or plaques and is most effective and best tolerated when used twice daily. The most common toxicity is irritation at the site of gel application, which occurs in the majority of patients with variable intensity. Because of the erythema from the irritant reaction, it may be necessary to withhold therapy for a few weeks to assess for residual active disease.

RADIATION THERAPY. Mycosis fungoides is an exquisitely radiosensitive neoplasm, and irradiation may be exploited in several ways for its management.[15] Individual plaques or tumors of mycosis fungoides may be treated with orthovoltage or electron beam radiation therapy (electron beam therapy) to total doses of 15 to 25 Gy in 1 to 3 weeks, with a high likelihood of achieving long-term local control. Electrons have an intrinsic advantage over photons in the treatment of mycosis fungoides since the depth of penetration of electrons can be controlled by the appropriate selection of electron energy, whereas the relative dose contribution to the subcutaneous and deeper tissues is greater with even low-energy photons. For indurated plaques, electron energies as low as 6 MeV are generally sufficient. Use of bolus may be indicated due to the relative "skin-sparing" effect of low energy electrons. For the unusual patient with unilesional or localized mycosis fungoides, local electron beam therapy achieves the most efficient and complete clearance of the disease.

Several centers have developed expertise in the use of total skin electron beam therapy.[47,48] OR rates are nearly 100%, with CR rates ranging from 40% to 98%, depending on the extent of skin involvement. As many as 50% of patients with limited plaque disease and 25% of patients with generalized plaque disease may remain free of disease for more than 5 years after completion of a single course of electron beam therapy. Although the curative potential of this treatment remains disputed, there is no doubt that it provides an important palliative benefit, especially for patients with extensive disease. Often, when disease recurs, it is in a more limited distribution and may be controlled more readily with localized topical therapies.

Total skin electron beam therapy should be considered as initial therapy for patients with very thickened plaques, since the effective depth of treatment of electron beam therapy is more substantial than either topical nitrogen mustard or phototherapy. It is also appropriate for patients with a recent history of rapid progression of disease and for those patients who failed topical nitrogen mustard, bexarotene gel, or phototherapy. Many of these patients would benefit from total skin electron beam therapy for efficient control of disease. Generally, following completion of total skin electron beam therapy, adjuvant treatment with topical nitrogen mustard is indicated and may be continued for up to 6 months.

Some patients may be candidates for a second course of total skin electron beam therapy.[49] Eligibility criteria should include a good response of reasonable duration to the initial course of treatment, failure of other subsequent therapies, and generalized symptomatic skin involvement. These patients will develop more pronounced skin changes secondary to treatment, including more prominent telangiectasia, skin dryness, atrophy, and hair loss.

In patients who have lymph node involvement or in some situations of localized visceral disease, megavoltage (4 to 15 MeV) photon irradiation may be helpful in providing important additional palliation. Doses of 30 to 36 Gy in 3 to 4 weeks are often sufficient to achieve local control of lymph nodes or other extracutaneous sites of disease. This is often combined with systemic chemotherapy or biologic therapy (interferon-alpha or bexarotene), depending on the extent of the extracutaneous involvement.

SYSTEMIC CHEMOTHERAPY. Systemic chemotherapy is most appropriate choice for patients with extracutaneous disease and has only limited indication for patients who have skin disease alone. With combination chemotherapy regimens, overall CR or PR rates can reach 80% to 100%; however, in most cases, the median duration of response is less than a year, and in many patients, less than several months.[50,51] Virtually all single agent and drug combinations that have proved useful in the management of patients with non-Hodgkin's lymphomas have been tested in patients with mycosis fungoides. The most effective and commonly used combinations include cyclophosphamide, vincristine, and prednisone with (CHOP) or without Adriamycin (CVP).[52] Other regimens used include cyclophosphamide, Adriamycin, vincristine, etoposide (CAVE), or CVP with methotrexate (COMP).[32,53,54] Chemotherapy may be used alone or in combination with topical therapy (e.g., radiation) or biologic response modifiers (e.g., IFN-alpha). A randomized trial comparing

electron-beam radiation plus chemotherapy with topical therapy in the initial treatment of mycosis fungoides failed to demonstrate an improved survival with the more aggressive management approach.[32]

Methotrexate, etoposide, bleomycin, vinblastine, or purine analogs (fludarabine, 2'-deoxycoformycin) are the most commonly used single-agent chemotherapy regimens in mycosis fungoides and Sézary syndrome.[50,51] The overall clinical response and response duration tend to be less than those observed with combination chemotherapy regimens. The newer purine analogs show promise in early clinical trials, but complications related to immunosuppression are significant. Fludarabine, which causes profound decreases in peripheral T-cell counts, has demonstrated clinical activity against mycosis fungoides, chronic lymphocytic leukemia, and the low-grade lymphomas.[55] Another drug that may be useful is 2'-deoxycoformycin, which inhibits adenosine deaminase, an enzyme with a high level of activity in T cells, and leads to inhibition of DNA synthesis. The response rate may be as high as 50%.[56,57] Recently, single agent gemcitabine has been reported to achieve CR and PR rates of 12% and 59%, respectively, with median durations of 15 and 10 months.[58] Another active single agent is liposomal doxorubicin.

In contrast to other non-Hodgkin's lymphomas, autologous bone marrow transplantation (ABMT) has not been actively investigated in mycosis fungoides and Sézary syndrome. In a study of six mycosis fungoides patients with advanced, extracutaneous disease, autologous bone marrow transplantation was successfully performed and managed without life-threatening complications.[59] Five of the six patients had complete clinical responses, although three of those responses lasted less than 100 days. In another series of nine patients, transplant-related mortality was 11%, eight of nine patients achieved a CR, but seven of the eight relapsed at a median interval of 7 months.[60]

The ablative regimen used in these autologous bone marrow transplants were combinations of total skin electron beam therapy, total body irradiation, and various combinations of cyclophosphamide, etoposide, carmustine, and cisplatin. Further studies are necessary to determine the role of autologous bone marrow transplantation in the treatment of this disease.

EXTRACORPOREAL PHOTOPHERESIS (ECPP). Photopheresis (ECPP or systemic photochemotherapy) is a method of delivering PUVA systemically via an extracorporeal technique.[61] The patient's white blood cells are collected (leukapheresis), exposed to a photoactivating drug, and then irradiated with UVA. Then the irradiated cells are returned to the patient. The mechanism of action of ECPP remains unclear. It is hypothesized that there may be a dual effect: a direct cytotoxic or antiproliferative effect on the neoplastic cells and an immune-enhancing effect on the competent lymphocytes against the neoplastic cells. Photopheresis is usually administered every 4 weeks, but in patients with severe disease, the frequency can be as often as every 2 to 3 weeks. Once complete clearance is achieved, the frequency can be gradually reduced and then discontinued.

Compared with other systemic therapies, ECPP has minimal adverse effects.[61] Some patients may experience nausea, mostly due to the ingested psoralen, and some have a transient low-grade fever or slight malaise after treatment. There are no reports of any significant organ damage or bone marrow/immune suppression.

In erythrodermic (T4) mycosis fungoides and Sézary syndrome, ECPP may be the initial treatment of choice.[62,63] Its effectiveness in T1, T2, and T3 diseases remains unclear. The largest study of erythrodermic patients revealed that the majority experienced some level of response to ECPP, with an OR rate of 83%.[64] The CR rate was only 21%, but 41% of patients showed at least a 50% improvement in their skin disease. If the response to ECPP alone is partial or slow, IFN-alpha can be added as a combined modality regimen.[65] The dose for IFN-alpha in the combined program is usually low, 1.5 to 5 million units three to five times weekly, not exceeding 10 million units per dose. The addition of other biologic therapies, such as bexarotene, may also enhance the response.

INTERFERON ALPHA. IFN-alpha is indicated primarily for the palliative management of refractory or advanced disease. It may be used alone or more often combined with topical or other systemic therapies. The dosage of IFN-alpha for mycosis fungoides is usually initiated at 3 to 5 million units daily or three times a week, and is gradually increased, depending on the clinical response and severity of adverse effects. Reported OR rates when used as monotherapy range from 53% to 74%, with CR rates of 21% to 35%.[66,67]

The clinical efficacy of combined IFN-alpha and PUVA has been demonstrated in mycosis fungoides and Sézary syndrome.[41] Patients in clinical stages IB to IVB have been treated, with an OR rate of 85% to 100% and CR rate of 33% to 80%, depending on disease severity.

SYSTEMIC RETINOIDS. Systemic therapy with retinoids, most commonly bexarotene, has been beneficial in the management of mycosis fungoides and Sézary syndrome. The reported response rate is approximately 45%, with a 20% CR rate.[68] Systemic retinoids are indicated for palliative therapy for refractory or advanced disease, often in combination with other topical or systemic therapies, including PUVA (Re-PUVA), IFN-alpha, or total skin electron beam therapy.[42,69-71]

The systemic retinoid most commonly used is bexarotene.[72] This agent is administered orally. The initial dose is 300 mg/m^2 per day, which can be adjusted according to clinical response and the severity of adverse effects. The most common adverse effects include photosensitivity, xerosis, myalgia, arthralgia, headaches, and impaired night vision. The well-known teratogenic effects of retinoids must be carefully addressed in female patients. Because of its potential hepatotoxic and hyperlipidemic effects, liver function and serum lipid levels should be monitored in each patient during treatment. In addition, central hypothyroidism is often induced, so patients are routinely started on levothyroxine (Synthroid) immediately before or simultaneously with bexarotene.

RECOMBINANT FUSION PROTEINS. Recombinant fusion protein therapy, such as the IL-2–diphtheria toxin fusion protein (Ontak, denileukin diftitox), involves the use of growth factor–diphtheria toxin fusion proteins designed specifically to kill defined neoplastic cell populations. Ontak has undergone a multicenter phase III trial in patients with IL-2 receptor (CD25+)-expressing mycosis fungoides.[73] Patients with stage IB to III mycosis fungoides who failed to respond to at least four prior therapies, or stage IVA mycosis fungoides who failed to respond to at least one prior therapy, were included in the phase III trial. The OR rate was 30%, with CR and PR rates of 10% and 20%, respectively. The main complication is related to a "capillary leak" syndrome, which may be ameliorated by pretreatment with corticosteroids.

COMBINED MODALITY THERAPY. Patients who fail to respond to a single-agent topical regimen can be treated with combined modality therapy. This may include combination topical therapies (e.g., total skin electron beam therapy, topical nitrogen mustard, PUVA, bexarotene gel), or combined topical and systemic biologic therapies (e.g., PUVA or total skin electron beam therapy with IFN-alpha or systemic bexarotene).[41,42,69]

Most patients with tumor stage IIB mycosis fungoides have generalized involvement with tumor and plaque disease, and the greatest likelihood of a response is with total skin electron beam therapy. However, in view of the high risk for relapse after irradiation, adjuvant therapy (e.g., topical nitrogen mustard) is generally employed after completion of electron beam therapy. Topical nitrogen mustard in Aquaphor provides the dual benefit of treatment for any residual disease and emolliation of the skin, often chronically dry after completion of electron beam therapy. Patients with a discrete number of tumors may be treated with topical nitrogen mustard or PUVA, combined with localized electron beam therapy to individual tumors. Although topical (nitrogen mustard or PUVA) or systemic (IFN-alpha or photopheresis) adjuvant therapy after skin clearance with total skin electron beam therapy may improve the disease-free interval, it does not improve survival.[74-76]

Patients with recalcitrant disease may require a combination of systemic therapies, either with biologic therapies or a combination of biologic therapies and chemotherapies, with or without topical therapy. IFN-alpha has been used in combination with systemic retinoids with variable results.[70,77] Various chemotherapy regimens have been used in combination with total skin electron beam therapy.[32,78] However, there is no evidence that an aggressive combination regimen employing systemic chemotherapy at the outset results in superior survival.[32] Focal resistant tumors can be boosted with local electron beam therapy or orthovoltage radiation.

PUVA can be given in combination with IFN-alpha. In one of the largest studies of this combination, a CR rate of 33% and PR rate of 50% was observed in patients with stage IIB disease.[41] Studies using PUVA alone for erythrodermic (stage III) patients have reported CR rates of 33% to 70%.[38-40,45,79] Despite these good response rates, the majority of the patients relapse during maintenance therapy. In another study, the CR and PR rates for a combination regimen of PUVA plus IFN-alpha in stage III disease were 62% and 25%, respectively.[41] It is thought that the combined regimen may improve clinical response or response duration beyond that observed with PUVA or interferon alone. However, there is no clear evidence that prolongation of response duration leads to improvement in the overall survival.

TECHNIQUES OF RADIOTHERAPY

Ionizing irradiation is the most effective single agent for the treatment of mycosis fungoides. Reports of dramatic responses to low doses of x-ray therapy (including photo-documentation) appeared within a decade of Roentgen's first discovery of x-irradiation.[80] Clinical dose-time fractionation studies indicate that permanent local control of lesions may be achieved with doses as low as 7 Gy. Reconstruction of data on a semi-log plot of cell survival indicates a Do = 0.90 Gy and *n* (extrapolation number) <2.[81]

For palliative treatment of individual lesions with 100 to 200 Kv x-rays or 6 to 9 MeV electrons, fractionated doses of as low as 15 Gy (e.g., 3 Gy × 5 or 5 Gy × 3) are often adequate to achieve long-term local control. Doses in excess of 30 Gy are rarely required.[82]

The ability to irradiate the entire skin was dependent upon the development of electron beam therapy. By the proper choice of electron energy, the depth dose characteristics of the electron beam make it possible to treat large surfaces of the skin in a single field, concentrating the dose of irradiation in the epidermis and upper dermis, while limiting the dose to the deep dermis and subcutaneous tissue. By using rotational, four-field, six-field, or eight-field techniques, it is possible to irradiate the entire cutaneous surface. The concept of total skin electron beam therapy for the management of mycosis fungoides was first described by Trump et al.[83] using a van de Graaff generator. The more widespread use of total skin electron beam therapy was facilitated by the development of the modern medical linear accelerator. At Stanford, the original Stanford Medical Linear Accelerator was modified to treat the entire skin, first using a four-field technique, and later a six-field technique.[84,85] Modifications of the Stanford technique have been adopted widely for the management of patients with mycosis fungoides.[86-91]

In general, the dosimetry of total skin electron irradiation improves as the number of fields of treatment increases.[92] With four-field treatment, there is significant overlap of adjacent fields, creating "hot spots" that may result in long-term telangiectasia, subcutaneous fibrosis, and even necrosis. These complications may be accentuated by fractionation programs that use larger doses per fraction or fewer fractions per week.

In a typical setup, patients are treated in the standing position at a distance of 3.5 meters from the isocenter (electron source). A 3/8 inch Lucite plate is placed as close as possible to the patient surface in order to degrade and scatter the electrons. During treatment, the machine is angled upward or downward at an angle of 18° to provide for better homogeneity of dose at the patient's

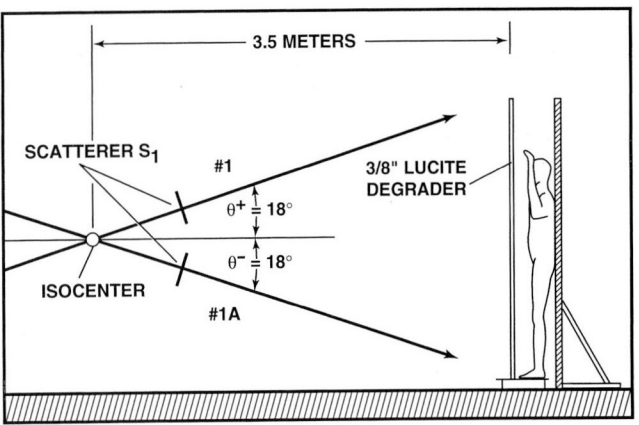

Figure 62–3. A schematic showing a patient in the anterior treatment position during total skin electron beam therapy. The electron beam field is angled upward and downward at an angle of 18 degrees to the horizontal.

surface and to minimize photon contamination, which is greatest in the central axis of the beam (Fig. 62-3).

Patients are treated with a six-field technique that includes anterior, posterior, and four opposed oblique fields (Fig. 62-4).[93] A full "cycle" of treatment is administered over a 2-day period. On day 1, the anterior and two posterior oblique fields are treated at each of the two accelerator angles. On day 2, the posterior and two anterior oblique fields are treated at each of the two accelerator angles. The total dose administered with each cycle is 1.5 to 2 Gy. Most patients will tolerate 2 Gy per cycle, but lower doses are used for patients with erythroderma, atrophic skin, or a previous course of electron beam therapy. The prescribed total dose is generally 36 Gy administered over a 10-week period, with a 1-week split after delivering a dose of 18 to 20 Gy to provide relief from the generalized skin erythema that usually accompanies treatment.

With this technique, certain portions of the body surface are "shadowed" and receive relatively lower total doses of irradiation. These areas include the top of the scalp, perineum, and soles of the feet. Other areas may be problematic in individual patients because of body habitus, such as underneath the breasts of some women and under the panniculus of obese individuals. To compensate for this effect, we routinely treat the perineum and soles of the feet using 6 MeV electrons (with 1 cm tissue-equivalent bolus) with daily fractions of 1 Gy to a total of 20 Gy. Supplemental treatment is provided to the vertex of the scalp only if there is scalp involvement, since permanent alopecia may result. Supplemental treatment also is administered underneath the breasts and panniculus of individual patients, as indicated. In addition, some patients with a discrete number of tumorous lesions will receive boost treatment to these tumors at the outset of electron beam therapy in order to reduce their thickness and permit better penetration by the electrons. Usually, doses of 15 Gy in 1.5 to 3 Gy fractions using 6 to 9 MeV electrons are adequate for this purpose.

In the standard course of treatment, only the eyes are shielded. Internal lead eye shields with an inner paraffin coating are used whenever disease is present on the face

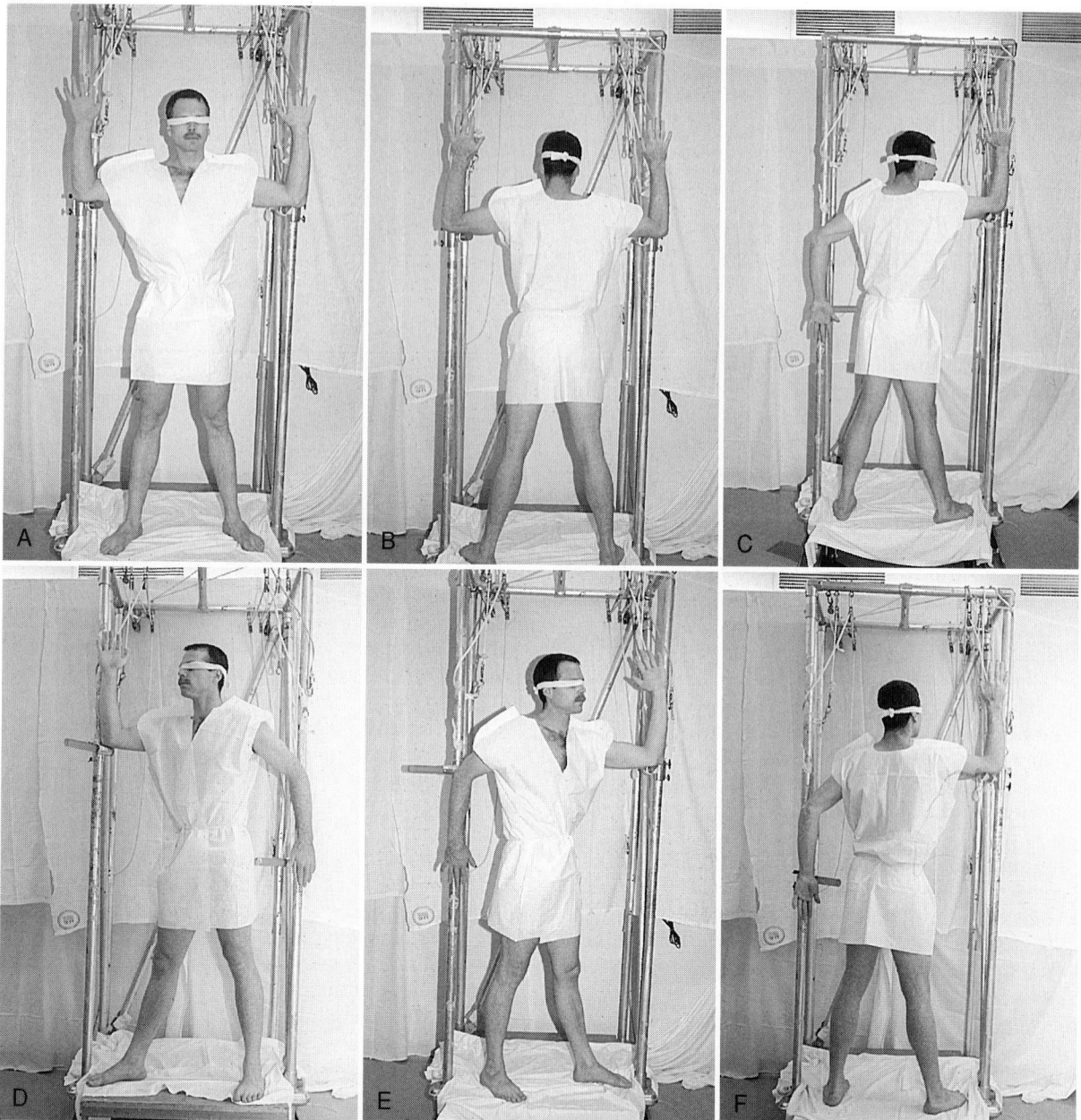

Figure 62–4. The six patient positions assumed for total skin electron beam therapy, including anterior, posterior, and four obliques. Arm and leg positions are designed to expose all body surfaces to some portion of the treatment.

or scalp. The shields are placed under the lids after the eyes have been anesthetized topically. If disease is absent from these areas, external lead eye shields, which are taped over the closed eyes, are used. In addition, in the absence of involvement of the scalp or face, a scalp shield is used after a dose of 25 Gy in order to facilitate adequate regrowth of scalp hair. Complete scalp shielding is contraindicated and may result in extension of disease to this area.[89]

Individualized shielding is used as clinical circumstances demand. For example, some patients develop a more intense skin reaction on the fingers than on other surfaces. This may be minimized by the use of modified lead-lined fluoroscopic gloves. When increased skin reactions are observed in the feet or toes, footboards several

inches in height may be placed behind the Lucite degrader to shield the feet from the electrons. The use of individualized shielding requires careful clinical judgment, taking into account the extent and location of the patient's disease, inherent inhomogeneity of dose on different body surfaces, and the intensity of the local reactions.

The composite depth dose distribution curve for total skin electron beam therapy with 9 MeV electrons using the six–dual field technique, is displayed in Figure 62-5. Using a 9 MeV beam and the six–dual field technique, the 80% dose is located at a depth of 0.7 cm. The 50% depth dose is at 1.25 cm. These depth dose characteristics are ideal for mycosis fungoides, where the malignant infiltrates are generally limited to the epidermis and upper portions of the dermis.

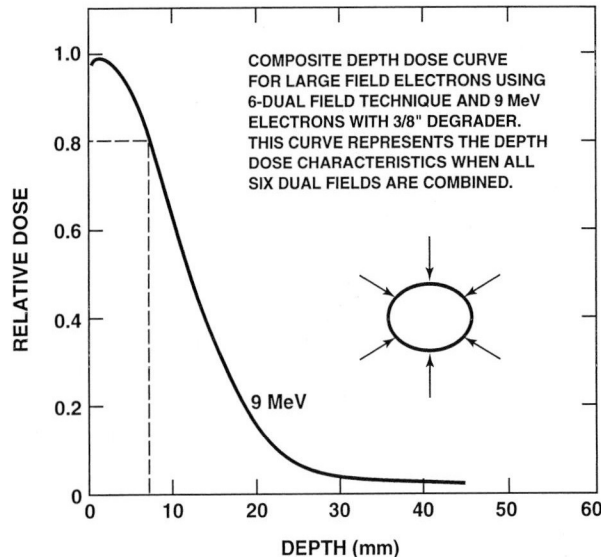

Figure 62–5. Composite depth dose data for 9 MeV total skin electron beam therapy using the six–dual field technique and a 3/8″ Lucite degrader near the patient surface.

Megavoltage photon treatment (energy ≥4 MeV), used judiciously, may provide a very important palliative benefit to patients with extracutaneous disease. Typically, involved lymph nodes may become symptomatic due to bulk. Pain and edema may be problems in this setting. Other patients may develop visceral manifestations, such as gastrointestinal tract involvement. In these situations, effective palliation may be achieved by external beam megavoltage photon irradiation. The fields used are typical of those employed for other lymphomas, including, for example, the mantle, whole abdomen, or pelvis. The dose may be titrated to response, but typically should be 24 to 36 Gy in 1.5 to 2 Gy fractions.

CRITICAL NORMAL TISSUES—RADIATION INJURY

The most common acute complications of this therapy are erythema and dry desquamation.[89,91,93] The severity of these problems can be minimized by proper fractionation techniques. In addition, a 1-week split may be given in the middle of the course of treatment in order to permit skin recovery. Intermediate-term complications include alopecia, which is incomplete and only temporary if the scalp dose is limited to 25 Gy.[91] Most patients will also suffer temporary loss of fingernails and toenails 2 to 4 months following completion of therapy. Most patients report the inability to sweat properly for 6 to 12 months following therapy[94] and chronically dry skin thereafter, which requires the regular use of emolliation. In long-term follow-up, evidence for chronic radiation dermatitis is uncommon in our experience.[95] Occasional patients may display scattered telangiectasia, and rarely these may be evident on casual examination. These skin changes may be more evident with irradiation techniques that employ fewer than six fields or use larger treatment fractions, administered only once weekly. Although secondary

Table 62–3 Survival (%) and Relative Risk of Death for 525 Patients with Mycosis Fungoides Treated at Stanford University

Stage	2 yr	5 yr	15 yr	RR
IA	100	97	75	0.7 (0.4–1.0)
IB/IIA	90	73	43	2.2 (1.8–2.6)
IIB/III	77	44	15	3.9 (3.2–4.6)
IV	43	27	10	12.8 (8.1–17.3)

RR, Relative risk of death (95% confidence interval).

malignancies such as squamous cell and basal cell cancers of the skin are increased after the use of total skin electron beam therapy, the only patients in whom these have become problematic are those who have received repeated treatment with multiple therapies including irradiation, topical nitrogen mustard, and PUVA.[43]

SELECTED OUTCOME

The T-classification and presence of extracutaneous disease are the most important predictors of survival in patients with mycosis fungoides.[30,96] Tables 62-3 and 62-4 display the survival and disease-specific survival as a function of disease stage. Figure 62-6 shows the disease-specific survival for 525 patients treated at Stanford.

STAGE IA (LIMITED PATCH/PLAQUE, T1) DISEASE. Most patients with limited patch/plaque (T1) involvement have stage IA disease. The primary therapies for patients with stage IA (T1) disease are topical. These include topical chemotherapy (mostly nitrogen mustard), phototherapy (UVB or PUVA), bexarotene gel, or localized radiation therapy (usually electron beam). The complete response rate to nitrogen mustard is 60% to 70%[97] and to total skin electron beam therapy is 85% to 95%.[98] However, there is no evidence that any one approach is superior to the others with respect to long-term disease control or survival. Treatment selection is often based on convenience and cost.

Patients with limited patch/plaque (T1, overall stage IA) disease who are treated with conventional therapies have an excellent prognosis with an overall long-term life expectancy that is similar to an age-, gender-, and race-matched control population. In a retrospective study of 122 patients with stage IA disease at Stanford, the median survival was not reached at 33 years.[25] Nearly all patients with stage IA disease who die will die from

Table 62–4 Disease-Specific Survival (%) of 525 Patients with Mycosis Fungoides Treated at Stanford University

Stage	2 yr	5 yr	15 yr
IA	100	100	98
IB	100	95	85
IIA	95	84	71
IIB	83	56	32
III	89	65	49
IV	43	30	14

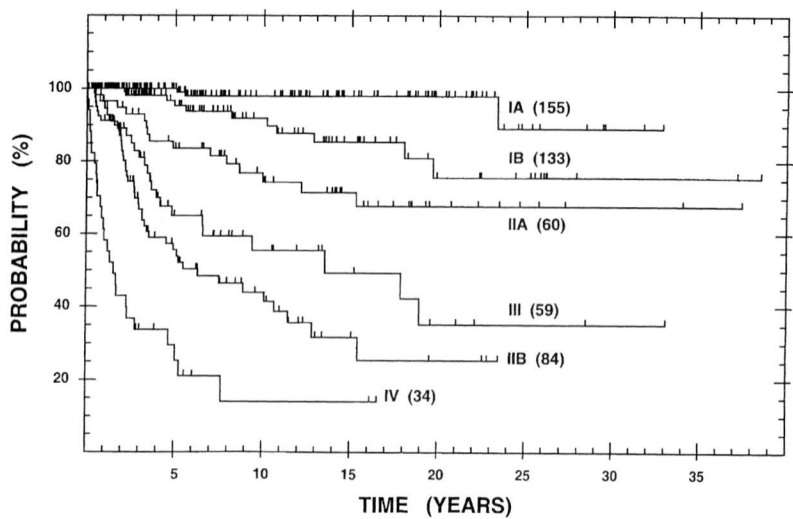

Figure 62–6. Disease-specific survival by initial disease stage for 525 patients with mycosis fungoides treated at Stanford University.

causes other than mycosis fungoides. Furthermore, only 9% of treated patients at this stage will ever progress to a more advanced stage of disease. Early, aggressive therapy with combination chemotherapy does not result in a more favorable survival outcome compared to patients managed more conservatively with sequential topical regimens.[32]

STAGE IB/IIA (GENERALIZED PATCH/PLAQUE, T2) DISEASE. Topical nitrogen mustard, PUVA, and total skin electron beam therapy are commonly used for patients with T2 disease. Complete response rates using topical nitrogen mustard are 50% to 70%,[26,34,99] whereas the CR rate for total skin electron beam therapy is 80% to 90%.[26,98] However, in a study at Stanford, patients treated with total skin electron beam therapy did not have an improved long-term survival compared to those who received topical nitrogen mustard as initial therapy, despite the superior CR rate.[26] In patients treated with PUVA, the CR rate ranges from 50% to 80%.[38,40,100]

Patients who fail to respond to one topical therapy, or who progress after an initial response, may be treated with an alternative topical therapy. There is no evidence that development of resistance to one modality affects subsequent response to an alternative topical therapy.[25,26] Combination topical or topical plus biologic therapies may also be used as initial therapy for patients with T2 disease. This may provide for better long-term control of disease, but the ultimate outcome is not usually affected.[45,74,76] Patients who have generalized patch/plaque disease without evidence of extracutaneous involvement and who are treated with these modalities have a median survival greater than 11 years and 25% of deaths in this group are attributable to mycosis fungoides.[26]

STAGE IIB (TUMOROUS) DISEASE. Patients who have a limited number of cutaneous tumors in the setting of generalized patch/plaque disease may be treated with local radiation to the tumors plus one of the topical therapies noted earlier. However, those who have generalized tumorous disease will be treated most effectively with total skin electron beam therapy followed by maintenance

therapy with nitrogen mustard[76] or combinations of PUVA with IFN-alpha[45] or PUVA plus oral bexarotene.

Secondary therapies for these patients include alternative topical or combination therapies, fusion proteins, or investigational treatment. Patients with cutaneous tumors have a median survival of 3.2 years and the majority of these patients will die of mycosis fungoides.

STAGE III (ERYTHRODERMIC, T4) DISEASE. Patients with erythrodermic (T4) mycosis fungoides usually have very inflamed and itchy skin that may be irritated by topical therapies. Common treatments for these patients include extracorporeal photopheresis, PUVA, oral bexarotene, IFN-alpha, and single agent methotrexate. With standard total skin electron beam therapy techniques, these patients may suffer severe desquamation with relatively low total doses. Therefore, total skin electron beam therapy is generally not considered appropriate as the initial treatment. Treatment intent in these patients is almost always palliative, and most will progress through several therapies or combinations of therapy during the course of their disease.

The long-term outcome for these patients is quite variable and dependent on patient age at presentation (younger than vs. older than 65 years), overall stage (III vs. IV), and peripheral blood involvement (B0 vs. B1).[101] The median survival varies widely, depending on the number of independent adverse prognostic factors present: three distinct prognostic subgroups may be identified (favorable, intermediate, and unfavorable), with median survivals of 10.2, 3.7, and 1.5 years, for patients with zero, one, or more than one unfavorable prognostic factor, respectively.

STAGE IV (EXTRACUTANEOUS) DISEASE. Patients with extracutaneous disease have a poor prognosis. Appropriate management for these patients includes topical therapy suitable to the extent of skin involvement and, in addition, systemic therapy that may include biologicals as well as chemotherapy. Given their poor prognosis and lack of any truly effective treatment, these patients are also candidates for investigational therapies such as monoclonal antibodies, vaccine trials, and stem cell transplants. Patients who have localized nodal disease as the only evidence of stage IV may benefit from treatment with involved field irradiation (30 to 36 Gy) in addition to systemic management.

In a Stanford series, 77 patients either presented with or later developed extracutaneous (stage IV) disease (56 stage IVA, 21 stage IVB). The median survival of the 77 patients was only 13 months and was similar, regardless of the extent of their skin involvement (T2 vs. T3 vs. T4, $P = 0.69$ to 0.88) or the site of extracutaneous disease (IVA vs. IVB).[30]

REFERENCES

1. Weinstock M: Mycosis fungoides in the United States-increasing incidence and descriptive epidemiology. *JAMA* 1988;260:42.
2. Crowley JJ, Nikko A, Varghese A, et al: Mycosis fungoides in young patients: Clinical characteristics and outcome. *J Am Acad Dermatol.* 1998;38:696.
3. Whittemore A, Holly E, Lee I, et al: Mycosis fungoides in relation to environmental exposures and immune response: A case-control study. *J Natl Cancer Inst.* 1989;81:1560.
4. Tuyp E, Burgoyne A, Aitchison T, et al: A case-control study of possible causative factors in mycosis fungoides. *Arch Dermatol.* 1987;123:196.
5. Poiesz B: Detection and isolation of type C retrovirus particles from fresh and cultures lymphocytes of a patient with cutaneous T-cell lymphoma. *Proc Am Soc Clin Oncol.* 1980;77:7415.
6. Safai B, Myskowski PL, Dupont B, Pollack MS: Association of HLA-DR5 with mycosis fungoides. *J Invest Dermatol.* 1983;80:39.
7. Rosen ST, Radvany R, Roenigk HJ, et al: Human leukocyte antigens in cutaneous T cell lymphoma. *J Am Acad Dermatol.* 1985;12:531.
8. Thangavelu M, Finn WG, Yelavarthi KK, et al: Recurring structural chromosome abnormalities in peripheral blood lymphocytes of patients with mycosis fungoides/Sézary syndrome. *Blood.* 1997;89:3371.
9. Karenko L, Hyytinen E, Sarna S, Ranki A: Chromosomal abnormalities in cutaneous T-cell lymphoma and in its premalignant conditions as detected by G-banding and interphase cytogenetic methods. *J Invest Dermatol.* 1997;108:22.
10. Vowels BR, Cassin M, Vonderheid EC, Rook AH: Aberrant cytokine production by Sézary syndrome patients: Cytokine secretion pattern resembles murine Th2 cells. *J Invest Dermatol.* 1992;99:90.
11. Bernengo MG, Fierro MT, Novelli M, et al: Soluble interleukin-2 receptor in Sézary syndrome: Its origin and clinical application. *Br J Dermatol.* 1993;128:124.
12. Wasik MA, Vonderheid EC, Bigler RD, et al: Increased serum concentration of the soluble interleukin-2 receptor in cutaneous T-cell lymphoma. Clinical and prognostic implications. *Arch Dermatol.* 1996;132:42.
13. Rook AH, Heald P: The immunopathogenesis of cutaneous T-cell lymphoma. *Hematol Oncol Clin North Am.* 1995;9:997.
14. Yoo EK, Cassin M, Lessin SR, Rook AH: Complete molecular remission during biologic response modifier therapy for Sézary syndrome is associated with enhanced helper T type 1 cytokine production and natural killer cell activity. *J Am Acad Dermatol.* 2001;45:208.
15. Hoppe RT, Wood GS, Abel EA: Mycosis fungoides and the Sézary syndrome: Pathology, staging, and treatment. *Curr Probl Cancer.* 1990;14:293.
16. Wood GS, Weiss L, Warnke R, et al: The immunopathology of cutaneous lymphomas: Immunophenotypic and immunogenotypic characteristics. *Semin Dermatol.* 1986;334.
17. Weiss L, Hu E, Wood GS, et al: Clonal rearrangements of T-cell receptor genes in mycosis fungoides and dermatopathic lymphadenopathy. *J Invest Dermatol.* 1985;85:199.
18. Ashton-Key M, Diss TC, Du MQ, et al: The value of the polymerase chain reaction in the diagnosis of cutaneous T-cell infiltrates. *Am J Surg Pathol.* 1997;21:743.
19. Sausville E, Worsha G, Matthews M, et al: Histologic assessment of lymph nodes in mycosis fungoides/Sézary syndrome (cutaneous T-cell lymphoma): Clinical correlations and prognostic import of a new classification system. *Am J Clin Pathol.* 1985;84:610.
20. Kern DE, Kidd PG, Moe R, et al: Analysis of T-cell receptor gene rearrangement in lymph nodes of patients with mycosis fungoides. Prognostic implications. *Arch Dermatol.* 1998;134:158.
21. Harmon C, Witzig T, Katzmann J, et al: Detection of circulating T cells with CD4+CD7-immunophenotype in patients with benign and malignant lymphoproliferative dermatoses. *J Am Acad Dermatol.* 1996;35:404.
22. Vonderheid EC, Sobel EL, Nowell PC, Finan JB: Diagnostic and prognostic significance of Sézary cells in peripheral blood smears from patients with cutaneous T cell lymphoma. *Blood.* 1985;66:358.
23. Bunn PA, Lambert SI: Report of the committee on staging and classification of cutaneous T-cell lymphomas. *Cancer Treat Rep.* 1979;63:725.
24. Kim YH, Hoppe RT: Mycosis fungoides and the Sézary syndrome. *Semin Oncol.* 1999;26:276.
25. Kim YH, Jensen RA, Watanabe GL, et al: Clinical stage IA (limited patch and plaque) mycosis fungoides. A long-term outcome analysis. *Arch Dermatol.* 1996;132:1309.
26. Kim YH, Chow S, Varghese A, Hoppe RT: Clinical characteristics and long-term outcome of patients with generalized patch and/or plaque (T2) mycosis fungoides. *Arch Dermatol.* 1999;135:26.
27. Wieselthier JS, Koh HK: Sézary syndrome: Diagnosis, prognosis, and critical review of treatment options. *J Am Acad Dermatol.* 1990;22:381.
28. de Coninck EC, Kim YH, Varghese A, Hoppe RT: Clinical characteristics and outcome of patients with extracutaneous mycosis fungoides. *J Clin Oncol.* 2001;19:779.
29. Epstein EH Jr, Levin DL, Croft JD Jr, Lutzner MA: Mycosis fungoides. Survival, prognostic features, response to therapy, and autopsy findings. *Medicine (Baltimore).* 1972;51:61.
30. Kim YH, Liu HL, Mraz-Gernhard S, et al: Long-term outcome of 525 patients with mycosis fungoides and Sézary syndrome. Clinical prognostic factors and risks for disease progression and second cancer. *Arch Dermatol.* 2003;139:857.
31. Salhany KE, Greer JP, Cousar JB, Collins RD: Marrow involvement in cutaneous T-cell lymphoma. A clinicopathologic study of 60 cases. *Am J Clin Pathol.* 1989;92:747.
32. Kaye FJ, Bunn PA Jr, Steinberg SM, et al: A randomized trial comparing combination electron-beam radiation and chemotherapy with topical therapy in the initial treatment of mycosis fungoides. *N Engl J Med.* 1989;321:1784.
33. Ramsey D, Halperin P, Zeleniuch-Jacquotte A: Topical mechlorethamine therapy for early stage mycosis fungoides. *J Am Acad Dermatol.* 1988;19:684.
34. Vonderheid EC, Tan ET, Kantor AF, et al: Long-term efficacy, curative potential, and carcinogenicity of topical mechlorethamine chemotherapy in cutaneous T cell lymphoma. *J Am Acad Dermatol.* 1989;20:416.
35. Zackheim HS, Epstein EH Jr, Crain WR: Topical carmustine (BCNU) for cutaneous T cell lymphoma: A 15-year experience in 143 patients. *J Am Acad Dermatol.* 1990;22:802.
36. Ramsay DL, Lish KM, Yalowitz CB, Soter NA: Ultraviolet-B phototherapy for early-stage cutaneous T-cell lymphoma. *Arch Dermatol.* 1992;128:931.
37. Resnik KS, Vonderheid EC: Home UV phototherapy of early mycosis fungoides: Long-term follow-up observations in thirty-one patients. *J Am Acad Dermatol.* 1993;29:73.
38. Honigsmann H, Brenner W, Rauschmeier W, et al: Photochemotherapy for cutaneous T cell lymphoma. A follow-up study. *J Am Acad Dermatol.* 1984;10:238.
39. Abel EA, Sendagorta E, Hoppe RT, Hu CH: PUVA treatment of erythrodermic and plaque-type mycosis fungoides. Ten-year follow-up study. *Arch Dermatol.* 1987;123:897.
40. Herrmann JJ, Roenigk HH Jr, Hurria A, et al: Treatment of mycosis fungoides with photochemotherapy (PUVA): Long-term follow-up. *J Am Acad Dermatol.* 1995;33:234.
41. Kuzel TM, Roenigk HH Jr, Samuelson E, et al: Effectiveness of interferon alpha-2a combined with phototherapy for mycosis fungoides and the Sézary syndrome. *J Clin Oncol.* 1995;13:257.
42. Thomsen K, Hammar H, Molin L, et al: Retinoids plus PUVA (RePUVA) in mycosis fungoides, plaque stage. A report from the

Scandinavian Mycosis Fungoides Group. *Acta Dermatol Venereol (Stockh).* 1989;69:217.

43. Abel EA, Sendagorta E, Hoppe RT: Cutaneous malignancies and metastatic squamous cell carcinoma following topical therapies for mycosis fungoides. *J Am Acad Dermatol.* 1986;14:1029.

44. Mostow EN, Neckel SL, Oberhelman L, et al: Complete remissions in psoralen and UVA (PUVA)-refractory mycosis fungoides-type cutaneous T-cell lymphoma with combined interferon alfa and PUVA. *Arch Dermatol.* 1993;129:747.

45. Roenigk HJ, Kuzel TM, Skoutelis A, et al: Photochemotherapy alone or combined with interferon alpha-2a in the treatment of cutaneous T-cell lymphoma. *J Invest Dermatol.* 1990;95:198S.

46. Breneman D, Duvic M, Kuzel T, et al: Phase 1 and 2 trial of bexarotene gel for skin-directed treatment of patients with cutaneous T-cell lymphoma. *Arch Dermatol.* 2001;138:325.

47. Hoppe R: Total skin electron beam therapy in the management of mycosis fungoides. In Vaeth J, Meyer J, eds, *Front Radiat Ther Oncol. The Role of High Energy Electrons in the Treatment of Cancer,* vol. 25. Basel, Switzerland: S Karger; 1991:80.

48. Jones GW, Tadros A, Hodson DI, et al: Prognosis with newly diagnosed mycosis fungoides after total skin electron radiation of 30 or 35 GY. *Int J Radiat Oncol Biol Phys.* 1994;28:839.

49. Becker M, Hoppe RT, Knox SJ: Multiple courses of high-dose total skin electron beam therapy in the management of mycosis fungoides. *Int J Radiat Oncol Biol Phys.* 1995;32:1445.

50. Bunn PA Jr, Hoffman SJ, Norris D, et al: Systemic therapy of cutaneous T-cell lymphomas (mycosis fungoides and the Sézary syndrome). *Ann Intern Med.* 1994;121:592.

51. Rosen ST, Foss FM: Chemotherapy for mycosis fungoides and the Sézary syndrome. *Hematol Oncol Clin North Am.* 1995;9:1109.

52. Grozoa P, Jones S, McKelvey E, et al: Combination chemotherapy for mycosis fungoides: A Southwest Oncology Group Study. *Cancer Treat Rep.* 1979;63:647.

53. Braverman IM, Yager NB, Chen M, et al: Combined total body electron beam irradiation and chemotherapy for mycosis fungoides. *J Am Acad Dermatol.* 1987;16:45.

54. Case DC Jr: Combination chemotherapy for mycosis fungoides with cyclophosphamide, vincristine, methotrexate, and prednisone. *Am J Clin Oncol.* 1984;7:453.

55. Von Hoff D, Dahlberg S, Hartsock R, et al: Activity of fludarabine monophosphate in patients with advanced mycosis fungoides: A Southwest Oncology Group study. *J Natl Cancer Inst.* 1990; 82:1353.

56. Mercieca J, Matutes E, Dearden C, et al: The role of pentostatin in the treatment of T-cell malignancies: Analysis of response rate in 145 patients according to disease subtype. *J Clin Oncol.* 1994; 12:2588.

57. Greiner D, Olsen EA, Petroni G: Pentostatin (2′-deoxycoformycin) in the treatment of cutaneous T-cell lymphoma. *J Am Acad Dermatol.* 1997;36:950.

58. Zinzani PL, Baliva G, Magagnoli M, et al: Gemcitabine treatment in pretreated cutaneous T-cell lymphoma: Experience in 44 patients. *J Clin Oncol.* 2000;18:2603.

59. Bigler RD, Crilley P, Micaily B, et al: Autologous bone marrow transplantation for advanced stage mycosis fungoides. *Bone Marrow Transplant.* 1991;7:133.

60. Olavarria E, Child F, Woolford A, et al: T-cell depletion and autologous stem cell transplantation in the management of tumour stage mycosis fungoides with peripheral blood involvement. *Br J Haematol.* 2001;114:624.

61. Edelson RL, Heald P, Perez M, et al: Photopheresis update. *Prog Dermatol.* 1991;25:1.

62. Holloway KB, Flowers FP, Ramos-Caro FA: Therapeutic alternatives in cutaneous T-cell lymphoma. *J Am Acad Dermatol.* 1992; 27:367.

63. Lim HW, Edelson RL: Photopheresis for the treatment of cutaneous T-cell lymphoma. *Hematol Oncol Clin North Am.* 1995;9:1117.

64. Heald P, Rook AH, Perez M, et al: Treatment of erythrodermic cutaneous T-cell lymphoma with extracorporeal photochemotherapy. *J Am Acad Dermatol.* 1992;27:427.

65. Gottlieb SL, Wolfe JT, Fox FE, et al: Treatment of cutaneous T-cell lymphoma with extracorporeal photopheresis monotherapy and in combination with recombinant interferon alfa: A 10-year experience at a single institution. *J Am Acad Dermatol.* 1996;35:946.

66. Olsen EA, Rosen ST, Vollmer RT, et al: Interferon alpha-2a in the treatment of cutaneous T cell lymphoma. *J Am Acad Dermatol.* 1989;20:395.

67. Vagna M, Papa G, Defazio D, et al: Interferon alpha-2a in cutaneous T-cell lymphoma. *Eur J Haematol.* 1990;52:32.

68. Duvic M, Martin AG, Kim Y, et al: Phase 2 and 3 clinical trial of oral bexarotene (Targretin capsules) for the treatment of refractory or persistent early-stage cutaneous T- cell lymphoma. *Arch Dermatol.* 2001;137:581.

69. Duvic M, Lemak NA, Redman JR, et al: Combined modality therapy for cutaneous T-cell lymphoma. *J Am Acad Dermatol.* 1996;34:1022.

70. Knobler RM, Trautinger F, Radaszkiewicz T, et al: Treatment of cutaneous T cell lymphoma with a combination of low-dose interferon alpha-2b and retinoids. *J Am Acad Dermatol.* 1991;24:247.

71. Jones G, McLean J, Rosenthal D, et al: Combined treatment with oral etretinate and electron beam therapy in patients with cutaneous T-cell lymphoma (mycosis fungoides and Sézary syndrome). *J Am Acad Dermatol.* 1992;26:960.

72. Miller V, Benedetti F, Rigas J, et al: Initial clinical trial of a selective retinoid X receptor (RXR) ligand, 3-methyl TTNEB (LGD1069). *Proc Am Soc Clin Oncol.* 1995;14:172.

73. Olsen E, Duvic M, Frankel A, et al: Pivotal phase III trial of two dose levels of denileukin diftitox for the treatment of cutaneous T-cell lymphoma. *J Clin Oncol.* 2001;19:376.

74. Quiros PA, Jones GW, Kacinski BM, et al: Total skin electron beam therapy followed by adjuvant psoralen/ultraviolet-A light in the management of patients with T1 and T2 cutaneous T-cell lymphoma (mycosis fungoides). *Int J Radiat Oncol Biol Phys.* 1997; 38:1027.

75. Wilson LD, Licata A, Braverman IM, et al: Systemic chemotherapy and extracorporeal photochemotherapy to T3 and T4 cutaneous T-cell lymphoma patients who have achieved a complete response to total skin electron beam therapy. *Int J Radiat Oncol Biol Phys.* 1995;32:987.

76. Chinn DM, Chow S, Kim YH, Hoppe R: Total skin electron beam therapy with or without adjuvant topical nitrogen mustard or nitrogen mustard alone as initial treatment of T2 and T3 mycosis fungoides. *Int J Radiat Oncol Biol Phys.* 1999;43:951.

77. Dreno B: Roferon-A (interferon alpha 2a) combined with Tigason (etretinate) for treatment of cutaneous T cell lymphomas. *Stem Cells.* 1993;11:269.

78. Winkler CF, Sausville EA, Ihde DC, et al: Combined modality treatment of cutaneous T cell lymphoma: Results of a 6-year follow-up. *J Clin Oncol.* 1986;4:1094.

79. Herrmann JJ, Roenigk HH Jr, Honigsmann H: Ultraviolet radiation for treatment of cutaneous T-cell lymphoma. *Hematol Oncol Clin North Am.* 1995;9:1077.

80. Scholtz W: Ueber den Einfluss der Röntgenstrahlen auf die Haut in gesunden und krankem Zustande. *Arch Dermat u Syph.* 1902; 59:421.

81. Kim JH, Nisce LZ, D'Anglo GJ: Dose-time fractionation study in patients with mycosis fungoides and lymphoma cutis. *Radiology.* 1976;119:439.

82. Cotter GW, Baglan RJ, Wasserman TH, Mill W: Palliative radiation treatment of cutaneous mycosis fungoides—A dose response. *Int J Radiat Oncol Biol Phys.* 1983;9:1477.

83. Trump JG, Wright KA, Evans WW: High energy electrons for the treatment of extensive superficial malignant lesions. *Am J Roentgenol.* 1953;69:623.

84. Karzmark CJ, Loevinger R, Steele RE, Weissbluth M: A technique for large-field, superficial electron therapy. *Radiology.* 1960;74:633.

85. Page V, Gardner A, Karzmark CJ: Patient dosimetry in the electron treatment of large superficial lesions. *Radiology.* 1970;94:635.

86. Spittle M: Electron-beam therapy in England. *Cancer Treat Rep.* 1969;63:639.

87. Nisce LZ, Safai B, Kim JH: Effectiveness of once weekly total skin electron beam therapy in mycosis fungoides and Sézary syndrome. *Cancer.* 1981;47:870.

88. Hamminga B, Noordijk EM, van Vloten WA: Treatment of mycosis fungoides: Total-skin electron-beam irradiation vs topical mechlorethamine therapy. *Arch Dermatol.* 1982;118:150.

89. Tadros AA, Tepperman BS, Hryniuk WM, et al: Total skin electron irradiation for mycosis fungoides: Failure analysis and prognostic factors. *Int J Radiat Oncol Biol Phys.* 1983;9:1279.

90. Van Vloten WA, DeVroome H, Noordijk EM: Total skin electron beam irradiation for cutaneous T-cell lymphoma (mycosis fungoides). *Br J Dermatol.* 1985;112:697.

91. Desai KR, Pezner RD, Lipsett JA, et al: Total skin electron irradiation for mycosis fungoides: Relationship between acute toxicities and measured dose at different anatomic sites. *Int J Radiat Oncol Biol Phys.* 1988;15:641.

92. Bjarngard BE, Chen GTY, Piontec RW, Svensson GK: Analysis of dose distributions in whole body superficial electron therapy. *Int J Radiat Oncol Biol Phys.* 1977;2:319.

93. Hoppe RT, Fuks Z, Bagshaw MA: Radiation therapy in the management of cutaneous T-cell lymphomas. *Cancer Treat Rep.* 1979;63:625.

94. Price NM: Electron beam therapy. Effect on eccrine gland function in mycosis fungoides patients. *Arch Dermatol.* 1979; 115:1068.

95. Price NM: Radiation dermatitis following electron beam therapy. An evaluation of patients ten years after total skin irradiation for mycosis fungoides. *Arch Dermatol.* 1978;114:63.

96. Sausville EA, Eddy JL, Makuch RW, et al: Histopathologic staging at initial diagnosis of mycosis fungoides and the Sézary syndrome. Definition of three distinctive prognostic groups. *Ann Intern Med.* 1988;109:372.

97. Kim YH, Martinez G, Varghese A, Hoppe R: Topical nitrogen mustard in the management of mycosis fungoides: Update of the Stanford experience. *Arch Dermatol.* 2003;139:165.

98. Jones GW, Hoppe RT, Glatstein E: Electron beam treatment for cutaneous T-cell lymphoma. *Hematol Oncol Clin North Am.* 1995;9:1057.

99. Ramsay DL, Zackheim HS: Topical treatment of early cutaneous T-cell lymphoma. *Hematol Oncol Clinics N Am.* 1995; 9:1031.

100. Abel EA, Deneau DG, Farber EM, et al: PUVA treatment of erythrodermic and plaque type mycosis fungoides. *J Am Acad Dermatol.* 1981;4:423.

101. Kim YH, Bishop K, Varghese A, Hoppe RT: Prognostic factors in erythrodermic mycosis fungoides and the Sézary syndrome [see comments]. *Arch Dermatol.* 1995;131:1003.

Plasma Cell Tumors: Multiple Myeloma and Solitary Plasmacytoma

Joachim Yahalom, MD

Multiple myeloma (MM) and solitary plasmacytoma are related entities, both included in the category of plasma cell tumors. Plasma cell tumors are characterized by neoplastic proliferation of a single clone of plasma cells producing a monoclonal immunoglobulin. MM is the disseminated and more prevalent neoplasm. The less common localized disease, solitary plasmacytoma, may arise in bone (solitary plasmacytomas of bone) or in soft tissue (extramedullary plasmacytoma). All plasma cell tumors are highly sensitive to ionizing radiation, but while radiation is the primary and a potentially curative treatment for both types of solitary plasmacytoma, it has only a palliative (yet effective) role in the management of MM.[1]

In MM, a clone of plasma cells proliferates in the bone marrow, often resulting in extensive skeletal destruction with osteolytic lesions, osteopenia, and high risk for pathologic fractures. Common clinical manifestations of multiple myeloma may also include anemia, hypercalcemia, and renal insufficiency. Bone marrow involvement results in recurrent bacterial infections and bleeding.

EPIDEMIOLOGY

In 2003, an estimated 14,600 new cases of plasma cell tumors (>90% were MM) accounted for 1.1% of new cancer cases.[2] In the United States, MM is responsible for approximately 10,800 cancer deaths per year (1.9% of total). Males are affected more frequently than females (1.4:1 ratio) and the incidence of MM in blacks is almost twice of that in whites. The median age at presentation for MM is between 62 and 65 years, and more than 75% of the patients are diagnosed when they are older than 70 years. Only 18% and 3% of patients are younger than 50 and 40 years, respectively.

ETIOLOGY AND RISK FACTORS

The cause of MM is unknown. Exposure to radiation, benzene, other organic solvents, herbicides, insecticides, and various other occupational exposures may play a role, but none of these have been proven to be statistically significant.[3]

Although MM has been reported in clusters of relatives and identical twins, the role of genetic factors is uncertain.[4] The finding of human herpes virus 8 (HHV8) in dendritic bone marrow cells of MM patients was interesting, since HHV8 expresses IL-6 homology and this cytokine is a major growth factor for MM.[5] Unfortunately, recent research did not support the earlier data.[6]

CLINICAL MANIFESTATIONS

The clinical features of MM are variable, and while approximately 20% of the patients are free of symptoms and are diagnosed by chance, most (two thirds) of patients will present with bone pain, particularly in the back or chest. At diagnosis, approximately 70% of patients have lytic lesions, and the pain often results from compression fractures of the vertebra or ribs. Bone lysis is caused by accelerated cytokine-induced osteoclast formation, leading to increased bone absorption in areas infiltrated by plasma cells.[7] Most patients have diffuse bone loss as well as vertebral fractures, and at presentation, hypercalcemia is found in about 20% of patients.

The most common neurologic complication of MM is radiculopathy, usually in the thoracic or lumbosacral area. It is a result of compression of the nerve by a vertebral lesion or by the collapsed bone itself. Spinal cord compression from MM or solitary plasmacytoma may present as one or more of the following: a severe back pain with weakness or paresthesias of the lower extremities or bladder/bowel dysfunction. Those symptoms require immediate imaging and treatment with corticosteroids, followed by radiation therapy or neurosurgery.

At diagnosis, anemia (normocytic, normochromic) is present in 60% of patients with MM. This is primarily due to the decreased production of red blood cells by marrow infiltrated with plasma cells. Patients may also have decreased levels of erythropoietin. Hypercalcemia is present in 20% of newly diagnosed patients and is secondary to progressive bone destruction and exacerbated by prolonged immobility. Symptoms that suggest hypercalcemia in MM patients are nausea, fatigue, confusion, polyuria, or constipation. Renal insufficiency is diagnosed in approximately 20% of patients with MM and another 20% will develop this complication in later phases of the disease. Patients with MM often develop bacterial infections resulting from their decreased immunocompetence and treatments with chemotherapy and steroids. *Streptococcus pneumoniae* and gram-negative organisms are the most frequent pathogens.

Pallor is the most common physical finding. The liver is palpable in approximately 20% of patients and the spleen in 5%.

INITIAL DIAGNOSTIC WORKUP

The initial diagnostic workup in patients with MM (Table 63-1) should include a history, physical examination, and the following baseline blood studies: a complete blood count (CBC) with differential and platelets, routine serum chemistry including serum creatinine, blood urea nitrogen (BUN), electrolytes, calcium, albumin, serum protein electrophoresis (SPEP), and immunofixation. Beta 2 microglobulin reflects the tumor mass and has become a standard measure of the tumor burden.

Other initial studies include 24-hour urine protein electrophoresis (UPEP), and immunofixation (for detection of Bence Jones proteins) and a skeletal survey (bone scans contribute little since isotope uptake is often low in purely lytic bone disease). Under some circumstances,

Table 63–1 Initial Diagnostic Workup

- H & P
- CBC, differential, platelets
- BUN/creatinine, electrolytes
- Calcium/albumin
- Quantitative immunoglobulins
- SPEP and immunofixation
- 24-hr UPEP and immunofixation
- Skeletal survey
- Unilateral bone marrow aspirate + biopsy
- 24-hr urine for Bence Jones quantitation
- β_2-microglobulin

Generally Useful Tests

- Labeling index
- C-reactive protein
- LDH
- Cytogenetics
- Bone marrow flow cytometry

Useful Under Some Circumstances

- MRI for suspected cord compression
- MRI of spine for suspicion of solitary plasmacytoma of bone
- CT scan for evaluation of suspected metastases
- Tissue biopsy to diagnose a solitary plasmacytoma
- Serum viscosity
- Erythropoietin level
- Bone marrow immunohistochemistry

BUN, blood urea nitrogen; CBC, complete blood count; CT, computed tomography; H & P, history and physical examination; LDH, lactate dehydrogenase; MRI, magnetic resonance imaging; SPEP, serum protein electrophoresis; UPEP, urine protein electrophoresis.

magnetic resonance imaging (MRI) is an excellent tool for evaluation of spinal cord compression or impingement. It is also useful for solitary plasmacytoma of the bone. Computed tomography (CT) scans are useful for evaluation of extradural extraosseous plasmacytomas.

Unilateral bone marrow aspirate and biopsy is always required, and in solitary plasmacytoma, a tissue biopsy is necessary to confirm the diagnosis. Cytogenetic tests may detect chromosomal abnormalities, particularly deletions, which may suggest a worse prognosis. Bone marrow flow cytometry, used to quantify the number of phenotypically abnormal cells, may help in elucidating a questionable diagnosis of MM.

Tests that are useful in most patients with MM include plasma cell labeling index; C-reactive protein (a surrogate marker for interleukin-6); and lactate dehydrogenase (LDH), which can serve as a measure of tumor burden in some situations. Erythropoietin levels may be obtained to help determine the need for erythropoietin therapy.

The most important diagnostic finding in MM is the presence of a monoclonal (M) protein in the serum or urine or both (98% of patients). Serum protein electrophoresis (SPEP) shows a localized band or peak in 80% of patients, and immunofixation of the urine discloses M protein in 75%. Hypogammaglobulinemia is seen in approximately one half of the 20% with no localized band on protein electrophoresis. The types of monoclonal protein produced are IgG (60%), IgA (20%), IgD (2%), IgE (<.1%), or only the light chains—kappa or delta (18%). Less than 5% of the patients are considered to have nonsecretory disease because their plasma cells do not secrete detectable levels of monoclonal immunoglobulin.

Bone marrow examination typically confirms the diagnosis of MM by revealing an increased number of plasma cells. For diagnosing MM, the bone marrow should contain more than 10% plasma cells. The plasma cells are strongly positive for CD38 and cytoplasmic immunoglobulins and are negative for CD5, CD20, and surface immunoglobulin expression.[8] Normal plasma cells express CD19, but malignant plasma cells lose this expression. CD10 expression is generally negative, but is occasionally found in advanced disease. Immunoperoxidase staining with kappa and lambda antibodies may demonstrate monoclonality. The pattern of bone marrow involvement may be macrofocal, and, as a result, the plasma cell count from an aspirate may be normal if an aggregate of plasma cells is missed. Overexpression of cyclin D1 was found in 30% of patients with MM, and in a multivariate analysis correlated significantly with reduced survival.[9]

STAGING AND PROGNOSTIC MARKERS

The diagnostic criteria for myeloma were defined by Durie and Salmon in 1975.[10] The Durie-Salmon clinical staging system that is based upon factors correlating with tumor cell mass is still the most commonly used system (Table 63-2).

The minimal criteria for diagnosis of MM include a bone marrow containing more than 10% of plasma cells

Table 63–2   Smoldering Multiple Myeloma

Criteria for Diagnosis

- Monoclonal gammopathy
  - ➤'M' component:
    - IgG >35 g/L and <50 g/L
    - IgA >20 g/L and <30 g/L
    - Bence Jones protein <1.0 g/24 hr
- Bone marrow infiltration with plasma cells >10% but <20%
- No anemia, renal failure, or hypercalcemia
- No bone lesions on skeletal survey

(or the presence of a plasmacytoma) plus at least one of the following:

1. M-protein in the serum (usually >3 gm/dl)
2. M-protein in the urine
3. lytic bone lesions

In addition, the patient must have some or all of the usual clinical features of MM (anemia, hypercalcemia, azotermia, hypoalbuminemia, bone demineralization). It should be noted that some connective tissue disorders, metastatic cancer, lymphoma, and leukemia may share some of the features of MM and must be excluded in the differential diagnosis.

Patients with plasma cell malignancies are generally classified into three categories with prognostic significance and treatment implications:

1. Smoldering myeloma (see Table 63-2) and Durie-Salmon stage I MM (Table 63-3)
2. Solitary plasmacytoma (osseous or extramedullary)
3. Advanced stages of MM (Durie-Salmon stage II to III)

In general, with smoldering myeloma and stage I MM, patients are observed and monitored for potential progression to more advanced MM that is likely to require systemic treatment. Solitary plasmacytomas, which are treated with radiation, are discussed separately. The most common presentation, MM in stages II or III, is treated with systemic chemotherapy.

The category of smoldering myeloma includes asymptomatic patients as defined in Table 63-2. In contrast to patients with overt myeloma, these patients have no lytic lesions, anemia, or hypercalcemia. Evolution to overt myeloma occurs at the rate of 3% to 4% per year.[11] Patients with Durie-Salmon stage I myeloma (see Table 63-3) also have a low amount of M protein without significant anemia, hypercalcemia, or bone disease. These patients do not need primary therapy because they can do well for many months to years before disease progresses.[12] In these patients, disease progression that may require therapy is defined as a sustained 25% or greater increase in M protein in the serum or urine, or development of new sites of lytic disease or hypercalcemia.

In the differential diagnosis plasma cell disorders, two other clinical situations should be mentioned, monoclonal gammopathy of unknown significance (MGUS) and primary amyloidosis. MGUS is characterized by the following findings: absence of symptoms, M component (IgA, IgG, or IgM) less than 3 gm/dL, less than 10% of plasma cells in the bone marrow, an absence of lytic lesions, anemia, hypercalcemia, and renal insufficiency.

Table 63–3   Durie-Salmon Staging System for Multiple Myeloma

Stage	Criteria	Myeloma Cell Mass ($\times 10^{12}$ cells/m²)

I	Hemoglobin >10 g/dL
	Serum calcium level ≤12 mg/dL (normal)
	Normal bone or solitary plasmacytoma on x-ray
	Low M-component production rate:
	    IgG <5 g/dL
	    IgA <3 g/dL
	    Bence Jones protein <4 g/24 hr
		<0.6 (low)

II	Not fitting stage I or III	0.6–1.2 (intermediate)

III	Hemoglobin <8.5 g/dL
	Serum calcium level >12 mg/dL
	Multiple lytic bone lesions on x-ray
	High M-component production rate:
	    IgG >7 g/dL
	    IgA >5 g/dL
	    Bence Jones protein >12 g/24 hr
		>1.2 (high)

Sub classification	Criterion
A	Normal renal function (serum creatinine level <2.0 mg/dL)
B	Abnormal renal function (serum creatinine level ≥2.0 mg/dL)

Primary amyloidosis has the same characteristics as MGUS plus evidence of amyloidosis on biopsy.

The following factors, which are not included in the Durie-Salmon staging system, were found to have prognostic implications:

1. Cytogenetic abnormalities—Chromosomal abnormalities, especially loss of chromosome 13 or deletions of parts of chromosome 13, have been associated with inferior survival after both standard chemotherapy and high-dose therapy. Multivariate analysis has shown these chromosomal changes to be the most important predictors of survival.[13]
2. β_2-microglobulin levels—Serum β_2 microglobulin is an important and easily available prognostic indicator. When cytogenetic changes are not included, β_2 microglobulin is consistently the most important prognostic indicator in multivariate analysis. It should be noted, however, that because β_2 microglobulin is excreted by the kidneys, high levels are present in patients with renal failure, which may complicate the interpretation of elevated values.
3. LDH level—High levels of LDH have also been associated with extraosseous disease, plasma cell leukemia, drug resistance, and shortened survival.

RADIATION THERAPY IN THE MANAGEMENT OF PLASMA CELL TUMORS

Solitary Plasmacytomas

Plasmacytomas are tumors composed of plasma cells of variable maturity that are histologically identical to those seen in MM. When they involve the bone, they are designated solitary plasmacytoma of bone (SPB) or osseous plasmacytoma. If they develop in soft tissues, they are called extramedullary plasmacytomas.[14,15] Table 63-4 compares the two types of plasmacytomas. Solitary plasmacytoma represents approximately 8% of all plasma cell tumors (5% osseous and 3% extramedullary). Males are more commonly affected than females (4:1), and the median age at diagnosis is between 50 and 55 years, which on average is 5 to 10 years younger than those diagnosed with MM (median age 60 years).[16,17]

The criteria for diagnosis of solitary plasmacytoma are: a histologically confirmed single lesion, normal bone marrow biopsy (<10% plasma cells), negative skeletal survey, no anemia, hypercalcemia, or impaired renal function. About one third to one half of all patients with solitary plasmacytoma have a myeloma protein (M-protein) detectable in the urine or on serum by plasma electrophoresis or both.[18-20]

Solitary Plasmacytoma of Bone (Osseous Plasmacytoma)

Solitary plasmacytoma of bone (SPB) is characterized by the presence of plasmacytoma in bone, in the absence of multiple osteolytic lesions, or other features of MM.[15]

Patients usually present with skeletal pain, neurologic compromise, or a pathologic fracture. Severe back pain or cord compression may be the presenting feature of solitary plasmacytoma involving the vertebra. Pathologic fractures or a soft tissue extension of the solitary plasmacytoma may result in a palpable mass.

SPB has a predisposition for the red marrow-containing axial skeleton, especially the pelvis and the spine.[17,21] Patients with solitary plasmacytoma should have similar diagnostic and staging procedures recommended for MM (see earlier). An additional radiologic evaluation by MRI of the spine has been recommended. It has been estimated that one third of patients diagnosed with solitary plasmacytoma

of bone based upon standard studies have evidence of other plasma cell tumors on MRI of the spine.[20,22-24] This information may have both prognostic and treatment implications as earlier systemic treatment may be considered.

Overt MM ultimately becomes evident in 50% to 80% of patients with SPB.[15,18,25,26] The median onset of conversion is between 2 and 5 years,[17,25,28] but progression may take up to 20 years.[28] With adequate follow-up, the majority of SPB cases progress inexorably to MM, at a rate of 58% to 84% at 10 years and 47% to 100% at 15 years (Table 63-5).[18,27] Overall median survival for SPB is 10 to 11 years from the diagnosis and 2 to 5 years after conversion to MM.[25,28] Several institutions have reported actuarial 10-year disease-free survival rates of 15% to 46% for patients with SPB.[17,18,25,28]

PROGNOSTIC FACTORS IN SOLITARY PLASMACYTOMA OF BONE

Prognostic features for conversion of SPB into MM remain controversial. According to Holland and co-workers, factors that predict for conversion of solitary osseous plasmacytoma include lesion size greater than or equal to 5 cm, age older than 40 years, and the presence of an M spike.[25] Bataille and colleagues showed that lesions located in the spine were more likely to progress to MM than were lesions in the extremities.[21]

The importance of persistence of an M-protein after radiation therapy as a predictor of subsequent conversion to MM is uncertain. Some studies have shown such a relationship.[21,22,25,29] In a recently updated MD Anderson Cancer Center series, persistence of the M-protein after treatment of SPB was an indicator for progression.[20] More than half (57%) of solitary osseous plasmacytoma patients with persistent M-protein progressed to MM, as compared with only 18% of patients in whom the protein disappeared after radiotherapy. In contrast, neither the presence of M-protein nor gender, age, or lesion site was prognostic in an analysis from Stanford University.[28] Frassica and coworkers also showed that regardless of whether the M-protein level remained elevated or returned to normal, 70% to 75% of patients with SPB progressed to MM.[17]

TREATMENT OF SOLITARY PLASMACYTOMA OF BONE

Radiation therapy is the treatment of choice for SPB. The recommended dose is between 40 to 50 Gy over a period of 4 to 5 weeks. This is, in principle, an involved field treatment, yet the optimal volume for radiotherapy has not been studied.[1] It has been customary to include the whole involved bone in the radiation port, but with modern imaging (such as MRI or PET scanning or both), it should be acceptable to treat the tumor volume alone with generous margins, particularly if it involves a long bone or the pelvis. Consideration for bone marrow volume should be exercised since more than half of these patients will eventually recur systemically with MM and may require high-dose therapy with stem cell transplantation. Radiotherapy localized to the tumor site should

Table 63–4   Characteristics of Solitary Plasmacytoma and Extramedullary Plasmacytoma*

Characteristic	Solitary Plasmacytoma	Extramedullary Plasmacytoma
Median age of onset	50-60 yr	50-60 yr
Main sites of presentation	Spine and pelvis	Upper aero-digestive tract
Percentage of patients with detectable M-protein	18%-58%	17%-60%
Percentage of patients with involved regional lymph nodes	Rare	31%-40%
Optimal radiation treatment dose	≥40 Gy	≥50 Gy
Long-term local control rate	88%-100%	80%-100%
Rate of progression to multiple myeloma†	54%-84%	11%-41%

*Adapted from Hu K, Yahalom J: Radiotherapy in the management of plasma cell tumors. *Oncology*. 2000;14:101.
†10-yr actuarial risk.

Table 63–5   Treatment Results of Solitary Plasmacytoma of Bone*

Study	Patients, n	Median Follow-up	M-Protein at Diagnosis, %	Local Control Rate, %	Rate of Progression to Multiple Myeloma, %†			Overall Survival Rate, %		
					5 yr	10 yr	15 yr	5 yr	10 yr	15 yr
Hospital St. Eloi	114	>10 yr	18	88	NS	58	NS	NS	68 (crude 10 yr)	NS
MDACC	57	1965-1966	58	96	NS	66 (crude 7 yr)	47 (20 yr)	77	58	29
Mayo Clinic	46	NS	NS	89	NS	NS	NS	74	45	NS
MIR	32	66 mo	38‡	94	NS	NS	NS	NS	NS	NS
University of Florida	27	1963-1993	52	96	40	54	100	86	52	23
PMH	25	39 mo	24	100	48	84	84	NS	7 yr (median)	NS
Stanford	20	72 mo	40	95	NS	NS	NS	83	55	28
Iowa	17	NS	NS	88	39	65	65	47	NS	NS

*Adapted from Hu K, Yahalom J: Radiotherapy in the management of plasma cell tumors. *Oncology.* 2000;14:101.
†Actuarial.
‡Combined extramedullary plasmacytoma and solitary plasmacytoma patient data.
MDACC, MD Anderson Cancer Center; MIR, Mallinckrodt Institute of Radiology; NS, not stated; PMH, Princess Margaret Hospital, Toronto.

be given even if the plasmacytoma appears to have been completely resected for diagnostic purposes. As demonstrated in Table 63-5, local control of SPB with radiation alone is in the range of 88% to 100%.

An analysis of 81 bone and extramedullary plasmacytoma by Mendenhall et al. showed the radiation dose-dependent improvement in crude local control in patients with SPB.[30] At a minimum follow-up of 2 years, local control was achieved in 94% of solitary osseous plasmacytoma patients treated with greater than or equal to 40 Gy, as compared with 64% of those receiving less than 40 Gy. An analysis of 43 plasmacytomas by Mill and coworkers demonstrated that local recurrence occurred only in lesions irradiated at doses less than 40 Gy.[31] Recent data by Tsang and colleagues from Princess Margaret Hospital in Toronto showed that tumor size preradiotherapy was of importance. All local failures, in their experience, were in tumors larger than 5 cm, suggesting that bulkier tumors should receive radiation at the higher end of the recommended dose range.[26]

It should be noted that following radiotherapy, radiologic residual abnormality often remained unchanged for a long time. Therefore, most authors define local control as the absence of disease progression in the irradiated field. In the long term, local control is evidenced by the absence of symptoms and imaging that indicates either no change in the lytic lesion or development of a sclerosis. Metabolic imaging such as PET scanning may allow better definition of response and may become an important tool in follow-up, but no studies have addressed this issue as yet.

Adjuvant chemotherapy in the setting of SPB that aims to reduce the high risk of progression to MM is theoretically appealing. Yet there is no convincing evidence that it will prevent the ultimate systemic progression of the disease, and data and the issue remain controversial. Some series indicated no benefit with adjuvant chemotherapy,[16,27,29] whereas others concluded that such

therapy prevents or delays the median time of progression into MM.[25,32,33] For example, in an uncontrolled study by Holland and coworkers, adjuvant chemotherapy did not affect the incidence of conversion but appeared to delay the median time to progression from 29 to 59 months.[25] In the randomized study reported by Aviles et al. from Mexico City, a group of 53 patients with SPB were randomized to receive either local radiotherapy followed by melphalan and prednisone for 3 years or radiotherapy alone.[33] After a median follow-up of almost 9 years, 22/25 patients remained alive and free of disease in the combined modality group compared to only 13/28 patients in the radiotherapy-alone group (P < 0.01). A major criticism of this work is its small size and the prolonged use of myelotoxic alkylating agents. Most myeloma experts (e.g., NCCN guidelines) do not recommend adjuvant chemotherapy as a standard approach in SPB.

Since more than 50% of patients with SPB progress to MM at the median of 2 to 3 years after treatment, careful follow-up is required. It is recommended that following primary treatment for SPB, patients should undergo laboratory testing with serum and urine immunofixation, complete blood count, serum calcium, and creatinine every 4 to 6 months for 1 year and annually thereafter. A bone survey or MRI should be performed annually or if the patient has symptoms, develops M-protein, or has a persistent M-protein that increases in magnitude.

EXTRAMEDULLARY PLASMACYTOMA

Extramedullary plasmacytoma is a plasma cell tumor that arises outside the bone marrow. Extramedullary plasmacytomas account for approximately 3% of plasma cell malignancies.[19,34] The median age at presentation is 50 to 60 years. Most patients present with a mass, and approximately 80% are located in the upper aerodigestive passages involving the paranasal sinuses, nasopharynx, or nasal cavity.[19,34] Symptoms of epistaxis, nasal discharge, or nasal obstruction are typical for these locations. Extramedullary plasmacytoma may involve other areas of the GI tract, liver, and lymph nodes; it is also reported in the testis and central nervous system. Primary plasmacytoma of the lung often presents as a pulmonary nodule or hilar mass.

The diagnosis of an extramedullary plasmacytoma requires the demonstration of a monoclonal plasma cell tumor at an extramedullary site with no evidence of MM based on imaging and bone marrow studies. The histologic diagnosis of extramedullary plasmacytoma can be difficult with the differential diagnosis being non-Hodgkin's lymphoma, particularly of MALT type, since marginal zone lymphoma may undergo an extensive degree of plasmacytic differentiation.[35] It should be mentioned that most of the experience with extramedullary plasmacytoma is from series collected before the recognition of MALT lymphoma as a separate entity. The histologic grading may influence outcome; in one study, local control after radiation therapy was achieved in 83% (15/18) of low-grade extramedullary plasmacytoma and was only 17% (1/6) in intermediate-grade to high-grade tumors.[36]

The treatment of choice for extramedullary plasmacytoma is radiotherapy with a dose ranging from 40 Gy to 50 Gy over a period of 4 to 5 weeks. The radiation dose required for optimal local control of EMP appears to be higher than that for solitary osseous plasmacytoma. Mill et al. showed that the optimal dose to control the majority of lesions is 50 Gy.[37] In a series of solitary bone and extramedullary plasmacytomas treated with radiation at the University of Florida, the only failures at radiation doses above 40 Gy were extramedullary plasmacytomas.[30] Yet other authors suggested that small tumors may be controlled with lower doses.[26,38] As in the case with SPB, local control rates of 80% to 100% are attainable in patients with extramedullary plasmacytoma

(Table 63-6).[17,18,20,21,27,28,32] In the Royal Marsden series of 202 patients, radiation therapy alone was equivalent to surgery alone with respect to local control rate (approximately 80% on crude analysis).[34] The most common sites of spread outside the primary tumor are the bone (80%) and soft tissue (20%), predominantly lymph nodes; less common sites of metastasis include the skin, subcutaneous tissues, and liver.[34]

Median overall survival for patients with extramedullary plasmacytoma in one study was 114 months.[19] In the Royal Marsden experience, the 10-year disease-specific survival rate was 50%,[34] whereas other groups had demonstrated rates ranging from 69% to 89%.[18-20,25,27,28,32,39]

Some reports indicated that the first echelon of lymph nodes is involved at initial presentation or at relapse in 30% to 40% of patients with extramedullary plasmacytoma and recommended inclusion of the adjacent lymph nodes in the radiation field.[18,19] Yet a recent extensive review of 800 cases[40] showed an incidence of lymph node involvement to be only 7.6% for upper aerodigestive locations and even lower for other sites. Therefore, it is no longer recommended that the immediate lymph node echelon be included in the radiation field.

The actuarial rate of progression to MM is significantly lower for extramedullary plasmacytoma than for SPB, ranging from 11% to 30% at 10 years. In a series by Wiltshaw et al., the overall risk for developing MM was 48% (on crude analysis).[34] In other studies, M-protein was found in 29% of patients with extramedullary plasmacytoma and was not associated with progression.[19,38] In a review of 400 publications on extramedullary plasmacytoma between 1905 and 1997 that included 800 cases,[40] patients who had combined surgery and radiation had better results (median survival >25 years) than those who had only surgical intervention (13 years) or only radiation therapy (12 years). The local recurrence rate was 22%. MM developed in 15% of patients and was independent of the primary tumor location.

Table 63–6   Treatment Results of Extramedullary Plasmacytoma*

Study	Patients, n	Median Follow-up	M-Protein at Diagnosis, %	Local Control Rate, %	Rate of Progression to Multiple Myeloma, %[†]			Overall Survival Rate, %		
					5 yr	10 yr	15 yr	5 yr	10 yr	15 yr
Royal Marsden	44	NS	42	79[‡]	NS	41 (crude)	NS	NS	40	NS
PMH	25	61 mo	32	100	NS	NS	NS	NS	NS	NS
Padua	25	94 mo	17	88	NS	NS	NS	75	49	NS
Oslo	18	NS	NS	NS	NS	NS	NS	90	90	55 (20 yr)
MIR	14	66 mo	38[§]	93	31	31	31	58	NS	NS
Iowa	13	NS	NS	92	NS	NS	NS	NS	NS	NS
MDACC	12	1965-1996	NS	83	NS	NS	NS	73	NS	NS
Stanford	10	NS	NS	80	10	18	18	50	NS	NS
University of Florida	10	1963-1993	60	100	11	11	33	80	80	80

*Adapted from Hu K, Yahalom J: Radiotherapy in the management of plasma cell tumors. *Oncology.* 2000;14:101.
[†]Actuarial.
[‡]Treated primarily with radiation, but also with surgery and/or chemotherapy.
[§]Combined extramedullary plasmacytoma and solitary plasmacytoma patient data.
MDACC, MD Anderson Cancer Center; MIR, Mallinckrodt Institute of Radiology; NS, not stated; PMH, Princess Margaret Hospital, Toronto.

After progression to MM, patients with extramedullary plasmacytoma may have different patterns of presentation and outcome compared to patients progressing following solitary plasmacytoma of bone. Bony lesions occur more often in nonaxial sites.[34] In the University of Florida series, patients with extramedullary plasmacytoma who progressed to MM had a 5-year survival rate of 100%, as compared with 33% for those with SPB who progressed.[30] These findings suggest a possible difference in the biologic aggressiveness of the extramedullary plasmacytoma compared to SPB. Mendenhall et al. recommended that patients who completed the treatment for extramedullary plasmacytoma be monitored with a paraprotein measurement every 3 months for 1 year and every other year thereafter. They also advocated CT or MRI every 6 months for 1 year and as clinically indicated later.

RADIATION THERAPY IN THE MANAGEMENT OF MULTIPLE MYELOMA

Palliative Radiotherapy

The main indication for radiation therapy in multiple myeloma is palliation of local bone pain.[1] Other indications for radiotherapy include: impending pathologic fracture, associated symptomatic soft-tissue mass, spinal cord compression, and pressure on cranial and peripheral nerves. The efficacy of radiotherapy in preventing impending pathologic fracture is unclear. It is important that lesions at risk of pathologic fracture, particularly in weight-bearing sites, will be referred for surgical stabilization first, and radiation for residual disease should be considered at a later stage.

Adequate treatment of long bone lesions was once thought to require irradiation of the entire bone. However, it has been shown that more limited, involved-field treatment (radiographic lesion with margin) does not compromise outcome.[41]

The radioresponsiveness of multiple myeloma allows for the use of a relatively low radiation dose for palliation of bone pain. While still effective in controlling pain, low-dose irradiation does not compromise bone marrow function and potential bone healing. In addition, the possibility of reirradiation either for local recurrence of symptoms or as part of a high-dose program (total-body irradiation for stem-cell transplantation) must be considered. Modern dose-response studies of radiation therapy for palliation of local lesions have been limited. An early study by Farhangi and Osterman suggested that the optimal total dose of radiation for local palliation of bone pain is between 10 and 20 Gy, delivered within 1 to 2 weeks.[42] Mill et al. confirmed this low dose range for effective palliation of bone pain.[3] Their study involved 278 radiation fields in 128 patients with multiple myeloma who were evaluated for responses to irradiation administered over a large dose range (from a few Gy up to 44 Gy in 2- to 3-Gy fractions). The primary indications for treatment included bone pain in 80% of the patients, cord compression in 9%, pathologic fracture in 9%, and soft-tissue mass in 2%. Of 116 patients available for pain relief assessment at the end of radiotherapy, 21% achieved a complete response while 70% had a partial

response. Only 6% of the sites required retreatment for recurrence of pain. The median dose at which subjective pain relief was first noted was between 10 and 15 Gy, with responses noted after irradiation with only 5 Gy. No correlation between dose and need for retreatment could be demonstrated. The authors recommended a dose of 10 to 20 Gy in 2- to 2.5-Gy fractions for palliation of pain in patients receiving chemotherapy. Higher radiation doses were suggested for patients with slower disease progression in order to potentially increase response duration.

Leigh et al. analyzed the University of Arizona experience with palliative local radiation for multiple myeloma.[43] The analysis included 306 symptomatic sites in 101 patients. The main indication for irradiation was bone pain (94% of patients). Other indications included neurologic impairment (6%), pathologic fracture (1%), and large plasma cell mass (2%). Overall, 97% of the patients experienced pain relief when treated with a mean tumor dose of 25 Gy (range, 3.0 to 60 Gy). A complete response was noted in 26% of patients and a partial response in 71%. No distinction in efficacy for relieving symptoms was noted between doses lower than 10 Gy (92% of 13 patients) and doses above 10 Gy (98% of 293 patients). No relationship was noted between the use of concurrent chemotherapy and the rate of complete response. A time-dose scattergram showed no correlation between radiation dose and time to relapse. Furthermore, the efficacy of palliation was not influenced by site or presenting symptom. Only 6% of patients had a local recurrence.

Although fractionated doses as low as 10 Gy may provide pain relief, the dose required to attain healing of lytic lesions may be larger. Norin's study of 53 irradiated lesions demonstrated no objective radiographic improvement with a cumulative dose below 10 Gy, and suggested that the optimal cumulative dose may be 15 Gy.[44] These results were supported by other studies[37,45] and are inconsistent with the study by Leigh et al.[43] The conflicting data may be due to differences in response parameters, follow-up quality, and patient selection.

It is conceivable that several processes underlie the response of multiple myeloma to radiation. It has been postulated that the lytic lesions created in multiple myeloma are due to paracrine-type pathways in which myeloma cells secrete cytokines that activate osteoclasts to generate bony destruction and pain.[46,47] Corticosteroids are important in inhibiting these pathways. It is possible that lower doses of radiation may also abrogate these pathways to alleviate pain. Yet higher doses may be required to kill myeloma cells, debulk the tumor, allow for bone healing, and provide longer duration of relief.

The multiple retrospective series support the notion that the palliative radiation dose to skeletal MM lesions should be markedly lower than the standard RT dose commonly practiced in the treatment of bony metastases from solid tumors (30 Gy in 10 fractions).

In our experience, most patients obtain pain relief and disease control at doses that range from 20 to 30 Gy using fractions of 1.5 to 2 Gy. Situations that may require radiation in the range of 30 to 36 Gy are cord compression, bulky soft tissue component, and incomplete palliation of symptoms in a radiation-responsive patient. The choice of dose and field is also influenced by the extent of critical lesions, potential normal tissue toxicity, bone marrow reserve, history of prior treatment, future treatment options, and overall disease and patient status and prognosis.[1]

HEMIBODY RADIATION

Hemibody and double hemibody irradiation for palliation or improvement in MM control was an attempt to use radiation as a systemic treatment in doses that would not be fully myeloablative and thus would not mandate stem cell transplantation. Although the idea appeared attractive in the 1970s and '80s, it has practically been abandoned over the past 2 decades and remains mostly of historic interest. In small phase II trials, hemibody irradiation relieved pain and reduced M-protein levels in advanced-stage MM patients refractory to chemotherapy,[48-51] but both acute toxicity and prolonged myelosuppression, particularly thrombocytopenia, limited its application in the commonly old and frail population with MM.[50-52] While the feasibility of using double hemibody irradiation following systemic chemotherapy in less heavily pre-treated patients was demonstrated in a prospective study, no additional therapeutic benefit could be attributed to adding large-field irradiation in this manner.[53]

A prospective randomized phase III trial conducted by the Southwest Oncology Group (SWOG) tested the efficacy of chemotherapy versus double hemibody irradiation as consolidation therapy after a complete remission was achieved with induction chemotherapy.[54] Consolidation chemotherapy consisted of vincristine, melphalan, cyclophosphamide, and prednisone (VMCP) for 1 year. Double hemibody irradiation consisted of 7.5 Gy over 5 daily fractions given first to the upper hemibody, followed (after a 6-week delay) by the same dose to the lower hemibody. The duration of relapse-free survival was significantly shorter in patients treated with double hemibody irradiation than in those given chemotherapy consolidation (20 vs. 26 months; P = .04); the same held true for overall survival time (29 vs. 43 months; P = .018). Moreover, median survival from the start of double hemibody irradiation consolidation did not differ in patients who did not achieve a complete response with induction chemotherapy from those who did attain a complete response (29 vs. 28 months, respectively). Myelosuppression was significantly worse in patients treated with double hemibody irradiation, with 25% of patients experiencing severe or life-threatening thrombocytopenia. Mortality from radiation-associated toxicity was 2.1% (3/147). Although the trial has been criticized on the grounds that it compared an 8-week consolidation regimen with a regimen that lasted 1 year, its results practically terminated the consideration of double hemibody irradiation as a treatment option for MM.

Total Body Irradiation in High-Dose Therapy Programs

Several high-dose therapy programs with autologous stem cell transplantation (ASCT) for MM incorporated total body irradiation (TBI) into the conditioning regimen, exploiting the high sensitivity of MM to radiation. A phase III study conducted by the Intergroupe Francophone du Myelome (IFM) showed that ASCT (melphalan 140 mg/m^2 + TBI 8 Gy in 4 daily fractions) resulted in a significantly better 5-year event-free survival rate (28%) compared to conventional chemotherapy (10%, P = 0.01).[55] In an attempt to substitute TBI with a higher melphalan dose, the IFM trial compared a higher dose of melphalan, 200 mg/m^2 (M200) versus TBI (8 Gy in 4 fractions) plus melphalan 140 mg/m^2 (M140/TBI).[56] In this trial, patients in the TBI-containing arm had more grade 3 to 4 mucosal toxicity, a heavier transfusion requirement, and a longer median hospitalization stay with the TBI-containing regimen. There was also a higher toxic death rate in the M140/TBI arm. Although the event-free survival was no different between the two treatment arms, the 45-month overall survival favored the M200 arm with borderline statistical significance (M200: 65.8%, M140/TBI: 45.5%, P = 0.05).[56] Similarly, another IFM protocol tested TBI in the tandem transplant setting by intensifying the conditioning regimen for the second transplant to melphalan 200 mg/m^2 without TBI and comparing it with the standard tandem regimen (M140 for the first, M140/TBI for the second). There was no benefit with TBI, and increased toxicity was again observed. Therefore, all subsequent IFM trials abandoned the use of TBI. The role of TBI in ASCT for MM and its potential contribution (in a lower dose) to the emerging experience with allogeneic nonmyoablative transplantation ("mini-allo") programs for MM remains to be evaluated.

ESSENTIALS OF CHEMOTHERAPY AND SUPPORTIVE CARE FOR MULTIPLE MYELOMA

Chemotherapy for Multiple Myeloma

Most patients with MM have symptomatic disease at diagnosis and require chemotherapy. Yet not all patients who fulfill the criteria for the diagnosis of multiple myeloma should be treated. In particular, treatment is not indicated in patients with smoldering multiple myeloma (See Table 63-1) or asymptomatic stage I, since some of these patients remain stable over extended periods of time.[57]

Chemotherapy with alkylating agents is the preferred initial treatment for overt, symptomatic multiple myeloma in patients older than 70 years and in younger patients in whom stem cell transplantation is not feasible.[58,59] Peripheral stem cells must be collected before the patient is exposed to alkylating agents, if transplantation is a possible consideration.

The chemotherapy combination of oral melphalan and prednisone (MP) remains the standard regimen for MM. Several analyses that compared MP to more multiple agent combinations failed to show a difference in outcome.[58,59] Approximately 40% of patients respond to MP, with an expected median remission of 2 years and overall median survival of 3 years. Melphalan and other alkylating agents are used sparingly or completely avoided if the patient is a candidate for autologous transplantation, since they may affect stem cell reserve and predispose the patient to myelodysplastic syndrome or acute myeloid leukemia. A commonly used effective regimen that spares the stem cells and with which responses occur more rapidly is VAD (vincristine, doxorubicin, dexamethasone). VAD is often used as an induction regimen before transplant. Pulsed dexamethasone has been useful in patients who need vertebral radiotherapy, as it is not myelosuppressive.

Conventional chemotherapy for MM results in different degrees of partial response, but only rarely complete remission. An objective response to chemotherapy has generally been defined as at least a 50 percent decrease in the serum or urine M-protein plus clinical improvement. Patient survival is greater in responders than in non-responders (43 vs. 19 months in one series).[62] Other drugs that are used in the treatment of myeloma are interferon alpha (as maintenance therapy),[63] and thalidomide (for relapsed or refractory disease).[64]

Complications and Supportive Therapy

In addition to treatment aimed directly at the myeloma cells, therapy must also be directed toward the complications of MM, including hypercalcemia, renal insufficiency, infection, and skeletal lesions.

Hypercalcemia is present in 15% of patients at diagnosis. Patients with hypercalcemia may be asymptomatic or complain of various symptoms such as anorexia, nausea, vomiting, polyuria, polydipsia, increased constipation, weakness, confusion, or stupor. Hypercalcemia can also contribute to the development of renal insufficiency. Hydration, preferably with isotonic saline plus steroids, is effective in most cases. If these measures fail, a bisphosphonate such as pamidronate or etidronate can be given.

Renal insufficiency (acute or insidious in onset) occurs in almost one half of patients with MM. Various etiologic mechanisms may be involved, including those related to the excess production of monoclonal light chains and hypercalcemia. Treatment is directed at the underlying cause. This includes hydration and, if indicated, plasmapheresis for acute renal failure, and treatment of hypercalcemia or hyperuricemia (if present).

Complications related to lytic skeletal lesions are not uncommon in patients with multiple myeloma. Patients with these lesions should be encouraged to be as active as possible and to avoid trauma. Fixation of fractures or impending fractures of long bones with an intramedullary rod and methyl methacrylate has produced good results.

An important approach to overall treatment in multiple myeloma is the administration of a bisphosphonate. The efficacy of this approach was evaluated in a study in which 377 patients with stage III multiple myeloma and at least one lytic lesion were treated with antimyeloma therapy plus either placebo or *pamidronate*.[65] The proportion of patients who had any skeletal events was significantly lower in the pamidronate group (24% vs. 41%, $P < 0.001$). Pamidronate therapy was also associated with significant reduction in bone pain.

Symptomatic anemia during the plateau phase is often improved by the administration of erythropoietin.[66] The response is best in patients with low serum erythropoietin concentrations in relation to the degree of anemia.

REFERENCES

1. Hu K, Yahalom J: Radiotherapy in the management of plasma cell tumors. *Oncology.* 2000;14:101.
2. Jemal A, Murray T, Samuels A, et al: *CA Cancer J Clin.* 2003;53:5.
3. Reidel DA, Pottern, LM: The epidemiology of multiple myeloma. *Hematol Oncol Clin North Am.* 1992;6:225.
4. Sobol H, Vey N, Sauvan R, et al: Re: Familial multiple myeloma: A family study and review of the literature. *J Natl Cancer Inst.* 2002;94:461.
5. Rettig MB, Ma HJ, Vescio RA, et al: Kaposi's sarcoma-associated herpes virus infection of bone marrow dendritic cells from multiple myeloma patients. *Science.* 1997;276:1851.
6. Tisdale JF, Stewart AK, Dickstein B, et al: Molecular and serological examination of the relationship of human herpesvirus 8 to multiple myeloma: orf 26 sequences in bone marrow stroma are not restricted to myeloma patients and other regions of the genome are not detected. *Blood.* 1998;92:2681.
7. Croucher PI, Apperley JF: Bone disease in multiple myeloma. *Br J Haematol.* 1998;103:902.
8. Harada H, Kawano MM, Huang N, et al: Phenotypic difference of normal plasma cells from mature myeloma cells. *Blood.* 1993; 81:2658.
9. Hoechtlen-Vollmar W, Menzel G, Bartl R, et al: Amplification of cyclin D1 gene in multiple myeloma: Clinical and prognostic relevance [In Process Citation]. *Br J Haematol.* 2000;109:30.
10. Durie BGM, Salmon SE: A clinical staging system for multiple myeloma. *Cancer.* 1975;36:842.
11. Cesana C, Klersy C, Barbarano L, et al: Prognostic factors for malignant transformation in monoclonal gammopathy of undetermined significance and smoldering multiple myeloma. *J Clin Oncol.* 2002;20:1625.
12. Kyle RA: Long-term survival in multiple myeloma. *N Engl J Med.* 1983;308:743.
13. Zojer N, Konigsberg R, Ackermann J, et al: Deletion on 13q14 remains an independent adverse prognostic variable in multiple myeloma despite its frequent detection by interphase fluorescence in situ hybridization [In Process Citation]. *Blood.* 2000;95:1925.
14. Jaffe ES, Harris NL, Stein H, Vardiman JW, eds: *World Health Organization Classification of Tumours. Pathology and Genetics of Tumours of Haematopoietic and Lymphoid Tissues.* Lyon, France: IARC Press; 2001.
15. Dimopoulos MA, Moulopoulos LA, Maniatis A, Alexanian R: Solitary plasmacytoma of bone and asymptomatic multiple myeloma. *Blood.* 2000;96:2037.
16. Shih LY, Dunn P, Leung WM, et al: Localised plasmacytomas in Taiwan: Comparison between extramedullary plasmacytoma and solitary plasmacytoma of bone. *Br J Cancer.* 1995;71:128.
17. Frassica DA, Frassica FJ, Schray MF, et al: Solitary plasmacytoma of bone: Mayo Clinic experience. *Int J Radiat Oncol Biol Phys.* 1989;16:43.
18. Knowling M, Harwood A, Bergsagel D: Comparison of extramedullary plasmacytomas with solitary and multiple plasma cell tumors of bone. *J Clin Oncol.* 1983;1:255.
19. Soeson M, Paccagnella A, Chiarion-Sileni V, et al: Extramedullary plasmacytoma: Clinical behavior and response to treatment. *Ann Oncol.* 1991;3:51.
20. Liebross R, Ha C, Cox J, et al: Solitary bone plasmacytoma: Outcome and prognostic factors following radiotherapy. *Int J Radiat Oncol Biol Phys.* 1998;41:1063.
21. Bataille R, Sany J: Solitary myeloma: Clinical and prognostic features of a review of 114 cases. *Cancer.* 1981;48:845.
22. Moulopoulos LA, Dimopoulos MA, Weber D, et al: Magnetic resonance imaging in the staging of solitary plasmacytoma of bone. *J Clin Oncol.* 1993;11:1311.
23. Wilder RB, HA CS, Cox JD, et al: Persistence of myeloma protein for more than one year after radiotherapy is an adverse prognostic factor in solitary plasmacytoma of bone. *Cancer.* 2002;94:1532.

24. Pertuiset E, Bellaiche L, Liote F, Laredo JD: Magnetic resonance imaging of the spine in plasma cell dyscrasias. *Rev Rhum Engl Ed.* 1996;63:837. Review.

25. Holland J, Trenkner DA, Wasserman TH, Fineberg B: Plasmacytoma. Treatment results and conversion to myeloma. *Cancer.* 1992; 69:1513.

26. Tsang RW, Gospodarowicz MK, Pintilie M, et al: Solitary plasmacytoma treated with radiotherapy: Impact of tumor size on outcome. *Int J Radiat Oncol Biol Phys.* 2001;50:113.

27. Bolek T, Marcus R, Mendenhall N: Solitary plasmacytoma of bone and soft tissue. *Int J Radiat Oncol Biol Phys.* 1996;36:329.

28. Chak L, Cox R, Bostwick D, et al: Solitary plasmacytoma of bone: Treatment, progression and survival. *J Clin Oncol.* 1987;5:1811.

29. Galieni P, Cavo M, Avvisati G, et al: Solitary plasmacytoma of bone and extramedullary plasmacytoma: Two different entities? *Ann Oncol.* 1995;6:687.

30. Mendenhall C, Thar T, Million M: Solitary plasmacytoma of bone and soft tissue. *Int J Radiat Oncol Biol Phys.* 1980;6:1497.

31. Mill W, Griffith R: The role of radiation therapy in the management of plasma cell tumors. *Cancer.* 1980;45:647.

32. Mayr NA, Wen BC, Hussey DH, et al: The role of radiation therapy in the treatment of solitary plasmacytomas. *Radiother Oncol.* 1990;17:293.

33. Aviles A, Huerta-Guzman J, Delgado S, et al: Improved outcome in solitary bone plasmacytoma with combined therapy. *Hematol Oncol.* 1996;14:111.

34. Wiltshaw E: The natural history of extramedullary plasmacytoma and its relation to solitary myeloma of bone and myelomatosis. *Medicine.* 1976;5:217.

35. Hussong JW, Perkins SL, Schnitzer B, et al: Extramedullary plasmacytoma. A form of marginal zone cell lymphoma? *Am J Clin Pathol.* 1999;111:111.

36. Susnerwala SS, Shanks JH, Banerjee SS, et al: Extramedullary plasmacytoma of the head and neck region: Clinicopathological correlation in 25 cases. *Br J Cancer.* 1997;75:921.

37. Mill W, Griffith R: The role of radiation therapy in the management of plasma cell tumors. *Cancer.* 1980;45:647.

38. Harwood AR, Knowling MA, Bergsagel DE: Radiotherapy of extramedullary plasmacytoma of the head and neck. *Clin Radiol.* 1981;32:31.

39. Brinch L, Hannisdal E, Foss A, et al: Extramedullary plasmacytomas and solitary plasma cell tumours of bone. *Eur J Haematol.* 1990;44:132.

40. Alexiou C, Kau RJ, Dietzfelbinger H, et al: Extramedullary plasmacytoma: Tumor occurrence and therapeutic concepts. *Cancer.* 1999;85:2305.

41. Catell D, Kogen Z, Donahue B, et al: Multiple myeloma of an extremity: Must the entire bone be treated? *Int J Radiat Oncol Biol Phys.* 1998;40:117.

42. Farhangi M, Osserman E: The treatment of multiple myeloma. *Semin Hematol.* 1973;10:149.

43. Leigh B, Kurtts T, Mack C, et al: Radiation therapy for the palliation of multiple myeloma. *Int J Radiat Oncol Biol Phys.* 1993; 25:801.

44. Norin T: Roentgen treatment of myeloma with special consideration to the dosage. *Acta Radiol.* 1986;13:291.

45. Bosch A, Frias Z: Radiotherapy in the treatment of multiple myeloma. *Int J Radiat Oncol Biol Phys.* 1988;15:1363.

46. Mundy G, Bertoloni D: Bone destruction and hypercalcemia in plasma cell myeloma. *Semin Oncol.* 1986;45:46.

47. Mundy G, Raisz L, Cooper R, et al: Evidence for the secretion of an osteoclast stimulating factor in myeloma. *N Engl J Med.* 1974;291:1041.

48. Singer C, Tobias J, Giles F, et al: Hemibody irradiation an effective second-line therapy in drug-resistant multiple myeloma. *Cancer.* 1989;63:2446.

49. Rostom A: A review of the place of radiotherapy in myeloma with emphasis on whole body irradiation. *Hematol Oncol.* 1988;6:193.

50. McSweeney E, Tobias J, Blackman G, et al: Double hemibody irradiation (DHBI) in the management of relapsed and primary chemoresistant multiple myeloma. *Clin Oncol.* 1993;378.

51. Jaffe J, Bosch A, Raich P, et al: Sequential hemi-body radiotherapy in advanced multiple myeloma. *Cancer.* 1979;43:124.

52. Tobias J, Richard J, Blackman G, et al: Hemibody irradiation in multiple myeloma. *Radiother Oncol.* 1985;3:11.

53. MacKenzie M, Wold H, George C, et al: Consolidation hemibody radiotherapy following induction combination chemotherapy in high-tumor-burden multiple myeloma. *J Clin Oncol.* 1992; 10:1769.

54. Salmon S, Tesh D, Crowley J, et al: Chemotherapy is superior to sequential hemibody irradiation for remission consolidation in multiple myeloma: A Southwest Oncology Group study. *J Clin Oncol.* 1990;8:1575.

55. Attal M, Harousseau JL, Stoppa AM, et al: A prospective, randomized trial of autologous bone marrow transplantation and chemotherapy in multiple myeloma. *N Engl J Med.* 1996;335:91.

56. Moreau P, Facon T, Attal M, et al: Comparison of 200 mg/m^2 melphalan and 8 Gy total body irradiation plus 140 mg/m^2 melphalan as conditioning regimens for peripheral blood stem cell transplantation in patients with newly diagnosed multiple myeloma: Final analysis of the Intergroupe Francophone du Myelome 9502 randomized trial. *Blood.* 2002;99:731.

57. Diagnosis and management of multiple myeloma. *Br J Haematol.* 2001;115:522.

58. Rajkumar SV, Gertz MA, Kyle RA, Greipp PR: Current therapy for multiple myeloma. *Mayo Clin Proc.* 2002;77:813.

59. Diagnosis and management of multiple myeloma. *Br J Haematol.* 2001;115:522.

60. Boccadoro M, Marmont F, Tribalto M, et al: Multiple myeloma: VMCP/VBAP alternating combination chemotherapy is not superior to melphalan and prednisone even in high-risk patients. *J Clin Oncol.* 1991;9:444.

61. Combination chemotherapy versus melphalan plus prednisone as treatment for multiple myloma: An overview of 6,633 patients from 27 randomized trials. Myeloma Trialists' Collaborative Group. *J Clin Oncol.* 1998;16:3832.

62. Blad J, Lopez-Guillermo A, Bosch F, et al: Impact of response to treatment on survival in multiple myeloma: Results in a series of 243 patients. *Br J Haematol.* 1994;88:117.

63. Interferon as therapy for multiple myeloma: an individual patient data overview of 24 randomized trials and 4012 patients. *Br J Haematol.* 2001;113:1020.

64. Rajkumar SV, Kyle RA: Thalidomide in the treatment of plasma cell malignancies. *J Clin Oncol.* 2001;19:3593.

65. Berenson JR, Lichtenstein A, Porter L, et al: Efficacy of pamidronate in reducing skeletal events in patients with advanced multiple myeloma. Myeloma Aredia Study Group. *N Engl J Med.* 1996;334:488.

66. Garton JP, Gertz MA, Witzig TE, et al: E-poetin alfa for the treatment of the anemia of multiple myeloma. A prospective, randomized, placebo-controlled, double-blind trial. *Arch Intern Med.* 1995; 155:2069.

Uveal Melanoma

64

*Jeanne Quivey, MD, Robert Takamiya, MD,
and Devron Char, MD*

EPIDEMIOLOGY, GENETICS, AND KNOWN CYTOGENETIC ABNORMALITIES

Uveal melanoma is the most common primary intraocular malignancy of adults. The incidence is estimated to be between 5 and 7 per million per year in the United States, Canada, and Scandinavia[1]; there are approximately 1500 to 2000 new cases diagnosed each year in the United States. The National Cancer Data Base (NCDB) between 1985 through 1994 includes a total of 4522 cases of ocular melanoma in the United States, representing 5.2% of all melanomas. Of ocular melanomas, 85% are uveal, 4.8% are conjunctival, and 10.2% occur at other sites.[2] Uveal melanoma occurs more frequently in light-skinned people, while the incidence rate among African-Americans is less than one eighth that found in whites[3]; it is also rare among Americans of Asian extraction.[4] Age-adjusted incidence rates of ocular melanoma reported by SEER, 1973 through 1986 (per 100,000 person-years), are 0.67 for white males, 0.09 for African-American males, 0.53 for white females, and 0.01 for African-American females; the relative risk of ocular melanoma among white males as compared with black males is 7.4, while it is 53 among white females as compared with black females.[3] The NCDB shows a steady increase in incidence with age, reaching a peak between 60 and 69 years with a mean age of 60.4 years, while less than 2% are younger than 20 years old at the time of diagnosis.[2,5] A similar age dependency is noted in Denmark.[6]

It is extremely rare to have bilateral tumors, multiple uveal melanomas, or familial uveal melanomas.[7] This malignancy is more prevalent in Caucasian patients with ocular or oculodermal melanocytosis (nevus of Ota), almost always arising in the affected eye.[8,9] The lifetime prevalence of uveal melanoma in patients with oculodermal melanocytosis is estimated to be 1 in 400.[10] Reports of cutaneous melanoma and uveal melanoma occurring as double primary malignancies, some in the presence of dysplastic nevi or atypical mole syndrome (AMS), and melanomas of both sites occurring among family members have led to speculation that cutaneous and uveal melanoma may have a common inheritable variant.[11,12] Other authors have been unable to detect an association between intraocular melanoma and cutaneous dysplastic nevi.[13,14]

The role of tumor suppressor genes in the pathogenesis of uveal melanoma has been studied. *P53*, the most common genetic alteration in human malignancies, is only rarely mutated in uveal melanoma.[15] Similarly, both archival and fresh tissue uveal melanomas show no evidence of mutations of *p16*, a putative link to hereditary cutaneous melanoma,[16] although cultured melanoma cell line DNAs may have deletions or rearrangements in this region.[17,18] Chromosomal alterations most often observed in uveal melanoma include deletion of chromosome 3 (a finding commonly associated with ciliary body involvement and poor prognosis), over-representation of 6p, and loss of 6q and multiplication of 8q.[18-22]

Loss of chromosome 3, loss of 6q, and gains of 8q are significant predictors of survival.[23,24] Abnormalities of chromosome 3 and 8 are present in approximately 50% of all cases.[25] Tumors with monosomy 3 also exhibit amplification of *c-myc* (encoded on chromosome 8q24.1), suggesting that both play a role in the pathogenesis of uveal melanomas.[26] In contrast, the most frequent abnormalities described in cutaneous malignant melanoma involve chromosomes 1 and 9.[27] Rearrangements of chromosomes 6, 7, and 10 are also reported with cutaneous melanomas.[28,29] Further, *c-myc* amplification, described in 70% of uveal melanomas, is associated with improved survival.[30,31] The opposite is found in cutaneous melanoma, where high levels of *c-myc* are associated with worse outcomes.

While the distinct cytogenetic characteristics of cutaneous and uveal melanomas support the hypothesis that different mechanisms are involved in the genesis and progression of these neoplasms,[19] some overlap in the pathogenesis of cutaneous and uveal melanomas may exist. In contrast to cutaneous melanoma, which has shown a fivefold to sixfold increase in incidence over the past several decades,[32] the frequency of uveal melanoma appears not to have changed.[6,33,34] Ultraviolet (UV) light exposure is thought to be the major mechanism of cutaneous tumor induction from sunlight exposure.[35] It is also a possible environmental risk factor for a number of ocular diseases including cataract and age-related macular degeneration (ARMD).[36,37] The highest incidence of uveal melanoma in the United States is in the southernmost region studied.[4] However, unlike cutaneous melanoma, there is no marked latitudinal gradient seen in uveal melanoma.[38,39] In Canada, altitude, not latitude, is positively correlated with the incidence of uveal melanoma,[40] while in Norway and Denmark, higher rates of uveal melanoma are found in more urbanized areas.[41,42] Perhaps most problematic with the putative link between sunlight exposure and uveal melanoma is that virtually no UV-A or UV-B is transmitted through the lens and cornea in adults. The juvenile lens may allow small amounts of UV radiation to reach the retina, but tissue overlying the uveal tract would still likely filter out the residual UV radiation.

ANATOMY

Melanomas develop in the uveal tract, the vascular support layer of the eye. Approximately 80% of uveal melanomas involve the choroid, which is the posterior portion of the uveal tract located under the retina; less than 10% involve the iris; approximately 10% to 15% involve the ciliary body (which contains the muscle responsible for accommodation and movement of the lens)[41] (Fig. 64-1). Choroidal lesions can penetrate through Bruch's membrane, the transparent inner membrane of the choroid, thereby creating the characteristic "collar button" or mushroom-shaped deformity by protrusion into the retina; this geometry is virtually pathognomonic for a uveal melanoma. Scleral penetration is often associated with tumor tracking along a vessel.

PATHOLOGY

Uveal melanoma cells are characteristically spindle shaped or epithelioid; these latter, plumper cells are associated with a worse prognosis. In addition to cellular characteristics, pathologists have quantitated pigment content, argyrophil fiber content, and the presence of tumor necrosis. This is the basis for the Callender classification initially described in 1931.[43] It has been modified to describe several pathologic patterns including spindle, mixed, necrotic, and epitheliod types. The American Joint Committee on Cancer (AJCC) 2002 histopathologic staging is shown in Table 64-1. It is likely that benign choroidal nevi were included in the "malignant" category

Table 64–1   Histopathologic Staging of Uveal Melanomas (AJCC, 2002)

Histopathologic Type	
Spindle cell melanoma	
Mixed cell melanoma	
Epithelioid cell melanoma	
Histologic Grade (G)	
GX	Grade cannot be assessed
G1	Spindle cell melanoma
G2	Mixed cell melanoma
G3	Epithelioid cell melanoma

AJCC, American Joint Committee on Cancer.
From Greene FL, Page DL, Fleming ID, et al, eds: *AJCC Cancer Staging Manual*, 6th ed. New York: Springer; 2002.

in early reported series[44]; virtually no tumor-related mortality is observed with the spindle A cell type,[45] although the spindle B variant is clearly malignant.

In patients undergoing enucleation, eye wall resection, or irradiation, several factors have been described as having prognostic significance. These include cell type, tumor size (largest tumor dimension), anterior location, (ciliary body invasion), high mitotic rate, alterations in DNA content, monosomy of chromosome 3, vascular pattern (microvascular loops and networks), and scleral penetration.[25,46-68] In most studies, several additional factors have no impact on survival with univariate or multivariate analysis, including duration of signs and symptoms, reticulin fiber content, location of the posterior tumor margin, or penetration through Bruch's membrane.[46] In many historic series, cell type is the most important single predictor of death following enucleation. The relative importance and relationship between various prognostic factors is uncertain. Probably the most important factors are monosomy chromosome 3, cell type, largest tumor diameter, cell cycling, and vascular content.

The potential predictive value of comparative genomic hybridization studies of melanoma genomes has recently been evaluated in the hopes of finding a more quantifiable and reproducible system of tumor classification. (DNA quantification is reported to be significantly correlated with treatment outcome for many tumor sites, including breast, prostate, endometrium, ovary, and rectum.) The relapse-free survival in 30 patients with monosomy 3 was 43% in contrast to 100% in 24 patients without this chromosomal loss.[25] Large tumor diameter and anterior location with involvement of the ciliary body are prognostic variables known to be significantly related to monosomy 3; all three factors remain excellent predictors of disease-free survival on multivariate analysis (Table 64-2 and Fig. 64-2).[25]

CLINICAL PRESENTATION

The history and presentation of uveal melanomas is variable. Approximately 33% of patients are asymptomatic at the time of initial clinical detection; they present to their local ophthalmologist/optometrist either for a

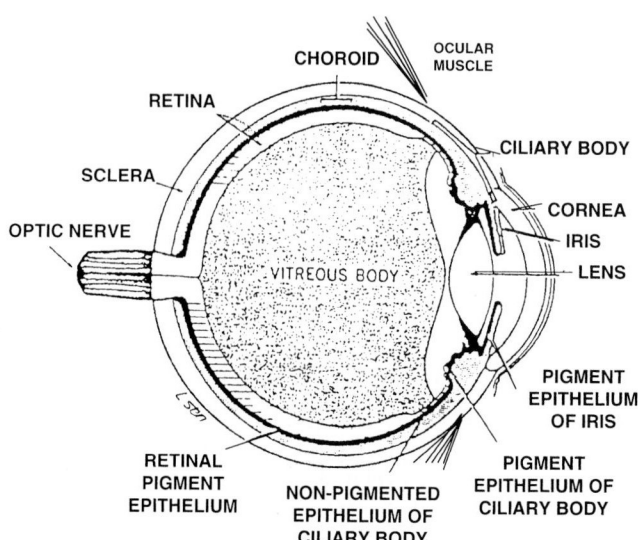

Figure 64–1. Anatomy of the eye.

Table 64-2 Prognostic Factors Associated with Increased Metastases

Epithelioid and mixed cell type[45,46,51,56]
↑ Largest tumor dimension[46,50,51,52]
Anterior location (ciliary body invasion)[46,95]
Monosomy of chromosomes 3[25]
Scleral penetration[46,51,64]
High mitotic rate[59]
Ki-67[58]
Pleomorphic nucleoli[63]
Vascular networks of closed vascular loops[59,60,67]
Mib-1 index[59]
Optic nerve invasion[46]

↑, increasing.

routine examination or refraction. Visual symptoms, if present, include distortion, visual field loss, floaters, scotomas, or flashing lights. Tumors located near the macula can physically distort the central vision while large tumors can produce an exudative retinal detachment. Anterior melanomas that involve the ciliary body occasionally produce an overlying episcleral area of vascular engorgement ("sentinel vessel"). Less commonly, large intraocular melanomas can produce enough inflammation and necrosis to produce a unilateral cataract or severe intraocular inflammation and pain.

The appearance of fundus lesions on indirect ophthalmoscopy is often diagnostic. Examination includes measurement of the tumor diameter and thickness, delineation of tumor location, geometry, and tumor coloration. Patients are also evaluated for associated subretinal fluid or exudative detachment. The pigmentation of uveal

melanomas is variable with as many as 25% of cases being amelanotic; most uveal melanomas are light to medium in pigmentation.

Lesions that most commonly simulate uveal melanoma include nevi, choroidal hemangiomas, rhegmatogenous retinal detachments, age-related disciform lesions, and choroidal metastases (most commonly from breast, lung, and gastrointestinal cancer).[69-71] Making the correct diagnosis in suspected uveal melanomas is a function of observer experience, media clarity, and tumor size.[72] Most ocular oncology units currently report a 99% accuracy,[73] although a generation ago, 20% of eyes enucleated with a clinical diagnosis of this malignancy had a simulating lesion on histopathologic examination.[44,74-78]

ROUTES OF SPREAD

Uveal melanoma is known to have an unpredictable clinical course in which fulminate metastatic disease may develop after a prolonged disease-free interval (up to 46 years).[79-81] In one study of 110 patients who developed metastatic disease, 92% were noted to have liver metastasis, 31% developed lung metastasis, and 23% had bone metastasis. Nodal (14%) and skin and subcutaneous metastasis (17%) are less frequent, while brain and adrenal metastasis are even less common.[82] In a smaller series reported by Kath, the main sites of metastases were liver (87%), lung (46%), bone (29%), and skin (17%).[83] At University of California in San Francisco (UCSF), the metastatic pattern of 41 patients initially referred with a primary choroidal melanoma who later developed metastatic disease also demonstrates the propensity of this tumor to metastasize to the liver as the initial manifestation (56%); skin and subcutaneous metastases are less frequent (24%) (Figure 64-3).[84]

DIAGNOSTIC AND STAGING STUDIES

The evaluation of patients with a possible uveal melanoma is straightforward. Clinical findings more frequent in larger tumor include the presence of subretinal fluid, orange pigmentation, and a collar button configuration. Ancillary tests include fundus photography, both immersion B-scan and Kretz A-scan ultrasonography, and visual field testing (Figure 64-4). Fluorescein angiography, which can identify tumor vessel leakage, is often not diagnostically useful except in differentiating uveal melanomas from hemorrhagic choroidal simulating lesions; in a masked study without other ancillary tests, this technique has a diagnostic accuracy of only 63%.[76] In contrast, experienced ultrasonographers can differentiate uveal melanomas from simulating lesions in approximately 89% to 96% of cases that require therapeutic intervention.[85] Ultrasound factors useful for diagnosing melanoma include choroidal excavation, orbital shadowing, acoustic quiet zone, and homogeneity on A-scan (Figure 64-5). Ultrasound is also useful and reproducible in measuring tumor height, although it is less reliable in tumors located anterior to the equator because of the difficulty in positioning of the A-scan

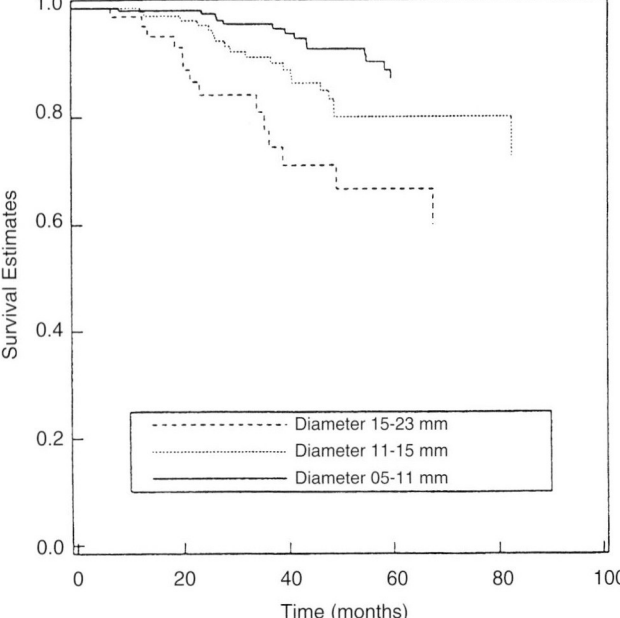

Figure 64-2. Kaplan-Meier survival estimate for time until metastasis following helium ion or iodine-125 plaque by largest tumor diameter. (From Char DH, Castro JR, Quivey JM, et al: Uveal melanoma radiation: 125-I brachytherapy versus helium ion irradiation. *Ophthalmology.* 1989;96:1708. Courtesy of *Ophthalmology.*)

Legend for figure:
- Diameter 15-23 mm
- Diameter 11-15 mm
- Diameter 05-11 mm

Axis labels: Survival Estimates (y-axis), Time (months) (x-axis)

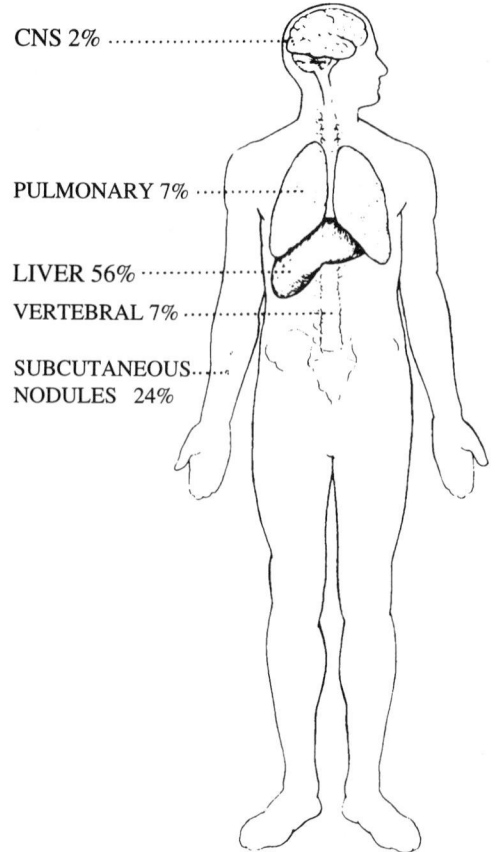

CNS 2%

PULMONARY 7%

LIVER 56%

VERTEBRAL 7%

SUBCUTANEOUS
NODULES 24%

Figure 64–3. Initial sites of metastatic uveal melanoma. (From Char DH: Metastatic choroid melanoma. *Am J Ophthalmol.* 1978;86:76.)

probe. Extensive subretinal fluid over the lesion can also lead to inaccuracy of A-scan with an overestimate of tumor height. Some observers have used ultrasound to estimate tumor diameter, although we note this to be less

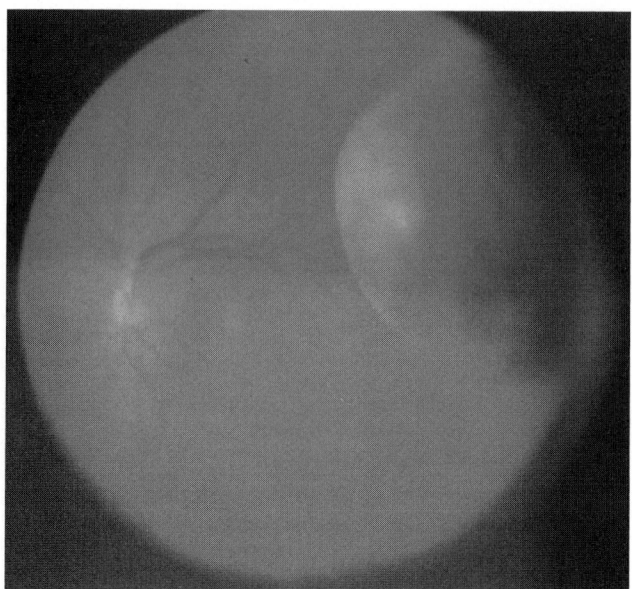

Figure 64–4. Fundus photo of a uveal melanoma. See also Color Figure 64-4.

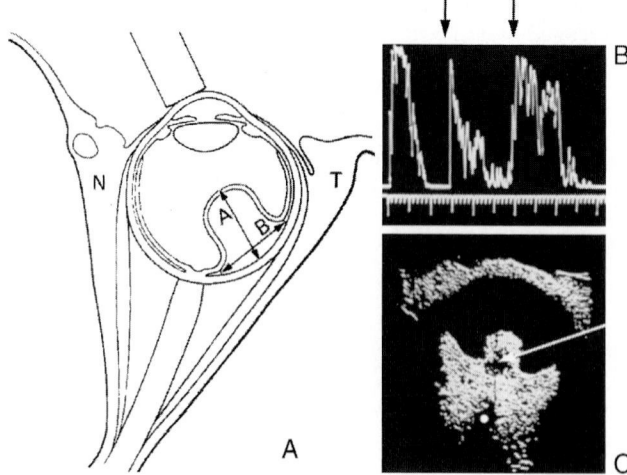

Figure 64–5. A, Diagrammatic view of globe with ultrasound probe in ideal position for quantitative A-scan; the sonolucent vitreous is interrupted by the tumor apex. **B,** Precise measurement in millimeters of tumor height *(black arrows)* is possible on the quantitative Kretz A-scan. **C,** The immersion B-scan show the typical "collar button" configuration of the tumor, as well as choroidal excavation and acoustic quiet beneath the tumor *(white arrow).*

accurate in lesions that have a large area of relatively flat tumor extension.

Additional imaging studies have been evaluated in this neoplasm. Magnetic resonance imaging (MRI) data has been reported in uveal melanomas and simulating lesions.[86-89] While the T1 and T2 pattern of pigmented uveal melanomas is relatively typical, a number of false-negative and false-positive cases have been reported. This is a relatively expensive test that usually does not increase diagnostic accuracy afforded by ultrasound. However, MRI can be diagnostically useful (although inaccuracies have been noted) in the detection of localized extraocular extension, and differentiation between a uveal melanoma and a peripheral choroidal hemorrhage due to an extramacular disciform lesion. These latter anteriorly located entities are sometimes not correctly diagnosed with ultrasound.

In smaller pigmented lesions, noninvasive diagnostic tests are less accurate.[75] It is usually not possible to distinguish an atypical benign melanocytic proliferation from a small melanoma. We have labeled patients who have indeterminate pigmented choroidal lesions with the neologism *nevoma*. This includes lesions that are too large to be clinically thought of as nevi (generally >7 mm in diameter and >1.5 mm thick) but which appear to be relatively inactive. The clinical approach to these lesions is usually close observation with serial fundus photography to assess changes in tumor borders, and ultrasound A-scan to assess changes in tumor thickness (height).

It is unusual (approximately 1% in contemporary series) to simultaneously present with metastatic disease and a primary uveal melanoma; the markedly shortened survival in this setting will significantly influence the treatment approach. The metastatic evaluation includes a thorough physical examination with liver function studies and a CT scan of the abdomen if serum abnormalities are detected. The most useful biochemical indicators of metastatic disease are serum LDH and GGT.[90] Chest x-rays have a very low yield for detecting metastasis, but are a useful baseline study.[91] The clinician must be mindful of other primary neoplasms including breast, lung, and genitourinary cancers, which may produce choroidal metastases that simulate uveal melanoma.

STAGING SYSTEM

The sixth edition of the AJCC staging manual modifies the TNM staging system to allow microscopic or macroscopic extraocular extension within the T1 through T2 categories.[92] The T classification defines uveal melanomas according to the tumor dimensions, including the largest basal diameter and the tumor thickness or height; these dimensions have also been modified from previous editions. A second staging system is recommended by the Collaborative Ocular Melanoma Study (COMS). The two systems, presented in Table 64-3, differ in the definition of stages, although the newer AJCC staging system is modified based on clinical observations in the COMS trials. Unfortunately, neither staging system takes primary tumor location or visual acuity into consideration. These latter factors greatly influence the optimization of treatment modalities. Most authors with large series have reported these factors and attempted to correlate them with tumor control and treatment complications.

STANDARD THERAPEUTIC APPROACHES

The optimum management of uveal melanomas is controversial, although recent publications from the COMS have provided some answers. In small, indeterminate, pigmented tumors (≤3 mm thick and ≤10 mm in diameter), data reported by our group and others have supported the concept that serial observation of these lesions is reasonable unless growth is documented.[93] The

survival in patients whose lesions subsequently grew and required treatment is no worse than has been reported with prompt, early therapy of small lesions. In addition, many such patients have been allowed to maintain good vision in an eye that would have had marked treatment sequelae.

Both prospective COMS and retrospective studies have demonstrated no difference in survival rates comparing enucleation with irradiation.[94-96] This data is detailed later in the "Outcome" section.

Finally, selecting the optimal method of radiation treatment, whether episcleral plaque or charged particle techniques, is dependent on tumor and patient parameters as well as accessibility to specialized treatment facilities. A randomized trial comparing helium ion therapy with 125-I plaques is discussed later in this chapter.[97]

Observation

As noted earlier, small (≤3 mm thick and ≤10 mm in diameter without detachment), apparently inactive lesions in patients with good vision are suitable for observation. We recently retrospectively reviewed approximately 300 such cases, many with long-term follow-up.[93] Approximately two thirds of these lesions did not grow. In several patients with long observation intervals, whose eyes became available at autopsy after dying of other causes, these tumors were found to be benign melanocytic proliferations. In patients without evidence of growth, none developed metastatic disease. In these small lesions that did grow, prompt institution of treatment led to a less than 5% five-year tumor-related mortality.

In the COMS "small tumor" study, patients who were ineligible for the "medium" or "large" tumor studies were managed with observation. These included tumors that were 1 to 3 mm in apical height and 5 to 16 mm in basal diameter, monitored with annual follow-up. Two hundred and four patients were enrolled, and mean follow-up was 92 months. The Kaplan-Meier estimate of 2-year and 5-year tumor growth is 21% and 31%, respectively. Greater initial tumor thickness (2.5 to 3 mm) and larger diameter (12.1 to 16 mm) are associated with higher recurrence and are the basis for the recent modifications in the AJCC staging system. The presence of orange pigment on color photography is also significantly associated with tumor growth on multivariate analysis, while the presence of drusen (hyaline or colloid bodies within the lesion) and area of change in the retinal pigment epithelium (RPE) adjacent to tumor are significantly associated with nongrowing tumors on multivariate analysis. Of 27 deaths in this study, only 6 were reported as melanoma related. The Kaplan-Meier estimates for 5-year and 8-year melanoma-specific mortality were 1% and 3.7%, respectively.[98,99]

Photocoagulation, Laser Treatment, and Thermotherapy

While photocoagulation and laser treatment have been used to treat small choroidal melanomas and high-risk nevomas for approximately 40 years, the efficacy of these

Table 64–3 AJCC and COMS Staging

AJCC 2002 Staging of Ciliary Body and Choroidal Melanomas		
	Height	Diameter
T1*	≤2.5 mm	≤10 mm
T2*	>2.5 to ≤10 mm	>10 to ≤16 mm
T3	>10 mm	>16 mm
T4	T3 and extraocular extension	
COMS Staging of Uveal Melanomas		
	Height	Diameter
Small	≤3 mm	≤5 to 16 mm
Medium	>3 to ≤10 mm	>5 to ≤16 mm
Large	>10 mm	>16 mm
Metastatic	Any N1 or M1	

*a, without microscopic extraocular extension; b, microscopic extraocular extension; c, macroscopic extraocular extension.
AJCC, American Joint Committee on Cancer; COMS, Collaborative Ocular Melanoma Study.

treatment modalities is limited. Newer laser approaches have used an 810 nm laser with long duration treatments. Although this treatment has been termed *transpupillary thermal therapy* (TTT), the exact cytotoxic mechanism of this infrared diode laser is uncertain. Most centers use thermotherapy to treat small posterior pole choroidal tumors, such as high-risk choroidal nevomas (based on clinical, ultrasound, and fluorescein angiographic criteria), small growing melanomas in close proximity to the optic nerve or fovea, or small growing tumors in the posterior pole that have produced sufficient subretinal fluid to decrease vision.[100]

Some investigators have combined infrared diode laser with radiation either to more promptly decrease subretinal fluid resorption[101] or for adjunctive therapy in posterior pole choroidal melanomas to improve the efficacy of brachytherapy.

The maximum depth of penetration of this modality is estimated to be about 4 mm, although several reports suggest it may routinely only reach a depth of 2 mm. In some centers, the use of transscleral (rather than transpupillary) infrared diode laser is being investigated.

Melanomas contiguous to the disc probably should not be treated by this technique. There is as much as a 30% late recurrence rate, and several centers have reported localized extraocular recurrences from the intrascleral extension of the tumor not effectively treated by this modality. In approximately one third of the treated eyes, there are other complications including retinal detachment, retinal vascular occlusions, hemorrhage, or internal limiting membrane contracture; all are associated with decreased vision.

Eyewall Resection

Surgical resection of uveal melanoma to salvage the eye has been described in several series.[102-104] The rationale for this approach is to preserve vision and eliminate the late visual changes associated with radiation. It is uncertain whether ocular complications in tumors not directly contiguous to the optic nerve or the fovea are due to direct radiation effects or cytokine-mediated effects from necrosing tumor. Presumably, surgical removal of the tumor would eliminate the exposure to these cytokines. The major problem with a local tumor resection is lack of predictability. In our experience we have treated tumors up to 18 mm in diameter and 12 mm thick with tumor resection. While some of the eyes were retained with 20/20 vision, others have been lost at the time of surgery and others have had what appeared to be good tumor resection but with major ocular complications. In a recent review of 125 patients followed for a mean of 6 years, 76% of eyes were successfully retained and 53% had a final visual acuity of at least 20/40.[105] Adjunctive radiation is an important part of this approach, using either protons or radioactive episcleral plaques.

Patients with large resected uveal melanomas appear to have a better ocular prognosis than those treated with radiation alone.

Enucleation

Although enucleation was the standard method for treating uveal melanomas as early as 1882,[106] the impact of this treatment on the natural history of uveal melanomas was called into question by Zimmerman,[107] who proposed an interesting hypothesis that the surgical manipulation at the time of enucleation might cause premature tumor dissemination. Several subsequent analyses pointed out the pitfalls inherent to his retrospective review and challenged this conclusion.[108] Nonetheless, the role of enucleation in the treatment of uveal melanoma has diminished with the availability of successful alternative therapies. Several indications still exist for enucleation, including: patient request after informed consent, failure of alternative therapy, tumor involving more than 40% of the intraocular volume, tumor in a blind or painful eye, and a melanoma in an eye with marked neovascularization. In multiple studies, patients who have known visceral metastases from uveal melanoma have a median survival of less than 7 months.[109] Patients with metastatic disease should not undergo enucleation unless the eye is painful.

Numerous techniques to enucleate the eye have been described. While some authors have supported cryo-enucleation techniques or paracentesis to decrease intraocular pressure during the procedure, we have favored a routine enucleation with placement of an integrated hydroxyapatite implant. If there is localized extrascleral extension, a local resection of Tenon's capsule and contiguous extraocular muscle is performed. The enucleated eye is carefully examined in the operating room and if there is transection of tumor at the time of enucleation, the gross residual tumor should be removed and no implant inserted into the orbital space.

Adjunctive pre-enucleation radiation therapy or postoperative radiation has been used in an attempt to minimize local recurrence and tumor-related mortality.[110-113] Preoperative irradiation was given to 42 patients in our institution in the hopes of exploiting the theoretic advantage of this approach (Figure 64-6). Unfortunately, when compared to 33 patients with similar tumors enucleated by the same surgeon without preoperative irradiation, no benefit could be measured.[110] The dose of radiation was 20 Gy given in 5 fractions of 4 Gy in this small series. This idea has also been subsequently studied by the COMS group using the same daily fractionation and total dose but done in a multi-institutional, prospective randomized setting. Between 1986 and 1994, 1003 patients were randomized to either receive enucleation alone or preceded by irradiation. This trial was powered to detect a 25% relative difference in mortality. Analysis of the data shows no statistically significant difference in overall survival between the two treatment arms (57% for enucleation vs. 62% for pre-enucleation radiation, $P = 0.32$).[114,115] There was a lower incidence of orbital recurrence in the irradiated patients (0 vs. 5, $P = 0.03$). Metastatic disease was most common in the liver (93%), lung (24%), and bone (16%).[116]

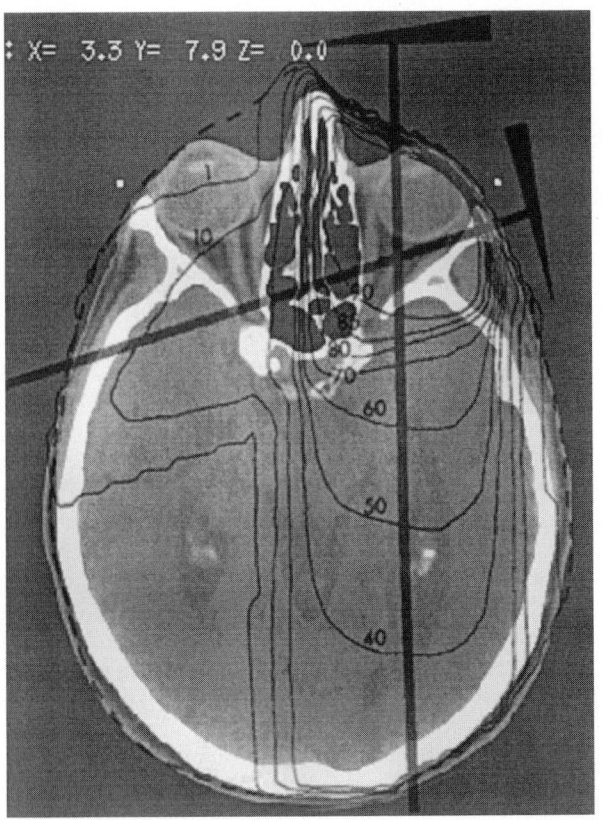

Figure 64–6. Wedged pair isodose lines for pre-enucleation irradiation.

Exenteration

If there is diffuse extraocular extension, exenteration is indicated provided there are no metastases.[117] Exenteration can be performed using either lid-sparing, or non–lid-sparing techniques (Figure 64-7A, B). An incision is made through the periosteum at the orbital rim to free orbital contents from the orbital bones. A temporalis muscle flap is often used to minimize the surgical defect and a partial thickness skin graft can cover the defect left by the eyelid resection.

Episcleral Radioactive Plaques

While brachytherapy has been used in uveal melanoma management since 1929,[118] there remain a number of unresolved issues regarding optimal treatment. Stallard has been credited with popularizing the use of Co-60 episcleral plaques.[119] He reported treatment results of the first 100 patients using Co-60 applicators or radon seeds between 1939 and 1964, outlining indications, surgical technique, and the radiation doses to the tumor base and apex over 7 to 14 days (70 to 140 Gy at the apex, and 200 to 400 Gy at the tumor base). The dose rate at the tumor base and apex was dependent on the thickness of the tumor, the source geometry, and the specific activity of the plaque selected. Excluding patients who died from

Figure 64–7. A, Orbital exenteration with lid-sparing approach. **B**, Orbital exenteration with lid resection. (Modified from Char DH: *Clinical Ocular Oncology.* Philadelphia: Lippincott-Raven; 1997:89.)

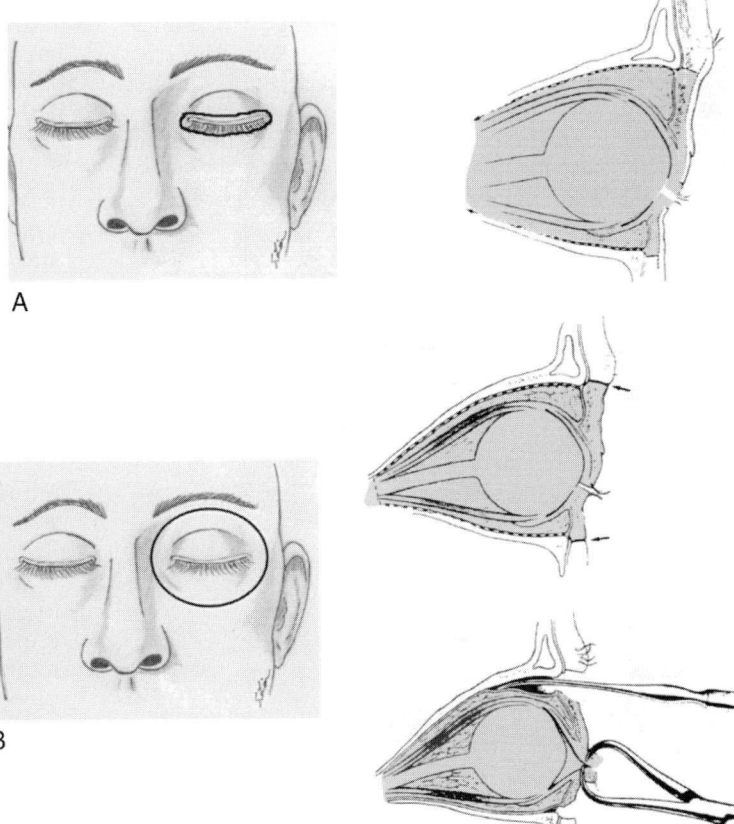

metastases, he described 69 successes (some after a repeated application), 16 failures, and 9 indeterminate responses. The majority of successes were small tumors measuring 5 to 8 mm in diameter, raising the issue of potentially benign lesions included in this analysis. He also described radiation complications including cataract, perimacular exudates, retinal hemorrhage, glaucoma, keratitis, and scleral necrosis. This initial experience, while somewhat empirical, provided a satisfactory alternative to enucleation. The Stallard applicator was subsequently used extensively in the United States. The local failure rate with Co-60 has been reported to be between 12% and 33%.[120-122]

Sealy described an ingenious adaptation of the episcleral technique using the lower energy isotope I-125 with intrinsic shielding in 1976.[123] The ability to shield the ocular adnexa including the eyelids and lacrimal apparatus and markedly decrease the radiation dose to the surgical team was a major advance. The early plaques were individually fabricated using a thin gold or lead foil to which an array of I-125 seeds was glued. Dose and dose rates were variable and dependent on the source strengths available, but in general mimicked the standardized Stallard applicators. A comparison of the dosimetry of plaques using different isotopes is elegantly described by Luxton, who notes that for tumors up to about 10 mm in thickness, there is a preponderance of the inverse square law effect, which is independent of the photon emission energy.[124]

Although it may be counter-intuitive, for a given dose to the tumor apex, the tumor base dose is similar for photon emitters from Co-60 (1.2 MeV) to I-125 (27 KeV) (Figure 64-8).[125] In contrast, beta emitters including Ru-106 deliver a very high dose to the sclera and are not suitable for the treatment of tumors thicker than 3 mm, although these applicators may be used to minimize the dose to other visually sensitive structures.[126,127] Ruthenium has been the most commonly employed isotope for brachytherapy in Europe.

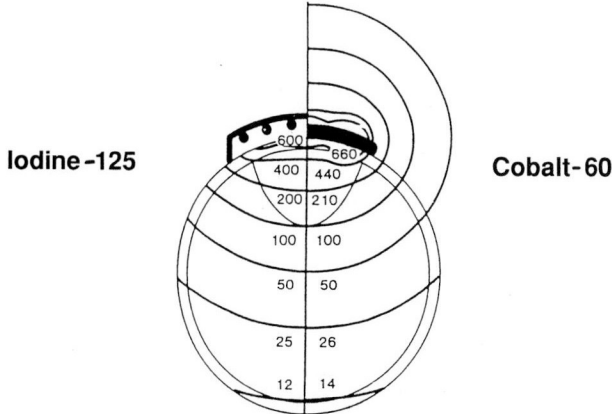

Figure 64–8. Schematic diagram of isodose line from iodine-125 and cobalt-60 episcleral plaques. Note the shielding by the gold plaque of the lower-energy iodine-125 sources and the spacer placed between the seeds and the sclera. Although the ocular adnexa is shielded with iodine-125, the dose to the globe and lens is similar to that with cobalt-60.

I-125 Plaque Brachytherapy

The most commonly used isotope for uveal melanoma therapy in the United States is I-125 because of its ease of shielding, availability in a wide range of seed strengths, and favorable half-life (59.6 days), which allows multiple usage. I-125 seeds exhibit considerable anisotropy, which requires that dose calculations be done with linear source modeling. Published computer algorithms have good agreement with measured values for depths from 0.5 to 1.5 cm along the central axis at angles near 90 degrees.[124,128] The gold backing of the applicator reduces the measured dose in the first 1.5 cm depth by 8%.[129] Further, Monte Carlo evaluations by Williamson suggest a specific dose constant 14% lower than previously recommended because of disparities between the dose measured in air and in water.[130] While the uncertainties of dose with I-125 dosimetry have frustrated attempts to standardize the clinical implementation of this technique, it is clear that the optimal seed array and activity is dependent on the tumor configuration and location. A sample dose distribution for a plaque is shown in Figure 64-9A, B. Several computerized treatment planning programs have been developed to include dose distribution to the tumor and the visually critical structures such as the fovea, optic nerve, and the lens. Although treatment planning programs using CT or MRI data have been proposed,[131] the lack of precision of these techniques to define the target volume, as well as the additional cost, has led most clinicians to rely on more pragmatic approaches. Some of these programs include fixed source positions into which seeds may be secured and may also include an algorithm to estimate the impact of the gold shielding applicator. The applicator is designed to follow the external curvature of the globe, perhaps with a notch or a cut-out to accommodate the optic nerve, or with a rim or a lip around the edge to "collimate" the beam (Fig. 64-10A, B). If a rimmed plaque is used, it must be 4 mm larger than the maximum tumor diameter to assure adequate dose at the tumor base margin (this allows a 2 mm circumferential margin to account for tumor extension and plaque placement uncertainties). It is important to note that while the gold plaque is clearly able to minimize the dose of radiation to the medical team and the periorbital tissues, it has not been demonstrated that the rim can limit radiation-induced visual loss, while achieving similar local control. In fact, concern about marginal tumor failures (approximately 50% of the local failures in most series) has led us to return to the use of unrimmed plaques in more recent years.

The brachytherapy treatment plan delivers a "tumor dose" of 70 to 100 Gy to the tumor apex with a margin to include the scleral thickness (1 mm), an additional mm of tumor thickness or height, and a 2 mm surround of the tumor diameter as defined by the ophthalmologist. The optimal dose rate is not clearly established, although most authors plan for an overall treatment time between 4 and 7 days. More recent analysis suggests that the optimal minimal tumor dose rate is likely between 0.7 and 1 Gy/hour using episcleral plaques.[132] The dose rate at the scleral surface is highly dependent on the seed

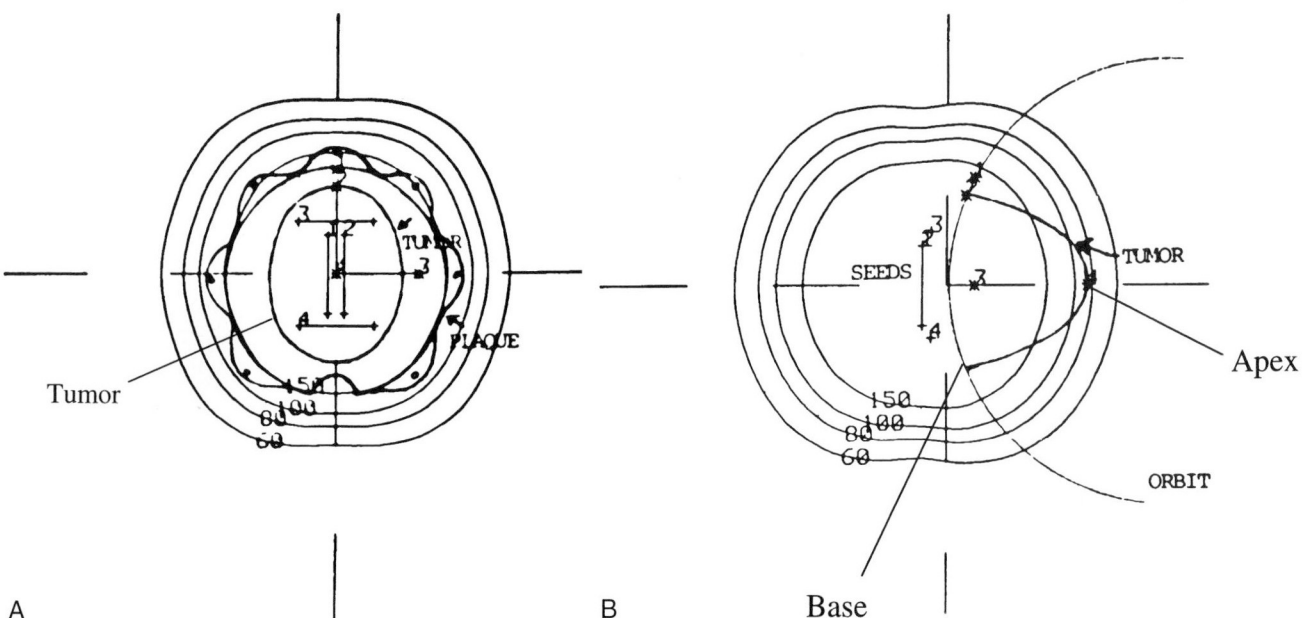

Figure 64–9. A, Base view of eye plaque with isodose contours designed to provide a dose rate at the tumor base plus a margin (150 cGy/h). **B**, Lateral view of eye plaque with isodose contours designed to provide a dose rate at the tumor apex of 80 cGy/h. (The shielding by the gold plaque is not reflected in those computer-generated plots.)

activity and the tumor thickness. A 1 mm spacer (or contact lens) is recommended to minimize hot spots over the individual seeds. In spite of very high doses to the sclera, scleral necrosis is a rare event, and often correlates with an anteriorly located tumor where the sclera is known to be thinner and inflammation more common from eroded or retracted conjunctiva. In general, radioactive seed selection and placement is dictated by the tumor geometry. Relatively flat or thin tumors are best treated with the seeds on the tumor perimeter, while thick tumors will require hot central sources to ensure a high central axis dose (Fig. 64-11).

Patient selection is critical for the successful application of brachytherapy techniques. Although tumors as thick as 10 or 12 mm have been treated using episcleral plaques, the optimal long-term visual results are for tumors with ultrasound height measurements less than 6 mm. The maximum basal tumor diameter is highly correlated with both local control and metastatic disease. Finally, the location of the tumor relative to the optic nerve, fovea, lens, and attachment of extraocular muscles must be understood if one is to plan the plaque design. While the plaque can theoretically be placed anywhere on the globe, the attachment of extraocular muscles or the

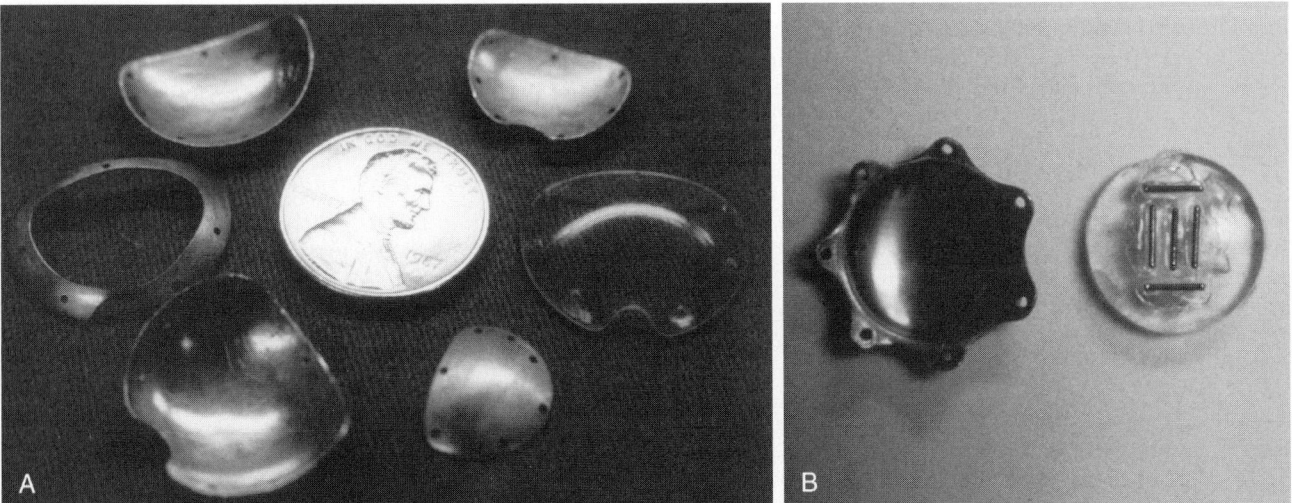

Figure 64–10. A, Gold plaque carriers, some with "cutouts" and "dummy plaques." **B**, Rimmed gold plaques with acrylic insert or spacer onto which iodine-125 seeds are glued.

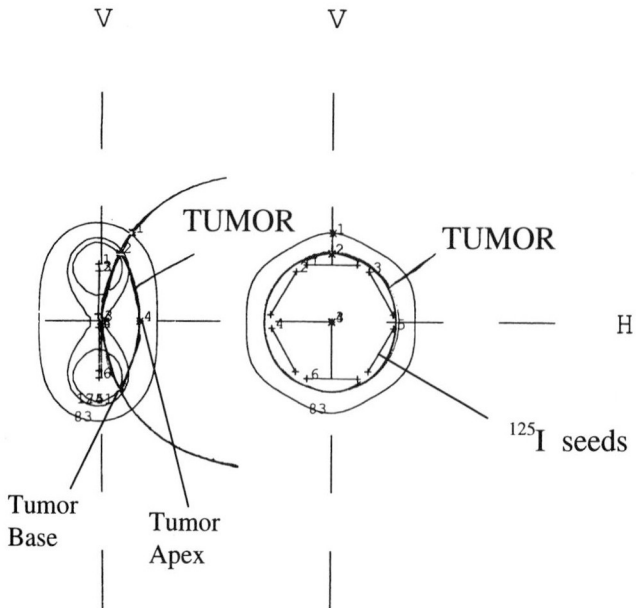

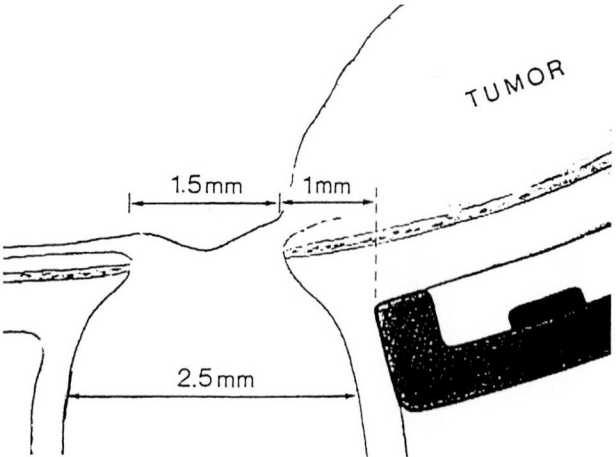

Figure 64–12. Rimmed plaques cannot be used next to the optic disc, because the larger exterior diameter of the nerve vis-à-vis the rim delivers insufficient radiation for a tumor that is contiguous to the optic nerve. (From Char DH: *Clinical Ocular Oncology.* Philadelphia: Lippincott-Raven; 1997:89.)

Figure 64–11. Base and lateral view of a tumor with a large diameter and shallow height. Note the seed placement around the perimeter rather than at hot centrally located sources, as for the thicker tumor illustrated in Figure 64–9.

optic nerve can displace the applicator (Fig. 64-12). To allow for the thickness of the optic nerve and its sheath, peripapillary tumors often require an eccentric seed array and a cutout or notched plaque.[47,120] Further, if the tumor is located close to a rectus muscle insertion, one can avoid the surgical detachment of the muscle by using a similar approach. The design of the plaque must be thoroughly understood by the ophthalmologist, as accurate placement is critical to tumor control. Great care must be taken to ensure that the surgeon understands the dose distribution relative to the physical plaque edge. Because this is not always symmetric, the orientation of the seed array can be indicated with a hatch mark on the plaque as well as the dummy plaque.

The surgical placement of the plaque is done with either general or local anesthesia. The eye is dilated before the procedure to ensure adequate tumor localization. A 360° perilimbal incision is made and Tenon's capsule is entered (Fig. 64-13A, B). The rectus muscles

are isolated and suture slings are placed to allow rotation of the globe. The melanoma is localized with diffuse corneal transillumination using diathermy marks to outline the scleral shadow cast by the tumor; the position is confirmed using point source transillumination with indirect ophthalmoscopy (Fig. 64-14A, B). This latter step is crucial to ensure that " shadowing" from the anteriorly placed diffuse transilluminator has not led to a misinterpretation of the tumor location. If necessary for the plaque placement, extraocular muscles can be detached. Intraoperative needle aspiration biopsy can be done if there are diagnostic uncertainties. A dummy plaque is sutured into place and the position verified before the placement of the radioactive plaque. The radiation oncologist should be present in the operating room with the isodose curves to ensure optimal plaque placement. After the radioactive plaque is secured, the eye is irrigated with antibiotic solution and the conjunctiva closed; the dressing is covered with a lead eye shield, which is left in place during the application. Verification of plaque placement can be accomplished with the use of intraoperative ultrasound. The patient can usually be discharged within

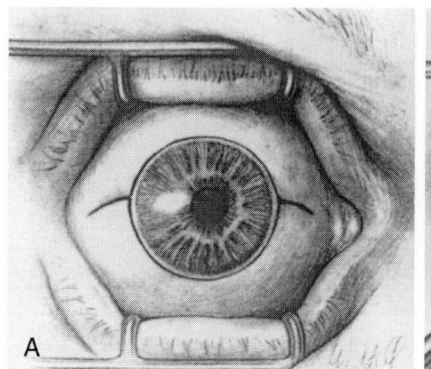

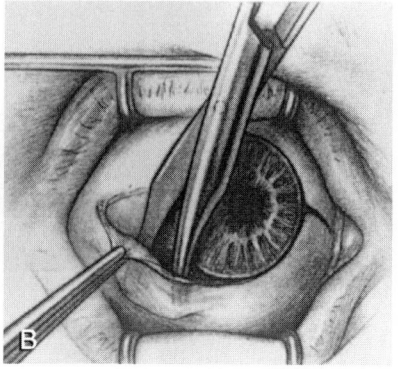

Figure 64–13. A, The conjunctival incision adjacent to the limbus around the entire circumference of the cornea. **B,** Tenon's capsule is entered by gently opening the membranous tissues beneath the conjunctiva and the sclera.

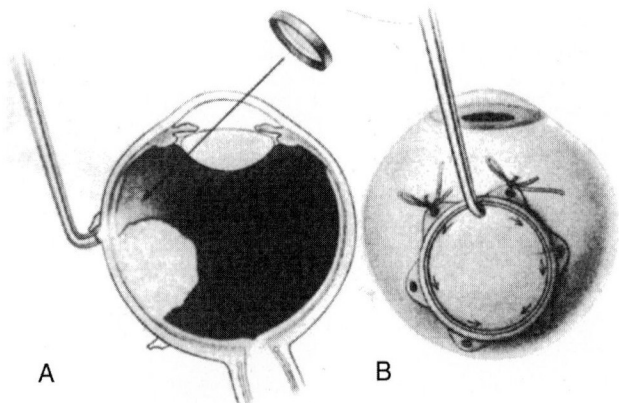

Figure 64–14. **A,** Indirect ophthalmoscopy and point-source transillumination are used to delineate the margins of the tumor. **B,** A rimmed radioactive plaque carrier is sutured in place over the tumor base. (Modified from Char DH: *Clinical Ocular Oncology.* Philadelphia: Lippincott-Raven; 1997:89.)

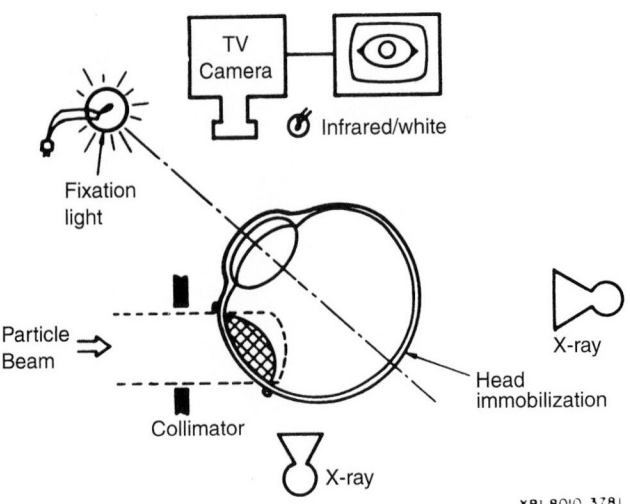

Figure 64–15. Schematic of treatment with charged particle beam. The optimal gaze angle is determined by preplanning; tantalum rings outlining the tumor base are localized on coplanar x-rays. The beam's eye view confirms the tantalum ring placement. An infrared television camera is used to ensure that the patient maintains eye fixation during treatment.

24 hours, dependent on state regulations, and return for plaque removal within 4 to 7 days, with reattachment of rectus muscles, if necessary. Brachytherapy guidelines for the treatment of uveal melanomas have recently been published with the goal of standardizing both treatment and dose reporting policies.[133]

Charged Particle Radiotherapy (Protons and Helium Ions)

The development of methodology to treat uveal melanomas with the Bragg peak of charged particle beams was described by Constable and others working at the Harvard cyclotron with a 160 MeV proton beam.[134,135] Accelerated charged particles can treat small targets with minimal lateral scatter and radiation dose beyond the end of the Bragg peak. Studies with modulated and collimated beams demonstrate a relative biologic efficiency (RBE) of close to unity when compared to 2 MeV photon beams. The adaptation of this technique for humans required the development of sophisticated tumor mapping using the surgical placement of tantalum rings, immobilization devices controlling for both head position and gaze angle, and a computerized treatment planning program.[136] A similar technique using helium ions was developed at the Lawrence Berkeley Laboratory in collaboration with the Department of Radiation Oncology and the Ocular Oncology Unit at the UCSF (Fig. 64-15). The RBE of the helium beam is slightly greater than the proton beam, and, accordingly, dose adjustments were made.[137] The *EYEPLAN* software used for the treatment planning schematically displays a drawing of the patient's eye including the lens, optic nerve, and fovea, and the surgeon's mapping of tumor and position of localizing tantalum rings, as well as the spatial coordinates of the tantalum rings localized on orthogonal radiographs. The optimal beam angle and gaze angle are selected so that the collimator shape and beam modulator are determined (Fig. 64-16*A-D*).

CRITICAL NORMAL TISSUES

Episcleral radioactive plaques and charged particle beams are used to treat uveal melanomas to control tumor while salvaging the globe and potentially preserving vision. Episcleral I-125 plaques can deliver a high tumor dose while usually shielding the ocular adnexa, including the lids and the lacrimal apparatus. These structures are not as easily shielded using charged particle techniques. Thus, acute epitheliitis of the eyelid, lash loss, dry eye, and epiphora (abnormal overflow of tears due to excess secretion of tears or to obstruction of the lacrimal duct) are more common with charged particle therapy (Fig. 64-17). The incidence of neovascular glaucoma (NVG) (caused by abnormal new blood vessel formation in and on the iris, with closure of angle drainage structures) is also higher in this latter group, presumably due to the higher radiation dose to the anterior filtration apparatus. An analysis of the development of NVG following helium-ion radiation shows a strong correlation with the percent of lens and anterior chamber in the treatment field, increasing tumor height, proximity of tumor to the fovea, a history of diabetes, and the development of vitreous hemorrhage.[138] Significant cataract, radiation maculopathy, and cystic macular edema are seen with equal frequency with plaques and particle techniques. However, vitreous hemorrhage and secondary strabismus are more frequently observed after I-125 plaques.

The long-term visual outcome is important to consider when evaluating irradiation techniques. The 1993 report of a randomized trial at UCSF comparing plaques with helium ions confirmed that visual acuities decreased by four or more Snellen lines in 69% of the patients in each group.[97] Visual acuity analysis show the impact of tumor location (>3 mm from the nerve or fovea, no ciliary body involvement) and tumor height (<6 mm) on good visual

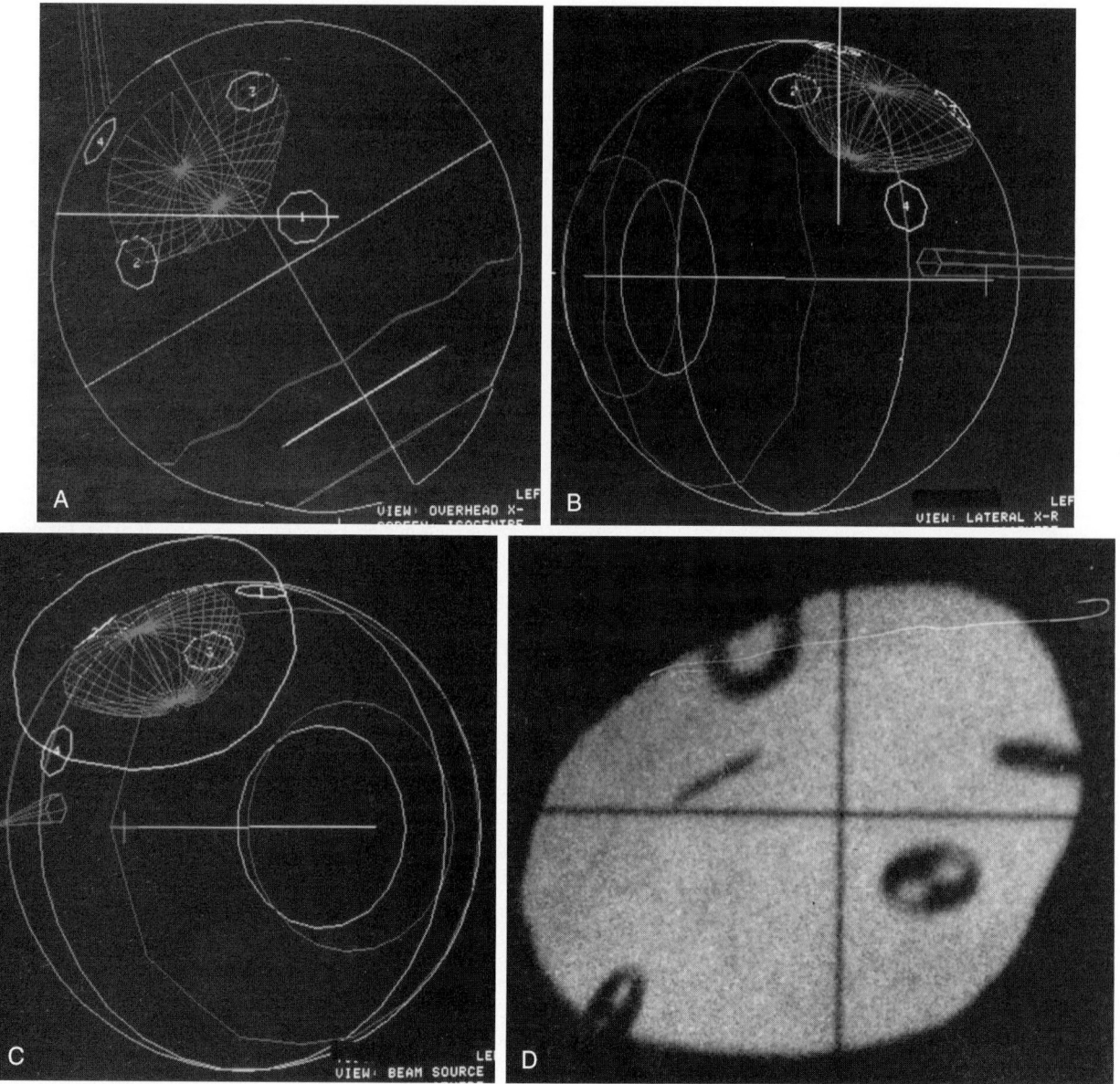

Figure 64–16. The EYEPLAN display of the tumor target with the tantalum ring placement as indicated by the surgeon and confirmed by coplanar x-rays. *See also Color Figure 64–16A–C* for identification of parts. **A**, Overhead view. **B**, Lateral view. **C**, Beam's-eye view. The port film confirms the tantalum ring placement indicated by the preplan (**D**). The most superior shadow on the port film is the eyelid retractor.

outcome. Nearly 60% of these more favorable patients have visual acuities of 20/50 or better at last follow-up. An update of the visual outcome analysis has identified several factors associated with the rate of visual loss and the post-treatment visual acuity. These include pretreatment visual acuity; tumor thickness; tumor location vis-á-vis the nerve, fovea, and ciliary body; patient age; and the degree of retinal detachment at the time of therapy.[139] Groups of patients with low and high probability of good visual outcome can be identified before treatment. The rate of visual loss can be shown using cumulative hazard plots (Fig. 64-18A, B). Transitory visual loss due to resolving retinal detachment, clearing vitreous hemorrhage, temporary macular edema, or post-radiation cataract followed by cataract extraction can be observed. Although no significant visual outcome differences between helium ion and I-125 irradiations are noted, some differences in the covariate effects between these two treatments are evident. Larger tumor location effects are present with helium ions while larger tumor size effects are present with episcleral plaques. Further follow-up is necessary to evaluate the late visual effects, although there is a suggestion that late onset visual loss may be greater with plaques.

The COMS randomized trial of I-125 brachytherapy for 657 patients with medium-sized choroidal melanomas confirmed the importance of long-term follow-up for visual outcome with visual acuity decreasing to 20/200 or worse in 17% of patients by 1 year, 33% by 2 years, and 43% by 3 years.[140] The loss of six lines of visual acuity

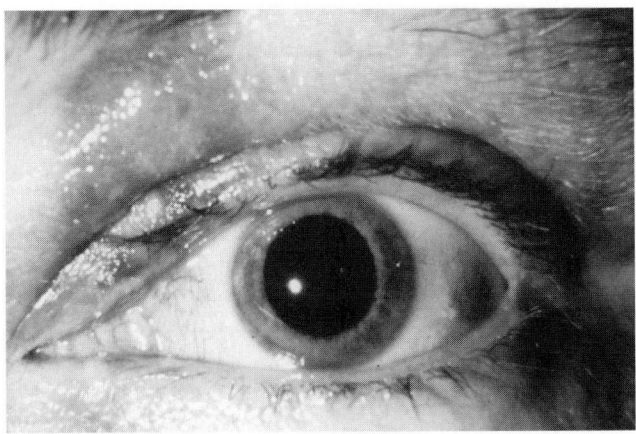

Figure 64–17. Acute lid epitheliitis following helium ion therapy.

after treatment was statistically associated with greater baseline tumor apical height and shorter distance between the tumor and the foveal avascular zone (FAZ). Patient history of diabetes, presence of tumor-associated retinal detachment, and tumors that were not dome shaped also were associated with greater risk for poor vision outcomes.[140]

OUTCOME

Episcleral Plaques

Analysis of high intensity I-125 plaque treatment of uveal melanoma at UCSF includes 449 patients treated between 1983 and 2000.[47,141] Fifty-eight of these lesions

Table 64–4 Multivariate Analysis of Factors Predicting Tumor Regrowth

	Estimates	Standard Errors	P Value
↓ Ultrasound height, mm	−0.333	0.121	0.0028
↓ Minimal radiation dose, Gy	−0.062	0.030	0.0532
↓ Distance from the fovea, mm	−0.311	0.108	0.0003
↓ Maximal tumor diameter, mm	0.244	0.070	0.0006
↑ Patient age, yr	−0.015	0.017	0.33835

↓ indicates decrease; ↑ indicates increase.
From Quivey JM, Char DH, Phillips TL, et al: High Intensity 125-iodine (125-I) plaque treatment of uveal melanomas. *Int J Radiat Oncol Biol Phys.* 1993;26:613.

recurred locally with a mean interval between treatment and detection of recurrence of 3.6 years (range 0.2 to 15.3 years). Eleven uveal melanoma patients had late intraocular tumor failures detected from 5.5 to 15.3 years after treatment. A multivariate analysis identified four factors that are associated with increased local failure: smaller tumor height, closer proximity to the fovea and disc, larger tumor diameter, and lower radiation dose (Table 64-4).[47] Interestingly, these factors were not observed in the late treatment failures.[141] The incidence of distant metastatic disease is only associated with larger tumor diameter (Table 64-5). Kaplan-Meier plots of the estimates of time to tumor response as measured by decrease in the ultrasound height displays the slow rate of tumor shrinkage (Fig. 64-19). Similar plots of the time to tumor regrowth are shown in Figure 64-20, and time until metastases is shown in Figure 64-21. The cumulative incidences of local recurrence at 5 and 10 years are 11.5% and 15.8%, respectively, while the estimated

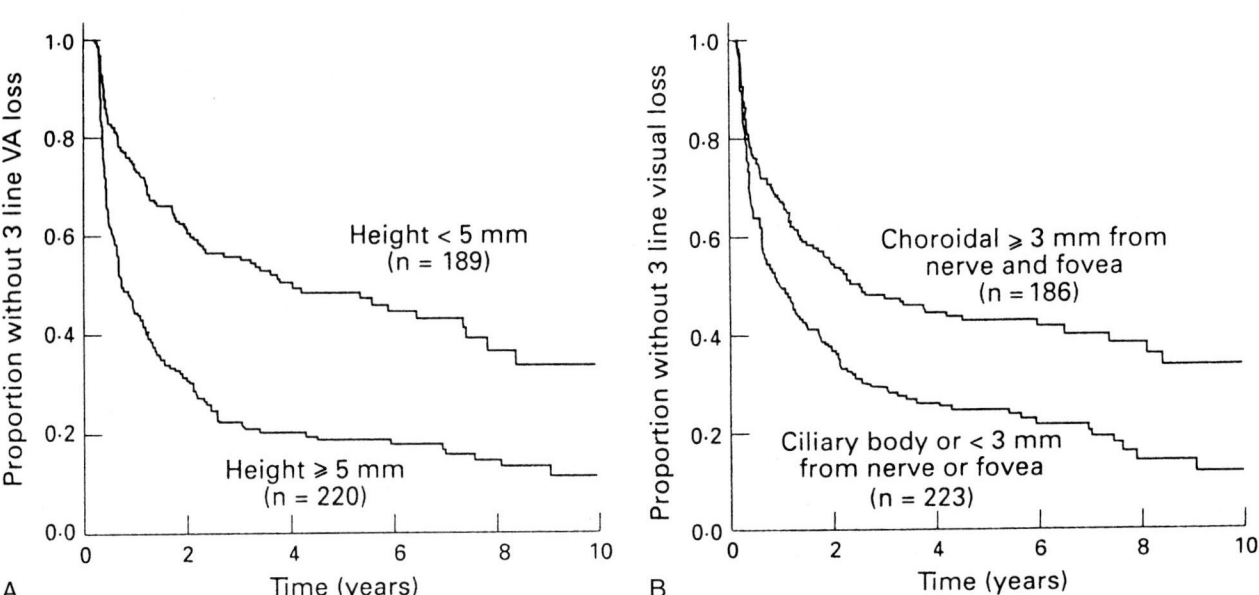

Figure 64–18. Visual loss following helium ion or iodine-125 treatment. Kaplan-Meier survival estimates for time until three or more lines are lost for 409 irradiated patients with pretreatment visual acuity (VA) of 6/120 or greater stratified by pretreatment ultrasound tumor height (**A**) and pretreatment tumor location with respect to the nerve, fovea, and ciliary body (**B**). (From Char DH, Kroll S, Quivey JM, Castro JR: Long term visual outcome of radiated uveal melanomas in eyes eligible for randomisation to enucleation versus brachytherapy. *Br J Ophthalmol.* 1996;80:117. With permission of the BMT Publishing Group.)

Table 64–5   Multivariate Analysis of Factors Predicting Metastases

	Estimates	Standard Errors	P Value
↓ Ultrasound height, mm	−0.333	0.116	0.9813
↓ Minimal radiation dose, Gy	−0.027	0.042	0.5288
↓ Distance from the fovea, mm	−0.115	0.085	0.1456
↓ Maximal tumor diameter, mm	0.211	0.095	0.027
↑ Patient age, yr	−0.010	0.020	0.607

↓ indicates decrease; ↑ indicates increase.
From Quivey JM, Char DH, Phillips TL, et al: High Intensity 125-iodine (125-I) plaque treatment of uveal melanomas. *Int J Radiat Oncol Biol Phys.* 1993;26:613.

incidence of metastasis at 5 years is 12%. The rate of metastasis is 0.457 per year for the epithelioid and mixed cell types, while it is 0.0 per year for the spindle cell type. The unexpected finding of a higher rate of local treatment failure with the I-125 plaques with thinner tumors located near the fovea led to speculation that either dose rate effects or technical factors might be coming into play. Analysis of the Wills Hospital experience with I-125 plaques also shows dose, dose rate, maximum tumor diameter, and tumor location (either ciliary body or in proximity to the nerve and fovea) to be statistically significant prognostic factors.[132] Higher recurrence rates were noted with tumors in close proximity to the fovea, optic nerve, and ciliary body. Although the prescribed dose was somewhat higher in this latter series (mean dose to tumor apex 94.8 Gy), the 5-year local control rate was 81% (Figs. 64-22 and 64-23).

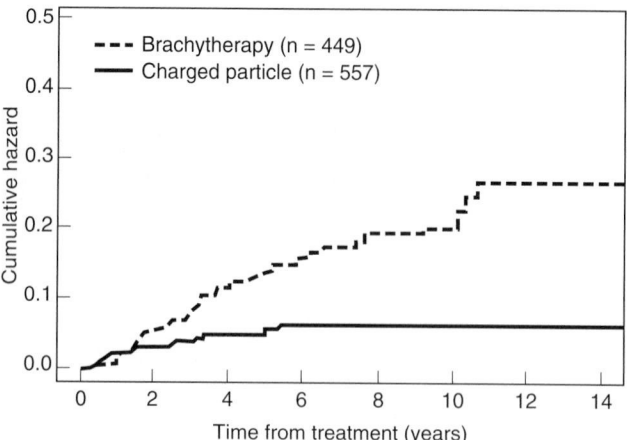

A

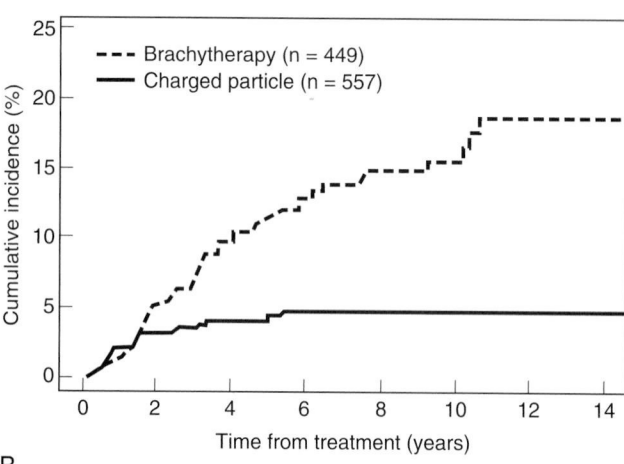

B

Figure 64–20. **A,** Cumulative hazard of local recurrence after radiation. **B,** Probability of local recurrence after radiation. (From Char DH, et al. *Opthalmology* 2002;109:1850–4.)

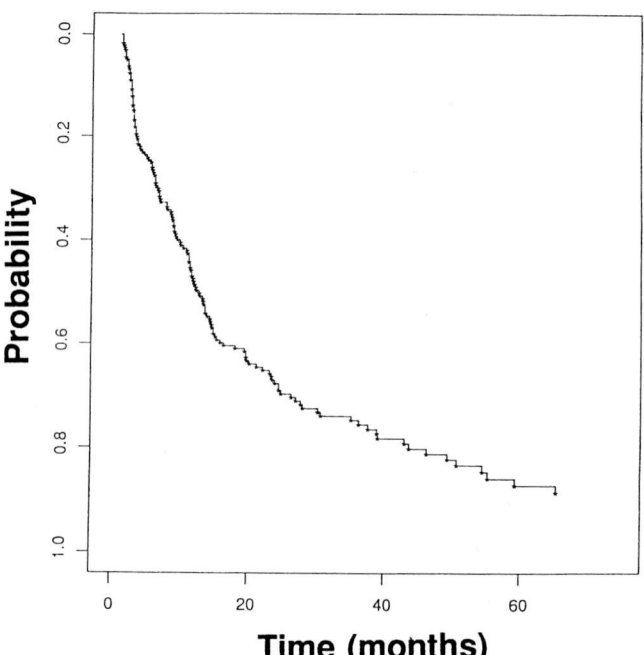

Figure 64–19. Kaplan-Meier probability of tumor height decrease by 1 mm following iodine-125 plaque therapy. (From Quivey JM, Char DH, Phillips TL, et al: High intensity 125-iodine (125I) plaque treatment of uveal melanoma. *Int J Radiat Oncol Biol Phys.* 1993;26:613.)

Charged Particle Beams: Protons and Helium Ions

More than 2000 patients with uveal melanoma have been treated with protons at the Harvard cyclotron. The prescribed dose in their series is 70 Cobalt Gray Equivalent (CGE) in 5 fractions over 7 to 10 days assuming CGE = proton Gy × RBE 1.1. Actuarial local control at 5 years is 97% and at 15 years is 95%.[142-144] The 5-year actuarial survival for the patients treated with protons is 78.5% for the entire group with 97.5%, 85.8%, and 58.1% survival for patients with small, intermediate, and large melanomas, respectively. Using the Cox proportional hazards model, the factors that predict survival on multivariate analysis include maximum tumor diameter greater than 15 mm, ciliary body involvement, age older than 59 years, and the presence of extrascleral tumor extension.[54] These results have been confirmed at the Paul Sherrer Institute by Egger et al.,[145] who reported 2435 patients treated between 1984 and 1998 with 54.5 CGE in 4 fractions. The 10-year local control rate was 95.8% at 5 years and 94.8% at 10 years

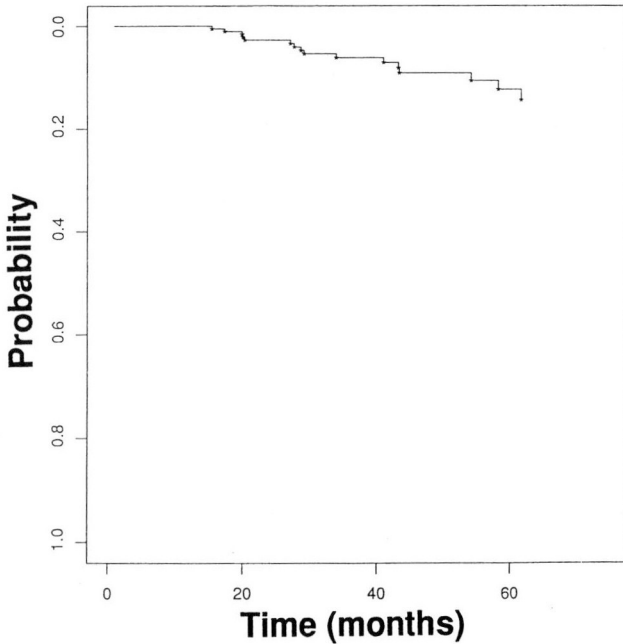

Figure 64–21. Kaplan-Meier plot of time to metastases following iodine-125 plaque treatment. (From Quivey JM, Char DH, Phillips TL, et al: High intensity 125-iodine (125I) plaque treatment of uveal melanoma. *Int J Radiat Oncol Biol Phys.* 1993;26:613.)

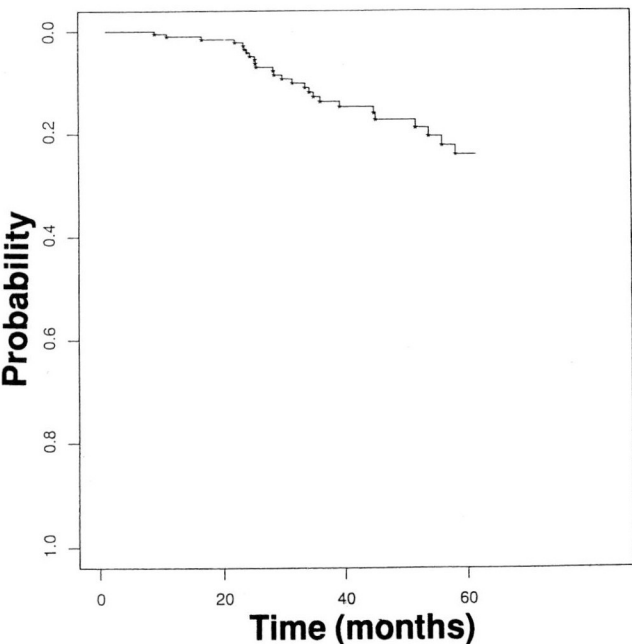

Figure 64–23. Kaplan-Meier plot of time to development of postradiation cataract. (From Quivey JM, Char DH, Phillips TL, et al: High intensity 125-iodine (125I) plaque treatment of uveal melanoma. *Int J Radiat Oncol Biol Phys.* 1993;26:613.)

(Kaplan-Meier estimate). Patients treated with a reduced safety margin due to proximity of the tumor to the fovea had a much higher local failure rate at 5 years, 28.7%. The overall 10-year cause-specific survival was 72.6% for patients with controlled tumors versus 47.5% for

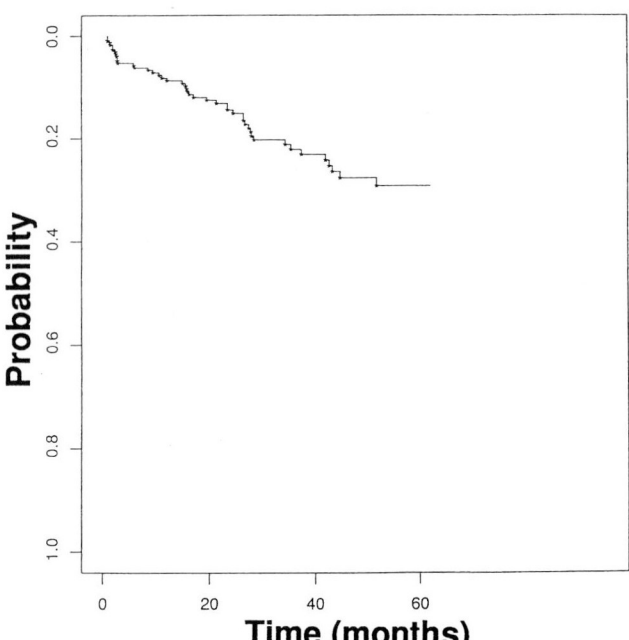

Figure 64–22. Kaplan-Meier plot of time to development of postradiation vitreous hemorrhage. (From Quivey JM, Char DH, Phillips TL, et al: High intensity 125-iodine (125I) plaque treatment of uveal melanoma. *Int J Radiat Oncol Biol Phys.* 1993;26:613.)

those with local recurrence. Additional factors affecting prognosis include age, amount of retinal detachment, ocular melanosis, large tumor diameter, increased tumor height, and extrascleral extension.

The results with helium ion therapy have been similar to those described for protons. The patients were treated with dose of 50, 60, 70, or 80 Gy equivalents (CGE = helium ion dose Gy × RBE 1.3) in a dose searching effort to establish the minimum dose necessary for optimal tumor control. The local control was 96% at 5 years for the 347 patients treated with helium ions. The actuarial 5-year survival for this group of patients was 80%.[97,146,147] The Kaplan-Meier survival was 76% at 10 years and 72% at 15 years.[148]

Prospective Randomized Trials

A prospective randomized trial of helium ions versus I-125 brachytherapy was conducted at UCSF and the Lawrence Berkeley Laboratory. To date, this is the only study comparing charged particles with episcleral plaques. A total of 184 patients with uveal melanoma were randomized with clinical parameters including the largest tumor diameter, ultrasound height, distance to the nerve or fovea, and preoperative visual acuity balanced between the two treatment arms. The treatment dose was 70 Gy in both arms, but there were profound differences in the dose rate in the particle arm (5 fractions over 5 to 7 days delivered in <2 minute fractions) versus continuous low dose rate radiation in the I-125 arm (0.7 to 0.75 Gy per hour at the tumor apex). The higher rate of local failure in the plaque-treated patients (13 patients vs. 0) led to increase in the dose and dose rate of subsequent patients treated with plaques. Long-term follow-up of the patients in this series shows no differences in tumor-related mortality between the two groups. However, there are clear differences in ocular morbidity with dry eye, epiphora, and neovascular glaucoma more common following helium ion therapy, while temporary strabismus due to the need to temporally disinsert a muscle to facilitate plaque placement is unique to I-125 treated patients (Table 64-6). Concerns about the development of NVG after helium ion irradiation has led to an in-depth analysis of factors that correlate with this complication.[149] Currently, we are using proton beams, with careful attention to minimize the radiation dose to the lens in an effort to maximize local control and minimize late visual complications. The incidence of NVG with these recent technical modifications is close to that observed with I-125 brachytherapy.

In the "medium" choroidal melanoma study, COMS addressed whether brachytherapy with I-125 is equal to enucleation with respect to mortality. This study addressed a long-time controversy regarding the efficacy of definitive irradiation. Patients with tumors between 2.5 and 10 mm in height and less than 16 mm diameter were randomized to receive I-125 plaques or enucleation. Brachytherapy was delivered using plaques with a 2 to 3 mm margin at the tumor base, delivering a dose of 85 Gy to the prescription point (the apex for tumors >5 mm in height or at 5 mm for tumors between 2.5 and 4.9 mm) using Task Group 43 guidelines.[150] Patient selection was similar to the UCSF randomized trial between I-125 plaques and helium ions. However, patients at highest risk for local recurrence following plaque therapy were excluded from this analysis. Thus, patients whose tumors were contiguous with the optic disc were ineligible, and those with peripapillary tumors (2 mm or closer to the optic disc) were eligible only when the tumor was limited within 90 degrees. Tumors located predominantly in the ciliary body were also excluded. More than 1300 patients were randomized over an 11-year period (1987

to 1998) with 657 patients assigned to brachytherapy. The mean apical height of the tumors was 4.8 mm, and mean largest diameter at the base was 11.4 mm. Only 16% of patients had tumors within 2 mm of the optic disc. Overall, 592 tumors were treated per protocol specifications. The 5-year actuarial survival rates are 81% and 82% for the enucleation and brachytherapy arms, respectively, firmly establishing the equivalency of these techniques. Fewer than half the decedents in each treatment arm were judged to have metastatic melanoma at the time of death. Only patient age, maximum tumor basal diameter, and location of the tumor relative to the optic disc were independent and statistically significant predictors of death with melanoma.[151] The subsequent publication of brachytherapy local treatment failure and enucleation results reports 69 patients with enucleation and 57 patients with local treatment failure (10.3%) in the first 5 years post treatment. Multivariate analysis indicated that older patient age, greater tumor height, and proximity to the FAZ were associated with treatment failure. The risk of failure in persons older than age 50 was nearly three times as high as in those younger than age 50.[152]

The outcome of the COMS studies of "small" and "large" melanomas has supported the safety and appropriateness of observation for small, nongrowing tumors and the lack of significant benefit from preoperative irradiation for large tumors. The equivalency of enucleation and definitive irradiation for medium-sized tumors is also supported by the COMS study. If the patient desires organ preservation, the selection of technique (brachytherapy or proton therapy) is highly dependent on the tumor location vis-à-vis the fovea, optic nerve, and ciliary body. Substantial retrospective data from many institutions show a significantly higher local failure rate when tumors in these latter areas are treated with episcleral plaques. In fact, these lesions were specifically excluded from the COMS "medium" melanoma trial. The available data from both randomized and nonrandomized prospective series clearly show a higher rate of local control with charged particle beams of helium

Table 64–6   Tumor Control and Complications: ^{125}I Plaque Versus Helium Ion

	^{125}I (98 Patients), %	Helium (86 patients), %	Relative Risk	95% Confidence Interval
Local tumor growth	13.3	0.0	Not defined	2.95*
Metastases	8.2	9.3	0.96	0.27, 2.78
Death by metastases	8.2	8.2	1.10	0.31, 3.40
Vitreous hemorrhage	29.6	19.8	1.76	0.82, 3.62
Radiation maculopathy	27.6	30.2	0.76	0.45, 1.74
Significant cataract	22.4	25.6	0.76	0.41, 1.75
Cystoid macular edema	19.4	16.3	1.17	0.55, 2.87
Radiation optic neuropathy	17.3	23.3	0.66	0.32, 1.52
Enucleation	17.3	9.3	1.99	0.78, 5.78
Neovascular glaucoma	11.2	29.1	0.32	0.13, 0.71
Dry eye	8.2	27.9	0.28	0.09, 0.57
Keratitis	5.1	5.8	0.65	0.20, 3.93
Epiphora	3.1	20.9	0.12	0.003, 0.43

*$P < 0.001$.

Modified from Char DH, Quivey JM, Castro JR, et al: Helium ion versus iodine 125 brachytherapy in the management of uveal melanoma: A prospective, randomized, dynamically balanced trial. *Ophthalmology*. 1993;100:1547. Courtesy of *Ophthalmology*.

ions or protons (95% to 98%) than has been observed with brachytherapy techniques. "Late" radiation failures (beyond 5 years after treatment) have also been more frequently observed after plaque therapy. Because of the limited number of proton facilities, many centers have preferred to use episcleral plaques, citing the equivalence of melanoma mortality across series. Certainly, for frail or elderly patients who are unable to travel for therapy, this is clinically appropriate. Visual outcome analysis remains somewhat disappointing, as the COMS observations regarding visual function closely parallels our own observations.

The treatment of uveal melanomas has been extensively and rigorously evaluated using observation only, surgery, photocoagulation, laser treatment and thermotherapy, episcleral plaques, and charged particle techniques. All of these approaches require specific expertise and great care in the application so that optimal local control and good long-term visual outcomes can be achieved. Both acute and late ocular morbidity are dependent on the treatment modality, and further clinical explorations of techniques to maximize good functional visual outcomes are needed. Nonetheless, it has been clearly shown that immediate enucleation is not necessary and that conservation approaches can successfully control tumor with the promise of preserving useful vision.

REFERENCES

1. Egan KM, et al: Epidemiologic aspects of uveal melanoma. *Surv Ophthalmol.* 1988;32:239.
2. Chang AE, Karnell LH, Menck HR: The National Cancer Data Base report on cutaneous and noncutaneous melanoma: a summary of 84,836 cases from the past decade. The American College of Surgeons Commission on Cancer and the American Cancer Society. *Cancer.* 1998;83:1664.
3. Neugut AI, Kizelnik-Freilich S: Black-white differences in risk for cutaneous, ocular, and visceral melanomas. *Am J Public Health.* 1994;84:1828.
4. Scotto J, Fraumeni JFJ, Lee JA: Melanomas of the eye and other noncutaneous sites: Epidemiologic aspects. *J Natl Cancer Inst.* 1976;56:489.
5. Barr CC, McLean IW, Zimmerman LE: Uveal melanoma in children and adolescents. *Arch Ophthalmol.* 1981;99:2133.
6. Jensen OA: Malignant melanomas of the human uvea: 25-year follow-up of cases in Denmark, 1943-1952. *Acta Ophthalmol (Copenh).* 1982;60:161.
7. Singh AD, et al: Familial uveal melanoma. Clinical observations on 56 patients (see comments). *Arch Ophthalmol.* 1996;114:392.
8. Gonder JR, et al: Uveal malignant melanoma associated with ocular and oculodermal melanocytosis. *Ophthalmology.* 1982;89:953.
9. Dutton JJ, et al: Orbital malignant melanoma and oculodermal melanocytosis: report of two cases and review of the literature. *Ophthalmology.* 1984;91:497.
10. Singh AD, et al: Lifetime prevalence of uveal melanoma in white patients with oculo(dermal) melanocytosis. *Ophthalmology.* 1998;105:195.
11. Abramson DH, Rodriguez-Sains RS, Rubman R: B-K mole syndrome. Cutaneous and ocular malignant melanoma. *Arch Ophthalmol.* 1980;98:1397.
12. Augsburger J, et al: Diffuse primary malignant melanoma of the choroid arising in a patient with primary cutaneous melanoma. *Arch Ophthalmol.* 1980;98:1261.
13. Greene MH, et al: The familial occurrence of cutaneous melanoma, intraocular melanoma, and the dysplastic nevus syndrome. *Am J Ophthalmol.* 1983;96:238.
14. Swerdlow AJ, Storm HH, Sasieni PD: Risks of second primary malignancy in patients with cutaneous and ocular melanoma in Denmark, 1943-1989. *Int J Cancer.* 1995;61:773.
15. Kishore K, et al: P53 gene and cell cycling in uveal melanoma. *Am J Ophthalmol.* 1996;121:561.
16. Hussussian CJ, et al: Germline p16 mutations in familial melanoma. *Nat Genet.* 1994;8:15.
17. Ohta M, et al: Rarity of somatic and germline mutations of the cyclin-dependent kinase 4 inhibitor gene, CDK4I, in melanoma. *Cancer Res.* 1994;54:5269.
18. Speicher MR: Chromosomal gains and losses in uveal melanomas detected by comparative genomic hybridization. *Cancer Res.* 1994;54:3817.
19. Wiltshire RN, et al: Cytogenetic analysis of posterior uveal melanoma. *Cancer Genet Cytogenet.* 1993;66:47.
20. Gordon KB, et al: Comparative genomic hybridization in the detection of DNA copy number abnormalities in uveal melanoma. *Cancer Res.* 1994;54:4764.
21. Prescher G, et al: Cytogenetics of twelve cases of uveal melanoma and patterns of nonrandom anomalies and isochromosome formation. *Cancer Genet Cytogenet.* 1995;80:40.
22. Horsman DE, White VA: Cytogenetic analysis of uveal melanoma. Consistent occurrence of monosomy 3 and trisomy 8q. *Cancer.* 1993;71:811.
23. Patel KA, et al: Prediction of prognosis in patients with uveal melanoma using fluorescence in situ hybridization. *Br J Ophthalmol.* 2001;85:1440.
24. Sisley K, et al: Association of specific chromosome alterations with tumour phenotype in posterior uveal melanoma. *Br J Cancer.* 2000; 82:330.
25. Prescher G, et al: Prognostic implications of monosomy 3 in uveal melanoma. *Lancet.* 1996;347:1222.
26. Parrella P, et al: Detection of c-myc amplification in uveal melanoma by fluorescent in situ hybridization. *Invest Ophthalmol Vis Sci.* 2001;42:1679.
27. Bale SJ, et al: Mapping the gene for hereditary cutaneous malignant melanoma-dysplastic nevus to chromosome 1p. *N Engl J Med.* 1989;320:1367.
28. Miele ME, et al: Metastasis suppressed, but tumorigenicity and local invasiveness unaffected, in the human melanoma cell line MelJuSo after introduction of human chromosomes 1 or 6. *Mol Carcinog.* 1996;15:284.
29. Ray ME, et al: Isolation and characterization of genes associated with chromosome-6 mediated tumor suppression in human malignant melanoma. *Oncogene.* 1996;12:2527.
30. Chana JS, et al: c-myc, p53, and Bcl-2 expression and clinical outcome in uveal melanoma. *Br J Ophthalmol.* 1999;83:110.
31. Chana JS, et al: The prognostic importance of c-myc oncogene expression in head and neck melanoma. *Ann Plast Surg.* 2001;47:172.
32. Armstrong BK, Kricker A: Cutaneous melanoma. *Cancer Surv.* 1994;19:219.
33. Strickland D, Lee JAH: Melanomas of the eye: Stability of rates. *Am J Epidemiol.* 1981;113:700.
34. Osterlind A: Trends in incidence of ocular malignant melanoma in Denmark: 1943-1982. *Int J Cancer.* 1987;40:161.
35. Armstrong BK, Kricker A: How much melanoma is caused by sun exposure? *Melanoma Res.* 1993;3:395.
36. Brilliant LB, et al: Associations among cataract prevalence, sunlight hours, and altitude in the Himalayas. *Am J Epidemiol.* 1983; 118:250.
37. Blumenkranz MS, et al: Risk factors in age-related maculopathy complicated by choroidal neovascularization. *Ophthalmology.* 1986;93:552.
38. Davidorf FH, et al: Epidemiology of ocular melanoma: Incidence and geographic relationship in Ohio (1967-1977). *Ohio State Med J.* 1979;75:561.
39. Swerdlow AJ: Epidemiology of eye cancer in adults in England and Wales, 1962-1977. *Am J Epidemiol.* 1983;118:294.
40. Gallagher RP, et al: Risk factors for ocular melanoma: Western Canada Melanoma Study. *J Natl Cancer Inst.* 1985;74:775.
41. Jensen OA: Malignant melanoma of the uvea in Denmark 1943-1952: A clinical, histopathological and prognostic study. *Acta Ophthalmol Scand.* 1963;65(suppl):17.
42. Mork T: Malignant neoplasms of the eye in Norway: Incidence, treatment and prognosis. *Acta Ophthalmol Scand.* 1961;39:824.

43. Callender G: Malignant melanotic tumors of the eye: A study of the histologic types on 111 cases. *Trans Am Acad Ophthalmol Otolaryngol.* 1931;36:131.

44. Gass DM: Problems in the differential diagnosis of choroidal nevi and malignant melanomas. *Am J Ophthalmol.* 1977;83:299.

45. Paul E, Parnell BI, Fraker M: Prognosis of malignant melanomas of the choroid and ciliary body. *Int Ophthalmol Clin.* 1962;2:387.

46. McLean IW, Foster WD, Zimmerman LE: Prognostic factors in small malignant melanomas of choroid and ciliary body. *Arch Ophthalmol.* 1977;95:48.

47. Quivey JM, et al: High intensity 125-iodine (125I) plaque treatment of uveal melanoma. *Int J Radiat Oncol Biol Phys.* 1993; 26:613.

48. Zimmerman LE, McLean IW: An evaluation of enucleation in the management of uveal melanomas. *Int Ophthalmol Clin.* 1980;20:1.

49. Shammas HF, Blodi FC: Prognostic factors in choroidal and ciliary body melanomas. *Arch Ophthalmol.* 1977;95:63.

50. Zimmerman LE, McLean IW, Foster WD: Statistical analysis of follow-up data concerning uveal melanomas, and the influence of enucleation. *Ophthalmology.* 1980;87:557.

51. Packard RBS: Pattern of mortality in choroidal malignant melanoma. *Br J Ophthalmol.* 1980;64:565.

52. Diener-West M, et al: A review of mortality from choroidal melanoma. II. A meta-analysis of 5-year mortality rates following enucleation, 1966 through 1988. *Arch Ophthalmol.* 1992; 110:245.

53. Seddon JM, et al: A prognostic factor study of disease-free interval and survival following enucleation for uveal melanoma. *Arch Ophthalmol.* 1983;101:1894.

54. Gragoudas ES, et al: Prognostic factors for metastasis following proton beam irradiation of uveal melanomas. *Ophthalmology.* 1986;93:675.

55. Gragoudas ES, et al: Metastasis from uveal melanoma after proton beam irradiation. *Ophthalmology.* 1988;95:992.

56. Char DH, Kroll SM, Miller T, et al: Irradiated uveal melanomas: Cytopathologic correlation with prognosis. *Am J Ophthalmol.* 1996;122:509.

57. Char DH, et al: Uveal melanoma radiation. 125I brachytherapy versus helium ion irradiation. *Ophthalmology.* 1989;96:1708.

58. Karlsson M, Boeryd B, Carstensen J, et al: Correlations of Ki-67 and PCNA to DNA ploidy, S-phase fraction and survival in uveal melanoma. *Eur J Cancer.* 1996;32A:357.

59. Mooy CM, et al: Immunohistochemical and prognostic analysis of apoptosis and proliferation in uveal melanoma. *Am J Pathol.* 1995; 147:1097.

60. Pe'er J, et al: Mean of the ten largest nucleoli, microcirculation architecture, and prognosis of ciliochoroidal melanomas. *Ophthalmology.* 1994;101:1227.

61. Coleman K, et al: Prognostic factors following enucleation of 111 uveal melanomas (see comments). *Br J Ophthalmol.* 1993; 77:688.

62. Gamel JW, McLean IW: Computerized histopathologic assessment of malignant potential. III. Refinements of measurement and data analysis. *Anal Quant Cytol.* 1984;6:37.

63. Gamel JW, McLean IW, McCurdy JB: Biologic distinctions between cure and time to death in 2892 patients with intraocular melanoma. *Cancer.* 1993;71:2299.

64. Seddon JM, Gragoudas ES, Egan KM, et al: Relative survival rates after alternative therapies for uveal melanoma. *Ophthalmology.* 1990;97:769.

65. Barr CC, Sipperley JO, Nicholson DH: Small melanomas of the choroid. *Arch Ophthalmol.* 1978;96:1580.

66. Flocks M, Gerende J, Zimmerman LE: The size and shape of malignant melanomas of the choroid and ciliary body in relation to prognosis and histologic characteristics. *Trans Am Acad Ophthamol Otolaryngol.* 1955;Nov.-Dec.:740.

67. Folberg R, et al: The prognostic value of tumor blood vessel morphology in primary uveal melanoma. *Ophthalmology.* 1993; 100:1389.

68. McLean IW, et al: Uveal melanoma: The importance of large nucleoli in predicting patient outcome—An automated image analysis study. *Cancer.* 1997;79:982.

69. Ferry AP: Lesions mistaken for malignant melanoma of the posterior uvea: A clinical pathologic analysis of 100 cases with ophthalmoscopically visible lesions. *Arch Ophthalmol.* 1964; 72:463.

70. Shields JA: Lesions simulating malignant melanoma of the posterior uvea. *Arch Ophthalmol.* 1973;89:466.

71. Shields JA, McDonald PR: Improvements in the diagnosis of posterior uveal melanomas. *Arch Ophthalmol.* 1974;91:259.

72. Char DH, Miller T: Accuracy of presumed uveal melanoma diagnosis before alternative therapy. *Br J Ophthalmol.* 1995;79:692.

73. Histopathologic characteristics of uveal melanomas in eyes enucleated from the Collaborative Ocular Melanoma Study. COMS report no. 6. *Am J Ophthalmol.* 1998;125:745.

74. Group COMS: Accuracy of diagnosis of choroidal melanomas in the Collaborative Ocular Melanoma Study. COMS Report No. 1. *Arch Ophthalmol.* 1990;108:1268.

75. Char DH: The management of small choroidal melanomas. *Surv Ophthalmol.* 1978;22:377.

76. Char DH, et al: Diagnostic modalities in choroidal melanoma. *Am J Ophthalmol.* 1980;89:223.

77. Davidorf FH, et al: Incidence of misdiagnosed and unsuspected choroidal melanomas. A 50-year experience. *Arch Ophthalmol.* 1983;101:410.

78. Robertson DM, Campbell RJ: Errors in the diagnosis of malignant melanoma of the choroid. *Am J Ophthalmol.* 1979;87:269.

79. Coupland SE, et al: Metastatic choroidal melanoma to the contralateral orbit 40 years after enucleation. *Arch Ophthalmol.* 1996;114:751.

80. Hall WEB: Malignant melanoma of the uveal tract. Report of a case with death 30 years after enucleation. *Arch Ophthalmol.* 1950; 44:381.

81. Kirk HQ: Delayed metastasis from choroidal melanoma. *Surv Ophthalmol.* 1966;11:651.

82. Lorigan JG, Wallace S, Mavligit GM: The prevalence and location of metastases from ocular melanoma: Imaging study in 110 patients. *Am J Roentgenology.* 1991;157:1279.

83. Kath R, et al: Prognosis and treatment of disseminated uveal melanoma (see comments). *Cancer.* 1993;72:2219.

84. Char DH: Metastatic choroidal melanoma. *Am J Ophthalmol.* 1978;86:76.

85. Coleman DJ: Reliability of ocular tumor diagnosis with ultrasound. *Trans Am Acad Ophthalmol Otolaryngol.* 1977;77:677.

86. Raymond WR, Char DH, Norman D, Protzko EE: Magnetic resonance imaging evaluation of uveal tumors. *Am J Ophthalmol.* 1991;111:633.

87. Mihara F, et al: Intraocular hemorrhage and mimicking lesions: role of gradient-echo and contrast-enhanced MRI. *Clin Imaging.* 1993;17:171.

88. De Potter P, et al: The role of fat-suppression technique and gadopentetate dimeglumine in magnetic resonance imaging evaluation of intraocular tumors and simulating lesions (see comments). *Arch Ophthalmol.* 1994;112:340.

89. Bloom PA, et al: Magnetic resonance imaging. Diverse appearances of uveal malignant melanomas. *Arch Ophthalmol.* 1992; 110:1105.

90. Albert DM, Niffenegger AS, Willson JK: Treatment of metastatic uveal melanoma: review and recommendations. *Surv Ophthalmol.* 1992;36:429.

91. Eskelin S, et al: Screening for metastatic malignant melanoma of the uvea revisited. *Cancer.* 1999;85:1151.

92. AJCC: *AJCC Cancer Staging Manual,* 6th ed. Greene FL, Page DL, Fleming ID, et al, eds. New York: Springer 2002:421.

93. Butler P, Char DH, Zarbin M, Kroll S: Natural history of indeterminate pigmented choroidal tumors. *Ophthalmology.* 1994; 101:710.

94. Seddon JM, et al: Comparison of survival rates for patients with uveal melanoma after treatment with proton beam irradiation or enucleation. *Am J Ophthalmol.* 1985;99:282.

95. Augsburger JJ, et al: Enucleation vs cobalt plaque radiotherapy for malignant melanomas of the choroid and ciliary body. *Arch Ophthalmol.* 1986;104:655.

96. Adams KS, et al: Cobalt plaque versus enucleation for uveal melanoma: Comparison of survival rates. *Br J Ophthalmol.* 1988; 72:494.

97. Char DH, et al: Helium ions versus iodine 125 brachytherapy in the management of uveal melanoma. A prospective, randomized, dynamically balanced trial. *Ophthalmology.* 1993;100:1547.

98. Factors predictive of growth and treatment of small choroidal melanoma: COMS Report No. 5. The Collaborative Ocular Melanoma Study Group. *Arch Ophthalmol.* 1997;115:1537.

99. Mortality in patients with small choroidal melanoma. COMS report no. 4. The Collaborative Ocular Melanoma Study Group. *Arch Ophthalmol.* 1997;115:886.

100. Shields CL, et al: Transpupillary thermotherapy in the management of choroidal melanoma. *Ophthalmology.* 1996;103:1642.

101. Char DH, Bove RM, Phillips TL: Laser and proton radiation to reduce uveal melanoma associated exudative retinal detachments. *Am J Ophthalmol.* 2003;136:180.

102. Shields JA, Shields CL: Surgical approach to lamellar sclerouvectomy for posterior uveal melanomas: The 1986 Schoenberg lecture. *Ophthalmic Surg.* 1988;19:774.

103. Shields JA, Shields CL, De Potter P: Local resection of posterior uveal tumors. *Int Ophthalmol Clin.* 1993;33:137.

104. Damato BE, Paul J, Foulds WS: Risk factors for residual and recurrent uveal melanoma after trans-scleral local resection. *Br J Ophthalmol.* 1996;80:102.

105. Char DH, Miller T, Crawford JB: Uveal tumour resection. *Br J Ophthalmol.* 2001;85:1213.

106. Fuchs E: *Das Sarcom des Uvealtractus.* Wien: Braumuller; 1882.

107. Zimmerman LE, McLean IW: An evaluation of enucleation in the management of uveal melanomas. *Am J Ophthalmol.* 1979;87:741.

108. Seigel D, et al: Survival rates after enucleation of eyes with malignant melanoma. *Am J Ophthalmol.* 1979;87:761.

109. Char DH: Therapeutic options in uveal melanoma (editorial). *Am J Ophthalmol.* 1984;98:796.

110. Char DH, Phillips TL: Pre-enucleation irradiation of uveal melanoma. *Br J Ophthalmol.* 1985;69:177.

111. Augsburger JJ, et al: The effect of pre-enucleation radiotherapy on mitotic activity of choroidal and ciliary body melanomas. *Ophthalmology.* 1987;94:1627.

112. Luyten GP, et al: No demonstrated effect of pre-enucleation irradiation on survival of patients with uveal melanoma. *Am J Ophthalmol.* 1995;119:786.

113. Char DH, Phillips TL: The potential for adjuvant radiotherapy in choroidal melanoma. *Arch Ophthalmol.* 1982;100:247.

114. The Collaborative Ocular Melanoma Study (COMS) randomized trial of pre-enucleation radiation of large choroidal melanoma III: local complications and observations following enucleation. COMS report no. 11. *Am J Ophthalmol.* 1998;126:362.

115. The Collaborative Ocular Melanoma Study (COMS) randomized trial of pre-enucleation radiation of large choroidal melanoma II: Initial mortality findings. COMS report no. 10. *Am J Ophthalmol.* 1998;125:779.

116. Assessment of metastatic disease status at death in 435 patients with large choroidal melanoma in the Collaborative Ocular Melanoma Study (COMS): COMS report no. 15. *Arch Ophthalmol.* 2001;119:670.

117. Kersten RC, Tse DT, Anderson RL, Blodi FC: The role of orbital exenteration in choroidal melanoma with extrascleral extension. *Ophthalmology.* 1985;92:436.

118. Moore R: Choroidal sarcoma treated by intra-ocular insertion of radon seeds. *Br J Ophthalmol.* 1930;14:145.

119. Stallard H: Radiotherapy for malignant melanoma of the choroid. *Br J Ophthalmol.* 1966;50:147.

120. Karlsson UL, et al: Recurrence of posterior uveal melanoma after 60Co episcleral plaque therapy. *Ophthalmology.* 1989;96:382.

121. Beitler JJ, McCormick B, Ellsworth RM, et al: Ocular melanoma: Total dose and dose rate effects with 60-Co plaque therapy. *Radiology.* 1990;176:275.

122. MacFaul PA: Local radiotherapy in the treatment of malignant melanoma of the choroid. *Trans Ophthalmol Soc UK.* 1977;97:421.

123. Sealy R, et al: The treatment of ophthalmic tumors with low energy sources. *Br J Radiol.* 1976;49:551.

124. Luxton G, Astrahan, Melvin A, et al: Dosimetric calculations and measurements of gold plaque ophthalmic irradiators using iridium-192 and iodine-125 seeds. *Int J Radiat Oncol Biol Phys.* 1988;15:167.

125. Straatsma BR, Fine SL, Earle JD, et al: The Collaborative Ocular Melanoma Study Research Group. Enucleation versus plaque irradiation for choroidal melanoma. *Ophthalmology.* 1988;95:1000.

126. Lommatzsch PK, Lommatzsch R: Treatment of juxtapapillary melanomas. *Br J Ophthalmol.* 1991;75:715.

127. Tjho-Heslinga RE, et al: Results of ruthenium irradiation of uveal melanoma. *Radiother Oncol.* 1993;29:33.

128. Ling CC, et al: Computer assisted treatment planning for 125-I ophthalmic plaque radiotherapy. *Int J Radiat Oncol Biol Phys.* 1989;17:405.

129. Weaver KA: The dosimetry of I-125 seed plaques. *Med Phys.* 1986;13:78.

130. Williamson J: Monte Carlo evaluation of specific dose constants in water for I-125 seeds. *Med Phys.* 1988;15:686.

131. Fiedler JA, et al: A magnetic resonance imaging-based treatment planning method for episcleral brachytherapy. *Endocurietherapy/Hyperthermia Oncol.* 1993;9:201.

132. Quivey JM, Augsburger J, Snelling L, Brady LW: I-125 plaque therapy for uveal melanoma: Analysis of the impact of time and dose factors on local control. *Cancer.* 1996;77:2356.

133. Nag S, et al: The American Brachytherapy Society recommendations for brachytherapy of uveal melanomas. *Int J Radiat Oncol Biol Phys.* 2003;56:544.

134. Constable IJ, Koehler AM, Schmidt RA: Proton irradiation of simulated ocular tumors. *Invest Ophthalmol.* 1975;14:547.

135. Gragoudas ES: The Bragg peak of proton beams for treatment of uveal melanoma. *Int Ophthalmol Clin.* 1980;20:123.

136. Goitein M, Miller T: Planning proton therapy of the eye. *Med Phys.* 1983;10:275.

137. Castro JR, Quivey JM: Clinical experience and expectations with helium and heavy ion irradiation. *Int J Radiat Oncol Biol Phys.* 1977;3:127.

138. Daftari IK, Char DH, Verhey LJ, et al: Anterior segment sparing to reduce charged particle radiotherapy complications in uveal melanoma. *Int J Radiat Oncol Biol Phys.* 1997;39:997.

139. Char DH, et al: Long term visual outcome of radiated uveal melanomas in eyes eligible for randomisation to enucleation versus brachytherapy. *Br J Ophthalmol.* 1996;80:117.

140. Melia BM, et al: Collaborative ocular melanoma study (COMS) randomized trial of I-125 brachytherapy for medium choroidal melanoma. I. Visual acuity after 3 years. COMS report no. 16. *Ophthalmology.* 2001;108:348.

141. Char DH, et al: Late radiation failures after iodine 125 brachytherapy for uveal melanoma compared with charged-particle (proton or helium ion) therapy. *Ophthalmology.* 2002;109:1850.

142. Suit H: The Gray Lecture 2001: Coming technical advances in radiation oncology. *Int J Radiat Oncol Biol Phys.* 2002;53:798.

143. Gragoudas ES, et al: Intraocular recurrence of uveal melanoma after proton beam irradiation. *Ophthalmology.* 1992;99:760.

144. Munzenrider JE, et al: Conservative treatment of uveal melanoma: Local recurrence after proton beam therapy. *Int J Radiat Oncol Biol Phys.* 1989;17:493.

145. Egger E, et al: Maximizing local tumor control and survival after proton beam radiotherapy of uveal melanoma. *Int J Radiat Oncol Biol Phys.* 2001;51:138.

146. Char D, Castro JR, Kroll SM, et al: Five-year follow-up of helium ion therapy for uveal melanoma. *Arch Ophthalmol.* 1990;108:209.

147. Linstadt D, Castro JR, Char DH, et al: Long-term results of helium ion irradiation of uveal melanoma. *Int J Radiat Oncol Biol Phys.* 1990;19:613.

148. Castro JR, et al: 15 years experience with helium ion radiotherapy for uveal melanoma. *Int J Radiat Oncol Biol Phys.* 1997;39:989.

149. Daftari IK, et al: Anterior segment sparing to reduce charged particle radiotherapy complications in uveal melanoma. *Int J Radiat Oncol Biol Phys.* 1997;39:997.

150. Nath R, et al: Dosimetry of interstitial brachytherapy sources: recommendations of the AAPM Radiation Therapy Committee Task Group No. 43. American Association of Physicists in Medicine. *Med Phys.* 1995;22:209.

151. Diener-West M, et al: The COMS randomized trial of iodine-125 brachytherapy for choroidal melanoma. III: initial mortality findings. COMS Report No. 18. *Arch Ophthalmol.* 2001;119:969.

152. Jampol LM, et al: The COMS randomized trial of iodine 125 brachytherapy for choroidal melanoma: IV. Local treatment failure and enucleation in the first 5 years after brachytherapy. COMS report no. 19. *Ophthalmology.* 2002;109:2197.

Retinoblastoma

David H. Abramson, MD, Beryl McCormick, MD, and Amy C. Schefler, MD

Retinoblastoma is the most common primary intraocular malignancy of infants and young children. Although it is rare, retinoblastoma is an important cancer because it has served as a conceptual model for other cancers with a genetic etiology.

Retinoblastoma was first described in the literature by Petras Pawius of Amsterdam as early as 1657. However, James Wardrop, an Edinburgh ophthalmologist, was officially credited for recognizing retinoblastoma in 1809, when he documented the first enucleation successfully performed to treat retinoblastoma.[1] Two centuries later, enucleation is still used to treat retinoblastoma, as well as other methods such as external beam radiation, brachytherapy, cryotherapy, and laser therapy. Newer modalities that have recently gained popularity include chemoreduction and transpupillary thermotherapy. In many cases, treatment can help preserve both patients' eyes and vision. In the United States, the current 5-year survival rate for children with retinoblastoma is 98%.[2]

INCIDENCE

Surveys suggest a relatively constant occurrence of retinoblastoma during the last century throughout the world. The frequency of retinoblastoma has been documented as 1 in 14,000 to 1 in 34,000 live births.[3] The incidence in the United States is relatively low, at 3.58 cases per million children under the age of 15 years, and is closely correlated with age. For ages 1 to 4 years, the incidence is 10.6 per million; for 5 to 9 years, 1.53 per million; and for 10 to 14 years, 0.27 per million.[4] Approximately 350 new cases are diagnosed in the United States each year, and retinoblastoma is the seventh most common cancer in the pediatric population in this country.

Retinoblastoma appears to have no predilection for any particular racial group or gender. It does appear to occur more commonly in poor patients worldwide. Preliminary evidence suggests that the reason for this predilection is that the presence of human papillomavirus (HPV) sequences in retinoblastoma tumor tissue may play a role in the development of some sporadic retinoblastoma.[5]

Retinoblastoma can affect one or both eyes. The right eye is affected as frequently as the left eye. Unilateral retinoblastoma occurs in 75% of all cases diagnosed, while bilateral disease occurs in 25% of cases. All patients with bilateral retinoblastoma have multifocal disease (more than one independent tumor focus in each eye) with 5 as the mean number of tumors distributed between the two eyes, and a possible range of 2 to 20 tumors. Of the patients with unilateral disease, only 15% have multifocal disease.[6]

GENETICS

Retinoblastoma was one of the disease models that served to demonstrate the genetic nature of cancer. Knudson proposed the now classic two-hit model in 1971 after noting that the timing of tumor development (younger age at diagnosis of bilateral tumors than of unilateral tumors) suggested a mechanism in which at least two events would be responsible for the development of the tumor.[7] He hypothesized that patients with multifocal bilateral disease were germline carriers for the first hit, with only one second hit necessary for the development of retinoblastoma. Unilateral unifocal patients, he determined, usually had a normal germline genome, but developed both hits in the progenitor tumor cell.

More recent molecular investigations of the gene have demonstrated that 40% of all retinoblastoma patients have the germinal form of the disease in which a germline mutation of the *RB1* gene on chromosome 13 is present. All patients with bilateral retinoblastoma are believed to carry the germinal form of the disease, and these patients make up 85% of the germinal cases. About 15% of patients with germinal retinoblastoma have only one eye involved, and in these cases, the disease is almost always multifocal. When patients with the germinal form of the disease reproduce, retinoblastoma presents in a Mendelian autosomal dominance pattern with 90% penetrance, but of note only 8% of all retinoblastoma patients have an antecedent family history of the disease. This low percentage reflects the fact that two thirds of cases of germinal retinoblastoma are the result of new mutations occurring in germ cells or mutations that occur very early during embryonic development.

In the more common nongerminal form of retinoblastoma, the disease is not inherited or passed on to subsequent generations. Nongerminal retinoblastoma is always unilateral and unifocal, although lack of tumor cohesiveness may cause the tumor to break apart, resulting in hundreds of tiny intraocular seeds.

Since the *RB* gene was isolated in 1986 by Friend et al., many studies have explored its location and function. The gene is located on the long arm of chromosome 13, band 14.2.[8] Further characterization of the gene has revealed that it spans 200 kilobase (kb) and is composed of 27 exons. The gene encodes a 4.7 kb mRNA transcript, which is expressed in all adult tissues. The 110 kilodalton (kD) nuclear phosphoprotein consists of 928 amino acids.

The protein encoded by the gene is a regulator at the cell cycle checkpoint between G1 and entry into the S-phase.[9] The phosphorylation pattern of p110 RB varies during the cell cycle and the current model suggests that the unphosphorylated normal RB1 protein binds transcriptional regulators that promote entry into the S-phase. When the normal RB1 protein is phosphorylated, it dissociates from E2F (one of these transcription factors), freeing it to bind to DNA and stimulate transcription of downstream genes that promote progression through the cell cycle. Loss of normal RB1 function, as in the case of the tumors, presumably allows for uncontrolled entry into the S-phase, more rapid cell cycling, and rapid cell division. The retinoblastoma protein is thus a dominant suppressor of tumor formation, making the *RB1* gene a member of the tumor suppressor class of genes.

Mutations in the *RB1* gene seem to occur throughout the gene. The majority of the mutations are nonsense, introducing a premature stop codon and therefore producing a truncated and presumably nonfunctional protein. While only limited amounts of data have been published to date, it seems that the majority of first hits are point mutations, while the remainder are small deletions.[10] Only about 2% to 3% of tumors demonstrate karyotypically visible larger deletions of material in the 13q14 band. Some of the children with this cytogenetic abnormality in their germline have a constitutional disease with severe developmental delay and dysmorphic features, while others are phenotypically normal other than their retinoblastoma. The second hit consists of loss of the normal allele (loss of heterozygosity) in 60% of cases, while the remainder of the

patients may have a second distinct point mutation, and an even smaller fraction of patients have a second distinct small deletion.[11]

Evidence suggests that retinoblastoma, like other cancers such as colon carcinomas and glial brain tumors, requires other genetic abnormalities to occur before transformation into malignancy. This finding has stimulated many studies focused on mutations other than those in the *RB1* gene. Although cytogenetic studies have revealed some consistent abnormalities that provide clues, it is still unclear exactly what these subsequent steps in the development of the retinoblastoma tumor are.

Genetic counseling for the families of retinoblastoma patients is complex and challenging (Table 65-1). A parent with bilateral retinoblastoma has a 45% chance of having a child with retinoblastoma, although the retinoblastoma may not be present at the child's birth in either eye. Of those parents with bilateral disease whose children develop unilateral disease, 96% of the children will have multifocal tumors and most of them will be diagnosed within the first 6 months of life. Since all of these children (of bilateral parents) have the germinal mutation, 45% of their children will also develop retinoblastoma.

Two of the most common and challenging types of families who require genetic counseling are: (1) families in which neither parent has a history of retinoblastoma but the couple already has one child with the disease and wants to know the chances that the next will also have retinoblastoma, and (2) families in which one parent has a history of unilateral retinoblastoma and the couple wants to know the risk to future children of developing the disease. In the first scenario, an ophthalmoscopic examination of both parents' eyes should be performed. The reason for this examination is that 1% to 2% of such parents on fundoscopic examination will demonstrate a rare benign clinical entity called a *retinoma*. A retinoma is thought to be a spontaneously regressed or arrested retinoblastoma (or "benign retinoblastoma"), which is the result of the loss of the *RB1* gene without the subsequent acquisition of other mutations that are required for progression to the malignant state. These parents should

Table 65–1   Genetic Counseling for Retinoblastoma

If Parent Was	Bilateral			Unilateral			Unaffected		
Chance of offspring having retinoblastoma	45% affected		55% unaffected	7-15% affected		85-93% unaffected	<<1% affected		99% unaffected
Laterality	85% bilateral	15% unilateral	0%	85% bilateral	15% unilateral	0%	33% bilateral	67% unilateral	0%
Focality	100% multifocal / 96% multifocal / 4% unifocal		0%	100% multifocal / 96% multifocal / 4% unifocal		0%	100% multifocal / 15% multifocal / 85% unifocal		0%
Chance of next sibling having retinoblastoma	45% 45% 45% 45%			45% 45% 45% 7-15%			5%* <1%* <1%*		<1%
							*If parent is a carrier, then 45%		

be counseled that although they have never been treated for retinoblastoma, they may harbor the germinal mutation, and if they have multifocal retinomas, each of their children will have a 45% chance of inheriting the mutation. Parents with no ophthalmoscopic evidence of retinoblastoma can be told that the chance that their next child will have retinoblastoma is between 1% and 5%. In the small percentage of cases in which the second child does develop the disease, it is presumed that one of the parents carries the germinal mutation although he or she is phenotypically normal. Ironically, some families have different mutations in different family members or have a family history of retinoblastoma but did not have the germinal form.

The second scenario also presents a complex situation. Most parents (85% to 93%) who have had unilateral retinoblastoma do not harbor the germinal mutation and will not pass the mutation on to their children. In 7% to 15% of cases, however, the parent has the germinal mutation and will pass it on to his or her children. Of the affected children, 85% will have bilateral disease and multifocal tumors. The remaining 15% of the children develop only unilateral disease, and of this group, 96% will have multifocal disease. Thus, heritable, unilateral, unifocal retinoblastoma is extremely rare, but it does occur.

In these scenarios as well as others, parents of children with retinoblastoma are often eager to undergo genetic analysis to determine the risk that siblings or future children will develop the disease. Karyotypical studies, which analyze the morphology of entire chromosomes, are generally not useful for the clinical diagnosis of retinoblastoma, as they can only identify large deletions spanning 2 to 5 million base-pairs and only 3% to 5% of retinoblastoma patients carry deletions this large. Instead, two other methods of genetic analysis are used.[12] The indirect method uses restriction fragment length polymorphisms (RFLP) analysis or variable number of tandem repeats (VNTR) analysis to detect the presence of a genetic marker that segregates along with the *RB1* gene. Particular RFLP markers can then be used to follow the inheritance of the mutant *RB1* gene within a family. However, both RFLP and VNTR analysis generally require the presence of two or more affected family members in order to be informative. Additionally, the accuracy of these analyses greatly increases with examination of tumor-derived DNA, which is not available if the proband is being treated with methods other than enucleation.

Direct detection methods are the second type of analyses that are performed for some of these families. These methods, including single-strand conformation polymorphism (SSCP) analysis and gel electrophoretic analysis of synthetically amplified axons of the *RB1* gene, are used to systematically analyze 200 base-pair-long regions of the *RB1* gene at a time. Once a region of the *RB1* gene containing the mutation is identified, the exact location and nature of the mutation is identified with further direct DNA sequencing. No preferential mutation or "hot spot" has been identified in the *RB1* gene, and the types of mutations detected in the gene have been highly variable, necessitating screening all 27 exons and

adjacent introns of the *RB1* locus. More recently, fluorescent in situ hybridization studies have provided additional information about the molecular structure of the retinoblastoma locus, including the identification of translocations and inversions undetectable using other methods. The direct detection methods are more sensitive than the indirect tests and can be performed on tumor tissue or blood samples of patients with germinal disease, but take 3 to 6 months to complete and are costly for families.[12] Future research that will increase the sensitivity of these tests will enable patients and their family members to undergo the analyses in a faster and more economic manner.

Finally, because the *RB1* gene is expressed in all adult tissues and the RB1 protein plays such a vital role in controlling cell proliferation, all patients who carry the germinal *RB1* mutation are at risk for the development of additional nonocular cancers. These cancers can occur as late as 40 years after the initial development of retinoblastoma. The incidence of these cancers is significantly increased in patients who receive external beam radiation. Patients should be educated about their risk factors for developing these cancers, as it is these cancers, not retinoblastoma, that are the leading cause of death in patients with the germinal *RB1* mutation.[13] See Select Results later in this chapter for more information on additional nonocular cancers.

ANATOMY

The eye is a spherical structure with anterior adaptations to admit and refract light. It sits in the bony orbit well protected in all directions except the anterior face, where the upper and lower lids open to admit light and close for protection. Six extraocular muscles are attached to the eye for movement in all directions.

Figure 65-1 illustrates the important anatomic structures of the eye. The inner layer is the retina, where the photoreceptors are located. Retinoblastoma is thought to originate from an unidentified progenitor cell in this layer. The normal retina extends from the posterior "pole" forward to a region just behind the lens, in cross-section called the *ora serrata*. The middle layer of

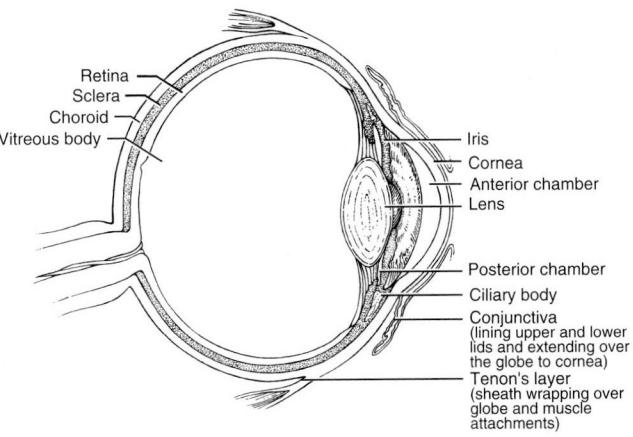

Figure 65–1. The anatomy of the eye.

the eye is the choroid; this pigmented structure is continuous anteriorly with the ciliary body and iris, and together these are considered to be the uveal tract. The outermost layer of the eye is the sclera, a tough and radioresistant structure that fuses with the cornea anteriorly. The anterior chamber of the eye is between the cornea and the iris; the posterior chamber is just behind it, between the iris and the lens. Both chambers are filled with aqueous humor, produced by the ciliary body. Behind the lens is the vitreous chamber, with vitreous humor, a thick gel-like substance. In advanced retinoblastoma, "seeding" of the tumor is noted in this chamber.

PATHOLOGY

The diagnosis of retinoblastoma is routinely made without pathologic confirmation. Needle biopsies are rarely, if ever, indicated, as puncturing the eye can lead to tumor seeding and orbital invasion. Aqueous taps, previously explored as a possible diagnostic tool, are inappropriate for the same reason.[14]

When enucleation is the treatment of choice, histopathologic examination of the globe can be useful in providing information about potential extraocular extension (Fig. 65-2). For optimal prognostic information, the globe should be fixed for at least 24 hours, with the optic nerve preserved for separate evaluation.[15]

Under the microscope, the appearance of the retinoblastoma cells can range from small, round, undifferentiated cells with frequent mitoses, as seen in Figure 65-3, to differentiated cells that form rosettes called Flexner-Wintersteiner rosettes.[15] Important observations in assessing the risk of the child for distant or local relapse include careful assessment of the degree of invasion of tumor cells beyond the retina and into the choroid and sclera, and assessment of the degree of tumor invasion into the optic nerve beyond the region of the lamina cribrosa.[16]

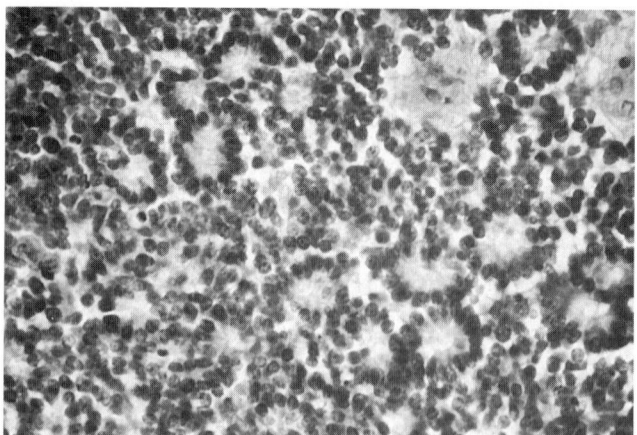

Figure 65–3. Retinoblastoma cells under a high-power view.

CLINICAL PRESENTATION

The presenting signs and symptoms of retinoblastoma vary depending on the geographic location in which the child presents. In developing countries, children have often developed extraocular disease by the time they are diagnosed, with proptosis and an orbital mass. In these cases, the retinoblastoma has often extended directly into the orbit, causing rupture of the globe (Fig. 65-4). Regional nodal metastasis may be found in the preauricular or submandibular regions or the children may have widespread metastatic disease. These children are older at diagnosis (age 4 to 6 years) than patients in the United States, and few survive. In the United States, when there is no family history of disease, the median age at presentation is 1 year for bilateral retinoblastoma and 2 years for unilateral disease. Most children in the United States present with only intraocular disease and are diagnosed with signs rather than symptoms.

In the United States, the most common presenting sign of retinoblastoma (60% of cases) is leukocoria or a white pupillary reflex that is sometimes referred to as a *cat's eye reflex*. Leukocoria can be the result of the tumor itself, a secondary retinal detachment associated with the tumor, or a reflection of light from the white mass at the posterior portion of the eye (Fig. 65-5).

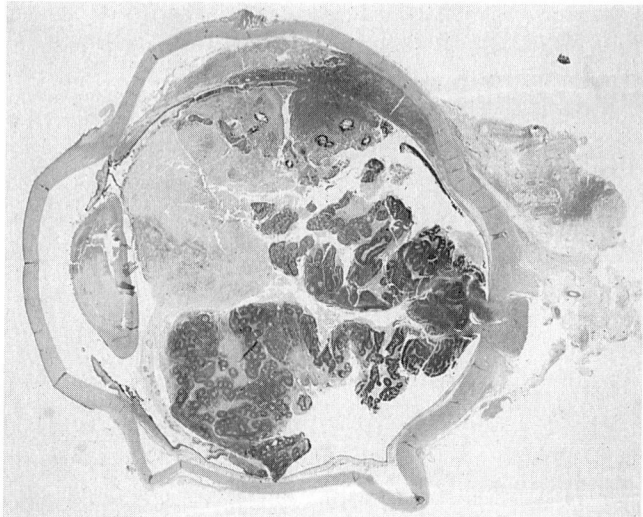

Figure 65–2. Gross section of a globe, showing extensive disease in the retina, vitreous body, choroid, and optic nerve.

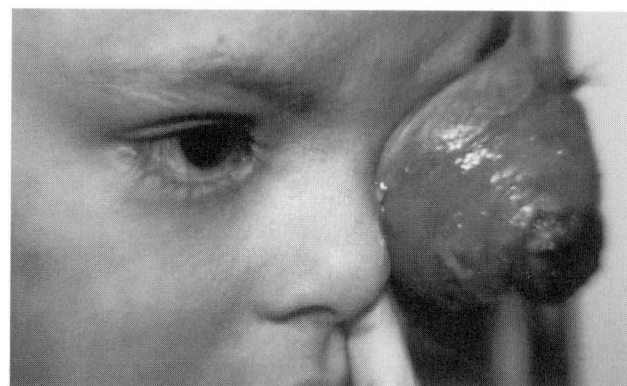

Figure 65–4. A child with extensive orbital disease: the most common presentation in the developing world.

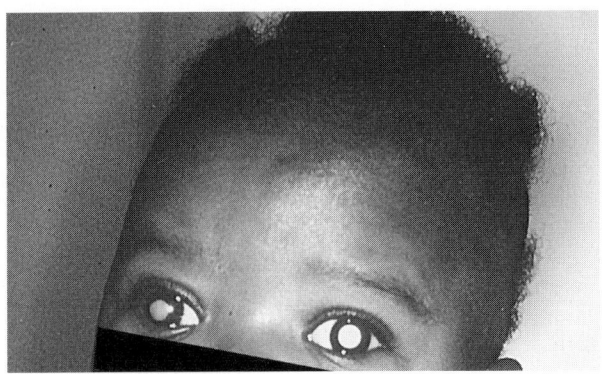

Figure 65–5. A child with the "cat's eye" reflex, with retinoblastoma visualized as the white material in the pupil.

The second most common sign is strabismus, misalignment of the two eyes. Of the 20% to 25% of patients who present with this sign, 10.5% have eyes crossed in (esotropia) and 5.2% out (exotropia).[17] Esotropia in children is generally more common than exotropia such that an infant with exotropia must be suspected to have retinoblastoma until proved otherwise. The strabismus in retinoblastoma patients is caused by tumor or retinal detachment located in the macula of the eye, the area of central vision. While patient survival is independent of whether patients present with strabismus or leukocoria, ocular survival rates are significantly lower for patients who present with leukocoria, as the disease tends to be more advanced at presentation in these cases.[18]

The third most common sign (6% to 10% of cases) is painful glaucoma with inflammatory signs. These children may present to the pediatric emergency room with a presentation that resembles orbital cellulitis. The patients appear systemically ill with irritability, failure to eat, and low-grade fever. Although the clinical examination and diagnostic imaging may suggest extraocular disease, the patients usually have only intraocular disease, frequently with massive necrosis and glaucoma.

Presenting signs in the United States that occur in less than 5% of cases include: anisocoria (different-sized pupils); heterochromia (different-colored irides); hyphema (blood in the anterior chamber); tumor hypopyon (tumor in the anterior chamber); nystagmus, a unilateral fixed and dilated pupil; and failure to thrive. In cases in which the patient has gross chromosomal abnormalities, children can present with other findings, such as absence or hyperplasia of the thumbs, mental retardation, prominent nasofrontal bones, large malformed ears, hypospadias, bifid scrotum, and extra digits. Only 7% of patients are detected on routine pediatric screening by a pediatrician, whereas 72% of cases are detected by a family member or friend.[18]

When there is a family history of retinoblastoma, diagnosis tends to occur earlier, with a median age at diagnosis of 5 months for patients with unilateral disease and 11 months for patients with bilateral disease.[19] Sixty percent of all retinoblastoma patients diagnosed under 6 months have no signs or symptoms, but are examined and diagnosed because of a family history of retinoblastoma.[20] At our center, children with a family history of retinoblastoma typically undergo frequent serial fundoscopic examinations beginning within 24 to 48 hours of birth and continuing until at least 28 months of age. Twenty-eight months is chosen as the earliest possible time to stop examining these patients because it is the oldest age at which a patient with a positive family history of retinoblastoma has developed his or her first tumor in a previously documented disease-free eye.[21] These serial examinations have a significant impact on ocular outcome. Patients who began undergoing screening examinations at our center as newborns because of a family history had a 68% ocular 5-year survival rate, whereas nonscreened patients with a family history had only a 38% ocular survival.[18]

There is a direct relationship between the age at which the patient is diagnosed and the likelihood of the patient's developing additional tumor foci. A child whose disease is diagnosed at birth, even with only one tumor, has a 96% chance of developing additional tumors in either eye. In contrast, a child who is diagnosed at 12 months of age has only a 12% chance of developing new tumors in either eye. By age 33 months, the likelihood of new tumor development is less than 1%, and it appears to be zero after the age of 6 to 7.5 years.

The anatomic location of these tumors within the retina and the age at which the lesions develop have been well studied (Fig. 65-6). Retinoblastoma may be present anywhere in the retina at birth, but as age at tumor development increases, tumors develop progressively farther into the periphery. Thus macular tumors present earliest and peripheral anterior tumors present later. In our center, the average macular tumor is diagnosed at 5.6 months and never presents after 15.5 months. In contrast, peripheral tumors are diagnosed at an average

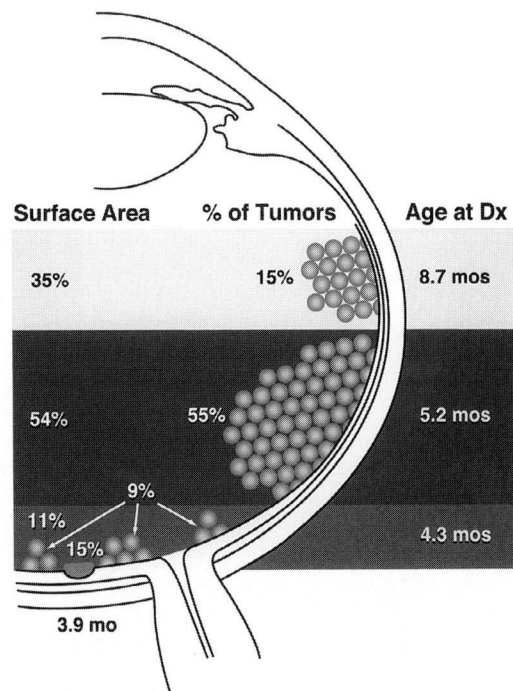

Figure 65–6. Artistic rendition of the relationship between the age at diagnosis, surface area of involved retina, and location of intraocular foci of retinoblastoma.

of 16.4 months and can present as late as 8 years of age. This pattern of ocular tumor development has important implications for the radiation oncologist. Since many young children will have no tumors in the anterior retina, there is no need to treat this area, thereby decreasing the incidence of radiation-induced cataracts. However, future development of new peripheral tumors should be expected and the family should be informed of this likelihood. The development of these tumors does not represent a failure of radiation, but rather the inevitable process of tumorigenesis in genetically altered cells. Furthermore, the family of a child with multifocal unilateral retinoblastoma can be assured that new tumors that develop in the fellow eye will not originate in the fovea, so the outlook for vision in the fellow eye is typically favorable.

ROUTES OF SPREAD

The natural course of untreated retinoblastoma follows one of five routes of progression: contiguous spread through the choroid, sclera, and orbit; extension along the optic nerve directly into the brain; invasion of the subarachnoid space and leptomeninges via the cerebrospinal fluid; hematogenous spread to bone marrow, bone, liver, and spleen; and dissemination via conjunctiva through the lymphatic system.[9] In the United States, the few patients with unilateral retinoblastoma who develop metastases usually have them at the time of diagnosis. All metastases occur within 5 years of diagnosis.[19]

DIAGNOSIS OF RETINOBLASTOMA

As mentioned earlier, the diagnosis of retinoblastoma is routinely made without pathologic confirmation and is based on a clinical examination by the ophthalmologist.

The fundus is examined via indirect ophthalmoscopy, performed with or without general anesthesia, depending on the age and level of cooperation of the child. The pupils of both eyes are dilated with phenylephrine (Neo-Synephrine) 2.5% and tropicamide (Mydriacyl) 1% before the examination. The child is placed in a supine position and is wrapped in a sheet in "mummy" fashion. Both eyes are examined, and scleral depression with a scleral indentor (a pen-shaped instrument with a flat tip) is used to view the anterior retina. Tumors as small as 1 mm in diameter can be detected with the indirect ophthalmoscope. Smaller tumors can appear white, pink, translucent, or clear and are hemispheric in shape. Retinal blood vessels may be seen on the surface of the tumors and sometimes the tumor's own blood supply can be seen within the mass. Larger tumors have a creamy appearance similar to cottage cheese, may contain calcium, and may produce an associated retinal detachment when growth of the tumor occurs.

All retinoblastoma tumors are drawn on an expanded concentric circle drawing of the globe called a fundus diagram, used to document the presence, location (in reference to the optic nerve and macula of the eye), and size of the retinoblastoma tumors. Some ophthalmologists document the presence of tumors in the posterior pole by taking color photographs with a hand-held fundus camera while the patient is under anesthesia. Figure 65-7 demonstrates both techniques in the same child. The original tumor drawing is referred to during follow-up visits, and new drawings are composed to document treatment response. Although the ophthalmoscopic examination should always be considered the primary method for evaluation of retinoblastoma, several ancillary tests can assist in the diagnosis, especially when there is no clear view of the fundus.

Ophthalmic ultrasonography is one of the most frequently performed ancillary tests for retinoblastoma.

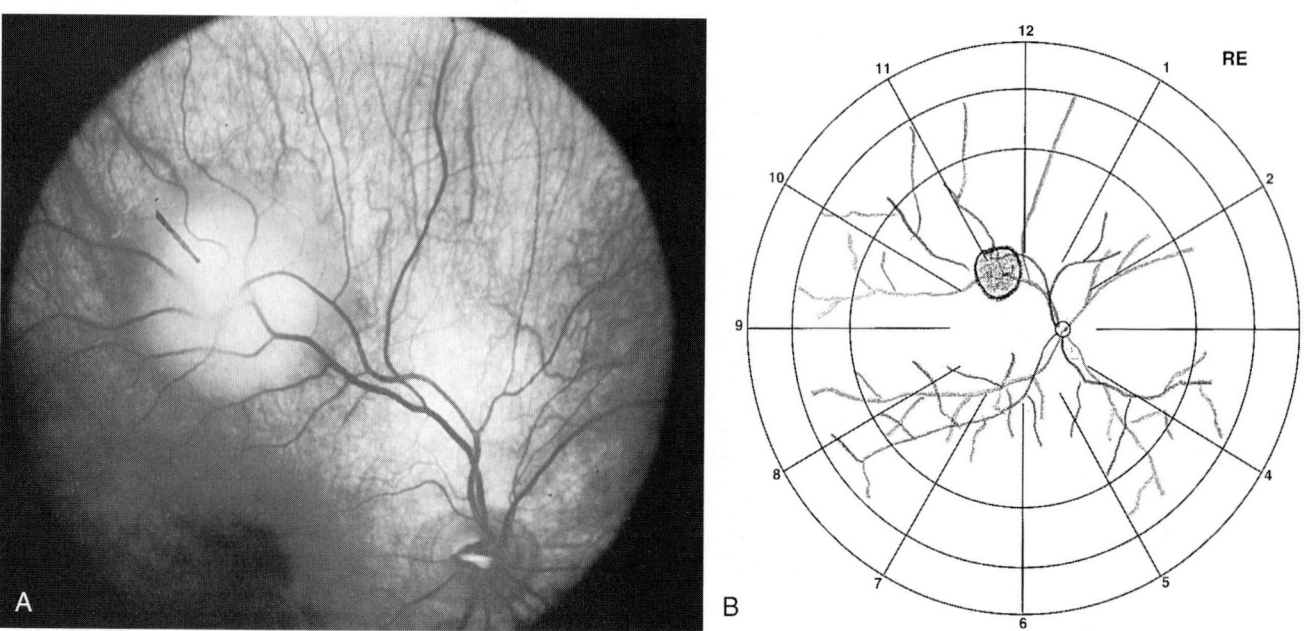

Figure 65–7. A fundus photograph of an eye with retinoblastoma (**A**) and the corresponding sketch of the disease in the eye diagram (**B**).

It is noninvasive, safe, repeatable, and immediately interpretable. Ultrasonography should be performed on both eyes and can be performed with or without general anesthesia. B-scan ultrasonography reveals a two-dimensional (2D) cross-sectional view of the eye, confirms the presence and the relationship of the solid tumor to other anatomical structures within the eye, and detects the size and shape of the tumors (Fig. 65-8). B-scan can detect orbital involvement, optic nerve invasion (sometimes), extrascleral extension, and calcification. Because there is calcium (which exhibits high reflectivity on ultrasonographic scans) in the majority of retinoblastoma tumors, high amplitude echoes will remain on the screen even if the gain or sensitivity is lowered. Shadowing defects posterior to the tumor may be present and are caused by the absorption of sound and high reflectivity. A-scan ultrasonography evaluates the internal characteristics and vascularity of the tumor and measures the height of the tumor.

Computed tomography (CT) scans may no longer be appropriate for retinoblastoma patients, as analysis has demonstrated an increased lifetime risk of other cancers in pediatric patients subjected to this imaging modality.[22] Instead, as part of an extent of disease workup, magnetic resonance imaging (MRI) is routinely performed (Fig. 65-9A and B). In addition to its excellent resolution in the diagnosis of extraocular soft tissue disease, MRI can readily distinguish between retinoblastoma and Coats' disease, as Coats' disease appears brighter than retinoblastoma on T2-weighted images due to proteinaceous exudate.[9] One disadvantage of MRI is that calcification, a key feature of retinoblastoma, is more easily demonstrated with CT than with MRI.

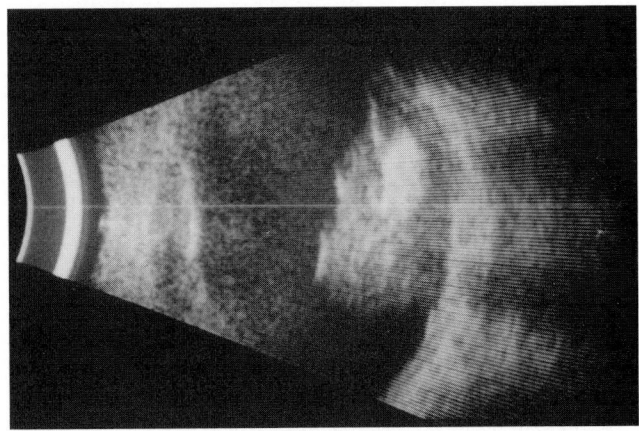

Figure 65–8. B-scan ultrasonography of an eye with retinoblastoma.

Differential Diagnosis of Retinoblastoma

Retinoblastoma can be simulated by several other ophthalmic tumors and ophthalmic disorders (Table 65-2). The lesion that most commonly simulates retinoblastoma is Coats' disease. Coats' disease is a nonheritable, primarily unilateral anomaly that affects mostly boys, with a later age at diagnosis than retinoblastoma (mean age at diagnosis is 6 years). Ophthalmic examination reveals telangiectatic vessels of the retina with intraretinal and subretinal exudates and an exudative retinal detachment. Presence of a yellow-green sheen on indirect ophthalmoscopic examination aids in differentiating Coats' from retinoblastoma. When rubeosis iridis, glaucoma, and corneal edema develop, the fundus may be impossible

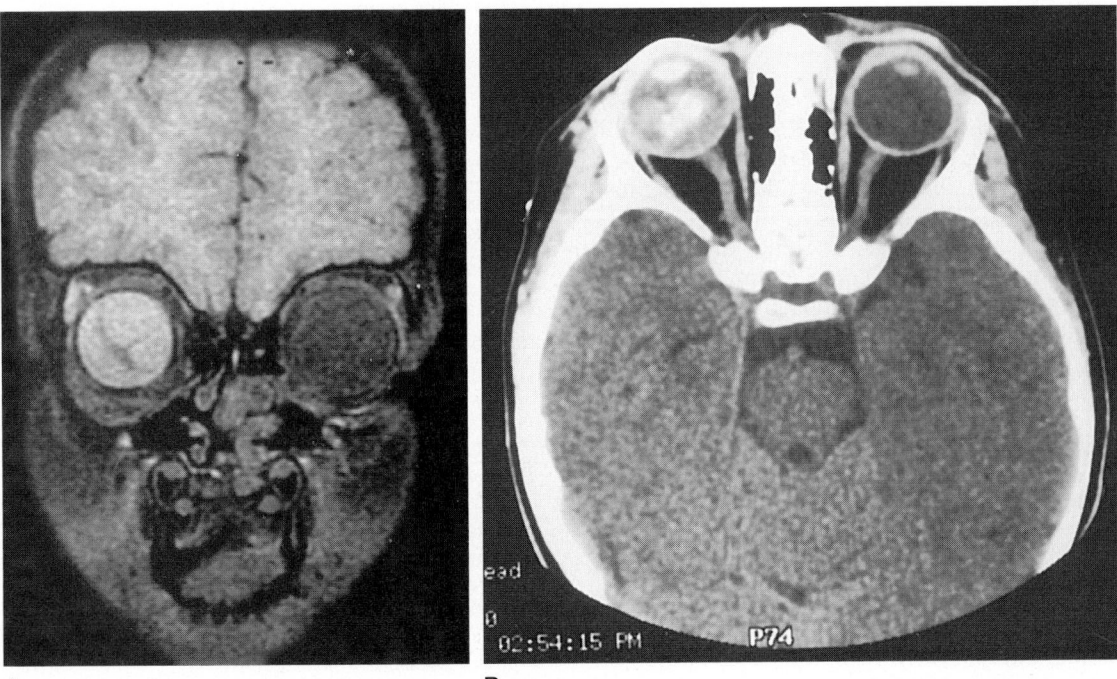

A   B

Figure 65–9. A, T2-weighted magnetic resonance imaging scans of Coats' disease. Note the bright signal of the proteinaceous exudate. **B,** A computed tomography scan of a large calcified retinoblastoma in the right eye.

Table 65–2   Lesions Simulating Retinoblastoma

Solitary Ocular Tumor

Astrocytic hamartoma
Toxocara canis

Total Retinal Detachment

Coats' disease
Retinopathy of prematurity
Persistent hyperplastic primary vitreous

to view. Under these circumstances, ultrasonography can be helpful.

Persistent hyperplastic primary vitreous is a congenital, nonheritable, predominantly unilateral disorder that may be present at birth or detected years later. Patients with this disorder can present with leukocoria, which results from an opaque, translucent, and sometimes vascularized membrane located behind the lens. This membrane can extend and pull down on the ciliary processes, making them visible through the dilated pupil. These eyes can be microphthalmic (small), causing enophthalmos or ptosis. Eyes with persistent hyperplastic primary vitreous can develop lens swelling, glaucoma, and phthisis bulbi (permanent shrinkage of the eye).

Retinopathy of prematurity (ROP) occurs in children who are born prematurely, have a low birth weight, and require oxygen for respiratory distress. However, ROP is also seen in term babies who do not require oxygen. ROP usually presents with bilateral involvement, microphthalmos, and myopia. Clinical ophthalmic examination of ROP reveals proliferation of the temporal retinal blood vessels, disorganization of the vitreous, and a detached retina. It is the vitreal fibrosis or white retrolental mass that simulates retinoblastoma. Ancillary tests can be of great assistance in differentiating ROP from retinoblastoma.

Astrocytic hamartomas can also mimic retinoblastoma. In patients who have the complete clinical syndrome of tuberous sclerosis with a positive family history of the disease, mental retardation, seizures, and central nervous system abnormalities aid in the diagnosis. However, many patients with astrocytic hamartoma have only the ophthalmic findings, making the diagnosis more challenging. On fundoscopic examination, early astrocytic hamartomas can be solitary or multifocal and can be located in the anterior fundus or in the optic nerve head. The lesions have a clear cellophane-like appearance above the retinal blood vessels. This lesion is more difficult to distinguish from retinoblastoma in its early stages of growth than during later stages. With time, astrocytic hamartomas calcify, develop distinct margins, and grow larger. These lesions can be detected as incidental findings in otherwise healthy adults.

Ocular toxocariasis also commonly mimics retinoblastoma. Nematode endophthalmitis and solitary granulomas are the two forms most often confused with retinoblastoma. Patients with nematode endophthalmitis present at an average age of 6 years with pain, photophobia, inflammatory signs including vascular injection, cataracts with cells and flare on the slit-lamp examination,

and sometimes posterior synechiae. Patients with solitary granulomas rarely have external ophthalmic inflammatory signs but present with a white, pearl, or yellow ball-shaped mass. Mild or severe vitreal traction may be seen.[6]

Staging of Retinoblastoma

The Reese-Ellsworth Classification scheme is the most commonly used classification system for describing intraocular tumors (Table 65-3).[23] It is not a true staging scheme, for untreated patients do not progress from group I to higher groups. It was originally developed to predict prognosis in eyes that were treated with lateral photons via external beam irradiation and other vision-preserving techniques. A higher numeric classification signifies that a tumor is located more anteriorly and that there is a decreased success rate treating the eye with lateral port external beam radiation. Despite its limited applicability, it has served as an excellent ocular

Table 65–3   Two Classifications for Retinoblastoma

Reese-Ellsworth—Intraocular

Group I
  a. Solitary tumor, <4 DD in size, at or behind the equator
  b. Multiple tumors, none >4 DD in size, all at or behind the equator
Group II
  a. Solitary tumor, 4-10 DD in size, at or behind the equator
  b. Multiple tumors, 4-10 DD in size, behind the equator
Group III
  a. Any lesion anterior to the equator
  b. Solitary tumors >10 DD behind the equator
Group IV
  a. Multiple tumors, some >10 DD
  b. Any lesion extending anteriorly to the ora seratta
Group V
  a. Massive tumors involving more than half the retina
  b. Vitreous seeding

Abramson/Grabowski—Extraocular

I. Intraocular disease
  a. Retinal tumor(s)
  b. Extension into choroid
  c. Extension up to lamina cribrosa
  d. Extension into sclerae
II. Orbital disease
  a. Orbital tumor
    1. Suspicious (pathology of scattered episcleral tumor cells)
    2. Proven (biopsy-proven orbital tumor)
  b. Regional nodes
III. Optic nerve disease
  a. Tumor beyond lamina but not up to cut section
  b. Tumor at cut section of optic nerve
IV. Intracranial metastases
  a. Positive CSF only
  b. Retinoblastoma mass in CNS
V. Hematogenous metastasis
  a. Positive marrow/bone lesions
  b. Other organ involvement

CNS, central nervous system; CSF, cerebrospinal fluid; DD, disc diameter.

reference for comparison of different series and treatment schemes. No single scheme that includes patients with extraocular retinoblastoma has been widely accepted among ophthalmologists. In our center, we use the Abramson-Grabowski Staging System for extraocular disease (see Table 65-3). The TNM system of the American Joint Committee on Cancer, shown for comparison in Table 65-4, is not commonly used (too complex; the Reese-Ellsworth Scheme has more history in the ophthalmic community, etc.).

TREATMENT OF RETINOBLASTOMA

The primary goal of retinoblastoma treatment is to ensure the survival of these children. Secondary but also

---

Table 65–4   Classification of Retinoblastoma

Primary Tumor (T)

TX	Primary tumor cannot be assessed
T0	No evidence of primary tumor
T1	Tumor confined to the retina (no vitreous seeding or significant retinal detachment) No retinal detachment or subretinal fluid >5 mm from the base of the tumor
T1a	Any eye in which the largest tumor is ≤3 mm in height and no tumor is located closer than 1 DD (1.5 mm) to the optic nerve or fovea
T1b	All other eyes in which the tumor(s) are confined to the retina regardless of location or size (up to half the volume of the eye). No vitreous seeding. No retinal detachment or subretinal fluid >5mm from the base of the tumor
T2	Tumor with contiguous spread to adjacent tissues or spaces (vitreous or subretinal space)
T2a	Minimal tumor spread to vitreous or subretinal space, or both. Fine local or diffuse vitreous seeding or serous, or both. Retinal detachment up to total detachment may be present, but no clumps, lumps, snowballs, or avascular masses are allowed in the vitreous or subretinal space. Calcium flecks in the vitreous or subretinal space are allowed. The tumor may fill up to 2/3 the volume of the eye.
T2b	Massive tumor spread to the vitreous or subretinal space, or both. Vitreous seeding or subretinal implantation, or both, may consist of lumps, clumps, snowballs, or avascular tumor masses. Retinal detachment may be total. Tumor may fill up to 2/3 the volume of the eye.
T2c	Unsalvageable intraocular disease. Tumor fills more than 2/3 the eye or there is no possibility of visual rehabilitation or one or more of the following are present: Tumor-associated glaucoma, either neovascular or angle closure Anterior segment extension of tumor Ciliary body extension of tumor Hyphema (significant) Massive vitreous hemorrhage Tumor in contact with lens Orbital cellulitis-like clinical presentation (massive tumor necrosis)
T3	Invasion of the optic nerve or optic coats, or both
T4	Extraocular tumor

Regional Lymph Nodes (N)

NX	Regional lymph nodes cannot be assessed
N0	No regional lymph node involvement
N1	Regional lymph node involvement (preauricular, submandibular, or cervical)
N2	Distant lymph node involvement

Distant Metastasis (M)

MX	Distant metastasis cannot be assessed
M0	No distant metastasis
M1	Metastasis to central nervous system or bone, or both; bone marrow; or other sites of pathologic classification (pTNM). There is 1 major difference in the pathologic classification from the last edition. No differentiation pathologic separation is proposed for those eyes in which the tumor may vary in size but is confined to the retina, vitreous, or subretinal space.

Primary Tumor (pT)

pTX	Primary tumor cannot be assessed
pT0	No evidence of primary tumor
pT1	Tumor confined to the retina, vitreous, or subretinal space. No optic nerve or choroidal invasion.
pT2	Minimal invasion of the optic nerve or optic coats, or both.
pT2a	Tumor invades optic nerve up to but not through the level of the lamina cribrosa
pT2b	Tumor invades choroid focally
PT2c	Tumor invades optic nerve up to but not through the level of the lamina cribrosa and invades the choroid focally
pT3	Significant invasion of the optic nerve or optic coats, or both.
pT3a	Tumor invades optic nerve through the level of the lamina cribrosa but not to the line of resection
pT3b	Tumor massively invades the choroid
pT3c	Tumor invades the optic nerve through the level of the lamina cribrosa but not to the line of resection and massively invades the choroid
pT4	Extraocular tumor extension that includes: Invasion on optic nerve to the line of resection Invasion of orbit both through the sclera Extension both anteriorly or posteriorly into the orbit Extension into the brain Extension into the subarachnoid space of the optic nerve Extension to the apex of the orbit Extension to but not through the chiasm Extension into the brain beyond the chiasm

Regional Lymph Nodes (pN)

pNX	Regional lymph nodes cannot be assessed
pN0	No regional lymph node metastasis
pN1	Regional lymph node metastasis

Distant Metastasis (pM)

pMX	Distant metastasis cannot be assessed
pM0	No distant metastasis
pM1	Distant metastasis
pM1a	Bone marrow
pM1b	Other sites

STAGE GROUPING

No stage grouping applies

HISTOPATHOLOGIC TYPE

This classification applies only to retinoblastoma

DD, disc diameter.
From Greene FL, Page DL, Fleming ID, et al., eds: *AJCC Cancer Staging Manual*. 6th ed. New York: Springer; 2002.

important goals include retention of the eyes and of vision. A final goal is the avoidance of facial bony deformities or other physical changes that can affect functional well-being.[24] Treatment approaches are guided by the presence of intraocular or extraocular disease. This section will concentrate on the treatment of intraocular disease. Because most of the children survive their retinoblastoma, long-term complications of treatment must be factored into initial treatment decisions.

The treatment modalities currently used for intraocular disease include enucleation, external beam radiation, cryotherapy, photocoagulation and transpupillary thermotherapy, episcleral brachytherapy, and systemic and periocular chemotherapy. Localized excision of the tumor from within the eye is never performed because of the risk of tumor seeding during the procedure (Fig. 65-10).

Enucleation

Enucleation is surgical removal of the eye, leaving untouched the lids and extraocular muscles. *Exenteration* is surgical removal of the eye and its orbital contents including the extraocular muscles, orbital fat, nerves, lids, lashes, lacrimal gland, and occasionally brow. Currently, exenteration is rarely used for retinoblastoma. Enucleation is a safe, effective, quick treatment for intraocular disease and is available worldwide. General anesthesia is used for children undergoing this procedure.

With the patient under anesthesia, both eyes are examined after having been dilated. The eye that will not be removed is taped shut, and the patient is prepped and draped in the usual sterile fashion. The conjunctiva is separated at the limbus, where the cornea meets the sclera and a 360-degree peritomy is made. Each of the four recti muscles and two oblique muscles are then isolated on a muscle hook and severed with cautery to minimize bleeding. In the past, a suture was passed through the stump of the medial rectus muscle to aid in traction, but today, the Brown-Addison forceps are preferred. Cases of inadvertent needle penetration into

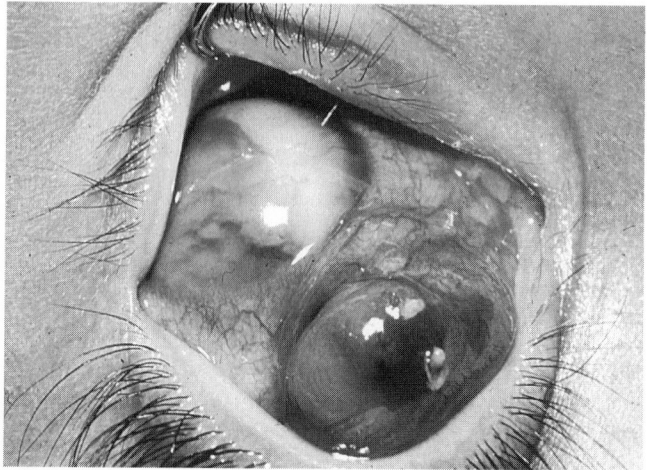

Figure 65-10. Extraocular growth of retinoblastoma cells following a biopsy.

the eye and rupture of the globe (the sclera adjacent to the muscle is <1 mm) have occurred with the previously used suture technique.

The optic nerve is usually approached from the nasal side of the eye because the longest stump of optic nerve is obtained this way. Just before severing the optic nerve, the lids are opened as widely as possible and anterior traction is applied from the forceps. The scissors should be straight and not sharply angulated, and the optic nerve should be cut in one motion. Long stumps of optic nerve are ideal for pathology and lengths of more than 10 mm in young children are commonly obtained with this technique. After removal, the surgeon inspects the globe for extraocular extension and optic nerve involvement while the assistant applies digital pressure for hemostasis by placing one finger in the socket extending to the orbital apex. Simultaneously, a digital search for extraocular tumor is made. A ball composed of inert material, such as silicone or plastic, which measures a few millimeters smaller than the eye, is then placed where the eye was within the muscle cone. The muscles and Tenon's layer are then pulled over the ball and the deeper layers are closed with a purse-string suture. The overlying conjunctiva is then closed and a conformer made of clear or opaque silicone or plastic is then placed between the lids. A firm Elastoplast dressing is applied for 24 hours.

The children are discharged on the same day. Postoperative pain is minimal and is easily controlled with acetaminophen (Tylenol). Parents are instructed on the daily changing of the dressing and application of topical antibiotic and steroid ointment. Three weeks after the enucleation, the conformer is removed and the permanent prosthesis is made by an ocularist. The ocularist makes a mold of the socket and transfers the mold into a plastic prosthesis, which is painted to match the fellow eye.

The artificial ball moves well but is not attached to the overlying prosthesis; movement of the final prosthesis is fair to poor but the cosmetic result is usually excellent. Over the years there have been many attempts to integrate the ball and prosthesis including magnets, male/female conforming shapes of the two structures, and connections between the two. These prostheses have all been abandoned because of high rates of recurrent local infections and rejection. Artificial balls of different materials have also been used including silicone, medpore, and hydroxyapatite. Hydroxyapatite, a synthetic implant made from sea coral, has been used over the past 10 years. Long-term data do not exist, but complications such as extrusion and infection are not uncommon. Surgically implanted balls of silicone or plastic never have to be replaced. The prosthesis requires no daily care and is removed from once per month to once or twice per year for cleaning. When children acquire upper respiratory infections, the prosthesis may need to be removed if the socket also gets infected. The prosthesis has a long life, but wear and tear mandates replacements every few years.

Enucleation is still widely used for retinoblastoma worldwide. Patients considered for enucleation include those with: unilateral or bilateral Reese-Ellsworth group V eyes, active tumor in a blind eye, and painful glaucoma from tumor invasion. Patients are also considered for enucleation if they have failed all other forms of treatment, or if they have active tumor and cannot be followed.[24] In the past, some centers have advocated in bilateral cases for enucleation of the eye with worse disease and treatment of the fellow eye with external beam radiation or other focal techniques.[24] In our center, however, we find that it is often difficult to predict which eye will have disease progression and which one will respond to treatment. An eye that appears worse at diagnosis may in fact result in better vision after treatment than the fellow eye. Therefore, we believe that in a case of bilateral disease in which neither eye meets the criteria for enucleation, but both eyes have disease too advanced for focal techniques, bilateral external beam radiation may be attempted if the family understands the short- and long-term risks.

Cryotherapy

Cryotherapy was first used for retinoblastoma by Lincoff in 1967 and has since been used extensively.[25-27] Cryoprobes, which look like blunted pencils, are applied to the sclerae outside the eye corresponding to the location of the intraocular tumor focus. Under direct visualization, the tumor to be treated is identified by pressing the probe on the sclera ("indenting") and a foot switch is pressed to commence the freezing. The tumor is completely covered by ice within 1 or 2 minutes. It has been shown that the tumors are frozen quickly (faster than –90°C a minute), forming intracellular ice crystals that expand and lead to cell death by causing protein denaturation, pH changes, and finally cell membrane rupture. There may also be a local vascular effect created by immediate slowing of blood flow, subsequent destruction of endothelial cells, and a possible local immunologic effect.

Cryotherapy may be used as the primary treatment for small peripheral retinoblastomas or as secondary treatment for recurrent tumors treated previously with external beam radiation. Size and location of the tumor are factors that determine success with cryotherapy. Retinoblastomas that are successfully treated with cryotherapy include small tumors (<3 to 4 disc diameter) not located at the vitreous base. The average tumor this size requires several treatments, and sessions are usually scheduled 3 to 6 weeks apart. Larger tumors require more treatments and have a poorer chance of success. Tumors with widespread vitreous seeding and tumors that settle at the vitreous base rarely respond to this treatment.[26,28,29] However, cryotherapy is uniquely useful for tumors with localized vitreous seeding overlying the tumor apex. In these cases, the freeze is extended in area to include the location of the seeds.[26]

Few side effects result from cryotherapy. Immediately following cryotherapy, edema of the conjunctiva and lids occurs, but is easily managed with topical steroids/antibiotic ointment. Retinal edema surrounding the tumor may also be noted immediately after treatment. Following freezing of the tumor, hemorrhages within the tumor may occur. Long-term complications such as prolonged retinal detachments are rare but do occur.

Tumors treated with cryotherapy will ultimately shrink and completely disappear if treatment is successful. In our center, 90% of tumors that are less than 3 mm in diameter are cured permanently.[26] The cryotherapy scars are flat and pigmented from the reaction of the overlying retinal pigment epithelium.

Photocoagulation

Light coagulation with the xenon arc photocoagulator was first described by Meyer-Schwickerath in 1957, who demonstrated that intense, focused, white light could be used to treat intraocular retinoblastomas.[21] Currently, patients are treated while under general anesthesia with their pupils dilated. One to three barriers of photocoagulation burns are aimed through the anterior chamber at the tumor's feeding vessels. The tumor itself is never treated because it does not absorb very much of the light energy due to its color. When the tumor's blood supply is destroyed, the tumor begins to involute within 1 week of treatment. Traditionally, xenon arc photocoagulation (wavelength 250 to 1500 nm) was used, but currently tumors can be treated with argon lasers in the visible range (wavelength 488 to 536 nm) or diode/infrared lasers in the invisible range (wavelength 810 nm) with success.[9]

Photocoagulation is employed as primary treatment for select, small retinoblastomas. The following tumor features correlate with the success of photocoagulation: small size (<3 disc diameter), anterior location, and low elevation (tumor ≤50% of the base diameter).[30] Photocoagulation is not used for tumors that involve the optic disc or fovea, as this technique would result in loss of central vision. In such cases, external beam radiation or chemoreduction are typically used.

More than 70% of tumors with the previously mentioned characteristics are cured with photocoagulation.[30] Success is attained when a flat scar develops, and long-term recurrence of photocoagulated tumors is extremely unusual. Potential complications of photocoagulation include cataracts, iris burns, vitreous hemorrhage, and traction effects.

Transpupillary Thermotherapy

Transpupillary thermotherapy (TTT) was first used as treatment for retinoblastoma by Lagendijk, although other researchers in the Netherlands had previously studied its use as treatment for choroidal melanoma.[31] Thermal energy is delivered from an 810 nm infrared ophthalmic laser with modifications to the laser's hardware and software. The mechanism by which TTT causes tumor cell death is different from the mechanism by which classic laser photocoagulation destroys tumors. With TTT, the temperature is thought to be lower (45°C to 60°C), and the thermal effect leads to apoptosis rather than burning. Because the effects of TTT rely on the direct killing of tumor cells, the laser beam is aimed directly at the tumor rather than at the feeding vessels as in photocoagulation.

Indications for TTT have not yet been established. In the largest series to date, patients with viable retinoblastoma within the retina or subretinal space with less than 1.0 mm of overlying subretinal fluid were included.[32] Larger tumors and tumors with vitreous seeding were excluded. Our group treats primarily tumors that are 3 mm or less in base diameter and are located in the posterior pole.

Limited studies demonstrating the effectiveness of TTT have been completed. Shields et al. have published the largest series of retinoblastomas treated with chemotherapy and TTT to date, in which 188 retinoblastomas in 80 eyes of 58 patients were treated.[32] One-hundred eight of the tumors were treated simultaneously with systemic chemotherapy and TTT, and mean follow-up was 12 months. While 86% of the tumors demonstrated regression, complications were significant and included focal iris atrophy, focal paraxial lens opacity, and sector optic disc atrophy.

Chemotherapy (Chemoreduction)

Systemic chemotherapy for intraocular retinoblastoma has been used since 1953, when Kupfer used intravenous nitrogen mustard as a primary treatment for retinoblastoma.[33] Then in 1955, Reese et al. used intracarotid triethylenemelamine (TEM) in combination with external beam radiation in order to decrease the required dose of radiation.[34] Currently, "chemoreduction" (using chemotherapy to reduce the size of tumors) is an area of active clinical and basic science research, motivated by the desire to avoid enucleation and external beam radiation in children at risk for developing nonocular cancers.[9]

The indications for chemoreduction are not yet well-established. In general, however, chemoreduction is currently employed for three purposes. Most commonly, this treatment is used for patients who have visual potential in eyes containing tumors that are too large to treat with focal methods. Chemoreduction is used to shrink these tumors so that focal treatments such as photocoagulation, cryotherapy, thermotherapy, or radioactive plaques can then be administered. It is the focal treatment methods that cause permanent inactivation of the tumors. Chemoreduction is also used for patients younger than 1 year of age with advanced bilateral disease who require external beam radiation to be cured. In these cases, chemotherapy is used just to control tumor growth until the patient is 1 year old and can safely undergo external beam radiation without an increased risk for developing nonocular cancers. Finally, chemotherapy has also been used in some studies as a potential single modality eye-preserving treatment. Permanent responses are rarely observed in these cases.

Most studies of chemoreduction for retinoblastoma have used vincristine, carboplatin, and an epipodophyllotoxin, either etoposide or teniposide. The addition of cyclosporine as a P-glycoprotein inhibitor has been suggested to decrease the ability of tumor cells to transport antineoplastic drugs from the intracellular space, thereby allowing the cells to develop multi-drug resistance.[35,36] Currently, choice of agents as well as number and frequency of cycles varies at different institutions.

The results of studies examining chemoreduction followed by focal therapies have been most promising for patients with Reese-Ellsworth group I to III eyes. For these patients, several authors have demonstrated that enucleation can be successfully avoided almost 100% of the time.[35-45] Results for patients with Reese-Ellsworth groups IV and V eyes have been more discouraging. A meta-analysis of studies demonstrated that only 30% of group IV and V eyes avoid both external beam radiation and enucleation. Forty-seven percent of eyes require external beam radiation but avoid enucleation, and 35% of eyes require enucleation (with or without prior external beam radiation).[9]

Another potential complication of chemoreduction is the development of secondary nonocular cancers. Several agents used in current chemoreduction studies for retinoblastoma have previously been demonstrated to increase the risk for secondary cancers either in retinoblastoma patients or in patients treated with these drugs for other primary malignancies. The follow-up periods of chemoreduction studies with retinoblastoma patients to date are inadequate to assess the development of second cancers in these patients. Studies with long-term follow-up are needed.

The Role of Radiation Therapy

External beam radiation therapy has been successfully employed for retinoblastoma since Hilgartner experimented with x-ray treatments in Austin, Texas in 1903.[46] Early experience demonstrated the efficacy of tumor regression with radiation therapy. However, significant complications were frequently observed due to the techniques employed.[47,48] Complications included keratitis sicca, keratinization of conjunctiva and sclera, lacrimal gland atrophy/fibrosis, loss of lashes, corneal ulcers/perforation, hyphema, rubeosis iridis, glaucoma, iritis/uveitis, cataract, vitreous hemorrhage, retinal vascular damage, optic nerve infarction, fat atrophy in the orbit, and arrest of orbital growth.[24] Currently most of these complications have been eliminated or minimized by reducing the total radiation dose, by changing the source of radiation and positioning of the portals, and by using fractionated doses.

External beam radiation is one means of preserving vision in a child with retinoblastoma. Unlike focal therapies including photocoagulation, cryotherapy, and episcleral plaque therapy, fractionated external beam radiation provides an excellent opportunity for useful vision in a macula undestroyed by tumor. External beam radiation is thus considered as a primary treatment option in children with small tumors located within the macula, as well as for multifocal tumors for which focal therapy is ineffective. In cases of bilateral advanced intraocular disease in which clinical judgment cannot predict which eye is more likely to have useful vision, radiation can be used bilaterally. In these cases, one or both eyes may eventually require salvage enucleation. External beam radiation also serves often as the salvage treatment of choice after focal therapies have failed. Finally, for children with advanced extraocular or metastatic disease, radiation therapy also plays a role in palliation and even potential cure of these sites along with chemotherapy.

SIMULATION

The simulation procedure begins with a visit to the mold room. Because of its inherent rigidity, a plaster of Paris mold over the entire head and neck region, molded directly onto a papoose board, is preferred over other immobilization techniques. For the rambunctious 1- to 3-year-old, anesthesia or sedation may be also necessary for this procedure. For most infants under the age of 1 year, anesthesia is not needed. The child's head is wrapped in plastic food wrap for easy removal of the molded plaster of Paris, and a thick steel band is placed coronally at the levels of the external auditory meatus and the vertex of the skull, to facilitate bivalving and removing the upper portion of the mold after it has set. The plaster of Paris is then applied, with special attention to the area over the mouth and chin for stability. After the mold has dried and has been sanded smooth for optimal patient comfort, the child returns to the simulator and is placed in the mold. Where plaster of Paris is not available, an Aquaplast mask or other immobilization system may be substituted.

At Memorial Sloan-Kettering Cancer Center, external beam treatment planning is a variation of the traditional lateral D-shaped field in all but exceptional cases. This reflects a philosophy of the group in avoiding, if at all possible, inducing a radiation-related cataract from an anterior field. Although the lensectomy itself is not a difficult surgical procedure to remove a cataract, small children are intolerant to both contact lenses and the prolonged use of eyeglasses. At present, intraocular lenses are approved in pediatric ophthalmology, but no long-term experience exists. Thus, if the child develops a cataract, a "lazy" eye often results, despite treatment designed to save vision.

A decade ago, we first analyzed our experience with a combination of lateral photon and anterior fields, employing a lens block and general anesthesia when the anterior electron field was treated. We found that because of the small size of the lens and the relationship of the posteriorly located tumor to the shadow cast by the lens block, local recurrences were higher in this group of children, and development of cataracts was similar to the lateral technique. Thus, we favor the lateral technique.[49]

The simulation procedure begins by placing the child straight in the mold, employing lateral lasers and lateral landmarks of the eye and orbit. A third laser is placed midline down the child's nose if both eyes are to be treated, or through the pupil of the treated eye if only one eye is to be treated. The gantry is then rotated 90 degrees, and, with the use of a CT or MRI scan of the globe to reference lens position, and a split beam or independent jaws, the central ray of the beam is placed 2 to 3 mm posterior to the surgical limbus, corresponding to the posterior pole of the lens (Fig. 65-11). This structure anatomically correlates with the anterior extent of the retina at the *ora serrata*. In a child under the age of 1 year, a field size measuring 3 cm wide and 4 cm high is an adequate field size, around which poured blocks

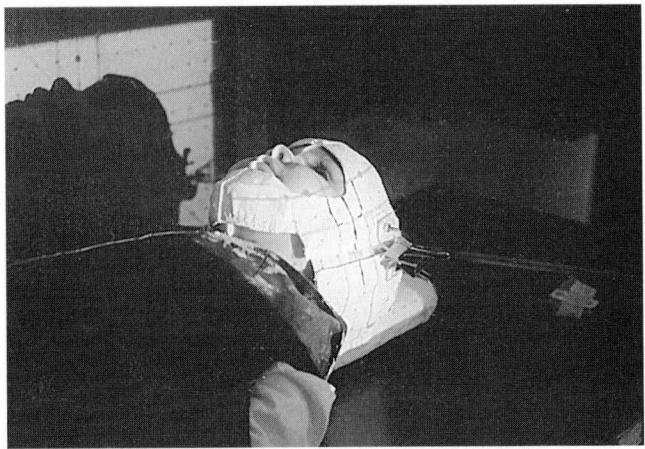

Figure 65–11. A child in a plaster of Paris mold lined up with lasers before simulation.

are designed, shaping the field to the bony orbit and including 1 cm of optic nerve as it exits the globe. Care must be taken to visualize the pituitary fossa and shield it from the primary beam. We use Cerrobend to define the entire field in all directions, minimizing the penumbra when compared to using the jaws (Fig. 65-12). Similar results can also be achieved using a CT-simulator.

For patients with bilateral disease, parallel opposing fields as described will deliver the prescription dose from the equator of the eye posteriorly, including the optic nerve. For patients with lesions between the equator and the *ora serrata*, the anterior edge of the field is brought forward, to include the lens but to spare the cornea. Although risk of a cataract increases, the lids, conjunctiva, and lacrimal gland are not treated, sparing the patient a dry eye. For the patient with unilateral disease, a combination of wedged superior and inferior lateral oblique fields are used for two thirds of the treatment using couch rotation after the patient is set up as described, and the last third of the treatment is done with a lateral electron field. This technique can be modified if dynamic multi-leaf

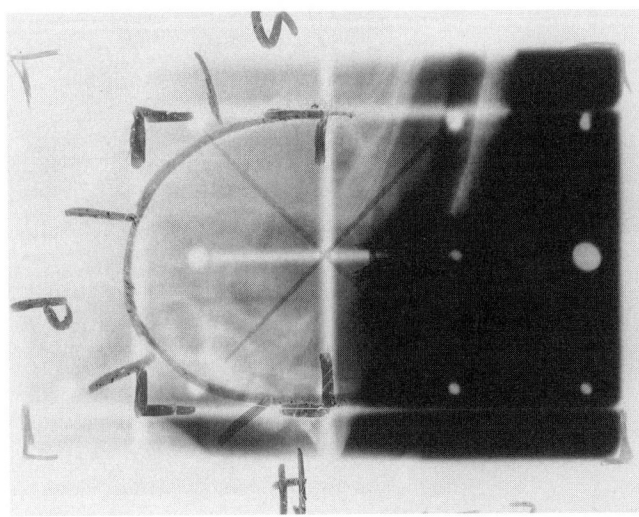

Figure 65–12. A simulation film showing the field and the design for the D-shaped block.

therapy is available, using intensity-modulation as compensation in place of the wedges.

To minimize permanent sequelae in these children from this treatment, we prefer to triangulate the patient using the pupil and the anterior lateral soft tissue canthi bilaterally. Tatoos are thus avoided.

RADIATION TREATMENT PLAN

Because of the marked variation in the relationship of the globe to the bony orbit, all treatment planning is done from CT or MRI images. A transaxial image that demonstrates the lens as well as soft tissue and bone landmarks is selected. Figure 65-13 illustrates a plan for patients with bilateral disease. The prescription isodoses cover the retina from the equator posteriorly. A dose gradient exists anteriorly toward the lens. As noted earlier, because of the philosophy of our group, every effort is made to spare the lens, and this sometimes results in less than the prescription dose to the most anterior portion of the retina. We find these areas are easy to monitor with post-treatment examinations under anesthesia and are amenable to cryotherapy should the need arise to treat new tumors in the region.

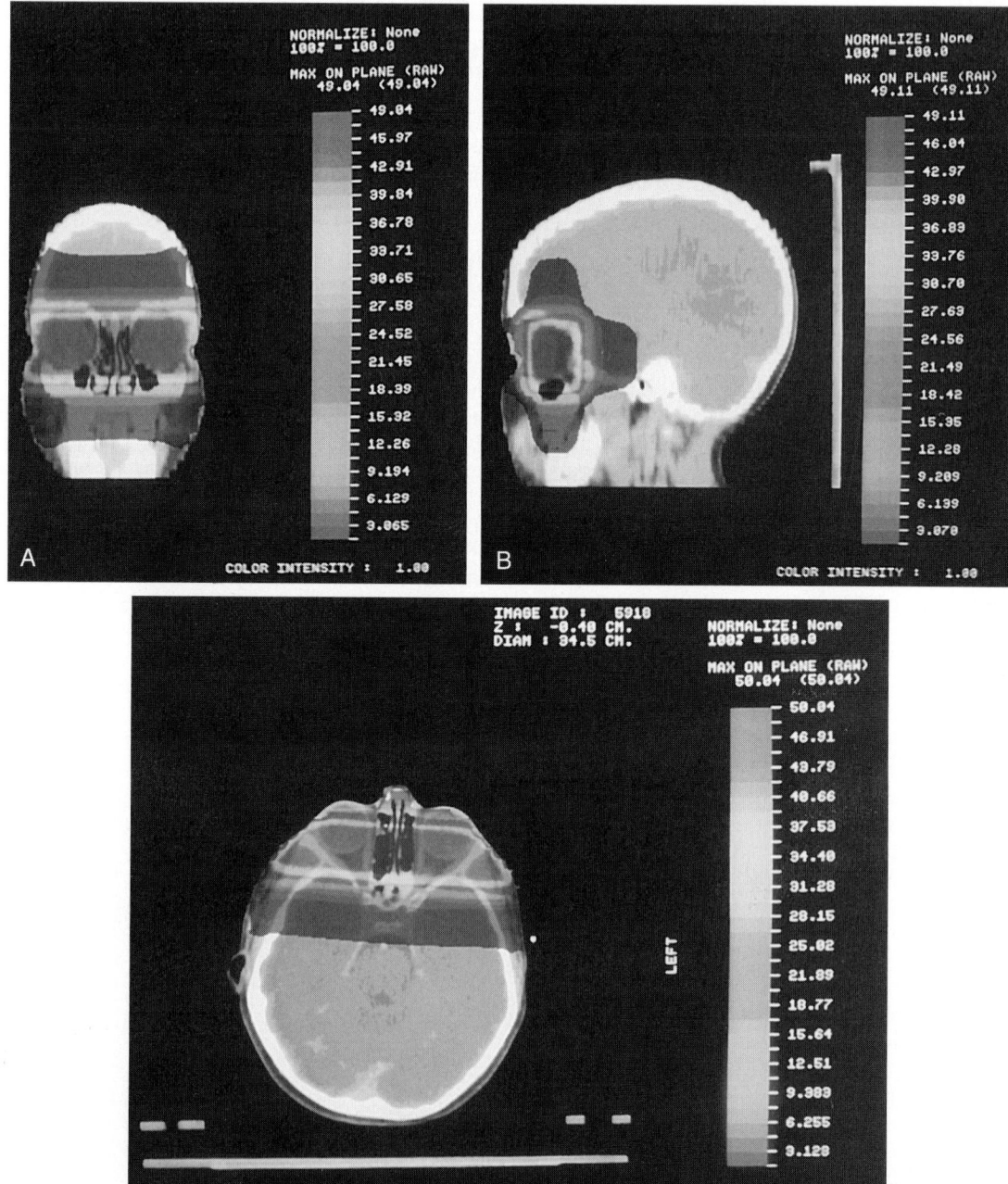

Figure 65–13. An isodose display for a patient with bilateral retinoblastoma located in each eye behind the equator. Parallel opposed fields with a D-shaped block are used to produce these isodose lines. The prescription is displayed in Gy in the coronal (**A**), sagittal (**B**), and transverse (**C**) directions. See also Color Figure 65-13.

While not necessary for the case illustrated, in very young infants, the bony rim of the orbit is so thin that bolus may be necessary to bring the prescription dose out to the lateral margin of the globe.

The dose prescribed is between 42 and 46 Gy, given as 1.8 to 2 Gy fractions, 5 days per week. Six MV photons are the preferred energy for the photon portion of the treatment. In all of the cases in which the last third of the treatment is given with the electron beam, the size and location of the globe within the bony orbit is measured on the CT or MRI scan and used as a determining factor in the electron beam energy selected. Also, a D-shaped cutout corresponding with a D-shaped photon field is used for this portion of the treatment.

Episcleral Brachytherapy

Episcleral brachytherapy was pioneered in medicine by the British eye surgeon Henry Stallard. He designed cobalt applicators that were curved to fit a child's eye with suture holes built in to attach the plaque to the sclerae. The plaques were left in place for 3 to 7 days and radiation was delivered at 40 Gy to the tumor apex; in recent years, this technique has been refined.[50]

Although cobalt plaques are still used, they have been widely replaced with iodine-125 plaques. Under general anesthesia, the conjunctiva is dissected from the limbus in the quadrant harboring the tumor. If an extraocular muscle overlies the tumor, the muscle is removed from its insertion. The tumor is carefully localized with the indirect ophthalmoscope, and either diathermy or ink marks are placed. A dummy plaque of exactly the same size with exactly the same suture holes is attached to the sclera. The plaque placement is confirmed by indirect ophthalmoscope and then the live plaque is inserted.

Many other radioactive sources have been used, including beta sources such as ruthenium and low-energy gamma sources such as palladium. Iodine plaques are safer for the medical and nursing staffs compared to the cobalt plaques. Yet because of their physical size, they are technically more difficult to implant, especially in very young infants with small orbits.

Following plaque treatment, tumors show a distinct response known as type IV radiation regression pattern.[51] A sharp demarcation distinguishes the profound radiation effect from an area where no effect is seen (this occurs in <1 mm of retina). The tumor, overlying retina, and choroid disappear (Fig. 65-14). Curiously, some overlying vessels may persist. Local tumor recurrence is rare.

Side effects from plaque therapy for retinoblastoma are far less common than from plaques for melanoma. The apical dose of a melanoma is usually 85 Gy, whereas for retinoblastoma it is 40 Gy. Melanomas range from 2.5 to 10 mm in height while retinoblastomas usually range from 2 to 4 mm in height. The difference in the doses delivered to the surrounding retina and underlying choroid are significant. Thus optic neuropathy and radiation retinopathy from treated retinoblastoma tumors is unusual. The incidence is so low that there are no publications adequately describing the incidence of these

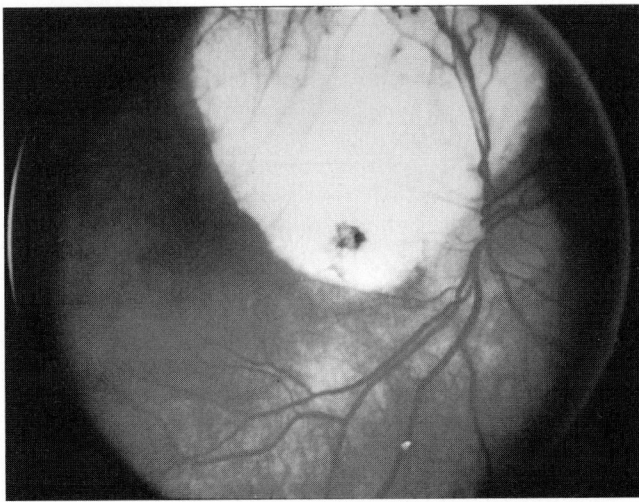

Figure 65–14. A type IV regression pattern after plaque therapy, illustrating the white sclera and calcium deposits.

complications in retinoblastoma eyes. Cataracts will occur when both iodine and cobalt plaques are placed over anterior retinoblastoma tumors. The cataracts may not be evident for years and usually do not require surgery.

Using plaques as primary therapy is a relatively recent development, and we have not yet analyzed our local failure data. When plaque therapy is used as a "salvage technique" in eyes that have failed other combinations of therapy, including external beam radiation, 50% to 89% of such eyes can be salvaged.[52,53] Plaques have not been shown to increase the incidence of second tumors in patients who have also received external beam radiation.

In an attempt to treat the entire eye while avoiding dose to the bony orbit and sinuses, a group in South Africa reported on using a custom-designed iodine-125 applicator with four "claws" that attach to a periorbital anchoring ring. Each "claw" is designed to fit between an extraocular muscle group and is loaded with three iodine-125 seeds. Promising early results were seen in patients with Reese-Ellsworth groups I to III disease, although considerable dose inhomogeneity was noted across the target volume.[54]

NORMAL TISSUE TOLERANCE

During the acute phase of treatment, the eye is quite tolerant of radiation therapy. Because the field is directed just posterior to the lens, the lids and lacrimal gland are not included in the beam and dry eye is not a problem, nor is conjunctivitis seen. Mild skin erythema is noted in the entrance and exit dose paths of the beam as the treatment progresses.

Late complications depend on both the choice of technique for delivery of the radiation and the age of the child when the treatment takes place. With the use of the modified lateral beam technique described, we have seen posterior lens cataracts develop in 20% of treated eyes, similar to findings associated with our anterior field techniques with lens shielding. In centers where an anterior port is used without lens shielding, the majority of children develop cataracts. With the use of an anterior port, keratoconjunctivitis becomes a problem; in addition, a significant exit dose is delivered to portions of the brain.

The late response of the tumor and the appearance of the retina itself have been well described by our group. With the use of indirect ophthalmoscopy when the treated tumor shrinks, the tumor loses its vascularity and picks up calcium; this is classified as a type I radiation regression pattern (Fig. 65-15). In contrast, a type II regression pattern is defined as less dramatic shrinkage of the tumor, ranging from 25% to 50%, with the lesion appearing a lucent gray color with no calcium. A type III regression pattern is a combination of type I and type II and is the type we see most frequently (Fig. 65-16). When plaque radiotherapy is used in the treatment, because of the increased sclera-to-tumor dose ratio, the regression pattern seen is described as a type IV regression pattern, notable for destruction of the overlying retina with a white appearance signifying visible sclera (see Fig. 65-14). In recent years, a fifth regression pattern has been observed, labeled type 0. This results when the post-treatment examination of the retina reveals no evidence at all of the previously existing retinoblastoma nest. It is uncommon to observe, except in the smallest-sized presenting tumors.[55]

Less commonly, the postradiation ophthalmic examination may also reveal vitreous hemorrhage and mild irradiation retinopathy.

Facial and temporal bone hypoplasia can occur following external beam radiation in very young children. It is most marked when both eyes are treated with parallel opposing fields and in children who are under the age of 6 months at diagnosis.[56] Because of the rapid head growth in the infant, this hypoplasia is noted to a lesser degree in older children. With the use of the three-field–modified lateral beam technique, the hypoplasia is minimized because of the smaller entrance dose at each of the three fields.

When the pituitary gland has been successfully excluded from the path of the primary beam, normal growth is almost never interrupted. Nonetheless, the child's pediatrician must be aware of the potential for this and should

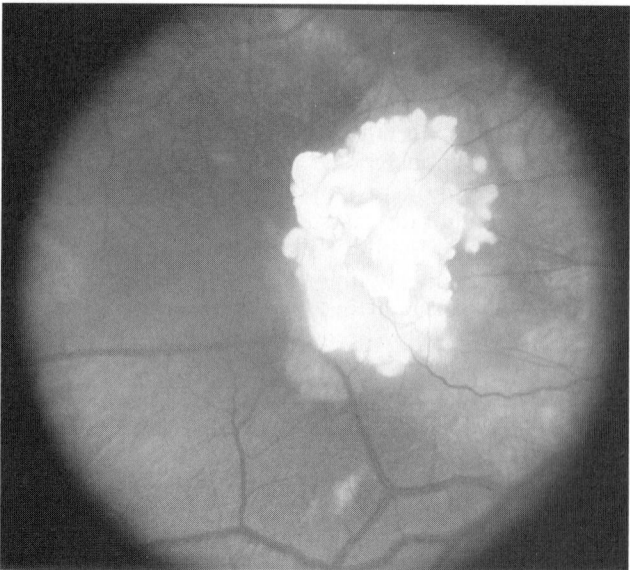

Figure 65–16. A type III regression pattern after external beam radiation to the globe, illustrating calcification as seen in type I, as well as the "fish-flesh" grayish appearance of the tumor at the edges of the treated area, which is more representative of type II regression pattern. The type III pattern is most commonly seen after external beam radiation and represents a combination of types I and II regression patterns.

chart the child's growth with a plan to interfere with the administration of a growth hormone should the child begin to "fall off" his or her growth curve.

Visual results depend on the size and location of the retinoblastoma tumors. Large or small lesions located in the macula region can result in poor central vision. Thus, "useful" or "satisfactory" vision is quoted as a treatment result, rather than visual activity in most papers. In our own material, defining this important treatment result has not been rewarding, because of young patient age and inability to better quantify visual acuity.

SELECT RESULTS

In the United States, retinoblastoma is a highly curable childhood cancer. Cancer registry reports in Europe and the United States have demonstrated 5-year survival rates of 90% and 98%, respectively.[2,57] Survival of children treated with external beam radiation, regardless of laterality, Reese-Ellsworth staging, or technique, ranges from 85% to 100%, excluding old orthovoltage series results.[58-64]

Local control in the irradiated eye, defined as preservation of the eye and based on seven large series, is shown in Table 65-5.[58-64] In many of these series, post-radiation therapy consisting of cryotherapy, photocoagulation, or further radiation was given; however, because of the difficulties in separating recurrence of previously treated tumors from new tumors located elsewhere in the retina, preservation of the eye is the definition of control that is used. Of note in the Stanford series, most eyes were enucleated because of complications from

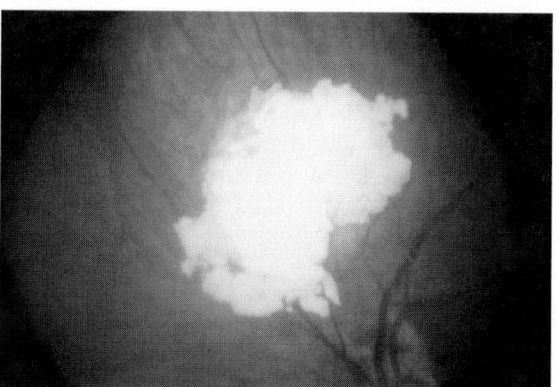

Figure 65–15. A type I regression pattern, displaying calcification and loss of vascularity.

Table 65–5   Ocular Preservation After Primary Radiation

Institution	Eyes, n	% Enucleated (n)	Radiation Dose, Gy
Stanford[58]	38	42 (16)*	35-60
U. Oregon[59]	12[†]	17 (2)	45-50
U. Indiana[60]	12	17 (2)	35-40[‡]
Wills Eye[61]	34	26 (9)	34-49
Mayo[62]	25	20 (5)	45
Militan Central (Buenos Aires)[63]	17	12 (2)	40-45[‡]
Memorial Sloan-Kettering Cancer Center[64]	182	22 (40)	42-46

*10 of the 16 eyes were enucleated because of complications, not recurrence.
[†]Orthovoltage cases excluded.
[‡]Children also received some chemotherapy.

the higher doses of radiation, not because of tumor recurrence.[58]

In our own series, preservation of the eye has been highest in eyes with Reese-Ellsworth stage I to III disease, where 95% of eyes treated with the lateral beam technique are preserved. In those eyes with stage IV to V disease, radiation is only successful in 50% of eyes so treated. Additional cryotherapy and photocoagulation are used frequently after treatment with external beam therapy.

Despite these excellent results, the potential late sequelae of external beam radiation for retinoblastoma patients are serious. As noted previously, patients carrying the germinal RB1 mutation are in danger of developing additional nonocular cancers, and the use of external beam radiation increases the risk for some of these cancers significantly (Table 65-6).[65-69] Cumulative incidence reports of second nonocular cancers among retinoblastoma survivors vary, but it is estimated that a rate of 1% per year of life approximates the risk.[70] Patients who develop a second cancer and then survive that cancer have an increased risk for the development of additional nonocular tumors of approximately 2% per year from the time of second tumor diagnosis.[71] The average latency period between subsequent tumor diagnoses becomes progressively shorter with each additional cancer that develops.

Second nonocular neoplasms observed in survivors of germinal retinoblastoma include, in order of most

Table 65–6   Risk Factors for Second Nonocular Cancer Development in Retinoblastoma Survivors

Factor	Increase in Incidence of Second Cancers
Presence of germinal mutation in RB1 gene	1000× increase[65,66]
External beam radiation	400-600× increase[66]
External beam radiation given at younger than 1 year of age	2-8× increase[67,68]
Dose of external beam radiation	12× increase @ 60 Gy[66]
Presence of lipomas	8× increase[69]

common to least: osteosarcomas (bone, nasal cavities, and nasopharynx), soft tissue sarcomas (connective and soft tissues, nasal cavities, orbit, and other sites), pineoblastomas, cutaneous melanomas, brain tumors, Hodgkin's disease, lung cancer, and breast cancer.[66,72] Survivors of hereditary retinoblastoma are also at increased risk for the development of lipomas throughout the body. Patients who develop lipomas are at an even higher risk of developing second cancers.[69]

In recent years, the effects of external beam radiation on the development of these cancers have been studied extensively. Children radiated during the first year of life are between two and eight times as likely to develop osteogenic sarcomas of the skull and face bones and soft tissue sarcomas of the head as those children radiated after the age of 1 year.[67,68] Patients treated with higher doses and older methods of radiation delivery that lead to increased superficial skin and bone exposure are at higher risk for subsequent tumor development in the radiation field.[71] The dose response curve for the development of soft tissue sarcomas in bilateral retinoblastoma patients has been described. The odds ratio at 0 to 4.9 Gy was 1.0, at 5 to 9.9 Gy was 1.91, at 10 to 29.9 Gy was 4.6, at 30 to 59.9 Gy was 6.4 and at greater than 60 Gy was 11.7.[66] Additional nonocular cancers develop both within and outside the field of radiation. Our group has reported that in radiated patients who develop second malignancies, the tumors are within the radiation field two thirds of the time and outside the field one third of the time. In nonirradiated patients who develop second tumors, the tumors are outside the hypothetic field two thirds of the time and within the hypothetic field one third of the time.[66,67]

Figure 65-17 demonstrates the timing of the development of each type of second cancer in retinoblastoma survivors. In general, external beam radiation treatment given before the age of 1 year both increases the risk that patients will develop certain nonocular cancers and causes the cancers to develop at an earlier age. For example, soft tissue sarcomas of the head, which occur at approximately age 30 in nonirradiated patients, can occur as early as the teenage years in patients radiated at younger than 1 year of age. Osteogenic sarcomas of the skull, for which nonirradiated patients carry a 1:1000 risk per year of developing, occur four times more commonly during the late teenage years in patients radiated under 1 year of age.

Our group published a report on the largest series of retinoblastoma survivors who developed a second cancer, survived, and went on to develop third, fourth, or fifth nonocular tumors.[71] Survivors of retinoblastoma who develop second malignancies and survive are at an even higher risk for the development of additional cancers than they were for the development of a second tumor. The distribution of tumor sites in the second-tumor group suggests a nonrandom pattern of third, fourth, and fifth tumor development. Of patients with skin cancers as their second tumors, skin cancers also represent most of the third, fourth, and fifth tumors that develop in this group. Of patients treated for a second tumor in the skull in whom a third tumor develops, most are diagnosed

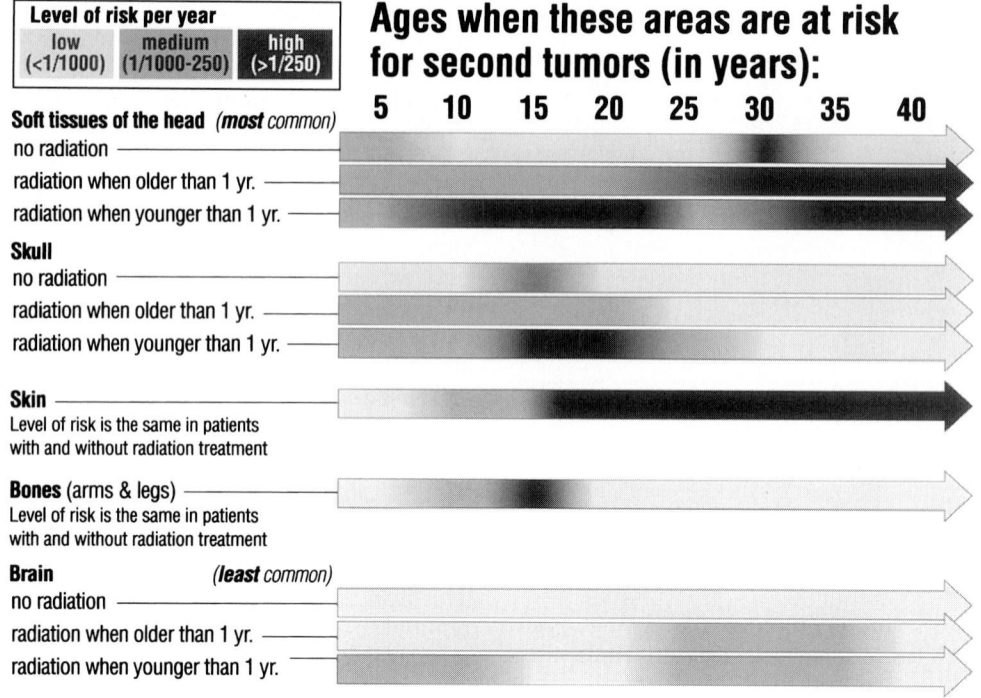

Figure 65–17. Risk of developing different types of second cancers for germinal retinoblastoma survivors from birth to age 40. ©1997, David H. Abramson, MD; Christopher M. Frank.

with a soft tissue sarcoma in the head as the third tumor. The locations and expected ages at which soft tissue sarcomas of the head and osteogenic sarcomas of the long bones develop are consistent with the patterns observed in second tumors (see Fig. 66-17).

REFERENCES

1. Spencer WH: *Ophthalmic Pathology.* Vol. 1. Philadelphia: WB Saunders; 1986.
2. Novakovic B: U.S. childhood cancer survival, 1973-1987. *Med Pediatr Oncol.* 1994;23:480.
3. Abramson DH: Retinoblastoma: Diagnosis and management. *CA Cancer J Clin.* 1982;32:130.
4. Abramson DH: Retinoblastoma. *Pediatr Emerg Casebook.* 1985;3:3.
5. Orjuela M, Castaneda VP, Ridaura C, et al: Presence of human papilloma virus in tumor tissue from children with retinoblastoma: An alternative mechanism for tumor development. *Clin Cancer Res.* 2000;6:4010.
6. Abramson DH: The diagnosis of retinoblastoma. *Bull N Y Acad Med.* 1988;64:283.
7. Knudson AG Jr: Mutation and cancer: Statistical study of retinoblastoma. *Proc Natl Acad Sci U S A.* 1971;68:820.
8. Friend SH, Bernards R, Rogelj S, et al: A human DNA segment with properties of the gene that predisposes to retinoblastoma and osteosarcoma. *Nature.* 1986;323:643.
9. Abramson DH, Dunkel IJ, McCormick B: Neoplasms of the eye. *Cancer Med.* 2000;1083.
10. Harbour JW: Overview of RB gene mutations in patients with retinoblastoma. Implications for clinical genetic screening. *Ophthalmology.* 1998;105:1442.
11. Zhu X, Dunn JM, Goddard AD, et al: Mechanisms of loss of heterozygosity in retinoblastoma. *Cytogenet Cell Genet.* 1992; 59:248.
12. Smith BJ, O'Brien JM: The genetics of retinoblastoma and current diagnostic testing. *J Pediatr Ophthalmol Strabismus.* 1996;33:120.
13. Eng C, Li FP, Abramson DH, et al: Mortality from second tumors among long-term survivors of retinoblastoma. *J Natl Cancer Inst.* 1993;85:1121.
14. Abramson DH: Lactate dehydrogenase and retinoblastoma. In Jakobiec FA, ed. *Ocular and Adnexal Tumors.* Birmingham, Ala.: Aesculaoius, 1978:454.
15. Messner EP: Histopathology of retinoblastoma. In Alberti WE, Sagerman RH, eds. *Radiotherapy of Intraocular and Orbital Tumors.* Berlin: Springer-Verlag; 1993:131.
16. Ellsworth RM: Retinoblastoma. In Duane TD, ed. *Clinical Ophthalmology.* Hagerstown, MD: Harper & Row; 1976:1.
17. Abramson DH, Frank CM, Susman M, et al: Presenting signs of retinoblastoma. *J Pediatr.* 1998;132:505.
18. Abramson DH, Beaverson K, Sangani P, et al: Retinoblastoma: Do the presenting signs have prognostic value for outcome? *J Pediatr.* in press 2003.
19. Abramson DH, Ellsworth RM, Grumbach N, et al: Retinoblastoma: Survival, age at detection and comparison 1914-1958, 1958-1983. *J Pediatr Ophthalmol Strabismus.* 1985;22:246.
20. Abramson DH, Servodidio CA: Retinoblastoma in the first year of life. *Ophthalmic Paediatr Genet.* 1992;13:191.
21. Abramson DH, Mendelsohn ME, Servodidio CA, et al: Familial retinoblastoma: Where and when? *Acta Ophthalmol Scand.* 1998;76:334.
22. Brenner D, Elliston C, Hall E, et al: Estimated risks of radiation-induced fatal cancer from pediatric CT. *Am J Roentgenol.* 2001;176:289.
23. Reese AB: *Tumors of the Eye.* New York: Harper & Row; 1963.
24. Abramson DH: Treatment of retinoblastoma. In Blodi FC, ed. *Retinoblastoma.* New York: Churchill Livingstone; 1985:3.
25. Lincoff H, McLean J, Long R: The cryosurgical treatment of intraocular tumors. *Am J Ophthalmol.* 1967;63:389.
26. Abramson DH, Ellsworth RM, Rozakis GW: Cryotherapy for retinoblastoma. *Arch Ophthalmol.* 1982;100:1253.
27. Abramson DH: Cryotherapy in retinoblastoma. In Jakobiec F, ed. *Advanced Techniques in Ocular Surgery.* Philadelphia: WB Saunders; 1984:433.
28. Hopping W, Bunke-Schmidt A: Light coagulation and cryotherapy in retinoblastoma. In Blodi FC, ed. *Retinoblastoma.* New York: Churchill Livingstone; 1985:95.
29. Shields JA, Parsons H, Shields CL, et al: The role of cryotherapy in the management of retinoblastoma. *Am J Ophthalmol.* 1989;108:260.

30. Abramson DH: The focal treatment of retinoblastoma with emphasis on xenon arc photocoagulation. *Acta Ophthalmol Suppl.* 1989;194:3.

31. Lagendijk JJ: A microwave heating technique for the hyperthermic treatment of tumours in the eye, especially retinoblastoma. *Phys Med Biol.* 1982;27:1313.

32. Shields CL, Santos MC, Diniz W, et al: Thermotherapy for retinoblastoma. *Arch Ophthalmol.* 1999;117:885.

33. Kupfer C: Retinoblastoma treated with intravenous nitrogen mustard. *Am J Ophthalmol.* 1953;36:1721.

34. Reese AB, Hyman GA, Merriam GR, et al: Treatment of retinoblastoma by radiation and triethylenemelamine. *Arch Ophthalmol.* 1955;53:505.

35. Gallie BL, Budning A, DeBoer G, et al: Chemotherapy with focal therapy can cure intraocular retinoblastoma without radiotherapy. *Arch Ophthalmol.* 1996;114:1321.

36. Chan HS, DeBoer G, Thiessen JJ, et al: Combining cyclosporin with chemotherapy controls intraocular retinoblastoma without requiring radiation. *Clin Cancer Res.* 1996;2:1499.

37. Murphree AL, Villablanca JG, Deegan WF III, et al: Chemotherapy plus local treatment in the management of intraocular retinoblastoma. *Arch Ophthalmol.* 1996;114:1348.

38. Shields CL, Shields JA, Needle M, et al: Combined chemoreduction and adjuvant treatment for intraocular retinoblastoma. *Ophthalmology.* 1997;104:2101.

39. Kingston JE, Hungerford JL, Madreperla SA, et al: Results of combined chemotherapy and radiotherapy for advanced intraocular retinoblastoma. *Arch Ophthalmol.* 1996;114:1339.

40. Greenwald MJ, Strauss LC: Treatment of intraocular retinoblastoma with carboplatin and etoposide chemotherapy. *Ophthalmology.* 1996;103:1989.

41. Shields CL, De Potter P, Himelstein BP, et al: Chemoreduction in the initial management of intraocular retinoblastoma. *Arch Ophthalmol.* 1996;114:1330.

42. Gunduz K, Shields CL, Shields JA, et al: The outcome of chemoreduction treatment in patients with Reese-Ellsworth group V retinoblastoma. *Arch Ophthalmol.* 1998;116:1613.

43. Friedman DL, Himelstein B, Shields CL, et al: Chemoreduction and local ophthalmic therapy for intraocular retinoblastoma. *J Clin Oncol.* 2000;18:12.

44. Wilson MW, Rodriguez-Galindo C, Haik BG, et al: Multiagent chemotherapy as neoadjuvant treatment for multifocal intraocular retinoblastoma. *Ophthalmology.* 2001;108:2106; discussion 2114–2115.

45. Beck MN, Balmer A, Dessing C, et al: First-line chemotherapy with local treatment can prevent external-beam irradiation and enucleation in low-stage intraocular retinoblastoma. *J Clin Oncol.* 2000;18:2881.

46. Hilgartner HL: Report of a case of a double glioma treated by x-ray. *Tex Med.* 1903;18:322.

47. Reese AB, Merriam GR, Martin HE: Treatment of bilateral retinoblastoma by irradiation and surgery. Report on 15-year results. *Am J Ophthalmol.* 1949;32:175.

48. Martin HE, Reese AB: Treatment of retinal gliomas by the fractionated or divided dose principal of roentgen radiation: Preliminary report. *Arch Ophthalmol.* 1936;16:733.

49. McCormick B, Ellsworth R, Abramson D, et al: Radiation therapy for retinoblastoma: Comparison of results with lens-sparing versus lateral beam techniques. *Int J Radiat Oncol Biol Phys.* 1988;15:567.

50. Stallard HB: Radiotherapy for malignant intraocular neoplasms. *Br J Ophthalmol.* 1948;32:681.

51. Buys RJ, Abramson DH, Ellsworth RM, et al: Radiation regression patterns after cobalt plaque insertion for retinoblastoma. *Arch Ophthalmol.* 1983;101:1206.

52. Abramson DH, Ellsworth RM, Haik BG: Cobalt plaques in advanced retinoblastoma. *Retina.* 1983;3:12.

53. Shields JA, Shields CL, De Potter P, et al: Plaque radiotherapy for residual or recurrent retinoblastoma in 91 cases. *J Pediatr Ophthalmol Strabismus.* 1994;31:242.

54. Stannard C, Sealy R, Hering E, et al: Localized whole eye radiotherapy for retinoblastoma using a ^{125}I applicator, "claws." *Int J Radiat Oncol Biol Phys.* 2001;51:399.

55. Abramson DH, McCormick B, Fass D, et al: Retinoblastoma. The long-term appearance of radiated intraocular tumors. *Cancer.* 1991;67:2753.

56. Imhof SM, Mourits MP, Hofman P, et al: Quantification of orbital and mid-facial growth retardation after megavoltage external beam irradiation in children with retinoblastoma. *Ophthalmology.* 1996;103:263.

57. Sant M, Capocaccia R, Badioni V: Survival for retinoblastoma in Europe. *Eur J Cancer.* 2001;37:730.

58. Egbert PR, Donaldson SS, Moazed K, et al: Visual results and ocular complications following radiotherapy for retinoblastoma. *Arch Ophthalmol.* 1978;96:1826.

59. Gagnon JD, Ware CM, Moss WT, et al: Radiation management of bilateral retinoblastoma: the need to preserve vision. *Int J Radiat Oncol Biol Phys.* 1980;6:669.

60. Shidnia H, Hornback NB, Helveston EM, et al: Treatment results of retinoblastoma at Indiana University Hospitals. *Cancer.* 1977;40:2917.

61. Hernandez JC, Brady LW, Shields JA, et al: External beam radiation for retinoblastoma: Results, patterns of failure, and a proposal for treatment guidelines. *Int J Radiat Oncol Biol Phys.* 1996;35:125.

62. Foote RL, Garretson BR, Schomberg PJ, et al: External beam irradiation for retinoblastoma: Patterns of failure and dose-response analysis. *Int J Radiat Oncol Biol Phys.* 1989;16:823.

63. Zelter M, Damel A, Gonzalez G, et al: A prospective study on the treatment of retinoblastoma in 72 patients. *Cancer.* 1991;68:1685.

64. Black L, McCormick B, Abramson DH: External beam radiation therapy and retinoblastoma: Long term results in the comparison of two techniques. *Int J Radiat Oncol Biol Phys.* 1995;35:45.

65. Abramson DH, Ellsworth RM, Kitchin FD, et al: Second nonocular tumors in retinoblastoma survivors. Are they radiation-induced? *Ophthalmology.* 1984;91:1351.

66. Wong FL, Boice JD Jr, Abramson DH, et al: Cancer incidence after retinoblastoma. Radiation dose and sarcoma risk. *JAMA.* 1997;278:1262.

67. Abramson DH, Frank CM: Second nonocular tumors in survivors of bilateral retinoblastoma: A possible age effect on radiation-related risk. *Ophthalmology.* 1998;105:573; discussion 579-580.

68. Moll AC, Imhof SM, Schouten-Van Meeteren AY, et al: Second primary tumors in hereditary retinoblastoma: A register-based study, 1945-1997: Is there an age effect on radiation-related risk? *Ophthalmology.* 2001;108:1109.

69. Li FP, Abramson DH, Tarone RE, et al: Hereditary retinoblastoma, lipoma, and second primary cancers. *J Natl Cancer Inst.* 1997;89:83.

70. Abramson DH: Second nonocular cancers in retinoblastoma: A unified hypothesis. The Franceschetti Lecture. *Ophthalmic Genet.* 1999;20:193.

71. Abramson DH, Melson MR, Dunkel IJ, et al: Third (fourth and fifth) nonocular tumors in survivors of retinoblastoma. *Ophthalmology.* 2001;108:1868.

72. Kleinerman RA, Tarone RE, Abramson DH, et al: Hereditary retinoblastoma and risk of lung cancer. *J Natl Cancer Inst.* 2000;92:2037.

Cancer of the Skin

Richard B. Wilder, MD, and Lawrence W. Margolis, MD

EPIDEMIOLOGY OF BASAL AND SQUAMOUS CELL CARCINOMAS

The most common malignancy in the United States is skin cancer, far exceeding prostate, breast, and lung cancer combined. Although the American Cancer Society estimated that there would be approximately 1,000,000 new basal and squamous cell carcinomas in the United States in 2003,[1] the actual incidence was much higher since cases often are not reported to cancer registries. Sixty-five percent of cutaneous carcinomas are basal cell carcinomas (also known as basal cell epitheliomas), 30% are squamous cell carcinomas, and 5% are adnexal carcinomas, such as sweat and sebaceous gland carcinomas.

Skin cancers typically develop in sun-exposed areas[2] and are more common in men than in women. Because damage from ultraviolet (UV) light is the most common (and preventable) predisposing factor,[3] there is a relatively low incidence of skin cancer in dark-skinned people, who are protected by the large amount of melanin in their skin.[4] On the other hand, there is a relatively high incidence in whites of Irish, Scottish, or English descent who have red or blond hair and blue or green eyes and who burn rather than tan when in the sun.[5] Damage to the skin from UV light is cumulative with time. Consequently, skin cancer usually develops after the age of 40 years.[6]

Trauma and chronic irritation also constitute predisposing factors. For example, cancers have been reported in scars resulting from a vaccination,[7] tattoo,[8] burn (Marjolin's ulcer),[9] or chickenpox[10]; at a colostomy site[11]; or in an area of chronic osteomyelitis[12] or chronic radiation dermatitis.[13] Occupational exposure to arsenic-based insecticides, mineral or shale oils, or coal tar can lead to the development of skin cancer.[14] Oncoviruses have also been suggested as etiologic agents.[15] Genetic disorders such as xeroderma pigmentosum, albinism, phenylketonuria, and basal cell nevus (Gorlin's) syndrome are associated with an increased incidence of skin cancer. Immunosuppressive therapy increases one's risk of developing skin cancer.[16] Similarly, patients with acquired immunodeficiency syndrome (AIDS), leukemia, lymphoma, or multiple myeloma have an increased risk of developing skin cancer.[17,18] The behavior of skin cancers in immunosuppressed patients is often aggressive, suggesting that both cell-mediated and humoral defenses are important.[18] Approximately 2100 people died from nonmelanoma skin cancer in the United States in 1996.[1]

ANATOMY OF THE SKIN

The skin is composed of three layers: the epidermis, the dermis, and the subcutaneous tissue.[19] The epidermis is made up of stratified squamous epithelium that, in most regions, is 0.05 to 0.15 mm thick. Cells in the basal layer of the epidermis regularly undergo mitotic division to replace epidermal cells lost from the surface. A thin basement membrane separates the epidermis from the dermis. The dermis, which is 1 to 2 mm thick, is composed of lymphatics, nerves, blood vessels, and sweat and sebaceous glands in a connective tissue stroma. The portion of the dermis in continuity with the epidermis is called the papillary layer because of its projecting papillae. The denser portion of the dermis, which contains bundles of collagenous and elastic fibers, is called the reticular layer. Subcutaneous tissue lies deep to the dermis and supports the lymphatics, blood vessels, and nerves in loose connective tissue containing variable amounts of fat.

PATHOLOGY AND CLINICAL PRESENTATION

Basal Cell Carcinoma Subtypes

There are several subtypes of basal cell carcinoma and they differ in clinical presentation, histologic appearance, and behavior.[20,21] The *noduloulcerative* ("rodent ulcer") subtype, which accounts for approximately one half of basal cell carcinomas, initially appears as a pink, waxy papule with prominent telangiectasia. As the carcinoma grows, it develops central ulceration and crusting. Histologically, the malignant cells form dermal nests.[22] At the periphery of the nests, the basaloid cells elongate in a parallel array, forming a palisading pattern. The malignant cells exhibit little pleomorphism, and mitoses are infrequent (Fig. 66-1). The differential diagnosis of noduloulcerative basal cell carcinomas includes rosacea, acne, folliculitis, and granulomatous disorders such as sarcoidosis and granuloma annulare. The *superficial* subtype, which accounts for one third of basal cell carcinomas, typically appears as a red, scaly macule located on the trunk. The differential diagnosis includes psoriasis, vascular abnormalities such as spider and cherry hemangiomas, nummular eczema, Bowen's disease, extramammary Paget's disease, and actinic keratosis. *Morphea* (sclerosing) basal cell carcinomas initially are

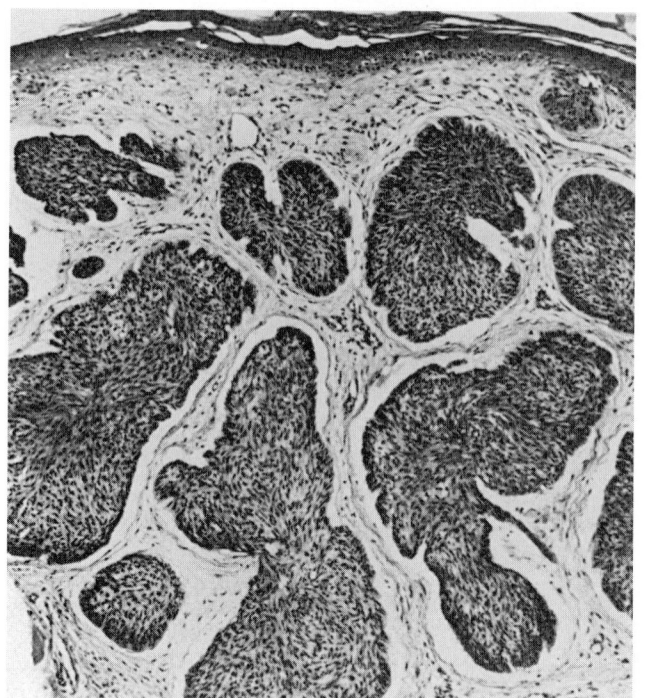

Figure 66–1. Noduloulcerative basal cell carcinoma, exhibiting nests of basaloid cells with parallel, palisading cells at the periphery of these nests and a dense, surrounding stroma. The malignant cells display little pleomorphism and infrequent mitoses. In this particular section, the origin of the tumor at the epidermis can be seen. (From Murphy GF, Kwan TH, Mihm MC Jr: The skin. In Robbins SL, Cotran RS, Kumar V, eds. *Pathologic Basis of Disease*. 3rd ed. Philadelphia: WB Saunders; 1984:1266.)

light-colored macules and later become smooth, shiny lesions. The margins of morphea basal cell carcinomas are difficult to assess clinically. The differential diagnosis includes granulomatous disorders and scleroderma. Similarly, *infiltrative* basal cell carcinomas have a light color and blend in with the surrounding normal skin. The morphea and infiltrative subtypes account for 10% of basal cell carcinomas. The *pigmented* subtype, which accounts for 1% of basal cell carcinomas, varies in color from blue to black and can be difficult to distinguish from melanoma. This subtype occurs more often in individuals with a dark complexion. *Fibroepithelial tumors of Pinkus*, which account for less than 1% of basal cell carcinomas, are flesh-colored papules that occur on the trunk or thighs. *Basosquamous* carcinomas (metatypical carcinomas or keratotic basal cell carcinomas) occur almost exclusively on the face. These are uncommon neoplasms that metastasize with a frequency similar to that of squamous cell carcinomas.

Squamous Cell Carcinoma Subtypes

Bowen's disease is a preinvasive squamous cell carcinoma (i.e., carcinoma in situ) that typically appears as a reddish-brown, sharply demarcated plaque located anywhere on the body. The lesion grows slowly and consequently may be present for years before penetrating the basement membrane that separates the epidermis from the dermis, thereby becoming an invasive squamous cell carcinoma. Bowen's disease is usually treated with surgical

excision, curettage and electrodesiccation, cryotherapy, or topical 5-fluorouracil, although radiation therapy with soft (50 kV) x-rays to a total dose of 40 Gy in 10 fractions over 5 weeks can also provide excellent results.[23] When a preinvasive squamous cell carcinoma involves the penis, it is referred to as erythroplasia of Queyrat. The lesion appears reddened, elevated, or ulcerated and is managed in a manner similar to that of Bowen's disease.

Verrucous carcinoma is a low-grade squamous cell carcinoma that grows slowly as an exophytic lesion. This variant of squamous cell carcinoma typically arises in the anogenital region or oral cavity or on the plantar surface of the foot. Spindle cell carcinoma, which is a rare subtype of squamous cell carcinoma, usually develops in sun-exposed areas in whites older than 40 years of age.[24] The prognosis is primarily dependent on the depth of invasion. Verrucous and spindle cell carcinomas are managed like the more common invasive squamous cell carcinomas. Histologically, squamous cell carcinomas (Fig. 66-2) have a pleomorphic appearance, have numerous and atypical mitoses, and show dyskeratosis and "horn pearl" formation (concentric layers of squamous cells with increasing keratinization centrally).

ROUTES OF SPREAD

During embryologic development from weeks 4 to 8, anatomic regions grow together and the covering epithelium migrates across junctional sites known as *embryologic fusion planes*. It used to be commonly

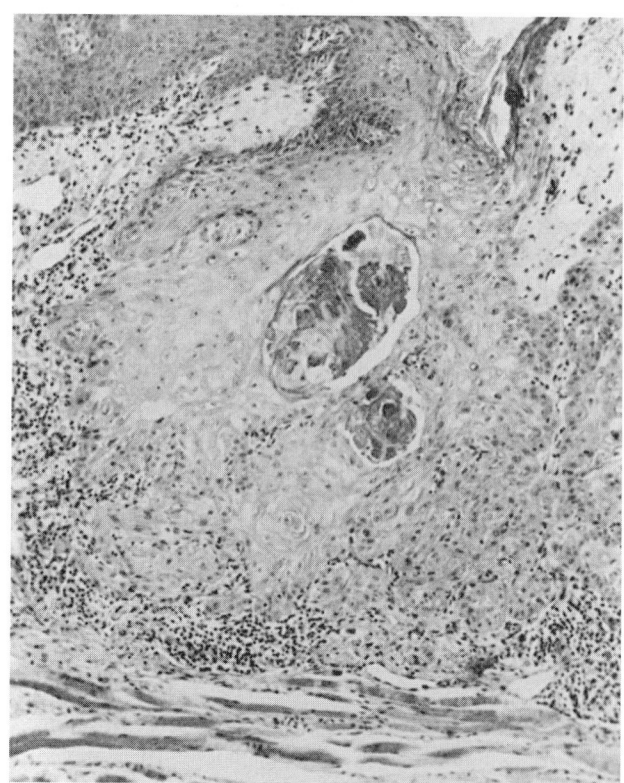

Figure 66–2. Well-differentiated squamous cell carcinoma of the skin invading to the skeletal muscle. The malignant cells are pleomorphic and exhibit many mitoses. (From Murphy GF, Kwan TH, Mihm MC Jr: The skin. In Robbins SL, Cotran RS, Kumar V, eds. *Pathologic Basis of Disease*. 3rd ed. Philadelphia: WB Saunders; 1984:1267.)

accepted that epithelial carcinomas were capable of spreading along embryologic fusion planes (e.g., the nasolabial groove or philtral rims).[25,26] However, controversy has arisen as to whether embryologic fusion planes persist in adults and influence the spread of skin cancers.[27]

The perineural space represents a cleavage plane between a nerve and its sheath, providing a route of spread for skin cancer.[28] Mohs[29] observed perineural invasion in 0.9% of 2488 basal cell carcinomas. Basal cell carcinomas are typically locally advanced or recurrent or both when perineural invasion is present.[30,31] Peripheral branches of the trigeminal and facial nerves are most commonly involved and provide direct access to the central nervous system.[32-34] "Skip areas," where no carcinoma is identified on the pathologic specimen, may exist along the nerve,[33] although inflammation is characteristically present in these regions.[35,36] From 60% to 70% of patients with pathologic evidence of nerve sheath invasion by a basal (or squamous) cell carcinoma are asymptomatic.[33,37-39] Compression of a nerve may develop over a period of years, causing a patient to eventually develop numbness; formication; burning, stinging, or shooting pain; facial weakness; ptosis; or blurred or double vision.[33,34,37,38,40] Intraneural invasion is rare.[28,37,41]

In individuals with normal immunity, the noduloulcerative, morphea, and infiltrative subtypes of basal cell carcinoma are slowly progressive, with a growth rate estimated at 5 mm per year.[42] These carcinomas invade locally by lateral and deep extension along the path of least resistance (e.g., fascial planes, the periosteum, the perichondrium, or nerve sheaths). The superficial, pigmented, and fibroepithelial tumor of Pinkus subtypes of basal cell carcinoma also tend to grow very slowly. However, if left untreated, basal cell carcinomas (or squamous cell carcinomas) can eventually cause significant disfigurement and, in rare cases, death.

Since the epidermis lacks lymphatics and blood vessels, less than 0.1% of basal cell carcinomas metastasize.[43] The rare basal cell carcinoma that does metastasize is typically a large, ulcerative tumor for which repeated treatments over the years have failed. The most common metastatic site for basal cell carcinomas is the regional lymph nodes, although the lungs, liver, or bones may also be involved.[44]

The incidence of regional lymph node metastases in patients with squamous cell carcinoma of the skin varies widely in the literature. In general, well-differentiated squamous cell carcinomas metastasize to lymph nodes in only 1% of cases.[42] However, poorly differentiated or recurrent squamous cell carcinomas; squamous cell carcinomas larger than 3 cm in the greatest dimension or 4 mm in thickness; or squamous cell carcinomas that arise on the lips metastasize to lymph nodes in approximately 10% of cases.[45-49] Squamous cell carcinomas that arise in burn scars or osteomyelitic foci metastasize to lymph nodes in 10% to 30% of cases.[45] When a squamous cell carcinoma metastasizes to regional (e.g., parotid) lymph nodes, surgery and postoperative radiation therapy provide better locoregional control than radiation therapy alone.[50] The 5-year survival rate for patients with lymph node metastases is 25%.[51] Like basal cell carcinomas, typical distant metastatic sites for squamous cell carcinomas are the lungs, liver, and bones.

Perineural invasion by squamous cell carcinomas occurs in 2% to 14% of cases.[29,38] Although perineural lymphatics do not exist,[28,52-54] some authors have reported that perineural invasion is associated with an increased incidence of regional (and distant) metastases.[29,38,55] Others, however, have not observed an increased incidence of regional metastases, even when a carcinoma had extended several centimeters along a nerve sheath.[29,36-38,52]

DIAGNOSTIC STUDIES AND STAGING

A careful history and physical examination, including questions regarding prior treatment along with inspection and palpation of the lesion, and a biopsy, usually constitute an adequate workup. The biopsy can occasionally be useful in elucidating not only the histologic appearance but also the depth of invasion. In the case of carcinomas involving the medial or lateral canthi of the eyes, one should consider obtaining either a computed tomography (CT) or magnetic resonance imaging (MRI) scan (with thin cuts) to assess the depth of invasion, since apparently superficial cancers sometimes extend along the wall of the orbit (Fig. 66-3). If perineural invasion is present, one should consider obtaining either a CT or MRI scan (with thin cuts) to determine if retrograde spread of the carcinoma has occurred; however, in some cases, abnormal radiographic findings, for example, nerve or foramen enlargement, may not develop until late in the course of the disease.[28,35,36] If there is suspicion that a locally advanced carcinoma has invaded underlying bone or metastasized to the regional lymph nodes, lungs, or liver, a CT scan should be obtained. Carcinomas of the skin should be staged according to the American Joint Committee on Cancer (AJCC) guidelines[56] presented in Table 66-1.

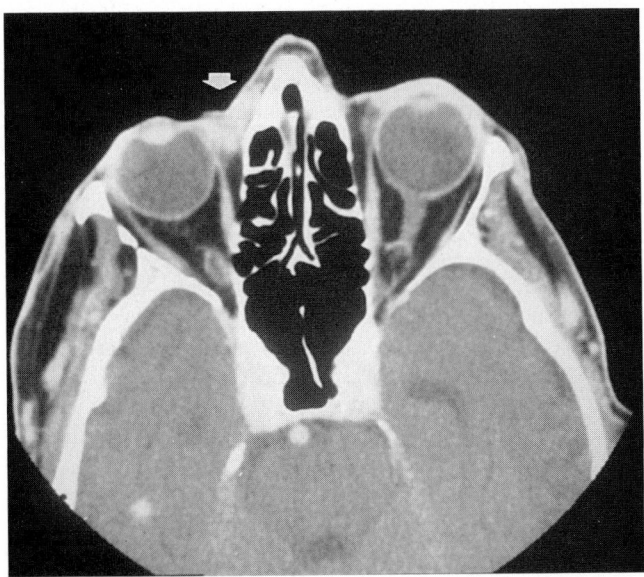

Figure 66–3. Computed tomographic scan demonstrating that a noduloulcerative basal cell carcinoma that by palpation appeared to involve the medial canthus of the right eye only superficially (arrow) actually extended to a depth of 1.5 cm along the wall of the orbit.

Table 66–1 Classification of Carcinoma of the Skin (Excluding Eyelid, Vulva, and Penis)

Primary Tumor (T)

TX	Primary tumor cannot be assessed
T0	No evidence of primary tumor
Tis	Carcinoma *in situ*
T1	Tumor 2 cm or less in greatest dimension
T2	Tumor more than 2 cm, but not more than 5 cm, in greatest dimension
T3	Tumor more than 5 cm in greatest dimension
T4	Tumor invades deep extradermal structures (i.e., cartilage, skeletal muscle, or bone)

Note: In case of multiple simultaneous tumors, the tumor with the highest T category will be classified and the number of separate tumors will be indicated in parentheses, e.g., T2 (5).

Regional Lymph Nodes (N)

NX	Regional lymph nodes cannot be assessed
N0	No regional lymph node metastasis
N1	Regional lymph node metastasis

Distant Metastasis (M)

MX	Distant metastasis cannot be assessed
M0	No distant metastasis
M1	Distant metastasis

Stage Grouping

Stage 0	Tis	N0	M0
Stage I	T1	N0	M0
Stage II	T2	N0	M0
	T3	N0	M0
Stage III	T4	N0	M0
	Any T	N1	M0
Stage IV	Any T	Any N	M1

From Greene FL, Page DL, Fleming ID, et al, eds: *AJCC Cancer Staging Manual*, 6/E. New York: Springer, 2002.

TREATMENT OPTIONS

Since most skin cancers can be treated with several different therapeutic approaches, it is important to select which treatment is most appropriate. A number of criteria are useful in making this decision. The cancer should be evaluated regarding its histologic appearance, size, location, and thickness; whether it is primary or recurrent; and whether single or multiple cancers are present.[57] The age and general health of the patient; cure and complication rates; cosmetic and functional results; convenience; and cost of the different therapeutic approaches should also be taken into consideration.[58]

There are six forms of treatment for basal and squamous cell carcinomas: cryotherapy; curettage and electrodesiccation; chemotherapy; surgical excision; Mohs' micrographic surgery (also known as chemosurgery); and radiation therapy.

Cryotherapy involves the application of liquid nitrogen to the skin to freeze the carcinoma along with a margin of normal tissue. The ice block is allowed to thaw, and the process is repeated one or two times to increase the likelihood of tumor necrosis. Normally, a thermocouple is inserted just beneath the carcinoma to ensure that a minimum temperature of −30°C is achieved. Cryotherapy is convenient and relatively inexpensive. Although well-suited to the treatment of small, superficial basal cell carcinomas and well-differentiated squamous cell carcinomas with clinically distinct margins, cryotherapy may result in a less than optimal cosmetic result with larger carcinomas where the resulting hypopigmentation is particularly noticeable.[59]

Curettage and electrodesiccation is commonly used for previously untreated superficial skin cancers. With a curet, the soft cancer-containing tissues are scraped away, leaving behind the firmer normal tissue. After each curettage, the wound is electrodesiccated to obtain hemostasis. Like cryotherapy, curettage and electrodesiccation is an effective method of managing small basal cell carcinomas and well-differentiated squamous cell carcinomas with clinically distinct margins; however, this approach is not recommended for recurrent morphea or infiltrative basal cell carcinomas or carcinomas involving scar tissue, cartilage, or bone.[57,59,60]

Although topical 5-fluorouracil chemotherapy can cure tumors confined to the epidermis, it is not recommended for invasive carcinomas since the carcinomas appear to heal on the surface but may continue to grow into the dermis and subcutaneous tissue.[61] Thus far, there have been few reports regarding the use of systemic chemotherapy for basal and squamous cell carcinomas. Overall, the results achieved with other therapeutic approaches have been excellent, so systemic chemotherapy has been unnecessary in most patients. However, advanced skin cancers do respond to 5-fluorouracil, cisplatin, bleomycin, doxorubicin, isotretinoin, or a combination of agents. For patients treated with chemotherapy alone, response rates have characteristically ranged from 70% to 80%, with a complete response rate of 30%.[62-64] These results are not surprising considering the high response rates that have been achieved when squamous cell carcinomas of the head and neck have been treated with two to three cycles of chemotherapy before radiation therapy.[65] Approximately half the responses have lasted longer than 1 year.[62] Hence, in the case of a locally advanced or metastatic carcinoma of the skin, one should consider administering cisplatin concurrently with radiation therapy[66] followed by cisplatin and 5-fluorouracil if the patient has a good performance status.

Advances in reconstructive techniques have helped to make surgical excision a more attractive therapeutic approach. Surgical excision allows pathologic assessment of the extent of a carcinoma but may be difficult in older patients with either a large solitary carcinoma or multiple small carcinomas in the same region.

With Mohs' micrographic surgery, horizontal layers of tissue are serially excised and systematically mapped. The peripheral and deep margins are then thoroughly examined. If carcinoma is detected at the margin, another horizontal layer of tissue is excised from the area and examined microscopically. The process is repeated until no cancer is detected at the margin. With Mohs' micrographic surgery, maximal sparing of normal tissue is accomplished. Frederic Mohs, the originator of this method, initially proposed that zinc chloride paste be applied to the skin as a fixative to facilitate the excision and sectioning of tissue (*fixed tissue technique*). Later, the fixative was omitted (*fresh tissue technique*) in order to do away with the pain associated with tissue fixation, to allow multiple stages of surgery to be performed in one day, and to leave a defect that could be repaired immediately if desired.[67] Mohs' micrographic surgery can be painful, even when the fresh tissue technique is used, and leaves a tissue defect that may require surgical repair; however, it represents an effective therapeutical approach for recurrent morphea or infiltrative basal cell carcinomas; basosquamous carcinomas; and carcinomas larger than 2 cm.[67] Basal and squamous cell carcinomas with perineural invasion should be treated with Mohs' micrographic surgery and postoperative radiation therapy.[35,36]

Like Mohs' micrographic surgery, radiation therapy constitutes an effective form of treatment for recurrent[68,69] carcinomas as well as large carcinomas involving the ears, forehead, or scalp.[70,71] Radiation therapy is generally recommended for carcinomas located in the central face and is particularly well suited to the treatment of cancers (≥0.5 cm) involving the eyelids; tip or ala of the nose; or commissure of the lips since these sites can be difficult to reconstruct surgically. Advantages of radiation therapy are that the treatment is relatively painless and, for the sites outlined earlier, less expensive than Mohs' micrographic surgery followed by reconstructive surgery.[68] Although morphea basal cell carcinomas normally are not managed with radiation therapy because the margins are difficult to assess clinically,[21,57] they are radioresponsive. When wide margins have been provided (see the section on field size), local control has been achieved with radiation therapy in patients who refused Mohs' micrographic surgery.[72,73]

In general, radiation therapy is not recommended for the treatment of skin cancer in patients younger than age 50 because the cosmetic results gradually worsen (telangiectasis, atrophy, and pallor) with time and the risk of a second cancer's developing in field increases with time.[21,74] In addition, skin cancers that recur postirradiation should not be retreated with radiation therapy because of the suboptimal salvage rate, poor long-term cosmetic results, and risk of complications in this select group of patients.

Skin cancers that recur after radiation therapy are best managed with Mohs' micrographic surgery.[75]

SIGNIFICANCE OF A POSITIVE MARGIN AFTER EXCISION

Studies with a minimum follow-up period of 5 years indicate that only approximately one third of basal cell carcinomas that extend to the margin of resection ultimately recur.[76-79] Consequently, the management of a positive margin is controversial. Since it may be difficult to detect early recurrences in cases where a basal cell carcinoma extends to the deep margin and is recurrent, and the area is fibrotic from prior treatment; where grafts have been used to close a surgical defect; or where close follow-up will not be possible, immediate retreatment with surgical excision, Mohs' micrographic surgery, or radiation therapy should be considered.[79-81] In cases involving a graft, radiation therapy should not be initiated until a good "take" has occurred, which usually requires 3 to 4 weeks. In addition, a treatment schedule that employs a relatively large number of fractions, such as in Table 66-2, should be used.[19] The entire graft should be included in the target volume (see the section on field size). In a study by Wilder and colleagues,[72] all 21 basal cell carcinomas that extended to the surgical margin were controlled with radiation therapy. Immediate retreatment should be considered when a squamous cell carcinoma extends to the surgical margin since this type of cancer is more likely to recur locoregionally than basal cell carcinoma, and less than half of the patients who develop lymph node metastases are salvaged.[80,81]

EXTERNAL BEAM RADIATION THERAPY TECHNIQUE

Energy and Filtration

Based on articles involving superficial (50 to 150 kV) and orthovoltage (160 to 300 kV) x-rays[82] that were published in the 1950s and 1960s,[83-85] a number of authors

Table 66–2   Dose Recommendations for Skin Cancer

Superficial or Orthovoltage X-rays					
Size of Skin Cancer, cm (Greatest Dimension)	Daily Dose, cGy* (5/wk)	Energy, kV	Filtration (Half-Value Layer)	Fractions, n	Total Dose cGy*
0.5–2.0	300	50–150	0.7 mm Al–0.52 mm Cu	15–17	4500–5100
>2.0 without bone involvement	250	180–300	0.87–3.7 mm Cu	20–22	5000–5500

Megavoltage Electrons or Photons or Both				
Size of Skin Cancer, cm (Greatest Dimension)	Energy (0.5–1.0 Bolus)	Daily Dose cGy* (5/wk)	Fractions, n	Total Dose, cGy*
0.5–2.0	6–9 MeV Electrons	330	15–17	4950–5610
>2.0 without bone involvement	9–16 MeV Electrons	275	20–22	5500–6050
>2.0 with bone involvement	4–6 MV photons or 9–20 MeV electrons or both	200	34–36	6800–7200

*Prescribed to the 100% isodose line, including buildup bolus in the case of electrons.

Table 66–3   Central Axis Percentage Depth-Doses as a Function of Energy, Buildup Bolus Thickness, Filtration, Field Size, and Source-to-Skin Distance

	Percentage Depth-Dose				
Centimeters	50 kV* (0.7 mm Al)§	100 kV† (0.19 mm Cu)§	150 kV† (0.52 mm Cu)§	6 MeV Electrons‡ (0.5 cm Bolus)	9 MeV Electrons‡ (1.0 cm Bolus)
0.0 (surface)	100	100	100	93	96
0.1	92	99	99	94	97
0.2	85	98	99	96	98
0.5	65	95	96	100	100
1.0	45	89	90	94	99
1.5	36	79	83	65	90
2.0	23	70	76	25	71

*2 cm² field, 10 cm source-to-skin distance.
†4 × 6 cm field, 40 cm source-to-skin distance.
‡10 × 10 cm field, 100 cm source-to-skin distance.
§Half-value layer.

have suggested that radiation therapy is contraindicated for carcinomas involving bone or cartilage because of the excessive risk of osteoradionecrosis and radiochondritis. However, more recent literature indicates that properly fractionated radiation therapy can be used in these cases and, in fact, is often the treatment of choice with or without surgery since the risk of radiation-induced complications is low when careful attention is paid to technical factors.[71,86]

Most carcinomas of the skin can be cured with superficial or orthovoltage x-rays or megavoltage electrons. Advantages of superficial or orthovoltage x-rays are that they require less of a margin on the skin surface around a carcinoma and are less expensive than electrons. In addition, when carcinomas of the eyelid are treated with orthovoltage x-rays rather than 6 MeV electrons, the cornea receives a lower dose of radiation.[87]

Because irradiation of deep subcutaneous tissue increases the likelihood of conspicuous scarring, energy selection is important. The most commonly used peak superficial and orthovoltage x-ray energies are 50, 100, 150, 200, 250, and 300 kV. With superficial and orthovoltage x-rays (and megavoltage electrons), an energy should be selected such that the 90% depth-dose encompasses the target volume (Table 66–3). Since most basal cell carcinomas extend to a depth of 2 to 5 mm,[88] 50 kV x-rays have been recommended in the dermatology literature. As presented in Table 66–4, a typical 50 kV beam delivers 85% of the surface dose at a depth of 2 mm and only 65% of the surface dose at a depth of 5 mm. Consequently, soft x-ray (50 kV) beams should be used only with very superficial lesions such as small eyelid tumors.[89]

The *f* factor, or roentgen-to-rad conversion factor, relates exposure in air to the absorbed dose of radiation in tissue.[82] The *f* factor depends on both radiation energy and tissue composition. For a tissue with an atomic number much greater than that of air, the *f* factor changes significantly as the radiation energy decreases below 300 kV (e.g., for compact bone, *f* factors equal 0.94 at 4 MV and 300 kV compared with 1.45 at 100 kV, whereas for skin, *f* factors equal 0.96 at 4 MV and 300 kV compared with 0.94 at 100 kV[90]). At energies below 300 kV, the

dose of radiation in a tissue with a high atomic number (e.g., compact bone) is greater than the dose in a tissue with a low atomic number (e.g., skin). As a result, if a carcinoma invades bone, megavoltage electrons or photons or both provide a more homogeneous dose of radiation in the target volume than superficial or orthovoltage x-rays.

Filtration "hardens" a superficial or orthovoltage x-ray beam, meaning it removes low-energy x-rays,[82] thereby reducing the dose in bone. The degree of hardening or beam quality can be expressed in terms of the half-value layer (HVL), or the thickness of a material that, when introduced into the path of an x-ray beam, reduces the exposure rate by one half. With older superficial and orthovoltage x-ray machines, one can select from among several filters after deciding on an energy. In general, one should select the thickest filter that will provide a dose rate greater than 50 cGy/min. Aluminum is commonly used to filter 50 to 100 kV x-rays, and copper with or without tin, both of which have a higher atomic number, is used to filter higher energies (1 mm of copper is approximately equal to 16 mm of aluminum).[91] Typical HVLs for 50, 100, and 150 kV x-rays are presented in Table 66–3. HVLs (and percentage depth-doses) for 75, 180, 200, 250, and 300 kV x-rays are presented in articles by Scrimger and Connors,[92] Niroomand-Rad and colleagues,[93] and McCullough.[91] More recently, manufacturers have

Table 66–4   Five-Year Local Control Rates for Previously Treated Basal Cell Carcinoma

Treatment Modality	5-Year Local Control, % (Controlled/Treated, n/n)
Mohs' micrographic surgery	94 (2841/3009)
Radiation therapy	87 (204/234)
Cryotherapy	—*
Surgical excision	83 (431/522)
Curettage and electrodesiccation	60 (69/115)

*The 5-year results have not been published for cryotherapy. The weighted mean of the local control rates for studies with fewer than 5 years of follow-up is 87% (227/261).
Data from Rowe DE, Carroll RJ, Day CL Jr: Mohs' surgery is the treatment of choice for recurrent (previously treated) basal cell carcinomas. *J Dermatol Surg Oncol.* 1989;15:424.

provided only one filter for each x-ray energy to ensure that proper filtration is used.

With megavoltage electrons, there is a rapid falloff of the dose with depth (see the percentage depth-doses for 6 MeV electrons in Table 66-3), allowing one to spare underlying tissue. When a skin cancer has invaded bone, megavoltage photons can provide a relatively homogeneous dose in the target volume. Consequently, with carcinomas that extensively invade soft tissue or bone or both, megavoltage electrons or photons or both are preferable to orthovoltage x-rays. Based on the skin-sparing property of megavoltage electrons and photons, 0.5 to 1.0 cm buildup bolus should be used.[82]

There is little variation in the dose of radiation delivered to cartilage by superficial or orthovoltage x-rays or megavoltage electrons or photons or both (for cartilage, the f factor equals 0.92 at both 4 MV and 100 kV).[94] Chondritis is rare after the administration of daily doses of radiation of 3 Gy or less and suggests tumor recurrence.[71,86,95,96]

To minimize normal-tissue toxicity, underlying structures such as the lens, cornea, nasal septum, and teeth should be protected by placing a lead shield under the eyelids (Fig. 66-4), over or in the nasal cavity (Fig. 66-5), or under the lips (Fig. 66-6). When an eyelid cancer is treated, a thin dental acrylic or wax coating should be applied to the superficial surface of the lead shield.[82] When skin cancers at other sites are treated, a thicker coating (e.g., 2 mm of aluminum) should be applied to the superficial surface of the lead shield.[82] The dental acrylic, Teflon, wax, or aluminum coating absorbs backscattered photons or electrons, thereby reducing the conjunctival or mucosal reaction.

Time, Dose, Fractionation

Time-dose relationships in skin cancer have been studied extensively. In his classic paper, Strandqvist[97] examined skin reactions for various fractionation schemes. His work was further expanded by von Essen,[98] who applied isoeffect lines for 99% probability of cure versus 3%

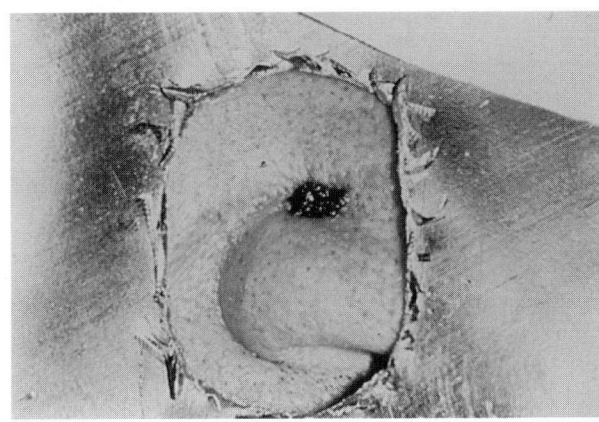

Figure 66–5. A 57-year-old woman with an ulcerative basal cell carcinoma involving the right ala of the nose. She is set up for superficial x-ray radiation therapy with a lead cutout that protects the nasal cavity but does not shield the nasolabial fold.

probability of skin necrosis and related these findings to the dose per fraction and total dose. He also demonstrated that larger volumes of tissue do not tolerate radiation as well and therefore require smaller daily doses. Total superficial and orthovoltage x-ray doses that resulted in an uncomplicated cure of basal and squamous cell carcinomas are presented in Figure 66-7. Ellis,[99] with the introduction of the nominal standard dose system, emphasized the importance of separating out overall time from the number of fractions. The nominal standard dose system allows one to select time-dose relationships that will produce similar acute skin reactions, provided that

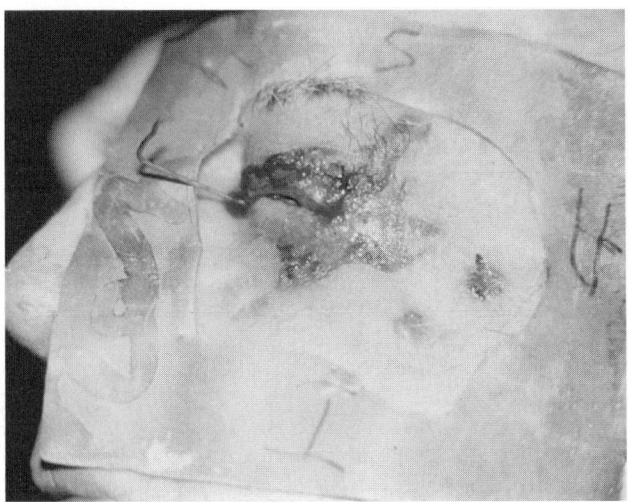

Figure 66–4. An 81-year-old man with a 4 × 6 cm periorbital basal cell carcinoma set up for radiation therapy with a lead cutout and internal eye shield.

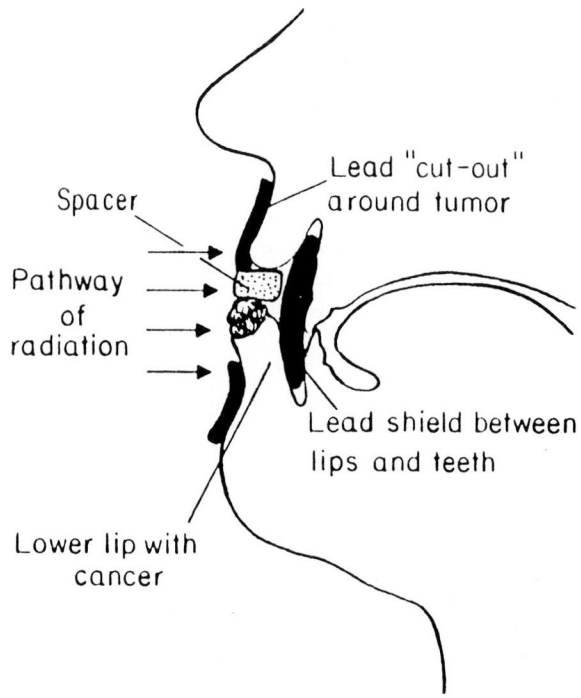

Figure 66–6. Diagram illustrating the proper setup for treating a carcinoma of the lower lip with superficial or orthovoltage x-ray therapy. A lead cutout should be placed around the tumor and a lead shield coated with wax or aluminum (see the section on energy and filtration) should be inserted between the lips and teeth. (From Buschke F, Parker RG: *Radiation Therapy in Cancer Management.* New York: Grune & Stratton; 1972:71.)

Labels in Figure 66-6: Spacer; Pathway of radiation; Lead "cut-out" around tumor; Lead shield between lips and teeth; Lower lip with cancer

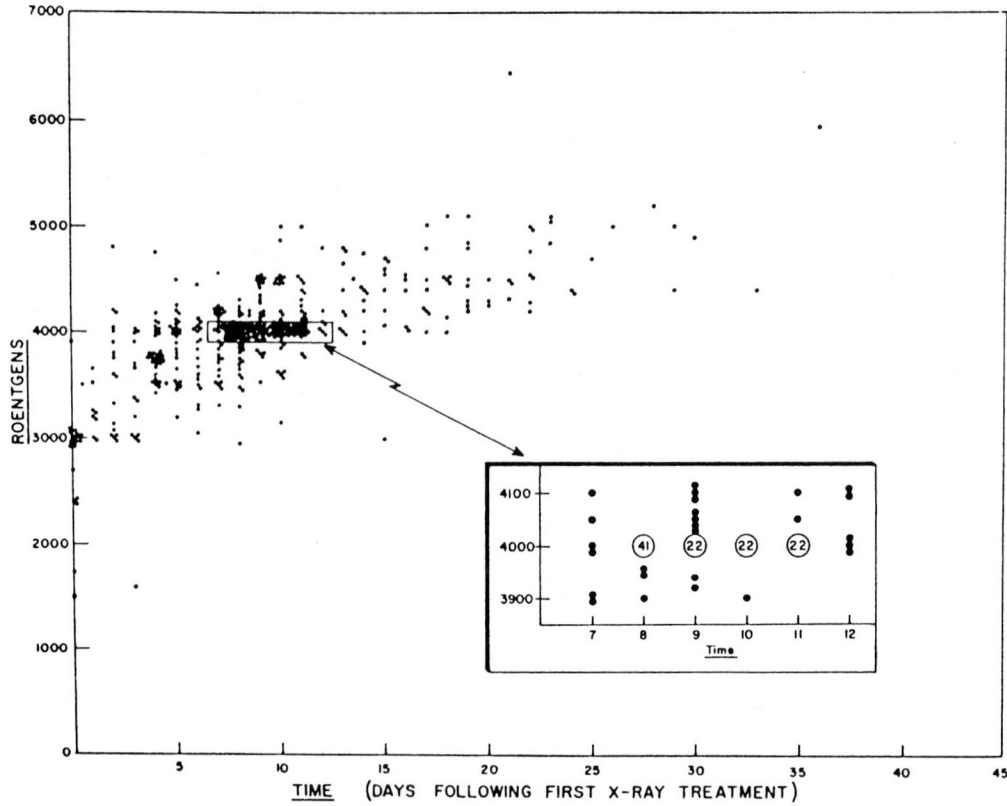

Figure 66–7. Uncomplicated cures in patients with basal and squamous cell carcinomas after the administration of superficial or orthovoltage x-rays. For skin treated with 120 to 140 kV x-rays (88% of the patients were treated with these energies), the roentgen-to-rad conversion factor equals 0.95. (From von Essen CF: Roentgen therapy of skin and lip carcinoma: Factors influencing success and failure. *Am J Roentgenol.* 1960;83:556.)

the range of time and difference in the number of fractions are not too great.[100]

Many studies have demonstrated that the late effects of radiation therapy on the skin (e.g., telangiectasia, atrophy, and hypopigmentation) can be minimized with the use of a more fractionated course of treatment. Turesson and Notter[101,102] examined late radiation changes of the skin in women with breast cancer treated to the internal mammary nodes. He observed less severe telangiectasia in patients who received five as opposed to one or two fractions each week. Traenkle and Mulay[103] studied the incidence of necrosis in 1751 patients with basal and squamous cell carcinomas treated with five different 100 kV (1.5 mm aluminum HVL) dose schedules. Patients treated with four or five 10 Gy fractions had a markedly higher incidence of necrosis (14% at 4½ years) than those who received nine 5 Gy fractions, thirteen 4 Gy fractions, or eighteen 3 Gy fractions (3% at 4½ years). Petrovich and colleagues[104] reported excellent cosmetic and functional results after the treatment of carcinomas of the skin with daily doses of 3 Gy or less (most of the 896 patients were managed with superficial x-rays). Since radiation therapy is typically recommended for carcinomas involving the pinna of the ear; eyelid; tip or ala of the nose; or lips based on its ability to provide excellent cosmetic and functional results, it seems prudent to select a time-dose relationship that will give not only the highest chance for tumor control but also the best cosmetic and functional outcome. To do otherwise may negate the

advantage of radiation therapy over surgery. Based on this premise, the time-dose relationships in Table 66-2 have been formulated. Doses in this table are prescribed to the 100% isodose line, including buildup bolus in the case of electrons.

The relative biological effectiveness (RBE) of superficial or orthovoltage x-rays is 10% to 15% higher than the RBE of megavoltage electrons or photons.[105,106] One way to account for this difference is to administer daily and total megavoltage doses that are 10% to 15% higher than the corresponding superficial or orthovoltage x-ray doses (see Table 66-2).

Field Size

Radiation has the advantage of being able to treat clinically detectable and subclinical disease as well as a margin of normal tissue without the creation of a tissue defect. With careful attention to technique, radiation therapy can produce high cure rates (see the section on results) and excellent cosmetic and functional results (Figs. 66-8 and 66-9).

When field sizes for superficial and orthovoltage x-rays and megavoltage electrons are discussed, it is important to distinguish the *target volume* from the *treatment volume*. The target volume consists of the palpable carcinoma and any adjacent tissue that may be infiltrated by carcinoma, taking prior treatment and histologic

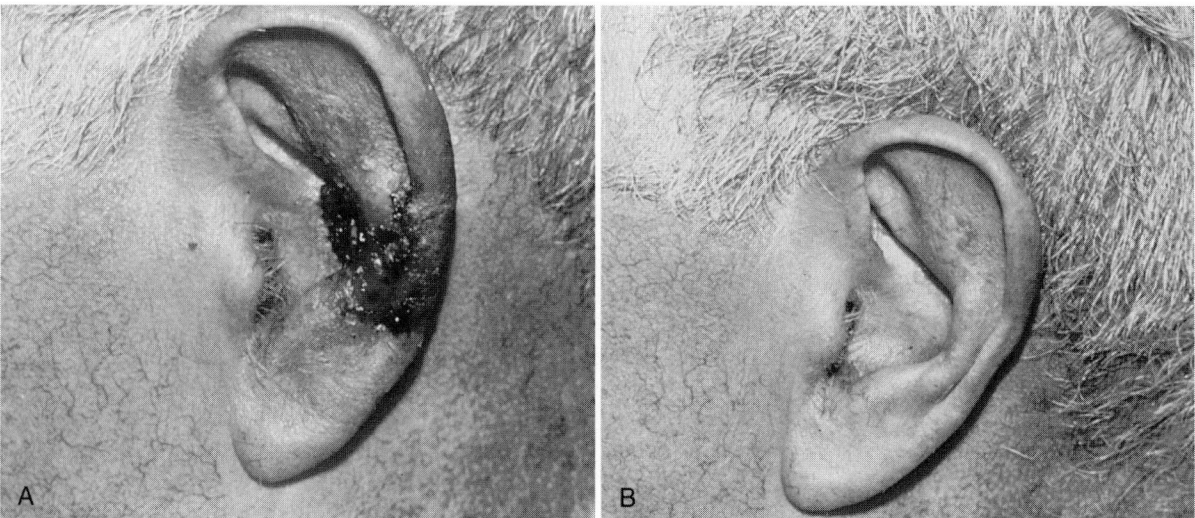

Figure 66–8. A 75-year-old man with a 2.5 cm squamous cell carcinoma of the left ear before (**A**) and 3 years after (**B**) superficial x-ray therapy to 55 Gy in 22 fractions over 32 days.

subtype into account. The treatment volume consists of an additional margin around the target volume that must be provided to allow for physical limitations of the technique.[82]

The margin of normal-feeling tissue included in the target volume is usually 0.5 to 1.0 cm for skin cancers of 2.0 cm or less and 1.5 to 2.0 cm for larger cancers. At least a 0.5 cm margin on the suspected depth of invasion should be included in the target volume. Since recurrent and morphea basal cell carcinomas tend to infiltrate more widely, the margins should be approximately 0.5 cm more generous to avoid a recurrence at the margin of the field.[107,108] As the field size decreases, the flatness of a superficial or orthovoltage x-ray beam decreases slightly.[93] With megavoltage electrons, there is lateral constriction of the isodose curves in the deep portion of the target volume (Fig. 66-10). As the field

size decreases, the lateral constriction of the isodose curves becomes more pronounced.[82] Consequently, if electrons are used rather than superficial or orthovoltage x-rays, a 0.5 cm wider margin should be provided at the skin surface, (i.e., the treatment volume should be larger). In one study of basal and squamous cell carcinomas, the local control rates achieved with electrons were less than the local control rates achieved with superficial x-rays.[109] In this study, the use of buildup bolus with electrons varied over time, and it is not stated whether the lateral constriction of electron isodose curves in the deep portion of the target volume and the decreased RBE of electrons relative to superficial x-rays were accounted for. The authors conclude that the poorer results obtained with electrons may have been "due to technical factors such as the use of bolus and the collimation of field sizes."[109] In most studies, equivalent results have

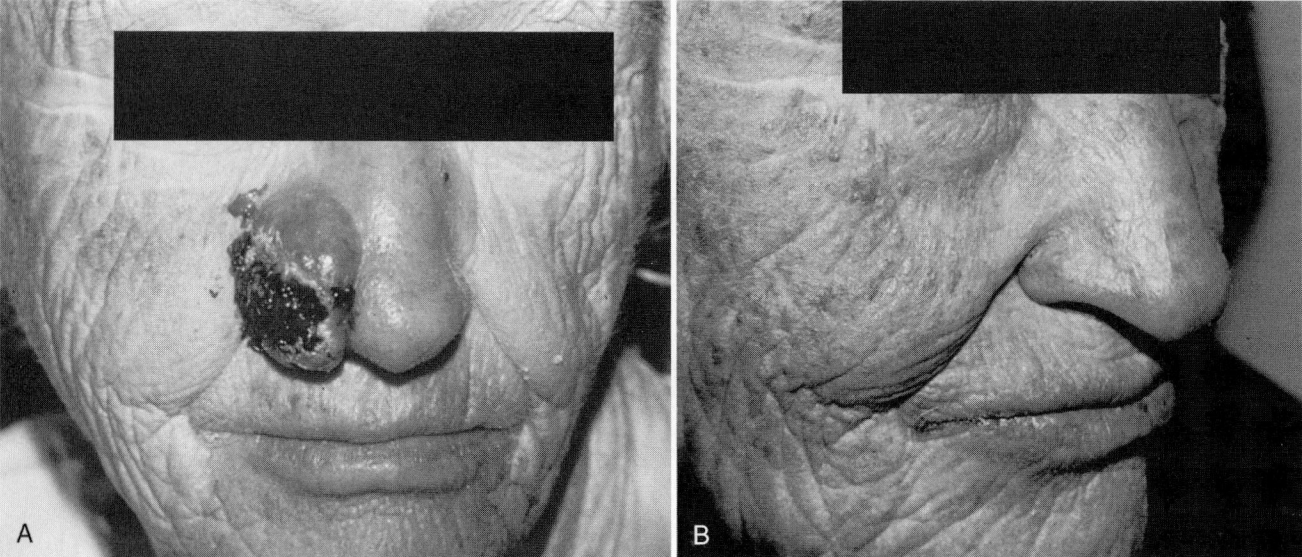

Figure 66–9. A 72-year-old woman with a 3.5 cm fixed basal cell carcinoma involving the ala of the nose before (**A**) and 5 years after (**B**) radiation therapy to 69.75 Gy in 31 fractions over 43 days using 12 MeV electrons and 1 cm buildup bolus.

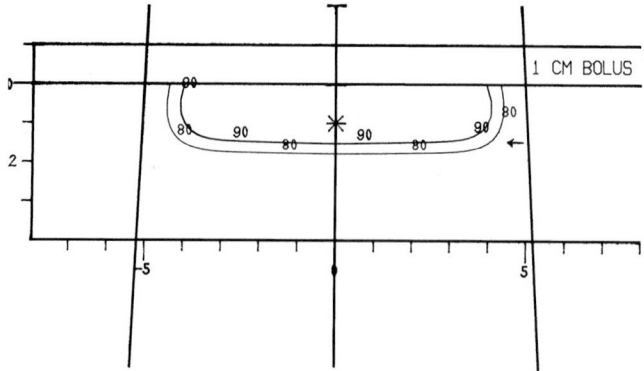

Figure 66–10. Lateral constriction of 90% and 80% isodose curves with depth *(arrow)* for 9 MeV electrons, 1 cm buildup bolus, a 10 × 10 cm field, and a 100 cm source-to-skin distance.

been achieved with either superficial x-rays or megavoltage electrons.[68,110,111]

Well-differentiated squamous cell carcinomas are generally treated in the same manner as basal cell carcinomas. However, in the case of high-risk squamous cell carcinomas (see the section on routes of spread), consideration should be given to the use of a 2.0 cm margin around the primary tumor[112] and the inclusion of regional lymph nodes (e.g., cervical or parotid nodes) in the target volume.

When perineural invasion is present, skin cancers typically extend 1 to 2 cm along the nerve sheath[113] but may occasionally extend up to 14 cm.[37] Consequently, the involved nerve retrograde toward the skull base foramen should be included in the target volume when perineural invasion is noted.[35,36,52,55]

BRACHYTHERAPY

There has been a decline in the treatment of skin cancer with interstitial brachytherapy and radioactive molds over the past few decades. Several reasons account for this, including the widespread availability of megavoltage electrons and the ability to deliver megavoltage electrons on an outpatient basis.[114]

Although skin cancers today are typically treated with external beam radiation therapy, interstitial brachytherapy is a treatment option for carcinomas smaller than 4 cm (larger carcinomas are technically difficult to implant).[115,116] In general, local anesthesia and systemic sedation are adequate for a skin cancer implant,[96,115] although some clinicians prefer to administer a regional nerve block.[116] Carcinomas that are 0.75 cm thick or less can be treated with a single-plane implant.[115] To improve the dose homogeneity, templates with predrilled, evenly spaced holes can be used to guide needle insertion. Steel hypodermic needles (e.g., 19.5-gauge [0.05 cm inner diameter]) or plastic tubes (e.g., 18-gauge angiocaths) can be used.[96,114-116] The optimal spacing between needles is typically 1.0 to 1.5 cm.[115,116] Two to five hypodermic needles or plastic tubes are usually required, depending on the size of the carcinoma. Stabilizing bars are commonly applied to the ends of needles to maintain parallelism

during treatment. Plain radiographs (orthogonal views) are taken so that computerized treatment planning can be performed. In the patient's shielded hospital room, iridium-192 is afterloaded and buttons are applied to secure the iridium-192 in place. When patients are treated with interstitial brachytherapy alone, the minimal tumor dose should be between 55 and 70 Gy (filtration by steel needles reduces the dose by less than 1%, and no correction is required).[115-117] Continuous low-dose-rate (LDR) irradiation is delivered over 5 to 8 days, depending on the activity of the iridium-192.

Skin cancers of 0.4 cm in thickness or less in regions that tolerate radiation poorly, such as the dorsum of the hand or the shin, may be treated with radioactive surface molds since the radiation dose falls off rapidly outside the target volume. Radium-226, radon-222, gold-198, and iridium-192 have typically been used in surface molds. Based on radiation safety concerns, gold-198 and iridium-192 have been used more often in recent years. Afterloading techniques for iridium-192 molds have been described in detail.[118,119] In summary, a treatment plan is constructed wherein iridium-192 seeds are positioned in a tissue-equivalent (e.g., wax) mold 1 cm from the surface of the skin to improve dose homogeneity. In the patient's shielded hospital room, 17-gauge hypodermic needles are passed through the mold. An iridium-192 ribbon is threaded into each hollow needle, the needles are removed, leaving the ribbons in place, and the mold is secured to the carcinoma with Micropore tape or a Velcro strap. For small, superficial carcinomas, Ashby and colleagues[120] recommend a minimal target dose of 40 Gy over 4 days, corresponding to a surface dose of 47 to 62 Gy.[120] High dose rate (HDR) delivered in multiple-daily or twice-daily fractions may be considered for replacement of LDR.

RESULTS

Rowe and colleagues[121] reviewed the literature on previously untreated basal cell carcinomas and reported 5-year local control rates of 90% (2342/2606) for surgical excision, 91% (4285/4695) for radiation therapy, 92% (3299/3573) for curettage and electrodesiccation, 93% (249/269) for cryotherapy, and 99% (7597/7670) for Mohs' micrographic surgery. Rowe and colleagues[69] also extensively reviewed the literature on recurrent basal cell carcinomas. Their findings, which have been updated with regard to radiation therapy,[68] are presented in Table 66-4. The 5-year local control rate for recurrent basal cell carcinomas managed with radiation therapy is 87% (204/234), which compares favorably with the results obtained with cryotherapy (<87%), surgical excision (83%; 431/522), and curettage and electrodesiccation (60%; 69/115).

Fitzpatrick and colleagues[122] reviewed 1166 eyelid carcinomas treated with radiation therapy. The 5-year local control rates were 95% for basal cell carcinomas and 93% for squamous cell carcinomas. The overall complication rate was 10%; however, most of the "complications" apparently represented normal tissue damage by the carcinomas before treatment, and less than half the cases were considered serious. In general, patients judged the cosmetic results to be excellent.

Petrovich and colleagues[123] reviewed 646 patients with carcinomas of the eyelids, ear, and nose. The 5-year actuarial local control rates achieved with radiation therapy were 93% for 464 basal cell carcinomas, 90% for 67 basosquamous cell carcinomas, and 83% for 115 squamous cell carcinomas. Including salvage treatment, the local control rates were 99% for basal cell carcinomas, 95% for basosquamous carcinomas, and 94% for squamous cell carcinomas. The 5-year local control rates obtained with radiation therapy were 93% for carcinomas less than 2 cm in the greatest dimension, 63% for carcinomas 2 to 5 cm in the greatest dimension, and 50% for advanced carcinomas. Bone or cartilage involvement was present in 23 patients, in whom the 3-year actuarial control rate was 83% with radiation therapy alone. No bone, cartilage, or soft tissue necrosis developed, and no serious complications were observed.

Petrovich and colleagues[104] reviewed an additional 3 basal and 247 squamous cell carcinomas of the lip treated over a 22-year period and reported an overall crude local control rate of 89%. The local control rates were 94% for AJCC stages I and II (221 patients), 90% for stage III (10 patients), and 47% for stage IV (19 patients). In 227 patients without nodal involvement, the local control rate was 93%. Nodal involvement was present in 23 patients; in these individuals, the control rate was 52%. The cosmetic and functional results were considered excellent in patients with smaller carcinomas and those who received daily superficial x-ray doses of 3 Gy or less. Five (2%) patients developed necrosis of the mandible; all of them had massive tumor involvement of the mandible before radiation therapy.

Locke and colleagues[109] analyzed 531 basal and squamous cell carcinomas treated with radiation therapy. For previously untreated cancers less than 2 cm, the local control rates were 96% (190/197) for basal cell carcinomas and 95% (39/41) for squamous cell carcinomas. For previously untreated cancers measuring 2 to 5 cm, the local control rates were 90% (36/40) and 86% (18/21), respectively, for basal and squamous cell carcinomas. For previously untreated cancers greater than 5 cm, 94% (15/16) of the basal cell carcinomas were controlled compared with 86% (6/7) of the squamous cell carcinomas. Recurrent cancers in all categories had slightly lower control rates. The cosmetic results were evaluated in 435 patients and judged to be good to excellent in 92%. As with the local control rates, the quality of the cosmetic results depended on the size of the carcinoma, with 99% of tumors less than 1 cm and 92% of tumors 1 to 3 cm, showing excellent or good cosmesis. Overall, 5% of the patients developed soft tissue necrosis. The authors point out that with attention to additional technical details as prescription depth, bolus, and margins, patients treated with electrons did not have higher local failure rates as compared to patients treated with superficial radiation therapy.

These studies indicate that previously untreated basal and squamous cell carcinomas are controlled more easily than recurrent lesions. The local control rates for basal cell carcinomas are slightly higher than those for basosquamous carcinomas or squamous cell carcinomas.

In summary, with careful attention to treatment volume, energy, and fractionation, radiation therapy can produce high cure rates with good to excellent cosmetic and functional results and a low risk of complications. Since radiation therapy is a relatively expensive form of treatment for skin cancer, it is most appropriate for carcinomas measuring 0.5 cm or more that involve the pinna of the ear; scalp; eyelid, tip or ala of the nose; or lip, particularly the commissure. In these cases, radiation therapy is less costly than Mohs' micrographic surgery followed by reconstructive surgery.[68] Hence, in properly selected patients with basal and squamous cell carcinomas, radiation therapy represents an excellent treatment option.

TREATMENT RECOMMENDATIONS BY SPECIFIC ANATOMICAL SITE

Dorsum of the Hand

The most common cancer of the dorsum of the hand is squamous cell carcinoma.[124] Small cancers at this site are typically treated with cryotherapy, curettage and electrodesiccation, surgical excision, or Mohs' micrographic surgery. In general, cancers involving the dorsum of the hand are not managed with radiation therapy because repeated trauma results in a higher risk of necrosis, though carcinomas of 0.4 cm or less in thickness have been successfully treated with radioactive surface molds (see the section on brachytherapy).[120,125] Mohs' micrographic surgery is generally the preferred method of treatment for carcinomas greater than 2 cm.[57]

Eyelid

Radiation therapy represents an effective method of treating eyelid carcinomas, with good cosmetic and functional results and a low risk of complications.[122,126] With orthovoltage x-rays, less of a margin needs to be provided at the skin surface, the cornea receives a lower dose of radiation, and the cost of treatment is less than with electrons.[87] For carcinomas measuring 0.5 to 2.0 cm in the greatest dimension, the delivery of a total dose of 48 Gy in 16 fractions over 3½ weeks using 100 kV x-rays and a 0.19 mm copper HVL (or similar technique) is recommended. Patients may develop mild conjunctivitis from the daily installation of the eye shields (see Fig. 66-4) and the acute effects of radiation on the conjunctiva. A decongestant solution or Lacri-Lube ophthalmic ointment helps to relieve the burning and pruritus. Bacterial conjunctivitis may be treated with 10% sodium sulfacetamide (Sodium Sulamyd) ophthalmic ointment four times daily and at bedtime. Although the eyelashes in the irradiated area fall out and do not grow back, this does not cause functional problems. Large carcinomas may produce ectropion, and carcinomas involving the lower eyelid, inner canthus, punctum lacrimale, or nasolacrimal duct may produce epiphora.[89] Ectropion or epiphora may also develop as a complication of treatment, regardless of the modality selected. These complications improve in approximately one half of patients who undergo corrective surgery.[122] Radiation-induced cataracts used to develop after radium plaque irradiation since it was not possible to shield the lens from the high-energy gamma-rays. However, with modern treatment techniques (e.g., superficial x-ray therapy with a lead shield placed under the eyelids), cataracts are uncommon. Surgery is preferred for carcinomas less than 0.5 cm in the greatest dimension and may be used to salvage radiation failures.[122]

Lip

The most common cancers of the upper and lower lips are basal cell carcinomas and squamous cell carcinomas, respectively. These carcinomas often involve the vermilion border between the red area of the lips and the surrounding facial skin and may be treated with surgical excision, radiation therapy, or Mohs' micrographic surgery.[57] When external beam radiation therapy is administered, a lead shield should be placed beneath the lip to reduce the absorbed dose of radiation in the teeth and mandible (see Fig. 66-6). For carcinomas measuring 0.5 to 2.0 cm in the greatest dimension, the delivery of a total dose of 48 Gy in 16 fractions over 3½ weeks using 150 kV x-rays and a 0.52 mm copper HVL (or similar technique) is recommended. If interstitial brachytherapy alone is used, a gauze roll containing a 2 mm lead shield should be placed under the lip to minimize the absorbed dose of radiation in the teeth and mandible.[116] From 55 to 70 Gy should be delivered over 5 to 8 days.[116,117] Carcinomas greater than 4 cm can be successfully treated with the delivery of external beam radiation therapy to the lip, chin, and neck to a total dose of 50 Gy in 25 fractions over 5 weeks followed by a 30 to 40 Gy iridium-192 interstitial brachytherapy boost over 3 to 4 days.[96,116] Rubber tubing containing an iridium-192 ribbon may be placed horizontally on top of a lower lip carcinoma to improve the dose distribution.[96] If a squamous cell carcinoma is poorly differentiated, recurrent, or more than 3 cm in the greatest dimension or 4 mm in thickness, the submandibular and upper jugular lymph nodes should be included in the target volume.

Nose and Ear

Similar results can be achieved with superficial x-rays, electrons, or interstitial brachytherapy.[111] A wax- or aluminum-coated lead strip should be placed in the nasal cavity to reduce the mucosal reaction. When carcinomas involving the ala of the nose are treated, the nasolabial fold should be included in the target volume (see Fig. 66-5). Wax can be used as bolus on irregular surfaces to improve the dose homogeneity in the target volume.[82] For carcinomas measuring 0.5 to 2.0 cm in the greatest dimension, the delivery of a total dose of 52.8 Gy in 16 fractions over 3½ weeks using 6 MeV electrons and 0.5 cm buildup bolus (or similar technique) is recommended.

SEQUELAE OF RADIATION THERAPY

Moist desquamation develops after the administration of the doses of radiation required to eradicate skin cancer. The skin reaction usually reaches a peak 3 to 6 weeks after the start of treatment and resolves spontaneously over approximately 6 weeks. The skin in field may gradually become telangiectatic, atrophic, and hypopigmented over a period of years and is more sensitive to trauma. The long-term cosmetic results depend on the fraction size, total dose, volume of tissue treated and anatomical location. Blood flow in the irradiated region decreases. As a result, healing may be delayed after surgery on an irradiated region. Hair loss and a loss of sweat gland function are usually permanent. Ectropion and epiphora may develop after the treatment of eyelid carcinomas (particularly ones involving the lower eyelid), though cataracts are uncommon. The incidence of soft tissue necrosis is typically less than 3%. Osteoradionecrosis occurs in approximately 1% of patients, and radiochondritis is rare, as previously discussed.

PREVENTION

Patients should be advised to wear a hat and sunscreen with a sun protection factor of at least 15 when outdoors. Regular follow-up is important so that premalignant lesions such as actinic keratoses can be treated. Successful chemoprophylaxis with oral isotretinoin has been reported in patients with basal cell nevus syndrome and xeroderma pigmentosum, but long-term, high-dose therapy is necessary.[127,128]

KERATOACANTHOMA

A keratoacanthoma is a benign tumor that develops in the sun-exposed skin of middle-aged and elderly people. Occasionally, it is associated with an internal malignancy.[129,130] A keratoacanthoma typically appears as a rapidly growing papule that reaches 1 to 2 cm in diameter over a 1- to 3-month period. During the initial growth phase, the lesion develops a central keratin plug surrounded by a raised border. The tumor subsequently undergoes gradual involution over a 2- to 6-month period and can produce an ugly scar. Treatment has been suggested to reduce the likelihood that an unsightly scar will develop.[131] Surgical excision is commonly performed; however, at sites such as the pinna of the ear; eyelid; tip or ala of the nose; or commissure of the lips, radiation therapy may provide better cosmetic and functional results.

Shimm and colleagues[129] described the treatment of 13 keratoacanthoma patients with radiation therapy. With a median follow-up of 41 months, the local control rate was 100% and the cosmetic results were excellent. For keratoacanthomas of 2 cm or less, Shimm and colleagues recommend a total dose of 25 Gy in 5 fractions on consecutive days, using superficial or orthovoltage x-rays. "Giant" (>2 cm) keratoacanthomas can be successfully managed with a total dose of 50 Gy in 15 fractions over 3 weeks using megavoltage electrons.[132,133]

MALIGNANT MELANOMA

The American Cancer Society estimated that in the United States in 1996, there would be 38,300 new cases and 7300 deaths secondary to cutaneous melanoma.[1] Over the past decade, the incidence of melanoma has increased faster than that of any other cancer except lung cancer in women. Like carcinomas of the skin, melanomas tend to develop in sun-exposed areas in fair-skinned people with red or blond hair who burn rather than tan when outdoors.[134] Blistering sunburns during childhood lead to an increased risk of melanoma later in life.[135] A patient with a melanoma has a 3% to 5% risk of developing a second melanoma, which is 900 times the risk that an individual in the general population will develop this type of cancer.[136-138] A patient with multiple dysplastic nevi or the uncommon familial form of melanoma has an even higher risk (4% to 10%) of developing melanoma.[137] Features that can help to distinguish melanomas from benign nevi are asymmetry, irregular borders, color variegation, and an increase in the diameter of the lesion. Melanomas can spread to any site, and metastases may not become apparent for years. The AJCC staging system for melanoma,[56] which is based on the thickness of the lesion as suggested by Breslow[139] and the level of invasion using the layers of the skin as a reference as suggested by Clark and colleagues,[140] is presented in Table 66-5.

The four major subtypes of melanoma are: superficial spreading, nodular, lentigo maligna, and acral lentiginous. *Superficial spreading melanomas* account for approximately 65% of melanomas. The cancer first appears as a deeply pigmented area in a brown junctional nevus. As it grows along the surface of the skin, it may assume a glossy appearance with indentations along the border. *Nodular melanomas* account for 23% of melanomas. These lesions commonly begin in uninvolved skin rather than preexisting nevi, tend to be darker and more uniform in coloration, and grow primarily into the dermis rather than along the surface. For superficial spreading and nodular melanomas, the main prognostic variables are tumor thickness, anatomic site, and ulceration.[141] Older patients tend to have thicker lesions and do not fare as well. Patients with superficial spreading or nodular melanomas on the face, ears, or arms tend to survive longer than individuals with these subtypes of melanoma on the scalp or neck. Since women have nonulcerative melanomas on the arms more often than men, they tend to have a more favorable prognosis. Lentigo maligna (Hutchinson's freckle) is characteristically located on the face of middle-aged to elderly white people, is flat (involves the epidermis only), and has a mottled light and dark brown appearance.[142] Once the tumor invades the dermis, it is known as *lentigo maligna melanoma*. Lentigo maligna melanomas, which constitute 7% of melanomas, grow slowly and metastasize to lymph nodes in only 10% of cases.[140] Consequently, the 10-year survival rate for lentigo maligna melanoma is 85% after wide local excision.[141] In areas of cosmetic and functional importance such as the pinna of the ear; eyelids; tip or ala of the nose; or lips, radiation therapy (e.g., 50 Gy in 20 fractions over a 4-week period using 100 to 250 kV x-rays and a 1.5 cm margin for a lentigo maligna melanoma

Table 66–5   Classification of Melanoma of the Skin (Excluding Eyelid)

Primary Tumor (T)

TX	Primary tumor cannot be assessed (e.g., shave biopsy or regressed melanoma)
T0	No evidence of primary tumor
Tis	Melanoma *in situ*
T1	Melanoma ≤1.0 mm in thickness with or without ulceration
T1a	Melanoma ≤1.0 mm in thickness and level II or III, no ulceration
T1b	Melanoma ≤1.0 mm in thickness and level IV or V or with ulceration
T2	Melanoma 1.01–2 mm in thickness with or without ulceration
T2a	Melanoma 1.01–2.0 mm in thickness, no ulceration
T2b	Melanoma 1.01–2.0 mm in thickness, with ulceration
T3	Melanoma 2.01–4 mm in thickness, with or without ulceration
T3a	Melanoma 2.01–4.0 mm in thickness, no ulceration
T3b	Melanoma 2.01–4.0 mm in thickness, with ulceration
T4	Melanoma greater than 4.0 mm in thickness with or without ulceration
T4a	Melanoma >4.0 mm in thickness, no ulceration
T4b	Melanoma >4.0 mm in thickness, with ulceration

Regional Lymph Nodes (N)

NX	Regional lymph nodes cannot be assessed
N0	No regional lymph node metastasis
N1	Metastasis in one lymph node
N1a	Clinically occult (microscopic) metastasis
N1b	Clinically apparent (macroscopic) metastasis
N2	Metastasis in two to three regional nodes or intralymphatic regional metastasis without nodal metastasis
N2a	Clinically occult (microscopic) metastasis
N2b	Clinically apparent (macroscopic) metastasis
N2c	Satellite or in-transit metastasis *without* nodal metastasis
N3	Metastasis in four or more regional nodes, or matted metastatic nodes, or in-transit metastasis or satellite(s) *with* metastasis in regional node(s)

Distant Metastasis (M)

MX	Distant metastasis cannot be assessed
M0	No distant metastasis
M1	Distant metastasis
M1a	Metastasis to skin, subcutaneous tissues or distant lymph nodes
M1b	Metastasis to lung
M1c	Metastasis to all other visceral sites or distant metastasis at any site associated with an elevated serum lactic dehydrogenase (LDH)

Clinical Stage Grouping

Stage 0	Tis	N0	M0
Stage IA	T1a	N0	M0
Stage IB	T1b	N0	M0
	T2a	N0	M0
Stage IIA	T2b	N0	M0
	T3a	N0	M0
Stage IIB	T3b	N0	M0
	T4a	N0	M0
Stage IIC	T4b	N0	M0
Stage III	Any T	N1	M0
	Any T	N2	M0
	Any T	N3	M0
Stage IV	Any T	Any N	M1

From Greene FL, Page DL, Fleming ID, et al, eds: *AJCC Cancer Staging Manual*, 6/E. New York: Springer, 2002.

greater than 5 cm) can be used rather than surgery and produce excellent results.[143] *Acral lentiginous melanomas* constitute only 5% of melanomas in fair-skinned people, although they are the most common form of melanoma in dark-skinned people. They generally occur on the palms or soles or underneath the nails. These cancers initially appear as flat, tan lesions but later may exhibit ulcerative or exophytic growth. As with the other subtypes of melanoma, acral lentiginous melanomas are usually managed with wide local excision. For stage I patients, the 10-year survival rate is 44%.[144]

Melanomas have traditionally been regarded as cancers that are unresponsive to radiation therapy. The origin of this concept is unclear, but it may be related to the fact that most melanomas can be readily excised. For melanomas less than 5 cm, the Radiation Therapy Oncology Group (RTOG) reported that radiation therapy alone produced a 31% complete response rate, which challenges the concept that melanomas are unresponsive to radiation.[145] In addition, Ang and colleagues[146] reported that preoperative or postoperative radiation therapy (24 to 30 Gy in four to five fractions over 2 to 2½ weeks) can improve locoregional control in patients with head and neck melanomas that are either thicker than 1.5 mm or metastatic to regional nodes (i.e., AJCC stages II or III). This approach is currently being evaluated in a phase III clinical trial (RTOG protocol 9302), in which patients with completely resected, pathologically node-positive melanoma of the head and neck (AJCC stage III) are randomly assigned to receive either postoperative radiation therapy (30 Gy in five fractions over 2½ weeks) or observation.

Although cutaneous melanoma is typically treated with surgery, radiation therapy should be considered in cases in which a patient is judged to be medically inoperable or refuses surgery. Hyperthermia can improve the complete response and 2-year local control rates obtained with radiation therapy.[147,148] Melanomas measuring 4 cm or less are more likely to respond to hyperthermia since a more uniform temperature distribution can be achieved.[148]

Radiobiology studies published in 1971 described an unusually large shoulder in the cell survival curve for several human melanoma cell lines,[149,150] suggesting a role for hypofractionation. Authors of nonrandomized studies have suggested that doses of 4 Gy or greater per fraction produce higher complete response rates,[151-153] although the size of the melanomas and the relationship between fraction size and total dose were not always addressed in these reports. To test the hypothesis that doses of 4 Gy or greater per fraction produce higher response rates, the RTOG conducted a prospective, randomized trial (protocol 8305) in which measurable melanomas (typically involving the skin, soft tissue, or lymph nodes) were treated with either four weekly 8 Gy fractions or 20 daily 2.5 Gy fractions.[145] For melanomas of all sizes, the 4 × 8 Gy arm produced a complete response rate of 24% and a partial response rate of 35%. Similarly, the 20 × 2.5 Gy arm produced a complete response rate of 23% and a partial response rate of 34%; that is, there was no difference in terms of the effectiveness of the two fractionation schemes. There also does not appear to be an association between fraction size and the ability of

radiation therapy to palliate visceral (e.g., brain[154,155]) metastases secondary to melanoma.[156-158] In support of these clinical findings, more recent radiobiological experiments have demonstrated that not all human melanoma cell lines have a broad, curvy shoulder.[159,160] These experiments suggest that melanomas may differ significantly in responsiveness to radiation from patient to patient, and even from lesion to lesion in a single patient.[161] Consequently, when a cutaneous melanoma is treated with radiation therapy with curative intent, the dose recommendations in Table 66-2 may be followed.

The most active chemotherapeutic agents against metastatic melanoma are dacarbazine (the most effective and one of the oldest agents), nitrosoureas, cisplatin, carboplatin, and paclitaxel (Taxol). Single-agent chemotherapy has yielded response rates of 20% or less, with responses typically lasting 6 months or less.[162] When melanoma extensively involves an extremity, palliation can sometimes be achieved with regional hyperthermic perfusion with melphalan.[163] Intralesional immunotherapy, for example, with bacillus Calmette-Guérin,[164] has also demonstrated activity against melanoma. Similarly, interferon-alpha has produced a response rate of 20%.[165] Combination chemotherapy has yielded response rates of approximately 40% but does not provide a significant survival advantage over single-agent chemotherapy and is more toxic.[162] McClay and colleagues[166] reported that tamoxifen can improve the response rate achievable with chemotherapy. Since conventional chemotherapy has produced low complete response rates (e.g., 5%), and the responses have been of limited duration, patients with stage IV melanoma should be entered into clinical trials whenever possible. Trials investigating interleukin 2; lymphokine-activated killer cells; tumor-infiltrating lymphocytes; tumor necrosis factor alpha; and gene therapy are currently ongoing.[162,167-171]

MERKEL CELL CARCINOMA

Merkel cell carcinoma (also known as trabecular carcinoma or neuroendocrine carcinoma of the skin) is a rare, aggressive neoplasm that was first described by Toker[172] in 1972. In general, 46% of Merkel cell carcinomas are located on the head and neck, 44% are located on the extremities, and 10% are located on the trunk.[173] Like other carcinomas of the skin, Merkel cell carcinomas usually develop in individuals who are in their sixth to eighth decade of life. These tumors characteristically appear as a firm nodule that is red, pink, or blue and varies in diameter from a few millimeters to several centimeters.[174] The differential diagnosis includes poorly differentiated squamous cell carcinoma, melanoma, sweat gland carcinoma, lymphoma, Langerhans' cell histiocytosis, and metastatic cancers including islet cell carcinoma, medullary carcinoma of the thyroid, and small-cell carcinoma of the lung.

There is no consensus on how to manage patients with Merkel cell carcinoma. Merkel cell carcinomas have traditionally been treated with wide local excision, which results in locoregional recurrences in 73% (43/59) of patients and distant metastases in 48% of patients.[175]

The average time to the development of metastases is 10 months. In contrast, locoregional recurrences have been described in only 15% (14/91) of patients treated with surgery and postoperative radiation therapy.[174,176-180] Since patients are usually referred for radiation therapy because they are judged to be at high risk for recurrence, it is unlikely that the individuals who were managed with surgery and postoperative radiation therapy in these studies had a more favorable prognosis than those who were managed with surgery alone.

Use of a wide margin in the radiation portals is important in achieving locoregional control. Morrison and colleagues[176] described 80% (4/5) regional recurrences in patients managed with small fields encompassing only the primary tumor bed. In the study by Goepfert and colleagues,[181] 67% (8/12) of patients without clinical evidence of lymph node metastases developed regional metastases when the draining lymph nodes were not electively irradiated. Consequently, inclusion of the regional lymphatics in continuity with the primary tumor bed is recommended.

In-field recurrences have been described in three of four patients with measurable disease who were treated palliatively to a total dose of 30 Gy.[177,182,183] On the other hand, Pacella and colleagues[178] reported that with a median follow-up of 14 months, in-field control was maintained in 13 of 13 patients with no measurable disease and 22 of 23 patients with measurable disease after the administration of a median dose of 45 Gy in 20 fractions over a 4-week period. In the study by Morrison and colleagues,[176] in-field control was maintained in 10 of 10 patients with macroscopic disease after the administration of 50 to 75 Gy using conventional fractionation with or without an interstitial boost. As a result, irradiation of the operative bed and regional lymphatics to a total dose of 50 to 55 Gy at 1.8 to 2 Gy per day is recommended in an adjuvant setting. In patients with gross disease 60 to 65 Gy is recommended. Local control has also been achieved with hyperthermia and radiation therapy,[177,182] although the follow-up period in these studies was brief.

In an effort to improve locoregional control, aggressive surgery has been advocated.[175] However, since radiation therapy is capable of sterilizing subclinical disease, the treatment of Merkel cell carcinoma with limited surgery (e.g., an excisional biopsy) and postoperative radiation therapy can obviate the need for extensive reconstructive procedures. Similarly, when the regional lymph nodes are clinically negative, they can be included in the radiation therapy portals, obviating the need for unilateral or bilateral lymph node dissections.

In certain patients with Merkel cell carcinoma, there appears to be an orderly progression of spread from the site of origin to regional lymphatics to distant organs.[177,184,185] In the study by Pacella and colleagues,[178] the only patient whose primary tumor was treated de novo with an excisional biopsy and radiation therapy remained disease-free 77 months later. Likewise, the two patients treated initially with surgery and postoperative radiation therapy in the study by Wilder and colleagues[177] remained disease-free 24 and 59 months later. Morrison and colleagues[176] reported that the 5-year actuarial disease-free survival rate was 11% for surgery alone versus 56% for surgery and postoperative radiation therapy (P = 0.002). Similarly, Meeuwissen and colleagues[180] reported that the 3-year actuarial disease-free survival rate was 0% for 38 patients treated with surgery alone versus 68% for 34 patients treated with surgery and postoperative radiation therapy. These results suggest that postoperative radiation therapy may be able to improve disease-free survival if it is incorporated into the initial treatment.[186]

The role of chemotherapy in the treatment of Merkel cell carcinoma remains controversial. In patients treated with chemotherapy alone, the partial and complete response rates have been 31% (8/26) and 15% (4/26), respectively.[173,177,185,187-191] Based on the neuroendocrine origin of Merkel cell carcinoma, drugs active against small-cell carcinoma of the lung (e.g., carboplatin and etoposide)[184] have typically been administered. Since distant metastases eventually develop in a relatively large number of patients, chemotherapy has been administered in combination with surgery or radiation therapy or both in an effort to improve cure rates. In a study by George,[192] locoregional disease responded to induction chemotherapy; however, the average duration of the responses was only 3 months. Similarly, Grosh and colleagues[188] reported that responses to chemotherapy lasted only 2 to 4 months. A recent literature review by Tai[193] revealed a total of 204 patients in the literature treated for locally recurrent or metastatic Merkel cell carcinoma. There was an overall 59% response rate. It is hoped that more active chemotherapeutic agents will be developed, leading to an improvement in cure rates. The role of chemotherapy in an adjuvant setting for localized disease remains uncertain, with no definite survival benefits reported thus far in the literature. There is increasing interest in the use of sentinel node mapping in Merkel cell carcinoma to help identify which patients may benefit from chemotherapy or elective radiation of the lymph nodes.[194-196] In the meantime, chemotherapy may offer palliation to Merkel cell carcinoma patients with locally advanced or metastatic disease, particularly those with predominantly nodal disease.[184]

REFERENCES

1. Jemal A, Murray T, et al: Cancer statistics, 2003. *CA Cancer J Clin.* 2003;55:5.
2. Blum HF: Sunlight as a causal factor in cancer of the skin of man. *J Natl Cancer Inst.* 1948;9:247.
3. Mackie BS, McGovern VJ: The mechanism of solar carcinogenesis. *Arch Dermatol.* 1958;78:218.
4. Mora RG, Burris R: Cancer of the skin in blacks: A review of 128 patients with basal-cell carcinoma. *Cancer.* 1981;47:1436.
5. Hall AF: Relationships of sunlight, complexion and heredity to skin carcinogenesis. *Arch Dermatol Syphilol.* 1950;61:589.
6. Kopf AW: Computer analysis of 3531 basal-cell carcinomas of the skin. *J Dermatol.* 1979;6:267.
7. Hazelrigg DE: Basal cell epithelioma in a vaccination scar. *Int J Dermatol.* 1978;17:723.
8. Wiener DA, Scher RK: Basal cell carcinoma arising in a tattoo. *Cutis.* 1987;39:125.
9. White SW: Basal-cell carcinoma arising in a burn scar: Case report. *J Dermatol Surg Oncol.* 1983;9:159.
10. Hendricks WM: Basal cell carcinoma arising in a chickenpox scar. *Arch Dermatol.* 1980;116:1304.

11. Didolkar MS, Douglass HO, Holyoke ED, et al: Basal-cell carcinoma originating at the colostomy site: Report of a case. *Dis Colon Rectum.* 1975;18:399.

12. Hejna WF: Squamous-cell carcinoma developing in the chronic draining sinuses of osteomyelitis. *Cancer.* 1965;18:128.

13. Anderson NP, Anderson HE: Development of basal cell epithelioma as a consequence of radiodermatitis. *Arch Dermatol Syphilol.* 1951; 63:586.

14. Simonato L: Occupational factors. In Higginson J, Muir CS, Muñoz N, eds. *Human Cancer: Epidemiology and Environmental Causes.* Cambridge: Cambridge University Press; 1992:97.

15. Ostrow RS, Bender M, Niimura M, et al: Human papillomavirus DNA in cutaneous primary and metastasized squamous cell carcinomas from patients with epidermodysplasia verruciformis. *Proc Natl Acad Sci U S A.* 1982;79:1634.

16. Gupta AK, Cardella CJ, Haberman HF: Cutaneous malignant neoplasms in patients with renal transplants. *Arch Dermatol.* 1986;22:1288.

17. Berg JW: The incidence of multiple primary cancers: I. Development of further cancers in patients with lymphomas, leukemias, and myeloma. *J Natl Cancer Inst.* 1967;38:741.

18. Sitz KV, Keppen M, Johnson DF: Metastatic basal cell carcinoma in acquired immunodeficiency syndrome–related complex. *JAMA.* 1987;257:340.

19. Rubin P, Casarett GW: *Clinical Radiation Pathology.* Philadelphia: WB Saunders; 1968:62.

20. Patterson JAK, Geronemus RG: Cancers of the skin. In DeVita VT Jr, Hellman S, Rosenberg SA, eds. *Cancer: Principles and Practice of Oncology.* 3rd ed. Philadelphia: JB Lippincott; 1989:1469.

21. Preston DS, Stern RS: Nonmelanoma cancers of the skin. *N Engl J Med.* 1992;327:1649.

22. Murphy GF, Kwan TH, Milm MC Jr: The skin. In Robbins SL, Cotran RS, Kumar V, eds. *Pathologic Basis of Disease.* 3rd ed. Philadelphia: WB Saunders; 1984:1257.

23. Blank AA, Schnyder UW: Soft-x-ray therapy in Bowen's disease and erythroplasia of Queyrat. *Dermatologica.* 1985;171:89.

24. Evans HL, Smith JL: Spindle cell squamous carcinomas and sarcoma-like tumors of the skin: A comparative study of 38 cases. *Cancer.* 1980;45:2687.

25. Mohs FE, Lathrop TG: Modes of spread of cancer of the skin. *Arch Dermatol Syphilol.* 1952;66:427.

26. Panje WR, Ceilley RI: The influence of embryology of the mid-face on the spread of epithelial malignancies. *Laryngoscope.* 1979;89:1914.

27. Wentzell JM, Robinson JK: Embryologic fusion planes and the spread of cutaneous carcinoma: A review and reassessment. *J Dermatol Surg Oncol.* 1990;16:1000.

28. Dodd GD, Dolan PA, Ballantyne AJ, et al: The dissemination of tumors of the head and neck via the cranial nerves. *Radiol Clin North Am.* 1970;8:445.

29. Mohs FE: *Chemosurgery: Microscopically Controlled Surgery for Skin Cancer.* Springfield, Ill: Charles C Thomas; 1978:261.

30. Von Domarus H, Stevens PJ: Metastatic basal cell carcinoma: Report of five cases and review of 170 cases in the literature. *J Am Acad Dermatol.* 1984;10:1043.

31. Binkley GW, Rauschkolb RR: Basal-cell epithelioma metastasizing to lymph nodes. *Arch Dermatol.* 1962;86:332.

32. Carlson KC, Roenigk RK: Know your anatomy: Perineural involvement of basal and squamous cell carcinoma on the face. *J Dermatol Surg Oncol.* 1990;16:827.

33. Hanke CW, Wolf RL, Hochman SA, et al: Chemosurgical reports: Perineural spread of basal-cell carcinoma. *J Dermatol Surg Oncol.* 1983;9:742.

34. Smith JB, Bishop VL, Francis IC, et al: Ophthalmic manifestations of perineural spread of facial skin malignancy. *Aust NZ J Ophthalmol.* 1990;18:197.

35. Barrett TL, Greenway HT Jr, Massullo V, et al: Treatment of basal cell carcinoma and squamous cell carcinoma with perineural invasion. *Adv Dermat.* 1993;8:277.

36. Cottel WI: Perineural invasion by squamous-cell carcinoma. *J Dermatol Surg Oncol.* 1982;8:589.

37. Ballantyne AJ, McCarten AB, Ibanez M: The extension of cancer of the head and neck through peripheral nerves. *Am J Surg.* 1963;106:651.

38. Goepfert H, Dichtel WJ, Medina JE, et al: Perineural invasion in squamous cell skin carcinoma of the head and neck. *Am J Surg.* 1984;148:542.

39. Mendenhall WM, Parsons JT, Mendenhall NP, et al: Carcinoma of the skin of the head and neck with perineural invasion. *Head Neck.* 1989;11:301.

40. Clouston PD, Sharpe DM, Corbett AJ, et al: Perineural spread of cutaneous head and neck cancer. Its orbital and central neurologic complications. *Arch Neurol.* 1990;47:73.

41. Mark GJ: Basal cell carcinoma with intraneural invasion. *Cancer.* 1977;40:2181.

42. Fitzpatrick PJ: Skin cancer of the head—treatment by radiotherapy. *J Otolaryngol.* 1984;13:261.

43. Cotran RS: Metastasizing basal cell carcinomas. *Cancer.* 1961; 14:1036.

44. Wermuth BM, Fajardo LF: Metastatic basal cell carcinoma. A review. *Arch Pathol.* 1970;90:458.

45. Møller R, Reymann F, Hou-Jensen K: Metastases in dermatological patients with squamous cell carcinoma. *Arch Dermatol.* 1979; 115:703.

46. Modlin JJ: Cancer of the skin: Surgical treatment. *Mo Med.* 1954;51:364.

47. Dinehart SM, Pollack SV: Metastases from squamous cell carcinoma of the skin and lip. An analysis of twenty-seven cases. *J Am Acad Dermatol.* 1989;21:241.

48. Binder SC, Cady B, Catlin D: Epidermoid carcinoma of the skin of the nose. *Am J Surg.* 1968;116:506.

49. Friedman HI, Cooper PH, Wanebo HJ: Prognostic and therapeutic use of microstaging of cutaneous squamous cell carcinoma of the trunk and extremities. *Cancer.* 1985;56:1099.

50. Shimm DS, Wilder RB: Radiation therapy for squamous cell carcinoma of the skin. *Am J Clin Oncol.* 1991;14:383.

51. Epstein E, Epstein NN, Bragg K, et al: Metastases from squamous cell carcinomas of the skin. *Arch Dermatol.* 1968;97:245.

52. Bourne RG: The Costello Memorial Lecture. The spread of squamous cell carcinoma of the skin via the cranial nerves. *Australas Radiol.* 1980;24:106.

53. Byers RM: The use of postoperative irradiation—Its goals and 1978 attainments. *Laryngoscope.* 1979;89:567.

54. Larson DL, Rodin AE, Roberts DK, et al: Perineural lymphatics: Myth or fact. *Am J Surg.* 1966;112:488.

55. Loeffler JS, Larson DA, Clark JR, et al: Treatment of perineural metastasis from squamous carcinoma of the skin with aggressive combination chemotherapy and irradiation. *J Surg Oncol.* 1985; 29:181.

56. American Joint Committee on Cancer: Carcinoma of the skin (excluding eyelid, vulva, and penis). In Fleming ID, Cooper JS, Henson DE, et al, eds. *AJCC Cancer Staging Manual.* 5th ed. Philadelphia: Lippincott-Raven; 1997:157.

57. Albright SD III: Treatment of skin cancer using multiple modalities. *J Am Acad Dermatol.* 1982;7:143.

58. Massullo V: The clinical and biological basis for radiation therapy of cutaneous carcinoma, melanoma, and lymphoma. *Adv Dermat.* 1995;10:201.

59. Levine H: Cutaneous carcinoma of the head and neck: Management of massive and previously uncontrolled lesions. *Laryngoscope.* 1983;93:87.

60. Menn H, Robins P, Kopf AW, et al: The recurrent basal cell epithelioma: A study of 100 cases of recurrent, re-treated basal cell epitheliomas. *Arch Dermatol.* 1971;103:628.

61. Mohs FE: Chemosurgery for basal cell and squamous carcinomas of the skin. M D Anderson Hospital and Tumor Institute, Houston. In *Neoplasms of the Skin and Malignant Melanoma.* Chicago: Year Book Medical; 1976:173.

62. Guthrie TH Jr, Porubsky ES, Luxenberg MN, et al: Cisplatin-based chemotherapy in advanced basal and squamous cell carcinomas of the skin: Results in 28 patients including 13 patients receiving multimodality therapy. *J Clin Oncol.* 1990;8:342.

63. Sadek H, Azli N, Wendling JL, et al: Treatment of advanced squamous cell carcinoma of the skin with cisplatin, 5-fluorouracil, and bleomycin. *Cancer.* 1990;66:1692.

64. Lippman SM, Meyskens FL Jr: Treatment of advanced squamous cell carcinoma of the skin with isotretinoin. *Ann Intern Med.* 1987;107:499.

65. Kish J, Drelichman A, Jacobs J, et al: Clinical trial of cisplatin and 5-FU infusion as initial treatment for advanced squamous cell carcinoma of the head and neck. *Cancer Treat Rep.* 1982;66:471.

66. Stell PM, Rawson NSB: Adjuvant chemotherapy in head and neck cancer. *Br J Cancer.* 1990;61:779.

67. Swanson NA, Grekin RC, Baker SR: Mohs surgery: Techniques, indications, and applications in head and neck surgery. *Head Neck Surg.* 1983;6:683.

68. Wilder RB, Shimm DS, Kittelson JM, et al: Recurrent basal cell carcinoma treated with radiation therapy. *Arch Dermatol.* 1991; 127:1668.

69. Rowe DE, Carroll RJ, Day CL Jr: Mohs' surgery is the treatment of choice for recurrent (previously treated) basal cell carcinoma. *J Dermatol Surg Oncol.* 1989;15:424.

70. Mendenhall WM, Parsons JT, Mendenhall NP, et al: T2-T4 carcinoma of the skin of the head and neck treated with radical irradiation. *Int J Radiat Oncol Biol Phys.* 1987;13:975.

71. Petrovich Z, Kuisk H, Langholz B, et al: Treatment of carcinoma of the skin with bone and/or cartilage involvement. *Am J Clin Oncol.* 1988;11:110.

72. Wilder RB, Kittelson JM, Shimm DS: Basal cell carcinoma treated with radiation therapy. *Cancer.* 1991;68:2134.

73. Bart RS, Kopf AW, Gladstein AH: Treatment of morphea-type basal cell carcinomas with radiation therapy. *Arch Dermatol.* 1977;113:783.

74. Janse GT, Westbrook KC: Cancer of the skin. In Suen JY, Myers EN, eds. *Cancer of the Head and Neck.* New York: Churchill Livingstone; 1981:212.

75. Smith SP, Grande DJ: Basal cell carcinoma recurring after radiotherapy: A unique, difficult treatment subclass of recurrent basal cell carcinoma. *J Dermatol Surg Oncol.* 1991;17:26.

76. Gooding CA, White G, Yatsuhashi M: Significance of marginal extension in excised basal-cell carcinoma. *N Engl J Med.* 1965; 273:923.

77. De Silva SP, Dellon AL: Recurrence rate of positive margin basal cell carcinoma: Results of a five-year prospective study. *J Surg Oncol.* 1985;28:72.

78. Pascal RR, Hobby LW, Lattes R, et al: Prognosis of "incompletely excised" versus "completely excised" basal cell carcinoma. *Plast Reconstr Surg.* 1968;41:328.

79. Richmond JD, Davie RM: The significance of incomplete excision in patients with basal cell carcinoma. *Br J Plast Surg.* 1987;40:63.

80. Koplin L, Zarem HA: Recurrent basal cell carcinoma. A review concerning the incidence, behavior, and management of recurrent basal cell carcinoma, with emphasis on the incompletely excised lesion. *Plast Reconstr Surg.* 1980;65:656.

81. Bieley HC, Kirsner RS, Reyes BA, et al: The use of Mohs' micrographic surgery for determination of residual tumor in incompletely excised basal cell carcinoma. *J Am Acad Dermatol.* 1992;26:754.

82. Khan FM: *The Physics of Radiation Therapy.* 2nd ed. Baltimore: Williams & Wilkins; 1994:42, 47, 135, 255, 291, 299, 365, 387, 397, 399.

83. Metcalf PB Jr: Carcinoma of the pinna. *N Engl J Med.* 1954;251:91.

84. Fredricks S: External ear malignancy. *Br J Plast Surg.* 1956;9:136.

85. Schewe EJ Jr, Pappalardo C: Cancer of the external ear. *Am J Surg.* 1962;104:753.

86. Avila J, Bosch A, Aristizabal S, et al: Carcinoma of the pinna. *Cancer.* 1977;40:2891.

87. Amdur RJ, Kalbaugh KJ, Ewald LM, et al: Radiation therapy for skin cancer near the eye: Kilovoltage x-rays versus electrons. *Int J Radiat Oncol Biol Phys.* 1992;23:769.

88. Atkinson HR: Skin carcinoma depth and dose homogeneity in dermatological x-ray therapy. *Aust J Dermatol.* 1962;6:208.

89. Levene MB: Radiotherapeutic management of carcinoma of the eyelid. In Brockhurst RJ, Boruchoff SA, Hutchinson BT, et al, eds. *Controversy in Ophthalmology.* Philadelphia: WB Saunders; 1977:390.

90. Hubbell JH: Photon mass attenuation and energy-absorption coefficients from 1 keV to 20 MeV. *Int J Appl Radiat Isot.* 1982;33:1269.

91. McCullough EC: Selection of techniques for orthovoltage radiation therapy. *Int J Radiat Oncol Biol Phys.* 1990;18:1237.

92. Scrimger JW, Connors SG: Performance characteristics of a widely used orthovoltage x-ray therapy machine. *Med Phys.* 1986;13:267.

93. Niroomand-Rad A, Gillin MT, Lopez F, et al: Performance characteristics of an orthovoltage x-ray therapy machine. *Med Phys.* 1987;14:874. Erratum: *Med Phys.* 1987;15:422.

94. White DR, Fitzgerald M: Calculated attenuation and energy absorption coefficients for ICRP Reference Man (1975) organs and tissues. *Health Phys.* 1977;33:73.

95. Fischbach AJ, Sause WT, Plenk HP: Radiation therapy for skin cancer. *West J Med.* 1980;133:379.

96. Wang CC: *Radiation Therapy for Head and Neck Neoplasms: Indications, Techniques, and Results.* 2nd ed. Chicago: Year Book Medical; 1990:76.

97. Strandqvist M: Studien über die kumulative Wirkung der Röngenstrahlen bei Fraktionierung. *Acta Radiol [Suppl].* 1944;55:1.

98. Von Essen CF: Roentgen therapy of skin and lip carcinoma: Factors influencing success and failure. *Am J Roentgenol.* 1960;83:556.

99. Ellis F: Nominal standard dose and the ret. *Br J Radiol.* 1971;44:101.

100. Hall EJ: *Radiobiology for the Radiologist.* 4th ed. Philadelphia: JB Lippincott; 1994:212.

101. Turesson I, Notter G: The influence of fraction size in radiotherapy on the late normal tissue reaction: II. Comparison of the effects of daily and twice-a-week fractionation on human skin. *Int J Radiat Oncol Biol Phys.* 1984;10:599.

102. Turesson I, Notter G: The influence of fraction size in radiotherapy on the late normal tissue reaction: I. Comparison of the effects of daily and once-a-week fractionation on human skin. *Int J Radiat Oncol Biol Phys.* 1984;10:593.

103. Traenkle HL, Mulay D: Further observations on late radiation necrosis following therapy of skin cancer. *Arch Dermatol.* 1960; 81:908.

104. Petrovich Z, Parker RG, Luxton G, et al: Carcinoma of the lip and selected sites of head and neck skin. A clinical study of 896 patients. *Radiother Oncol.* 1987;8:11.

105. Williams PC, Hendry JH: The RBE of megavoltage photon and electron beams. *Br J Radiol.* 1978;51:220.

106. Boland J: Human skin reaction. *Br J Radiol.* 1957;30:351.

107. Burg G, Hirsch RD, Konz B, et al: Histographic surgery: Accuracy of visual assessment of the margins of basal-cell epithelioma. *J Derm Surg.* 1975;1:21.

108. Breuninger H, Dietz K: Prediction of subclinical tumor infiltration in basal cell carcinoma. *J Dermatol Surg Oncol.* 1991;17:574.

109. Locke J, Karimpur S, Young G, et al: Radiotherapy for epithelial skin cancer. *Int J Radiat Oncol Biol Phys.* 2001;51:748.

110. Griep C, Davelaar J, Scholten AN, et al: Electron beam therapy is not inferior to superficial x-ray therapy in the treatment of skin carcinoma. *Int J Radiat Oncol Biol Phys.* 1995;32:1347.

111. Mazeron JJ, Chassagne D, Crook J, et al: Radiation therapy of carcinomas of the skin of nose and nasal vestibule: A report of 1676 cases by the Groupe Européen de Curiethérapie. *Radiother Oncol.* 1989;13:165.

112. Brodland DG, Zitelli JA: Surgical margins for excision of primary cutaneous squamous cell carcinoma. *J Am Acad Dermatol.* 1992; 27:241.

113. Carter RL, Foster CS, Dinsdale EA, et al: Perineural spread by squamous carcinomas of the head and neck: A morphological study using antiaxonal and antimyelin monoclonal antibodies. *J Clin Pathol.* 1983;36:269.

114. Paine CH: Modern after-loading methods for interstitial radiotherapy. *Clin Radiol.* 1972;23:263.

115. Crook JM, Mazeron JJ, Marinello G, et al: Interstitial iridium 192 for cutaneous carcinoma of the external nose. *Int J Radiat Oncol Biol Phys.* 1990;18:243.

116. Pigneux J, Richaud PM, Lagarde C: The place of interstitial therapy using ^{192}iridium in the management of carcinoma of the lip. *Cancer.* 1979;43:1073.

117. Durrant KR, Ellis F: The treatment of squamous-cell carcinoma of the lower lip by rigid implants. *Clin Radiol.* 1973;24:502.

118. Rosen I, Gordon W Jr, Loyd M: A surface mold using iridium-192 seeds. *Int J Radiat Oncol Biol Phys.* 1986;12:2203.

119. Rustgi SN, Cumberlin RL: An afterloading ^{192}Ir surface mould. *Med Dosim.* 1993;18:39.

120. Ashby MA, Pacella JA, de Groot R, et al: Use of a radon mould technique for skin cancer: Results from the Peter MacCallum Cancer Institute (1975-1984). *Br J Radiol.* 1989;62:608.

121. Rowe DE, Carroll RJ, Day CL Jr: Long-term recurrence rates in previously untreated (primary) basal cell carcinoma: Implications for patient follow-up. *J Dermatol Surg Oncol.* 1989;15:315.

122. Fitzpatrick PJ, Thompson GA, Easterbrook WM, et al: Basal and squamous cell carcinoma of the eyelids and their treatment by radiotherapy. *Int J Radiat Oncol Biol Phys.* 1984;10:449.

123. Petrovich Z, Kuisk H, Langholz B, et al: Treatment results and patterns of failure in 646 patients with carcinoma of the eyelids, pinna, and nose. *Am J Surg.* 1987;154:447.

124. Bean DJ, Rees RS, O'Leary JP, et al: Carcinoma of the hand: A 20-year experience. *South Med J.* 1984;77:998.

125. Solan MJ, Brady LW, Binnick SA, et al: Skin. In Perez CA, Brady LW, eds. *Principles and Practice of Radiation Oncology.* Philadelphia: JB Lippincott; 1992:479.

126. Cobb GM, Thompson GA, Allt WEC: Treatment of basal cell carcinoma of the eyelids by radiotherapy. *Can Med Assoc J.* 1964;91:743.

127. Cristofolini M, Zumiani G, Scappini P, et al: Aromatic retinoid in the chemoprevention of the progression of nevoid basal-cell carcinoma syndrome. *J Dermatol Surg Oncol.* 1984;10:778.

128. Kraemer KH, DiGiovanna JJ, Moshell AN, et al: Prevention of skin cancer in xeroderma pigmentosum with the use of oral isotretinoin. *N Engl J Med.* 1988;318:1633.

129. Shimm DS, Duttenhaver JR, Doucette J, et al: Radiation therapy of keratoacanthoma. *Int J Radiat Oncol Biol Phys.* 1983;9:759.

130. Caccialanza M, Sopelana N: Radiation therapy of keratoacanthomas: Results in 55 patients. *Int J Radiat Oncol Biol Phys.* 1989;16:475.

131. Ghadially FN: Keratoacanthoma. In Fitzpatrick TB, Eisen AZ, Wolff K, et al, eds. *Dermatology in General Medicine.* New York: McGraw-Hill; 1987:766.

132. Goldschmidt H, Sherwin WK: Radiation therapy of giant aggressive keratoacanthomas. *Arch Dermatol.* 1993;129:1162.

133. Donahue B, Cooper JS, Rush S: Treatment of aggressive keratoacanthomas by radiotherapy. *J Am Acad Dermatol.* 1990; 23:489.

134. Beral V, Evans S, Shaw H, et al: Cutaneous factors related to the risk of malignant melanoma. *Br J Dermatol.* 1983;109:165.

135. Lew RA, Sober AJ, Cook N, et al: Sun exposure habits in patients with cutaneous melanoma: A case control study. *J Dermatol Surg Oncol.* 1983;9:981.

136. Scheibner A, Milton GW, McCarthy WH, et al: Multiple primary melanoma—A review of 90 cases. *Australas J Dermatol.* 1982; 23:1.

137. Bellet RE, Vaisman I, Mastrangelo MJ, et al: Multiple primary malignancies in patients with cutaneous melanoma. *Cancer.* 1977; 40:1974.

138. Veronesi U, Cascinelli N, Bufalino R: Evaluation of the risk of multiple primaries in malignant cutaneous melanoma. *Tumori.* 1976;62:127.

139. Breslow A: Prognosis in cutaneous melanoma: Tumor thickness as a guide to treatment. *Pathol Annu.* 1980;15:1.

140. Clark WH Jr, From L, Bernardino EA, et al: The histogenesis and biologic behavior of primary human malignant melanomas of the skin. *Cancer Res.* 1969;29:705.

141. Urist MM, Balch CM, Soong SJ, et al: Head and neck melanoma in 534 clinical stage I patients. A prognostic factors analysis and results of surgical treatment. *Ann Surg.* 1984;200:769.

142. Wayte DM, Helwig EB: Melanotic freckle of Hutchinson. *Cancer.* 1968;21:893.

143. Harwood AR: Conventional fractionated radiotherapy for 51 patients with lentigo maligna and lentigo maligna melanoma. *Int J Radiat Oncol Biol Phys.* 1983;9:1019.

144. Sutherland CM, Mather FJ, Muchmore JH, et al: Acral lentiginous melanoma. *Am J Surg.* 1993;166:64.

145. Sause WT, Cooper JS, Rush S, et al: Fraction size in external beam radiation therapy in the treatment of melanoma. *Int J Radiat Oncol Biol Phys.* 1991;20:429.

146. Ang KK, Byers RM, Peters LJ, et al: Regional radiotherapy as adjuvant treatment for head and neck malignant melanoma. Preliminary results. *Arch Otolaryngol Head Neck Surg.* 1990; 116:169.

147. Sneed PK, Phillips TL: Combining hyperthermia and radiation: How beneficial? *Oncology.* 1991;5:99.

148. Overgaard J, Gonzalez DG, Hulshof MCCM, et al: Randomized trial of hyperthermia as adjuvant to radiotherapy for recurrent or metastatic malignant melanoma. *Lancet.* 1995;345:540.

149. Barranco SC, Romsdahl MM, Humphrey RM: The radiation response of human malignant melanoma cells grown in vitro. *Cancer Res.* 1971;31:830.

150. Dewey DL: The radiosensitivity of melanoma cells in culture. *Br J Radiol.* 1971;44:816.

151. Overgaard J, Overgaard M, Hansen PV, et al: Some factors of importance in the radiation treatment of malignant melanoma. *Radiother Oncol.* 1986;5:183.

152. Habermalz HJ, Fischer JJ: Radiation therapy of malignant melanoma: Experience with high individual treatment doses. *Cancer.* 1976;38:2258.

153. Hornsey S: The relationship between total dose, number of fractions and fractions size in the response of malignant melanoma in patients. *Br J Radiol.* 1978;51:905.

154. Ziegler JC, Cooper JS: Brain metastases from malignant melanoma: Conventional vs. high-dose-per-fraction radiotherapy. *Int J Radiat Oncol Biol Phys.* 1986;12:1839.

155. Rate WR, Solin LJ, Turrisi AT: Palliative radiotherapy for metastatic malignant melanoma: Brain metastases, bone metastases, and spinal cord compression. *Int J Radiat Oncol Biol Phys.* 1988; 15:859.

156. Konefal JB, Emami B, Pilepich MV: Analysis of dose fractionation in the palliation of metastases from malignant melanoma. *Cancer.* 1988;61:243.

157. Lobo PA, Liebner EJ, Chao JJ, et al: Radiotherapy in the management of malignant melanoma. *Int J Radiat Oncol Biol Phys.* 1981;7:21.

158. Katz HR: The results of different fractionation schemes in the palliative irradiation of metastatic melanoma. *Int J Radiat Oncol Biol Phys.* 1981;7:907.

159. Fertil B, Malaise EP: Intrinsic radiosensitivity of human cell lines is correlated with radioresponsiveness of human tumors: Analysis of 101 published survival curves. *Int J Radiat Oncol Biol Phys.* 1985;11:1699.

160. Rofstad EK: Radiation biology of malignant melanoma. *Acta Radiol Oncol.* 1986;25:1.

161. Swift PS, Fu KK: Radiation therapy for melanoma. In Leong SPL, ed. *Malignant Melanomas: Advances in Treatment.* Boca Raton, Fla: CRC Press; 1992:64.

162. Ho RC: Medical management of stage IV malignant melanoma. Medical issues. *Cancer.* 1995;75:735.

163. Hafstrom L, Rudenstam CM, Blomquist E: Regional hyperthermic perfusion with melphalan after surgery for recurrent malignant melanoma of the extremities. *J Clin Oncol.* 1991;9:2091.

164. Seigler HF, Shingleton WW, Pickrell KL: Intralesional BCG, intravenous immune lymphocytes, and immunization with neuraminidase-treated tumor cells to manage melanoma: A clinical assessment. *Plast Reconstr Surg.* 1975;55:294.

165. Legha SS: Current therapy for malignant melanoma. *Semin Oncol.* 1989;16:34.

166. McClay EF, Mastrangelo MJ, Berd D, et al: Effective combination chemo-hormonal therapy for malignant melanoma: Experience with three consecutive trials. *Int J Cancer.* 1992;50:553.

167. Lejeune F, Lienard D, Eggermont A, et al: Clinical experience with high-dose tumor necrosis factor alpha in regional therapy of advanced melanoma. *Circ Shock.* 1994;43:191.

168. Whittington R, Faulds D: Interleukin-2. A review of its pharmacological properties and therapeutic use in patients with cancer. *Drugs.* 1993;46:446.

169. Vaglini M, Belli F, Santinami M, et al: Isolation perfusion in extracorporeal circulation with interleukin-2 and lymphokine-activated killer cells in the treatment of in-transit metastases from limb cutaneous melanoma. *Ann Surg Oncol.* 1995;2:61.

170. Stevens EJ, Jacknin L, Robbins PF, et al: Generation of tumor-specific CTLs from melanoma patients by using peripheral blood stimulated with allogeneic melanoma tumor cell lines. Fine specificity and MART-1 melanoma antigen recognition. *J Immunol.* 1995;154:762.

171. Foa R, Guarini A, Cignetti A, et al: Cytokine gene therapy: A new strategy for the management of cancer patients. *Nat Immun.* 1994;13:65.

172. Toker C: Trabecular carcinoma of the skin. *Arch Dermatol.* 1972;105:107.

173. Sibley RK, Dehner LP, Rosai J: Primary neuroendocrine (Merkel cell?) carcinoma of the skin: I. A clinicopathologic and ultrastructural study of 43 cases. *Am J Surg Pathol.* 1985;9:95.

174. Cotlar AM, Gates JO, Gibbs FA Jr: Merkel cell carcinoma: Combined surgery and radiation therapy. *Am Surg.* 1986;52:159.

175. Rice RD Jr, Chonkich GD, Thompson KS, et al: Merkel cell tumor of the head and neck. Five new cases with literature review. *Arch Otolaryngol Head Neck Surg.* 1993;119:782.

176. Morrison WH, Peters LJ, Silva EG, et al: The essential role of radiation therapy in securing locoregional control of Merkel cell carcinoma. *Int J Radiat Oncol Biol Phys.* 1990;19:583.

177. Wilder RB, Harari PM, Graham AR, et al: Merkel cell carcinoma. Improved locoregional control with postoperative radiation therapy. *Cancer.* 1991;68:1004.

178. Pacella J, Ashby M, Ainslie J, et al: The role of radiotherapy in the management of primary cutaneous neuroendocrine tumors (Merkel cell or trabecular carcinoma): Experience at the Peter MacCallum Cancer Institute (Melbourne, Australia). *Int J Radiat Oncol Biol Phys.* 1988;14:1077.

179. O'Brien PC, Denham JW, Leong AS: Merkel cell carcinoma: A review of behaviour patterns and management strategies. *Aust NZ J Surg.* 1987;57:847.

180. Meeuwissen JA, Bourne RG, Kearsley JH: The importance of postoperative radiation therapy in the treatment of Merkel cell carcinoma. *Int J Radiat Oncol Biol Phys.* 1995;31:325.

181. Goepfert H, Remmler D, Silva E, et al: Merkel cell carcinoma (endocrine carcinoma of the skin) of the head and neck. *Arch Otolaryngol.* 1984;110:707.

182. Knox SJ, Kapp DS: Hyperthermia and radiation therapy in the treatment of recurrent Merkel cell tumors. *Cancer.* 1988;62:1479.

183. Bart RS, Kopf AW: Tumor conference #46: Merkel-cell carcinoma of the skin. *J Dermatol Surg Oncol.* 1983;9:130.

184. Boyle F, Pendlebury S, Bell D: Further insights into the natural history and management of primary cutaneous neuroendocrine (Merkel cell) carcinoma. *Int J Radiat Oncol Biol Phys.* 1994;31:315.

185. Raaf JH, Urmacher C, Knapper WK, et al: Trabecular (Merkel cell) carcinoma of the skin. Treatment of primary, recurrent, and metastatic disease. *Cancer.* 1986;57:178.

186. Westgate SJ: Radiation therapy for skin tumors. *Otolaryngol Clin North Am.* 1993;26:295.

187. Feun LG, Savaraj N, Legha SS, et al: Chemotherapy for metastatic Merkel cell carcinoma. Review of the M D Anderson Hospital's experience. *Cancer.* 1988;62:683.

188. Grosh WW, Giannone L, Hande KR, et al: Disseminated Merkel cell tumor. Treatment with systemic chemotherapy. *Am J Clin Oncol.* 1987;10:227.

189. Pollack SV, Goslen JB: Small-cell neuroepithelial tumor of skin: A Merkel-cell neoplasm? *J Dermatol Surg Oncol.* 1982;8:116.

190. Wick MR, Goellner JR, Scheithauer BW, et al: Primary neuroendocrine carcinomas of the skin (Merkel cell tumors). A clinical, histologic, and ultrastructural study of thirteen cases. *Am J Clin Pathol.* 1983;79:6.

191. George TK, di Sant'agnese PA, Bennett JM: Chemotherapy for metastatic Merkel cell carcinoma. *Cancer.* 1985;56:1034.

192. Fenig E, Lurie H, Klein B, et al: The treatment of advanced Merkel cell carcinoma. A multimodality chemotherapy and radiation therapy treatment approach. *J Dermatol Surg Oncol.* 1993;19:860.

193. Tai Patricia TH, Yu E, Winquist E, et al: Chemotherapy in neuroendocrine/Merkel cell carcinoma of the skin: Case series and review of 204 cases. *J Clin Oncol.* 2000;18:2493.

194. Hill ADJ, Brady MS, Coit DG: Intraoperative lymphatic mapping and sentinel lymph node biopsy for Merkel cell carcinoma. *Br J Surg.* 1999;86;518.

195. Messina JL, Reintgen DS, Cruse CW, et al: Selective lymphadenopathy in patients with Merkel cell (cutaneous neuroendocrine) Carcinoma. *Ann Surg Oncol.* 1997;4;389.

196. Ames SE, Krag DN, Brady MS: Radiolocalization of the sentinel lymph node in Merkel cell carcinoma: A clinical analysis of seven cases. *J Surg Oncol.* 1998;67:251.

HIV-Related Malignancies

Patrick S. Swift, MD

THE SCOPE OF THE PROBLEM

In July 2002, the Joint United Nations Programme on HIV/AIDS estimated that 40 million people were living with the human immunodeficiency virus (HIV) in the world, with 5 million new infections occurring in 2001 alone.[1] During that same year, HIV-associated illnesses caused death in approximately 3 million people worldwide. The Global AIDS Policy Coalition postulated that more than 60 million people had been infected with HIV through the end of 2001, one third of whom were 15 to 24 years old. In North America, 940,000 people were believed to be living with the virus, while 45,000 new infections and 20,000 deaths occurred in 2001. The impact in terms of loss of life, decreased life expectancy, and financial burden for major sections of the world is staggering.

In the United States and other first-world nations, the widespread introduction of a new class of drugs called the protease inhibitors in 1996 marked a transition point in the outlook for people living with HIV.[2] As part of an approach termed highly active anti-retroviral therapy (HAART) (Tables 67-1 and 67-2), these and subsequent classes of drugs have led to a major reconstitution of some portion of the immune function of most patients. Unfortunately, the great expense of these medications and the complexity of the dosing regimens places them beyond the reach of much of the affected population worldwide.

Among those with access to HAART, the median time from seroconversion to the development of an AIDS-defining illness increased from 8 years (before 1995) to 20 years (after mid-1997).[2-4] Mortality rates declined steeply from late 1995 to early 1997 due to the introduction

of the newer classes of anti-retroviral agents and the institution of triple drug regimens.[3] Similar decreases were seen in the incidence of serious opportunistic infections and new cases of frank AIDS, with those patients treated most aggressively showing the greatest degree of benefit.

From the earliest days of the epidemic, several malignancies were found to occur more commonly in HIV-infected patients than in the general population, most notably Kaposi's sarcoma (KS) and non-Hodgkin's lymphoma (NHL).[5,6] Cervical cancer concurrent with HIV infection was also officially designated a criterion for diagnosis of AIDS,[7,8] and other diseases such as anal carcinoma, Hodgkin's disease, squamous cell cancer of the skin, and conjunctive and non–small-cell cancer of the lung[9] are considered by some as associated malignancies in this setting. Of great interest is the fact that four of these malignancies (KS, NHL, and cervical and anal cancer) are associated with specific viral infections in addition to HIV (human herpesvirus type 8 [HHV8], also known as Kaposi's sarcoma-associated herpesvirus [KSHV]; Epstein-Barr virus [EBV]; and human papillomavirus [HPV]).[10,11]

The scope of the oncological problem could potentially increase over time because of three major factors. First, as the number of infected patients continues to rise, the incidence of some established HIV-related malignancies

Table 67–1   Definition of Highly Active Antiretroviral Therapy Used by the Multi-Center AIDS Cohort Study

One of the Following Combinations:
2 or more NRTIs + 1 PI or 1 NNRTI
1 NRTI + 1 PI + 1 or more NNRTI
Ritonavir + Saquinavir + 1 NRTI
Abacavir + 3 or more NRTIs

NNRTI, non-nucleoside reverse transcriptase inhibitor; NRTI, nucleoside or nucleotide reverse transcriptase inhibitors; PI, protease inhibitor.
From DHHS/Henry J Kaplan Foundation Panel on Clinical Practices for the Treatment of HIV Infection, "Guidelines for the use of anti-retroviral agents in HIV-infected adults and adolescents," http://hiv.atis.org, 2002.

Table 67–2   Classes of Drugs in Highly Active Antiretroviral Therapy

Nucleoside or Nucleotide Reverse Transcriptase Inhibitors (NRTI)		
AZT	DdC	DAPD
D4T	DdI	
3TC	Abacavir	
FTC	Tenofavir	
Non-Nucleoside Reverse Transcriptase Inhibitors (NNRTI)		
Nevirapine	Efavirenz	TMC-125
Delavirdine	Capravirine	
Protease Inhibitors (PI)		
Saquinivir	Lopinavir	Amprenavir
Ritonavir	Indinavir	Nelfinavir
Atazanavir	Tipranavir	
Fusion Inhibitors		
Pentafuside		

From http://www.projectinform.com.

will continue to rise.[6,12-14] On a worldwide level, for instance, KS is very common. Second, as patients survive longer with the development of effective therapeutic interventions such as HAART, they can be expected to develop malignancies commonly found in the general population.[5,9,15,16] Currently, the average age group infected with HIV in the United States is the 25- to 45-year-old group, but a significant portion of those infected are surviving to reach older age. These older patients are at risk for the development of such common diseases as prostate, colon, and lung cancer. Patients who present with malignancies unrelated to HIV infection in the setting of inadequately managed HIV disease tend to have more aggressive presentations and more rapidly progressive courses, combined with a decreased ability to tolerate full-scale intervention. A longer period of life with some degree of immunosuppression may ultimately result in a greater incidence of these malignancies later in life, compared to the general population. Third, as it has been shown that the main HIV-related tumors may have as a common element initiation by concomitant viral mechanisms, such as EBV, KSHV, and HPV,[17-21] other virally initiated malignancies with longer latency periods may become evident.[22] Rising rates of co-infection with hepatitis C, for example, are associated with increasing incidence of hepatocellular carcinoma and hepatoblastoma.[23]

DEVELOPING A STRATEGY

Developing a strategy for the optimal radiotherapeutic management of malignancies in the setting of HIV disease requires the oncologist to become aware of a number of factors: the patient's immune status at the time of diagnosis; history of prior opportunistic insults; current viral burden; antiretroviral interventions previously attempted or currently in use; presence of a polyresistant strain or strains of HIV; potential interactions between antiretroviral drugs and oncological interventions; and the patient's willingness to risk significant morbidity and further stress on the immune system associated with systemic chemotherapy or large-field irradiation in the setting of an already reduced life expectancy (Table 67-3). Treatments that might have been appropriate in 1995 may be less so in 2004.

A key event in the immunopathogenesis of HIV immunosuppression is the attachment of the virus to the external envelope protein gp120 and CD4 molecule that is present on the CD4+ T lymphocyte.[24] These lymphocytes are crucial for the immunologic response to various pathogens through interactions with B cells, NK cells, cytotoxic T cells, and monocyte/macrophages through the release of cytokines. In addition, CD4+ T lymphocytes influence the growth of lymphoid and hematopoietic cells. These actions add up to the critical role that the CD4+ cell plays in maintaining a healthy immune response to pathogens in the immunocompetent individual. In the healthy non–HIV-infected person, the CD4+ count is between 600 and 1200 cells/mm^3. Infection with HIV results in a quantitative drop, and perhaps a qualitative decline, in CD4+ T cells in the initial postinfection period,

which tends to be temporary. After a latency period that lasts from months to more than 10 years, during which viral replication continues at a variable rate from individual to individual, the viral burden gradually begins to rise and the CD4+ T cell count declines. Measurements of these levels are used as surrogate markers for the state of the immunocompetence of the patient and the risk for various HIV-related illnesses. As the count drops below 500, certain diseases such as thrush or KS can be seen. With further decline below 200 cells/mm^3, the incidence of *P. carinii* pneumonia and other life-threatening infections increases.

The nadir that the CD4+ count reached before effective institution of HAART is an important level. It is not yet clear that the reconstitution of the immune system via HAART, as evidenced by a climbing CD4+ count, truly represents a resurrection of the full complement of immune surveillance cell lines. The lower the nadir, the greater the possibility that some degree of immunodeficiency will persist.[25,26]

Patients who develop malignancies in the setting of HIV disease may present at any point during their postinfection period and would be expected to have a different tolerance to intervention, depending on the degree of their immune decline. There is a clear relationship between the CD4 level and the risk of aggressive opportunistic infections in patients with HIV disease. As an example, a 50-year-old HIV-positive patient with stage T2a prostate cancer, a CD4 count of 550 cells/mm^3, an undetectable viral load on his first regimen of HAART, and no prior infections should obviously not be approached in the same way as a similar man with a CD4 count of less than 10 cells/mm^3, a high viral burden, a viral strain that has been shown to be resistant to a number of drug regimens, and a history of two bouts of pneumocystic and cryptococcal meningitis. But what of a man with a CD4 count of 150 cells/mm^3, no prior use of antiretroviral agents, and one episode of pneumocystic pneumonia? Therapeutic nihilism is not justifiable in such cases, as there is a significant chance that such a patient would live long enough to succumb to progressive prostate cancer rather than to AIDS.

In addition to the standard past medical history of the patient, factors unique to HIV disease must be taken into account. By analyzing the past infectious history, known

Table 67–3   Factors Affecting Radiotherapeutic Decisions

Patient-Related

Time since seroconversion
Prior opportunistic diseases
Prior antiretroviral history
CD4+ count, trend over time
Current viral burden
CD4+ nadir
Presence of polyresistant strains

Treatment-Related

Extent of radiation (dose, field size)
Definitive versus prophylactic intent
Concurrent chemotherapy
Proven benefit versus experimental

duration of disease (time since seroconversion), immune status (indicator: CD4 count), history of the success or failure of prior antiretroviral regimens, and current viral burden, the treating clinician can get an idea of the rapidity of decline of the overall immune system and a rough estimate of the expected life duration.[15,27-29] This information is critical in defining the optimal treatment path for the patient, regardless of the particular malignancy being addressed (HIV-related or unrelated tumors). A decision is made to treat with curative or palliative intent. If the latter, an estimation must be made of the expected length of time that palliation may be required to assure maximal quality of life. Once a course of treatment is chosen, the initiation of antiretroviral therapy should be strongly considered for those patients who have not previously been treated with such agents or who have received minimal therapy. The initiation of systemic chemotherapy or extensive radiation is a major stress that may redirect critical immune resources from maintaining a balance with the prime offender, HIV, allowing a rapid increase in overall viral burden.

Added to this equation is information regarding the relative benefits of the proposed treatment. The selection of initial whole pelvic irradiation for T_3 prostate cancer in the absence of measurable adenopathy, for instance, may be defensible in the HIV-negative patient, but such a challenge might prove imprudent in the patient with a CD4 count below 100 cells/mm^3. Likewise, the routine use of combined chemoradiotherapy, although preferred for HIV-negative patients with cervical carcinoma, may have devastating consequences in the patient with advanced HIV-infection that is drug resistant. Treatment selection must weigh the potential benefits (local control, improved survival, quality of life) against the risk of causing further deterioration of the immune system in the face of HIV disease. With median life expectancies of 20 years after seroconversion and treatment with HAART, substantial time exists during which the patient can develop considerable degradation of life quality due to under- or over-treated malignancies.

KAPOSI'S SARCOMA

Epidemiology

Since the first description of the lesions of KS in 1872 by Moritz Kaposi,[30] four separate subgroups of patients with the disease have been identified.[31] The classic disease, seen in elderly men of Eastern European and Middle Eastern extraction, particularly Ashkenazic Jews, is an indolent disease that usually involves the lower extremities, is gradually progressive, is very sensitive to radiation, and is rarely fatal. A second group, identified in the 1960s, is made up of young men and children with nodular disease and no evidence of underlying immuno-suppression in the countries of sub-Saharan Africa, particularly Uganda and Zaire. This disease disseminates more widely than the classic form, may involve the viscera, and not infrequently progresses to a more critical condition with resultant death after several years.[32,33] The third group comprises patients undergoing chronic

immunosuppression after organ transplantation. KS appears at a median of 22 months after transplantation and tends to regress with cessation of the deliberate immunosuppression.[34-36]

Since the first reports of KS in homosexual men in 1981,[37-39] the sheer numerical increase in incidence has been due to a fourth group: patients with HIV disease who either present with KS as their first AIDS-defining illness or develop the disease in the course of the gradual deterioration of their immune systems. A fifth group must also be mentioned: homosexual men with no evidence of HIV disease but with pathologically identified KS.[40-46]

KS accounts for the largest number of AIDS-related malignancies reported to the Centers for Disease Control and Prevention (CDC).[47] Early in the epidemic, KS was one of the two most common presenting illnesses of AIDS, along with *P. carinii* pneumonia, but its appearance differed significantly among risk groups. Between 1981 and 1983 in New York City, 51% of homosexual males with AIDS as well as 32% of homosexual males with a history of IV drug abuse presented with KS, but only 5% of heterosexual drug abusers and close to 0% of partners of heterosexual drug users developed KS.[19,48] From 1984 to 1987, the incidence of KS at presentation had declined to 30% among all homosexual men with AIDS and 15% of homosexual IV drug abusers, but remained constant at about 3% in the heterosexual group of IV drug abusers. In a 1993 report from the CDC,[20] KS was being reported in 17% to 19% of homosexual patients, 3% to 5% of heterosexual IV drug abusers, and only 1% to 2% in cases of transfusion or hemophilia-related AIDS. In a report from 17 Western European nations based on the European Non-Aggregate AIDS Data Set, the appearance of KS as the initial AIDS-defining illness fell steadily from 13% in 1988 to 6.4% in 1998.[49] In a meta-analysis of more than 47,000 patients, the incidence of KS as either a first defining illness or subsequent AIDS diagnosis fell from 15.2 per 1000 patient years before the HAART era to 4.9 per 1000 patient years during the HAART era.[50] The CDC's report on more than 37,000 patients in the Adult/Adolescent Spectrum of Disease project showed a 50% reduction in the incidence of KS with the use of a three-drug antiviral regimen.[51] This represents a dramatic reduction in the incidence of a disease that in the early 1990s affected 50% of HIV-positive patients eventually.[25,26] In Africa, however, KS remains the most common form of cancer diagnosed in men, and is second most common in women, with a relative risk of 35 for sero-positive patients.

Pathogenesis

HHV-8, also known as KSHV, was identified in 1994 and has subsequently been identified in almost all HIV-related and HIV-unrelated KS tissue.[25,26] Chang and associates[21] of Columbia identified unique DNA sequences in more than 90% of samples of KS tissue from HIV-infected adults, sequences that were not present in the DNA of HIV-negative patients and found in only 15% of non-KS tissue from HIV-infected patients. These DNA sequences showed a homology to two previously identified herpesviruses (EBV and saimiri virus), but differed enough to suggest the presence of a new human herpesvirus. In a separate analysis of 21 tissue samples of KS, the herpes-like DNA sequence was identified in 95%: 10 of 11 patients with AIDS-associated KS, all 6 patients with classic KS, and all 4 HIV-negative homosexual patients with KS.[52] These findings suggested that this agent was responsible for all three forms of KS. In 14 samples of uninvolved skin from patients with KS, the sequence was found in only 3, and in only 1 of 21 control samples tested. The HHV-8 virus has a 100% association with the KS seen in HIV disease, but although it has been identified in saliva, mucous membranes, semen, and gastrointestinal membranes, its mode of transmission remains unclear.

In its earliest manifestations, KS does not appear to be a true sarcoma but rather a reactive process resulting from an interaction of the latent forms of HHV-8 and HIV. This fits with the clinical observation of multiple sites of involvement at initial diagnosis, often with symmetrical or dermatomal distributions. By itself, infection with HHV-8 is not sufficient to lead to the development of KS. In areas where non–HIV-related KS is endemic, for instance, HHV-8 is found in high penetrance, yet few go on to develop the lesions. Likewise, in patients who develop KS while receiving immunosuppressive drugs after organ transplant, KS often spontaneously regresses after withdrawal of the immunosuppressive agents. In the setting of AIDS, HIV is felt to play an integral role in the development of the KS lesion through an initiation process of chronic antigenic stimulation and CD8+ activation. Activated CD8+ cells release a series of cytokines (T helper type 1, Th-1) that include γ-IFN, TNF-α, IL-1-β, IL-2, and IL-6. These inflammatory cytokines carry out a series of actions that lead to the early reactive form of the KS lesion. Activated endothelial cells in the area are induced to release adhesion molecules and secondary cytokines that recruit circulating cells into the area, including HHV-8–infected macrophages. Cytokines induce the transformation of endothelial cells into the spindle cells characteristic of the early lesions, cells that respond to the release by HIV of the Tat-1 protein with increased growth and aggressive behavior with invasive capability. These inflammatory cytokines induce the process of angiogenesis by causing the spindle cells to release substantial quantities of bFGF and VEGF. This process is a complex interplay of inflammatory cells, cytokines, and endothelial cells that results in neoangiogenesis, edema, extravasation of red blood cells, and spindle cell growth.[53] During periods of immune decline with new opportunistic infections, additional inflammatory cytokines are released, explaining why new diffuse lesions are often observed shortly after a patient develops such an infection. Up to this point, however, the typical lesion is usually still composed of a polyclonal array of spindle cells. Persistent expression of the HHV-8 latency gene products over time may result in the overexpression of antiapoptotic mechanisms, such as bcl-2, and upregulation of oncogenes. This deregulation can eventually result in the formation of monoclonal cell lines that go on to form the nodular form of KS and become a full-scale sarcoma.

Clinical Presentation

Clinically, KS presents in a vast array of forms, including macular, nodular, or plaque-like lesions, lymphadenopathic involvement, and visceral spread. In the earliest stage of the disease, macular lesions arise in the reticular dermis. Clusters of small, irregular, jagged spaces lined with endothelium surround normal dermal vessels and adnexal structures, with an inflammatory component of variable intensity. As it progresses into a plaque form, the disease infiltrates the entire dermis into the subcutaneous fat. Kaposi's spindle cells are seen, forming irregular vascular channels throughout the dermal collagen bundles. These spindle cells form sheets and fascicles with cytological atypia, necrosis, and trapped red blood cells, with blockage of normal lymphatic channels. Involvement of lymph nodes is common, with replacement of normal lymph node architecture by diffuse spindle cells and plasma cell infiltrates. Biopsies of these lesions are important because the differential diagnosis includes various other conditions, including bacillary angiomatosis (Bartonella species), hemangioma, lymphangioendothelioma, acroangiodermatitis, angiosarcoma, angiolipoma, and scar tissue.[31]

The earliest lesion is a small flat painless purplish lesion, varying in size from several millimeters to several centimeters, arising anywhere on the skin or mucosal surfaces. These are often initially mistaken for insect or flea bites. KS may occur either singly or as multiple lesions scattered on the skin surface. Preferred skin sites include the nose and face, pinnae and retroauricular regions, trunk, groin, penis, buttocks, extremities, toes, and soles of feet, usually sparing the palms of the hands. One particularly common feature is a symmetrical distribution of lesions (such as the arches of both soles or similar locations on each extremity). Other surfaces frequently involved and easily examined include the conjunctivae, palate, tonsils, alveolar ridges, posterior pharynx, and low rectum. Superinfection with fungi or bacteria may be present, changing the characteristic appearance of lesions. Biopsy confirmation of the diagnosis is strongly recommended before initiation of any aggressive therapy, as the diagnosis carries with it a tremendous psychological burden for the patient. Although KS may appear at any time in the course of HIV disease, less than one sixth of cases occur when the patient's CD4 count is above 500 cells/mm^3.[31] The majority of patients present after their CD4 count has fallen below 100 cells/mm^3.

Isolated lesions may remain stable for months to years, with an occasional new lesion discovered on a weekly or monthly basis as long as the person is in reasonably good health. Lesions initially identified before the institution of antiretroviral therapy often regress substantially as immunocompetence is restored. In the patient with refractory HIV, however, the progression may be rapid. Although the amount of disease may appear small at first and the physical discomfort minimal, the psychological burden of the disease cannot be overstated. As HIV disease progresses, and the immune system declines, new infectious complications occur, such as pneumocystis or toxoplasmosis. With the resolution or progression of each of these insults, KS tends to seize the opportunity and advance, as evidenced by a shower of new lesions, decreasing time interval between new lesions, growth of existing lesions with associated ecchymosis, and coalescence of nearby lesions into a larger plaque form. The lesions may take on a more nodular appearance, are often painful, and become more extensive subcutaneously. Involvement of the regional lymph nodes and lymphatic spaces occurs, leading to progressive edema, most commonly seen in the legs, groins, and genitalia or in the facial and periorbital regions. Massive edema develops because of complete obstruction of the lymphatic channels, interfering with ambulation, urination, and vision. Edema in the lower extremities may eventually lead to breakdown of the skin, with severe pain and superinfection.

Internal involvement with KS (present in up to 80% of cases at autopsy[54]) is usually quiet in the early stages of disease, but may become life-threatening in 10% to 20% of patients with KS.[31,55] Autopsy studies reveal that gastrointestinal tract involvement is seen in up to 50% of patients with KS, and lung involvement in 41%.[56] Patients with gastrointestinal tract involvement may develop substantial bleeding, particularly with stomach and rectal lesions, that requires intervention. Pulmonary involvement may progress rapidly to florid respiratory compromise and death, with a median life expectancy of 3 to 4 months.[57] Because many different pulmonary infections may be indistinguishable from KS on plain chest x-rays, bronchoscopy with visual or pathologic verification is necessary. Gallium-negativity and thallium-positivity may help establish the diagnosis.[54]

Staging

The AIDS Clinical Trial Group developed a staging system for AIDS-related KS that incorporates information about the clinical extent of KS, the current status of the immune system, and the presence or history of other HIV-related illnesses (Table 67-4).[58] The value of this staging system has been proved prospectively to predict survival.[59] It offers some guidance to the radiation oncologist in the process of devising a treatment strategy.

Management: General Approach

The impact of HAART on KS is difficult to overstate. Multiple studies have shown a remarkable decline in the incidence of KS after institution of effective antiretroviral therapy, as well as objective regression and prolongation of times to progression.[25,26,50,60-62] Therefore, the initial approach to this disease should be an active discussion regarding the institution of HAART in the naïve patient, or the optimization of the antiretroviral regimen of a patient who is progressing on an earlier regimen with a rising viral burden. Patients who are failing their antiretroviral regimen will go on to require additional treatment. Occasionally, patients may see their KS progress even while their viral burden is low and their CD4+ counts are high, but usually at a much slower pace.

Patients can initially be divided into three categories based on the amount of KS present: those with only a few

Table 67–4 AIDS Clinical Trial Group Staging System for Kaposi's Sarcoma (KS)

	Good Risk All of the Following	Poor Risk Any of the Following
Tumor (T)	Confined to skin, lymph nodes, minimal oral disease, or more than one	Tumor-associated edema or ulceration
		Extensive oral KS
		Gastrointestinal KS
		KS in other non-nodal sites
Immune system (I)	CD4+ count ≧200	CD4+ count <200
Systemic illness (S)	No history of thrush or OI No B symptoms KPS ≧70	History of thrush or OI B symptoms present KPS <70 Other HIV-related illness

KPS, Karnofoky performance score; OI, opportunistic infections
From Dezube BJL: Acquired immunodeficiency syndrome-related Kaposi's sarcoma: Clinical features, staging, and treatment. *Semin Oncol.* 2000;27:424.

lesions that are relatively stable or associated with minor symptoms; those with advanced disease including lesions too numerous to count, lymphadenopathic or visceral involvement, and large plaque-like areas of involvement; and those with an intermediate burden who have many lesions, mostly asymptomatic and not associated with appreciable edema. The first group can be further subdivided based on their immune status: CD4 count greater than 200 cells/mm³ with no major prior opportunistic infections; CD4 count less than 200 cells/mm³ with a limited history of opportunistic infections; CD4 count close to 0 cells/mm³ with multiple opportunistic infections. The rapidity of the downward trend in the CD4 count is more useful than the absolute number itself, as the trend indicates the stability of the overall immune status.[63-67]

Patients with minimal disease and relatively intact immune systems should be treated with minimal interventions. These patients have long life expectancies (in the range of years), and care should be taken not to treat them in such a way as to hasten the progression of the HIV disease. Since many of these patients are continuing to work and carry on fully active lives, however, cosmetic concerns must be addressed. Local therapies for KS are available (see later discussion). Watchful waiting is also an acceptable approach in this cohort.

Patients with minimal stable disease but a collapsed immune system, as evidenced by a low CD4 count or recent opportunistic infections, should also be treated with local therapies for symptomatic disease. This group, as well as those with minimal but noticeably progressive disease, should be considered for entry into trials of nonchemotherapeutic biological modifiers.

Patients who present with advanced disease, including those with significant areas of painful and growing KS, lymphatic spread, and sludging with resultant edema or visceral involvement, should be considered for systemic therapy. Radiation should be used for relief of local symptoms that are unresponsive to the systemic therapy, or more liberally in the patient who either refuses systemic approaches or who is too neutropenic to tolerate them. In some circumstances, patients may be undergoing therapy with agents such as ganciclovir for active cytomegalovirus retinitis, which will prevent the immediate initiation of chemotherapy, thereby necessitating the use of radiation in the interim.

Local Therapies

Aside from radiotherapy, a number of modalities are available for local therapy of KS. The choice is based on the location of the lesion, prior responsiveness to each modality, and the expected side effects of the modality. Alitretinoin gel, a patient-administered topical gel, is a naturally occurring retinoid that binds to both retinoic acid receptors and retinoid X receptors, as a regulator of both cell proliferation and apoptosis. In phase III trials, comparing isotretinoin gel 0.1% with the vehicle gel alone, isotretinoin resulted in 49% to 67% response rates, with a duration of response of up to 65 weeks. The applications took 4 to 8 weeks for most patients to achieve best results. It was well tolerated, with some dermal irritation noted at the application site.[54,68,69]

Intralesional injections with 0.01 to 0.02 mg of vinblastine to a maximum of three injections per lesion have resulted in a response rate of 92% in 190 lesions in 15 patients injected by Newman,[70] with a median duration of 4.5 months. Local pain and irritation are the main side effects.[71-73] Intra-oral lesions have also been successfully treated with this approach,[73] although lesions larger than 3 cm usually are considered too large to treat with injections. Tetradecyl sulfate has also been used as an effective intralesional agent.[74] Cryotherapy, with liquid nitrogen, is used by dermatologists for small lesions of the face, neck, and hands. In a phase II efficacy study from San Francisco General Hospital, Tappero and associates[75] reported 88% major responses, lasting from 6 weeks to 6 months, with the best results seen in lesions smaller than 1 cm. Local inflammation with minor blistering and pain occurs after treatment, with residual hypopigmentation seen occasionally after treatment of larger lesions. Due to the ease of administration and small expense, treatment by intralesional injections or cryotherapy is preferred for lesions smaller than 1 cm, with the exception of sensitive sites such as the penis, soles of feet, and conjunctivae.

None of these local approaches has been proven superior to any other. Residual evidence of the disease process generally remains, whether it be a scar associated with laser therapy or cryotherapy or persistent pigmentation after radiation or intralesional injections. The aim of each modality is to limit progression in the local site.

Systemic Therapies

For patients with rapidly progressive disease, extensive disease at presentation, or visceral and lymphadenopathic disease, consideration must be given to systemic chemotherapy. Local therapies such as radiation may be carefully interdigitated with chemotherapy for particularly bothersome sites of involvement, but systemic therapy is the mainstay. The main two chemotherapeutic approaches involve the administration of either liposomal doxorubicin or paclitaxel. Liposomal doxorubicin at 20 mg/m^2 every 2 to 3 weeks has a response rate of 46% to 59%, with a duration of response of 3 to 6 months,[76] and is generally well tolerated. Paclitaxel at 100 mg/m^2 every 2 weeks has a response rate of 56%, with a duration of response of 9 months, but with higher toxicity.[77] Vinorelbine at 30 mg/m^2 every 2 weeks results in a 43% response rate and low levels of toxicity.[25,26]

Oral 9-cis-retinoic acid has undergone phase II testing in 60 patients with cutaneous KS, simultaneously with the best available antiretroviral regimens.[78] A 37% response rate was reported regardless of the extent of the disease or the baseline CD4+ and viral levels, with a median time to response of 9 weeks, and a median duration of response that had not been reached by 37 weeks. Toxicity (headaches, skin toxicity) led to withdrawal of the medicine by 28 of the 60 patients, however.

Interferon-alpha has been extensively tested in the treatment of KS, with some success seen in patients with CD4+ counts greater than 200 and no prior history of major opportunistic infection.[79] Its efficacy is increased when used in conjunction with antiretrovirals and when used at higher doses, but its use has been limited by substantial toxicity and the need for frequent subcutaneous injections. The potential mechanisms of action (inhibition of replication of HIV, inhibition of reactivation of HHV-8, inhibition of bFGF, and downregulation of c-*myc* expression by KS spindle cells) make it worthy of further study.

Radiation Therapy

The main indications for radiation treatment for cutaneous KS are to relieve pain associated with progressive lesions, reduce edema (mainly in the face, genitalia, and extremities), and improve cosmesis of visible lesions, notably those on the face and arms (although any lesions may be identified as "cosmetically bothersome" by the patient). No attempt is made to treat all lesions seen on the skin surface, since most are asymptomatic, readily concealed by clothing, and unlikely to disappear completely with the radiation and may progress in the future. In the oral cavity, radiation can be used to treat lesions causing bleeding, loosening of teeth, pain, and interference with eating, swallowing, or speech. Lesions in the pharynx, larynx, trachea, and pulmonary parenchyma may impede respiration and are responsive to radiation. Treatment is appropriate to stop bleeding or pain associated with lesions anywhere in the gastrointestinal tract.

TECHNICAL FACTORS

Small superficial lesions are best treated with superficial electrons of an energy sufficient to ensure treatment of the deepest extent of tumor, or with an orthovoltage unit for thin lesions. Care should be taken to select an orthovoltage beam with a sufficient energy and half-value layer to ensure adequate penetration for treatment of thick tumors. Dose falls off rapidly from the surface and may lead to significant underdosing of all but the thinnest lesions. The treating clinician must be very familiar with the depth dose curves of the energy being used and the variance with field size. Fields should encompass not only the visible extent of disease but the subcutaneous extent as well, with at least a 1-cm margin. When small electron fields are used, attention must be paid to the dose falloff toward the edge of the field. The use of electrons must also take into account the superficial skin sparing seen with low-energy electrons, using enough bolus to adequately bring up the surface dose.

Larger plaque-like areas of disease, with diffuse nodularity, multiple satellite lesions, or considerable edema may require coverage with megavoltage photons. If large-field irradiation is to be used, it must be used cautiously, especially in the lower extremities such as in the treatment of an edematous leg or groin region. Even with low doses, considerable brawny induration may develop within months in the treatment field. This phenomenon occurs at a much lower dose than would be expected in the HIV-negative patient. Since these patients may go on to receive multiple courses of medications such as liposomal doxorubicin, the development of radiation recall may be seen. In setting up the original field, precautions commonly used in the treatment of sarcomas of the limb should be followed, with sparing of as much of the circumference of the extremity as possible. If disease is predominantly located on one surface, a single field rather than an opposed pair would be preferred, to reduce the dose to the opposite side. Adjacent fields need to be adequately gapped to prevent areas of overlap, but every attempt should be made to encompass all disease in the contiguous fields, since missed areas will eventually regrow into the field.

DOSE

Various radiation dosing schemes have been reported for the treatment of KS, from single doses of 800 cGy to fractionated schemes with total doses up to greater than 4000 cGy.[80-97] A prospective randomized study of 54 patients comparing 8 Gy in a single fraction to 16 Gy over four fractions in 596 lesions showed response rates of 77% to 80% with either fractionation scheme.[98] A retrospective review of 6777 lesions treated at a single institution with doses from 10 Gy to 30 Gy to various sites resulted in a 92% response rate, with acceptable toxicity.[99] In another prospective randomized study, confined to the pre-HAART era, in which each patient served as an internal control, 14 patients had a total of 71 cutaneous lesions treated with one of three regimens: 8 Gy in a single fraction, 20 Gy in 10 fractions of 2 Gy, or 40 Gy in 20 fractions of 2 Gy.[87] Complete response rates and duration of control were better in the two higher-dose arms than in the single-fraction arm. Lesions treated to 20 to 40 Gy had a 79% to 83% CR rate (defined as complete resolution of palpable disease regardless of residual pigmentation), whereas the single-fraction CR rate was only 50%. Only 8% of both the 20 and 8 Gy arms were without residual pigmentation, compared to 43% of the 40 Gy group. The 40-week actuarial failure rate was 48% with 40 Gy, 62% with 20 Gy, and 84% with 8 Gy.

No differences were noted in the acute toxicity of the three regimens, but late toxicity was reported only in the high-dose arm. A retrospective review of 187 patients treated to 375 sites at the University of California, San Francisco (UCSF) showed no difference in duration of response for patients treated with a single fraction compared with those treated with higher doses in fractionated schemes. It did, however, find a reduction in acute toxicity with the single fraction.[82] Response, defined as a reduction to 50% of the pretreatment size, regardless of residual pigmentation, occurred in 93% of those treated with 8 Gy, with an actuarial local control rate of 69% at 6 months. This study included oral, visceral, and nodal disease as well as cutaneous disease. A separate study of 74 treatments with 8 Gy resulted in 90% subjective cosmetic improvement, pain relief in 100%, and improved lymphatic drainage in 75%.[80] Duration of control was, however, short, with two thirds of patients showing progression of disease at 4 months.

No single dosing schedule is appropriate for all patients with KS. The final recommendation must take into account the site to be treated, the size of the lesion, the prior treatment (both local and systemic), the particular symptom being addressed, and most importantly, the overall medical condition and life expectancy of the patient. Optimization of the antiviral regimen remains the cornerstone of management, and radiation is reserved for progressive disease in the setting of a declining immune status. Long-term toxicity of radiation should be kept in mind and avoided, however, as the introduction of new classes of antivirals, such as the inhibitors of HIV entry and viral fusion, may rescue patients who have failed current best available HAART.[100]

With those facts in mind, the clinician can make dosing recommendations. Patients with a long history of severe opportunistic infections or diseases such as lymphoma or progressive multifocal leukoencephalopathy and with life expectancies less than 4 months are best approached with a single dose of 8 Gy to small areas of involvement, including oral cavity lesions or bleeding rectal lesions. Such treatment is easy on the patient, eliminates the need for multiple trips to the radiation department, and is likely to provide significant palliation for the duration of life. Larger areas may be treated with short fractionated courses to improve tolerance if bowel or oropharyngeal exposure is of concern, but in our experience, 800 cGy is well tolerated for any body site. If disease recurs or progresses before death, retreatment with the same approach for small regions or with a fractionated course in larger areas is possible with minimal morbidity in most sites.

At the other extreme, patients with high CD4 counts (>100 cells/mm^3), few or no opportunistic infections, and a good overall condition should be treated with a protracted course, in an attempt to prolong the duration of local control for as long as possible, bearing in mind that with disease progression, these patients will be exposed to agents with recall potential, such as doxorubicin. A reasonable approach is to use 200 cGy fractions to a total dose of 2400 cGy, with frequent assessment of level of reaction. This dose is lower than the highest dose regimen in the Washington study[87] but is chosen to reduce late toxicity and to allow for retreatment at the time of disease progression, if necessary.

The intermediate group represents a more difficult decision. These patients, with declining immune systems but prognoses measured still in many months to years, are often under the care of multiple clinicians, with a number of ongoing problems requiring frequent visits to specialists. Prolonging their course of treatment is often an undue burden. One option is the fractionated approach similar to that used routinely in healthier patients; another is treatment with a single dose with close follow-up. As evidenced by the UCSF data,[82] many of these patients will have controlled symptoms until the time of death or will go on to receive systemic chemotherapy for their KS when it progresses generally. At the time of local progression, retreatment can be administered using either another single dose (if the patient is terminally ill or had a prolonged period of control >1 year with the prior treatment) or with a fractionated course. Several reports of retreatment have shown that it is safe as long as original doses were kept low.[82,87,101] Third treatments are strongly discouraged unless the patient is in extremis and immediate pain relief is the goal.

HEAD AND NECK SKIN SITES

Small lesions without associated edema may occur anywhere on the skin of the head, including the scalp and retroauricular region. These lesions are easily treated with small margins around the subcutaneous extent of disease for cosmetic purposes. In terms of cosmetic outcomes, KS lesions rarely completely disappear after radiation. The usual response is a rapid reduction in any associated pain and ecchymosis, a gradual reduction in the size and thickness of the lesion, and a change in color from a violaceous hue to a calmer brownish lesion, which may last from months to years. The aim of treatment in cosmetic cases is to stop the growth of the lesion and to cause it to fade as much as possible, so that it becomes less obvious or can be more easily concealed with makeup. On close inspection, the lesion remains visible and may regrow in the future as generalized KS progresses. Therefore, if lesions are already easily concealed by the hairline or beard, cosmetic treatment may not be recommended since hair loss may increase the visibility of the lesion. In some fair-complected as well as darker individuals, such irradiation may result in geographical erythema of the skin in the field that can persist for several months. This effect of irradiation, although uncommon, may be cosmetically more displeasing than the original KS itself, which must be considered when treatment is solely for cosmetic purposes. Treating a less obvious site on the head initially may help select those patients likely to have a significant reaction before treatment of more extensive and visible lesions is attempted.

The retroauricular region and pinnae may be involved with bulky, painful KS, especially bothersome with pressure during sleeping. Radiation quickly reduces this pain and tumor size. The pinnae are safely treated with the same dosing schedule used for skin lesions.

Lesions on the nose, where the skin is quite thin, are preferably treated with radiation or alitretinoin rather than with injections or cryotherapy, since radiation is associated with less scarring in this site than other modalities. Treatment while the lesions are small is preferred, since these lesions will become quite bulky if their development is unchecked.

EYELID AND CONJUNCTIVAL LESIONS

Involvement of the conjunctivae or eyelids occurs in 20% to 24% of AIDS-related KS cases.[102] Lesions involving the conjunctivae are often associated with subconjunctival hemorrhage and gritty discomfort but do not usually interfere with vision.[86,102-104] They may extend from the scleral surface onto the tarsal conjunctiva. Treatment can be administered using either superficial radiation with orthovoltage or electrons, sparing the cornea and lens in the process. Very small lesions have been treated using strontium with fair to good response.[105] If strontium is used, doses comparable to those used for pterygia are safe (e.g., 800 to 1000 cGy × 2 to 3 at weekly intervals).

Disease involving the eyelids is also safely approached with superficial irradiation. Internal lead eye shields coated in a thin layer of wax to reduce back scatter to the internal surface of the lid are routinely used to protect the cornea and lens. Loss of the eyelashes can be expected.

ORAL AND PHARYNGEAL LESIONS

In the majority of patients with extensive skin involvement, disease will be found in the oral cavity.[82,86,90,106-108] The hard palate may show small focal or diffuse flat areas of disease that are asymptomatic or bulky lesions. Bulkier lesions are frequently associated with the teeth and may extend onto the anterior gingival surfaces, surrounding the base of the teeth, with loosening and loss of teeth possible. The soft palate, uvula, tonsillar pillars and fossae, and posterior wall of the pharynx, as well as the surfaces of the tongue, should be examined for disease. Bleeding, pain, and interference with chewing may be seen in advanced disease.

Flat asymptomatic palatal lesions are generally not treated with radiation, since they may remain quiescent for months to years. Since radiation at any dosing schedule is associated with significant painful mucositis, the preference is to wait until symptoms develop before subjecting the patient to the pain of radiation treatment. These lesions may subside with proper antiviral therapy and appropriate treatment of other opportunistic infections.

Patients treated with either 150 cGy × 10 or 800 cGy × 1 have developed mucositis requiring mild narcotic administration for approximately 1 week.[86,106-109] The appearance of such mucositis at lower doses than those that cause mucositis in the HIV-negative patient suggests that there is impaired ability to repair radiation damage associated either with the HIV infection, the KS, or some other unidentified factor.[81-83,110] To minimize morbidity, patients are aggressively treated for any thrush or herpetic lesions before irradiation. Prophylaxis is given with fluconazole (200 mg per day) plus or minus acyclovir (200 mg five times a day) for 2 days prior and 7 to 10 days after treatment. Fields are kept small (Fig. 67-1),

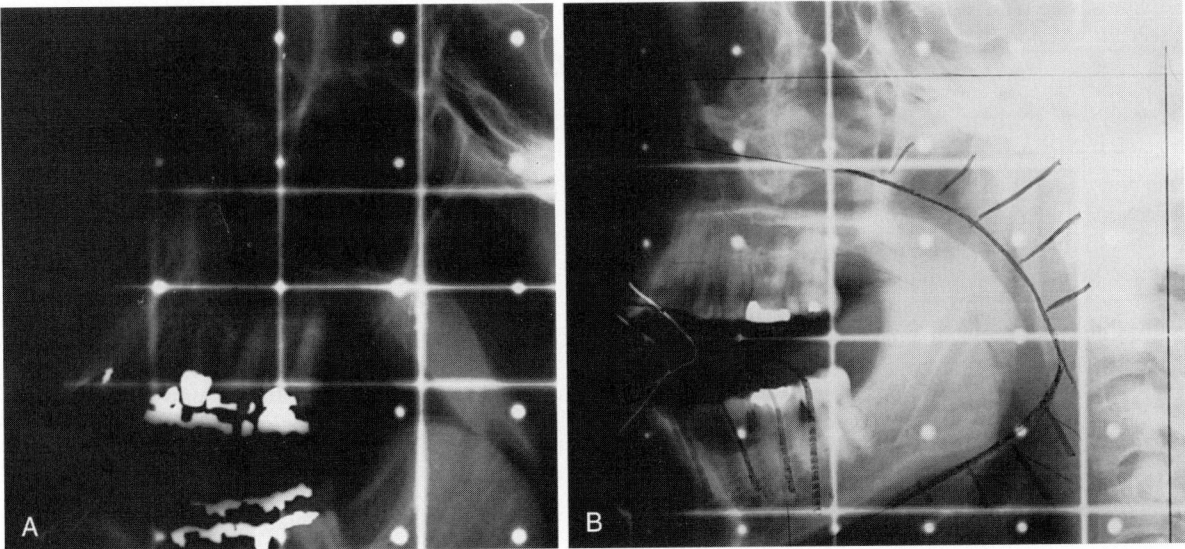

Figure 67–1. Two examples of fields for patients with oral Kaposi's sarcoma treated with photon irradiation. **A,** Disease confined to the anterior hard palate. **B,** Disease involving entire hard and soft palate, anterior superior gingival ridge, and tonsillar fossa.

covering only the areas of visible involvement, with customized shielding used to reduce toxicity. If disease is confined to the palate in patients with advanced HIV disease (life expectancy is short), a single dose of 800 cGy has been effective in reducing acute symptoms associated with the KS. For patients with more extensive disease and a longer life expectancy, a fractionated course is generally selected. Typically, pain associated with patchy mucositis occurs about 10 days after the initiation of treatment, whether a single or fractionated approach is used. This necessitates the short-term use of narcotics for relief. Attention should be paid to proper hydration and nutrition during this period.

Patients with a history of sterile aphthous ulcers in the oral cavity, either separate from or associated with the KS, are at a high risk of developing deep ulcerations with bone or cartilage exposure after treatment with either radiation or other local measures.[111-119] These patients should not be irradiated until the ulcers have completely resolved. Agents such as thalidomide are associated with a reduction in the time course of these recurrent ulcers.

Less commonly, bulky disease may arise in the base of tongue, larynx, and supraglottic region, causing pain, choking, or difficulty swallowing. Rarely, disease may interfere with breathing because of laryngeal edema or epiglottic involvement. In the presence of such symptoms, indirect laryngoscopy or fiberoptic endoscopy is necessary to define the true extent of disease before treatment. As with other sites in the oropharynx, laryngeal irradiation is effective in reducing symptoms caused by KS.

GROIN AND GENITALIA

Small lesions may arise on the scrotum and penis in 20% of cases[101] and may remain stable for prolonged periods. Lesions on the shaft or glans of the penis are not treated unless symptomatic (pain, interference with urination or erection, bleeding, recurrent infection).[93,101,120]

If lesions are symptomatic, both single-dose and fractionated sequences are successful in alleviating problems without appreciable side effects. For small lesions on the glans or shaft, orthovoltage or electrons are sufficient. For larger circumferential lesions, a wax mold is used to surround the penis in an upright position, and the field is treated with opposed lateral photon ports, encompassing as much of the shaft as necessary. Alternatively, mesh is used to surround the penis and suspend it upright, in conjunction with bolus to assure adequate surface dosing. A response rate of 92% was reported in a study of 19 men irradiated for genital KS.[101]

FEET

Minimal disease involving the toes and arch of the foot can cause severe pain, which interferes with ambulation or prevents the use of shoes.[82,85,92,93,121-123] Injections in these areas are exquisitely painful and generally avoided. These areas are easily treated with superficial radiation, with an excellent response rate in terms of reduction of pain. Pain relief occurs generally within 1 week to 10 days of the administration of a single superficial dose of 800 cGy in orthovoltage therapy. Expected side effects of treatment include a temporary increase in the discomfort occurring approximately 3 to 5 days after treatment and lasting about 1 week. Rarely, a sterile blister may form in the radiation field, which may require drainage and careful cleaning with povidone-iodine (Betadine). Cellulitis may develop in a foot with bad hygiene before treatment or trauma after treatment. Whole foot irradiation should be avoided except in the patient with a short life expectancy.

To minimize symptoms, the patient is instructed to remain off the foot for as much time as possible in the week after treatment, keeping it elevated when sitting or lying down. The foot should be kept clean and dry, and trauma should be avoided. If painful areas are present on both feet and the patient has to remain ambulatory, only one foot should be treated initially and the reaction should be allowed to subside before treatment of the second foot.

EDEMA

Progressive lymphatic infiltration with KS can occur in multiple body sites, with major morbidity. Any evidence of significant edema should be cause for consideration of initiating systemic therapy, since lymphatic obstruction can quickly progress to a major reduction in quality of life for the patient. Radiation should be considered in the patient unable to tolerate or unresponsive to chemotherapy. The effectiveness of the treatment is directly related to the duration of the problem; long-standing edema (>3 months) that is progressive is less likely to show appreciable reduction after radiation than newly developing swelling. Dramatic, albeit short-lived, reductions in edema have been reported after such an approach.[80,82,89] Preference should be given to systemic approaches if possible, since even low-dose chemotherapy may lead to substantial reductions in edema.

In the cheek, preauricular region, and upper neck, KS frequently results in periorbital or diffuse facial edema and ecchymosis, with or without visible lesions in the skin of the cheek. The edema may be severe enough to interfere with vision. Radiation treatment of the nodal drainage and intervening lymphatics often is quite successful in reducing this edema.[80,82,89]

Disease involvement of the inguinal nodes frequently causes edema in the suprapubic and inguinal areas, as well as the scrotum and penis. The edema may be enormous, with the scrotum expanding to the size of a large grapefruit. KS lesions may not be visible in the edematous areas, although subcutaneous induration is palpable. In the past, routine computed tomography scans of the pelvis and abdomen were performed to define the amount of pelvic lymphadenopathy, but these were rarely enlightening and are no longer routinely obtained.

Lesions on the upper extremities are rarely a problem, unlike those seen in the lower extremities. Small macular lesions may form a string of lesions that appear to be following the lymphatic channels. Although initially not bothersome, they may gradually become associated with significant edema, either locally over the patch of disease (thighs, calves) or diffusely distal to the disease (foot, ankle, calf, thigh).[80,89] Edema interferes with ambulation, causes pain, and may lead to the development of skin breakdown and stasis ulcers with superinfection. Interventions that could potentially aggravate the obstruction to lymphatic flow should be avoided. Initially in the AIDS epidemic, wide-field irradiation was routinely administered for this condition, with photon fields that often encompassed the entire circumference of the extremity because of solid disease. Although an initial reduction in edema was commonly seen, the disease continued to progress, with recurrence of the edema as well as brawny induration and thickened KS in the previously irradiated field, which complicated the issue. Reirradiation was often undertaken for short-term benefit, but a significant price was paid by those who survived more than a few months in the form of skin breakdown, ulceration, and infection distal to and within the irradiated field. These complications were due to progressive disease, radiation insult and, occasionally, direct effects of chemotherapeutic agents.[124,125]

The current approach is to proceed if possible with systemic therapy at the onset of significant edema in the lower extremity, reserving radiation for small areas of painful, unresponsive disease. Fields are kept small, with superficial energies preferred, and strict avoidance of circumferential coverage. The use of careful hygiene, support stockings, and intermittent compression devices, and the judicious use of diuretics may help retard the problem but will not stop its progression. In the person with very advanced KS, multiple opportunistic infections, and an inability to tolerate systemic therapy, wide-field irradiation may be used temporarily to palliate pain and edema, since the life expectancy is quite short.

VISCERAL INVOLVEMENT

In the presence of cutaneous disease, KS is frequently found in the gastrointestinal tract at autopsy.[56,126-128] In the autopsy study by Klatt and associates,[56] 138 patients were found to have KS. Of this group, the esophagus was involved in 20%, stomach in 33%, small intestine in 44%, colorectum in 33%, hepatobiliary region in 28%, pancreas in 9%, and spleen in 11%. Overall, however, with the declining incidence of KS in the HIV-infected population, the presence of internal KS at autopsy has fallen significantly.[129] Symptoms are uncommon but when present may be quite severe, including bleeding, pain, and obstruction. Although systemic therapy is preferred, radiation therapy is effective in rapidly reducing symptoms and should be considered in the patient unresponsive to systemic therapy or unable to tolerate it. Specific areas of concern are the rectum and stomach, where ulcers may be particularly troublesome. Care should be taken to keep the field as small as possible while encompassing disease described via endoscopy. Large-field irradiation of the bowels is very unwise in patients who already have malabsorption problems and significant diarrhea. In these areas, fractionated radiation is preferred to minimize the acute symptoms associated with treatment.

Clinically detectable lung involvement occurs late in the course of the disease and has a poor prognosis,[55-57,82,130-133] although recent reports of an aggressive approach with HAART in conjunction with chemotherapy have shown a major improvement in outcome.[134] After failure of systemic agents, radiation has been attempted with some palliative success. Meyer[57] reported on 25 patients treated with doses of 1050 to 1500 cGy in 150 cGy fractions, with subjective improvement seen in 89% of patients and radiographic improvement in 78%. Overall, however, life expectancy is short, with only 9 of the 25 surviving beyond 12 weeks after therapy and a mean survival of only 15 weeks for patients who completed the radiation.

NON-HODGKIN'S LYMPHOMA

NHL is the second most common malignancy reported in the setting of AIDS. The impact of HAART on the incidence and outcome of non-Hodgkin's lymphoma in this setting is less clear than what was seen for KS. Before the onset of the AIDS epidemic, the incidence of non-Hodgkin's lymphoma (NHL) had been on the rise in the United States, increasing by 3% to 4% per year from the early 1970s.[135] With the appearance of HIV disease in the 1980s, NHL incidence rates began rising more rapidly.[136] Of 1115 men in the San Francisco City Clinic Cohort Study who died of AIDS before 1992, 4.2% had NHL as their initial AIDS-defining illness, and 12.6% had developed the disease before death.[5] On a national level, the CDC reported that 3.4% of patients with HIV had NHL as their AIDS-defining illness.[137] In a separate study, NHL was listed as the cause of death in 8% of men who underwent autopsy for AIDS in Los Angeles from 1982 to 1993.[56] Sixteen percent of these patients had lymphoma, and in 60% of those with lymphoma, the disease was listed as the cause of death.

The changes in incidence in NHL in AIDS since the introduction of HAART differ for the three main types of lymphomas reported (primary central nervous system lymphoma [PCNSL], systemic NHL, and primary effusion lymphomas [PELs]).[49] PCNSL incidence has declined the most,[50] whereas the change in percentage of patients with HIV disease that develop systemic NHL is controversial.[25,26,49,50] The appearance of PEL is still so rare that it is difficult to assess the true change in incidence.[25,26] According to the meta-analysis by Appleby et al.,[50] the overall incidence of NHL declined from 6.2 cases per 1000 patients per year from 1992 to 1996 to 3.6 from 1997 to 1999, a rate ratio of 0.58 for the latter years compared to the former.

Systemic Non-Hodgkin's Lymphoma

It is estimated that the HIV-infected patient has a 200-fold greater risk of developing NHL than the general population[138] and a 1000-fold greater risk of developing Burkitt's lymphoma.[139] The large majority of lymphomas in AIDS are of B-cell origin. T-cell varieties constitute only 1.5% to 5% of the load, but an HIV-infected patient exhibits a 15-fold increased risk of developing T-cell lymphoma compared to the general population.[140,141] The systemic presentations are composed of approximately 40% Burkitt's lymphoma, 25% immunoblastic lymphoma, and 25% large cell, anaplastic lymphoma.[139] Approximately 80% of the Burkitt's and immunoblastic lymphomas are Epstein-Barr virus (EBV)-positive, whereas few of the large cell, anaplastic lymphomas are.[25,26,139]

The exact mechanism by which the lymphomas develop is unclear. In a model proposed by Levine,[6] chronic B-cell proliferation and stimulation occurs in the setting of HIV disease, caused by HIV itself, HIV-infected lymphocyte cytokine release, and possibly EBV. This is seen as the generalized lymphadenopathy common in the early course of HIV disease. With ongoing B-cell proliferation in the setting of immunodeficiency, abnormal DNA rearrangements are prone to occur because of chance recombinase errors. These errors can lead to dysregulation of c-*myc* and other unidentified oncogenes, as evidenced by an increase in translocations (t8;14), (t8;22), and (t8;2). Monoclonal or polyclonal

proliferation eventually leads to the development of an array of lymphomas.[11] Another model suggests that HIV-infected macrophages proliferate and overexpress cytokines, leading to proliferation of surrounding lymphocytes that subsequently develop a malignant phenotype.[142]

Systemic lymphoma appears as widespread disease with extranodal presentation in up to 95% of cases.[143-150] Common extranodal sites of involvement include the gastrointestinal tract (27%) and central nervous system (CNS) (25%),[140,149] although any site may be involved and frequently there is no evidence of nodal involvement. Unusual presentations such as cutaneous soft tissue masses, paranasal sinuses, pericardial involvement, and epidural space have been reported as well.[149] In a review of cases from San Francisco General Hospital, two thirds presented with stage IV disease.[149]

The disease may occur at any point in the course of the immunosuppression. Before the introduction of HAART, patients presented with a mean CD4 count of 100 to 180 cells/mm³, with 30% having D4+ counts greater than 200 at diagnosis.[150] Since 1996, more than half have not had a prior AIDS-defining illness, and the CD4+ count at diagnosis tends to be higher.[25,26] Presenting symptoms are protean, including fevers, night sweats, gastrointestinal disturbances, and pain. NHL should be suspected in the presence of a rapidly expanding nodal or nonnodal mass in any site, chronic progressive gastrointestinal discomfort, hepatic obstruction, or worsening systemic symptoms. Due to its diffuse presentation, extensive radiographic imaging is necessary to determine the extent of disease before treatment, as is examination of the bone marrow.

The approach to patients with systemic lymphoma is dictated by the overall status of the immune system, since aggressive intervention often exacerbates the immunodeficient state, with resultant increase in opportunistic infection and shortened survival. A number of different treatment regimens (CHOP, MACOP-B, m-BACOD, Pro-MACE-MOPP*) were used before 1995, with CR rates varying from 33% to 63%. Later studies, such as that using an aggressive chemotherapy regimen (EPOCH—VP-16, prednisone, vincristine, doxorubicin, and cyclophosphamide) resulted in a 79% CR rate.[151] In this study, HAART was discontinued during the chemotherapy and restarted immediately after cessation of chemotherapy. Prospective studies of the addition of HAART to chemotherapy have, for the most part, shown acceptable toxicity with the combination and improved duration of survival,[25,26,152] although a retrospective report on 8000 patients with HIV-related lymphomas showed no benefit to the addition of the anti-retroviral therapy.[153] Relapse occurs in 25% to 50% within 6 months, and median survivals are only 4 to 7 months, regardless of the

---

*CHOP: cyclophosphamide, doxorubicin, vincristine, prednisone; MACOP-B: cyclophosphamide, doxorubicin, vincristine, methotrexate, bleomycin, prednisone, cotrimoxazole; m-BACOD: methotrexate, bleomycin, doxorubicin, cyclophosphamide, vincristine, dexamethasone; HD AraC/HD MTX: high-dose cytosine arabinoside, high-dose methotrexate; Pro-MACE-MOPP: doxorubicin, etoposide, cytosine arabinoside, prednisone, cyclophosphamide, vincristine, procarbazine, prednisone.

combination used.[149] The most common cause of death in these patients is opportunistic infections, with uncontrolled disease a close second. Factors that are usually quite important in determining prognosis in NHL in the HIV-negative patient (stage, number of extranodal sites, meningeal involvement, LDH) have little or no prognostic value in this setting. Kaplan and associates[154] have, however, defined a group with an improved life expectancy after diagnosis of HIV-related lymphoma who are appropriately considered for aggressive therapy. Patients with CD4 counts of more than 100 cells/mm³, absence of prior AIDS-defining illnesses, Karnofsky performance status (KPS) score greater than 70, and absence of extranodal disease had a median survival after therapy of 24 months, as opposed to a median survival of only 5.5 months for all other patients.

New approaches are desperately needed. Novel agents, such as the use of anti-CD-20 therapy, rituximab, and IL-12, are undergoing clinical testing.[25,26] Up to 95% of HIV-NHL are CD20+, and combinations of rituximab and chemotherapy regimens are showing promising results as tested by the AIDS Malignancy Consortium.[25,26]

PRIMARY EFFUSION LYMPHOMAS

A particular subset of NHL that appears in the peritoneal, pericardial, and pleural spaces and was formerly called body cavity lymphoma has been renamed *primary effusion lymphoma* (PEL).[25,26,155-158] This particular lymphoma has a 100% correlation with HHV-8, is confined to these body cavities as a lymphomatous effusion, and displays an immunoblastic cytology. It composes approximately 3% of all HIV-related NHLs and is defined by a number of characteristics.[139] Clinically, it is confined to the cavity of origin, has no associated solid mass, and has a patient distribution that epidemiologically mimics that of KS. Genotypically, it has a B-cell origin, always has the presence of HHV-8, and frequently has the presence of the EBV genome, in the absence of *myc* gene rearrangements, is CD45+, and shows expression of the activation-associated antigen. The outcome for these patients is quite poor, with median survivals of 3 to 5 months. Given their correlation with HHV-8 and EBV, the possibility exists that the incidence will decline with the routine use of HAART, but this remains to be seen. Rapid initiation of HAART remains the prime therapy for this aggressive disease.

Primary Central Nervous System Lymphoma

Primary CNS disease in the absence of HIV disease affects only 1% to 2% of patients with non–HIV-related lymphoma,[159-161] as opposed to 25% of patients with AIDS-related lymphoma.[150,162] There was a 3600-fold greater incidence of PCNSL in HIV-infected patients compared to the general population[63] before the introduction of HAART, but a significant decline has since been reported.[50,51] Before 1996, the mean incidence rate of PCNSL in the Multicenter AIDS Cohort Study of 2734 HIV-positive men in four major U.S. metropolitan centers was 4.3 but has subsequently declined to 0.4.[164]

As patients develop resistance to antiretroviral medications, or as multiple-drug-resistant strains develop, it is possible that these rates will once again rise.

The majority of CNS lymphomas are large cell, are immunoblastic, and show little evidence of c-*myc* rearrangement. EBV DNA is found almost universally in association with CNS lymphoma in AIDS, suggesting that EBV infection plays a major role in the B-cell proliferation and development of primary CNS lymphoma in the late stages of AIDS.[140,165] EBV can be detected in the cerebrospinal fluid of these patients,[163] and may, if detected, obviate the need for biopsy.

Primary CNS lymphoma presents much later in the course of immune decline than does systemic NHL, with mean CD4 counts of less than 50 cells/mm³.[150,162] Common presenting symptoms include nonfocal findings such as headache, lethargy, confusion, and memory loss or findings suggestive of mass lesions such as aphasia, seizures, hemiparesis, and cranial nerve palsies. In the UCSF study of 41 HIV-related CNS lymphomas, 56% presented with focal symptoms or seizures.[162] The average KPS score before initiation of therapy was 50.

Radiographically, PCNSL may present as either focal (35%) or multifocal (65%) disease,[162] findings that are generally indistinguishable from those of toxoplasmosis (Fig. 67-2). Thallium-201 SPECT scan may be helpful in differentiating lymphoma from an infectious etiology. For the patient in whom PCNSL is suspected based on MRI results, cerebrospinal fluid should be tested for EBV DNA by polymerase chain reaction (sensitivity 80%, specificity 100%),[155] toxoplasmosis titers, and cytology. Serum toxoplasmosis titers should be sent off as well and antitoxoplasmosis therapy should be instituted immediately. In those patients who either cannot undergo cerebrospinal fluid tap or fail to reveal an answer through the tap, antitoxoplasmosis therapy should be carried out, with close follow-up evaluation including repeat MRI in 1 to 3 weeks. With the presence of negative serum titers or progressive neurologic decline despite antitoxoplasmosis measures, the clinician should proceed to stereotactic biopsy of lesions to establish or eliminate the diagnosis of lymphoma.

Because primary CNS lymphomas appear very late in the course of immunosuppression in AIDS, the use of chemotherapy has been uncommon.[166] Recent reports have, however, shown a number of responses to the initiation of aggressive antiretroviral therapy,[167] and the AIDS Malignancy Consortium is studying a regimen that includes HAART along with IV zidovudine, ganciclovir, and IL-12.[25,26] The current management of these patients should, if possible, center around the optimization of antiretroviral therapy, with other therapeutic interventions chosen depending on the overall status of the patient. The use of HAART may allow more patients to be treated with regimens that have shown benefit in the HIV-negative population with PCNSL. Protocols using high-dose methotrexate with or without radiation have shown CR rates of 65% with 2-year survivals in excess of 60%.[168] The majority of AIDS-afflicted patients, however, have historically been referred for radiation management of symptoms.

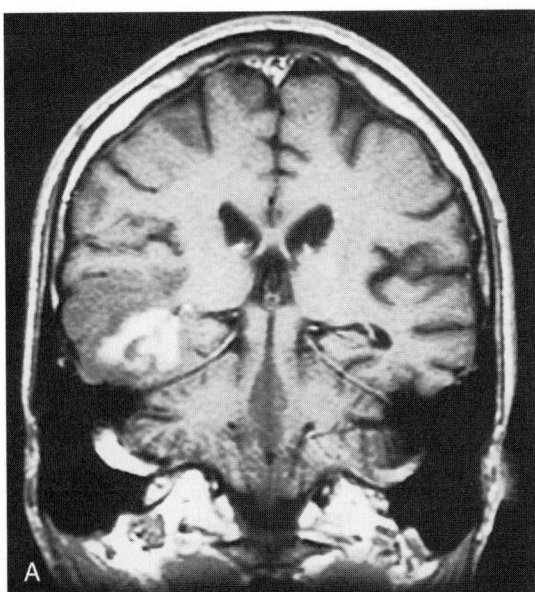
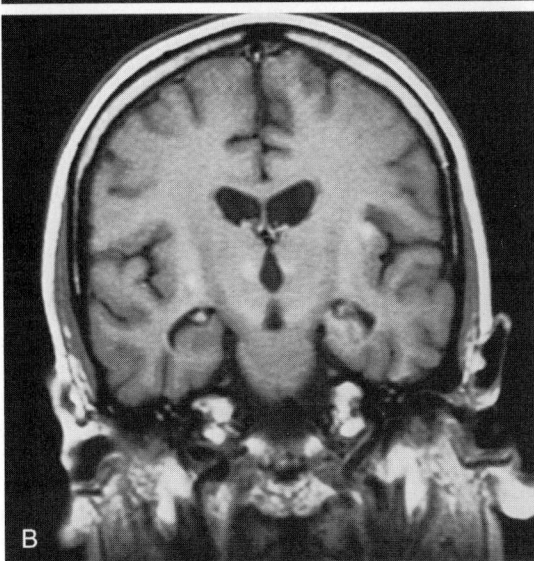

Figure 67–2. Brain magnetic resonance scans of two patients with primary central nervous system lymphoma, originally treated presumptively for toxoplasmosis before stereotactic biopsy. **A,** Solitary mass lesion. **B,** Multifocal lesions.

Radiation Therapy Recommendations and Results

Little has been reported on the routine use of radiation in the setting of HIV-related lymphomas other than for CNS disease. As mentioned earlier, chemotherapy is the mainstay of therapy for systemic disease, and radiation is the mainstay for CNS disease.[84,146,148-150,162,169-174] Ling and associates[162] reported on the results of radiation therapy in 41 patients with HIV-related primary cerebral non-Hodgkin's lymphoma over a 10-year period. Mean CD4 count at diagnosis in this group was 50 cells/mm³, 78% had a history of prior opportunistic infections, and 68% had received prior treatment with antiretroviral therapy of varying duration. Doses of radiation varied from 38 to 60 Gy and were delivered with initial opposed lateral whole brain fields. Of 38 evaluable patients, 71% had mild to excellent

symptomatic response to the radiation, with no significant morbidity noted. The mean length of survival from initiation of therapy was only 3.2 months, including the two longest survivors at 13 and 15 months. A prior report from the same institution stated that deaths were due to opportunistic infections and not uncontrolled CNS disease.[170] Studies looking at the addition of chemotherapy do not reveal an increase in survival over radiation alone.[155,166,169]

The current recommendation for the treatment of primary CNS lymphoma in the setting of AIDS is aggressive optimization of the antiretroviral program, with whole brain radiation used for the palliation of symptoms. No particular dosing schedule has proven superior in this disease, with schedules varying from 180 to 200 cGy per day to 5000 cGy,[155] 200 to 267 cGy per day to 4000 cGy,[162] or 300 cGy to 3000 cGy. Boosts are not routinely delivered but are considered in patients with good KPS scores before treatment, unifocal disease on scan, and no major opportunistic infections. This approach has a good chance of improving symptoms associated with lymphoma, is well tolerated, and is likely to control disease until the time of death. Consideration should, however, also be given to novel trials, such as that of the AIDS Malignancy Consortium (HAART along with IV zidovudine, ganciclovir, and IL-12[25,26]).

For systemic disease, patients with the good prognostic categories mentioned earlier (CD4 >100 cells/mm³, KPS >70, no extranodal disease, no prior opportunistic infections), should be approached aggressively. For those with localized disease, three cycles of CHOP followed by localized radiation (200 cGy per fraction to 4000 cGy as in the prospective randomized SWOG trial) to all original sites of disease is a reasonable approach,[175-177] although this represents only a very small subgroup of patients. In other patients with localized disease, local radiation to doses of 36 to 44 Gy may be considered as a consolidative boost in those patients with areas of bulky disease who, after initial chemotherapy, demonstrate a partial or slow response to chemotherapy. Attempts are made to minimize the amount of marrow that is irradiated, given the underlying immunosuppression and the myelosuppression common with the drug regimens selected. Prophylactic craniospinal irradiation is not routinely recommended, even in patients with T-cell disease and marrow involvement, since the myelosuppression is tremendous. Craniospinal irradiation is reserved for those patients with proven leptomeningeal spread, and then only as a palliative measure. Radiation is also an excellent palliative for patients with recurrent or unresponsive disease and for patients who are unable to tolerate systemic chemotherapy. The use of radiolabeled monoclonal antibodies, such as 90Y-ibritumomab tiuxetan, specific for CD20+ cells, has not yet been tested in the setting of HIV disease but may play a role in the future.

CERVICAL CARCINOMA

Epidemiology

There has not been a reported increase in the incidence of frankly invasive cervical carcinoma in the setting of HIV disease.[7,8,47,137,178-184] Despite this fact, as of January 1,

1993, the CDC revised the AIDS case definition to include those patients with cervical carcinoma in the setting of HIV infection for several reasons.[7,8] Studies have shown that patients infected with HIV are at an increased risk of having cervical or anal intraepithelial lesions in conjunction with detectable human papillomavirus (HPV) infections, compared with HIV-negative patients from similar risk groups.[182,183,185-188] Neoplastic changes are also more frequently encountered in patients with lower CD4 counts than in HIV-infected patients with higher CD4 counts.[185,189] Cervical cancer is a preventable disease, if detected at an early, preinvasive stage, so its inclusion in the CDC criteria was meant to emphasize the importance of close gynecological care and surveillance in the HIV-infected woman. The use of HAART has been shown to reduce the rate of persistence of cervical intraepithelial neoplasia and to prevent its progression to more aggressive clinical manifestations.[190]

Pathogenesis

Women with HIV infection are approximately four times more likely to be infected with HPV than HIV-negative women, and the incidence of squamous intraepithelial lesions (SIL) is dramatically higher, ranging from 11% to 40%.[191] HPV is strongly associated with the development of intraepithelial neoplasia in the cervical and anal mucosal regions.[185,189,191-196] Low-grade intraepithelial dysplastic changes are associated with a wide variety of strains of HPV, while high-grade changes (high-grade squamous intraepithelial lesions), precursors to invasive carcinomas, are associated with strains 16, 18, 31, and 45[191] and, to a lesser extent, 33, 35, 39,51, 52, 56, 58, 59, and 68.[193] After infection of the epithelial cell, the viral genome generally remains episomal, that is, it exists as a circular plasmid within the cell, separate from the host DNA. At some point, the viral genome is integrated into the host chromosome, and increased expression of two early region gene sequences occurs. These proteins, E6 and E7, may be key elements in the induction of malignant transformation.[196] E6 is believed to bind and inactivate the p53 gene product, while E7 inactivates the retinoblastoma gene product, both of which are negative growth regulators. Loss of p53 function causes disruption of the normal process of growth arrest in cells with DNA damage, potentially making cells more susceptible to accumulation of genetic mutations.

Through careful screening, it is hoped that cervical dysplasia in the HIV-infected population can be effectively eliminated before it has time to progress to invasive disease.[179,190,197] Several reports of the clinical presentation of cervical carcinoma in HIV disease make it evident that, if allowed to progress, cervical cancer has a more aggressive course in the immunocompromised patient.[198-200] In a population of 84 women with cervical cancer and known HIV status, Maiman and associates[201] found 16 to be HIV-positive; 14 of these did not have evidence of other opportunistic diseases. Fifty percent of the HIV-positive women presented with stage III/IV disease, as opposed to only 19% of the HIV-negative women. Their mean CD4 count was 360 cells/mm³ (range, 129 to 616). Eleven of the 16 died at a mean interval of 9.2 months from diagnosis. Nine of the 11 died from cervical cancer, and the other two from other manifestations of AIDS.

Management

As with all other malignancies in the setting of AIDS, treatment plans should take into account the patient's overall immune status. With detailed assessment of the patient's past history of opportunistic disease, current viral burden, rate of CD4 decay, and performance status, patients can be divided into three general categories. At one extreme are those with relatively intact immune systems (CD4 >200 cells/mm³, no major opportunistic disease), who have a reasonable chance of surviving several years with appropriate medical care and prophylaxis. At the other extreme are those with significant impairment of the immune system (CD4 <50 cells/mm³) despite aggressive antiretroviral therapy, one or more life-threatening opportunistic diseases such as progressive multifocal leukoencephalopathy (PML), mycobacterium avium intracellulare, CNS toxoplasmosis, cytomegalovirus esophagitis, and a poor performance status, whose life expectancy is measured in months. In between lies the group of patients on the verge of decline, for whom overly aggressive intervention holds the greatest risk: those with CD4 counts from 50 to 200 cells/mm³, in reasonably good condition but with a downward trend evidenced by a decreasing CD4 count.

The first and healthiest group should be managed much as they would be in the absence of HIV disease, using surgical and radiotherapeutic techniques described in Chapter 48, Cancer of the Uterine Cervix. The use of prophylactic paraortic irradiation, however, or the addition of chemotherapy should be used judiciously in these patients, as these treatments might unduly stress the marrow and the small intestine. The maintenance of HAART is important during this process. In the patient with early-stage disease (nonbulky stage I/IIA) amenable to a radical hysterectomy, surgery would be preferred over radiation, as it would be expected to have less impact on already stressed marrow. Although radiation may be well tolerated in such a patient, it is not clear that this would be a prudent approach. Patients with stage IB/IIA (bulky), IIB, or III/IVA disease should be treated aggressively with standard radiotherapeutic approaches, since death due to progressive cervical disease is a more immediate risk than progression of AIDS. The use of antiretroviral agents and continuation of appropriate prophylaxis against opportunistic infections is recommended during this period of potentially iatrogenic immunosuppression.[202]

In the intermediate group, those with an immune status beginning to decline, aggressive local therapy is still warranted, but it must be tempered by an awareness of the risks of increased intolerance to radiation as well as the profound risk of development of concomitant opportunistic infections. Once again, antiretroviral use and prophylaxis measures should be maintained. Radiation fields should be kept as tight as possible to reduce irritation of bowels that may already be plagued by such offenders as cryptosporidiosis, mycobacterium avium intracellulare, or cytomegalovirus. The decision to treat clinically uninvolved nodes must, therefore, be individualized. Brachytherapy alone should be considered for stage I patients since it minimizes immunosuppression. Surgical approaches for early-stage disease are preferred, and the use of chemotherapy for advanced disease should be used judiciously and with the support of colony-stimulating factors to reduce the degree of iatrogenic immunosuppression.

The final group, those with devastated immune systems and a brief life expectancy, should be treated with palliation of symptoms as the main goal. Reduction of pain and cessation of bleeding for the last remaining months is important in allowing patients to be managed at home with some maintenance of quality of life and dignity. For the patient with a very short life expectancy, the use of the schema from the Radiation Therapy Oncology Group study for advanced pelvic malignancies[203,204] (370 cGy twice a day for 2 days, followed by a 2 to 3 week break, then repeated for another 2 days, an additional break, and a third course) has been well tolerated by patients. Some of these patients will die of other diseases before completion of all three courses, but significant improvement in symptoms is usually seen after the first course. Great care is taken not to unnecessarily irradiate the bowel.

ANAL CARCINOMA

Several reports point to a slight increase in the incidence of squamous cell carcinoma of the anus associated with the HIV epidemic,[5,22,185,196,205] whereas others have failed to show such an increase.[47,206] In 1992, a linkage was established between the AIDS registries and cancer registries of nine regions of the United States, including information on 859,398 reports of cancer and 50,050 cases of AIDS.[22] Epidermoid anal cancer was found in 39 cases, with a relative risk of 63.4 after a diagnosis of AIDS compared to the general population. The risk was highest in the time period immediately before diagnosis of AIDS or in the pursuant years. It is important to note that anal cancer was on the rise among homosexual males before the AIDS epidemic, due to increased transmission of HPV via anal intercourse.[6,207-211]

As with cervical carcinoma, HIV-related immunosuppression facilitates the development of perianal epithelial abnormalities in the presence of HPV infection.[185,196] The prevalence of anal SIL ranges from 20% to 45% in homosexual and bisexual men with HIV infection.[212] In a cohort of 114 women with a history of IV drug abuse studied at San Francisco General Hospital, 48% were HIV-positive. The frequency of perianal dysplastic change was greater than the incidence of cervical dysplastic change in the entire cohort, as well as in both subsets of HIV-positive and HIV-negative women.[185] As patients continue to live longer due to improved antiretroviral and prophylactic therapy, a rise in invasive anal carcinoma is expected, which argues for a heightened surveillance to detect early changes in this population as is recommended for cervical dysplasia.[7,22,179,193] The routine use of annual screening for anal dysplasia in

HIV-infected homosexual and bisexual men has been associated with a substantial clinical benefit.[212] While the introduction of HAART has dramatically increased the CD4+ counts of many patients, it is not clear that HAART has had a substantial impact on the natural progression of anal SIL.[213] In a study of 98 HIV-infected men followed in the Anal Dysplasia Clinic at UCSF, who were followed for 6 months before and after initiation of HAART, similar rates of disease progression were seen. This raises the possibility that, as HIV- and HPV-infected men live longer, they may actually develop a greater incidence of invasive squamous cell carcinoma, since most of the anal SIL lesions persist after initiation of HAART.

In a retrospective review of 17 patients with anal carcinoma in the setting of HIV infection treated at UCSF between 1991 and 1997, 9 patients had CD4+ counts greater than 200, and the other 8 had counts less than 200.[214] The nine with higher CD4+ counts were treated with chemoradiotherapy, using the standard regimen used for HIV-negative patients. All nine had disease control at a median follow-up of 2 years, none required colostomy for salvage, and only two required major breaks in therapy due to substantial moist desquamation. Of the eight with lower CD4+ counts, one received radiation alone and seven had some modification of their chemotherapy in consideration of their immunosuppression. Seven of the eight developed major complications of therapy, four of whom had colostomies (two for therapy-related complications, two for recurrent disease). Six of these eight were disease free at time of death due to AIDS or at last follow-up. In a report on 11 HIV-positive patients (average CD4+ count of 209) treated between 1989 and 1999 with standard combinations of radiation, 5-FU, and mitomycin-C, 9 had complete remissions, 2 of whom ultimately relapsed.[215] There was one case of fatal bowel obstruction, 25% had grade 3 or greater hematological toxicity, 17% grade 3 to 4 diarrhea, and 8% grade 3 to 4 skin toxicity.

The management of patients with high-grade anal SIL is surgical, guided by high-resolution direct anoscopy, and close follow-up.[216] Those who go on to develop invasive disease are managed according to their overall current immune status as measured by their CD4+ counts and viral loads. Patients with anal carcinoma and HIV disease but no diagnostic criteria of AIDS should receive standard therapy with combined 5-FU and mitomycin-C plus radiation, as in the HIV-negative patient. Consideration is given to the substitution of cisplatin for mitomycin-C, an approach that is being evaluated in an RTOG trial of anal cancer in the HIV-negative population. Maintenance of the antiretroviral program during the course of therapy is essential and may actually lead to a reduction in morbidity. Radiation fields are designed to cover the main lesion, inguinal nodes, and low pelvic nodes in most cases. Decisions to avoid prophylactic nodal irradiation may be made on an individualized basis.

In patients with frank AIDS and a failing immune system despite aggressive antiretroviral therapy, the decision to treat is tempered by the short life expectancy and the fact that combination therapy in this group is associated with significant toxicity, which may hasten the progress of the HIV disease. The prudent use of debulking surgery with *limited-field postoperative radiation*, or radiation alone to areas of known disease, is the preferred approach. The dose delivered and fractionation scheme depend on the overall condition of the patient. For patients in reasonable condition, with very low CD4+ counts but no active opportunistic disease, definitive doses of radiation with reduced doses of concurrent chemotherapy may be attempted, with careful observation during treatment. Since the failure rate is significant in this group (three of four patients at UCSF with anal cancer and frank AIDS died with locally uncontrolled disease),[217] high doses are necessary to control disease for as long as possible. For the patient with advanced disease, the palliative approach outlined for cervical carcinoma is also appropriate.

HODGKIN'S DISEASE

It is still unclear whether there is an actual increase in the incidence of Hodgkin's disease (HD) in the setting of HIV infection.[13,17,206,218-222] An analysis of the Surveillance, Epidemiology and End Results (SEER) database of cases of HD in San Francisco County found a slight increase in the mid-1980s compared with the late 1970s.[222] The AIDS-Cancer Match Registry revealed 140 cases of HD among patients with HIV infection, 7.6-fold higher than expected for the general population.[138] There is ample evidence, however, that the presentation of HD is different in the HIV-infected patient than in the HIV-negative individual. Information from cohorts of patients in France,[221] Spain,[223] Italy,[224-226] and San Francisco[219] reveal that HIV-positive patients are more likely to present with HD in the advanced stages: 75% to 89% present in stage III or IV, compared to less than 33% of HIV-negative patients). These cases have a higher percentage of mixed cellularity or lymphocyte-depleted disease (53% to 63%), a greater incidence of B symptoms (83%), and a variable complete response rate to therapy (44% to 79%). The introduction of HAART is expected to have a major impact on the outcome in these patients, since such a high percentage of patients died due to AIDS-related complications during treatment for HD in the pre-HAART era, but little has been reported to date. Preference is given to instituting standard approaches with combined modality therapy as in the HIV-negative population, with aggressive HAART support included.

OTHER MALIGNANCIES

In the HIV Setting

Epidemiologic reviews have failed to show a significant rise in the incidence of most other malignancies in the setting of HIV disease or frank AIDS.[6,13,47,206,220] Squamous cell carcinoma of the conjunctiva has been associated with HPV and HIV infection, especially in Rwanda and Uganda.[138] Common cancers such as lung, prostate, and colon continue to occur at an expected rate in the HIV-positive population and present a therapeutic dilemma to radiation and medical oncologists. As with each of the previously mentioned diseases, therapeutic decisions should be based on an understanding of the

patient's current location on the timeline of their HIV disease. The institution of HAART, and manipulations of the regimen used based on changes in viral load, may continue to prolong the life expectancy of the HIV-infected individual. The ability to integrate standard chemotherapeutic strategies with HAART will continue to be a dilemma. Patients with CD4+ counts in excess of 200 cells/mm³ tolerate radiation therapy acutely as well as HIV-negative patients do, but they may suffer in the long term from prolonged marrow or bowel toxicity not normally seen in the HIV-negative population. Strong consideration should be given to the use of antiretroviral therapy during the course of radiation for any of these diseases, since the treatment itself represents a major stress that might afford a window of opportunity for increased viral replication and progression of the HIV disease.[25,26,152,202] Likewise, the use of extensive radiation fields for prophylaxis of nodal spread or combined chemoradiation in an unproven setting should be analyzed in terms of its expected risk-to-benefit ratio. The patient has not necessarily been helped if overly aggressive treatment results in rapid progression to full-blown AIDS.

REFERENCES

1. Joint United Nations Programme on HIV/AIDS (2002). http://www.unaids.org.
2. Tassie J, Grabar S, Lancar R, et al: Time to AIDS from 1992 to 1999 in HIV-1-infected patients with known date of infection. *J Acquir Immune Defic Syndr.* 2002;30:81.
3. Palella F, Delaney KM, Moorman AC, et al: Declining morbidity and mortality among patients with advanced HIV infection. *N Engl J Med.* 1998;338:853.
4. Weidle P, Holmberg SD, DeCock KM: Changes in HIV and AIDS epidemiology from new generation antiretroviral therapy. *AIDS.* 1999;13:S61.
5. Katz MH, Hessol NA, Buchbinder SP, et al: Temporal trends of opportunistic infections and malignancies in homosexual men with AIDS. *J Infect Dis.* 1994;170:198.
6. Levine AM: AIDS-related malignancies: The emerging epidemic. *J Natl Cancer Inst.* 1993;85:1382.
7. 1993 revised classification system for HIV infection and expanded surveillance case definition for AIDS among adolescents and adults. *MMWR Morb Mortal Wkly Rep.* 1992;41(RR-17):1.
8. Centers for Disease Control and Prevention: 1993 revised classification system for HIV infection and expanded surveillance case definition for AIDS among adolescents and adults. *JAMA.* 1993;269:729.
9. Engels EA: Human immunodeficiency virus infection, aging, and cancer. *J Clin Epidemiol.* 2001;54:S29.
10. Carbone A, Gaidano G: AIDS-related cancer: A study model for the mechanisms contributing to the genesis of cancer. *Eur J Cancer.* 2001;37:1184.
11. Gaidano G, Capello D, Carbone A, et al: The molecular basis of acquired immunodeficiency syndrome–related lymphomagenesis. *Semin Oncol.* 2000;27:431.
12. Levine A: Cancer in AIDS. *Curr Opin Oncol.* 1992;4:863. Editorial.
13. Levine AM: Cancer in AIDS. *Curr Opin Oncol.* 1993;5:819. Editorial.
14. Beral V, Jaffe H, Weiss R: Overview: Cancer, HIV and AIDS. *Cancer Surv.* 1991;10:1.
15. Saah AJ, Hoover DR, He Y, et al: Factors influencing survival after AIDS: Report from the Multicenter AIDS Cohort Study (MACS). *J Acquir Immune Defic Syndr.* 1994;7:287.
16. Graham NM, Zeger SL, Park LP, et al: Effect of zidovudine and *Pneumocystis carinii* pneumonia prophylaxis on progression of HIV-1 infection to AIDS. The Multicenter AIDS Cohort Study. *Lancet.* 1991;338:265.

17. Tirelli U, Francheschi S, Carbone A: Malignant tumors in patients with HIV infection. *BMJ.* 1994;308:1148.
18. Kaplan MH: Human retroviruses and neoplastic disease. *Clin Infect Dis.* 1993;17:S400.
19. Wahman A, Melnick SL, Rhame FS, et al: The epidemiology of classic, African, and immunosuppressed Kaposi's sarcoma. *Epidemiol Rev.* 1991;13:178.
20. Peterman TA, Jaffe HW, Beral V: Epidemiologic clues to the etiology of Kaposi's sarcoma. *AIDS.* 1993;7:605. Editorial.
21. Chang Y, Cesarman E, Pelissa MS, et al: Identification of herpesvirus-like DNA sequences in AIDS-associated KS. *Science.* 1994;266:1865.
22. Melbye M, Cote TR, Kessler L, et al: High incidence of anal cancer among AIDS patients. The AIDS/Cancer Working Group. *Lancet.* 1994;343:636.
23. Bonacini M, Puoti M: Hepatitis C in patients with human immunodeficiency virus infection: Diagnosis, natural history, meta-analysis of sexual and vertical transmission, and therapeutic issues. *Arch Intern Med.* 2000;160:3365.
24. Fauci AS, Rosenberg ZF: Immunopathogenesis. In Broder S, Merigan TC, Bolognesi D, eds. *Textbook of AIDS Medicine.* Baltimore: Williams & Wilkins; 1994:55.
25. Gates AE, Kaplan LD: AIDS malignancies in the era of highly active antiretroviral therapy part 1. *Oncology (Huntingt).* 2002;16:441, 456, 459.
26. Gates AE, Kaplan LD: AIDS malignancies in the era of highly active antiretroviral therapy part 2. *Oncology (Huntingt).* 2002;16:657; discussion 665, 668.
27. Hanson DL, Horsburgh CJ, Fann SA, et al: Survival prognosis of HIV-infected patients. *J Acquir Immune Defic Syndr.* 1993;6:624.
28. Saah AJ, Munoz A, Kuo V, et al: Predictors of the risk of development of acquired immunodeficiency syndrome within 24 months among gay men seropositive for human immunodeficiency virus type 1: A report from the Multicenter AIDS Cohort Study. *Am J Epidemiol.* 1992;135:1147.
29. Sabin CA, Phillips AN, Lee CA, et al: Beta-2 microglobulin as a predictor of prognosis in HIV-infected men with haemophilia: A proposed strategy for use in clinical care. *Br J Haematol.* 1994;86:366.
30. Kaposi M: Idiopathisches multiples Pigmentsarkom der Haut. *Arch Dermatol Syph.* 1872;4:265.
31. Tappero JW, Conant MA, Wolfe SF, et al: Kaposi's sarcoma: Epidemiology, pathogenesis, histology, clinical spectrum, staging criteria and therapy. *J Am Acad Dermatol.* 1993;28:371.
32. Kestons L, Melbye M, Bigger RJ: Endemic African Kaposi's is not associated with immunodeficiency. *Int J Cancer.* 1985;36:49.
33. Taylor JF, Templeton AC, Vogel CL: Kaposi's sarcoma in Uganda: A clinico-pathologic study. *Int J Cancer.* 1971;3:122.
34. Penn I: Depressed immunity and the development of cancer. *Cancer Detect Prev.* 1994;18:241. Review.
35. Penn I: Kaposi's sarcoma in immunosuppressed patients. *J Clin Lab Immunol.* 1983;12:1.
36. Harwood AR, Osoba D, Hofstadter SL: Kaposi's sarcoma in recipients of renal transplants. *Am J Med.* 1979;67:759.
37. Masur H, Michilis MA, Green JB: An outbreak of community acquired *Pneumocystis carinii* pneumonia: Initial manifestations of cellular immune dysfunction. *N Engl J Med.* 1981;305:1431.
38. Hymes KB, Cheung TL, Green JB: Kaposi's sarcoma in homosexual men: A report of 8 cases. *Lancet.* 1981;2:598.
39. Friedman-Kein A, Laubenstein L, Marmor M: Kaposi's sarcoma and pneumocystis pneumonia among homosexual men: NYC and Calif. *MMWR Morb Mortal Wkly Rep.* 1981;30:305.
40. Zucker FD, Huang YQ, Grusky GE, et al: Kaposi's sarcoma in a human immunodeficiency virus–negative patient with asymptomatic human T lymphotropic virus type I infection. *J Infect Dis.* 1993;167:987. Letter.
41. Wang JC, Rosen Y, Goel PC, et al: Kaposi's sarcoma presenting as lymphadenopathy in two HIV-negative elderly patients. *Am J Med.* 1993;94:342.
42. Huang YQ, Buchbinder A, Li JJ, et al: The absence of Tat sequences in tissues of HIV-negative patients with epidemic Kaposi's sarcoma. *AIDS.* 1992;6:1139.
43. Castro A, Pedreira J, Soriano V, et al: Kaposi's sarcoma and disseminated tuberculosis in HIV-negative individual. *Lancet.* 1992;339:868. Letter.
44. Marguart EH, Engst R, Oehlschlaegel G: An 8-year history of Kaposi's sarcoma in an HIV-negative bisexual man. *AIDS.* 1991;5:346. Letter.
45. García-Muret MP, Pujol RM, Puig L, et al: Disseminated Kaposi's sarcoma not associated with HIV infection in a bisexual man. *J Am Acad Dermatol.* 1990;5:1035.
46. Friedman KA, Saltzman BR, Cao YZ, et al: Kaposi's sarcoma in HIV-negative homosexual men. *Lancet.* 1990;335:168. Letter; see comments.
47. Rabkin CS: Epidemiology of AIDS-related malignancies. *Curr Opin Oncol.* 1994;6:492. Review.
48. Des Jarlais DC, Stoneburner R, Thomas P: Declines in proportion of Kaposi's sarcoma among cases of AIDS in multiple risk groups in NYC. *Lancet.* 1987;2:1024.
49. Dal Maso L, Serraino D, et al: Epidemiology of AIDS-related tumours in developed and developing countries. *Eur J Cancer.* 2001;37:1188.
50. Appleby P, Beral V, Newton R: HAART and incidence of cancer in HIV-infected adults. *J Natl Cancer Inst.* 2000;92:1823.
51. Jones J, Hanson DL, Dworkin MS, Jaffe HW: Incidence and trends in Kaposi sarcoma in the era of effective antiretroviral therapy. *J Acquir Immune Defic Syndr.* 2000;24:270.
52. Moore PS, Chang Y: Detection of herpesvirus-like DNA sequences in Kaposi's sarcoma in patients with and those without HIV infection. *N Engl J Med.* 1995;332:1181.
53. Ensoli B, Sgadari C, Barillari G, et al: Biology of Kaposi's sarcoma. *Eur J Cancer.* 2001;37:1251.
54. Dezube BJ: Acquired immunodeficiency syndrome–related Kaposi's sarcoma: Clinical features, staging, and treatment. *Semin Oncol.* 2000;27:424.
55. McKenzie R, Travis WD, Solan SA: The causes of death in patients with HIV infection: A clinical and pathologic study with emphasis on the role of pulmonary diseases. *Medicine (Baltimore).* 1991;70:326.
56. Klatt EC, Nichols L, Noguchi TT: Evolving trends revealed by autopsies of patients with the acquired immunodeficiency syndrome. 565 autopsies in adults with the acquired immunodeficiency syndrome, Los Angeles, Calif., 1992-1993. *Arch Pathol Lab Med.* 1994;118:884.
57. Meyer JL: Whole-lung irradiation for Kaposi's sarcoma. *Am J Clin Oncol.* 1993;16:372.
58. Krown SE, Metroka C, Wernz JC: KS in the acquired immunodeficiency syndrome: A proposal for uniform evaluation, response and staging criteria. *J Clin Oncol.* 1989;7:1201.
59. Krown S, Testa MA, Huang J: AIDS-Related KS: Prospective validation of the AIDS clinical trial group staging classification. *J Clin Oncol.* 1997;15:3085.
60. Jacobson L, Yamashita TE, Detels R: Impact of potent antiretroviral therapy on the incidence of KS and NHL among HIV-infected individuals. *J Acquir Immune Defic Syndr.* 1999;21:S34.
61. Ledergerber B, Telenti A, Egger M: Risk of HIV-related KS and NHL with potent anti-retroviral therapy: A prospective cohort. *BMJ.* 1999;319:23.
62. Tam HK, Zhang ZF, Jacobson LP, et al: Effect of highly active anti-retroviral therapy on survival among HIV-infected men with Kaposi sarcoma or non-Hodgkin lymphoma. *Int J Cancer.* 2002;98:916.
63. Fischl MA, Stanley K, Collier AC, et al: Combination and monotherapy with zidovudine and zalcitabine in patients with advanced HIV disease. The NIAID AIDS Clinical Trials Group. *Ann Intern Med.* 1995;122:24.
64. Zeger SL, Diggle PJ: Semiparametric models for longitudinal data with application to CD4 cell numbers in HIV seroconverters. *Biometrics.* 1994;50:689.
65. Munoz A, Schrager LK, Bacellar H, et al: Trends in the incidence of outcomes defining acquired immunodeficiency syndrome (AIDS) in the Multicenter AIDS Cohort Study: 1985-1991. *Am J Epidemiol.* 1993;137:423.
66. el-Sadr W, Goetz RR, Sorrell S, et al: Clinical and laboratory correlates of human immunodeficiency virus infection in a cohort of intravenous drug users from New York, NY. *Arch Intern Med.* 1992;152:1653.
67. Lau RK, Hill A, Jenkins P, et al: Eight year prospective study of HIV infection in a cohort of homosexual men: Clinical progression, immunological and virological markers. *Int J STD AIDS.* 1992;3:261.
68. Bodsworth NJ, Bloch M, Bower M, et al: Phase III vehicle-controlled, multi-centered study of topical alitretinoin gel 0.1% in cutaneous AIDS-related Kaposi's sarcoma. *Am J Clin Dermatol.* 2001;2:77.

69. Walmsley S, Northfelt DW, Melosky B, et al: Treatment of AIDS-related cutaneous Kaposi's sarcoma with topical alitretinoin (9-cis-retinoic acid) gel. Panretin Gel North American Study Group. *J Acquir Immune Defic Syndr.* 1999;22:235.

70. Newman S: Treatment of epidemic Kaposis's sarcoma with intralesional vinblastine injection. *Proc Am Soc Clin Oncol.* 1988;7:19. Abstract.

71. Boudreaux AA, Smith LL, Cosby CD, et al: Intralesional vinblastine for cutaneous Kaposi's sarcoma associated with acquired immunodeficiency syndrome. A clinical trial to evaluate efficacy and discomfort associated with infection. *J Am Acad Dermatol.* 1993;28:61.

72. Gascon P, Schwartz RA: Treatment of Kaposi's sarcoma. *Dermatol Clin.* 1994;12:451.

73. Moyle G, Youle M, Barton S: Intralesional vinblastine in the treatment of oral Kaposi's sarcoma. *Br J Clin Pract.* 1993;47:79.

74. Ramirez-Amador V, Esquivel-Pedraza L, Lozada-Nur F, et al: Intralesional vinblastine vs. 3% sodium tetradecyl sulfate for the treatment of oral Kaposi's sarcoma. A double blind, randomized clinical trial. *Oral Oncol.* 2002;38:460.

75. Tappero JW, Berger TG, Kaplan LD, et al: Cryotherapy for cutaneous Kaposi's sarcoma (KS) associated with acquired immune deficiency syndrome (AIDS): A phase II trial. *J Acquir Immune Defic Syndr.* 1991;4:839.

76. Stewart S, Jablonowski H, et al: Randomized comparative trial of pegylated liposomal doxorubicin versus bleomycin and vincristine in the treatment of AIDS-related Kaposi's sarcoma. International Pegylated Liposomal Doxorubicin Study Group. *J Clin Oncol.* 1998;16:683.

77. Tulpule A, Groopman J, et al: Multicenter trial of low-dose paclitaxel in patients with advanced AIDS-related Kaposi sarcoma. *Cancer.* 2002;95:147.

78. Miles SA, Dezube BJ, Lee JY, et al: Antitumor activity of oral 9-cis-retinoic acid in HIV-associated Kaposi's sarcoma. *AIDS.* 2002;16:421.

79. Krown S: Management of Kaposi sarcoma: The role of interferon and thalidomide. *Curr Opin Oncol.* 2001;13:374.

80. de Wit R, Smit WG, Veenhof KH, et al: Palliative radiation therapy for AIDS-associated Kaposi's sarcoma by using a single fraction of 800 cGy. *Radiother Oncol.* 1990;19:131.

81. Geara F, Le Bourgeois JP, Piedbois P, et al: Radiotherapy in the management of cutaneous epidemic Kaposi's sarcoma. *Int J Radiat Oncol Biol Phys.* 1991;21:1517.

82. Berson AM, Quivey JM, Harris JW, et al: Radiation therapy for AIDS-related Kaposi's sarcoma. *Int J Radiat Oncol Biol Phys.* 1990;19:569. See comments.

83. Raju PI, Roy T, Knight W III, et al: Palliative radiation therapy for Kaposi's sarcoma in patients with AIDS. *Mo Med.* 1990;87:26.

84. Krown SE: Treatment of AIDS-associated malignancy. *Cancer Detect Prev.* 1990;14:405.

85. Piedbois P, Frikha H, Martin L, et al: Radiotherapy in the management of epidemic Kaposi's sarcoma. *Int J Radiat Oncol Biol Phys.* 1994;30:1207.

86. Le Bourgeois JP, Frikha H, Piedbois P, et al: Radiotherapy in the management of epidemic Kaposi's sarcoma of the oral cavity, the eyelid and the genitals. *Radiother Oncol.* 1994;30:263.

87. Stelzer KJ, Griffin TW: A randomized prospective trial of radiation therapy for AIDS-associated Kaposi's sarcoma. *Int J Radiat Oncol Biol Phys.* 1993;27:1057.

88. Chang LF, Reddy S, Shidnia H: Comparison of radiation therapy of classic and epidemic Kaposi's sarcoma. *Am J Clin Oncol.* 1992;15:200.

89. Geara F, Le Bourgeois JP, Piedbois P, et al: Radiotherapy in the management of cutaneous epidemic Kaposi's sarcoma. *Int J Radiat Oncol Biol Phys.* 1991;21:1517.

90. Andriolo MJ, Lazarus TS: Radiation therapy for the treatment of palatal Kaposi's sarcoma: Report of case. *J Am Dent Assoc.* 1989;(suppl):40S.

91. Rodriguez R, Fontanesi J, Meyer JL, et al: Normal-tissue effects of irradiation for Kaposi's sarcoma/AIDS. *Front Radiat Ther Oncol.* 1989;23:150.

92. Chak LY, Gill PS, Levine AM, et al: Radiation therapy for acquired immunodeficiency syndrome-related Kaposi's sarcoma. *J Clin Oncol.* 1988;6:863.

93. Hill DR: The role of radiotherapy for epidemic Kaposi's sarcoma. *Semin Oncol.* 1987;14:19.

94. Cooper JS, Fried PR: Defining the role of radiation therapy in the management of epidemic Kaposi's sarcoma. *Int J Radiat Oncol Biol Phys.* 1987;13:35.

95. el-Akkad S, Bull CA, el-Senoussi M, et al: Kaposi's sarcoma and its management by radiotherapy. *Arch Dermatol.* 1986;122:1396.

96. Hamilton CR, Cummings BJ, Harwood AR: Radiotherapy of Kaposi's sarcoma. *Int J Radiat Oncol Biol Phys.* 1986;12:1931.

97. Harris JW, Reed TA: Kaposi's sarcoma in AIDS: The role of radiation therapy. *Front Radiat Ther Oncol.* 1985;19:126.

98. Harrison M, Harrington KJ, Tomlinson DR, et al: Response and cosmetic outcome of two fractionation regimens for AIDS-related Kaposi's sarcoma. *Radiother Oncol.* 1998;46:23.

99. Kirova YM, Belembaogo E, Frikha H, et al: Radiotherapy in the management of epidemic Kaposi's sarcoma: A retrospective study of 643 cases. *Radiother Oncol.* 1998;46:19.

100. Laurence J: 9th National Retrovirus Conference: New treatments, new choices. *AIDS Patient Care STDS.* 2002;16:193.

101. Vapnek JM, Quivey JM, Carroll PR: Acquired immunodeficiency syndrome-related Kaposi's sarcoma of the male genitalia: Management with radiation therapy. *J Urol.* 1991;146:333.

102. Ghabrial R, Quivey JM, Dunn JJ, et al: Radiation therapy of acquired immunodeficiency syndrome-related Kaposi's sarcoma of the eyelids and conjunctiva. *Arch Ophthalmol.* 1992;110:1423.

103. Cooper JS, Fried PR: Case report. Treatment of aggressive epidemic Kaposi's sarcoma of the conjunctiva by radiotherapy. *Arch Ophthalmol.* 1988;106:20.

104. Shuler JD, Holland GN, Miles SA, et al: Kaposi sarcoma of the conjunctiva and eyelids associated with the acquired immunodeficiency syndrome. *Arch Ophthalmol.* 1989;107:858.

105. Brunt AM, Phillips RH: Strontium-90 for conjunctival AIDS-related Kaposi's sarcoma: The first case report. *Clin Oncol (R Coll Radiol).* 1990;2:118.

106. Regezi JA, MacPhail LA, Daniels TE, et al: Human immunodeficiency virus–associated oral Kaposi's sarcoma. A heterogeneous cell population dominated by spindle-shaped endothelial cells. *Am J Pathol.* 1993;143:240.

107. Silverman SJ: Oral cancer education and HIV-associated malignancies. *J Cancer Educ.* 1994;9:152.

108. Cooper JS, Fried PR: Toxicity of oral radiotherapy in patients with acquired immunodeficiency syndrome. *Arch Otolaryngol Head Neck Surg.* 1987;113:327.

109. Watkins EB, Findlay P, Gelmann E, et al: Enhanced mucosal reactions in AIDS patients receiving oropharyngeal irradiation. *Int J Radiat Oncol Biol Phys.* 1987;13:1403. See comments.

110. Macklis RM: Atypical radiation toxicity in patients with classical Kaposi's sarcoma. *Tumori.* 1991;77:491.

111. Oldfield E III: Thalidomide for severe aphthous ulceration in patients with human immunodeficiency virus (HIV) infection. *Am J Gastroenterol.* 1994;89:2276.

112. Friedman M, Brenski A, Taylor L: Treatment of aphthous ulcers in AIDS patients. *Laryngoscope.* 1994;104:566.

113. Muzyka BC, M Glick: Major aphthous ulcers in patients with HIV disease. *Oral Surg Oral Med Oral Pathol.* 1994;77:116.

114. Reyes-Teran G, Ramirez-Amador V, De la Rosa E, et al: Major recurrent oral ulcers in AIDS: Report of three cases. *J Oral Pathol Med.* 1992;21:409.

115. Harindra V, Roy RB: Papulo-pruritic eruption and giant ulceration of the mouth: A difficult clinical feature to treat in the patient infected with human immunodeficiency virus. *Arch Intern Med.* 1992;152:1924. Letter; comment.

116. MacPhail LA, Greenspan D, Greenspan JS: Recurrent aphthous ulcers in association with HIV infection. Diagnosis and treatment. *Oral Surg Oral Med Oral Pathol.* 1992;73:283. See comments.

117. Silverman SJ, Gallo J, Stites DP: Prednisone management of HIV-associated recurrent oral aphthous ulcerations. *J Acquir Immune Defic Syndr.* 1992;5:952. Letter.

118. MacPhail LA, Greenspan D, Feigal DW, et al: Recurrent aphthous ulcers in association with HIV infection. Description of ulcer types and analysis of T-lymphocyte subsets. *Oral Surg Oral Med Oral Pathol.* 1991;71:678.

119. Phelan JA, Eisig S, Freedman PD, et al: Major aphthous-like ulcers in patients with AIDS. *Oral Surg Oral Med Oral Pathol.* 1991;71:68.

120. Lands RH, Ange D, Hartman DL: Radiation therapy for classic Kaposi's sarcoma presenting only on the glans penis. *J Urol.* 1992;147:468.

121. Montes C, Luepschen OM, Schmall L, et al: Kaposi's sarcoma of the foot in the HIV patient. *J Foot Ankle Surg.* 1994;33:341.

122. Steinfeld AD, Cooper JS: Epidemic and classic Kaposi's sarcoma of the feet. A comparative study. *J Am Podiatr Med Assoc.* 1990;80:469.

123. Berlin SJ, Jurd JA: Kaposi's sarcoma in the foot. A retrospective study. *Clin Podiatr Med Surg.* 1992;9:849.

124. Stelzer KJ, Griffin TW, Koh WJ: Radiation recall skin toxicity with bleomycin in a patient with Kaposi sarcoma related to acquired immune deficiency syndrome. *Cancer.* 1993;71:1322.

125. Nemechek PM, Corder MC: Radiation recall associated with vinblastine in a patient treated for Kaposi sarcoma related to acquired immune deficiency syndrome. *Cancer.* 1992;70:1605.

126. Laine L, Amerian J, Rarick M, et al: The response of symptomatic gastrointestinal Kaposi's sarcoma to chemotherapy: A prospective evaluation using an endoscopic method of disease quantification. *Am J Gastroenterol.* 1990;85:959.

127. Parente F, Cernuschi M, Orlando G, et al: Kaposi's sarcoma and AIDS: Frequency of gastrointestinal involvement and its effect on survival. A prospective study in a heterogeneous population. *Scand J Gastroenterol.* 1991;26:1007.

128. Perciballi JA, Etienne HB, BC Ghosh: Kaposi's sarcoma with emphasis on gastrointestinal manifestations. *Mil Med.* 1990;155:23.

129. Morgello S, Mahboob R, et al: Autopsy findings in a human immunodeficiency virus–infected population over 2 decades: Influences of gender, ethnicity, risk factors, and time. *Arch Pathol Lab Med.* 2002;126:182.

130. Mitchell DM, McCarty M, Fleming J, et al: Bronchopulmonary Kaposi's sarcoma in patients with AIDS. *Thorax.* 1992;47:726.

131. Miller RF, Tomlinson MC, Cottrill CP, et al: Bronchopulmonary Kaposi's sarcoma in patients with AIDS. *Thorax.* 1992;47:721.

132. Doyle M, Johnstone PA, Watkins EB: Role of radiation therapy in management of pulmonary Kaposi's sarcoma. *South Med J.* 1993;86:285.

133. Nobler MP: Pulmonary irradiation for Kaposi's sarcoma in AIDS. *Am J Clin Oncol.* 1985;8:441.

134. Holkova B, Takeshita K, et al: Effect of highly active antiretroviral therapy on survival in patients with AIDS-associated pulmonary Kaposi's sarcoma treated with chemotherapy. *J Clin Oncol.* 2001;19:3848.

135. Devesa SS, Fears T: Non-Hodgkin's lymphoma time trends: United States and international data. *Cancer Res.* 1992;52 (suppl):5432S.

136. Gail MH, Pluda JM, Rabkin CS, et al: Projections of the incidence of non-Hodgkin's lymphoma related to acquired immunodeficiency syndrome. *J Natl Cancer Inst.* 1991;83:695. See comments.

137. Rabkin CS, Biggar RJ, Baptiste MS, et al: Cancer incidence trends in women at high risk of human immunodeficiency virus (HIV) infection. *Int J Cancer.* 1993;55:208.

138. Goedert J, Cote TR, Virgo P: Spectrum of AIDS-associated malignant disorders. *Lancet.* 1998;351:1833.

139. Knowles D, Pirog EC: Pathology of AIDS-related lymphomas and other AIDS-defining illnesses. *Eur J Cancer.* 2001;37:1236.

140. Herndier BG, Kaplan LD, McGrath MS: Pathogenesis of AIDS lymphomas. *AIDS.* 1994;8:1025.

141. Biggar R, Engels EA, Frisch M, Goedert JJ: Risk of T-cell lymphomas in persons with AIDS. *J Acquir Immune Defic Syndr.* 2001;26:371.

142. Shiramizu B, Herndier BG, McGrath MS: Identification of a clonal human immunodefieiciency virus integration site in HIV-associated lymphomas. *Cancer Res.* 1994;54:2069.

143. Ziegler JL: Lymphomas and other neoplasms associated with AIDS. *Immunol Ser.* 1989;44:359.

144. Kaplan LD: AIDS-associated lymphomas. In Volberding P, Jacobson MA, eds. *AIDS Clinical Review 1991.* New York: Marcel Dekker Inc.; 1991:181.

145. Rabkin CS, Hilgartner MW, Hedberg KW, et al: Incidence of lymphomas and other cancers in HIV-infected and HIV-uninfected patients with hemophilia. *JAMA.* 1992;267:1090.

146. Lamb R, Gonzalez R, Myers A, et al: Aggressive non-Hodgkin's lymphomas in AIDS: The University of Colorado experience. *Am J Med Sci.* 1990;300:345.

147. Stanley H, Fluetsch BM, Bunce CM: HIV-related non-Hodgkin's lymphoma. *Oncol Nurs Forum.* 1991;18:875.

148. Irwin D, Kaplan L: Clinical aspects of HIV-related lymphoma. *Curr Opin Oncol.* 1993;5:852.

149. Kaplan LD: HIV-associated lymphoma. *Aids Clin Rev.* 1993;94:145.

150. Levine AM: AIDS-associated malignant lymphoma. *Med Clin North Am.* 1992;76:253.

151. Little R, Pearson D, Steinberg S: Dose-adjusted EPOCH chemotherapy in previously untreated HIV-associated NHL. *Proc Am Soc Clin Oncol.* 1999;18:16a.

152. Levine AM: Acquired immunodeficiency syndrome–related lymphoma: Clinical aspects. *Semin Oncol.* 2000;27:442.

153. Matthews B, Bower M, Mandalia S: Changes in AIDS-related lymphoma since the introduction of highly active anti-retroviral therapy. *Blood.* 2000;96:2730.

154. Kaplan LD, Abrams DI, Feigal E, et al: AIDS-associated non-Hodgkin's lymphoma in San Francisco. *JAMA.* 1989;261:719.

155. Sparano JA: Clinical aspects and management of AIDS-related lymphoma. *Eur J Cancer.* 2001;37:1296.

156. Cesarman E: The role of Kaposi's sarcoma-associated herpesvirus (KSHV/HHV-8) in lymphoproliferative diseases. *Recent Results Cancer Res.* 2002;159:27.

157. Hengge UR, Ruzicka T, Tyring SK, et al: Update on Kaposi's sarcoma and other HHV8 associated diseases. Part 1: Epidemiology, environmental predispositions, clinical manifestations, and therapy. *Lancet Infect Dis.* 2002;2:281.

158. Oksenhendler E, Boulanger E, Galicier L, et al: High incidence of Kaposi sarcoma–associated herpesvirus-related non-Hodgkin lymphoma in patients with HIV infection and multicentric Castleman disease. *Blood.* 2002;99:2331.

159. Loeffler JS, Ervin TJ, Mauch P, et al: Primary lymphomas of the central nervous system: Patterns of failure and factors that influence survival. *J Clin Oncol.* 1985;3:490.

160. Freeman CR, Shustik C, Brisson ML, et al: Primary malignant lymphoma of the central nervous system. *Cancer.* 1986;58:1106.

161. Mendenhall NP, Thar TL, Agee OF, et al: Primary lymphoma of the central nervous system. Computerized tomography scan characteristics and treatment results for 12 cases. *Cancer.* 1983;52:1993.

162. Ling SM, Roach M III, Larson DA, et al: Radiotherapy of primary central nervous system lymphoma in patients with and without human immunodeficiency virus. Ten years of treatment experience at the University of California San Francisco. *Cancer.* 1994;73:2570.

163. Ambinder RF, Sparano JA: Primary central nervous system lymphoma. *Cancer Treat Res.* 2001;104:231.

164. Sacktor N, Lyles RH, Skolasky R et al: HIV-associated neurologic disease incidence changes: Multicenter AIDS Cohort Study, 1990-1998. *Neurology.* 2001;56:257.

165. Shiramizu B, McGrath MS: Molecular pathogenesis of AIDS-associated non-Hodgkin's lymphoma. *Hematol Oncol Clin North Am.* 1991;5:323.

166. Forsyth PA, Yahalom J, DeAngelis LM: Combined-modality therapy in the treatment of primary central nervous system lymphoma in AIDS. *Neurology.* 1994;44:1473.

167. Raez L, Cabral L, Cai JP: Treatment of AIDS-related primary CNS lymphoma with zidovudine, ganciclovir and IL-2. *J AIDS Hum Retroviruses.* 1999;15:713.

168. Ferreri A, Reni M, Villa E: Therapeutic management of primary CNS lymphoma: Lessons from prospective trials. *Ann Oncol.* 2000;11:927.

169. Kaplan LD: AIDS-related non-Hodgkin's lymphoma. In UCSF 15th Annual Conference: Current Approaches to Radiation Oncology, Biology, and Physics; March 13-15, 1995; San Francisco. Paper number 12.

170. Baumgartner JE, Rachlin JR, Beckstead JH, et al: Primary central nervous system lymphomas: Natural history and response to radiation therapy in 55 patients with acquired immunodeficiency syndrome. *J Neurosurg.* 1990;73:206.

171. Errante D, Vaccher E, Tirelli U, et al: Management of AIDS and its neoplastic complications. *Eur J Cancer.* 1991;27:380.

172. Pluda JM, Broder S, Yarchoan R: Therapy of AIDS and AIDS-related tumors. *Cancer Chemother Biol Response Modif.* 1991;12:395.

173. Remick SC, McSharry JJ, Wolf BC, et al: Novel oral combination chemotherapy in the treatment of intermediate-grade and high-grade AIDS-related non-Hodgkin's lymphoma. *J Clin Oncol.* 1993;11:1691.

174. Sparano JA, Wiernik PH, Strack M, et al: Infusional cyclophosphamide, doxorubicin, and etoposide in human immunodeficiency virus- and human T-cell leukemia virus type I-related non-Hodgkin's lymphoma: A highly active regimen. *Blood.* 1993;81:2810.

175. O'Reilly SE, Connors JM: Non-Hodgkin's lymphoma: II. Management problems. *BMJ.* 1992;305:39.

176. O'Reilly SE, Connors JM: Non-Hodgkin's lymphoma: I. Characterisation and treatment. *BMJ.* 1992;304:1682.

177. Miller T, Dahlberg S, Cassady JR, et al: Chemotherapy alone compared with chemotherapy plus radiotherapy for localized intermediate- and high-grade non-Hodgkin's lymphoma. *N Engl J Med.* 1998;339:21.

178. Rabkin CS, Yellin F: Cancer incidence in a population with a high prevalence of infection with human immunodeficiency virus type 1. *J Natl Cancer Inst.* 1994;86:1711.

179. Buehler JW, Ward JW: A new definition for AIDS surveillance. *Ann Intern Med.* 1993;118:390. Editorial.

180. Reardon D, Johnson D, Alderete E, et al: Review of invasive cervical cancer cases for AIDS surveillance. *J Acquir Immune Defic Syndr.* 1994;7:631. Letter.

181. McKenna MT, Buehler JW, Qualters JR, et al: HIV and trends in cervical cancer death rates among young women. *Am J Public Health.* 1993;83:1792. Letter; comment.

182. Smith JR, Kitchen VS, Botcherby M, et al: Is HIV infection associated with an increase in the prevalence of cervical neoplasia? *Br J Obstet Gynaecol.* 1993;100:149.

183. Centers for Disease Control: Risk for cervical disease in HIV-infected women–New York City. *JAMA.* 1991;265:23.

184. Risk for cervical disease in HIV-infected women–New York City. *MMWR Morb Mortal Wkly Rep.* 1990;39:846.

185. Williams AB, Darragh TM, Vranizan K, et al: Anal and cervical human papillomavirus infection and risk of anal and cervical epithelial abnormalities in human immunodeficiency virus-infected women. *Obstet Gynecol.* 1994;83:205.

186. Tweddel G, Heller P, Cunnane M, et al: The correlation between HIV seropositivity, cervical dysplasia, and HPV subtypes 6/11, 16/18, 31/33/35. *Gynecol Oncol.* 1994;52:161.

187. Maggwa BN, Hunter DJ, Mbugua S, et al: The relationship between HIV infection and cervical intraepithelial neoplasia among women attending two family planning clinics in Nairobi, Kenya. *AIDS.* 1993;7:733.

188. Mandelblatt JS, Fahs M, Garibaldi K, et al: Association between HIV infection and cervical neoplasia: Implications for clinical care of women at risk for both conditions. *AIDS.* 1992;6:173.

189. Northfelt DW, Palefsky JM: Human papillomavirus–associated anogenital neoplasia in persons with HIV infection. *AIDS Clin Rev.* 1992;1992:241.

190. Robinson WR, Freeman D: Improved outcome of cervical neoplasia in HIV-infected women in the era of highly active antiretroviral therapy. *AIDS Patient Care STDS.* 2002;16:61.

191. Del Mistro A, Chieco Bianchi L: HPV-related neoplasias in HIV-infected individuals. *Eur J Cancer.* 2001;37:1227.

192. Dorrucci M, Suligoi B, et al: Incidence of invasive cervical cancer in a cohort of HIV-seropositive women before and after the introduction of highly active antiretroviral therapy. *J Acquir Immune Defic Syndr.* 2001;26:377.

193. Northfelt DW: Cervical and anal neoplasia and HPV infection in persons with HIV infection. *Oncology (Huntingt).* 1994;8:33.

194. Palefsky J: Human papillomavirus infection among HIV-infected individuals. Implications for development of malignant tumors. *Hematol Oncol Clin North Am.* 1991;5:357.

195. Palefsky JM, Holly EA, Gonzales J, et al: Natural history of anal cytologic abnormalities and papillomavirus infection among homosexual men with group IV HIV disease. *J Acquir Immune Defic Syndr.* 1992;5:1258.

196. Palefsky JM: Anal human papillomavirus infection and anal cancer in HIV-positive individuals: An emerging problem. *AIDS.* 1994;8:283. Editorial.

197. Schafer A, Friedmann W, Mielke M, et al: The increased frequency of cervical dysplasia-neoplasia in women infected with the human immunodeficiency virus is related to the degree of immunosuppression. *Am J Obstet Gynecol.* 1991;164:593.

198. McDermott VG, Langer JE, Schiebler ML: Case report: HIV-related rapidly progressive carcinoma of the cervix AIDS-CT and MRI findings. *Clin Radiol.* 1994;49:896.

199. Schwartz LB, Carcangiu ML, Bradham L, et al: Rapidly progressive squamous cell carcinoma of the cervix coexisting with human immunodeficiency virus infection: Clinical opinion. *Gynecol Oncol.* 1991;41:255.

200. Rellihan MA, Dooley DP, Burke TW, et al: Rapidly progressing cervical cancer in a patient with human immunodeficiency virus infection. *Gynecol Oncol.* 1990;36:435.

201. Maiman M, Fruchter RG, Guy L, et al: Human immunodeficiency virus infection and invasive cervical carcinoma. *Cancer.* 1993;71:402.

202. Mueller BU, Pizzo PA: Cancer in children with primary or secondary immunodeficiencies. *J Pediatr.* 1995;126:1.

203. Spanos WJ, Clery M, Perez CA, et al: Late effect of multiple daily fraction palliation schedule for advanced pelvic malignancies (RTOG 8502). *Int J Radiat Oncol Biol Phys.* 1994;29:961.

204. Spanos WJ, Perez CA, Marcus S, et al: Effect of rest interval on tumor and normal tissue response—A report of phase III study of accelerated split course palliative radiation for advanced pelvic malignancies (RTOG-8502). *Int J Radiat Oncol Biol Phys.* 1993;25:399. See comments.

205. Melbye M, Rabkin C, Frisch M, et al: Changing patterns of anal cancer incidence in the United States, 1940-1989. *Am J Epidemiol.* 1994;139:772.

206. Biggar RJ, Curtis RE, Cote TR, et al: Risk of other cancers following Kaposi's sarcoma: Relation to acquired immunodeficiency syndrome. *Am J Epidemiol.* 1994;139:362.

207. Holly EA, Whittemore AS, Aston DA, et al: Anal cancer incidence: Genital warts, anal fissure or fistula, hemorrhoids, and smoking. *J Natl Cancer Inst.* 1989;81:1726.

208. Sonnex C, Mindel A: Sexual practices, sexually transmitted diseases, and the incidence of anal cancer. *N Engl J Med.* 1988;318:990. Letter.

209. Daling JR, Weiss NS, Hislop TG, et al: Sexual practices, sexually transmitted diseases, and the incidence of anal cancer. *N Engl J Med.* 1987;317:973.

210. Melbye M, Rabkin C, Frisch M, et al: Changing patterns of anal cancer incidence in the United States, 1940-1989. *Am J Epidemiol.* 1994;139:772.

211. Frisch M, Melbye M, Moller H: Trends in incidence of anal cancer in Denmark. *BMJ.* 1993;306:419.

212. Goldie S, Kuntz KM, Weinstein MC, et al: The clinical effectiveness and cost-effectiveness of screening for anal squamous intraepithelial lesions in homosexual and bisexual HIV-positive men. *JAMA.* 1999;281:1822.

213. Palefsky JM, Holly EA, Ralston ML, et al: Effect of highly active antiretroviral therapy on the natural history of anal squamous intraepithelial lesions and anal human papillomavirus infection. *J Acquir Immune Defic Syndr.* 2001;28:422.

214. Hoffman R, Welton ML, Klencke B, et al: The significance of pretreatment CD4 count on the outcome and treatment tolerance of HIV-positive patients with anal cancer. *Int J Radiat Oncol Biol Phys.* 1999;44:127.

215. Cleator S, Fife K, Nelson M, et al: Treatment of HIV-associated invasive anal cancer with combined chemoradiation. *Eur J Cancer.* 2000;36:754.

216. Chang GJ, Berry JM, et al: Surgical treatment of high-grade anal squamous intraepithelial lesions: A prospective study. *Dis Colon Rectum.* 2002;45:453.

217. Holland JM, Swift PS: Tolerance of patients with human immunodeficiency virus and anal carcinoma to treatment with combined chemotherapy and radiation therapy. *Radiology.* 1994;193:251.

218. Wabinga HR, Parkin DM, Wabwire MF, et al: Cancer in Kampala, Uganda, in 1989-91: Changes in incidence in the era of AIDS. *Int J Cancer.* 1993;54:26.

219. Hessol NA, Katz MH, Liu JY, et al: Increased incidence of Hodgkin disease in homosexual men with HIV infection. *Ann Intern Med.* 1992;117:309. See comments.

220. Reynolds P, Saunders LD, Layefsky ME, et al: The spectrum of acquired immunodeficiency syndrome (AIDS)-associated malignancies in San Francisco, 1980-1987. *Am J Epidemiol.* 1993;137:19.

221. Andrieu JM, Roithmann S, Tourani JM, et al: Hodgkin's disease during HIV1 infection: The French registry experience. French Registry of HIV-associated Tumors. *Ann Oncol.* 1993;4:635.

222. Medeiros LJ, Greiner TC: Hodgkin's disease. *Cancer.* 1995;75(suppl):357.

223. Rubio R: Hodgkin's disease associated with human immunodeficiency virus infection. A clinical study of 46 cases. Cooperative Study Group of Malignancies Associated with HIV Infection of Madrid. *Cancer.* 1994;73:2400.

224. Errante D, Zagonel V, Vaccher E, et al: Hodgkin's disease in patients with HIV infection and in the general population: Comparison of clinicopathological features and survival. *Ann Oncol.* 1994;2:37.

225. Spina M, Vaccher E, et al: Human immunodeficiency virus-associated Hodgkin's disease. *Semin Oncol.* 2000;27:480.

226. Dolcetti R, Boiocchi M, et al: Pathogenetic and histogenetic features of HIV-associated Hodgkin's disease. *Eur J Cancer.* 2001;37:1276.

Benign Disease

68

Seth A. Rosenthal, MD

The use of radiation in the treatment of benign diseases has a long and not entirely honorable history. Soon after the discovery of x-rays by Röntgen in 1895, the therapeutic potential of radiation was recognized. In the first half of the 20th century, radiation therapy was used empirically for a host of conditions, both benign and malignant. In many situations in which no effective therapeutic alternatives existed, radiation therapy may have been one of the few treatment options available. In the pre–World War II era, few controlled studies that would pass muster by today's standards were performed. It is likely that the true efficacy of radiation treatment in relation to contemporary standard therapies for a host of conditions will never be known.[1-3]

Radiation treatment for benign conditions has declined for two major reasons. One is awareness of the deleterious late effects of radiation including the potential for the induction of malignancy. In addition, advances in surgical technique and the development of effective medical therapies such as corticosteroids and antibiotics have provided effective alternatives to the use of ionizing radiation for benign conditions in most instances. With today's knowledge there is a tendency for prima facie condemnation of the prior widespread use of radiation for benign conditions. However, when critiquing past uses of radiation therapy for benign conditions, one must remember the limited alternative therapies available at the time the treatment was delivered, as well as the state of knowledge regarding the late effects of radiation.

Nonetheless, the radiation oncologist remains the clinician with primary expertise in the use of ionizing radiation to treat disease, both benign and malignant. There are situations in which ionizing radiation remains a commonly accepted therapeutic alternative or even the treatment of choice for nonmalignant conditions. In these situations, the radiation oncologist's knowledge of the effects of radiation on normal tissues can assist the patient and referring clinician in selecting the treatment regimen with the highest therapeutic ratio for a particular individual. In many cases, the use of radiation therapy for benign disorders may be able to spare the patient morbidity associated with the progression of the disease, or additional medical or surgical therapy. Although radiation can have significant morbidity, in many cases the morbidity of radiation is low when compared with the morbidity (or even mortality) associated with alternative therapies, or with the complications associated with progressive or recurrent disease. Radiation carcinogenesis, although always a concern when ionizing radiation is used, appears to be a greater risk for pediatric patients and young adults than for older adults and must be weighed in relation to the consequences of progressive disease and the side effects associated with alternative therapies.[4]

There are certain benign tumors for which radiation therapy has continued to be standard treatment, such as pituitary tumors, meningiomas, keratoacanthoma, craniopharyngiomas, and so forth, that are discussed elsewhere in the book. However, the therapeutic use of radiation for benign disorders is not static, nor is it limited to conditions for which radiation was used in the past and is now "grandfathered" into the standard of care. For example, stereotactic radiation therapy for the treatment of intracranial arteriovenous malformations (AVMs) has become accepted as a standard treatment in recent years. The use of intravascular brachytherapy to reduce the risk of restenosis after angioplasty has become standard practice in a short period of time. The use of radiation to prevent heterotopic ossification (HO) has begun and expanded in the last 2 decades, as HO was not a significant clinical problem before the routine use of total hip arthroplasty. These examples should remind the reader that radiation treatment of benign diseases represents an important part of the mainstream practice of radiation oncology in the new millenium.

This chapter reviews the rationale, indications, and treatment of benign conditions commonly encountered in contemporary practice. Monographs written on the subject of radiation therapy for benign diseases provide more detailed and comprehensive reviews, as well as reference lists, than can be contained here.[5-7,7a] Literature reviews or computerized searches of medical databases may be useful in approaching a consultation on an unusual clinical problem.

The topics covered in this chapter include those that are most likely to be commonly encountered in contemporary radiation oncology practice and are not covered elsewhere in the book. They include eye and orbital conditions (pterygium, thyroid ophthalmopathy, orbital lymphoid hyperplasia, and pseudotumor), certain benign tumors of the head and neck (juvenile nasal angiofibroma, chemodectomas), proliferations of tissue in response to injury that cause functional or cosmetic impairment (pterygia, keloids, heterotopic ossification), and several miscellaneous uses of radiation for benign diseases (gynecomastia, Peyronie's disease). In these situations, a role for radiation therapy in the contemporary management of a benign disorder continues to exist. The use of total lymphoid irradiation (TLI) as treatment for diseases such as rheumatoid arthritis, multiple sclerosis, and amyotrophic lateral sclerosis (ALS), and in conjunction with organ transplantation, is discussed at the end of the chapter. More comprehensive lists of benign diseases for which radiation has been used therapeutically can be found in other sources.[7]

The need for informed consent exists everywhere in radiation oncology, and certainly in the use of radiation therapy for benign diseases. Patients should be informed of the rationale, potential side effects, and treatment alternatives to radiation treatment before it is delivered. Special caution should be used before radiation is delivered to pediatric patients and young adults for benign conditions, as they may be at increased risk of second malignancy induction, as well as late atrophy, especially if the area to be treated is in proximity to the breasts or thyroid, tissues that may be sensitive to carcinogenesis. As in all aspects of radiation therapy, care should be taken to use beams of appropriate energy and to shield adjacent normal structures.[3,5,7]

KELOIDS

Keloids are hypertrophic scars in which collagenous tissue is overproduced and grows beyond the original dimensions of the wound. The etiology of keloids is unknown, but increased rates of collagen metabolism have been noted in keloids. For unknown reasons, certain individuals are predisposed to keloid formation after surgery or other skin injury. Lesions appear to occur more frequently among black people and Asian people. In addition to cosmetic problems, keloids can become painful, pruritic, or fibrotic and can produce significant morbidity.[8]

Various treatment options have been described. Surgical re-excision of the keloid alone is sufficient in some cases. The use of pressure postoperatively has been effective in some cases, but it is inconvenient because it must be applied for many months postoperatively to be effective. Injections of a corticosteroid (triamcinolone) have been used and can produce a reduction in the size of established keloids, although it is not effective in all cases.[9] Pulsed-dye laser treatment has been reported to be successful in one series.[9a] Various other drugs and surgical methods have been used in small series of patients with variable results.

Radiation therapy has been employed successfully in the treatment of keloids since the early 20th century.[10] In most series, external kilovoltage or electron beam radiation is directed at the surgical bed within 24 to 72 hours after re-excision of the keloid. Interstitial iridium (Ir)-192 treatment has been reported in a large contemporary series from France.[11] Treatment of established lesions without re-excision may relieve symptoms in some cases, but results appear to be significantly less satisfactory than when radiation treatment is performed promptly after re-excision.[12] Large lesions may be treated with a combination of re-excision and skin grafting followed by

postoperative irradiation.[13] Typical dose-fractionation schemes range from 9 to 16 Gy in 3 to 4 Gy fractions. There does not appear to be a significant dose-response relationship in this dose range.

Results with the combination of re-excision and irradiation for keloids have been excellent. Borok and colleagues[12] reported a recurrence rate of only 2% in a series of 393 lesions in 250 patients; doses in the range of 9 to 12 Gy were most commonly used. Doornbos and colleagues[14] reported on 278 keloids treated with 120 kV x-rays and reported a 26% recurrence rate; an increased rate of recurrence has been reported when doses of 6 Gy or less have been used. Kovalic and colleagues[15] analyzed results of 107 patients treated at the Mallinckrodt Institute of Radiology from 1966 to 1987. Of these, 74% were earlobe lesions and were most commonly treated with 12 Gy in three fractions of 4 Gy over 3 days, with initiation of radiation within 72 hours of surgery. With a mean follow-up of 117 months, 27% of lesions recurred, with a mean time to recurrence of 12.8 months. Factors associated with significantly increased risk of recurrence included male sex, lesion size greater than 2 cm, and previous antikeloid therapy. No advantage to beginning therapy within 24 hours was reported. Excellent cosmetic results were reported in 95% of the patients.

The technique for the treatment of keloids is relatively straightforward. The re-excision incision, plus a 1 to 2 cm margin, is treated. All suture sites should be included. Superficial 100 to 250 kV x-rays can be used, or 6 to 10 MeV electrons with 0.5 to 1.0 cm of bolus so that the most superficial tissues are not underdosed. Doses of 9 to 16 Gy in three to four fractions of 3 to 4 Gy each are adequate if treatment is begun within 72 hours of excision.

Overall cosmetic results after re-excision and radiation are excellent, and acute morbidity is minimal. The overall profile of morbidity and efficacy compares favorably with that of other treatments for keloids. For patients with keloids that have recurred after a trial of other therapeutic modalities, re-excision followed by irradiation should be considered.

PTERYGIA

Pterygia are triangular, fleshy-colored proliferations of fibrovascular tissue that can obscure vision if they progress onto the visual axis of the cornea. They occur most frequently in fair-skinned individuals between 20 and 50 years of age, and an association with exposure to ultraviolet light and dust has been postulated. Surgical excision is performed if the lesions become symptomatic with respect to visual impairment or decreased ocular mobility, or if they cause cosmetic problems.

Approximately 20% to 30% of primarily excised pterygia recur if no adjuvant treatment is employed. The recurrence rates increase to 30% to 60% after the excision of recurrent lesions. Various surgical (keratectomy, conjunctival grafts) and medical (e.g., topical mitomycin C, thiotepa, or steroids) therapies have been used to reduce recurrence rates, and postoperative radiation treatment has also been widely used.

Radiation is applied postoperatively using a strontium-90 applicator, which replaced earlier generations of beta-ray applicators when strontium-90 became available in the 1950s. Strontium-90 (half-life, 28.1 years; maximal beta energy, 0.54 MeV) is in secular equilibrium with yttrium-90 (half-life, 64 hours; maximal beta energy, 2.27 MeV). The dose is rapidly attenuated, with approximately 38% of the dose at 2 mm depth, and 10% at the 4 mm depth of the lens.[16]

Radiation is delivered by the direct application of the strontium-90 applicator to the surgical bed, with a 1 to 2 mm margin. Lid retractors are often used to facilitate visualization and placement of the source (Fig. 68-1). The dose is determined by controlling the time the applicator is in contact with the eye. The time interval from surgery to the first strontium-90 application is important. Treatment is generally initiated within 48 hours of excision, with some authors recommending the initiation of radiation on the day of excision. Wilder and colleagues[17] reported an improved local control rate (87% vs. 62%; $P = 0.005$) for those patients in whom radiation began 1 to 8 versus 16 to 24 hours after excision.

Various dose-fractionation schemes have been used, ranging from 18 Gy in a single fraction[18] to 60 Gy in 6×10 Gy fractions.[19] A common dose-fractionation scheme is 3×8 Gy, with the first fraction delivered on the day of excision and the second and third doses 1 and 2 weeks later. Although there is not a clearly demonstrable dose-response relationship, a number of authors have reported improved results in patients who received three fractions (8 to 12 Gy) compared with only one or two fractions (8 to 12 Gy).[17,20,21] Recurrence rates after the use of radiation have been low, ranging from approximately 2%[19,20] to approximately 12%[17,21-23] across a range of major reported series. Differences in results among series may be due to patient selection and the intensity and duration of follow-up, as well as the dose-fractionation schemes, time between surgery and radiotherapy, and technique employed.

Complications are reported after radiation treatment. It is not uncommon for patients to have conjunctival irritation, which can persist for several weeks to months after treatment in rare cases. Other complications, such as corneal ulceration, scleral thinning, granuloma formation, and telangiectasia formation, have been reported. The exact incidence of significant complications is difficult to define, but MacKenzie and colleagues[23] estimated a 4.5% incidence of severe scleral thinning in a large Australian cohort that had been followed for at least 10 years.

Concern regarding cataractogenesis surrounds the role of radiation treatment for pterygia, but it is not clear that it occurs. Van den Brenk[20] reported an absence of radiation-induced cataracts in a series of more than 1000 cases treated, and several studies[17,24] have reported no difference in the number of cataracts in irradiated versus nonirradiated eyes if dose-fractionation schemes such as 8 Gy $\times 3$ are used. In this fractionation scheme, the dose to the lens would be approximately 0.8 Gy $\times 3$, below the threshold for cataractogenesis.

In patients who have undergone reirradiation of recurrent pterygia, both higher recurrence rates and more severe complications have been observed.[17,25] Reirradiation of pterygia should be approached with caution, but the rate of serious complications after primary treatment is low.

The use of beta irradiation from strontium-90 plaques as an adjunctive therapy to surgical removal of pterygia is simple, well-tolerated, and effective. Patients in whom pterygia recur after primary surgical therapy may be at higher risk of subsequent recurrence and may be especially good candidates for radiation. After irradiation, the subsequent recurrence rate is reduced, and the patient can avoid the morbidity of recurrence as well as the need for an additional surgical procedure.

THYROID OPHTHALMOPATHY

Thyroid ophthalmopathy occurs most frequently in association with Graves' disease but can arise in association with other conditions such as Hashimoto's thyroiditis. Euthyroid Graves' ophthalmopathy may also occur. The cause of Graves' disease is not certain, but thyroid ophthalmopathy arises when circulating T cells directed at an antigen on thyroid cells recognize a similar or closely related antigen on orbital fibroblasts and/or extraocular myocytes. These T cells then infiltrate orbital connective tissues, producing an autoimmune reaction whereby glycosaminoglycan production by fibroblasts is increased. This produces an increase in connective tissue volume and the resultant clinical manifestations of reduced extraocular muscle mobility, diplopia, exophthalmos, and periorbital edema. Histopathologically, these changes are characterized by lymphocytic infiltration of orbital tissues (primarily by T cells) and by the accumulation of glycosaminoglycans in orbital fat and extraocular muscles.[26,27]

Although most patients with Graves' disease have some measure of exophthalmos or increased size of extraocular muscles when compared with normal subjects, clinically evident ophthalmopathy is present in approximately 40% of patients. Use of an exophthalmometer can assist in the assessment and follow-up of patients with thyroid

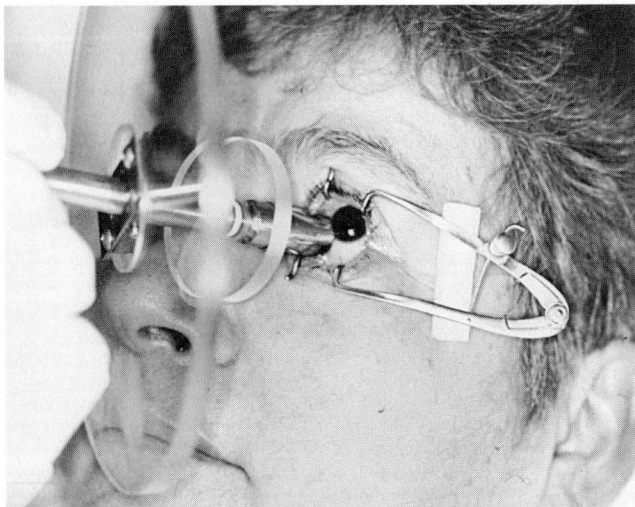

Figure 68–1. Strontium plaque being applied as postoperative treatment for pterygium.

ophthalmopathy. Clinical manifestations range from subtle changes of periorbital edema or exophthalmos, sometimes associated with lid retraction and stare, which may be primarily a cosmetic concern, to situations in which the eye or vision may be threatened. Severe exophthalmos can leave the cornea exposed to inflammation and potential injury. Decreased motion of extraocular muscles and orbital compression can lead to diplopia, pain, optic neuropathy, and the potential for permanent loss of vision.[28]

Except in circumstances in which there is the threat of impending visual loss, management of ophthalmopathy should begin with treatment of the underlying thyroid disorder by appropriate means (i.e., thyroidectomy, antithyroid drugs, radioactive iodine). For better or worse, there seems to be greater consensus and success surrounding the management of the thyroid condition than the associated ophthalmopathy.[28] A wide range of therapeutic options have been proposed and advocated for the treatment of thyroid ophthalmopathy. For some patients with mild ophthalmopathy, no treatment at all, or simple symptomatic remedies such as eye drops and sleeping with the head of the bed elevated to reduce periorbital edema may be sufficient, whereas for patients in whom there is rapid progression, neuropathy, and imminent loss of vision, emergency decompressive surgery may be appropriate.[29] Between those extremes of therapy are the options for medical management with corticosteroids, cyclosporine, or other immunosuppressive agents[30,31] and orbital radiation therapy.

Results of the use of orbital radiation therapy in the treatment of thyroid ophthalmopathy have been reported in many retrospective single-institution studies.[32-36] The rationale for radiotherapy in this disorder is straightforward: Ophthalmopathy is produced by, or in association with, a local autoimmune infiltration of lymphocytes. Lymphocytes are sensitive to radiation; radiation beams can be collimated so that an adequate dose can be precisely delivered to the orbits without significant sequelae and without the potential side effects associated with systemic therapies.

Petersen and colleagues[35] reported on the Stanford experience in 311 patients treated with megavoltage radiation therapy from 1968 to 1988. The majority of patients were treated to doses of 20 Gy in 10×2 Gy fractions. A cohort of 69 patients were treated from 1979 to 1983 with a higher dose, 30 Gy in 15×2 Gy fractions, and although no increased complications were reported,

there was no additional benefit to higher dose levels, and the treatment policy returned to 20 Gy in 10 fractions. Techniques were used to minimize the dose to the contralateral lens, initially using lateral fields angled 5 degrees posteriorly; later, a half-beam block (beam-split technique) was used to eliminate divergence anteriorly. Before treatment more than 90% of patients had soft tissue changes and involvement of extraocular muscles, approximately 66% had proptosis, approximately 50% had decreased visual acuity, and approximately 20% had corneal involvement.

Results obtained in the Stanford series showed a high rate of symptom response and a low rate of symptom progression after radiation therapy, as shown in Table 68-1.[35] Worsening of symptoms occurred in only 1% to 6% of patients, with rates of complete resolution or improvement of symptoms ranging from 51% for proptosis, 61% for visual acuity and impairment of eye muscles, 77% for corneal involvement, and 80% for soft tissue changes. Of the one third of patients who were on steroids when beginning radiation, 76% were able to discontinue corticosteroid use within several months of completing radiation therapy.

Side effects from radiation therapy for ophthalmopathy are minimal, and the time course to symptomatic improvement can be rapid. In the Stanford experience, about 10% of patients developed acute side effects, primarily transient soft tissue inflammation.[35] No long-term side effects were reported. In a series from the University of Pennsylvania, Sandler and colleagues[34] reported acute symptoms of conjunctival irritation in 12 of 35 patients. Early symptomatic improvement often occurs, with objective signs of response to radiation occurring as early as 2 days into treatment, with a mean time to the first objective response of 14 days after the first fraction of radiation. However, the time to maximal clinical response is variable and can be prolonged, with a range of 1 to 24 months (mean 5.6) after the initiation of therapy.[36]

Although radiotherapy is safe and efficacious in the treatment of thyroid ophthalmopathy, controversy exists regarding the appropriate initial treatment. Many patients are treated initially with steroids and are referred for radiation only after they have not responded to or had progression of symptoms on steroids or have developed unacceptable side effects. Prummel and colleagues[37] reported a double-blind, prospective, randomized study in which patients were assigned to receive either oral prednisone or radiotherapy (20 Gy using opposed lateral fields).

Table 68-1   Response of Symptoms to Orbital Radiotherapy for Thyroid Ophthalmopathy: Stanford Experience with 311 Patients, 1968-1988

Symptom	Complete Resolution, %	Improved, %	Unchanged, %	Worse, %
Soft tissue changes	58	22	19	2
Proptosis	32	19	42	6
Eye muscle impairment	32	29	38	1
Corneal involvement	73	4	20	4
Visual acuity	45	16	34	4

Data from Petersen IA, Kriss JP, McDougall IR, Donaldson SS: Prognostic factors in the radiotherapy of Graves' ophthalmopathy. *Int J Radiat Oncol Biol Phys.* 1990;19:259.

Table 68–2   Double-Blind Randomized Trial of Prednisone versus Radiotherapy for Thyroid Ophthalmopathy*

	Side Effects, n (%)		Response at 24 Weeks, n (%)		
	Major or Moderate	*Minor or None*	*Responders*	*No Change*	*Progression*
Prednisone	20 (71)	8 (29)	14 (50)	10 (36)	4 (14)
Radiotherapy	5 (18)	23 (82)	13 (46)	11 (40)	4 (14)

*Total patients, *n* = 28.
Data from Prummel MF, Mourits MP, Blank L, et al: Randomised double-blind trial of prednisone versus radiotherapy in Graves' ophthalmopathy. *Lancet*. 1993;342.

Patients received either placebo or sham irradiation in addition to the prescribed therapy. Results are summarized in Table 68-2. The response rate to treatment was similar in both arms of the study (50% vs. 46%). However, there was a much higher incidence of moderate to severe complications in the prednisone arm (e.g., weight gain, cushingoid facies, pyrosis requiring treatment with ranitidine, behavioral changes) than in the radiotherapy arm. Based on these findings, the authors concluded that "the efficacy of retrobulbar radiotherapy and of oral prednisone in the management of patients with moderately severe Graves' ophthalmopathy appears to be similar. Because radiotherapy is better tolerated, it should replace the standard corticosteroid regimen as the initial treatment in these patients."[37]

Long-term complications are rare after radiation therapy for ophthalmopathy. Although cataractogenesis is a concern when orbital radiation is used and it is prudent to advise the patient that cataracts may develop, the threshold for cataractogenesis from fractionated radiation therapy is about 4 Gy,[24] and in most cases with the use of either beam-split or posteriorly angled fields, the dose to the lens is about 5%.[33] Fortunately, the thresholds for other optic complications of radiation, such as optic neuropathy, retinal injury, or severe dry eye due to lacrimal gland injury, are above 20 Gy,[38] and these injuries have not been reported after doses of 20 Gy for thyroid ophthalmopathy or orbital pseudotumor (lymphoid hyperplasia) (see next section). As with all situations in which ionzing radiation is used, there is a theoretical risk of carcinogenesis that must be considered.[38a]

Radiation therapy for thyroid ophthalmopathy is generally delivered using 20 Gy in 10 × 2 Gy fractions with photon energies of 4 to 6 MV. Lateral opposed fields are generally used. Treatment fields should extend from the posterior aspect of the globe to the anterior clinoids, with superior and inferior margins defined by the bony orbit. Field sizes are generally in the range of 4 × 4 to 5.5 × 5.5 cm. Care should be taken to place the anterior field border behind the lens; clinical correlation in addition to the use of bony landmarks is important, especially in those patients with severe proptosis. If the port extends to 10 mm behind the limbus, the orbital tissues that must be irradiated are covered and the lens is spared. At some institutions a radiopaque contact lens may be used to help define the anterior field border.

Two techniques to minimize divergence into the contralateral lens are commonly used. The lateral fields can be angled 5 degrees posteriorly. Alternatively, a nondivergent beam edge can be created using either a half-beam block or the asymmetrical collimation capabilities of certain linear accelerators, avoiding increased posterior divergence.[39] In most cases, there is some degree of bilateral involvement, so both orbits are treated. A representative simulation film is shown in Figure 68-2.

In summary, thyroid ophthalmopathy, when symptomatic, responds well to low-dose (20 Gy) radiotherapy. Symptom response rates of about 50% to 80% are reported, with symptoms of soft tissue involvement among the most responsive. Corticosteroids are frequently used as first-line management, with patients who do not respond to or do not tolerate steroids subsequently referred for radiotherapy. However, randomized data indicate that radiotherapy may be as effective as corticosteroids with fewer side effects when used as primary treatment.

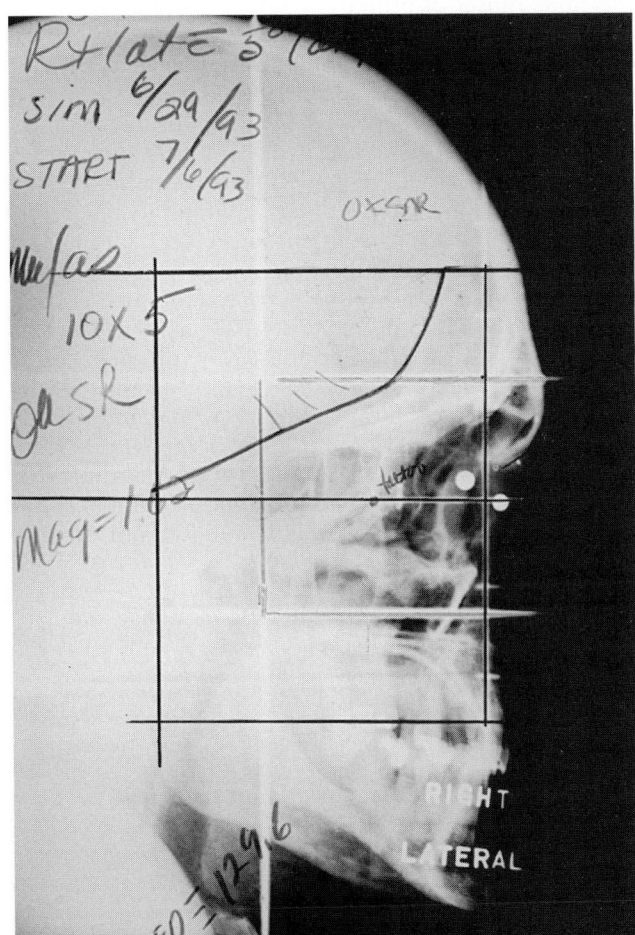

Figure 68–2. Simulation film showing fields used in the treatment of thyroid ophthalmopathy.

ORBITAL PSEUDOTUMOR (ORBITAL LYMPHOID HYPERPLASIA; ORBITAL PSEUDOLYMPHOMA)

Orbital pseudotumor, orbital lymphoid hyperplasia, and *orbital pseudolymphoma* are terms used to describe benign orbital mass lesions in which mature lymphocytes are noted to infiltrate orbital structures such as orbital fat, extraocular muscles, lacrimal glands, or other extraocular orbital structures. Some authors[40] have attempted to distinguish orbital pseudotumor from orbital lymphoid hyperplasia, but these distinctions are difficult and of uncertain prognostic or therapeutic importance. However, in general, lymphoid hyperplasia arises in anterior ocular structures, and pseudotumor arises more posteriorly in the bony orbit. In practice and in many reports, the terms for these benign entities are used interchangeably and the cases intermingled. However, it is important to distinguish between the benign conditions, which are referred to as orbital pseudotumor in this section, and malignant orbital lymphomas, which can have similar clinical presentations and histopathological appearance. Recent developments in immunology, electron microscopy, and flow cytometry have made it easier to differentiate benign (polyclonal) from malignant (generally monoclonal) orbital lymphoid disorders with the use of special studies.[41] It is also important to rule out infectious causes of orbital inflammation (e.g., spread of an adjacent sinus infection, trichomonal infection), as well as endocrine and autoimmune disorders (e.g., thyroid ophthalmopathy, discussed previously), which can have similar clinical presentations. Because of the difficult differential diagnosis associated with this disorder, a thorough and careful complete history and physical examination, along with the use of appropriate laboratory and radiologic studies, is important before radiotherapy for orbital pseudotumor is initiated.

Clinical presentation of orbital pseudotumor is characterized by symptoms of soft tissue swelling, orbital pain, proptosis, extraocular muscle involvement, and, occasionally, decreased visual acuity (Table 68-3). Bilateral involvement is much less frequent than with thyroid ophthalmopathy. Computed tomography (CT) scans may demonstrate mass lesions anywhere in the orbit, often multiple, with the posterior globe a common site of involvement.[42,43] Overall, orbital pseudotumor is quite rare. Although precise figures are not available, some authors estimate that the combination of orbital pseudotumor and primary orbital lymphomas make up about 1% of both primary orbital neoplasms and primary lymphoid neoplasms.[44,45] Some controversy exists regarding the need for biopsy before therapy is initiated, with some authors believing that the diagnosis can be made on clinical grounds, after radiographic, ophthalmologic, and laboratory evaluation.[43] However, given the unusual nature of this disorder and the similarity in clinical presentation to malignant orbital lymphomas, it is prudent to obtain a biopsy if this can be performed without significant morbidity.

In most cases, orbital pseudotumor responds to treatment with corticosteroids, with about 50% of patients having a durable complete response, and steroids are generally used as first-line therapy.[46] However, radiation therapy has been used successfully and with low morbidity for those patients who have contraindications to steroid therapy, develop unacceptable complications while on steroids, or relapse after steroid therapy. Results of radiation therapy for orbital pseudotumor have often been combined with results of the radiation treatment of orbital lymphomas. As orbital lymphomas commonly occur localized to the orbit, the primary difference in management with radiation therapy is dose. Doses of 20 Gy in 10 fractions are commonly used in the treatment of pseudotumor, with higher doses generally used for malignant lymphomas. Overall durable complete response rates range from 75% to 100%.[43-45,47-49]

Lanciano and colleagues[43] reported a series of 26 orbits in 23 patients treated with radiation for orbital pseudotumor. The mean follow-up was 53 months. In that series, 20 patients (87%) had a trial of corticosteroids before radiotherapy, with 15 (75%) having a complete response, 1 (5%) a partial response, and 4 (20%) no response. However, 16 patients (70%) were referred because clinical relapse was noted with steroid taper. Twelve patients (52%) had developed significant morbidity to steroids including aseptic necrosis, cushingoid facies, psychiatric disorders, gastritis, and pseudotumor cerebri. All patients were treated to 20 Gy in 10 × 2 Gy fractions. Symptomatic response is shown in Table 68-3. At the time of last follow-up, 66% had a durable complete response and required no further steroid treatment; 11% had local relapse 30 to 34 months after radiation therapy but subsequently achieved complete response again either spontaneously or with additional steroid treatment; 11% had partial responses to radiation; and three patients (11%) had no response to radiation. There were no cases of progression during or after radiotherapy. Acute side effects of irradiation were minimal, with 35% of patients having minor signs or symptoms; there were no radiation-related cataracts or other significant late morbidities related to the radiation treatment.

Various radiation treatment techniques have been used for orbital pseudotumor. In some cases, techniques similar to those used for thyroid ophthalmopathy are used, but as fewer patients have bilateral disease and the location of disease within the orbit is more variable than in thyroid ophthalmopathy, treatment must be individualized. CT or magnetic resonance imaging (MRI) of the

Table 68–3 Symptoms of Orbital Pseudotumor and Response to Radiation Therapy

Symptom	Percentage Presenting with Symptom	Percentage with Complete Response After Radiotherapy
Soft tissue swelling	92	87
Pain	92	75
Proptosis	85	82
Extraocular muscle dysfunction	69	78
Decreased visual acuity	19	60

Data from Lanciano RM, Fowble B, Sergott RC, et al: The results of radiotherapy for orbital pseudotumor. *Int J Radiat Oncol Biol Phys.* 1990;18:407.

orbit are necessary in most cases to adequately define the extent of disease, and CT planning can be helpful in evaluating and selecting treatment plans. Single and opposed lateral photon fields, anterior electron fields, and wedged-pair techniques have all been used. Patients with conjunctival or other anterior disease and no posterior disease may be well treated with an anterior electron field, whereas patients with disease in the retrobulbar region may be best treated with lateral photon fields. If anterior photon or electron fields are used, lens blocks may be added to reduce the dose to the lens and the chance of subsequent cataract formation.[50]

Progression to systemic lymphoma occurs in a small number of patients and must be a concern in continued follow-up of these patients. In individual series, progression has been noted in zero to 25% of patients.[51] In a literature review, Lanciano and colleagues[43] reported that 12 of 101 (12%) patients subsequently developed systemic disease. In addition, a total of 14 of 101 (14%) had bilateral disease at presentation, with an additional 6 of 101 (6%) developing bilateral disease after therapy.[43]

In summary, orbital pseudotumor and orbital lymphoid hyperplasia are benign lymphoid infiltrates of orbital tissues, closely related in clinical presentation to orbital lymphomas. When steroids are not tolerated or are ineffective, durable complete responses after radiation therapy (20 Gy in 10 fractions) can be obtained in 75% to 100% of cases. Relapse in the treated orbit is rare. Twenty percent of patients demonstrate some degree of bilaterality, and progression to systemic lymphoma occurs in some cases.

LYMPHOID HYPERPLASIA

Areas of benign lymphoid hyperplasia can arise outside the orbits, especially in Waldeyer's ring and the skin. Cases of cutaneous lymphoid hyperplasia have been reported in conjunction with acquired immunodeficiency syndrome (AIDS), and progression to malignant lymphoma occurs in some cases. Pathologically, the disease is characterized by a cutaneous infiltrate of lymphocytes in the upper dermis associated with germinal centers underlying a typically normal epidermis. The appearance is similar to that of Spiegler-Fendt sarcoid and malignant lymphoreticular neoplasms. Treatment alternatives included corticosteroid treatment and excision. For cases refractory to conventional therapy, persistent local control has been reported with doses of 12 to 20 Gy with minimal morbidity.[52-54]

HETEROTOPIC OSSIFICATION

HO, also known as heterotopic or ectopic bone formation, has long been recognized as a complication of total hip replacement (total hip arthroplasty; THA). The use of THA began in the late 1960s, and by the 1970s, a significant number of cases of HO had been described. The presence of HO can be demonstrated radiographically and can cause significant symptoms, such as pain, impaired joint mobility, or complete ankylosis of

the joint. The exact incidence of HO is not known; incidence figures ranging from 8% to 90% have been reported, depending in large part on the risk factors (see later discussion) in each series, as well as the intensity of postoperative surveillance. Brooker and colleagues[55] proposed an HO classification that is in general use (Table 68-4).

A number of risk factors for HO have been described. These include male sex, age older than 60 years, previous HO in either hip, post-traumatic arthritis, hypertrophic osteoarthritis, or active ankylosing spondylitis. Surgical technique, or perioperative complications such as hemorrhage, do not appear to be a significant predisposing factor.[56-58]

As the variety of risk factors for HO suggests, the etiology of this disorder is not well understood. However, it has been theorized that in the setting of significant trauma or surgery, pluripotent mesenchymal cells are induced to differentiate into osteogenic progenitor cells. These cells subsequently develop osteoblastic tissue, resulting in the production of heterotopic bone.[59]

The time course to formation of heterotopic bone after surgery has been characterized. Postoperatively, ectopic bone generally becomes visible radiographically by 3 to 6 weeks. By 8 weeks the bone mass may be complete, but not matured. Maturation of bone occurs within 6 to 12 months, with little change noted subsequently. Once the heterotopic bone has formed, there is little in the way of effective therapy short of reoperation.[56,57]

The difficulties presented by heterotopic bone formation led to an active interest in effective means of prophylaxis. In 1977, Ritter and Vaughan[56] wrote, "To our knowledge, there is no way to prevent the formation of heterotopic bone or its recurrence after surgical resection." Since that time, a wide variety of therapies have been proposed, including transplantation of fat into the operative bed, and the use of diphosphonates, which may have significant systemic side effects on calcium and phosphate metabolism. In a recent review, the only methods of prophylaxis recognized as being effective were radiation therapy and the use of anti-inflammatory drugs.[58]

Anti-inflammatory agents, most frequently nonsteroidal anti-inflammatory drugs (NSAIDs) rather than corticosteroids, and the drug indomethacin in particular, have been used effectively to prevent HO. The mechanism of action is not well defined, but initiation of therapy within the first 5 days of surgery may be important. In a randomized study, Schmidt and colleagues[60] found that patients receiving indomethacin 25 mg three times daily

Table 68–4   Brooker Classification of Heterotopic Ossification

Class	Findings
I	Isolated bone islands
II	Bone spurs; separated by >1 cm
III	Bone spurs; separated by <1 cm
IV	Apparent bony ankylosis

Data from Brooker AF, Bowerman JW, Robinson RA, Riley LH: Ectopic ossification following total hip replacement: Incidence and a method of classification. *J Bone Joint Surg Am.* 1973;55:1629.

for 6 weeks postoperatively had decreased rates of HO compared with patients treated with placebo. However, NSAIDs such as indomethacin do have significant gastrointestinal, hematologic, and neurologic side effects, and there is some concern that they may promote loosening of the noncemented components of hip prostheses.[58] In a series of 74 high-risk patients who received indomethacin after THA, Cella and colleagues[61] reported that 37% were unable to complete the prescribed course of NSAID therapy.

Radiation therapy has been shown to be a safe and effective prophylactic treatment for HO. In the 1970s, prophylactic treatment with radiation began. At the Mayo Clinic, 20 Gy in 10 fractions was chosen somewhat arbitrarily as a dose likely to impede bone formation (based on experience with radiation-induced bone growth retardation in pediatric patients), yet not high enough to be associated with significant morbidity. From 1970 to 1977, 48 hips in 42 patients were treated in this manner, using megavoltage equipment and large (12 to 18 × 14 to 20 cm) radiation portals. In general, care was taken to exclude the lateral skin incision from the radiation portals. Patients who started radiation treatment early (within the first 2 to 10 postoperative days) had effective prophylaxis against HO. However, patients in whom the initiation of radiation was delayed until after radiographical evidence of heterotopic bone formation appeared (21 to 69 postoperative days) had regression noted in only 1 of 12 cases. No significant complications attributable to radiotherapy were noted.[57]

Since the initial report by Coventry and Scanlon,[57] many reports documenting the efficacy of radiotherapy as a prophylactic measure have appeared. Select series are listed in Table 68-5. There has been an evolution in technique and doses in the past 10 to 15 years (see later discussion), but several general principles remain unchanged: (1) radiotherapy is effective if delivered prophylactically, but not once heterotopic bone has been established; (2) radiotherapy should be begun early postoperatively (0 to 96 hours); and (3) radiotherapy is associated with a low level of complications.

Radiation dose and fractionation schemes have changed since early reports. In an early series, MacLennan and colleagues[62] from the University of Rochester, N.Y., obtained good results using 20 Gy in 10 × 2 Gy fractions. Subsequently, using the cohort of patients treated with 20 Gy as historical controls, Anthony and colleagues[63] from the same institution demonstrated that 10 Gy in five fractions produced equivalent results. Similar findings have been reported by investigators from the University of California, Los Angeles, where no increased failure rate was observed with 10 Gy compared with 20 Gy, and total doses of 7 to 8 Gy in one to two fractions were also found to be effective.[64,65]

Low-dose fractionated radiation therapy has since been replaced at many institutions with single-fraction radiotherapy. This has the main advantage of being easier logistically. Only one trip to the radiation oncology department may be required, and the number of times a patient has to be moved (transport, on/off treatment couch, etc.) is dramatically reduced. Furthermore, with single-fraction therapy, the entire treatment course can be completed while the patient remains hospitalized in the postoperative period. Doses used are generally 7 to 8 Gy in a single fraction. Lo and colleagues[66] have reported good results with a single fraction of 7 Gy delivered within 72 hours postoperatively, with only 4% of patients developing recurrent disease. In a randomized trial, Konski and colleagues[67] found no significant difference in recurrence rates between patients treated with 8 Gy in a single fraction and 10 Gy in five fractions. No significant side effects were reported in either patient group. The lower limit of effective radiotherapy dose remains to be determined. In Lo's series, one patient received 2.8 Gy in a single fraction, and the HO recurred. A preliminary report of a randomized trial from Rush-Presbyterian by Graybill and colleagues[68] suggests that a total dose of 5 Gy in two fractions may be as effective as a total dose of 10 Gy in five fractions.

Although most experience with the use of radiotherapy for heterotopic bone prophylaxis comes from older patients, there is evidence that prophylactic radiation is also of value in young adults who suffer traumatic hip fractures. Slawson and colleagues[69] from the University of Maryland reported on 50 patients who presented to the trauma unit at their institution with acetabular fractures. Thirty consecutive patients (mean age 34 years) were treated with postoperative radiation (total dose of 10 Gy in five fractions), and 20 consecutive patients (mean age 28 years) treated immediately before the institution of postoperative radiation were selected as historical controls. There was a significant difference in

Table 68–5 **Select Series of Postoperative Radiation Therapy for Prophylaxis Against Heterotopic Ossification**

First Author (Institution) Year	Patients, n	Hips, n	Dose, Gy/Fractions, n	Postoperative Progression, %
MacLennan et al[62] (Rochester) 1984	58	67	20/10	5
Anthony et al[63] (Rochester) 1987	54	62	20/10	3
	41	46	10/5	5
Lo et al[66] (Lahey Clinic) 1988	23	24	7/1	4
Sylvester et al[64] (UCLA) 1988	28	29	20/10	11
			10/5	
Konski et al[67] (Medical College of Ohio)	17	17	8/1	6
	20	20	10/5	15
Seegenschmiedt et al[76] (Erlangen) 1993	137	68	17.5/5	4
	77	73	10/5	12

the number of patients who developed severe (Brooker grade III to IV) HO in the two groups. Only 3 of 30 (10%) patients treated with radiotherapy developed significant HO compared with 10 of 28 (36%) who did not receive irradiation (P <0.01). Complication rates were similar in both cohorts, and the authors concluded that radiation is useful and effective in the setting of traumatic acetabular fractures.

The nature of radiation treatment fields used for prophylaxis of heterotopic bone formation has changed as the nature of hip prostheses has changed. In the 1970s and early 1980s, cemented hip prostheses were primarily used, and large fields were often treated. However, loosening of hip implants remained a significant indication for revision surgery, and for securing implants, alternative methods to cement were sought. In recent years, porous coated hip implants have been more frequently used. In these procedures, the porous implant is anchored physiologically by bone ingrowth (biological fixation). This process has physiologic similarities to the process of heterotopic bone formation. This led to concern that postoperative radiation for HO would not only prevent ectopic bone formation but might also prevent secure fixation of the prostheses. This hypothesis was tested in a rabbit model by Konski and colleagues[70] from Rochester, and decreased strength of prosthetic devices was demonstrated in the initial 2- to 3-week period after surgery, although not in the longer term. However, because of these concerns, treatment fields have been modified, and reduced field sizes have been successfully used in patients with porous prostheses. Although the fields used with cemented prostheses were large (about 14 × 16 cm),[57] the fields used with porous prostheses are much smaller, with care taken to shield the porous components of both the femoral and the acetabular prosthesis. A typical field used in our department is on the order of 8 × 4 cm. An example is shown in Figure 68-3. No significant complications or decreases in efficacy have been demonstrated with the use of restricted fields.[63,64,67]

Radiotherapy has been used as prophylactic treatment for HO in joints other than the hip. Use of radiation in the temporomandibular joint (TMJ) has been described by Durr and colleagues[71] in a series of 15 TMJs in 10 patients who underwent arthroplasty or debridement of heterotopic bone in the TMJ. Patients received a modal dose of 10 Gy in five fractions, with irradiation generally beginning within 2 days of surgery. Treatment was effective, with improvement over preoperative levels of ectopic ossification noted in 13 of 15 (87%) TMJs. Acute toxicity was acute parotitis reported in three patients, with no long-term complications reported.

Radiation therapy to prevent HO of the elbow has been reported by Wolfson and colleagues.[72] A series of 19 elbows at high risk for HO was treated with 10 Gy in five fractions postoperatively after excision of HO. Only 1 in 19 (5.3%) recurred, and no complications were observed. The successful use of radiation (10 Gy in five fractions) as prophylaxis against HO in the elbow, as well as in the wrist and shoulder, has also been reported by Rubenstein and colleagues.[73] Recently, the use of single fraction radiotherapy (7 to 8 Gy) has been used as prophylactic treatment for HO of the elbow.[73a,73b]

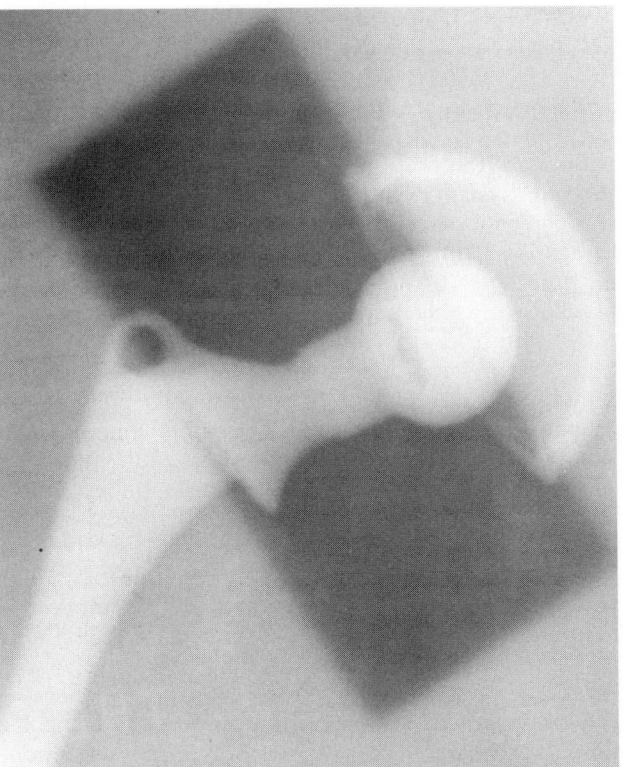

Figure 68–3. Megavoltage film of a treatment field for heterotopic ossification prophylaxis in a patient with a porous prosthesis.

The role of radiation in HO prophylaxis continues to evolve. Work to optimize the dose-fractionation schemes used continues, and other innovations are also developing. For example, Kantorowitz and colleagues[74] experimented with the use of preoperative radiation. In a rat model, they found that 8 Gy given 1 hour preoperatively was as effective as a similar dose given 2 days postoperatively. This concept has subsequently been tested in a clinical trial, with patients randomized to receive a single 7 to 8 Gy fraction of radiation either within 4 hours before surgery or within 72 hours after surgery.[75] Preliminary results indicate that the preoperative approach may be as effective as postoperative radiotherapy, without any increased risk of complications. Preoperative treatment would have potential advantages with respect to patient comfort, avoiding the need to transport and transfer the patient for radiation treatment in the immediate postoperative period.

The potential that radiation combined with NSAID use may be better than either modality alone as a prophylactic measure has been suggested by a group from Erlangen.[76] They found a failure rate of 3% for patients treated with radiation and NSAIDs for 6 weeks postoperatively compared with 12% for patients treated with radiotherapy alone (P <0.05). It is not certain if this approach will prove efficacious and safe in further studies.

In summary, HO is a significant source of morbidity after THA. Single-dose radiotherapy to restricted fields has been found to be a safe and effective means of prophylaxis, with minimal levels of acute and long-term morbidity reported. Doses of 7 to 8 Gy are used, and therapy should begin within 96 hours of surgery.

PARAGANGLIOMAS (GLOMUS TUMORS; CHEMODECTOMAS)

Paragangliomas are tumors that arise from the paraganglia, collections of cells of neural crest origin dispersed throughout the body in association with the autonomic nervous system. They are histologically related to pheochromocytomas (which are chromaffin-positive). Nonchromaffin paragangliomas often arise from chemoreceptor tissues in the head and neck area and are also known as chemodectomas, or glomus tumors. The nomenclature can be confusing and imprecise, with the related terms often used interchangeably. Glomus jugulare tumors arise in the area of the jugular bulb, glomus tympanicum tumors in the middle ear, and glomus vagale tumors in the area of the ganglion nodosum adjacent to the vagal nerve. Paragangliomas that arise in the chemoreceptor cells near the carotid bifurcation are also called carotid body tumors. Although these sites in the neck, base of skull, and temporal bone are the most common, paragangliomas have been reported at a multitude of anatomic sites throughout the body. Paragangliomas arising in the head and neck are of the greatest concern to radiation oncologists.[77-79]

Glomus tumors are generally considered to be benign, although rare (<5%) cases of metastases, most commonly to the lungs, have been reported. Occasionally, patients may secrete catecholamines, serotonin, or similar substances, producing severe hypertension, flushing, and associated symptoms. If the history suggests, appropriate laboratory studies should be ordered. There may be some association with multiple endocrine neoplasia (MEN) syndromes. A family history is present in approximately 10% of cases, and there is a significant incidence of bilaterality in familial cases.[80,81] Glomus tumors are rare, but the peak incidence is between 40 and 60 years, with a higher incidence noted in patients suffering from chronic hypoxia or living at high altitudes. Although glomus tumors are generally highly vascular, they are made up of cells that are histologically similar to normal paraganglia associated with epithelioid tissue in a multitude of thin-walled blood vessels.[77-79]

Glomus tumors grow slowly, and in retrospect there may be a history of years or decades of symptoms before the tumor is brought to clinical attention. Tumors are often 2 to 3 cm at the time of presentation. Presenting symptoms vary with the site of origin, although all tumors may manifest with cranial nerve symptoms, especially those relating to nerves VIII to XII. Carotid body tumors commonly appear with a neck mass or carotid sinus syndrome. Middle ear lesions may appear with hearing loss, pulsatile tinnitus, or headache, and glomus vagale tumors may appear with hoarseness.

If the diagnosis of a glomus tumor is suspected, workup should proceed with a careful history and physical examination. Middle-ear lesions may be characterized by a bluish mass visible behind the tympanic membrane. CT or MRI imaging of the neck and base of skull should be performed. Angiography is helpful in establishing a diagnosis and is essential as part of the preoperative evaluation if surgery is to be contemplated as a treatment option. An angiogram showing the characteristic appearance of a glomus jugulare tumor is shown in Figure 68-4. The radiographic picture is generally sufficiently characteristic to establish a definitive diagnosis; histologic proof is not necessary except in unusual cases, especially as biopsy of these very vascular lesions can involve significant morbidity.

Although these lesions are slow-growing and histologically benign, they can cause significant symptoms and demonstrate malignant behavior by local spread, causing cranial nerve palsies, bony erosion, hearing loss, and intracranial extension. Treatment options have generally involved surgery, often in association with embolization, and radiation therapy.

There can be sharp divisions between surgeons and radiation oncologists regarding optimal management of paragangliomas. Contemporary papers written by surgeons often refer to surgical excision as the treatment of choice,[81,82] but there is a long experience showing that radiation therapy (see later discussion) can also be effective.[83] An extensive literature review comparing results and complications associated with radiation therapy versus surgery for temporal bone chemodectomas was conducted by Springate and colleagues.[84,85] Results from 8 surgical series and 19 radiotherapy series were reviewed (Table 68-6). Local control was 86% (349 of 405) in those patients treated with surgery alone, 91% (344 of 379) for those patients treated with radiotherapy before or after surgery, and 93% (182 of 195) for the subset of patients treated with radiotherapy alone (surgery no more extensive than biopsy).

Complication rates were also compared. Serious sequelae of radiation therapy occurred in 2% to 3% of patients, including bone necrosis, brain necrosis, and a

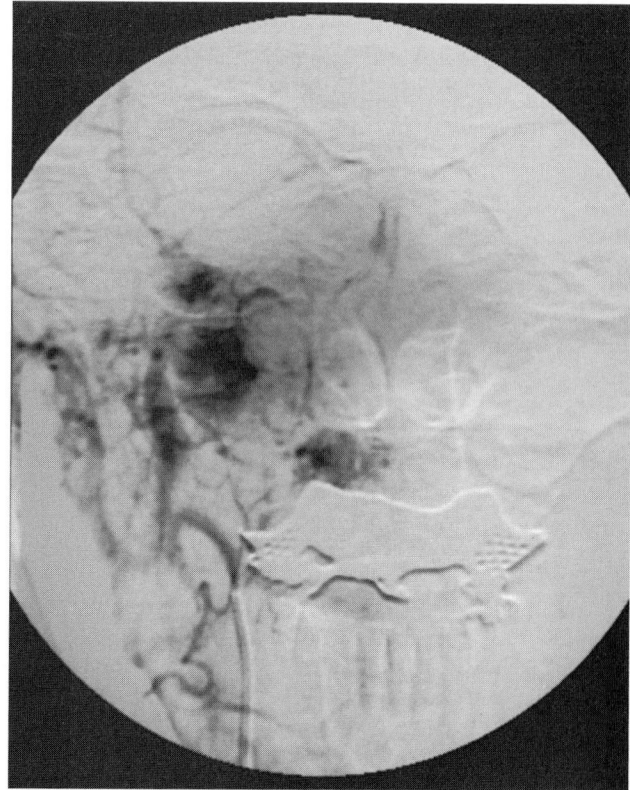

Figure 68–4. Angiogram showing typical appearance of a glomus tumor.

Table 68–6   Paraganglioma: Literature Review

	Local Control, *n*	Percentage
Surgery alone	349/405	86
Radiotherapy + surgery	344/379	91
Radiotherapy alone	182/195	93

Data from Springate SC, Weichselbaum RR: Radiation or surgery for chemodectoma of the temporal bone: A review of local control and complications. *Head Neck.* 1990;12:303. Springate SC, Haraf D, Weichselbaum RR: Temporal bone chemodectomas—Comparing surgery and radiation therapy. *Oncology.* 1991;5:131.

single case of a radiation-induced second malignancy (fibrosarcoma). The severe complications observed in the radiotherapy series were generally found in the 54 to 70 Gy dose range, higher than that recommended by most contemporary authors. Surgical series have reported a significant incidence of postoperative complications, including postoperative deaths, cerebrospinal fluid leaks, and cerebrovascular accidents. In addition, new postoperative cranial nerve palsies were noted in significant numbers of patients. Cece and colleagues[82] reported either new cranial nerve palsies or exacerbation of preexisting palsies in all 17 of their patients after surgery for large glomus jugulare tumors. Although treatment decisions must be individualized, the equivalent local control rates obtained with surgery and radiation and the higher rate of treatment-related morbidity associated with surgical management makes primary radiation treatment an attractive option for many chemodectomas. The finding that results with radiotherapy alone are not appreciably different from those obtained with radiotherapy combined with surgery suggests that initial management should probably be with a single modality except in unusual circumstances to avoid exposing the patient to the unnecessary morbidity of combined therapy.[84,85]

Long-term control of head and neck paragangliomas treated with radiotherapy without significant late morbidity has been reported from a number of institutions. With mean follow-up of 11 years and follow-up extending to 23 years, Pryzant and colleagues[86] reported local control in 18 of 18 (100%) patients with temporal bone chemodectomas treated with radiation with no significant late morbidity. Hansen and Thomsen[87] reported on a series of 39 patients treated with radiation for paraganglioma in Copenhagen, with local control obtained in 36 of 39 (92%); there was a mean follow-up of 8 years and a follow-up period extending over 25 years. The side effects and results obtained with irradiation compared favorably with those of surgical results at their institution, and they recommend radiation as treatment for all but early tumors limited to the tympanic cavity. In the Royal Mardsen Hospital experience, with follow-up extending to 32 years, the 10- and 25-year actuarial local control rates for patients treated with radiation alone for glomus jugulare and glomus tympanicum tumors were 90% and 73%, respectively.[88] Long-term morbidity was less for patients treated with radiation than for those treated with surgery alone at the same institution.

Consensus regarding appropriate radiation doses and treatment techniques has been developing over the past

15 years. In 1980, Kim and colleagues,[89] reviewing the available literature, found a recurrence rate of 22% in patients treated to doses of less than 40 Gy but only 2% for patients treated to doses of greater than 40 Gy. They suggested that doses up to 50 Gy might be appropriate for patients with advanced lesions. From Iowa, Wang and colleagues[90] observed no improved local control with higher doses in the 55 to 66 Gy range but did report an increased rate of complications with higher doses. Most reports since 1980 have generally endorsed the use of doses in the 45 to 50 Gy range as providing a good balance between adequate local control and a low rate of severe complications such as cranial nerve, brainstem, or temporal bone injury. Wedged-pair techniques are generally used, although lateral mixed photon-electron beam arrangements have been reported, and opposed lateral fields may be necessary for advanced lesions. CT treatment planning is helpful in adequately defining target volume and evaluating treatment plans. "Hot spots" that may arise with the use of wedged-pair plans must be considered in relation to the location of adjacent normal structures.[91-93]

The optimal management of chemodectomas remains in dispute. Some, especially advocates of skull base surgery, may advocate a primary surgical approach for all lesions. However, the morbidity of these approaches may be high for advanced lesions. Consultation with both a surgeon and a radiation oncologist or presentation at a combined-modality tumor board before the selection of therapy assists in the selection of appropriate therapy for the individual patient. For lesions in which the surgical approach carries low morbidity, as in small lesions of the middle ear, especially in young, fit patients, surgery is the preferred approach. However, for larger or more extensive lesions, or in patients with concurrent medical problems, radiation doses of approximately 45 Gy provide good local control with low morbidity. During the follow-up period, it should be understood that paragangliomas often respond slowly after irradiation, with stabilization more typical than rapid involution and complete resolution. However, in these tumors, which grow slowly, rarely metastasize, and cause symptoms by local growth, arrest of progression is generally sufficient to provide long-term local control.

In summary, paragangliomas are rare benign tumors that may arise at multiple locations in the head and neck and cause significant morbidity by local extension and invasion. The diagnosis can often be made on the basis of a characteristic radiographic appearance. Treatment decisions must be individualized. Surgical extirpation is appropriate as primary management in certain cases. Radiation therapy doses of approximately 45 Gy provide excellent rates of long-term local control with acceptable levels of morbidity.

JUVENILE NASOPHARYNGEAL ANGIOFIBROMA

Juvenile nasopharyngeal angiofibroma (JNA) is a histologically benign vascular tumor that arises in boys between the ages of 12 and 15 years, with only rare cases reported in patients younger than 10 or older than 25. Although rare cases have been reported in females, the tumor has such a strong male predilection that the diagnosis has been questioned in those instances. The cell of origin is uncertain. Paraganglionic tissue, ectopic rests of hormone-sensitive vascular tissue, and others have been proposed as candidates. Pathologically, it is not certain if the tumor is of vascular or fibrous origin. JNA is characterized microscopically by dense fibrous tissue interspersed with thin-walled vasculature of differing caliber, often associated with metaplasia or ulceration, or both, of the overlying mucosa.[94-96]

Clinically, JNA is rare, comprising less than 1% of head and neck neoplasms. The most common presenting symptoms are of nasal obstruction and recurrent or severe epistaxis, although other symptoms, such as headaches, facial deformities ("frog face"), and visual and neurologic disturbances, can be seen, especially with advanced lesions. On physical examination, a polypoid or lobulated red or reddish blue mass arising in the nasopharynx is evident. The diagnosis of JNA can be made by a combination of clinical and radiographic means. The radiographic picture obtained by contrast-enhanced CT, MRI, and angiography in the appropriate clinical setting is diagnostic. MRI images of a typical JNA are shown in Figures 68-5 and 68-6. Biopsy can produce severe hemorrhage and is not necessary to establish the diagnosis before therapy is begun.

Although JNA is histologically benign, it has the potential to cause serious morbidity or death if untreated. The tumor can expand to fill the entire nasopharynx and erode into the hard palate, maxillary sinus, base of skull, or intracranial structures. Morbidity or mortality can arise either from invasion of tumor or bleeding associated with the tumor.

There is controversy regarding the optimal initial therapy for JNA, with advocates for surgical resection and radiation as primary therapy; both options have different

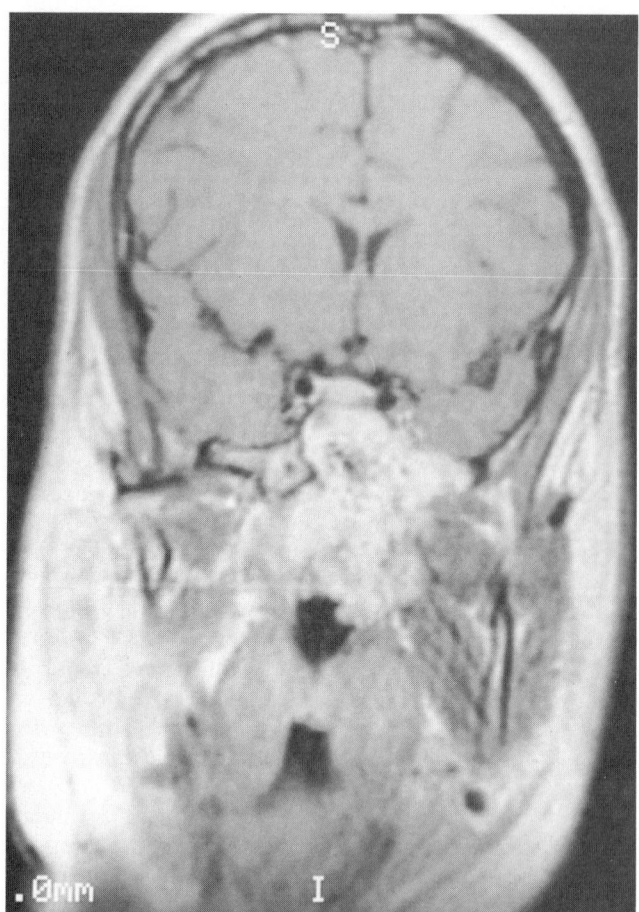

Figure 68–6. Coronal magnetic resonance image showing juvenile nasopharyngeal angiofibroma.

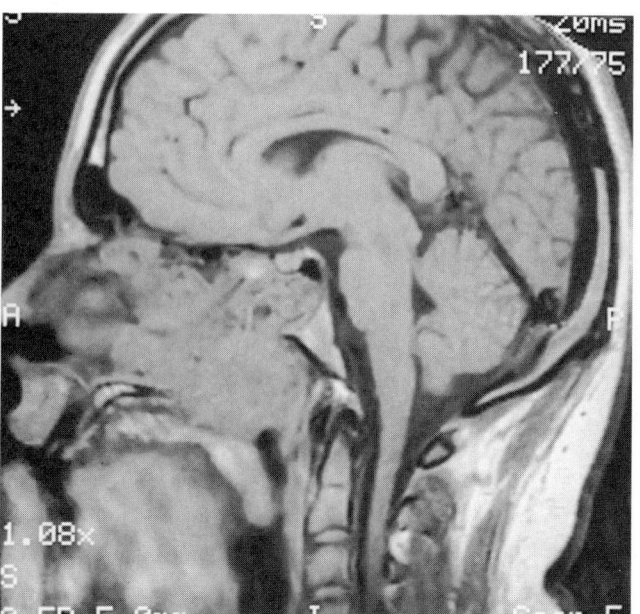

Figure 68–5. Sagittal magnetic resonance image showing juvenile nasopharyngeal angiofibroma.

risks (see later discussion).[97,98] However, whenever possible, a single modality should be selected to minimize the risks. In general, early lesions limited to the nasopharynx or nasal cavity, or lesions with lateral extension, are more amenable to primary surgical therapy than are lesions with major intracranial extension. With surgical resection of extracranial tumors, cure rates ranging from 78% to 100% have been reported. Although successful resections of intracranial lesions have been reported, the risks are greater, and radiotherapy may be preferred as primary treatment in these cases. Angiography is essential, and preoperative embolization may be helpful in reducing intraoperative bleeding.[94,96,99,100]

A number of authors have reported favorable results after radiation therapy for JNA, with local control rates ranging from 73% to 100% (Table 68-7). Many patients in all series were referred after surgical failure or because of advanced or intracranial lesions. Most authors suggest the use of doses between 30 and 36 Gy. However, in the Baylor experience, four of five patients treated with 32 Gy failed, whereas none of 11 patients treated with higher doses (36 to 46 Gy) failed.[101] However, although other institutions have used doses greater than 36 Gy, the high success rate obtained with doses of 30 to 36 Gy in many series suggests that there is not a clear dose-response relationship above this level. Some failures are probably due to geographic miss of the tumor,[98] underlying

Table 68–7   Results of Radiation Therapy for Juvenile Nasopharyngeal Angiofibroma

First Author	Radiotherapy Dose, Gy	Fraction Size, Gy	Patients, n	Local Control, n (%)
Kasper et al[102]	30-35 (8/9 pts rec'd 30 Gy)	1.37	9	9 (100)
Fields et al[104]	36-52 (med dose = 48 Gy)	1.8-2	13	11 (85)
Robinson et al[103]	30-40	2	10	10 (100)
Cummings et al[98]	30-35 (40 pts, 30 Gy; 15 pts, 35 Gy)	2-2.25	55	44 (80)
McGahan et al[101]	32-46 (5 pts, 32 Gy; 9 pts, 40-46 Gy)	2	15	11 (73)

pts, patients; med, median.

the need for CT-based three-dimensional treatment planning for this disorder. A representative three-field plan is shown in Figures 68-7 and 68-8.

Kasper and colleagues[102] analyzed the University of Florida experience with JNA. Nine patients were treated with radiation from 1975 to 1987. All were male, with a median age of 15. Two patients were treated with primary irradiation because of the difficulty of surgical resection, and the other seven were treated initially with surgery (total of 15 procedures) and received radiotherapy for recurrent disease. One of these patients had cryosurgery as a portion of his prior management; another had hemorrhage requiring a 21-unit transfusion. The base of the skull was involved in eight patients, with seven having evidence of intracranial extension. The dose of radiation used was 30 Gy in eight patients, with six of eight treated with 22 × 1.37 Gy fractions. One patient received 35 Gy. A three-field (anterior and opposed laterals) technique was used in seven of nine patients, with an average field size of 12 × 12 cm. Local control was achieved in all patients clinically, although five of seven patients with follow-up imaging studies had residual abnormalities. Clinical assessment of tumor regression greater than 25% was noted during treatment in eight of nine patients. Acute morbidity was mild, with no patients requiring a treatment break. No late complications have been observed.

Although rapid response of JNA during radiotherapy has been observed, delayed responses can also occur. Cummings and colleagues[98] found residual masses on examination of the nasopharynx in 50% of patients 12 months from treatment. Robinson and colleagues[103] from the Christie Hospital reported residual masses on examination in 6 of 10 patients at 6 months and observed that radiographic findings of response lagged behind clinical findings, with 4 of 4 patients examined with CT 12 to 24 months after radiotherapy having persistent CT abnormalities.

Various late complications have been reported after radiotherapy for JNA in other series, most frequently nasal-mucosal dryness and xerostomia, although cases of cataract formation have been reported.[103,104] However, although the disease may be life-threatening, treatment of a benign disease such as JNA, which occurs primarily in a pediatric population, raises concerns regarding the potential for induction of malignant disease in the patient. A detailed analysis of the relative risks of surgery and radiation therapy for JNA was conducted by Cummings in 1980.[105] At that time, he estimated that the risks of mortality from primary JNA therapy with surgery or radiation were similar, about 1%. The primary difference was that the surgical risks were largely perioperative and immediate (e.g., anesthesia, hemorrhage, transfusion), whereas the risks of radiation were delayed (e.g., radiation-induced sarcoma or thyroid neoplasm). Others have estimated the risk for a radiation-induced neoplasm to be about 1 in 150 for a patient 10 to 20 years old, and 1 in 400 for a patient older than 20.[96]

Fortunately, recurrences after radiotherapy for JNA are uncommon, so experience with salvage therapy is limited.

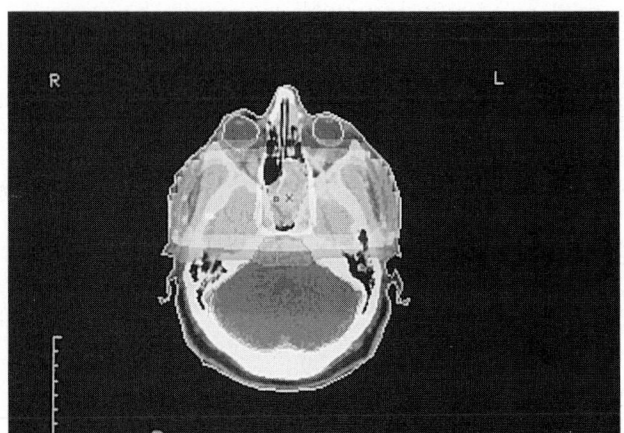

Figure 68–7. Computed tomographic treatment plan for juvenile nasopharyngeal angiofibroma. Axial image, color-wash display: three-field plan.

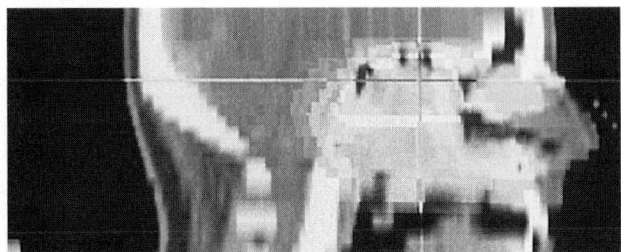

Figure 68–8. Computed tomographic treatment plan for juvenile nasopharyngeal angiofibroma. Sagittal reconstructed image, color-wash display: three-field plan.

Depending on the individual situation, surgery may be appropriate. Goepfert and colleagues[106] reported tumor remissions in five of five patients with recurrent JNA treated with combination chemotherapy with vincristine, dactinomycin, and cyclophosphamide. Clinicians at the Princess Margaret Hospital in Toronto described the efficacy and feasibility of delivering a second course of radiotherapy without significant untoward effects.[98,107]

In summary, JNA is a unique neoplasm, because of its peculiar predilection for a particular age, sex, and site of origin, as well as for the difficulties in management posed by this vascular neoplasm. Primary treatment should be either surgery or radiotherapy: resection if feasible with acceptable morbidity; radiation for advanced lesions not amenable to surgery or for surgical failures. Doses of 30 to 36 Gy are probably adequate for most patients, and local control rates of 75% to 100% can be obtained.

PEYRONIE'S DISEASE

Peyronie's disease has been described since the 18th century. It is characterized by the development of penile plaques, arising from fibrosis of the corpus cavernosum. The disorder is characterized by penile curvature during erection and the presence of penile plaques or induration, often leading to pain on erection or during intercourse. Pathologically, the disorder is characterized in its early stages (<3 months' duration) by an inflammatory cellular infiltrate and in its later stages by the development of fibrous connective tissue and rarely even ossification.[108] Various therapeutic modalities have been used in the management of this disorder, including steroid injections, vitamin E, surgery, and radiation therapy. A comparison of treatments is confounded by the fact that the condition is self-limited in many cases, with as many as 50% of cases resolving spontaneously within 12 to 18 months.[109]

Radiotherapy has been used as a treatment for Peyronie's disease since at least the 1920s. Initially, radium molds were frequently used; however, external beam radiotherapy has been used virtually exclusively in recent decades. Indications and rationale for radiotherapy, as reviewed and summarized by Mira and colleagues,[110,111] include the following:

1. There is a high rate of success when compared with other treatments:

   - Palliation of pain in approximately 80% of patients.
   - Decreased size of plaque in approximately 61% of patients.

   - Improvement of curvature in approximately 57% of patients.

2. Treatment is painless, localized to the penis, without systemic side effects, and completed in 1 to 2 weeks, with only rare complications if external beam radiotherapy is used.

3. Failure of other therapies does not preclude a response to radiotherapy, and failure of radiotherapy does not preclude the use of other modalities.

Mira and colleagues[110,111] reported on 56 evaluable patients treated at the Penrose Cancer Hospital from 1949 to 1972, with follow-up ranging from 6 months to 23 years. Ages ranged from 23 to 74 with a mean age of 53, and 62% of patients in their 50s or 60s. Doses of 600 to 2100 roentgens (R) delivered with 140 to 300 kV orthovoltage x-rays were used. The most common regimen used was 1000 to 1400 R administered in 200 R per day increments, 3 days per week, in 9 to 17 elapsed days. The testes were shielded with lead, with a second lead cutout placed over the penis so that uninvolved areas could be shielded. Martin[112] has suggested that the glans be shielded if uninvolved with plaque.

Results of treatment by Mira and colleagues[110,111] are summarized in Table 68-8. Pain is the most reliably palliated symptom, with lesser rates of palliation achievable for induration and curvature. A series from Duke demonstrated similar results; 79% of patients reported decreased pain, with an interval to improvement averaging 2.4 months; lesser response rates were reported for plaques and curvature.[110] Based on their findings, a trial of radiation was recommended for patients presenting with pain, with surgery reserved for radiotherapy failures.

The duration of symptoms was an important predictor of response in the series of Mira and colleagues.[110,111] Seventy-six percent of patients with a duration of symptoms less than the mean of 5.1 months responded to radiation, whereas only 44% of those with a longer duration of symptoms responded (P <0.05). This suggests that an early trial of radiotherapy, rather than observation, may be important if optimal results are to be achieved. This would correlate with the pathologic findings that for early cases, an inflammatory cellular infiltrate is predominant. There was no clear dose-response demonstrable in the 600 to 1400 R dose range commonly employed.

In summary, radiation treatment is a well-tolerated and noninvasive form of therapy for Peyronie's disease, especially when pain is the dominant symptom. Doses of 8 to 12 Gy, in 2 to 3 Gy fractions delivered two to three times per week to the penis, are adequate. Superficial

Table 68–8   Peyronie's Disease: Symptoms and Response to Radiation Therapy

Symptom	Incidence, %	Percentage Responding	Percentage Not Responding	Treatment-Response Interval, mo
Induration	100	44	56	9.1
Curvature	87	38	62	6.5
Pain	70	79	21	2.8

Data from Mira JG, Chabazian CM, del Regato JA: The value of radiotherapy for Peyronie's disease: Presentation of 56 new case studies and review of the literature. *Int J Radiat Oncol Biol Phys.* 1980;6:161.

(100 to 250 kV) x-rays, or 6 to 12 MeV electrons with bolus, may be used, with appropriate shielding for the glans and testes. A bolus mold may be constructed and 4 to 6 MeV x-rays used as well.

GYNECOMASTIA

Gynecomastia (enlarged breasts) and mammalgia (painful breasts) are common side effects that may accompany estrogenic hormonal therapy for prostate cancer with agents such as diethylstilbestrol (DES). The risk of estrogen-associated breast changes has been estimated at about 70%. Physical changes in the male breast are associated with histologic proliferative changes in ductal epithelium and connective tissue stroma, associated with edema in the normally quiescent male breast. These changes can be tender, painful, and embarrassing for patients and can represent a significant source of morbidity.[113] In patients treated with gonadotropin-releasing hormone (GnRH) agonists (e.g., leuprolide, goserelin), side effects of gynecomastia are significantly less common, occurring in less than 10% of patients.[114] The incidence of gynecomastia decreased when GnRH agonists replaced DES for androgen suppression. However, some novel antiandrogenic regimens, and some regimens of prolonged androgen suppression have been associated with significant incidences of gynecomastia, so it is likely to persist as a concern for prostate cancer patients.

Breast irradiation before the initiation of androgen suppression therapy is effective at preventing gynecomastia with minimal morbidity. For optimum efficacy, treatment should be delivered at least 2 days before DES or other androgen suppression therapy is begun. Doses of 9 to 15 Gy delivered in 3 to 4 Gy fractions have commonly been employed, with results indicating that about 80% of patients treated in this manner do not develop any significant gynecomastia. Circular 5 to 7 cm cones generally provide an adequate treatment volume. Treatment may be delivered with either kilovoltage units (100 to 300 kV; 2 mm A1 to 1 mm Cu half-value layer) or with 6 to 9 MeV electrons, although megavoltage photons and cobalt units have also been used. Morbidity is minimal, with an occasional patient developing erythema and a rare patient, desquamation. Significant late effects have not been reported.[115-117]

When patients who did not receive prophylactic breast irradiation subsequently develop breast symptoms, there is limited experience with the use of radiotherapy. Chou and colleagues[118] found that total doses of 20 Gy in 5 fractions to 40 Gy in 20 fractions palliated symptoms of mammalgia in 11 of 11 patients. However, gynecomastia was palliated in only three of eight patients.

TOTAL LYMPHOID IRRADIATION FOR NONMALIGNANT CONDITIONS

TLI has been used in the treatment of conditions for which an autoimmune cause is known or hypothesized. In these conditions, the immunosuppressive effects of TLI may serve as an alternative to drugs such as prednisone, cyclophosphamide, and azathioprine. TLI offers the potential to improve the therapeutic ratio by proving either more effective or less toxic, or both, than pharmacological immunosuppression.[119] Although a well-defined role for TLI in the clinical setting in the routine practice of radiation oncology does not exist at present, investigation into its potential use continues. Conditions for which TLI has been used include organ transplantation, rheumatoid arthritis, lupus nephritis, multiple sclerosis, and ALS (see following sections).

Rheumatoid Arthritis and Lupus Nephritis

Both rheumatoid arthritis and lupus nephritis are diseases that share an autoimmune cause. TLI has been used for severe rheumatoid arthritis refractory to conventional therapy. Doses of approximately 20 Gy have produced favorable symptomatic responses in small series.[120,121] In a double-blind, randomized trial, a dose of 20 Gy was found to produce a significant improvement in symptoms ($P < 0.05$) when compared with a control group that received fractionated TLI to a total of only 2 Gy in 0.2 Gy fractions.[122] However, side effects such as cytopenias, pericarditis, and pneumonitis were reported more frequently in the cohort receiving 20 Gy. Improvement after TLI was also demonstrated in a series of 10 patients with severe lupus nephritis refractory to conventional therapy.[123]

Organ Transplantation

Allograft rejection after organ transplantation is a significant problem. In animal models, TLI was found to produce improved allograft survival.[124] In recent years, TLI has continued to play a role in cardiac transplantation, both as an adjunct to conventional immunosuppressive therapy and as salvage therapy before retransplantation for patients with persistent rejection on conventional immunosuppressive therapy.[125,126] TLI doses in the range of 8.0 Gy in twice-weekly 0.8 Gy fractions have been used.[127]

Multiple Sclerosis and Amyotrophic Lateral Sclerosis

Both multiple sclerosis and ALS are progressive neurological disorders for which satisfactory therapies are not available. Although the causes are not known, a role for autoimmunity in the pathogenesis of these disorders has been hypothesized. In a double-blind randomized trial, 20 patients with multiple sclerosis received 19.8 Gy TLI, and 20 received sham radiotherapy.[128,129] A significantly lower rate of functional decline was observed in the patients receiving TLI ($P < 0.01$), with the therapeutic benefit correlating with decreased lymphocyte counts after radiation. A subsequent trial, however, in which only 24 multiple sclerosis patients were randomized, did not show a significant benefit with TLI. In that trial, however, the small sample size allowed a significant chance of a false-negative result.[130] A double-blind randomized trial of TLI (30.6 Gy in 1.8 Gy fractions) versus sham radiotherapy for ALS was conducted in 61 patients.[131] No significant improvement in neurological or motor function was observed. The role of TLI for neurological conditions such as multiple sclerosis and ALS remains investigational.

INTRAVASCULAR BRACHYTHERAPY FOR PREVENTION OF RESTENOSIS

One of the newest areas where radiation therapy for a benign condition has come into widespread clinical practice has been the use of intravascular radiotherapy to reduce the risk of intravascular restenosis. This procedure has had its greatest clinical application in the coronary arteries, to reduce the risk of coronary artery restenosis following angioplasty. The use of intravascular brachytherapy has also been investigated in peripheral vessels,[132] and to maintain the patency of arteriovenous shunts required by renal dialysis patients for vascular access.[133]

Restenosis following coronary angioplasty is a significant limitation to the long-term efficacy of the procedure. Pathologic correlates to restenosis include persistent and recurrent plaque formation, thrombus formation, and inflammatory cell infiltration and proliferation. After animal studies had shown that intravascular radiotherapy was technically feasible and produced reduced restenosis rates in animal models, clinical trials in human subjects were initiated.[134]

In a trial conducted by Teirstein, Massullo, and colleagues at the Scripps Clinic, patients with restenosis underwent balloon dilation and then received intracoronary catheter treatment with either placebo or a gamma-emitting Ir-192 source. Fifty-five patients were enrolled. The rate of restenosis was reduced from 54% in the placebo group to 17% in the Ir-192 cohort ($P = 0.01$).[135] Subsequently, a larger, multicenter trial (Gamma-One trial) enrolled 252 patients. In this trial, a reduction in restenosis rates was also noted.[136]

An alternative to the use of the gamma-emitting Ir-192 source has been the use of beta-emitting sources, which have also been found effective at reducing the rates of restenosis.[137,138] Beta irradiation is less penetrating than gamma radiation and, at present, can be delivered with shorter dwell times and a lower level of radiation safety precautions. At present, however, the Ir 192 sources have the advantage of being able to treat longer vessel segments. Regardless of the radioactive source used, it is important that the radiation oncologist be actively involved in patient selection and treatment.

CONCLUSIONS

Radiation therapy continues to be used in the treatment of various benign disorders because the profile of efficacy and morbidity compares well with the available treatment alternatives. There is a well-established role for radiotherapy in the management of benign neoplasms when surgical therapy is medically contraindicated or would carry undue morbidity. In addition, there are situations in which anatomically limited proliferations of lymphoid, epithelial, or mesenchymal tissue can cause significant morbidity that can be avoided or mitigated with local radiation treatment rather than systemic medical therapy or repeated surgical procedures.

REFERENCES

1. DiSantis DJ, DiSantis DM: Wrong turns on radiology's road of progress. *Radiographics.* 1991;11:1121.
2. Berk LB, Hodes PJ: Roentgen therapy for infections: An historical review. *Yale J Biol Med.* 1991;64:155.
3. Kaplan II: *Clinical Radiation Therapy.* 2nd ed. New York: Paul B Hoeber; 1949.
4. Hall EB: Radiation carcinogenesis. In Hall EB, ed. *Radiobiology for the Radiologist.* 4th ed. Philadelphia: JB Lippincott; 1994:323.
5. Bureau of Radiologic Health, US Department of Health, Education and Welfare (HEW): *A Review of the Use of Ionizing Radiation for the Treatment of Benign Diseases,* Vol I. HEW Publication 78-8043. Rockville, Md: HEW; 1977.
6. Dewing SB: *Radiotherapy of Benign Disease.* Springfield, Ill: Charles C Thomas; 1965.
7. Order SE, Donaldson SS: *Radiation Therapy of Benign Diseases. A Clinical Guide.* New York: Springer-Verlag; 1990.
7a. Meyer JL: *The Radiation Therapy of Benign Diseases: Current Indications and Techniques.* New York: Karger; 2001.
8. Enzinger FM, Weiss SW: Benign tumors and tumorlike conditions of fibrous tissue. In Enzinger FM, Weiss SW, eds. *Soft Tissue Tumors.* 2nd ed. St Louis: CV Mosby; 1988:129.
9. Ketchum LD, Cohen IK, Masters FW: Hypertrophic scars and keloids. A collective review. *Plast Reconstr Surg.* 1974;31:140.
9a. Alster TS, Williams CM: Treatment of keloid sternotomy scars with 585 nm flashlamp-pumped pulsed-dye laser. *Lancet.* 1995;345:1198.
10. DeBeurmann R, Gougerot H: Cheloides des muqueuses. *Ann Derm Syph.* 1906;7:151.
11. Escarmant P, Zimmermann S, Amar A, et al: The treatment of 783 keloid scars by iridium-192 interstitial irradiation after surgical excision. *Int J Radiat Oncol Biol Phys.* 1993;26:245.
12. Borok TL, Bray M, Sinclair I, et al: The role of ionizing radiation for 393 keloids. *Int J Radiat Oncol Biol Phys.* 1988;15:865.
13. Ship AG, Weiss PR, Mincer FR, Wolkstein W: Sternal keloids: Successful treatment employing surgery and adjunctive radiation. *Ann Plast Surg.* 1993;31:481.
14. Doornbos JF, Stoffel TJ, Hass AC, et al: The role of kilovoltage irradiation in the treatment of keloids. *Int J Radiat Oncol Biol Phys.* 1990;18:833.
15. Kovalic JJ, Perez CA: Radiation therapy following keloidectomy—A 20 year experience. *Int J Radiat Oncol Biol Phys.* 1989;17:77.
16. Johns HE, Cunningham JR: *The Physics of Radiology.* 4th ed. Springfield, Ill: Charles C Thomas; 1983:493.
17. Wilder RB, Buatti JM, Kittelson JM, et al: Pterygium treated with excision and postoperative beta irradiation. *Int J Radiat Oncol Biol Phys.* 1992;23:533.
18. Bahrassa F, Datta R: Postoperative beta radiation treatment of pterygium. *Int J Radiat Oncol Biol Phys.* 1983;9:679.
19. Paryani SB, Scott WP, Wells JW, et al: Management of pterygium with surgery and radiation therapy. *Int J Radiat Oncol Biol Phys.* 1994;28:101.
20. Van den Brenk HAS: Results of prophylactic postoperative irradiation in 1300 cases of pterygium. *Am J Roentgenol.* 1968;103:723.
21. Cooper JS: Postoperative irradiation of pterygia: Ten more years of experience. *Radiology.* 1978;128:753.
22. Campbell OR, Amendola BE, Brady LW: Recurrent pterygia: Results of postoperative treatment with Sr-90 applicators. *Radiology.* 1990;174:565.
23. MacKenzie FD, Hirst LW, Kynaston B, Bain C: Recurrence rate and complications after beta irradiation for pterygia. *Ophthalmology.* 1991;98:1776.
24. Hall EB: Radiation cataractogenesis. In Hall EB, ed. *Radiobiology for the Radiologist.* 4th ed. Philadelphia: JB Lippincott; 1994:379.
25. Dusenbery KE, Alul IH, Holland EJ, et al: Beta-irradiation of recurrent pterygia: Results and complications. *Int J Radiat Oncol Biol Phys.* 1992;24:315.

26. Bahn RS, Heufelder AE: Pathogenesis of Graves' ophthalmopathy. *N Engl J Med.* 1993;329:1468.

27. Kendler DL, Lippa J, Rootman J: The initial clinical characteristics of Graves' orbitopathy vary with age and sex. *Arch Opthalmol.* 1993;111:197.

28. Utiger RD: Treatment of Graves' ophthalmopathy. *N Engl J Med.* 1989;321:1403.

29. Larkins R: Treatment of Graves' ophthalmopathy. *Lancet.* 1993;342:941.

30. Bartalena L, Marcocci C, Bogazzi F, et al: Use of corticosteroids to prevent progression of Graves' ophthalmopathy after radioiodine therapy for hyperthyroidism. *N Engl J Med.* 1989;321:1349.

31. Prummel MF, Mourits MP, Berghout A, et al: Prednisone and cyclosporine in the treatment of severe Graves' ophthalmopathy. *N Engl J Med.* 1989;321:1353.

32. Palmer D, Greenberg P, Cornell P, Parker RG: Radiation therapy for Graves' ophthalmopathy: A retrospective analysis. *Int J Radiat Oncol Biol Phys.* 1987;13:1815.

33. Olivotto IA, Ludgate CM, Allen LH, Rootman J: Supervoltage radiotherapy for Graves' ophthalmopathy: CCABC technique and results. *Int J Radiat Oncol Biol Phys.* 1985;11:2085.

34. Sandler HM, Rubenstein JH, Fowble BL, et al: Results of radiotherapy for thyroid opthalmopathy. *Int J Radiat Oncol Biol Phys.* 1989;17:823.

35. Petersen IA, Kriss JP, McDougall IR, Donaldson SS: Prognostic factors in the radiotherapy of Graves' ophthalmopathy. *Int J Radiat Oncol Biol Phys.* 1990;19:259.

36. Hurbli T, Char DH, Harris J, et al: Radiation therapy for thyroid eye diseases. *Am J Opthalmol.* 1985;99:633.

37. Prummel MF, Mourits MP, Blank L, et al: Randomised double-blind trial of prednisone versus radiotherapy in Graves' ophthalmopathy. *Lancet.* 1993;342:949.

38. Parsons JT, Fitzgerald CR, Hood CI, et al: The effects of irradiation on the eye and optic nerve. *Int J Radiat Oncol Biol Phys.* 1983;9:609.

38a. Snijders-Keilholz A, De Keizer RJW, Goslings BM, et al: Probable risk of tumor induction after retro-orbital irradiation for Graves' opthalmopathy. *Radiother Oncol.* 1996;38:69.

39. Stern RL, Rosenthal SA, Doggett EC, et al: Applications of asymmetric collimation with linear accelerators in a radiation oncology department. *Radiology (RSNA Proceedings).* 1993;189:183. Abstract.

40. Knowles DM, Jakobiec FA: Orbital lymphoid neoplasms: A clinicopathologic study of 60 patients. *Cancer.* 1980;46:576.

41. Jakobiec FA, Neri A, Knowles DM: Genotypic monoclonality in immunophenotypical polyclonal orbital lymphoid tumors: A model for tumor progression in the lymphoid system. *Ophthalmology.* 1987;94:980.

42. Enzmann D, Donaldson SS, Marshall WH, Kriss JP: Computed tomography in orbital pseudotumor (idiopathic orbital inflammation). *Radiology.* 1976;120:597.

43. Lanciano RM, Fowble B, Sergott RC, et al: The results of radiotherapy for orbital pseudotumor. *Int J Radiat Oncol Biol Phys.* 1990;18:407.

44. Gordon PS, Juillard GJF, Selch MT, et al: Orbital lymphomas and pseudolymphomas: Treatment with radiation therapy. *Radiology.* 1986;159:797.

45. Keleti D, Flickinger JC, Hobson SR, Mittal BB: Radiotherapy of lymphoproliferative diseases of the orbit. *Am J Clin Oncol.* 1992;15:422.

46. Leone C, Lloyd W: Treatment protocol for orbital inflammatory disease. *Ophthalmology.* 1985;92:1325.

47. Donaldson SS, McDougall IR, Egbert PR, et al: Treatment of orbital pseudotumor (idiopathic orbital inflammation) by radiation therapy. *Int J Radiat Oncol Biol Phys.* 1980;6:79.

48. Fizpatrick PJ, Macko S: Lymphoreticular tumors of the orbit. *Int J Radiat Oncol Biol Phys.* 1984;10:333.

49. Austin-Seymour M, Donaldson SS, Egbert PR, et al: Radiotherapy of lymphoid diseases of the orbit. *Int J Radiat Oncol Biol Phys.* 1985;11:371.

50. Smitt MC, Donaldson SS: Radiotherapy is successful treatment for orbital lymphoma. *Int J Radiat Oncol Biol Phys.* 1993;26:59.

51. Mittal BB, Deutsch M, Kennerdell J, et al: Paraocular lymphoid tumors. *Radiology.* 1986;159:793.

52. Duray PH, Burgdorf WHC, Goltz RW: Persistent cutaneous lymphoid hyperplasia of the face with conjunctival involvement. *Arch Ophthamol.* 1985;103:555.

53. Olson LE, Wilson JF, Cox JD: Cutaneous lymphoid hyperplasia. Results of radiation therapy. *Radiology.* 1985;155:507.

54. Order SE, Donaldson SS: *Lymphoid Hyperplasia—Pseudotumor in Radiation Therapy for Benign Diseases.* New York: Springer-Verlag; 1990:156.

55. Brooker AF, Bowerman JW, Robinson RA, Riley LH: Ectopic ossification following total hip replacement: Incidence and a method of classification. *J Bone Joint Surg.* 1973;55:1629.

56. Ritter MA, Vaughan RB: Ectopic ossification after total hip arthroplasty. Predisposing factors, frequency, and effect on results. *J Bone Joint Surg Am.* 1977;59:345.

57. Coventry MB, Scanlon PW: The use of radiation to discourage ectopic bone. *J Bone Joint Surg Am.* 1981;63:201.

58. Kjaersgaard-Andersen P, Ritter MA: Prevention of formation of heterotopic bone after total hip arthroplasty. *J Bone Joint Surg Am.* 1991;73:942.

59. Thomas BJ: Heterotopic bone formation after total hip arthroplasty. *Orthop Clin North Am.* 1992;23:347.

60. Schmidt SA, Kjaersgaard-Andersen P, Pedersen NW, et al: The use of indomethacin to prevent the formation of heterotopic bone after total hip replacement. A randomized, double-blind, clinical trial. *J Bone Joint Surg Am.* 1988;70A:834.

61. Cella JP, Salvati EA, Sculco TP: Indomethacin for the prevention of heterotopic ossification following total hip arthroplasty: Effectiveness, contraindications, and adverse effects. *J Arthroplasty.* 1988;3:229.

62. MacLennan I, Keys HM, Evarts CM, Rubin P: Usefulness of postoperative hip irradiation in the prevention of heterotopic bone formation in a high risk group of patients. *Int J Radiat Oncol Biol Phys.* 1984;10:49.

63. Anthony P, Keys H, Evarts CM, et al: Prevention of heterotopic bone formation with early postoperative irradiation in high risk patients undergoing total hip arthroplasty: Comparison of 10 Gy vs. 20 Gy schedules. *Int J Radiat Oncol Biol Phys.* 1987;13:365.

64. Sylvester JE, Greenberg P, Selch MT, et al: The use of postoperative irradiation for the prevention of heterotopic bone formation after total hip replacement. *Int J Radiat Oncol Biol Phys.* 1988;14:471.

65. Blount LH, Thomas BJ, Tran L, et al: Postoperative irradiation for the prevention of heterotopic bone: Analysis of different dose schedules and shielding considerations. *Int J Radiat Oncol Biol Phys.* 1990;19:577.

66. Lo TC, Healy WL, Corall DJ, et al: Heterotopic bone formation after hip surgery; prevention with single dose postoperative hip irradiation. *Radiology.* 1988;168:851.

67. Konski A, Pellegrini V, Poulter C, et al: Randomized trial comparing single dose vs. fractionated irradiation for prevention of heterotopic bone: A preliminary report. *Int J Radiat Oncol Biol Phys.* 1990;18:1139.

68. Graybill JC, Padgett DE, Hartsell WF, et al: Prevention of heterotopic ossification with 500 cGy postoperative RT: A report of a randomized trial. *Int J Radiat Oncol Biol Phys.* 1993;27(suppl 1):310. Abstract.

69. Slawson RG, Poka A, Bathon H, et al: The role of postoperative radiation in the prevention of heterotopic ossification in patients with traumatic acetabular fracture. *Int J Radiat Oncol Biol Phys.* 1989;17:669.

70. Konski A, Weiss C, Rosier R, et al: The use of postoperative irradiation for the prevention of heterotopic bone after total hip replacement with biologic fixation (porous coated) prosthesis: An animal model. *Int J Radiat Oncol Biol Phys.* 1990;18:861.

71. Durr ED, Turlington EG, Foote RL: Radiation treatment of heterotopic bone formation in the temporomandibular joint articulation. *Int J Radiat Oncol Biol Phys.* 1993;27:863.

72. Wolfson AH, McAuliffe JA, Ouelette EA, et al: Role of postoperative radiation therapy of the elbow as prophylaxis against heterotopic ossification. *Radiology (RSNA Proceedings).* 1993;189:267. Abstract.

73. Rubenstein JH, Salenius SA, Blitzer PH, et al: Prevention of heterotopic bone formation with low dose radiation therapy. *J Fla Med Assoc.* 1992;79:828.

73a. Poggi MM, Thomas BE, Johnstone PAS: Excision and radiotherapy for heterotopic ossification of the elbow. *Orthopedics.* 1999;22:1059.

73b. Viola RW, Hastings H: Treatment of ectopic ossification about the elbow. *Clin Orthop.* 2000;370:65.

74. Kantorowitz DA, Miller GJ, Ferrara JA, et al: Preoperative versus postoperative irradiation in the prophylaxis of heterotopic bone formation in rats. *Int J Radiat Oncol Biol Phys.* 1990;19:1431.

75. Gregoritch S, Chadha M, Pelligrini V, et al: Pre-operative irradiation for prevention of heterotopic ossification following prosthetic total hip replacement—Preliminary results. *Int J Radiat Oncol Biol Phys.* 1993;27(suppl 1):157. Abstract.

76. Seegenschmidt MH, Goldman AR, Martus P, et al: Prophylactic radiation therapy for prevention of heterotopic ossification after hip arthroplasty: Results in 141 high-risk hips. *Radiology.* 1993;188:257.

77. Enzinger FM, Weiss SW: Paraganglioma. In Enzinger FM, Weiss SW, eds. *Soft Tissue Tumors.* 2nd ed. St Louis: CV Mosby; 1988:836.

78. Million RR, Cassisi NJ, Mancuso AA, Stringer SP: Chemodectomas (glomus body tumors). In Million RR, Cassisi NJ, eds. *Management of Head and Neck Cancer.* 2nd ed. Philadelphia:JB Lippincott; 1994:765.

79. Wang CC: Paraganglioma of the head and neck. In Williams CJ, Krikorian JG, Green MR, Raghavan D, eds. *Textbook of Uncommon Cancer.* New York: John Wiley; 1988:725.

80. Coia LR, Fazekas JT, Farb SN: Familial chemodectoma. *Int J Radiat Oncol Biol Phys.* 1981;7:949.

81. Shedd DP, Arias JD, Glunk RP: Familial occurrence of carotid body tumors. *Head Neck.* 1990;12:496.

82. Cece JA, Lawson W, Biller HF, et al: Complications in the management of large glomus jugulare tumors. *Laryngoscope.* 1988;97:152.

83. Cummings BJ, Beale FA, Garrett PG, et al: The treatment of glomus tumors in the temporal bone by megavoltage radiation. *Cancer.* 1984;53:2635.

84. Springate SC, Weichselbaum RR: Radiation or surgery for chemodectoma of the temporal bone: A review of local control and complications. *Head Neck.* 1990;12:303.

85. Springate SC, Haraf D, Weichselbaum RR: Temporal bone chemodectomas—Comparing surgery and radiation therapy. *Oncology.* 1991;5:131.

86. Pryzant RM, Chou JL, Easley JD: Twenty year experience with radiation therapy for temporal bone chemodectomas. *Int J Radiat Oncol Biol Phys.* 1989;27:1303.

87. Hansen HS, Thomsen KA: Radiotherapy in glomus tumors (paragangliomas). A 25 year review. *Acta Otolaryngol (Stockh).* 1988;449:151.

88. Powell S, Peters N, Harmer C: Chemodectoma of the head and neck: Results of treatment in 84 patients. *Int J Radiat Oncol Biol Phys.* 1992;22:919.

89. Kim J-A, Elkon D, Lim M-L, Constable WC: Optimum dose of radiotherapy for chemodectomas of the middle ear. *Int J Radiat Oncol Biol Phys.* 1980;6:815.

90. Wang M-L, Hussey DH, Doornbos JF, et al: Chemodectoma of the temporal bone: A comparison of surgical and radiotherapeutic results. *Int J Radiat Oncol Biol Phys.* 1988;14:643.

91. Wang CC: What is the optimum dose of radiation therapy for glomus tumors? *Int J Radiat Oncol Biol Phys.* 1980;6:945.

92. Konefal JB, Pilepich MV, Spector GJ, Perez CA: Radiation therapy in the treatment of chemodectomas. *Laryngoscope.* 1987;97:1331.

93. Larner JM, Hahn SS, Spaulding CA, Constable WC: Glomus jugulare tumors. Long term control by radiation therapy. *Cancer.* 1992;69:1813.

94. Grybauskas V, Parker J, Friedman M: Juvenile nasopharyngeal angiofibroma. *Otolaryngol Clin North Am.* 1986;19:647.

95. Enzinger FM, Weiss SW: Benign tumors and tumorlike lesions of fibrous tissue. In Enzinger FM, Weiss SW: *Soft Tissue Tumors.* 2nd ed. St Louis: CV Mosby; 1988;127.

96. Million RR, Cassisi NJ, Stringer SP, Mancuso AA: Juvenile angiofibroma. In Million RR, Cassisi NJ, eds. *Management of Head and Neck Cancer: A Multidisciplinary Approach.* 2nd ed. Philadelphia: JB Lippincott; 1994.

97. Gantz B, Seid AB, Weber RS: Controversies: Nasopharyngeal angiofibroma. *Head Neck.* 1992;14:67.

98. Cummings BJ, Blend R, Keane T, et al: Primary radiation therapy for juvenile nasopharyngeal angiofibroma. *Laryngoscope.* 1984; 94:1599.

99. Ward PH, Thompson R, Calcaterra T, Kadin MR: Juvenile angiofibroma: A more rational therapeutic approach based upon clinical and experimental evidence. *Laryngoscope.* 1974;84:2181.

100. Krekorian EA, Kato RH: Surgical management of nasopharyngeal angiofibroma with intracranial extension. *Laryngoscope.* 1977;87:154.

101. McGahan RA, Durrance FY, Parke RB, et al: The treatment of advanced juvenile nasopharyngeal angiofibroma. *Int J Radiat Oncol Biol Phys.* 1989;17:1067.

102. Kasper ME, Parsons JT, Mancuso AA, et al: Radiation therapy for juvenile angiofibroma: Evaluation by CT and MRI, analysis of tumor regression, and selection of patients. *Int J Radiat Oncol Biol Phys.* 1993;25:689.

103. Robinson ACR, Khoury GG, Ash DV, Daly BD: Evaluation of response following irradiation of juvenile angiofibromas. *Br J Radiol.* 1989;62:245.

104. Fields JN, Halverson KJ, Devineni VR, et al: Juvenile nasopharyngeal angiofibroma: Efficacy of radiation therapy. *Radiology.* 1990;176:263.

105. Cummings BJ: Relative risk factors in the treatment of juvenile nasopharyngeal angiofibroma. *Head Neck Surg.* 1980;3:21.

106. Goepfert H, Cangir A, Lee YY: Chemotherapy for aggressive juvenile nasopharyngeal angiofibroma. *Arch Otolaryngol.* 1985;111:285.

107. Fitzpatrick PJ, Rider WD: The radiotherapy of nasopharyngeal angiofibroma. *Radiology.* 1973;109:171.

108. Smith BH: Peyronie's disease. *Am J Clin Pathol.* 1966;45:670.

109. Carson CC, Coughlin PWF: Radiation therapy for Peyronie's disease: Is there a place? *J Urol.* 1985;134:684.

110. Mira JG: Is it worthwhile to treat Peyronie's disease? *Urology.* 1980;16:1.

111. Mira JG, Chabazian CM, del Regato JA: The value of radiotherapy for Peyronie's disease: Presentation of 56 new case studies and review of the literature. *Int J Radiat Oncol Biol Phys.* 1980;6:161.

112. Martin CL: Long-time study of patients with Peyronie's disease treated with irradiation. *Am J Roentgenol.* 1972;114:492.

113. Gagnon JD, Moss WT, Stevens KR: Pre-estrogen breast irradiation for patients with carcinoma of the breast: A critical review. *J Urol.* 1979;121:182.

114. Physicians' Desk Reference. 48th ed. Montvale, N.J.: Medical Economics Data; 1994:2382, 2638.

115. Malis I, Cooper JF, Wolever THS: Breast radiation in patients with carcinoma of the prostate. *J Urol.* 1969;102:326.

116. Corvalan JG, Gill WM, Egelston TA, Rodriguez-Antunez A: Irradiation of the male breast to prevent hormone induced gynecomastia. *Am J Roentgenol.* 1969;106:839.

117. Fass D, Steinfeld A, Brown J, Tessler A: Radiotherapeutic prophylaxis of estrogen-induced gynecomastia: A study of late sequela. *Int J Radiat Oncol Biol Phys.* 1986;12:407.

118. Chou L, Easley JD, Feldmeier JJ, et al: Effective radiotherapy in palliating mammalgia associated with gynecomastia after DES therapy. *Int J Radiat Oncol Biol Phys.* 1988;15:749.

119. Fuks Z, Slavin S: The use of total lymphoid irradiation (TLI) as immunosuppressive therapy for organ allotransplantation and autoimmune diseases. *Int J Radiat Oncol Biol Phys.* 1981;7:79.

120. Kotzin BL, Strober S, Engleman EG, et al: Treatment of intractable rheumatoid arthritis with total lymphoid irradiation. *N Engl J Med.* 1981;305:969.

121. Herbst M, Fritz H, Sauer R: Total lymphoid irradiation of intractable rheumatoid arthritis. *Br J Radiol.* 1986;59:1203.

122. Strober S, Tanay A, Field E, et al: Efficacy of total lymphoid irradiation in intractable rheumatoid arthritis: A double-blind, randomized trial. *Ann Intern Med.* 1985;102:441.

123. Strober S, Field E, Hoppe RT, et al: Treatment of intractable lupus nephritis with total lymphoid irradiation. *Ann Intern Med.* 1985;102:450.

124. Slavin S, Reitz B, Bieber CP, et al: Transplantation tolerance in adult rats using total lymphoid irradiation: Permanent survival of skin, heart, and marrow allografts. *J Exp Med.* 1978;147:700.

125. Salter MM, Kirklin JK, Bourge RC, et al: Total lymphoid irradiation in the treatment of early or recurrent heart rejection. *J Heart Lung Transplant.* 1992;11:902.

126. Kirklin JK, George JF, McGiffin DC, et al: Total lymphoid irradiation: Is there a role in pediatric heart transplantation? *J Heart Lung Transplant.* 1993;12:S293.

127. Hunt SA, Strober S, Hoppe RT, Stinson EB: Total lymphoid irradiation for treatment of intractable cardiac allograft rejection. *J Heart Lung Transplant.* 1991;10:211.

128. Cook SD, Devereux C, Troiano R, et al: Effect of total lymphoid irradiation in chronic progressive multiple sclerosis. *Lancet.* 1986;1:1405.

129. Devereux CK, Vidaver R, Hafstein MP, et al: Total lymphoid irradiation for multiple sclerosis. *Int J Radiat Oncol Biol Phys.* 1988;14:197.

130. Wiles WM, Omar L, Swan AV, et al: Total lymphoid irradiation in multiple sclerosis. *J Neurol Neurosurg Psych.* 1994;57:154.

131. Drachman DB, Chaudhry V, Cornblath D, et al: Trial of immunosuppression in amyotrophic lateral sclerosis using total lymphoid irradiation. *Ann Neurol.* 1994;35:142.

132. Tripuraneni P, Giap H, Jani S: Endovascular brachytherapy for peripheral vascular disease. *Semin Radiat Oncol.* 1999;9:190.

133. Parikh S, Nori D: Radiation therapy to prevent stenosis of peripheral vascular access. *Semin Radiat Oncol.* 1999;9:144.

134. Crocker I: Radiation therapy to prevent coronary artery restenosis. *Semin Radiat Oncol.* 1999;9:134.

135. Teistein PS, Massullo V, Jani S, et al: Catheter-based radiotherapy to inhibit restenosis after coronary stenting. *N Eng J Med.* 1997;336:1697.

136. Leon MB, Teirstein PS, Moses JW, et al: Localized intracoronary gamma-radiation therapy to inhibit the recurrence of restenosis after stenting. *N Eng J Med.* 2001;344:250.

137. Waksman R, Bhargava B, White L, et al: Intracoronary beta-radiation therapy inhibits recurrence of in-stent restenosis. *Circulation.* 2000;101:1895.

138. Verin V, Popowski Y, De Bruyne B, et al: Endoluminal beta-radiation therapy for the prevention of coronary restenosis after balloon angioplasty. *N Eng J Med.* 2001;344:243.

Emerging Radiation Modalities

Particle Radiation Therapy

Joseph R. Castro, MD, Paula L. Petti, PhD,
Eleanor A. Blakely, PhD, and Inder K. Daftari, PhD

Particle beams have potential for therapeutic application because of the precise dose localization possible with charged particles such as protons (due to the sharp dose falloff of the Bragg peak, Fig. 69-1A) and the biological attributes of high linear energy transfer (LET) particles (including uncharged neutrons or heavy ions such as carbon, neon, and silicon (Table 69-1) or both. The first clinical use of particle radiotherapy was in the pioneering *neutron* studies of R. Stone[1,2] and J. Lawrence in the late 1930s. *Charged-particle* therapy was first proposed in 1946 by Wilson[3] and begun in the 1950s by Tobias, Lawrence, and colleagues.[4,5] In the late 1950s and early '60s, proton beams were in use at Uppsala, Sweden, for small field cranial radiosurgery and large field radiotherapy[6] and at proton beam facilities in Russia in Moscow, Dubna, and St. Petersburg.

Charged-particle therapy of cancer was only made practical, however, with the advent of computed tomography (CT), which could accurately determine the beam path in a patient. Studies of fractionated charged particle therapy were initiated by Suit et al.[7] at the Massachusetts General Hospital–Harvard Cyclotron Laboratory (MGH-HCL) in 1974, and by Castro et al.[8] at the University of California's Lawrence Berkeley Laboratory and The Medical Center at San Francisco (UCSF-LBL) in 1975. Proton therapy began in Japan at the National Institute of Radiological Sciences (NIRS), Chiba in 1979 and at the Proton Medical Research Center (PARMS), Tsukuba in 1983. The first particle facility to be built expressly for medical radiotherapy use was the Loma Linda University proton beam facility[9] in Loma Linda, Calif. (LLUPAF), which began patient treatments in 1990.

As interest in proton therapy increased, additional clinical programs using existing physics accelerators were established in several countries including Switzerland (the Paul Scherrer Institute [PSI]); the United Kingdom (Clatterbridge); France (Centre A. Lacassagne [CAL], Nice, and the Centre for Protontherapie, Orsay [CPO]); Belgium (Louvain-la-Neuve); South Africa (National Accelerator Centre); and Canada (University of Vancouver–TRIUMF). In the United States, the UC Davis Crocker Cyclotron—UCSF and the Midwest Proton Therapy Institute (MPRI) at the Indiana University Cyclotron have begun clinical therapy for eye tumors (Table 69-2).

Three new dedicated accelerators have begun patient treatments: the National Cancer Center Hospital East (NCCHE) in Kashiwa, Japan (1998); the Northeast Proton Therapy Center (NEPTC) at MGH-Harvard, replacing the MGH-HCL proton therapy facility (2001); and the Hyogo Ion Beam Medical Center (HIBMC)[10] facility in Harima, Japan (2001). Worldwide, more than 27,000 patients have been treated with proton beams, and long-term follow-up results are available for several treatment sites.

Heavy charged particle trials in cancer therapy[11] were initiated at UCSF-LBL in 1975. At UCSF-LBL, ions ranging from helium ions through silicon were available with sufficient intensity for 28 cm penetration in tissue. In a wide array of tumors, helium ions were used for their dose-distribution advantages and neon ions mainly for their high-LET biologic advantages. The phase I-II trials at LBL were terminated in 1992 due to lack of Department of Energy funding for accelerator operations.

In Japan and Germany, attention has been directed to continued study of carbon ions in clinical trials, both for their excellent depth dose distribution and for their high-LET biologic potential. Currently there are three operating heavy ion facilities treating cancer patients. In 1994 the first patient was treated with carbon ions at the Heavy Ion Medical Accelerator in Chiba, Japan (HIMAC)[12]; 1601 patients were entered in protocol studies through August 2003. A second carbon ion facility is at the Gesellschaft für Schwerionen Forschung (GSI), Darmstadt, Germany,[13,14] in collaboration with the Heidelberg University Strahlenklinik, where patient treatments began in 1997. In Japan, another therapy (HIBMC) facility has recently been commissioned to treat patients with carbon ion beams. About 2000 patients have been treated worldwide with carbon, neon, or heavier ion beams.

BIOLOGIC PROPERTIES OF HIGH-LET CHARGED-PARTICLE BEAMS AND NEUTRONS

Radiobiologic studies have shown experimental evidence that both qualitative and quantitative differences exist between the biologic effects of low-LET photons and

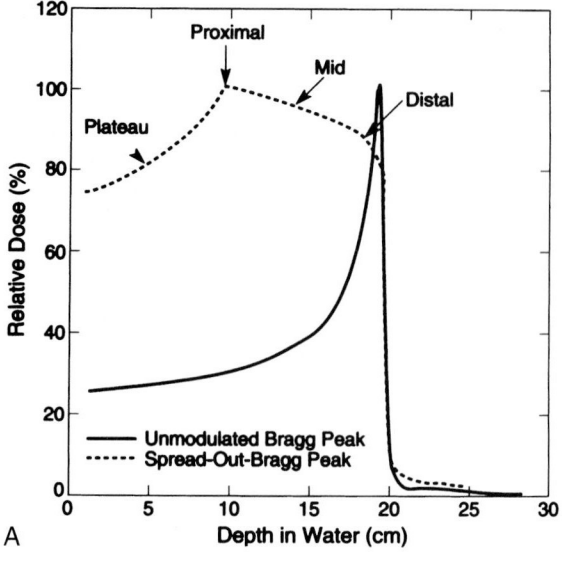

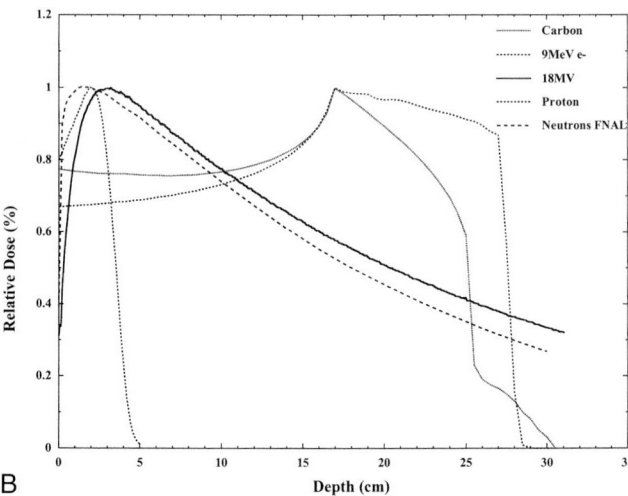

Figure 69–1. Depth dose distribution for 215 MeV/amu helium ion beam. **A,** Example of an unmodulated (monoenergetic) Bragg curve (sharp peak) and a Bragg curve (spread peak) modulated as appropriate for clinical radiotherapy. In this case a helium beam is illustrated, although protons and carbon and neon beams are similar except for a larger fragmentation tail for heavier ions such as neon and silicon. The slope in the spread-Bragg curve compensates for increasing linear energy transfer by decreasing the physical dose across the Bragg curve. A family of spread peaks from 1 to 15 cm is needed for clinical therapy of tumors of differing sizes. **B,** Comparison of clinical depth-dose profiles for carbon ions, protons, 9 MeV electrons, 18 MV photons, and neutrons used for radiotherapy at Fermi National Accelerator Laboratory (FNAL), Batavia, Ill. which are produced by 66 MeV protons incident on a beryllium target. The buildup region of the FNAL neutron beam is similar to 4 MV x-rays, whereas the dose falloff at depth resembles 8 MV x-rays. Note the sharp falloff of dose at depth for the proton and carbon beams. The high dose zone of the charged particle beams can be varied in size and depth of penetration, but maintains its sharp distal falloff at depth, in contrast with electrons of energy greater than 20 MeV.

those of high-LET radiations. These techniques are used to screen for differences in biologic effects due to ion beam characteristics or different modes of beam delivery. Radiobiologic measurements have also been used to predict optimal patient selection for individual response of

both tumor and normal tissues to radiations of different qualities.[15-17]

PARTICLE FIELD CHARACTERIZATION. Particle radiation fields become complex as the individual ions traverse absorbing material. *Linear energy transfer* (LET) is a physical parameter that is a measure of the mean rate of energy deposited locally along the track of a charged particle by electromagnetic interactions. LET is an important quantity because the amount of radiation damage incurred by a cell depends on the number of ionizing events produced by the radiation presumed to be in the vicinity of the cell's DNA. Radiation damage along a particle track is caused by direct mechanisms in which DNA molecules are ionized by the particle and by indirect mechanisms in which free radicals, such as e⁻aq, OH• and H•, produced by the ionizing particle react with the DNA. However, this paradigm for both low-LET and high-LET radiation effects has been modified at low doses (e.g., <10 cGy) by experimental evidence for bystander effects in unirradiated neighboring cells.[18-21] Yet the clinical significance of these and other low-dose effects is not clear. Despite these new observations it is generally accepted that changes in the genetic code, or changes in gene expression, of individual cells of the tumor and of the surrounding normal tissues, lead to local tumor control and are also responsible for undesirable normal-tissue effects. One clear advantage of the use of charged particles over x-rays is the control achievable in the mapping of the radiation fields to the tumor target.

Values of LET increase as charged particles slow down. The LET for 1 MeV electrons is 0.25 keV/μm. For neutrons produced in the reaction 50 MeV d + Be, the LET distribution ranges from 1.5 to 500 keV/μm with peaks near 8 keV/μm and 100 keV/μm.[22] Particles with an LET value of less than 30 to 50 keV/μm are called low-LET particles, whereas those with higher LET values are categorized as high-LET particles. High-LET particles are more biologically damaging (Table 69-3) primarily

Table 69–1   Attributes of Particle Beams

Particle	Charge	Mass	Range of Average RBE Values
Electron	−1	1 m$_e$	1
Proton	+1	1832 m$_e$	1.1–1.6*
Neutron	0	1835 m$_e$	3.0–3.3†
Pions	−1	276 m$_e$	1.0–1.8‡
Helium ion	+2	4 amu	1.2–1.4§
Carbon ion	+6	12 amu	1.4–3.5‖
Neon ion	+10	20 amu	2.0–3.0¶

*Data from references 28,107,111,192,194,195. RBE used in clinical practice: 1.1–1.2, but up to 1.6 in distal edge of extended beams.
†Data from references 37,111,191,193.
‡Data from Raju.[111]
§Data from Blakely et al.[16] and Raju.[111] Helium RBE used in clinical practice with 8 cm Bragg peak at 2.0 GyEq fraction.
‖Data from references 13,14,16,111,164,196–204. Carbon RBE used in clinical practice adjusted for energy, depth, RBE, and fraction size.
¶Data from Blakely et al.[16] and Raju.[111] Neon RBE used in clinical practice with 8 cm Bragg peak at 3.0 GyEq fraction.
RBE, relative biologic effectiveness.

Table 69–2   Active Charged Particle Centers

Site	Particles	Accelerator	Max Energy (MeV)	First Rx	Patients Treated
MGH-HCL, NEPTC, USA	Protons	Cyclotron	160-230	1961	8906
Dubna, Russia	Protons	Synchro cyclo	680	1967	172
Moscow, Russia	Protons	Synchrotron	200	1969	3414
St. Petersburg, Russia	Protons	Synchro cyclo	1000	1975	1029
Chiba, Japan	Protons	Cyclotron	90	1979	133
Tsukuba, Japan	Protons	Synchrotron	250	1983	700
PSI, Switzerland	Protons	Cyclotron	250	1984	3432
Clatterbridge, UK	Protons	Cyclotron	62	1989	1033
Loma Linda, USA	Protons	Synchrotron	250	1990	6174
Louvain-la-Neuve, Belgium	Protons	Cyclotron	90	1991	21
Nice, France	Protons	Cyclotron	65	1991	1590
Orsay, France	Protons	Synchro cyclo	200	1991	1894
N.AC S. Africa	Protons	Cyclotron	<200	1993	398
MPRI, IUCF, USA	Protons	Cyclotron	200	1993	34
UCSF–CNL, USA	Protons	Cyclotron	65	1994	430
HIMAC, Japan	Ion	Synchrotron	800(/u)	1994	1601
TRIUMF, Canada	Protons	Cyclotron	70	1995	57
GSI, Germany	Ion	Synchrotron	2000	1997	100
Berlin, Germany	Protons	Cyclotron	65	1998	166
Kashiwa, Japan	Protons	Cyclotron	235	1998	75
Hyogo, Japan	Protons/Ion	Synchrotron	230/320/u	2001	1

Adapted from Sisterson J, ed: Particles. *PTCOG Newsletter*. July, 2001; vol 28.

because they cause more severe, less reparable damage per unit track length than low-LET radiations.[23,24]

RELATIVE BIOLOGIC EFFECTIVENESS. The concept of *relative biologic effectiveness* (RBE) arose from observations that ionizing particulate radiations can be several times more effective per unit dose in producing biologic effects than x-rays or gamma-rays.[25] RBE is defined as the ratio of absorbed doses of two radiations required to produce the same biologic effect. One extension of this concept has been the clinical use of the terminology gray-equivalent (GyEq) dose. This is the dose of a particle modality that yields an equivalent biologic response to a dose of megavoltage x-ray or cobalt-60 gamma-rays. The RBE for therapeutic neutron beams at a 2 GyEq dose fraction ranges from 3.0 to 3.3 relative to ^{60}Co. For 160 to 230 MeV proton beams, the RBE[26-30] is generally considered to be about 1.1 to 1.2, and for heavier particles (helium, carbon, neon, silicon), the RBE ranges from 1.2 to 4.5. RBE depends on dose fraction size as well as the type of tissue irradiated and the position on the depth

dose curve at which it is measured. For example, at UCSF-LBL, the clinical RBE was referenced to the proximal portion of the Bragg peak unless otherwise noted. Successful use of high-LET charged particle therapy requires understanding of the complicated dependency of RBE on these variables.

OXYGEN ENHANCEMENT RATIO. The *oxygen enhancement ratio* (OER) is the ratio of dose needed to inactivate severely hypoxic or anoxic tumor cells relative to the dose needed to inactivate well-oxygenated tumor cells. It has a value of about 3 for low-LET photons, electrons, or protons but is diminished with the use of high-LET irradiations to about 1.6 to 1.7 at LET values of about 100 keV/μm. The degree to which the OER is reduced is an indication of high-LET biologic effectiveness.

Radiobiologic Advantages of High-Let Radiotherapy

DECREASED RADIORESISTANCE OF HYPOXIC TUMOR CELLS TO HIGH-LET RADIATION. Although factors other than hypoxia are important in tumor control, most tumors have significant numbers of hypoxic cells that are preferentially killed with high-LET irradiations. The RBE for high-LET radiation is also increased for normal tissues as well as for tumors. Whether or not high-LET radiotherapy is effective in treating a given disease depends on the relative values of the tumor and normal-tissue RBEs, as well as reduction in the OER. For example, the neon-ion RBE for late effects in central nervous system (CNS) tissues is between 4 and 5 at a dose fraction of 0.7 Gy[31]; RBEs for hypoxic tumors are probably

Table 69–3   Relative Advantages of Charged-Particle and Neutron Beams

	Dose Localization	Biologic Effect
Protons	+ + + +	+
Helium ions	+ + + + +	+
Carbon ions	+ + + + + +	+ + +
Neon ions	+ + +	+ + + +
Silicon ions	+ +	+ + + + +
Neutrons	+	+ + + +

similar. Thus, care must be taken to protect normal tissues in neon-ion or neutron therapy of CNS structures. High-LET charged particles have dose-localizing advantages compared to neutrons, which aids selective deposition of a biologically effective dose in the tumor relative to normal CNS tissue.

DECREASED REPAIR OF RADIATION INJURY. Decreased repair of radiation injury imparted by high-LET particles is evidenced by the absence of a shoulder on the cell-survival dose response curve for high-LET radiation, also implying that the RBE for high-LET particles is larger for smaller fraction sizes than it is for larger doses per fraction. Thus, it is important to recognize that using smaller doses per fraction of high-LET irradiation will not help spare normal tissues as in low-LET radiation. Fowler[32] has recommended that large numbers of small dose fractions of neutrons be avoided because such treatment schedules may lead to severe late injury. Shortening the overall treatment schedule for high-LET radiation therapy to 2 to 4 weeks also minimizes the proliferation of tumor cells during treatment.

LESS VARIATION IN RADIORESISTANCE THROUGHOUT THE CELL CYCLE. For several cell types tested in vitro, the late S phase has been shown to be most resistant to low-LET radiation.[32] In addition, Sinclair[33] reported that for HeLa cells, there is a second phase of radioresistance in the relatively long G1 phase. High-LET radiation can overcome cell cycle–dependent resistance and is advantageous in either fast-growing tumors with a large proportion of cells in the S phase or slowly proliferating tumors with a large fraction of cells in G1 or G0.

Other High-Let Radiobiologic Results of Potential Therapeutic Significance

ACCELERATED TUMOR REOXYGENATION. Carbon ion irradiation has been shown experimentally to accelerate the reoxygenation of murine fibrosarcoma compared to x-irradiation.[34] This is due to the smaller OER value for carbon ions compared to x-irradiation, as has also been reported for neutrons, and would suggest that high-LET radiations would be effective with shortened treatment durations compared to low-LET radiotherapy.[35,36]

TISSUE-SPECIFIC RESPONSES DEPENDENT ON RADIATION TYPE, PARTICLE ATOMIC NUMBER, AND ENERGY. The RBE varies to a large extent with the biologic system and the criteria evaluated.[37-39] For example, even in a given tissue like the spinal cord, Van der Kogel[40,41] has reported different RBE values for late neutron damage to blood vessels, to white matter, or for functional performance. Using variable lengths (<8 mm) of rat cervical spinal cord with a high-precision 150 to 190 MeV proton beam at the plateau of the Bragg curve allowed Bijl et al.[42] to determine the steep dose-effect relationships. The results showed steeply increasing ED50 values

for lengths of less than 8 mm, and decreased latencies at the higher doses of the shortened exposure lengths, which suggested the presence of a critical migration distance of 2 to 3 mm for cells involved in regeneration processes.

GENETIC SUSCEPTIBILITY. There are several genetic autosomal recessive syndromes that render patients susceptible to enhanced acute and late radiation effects; in fact, these patients are frequently cancer prone. Mutations in the ATM (ataxia telangiectasia mutated) gene in female breast cancer patients predict for an increase in radiation-induced late effects.[43] It has been reported that some prostate cancer patients who have late sequelae after high-dose radiation therapy are heterozygous for mutations in the ATM gene.[44] ATM homozygosity or heterozygosity could be associated with severe radiotoxicities to high-LET radiations.[39]

POSSIBLE INCREASED RISK OF CARCINOGENESIS AND OTHER LATE RADIATION EFFECTS. In using high-LET radiotherapy the cost-benefit analysis must include an awareness of enhanced late sequelae, including undesirable tissue fibrosis,[45] vascular damage,[46] central nervous system (CNS) toxicities, genomic instability,[47] and secondary cancers.[48] In the clinical trial at LBL-UCSF, relatively short-term follow-up (24 to 173 months; mean, 67 months) of neon ion–treated patients at UCSF-LBL suggested an increased radiation-induced tumor rate of about 2%. There was no increase over conventional x-ray rates for the helium patients.[49]

Biologic Dosimetry for Differing Modes of Beam Delivery

The type of charged-particle beam delivery system used can significantly affect the beam quality and consequent biologic effects. The first delivery systems used clinically broadened the pencil particle beams that are extracted from accelerators with a simple array of metal scattering foils to produce larger field sizes. As biologic evidence indicated that the primary beam fragmentation processes occurring in the scattering foils contributed to a loss of beam quality and biologic effectiveness, alternative methods of beam delivery were developed. Dynamic conformal therapy with a scanning system allows the most effective distribution of particle dose in the tumor while sparing the normal tissues (Fig. 69-2).[50,51] Particle atomic number and energy, as well as the techniques used to enlarge the beam field, can change the effective LET value of the charged-particle beam. Biologic systems such as human fibroblasts in culture are sensitive to the LET differences. Although the single-dose RBE data for clonal survival are not absolutely correct quantitatively for human tissue, they appear to be proportional to human skin and mucosal RBE data for acute dose reactions. Relative changes in cell killing determined with in vitro techniques provide a quantitative basis for beam modulation design and input into the treatment planning model.

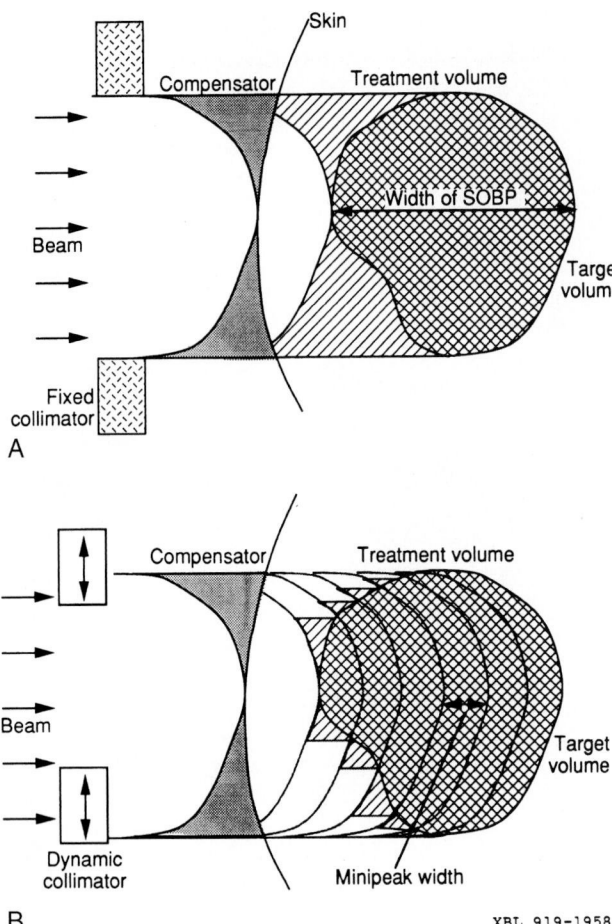

A

B

XBL 919-1958

Figure 69–2. Fixed (*A*) and variable (*B*) modulation dynamic charged-particle conformal therapy. **A,** The technique employed at Lawrence Berkeley Laboratory was a static charged particle therapy with stopping of the beam along the distal edge of the target volume. **B,** A new technique uses a dynamic collimator and variable energy absorber to irradiate in a stepwise fashion. The most distal layer in the target volume is irradiated first. The range of the beam is then shortened and the field shape is adjusted with the dynamic multileaf collimator to irradiate subsequent layers. This technique gives added sparing of normal tissues proximal to the target volume as well as stopping the beam along the distal edge of the target volume and should lead to an even higher therapeutic ratio than current techniques. (From Chu WT, Ludewigt BA, Renner TR: Instrumentation for treatment of cancer using proton and light-ion beams. *Rev Sci Instrum.* 1993;64:2055.)

PHYSICS AND TREATMENT PLANNING OF CHARGED PARTICLES AND NEUTRONS

Basic Physical Properties of Charged-Particle Beams

Low-LET charged particles derive their therapeutic advantage from their physical properties. In the therapeutic energy range (for protons, between 60 and 250 MeV), charged particles lose energy primarily by ionizing and exciting electrons as they penetrate a medium. The energy deposited at a given depth is inversely proportional

to the square of the particle's velocity. This leads to a sharp increase in dose, called the Bragg peak, at the maximum depth of penetration (Fig. 69-1*A*) with abrupt falloff of dose in a short distance. The maximum depth of penetration (range) of a charged-particle beam is a function of the initial beam energy and can be adjusted by varying the energy or adding or removing absorbing material upstream from the patient. Absorbers or compensators of variable thickness can be constructed to precisely control the beam penetration in three dimensions. The resulting isodose distributions (Figs. 69-3 and 69-4) can be made to conform closely to the target volume, allowing higher doses to be delivered to the target without exceeding the tolerance doses of surrounding healthy tissues. Multiple-coulomb scattering between charged particles and atomic nuclei changes the direction of motion of the incoming particles without significantly affecting their energy. The net result of a large number of these interactions is to increase the angular spread of the beam and, in complex heterogeneous regions, to degrade the sharpness of the Bragg peak.[52-54] The effects of multiple scattering increase as a function of decreasing particle mass. Electrons, for example, exhibit no Bragg peak due to multiple scattering. For protons and heavier charged particles, multiple scattering increases the penumbra width as a function of depth and increases the distance over which the Bragg peak falls from the maximum dose to a few percent of the maximum dose.

Heavy ions, but not protons, can also undergo inelastic nuclear interactions with atomic nuclei, resulting in the fragmentation of either the incoming ion or the atomic nucleus. These fragments cause dose to be

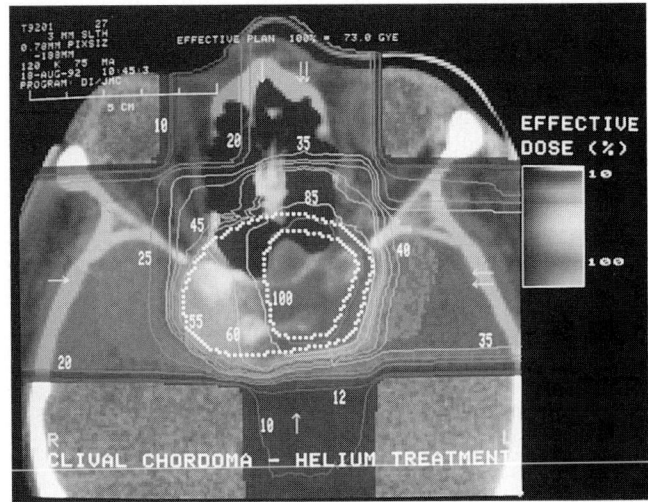

Figure 69–3. Clival chordoma isodose plan: a single slice through the tumor from a helium ion isodose plan for treatment of clival chordoma. Multiple coplanar portals are used. Isodose lines are in equivalent doses and corrected for relative biologic effectiveness (RBE) to compensate for biologic effects from the small amount of high linear energy transfer (LET) present in the helium beam. *Dotted lines* represent initial and cone-down tumor volumes as determined from magnetic resonance imaging and computed tomography scans. A total of 72 GyEq was given to the smaller target volume. Critical nearby normal tissues are also evaluated by use of three-dimensional dose-volume histograms, as are the target volumes. See also Color Figure 69-3.

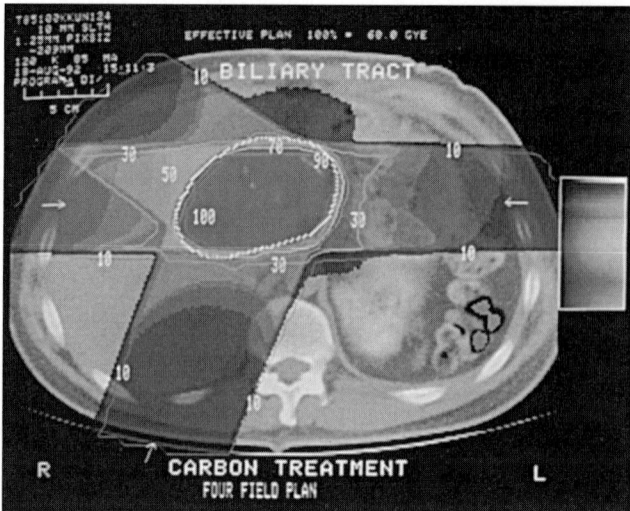

Figure 69–4. Heavy ion (carbon) treatment plan for biliary tract cancer consisting of four coplanar portals. The total dose was 60 GyEq. Isodose lines represent biologically (RBE) corrected doses. Three-dimensional dose-volume histograms were used to assess the dose to liver and stomach, as an aid in planning for this type of therapy, and to be certain that doses remain below the tolerance level to critical adjacent organs. See also Color Figure 69–4.

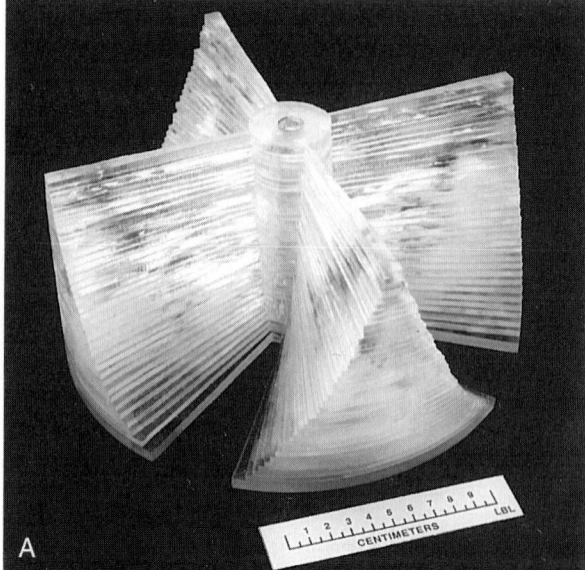

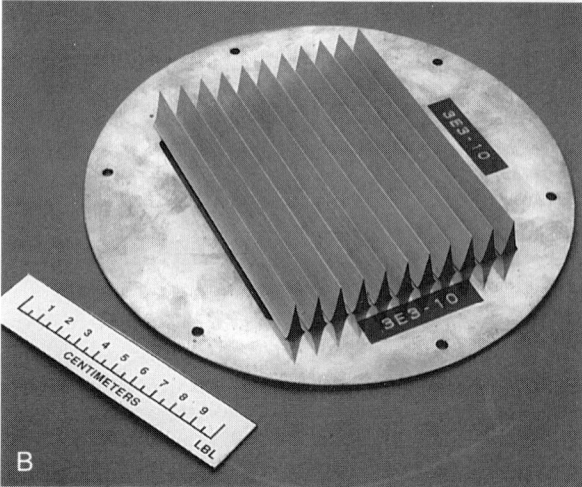

Figure 69–5. Ridge filter or Lucite propeller to spread the Bragg peak. Insertion of some type of variable-thickness absorber such as a Lucite propeller (**A**) or brass ridge filter (**B**) has the effect of modulating or spreading the Bragg peak from a narrow width to a clinically useful width that will cover the desired target volume (see spread-Bragg peak as shown in Figure 69-1*A and B*). Particles penetrating different portions of the propeller or ridge filter have different ranges in tissue, depending on the thickness of the material they traverse.

deposited beyond the Bragg peak in a fragmentation tail, which must be considered in planning treatment.

Treatment Planning for Charged-Particle Beams

Treatment planning always begins with a careful history and physical examination. Simulation for charged particle therapy is usually done with the CT scanner. Integration of clinical, radiographic, CT, positron emission tomography, ultrasound, and magnetic resonance imaging (MRI) information must be done by the clinician and physicist to properly plan treatment for the patient.

To treat large lesions, it is necessary to modulate the beam's range to spread out the Bragg peak, as shown in Fig. 69-1*B*. This is most commonly done with variable thickness absorbers such as a propeller or ridge filter (Fig. 69-5).[55-58] As the blades of a propeller (or ridges of a brass filter) move through the beam, particles penetrating different thicknesses of plastic have their ranges correspondingly shortened. The resulting beam is the superposition of Bragg peaks with different ranges. Propellers are made of low-Z materials (e.g., Lucite) to minimize multiple scattering. Ridge filters[59,60] are made of heavy metals (e.g., brass) and consist of a series of closely spaced wedges. The mixing of particles with different ranges occurs through multiple scattering.

With passive beam-modulation techniques such as propellers or brass ridge filters, the spread-Bragg peak width is constant over the entire tumor volume. Because most tumors have a variable thickness across the radiation field, some normal tissues immediately proximal to the target will receive the full dose delivered with that beam. This dose can be minimized by using several beam portals in the treatment plan. A more challenging approach is to dynamically modulate the beam during the treatment using raster-scanning to produce a beam with a variable spread-Bragg peak width across the radiation field.[50,51,60] The potential advantages of dynamic conformal therapy (Figs. 69-6 and 69-7, and see Fig. 69-2) with charged particles are diminished dose to normal tissues, reduction in the number of beam direction required, and potential ability to distribute the high-LET where desired.[60-63] Dynamic charged particle conformal therapy is currently being studied at PSI in Switzerland[64,65] and GSI in Germany.[13,14]

Treatment planning for charged particles is inherently three-dimensional (3D), and many 3D treatment planning concepts were first introduced in charged-particle

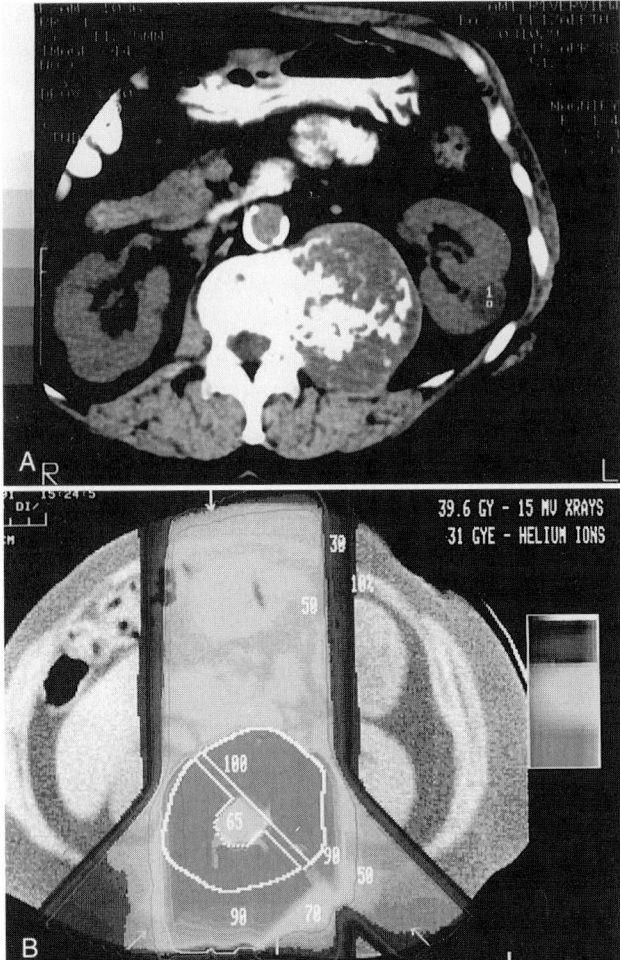

Figure 69–6. Divided target technique for irradiation of tumors of the para-central nervous system (CNS). Charged particles are used to irradiate a target volume wrapped around a critical structure such as the spinal cord. **A,** A large chondrosarcoma was present abutting and encircling the spinal cord and cauda equina and invading the vertebrae. **B,** After subtotal resection, a combined photon and charged-particle plan was devised to irradiate the target volume and minimize dose to the CNS. The target volume, indicated by the *heavy dotted line*, received a total of 70.6 GyEq, except for the inner region around the spinal cord, which received less than 46 GyEq. Computerized three-dimensional treatment planning based on metrizamide-enhanced CT scanning, together with precise immobilization and treatment delivery, is needed to accomplish this technique without CNS injury. A number of patients have been treated with this technique at Lawrence Berkeley Laboratory, with safe protection of the brainstem, spinal cord, and cauda equina. See also Color Figure 69-6B.

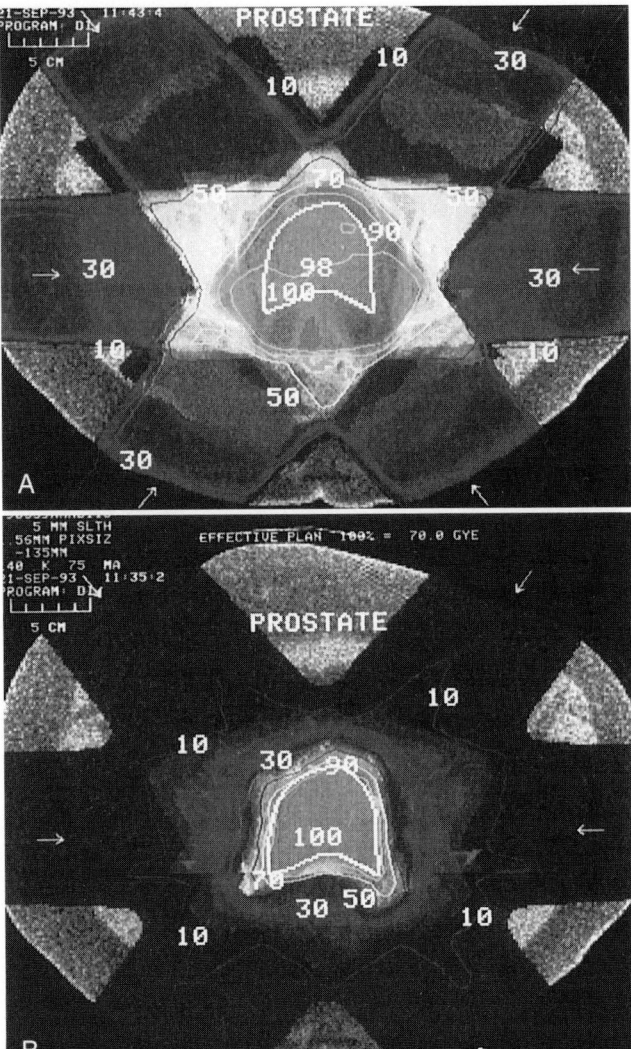

Figure 69–7. Prostate treatment plan comparison. **A,** Six-field coplanar 18 MeV x-ray conformal plan for irradiation of the prostate gland. **B,** A computer simulation of a plan using dynamic conformal proton therapy. Better conformation of the high-dose zone to the target volume is observed with conformal proton therapy. Evaluation of several target sites for proton and heavy ion therapy has suggested clinical gains when moving from static charged particle therapy to dynamic conformal charged particle therapy (Courtesy of I. Daftari, PhD.). See also Color Figure 69-7.

therapy. To exploit the sharp distal edge of the Bragg peak, it is necessary to have an accurate 3D density map (provided by CT) of the tumor in relation to adjacent critical structures. MRI studies are also important in outlining tumors and normal tissues and are a vital part of the treatment planning process.[66] Techniques to merge the CT and MRI data sets were first used in particle therapy and are now standard in modern 3D planning systems. Detailed tissue-density information is inferred from the CT numbers[67] and used to design compensators that stop the beam at the distal surface of the tumor. Because these compensators must be carefully registered

with respect to the patient, the relation of the internal organs to each other during the treatment-planning CT scan must be as close as possible to their relation during actual treatment. This is achieved by immobilizing the patient in the treatment position during CT scanning.

PATIENT IMMOBILIZATION AND SCANNING. Precise daily positioning is obtained by use of an immobilization device that is individually constructed for each patient, generally from thermoplastic splinting material (Fig. 69-8). Many types of immobilization techniques have been developed; for example, at the LLUPAF, a specially constructed whole-body pod is used. This technique was adapted from the pion therapy project at PSI.[68-70] The planning CT scan

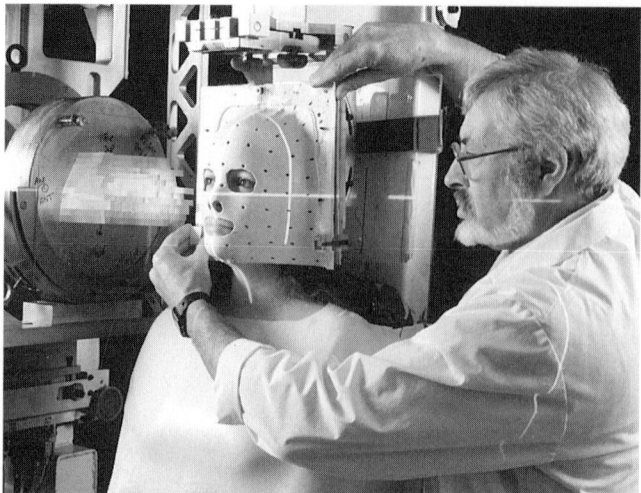

Figure 69–8. Immobilization device for charged particle therapy: an example of a typical patient setup for head and neck treatment at the University of California, San Francisco-Lawrence Berkeley Laboratory. An individual thermoplastic head mask or body cast is constructed for each patient in the treatment position, with material that allows computed tomography or magnetic resonance imaging treatment planning scans.

and MRI are performed when possible with the patient in the immobilization device and in treatment position; special image correlation techniques may be needed to transfer data sets and reformulate other scans in the treatment orientation.

TARGET AND CRITICAL STRUCTURE DEFINITION. Using the MRI and CT scans, the clinician outlines the tumor and critical structures on all relevant slices of the CT scan. Volumes-of-interest defined on MRI must be transformed to CT because tissue densities derived from CT numbers are required for both dose calculations and compensator design.[71] Image-correlation techniques[72-74] are used, based on matching external markers or anatomical structures and surfaces to determine the relative rotation, linear scaling, and translation between the CT and MRI coordinate systems.

BEAM ANGLE SELECTION AND COLLIMATOR DESIGN. Suitable beam entry angles are chosen, and customized beam collimators are designed by projecting the tumor volume and critical structure volumes in the "beam's-eye-view."[67,75] In this technique, experienced physicists and dosimetrists select possible beam angles with input from the clinician, but an increasingly used technique makes use of "inverse" system algorithms that iteratively examine many angles to arrive at the best solution to the desired dose distribution.[76-78]

TISSUE COMPENSATOR DESIGN. After the beam orientations have been chosen and collimator margins defined, tissue compensators are designed for each treatment angle. These devices are usually fabricated from wax or Lucite (see Fig. 69-5), generally by computer-driven milling machines, using output from the treatment planning code. To design a compensator, the water-equivalent

distance along the beam trajectory to each point on the distal surface of the target volume is determined from the CT data. The *nominal* thickness of the compensator at each of these points is calculated by subtracting this water-equivalent distance from the beam range. The *actual* compensator thickness is then determined at each point by selecting the minimum thickness within some specified radius, usually between 0.1 and 0.3 cm, of that point.[79] This assures that the target receives the minimum prescribed dose even if the patient moves during treatment by that amount.

INTENSITY-MODULATED PHOTONS VS. CHARGED PARTICLES

Intensity-modulated radiation therapy (IMRT) with photons has generated much interest over the past several years as a means of obtaining increasingly conformal dose distributions. Several different methods of IMRT have been proposed,[78,80-82] all requiring the delivery of a series of nonuniform intensity fields that ultimately add up to a fairly uniform dose distribution within the target. Charged-particle radiation therapy, as described here, is *inherently* intensity modulated.[83] Tissue compensators modulate the depth of penetration of the beam such that the dose falls to zero just beyond the distal edge of the target. Fixed modulation devices such as ridge filters or propellers modulate the width of the spread-Bragg peak so that it conforms to the largest width of the target. Further reduction in dose to non–target tissues can be achieved if, instead of these fixed-modulation devices, a variable-modulation system such as raster scanning is used.[61-63] The proximal end of the spread-Bragg peak can then be matched to the proximal surface of the target (see Fig. 69-2). Perhaps the most general form of charged-particle IMRT is the spot-scanning method in which individual Bragg peaks are distributed throughout the target volume. This technique has been employed for protons at PSI[85,86] and for pions by Pedroni.[87] Brahme et al.[88] and Carlsson et al.[89] have described similar techniques. Due to their complexity, raster-scanning and spot-scanning beam delivery systems require that some type of inverse-treatment planning system is used to determine the optimal beam intensities for each beamlet.

It should be noted that with spot-scanning and raster-scanning techniques, tissue compensators are not necessarily needed, provided it is possible to vary the beam energy (and hence the beam penetration) on a pixel-by-pixel basis. GSI has implemented a raster-scanning device for carbon ions and developed treatment planning software (called TRiP) that uses biological effectiveness in the objective function to optimize the intensities and positions of the scanned beam.[84] The TRiP program has been used clinically at GSI for all patients treated with carbon ions since 1997 and may be the first clinical implementation of an inverse-treatment-planning code that uses biological effectiveness as the desired endpoint.

Conformal proton treatment plans have been compared to IMRT photon plans for various sites.[90,91] Cella et al.[92] compared IMRT photon plans to both fixed-modulation and variable-modulation proton plans for prostate cancer. Zurlo et al.[93] performed similar comparisons for pancreatic and biliary tumors, and Lomax et al.[94,95] considered nine different cases including meningioma, malignant melanoma, cervical cancer, and medulloblastoma. In all of these comparisons, the variable-modulation proton plans were generated using the spot scanning technique. The general conclusions of these studies were as follows: (1) The total integral dose was always lower for the proton plans than for the IMRT photon plans, with the integral dose reduced by a factor of two for the variable-modulation proton plans as compared to the IMRT photon plans. (2) The mean dose delivered to organs at risk was significantly lower for the proton plans than for the IMRT photon plans, as was the volume of these structures receiving at least 50% of the mean target dose. The volume of organs at risk that was irradiated to at least 70% of the mean target dose was similar for the proton plans and intensity-modulated photon plans. (3) It was possible to deliver high doses to the target volume with both protons and intensity-modulated photons, but the proton dose distributions within the target tended to be more homogeneous. (4) Acceptable dose conformation with protons was achieved with four fields or less as compared to nine fields or more for the intensity-modulated photon plans.

Dose Calculations

An accurate assessment of the dose distribution on all CT planes through the tumor volume and surrounding critical structures is required for charged-particle therapy. Dose-volume histograms (DVHs) are also useful in evaluating the dose to the target and critical structures.[96-98]

At UCSF-LBL, charged-particle treatment planning and isodose calculations were performed using a computerized treatment planning system developed at LBL.[67] Similarly, treatment planning programs were developed at MGH-HCL, PSI, LLUPAF, CPO, the National Institute of Radiological Sciences (NIRS) in Japan, and others. At least one commercial company has incorporated proton dose calculation modules into its treatment-planning systems[99] using pencil-beam algorithms as well as broad-beam ray tracing.

Three-dimensional dose distributions (see Figs. 69-3 and 69-4) are most easily calculated by computing the water-equivalent distance to each point using CT data and extracting the dose at these depths from a lookup table compiled from measurements made in a water-equivalent phantom. This method neglects multiple-coulomb scattering effects in complex heterogeneous regions but is sufficient for most clinical applications. Dose calculation techniques relying on the Molière theory of multiple scattering or on the Fermi-Eyges algorithm have been proposed by several investigators to account for multiple-scattering effects.[100-102] Pencil-beam dose calculation algorithms that accurately model multiple-scattering effects have also been developed.[53,102] Using these techniques, the dose from primary and scattered particles is determined by superimposing the contributions from pencil beams summed over the entire beam area. The more accurate pencil-beam method is better at predicting dose inhomogeneities within the target, the degradation in the distal falloff in dose, and the widening of the penumbra as a function of beam penetration due to multiple scattering in complex tissue heterogeneities.

For charged-particle beams, which have different biological effects than low-LET beams such as x-rays or electrons,[55] the effects of high-LET must be accounted for in planning therapy, either by RBE corrections to create isodoses "equivalent" to low-LET irradiations or by using particle fluence to account for biological effects of individual particles. Tumor doses may be expressed in GyEq by multiplying the charged-particle physical dose by the RBE representing the ratio of the photon beam dose to the charged-particle dose required for similar late effects. At UCSF-LBL, dose was tabulated in both physical gray (Gy) and GyEq,[55,67] although both have limitations in describing the treatment plan.

G. Kraft and associates[14,103,104] at GSI-Darmstadt have extended the scanning-beam techniques begun at UCSF-LBL and developed an elegant technique for treatment delivery of heavy charged particles, using intensity-controlled raster scanning with pulse-to-pulse energy variation. Biological plan optimization is part of their 3D treatment planning, accounting for biological effects assessed pixel-by-pixel in depth.[105]

Variation in Relative Biologic Effect Across the Spread-Bragg Peak

Since the RBE depends on the LET of the particle, and the LET of a charged-particle beam varies as a function of energy and hence depth of penetration, the RBE for charged-particle beams varies across the spread-Bragg peak. Generally, for particle beams of silicon or lower atomic number, which are the ion beams of clinical interest, the RBE is highest at the distal end of the peak where the LET is highest. To compensate for the variation in RBE across the spread-Bragg peak and to try to deliver a uniformly effective dose across the tumor volume, spread-Bragg peaks for heavy ion radiotherapy are sloped as illustrated in Fig. 69-1A. For the high-LET treatments undertaken at UCSF-LBL, the slope of these curves was determined by requiring that the biological effect, as predicted by the linear-quadratic cell survival model (i.e., $S = S_0 e^{-\alpha D - \beta D^2}$), be uniform across the spread-Bragg peak.[55,58] The variation in the linear-quadratic variables alpha and beta with LET was taken from the publication by Chapman and associates.[106]

Treatment Delivery and Verification

Positioning the patient for treatment and ascertaining that the patient remains in the same position throughout the treatment is critical for charged-particle radiotherapy. This is most commonly done by comparing radiographic images taken with a back-pointing x-ray unit of the patient in the treatment position with digitally reconstructed radiographs (DRRs). Projections of bony anatomy outlined on the CT scan may also be transferred to a transparent sheet and overlaid on the portal alignment film to verify the patient's position. The patient alignment process at LBL required 10 to 30 minutes for each charged-particle treatment. New immobilization and electronic portal imaging techniques have the potential to improve on this.

Clinical Factors in Selection of Charged Particles

Helium ions were used instead of protons at UCSF-LBL because they were easier to produce in the LBL accelerators. They deposit a small amount of high-LET, which must be accounted for in treatment planning. The OER of helium ions[15-17] has been measured around 2.5 to 3.0. Their clinical effects are similar to protons, although they do exhibit tissue RBE values of 1.2 to 1.4 compared with megavoltage x-rays (except in CNS, where the RBE is ~1.6). For comparison, the proton RBE[26,28,107] used clinically is about 1.1 to 1.2. The physical properties of protons (and helium ions) are well suited to precise localization of radiation dose (see Fig. 69-3), with reduction of unwanted dose to adjacent critical structures such as brain, cranial nerves, and spinal cord.[108-110]

Heavy ions that have an atomic weight between carbon and silicon are of interest for clinical use (see Table 69-3).[4,16,17,39] Slowly growing tumors seem to be effectively treated by high-LET particles, both charged particles and neutrons.

The carbon ion beam has both biologic and dose localization advantages over lighter ions such as protons and neutrons and the best biologically corrected depth dose distribution of all particles. The ratio of dose in the tumor to that in the entrance region is maximized, and the beam penumbra is sharper. Enough high-LET is present to provide significant differences in DNA damage and suppression of radiation repair.

The use of heavier ions such as neon and silicon leads to complexity in treatment planning because of the high-LET in the entrance region and the fragmentation tail. Normal tissues in these regions need to be carefully assessed and treatment plans designed that avoid significant late effects, especially in CNS, gastrointestinal tract, and soft tissue. Heavy ions such as neon or silicon may be associated with an increased rate of radiation-induced tumors.

Basic Physical Properties of Neutron Beams

Fast neutrons undergo two basic types of interactions in tissue, elastic collisions and inelastic interactions. In elastic collisions, the incident neutron collides with a target nucleus, imparting energy to it in much the same way one billiard ball imparts energy to another. If the mass of the nucleus is comparable to the neutron mass, a large amount of energy is transferred. If, however, the nucleus is much more massive than the incoming neutron, the recoil nucleus travels only a small distance. For example, the maximum range of a recoil hydrogen nucleus (consisting of a single proton) produced in an elastic collision with a 15 MeV neutron is approximately 2.5 mm,

whereas the maximum range of a heavy nucleus (e.g., carbon or oxygen) produced in the same collision is smaller by a factor of about 200. The LET of recoil heavy nuclei, however, is much greater than that of recoil protons (on the order of 800 keV/mm as compared to about 30 keV/mm).[111]

Whereas in elastic collisions the target nuclei remain intact, in inelastic interactions the target nuclei disintegrate, producing fragment particles. This type of interaction results in the emission of alpha particles, protons, neutrons, and gamma-rays. However, most of the dose deposited in tissue by therapeutic neutron beams is a result of elastic rather than inelastic interactions. In particular, for 14 MeV neutrons, approximately 70% of the dose is deposited by recoil protons, less than 10% of the dose is a result of recoil heavy nuclei, and as much as 30% is deposited by the products of nuclear disintegrations.

Treatment Planning for Neutron Beams

Depth-dose distributions for therapeutic neutron beams resemble photon depth-dose curves (see Fig. 69-1B). The dose due to recoil protons builds up to a maximum beneath the skin surface in much the same way that electrons produce a build-up region in photon depth-dose curves. The skin-sparing effect for therapeutic neutron beams is greater for higher energy neutrons because recoil protons produced by these neutrons have higher energies and travel farther in tissue. Higher energy neutron beams are preferred for radiotherapy because of their superior depth-dose distributions. The depth-dose curve for a 14 MeV neutron beam produced by a D-T generator resembles a ^{60}Co depth-dose curve, whereas the depth-dose curve for a neutron beam generated by bombarding a beryllium target with high-energy protons of 50 to 70 MeV is similar to that of a clinical photon beam of 6 to 8 MeV. Treatment planning for neutron therapy is similar to photon treatment planning. Tissue heterogeneities do not perturb neutron dose distributions significantly and are usually not taken into account in treatment planning. Multi-port plans, including wedge filter plans, can be used to improve dose distributions.

CLINICAL RESULTS WITH PROTONS AND HELIUM IONS

Initial studies of proton therapy began in the 1950s at LBL by Tobias and Lawrence and associates[4,5] and in Sweden at the University of Uppsala by Larsson and Leksell and associates.[6] At LBL, the emphasis was on high dose–small fraction number treatment of pituitary diseases, including pituitary tumors, diabetic retinopathy, and suppression of pituitary function in metastatic breast cancer.[112,113] At Uppsala, functional neurological diseases were of initial interest, with cancer therapy started later.[6] At MGH-HCL, protons became available for clinical work in the 1960s, leading initially to treatment of pituitary diseases and arteriovenous malformations (AVMs) by Kjellberg.[114] In 1974, Suit and others at MGH-HCL began long-term studies of the dose-localizing properties of Bragg peak fractionated proton therapy in select human tumors.[7,115,116] Limitations of beam energy (160 MeV) and depth of penetration (16 cm) at MGH-HCL directed most clinical work to the head and neck, and other relatively superficial sites such as paraspinal and prostate gland tumors.

A clinical trial also began at UCSF-LBL in 1975 by Castro and colleagues to determine the efficacy of heavy charged particles in the treatment of human cancers.[8,11,117] This study was predicated on the physical and biological advantages of heavy ions and aimed at defining whether dose localization or biologic effectiveness or both would be most important clinically. The MGH-HCL and UCSF-LBL trials were the first extended studies of fractionated Bragg peak therapy in the treatment of cancer. Their experience confirmed the efficacy of charged particles in increasing the tumor dose relative to normal tissue dose[108,109,116] and the resultant significant increases in local control and survival for a number of tumor sites.

Irradiation of Skull-Base Tumors with Charged Particles

The use of charged-particle radiation in skull-base tumors has progressively improved over the past 25 years with increasingly precise treatment planning and delivery (Table 69-4).[108,116,118-120] Improved surgical techniques for debulking difficult-to-reach tumors[109,121] and treatment planning based on both CT and MRI have helped. As these tumors tend to remain localized, improved local control directly translates into improved survival. Among the important factors in irradiation of skull-based tumors are histology, tumor extent, and whether treatment is for primary or recurrent disease.

At UCSF-LBL, 126 patients were irradiated with charged particles for tumors arising in the skull base.[108] Of these, 109 patients were treated with helium ions, often combined with photon treatment for 30% to 70% of the total dose, owing to limitations of beam availability. Follow-up ranged from 4 to 201 months, median 53 and mean 61 months. Of these patients, 53 had chordoma, 27 had chondrosarcoma, 27 had paraclival meningioma, and 19 patients had other histologies such as osteosarcoma or neurofibrosarcoma. The daily dose

was 2.0 GyEq, given in four fractions per week to total doses of 60 to 80 GyEq (mean, 68 GyEq). The limiting dose to the brainstem was 60 GyEq; to the optic chiasm, 55 GyEq; and to the edge of the cervical spinal cord, 45 GyEq, using CNS RBE values of 1.6 for helium and 4.5 for neon. Local control and survival rates appeared improved compared with historical data in all tumor histologies. The 5- and 10-year Kaplan-Meier (K-M)[122] local control rates for all histologies were 78% and 62%; the K-M survival rates for 5 and 10 years were 84% and 70%. By histology, the 5-year K-M local control rate was 88% for 23 patients with chondrosarcoma, 60% for 48 patients with chordoma, and 89% for 26 patients with meningioma. A local control rate of 58% was seen in other histologies (including osteosarcoma), with a 71% K-M survival rate at 5 years.

Patients with skull-base and cervical spine tumors have been a major group irradiated with protons at MGH-HCL.[115] Munzenrider et al.[116] reported on 194 patients irradiated for chordoma and low-grade chondrosarcoma. The tumor doses ranged from 57 to 76 GyEq, with a median of 68 GyEq, using a proton RBE value of 1.1. Daily doses were 1.8 GyEq given 5 days per week, usually in four fractions of protons and one of megavoltage x-rays. Excellent results were obtained with a local recurrence-free survival rate of 76% at 5 years and overall survival rate of 90% at 5 years for the entire group. In a later review,[123] they reported a 10-year local recurrence-free survival rate of 94% for chondrosarcoma. For nonchondroid chordoma, local recurrence-free survival at 10 years dropped to 65% in males and 42% in females. Those patients with tumors arising in the cervical spine had worse outcomes than those with skull-base tumors, with 10-year local control rates of 54% for chordoma and 48% for chondrosarcoma, no sex differences noted.[123]

Confirmatory data for these results are seen at CPO, which has reported a high rate of local control and survival in 45 patients treated with proton therapy for skull-base chordoma and chondrosarcoma,[120] and PSI who have recently begun therapy of skull-base tumors with spot scanned protons.[124] Other cranial tumor sites advantageously treated with protons or helium ions include meningioma and carcinoma of the paranasal sinuses, nasopharynx, and salivary gland involving the skull base.[108,109]

Table 69–4   Percent 5-Year Local Control in Skull-Base Tumors with Charged Particles*

	UCSF-LBL	MGH-HCL[†]	GSI-Heidelberg[§]
Meningioma	89	100	
Chondrosarcoma	88	94 (10 yr)	90 (2 yr)
Chordoma	60	65, 42[‡] (10 yr)	
Other sarcoma	58	59	

*Protons at MGH-HCL, helium ions at UCSF-LBL, carbon ions at GSI-Heidelberg.
[†]Data from Munzenrider et al.[115,116,123]
[‡]65% for males, 42% for females, nonchondroid chordoma.
[§]Data from Debus et al.[118]
UCSF-LBL, University of California, San Francisco–Lawrence Berkeley Laboratory; MGH-HCL, Massachusetts General Hospital–Harvard Cyclotron Laboratory; GSI, Gesellschaft für Schwerlonen Forschung, Darmstadt, Germany.

Complications of Charged-Particle Irradiation of the Skull Base

The complication rate for the use of charged particles in the skull base has proven to be acceptably low, given the levels of dose required for control of these lesions.[108,125,126] Treatment-related morbidity has included endocrine, auditory, visual, and brain complications with a serious (grades 3 to 4) rate of 5% to 8%. The major events in the patients at UCSF-LBL with severe complications were brain necrosis, osteoradionecrosis of the skull base, and severe temporal lobe injury. Males appear to have a higher predilection for temporal lobe injury.[125] The use of high-LET ions heavier than carbon ions is not advised for skull-base lesions, because of the high RBE for late damage to CNS structures. Preliminary data from the GSI-Heidelberg facility using carbon beams suggests that skull-base tumors can be safely treated with high rates of local control.[105,118]

Juxtaspinal and Sacral Tumors

Charged-particle therapy has been useful in the treatment of residual or unresectable tumors of the spine and sacrum,[109,126,127] which often requires a specialized technique developed at UCSF-LBL for tumors partially or completely encircling the brainstem or spinal cord.[127] By dividing the target volume into two or more portions and using a combination of beams, a reasonably homogeneous irradiation of the target volume can be obtained, thus protecting critical CNS structures from over-irradiation (see Fig. 69-6). The physical and biologic effects of the charged-particle beams must be known; patient immobilization must be reproducible to less than or equal to 2 mm; the treatment must be carefully planned, based on metrizamide-contrast CT or MRI or both; compensation must be made for tissue inhomogeneities; radiation delivery must be accurate and verifiable; and uncertainties in the dose distribution must be taken into account. This method has been used to safely irradiate lesions encircling the brainstem or spinal cord to tumor doses of 60 GyEq or more, generally higher than can be achieved with current low-LET irradiation techniques, with the possible exception of IMRT. At UCSF-LBL, local control in the spine was poorer than in the skull base: 50% (11/22 patients) for chondrosarcoma, with a follow-up of 7 to 141 months, median of 31 months; and 45% (18/40 patients) for chordoma, with a follow-up of 6 to 167 months, median of 40 months. There was a trend for higher local control when neon ions were used with six of eight chordoma patients whose disease was controlled with neon ions versus 12 of 32 patients for whom helium ions were used. For patients with juxtaspinal sarcoma of other histologic type (e.g., osteosarcoma, neurofibrosarcoma, malignant fibrous histiocytoma), local control was obtained in 16 of 29 patients. Follow-up ranged from 4 to 128 months, with a median of 32 months.

Hug and coworkers[128] reported 47 patients with axial skeletal tumors treated with proton therapy at MGH-HCL. The 5-year actuarial local control and survival rates were 53% and 50%, respectively, for chordoma and 100% each for chondrosarcoma. For osteogenic sarcoma, a 5-year local control rate of 59% was obtained, although overall survival fell to 44% in 5 years, mainly because of metastatic disease.

Prostate Carcinoma

Protons have been used in the treatment of locally advanced prostatic carcinoma at MGH and LLUPAF, investigating the use of conformal proton therapy to raise the dose to the prostate gland. Higher doses to prostate tumors have been shown to be associated with improved local control and survival.[129] More than 600 patients were treated at LLUPAF by 1998 with an overall clinical disease-free survival rate of 89% at 5 years. Toxicity was acceptably low at doses of 74 to 75 GyEq.[130,131] MGH and LLUPAF have combined in a randomized dose escalation trial comparing doses of 70.2 and 79 GyEq, and are planning additional studies in prostate cancer.

OCULAR PROTON THERAPY

Proton and helium ion irradiation of uveal melanoma have now been studied for more than 25 years with a remarkable consistency of results. Because of the ability to deliver a high dose to a sharply confined target volume, there is a very high local control rate ($\approx$96%), high rate of retention of the eye ($\approx$85% to 94%), and preservation of useful vision in about 50% of patients. These treatments have been steadily refined by new treatment planning methods and are now carried out in many countries around the world[132-135] after being pioneered by Constable, Gragoudas, Suit, et al. at MGH-MEEI-HCL[136-138] and Char, Castro, Chen, et al. at UCSF-LBL.[139] Proton therapy is also being used for other lesions in the eye including iris and conjunctival melanoma, age-related macular degeneration[134,140] and retinoblastoma.[141]

At UCSF-LBL, 347 patients with uveal melanoma[139] were treated with helium ions from 1978 to 1992. Tumor dose levels from 48 to 80 GyEq were given in four to five fractions over 4 to 16 days. A high local control rate of 96% was seen overall for large as well as small tumors, but there was a deterioration of the local control rate to 87% at the lowest dose level of 48 GyEq in four fractions of 12 GyEq each. The median follow-up period was 90 months (range, 3 to 206 months) at closing of the LBL study. Fifteen patients (4%) had local failure (LFR) in the eye, requiring enucleation or reirradiation. Eight of the 15 patients (53%) with LFR died of distant metastases (DM), compared with 19% of patients with local control in the eye. Of patients who had 20/200 vision or better in the affected eye before treatment, 41% retained at least 20/200 vision in the treated eye. Multivariate analysis revealed that the strongest independent risk factors influencing vision outcome ($P < 0.05$) were tumor size, pretreatment visual acuity, tumor-fovea distance, and maximum tumor dose. Fifteen percent of patients were enucleated because of complications, mostly secondary to severe neovascular glaucoma.[139]

In reviews of MGH-MEEI proton-treated uveal melanoma patients and UCSF-LBL helium ion–treated patients,[139,142,143] the liver was the most common site of metastases (DM). DM were detected as long as 12 years after therapy; unfortunately, less than 15% of these patients survived 1 year after the appearance of DM. Multivariate analysis identified that anterior location of tumor (*P* = 0.02), and tumor diameter greater than 10 mm (*P* = 0.0075) independently predicted the development of DM and lack of survival.[143] Melanoma involving the ciliary body carries a poor prognosis.[139] Adjuvant therapy is needed for patients with large or anterior tumors who are at high risk for metastatic disease.

Following closure of the LBL facility for charged particle therapy in 1992, 246 patients with uveal melanoma were treated with protons at the Crocker Cyclotron at the University of California, Davis (UCD) between 1994 and 2001.[144,145] Among 43 patients treated with 48 GyEq/4 fractions, the LFR was 6/43, neovascular glaucoma (NVG) occurred in 10/43, and the DM rate was 6/43. Enucleation was required in 5/9 patients who had NVG without LFR. The overall enucleation rate was 9/43. Among 203 patients treated with 56 GyEq in 4 fractions and a greater effort at sparing of the ciliary body, 4 failed locally, requiring enucleation; and 4 additional patients had marginal recurrences and received additional laser treatment without enucleation. Five of 203 patients developed NVG; one of these required enucleation. The overall enucleation rate was 5/203. The DM rate was 6/203. The LFR was similar between 56 GyEq of protons (≈4 %) and helium ion treatment (≈4%) but higher in the 48 GyEq group (≈12% to 13%). Specific treatment planning in the proton group to spare the anterior chamber appears superior to the helium ion results in terms of decreased NVG and enucleation. The lesser amount of high-LET in the proton beam likely also contributed to the lesser rate of NVG and enucleation compared to the helium ion study.

Particle radiation–induced cataracts have been reported in eye tumor patients treated with helium ion or protons.[139,145] Where possible to do so, the lens should be avoided.

STEREOTACTIC PROTON TREATMENT OF ARTERIOVENOUS MALFORMATIONS (AVMs) AND PITUITARY LESIONS

The dose localizing properties of protons and helium ions have been used for the stereotactic treatment of AVMs. Proton treatments of AVMs were begun by Kjellberg and associates[114] at MGH-HCL, where more than 1300 patients were treated. More than 400 patients with surgically inaccessible intracranial vascular malformations were treated with helium ions at LBL.[146] Large numbers of patients with AVMs were also treated with protons at the Burdenko Neurosurgical Institute for Theoretical and Experimental Physics in Moscow and at the Leningrad Institute of Nuclear Physics, with a total obliteration rate of 60%.[147]

Kjellberg[114] reported a 20-year follow-up on 709 patients in 1988, with partial or complete obliteration in most patients. With careful attention for volume of brain treated and dose, complications were acceptable. He concluded that proton beam radiosurgery was useful for inoperable or inaccessible AVMs. In the LBL trial, doses up to 45 GyEq were delivered to volumes ranging from 0.1 cm³ to 70 cm³. In the first 230 patients treated, the complete angiographic obliteration rate 3 years after treatment was between 90% and 95% for volumes less than 14 cm³ and between 60% and 70% for volumes larger than 14 cm³. The overall obliteration rate for all volumes (up to 70 cm³) is approximately 80% to 85%. No complications occurred in patients who received doses less than 25 GyEq. In patients who received higher doses, the rate of serious complications, including symptomatic vasogenic edema (white matter changes) and vasculopathy, was 11%. Protons may be of special value in large, irregular lesions that are difficult to treat with x-ray or gamma knife techniques.[148]

Many years after the pioneering studies of high dose, low fraction number proton therapy for pituitary tumors by Lawrence,[5] stereotactic use of protons is again being used to treat pituitary adenoma and acromegaly[149] and other skull-base lesions such as meningioma.[150]

CLINICAL EXPERIENCE WITH NEUTRONS AND HIGH-LET CHARGED PARTICLES

Particle beams have been used to treat cancer since 1938, when R. Stone and J. Lawrence[1,2] first used *fast neutrons* to treat advanced malignancies at the University of California, Berkeley. At that time, the radiobiological differences between low-LET and high-LET radiation were not clearly appreciated, single-dose RBEs were being used to predict RBE for fractionated treatment, and surviving patients experienced significant late effects on normal tissues. Because of this, clinical use of particles went into hiatus in 1943. In the 1950s and 1960s, radiobiologic studies better defined the characteristics of high-LET beams, and there was a reassessment of the Stone data.[151] Neutron clinical trials resumed in the United Kingdom and Holland in the 1960s. Initially, encouraging results were obtained for some tumors that respond poorly to conventional treatment, especially in the head and neck.[152] Facilities based in physics laboratories in the United States began phase I and II clinical trials with neutrons in the 1970s, and hospital-based neutron facilities became available in a few locations in the 1980s. As a result, phases I, II, and III clinical trials with neutrons were completed for several types of tumors.

The results of these studies suggest that neutron beams are useful for treating selected malignancies, particularly unresectable salivary gland cancers[153] and unfavorable soft tissue sarcoma (Table 69-5).[154] Possible advantages have also been observed for locally advanced prostate cancer.[155,156] On the other hand, results for primary tumors arising in the head and neck, brain, lung, and pancreas were not improved in these trials.[157-161] Late effects have been troublesome.[162]

In 1979 a phase I to II clinical trial was started at UCSF-LBL using high-LET charged particles to irradiate patients for tumors in which conventional treatment

Table 69–5   Results of High-LET Therapy

	5-Year Local Control, %* Neutrons[†]	5-Year Local Control, %*		5-Year Survival, %* Neutrons	5-Year Survival, %* Neon Ions[†]
		Neon Ions	Carbon Ions		
Salivary gland	57	50		72	52
Prostate gland	89	87	97 (2 yr)[‡]	68	85
Soft tissue sarcoma	53	42	75 (2 yr)[‡]	—	59
Bone sarcoma	54	45	75 (2 yr)[‡]	—	59
Paranasal sinus	—	69		—	69
Biliary tract	—	28		—	44
Skull base tumors			90 (2 yr)[§]		

*Kaplan-Meier rates.
[†]Data from references 153-155,157,165,195.
[‡]Data from Tsujii H[12] and Tsujii H, Koto M, Morita S, et al.[164]
[§]Data from Nagasawa H, Little J[18] and Schulz-Ertner D, Haberer T, Jakel O, et al.[105]

modalities were likely to be ineffective.[109,163] By May 1992, when the Bevalac accelerator operation at LBL was terminated by the Department of Energy for budgetary reasons, 299 patients had received at least 10 Gy of neon ions, representing at least 40% of their total equivalent dose. Compared with historical results, the 5-year K-M survival and local control rates (see Table 69-5) in this preliminary trial suggested potential for heavy ion treatment in several types of tumors: advanced or recurrent macroscopic salivary gland carcinoma, paranasal sinus tumors, advanced soft tissue sarcoma, macroscopic sarcoma of bone, locally advanced prostate carcinoma, and biliary tract carcinoma. Treatment of malignant glioma, pancreatic, gastric, esophageal, lung, and advanced or recurrent head and neck cancer did not show results improved over conventional therapy, although only limited numbers of patients were treated. Late effects were of concern in CNS, gastrointestinal tract, and soft tissue for neon and silicon ion–treated patients. Current heavy ion trials are centered on use of carbon ions with a lower number of fractions and a shorter overall treatment time.[12,105,118,164]

Salivary Gland Carcinoma

Patients treated with high-LET beams for unresectable salivary gland cancer appeared to do better than conventionally irradiated patients.[153] In an abbreviated phase III RTOG/MRC neutron trial,[153] 12 patients were treated with conventional photon or electron irradiation, while 13 were treated with neutrons. The 10-year results showed a significant local control advantage for neutrons (56% vs. 17%), although there was no overall survival difference. At LBL a small group of patients who were treated for unresectable primary or recurrent salivary gland malignancies with high-LET neon ions continued to show a significant local control and survival rate of about 50% at 5 years post treatment.[109,117,163] A larger series of 151 patients with locally advanced or recurrent adenoidcystic salivary gland tumors treated with neutrons has been reported from the University of Washington to show an impressive 5-year actuarial local-regional control rate of 57% and a 5-year survival rate of 72%.[165]

The results have been sufficient to establish high-LET beams, either charged particles or neutrons, as the treatment of choice for unresectable, locally advanced, or gross residual salivary malignancies.

Prostate Cancer

High-LET therapy may be beneficial for slowly growing tumors such as prostatic carcinoma, because of decreased repair of radiation injury and decreased radioresistance of hypoxic tumor cells associated with high-LET radiation.

Two phase III Radiation Therapy Oncology Group (RTOG)/Neutron Therapy Clinical Working Group studies were completed comparing neutron versus proton treatment for locally advanced prostate cancer.[156,157] The first study, conducted from 1977 to 1983, analyzed 91 patients with either stage T3N0 or N1 (stage "C" and "D1") prostate cancers who were treated with either megavoltage irradiation (36 patients) or mixed photon/ neutron beams (55 patients). There was no difference in terms of developing distant metastases, with 36% of the neutron-treated patients and 44% of the photon-treated patients developing disseminated disease at the time of initial analysis. Ten-year actuarial results showed a significant advantage to the neutron arm in terms of locoregional control (70% neutron vs. 58% photon) as well as overall survival (46% vs. 29%).[156]

A second trial using hospital-based neutron beams was implemented in 1986 for patients with stage T2-4N0-1 ("B2," "C," "D1") disease.[157] Eighty-seven patients were treated with neutrons and 85 with photons. Five-year actuarial results were again significantly better for neutron patients in terms of locoregional failure (11% vs. 32% for photons). There were no differences in terms of overall or disease-specific survival. Severe late complications were more common in the neutron treatment arm (11% vs. 3%).

The superiority of neutron therapy for prostate treatment has not been shown in view of the small study size, the limited availability of neutron therapy centers, the lack of prostate-specific antigen data, and lack of a clear-cut disease-free survival advantage. Neutrons continue to be successfully used to treat prostate cancer in some centers.[166]

At UCSF-LBL, neon ions were used for the cone-down "boost" portion of prostate cancer therapy in 23 patients with B2-C tumors, following pelvic irradiation with photons. Follow-up ranged from 5 to 91 months, with a median of 51 months. K-M local control and survival were projected at the 85% and 64% level at 7.5 years after treatment.[117] However, 3/23 patients had rectal injuries, an unacceptably high rate. If high-LET beams are to be used in prostate cancer therapy, carbon ions would be a better choice; avoidance of the rectum and bladder is a must. Excellent results in treatment of prostate carcinoma with carbon ions has recently been reported from HIMAC.[12]

Soft Tissue Sarcoma

Phase II trials involving 297 neutron-treated patients with unfavorable soft tissue sarcoma[154] reported local control rates on the order of 50%. Similar results using neutrons have also been reported for osteogenic sarcoma and chondrosarcoma. Between 1978 and 1989 at UCSF-LBL, 32 patients with unfavorable soft tissue sarcoma underwent heavy charged-particle irradiation (helium or neon ions or both) with curative intent. Follow-up times for surviving patients ranged from 4 to 121 months (median 27 months). The 3-year K-M local control rate was 62%; the corresponding survival rate was 50%. Patients with retroperitoneal sarcoma did notably well, with local control and survival rates of 64% and 62%, respectively. Complications were acceptable and there were no radiation-related deaths. Subsequently, follow-up of all patients treated through May 1992 continued to show promising results,[117] with a K-M 5-year survival rate of 42% and a K-M local control rate of 59%. Conclusions regarding the role of high-LET beams for sarcoma cannot yet be made, but these data merit further investigation, especially for retroperitoneal and pelvic lesions close to the gastrointestinal tract, the genitourinary tract, or the CNS.

Bone Sarcoma

Between 1979 and 1989, 17 patients with bone sarcoma were treated wholly or in part with helium or neon ions or both at UCSF-LBL.[167] The majority of tumors were located near critical structures such as the spinal cord or brain. Gross tumor was present in all but two patients at the time of irradiation. The follow-up ranged from 7 to 118 months (median 40 months). The 5-year K-M survival rate was 41% because many patients succumbed to distant metastases. At the latest review of these patients[117] plus additional patients treated between 1989 and 1992, the results showed a 5-year K-M local control rate of 59% and a 5-year K-M survival rate of 45%. From the results of this preliminary study, we believe that heavy charged-particle irradiation can be effectively used for control of locally advanced or unresectable bone sarcoma.

Head and Neck Cancer

Despite initial optimism, the results with high-LET neutron beams for head and neck cancer were not encouraging. Two phase III RTOG trials that compared neutrons versus photons and mixed beam (neutron + photons) versus photons alone were completed. The first trial showed an advantage for neutrons in terms of complete response (52% vs. 17%), but there was no overall survival difference between the two groups.[159] The second trial found no advantage to the high-LET arm in terms of control of the primary tumor or of overall survival.[160] Control of metastatic cervical lymph nodes was statistically superior for the mixed-beam arm (complete response rate 69% vs. 55%; 2-year adenopathy control rate 46% vs. 33%), but this did not translate into a survival advantage.

The last international head and neck cancer fast neutron trial was completed in 1991, a collaboration among several hospital-based cyclotrons in the United States and the United Kingdom.[161] This trial compared 20.4 Gy of neutrons in 12 fractions over 4 weeks against 70 Gy of photons in 35 fractions over 7 weeks for treatment of locally advanced squamous carcinoma of the oral cavity, oropharynx, and laryngopharynx. There was an increased complete response rate for neutrons, but ultimate local-regional control and survival rates were not significantly different. The neutron arm had a higher late complication rate.

Other Tumor Sites Treated with High-LET Particles

A trial[105] of carbon ion therapy for *skull-base chordoma* (24 patients) *and low grade chondrosarcoma* (13 patients) has shown good preliminary results at GSI-Heidelberg. Although follow-up is short, (mean = 13 months), local control was better than 90% in these patients. Two failures were noted outside the target volume in the chordoma group, but none in chondrosarcoma. More importantly, for this preliminary study, no severe treatment toxicity was encountered. The mean tumor dose was 60 GyEq with dose escalation to 70 GyEq being undertaken.

The NIRS in Chiba, Japan, began preliminary phase I to II clinical studies in 1994 with carbon ions.[12,164] By August 2003, more than 1600 patients had been treated in dose escalation studies with favorable response in adenocarcinoma, adenoid cystic caranoma, melanoma, hepatoma and bone/soft tissue sarcoma.[12,164,168] Treatment schedules have been shortened to 4-12 fractions in 1-3 weeks for lung cancer and hepatoma with acceptable morbidity.[12] This is an important advantage for carbon ions, as it reduces the time for tumor proliferation during therapy and is easier and more practical for patients.

A retrospective (nonrandomized) study[169] analyzed patients with *bile duct adenocarcinoma* who received radiotherapy at UCSF-LBL between 1977 and 1987. The overall 2-year actuarial survival rate was 28%: 44% for particle-treated patients and 18% for patients treated with photons ($P = 0.048$). Local control was also improved, although less significantly, in patients treated with particles. Many of these patients have had problems with late effects on bowel.

Pancreatic cancer was examined in two randomized prospective neutron trials.[156] An RTOG study (49 patients) compared photons, mixed neutrons and photons, and neutrons alone. The median survival rates were 5.6 months (neutrons), 7.8 months (mixed beam), and 8.3 months (photons). Differences were not significant.[156] An NCOG study (49 patients) compared helium ions with photons; concurrent fluorouracil was given in both arms. Median survival was 7.8 months for helium and 6.5 months for photons ($P = NS$). Neon ions were used in 64 patients in a phase I to II trial.[163] The median survival was 7 months, with one long-term survivor. Similar findings were noted in *gastric and esophageal cancer. Malignant glioma* has also been examined extensively using high-LET beams. An RTOG dose-searching study using mixed photons and neutrons enrolled 190 evaluable patients. Median survival was 9.9 months for glioblastoma multiforme and 22 months for anaplastic astrocytoma; there was no difference between neutron doses.[158] A poorer outcome was actually observed for anaplastic astrocytoma patients who received higher doses of neutrons, reflecting the toxicity of high-LET radiation on normal brain tissue. A trial of high-dose neon ion therapy at UCSF-LBL in 14 patients with glioblastoma did not show a significant survival benefit, with a median survival of 12 months.

PION THERAPY

Negative pi mesons (pions) represent a special case of charged particles and were tried clinically at the Los Alamos National Laboratory–University of New Mexico (UNM-LAMPF), the Paul Scherrer Institute (PSI), formerly the Swiss Institute of Nuclear Research (SIN), and TRIUMF in Vancouver, Canada, after first being proposed by Fowler and Perkins[170] and Kaplan and colleagues.[171] Pions are unstable charged particles with a mass intermediate between the electron and the proton. In addition to the Bragg peak, negative pions also exhibit a unique phenomenon called *stars*, which makes them particularly attractive for treating radioresistant tumors. As a negative pion slows down near the end of its trajectory in tissue, it can be captured by one of the constituent atoms such as carbon, oxygen, or nitrogen, cascade down the atomic levels, and then be absorbed by the nucleus. The 140 MeV pion rest mass energy then appears as kinetic energy of the fragments produced when the nucleus disintegrates into a star of alpha particles, neutrons, and protons.[172] It was thought that the combination of high-LET plus dose distribution would result in improved local and regional control of tumors.

Clinical trials were carried out at UNM-LAMPF by Kligerman and von Essen[173,174] without significant improvement in results compared to historical photon results. At PSI, pions did exhibit some promise in the treatment of unresectable soft tissue sarcoma. Greiner and associates[175] reported an actuarial local control rate of 64% at 5 years in 35 patients with lesions in the retroperitoneum, pelvis, groin, or thigh. At the TRIUMF facility, randomized trials in glioblastoma and prostate cancer were completed without showing an advantage for pion therapy.[176]

In practice, pions do not exhibit the sharp physical parameters of protons or heavier ions, nor do they have as much deposition of high-LET as neon ions or neutrons. As a result, their realized potential has not been as great as initially hoped for, and they have been discontinued in clinical work.

NEUTRON BRACHYTHERAPY WITH CALIFORNIUM 252

Californium 252 (^{252}Cf) is a manufactured radionuclide that emits a mixture of neutrons and gamma rays. With a half-life of 2.64 years, it is practical for use in brachytherapy, emitting a fission energy spectrum of neutrons with an average energy of 2.35 MeV and modal energy of about 1.5 MeV. ^{252}Cf decays by alpha particle emission and spontaneous fission. Beta particles result from the decay of the fission products, as does gamma radiation in the range of 0.5 to 1.0 MeV. The metallic wall of the seeds stops the alpha particles and partially attenuates the beta and gamma dose rate to one half the neutron dose rate at 0.5 cm distance from the source. Because of the increased RBE of the neutrons (about 6 to 7 at dose rates of 30 to 60 rads per hour), the greatest portion of the biological effect is due to neutrons, for tissues close to the implant. The OER is approximately 1.6 when compared to ^{226}Ra or ^{137}Cs at dose rates of 30 to 60 rads per hour. The OER for radium at these dose rates ranges from 2 to 2.5. At higher dose rates (more than 100 rads/hour), such as might be obtained if high intensity ^{252}Cf is used in a specially shielded room for gynecologic therapy, the OER is about 1.9. At the University of Texas MD Anderson Hospital, an RBE of 5 for the combined neutron and gamma dose was used for ^{252}Cf interstitial implants.[177,178]

The first clinical brachytherapy with ^{252}Cf was carried out by Castro et al.[177] at the MD Anderson Hospital in 1969, but subsequent studies have been carried out by Maruyama et al.[179,180] in the United States, Russia,[181] and Japan. Interesting results were reported by Maruyama in the use of ^{252}Cf in irradiation of advanced tumors of the cervix uteri and endometrium.[179,182] He noted more rapid regression of tumors when ^{252}Cf implants were used before external irradiation, possibly because initial neutron therapy from ^{252}Cf had a greater effect on poorly vascularized, hypoxic tumors such as locally advanced carcinoma of the cervix uteri. The possibility of using ^{252}Cf as a source of epithermal and thermal neutrons in boron neutron capture therapy of brain tumors has also been proposed.

CURRENT CLINICAL INDICATIONS AND FUTURE DIRECTIONS

Protons

The use of protons in the treatment of unresectable or partially resectable neoplasms in critical locations such as the orbit, eye, skull base, juxtaspinal area, retroperitoneum, biliary tract, and pelvis has been clearly demonstrated to be of value. Higher rates of local control and survival have been achieved compared with previous results with megavoltage x-ray or electron beam therapy. At new proton facilities around the world, clinical data confirming the usefulness of protons has emerged. MGH-HCL and LLUPAF[183-185] have used protons in treating prostate cancer with successful results, although not clearly more advantageously than modern megavoltage conformal therapy.

The hallmark of charged particle therapy with protons is precise dose localization with tight margins to spare normal tissues. With proper techniques, high doses can be delivered successfully with excellent local control. Proton therapy is being tried in other tumor sites now that improved medical accelerators are coming into use. The availability of gantry proton beams at the NEPTC, LLUPAF, NCCHE, PSI, and future facilities, together with improvements in tumor localization and treatment planning, should lead to successful use of protons in a wider array of clinical sites. Protons appear especially valuable in children, where preservation of normal tissues is of paramount importance.[186-189,205]

The cost of proton therapy should be judged fairly against other techniques of cancer therapy. The higher initial costs are amortized over 30 to 40 years of useful life, with several treatment rooms being served from a single accelerator. Outfitting of treatment rooms, treatment planning, and immobilization costs will be similar for protons, IMRT, and 3D conformal photon therapy. Protons require a higher capital cost for accelerator construction and are likely to remain regional centers requiring patient travel for access. IMRT, 3D conformal photon therapy, and stereotactic radiation techniques have become accessible in virtually all radiotherapy centers in the United States, and, despite the inherent physical advantages of charged particles, may offer sufficient dose distributions for nearly all clinical tumor sites. The excellent results achieved with protons must be compared with these techniques to determine the best application of these modalities for each tumor and patient.

High-LET Particles

Neutrons have demonstrated advantages for certain types of tumors (salivary gland, prostate, sarcoma, and possibly head and neck tumors), but their clinical role is limited in view of their limited availability, reported increased late effects, and less favorable dose distributions than charged particles.

Sufficient study of high-LET charged particles such as carbon, neon, and silicon ions has not yet been performed to prove or disprove the merits of such particles in clinical therapy. Neon ions, while giving promising initial results, have caused significant late effects in normal tissues. The use of carbon ions may eliminate this problem because of their excellent dose-localization and lesser high-LET deposition in the entrance region. Their optimal use requires state-of-the art beam delivery scanning techniques plus sophisticated tumor localization and treatment planning. A C^{11} beam may be used to image the high dose deposition region through positron emission scanning as an aid to assuring coverage of the tumor target volume.

The HIMAC in Chiba, Japan, began preliminary phase I to II clinical studies[12,164] in 1994 with carbon ions. By August 2003, 1601 patients had been entered on dose escalation studies in various tumor sites: advanced head and neck tumors, stage I non–small-cell lung cancer, hepatocellular carcinoma, prostate carcinoma, uterine cervix carcinoma, and unresectable bone/soft tissue sarcoma. A concerted effort has been made to shorten overall treatment time and reduce the number of fractions given, to as low as four fractions in small lung tumors. This important hypofractionation advantage is possible with tight dose delivery to the target volume; toxicity has been acceptable.[12]

An excellent physics accelerator at GSI in Darmstadt, Germany has begun clinical studies with carbon ions in conjunction with the University of Heidelberg Strahlenklinik. By 2003, more than 100 patients had been treated in their preliminary study, mostly for tumors at the base of skull. A high level of local control with low toxicity has been observed in early follow-up.[105,118,206,207] This project is planned to move to the Clinical Center at the University of Heidelberg with the construction of a dedicated medical accelerator.

The preliminary results in the first two carbon centers have established that carbon ion therapy can be safely and effectively delivered. The results also demonstrate the potential of carbon ion therapy for high dose delivery in a short course of treatment to tumors located at depth in all regions of the body. Other carbon ion therapy units are under development in Japan and Europe,[10] although none are as yet planned for the United States!

While much has been learned regarding the clinical potential of high-LET charged particles in radiotherapy, sufficient numbers of patients have not been accrued in rigorously conducted trials to fully assess the role of high-LET charged particles in clinical practice. Questions remain regarding the molecular nature of high-LET effects and whether molecular studies can aid in predicting which patients will benefit most from high-LET therapy. The late normal tissue effects of high-LET therapy must be minimized and the effects of shortened fractionation regimens studied. Clinical results from carbon ion therapy should be compared to results from the most up-to-date low-LET therapy and other modalities in order to assess their place in cancer therapy.

REFERENCES

1. Stone RS, Larkin JC: Treatment of cancer with fast neutrons. *Radiology.* 1942;39:608.
2. Stone RS: Neutron therapy and specific ionization. *Am J Roentgen Rad Ther Nucl Med.* 1948;59:771.
3. Wilson RR: Radiological use of fast protons. *Radiology.* 1946; 47:487.
4. Tobias CA, Anger HO, Lawrence JH: Radiological use of high energy deuterons and alpha particles. *Am J Roentgen Rad Ther Nucl Med.* 1952;67:1.
5. Lawrence JH: Proton irradiation of the pituitary. *Cancer.* 1957; 10:795.

6. Larsson B, Leksell L, Rexed B, et al: The high-energy proton beam as a neurosurgical tool. *Nature* (London). 1958;182:1222.

7. Suit HD, Goitein M, Munzenrider J, et al: Definitive radiation therapy for chordoma and chondrosarcoma of the base of the skull and cervical spine. *J Neurosurg.* 1982;56:377.

8. Castro JR, Quivey JM, Lyman JT, et al: Current status of heavy charged particle radiotherapy at Lawrence Berkeley Laboratory. *Cancer.* 1980;46:63.

9. Slater JM, Archambeau J, Miller D, et al: The proton treatment center at Loma Linda University Medical Center: Rationale for and description of its development. *Int J Radiat Oncol Biol Phys.* 1992; 22:383.

10. Kagawa K, Murakami M, Hishigawa Y, et al: Preclinical biological assessment of proton and carbon ion beams at Hyogo ion beam medical center. *Int J Radiat Oncol Biol Phys.* 2001;51:239.

11. Castro JR, Chen GTY, Blakely EA: Current considerations in heavy charged particle radiotherapy. *Radiat Res.* 1985;104:s263.

12. Tsujii H: Overview of clinical experience on carbon ion radiotherapy at NIRS. *Personal communication.* 2003;9.

13. Eickhoff H, Haberer T, Kraft G, et al: The GSI Cancer Therapy Project. *Strahlenther Onkol.* 1999;175:suppl. 2:21.

14. Kraft G: Tumor therapy with heavy charged particles. Progress in Particle and Nuclear Physics. 2000;45:5473.

15. Blakely EA, Tobias CA, Ludewigt BA, et al: Some physical and biological properties of light ions. In Proceedings of PTCOG V and International Workshop on Biomedical Accelerators; 1987. LBL#22962.

16. Blakely E, Ngo F, Curtis S, et al: Heavy-ion radiobiology: Cellular studies. *Adv Radiat Biol.* 1984;11:195.

17. Blakely E: Cell inactivation by heavy charged particles. *Radiat Environ Biophys.* 1992;31:181.

18. Nagasawa H, Little J: Induction of sister chromatid exchanges by extremely low doses of alpha-particles. *Cancer Res.* 1992;52:6394.

19. Ballarini F, Biaggi M, Ottolenghi A, et al: Cellular communication and bystander effects: A critical review for modeling low-dose radiation action. *Mutation Research.* 2002;501:1.

20. Iyer R, Lehnert B: Alpha-particle-induced increases in the radioresistance of normal human bystander cells. *Radiat Res.* 2002; 157:3.

21. Mothersill C, Seymour C: Radiation-induced bystander effects: Past history and future directions. *Radiat Res.* 2001;155:759.

22. Petti PL, Lennox AJ: Hadronic radiotherapy. *Ann Rev Nucl Part Sci.* 1994;44:155.

23. Barendsen GW: Responses of different linear energy transfer. In Ebert M and Howard A, eds. *Current Topics of Radiation Research.* Vol 4. Amsterdam: North-Holland; 1968:293.

24. Belli M, Cherubini R, Ianzini F, et al: RBE-LET relationship for the survival of V79 cells irradiated with low energy protons. *Int J Radiat Oncol Biol Phys.* 1989;55:93.

25. Zirkle RE, Tobias CA: Effects of ploidy and LET on radiobiological survival curves. *Arch Biochem Biophys.* 1953;47:282.

26. Tepper J, Verhey L, Goitein M, et al: In vivo determinations of RBE in a higher energy modulated proton beam using normal tissue reactions and fractionated dose schedules. *Int J Radiat Oncol Biol Phys.* 1977;2:1115.

27. Coutrakon G, Cortese J, Ghebremedhin A, et al: Microdosimetry spectra of the Loma Linda proton beam and relative biological effectiveness comparisons. *Med Phys.* 1997;24:1499. (1997).

28. Paganetti H, Niemierko A, Ancukiewicz M, et al: Relative biological effectiveness (RBE) values for proton beam therapy. *Int J Radiat Oncol Biol Phys.* 2002;53:407.

29. Gueulette J, Gregoire V, Octave-Prignot M, et al: Measurements of radiobiological effectiveness in the 85 MeV proton beam produced at the cyclotron CYCLONE of Louvain-la-Neuve, Belgium. *Radiat Res.* 1996;145:70.

30. Gueulette J, Bohm L, De Coster B, et al: RBE variation as a function of depth in the 200-MeV proton beam produced at the National Accelerator Centre in Faure (South Africa). *Radiother Oncol.* 1997;42:303.

31. Leith JT, Ainsworth EJ, Alpen EA: Heavy-ion radiobiology: Normal tissue studies. *Adv Radiat Biol.* 1983;10:192.

32. Fowler JF: Rationales for high linear energy transfer radiotherapy. In Steel G, Adams GE, Peckham, MJ, eds. *The Biological Basis for Radiotherapy.* New York: Elsevier; 1983:261.

33. Sinclair WK: Cell cycle dependence of the lethal radiation response in mammalian cells. *Curr Top Radiat Res Q.* 1972;7:264.

34. Ando K, Koike S, Ohira C, et al: Accelerated reoxygenation of a murine fibrosarcoma after carbon ion irradiation. *Int J Radiat Biol.* 1999;75:505.

35. Fowler J: What to do with neutrons in radiotherapy: A suggestion. *Radiother Oncol.* 1988;13:233.

36. Raju M: Particle radiotherapy: Historical developments and current status. *Radiat Res.* 1996;145:391.

37. Field S, Hornsey S: Neutron RBE for normal tissues. In Barendsen GW, Broerse JJ, Breur K, eds. *High-LET Radiations in Clinical Radiotherapy.* Oxford: Pergamon Press; 1979:181.

38. Leith J: Heavy-ion radiobiology: Normal tissue studies. In *Advances in Radiation Biology.* (Ainsworth J, Alpen E, eds.) San Diego, Calif.: Academic Press; 1983:191.

39. Tobias C, Blakely E, Chang P, et al: Response of sensitive human ataxia and resistant T-1 cell lines to accelerated heavy ions. *Br J Cancer.* 1984;49 (Suppl. VI):175.

40. van der Kogel, A: *Late Effects of Radiation on the Spinal Cord.* Rijswijk, Holland; Radiobiological Institute TNO: 1979.

41. van der Kogel A, Sissingh H, Zoetelief J: Effect of X rays and neutrons on repair and regeneration in the rat spinal cord. *Int J Radiat Oncol Biol Phys.* 1982;8:2095.

42. Bijl H, van Luick P, Coppes R, et al: Dose volume effects in rat cervical spinal cord after proton irradiation. *Int J Radiat Oncol Biol Phys.* 2002;52:205.

43. Iannuzzi C, Atencio D, Green S, et al: ATM mutations in female breast cancer patients predict for an increase in radiation-induced late effects. *Int J Radiat Oncol Biol Phys.* 2002;52:606.

44. Hall E, Schiff P, Hanks G, et al: A preliminary report: Frequency of A-T heterozygotes among prostate cancer patients with severe late responses to radiation therapy. *Cancer J Sci Am.* 1998;4:385.

45. Fournier C, Scholz M, Weyrather W, et al: Changes of fibrosis-related parameters after high- and low-LET irradiation of fibroblasts. *Int J Radiat Biol.* 2001;77:713.

46. Griem M, Robotewskyj A, Nagel R: Potential vascular damage from radiation in the space environment. *Adv Space Res.* 1994; 14:555.

47. Barcellos-Hoff M, Brooks A: Extracellular signaling through the microenvironment: A hypothesis relating carcinogenesis, bystander effects, and genomic instability. *Radiat Res.* 2001;156(5 Pt 2):618.

48. Schneider U, Lomax A, Lombriser N: Comparative risk assessment of secondary cancer incidence after treatment of Hodgkin's disease with photon and proton radiation. *Radiat Res.* 2000;154:382.

49. Castro JR: Unpublished data.

50. Chu W, Renner T, Ludewigt B: Dynamic beam delivery for three-dimensional conformal therapy. In Chauvel P, Wambersie A, eds. *Proceedings of the EULIMA Workshop on the Potential Value of Light Ion Beam Therapy; Nice, France;* Nov. 3-5, 1988; EUR #12165; pp EN:295-328.

51. Chu WT, Ludewigt BA, Renner TR: Instrumentation for treatment of cancer using proton and light-ion beams. *Rev Sci Instrum.* 1993; 64:2055.

52. Goitein M: A technique for calculating the influence of thin inhomogeneities on charged particle beams. *Med Phys.* 1978; 5:258.

53. Petti PL: Differential-pencil-beam dose calculations for charged particles. *Med Phys.* 1992;19:137.

54. Urie M, Goitein M, Holley WR, et al: Degradation of the Bragg peak due to inhomogeneities. *Phys Med Biol.* 1986;31:1.

55. Lyman JT: Heavy charged particle beam dosimetry. In *Advances in Dosimetry for Fast Neutrons and Heavy Charged Particles for Therapy Applications.* Vienna, Austria: International Atomic Energy Agency; 1984:267.

56. Wilson RR: Range, straggling and multiple scattering of fast protons. *Phys Rev.* 1947;71:385.

57. Koehler AM, Schneider RJ, Sisterson JM: Range modulators for protons and heavy ions. *Nucl Instrum Meth.* 1975;131:437.

58. Petti PL, Lyman JT, Castro JR: Sensitivity of helium beam-modulator designs to uncertainties in biological data. *Med Phys.* 1991; 18:506.

59. Petti PL, Lyman JT, Renner TR, et al: Design of beam-modulating devices for charged-particle therapy. *Med Phys.* 1991;18:513.

60. Castro JR, Petti PL, Daftari IK, et al: Clinical gain from improved beam delivery systems. *Radiat Envir Phys.* 1992;31:233.

61. Daftari IK, Petti PL, Collier JM, et al: Evaluation of fixed- versus variable-modulation treatment modes for charged-particle irradiation of the gastrointestinal tract. *Med Phys.* 1993;20:1387.

62. Goitein M, Chen GTY: Beam scanning for heavy charged particle radiotherapy. *Med Phys.* 1983;10:831.

63. Urie M, Goitein M: Variable versus fixed modulation of proton beams for treatment in the cranium. *Med Phys.* 1989;16:593.

64. Pedroni E, Bohringer T, Coray A, et al: Initial experience of using an active beam delivery technique at PSI. *Strahlenther Onkol.* 1999; 175(suppl 2):18.

65. Pedroni E, Bacher R, Blattmann H, et al: The 200-MeV proton therapy project at the Paul Scherrer Institute: Conceptual design and practical realization. *Med Phys.* 1995;22:37.

66. Fraass BA, McShan DL, Diaz RF, et al: Integration of magnetic resonance imaging into radiation therapy treatment planning: Technical considerations. *Int J Radiat Oncol Biol Phys.* 1987; 13:1897.

67. Chen GTY, Singh RP, Castro JR, et al: Treatment planning for heavy ion radiotherapy. *Int J Radiat Oncol Biol Phys.* 1979;5:1809.

68. von Essen CF, Blattman H, Bodendoerfer G, et al: The Piotron: II. Methods and initial results of dynamic pion therapy in Phase II studies. *Int J Radiat Oncol Biol Phys.* 1985;11:217.

69. Coray A, Blattman H, Pedroni E: Patient preparation, treatment planning, and dose verification for dynamic radiotherapy with pions. In *Proceedings of 5th Annual Meeting of ESTRO*; Sept. 8-10, 1986; Baden-Baden, Germany. Abstract, p 200.

70. Greiner R, von Essen CF, Blattmann H, et al: Pion therapy at Swiss Institute for Nuclear Research (SIN). *Int J Radiat Oncol Biol Phys.* 1986;12(suppl 1):98.

71. Chen GTY, Kessler ML, Pitluck S: *Structure Transfer in Three-Dimensional Medical Imaging Studies.* Dallas: Proceedings of the National Computer Graphics Association; 1985:171.

72. Kessler ML, Pitluck S, Petti PL, et al: Integration of multimodality imaging data for radiotherapy treatment planning. *Int J Radiat Oncol Biol Phys.* 1991;21:1653.

73. Petti PL, Kessler ML, Fleming T, et al: An automated image-registration technique based on multiple structure matching. *Med Phys.* 1994;21:1419.

74. Phillips M, Kessler M, Chuang F, et al: Image correlation of MRI and CT in treatment planning of intracranial vascular malformations. *Int J Radiat Oncol Biol Phys.* 1991;20:881.

75. Goitein M, Abrams M, Rowell D, et al: Multi-dimensional treatment planning: II. Beam's-eye-view back projection, and projection through CT sections. *Int J Radiat Oncol Biol Phys.* 1983;9:789.

76. Brahme A, Kallman P, Lind B: Optimization of the probability of achieving complication free tumor control using a 3D pencil beam scanning technique for proton and heavy ions. In Itano A, Kanai T, eds. *Proceedings of the NIRS International Workshop on Heavy Charged Particle Therapy and Related Subjects.* Chiba, Japan: Proceedings of the NIRS International Workshop on Heavy Charged Particle Therapy and Related Subjects; 1991;124.

77. Brahme A, Kallman P, Tilikidis A: Developments in ion beam therapy planning and optimization. In Linz U, ed. *Ion Beams in Tumor Therapy.* New York: Chapman & Hall; 1995:290.

78. Mohan R, Wang X, Lackson A, et al: The potential and limitations of the inverse radiotherapy technique. *Radiother Oncol.* 1994; 32:232.

79. Urie M, Goitein M, Wagner M: Compensating for heterogeneities in proton radiation therapy. *Phys Med Biol.* 1983;29:553.

80. Bortfeld T, Boyer AL, Schlegel W, et al: Realization and verification of three-dimensional conformal radiotherapy with modulated fields. *Int J Radiat Oncol Biol Phys.* 1994;30:899.

81. Chui C-S, Chan MF, Yorke E, et al: Delivery of intensity-modulated radiation therapy with a conventional multileaf collimator: Comparison of dynamic and segmental methods. *Med Phys.* 2001;28:2441.

82. Vijayakumar S, Chen G: Implementation of three dimensional conformal radiation therapy: Prospects, opportunities and challenges. *Int J Radiat Oncol Biol Phys.* 1995;33:979.

83. Lomax A: Intensity modulation methods for proton radiotherapy. *Phys Med Biol.* 1999;44:185.

84. Kraemer M, Jaekel O, Geiss O, et al: Inverse treatment planning for intensity modulated scanned ion beams. Abstracts of PTCOG XXXII meeting, HMI, Berlin, Germany, Sept 25-27, 2000: J. Sisterson, ed. NEPTC, 30 Fruit St, Boston, Mass.

85. Lomax A, Pedroni E, Schaffher B, et al: Treatment planning for conformal proton therapy by spot scanning. In Faulkner K, Carey B, Crellin A, et al, eds. *Quantitative Imaging in Oncology.* London: BIR publishing; 1999:67.

86. Scheib S, Pedroni E: Dose calculations and optimisation for 3D conformal voxel scanning. *Radiat Environ Biophys.* 1996;31:251.

87. Pedroni E: Therapy planning system for the SIN-pion therapy facility. In Burger G, Breit A, Broerse JJ, eds. *Treatment Planning for External Beam Therapy with Neutrons.* Munich: Urban and Schwarzenberg; 1981:60.

88. Brahme A, Kallman P, Lind B: Optimization of proton and heavy ion therapy using an adaptive inversion algorithm. *Radiother Oncol.* 1989;15:189.

89. Carlsson A, Andreo P, Brahme A: Monte Carlo and analytical calculation of proton pencil beams for computerized treatment plan optimization. *Phys. Med. Biol.* 1997;42:1033.

90. Cella L, Lomax A, Miralbell R: New techniques in hadrontherapy: Intensity modulated proton beams. *Phys Med.* 2001;17 (suppl 1):100.

91. Miralbell R, Cella L, Weber W, et al: Optimizing radiotherapy of orbital and paraorbital tumors: Intensity-modulated X-ray beams vs. intensity-modulated proton beams. *Int J Radiat Oncol Biol Phys.* 2000;47:1111.

92. Cella L, Lomax A, Miralbell R: Potential role of intensity modulated proton beams in prostate cancer radiotherapy. *Int J Radiat Oncol Biol Phys.* 2001;49:217.

93. Zurlo A, Lomax A, Hoess A, et al: The role of proton therapy in the treatment of large irradiation volumes: A comparative planning study of pancreatic and biliary tumors. *Int J Radiat Oncol Biol Phys.* 2000;48:277.

94. Lomax A, Bortfeld T, Goitein G, et al: A treatment planning inter-comparison of proton and intensity modulated photon radiotherapy. *Radiother Oncol.* 1999;51:257.

95. Lomax A, Boehringer T, Coray A, et al: Intensity modulated proton therapy: A clinical example. *Med Phys.* 2001;28:317.

96. Lyman JT: Complication probability as assessed from dose volume histograms. *Radiat Res.* 1985;104:s13.

97. Austin-Seymour M, Chen G, Castro J, et al: Dose volume histogram analysis of liver radiation tolerance. *Int J Radiat Oncol Biol Phys.* 1986;12:31.

98. Fuss M, Poljanc K, Miller D et al: Normal tissue complication probability (NTCP) calculations as a means to compare proton and photon plans and evaluation of clinical appropriateness of calculated values. *Int J Cancer.* 2000;90:351.

99. Focus 9200 3-D RTP Computerized Medical Systems, Inc. St. Louis, 63132.

100. Deasy J: A proton dose calculation algorithm for conformal therapy simulations based on Molière's theory of lateral deflections. *Med Phys.* 1998;25:476.

101. Russell KR, Grussell E, Montelius A: Dose calculations in proton beams: Straggling corrections and energy scaling. *Phys Med Biol.* 1993;40:1031.

102. Hong L, Goitein M, Bucciolini M, et al: A pencil beam algorithm for proton dose calculations. *Phys Med Biol.* 1996;41:1305.

103. Jakel O, Kramer M, Karger C, et al: Treatment planning for heavy ion radiotherapy: Clinical implementation and application. *Phys Med Biol.* 2001;46:1101.

104. Kramer M, Jakel O, Haberer T, et al: Treatment planning for heavy-ion radiotherapy: Physical beam model and dose optimization. *Phys Med Biol.* 2000;45:3299.

105. Schulz-Ertner D, Haberer T, Jakel O, et al: Radiotherapy for chordoma and low-grade chondrosarcoma of the skull base with carbon ions. *Int J Radiat Oncol Biol Phys.* 2002;53:36.

106. Chapman JD, Blakely EA, Smith KC, et al: Radiobiological characterization of the inactivating events produced in mammalian cells by helium and heavy ions. *Int J Radiat Oncol Biol Phys.* 1977;3:97.

107. Vatnitsky S, Moyers M, Miller D, et al: Proton dosimetry inter-comparison based on the ICRU report 59 protocol. *Radiother Oncol.* 1999;51:273.

108. Castro JR, Linstadt DE, Bahary JP, et al: Experience in charged particle irradiation of tumors of the skull base: 1977-1992. *Int J Radiat Oncol Biol Phys.* 1994;29:647.

109. Lillis-Hearne PK, Castro JR: Indications for heavy ions: Lessons from Berkeley. In Linz U, ed. *Ion Beams in Tumor Therapy.* New York: Chapman & Hall; 1995:133.

110. Lin R, Hug E, Schaefer R, et al: Conformal proton radiation therapy of the posterior fossa: A study comparing protons to 3-D planned photons in limiting dose to the auditory structures. *Int J Radiat Oncol Biol Phys.* 2000;Vol 48:1219.

111. Raju M: *Heavy Particle Radiotherapy.* New York; Academic Press: 1980.

112. Tobias CA, Lawrence JH, Born JL, et al: Pituitary irradiation with high energy proton beams: A preliminary report. *Cancer Res.* 1958; 18:121.

113. Linfoot J: Heavy ion therapy: Alpha particle irradiation of pituitary tumors. In Linfoot JA, ed. *Recent Advances in the Diagnosis and Treatment of Pituitary Tumors.* New York: Raven Press; 1979:245.

114. Kjellberg R: Proton beam therapy for arteriovenous malformation of the brain. In Schmidek HH, Sweet WH, eds. *Operative Neurological Techniques.* Vol 1. New York: Grune & Stratton; 1988:911.

115. Austin-Seymour M, Munzenrider J, Goitein M, et al: Fractionated proton radiation therapy of chordoma and low grade chondrosarcoma of the base of the skull. *Neurosurgery.* 1989;70:13.

116. Munzenrider JE, Liebsch NJ, Efird JT: Chordoma and chondrosarcoma of the skull base: Treatment with fractionated x-ray and proton radiotherapy. In Johnson JT, Didolkar MS, eds. *Head and Neck Cancer.* Vol III. Amsterdam: Elsevier Science Publishers; 1993.

117. Castro JR: Future research strategy for heavy ion radiotherapy. Progress in radio-oncology V. In Kogelnik HD, ed. *Proceedings of the 5th International Meeting on Progress in Radio-Oncology, ICRO/OGRO 5; May 10-14, 1995; Salzburg, Austria.* Bologna, Italy: Monduzzi Editore; 1995:643.

118. Debus J, Haberer T, Schulz-Ertner D, et al: Carbon ion irradiation of skull base tumors at GSI. First clinical results and future perspectives. *Strahlenther Onkol.* 2000;176:211.

119. Hug E, Loredo L, Slater JD, et al: Proton radiation therapy for chordoma and chondrosarcoma of the skull base. *J Neurosurg.* 1999;91:432.

120. Noel G, Habrand JL, Mammar H, et al: Combination of photon and proton therapy for chordoma and chondrosarcoma of the skull base: The Centre de Protontherapie d'Orsay experience. *Int J Radiat Oncol Biol Phys.* 2001;51:392.

121. Gutin P, Crumley R, Castro J: Treatment of cranial chordoma. Surgery for skull base tumors. In Long D, ed.: *Contemporary Issues in Neurological Surgery.* Oxford: Blackwell Scientific Publications; 1992:254.

122. Kaplan EL, Meier P: Nonparametric estimation from incomplete observations. *J Am Stat Assoc.* 1958;53:457.

123. Munzenrider JE, Liebsch NJ: Proton therapy for tumors of the skull base. *Strahlenther Onkol.* 1999;175:57.

124. Goitein G: Skull base sarcoma. Abstracts of the 34th PTCOG Mtg June 2001 Particle Therapy Cooperative Oncology Group Newsletter Ed J Sisterson NEPTC 30 Fruit St, Boston.

125. Santoni R, Liebsch N, Finklestein D, et al: Temporal lobe damage following surgery and high dose photon and proton in 96 patients affected by chordoma and chondrosarcoma of the base of the skull. *Int J Radiat Oncol Biol Phys.* 1998;41:59.

126. Urie M, Fullerton B, Tatsuzaki H, et al: A dose response analysis of injury to cranial nerves and/or nuclei following proton beam radiotherapy. *Int J Radiat Oncol Biol Phys.* 1992;23:27.

127. Castro JR, Collier JM, Petti PL, et al: Charged particle radiotherapy for lesions encircling the brain stem or spinal cord. *Int J Radiat Oncol Biol Phys.* 1989;17:477.

128. Hug EB, Fitzek MM, Liebsch NJ, et al: Locally challenging osteo- and chondrogenic tumors of the axial skeleton: Results of combined proton and photon radiation therapy using 3-D treatment planning. *Int J Radiat Oncol Biol Phys.* 1995;31:467.

129. Zelefsky M, Leibel S, Gaudin P, et al: Dose-escalation with three-dimensional conformal radiation therapy affects the outcome in prostate cancer. *Int J Radiat Oncol Biol Phys.* 1998;41:491.

130. Slater J, Yonemoto L, Rossi C, et al: Conformal proton therapy for prostatic carcinoma. *Int J Radiat Oncol Biol Phys.* 1998; 42:299.

131. Rossi C, Slater JD, Slater JM: Conformal proton beam therapy of prostate cancer—Report of long-term PSA-based outcomes in over 1200 patients. Proceedings of ASTRO 42nd Annual Meeting, Boston. *Int J Radiat Oncol Biol Phys.* 2000;(suppl 48):227.

132. Egger E, Schalenbourg A, Zografos L, et al: Maximizing local tumor control and survival after proton beam radiotherapy of uveal melanoma. *Int J Radiat Oncol Biol Phys.* 2001;51:138.

133. Chauvel P: Treatment of eye tumors. In Linz U, ed. *Ion Beams in Tumor Therapy.* New York: Chapman & Hall; 1995:116.

134. Kacpek A, Briggs M, Sheen MA, et al: Clinical treatments at Clatterbridge: ARMD and Iris Melanoma. Abstracts of PTCOG XXXII, HMI, Berlin, Germany, Particle Therapy Cooperative Oncology Group Newsletter Ed J Sisterson NEPTC 30 Fruit St, Boston. September 2000.

135. Fuss M, Loredo L, Blacharski P, et al: Proton radiation therapy for medium and large choroidal melanoma: Preservation of the eye and its functionality. *Int J Radiat Oncol Biol Phys.* 2001; 49:1053.

136. Constable IJ, Koehler AM: Experimental ocular irradiation with accelerated protons. *Invest Ophthal.* 1974;13:280.

137. Gragoudas ES, Goitein M, Koehler AM, et al: Proton irradiation of small choroidal malignant melanoma. *Am J Ophthalmol.* 1977; 83:665.

138. Gragoudas ES, Seddon JM, Egan K, et al: Long term results of proton beam irradiated uveal melanoma. *Ophthalmology.* 1987; 94:349.

139. Castro JR, Char DH, Petti PL, et al: 15 years experience with helium ion radiotherapy for uveal melanoma, *Int J Radiat Oncol Biol Phys.* 1997;39:989.

140. Moyers M, Galindo R, Yonemoto L, et al: Treatment of macular degeneration with proton beams. *Med Phys.* 1999;26:777.

141. Mukai S, Munzenreider J, Hug E, et al: Proton radiotherapy of Intraocular Retinoblastoma. Abstracts of PTCOG XXXII, HMI, Berlin, Germany, September 2000. Particle Therapy Cooperative Oncology Group Newsletter Ed J Sisterson NEPTC 30 Fruit St, Boston.

142. Gragoudas ES, Egan KM, Seddon JM, et al: Survival of patients with metastases from uveal melanoma. *Ophthalmology.* 1991; 98:383.

143. Nowakowski V, Ivery G, Castro JR, et al: Metastases in uveal melanoma treated with helium ion irradiation. *Radiology.* 178: 277,1991.

144. Daftari IK: Personal communication (Abstract submitted to ASTRO).

145. Gragoudas E, Egan K, Walsh S, et al: Lens changes after proton beam irradiation for uveal melanoma. *Am J Ophthalmol.* 1995; 119:157.

146. Fabrikant J, Levy R, Steinberg G, et al: Charged-particle radiosurgery for intracranial vascular malformations. *Neurosurg Clin North Am.* 1992;3:99.

147. Minakova E: Clinical results of proton therapy in Russia. In Linz U, ed. *Ion Beams in Tumor Therapy.* Germany: Chapman & Hall; 1995:106.

148. Levy R, Schulte R, Slater JD, et al: Stereotactic radiosurgery—The role of charged particles. *Acta Oncol.* 1999;38:165.

149. Coen J, Yock T, Swearingen B, et al: Stereotactic proton radiosurgery in the management of persistent acromegaly. *Int J Radiat Oncol Biol Phys.* 2001;51:161.

150. Vernimmen F, Harris J, Wilson J, et al: Stereotactic proton therapy of skull base meningioma. *Int J Radiat Oncol Biol Phys.* 2001;49:99.

151. Sheline G, Phillips T, Field S, et al: Effects of fast neutrons on human skin. *Am J Roentgenol.* 1971;3:31.

152. Catterall M, Bewley D, Sutherland I: Second report on a randomized clinical trial of fast neutrons compared with x- or gamma-rays in treatment of advanced head and neck cancers. *Br Med J.* 1977;1:1942.

153. Laramore G, Krall J, Griffin T, et al: Neutron versus photon irradiation for unresectable salivary gland tumors: Final report of an RTOG/MRX randomized clinical trial. *Int J Radiat Oncol Biol Phys.* 1993;27:235.

154. Laramore G, Griffin T: Fast neutron therapy: Where have we been and where are we going? *Int J Radiat Oncol Biol Phys.* 1995:32:879.

155. Laramore G, Krall J, Thomas F, et al: Fast neutron radiotherapy for locally advanced prostate cancer: Final report of an RTOG randomized clinical trial. *Am J Clin Oncol.* 1993;16:164.

156. Thomas F, Krall J, Hendrickson F, et al: Evaluation of neutron irradiation of pancreatic cancer. Results of a randomized Radiation Therapy Oncology Group clinical trial. *Am J Clin Oncol.* 1989;12:283.

157. Russell K, Caplan R, Laramore G, et al: Photon versus fast neutron external beam radiotherapy in the treatment of locally advanced prostate cancer: Results of a randomized prospective trial. *Int J Radiat Oncol Biol Phys.* 1993;28:47.

158. Laramore G, Diener-West M, Griffin T, et al: Randomized neutron dose searching study for malignant glioma of the brain: Results of an RTOG study. *Int J Radiat Oncol Biol Phys.* 1988; 14:1093.

159. Griffin TW, Davis R, Hendrickson FR, et al: Fast neutron radiation therapy for unresectable squamous cell carcinoma of the head and neck: The results of a randomized RTOG study. *Int J Radiat Oncol Biol Phys.* 1984;10:2217.

160. Griffin TW, Davis R, Laramore GE, et al: Mixed beam radiation therapy for unresectable squamous cell carcinoma of the head and neck: The results of a randomized RTOG study. *Int J Radiat Oncol Biol Phys.* 1984;10:2211.

161. Maor MH, Errington RD, Caplan RJ, et al: Fast-neutron therapy in advanced head and neck cancer, a collaborative international randomized trial. *Int J Radiat Oncol Biol Phys.* 1995;32:599.

162. Cohen L, Saroja K, Hendrickson F, et al: Neutron irradiation of human pelvic tissues yields a steep dose-response function for late sequelae. *Int J Radiat Oncol Biol Phys.* 1995;32:367.

163. Linstadt D, Castro J, Phillips T: Neon ion radiotherapy. Results of the phase I-II clinical trial. *Int J Radiat Oncol Biol.* 1991;20:761.

164. Tsujii H, Koto M, Morita S, et al: Present status and perspective of carbon ion therapy at NIRS. Abstracts of the Low-Dose Particle Biology and Emerging Issues in Hadron Therapy Conference June 8-9, 2001, Lawrence Berkeley National Laboratory, W. Chu and E. Blakely, eds., LBNL, Berkeley, 94720, Ca.

165. Douglas J, Laramore G, Austin-Seymour M, et al: Treatment of locally advanced adenoidcystic carcinoma of the head and neck with neutron radiotherapy. *Int J Radiat Oncol Biol Phys.* 2000; 46:551.

166. Kaufman N, Frazier A, Cher M, et al: Toxicity and PSA outcome for patients with intermediate risk prostate cancer after permanent brachytherapy boost and conformal photon or neutron radiotherapy. *Int J Radiat Oncol Biol Phys.* 2001;51:325.

167. Uhl V, Castro J, Knopf K, et al: Preliminary results of heavy charged particle irradiation of bone sarcoma. *Int J Radiat Oncol Biol Phys.* 1992;24:775.

168. Kamada T, Tsujii H, Tsuji H, et al: A phase I/II trial of carbon-ion therapy for patients with bone and soft tissue sarcoma not suited for surgical resection. *Eur J Cancer.* 2001;37(suppl.6):84.

169. Schoenthaler R, Castro J, Halberg F, et al: Definitive postoperative irradiation of bile duct carcinoma with charged particles and/or photons. *Int J Radiat Oncol Biol Phys.* 1993;27:75.

170. Fowler P, Perkins D: The possibility of therapeutic applications of beams of negative pi-mesons. *Nature.* 1961;189:524.

171. Kaplan H, Schwettman H, Fairbank W, et al: A hospital-based superconducting accelerator for negative pi-meson beam radiotherapy. *Radiology.* 1973;108:159.

172. Petti P, Lennox A: Hadronic radiotherapy. *Ann Rev Nucl Part Sci.* 1994;44:155.

173. Kligerman M, West G, DeCello J, et al: Initial comparative response to peak pions and x-rays of normal skin and underlying tissue surrounding superficial metastatic nodules. *Am J Roentgen.* 1976;126:261.

174. von Essen C, Bagshaw M, Bush S, et al: Long-term results of pion therapy at Los Alamos. *Int J Radiat Oncol Biol Phys.* 1987; 13:1389.

175. Greiner R, Munkel G, Kann R, et al: Pion irradiation at Paul Scherrer Institute. Results of dynamic treatment of unresectable soft tissue sarcoma. *Strahlenther Onkol.* 1990;166:30.

176. Pickles T, Goodman G, Fryer C, et al: Pion conformal radiation of prostate cancer: Results of a randomized study. *Int J Radiat Oncol Biol Phys.* 1999;43:47.

177. Castro JR: Experimental brachytherapy: Californium 252. In Pierquin B, Wilson JF, Chassagne D, eds. *Modern Brachytherapy.* New York: Masson Publishing USA; 1987:317.

178. Castro J, Oliver G, Withers R, et al: Experience with californium 252 in clinical radiotherapy. *Am J Roentgen Rad Ther Nucl Med.* 1973;117:182.

179. Maruyama Y, Van Nagell J, Yoneda J, et al: Clinical evaluation of ^{252}Cf neutron intracavitary therapy for primary endometrial adenocarcinoma. *Cancer.* 1993;71:3932.

180. Wierzbicki J, Maruyama Y, Alexander C: Cf-252 for teletherapy and thermalized Cf-252 neutrons for brachytherapy. *Nucl Sci Appl.* 1991;a4:361.

181. Vtyurin B, Tsyb A: Therapy with Cf-252 in USSR: Head and neck, gynecologic, and other tumors. In press.

182. Maruyama Y, Bowen MG, Van Nagell JR, et al: A feasibility study of ^{252}Cf neutron brachytherapy, cisplatin + 5-FU chemoadjuvant and accelerated hyperfractionated radiotherapy for advanced cervical cancer. *Int J Radiat Oncol Biol Phys.* 1994; 29:529.

183. Slater JD, Rossi C, Yonemoto L, et al: Conformal proton therapy for early-stage prostate cancer. *Urology.* 1999;53:978; discussion 984.

184. Yonemoto LT, Slater JD, Rossi CJ Jr., et al: Combined proton and photon conformal radiation therapy for locally advanced carcinoma of the prostate: Preliminary results of a phase I/II study. *Int J Radiat Oncol Biol Phys.* 1997;37:21.

185. Shipley W, Verhey L, Munzenrider J, et al: Advanced prostate cancer: The results of a randomized comparative trial of high dose irradiation boosting with conformal protons compared with conventional dose irradiation using photons alone. *Int J Radiat Oncol Biol Phys.* 1995;32:3.

186. Hug E, Muenter M, Archambeau J, et al: Conformal proton radiation therapy for pediatric low-grade astrocytoma. *Strahlenther Onkol.* 2002;178:10.

187. McAllister B, Archambeau J, Nguyen M, et al: Proton therapy for pediatric cranial tumors: Preliminary report on treatment and disease-related morbidities. *Int J Radiat Oncol Biol Phys.* 1997; 39:455.

188. Hug E, Nevinny-Stickel M, Fuss M, et al: Conformal proton radiation treatment for retroperitoneal neuroblastoma: Introduction of a novel technique. *Med Pediatr Oncol.* 2001;37:36.

189. Hug E, Sweeney R, Nurre P, et al: Proton radiotherapy in management of pediatric base of skull tumors. *Int J Radiat Oncol Biol Phys.* 2002;52:1017.

190. Tsujii H, Tsuji H, Okunura T, et al: Proton therapy of thoracoabdominal tumors. In Linz U, ed. *Ion Beams in Tumor Therapy.* Weinheim, Germany: Chapman & Hall; 1995:127.

191. Beauduin M, Gueulette J, de Coster M, et al: Radiobiological intercomparisons of fast neutron beams used in therapy. *Strahlenther Onkol.* 1989;165:263.

192. Belli M, Campa A, Ermolli I: A semi-empirical approach to the evaluation of the relative biological effectiveness of therapeutic proton beams: The methodological framework. *Radiat Res.* 1997; 148:592.

193. Hall E, Astor M, Brenner D: Biological intercomparisons of neutron beams used for radiotherapy generated by p$^{(+)}$→Be in hospital-based cyclotrons. *Br J Radiol.* 1992;65:66.

194. Paganetti H: Calculation of the spatial variation of relative biological effectiveness in a therapeutic proton field for eye treatment. *Phys Med Biol.* 1998;43:2147.

195. Wambersie A, Richard F, Breteau N: Development of fast neutron therapy worldwide. Radiobiological, clinical and technical aspects. *Acta Oncol.* 1994;33:261.

196. Weyrather W, Ritter S, Scholz M, et al: RBE for carbon track-segment irradiation in cell lines of differing repair capacity. *Int J Radiat Biol.* 1999;75:1357.

197. Jakel O, Kramer M, Karger C, et al: Treatment planning for heavy ion radiotherapy: Clinical implementation and application. *Phys Med Biol.* 2001;46:1101.

198. Kraft G: RBE and its interpretation. *Strahlenther Onkol.* 1999; 175(suppl 2):44.

199. Suzuki M, Kase Y, Kanai T, et al: Correlation between cell killing and residual chromatin breaks measured by PCC in six human cell lines irradiated with different radiation types. *Int J Radiat Biol.* 2000;76:1189.

200. Suzuki M, Kase Y, Kanai T, et al: Change in radiosensitivity with fractionated-dose irradiation of carbon-ion beams in five different human cell lines. *Int J Radiat Oncol Biol Phys.* 2000; 48:251.

201. Suzuki M, Kase Y, Yamaguchi H, et al: Relative biological effectiveness for cell-killing effect on various human cell lines irradiated with heavy-ion medical accelerator in Chiba (HIMAC) carbon-ion beams. *Int J Radiat Oncol Biol Phys.* 2000;48:241.

202. Kanai T, Endo M, Minohara S, et al: Biophysical characteristics of HIMAC clinical irradiation system for heavy-ion radiation therapy. *Int J Radiat Oncol Biol Phys.* 1999;44:201.

203. Fukutsu K, Kanai T, Furusawa Y, et al: Response of mouse intestine after single and fractionated irradiation with accelerated carbon ions with a spread-out Bragg peak. *Radiat. Res.* 1997; 148:168.

204. Furusawa Y, Fukutsu K, Aoki M, et al: Inactivation of aerobic and hypoxic cells from three different cell lines by accelerated (3)He-, (12)C- and (20)Ne-ion beams. *Radiat Res.* 2000;154:485.
205. Benk V, Liebsch NJ, Munzenrider JE, et al: Base of skull and cervical spine chordomas in children treated by high-dose irradiation. *Int J Radiat Oncol Biol Phys.* 1995;31:577.
206. Ertner D, Haberer T, Scholz M, et al: Acute radiation-induced toxicity of heavy ion radiotherapy delivered with intensity modulated pencil beam scanning in patients with base of skull tumors. *Radioth and Oncol.* 2002;64:189.
207. Debus J, Kraft G: Hadronentherapie GSI, Preprinted 2003-01, Darmstadt, Germany.

Hyperthermia

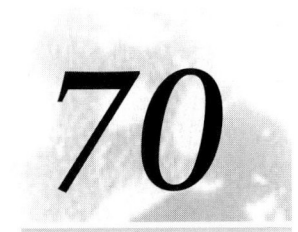

70

Penny K. Sneed, MD, Paul R. Stauffer, MSEE, and Gloria C. Li, PhD

yperthermia (HT) is the use of elevated temperature for the treatment of cancer, in this case, typically using temperatures in the range of 41°C to 45°C for 1 hour or more. Tumor regression after a high fever due to erysipelas was first reported in the medical literature in 1866 by the German clinician W. Busch.[1] This case and others led a New York surgeon, W. B. Coley, to treat cancer patients with bacterial pyrogens *(Coley's toxin)*.[2] In 1910 Müller described the potential of hyperthermia as an adjuvant to radiotherapy (RT).[3] However, the biological rationale for applying HT with RT in cancer therapy was not investigated in depth until the 1970s.[4-6] Exciting laboratory studies demonstrating the activity of heat against tumor cells in tissue culture and animal models encouraged numerous non-randomized clinical trials of RT plus HT in small superficial human tumors.[7] Promising results of these early trials led to premature randomized trials, before adequate thermometry or hyperthermic delivery systems were available, with disappointing results.[8,9] Since then, multiple prospective, randomized trials have shown a benefit of adjuvant HT,[10-15] and thermal dose-response analyses have predicted appropriate thermal dose prescriptions for superficial and deep tumors.[16] New protocols that prescribe higher minimum thermal doses or combine HT simultaneously with RT for increased thermal radiosensitization are nearing completion. Encouraging trials of HT combined with chemotherapy or liposomal chemotherapy have been performed. There is also recent interest in using HT as a modulator for gene therapy or immunotherapy. However, for HT to become an established treatment modality, much work is needed to (1) better understand and exploit the biology of heat in combination with RT or chemotherapy or novel therapies; (2) improve the equipment used for performing, monitoring, and planning hyperthermic treatments; and (3) further define appropriate thermal dose goals and clinical applications. This chapter reviews the biological rationale for HT, physical principles of techniques used to heat tissues, clinical results, and future directions of HT research.

BIOLOGICAL RATIONALE

Heat kills cells as a function of time and temperature and also sensitizes cells to radiation damage. Evidence suggests that protein denaturation is involved in this process,

whereas direct damage to DNA is not.[17] Although the exact mechanisms of hyperthermic cell killing are still not clear, much progress has been made in the past decade in understanding the molecular, biochemical, and cellular consequences of thermal stress. Heating induces various intracellular changes: activation of heat shock transcription factors; enhanced synthesis of heat shock proteins; and alterations in nuclear and cytoskeletal structures, cellular metabolism, macromolecular synthesis, intracellular signal transduction, and hormone-receptor interactions.[18]

This section summarizes our current knowledge of the response of cells to heat, the concept of thermal dose, the mechanisms of heat action, thermotolerance and the heat shock proteins, the regulation of the heat shock response, the interaction between heat and RT including continuous long-duration HT, the interaction between heat and chemotherapeutical agents, hyperthermia and liposomes, and heat shock proteins and cancer immunotherapy and gene therapy.

Cellular Response to Heat

Exposure of mammalian cells to temperatures above 40°C leads to reproductive cell death. This effect of hyperthermic treatment on cells' reproductive capacity depends on both the applied temperature and the duration of the exposure and can be represented as survival curves resembling x-ray survival curves (Fig. 70-1). When the surviving cell fraction (capable of reproduction) is plotted on a logarithmic scale versus the duration of heating on a linear scale, the survival curve is characterized by an initial shoulder region followed by an exponential decrease in the surviving fraction.[5] The time required to reduce the survival in the exponential region to 37% of its initial value is defined as D_0.

Several mathematical models have been postulated to describe heat-induced cell killing. The most uncomplicated model assumes a one-step reaction:

$$S = e^{-kt}$$

where S is survival, t is the treatment time, and k is the inactivation rate at the treatment temperature.[19] The term k may also be replaced by $1/D_0$ as used in RT biology.[6] This model does not account for the survival curve "shoulder."

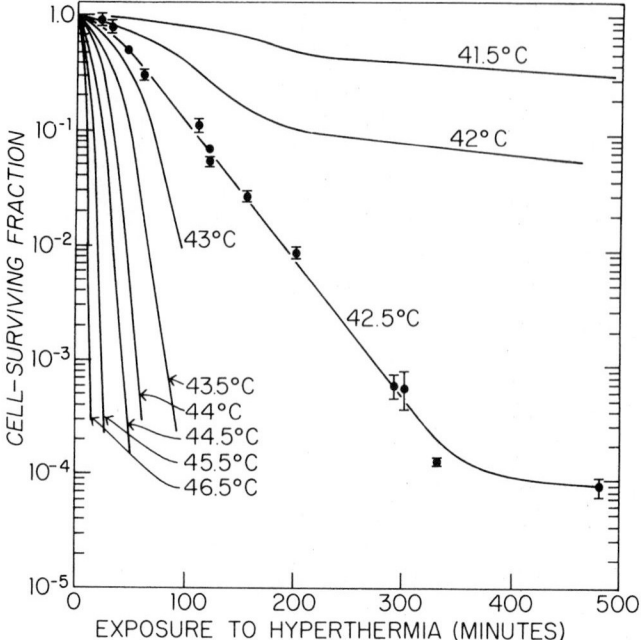

Figure 70–1. Survival curves for asynchronous Chinese hamster ovary cells heated at different temperatures for varying time. (Reproduced with permission from Hall EJ: *Radiobiology for the Radiologist*. Philadelphia: JB Lippincott; 1994:260.)

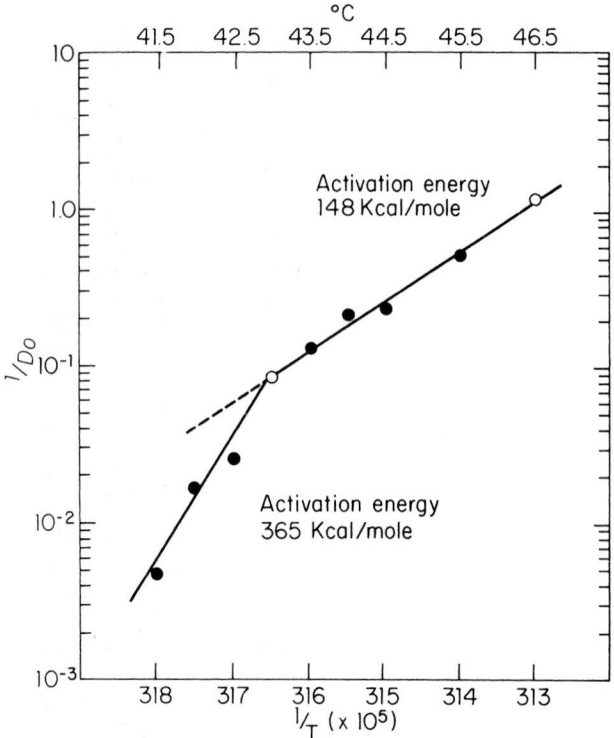

Figure 70–2. An Arrhenius plot for heat inactivation of Chinese hamster ovary cells plotting the reciprocal of D_0 (the inactivation rate) versus the reciprocal of the absolute temperature. Note the breakpoint at about 43°C. (Reproduced with permission from Hall EJ: *Radiobiology for the Radiologist*. Philadelphia: JB Lippincott; 1994:261.)

The most commonly used model to describe survival curves for heat killing is the *multitarget single hit* model

$$S = 1 - (1 - e^{-D/D_0})^n$$

where n is the number of targets to be inactivated before the cell is killed.[6,20] The survival curves for this model are characterized by the parameters n, D_0, and D_q (the quasithreshold dose) where $D_q = (\ln n)D_0$. Using this model, one can construct Arrhenius plots to demonstrate the kinetics of heat killing, where $1/D_0$ is plotted against the inverse of the absolute temperature (Fig. 70-2). For most cell lines studied, the Arrhenius plots of cell inactivation seem to be composed of two segments, with a break at or near 43°C.[4] Above the break point, the activation energy is between 110 and 150 kcal/mol, which is the energy required for protein denaturation,[21] suggesting that protein damage is mainly responsible for cell death due to HT. At lower temperatures, the activation energy is higher, around 300 to 400 kcal/mol. On the basis of the difference in activation energies, it has been suggested that there may be different primary modes of heat-induced cell death, one dominant above 43°C and the other below 43°C. However, the change in the slope of Arrhenius plots below 43°C could simply be a manifestation of the ability of the cells to develop thermotolerance, the transient resistance of cells to heat killing.[22] The Arrhenius plot for a given cell line can be modulated by thermotolerance or environmental parameters such as pH.

Using the activation enthalpy and entropy for hyperthermic cell killing (determined from Arrhenius plots based on D_0s), Lepock and colleagues[23] introduced a thermodynamic model for hyperthermic cell killing based on the existence of a *critical target*. The rate of cell killing is thought to correspond with the rate of inactivation

and denaturation of this hypothetical critical target. The calculated transition temperature of this critical target appeared to be 46.0°C for V79-WNRE cells when the temperature was raised by 1°C/minute. When the scan rates 0.1°C/minute or 10°C/minute were used for differential scanning calorimetry (DSC), the calculated transition temperature was 43.5°C or 48.5°C, respectively. Thus, transition temperatures are only meaningful when the scan rate used in the measurements is specified.[23] Cellular fractionation to localize the critical target showed that protein denaturation occurred at 46°C in all subcellular fractions.

A fourth model, which nicely describes heat killing under various conditions (single heating, thermotolerance, and step-down heating), was proposed by Jung.[24] This model assumes a two-step process. The first step is the production of nonlethal lesions that can be converted into lethal lesions upon further heating in the second step. After the cells are heated for a time period t at a certain temperature, the surviving fraction S is given by the equation

$$S = e^{(p/c)(1 - ct - e^{-ct})}$$

where p is the rate constant for the production of nonlethal lesions per cell per unit of time and c is the rate constant for the conversion of a nonlethal lesion into a lethal lesion per unit of time. One lethal lesion is sufficient to kill a cell. Jung assumed that the production and conversion of nonlethal lesions were random and the rate constants only depended on the temperature of the heat treatment.

The intrinsic thermal sensitivity of different cell lines varies significantly. So far, no consistent difference has been demonstrated between normal and malignant cells. On the other hand, the extracellular milieu can modify cells' thermal sensitivity. In general, cells that are at low pH or nutrient-deprived or both are more sensitive to heat. They may be hypoxic cells that are three times more resistant to radiation than are normally oxygenated cells. However, cells exposed to low pH for long periods of time adapt to pH changes and lose their increased heat-sensitivity.[25,26] Sensitivity to heat shock as a function of cell cycle has also been extensively studied. It is well established that the age response of thermal sensitivity complements that for x-irradiation. The phase of the cell cycle most resistant to x-rays (late S phase) is most sensitive to heat shock response.[27]

When more than one heat treatment is given, cellular thermal sensitivity to the combined treatments can be modified depending on the order of the heat shock temperatures involved. *Step-up heating* occurs when the second heat shock is at a higher temperature than the first heat exposure at 39°C to 42°C. Conversely, *step-down heating* occurs when the first treatment is a short exposure at a high temperature, greater than 43°C, immediately followed by a subsequent exposure to less than 43°C. During step-up heating, thermotolerance may be induced if the first treatment temperature is less than 43°C. Therefore, the cytotoxic effect of combined heat treatments is much less than the effect without preheat treatment. On the other hand, during step-down heating, preheat treatment at greater than 43°C for a short period of time can sensitize cells to a subsequent heat shock treatment at a lower temperature, which may have been nonlethal by itself without the preheat treatment. However, a high temperature pulse does not abolish any thermotolerance developed earlier.[6]

Thermal Dose

Because heat killing is a function of both time and temperature, a thermal dose unit is needed to combine both factors and account for the different effect of heat above and below 43°C. Equivalent minutes at 43°C (EM 43°) was proposed as the thermal dose unit by Sapareto and Dewey in 1984[28]:

$$EM\ 43° = t \cdot R^{(43-T)}$$

where t is the time at temperature T, the constant $R = 0.5$ for temperatures above 43°C, and $R = 0.25$ below 43°C. Thermal dose for a given treatment can be obtained by summing thermal doses for each minute of treatment, and the thermal dose from multiple treatments can be summed to obtain the cumulative equivalent minutes at 43°C (CEM 43°) for an entire treatment course, assuming that the interval between heat treatments is long enough to allow for decay of thermotolerance. To describe the variations in thermal dose throughout a tumor, minimum, maximum, and average values can be given as well as thermal dose values for the T_{90} and T_{50}

temperatures (the temperatures exceeded by 90% or 50% of the measured intratumoral points, respectively), and so on.

This concept of thermal dose has been validated in multiple pet animal and human clinical trials. Multivariate analysis of a randomized trial in pet animals with spontaneous tumors treated with RT alone or RT plus HT showed that, along with tumor volume, the non–site-specific average minimum EM 43° was the most important predictor of complete response (CR) ($P < 0.001$) and local control ($P < 0.05$). The CR rate was only 32% for 28 tumors with an average minimum CEM 43° (CEM 43° T_{min}) of 1.0 minute or less but 68% for 79 tumors with greater than 1.0 average CEM 43° T_{min}.[29] A thermal dose analysis of a prospective, randomized trial in patients with recurrent breast cancer showed a significant association between CEM 43° T_{min} and response, with CR rates of 43% for CEM 43° T_{min} less than or equal to 10 minutes versus 77% for CEM 43° T_{min} greater than 10 minutes.[30] Retrospective analyses of HT patients treated at Duke University showed that the cumulative minutes of treatment for which T_{90} exceeded 39.5°C was highly associated with CR of superficial tumors[31] and that the cumulative minutes of treatment for which T_{50} exceeded 41.5°C was highly associated with greater than 80% necrosis of soft tissue sarcomas treated preoperatively with thermoradiotherapy.[32] Thermal dose-response formulas based on these data showed that T_{90} and T_{50} temperatures routinely achieved need to be improved by 1.2°C to 1.5°C, or treatment duration increased threefold to fivefold, in order to increase thermal dose sufficiently to justify phase III trials.[16] There were also significant associations between CEM 43° T_{90} and response in a study of preoperative regional HT combined with conventional RT and low-dose 5-fluorouracil chemotherapy and leucovorin for 37 locally advanced primary rectal cancers ($P = 0.006$)[33] and between CEM 43° T_{90} and CR and local control in patients with recurrent breast adenocarcinoma treated at Stanford with RT and HT.[34] These parameters, CEM 43° T_{min} and CEM 43° T_{90}, have become standard thermal dose descriptors for superficial HT.

Mechanisms of Heat Action

Unlike ionizing radiation, HT does not result in the localized deposition of high levels of energy in cells. The thermal energy is more or less evenly absorbed by all molecules in the cell. As mentioned previously, the activation energy obtained for cultured cell lines and transplantable tumors in the temperature range from 42.5°C to 47°C is around 150 kcal/mol,[6,27] suggesting that protein denaturation is the main cause of hyperthermic cell killing.

More direct evidence that protein denaturation is responsible for thermal killing was provided using DSC (differential scanning calorimetry).[23] In eukaryotes, the onset for protein denaturation was found to be around 40°C. Thermotolerance, cycloheximide, and D_2O all increased the thermostability of proteins and also resulted in increased survival levels after HT.[35] These results were further confirmed by studies of Burgman and colleagues[36] using electron spin resonance (ESR) measurements and thermal gel analysis, showing that a correlation existed between protein denaturation and heat killing.

Protein denaturation and subsequent aggregation appear to occur throughout the entire cell, including cytoplasmic, nuclear, and membrane proteins.[36] It is unlikely that a single type of protein is the critical target for cell killing by heat. All subcellular structures contain temperature-sensitive proteins that denature and may subsequently aggregate.[37] Small changes in temperature can drastically alter the structure of plasma membranes and impair many membrane-related functions that, by themselves or in combination with other protein damage in the cell, could lead to cell death.[38,39] Heat has also been shown to alter the mitotic spindle and centrosome organization, resulting in the formation of multinucleated, nonclonogenic cells,[40] and to damage mitochondria,[41] with heat-induced inhibition of metabolic functions such as glycolysis and respiration. Heat damages polysomes and microsomes and inhibits the synthesis of proteins, RNA, and DNA in a thermal dose-dependent manner.[39,41] The inhibition of RNA and DNA synthesis appears to be due to heat-induced changes in chromatin structure caused by the denaturation and aggregation of nuclear proteins. Heat-induced changes in the nuclei of eukaryotic cells include the appearance of actin bundles; increased vesiculation; the reduction of intact nucleoli[41]; and a dramatic, dose-dependent increase in protein content in isolated chromatin, nuclei, nuclear matrices, and nucleoids.[35,42,43] This appears to be at least partially due to decreased leakage of proteins such as DNA and RNA polymerases from the nucleus during isolation as the heat-denatured proteins become aggregated and thus insoluble. This phenomenon is referred to as *heat-induced nuclear protein aggregation.* It is likely that nuclear protein aggregation, which occurs largely at the nuclear matrix, interferes with DNA replication, transcription complex interactions, and DNA unwinding needed for DNA replication and DNA repair.[44]

Interestingly, upon exposure to heat, a group of proteins called *heat shock proteins* (HSPs) translocate from the cytoplasm to the nucleus.[41,44,45] It has been shown that HSPs protect against protein aggregation or facilitate disaggregation of heat-induced insoluble protein complexes in cell lines and yeast.[46-48]

Thermotolerance and Heat Shock Proteins

One of the most interesting aspects of thermal biology in the mammalian system is the response of heated cells to subsequent heat challenges. Mammalian cells, when exposed to a nonlethal heat shock, have the ability to acquire a transient and nonheritable resistance to subsequent exposures at elevated temperature. This phenomenon, first shown by Henle and Leeper[49] and Gerner and Schneider,[50] has been described as *induced thermal resistance, thermal tolerance,* or, most commonly, *thermotolerance.* Several excellent reviews have discussed this phenomenon in considerable detail.[51-53]

In vitro, *acute* thermotolerance can be induced by a short initial heat treatment at temperatures above 43°C followed by a 37°C incubation before the second heat challenge. Thermotolerance can also be induced during a continuous and long exposure (1 to 20 hours) at temperatures below 43°C (*chronic* thermotolerance).[54-56] The degree of thermotolerance developed can be dramatic; increases in survival levels by several orders of magnitude are commonplace. The thermal history, heat fractionation interval, and recovery conditions all significantly modify the kinetics of thermotolerance.[52,53]

Thermotolerance can also be induced by treatment of cells with various chemicals followed by a drug-free period before the heat challenge. Some examples of the thermotolerance-inducing chemicals are heavy metals, ethanol, sodium arsenite, procaine, lidocaine, aliphatic alcohols (C_5-C_8), dinitrophenol, carbonyl cyanide m-chlorophenyl hydrazone, puromycin, and prostaglandins.[56-58] Pretreatment with heat or chemicals induces both thermotolerance and resistance against the cytotoxicity of the tolerance-inducing chemicals. This development of cross-resistance suggests overlap in the mechanisms of induction of tolerance by heat and chemicals.

The amount of thermotolerance expressed depends on the temperature and duration of the first heat treatment and the interval between the two heat treatments (Fig. 70-3).[59] At temperatures of 43°C or higher, thermotolerance does not develop during the first heat exposure; a subsequent incubation at 37°C is required for its expression. In contrast, for initial treatment at 41°C, thermotolerance is almost completely developed at the end of the first heat treatment. Based on these data, an operational model for the development of thermotolerance was formulated with three phases: an initial event (*trigger*), the expression of resistance (*development*), and the gradual disappearance of resistance (*decay*).[59] First, the triggering event converts normal cells to the triggered state with a rate constant k_1. This process very likely involves the activation of the heat shock transcription factor HSF1[60,61] and probably an additional regulatory factor or factors.[62] Second, these triggered cells are converted to thermotolerant cells with a rate constant k_2. Above 43°C, $k_2 = 0$; the triggered cells remain sensitive, and only after being transferred to 37°C do they convert to their thermotolerant state. This thermotolerant state, in general, is associated with the elevated expression of HSPs, and enhanced protection against and faster recovery from thermal damage. Finally, thermotolerant cells all reconvert to their sensitive state at a slower rate governed by rate constant k_3.

The mechanisms for the development of thermotolerance are not well understood, but it is known that heat shock activates a specific set of "heat shock" genes, resulting in the preferential synthesis of HSPs. Heat shock response—specifically regulation, expression, and functions of HSPs—has been extensively studied in the past decades and has attracted the attention of a wide spectrum of investigators ranging from molecular and cell biologists to radiation and HT oncologists. There is a large body of data supporting the hypothesis that HSPs play important roles in modulating the cellular response

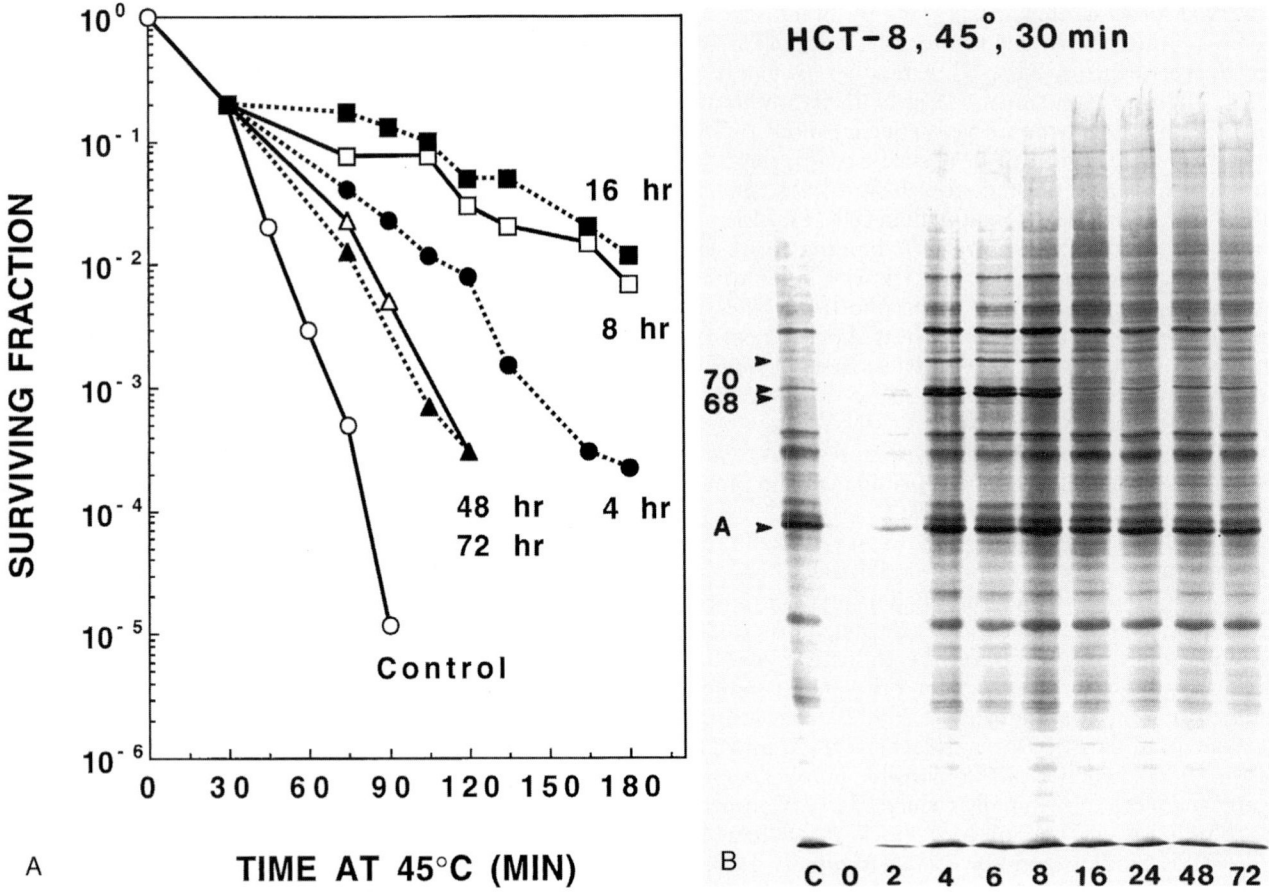

Figure 70–3. A, Survival fractions of HCT-8 cells given two 45°C treatments separated by a time period of 0 to 72 hours at 37°C. The first heating period was 30 minutes. Control cells received a single heat treatment at 45°C. **B**, One-dimensional electrophoretic analysis of cellular proteins of HCT-8 cells at various times after a heat dose of 45°C for 30 minutes. Indicated at the bottom are the times at 37°C (0 to 72 hours) after the treatment and before labeling (S35-methionine for 1 hour). The heat shock proteins of 68 (HSP70) and 70 kD (HSC70) are indicated; actin is denoted by the symbol *A*.

to heat shock and other types of environmental stress and are involved in the development of thermotolerance.

HSPs are usually identified by their molecular mass; for example, HSP70 is an HSP with a molecular mass of 70,000 daltons. In mammalian systems, HSP110, HSP90, HSP70, HSP60, HSP56, HSP47, HSP40, and HSP27 have been identified. The most extensively studied HSPs with respect to their role in thermotolerance and cellular heat sensitivity are HSP27, HSP70, and HSP90. In mammalian cells, good correlations have been reported for thermotolerance development and (1) HSP70 synthesis, (2) HSP27 synthesis, and (3) HSP27 phosphorylation. Enhanced thermosensitivity has been shown to result from reduction of the level of HSP70, whether by competitive inhibition of HSP70 gene expression or by microinjection of cells with antibodies against HSP70. Reduction of the cellular HSP90 levels has also been shown to increase thermosensitivity in mouse L cells, whereas an increased HSP90 expression resulted in stable heat resistance in Chinese hamster ovary (CHO) cells.[63] Transfection of cells with genes coding for HSP27[64] or HSP70,[65,66] resulting in constitutive expression of the genes, confers stable heat resistance. Transfection of rat cells with a gene coding for a homologue of the mammalian HSP60 also confers heat resistance to the transfected cells (Burgman and colleagues, unpublished results). These data provide direct evidence for a causal relation between the expression of HSPs and heat resistance.

Chronic thermotolerance (thermotolerance that develops during long-duration, mild HT at about 41°C) may be different from acute thermotolerance, which occurs after heat shock and incubation before heating at high hyperthermic temperatures, at or above 43°C). Chronic-type thermotolerance is not always observed in all mammalian cell lines. Studies with a range of human cell lines have shown that, unlike rodent cells, the human cells did not develop chronic thermotolerance during mild HT. In HeLa cells, this absence of thermotolerance may be related to cell cycle progression.[67] In other studies, the lack of thermotolerance did not appear to be linked directly to cell cycle progression, as shown by cell cycle analysis and the use of plateau-phase cultures.[68,69] More research is needed to better understand the development and decay of acute and chronic thermotolerance in human tumors.

Regulation of Heat Shock Response

As described earlier, the heat shock response refers to the increased transcription of a set of genes, the heat shock genes, when cells are subjected to heat stress. It is a highly conserved process that occurs in all organisms from bacteria to human. In eukaryotes, the response is mediated by a sequence-specific DNA binding protein termed HSF1.[70] In its trimeric form, HSF1 binds tightly to multiple copies of a highly conserved sequence motif (nGAAn) in the promoter region of heat shock genes; these HSF-binding sites are termed the heat shock elements (HSEs).[71,72] In unstressed mammalian cells, HSF1 is maintained in a monomeric, non–DNA binding form. Upon heat shock, HSF1 assembles into trimers, binds to HSEs with high affinity, becomes hyperphosphorylated, and activates the transcription of the heat shock genes. Transcriptional activation of these genes, in turn, increases the synthesis of HSPs. During post-heat-shock recovery, the HSF1 trimers dissociate from the DNA and are eventually converted to the inactive, non–DNA binding monomers. Several other models, similar to the previous model, have also been proposed.[18,73]

Although the importance of HSF1 in the regulation of mammalian heat shock genes is well-established,[70] data from multiple laboratories, obtained using various rodent and human cell lines, indicate that the activation of HSF1 by itself is not sufficient for the induction of HSP70 mRNA synthesis,[62,74-80] and that other factors may be involved in the regulation of HSP70 transcription. Subsequent studies of Rat-1, hamster HA-1, and HeLa cells provided evidence of the plausible involvement of a negative regulator,[62,81] initially termed CHBF (Constitutive HSE Binding Factor). Upon heat shock, the cellular level of the HSE binding activity of HSF1 rapidly increases ("activation of HSF1") and that of CHBF rapidly decreases ("inactivation of CHBF"). When HSP70 transcription returns to its pre-heat-shock level during post-heat-shock recovery, the disappearance of the HSF1-HSE binding activity again parallels the reappearance of the CHBF-HSE binding activity.[62,82] Interestingly, in rat, mouse, and human cells treated with sodium salicylate or sodium arsenite, which elicit considerable HSF1-HSE binding activity but show no reduction in CHBF-HSE binding activity, the induction of HSP70 mRNA synthesis was not observed.[62,77,80,83] Thus, data from studies of a wide variety of rodent and human cells all support the notion of a negative regulatory role of CHBF in HSP70 induction.

Subsequently, CHBF was purified and identified as the Ku protein, a heterodimer of Ku70 and Ku80,[81] allowing more direct testing of the hypothesis that CHBF/Ku acts as a negative regulator in the heat induction of HSP70. To carry out such experiments, Li and colleagues established Rat-1 cells that stably and constitutively express human Ku70 or Ku80 or both and found that overexpression of the human Ku70 by itself, or Ku70 and Ku80 jointly, specifically inhibits heat-induced HSP70 expression without affecting induction of other HSPs or activation of HSF1.[84,85] How does Ku70 specifically suppress HSP70 expression? There are at least four nonmutually exclusive possibilities: (1) Ku70 may bind directly to sites located in the HSP70 promoter and repress transcription; (2) Ku may regulate HSF1 binding to the HSP70 promoter; (3) Ku may affect the interaction among other transcription factors and their binding to the HSP70 promoter; (4) overexpression of

Ku70 could result in altered chromatin structure, inhibiting the access of positive factors to their respective regulatory elements in the HSP70 promoter. Related to (2) earlier is the recent finding that in vitro-translated Ku70/Ku can bind to HSF1 and displace it from HSE.[86,87] Thus the existing evidence strongly supports a role of Ku in HSP70 gene regulation.

Interaction of Heat with Radiation

Heat interacts with radiation in a more than additive way. This synergistic interaction of heat and radiation is interpreted as a heat-induced sensitization of cells to radiation, termed *heat radiosensitization*, or *thermal radiosensitization*. Heat radiosensitization can be quantified using a thermal enhancement ratio (TER), defined as the ratio of radiation doses with and without heat to produce the same biological effect (isoeffect TER). In some cases, TERs are expressed as a ratio of the biological effects for the same radiation dose, with and without heat (isodose TER), or as a ratio of the D_0s of the radiation survival curves. Usually, TER increases with increasing heat dose. The maximal interaction is observed when heat and radiation are given simultaneously. The TER decreases with an increasing time interval between heat and radiation (Fig. 70-4). When radiation precedes HT, sensitization is no longer detectable 2 to 3 hours after radiation. When HT precedes radiation, cells can be sensitized for up to several hours.

The therapeutic gain factor (TGF) is defined as the ratio of the TER in the tumor to the TER in surrounding normal tissue. Maximal heat radiosensitization is achieved when heat and radiation are applied simultaneously, but a therapeutic gain (more damage to tumor than to normal tissue) may not always be obtained under these

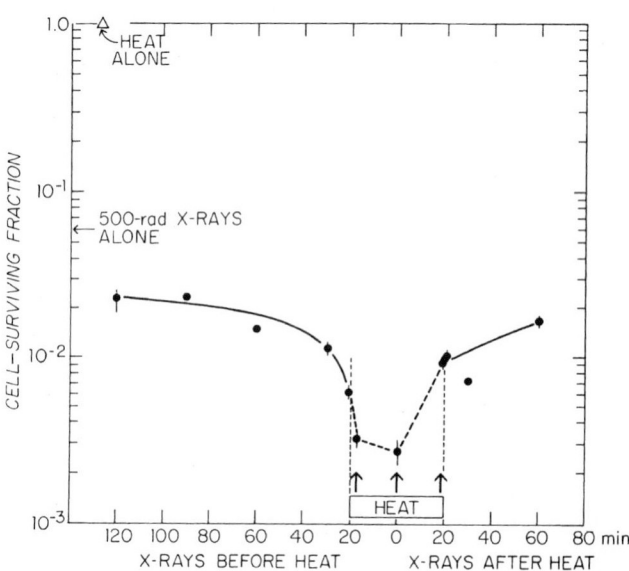

Figure 70–4. Survival of Chinese hamster ovary cells irradiated with 5 Gy during or at varying intervals before or after a heat treatment at 42.5°C for 40 minutes. The maximum effect occurs for simultaneous heat and radiation. (Reproduced with permission from Hall EJ: *Radiobiology for the Radiologist*. Philadelphia: JB Lippincott; 1994:272.)

conditions, especially if tumor and normal tissue are heated to the same degree.[88,89] In some cases, the TGF may increase when time intervals are introduced between radiation and heating.

The combination of heat and radiation does not result in an enhancement of *heat lesions*; thus, no radiation-induced heat sensitization takes place and the synergistic effect is most likely due to radiosensitization by heat.[56] The primary target for radiation is believed to be DNA, whereas protein denaturation and aggregation seem to be involved in thermal cell killing.[42,90] DNA damage (e.g., breaks) can be detected at low lethal doses of x-rays (≤1 Gy), whereas no DNA breaks are found at low lethal heat doses.[91] The combination of radiation and HT generally does not result in more initial DNA breaks than are observed for radiation alone.[90,91] Instead, HT appears to inhibit the rejoining of radiation-induced DNA strand breaks[91-93] and the excision of damaged bases[94] in a heat-dose dependent manner.[91,93] This effect may be caused by (1) heat-induced inactivation of DNA repair enzymes,[88,95] (2) alteration of the chromatin structure due to protein denaturation and aggregation, which causes decreased accessibility of the damaged sites to the repair machinery,[44,92,94,96] or (3) both. Using cell lines in tissue culture, researchers found a good correlation between the amount of heat-induced nuclear protein aggregates and the extent of thermal radiosensitization.[95,97]

The impact of thermotolerance on heat radiosensitization has also been a topic of extensive investigation. Studies using tissue-cultured cell lines have shown that thermoradiosensitization could be affected by thermotolerance development.[98,99] Since it has been reported that HSPs might be involved in the protection against nuclear protein aggregation as well as in facilitated disaggregation,[46,48] the presence of these proteins might indirectly be responsible for the thermotolerance effect on protein aggregation and as such affect DNA repair and cellular radiosensitivity. Rodent cells transfected with human HSP70 showed protection against heat-induced nuclear protein aggregation that was reflected in the extent of thermal radiosensitization.[95] Transfection with HSP27 resulted in an accelerated nuclear protein disaggregation and was paralleled by an accelerated decline of thermal radiosensitization. These observations point to the importance of HSPs as a regulator in protein denaturation, aggregation, and disaggregation, thereby modulating the heat effects on DNA repair. As such, the expression of HSPs may explain the impact of thermotolerance on the extent and disappearance of thermal radiosensitization and could have a major impact on the choice of sequence and spacing of heat and radiation in clinical practice. Elevated HSP expression should either be avoided, if occurring in the tumor, or exploited, if occurring in the normal tissue at risk during treatment.

Chronic thermotolerance has been found to affect heat radiosensitization in some cell lines,[17,93,99,100] although for other cell lines no effect of thermotolerance was observed at the level of heat radiosensitization.[99,101] For example, chronic thermotolerance development in CHO cells inhibited further sensitization to radiation.[100] This lack of further radiosensitization was also found in HeLa cells when no chronic thermotolerance developed.[67]

Interestingly, long-duration, mild HT (as low as 41°C) given concurrently with low-dose-rate irradiation can cause extensive radiosensitization and eliminate the low-dose-rate irradiation sparing effect.[69,88,102,103] This thermoradiosensitization to low-dose-rate irradiation occurred for protracted heating times and did not appear to be inhibited for prolonged heating times, supporting the absence of a thermotolerance process in radiosensitization.[69,102] The mechanism underlying this low-temperature radiosensitization may very well be different from the one discussed in the previous section on the mechanism of heat radiosensitization because DNA repair rates are often found to be higher at 41°C[104-106] and heat-induced protein aggregation in the nucleus is limited (Stege and associates, unpublished results). Effects of heat on cell cycle progression or changes in fidelity of repair may be possible explanations of radiosensitization by long-duration low-temperature HT.

Heat and Chemotherapy

Although the combination of HT with radiation has been the focus of more attention, there is an equally strong rationale for combining HT with chemotherapy. Moderate or even mild HT (such as 39°C) enhances cell killing in vivo of a number of chemotherapeutical agents, such as cyclophosphamide, melphalan, mitomycin C, cisplatin, doxorubicin, bleomycin, and the nitrosoureas. Various mechanisms may account for increased chemotherapeutical effect at elevated temperatures, including altered pharmacokinetics or pharmacodynamics, increased DNA damage, decreased DNA repair, reduced oxygen radical detoxification, and increased membrane damage.[107] Concentrations of agents that are not normally toxic at normal body temperature can become cytotoxic at 39°C, and in some cases, HT may partially overcome some types of drug resistance.

Heat and Liposomes

It is well recognized that when systemic chemotherapy is used for the treatment of solid tumors, significant normal tissue toxicities commonly occur when therapeutical levels of drug at the tumor site are achieved.[108] Liposomes have been identified as one of the promising carriers for therapeutical agents to improve drug delivery in the treatment of cancer.[109,110] Conventional liposomes have been clinically evaluated and approved in various diseases[111-113] and hyperthermia has been shown to increase extravasation of conventional liposomes within tumor tissue.[114] Early in 1978, Yatvin and colleagues proposed the use of hyperthermia with temperature-sensitive liposomes to allow increased control over the release of encapsulated drugs at the diseased site,[115] and their efforts have stimulated many additional studies.[116] In recent years, Dewhirst and collaborators have focused on developing a new thermosensitive, doxorubicin-containing lipid formulation optimized for rapid drug release under mild hyperthermic temperatures (39°C to 40°C) readily achievable in the clinic.[113,117] Their in vitro studies clearly demonstrate advantages that the new lipid composition has compared with existing liposome formulation; the characteristics of attainable and narrow triggering temperature, rapid release of drug, and high accumulative drug release would appear to offer potential advantages that could lead to an increased therapeutic effect over traditional chemotherapy and current liposomal and other drug carrier/delivery systems. Furthermore, in vivo studies demonstrated that this new liposome, in combination with mild hyperthermia, was significantly more effective than free drug or current liposome formulations at reducing tumor growth in a human squamous cell carcinoma xenograft line (FaDu), producing 100% complete regressions in 11 tumors lasting up to 60 days post treatment.[113,117]

Heat Shock Proteins and Cancer Immunotherapy

While HSPs have been intensively studied at the level of transcription and translation for mammalian cells for more than 2 decades, a novel and physiologically important role for these highly conserved gene products has only become evident in the past several years. In the early 1990s, Srivastava and colleagues found that a tumor rejection antigen, isolated by biochemical fractionation of tumor cells, was an HSP (grp94/gp96).[118-121] Since then, convincing evidence has accumulated that the HSPs derived from a given cancer, including HSP70, HSP90, and grp94/gp96, can elicit protective immunity specific to that particular cancer. Heat shock proteins derived from normal tissues do not have such effect against any cancer tested. In recent years, the immunogenicity of HSP preparations from tumors has been seen in different experimental tumor systems of distinct histological origins, ranging from chemical- or UV-induced tumors to spontaneous tumors.[122-124] Immunization of mice and rats with HSP-peptide complexes leads to protective and specific immunity against cancer from which the HSP-peptide complexes are derived.[120] This phenomenon has been shown in mice[120] and rats[125] in a wide array of tumor types including fibrosarcoma,[118] hepatocarcinoma,[125] lung carcinoma, melanoma, colon carcinoma,[123] squamous carcinoma,[126] and in prophylaxis[118,125] as well as in therapy of preexisting diseases.[123] Two high-molecular weight HSPs, HSP110 and grp170 derived from CT26 and Meth A tumors, were found to induce an anti-tumor response against these tumors.[127-129] Furthermore, it has been demonstrated that the immunization of mice resulted in the induction of memory T cells.[126] Taken together, these data suggest that HSPs prepared from tumors can serve as tumor vaccines, and that HSPs may play a central role in the host's immune system.

Hyperthermia and Gene Therapy

Another new application of hyperthermia is its use in gene therapy to provide both spatial and temporal control over gene expression governed by heat shock or other stress-inducible promoters.[130-133] As one example,

Huang and colleagues transfected cells with adenovirus vectors containing an HSP70 promoter and genes for green fluorescence, interleukin 12, or tumor necrosis factor alpha.[134] Experiments with heat-induced green fluorescence protein showed detectable expression at 3 hours reaching a peak at 18 to 24 hours and disappearing by 72 hours after heating. A modest heat shock of 42°C for 30 minutes increased interleukin-12 gene expression by more than 13,000-fold over baseline and increased tumor necrosis alpha gene expression by 6.8×10^5-fold.[134]

PHYSICAL PRINCIPLES

Mechanisms of Heating

Heating of biological tissue may be accomplished by one of three primary mechanisms: (1) thermal conduction of heat away from a source at higher temperature; (2) a combination of resistive and dielectric losses in tissue from an applied electromagnetic (EM) field; or (3) mechanical losses from molecular oscillations caused by an ultrasonic pressure wave. The underlying physical principles of each of these three modalities are reviewed briefly.

THERMAL CONDUCTION

In the simplest form of hyperthermia, tissue may be heated by circulating externally preheated blood through the tissue; by placing a heated surface on the skin or in natural body cavities; or by interstitially implanting hot sources in wires, needles, or catheters into the target tissue. It is generally not possible to heat well-perfused normal tissue more than a few millimeters from a hot surface.[135]

A good approximation for describing heat transfer in biological tissue is given by the bioheat transfer equation (BHTE), derived in 1948 by Pennes[136]:

$$APD + M + \nabla(k_t \cdot \nabla T) - \omega_b\, c_b\, (T - T_a) = \rho c_t\, \partial T/\partial t$$

where ∇ is the vector gradient operator; tissue thermal conductivity (k_t) quantifies the tissue's ability to conduct heat; ω_b and c_b quantify the perfusion rate and specific heat capacity of blood; c_t and ρ are the specific heat and mass density of tissue; APD represents the absorbed power density or external heat input to the tissue; M is the heat generated from tissue metabolism (generally negligible compared with other heat inputs); and T and T_a are the tissue and arterial blood temperatures, respectively, at time t. The first two terms represent heat inputs to the tissue volume, the third and fourth terms describe heat transfer kinetics due to thermal conduction and convection (blood flow), respectively, and the right side of the equation specifies the net heating effect in terms of the rate of change of temperature with time ($\partial T/\partial t$). Alternative theoretical models have been studied to describe the heat transfer characteristics of tumors more accurately by accounting for "thermally significant" blood vessels,[135,137] but the BHTE serves as a good starting point. Review articles are available on thermal modeling and hyperthermia treatment-planning issues.[138-140]

ELECTROMAGNETIC POWER DEPOSITION

All living tissues contain electrical charges, some free and some bound, that are available for interaction with externally applied EM fields. Tissues with high water content and blood circulation such as muscle, skin, brain, and internal body organs have a high percentage of polar water molecules and thus conduct electric current well. Tissues with low water content such as fat and bone have mostly bound charges that do not conduct current well. Over the frequency range of interest for hyperthermia, all tissues may be considered as *lossy dielectrics*—somewhere between poor electric conductors and poor insulators. The electric properties of human tissues vary considerably and may be characterized by the relative dielectric constant (ε_r) and electrical conductivity (σ). The primary mechanism of EM heating of tissue also varies with frequency. In the radiofrequency (RF) range below about 10 MHz, the alternating field induces a net movement of free electrons and power deposition results from resistive (ohmic) losses due to the electric currents in lossy tissue. At microwave (MW) frequencies above about 100 MHz, the dielectric losses in tissue predominate and heating results primarily from friction caused by interactions between polar water molecules that rotate and oscillate to maintain alignment with the time-varying EM field. In either case, the time-averaged absorbed power density

$$\text{APD} = (1/2\sigma)\,|\mathbf{J}|^2 = (\sigma/2)\,|\mathbf{E}|^2$$
$$\text{in watts per cubic meter}$$

where $\mathbf{J} = \sigma\mathbf{E}$ is the induced current density. This absorbed power density is closely related to the more commonly used specific absorption rate (SAR) by the formula SAR = APD/ρ where ρ is the mass density of tissue in kilograms per cubic meter.

For both RF and MW radiation, APD decreases with depth in tissue. The APD for the simplest case of plane wave radiation is plotted as a function of penetration depth into muscle tissue in Figure 70-5. At higher frequencies, power is deposited very superficially, whereas lower frequencies provide deeper penetration. However, for practical hyperthermia applicators, the tissue penetration may be much less due to coupling problems at the applicator-tissue interface, tissue heterogeneities, and nonuniform beam profile in the near-field region of hyperthermia applicators that are small compared to the wavelength or at the wrong distance from the target.

For frequencies used in hyperthermia, the wavelength (λ) of EM energy in soft tissue varies from about 300 m at 1 MHz to less than 5 cm at 1000 MHz. The minimum spot size for focusing power deposition is approximately $\lambda/2$, or over 1 m at the lowest RF frequencies typically used (100 MHz) and about 2 cm at the higher MW frequencies. Thus, lower RF frequencies penetrate well but affect large regions of the body whereas higher MW frequencies may be localized effectively in tumor-sized volumes located close to the tissue surface. Compilations of electrical conductivity, dielectric constants, wavelengths,

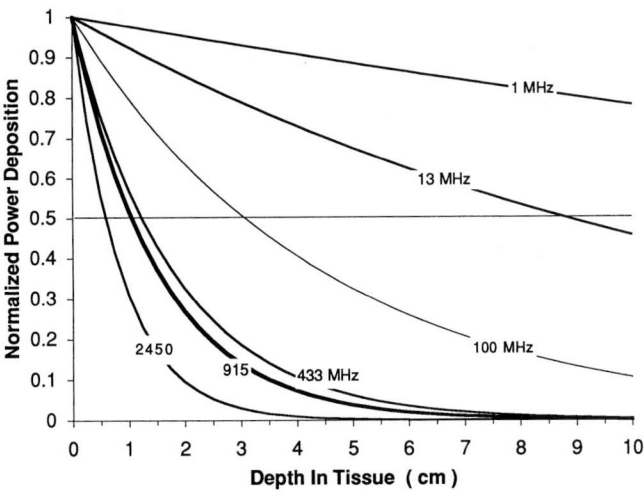

Figure 70–5. Electromagnetic plane wave penetration in muscle tissue as a function of frequency, showing deeper penetration with lower frequency.

and penetration depths of EM waves in air, muscle, and fat are readily available.[140,141]

ULTRASOUND POWER DEPOSITION

Unlike EM radiation, ultrasound (US) energy propagates through tissue as a traveling pressure wave. Variations in pressure from the alternating compressive and expansive forces cause tissue molecules to vibrate and collide, producing heat from mechanical friction within the molecular structure. As a result of these losses, US energy within the pressure wave is attenuated exponentially as it propagates through homogeneous tissue such that the acoustic pressure $P = P_0 e^{-\alpha x}$, where α is the amplitude attenuation coefficient, x is the distance into tissue, and P_0 is the initial pressure at the surface. The acoustic intensity (the rate of energy flow through a unit area) $I = P^2/(2\rho c_s)$ where ρ is the tissue mass density and c_s is the acoustic wave velocity, or speed of sound in tissue. Thus, the acoustic power deposition, or absorbed power density

$$\text{APD} = -dI/dx = 2\alpha I = \alpha P^2/(\rho c_s)$$
$$\text{in watts per cubic meter}$$

and

$$\text{SAR} = \text{APD}/\rho \text{ in watts per kilogram.}$$

Figure 70-6 shows the penetration depth characteristics of US in homogenous muscle tissue as a function of frequency, assuming well-behaved plane wave radiation. Higher frequencies result in more superficial localization of power and lower frequencies result in deeper penetration. For practical hyperthermia transducers, the target volume usually appears in the transducer near field, where there are marked fluctuations in beam intensity both longitudinally in the direction of propagation as well as across the wavefront as opposed to much smoother inverse-square-law longitudinal decay of intensity in the far field. Reflections, scattering, and thermal conduction within the tissue are relied upon to smooth the temperature distribution that results from the peaky SAR. Nonfocused applicators operating at about 3.5 MHz

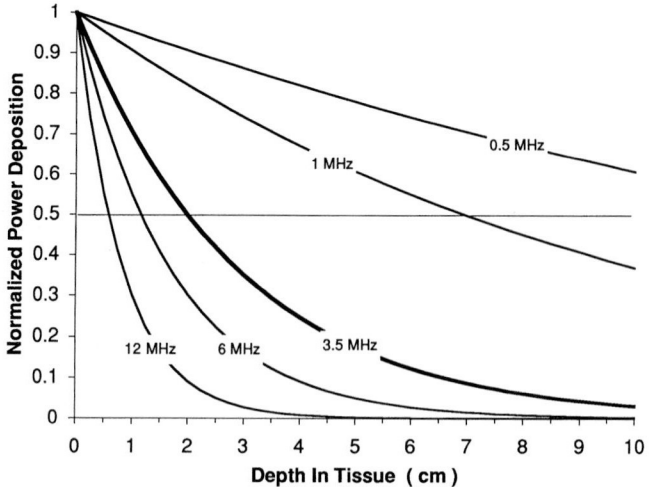

Figure 70–6. Ultrasound plane wave penetration in muscle tissue as a function of frequency, showing deeper penetration with lower frequency.

can heat tumors up to 4 to 6 cm in depth.[142] Nonfocused applicators operating at lower frequencies generally produce increased pain due to unavoidable absorption in underlying bone. Deeper penetration is made possible by directing the US beams to avoid bone and air interfaces, using a larger acoustic window at the surface, and focusing the US beams to increase the power density at depth, relative to that at the skin surface.

Because the speed of sound (c_s) is orders of magnitude lower than the speed of light, the wavelength (λ) of US radiation $\lambda = c_s/f$ in tissue over the frequency (f) range of interest (0.5 to 10 MHz) is 0.1 to 3 mm. With such small wavelengths, US beams are easily focused into very small volumes at depth. With care, treatment of larger volumes may be accomplished by using mechanically or electrically scanned focal spots or by using multiple beams aimed at different locations within the target volume.

The characteristic acoustic impedance $Z = \rho c_s$ is an important parameter in determining the behavior of US at tissue interfaces. The Zs of most soft tissues are quite similar, so there is little reflective loss during the propagation of US from one soft tissue to another. However, the Z values for bone, air, and lung are considerably different from those of soft tissues, causing almost complete reflection at soft tissue–gas interfaces and both reflection and rapid absorption of the transmitted portion of the wave at soft tissue–bone interfaces.[143] A tabulation of acoustic properties of tissues and more in-depth coverage of US interactions with tissue are available.[140,141,144]

Because of the problem of reflection of US energy at air interfaces, it is critical to carefully couple US energy into the body through degassed water and a thin layer of US coupling gel, with elimination of all air pockets and bubbles between the source and tumor. For US frequencies below about 1.5 MHz, a second water bag coupled with gel to the skin at the exit beam site may be necessary. Ultrasound reflection at air interfaces may be turned to an advantage to block out critical normal tissues located close to the desired target (e.g., the mandible adjacent to a neck mass) by intentionally drying off the skin surface and placing a 3 to 5 mm layer of closed cell foam (e.g., common plastic packing material) on the skin surface under the applicator and over areas to be protected.

Heating Equipment and Techniques

Over the past 2 decades, hyperthermia equipment has evolved with a consistent trend toward more complex systems with expanded treatment flexibility. Many unique devices have resulted and may be classified as local (external, interstitial, or intracavitary), regional, or whole body heating techniques. Select representative devices are mentioned in the following section.

EXTERNAL LOCAL HEATING

The largest development effort has gone into producing local heating devices. Electromagnetic techniques have generally been used for superficial tumors less than or equal to 3 cm in depth, such as chest wall recurrence of breast carcinoma, whereas US beams are useful for tumors up to about 6 cm deep.[140,145-148]

Electromagnetic Techniques

The most basic applicator design used in clinical hyperthermia has been the single-aperture MW waveguide. An MW radiator mounted within a waveguide (a tubular or rectangular structure for guiding EM waves) radiates EM waves out the waveguide opening *(aperture)*. Commercial applicators have been available in various sizes from 7.5 to 24 cm on a side, normally operated at 915 MHz or around 430 MHz. The effective heating area, expressed as the area at 50% or greater of the maximal SAR, typically covers only 30% to 60% of the applicator face, with the high-SAR "hot spots" located centrally surrounded by a "cool" periphery.[149,150] These single-aperture waveguide devices are useful for only small superficial tumors up to about 3 cm in diameter.[8] One group has placed variable absorption bolus pads in front of the aperture to reduce SAR centrally and achieve a larger area of effective heating.[151] The HTS-100 Lens Applicator has movable metal plate "vanes" within the concave opening of a single aperture to form convergent 430 MHz beams for heating small tumors up to 3 to 5 cm deep.[152]

Various approaches have been taken to build applicators capable of heating larger areas, such as computer-controlled motorized scanning of one or two spiral microstrip MW antennas repetitively over the target surface[153] or robotically scanned air-coupled MW antennas[154] with thermal feedback control systems. Alternatively, several groups have developed multiaperture array applicators for large-area superficial disease such as the Microtherm 1000, a 16-element planar 915 MHz waveguide array (Fig. 70-7)[155]; and a slightly deeper heating array of 433 MHz Lucite Cone Applicators.[156] Other more flexible large-area MW array applicators have been constructed and used clinically, including hinged 433 MHz Current Sheet Applicators,[157] the 915 MHz 25-element "microwave blanket" spiral microstrip conformal array,[158] and the 915 MHz Conformal Microwave Array

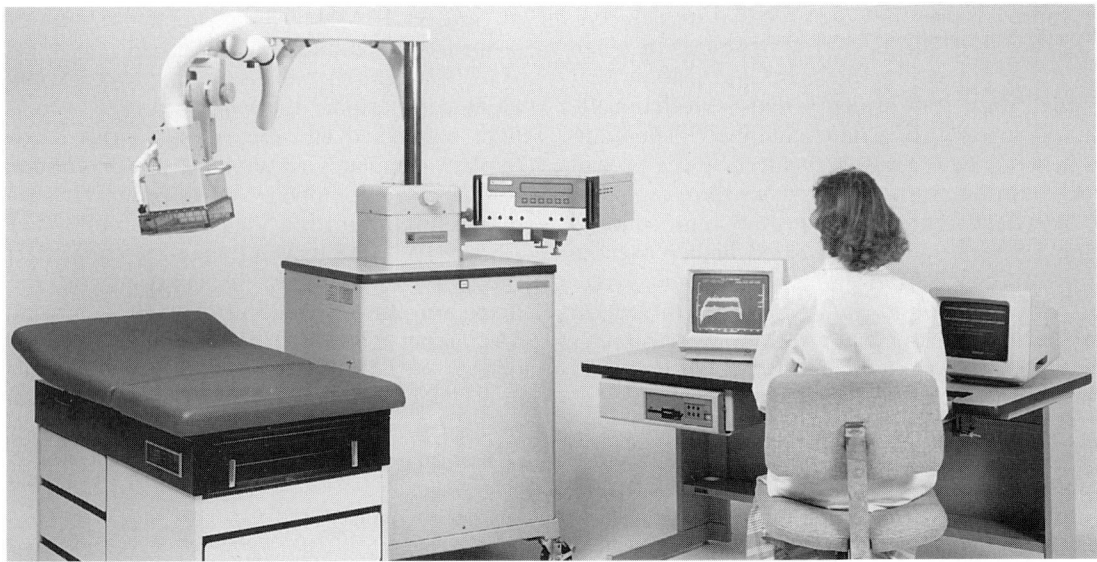

Figure 70–7. The "Microtherm 1000" superficial microwave heating device with a 16-aperture 4 × 4 array applicator to vary power deposition over a 15 × 15 cm area. The applicator is coupled to the patient through a temperature-controlled water bolus. (Photo courtesy of Labthermics Technologies, Inc.)

applicator.[148,159] Figure 70-8 shows a 6 mm thick custom water bolus vest and printed circuit board Conformal Microwave Array applicator being set up on a patient with chest wall recurrence of breast carcinoma extending across the left upper back and shoulder. The patient is shown at right with an elastic overgarment to secure the applicator in place, allowing the patient to stand, sit, or lie down during treatment. This applicator is essentially transparent to photon and electron radiation and thus may be used to apply heat simultaneously with radiation. Recent developments are beginning to produce EM applicators with the capability of noninvasive thermal monitoring of subsurface temperature for feedback control of the multiple apertures.[160-163]

Ultrasound Techniques

Early efforts to apply US for superficial heating applications used single round disk "piston" style transducers operating at 0.5 to 3.5 MHz.[164] These devices were capable of heating only small superficial lesions less than 3 cm in diameter.[8] Later, multitransducer arrays were constructed to increase the lateral extent and control of heating. The Sonotherm 1000 is one such device with 16 individual transducers arranged in a 15 cm square 4 × 4 element planar array coupled to the patient with an attached degassed water bolus bag.[142] This device has been used successfully to heat tumors up to 4 to 6 cm in depth.

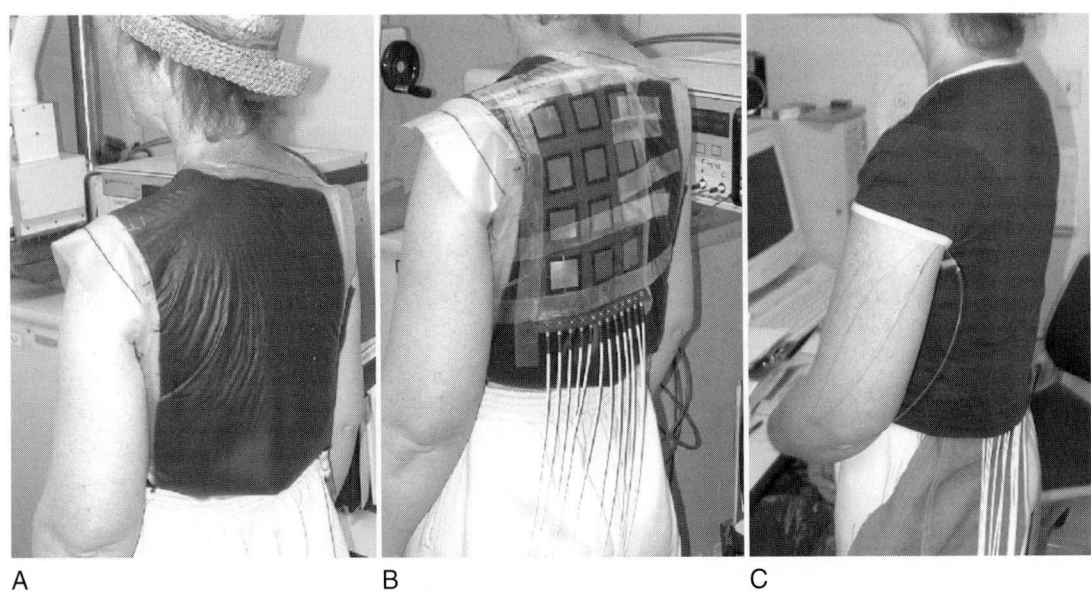

A   B   C

Figure 70–8. Custom CMA applicator treatment setup showing 6 mm thick 42.5°C circulating water bolus vest **(A)**, 12-aperture flexible printed circuit board CMA applicator over large area back lesion **(B)**, and patient undergoing hyperthermia treatment with CMA applicator as monitored with fiberoptic sensors mapped through catheters on the skin surface **(C)**.

Another approach uses arrays of focused transducers. The Scanned Focused Ultrasound system uses a small number of low-frequency transducers (≤1 MHz) that produce a small focal spot at depth that is mechanically scanned rapidly around the tumor volume.[165] The addition of less penetrating 4 MHz transducers and a patient pain feedback button to turn off power for short segments of the scan path have improved the heating uniformity of this scanning US technique and yielded higher average tumor temperatures.[166] In order to heat even larger regions up to 8 cm wide and up to 12 to 15 cm deep in the body, systems have been built with a larger number of transducers having spatially close but offset focal spots, such as the 30-transducer Helios[167] and the 56-transducer Focused Segmented Ultrasound Machine,[168] and the Cylindrical-Section Array[169] and Spherical Section Array[170] applicators, which can synthesize and electronically scan multiple focused beams simultaneously. These large transducer arrays require a large entrance window with minimal air or bone in the US beam paths. Another innovative US system has a computer-controlled scanning reflector for distributing US energy at two different frequencies over large surface areas.[171] With only water and Plexiglas over the tumor surface, this system allows simultaneous HT and RT.[172]

INTERSTITIAL LOCAL HEATING

For applications requiring precise localization of heat in regions that are too difficult to access externally, there are at least nine distinctly different interstitial heating techniques. Excellent reviews are available.[140,145,147,173]

Interstitial Microwave Antennas

Interstitial MW antennas are usually constructed from flexible or semi-rigid coaxial cable less than 1.5 mm in diameter that fits snugly inside afterloading plastic implant catheters. The most common types are *dipole* antennas, which can be used in phased arrays to enlarge the heated volume,[173-175] and *helical coil* antennas, which tend to restrict heating more effectively to the region immediately surrounding the active coil length of the antenna.[176,177] Frequencies between 433 and 2450 MHz are normally used for interstitial MW heating of tumors up to 5 cm across. Radial penetration of heating may be extended by several millimeters with air or water cooling of the implanted antenna surface, but generally the antennas should be placed within 1.5 to 2 cm from each other. Implantable MW antennas have been most useful in high-perfusion tissues or when nonparallel or flexible catheter implants are required. Recent developments have produced interstitial MW antennas with integrated MW radiometry for real-time monitoring of temperature around each antenna.[178,179]

Radiofrequency Electrode Systems

Radiofrequency electrode systems heat tissue with resistively or capacitively coupled electric currents between implanted metal electrodes. Initial work used arrays of implant needles up to 20 cm long spaced 1 to 1.25 cm apart connected to a single RF power amplifier operating at under 1 MHz. Subsequent systems used time-sequenced, computer-controlled *localized current field* (LCF) sources that distributed power to multiple electrode pairs around the implant array.[147] Newer systems with segmented RF electrodes,[180] printed circuit board implant templates to simplify power connections, and sophisticated computer-control programs allow simultaneous long-duration heat and brachytherapy.[147,181] Above 10 MHz, current may be coupled capacitively through a thin layer of insulating plastic, resulting in a more uniform distribution of heating current, as in the 64-channel 27.12 MHz capacitively coupled radiofrequency (CC-RF) electrode system.[137,182] For both LCF and CC-RF systems, the radial falloff of power deposition is extremely sharp so that implant spacing is limited to less than 1.25 to 1.5 cm.[183]

Hot Source Techniques

Because the penetration of thermally conducted heat energy is limited, hot source techniques are appropriate only for tissues with low to moderate perfusion that can be implanted with closely spaced arrays of implants—generally no more than 1.0 to 1.25 cm apart. However, heating length is almost unlimited. Hot source techniques include hot water perfusion (HWP) through implanted catheters,[147,181] resistive wire (RW) implants heated by computer-controlled direct current voltage sources,[184] and ferromagnetic implants (FMI) (special high-permeability alloys that are heated by an externally applied magnetic field at less than 1 MHz and that automatically thermoregulate over a narrow range of temperature due to steep Curie point transitions from a magnetic to a nonmagnetic state.[185-187] The HWP and RW techniques have been adapted to allow simultaneous hyperthermia and brachytherapy. The FMI technique simplifies reheating of permanent implants because no externalized connections are required for either power or thermal monitoring of the thermoregulating ferroseeds.[188]

Interstitial Ultrasound Applicators

Interstitial US applicators appear close to revolutionizing interstitial HT delivery for many sites. Linear arrays of 0.5 to 1 cm long tubular transducers have been constructed either with water cooling[189,190] or direct coupled sources with an open central lumen to accommodate brachytherapy sources for simultaneous thermobrachytherapy.[191] Implant spacing up to 2.5 cm apart should be possible for the water-cooled version. These applicators allow precise power control along the implant length as well as radially directional heating capability. Recently, implantable US arrays have been used for treatment with real-time noninvasive MRI monitoring of both temperature and tissue property changes during heating.[192]

INTRACAVITARY LOCAL HEATING

A number of site-specific EM- and US-powered devices have been developed for inducing local HT around natural body cavities such as the esophagus, vagina, urethra, and rectum for esophageal and pelvic tumors using dipole MW antennas,[193] tapered diameter dipole antennas,[194] helical coil antennas,[195] and segmented multi-element intracavitary US applicators such as the 8-element transrectal ultrasound (TRUS) applicator[196] and cylindrical phased array intracavitary applicators with up to sixty-four 0.5 to 1 MHz US transducers.[197,198]

REGIONAL HEATING

The most common regional heating approaches involve the use of radiated EM fields in the frequency range of 10 to 100 MHz where the wavelength in tissue is large compared to the height of the human body, so that focusing of heat to a small region within the torso is generally not possible. These techniques are intended to heat a large region and usually produce temperatures of about 39°C to 41°C throughout the tumor, limited by power deposition in surrounding normal tissues.

Early regional heating devices included the single large 27 MHz Ridged Waveguide aperture[199] and the single 82 MHz torso-sized Helix coil.[200] With the newer 70 MHz Coaxial TEM Applicator, the entire patient is positioned inside a hollow 60 cm diameter chamber filled with coupling water, and partial steering of SAR is possible by shifting the patient's position within the chamber.[201,202] Another single-channel deep-heating technique uses 8 to 27 MHz RF capacitive heating, such as the Thermotron RF-8.[203] This device creates an electric field between two saline bolus-coupled metal plate electrodes on opposite sides of the patient. Heating is maximum in the fat layer, but this problem can be overcome with aggressive skin cooling in patients with a fat layer less than 1 to 2 cm thick.[204] Limited steering of power deposition is possible through electrode placement and by using a smaller electrode on one side to concentrate heating.

It is possible to increase heating at depth by using an array of phase-focused radiating apertures. The first commercial device built for this approach was the Annular Phased Array, which consisted of an array of eight equal-power, equal-phase radiators mounted on the surface of a large cylinder coupled tightly around the body torso with a refillable distilled water bolus.[205] Subsequent development of the 60 to 120 MHz Sigma 60 applicator shown in Figure 70-9 improved the patient interface and increased control flexibility via four independent relative phase and amplitude controls for the eight radiators.[206] A similar device, the Matched Phased Array system, has four large 70 MHz waveguide sources with flexible positioning as well as phase and amplitude steering of power deposition in the body.[207] Treatment-planning systems have been developed to take advantage of this control flexibility and improve regional heating.[208] Although these regional heating devices are still in clinical use, newer systems are now available such as the 100 MHz Sigma Eye applicator with 12 independently controlled radiator pairs in three rings to allow phase and amplitude steering both longitudinally and radially within the body.[209] At the Charité Medical School in Berlin, a hybrid system integrating the Sigma Eye applicator with both magnetic resonance imaging (MRI) and treatment planning systems began clinical operation in late 2001. This hybrid system allows MRI-based preplanning as well as noninvasive monitoring of thermal estimations

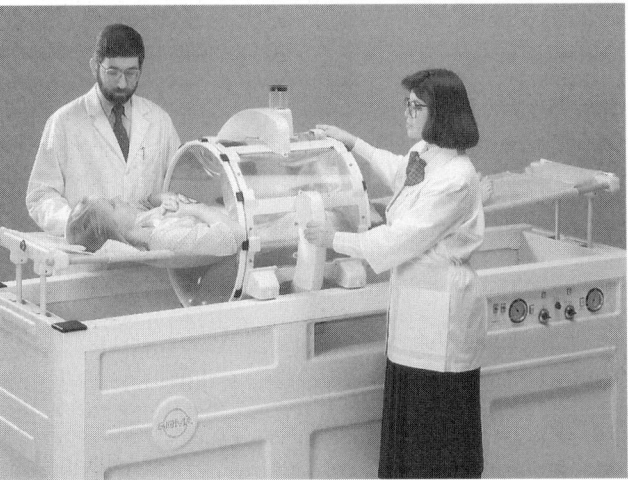

Figure 70–9. The "Sigma 60" deep regional heating device with eight dipole antennas mounted concentrically around a 60-cm diameter cylinder and driven at about 80 MHz. Phase and amplitude can be adjusted independently for each quadrant (pair of dipoles) to steer power deposition at depth. (Photo courtesy of BSD Medical Corp.)

during HT, where the quantity measured represents a mixture of temperature and perfusion.[210]

WHOLE BODY HEATING

Whole-body heating produces the most uniform tumor heating, regardless of tumor location within the body. The disadvantages are the significant systemic stress exerted by whole-body heating, the lack of preferential tumor heating, and the fact that temperatures are limited to about 41.8°C to 42°C[211,212] because of thermosensitivity of critical tissues such as heart, lung, liver, and brain. Systemic heating has generally been accomplished by noninvasive means such as immersion in hot fluids like water or molten wax, enclosure of the patient in a radiant heat chamber with infrared or water-RF heat input, or entirely wrapping the patient in hot water blankets. Several groups have used supplemental RF regional heating devices. Invasive heating methods include extracorporeal circulation of heated blood through an exteriorized arterial-venous shunt or intraperitoneal irrigation with heated fluid. For all of these techniques, normal body-cooling mechanisms such as respiration and contact of skin with room temperature air must be blocked by preheating the patient's breathing circuit and thermally insulating the patient. The patient is often anesthetized or sedated and physiological conditions must be carefully monitored and controlled throughout the treatment, which often extends over many hours.[140,145]

Thermometry and Quality Assurance

Appropriate monitoring of tissue temperature during hyperthermia is an essential component of therapy, and successful analyses correlating tumor response with thermal parameters require detailed knowledge of tumor temperature distributions. Three excellent reviews of thermometry techniques are available.[145,146,213]

INVASIVE THERMOMETRY TECHNIQUES

Thermocouple probes are one of the primary monitoring techniques for clinical hyperthermia because of their low cost, simple operation, interchangeability, small size, and accuracy of ± 0.2°C to 0.3°C, which remains stable over many years. The most common copper-constantan probes produce significant (>2°C) thermal conduction smearing of high thermal gradients, so that many users have switched to manganin-constantan thermocouples that have lower thermal smearing errors.[140,214,215] Small-diameter bare wire, fused silica, or metal needle-encased thermocouples are preferred for thermometry in US fields due to minimal self-heating and field perturbation effects. With appropriate filtering, shielding, and orientation of wires perpendicular to the electric field, thermocouples may be used with caution in RF fields but are generally not recommended for use in MW fields.[216]

Fiberoptic probes consist of plastic or glass fibers with a nonmetallic temperature-sensing element at one to seven locations along the fibers. Current systems provide essentially artifact-free readout of temperature even in the most intense EM fields but are prone to drifting (0.5°C to 1°C/day) and must be calibrated before each heat treatment to maintain accuracy within ± 0.2°C to 0.3°C over a 2- to 3-hour interval. Because the fiberoptic probes are fragile, they are generally inserted into soft plastic catheters that may be left in the tumor between heat treatments. For use in US fields, fiberoptic probes can be inserted inside small-gauge metal needles to minimize probe self-heating.[142]

After careful calibration, high-resistance lead thermistor sensors exhibit very good accuracy and precision and longer-term stability than fiberoptic sensors. Calibration is unique to each sensor so that probes are not interchangeable. These probes have good immunity to electric readout artifacts but produce some minor perturbation of MW fields. They are not recommended for US thermometry because of self-heating artifacts and perturbation of the US field. Other probes can directly measure electric field strength, US intensity, or tissue parameters such as thermal conductivity and effective blood perfusion.

Although predominantly fixed-position 1- to 4-sensor implanted temperature probes were used in the early HT trials, later studies generally report a much larger number of temperatures recorded from *thermal maps* of temperature measured at 0.25 to 1 cm spaced increments along catheters located both at depth in tumor and on the skin surface.[140] These temperature profiles are obtained manually or via automated thermal mapping systems.[217] Radiation Therapy Oncology Group (RTOG) thermometry guidelines recommend that temperatures be mapped along each probe track at least once every 10 minutes, in increments of no more than 5 mm for tumors less than 5 cm and 1 cm for tumors greater than 5 cm across.[218] Additional quality assurance guidelines specific to interstitial,[219] US,[220] and deep regional heating[203,221,222] provide guidance for recommended number and locations of thermometry probes.

NONINVASIVE THERMOMETRY TECHNIQUES

A number of noninvasive thermometry techniques are under investigation to allow both improved patient comfort and quantification of more complete temperature distributions. Infrared thermography has been available for years for monitoring complete surface temperature distributions.[154] Methods under development to determine temperatures within tissue include computerized tomography, US time-of-flight tomography, applied potential tomography (sometimes called *electrical impedance tomography*),[213] microwave radiometry,[160,162,178,223] and real-time multi-slice MRI.[224,225] Recent investigations indicate that MRI should be capable of 0.5°C resolution in regions less than or equal to 1 cm³ with scan acquisition times less than 1 minute throughout small or large tumor volumes at depth in the body.[210,226]

CLINICAL RESULTS

Hyperthermia is applied to tumors in combination with RT or chemotherapy or both to improve local control and thereby improve survival or palliation of patients with recurrent or advanced cancers unlikely to be controlled by conventional therapy. Hyperthermia has been used in a wide variety of tumor types and anatomical locations. Local HT has been used extensively for superficial lymph nodes, recurrent or advanced breast cancer, and cutaneous or subcutaneous melanoma metastases. Interstitial HT has been applied to essentially all technically implantable sites, especially gynecological malignancies, prostate cancer, other pelvic tumors, head and neck cancers, breast cancers, and brain tumors. Regional HT has been used primarily for advanced pelvic tumors and for sarcomas of the trunk or extremities. There is a limited but growing experience with whole body HT combined with chemotherapy.

This section reviews clinical experience with HT alone, HT combined with RT, HT combined with chemotherapy, and trimodality therapy. Select studies are described individually in the text; Tables 70-1 to 70-2 provide a more complete listing.

Hyperthermia Alone

Early clinical studies using HT alone for the treatment of small, superficial neoplasms showed that HT alone (using multiple 30 to 60 minute HT sessions) has very limited efficacy. Overgaard[227] summarized the results of 18 such studies including 380 tumors treated with 2 to 22 heat sessions with a CR rate of 13% and a partial response (PR) rate of 36%. The duration of HT responses was generally brief.

Hyperthermia and Radiation

SUPERFICIAL HYPERTHERMIA

Miscellaneous Sites

In the 1970s and 1980s, numerous nonrandomized studies in superficial malignancies showed higher CR rates for RT plus HT in comparison with RT alone (see Table 70-1).[164,228-247] These trials typically used 30- to 60-minute HT sessions one, two, or three times

Table 70–1   Nonrandomized Trials Comparing Radiotherapy to Radiotherapy + Hyperthermia in Superficial Malignancies

First Author	Yr	Lesions, n	Complete Response, n/n (%)	
			RT alone	RT + HT
Miscellaneous Sites				
Arcangeli[228]	1984	52*	11/26* (42)	19/26* (73)
		40*	6/17* (35)	16/23* (70)
		41*	6/16* (38)	18/25* (72)
		30*	5/15* (33)	13/15* (87)
Bey[229]	1984	90*	4/45* (9)	19/45* (42)
Corry[164]	1982	34 (26*)	0/13 (0)	13/21 (62)
Dunlop[230]	1986	77 (52*)	16/32 (50)	27/45 (60)
Hiraoka†[231]	1984	48 (16*)	2/8* (25)	5/8* (63)
				16/32 (50)
Howard[232]	1987	41 (35*)	7/21 (33)	9/20 (45)
Li[233]	1984	124 (62*)	9/31* (29)	21/31* (68)
				29/62 (47)
Lindholm[234]	1987	85 (56*)	7/28* (25)	16/28* (57)
				10/29 (34)
Scott[235]	1984	90 (62*)	12/31* (39)	27/31* (87)
				26/28 (93)
Steeves[236]	1986	90*	11/36* (31)	35/54* (65)
U[237]	1980	25 (14*)	1/7* (14)	6/7* (86)
				8/11 (73)
Neck Lymph Nodes				
Arcangeli[238]	1985	81	18/43 (42)	30/38 (79)
Perez[239]	1989	212	15/88 (17)	45/124 (36)
Valdagni[240]	1986	72	16/45 (36)	16/27 (59)
Chest Wall Recurrence				
González González[241]	1988	54 (18*)	3/9* (33)	7/9* (78)
				20/36 (56)
Kjellén[242]	1989	88 (44*)	6/22* (27)	15/22* (68)
				29/45 (64)
Perez[239]	1989	215	59/116 (51)	69/99 (70)
van der Zee[243]	1984	113 (62*)	17/31 (55)	74/82 (90)
Metastatic Malignant Melanoma				
Arcangeli[244]	1987	38	9/17 (53)	16/21 (76)
González González[245]	1986	46 (20*)	3/8* (38)	10/12* (83)
				9/26 (35)
Kim[246]	1982	99	25/54 (46)	31/45 (69)
Overgaard[247]	1987	99 (25*)	2/10* (20)	11/15* (73)
				18/28 (64)
Perez[239]	1989	116	16/67 (24)	29/49 (59)
TOTAL			339/963 (35)	779/1293 (60)
Same-Patient Comparisons			88/309* (28)	238/351* (68)

*Indicates lesions included in same-patient comparisons.
†Most tumors within 3 to 5 cm deep but 8/40 greater than 5 cm deep.
CR, complete response; RT, radiotherapy; HT, hyperthermia.

weekly. Some of the lesions included in these early studies were paired lesions used for same-patient comparisons (indicated with asterisks in Table 70-1). Results were surprisingly similar among these studies despite a broad range of histologies, RT dose and fractionation, and number of HT treatments. Overall, the CR rate was 35% for 963 lesions treated with RT alone compared with 60% for 1293 lesions treated with RT plus HT. In the same-patient comparisons, the CR rate was 28% for 309 lesions treated with RT alone compared with 68% for

351 lesions treated with RT plus HT, representing more than a doubling of the CR rate. The most frequent toxicity of HT was blisters in about 10% to 23% of patients and rare thermal burns.[239,248] Most studies showed no increase in late radiation effects.

Encouraging results of early nonrandomized trials prompted the RTOG to mount a randomized phase II trial (RTOG 81-04) comparing RT alone (32 Gy in eight fractions over 4 weeks) with RT plus twice-weekly HT (nominally 43°C for 60 minutes) in measurable advanced

Table 70–2 Prospective Randomized Trials Comparing Radiotherapy to Radiotherapy + Hyperthermia

Trial or First Author	Yr	Evaluable Lesions, n	Complete Response, n/n (%)		P Value
			CR Rate for RT Alone	CR Rate for RT + HT	
Miscellaneous Sites					
Egawa[249]	1989	92	18/48 (38)	20/44 (46)	—
RTOG 81-04[8]	1989	218	32/107 (30)	37/111 (33)	NS
	(33% vs. 54% for 48 lesions <3 cm diameter)				
RTOG 84-19[9]	1996	174	47/87 (54)	50/87 (57)	NS
Advanced Head and Neck Cancer					
Datta[10]	1990	52 stage III/IV	3/24 (13)	13/28 (46)	<0.05
Valdagni[13]	1994	40	9/22 (41)	15/18 (83)	0.016
ESHO-2[250]	1995	62	17/32 (53)	15/30 (50)	NS
Advanced Breast Cancer					
ESHO-1/MRC[250]	1995	143	43/67 (64)	54/76 (71)	NS
Chest Wall Recurrence/Advanced or Recurrent Breast Cancer					
ESHO-5/MRC/ DHG/PMH[15]	1996	306	55/135 (41)	101/171 (59)	<0.001
Recurrent or Metastatic Malignant Melanoma					
ESHO-3[11]	1995	128	23/65 (35)	39/63 (62)	<0.05
Advanced Cervix/Rectal/Bladder Cancers					
DDHG[14]	2000	143 (rectal)	11/71 (15)	15/72 (21)	NS
		114 (cervix)	32/56 (57)	48/58 (83)	0.003
		101 (bladder)	25/49 (51)	38/52 (73)	0.01
Harima[270]	2001	40	10/20 (50)	16/20 (80)	0.048
Sharma[274]	1991	42	11/22 (50)	14/20 (70)	—
Berdov[275]	1990	115	9/56 (16)	1/59 (2)	<0.05
TOTAL		1770	345/861 (40)	476/909 (52)	

CR, complete response; RT, radiotherapy; HT, hyperthermia; NS, not significant.

primary, recurrent, or metastatic epithelial or mesenchymal malignancies. Overall, there was no difference in the CR rate for the 107 single lesions treated with RT alone (30%) and for the 111 single lesions treated with RT plus HT (33%) (see Table 70-2).[8] For 48 lesions less than 3 cm in diameter, amenable to adequate HT with the heating equipment available at the time, there was a trend toward improved CR rate for RT plus HT in comparison with RT alone (54% vs. 33%), and the actuarial probability of local control at 1 year was 80% for RT plus HT compared with 15% for RT alone (*P* = 0.02). However, with 78% of lesions entered on the study measuring 3 cm or greater in diameter, the study was negative overall. The resulting report cited poor thermometry and inadequate quality assurance as major factors influencing the outcome of the trial. A large number of the lesions entered were too large or too deep, or both, to be adequately heated

by the existing HT equipment. Furthermore, the thermometry was too limited in many cases to allow for adequate control of treatment delivery or for meaningful subsequent evaluation of the temperature distributions achieved.[8] One positive outcome was the formulation of RTOG quality assurance guidelines for future clinical trials.[218]

In another non–site-specific, prospective, randomized trial comparing RT with RT plus HT for 92 evaluable superficial lesions, the CR rates were 38% versus 45%, and overall response rates 63% versus 82% (*P* < 0.05) for RT versus RT plus HT, respectively. No improvement in the CR rate was observed for patients with head and neck cancer (45% vs. 44%), whereas HT was associated with a doubling of the CR rate for patients with chest wall recurrence of breast cancer (67% vs. 33%).[249]

A trial incorporating careful quality assurance guidelines was recently completed at Duke University in which patients underwent a low-thermal-dose test HT treatment before randomization. Only patients whose tumors were deemed to be adequately heatable were allowed to proceed to randomization into RT-alone or RT-plus-HT arms. Results of this study will be valuable to assess the efficacy of adjuvant HT in the setting of a well-controlled trial with adequate thermal dose.

Advanced or Recurrent Neck Nodes

Results of RT with or without HT for superficially located large, fixed, or recurrent lymph nodes have been reported by Perez and Emami,[239] Valdagni and colleagues,[240] and Arcangeli and colleagues,[238] with CR rates of 17%, 36%, and 42% for RT alone versus 36%, 59%, and 79% for RT plus HT, respectively (see Table 70-1). By plotting dose-response curves for RT and RT plus HT from available published and unpublished observations, Overgaard[7] estimated a TER of 1.6 for advanced neck nodes.

Several prospective, randomized trials have been performed for head and neck cancers (see Table 70-2). Datta and colleagues[10] reported on 65 patients with head and neck carcinomas treated with 60 to 65 Gy at 2.0 Gy per daily fraction with or without twice-weekly HT. Overall, the CR rate was 10 of 32 (31%) for RT versus 18 of 33 (55%) for RT plus HT. Hyperthermia appeared to benefit only stage III and stage IV patients, in whom the CR rate was 3 of 24 (13%) for RT alone versus 13 of 28 (46%) for RT plus HT. Another prospective, randomized trial compared RT alone (64 to 70 Gy at 2 to 2.5 Gy per fraction) to RT plus HT in 44 fixed, inoperable squamous cell carcinoma neck nodes. The CR rate at 3 months was 9 of 22 (41%) for RT alone versus 15 of 18 (83%) for RT plus HT, without increased toxicity.[12,13] Long-term follow-up of the study showed significantly improved 5-year actuarial nodal control ($P = 0.015$) and 5-year survival ($P = 0.02$).[13] On the other hand, the later European Society for Hyperthermic Oncology (ESHO) trial for advanced neck nodes showed no difference in CR rate or local control for RT versus RT plus HT (53% vs. 50% and 33% vs. 31%, respectively).[250]

Chest Wall Recurrence and Locally Advanced Breast Cancer

Local control of chest wall recurrences of breast cancer probably does not affect survival, but it can profoundly improve quality of life. Promising results were obtained in nonrandomized trials by combining HT with RT for the treatment of chest wall lesions with or without prior RT (see Table 70-1). González González and colleagues,[241] Kjellén and colleagues,[242] Lindholm and colleagues,[234] Perez and Emami,[239] Scott and colleagues,[235] and van der Zee and colleagues[243] reported CR rates of 27% to 55% for RT versus 60% to 94% for RT plus HT. By plotting dose-response curves for RT versus RT plus HT from available published and unpublished observations, Overgaard[7] estimated the TER to be 1.5 for breast cancer chest wall recurrence.

A multi-institutional, prospective, randomized experience has been reported from the Medical Research Council (MRC) of Great Britain, ESHO, the Dutch Hyperthermia Group (DHG), and Princess Margaret Hospital in Toronto (see Table 70-2).[15] Each institution had planned independent, prospective, randomized trials for patients with chest wall recurrence of breast cancer or T3 to T4 primary breast cancer, but because the goals were similar and better accrual was desired, the studies were combined into one joint trial. The RT schemes used included 28.8 Gy at 3.6 Gy per fraction over 2 weeks with HT weekly, 32 Gy at 4 Gy per fraction over 4 weeks with HT once or twice weekly, 32 Gy at 1.8 Gy per fraction with two HT treatments, and 40 to 50 Gy at 2 to 3 Gy per fraction with a total of two to eight HT treatments. Of 306 evaluable lesions in 306 patients, 216 (71%) were on the chest wall, 79 (26%) were in breast tissue, and 11 were in lymph nodes. Thirty were primary breast cancers, 66 were recurrences without prior RT, and 210 were recurrences in the setting of previous RT. Adjuvant HT resulted in significantly improved response, with a CR rate of 41% in 135 lesions treated with RT alone versus 59% in 171 lesions treated with RT plus HT, and an odds ratio for CR of 2.3 overall after stratification by trial. Patients with recurrent lesions in previously irradiated areas appeared to benefit the most from HT.[15] An analysis of 120 of the HT patients with recurrent breast cancer demonstrated a significant association between response and the cumulative minimum thermal dose over all HT treatments; the CR rate was 77% for CEM 43° T_{min} greater than 10 minutes versus 43% for CEM 43° T_{min} less than or equal to 10 minutes.[30] A separate multivariate analysis of 101 patients treated on the MRC trials for intact or recurrent breast cancers showed that the most important nonthermal parameters associated with a decreased probability of CR included greater tumor depth ($P = 0.001$), the use of a palliative as opposed to a curative radiotherapy regimen ($P = 0.005$), and presence or history of disease outside the treated area ($P = 0.010$).[251] Tumor area was not a significant prognostic covariate. Higher CEM 43° T_{min} over the first, second, and third HT treatments was consistently significantly associated with a greater probability of CR in various models tested. Among 74 recurrent tumors, the CR rates were 44%, 69%, 75%, and 80% for CEM 43° T_{min} less than 10, 10 to 20, 20 to 30, and at least 30 minutes, respectively.

Metastatic Malignant Melanoma

Melanoma recurrences in the skin or metastases to skin, subcutaneous sites, or superficial lymph nodes are often amenable to HT, and control rates are generally inadequate with RT alone. Results of nonrandomized trials are shown in Table 70-1. Arcangeli and associates,[244] González González and associates,[245] Kim and associatess,[246] Overgaard and Overgaard,[247] and Perez and Emami[239] reported CR rates of 24% to 53% for RT alone versus 50% to 76% for RT plus HT. Overgaard[7] estimated the TER to be 1.6 for malignant melanoma.

A prospective, randomized trial comparing RT to RT plus HT for metastatic or recurrent melanoma (ESHO-3) randomized 134 lesions to receive 24 or 27 Gy in three fractions over 8 days with or without HT (with a goal of 43°C for 60 minutes) after each RT fraction. Of the 128 evaluable lesions, the CR rate was 35% for RT alone versus 62% for RT plus HT ($P < 0.05$) (see Table 70-2), and the 2-year actuarial local control was 28% for RT versus 46% for RT plus HT ($P = 0.008$). A stepwise logistic regression analysis showed that HT ($P = 0.0015$), smaller tumor size ($P = 0.0048$), and higher RT dose ($P = 0.049$) were significantly associated with CR.[11]

INTERSTITIAL HYPERTHERMIA

Miscellaneous Sites

For the major nonrandomized interstitial hyperthermia (IHT) trials for head and neck, breast, pelvic, and other sites, CR rates have ranged from 38% to 88%.[252] The IHT was generally given for 1 hour immediately before brachytherapy, and usually immediately after brachytherapy, as well. An excellent review article on IHT is available.[253]

A prospective, randomized RTOG trial (RTOG 84-19) for recurrent or advanced tumors comparing interstitial radiotherapy (IRT) with IRT plus IHT accrued 173 evaluable patients from 1986 to 1992. No differences between the two arms were observed in terms of CR rates (54% vs. 57%) (see Table 70-2) or survival (2-year survival 34% vs. 35%). It was noted that only one patient met minimal criteria for "adequate" HT and that substantial technical advances to improve heat delivery were needed.[9] Lesions less than 4 cm in diameter showed a trend toward improved CR rate in the HT arm (74% for IRT plus IHT vs. 58% for IRT; $P = 0.11$). The trial did have a positive impact in terms of prompting the RTOG to develop quality assurance guidelines for IHT.[219]

Malignant Gliomas

For a long time, there was considerable interest in combining IHT with brachytherapy to improve local control of malignant gliomas. Although normal brain tolerance to HT is very limited, patient tolerance to HT is excellent due to the lack of pain sensation in the brain. Phase I/II brain HT trials are summarized elsewhere.[254] Because of the difficulty in distinguishing radiation necrosis from tumor, survival results are often reported rather than response rates.

Sneed and colleagues[255,256] performed multivariate analyses to determine parameters associated with improved freedom from local tumor progression and survival among 25 patients with recurrent glioblastoma and 16 with recurrent anaplastic astrocytoma treated with thermoradiotherapy. They found that minimum tumor temperature and T_{90} were the only significant factors predicting freedom from local tumor progression. The median freedom from local tumor progression was 38 weeks for gliomas heated to a T_{90} of at least 41.5°C versus 18 weeks for those heated to a T_{90} less than 41.5°C ($P < 0.001$). A multivariate analysis stratifying by histological type showed that age ($P = 0.04$) and T_{90}

($P = 0.04$) were also significant prognostic factors for survival. For patients with glioblastoma, the median survival was 63 weeks for a T_{90} of at least 41.2°C versus 38 weeks for a T_{90} less than 41.2°C ($P = 0.008$).

Stea and colleagues retrospectively compared implant alone to implant with IHT in patients with primary or recurrent malignant gliomas treated with brachytherapy boost or brachytherapy for recurrence.[257] On multivariate analysis, three parameters were significantly associated with improved survival: lower patient age ($P < 0.0001$), anaplastic astrocytoma versus glioblastoma ($P = 0.023$), and adjuvant HT ($P = 0.0487$). The median survival from the date of diagnosis was 35.1 months for patients who received HT versus 22.3 months for those who did not.

A prospective, randomized phase II/III trial was performed at the University of California San Francisco for 112 patients with newly diagnosed glioblastoma.[258] Patients were registered postoperatively, treated with focal RT (59.4 Gy at 1.8 Gy per daily fraction) with oral hydroxyurea, and then randomized to a 60 Gy brachytherapy boost with or without IHT (42.5°C for 30 minutes immediately before and after brachytherapy). Primarily owing to tumor progression, 33 patients were never randomized and 11 randomized patients never underwent brachytherapy. Comparing the 33 brachytherapy and 35 brachytherapy plus IHT patients, the median time to progression was 33 versus 49 weeks ($P = 0.045$), the median survival times were 76 versus 85 weeks ($P = 0.02$), and the 2-year survival probabilities were 15% versus 31%, respectively. A multivariate analysis adjusting for age and Karnofsky performance status showed significantly improved survival probability for the IHT arm ($P = 0.008$ with a hazard ratio of 0.51). Toxicity was acceptable, with six grade 3 toxicities on the IHT arm, one grade 3 toxicity on the brachytherapy-alone arm, and one grade 4 toxicity on each arm.

Long-Duration, Simultaneous Thermoradiotherapy

Because the greatest radiosensitization occurs when HT and RT are delivered simultaneously, several groups are investigating simultaneous external beam RT and superficial HT[172] or simultaneous brachytherapy and IHT. Forty-four patients with recurrent superficial tumors were treated on phase I/II studies with simultaneous superficial 41°C HT and RT at Mallinckrodt Institute of Radiology.[259] The CR rate was 51% and slow-healing soft tissue ulcers were noted in 10 of 47 sites treated (21%), perhaps suggesting increased toxicity compared with sequential HT and RT. In vitro studies suggest that low-temperature (41°C), continuous, long-duration heat applied simultaneously with continuous low-dose-rate radiation or pulsed high-dose-rate radiation may maximize radiosensitization.[103,260] Preliminary results for long-duration interstitial thermoradiotherapy of advanced, bulky pelvic malignancies have been promising. At William Beaumont Hospital, 20 patients with persistent or recurrent pelvic tumors had simultaneous low-dose-rate brachytherapy with long-duration continuous 41°C interstitial HT using a computer-controlled RF-LCF system. The CR and overall response rates were 74% and

95% (vs. 50% and 57% in patients at the same institution who had standard sequential interstitial RT plus HT) (Corry, personal communication).

REGIONAL HYPERTHERMIA

Regional HT treatments are often limited by local pain or systemic stress or both, frequently resulting in tumor temperatures below the desired range, although treatment tolerance improves with each successive generation of regional heating devices. In 119 patients treated with RT and 8 MHz RF capacitive heating, the average T_{min} and T_{max} were 39.3°C and 41.4°C, respectively. With the Annular Phased Array and the Sigma 60 applicators, the T_{min}, T_{90}, and T_{max} tumor temperatures achieved averaged 39.3°C to 39.5°C, 39.9°C to 40.1°C, and 42.5°C to 42.9°C, respectively.[261,262] For 772 BSD 2000 regional HT sessions in 190 patients with pelvic tumors, the mean T_{90} and T_{max} were 40.2°C and 41.6°C, respectively.[263]

Response rates have varied widely in the major nonrandomized regional HT trials. One large multi-institutional series reported 10% CRs and 17% PRs.[264] A later RTOG trial of radiotherapy plus regional HT including 66 patients treated predominantly with the BSD 2000 system achieved CR in 34% of patients and PR in 16% of patients.[265] Response was strongly associated with radiation dose but not with maximum tumor temperature.

In general, regional HT is better tolerated and produces better response rates for pelvic than abdominal tumors, although it has also been applied with some apparent success for advanced lung cancers,[266] especially those in contact with the chest wall.[267] Major improvements, including a larger number of heating elements, better phase and amplitude control of the heating elements,[209] flexible patient positioning, and sophisticated three-dimensional computed tomography-based[208] or MRI-based[210] HT treatment-planning software, should allow higher tumor temperatures and even better patient tolerance in the future. Comprehensive quality assurance guidelines have also been published covering treatment planning, the treatment process, treatment documentation, equipment, and safety.[268]

Despite heating limitations, regional HT significantly improved local control and survival in patients with advanced cervical cancer in a phase III prospective, randomized multi-center trial performed by the Dutch Deep Hyperthermia Group.[14] From 1990 through 1996, 358 evaluable patients with T2 to T4 bladder cancer; stage IIB, IIIB, or IV cervical cancer; or locally advanced or recurrent rectal cancer were randomized to conventional RT (including brachytherapy boost for cervical cancer patients when feasible) with or without weekly regional HT for a total of five HT treatments. The respective CR rates for RT compared with RT plus HT were 39% versus 55% overall ($P = 0.0003$), 15% versus 21% among 143 rectal cancer patients (not significant), 57% versus 83% among 114 cervical cancer patients ($P = 0.003$), and 51% versus 73% among 101 bladder cancer patients ($P = 0.01$). The 3-year local control rates for RT versus RT plus HT were 26% and 38% overall, 8% and 16% for rectal cancer, 41% and 61% for cervical cancer, and 33% and 42% for bladder cancer, respectively. Survival was not significantly different between RT and RT plus HT groups except in the case of cervical cancer, for which 3-year survival probabilities were 27% after RT alone versus 51% after RT plus HT ($P = 0.009$). An associated economic evaluation of the Rotterdam experience indicated that adjuvant HT was cost-effective in cervical cancer patients.[269]

A smaller prospective, randomized trial showed that regional HT using 8 MHz RF capacitive regional HT significantly improved local control in patients with stage IIIB cervical cancer treated with external beam radiotherapy plus high-dose-rate brachytherapy.[270] The CR rate was 50% for 20 patients treated with RT alone versus 80% for 20 patients treated with RT plus HT. The 3-year local relapse-free survival and overall survival probabilities for RT versus RT plus HT were 58% versus 64% (not significant) and 50% versus 80% ($P = 0.048$), respectively.

WHOLE BODY HYPERTHERMIA

Whole body temperatures of about 41.8°C to 42.0°C for 2 hours can be tolerated by mildly sedated patients with acceptable toxicity, commonly including acute thrombocytopenia and granulocytosis, mild hypotension, and occasional pulmonary edema.[271] There has also been recent interest in fever-range whole body hyperthermia (WBH) using temperatures of 39°C to 40°C for 3 to 6 hours.[272] In either case, WBH is generally combined with chemotherapy for treatment of advanced systemic disease, as discussed in the section on "Hyperthermia and Chemotherapy," and there is rationale for combining WBH with immunotherapy.[273]

SUMMARY OF RANDOMIZED HUMAN STUDIES OF RT AND HT

Table 70-2 summarizes major published prospective, randomized human hyperthermia trials of RT with or without HT.[8-12,14,15,249,250,270,274,275] More than 1700 patients were treated with a CR rate of 40% for RT alone versus 52% for RT plus HT. Overgaard[276] performed a meta-analysis of 22 known trials, comparing the risk of failure for patients treated with RT plus HT versus RT alone. Although individual trials may have been inconclusive, the combined data indicated a significantly reduced risk of failure in patients who received adjuvant HT, with an odds ratio of 1.77 ± 0.20 (95% confidence interval) and a P value of <0.00001. These data are grouped by disease site and presented in graphical form in Figure 70-10, showing clear evidence for a benefit of adjuvant HT for melanomas and head and neck, chest wall, cervical, rectal, and bladder cancers but no benefit for prostate or intact breast cancers.

Hyperthermia and Chemotherapy

Multiple, mostly small, phase II trials have been performed combining local, endoluminal, regional, or whole-body HT with chemotherapy for treating esophageal cancer preoperatively, stomach cancer, pancreatic cancer,

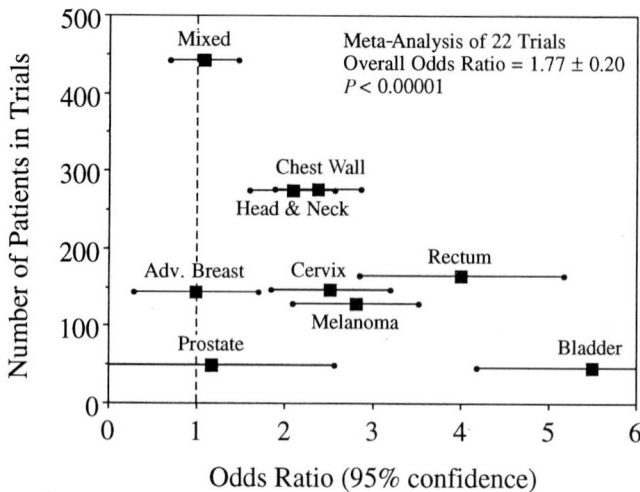

Figure 70–10. Graphical representation of a meta-analysis of risk of failure in 22 prospective, randomized trials comparing radiotherapy alone to radiation plus hyperthermia. The number of patients included in the trials is plotted versus the odds ratio with the 95% confidence interval, grouped by disease site. There is clear evidence for a benefit of adjuvant hyperthermia for melanomas and head and neck, chest wall, cervix, rectum, and bladder cancers. (Redrawn with permission from Jens Overgaard, unpublished.)

metastatic or high-risk soft tissue sarcomas, recurrent cervical cancer, advanced rectal cancer, miscellaneous advanced or metastatic cancers,[277,278] small-cell lung cancer,[279] disseminated melanoma,[280] and ovarian cancer.[281,282] A phase III randomized trial comparing preoperative chemotherapy to preoperative chemotherapy plus hyperthermia was performed in 40 esophageal cancer patients showing higher rates of subjective and radiographic improvement (70% vs. 40% and 50% vs. 25%, respectively) and a higher proportion of necrosed cancer cells on histological examination in the combined therapy arm.[283] Following up on promising phase II chemothermotherapy trials in patients with high-risk soft tissue sarcomas, ESHO and the European Organization for Research and Treatment of Cancer are conducting a phase III trial of neoadjuvant chemotherapy (etoposide, ifosfamide, and doxorubicin) with or without RHT (Regional Hyperthermia) before resection and radiotherapy.[284]

Preoperative hyperthermic isolated limb perfusion (HILP) with melphalan, tumor necrosis factor, or other agents has been used extensively in patients with high-risk or recurrent extremity melanomas. One prospective, randomized trial was closed early because of significantly higher local control and survival in patients treated with preoperative melphalan HILP compared with those who underwent surgery alone.[285] A large phase III, multi-center, multi-continent randomized trial in 832 assessable patients showed a trend toward longer disease-free interval but no benefit in terms of survival or time-to-distant metastasis for HILP before surgery compared with surgery alone.[286]

Hyperthermia has also been used in combination with drug-containing liposomes to improve drug delivery. Kong and Dewhirst have provided an excellent review of preclinical data[116] and Park has reviewed early clinical data and rationale for liposome-based breast cancer

treatment.[287] A phase I/II trial was performed in 2 patients with chest wall recurrence of breast cancer using superficial HT immediately before intravenous administration of doxorubicin-containing liposomes (Doxil) at 45 mg/m^2 every 28 days for 4 to 6 cycles.[288] The response rate in heated fields was 57% with 1 CR and 12 PRs. Furthermore, HT was associated with significantly improved response in 18 patients with both heated and nonheated disease ($P < 0.04$). Another phase I/II trial was performed in 15 patients with advanced, chemotherapyresistant cancers using fever-range WBH with Doxil, 5-fluorouracil, and low-dose metronomic interferon-α repeated every 28 days for 1 to 9 cycles (median, 3 cycles).[289] Six patients had objective responses, five had stable disease for more than 12 weeks, and four had progressive disease.

Hyperthermia, Radiation, and Chemotherapy

There is also growing literature on trimodality studies combining HT, RT, and chemotherapy for head and neck, breast, esophageal, and rectal cancers, including promising phase III studies for resectable or unresectable esophageal cancer.[277] In one trial, 66 patients with resectable squamous cell carcinoma of the esophagus were randomized to preoperative chemoradiotherapy or thermochemoradiotherapy using twice-weekly RF capacitive HT with an endoluminal applicator, cisplatin or bleomycin, and 30 Gy in 15 fractions over 3 weeks.[290] Operative specimens showed absence of viable cancer cells in 25% of the trimodality patients versus 6% of the chemoradiotherapy patients and 3-year survival rates were 50% versus 24%, respectively.

To date, experience with thermochemotherapy and thermochemoradiotherapy is too limited to draw conclusions, although preliminary results are encouraging.

Heat Shock Proteins and Immunotherapy

The fact that vaccines against tumor HSPs are applicable to the treatment of cancer has opened up a new perspective in cancer immunotherapy. A number of preliminary clinical trials have been carried out to test the use of HSPs derived from autologous human tumors in immunotherapy of human cancer: Janetzki and colleagues prepared individual gp96 vaccines derived from the tumors of 16 patients with advanced malignancies[291]; Amato and colleagues have treated patients with renal cell carcinoma with gp96 vectors.[292] Eton and colleagues also used gp96 vaccines in metastatic melanoma using similar dosing regimen as described for renal cancers.[293] However, all of these clinical trials are nonrandomized and the clinical data generated thus far can only be suggestive. To the extent that one may draw any inferences from them, the results so far are consistent with the murine data, which showed that the autologous gp96 vaccine was effective in the adjuvant setting where most treated animals remained disease-free for their entire life span, and less effective in animals with progressive tumors, where only disease stabilization was achieved.[123] Most recently, double-blind phase III clinical trials using gp96-peptide complex for the treatment of stage III renal cell carcinoma in the adjuvant setting are being conducted at numerous centers worldwide.[294]

The advantages and disadvantages of various vaccination approaches are discussed in a review article by Manjili and colleagues.[295] In addition, several other excellent reviews of this field emphasize the development, analysis, and application of HSP-related vaccination approaches.[123,296-300]

Randomized Animal Studies

In comparison with human trials, studies in pet animals often allow for better acceptance of novel therapies and randomization, more detailed thermometry, better control over the heat treatment, and better tolerance due to the use of general anesthesia, resulting in higher minimum tumor temperatures. Four prospective, randomized trials performed in pet animals with spontaneous tumors all demonstrated significant benefit for HT in combination with RT over RT alone.[29,301-303] A University of Arizona trial included 236 dogs and cats with various spontaneous cancers stratified by histological type and randomized to receive RT alone (36.8 Gy in eight fractions over 4 weeks) or RT plus once-weekly HT for 30 minutes. For 217 evaluable animals, the CR rate was 35% in the RT arm and 59% in the RT plus HT arm, with no increase in acute or late effects.[29]

Denman and colleagues[301] performed a phase III randomized trial in spontaneous canine malignancies stratified by histological type and anatomical site and randomized to receive RT (49.0 Gy in 14 fractions given on Mondays, Wednesdays, and Fridays) with or without once-weekly HT for 30 minutes. Hyperthermia significantly increased the CR rate for sarcomas (33% for RT alone vs. 73% for RT plus HT), tumors of the trunk and extremities (45% vs. 83%), and tumors less than 10 cm^3 in volume (50% vs. 84%).

Gillette and associates[302] randomized oral carcinomas in 38 dogs to graded radiation doses (25 to 45 Gy in 10 fractions over 22 days) with or without seven 30-minute HT treatments to determine the dose that would result in a 50% probability of tumor control (TCD$_{50}$) and then to determine the TER as the ratio of the TCD$_{50}$ for RT alone to the TCD$_{50}$ for RT plus HT. To limit normal tissue temperatures, the tumor margins did not exceed 41.5°C. The TER was 1.15 and the slope of the dose-response curve was much steeper for RT and HT than for RT alone. Late complications were not increased in the animals receiving heat.

A similar study was performed in 64 canines with spontaneous soft tissue sarcomas.[303] The animals were stratified by tumor volume and randomized to receive graded doses of RT (35.0 to 55.0 Gy in 10 fractions on a Monday-Wednesday-Friday schedule) with or without US HT for 30 minutes 3 hours after RT twice weekly on a Monday-Friday schedule. The HT goal was a minimum tumor temperature of 42°C. Freedom from local tumor progression was significantly increased in animals treated with RT plus HT (Wilcoxon $P = 0.046$; log rank $P = 0.064$). There was no significant difference between the two study arms in terms of late normal tissue complications or distant metastatic rate.

A fifth phase III study of RT (36 Gy at 9 Gy per fraction) with or without local HT for spontaneous head and neck tumors in 145 dogs showed no difference between the treatment arms in terms of CR rate (47% for RT versus 43% for RT and HT)[304] or progression-free survival (median, 26 weeks for RT versus 27 weeks for RT and HT). The authors cited inadequate thermal dose as a probable cause.

These well-controlled, randomized studies show convincingly that adjuvant HT enhances the response and control rates of spontaneous malignancies in anesthetized animals, in which adequate minimum thermal doses are more often achievable than in nonanesthetized human patients.

Whole body hyperthermia has also been investigated in combination with RT or chemotherapy in dogs. A phase III trial of RT with or without WBH performed in 45 dogs with spontaneous brain tumors resulted in 1-year survival probabilities of 44% for RT versus 40% for RT and WBH and six dogs had severe toxicity from WBH.[305] In another study, 64 dogs with spontaneous soft tissue sarcomas were randomized to RT with localized HT with or without WBH to improve T_{min} and T_{90} temperatures. The addition of WBH significantly increased CEM 43° T_{90} but also resulted in more toxicity and significantly shorter time to metastasis ($P = 0.02$).[306] However, WBH was associated with a trend toward improved disease-free survival among 46 dogs with high-grade lymphoma achieving a CR with doxorubicin and then randomized to five additional doxorubicin treatments with or without WBH.[307,308]

CONCLUSIONS AND FUTURE DIRECTIONS

There is a strong radiobiologic rationale for combining heat and RT: heat radiosensitizes cells and kills cells as a function of time and temperature. Heat appears to be especially effective against cells that are radioresistant, and mild or moderate HT may allow increased reoxygenation of tumors during the course of RT.[309,310] As we come to better understand the mechanisms and kinetics of thermal effects, we should be able to devise strategies to enhance the therapeutic gain for adjuvant HT, taking advantage of pH, response modifiers, and the relative thermotolerance of normal tissues and tumors. Further phase I/II trials are needed to help define the optimal thermal dose and sequencing of HT with RT, including investigation of long-duration, simultaneous RT plus HT, and to evaluate HT with chemotherapy, conventional liposomes, or thermosensitive liposomes, with or without RT. Phase I/II trials are also in progress exploring entirely new applications of HT in immunotherapy or as a promoter for gene therapy.

Clinically, for both human and spontaneous animal tumors, adjuvant HT has been shown to improve response rates and local control of accessible malignancies treated with RT. A major stumbling block for clinical HT has been the inability to adequately heat the designated target volume of tissue. Limitations of initial heating equipment were not fully recognized until after the failure of early randomized trials. Dramatic improvements in HT technology have been made over the past several decades. Using "second generation" HT equipment, phase III trials for recurrent breast cancer and metastatic malignant melanoma have proven a benefit of adjuvant superficial HT combined with RT. Prospective randomized trials have also shown a benefit of adjuvant interstitial HT for glioblastomas and regional HT for advanced cervical and bladder cancers. Further trials are in progress using careful thermometry and "third generation" equipment to confirm these results and establish the safety and efficacy of HT in other sites. Future studies will need to compare optimal radiation doses alone to the same doses with HT.

REFERENCES

1. Busch W: Uber den Einfluss, welchen heftigere Erysipelin zuweilig auf organisierte Neubildungen ausüben. *Verhandlugen des naturhistorischen Vereines der preussischen Rheinlande und Westphalens.* 1866;23:28.
2. Coley WB: The treatment of malignant tumors by repeated inoculations of erysipelas: With a report of ten original cases. *Am J Med Sci.* 1893;105:486.
3. Müller C: Eine neue Behandlungsmethode bosartiger Geschwulste. *Munchener Medizinische Wochenschrift.* 1910;28:1490.
4. Dewey WC, Hopwood LE, Sapareto SA, et al: Cellular responses to combinations of hyperthermia and radiation. *Radiology.* 1977;123:463.
5. Dewey WC, Freeman ML, Raaphorst GP, et al: Cell biology of hyperthermia and radiation. In Meyn RE, Withers HR, eds. *Radiation Biology in Cancer Research.* New York: Raven Press; 1980:589.
6. Hahn GM: *Hyperthermia and Cancer.* New York: Plenum Press; 1982:285.
7. Overgaard J: The current and potential role of hyperthermia in radiotherapy. *Int J Radiat Oncol Biol Phys.* 1989;16:535.
8. Perez CA, Gillespie B, Pajak T, et al: Quality assurance problems in clinical hyperthermia and their impact on therapeutic outcome: A report by the Radiation Therapy Oncology Group. *Int J Radiat Oncol Biol Phys.* 1989;16:551.
9. Emami B, Scott C, Perez CA, et al: Phase III study of interstitial thermoradiotherapy compared with interstitial radiotherapy alone in the treatment of recurrent or persistent human tumors: A prospectively controlled randomized study by the Radiation Therapy Oncology Group. *Int J Radiat Oncol Biol Phys.* 1996;34:1097.
10. Datta NR, Bose AK, Kapoor HK, et al: Head and neck cancers: Results of thermoradiotherapy versus radiotherapy. *Int J Hyperthermia.* 1990;6:479.
11. Overgaard J, González González D, Hulshof MCCM, et al: Randomized trial of hyperthermia as adjuvant to radiotherapy for recurrent or metastatic malignant melanoma. *Lancet.* 1995;345:540.
12. Valdagni R, Amichetti M, Pani G: Radical radiation alone versus radical radiation plus microwave hyperthermia for N3 (TNM-UICC) neck nodes: A prospective randomized clinical trial. *Int J Radiat Oncol Biol Phys.* 1988;15:13.
13. Valdagni R, Amichetti M: Report of long-term follow-up in a randomized trial comparing radiation therapy and radiation therapy plus hyperthermia to metastatic lymph nodes in stage IV head and neck patients. *Int J Radiat Oncol Biol Phys.* 1994;28:163.
14. van der Zee J, González González D, van Rhoon GC, et al: Comparison of radiotherapy alone with radiotherapy plus hyperthermia in locally advanced pelvic tumors: A prospective, randomized, multicentre trial. *Lancet.* 2000;355:1119.
15. Vernon CC, Hand JW, Field SB, et al: Radiotherapy with or without hyperthermia in the treatment of superficial localized breast cancer: Results from five randomized controlled trials. *Int J Radiat Oncol Biol Phys.* 1996;35:731.
16. Oleson JR, Samulski TV, Leopold KA, et al: Sensitivity of hyperthermia trial outcomes to temperature and time: Implications for thermal goals of treatment. *Int J Radiat Oncol Biol Phys.* 1993;25:289.
17. Jorritsma JBM, Burgman P, Kampinga HH, et al: DNA polymerase activity in heat killing and hyperthermia radiosensitization of mammalian cells as observed after fractionated heat treatments. *Radiat Res.* 1986;105:307.
18. Morimoto RI, Tissieres A, Georgopoulos C: *The Biology of Heat Shock Proteins and Molecular Chaperones.* Plainview, New York: Cold Spring Harbor Laboratory Press; 1994.
19. Landry J, Marceau N: Rate limiting events in hyperthermic cell killing. *Radiat Res.* 1978;75:573.
20. Alper T: *Cellular Radiobiology.* Cambridge, England; Cambridge University Press: 1979.
21. Privalov P: Stability of proteins: Small globular proteins. *Adv Protein Chem.* 1979;33:167.
22. Lepock JR, Kruuv J: Thermotolerance as a possible cause of the critical temperature at 43°C in mammalian cells. *Cancer Res.* 1980;40:4485.
23. Lepock JR, Frey HE, Heynen MP, et al: Increased thermostability of thermotolerant CHL V79 cells as determined by differential scanning calorimetry. *J Cell Physiol.* 1990;142:628.
24. Jung HA: A generalized concept for cell killing by heat. Effect of chronically induced thermotolerance. *Radiat Res.* 1991;127:235.
25. Hahn GM, Shiu EC: Adaptation to low pH modifies thermal and thermo-chemical responses of mammalian cells. *Int J Hyperthermia.* 1986;2:379.
26. Hofer KG, Mivechi NF: Tumor cell sensitivity to hyperthermia as a function of extracellular and intracellular pH. *J Natl Cancer Inst.* 1980;65:621.
27. Westra A, Dewey WC: Variation in sensitivity to heat shock during the cell cycle of Chinese hamster cells in vitro. *Int J Radiat Biol.* 1971;19:467.
28. Sapareto SA, Dewey WC: Thermal dose determination in cancer therapy. *Int J Radiat Oncol Biol Phys.* 1984;10:787.
29. Dewhirst MW, Sim DA: The utility of thermal dose as a predictor of tumor and normal tissue responses to combined radiation and hyperthermia. *Cancer Res.* 1984;44(suppl 10):4772s.
30. Sherar M, Liu F-F, Pintilie M, et al: Relationship between thermal dose and outcome in thermoradiotherapy treatments for superficial recurrences of breast cancer: Data from a phase III trial. *Int J Radiat Oncol Biol Phys.* 1997;39:371.
31. Leopold KA, Dewhirst MW, Samulski TV, et al: Cumulative minutes with T_{90} greater than Temp$_{index}$ is predictive of response of superficial malignancies to hyperthermia and radiation. *Int J Radiat Oncol Biol Phys.* 1993;25:841.
32. Leopold KA, Dewhirst M, Samulski T, et al: Relationships among tumor temperature, treatment time, and histopathological outcome using preoperative hyperthermia with radiation in soft tissue sarcomas. *Int J Radiat Oncol Biol Phys.* 1992;22:989.
33. Rau B, Wust P, Tilly W, et al: Preoperative radiochemotherapy in locally advanced or recurrent rectal cancer: Regional radiofrequency hyperthermia correlates with clinical parameters. *Int J Radiat Oncol Biol Phys.* 2000;48:381.
34. Kapp DS, Cox RS: Thermal treatment parameters are most predictive of outcome in patients with single tumor nodules per treatment field in recurrent adenocarcinoma of the breast. *Int J Radiat Oncol Biol Phys.* 1995;33:887.
35. Borrelli MJ, Stafford DM, Rausch CM, et al: Reduction of levels of nuclear-associated protein in heated cells by cycloheximide, D_2O, and thermotolerance. *Radiat Res.* 1992;131:204.
36. Burgman PWJJ, Kampinga HH, Konings AWT: Possible role of localized protein denaturation in the induction of thermotolerance by heat, sodium-arsenite, and ethanol. *Int J Hyperthermia.* 1993;9:151.
37. Kampinga HH, Brunsting JF, Stege GJJ, et al: Thermal protein denaturation and protein aggregation in cells made thermotolerant by various chemicals: Role of heat shock proteins. *Exp Cell Res.* 1995;219:536.
38. Konings AWT: Membranes are targets for hyperthermic cell killing. *Recent Results Cancer Res.* 1988;109:9.
39. Laszlo A: The effects of hyperthermia on mammalian cell structure and function. *Cell Prolif.* 1992;25:59.
40. Vidair CA, Doxsey SJ, Dewey WC: Heat shock alters centrosome organization leading to mitotic dysfunction and cell death. *J Cell Physiol.* 1993;154:443.

41. Welch WJ, Suhan JP: Morphological study of the mammalian stress response: Characterization of changes in cytoplasmic organelles, cytoskeleton, and nucleoli, and appearance of intranuclear actin filaments in rat fibroblasts after heat-shock treatment. *J Cell Biol.* 1985;101:1198.

42. Kampinga HH, Turkel-Uygur N, Roti Roti JL, et al: The relationship of increased nuclear protein content induced by hyperthermia to killing of HeLa S3 cells. *Radiat Res.* 1989;117:511.

43. Roti Roti JL, Henle KJ, Winward RT: The kinetics of increase in chromatin protein content in heated cells: A possible role in cell killing. *Radiat Res.* 1979;78:522.

44. Kampinga HH, Wright WD, Konings AWT, et al: The interaction of heat and radiation affecting the ability of nuclear DNA to undergo supercoiling changes. *Radiat Res.* 1988;116:114.

45. Hayashi Y, Tohnai I, Kaneda T, et al: Translocation of hsp-70 and protein synthesis during continuous heating at mild temperatures in HeLa cells. *Radiat Res.* 1991;125:80.

46. Kampinga HH, Brunsting JF, Stege GJJ, et al: Cells overexpressing hsp27 show accelerated recovery from heat-induced nuclear protein aggregation. *Biochem Biophys Res Commun.* 1994;204:1170.

47. Parsell DA, Kowal AS, Singer MA, et al: Protein disaggregation mediated by heat-shock protein hsp104. *Nature.* 1994;372:475.

48. Stege GJJ, Li GC, Li L, et al: On the role of hsp72 in heat-induced intranuclear protein aggregation. *Int J Hyperthermia.* 1994;10:659.

49. Henle KJ, Leeper DB: Interaction of hyperthermia and radiation in CHO cells: Recovery kinetics. *Radiat Res.* 1976;66:505.

50. Gerner EW, Schneider MJ: Induced thermal resistance in HeLa cells. *Nature.* 1975;256:500.

51. Field SB, Anderson RL: Thermotolerance: A review of observations and possible mechanisms. Cancer therapy by hyperthermia, drugs and radiation. *Natl Cancer Inst Monogr.* 1982;61:193.

52. Gerner EW: Thermotolerance. In Storm FK, ed: *Hyperthermia in Cancer Therapy.* Boston: GK Hall; 1983:141.

53. Henle KJ, Dethlefsen LA: Heat fractionation and thermotolerance: A review. *Cancer Res.* 1978;38:1843.

54. Sapareto SA, Hopwood LE, Dewey WC, et al: Effects of hyperthermia on survival and progression of Chinese hamster ovary cells. *Cancer Res.* 1978;38:393.

55. Gerweck LE: Modification of cell lethality at elevated temperatures: The pH effect. *Radiat Res.* 1977;70:224.

56. Henle KJ: Thermotolerance in cultured mammalian cells. In Henle KJ, ed. Thermotolerance. Boca Raton, Fla.: CRC Press; 1987:13.

57. Hahn GM, Shiu EC, West B, et al: Mechanistic implications of the induction of thermotolerance in Chinese hamster cells by organic solvents. *Cancer Res.* 1985;45:4138.

58. Lee YJ, Dewey WC: Induction of heat shock proteins in Chinese hamster ovary cells and development of thermotolerance by intermediate concentrations of puromycin. *J Cell Physiol.* 1987;132:1.

59. Li GC, Hahn GM: A proposed operational model of thermotolerance based on effects of nutrients and the initial treatment temperature. *Cancer Res.* 1980;40:4501.

60. Lis J, Wu C: Protein traffic on the heat shock promoter: Parking, stalling, and trucking along. *Cell.* 1993;74:1.

61. Morimoto RI, Sarge KD, Abravaya K: Transcriptional regulation of heat shock genes: A paradigm for inducible genomic responses. *J Biol Chem.* 1992;267:21987.

62. Liu RY, Kim D, Yang S-H, et al: Dual control of heat shock response: Involvement of a constitutive heat shock element-binding factor. *Proc Natl Acad Sci USA.* 1993;90:3078.

63. Burgman P, Nussenzweig A, Li GC: Thermotolerance. In Seegenschmiedt MH, Fessenden P, Vernon CC, eds. *Principles and Practice of Thermoradiotherapy and Thermochemotherapy, vol 1.* Berlin, New York: Springer-Verlag; 1995:75.

64. Landry J, Chretien P, Lambert H, et al: Heat shock resistance conferred by expression of the human HSP27 gene in rodent cells. *J Cell Biol.* 1989;109:7.

65. Li GC, Li LG, Liu Y-K, et al: Thermal response of rat fibroblasts stably-transfected with the human 70 kDa heat shock protein-encoding gene. *Proc Natl Acad Sci USA.* 1991;88:1681.

66. Angelidis CE, Lazaridis I, Pagoulatos GN: Constitutive expression of heat-shock protein 70 in mammalian cells confers thermoresistance. *Eur J Biochem.* 1991;199:35.

67. Mackey MA, Anolik SL, Roti Roti JL: Cellular mechanisms associated with the lack of chronic thermotolerance expression in HeLa S3 cells. *Cancer Res.* 1992;52:1101.

68. Armour EP, McEachern D, Wang Z, et al: Sensitivity of human cells to mild hyperthermia. *Cancer Res.* 1993;53:2740.

69. Raaphorst GP, Bussey A, Heller DP, et al: Comparison of thermoradiosensitization in two human melanoma cell lines and one fibroblast cell line by concurrent mild hyperthermia and low-dose-rate irradiation. *Radiat Res.* 1994;137:338.

70. Morimoto RI, Tissieres A, Georgopoulos C: *Stress Proteins in Biology and Medicine.* Plainview, New York: Cold Spring Harbor Laboratory Press; 1990.

71. Maresca B, Lindquist S: *Heat Shock.* New York: Springer-Verlag; 1991.

72. Wu C, Zimarino V, Tsai C, et al: Transcriptional regulation of heat shock genes. In Morimoto RI, Tissierres A, Georgopoulos C, eds. *Stress Proteins in Biology and Medicine.* Plainview, New York: Cold Spring Harbor Laboratory Press; 1990:429.

73. Sorger PK: Heat shock factor and the heat shock response. *Cell.* 1991;65:363.

74. Hensold JO, Hunt CR, Calderwood SK, et al: DNA binding of heat shock factor to the heat shock element is insufficient for transcriptional activation in murine erythroleukemia cells. *Mol Cell Biol.* 1990;10:1600.

75. Gorzowski JJ, Eckerley CA, Halgren RG, et al: Methylation-associated transcriptional silencing of the major histocompatibility complex-linked hsp70 genes in mouse cell lines. *J Biol Chem.* 1995;270:26940.

76. Bruce JL, Price BD, Coleman CN, et al: Oxidative injury rapidly activates the heat shock transcription factor but fails to increase levels of heat shock proteins. *Cancer Res.* 1993;53:12.

77. Liu RY, Corry PM, Lee YJ: Regulation of chemical stress-induced hsp70 gene expression in murine L929 cells. *J Cell Sci.* 1994;107 (Pt 8):2209.

78. Leppa S, Kajanne R, Arminen L, et al: Differential induction of hsp70-encoding genes in human hematopoietic cells. *J Biol Chem.* 2001;276:31713.

79. Mathur SK, Sistonen L, Brown IR, et al: Deficient induction of human hsp70 heat shock gene transcription in Y79 retinoblastoma cells despite activation of heat shock factor 1. *Proc Natl Acad Sci USA.* 1994;91:8695.

80. Jurivich DA, Sistonen L, Kroes RA, et al: Effect of sodium salicylate on the human heat shock response. *Science.* 1992;255:1243.

81. Kim D, Ouyang H, Yang S-H, et al: A constitutive heat shock element-binding factor is immunologically identical to the Ku-autoantigen. *J Biol Chem.* 1995;270:15277.

82. Kim D, Ouyang H, Li GC: Heat shock protein hsp70 accelerates the recovery of heat-shocked mammalian cells through its modulation of heat shock transcription factor HSF1. *Proc Natl Acad Sci USA.* 1995;92:2126.

83. Liu RY, Corry PM, Lee YJ: Potential involvement of a constitutive heat shock element binding factor in the regulation of chemical stress-induced hsp70 gene expression. *Mol Cell Biochem.* 1995;144:27.

84. Li GC, Yang S-H, Kim D, et al: Suppression of heat-induced hsp70 expression by the 70-kDa subunit of the human Ku-autoantigen. *Proc Natl Acad Sci USA.* 1995;92:4512.

85. Yang S-H, Nussenzweig A, Li L, et al: Modulation of thermal induction of hsp70 expression by Ku autoantigen or its individual subunits. *Mol Cell Biol.* 1996;16:3799.

86. Tang D, Xie Y, Stevenson MA, et al: Repression of the HSP70B promoter by NFIL6, Ku70, and MAPK involves three complementary mechanisms. *Biochem Biophys Res Commun.* 2000; 280:280.

87. Huang J, Nueda A, Yoo S, et al: Heat shock transcription factor 1 binds selectively in vitro to Ku protein and the catalytic subunit of the DNA-dependent protein kinase. *J Biol Chem.* 1997; 272:26009.

88. Konings AWT: Interaction of heat and radiation in vitro and in vivo. In Seegenschmiedt MH, Fessenden P, Vernon CC, eds. *Thermoradiotherapy and Thermochemotherapy, vol 1: Biology, Physiology and Physics.* Heidelberg, Germany: Springer-Verlag; 1995;89.

89. Overgaard J, Nielsen OS, Lindegaard JC: Biological basis for rational design of clinical treatment with combined hyperthermia and radiation. In Field SB, Franconi C, eds. *Physics and Technology of Hyperthermia.* Amsterdam: Martinus Nijhoff; 1987:54.

90. Warters RL, Roti Roti JL: Hyperthermia and the cell nucleus. *Radiat Res.* 1982;92:458.

91. Jorritsma JBM, Konings AWT: Inhibition of repair of radiation-induced strand breaks by hyperthermia and its relation to cell survival after hyperthermia alone. *Int J Radiat Biol.* 1983;43:506.

92. Mills HD, Meyn RE: Hyperthermic potentiation of unrejoined DNA strand breaks following irradiation. *Radiat Res.* 1981; 87:314.

93. Dikomey E, Franzke J: Effect of heat on induction and repair of DNA strand breaks in X-irradiated CHO cells. *Int J Radiat Biol.* 1992;61:221.

94. Warters RL, Roti Roti JL: Excision of X-ray-induced thymine damage in chromatin from heated cells. *Radiat Res.* 1979;79:113.

95. Stege GJJ, Kampinga HH, Konings AWT: Heat-induced intranuclear protein aggregation and thermal radiosensitization. *Int J Radiat Biol.* 1995;67:203.

96. Wynstra JH, Wright WD, Roti Roti JL: Repair of radiation-induced DNA damage in thermotolerant and nonthermotolerant HeLa cells. *Radiat Res.* 1990;124:85.

97. Kampinga HH, Keij JF, van der Kruk G, et al: Interaction of hyperthermia and radiation in tolerant and nontolerant HeLa S3 cells: Role of DNA polymerase inactivation. *Int J Radiat Biol.* 1989;55:423.

98. Henle KJ, Nagle WA, Moss AJ: Effect of thermotolerance on the cellular heat-radiation response. In Urano M, Douple E, eds. *Hyperthermia and Oncology, vol 2.* Boca Raton, Fla: VSP; 1989:53.

99. Raaphorst GP, Azzam EI: Thermal radiosensitization in Chinese hamster (V79) and mouse C3H 10T 1/2 cells. The thermotolerance effect. *Br J Cancer.* 1983;48:45.

100. Freeman ML, Raaphorst GP, Dewey WC: The relationship of heat killing and thermoradiosensitization to the duration of heating at 42°C. *Radiat Res.* 1979;78:172.

101. Konings AWT: Effects of heat and radiation on mammalian cells. *Radiat Phys Chem.* 1987;30:339.

102. Heller DP, Raaphorst GP: Low dose-rate irradiation of human glioma cells and thermoradiosensitization by mild hyperthermia. *Radiat Oncol Invest.* 1993;1:218.

103. Armour EP, Wang ZH, Corry PM, et al: Sensitization of rat 9L gliosarcoma cells to low dose rate irradiation by long duration 41°C hyperthermia. *Cancer Res.* 1991;51:3088.

104. Dikomey E: Effect of hyperthermia at 42 and 45°C on repair of radiation-induced DNA strand breaks in CHO cells. *Int J Radiat Biol.* 1982;41:603.

105. Ben Hur E, Elkind MM: Thermally enhanced radioresponse of cultured Chinese hamster cells: damage and repair of single-stranded DNA and a DNA complex. *Radiat Res.* 1974;59:484.

106. Warters RL, Lyons BW, Axtell-Bartlett J: Inhibition of repair of radiation-induced DNA damage by thermal shock in Chinese hamster ovary cells. *Int J Radiat Biol.* 1987;51:505.

107. Dahl O, Mella O: Hyperthermia and chemotherapeutic agents. In Field SB, Hand JW, eds. *An Introduction to the Practical Aspects of Clinical Hyperthermia.* London, New York: Taylor & Francis; 1990:108.

108. Jain RK: Barriers to drug delivery in solid tumors. *Sci Am.* 1997;271:58.

109. Lasic DD: Liposomes from Physics to Applications. Amsterdam: Elsevier; 1993:269.

110. Massing U: Cancer therapy with liposomal formulations of anticancer drugs. *Int J Clin Pharmacol Ther.* 1997;35:87.

111. Campos D, Shapiro C: Clinical evaluation of liposomal anthracyclins. In Janoff A, ed. *Liposomes: Rational Design.* New York: Marcel Dekker; 1999:363.

112. Gabizon A, Barenholtz Y: Liposomal anthracyclins. From basics to clinical approval of PEGylated liposomal doxorubicin. In Janoff A, ed. Liposomes: Rational Design. New York: Marcel Dekker; 1999:343.

113. Needham D, Anyarambhatla G, Kong G, et al: A new temperature-sensitive liposome for use with mild hyperthermia: Characterization and testing in a human tumor xenograft model. *Cancer Res.* 2000;60:1197.

114. Ning S, Macleod K, Abra RM, et al: Hyperthermia induces doxorubicin release from long-circulating liposomes and enhances their anti-tumor efficacy. *Int J Radiat Oncol Biol Phys.* 1994;29:827.

115. Yatvin MB, Weinstein JN, Dennis WH, et al: Design of liposomes for enhanced local release of drugs by hyperthermia. *Science.* 1978;202:1290.

116. Kong G, Dewhirst MW: Review: Hyperthermia and liposomes. *Int J Hyperthermia.* 1999;15:345.

117. Kong G, Anyarambhatla G, Petros WP, et al: Efficacy of liposomes and hyperthermia in a human tumor xenograft model: importance of triggered drug release. *Cancer Res.* 2000; 60:6950.

118. Srivastava PK, DeLeo AB, Old LJ: Tumor rejection antigens of chemically induced sarcomas of inbred mice. *Proc Natl Acad Sci USA.* 1986;83:3407.

119. Srivastava PK, Maki RG: Stress-induced proteins in immune response to cancer. *Curr Top Microbiol Immunol.* 1991;167:109.

120. Srivastava PK: Peptide-binding heat shock proteins in the endoplasmic reticulum: role in immune response to cancer and in antigen presentation. *Adv Cancer Res.* 1993;62:153.

121. Ullrich SJ, Robinson EA, Law LW, et al: A mouse tumor-specific transplantation antigen is a heat shock-related protein. *Proc Natl Acad Sci USA.* 1986;83:3121.

122. Udono H, Srivastava PK: Comparison of tumor-specific immunogenicities of stress-induced proteins gp96, hsp90, and hsp70. *J Immunol.* 1994;152:5398.

123. Tamura Y, Peng P, Liu K, et al: Immunotherapy of tumors with autologous tumor-derived heat shock protein preparations. *Science.* 1997;278:117.

124. Basu S, Srivastava PK: Calreticulin, a peptide-binding chaperone of the endoplasmic reticulum, elicits tumor- and peptide-specific immunity. *J Exp Med.* 1999;189:797.

125. Srivastava PK, Das MR: The serologically unique cell surface antigen of Zajdela ascitic hepatoma is also its tumor-associated transplantion antigen. *Int J Cancer.* 1984;33:417.

126. Janetzki S, Blachere NE, Srivastava PK: Generation of tumor-specific cytotoxic T lymphocytes and memory T cells by immunization with tumor-derived heat shock protein gp96. *J Immunother.* 1998;21:269.

127. Wang X-Y, Kazim L, Repasky EA, et al: Characterization of heat shock protein 110 and glucose-regulated protein 170 as cancer vaccines and the effect of fever-range hyperthermia on vaccine activity. *J Immunol.* 2001;166:490.

128. Wang X-Y, Li Y, Manjili MH, et al: Hsp110 over-expression increases the immunogenicity of the murine CT26 colon tumor. *Cancer Immunol Immunother.* 2002;51:311.

129. Manjili MH, Henderson R, Wang X-Y, et al: Development of a recombinant HSP110-HER-2/neu vaccine using the chaperoning properties of HSP110. *Cancer Res.* 2002;62:1737.

130. Gerner EW, Hersh EM, Pennington M, et al: Heat-inducible vectors for use in gene therapy. *Int J Hyperthermia.* 2000;16:171.

131. Lohr F, Hu K, Huang Q, et al: Enhancement of radiotherapy by hyperthermia-regulated gene therapy. *Int J Radiat Oncol Biol Phys.* 2000;48:1513.

132. Vekris A, Maurange C, Moonen C, et al: Control of transgene expression using local hyperthermia in combination with a heat-sensitive promoter. *J Gene Med.* 2000;2:89.

133. Borrelli MJ, Schoenherr DM, Wong A, et al: Heat-activated transgene expression from adenovirus vectors infected into human prostate cancer cells. *Cancer Res.* 2001;61:1113.

134. Huang Q, Hu JK, Lohr F, et al: Heat-induced gene expression as a novel targeted cancer gene therapy strategy. *Cancer Res.* 2000; 60:3435.

135. Lagendijk JJW: Thermal models: Principles and implementation. In Field SB, Hand JW, eds. *An Introduction to the Practical Aspects of Clinical Hyperthermia.* London, New York: Taylor & Francis; 1990:478.

136. Pennes HH: Analysis of tissue and arterial blood temperatures in the resting human forearm. *J Appl Physiol.* 1948;85:5.

137. Lagendijk JJW, Visser AG, Kaatee RSJP, et al: Interstitial hyperthermia & treatment planning: The 27 MHz multi-electrode current source method. *Nucletron-Odelft Activity Report No 6.* 1995;83.

138. Arkin H, Xu LX, Holmes KR: Recent developments in modeling heat transfer in blood perfused tissues. *IEEE Trans Biomed Eng.* 1994;41:97.

139. Gautherie M: *Thermal Dosimetry and Treatment Planning. Clinical Thermology: Subseries Thermotherapy.* Berlin: Springer-Verlag; 1990.

140. Seegenschmiedt MH, Fessenden P, Vernon CC: *Thermoradiotherapy and Thermochemotherapy, vol. 1: Biology, Physiology, and Physics.* Berlin: Springer-Verlag; 1995.

141. Fessenden P, Hand JW: Hyperthermia therapy physics. In Smith AR, ed. *Medical Radiology: Radiation Therapy Physics.* Berlin: Springer-Verlag; 1995:315.

142. Samulski TV, Grant WJ, Oleson JR, et al: Clinical experience with a multi-element ultrasonic hyperthermia system: Analysis of treatment temperatures. *Int J Hyperthermia.* 1990;6:909.

143. Hynynen K: Hot spots created at skin-air interfaces during ultrasound hyperthermia. *Int J Hyperthermia.* 1990;6:1005.

144. Goss SA, Johnston RL, Dunn F: Comprehensive compilation of empirical ultrasonic properties of mammalian tissues. *J Acoust Soc Am.* 1978;64:423.

145. Field SB, Hand JW: *An Introduction to the Practical Aspects of Clinical Hyperthermia.* London: Taylor & Francis; 1990:572.

146. Gautherie M: *Methods of External Hyperthermic Heating. Clinical Thermology: Subseries Thermotherapy.* Berlin, Heidelberg: Springer-Verlag; 1990:143.

147. Seegenschmiedt MH, Sauer R: *Interstitial and Intracavitary Thermoradiotherapy. Medical Radiology.* Berlin, Heidelberg: Springer-Verlag; 1993.

148. Stauffer PR: Thermal therapy techniques for skin and superficial tissue disease. In Ryan TP, ed. *Critical Reviews: Matching the Energy Source to the Clinical Need.* Bellingham, Wash: SPIE Optical Engineering Press; 2000;327.

149. Chou CK, McDougall JA, Chan KW, et al: Evaluation of captive bolus applicators. *Med Phys.* 1990;17:705.

150. Straube WL, Myerson RJ, Emami B, et al: SAR patterns of external 915 MHz microwave applicators. *Int J Hyperthermia.* 1990; 6:665.

151. Sherar MD, Liu FF, Newcombe DJ, et al: Beam shaping for microwave waveguide hyperthermia applicators. *Int J Radiat Oncol Biol Phys.* 1993;25:849.

152. Nishimura Y, Hiraoka M, Mitsumori M, et al: Thermoradiotherapy of superficial and subsurface tumors: Analysis of thermal parameters and tumor response. *Int J Hyperthermia.* 1995;11:603.

153. Fessenden P, Lee ER, Kapp DS, et al: Review of the Stanford experience developing non-focusing scanning and array surface microwave (MW) applicators. In Gerner EW, Cetas TC, eds. *Hyperthermic Oncology, 1992, vol 2.* Tucson, Ariz. Board of Regents; 1993:183.

154. Tennant A, Conway J, Anderson AP: A robot-controlled microwave antenna system for uniform hyperthermia treatment of superficial tumors with arbitrary shape. *Int J Hyperthermia.* 1990;6:193.

155. Diederich CJ, Stauffer PR: Pre-clinical evaluation of a microwave planar array applicator for superficial hyperthermia. *Int J Hyperthermia.* 1993;9:227.

156. van Rhoon GC, Rietveld PJ, van der Zee J: A 433 MHz Lucite cone waveguide applicator for superficial hyperthermia. *Int J Hyperthermia.* 1998;14:13.

157. Gopal MK, Hand JW, Lumori MLD, et al: Current sheet applicator arrays for superficial hyperthermia of chestwall lesions. *Int J Hyperthermia.* 1992;8:227.

158. Lee ER, Wilsey TR, Tarczy-Hornoch P, et al: Body conformable 915 MHz microstrip array applicators for large surface area hyperthermia. *IEEE Trans Biomed Eng.* 1992;39:470.

159. Stauffer PR, Diederich CJ, Bozzo D: Conformal array microwave applicator for superficial hyperthermia of large contoured surfaces. *1994 IEEE MTT-S International Microwave Symposium Digest.* 1994;1:531.

160. Stauffer PR, Jacobsen S, Neuman DG: Microwave array applicators for radiometry controlled superficial hyperthermia. In Ryan TP, ed. *Thermal Treatment of Tissue: Energy Delivery and Assessment.* Bellingham, Wash.: SPIE Press; 2001;19.

161. Chive M: Use of microwave radiometry for hyperthermia monitoring and as a basis for thermal dosimetry. In Gautherie M, ed. *Methods of Hyperthermia Control.* Heidelberg, Germany: Springer-Verlag; 1990:113.

162. Jacobsen S, Stauffer PR, Neuman DG: Dual-mode antenna design for microwave heating and noninvasive thermometry of superficial tissue disease. *IEEE Trans Biomed Eng.* 2000;47:1500.

163. Novak P, Zuna I, Pousek L, et al: Ultrasonic approach to noninvasive temperature monitoring during microwave thermotherapy. *Radioengr.* 2001;10:32.

164. Corry PM, Spanos WJ, Tilchen EJ, et al: Combined ultrasound and radiation therapy treatment of human superficial tumors. *Radiology.* 1982;145:165.

165. Hynynen K, Shimm D, Anhalt D, et al: Temperature distributions during clinical scanned, focused ultrasound hyperthermia treatments. *Int J Hyperthermia.* 1990;6:891.

166. Anhalt DP, Hynynen K, Roemer RB, et al: Scanned ultrasound hyperthermia for treating superficial disease. In Gerner E, Cetas T, eds. *Hyperthermic Oncology 1992, vol 2.* Tucson, Ariz. Board of Regents; 1993:191.

167. Lindsley K, Stauffer PR, Sneed P, et al: Heating patterns of the Helios ultrasound hyperthermia system. *Int J Hyperthermia.* 1993;9:675.

168. Svensson GK, Hansen JL, Delli Carpini D, et al: Interstitial radiofrequency-induced hyperthermia. In Gerner EW, ed. *Hyperthemic Oncology 1992, vol 1.* Tucson, Ariz. Board of Regents; 1992:335.

169. Ebbini ES, Cain CA: Optimization of the intensity gain of multiple-focus phased-array heating patterns. *Int J Hyperthermia.* 1991; 7:953.

170. McGough RJ, Ebbini ES, Cain CA: Optimization of apertures and intensity patterns for hyperthermia with ultrasound phased array systems. In Gerner EW, Cetas TC, eds. *Hyperthermic Oncology 1992, vol 2.* Tucson, Ariz. Board of Regents; 1993:205.

171. Moros EG, Fan X, Straube WL: Experimental assessment of power and temperature penetration depth control with a dual frequency ultrasonic system. *Med Phys.* 1999;26:810.

172. Moros EG, Straube WL, Klein EE, et al: Simultaneous delivery of electron beam therapy and ultrasound hyperthermia utilizing scanning reflectors: A feasibility study. *Int J Radiat Oncol Biol Phys.* 1995;31:893.

173. Strohbehn JW: Interstitial techniques for hyperthermia. In Field SB, Franconi C, eds. *Physics and Technology of Hyperthermia.* Dordrecht: Martinus Nijhoff Publishers; 1987:211.

174. Camart JC, Dubois L, Fabre JJ, et al: 915 MHz microwave interstitial hyperthermia. Part II: Array of phase-monitored antennas. *Int J Hyperthermia.* 1993;9:445.

175. Trembly BS, Douple EB, Ryan TP, et al: The effect of phase modulation on the temperature distribution of a microwave hyperthermia antenna array in vivo. *Int J Hyperthermia.* 1994; 10:691.

176. Satoh T, Stauffer PR, Fike JR: Thermal distribution studies of helical coil microwave antennas for interstitial hyperthermia. *Int J Radiat Oncol Biol Phys.* 1988;15:1209.

177. Ryan TP: Comparison of six microwave antennas for hyperthermia treatment of cancer: SAR results for single antennas and arrays. *Int J Radiat Oncol Biol Phys.* 1991;21:403.

178. Fabre JJ, Chive M, Dubois L, et al: 915 MHz microwave interstitial hyperthermia. Part I: Theoretical and experimental aspects with temperature control by multifrequency radiometry. *Int J Hyperthermia.* 1993;9:433.

179. Camart JC, Despretz D, Prevost B, et al: New 434 MHz interstitial hyperthermia system monitored by microwave radiometry: Theoretical and experimental results. *Int J Hyperthermia.* 2000;16:95.

180. Prionas SD, Kapp DS, Goffinet DR, et al: Interstitial radiofrequency-induced hyperthermia. In Gerner EW, Cetas TC, eds. *Hyperthemic Oncology 1992, vol 2.* Tucson, Ariz. Board of Regents; 1993:249.

181. Handl-Zeller L: *Interstitial Hyperthermia.* Wien: Springer-Verlag; 1992.

182. Visser AG, Deurloo IKK, Levendag PC, et al: An interstitial hyperthermia system at 27 MHz. *Int J Hyperthermia.* 1989;5:265.

183. Marchal C, Nadi M, Hoffstetter S, et al: Practical interstitial method of heating operating at 27.12 MHz. *Int J Hyperthermia.* 1989;5:451.

184. DeFord JA, Babbs CF, Patel UH, et al: Effective estimation and computer control of minimum tumor temperature during conductive interstitial hyperthermia. *Int J Hyperthermia.* 1991;7:441.

185. Matsuki H, Murakami K, Satoh T, et al: High quality soft heating method utilizing temperature dependence of permeability and core loss of low curie temperature ferrite. *IEEE Trans Magnetics.* 1987;23:2440.

186. Stauffer PR, Cetas TC, Jones RC: Magnetic induction heating of ferromagnetic implants for inducing localized hyperthermia in deep seated tumors. *IEEE Trans Biomed Eng.* 1984;31:235.

187. Stauffer PR, Sneed PK, Hashemi H, et al: Practical induction heating coil designs for clinical hyperthermia with ferromagnetic implants. *IEEE Trans Biomed Eng.* 1994;41:17.

188. Shinohara K, Master V, Carroll P: Preliminary report of thermal ablation therapy using ferromagnetic rod (ThermoRod) in locally recurrent prostate cancer following external beam radiation therapy (abstract). The forty-ninth annual meeting of the Radiation Research Society and the twentieth annual meeting of the North American Hyperthermia Society, Reno, Nev., April 20-24, 2002, p 77.

189. Hynynen K, Davis KL: Small cylindrical ultrasound sources for induction of hyperthermia via body cavities. *Int J Hyperthermia.* 1993;9:263.

190. Diederich CJ: Ultrasound applicators with integrated catheter-cooling for interstitial hyperthermia: Theory and preliminary experiments. *Int J Hyperthermia.* 1996;12:279.

191. Diederich CJ, Khalil IS, Stauffer PR, et al: Direct-coupled interstitial ultrasound applicators for simultaneous thermo-brachytherapy: A feasibility study. *Int J Hyperthermia.* 1996; 12:401.

192. Diederich CJ, Stafford RJ, Price RE, et al: Minimally-invasive ultrasound thermal therapy with MR thermal monitoring and guidance. In Ryan T, ed. *Thermal Treatment of Tissue: Energy Delivery and Assessment, Proceedings of the SPIE, vol. 4247.* San Jose, Calif.: SPIE Press; 2001:166.

193. Li DJ: Present status on treatment of esophageal cancer in China. *Int J Radiat Oncol Biol Phys.* 1990;18:477.

194. Sorbe B, Roos DI, Karlsson LG: The use of microwave-induced hyperthermia in conjunction with afterloading irradiation of vaginal carcinoma. A preliminary report. *Acta Oncol.* 1990; 29:1029.

195. Liu RL, Zhang EY, Gross EJ, et al: Heating pattern of helical microwave intracavitary oesophageal applicator. *Int J Hyperthermia.* 1991;7:577.

196. Fosmire H, Hynynen K, Drach GW, et al: Feasibility and toxicity of transrectal ultrasound hyperthermia in the treatment of locally advanced adenocarcinoma of the prostate. *Int J Radiat Oncol Biol Phys.* 1993;26:253.

197. Buchanan MT, Hynynen K: Design and experimental evaluation of an intracavitary ultrasound phased array system for hyperthermia. *IEEE Trans Biomed Eng.* 1994;41:1178.

198. Smith NB, Buchanan MT, Hynynen K: Transrectal ultrasound applicator for prostate heating monitored using MRI thermometry. *Int J Radiat Oncol Biol Phys.* 1999;43:217.

199. Paglione R, Sterzer F, Mendecki J, et al: 27 MHz ridged waveguide applicators for localized hyperthermia treatment of deep-seated malignant tumors. *Microwave J.* 1981;24:71.

200. Croghan MK, Shimm DS, Hynynen KH, et al: A phase I study of the toxicity of regional hyperthermia with systemic warming. *Am J Clin Oncol.* 1993;16:354.

201. De Leeuw AA, Mooibroek J, Lagendijk JJ: Specific absorption rate steering by patient positioning in the "Coaxial TEM" system: Phantom investigation. *Int J Hyperthermia.* 1991;7:605.

202. van Es CA, Wyrdeman HK, de Leeuw AA, et al: Regional hyperthermia of pelvic tumors using the Utrecht "Coaxial TEM" system: A feasibility study. *Int J Hyperthermia.* 1995;11:173.

203. Kikuchi M, Amemiya Y, Egawa S, et al: Guide to the use of hyperthermic equipment. 1. Capacitively-coupled heating. *Int J Hyperthermia.* 1993;9:187.

204. van Rhoon GC, van der Zee J, Broekmeyer-Reurink MP, et al: Radiofrequency capacitive heating of deep-seated tumors using pre-cooling of the subcutaneous tissues: Results on thermometry in Dutch patients. *Int J Hyperthermia.* 1992;8:843.

205. Turner PF: Regional hyperthermia with an annular phased array. *IEEE Trans Biomed Eng.* 1984;31:106.

206. Samulski TV, Kapp DS, Fessenden P, et al: Heating deep seated eccentrically located tumors with an annular phased array system: A comparative clinical study using two annular array operating configurations. *Int J Radiat Oncol Biol Phys.* 1987;13:83.

207. González González D, van Dijk JDP, Oldenburger F, et al: Results of combined treatment with radiation and hyperthermia in 111 patients with large or deep seated tumors. In Gerner EW, ed. *Hyperthermic Oncology 1992, vol 1.* Tucson, Ariz. Board of Regents, 1992:415B.

208. Sullivan DM, Ben-Yosef R, Kapp DS: Stanford 3-D hyperthermia treatment planning system. *Int J Hyperthermia.* 1993;9:627.

209. Wust P, Beck R, Berger J, et al: Electric field distributions in a phased-array applicator with 12 channels: Measurements and numerical simulations. *Med Phys.* 2000;27:2565.

210. Carter D, MacFall JR, Clegg ST, et al: Magnetic resonance thermometry during hyperthermia for human high-grade sarcoma. *Int J Radiat Oncol Biol Phys.* 1998;40:815.

211. Pettigrew RT, Galt JM, Ludgate CM, et al: Clinical effects of whole-body hyperthermia in advanced malignancy. *Br Med J.* 1974;4:679.

212. Gerad H, van Echo DA, Whitacre M, et al: Doxorubicin, cyclophosphamide and whole body hyperthermia for treatment of advanced soft tissue sarcoma. *Cancer.* 1984;53:2585.

213. Gautherie M: *Methods of Hyperthermia Control. Clinical Thermology: Subseries Thermotherapy.* Berlin: Springer-Verlag; 1990.

214. Anhalt D, Hynynen K: Thermocouples—The Arizona experience with in-house manufactured probes. *Med Phys.* 1992;19:1325.

215. Hoh LL, Waterman FM: Use of manganin-constantan thermocouples in thermometry units designed for copper-constantan thermocouples. *Int J Hyperthermia.* 1995;11:131.

216. Chan KW, Chou CK: Use of thermocouples in the intense fields of ferromagnetic implant hyperthermia. *Int J Hyperthermia.* 1993; 9:831.

217. Tarczy-Hornoch P, Lee ER, Sokol JL, et al: Automated mechanical thermometry probe mapping systems for hyperthermia. *Int J Hyperthermia.* 1992;8:543.

218. Dewhirst MW, Phillips TL, Samulski TV, et al: RTOG quality assurance guidelines for clinical trials using hyperthermia. *Int J Radiat Oncol Biol Phys.* 1990;18:1249.

219. Emami B, Stauffer P, Dewhirst MW, et al: RTOG quality assurance guidelines for interstitial hyperthermia. *Int J Radiat Oncol Biol Phys.* 1991;20:1117.

220. Waterman FM, Hoh LL: A recommended revision in the RTOG thermometry guidelines for hyperthermia administered by ultrasound. *Int J Hyperthermia.* 1995;11:121.

221. Sapozink MD, Corry PM, Kapp DS, et al: RTOG quality assurance guidelines for clinical trials using hyperthermia for deep-seated malignancy. *Int J Radiat Oncol Biol Phys.* 1991; 20:1109.

222. Schneider CJ, van Dijk JD, De Leeuw AA, et al: Quality assurance in various radiative hyperthermia systems applying a phantom with LED matrix. *Int J Hyperthermia.* 1994;10:733.

223. Dubois L, Sozanski JP, Tessier V, et al: Temperature control and thermal dosimetry by microwave radiometry in hyperthermia. *IEEE Trans Micro Theory Tech.* 1996;44:1755.

224. Hynynen K, Darkazanli A, Unger E, et al: MRI-guided noninvasive ultrasound surgery. *Med Phys.* 1993;20:107.

225. Samulski TV, Clegg ST, Das S, et al: Application of new technology in clinical hyperthermia. *Int J Hyperthermia.* 1994;10:389.

226. Hynynen K, Pomeroy O, Smith DN, et al: MR imaging-guided focused ultrasound surgery of fibroadenomas in the breast: A feasibility study. *Radiology.* 2001;219:176.

227. Overgaard J: The design of clinical trials. In Field SB, Franconi C, eds. *Hyperthermic Oncology: Physics and Technology of Hyperthermia.* Amsterdam: Martinus Nijhoff Publishers; 1982.

228. Arcangeli G, Nervi C, Cividalli A, et al: Problem of sequence and fractionation in the clinical application of combined heat and radiation. *Cancer Res.* 1984;44(suppl 10):4857s.

229. Bey P, Marchal C, Forcard JJ, et al: Potentialisation de la radiothérapie par hyperthermie locale. A propos de 90 tumeurs superficielles comparables (abstract). *Bull Cancer.* 1984;71:263.

230. Dunlop PRC, Hand JW, Dickinson RJ, et al: An assessment of local hyperthermia in clinical practice. *Int J Hyperthermia.* 1986; 2:39.

231. Hiraoka M, Jo S, Dodo Y, et al: Clinical results of radiofrequency hyperthermia combined with radiation in the treatment of radioresistant cancers. *Cancer.* 1984;54:2898.

232. Howard GCW, Sathiaseelan V, Freedman L, et al: Hyperthermia and radiation in the treatment of superficial malignancy: An analysis of treatment parameters, response and toxicity. *Int J Hyperthermia.* 1987;3:1.

233. Li RY, Zhang TZ, Lin SY, et al: Effect of hyperthermia combined with radiation in the treatment of superficial malignant lesion in 90 patients. In Overgaard J, ed. *Hyperthermic Oncology 1984, vol 1.* London: Taylor & Francis; 1984:395.

234. Lindholm CE, Kjellén E, Nilsson P, et al: Microwave-induced hyperthermia and radiotherapy in human superficial tumors: Clinical results with a comparative study of combined treatment versus radiotherapy alone. *Int J Hyperthermia.* 1987;3:393.

235. Scott RS, Johnson RJ, Story KV, et al: Local hyperthermia in combination with definitive radiotherapy: Increased tumor clearance, reduced recurrence rate in extended follow-up. *Int J Radiat Oncol Biol Phys.* 1984;10:2119.

236. Steeves RA, Severson SB, Paliwal BR, et al: Matched-pair analysis of response to local hyperthermia and megavoltage electron therapy for superficial human tumors. *Endocurie Hypertherm Oncol.* 1986;2:163.

237. U R, Noell KT, Woodward KT, et al: Microwave-induced local hyperthermia in combination with radiotherapy of human malignant tumors. *Cancer.* 1980;45:638.

238. Arcangeli G, Guerra A, et al: Tumor response to heat and radiation: Prognostic variables in the treatment of neck node metastases from head and neck cancer. *Int J Hyperthermia.* 1985;1:207.

239. Perez CA, Emami B: Clinical trials with local (external and interstitial) irradiation and hyperthermia. *Radiol Clin North Am.* 1989;27:525.

240. Valdagni R, Kapp DS, Valdagni C: N3 (TNM-UICC) metastatic neck nodes managed by combined radiation therapy and hyperthermia: Clinical results and analysis of treatment parameters. *Int J Hyperthermia.* 1986;2:189.

241. González González D, van Dijk JDP, Blank LECM: Chestwall recurrences of breast cancer: Results of combined treatment with radiation and hyperthermia. *Radiother Oncol.* 1988;12:95.

242. Kjellén E, Lindholm C-E, Nilsson P: Radiotherapy in combination with hyperthermia in recurrent or metastatic mammary carcinomas. In Sugahara T, Saito M, eds. *Hyperthermic Oncology 1988, vol 2.* London: Taylor & Francis; 1989:426.

243. van der Zee J, van Rhoon GC, Wike-Hooley JL, et al: Thermal enhancement of radiotherapy in breast carcinoma. In Overgaard J, ed. *Hyperthermic Oncology 1984, vol 1.* London: Taylor & Francis; 1984:345.

244. Arcangeli G, Benassi M, Cividalli A, et al: Radiotherapy and hyperthermia: Analysis of clinical results and identification of prognostic variables. *Cancer.* 1987;60:950.

245. González González D, van Dijk JDP, Blank LECM, et al: Combined treatment with radiation and hyperthermia in metastatic malignant melanoma. *Radiother Oncol.* 1986;6:105.

246. Kim JH, Hahn EW, Ahmed SA: Combination hyperthermia and radiation therapy for malignant melanoma. *Cancer.* 1982;50:478.

247. Overgaard J, Overgaard M: Hyperthermia as an adjuvant to radiotherapy in the treatment of malignant melanoma. *Int J Hyperthermia.* 1987;3:483.

248. Kapp DS, Fessenden P, Samulski TV, et al: Stanford University institutional report. Phase I evaluation of equipment for hyperthermia treatment of cancer. *Int J Hyperthermia.* 1988;4:75.

249. Egawa S, Tsukiyama I, Watanabe S, et al: A randomized clinical trial of hyperthermia and radiation versus radiation alone for superficially located cancers. *J Jpn Soc Ther Radiol Oncol.* 1989;1:135.

250. Overgaard J, van der Zee J, Vernon C, et al: Thermoradiotherapy of malignant tumors. European randomized multicenter trials evaluating the effect of adjuvant hyperthermia in radiotherapy. In Kogelnik HD, ed. Progress in Radio-Oncology V. Bologna, Italy: Monduzzi Editore; 1995:507.

251. Hand JW, Machin D, Vernon CC, et al: Analysis of thermal parameters obtained during Phase III trials of hyperthermia as an adjunct to radiotherapy in the treatment of breast carcinoma. *Int J Hyperthermia.* 1997;13:343.

252. Sneed PK: Clinical interstitial hyperthermia: Where have we been? where are we going? In Hagen U, Harder D, Jung H, et al., eds. *Radiation Research 1895-1995, vol 2.* Würzburg, Germany: 10th ICRR Society; 1995:1009.

253. Seegenschmiedt MH, Brady LW, Sauer R: Interstitial thermoradiotherapy: Review on technical and clinical aspects. *Am J Clin Oncol.* 1990;13:352.

254. Seegenschmiedt MH, Klautke G, Grabenbauer GG, et al: Thermoradiotherapy for malignant brain tumors: Review of biological and clinical studies. *Endocurie Hypertherm Oncol.* 1995;11:201.

255. Sneed PK, Gutin PH, Stauffer PR, et al: Thermoradiotherapy of recurrent malignant brain tumors. *Int J Radiat Oncol Biol Phys.* 1992;23:853.

256. Sneed PK, Larson DA, Gutin PH: Brachytherapy and hyperthermia for malignant astrocytoma. *Semin Oncol.* 1994;21:186.

257. Stea B, Rossman K, Kittelson J, et al: Interstitial irradiation versus interstitial thermoradiotherapy for supratentorial malignant gliomas: A comparative survival analysis. *Int J Radiat Oncol Biol Phys.* 1994;30:591.

258. Sneed PK, Stauffer PR, McDermott MW, et al: Survival benefit of hyperthermia in a prospective, randomized trial of brachytherapy boost ± hyperthermia for glioblastoma multiforme. *Int J Radiat Oncol Biol Phys.* 1998;40:287.

259. Myerson RJ, Straube WL, Moros EG, et al: Simultaneous superficial hyperthermia and external radiotherapy: Report of thermal dosimetry and tolerance to treatment. *Int J Hyperthermia.* 1999;15:251.

260. Armour EP, Wang Z, Corry PM, et al: Hyperthermic enhancement of high dose-rate irradiation in 9L gliosarcoma cells. *Int J Radiat Oncol Biol Phys.* 1994;28:171.

261. Feldmann HJ, Molls M, Krümpelmann S, et al: Deep regional hyperthermia: Comparison between the annular phased array and the Sigma-60 applicator in the same patients. *Int J Radiat Oncol Biol Phys.* 1993;26:111.

262. Feldmann HJ, Molls M, Heinemann H-G, et al: Thermoradiotherapy in locally advanced deep seated tumors-thermal parameters and treatment results. *Radiother Oncol.* 1993;26:38.

263. Tilly W, Wust P, Rau B, et al: Temperature data and specific absorption rates in pelvic tumors: Predictive factors and correlations. *Int J Hyperthermia.* 2001;17:172.

264. Petrovich Z, Langholz B, Gibbs FA, et al: Regional hyperthermia for advanced tumors: A clinical study of 353 patients. *Int J Radiat Oncol Biol Phys.* 1989;16:601.

265. Myerson RJ, Scott CB, Emami B, et al: A phase I/II study to evaluate radiation therapy and hyperthermia for deep-seated tumors: A report of RTOG 89-08. *Int J Hyperthermia.* 1996;12:449.

266. Karasawa K, Muta N, Nakagawa K, et al: Thermoradiotherapy in the treatment of locally advanced non–small-cell lung cancer. *Int J Radiat Oncol Biol Phys.* 1994;30:1171.

267. Hiraoka M, Masunaga S, Nishimura Y, et al: Regional hyperthermia combined with radiotherapy in the treatment of lung cancers. *Int J Radiat Oncol Biol Phys.* 1992;22:1009.

268. Lagendijk JJW, van Rhoon GC, Hornsleth SN, et al: ESHO quality assurance guidelines for regional hyperthermia. *Int J Hyperthermia.* 1998;14:125.

269. van der Zee J, González González D: The Dutch Deep Hyperthermia Trial: Results in cervical cancer. *Int J Hyperthermia.* 2002;18:1.

270. Harima Y, Nagata K, Harima K, et al: A randomized clinical trial of radiation therapy versus thermoradiotherapy in stage IIIB cervical cancer. *Int J Hyperthermia.* 2001;17:97.

271. Robins HI, Neville AJ, Cohen JD: *Whole Body Hyperthermia: Biological, Physical and Clinical Aspects.* Berlin: Springer-Verlag; 1992.

272. Kraybill WG, Olenki T, Evans SS, et al: A phase I study of fever-range whole body hyperthermia (FR-WBH) in patients with advanced solid tumors: Correlation with mouse models. *Int J Hyperthermia.* 2002;18:253.

273. Ostberg JR, Gellin C, Patel R, et al: Regulatory potential of fever-range whole body hyperthermia on Langerhans cells and lymphocytes in an antigen-dependent cellular immune response. *J Immunol.* 2001;167:2666.

274. Sharma S, Singhal S, Sandhu AP, et al: Local thermo-radiotherapy in carcinoma cervix: Improved local control versus increased incidence of distant metastases. *Asia-Oceania J Obstet Gynaecol.* 1991;17:5.

275. Berdov BA, Menteshashvili GZ: Thermoradiotherapy of patients with locally advanced carcinoma of the rectum. *Int J Hyperthermia.* 1990;6:881.

276. Overgaard J: Personal communication, 1995.

277. Falk MH, Issels RD: Hyperthermia in oncology. *Int J Hyperthermia.* 2001;17:1.

278. Bull JMC, Cronau LH, Mansfield Newman B, et al: Chemotherapy resistant sarcoma treated with whole body hyperthermia (WBH) combined with 1-3-Bis(2-chloroethyl)-1-nitrosourea (BCNU). *Int J Hyperthermia.* 1992;8:297.

279. Engelhardt R, Neumann H, von der Tann M, et al: Preliminary results in the treatment of oat cell carcinoma of the lung by combined application of chemotherapy (CT) and whole-body hyperthermia. *Prog Clin Biol Res.* 1982;107:761.

280. Engelhardt R, Müller U, Weth-Simon R, et al: Treatment of disseminated malignant melanoma with cisplatin in combination with whole-body hyperthermia and doxorubicin. *Int J Hyperthermia*. 1990;6:511.

281. Leopold KA, Oleson JR, Clarke-Pearson D, et al: Intraperitoneal cisplatin and regional hyperthermia for ovarian carcinoma. *Int J Radiat Oncol Biol Phys*. 1993;27:1245.

282. Westermann AM, Grosen EA, Katschinski DM, et al: A pilot study of whole body hyperthermia and carboplatin in platinum-resistant ovarian cancer. *Eur J Cancer*. 2001;37:1111.

283. Sugimachi K, Kuwano H, Ide H, et al: Chemotherapy combined with or without hyperthermia for patients with oesophageal carcinoma: A prospective randomized trial. *Int J Hyperthermia*. 1994;10:485.

284. Issels RD, Schlemmer M: Current trials and new aspects in soft tissue sarcoma of adults. *Cancer Chemother Pharmacol*. 2002; 49(suppl 1):S4.

285. Ghussen F, Kruger I, Smalley RV, et al: Hyperthermic perfusion with chemotherapy for melanoma of the extremities. *World J Surg*. 1989;13:598.

286. Koops HS, Vaglini M, Suciu S, et al: Prophylactic isolated limb perfusion for localized, high-risk limb melanoma: Results of a multicenter randomized phase III trial. *J Clin Oncol*. 1998;16:2906.

287. Park JW: Liposome-based drug delivery in breast cancer treatment. *Breast Cancer Res*. 2002;4:95.

288. Park JW, Stauffer PR, Diederich CJ, et al: Hyperthermia significantly enhances drug delivery and efficacy of pegylated liposomal doxorubicin in metastatic breast cancer of the chest wall: A phase I/II study (abstract). The 49th annual meeting of the Radiation Research Society and the 20th annual meeting of the North American Hyperthermia Society, Reno, Nev., April 20-24, 2002, p 66.

289. Bull JMC, Scott GL, Strebel FR, et al: A phase I-II clinical trial of fever-range whole-body hyperthermia combined with liposomal doxorubicin (Doxil), 5-fluorouracil (5-FU), & metronomic interferon-α (IFN-α): an interim report (abstract). The 49th annual meeting of the Radiation Research Society and the 20th annual meeting of the North American Hyperthermia Society, Reno, Nev., April 20-24, 2002, p 66.

290. Kitamura K, Kuwano H, Watanabe M, et al: Prospective randomized study of hyperthermia combined with chemoradiotherapy for esophageal carcinoma. *J Surg Oncol*. 1995;60:55.

291. Janetzki S, Palla D, Rosenhauer V, et al: Immunization of cancer patients with autologous cancer-derived heat shock protein gp96: A pilot study. *Int J Cancer*. 2000;88:232.

292. Amato RJ, Murray L, Wood LA, et al: Active specific immunotherapy in patients with renal cell carcinoma (RCC) using autologous tumor derived heat shock protein-peptide complex-96 (HSPPC-96) vaccine (abstract). The 35th annual meeting of the American Society of Clinical Oncology, Atlanta, May 15-18, 1999, p. 332a.

293. Eton O, East MJ, Ross M, et al: Autologous tumor-derived heat-shock protein peptide complex-96 (HSPPC-96) in patients (PTS) with metastatic melanoma (abstract). Proceedings of the American Association for Cancer Research. 2000;41:543.

294. Caudill MM, Li Z: HSPPC-96: A personalised cancer vaccine. *Exp Opin Biol Ther*. 2001;1:539.

295. Manjili MH, Wang X-Y, Park J, et al: Immunotherapy of cancer using heat shock proteins. *Front Biosci*. 2002;7:d43.

296. Srivastava PK, Menoret A, Basu S, et al: Heat shock proteins come of age: Primitive functions acquire new roles in an adaptive world. *Immunity*. 1998;8:657.

297. Blachere NE, Srivastava PK: Heat shock protein-based cancer vaccines and related thoughts on immunogenicity of human tumors. *Semin Cancer Biol*. 1995;6:349.

298. Nicchitta CV: Biochemical, cell biological and immunological issues surrounding the endoplasmic reticulum chaperone GRP94/gp96. *Curr Opin Immunol*. 1998;10:103.

299. Przepiorka D, Srivastava PK: Heat shock protein-peptide complexes as immunotherapy for human cancer. *Mol Med Today*. 1998;4:478.

300. Basu S, Srivastava PK: Heat shock proteins: The fountainhead of innate and adaptive immune responses. *Cell Stress Chaperones*. 2000;5:443.

301. Denman DL, Legorreta RA, Kier AB, et al: Therapeutic responses of spontaneous canine malignancies to combinations of radiotherapy and hyperthermia. *Int J Radiat Oncol Biol Phys*. 1991; 21:415.

302. Gillette EL, McChesney SL, Dewhirst MW, et al: Response of canine oral carcinomas to heat and radiation. *Int J Radiat Oncol Biol Phys*. 1987;13:1861.

303. Gillette SM, Dewhirst MW, Gillette EL, et al: Response of canine soft tissue sarcomas to radiation or radiation plus hyperthermia: A randomized phase II study. *Int J Hyperthermia*. 1992; 8:309.

304. Frew DG, Dobson JM, Stenning SP, et al: Response of the 145 spontaneous canine head and neck tumours to radiation versus radiation plus microwave hyperthermia: Results of a randomized phase III clinical study. *Int J Hyperthermia*. 1995;11:217.

305 Thrall DE, LaRue SM, Powers BE, et al: Use of whole body hyperthermia as a method to heat inaccessible tumors uniformly: A phase III trial in canine brain masses. *Int J Hyperthermia*. 1999;15:383.

306. Thrall DE, Prescott DM, Samulski TV, et al: Radiation plus local hyperthermia versus radiation plus the combination of local and whole-body hyperthermia in canine sarcomas. *Int J Radiat Oncol Biol Phys*. 1996;34:1087.

307. Novotney CA, Page RL, Macy DW, et al: Phase I evaluation of doxorubicin and whole-body hyperthermia in dogs with lymphoma. *J Vet Intern Med*. 1992;6:245.

308. Page RL, Macy DW, Ogilvie GK, et al: Phase III evaluation of doxorubicin and whole-body hyperthermia in dogs with lymphoma. *Int J Hyperthermia*. 1992;8:187.

309. Oleson JR: Hyperthermia from the clinic to the laboratory: A hypothesis. *Int J Hyperthermia*. 1995;11:315.

310. Vujaskovic Z, Poulson JM, Gaskin AA, et al: Temperature-dependent changes in physiologic parameters of spontaneous canine soft tissue sarcomas after combined radiotherapy and hyperthermia treatment. *Int J Radiat Oncol Biol Phys*. 2000;46:179.

Gene-Targeted Therapy

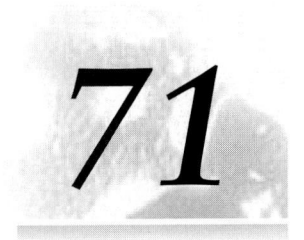

Daphne A. Haas-Kogan, MD and
Alexander R. Gottschalk, MD, PhD

Conventional chemotherapeutic cytotoxic agents offer a therapeutic index based on their propensity to kill rapidly dividing cells. The toxicities of these agents, similarly, result from their effects on rapidly dividing normal tissues, with prominent bone marrow and gastrointestinal side effects. The narrow therapeutic windows of traditional chemotherapies limit their effectiveness.

Over the past several years our understanding of the molecular abnormalities that underlie the development and progression of cancer has advanced greatly. As these genetic alterations are elucidated, scientists have developed new therapies that specifically target mutations seen in cancer. This gene-targeted therapy includes small molecule inhibitors, monoclonal antibodies, and viral therapies. Many gene-targeted therapies have cytostatic effects on tumor cells rather than the cytotoxic effects commonly seen with traditional chemotherapy agents. Because these gene-targeted therapies are cancer specific, based on molecular aberrations present only in tumor cells, they have limited toxicities to normal tissues.

The limited toxicities of molecularly targeted agents have shifted the paradigm of clinical trials. Whereas phase I studies of traditional chemotherapies have focused on dose escalations to maximum tolerated doses, initial phase I trials of gene-targeted therapies incorporate not only maximum tolerated doses but also assessment of biochemical function. For example, the choice of dosing for a tyrosine kinase inhibitor will likely rely on laboratory assays of tumor and normal tissues that document biological readouts of *in vivo* activity.

The effectiveness of such novel therapies must be measured differently from classical chemotherapeutic agents. Measurements of tumor size reflect response to traditional antineoplastic agents. However, since new molecular-targeted therapies are commonly cytostatic rather than cytocidal, measurements of tumor responses must be refined. Following treatment with gene-targeted therapies, assessment of tumor size may not reflect antitumoral efficacy. Often these therapies must be combined with a cytotoxic therapy such as radiation or chemotherapy.

Table 71-1 lists the types of gene-targeted therapies discussed in this chapter. New small molecule inhibitors, monoclonal antibodies, and viral therapies evolve rapidly and continuously. This chapter is not intended to delineate a complete list of all agents under development.

Table 71–1   Types of Gene-targeted Therapies

Molecularly Targeted Approach		Agent
Tyrosine kinase inhibitors	ErbB family inhibitors	ZD 1839
		OSI-774
		C225
		Trastuzumab
	PDGF receptor inhibitors	STI-571
	VEGF receptor inhibitors	SU5416
		SU6668
Farnesyltransferase inhibitors (FTIs)		R115777
Nonreplicating viral therapy	Gene replacement	p53
	Suicide gene therapy	HSV-tk
	Radiation-inducible viral therapy	Egr-TNFα
Replicating viral therapy	Oncolytic adenoviral therapy	Onyx-015
		CV707
		CV787
	Oncolytic herpes virus therapy	G207
		G92a

EGF, epidermal growth factor; PDGF, platelet-derived growth factor receptor; VEGF, vascular endothelial growth factor.

Instead, we will try to provide an overview of the different strategies available, paying particular attention to the better-known agents that are likely to affect the clinical approach to cancer.

MOLECULAR TARGETS FOR RADIOSENSITIZATION

Tyrosine Kinase Receptors

Receptor tyrosine kinases (RTKs) play pleiotropic roles in maintaining homeostasis of individual cells, specific tissues, and entire organisms. The function of RTKs must be tightly regulated since they mediate fundamental cellular functions including proliferation, survival, adhesion, and differentiation. RTK molecules share a ligand-binding extracellular portion, a transmembrane section, and an intracellular portion that contains the tyrosine kinase catalytic domain.[1-3] The family of RTKs includes the epidermal growth factor receptor (EGFR), platelet-derived growth factor receptor (PDGFR), vascular endothelial growth factor receptor (VEGFR), fibroblast growth factor receptor (FGFR), stem-cell factor receptor (SCFR), and nerve growth factor receptor (NGFR). Inactivating mutations in various domains of the protein, including cytoplasmic juxtamembrane and extracellular and kinase domains, confer ligand-independent phosphorylation and kinase activation.[4] Activation of RTKs directly contributes to the initiation, progression, and prognosis of several human malignancies.[5,6]

Activating mutations occur in distinct domains of RTKs. These RTK domains are also targets of pharmacologic inhibitors that are directed at either the extracellular or intracellular domain. Agents that inhibit protein tyrosine kinases fall into two main categories: monoclonal antibodies and small molecule inhibitors.

Monoclonal antibodies can prevent binding of ligands to their receptors, impede the subsequent phosphorylation loop, and thus block signaling through growth factor receptors.[7,8] Technical difficulties such as detrimental antibodies that patients develop against rodent antibodies have been addressed by advances in antibody construction.[9]

Small molecule inhibitors compete with adenosine triphosphate (ATP) for binding sites in the receptor, thus blocking signaling through RTKs.[2] Both strategies of RTK inhibition, monoclonal antibodies and small pharmacologic agents, impact significantly on the antineoplastic effects of ionizing radiation. Inhibitors of several RTKs result in radiosensitization of cancer cells, and their incorporation into radiation regimens, is both imminent and promising.

EPIDERMAL GROWTH FACTOR RECEPTOR INHIBITORS

The ErbB family includes four different receptors: ErbB-1 (also known as EGFR), ErbB-2 (also known as HER2/neu), ErbB-3 (also known as HER3), and ErbB-4 (also known as HER4).[10-12] EGFR is located on chromosome 7p12, and its activation occurs via several mechanisms including amplification, overexpression, and expression of a truncated constitutively active form. EGFR plays a key role in the pathogenesis of many human malignancies, including non–small-cell lung, breast, head and neck, gastric, colorectal, esophageal, prostate, bladder, renal, pancreatic, ovarian, and brain malignancies. For example, EGFR is the most commonly amplified oncogene in glioblastoma multiforme (GM), with amplification seen in 40% of tumors.[13-15] One third of GMs in which EGFR is amplified contain a mutant form, most commonly the EGFRvIII mutant, in which deletion in the extracellular domain results in constitutive tyrosine kinase activity.[16,17]

EGFR offers a promising and exciting target for therapeutic intervention. Several small molecule inhibitors of EGFR signaling have entered clinical trials for gliomas. ZD1839 and OSI-774 are two such oral drugs that inhibit EGFR signaling by targeting the ATP-binding site of the receptor.[18,19]

Inhibition of EGFR signaling has been accomplished not only with pharmacologic agents but also with monoclonal antibodies (mAbs) directed against the extracellular domain of EGFR. Human/murine chimeric antibodies offer the advantage of reduced immunogenicity while preserving potency. mAb-C225 is such an antibody, whose administration in animal models delays growth of xenograft tumors overexpressing ErbB-1.[20]

PLATELET-DERIVED GROWTH FACTOR RECEPTOR INHIBITORS

Whereas some novel signaling inhibitors exhibit specificity toward a given receptor, other drugs can inhibit a number of RTKs. STI571 is a small molecule drug that inhibits the tyrosine kinases Abl, PDGFR, and Kit.[21] Clinical trials have documented efficacy of STI571 in the treatment of chronic myeloid leukemia, a malignancy driven by constitutive activation of Abl resulting from a chromosomal translocation called Bcr-Abl. Clinical trials are incorporating treatment with STI571 in the approach to several adult and pediatric malignancies. For example, studies of gliomas are capitalizing on the inhibitory function of STI571 against PDGFR. The relevance of STI571 for glioma therapy rests in molecular aberrations involving PDGF and PDGFR. PDGFR-α and PDGFR-β are two distinct receptors that bind PDGF ligand, which in turn consists of various dimers of PDGFA and PDGFB chains. Overexpression of the PDGF ligand and receptor are seen in all grades of gliomas, suggesting activation of an autocrine loop that drives glioma proliferation.[24,25] In the minority of cases, amplification of the PDGFR-α gene underlies overexpression; however, in the majority of cases the mechanism of overexpression remains unknown.[22-24]

Molecular abnormalities such as aberrations in PDGFR signaling establish the rationale for treating gliomas of all grades with PDGFR inhibitors and have provided the impetus for ongoing trials evaluating STI571 in the treatment of various human tumors.

VASCULAR ENDOTHELIAL GROWTH FACTOR RECEPTOR INHIBITORS

Initiation and maintenance of gliomas rely not only on cell proliferation and survival but also on the concomitant development of a blood supply to support the enlarging tumor. Therefore, much effort has focused on developing molecules that block proangiogenic factors and therefore inhibit angiogenesis. The best-described proangiogenic factors are VEGFs that transmit their signals through Flt-1 (also known as VEGF-R1) and Flk-1/KDR (also known as VEGF-R2) receptors.[26] Whereas VEGF ligands are secreted by tumor and stromal cells, VEGF receptors are expressed mostly by endothelial cells.

Strategies to block signaling through VEGFR follow the familiar dual paths of small molecule inhibitors and antibodies directed against receptors or ligands. This theme applies to all RTKs targeted to date. SU5416 selectively inhibits Flk-1/KDR and Flt-1.[27] A second pharmacologic molecule, SU6668, exhibits wider specificity toward potentially proangiogenic RTKs, including Flk-1/KDR, PDGF, and FGF receptors.[28] In addition to small molecule inhibitors, antibodies directed against VEGF or its receptors have entered clinical trials.[29] Studies of anti-VEGF agents have focused on human solid tumors since solid malignancies rely on a robust blood supply. Phase I clinical trials employing VEGF inhibitors as single agents report disease stabilization but not objective tumor responses. Many human tumors exhibit robust neovascularity and endothelial proliferation and thus represent excellent potential targets for anti-angiogenic therapy.

Farnesyltransferase Inhibitors

Intermediate molecules transmit downstream signals that emanate from engagement of growth factor receptors. The Ras proteins are such intermediaries that help propagate downstream signaling cascades. Ras is a GTPase that cycles between its active guanosine 5′-triphosphate (GTP)-bound state and its inactive guanosine 5′-biphosphate (GDP)-bound state. Ras regulates many physiologic, cellular functions. Biologic functions of Ras, including proliferation, survival, cytoskeletal organization, differentiation, and membrane trafficking, rely on its association with the inner surface of the plasma membrane.[30-32] Ras proteins are synthesized as cytosolic precursors and are converted to membrane-bound forms through post-translational modifications. Such post-translational modifications begin with the addition of a 15-carbon farnesyl moiety (an isoprene lipid) to a specific motif at the carboxyl-terminus of Ras proteins. Farnesyltransferase catalyzes the transfer of a farnesyl group from farnesyl diphosphate to a cystein residue within the CAAX box (A is an aliphatic amino acid and X is methionine or serine) of Ras.[33]

By blocking farnesylation of Ras and inhibiting its function, farnesyltransferase inhibitors (FTIs) can interrupt the effects of tyrosine kinase receptors that signal through Ras. Thus, FTIs may demonstrate antineoplastic activity not only against tumors that contain oncogenic Ras mutations but also against malignancies that are driven by aberrant signaling through receptor tyrosine kinases. For example, although gliomas rarely possess mutated, oncogenic forms of Ras, common genetic aberrations such as EGFR overexpression may be susceptible to therapeutic targeting by FTIs. However, the precise mode of FTI action remains unclear, as the mutational status of Ras does not consistently correlate with response of cells to FTI treatment. Furthermore, an enlarging body of evidence suggests that FTI activity is mediated in part through inhibition of farnesylation of other Ras family members, such as RhoB.[34-36] As a result, it remains difficult to use biochemical characteristics of individual tumors to predict which malignancies will prove most susceptible to FTI therapy. These ambiguities notwithstanding, FTI treatment has resulted in objective tumor responses in early clinical trials of various human malignancies.

Combining Molecularly Targeted Therapies with Conventional Antineoplastic Treatment

Novel inhibitors of signaling cascades hold great promise in the treatment of human malignancies. Inhibitors of cell signaling, whether antibodies or small molecule drugs, are most likely to affect the treatment of human cancers when combined with standard forms of antineoplastic therapy such as chemotherapy and radiation. Clinical impact will be maximized for combinations of signaling inhibitors and standard cytotoxic agents that result in synergistic effects. Many studies of cell lines *in vitro* and xenograft tumor models *in vivo* indicate that treatment with signaling inhibitors augments tumor response to radiation and chemotherapy.[37] Effects on cell proliferation, survival, migration, invasion, angiogenesis, and DNA repair constitute molecular mechanisms that may underlie radiosensitization associated with signaling inhibitors. The precise molecular mechanisms, however, remain elusive.

Consistent results in multiple published studies demonstrate that blocking EGFR signaling sensitizes tumor cells to ionizing radiation. In several tumor types, overexpression of EGFR correlates with resistance to radiation *in vitro* and *in vivo*.[38-41] Furthermore, EGFR overexpression correlates with radiographically measured radiation response in tumors such as GMs *in vivo*.[42] In a model of human squamous cell carcinoma cells grown in mice, administration of mAb-C225 together with radiation resulted in complete regression of established xenograft tumors.[43,44] Impressive efficacy of concurrent mAb-C225 and radiation has also been documented in intracranial tumors of human glioma cells grown as xenografts in athymic mice. Small molecule inhibitors of EGFR similarly sensitize human malignancies to radiation in cell lines *in vitro* and in animal models of human malignancies *in vivo*. ZD1839 sensitizes several human cell lines to radiation, as does an additional pharmacologic tyrosine kinase inhibitor, CI-1033, which blocks activities of all four types of ErbB receptors.[11] These studies have established the rationale for current clinical trials in which ZD1839 is administered concurrently with radiation in the treatment of adult as well as pediatric malignancies.

Agents that inhibit EGFR signaling offer the dual benefit of potentially inhibiting tumor growth as well as sensitizing resistant tumors to radiation. Similarly, promising results indicate that treatment with FTIs sensitizes human cancer cell lines to irradiation. FTIs reverse the radiation resistance of cell lines containing mutant Ras without affecting the radiosensitivity of cells expressing wild-type Ras.[37] A critical unanswered question is whether FTIs will also preferentially radiosensitize cells with aberrant signaling cascades that rely on Ras as an intermediary.

Novel agents that inhibit signaling through other RTKs such as PDGF and VEGF receptors are not yet established radiosensitizers. However, laboratory investigations offer encouraging evidence that additional signaling inhibitors will augment the radiation response. For example, studies in which VEGF mediates resistance to radiation predict that blocking VEGF signaling will augment the cytotoxic effects of radiation. Furthermore, anti-angiogenic drugs synergize with radiation to block tumor growth *in vivo*.[45] Such promising preliminary studies provide the impetus for designing innovative studies in which molecularly targeted agents are administered concurrently with radiation or chemotherapy.

NONREPLICATING VIRAL THERAPY

Gene Replacement

The theory of gene replacement therapy, also called corrective gene therapy, is simple to comprehend but limited in practicality. The idea behind gene replacement therapy is to identify a specific gene mutation in a tumor and use a virus, as a vector, to introduce the normal copy of the gene back into the tumor. Replacing the mutated copy of a gene with its wild type counterpart is an attempt to "normalize" the cell and, subsequently, the tumor. This approach is filled with many pitfalls. First, tumors are very heterogeneous; hence, the mutations found within a tumor are also heterogeneous. While gene replacement may have an effect on tumor cells that contain that particular mutation, it will be ineffective on other tumor cells that do not. Second, gene replacement therapy uses nonreplicating viruses out of concern for the effects on normal cells, therefore requiring that every single cell be infected with the virus and express the gene of interest. The technology currently available for viral therapy does not allow for infection of every tumor cell and is often limited by the route by which the virus is administered.

Initial interest in gene replacement therapy has focused on the tumor suppressor gene *p53*. This gene is an attractive option for gene replacement therapy because *p53* is mutated in a majority of human tumors and plays a central role in growth arrest, apoptosis, and subsequent response to radiation or chemotherapy or both. Using a replication-defective adenovirus carrying wild type *p53*, scientists have shown that this therapy can sensitize many tumor types to radiation therapy.[52,53] Phase I clinical trials have demonstrated feasibility and safety of delivering adenoviral vectors expressing *p53* through repeated endobronchial injections for non–small-cell lung cancer.[54,55] Current trials are investigating the combination of this approach with radiation therapy. Unfortunately, this gene therapy approach only affects a small number of tumor cells near the injection site of the virus. There is no effect on disease at distant sites and, therefore, no effect on the ultimate outcome of the patient.

p53 Tumor Suppressor Protein

p53 stands at the crossroads of cell death, growth, and differentiation and therefore sustains homeostasis of individual cells, specific tissues, and entire organisms. *p53* regulates apoptosis, proliferation, differentiation, angiogenesis, and cell-matrix interactions.[46-48] Each individual tissue and cell lineage incorporates a distinct balance among the various biological processes mediated by *p53*.[49] For example, *p53*-dependent apoptosis dominates the behavior of hematologic cells; therefore, irradiation of hematologic malignancies, such as leukemia and lymphoma, produces rapid apoptosis. A clinical corollary of this laboratory observation is that irradiation of hematologic malignancies produces rapid and durable responses. Similarly, in many pediatric tissues, apoptosis plays a key role during organogenesis, and pediatric solid tumors such as Wilms' tumor and neuroblastoma exhibit significant apoptosis and excellent cure rates when treated with radiation. In contradistinction, in many adult solid tumors apoptosis plays a minor role and the balance of *p53*-mediated functions tilts toward proliferation and differentiation. Thus, documentation of *p53*-mediated apoptosis *in vivo* following irradiation of adult solid tumors such as GMs and sarcomas has remained elusive.

Despite these complex considerations, the presence of *p53* mutations in more than half of human cancers has provided enthusiasm for harnessing *p53* to overcome tumor resistance to conventional therapies such as radiation.[50] *p53* expression in cells lacking wild type *p53* enhances cellular sensitivity to ionizing radiation.

In the quest to restore wild type *p53* function and overcome resistance to radiation, two main approaches have been used: gene therapy and pharmacologic molecules that confer wild type *p53* function on mutant forms of *p53*.[51] Genetic introduction of wild type *p53* with viral or nonviral vectors may restore physiologic roles of *p53*, and such functions, particularly *p53*-mediated apoptosis, may radiosensitize human tumors. However, many impediments to gene therapy have arisen, including inefficient delivery and detrimental immune responses.

Pharmacologic agents that impinge on *p53* functions hold great promise for translational clinical practice. Some mutated forms of *p53* are amenable to treatment with either synthetic peptides or monoclonal antibodies that can restore wild type *p53* function. Furthermore, large libraries of pharmacologic compounds can be rapidly screened for their ability to reinstate transcriptional transactivating abilities of mutant *p53*. As such novel agents enter clinical trials, the prospect of overcoming radiation resistance of gliomas and other resistant tumors appears within reach.

Suicide Gene Therapy

Another therapeutic approach is to use viral vectors to introduce an enzyme that converts an inactive prodrug to a toxic antimetabolite, aiming to increase intratumoral concentration and efficacy of the drug. One such strategy uses adenovirus to introduce the herpes simplex virus tyrosine kinase (*HSV-tk*) gene into tumor cells followed by administration of acyclovir or ganciclovir. *HSV-tk* phosphorylates the prodrug, acyclovir or ganciclovir, to an active metabolite. The active drug can diffuse to neighboring, uninfected cells through cellular gap junctions, causing toxicity in cells that do not contain the *HSV-tk* gene. This bystander effect increases tumor kill beyond that observed due to direct infection of tumor cells. A second example of this approach is the use adenoviral vectors to introduce the bacterial gene cytosine deaminase (CD) followed by 5-fluorocytosine (5-FC) administration. CD converts 5-FC to the toxic metabolite 5-fluorouracil (5-FU). Active 5-FU may diffuse throughout the tumor, thereby causing direct cytotoxicity or radiosensitization or both of tumor cells in vitro.[56-58] Clinical trials are currently under way with and without radiation therapy in several human tumors.[59-64]

Radiation-Inducible Viral Therapy

A large number of genes are involved in the response to ionizing radiation: *p53*, *p21*, *ATM*, *c-jun*, *egr-1*, *c-fos*, *GADD45*, and *NF-κB*. The induction of genes in response to radiation has led to the engineering of viral vectors to deliver gene therapy within the radiation field, hoping to improve local tumor control while minimizing systemic toxicity. By investigating the genes induced by radiation, radiation response elements (promoters and enhancers) have been identified. These radiation response elements can be inserted upstream from a gene of interest and introduced into a viral vector, creating a radiation-inducible viral therapy. Using this principle, the *egr-1* promoter was linked to tumor necrosis factor alpha (TNFα). TNFα is directly cytotoxic to some tumors, activates the immune response, and can increase sensitivity to radiation,[65,66] but it is limited in its clinical application because of systemic toxicity. A replication-deficient adenovirus carrying the egr-TNFα construct in combination with radiotherapy has shown dramatic effects on animal models.[67,68] Phase I clinical trials with this virus in combination with radiation are currently under way at multiple institutions, with preliminary results demonstrating gene expression in human tumors.[69,70]

REPLICATING VIRAL THERAPY

Oncolytic Adenoviral Therapy

Replicating adenoviruses is being investigated as a new method of delivering targeted therapy. Adenoviruses are nonenveloped, linear, double-stranded DNA viruses with a genome size of 38 kb. Adenoviruses can infect dividing and nondividing epithelial cells. Once inside the cell, the virus uses the cell's normal proteins to produce and package more virus particles. The virus then lyses and kills the cell, exposing neighboring cells to new virus particles. When adenovirus infects normal cells, *p53* levels are increased and the cell undergoes either apoptosis or growth arrest, attempting to prevent viral replication. Wild type adenovirus evades apoptosis and growth arrest by expressing the *E1B-55 kD* gene, which encodes

a protein that binds to and inactivates *p53* and thus allows viral replication to proceed.[71] One strategy of generating a tumor-specific adenovirus is to mutate the *E1B-55 kD* gene. ONYX-015 is an adenovirus that lacks the *E1B* gene; therefore, viral replication is prevented in cells with normal *p53* for the previously mentioned reasons.[72] Many tumor cell types lack functional *p53*, which accounts for the tumor-specific replication of the ONYX-015 virus. Loss of *p14(arf)*, a tumor suppressor gene whose product functionally stabilizes *p53*, also allows for replication of ONYX-015.[73] Put together, the ONYX-015 virus is able to replicate and kill tumor cells that have mutation in the *p53* pathway as a whole.

ONYX-015 is now under study for the treatment of *p53*-deficient malignancies. Recurrent squamous cell carcinomas of the head and neck region have been treated with the combination of ONYX-015 and chemotherapy.[74,75] Head and neck cancers often have mutation in the *p53* gene. This fact, in combination with easy access for direct injection of the virus, has made head and neck tumors an ideal place to start investigating the effect of ONYX-015. This phase II trial of ONYX-015 and chemotherapy has demonstrated limited toxicity and significant antitumor activity.[74] A phase III randomized trial of chemotherapy ± ONYX-015 is currently under way for recurrent squamous cell carcinoma of the head and neck region. ONYX-015 in combination with 5-FU is also under investigation in a phase I/II trial of intraarterial administration to patients with liver metastases from colorectal adenocarcinoma.[76] This virus is also being investigated in primary liver, ovarian, and unresectable pancreatic tumors.[77-79]

A similar approach in developing a tumor-specific adenovirus involves deletion of the *E1A* gene from the adenoviral genome. *E1A* binds to and inhibits the action of the tumor suppressor gene *pRB*.[80] This serves to release *pRB* from the transcription factor E2F and facilitate entry into the G1 phase of the cell cycle. E2F mediates the transcription of several cellular enzymes necessary for DNA synthesis. The ultimate effect of *E1A* expression is to create a cellular environment favorable for the synthesis of multiple copies of the viral genome. An adenovirus containing a deletion in the *E1A* gene will, therefore, replicate in and lyse cells containing mutations in *pRB*. The *E1A*-deleted virus can also replicate in cells mutant in p16, indicating that a deficiency in the *pRB* pathway as a whole is sufficient to allow for viral replication.[81] The clinical studies using the *E1A*-deleted virus have not been reported.

A second approach to achieve tumor-selective adenoviral replication is the use of tumor- or tissue-specific promoters to drive the expression of an adenoviral gene that is critical for efficient replication, such as *E1A*. One example of this strategy is CV706, an engineered virus that is specific for prostate cancer. By placing the prostate-specific antigen (PSA) promoter-enhancer region upstream of the *E1A* gene, scientists have developed an adenovirus that will replicate only within PSA-producing cells.[82] This virus has been used in a phase I trial of intraprostatic injection of patients with locally recurrent prostate cancer following definitive radiation therapy.[83] A more potent oncolytic virus, CV787, has been generated using the prostate-specific rat probasin promoter driving the *E1A* expression and the human PSA enhancer/promoter driving the *E1B* gene. Currently CV787 is being investigated in patients with either organ-confined disease or hormone-refractory metastatic prostate cancer. In addition, laboratory experiments have shown synergy between radiation therapy and this prostate-specific adenovirus.[84] In future studies, this virus may be used in conjunction with more traditional therapies such as surgery or radiation therapy.

Oncolytic Herpes Virus Therapy

Herpes simplex virus 1 (HSV-1) is an enveloped double-stranded DNA virus with a genome size of 152 kb. As with the oncolytic adenoviruses, deletion or inactivation of essential viral genes may lead to tumor specificity. A deletion in the *HSV tyrosine kinase* (*tk*) gene prevents replication of the virus in normal cells. Malignant glioma cells are actively dividing and therefore have high endogenous levels of tk, allowing replication of the virus and destruction of the tumor cells. This tk-mutant HSV has not been used in clinical trials because of neurotoxicity and resistance to antiviral therapies (acyclovir and ganciclovir). Investigators have looked instead at developing HSV-1 mutants that maintain sensitivity to acyclovir and ganciclovir and exhibit less neurovirulence by deletion of the $\gamma_1 34.5$ gene. The protein product of $\gamma_1 34.5$ blocks the inhibition of host protein synthesis in infected cells by interacting with cellular phosphatase 1α to dephosphorylate eIF2α. This leads to production of more progeny virion from each infected cell. Replication of the $\gamma_1 34.5$-null mutant is attenuated in normal cells, such as adult neurons, thereby minimizing the risk of viral encephalitis. However, $\gamma_1 34.5$-null mutants replicate in actively dividing tumor cells. Without disruption of the *HSV-tk* gene, these mutants remain sensitive to acyclovir and ganciclovir.[85,86]

G207 is an HSV-1 mutant in $\gamma_1 34.5$ with an additional inactivation of the ICP6 gene that encodes for a subunit of the viral ribonucleotide reductase. The presence of two mutations makes spontaneous reversion to a wild-type virus nearly impossible, therefore providing an added level of safety. Mammalian ribonucleotide reductase is elevated in tumor cells relative to normal cells, so HSV-1 mutants defective in ribonucleotide reductase replicate preferentially in tumor cells. G207 HSV is being used in clinical trials for recurrent glioma with no toxicity seen.[87] The $\gamma_1 34.5$-null mutant HSV is also being combined with transgene expression of IL-4 and IL-12 to combine the oncolytic property of the virus with enhancement of the host's endogenous T cell immunity.

Another approach to achieve preferential viral replication in tumor cells is to use tumor- or tissue-specific promoters to drive expression of a critical viral gene. G92a is one such vector in which the *ICP4* gene is under transcriptional control of the albumin promoter/enhancer.[88] Replication of G92a is several logs more efficient in albumin-expressing hepatoma cells. So far, this virus has only been used in animal models.[89]

CONCLUSION

As molecular abnormalities involved in the pathogenesis and progression of cancer are elucidated, more molecular targeted therapies will emerge. Due to well-described heterogeneities in molecular abnormalities within individual tumors, any one gene-targeted therapy is unlikely to cure a specific type of cancer. Combinations of targeted therapies integrated with traditional treatments of surgery, radiotherapy, and chemotherapy will soon represent standard therapy for many cancers.

REFERENCES

1. Porter AC, Vaillancourt RR: Tyrosine kinase receptor–activated signal transduction pathways which lead to oncogenesis. *Oncogene.* 1998;17:1343.
2. Levitzki A, Gazit A: Tyrosine kinase inhibition: An approach to drug development. *Science.* 1995;267:1782.
3. Hunter T: Signaling—2000 and beyond. *Cell.* 2000;100:113.
4. Demetri GD: Targeting c-kit mutations in solid tumors: Scientific rationale and novel therapeutic options. *Semin Oncol.* 2001;28:19.
5. Taniguchi M, Nishida T, Hirota S, et al: Effect of c-kit mutation on prognosis of gastrointestinal stromal tumors. *Cancer Res.* 1999; 59:4297.
6. Lasota J, Jasinski M, Sarlomo-Rikala M, et al: Mutations in exon 11 of c-Kit occur preferentially in malignant versus benign gastrointestinal stromal tumors and do not occur in leiomyomas or leiomyosarcomas. *Am J Pathol.* 1999;154:53.
7. Drebin JA, Link VC, Stern DF, et al: Down-modulation of an onco-gene protein product and reversion of the transformed phenotype by monoclonal antibodies. *Cell.* 1985;41:697.
8. Drebin JA, Link VC, Weinberg RA, et al: Inhibition of tumor growth by a monoclonal antibody reactive with an oncogene-encoded tumor antigen. *Proc Natl Acad Sci U S A.* 1986;83:9129.
9. Fan Z, Mendelsohn J: Therapeutic application of anti-growth factor receptor antibodies. *Curr Opin Oncol.* 1998;10:67.
10. Klapper LN, Kirschbaum MH, Sela M, et al: Biochemical and clinical implications of the ErbB/HER signaling network of growth factor receptors. *Adv Cancer Res.* 2000;77:25.
11. Mendelsohn J, Baselga J: The EGF receptor family as targets for cancer therapy. *Oncogene.* 2000;19:6550.
12. Olayioye MA, Neve RM, Lane HA, et al: The ErbB signaling network: Receptor heterodimerization in development and cancer. *EMBO J.* 2000;19:3159.
13. Wong AJ, Bigner SH, Bigner DD, et al: Increased expression of the epidermal growth factor receptor gene in malignant gliomas is invariably associated with gene amplification. *Proc Natl Acad Sci U S A.* 1987;84:6899.
14. Ekstrand AJ, James CD, Cavenee WK, et al: Genes for epidermal growth factor receptor, transforming growth factor alpha, and epidermal growth factor and their expression in human gliomas in vivo. *Cancer Res.* 1991;51:2164.
15. von Deimling A, Louis DN, von Ammon K, et al: Association of epidermal growth factor receptor gene amplification with loss of chromosome 10 in human glioblastoma multiforme. *J Neurosurg.* 1992;77:295.
16. Ekstrand AJ, Sugawa N, James CD, et al: Amplified and rearranged epidermal growth factor receptor genes in human glioblastomas reveal deletions of sequences encoding portions of the N- and/or C-terminal tails. *Proc Natl Acad Sci U S A.* 1992;89:4309.
17. Wikstrand CJ, McLendon RE, Friedman AH, et al: Cell surface localization and density of the tumor-associated variant of the epidermal growth factor receptor, EGFRvIII. *Cancer Res.* 1997; 57:4130.
18. Fry DW, Kraker AJ, McMichael A, et al: A specific inhibitor of the epidermal growth factor receptor tyrosine kinase. *Science.* 1994;265:1093.
19. Klohs WD, Fry DW, Kraker AJ: Inhibitors of tyrosine kinase. *Curr Opin Oncol.* 1997;9:562.

20. Goldstein NI, Prewett M, Zuklys K, et al: Biological efficacy of a chimeric antibody to the epidermal growth factor receptor in a human tumor xenograft model. *Clin Cancer Res.* 1995;1:1311.

21. Sawyers CL: Rational therapeutic intervention in cancer: Kinases as drug targets. *Curr Opin Genet Dev.* 2002;12:111.

22. Maxwell M, Naber SP, Wolfe HJ, et al: Coexpression of platelet-derived growth factor (PDGF) and PDGF-receptor genes by primary human astrocytomas may contribute to their development and maintenance. *J Clin Invest.* 1990;86:131.

23. Hermanson M, Funa K, Hartman M, et al: Platelet-derived growth factor and its receptors in human glioma tissue: Expression of messenger RNA and protein suggests the presence of autocrine and paracrine loops. *Cancer Res.* 1992;52:3213.

24. Hermanson M, Funa K, Koopmann J, et al: Association of loss of heterozygosity on chromosome 17p with high platelet-derived growth factor alpha receptor expression in human malignant gliomas. *Cancer Res.* 1996;56:164.

25. Westermark B, Heldin CH, Nistér M: Platelet-derived growth factor in human glioma. *Glia.* 1995;15:257.

26. Carmeliet P, Jain RK: Angiogenesis in cancer and other diseases. *Nature.* 2000;407:249.

27. Fong TA, Shawver LK, Sun L, et al: SU5416 is a potent and selective inhibitor of the vascular endothelial growth factor receptor (Flk-1/KDR) that inhibits tyrosine kinase catalysis, tumor vascularization, and growth of multiple tumor types. *Cancer Res.* 1999;59:99.

28. Laird AD, Vajkoczy P, Shawver LK, et al: SU6668 is a potent antiangiogenic and antitumor agent that induces regression of established tumors. *Cancer Res.* 2000;60:4152.

29. Presta LG, Chen H, O'Connor SJ, et al: Humanization of an anti-vascular endothelial growth factor monoclonal antibody for the therapy of solid tumors and other disorders. *Cancer Res.* 1997;57:4593.

30. Bourne HR, Sanders DA, McCormick F: The GTPase superfamily: A conserved switch for diverse cell functions. *Nature.* 1990;348:125.

31. Downward J: Control of ras activation. *Cancer Surv.* 1996;27:87.

32. Lowy DR, Willumsen BM: Function and regulation of ras. *Annu Rev Biochem.* 1993;62:851.

33. Rowinsky EK, Windle JJ, Von Hoff DD: Ras protein farnesyltransferase: A strategic target for anticancer therapeutic development. *J Clin Oncol.* 1999;17:3631.

34. Du W, Lebowitz PF, Prendergast GC: Cell growth inhibition by farnesyltransferase inhibitors is mediated by gain of geranylgeranylated RhoB. *Mol Cell Biol.* 1999;19:1831.

35. Reuter CW, Morgan MA, Bergmann L: Targeting the Ras signaling pathway: A rational, mechanism-based treatment for hematologic malignancies? *Blood.* 2000;96:1655.

36. Lebowitz PF, Prendergast GC: Non-Ras targets of farnesyltransferase inhibitors: Focus on rho. *Oncogene.* 1998;17:1439.

37. Jones HA, Hahn SM, Bernhard E, et al: Ras inhibitors and radiation therapy. *Semin Radiat Oncol.* 2001;11:328.

38. Pillai MR, Jayaprakash PG, Nair MK: Tumor-proliferative fraction and growth factor expression as markers of tumor response to radiotherapy in cancer of the uterine cervix. *J Cancer Res Clin Oncol.* 1998;124:456.

39. Miyaguchi M, Takeuchi T, Morimoto K, et al: Correlation of epidermal growth factor receptor and radiosensitivity in human maxillary carcinoma cell lines. *Acta Otolaryngol.* 1998;118:428.

40. Sheridan MT, O'Dwyer T, Seymour CB, et al: Potential indicators of radiosensitivity in squamous cell carcinoma of the head and neck. *Radiat Oncol Investig.* 1997;5:180.

41. Wollman R, Yahalom J, Maxy R, et al: Effect of epidermal growth factor on the growth and radiation sensitivity of human breast cancer cells in vitro. *Int J Radiat Oncol Biol Phys.* 1994;30:91.

42. Barker FG II, Simmons ML, Chang SM, et al: EGFR overexpression and radiation response in glioblastoma multiforme. *Int J Radiat Oncol Biol Phys.* 2001;51:410.

43. Huang SM, Bock JM, Harari PM: Epidermal growth factor receptor blockade with C225 modulates proliferation, apoptosis, and radiosensitivity in squamous cell carcinomas of the head and neck. *Cancer Res.* 1999;59:1935.

44. Milas L, Mason K, Hunter N, et al: In vivo enhancement of tumor radioresponse by C225 antiepidermal growth factor receptor antibody. *Clin Cancer Res.* 2000;6:701.

45. Gorski DH, Beckett MA, Jaskowiak NT, et al: Blockage of the vascular endothelial growth factor stress response increases the antitumor effects of ionizing radiation. *Cancer Res.* 1999;59:3374.

46. Lane DP: Cancer. *p53*, Guardian of the genome. *Nature.* 1992; 358:15.

47. Kastan MB, Zhan Q, el-Deiry WS, et al: A mammalian cell cycle checkpoint pathway utilizing *p53* and GADD45 is defective in ataxia-telangiectasia. *Cell.* 1992;71:587.

48. Sionov RV, Haupt Y: The cellular response to *p53*: The decision between life and death. *Oncogene.* 1999;18:6145.

49. Schmitt CA, Fridman JS, Yang M, et al: Dissecting *p53* tumor suppressor functions in vivo. *Cancer Cell.* 2002;1:289.

50. Brown JM, Wouters BG: Apoptosis, *p53*, and tumor cell sensitivity to anticancer agents. *Cancer Res.* 1999;59:1391.

51. Pruschy M, Rocha S, Zaugg K, et al: Key targets for the execution of radiation-induced tumor cell apoptosis: The role of *p53* and caspases. *Int J Radiat Oncol Biol Phys.* 2001;49:561.

52. Cowen D, Salem N, Ashoori F, et al: Prostate cancer radiosensitization in vivo with adenovirus-mediated *p53* gene therapy. *Clin Cancer Res.* 2000;6:4402.

53. Kawabe S, Munshi A, Zumstein LA, et al: Adenovirus-mediated wild-type *p53* gene expression radiosensitizes non–small-cell lung cancer cells but not normal lung fibroblasts. *Int J Radiat Biol.* 2001;77:185.

54. Weill D, Mack M, Roth J, et al: Adenoviral-mediated *p53* gene transfer to non–small-cell lung cancer through endobronchial injection. *Chest.* 2000;118:966.

55. Swisher SG, Roth JA, Nemunaitis J, et al: Adenovirus-mediated *p53* gene transfer in advanced non–small-cell lung cancer. *J Natl Cancer Inst.* 1999;91:763.

56. Khil MS, Kim JH, Mullen CA, et al: Radiosensitization by 5-fluorocytosine of human colorectal carcinoma cells in culture transduced with cytosine deaminase gene. *Clin Cancer Res.* 1996; 2:53.

57. Pederson LC, Buchsbaum DJ, Vickers SM, et al: Molecular chemotherapy combined with radiation therapy enhances killing of cholangiocarcinoma cells in vitro and in vivo. *Cancer Res.* 1997; 57:4325.

58. Hanna NN, Mauceri HJ, Wayne JD, et al: Virally directed cytosine deaminase/5-fluorocytosine gene therapy enhances radiation response in human cancer xenografts. *Cancer Res.* 1997;57:4205.

59. Klatzmann D, Valery CA, Bensimon G, et al: A phase I/II study of herpes simplex virus type 1 thymidine kinase "suicide" gene therapy for recurrent glioblastoma. Study Group on Gene Therapy for Glioblastoma. *Hum Gene Ther.* 1998;9:2595.

60. Klatzmann D, Cherin P, Bensimon G, et al: A phase I/II dose-escalation study of herpes simplex virus type 1 thymidine kinase "suicide" gene therapy for metastatic melanoma. Study Group on Gene Therapy of Metastatic Melanoma. *Hum Gene Ther.* 1998; 9:2585.

61. Eck SL, Alavi JB, Alavi A, et al: Treatment of advanced CNS malignancies with the recombinant adenovirus H5.010RSVTK: A Phase I trial. *Hum Gene Ther.* 1996;7:1465.

62. Schwarzenberger P, Harrison L, Weinacker A, et al: The treatment of malignant mesothelioma with a gene modified cancer cell line: A phase I study. *Hum Gene Ther.* 1998;9:2641.

63. Rainov NG: A phase III clinical evaluation of herpes simplex virus type 1 thymidine kinase and ganciclovir gene therapy as an adjuvant to surgical resection and radiation in adults with previously untreated glioblastoma multiforme. *Hum Gene Ther.* 2000;11:2389.

64. Kun LE, Gajjar A, Muhlbauer M, et al: Stereotactic injection of herpes simplex thymidine kinase vector producer cells (PA317-G1Tk1SvNa.7) and intravenous ganciclovir for the treatment of progressive or recurrent primary supratentorial pediatric malignant brain tumors. *Hum Gene Ther.* 1995;6:1231.

65. Sersa G, Willingham V, Milas L: Anti-tumor effects of tumor necrosis factor alone or combined with radiotherapy. *Int J Cancer.* 1988; 42:129.

66. Old LJ: Tumor necrosis factor (TNF). *Science.* 1985;230:630.

67. Staba MJ, Mauceri HJ, Kufe DW, et al: Adenoviral TNF-alpha gene therapy and radiation damage tumor vasculature in a human malignant glioma xenograft. *Gene Ther.* 1998;5:293.

68. Chung TD, Mauceri HJ, Hallahan DE, et al: Tumor necrosis factor-alpha-based gene therapy enhances radiation cytotoxicity in human prostate cancer. *Cancer Gene Ther.* 1998;5:344.

69. Sharma A, Mani S, Hanna N, et al: Clinical protocol. An open-label, phase I, dose-escalation study of tumor necrosis factor-alpha (TNFerade Biologic) gene transfer with radiation therapy for locally advanced, recurrent, or metastatic solid tumors. *Hum Gene Ther.* 2001;12:1109.

70. Hallahan DE, Vokes EE, Rubin SJ, et al: Phase I dose-escalation study of tumor necrosis factor-alpha and concomitant radiation therapy. *Cancer J Sci Am.* 1995;1:204.

71. Yew PR, Berk AJ: Inhibition of *p53* transactivation required for transformation by adenovirus early 1B protein. *Nature.* 1992; 357:82.

72. Bischoff JR, Kirn DH, Williams A, et al: An adenovirus mutant that replicates selectively in *p53*-deficient human tumor cells. *Science.* 1996;274:373.

73. Ries SJ, Brandts CH, Chung AS, et al: Loss of p14ARF in tumor cells facilitates replication of the adenovirus mutant dl1520 (ONYX-015). *Nat Med.* 2000;6:1128.

74. Nemunaitis J, Khuri F, Ganly I, et al: Phase II trial of intratumoral administration of ONYX-015, a replication-selective adenovirus, in patients with refractory head and neck cancer. *J Clin Oncol.* 2001; 19:289.

75. Lamont JP, Nemunaitis J, Kuhn JA, et al: A prospective phase II trial of ONYX-015 adenovirus and chemotherapy in recurrent squamous cell carcinoma of the head and neck (the Baylor experience). *Ann Surg Oncol.* 2000;7:588.

76. Reid T, Galanis E, Abbruzzese J, et al: Intra-arterial administration of a replication-selective adenovirus (dl1520) in patients with colorectal carcinoma metastatic to the liver: A phase I trial. *Gene Ther.* 2001;8:1618.

77. Mulvihill S, Warren R, Venook A, et al: Safety and feasibility of injection with an E1B-55 kDa gene-deleted, replication-selective adenovirus (ONYX-015) into primary carcinomas of the pancreas: A phase I trial. *Gene Ther.* 2001;8:308.

78. Habib NA, Sarraf CE, Mitry RR, et al: E1B-deleted adenovirus (dl1520) gene therapy for patients with primary and secondary liver tumors. *Hum Gene Ther.* 2001;12:219.

79. Heise C, Ganly I, Kim YT, et al: Efficacy of a replication-selective adenovirus against ovarian carcinomatosis is dependent on tumor burden, viral replication and p53 status. *Gene Ther.* 2000; 7:1925.

80. Whyte P, Buchkovich KJ, Horowitz JM, et al: Association between an oncogene and an anti-oncogene: The adenovirus E1A proteins bind to the retinoblastoma gene product. *Nature.* 1988; 334:124.

81. Johnson L, Shen A, Boyle L, et al: Selectively replicating adenoviruses targeting deregulated E2F activity are potent, systemic antitumor agents. *Cancer Cell.* 2002;1:325.

82. Rodriguez R, Schuur ER, Lim HY, et al: Prostate attenuated replication competent adenovirus (ARCA) CN706: A selective cytotoxic for prostate-specific antigen-positive prostate cancer cells. *Cancer Res.* 1997;57:2559.

83. DeWeese TL, van der Poel H, Li S, et al: A phase I trial of CV706, a replication-competent, PSA selective oncolytic adenovirus, for the treatment of locally recurrent prostate cancer following radiation therapy. *Cancer Res.* 2001;61:7464.

84. Chen Y, DeWeese T, Dilley J, et al: CV706, a prostate cancer-specific adenovirus variant, in combination with radiotherapy produces synergistic antitumor efficacy without increasing toxicity. *Cancer Res.* 2001;61:5453.

85. Mullen JT, Tanabe KK: Viral oncolysis. *Oncologist.* 2002;7:106.

86. Martuza RL: Conditionally replicating herpes vectors for cancer therapy. *J Clin Invest.* 2000;105:841.

87. Markert JM, Medlock MD, Rabkin SD, et al: Conditionally replicating herpes simplex virus mutant, G207 for the treatment of malignant glioma: Results of a phase I trial. *Gene Ther.* 2000; 7:867.

88. Miyatake S, Iyer A, Martuza RL, Rabkin SD: Transcriptional targeting of herpes simplex virus for cell-specific replication. *J Virol.* 1997;71:5124.

89. Miyatake SI, Tani S, Feigenbaum F, et al: Hepatoma-specific antitumor activity of an albumin enhancer/promoter regulated herpes simplex virus in vivo. *Gene Ther.* 1999;6:564.

72

Tumor-Targeted Radioisotope Therapy

Sally J. DeNardo, MD, and Ignacio Azinovic, MD

HISTORY OF RADIOIMMUNOTHERAPY

In the late 1940s, a method was developed for linking ^{131}I to proteins including antibodies (Abs) in vitro without significantly altering biologic function such as Ab immunologic specificity.[1] Using this technique, Pressman and Komgold[2] demonstrated in 1953 that intravenously administered Ab accumulated to a slightly greater extent in tumors than in normal tissue.[3]

Clinical trials involving radioimmunotherapy (RIT), tumor-targeted systemic radiotherapy, began in the 1950s with polyclonal Abs when Beierwaltes[4] administered ^{131}I-labeled rabbit Ab to 14 patients with metastatic melanoma and achieved a pathologically documented complete response (CR) in one patient. In the 1960s, Spar and coworkers[5] administered ^{131}I-antifibrinogen polyclonal Abs to cancer patients and observed symptomatic improvement in some cases. In 1965, polyclonal Abs began to be developed against more specific tumor-associated antigens (e.g., carcinoembryonic antigen). This was associated with greater Ab uptake in tumors. In the 1970s, Ettinger et al.[6,7] began to treat patients with cholangiocarcinomas and hepatomas with ^{131}I-anti-carcinoembryonic antigen and ^{131}I-antiferritin polyclonal Abs in combination with external beam radiation therapy, doxorubicin, and 5-fluorouracil chemotherapy. A 30% or greater decrease in tumor size was observed in six of nine evaluable patients. Order et al.[8] pursued an aggressive combined modality approach to hepatoma, with one trial arm including radiolabeled polyclonal Abs. Because of their polyclonal nature, these tumorphilic radiolabeled Ab mixtures were heterogeneous in their pharmacokinetics and tumor binding.

When Kohler and Milstein, in 1975, published a technique[9] for the production of monoclonal antibodies (mAbs), where each clone selected could produce one molecular Ab species of a predefined specificity, the technology provided the critical keystone for the development of RIT. With this hybridoma approach, mAbs to predefined cancer-associated antigens could be produced in gram quantities, thus revolutionizing the field. Although no mAb is yet considered absolutely specific for tumor, tumor to normal tissue radiation dose ratios (therapeutic index, TI) ranging from 2:1 to greater than 30:1 have been achieved with tumor-targeting radiolabeled mAbs in cancer patients.[10,11]

MAbs have been conjugated with chemotherapeutic agents, biologic toxins, or radioisotopes in an attempt to use them to selectively target malignant cells while sparing normal tissues.[12] Treatment of cancer with mAbs conjugated with chemotherapeutic agents or toxins has faced a number of obstacles, including (1) the requirement that every malignant cell express the target antigen; (2) the development of multidrug resistance; (3) the degradation of the drug or toxin by lysosomes following endocytosis; (4) the formation of Abs against the toxin; and (5) a dose-limiting capillary leak syndrome, manifested by hypoalbuminemia and edema.[13,14] Tumor-targeted radioisotopes have several advantages over drugs or toxins: (1) beta particles emitted by radionuclides such as iodine-131 (^{131}I), yttrium-90 (^{90}Y), or copper-67 ([67]Cu) can kill adjacent tumor cells (crossfire) (Table 72-1), partially overcoming heterogeneous antigen expression and poor tumor penetration; (2) radioisotopes are not subject to multidrug resistance; and (3) pharmacokinetics and dosimetry can be obtained from scintigraphic imaging, helping to develop and prescribe therapy.

Radioimmunoconjugates, however, have usually been made with the entire 150 kD mAb, resulting in large molecules that have slow blood clearance; retention in normal organs involved in Ab metabolism; and slow, incomplete tumor penetration. Combined with antigenic heterogeneity, only 0.0001% to 0.1% of the injected dose of Abs binds to each gram of tumor.[15] Consequently, RIT has typically produced tumor doses of less than 20 Gy unless bone marrow support allowed larger injected doses. Challenges facing RIT along with possible solutions[16] are presented in Table 72-2.

Over the past few years, steady progress has been made in the multidisciplinary field of RIT. The studies in non-Hodgkin's lymphoma (NHL) from expert institutions and multi-institutional trials, as well as FDA approval of RIT drugs for standard clinical use, have opened this treatment modality to more widespread care of cancer patients. In this chapter, Ab structure; suitable radioisotopes; challenges facing current RIT trials; reported

Table 72–1   Radionuclides Suitable for Radioimmunotherapy

Radionuclide	Decay Mode	Physical Half-Life	Max. Particulate Energy (%)	Max. Range of Particulate Energy in Tissue, mm	γ energy, keV (% of total energy)	Advantages	Disadvantages
I-131	β, γ	8d	807 keV (1)* 606 keV (86)* 336 keV (13)*	2.4	364 (81)	Iodine chemistry, inexpensive	Dehalogenation radiation safety concerns
Cu-67	β, γ	62h	577 keV (20)* 484 keV (35)* 395 keV (45)*	2.2	184 (47)	Images, metal chemistry, long retention in tumor	Scarce
Lu-177	β, γ	6.7d	497 keV (90)* 384 keV (3)* 175 keV (7)*	2.2	208 (11) 113 (7)	Images	Scarce, bone seeker
Re-186	β, γ electron capture	91h	1.07 MeV (77)* 934 keV (23)*	5.0	137 (9)	^{99m}Tc chemistry	Scarce
Y-90	β	64h	2.29 MeV (100)*	11.9	—	Metal chemistry	Doesn't image, bone seeker
Re-188	β	17h	2.13 MeV (100)*	11.1	—		Scarce, short ½ life
Bi-212	α, β	1h	6.09 MeV (27)† 6.05 MeV (70)† 5.77 MeV (2)† 5.61 MeV (1)†	0.09	—		Doesn't image, short ½ life, unstable daughter product
At-211	α, electron capture	7h	5.87 MeV (100)†	0.09	—	High RBE, hypoxia less important, short range	Doesn't image, short ½ life, unstable daughter product
I-125	Electron capture	60d	35 keV (100)	0.02	—	Short range	Doesn't image, long ½ life

*Beta irradiation.
†Alpha irradiation.
RBE, relative biologic effectiveness.

Table 72–2   Challenges to Improve the Therapeutic Index for Radioimmunotherapy

Problems Facing the Therapeutic Index	Possible Solution
Marrow toxicity	Small targeting molecules Pretargeting approach
Normal tissue antigen	Preinfusion of cold Ab Pretargeting approach
Non-specific Fc receptor binding	Saturate receptors with cold Ab Intracavitary (e.g., intraperitoneal administration) Ab fragments: F(ab′)₂, svFc, diabody… Pretargeting
Tumor penetration	Ab fragments: F(ab′)₂, svFc, diabody… Multimodality approach: chemotherapy, external beam… Pretargeting Inject Ab directly into the tumor
Antigenic heterogeneity and insufficient antigen expression	Isotopes: beta-emitters (cross-fire effect) Cocktail of Ab recognizing different antigens Enhance antigen expression: interferon, hyperthermia
Antigenic modulation	Administer subsequent Ab infusions after re-expression of the target antigen
HAMA	mAb modifications: chimeric, humanize, fragments Temporary immune suppression (Cyclosporin A, Fludaribine) Complex circulating HAMA with mAb

Ab, antibody; HAMA, human anti-mouse antibodies; mAb, monoclonal antibody.

clinical results; expected toxicities; and new strategies in current clinical trials, including pretargeted RIT approaches, are addressed.

ANTIBODY STRUCTURE AND FUNCTION

The majority of Abs produced in mammals are composed of two pairs of polypeptide chains, light and heavy, which are linked by disulfide bridges. They represent the five major classes: IgG, IgA, IgE, IgD, and a pentameric version IgM.

These contain variable and constant regions with the variable regions of the heavy and light chains (V_H and V_L)

containing the antigen-binding site (Fig. 72-1A). The major constant portion (Fc) of the Ab molecule contains a number of molecular signals that mediate biologic functions such as complement binding, hepatocyte binding, and recruitment or activation of effector cells, such as monocytes and natural killer cells. Pepsin digests of Abs result in a short divalent ($F(ab')_2$) antigen-binding molecule without most of the Fc fraction, and papain digestion results in an even smaller antigen-binding monovalent fragment (Fab) (Fig. 72-1B).[17,18] Genetic engineering, using the V_H and V_L MAb DNA, has fashioned smaller binding units, fragment (Fv), as well as the linked single chain fragments (scFvs). These may provide the targeting molecules of the future (Fig. 72-1B).

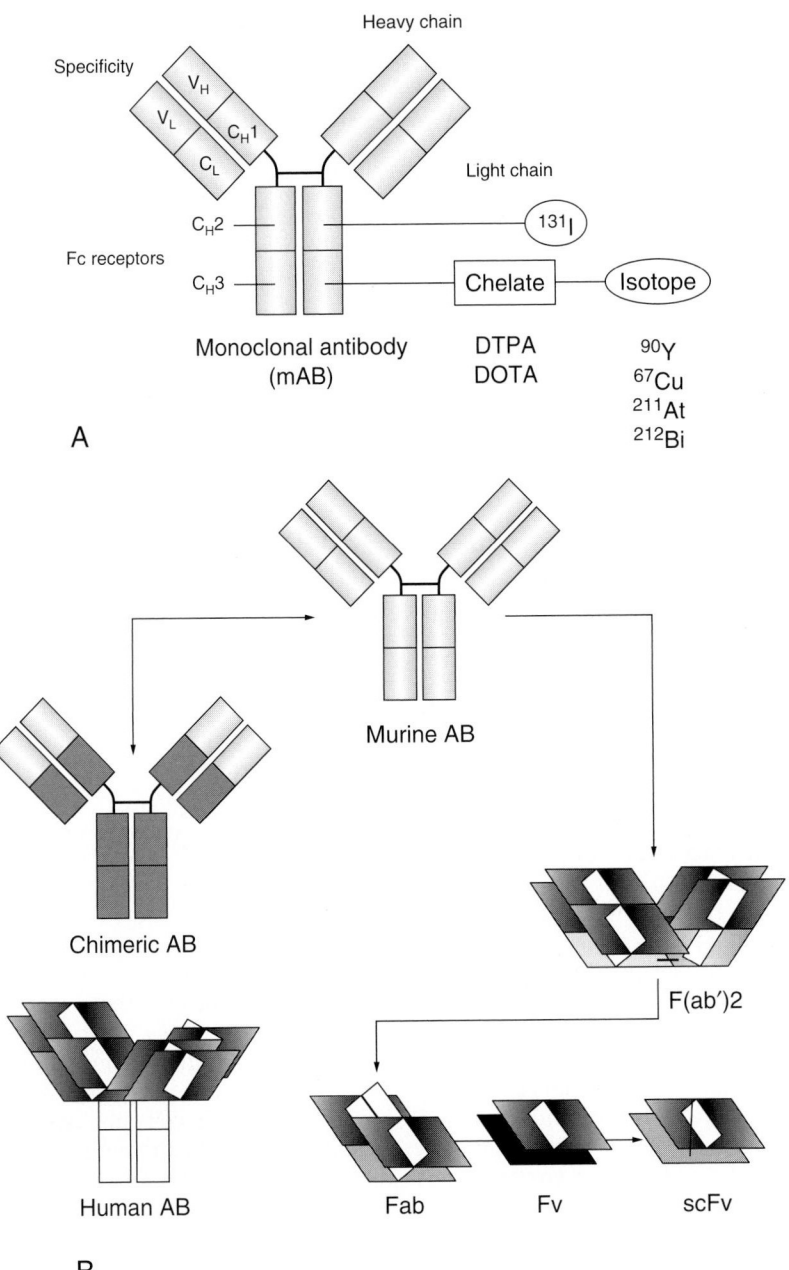

Figure 72–1. A, Schematic diagram of antibody structure and radioimmunoconjugate (± chelator agent), with light (L) and heavy (H) chains containing constant (C) and variable regions (V). **B,** Schematic diagram of different types of monoclonal antibodies and fragments used in current clinical trials or as molecules for new targeting and pretargeting radiopharmaceuticals.

Many tumor-binding mAbs can produce antitumor effects: (1) complement-mediated cytotoxicity[19]; (2) Ab-dependent cellular cytotoxicity[20,21]; (3) receptor-mediated apoptosis[22,23]; (4) interference with growth-related receptors[24-28]; (5) stimulation of the humoral immune system producing a vaccine-like response[29-31]; or (6) trigger apoptosis by appropriate intracellular signal transduction. Smaller binding units (scFv) seldom have these functions but can be linked into molecular formats developed to improve the TI, such as small high-affinity rapid-targeting radioactive molecules or larger multidentate and multifunctional pretargeted RIT drugs.

ANTIBODY PRODUCTION

The immunization of mice with foreign proteins or tumor cells creates a response from diverse B lymphocytes and the production of heterogeneous Abs to multiple antigenic determinants, or *epitopes*. Abs isolated from the serum are therefore polyclonal. Since 1978, sensitized lymphocytes have been removed, fused with mouse myeloma cells using polyethylene glycol. The surviving hybrid myeloma cells that had incorporated lymphocyte genes (hybridomas), when isolated as single cells, develop clones that produced single Ab molecules binding the desired target antigen. These cells can be expanded and frozen. Aliquots can be used to produce gram quantities of a single mAb molecule or provide genes for recombinant production of a selected portion of the molecule for future molecular formats.[9,32,33]

RADIOISOTOPES

Many radioisotopes suitable for systemic tumor-targeted radionuclide therapy are presented in Table 72-1. Radioisotopes undergo decay because of inherent instability of their nucleus. The most important types of decay for medical use lead to gamma emission, beta and alpha particles, and electron capture resulting in auger electrons. [131]I has both beta and gamma emissions, the latter being less absorbed by the body, allowing scintigraphic imaging to determine the pharmacokinetics and calculate the dosimetry of the radiopharmaceutical. In contrast, beta particles travel only millimeters to centimeters in tissue and deposit their energy in the vicinity of the point of decay. Beta emissions from radioisotopes such as ^{131}I, ^{90}Y, or [67]Cu in targeting antigen-positive tumor cells can kill nearby antigen-negative tumor cells through a "crossfire" effect, which increases the homogenicity of tumor radiation.[34-37]

Iodine-131 is selected in many clinical trials because of well-known radiochemistry, availability, and low cost. However, if the radioiodinated MAb is taken into the tumor cells (internalized), the ^{131}I can be enzymatically removed and excreted from the tumor (and the body) before it can deposit all of its particulate energy, thus lowering tumor dose; the same process, however, can result in a lower dose to the liver and kidneys since these products, small iodinated peptides and free iodine, are rapidly excreted via the kidneys. It should be noted that free iodine in the blood can be concentrated in the thyroid gland if not blocked in advance by an oral potassium iodine solution. Since the gamma rays emitted by ^{131}I have a relatively high energy (364 keV),[38] practical considerations are needed to minimize the dose of radiation that is delivered to family members and health care personnel. Patients receiving high doses who are unable to be properly managed at home may need hospitalization to limit the irradiation of others.

Yttrium-90, a pure beta emitter, has three properties that make it an attractive choice for RIT[39-41]: (1) a high beta energy ($E_{\beta max}$ = 2.29 MeV; maximum range of particulate energy in tissue = 12 mm), which enables it to kill adjacent tumor cells and thus increase the homogenicity of tumor radiation[34,35]; (2) metal chemistry, which facilitates the pre-synthesis of storable Ab chelate conjugates that can be quickly and easily radiolabeled in RIT form when needed; and (3) a half-life (2.67 days) useful with both intact mAbs, that may take 1 to 3 days to concentrate in tumors or smaller fragments and peptides, with maximal concentration within a day. However, ^{90}Y needs well-selected chelation chemistry since, if it escapes the chelate, the ^{90}Y will accumulate in cortical bone, increasing the radiation to bone marrow. Further, although ^{90}Y-labeled Abs allow easy patient management because they have no primary gamma emissions, pharmacokinetics and thus dosimetry cannot be accurately quantitated by imaging the secondary ^{90}Y emissions. Thus, gamma-emitting indium-111 (^{111}In) in the same chelated mAb, when concurrently administered, acts as an effective surrogate to provide pharmacokinetic information for its ^{90}Y counterpart (Fig. 72-2).

Other radioisotopes have been studied in RIT. Generally their availability, cost, labeling, or chemistry characteristics have outweighed the suitability of their physical characteristics for therapy. An example is [67]Cu, suitable for RIT because it emits ^{99m}Tc-like photons for imaging, has a sufficiently long physical half-life for use with intact murine mAb (62 hours), emits beta particles similar to ^{131}I, and does not accumulate in bone. Preliminary studies demonstrate [67]Cu may provide a better TI than ^{131}I, based in part on its relatively long retention in tumors,[42,43] resulting in 1.5- to 5-fold higher tumor doses when equivalent radioactivities (mCi) are administered.[44,45] The disadvantage of [67]Cu is availability and cost.

Alpha particles deposit energy over a much shorter range than beta particles, typically 50 to 100 μm, targeting lesions of 1 to 2 mm diameters (micrometastasis). Thus radioisotopes that undergo alpha decay, such as astatine-211 ([211]At) and bismuth-212 ([212]Bi) must be on or in a tumor cell to kill it.[46,47] Although nearby normal cells are spared by alpha emitters, adjacent non-targeted tumor cells are spared as well. These radionuclides are ideal candidates to target microscopic residual disease or leukemia, where beta particles are relatively inefficient, depositing much of their energy outside their small tumor volume. [211]At and [212]Bi have been used in clinical RIT trials of leukemia and brain tumors. Their short physical half-lives and complex decay cascades makes routine clinical use more difficult (see Table 72-1).[46,48-50]

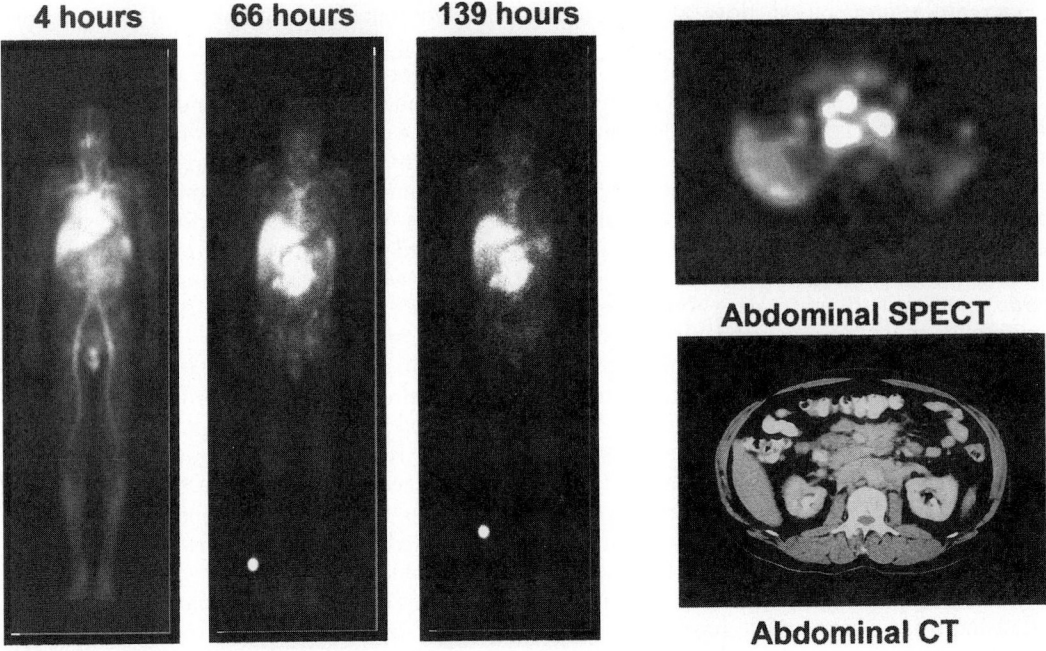

Figure 72–2. Indium-111-Zevalin (IDEC Pharmaceuticals Corporation, San Diego, Calif.) dosimetry study in a patient with non-Hodgkin's lymphoma was performed before therapy to estimate the absorbed radiation dose to normal organs and bone marrow from yttrium-90-Zevalin (IDEC Pharmaceuticals Corporation). Calculated marrow absorbed radiation dose from the information derived from imaging of sacral or lumbar areas was hindered by the abdominal disease clearly demonstrated. SPECT, single photon emission computed tomography; CT, computed tomography. (Provided courtesy of Gregory A. Wiseman, MD, and IDEC Pharmaceuticals Corporation. From DeNardo SJ, Williams LE, Leigh BR, et al: Choosing an optimal radioimmunotherapy dose for clinical response. *Cancer.* 2002;94(suppl):1275.)

Chelates

Isotopes are attached to mAbs by different methods. The stability of isotope on the mAb is crucial for RIT to maximize the TI. ^{131}I is covalently linked to the Fc portion by iodination of tyrosine residues, whereas radioisotopes of metals such as ^{90}Y, ^{67}Cu, lutetium-177 (^{177}Lu), rhenium-188 (^{188}Re) are more firmly attached by an intermediary molecule known as a chelate. Diethylenetriaminepentaacetic acid (DTPA) was initially used for ^{111}In and ^{90}Y.[51] Macrocyclic bifunctional agents[52] such as DOTA (1,4,7,11-tetrazacyclododecane-N,N′,N″,N‴-tetraacetic acid)[53] or TETA (1,4,7,11-tetraazacyclotetradecane-N,N′,N″,N‴-tetraacetic acid) have increasingly been used as they hold useful radiometals in a more stable manner in vivo[52,54] (e.g., stability of yttrium-DOTA minimizes the loss of ^{90}Y to the bone).[55]

RADIOBIOLOGY

RIT differs in three important ways from conventional external beam radiation therapy, wherein a high ($\cong$150 Gy/hour) constant dose rate is intermittently delivered to a limited region of the body: (1) radiation is continuously delivered to tumors at a low dose rate that initially increases with time as radiolabeled Abs accumulate in a tumor (maximal tumor dose rates approximate $\leq$0.40 Gy/hour for ^{90}Y-labeled and ^{67}Cu-labeled Abs and <0.10 Gy/hour for ^{131}I-labeled Abs[56]) and then decreases because of physical decay and biologic clearance[36]; (2) a low dose of radiation is delivered to the whole body; and (3) Abs themselves may, in some cases, exert antitumor effects through biologic mechanisms. For most tumors, one would expect the relative effectiveness of RIT to be approximately 20% less than that of dose-equivalent external beam radiation therapy since the low dose rates characteristic of RIT allow time for repair of sublethal damage.[57-59] This has not necessarily been the case.

Most studies on tumor effects of 0.40 Gy/hour or less have used nearly constant dose rates.[57] In general, these studies have indicated that dose rates of 0.23 Gy/hour or more are required to stop the growth of malignant epithelial cells in vitro,[60,61] although lower dose rates such as 0.09 to 0.11 Gy/hour can halt the growth of HeLa and Morris hepatoma cells[62] (dose rates as low as 0.05 Gy/hour can stop the growth of lymphoma cells in vitro).[63]

Although radiolabeled Abs emit radiation at a low dose rate, several studies of human tumor xenografts in mice have suggested that RIT can, in certain instances, exert greater antitumor activity than dose-equivalent external beam radiation therapy.[64-66] A number of explanations have been proposed to account for an inverse relationship between dose rate and cell killing: (1) reoxygenation occurs during the protracted course of irradiation delivered by RIT, increasing the radiosensitivity of tumor cells[67]; (2) RIT may target a rapidly proliferating subpopulation of tumor cells (growth fraction) that is largely responsible for tumor doubling[68]; (3) low dose rate irradiation may, in some cases, cause tumor cells to accumulate in the radiosensitive G2 phase of the cell cycle (G2 block) to a greater extent than conventional dose rate irradiation[69]; (4) the importance of sublethal damage repair mechanisms may be minimal for tumors (e.g., lymphomas that radiobiologically have a small shoulder and large α/β ratio[58]; (5) the biologic effects of some mAbs may acutely increase tumor blood flow and elicit an inflammatory response[70]; and (6) low dose rate irradiation may induce apoptosis, to a much greater extent than high-dose-rate irradiation,[71,72] and this event may be enhanced in a synergistic manner by various biologic effects of some tumor targeting mAbs.

There is evidence that apoptosis is the major response of tumors to RIT. In experimental human lymphoma tumors (Raji) treated with ^{67}Cu-1-2IT-BAT-Lym-1, apoptosis preceded tumor regression by 4 to 6 days. In these therapy-resistant human lymphoma tumors, apoptosis was convincingly demonstrated to be a major mechanism for the effectiveness of RIT and occurred by p53-independent mechanisms.[73] Other experimental tumors (human breast carcinoma xenograft, HBT3477) demonstrate increased apoptotic activity independent of p53 after RIT.[74]

Linear energy transfer (LET) represents the average energy (keV) locally imparted to a medium by radiation in traversing one micrometer along its path (track).[67] Because energy exchanges with matter are widely spaced with low LET radiation, a beta particle has only a small probability of releasing enough energy along its track to produce DNA breaks. Approximately 200 DNA double-strand breaks per cell are required to sterilize 99% of a tumor-cell population when low LET radiation is administered.[35] The cytotoxicity of low LET radiation may also be diminished by tumor hypoxia.[75] In addition, low LET radiation may not be completely tumoricidal because repair of sublethal damage occurs at low dose rates.[75]

By using a radionuclide that emits beta particles with a high energy (e.g., ^{90}Y rather than ^{131}I), dose rates can be increased up to 10-fold because of the higher energy deposited by each disintegration of ^{90}Y relative to ^{131}I (see Table 72-1).[76,77] High LET irradiation (alpha emitters) is densely ionizing along particle tracks and consequently is more efficient at producing DNA breaks than low LET radiation. The cell killing produced by high LET radiation is less dependent upon hypoxia[78] since it directly produces irreparable DNA breaks, whereas low LET radiation forms highly reactive molecules that produce repairable DNA breaks and relies upon oxygen to prevent repair of these breaks.[67] In conclusion, a better understanding of mechanisms and timing in RIT-induced tumor cell death may lead to the selection of combined therapies that enhance tumor responses without increased toxicities.

DOSIMETRY AND THERAPEUTIC INDEX (TI)

The concept of dosimetry is important for treatment planning and the assessment of results. In contrast to dosimetry for external beam radiation therapy, dosimetry for RIT is dependent on (1) the kinetics of uptake and clearance of radiolabeled Abs; (2) the distribution of radiolabeled Abs; and (3) the radioisotope attached to the Abs.[79-81]

Serial quantitative studies with gamma camera imaging (see Fig. 72-2) have traditionally been used to measure radioactivity, determine pharmacokinetics, and derive calculated dosimetry. Magnetic resonance (MR) and computed tomography (CT) imaging provide normal tissue and tumor volumes.[82,83] However, accurate measurement of the radioactivity in small, deep-seated tumors, surrounded by background radioactivity, is difficult. Several excellent overviews of quantitative imaging techniques and approaches to treatment planning in RIT have been published.[81,83-86] The medical internal radiation dose (MIRD) method has traditionally been used to calculate absorbed doses of radiation to normal organs, tumor, and the whole body following the administration of radiopharmaceuticals.[87] The MIRD method makes a number of assumptions, including: (1) radioactivity is uniformly distributed in that entity, and (2) nonpenetrating, (e.g., beta) emissions from radionuclides are completely absorbed in a tumor or organ. This assumption is reasonable provided that the range of beta emissions does not exceed the diameter of the target. Specific absorbed fractions (S factors) for penetrating emissions have been calculated for many organs using mathematical anthropomorphic phantoms for a "standard" man, woman, child, and infant that approximate human anatomy. Actual patient organ volumes provide the best alternative.[88] For radionuclides that undergo alpha decay (or electron capture), energy deposition needs to be considered at the cellular and subcellular level,[89] which entails the use of a Monte Carlo model[90] or analytical microdosimetry with Fourier transform techniques.[91]

The dosimetric process currently employed consists of the pretherapy administration of a tracer dose of RIT (or its gamma-emitting surrogate) followed by serial planar conjugate view imaging using a gamma camera to determine the quantitative spatial distribution of the radionuclide (Fig. 72-3A). Three-dimensional images from gamma camera tomographic scintigraphy (SPECT) provide more detailed pictorial information about deep-seated tumors but have inherent problems with providing quantitative data (Fig. 72-3B). Using appropriate standards and planar imaging data, cumulated activity (area under the curve, AUC), that is, the amount of radioactivity integrated over time or residence time, can be calculated for organs or tumor and related to the organ or tumor volume. MIRD "S" values provide the tissue-absorbed fraction for final calculation of absorbed dose to specific organs and tumors.[92]

Various dosing methods for prescribing treatment doses for RIT have been used (Table 72-3).[92] Most clinical trials present their results by reporting the injected activity in millicuries (mCi) or Becquerels (Bq) per body surface area (m^2) or weight (kg). One mBq is equal to 2.7 × 10^{-2} mCi (0.027 mCi). The tumor-absorbed doses are reported either in absolute numbers (cGy or rads) or relative to the injected activity (e.g., cGy/mBq, rads/mCi). Except for intratumoral administration, the average tumor doses delivered over several days in most RIT using nonmyeloablative therapy are 7 to 30 Gy and in myeloablative regimens, 30 to 60 Gy.

Enhancing the TI (tumor dose to most sensitive normal tissue dose) is critical to the future success of systemic tumor-targeted radiation therapy. Circulating radiolabeled mAb irradiates the most sensitive tissue, marrow. Marrow toxicity is thus the most frequent dose-limiting toxicity from non–marrow-supported RIT.

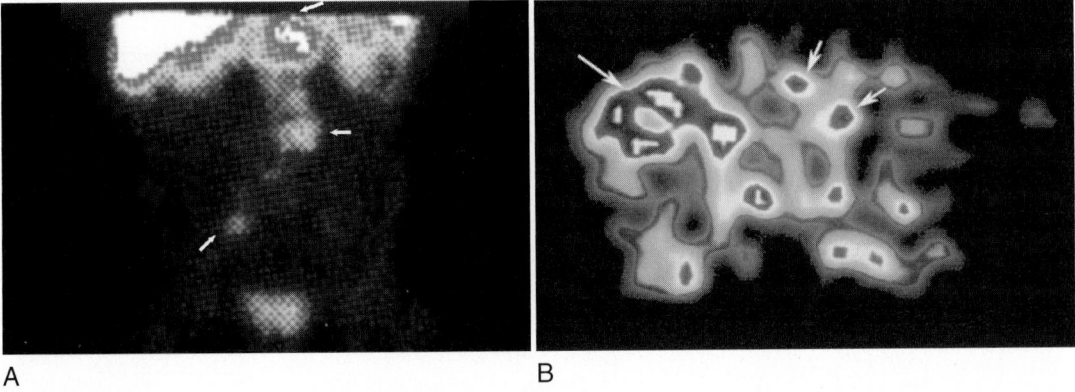

A   B

Figure 72–3. A, Gamma-camera image of the anterior pelvis of a patient with B cell lymphoma. The image was obtained 3 days after administration of ^{111}In-Lym-1 in order to derive pharmacokinetic data that can be used to calculate dosimetry for therapy with ^{90}Y-Lym-1. Excellent uptake in all known areas of lymphoma is demonstrated in the upper- and mid-abdomen and right iliac lymph nodes (*arrows*). Radioactivity in the bladder and liver demonstrates ^{111}In-Lym-1 metabolism and ^{111}In metabolite excretion. **B,** Gamma-camera image of patient with metastatic breast cancer. Anterior (A) and posterior (P) aspects of the patient are indicated. The image was obtained 3 days after RIT with ^{111}In/^{90}Y-DOTA-peptide-mAb. DOTA-peptide-mAb is a novel immunoconjugate with a catabolizable peptide linker. This three-dimensional, cross-sectional chest image was obtained by SPECT (single photon emission computerized tomography) and demonstrates uptake in metastatic disease in the right anterior chest wall, mediastinal lymph nodes, and lungs (*arrows*). No uptake is seen in normal tissues. The high therapeutic index for radiation dose in the tumor (compared with normal tissue) is evident. White is the most intense radiation, followed by red, yellow, and green. Blue/black indicates no radiation. (**A** from DeNardo GL, O'Donnell RT, Shen S, et al: Radiation dosimetry for 90Y-2IT-BAD-Lym-1 extrapolated from pharmacokinetics using [111]In-2IT-BAD-Lym-1 in patients with non-Hodgkin's lymphoma. *J Nucl Med.* 2000;41:952. **B** from DeNardo SJ, Richman CM, Goldstein DS, et al: Yttrium-90/Indium-111-DOTA-peptide-chimeric L6: Pharmacokinetics, dosimetry and initial results in patients with incurable breast cancer. *Anticancer Res.* 1997;17:1735 and DeNardo SJ, Kroger LA, DeNardo GL: A new era for radiolabeled antibodies in cancer? *Curr Opin Immunol.* 1999;11:563.) See also Color Figure 72-3.

In an effort to reduce marrow radiation from its exposure to hours of circulating radioactive drug, pretargeting or multi-step strategies that demonstrate exciting potential have been developed. These pretargeting approaches increase the TI in both NHL and solid tumors and are discussed later in the section Approaches to Improve the Therapeutic Index.[11,93,94]

CLINICAL STUDIES

Lymphoma

Since 1985, the more promising results for RIT have been described in NHL. A description of the main mAbs (anti CD20, CD22, Lym-1) used in different clinical trials, isotopes, and commercial names are described in Table 72-4. RIT for NHL varies from the use of a single dose of a radionuclide at either nonmyelosuppressive doses or at myeloablative dose levels, to the use of multiple (fractionated) doses, consisting of dose spacing either by days or weeks.

LYM-1. After developing pharmacokinetic data in patients for ^{131}I-mAb on fragments (1982-1984), DeNardo et al.[95] treated a moribund woman with a Richter's lymphomatous transformation of CLL in 1985, using ^{131}I-Lym-1 mAb on a compassionate basis. When she responded favorably to the initial low dose of ^{131}I-Lym-1 without toxicity, a protocol was developed not only to continue her treatment but also to more generally study that approach in patients with advanced lymphoma (Fig. 72-4). Substantial responses in most of the first 10 patients reported[96] led to studies by others. DeNardo et al.[97] have summarized their results in patients with B-cell malignancies from the past 2 decades. Two consecutive trials

Table 72–3   Dosing Methods in Radioimmunotherapy Trials

Dosing methods	Example
Radiation dose (cGy)-based methods/prior dosimetry study	
Marrow radiation dose (nonmyeloablative)	^{131}I-tositumomab
Total body surrogate	
Blood/body surrogate	
Marrow imaging	^{131}I-tositumomab
Critical (dose-limiting) organ radiation (myeloablative)	
Radionuclide dose (radioactivity, gBq or mCi)-based methods	
Fixed total gBq (mCi)	^{131}I-antitenascin, ^{90}Y-antitenascin
gBq (mCi) per unit body weight (kg)	^{90}Y-tiuxetan ibritumomab, ^{90}Y-CC49
gBq (mCi) per unit body surface area (m²)	^{131}I-Lym-1, ^{131}I-hMN14

Adapted from DeNardo GL, Juweid ME, White CA, et al: Role of radiation dosimetry in radioimmunotherapy planning and treatment dosing. *Crit Rev Oncol Hematol* 2001;39:203.

Table 72–4   Monoclonal Antibodies Used in Clinical Trials for Non-Hodgkin's Lymphoma

Antibody	Antigen	Type	Isotope or toxin	Generic/Commercial name
Lym-1	HLA-DR10	M	^{67}Cu, ^{90}Y	
Lym-1	HLA-DR10	M	^{131}I	Lym-1/Oncolym
B-1	Anti-CD20	M	^{131}I	Tositumomab/Bexxar
2B8	Anti-CD20	M	^{90}Y	Ibritumomab/Zevalin
C2B8	Anti-CD20	Ch	—	Rituximab/Rituxan
IF5	Anti-CD20	M	^{131}I	
LL2	Anti-CD22	M	^{131}I, ^{90}Y	
hLL2	Anti-CD22	H	^{90}Y	Epratuzumab/Lymphocide
MB-1	Anti-CD37	M	^{131}I	
Anti-idiotype	B-cell surface Ig	H	^{90}Y	
OKB7	Anti-CD21	M	^{131}I	
RFBR	Anti-CD22		Deglycosylated ricin A Chain	
Anti-B4-blocked ricin	Anti-CD19		Blocked ricin	

Ch, chimeric; H, humanized; M, mouse.

have been reported using fractionated RIT. Thirty patients with relapsed B-cell malignancies were treated with repeated cycles (10 to 100 mCi) of ^{131}I-Lym-1 as part of a "low-dose fractionated" phase I/II study. Partial response (PR) was achieved in 17 (57%) patients; 13 NHL patients and 4 CLL patients. Advanced disease often interrupted therapy prematurely. However, in 18 patients who received at least 180 mCi of ^{131}I-Lym-1, 94% responded to the therapy.[98] No responses had previously been obtained when patients with NHL were treated with unconjugated Lym-1, which binds the beta subunit on HLA-DR10.[99] In a second phase II trial to assess the maximum tolerated dose (MTD) from fractionated RIT, 20 patients (21 entries) with relapsed or refractory NHL were treated in a dose-escalating study with ^{131}I-Lym-1 (one to five 40 to 100 mCi/m^2 infusions at 4-week intervals). The response rate was 52% (11 of 21 entries) and was 71% (10 of 14 entries) for those who received at least two doses of ^{131}I-Lym-1. Seven of the responses were complete, with a mean duration of 14 months. All three entries in the 100 mCi/m^2 cohort had complete remissions. Responses were observed in all histologic grades and were more rapid and complete when higher radioactivities of ^{131}I-Lym-1 were delivered; however, myelosuppression occurred earlier and was more severe.[100] In general, two or more 80 mCi/m^2 intravenous infusions of ^{131}I-Lym-1 at 4-week-intervals were well tolerated.

A phase I study for NHL patients with ^{67}Cu-2IT-BAT-Lym-1 resulted in a 58% (7 of 12) overall response rate (ORR).[101] For a given level of administered radioactivity, higher absorbed doses of radiation were achieved in the tumors with ^{67}Cu-2IT-BAT-Lym-1 than ^{131}I-Lym-1. Combination of Lym-1 with ^{90}Y has been presented in a small study using ^{90}Y-2IT-BAD-Lym-1, reporting five of eight patients that failed prior chemotherapy had a PR or stabilization of NHL after RIT.[102]

ANTI-B1 (^{131}I-TOSITUMOMAB, BEXXAR). Tositumomab is a murine mAb directed against the CD20 antigen expressed on the surface of normal and malignant B-lymphocytes. The preliminary experience was reported by Kaminski et al. treating nine patients with recurrent B-cell NHL with one to two intravenous infusions of 34 to 66 mCi ^{131}I-anti-B1 (anti-CD20).[103] Tumor doses ranged

from 3 to 24 Gy. Four CRs (44%) and two PRs (22%) were observed.

Several phase I/II studies have assessed the efficacy and safety of ^{131}I-tositumomab. Kaminski et al. treated 59 patients with refractory/relapsed NHL in a phase I/II single-center study.[104] Fifty-three patients received individualized therapeutic doses, delivering a specified total-body radiation dose based on the clearance rate of a preceding dosimetric dose. Unlabeled Ab (300 mg) was given before labeled dosimetric and therapeutic doses to improve biodistribution. Forty-two (71%) of 59 patients responded and 20 patients (34%) had CR. Thirty-five (83%) of 42 with low-grade or transformed NHL responded versus 7 (41%) of 17 with de novo intermediate-grade NHL (P = .005). The median progression-free survival for the 42 responders was 12 months and 20.3 for those with CR. Reversible hematologic toxicity was dose limiting. Only 10 patients (17%) had human anti-mouse Abs detected. Over the long term, five patients developed elevated thyroid-stimulating hormone levels, five were diagnosed with myelodysplasia, and three with solid tumors. Similar information was provided in a multicenter trial reporting a 57% response rate and 32% CR.[105] Both studies prove that a single dose with iodine ^{131}I-tositumomab produce frequent and durable responses in NHL, especially in low-grade or transformed NHL with low adverse events.

A pivotal multicenter clinical trial compared responses and duration in each patient with the last chemotherapy regimen (LCR).[106] After ^{131}I-tositumomab, a response was observed in 39 patients (65%), compared with responses in 17 patients (28%) after their last chemotherapy regimen (P < .001). The median duration and CR rates (6.5 months after ^{131}I-tositumomab, 3.4 months after the LCR (P < .001), and 20% CR after ^{131}I-tositumomab (P < .001) with 3% after LCR. The median duration of response for CR was 6.1 months after the LCR and had not been reached with follow-up of more than 47 months after ^{131}I-tositumomab. In a recent phase II study including 76 patients with previously untreated low grade or transformed NHL, the PR rate was 97% with 63% of the patients achieving a CR.

Using a nonmarrow normal organ dosimetry-driven approach with myeloablative doses, Press et al.[107,108]

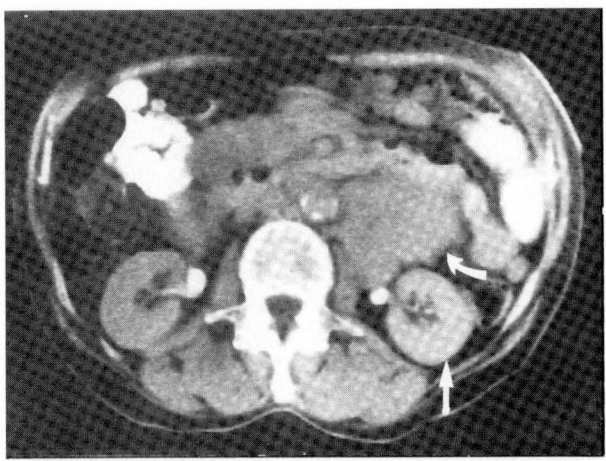

Top

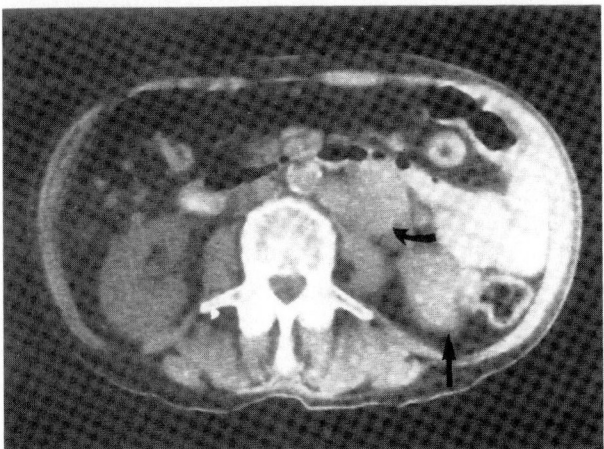

Middle

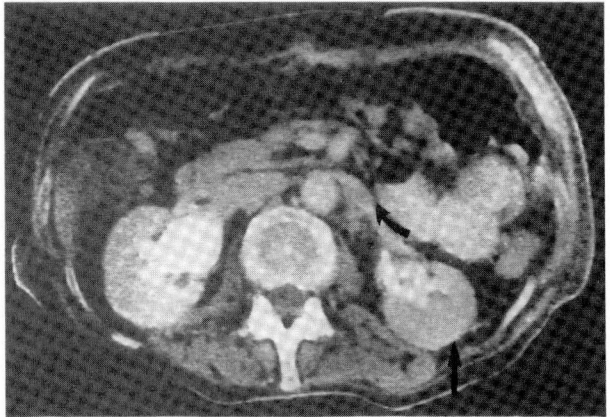

Bottom

Figure 72–4. Regression of tumor (→) in response to treatment with radiolabeled Ab is illustrated by abdominal CT sections at the level of the distal kidney (↑), pretreatment (Top), 2 months (Middle), and 6 months (Bottom) later. Current CT 10 months later is not significantly different from that obtained at 6 months. (From DeNardo SJ, DeNardo GL, O'Grady LF, et al: Treatment of a patient with B-cell lymphoma by I-131 Lym-1 monoclonal antibodies. *Int J Biol Markers*. 1987;2:49.)

administered 234 to 777 mCi ^{131}I-anti-CD20 or ^{131}I-anti-CD37 to 19 patients with NHL. Tumor doses ranged from 10 to 91 Gy. The high-dose RIT was followed by autologous bone marrow reinfusion. A CR was achieved in 16 cases (84%), a PR was achieved in two cases (11%),

and a minor response (40% tumor reduction without regrowth for 18 months) was achieved in the remaining patient (5%). The median response duration was more than 18 months for all patients.[109] Nine patients remain in complete remission without further therapy, including one patient treated more than 5 years ago. Median survival is more than 35 months.[109] Toxicity included myelosuppression, nausea, diarrhea, three serious infections, and two cases of cardiopulmonary toxicity at the MTD. Update results from the phase I and II trials showed,[110] with a median follow-up time of 42 months, the estimated overall and progression-free survival rates are 68% and 42%, respectively, and 14 of 29 patients remained in unmaintained remissions that range from 27+ to 87+ months after RIT. Late toxicities observed were uncommon except for elevated thyroid-stimulating hormone levels found in approximately 60% of the subjects. Two patients developed second malignancies, and there were no reported cases of myelodysplasia. A study then defined the MTD of this RIT with high-dose chemotherapy and ASCT. Fifty-two patients received a trace-labeled infusion of ^{131}I-tositumomab followed by serial quantitative gamma-camera imaging and estimation of absorbed doses of radiation to tumor sites and normal organs. Twenty-four Gy to critical normal organs from ^{131}I-tositumomab was considered the MTD that could be safely combined with 60 mg/kg etoposide and 100 mg/kg cyclophosphamide. The estimated overall survival and progression-free survival of all treated patients at 2 years was 83% and 68%, respectively. These findings were favorable when compared with those in a nonrandomized control group of patients who underwent transplantation, external-beam total-body irradiation, and etoposide and cyclophosphamide therapy during the same period (overall survival of 53% and progression-free survival of 36% at 2 years), even after adjustment for confounding variables in a multivariable analysis.[111]

Myeloablative regimens using the C2B8 Ab have also been reported. Behr et al. treated seven patients with relapsed mantle cell lymphoma after high dose chemotherapy with ASCT using ^{131}I-labeled C2B8, reporting six CRs and one PR delivering up to 100 Gy to the tumors after 261 to 495 mCi of injected activity.[112]

2B8 (^{90}Y-ANTI-CD20, IBRITUMOMAB, ZEVALIN). Ibritumomab is the mouse parent of rituximab (anti CD20). When radiolabeled using the chelate MX-DTPA (tiuxetan) to the mAb, it forms Zevalin. Knox et al. used cold ibritumomab before each administration in 18 patients treated with ^{90}Y-ibritumomab from 13.5 to 50 mCi. The ORR was 72% (13 of 18) and there was a 33% CR rate (6 of 18). They observed that doses less than or equal to 40 mCi were found to be nonmyeloablative.[113] In a phase I/II dose escalation trial of ^{90}Y-ibritumomab, patients received [111]I-Ibritumomab (for dosimetry) on day 0 followed by a therapeutic dose of ^{90}Y-Ibritumomab on day 7, in a dose escalation fashion, starting at 0.2 mCi/kg. Both radioimmunoconjugates were preceded by two doses of the unlabeled rituximab alone. MTD was 0.4 mCi/kg, reaching an estimated tumor dose of 17 Gy, with transient or mild hematological toxicity. Adverse events were primarily hematologic and correlated with baseline extent of marrow involvement with NHL and baseline platelet count, suggesting a dependence of the bone marrow reserve.[114] Witzig et al. treated 68 patients, observing that the MTD was 0.4 mCi/kg IDEC-Y2B8 and 0.3 mCi/kg for patients with baseline platelet counts 100 to 149,000/l (see Fig. 72-2). The ORR for the intent-to-treat population (n = 51) was 67% with 26% CR. Response rates were 82% for low-grade disease (n = 34); 43% for intermediate-grade disease (n = 14); and 0% for mantle-cell disease (n = 3). Responses occurred in 41% of patients with bulky disease ($\geq$7 cm) and 50% of the patients with splenomegaly. Time to progression in responders and duration of response is 12.9+ months and 11.7+ months, respectively. One patient (2%) developed an anti-Ab response (human antichimeric Ab/human antimouse Ab.[115]

A prospective randomized trial was designed to evaluate the efficacy of ^{90}Y-ibrutumomab compared to rituximab alone.[116,117] A total of 143 patients were randomized in IDEC106-04. ORR rate was 80% for the ^{90}Y-ibritumomab tiuxetan group versus 56% for the rituximab group (P = .002). CR rates were 30% and 16% in the ^{90}Y-ibritumomab tiuxetan and rituximab groups, respectively (P = .04).[117] This clearly demonstrated additional therapeutic value by adding the isotope ^{90}Y to rituximab. ^{90}Y-ibritumomab tiuxetan is the first radioimmunoconjugate to receive U.S. FDA approval for clinical use, and treatment is performed in an outpatient setting.

hLL2. ^{90}Y-epratuzumab targets the CD22 antigen and then internalizes into the cell.[118] The interest of LL2 as a possible tool for RIT comes from the apparent efficacy with very low doses of irradiation.[119-121] Dosimetric studies have evaluated the advantage of ^{90}Y with this Ab.[122] Other mAbs used in RIT for NHL are MB-1 (anti CD37) and OKB7 (anti CD21). Anti-idiotype Abs achieved mixed results.[111,123,124]

Early studies in other lymphomas included seven patients with cutaneous T-cell lymphoma who were treated with 100 to 150 mCi ^{131}I-T101.[125] Two PRs lasting 2 months and four minor responses lasting 3 weeks to 3 months were observed. Toxicity consisted of fever, pruritus, dyspnea, urticaria, neutropenia, and thrombocytopenia. All of the patients developed a human anti-mouse antibodies (HAMA) response. Lenhard et al.[126] treated 37 patients with progressive, advanced Hodgkin's disease with three 50 mCi cycles of ^{131}I-antiferritin polyclonal Abs and reported a 3% CR rate and a 38% PR rate. Leukopenia and thrombocytopenia were the primary toxicities. In a subsequent study,[127] 12 patients with poor-prognosis Hodgkin's disease were treated with ^{90}Y-antiferritin polyclonal Abs followed by high-dose cyclophosphamide, carmustine, and etoposide chemotherapy and autologous bone marrow transplantation. The progression-free survival rate at 1 year was estimated to be 21%. Four patients (33%) experienced early, transplant-related mortality.

A review of the literature indicates that RIT has produced CR and PR in approximately two thirds of patients with recurrent B-cell NHL and preliminary outstanding responses in previously untreated patients.[128] As advances are made in the field, response rates and the duration of the responses will continue to improve. NHL appears to be particularly susceptible to RIT for several reasons, including: (1) the tumors are relatively radioresponsive[129,130] and (2) lymphoma cells may be more accessible to Abs than are the cells of solid tumors.[131]

LEUKEMIA

CLL. Although chronic lymphocytic leukemia (CLL) is usually indolent and responsive to treatment early in its course, later stages are characterized by inexorable progression despite conventional treatment. DeNardo et al.[131,132] treated five CLL patients who had failed to respond to intensive multidrug chemotherapy with ^{131}I-Lym-1 (a murine IgG2a MAb recognizing a tumor-associated antigen that is an HLA-DR variant). CR occurred in one patient, greater than 70% reduction of lymphadenopathy was observed in the remaining four patients, and normalization of the leukocyte counts was observed in two of those patients. The responses, however, were of short duration. Since CLL patients have heavy marrow infiltration with malignant cells, radiation-induced thrombocytopenia from a "bystander" irradiation limited the amount of ^{131}I-Lym-1 that could be administered.

AML. For acute nonlymphocytic leukemia (AML) patients who have relapsed after bone marrow transplantation or are refractory to chemotherapy, or who have acute nonlymphocytic leukemia secondary to prior chemotherapy, no curative therapy exists.[133] Schwartz et al.[134] reported the results achieved with ^{131}I-M195, a murine IgG2a mAb that binds CD33, a cell-surface glycoprotein present on committed erythroid and myelomonocytic progenitor cells but not on the earliest pluripotent stem cells, in patients with myeloid leukemias. Twenty-four patients, including seven who had failed to respond before bone marrow transplantation, received 50 to 210 mCi/m^2 ^{131}I-M195 in divided doses. Twenty-three patients (96%) demonstrated decreases in peripheral blood counts, and 20 patients (83%) demonstrated fewer bone marrow blasts. Eight patients had sufficient marrow cytoreduction to proceed to bone marrow transplantation. Three of these achieved marrow remission, one of more than 6 and one of 9 months' duration. Two patients in blastic phase temporarily reverted to their original myelodysplastic states. Thirty-seven percent developed human anti-mouse Abs, limiting retreatment. A humanized IgG1 M195 (HuM195)[135] capable of inducing Ab-dependent cellular cytotoxicity[21] without significant immunogenicity[136] is now in clinical trials.

These studies use targeted radiotherapy to eliminate minimal residual disease after relapse or as part of the conditioning regimen before stem cell transplantation.[133] The latter approach allows the delivery of higher bone marrow doses than total body irradiation alone. Myeloablative therapy using ^{131}I-anti-labeled CD33 with M195 or HuM195 was added to busulfan and cyclophosphamide followed by infusion of HLA-compatible bone marrow. Patients received 120 to 380 mCi of ^{131}I, delivering up to 16 Gy to the bone marrow. Results showed that 27 of 30 patients obtained complete remissions.

Reske et al.,[137] in a phase I study, added rhenium-188-labeled CD66a, b, c, e specific for normal bone marrow in addition to the conventional conditioning with high-dose chemotherapy and 12 Gy total body irradiation. They reported a death rate of 15% after relapse, 9 of the 27 patients (33%) from transplantation-related complications and 14 patients (52%) were alive in complete clinical remission.

On the other hand, alpha emitters are promising candidates for therapy of hematological malignancies with minimal residual disease[133] due to the physical properties of the irradiation. Eighteen patients with relapsed AML (14 patients), refractory AML (3 patients), and CML were treated with the alpha emitter [213]Bi-HuM195 in a phase I trial receiving 16 to 95 mCi in 3 to 6 fractions over 2 to 4 days. Ten of the 12 evaluable patients had reductions in peripheral blood leukemia cells, and 13 of the 18 patients had decreases in the percentages of bone marrow blasts.[133]

SOLID TUMORS

MALIGNANT MELANOMA. Carrasquillo et al., between 1982 and 1984, administered multiple 3-342 mCi infusions of ^{131}I-labeled Fab fragments to 10 patients with malignant melanoma. There was one PR (10%) lasting 3 months. The main toxicities were neutropenia and thrombocytopenia.[138]

GLIOMA. There is special interest in RIT of glioma patients since higher doses may be achieved due to the intratumoral or compartmental administration of the radioimmunoconjugates.[139] Using a systemic route of administration, Brady et al.[140] treated 14 recurrent malignant glioma patients (7 had an anaplastic astrocytoma and 7 had glioblastoma multiforme) with multiple 7 to 50 mCi intra-arterial infusions of ^{125}I-anti-epidermal growth factor receptor mAb. One CR (7%) and two PRs (14%) of brief duration were observed. Median survival from the date of initial diagnosis was 14 months. In primary disease, 59 patients with primary high-grade gliomas of the brain, (13 astrocytomas with anaplastic foci and 46 with glioblastoma multiforme) were treated after tumor resection and postoperative radiation therapy also using multiple intravenous administration of ^{125}I-anti-epidermal growth factor receptor. Cumulative injected dose ranged from 40 to 296 mCi with no significant life-threatening toxicities. At 1 year, 34 (58%) of the 59 patients were alive with a median overall survival of 13.5 months.[141]

Anti-tenascin mAbs provide another option for targeting brain tumors.[139] Tenascin is present in the extracellular matrix of malignant glioma tissue and it cannot be found in normal brain tissue. Both mAb BC-2 and mAb 81C6 have been used in clinical trials; 81C6 offers the advantage that several normal tissue-associated variants are not recognized by the mAb.[139] Riva et al. treated 24 recurrent malignant glioma patients with one to three intratumoral infusions of ^{131}I-anti-tenascin mAb.

Seventeen patients were evaluable. Three CRs (18%) and three PRs (18%) were observed, typically lasting 13 months. Median survival from the date of initial diagnosis was 16 months.

Both Riva et al.[142] and Coknor and Bigner[143] reported compartmental administration in recurrent and primary gliomas of the brain, using a single dose ^{131}I-labeled mAb 81C6. Thirty-four previously irradiated patients with recurrent malignant gliomas were treated with ^{131}I-labeled 81C6. The MTD was 100 mCi. The median survival for patients with glioblastoma was 56 weeks and for the entire series, 60 weeks.[143] A subsequent dose escalation study (42 patients) and phase II trial (33 patients) with primary gliomas using a combined modality approach with surgery, postoperative radiotherapy, and ^{131}I-labeled 81C6. The MTD was 120 mCi. At greater doses delayed neurotoxicity was dose limiting.[144] The median survival for all patients was 86.7 and 79.4 weeks for those with glioblastoma multiforme (GBM). Eleven patients remain alive at a median follow-up of 93 weeks (range, 49 to 220 weeks). Nine patients (27%) developed reversible hematologic toxicity, and histologically confirmed, treatment-related neurologic toxicity occurred in five patients (15%).[145]

ANDROGEN-INDEPENDENT PROSTATE CARCINOMA. Conceptually, tumor-targeted high-dose RIT with marrow support or RIT as part of combined multimodality therapy (CMRIT), can offer effective therapy for this lethal disease. Meredith et al. used 75 mCi/m^2 ^{131}I-CC49 (anti-TAG-72) mAb in 15 patients with metastatic hormone-resistant prostate cancer.[146] Tumor doses ranged from 2 to 11 Gy. Six of 10 evaluable symptomatic patients had bone pain relief, but no patients met radiographic or prostate-specific antigen criteria for an objective response. O'Donnell et al. reported ^{111}In/^{90}Y-m170 mAb therapy in a phase I dose escalation study in 17 patients from 5 to 20 mCi/m^2 in similar prostate cancer patients.[147] Tumor doses ranged from 2 to 20 Gy, with similar response. Ongoing CMRIT studies with Taxol have shown more evidence of PSA and tumor response (DeNardo et al., data not published).

NEUROENDOCRINE TUMORS. Targeted irradiation with the radiolabeled somatostatin analogue ^{90}Y-DOTATOC was assessed for palliation in 41 patients with neuroendocrine gastroenteropancreatic and bronchial tumors. Eighty-two percent of the patients had therapy-resistant and progressive disease. Four intravenous injections (6000 mBq/m^2) of ^{90}Y-DOTATOC, administered at intervals of 6 weeks, resulted in an overall response of 24% and 36% for endocrine pancreatic tumors. CRs were found in 2% (1 of 41), PRs in 22% (9 of 41). The median duration of response was not reached by 26 months. The 2-year survival time was 76 ± 16%. Excellent palliation was achieved as 83% of the patients suffering from the malignant carcinoid syndrome obtained a significant reduction of symptoms. The treatment was well tolerated. Side effects included grade III pancytopenia in 5%, but no grade III to IV renal toxicity was observed.[148]

In 30 patients with cancers expressing somatostatin receptors, ^{90}Y-DOTATOC was given in a dose escalation study with six patients per group receiving equivalent-activity doses in each of three cycles over 6 months (1.11 to 3.3 gBq per cycle). After a total dose of 3.33 gBq, one patient developed grade II renal toxicity 6 months later. Total injected activity is limited by the tolerated kidney dose, estimated to be 20 to 25 Gy. CRs or PRs occurred in 23% of patients. ^{90}Y-DOTATOC is thus a very interesting radioligand for somatostatin-expressing tumors—doses can be administered safely with a low risk of myelotoxicity, although the cumulative radiation dose to the kidneys requires careful evaluation.[149]

BREAST. DeNardo et al.[150-152] administered multiple 60 to 70 mCi/m^2 infusions of ^{131}I-chimeric L6 to 10 women with metastatic breast cancer. ChL6 was noted to have in vivo biologic activities resulting in a fall in serum complement and IL2R[151] but did not have clinical effects in the nonradioactive form.[153] A PR lasting up to 5 months was achieved in 4 patients with advanced breast cancer (40%) and a minor response was observed in 2 patients (20%). A phase I trial then explored the use of single high-dose ^{90}Y-MX-DTPA-BrE-3 and autologous hematologic cell support.[154] Nine women with heavily pre-treated disease were enrolled.[154] Objective PRs were noted in 4 of 8 (50%) patients with measurable tumors.[154] Eleven patients were treated (30 to 60 mCi of ^{90}Y-m170). Three had a PR (70% tumor reduction), three had a minor response (measurable tumor reduction but <70%), and two had stable disease for more than 1 month. Cyclosporin was administered to suppress HAMA[155-157] and PBSC prevented prolonged myelosuppression. Ongoing phase I dose escalation studies with ^{90}Y-DOTA-peptide-m170 include combination therapy with Taxol.

GASTROINTESTINAL MALIGNANCIES. Intensive research has occurred in colon cancer. However, response rates in most clinical trials are below 10%, and the best reported rates are in the subgroup of patients with minimal metastatic disease. Behr et al. have treated 21 patients refractory to 5-fluorouracil with small volume metastatic disease (≤3 cm) and 9 patients as an adjuvant setting after metastatic liver resection. Treatment consisted of a single injection of 60 mCi/m^2 of ^{131}I-hMN-14 (humanized anti-CEA Ab). The objective response rate in 19 assessable patients was 16%, and the ORR was 58% (partial, minor responses) with a mean duration of 9 months. Seven of nine patients with adjuvant treatment remained free of disease in up to 36 months of follow-up. Five patients with stabilized disease were re-treated at the same dose level and two of four assessable patients obtained a PR.[158]

OTHER TUMORS. In Stewart et al.'s phase I/II study,[159-161] encouraging preliminary results were observed in ovarian cancer patients (stage IIB or greater), with no evidence of gross residual disease after cytoreductive surgery and cisplatin or carboplatin-based chemotherapy, who subsequently received a single 5 to 30 mCi intraperitoneal infusion of ^{90}Y-labeled mAb. Long-term results from the same group included 52 patients—31 had residual disease following chemotherapy and 21 were in complete remission. In the group of 21 patients who had achieved complete remission following surgery, conventional chemotherapy, and intraperitoneal RIT, the median survival has

not been reached. The maximum follow-up of 12 years with a survival rate at greater than 10 years of 78%.[162]

Cheung et al. treated nine neuroblastoma patients with multiple 30 to 300 mCi infusions of ^{131}I-3F8.[163] Autologous bone marrow was reinfused into seven patients. Two PRs (22%) and two minor responses (22%) lasting several months were observed.[163]

HUMAN ANTI-MOUSE ANTIBODIES

After exposure to murine Abs, patients may develop HAMAs. A HAMA response usually results in rapid clearance of the therapeutic mAb from the circulation, thereby reducing tumor uptake. On rare occasions, a HAMA response has also produced serum sickness and anaphylactoid reactions. There is considerable variability in the development of a HAMA response among patients. Despite the adverse effects of HAMA, some investigators have reported improved survival after unlabeled or labeled mAb as a consequence of a better immune system.[164] In general, there is a lower frequency of HAMA in patients who are immunosuppressed, such as individuals with leukemia, NHL, or Hodgkin's disease (3% to 35%). HAMAs develop in approximately half of immunocompetent patients following a single infusion of intact murine Abs; this increases to approximately 90% in patients receiving three or more infusions.[165] In contrast, HAMAs develop in approximately half of immunodeficient patients following three or more infusions of Ab fragments.[166] HAMAs can be detected in some patients as soon as 1 week after the infusion of murine Abs[167] and may persist for months or years, precluding tumor targeting with subsequent Ab infusions. Cyclosporin given orally from 2 days before until 2 weeks after the infusion of murine Abs can suppress HAMA formation.[156,157] Lower levels of HAMA have been reported after fludarabine in combination with tositumomab.[168] It should be noted that the cold preinfusion of Rituxan (rituximab) (anti-CD20), which results in several weeks of asymptomatic loss of circulating B lymphocytes, also is associated with almost no HAMA to the co-treatment of murine mAb as radioactive Zevalin (ibritumomab).[115] The amount of previous chemotherapy received before RIT may influence the development of HAMA as the reported rates in naïve treated patients for low grade NHL of 65%[169] are reduced to 17% in refractory/relapsed disease.[104]

TOXICITY

Overall, the acute side effects to RIT are minimal and vary with the amount of mAb given and its biologic properties. However, Dillman et al.[170] described any toxic reactions that occurred in 82 cancer patients who received 0.5 to 500 mg intravenous infusions of murine mAbs. Approximately one fifth of the patients in this study developed fever, chills, and diaphoresis 2 to 8 hours postinfusion. Although this is more than usually seen, the reactions typically lasted no more than a few hours. Acute allergic reactions were observed in less than 1% of the patients in this study and rapid infusions of a large quantity of mAbs increased the likelihood. To reduce the risk of an allergic response, patients are commonly medicated with acetaminophen and diphenhydramine before the delivery of Abs, particularly when large quantities of intact murine IgG2a or chimeric IgG1 Abs are given.

MYELOSUPPRESSION. Myelosuppression has been the dose-limiting toxicity of almost all systemic RIT not receiving marrow support.[171] Most groups have chosen to avoid severe neutropenia and thrombocytopenia by limiting the amount of radioactivity administered per infusion. Alternatively, myeloablative doses of RIT may be delivered if peripheral blood stem cells (PBSC)[172,173] or bone marrow cells[174] are reinfused once radioactivity in the body has adequately cleared.

NONMARROW NORMAL ORGAN TOXICITY. Usually no nonmarrow organ toxicity is seen, since marrow provides the major dose-limiting toxicity. However, in a dose escalation trial, with marrow transplant, Press et al.[174] reported that the MTD was for a single infusion of ^{131}I-labeled mAb defined by severe postural hypotension when 31 Gy was delivered to the lungs. Life-threatening congestive cardiomyopathy and hemorrhagic pneumonitis developed in another patient 2 months after a single infusion of ^{131}I-labeled mAb that delivered a similar 27 Gy to the lungs. When dose escalation is performed, hepatic toxicity has been observed in beagle dogs.[175] Although serious hepatic toxicity was not noted in systemically given RIT trials, in patients in whom high doses of radioactivity have been delivered, hyperbilirubinemia and transient elevation of a patient's serum alanine aminotransferase level may develop.[21,174]

NEUROLOGIC COMPLICATIONS. Neurotoxic events in brain tumors have been reported with doses greater than 100 to 120 mCi treated with ^{131}I-labeled mAb.[143,144] At the dose of 100 mCi, the radiation absorbed estimated dose by the brain is 6 to 7 Gy,[176] and doses of 120 mCi develop neurologic toxicity rates in 15% of the patients with a 3% reoperation rate.[145] Cumulative doses from previous or concurrent brain irradiation may have to be taken into account before designing new protocols.

RENAL COMPLICATIONS. Renal adverse events are reported after ^{90}Y-DOTATOC; Paganelli et al. reported renal doses as high as 11 to 25 Gy. This is in the upper high limits of tolerance after external beam irradiation.[177] Moll et al. reported that five of seven patients with cumulative doses greater than 200 mCi/m^2 developed renal failure. End-stage renal failure occurred in three within 6 months, chronic renal failure in two. Renal biopsies performed in three patients showed typical signs of thrombotic microangiopathy involving glomeruli, arterioles, and small arteries. The histopathologic lesions were identical to those found after external radiotherapy, which suggests a causal relationship between ^{90}Y-DOTATOC and renal thrombotic microangiopathy.[178]

Information about long-term renal effects from RIT irradiation are lacking due to the few patients receiving high renal levels and the short-term follow-up available in these advanced cancer patients. Work with bones seeking radioactive drugs for bone pain or aggressive CMRIT for myeloma with Ho[166] has suggested both

radiation dose and dose rate must be considered in the renal toxicity.[179]

Myelodisplasic syndromes have been reported after RIT in NHL. These adverse events may not be associated with a single modality in a population heavily pretreated with different chemotherapy regimens or radiation therapy, or both, and in a disease with an associated statistical incidence. This integration of newer strategies stresses the importance of careful and well-designed protocols with dosimetric studies on normal and tumor tissues to estimate and subsequently predict short-term and long-term effects of RIT.

APPROACHES TO IMPROVE THERAPEUTIC INDEX

Organs such as the liver or kidneys are involved in the metabolic pathway of proteins and thus concentrate radiolabeled mAb (liver) or small fragments (kidney tubule). Several strategies have been described to accelerate clearance of radioactivity from these organs and thus to enhance TI.[180] These include cleavable linkers, the pretargeting approach previously mentioned to lower blood and marrow dose, and Ab Fvs.

As an example, ^{90}Y DOTA linked to m170 mAb by a peptide preferentially catabolized in the liver resulted in a one third reduction in liver concentration and thus radiation doses in prostate and breast cancer patients, compared to the more conventional DOTA-mAb linkage.[181] Tumor targeting was not diminished (see Fig. 72-3). The results of this study were consistent with in vitro data, which indicated that the peptide linker of DOTA-peptide-mAb is catabolized by cathepsin B, releasing the small radioactive molecule that should be rapidly excreted.[180] Small Fvs of mAb have little hepatic uptake and more rapid blood clearance but usually demonstrate high localization in the kidneys. Both similar and different concepts have been used to develop linkers to lower this retention of radioactivity in the renal tubule. Zimmermann and Novak-Hofer et al.[182] evaluated the peptide-linked copper chelators CPTA-triglycyl-L-p-isothiocyanato-phenylalanine (CPTA-R1-NCS) and the DOTA-triglycyl-L-p-isocyanato-phenylalanine (DOTA-R1-NCS) coupled to F(ab')2 Fvs. DOTA-R1-F(ab')2 achieved the best tumor/tissue ratios. Arano et al.[183-185] took advantage of lysine-specific carboxypeptidase activity in the tubular cell brush border to develop linkages that appear effective in reducing renal concentration of radiometal from radiolabeled Ab fragments and peptides.

PRETARGETED RIT. This drug delivery system separates the specific localization of the larger tumor-targeting mAb and the smaller radioactive molecule, which is quickly bound at the tumor site or rapidly excreted in the kidney. The procedure was first described by Goodwin et al.[186] and provides an alternative to increase the therapeutic ratio by selectively targeting the tumor tissue and minimizing the radiation-absorbed dose to normal tissues, particularly blood and marrow. Different systems have been described depending on the first step conjugates[94]: biotinylated,[187] streptavidin conjugated,[188] bifunctional Abs,[189] and oligonucleotide conjugates.[190] An important proof of principle pretargeting study for delivering systemic radiation therapy to metastatic cancers has been shown by Breitz et al.[191] using available molecules (i.e., streptavidin/biotin) in a three-step pretargeting approach with an anti-CD20 mAb in patients with NHL. Tumor-to-whole body-ratios were obtained that were substantially higher than those achieved with conventional anti-CD20 RIT. In these pretargeting studies using scFv with streptavidin conjugate, the clearing agent biotin-galactose–human serum albumin has been used before injection of radiolabeled DOTA-biotin,[192,193] with resultant reduction in circulating Ab by greater than 95%. However, high cure rates and high tumor-to-normal ratios in mice,[93,194] as well as promising clinical results[195] using bispecific Abs (F(ab')$_2$ fragment) followed by radiolabeled bivalent hapten, have been achieved without clearing agents.

Preliminary RIT results in patients by Barbet et al.,[93] using bispecific Abs as the pretargeting agent and subsequent radioiodinated bivalent haptens to bind cooperatively (crosslink) on target cells, demonstrated useful effects of modestly increasing radioactive hapten circulation time. Greatly increased tumor retention by creating crosslinking of that bivalent second agent on the tumor has been shown. This bivalent radiolabeled hapten approach increased the tumor-to-blood ratio eight times over previous methods.[196]

Weiden et al.[11] reported a three-step procedure in patients with NHL. The anti-CD20, C2B8 Ab conjugated to streptavidin (C2B8/SA), followed after a clearing agent and ^{90}Y-DOTA-biotin were able to administrate doses of 29 ± 23 cGy/mCi and mean tumor to whole body ratios of 38:1. In six of seven patients with injected activities of 30 to 50 mg/m^2 ^{90}Y, three CRs and one PR were observed.

Paganelli et al. enrolled 37 high-grade glioma patients, 20 with glioblastoma, in a controlled, open, nonrandomized study using a three-step avidin-biotin pretargeting approach to target ^{90}Y-biotin to the tumor. All patients received surgery and radiotherapy and were disease free. Nineteen patients received adjuvant treatment with RIT. The median survival for the glioblastoma patients was 33.5 months, and all 12 control glioblastoma patients died after a median survival from diagnosis of 8 months. In the treated grade III glioma patients, median disease-free interval was 56 months (range = 15 to 60) and survival cannot be calculated as only two, within this group, died.

RADIOSENSITIZATION AND COMBINED MODALITY RIT

As RIT is ultimately a very specific form of administering irradiation to tumors, all proposed radiosensitizers for conventional external beam irradiation are possible candidates to be combined with RIT. Combined modality using chemotherapy and radiotherapy has shown improved results in most solid tumors.[197,198] The rationale for combining chemotherapy and RIT is based on the potential benefits in combining two systemic therapies as radiosensitizing agents related to interaction of both

modalities at different biologic levels.[199] Experimental studies with RIT have shown the potential of Taxol,[200,201] taxotere,[200] topotecan,[202] dacarbazine,[203] and gemcitabine[204] in animal models. As with external beam, the timing, dose schedule, and route of administration will be critical. Myeloablative RIT doses with high-dose chemotherapy plus ASCT have shown promising results in NHL.[111] There is evidence in a recent randomized phase II trial that isotope therapy with strontium-89 increases survival in advanced carcinoma of the prostate as consolidation therapy after response to chemotherapy.[205] Future CMRIT trials may include this approach.[159]

In CMRIT studies with external beam radiation, Msirikale et al.[206] reported that patients with hepatoma receiving 6 to 9 Gy in two to three treatments before RIT had approximately threefold improvement in RIT tumor uptake. This finding is consistent with reports that low-dose external beam radiation therapy increases tumor vascular permeability and Ab uptake in human breast[207] and melanoma[208] xenografts in nude mice. At higher radiation doses (10 to 30 Gy), external beam decreased the interstitial fluid pressure and a single dose of 30 Gy decreased by 35% the interstitial pressure. This could have been, in part, responsible for the increased uptake of mAb following single or fractionated radiation.[209]

ANGIOGENESIS. Tumor vasculature is highly heterogeneous in most solid tumors, resulting in underperfused areas leading to abnormal tumor blood flow. Combined with the lack of lymph drainage in tumors, this produces an abnormal high interstitial pressure jeopardizing the normal transport of macromolecules to the stroma and tumor cell compartment.[210] Targeting neovessels with agents that selectively increase permeability may contribute to optimize RIT.[211] The αvβ3-integrin receptor may be used to target tumor vasculature for enhancing tumor permeability because it is highly and preferentially expressed in tumors. Antagonists to αvβ3 receptor have shown apoptosis of endothelial neovascular cells. The cyclic RGD pentapeptide is an antagonist of the αvβ3-integrin receptor and when given 1 hour before[111] In-ChL6, resulted in a 40% to 50% increase in tumor uptake, compared to the control tumor uptake 24 hours after administration.[212,213] Hallahan et al., using ^{99m}Tc-biapcitide (RGD peptidomimetic), showed selective binding to all neoplasms irradiated after peptide administration but not untreated neoplasms or those irradiated before administration.[214] These studies demonstrate the possibility to guide drugs selectively to tumors with the use of radiation-induced receptors.[214]

FRACTIONATED RADIOIMMUNOTHERAPY

Dose distribution after RIT is known to be highly inhomogeneous, due to the inability of mAb to penetrate uniformly throughout the tumor.[215,216] Vascular density, inhomogeneous tumor blood flow, or interstitial pressure are among the related factors that affect an uneven tumor distribution.[215,217,218] Single administration of low-dose-rate irradiation may lead to cold spots in the tumor and subsequently to tumor recurrence.[219] Several strategies have been proposed to overcome this biologic problem related to mAb.[220] The rationale to multiple fractions in RIT are based on delivering a more homogeneous distribution into the tumor, higher cumulative radiation doses, and lower side effects.[220,221]

There is experimental and clinical evidence that fractionated RIT is effective in different tumor systems. Schlom et al. demonstrated the effect of fractionation in a human colon xenograft using ^{131}I-B72.3 against the TAG-72 antigen. Lethal doses in mice were fractionated to assess the toxicity and the tumor growth effect. One single 600 mCi dose produced a mortality rate of 60% of the mice whereas two 300 mCi weekly doses produced 90% response rates and 10% of toxic deaths.[222] Dose fractionation permitted further dose escalation in this model. Three weekly doses were allowed with improved results. The same effect was observed by Buchsbaum et al.[223]

Clinical experiences with multiple doses of RIT are described earlier in this chapter.[98,100] Several issues must be addressed for fractionated RIT: (1) decreased immunogenicity of mAb; (2) number of radionuclide doses; (3) dose amount per cycle; (4) interval between doses; and (5) optimal radionuclide physical half-life for a specific treatment interval.[220]

CONCLUSION

B-cell NHLs, which are particularly susceptible to radiation-induced apoptosis and radiobiologically have a small shoulder, large α/β ratio, and reduced sublethal damage repair capacity, have shown the best single-agent efficacy of RIT. A number of challenges face RIT for solid tumors including insufficient tumor penetration, antigenic modulation, antigenic heterogeneity, and HAMA. Many possible approaches to these challenges, including high-dose RIT, pretargeting strategies and the use of radionuclides such as ^{90}Y, [67]Cu, and alpha emitters, and the development of humanized or bifunctional Abs, are under clinical investigation. High-dose therapy with bone marrow support has also demonstrated a high tumor response rate and nonmarrow normal organ toxicities that correlate with calculated dose to those organs from imaging. Although the field of RIT is relatively young, a great deal of progress has been made. RIT is ready for clinical use in lymphomas, and considerable advances have been made in solid tumors, showing the most potential when integrated in multidisciplinary approaches or low tumor burden scenarios. In the future, the real challenge facing RIT is to increase the tumor radiation absorbed dose while minimizing normal tissue exposure. Variations in clinical RIT choices, dosing methods, and dosimetry methods emphasize the need for clinical trial designs, with sophistication in dosimetry, treatment planning, and clinical treatment questions.

ACKNOWLEDGMENTS

This work was sponsored by the National Cancer Institute grant PO1 CA47829 and Department of Energy grant DE-FG03-84ER60233. The authors thank Nona L. Simons for substantial assistance in preparing this chapter.

REFERENCES

1. Eisen HN, Keston AS: The immunologic reactivity of bovine serum albumin labeled with trace-amounts of radioactive iodine (I-131). *J Immunol.* 1950;63:71.
2. Pressman D, Korngold L: The in vivo localization of anti-Wagner-osteogenic sarcoma antibodies. *Cancer.* 1953;6:619.
3. Pressman D, Day ED, Blau M: The use of paired labeling in the determination of tumor-localizing antibodies. *Cancer Res.* 1957; 17:845.
4. Beierwaltes WH: Radioiodine-labeled compounds previously or currently used for tumor localization. In *Proceedings of an Advisory Group Meeting on Tumor Localization with Radioactive Agents. Panel Proceedings Series.* Vienna, Austria: International Atomic Energy Agency: 1974. p 47.
5. Spar IL, Bale WF, Marrack D, et al: ^{131}I-labeled antibodies to human fibrinogen. Diagnostic studies and therapeutic trials. *Cancer.* 1967;20:865.
6. Ettinger DS, Order SE, Wharam MD, et al: Phase I-II study of isotopic immunoglobulin therapy for primary liver cancer. *Cancer Treat Rep.* 1982;66:289.
7. Ettinger DS, Dragon LH, Klein J, et al: Isotopic immunoglobulin in an integrated multimodal treatment program for a primary liver cancer. A case report. *Cancer Treat Rep.* 1979;63:131.
8. Order S, Pajak T, Leibel S, et al: A randomized prospective trial comparing full dose chemotherapy to ^{131}I antiferritin: An RTOG study. *Int J Radiat Oncol Biol Phys.* 1991;20:953.
9. Kohler G, Milstein C: Continuous culture of fused cells secreting antibody of predefined specificity. *Nature.* 1975;256:495.
10. Esteban JM, Colcher D, Sugarbaker P, et al: Quantitative and qualitative aspects of radiolocalization in colon cancer patients of intravenously administered MAb B72.3. *Int J Cancer.* 1987; 39:50.
11. Weiden PL, Breitz HB: Pretargeted radioimmunotherapy (PRIT) for treatment of non-Hodgkin's lymphoma (NHL). *Crit Rev Oncol Hematol.* 2001;40:37.
12. Carter P: Improving the efficacy of antibody-based cancer therapies. *Nat Rev Cancer.* 2001;1:118.
13. Goldenberg DM: Monoclonal antibodies in cancer detection and therapy. *Am J Med.* 1993;94:297.
14. Roninson IB: The role of the MDR1 (P-glycoprotein) gene in multidrug resistance in vitro and in vivo. *Biochem Pharmacol.* 1992;43:95.
15. Mach JP, Forni M, Ritschard J, et al: Use and limitations of radiolabeled anti-CEA antibodies and their fragments for photoscanning detection of human colorectal carcinomas. *Oncodev Biol Med.* 1980;1:49.
16. DeNardo GL, DeNardo SJ: Overview of obstacles and opportunities for radioimmunotherapy of cancer. In Goldenberg DM, ed. *Cancer Therapy with Radiolabeled Antibodies.* Boca Raton, Fla: CRC Press; 1994:141.
17. Larson SM, Carrasquillo JA, Krohn KA, et al: Localization of ^{131}I-labeled p97-specific Fab fragments in human melanoma as a basis for radiotherapy. *J Clin Invest.* 1983;72:2101.
18. Moldofsky PJ, Powe J, Mulhern CB, et al: Metastatic colon carcinoma detected with radiolabeled F(ab')2 monocolonal antibody fragments. *Radiology.* 1983;149:549.
19. Oettgen H, Old LJ: In Oetgen H, Old LJ, eds. *The History of Cancer Immunotherapy.* Philadelphia: JB Lippincott; 1991.
20. Eisenthal A, Shiloni E, Rosenberg SA: Characterization of IL-2-induced murine cells which exhibit ADCC activity. *Cell Immunol.* 1988;115:257.
21. Caron PC, Co MS, Bull MK, et al: Biological and immunological features of humanized M195 (anti-CD33) monoclonal antibodies. *Cancer Res.* 1992;52:6761.
22. Takahashi S, Maecker HT, Levy R: DNA fragmentation and cell death mediated by T cell antigen receptor/CD3 complex on a leukemia T cell line. *Eur J Immunol.* 1989;19:1911.
23. Trauth BC, Klas C, Peters AM, et al: Monoclonal antibody-mediated tumor regression by induction of apoptosis. *Science.* 1989;245:301.

24. Sauvage CA, Mendelsohn JC, Lesley JF, et al: Effects of monoclonal antibodies that block transferrin receptor function on the in vivo growth of a syngeneic murine leukemia. *Cancer Res.* 1987;47:747.

25. Cuttitta F, Carney DN, Mulshine J, et al: Bombesin-like peptides can function as autocrine growth factors in human small-cell lung cancer. *Nature.* 1985;316:823.

26. Waldmann TA, Goldman CK, Bongiovanni KF, et al: Therapy of patients with human T-cell lymphotrophic virus I-induced adult T-cell leukemia with anti-Tac, a monoclonal antibody to the receptor for interleukin-2. *Blood.* 1988;72:1805.

27. Trowbridge IS, Lopez F: Monoclonal antibody to transferrin receptor blocks transferrin binding and inhibits human tumor cell growth in vitro. *Proc Natl Acad Sci U S A.* 1982;79:1175.

28. Masui H, Kawamoto T, Sato JD, et al: Growth inhibition of human tumor cells in athymic mice by anti-epidermal growth factor receptor monoclonal antibodies. *Cancer Res.* 1984;44:1002.

29. Fagerberg J, Frodin JE, Ragnhammar P, et al: Induction of an immune network cascade in cancer patients treated with mono-clonal antibodies (ab1). II. Is induction of anti-idiotype reactive T cells (T3) of importance for tumor response to MAb therapy? *Cancer Immunol Immunother.* 1994;38:149.

30. Herlyn D, Wettendorff M, Schmoll E, et al: Anti-idiotype immu-nization of cancer patients: Modulation of the immune response. *Proc Natl Acad Sci U S A.* 1987;84:8055.

31. Mittelman A, Chen ZJ, Kageshita T, et al: Active specific immunotherapy in patients with melanoma. A clinical trial with mouse antiidiotypic monoclonal antibodies elicited with syngeneic anti-high-molecular-weight-melanoma-associated antigen mono-clonal antibodies [published erratum appears in *J Clin Invest* 1991 Feb;87(2):757]. *J Clin Invest.* 1990;86:2136.

32. Keenan AM, Harbert JC, Larson SM: Monoclonal antibodies in nuclear medicine. *J Nucl Med.* 1985;26:531.

33. Milstein C: Monoclonal antibodies. *Sci Am.* 1980;243:66.

34. Nourigat C, Badger CC, Bernstein ID: Treatment of lymphoma with radiolabeled antibody: Elimination of tumor cells lacking target antigen. *J Natl Cancer Inst.* 1990;82:47.

35. Cobb LM, Humm JL: Radioimmunotherapy of malignancy using antibody targeted radionuclides. *Br J Cancer.* 1986;54:863.

36. O'Donoghue JA: The impact of tumor cell proliferation in radio-immunotherapy. *Cancer.* 1994;73:974.

37. Wheldon TE, O'Donoghue JA: The radiobiology of targeted radiotherapy. *Int J Radiat Biol.* 1990;58:1.

38. Griffiths GL: Radiochemistry of therapeutic radionuclides. In Goldenberg DM, ed. *Cancer Therapy with Radiolabeled Antibodies.* Boca Raton, Fla: CRC Press; 1995:47.

39. Order SE, Klein JL, Leichner PK, et al: Yttrium antiferritin—A new therapeutic radiolabeled antibody. *Int J Radiat Oncol Biol Phys.* 1986;12:277.

40. Parker BA, Vassos AB, Halpern SE, et al: Radioimmunotherapy of human B-cell lymphoma with Y-90-conjugated antiidiotype monoclonal antibody. *Cancer Res [suppl].* 1990;50:1022s.

41. Vriesendorp HM, Herpst JM, Germack MA, et al: Phase I-II studies of yttrium-labeled antiferritin treatment for end-stage Hodgkin's disease, including radiation therapy oncology group 87-01. *J Clin Oncol.* 1991;9:918.

42. DeNardo SJ, DeNardo GL, Kukis DL, et al: Pharmacology of ^{67}Cu-TETA-Lym-1 antibody in patients with B cell lymphoma. *Antibody Immunoconj Radiophar.* 1991;4:36.

43. DeNardo GL, DeNardo SJ, O'Donnell RT, et al: Are radiometal-labeled antibodies better than iodine-131-labeled antibodies: Comparative pharmacokinetics and dosimetry of copper-67-, iodine-131-, and yttrium-90-labeled Lym-1 antibody in patients with non-Hodgkin's lymphoma. *Clin Lymphoma.* 2000;1:118.

44. DeNardo GL, DeNardo SJ, Levy NB: Treatment of B cell malignancies with ^{131}I-Lym-1 and mechanisms for improvement. In Epenetos A, ed. *Monoclonal Antibodies 2, Applications in Clinical Oncology.* New York: Chapman & Hall Medical; 1993:355.

45. DeNardo GL, Kukis DL, Shen S, et al: Copper-67 versus iodine-131 labeled Lym-1 antibody: Comparative pharmacokinetics and dosimetry in patients with non-Hodgkin's lymphoma. *Clin Cancer Res.* 1999;5:533.

46. Mattes MJ: Radionuclide-antibody conjugates for single-cell cytotoxicity. *Cancer.* 2002;94:1215.

47. Imam SK: Advancements in cancer therapy with alpha-emitters: A review. *Int J Radiat Oncol Biol Phys.* 2001;51:271.

48. Hadley SW, Wilbur DS, Gray MA, et al: Astatine-211 labeling of an antimelanoma antibody and its Fab fragment using N-succinimidyl p-astatobenzoate: Comparisons in vivo with the p-[125I]iodobenzyl conjugate. *Bioconjug Chem.* 1991;2:171.

49. Zalutsky MR, Garg PK, Friedman HS, et al: Labeling monoclonal antibodies and F(ab')2 fragments with the alpha-particle-emitting nuclide astatine-211: Preservation of immunoreactivity and in vivo localizing capacity. *Proc Natl Acad Sci U S A.* 1989;86:7149.

50. McDevitt MR, Ma D, Lai LT, et al: Tumor therapy with targeted atomic nanogenerators. *Science.* 2001;294:1537.

51. Hnatowich DJ, McGann J: DTPA-coupled proteins—Procedures and precautions. *Int J Rad Appl Instrum [B].* 1987;14:563.

52. Moi MK, DeNardo SJ, Meares CF: Stable bifunctional chelates of metals used in radiotherapy. *Cancer Res.* 1990;50(suppl):789.

53. Stimmel JB, Stockstill ME, Kull FC: Yttrium-90 chelation properties of tetraazatetraacetic acid macrocycles, diethylenetriaminepentaacetic acid analogues, and a novel terpyridine acyclic chelator. *Bioconjug Chem.* 1995;6:219.

54. Harrison A, Walker CA, Parker D, et al: The in vivo release of 90Y from cyclic and acyclic ligand-antibody conjugates. *Int J Rad Appl Instrum [B].* 1991;18:469.

55. DeNardo GL, Kroger LA, DeNardo SJ, et al: Comparative toxicity studies of yttrium-90 MX-DTPA and 2-IT-BAD conjugated mono-clonal antibody (BrE-3). *Cancer.* 1994;73:1012.

56. Dillehay LE, Williams JR: Radiobiology of dose-rate patterns achievable in radioimmunoglobulin therapy. *Front Rad Ther Oncol.* 1990;24:96.

57. Hall EJ: Radiation dose rate: A factor of importance in radiobiology and radiotherapy. *Br J Radiol.* 1972;45:81.

58. Fowler JF: Radiobiological aspects of low dose rates in radio-immunotherapy. *Int J Radiat Oncol Biol Phys.* 1990;18:1261.

59. Shipley WU, Peacock JH, Steel GG, et al: Continuous irradiation of the Lewis lung carcinoma in vivo at clinically-used "ultra" low dose-rates. *Int J Radiat Oncol Biol Phys.* 1983;9:1647.

60. Mitchell JB, Bedford JS, Bailey SM: Dose-rate effects on the cell cycle and survival of S3 HeLa and V79 cells. *Radiat Res.* 1979;79:520.

61. Mitchell JB, Bedford JS, Bailey SM: Dose-rate effects on the cell cycle and survival of S3 HeLa and V79 cells. *Radiat Res.* 1979;79:520.

62. Szechter A, Schwartz G, Barsa JM: Continuous and fractionated irradiation of mammalian cells in culture—1. The effect of growth rate. *Int J Radiat Oncol Biol Phys.* 1978;4:991.

63. Courtenay VD: Radioresistant mutants of L5178Y cells. *Radiat Res.* 1969;38:186.

64. Knox SJ, Levy R, Miller RA, et al: Determinants of the antitumor effect of radiolabeled monoclonal antibodies. *Cancer Res.* 1990;50:4935.

65. Wessels BW, Vessella RL, Palme DF, et al: Radiobiological comparison of external beam irradiation and radioimmunotherapy in renal cell carcinoma xenografts. *Int J Radiat Oncol Biol Phys.* 1989;17:1257.

66. Ning S, Trisler K, Wessels BW, et al: Radiobiologic studies of radioimmunotherapy and external beam radiotherapy in vitro and in vivo in human renal cell carcinoma xenografts. *Cancer.* 1997;80:2519.

67. Hall EJ: *Radiobiology for the Radiologist.* Philadelphia: JB Lippincott; 1994:29-43,107-131.

68. Rostock RA, Klein JL, Leichner PK, et al: Distribution of and physiologic factors that affect 131I-antiferritin tumor localization in experimental hepatoma. *Int J Radiat Oncol Biol Phys.* 1984;10:1135.

69. Knox SJ, Sutherland W, Goris ML: Correlation of tumor sensitivity to low-dose-rate irradiation with G2/M-phase block and other radiobiological parameters. *Radiat Res.* 1993;135:24.

70. Sands H, Jones PL, Shah SA, et al: Correlation of vascular permeability and blood flow with monoclonal antibody uptake by human Clouser and renal cell xenografts. *Cancer Res.* 1988;48:188.

71. Macklis RM, Lin JY, Beresford B, et al: Cellular kinetics, dosime-try, and radiobiology of alpha-particle radioimmunotherapy: Induction of apoptosis. *Radiat Res.* 1992;130:220.

72. Macklis RM, Beresford BA, Palayoor S, et al: Cell cycle alterations, apoptosis, and response to low-dose-rate radioimmunotherapy in lymphoma cells. *Int J Radiat Oncol Biol Phys.* 1993;27:643.

73. Kroger LA, DeNardo GL, Gumerlock PH, et al: Apoptosis related gene and protein expression in human lymphoma xenografts (Raji) after low dose rate radiation using [67]Cu-2IT-BAT-Lym-1 radioimmunotherapy. *Cancer Biother Radiopharm.* 2001;16:213.

74. Winthrop MD, DeNardo SJ, Muenzer JT, et al: *p53*-independent response of a human breast cancer xenograft to radioimmunotherapy. *Cancer.* 1997;80(suppl):2529.

75. Kurtzman SH, Russo A, Mitchell JB, et al: [212]Bismuth linked to an antipancreatic carcinoma antibody: Model for alpha-particle-emitter radioimmunotherapy. *J Natl Cancer Inst.* 1988;80:449.

76. Order SE, Stillwagon GB, Klein JL, et al: Iodine 131 antiferritin, a new treatment modality in hepatoma: A Radiation Therapy Oncology Group study. *J Clin Oncol.* 1985;3:1573.

77. Wessels BW, Rogus RD: Radionuclide selection and model adsorbed dose calculations for radiolabeled tumor associated antibodies. *Med Phys.* 1984;11:638.

78. Brown I: Astatine-211: Its possible applications in cancer therapy. *Int J Rad Appl Instrum. [A]* 1986;37:789.

79. Buchsbaum DJ, Wessels BW: Radiolabeled antibody tumor dosimetry. In Goldenberg DM, ed. *Cancer Therapy with Radiolabeled Antibodies.* Boca Raton, Fla: CRC; 1995:21.

80. Buchsbaum DJ, Wessels BW: Introduction: Radiolabeled antibody tumor dosimetry. *Med Phys.* 1993;20:499.

81. DeNardo GL, Raventos A, Hines HH, et al: Requirements for a treatment planning system for radioimmunotherapy. *Int J Radiat Oncol Biol Phys.* 1985;11:335.

82. Scott AM, Macapinlac HA, Divgi CR, et al: Clinical validation of SPECT and CT/MRI image registration in radiolabeled monoclonal antibody studies of colorectal carcinoma. *J Nucl Med.* 1994;35:1976.

83. Sgouros G, Chiu S, Pentlow K, et al: Three-dimensional dosimetry for radioimmunotherapy treatment planning. *J Nucl Med.* 1993;34:1595.

84. Leichner PK, Koral KF, Jaszczak RJ, et al: An overview of imaging techniques and physical aspects of treatment planning in radioimmunotherapy. *Med Phys.* 1993;20:569.

85. Stabin MG: Internal dosimetry in the use of radiopharmaceuticals in therapy—Science at a crossroads? *Cancer Biother Radiopharm.* 1999;14:81.

86. DeNardo SJ, Williams LE, Leigh BR, et al: Radioimmunotherapy: Choosing an optimal dose for clinical response. *Cancer.* 2002; 94(suppl):1275.

87. Watson EE, Stabin MG, Siegel JA: MIRD formulation. Review. *Med Phys.* 1993;20:511.

88. Fisher DR: Radiation dosimetry for radioimmunotherapy. *Cancer.* 1994;73:905.

89. Humm JL, Roeske JC, Fisher DR, et al: Microdosimetric concepts in radioimmunotherapy. *Med Phys.* 1993;20:535.

90. Humm JL: A microdosimetric model of At-211 labeled antibodies for RIT. *Int J Radiat Oncol Biol Phys.* 1987;13:1767.

91. Stinchcomb TG, Roeske JC: Analytic microdosimetry for radioimmunotherapeutic alpha emitters. *Med Phys.* 1992;19:1385.

92. DeNardo GL, Juweid ME, White CA, et al: Role of radiation dosimetry in radioimmunotherapy planning and treatment dosing. *Crit Rev Oncol Hematol.* 2001;39:203.

93. Barbet J, Kraeber-Bodere F, Vuillez JP, et al: Pretargeting with the affinity enhancement system for radioimmunotherapy. *Cancer Biother Radiopharm.* 1999;14:153.

94. Chinol M, Grana C, Gennari R, et al: Pretargeted radioimmunotherapy of cancer. In Abrams PG, Fritzberg AR, eds. *Radioimmunotherapy of Cancer.* New York: Marcel Dekker; 2000:169.

95. DeNardo SJ, DeNardo GL, O'Grady LF, et al: Treatment of a patient with B cell lymphoma by I-131 Lym-1 monoclonal antibodies. *Int J Biol Markers.* 1987;2:49.

96. DeNardo SJ, DeNardo GL, O'Grady LF, et al: Treatment of B cell malignancies with I-131 Lym-1 monoclonal antibodies. *Int J Cancer.* 1988;3(suppl):96.

97. DeNardo GL, DeNardo SJ: Treatment of B-lymphocyte malignancies with ^{131}I-Lym-1 and [67]Cu-2IT-BAT-Lym-1 and opportunities for improvement. In Goldenberg DM, ed. *Cancer Therapy with Radiolabeled Antibodies.* Boca Raton, Fla: CRC Press; 1994:217.

98. DeNardo GL, DeNardo SJ, Lamborn KR, et al: Low-dose fractionated radioimmunotherapy for B-cell malignancies using ^{131}I-Lym-1 antibody. *Cancer Biother Radiopharm.* 1998;13:239.

99. Hu E, Epstein AL, Naeve GS, et al: A phase 1a clinical trial of Lym-1 monoclonal antibody serotherapy in patients with refractory B cell malignancies. *Hematol Oncol.* 1989;7:155.

100. DeNardo GL, DeNardo SJ, Goldstein DS, et al: Maximum tolerated dose, toxicity, and efficacy of ^{131}I-Lym-1 antibody for fractionated radioimmunotherapy of non-Hodgkin's lymphoma. *J Clin Oncol.* 1998;16:3246.

101. Smith A, Alberto R, Blaeuenstein P, et al: Preclinical evaluation of [67]Cu-labeled intact and fragmented anti–colon carcinoma monoclonal antibody MAb351. *Cancer Res.* 1993;53:5727.

102. O'Donnell RT, Shen S, DeNardo SJ, et al: A phase I study of [90]Y-2IT-BAD-Lym-1 in patients with non-Hodgkin's lymphoma. *Anticancer Res.* 2000;20:3647.

103. Kaminski MS, Zasadny KR, Francis IR, et al: Radioimmunotherapy of B-cell lymphoma with [131I] anti-B1 (anti-CD20) antibody. *N Engl J Med.* 1993;329:459.

104. Kaminski MS, Estes J, Zasadny KR, et al: Radioimmunotherapy with iodine [131]I Tositumomab for relapsed refractory B-cell non-Hodgkin lymphoma: Update results and long-term follow-up of the University of Michigan experience. *Blood.* 2000; 96:1259.

105. Vose JM, Wahl RL, Saleh M, et al: Multicenter phase II study of iodine-131 tositumomab for chemotherapy-relapsed/refractory low-grade and transformed low-grade B-cell non-Hodgkin's lymphoma. *J Clin Oncol.* 2000;18:1316.

106. Kaminski MS, Zelenetz AD, Press OW, et al: Pivotal study of iodine I 131 tositumomab for chemotherapy-refractory low-grade or transformed low-grade B-cell non-Hodgkin's lymphomas. *J Clin Oncol.* 2001;19:3918.

107. Press OW, Eary JF, Badger CC, et al: Treatment of refractory non-Hodgkin's lymphoma with radiolabeled MB-1 (anti-CD37) antibody. *J Clin Oncol.* 1989;7:1027.

108. Press OW, Eary JF, Badger CC, et al: High-dose radioimmunotherapy of B cell lymphomas. *Front Radiat Ther Oncol.* 1990;24:204.

109. Press OW, Eary JF, Appelbaum FR, et al: Treatment of relapsed B cell lymphomas with high-dose radioimmunotherapy and bone marrow transplantation. In Goldenberg DM, ed. *Cancer Therapy with Radiolabeled Antibodies.* Boca Raton, Fla: CRC Press; 1995:229.

110. Liu SY, Eary JF, Petersdorf SH, et al: Follow-up of relapsed B-cell lymphoma patients treated with iodine-131-labeled anti-CD20 antibody and autologous stem-cell rescue. *J Clin Oncol.* 1998; 16:3270.

111. Press OW, Eary JF, Gooley T, et al: A phase I/II trial of iodine-131-tositumomab (anti-CD20), etoposide, cyclophosphamide, and autologous stem cell transplantation for relapsed B-cell lymphomas. *Blood.* 2000;96:2934.

112. Behr TM, Griesinger F, Riggert J, et al: High-dose myeloablative radioimmunotherapy of mantle cell non-Hodgkin lymphoma with the iodine-131-labeled chimeric anti-CD20 antibody C2B8 and autologous stem cell support. Results of a pilot study. *Cancer.* 2002;94:1363.

113. Knox SJ, Goris ML, Trisler K, et al: Yttrium-90-labeled anti-CD20 monoclonal antibody therapy of recurrent B-cell lymphoma. *Clin Cancer Res.* 1996;2:457.

114. Wiseman GA, White CA, Stabin M, et al: Phase I/II ^{90}Y-Zevalin (yttrium-90 ibritumomab tiuxetan, IDEC-Y2B8) radioimmunotherapy dosimetry results in relapsed or refractory non-Hodgkin's lymphoma. *Eur J Nucl Med.* 2000;27:766.

115. Witzig TE, White CA, Wiseman GA, et al: Phase I/II trial of IDEC-Y2B8 radioimmunotherapy for treatment of relapsed or refractory CD20+ B-cell non-Hodgkin's lymphoma. *J Clin Oncol.* 1999; 17:3793.

116. Witzig TE: Radioimmunotherapy for patients with relapsed B-cell non-Hodgkin lymphoma. *Cancer Chemother Pharmacol.* 2001; 48:S91.

117. Witzig TE, Gordon LI, Cabanillas F, et al: Randomized controlled trial of yttrium-90-labeled ibritumomab tiuxetan radioimmunotherapy versus rituximab immunotherapy for patients with relapsed refractory low-grade, follicular, or transformed B-cell non-Hodgkin's lymphoma. *J Clin Oncol.* 2002;20:2453.

118. Shih LB, Lu HH, Xuan H, et al: Internalization and intracellular processing of an anti-B-cell lymphoma monoclonal antibody, LL2. *Int J Cancer.* 1994;56:538.

119. Goldenberg DM, Horowitz JA, Sharkey RM, et al: Targeting, dosimetry, and radioimmunotherapy of B-cell lymphomas with iodine-131-labeled LL2 monoclonal antibody. *J Clin Oncol.* 1991;9:548.

120. Juweid M, Sharkey RM, Markowitz A, et al: Treatment of non-Hodgkin's lymphoma with radiolabeled murine, chimeric, or humanized LL2, an anti-CD22 monoclonal antibody. *Cancer Res.* 1995;55:5899s.

121. Vose JM, Colcher D, Gobar L, et al: Phase I/II trial of multiple dose ^{131}I-MAb LL2 (CD22) in patients with recurrent non-Hodgkin's lymphoma. *Leuk Lymphoma.* 2000;38:91.

122. Juweid ME, Stadtmauer E, Hajjar G, et al: Pharmacokinetics, dosimetry and initial therapeutic results with [131]I- and [111]In-/^{90}Y-labeled humanized LL2 anti-CD22 monoclonal antibody (MAb) in patients with relapsed/refractory non-Hodgkin's lymphoma (NHL). *Clin Cancer Res.* 1999;5:3292s.

123. Czuczman MS, Straus DJ, Divgi CR, et al: Phase 1 dose-escalation trial of iodine 131–labeled monoclonal antibody OKB7 in patients with non-Hodgkin's lymphoma. *J Clin Oncol.* 1993;11:2021.

124. White CA, Halpern SE, Parker BA, et al: Radioimmunotherapy of relapsed B-cell lymphoma with yttrium 90 anti-idiotype monoclonal antibodies. *Blood.* 1996;87:3640.

125. Rosen ST, Zimmer AM, Goldman-Leikin R, et al: Radioimmunodetection and radioimmunotherapy of cutaneous T cell lymphomas using an ^{131}I-labeled monoclonal antibody: An Illinois Cancer Council study. *J Clin Oncol.* 1987;5:562.

126. Lenhard RE Jr, Order SE, Spunberg JJ, et al: Isotopic immunoglobulin: A new systemic therapy for advanced Hodgkin's disease. *J Clin Oncol.* 1985;3:1296.

127. Bierman PJ, Vose JM, Leichner PK, et al: Yttrium 90–labeled antiferritin followed by high-dose chemotherapy and autologous bone marrow transplantation for poor-prognosis Hodgkin's disease. *J Clin Oncol.* 1993;11:698.

128. DeNardo GL, O'Donnell RT, DeNardo SJ: Radiolabeled anti-lymphoma antibodies. In Harrison PW, ed. *Cancer Chemotherapy & Biological Response Modifiers Annual 19.* Amsterdam: Elsevier Science; 2001:297.

129. Safwat A: The role of low-dose total body irradiation in treatment of non-Hodgkin's lymphoma: A new look at an old method. *Radiother Oncol.* 2000;56:1.

130. Girinsky T, Guillot-Vals D, Koscielny S, et al: A high and sustained response rate in refractory or relapsing low-grade lymphoma masses after low-dose radiation: analysis of predictive parameters of response to treatment. *Int J Radiat Oncol Biol Phys.* 2001;51:148.

131. DeNardo SJ, DeNardo GL, O'Grady LF, et al: Pilot studies of radioimmunotherapy of B cell lymphoma and leukemia using I-131 Lym-1 monoclonal antibody. *Antibody Immunoconj Radiophar.* 1988;1:17.

132. DeNardo GL, Lewis JP, DeNardo SJ, et al: Effect of Lym-1 radioimmunoconjugate on refractory chronic lymphocytic leukemia. *Cancer.* 1994;73:1425.

133. Jurcic JG: Antibody therapy for residual disease in acute myelogenous leukemia. *Crit Rev Oncol Hematol.* 2001;38:37.

134. Schwartz MA, Lovett DR, Redner A, et al: Dose-escalation trial of M195 labeled with iodine 131 for cytoreduction and marrow ablation in relapsed or refractory myeloid leukemias. *J Clin Oncol.* 1993;11:294.

135. Co MS, Avdalovic NM, Caron PC, et al: Chimeric and humanized antibodies with specificity for the CD33 antigen. *J Immunol.* 1992;148:1149.

136. Caron PC, Jurcic JG, Scott AM, et al: A phase 1B trial of humanized monoclonal antibody M195 (anti-CD33) in myeloid leukemia: Specific targeting without immunogenicity. *Blood.* 1994;83:1760.

137. Reske SN, Bunjes D, Buchmann I, et al: Targeted bone marrow irradiation in the conditioning of high-risk leukemia prior to stem cell transplantation. *Eur J Nucl Med.* 2001;28:807.

138. Carrasquillo JA, Krohn KA, Beaumier P, et al: Diagnosis of and therapy for solid tumors with radiolabeled antibodies and immune fragments. *Cancer Treat Rep.* 1984;68:317.

139. Wikstrand CJ, Cokgor I, Sampson JH, et al: Monoclonal antibody therapy of human gliomas: Current status and future approaches. *Cancer Metastasis Rev.* 1999;18:451.

140. Brady LW, Woo DV, Markoe AM, et al: Treatment of malignant gliomas with ^{125}I-labeled monoclonal antibody against epidermal growth factor receptor. *Antibody Immunoconj Radiophar.* 1990; 3:169.

141. Snelling L, Miyamoto CT, Bender H, et al: Epidermal growth factor receptor 425 monoclonal antibodies radiolabeled with iodine-125 in the adjuvant treatment of high-grade astrocytomas. *Hybridoma.* 1995;14:111.

142. Riva P, Franceschi G, Riva N, et al: Role of nuclear medicine in the treatment of malignant gliomas: The locoregional radioimmunotherapy approach. *Eur J Nucl Med.* 2000;27:601.

143. Bigner DD, Brown MT, Friedman AH, et al: Iodine-131-labeled antitenascin monoclonal antibody 81C6 treatment of patients with recurrent malignant gliomas: Phase I trial results. *J Clin Oncol.* 1998;16:2202.

144. Cokgor I, Akabani G, Kuan CT, et al: Phase I trial results of iodine-131-labeled antitenascin monoclonal antibody 81C6 treatment of patients with newly diagnosed malignant gliomas. *J Clin Oncol.* 2000;18:3862.

145. Reardon DA, Akabani G, Coleman RE, et al: Phase II trial of murine ^{131}I-labeled antitenascin monoclonal antibody 81C6 administered into surgically created resection cavities of patients with newly diagnosed malignant gliomas. *J Clin Oncol.* 2002; 20:1389.

146. Meredith RF, Bueschen AJ, Khazaeli MB, et al: Treatment of metastatic prostate carcinoma with radiolabeled antibody CC49. *J Nucl Med.* 1994;35:1017.

147. O'Donnell RT, DeNardo SJ, Yuan A, et al: Radioimmunotherapy with ^{111}In/[90]Y-2IT-BAD-m170 for metastatic prostate cancer. *Clin Cancer Res.* 2001;7:1561.

148. Waldherr C, Pless M, Maecke HR, et al: The clinical value of [^{90}Y-DOTA]-D-Phe1-Tyr3-octreotide (^{90}Y-DOTATOC) in the treatment of neuroendocrine tumours: A clinical phase II study. *Ann Oncol.* 2001;12:941.

149. Cybulla M, Weiner SM, Otte A: End-stage renal disease after treatment with ^{90}Y-DOTATOC. *Eur J Nucl Med.* 2001; 28:1552.

150. DeNardo SJ, O'Grady LF, Richman CM, et al: Radioimmunotherapy for advanced breast cancer using I-131-ChL6 antibody. *Anticancer Res.* 1997;17:1745.

151. DeNardo SJ, Mirick GR, Kroger LA, et al: The biologic window for chimeric L6 radioimmunotherapy. *Cancer.* 1994;73(suppl):1023.

152. DeNardo SJ: Radioimmunotherapy in the treatment of metastatic breast cancer: An overview. In Goldenberg DM, ed. *Cancer Therapy with Radiolabeled Antibodies.* Ann Arbor, Mich: CRC Press; 1995:189.

153. Goodman GE, Hellstrom I, Yelton DE, et al: Phase I trial of chimeric (human-mouse) monoclonal antibody L6 in patients with non–small-cell lung, colon, and breast cancer. *Cancer Immunol Immunother.* 1993;36:267.

154. Schrier DM, Stemmer SM, Johnson T, et al: High-dose [90]Y Mx-diethylenetriaminepentaacetic acid (DTPA)-BrE-3 and autologous hematopoietic stem cell support (AHSCS) for the treatment of advanced breast cancer: A phase I trial. *Cancer Res.* 1995;55:5921s.

155. Richman CM, DeNardo SJ, O'Donnell RT, et al: Dosimetry-based therapy in metastatic breast cancer patients using ^{90}Y monoclonal antibodies 170H.82 with autologous stem cell support and cyclosporin A. *Clin Cancer Res.* 1999;5:3243s.

156. Ledermann JA, Begent RH, Massof C, et al: A phase I study of repeated therapy with radiolabelled antibody to carcinoembryonic antigen using intermittent or continuous administration of cyclosporin A to suppress the immune response. *Int J Cancer.* 1991;47:659.

157. Weiden PL, Wolf SB, Breitz HB, et al: Human anti-mouse antibody suppression with cyclosporin A. *Cancer.* 1994;73:1093.

158. Behr TM, Liersch T, Greiner-Bechert L, et al: Radioimmunotherapy of small-volume disease of metastatic colorectal cancer. *Cancer.* 2002;94:1373.

159. Stewart JSW, Hird V, Snook D, et al: Intraperitoneal radioimmunotherapy of ovarian cancer: Pharmacokinetics, toxicity, and efficacy of I-131 labeled monoclonal antibodies. *Int J Radiat Oncol Biol Phys.* 1989;16:405.

160. Stewart JS, Hird V, Snook D, et al: Intraperitoneal radioimmunotherapy for ovarian cancer: Pharmacokinetics, toxicity, and efficacy of I-131 labeled monoclonal antibodies. *Int J Radiat Oncol Biol Phys.* 1989;16:405.

161. Hird V, Maraveyas A, Snook D, et al: Adjuvant therapy of ovarian cancer with radioactive monoclonal antibody. *Br J Cancer.* 1993;68:403.

162. Epenetos AA, Hird V, Lambert H, et al: Long term survival of patients with advanced ovarian cancer treated with intraperitoneal radioimmunotherapy. *Int J Gynecol Cancer.* 2000;10:44.

163. Cheung NKV, Yeh SDJ, Gulati S, et al: ^{131}I-3F8 targeted radiotherapy of neuroblastoma (NB): A phase I clinical trial. *Proc Am Assoc Cancer Res.* 1990;31:284.

164. Lamborn KR, DeNardo GL, DeNardo SJ, et al: Treatment-related parameters predicting efficacy of Lym-1 radioimmunotherapy in patients with B-lymphocytic malignancies. *Clin Cancer Res.* 1997; 3:1253.

165. Reynolds JC, Del Vecchio S, Sakahara H, et al: Anti-murine response to mouse monoclonal antibodies: Clinical findings and implications. *Int J Rad Appl Instrum [B].* 1989;16:121.

166. Sears HF, Atkinson B, Mattis J, et al: Phase I clinical trial of monoclonal antibody in treatment of gastrointestinal tumors. *Lancet.* 1982;762.

167. Pimm MV, Perkins AC, Armitage NC, et al: The characteristics of blood-borne radiolabels and the effect of anti-mouse IgG antibodies on localization of radiolabeled monoclonal antibody in cancer patients. *J Nucl Med.* 1985;26:1011.

168. Leonard JP, Coleman M, Kostakoglu L, et al: Fludarabine monophosphate followed by iodine I-131 tositumomab for untreated low-grade and follicular non-Hodgkin's lymphoma (NHL). *Blood.* 1999;94:90a.

169. Kaminski MS, Estes J, Tuck M, et al: Iodine I131 Tositumomab therapy for previously untreated follicular lymphoma. *Proc Am Soc Clin Oncol.* 2000;19:11.

170. Dillman RO, Beauregard JC, Halpern SE, et al: Toxicities and side effects associated with intravenous infusions of murine monoclonal antibodies. *J Biol Resp Mod.* 1986;5:73.

171. DeNardo GL, DeNardo SJ, Macey DJ, et al: Overview of radiation myelotoxicity secondary to radioimmunotherapy using ^{131}I-Lym-1 as a model. *Cancer.* 1994;73(suppl):1038.

172. Richman CM, Schuermann TC, Wun T, et al: Peripheral blood stem cell mobilization for hematopoietic support of radioimmunotherapy in patients with breast carcinoma. *Cancer.* 1997;80:2728.

173. Richman CM, DeNardo SJ: Systemic radiotherapy in metastatic breast cancer using ^{90}Y-linked monoclonal MUC-1 antibodies. *Crit Rev Oncol Hematol.* 2001;38:26.

174. Press OW, Eary JF, Appelbaum FR, et al: Radiolabeled-antibody therapy of B cell lymphoma with autologous bone marrow support. *N Engl J Med.* 1993;329:1219.

175. Vriesendorp HM, Shao Y, Blum JE, et al: Fractionated intravenous administration of ^{90}Y-labeled B72.3 GYK-DTPA immunoconjugate in beagle dogs. *Nucl Med Biol.* 1993;20:571.

176. Akabani G, Reist CJ, Cokgor I, et al: Dosimetry of ^{131}I-labeled 81C6 monoclonal antibody administered into surgically created resection cavities in patients with malignant brain tumors. *J Nucl Med.* 1999;40:631.

177. Cassidy JR: Clinical radiation neuropathy. *Int J Radiat Oncol Biol Phys.* 1995;31:1249.

178. Moll S, Nickeleit V, Mueller-Brand J, et al: A new cause of renal thrombotic microangiopathy: Yttrium 90-DOTATOC internal radiotherapy. *Am J Kidney Dis.* 2001;37:847.

179. Breitz H, Wendt R, Stabin M, et al: Dosimetry of high dose skeletal targeted radiotherapy (STR) with ^{166}Ho-DTMP. *Cancer Biother Radiopharm.* 2003;18:225.

180. Kukis DL, Novak-Hofer I, DeNardo SJ: Cleavable linkers to enhance selectivity of antibody-targeted therapy of cancer. *Cancer Biother Radiopharm.* 2001;16:457.

181. DeNardo SJ, Yuan A, Richman C, et al: Therapeutic index enhancement by DOTA peptide linkage in ^{111}In/^{90}Y DOTA-Lym-1 and m170 MAbs in clinical trials. *J Nucl Med.* 2002;43:117P.

182. Zimmermann K, Gianollini S, Schubiger PA, et al: A triglycine linker improves tumor uptake and biodistributions of ^{67}Cu-labeled anti-neuroblastoma MAb chCE7 F(ab')$_2$ fragments. *Nucl Med Biol.* 1999;26:943.

183. Arano Y, Fujioka Y, Akizawa H, et al: Chemical design of radiolabeled antibody fragments for low renal radioactivity levels. *Cancer Res.* 1999;59:128.

184. Arano Y: Strategies to reduce renal radioactivity levels of antibody fragments. *Q J Nucl Med.* 1998;42:262.

185. Li L, Olafsen T, Anderson AL, et al: Reduction of kidney uptake in radiometal labeled peptide linkers conjugated to recombinant antibody fragments. Site-specific conjugation of DOTA-peptides to a Cys-diabody. *Bioconjug Chem.* 2002;13:985.

186. Goodwin DA, Meares CF, McCall MJ, et al: Pre-targeted immunoscintigraphy of murine tumors with indium-111-labeled bifunctional haptens. *J Nucl Med.* 1988;29:226.

187. Paganelli G, Magnani P, Zito F, et al: Three-step monoclonal antibody tumor targeting in carcinoembryonic antigen-positive patients. *Cancer Res.* 1991;51:5960.

188. Sung C, van Osdol WW: Pharmacokinetic comparison of direct antibody targeting with pretargeting protocols based on streptavidin-biotin binding. *J Nucl Med.* 1995;36:867.

189. Le Doussal JM, Barbet J, Delaage M: Bispecific-antibody-mediated targeting of radiolabeled bivalent haptens: Theoretical, experimental and clinical results. *Int J Cancer.* 1992;7(suppl):58.

190. Bos ES, Kuijpers WH, Meesters-Winters M, et al: In vitro evaluation of DNA–DNA hybridization as a two-step approach in radioimmunotherapy of cancer. *Cancer Res.* 1994;54:3479.

191. Breitz HB, Weiden PL, Appelbaum JW, et al: Pretargeted radioimmunotherapy (PRIT) for treatment of non-Hodgkin's lymphoma: Preliminary results. *J Nucl Med.* 1999;40:19P.

192. Breitz HB, Weiden PL, Beaumier PL, et al: Clinical optimization of pretargeted radioimmunotherapy with antibody-streptavidin conjugate and ^{90}Y-DOTA-biotin. *J Nucl Med.* 2000;41:131.

193. Axworthy DB, Reno JM, Hylarides MD, et al: Cure of human carcinoma xenografts by a single dose of pretargeted yttrium-90 with negligible toxicity. *Proc Natl Acad Sci U S A.* 2000;97:1802.

194. Gautherot E, Rouvier E, Daniel L, et al: Pretargeted radioimmunotherapy of human colorectal xenografts with bispecific antibody and ^{131}I-labeled bivalent hapten. *J Nucl Med.* 2000;41:480.

195. Weichselbaum R, Beckett MA, Vokes EE, et al: Cellular and molecular mechanisms of radioresistance. *Cancer Treat Res.* 1995;74:131.

196. Leung SO, Qu Z, Sharkey RM, et al: Pretargeting colonic tumors with engineered bispecific antibodies for improved radioimmunotherapy (RAIT). *J Nucl Med.* 2000;41:270.

197. O'Connell MJ, Martenson JA, Wieand HS, et al: Improving adjuvant therapy for rectal cancer by combining protracted-infusion fluorouracil with radiation therapy after curative surgery. *N Engl J Med.* 1994;331:502.

198. Herskovic A, Martz K, al-Sarraf M, et al: Combined chemotherapy and radiotherapy compared with radiotherapy alone in patients with cancer of the esophagus. *N Engl J Med.* 1992;326:1593.

199. Hennequin C, Favaudon V: Biological basis for chemo-radiotherapy interactions. *Eur J Cancer.* 2002;38:223.

200. O'Donnell RT, DeNardo SJ, Miers L, et al: Combined modality radioimmunotherapy for human prostate cancer xenografts with taxanes and ^{90}Yttrium-DOTA-peptide-ChL6. *Prostate.* 2002;50:27.

201. DeNardo SJ, Kukis DL, Kroger LA, et al: Synergy of Taxol and radioimmunotherapy with yttrium-90-labeled chimeric L6 antibody: Efficacy and toxicity in breast cancer xenografts. *Proc Natl Acad Sci U S A.* 1997;94:4000.

202. Ng B, Kramer E, Liebes L, et al: Radiosensitization of tumor-targeted radioimmunotherapy with prolonged topotecan infusion in human breast cancer xenografts. *Cancer Res.* 2001;61:2996.

203. Stein R, Chen S, Reed L, et al: Combining radioimmunotherapy and chemotherapy for treatment of medullary thyroid carcinoma: Effectiveness of dacarbazine. *Cancer.* 2002;94:51.

204. Cardillo TM, Blumenthal RD, Ying Z, et al: Combined gemcitabine and radioimmunotherapy for the treatment of pancreatic cancer. *Int J Cancer.* 2002;97:386.

205. Tu S, Millikan RE, Mengistu B, et al: Bone-targeted therapy for advanced androgen-independent carcinoma of the prostate; a randomised phase II trial. *Lancet.* 2001;357:336.

206. Msirikale JS, Klein JL, Schroeder J, et al: Radiation enhancement of radiolabeled antibody deposition in tumors. *Int J Radiat Oncol Biol Phys.* 1987;13:1839.

207. Warhoe KA, DeNardo SJ, Wolkov HB, et al: Evidence for external beam irradiation enhancement of radiolabeled monoclonal antibody uptake in breast cancer. *Antibody Immunoconj Radiophar.* 1992;5:227.

208. Stickney DR, Gridley DS, Kirk GA, et al: Enhancement of monoclonal antibody binding to melanoma with single dose radiation or hyperthermia. *NCI Monogr.* 1987;3:47.

209. Znati CA, Rosenstein M, Boucher Y, et al: Effect of radiation on interstitial fluid pressure and oxygenation in a human tumor xenograft. *Cancer Res.* 1996;56:964.

210. Dvorak HF, Nagy JA, Feng D, et al: Tumor architecture and targeted delivery. In Abrams PG, Fritzberg AR, eds. *Radioimmunother Cancer.* New York: Marcel Dekker; 2000:107.

211. Burke PA, DeNardo SJ: Antiangiogenic agents and their promising potential for combined therapy. *Crit Rev Oncol Hematol.* 2001;39:155.

212. DeNardo SJ, Burke PA, Leigh BR, et al: Neovascular targeting with cyclic RGD peptide (cRGDf-ACHA) to enhance delivery of radioimmunotherapy. *Cancer Biother Radiopharm.* 2000;15:71.

213. Burke PA, DeNardo SJ, Miers LA, et al: Cilengitide targeting of $\alpha_v\beta_3$ integrin receptor synergizes with radioimmunotherapy to increase efficacy and apoptosis in breast cancer xenografts. *Cancer Res.* 2002;62:4263.

214. Hallahan DE, Qu S, Geng L, et al: Radiation-mediated control of drug delivery. *Am J Clin Oncol.* 2000;24:473.

215. Jain RK: Vascular and interstitial barriers to delivery of therapeutic agents in tumors. *Cancer Metastasis Rev.* 1990;9:253.

216. Humm JL: Dosimetric aspects of radiolabeled antibodies for tumor therapy. *J Nucl Med.* 1986;27:1490.

217. Jain RK, Baxter LT: Mechanisms of heterogenous distribution of monoclonal antibodies and other macromolecules in tumors: Significance of elevated interstitial pressure. *Cancer Res.* 1988;48:7022.

218. Shockley TR, Lin K, Nagy JA, et al: Spatial distribution of tumor-specific monoclonal antibodies in human melanoma xenografts. *Cancer Res.* 1992;52:367.

219. O'Donoghue JA: The implications of nonuniform tumor doses for radioimmunotherapy. *J Nucl Med.* 1999;40:1337.

220. DeNardo GL, Schlom J, Buchsbaum DJ, et al: Rationales, evidence and design considerations in multiple dose (fractionated) radioimmunotherapy. *Cancer.* 2002;94:1332.

221. Withers HR, Taylor JM, Maciejewski B: The hazard of accelerated tumor clonogen repopulation during radiotherapy. *Acta Oncol.* 1988;27:131.

222. Schlom J, Molinolo A, Simpson JF, et al: Advantage of dose fractionation in monoclonal antibody-targeted radioimmunotherapy. *J Natl Cancer Inst.* 1990;82:763.

223. Buchsbaum DJ, Khazaeli MB, Liu TP, et al: Fractionated radioimmunotherapy of human colon carcinoma xenografts with I-131-labeled monoclonal antibody CC49. *Cancer Res.* 1995;55 (suppl):5881.

Clinical Applications of Photodynamic Therapy

73

Roberto Santiago, Stephen Hahn, and Eli Glatstein

BACKGROUND

Photodynamic therapy (PDT) involves a classic binary system that combines the use of a photosensitizer and light of a wavelength specific to the absorption characteristics of the photosensitizer.[1] Both the sensitizer and the light must be at the same place at the same time for biological impact to result. The activation of a photosensitizer by light involves a photooxidative reaction and thus also requires the presence of oxygen.[2]

The origin of PDT can be traced back to the turn of the century, when Raab described the lethal effect of light on paramecia treated with an acridine dye.[3] Lipson and colleagues[4] reported on the use of hematoporphyrin derivative (HPD) for the fluorescent detection of tumor tissue. In 1975, Dougherty[3] first reported on the use of HPD and red light to eradicate transplanted animal tumors without excessive damage to surrounding uninvolved skin. What makes the treatment of particular clinical interest is that several of the photosensitizers available are reported to have preferential distribution and retention in tumors compared to other normal tissues.[5-8]

The mechanism by which photosensitizers are selectively assimilated or retained has not been completely elucidated. However, there may be a window of time during which the biologic effects of PDT are greater in tumors compared to normal tissues. If this selectivity can be confirmed in human tumors, it would represent a significant advantage for PDT compared to other cancer treatment modalities. However, the treatment is limited in scope because it is dependent on the penetration of light into tissues. These observations, along with the development of lasers and fiberoptic systems for light delivery, propel the current therapeutical interest in this field.

With these advantages and limitations in mind, PDT has been employed in the treatment of various malignant and premalignant processes. With ingenuity, PDT researchers have recognized clinical situations where the location of the disease process as well as the geometry and pigmentation of the area involved are technically amenable to light delivery. Moreover, investigators have identified suitable stages in the natural history of diseases where PDT, either alone or in combination with other therapies, has the potential to favorably impact clinical outcome.

Currently, there are two Federal Drug Administration (FDA)-approved photosensitizers in the United States, Photofrin and Levulan. Photofrin is a systemic photosensitizer that, in combination with 630-nm light, is approved for the treatment of obstructing esophageal cancer, obstructing bronchial non–small cell lung cancer (NSCLC), microinvasive bronchial lung cancer, and recently, Barrett's esophagus with high grade dysplasia. Levulan is a topical photosensitizer that, in combination with blue light, is approved for the treatment of actinic keratosis.

LIGHT AND LASERS

The delivery of light of a specific wavelength to activate a particular photosensitizer is essential for photodynamic action. PDT has a superficial treatment effect because, in general, the available photosensitizers require light in the visible or near-infrared light range. The penetration of light in tissues is hindered by the absorption of light by hemoglobin and other endogenous chromophores. The absorption of light by these chromophores decreases as the wavelength of light in the visible and near infrared range increases. Correspondingly, the depth of penetration of light in tissues increases with increased wavelength of light. Therefore, the use of light of higher wavelength to activate a photosensitizer facilitates the treatment of tissues at greater depths and also tissues with greater pigmentation.[9-11] In addition, the penetration of light is affected by other factors including the geometry and the optical properties of the tissues as well as the mode of light delivery (e.g., interstitial delivery vs. external delivery).

Light dose or fluence is expressed in joules (J) or energy density, such as joules per square centimeter (J/cm²). Light dose may also be expressed as energy output per centimeter of light-diffusing fiber (J/cm) for interstitially placed fibers. The total fluence deposited is a function of both the incident light delivered and scattered light. The rate of light delivery or fluence rate is expressed in mW/cm² or mW/cm. The light fluence delivered from a laser can be calculated by multiplying the fluence rate (in W/cm² or W/cm) by the total treatment time (in seconds). For example, a fluence rate of 0.4 W/cm (400 mW/cm) for 500 seconds would deliver a light fluence of 200 J/cm. For the most part, PDT has been prescribed in terms of the incident light delivered from a laser (as described earlier) rather than the total fluence of light the tissues receive, which is a combination of incident and scattered light. Difficulty in measuring scatter dose has led many simply to neglect it from consideration. Dosage based only on incident light can be limited by substantial differences in total fluence in the tissues among different patients.[12-14] The use of incident fluence to prescribe PDT may, therefore, lead to large discrepancies in light doses that patients actually receive. This could lead, in turn, to large differences in tumor and normal tissue responses to PDT. Dosimetry systems using isotropic light detectors have been developed to measure both incident and scattered light in patients.[15-16] These systems should allow clinical researchers to measure and therefore prescribe a consistent total fluence to the tissues.

Lasers and optical fibers allow light delivery of a specific wavelength to deep-seated tumors using endoscopic, interstitial, or intracavitary techniques. Light delivery systems have been developed to illuminate uniformly the desired site and to prevent thermal injury to tissues. These systems include flat-cut optical fibers and microlenses for illumination of external surfaces like the skin, balloon-type systems for intra-operative light delivery, and diffusing fibers that emit light longitudinally and circumferentially for illumination of interstitial situations as well as cylindrical surfaces such as the aerodigestive tract.[17]

Lasers provide light of an appropriate wavelength at sufficiently high power to excite the photosensitizer retained in the tumor. Clinical PDT lasers include argon-pumped dye lasers or pulsed metal vapor lasers, which can yield up to 5 W of usable light.[18] The gold vapor or pulsed argon dye laser emits in the visible light spectrum, generally under 700 nm. At such wavelengths, the light by itself does not cause any recognizable biological effect in tissues. Light in this range must be combined with a photosensitizer and oxygen in order to cause any injury to tissues. The advantage of dye lasers is that they can be tuned to produce monochromatic light of various wavelengths and thus are versatile sources of light for clinical PDT.[19] Diode lasers have been developed for PDT that[20] produce a single wavelength of light. The advantages of diode lasers compared to dye lasers are their small size, ease of use, and affordability. The disadvantage of diode lasers is that they do not provide multiple wavelengths of light; therefore, they are typically used with only one photosensitizer. Currently, there is no clear evidence to suggest that light produced from a diode laser produces a different tissue or cellular effect compared to a dye laser.[21]

PHOTOBIOLOGY

The activation of a photosensitizer by light involves photooxidation reactions.[22] Light causes excitation of the photosensitizer, which then reacts directly or indirectly with molecular oxygen-producing singlet oxygen ($^1O_2$) and other reactive oxygen species. Reactive oxygen species are the proposed mediators of photodynamic cytotoxicity.[1-2] Still, the exact mechanisms of action have not been fully elucidated (Fig. 73-1). An activated sensitizer also has the potential to fluorescence when returning to

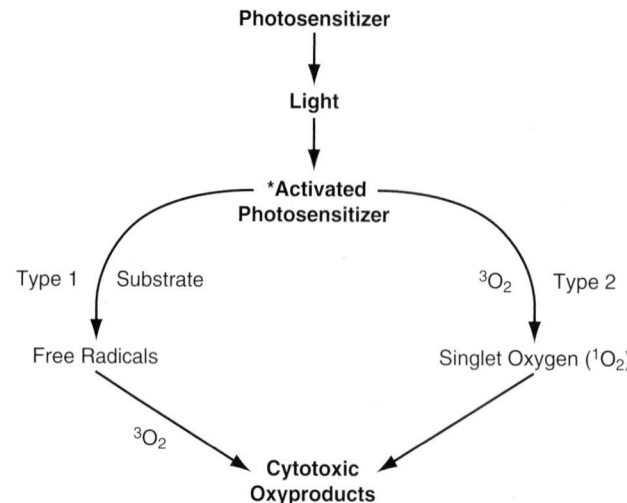

Figure 73–1. Diagram showing the interaction of oxygen, photosensitizer, and light in photodynamic therapy. $^3O_2$, triplet O_2; $^1O_2$, singlet O_2. (From Delaney T: Photodynamic Therapy. In Moosa AR, Schrimpff SC, Robson MC, eds. *Comprehensive Textbook of Oncology.* 2nd ed. Baltimore: Williams & Wilkins; 1990.)

the ground state, thus permitting the fluorescent detection of tumors.

An alluring feature of this therapy, especially for clinical oncology, is that several of the photosensitizers available are reported to have selective distribution in tumors compared to other normal tissues.[5-8] The precise mechanism by which photosensitizers are preferentially assimilated or retained in experimental tumor systems has not been completely elucidated. There is little difference in the effect of PDT on *in vitro* cell lines derived from tumors versus normal tissue.[23] Tumors and their surrounding stroma have a number of unique characteristics compared to normal tissues that may increase their affinity for photosensitizers. Among these characteristics are increased lipid content[24] and higher concentration of low-density lipoprotein (LDL) receptors,[25-28] as well as more acid microenvironments[29] with abnormal vasculature.[30-31] Tumor stroma retains more labeled HPD than tumor cells, suggesting that a higher vascular permeability and inefficient lymphatic clearance may account for some of the differential retention in tumor tissues.[32] In addition, the most hydrophobic HPD components appear to be involved in tumor localization.[33] Porphyrins bind to LDLs in the serum, and it has been proposed that LDL receptors may play an important role in porphyrin localization in or on tumor cells.[34]

Much of the data to support this tumor selectivity have been derived from murine tumor systems.[5-6] Tumor selectivity has not been completely confirmed in human tumors. Ris et al. reported one of the first studies regarding photosensitizer uptake in human tumors. They described concentrations of the photosensitizer mTHPC that were up to 14 times higher in tumors compared to normal tissues in patients with malignant mesothelioma.[7] Peng et al. demonstrated selective distribution of porphyrins within basal cell carcinomas compared to normal skin following topical application of lipophilic esters of 5-ALA.[8] Similarly, porphyrin fluorescence of tumors after topical application of 5-ALA was reported in patients with squamous cell intraepithelial neoplasia of the cervix (CIN). Interestingly, increasing fluorescence relative to surrounding normal epithelium was noted with worsening grade of CIN.[35] However, one study suggests that tumor selectivity may not be present in some patients.[36] More studies are required to evaluate the distribution of photosensitizers in tissues, and ultimately at the cellular level.

Many investigators believe that the photodynamic damage in tumor cells represents a secondary effect produced by the photodynamic destruction of tumor microvasculature.[41] However, there is almost certainly a direct anti-tumor cell effect as well, since this binary system is very effective in vitro, where there are no vessels. In addition, when treatment is administered clinically, effects are usually seen within a matter of minutes to a few hours, which is a much faster course than is associated with other cancer treatments (i.e., chemotherapy or radiation therapy). Thus, the hypothesis has evolved that the mechanism of PDT cytotoxicity is related to membrane damage of the cell or mitochondrion, as opposed to a direct DNA target. Today, membranes, especially in mitochondria, are considered likely sites of cellular killing by PDT.[42]

The activation of a photosensitizer by light involves a photooxidative reaction.[2] In this reaction, the photosensitizer absorbs a photon and is activated to a triplet state. The excited photosensitizer then either reacts with a nearby molecule (such as lipids in the membrane), which then may react with oxygen, which leads to formation of peroxyl radicals and other oxygen radicals (type I reaction), or reacts directly with molecular O_2 producing highly reactive singlet oxygen (type II reaction). Thus, oxygen is a critical component in these reactions. The necessity of adequate oxygen for porphyrin-mediated PDT cytotoxicity has been demonstrated in vitro[37-38] and in vivo.[39-40]

Baseline tumor hypoxia may affect the efficacy of PDT[40] similar to the adverse effect reported for hypoxia on the response to surgery and radiotherapy.[42-48] Despite the data demonstrating an important role for oxygen in photodynamic action, no clinical studies that systematically evaluate baseline tumor hypoxia in patients undergoing PDT are available. Baseline hypoxia has been identified in sarcomas, cervical cancer, and other human tumors.[49-56] These data demonstrate substantial heterogeneity in human tumor hypoxia within tumor types and support the need to evaluate tumor oxygenation in individual patients.[43,53-54] Clinical trials of strategies to improve tumor oxygenation in combination with PDT are in progress.[57-60]

Another factor affecting oxygen concentrations necessary for PDT cytotoxicity is the photodynamic process itself. PDT has been observed to cause regional hypoxia either through vascular collapse[61] or through oxygen consumption by the photochemical process.[62-64] It is possible that the depletion of oxygen during the photodynamic process could limit the effectiveness of PDT. Preclinical studies have demonstrated the induction of hypoxia in human tumors by PDT.[63,65] Furthermore, Henderson and colleagues reported a study using Eppendorf electrode measurements in patients with basal cell carcinomas during PDT treatment.[66] PDT-induced hypoxia was detected during the initial treatment period in the majority of skin lesions treated.[66]

Schemes to reduce the effect of oxygen depletion during PDT have focused on altering the fluence rate of light delivery.[67-68] Lower fluence rates decrease the consumption of oxygen and may lead to improved PDT efficacy.[66,68-69] The difficulty of decreasing fluence rates in the clinical setting is that this increases the patient's treatment time, which has obvious technical and practical constraints. The most efficacious and practical fluence rate has not been established definitively.

PHOTOSENSITIZING COMPOUNDS AND LIGHT PENETRATION

Photosensitizing drugs can be administered via a topical, oral, or parenteral route. In general, all of these agents are well tolerated with their major side effect being cutaneous photosensitivity. Photosensitizers have typically been porphyrins or porphyrin-like compounds.[1-2] The HPD compound is a complex mixture of porphyrins produced by the acid treatment of hematoporphyrin. Although HPD absorbs light most strongly in the UV and blue region around 400 nm,[70] 630 nm red light is generally used in the clinic because of its superior penetration through tissues. HPD-mediated PDT with 630 nm of light can produce tumor necrosis to a depth of 5 mm and rarely as deep as 10 mm. Though some carcinomas in situ, certain early-stage invasive cancers, some dermatological malignancies, and even some intraperitoneal carcinomatoses may be confined to such dimensions, externally directed red light will not penetrate deeply enough to sterilize many gross tumors with a single treatment. Hence, the effective use of HPD with red light may require several treatments or the placement within the tumor of interstitial optical fibers or combined-modality therapy using surgery, radiotherapy, or chemotherapy to reduce the bulk of the tumor followed by PDT to sterilize superficial residual tumor within a tumor bed. For multiple exposures, the period of risk for the cutaneous reactions must be short enough that multiple injections over a finite period are safe.

Dougherty[3] purified from HPD a more active fraction of porphyrin oligomers and monomers with a high proportion of the active moiety, which has been proposed to be a dihematoporphyrin ether[3] or ester.[71] This enriched fraction (termed polyporphyrin or dihematoporphyrin ether, DHE) provided a higher therapeutical ratio (tumor compared with skin reaction) in animal testing than the previously employed HPD.[1,72] DHE (Photofrin) was the first drug approved by the FDA for photodynamic therapy. Photofrin is approved by the FDA for the palliative treatment of obstructing esophageal cancer and obstructing lung cancer, the definitive treatment of microinvasive endobronchial cancer, and the treatment of Barrett's esophagus with high grade dysplasia. Most of the work with Photofrin has been performed at a wavelength of 630 nm. At this wavelength, red light reliably penetrates into 0.5 cm of most tissues. Photofrin is administered

Table 73–1 Clinical Characteristics of FDA-Approved Photosensitizers for Oncologic Photodynamic Therapy

Photosensitizer	Excitation Wavelength	Duration of Photosensitivity	Method of Administration	FDA-Approved Oncologic Indications
Photofrin	630 nm	4 to 6 Wk	Intravenous	1. Obstructing esophageal cancer 2. Obstructing lung cancer 3. Microinvasive endobronchial cancer 4. Barrett's esophagus with high grade dysplasia
Levulan	Blue light	24 Hr	Topical	Actinic keratosis

intravenously 48 hours before light administration. The cutaneous photosensitivity associated with Photofrin lasts approximately 4 to 6 weeks. Prolonged cutaneous photosensitivity beyond 6 weeks has been noted in approximately 20% of patients.

5-Aminolevulenic acid (5-ALA) is a photosensitizer that employs the heme synthesis pathway to produce porphyrins within tissues.[2] Topical 5-ALA is manufactured as Levulan, which, in combination with blue light, has been approved by the FDA for the treatment of actinic keratosis. Induction of endogenous porphyrins by 5-ALA appears to be greater in more rapidly dividing cells such as tumors.[2] This provides another basis for potential tumor selectivity with ALA-mediated PDT.

The second-generation chlorin photosensitizer mTHPC (also known as Foscan) has been approved in Europe for the palliative treatment of patients with refractory head and neck squamous cell carcinoma. As approved in Europe, mTHPC is administered intravenously at a dose of 0.15 mg/kg 96 hours before illumination. Following activation with 652 nm light, the clinically effective depth range of mTHPC has been reported to be up to 1 cm.[15] This makes Foscan one of the most active and efficient photosensitizers currently available.[73-74] mTHPC-induced cutaneous photosensitivity lasts approximately 15 days.

Motexafin-lutetium (also known as Lutrin or Lutetium texaphyrin) is another second-generation photosensitizer.[6,75] Motexafin lutetium is a pentadentate aromatic metalloporphyrin, which has an absorption band at 732 nm. Treatment at this wavelength has the advantage of deeper penetration into tissues compared to the light used to activate other photosensitizers. Motexafin-lutetium has not been approved for human use in the United States but is actively being studied for various malignancies.[76] This photosensitizer is administered intravenously 6 to 24 hours before illumination. The duration of cutaneous photosensitivity with Motexafin-lutetium is 1 to 2 days.

The second-generation chlorin photosensitizer SnET2 (also known as Purlytin)[77-78] is being evaluated for oncological indications and has not been approved for routine human use in the United States. Purlytin is administered intravenously 24 hours before illumination with 660 to 664 nm light. Cutaneous photosensitivity is reported to last 2 to 3 weeks, although prolonged photosensitivity of 1 or more months has been reported in 10% to 15% of patients.[2]

Phototoxicity can be avoided by having the patient shielded from the sunlight. Sunscreen is not effective as a protective measure. Table 73-1 lists clinical characteristics of FDA-approved photosensitizers for oncologic PDT.

CLINICAL INDICATIONS FOR PHOTODYNAMIC THERAPY

Esophageal Cancer

OBSTRUCTING ESOPHAGEAL CANCER

Many patients with advanced esophageal cancer suffer from dysphagia. Patients with tumors that are unresectable, refractory to chemotherapy or radiation, or have recurrent disease often require palliative therapy to help manage symptoms.[98-100] PDT has been demonstrated to achieve effective palliation of dysphagia in such patients.[79]

A randomized trial of 236 patients directly compared Photofrin-mediated PDT to Nd:YAG laser thermal ablation for the palliation of dysphagia from esophageal cancer.[80] In the PDT-treated group, 44% of patients had symptom improvement at 1 week and 35% had improvement at 1 month, which was similar to the Nd:YAG-treated group. Objective tumor responses (complete response + partial response) were longer lasting in the PDT arm (32% at 1 month for PDT vs. 20% for Nd:YAG). Also, there were more complete responses in the PDT group, nine versus two in the Nd:YAG arm. The conclusions were that PDT was as efficacious for palliation of dysphagia compared to Nd:YAG laser therapy with a higher objective tumor response rate and similar levels of toxicity.

Combining PDT with radiotherapy for patients with advanced esophageal cancer is another potential treatment strategy. A nonrandomized trial compared HPD-mediated PDT combined with high dose rate intraluminal brachytherapy to brachytherapy alone.[81] In both groups, external beam radiation (30 to 60 Gy) was delivered to some patients. The patients who received PDT and radiation had significantly better improvement in luminal diameter and dysphagia scores compared to the radiation-alone group. The major complication rate in the PDT group was 14% and limited to patients with T4 tumors. The authors concluded that PDT is an effective palliative tool, but that proper patient selection was needed.[81]

Scheider et al. have reported the use of Photofrin-mediated PDT in esophageal cancer patients who have tumor ingrowth after the placement of expandable stents.[82] PDT produced a large improvement in mean dysphagia scores, and a mean dysphagia-free interval of 92 days with no major complications.

In general, PDT for obstructing esophageal cancer is safe. However, major, life-threatening complications can occur and patient selection is important. In particular, patients with tumors that have eroded into the tracheobronchial tree[81] or a major vessel,[83] patients with esophageal varices, and patients who have received a combination of external beam and high dose rate brachytherapy[83] are at risk for major complications. In these clinical circumstances, it is probably wise to avoid PDT as a palliative treatment.

The FDA has approved Photofrin-mediated PDT for the palliation of patients with completely obstructing esophageal cancer, or for patients with partially obstructing esophageal cancer who cannot be satisfactorily treated with Nd:YAG laser therapy. The FDA-approved regimen is the intravenous injection of Photofrin 2 mg/kg, intravenously 40 to 50 hours before 630 nm light delivery. The light is delivered with a cylindrical diffuser passed through the endoscope. A dose of 300 J/cm is delivered at a fluence rate of 400 mW/cm (total treatment time 750 seconds). Patients may develop odynophagia, dysphagia, nausea, or vomiting after the initial light treatment. A second light treatment may be given 96 to 120 hours after Photofrin administration.

BARRETT'S ESOPHAGUS AND EARLY-STAGE ESOPHAGEAL CANCER

Barrett's esophagus is the development of intestinal-type metaplasia in the esophagus.[84-87] Dysplasia may arise in the setting of Barrett's and can lead to the development of carcinoma. Medical management has little effect on the development of malignancy in Barrett's esophagus and the current standard treatment approach for patients with high-grade dysplasia is surgical resection.[88] Given the potential for morbidity associated with esophagectomy, the development of less invasive treatments such as PDT for Barrett's esophagus is warranted.

One randomized study compared Photofrin-mediated PDT plus the proton-pump inhibitor omeprazole to omeprazole alone for the treatment of high-grade dysplasia associated with Barrett's esophagus.[89] At the 6-month follow-up endoscopy, high-grade dysplasia was ablated in 80% of the PDT-plus-omeprazole group compared to 40% of the omeprazole-alone group ($P < .0001$). After a mean follow-up of 12 months, 17% of patients had disease progression in the PDT group compared to 39% in the omeprazole-alone group. There was also a trend toward reduction in the development of cancer in the PDT group (9% vs. 19%). The main adverse event from PDT was esophageal stricture, which developed in 12% of patients who received one course of PDT and 38% of patients who received two courses.

These clinical trials suggest that Photofrin-mediated PDT is reasonably effective for the treatment of Barrett's esophagus with high-grade dysplasia. The FDA has recently approved PDT using any photosensitizer for the treatment of this condition.

Similarly, PDT is a potential, nonoperative treatment for small, superficial, early esophageal cancers. Savary et al. evaluated PDT in 24 patients with 31 early squamous cell carcinomas (Tis or T1a) of the esophagus.[90] Several photosensitizers were used, including HPD, Photofrin, and mTHPC. Complete responses were seen in 29 cancers in 22 patients. Twenty-six of the 31 cancers (84%) did not recur in a median follow-up of 2 years.

Corti et al. reported on the treatment of 62 patients with esophageal cancer who were treated with HPD-mediated PDT.[91] Eighteen of these patients had in situ cancer (Tis), 30 had T1 tumors, 7 had T2 tumors, and 7 had recurrence of tumors at the surgical anastomotic site from prior esophagectomy. Patients were treated with radiation therapy if disease persisted after two courses of PDT. The complete response rate after PDT alone was 37% (23 out of 62 patients) and 82% (51 out of 62 patients) after PDT and radiation. The complete response rate to PDT alone was the highest in Tis/T1 patients (44%) compared to T2 patients (28%) or patients with recurrence at the anastomotic site (0%). Median local progressive-free survival was 49 months for patients with Tis/T1 lesions, 30 months for patients with T2 lesions, and 14 months for patients with recurrent tumors. The authors concluded that PDT for early superficial (Tis/T1)-stage esophageal cancer was effective and that radiotherapy could be used in those patients who did not respond completely to PDT.[91]

Although some efficacy has been reported for PDT in the treatment of Barrett's esophagus and early-stage esophageal cancer, toxicities associated with this treatment must be considered. The frequency of esophageal stricture with Photofrin-mediated PDT is aproximately 30%. Attempts to modulate this complication with corticosteroids have not been successful.[92] In addition, cutaneous photosensitivity, esophageal perforation, tracheoesophageal fistulae, and transient cardiac arrhythmias are potential complications of PDT.[93]

There are concerns that Barrett's mucosa, dysplasia, or even frank carcinoma could be present under the regenerating squamous mucosa after the treatment of Barrett's with PDT. The risk for cancer development in patients with Barrett's is debatable but appears to be highest in patients with high-grade dysplasia.[94] Therefore, the treatment strategy targeting patients with high-grade dysplasia seems to be reasonable. Photofrin-mediated PDT could be offered to patients with Barrett's esophagus and high-grade dysplasia who are not surgical candidates or who refuse surgery. We recommend multiple biopsies and careful pathological assessment to exclude cancer in cases of Barrett's before making a treatment decision. Likewise, we recommend endoscopic ultrasound and computerized tomography of the chest and upper abdomen to exclude metastatic disease in cases of early carcinomas.

Non–Small Cell Lung Cancer

ADVANCED LUNG CANCER–PALLIATION OF OBSTRUCTING LESIONS

Obstructing endobronchial lesions can cause significant symptoms including shortness of breath, fatigue, cough, and postobstructive pneumonia.[95] For patients who are not candidates for surgical resection, several treatment modalities are available for alleviation of airway obstruction. These include radiation therapy, laser ablation, and stent placement.[96] Studies have also shown that PDT is an effective treatment of lung cancer causing airway obstruction.[97-100]

Moghissi et al. performed a larger study of 100 patients with stage III-IV NSCLC and an obstructing endobronchial lesion.[98] Eighty-two percent of the patients on this study had prior chemotherapy or radiation therapy. After Photofrin-mediated PDT, the mean endoluminal obstruction decreased from 86% to 18% with subsequent improvement in FEV1 and FVC. Median survival was 5 months. This study demonstrated that PDT could be an effective palliative maneuver for endoluminal obstruction in inoperable NSCLC.

A randomized trial has been performed comparing Photofrin-mediated PDT to the more traditional Nd:YAG laser resection in 31 patients with NSCLC and luminal obstruction.[99] Five patients in the PDT group required a second treatment compared to one patient in the Nd:YAG group. Response to treatment was similar between the two groups, but the response was more durable in the PDT group.

Although PDT is efficacious in the palliation of endobronchial obstruction, serious toxicities such as life-threatening hemoptysis have been reported.[83] Care should be taken to avoid treating patients with evidence of invasion of major vessels and patients who have received prior combined external beam radiation and high dose rate brachytherapy.[83]

The FDA has approved Photofrin-mediated PDT for the treatment of obstruction and palliation of symptoms in patients with completely or partially obstructing endobronchial NSCLC. The FDA-approved regimen is the intravenous injection of Photofrin 2 mg/kg, intravenously 40 to 50 hours before 630 nm light delivery. The light is delivered with a cylindrical diffuser passed through the bronchoscope. A dose of 200 J/cm is delivered at a fluence rate of 400 mW/cm (total treatment time 500 seconds). Necrotic tissue is often found in the bronchial tree after light administration. A repeat bronchoscopy to debride the airway is second light treatment may be given 96 to 120 hours after Photofrin administration.

EARLY-STAGE LUNG CANCER

The standard of care for early-stage lung cancer is surgical resection, with a reported 5-year survival rate for patients with stage I disease of up to 75%.[101] However, in a disease where the largest risk factor is smoking, many patients do not have adequate lung function to tolerate surgery. Radiation therapy is an alternative treatment to surgery, but compromised pulmonary function may also limit the ability to deliver this treatment.[96] Therefore, there has been an increasing interest in developing PDT for the treatment of superficial endobronchial tumors.

In an early pilot study by Sutedja et al., 26 patients with NSCLC were treated with Photofrin-mediated PDT.[148] In 11 patients with stage I cancer, 10 achieved a complete response. The objective response in all 26 patients was 85% (22 out of 26).

Furuse et al. reported a phase II study investigating the use of Photofrin-mediated PDT in centrally located early-stage lung cancer.[151] Of 49 assessable patients, a complete response was seen in 90% after initial PDT, with a median duration of complete response of 14 months.

In the largest study of PDT for early-stage lung cancer published, Kato et al. report treating 283 lesions in 240 patients.[153] Of the 95 patients with early-stage disease, 83% had a complete response after PDT.

The FDA has approved Photofrin-mediated PDT for the treatment of microinvasive endobronchial NSCLC in patients for whom surgery or radiotherapy is not indicated. The FDA-approved regimen is the intravenous injection of Photofrin 2 mg/kg intravenously 40 to 50 hours before 630 nm light delivery. The light is delivered with a cylindrical diffuser passed through the bronchoscope. A dose of 200 J/cm is delivered at a fluence rate of 400 mW/cm (total treatment time 500 seconds). A second bronchoscopy for debriding is performed 2 days after light treatment. A second light treatment may be given 96 to 120 hours after Photofrin administration.

NON–SMALL CELL LUNG CANCER WITH MALIGNANT PLEURAL SPREAD

Malignant spread of NSCLC to the pleura can be manifested by the development of a pleural effusion or by studding of the pleura, usually found incidentally at the time of surgery. The presence of a malignant pleural effusion in NSCLC is associated with a poor prognosis with survival rates similar to patients with stage IV disease.[105-108] The standard treatment for these patients in the United States has been chemotherapy. Conflicting results have been reported concerning the role of radical surgical resection in this group of patients,[107,109] but in general, surgery is not recommended.

One of the major conceptual problems with treating NSCLC patients who have malignant pleural spread with surgery is that radical surgical resection is unlikely to remove all microscopic disease from the thoracic cavity. Adjuvant intraoperative PDT is one potential method for treating residual microscopical disease after surgical resection. A phase I study by Pass et al. evaluated Photofrin-mediated PDT in patients with isolated hemithorax pleural malignancies who had undergone maximal surgical debulking.[110] The maximally tolerated dose (MTD) of Photofrin-mediated PDT was determined and the authors later reported that the dose limiting toxicity was esophago-pleural fistula.[111] This study showed that intrapleural PDT could be delivered safely in combination with radical surgery.

Friedberg et al. reported the results of a phase II study of intraoperative pleural Photofrin-mediated PDT in 16 patients with stage III NSCLC that had spread to the pleura.[112] The majority of patients were treated with chemotherapy before surgical resection and PDT. Surgical procedures included segmentectomy, lobectomy, and pneumonectomy combined with resection of gross pleural disease. When clinically indicated, radiation therapy was delivered to the mediastinum. Local control at 6 months was achieved in 10 patients and the median survival of all treated patients was reported to be 21.7 months. Two patients died postoperatively from adult respiratory distress syndrome and sepsis, respectively. These encouraging results form the basis for continued investigation of PDT in NSCLC with malignant pleural spread.

Mesothelioma

Malignant pleural mesothelioma is a cancer of the pleural surface that has an extremely poor prognosis with a median survival of 6 to 15 months.[113] Cure is rare and local failure is a common problem in patients with mesothelioma. PDT has been investigated as an adjuvant treatment to maximal surgical debulking for many years.[15,114-117]

One of the first trials evaluating Photofrin-mediated PDT for mesothelioma was updated in 1998.[118] A phase II trial was performed in 40 patients with mesothelioma. Patients with stage III to IV disease ($n = 24$) had a median survival of 10 months with no survivors beyond 2 years. However, patients with stage I and II disease ($n = 13$) had a median survival of 36 months and a 61% two-year overall survival. The conclusion drawn from this study is that patients with early-stage disease benefited from the adjuvant use of PDT, but that other treatment modalities are needed for patients with more advanced stages of disease.[115,118]

Based upon the phase I trial by Pass et al.,[107] a randomized phase III study[117] was initiated in patients with mesothelioma. Out of 63 patients enrolled, 15 (24%) were taken off study due to inadequate debulking or disease progression before surgery. Randomization was between surgery plus PDT versus surgery alone, with all patients receiving immunochemotherapy consisting of Tamoxifen, interferon α 2b, and cisplatin. Median recurrence-free survival for patients in the PDT group was 8.5 months versus 7.7 months in the control group. Median survival in the PDT group was 14.1 months versus 14.4 months in the control group. Median survival in those patients that were randomized was 14.4 months compared to 7.2 months in those who could not be surgically resected. The results of this study demonstrated no survival or local control benefit from the addition of adjuvant PDT to debulking surgery.

Attempts to improve upon the results of Photofrin led to the use of mTHPC in mesothelioma. Bass et al. reported early results with mTHPC-mediated PDT in five patients with mesothelioma.[15] Four out of the five patients were alive with no evidence of disease 9 to 11 months after treatment; the fifth patient developed a scar recurrence as well as metastatic disease. Recently, this group provided an update of their work with mTHPC.[114] All patients underwent an extrapleural pneumonectomy. The authors concluded that mTHPC-mediated PDT in combination with extrapleural pneumonectomy provided good local control (13 of 26 patients) but noted considerable toxicity, thereby limiting its use. The median survival was 10 months.

Freidberg and colleagues reported the results of a phase I clinical trial combining surgical debulking with Foscan-mediated PDT in patients with malignant pleural mesothelioma. Patients were enrolled regardless of tumor subtype or nodal status. Twenty-six patients received intrapleural pnemonectomy (7/26) or lung-sparing pleuretomy-decortication (19/26). The Foscan dose was fixed at 0.1 mg/kg. The dose of 652 nm light and the drug-light interval were escalated (5 J/cm² after a 6-day interval, 5 J/cm² after a 4-day interval, 10 J/cm² after a 6-day inerval; and 10 J/cm² after a 4-day interval). The dose of 652 nm light was measured with intrathoracic light sensors. The MTD was 0.1 mg/kg of Foscan injected 6-days before surgery in combination with 10 J/cm² 652 nm light. Fourteen patients treated at this dose had no significant complications. Two out of three patients who received the next dose level died of a systemic capillary leak syndrome. The median progression-free survival and overall survival for patients enrolled at the MTD was 12.4 months. The researchers concluded that the survival rates observed are comparable with those afforded by other treatments for mesothelioma. Furthermore, Foscan-mediated PDT may allow patients to undergo a lung-sparing procedure, as was performed in the last 17 of 19 patients enrolled.[118a]

Although several studies have investigated the efficacy of PDT in mesothelioma, none have convincingly proven that PDT is superior to other adjuvant therapies or surgery alone. Further study is necessary to determine the role of PDT in the treatment of this disease.

Head and Neck Cancer

The treatment of head and neck cancer with PDT has been actively investigated with promising results. In the majority of studies, early-stage disease has been treated.

Biel has reported on a series of patients with early-stage head and neck cancer who were treated with Photofrin-mediated PDT.[119-122] Of the patients with Tis/T1 tumors of the larynx, 100% had a complete response to PDT with a 95% cure rate at a mean follow-up of 37 to 44 months. Of patients with Tis/T1 tumors of the oral cavity, 100% had a complete response rate with an 80% cure rate at a mean follow-up of 40 months.

More advanced carcinomas of the head and neck have also been treated with PDT. Biel treated eight patients with more advanced T2 and T3 tumors with Photofrin-mediated PDT with disappointing results.[119] All eight patients had an initial complete response to PDT; however, all developed local recurrences. In a review of the literature of PDT for head and neck cancer, Biel reported that most advanced lesions respond to PDT, although recurrence is common.[121] Therefore, PDT used alone in the setting of advanced or bulky head and neck cancer is usually considered palliative and the risk/benefit profile of the treatment should be considered with this in mind.

PDT may also be useful for local recurrence of head and neck cancer after prior definitive therapy. The salvage rate in this group of patients with traditional therapies is poor. Tong et al. used HPD-mediated PDT in 12 patients with recurrent nasopharyngeal cancer who had previously been treated with definitive radiotherapy.[123] The authors reported that all 12 had radiographical responses to PDT. In eight patients, PDT was given with curative intent. Three of these patients were disease free at 9 to 12 months after treatment. Of the four patients treated with palliative intent, three had palliation of symptoms.

A different approach for treating patients with recurrent disease is to deliver adjuvant PDT intraoperatively to destroy any remaining cancer cells within the surgical bed. Biel has treated 10 patients with neck recurrences with intraoperative Photofrin-mediated PDT following resection.[122] Recurrences developed in only 3 of the 10 patients treated with surgery and PDT.

Treatment of premalignant lesions or carcinoma in situ of the head and neck region with PDT has also been evaluated. Grosjean et al. reported using mTHPC in 27 patients with Tis or microinvasive carcinoma and 4 patients with T1 or T2 cancers.[124] Eighty-three percent of Tis or microinvasive carcinomas showed no recurrence after a median follow-up of 15.3 months. In those with T1 or T2 cancers, only one complete response was observed.

PDT is a promising modality for the treatment of head and neck cancers. The best results with PDT appear to be in patients with premalignant or early cancers. The use of adjuvant intraoperative PDT after surgical resection for recurrent head and neck cancer also deserves further investigation.

Skin Cancer

PDT for cutaneous cancers (both primary and metastatic) and premalignant lesions has been well investigated. 5-ALA has been used extensively to treat actinic keratosis, in situ squamous cell carcinoma (Bowen's disease), and basal cell carcinoma.[125-128] The topical application of ALA with external light illumination is highly effective and associated with minimal toxicity. The FDA has approved one topical formulation of 5-ALA, Levulan (containing 20% ALA), with blue light for the treatment of nonhyperkeratotic actinic keratoses of the face or scalp. Levulan solution is directly applied to the lesions avoiding the perilesional skin.

Photofrin-mediated PDT has also been used effectively to treat skin cancers.[129] Schweitzer used low-dose Photofrin, 1 mg/kg with 630 nm light for the treatment of 12 patients with nonmelanomatous skin tumors. Five patients were treated with intraoperative PDT after surgical resection using a light dose of 50-100 J/cm². Seven patients were treated with PDT alone using a light dose of 100-300 J/cm². A complete response was achieved in 10 of the 12 patients. Excellent wound healing and cosmetic outcome was reported.

Baas et al. have used mTHPC-mediated PDT for the treatment of patients with multiple basal cell carcinomas.[130] Long-term cures with mTHPC have been observed with good cosmetic outcome.

Motexafin lutetium has been evaluated clinically in a phase I trial of patients with unresectable or metastatic cancers located in skin.[131-132] Yuen et al. reported on 35 patients with breast cancer, malignant melanoma,

Kaposi's sarcoma, basal cell carcinoma, and squamous cell carcinoma of the skin treated with lutetium texaphyrin-mediated PDT. The dose-limiting toxicities were pain in the treatment field and dysesthesias in light-exposed areas. The maximally tolerated dose of then drug in this study was 5.5 mg/kg. Skin photosensitivity was of short duration (approximately 24 hours). The overall response was 44% with 26% complete response and 18% partial response. Responses were seen at all dose levels.

ALA-mediated PDT is a safe and effective treatment for actinic keratosis, and Levulan has been approved by the FDA for this indication. The role of PDT in the treatment of skin cancer has not been completely defined, however. PDT is efficacious for superficial nonmelanomatous skin cancers such as Bowen's disease and basal cell carcinoma. However, there are many effective treatments for skin cancers and it is not clear how PDT fits into the current treatment schemes. Invasive squamous cell cancers of the skin are not typically treated with Photofrin or ALA-mediated PDT because of the limited treatment depths with these therapies. The development of PDT with newer photosensitizers, which have greater depths of penetration, may broaden the indications for PDT in skin cancer.

Intraperitoneal Malignancies

Cancers that spread to or originate in the serosal surfaces of the abdomen include primary peritoneal cancer, ovarian cancer, sarcoma, gastrointestinal malignancies, and mesothelioma. Although the natural history and systemic therapy of these cancers differ, one common feature is that, generally, curative therapy is not available when the peritoneum is diffusely involved with cancer. Traditional therapies such as surgery, radiotherapy, and chemotherapy can lead to tumor response, but local recurrence is the rule. PDT is potentially an ideal treatment for peritoneal carcinomatosis or sarcomatosis because of the superficial treatment effect.[133]

A phase I study of surgery and intraperitoneal PDT (IP PDT) with laser light and Photofrin was conducted by the Surgery and Radiation Oncology Branches of the NCI for disseminated intraperitoneal (IP) malignancies.[17,134] Fifty-four patients with a variety of IP malignancies including ovarian cancer, sarcoma, and gastrointestinal cancer were enrolled in the study. A surgical attempt was made to debulk tumor deposits to less than 5 mm of residual disease. Initially 630 nm red light alone was used but was associated with small bowel edema and occasional perforations. Less penetrating 514 nm green light was used thereafter for the large field exposures to the bowel and mesentery. This allowed further light dose escalation locally, and no further small bowel complications were seen.[135-136] The follow-up of these patients was updated by Sindelar in 1995.[137] An overall peritoneal cytological response rate of 76% was reported in evaluable patients. More importantly, long-term disease-free survivors were reported in the subgroup of patients with ovarian cancer. Three out of 25 ovarian cancer patients were disease free more than 36 months after treatment.

A phase II trial of Photofrin-mediated IP PDT to determine the efficacy of this treatment in IP malignancies is being conducted at the University of Pennsylvania.[135-136] Fifty-six patients have been enrolled and IP PDT was delivered to 42 patients. The actuarial median survival was reported to be 21 months, although the median time to recurrence was only 3 months. Toxicities included postoperative fluid shifts, volume overload, transient thrombocytopenia, elevated liver function tests, and gastrointestinal toxicities. This study is ongoing.

Central Nervous System Tumors

Tumors of the central nervous system, especially malignant gliomas, have a propensity for local failure despite surgery and radiotherapy.[138-139] PDT has been investigated in patients with these tumors as a means of reducing local failure after surgery.

Kaye et al. performed a phase 1 to 2 study of HPD-mediated (5 mg/kg) PDT for cerebral tumors.[140] HPD was administered in 22 patients with high-grade gliomas and 1 patient with a frontal metastasis from a carcinoma of the lung. They all underwent a craniotomy with radical excision of the tumor. The tumor bed was then irradiated with 630 nm light, receiving total doses of 70 to 230 J/cm^2. There was no evidence of increased cerebral edema and no other toxicity from the therapy. Fifteen patients who developed new tumors underwent postoperative radiotherapy. Overall, 6 of the 22 patients with gliomas suffered a recurrence at the PDT site. Fifteen patients have had no recurrence of their tumor at a median follow-up period of 7 months. It was concluded that PDT could be used as an adjuvant to surgery and radiotherapy with no additional complications.

Muller and Wilson have had extensive experience in the treatment of supratentorial gliomas with Photofrin-mediated PDT.[141-144] Fifty-six patients with recurrent gliomas underwent resection and PDT.[143] Illumination was performed via an intracavitary or interstitial approach. Median survival for patients with recurrent glioblastoma multiforme and malignant astrocytoma was 30 and 44 weeks, respectively. The authors report that the survival of patients with malignant astrocytoma was related to the light dose delivered to the tumor bed. These authors also reported treating 20 patients with newly diagnosed supratentorial malignant gliomas using intraoperative Photofrin-mediated PDT.[144] In 18 of the 20 patients the PDT was supplemented with postoperative radiotherapy. The median survival for GBM and MA patients was 37 and 44 weeks, respectively. The authors concluded that PDT is safe in this setting and appeared to prolong survival in select patients.

Kostron et al. reviewed the status of the literature for HPD-mediated PDT in brain tumors and included 58 patients treated at their own institution.[145] The major side effects of PDT were cutaneous photosensitivity and increased intracranial pressure. They reported that PDT for brain tumors after surgical resection was safe and was associated with a trend toward increased median survival. Definitive statements regarding the use of PDT in malignant brain tumors cannot be made until the results of ongoing, randomized phase III trials are complete.[2]

SUMMARY AND FUTURE DIRECTIONS

PDT is an emerging treatment for cancer that requires the presence of a photosensitizer, oxygen, and light. Several of the photosensitizers available are reported to have preferential distribution and retention in tumors compared to other normal tissues. The treatment is dependent on the penetration of light into tissues. The superficial therapeutic effect of PDT is a potential advantage for the treatment of superficial neoplasms such as skin cancers,[130a] early cancers of the respiratory or digestive tracts, or malignancies that spread to serosal surfaces.[110,133-134,146-147] However, this is a disadvantage when considering PDT for large, bulky cancers or for deep-seated tumors. Recent studies, however, demonstrate that the interstitial delivery of light may permit PDT to become effective for larger or more deeply seated tumors.[148-150] Furthermore, unlike radiotherapy, PDT can be administered more than once.

Several clinical situations have been identified in which PDT may become effective therapy for malignant or premalignant conditions. The curative treatment of such conditions with PDT alone has been studied extensively. Another clinical situation that holds much promise is the incorporation of PDT as an adjuvant treatment with surgery. The major advantage of this approach is that bulky cancers that cannot be completely eradicated by surgery may be sterilized by the addition of intraoperative PDT. Furthermore, other cancer treatments such as radiation and chemotherapy can be added to the treatment regimen and are often complementary to PDT.[133]

Currently, two photosensitizers are approved for clinical use in the United States, Photofrin and Levulan. Photofrin is a systemic photosensitizer that, in combination with 630 nm light, is approved for the treatment of obstructing esophageal cancer, obstructing bronchial NSCLC, microinvasive bronchial lung cancer, and Barrett's esophagus with high grade dysplasia. Levulan is a topical photosensitizer that, in combination with blue light, is approved for the treatment of actinic keratosis. New photosensitizers with deeper activity profiles and a shorter period of enhanced skin reaction to sunlight are being developed, making deeper and more frequent treatments feasible. PDT is currently being studied for many conditions including peritoneal carcinomatosis, pleural carcinomatosis, central nervous system tumors, and head and neck cancers.

The investigation of oncologic PDT on a basic level has focused on understanding the interaction of photosensitizers, light, and oxygen on a molecular, cellular, and tissue level.[62,151-156] Advances in the use of PDT for cancers will result from increased preclinical research on the basic mechanisms of photodynamic action and with a better understanding of light and photosensitizer dosimetry.

REFERENCES

1. Oleinick NL, Evans HH: The photobiology of photodynamic therapy: Cellular targets and mechanisms. *Radiat Res.* 1998;150 (5 suppl):S146.
2. Dougherty TJ, et al: Photodynamic therapy. [Review]. *J Natl Cancer Instit.* 1998;90:889.
3. Dougherty TJ: Photosensitization of malignant tumors. *Semin Surg Oncol.* 1986;2:24.
4. Lipson RL, Baldes EJ, Olsen EM: Hematoporphyrin derivative for detection, and management of cancer. In: Proceedings of the Ninth International Cancer Congress. 1966. Abstract 393.
5. Gomer C, Dougherty T: Determination of [3H]- and [14C] hematoporphyrin derivative distribution in malignant and normal tissue. *Cancer Res.* 1979;39:146.
6. Young SW, et al: Lutetium texaphyrin (PCI-0123): a near-infrared, water-soluble photosensitizer. *Photochem Photobiol*, 1996;63:892.
7. Ris HB, et al: Photodynamic therapy with chlorins for diffuse malignant mesothelioma: Initial clinical results. *Br J Cancer.* 1991; 64:1116.
8. Peng Q, et al: Selective distribution of porphyrins in skin thick basal cell carcinoma after topical application of methyl 5-aminolevulinate. *J Photochem Photobiol B.* 2001;62:140.
9. Karrer S, et al: Role of lasers and photodynamic therapy in the treatment of cutaneous malignancy. *Am J Clin Dermatol.* 2001; 2:229.
10. Woodburn KW, et al: Photodynamic therapy of B16F10 murine melanoma with lutetium texaphyrin. *J Invest Dermatol.* 1998; 110:746.
11. Koderhold G, et al: Experiences of photodynamic therapy in dermatology. *J Photochem Photobiol B.* 1996;36:221.
12. Star WM: Light dosimetry in vivo. *Phys Med Biol.* 1997;42:763.
13. Marijnissen JP, et al: Pilot study on light dosimetry for endobronchial photodynamic therapy. *Photochem Photobiol B.* 1993; 58:92.
14. Marijnissen JP, et al: In situ light dosimetry during whole bladder wall photodynamic therapy: clinical results and experimental verification. *Phys Med Biol.* 1993;38:567.
15. Baas P, et al: Photodynamic therapy as adjuvant therapy in surgically treated pleural malignancies. *Br J Cancer.* 1997;76:819.
16. Vulcan TG, et al: Comparison between isotropic and nonisotropic dosimetry systems during intraperitoneal photodynamic therapy. *Lasers Surg Med.* 2000;26:292.
17. Sindelar WF, et al: Technique of photodynamic therapy for disseminated intraperitoneal malignant neoplasms. Phase I study. *Arch Surg.* 1991;126:318.
18. Wilson BC, Patterson MS: The physics of photodynamic therapy. *Phys Med Biol.* 1986;31:7.
19. Pass HI: Photodynamic therapy in oncology: Mechanisms and clinical use. *J Natl Cancer Inst.* 1993;85:443.
20. DeJoe M, et al: A comparison of novel light sources for photodynamic therapy. *Lasers Med Sci.* 1997;12:260.
21. Hammer-Wilson MJ, et al: In vitro and in vivo comparison of argonpumped and diode lasers for photodynamic therapy using second-generation photosensitizers. *Lasers Surg Med.* 1998;23:274.
22. Foote CS: Mechanisms of photooxygenation. *Prog Clin Biol Res.* 1984;170:3.
23. Henderson BW, Bellnier DA, Ziring B, Dougherty J: Aspects of the cellular uptake and retention of hematoporphyrin derivative and their correlation with the biological response to PRJ in vitro. In Kessel D, Dougherty TJ, eds. *Porphyrin Photosensitization.* New York: Plenum Press; 1983:129.
24. Freitas I: *Lipid accumulation: The common feature to photosensitizer-retaining normal and malignant tissues. J Photochem Photobiol B.* 1990;7:359.
25. Polo L, et al: Low-density lipoprotein receptors in the uptake of tumor photosensitizers by human and rat transformed fibroblasts. *Int J Biochem Cell Biol.* 2002;34:10.
26. Hamblin MR, Newman EL: Photosensitizer targeting in photodynamic therapy. II. Conjugates of haematoporphyrin with serum lipoproteins. *J Photochem Photobiol B.* 1994;26:147.
27. Schmidt-Erfurth U, et al: Photodynamic targeting of human retinoblastoma cells using covalent low-density lipoprotein conjugates. *Br J Cancer.* 1997;75:54.
28. Korbelik M: Low density lipoprotein receptor pathway in the delivery of Photofrin: how much is it relevant for selective accumulation of the photosensitizer in tumors? *J Photochem Photobiol B.* 1992;12:107.
29. Bohmer RM, Morstyn G: Uptake of hematoporphyrin derivative by normal and malignant cells: effect of serum, pH, temperature, and cell size. *Cancer Res.* 1985;45:5328.
30. Kurohane K, et al: Photodynamic therapy targeted to tumor-induced angiogenic vessels. *Cancer Lett.* 2001;167:49.
31. Hamblin MR, et al: In vivo fluorescence imaging of the transport of charged chlorin e6 conjugates in a rat orthotopic prostate tumor. *Br J Cancer.* 1999;81:261.
32. Bugelski PJ, Porter CW, Dougherty TJ: Autoradiographic distribution of HPD in normal and tumor tissue of the mouse. *Cancer Res.* 1982;41:4606.
33. Kessel D, Chow T: Tumor-localizing components of the porphyrin preparation hematoporphyrin derivative. *Cancer Res.* 1983; 43:1994.
34. Barel A, Jaro G, Penn A, et al: Role of high, low, and very low density lipoproteins in the transport and tumor delivery of hematoporphyrin in via. *Cancer Lett.* 1986;32:145.
35. Pahernik SA, et al: Pharmacokinetics and selectivity of aminolevulinic acid-induced porphyrin synthesis in patients with cervical intra-epithelial neoplasia. *Int J Cancer.* 1998;78:310.
36. Andrejevic Blant S, et al: Localization of tetra(m-hydroxyphenyl) chlorin (Foscan) in human healthy tissues and squamous cell carcinomas of the upper aero-digestive tract, the esophagus and the bronchi: A fluorescence microscopy study. *J Photochem Photobiol B.* 2001;61:1.
37. Mitchell J, et al: Oxygen dependence of hematoporpyrin derivative-induced photoinactivation of Chinese hamster cells. *Cancer Res.* 1985;45:2008.
38. Chapman J, et al: Oxygen dependency of tumor cell killing in vitro by light-activated Photofrin II. *Radiat Res.* 1991;126:73.
39. Henderson BW, Fingar VH: Relationship of tumor hypoxia and response to photodynamic treatment in an experimental mouse tumor. *Cancer Res.* 1987;47:3110.
40. Fingar VH, et al: Implications of a pre-existing tumor hypoxic fraction on photodynamic therapy. *J Surg Res.* 1992;53:524.
41. Henderson BW, Waldow SM, Mang JS, et al: Tumor destruction and kinetics of tumor cell death in two experimental mouse tumors following photodynamic therapy. *Cancer Res.* 1985; 45:572.
42. Kessel D: Effects of photoactivated porphyrins at the cell surface of leukemia L-1210 cell. *Biochemistry.* 1977;16:3343.
43. Hockel M, et al: Intratumoral pO2 predicts survival in advanced cancer of the uterine cervix. *Radiother Oncol.* 1993;26:45.
44. Brizel DM, et al: Oxygenation of head and neck cancer: changes during radiotherapy and impact on treatment outcome. *Radiother Oncol.* 1999;53:113.
45. Rofstad EK, et al: Hypoxia-induced treatment failure in advanced squamous cell carcinoma of the uterine cervix is primarily due to hypoxia-induced radiation resistance rather than hypoxia-induced metastasis. *Br J Cancer.* 2000;83:354.
46. Vanselow B, et al: Oxygenation of advanced head and neck cancer: prognostic marker for the response to primary radiochemotherapy. *Otolaryngol Head Neck Surg.* 2000;122:856.
47. Knocke TH, et al: Intratumoral pO2-measurements as predictive assay in the treatment of carcinoma of the uterine cervix. *Radiother Oncol.* 1999;53:99.
48. Brizel DM, et al: Tumor hypoxia adversely affects the prognosis of carcinoma of the head and neck. *Int J Radiat Oncol Biol Phys.* 1997;38:285.
49. Evans SM, et al: Hypoxic heterogeneity in human tumors: EF5 binding, vasculature, necrosis, and proliferation. *Am J Clin Oncol.* 2001;24:467.
50. Evans S, et al: Detection of hypoxia in human squamous cell carcinoma by EF5 binding. *Cancer Res.* 2000;60:2018.
51. Evans SM, et al: Hypoxia in human intraperitoneal and extremity sarcomas. *Int J Radiat Oncol Biol Phys.* 2001;49:587.
52. Hockel M, et al: Tumor oxygenation: a new predictive parameter in locally advanced cancer of the uterine cervix [see comments]. *Gynecol Oncol.* 1993;51:141.
53. Brizel DM, et al: Pretreatment oxygenation profiles of human soft tissue sarcomas. *Int J Radiat Oncol Biol Phys.* 1994;30:635.

54. Hockel M, et al: Association between tumor hypoxia and malignant progression in advanced cancer of the uterine cervix. *Cancer Res.* 1996;56:4509.

55. Fyles A, et al: Oxygenation predicts radiation response and survival in patients with cervix cancer. *Radiother Oncol.* 1998; 48:149.

56. Movsas B, et al: Hypoxic regions exist in human prostate carcinoma. *Urology.* 1999;53:11.

57. Tomaselli F, et al: Acute effects of combined photodynamic therapy and hyperbaric oxygenation in lung cancer—A clinical pilot study. *Lasers Surg Med.* 2001;28:399.

58. Maier A, et al: Effect of photodynamic therapy in a multimodal approach for advanced carcinoma of the gastro-esophageal junction. *Lasers Surg Med.* 2000;26:461.

59. Maier A, et al: Hyperbaric oxygen and photodynamic therapy in the treatment of advanced carcinoma of the cardia and the esophagus. *Lasers Surg Med.* 2000;26:308.

60. Maier A, et al: Does hyperbaric oxygen enhance the effect of photodynamic therapy in patients with advanced esophageal carcinoma? A clinical pilot study. *Endoscopy.* 2000;32:42.

61. Engbrecht BW, et al: Photofrin-mediated photodynamic therapy induces vascular occlusion and apoptosis in a human sarcoma xenograft model. *Cancer Res.* 1999;59:4334.

62. Busch TM, et al: Depletion of tumor oxygenation during photodynamic therapy: detection by the hypoxia marker EF3 [2-(2-nitroimidazol-1[H]-yl)-N-(3,3,3-trifluoropropyl)acetamide]. *Cancer Res.* 2000;60:2636.

63. Sitnik TM, Hampton JA, Henderson BW: Reduction of tumor oxygenation during and after photodynamic therapy in vivo: effects of fluence rate. *Br J Cancer.* 1998;77:1386.

64. Chen Q, Chen H, Hetzel FW: Tumor oxygenation changes post-photodynamic therapy. *Photochem Photobiol.* 1996;63:128.

65. Pogue BW, et al: Analysis of the heterogeneity of pO2 dynamics during photodynamic therapy with verteporfin. *Photochem Photobiol.* 2001;74:700.

66. Henderson BW, et al: Photofrin photodynamic therapy can significantly deplete or preserve oxygenation in human basal cell carcinomas during treatment, depending on fluence rate. *Cancer Res.* 2000;60:525.

67. Schouwink H, et al: Photodynamic therapy for malignant mesothelioma: Preclinical studies for optimization of treatment protocols. *Photochem Photobiol.* 2001;73:410.

68. Sitnik TM, Henderson BW: The effect of fluence rate on tumor and normal tissue responses to photodynamic therapy. *Photochem Photobiol.* 1998;67:462.

69. Langmack K, et al: Topical photodynamic therapy at low fluence rates—Theory and practice. *J Photochem Photobiol B.* 2001; 60:37.

70. Moan J, Sommer S: Action spectra for hematoporphyrin derivative, and photo II with respect to Sensitization of human cells in vitro to photo inactivation. *Photochem Photobiol.* 1984; 40:631.

71. Kessel O, Thompson P, Musselman B, Chang CK: Chemistry of hematoporphyrin-derived photosensitizers. *Photochem Photobiol.* 1987:46:563.

72. Pandey RK, Dougherty TJ: Syntheses and photosensitizing activity of porphyrins joined with ester linkages. *Cancer Res.* 1989; 49:2042.

73. Ma L, Moan J, Berg K: Evaluation of a new photosensitizer, meso-tetra-hydroxyphenyl-chlorin, for use in photodynamic therapy: A comparison of its photobiological properties with those of two other photosensitizers. *Int J Cancer.* 1994;57:883.

74. van Geel IP, et al: Photosensitizing efficacy of MTHPC-PDT compared to photofrin-PDT in the RIF1 mouse tumor and normal skin. *Int J Cancer.* 1995;60:388.

75. Sessler JL, Miller RA: Texaphyrins: New drugs with diverse clinical applications in radiation and photodynamic therapy. *Biochem Pharmacol.* 2000;59:733.

76. Ivy SP, Blatner G, Cheson BD: Clinical trials referral resource. Clinical trials with gadolinium-texaphyrin and lutetium-texaphyrin. *Oncology (Huntingt).* 1999;13:671, 674.

77. Mang TS, et al: A phase II/III clinical study of tin ethyl etiopurpurin (Purlytin)-induced photodynamic therapy for the treatment of recurrent cutaneous metastatic breast cancer. *Cancer J Sci Am.* 1998;4:378.

78. Kaplan MJ, et al: Photodynamic therapy in the management of metastatic cutaneous adenocarcinomas: case reports from phase 1/2 studies using tin ethyl etiopurpurin (SnET2). *J Surg Oncol.* 1998;67:121.

79. Narayan S, Sivak MV Jr: Palliation of esophageal carcinoma. Laser and photodynamic therapy. *Chest Surg Clin N Am.* 1994; 4:347.

80. Lightdale CJ, Zimbalist E, Winawer SJ: Outpatient management of esophageal cancer with endoscopic Nd:YAG laser. *Am J Gastroenterol.* 1987;82:46.

81. Maier A, et al: Palliation of advanced esophageal carcinoma by photodynamic therapy and irradiation. *Ann Thorac Surg.* 2000;69:1006.

82. Scheider DM, et al: Photodynamic therapy for the treatment of tumor ingrowth in expandable esophageal stents. *Endoscopy.* 1997;29:271.

83. Sanfilippo NJ, et al: Toxicity of photodynamic therapy after combined external beam radiotherapy and intraluminal brachytherapy for carcinoma of the upper aerodigestive tract. *Lasers Surg Med.* 2001;28:278.

84. Webb DD: Introduction. GERD warrants increased physician appreciation and improved treatment. *Postgrad Med.* 2001; Spec No: 5.

85. Spechler SJ: Clinical practice. Barrett's Esophagus. *N Engl J Med.* 2002;346:836.

86. van Sandick JW, et al: Barrett oesophagus and adenocarcinoma: An overview of epidemiologic, conceptual and clinical issues. *Scand J Gastroenterol Suppl.* 2001;234:51.

87. Ofman JJ: The relation between gastroesophageal reflux disease and esophageal and head and neck cancers: A critical appraisal of epidemiologic literature. *Am J Med.* 2001;111(suppl 8A):124S.

88. Dent J: Approaches to oesophageal columnar metaplasia (Barrett's oesophagus). *Scand J Gastroenterol Suppl.* 1989;168:60.

89. Overholt BF: A multicenter, partially blinded, randomized study of the efficacy of photodynamic therapy (PDT) using porfimer sodium (POR) for the ablation of high-grade dysplasia (HGD) in Barrett's esophagus (BE): Results of 6-month follow-up. *Gastroent Suppl.* 2001;120:A-79.

90. Savary JF, et al: Photodynamic therapy of early squamous cell carcinomas of the esophagus: a review of 31 cases. *Endoscopy.* 1998;30:258.

91. Corti L, et al: Outcome of patients receiving photodynamic therapy for early esophageal cancer. *Int J Radiat Oncol Biol Phys.* 2000;47:419.

92. Panjehpour M, et al: Results of photodynamic therapy for ablation of dysplasia and early cancer in Barrett's esophagus and effect of oral steroids on stricture formation. *Am J Gastroenterol.* 2000;95:2177.

93. Overholt BF, Panjehpour M, Ayres M: Photodynamic therapy for Barrett's esophagus: cardiac effects. *Lasers Surg Med.* 1997;21:317.

94. Clouston AD: Timely topic: Premalignant lesions associated with adenocarcinoma of the upper gastrointestinal tract. *Pathology.* 2001;33:271.

95. Lam S: Photodynamic therapy of lung cancer. *Semin Oncol.* 1994;21(6 suppl 15):15.

96. Metz JM, Friedberg JS: Endobronchial photodynamic therapy for the treatment of lung cancer. *Chest Surg Clin N Am.* 2001;11:829.

97. LoCicero J III, Metzdorff M, Almgren C: Photodynamic therapy in the palliation of late stage obstructing non-small cell lung cancer. *Chest.* 1990;98:97.

98. Moghissi K, et al: The place of bronchoscopic photodynamic therapy in advanced unresectable lung cancer: experience of 100 cases. *Eur J Cardiothorac Surg.* 1999;15:1.

99. Diaz-Jimenez JP, et al: Efficacy and safety of photodynamic therapy versus Nd-YAG laser resection in NSCLC with airway obstruction. *Eur Respir J.* 1999;14:800.

100. Maier A, et al: Comparison of 5-aminolaevulinic acid and porphyrin photosensitization for photodynamic therapy of malignant bronchial stenosis: A clinical pilot study. *Lasers Surg Med.* 2002;30:12.

101. Martini N, et al: Incidence of local recurrence and second primary tumors in resected stage I lung cancer. *J Thorac Cardiovasc Surg.* 1995;109:120.

102. Sutedja T, et al: A pilot study of photodynamic therapy in patients with inoperable non-small cell lung cancer. *Eur J Cancer.* 1992; 28A:1370.

103. Furuse K, et al: A prospective phase II study on photodynamic therapy with photofrin II for centrally located early-stage lung cancer. The Japan Lung Cancer Photodynamic Therapy Study Group. *J Clin Oncol.* 1993;11:1852.
104. Kato H, Okunaka T, Shimatani H: Photodynamic therapy for early stage bronchogenic carcinoma. *J Clin Laser Med Surg.* 1996; 14:235.
105. Sugiura S, et al: Prognostic value of pleural effusion in patients with non-small cell lung cancer. *Clin Cancer Res.* 1997;3:47.
106. Werner-Wasik M, et al: Recursive partitioning analysis of 1999 Radiation Therapy Oncology Group (RTOG) patients with locally-advanced non-small-cell lung cancer (LA-NSCLC): identification of five groups with different survival. *Int J Radiat Oncol Biol Phys.* 2000;48:1475.
107. Sawabata N, et al: Malignant minor pleural effusion detected on thoracotomy for patients with non-small cell lung cancer: Is tumor resection beneficial for prognosis? *Ann Thorac Surg.* 2002;73:412.
108. Fukuse T, et al: The prognostic significance of malignant pleural effusion at the time of thoracotomy in patients with non-small cell lung cancer. *Lung Cancer.* 2001;34:75.
109. Yokoi K, Matsuguma H, Anraku M: Extrapleural pneumonectomy for lung cancer with carcinomatous pleuritis. *J Thorac Cardiovasc Surg.* 2002;123:184.
110. Pass HI, et al: Intrapleural photodynamic therapy: Results of a phase I trial. *Ann Surg Oncol.* 1994;1:28.
111. Temeck BK, Pass HI: Esophagopleural fistula: A complication of photodynamic therapy. *South Med J.* 1995;88:271.
112. Freidberg JS, et al: Multimodality treatment including pleural photodynamic therapy (PDT) for non-small cell lung cancer (NSCLC) patients with pleural carcinomatosis. *Proceedings of ASCO,* 2001;20(Abstract #1303):327a.
113. Antman K, Pass H, Schiff P: Benign and malignant mesothelioma. In: Devita VT, Hellman S, Rosenberg SA, eds., 5th ed. *Cancer: Principles and Practice of Oncology.* Philadelphia: Lippincott-Raven; 1997:1853.
114. Schouwink H, et al: Intraoperative photodynamic therapy after pleuropneumonectomy in patients with malignant pleural mesothelioma: Dose finding and toxicity results. *Chest.* 2001; 120:1167.
115. Takita H, et al: Operation and intracavitary photodynamic therapy for malignant pleural mesothelioma: A phase II study. *Ann Thorac Surg.* 1994;58:995.
116. Takita H, Dougherty TJ: Intracavitary photodynamic therapy for malignant pleural mesothelioma. *Semin Surg Oncol.* 1995; 11:368.
117. Pass HI, et al: Phase III randomized trial of surgery with or without intraoperative photodynamic therapy and postoperative immunochemotherapy for malignant pleural mesothelioma. *Ann Surg Oncol.* 1997;4:628.
118. Moskal TL, et al: Operation and photodynamic therapy for pleural mesothelioma: 6-year follow-up. *Ann Thorac Surg.* 1998; 66:1128.
118a. Friedberg JS, Mick R, Stevenson J, Metz J, et al: A phrase I study of Foscan-mediated photodynamic therapy and surgery in patients with mesothelioma. *Ann Thorac Surg.* 2003;75:952.
119. Biel MA: Photodynamic therapy of head and neck cancers. *Semin Surg Oncol.* 1995;11:355.
120. Biel MA: Photodynamic therapy and the treatment of neoplastic diseases of the larynx. *Laryngoscope.* 1994;104:399.
121. Biel MA: Photodynamic therapy and the treatment of head and neck neoplasia. *Laryngoscope.* 1998;108:1259.
122. Biel MA: Photodynamic therapy and the treatment of head and neck cancers. *J Clin Laser Med Surg.* 1996;14:239.
123. Tong MC, van Hasselt CA, Woo JK: Preliminary results of photodynamic therapy for recurrent nasopharyngeal carcinoma. *Eur Arch Otorhinolaryngol.* 1996;253:189.
124. Grosjean P, et al: Photodynamic therapy for cancer of the upper aerodigestive tract using tetra(m-hydroxyphenyl)chlorin. *J Clin Laser Med Surg.* 1996;14:281.
125. Ormrod D, Jarvis B: Topical aminolevulinic acid HCl photodynamic therapy. *Am J Clin Dermatol.* 2000;1:133; discussion 140.
126. Dijkstra AT, et al: Photodynamic therapy with violet light and topical 6-aminolaevulinic acid in the treatment of actinic keratosis, Bowen's disease and basal cell carcinoma. *J Eur Acad Dermatol Venereol.* 2001;15:550.
127. Wang I, et al: Photodynamic therapy vs. cryosurgery of basal cell carcinomas: results of a phase III clinical trial. *Br J Dermatol.* 2001;144:832.
128. Jeffes EW, et al: Photodynamic therapy of actinic keratosis with topical 5-aminolevulinic acid. A pilot dose-ranging study. *Arch Dermatol.* 1997;133:727.
129. Gayl Schweitzer V: Photofrin-mediated photodynamic therapy for treatment of aggressive head and neck nonmelanomatous skin tumors in elderly patients. *Laryngoscope.* 2001;111:1091.
130. Baas P, et al: Photodynamic therapy with meta-tetrahydroxyphenylchlorin for basal cell carcinoma: a phase I/II study. *Br J Dermatol.* 2001;145:75.
130a. Yuen AR, Panella TJ, Julius C, et al: Phase I trial of photodynamic therapy with lutetium-texaphyrin. *Proc Am Soc Clin Oncol.* 1997;16:219a.
131. Panella TJ, et al: Lutetium texaphyrin (Lu-Tex) photodynamic therapy (PDT) of patients with refractory locally recurrent breast cancer. *Proceedings of ASCO,* 1998;17(Abstract # 632):165a.
132. Wieman TJ, et al: Photodynamic therapy (PDT) of locally recurrent breast cancer (LRBC) with lutetium texaphyrin (Lutrin): a phase IB/IIA trial. *Proceedings of ASCO,* 1999;18(Abstract # 418):111a.
133. Hahn S, Glatstein E: The Emergence of Photodynamic Therapy as a Major Modality in Cancer Treatment. *Rev Contemp Pharmocother.* 1999;10:69.
134. DeLaney TF, et al: Phase I study of debulking surgery and photodynamic therapy for disseminated intraperitoneal tumors. *Int J Radiat Oncol Biol Phys.* 1993;25:445.
135. Bauer TW, et al: Preliminary report of photodynamic therapy for intraperitoneal sarcomatosis. *Ann Surg Oncol.* 2001;8:254.
136. Hendren SK, et al: Phase II trial of debulking surgery and photodynamic therapy for disseminated intraperitoneal tumors. *Ann Surg Oncol.* 2001;8:65.
137. Sindelar W, et al: Intraperitoneal Photodynamic Therapy shows efficacy in Phase I Trial. *Proc Am Soc Clin Oncol.* 1995;14:447.
138. Garden AS, et al: Outcome and patterns of failure following limited-volume irradiation for malignant astrocytomas. *Radiother Oncol.* 1991;20:99.
139. Sneed PK, et al: Patterns of recurrence of glioblastoma multiforme after external irradiation followed by implant boost. *Int J Radiat Oncol Biol Phys.* 1994;29:719.
140. Kaye AH, et al: Adjuvant high-dose photoradiation therapy in the treatment of cerebral glioma: a phase 1-2 study. *J Neurosurg.* 1987;67:500.
141. Muller PJ, Wilson BC: Photodynamic therapy of malignant primary brain tumors: clinical effects, post-operative ICP, and light penetration of the brain. *Photochem Photobiol.* 1987; 46:929.
142. Muller PJ, Wilson BC: Photodynamic therapy of malignant brain tumors. *Can J Neurol Sci.* 1990;17:193.
143. Muller PJ, Wilson BC: Photodynamic therapy for recurrent supratentorial gliomas. *Semin Surg Oncol.* 1995;11:346.
144. Muller PJ, Wilson BC: Photodynamic therapy for malignant newly diagnosed supratentorial gliomas. *J Clin Laser Med Surg.* 1996;14:263.
145. Kostron H, Obwegeser A, Jakober R: Photodynamic therapy in neurosurgery: A review. *J Photochem Photobiol B.* 1996;36:157.
146. Pass HI, et al: Intraoperative photodynamic therapy for malignant mesothelioma. *Ann Thorac Surg.* 1990;50:687.
147. Hahn S, et al: Intraperitoneal photodynamic therapy for peritoneal carcinomatosis and sarcomatosis. In Dougherty TJ, ed: *Optical Methods for Tumor Treatment and Detection: Mechanisms and Techniques in Photodynamic Therapy IX.* San Jose, Calif: SPIE-The International Society for Optical Engineering; 2000; 3909:2.
148. Hsi RA, et al: Photodynamic therapy in the canine prostate using motexafin lutetium. *Clin Cancer Res.* 2001;7:651.
149. Fielding DI, et al: Fine-needle interstitial photodynamic therapy of the lung parenchyma: photosensitizer distribution and morphologic effects of treatment. *Chest.* 1999;115:502.
150. Fielding DI, et al: Interstitial laser photocoagulation and interstitial photodynamic therapy of normal lung parenchyma in the pig. *Lasers Med Sci.* 2001;16:26.
151. Gomer CJ, et al: Cellular targets and molecular responses associated with photodynamic therapy. *J Clin Laser Med Surg.* 1996; 14:315.

152. Fisher AM, et al: Photodynamic therapy sensitivity is not altered in human tumor cells after abrogation of p53 function. *Cancer Res.* 1999;59:331.

153. Ferrario A, et al: Antiangiogenic treatment enhances photodynamic therapy responsiveness in a mouse mammary carcinoma. *Cancer Res.* 2000;60:4066.

154. Luna MC, Wong S, Gomer CJ: Photodynamic therapy mediated induction of early response genes. *Cancer Res.* 1994;54:1374.

155. Patterson MS, Wilson BC, Graff R: In vivo tests of the concept of photodynamic threshold dose in normal rat liver photosensitized by aluminum chlorosulphonated phthalocyanine. *Photochem Photobiol.* 1990;51:343.

156. Molckovsky A, Wilson BC: Monitoring of cell and tissue responses to photodynamic therapy by electrical impedance spectroscopy. *Phys Med Biol.* 2001;46:983.

74

Extracranial Stereotactic Radioablation

Richard L. Crownover, MD, PhD
and Dan P. Garwood, MD

"Radiosurgery," first with the GammaKnife and subsequently with modified linear accelerators (LINACs), has gradually gained credibility as an alternative to surgery or conventional external beam radiotherapy for many patients with lesions in the brain. A confluence of recent developments in computer science, medical imaging, and robotics has contributed to a new generation of radiation treatment devices capable of delivering highly conformal dose distributions anywhere in the body, generating the attractive prospect that radiosurgery can be applied to suitable extracranial sites as well. "Radiosurgery" refers specifically to the application of a single large dose of radiation with precise stereotactic target localization; the more general term "radioablation" encompasses highly conformal hypofractionated schedules that are also intended to achieve an ablative effect within the target volume. Employing diverse techniques, a few centers have already taken the pioneering steps of treating with extracranial stereotactic radioablation (ESR) in the spine, liver, lung, and pancreas.[1-16]

In the brain, radiosurgery is typically administered by a team that includes a neurosurgeon, a radiation oncologist, and a medical physicist. The medical physicist, whose training emphasizes the technical, physical, and operational aspects of treatment planning and radiation delivery, assures that the plan is optimal; the delivery equipment functions correctly; and the treatment is delivered as prescribed. The neurosurgeon provides a detailed knowledge of functional neuroanatomy, which is crucial. Together, the team determines whether the procedure is technically feasible and whether the procedure "makes sense" in the context of the patient's overall status; for instance, palliative radiosurgery for central nervous system lesions is usually only justifiable if the patient has at least a 3-month life expectancy. The radiation oncologist, whose training emphasizes the natural history of and a multimodality approach to malignancies arising anywhere in the body, is well equipped to assess the patient's intercurrent treatment needs and prognosis. The expertise of the various clinical specialties are most important in the consultation process rather than during the actual procedure. When treatment is confined to single fractions within the brain, the limited knowledge relevant to prescribing radiation is easily mastered by the neurosurgeon, as demonstrated in other nations where radiosurgery is often performed by a neurosurgeon or a radiation oncologist working independently.

When treating below the foramen magnum, the functional role of the organs is familiar to all clinicians, and structure identification, as opposed to the nuances of functional neuroanatomy, is relatively straightforward. In defining target lesions, there are situations where image interpretation still becomes subtle; for instance, contouring lesions in the lung may require differentiation of tumor from transiting vessels, postobstructive atelectasis, granulomatous adenopathy, and so on. In the body, image interpretation is facilitated by the diagnostic radiologist, and decisions hinge on the radiation oncologist's working knowledge of whole- and partial-organ radiation tolerance. As always, treatment recommendations should derive from a multidisciplinary discussion; however, billing arguments aside, once a decision has been reached to treat with ESR, there is no more use to having the surgeon directly participate in extracranial procedures than there is to having a radiation oncologist assist in a resection if surgery is selected as the best management. We have found in our practice that the recognized availability of both high-quality conformal radiotherapy and exceptional surgical expertise draws outside consultations that contribute an increased number of cases to both programs.

PHYSICAL GRADIENTS

Conventional doses and treatment schedules in radiotherapy have been titrated to the clinical tolerance of normal tissues. Protracted treatment courses delivered over several weeks, "fractionated schedules," are a radiobiologic compromise employed to permit normal tissue repair between multiple small doses of radiation, with the goal of reducing morbid late effects of treatment. This approach is often successful in dealing with microscopic disease or particularly radiosensitive tumors; however, for bulky disease or radioresistant tumors, sterilizing tumoricidal doses may never be reached due to limitations imposed by nearby critical structures.

Conformal radiotherapy, in which the high-dose region is shaped to fit the target lesion and the incidental dose to adjacent normal tissues is limited, can be employed in strategies that vary depending on the clinical situation. When treating lesions with an established effective dose, conformal techniques can permit reduction of dose to adjacent tissues, with a resultant decrease in acute and late morbidity. In cases where tumors have not been reliably controlled by conventional doses, the localized dose applied to the tumor can be increased, or "escalated," to a higher total while doses nearby are held constant to maintain normal tissue effects at the level previously considered acceptable. Both approaches would represent an improvement in therapeutic ratio for radiotherapy. ESR aims to accomplish both goals simultaneously.

The earliest way of delivering localized treatments was "by treating from the inside out" with implanted radioactive sources: a technique formally known as *brachytherapy*. Years of clinical experience with these techniques have demonstrated the efficacy of localized high-dose radiation treatments, even in dealing with bulky tumors. From brachytherapy, much has been learned about the doses required to consistently sterilize tumors and the optimal target volumes at risk of tumor involvement; these insights provide guidance for initial trials with the new conformal technologies. With the exception of cervix and prostate implants, brachytherapy is practiced in only a few specialized centers because implant techniques require special skills in the clinician and medical physicist. General application of brachytherapy is also hampered by results that are markedly user dependent.

Conventional radiation treatments are delivered through a small number of beams: typically one to four. With these techniques, dose is prescribed to a crudely shaped volume encompassing the target. When a small number of beams are used, each beam carries a significant fraction of the dose, and tissue damage occurs along the path of each beam. The rate of change in dose falloff at the edge of a treatment plan is known as the *dose gradient*. A *steep gradient* would indicate that the delivered dose decreases sharply at the edge of a treatment plan; conversely, a *shallow gradient* means that the dose gradually falls off over a significant distance. Conventional external-beam treatments have shallow gradients, often delivering substantial doses even several centimeters from the intended target.

In conformal treatments, a large number of precisely directed beams converge on a target so that no single beam carries much of the radiation dose. In this situation, very little damage is done to tissues as an individual beam traverses the body, but at the point where the beams intersect, a very high localized dose of radiation is delivered. By clever positioning and weighting of the beams, the high-dose region can be shaped to match the target lesion "like a glove." This can be accomplished in various ways, such as an array of fixed isocentric beams, rotational arcs, or multiple noncoplanar beams. Radiosurgery represents the extreme situation in which a very large number of beams are used to almost completely exclude normal tissues from the treatment volume so that a large ablative dose of radiation can be delivered in a single fraction.

Intensity-modulated radiotherapy (IMRT) is a simple concept. When a metal wedge is placed in the path of a radiation beam, it causes the intensity of the beam to vary from one area to another by attenuating the beam more where the metal is thicker and less where the metal is thinner; the metal wedge modulates the intensity of the beam across its profile. Varying the intensity across a beam profile can improve dose homogeneity, minimizing hot and cold spots when treating a part of the body that varies in thickness, such as the breast or neck. This simplest case is so trivial that the term IMRT would not be used to describe it, though the core principles are relevant.

More complex intensity modulation can be accomplished using a multi-leaf collimator, which consists of a number of parallel metal fingers positioned to move in and out of a treatment beam under computer control, producing intricate variations in a beam's intensity profile. With multiple-shaped intensity-modulated beams, dose can be shaped to fit targets that are highly irregular or even concave. For ESR, milled blocks or micromultileaf collimators are used to deliver high-resolution IMRT plans. Until quite recently, it was a quirk of U.S. billing codes that medically equivalent treatments were reimbursed at dramatically different rates depending on the treatment platform: GammaKnife radiosurgery versus LINAC radiosurgery. A similar artificial distinction is currently developing in proprietary claims for IMRT versus other forms of conformal radiation that deliver equivalent dose distributions by alternative methods of similar complexity. The financial ramifications of this debate will greatly affect the availability of ESR techniques in coming years.

Therapeutic proton beams have fundamentally different physical properties than photon beams and deposit energy in a pattern that is quite distinctive. Proton beams have a sharp peak in energy deposition at depth in tissue, which is followed by an abrupt drop. This exotic pattern can be exploited to deliver very high doses abutting critical structures. Unfortunately, proton machines are prohibitively expensive and only two facilities in the United States are able to treat deep sites within the body.

NORMAL TISSUE TOLERANCE

Because dose falloff at the edge of a radiosurgical treatment volume is not perfectly sharp, a few millimeters' separation between the target lesion and critical structures has been a typical requirement for consideration of radiosurgery in the brain. Due respect has been shown for structures such as the optic chiasm, brainstem, speech areas, and sensorimotor strip, where induced deficits would have an obvious deleterious impact; this appropriately conservative approach has resulted in a low incidence of complications, which obscures true dose-response relationships.

In moving radioablation to the body, common sense dictates that lesions in or near the spinal cord should be approached cautiously; additional structures within the body must also be treated with respect. For instance, the esophagus, trachea, bronchi, heart, and major vessels are all demonstrated sites of life-threatening late complications in the thorax.[17-32] Initial guidance can be obtained from the radiotherapy experience with radioactive implants (brachytherapy, BRT) and intraoperative electron beam radiotherapy (IORT), which treats with a single large fraction applied directly to the resection bed during surgery; however, the extrapolated tolerance doses for thoracic structures, and others in the peritoneal cavity and retroperitoneum, must be recognized as tentative in a setting where unprecedented large doses are being applied.

Perhaps the least defined aspect of tolerance concerns "volume effects." Radiation oncologists are used to evaluating plans with the aid of a dose-volume histogram (DVH), which plots the percentage of a structure that receives a given dose as a function of the dose. This is helpful in predicting results for organs with "parallel architecture," such as the liver or lung, where all portions of the organ function independently and redundantly; in a parallel organ the goal is to keep enough of the organ below a tolerance threshold that adequate function will be retained. Another subtlety is that the threshold dose is a moving target that is also understood as a function of volume—small volumes tolerate higher doses than large volumes do.

The DVH concept is less helpful in considering organs with "serial architecture" such as the spinal cord or esophagus, where damaging even a small segment may interrupt function of the whole. Serial organs are best evaluated in terms of doses to quantified volumes rather than as a percentage of the structure. In BRT, high localized doses are unavoidable near the radiation sources. Brachytherapy plans are scrutinized to assure that large confluent high-dose volumes do not occur in normal tissues; however, small "hot spots" in such plans are safely ignored. Reviewing plans with the mindset of BRT provides a sanity check on the intended treatment; in fact, radioablation seems a natural extension of the BRT experience and that literature is probably the most relevant to these new techniques.

BIOLOGICAL GRADIENTS

Even with sophisticated delivery and treatment planning systems, when a lesion is located in extensive contact with a critical structure, it may be impossible to achieve a physical dose gradient that adequately discriminates between the target and adjacent tissue. In these cases, the biological gradient can be improved by use of fractionation. When small doses of radiation are delivered to a tissue each day, significant repair has time to occur between doses, which reduces the cumulative damage; the amount of repair between fractions increases rapidly as the size of the daily dose is decreased.

As an illustrative example of how fractionation can help localize radiation effects, suppose that a 1.5 cm metastatic adenocarcinoma in the spine has epidural extension within 2 mm of the spinal cord. Based on historical results with similar tumors in the brain, a reasonable objective would be to deliver a minimum of 24 Gy in a single fraction to the entire tumor. A radiosurgical plan that has a high peaking dose inside the tumor and that covers the entire lesion with at least 24 Gy is developed; however, even with the best planning efforts, a portion of the spinal cord will still receive 14 Gy, which would exceed the nominal tolerance dose of 8 Gy in a single fraction. An unattractive option would be to reduce the dose to that portion of the tumor immediately adjacent to the cord, knowing that this will compromise the probability of durable tumor control; instead, fractionated schedules are explored as an alternate approach. The linear-quadratic model (LQ model) developed by Fowler can provide some guidance in comparing schedules but still requires skilled clinical judgment to apply safely.[33,34] If the total dose is divided over 5 days, then the daily cord dose falls from 14 Gy to 2.8 Gy. Calculations based on reasonable assumptions regarding tumor kinetics and rates of normal tissue repair reveal that the biologic impact on the cord would be reduced by approximately two thirds, though the physical dose delivered to the cord is still 14 Gy. For comparison, a common palliative regimen used "safely" for spinal cord compression is 20 Gy in 5 fractions of 4 Gy daily, demonstrating that the calculation is consistent with clinical experience. Because the daily doses to the tumor remain quite large, greater than or equal to 4.8 Gy each day, there is minimal reduction in efficacy for tumor control; if a larger number of fractions were required, then the total physical dose might have to be increased slightly to compensate for the protracted duration of the overall course.

TARGET DEFINITION

If treatments are tightly localized, then the gross target volume, which specifies the visualized lesion, must be drawn accurately to avoid geographic misses and collateral ablative damage to normal structures. This requires careful attention to imaging technique and consideration of fusing image sets obtained with complementary modalities: magnetic resonance imaging, computed tomography (CT), positron emission tomography, and angiography. At least one data set will be obtained with the target in the "treatment position." The clinical target volume, which incorporates areas at risk of occult microscopic extension, is typically addressed with external beam radiotherapy rather than being included in a radiosurgical target. In an ideal radiosurgical case, the gross target volume would be equivalent to the planning target volume (PTV), which includes a margin accounting for uncertainty in localization and tumor motion. The size of the PTV expansion is technique dependent and requires that the treatment team have a clear understanding of their system's limitations in targeting and dose calculations.

TREATMENT PLANNING

With the exception of isocentric "shot placement," treatment planning with large numbers of beams was not feasible before the advent of inexpensive high-performance computers capable of "inverse treatment planning." Traditional treatment planning proceeds *forward* in the sense that a human operator (dosimetrist, medical physicist, or clinician) designs a set of treatment fields that are all in one plane for geometric simplicity, then calculates the resultant dose distribution and makes small modifications as needed until an acceptable plan is generated. The forward approach has been carried to its practical limit with three-dimensional conformal radiotherapy (3DCRT). In 3DCRT, the target volume is delineated on an imaging study such as a CT or magnetic resonance imaging scan, then "beam's-eye views" are generated for up to 12 noncoplanar beams. In each beam's-eye view, shaping blocks are drawn to make the beam fit the tumor cross section as projected from that particular direction. As the name suggests, "inverse planning" proceeds in reverse order; the clinician supplies information about what the final plan should look like in terms of desired dose to the target and dose limitations for other structures, then software searches for a beam arrangement that would achieve the desired goals. Inverse planning is frequently compared to the method of image reconstruction using CT scanners; instead of interpreting CT beam data to generate an image, the desired "picture," in this case the requested dose distribution, is known and the beams to produce it are back-calculated.

A serious limitation of inverse treatment planning is determining when a plan is "good enough." Objective tools for quantitative comparison of plans are lacking; currently, such decisions are still based on the clinician's subjective interpretation. The calculations that have been used for many years in radiotherapy are only "adequate" for conventional techniques; radiation oncologists are trained to be skeptical of dose calculations where dissimilar tissues are abutting or where air cavities are present. In conformal treatments, the calculation algorithms must be more subtle, appropriately accounting for variations in tissue density and "second-order" physical effects that were beyond the computational scope of prior software. Sophisticated Monte Carlo calculation techniques developed by the national weapons laboratories are now appearing in treatment planning systems; the resulting "correct" dose calculations must be evaluated carefully by clinicians since the calculated values cannot be compared directly with historical experience. This represents a place where unintentional and potentially harmful "clinical trials" could occur.

The final point regarding physical dose is that in reaching a target, even a lightly weighted radiation beam must pass through tissue and deposit some energy along the path. This is a subtle cost of conformal treatments, that numerous low-dose beams may actually deposit a larger "integral dose," or total distributed dose, to the body than a small number of conventional beams. Distributing dose at low levels over large volumes of the body has raised concerns of induced malignancies in the future; this issue is of particular importance in pediatric patients. Caution must also be used to avoid "dose dumping" into particularly sensitive tissues such as the lungs, where a widely distributed low dose of radiation may have functional consequences.

IMMOBILIZATION TECHNIQUES

Effective and safe administration of conformal plans requires precise knowledge of target position throughout the duration of radiation delivery; for the high doses used in radiosurgery or hypofractionated radioablation, each treatment session may last an hour or more. Targets in the brain can be localized in space by means of a stereotactic frame bolted to the outer table of the skull. The frame establishes a reference coordinate system that is consistent throughout the imaging scans, planning, and treatment. During a radiosurgical procedure, the frame is fixed to the treatment couch, rigidly immobilizing the head. Since the planning images and treatment must both occur while the frame is in place, fractionated treatments become impractical because the patient must either wear the frame for an extended period or go through the entire procedure of frame placement, imaging, and planning for each fraction delivered. Devices that clamp firmly to external bony structures of the head exist. They allow repeated sessions of imaging and treatment but have not gained wide acceptance.[35] Image-guided strategies have also been employed for reproducible positioning and to obviate the need for rigid immobilization; these systems find use in the brain and at extracranial sites.

For extracranial IMRT treatments, the Cleveland Clinic has used an Aquaplast mold encompassing approximately one third of the patient's body centered on the treatment site (Fig. 74-1). The mold locks down to the edges of the treatment table and also snaps down to the table between the patient's legs. Alignment tattoos are placed on the patient's skin where they can be visualized through holes punched in the immobilization device. This arrangement has been used to deliver conventional or hypofractionated schedules of radiation to well-defined targets within the vertebral bodies or spinal canal at all levels of the spine: cervical, thoracic, lumbar, and sacral. Particularly in the thoracic region, it is important to restrict this technique to relatively thin patients. With a snugly fitting body mold, respiratory motions are

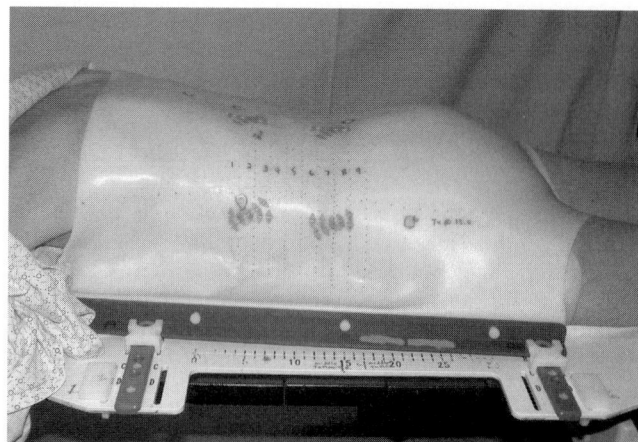

Figure 74–1. Aquaplast body mold for extracranial stereotactic radioablation. The mold attaches rigidly to the CT table and treatment couch. Tattoos are visualized through holes punched in the mold. Setup marks are drawn on the mold to facilitate setup. (Photo courtesy of Gayle Harnisch, Cleveland Clinic Foundation.)

directed primarily toward the diaphragm and have not hampered accurate delivery of conservatively designed treatment plans. When the Cleveland Clinic applied the same immobilization strategy to spinal radiosurgery with the CyberKnife, position confirmation of fiducials in the lumbar spine taken at approximately 1-minute intervals during two treatments showed anatomic displacements that were consistently less than 2 mm.

A group at the University of Heidelberg described a more elaborate noninvasive fixation device for extracranial stereotactic radiotherapy.[36-40] In their system a body cast/head mask combination enclosed the head and extended to the mid-thigh level. During treatments, the body cast was rigidly attached to a stereotactic body frame. Based on five patients treated to sites in the thoracic and lumbar spine, they estimated that the overall accuracy "can be safely estimated to be less than or equal to 3.6 mm." In their most recent update on a series of patients treated for metastatic or primary disease in the liver, they described treatment of 60 lesions using single fractions of 14 to 26 Gy maximum dose with the 80% isodose line (IDL) encompassing the target lesion. Their patients experienced no major side effects. In patients treated subsequent to their dose-escalation phase, the Heidelberg group reported 81% lesion control at 18 months.

The Heidelberg group has also reported its experience treating stage I non–small cell lung cancer.[41] The first five patients were treated using jet ventilation to completely immobilize the lung. Patients were treated with single fractions from 19 to 26 Gy. In 10 patients followed to a median of 14.9 months, they observed 89% local control at 1 year and 71% at 2 years without significant toxicity. Actuarial overall survival was 64% at 2 years.

At the University of Arizona, an attempt was made to circumvent anatomic flexibility and internal motions by using an invasive technique to immobilize a segment of the spine for radiosurgery.[42,43] This approach involved surgically exposing the spinous processes of vertebral bodies immediately above and below the target level, which are then clamped to a rigid external frame. From phantom measurements, a localization accuracy of 1.4 mm was reported.

The group at Karolinska Hospital in Stockholm implemented a stereotactic body frame consisting of a wooden box lined with a form-fitting vacuum bag (Fig. 74-2).[44-46] Serial scans obtained over several days demonstrated that most tumors could be repositioned within 5 to 8 mm during a hypofractionated course of treatment. In their technique, gentle upward pressure is applied to the abdomen with the effect of reducing tumor motion. They report that most tumors in the lung and liver can be restricted to displacements of 5 to 10 mm in the craniocaudal direction and 5 mm in the axial plane. Their PTV takes the motion into account with an expansion of 1 cm in the craniocaudal direction and 5 mm radially; they suggest that this delivers the minimum target dose to the entire tumor in approximately 90% of cases. A commercial version of their device, Stereotactic Body Frame (Elekta Oncology, Norcross, Ga.), has found use at numerous institutions.

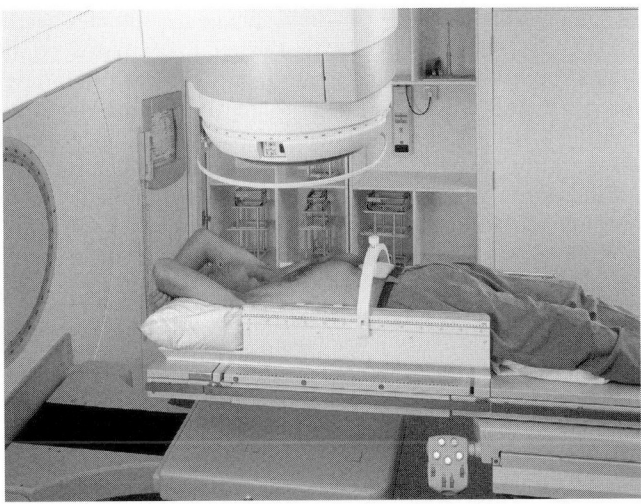

Figure 74–2. Commercially available Stereotactic Body Frame, which consists of a form-fitting vacuum bag, box with Cartesian reference system, and abdominal compression paddle to limit excursions of the diaphragm. (Photo courtesy of Elekta Oncology, Inc.)

In a published report, the Karolinska group described its early results with 31 patients who had lesions in the liver, lung, or retroperitoneum. Daily doses from 7.7 to 30 Gy were delivered in total courses, reaching 8 to 66 Gy in 1 to 4 fractions. They indicated that 50% of the lesions decreased in size or disappeared. Current treatments at Karolinska are typically delivered with 5 to 10 beams prescribed to the 65% IDL, covering the planned target volume as described earlier. Schedules have evolved from a single fraction initially to hypofractionated courses with 45 Gy in 3 fractions delivered every other day as their typical schedule now. At a conference in 2002, Dr. Lax reported that the Karolinska series had grown to include 1540 treated tumors: 48% lung, 27% liver, 9% pancreas, and 16% other.[47]

At the Indiana University School of Medicine, a phase I study of ESR has been completed for selected adult patients with biopsy-proven non–small cell lung cancer American Joint Committee on Cancer stage I (T1/2N0) with tumors up to 7 cm in greatest dimension, and Karnofsky performance status (KPS) greater than or equal to 60.[48] Eligible patients were medically inoperable but had tumors that were otherwise technically resectable for cure—as determined by a thoracic surgeon and standard pulmonary function guidelines. Patients who refused surgery were not eligible for protocol treatment.

Patients were immobilized with the commercially available Stereotactic Body Frame described earlier. Repositioning was accomplished by aligning two tattoo marks on the sternum and bilateral tibial tattoo marks with the body frame. Planning was based on contrast-enhanced CT of the chest and upper abdomen, which was obtained in the body frame. The gross target volume was defined as solid tumor plus ground glass density on lung windows, and the clinical target volume was identical to the gross target volume. The PTV included a 0.5 cm axial expansion and 1 cm expansions in the craniocaudal directions. Seven noncoplanar, nonopposing beams were used, with each delivering an approximately equal portion of the total dose. Beam trajectories were arranged to avoid delivering more than 6 Gy to any point in the spinal cord in a single treatment. Forward-planning intensity modulation was used to create a parabolic dose profile across each beam with the effect of increasing dose to the central region of the tumor; the intensity modulation was accomplished by using milled beam attenuation compensators. Shaping focus blocks cut for each beam also contributed to conformality. The average duration of each treatment session was 45 minutes.

Prescriptions covered at least 95% of the PTV with the 80% IDL. The starting dose was 24 Gy divided into three fractions of 8 Gy delivered with minimum separation between fractions of 2 days, and a maximum of 8 days. According to study design, the dose was escalated in 6 Gy increments (2 Gy per fraction), until the maximum tolerated dose was established. At the 14 Gy per fraction level, a decision was made to escalate doses separately for patients with tumors less than or equal to 3 cm versus greater than 3 cm in greatest dimension: separate cohorts for T1 and T2 tumors. Tumor response was considered complete if all anatomic abnormalities related to the tumor disappeared, and partial if the maximum dimension decreased by at least 50%. Tumor progression was recorded if soft-tissue abnormalities increased on serial CT scans with a spatially correlated abnormality on positron emission tomography scan.

All 37 patients enrolled on the protocol received all intended radiation. Abdominal compression caused chest wall tenderness, which was managed with over-the-counter analgesics. The investigators observed fatigue in every patient. Six patients had worsened breathing and nonproductive coughing. There were no statistically significant declines in pulmonary function tests. Localized fibrotic changes occurred in twenty-five patients. No esophageal toxicity was observed. One patient developed an asymptomatic pericardial effusion demonstrated on follow-up CT scan. One T1 patient treated at 16 Gy per fraction developed transient grade 3 hypoxemia; one T2 patient treated at 14 Gy per fraction required hospitalization for symptomatic pneumonitis. Dose escalation proceeded until the investigators ended the trial at 60 Gy total dose: 20 Gy per fraction. Maximum tolerated dose was never reached for either T-stage cohort. Local fibrosis could obscure tumor response, and in cases where those changes could not be distinguished from residual tumor, the response was scored as incomplete; with this conservative interpretation, partial and complete responses were 60% and 27%, respectively. Local recurrences have been observed more frequently in patients treated in the lower-dose cohorts, and local control has been better in the T1 cohort.

Since 1997, ESR has been offered at the University of Wurzburg for treatment of lung and liver tumors.[49,50] Their term for this type of treatment is *extracranial stereotactic radiotherapy* (ESRT). They report their results treating 39 patients: 21 patients with 22 targets in the lung, 17 patients with 21 targets in the liver. They also use the Stereotactic Body Frame for immobilization. The clinical target volume consisted of the macroscopic tumor with margins of 2 to 3 mm. Contrast-enhanced treatment planning CT scans were obtained in the body frame.

Pulmonary tumors were segmented using lung windows; hepatic lesions were segmented in arterial or portal venous phases, or both. Breathing control via diaphragm compression was used only if target mobility, determined by repeated slices on dynamic CT scan with intervals of 2 seconds, was larger than 5 mm in any direction as a result of diaphragm movements. The planned target volume was created by expanding the clinical target volume 5 mm axially and 5 to 10 mm longitudinally. In cases where the patient did not tolerate compression, maximal tumor excursions were measured and the PTV was enlarged accordingly. Breathing control was used for all liver treatments, and 8/22 lung treatments—when tumors were located in the lower lobes. Five to nine static fields or rotational fields, or both, were delivered with a multi-leaf collimator (10 mm leaf width). Before each fraction, a CT scan was repeated through the target volume and a longitudinal offset correction was calculated for use on that day; no transverse corrections were applied.[51] Prescriptions were 30 Gy in three fractions of 10 Gy to a 65% IDL encompassing the planning target volume.

A group using the Stereotactic Body Frame at the University of Kyoto has reported its initial experience with 40 patients undergoing pulmonary radioablation: 31 with primary lung cancer and 9 with metastatic lesions.[52,53] Respiratory motions were regulated if they were more than 8 mm in the craniocaudal direction. They delivered a hypofractionated course of 40 to 48 Gy in 4 fractions over approximately 2 weeks. Treatments consisted of either 6 to 10 noncoplanar static fields or 7 dynamic arcs. For 33 tumors evaluable beyond 6 months, they observed a 94% rate of local response defined as at least a 30% decrease in volume, and an 18% complete response rate. They saw nothing more than National Cancer Institute Common Toxicity grade 2 reactions.

IMAGE-GUIDED APPROACHES

A frameless image-guided system, Novalis Body, is marketed for reproducible positioning (Fig. 74-3). In this technique, the patient is immobilized with a vacuum bag or alternate device, then a CT scan is obtained in the treatment position with infrared reflective markers placed on the patient's skin. Novalis Body consists of two infrared cameras and a computerized control system, which detect the skin markers and move the treatment couch to a preplanned reference position. Novalis Body then compares diagnostic x-rays obtained in the treatment room with a digitally reconstructed library of images based on the planning CT and further refines the patient positioning before treatment. This image-guided system has been used to deliver gated ablative treatments as described in the next section.

The noninvasive CyberKnife radiosurgical platform is available at a small number of sites in the United States and Japan (Fig. 74-4). The CyberKnife consists of a robotic manipulator wielding a compact linear accelerator. As with other radiosurgical platforms, numerous convergent beams are used to produce a highly conformal dose distribution. Before delivery of each beam, a pair of

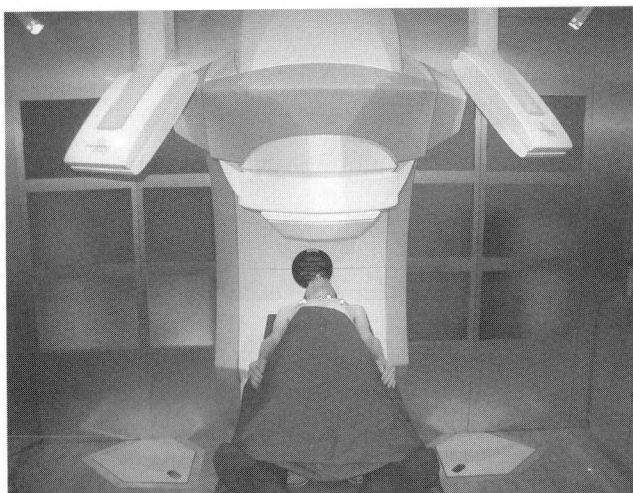

Figure 74–3. Novalis Body system for automated reproducible positioning. Two diagnostic x-ray units are embedded in the floor with ceiling-mounted amorphous silicon imaging panels. Infrared cameras (not shown) are used to track the passive reflective markers visible on the patient's chest. (Photo courtesy of Novalis, Inc.)

orthogonal diagnostic radiographs are obtained. From these stereoscopic views, the current location of the target can be deduced rapidly and precisely; this is accomplished by triangulation from implanted metal fiducials or directly from image correlations based on skeletal anatomy. The robotic manipulator adjusts the position of the radiation source to produce idealized geometry that conforms to the original treatment plan.

Stanford University published initial results treating spinal lesions with the CyberKnife.[54-56] They described 16 patients treated with doses of 11 to 25 Gy delivered in 1 to 5 fractions. No acute toxicity was reported. The paper from Stanford indicates "alignment of the treatment dose with the target volume within ±1 mm."

The University of Pittsburgh has published a series of 56 spinal lesions in 46 patients treated with the

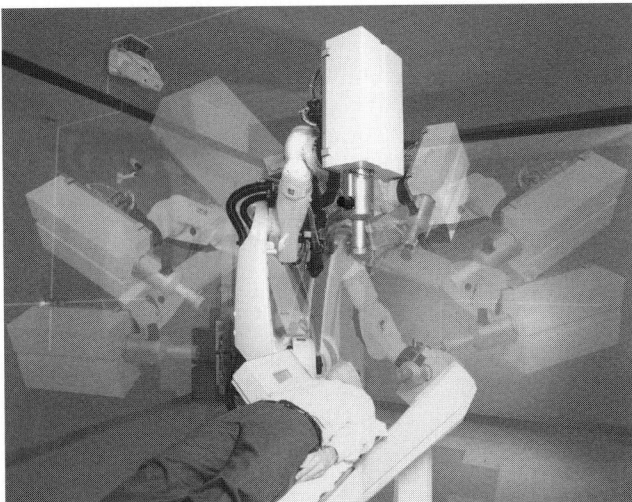

Figure 74–4. Accuray CyberKnife displaying flexibility of the robotic arm wielding a compact linear accelerator, one of the two ceiling-mounted diagnostic x-ray sources, amorphous silicon imaging pedestals beside the patient, and the in-room laser system for initial crude positioning. (Photo courtesy of Accuray, Inc.)

CyberKnife.[54] Thirty-one of their patients had received conventional external beam radiotherapy previously. Prescriptions consisted of a single fraction of 12 to 18 Gy prescribed to the 80% IDL. They reported symptomatic improvement in all patients who were symptomatic before treatment, had no new neurologic deficits, and had no acute toxicity. They have continued an active program treating spinal lesions and recently treated their 100th patient.[55]

A team at the National Defence Medical College in Japan has developed a CT-guided frameless technique for stereotactic radiotherapy.[56-59] Their approach places a LINAC, a CT scanner, and a fluoroscopic x-ray simulator in a single room with a shared treatment couch that can be rotated into alignment with any one of the component machines. They have used this composite system to treat tumors in the lung and liver with noncoplanar arcs. During the procedure, patients are provided with supplemental oxygen and instructed to breathe shallowly. If the tumor motions still exceed 1 cm, then a restraining abdominal belt is applied. Treatment planning is based on slowly acquired CT scans (4 seconds per slice) that intentionally blur the images to create a more complete representation of the tumor without the paradoxical images that can be induced by partial-volume effects. Their PTV consists of the imaged lesion with a 5 to 10 mm expansion. The couch is then shifted to the fluoroscopic simulation unit, where tumor displacements are confirmed to be less than 1 cm, and the centroid of the tumor is determined visually; lateral and horizontal fiducials are placed to indicate the tumor's center and then the couch is returned to the CT scanner for verification. After confirming, follow-up was 36 months. Twenty-one of their patients were medically inoperable and the remainder had refused surgery. Treatment was typically 50 to 60 Gy in 5 to 10 fractions delivered over 1 to 2 weeks. Eighteen of the patients received conventional external beam treatments as well. They report local control of disease in 94%, and 3-year overall survival was 66% for the entire group, but 86% in the operable patients. Two patients who had bones encompassed by the 80% IDL developed fractures, which subsequently healed.

Nakagawa et al. at the University of Tokyo have developed a megavoltage CT scanner for precise patient positioning and real-time delivery verification for radiosurgery in the lung.[60-62] Patients were selected to have "calm respirations," and patients with poor pulmonary function were excluded. They treated 22 tumors in 15 patients; 10 tumors were in the chest wall or pleura, 12 tumors were in the lung parenchyma. Patients were instructed to maintain shallow respiration and two patients with tumor motion exceeding 1 cm were given an oxygen mask and were confined with a chest/abdomen belt to restrain respiratory excursions. Tumor motions were assessed under fluoroscopy for each patient, but the authors generalize that their typical PTV consisted of the target plus 5 to 10 mm transversely plus 10-15 mm in the craniocaudal direction. Static multiport conformal radiotherapy was used to treat 9/10 chest wall and pleural tumors. Rotational arcs with the dynamic multi-leaf were used to treat 11/12 parenchymal lesions. Tumor volumes were larger for the chest wall lesions, reflecting the decreased amount of lung tissue encompassed at those locations: median 40 cc for chest wall and 4.5 cc for pulmonary lesions. Peripheral doses were 20 to 25 Gy but the IDL is not stated. Total treatment time was approximately 40 minutes. Among 21 evaluable tumors representing a wide variety of metastatic histologies, they observed 13 complete responses and 6 partial responses. Pulmonary fibrosis was minimal and localized to the site of treatment.

GATING TECHNIQUES

An alternate method of localizing dose to a moving target is to switch the beam on at times when the tumor would be passing through the treatment field, and off when it is elsewhere.[63-66] One limitation of this approach is wasted time when the beam is off because the tumor is outside the treatment field; the fraction of the time that dose is actually being delivered is known as the *duty cycle*. If the beam were on 30% of the time, the duty cycle would be 0.3. At William Beaumont Hospital, a device for "active breathing coordination" has been developed to increase treatment efficiency.[67] This valve mechanism and monitoring computer can repetitively pause respiration at a predetermined point in the breathing cycle and trigger the LINAC on or off in a coordinated way. The Active Breathing Coordinator is commercially available for this purpose (Elekta Oncology).

In collaboration with Mitsubishi Electronics, Hokkaido University has developed a gating technique that synchronizes LINAC output with continuous fluoroscopic visualization of a gold fiducial implanted in lung tumors.[68] As an early step in treatment planning, they obtain multiple CT scans of the chest and investigate the tumor's relationship to other anatomic structures during various phases of respiration. They determine an optimal portion of the respiratory cycle that will maximize target dose and minimize dose to any critical structures in the vicinity; the treatment isocenter is positioned where the tumor will be located at that favorable point in the respiratory cycle; they refer to this technique as *four-dimensional treatment planning*. The beam is gated on 10% to 30% of the time, when the fiducial is within a few millimeters of the beam isocenter. They report that their system determines fiducial position within 1 mm and that the LINAC can be gated on or off within 0.03 seconds. They report treating 14 patients with "a tight PT." Tumors were located in the liver, lung, bladder, prostate, rectum, and spinal cord. At 6-month follow-up, no tumor had progressed and no complications were observed.

The radiosurgery program at Henry Ford Hospital in Detroit has reported initial results treating 10 patients with metastatic lesions in the spine.[54-56] They initially treated spinal lesions with 25 Gy external beam radiotherapy in 10 fractions to a field covering one or two involved vertebral levels plus two additional vertebral levels above and below. They then delivered a single-fraction 6 to 8 Gy radiosurgical boost restricted to the gross lesion. Radiosurgical prescriptions were to the 80% IDL. Their approach used the Novalis IMRT radiosurgery system, which employs micro–multi-leaf collimators on a Varian 6 MVX linear accelerator. They used the passive infrared positioning system, Novalis ExacTrac, to automate initial patient alignment and Novalis Body for precise image-guided target localization. With this system, the accuracy of isocenter positioning was measured at 1.36 ± 0.11 mm. They reported prompt pain relief in the majority of patients and complete or partial recovery of motor deficits in the patients who had cord compression. They observed no acute radiation toxicity with a mean follow-up of 6 months.

Dr. Whyte at Stanford has used the CyberKnife to perform gated radiosurgery in the lung. His protocol was offered to adult patients with biopsy-proven non–small cell lung cancer or metastatic disease in the lungs from a biopsy-proven primary tumor, who were medically inoperable or refused surgery. Tumors could be up to 5 cm in greatest dimension at the time of enrollment. The trial was a phase I dose escalation study beginning at 15 Gy in a single fraction delivered to the 50% IDL covering at least 95% of the tumor. At Stanford, nine patients were treated using this technique; an additional 18 patients were treated on this protocol at the Cleveland Clinic using dynamic tracking as described in the next section. Their approach used respiratory gating in which the patient repeatedly held their breath while the treatment beam was on, then the beam was stopped when the patient took a breath and restarted when they had recovered sufficiently to hold their breath again. Treatment was delivered in "bursts" that lasted approximately 20 seconds. Targeting was based on gold seed fiducials measuring 1×3 mm, which were placed into the tumor percutaneously. For the overall series at both institutions, radiographic response was complete in 2 patients, partial in 15, stable in 4, and progressive in 2. The only complications observed were related to pneumothoraces induced at the time of fiducial placement.

DYNAMIC TRACKING

At the Cleveland Clinic, a modified version of the CyberKnife has been used to deliver an ablative radiosurgical dose to moving lung tumors during relaxed breathing. In the complicated radiographic environment of the chest, where many structures are moving and a soft tissue tumor is not dissimilar to the other tissues present, there was no expectation that software would be able to quickly identify the target lesion (Fig. 74-5). For this reason, a small gold pellet (fiducial marker) was implanted into the tumor so that it would stand out distinctly in images. The gold fiducial was a cylinder measuring 4 mm in length and 0.5 mm in diameter. Fiducials were placed by a method of "inverse biopsy" in which a diagnostic radiologist passed a 16-gauge needle through the chest wall under CT guidance and penetrated the tumor at a location that was not necrotic. Several patients developed a clinically insignificant pneumothorax from this procedure, as would be expected based on experience with stereotactic biopsy of lung tumors.

A few days later, a foam alpha cradle was made, and positioning references were drawn on the cradle and the patient to facilitate reproducible positioning between the planning CT and treatment. The alpha cradle was not formed in a way that would inhibit respiratory motion.

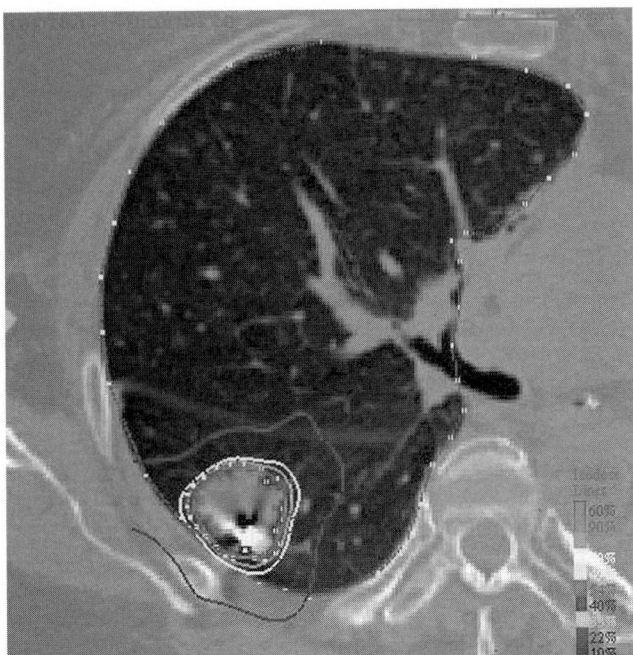

Figure 74–5. Radiosurgical dose distribution delivered using the CyberKnife with dynamic target tracking. *Red* outlines the gross target volume. *Yellow* is the prescription isodose line (IDL): 20 Gy in a single fraction at 49% IDL. *Blue* is the envelope that received 6 Gy or greater. Artifacts from the implanted gold fiducial are apparent. (Photo courtesy of Raymond Rodebaugh, Cleveland Clinic Foundation.) See also Color Figure 74-5.

Patients were positioned either prone or supine depending on the location of their tumor. Each patient was observed under fluoroscopy in the alpha cradle so that target motion could be understood. If a high-frequency component of motion was identified, such as might be induced by proximity to the heart, then the PTV was slightly expanded in the direction of that motion, acknowledging the fact that cardiac effects were independent of the respiratory motions. The patient underwent a breath-hold CT scan in the alpha cradle using a multi-slice spiral CT. Because beams entered from a wide variety of oblique angles, it was necessary to scan from approximately the umbilicus to the nose.

Once the imaging studies had been transferred to the treatment planning computer, the patient surface was automatically segmented from the environment. The lungs, target lesion, and sensitive structures in proximity to the target were manually contoured. Planning proceeded inversely based on goals specifying dose to the tumor and dose limits for normal tissues. An acceptable plan, depending on which level in the dose-escalation schedule had been achieved, would deliver either 15 or 20 Gy to the 50% IDL, covering at least 95% of the target lesion.

Before treatment, five infrared light-emitting diodes (LEDs) were taped to the chest and abdomen. LEDs were positioned in locations that demonstrated maximal motion during the respiratory cycle and in locations that captured independent information; for instance, one LED might rise and fall as the patient breathed, while another might be displaced laterally by expansion of the chest wall. After a brief period of observation, the most informative LEDs were selected for monitoring during treatment.

On the day of treatment, the patient was positioned in the alpha cradle and located with the tumor approximately centered at an ideal position for treatment delivery. The robot was capable of treating the tumor as long as it remained within 5 cm of the starting location. While the external LEDs were being monitored continuously, several orthogonal x-ray pairs were obtained and a correlation model developed that predicted where the tumor would be located given a particular constellation of LED positions. In acquiring the radiographs, an attempt was made to sample various portions of the respiratory cycle, with the goal of making the majority of the model an interpolation from the data points, rather than extrapolation from a few clustered observations. It typically required four or five x-ray pairs to establish the model. When the model appeared stable as determined by a few additional radiographs confirming that the tumor was observed at the predicted location, then treatment was initiated.

Robot targeting was driven by predictions from the model. The LEDs were monitored continuously. Based on their positions, the position of the tumor 0.8 seconds in the future was predicted; this lead time, which is long relative to the respiratory cycle, was necessary due to engineering constraints on the robot response time. Further development of this technique will be greatly facilitated by introduction of a more rapidly responsive treatment platform. Approximately once each minute, a pair of radiographs were obtained and tumor location was compared with the predicted location. If the offset in the tumor position was within 5 mm of the prediction, treatment continued without interruption. If at any time the tumor was observed to be displaced by more than 5 mm from the prediction, then a software interlock interrupted treatment on the presumption that the correlation model was no longer valid. Examples of situations where this might occur would be a patient moving an arm or a leg, or coughing, with resultant shift of the LED positions on the body surface. In these instances, the model would be rebuilt and treatment resumed. The treatment times ranged from slightly more than 2 hours to more than 8 hours for a patient treated to several targets in one session. Most patients with multiple tumors were treated on separate days in recognition of the lengthy time of this procedure. The treatment time can be justified by comparison with fractionated courses delivered over several weeks, particularly when daily travel time is considered. There is no fundamental reason why treatment times cannot be shortened by the introduction of higher output sources and more responsive robotics. It should be emphasized that patients treated with this technique were allowed to breathe comfortably, and often they slept through the procedure. This technique is now also available at Osaka University in Japan, where it has been applied in treatment of hepatic lesions (H. Shiomi, personal communication).

At the Cleveland Clinic a series of 35-kg pigs have been treated with extra-cranial radiosurgery targeted to the kidney.[57] A gold pellet was implanted percutaneously and the animal was maintained under general anesthesia during radiosurgery using the CyberKnife. Over the course of a year, doses were escalated from 24 to 40 Gy with the

50% IDL defining a 2 cm diameter volume. Animals were sacrificed at 4, 6, and 8 weeks for pathologic examination of the kidneys. Tightly localized fibrosis with well-demarcated sparing of adjacent tissues was observed, with progression to complete fibrosis by 8 weeks. Clinical trials are planned to follow up on this encouraging feasibility study.

REFERENCES

1. Blomgren H, Lax I, Naslund I, et al: Stereotactic high dose fraction radiation therapy of extracranial tumors using an accelerator. *Acta Oncologica*. 1995;34:861.
2. Blomgren H, Lax I, Goranson H, et al: Radiosurgery for tumors in the body: Clinical experience using a new method. *J Radiosurgery*. 1998;1:63.
3. Crownover RL, Rodebaugh R, Weinhous MS, et al: Dynamic radiosurgery by tracking moving lung tumors during relaxed breathing. *Int J Radiat Oncol Biol Phys*. 2002;54S:194.
4. Crownover RL, Rodebaugh R, Weinhous MS, et al: First report of dynamic radiosurgery to primary and metastatic lung tumors using an image-guided robotic delivery platform (Submitted to *Cancer*, 2003).
5. Uematsu M, Shioda A, Suda A, et al: Computed tomography–guided frameless stereotactic radiotherapy for stage I non–small cell lung cancer: A 5-year experience. *Int J Radiat Oncol Biol Phys*. 2001;51:666.
6. Wulf J, Hadinger U, Oppitz U, et al: Stereotactic radiotherapy of targets in the lung and liver. *Strahlentherapy Onkol*. 2001;177:645.
7. Takai Y, Mituya M, Nemoto K, et al: Simple method of stereotactic radiotherapy without stereotactic body frame for extracranial tumors. *Nippon Igaku Hoshasen Gakkai Zasshi*. 2001;61:403.
8. Hara R, Itami J, Kondo T, et al: Stereotactic single high dose irradiation of lung tumors under respiratory gating. *Radiother Oncol*. 2002;63:159.
9. Nagata Y, Yoshiharu N, Tetsuya A, et al: Clinical outcomes of 3D conformal hypofractionated single high-dose radiotherapy for one or two lung tumors using a stereotactic body frame. *Int J Radiat Oncol Biol Phys*. 2002;52:1041.
10. Hara R, Itami J, Kondo T, et al: Stereotactic single high dose irradiation of lung tumors under respiratory gating. *Radiother Oncol*. 2002;63:159.
11. Gerstzen PC, Ozhasoglu C, Burton SA, et al: Feasibility of frameless single-fraction stereotactic radiosurgery of spinal lesions. *Neurosurg Focus*. 2002;13:1.
12. Ryu SI, Chang SD, Kim DH, et al: Image-guided hypo-fractionated stereotactic radiosurgery to spinal lesions. *Neurosurgery*. 2000;49:838.
13. Ryu S, Yin FF, Rock J, et al: Image-guided and intensity-modulated radiosurgery for spinal metastasis. *Cancer*. 2003;97:2013.
14. Wulf J, Hadinger U, Oppitz U, et al: Stereotactic radiotherapy of targets in the lung and liver. *Strahlentherapy Onkol*. 2001;177:645.
15. Hamilton AJ, Lulu BA, Fosmire H, et al: Preliminary clinical experience with linear accelerator-based spinal stereotactic radiosurgery. *Neurosurgery*. 1995;36:311.
16. Whyte RI, Crownover R, Murphy MJ, et al: Stereotactic radiosurgery for lung tumors—Preliminary report of a phase I trial. *Ann Thorac Surg*. 2003;75:1097.
17. de Boer WJ, Mehta DM, Timens W, et al: The short and long term effects of intraoperative electron beam radiotherapy (IORT) on thoracic organs after pneumonectomy an experimental study in the canine model. *Int J Radiat Oncol Biol Phys*. 1999;45:501.
18. Abe M, Yabumoto E, Nishidai T, et al: Trials of new forms of radiotherapy for locally advanced bronchogenic carcinoma. *Strahlentherapie*. 1977;159:149.
19. Arian-Schad KS, Juettner FM, Ratzenhofer B, et al: Intraoperative plus external beam irradiation in nonresectable lung cancer: Assessment of local response and therapy-related side effects. *Radiother Oncol*. 1990;19:137.
20. Arimoto T, Takamura A, Tomita M, et al: Intraoperative radiotherapy for esophageal carcinoma—Significance of IORT dose for the incidence of fatal tracheal complications. *Int J Radiat Oncol Biol Phys*. 1993;27:1063.
21. Barnes M, Pass H, DeLuca A, et al: Response of the mediastinal and thoracic viscera of the dog to intraoperative radiation therapy (IORT). *Int J Radiat Oncol Biol Phys*. 1987;13:371.
22. Calvo FA, Ortiz De Urbina D, Abuchaibe O, et al: Intraoperative radiotherapy during lung cancer surgery: Technical description and early clinical results. *Int J Radiat Oncol Biol Phys*. 1990;9:103.
23. Cromack DT, Maher MM, Hoekstra H, et al: Are complications in intraoperative radiation therapy more frequent than in conventional treatment? *Arch Surg*. 1989;124:229.
24. Gaspar LE: Brachytherapy in lung cancer. *J Surg Oncol*. 1998;67:60.
25. Hoekstra HJ, Sindelar WF, Kinsella TJ, et al: History, preliminary results, complications, and future prospects of intraoperative radiotherapy. *J Surg Oncol*. 1987;36:175.
26. Juettner FM, Arian-Schad K, Porsch G, et al: Intraoperative radiation therapy combined with external irradiation in nonresectable non–small cell lung cancer: Preliminary report. *Int J Radiat Oncol Biol Phys*. 1990;18:1143.
27. Pass HI, Sindelar WF, Kinsella TJ, et al: Delivery of intraoperative radiation therapy after pneumonectomy: Experimental observations and early clinical results. *Ann Thor Surg*. 1987;44:14.
28. Raben A, Mychalczak B: Brachytherapy for non–small cell lung cancer and selected neoplasms of the chest. *Chest*. 1997;112 (suppl 4):276.
29. Schneidrzik WEJ: Intrathoracic irradiation of the hilum after resection of bronchial carcinoma. *J Thor Surg*. 1953;25:327.
30. Sindelar WF, Tepper JE, Kinsella TJ, et al: Pathological tissue changes following intraoperative radiotherapy. *Am J Clin Oncol*. 1986;6:504.
31. Smolle-Juettner FM, Geyer E, Kapp KS, et al: Evaluating intraoperative radiation therapy (IORT) and external beam radiation therapy (EBRT) in non–small cell lung cancer (NSCLC). Five years experience. *Eur J Cardiothorac Surg*. 1994;8:511.
32. Tochner ZA, Pass HI, Sindelar WF, et al: Long term tolerance of thoracic organs to intraoperative radiotherapy. *Int J Radiat Oncol Biol Phys*. 1992;22:65.
33. Fowler JF: The linear-quadratic formula and progress in fractionated radiotherapy—A review. *Br J Radiol*. 1989;62:679.
34. Jones B, Dale RG, Deehan C, et al: The role of biologically effective dose (BED) in clinical oncology. *Clin Oncol*. 2001;13:71.
35. Kalapurakal JA, Ilahi Z, Kepka AG, et al: Repositioning accuracy with the Laitinen frame for fractionated stereotactic radiation therapy in adult and pediatric brain tumors: Preliminary report. *Radiology*. 2001;218:157.
36. Herfarth KK, Debus J, Lohr F, et al: Extracranial stereotactic conformal radiation treatment of tumors in the liver and the lung. *Int J Radiat Oncol Biol Phys*. 1998;42S:214.
37. Lohr F, Debus J, Frank C, et al: Noninvasive patient fixation for extracranial stereotactic radiotherapy. *Int J Radiat Oncol Biol Phys*. 1999;45:521.
38. Herfarth KK, Debus J, Lohr F, et al: Stereotactic single-dose radiation therapy of liver tumors: Results of a phase I/II trial. *J Clin Oncol*. 2001;19:164.
39. Herfarth KK, Debus J, Lohr F, et al: Extracranial stereotactic radiation therapy: Set-up accuracy of patients treated for liver metastases. *Int J Radiat Oncol Biol Phys*. 2000;46:329.
40. Hof H, Herfarth KK, Munter M, et al: Stereotactic single-dose radiotherapy of stage I non–small-cell lung cancer (NSCLC). *Int J Radiat Oncol Biol Phys*. 2003;56:335.
41. Hof H, Herfarth KK, Munter M, et al: Stereotactic single-dose radiotherapy of stage I non–small-cell lung cancer (NSCLC). *Int J Radiat Oncol Biol Phys*. 2003;56:335.
42. Hamilton AJ, Lulu BA, Fosmire H, et al: LINAC-based spinal stereotactic radiosurgery. *Stereotact Funct Neurosurg*. 1996;66:1.
43. Takacs I, Hamilton AJ: Extracranial stereotactic radiosurgery. *Neurosurg Clin N Am*. 1999;10:257.
44. Lax I: Target dose versus extra-target dose in stereotactic radiosurgery. *Acta Oncol*. 1993;32:453.
45. Lax I, Blomgren H, Naslund I, et al: Stereotactic radiotherapy of malignancies in the abdomen. *Acta Oncologica*. 1994;33:677.
46. Lax I, Blomgren H, Naslund I, et al: Extracranial stereotactic radiosurgery of localized targets. *J Radiosurgery*. 1998;1:135.
47. Lax I: Extracranial stereotactic radioablation: Future directions. *Niagara Ontario*. 2002;May.
48. Timmerman R, Papiez L, McGarry R, et al: Extracranial stereotactic radioablation: Results of a phase I study in medically inoperable stage I non–small cell lung cancer. *Chest*, 2003;124:1946.

49. Wulf J, Hadinger U, Oppitz U, et al: Stereotactic radiotherapy of extracranial targets: CT-simulation and accuracy of treatment in the stereotactic body frame. *Radiother Oncol.* 2000;57:225.

50. Wulf J, Hadinger U, Oppitz U, et al: Impact of target reproducibility on tumor dose in stereotactic radiotherapy of targets in the lung and liver. *Radiother Oncol.* 2003;66:141.

51. Wulf J, Hadinger U, Oppitz U, et al: Stereotactic radiotherapy of extracranial targets: CT-simulation and accuracy of treatment in the stereotactic body frame. *Radiother Oncol.* 2000;57:225.

52. Nagata Y, Negoro Y, Araki N, et al: Initial clinical findings of 3-D-conformal radiotherapy for solitary lung tumor using a stereotactic body frame part 2. Treatment planning and clinical outcome. *Int J Radiat Oncol Biol Phys.* 1999;45S:411.

53. Negoro Y, Nagata Y, Aoki T, et al: The effectiveness of an immobilization device in conformal radiotherapy for lung tumor: Reduction of respiratory movement and evaluation of daily set-up accuracy. *Int J Radiat Oncol Biol Phys.* 2001;50:889.

54. Ryu S, Yin FF, Rock J, et al: Image-guided and intensity-modulated radiosurgery for spinal metastasis. *Cancer.* 2003;97:2013.

55. Yin FF, Zhu J, Guan H, et al: Dosimetric characteristics of Novalis shaped beam surgery unit. *Med Phys.* 2002;29:1729.

56. Rock J, Kole M, Yin F-F, et al: Radiosurgical treatment for Ewing's sarcoma of the lumbar spine. *Spine.* 2002;27:E471.

57. Ponsky LE, Crownover RL, Rosen MJ, et al: Initial evaluation of CyberKnife technology for extracorporeal renal tissue ablation. *Urology.* 2003;61:498.

Index

Note: Page numbers followed by f indicate figures; page numbers followed by t indicate tables.

1651